Twenty-Second Edition

The Principles and Practice of Medicine

Twenty-Second Edition

The Principles and Practice of Medicine

APPLETON & LANGE
Norwalk, Connecticut/San Mateo, California

EDITED BY

A. McGehee Harvey, M.D., D.Sc. (Hon.)
Distinguished Service Professor of Medicine
The Johns Hopkins University School of Medicine
Physician-in-Chief Emeritus, The Johns Hopkins Hospital
Baltimore, Maryland

Richard J. Johns, M.D.
Professor of Medicine
Massey Professor of Biomedical Engineering and
Director of the Department of Biomedical Engineering
The Johns Hopkins University School of Medicine
Baltimore, Maryland

Victor A. McKusick, M.D., D.Sc. (Hon.)
University Professor of Medical Genetics
and Former Director of the Department of Medicine
The Johns Hopkins University School of Medicine
and Former Physician-in-Chief, The Johns Hopkins Hospital
Baltimore, Maryland

Albert H. Owens, Jr., M.D.
Professor of Medicine
Professor of Oncology
The Johns Hopkins University School of Medicine
President
The Johns Hopkins Hospital
Baltimore, Maryland

Richard S. Ross, M.D.
Professor of Medicine
Dean of the Medical Faculty and
Vice President for Medicine
The Johns Hopkins University School of Medicine
Baltimore, Maryland

Notice: Our knowledge in the clinical sciences is constantly changing. As new information becomes available, changes in treatment and in the use of drugs become necessary. The author(s) and the publisher of this volume have taken care to make certain that the doses of drugs and schedules of treatment are correct and compatible with the standards generally accepted at the time of publication. The reader is advised to consult carefully the instruction and information material included in the package insert of each drug or thera- peutic agent before administration. This advice is especially important when using new or infrequently used drugs.

88 89 90 91 / 10 9 8 7 6 5 4 3 2 1

Prentice-Hall of Australia, Pty. Ltd., Sydney
Prentice-Hall Canada, Inc.
Prentice-Hall Hispanoamericana, S.A., Mexico
Prentice-Hall of India Private Limited, New Delhi
Prentice-Hall International (UK) Limited, London
Prentice-Hall of Japan, Inc., Tokyo
Prentice-Hall of Southeast Asia (Pte.) Ltd., Singapore
Whitehall Books Ltd., Wellington, New Zealand
Editora Prentice-Hall do Brasil Ltda., Rio de Janeiro

Library of Congress Cataloging-in-Publication Data
The Principles and practice of medicine. —22nd ed. / edited by A.
  McGehee Harvey . . . [et al.]
    p. cm.
  Includes bibliographies and index.
  ISBN 0-8385-7944-2
  1. Internal medicine.   I. Harvey, A. McGehee (Abner McGehee),
1911–
  [DNLM: 1. Medicine.   WB 100 P957]
RC46.089 1988
616—dc19
DNLM/DLC
for Library of Congress   88-981
                                                          CIP

A&L: 0-8385-7944-2
PHI: 0-8385-7946-9

Design: M. Chandler Martylewski

PRINTED IN THE UNITED STATES OF AMERICA

This volume is dedicated to the physicians
of the Medical Service of the past
for their precept and guidance,
to our colleagues of today
for their support and encouragement,
and to the students,
our colleagues of tomorrow,
for their stimulation and criticism.

Contents

Contributors

Martin D. Abeloff
Professor of Oncology
Associate Professor of Medicine

Stephen C. Achuff
Associate Professor of Medicine

Elaine L. Alexander
Assistant Professor of Medicine

Arnold E. Andersen
Associate Professor of Psychiatry

Frank C. Arnett, Jr.
Professor of Medicine
University of Texas Medical School at Houston

Wilmot C. Ball, Jr.
Associate Professor of Medicine

John G. Bartlett
Stanhope Bayne-Jones Professor of Medicine

Kenneth L. Baughman
Associate Professor of Medicine

Theodore M. Bayless
Professor of Medicine

Stephen B. Baylin
Professor of Oncology
Associate Professor of Medicine

William R. Bell
Professor of Medicine

Bradley Bender
Assistant Professor of Medicine
University of Florida College of Medicine

Walter L. Bender, Jr.
Assistant Professor of Medicine

Eugene R. Bleecker
Associate Professor of Medicine

A. Michael Borkon
Assistant Professor of Cardiac Surgery
University of Kansas School of Medicine

Hayden G. Braine
Associate Professor of Oncology
Associate Professor of Medicine
Joint Appointment in Laboratory Medicine

Jason Brandt
Assistant Professor of Psychiatry and Behavioral Sciences

Barbara L. Braunstein
Assistant Professor of Dermatology

Henry Brem
Assistant Professor of Neurosurgery
Assistant Professor of Oncology
Joint Appointment in Ophthalmology

E. James Britt
Assistant Professor of Medicine

Roy G. Brower
Assistant Professor of Medicine

David Buchholz
Assistant Professor of Neurology

Gregory B. Bulkley
Professor of Surgery

Philip J. Burke
Associate Professor of Oncology
Associate Professor of Medicine

John R. Burton
Associate Professor of Medicine

Nisha Chibber Chandra
Associate Professor of Medicine

Samuel Charache
Professor of Medicine
Professor of Laboratory Medicine

Michael Colvin
Professor of Oncology
Professor of Medicine
Joint Appointment in Pharmacology and Molecular Sciences

David S. Cooper
Associate Professor of Medicine

David R. Cornblath
Assistant Professor of Neurology

Joseph T. Coyle
Professor of Psychiatry and Behavioral Sciences
Professor of Neuroscience
Professor of Pediatrics
Professor of Pharmacology and Molecular Sciences

Catherine DeAngelis
Professor of Pediatrics

Mahlon R. DeLong
Professor of Neurology
Professor of Neuroscience

Daniel B. Drachman
Professor of Neurology
Professor of Neuroscience

Robert S. Fisher
Assistant Professor of Neurology

Marshal Folstein
Eugene Meyer Professor of Psychiatry
Professor of Medicine

Nicholas J. Fortuin
Professor of Medicine

William R. Furman
Assistant Professor of Anesthesiology and Critical Care Medicine

Angeliki Georgopoulos
Assistant Professor of Medicine

Francis M. Giardiello
Instructor in Medicine
Instructor in Oncology

Barry Gordon
Assistant Professor of Neurology

Vincent L. Gott
Darnall Professor of Cardiac Surgery

Unless otherwise indicated, faculty appointments are at The Johns Hopkins University School of Medicine, Baltimore, Maryland.

Diane E. Griffin
Professor of Medicine
Professor of Neurology

John W. Griffin
Professor of Neurology
Professor of Neuroscience

Lawrence S.C. Griffith
Associate Professor of Medicine
Joint Appointment in Radiology and Radiological Science

Stuart A. Grossman
Assistant Professor of Oncology
Assistant Professor of Medicine
Assistant Professor of Neurosurgery

Thomas Guarnieri
Assistant Professor of Medicine

Alan D. Guerci
Assistant Professor of Medicine

Bruce Hamilton
Assistant Professor of Medicine

Daniel F. Hanley
Assistant Professor of Neurology
Assistant Professor of Anesthesiology and Critical Care Medicine
Joint Appointment in Neurosurgery

A. McGehee Harvey
Distinguished Service Professor
of Medicine

William R. Hazzard
Professor of Medicine
Bowman Gray School of Medicine of Wake Forest University

Thomas R. Hendrix
Professor of Medicine
Moses & Helen Golden Paulson Professor of Gastroenterology

H. Franklin Herlong
Associate Professor of Medicine

Marc C. Hochberg
Associate Professor of Medicine

Richard L. Humphrey
Associate Professor of Oncology
Associate Professor of Medicine
Associate Professor of Immunology
Associate Professor of Laboratory Medicine

John B. Imboden
Associate Professor of Psychiatry and Behavioral Sciences
Instructor in Medicine

Douglas A. Jabs
Assistant Professor of Ophthalmology
Joint Appointment in Medicine

Dudley P. Jackson
Professor of Medicine
Georgetown University School of Medicine

Donald Jasinski
Associate Professor of Medicine
Joint Appointment in Anesthesiology and Critical Care Medicine

Richard S. Johannes
Assistant Professor of Medicine
Assistant Professor of Biomedical Engineering

Carol J. Johns
Associate Professor of Medicine

Richard J. Johns
Massey Professor of Biomedical Engineering
Professor of Medicine

David R. Kafonek
Instructor in Medicine

Thomas S. Kickler
Associate Professor of Laboratory Medicine
Associate Professor of Medicine

Allan Krumholz
Associate Professor of Neurology

Paul W. Ladenson
Assistant Professor of Medicine

Michael A. Levine
Associate Professor of Medicine

Paul S. Lietman
Professor of Medicine
Professor of Pediatrics
Professor of Pharmacology and Molecular Sciences
Wellcome Professor of Clinical Pharmacology

James J. Lipsky
Associate Professor of Medicine
Associate Professor of Pharmacology and Molecular Sciences

Gordon D. Luk
Professor of Medicine
Wayne State University School of Medicine

John J. Mann
Associate Professor of Medicine

Simeon Margolis
Professor of Medicine
Professor of Biological Chemistry

W. Lowell Maughan
Associate Professor of Medicine

Andrew R. Mayrer
Assistant Professor of Medicine

Justin C. McArthur
Assistant Professor of Neurology

Guy M. McKhann
Kennedy Professor of Neurology

Victor A. McKusick
Professor of Medicine
University Professor of Medical Genetics

Harold A. Menkes[†]
Professor of Enviromental Health Sciences
Joint Appointment in Medicine

Esteban Mezey
Professor of Medicine

John R. Michael
Associate Professor of Medicine
Assistant Professor of Anesthesiology and Critical Care Medicine

Neil R. Miller
F. B. Walsh Professor of Ophthalmology
Professor of Neurology
Professor of Neurosurgery

Robert E. Miller
Associate Professor of Laboratory Medicine
Associate Professor of Biomedical Engineering

William E. Mitch
Professor of Mcdicine
Emory University School of Medicine

Mack C. Mitchell
Assistant Professor of Medicine

[†]Deceased.

John Modlin
Associate Professor of Pediatrics

Hamilton Moses III
Associate Professor of Neurology

Patrick A. Murphy
Professor of Medicine
Professor of Molecular Biology and Genetics

Robert P. Murphy
Associate Professor of Ophthalmology

Paul M. Ness
Associate Professor of Laboratory Medicine
Associate Professor of Medicine
Joint Appointment in Oncology

David S. Newcombe
Professor of Environmental Health Sciences
Joint Appointment in Medicine

Cheryl L. Newman
Fellow in Medicine

Philip S. Norman
Professor of Medicine

Albert H. Owens, Jr.
E. K. Marshall, Jr. Professor of Oncology
Professor of Medicine

Godfrey Pearlson
Associate Professor of Psychiatry and Behavioral Sciences

David B. Pearse
Assistant Professor of Medicine

Thomas A. Pearson
Associate Professor of Medicine
Assistant Professor of Pathology

Stephen P. Peters
Associate Professor of Medicine
Jefferson Medical College of the Thomas Jefferson University

Brent G. Petty
Assistant Professor of Medicine

Nathaniel F. Pierce
Professor of Medicine

Marshall Plaut
Associate Professor of Medicine

B. Frank Polk
Associate Professor of Epidemiology
Joint Appointment in Medicine
Joint Appointment in Gynecology and Obstetrics

Thomas Pozefsky
Assistant Professor of Medicine

Thomas J. Preziosi
Associate Professor of Neurology

Leonard R. Proctor
Associate Professor of Otolaryngology, Head and Neck Surgery

Thomas T. Provost
Professor of Dermatology

Thomas C. Quinn
Associate Professor of Medicine

William J. Ravich
Assistant Professor of Medicine

Peter Rock
Assistant Professor of Anesthesiology and Critical Care Medicine
Assistant Professor of Medicine

Robert C. Rock
Associate Professor of Laboratory Medicine

Mark C. Rogers
Professor of Anesthesiology and Critical Care Medicine
Professor of Pediatrics

Richard S. Ross
Professor for Medicine

Barry W. Rovner
Assistant Professor of Psychiatry and Behavioral Sciences

R. Patterson Russell
Associate Professor of Medicine

John Rybock
Assistant Professor of Neurosurgery

R. Bradley Sack
Professor of Medicine
Associate Professor of Molecular Biology and Genetics

Daniel G. Sapir
Associate Professor of Medicine

Christopher D. Saudek
Associate Professor of Medicine

Chester W. Schmidt, Jr.
Associate Professor of Psychiatry and Behavioral Sciences

Marvin M. Schuster
Professor of Medicine
Joint Appointment in Psychiatry and Behavioral Sciences

Stephen R. Selinger
Assistant Professor of Medicine

Lyle L. Sensenbrenner
Associate Professor of Oncology
Associate Professor of Medicine
Wayne State University School of Medicine

James V. Sitzmann
Associate Professor of Surgery

Keith T. Sivertson
Assistant Professor of Emergency Medicine

Craig R. Smith
Associate Professor of Medicine

Philip L. Smith
Associate Professor of Medicine

Kim Solez
Professor of Pathology
University of Alberta, Canada
Lecturer, Pathology

William G. Speed III
Associate Professor of Medicine

Jerry L. Spivak
Associate Professor of Medicine
Associate Professor of Oncology

Barney J. Stern
Assistant Professor of Neurology

Mary Betty Stevens
Professor of Medicine

J.T. Sylvester
Associate Professor of Medicine
Assistant Professor of Anesthesiology and Critical Care Medicine

Mark Teitelbaum
Assistant Professor of Psychiatry and Behavioral Sciences
Assistant Professor of Medicine

Peter B. Terry
Associate Professor of Medicine
Associate Professor of Anesthesiology and Critical Care Medicine
Associate Professor of Environmental Health Sciences

Melvyn S. Tockman
Associate Professor of Environmental Health Sciences
Joint Appointment in Medicine
Joint Appointment in Epidemiology

Thomas A. Traill
Associate Professor of Medicine

Larry E. Tune
Associate Professor of Psychiatry and Behavioral Sciences
Assistant Professor of Medicine

John Chapman Urbaitis
Assistant Professor of Psychiatry and Behavioral Sciences

Martin D. Valentine
Professor of Medicine

Sandra M. Walden
Assistant Professor of Medicine

Gary D. Walford
Assistant Professor of Medicine

W. Gordon Walker
Professor of Medicine

Patrick C. Walsh
Professor of Urology

Gary S. Wand
Assistant Professor of Medicine

Ko-Pen Wang
Associate Professor of Medicine
Associate Professor of Otolaryngology, Head and Neck Surgery

Andrew C. Warren
Fellow in Psychiatry and Behavioral Sciences

Gail G. Weinmann
Assistant Professor of Environmental Health Sciences
Joint Appointment in Medicine

Myron L. Weisfeldt
Professor of Medicine
Robert L. Levy Professor of Cardiology

Paul S. Wheeler
Associate Professor of Radiology

Andrew Whelton
Associate Professor of Medicine

Paul K. Whelton
Associate Professor of Medicine

Frederick M. Wigley
Associate Professor of Medicine

G. Melville Williams
Professor of Transplantation Surgery

Robert A. Wise
Associate Professor of Medicine
Instructor in Radiology and Radiological Science

Thomas N. Wise
Associate Professor of Psychiatry and Behavioral Sciences
Assistant Professor of Medicine

Howard A. Zacur
Associate Professor of Gynecology and Obstetrics

David S. Zee
Professor of Neurology
Professor of Neuroscience
Professor of Ophthalmology

Carol M. Ziminski
Assistant Professor of Medicine

Thomas M. Zizic
Associate Professor of Medicine

Preface to the Twenty-Second Edition

This edition of *The Principles and Practice of Medicine* is the sixth that we have edited in the past 20 years.

In preparation for this edition each section of the Twenty-First Edition was sent to two external reviewers for their comments and expert criticism. This detailed outside review was helpful to us in planning our revisions for this new edition. It prompted us to address issues which they raised as well as a host of related issues.

This textbook continues to reflect the coherent view of a single institution—Johns Hopkins. Nevertheless, institutions change and evolve from edition to edition and certainly the *practice* of medicine advances rapidly between editions. There are also fresh approaches to clinical problem-solving and new insights into patient management, that is, there are advances in *principles* as well. This edition has been extensively revised in response to these advances and changes. In addition, the sequence of sections has been changed to reflect newly developed connections between clinical problem areas.

In this edition we have a number of new section editors: Joseph T. Coyle, Jr., H. Franklin Herlong, Dudley P. Jackson, Paul W. Ladenson, Simeon Margolis, John R. Michael, William E. Mitch, Mack C. Mitchell, Mark C. Rogers, J.T. Sylvester, and Peter B. Terry.

We also welcome 59 new contributors to this edition. They include: Elaine L. Alexander, A. Michael Borkon, Jason Brandt, Barbara L. Braunstein, Henry Brem, Roy G. Brower, Philip J. Burke, John R. Burton, David S. Cooper, David R. Cornblath, Robert S. Fisher, William R. Furman, Francis M. Giardiello, Vincent L. Gott, Stuart S. Grossman, Thomas Guarnieri, Alan D. Guerci, Bruce Hamilton, Douglas A. Jabs, Dudley P. Jackson, Donald R. Jasinski, David B. Kafonek, Allan Krumholz, Paul W. Ladenson, W. Lowell Maughan, Andrew R. Mayrer, Justin C. McArthur, Esteban Mezey, William E. Mitch, John F. Modlin, Cheryl L. Newman, Godfrey D. Pearlson, David B. Pearse, Thomas A. Pearson, Stephen P. Peters, Marshall Plaut, Leonard R. Proctor, Peter Rock, Mark C. Rogers, Barry W. Rovner, Chester W. Schmidt, Jr., Marvin M. Schuster, Stephen S. Selinger, James V. Sitzmann, Keith T. Sivertson, Barney J. Stern, Mark L. Teitelbaum, Melvyn S. Tockman, Larry E. Tune, Martin D. Valentine, Sandra M. Walden, Gary D. Walford, Patrick C. Walsh, Gary S. Wand, Andrew C. Warren, Gail G. Weinmann, Paul S. Wheeler, Howard A. Zacur, and Carol M. Ziminski.

We also wish to thank the section editors and authors who have contributed not only to this edition but to previous editions as well. Their experience is invaluable, and their continued interest, effort, and tolerance are warmly appreciated.

As in the last edition Ms. Christine D. Young prepared the illustrative material. We appreciate her skill in communicating complex topics clearly and artistically.

Finally, we are grateful to those who assisted us so ably in the preparation of this edition, particularly Mrs. Sandra M. Sann.

THE EDITORS

Preface to the Twenty-Second Edition

Preface to the Seventeenth Edition

In 1892 the first edition of Sir William Osler's textbook was published, in which he covered single-handedly the entire field of medicine. His book was well received both as a scientific work and as a contribution to literature. When the time came for the seventh edition, he wrote the following in a letter to Dr. Lewellys Barker: "This new edition will not be a very serious revision, as they will not break up the plates, but in the next edition we can do as we like. It would be very nice if you and Thayer came in with me as joint authors. It would be possible, I think, to arrange to have the work kept up as a Johns Hopkins Textbook of Medicine." This never came about. After Dr. Osler's death, the textbook was edited by Dr. Thomas McCrae until the completion of the twelfth edition in 1935. After the death of Dr. McCrae, Dr. Henry Christian continued as editor through the sixteenth and last edition published in 1947.

This current revision was conceived as a Johns Hopkins Textbook of Medicine as proposed by Osler. There was hesitancy to assume this task in view of the several excellent, comprehensive textbooks of medicine already available. However, it was decided that there was a need for a different type of textbook, one which would complement the existent encyclopedic texts. This text emphasizes clinical problems rather than disease entities. It attempts to describe and define the way in which the experienced physician approaches the solution and management of such problems.

This is clearly not a revision of Dr. Osler's great book. Nor is it the product of a single author. Rather, it is the product of a single department in which the preservation of a heritage of clinical excellence has been a major goal. We hope this volume reflects the tradition of excellence which this Department of Medicine received from Dr. Osler.

THE EDITORS

A Note from the Editors

In the practice of medicine the physician is confronted by three basic questions:

1. What is the matter with the patient?
2. What can I do for him?
3. What will be the outcome?

A fourth question, Why did it happen? will also arise in the mind of the inquiring physician who feels that each patient affords an opportunity and imposes a responsibility to contribute to a better understanding of causation and prevention.

The usual textbook of medicine does not prepare the practitioner to deal systematically with these questions. Its focus is upon the disease rather than the patient. It presents its subject matter in a series of essays each devoted to a description—as simple and straightforward as possible—of the disease entity. Some general information may be provided but rarely is sufficient emphasis placed upon the confusing complexities which arise in the day-to-day investigation and management of clinical problems.

The answer to the first of the questions enumerated above is the key to the answers to the second and third. The first question is the only one that requires an analytical approach, and obviously the analysis must begin with a study of the patient and must continue to be focused upon the patient until a solution is reached.

It is our purpose to produce a book which is built around the patient rather than the disease— the patient and the problems which he presents in diagnosis, management, and prognosis. Consideration will be given to the methods employed in acquiring factual data, the discriminating use of ancillary diagnostic techniques, and the systematic analysis of the accumulated information. This book also presents the essential information necessary for an understanding of the basic mechanisms involved in the various manifestations of disease, the important features of the natural history of the major diseases, the principles involved in the management of the patient, and the estimation of the probable outcome. In order to devote more space to the sequential steps which should be taken by the physician seeking the answers to his three basic questions, we have avoided as far as possible duplication of the type of presentation so successfully employed in texts already available. Since much of the material contained in current texts is to be sacrificed, the physician may have to turn elsewhere to fill the gaps in his knowledge of the subject in hand. To meet this need for quick access to more detailed information on specific topics, particular attention has been devoted to the selection of the bibliography.

William Osler, having recognized a clear need for a fresh endeavor in the textbook field, assumed responsibility for the task, and in 1892 published the first edition of *The Principles and Practice of Medicine*. The book had gone through six editions by the time Osler left Hopkins for Oxford in 1905. Soon after his arrival at Oxford he began to give thought to the disposition of the authorship of the book. In 1908, while in the throes of preparing the seventh edition, he wrote to Lewellys F. Barker, his successor in the Chair of Medicine at Hopkins, suggesting that he and William S. Thayer, one of Osler's former chief medical residents at Hopkins, join him (Osler) as joint authors. He expressed the belief that it should be possible to arrange to have the work kept up as a Johns Hopkins Hospital textbook of medicine. Osler expressed the view that some arrangement could be made with the publishers and a plan devised by which the head of the medical department would have ex-officio rights in it.

Osler's proposal appears to have had a cool reception from Barker and Thayer because with the eighth edition Thomas McCrae, a former Osler resident and later Professor of Medicine at Jefferson Medical College, joined Osler in editing the textbook. After Osler's death in 1919 and until his own death in 1935, McCrae continued the book (the ninth through the twelfth editions), taking sole responsibility. Henry A. Christian (1876–1951), professor of medicine at Harvard Medical School and Physician-in-Chief of the Peter Bent Brigham Hospital, took over the editorship with the 13th edition (1938). The last edition edited by Christian, the 16th, appeared in 1947. Thus, through its existence up to this 1947 edition, it continued as a one man book throughout.

In 1963 Mr. George McDermott of Appleton-Century-Crofts proposed that the book be taken over by the Department of Medicine at Hopkins as a Johns Hopkins textbook of Medicine. This suggestion was implemented and the 17th edition of *The Principles and Practice of Medicine* appeared in 1968 with A. McGehee Harvey, Leighton E. Cluff, Richard J. Johns, Albert H. Owens, Jr., David Rabinowitz, and Richard S. Ross as editors. For the 18th edition in 1972 and the 19th in 1976 the editors were Harvey, Johns, Owens, and Ross. For the 20th edition in 1980 these editors were joined by Victor A. McKusick and the same authors were responsible for the 21st edition which appeared in 1984.

Edition	Author(s)	Year
First	William Osler	1892
Second	William Osler	1895
Third	William Osler	1898
Fourth	William Osler	1901
Fifth	William Osler	1904
Sixth	William Osler	1905
Seventh	William Osler	1909
Eighth	William Osler Thomas McCrae	1914
Ninth	William Osler Thomas McCrae	1920
Tenth	Thomas McCrae	1926
Eleventh	Thomas McCrae	1930
Twelfth	Thomas McCrae	1935
Thirteenth	Henry A. Christian	1938
Fourteenth	Henry A. Christian	1942
Fifteenth	Henry A. Christian	1944
Sixteenth	Henry A. Christian	1947
Seventeenth	A. McGehee Harvey Leighton E. Cluff Richard J. Johns Albert H. Owens, Jr. David Rabinowitz Richard S. Ross	1968
Eighteenth	A. McGehee Harvey Richard J. Johns Albert H. Owens, Jr. Richard S. Ross	1972
Nineteenth	A. McGehee Harvey Richard J. Johns Albert H. Owens, Jr. Richard S. Ross	1976
Twentieth	A. McGehee Harvey Richard J. Johns Victor A. McKusick Albert H. Owens, Jr. Richard S. Ross	1980
Twenty-First	A. McGehee Harvey Richard J. Johns Victor A. McKusick Albert H. Owens, Jr. Richard S. Ross	1984

Twenty-Second Edition

The Principles and Practice of Medicine

To anyone who has chosen a career in medicine there can be no better motto than to strive to be a person with technical skill, broad scientific knowledge and wisdom, and those personal characteristics of warmth and humility that serve to cement the art with the science of medicine. Such a person exemplifies the inscription on the statue of Edward Livingston Trudeau: "To cure sometimes, to relieve often, to comfort always."

Every student and practitioner of medicine should familiarize himself with the classic essay on *The Care of the Patient*, by Francis Peabody.[1]

The practice of medicine in its broadest sense includes the whole relationship of the physician with his patient. It is an art, based to an increasing extent on the medical sciences but comprising much that still remains outside the realm of any science. The art of medicine and the science of medicine are not antagonistic but supplementary to each other. There is no more contradiction between the science of medicine and the art of medicine than between the science of aeronautics and the art of flying. Good practice presupposes an understanding of the sciences that contribute to the structure of modern medicine, but it is obvious that sound professional training should include a much broader equipment.

The treatment of disease may be entirely impersonal; the care of a patient must be completely personal. The significance of the intimate personal relationship between physician and patient cannot be too strongly emphasized, for in an extraordinarily large number of cases both diagnosis and treatment are directly dependent on it, and failure of the young physician to establish this relationship accounts for much of his ineffectiveness in the care of patients.

What is spoken of as a "clinical picture" is not just a photograph of a man sick in bed; it is an impressionistic painting of the patient surrounded by his home, his work, his relations, his friends, his joys, sorrows, hopes, and fears.

Thus the physician who attempts to take care of a patient while he neglects those factors that contribute to the emotional life of his patient is as unscientific as the investigator who neglects to control all the conditions that may affect his experiment. The good physician knows his patients through and through, and his knowledge is bought dearly. Time, sympathy, and understanding must be lavishly dispensed, but the reward is to be found in that personal bond which forms the greatest satisfaction of the practice of medicine. One of the essential qualities of the clinician is interest in humanity, for the secret of the care of the patient is in caring for the patient.

These beautifully expressed thoughts about the physician and his relationship to the patient are even more important today than when they were written over 50 years ago. Medicine has become, and will continue to become, much more a science, not less, so that the physician of tomorrow will have to be more a scientist, not less. Nevertheless, the art of medicine remains, and the physician must continue to be wise and understanding, with a deep respect for the patient as a human being. The secret of success in the care *of* the patient is still in caring *for* the patient.

REFERENCE

1. Peabody FW: The care of the patient. JAMA 88:877, 1927

CHAPTER 1.1
Clinical Information and Clinical Problem Solving

Richard J. Johns and Nicholas J. Fortuin

The kind of patient care described in the quotation of Peabody in the introduction is the goal of all conscientious physicians. Although effective patient care is determined by many factors, we shall emphasize two in particular: (1) the quality of the diagnostic management and (2) the quality of therapeutic management. Diagnostic management encompasses all of the steps that lead from the patient's complaints to a clear understanding of the patient's problems. Therapeutic management encompasses all of the measures directed toward correcting or alleviating the patient's problems. Taken together, these aspects are the core of clinical problem solving.

The basic precepts of medical practice cannot be communicated by books alone. Clinical teaching at the patient's bedside is an essential element. As Osler said, "To study medicine without textbooks is to sail an uncharted sea; to study medicine without patients is to not go to sea at all." Many of the aspects of management that are poorly communicated in writing are the very elements Peabody emphasized—the caring, the sensitivity to the pa-

tient's feelings and concerns, the humanistic aspects of medical practice. The fact that these aspects of the practice of medicine often seem neglected in textbooks is in no way intended to deemphasize their importance. It is simply an acknowledgment of a reality: the burden for imparting these precepts falls more heavily on clinical teachers than on textbooks. Wherever such material can be meaningfully rendered into print, we have attempted to include it in this book.

This initial chapter is designed to summarize this process of solving a patient's clinical problem. The subsequent chapters address the process in more detail: the collection and the evaluation of clinical information, the ways in which information is analyzed and synthesized, and the basis of clinical decision making. The final chapter is devoted to the difficult issues in patient management.

CLINICAL PROBLEM SOLVING

Experienced clinicians appear to approach and solve the problems of their patients with ease. The novice, in contrast, may have difficulty eliciting even the basic information about the patient's problem. This paradox has led some to ascribe this skill in problem solving to "experience," the "art of medicine," clinical "insight,"

Contributors to this section in previous editions included Rex B. Conn, Martin W. Donner, William R. Hazzard, John B. Imboden, Louis C. Lasagna, Robert E. Miller, Anthony J. Reading, Roger C. Sanders, Philip A. Tumulty, and Henry N. Wagner, Jr.

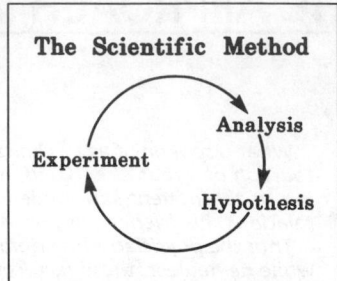

Figure 1.1–1. An illustration of the recursive nature of the scientific method: the analysis of experimental data leads to the formulation of an hypothesis. This hypothesis, in turn, suggests further experimental studies that will test the hypothesis.

or "judgment." To be sure, problem-solving ability improves with experience, and there are important humanistic elements in obtaining clinical information which are artful. Nevertheless, such formulations are not instructive to the novice who wishes to learn these skills or to the practitioner who wishes to improve his clinical ability.

Clinical problem solving is neither an arcane art nor a mysterious process. It is a method that parallels the scientific problem-solving process, as will be described below. It is a method that can be both taught and learned. It requires both knowledge and skill, and these skills can be refined only through practice.

Clinical problem solving is the cornerstone of clinical medicine.

THE SCIENTIFIC METHOD

The analytic process by which clinical information leads to the diagnosis is closely akin to the scientific method—the process whereby experimentation leads to the discovery of new knowledge.

As shown in Figure 1.1–1, experimental observations yield data. By analyzing and extracting meaning from these data, a hypothesis is formulated that will explain the observed facts. The process does not stop at that point. The scientist then designs a further experiment that will test (support or refute) the current hypothesis. The scientist may also have formulated alternative hypotheses and will design an experiment to distinguish between them.

In the clinical setting, experimental observations may be obtained by interrogation of the patient, the examination of the patient, or the performance of some laboratory test (Fig. 1.1–2). The resulting information is analyzed by differential diagnosis (consideration of all reasonable possibilities) to yield a tentative hypothesis (tentative diagnosis or diagnoses). These, in turn, prompt the clinician to ask further questions, make further observations, or order tests that will support, refute, or distinguish between the diagnoses

under consideration. Figure 1.1–2 also illustrates the cyclic or iterative, nature of this process.

The discussion of these similarities is not mere pedantry. It leads to a number of practical points:

1. The collection and analysis of clinical information are essentially the application of the scientific method to the solution of a clinical problem.
2. This process can be taught and learned; it is not an art in which one is either gifted or not. Proficiency can be improved by consciously considering the meaning of each piece of information as it is received.
3. The process is rapidly iterative. The cycle is repeated *within* the time interval of asking a few questions or making physical observations. This explains the mystery of why the novice fails to ask the key question or seek the key physical finding.
4. The process is an ongoing one. There are no irrefutable hypotheses, only unrefuted hypotheses. In clinical terms the physician should not arrive at a diagnosis and abandon any further consideration of alternative explanations. He must remain alert for information that does not fit with his current hypothesis and for sources of new information that might make him alter his considerations. When uncertain, he should continue to seek ways of testing the tentative diagnosis.
5. Consideration of a diagnosis that can neither be confirmed nor excluded fails to advance the decision-making process. Such a diagnosis is directly parallel to a scientific hypothesis that cannot be tested.
6. Finally, clinical problem solving is as sensitive to flawed or missing information as are scientific experiments. A major difference lies in the fact that clinical decisions must often be made on what is acknowledged to be incomplete evidence.

In summary, the diagnostic process is a dynamic one that begins with the initial contact with the patient. Each piece of information obtained from or about the patient prompts the physician to consider new hypotheses and to test or to discard others. Studies indicate that skilled physicians may consider 15 or 20 diagnostic possibilities during the initial contact with the patient, but they rarely have more than 5 or 6 possibilities under active consideration at any one time.

Many students are taught that differential diagnosis is limited to an orderly, formal consideration of all of the diagnostic possibilities that is performed only after all of the clinical information has been acquired. This is a counterproductive notion. A review of the diagnostic possibilities at this point is helpful, but it is the rapid iteration of the diagnostic process throughout the encounter with the patient that enables the physician to obtain the information that will lead him to the appropriate conclusion.

Figure 1.1–2. An illustration of the clear parallel between the general scientific method (Fig. 1.1–1) and the scientific method applied in the clinical setting. In the left portion of this illustration, experimental data are obtained through examination; analysis of these data is called differential diagnosis; the formulation of a hypothesis is stated as a tentative diagnosis. This tentative diagnosis, or hypothesis, is tested by obtaining further data through further examination. The clinical example shown in the right portion is drawn from history taking.

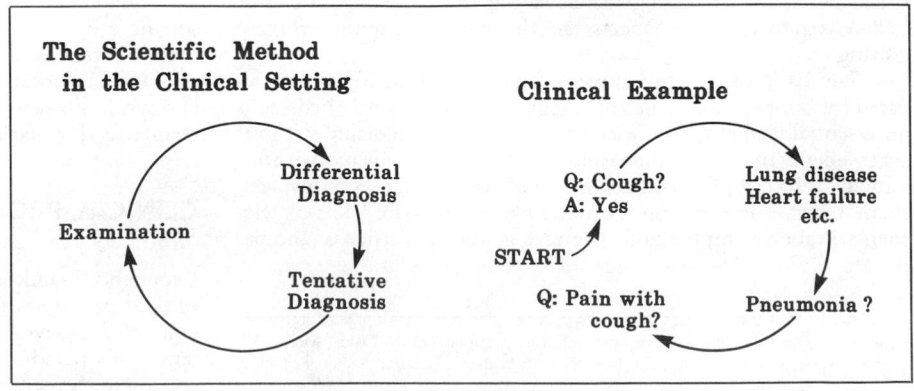

INFORMATION VERSUS DATA

Clinical information can be obtained from the patient himself through dialogue (the history) or through observation (the physical examination). Information may also be obtained from laboratory or radiographic examinations. These sources of information (dialogue, observation, the laboratory) are separate and distinct. These distinctions, however, obscure the similar way in which the experienced physician uses clinical data, regardless of the source.

In each instance this collection of clinical information is not simply data collection. Data are a group of facts, whereas information implies the communication of knowledge. Thus clinical information imparts meaning; it represents meaningful data, not just an ensemble of facts. Furthermore, useful information will prompt the physician to take certain actions, actions that may include seeking further information. As will be discussed later, clinical information that has no action-oriented implications is of limited value in patient management.

This distinction between data and information can be exemplified. A patient complains of weakness and breathlessness and is found to have a blood pressure of 135/80 mm Hg. The information content of this datum, 135/80, is usually taken to be that this patient's blood pressure is normal; however, the information, or its meaning, is decidedly different if the data from the previous week included a blood pressure of 190/110 mm Hg. Now the physician knows the patient was hypertensive and is presently normotensive. This prompts the collection of more information regarding the possibility of recent myocardial infarction, blood loss, and the like.

This distinction between data and information explains one of the mysteries of history taking. For example, the complete novice can ask all the "usual" questions and record the patient's answers with fidelity. Such an interview (data collection) may not impart much knowledge about the patient's problem even when these data are subsequently reviewed by an expert. The communication of clinical information imparts meaning to the experienced interviewer that guides and directs his further dialogue with the patient. Thus each datum communicates information to the experienced person. It is thus apparent that some important analysis occurs during the course of the collection of clinical information. Analysis is not simply a separate, subsequent event.

This leads to the following dicta: (1) The experienced clinician weighs each piece of clinical data as he elicits it for its meaning, for its information content. (2) He also analyzes it in the context of other information about the patient to determine whether there is still more information that should be acquired. (3) The collection and analysis of clinical information proceed in parallel, not as separate, sequential steps.

HUMANISTIC ASPECTS

None of the foregoing emphasis on the scientific aspects of the collection and analysis of clinical information should be interpreted as deprecation of the importance of the humanistic aspects of dealing with patients. Indeed, disregard of these aspects can even prevent the collection of clinical information. The physician who appears impatient, or bored, or insensitive may be unable to elicit important information from the patient. The physician must be aware that the patient, especially the new patient, is scrutinizing him every bit as carefully and critically as he is examining the patient. The physician who is rough and uninterested in the patient's comfort may be unable to feel an abdominal mass. Thus, inattention to these important aspects may defeat the whole purpose of clinical information analysis—the solution of a patient's problem.

There can be little doubt that the most humane act a physician can perform for the patient is to establish a proper diagnosis and initiate correct treatment. The physician's responsibility, however, goes far beyond these two seminal events, for he must minister to the patient's emotional needs as well. A physician's exultation at establishing a brilliant diagnosis or management scheme is often dashed with the later realization that the patient is unhappy, unappreciative, or even hostile because proper rapport has not been established. Central to every medical encounter from the patient's perception is fear or apprehension that may be manifest in many ways. The prospect of illness engenders fear of death, fear of pain, fear of change in life-style, fear of economic loss, or fear of medical procedures. The physician must deal with this aspect of the patient's illness by demonstrating professional competence, a calm demeanor, a reassuring and positive manner, and an interest in the patient as an individual. Illness tends to behave in predictable patterns, but each individual's interaction with an illness is unique. The physician's challenge is to recognize and manage the illness by employing the best scientific tools available and dealing effectively with the patient's reaction to the illness, its diagnosis, and management. This "caring" function, which Peabody also addressed, means that the physician will always act as the patient's advocate and friend. The potent therapeutic modalities available to the modern physician may seem to diminish the importance of the role of the individual physician in the healing process, but personal interaction between patient and physician is an essential component of a proper therapeutic outcome.

ECONOMIC ASPECTS

A major complaint of the lay public concerning modern medical care is its "excessive" cost. Many believe that the clinical problem-solving process, both diagnostic and therapeutic, is too costly. Yet the individual patient insists on and is entitled to high-quality medical care. Are these positions antithetical?

The direct answer is that these views are not antithetical. Every physician has as a part of his responsibility to his patients the obligation not to waste clinical resources. Irrelevant or redundant laboratory data do not improve the quality of care, but they do contribute substantially to the cost of care. This topic is addressed later in this section in a discussion of the prudent use of ancillary studies in both diagnostic management and prudent therapeutic management. It is also addressed throughout the book in outlines of the optimal sequence in the diagnostic management of specific clinical problems. Inept sequences are a major source of waste. For example, when one is dealing with the problem of anemia, it is wasteful and pointless to obtain serum iron, folate, and B$_{12}$ determinations simultaneously before determining whether the patient's red blood cells are normocytic, macrocytic, or microcytic. We shall outline a series of questions that a clinician can ask when selecting ancillary tests and procedures in the investigation of a problem in which he is not experienced (see Chapter 1.2).

Other aspects contributing needlessly to the expense of medical care include (1) hospitalizing patients for problems that can readily be managed on an ambulatory basis, (2) failing to use effectively the time during which the patient is hospitalized, and (3) failing to plan in advance for the patient's discharge from hospital. These, too, are items of expense that detract from rather than contribute to the quality of care given to the patient.

It is well recognized that an inverse relationship exists between the competence of a physician and the use of laboratory studies. The best physicians require fewer and less costly laboratory tests to establish a diagnosis or follow up a patient than do less competent physicians. The reason is that experienced clinicians have greater confidence in their basic clinical skills. They require less confirmation of diagnoses by expensive testing and less testing to exclude diagnoses that were not reasonable in the first place. There is another important reason for this—expert physicians who care for their patients will also care about their patient's economic welfare and the financial impact of their medical care. It is not proper to abrogate responsibility for medical costs by assuming that some

third-party payer will provide coverage. It is the physician's responsibility not only to hold down costs for society overall but also to know what the cost of tests and treatments are for individual patients and how much of the cost the patient will have to bear. Selecting the least costly diagnostic or therapeutic plan without sacrificing quality is an important responsibility for the modern physician.

SUMMARY

This chapter supports the view that the collection and analysis of clinical information, whatever its source, are the cornerstone of patient care. The skills involved can be taught and learned. The approach is similar to any scientific problem-solving endeavor, but the effective physician must have an understanding of the humanistic elements involved in the care of the sick.

In the subsequent chapters of this section the various ways of acquiring and analyzing clinical information are discussed. Furthermore, attention is given to the use of this information in the diagnostic and therapeutic management of patients.

REFERENCES

1. Dudley HAF: The clinical task. Lancet 2:1352, 1970
2. Dudley HAF: The clinical method. Lancet 1:35, 1971
3. Elstein AS, Shulman LS, Sprafka SA: Medical Problem Solving: An Analysis of Clinical Reasoning. Cambridge, Mass, Harvard University Press, 1978
4. Enelow AJ, Swisher SN: Interviewing and Patient Care. New York, Oxford University Press, 1972
5. Engel GR, Morgan WL Jr: Interviewing the Patient. Philadelphia, WB Saunders, 1973
6. Feinstein AR: Clinical Judgment. Baltimore, Williams & Wilkins, 1967
7. Feinstein AR: Clinical Biostatistics. St. Louis, CV Mosby, 1977
8. Feinstein AR: An additional basic science for clinical medicine. I. The constraining fundamental paradigms. Ann Intern Med 99:393, 1983
9. Galen RS, Gambino SR: Beyond Normality: The Predictive Value and Efficiency of Medical Diagnoses. New York, John Wiley & Sons, 1975
10. Groen GJ, Patel VL: Medical problem-solving: Some questionable assumptions. Med Education 19:95, 1985
11. Kassirer JP, Knipers BJ, Gorry GA: Toward a theory of clinical expertise. Am J Med 73:251, 1982
12. Lipkin M Jr, Quill TE, Napudano RJ: The medical interview: A core curriculum for residencies in internal medicine. Ann Intern Med 100:277, 1984
13. McCormick JS: Diagnosis: The need for demystification. Lancet 2:1434, 1986
14. Morgan WL Jr, Engel GL: The Clinical Approach to the Patient. Philadelphia, WB Saunders, 1969
15. Murphy EA: The Logic of Medicine. Baltimore, Johns Hopkins University Press, 1976
16. Popper K: The Logic of Scientific Discovery, 3d ed. London, Hutchinson, 1972
17. Whitehorn JC: Guide to interviewing and clinical personality study. Arch Neurol (Chicago) 52:197, 1944

CHAPTER 1.2

The Collection and Evaluation of Clinical Information

Richard J. Johns, Nicholas J. Fortuin, and Paul S. Wheeler

Clinical information may be obtained by conversing with the patient and his relatives (the history), by observing and examining the patient (the physical examination), as well as through laboratory examinations of the patient or specimens obtained from the patient (laboratory tests) and through special procedures such as endoscopy. Different techniques are required for the collection and evaluation of these different kinds of information. Before discussing these specific examples, we should consider certain common features that influence the determination of what information should be obtained and how it should be evaluated, whatever its source.

ATTRIBUTES OF CLINICAL INFORMATION

It is neither possible nor desirable to obtain *all* clinical information on *every* patient. There must be selectivity in choosing what information to obtain. How does one make this decision? A number of attributes are important in making this selective judgment. These include the information's (1) accuracy, (2) precision, (3) variance, (4) specificity, (5) sensitivity, (6) validity, (7) risk, (8) cost, and (9) benefit. For example, it is obvious that one would not choose to obtain information of dubious validity, particularly if its collection were associated with some risk.

Physicians tend to believe that these attributes apply only to laboratory tests. However, they apply to all types of clinical information, including historical facts and physical findings. Does the absence of a history of rheumatic fever exclude the possibility of rheumatic mitral insufficiency? Does a lid-lag specifically mean hyperthyroidism? Is a liver edge palpable 1 cm below the costal margin normal? These questions are as amenable to assessment as the question, Does a fasting blood glucose concentration of 124 mg/dl mean diabetes mellitus?

A clear understanding of these attributes is fundamental to the selection and evaluation of all kinds of clinical information. In the discussion that follows, we shall draw on nonlaboratory examples wherever possible to emphasize the breadth of applicability of these concepts.

ACCURACY

Accuracy is the measure of how closely the given piece of clinical information represents the correct and true state. The usual examples drawn from clinical chemistry indicate that the accuracy of blood glucose concentrations are assessed by analyzing replicates of an authentic glucose standard. The test is deemed to be accurate if there is close agreement between the observed and the true value.

This concept of accuracy is equally applicable to historical information.[2] When the physician asks about alcohol consumption, the patient may admit to only one or two cocktails before dinner. This information is accurate if it reflects the true state. It is not accurate if, in fact, the patient has two cocktails before lunch, three before dinner, and several more drinks after dinner. Thus, if a piece of information is of particular importance (or if there is reason to question its accuracy), the physician should take steps to authenticate it before using it in his analysis of a problem. This principle of authentication applies to historical information and physical findings as well as to laboratory tests and special procedures. Failure

to appreciate the importance of this principle is a major source of error and inefficiency in clinical management.

PRECISION

Precision is a measure of the reproducibility of a piece of information. A common measure of precision is to note the variability, or variance, in the results when the observation is repeated on replicates or on successive occasions. Blood pressure measurements by auscultation may be consistent and reproducible in an hypotensive patient, but they may not accurately reflect the true intra-arterial pressure. In this example the measurement would be precise but inaccurate. It is a common error to consider information that is highly reproducible (precise) to be accurate. Precise information may or may not be accurate. (It is not possible to have information that is accurate but imprecise.)

VARIANCE

The variability in observations, including clinical observations, comes from several sources.[2,18] Some are attributable to the observational method itself, some to the observer, and some to the feature being observed. A simple example—determining the location of the liver edge by palpation—can illustrate these points.

Suppose one observer reports the liver edge to be two fingerbreadths below the right costal margin and another reports it to be 4 cm below. One source of variance stems from using a variable unit of measurement of size, distance, and the like (fingerbreadths, hen's eggs, golf balls); this source of variance is easily avoided. Apart from this, there is variance from quantitative estimation: On one occasion a 3.5 cm measurement might be rounded up to 4 cm and on another down to 3 cm. Even greater variance can be introduced by the methodology. Was the measurement made with the patient fully supine? Was it in full inspiration? These all contribute to the *variance of the method*.

There may be differences in the ways an observer performs a measurement from one time to another, resulting in *intraobserver variance*. There are also differences in the ways different observers perform a measurement, *interobserver variance*.

Still another kind of variance relates to differences in, as an example, the location of the liver edge from one person to another. This kind of variance will be discussed in the context of normality and the normal range.

DIAGNOSTIC SPECIFICITY AND SENSITIVITY[3,18,21,25]

The specificity of clinical information and its sensitivity are important in assessing its meaning; yet these terms are often only vaguely or imperfectly understood. Specificity and sensitivity relate to the inferences that may be drawn about the patient's *condition* based on the presence or absence of a certain *finding*. The condition may be a disease (e.g., diabetes mellitus) or an abnormality (e.g., pulmonary consolidation), and the finding may be a laboratory test result, historical fact, or physical finding.

Table 1.2–1 indicates the four possible relationships between a finding and a condition and defines "sensitivity," "specificity," and "predictive value." "Sensitivity" describes the diagnostic power of a finding. A finding present in all patients with a condition would have perfect sensitivity; that is, there would be no false-negative results. One would use such a finding to confirm the presence of a condition. "Specificity" describes the diagnostic error of a finding resulting from a false-positive diagnosis. A finding that was never present in patients who did not have the condition (no false-positive results) would have perfect specificity. One could use the absence of a finding with perfect specificity to exclude or rule out a condition with accuracy. Such perfection of clinical findings does not exist in clinical medicine. Some findings may be sensitive but lack specificity. For example, rales heard over the right lower lobe of the lung are present in most patients with bacterial pneumonia (high sensitivity), but this finding alone cannot establish the diagnosis, because there are many other conditions that may be responsible for this physical finding (low specificity). Because all patients with pneumonia do not have rales, the absence of this finding does not exclude this diagnosis. As an example, most patients with bacterial endocarditis have fever. The absence of fever in a patient in whom this diagnosis is suspected would be a highly specific finding that would be useful in excluding this diagnosis. Many clinical findings lack both sensitivity and specificity and thus are of little value, by themselves, in diagnosis. For example, splinter hemorrhages in the nail beds are found in a small percentage of patients with bacterial endocarditis (low sensitivity), but they are most frequently caused by trauma (low specificity). Thus, finding a splinter hemorrhage would not inevitably lead to the diagnosis of bacterial endocarditis, and the absence of this finding would be of no value in excluding the possibility.

Clinical findings can also be described in terms of predictive value, both positive and negative, which describes the probability that a condition is present or absent if a given finding is present or absent. Thus a positive predictive value is related to the specificity of a finding, and a negative predictive value to its sensitivity. Data are not available to define the sensitivity, specificity, and predictive value of most clinical findings. Experienced clinicians learn these things intuitively by exposure to many clinical situations. The clinician also recognizes that the specificity of certain findings changes depending on the clinical picture with which the findings are associated. For example, stiffness of the neck is a nonspecific finding for which there may be many causes. It is a sensitive finding in the diagnosis of meningitis, because most patients with meningitis will

TABLE 1.2–1. RELATIONSHIP BETWEEN FINDINGS AND CONDITIONS

	Finding	
Condition	*Positive*	*Negative*
Present	True positive (TP)	False negative (FN)
Absent	False postive (FP)	True negative (TN)

$$\text{Sensitivity} = \frac{TP}{TP + FN} \quad \begin{array}{l}\textit{(No. of patients with condition with positive finding)}\\ \textit{(Total no. of patients with condition)}\end{array}$$

$$\text{Specificity} = \frac{TN}{TN + FP} \quad \begin{array}{l}\textit{(No. of patients without condition with negative finding)}\\ \textit{(No. of patients without condition)}\end{array}$$

$$\text{Positive predictive value} = \frac{TP}{TP + FP} \quad \textit{(Probability of condition if finding is present)}$$

$$\text{Negative predictive value} = \frac{TN}{TN + FN} \quad \textit{(Probability that condition is absent if finding is absent)}$$

have nuchal rigidity. Thus the finding of a stiff neck in the context of fever and headache would readily lead to the diagnosis of meningitis, but such a finding in an otherwise healthy individual would not. In the latter situation, local musculoskeletal factors would probably be responsible. Stated another way, the predictive value of nuchal rigidity for the diagnosis of meningitis is low, so that further diagnostic evaluation (e.g., lumbar puncture) would not be performed unless other clinical findings were present.

The performance of laboratory tests with respect to sensitivity, specificity, and predictive value can be defined more easily than clinical findings, but for most such tests, proper information does not exist.[8,25] Furthermore, for most tests, particularly early in their use, the information available may be too optimistic because their performance on very ill individuals cannot be extrapolated to patients with milder forms of the disease or to populations in which the disease is uncommon. This points out another important variable in assessing the diagnostic impact of a test, namely, that the performance of the test, in terms of its ability to predict the presence of a condition, will vary depending on the prevalence of the condition in the population under study (Bayes theorem). A clinical example will help to illustrate this point. The exercise electrocardiogram (ECG) has been applied to the study of coronary artery disease.[22] Many studies have established that the sensitivity of this test is 80 percent (0.8) and the specificity 90 percent (0.9). If we evaluate 1000 men with the clinical diagnosis of angina pectoris, studies employing coronary arteriography have documented that 90 percent of them will have coronary atherosclerosis and 10 percent will not. If we use the exercise test in this population, there would be 720 true-positive test results (900×0.8) from the group with disease and 9 false-positive test results in the group without coronary disease (100×0.9). The predictive value of an abnormal test result in this population would be high: $720/(720 + 9) = 0.98$, or 98 percent of the abnormal test results in this population, would accurately predict the presence of disease. Consider next the performance of the test in a population of 1000 healthy young men aged 30 to 40 years who are being screened for the presence of coronary artery disease. The prevalence of the disease in this population might be 10 percent; thus 900 men would be normal, and 100 would have the disease. Of these 100 patients 80 would have abnormal results on a stress test (true-positive results), but of the 900 normal young men, 90 would have abnormal test results (false-positive results). The predictive value of an abnormal test result in this group would be

$$80/(80 + 90) = 0.47$$

or 47 percent. In this population there would be more false-positive than true-positive diagnoses, and the test would give more misleading than useful information. This example points out another useful point about diagnostic testing: the test provides little useful diagnostic information when the condition under evaluation is highly prevalent or of low prevalence. In the group of patients with the clinical diagnosis of angina pectoris, the probability of disease is known to be 90 percent on the basis of the history alone; an abnormal test result does little to increase this probability. A negative test result in this group does not exclude the condition, since the test does not have perfect sensitivity. The problems with low-prevalence populations have been noted. Generally most tests have their greatest impact on diagnosis when the prevalence of the condition is intermediate (i.e., has a probability of 50 percent, a situation in which there is true diagnostic uncertainty).

Strategic Errors[12,13,20]

The first kind of strategic error is to fail to weigh the consequences of being wrong. For example, the consequences of failing to treat acute bacterial meningitis are grave. Accordingly, in a patient with fever, headache, and mental confusion one would pursue the diagnosis of meningitis with a sensitive test, such as lumbar puncture, even if there were no stiffness of the neck. Where the cost of error is high, even a slight risk of a false-negative result is unacceptable.

Another strategic error is to fail to evaluate thoroughly an important finding. For example, the failure to pursue the incidental finding of a mild microcytic anemia may jeopardize the chance of recognizing an early carcinoma of the large bowel. The obverse also represents a common strategic error, namely, the exhaustive evaluation of an isolated, nonspecific finding. This type of error is frequent when normal individuals undergo multiple screening tests that detect abnormalities of low predictive value for disease in healthy populations. It also occurs when patients are evaluated for one type of medical problem and are incidentally found to have an unrelated problem suggesting serious disease. This leads to what has been termed the "cascade effect" of medical encounters.[17] For example, an elderly patient who has been hospitalized for repair of an inguinal hernia is found to have ventricular ectopic beats on an admission ECG. This finding may lead to specialty consultation, sophisticated ambulatory ECG monitoring, stress testing, and even the introduction of potentially dangerous treatment, with delay in surgery for the simple presenting problem. Much of this may be inappropriate, since ventricular ectopy is found in many normal individuals.

A final strategic error is to act on the basis of a finding of low predictive value without establishing that a disorder is present. For example, all too frequently, patients have been told that they have "heart disease" as a result of minor changes on the ECG, when further evaluation of the finding with more specific tests might exclude this possibility.

RISK, COST, AND BENEFIT

Risk and cost relate to the *collection* of clinical information, not to the information itself. The benefits, if any, accrue from the *use* to which the information is put, not from simply possessing the information. Consideration of risk, cost, and benefit is important in determining what clinical information to collect. As will be shown, these considerations are not limited to high-risk or high-cost decisions, nor should consideration be limited to persons interested in medical ethics (risk versus benefit) or medical economics (cost versus benefit).

Benefits from clinical information may be diagnostic, therapeutic, or prognostic. Since the collection of information is almost always associated with some cost, and perhaps even some minimal risk, there is no merit in collecting a piece of clinical information if it is of no benefit to the patient.

There are three common problems concerning benefit. The first is the problem of clinical information obtained by habit. For example, there may be a reason to repeat a patient's white blood cell count, but was the differential count beneficial or was it simply requested by habit? Is 12 months the appropriate interval for "checkups" for an asymptomatic, apparently disease-free person? What information should be collected in such a checkup? Even acknowledging that sometimes it is cheaper and more efficient to collect certain information than it is to decide whether or not to obtain it, we should periodically pause to question the benefit of some of our "routine procedures."

Second, physicians sometimes fail to distinguish between clinical interest and patient benefit. It may be of considerable interest to repeat a liver biopsy in a patient with hepatitis, but the procedure is not justifiable unless the information would alter the patient's management. A good test is to ask, What will I do differently if the result is A versus B versus C? If the course of action is the same whatever the result, usually no clinical benefit is derived from the information.

Prognostic information may or may not alter the patient's management. Nevertheless, this information *is* of benefit to the patient. Indeed, patients are more concerned with prognosis than diagnosis.

This issue of clinical interest should not be confused with clinical investigation. In that latter circumstance it may be justified to obtain information that is of no benefit to that particular patient (if the legal and ethical requirements are met). The justification is

based on the fact that a nontrivial question has been asked and that the information being sought will contribute to the answer. Furthermore, the expense of the investigation is not borne by the patient but by research support.

The third problem, the notion of marginal benefit, is the most difficult. This issue arises most often in obtaining information to exclude a diagnostic possibility. Take the case of a patient in whom there is reason to suspect infective endocarditis. There is clearly potential benefit from obtaining several blood cultures. If the first five cultures are negative, what is the benefit (the marginal, or incremental, benefit) of obtaining one more? If ten are negative, what is the benefit of obtaining yet another one? Since the patient may *not* have infective endocarditis, and since in some patients *with* endocarditis the bacteria cannot be demonstrated on culture, when should one stop collecting information? Put another way, the probable benefit to be derived from additional information is steadily decreasing. Similar questions may arise when one is seeking the site of occult gastrointestinal bleeding or the primary site of a metastatic carcinoma. In each, the issue is how far to go in the face of negative results and a declining marginal benefit. In the example of suspected endocarditis, the data suggest the prudent course, but in most instances we have no data on marginal benefit.[8,19,24]

Another wasteful habit is to order or repeat tests out of frustration or to give the appearance of "doing something." This behavior commonly occurs in the setting of uncertainty about the diagnosis. When the reasonable diagnostic studies have been performed, the experienced clinician will accept this uncertainty and make his diagnostic or therapeutic decisions on the basis of the most likely possibility. When there is uncertainty and there is no likely possibility, consultation is in order.

Risk assessment in medicine is not an exact science, and the assessment of risk versus benefit, or risk/benefit ratio, is even less exact, since benefit must also be quantified. The difficulties in assessing risk are several: (1) The probability of a given untoward outcome is often not known. (2) There are difficulties in weighing the severity of unfavorable outcomes. (Which is worse, a 0.1 probability of thrombocytopenia or a 0.0001 probability of respiratory arrest?) (3) There are important variations in risk factors among different patients with different diseases. Balancing risks and benefits, although poorly understood, is generally done conscientiously and comfortably. A common shortcoming, as mentioned previously, results from undertaking procedures that have low (but not zero) risk and no benefit.

Physicians are primarily concerned with the benefits of clinical information. Although they are also concerned with the associated risks, they are often much less concerned about the costs. Concerns about costs usually focus on high-cost tests and procedures and extend to being certain that they are clinically indicated. It is appropriate that cost not be considered to be a deterrent to obtaining needed information. Nonetheless, more attention should be given to the total cost of the high-volume, low-cost tests that may be of no benefit to the patient. These are the tests and studies ordered by habit that were mentioned previously.

Finally, it is becoming clear that the resources available for medical care are limited. It is important that physicians use these resources prudently, as noted above. Furthermore, it is important that physicians recognize their role in the allocation of clinical resources, that they accept responsibility for balancing the use of clinical resources both for their individual patients and for patients collectively. If physicians do not undertake this responsibility, others, less able to make these sensitive decisions, will.

mal. The term "normal" is subject to varied interpretations.* In the context of clinical decision making, we shall define a normal finding as one that is innocuous and warrants no diagnostic or therapeutic action. An abnormal finding, then, is one that is not innocuous and may warrant action. Such evaluations of normality are not limited to comparing the patient's fasting blood glucose concentration with the "normal range" of blood glucose concentration. Historical information is similarly evaluated: How many tampons per day represent a normal menstrual flow versus menorrhagia? Similar issues are raised in assessing physical findings such as retinal arteriolar narrowing, pallor of mucous membranes, obesity, and findings that imply abnormality.

In principle, assessment of normality is straightforward. One compares the given observation in the patient with similar observations in a group of comparable persons known to be normal and free of disease. This implies that we know (1) that the persons in the normal group are normal and disease-free, (2) that they are comparable to the patient (in age, sex, ethnic origin, and the like), (3) the range of variation with the normal group, and (4) the criteria for defining abnormality.

In practice, we usually do not have valid information on these points. The control group may be a nonrandom sample of apparently healthy persons. Their age and sex distribution may not be known. The assessment of the range and limits of normality may be based on statistical assumptions that are unproved or invalid.[3]

The findings of many clinical observations are clearly either normal or abnormal, and there is no difficulty in making the decision. Although the physician's task is therefore easier, we can anticipate that better medical care and health surveillance will reduce the incidence of obvious, gross abnormalities. In some instances the patient's findings are borderline, and the aforementioned problems arise. A brief example will serve to illustrate them.

It is relatively simple to obtain an accurate measurement of a patient's body weight. Having obtained this information, how do you determine whether the patient's weight is normal? When the patient is grossly overweight, the answer is obvious and no refined comparison is needed. Indeed, one need not have weighed the patient. In less obvious cases, one must have data on the body weight of normal subjects and a criterion for abnormality.

The usual approach to this problem is to consult a table listing average weight and range by height, sex, and body build. For example, adult males with a height of 5 feet 11 inches and medium build are listed as having an average weight of 158 pounds with a normal range of 144 to 179. Thus, if the patient weighed 180 pounds, he would be evaluated as being slightly overweight. These commonly used tables, however, do not contain data obtained from surveying a sample of a normal population. They are derived from life insurance information and reflect the average body weight associated with the minimum mortality rate.[15] Ideal weights probably form a better basis for comparison than population-derived norms, because independent measures suggest that our population is overweight, i.e., population mean weights are higher than the ideal weights.

Body weight also illustrates the added information content of individual norms or individual time trends. A weight of 180 pounds today has additional meaning if the patient weighed 190 pounds 2 months ago. That is, knowing that there has been a weight gain, or loss, has greater value than knowing the weight at one point in time. The importance of time-trend information is often unappreciated. Its importance is most often neglected in the hospital setting if the physician feels driven to resolve all abnormal findings within the time constraints of a single admission.

In summary, each piece of clinical information should prompt

EVALUATION

NORMALITY

In the assessment of clinical information, the most common evaluation is to determine whether a given finding is normal or abnor-

*Murphy[18] points out that "normal serum cholesterol level" may mean (1) a bell-shaped probability distribution of cholesterol values, (2) the most representative cholesterol value as defined by a mean, (3) the most commonly encountered cholesterol values as defined by a range—the usual "laboratory normal range," (4) cholesterol values most suited for reproduction and survival, (5) cholesterol values unlikely to cause harm, (6) a committee's consensus, that is, "approved" cholesterol values, or (7) the ideal cholesterol value.

the question, Is this normal or abnormal? In making this evaluation, it is necessary to know the range observed in normal subjects and whether these subjects are comparable to the patient. Finally, additional information can be gleaned from comparisons of current and past observations in the same individual, because in many instances the variance in a given person is far less than the variance in the population, and time trends may provide added insights.

CLINICAL IMPORT

Once it has been established that a finding is abnormal, a second level of evaluation occurs almost imperceptibly. How important is this abnormal finding? Some findings are always important, that is, they require explanation. The history of hematemesis, the finding of a hard lymph node, and an elevated serum calcium concentration are always important. Other clinical information may be conditionally important. For example, the history of a nosebleed may be important in the context of a bleeding disorder but is otherwise inconsequential. Finding a broken tooth may be important in the context of a pulmonary abscess (possible aspiration) but is otherwise trivial.

Information that is either intrinsically or conditionally important must be carefully verified. Chapter 1.3 emphasizes the analysis that important clinical findings demand. When a patient states that he has been "spitting up blood," it is essential to determine whether he coughed up blood, vomited blood, or simply expectorated blood from a nosebleed.

CONVERSING WITH PATIENTS AND OBTAINING A HISTORY

GENERAL CONSIDERATIONS[1]

Vital clinical information is derived from conversation with the patient. This process, often called history taking, is not simply a question-and-answer session; it is a dialogue. The physician must listen with care to what the patient is saying, he must interpret what the patient is trying to say, and he must be attuned to what the patient does not say—topics and issues the patient avoids.

The principal complaint that patients make about "modern scientific medicine" is the failure of physicians to communicate adequately. A physician should recognize this problem and be aware that conversations with the patient can accomplish a great deal of good. Indeed, the therapeutic benefit to the patient begins with the initial interview, not with the prescribed treatment. Thus the physician should also realize that ill-conceived or misinterpreted conversations can result in great, even irreparable, harm to the patient.

Finally, not all communication is verbal. Posture, gestures, tone of voice, and facial expressions transmit powerful messages to patients. Patients and their families are carefully attentive to these aspects. Discordant verbal and nonverbal messages are interpreted as empty reassurance, bravado, insincerity, and the like.

This section is first concerned with the information-gathering aspects of conversing with patients. Finally, some of the other aspects of communicating with patients (explaining, answering questions, counseling) are discussed.

OBTAINING THE HISTORY

History taking involves several distinct elements. One aspect involves the elicitation of straightforward, factual information. For example, the physician may ask, "Does anyone in your family have diabetes?" If provision is made for further explanation of the question, the expert, the novice, or even a simple questionnaire can obtain this type of information with equal facility.

A second aspect involves branching to other questions depending on the patient's response to an earlier question. Here, one sees differences between the expert and the novice. For example, the patient who is asked whether he has headaches may reply, "Occasionally." The novice examiner may simply record "occasional headaches," but the more experienced clinician will want to explore further the nature of these headaches: Are they caused by emotional tension, hypertension, sinusitis, or brain tumor? Questions will be asked in an attempt to distinguish among these possibilities. Thus the skilled physician will analyze the historical data while acquiring them and, furthermore, will act on this analysis by asking other questions to develop the data further. The physician traverses the cycle shown in Figure 1.1–1 with each response.

A third aspect relates to the rich and relatively unstructured information about the patient's complaint, the history of the present illness. Obtaining this information embodies the elements discussed above, but it also requires flexibility, analysis, interpretation, assessment of nuances, and nonverbal communication. In these areas the expert clinician excels.

Finally, it must be emphasized that taking a history is not an isolated, circumscribed procedure. Further historical information may be gathered during the physical examination, on examining laboratory results, or later in the course of the patient's illness. For example, finding a murmur of mitral stenosis demands questioning the patient again about sore throats, manifestations of rheumatic fever, and congestive heart failure. Similarly, finding an apical infiltrate on a chest film requires reexploration of symptoms referable to tuberculosis.

Practical Considerations
Since the initial taking of a history is usually the physician's introduction to the patient, it is important that this relationship get off to a good start. Some practical considerations to successful history taking are described in the following paragraphs.

1. Make the patient comfortable, both physically and mentally. A few moments spent in friendly conversation will allow the patient to settle down before proceeding to the business at hand. Furthermore, the physician gains insight into the patient's social, occupational, and physical environment.
2. Make certain the patient knows who you are and understands your role in his care. With team approaches to patient care there is increasing opportunity for confusion, which leads to uncertainty and resentment.
3. Make certain that there is good two-way communication. Patients who are elderly, who are not facile in English, or who have impaired vision or hearing may not acknowledge their difficulties in understanding the physician.
4. In general, interview the patient alone. At times, a parent or spouse may insist on being present. Try to avoid this, but do not force the issue against strong opposition. On the other hand, family members may be a source of valuable information, which should be sought at an appropriate time. This is obvious when the patient is unable to communicate adequately because of the nature of his illness or its severity. In other instances the family may possess information not known by the patient or that the patient is unwilling to disclose (e.g., failure to take prescribed medications, personality deterioration, change in appearance, or alcoholism). Finally, family discussions give insight into the strength of the family support during illness and convalescence.
5. Give the patient the conviction that he has a warm and understanding listener and adequate time in which to tell his whole story. The patient must feel that the physician has no distracting concerns or commitments. Avoid writing detailed notes while the patient is talking. The atmosphere should be one of thoughtful conversation, not the dictation of a diary.
6. Meaningful questions cannot be asked without an understanding of the general nature of the patient's problem.

Hence, at the outset afford the patient enough time to express in his own terms, without interruption, his basic reasons for visiting you. Otherwise, questioning of the patient may be routine, haphazard, and unrevealing.

7. The sequence in which the history is obtained is dictated by the specific circumstances. Thus, if the patient is severely ill, infirm, or emotionally upset, it is wise to inquire about the present illness before reviewing the past health and the family history. Since the patient is most interested in his current problem, beginning the sequence with the present illness is generally preferable.

8. Assure the patient that you appreciate that he may have forgotten much of his past history but not to be concerned if he has. This is of particular importance when one is talking to elderly patients who may feel inadequate and embarrassed by their difficulties with memory.

9. Encourage the patient to use his own words and not simply to recite diagnoses and interpretations of other physicians.

10. Never make the patient feel inadequate, dull, or distraught. If a particular line of questioning makes the patient embarrassed or anxious, move on to another topic without pressing too far at the time of the initial encounter. However, it is wise to explore that topic later, once rapport has been established, because such behavior may indicate that significant information lies in that area.

11. Do not spend so much time and effort extracting specific details about less consequential points in the history that the patient's temper and the physician's energies are exhausted before the crucial items are reached.

12. As a corollary, do not let the patient's narrative bog down in needless detail or drift off into irrelevancies. The reminder must be gentle, "I believe you were telling me about . . ." lest the patient feel he has been chastised.

13. The patient must be requestioned as the illness proceeds and new information evolves. Neglect of this important point is a common cause of failure to make a correct diagnosis. Requestioning may also be necessary because the patient is too ill, tired, confused, or frightened at the time of the initial interview. This is particularly important in the care of elderly persons.

Begin at the Beginning

It is essential to delineate the exact manner in which the illness began. What were the precise circumstances of its onset? Where was the patient? What was he doing? One must be certain that the patient is actually starting his story at the beginning. Patients often date the onset of their illness by some dramatic occurrence, forgetting to mention the events that led up to it. These are frequently highly significant. Thus the insidious onset of fatigue and mild weight loss may give important insight into the nature of an acute upper abdominal pain that started 6 months later. The physician must push the patient's recall back to the earliest beginnings of his illness. It may be helpful to ask, Are you certain your health was entirely normal before this particular symptom began? Often a reference to a date or season will prompt recollection. For example, one might ask, Were you feeling perfectly well last Christmas?

Chronic, Recurrent Illness

When dealing with a complicated illness in which the basic pattern is recurrence of episodes of similar manifestations (e.g., fever and joint pains), one should acquire a detailed account of typical episodes. Often the initial and the most recent episodes are the most revealing and give insight into changes that may have occurred over time.

Importance of Details

Patients sometimes tell small details about their illnesses that are disregarded by the physician because at the time they do not seem pertinent to the rest of the story. For example, a patient insisted that he got chills, fever, and jaundice each time he took a cathartic,

and only then. This detail did not make much sense and was ignored. Search for the usual causes of intermittent fever were unrevealing until the patient was given a cathartic and subsequently developed a temperature of 105F, chills, and jaundice. He was later found to have diverticulitis of the colon with abscess formation. Cathartics precipitated acute episodes by showering his liver with septic emboli.

Avoid Bias

In taking a medical history, the physician must weigh and analyze the information as it is being acquired. As mentioned before, this formulation and testing of hypotheses as to what may be the cause of the patient's illness is a major element in the gathering of meaningful information. The physician must exercise self-discipline, however, to avoid bias or, at least, recognize bias. The physician must not disregard or ignore information that does not fit with a current hypothesis under consideration. Furthermore, one should not ask leading questions in a manner that makes it difficult for the patient to disagree: You do find that greasy foods give you indigestion, don't you? The history should be an unbiased statement of *all* the facts presented by the patient.

Be Critical

Do not accept uncritically such expressions as "arthritis," "eczema," "pneumonia," or "indigestion." An episode of "pneumonia" may, in reality, have been a pulmonary infarction, or "indigestion" may have been coronary insufficiency. Acquire the details and interpret the facts. Do not simply record the patient's own diagnosis; do not be biased by other physicians' diagnoses. Conservative skepticism is a desirable trait.

Similarly, be cautious in evaluating such major symptoms as fever, weight loss, hemoptysis, hematemesis, black stools, chills, convulsions, hematuria, pain, and lapse of consciousness. These often herald serious underlying disease and demand explanation.

Quantify Symptoms

Whenever possible, have the patient quantify the symptoms in simple terms. Thus sputum production can be expressed in terms of cups, diarrhea in number of stools, dyspnea in flights of stairs, and orthopnea in number of pillows required for comfort in sleeping. Such manifestations take on increased significance when thus quantified.

Environmental Factors

Inquire whether the present illness was associated with alterations in the patient's environment. This could include any incident, such as going on a picnic in the country or getting a job in a chemical plant. Has anyone or anything (such as a dog or a pet bird) in the patient's home or work environment been ill recently? Have any of the patient's relatives ever had a similar illness?

Drugs

If possible, list all drugs the patient may have been taking, with the approximate dates on which they were administered. Describe any untoward reactions that the patient may have had to these agents. Delineate what effect, if any, they may have had on the manifestations of the illness. Thus, in the differential diagnosis of acute polyarthritis, it is important to know that adequate salicylate therapy failed to affect the degree of joint involvement.

It is often difficult to get an accurate history of drug usage, even when a drug reaction is suspected. Patients often regard as "drugs" only those medications that are expensive, prescribed, or given by injection. They may not realize that you want to know about *all* tablets, capsules, pills, and liquids. Commonly overlooked but potentially important agents are sedatives, laxatives, tonics, "nerve medicines," "vitamins," birth control pills, and menstrual cramp remedies. It is useful to ask the patient to bring in all drugs and medications being taken.

In addition to medicinal agents, it is important to inquire about the use of other drugs, specifically alcohol, caffeine, nico-

tine, and recreational drugs. Alcohol plays an important role in many diseases. Since patients characteristically underreport their use of this drug, it is important to ask specific questions about quantities consumed. Patients may report that they have two drinks each night before dinner, failing to mention that each drink contains 4 ounces of liquor and is followed by wine and after-dinner drinks. Alcoholism is often an occult condition not readily recognized by the patient. Sometimes the clues uncovered only lead to the suspicion of excessive alcohol consumption. These clues include deterioration in job performance, frequent missed days from work for minor illness, marital or family discord, sloppy appearance, repeated involvement in traffic accidents, social withdrawal, depression, obesity, or impotence. Other family members may provide important insights into drinking habits (see Chapter 17.5). Caffeine, which is a constituent of many commonly ingested substances such as chocolate and cola drinks as well as coffee or tea, may be ingested in large quantities and produce symptoms such as tremor, panic reactions, and palpitations. The use of drugs such as cocaine and marijuana and of injected agents such as heroin is increasing in our society, and the medical consequences may be serious. Patients will not often admit to the use of these agents unless they are reassured that the physician is in a supportive, not an antagonistic or accusatory, role (see Chapter 16.9).

Other Information Sources

Valuable information contained in the records of previous hospitalizations is often allowed to lie fallow. A telephone call to a former physician, hospital history department, or corner drugstore may answer a perplexing question. Thus finding a coin lesion on a 10-year-old chest film may be the deciding factor in excluding cancer as its cause. A patient suspected of having ingested poison may be found, when the druggist is called, to have taken a harmless substance. Failure to explore these ancillary sources of information is a common and serious shortcoming. Time spent in pursuit of such information is often rewarded many times over.

Evaluate the Person

It is as important to understand the person afflicted by the disease as it is to understand the disease afflicting the person. Information about both are obtained at the same time. The patient's attitude, demeanor, and appearance all give the perceptive physician insights into the patient, as does the way in which the patient relates to the physician.

The patient should be given an opportunity to discuss the way in which the illness has affected him. This allows the physician to evaluate the patient's reaction to the illness. Direct questions may be helpful: "How has all this affected you—your family, your job, your finances, your pursuit of pleasures?" "Has this illness gotten you down?"

It is also important to explore the patient's perception of his illness: What do you make of this? What do you think is wrong? Do you feel you are getting better or worse? What is especially worrisome to you? Often the physician is surprised to learn of the patient's misapprehensions. For example, it is important to know whether a worried patient with back pain is concerned about having cancer or about losing his job.

Only if the physician understands the patient can effective treatment be given. In this regard, empathy is a useful diagnostic tool: by putting oneself in the patient's position, one can be guided to areas that are of concern to the patient. The physician needs to know much about both the personal habits and the personal relationships of the patient, since relationships may be a source of either support or stress, and habits, such as dietary, recreational, and sleep habits, as well as matters related to sexual function, greatly affect health. For example, homosexuality must be dealt with in a straightforward, nonjudgmental fashion. Learning that a patient is homosexual opens up a wide array of diagnostic possibilities, mostly related to AIDS, which might not be considered in the heterosexual patient.

Encourage Communication

At the conclusion of the interview, it is helpful to say in an unhurried way, "Is there anything more you want to tell me—about anything at all?" Explain to the patient that you hope he will regard your office as a place to feel free to discuss fully any and all matters that may be causing concern.

The Value of the History

The harried physician may be tempted to take shortcuts in eliciting a history, perhaps feeling that the limited time might better be spent in physical examination or in the selection of laboratory studies. Objective analysis, however, shows the history to be the linchpin of the diagnostic process. Essential information lost from the history often cannot be recovered through other studies. Indeed the entire diagnostic process may proceed down the wrong path.

PAIN AS A SYMPTOM

Pain merits special consideration because it is frequently the predominant or only clinical manifestation of a wide variety of disease processes. Pain illustrates the proper analysis of an aspect of the patient's history because, being a subjective manifestation of disease, it can be evaluated only through careful questioning of the patient. Carefully assessed, it stands preeminent among the manifestations of disease that lead to a correct diagnosis.

Clinical Aspects

Several types of pain can be distinguished clinically. Superficial pain derived from injury to skin and superficial somatic structures has two components. There is the sharp, pricking sensation that elicits a startle response, withdrawal, and tachycardia. The second, slower, aching component may persist for extended periods after the initial injury. These pains are felt superficially and can be localized with precision. In most instances the lesion producing the superficial pain is readily apparent. There are, however, two general exceptions. The first is pain caused by nerve or nerve root involvement, such as arm pain with cervical disc disease. The second is superficial pain referred from a deeper structure, such as wrist pain as a manifestation of angina pectoris.

Visceral pain is dull or aching; it is associated with quiescence, slowing of the pulse, often with some fall in blood pressure, and sweating and nausea. This last manifestation is responsible for the common designation of "sickening" when referring to deep pain. These vasovagal responses may be associated with all of the major visceral pain syndromes (angina pectoris; biliary, renal, and bowel colic; bladder pain; pancreatitis; peptic ulcer), especially when the pain is severe. These responses can also occur with injury to muscle, fascia, periosteum, or arteries.

Deep pain is often poorly localized and is felt to arise from an area beneath the surface rather than from a point. Vague localization and misleading referral of deep pain are two important problems in analyzing pain. For example, diaphragmatic peritonitis produces pain referred to the shoulder.

Factors that alter pain perception are of clinical importance. It is clear that in the heat of an athletic event or of physical combat, a serious injury may be sustained without experiencing any pain whatsoever. Pain may not be perceived until the danger and excitement are over. In contrast, fear, anxiety, and apprehension all serve to heighten the perception of pain. These factors are of importance not only in evaluating pain but also in alleviating pain. A different phenomenon is exhibited by patients with frontal lobe lesions. They perceive the pain, but it induces no emotional response. In contrast, there are some patients who hyperreact to pain.

Pain should always be methodically analyzed as follows: localization, radiation, character, exacerbating and ameliorating factors, associated phenomena, and time relationships. These will be discussed in turn.

Sequential Steps in the Analysis of Pain

Localization. It is essential that the patient localize the point of origin of his discomfort as precisely as possible. The localization of pain is usually obvious when the lesion is superficial, but with deep pain the patient may confuse the area of radiation with its point of origin and hence mislead the physician. It is best to request that the patient indicate with his index finger the area from which the discomfort seems to stem, and then to indicate the extent of diffusion of the pain around this point. Ask the patient to describe the depth at which the pain seems to be located. The pattern in which pain arises from any given structure may be extremely variable. Thus the pain of angina pectoris may be felt substernally, in the interscapular area, in the shoulder, down the arms, in the wrist or fingers, or in the neck or jaw.

Radiation. It is also imperative that the patient trace with his finger the pattern of radiation of his distress in response to the question, "Where does your pain move?" It should be emphasized again that, when the point of origin of the pain is silent, the area of radiation may be assumed to be the site of origin. For example, angina pectoris may be present only as a peculiar sensation felt in the left hand when the patient hurries for the bus, or a peptic ulcer may be mistaken for an orthopedic condition because the patient has recurrent severe pain in the midportion of the back.

Character. Questions to elicit information about pain must be carefully phrased. Patients are frequently unfamiliar with pain as an experience in life, and their concept of what the word "pain" connotes may be limited. To some it may simply mean the sensation they had when they slammed a door on a finger or when they burned themselves in the kitchen. Many patients, therefore, will not be aware that they are experiencing what the physician calls pain. It is well to avoid use of the narrow question "Do you have pain?" and to employ broader expressions such as "distress," "discomfort," or "unpleasant feelings." Some patients, for a variety of personal reasons, such as fear, shame, or denial, will conceal their true symptoms.

In describing the quality of a pain, the patient's choice of words will be colored by both his vocabulary and his interpretation of what is happening. However, there are certain basic characteristics that may serve to guide the physician in his effort to identify the source of pain. For example, anginal pain may be described as "crushing," "squeezing," "burning," "searing," "tight," "constricting," "heavy," or "cutting off of breath," but basically it has a midline component and is steady, without appreciable fluctuation. The nonverbal gesture of the fist clenched over the sternum is a classic accompaniment of the description. The pain of a peptic ulcer may be "gnawing," "burning," "eating," "hungry," "tightfisted," or "like a dull toothache," but it is also steady and is localized below the surface of the abdomen. "Bloated," "distended," or "dyspeptic" feelings are the hallmarks of gallbladder disease. The pain of gallstones or of renal colic is paroxysmal in its degree of severity, but it also has a steady component, in contrast to the truly colicky pain associated with obstruction of a hollow viscus such as the gut. Specific questioning may be required to bring out the fact that the patient is having true colic: Does it grab and let go intermittently? Is it like the sensation you have when you urgently need to move your bowels but are unable to do so? A tearing pain may be described by the patient with a dissecting aneurysm. A throbbing pain suggests that arterial pulsation is an important factor, whereas a sharp, burning, transitory pain is more characteristic of a nerve root origin.

Precipitating and Aggravating Factors. Extract from the patient a detailed description of the exact setting in which his pain occurs. A general description will not suffice. The particulars of the story frequently supply the key. Precisely what was the patient doing when the pain began? What were the specific circumstances surrounding the occurrence of the pain? What factors seem to precipitate or exaggerate the pain? Is it affected by activity, coughing, breathing, eating, or time of day? If the pain is episodic, ask the patient to describe a typical "spell" in full detail.

Lack of clear-cut answers to this kind of probing is sometimes an indication of functional illness, although one has to be careful, since some important organic diseases may be characterized initially by a vague discomfort that is hard to put into words. Carcinomatosis, for example, frequently presents such symptoms.

Factors Bringing Relief. Again, the physician must insist on a complete listing of all factors that seem to diminish the discomfort. These factors generally will have to be suggested to the patient by the physician, so that no important categories are omitted.

One cannot discount any of the factors that the patient claims play a role in his discomfort, even though they may sound inconsequential or even bizarre. The diagnosis may be overlooked if the physician concludes that what the patient says does not make sense. The key to the diagnosis may be contained in the very peculiarity of the patient's story. It is prudent to accept the patient's story at face value. It is an error to censor the patient's account to accommodate one's own thinking.

To evaluate the character of a patient's pain and related changes, the observer must be familiar with whatever medications the patient has been receiving. Drugs may ameliorate or alter the key symptoms or manifestations of an illness. Thus morphine may profoundly change the pain and muscle spasm associated with a ruptured appendix. Drugs may also induce symptoms or changes that have nothing to do with the underlying disease process. For example, the development of polyarthritis after acute tonsilitis may suggest rheumatic fever, when it is, in fact, caused by allergy to the penicillin used to treat the tonsillitis.

Dependency on drugs of various sorts may significantly color the patient's description of symptoms and make the differential diagnosis of chronic or recurrent discomfort particularly difficult.

Associated Phenomena. In this category are included all of the clinical manifestations associated with the patient's pain, such as anxiety, dyspnea, sweating, nausea, and vomiting. The physician must insist on an unabridged listing and must act as a prompter.

Time Relationships. The average duration of discomfort has great significance in understanding its source. The pain of angina pectoris lasts for only a few minutes and is relieved by the immobility that it imposes on the patient. The intermittent pain of intestinal colic and its causative peristaltic overactivity lasts only a few seconds. On the other hand, the discomfort of a peptic ulcer may last an hour or more, unless some food or an alkali is taken.

The frequency and specific time at which a pain occurs are also of importance. Epigastric pain that occurs daily with a constant relationship to meals is characteristic of a peptic ulcer, whereas the pain of gallbladder disease comes at unexpected times and is independent of eating or exercise. The pain of osteoarthritis may be most severe during the period of early activity after a night's sleep. Peptic ulceration is one of the few conditions that cause chronic, recurrent abdominal discomfort at night. Nocturnal intensification of skeletal pain is frequently observed in metastatic carcinoma, and repetitive episodes of chest discomfort at night suggest angina decubitus or hiatal hernia. Environmental factors, at home or on the job, should be investigated because of the role they often play.

It is helpful to ask, "Have you ever previously had a pain at all similar to this one?" Patients have a way of describing an episode of pain as a unique experience. The physician is thus misled into thinking it is an acute and newly formed process, only to discover to his chagrin that this illness can be traced to one of several similar episodes dating back many years. Since the knowledge that an episode of pain is part of a recurrent process vitally affects one's thinking about the nature of the pain, this point must be pursued forcefully.

OTHER COMMUNICATION

To this point, emphasis has been on obtaining information *from* patients. Of equal importance is the ability to impart information *to* patients. This is fundamental to obtaining the patient's confidence and cooperation in both diagnostic and therapeutic management. It is a key element in fostering patient satisfaction. Certain features involving both the special nature of the physician-patient relationship and the special attitudes of people who are sick merit discussion.

Stated negatively, poor communication between physician and patient is an important cause of the increasing frequency of malpractice suits. The physician who makes hurried explanations is often assumed to be making hurried judgments. Failure to understand and cope with a patient's unrealistic expectations can lead to disappointment, anger, and litigation even when the outcome is as good as could reasonably be expected. Hasty dismissal of realistic patient concerns by hearty and unwarranted reassurances can lead to the development of unrealistic expectations.

Physicians must be aware of the nature of the psychologic relationship that usually exists between patient and doctor. The patient expects to be able to trust and believe in his physician. Frequently, this belief and trust is amazingly uncritical and naive. What the physician says is regarded as infallible, even though the patient may actually know very little about his physician's professional qualifications.

Conversely, patients can lack confidence and trust in a physician over aspects that are unrelated to professional competence. For example, the physician's attire or demeanor may not fit with the patient's expectations of how a physician should dress or act. Physicians who choose to ignore such expectations are no less competent clinicians, but they do create problems for themselves in establishing the mutual trust that is so important.

Thus, in conversing with patients, the physician can be guided by certain general principles:

1. Avoid careless, haphazard conversation and give considered thought to everything the patient is told. The passing mention that the patient has a slight heart murmur serves no useful purpose and will likely produce needless worry.
2. At the outset, assay the intellectual, emotional, and social capacities of the patient and pitch the content of the conversation accordingly. It is important to avoid a patronizing air, whatever the patient's intellectual level.
3. Be certain you understand the patient's question and its implications to him before attempting to answer. For example, an ulcer patient may ask, Why am I still having pain? He may not be interested in an explanation of the pathophysiology but may really be asking, Does this pain mean that my ulcer is not healing, or do I have cancer?
4. Employ simple expressions that are easily understood. Terms that are often misinterpreted are "tumor" (interpreted as cancer), "functional" (malingering), "chronic" (hopeless), and "nervous" (psychotic).
5. Never frighten the patient, but foster optimism, self-confidence, and security. Not frightening the patient does not mean that he is to be misled, because only the truth will sustain the patient's faith. He should be told the truth, however, in a manner that creates understanding of his problem, dissipates fear, and leads to confidence in the future. Sometimes it is the physician's responsibility to soften the truth to accomplish these goals.
6. Be aware of your own anxieties and biases and adjust accordingly. Physicians have important emotional needs. These should not, however, be allowed to have an adverse effect on the attention given to the patient's needs.
7. By thoughtfulness, thoroughness, and personal dignity, increase the patient's confidence.

OUTLINE OF THE HISTORY

It is essential that the physician have a firmly established habit pattern in what has been described as the fact-gathering aspect of history taking. This includes the family history, the history of past illnesses, the review of systems, and personal and social matters. The advantages of a rote pattern are (1) that no intellectual effort is devoted to what topic is next, so that full attention can be devoted to interpreting the meaning of each response and (2) that it is much less likely for a topic to be overlooked.

A variety of outlines or formats for recording the patient's history are available. There may be personal or institutional preferences for one or another. It is essential, however, to adopt one format and adhere to it until it becomes a habit.

THE PHYSICAL EXAMINATION

Some aspects of a patient's illness are revealed only by physical examination.[1,23] Inadequacies in the appraisal of these aspects cannot be corrected by excellence in taking and evaluating the history or by generous selection of laboratory studies.

Physical examination is often considered only as an initial appraisal of the patient; however, the other areas in which it provides essential information should also be recognized. In the diagnostic process (see Chapter 1.3) it is important that the patient be reexamined periodically. New signs may have developed, or physical signs may be sought and discovered on the basis of ancillary findings. Furthermore, changes in physical signs may provide crucial information on the course of the illness or on the patient's response to therapy. It is essential, therefore, to consider the physical examination as a continuing, dynamic process that is carried out, not at just one point in time, but throughout the period of observation of the patient.

Proficiency in physical examination depends on three related factors:

1. Thoroughness in the routine examination
2. Skill in techniques of physical examination
3. Understanding of the sequential logic used in the examining process

The importance of thoroughness is obvious. For example, unless the skin is carefully inspected, the physician will not discover a melanoma on the patient's back. Similarly, the physician who does not have sufficient skill in auscultation will miss the diastolic rumble of mitral stenosis.

The importance of the third factor, understanding the logic involved, is more subtle. A novice may be as thorough as an expert on routine examination, and as skilled in techniques of examination, but he may be unable to extract as much information from a physical examination as the expert can. The proficiency of the expert is related to his ability to branch out from his routine examination. This branching out is similar to that described in history taking. For example, on finding signs of pulmonary consolidation, the expert will consider the possibility of pulmonary infarction and will measure and compare the circumferences of the patient's legs. These actions are based in part on greater experience and in part on the habit of analyzing the meaning of each physical finding and searching for other findings that may be related.

This section is designed to supplement and extend, rather than to supplant, standard texts on physical diagnosis. In keeping with the format of this book, much of the specific information on physical signs and their interpretation is presented in relation to the relevant clinical problem. The areas to be emphasized here are (1) the thorough examination, (2) the practical considerations in examining patients, and, finally (3) the sequential logic used in physical examination.

THE THOROUGH EXAMINATION

There is often confusion between thoroughness and completeness. It is neither possible nor desirable to perform a complete examination. A succession splash need not be sought in every patient, nor should every patient be subjected to caloric vestibular stimulation. However, there are occasions when it is essential to branch off the mainstream of the examination into a special routine. It may be important in one of these special routines to listen for a bruit over the popliteal artery or, in another, to perform vestibular stimulation tests. The recognition of these occasions will be discussed in a later section.

The thorough routine examination contains certain elements that should never be omitted. They are discussed below. The necessity for diligence in performing these examinations is illustrated by the case of a woman whose chills, fever, and lung abscesses were a diagnostic problem until a pelvic examination (deferred because she was "too sick") was performed. Examination revealed a soft cervix and a boggy, tender uterus. On further questioning she acknowledged having induced an abortion. Pelvic thrombophlebitis was producing septic emboli. Although thoroughness is important in all areas, there are some in which it is essential.

Areas in Which Physical Examination Is Indispensable

As mentioned initially, there are abnormalities that, if missed, can never come to the physician's attention. As a consequence, the physician must exercise particular diligence in performing these portions of the examination. For example, a testicular nodule will not be revealed except by careful palpation, whereas a routine chest radiograph will readily reveal cardiac enlargement. Nevertheless, some physicians will, in error, examine the genitalia in a cursory fashion but percuss the heart borders with meticulous care.

Table 1.2–2 lists some of the physical findings that provide information not obtained by other means. A few of those meriting special attention are discussed in more detail.

Of equal importance is the realization that physical examination has certain shortcomings. For example, when a mediastinal mass is suspected on the basis of venous congestion limited to the head and arms, the physician should percuss the width of the mediastinum but should not rely on negative findings. He should obtain radiographic studies, because only the largest lesions can be detected by percussion. Table 1.2–3 lists the areas in which other techniques should be employed to supplement physical examination.

Severity of Illness. The most important single observation to make about a patient is the severity of his illness, because the answer often indicates what must be done for the patient, and how rapidly. In a sense, this is an interpretation, a judgment, rather than an observation. Yet some patients who are only slightly pallid, slightly restless, and slightly sweaty appear severely ill to the experi-

TABLE 1.2–3. FINDINGS BEST DEFINED BY TECHNIQUES OTHER THAN PHYSICAL EXAMINATION

- Masses (pulmonary, mediastinal, retroperitoneal, intracranial, nasopharyngeal, intrahepatic)
- Intraocular pressure, visual fields
- Cardiac size
- Cardiac arrhythmias
- Lesions within the gastrointestinal tract
- Diminished alveolar ventilation

enced observer. The ability to recognize this poorly defined picture of severe illness comes largely with experience. It is, however, good practice to ask oneself at the outset of the examination: How sick is this patient?

Fortunately for the less experienced observer, severe illness is often accompanied by alterations in the vital signs: temperature, pulse rate, respiratory rate, and blood pressure. Certain pitfalls should be kept in mind when considering the vital signs. Oral temperatures may be erroneously low with mouth breathing, drinking of cool liquids, and shock. An elevated thermometer reading in the presence of a cool skin may indicate failure to shake down the thermometer, fever together with shock, or factitious fever. Errors in peripheral pulse rate measurements often arise in tachyarrhythmias in which each heartbeat does not produce a systolic ejection. Respiratory rate measurement may be inaccurate, especially in periodic breathing. Furthermore, a normal rate need not indicate adequate ventilation. A previously hypertensive patient with shock may have normal blood pressure, and there may be variation in the blood pressure in the limbs with coarctation or dissecting aneurysm of the aorta.

Some additional findings should alert the physician to the urgency of the problem (Table 1.2–4). Some of these manifestations may be produced by less ominous causes, such as increased intracranial pressure caused by pseudotumor cerebri, but the findings must be taken seriously until it is proved that the condition is benign.

General Observation. Apart from indicating the severity of the patient's illness, the general appearance of the patient gives information about his personality, distress, and reaction to his disease. This information can be obtained only by observation; yet all too often the physician pushes ahead with the specific aspects of physical examination without stopping to ask, "Is there anything unusual about this patient's attitude, mental status, appearance, or body build?"

Certain precise information about the nature of the patient's distress can best be obtained by careful evaluation of dyspnea, evident pain, or tenderness. For example, rapid, deep respiration sug-

TABLE 1.2–2. FINDINGS BEST DEFINED BY PHYSICAL EXAMINATION

- Vital signs (temperature, pulse rate, respiratory rate, blood pressure)
- Evidence of severity of illness
- General appearance (including mental status)
- Visible lesions (including integument, eyes and fundi, ears, nose, throat, joints)
- Palpable lesions (including masses, local tenderness, deformities, pulsations or their absence, genitalia)
- Respiratory difficulty (including signs of obstruction, weakness, splinting, cyanosis)
- Murmurs, bruits, friction rubs, and bowel sounds
- Neurologic signs

TABLE 1.2–4. COMMON SIGNS OF SEVERE ILLNESS

- Excessively high or low temperature
- Excessively high or low pulse rate
- Excessively high or low respiratory rate
- Excessively high or low blood pressure
- Altered state of consciousness (anxiety, lethargy, confusion, delirium, coma)
- Respiratory distress (noisy, labored, or ineffective)
- Central cyanosis
- Profuse sweating
- Evidence of intense pain
- Signs of pulmonary edema
- Signs of increased intracranial pressure
- Nuchal rigidity

gests acidosis, whereas labored respiration with crowing inspiration suggests large-airway obstruction as the cause of dyspnea.

General observation may cast doubt on the history. A stoic may deny exertional dyspnea while observation reveals that the effort of getting undressed produces panting. Conversely, claims of disability from back pain may be questioned if the patient bends to tie his shoes without difficulty.

The patient's position may be of diagnostic significance. Pericarditis is suggested if the patient finds relief of chest pain by sitting up and leaning forward; psoas irritation may be present if he lies with his hip flexed to relieve pain.

Changes in facial appearance may give early clues in the diagnosis of such diverse entities as myxedema, hyperthyroidism, parkinsonism, and depression. Furthermore, the body habitus may suggest one or another heritable disorder, such as the long limbs of S-S hemoglobinopathy or Marfan syndrome. Personal appearance may be important. For example, a slovenly appearance may indicate that the patient has had some deterioration of his intellectual faculties or he is too sick to care about his appearance. Similarly, general observation of the environment may be helpful. Is the room neat? Are the relatives attentive, anxious, or indifferent?

PRACTICAL CONSIDERATIONS

Thus far, attention has been directed toward the principles that should guide the physician in performing the physical examination. A number of practical matters are equally important to the success of the examination.

Be Systematic
There is a need to be systematic in the usual sequence of procedures performed in the routine physical examination. Although there is no "best" order in which to perform the examination, an orderly sequence is essential to prevent inadvertent omissions. One such sequence, developed by Hillman and Funk,[10] is listed on pages 16 to 18. It was developed to maximize efficiency.

It is likewise essential that the physician be systematic and consistent in recording physical findings. It is clear that the optimal order for *performing* the elements of a physical examination does not coincide with the most logical order for *recording* these findings.

Be Considerate
The physician should always pay heed to the patient's modesty and need for privacy. He should make the patient as comfortable as possible; the thoughtless application of cold hands or of a cold stethoscope can damage the doctor-patient relationship. Care should be taken in palpating tender areas; the rough and heavy-handed palpation of a tender abdomen may induce such guarding that important findings are missed. Thus it is better to start palpating in a nontender area and to be as gentle as possible.

The Environment
The environment in which the patient is examined should be quiet and well lighted, preferably by daylight. The physician should neither stand in his own light nor face the glare. The examining area should be free of distractions and interruptions. All of the patient's clothing should be removed and replaced by a drape or gown. Nothing deters thoroughness so much as attempting to examine over and around undergarments.

Observe Quantitatively
Both in observing and in recording observations, the physician should be quantitative. The descent of the liver edge should be measured in centimeters, not fingerbreadths; masses should be measured, rather than described in terms of fruit, eggs, golf balls, or baseballs.

Be Objective
It is important that the physician think of the abnormal physical finding in terms of the objective observation, not in terms of an interpretation of these observations or in terms of the diagnosis derived therefrom. It is acceptable to think of a stuporous patient as smelling uremic if he, in fact, has uremia. However, if the uriniferous odor is due to incontinence and the patient is actually hypoglycemic, the physician may have started down an erroneous path through imprecise thinking.

Such imprecise thinking often leads to erroneous conclusions. For example, a 60-year-old man was seen because of progressive weakness and weight loss. The initial examiner found pallor and an enlarged spleen. After initial studies for causes of splenomegaly and anemia were unproductive, a consultant demonstrated that both the upper and the lower border of the "spleen" could be demarcated. The initial observer had lost his objectivity by palpating the left upper quadrant in search of splenomegaly and "finding" it. The consultant recognized a left upper quadrant mass and went on to determine whether it was the spleen or not. In this case the mass was found to be a carcinoma of the splenic flexure of the colon.

Use Flexible Norms
A liver edge felt 5 cm below the costal margin in a patient with emphysema and low diaphragms would be regarded as normal, whereas the same finding in a young adult would be distinctly abnormal. Similarly, the experienced examiner realizes that lymph nodes are easily felt in thin patients and in children. Thus the physician must constantly adjust examining standards to the situation at hand.

This flexibility does not imply a permissive attitude toward the significance of slight abnormalities. The small mass in the breast is not trivial; the faint, diastolic, decrescendo, blowing murmur along the left sternal border is not insignificant.

THE SEQUENTIAL LOGIC USED IN PHYSICAL EXAMINATION

Definition
The logical process that the physician follows in examining a patient involves not only performing the thorough, routine examination but also recognizing when and how to branch out from this routine.

Importance
Despite the recognized importance of the physical examination, the examination process is much misunderstood by students and physicians alike. Most of this misunderstanding arises from the disparity between what the physician believes he does (and seems to do) and what he does in fact. Students, for example, are puzzled that experienced physicians can discover more abnormalities than the students can when both use the same techniques and apparently follow the same format in examining a given patient. Physicians themselves are not always consciously aware of the process by which they achieve their success. They are puzzled by the student's failure to observe the palmar erythema in the alcoholic patient or to elicit the plastic rigidity in the patient with early parkinsonism. Analysis of this process makes it apparent that the novice and the expert do *not* follow the same format in examining a patient. Appreciation of these differences is helpful in guiding the novice toward success and in encouraging the expert to improve his expertise.

Example
The basic difference between the novice and the expert is that the expert branches off from his routine, often quite unconsciously, during the course of his routine examination. When, for example, the examination has reached the point where the skin is being inspected, a specific question is asked: Is the color normal? If the

answer is yes, the physician proceeds to the next question: Is the skin free of lesions? If the answer is no, the physician's mental questioning follows another branch, one that pursues the nature of the color change (Fig. 1.2–1).

In this example, jaundice is the first condition considered as a cause of the yellowish brown discoloration. If jaundice seems likely, the expert consciously or unconsciously enters his "jaundice routine." The novice, on the other hand, simply proceeds to the next major question.

In his jaundice routine, the expert first verifies his observation by looking for scleral icterus. He next considers possible causes for jaundice, prompting him to look for excoriations that may indicate the itching of obstructive jaundice. He seeks evidence of cirrhosis. He may revert to the history to ask about drugs or to inquire in further detail about alcohol intake. He thinks ahead and will be certain to note a Kayser-Fleischer ring or splenomegaly, if present. He makes a mental note to determine urine bilirubin and urobilinogen values on completion of his examination.

To the bystander, the novice and the expert performed an identical physical examination. Yet the expert would note the xanthomas about the patient's ankles, and the novice might miss them. The expert would then be certain the patient had chronic obstructive jaundice, whereas the novice would know only that the patient was jaundiced.

Knowledge of Special Routines

With increasing experience and increasing knowledge of medicine, the physician develops an increasing repertoire of special routines. He comes to know what other information to seek when he encounters unequal pupils, a prominent venous pattern over the abdomen, a narrow pulse pressure, or an absent apical impulse. Although the experienced physician employs these techniques unconsciously, the novice can improve his ability to examine patients by consciously considering the diagnostic implication of each abnormality that he finds in his routine examination.

It is clear, then, that the novice cannot "learn" these special routines, because they encompass all of medicine. One can learn, however, to be alert to the clues that indicate the need for further investigation.

INDICATIONS FOR A SPECIAL ROUTINE

Jaundice has already been cited as an example of an abnormality that prompts the experienced examiner to modify his basic examination to ensure full exploration of this finding. He should not perform his usual physical examination and *then* review the abnormal findings. He should consider the implications of any abnormalities *while* performing the examination. The perceptive examiner, then, is one who is alert to signals that he should branch off from his usual routine. These signals may arise from the history, from other physical findings, from the results of laboratory studies, from the differential diagnosis, or even from knowledge of the primary diagnosis. Illustrative examples of each are given.

History

Any part of the history may provide clues that alert the physician to devote extra attention to various portions of the examination. For example, a complaint of left pleuritic pain will alert the physician to palpate and compress each rib in search of a fracture, as well as to listen carefully over the spleen for a friction rub.

Physical Findings

The discovery of any abnormal finding should make the examiner ask two related questions: What might have caused this? What should I do to distinguish between these causes? An early diastolic sound may represent an opening snap and should prompt an intensive search for other signs of mitral stenosis, not only at rest but also after exercise and in different positions. Similarly, vascular spiders will prompt a search for liver disease, and clubbing of the fingers will suggest cyanotic heart disease, tumor of the lung or pleura, pulmonary suppuration, colitis, or enteritis.

Laboratory Results

Positive findings in the laboratory procedures should prompt the appropriate reappraisal of the physical findings, just as physical findings may suggest further laboratory studies. For example, the unexpected observation of the formation of rouleaux in the blood would suggest the possibility of myeloma; careful palpation in search of bony tenderness should be the response.

Whenever abnormal laboratory findings are reported, the physician should specifically consider what physical findings might be helpful in their interpretation. It must be emphasized that physical and laboratory examinations complement rather than supplant one another in the diagnostic process. This is illustrated clearly in the relationship between physical examination and radiographic examination of the pulmonary system. Physical examination may be unable to distinguish between emphysema and pneu-

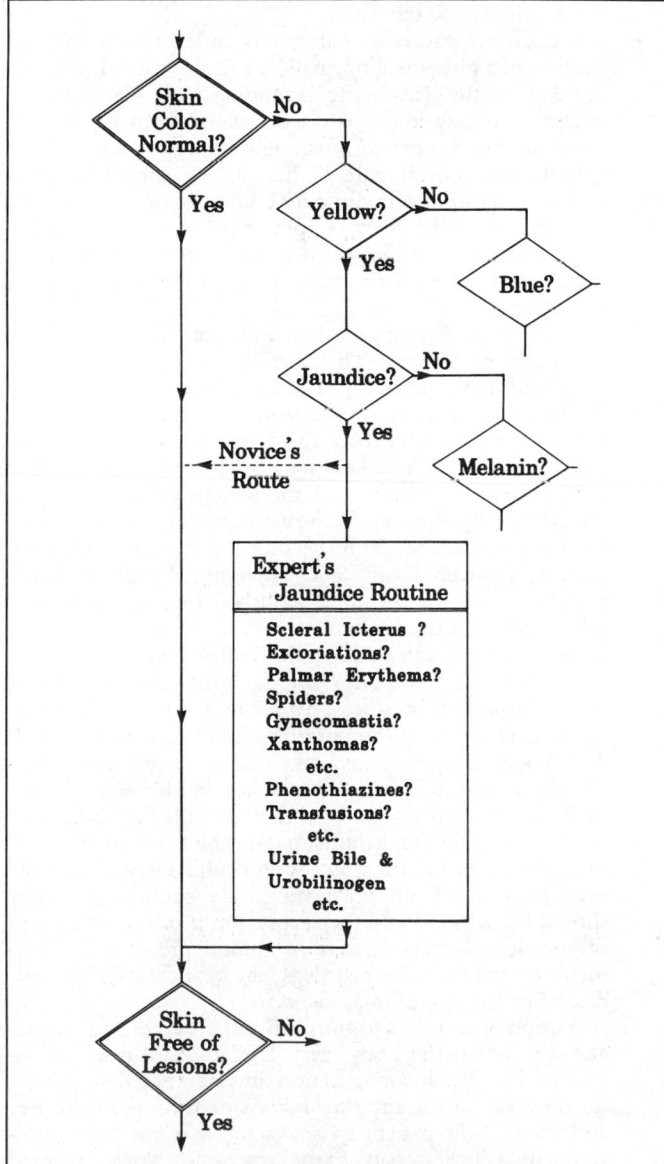

Figure 1.2–1. Schematic view of questions asked by the experienced clinician while examining the skin. The clinician is not satisfied with merely establishing the presence of jaundice but will probe further to narrow down the differential diagnosis.

mothorax. When an emphysematous patient becomes acutely dyspneic, one should promptly obtain a chest radiograph. On the other hand, the radiograph may not be able to differentiate pleural effusion from pulmonary consolidation. These are conditions that have distinctive physical signs.

Differential Diagnosis

Indications for further or more intensive examination may arise from consideration of the differential diagnosis. In all patients with bleeding from the gastrointestinal tract, for instance, careful search should be made for physical evidence of a bleeding tendency (petechiae, ecchymoses, or positive results on a tourniquet test) or telangiectasia. The characteristic lesions of Osler-Weber-Rendu disease may be found in the oral mucous membranes of these patients.

It is common practice to select laboratory tests on the basis of the diagnostic possibilities under consideration. It is of equal importance to select portions of the physical examination for repeated evaluation on the same basis. For example, a common problem is distinguishing infective endocarditis from rheumatic activity in the febrile patient with rheumatic heart disease. Here, the frequent inspection of skin, mucous membranes, and fundi for emboli is as important as making frequent blood cultures. Similarly, serial examination for hot, red, swollen, or tender joints is as important as serial antistreptolysin O titers.

Another common example is the differential diagnosis of hypertension. Here the physician will look for the presence or absence of signs indicating coarctation of the aorta. Unilateral renal vascular disease will come to mind, and the expert examiner will listen over the lumbar region and epigastrium for bruits that might indicate arterial stenosis.

Diagnosis

Often, the physician knows the primary diagnosis before he examines the patient. He may know the patient has diabetes mellitus or chronic myelogenous leukemia, for example. The physician's knowledge of the disease and its complications may direct him to take particular pains with certain aspects of the examination. In the instance of the diabetic patient in acidosis, the physician will look carefully at the periorbital and nasal tissues for evidence of inflammation, which might indicate mucormycosis. He will also palpate the insulin injection sites to determine whether the acidosis might be caused by poor insulin absorption associated with injection into an area of subcutaneous fibrosis, or whether there is evidence of cellulitis at the injection site. Thus it is clear that the knowledge of the physician about the disease enables him to perform a better physical examination.

OUTLINE FOR PERFORMING ROUTINE PHYSICAL EXAMINATION*

1. In preparation for a routine physical examination, the patient is asked to remove his or her clothing, except for underpants, and put on a short paper or cloth gown, which permits easy access to the chest and back. This type of gown is commonly available in most hospitals and outpatient facilities. In the examination of a woman it is also important to have available a half sheet to use as a drape while the patient is in the supine position.
2. The collection of physical examination data may begin before the physician's examination, when the nurse or physician's assistant performs measurements of height, weight, blood pressure, pulse, respiration, and visual acuity using the Snellen chart. In addition, such procedures as tonometry, dilation of pupils with Neo-Synephrine, audiometry, and

---

*Adapted from Hillman and Funk.[10] Courtesy of the Health Sciences Learning Resources Center of the University of Washington.

the performance of an electrocardiogram may be carried out by the nurse as part of a systematic health profile.

3. Before the physical examination the required equipment is laid out in an organized fashion within easy reach of the examining table or bed. Depending on personal preference, instruments such as the stethoscope, penlight, tongue blades, and pocket visual screener may be carried in a jacket pocket. For the routine physical examination, a full complement of equipment should include the following:
   - Stethoscope
   - Penlight
   - Tongue blades
   - Oto-ophthalmoscope
   - Reflex hammer
   - Sphygmomanometer
   - Tuning fork
   - Pocket visual screener
   - Phenylephrine hydrochloride
   - Glove and lubricating jelly
   - Guaiac test reagents
   - Pelvic speculum
   - Tonometer and tetracaine
4. The examiner washes his hands and, unless contraindicated because of a physical abnormality, asks the patient to sit on the edge of the bed or the examining table. Considerable information may immediately be gained from the general appearance of the patient, including impressions as to body habitus and general state of health. An almost instantaneous recognition of a distinctive body position associated with disease of the chest or spine may come from his first inspection, and with experience, a number of clues to disease, mood, or even the patient's personal image may be appreciated.
5. The patient is then approached and a careful inspection of his hands performed. This includes observation for the color and conformation of the nails, joint symmetry, and the status of the hand musculature. It is best done by supporting the patient's hands with your own at chest level, so that each aspect of the hand may be closely scrutinized and compared to its fellow. Next the patient's right arm is explored by palpating the forearm and upper arm for muscle tone and tenderness, by inspecting the skin for lesions and then by passively flexing and extending the elbow, wrist, and metacarpal joints simultaneously. The same maneuvers are repeated on the left arm.
6. Radial pulses are compared so that a major difference in amplitude can be detected. With the wristwatch, one radial pulse is counted for at least 10 seconds. During this time, the characteristics of the pulse should be further observed. The blood pressure is next taken on the right arm with a blood pressure cuff of appropriate size. With the diaphragm of the stethoscope, good Korotkoff sounds may usually be heard by placing the diaphragm over the approximate position of the brachial artery in the antecubital fossae. If, however, there is difficulty in hearing these sounds, the artery should be palpated and the diaphragm placed over a point of strong pulsation. Additional blood pressure measurements on the left arm or the legs may be included if vascular disease or hypertension is suspected.
7. Attention now moves to the head and proceeds in a systematic way down the body. First the face and head are inspected for overall configuration and symmetry, with careful observation for any skin lesions or tumors of the face and scalp. If the patient's visual acuity has not been evaluated with a Snellen chart, a rapid test of near vision is carried out with a pocket visual screener or a sample of printed material. This is not a test of refractive error or distance vision and should therefore be performed while the patient uses his glasses and the card or printed material is held at a distance of approximately 14 inches.

8. With a good light source, such as a penlight, the conjunctiva and sclera of the eye are inspected for changes in color or the appearance of vascular abnormalities such as petechial hemorrhages. If there is suspicion of extraocular muscle weakness, the penlight is also used as a light source to test for any displacement of the light reflex. While the patient looks directly at the light, the symmetry of the position of the reflected light image is observed. Next, direct and consensual pupillary reaction to light is tested. If it is considered important to dilate the patient's pupils before funduscopy, phenylephrine may be instilled at this time. A 10 percent ophthalmic phenylephrine solution will generally dilate the pupils with little interference, if any, with the patient's ability to focus.

9. The examination now moves to the ear. The ear is first examined externally by pulling on the pinna and pushing on the tragus, while one looks for tenderness related to the soft tissues and cartilage of the external auditory canal. Then, with gentle traction in an upward and backward direction, the otoscope is introduced into the external auditory canal and the tympanic membrane inspected. A change in speculum size may be necessary depending on the diameter of the patient's auditory canal. Once both ears have been inspected, the otoscope light source may be used to carry out a brief inspection of the nose, specifically an observation of the lower portion of the nasal septum and turbinate bone.

10. The otoscope is now put aside and the mouth inspected with penlight and tongue blade. A systematic look at the buccal mucosa, teeth, gums, tongue, tonsillar fossae, and pharynx is important. In addition, the patient should be asked to phonate a vowel sound such as "ah" so that the movement of the uvula and palate can be observed.

11. The final step in the examination of the head is the test of hearing with either a wristwatch, a whispered number, or, in some cases, a 256-hertz tuning fork. Since this is a superficial screening test, any patient with a suspected hearing deficit should be evaluated further with an audiometer.

12. The physician now moves behind the patient to carry out an examination of the neck and spine and the posterior portion of the lung fields. Neck range of motion is tested by having the patient touch his chin to his chest and to each shoulder and then tilt the head as far back as possible. Shoulder girdle strength and mobility are tested by first asking the patient to shrug while the examiner exerts downward pressure on both shoulders and then by asking the patient to extend both arms as far above his head as possible, with palms together and biceps touching the ears. For each of these maneuvers, the normal range of joint mobility will vary according to the patient's age.

13. The patient's gown is loosened, and the examiner performs a systematic examination of the neck, looking for lymph node enlargement or abnormal masses. The mandibular, anterior cervical, posterior cervical, and supraclavicular areas are carefully explored. The thyroid is examined bimanually as the patient swallows.

14. The patient is next asked to take a deep breath while the symmetry of chest wall movement is observed. The use of accessory muscles of respiration and the length of time required for expiration are noted. The spine is percussed with the fist or by striking sharply with the fingertips on the vertebral spines while looking for any tenderness. Next, percussion of the posterior lung fields is performed, with right and left sides compared and the descent of the lung bases with a deep inspiration noted. This is followed by auscultation in the same position while the patient breathes through the mouth. The same procedure is followed in the assessment of the axillary and anterior portions of the lung fields.

15. The patient is next asked to lie down for the examination of the anterior part of the neck and of the chest and abdomen. This begins with a systematic palpation of the breast, including each quadrant and areolar tissue. When a female patient is examined, care should be taken to arrange the gown or half-sheet to protect the patient's modesty. Each axillary area should also be palpated for lymph node enlargement.

16. Next the pillow is removed in preparation for inspection of neck veins. Although a well-filled external jugular vein is commonly seen when a patient is in the fully supine position, occlusion of the vein at the angle of the jaw should result in incomplete filling from below, once the vein is stripped. Rapid refilling from below, with distention to the occluding finger, suggests increased venous pressure. Carotid pulses are then palpated and compared.

17. The cardiac portion of the examination continues with inspection of the precordium for the position and character of the apex impulse and any abnormal pulsations. The apex impulse is palpated by placing the middle finger over the point of visible impulse, with the index and fourth fingers placed in the rib spaces on either side. The force, duration, and extent of the apex impulse are noted. With the heel of the hand, the examiner explores the precordium for any heaves, thrusts, or thrills. The heart borders are then percussed to detect gross abnormalities. Next, auscultation with the diaphragm of the stethoscope is carried out by beginning at the apex and moving up the left sternal border to the pulmonic area, the aortic area, and finally along the right sternal border. The timing of systole and diastole can be verified by simultaneously feeling the carotid pulse. The appreciation of any abnormality in the rhythm or in the quality of heart sounds should stimulate further exploration of the precordium for detection of murmur radiation and variations with phase of respiration. Then, before taking off the stethoscope, the examiner listens for bruits in each carotid artery, the epigastrium, and each femoral area.

18. Once the examination of the chest is complete, the female patient should be assisted in replacing her gown. The abdomen is then uncovered for detailed inspection and superficial and deep palpation for any abnormalities in contour, tenderness, or palpable masses. This part of the examination should be performed gently and slowly. With one hand lifting from behind the lower ribs on the right, the examiner searches for the liver edge as the patient takes a deep breath. If the liver is palpated, the edge is explored to define consistency, conformation, and tenderness. To confirm a suspicion of hepatic enlargement, the upper border of the liver is percussed and the overall length of the liver is estimated. Next, the spleen is palpated by the same technique of lifting the rib cage with one hand while palpating with the other. The patient is asked to take one or more deep breaths while the palpating hand is held firmly against the left upper quadrant of the abdomen. Finally, both femoral areas are palpated both for node enlargement and for the amplitude of the femoral pulses.

19. When the examination of the abdomen has been completed, the legs are uncovered. Inspection of the skin, palpation of musculature, and flexion of the knee and hip joints are carried out. Edema is searched for by pressing the index finger firmly against the lower tibia. The dorsalis pedis pulse is palpated and compared to its fellow. Finally, with a reflex hammer or other pointed object, the plantar flexion reflex is tested bilaterally.

20. At this point the patient is asked to return to the sitting position. In the examination of the female patient the gown is once again removed and both breasts carefully inspected for skin retraction, dimpling, or any asymmetry suggesting a tumorous growth. This examination is assisted by asking the patient to arch her back, with hands first on hips and then behind her head. The gown is then replaced.

21. Next, the funduscopic examination is carried out. Initially,

the red reflex is checked with plano lens in place and the ophthalmoscope held 1 to 2 feet from the patient's eye. A +8 to +12 lens is used to approach the eye, and then the lens power is reduced while the physician watches for any lesions of the cornea, lens, or vitreous until the retina comes into focus. An attempt is made to view as much of the retina as possible by moving the ophthalmoscope and, with patients whose eyes have been dilated with phenylephrine, by having the patient move one eye on command in all directions. The other eye is examined in the same manner.

22. To finish neurologic testing, the physician asks the patient to wrinkle his forehead, show his teeth, and stick out his tongue while the physician watches for any muscle movement disorders. Biceps, knee, and ankle reflexes are tested, and the patient is asked to extend his arms and close his eyes while the physician looks for arm drift or tremor. Then the patient is asked to stand up and walk across the room. As he walks, the position of his feet, his gait, and his arm swing are observed.

23. The last part of any routine physical examination involves the examination of the genitalia and rectum. The male patient is asked to stand and remove his underpants. The penis and meatus are inspected for ulceration or discharge; the epididymis and testes are carefully palpated for tenderness, masses, or evidence of testicular atrophy. The physician's index finger is introduced into the external inguinal canal, and the patient is asked to cough or bear down while the physician feels for evidence of an inguinal hernia. Finally, the patient is asked to bend over the bed or assume the knee-chest position for inspection and palpation of the rectum. After the anus is lubricated, the physician's index finger is introduced into the rectum, and careful palpation of the rectal ampulla and prostate gland is performed. Similarly, with the examination of the female patient the last step in a routine physical is the performance of the pelvic and rectal examination.

USE OF THE CLINICAL LABORATORY IN PATIENT CARE

Ability to use laboratory data in patient care has become an essential skill required of every physician. Effective use of the laboratory should be developed as carefully as other clinical skills required in the practice of medicine.

To use the laboratory advantageously one must understand its functions and its limitations. Laboratory tests cannot be substituted for a careful history and examination of the patient, yet properly selected tests can give the physician information that can be obtained through no other means. Thus the function of the laboratory is to extend the physician's powers of observation. Skillful use of the laboratory requires an ability to integrate laboratory data with other clinical information, but it is a logical error to consider laboratory information as being of a different order than that obtained through the history or physical examination. All laboratory data are objective data (in contrast to the patient's complaint of headache, for example), and they usually are expressed in quantitative terms. However, each laboratory measurement merely represents an observation of the same disordered physiology that is the object of the physician's attention during examination of the patient.

USES OF LABORATORY DATA

Screening (Detection of Disease)

Laboratory tests may be carried out on an apparently healthy individual as part of a comprehensive examination or as part of the initial evaluation of a patient, even though the history and physical examination do not suggest the need for such tests. Just as the physician measures the blood pressure in the absence of symptoms of hypertension, he may order a serologic test for syphilis without any clinical indication. Such screening tests are usually limited to simpler, less expensive procedures that can detect medically significant abnormalities with a high prevalence in the general population. The blood cell count (hemoglobin or hematocrit, white cell count, differential count, and examination of the blood film) and the urinalysis (appearance, pH, specific gravity, protein, reducing substances, and microscopic examination) are done so frequently to supplement the history and physical examination that they may be considered essential components of an initial evaluation. This type of laboratory information is considered part of the "data base," in the terminology of the problem-oriented medical record.

The problems that arise in screening for disorders with a low prevalence were discussed earlier.

Diagnosis

During the initial evaluation of a patient, laboratory studies are usually selected on the basis of information obtained during the history and physical examination. A laboratory procedure may be used to assist the physician in establishing the presence of a suspected illness; for example, serum thyroxine may be measured to confirm a suspicion of hypothyroidism, or serum creatine phosphokinase may be measured to substantiate a clinical diagnosis of myocardial infarction. In this situation, a positive laboratory result increases the probability that the clinical diagnosis is correct, and the function of the laboratory information is to enhance the reliability of that diagnosis. Conversely, laboratory tests may be used to exclude the presence of disease; for example, normal values for serum aspartate aminotransferase and alanine aminotransferase can effectively rule out the presence of acute hepatitis. This use of laboratory data also serves to increase the reliability of the diagnostic process, since exclusion of some diagnoses increases the probability that one of the other suspected diagnoses is correct. These two applications of laboratory data are frequently used to aid the physician in selecting the most likely diagnosis from a list of several possibilities (i.e., differential diagnosis).

Following the Course of Disease

Because laboratory tests are objective and quantitative, they often provide a useful initial measure of the severity of the disease process, and in many clinical situations they also provide the most reliable indication that therapy is having its desired effect. The erythrocyte sedimentation rate is a simple but useful indicator of improvement or exacerbation in giant cell arteritis. Initial measurement of the reticulocyte count, and then of either the hemoglobin level or hematocrit, provides invaluable information regarding the effectiveness of treatment of anemia.

Selecting and Monitoring Therapy

Laboratory studies, by improving the precision of diagnosis, may be of assistance in selection of appropriate therapy, for example, antimicrobial susceptibility tests in selection of the most effective antibiotic for a patient with bacterial infection. In other instances, dosage regimens of a selected therapeutic agent may be determined largely on the basis of laboratory tests; for example, anticoagulant therapy with warfarin derivatives is hazardous without frequent measurement of prothrombin time. In circumstances where no quantitative clinical or laboratory measurements of the effects of a drug can be made, and particularly when there is reason to suspect that the dosage is too high or too low, it is often useful to measure the blood level of the agent itself. Therapeutic monitoring by measurement of blood levels of anticonvulsant drugs, cardiac glycosides, and antibiotics can indicate to the physician that the dosage schedule chosen is resulting in the desired concentration of drug in body fluids.

Other Uses

Laboratory tests are used in numerous other aspects of patient care: compatibility testing before blood transfusion or other types

of tissue transplantation, detection of carrier states for purposes of genetic counseling, and detection of hereditary enzyme deficiencies that might be harmful under certain circumstances, for example, erythrocyte glucose-6-phosphate dehydrogenase deficiency, which may result in hemolytic anemia if affected patients take certain drugs.

Laboratory tests are used also for such diverse purposes as environmental microbiological surveillance and provision of legal evidence in paternity litigation.

LABORATORY DATA IN THE MEDICAL DECISION-MAKING PROCESS

As explained in a previous section, medical diagnosis consists of an iterative process through which information is collected, evaluated, and utilized to determine further appropriate action.[6,8,9,11,25] Laboratory data are used in this process in exactly the same manner as data obtained during the history taking or physical examination. Because collecting laboratory information in this iterative process is more time-consuming than taking the patient's history and giving the physical examination, it is usually more efficient for the physician to anticipate the possible outcomes of the iterative process and to order as promptly as possible all laboratory procedures that have a high probability of being required. Of course, the cost of the laboratory tests, any risk or inconvenience to the patient, an unnecessarily prolonged hospital stay, the inconvenience to the patient asked to return repeatedly for sequential testing, and the risk to the patient posed by any delay in diagnosis must be balanced against the possible benefits of the tests.

COMMON ERRORS IN LABORATORY TESTING

Serious pitfalls in the use of the clinical laboratory can occur at three points: first, in choosing which test to perform; second, in collecting the specimen and in the actual performance of the determination; and finally, in interpreting the result. Physicians should strive to avoid redundant laboratory testing because this is expensive and often results in conflicting results, promoting yet more testing. It is important to formulate a clinical question before ordering any laboratory test and then to decide what is the most expeditious and inexpensive test that will answer that question. For example, if the clinical problem is upper abdominal pain, it is not good practice to order both an upper gastrointestinal series and an endoscopic examination, because either test may answer the question of whether an ulcer is present.

Selection
Failure to select the appropriate laboratory test usually stems from a lack of understanding of specific analytic methods used and how they relate to the patient's functional abnormality. Laboratory techniques are rapidly evolving, and tests are often methodologically complex. Lack of appreciation of the inherent limitations of a test method may mean that misleading or diagnostically valueless information will be obtained from the laboratory procedure requested. The former use of the red blood cell count as a test for anemia resulted in frequent misdiagnosis in those cases of anemia accompanied by normal red cell counts. The use of the T_3 resin uptake test as the sole means of assessing thyrometabolic status of a pregnant patient may result in an erroneous diagnosis of hypothyroidism. An understanding of the basic principles of test methods is critical, and appropriate consultation should be sought from the laboratory whenever there is concern that test limitations may preclude a satisfactory answer to the diagnostic question at hand.

Collection
The second point where pitfalls occur in laboratory testing is during the collection of the specimen and the actual performance of the test in the laboratory. Incorrect choice or handling of the submitted specimen frequently causes erroneous or misleading results,

with the cause often not apparent to either the physician or the laboratory staff. For example, the wrong choice of a bacterial transport medium for fastidious pathogens or the exposure of strict anaerobic organisms to the atmosphere may prevent their recovery in the laboratory, with a "negative" result then reported to the physician. Incorrect anticoagulants in tubes for blood specimens may give rise to gross errors in coagulation tests and chemical determinations. Improper or inadequate specimens constitute a major technical problem in laboratory testing; hence as much care should be given to collection of the specimen as to each of the other steps in the entire process.

Technical and clerical steps within the laboratory may be an additional source of error in the performance of laboratory tests. This possibility has resulted in the development of comprehensive specimen accessioning and quality control procedures that are now used almost universally in the clinical laboratory. It should be emphasized, however, that most of these quality control procedures are designed to detect systematic rather than random errors, and they are usually incapable of identifying improperly handled or deteriorated specimens. Although technical and clerical mistakes still occur, caution should be used in summarily attributing all unanticipated results to "lab error." The unexpected test result, if valid, may contain important diagnostic information, and it should be viewed no differently from a physical finding that was not suggested by the history. In both instances the finding should be pursued in depth if it could be of import.

Interference with test methods by medications, the nonfasting state, recumbency, or exercise, and so forth is a type of technical "error" that deserves special mention. Numerous types of chemical interference by medications have been documented for a variety of laboratory tests, and there is increasing awareness of the effects of both exercise and the postabsorptive state on the results obtained with some laboratory determinations. The laboratory staff, having no information regarding the patient's drug therapy, cannot detect or circumvent these chemical interferences, which may cause significant quantitative differences in the results obtained. It is hoped that misleading results caused by drug interference will diminish as new analytic methods are developed that are more specific for the substances in question, and as computer systems allow detection of potential interference by automatic review of patients' therapeutic regimens.

Interpretation
The final point at which pitfalls can occur is in the physician's interpretation of the laboratory test results. Problems frequently arise from use of incorrect normal ranges or from overestimating the precision of the result reported. Differences in the technical methods of performing a test can have a profound effect on the normal range for that test. For example, the various methods of performing an erythrocyte sedimentation rate yield substantially different values in health and disease, and the use of the wrong range for the test may result in an erroneous diagnostic impression. Normal ranges are too often taken from the literature with the assumption that they apply to all test methods with that name. Age, race, and sex variations in values for tests such as blood cell counts and immunoglobulin concentrations may result in diagnostic errors if a single normal range is assumed.

The statistical precision of the test method provides a second potential pitfall in interpretation of laboratory results. For example, the inherent error in the usual 100-cell leukocyte differential count limits the significance of changes in proportions of the various cell types on repeated determinations for the same patient. Because of the statistical sampling error a patient with a "true" value of 50 percent neutrophils may have percentages ranging from 40 to 60 on repeated determinations; hence little significance can be attached to an apparent "increase" of this magnitude on successive determinations.

The ultimate value of a laboratory test result is determined entirely by the use the physician makes of it. This, in turn, is dependent on the physician's appreciation of the limits and capabili-

ties of the clinical laboratory in identifying the abnormality responsible for the patient's disease.

DIAGNOSTIC IMAGING

Diagnostic imaging has evolved rapidly and now includes five major modalities: radiography, nuclear medicine, ultrasonography, computed tomography (CT), and magnetic resonance imaging (MRI). They provide increasingly exact details of anatomy and abnormality. MRI and positron emission tomography (PET) provide physiologic information.

Imaging progress has brought increased complexity and cost. Each modality has distinct advantages and limitations. Routine radiography may provide a useful initial overview (like low-power microscopy), but CT, ultrasonography, and endoscopy increasingly give the exact diagnoses. The preferred approach will change as MRI becomes more generally available.

This chapter covers general features of the major imaging modalities together with their strengths and limitations (Table 1.2–5). Diagnostic images are abstract two-dimensional representations of a three-dimensional form. Some findings, such as skeletal fractures or air in abnormal locations, are specific. Others, such as masses and lytic lesions, are nonspecific, and in many instances the main value of the imaging is to locate a lesion for biopsy. The increasing use of digital imaging techniques means that some lesions will be demonstrated only by precise technical procedures. This mandates useful communication between the clinician and the radiologist about specific clinical problems before imaging occurs.

Efficient and cost-effective medical care requires logical use of high-yield diagnostic methods and avoidance of ones that provide inexact or confusing results. This is another reason for close coordination between clinicians and imaging specialists. Feedback on the value of an examination will progressively revise and improve the process of diagnosis.

Imaging Principles

Diagnostic images are made by equipment that exploits principles of physics that may be relatively simple in concept. The technology, in contrast, is complex and ranges from portable x-ray and ultrasound units to the large and complex MRI installation with its superconducting magnet, cryogenics, radio frequency devices, and powerful computers.

All imaging involves sending some form of energy into the body, detecting the energy that comes out, and converting the detected signal into a useful image.

The energy used for radiography, CT scanning, nuclear medicine, and MRI is electromagnetic radiation, which penetrates tissues. X-rays and gamma rays are part of the electromagnetic spectrum, which includes heat, light, and radio frequencies. X-rays are created when fast-moving electrons collide with the anode of an x-ray tube, whereas the gamma rays used in nuclear medicine result from decay of certain unstable atomic nuclei. The shorter the wavelength of the radiation, the farther it can penetrate tissues. These rays are absorbed and scattered by tissue. The thicker the tissue and the higher the atomic number of its atoms, the greater the absorption. A variety of "densities" can be distinguished. Transmitted x-rays can be detected by photographic means, by fluorescent screens in combination with image intensifiers as in fluoroscopes, or by solid-state detectors as in CT. The more-penetrating gamma rays are detected by large crystals usually containing iodides. The light that results when some of the gamma rays are captured in the crystal are counted, and a spatial image is constructed to show the site from which the radioactivity was emitted in the body.

The energy involved in ultrasonography is acoustic. High-frequency sound waves are sent into the body by a transducer, which also acts as a receiver of the echoes reflected from tissue interfaces. A transducer transmits acoustic waves 5 percent of the time and is receiving ("listening") 95 percent of the time. As in sonar, it times the return of echoes and computes the distances to map the underlying zone.

MRI uses two different forms of energy. Each hydrogen atom (proton) spins and behaves like a small magnet. When placed in a magnetic field, the protons line up and precess like gyroscopes at a characteristic frequency. Radio waves can be used to pull them away from this magnetic axis and get them cycling in phase. When the radio frequency input stops, the protons give back a detectable radio wave of the characteristic frequency. The device includes a powerful magnet to align the protons and radio-frequency coils to pulse them into phase and also to measure the radio-frequency signal given back.

The key to imaging the body is to modify the magnetic field with special gradient coils so that protons at each point will resonate at a slightly different characteristic frequency, analogous to the different pitches on a set of guitar strings, and then define where the sound is coming from by the pitch.

The present imaging equipment is used for hydrogen, but in theory the technique can work for any nucleus with an odd atomic number.

Tissue Density Discrimination

Imaging of transmitted x-rays by means of photographic emulsions is the simplest, least expensive, and most widely available modality. It is poor in distinguishing between various soft-tissue densities

TABLE 1.2–5. MAJOR IMAGING MODALITIES: ADVANTAGES AND LIMITATIONS

	Advantages	Limitations
Routine radiography	Availability Relatively low cost Big picture Excellent for fractures, obstructions Real-time imaging with fluoroscopy and cineradiography	Poor soft-tissue detail Needs contrast agents Overlapping shadows cause confusion Obesity limits detail Radiation dose must be low
Computed tomography (CT)	Precise cross-sectional anatomy Good soft-tissue detail Obesity and injected contrast agents enhance detail	High cost Thin patients have poor unenhanced soft-tissue contrast Difficult to get axial coronal displays Radiation dose must be low
Ultrasonography	Good soft-tissue detail Cyst versus solid distinction Safety Real-time imaging	Bone and air block the sound waves Obesity limits detail
Nuclear medicine	Excellent for bone metastasis Early osteomyelitis Stress fractures Excellent physiologic information (PET scan)	Limited anatomic detail Limited availability Radiation dose must be very low
Magnetic resonance imaging	Best soft-tissue contrast Sections made in any plane Excellent cardiovascular and neuroanatomic detail Usually no need for contrast agents Safe	High cost and limited availability Relatively long imaging time No real-time imaging

but can easily identify metals and calcium (with their high atomic numbers), water and soft-tissue organs, fat, and air.

Because routine radiography has limited soft-tissue discrimination, various methods are employed to increase its usefulness. Hollow organs can be opacified by radiopaque materials: barium for the gastrointestinal tract and iodine-containing contrast agents for injection into blood vessels, the subarachnoid space, wounds, and sinus tracts. The liver and kidneys excrete certain contrast agents extracted from the blood, allowing the biliary and urinary tracts to be seen. Air is a useful contrast agent for intestinal studies.

CT scanning is 10 to 20 times more sensitive than conventional radiography in distinguishing tissue densities, and MRI is 4 to 5 times better than CT.

The Gray Scale

Routine radiography creates an image on photographic emulsion with a wide scale of gray tones between black and white, depending on how many photons reach the film. All other imaging methods involve digitization of the image. The digital images are converted back into a gray scale because our eyes prefer images with contrasting shades of gray (or color). In practice we can distinguish about 16 to 20 shades of gray. The CT scan takes 4000 different tissue densities and makes a useful image by sorting them into 16 groups and assigning each a shade of gray (or color). The image can be manipulated in a variety of ways to emphasize soft tissue or bone detail. Programs can be employed to enhance edges of organs, and often several sets of images must be used in CT scanning depending on the organ of interest.

Safety

X-rays and gamma rays are ionizing radiations that can cause mutations and cell death. The true risks of low-level diagnostic radiation are difficult to prove. Ultrasound causes no damage, and its use has become the preferred diagnostic technique for obstetrics for that reason. MRI at current field strength is also safe biologically.

Image Plane, Movement, and Gating

Routine radiographs are recognizably human in outline and shape. The other images are slices of varying thickness and thus require precise knowledge of where the plane, or "cut," was made through the body. The imaging place in ultrasonography and MRI can be in any direction, whereas CT is generally limited to transaxial cross sections because multiplane reconstruction is time consuming. An exciting aspect of CT is the use of thin-section (1.5 to 2 mm), high-resolution techniques that offer anatomic detail approaching 1 mm in resolution.

Only ultrasonography and fluoroscopy allow the imaging of moving structures. Echocardiography gives detail of the beating heart, and fluoroscopy shows excellent intestinal anatomy. MRI and nuclear medicine can evaluate the beating heart even with a relatively long scan time by using a gated technique. This involves using data collected over a period of time at the same phase of the cardiac cycle.

Special Procedures and Subtraction

Angiography is a special technique that involves injection of contrast agents into blood vessels. Rapid filming demonstrates arterial, capillary, and venous phases of the circulation, as well as the chambers of the heart. Confusing overlying shadows can now be eliminated by electronic "subtraction," and this process permits significant reduction of the amount of contrast agent needed for visualization of the vessel.

REFERENCES

1. Bates B: A Guide to Physical Examination and History Taking. Philadelphia, JB Lippincott, 1987
2. Cochrane AL, Chapman PJ, Oldham PD: Observers' errors in taking medical histories. Lancet 1:1007, 1951
3. Elveback LR, Guillies CL, Keating FR Jr: Health, normality, and the ghost of Gauss. JAMA 211:69, 1970
4. Feinstein AR: Scientific methodology in clinical medicine, I, II, IV. Ann Intern Med 61:564, 757, 1162, 1964
5. Feinstein AR: Clinical Judgment. Baltimore, Williams & Wilkins, 1967
6. Feinstein AR: The problems of the "problem-oriented medical record." Ann Intern Med 78:751, 1973
7. Feinstein AR: Clinical Biostatistics. St. Louis, CV Mosby, 1977
8. Griner PF, Mayewski RJ, et al: Selection and interpretation of diagnostic tests and procedures: Principles and applications. Ann Intern Med 94:553, 1981
9. Henry RJ, Reed AH: Normal values. In Henry RJ, Cannon DC, Winkleman JW (eds): Clinical Chemistry, Principles and Techniques. Hagerstown, Md, Harper & Row, 1974
10. Hillman RS, Funk DC: Routine Examination of the Adult. Seattle, Health Sciences Learning Resources Center of the University of Washington, 1973
11. Jelliffe RW: Quantitative aspects of clinical judgment. Am J Med 55:431, 1973
12. Kassirer JP, Moskowitz AJ, et al: Decision analysis: A progress report. Ann Intern Med 106:275, 1987
13. Kong AM, Barnett GO, Mosteller F, Youtz C: How medical professionals evaluate probability. N Engl J Med 315:740, 1986
14. Koran LM: The reliability of clinical methods, data and judgments. N Engl J Med 293:642, 695, 1975
15. Metropolitan Life Insurance Co: Statistical Bulletin 40, November–December, 1959; Bulletin 41, February–March, 1960
16. Miller GA: The magical number seven, plus or minus two: Some limits on our capacity for processing information. Psychol Rev 63:81, 1956
17. Mold JW, Stein HF: The cascade effect in the clinical care of patients. N Engl J Med 314:512, 1986
18. Murphy EA: The Logic of Medicine. Baltimore, Johns Hopkins University Press, 1976
19. Neuhauser D, Lewici AM: What do we gain from the sixth stool guaiac? N Engl J Med 293:226, 1975
20. Pauker SB, Kassirer JP: Decision analysis. N Engl J Med 316:250, 1987
21. Riegelman RK: Studying a Study and Testing a Test. Boston, Little, Brown, 1981
22. Rifkin RD, Hood WB Jr: Bayesian analysis of electrocardiographic exercise stress testing. N Engl J Med 297:681, 1977
23. Seidel HM, Ball JW, et al: Mosby's Guide to Physical Examination. St. Louis, CV Mosby, 1987
24. Sisson JC, Schoomaker EB, Ross JC: Clinical decision analysis: The hazard of using additional data. JAMA 236:1259, 1976
25. Sox HC: Probability theory in the use of diagnostic tests. Ann Intern Med 104:60, 1986
26. Sox HC: Decision analysis: A basic clinical skill? N Engl J Med 316:271, 1987

The Analysis and Synthesis of Clinical Information

Richard J. Johns and Nicholas J. Fortuin

Clinical information is collected and manipulated in order to solve a patient's clinical problem. Usually the problem is solved through diagnosis and therapeutic management. Sometimes the problem disappears during the procedure, and sometimes the diagnosed problem is not amenable to treatment. Nevertheless, the initial objective of the analysis and synthesis of clinical information is to arrive at a diagnosis.

In recent years this clinical diagnostic process has come under investigation.[1,2,5,6] Although these studies do not provide clear insight into the inner workings of the diagnostic process of experienced physicians, they have been valuable in demonstrating what the process is *not*. First, it has been shown that the physician does not separate or compartmentalize the collection of information from the analysis of information—the two processes are intermingled. Second, the diagnostic process is more akin to progression down a logical decision tree than it is to a pattern-matching *Gestalt*.

INITIAL INFORMATION ANALYSIS

In Chapter 1.2 it was emphasized that each piece of information should be analyzed as it is received: What does it mean? What diagnostic possibilities (hypotheses) does it suggest? What further information will be helpful in sorting out these hypotheses? This initial analysis serves two important functions. First, it guides the course of further information gathering in a rational way. Second, it permits the physician to organize, store, recall, and manipulate the clinical information. It would be impossible to deal with the informational content of the history of a present illness and the abnormal physical findings if they were treated as a list of unrelated facts. Consciously or unconsciously, physicians aggregate the facts in a meaningful way. For example, the history of chills and fever, the history of dysuria, the finding of a temperature of 39C, and the finding of right costovertebral angle tenderness become organized by the hypothesis that the patient may have an upper urinary tract infection. Four separate pieces of information have been compressed into one concept. The importance of this aspect can be seen in the novice's difficulty in "remembering" the clinical information about a patient or in the experienced physician's difficulty in dealing with the information concerning a patient in which the manifestations "do not make sense." In both examples, there is a lack of organizing and unifying concepts.

Thus the initial analysis of clinical information has a beneficial effect on the information-gathering process, and it is essential to the mental processing of the information.

FURTHER ANALYSIS

Although the initial analysis is necessary, it is not sufficient. To rely exclusively on the analysis carried out during the information-gathering phase can lead to two possible errors.

First, if you obtain information only to test your current hypotheses, you may miss important pieces of information. This is the basic reason that one performs a system review, conducts a routine physical examination, and obtains screening laboratory studies. You seek certain basic items of information whether or not your concurrent analysis suggests that it might be worthwhile.

Second, the initial analysis is of necessity a serial process. Various hypotheses are considered and then are either abandoned or explored further. In the light of subsequent information, some of these hypotheses may have been abandoned prematurely. Furthermore, in the review of all the information, additional hypotheses must be considered. For example, if the patient described above also has cough with purulent sputum, one must also give consideration to the possibility that the problem is pneumonia at the right lung base.

This chapter is devoted to discussing this second step, the further analysis that is performed when the initial information has been collected. It also addresses the synthesis of this information with knowledge of disease. It addresses the questions of which disease best explains the patient's problems and whether one disease explains all the problems.

ANALYZE THE FACTS

The steps in the further analysis of a clinical problem can be illustrated by applying them to a specific case.

ILLUSTRATIVE EXAMPLE

A 74-year-old man was seen in the outpatient department with complaints of ankle and abdominal swelling.

His past history was one of good general health except for diabetes mellitus of 15 years' duration controlled by diet and tolbutamide. He had consumed 4 ounces of alcohol daily for many years and had smoked in excess of one pack of cigarettes per day since his youth.

For 6 months he had noted fatigue and weakness. Swelling of the ankles had been present for 3 months and abdominal swelling for 2. He complained of early satiety and a poor appetite but had gained 20 pounds in 2 months. He denied dyspnea or orthopnea.

On examination the patient's temperature was 99F, blood pressure 100/80 mm Hg, pulse 104/min and regular, and respirations 24/min. He appeared chronically ill but was comfortable while lying flat. Funduscopic examination showed a few scattered microaneurysms. The neck veins were distended to the angle of the jaw at a 45-degree elevation. Chest examination revealed an increased anteroposterior diameter, low diaphragm, and dullness at the right lung base to the scapular tip. Breath sounds were coarse, with prolonged expiratory phase; fine rales were noted at both lung bases. The cardiac apex impulse was not palpable, and the carotid pulses showed reduced volume; the heart sounds were distant, with a soft sound in early diastole. The liver was palpable 4 fingerbreadths below the costal margin, and there was moderate ascites. The extremities showed pitting edema to the knees. Neurologic examination revealed decreased vibratory sense in the feet and absent ankle jerks. The prostate was enlarged.

Initial laboratory studies revealed normal complete blood cell count, glucose 220 mg/dl, creatinine 2.4 mg/dl, urea 45 mg/dl, bilirubin 2.3 mg/dl, aspartate aminotransferase 65 U, alanine aminotransferase 57 U, alkaline phosphatase 135 U, and normal serum protein values. Urinalysis showed 2+ protein and a few granular casts. The ECG showed low-voltage and nonspecific T-wave flattening. Radiographic examination of the chest showed signs of chronic obstructive lung disease, a right pleural effusion, and a normal cardiac silhouette.

LIST THE FACTS

The first step in the analysis is to list the facts in chronologic order. In this example the list would include the following:

- Diabetes mellitus
- Alcohol and cigarette consumption
- Ankle edema and ascites
- Fatigue and weakness
- Anorexia
- Retinal microaneurysms
- Signs of chronic obstructive pulmonary disease
- Pleural effusion and pulmonary rales
- Distended neck veins
- Small heart with diastolic sound
- Hepatomegaly and abnormal liver function test results
- Proteinuria and mild renal insufficiency
- Prostatic enlargement
- Decreased vibratory sense and absent ankle jerks

RANK IN ORDER OF IMPORTANCE

Before one can arrange these findings in the order of their importance, each must be evaluated as to its possible significance with regard to the patient's presenting problem. In this example there are several chronic conditions that may not be of relevance. These include diabetes, chronic lung disease caused by smoking, and enlargement of the prostate. Other findings, such as anorexia, fatigue, and weakness, are so nonspecific as to be of little help in moving toward a diagnostic formulation. Decreased vibratory sense and absent ankle jerks could be reasonably ascribed to the diabetes as a manifestation of peripheral neuropathy, and retinal microaneurysms are also due to diabetes. Some findings, such as the history of moderate alcohol consumption, are of uncertain significance with regard to the presenting problem and should therefore be kept high on the list of important findings. As one moves through a diagnostic plan, findings such as this may achieve greater or lesser importance. The same could be said for the chronic conditions that at the outset may be ranked as of lesser importance.

After a careful examination of the findings, they can be rearranged in the order of their importance as follows:

- *Ankle edema and ascites*
- *Pleural effusion and pulmonary rales*
- *Distended neck veins*
- *Small heart with diastolic sound*
- *Hepatomegaly and abnormal liver function test results*
- *Proteinuria and mild renal insufficiency*
- *Moderate alcohol consumption*
- Diabetes mellitus
- Retinal microaneurysms
- Decreased vibratory sense and absent ankle jerks
- Signs of chronic obstructive pulmonary disease
- Cigarette smoking
- Prostatic enlargement
- Anorexia
- Fatigue and weakness

The findings italicized in the above list are those that appear to be so intimately associated with the illness that the final diagnosis should account for them. Later in the analysis it is important to verify that the diagnosis selected does explain these findings.

After the facts have been critically evaluated and listed according to their apparent importance, one may find in the list a disease manifestation that unequivocally provides a diagnosis. Calcification in the pericardium on a chest radiograph would be such a finding, pointing clearly to the diagnosis of constrictive pericarditis. If the remaining findings on the list were adequately explained by a diagnosis of constrictive pericarditis, the analysis would not need to

proceed further, and appropriate confirmatory studies, such as cardiac catheterization, would be obtained. As in the case example given above, however, one usually finds that the accumulated facts are common to several diseases.

SELECT A CENTRAL FEATURE

The next step is to select some outstanding feature of the illness about which one can orient the diagnostic analysis. Examples of such orienting, or central, features are fever, jaundice, hepatomegaly, ascites, renal failure, and heart failure, among others. It is preferable that the feature selected is an objective finding and, if possible, one that can be at least roughly quantified. However, in some cases the major complaint is subjective, such as pain in a particular area, and is the only feature that can serve as the basis for the systematic analysis of the problem. The selection of a feature as the focal point about which the differential diagnosis will be centered requires practice and a wide knowledge of the important hallmarks and of the natural course of the various diseases. As one reads through this text, many examples illustrating this type of analysis will be found in the discussions of the clinical problems presented.

When the case presents two or more features that appear to have the same potential value, one should not be content to base this analysis on only one of them. Two or more analyses should be made, each based on one of the features. By pursuing this course, one may find two or more avenues that lead to the same diagnosis, thus reinforcing one's confidence in its validity. As a general rule it is best to find a single explanation for the patient's illness, even when there are manifestations in several organ systems, as in the example presented here.

In the example under consideration, fluid retention was selected as the central feature. In many cases a single finding from the history or physical examination may provide more specific insight into the nature of the patient's problems. In this example, fluid retention could be attributed to abnormality of cardiac, hepatic, or renal function. The finding of distended neck veins clearly suggests, however, that the heart is the likely cause, thus focusing the diagnostic evaluation on a consideration of congestive heart failure. Failure to heed this important physical finding could lead the physician into laborious, costly, and potentially dangerous evaluation of the liver or kidneys.

LIST THE DIAGNOSTIC POSSIBILITIES

The diagnosis of congestive heart failure in this patient is merely the start of a more precise diagnostic evaluation, because this diagnosis is only a syndrome. Proper understanding, prognostication, and ultmately management of this problem requires a specific etiologic diagnosis. The causes of congestive heart failure (see Chapter 2.2) are too numerous to list as diagnostic possibilities in this case. One needs to search for other clues in the presentation that might refine the list of possibilities. Of importance here is the finding of normal cardiac size on a chest radiograph. The causes of congestive heart failure with normal cardiac size are few:

- Constrictive pericarditis
- Mitral stenosis
- Infiltrative cardiomyopathy (i.e., amyloidosis)
- Acute valvular regurgitation
- Myocardial infarction
- Myocarditis
- Atrial myxoma

In listing the diagnostic possibilities, one should make an effort to be comprehensive. Some of the possibilities on the comprehensive list can be eliminated on the basis of the evaluation to date. Acute valvular regurgitation is unlikely in the absence of a

murmur; myocardial infarction is unlikely with nonspecific ECG changes; and myocarditis is unlikely because of the chronic course of the patient's illness. Atrial tumors are rare but cannot be excluded on this basis alone.

DISTINGUISH BETWEEN THESE POSSIBILITIES

On the basis of the information at hand it is difficult to choose between the remaining diagnostic possibilities. The early diastolic sound could be an opening snap of mitral stenosis, a third heart sound of infiltrative disease, a pericardial knock, or a "tumor plop" of atrial myxoma. The history, physical examination, and laboratory survey do not allow one to select the proper diagnosis. Further testing is in order. It is important to select the simplest test that will distinguish between these possibilities. Ordering a barrage of noninvasive studies simply because they can be performed easily is not a good approach. Nor is it proper to proceed directly to sophisticated testing such as cardiac catheterization, which would entail hospitalization and extra cost and would carry some risk to the patient. The simplest approach to this man's diagnosis is to obtain an echocardiogram. This test will readily distinguish between the possibilities under consideration and can be performed on an outpatient basis. In this patient the study showed normal cardiac valves and no evidence of atrial mass. The left ventricular cavity was small, the walls of the left ventricle were markedly thickened, and contractility of the ventricle was reduced. These findings point to the diagnosis of amyloidosis. Confirmation could be obtained by biopsy of a distal site, such as the rectum or gingiva, or directly by myocardial biopsy.

SYNTHESIS

The next step is to determine whether the diagnosis of cardiac amyloidosis can account for all the findings in this case. Fluid retention is a prominent feature of this disorder and explains the distended neck veins, pleural effusion, ascites, and peripheral edema. Elevated pressures of the right side of the heart cause hepatic enlargement, and the liver function abnormalities can be ascribed to chronic passive congestion of the liver. Renal dysfunction may re-sult from inadequate renal blood flow or elevated renal venous pressure, or it may be due to amyloid infiltration in the kidneys. Anorexia is common when the liver is distended. Thus all the features of this man's illness can be explained adequately by this diagnosis. Treatment can now be planned. Knowing that cardiac amyloidosis is the cause of the patient's heart failure allows the physician to avoid the use of digitalis, which may be poorly tolerated in this setting, or afterload-reducing agents, which are ineffective. Finally, a prognosis can be determined, in this case a poor one because there is no effective long-term treatment that will improve the condition.

If the presumptive diagnosis does not explain all the findings, the physician must decide whether the findings are significant or whether they may be discounted as normal variations. If the findings are significant, the physician must then decide whether it is necessary to make a second diagnosis to account for them.

At this stage of the analysis, attention must also be given to negative findings. For example, does a normal ECG exclude a myocardial infarction? What value may be attached to a negative result on a serologic test for syphilis when the other findings point to a diagnosis of syphilitic aortitis?

REFERENCES

1. Elstein AS, Shulman LS, Sprafka SA: Medical Problem Solving: An Analysis of Clinical Reasoning. Cambridge, Mass, Harvard University Press, 1978
2. Feinstein AR: An analysis of diagnostic reasoning. II. The strategy of intermediate decisions. Yale J Biol Med 46:264, 1973
3. Folstein MR, Folstein SE, McHugh PR: "Minimental state": A practical method for grading the cognitive state of patients for the clinician. J Psychiatr Res 12:189, 1975
4. Harvey AM, Bordley J III, Barondess JA: Differential Diagnosis: The Interpretation of Clinical Evidence. 3d ed. Philadelphia, WB Saunders, 1979.
5. Kassirer JP, Moskowitz AJ, et al: Decision analysis: A progress report. Ann Intern Med 106:275, 1987
6. Sox HCJ: Decision analysis: A basic clinical skill. N Engl J Med 316:271, 1987

CHAPTER 1.4
Issues in Diagnostic and Therapeutic Management

Richard J. Johns, Nicholas J. Fortuin,
and Thomas A. Pearson

Patient management involves far more than treatment. Indeed, it involves more than managing the patient's illness. *Treatment* implies the application of one or several therapeutic measures. *Management* is directed toward designing and implementing the most effective program of care for the particular patient's total problem. Management encompasses an orderly analysis of the patient's problems (including those that may or may not relate to his illness), the thoughtful planning of a solution or an approach to these problems, and an effective implementation of these plans. Management implies accepting the responsibility for performing these professional tasks, but it also includes the responsibility for communicating the rationale, the meaning, and the implications of the diagnostic and therapeutic procedures to the patient and to the family.

Pneumococcal lobar pneumonia, for example, is adequately treated by administering penicillin. Management, however, includes investigation of alternative diagnostic possibilities (tumor, *Klebsiella* pneumonia, and the like); assessment of possible complications (meningitis, septicemia, pericarditis); treatment of hypoxia, fluid deficit, or paralytic ileus; as well as the treatment of the infection. Management also takes cognizance of personal and social factors, such as the role of the patient's chronic alcoholism or the impact of hospitalization on his employment. Furthermore, management includes recognition of a home environment that may preclude effective implementation of a therapeutic plan outside the hospital.

The scope of management is illustrated in Figure 1.4–1. Physicians commonly focus their attention on management of the patient's illness (A). As was discussed in Chapter 1.2, these interactions have, in addition, a profound and direct effect on the patient (B). Nurses, other physicians, and other health professionals have an important role in management of the patient and his illness (C). This is especially true in hospitals, where many aspects of management must be shared and delegated. It is equally true in the man-

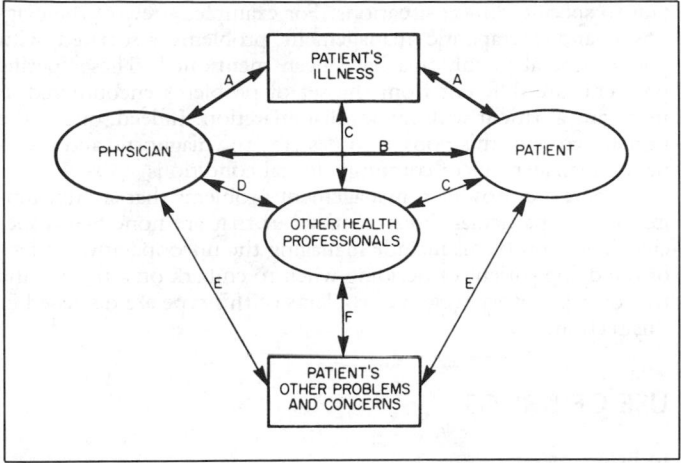

Figure 1.4–1. The multiple interactions that occur between the various people (*ellipses*) and problems (*rectangles*). There is a tendency to focus on the interactions shown by the bold arrows. Good management, as indicated in the text, requires attention to all of the interactions.

agement of chronically ill patients, for whom the support of family, friends, clergy, and social workers is important. Under such circumstances the responsible physician must always be aware of the example he sets and of the need for clear and effective communication (D). Management includes attention to other problems and concerns of the patient (E). Here, too, the physician must incorporate the efforts of other health professionals, such as social workers, in discovering problems and in contributing to their solution (F and C).

This chapter focuses on the principles of good management. It will also discuss common management problems that are not related to specific disease entities, for example, the management of the dying patient. In the discussion in this chapter it is assumed that the physician has collected and analyzed the clinical information as described in the preceding chapters.

ORGANIZE AND RECORD THE FACTS

Ideally, all the facts should be organized in the form of etiologic diagnoses, such as (1) diabetes mellitus, (2) pyelonephritis caused by *Escherichia coli,* or (3) atherosclerotic heart disease with congestive failure. As Weed[12] points out, since this is rarely possible, it is better to start with a complete list of problems. Some of these may be diagnoses, and others may be signs or symptoms. For example, the list presented above might initially be (1) diabetes mellitus, (2) dysuria, (3) pyuria, (4) proteinuria, (5) exertional dyspnea, and (6) edema. The problems on this list must be investigated, explained (diagnosed), and treated.

This approach has several advantages. First, it provides a framework on which to organize laboratory studies, progress notes, and therapeutic measures, each of which should be directed toward one or another of the specific problems. Second, it avoids the pitfall of "ruling out" a given condition. For example, one might have assumed that problems 2 to 5 were manifestations of the nephrotic syndrome. A diagnostic program designed to "rule out the nephrotic syndrome" would not be as productive as one that investigates each problem. Third, it provides an effective means of communicating with others (nurses, consultants, house staff) involved in the patient's management. Fourth, it serves to remind the physician of problems that are unexplained or untreated and that may require attention. Fifth, it provides a convenient way to monitor the patient's progress over the course of weeks and months.

HAVE A PLAN

After the problem list has been constructed, the physician should list in detail all the tests and consultative opinions considered necessary to achieve a final diagnosis. Such a work sheet should outline all, not just some, of the necessary diagnostic and therapeutic steps. Some will require immediate completion, whereas others may be delayed pending the results of other initial studies.

In planning studies, set a pace that is compatible with the patient's physical and emotional state. Patients are sometimes made seriously ill by poorly conceived diagnostic programs. Thus an elderly person with advanced arteriosclerosis may have a vascular accident when injudiciously given a series of enemas and cathartics or when placed on a fast and dehydrated for a lengthy period. Set the pace to fit the particular patient.

In planning the diagnostic and therapeutic program, pay particular attention to treatable possibilities. Thus, if an elderly patient is believed to have either miliary tuberculosis or a disseminated tumor, the major effort should be aimed at establishing or eliminating the diagnosis of tuberculosis, which can be cured with effective treatment.

COMMUNICATE WITH THE PATIENT

One of the most important skills of a physician is the ability to communicate effectively with the patient and his family. The communication of information from patient to physician should not stop with the taking of the history, nor is communication between physician and patient limited to discussions of tests, diagnoses, and drugs. The patient and his family should have the opportunity to ask any questions—both reasonable and unreasonable—that they may have and to express any doubts, fears, or confusion that may have arisen. The patient is often troubled by an aspect of his illness which does not concern the physician. For example, an ulcer patient may be concerned because his near vision is blurred (from the parasympatholytic drug) and because of constipation (caused by the antacid). The physician, in his concern that the patient is still passing occult blood, may be unaware of the patient's symptoms.

During the course of diagnostic studies the plan of management should be explained to the patient in understandable terms. This should be done without creating anxiety but in a way that will generate confidence and a feeling of security. It is a mistake to surprise a patient with any test or consultation. Thus it is inconsiderate to have the patient learn from the nurse that he is on the way to have a bronchoscopic examination, nor should the patient learn only on arrival at the consultant's office that the consultant is a psychiatrist. The patient's primary physician must lay the groundwork in such a way that understanding will be achieved, cooperation won, and anxieties dissipated.

When diagnostic investigations have been completed and the physician has reached a conclusion regarding optimal management, a summarizing conference should be held with the patient and, if indicated, a relative. Such a conference reflects one of the most significant and important relationships of the physician to the patient, because it will almost surely determine the degree of effectiveness of the physician's advice and guidance. During this conference the physician has several responsibilities. First, he should review each of the studies, explaining in meaningful terms why the test was done and what it indicates. The drawing of a few simple diagrams may be helpful in explaining to the patient the nature of his illness. Next, the physician should outline what needs to be done in order to take care of the problem in the most effective way. Adequate time must be afforded to answer questions and to prepare and explain prescriptions. The therapeutic program must be a practical one that the patient can follow without unreasonable effort or sacrifice. Throughout this discussion the physician should anticipate the probable fears and anxieties of the patient, and his conversation should be directed toward eliminating them.

The physician should take nothing for granted in making cer-

tain that the patient or his relatives understand precisely what drug and other forms of treatment are to be administered. One should not simply hand the patient several prescriptions with the instruction that "the directions will be on the bottle." The knowledgeable physician will list in brief outline on a piece of paper the treatment to be followed, stating specific dosages and directions. Such specificity does away with confusion in the patient's mind. To be certain that the patient understands fully, he should be asked to reiterate the directions given to him. On subsequent visits the patient or his relatives should be asked to repeat the program being followed. It is frequently surprising to see how grossly distorted a carefully presented therapeutic plan has become. Only repetition of directions brings ultimate understanding.

Be sure to explain to the patient the significance of important side effects a given drug may induce and how to proceed should these develop. If serious effects are at all likely, the patient should be told to stop the drug immediately on their appearance and to call the physician. In thus indoctrinating the patient regarding potential side effects of various drugs, one must be circumspect and not generate needless fears or actually produce the very reactions warned against. If, in giving a patient iron, the physician says, "This may upset your stomach," there is an excellent likelihood that the prediction will come true.

Certain drugs have acquired public notoriety, and although the patient may not voice his anxieties to the physician, he may view with inward alarm the physician's admonition that such an agent is essential for the patient's well-being. He will be torn by ambivalence, believing that he must take the medicine and, at the same time, being frightened to do so. He may conjure up all sorts of bizarre notions about the drug. An example of such a drug is prednisone: "Is it true it grows hair on your face, causes diabetes, and all your bones collapse?" Others may feel that sex hormones "make you feel queer." Such misconceptions must be anticipated, inquired about, and eradicated with a few simple words of explanation.

THE PHYSICIAN MUST DECIDE

Because patients lack theoretic and technical knowledge, it is unfair for the physician to expect or to ask the patient to decide important clinical issues. On the other hand, when a diagnostic or therapeutic procedure involves a risk to health or life (e.g., coronary arteriography or extensive surgery), the patient's consent must be informed consent.

In such instances the physician must weigh the risks and benefits and then advocate a course of action based on his best judgment. In presenting the plan to the patient and family, it is important that the matter be explained clearly, honestly, and in a well-balanced fashion. The physician should provide ample opportunity for both questions and comments.

When one is advocating a course of action that involves risk, it may be difficult to achieve a balance between offering an overly optimistic view, which would protect the patient from anxiety, and an overly pessimistic view, which would protect one's own position. This balance is achieved by fully informing the patient without terrifying him with a recitation of every possible misadventure that can occur. When both alternatives (action or inaction) may be associated with a grave risk—for example, when massive gastrointestinal bleeding needs investigation—this balance is especially difficult to achieve.

The physician should not defer the decision making to the patient or his family but should present the plan fairly and openly in soliciting consent. Even if the patient withholds consent, the physician must continue to provide diligent care.

COMMON MANAGEMENT PROBLEMS

The foregoing general considerations apply to many clinical situations. There are, however, specific management problems that pertain to specific clinical situations. For example, a few of the diagnostic and therapeutic management problems associated with pneumococcal pneumonia have been mentioned. These specific problems are different from the set of problems encountered in managing a patient with myocardial infarction. Indeed, one of the primary goals of this book is to describe the diagnostic and therapeutic management of common clinical conditions.

There are, however, management problems that are not limited to any particular disease entity but that are nonetheless specific. These problems include managing the uncooperative patient or the dying patient or deciding when to embark on a therapeutic trial or exploratory surgery. Problems of this type are discussed in this section.

USE OF DRUGS

Indications
The physician must always have a reasonably clearcut indication for the administration of any drug. This implies that he knows what is wrong with the patient and which drug is the most effective. There is little room in therapeutic technique for the shotgun approach to drug administration. The haphazard administration of a large number of drugs is more likely to harm the patient than to benefit him. If the physician does not know what is going on, he is better advised to follow a course of watchful waiting. There are certain exceptions, usually related to life-threatening diseases, that do not permit sufficient time to reach a final diagnosis. For example, the patient with findings suggesting septic meningitis is treated with several antibiotics while awaiting bacteriologic confirmation of the presumptive diagnosis.

Contraindications
No drug should ever be given until the physician has determined whether or not the patient is hypersensitive to it. If a drug sensitivity exists, the fact should be noted prominently. If a patient develops a drug hypersensitivity while under treatment, this fact should be clearly explained to him, and he should be encouraged to carry on his person a notation to that effect.

Other contraindications must be carefully weighed. This implies that the physician knows both the general contraindications of the drug and the specific drug-drug and drug-disease contraindications that may affect his patient. Barbiturates, for example, may precipitate a fatal attack in a patient with acute porphyria. The drug-drug interaction can be avoided only if the prescribing physician knows what medicines the patient is taking. When a patient is being seen by a number of physicians simultaneously, errors of this sort may easily occur.

The careful physician also avoids drugs that might further complicate his patient's problem. Thus, if a patient with viral hepatitis is nauseated, it may only complicate the illness to order a phenothiazine for nausea, because if the jaundice becomes worse, it may be difficult to tell whether the hepatitis or a drug reaction is responsible. One must know when *not* to give drugs as well as when to use them.

Choice of Drug
There are several important principles in the selection of drugs. First, the physician should employ drugs with which he is familiar, both in terms of beneficial effects and possible side effects or reactions. A physician should select a relatively small number of agents to handle the various therapeutic problems, read about them, and then use them primarily. Thus over a period of time he can develop a broad background of experience with a small number of drugs, rather than a fragmentary knowledge of many drugs.

Dosage and Administration
Drugs should be given on the basis of sound physiologic and pharmacologic principles, but this rule is easily broken. Thus one finds L-thyroxine being given three times a day instead of once, or corticosteriods being administered over long periods when short

courses might suffice; a very ill patient may awaken repeatedly during the night to void because a diuretic was given late in the evening. The physician must understand the actions of the drugs being employed and use them to the best advantage of each particular patient.

Once a given drug is chosen, it is important to be flexible in regard to dosage. There is no such thing as an average dose of a drug; one must tailor the dose to the individual patient, taking into account his general health, age, size, and clinical response. At times, to produce the desired effects one may need to halve or double the dose originally tried.

Selecting the route of administration is as important as choosing the drug itself. For example, the patient with nausea, vomiting, or distension may not absorb oral drugs effectively. The patient with congestive heart failure who has hepatomegaly and nausea should receive digitalis parenterally. Patients in shock will not dependably absorb drugs injected intramuscularly. Thus the patient with pneumococcal pneumonia who is in shock should receive penicillin intravenously. Finally, some oral medications should be given well before a meal, whereas others should be given after meals.

New Drugs

The physician should develop a healthy skepticism about claims regarding new drugs and should always seek out objective sources describing a drug's efficacy, rather than relying on promotions by the drug industry. These promotions, which are omnipresent and seductive, may be in the form of direct product advertising, statements by pharmaceutical "detail" representatives, or the more subtle advertising in articles written by experts in the many non-peer-reviewed journals ("throwaways") that are provided to physicians without charge. The history of medicine indicates that some doctors eagerly embrace new therapies without asking critical questions about the proof of efficacy.

If a new preparation clearly provides a therapeutic effect that has not been obtainable with drugs already available, its use is indicated at an early date. On the other hand, if the drug appears to do no more than older medications, it is good judgment to use the older preparations, which are likely to be both less expensive and safer. With most drugs the therapeutic claims become more modest as experience accumulates and as various toxic effects, previously unsuspected, become manifest. One legitimate time for using a new drug, however, is when older preparations have failed to produce the desired results in a given patient.

The physician must satisfy himself that a drug's claims of superiority to other drugs already available are justified by the evidence at hand. In evaluating reports on the efficacy of new drugs, the physician will find the following questions helpful[7]:

1. Has the agent or technique been compared against a placebo or standard therapy?
2. How has the author randomly allocated patients to receive the treatments under comparison?
3. Has the author controlled bias in the evaluation of results?
4. Have dose-response relationships been studied, or does the article deal only with single dose levels?
5. Is there information on the relative efficacy of different routes of administration?
6. Is there information on efficacy and toxicity of the agent when it is given on a long-term basis?
7. Is the experimental population studied of sufficient size to justify either favorable or unfavorable statements about the drug?
8. Is this patient comparable to the experimental population in which efficacy was demonstrated?

Noncompliance

The most carefully planned therapeutic regimen will be of no benefit if the patient fails to comply with it.[5,10] Noncompliance is obviously an important complication in management, and it is far more common than most physicians realize. Furthermore, physicians often do not recognize the patients who are likely candidates for noncompliance. Finally, the common reaction to noncompliance once it is discovered is to tell the patient that both the physician's time and the patient's money are being wasted.

The factors contributing to noncompliance can be grouped according to those related to (1) the psychologic status of the patient, (2) his social and familial environment, (3) characteristics of the illness, (4) the therapeutic regimen, and (5) the physician-patient relationship.

Patient's Psychologic Status. The patient who is skeptical about the seriousness of his illness may be too unconcerned to follow the prescribed treatment. Such a patient may also have little confidence in the general efficacy of modern medicine, which further supports his noncompliance. On the other hand, the illness may evoke such intense anxiety that the patient resorts to denial of his problems and, indeed, may not have been able to pay adequate attention to the physician's instructions; in this situation, intense anxiety may be obscured by a defensive attitude of coldness, hostility, or aggressiveness.

Therefore either lack of concern or cold, critical, or aggressive behavior should arouse suspicion of impending noncompliance. In the former instance the problem may be essentially an educational one and may be remedied by clear, factual communication with the patient in understandable terms. If the patient's behavior suggests, however, a negative rejection of medical advice (serving to allay anxiety), the physician's task is much more difficult. The patient should be encouraged to discuss his feelings about the illness and treatment; occasionally it may be necessary to modify the treatment plan, at least temporarily, to secure some level of cooperation.

Social and Family Background. The physician should always pay careful attention to the patient's family situation and socioeconomic background. Lack of money or transportation and preoccupation with pressing family or occupational demands may gravely interfere with the patient's ability and willingness to comply with the management plan. In this situation it is sometimes tempting for the physician himself to ignore these aspects and to rationalize this posture by claiming responsibility only for prescribing treatment: the patient must carry out the prescription. Tactful but frank discussion of the home and job situation, however, may well lead to the discovery of practical aids to facilitate participation in treatment. A skilled social worker is often invaluable in the assessment of these problems and in the mobilization of community resources in their solution.

Nature of the Illness. It is likely that when the illness produces considerable discomfort, such as pain, shortness of breath, or weakness, which is substantially improved by the prescribed drug and recurs when the medicine is not taken, the patient will comply with treatment. In the case of a relatively "silent" illness, however, such as uncomplicated essential hypertension, the likelihood of noncompliance is enhanced. In these instances, noncompliance should be anticipated and counteracted by a clear explanation of the benefits of treatment.

Sometimes the converse is true; the patient is too ill to comply and may not be able to obtain or take the medication on the prescribed schedule. He may be too sick to understand a complicated regimen. Hospitalization or professional home care may be needed for such a patient.

Nature of the Therapy. More complex therapeutic regimens, especially those requiring substantial changes in daily habits, are more likely to evoke noncompliant behavior than are simple treatment plans. Here, too, it is important to encourage the patient to express his feelings, ask questions, and sometimes to "negotiate" a treatment plan that, although it may fall short of the ideal, has a better chance of being carried out.

Similarly, in programs in which the benefits of the treatment

are slow to appear, the tendency toward noncompliance is great. The dietary management of obesity is a common example.

The Patient-Physician Relationship. In the last analysis, the physician-patient relationship may well be the most crucial variable in determining compliance with treatment plans. In the daily work of the busy practitioner, failure to take the time for truly adequate communication is probably the most common and damaging deficiency of modern medicine. To maximize effectiveness, the physician must cultivate a relationship of mutual respect, offer explanations in a clear manner, invite questions and expressions of feelings and ideas, and be sensitive to psychologic and other obstacles that may stand in the way of full patient cooperation. This topic is discussed further in Chapter 16.2.

THERAPEUTIC TRIAL

The physician should not prematurely discontinue his step-by-step, considered attack on the patient's problem until a reasonable diagnosis is obtained. Nevertheless, it is sometimes necessary to begin specific therapy without knowing the actual cause of the patient's illness. There are other instances where a therapeutic trial must be begun on the basis of the most probable diagnosis.

Although the nature of the illness is still obscure, if the patient is seriously ill or if essential organ function seems threatened, the program of therapy chosen should cover all of the reasonable therapeutic possibilities. Even in these circumstances, however, one should try to avoid a shotgun approach. If the condition of the patient seems to warrant it, a progressive type of therapeutic trial may be begun in which first one, and then another, agent is added to the treatment program in an effort to determine its effect on the disease's course. The drugs chosen should be safe, specific in action, and unlikely to cause further complications.

Once it is decided that a therapeutic trial is the wisest course of action, the treatment should be maintained long enough to test its effectiveness. In this regard, it is advisable to select criteria of improvement that can be subjected to objective analysis (e.g., fever and spleen size). The indecisive approach, in which regimens are started and then abandoned, too often leads to dangerous confusion.

EXPLORATORY SURGERY

Surgical procedures are sometimes necessary to achieve a diagnosis. Laparotomy and thoracotomy, major procedures requiring careful consideration, are discussed in this section. In contrast, skin, muscle, and lymph node biopsies are considered simple procedures involving little risk, if any. Intermediate, in terms of risk, are a group of procedures that are discussed elsewhere. These include pleural biopsy, needle biopsy of lung lesions, scalene node biopsy, and mediastinoscopy (see Chapter 3.1), liver biopsy (see Chapter 13.1), and renal biopsy (see Chapter 11.1).

Laparotomy

Since exploratory laparotomy is of value in determining the cause of illness in some instances, it is important to consider when such a procedure is indicated. If the clinical evidence clearly points to localized intra-abdominal disorder, laparotomy is obviously in order. Considerable judgment is required when there is little or no evidence pointing to intra-abdominal disease. On the one hand, all operations carry some risk, especially in a seriously ill patient; on the other, surgical exploration may reveal the cause of disease even in the absence of local symptoms and signs.

Exploratory laparotomy should not be pursued until all indirect methods that afford a reasonable chance of establishing the cause of the disease have been exhausted. Included in this category are not only history taking and physical examination, laboratory and radiographic studies, endoscopy, CT scan, and other special procedures, but also, and especially, a period of searching clinical

observation, during which the patient is thoughtfully re-questioned and re-examined. Such a period must not become one in which the patient is allowed to drift or in which conflicting forms of therapy are added.

In deciding when to terminate such an observation period, one should neither be premature nor delay too long. One must assay the degree to which the disease has already importantly affected the patient—or is likely to do so in the near future. Such an inventory must encompass not only the physical effects of the illness but also the personal ones. The inability to work, the periodic suspension of normal living, the psychologic effects of being considered ill, and the financial drain of chronic or recurrent illness are all factors that must be weighed. From the physical standpoint, evidence that any of the organ systems are being seriously affected in a deleterious manner is the most important determinant. Clearly, significant progressive alterations would call for an immediate decision. Another consideration is the likelihood that by prolonged waiting a condition that is now curable may progress to an uncontrollable stage. A decision on this point is, of course, dependent on the diagnostic possibilities being considered.

The risks entailed in an exploratory operation will be determined not only by the patient's general physical status but also by what may be required surgically should a suspected abnormality be discovered. It is not enough to decide that the patient can withstand an exploration. Of equal significance is a decision regarding the patient's ability to survive surgical correction of whatever may be discovered. For example, if the clinical evidence indicates that a patient has right-sided colitis but that his general condition interdicts surgical treatment of this condition, it may be inadvisable to prove the diagnosis by a laparotomy; further medical treatment may be preferable.

When the physician has decided on an exploratory operation, how should this procedure be accomplished so that the necessary information will be forthcoming? It would be unfortunate for the operation to be performed in such a way that valuable information is overlooked or discarded. Two points are worthy of emphasis. First, biopsy specimens should be taken from all suspicious lesions because it is impossible to distinguish tumor from inflammation with certainty without histologic study. Second, biopsy material should be studied adequately and properly. For example, cultures for tubercle bacilli, fungi, and anaerobic bacteria should be made when appropriate. Similarly, a biopsy of the skin, subcutaneous tissue, and muscle can easily be accomplished while doing a laparotomy. It is regrettable if the patient must undergo a muscle biopsy at a later date to establish the diagnosis of polyarteritis.

Thoracotomy

The principles discussed for exploratory laparotomy also apply in general to exploration of the chest, mediastinum, or pericardium. There are, however, several matters deserving special note.

First, thoracotomy for a mass lesion in the lung may require a segmental resection or even a lobectomy. Hence, if the plan is to open the chest, the physician must be certain that the patient is able to withstand whatever procedures are necessary. In addition, he must ascertain that the patient and family fully understand how extensive the exploration may ultimately be.

Second, a specific diagnosis may not be made even when adequate tissue samples are obtained and studied thoroughly, both histologically and biologically. This is especially true of granulomatous lesions of the lung, pleura, pericardium, and mediastinum. A wide variety of infectious agents, including tuberculosis, syphilis, fungi, parasites, and certain malignant tumors, in addition to some chemical agents, may cause a granulomatous inflammatory response that is totally nonspecific and that may become so widespread as to obscure the parent process.

Exploratory laparotomy may occasionally be undertaken on the basis of symptoms alone. In contrast, thoracotomy is almost never undertaken unless clear signs of disease are shown in the results of physical or radiographic examination or another diagnostic test.

SURGERY TO IMPROVE PROGNOSIS

Increasingly, surgical procedures are advocated to improve the patient's prognosis, not to relieve symptoms or provide diagnostic information. A good example of this kind of surgery is the resection of an abdominal aortic aneurysm. In this situation the evidence is clear that most aneurysms will rupture with fatal consequences within 3 years once the aneurysm is more than 5 cm in diameter. Surgery to prevent rupture can be done with low risk and should be performed once the aneurysm is recognized.

In some cases prophylactic surgery will improve the problem but will not alter the natural history of the disease. For example, portacaval shunt surgery for patients with cirrhosis of the liver who have had bleeding from esophageal varices will prevent recurrent bleeding, but the longevity of patients is not prolonged because they die of other complications of liver failure and are more prone to portal-systemic encephalopathy after surgery. Surgery may be recommended for chronic conditions where proper randomized trials have not been done or have not provided proof of efficacy. The role of coronary artery bypass surgery in improving the prognosis in patients with chronic ischemic heart disease is a case in point. Early claims that such surgery would prevent myocardial infarction and prolong life have not been substantiated by long-term follow-up studies except in a few select patient subgroups.

MALPRACTICE

Malpractice suits and the threat of malpractice suits represent significant and difficult issues in patient management today. Legally, medical malpractice is negligence on the part of the physician or his agent that leads to injury of the patient. The problems concerning malpractice are real, and there is no reason to expect that they will diminish.

Unfortunately, malpractice does occur. For example, the physician forgets that the patient is allergic to penicillin and administers it, or he fails to note a coin lesion on a routine chest film. This is negligence, and the patient may be injured. Physicians aim to manage their patients in a conscientious fashion, and they intend to avoid this type of negligent error.

In current medical practice, although avoiding negligence is necessary, it is not sufficient to guard against being sued for malpractice. It is estimated that only one fifth of malpractice claims reflect actual negligence on the part of the physician. Why do the other four fifths of patients who file malpractice claims believe they have been injured through physician negligence? A clear understanding of the basis for these claims is necessary if one is to avoid them.

Societal Factors

There is a widespread belief today that if something goes wrong and you are injured, "somebody should pay." This is seen in product liability suits as well as in medical malpractice claims. The public expects to be compensated by the automobile manufacturer if injury results from a steering gear failure. The public expects to be compensated by the physician if there is residual disability after reduction of a fracture. There is no question about the injury, but the steering gear failure may not be caused by the manufacturer's negligence and the residual disability may not be related to negligence on the part of the physician. The view that the injured party is entitled to compensation whether or not there was negligence is called *strict liability in tort* by the legal profession. Although it is not accepted in many jurisdictions, it reflects a common belief—a change in belief by our society. Much of the increase in malpractice litigation is explained by this widespread belief that one is entitled to compensation for injury (whatever its cause) in combination with the factors discussed below.

Unfavorable Outcome

Almost all claims arise from patients who experience an unfavorable medical outcome. Although this is a necessary condition, it, too, is usually not sufficient. There is often another factor that prompts such a patient to claim malpractice.

Unrealistic Expectations

The most common combination of factors in precipitating malpractice claims is an unfavorable outcome in a patient who had unrealistic expectations about the outcome. Some patients die despite the best possible medical management, and others make substantially less than a full recovery. Physicians have a great propensity for wanting to spare patients and their families from anxiety. They may persuade them that everything will turn out well even when it is clear that the situation is grave or the proposed course of action is risky.

Thus the physician himself contributes to unrealistic expectations on the part of patients and families. When the results fall far short of what the patient and family were led to believe, it is understandable that they conclude that something went wrong. The following sequence accounts for many malpractice claims: (1) everything was supposed to be fine, (2) it was not, (3) therefore something must have gone wrong, and (4) therefore somebody should pay for this unfavorable and unexpected outcome.

The physician need not burden patients or their families with the most pessimistic outcome to ensure that they will be pleased with anything short of disaster. Nevertheless, the prudent physician must give the patient or at least responsible family members a realistic appraisal of the situation. Ironically, it is the physician whose manner with patients is the most persuasive who can impart the most unrealistic expectations.

Anger

The patient who is angry for any reason may seize on an unfavorable outcome to gain retribution. Unfortunately for the physician the anger may arise from shortcomings of the hospital billing system, the nursing service, the physician's receptionist, or even frustrations with the illness itself. The physician may become the target of this anger even though not directly responsible for it. There are many reasons to be alert to anger on the part of patients, and physicians should take responsibility in seeing that the vexing issues are resolved. A considerable degree of sensitivity is required, because patients frequently have difficulty in expressing their anger to physicians, especially if the anger is directed toward the physician himself.

The Litigious Patient

More patients are made litigious by circumstances than are litigious by nature. There are, however, some patients who are frankly litigious. Such patients often move from physician to physician, deprecate their past medical care, and are unreasonably demanding. This behavior tends to evoke hostility, anger, and defensiveness on the part of the physician. Even when the physician does not allow these feelings to affect his management of the patient, the scene is set for contention.

Defensive Medicine

One must practice defensive medicine. This does not imply ordering unnecessary tests or obtaining unnecessary consultations. The best defense against malpractice claims is simply good management: (1) establish an attitude of mutual trust with the patient; (2) communicate realistically with the patient; (3) be sensitive to his needs, fears, concerns (whether well founded or not); (4) be aware of your own limitations; and (5) keep good records of what was done and why it was done.

NEED FOR CONSULTATION

The physician should always be willing to ask for consultative help when it is needed. To practice first-rate medicine one must always be prepared to seek the opinion and judgment of those whose experience is greater. Even if the medical necessity is nonexistent, the

physician should be alert to anxiety and restiveness in the patient or in members of his family and respond by suggesting that the fresh viewpoint of a consultant be secured. To be fully productive, the physician and the consultant should meet and discuss the problem. Consultations carried out through an exchange of notes are often of very little value.

It is important to recognize, however, that the physician in charge of a patient cannot abdicate responsibility for management. Management by a committee of consultants never ensures that the best opinion is brought to bear on a problem.

MEDICAL EMERGENCIES

The usual orderly steps in management may need to be altered in dealing with emergencies. The details of managing these problems are discussed in Section 4.

MANAGEMENT OF EMOTIONAL DISORDERS

The management of emotional disorders[5] is of considerable importance to the practicing physician, because a number of studies show that a substantial percentage of patients seen in diagnostic clinics have no demonstrable organic abnormalities that can be related to their symptomatic complaints. The large numbers of these patients make it impractical to refer all of them to psychiatrists, even if such large-scale referrals were considered to be desirable.

Thus the appropriate management of emotional problems is important to all physicians. Although this subject is treated in some depth in Section 16, it is worth outlining several aspects of the management problem here.

The recognition that an emotional problem exists is the first step in management. In general, patients whose problems are exclusively of a "mental" or emotional nature will have initial complaints concerned with subjective discomfort or functional disturbance, or they will have exhibited aberrant behavior that has aroused concern in others. It is important to keep in mind that apparent symptoms of emotional disturbances may in fact represent an organic entity such as thyroid dysfunction. Therefore it is also necessary in this situation to regard symptoms and behavioral disturbances as problems that, with further fact gathering and analysis, may later become grouped under a single diagnostic entity, psychiatric or other.

It is common for an emotionally disturbed patient to complain of a physical symptom such as chronic fatigue, headache, or insomnia, and often a whole host of physical complaints will be elicited in the history taking. Among the reasons for this, two may be mentioned here: (1) The patient may be focusing on physical discomforts as a means of minimizing painful feelings that might accompany an awareness of his emotional difficulty. (2) His preconception of what the physician's interest may be could lead him to use a physical complaint as an "admission ticket" to the doctor's office.

It is apparent that in this situation, as elsewhere in medicine, treatment of the symptoms, such as prescribing aspirin for headache, is doomed to failure unless it is accompanied by recognition and adequate management of the total problem. This symptomatic approach often occurs, however, and contributes to the fact that such patients frequently have had disappointing experiences with prior medical contacts and may become resentful, difficult, and demanding. Occasionally a physical symptom may be of such psychologic importance that a radical approach to it alone, without appropriate evaluation and management of the whole problem, may precipitate rapid psychologic decompensation. On rare occasions the result may be the development of a paranoid accusation directed at the physician. Many patients find it hard to accept the fact than an emotional disorder underlies their symptoms. They may seek repeated evaluation by a succession of physicians in order to prove that their complaints are due to organic disease. Even though the physician may recognize that emotional problems underlie the complaints early in the encounter with the patient, it is important to satisfy the patient that a thorough search has been made for disease processes that might produce symptoms. Taking a cursory history and giving a brief examination, followed by prescribing a tranquilizer or an antidepressant, are not satisfactory. Rather the physician should take a meticulous history and perform a careful physical examination; many laboratory studies may also have to be ordered before the patient will be convinced that no organic illness exists. Only then will some patients accept psychologic management of the problem. Often, reassuring the patient that he is physically well will have a major salutary effect on symptoms.

The next question to arise after recognition of the true nature of the problem is whether the physician chooses to manage the problem, with or without psychiatric consultation, or to refer the patient to a psychiatrist. Parallel issues are *how* to manage the problem if the physician elects to do so and how to facilitate the patient's acceptance of psychiatric consultation or referral. On each of these questions it is often helpful for the physician to discuss the issue with a psychiatric consultant.

Both general principles of management and management of specific problems such as suicidal behavior and anxiety states are discussed in detail in Section 16.

DIAGNOSIS OF MALIGNANCY

The physician must make it an unbroken rule never to conclude that a patient has a malignant disease without histologic proof of the diagnosis. In these matters, the physician should neither trust hearsay evidence nor be willing to take anything for granted. Serious mistakes may be made by assuming that the patient has a malignant disease on the basis of an exploration of the chest or abdominal cavity in the absence of objective evidence based on the histologic study of a biopsy specimen. These mistakes can take the form of irrevocable action (e.g., irradiation of a granuloma in the lung) or the form of inaction (e.g., the failure to treat ameboma of the colon).

When the diagnosis has been established, the question always arises as to whether the patient should be told. Although it is impossible to generalize, it is safe to say that most patients realize the nature of their illness sooner or later. If the patient has been assured by his physician that his condition is benign, he may feel betrayed. More important, the physician has then lost much of his power to support and sustain the patient through a difficult situation. Often a gentle, honest explanation will convey the information. At the same time, the physician should offer hope in the form of a specific program of management.

HOPELESS ILLNESS

Much of what has been said of malignant tumor applies to hopeless illnesses as well. The physician must be certain to have excluded all treatable conditions, even if they are much less common. For example, reasonable steps must be taken to exclude frontal lobe tumor in the patient thought to have senile dementia of the Alzheimer type.

Similarly, it is important that the physician remain alert to the appearance of unassociated treatable complications. There is an understandable tendency to ascribe an unfavorable clinical course to the underlying disease without adequate investigation.

The only prudent philosophy for a physician to adopt is always to support life as long as it is present. It is dangerous to do otherwise. However, if the reasoned judgment of the physician and his colleagues is that a patient's illness is entirely hopeless and that the patient is undergoing significant mental or physical suffering, the use of extraordinary means to support life is certainly not

expected or even desired. A cardinal principle is not to prolong the dying process, especially when the patient is clearly suffering.

THE DYING PATIENT

The patient who is dying represents a special management problem. Most patients, their families, physicians, and nurses are uncomfortable in dealing with death or in discussing its prospect. Because most persons now die in a medical institution rather than at home, physicians are centrally involved. Furthermore, because death is such an emotionally charged issue for everyone involved, it is essential that the physician be able to manage the problem effectively and with understanding.

The discomfort involved in managing a dying patient leads both physicians and nurses to avoid patient contact, to be brief and cursory when in contact with the patient, and to be evasive if the patient directs the conversation toward prognosis, outcome, and the like. At the same time the family is upset and may be struggling to suppress grief or guilt. As a result, the patient, in a time of great need, may feel cut off from counsel, emotional support, and perhaps even conversation and full attention to physical needs.

Thus this important clinical management problem has not been handled well by physicians or health-care professionals in general, and little has been taught or learned about management of the dying patient in our educational programs. In recent years, however, this problem of the dying patient has been subjected to clinical study. Kübler-Ross[6] has identified a common pattern of emotional stages through which patients pass after recognizing the fact that they are dying. These stages are (1) shock and denial, (2) anger, (3) bargaining, (4) depression, (5) preparatory grief, and finally (6) a peaceful acceptance. These feelings occur with some overlap and some shifting back and forth, and it is a sense of hope that sustains the patient throughout.

The physician's role is to support the patient and provide understanding. Insight into these stages permits the physician to deal with the real issues better. For example, the patient's anger may appear to be directed toward some trivial aspect of his care. His need is not simply to have the triviality corrected, and it is certainly not to have the triviality of the issue emphasized. He needs an opportunity to express his anger and resentment about the outrageous situation in which he finds himself.

It is not necessary for the physician to *tell* the patient he is terminally ill. The physician should, however, be attuned to the patient's efforts to communicate his awareness of the terminal nature of the illness to the physician. Often the patient does this obliquely by making comments such as "I don't think there is much more that you can do for me" or "I don't really think I am going to get better." These are not cues for hearty reassurance by the physician; they are requests for discussion of the problem. Reassurance, denial, and disclaimers by the physician promptly bar further discussion of the topic, a message that the patient clearly perceives. Inquiry into areas of particular concern to the patient, on the other hand, opens the way to a meaningful conversation about issues important to the patient. Such conversations can lead to more openness between the patient and his family as well.

HEALTH PROMOTION AND DISEASE PREVENTION

PREVENTIVE HEALTH CARE IN THE ASYMPTOMATIC ADULT

An important role exists for the clinician, not only in the diagnosis and treatment of acute conditions but also in the prevention of chronic conditions for which no effective treatment is available and in the identification of other diseases at a stage where treatment is effective. This requires a different type of approach to asymptomatic patients or to patients who are under the physician's care for other unrelated conditions. Certainly the routine "checkup" is one of the most common reasons for visiting a physician, including a physician practicing in a subspecialty. The preventive approach to the asymptomatic patient thus requires several steps: (1) the orderly collection of information on conditions, so-called risk factors, that predispose the patient to the development of disease, (2) the ordering of screening tests to detect disease that is clinically silent, and (3) intervention to correct or modify risk factors and treat disease at an early stage to prevent illness, disability, or premature death.

The identification of risk factors and the detection of asymptomatic disease both require the judicious use of screening tests. It is obvious that a vast array of tests are available to the clinician, but relatively few are appropriate for use with the asymptomatic patient. Several organizations, such as the World Health Organization and the Canadian Task force on the Periodic Health Examination, have developed criteria to select tests for screening asymptomatic patients.[3] The disease should be a significant cause of illness, death, or disability. There should be a period in which the disease is asymptomatic. An effective treatment should be available for the disease. The treatment of the disease in the asymptomatic stage should give a better result or prognosis than treatment in the symptomatic stage. The screening test should be accurate, simple, and acceptable to the population. Finally, the disease sought should have sufficient prevalence to justify screening and follow-up costs.

Thus one goal is to provide *all* patients with a minimum of preventive health services. A second goal is to assess whether the patient may be at high risk for certain chronic conditions and therefore require more extensive preventive services than would ordinarily be necessary. Such high-risk groups include patients with family history of diseases known to have a genetic predisposition, patients whose occupations carry an increased risk of certain diseases, and patients who have been cured of chronic diseases but who carry a high risk of recurrence. For example, if a woman has a mother or sister with breast cancer or has had a cancer successfully treated in one breast, she would require more frequent screening for breast cancer than women without these histories. A variety of high-risk conditions exist and are discussed as they relate to specific diseases.

SCREENING PROGRAM FOR THE OTHERWISE HEALTHY ADULT

The comprehensive physical examination is no longer considered cost effective when performed on an annual basis. Rather most authorities recommend an individualized preventive care program based on the age, sex, and risk category of the patient. Recommendations for a *minimum* program are presented in Table 1.4–1, to be used as a rapid reference for determination of the appropriate screening tests.

Several points must be emphasized regarding these routine screening tests. First, the history and physical examination remain important screening tests and should not be totally replaced by laboratory testing. This is particularly true for those life-style and other risk behaviors requiring counseling. Second, the test recommendations vary considerably with the age and sex of the patient. These age-specific recommendations are based on the relative prevalence and preventability of disease at each age. Third, it is likely that considerable change will occur in these recommendations with the advent of new cost-benefit studies and with the development of new technologies. For example, screening for serum cholesterol levels has recently been recommended for all adults, beginning at age 18 years, with new definitions of "abnormal" values. In addition, whereas the American Cancer Society had previously recom-

TABLE 1.4–1. PREVENTIVE SERVICES FOR ASYMPTOMATIC PATIENTS

Service	Age Groups (yr)				
	Adult Entry (18–24[a])	Young Adult (25–39[b])	Middle Adult (40–59[c])	Older Adult (60–74[d])	Old Age (75+[e])
History and physical examination with referrals as necessary					
Height and weight	+	+	+[b]	+	+
Blood pressure	+	+	+[b]	+	+
Vision			+[b]	+	+
Hearing			+[b]	+	+
Breast examination (women)	+	+	+[b]	+	+
Rectal examination			+[b]	+	+
Laboratory examination					
Mammography			+	+	+
ECG (one baseline at age 40 or 45 yr)			+		
Serum cholesterol (every 5 yr if baseline normal)	+	+	+		
VDRL (if not otherwise obtained)	+				
Papanicolaou smear (women)	+	+	+	+	
Gonococcal culture (women)	+				
Rubella titer (women)	+				
Blood glucose			+[b]	+	+
Hematocrit			+[b]	+	+
Urinalysis for protein, sugar			+[b]	+	+
Stool guaiac			+[b]	+	+
Immunizations					
Tetanus (booster, every 10 yr)	+	+	+	+	+
Influenza (especially over 65 yr)				+	+
Pneumococcus (high risk only)	+	+	+	+	+
Rubella (nonimmunized pregnant women)	+	+			
Counseling with referrals as necessary					
Nutrition	+	+	+	+	+
Accident prevention	+	+	+	+	+
Physical activity and exercise	+	+	+	+	+
Alcohol, drug use	+	+	+	+	+
Cigarette smoking	+	+	+	+	+
Family relations, social problems, sexual adjustment	+	+	+	+	+
Family planning	+	+	+	+	+
Sleep	+	+	+	+	+
Obesity	+	+	+	+	+
Teaching breast and skin self-examination	+	+	+	+	+
Retirement				+	+
Living arrangements				+	+
Individual concerns	+	+	+	+	+

[a]One health visit
[b]Three health visits, about age 25, 30, and 35 yr
[c]Four health visits, about age 40, 45, 50, and 55 yr
[d]Health visit at age 60 yr and every 2 yr thereafter
[e]Annual health visits
[f]To be performed once during interim between examinations
Modified from the American College of Physicians Medical Practice Committee.[1]

mended mammography for women 50 years of age and older, it is now recommended for women aged 40 to 49 years at 1- to 2-year intervals.

PREVENTIVE INTERVENTIONS

The third step in disease prevention is the intervention based on the risk factors or the asymptomatic disease process. This, of course, requires the follow-up of all abnormal results of the screening program. Certainly one necessary step is to repeat the screening test or, if a single positive test result causes enough concern, to proceed with diagnostic or therapeutic measures. These are described for the specific conditions in later chapters.

To be effective in the prevention of disease, the physician must often persuade the patient to modify the life-style. This is a traditionally discouraging enterprise, as exemplified by low success rates with smoking cessation, weight loss, and physical exercise programs. However, some general guidelines may be provided to maximize the effect of such counseling. First, obtain a thorough history of the patient's life-style behavior, including when the behavior began, past attempts to modify the behavior, which methods were most successful, and perceived barriers to success of life-style modification. For example, a history of cigarette smoking should include not only the number of years of smoking and the number of cigarettes smoked per day but also the age at which smoking began, whether the patient has ever tried to quit smoking and

what caused him to return to smoking, types of programs tried, and symptoms of nicotine addiction. Second, emphasize to the patient the benefits of changing the life-style, in addition to decreasing the risks of continuing the deleterious life-style. Using scare tactics by describing the diseases related to smoking has never been very successful in getting smokers to quit. Reviewing the financial benefits, the ability to continue to exercise vigorously, and the avoidance of smoking in one's children if a better role model is provided may be more effective arguments. Third, identify whether the patient is committed to changing the life-style and, if so, provide continued support for that commitment, even if the patient is initially unsuccessful. Fourth, develop a specific plan for modification of the behavior with the patient, such as a "quit date" for the cigarette smoker or the amount of weight loss for the obese patient. Finally, identify others, such as family members, to help the patient modify the behaviors, including changing the entire family's behavior if necessary. It is important to provide consistent support and encouragement to the patient; the expression of anger and frustration is deleterious to the effort and should be avoided.

The modification of patient behavior often requires referral of the patient to another health professional, such as a nutritionist, behavioral scientist, or exercise therapist. The physician plays an important role in ensuring the success of the efforts of these professionals. The physician should clearly inform the patient as to the reasons why he or she is being referred. The importance of the visit should be emphasized as part of the behavior modification program. Similarly, the condition for which the referral was requested should be clearly communicated to the other health professional, including any other information that could help or interfere with the intervention. A close interaction with these other professionals is essential to the effective intervention in health behaviors at the cost of relatively little additional time and effort.

REFERENCES

1. American College of Physicians Medical Practice Committee. Periodic health examination: A guide for designing individualized preventive health care in the asymptomatic patient. Ann Intern Med 95:729, 1981
2. Brim OG Jr, Freeman HE, Levine S, Scotch NA (eds.): The Dying Patient. New York, Russell Sage Foundation, 1970
3. Canadian Task Force on the Periodic Health Examination: The periodic health examination. II (1984 update). Can Med Assoc J 130:1278, 1984
4. Gillum RF, Barsky AJ: Diagnosis and management of patient noncompliance. JAMA 288:1563, 1974
5. Imboden JB, Urbaitis JC: Practical Psychiatry in Medicine. New York, Appleton-Century-Crofts, 1978
6. Kübler-Ross E: Questions and Answers on Death and Dying. New York, Macmillan, 1974
7. Lasagna L: On evaluating drug therapy: The nature of the evidence. In Talalay P (ed): Drugs in Our Society. Baltimore, Johns Hopkins University Press, 1964
8. Medical Practice Committee, American College of Physicians: Periodic health examination: A guide for designing individualized preventive health care in the asymptomatic patient. Ann Intern Med 95:729, 1981
9. Rose SD: The periodic health examination. Primary Care 7:653, 1980
10. Rosenstock IM: Patients' compliance with health regimens. JAMA 234:402, 1975
11. Tumulty PA: The Effective Clinician. Philadelphia, WB Saunders, 1973
12. Weed LL: Medical Records, Medical Education, and Patient Care. Cleveland, Case Western Reserve University Press, 1969

Patients with heart disease are discovered in many ways—from the patient with severe, unbearable chest pain indicative of life-threatening illness, to one with an asymptomatic abnormality detected on routine physical examination, chest radiograph or electrocardiogram (ECG). In both cases the physician must arrive at a precise etiologic, anatomic, and physiologic diagnosis, which usually requires the analysis of information from many sources. The sources of information and tools used in evaluation will be presented in the first chapter; the problem situations or patterns of presentation occurring in practice will be discussed in the subsequent chapters.

The clinical evaluation of the cardiovascular system, the symptoms and signs of the diseases of the heart, and the use of laboratory studies in the assessment of cardiovascular disease are outlined in Chapter 2.1. Congestive heart failure is a common manifestation of disordered cardiac function, and Chapter 2.2 is devoted to the pathophysiology of this condition, the approach to the patient with congestive failure, and the management of congestive failure. The interpretation of murmurs and the specific problems related to valvular heart disease and its surgical treatment are discussed in Chapter 2.3. The heart murmur may have been detected on routine physical examination. Although a heart murmur may not have been the original reason to suspect cardiac disease, it may be the most reliable manifestation on which to base a differential diagnosis. Disorders of cardiac rhythm may be responsible for the patient's seeking medical attention, as in the case of palpitation due to frequent premature contrac-

tions. Under other circumstances an arrhythmia may be a manifestation of disease of the valves, myocardium, or coronary arteries, or it may be responsible for congestive failure or circulatory collapse (Chapter 2.9).

Chest pain may be a symptom of potentially fatal heart disease, and the differentiation of chest pain of cardiac origin from that due to other causes is a common and important problem (Chapter 2.7). Myocardial infarction and pericarditis, common cardiovascular conditions associated with pain in the chest, are covered in Chapters 2.4 and 2.8.

A high systemic arterial blood pressure may be detected on routine examination in the absence of symptoms, or it may be the cause of congestive heart failure. In either case, it is an important finding and worthy of individual attention (Chapter 2.10). Another important abnormality, the cause of which must be clearly established, is pulmonary hypertension. Usually there are symptoms that, when considered with physical signs and laboratory data, lead to the recognition of the problem as one of increased pulmonary vascular resistance (Chapter 2.6).

Congenital heart disease is the subject of Chapter 2.5. Diseases of the aorta and the peripheral circulation also are discussed from the point of view of the presenting complaint (Chapters 2.11 and 2.12). Acute circulatory collapse (shock) and pulmonary edema often indicate serious heart disease, and prompt emergency therapy can save life. Therefore these particular problems are discussed in the section on critical care (Chapters 4.3 and 4.4).

CHAPTER 2.1
Clinical and Laboratory Evaluations of the Cardiovascular System

Richard S. Ross and Nicholas J. Fortuin

CLINICAL EVALUATION

Information useful in the clinical assessment of the cardiovascular system is derived from (1) history, (2) physical examination, (3) roentgenography, (4) electrocardiography, and (5) special laboratory studies.[1,4,6,8] The patient's cardiac abnormality may be detected on history, physical examination, or laboratory study, but information from all sources is often required to establish a diagnosis and to plan management. Most patients with heart disease come to medical attention because of symptoms that may be sudden in onset, as in acute pulmonary edema or myocardial infarction, or that may evolve gradually over days to weeks, as in angina pectoris or chronic congestive heart failure. Occasionally heart disease may be suspected in the asymptomatic person because of an abnormal physical or laboratory finding detected during routine medical screening. In most patients, hypertension and heart murmurs are detected in this way. Abnormalities of the resting or exercise electrocardiogram (ECG), the cardiac silhouette on the chest radiograph, or echocardiogram may also be the first indication of a cardiac abnormality.

The physiologic basis for the major cardiac manifestations can be appreciated by consideration of the function of the heart as a

pump interposed between two interlocking circuits. The overall function of the circulation depends on the satisfactory performance of both cardiac muscle and heart valves. The myocardium provides energy for blood flow, and the valves ensure that the flow is unidirectional. Dysfunction of either the myocardium or the valves leads to circulatory failure and the development of symptoms.

CARDIOVASCULAR SYMPTOMS

The major cardiovascular symptoms are described and tabulated and the generally accepted physiologic interpretation given in Table 2.1–1. All these symptoms and their physiologic mechanisms are discussed in greater detail in later chapters. This and subsequent tables are concerned only with the role of heart disease in the production of a given symptom or sign and do not include all possible causes of the manifestations listed.

Eliciting the Cardiovascular History

The general principles of history taking apply to the patient with cardiovascular disease, but certain points deserve special emphasis (see Chapter 1.2). The patient may be short of breath (especially while talking) and therefore should be seated comfortably at the

TABLE 2.1–1. MAJOR CARDIOVASCULAR SYMPTOMS

Symptom	Description	Mechanism
Dyspnea on exertion	Difficult breathing, shortness of breath on exertion, or air hunger on exertion that is excessive relative to patient's age, state of physical fitness, and severity of exercise	Pulmonary vascular congestion. Cardiac output unable to rise. Left side of heart unable to transfer pulmonary venous return to systemic circulation because of myocardial disease or inflow obstruction. Congested lungs turgid, rigid, and stiff. Work of breathing increased
Orthopnea	Patient unable to lie down flat and becomes short of breath if he does	Shift of blood to heart and pulmonary circulation from veins in lower part of body
Paroxysmal nocturnal dyspnea	Patient awakens from sound sleep with extreme shortness of breath and must stand or sit up to become comfortable	Increased plasma volume in recumbent posture, secondary to movement of fluid from extravascular to vascular space and shift of blood from peripheral veins to heart and lungs
Edema of ankles	Patient complains of swelling of the ankles, usually at end of day	Increased volume of extracellular fluid distributed in dependent parts (i.e., ankles)
Abdominal pain	Aching pain in upper abdomen. Sometimes acute and may be confused with acute cholecystitis	Hepatic congestion and swelling with stretching of liver capsule
Palpitation	Patient aware of forceful, rapid, or irregular heartbeat	Cardiac arrhythmia, such as multiple premature systoles, tachycardia, or atrial fibrillation
Angina pectoris	Patient complains of substernal tightness or distress that comes on with exertion and disappears with rest	Relative inadequacy of myocardial blood flow, usually because of atherosclerosis of coronary arteries, but also present in aortic valve disease, hypertrophic cardiomyopathy, and pulmonary hypertension
Fatigue or decreased exertional tolerance	Patient tires easily or cannot keep up with contemporaries	Inability of cardiac output to increase in proportion to metabolic demands, or arterial oxygen unsaturation
Syncope or lightheadedness	Sudden loss of consciousness or feeling of impending faint	Sudden loss of cerebral blood flow because of arrhythmia, left ventricular dysfunction, cerebral vessel occlusion

beginning of the interview. He should be encouraged to discuss his present illness first, but the family and past histories must not be neglected. The past history is often important in determining whether a heart murmur represents congenital or acquired heart disease. A history of acute rheumatic fever is helpful, if present, but does not exclude rheumatic heart disease if it is absent. Special questioning about previous physical examinations for athletic teams, military service, or life insurance is often rewarding. The patient may remember that the auscultation of his heart received special attention on one of these occasions.

Dyspnea and chest pain may indicate major abnormalities of cardiovascular function, and the identification and quantitation of these symptoms can be accomplished only by history taking. The questioning of a patient with dyspnea or chest pain should be specific with regard to the relation of the symptoms to exertion. His exercise tolerance can be quantified by asking how many blocks he can walk or how many stairs he can climb before experiencing symptoms. Variability in the degree of exercise required to produce dyspnea or in dyspnea at rest with preserved effort capacity suggests that organic valvular or myocardial disease is not responsible. Sudden isolated episodes of severe dyspnea or pulmonary edema in a patient with normal exercise tolerance indicate that the precipitating condition is inconstant, as in the case of repeated episodes of pulmonary embolism or intermittent obstruction to pulmonary venous return by a left atrial thrombus or tumor.

The evaluation of chest pain is considered in detail in Chapters 2.7 and 2.8. It is important to emphasize that patients with angina pectoris often respond negatively when asked whether they have chest pain because this symptom is not perceived so much as pain as an uncomfortable sensation in the chest, often described as smothering, pressing, suffocating, burning, or a breathless feeling. When one is eliciting the history of chest pain, it is important to determine the precise circumstances that precipitate and relieve the symptom, as well as the duration, quality, and radiation of the discomfort.

Paroxysmal nocturnal dyspnea is an important symptom of pulmonary vascular congestion. The patient with true paroxysmal nocturnal dyspnea usually has no difficulty going to sleep but is awakened by dyspnea. The patient who reports difficulty "drawing a deep breath" when he goes to bed and, hence, has a problem getting to sleep does not have paroxysmal nocturnal dyspnea. This type of complaint is more common in anxiety. Orthopnea is shortness of breath that occurs within a few minutes after the patient lies down; the patient learns to prevent this symptom by sleeping with the head elevated on three or more pillows. Sometimes nocturnal cough and restlessness may be subtle early signs of left ventricular failure and may be approached by asking the patient how he or she sleeps.

Fatigue is a common symptom of heart failure, but it often develops so gradually that the patient may be unaware of its presence. Questioning about daily habits, especially the activities after work, may be revealing. The patient may report going to bed after dinner, whereas formally he or she walked, worked on a hobby, or engaged in other daily activity.

The symptoms of right-sided heart failure are attributable to the pooling of blood in the systemic venous circulation and the extravasation of fluid into the extravascular space. These are discussed in more detail in Chapter 2.2. The history of ankle edema is elicited by inquiring about difficulty in putting shoes back on at the end of the day after they have been removed.

CARDIAC RISK FACTORS

Special attention should be given to the presence of the major "risk factors" for coronary artery disease: cigarette smoking, hy-

pertension, and elevated serum cholesterol levels. Numerous studies have shown that the patient who smokes more than one pack of cigarettes a day has a risk of having a heart attack that is three times that of a nonsmoker. Similar but less strong relationships exist for hypertension and elevation of serum cholesterol levels. If all three risk factors are present, the incidence of heart attack is approximately eight times that in subjects with none of the three.

This strong relationship between smoking and risk makes it imperative that the patient's smoking history be recorded quantitatively in terms of pack-years of smoking. The patient who has smoked an average of two packs a day for 25 years is said to have smoked for 50 pack-years (2 × 25).

A history of hypertension can be obtained by asking whether blood pressure has ever been found to be elevated on physical examination or whether the patient has ever been instructed to take medicine for his blood pressure.

A history of hypercholesterolemia is usually obtained by asking the patient whether he or other members of his family have ever been told by a physician that the cholesterol level was elevated. A history of premature death or myocardial infarction in relatives is another indication that there may be an inherited predisposition to premature coronary artery disease.

Other risk factors with a less strong relationship and therefore of less importance from the point of view of history are diabetes, gout, obesity, sedentary life, and a certain personality type.

The physician should take advantage of every contact to educate his patient about the importance of risk factors. The physician's responsibility to his patient should be extended to the prevention of disease as well as to its treatment, and therefore the patient should be persuaded to alter behavior in such a way as to minimize the risk of developing heart disease.

CARDIOVASCULAR PHYSICAL SIGNS[4,10]

Physiologic Basis

Cyanosis. Cyanosis is the bluish discoloration of the skin, the mucous membranes, and nail beds resulting from an increased amount of unsaturated hemoglobin in the blood and in the tissue under inspection. About 5 g of unsaturated hemoglobin per 100 ml blood is the threshold for the clinical recognition of cyanosis.

The commonest causes of cyanosis are those related to low blood flow in the peripheral vascular bed (peripheral cyanosis). The arterial oxygen saturation is normal but the flow is slow; each red cell remains in contact with the tissue for a longer period, more oxygen is lost from the cells, and more unsaturated hemoglobin is present in the venous blood. Peripheral cyanosis, due to reduced flow, will usually be more pronounced in peripheral tissues and less pronounced or even absent in central tissues, such as the mucous membranes of the mouth and the conjunctiva. The most common cause of cyanosis of the extremities is a cold environment, but it may accompany any condition associated with reduced peripheral blood flow. Peripheral cyanosis is present in shock and heart failure because the cardiac output is decreased and hence the flow to the skin is slow. The impaired circulation associated with disease of the arteries and veins also results in peripheral cyanosis in the involved extremity. If cyanosis is present when the patient is warm, it is more likely to be of central origin and not the result of reduced flow. The presence of pulmonary osteoarthropathy, or clubbing, usually means that cyanosis is of a central type due to arterial unsaturation of long standing; its absence does not, however, guarantee that the cyanosis is peripheral.

The term "central cyanosis" has been applied to the situation in which there is arterial oxygen unsaturation. Central cyanosis occurs when blood passes from the venous circulation to the aorta without coming into contact with oxygen in the lungs. This occurs in the following situations: (1) hypoventilation and (2) right-to-left shunts, which may be (a) intrapulmonary (ventilation-perfusion abnormality) or (b) cardiac (including the great vessels). The

pulmonary conditions are described in Section 3 and the cardiac conditions in Chapter 2.5.

Skin Pallor and Temperature. Pallor of the skin or mucous membranes suggests anemia, which may be a cause of heart failure or responsible for murmurs that are secondary to excessive blood flow. Anemia may be secondary to infective endocarditis, especially in a patient with valvular or congenital heart disease. Skin temperature and moisture are important. Cool, damp skin in a warm environment usually indicates that the cardiac output is low and that maximum vasoconstriction is present.

Evidence of Fluid Retention. Certain aspects of the general physical examination may indicate the presence of early heart failure. Percussion of the thorax may reveal evidence of pleural effusion, and fine, moist rales in the lungs may be the earliest sign of pulmonary congestion. Hepatic enlargement and tenderness are signs of right-sided heart failure. A careful search for edema about the ankles and over the sacrum should also be carried out.

Heart Sounds. Correct interpretation of cardiovascular signs, as well as symptoms, depends on clear understanding of the physiologic processes responsible. Information obtained from cardiac catheterization, angiocardiography, echocardiography, and phonocardiography has led to a better understanding of the origin of physical signs, and therefore the physical examination has assumed new significance. These new techniques have not replaced the old but rather have enhanced their value.

The events of the cardiac cycle are shown in relation to the common auscultatory signs in Figure 2.1–1. These relationships

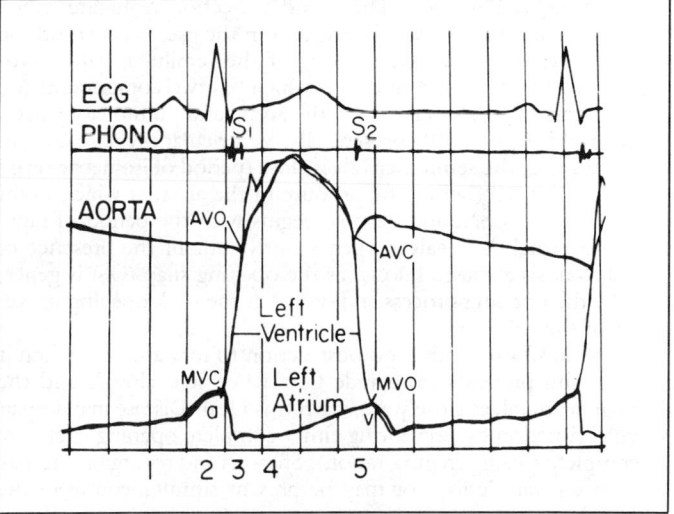

Figure 2.1–1. The hemodynamic and phonocardiographic events are related to mechanical events in the left atrium and ventricle. The temporal relation of the pressure recording to the events of the cardiac cycle is indicated by the position of the numbers. **1.** Passive ventricular filling. The pressures in the left atrium and left ventricle are identical and are rising slowly. **2.** Atrial systole. The atrium contracts forcing blood into the ventricle. The mitral valve approaches the closed position. The pressure in the left atrium and left ventricle rises to form the *a* wave. **3.** Isometric ventricular contraction. The ventricle contracts and the mitral valve is firmly closed (MVC). The aortic valve has not opened, and pressure in the left ventricle rises. The first heart sound (S₁) is generated. **4.** Rapid ventricular ejection. Ventricular contraction continues. The aortic valve opens (AVO) and aortic pressure rises. **5.** Isometric ventricular relaxation. Left ventricular pressure falls, the aortic valve closes (AVC), but the mitral valve has not yet opened. The second heart sound (S₂) corresponds with the closure of the aortic valve. When the mitral valve opens (MVO), the period of rapid ventricular filling—stage 1—begins.

should be kept in mind during the examination of the heart. Throughout the cardiac cycle, blood returns to the right atrium from the venae cavae and to the left atrium from the pulmonary veins. When the mitral and tricuspid valves open, the blood contained in the atria flows into the ventricles, as does the blood that continues to enter from the veins. During most of diastole, ventricular filling is passive, the driving force being the venous pressure. Filling is rapid during the early part of diastole, just after the atrioventricular (A-V) valves open, and the third heart sound (S_3) is temporally related to the culmination of this period of rapid ventricular filling. The flow of blood into the ventricle slows down later in diastole, as the ventricles become nearly full. The pressures in atria and ventricles are equal throughout diastole. Atrial systole marks the end of the period of passive filling and completes ventricular filling by the transfer of a final increment of blood from the atrium to the ventricle. The fourth heart sound (S_4) arises in the ventricle as the chamber receives the contribution of atrial systole.

Ventricular systole begins with the onset of ventricular muscle contraction and the development of pressure in the ventricle. The leaflets of the atrioventricular valves have already approached the closed position and are now firmly approximated by the rise in ventricular pressure. The first heart sound (S_1) is generated by the onset of contraction of the ventricular myocardium and the closure of the mitral and tricuspid valves. During the first part of systole, all valves are closed, and pressure develops in the ventricle without a change in volume: this is the period of isometric contraction. When the pressure in the ventricle exceeds that in the corresponding great vessels, the semilunar valves open and the period of ejection begins. The opening of the semilunar valves and the onset of ejection do not normally produce audible sound but may cause an ejection click (EC) in the presence of disease. The pressures in the ventricles and great vessels (aorta and pulmonary artery) are the same throughout ejection. The period of ejection terminates when the ventricular pressure falls below that in the great vessels and the semilunar valves close. The closure of the semilunar valves produces the second heart sound (S_2), which has two components (A_2 and P_2) attributable to closure of the aortic and pulmonary valves, respectively. A_2 normally precedes P_2. Ventricular pressure continues to fall after the semilunar valves close (period of isometric relaxation) until it falls below the pressure in the atria, at which point the A-V valves open and diastole begins with the period of rapid filling. Normal A-V valves open silently, but in the presence of mitral stenosis a sound known as the opening snap (OS) is generated by the opening process and occurs at the peak opening movement of the valve.

The ideal valve offers no obstruction to forward flow when it is open and prevents retrograde flow when it is closed, and the normal heart valves closely approach this ideal. Disease may impair valvular function by preventing either complete opening (stenosis) or complete closing (regurgitation). Stenosis and regurgitation may exist as separate lesions or may be present simultaneously in the same valve.

Cardiac Abbreviations. The condensation of material into tables is made possible by abbreviations commonly used in cardiologic practice.

Chambers of the Heart

SVC	Superior vena cava
IVC	Inferior vena cava
RA	Right atrium
RV	Right ventricle
PA	Pulmonary artery
PV	Pulmonary vein
LA	Left atrium
LV	Left ventricle
Ao	Aorta

Heart Valves

TV	Tricuspid valve
PV	Pulmonary valve
MV	Mitral valve
AoV	Aortic valve

Valvular Lesions

AR	Aortic regurgitation
AS	Aortic stenosis
MR	Mitral regurgitation
MS	Mitral stenosis
TR	Tricuspid regurgitation
TS	Tricuspid stenosis
PR	Pulmonary regurgitation
PS	Pulmonary stenosis

Congenital Lesions

ASD	Atrial septal defect
VSD	Ventricular septal defect
PDA	Patent ductus arteriosus
TGV	Transposition of great vessels
AVR	Anomalous venous return

Other

AF	Atrial fibrillation
PH	Pulmonary hypertension
RVH	Right ventricular hypertrophy
LVH	Left ventricular hypertrophy
LLSB	Left lower sternal border
i.s.	Interspace—between ribs
RBBB	Right bundle-branch block
LBBB	Left bundle-branch block
OS	Opening snap
EC	Ejection click

Interpretation of Cardiovascular Signs

The salient features of the cardiovascular physical examination are listed in Table 2.1–2. Opposite a given physical finding are listed the physiologic or pathologic mechanism and the usual interpretation. The mechanisms of production of some of the physical signs remains uncertain, and the explanations selected appear to be the best available.

TECHNIQUE OF THE CARDIOVASCULAR PHYSICAL EXAMINATION

The physical examination begins with the physician's first meeting with the patient, continues during the elicitation of the history, and ends when the patient leaves. The astute examiner also often elicits essential history while he is examining the patient, the stimulus for the additional questioning being provided by a particular physical finding. Observation of the patient's manner of moving and speaking yields information about his exercise tolerance. He may catch his breath in the midst of a long sentence or rest for a moment after entering the consultation room. In contrast, the patient whose dyspnea is due to anxiety may exhibit gasping respiration when the complaint is under discussion but breathe quietly when attention is directed elsewhere. Counting the respirations when the patient first lies down on the examining table gives some indication of the magnitude of the circulatory load imposed by disrobing. Cyanosis or pallor may be apparent when the patient first enters the room and may disappear after he rests and becomes warm.

During the formal part of the physical examination, one must be certain that the patient is comfortable. A common error is failure to recognize that the patient is orthopneic and, therefore, fail-

TABLE 2.1–2. CARDIOVASCULAR PHYSICAL SIGNS

Physical Findings	Mechanism	Interpretation
Venc Pulse (JVP)		
Distention of neck veins	Elevated RA mean pressure	Right heart failure, pericardial constriction or tamponade, obstruction of superior vena cava
a wave dominant	Forceful RA systole	TS, TR, or elevated RV end-diastolic pressure as in PH or PS
v wave dominant	Transmission of RV systole to RA	TR or AF
Cannon waves—extraordinarily large waves	Simultaneous RA and RV contraction	Arrhythmia, e.g., A-V dissociation
Arterial Pulse		
Quick upstroke—wide pulse pressure	Large stroke output Increased diastolic runoff Decreased peripheral resistance	AR, A-V communication (e.g., peripheral artery-vein fistula, patent ductus arteriosus, thyrotoxicosis, fever, anemia)
Slow upstroke—narrow pulse pressure	High resistance to ejection Small stroke output	AS MS
Pulsus biferiens—double peak pulse	Rapid left ventricular ejection	AR or hypertrophic cardiomyopathy
Pulsus alternans—alternate pulse beats less forceful	Variation in force of ventricular systole	Myocardial disease
Pulsus paradoxus—inspiratory decrease in arterial pressure >10 mm Hg	Impaired filling or excessively forceful respiration	Pericardial, myocardial, or respiratory disease
Precordial Examination		
Parasternal lift (RV lift)	RV hypertrophy	PS or PH Increased pulmonary blood flow
Apical lift (LV lift)	LV hypertrophy	AS, AR, or MR Systemic hypertension, hypertrophic cardiomyopathy
Systolic bulge (adjacent to apex)	Akinetic area	Myocardial infarction and/or aneurysm
Auscultation: Sounds		
First heart sound (S₁)		
Normal intensity	Closure of A-V valves	—
Decreased intensity	Absence of pliable valve tissue	MR or calcified mitral stenosis
	Impaired myocardial contraction	Myocardial infarction or cardiomyopathy
	Mitral valve closed at onset of systole	Long P-R interval—first degree heart block Severe AR—premature closure
Increased intensity	Forceful closure of stenotic valve	Pliable but stenotic mitral valve
	Mitral valve wide open at onset of systole	Short P-R interval Short R-R interval, e.g., atrial fibrillation or tachycardia Ventricular premature systole
Variation in intensity	Variation in position of the mitral valve at onset of ventricular systole	A-V dissociation, ventricular tachycardia, AF, ventricular premature systoles
Second heart sound (S₂)		
A₂		
Normal intensity	Aortic valve closure normally precedes pulmonary closure	—
Decreased intensity	Diseased aortic valve Low aortic pressure	Calcific aortic stenosis—rigid valve Hypotension
Increased intensity	Forceful closure of aortic valve	Systemic hypertension
Ringing, tambour quality	Disease of aorta and valve ring	Syphilitic aortitis
P₂		
Normal intensity	Pulmonary valve closure normally follows aortic closure	—
Decreased intensity	Absent pulmonary valve No flow through pulmonary valve	Destroyed by surgery or infection Pulmonary atresia
Increased intensity	Forceful closure of pulmonary valve	Pulmonary hypertension

(continued)

TABLE 2.1–2. CARDIOVASCULAR PHYSICAL SIGNS (Continued)

Physical Findings	Mechanism	Interpretation
Second heart sound (S_2) (Cont.)		
Physiologic splitting (S_2)—A_2–P_2 interval increases with inspiration	Inspiratory increase in RV filling	Intact atrial septum
Fixed splitting Absence of normal inspiratory increase in A_2–P_2 interval	Inspiratory increase in filling of both RV and LV via abnormal communication	Atrial septal defect
Paradoxical splitting Widening of split S_2 with expiration	Delayed LV ejection A_2 follows P_2	Left ventricular myocardial disease, aortic stenosis, systemic hypertension, LBBB
Variable wide splitting	Variation in ventricular activation and ejection	RBBB, PS, MR
Third heart sound (S_3)		
Physiologic S_3—no other signs of heart disease	Ventricular filling	Normal in the young (especially after exercise), pregnancy, anemia, and thyrotoxicosis
Pathologic S_3—other signs of heart disease	Sudden termination of filling of dilated heart Excessive or unusually rapid filling	Myocardial weakness VSD or PDA, MR, TR
Fourth heart sound (S_4)		
Physiologic S_4—no other signs of heart disease	Atrial systole	Occasionally in normal children, pregnancy, anemia, and thyrotoxicosis May be heard with long P-R interval as only other abnormality
Pathologic S_4—atrial gallop, other signs of heart disease	Atrial systole plus decreased compliance of left ventricle	Systemic hypertension AS or PH Hypertrophic cardiomyopathy Acute myocardial infarction Chronic coronary artery disease
Abnormal sounds		
Opening snap (OS) of mitral valve	Sudden arrest of LA-to-LV flow because fusion of mitral commissures prohibits complete opening of valve Normal mitral valve opens silently	MS—pliable, movable valve tissue must be present. Absence of OS suggests valve calcified, fixed and immobile or destroyed as in MR Rarely ASD, VSD, MR
Ejection click (EC) (early systolic)	Related to ejection of blood into great vessels and, in other situations, to the motion of valves	PS and AS Dilated pulmonary artery or aorta High pulmonary flow Pulmonary and systemic hypertension
Midsystolic click	Related to motion of A-V valves or to extracardiac events	Abnormal chordae or prolapse of the mitral valve, old pericarditis
Friction rub	Contact between visceral and parietal pericardium. Usually three components because of atrial systole, ventricular systole, and ventricular relaxation	Pericarditis

ure to elevate his head during the examination. He must be kept warm. Minor degrees of shivering produce muscle noise, making a cardiac auscultation difficult.

The examination should begin with inspection of the skin and mucous membranes for pallor, cyanosis, or petechial lesions, then of the nails for clubbing, followed by the examination of the arterial pulse.

Arterial Pulse[4,10]

The experienced observer derives valuable information from palpation of the arterial pulse, which should be examined at a peripheral site, such as the brachial artery, and also at a more central location, such as in the carotid artery. The contour of the pulse is best appreciated in the more central vessels. The brachial artery pulse is best examined by raising the patient's arm vertically from the examining table and compressing the brachial artery with the fingers at a point midway between the shoulder and the elbow. Attention should be directed to the rate of rise and amplitude, both of which are decreased in the patient with aortic stenosis or myocardial disease (pulsus parvus) and are greater than normal when aortic regurgita-

tion is present (Corrigan pulse). The significance of other alterations in the arterial pulse can be determined from Table 2.1–2. Abnormalities of rhythm, such as atrial fibrillation and multiple premature contractions, can be detected from the arterial pulse. The consulting cardiologist often stands by the patient's bedside, with his hand on the patient's radial or brachial artery throughout the presentation of the history, so that he samples a large number of beats and may detect short runs of arrhythmia that have not been noted previously. At some point, the pulses in other major arteries should be examined. Coarctation of the aorta may be suspected when the femoral pulse is absent or when there is a delay in the femoral pulse wave. The significance of an absent dorsalis pedis pulse at a later examination can be appreciated only if it was known to be present initially. Palpation of peripheral arteries such as the radial artery may disclose evidence of atherosclerosis, which is manifest as thickening and tortuosity of the vessel. Bruits over large arteries are an important sign of obstruction, usually as a result of atherosclerosis. They should be sought by careful auscultation over the course of the carotid arteries, the supraclavicular fossae (subclavian arteries), the abdomen (renal arteries and aorta), and the femoral arteries in the groin.

The Venous System[4,10]

The examiner then directs his attention to the venous system with two objectives in mind: the determination of the level of venous pressure and the delineation of the character of the venous pulse wave. The venous pressure can be estimated at the bedside by adjusting the head of the patient's bed until pulsations are seen in his jugular veins. If the veins are collapsed, the head of the bed should be lowered until the veins are seen to fill, but if they are filled initially, the head of the bed should be elevated gradually to 90 degrees to search for the point of collapse. A position will usually be found somewhere between the recumbent position and 90 degrees (sitting up straight), at which the point of collapse lies above the clavicle but below the jaw. This is the position in which the neck veins should be examined. The height of the venous pressure can be estimated by measuring the vertical distance between the level of collapse of the veins and the second costosternal junction and then adding 5 cm to this value. The 5 cm addition represents a reasonably accurate measure of the distance between the surface of the chest at the level of the second rib and the center of the right atrium, which is constant in all positions. If the neck veins cannot be visualized, venous pressure can be determined by elevating the patient's arm and noting the elevation above the level of the heart at which the veins collapse.

Useful information about hemodynamics of the right side of the heart can be obtained from an accurate examination of the venous pulse. The head of the patient's bed should be adjusted, the patient's head turned, and the light adjusted to provide optimal conditions for the evaluation of the venous waves. Venous pulsations can be differentiated from arterial pulsations by palpation of the arterial pulse on the opposite side of the neck. Venous pulsations are visible, but usually they either cannot be felt or are obliterated by light pressure.

The goal is to identify the *a* and *v* waves and to determine which is larger. The *a* wave is produced by atrial systole, which immediately precedes ventricular systole. The venous waves are timed by the palpation of the carotid pulse on the opposite side of the neck, and the *a* wave is recognized in the neck by the fact that it appears to precede or coincide with the upstroke of the carotid pulse (Fig. 2.1–2). The *a* wave is a quick-up, quick-down wave of very short duration. It often appears as an almost instantaneous "flicker" in the supraclavicular fossa. The *v* wave is caused by the buildup of pressure in the right atrium as a result of its distension by the inflow of blood from the great veins during ventricular sys-

tole while the tricuspid valve is closed. The *v* wave rises slowly and decays rapidly after the fall of the carotid pulse. It is the descent of the *v* wave that is usually noted, and this is referred to as the "*y* descent." The *v* wave sometimes disappears when the patient sits up, but the *a* wave remains visible.

The *a* wave is larger than normal when the force of atrial systole is exerted against increased resistance. If the tricuspid valve has been closed before atrial systole by a ventricular premature contraction, the force of atrial systole cannot force blood into the ventricle; hence a large *a* wave appears in the jugular pulse. Similarly, the *a* wave is large in patients with tricuspid stenosis because the resistance to inflow through the tricuspid valve is increased. The *a* wave is also increased in the presence of right-ventricular hypertension due to pulmonary stenosis or increased pulmonary vascular resistance, as in primary pulmonary hypertension. In this situation, there is increased resistance to atrial emptying, but it is caused by the elevated end-diastolic pressure in the right ventricle, which faces atrial systole.

The *v* wave of the jugular venous pulse is increased in amplitude when the tricuspid valve is incompetent. In this situation, the force of ventricular systole is transmitted into the right atrium and hence into the great veins. If tricuspid regurgitation is severe, the liver may also exhibit systolic pulsation synchronous with the *v* wave in the neck vein.

An unusually rapid decay of the *v* wave, or rapid *y* descent, is seen in constrictive pericarditis. Filling is impaired throughout most of the cardiac cycle and is very rapid early in diastole. The veins appear to collapse during this phase of rapid filling.

It is useful to compress the liver during the examination of the neck veins. In the presence of congestive failure, a large volume of blood may be pooled in the liver, and when it is expressed into the vena cava by firm pressure on the upper abdomen, the venous pressure in the neck will rise, resulting in jugular venous distension. This response is termed the hepatojugular reflux and merely indicates that there is pooling of an excessive quantity of blood in the abdomen. The elevation of intrathoracic pressure by abdominal compression may also contribute to the production of this sign.

Configuration of the Chest

The configuration of the chest is important in the interpretation of physical findings. Asymmetric enlargement of the left side of the chest indicates that the cardiac condition developed before chest growth was complete and may help to differentiate congenital from acquired forms of heart disease. Pectus excavatum may explain displacement of the apex beat to the left. A shallow chest resulting from a straightening of the thoracic spine may be associated with a systolic murmur in the left second interspace because of the proximity of the pulmonary artery to the chest wall.

Inspection and Palpation of the Precordium

The procedure of inspecting and palpating the precordium yields information about the heart that cannot be obtained in any other way. The first step is to identify the apex impulse, which is defined as the point of maximum mechanical activity. This is sometimes accomplished more easily by inspection than by palpation. The examiner must adjust the light and move his head so that the fourth, fifth, and sixth interspaces are scanned from the axilla to the sternum. The position of the apex beat is recorded by noting the interspace in which it is located and also the distance, measured in centimeters, from the midsternal line. The location of the apex impulse is the best index of the size of the heart, provided that the heart is not displaced.

A prominent presystolic impulse can sometimes be identified by inspection or palpation and suggests careful auscultation for an S_4, which is indicative of an unusually forceful atrial systole. Systolic pulsations between the apex and the sternal border occur when a portion of the left ventricle fails to contract with systole. The extent, character, and force of the apical impulse should be noted. Sometimes these are best demonstrated when the patient

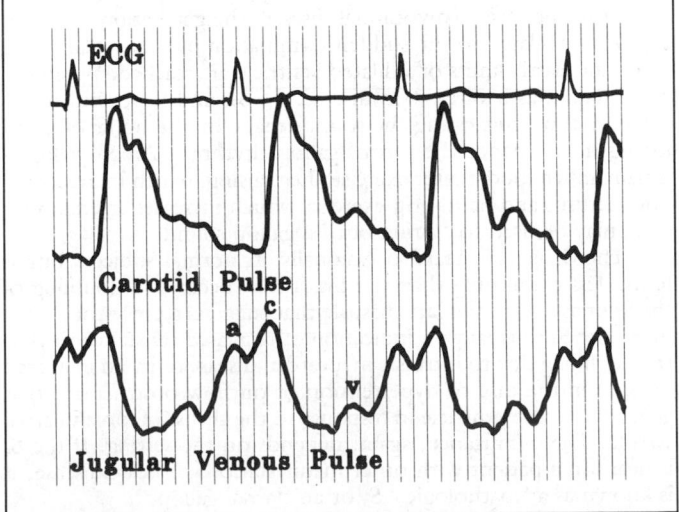

Figure 2.1–2. Venous pulse. Carotid pulse and jugular venous pulse are recorded by an external capsule on the neck of a normal subject. The *a* wave precedes and the *v* wave follows the upstroke of the carotid pulse.

is in the left lateral decubitus position. The left ventricle is chiefly responsible for the mechanical activity in the region of the apex beat, and with left ventricular hypertrophy the apical impulse is sustained and forceful. In addition, left ventricular hypertrophy is sometimes associated with retraction of the precordium in the third and fourth interspaces near the sternum. Apical expansion and parasternal retraction lead to a rocking motion. It is possible to predict whether the left ventricular hypertrophy is a result of a pressure or of a volume overload. If there is pressure overload—as in aortic stenosis or essential hypertension—the apical impulse is a sustained lift that seems to hold the examiner's hand up for a finite period before collapsing. In contrast, when there is a volume overload—as in aortic or mitral regurgitation—the apex impulse may have a greater amplitude but a shorter duration.

When the right ventricle is the site of hypertrophy, the maximum activity is located in the parasternal area. The right ventricular lift is a systolic expansion in the third and fourth interspaces adjacent to the sternum. The examiner may have difficulty appreciating precordial activity due to right ventricular enlargement if his hand is applied only lightly to the patient's parasternal region. A right ventricular lift or heave often is best felt by applying firm pressure with the base of the hand or by applying the fingers of the left hand lightly and adding pressure with the right hand on top of the left. Systolic expansion in this area is sometimes associated with retraction in the area of the apex, yielding a rocking motion to the precordium that is similar but opposite in direction to that associated with left ventricular hypertrophy. Systolic expansion in the second left interspace near the sternum indicates enlargement of the pulmonary artery and can often be better seen than felt. Systolic expansion in the right second interspace near the sternum usually indicates that the ascending aorta is enlarged.

Systematic palpation of the precordium at the apex and along both sternal borders is indicated to detect thrills. The thrill of aortic stenosis is best felt along the right sternal border when the patient is sitting and during full expiration. The presystolic thrill of mitral stenosis is best felt with the patient in the left lateral decubitus position. Any murmur may be associated with a thrill if it is loud enough. Heart sounds can be felt, especially if they are accentuated, and are referred to as "taps." The snapping S_1 of mitral stenosis and the pulmonary valve closure sound in pulmonary hypertension are frequently palpable; a gallop is sometimes first detected by inspection and palpation and its presence confirmed by auscultation.

Percussion of the Heart

Percussion is far less important than inspection, palpation, and auscultation, but it may be helpful in certain situations. When the apical impulse cannot be identified, the size of the heart can sometimes be determined by percussing the left border of cardiac dullness. The presence of a pericardial effusion can be confirmed by finding the apical impulse inside the left border of cardiac dullness. *A good radiologic examination of the heart provides far more accurate information about the size and shape of the heart than can be obtained by percussion.*

Auscultation[1,4,8,10]

Auscultation is the final step in the physical examination of the heart and must be performed in a quiet room with the patient and the physician in comfortable and relaxed circumstances. Air conditioners and fans should be turned off, and doors and windows closed to reduce background noise to a minimum. The examination usually begins with the patient in the recumbent position and always includes examination in the sitting position as well. Depending on the findings in these primary positions, the patient may also be examined in the left lateral decubitus position or after exercise. There are four prime areas for auscultation on the chest wall: apex, left lower sternal border, left second interspace, and right second interspace. It is often helpful, however, to move the stethoscope by small steps from one of these areas to the next to note changes in the amplitude and character of various auscultatory phenomena. The stethoscope should be applied over the carotid arteries in the neck, especially in the presence of a systolic murmur at the base of the heart, because murmurs generated in the great vessels may be heard over the upper part of the chest and those of aortic valve disease may be heard in the neck. It is advisable to listen for murmurs over the back of the chest while the patient is sitting up.

At each area, attention should first be directed to the normal sounds and rhythm, then to the abnormal sounds, and last to the murmurs. The normal S_1 and S_2 can usually be easily identified by their differing character, but in disease this difference may be difficult to determine; therefore auscultation should be carried out with a finger on the carotid pulse. The S_1 can be identified by its occurrence coincident with the upstroke of the carotid pulse. The S_1 sound is best heard at the apex, and the S_2 will be found to be loudest in the second interspaces both to the right and to the left of the sternum. The S_2 consists of two parts: A_2, due to closure of the aortic valve; and P_2, due to the closure of the pulmonary valve. Both components can be heard on both sides of the sternum in the second interspace, but A_2 is the loudest component of S_2 on the right side, and P_2 is the major component of S_2 heard on the left. The two components of S_2 are identified by their temporal relationships and not by the point of maximum audibility; therefore it is misleading to use the terms "aortic area" and "pulmonic area." With inspiration, the pulmonary closure sound is delayed, S_2 splits, and P_2 can be identified as the second component. Observation of the effects of respiration on the second sound is an important part of auscultation and is discussed in more detail later. The third and fourth heart sounds (S_3 and S_4) are both heard at the apex with the patient in the left lateral decubitus position. These are low-frequency, low-energy sounds heard best with the bell of the stethoscope lightly applied to the cardiac apex.

The significance of an S_3 depends on the clinical setting in which it is heard. The S_3 is frequently heard in children and adolescents, in whom it is termed a "physiologic" third heart sound and has no significance. The S_3 may be heard in situations in which blood flow is increased, as in anemia, thyrotoxicosis, and pregnancy. The sound is apparently generated by the termination of rapid inflow of blood into the ventricle in early diastole. The S_3 is heard with decreasing frequency with advancing age and is a rare finding in adults who have normal hearts.

An S_3 in a patient with heart disease has special significance. In this setting, the S_3 is termed a "pathologic" S_3 or a "ventricular gallop" and indicates an abnormally large diastolic inflow, as in mitral regurgitation, or ventricular dysfunction. The timing, character, and intensity are the same as in the case of the physiologic S_3, but in the case of myocardial disease, the generation of sound is probably related to the sudden termination of ventricular filling when the elastic limits of a dilated ventricle are reached. When the rate is rapid, as it often is in disease, S_1, S_2, and S_3 are heard as a triple rhythm, suggesting the sounds made by the hoofs of a galloping horse—hence the term "gallop rhythm." An S_3 gallop is usually much louder after exercise. Leg raising, which increases venous return, and hand-grip exercise, which increases arterial pressure, may be used to "bring out" a gallop sound.

The S_4 is also heard occasionally in normal subjects but is found less commonly than the S_3. It may occur as a doubling of the S_1 or as a sound in late diastole that suggests a presystolic murmur. The S_4 is usually an indication of increased resistance to ventricular filling due to intrinsic myocardial disease or by an increased load, as in the case of hypertension or outflow obstruction. It is generated in the ventricle in response to the thrust of forceful atrial systole. The significance, again, depends on the setting. If the S_4 is heard in a patient with other manifestations of heart disease, it is known as a "pathologic" S_4 or an "atrial gallop."

After these sounds have been identified, attention is turned to a search for abnormal sounds such as clicks and friction rubs. This is best done by listening in all four areas while concentrating on systole and then on diastole. Systole and diastole are normally silent, and abnormal sounds and murmurs are best identified by

asking oneself whether the period between S_1 and S_2 is completely silent and then asking the same question about the period between S_2 and S_1.

CARDIAC MURMURS

Heart murmurs, which are subject to precise description with regard to timing and location of maximal audibility, frequently form a starting point in the diagnosis of cardiovascular disease. A murmur may serve as a basis for differential diagnosis in a patient ill with congestive failure, or it may be an incidental finding on routine examination.

Origin and Significance
Not all heart murmurs are indicative of organic heart disease, a fact emphasized by their classification into three groups on the basis of the mechanism of production: (1) organic murmurs due to anatomic abnormalities within the heart or central circulation, the identification of which constitutes evidence for organic heart disease, (2) physiologic murmurs related to altered function within anatomically normal hearts, as with the systolic murmurs of anemia, thyrotoxicosis, and fever, and (3) innocent murmurs that cannot be related to either altered anatomy or altered function. The mechanisms of production of the third type are unknown, but it is known that such murmurs are not associated with organic heart disease.

The importance of distinguishing between these three types of murmurs is obvious. It is sometimes necessary to employ echocardiography, cardiac catheterization, and angiocardiography to solve the problem, but innocent murmurs can usually be differentiated from those of organic origin at the bedside.

Innocent murmurs are usually systolic. Diastolic murmurs are rarely heard in the absence of organic heart disease. The innocent systolic murmurs are usually confined either to the first or to the middle part of systole, are not loud, are rarely accompanied by a thrill, and show variability with respiration or position or both. Final judgment about the significance of a particular murmur depends on the evaluation of that finding in relation to variation within the normal population and the presence or absence of other abnormal cardiac findings.

Timing and Location
Standardization of classification and description is necessary if heart murmurs are to be of maximum value in differential diagnosis, if communication between one physician and another is to be effective, and if meaningful comparison is to be made between findings recorded at different times by the same physician. Classification of murmurs on the basis of timing forms the basis for Figure 2.1–3. Further description with regard to intensity, character, and radiation also is possible and valuable.

The division of murmurs on the basis of timing into systolic and diastolic is indicated across the top of Figure 2.1–3. Each of these periods can be subdivided into thirds and murmurs classified according to their onset as early, mid, or late. Early diastole is sometimes referred to as protodiastole, and late diastole as presystole. If a murmur lasts throughout systole, it is called pansystolic or holosystolic.

Intensity
The loudness of a murmur should be described on a scale of 1 to 6, with 1 representing a very soft murmur appreciated only after careful auscultation and with 6 representing a loud murmur with an associated thrill. The intensity of murmurs does not necessarily correlate with the severity of the lesion. For example, the smallest ventricular septal defect (VSD) often produces a grade 6/6 murmur, whereas a large VSD may have no associated murmur. External factors such as an emphysematous chest configuration, previous chest surgery, pericardial effusion, or obesity may blunt the intensity of a murmur, as may cardiac factors such as low stroke volume or loss of pliability of a valve.

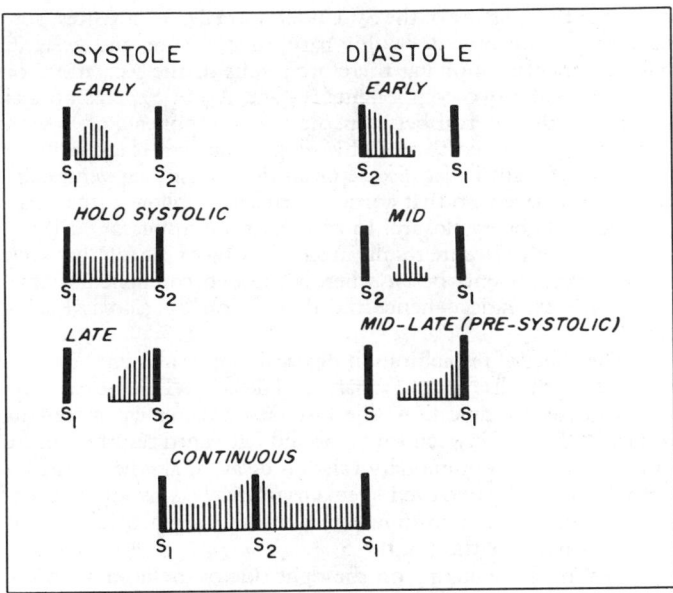

Figure 2.1–3. Timing and configuration of common murmurs in relation to the first (S_1) and second (S_2) heart sounds.

Character
The character of the murmur is sometimes described as crescendo or decrescendo to indicate progressive increase or decrease in intensity. The early-diastolic murmur of aortic regurgitation is classically decrescendo and the late-diastolic murmur of mitral stenosis is crescendo. The systolic murmur of aortic or pulmonary stenosis is best described as a crescendo-decrescendo murmur. The term "ejection systolic murmur" is applied to these and all other murmurs related to the ejection of blood into the great vessels. The terms "diamond shaped" and "Christmas tree" are applied to the early-systolic crescendo-decrescendo murmur and refer to its phonocardiographic appearance. The quality of a murmur is described as "harsh," "blowing," or "musical." Although lacking in quantitative precision, these terms serve a useful purpose. Furthermore, the term "musical" used to describe a decrescendo diastolic murmur indicates the possibility of an unusual cause of aortic regurgitation, such as rupture of an aortic leaflet.

The radiation of a murmur is of limited help, since it is, at least in part, a function of intensity. A loud murmur may be heard all over the chest, a faint one only at one spot.

Effect of Respiration
More can be learned about the physiology of any organ system by observing its response to changing conditions or stress than by prolonged observation at rest. This general physiologic principle underlies the importance of careful observation of the effects of respiration on the heart. Normal, quiet respiration results in phasic alterations in venous return, cardiac output, venous pressure, and arterial blood pressure. The response is often altered by disease.

All the hemodynamic changes depend on the negative intrathoracic pressure, which initiates inspiration. When the pressure within the chest becomes negative with respect to that in the atmosphere and in the extrathoracic airways, air flows into the chest through the respiratory tree. The veins are similar to the trachea and bronchi in that they are conduits running into the thoracic cavity from outside. The decrease in intrathoracic pressure that initiates airflow into the trachea also initiates blood flow into the thorax from the extrathoracic portions of the superior and inferior venae cavae. Venous pressure in the neck veins falls with inspiration. The return to the right atrium and right ventricle is therefore *increased* by the act of inspiration, and the output of the right ventricle into the lung is increased.

An important effect of respiration on physical signs is the

change in the splitting of the S_2. Under normal circumstances, aortic valve closure precedes pulmonary valve closure, and delay in right ventricular emptying therefore results in the separation, or splitting, of the two components (P_2 and A_2) of S_2. This normal increase in the interval between the two components of S_2 with inspiration is referred to as a physiologic splitting. If the splitting is due to left ventricular disease or aortic stenosis, left ventricular ejection is delayed, so that aortic valve closure follows rather than precedes pulmonary closure. In this situation, inspiratory delay in pulmonary valve closure results in a narrowing of the split between the two components of S_2, whereas the two components move apart with expiration—hence the designation "paradoxical splitting."

The effect of respiration on physical signs is also important in establishing the diagnosis of atrial septal defect. When the two atria are in free communication, the inspiratory increment in venous return is divided between the right and left ventricles; the closure of both aortic and pulmonary valves is delayed, and hence the interval between the two events remains relatively constant. The majority of patients with ostium secundum atrial septal defect exhibit this sign—fixed splitting of the S_2.

Murmurs originating on the right side of the heart are made louder by inspiration, a fact that is useful in differentiating tricuspid from mitral regurgitation. The systolic murmur of tricuspid regurgitation becomes louder, and that of mitral regurgitation changes very little. This inspiratory increase is best observed in cases of minimal tricuspid regurgitation. In severe lesions, the murmur may be heard throughout both phases of the respiratory cycle.

Other Stress Maneuvers

There are several measures other than respiration that can be used to stress the heart during physical examination. Hand-grip exercise is performed by asking the patient to squeeze the examiner's fingers firmly during auscultation of the heart. This maneuver increases arterial blood pressure and therefore increases the "afterload" on the left ventricle. A gallop sound of either the S_3 or S_4 type may be precipitated by this procedure. Left ventricular afterload may also be increased by asking the patient to squat down beside the examiner. This procedure increases venous return to the heart and is especially valuable in differentiating the systolic murmur of hypertrophic cardiomyopathy from that due to other abnormalities of the mitral valve. The murmur of hypertrophic cardiomyopathy decreases in intensity in this situation, whereas that of other forms of mitral regurgitation becomes louder or remains unchanged.

Venous return to the right side of the heart can also be increased by raising the patient's legs, and this will sometimes make it possible to hear an S_3 that is absent or only intermittently present while the patient is at rest. Exercise, either by passive bicycling while recumbent or hopping on one leg by the bedside, is also useful as a tool for stressing the heart by increasing oxygen consumption and hence the demand for cardiac output.

LABORATORY EVALUATION

Laboratory tests supplement but never replace history taking and physical examination in the evaluation of a patient with cardiac disease. No cardiovascular assessment is complete without a standard chest roentgenogram and a 12-lead ECG, but other studies are ordered only to answer specific questions. In some instances a laboratory test will establish a diagnosis, as in the case of the ECG in the patient with atrial fibrillation. In other situations the same test may have nonspecific results, as in the case of mitral stenosis. Some tests are necessary to quantify or determine the extent of cardiac disease, as in the case of coronary arteriography. The amount of information available from laboratory tests has been increased greatly by the availability of noninvasive techniques, such as echocardiography and radionuclide studies.

NONINVASIVE TECHNIQUES

Radiologic Examination of the Heart

The posteroanterior and lateral chest radiographs are the standard examinations and are used to determine overall heart size and configuration and enlargement of the aorta, pulmonary artery, and left atrium. Rib notching, characteristic of coarctation of the aorta, can also be detected on the chest roentgenogram. Intracardiac calcification can sometimes be identified on the plain roentgenogram, but image-intensified fluoroscopy is usually required for precise localization. Calcification in valves can be seen to move, whereas that in the pericardium and lung remains motionless. Calcification of coronary arteries can sometimes be seen and when present indicates that the coronary atherosclerosis is severe. Fluoroscopic examination may be used to evaluate mass lesions in the region of the heart. It is often difficult, however, to distinguish between a solid tumor, cyst, or aneurysm because cardiac pulsations may be transmitted to lesions in contact with a vascular structure.

Occasionally, a routine chest roentgenogram may lead to the detection of heart disease in a totally asymptomatic patient. Pericardial cysts, benign cardiac tumors, and even atrial septal defects may be discovered in this way before the development of symptoms.

In addition to the examination of the cardiac silhouette, evaluation of the pulmonary vasculature is equally important in a variety of cardiac disorders. Signs of pulmonary arterial and pulmonary venous hypertension and pulmonary hyperperfusion (e.g., left-to-right shunt) can be detected by careful examination of the vessels in the lung fields. The size of the central and peripheral pulmonary vessels provides information about pressure and flow in pulmonary arteries. Large central pulmonary arteries with attenuated vessels in the periphery of the lung suggest pulmonary arterial hypertension, whereas large central and peripheral pulmonary arteries indicate increased blood flow, as in left-to-right shunts. Normally the lower lobes receive more blood supply than the upper lobes, and the chest roentgenogram shows prominence of lower lobe vessels leading to the hilum, in comparison with those from the upper lobes. With increased pulmonary venous pressure there is relatively less flow to the lower lobes due to regional hypoxia, and flow is shifted to the upper lobe vessels, which appear more prominent than normal. Interstitial edema may produce diffuse haziness or occasionally a reticular or nodular infiltrative appearance. Alveolar edema causes lung opacification and "fluffy" infiltrates. Kerley B lines are horizontal densities at the lung bases, best seen at the lateral margins in the posteroanterior projection. They are important to recognize, because they reliably indicate severe pulmonary venous hypertension. In chronic states (e.g., mitral stenosis) Kerley B lines may be present without evidence of interstitial or alveolar edema.

One useful adjunct to the plain chest film is the barium swallow. With this technique the esophagus is filled with barium paste, thus permitting the posterior contour of the heart to be outlined where it is in direct relation to the esophagus. The use of this technique has declined in recent years because of the advent of other noninvasive techniques, such as ultrasonography and radionuclide angiography, which allow more direct measurement of chamber size.

The development of computed tomography (CT scanning) and magnetic resonance imaging (MRI) has aided the noninvasive evaluation of the heart and associated structures in a number of important ways. These include the evaluation of masses extrinsic to or within the heart itself. Pericardial masses, including metastatic deposits, as well as abnormal pericardial thickening can be detected by these techniques with a high degree of reliability. The evaluation of intracardiac masses requires devices that are "gated," or synchronized to the ECG. CT scanning of the aorta is commonly used as a reliable and important screening tool for both aortic size and the presence of aortic dissection. MRI has unique applications in congenital heart disease because it can depict accurately the ab-

normal position of intracardiac structures and describe defects in these structures.

Electrocardiography[2,9]

Twelve-Lead Recording. ECG abnormalities may accompany all types of heart disease but may also be caused by many other factors, such as electrolyte disturbances or drugs. The resting ECG may be completely normal in many patients with cardiac conditions, including significant coronary artery disease. On the other hand, it may be abnormal in patients with no evidence of cardiac disease whatever. The practice of making a diagnosis of cardiac disease on the basis of minor, nonspecific ECG abnormalities has needlessly created many "cardiac cripples" and is to be condemned strongly. The ECG is especially valuable in the diagnosis and management of arrhythmias and conduction disturbances (see Chapter 2.9). In addition, it provides useful but less specific information about hypertrophy of the right and left ventricles, patients with valvular or congenital heart disease, and hypertensive heart disease. The diagnosis of myocardial infarction can usually be confirmed electrocardiographically (see Chapter 2.8). The reader is referred to the many excellent texts on electrocardiography for detailed descriptions of specific ECG abnormalities.

Occasionally the clinician is confronted with a patient who has serious arrhythmias that defy interpretation by standard ECG techniques. In this circumstance, definition of the mechanism of the arrhythmias—for example, ventricular as opposed to supraventricular origin of a tachycardia—may provide important information that can direct therapeutic maneuvers. This kind of information may be obtained by recording the electrical activity of the cardiac conduction system. This type of electrophysiologic study is accomplished in the laboratory by selectively positioning one or several electrode catheters within the chambers of the right heart and recording the electrical activity at different sites, including several areas of the right atrium, the bundle of His, and the right ventricle. In addition to study of impulse conduction, arrhythmias may be stimulated under controlled conditions, and the effects of drugs on these arrhythmias studied (see Chapter 2.9).

Twenty-Four-Hour Holter (Ambulatory) Monitoring. Monitoring the ECG for a 24-hour period with a portable tape recorder (Holter monitor) can be of value in the identification of both symptomatic and asymptomatic arrhythmias and, to a lesser extent, ischemia. The patient carries a small portable tape recorder to which one or two electrocardiographic leads are connected. Some monitors have an event marker by which the patient himself can denote the presence of symptoms on the tape to enable correlation of symptoms with electrocardiographic changes. The 24-hour tape is later processed on a high-speed computer-aided system that quantifies disturbances of rhythm and of ST segment abnormalities indicative of ischemia. Holter monitoring is especially useful in the evaluation of the patient with presyncope or syncope or with unexplained palpitations. It is also of value in monitoring the efficacy of antiarrhythmic drug therapy.

Graded Exercise Testing.[1,8] Exercise testing serves two major functions. One is to determine whether the coronary circulation can increase oxygen delivery to the myocardium in response to increased demands. The other is to assess exercise capacity. In the absence of ischemia, disabling skeletal or muscular abnormalities, lung disease, or peripheral vascular or nervous system disability, the major determinant of exercise capacity is cardiac output.

Exercise testing is employed frequently to evaluate the presence of ischemia in the patient with chest pain. In many patients with chest pain, it is not possible to be certain on the basis of history or other clinical findings about the presence or absence of coronary artery disease, and in this group the observation of the patient's subjective and electrocardiographic response to exercise is an important diagnostic tool. In patients with established coronary artery disease, stress testing is of value in determining both the

functional exercise capacity and the exercise level and heart rate at which ischemia occurs. Efficacy of therapeutic antianginal interventions can also be assessed with exercise testing, with expected improvement in the duration of exercise before ischemia. The exercise test may also be helpful in the evaluation of cardiac arrhythmias. Complex ventricular arrhythmias are seen more frequently during exercise than at rest in patients with a history of arrhythmias or coronary artery disease.

For the above-mentioned indications the exercise technique of choice is the graded exercise test. The patient walks on a treadmill at gradually increasing grade and speed while heart rate, blood pressure, and the ECG are monitored. Alternatively a bicycle may be used by increasing the resistance to pedaling in a stepwise fashion. Graded exercise allows the physician to terminate the test at any stage. During, before, and for several minutes after the exercise period, a multilead ECG is obtained. In this way, ST segment depression, the hallmark of myocardial ischemia, can be detected at any time during the test. The end points for the test include exhaustion (maximal test), chest pain, ischemic ECG changes, severe ventricular arrhythmias, a fall in blood pressure, and reaching a predetermined percentage (usually 90 percent) of the age-predicted maximal heart rate (submaximal test).

The most commonly accepted criterion of an "ischemic" response, or a "positive" exercise test, is horizontal or downsloping ST segment depression of at least 1 mm, lasting for at least 80 msec after the J-point (junction between the QRS complex and the ST segment, Fig. 2.1–4). This criterion, although valid in many situations, has major limitations regarding the ability of the exercise test to predict either coronary artery disease or its absence. The most accurate possible use of the ST segment information derived from exercise testing requires that the clinician establish some estimate of the pretest risk of coronary artery disease in a given patient and then apply the results of the stress test to that patient on the basis of such an estimate. For example, although the ability of an abnormal stress test to predict future coronary events in various populations has been validated by numerous epidemiologic studies, the potential for making more false-positive than true-positive diagnoses exists in populations with relatively low prevalence rates of coronary artery disease, such as in asymptomatic young women. Here, there is danger that a false-positive diagnosis will be made if the ST segment criteria are considered as an isolated phenomenon in the absence of an appropriate pretest estimate of the risk of coronary artery disease. In populations with a high prevalence of coronary disease, a "positive" test result has far more predictive value for the presence of disease than does a similar test result in populations with a low prevalence of disease. Hence the uncritical use of graded exercise testing for screening asymptomatic populations for coronary artery disease is to be eschewed. By taking a "probability" approach, rather than merely applying rigid criteria for "positivity" or "negativity," the clinician has the best chance of making an accurate diagnosis based on a combination of the exercise test results and his estimate of the pretest risk of disease.

In some patients, radionuclide imaging during and after exercise may provide additional evidence for or against the presence of myocardial ischemia. Thallium testing may show evidence of exercise-related abnormalities of regional myocardial perfusion, or gated blood pool scanning may show evidence of global or regional left ventricular dysfunction during exercise (see below).

Echocardiography[3,5]

Echocardiography plays an important role in cardiac diagnosis because the technique provides direct information about the structure and motion of intracardiac structures, is noninvasive, carries no risk to the patient, and has relatively low cost. The technique is based on the principle of sonic reflection. Some of the energy of ultrasonic waves (2 to 5 MHz), which are directed through the chest wall and into the heart, are reflected backward, or echoed, when they encounter a medium of different acoustic impedance. Blood and cardiac tissues provide such an acoustic interface, caus-

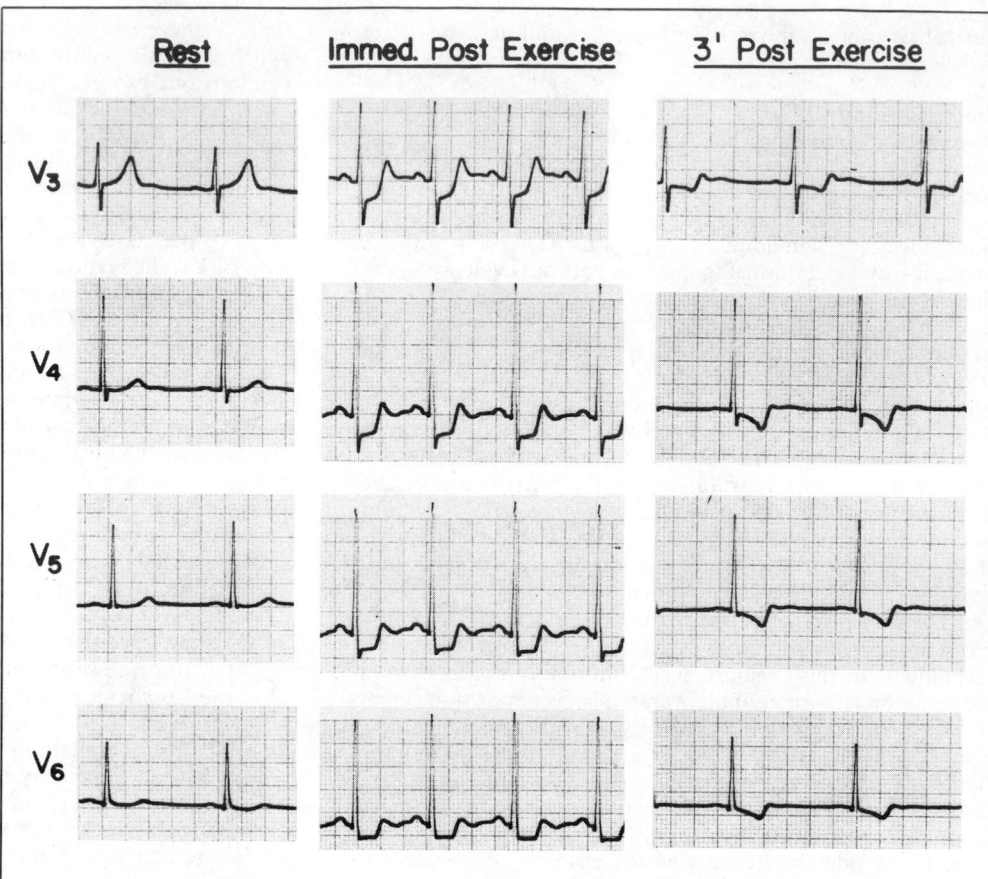

Figure 2.1–4. Exercise ECG with typical ischemic response. Resting tracing shows T-wave flattening, but normal ST segments. Immediately after exercise there is a 3.0-mm flat ST segment depression in V_5–V_6, deep junctional depression with slow rising ST segment V_3–V_4. By 3 minutes after exercise, ST depression is downsloping and T waves have become inverted.

ing echoes to be reflected from many intracardiac structures. Because the speed of sound in tissue is known, the distance between structures can be measured accurately. In this way the size of each cardiac chamber can be determined, as can the thickness of myocardium. The echocardiographic examination is performed simply and painlessly by placing a transducer on the chest wall. This transducer both transmits ultrasonic waves and receives the resultant echoes. Echocardiographic imaging can be either single dimensional (M-mode technique) or two dimensional. Single dimensional echocardiography employs a single beam of ultrasonic energy. Reflected echoes are recorded on a strip chart recorder as a time-versus-distance display (Fig. 2.1–5). The sampling frequency of 1000/sec permits analysis of motion of rapidly moving cardiac structures such as valves, and the hardcopy recording allows accurate measurement of chamber sizes and wall thickness. Single dimensional echocardiography provides only a limited view of the heart, so that it is done in conjunction with two dimensional study. This technique employs either a rotating single transducer or an array of many transducers that produces a wedge-shaped view of adjacent cardiac structures. These images, which are recorded on videotape, provide a "real time" tomographic view of cardiac structures in motion (Fig. 2.1–6).

Doppler echocardiography is the third component of the ultrasound examination. It is based on the familiar Doppler effect, in which the frequency, or pitch, of a reflected ultrasonic signal is altered by movement of the reflecting surface toward or away from the source of sound waves. The shift in frequency, which can be measured, is proportional to the velocity of motion of the reflecting surface. In the cardiovascular system, red blood cells provide a reflecting surface. Velocity measurements of red cells in the heart can be correlated with blood flow and pressure gradients across valves and can also be employed to recognize valvular regurgitant lesions and movement of blood through intracardiac shunts.

Applications of echocardiography are numerous and expand yearly. They include the following:

1. Mitral valve disease. Echocardiography can establish the diagnosis of mitral stenosis without recourse to other studies. The degree of fibrosis and calcification of the valve can be assessed and some indication of the severity of obstruction obtained by measurement of the valve orifice on two-dimensional images and of the time course of decay of the Doppler frequency shift in the left ventricle. Mitral valve prolapse, rupture of the valve apparatus, and vegetations on the valve are recognized easily.
2. Aortic disease. The echocardiographic technique describes the degree of fibrosis, immobilization, and calcification of the valve in stenotic lesions, and the Doppler method gives an indication of the gradient. Bicuspid aortic valve, valve rupture, proximal aortic root dissection, and vegetations from infective endocarditis can be recognized. Dilation of the proximal aortic root, as seen in Marfan syndrome, can be measured and followed.
3. Pericardial effusion. This is a preferred method for recognizing and quantitating pericardial effusion.
4. Hypertrophic cardiomyopathy. The characteristic pathophysiologic features of this condition can be described by this method.
5. Ventricular size and function. The echocardiographic technique can provide information about the size of the left ventricle, its overall function (estimated ejection fraction), regional dysfunction caused by myocardial infarction, and the presence of a ventricular aneurysm.
6. Cardiac tumors, clots, and masses. Echocardiography is the most sensitive technique to detect atrial myxomas (Fig. 2.1–5), but other tumors of the heart and pericar-

dium, both primary and secondary, and thrombi in various chambers of the heart can also be seen.

7. Congenital heart disease. The applications in this area are too numerous to list. Examples include visualization of defects of both ventricular and atrial septum, the abnormal position of the tricuspid valve in Ebstein anomaly, and recognition of volume overload of the right ventricle, which results from atrial septal defect.

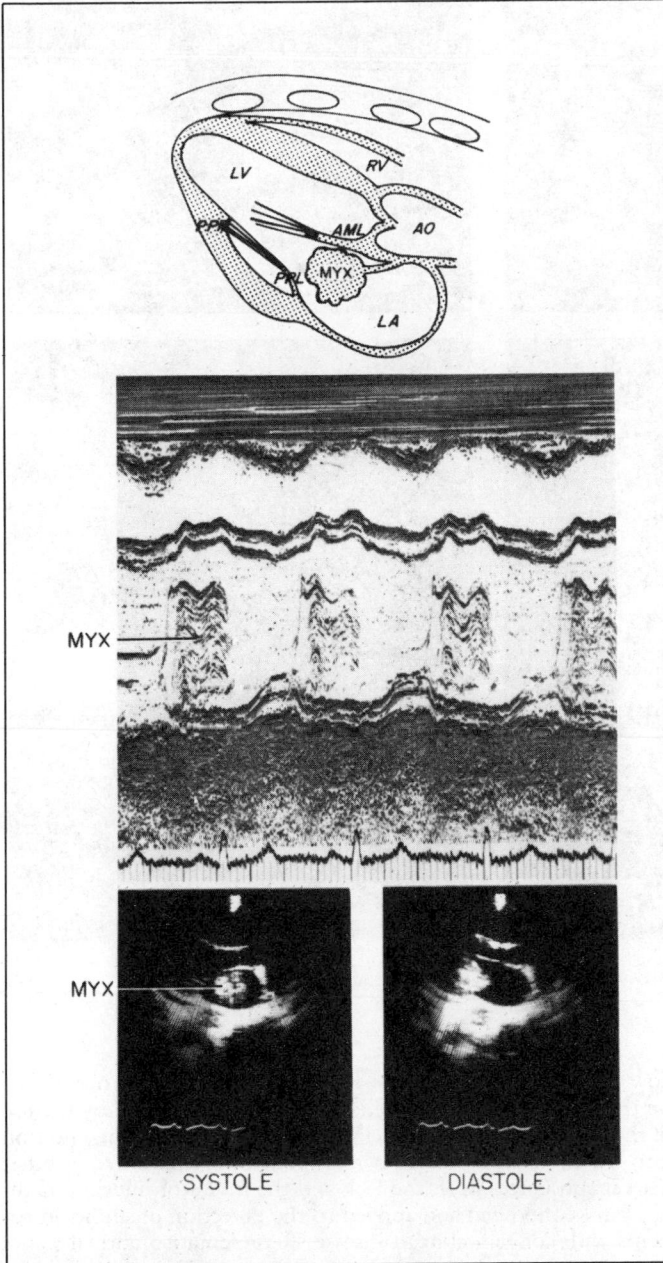

Figure 2.1–5. Left atrial myxoma (MYX). **Top panel:** Diagram of sagittal section of heart with myxoma on stalk attached to interatrial septum, prolapsing into mitral valve apparatus. RV = right ventricle; LV = left ventricle; PPM = posterior papillary muscle; AML, PML = anterior and posterior mitral leaflets, respectively; LA = left atrium; AO = aorta. **Middle panel:** M-mode echocardiogram of myxoma, showing mass of echoes behind the mitral valve echogram during each diastole. **Bottom panel:** Two-dimensional echocardiogram of above-depicted left atrial myxoma during both systole, when mass is in left atrium, and diastole, when mass can be seen prolapsing into mitral valve apparatus.

Radionuclide Imaging of the Circulation[1,3,8]

Important structural and functional information about the heart can be obtained by imaging the circulation with a scintillation camera after injection of an appropriate radioactive tracer.

Blood Pool Imaging and Radionuclide Angiography. Left and right ventricular function can be assessed with a tracer that stays in the intravascular compartment, such as Tc-99m-tagged red blood cells. Multiple images are entered into a computer during the cardiac cycle by synchronizing ("gating") the camera with the ECG. Data from a number of heartbeats are summed to generate a repetitive cinematic display of an average cardiac cycle. This technique has proved useful for evaluating left and right ventricular size and shape, global ventricular function (ejection fraction), and the presence of segmental left ventricular wall motion abnormalities, including aneurysms. Comparison of right and left ventricular stroke counts (analogous to stroke volume) can be used to quantify left-sided valvular regurgitant lesions. Left and right ventricular function can also be evaluated with the "first pass" technique, wherein an intravenously injected bolus of isotope is monitored during its initial passage through the central circulation. Information can be derived concerning the anatomic relationships between the various cardiac chambers and great vessels, especially important in the study of congenital cardiac lesions, and the severity of left-to-right cardiac shunts can be measured by computer analysis of the changes in lung radioactivity during the first minute.

Both gated and first-pass techniques can be combined with exercise testing to determine the changes in cardiac performance during peak stress. A decline in left ventricular ejection fraction or the appearance of regional wall motion abnormalities during exercise is generally an indication of exercise-induced myocardial ischemia related to coronary artery disease.

Myocardial Perfusion Imaging. The distribution of blood flow to the left ventricular myocardium can be imaged with Tl-201, which, like other potassium analogues, is taken up by cells throughout the body in proportion to flow after an intravenous injection. Areas of diminished left ventricular radioactivity represent regions of reduced flow, due to either scar or ischemia. Perfusion defects are generally related to coronary artery disease, although cardiomyopathies that produce regional scarring may also be associated with areas of diminished radionuclide uptake. Images obtained at rest are useful for evaluating the extent of abnormality in patients with acute myocardial infarction, but thallium perfusion imaging is most often used in conjunction with graded exercise stress testing (see above). Thallium is injected intravenously at peak exercise, and images are obtained 5 minutes later, after the patient has stopped. Since the distribution of radionuclide in the left ventricle at this time reflects the distribution of blood flow that was present at peak exercise, the appearance of perfusion defects may be used to determine the presence and location of coronary artery narrowings (Fig. 2.1–7). Defects that disappear or "fill in" on delayed images (obtained several hours later), or that are not present on resting images, usually represent areas of ischemic but viable myocardium, whereas those that are unchanged generally represent areas of scar tissue.

Both types of exercise radionuclide procedures—perfusion imaging and left ventricular function studies—appear to be more sensitive and specific than the exercise ECG alone for the diagnosis of coronary artery disease. In addition, the degree of abnormality induced by exercise appears to be related to the severity of coronary artery disease and may therefore be useful for selecting high-risk patients for further invasive studies, such as coronary arteriography. However, these procedures are also considerably more expensive than the exercise ECG, and at the present time they are recommended mainly for patients with equivocal or uninterpretable exercise ECGs or for those for whom there is a strong suspicion of coronary disease despite an apparently negative standard exercise test result.

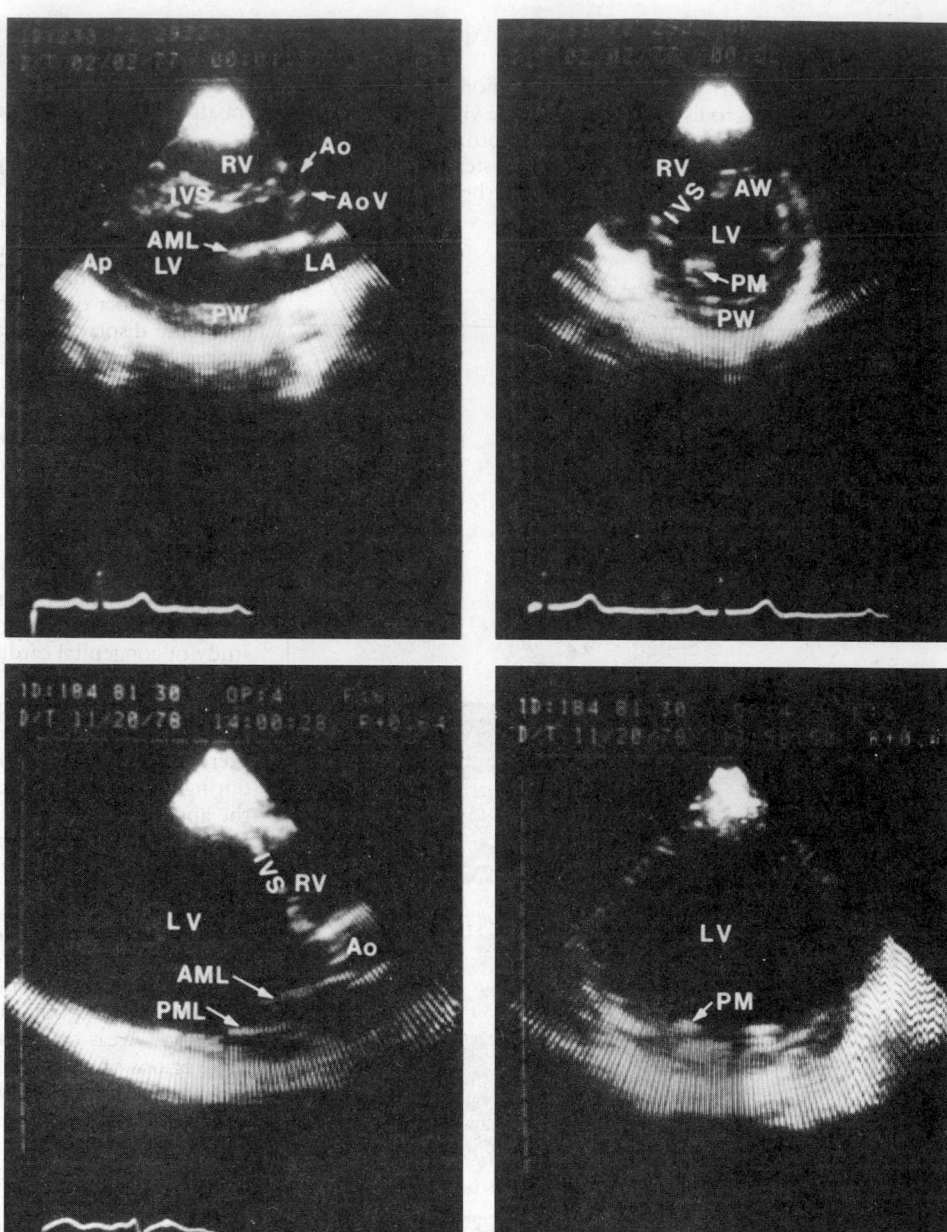

Figure 2.1–6. Two dimensional echocardiogram of a normal heart (*top*) and a severely dilated myopathic heart (*bottom*). **Left:** Longitudinal or long axis view. **Right:** Cross-sectional view. RV = right ventricle; LV = left ventricle; Ao = aorta; AoV = aortic valve; AML, PML = anterior and posterior mitral leaflets, respectively; IVS = interventricular septum; Ap = apex; PW = posterior LV wall; AW = anterior LV wall; PM = papillary muscle.

INVASIVE TECHNIQUES[7]

Hemodynamics

Most medical centers have a laboratory where the specialized techniques of cardiac catheterization and angiography can be applied to the study of the physiology and anatomy of the circulation. These laboratories are essential for the solution of certain clinical problems and have contributed significantly to understanding the pathophysiology of valvular heart disease, congenital heart disease, and myocardial dysfunction.

The basic technique used is cardiac catheterization. Catheters are introduced into the peripheral veins or arteries either by surgical exposure of the vessel or by percutaneous puncture, and it is possible to position a catheter in any chamber of the heart and all the great vessels. The basic measurements are those of pressure and flow, and from these the resistance to blood flow through a vascular bed or a valvular orifice can be derived. Cardiac output or total

flow can be measured by the Fick principle, which is dependent on the oxygen transport function of the circulation, or by the use of the indicator dilution principle, which depends on the injection into the circulation of a known amount of harmless dye or other marker substance. Both the Fick and the indicator dilution methods can be modified and applied to the detection of shunts in patients with congenital heart disease. Representative normal values for intracardiac pressures, cardiac output, and other derived values pertinent to the catheterization laboratory evaluation of cardiac disease are given in Table 2.1–3.

Angiography

Anatomic information concerning the heart and great vessels is obtained by contrast radiography, which involves the injection of radiopaque material through a catheter into the heart chamber. The flow of this material through the chambers of the heart and great vessels is recorded radiographically. Large-film roentgenograms ob-

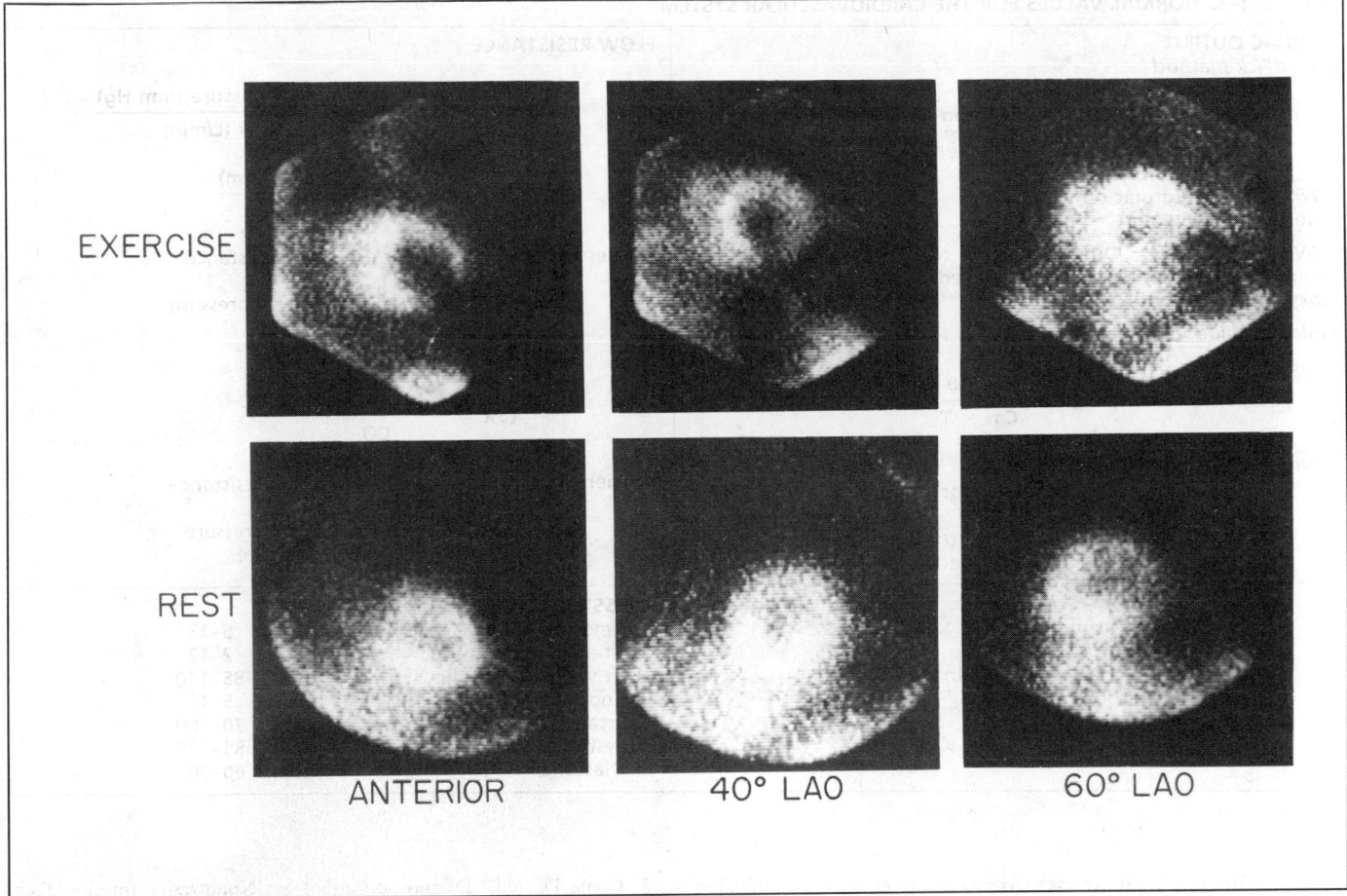

EXERCISE

REST

ANTERIOR   40° LAO   60° LAO

Figure 2.1–7. Rest and exercise thallium study. Images immediately after exercise (*top row*) show moderate to severe perfusion defects involving the anterolateral, apical, and posterolateral regions of the left ventricle. Resting study performed several days later (*bottom row*) is normal. These scintigraphic findings suggest severe three-vessel coronary artery disease without significant areas of myocardial scar.

tained 6 to 20 times per second after injection of the contrast material provide the greatest anatomic detail. Cineangiograms recorded at 60 to 120 frames per second on movie films by coupling a motion picture camera to the fluoroscope provide more information about the dynamic aspects of the heart and about normal and abnormal flow patterns.

Indications for Study in a Cardiovascular Diagnostic Laboratory

No laboratory procedure should be used indiscriminately, and this is especially true of cardiac catheterization and angiocardiography. These procedures should be undertaken only to provide an answer to a specific question formulated by the physician on the basis of clinical facts. Cardiac catheterization is seldom indicated or helpful in the patient whose condition presents a diagnostic problem because symptoms, physical signs, and laboratory evidence of heart disease are absent. The techniques of the cardiovascular laboratory are best used if the physicians performing the study are thoroughly informed of the patient's problem. This is important because the same procedure is not followed with each patient, as in the electrocardiographic laboratory. Methods and techniques are selected to provide an answer to a specific problem in the best possible way.

Coronary arteriography is usually performed to determine the location and severity of coronary atherosclerosis, and in man it is the only method that will precisely define the coronary artery anatomy. The coronary arteries are best visualized by selective techniques whereby a catheter is positioned in the orifice of the coronary artery and an injection of contrast material is made directly into the vessel. The two most commonly used methods are (1) percutaneous femoral technique (Judkins) and (2) brachial technique (Sones). The indications for coronary arteriography (apart from the purely diagnostic study) are closely linked to the indications for myocardial revascularization surgery (see Chapter 2.7).

The determination of left ventricular function or, more precisely, the localization of left ventricular damage, with determination of its extent, is an essential part of the arteriographic procedure because of the importance of ventricular function in the determination of prognosis and surgical results. This information is best obtained by careful inspection of the left ventriculogram in two planes; in many cases a high-quality two-dimensional echocardiogram will provide similar information noninvasively. The vigor of left ventricular contraction and the motion of specific portions of the ventricular wall are noted. This visual assessment of ventricular performance is usually supplemented by the measurement of end-diastolic volume, end-systolic volume, angiographic stroke volume, and ejection fraction. The level of left ventricular end-diastolic pressure is also of some value, as is the ability of the cardiac

TABLE 2.1–3. NORMAL VALUES FOR THE CARDIOVASCULAR SYSTEM

CARDIAC OUTPUT
Direct Fick method

$$CO = \frac{O_2 \text{ Consumption (ml/min)}}{AV\ O_2 \text{ Difference (vol \%)} \times 10}$$

Where CO = Cardiac output (L/min)
Normal = 5–6 L/min

AV O_2 difference = Difference in O_2 content of the arterial and mixed venous blood, usually expressed in volume percent (ml of oxygen/dl of blood)

Indicator dilution method

$$CO = \frac{I \times 60}{Cm \times T}$$

Where CO = Cardiac output (L/min)
I = Amount of the indicator injected (mg)
60 = 60 sec/min
Cm = Mean indicator concentration (mg/L)
t = Total curve duration (sec)

FLOW RESISTANCE

$$\text{Resistance} = \frac{\text{Mean driving pressure (mm Hg)}}{\text{Mean Flow (L/min)}}$$

$$PAR = \frac{(PAm - LAm)}{CO}$$

Where PAR = Pulmonary arteriolar resistance
Normal = <4 U
PAm = Mean pulmonary artery pressure
LAm = Mean left atrial pressure
CO = Cardiac output

$$TSR = \frac{(SAm - RAm)}{CO}$$

Where TSR = Total systemic vascular resistance
Normal = 30 ± 5 U
SAm = Mean systemic arterial pressure
RAm = Mean right atrial pressure

NORMAL INTRACARDIAC PRESSURES (mm Hg)

Right atrium mean	=	1–5	Pulmonary capillary wedge mean	=	5–13
Right ventricle systolic	=	10–25	Left atrium mean	=	2–12
Pulmonary artery mean	=	5–15	Left ventricle systolic	=	85–140
• Systolic	=	10–25	• End-diastolic	=	5–12
			Aorta mean	=	70–100
			• Systolic	=	85–140
			• Diastolic	=	60–90

output to increase with exercise. Angiocardiography is also of value in assessing the severity of valvular regurgitant lesions, localizing shunts, and describing altered anatomic relationships of cardiac structures in patients with congenital heart disease.

REFERENCES

1. Braunwald E (ed): A Textbook of Cardiovascular Medicine, 2d ed. Philadelphia, WB Saunders, 1984
2. Chou TC: Electrocardiography in Clinical Practice, 2d ed. Baltimore, Williams & Wilkins, 1983
3. Come PC (ed): Diagnostic Cardiology: Noninvasive Imaging Techniques. Philadelphia, JB Lippincott, 1985
4. Constant J: Bedside Cardiology, 3d ed. Boston, Little, Brown, 1985
5. Feigenbaum H: Echocardiography, 4th ed. Philadelphia, Lea & Febiger, 1985
6. Fozzard HA, Haber E, et al (eds): The Heart and Cardiovascular System: Scientific Foundations. New York, Raven Press, 1986
7. Grossman W (ed): Cardiac Catheterization and Angiography, 3d ed. Philadelphia, Lea & Febiger, 1986
8. Hurst JW (ed): The Heart, 6th ed. New York, McGraw-Hill, 1986
9. Marriott H: Practical Electrocardiography, 7th ed. Baltimore, Williams & Wilkins, 1983
10. Tavel ME: Clinical Phonocardiography and External Pulse Recording, 4th ed. Chicago, Yearbook Medical Publishers, 1985

CHAPTER 2.2
Congestive Heart Failure: Pathophysiology, Evaluation, and Approach to Management

Kenneth L. Baughman

The term "congestive heart failure" does not refer to a discrete disease entity but rather to a functional state in which the heart either is unable to meet the needs of the peripheral organs for blood flow or cannot meet those needs without the use of compensatory mechanisms. The major clinical manifestations of congestive heart failure reflect the reduced cardiac output and high diastolic filling pressures that often lead to fluid retention.

NORMAL CARDIAC PHYSIOLOGY

It is impossible to understand the pathophysiology of heart failure without first appreciating the physiologic principles under which the heart operates normally. With appropriate high-fidelity catheters, the function of the heart as a pump can be analyzed by mak-

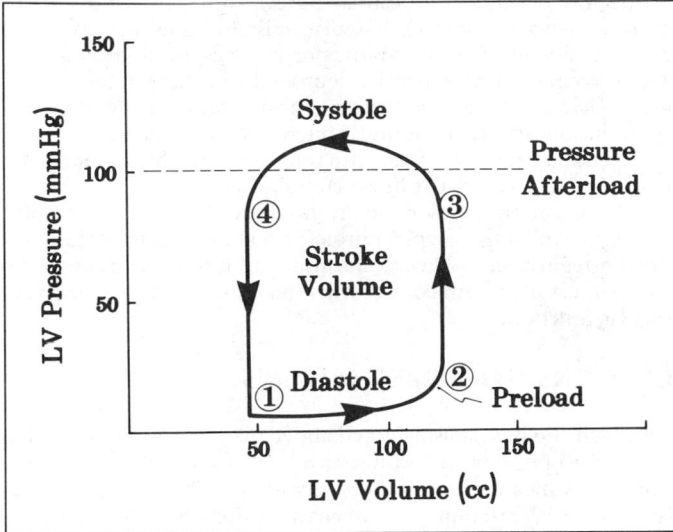

Figure 2.2–1. ① With completion of isovolumetric relaxation, left ventricular pressure falls below left atrial pressure, forcing mitral valve open and allowing diastolic filling of ventricle. This filling results in a gradual increase in ventricular volume. End-diastolic pressure and volume just before systolic contraction is termed "preload." ② At initiation of systole, ventricular pressure rises rapidly, forcing the mitral valve shut. It continues to rise until ventricular pressure exceeds aortic pressure. ③ This pressure elevation forces the aortic valve open and allows discharge of ventricular volume into aortic outflow tract. Throughout systole, ventricular volume declines. The difference between the volume present in the ventricle at end-systole relative to end-diastole is the stroke volume. The stroke volume multiplied by the heart rate is the cardiac output. The mean aortic pressure in systole can be termed "afterload." ④ After contraction the ventricle relaxes, which results in a rapid fall in intraventricular pressure. When ventricular pressure falls below aortic pressure, the aortic valve is closed. Ventricular pressure declines until it falls below left atrial pressure, allowing opening of mitral valve.

Every ventricle inscribes a pressure-volume loop unique to its individual characteristics. Normal ventricular function can be defined as the ability of the ventricle to maintain its cardiac output within the confines of physiologic pressure limits. Excessive diastolic pressures may result in venous congestion and low systolic pressures or cardiac output in inadequate organ perfusion. Each ventricle will display a "family" of pressure-volume loops determined by variations in ventricular volume or systemic pressure (Fig. 2.2–2). The creation of a family of pressure-volume loops allows the identification of two lines that additionally characterize ventricular function, the lines of *compliance* and *contractility*. Compliance reflects the change in ventricular pressure during diastole. A more compliant ventricle will increase end-diastolic pressure less for a given influx of volume than will a stiff, or noncompliant, ventricle. Even a normal ventricle can exceed its distensible limits and develop an abnormally high diastolic pressure if the volume challenge is sufficient. The second characteristic ventricular function line connects the end-systolic pressure of the family of pressure-volume loops. This end-systolic pressure line reflects the contractility of the ventricle and therefore characterizes the strength of the ventricle virtually independently of the diastolic load placed on it.

The volume and pressure conditions placed on the heart are termed *preload* and *afterload*. Preload represents the pressure and volume present in the ventricle at end-diastole. End-diastolic pressure alone is readily measured with fluid-filled catheters and is used as an estimate of the preload conditions present. Afterload describes the vascular resistance and impedance that the ejecting ventricle faces. This is clinically estimated by the mean systemic systolic pressure and is influenced primarily by peripheral vascular resistance.

An understanding of pressure-volume loops and the loading conditions under which the heart operates provides a useful conceptual framework for evaluating cardiac performance. This is particularly helpful when one is choosing among various options in therapy for heart failure. In clinical practice, however, the most straightforward method of assessing pump function is the determination of left ventricular ejection fraction (EF), which is the percentage of the end-diastolic volume ejected during systole. End-diastolic and end-systolic volumes are calculated from contrast left

ing measurements of pressure, volume, and flow and combining these measurements into a single graphic presentation—the pressure-volume loop. This loop traces the instantaneous relationship (Fig. 2.2–1). The pressure-volume loop is continuous, but for descriptive purposes we can choose to interrupt it at the end of isovolumetric relaxation. At this point the pressure inside the ventricle falls below the pressure in the left atrium and the mitral valve opens. The ventricle then gradually increases its volume as it is passively filled by the influx of blood from the atrium. Near the end of diastole, atrial contraction forces additional blood into the ventricular cavity. Electrical stimulation of the ventricle then initiates ventricular systole. The initial phase of systole is isovolumetric after rising ventricular pressure closes the mitral valve, preventing further volume influx. Once ventricular pressure rises above aortic systolic pressure, the aortic valve opens and blood is ejected into the aorta. This decreases the left ventricular volume, and ejection continues until electrical-mechanical systole is complete and the ventricular pressure falls below aortic diastolic pressure. The falling left ventricular pressure results in closure of the aortic valve and marks the initiation of isovolumetric relaxation. Left ventricular relaxation produces a rapid fall in pressure until the left ventricular cavitary pressure is exceeded by left atrial pressure and the mitral valve opens to reinitiate the cycle. Stroke volume is the difference between the end-diastolic and end-systolic volumes. Cardiac output is the stroke volume per contraction multiplied by the number of contractions per minute (heart rate). Stroke work, another measure of ventricular function, is defined as the stroke volume multiplied by the difference between left ventricular and end-diastolic pressures.

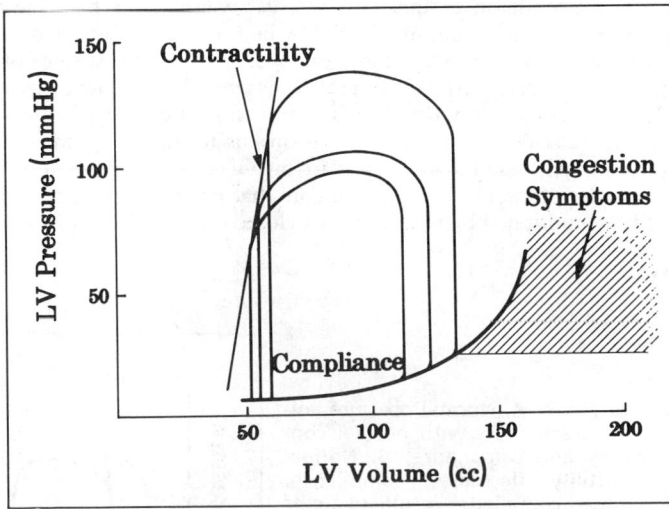

Figure 2.2–2. A "family" of pressure-volume loops is created by alterations in ventricular filling volume. Two lines are created by connecting end-diastolic pressure and end-systolic pressure point, defining ventricular function as "diastolic compliance and systolic contractility." Diastolic filling pressures above 25 mm Hg result in symptoms of fluid congestion. Symptoms may also be produced by a decrease in pressure-volume loop size, which correlates with reduced stroke volume and cardiac output.

ventriculography at cardiac catheterization. The following formula is applied, yielding a percent number (normal range, 60 to 70 percent):

$$EF = \frac{\begin{array}{c}\text{End-diastolic} \\ \text{volume}\end{array} - \begin{array}{c}\text{End-systolic} \\ \text{volume}\end{array}}{\begin{array}{c}\text{End-diastolic} \\ \text{volume}\end{array}} \times 100$$

The accuracy of this assessment of cardiac performance can be enhanced by simultaneously measuring end-diastolic pressure, since injection of the radiographic dye requires placement of a catheter into the left ventricular cavity. Although cardiac catheterization and quantitative angiography are the "gold standard" methods for evaluating left ventricular function, the ejection fraction may also be determined from noninvasive techniques such as echocardiography and radionuclide ventriculography (see Chapter 2.1).

PATHOPHYSIOLOGY OF HEART FAILURE[6]

Regardless of etiology, the pathophysiology of heart failure ultimately reflects an abnormality of contractility, compliance, or both (Fig. 2.2–3). Alterations in ventricular compliance or excessive preload result in elevated ventricular diastolic pressures, which increase the venous pressure. This excessive venous pressure exceeds intravascular oncotic pressure and results in transudation of fluid in the venous system feeding the affected ventricle (pulmonary or systemic). Both decreased contractility and decreased compliance reduce the size of the pressure-volume loop and cardiac output. Unless compensatory mechanisms correct the decrease in cardiac output, a subsequent systemic and vascular response provokes an increase in salt and water retention, an increase in vascular stiffness, and ultimately a further decrease in heart contractility (Fig. 2.2–4).

Diminished renal perfusion from a low cardiac output results in decreased filtration of sodium and subsequent increased renin release, which in turn leads to increased aldosterone and angiotensin levels. Aldosterone acts at the distal tubule of the kidney to cause retention of salt and subsequently water. Salt and water retention is also affected by a third factor, probably an atrial natriuretic factor, which is influenced by atrial distensibility (see Chapter 10.1). This sequence results in an increased vascular volume, which is transmitted to the heart and manifested by increased end-diastolic pressure and volume or by increased preload. A decrease in stroke volume and cardiac output may reduce systemic blood flow as well. This decrease in flow threatens the function of every vital organ, and the compensatory vascular response is to maintain perfusion pressure. Although many organs are capable of autoregulation, the principles of vascular physics mandate that pressure is the product of flow multiplied by resistance in a closed system. Blood pressure

is therefore dependent on cardiac output (flow) and systemic vascular resistance (resistance). Vascular resistance must increase in order to maintain organ perfusion pressure despite decreased flow. This is accomplished in part by neuroendocrine alterations, particularly increased release of norepinephrine. Additionally, renal underperfusion and renin stimulation result in increased release of angiotensin, a potent vasoconstrictor. Norepinephrine and angiotensin increase vascular stiffness cumulatively.

Constant stimulation of the myocardial adrenergic-receptor sites by circulating norepinephrine results in receptor fatigue, or "down-regulation." This receptor fatigue ultimately causes a decrease in cardiac contractility, which may further depress left ventricular function.

COMPENSATORY MECHANISMS

Although the mechanisms noted above may ultimately prove detrimental to patients with congestive heart failure, there remains a degree to which these responses are salutary. The heart and vascular system may attempt to compensate acutely by ventricular dilation (Starling effect) or by increased sympathetic stimulation. Chronic compensatory mechanisms include ventricular hypertrophy as well as dilation.

The Frank-Starling mechanism indicates that within limits, the performance of the heart is a function of the length of the myocardial fibers at the onset of contraction. A longer initial fiber length because of a larger diastolic volume results in improved systolic performance. This acute compensatory mechanism is likely due to increased actin-myosin interaction and increased calcium flux. The Frank-Starling mechanism is an acute process and can be overwhelmed by ventricular volumes that distend myofibers beyond the limits that allow effective actin-myosin interaction.

The second acute compensatory process is increased sympathetic stimulation. Sympathetic stimulation increases the inotropic (contractility) and chronotropic (heart rate) state of the myocardium. The simplest mechanism to increase cardiac output is to increase heart rate. Additionally, sympathetic stimulation of myocardial adrenergic receptors results in increased adenylate cyclase and cyclic adenosine monophosphate levels and subsequently in increased myocardial contractility. There is now evidence that worsening heart failure increasingly stimulates the sympathetic nervous system to maintain vascular tone and myocardial contractility, but as noted previously, chronic sympathetic stimulation results in adrenergic receptor fatigue, or "down-regulation." This down-regulation process may negate or lessen the beneficial sympathetic response in patients with chronic heart failure.

In chronic congestive heart failure the heart has two important adaptive mechanisms, hypertrophy and dilation, that attempt to maintain normal cardiac output despite increased demands for work. These mechanisms may allow the heart to perform almost normally for years and keep the patient free of symptoms. They

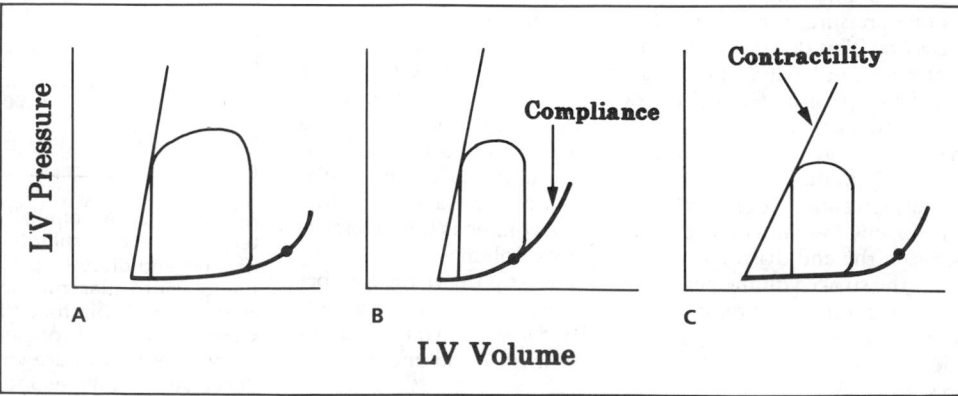

Figure 2.2–3. A. Normal pressure volume characteristics with normal contractility and compliance. B. Normal contractility, decreased compliance. Decreased compliance results in a stiff ventricle with a marked increase in ventricular pressure with increases in diastolic volume. C. Decreased contractility and normal compliance. If the ventricular diastolic filling volume is maintained at a constant level, the decrease in contractility markedly decreases stroke volume and effectively limits cardiac output.

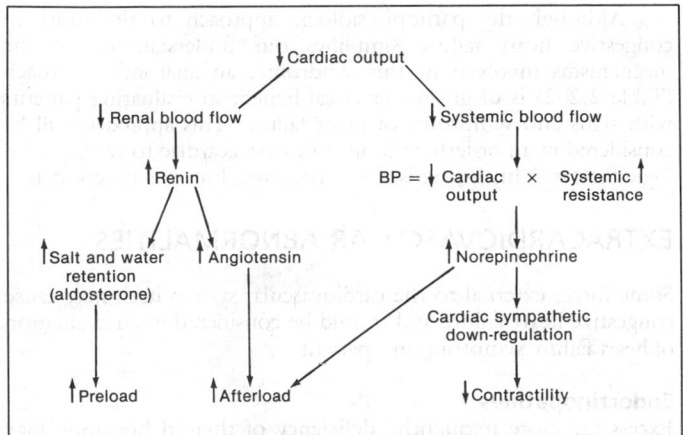

Figure 2.2–4. The deleterious effects of decreased cardiac output include increased ventricular preload and afterload. Persistent sympathetic stimulation of the myocardial beta-sympathetic receptor results in receptor fatigue, or "down-regulation," and further depression of left ventricular contractility. BP = Blood pressure.

will be less effective if the increased work demand on the heart worsens with time or if other disease processes supervene.

Ventricular hypertrophy occurs when the heart is required to generate increased wall stress for a prolonged period. Wall tension, or wall stress, is defined by the Laplace relationship and is equal to the pressure in the ventricle multiplied by the simultaneously determined radius of the ventricular cavity divided by the wall thickness. Heart failure results in an increase in left ventricular cavity diameter, both acutely and chronically. Similarly, heart failure may be associated with increased ventricular afterload, as in aortic stenosis or hypertension. Heart failure therefore induces a marked increase in wall stress. An increase in wall thickness, or hypertrophy, will normalize wall stress and will therefore decrease the demand on each myofiber. Additionally, the total overall pump capabilities of the hypertrophied left ventricle are greater than those of the normal ventricle. The disadvantages of ventricular hypertrophy relate to the increased stiffness, or decreased compliance, and the increased demand for myocardial oxygen. This shift in the diastolic compliance curve results in a higher diastolic pressure for a given left ventricular volume and may produce symptoms caused by venous hypertension and fluid transudation. The major determinants of myocardial oxygen consumption and coronary perfusion are heart rate, contractility, and wall stress. Increased wall thickness, associated with a decrease in cardiac output, lower diastolic coronary perfusion pressure, and increased ventricular cavity diastolic pressure all contribute to diminished subendocardial coronary perfusion in the patient with chronic heart failure.

A prolonged increase in left ventricular diastolic pressure or volume will result in cavity dilation. As long as the ventricle maintains normal function, increases in end-diastolic volume will result in proportional increases in stroke volume. Ultimately the distensibility of the ventricular fibers may be overcome, even if allowed to compensate over time, and compliance may then decrease, resulting in elevation of diastolic pressures into the range at which transudation of fluid results in pulmonary or systemic symptoms. Chronic dilation of the ventricular cavity increases wall stress and myocardial oxygen demands, placing the ventricle in a tenuous position.

CLINICAL MANIFESTATIONS

Heart failure may be characterized pathophysiologically as an alteration in ventricular contractility, in compliance, or both, resulting in a low cardiac output, in high diastolic pressures with secondary fluid retention, or both. The clinical manifestations of a low cardiac output include weakness, fatigue, malaise, lightheadedness, diaphoresis, nausea, and diarrhea. High diastolic filling pressures may affect the pulmonary venous system (left ventricular failure), the systemic venous system (right ventricular failure), or both. Pulmonary congestion may result in cough, dyspnea on exertion, shortness of breath, orthopnea, paroxysmal nocturnal dyspnea, or rarely hemoptysis. Systemic congestion causes jugular venous distension, hepatomegaly, and extravasation of fluid in the lower extremities or abdomen.

The distribution of the increased extravascular fluid resulting from increased total body sodium and water varies from patient to patient. Venous pressure is the major factor determining distribution, and its effect is emphasized by the influence of posture. An ambulatory patient will accumulate edema in the feet and ankles because gravity makes the venous capillary pressure highest in the lower extremities. If the patient is put to bed, edema appears over the sacrum. The colloid osmotic pressure of the plasma proteins tends to counteract the effects of the venous hydrostatic pressure, which favors the movement of fluid into the extravascular spaces. Edema formation therefore occurs more readily in the patient with a subnormal concentration of plasma proteins. Tissue pressure is important in determining the distribution of edema, which forms more readily in loose tissue, such as that around the posterior part of the ankle.

Pulmonary vascular congestion is the major abnormality in left ventricular failure and presents clinically as dyspnea on exertion and, in later stages, at rest. A characteristic manifestation is paroxysmal nocturnal dyspnea, in which the patient awakens from sound sleep with extreme shortness of breath. A closely related symptom is orthopnea, which requires the patient to sleep with the head and trunk elevated. On occasion, pulmonary congestion is manifest only by cough or hemoptysis.

Early in the course of left-sided heart failure, the volume of blood contained in the pulmonary vasculature is increased and the pressure in both the arteries and the veins is elevated. The turgid, congested lung becomes relatively inelastic and ventilation is impaired. The work of breathing is increased by reduced compliance of the lung, and this may be responsible, in part, for the symptom of dyspnea, a term that literally means "difficult breathing." Reflex mechanisms originating in the distended vessels or compromised alveoli probably contribute to the tachypnea and sensation of air hunger. If the pulmonary venous pressure is increased, the equilibrium between hydrostatic pressure and colloid osmotic pressure becomes unbalanced and fluid is extravasated into the alveolar spaces. Minor extravasation produces moist rales at the lung bases. If it is more massive and sudden in onset, pulmonary edema results.

Orthopnea and paroxysmal nocturnal dyspnea are closely related and probably depend on the same physiologic mechanism. When the body changes from the erect to the supine position, the hydrostatic pressure in the veins of the legs falls, and the portion of the total blood volume that had been pooled there returns to the right side of the heart to be delivered to the lungs. If the function of the left side of the heart is inadequate, the flow of blood out of the pulmonary vascular bed is impaired and the lungs become congested. A second, more gradual change may play a role in the development of paroxysmal nocturnal dyspnea. The reduction of venous pressure in the extremities resulting from the assumption of the supine position leads to a shift in the fluid equilibrium across the capillary membranes, and fluid enters the vascular space from the extravascular compartment. The result is an overall increase in circulating blood volume, which acts, along with the redistribution, to produce pulmonary vascular congestion. A patient with impaired left ventricular function tends to keep his head and trunk elevated, and if he awakens from a sound sleep with severe shortness of breath, he usually seeks relief by assuming the erect posture, thereby utilizing the effect of gravity to reduce the pulmonary congestion. The congestion of the pulmonary vascula-

ture probably initiates reflexes that result in bronchoconstriction; wheezes are usually present, along with moist rales.

It is traditional to express the cardiac patient's functional capacity in terms of the classification system of the New York Heart Association. Such classification is valuable in transmitting information from one physician to another and also in categorizing patients with regard to their suitability for operation or to indicate the degree of improvement after therapy.

Functional Classification

Class I   Patients with cardiac disease but without resulting limitations of physical activity. Ordinary physical activity does not cause undue fatigue, palpitation, dyspnea, or anginal pain.

Class II   Patients with cardiac disease resulting in slight limitation of physical activity. They are comfortable at rest. Ordinary physical activity results in fatigue, palpitation, dyspnea, or anginal pain.

Class III Patients with cardiac disease resulting in marked limitation of physical activity. They are comfortable at rest. Less than ordinary physical activity causes fatigue, palpitation, dyspnea, or anginal pain.

Class IV   Patients with cardiac disease resulting in inability to carry on any physical activity without discomfort. Symptoms of cardiac insufficiency or of the anginal syndrome may be present even at rest. If any physical activity is undertaken, discomfort is increased.

ETIOLOGY OF CONGESTIVE HEART FAILURE[6,7]

The most important task in evaluating patients with congestive heart failure is to define accurately the cause of the heart failure syndrome. This can be approached according to pathophysiology or abnormal anatomy.

All causes of heart failure can be classified pathophysiologically in one of the three categories listed in Table 2.2–1: increased work load (pressure or volume), restrictive filling (inflow valvular obstruction or decreased ventricular compliance), or decreased contractility. An increased systolic-pressure work load (hypertension, aortic stenosis) may exceed the stroke work capabilities of the ventricle, resulting in cardiac decompensation. Similarly, an excessive volume work load (aortic or mitral regurgitation, arteriovenous fistulae) may distend the ventricle so that even with normal diastolic compliance, excessively high end-diastolic pressures are reached that produce venous fluid transudation. Restrictive ventricular filling may be due to inflow valvular obstruction (mitral stenosis) or decreased ventricular compliance. Ventricular compliance alterations may be due to changes in the myocardium itself (hypertrophy or infiltrative disease) or to changes in the pericardium (constriction or tamponade). Finally, decreased contractility (dilated cardiomyopathy) may cause, first, congestive heart failure as a result of the ventricles' inability to maintain an adequate cardiac output and, second, an eventual increase in diastolic filling pressure as a result of excessive fluid retention and increased intravascular volume.

TABLE 2.2–1. PATHOPHYSIOLOGIC CAUSES OF HEART FAILURE

Increased work load
• Volume
• Pressure

Restrictive filling
• Inflow valvular obstruction
• Decreased myocardial or pericardial compliance

Decreased contractility

Although the pathophysiologic approach to the cause of congestive heart failure simplifies our understanding of the mechanisms involved in this syndrome, an anatomic approach (Table 2.2–2) is of greater practical benefit in evaluating patients with signs and symptoms of heart failure. This approach will be considered in an orderly fashion, from extracardiac to cardiac etiologic factors. This listing is not exhaustive, but it is functional.

EXTRACARDIOVASCULAR ABNORMALITIES

Some forces external to the cardiovascular system itself may cause congestive heart failure and should be considered in an evaluation of heart failure symptoms in a patient.

Endocrinopathies

Excess or, more frequently, deficiency of thyroid hormone may result in myocardial dysfunction. Hypothyroidism decreases heart rate, decreases contractility, and results in myocyte edema and disruption. Cardiac performance is shifted to a lower level of function associated with mildly elevated diastolic filling pressures and a low output state. A pheochromocytoma may also cause congestive heart failure because of excessive norepinephrine stimulation, provoking receptor down-regulation and focal myocardial necrosis with associated inflammatory infiltration. Hypothyroidism and pheochromocytoma result in diffuse hypofunction of the left ventricle.

Anemia

Decreased effective hemoglobin results in a diminished oxygen-carrying capacity for a given volume of blood. Therefore, greater volumes of blood must be pumped to maintain the demands of the body for oxygen. Sustained anemia results in a persistent volume challenge to the ventricle, often with decreased myocardial oxygen

TABLE 2.2–2. ANATOMIC APPROACH TO THE CAUSE OF CONGESTIVE HEART FAILURE

Extracardiovascular
• Endocrinopathies (thyroid, adrenal)
• Anemia
• Toxic
• Hypersensitivity
• Metabolic

Vascular
• Hypertension: systemic or pulmonary
• Pulmonary emboli
• Arteriovenous fistulae

Pericardial
• Effusion
• Effusive constrictive
• Constriction

Coronary
• Transient ischemia
• Ischemic myopathy
• Completed ischemic myocardial damage

Myocardial
• Cardiomyopathy
   Dilated
   Hypertrophic
   Restrictive
• Myocarditis
• Postpartum cardiomyopathy

Endocardial
• Fibrosis
• Löffler syndrome (hypereosinophilia, fibrosis)

Valvular
• Stenosis
• Regurgitation

supply. This demand may cause diffuse global myocardial dysfunction, particularly in patients with coexisting coronary atherosclerosis.

Toxins[12]
A multitude of drugs, including phenothiazines, corticosteroids, and chloroquine, may be toxic to the myocardium. The two most common toxic agents encountered in clinical practice are alcohol and doxorubicin.

Alcohol and its major metabolites alter many components of myocardial cellular function, including calcium metabolism, lipid metabolism, mitochondrial respiration, protein synthesis, and catecholamine release. Alcohol causes acute depression even of the normal left ventricle, and this is even more marked if the catecholamine release associated with alcohol intake is blocked. Patients with clinically evident alcoholic cardiomyopathy usually have consumed moderate quantities of alcohol over an extended period on nearly a daily basis.

Doxorubicin may cause an acute idiosyncratic cardiomyopathy or a chronic dose-related deterioration in left ventricular function. Although fewer than 1 percent of patients receiving 500 mg/m^2 or less of doxorubicin display abnormal left ventricular function, this proportion rises to over 30 percent of those receiving over 600 mg/m^2. The risk of doxorubicin toxic effects is increased in patients who are elderly or who have received previous radiation or cyclophosphamide therapy.

Hypersensitivity
Myocarditis with associated left ventricular dysfunction may result from drugs such as penicillin, sulfonamides, α-methyldopa, or chloroquine. Therefore, patients with congestive heart failure should have their medication history reviewed for clues as to the cause of heart failure.

Metabolic Abnormalities
A number of inherited and acquired metabolic abnormalities may cause global ventricular hypofunction. Two examples are thiamine deficiency (beriberi) and carnitine deficiency.

Thiamine (vitamin B$_1$) is important to cellular aerobic and anaerobic metabolism and has both myocardial and vascular effects. Thiamine deficiency results in vasodilation, and this lower vascular resistance may allow an increase in cardiac output (high-output heart failure). Thiamine deficiency may result in a diffuse cardiomyopathy, vasodilation, and high-output heart failure, or myopathy with marked hypotension may occur. Thiamine deficiency is found frequently in alcoholic patients but should be considered also in patients on fad diets that eliminate thiamine intake or in patients on a long-term regimen of diuretics without adequate oral intake.

Carnitine is a quarternary ammonium compound necessary for transporting long-chain fatty acids into the mitochrondria for metabolism. A few families have been recognized with systemic and/or myocardial deficiencies of carnitine who responded to oral carnitine replacement. Although this particular disorder is rare, it is important to obtain a family history from all patients with congestive heart failure and diffuse left ventricular dysfunction, because research is increasingly identifying metabolic causes for heart failure.

VASCULAR ABNORMALITIES

Abnormalities of the systemic or pulmonary vascular system may produce sufficient strain on the myocardium that dysfunction of the left or right ventricle may result.

Hypertension[8]
Systemic hypertension and pulmonary hypertension, either primary or secondary, are the most likely causes of left and right ventricular failure, respectively (see Chapter 2.10). Persistent hypertension or any chronic afterload increase may cause ventricular hypertrophy and secondary abnormalities in diastolic compliance. The level and duration of systemic blood pressure elevation necessary to produce ventricular dysfunction is unclear, but patients often have other manifestations of hypertensive end-organ damage, including retinopathy or renal insufficiency. Malignant hypertension may induce myocardial necrosis with a rapid deterioration in left ventricular function. Successful long-term control of blood pressure will likely prevent left ventricular dysfunction, and successful treatment of systemic hypertension or removal of its cause may actually cause regression of left ventricular hypertrophy. In advanced states of ventricular dysfunction, the blood pressure may normalize without antihypertensive therapy because the left ventricle is unable to generate an adequate cardiac output.

Pulmonary Emboli
Acute pulmonary embolization capable of producing right ventricular dysfunction is rarely compatible with life. Chronic recurrent pulmonary emboli, however, may cause a progressive increase in pulmonary artery pressure and sufficient obstruction to forward blood flow to produce right ventricular dysfunction and right-sided congestive heart failure.

Arteriovenous Fistulas
Rarely, peripheral arteriovenous communications may be of such size or number that a volume load is placed on the heart that it is unable to manage. These vascular communications are usually obvious on examination or occur in patients with inherited conditions such as Rendu-Osler-Weber syndrome (hereditary hemorrhagic telangiectasia).

PERICARDIAL DISEASE

Acute and chronic pericardial disease may produce congestive heart failure (see Chapter 2.4). In subacute and chronic pericardial disease states, the symptoms and signs of heart failure are more prominent from the right than the left ventricle. This greater right- than left-sided heart failure despite equalization of diastolic filling pressures is due to the greater ability of the pulmonary venous system, as opposed to the systemic venous system, to accommodate to moderately high venous pressure. Recognition of this syndrome is of great importance because it is a treatable cause of congestive failure, the discovery of which is often preceded by a prolonged period of incorrect diagnosis and unsuccessful treatment.

CORONARY ARTERY DISEASE

Atherosclerosis is the most common form of coronary artery–related ventricular dysfunction, although vasospastic or immune system–related coronary artery conditions may rarely adversely affect left ventricular performance. Only atherosclerosis will be considered in this section.

Transient Ischemia
In the early stages of the disease, patients with coronary artery atherosclerosis may occasionally have an angina equivalent characterized by heart failure during episodes of transient ischemia. Additionally, profound heart failure may develop either because of severe global ventricular dysfunction during ischemic episodes or because of focal ventricular dysfunction with mitral regurgitation. Function returns as the ischemia is resolved. Transient global left ventricular dysfunction indicates severe and diffuse coronary artery disease.

Ischemic Myopathy
The existence of an ischemic cardiomyopathy remains controversial. Nonetheless, rare patients have global left ventricular dysfunction associated with diffuse, severe coronary artery disease and with diffuse, as opposed to focal, left ventricular damage.

Completed Focal Ischemic Myocardial Damage

Because of extensive regional myocardial damage (ventricular aneurysm) or strategic location (ventricular septal defect, papillary muscle rupture), patients with ischemic heart disease develop congestive heart failure. These ischemic causes of heart failure follow recognized myocardial infarction (see Chapter 2.8). Mechanical causes of heart failure after myocardial infarction usually appear within 2 weeks of the initial ischemic event, although symptoms from a left ventricular aneurysm may be delayed for several weeks or months.

MYOCARDIAL ABNORMALITIES

In many patients, temporary or permanent abnormalities of the myocardium result in congestive heart failure.

Cardiomyopathy[5,7]

Primary abnormalities of ventricular muscle are characterized as cardiomyopathies. The most popular classification uses gross anatomic and hemodynamic descriptors to segregate cardiomyopathies into (1) dilated, (2) hypertrophic, and (3) restrictive categories (Table 2.2–3).

***Dilated Cardiomyopathy.*[4]** Patients with dilated cardiomyopathy have enlarged hearts as defined by physical examination, chest radiograph, or echocardiogram. The cardiomegaly is due to left ventricular cavity enlargement, and there is usually normal or reduced left ventricular wall thickness. The left ventricular contractility, as judged by ejection fraction, is reduced to below 40 percent, and diastolic relaxation becomes abnormal as myocyte dysfunction and fibrosis develop. Among patients with congestive heart failure who have a dilated cardiomyopathy, in less than 10 percent is a cause established. The remainder of cases are termed idiopathic in origin. Only if a specific cause can be found (e.g., endocrinopathy, metabolic dysfunction, toxic effects, myocarditis) can specific therapy be used to improve left ventricular function. Otherwise, patients with dilated cardiomyopathy have a poor prognosis, with 15 to 20 percent dying in 1 year and over 80 percent succumbing to progressive heart failure or sudden death in 5 years. Systemic embolization occurs in 10 to 15 percent of patients as a result of cardiomegaly, decreased contractility, sluggish blood flow, and atrial or ventricular arrhythmias.

***Hypertrophic Cardiomyopathy.*[10]** Patients with hypertrophic cardiomyopathy display markedly increased ventricular wall thickness and decreased left ventricular cavity size. The abnormal wall thickness may be symmetric or asymmetric, affecting the septum more severely than the posterior wall. The hypertrophic heart is hyperdynamic in contractility, ejecting the major portion of the stroke volume early in systole. Diastolic relaxation, however, is slow and often incomplete, and diastolic filling pressures are elevated. Hypertrophic cardiomyopathy infers a primary muscle disorder, and not hypertrophy, in response to hypertension or valvular outflow obstruction. Hypertrophic cardiomyopathy has also been called idiopathic hypertrophic subaortic stenosis (IHSS), hypertrophic obstructive cardiomyopathy (HOCM), or asymmetric septal hypertrophy (ASH). Many cases are inherited in an autosomal dominant pattern, and family investigation and counseling are mandatory when the diagnosis is established in a patient. There is, however, variable penetrance, and sporadic cases do appear.

The prognosis is highly variable for patients with hypertrophic cardiomyopathy. There is no correlation with the left ventricular outflow gradient demonstrable at catheterization in some patients. The prognosis may be adversely affected by complex ventricular ectopy.

The age at recognition of patients with hypertrophic cardiomyopathy varies from childhood to greater than 60 years. The average age of diagnosis is the mid twenties. In addition to complaints of pulmonary congestion due to diastolic abnormalities, these patients may also complain of symptoms suggesting a low output state due to the small left ventricular cavity and incomplete relaxation. This is exacerbated by the loss of atrial systole and a rapid ventricular rate when these patients develop atrial fibrillation. The excessively thick left ventricular wall and low output may result in symptoms of myocardial ischemia even without atherosclerotic coronary artery disease. Hyperdynamic contractility, restricted filling, and arrhythmias may predispose to syncope.

Some patients, particularly elderly women, may develop an inappropriately hypertrophied heart in response to hypertension or other unknown stimuli. This disorder represents a different form of hypertrophic cardiomyopathy from the familial variety, but the hemodynamic abnormalities are the same.

Restrictive Cardiomyopathy. A number of infiltrative diseases cause restrictive cardiomyopathy, although rare patients with hypertrophy alone also display this pattern. Both the thickness of the cardiac muscle and cavity size are usually normal until late in the course of disease, when both may increase. Impaired diastolic relaxation is the primary hemodynamic abnormality. Ventricular compliance is markedly decreased, resulting in an elevation in diastolic filling pressures and limited ventricular filling. Ultimately, as the disease progresses, systemic contractility is decreased and heart failure symptoms worsen. The condition of patients with a restrictive cardiomyopathy pattern must be completely evaluated for a possibly treatable infiltrative process and to rule out constrictive pericarditis, which can have very similar clinical and hemodynamic abnormalities.

Causes of restrictive cardiomyopathy include amyloidosis, hemochromatosis, and sarcoidosis. Any form of amyloidosis may result in infiltration of the myocardium with beta-pleated protein chains. Occasionally the cardiac involvement produces more symptoms than amyloid infiltration elsewhere, although usually the opposite is the case. Similarly, hemochromatosis with cardiac involvement is usually preceded by hepatic dysfunction, skin pigmentation changes, and diabetes. Although up to 25 percent of patients dying from sarcoidosis have cardiac involvement, this involvement is clinically apparent in less than 10 percent. Sarcoid cardiac involvement may precede symptomatic systemic involvement and may result in conduction abnormalities, arrhythmias, valvular disease, a diffuse cardiomyopathy, or any combination of these conditions. These infiltrative disease states can be proved by biopsy of any clinically involved organ, and endomyocardial biopsy

TABLE 2.2–3. PRIMARY CARDIOMYOPATHY[a]

	LV Wall	LV Cavity	Systolic Contractility	Diastolic Compliance
Dilated cardiomyopathy	Thin	Large	↓	NL → ↓
Hypertrophic cardiomyopathy	Thick	Small	↑	↓
Restrictive cardiomyopathy	NL	NL	NL → ↓	↓↓

NL = Normal.
[a]Primary cardiomyopathies are defined by anatomic variation in ventricular cavity size and ventricular wall thickness, in addition to the ventricular systolic and diastolic characteristics. Contractility or compliance may be normal early in the disease state but may become abnormal subsequently.

can be used to establish the diagnosis or document cardiac involvement.

Myocarditis[1]

Inflammation of the myocardium can result in ventricular dysfunction. The mechanism by which the heart damage occurs is unclear but may relate to actual myocyte injury by phagocytic and inflammatory cells, alteration in calcium transport, or interference with membrane-bound adenylate cyclase. A postviral cause is hypothesized for most patients with myocarditis, although autoimmune diseases such as systemic lupus erythematosus may also be associated with myocarditis. Several lines of evidence suggest that a postviral process may induce chronic cardiomyopathy: (1) an animal model of postviral autoimmune myocarditis resulting in ventricular dysfunction exists; (2) many patients with dilated cardiomyopathy had a serious viral illness before the onset of heart failure symptoms; (3) a greater number of patients with dilated cardiomyopathy than expected have antibodies to viral agents; (4) viral infections with associated myocarditis induce antibodies to heart tissue; (5) patients with dilated cardiomyopathy often have an altered immune response incapable of suppressing antibody production; and, finally (6), in patients with endomyocardial biopsy–proved myocarditis and depressed left ventricular function, left ventricular function may improve with treatment with immunosuppressive agents. The incidence of myocarditis remains low in patients with global left ventricular dysfunction (5 to 10 percent), and treatment with immunosuppressive agents entails some risk. The diagnosis of myocarditis can be established only by endomyocardial biopsy demonstrating an inflammatory infiltrate and myocyte necrosis. Patients with dilated cardiomyopathy should be evaluated by endomyocardial biopsy if they are young, have had congestive heart failure symptoms for less than 6 months, and are candidates for treatment with immunosuppressive therapy.

Peripartum Cardiomyopathy

Global left ventricular dysfunction occurring in the last month of pregnancy or in the first 5 months post partum is termed peripartum cardiomyopathy. No other cause of heart failure is apparent in women affected with this disorder. The cause of this sudden deterioration in left ventricular function is unclear; however, in some patients, myocarditis has been demonstrated by endomyocardial biopsy. Affected patients are usually multiparous and over age 30 years; in addition, the condition is seen more frequently in twin births. Regardless of the presence or absence of myocarditis, in approximately half of the affected patients, ventricular function returns spontaneously to normal or nearly normal levels. Patients who continue to display cardiomegaly share the same poor prognosis as patients with dilated cardiomyopathy. Attempted subsequent pregnancies result in recurrence of congestive heart failure or death in many patients who have previously suffered from peripartum cardiomyopathy; sterilization is therefore suggested after resolution of the initial bout of congestive heart failure.

ENDOCARDIAL FIBROSIS

Fibrosis of the endocardial surface can effectively result in restricted filling of the left or right ventricle, eventually compromise valvular function, and serve as a nidus for thrombus formation and subsequent embolization.

Endocardial fibrosis is an endemic disease of the tropics characterized by extensive fibrosis, sometimes in excess of 1 cm, extending over specific areas of the left or right ventricle. The primary functional abnormality is decreased diastolic compliance rather than impaired systolic contractility.

Endocardial Fibroelastosis

Primary endocardial fibroelastosis is a disease of childhood, with presentation between 4 and 12 months of age. Endocardial fibroelastosis may be "secondary" and is occasionally associated with other cardiac disorders, including coarctation of the aorta, congenital aortic stenosis, and hypoplastic left heart syndrome. Primary endocardial fibroelastosis may resolve, or may result in congestive heart failure or death.

Löffler Syndrome

This syndrome is an entity characterized by eosinophilia, eosinophilic infiltration of extracardiac organs (including the liver and spleen), and endomyocardial fibrosis. The eosinophilia may be idiopathic or associated with a number of other disease entities, including collagen vascular disorders, tumors, and parasitic infection.

VALVULAR ABNORMALITIES

Significant stenosis of, or regurgitation through, the aortic and mitral valves may cause severe left-sided and subsequently right-sided heart failure, whereas stenosis of, or regurgitation through, the pulmonic or tricuspid valves may cause right-sided heart failure. These lesions are discussed in Chapter 2.3. Often in patients with congestive heart failure and left or right ventricular dilation, murmurs of mitral or tricuspid regurgitation appear secondarily. It is important in the treatment of patients with heart failure to ensure that the auscultatory abnormalities are not due to primary valvular disease. A history of rheumatic heart disease or endocarditis, together with the appearance of a murmur before the onset of heart failure, suggests that the valvular disease may be primary. The murmurs from many primary valvular lesions become less apparent in the presence of heart failure due to the associated decreased cardiac output or decreased pressure gradient across the affected valve. Echocardiography may be helpful in differentiating primary from secondary valvular lesions; rarely is cardiac catheterization necessary.

EVALUATION OF PATIENTS WITH CONGESTIVE HEART FAILURE

The evaluation of patients with congestive heart failure proceeds from a general, noninvasive examination to specifically directed invasive studies such as cardiac catheterization and endomyocardial biopsy. Appropriate therapy mandates knowledge of the pathophysiology of the patient's condition, although occasionally the degree of heart failure will be so severe that therapy must precede thorough evaluation. Once the patient's condition is stable, however, the cause and pathophysiology of the patient's heart failure must be clarified. Every patient should have certain studies when the heart failure syndrome is diagnosed; the more directed studies should be used selectively (Table 2.2–4).

GENERAL EVALUATION

On initial presentation of congestive heart failure, patients should undergo the following investigations:

History Taking

In this era of high technology a historical evaluation is often overlooked. Because of the multitude of causes of heart failure, historical clues to direct one's attention to a cause are of utmost importance (see Table 2.2–2). Patients and their families should be questioned as to the exact duration of symptoms, the presence or absence of prior evidence of heart disease, and events immediately preceding the deterioration of the patient's condition.

Physical Examination

This examination allows confirmation of the presence of heart failure and may point to its cause. The degree of jugular venous distension offers a noninvasive measure of mean right atrial pressure.

TABLE 2.2–4. EVALUATION OF PATIENTS WITH CONGESTIVE HEART FAILURE

General Evaluation	
• History	• CXR
• Physical examination	• Echocardiogram
• ECG	• Holter monitor

Specific Evaluation		
Dilated Heart	*Hypertrophic Heart*	*Restrictive Heart*
TFTs, VMA, hGH	TFTs, hGH	Fluoroscopy U & SPEP Fe/TIBC, transferrin, desferrioxamine, Fe excretion test
Thiamin, RBC trans-ketolase, carnitine		Eosinophil count
Thallium scan, coronary angiography		Gallium scan, α_1-anti-trypsin level
EMB		EMB

CXR = chest radiograph; TFTs = thyroid function tests; VMA = vanillylmandelic acid; hGH = human growth hormone; EMB = endomyocardial biopsy; U & SPEP = urine and serum protein electrophoresis; Fe/TIBC = iron/total iron binding capacity.

In addition, the jugular venous waves may assist in the diagnosis of tricuspid valve disease, high right ventricular end-diastolic pressure, and restrictive or constrictive physiology. Tricuspid regurgitation results in a giant *v* wave of venous engorgement at the same time as the carotid upstroke. Tricuspid stenosis or diseases resulting in a high right ventricular end-diastolic pressure produce a large venous *a* wave at the time of atrial systole. The *a* wave of tricuspid stenosis is slow to recede, whereas restrictive or constrictive physiology demonstrates large *a* and *v* waves with rapid descent.

The arterial pulse allows an assessment of the degree of arterial tone. Patients with anemia, thyrotoxicosis, high output states, aortic reflux, or arteriovenous communication have bounding pulses of generous volume. Patients with hypertrophic hyperdynamic hearts have a brisk, rapid, "percussion" pulse wave often followed by a secondary "tidal" wave. Patients with low output states have low pulse volumes and evidence of underperfusion, including diaphoresis and peripheral or central cyanosis.

In addition to jugular venous engorgement, other evidence of right-sided heart failure may include hepatic enlargement, peripheral edema, or ascites. Left-sided venous congestion is evidenced by pulmonary rales, pleural effusions, or cardiac "asthma" due to peribronchial edema.

Patients with dilated hearts have a displaced point of maximal impulse (PMI) with a weak apical beat, usually with an S₃ gallop. The hypertrophic heart may have a displaced PMI; however, the apex is active and may or may not have a palpable S₄ gallop. Constrictive or restrictive hearts are usually quiet, and in the case of pericardial disease a "knock" may be heard in early diastole. In all forms of left ventricular dysfunction resulting in heart failure the patient may have murmurs of mitral or tricuspid regurgitation.

Patients should be thoroughly examined for any other clues to the cause of their heart failure. These clues may include evidence of an endocrinopathy, auscultation of arteriovenous fistulae, skin coloration, or skin nodules.

Electrocardiography

Most patients with heart disease have an abnormal ECG, but seldom are the electrocardiographic changes diagnostic. The ECG can be used to diagnose rhythm disturbances and assess atrial enlargement. Patients with a prior myocardial infarction may display appropriate Q waves; however, pseudoinfarct patterns are common in amyloidosis, and large Q waves may represent septal depolariza-

tion in hypertrophic cardiomyopathy. Increased QRS complex voltage may characterize the hypertrophic, hypertensive population, whereas low voltage is seen in amyloidosis or pericardial disease. Intraventricular conduction delay (IVCD) and ST segment and T wave changes are frequent but nonspecific abnormalities.

Chest Radiograph

The chest radiograph allows an evaluation of overall cardiac size and, in some patients, an assessment of particular chamber enlargement. Additionally, the chest radiograph permits an evaluation of vascular abnormalities, including coarctation, arteriovenous communication, and pulmonary hypertension. Heart failure may appear as pulmonary vascular redistribution with increased flow to the upper lobes, pleural effusions, or pulmonary edema with alveolar transudation of fluid.

Echocardiography

The most helpful noninvasive study for evaluating patients with congestive heart failure is echocardiography. The technique allows a patient's condition to be categorized, by ventricular size and function, into dilated, hypertrophic, or restrictive-constrictive heart disease. Segmental left ventricular contraction abnormalities suggestive of ischemic disease can usually be determined by echocardiography. Additionally, wall thickness can be accurately measured. M-mode and two-dimensional echocardiography permits evaluation of the cardiac valves for intrinsic disease, and Doppler echocardiography may assist in the determination of the degree of valvular regurgitation or stenosis. Echocardiography is the most sensitive test for diagnosis of pericardial effusions and usually can demonstrate pericardial thickening or calcification. Right ventricular size and function can also be evaluated, and changes suggestive of right ventricular pressure or volume overload may lead to further diagnostic evaluation of the right side of the heart.

Holter Monitor

This device adds little to the evaluation of the cause of heart failure unless extreme bradycardia or ventricular arrhythmias are suspected as precipitating factors. However, since nearly half of all deaths in congestive heart failure patients are sudden and presumably arrhythmic, the recognition and treatment of ventricular arrhythmias may be important.

SPECIFIC EVALUATION

Once the generic problem of heart muscle abnormality has been recognized, specific etiologic analysis can be undertaken (Table 2.2–4). Not every study should be performed in every patient, but this incomplete list of diagnostic tests should be considered, together with clues from the history and physical examination, to direct the search for the cause of the patient's heart failure.

Dilated Heart

As examples of this approach, the clinical clues and physical findings suggesting thyroid disease or pheochromocytoma are often masked by heart failure itself. Thyroid function tests and urinary vanillylmandelic acid (VMA) determinations should therefore be obtained in patients with diffuse cardiac dysfunction and without an obvious source for heart failure. Nutritional deficiencies are uncommon in the United States; however, thiamine levels or red blood cell transketolase levels should be assessed in certain patient populations, including alcoholics, fad dieters, and hospitalized patients on a long-term regimen of diuretics without nutritional supplementation. Carnitine deficiency is exceedingly rare, and levels should be measured only in patients with a familial myopathy. For patients in whom coronary artery disease is suspected, or for those more than 35 years of age without an obvious cause of congestive heart failure, a resting thallium scan or coronary angiography, or both, should be considered. Coronary atherosclerosis should be of

sufficient magnitude to explain the left ventricular dysfunction and not be an incidental finding. For patients with a short history of heart failure and without another cause of dilated cardiomyopathy, endomyocardial biopsy may demonstrate inflammation or another infiltrative cause of cardiac enlargement.

Hypertrophic Heart

Patients with classic asymmetric septal hypertrophy as demonstrated by echocardiogram need no further diagnostic studies. Family members of these patients and others with proved hypertrophic cardiomyopathy should, however, have echocardiographic screening. Patients without familial hypertrophy may have a hypertrophic response to hypertension, hyperthyroidism, or ventricular hypertrophy as a result of excess growth hormone. Thyroid function tests and growth hormone measurement should be considered in patients with hypertrophic or hyperdynamic hearts if no other cause is obvious.

Restrictive Heart

A restrictive cardiomyopathy is the most difficult to diagnose by noninvasive means, and left- and right-sided heart catheterization may be necessary to confirm the diagnosis. Additionally, patients with restrictive disease often develop features of dilated cardiomyopathy as the disease process progresses, with an overlap state resulting. Fluoroscopy should be considered initially to rule out pericardial calcification. If amyloidosis is suspected, appropriate serum and urine electrophoresis studies should be performed and biopsy specimens taken from other involved organs. Hemochromatosis can usually be diagnosed with iron, total iron-binding capacity (TIBC), and transferrin levels; more complicated studies, such as a desferrioxamine infusion test and a liver biopsy, can be reserved for equivocal situations. An eosinophil count should be obtained to rule out Löffler syndrome. If sarcoidosis is suspected, determination of the α_1-antitrypsin level, a whole-body gallium scan, or a Kveim test may be beneficial; however, tissue diagnosis is also necessary. For all restrictive disorders, endomyocardial biopsy may be definitive and should be done if the diagnosis cannot be established easily by other means.

THERAPY FOR PATIENTS WITH CONGESTIVE HEART FAILURE

The most effective therapy for congestive heart failure is that which corrects the primary etiologic basis of the heart failure (e.g., replacement of thyroid hormone, removal of pheochromocytoma, supplemental thiamine or carnitine therapy, or correction of anemia). In most patients, however, a specific cause is not recognized, and one must resort to treatment with supportive therapy. This supportive therapy should reflect an understanding of the pathophysiology involved in the dilated, hypertrophic, or restricted heart.

Restrictive and hypertrophic heart disease are the least common forms of cardiac dysfunction and require specific therapy. Therapeutic measures will be discussed initially, and more general comments about therapy for heart failure will be addressed under the section on dilated cardiomyopathy, below.

RESTRICTIVE HEART DISEASE

Restrictive-constrictive heart failure is the most difficult form to treat. Inotropic agents, diuretics, and vasodilators may be detrimental. Patients with infiltrative disease are particularly prone to the toxic effects of digitalis; if it is used, it should be given in low dosage. The most effective treatment for this type of heart failure is diuresis. Diuretics are used to remove excess fluid and decrease symptoms of pulmonary or systemic venous congestion. Excessive diuresis, however, may reduce the cardiac output and compromise organ perfusion. Careful assessment of cerebral and renal function should therefore be undertaken while these agents are administered.

HYPERTROPHIC HEART DISEASE

In contrast to the restrictive forms of heart disease, diastolic abnormalities in hypertrophic cardiomyopathy can be influenced favorably by drug therapy. Beta-blocking drugs and calcium-channel blocking agents may increase diastolic compliance and lower diastolic filling pressures. Beta-blocking drugs also lower the heart rate and allow greater time for ventricular filling, which may improve cardiac output. Both beta-blocking drugs and calcium antagonists have a negative inotropic effect and decrease hypercontractility and cavity obliteration. Caution should be exercised when one is using calcium antagonists in patients with hypertrophic myopathy who have had severe congestive heart failure, because these agents may occasionally induce profound low cardiac output that is poorly responsive to other drug therapy.

Digitalis or other inotropic agents are not used in patients with hypercontractile left ventricular function. Digitalis may be given to control the ventricular response to atrial fibrillation; however, in all but "burnt out" cases of hypodynamic hypertrophic hearts, a beta blocker or a calcium antagonist would be more beneficial.

Vasodilator therapy may worsen symptoms in patients with a hypertrophic, hyperdynamic heart by further enhancing left ventricular contractility and cavity obliteration.

Diuretics are occasionally necessary to remove excess volume and reduce symptoms due to fluid retention. Caution should again be exercised, inasmuch as it is possible for overdiuresis to occur in patients with hypertrophic cardiomyopathy, with lower cardiac output or greater cavity obliteration resulting.

DILATED CARDIOMYOPATHY

The patient with a dilated heart and congestive heart failure has decreased contractility and reduced cardiac output, resulting in increased preload and increased afterload. Medical therapy is tailored to improve each of these hemodynamic abnormalities singly or in combination.

Digitalis[9] or other oral or intravenous inotropic agents may improve contractility and therefore may also improve cardiac output. Digitalis has a narrow therapy/toxicity ratio, and because patients with myocardial disease are prone to toxic effects, the drug is used in the lowest dose possible to achieve a demonstrable effect. Increased preload can effectively be reduced with diuretics or nitrate therapy. Narcotics have a similar venous pooling effect and may be used in acute situations. Patients with congestive heart failure and dilated cardiomyopathy often have an inappropriate increase in systemic vascular resistance relative to the decrease in cardiac output. A decrease in this systemic resistance (or afterload) may therefore improve cardiac output and increase blood pressure and organ perfusion.

Anticoagulant therapy should be strongly considered for all patients with dilated cardiomyopathy and heart failure in view of the high risk of systemic embolization. The risk is increased in patients with valvular disease, arrhythmias, or both.

All patients with recurrent heart failure despite a stable medical regimen should have an appropriate investigation of the precipitating cause (e.g., dietary indiscretion, medication noncompliance, or infection), and that problem should be addressed. Similarly, all patients with heart failure should receive appropriate rest and appropriate dietary restriction, as noted below.

Rest

Rest is an often overlooked and effective form of treatment. Regardless of what has upset the balance between cardiac performance

and the metabolic requirements of the body, a reduction in activity is always possible, whereas an increase in cardiac performance may not be. In some situations, rest may do more than just reduce the cardiac work load. When the patient has edema or dyspnea, he should be placed on a regimen of bed rest, with the head of the bed elevated to 45 degrees. It is also advisable to employ a "cardiac" bed, which allows the patient's legs to be below the pelvis while the patient is recumbent. If this is not done, fluid present in the legs may be returned to the vascular system and may precipitate pulmonary edema. This shift in fluid associated with recumbency may lead to the incorrect impression that the patient is improving, because the ankle edema may decrease, but an increase in sacral edema will be noted if the latter area is examined carefully.

If the patient has difficulty using a bedpan, it may be better to let him use a bedside commode. If he is properly assisted, the energy thus expended is minimal. A mild laxative or stool softener is indicated to reduce straining at stool.

Venous thrombosis and embolism are hazards of bed rest in patients with congestive failure. The circulation to the extremities is decreased by virtue of the basic disease, and venous return is further compromised by the pressure of the edema fluid itself. For these reasons, the period of bed rest should not be longer than is necessary to initiate a good diuresis. Three measures may prevent thromboembolism. The first and simplest is regular leg exercise. The patient is instructed to flex his feet against a footboard. The patient may also wear snugly fitting elastic stockings to reduce the volume of blood pooled in the venous channels. Last, anticoagulants may be employed. Low-dose heparin therapy may prevent thromboembolism without causing bleeding in patients who are not candidates for warfarin therapy.

As soon as diuresis has occurred and weight is stable, the patient should be moved to a bedside chair and encouraged to walk to the bathroom; only in the most severe situation is it necessary to maintain complete bed rest after the patient's discharge from the hospital, and a satisfactory semiambulatory regimen should be formulated whenever possible.

Diet

Diet is another critical component of therapy for congestive heart failure. The basic feature is restriction of salt or, more specifically, sodium. The degree of restriction required depends on the severity of the heart failure. The normal hospital diet contains 10 to 15 g of sodium chloride, or 4000 to 6000 mg of sodium per day. In the treatment of heart failure, we are concerned with sodium, not sodium chloride; therefore, it is preferable to designate diets by their sodium content. If the patient omits salty food and adds no salt to his food at the table, he can reduce the sodium intake to between 2000 and 4000 mg per day. If restriction to 1000 mg of sodium or less is necessary, specifically prepared salt-poor milk and bread can be ordered. Diets of this type are maintained outside the hospital only with great difficulty. The patient is more likely to adhere to a low-salt diet if he is provided with a salt substitute that will make food more palatable.

It is generally true that the patient with congestive heart failure cannot retain fluid without sodium, and therefore it usually is unnecessary to control fluid intake when sodium is being restricted. If, however, the serum sodium level is below the normal range, fluid restriction may be beneficial.

Medication

Diuretics, inotropic agents, and vasodilators are used in the treatment of heart failure in the vast majority of these patients. Each category of agents will be addressed.

Diuretics. Diuretics are the mainstay of therapy for congestive heart failure, and no therapy has been proved to be safer or more effective. The potency of a diuretic is determined by its site of action in the nephron and the sodium reabsorption capability at the site of action. There are four anatomic sites of action of diuretic agents: the proximal tubule, the ascending limb of Henle loop,

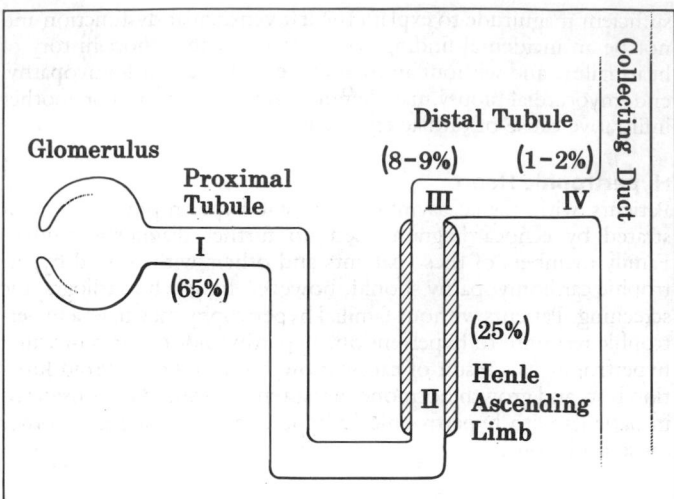

Figure 2.2–5. Anatomic sites of action of the classes of diuretic agents available. Percentages indicate percent sodium reabsorption occurring at each site.

and the early and late distal tubules (Fig. 2.2–5). The diuretics effective at these sites and the maximal fractional excretion of sodium are shown in Table 2.2–5, and the names and dosages of diuretics are shown in Table 2.2–6.

Proximal Tubular Agents. Although a large portion of filtered sodium is reabsorbed in the proximal tubular site, there is no effective diuretic that influences this portion of the nephron. Additionally, renal tubular compensatory mechanisms correct for increased proximal tubular sodium absorption, and the result is diminished distal sodium excretion. Osmotic agents are considered impractical except to ensure adequate intravascular volume before more potent loop diuretics are administered. Acetazolamide inhibits carbonic anhydrase, resulting in decreased sodium and bicarbonate absorption. The amount of enzymatic carbonic anhydrase available to inhibit is limited, and failure of acetazolamide as a diuretic usually implies depletion of carbonic anhydrase or depletion of bicarbonate. Acetazolamide is considered a mild diuretic.

Henle Loop Agents. This group of agents are the most powerful diuretics available. They inhibit chloride transport, resulting in sal-

TABLE 2.2–5. EFFECT OF DIURETICS ACCORDING TO SITE OF ACTION IN THE NEPHRON AND MAXIMAL FRACTION OF SODIUM EXCRETION

Site	Agent	Maximal Fraction of Na+ Excretion
Proximal tubule	Osmotic (mannitol) Carbonic anhydrase inhibitor (acetazolamide)	<5%
Henle ascending limb	Ethacrynic acid Furosemide Bumetanide	>15%
Early distal tubule	Thiazide Chlorthalidone Metolazone	5–10%
Late distal tubule	Aldosterone antagonist (spironolactone) Pteridines (triamterene, amiloride)	<5%

TABLE 2.2–6. COMMONLY USED DIURETICS

Site	Generic Drug	Brand Name	Usual Dose/Day (mg)	Frequency of Administration
Proximal tubule	Acetazolamide	Diamox	250	qd, qod
Henle loop	Ethacrynic acid	Edecrin	50–200	qd, bid
	Furosemide	Lasix	40–80	qd, bid
	Bumetanide	Bumex	0.5–2.0	qd, bid
Early distal tubule	Thiazide	Diuril	500	qd
	Hydrochlorothiazide	Hydrodiuril	50	qd, bid
	Chlorthalidone	Hygroton	50–100	qod, qd
	Metolazone	Zaroxolyn	2.5–5.0	qd, bid
Late distal tubule	Spironolactone	Aldactone	25–100	qd, bid
	Triamterene	Dyrenium	50–150	qd, bid
	Amiloride	Moduretic	5	qd

uresis, have a rapid intravenous and oral effect, and share similar toxic manifestations. Because of the potency of these agents, intravascular depletion, hypochloremia, and hypokalemia can occur. All loop diuretics have ototoxic effects, although ethacrynic acid is the agent most prone to affect hearing. All loop diuretics should be used cautiously with other ototoxic and nephrotoxic drugs, such as aminoglycosides. Because ethacrynic acid is not a sulfonamide derivative, it is the only loop diuretic that can be used for patients with sulfonamide allergy. Loop diuretics display a threshold phenomenon. Only doses of the drug above the patient's renal threshold will result in an effective diuresis. Intravenous therapy should be reserved for patients in whom oral administration is impossible or in whom a rapid onset of action is required.

Early Distal Tubular Agents. These agents promote saluresis through a yet undefined mechanism, but it is known that they are secreted into the distal tubule by an active secretory process and that they also have a minor effect as an inhibitor of carbonic anhydrase. The thiazide agents differ primarily only in their duration of action. Metolazone is the only early distal tubular agent that retains diuretic properties in patients with glomerular filtration rates below 20 ml/min.

Late Distal Tubular Agents. The late distal tubular agents are mild diuretics, and yet all have potassium-sparing properties. Spironolactone is an aldosterone antagonist, and triamterene and amiloride have a direct tubular effect independent of aldosterone function. Because of their potassium-sparing properties, potassium supplementation and hyperkalemia must be evaluated closely in the 3 to 5 days after treatment with these agents is initiated.

Combination Diuretic Therapy. Patients with refractory heart failure may require combination diuretic therapy. Diuretic agents sharing the same site of action should not be used together. The most common combinations use potassium-sparing drugs with either loop diuretics or early distal tubular agents. The combination of a loop diuretic and an early distal tubular agent results in marked hypokalemia and is therefore impractical without a potassium-sparing drug or massive quantities of potassium replacement. Potassium-sparing drugs should never be used in combination with one another.

Diuretic Use in Congestive Heart Failure. It is of great importance to match the power of the diuretic agent with the severity of the heart failure. Patients should be treated initially with dietary salt restriction and then progressively more powerful diuretics as persistent failure demands. Patients with refractory congestive heart failure or those with pulmonary edema should receive intravenous therapy with loop diuretics. Intravenously administered diuretics should be monitored with hourly urine output determinations. Once the threshold dose of diuretic has been established, this dose

should be used repeatedly to maintain an effective diuresis. Intravenous therapy increases the risk of toxic effects, particularly excessive intravascular volume depletion, hypokalemia, and ototoxic effects.

Hospitalized patients with heart failure not requiring intravenous loop diuretics should receive orally administered loop diuretics. Once effective diuresis is established, a progressive weight loss of approximately 1 pound per day is ideal. Diuretic therapy should be adjusted for home administration by giving diuretics no more frequently than twice per day and giving the last diuretic dose at a time when its saluretic effect can dissipate before the patient retires.

Patients with renal insufficiency and heart failure should receive a loop diuretic or metolazone. Larger doses of loop diuretics may be necessary, since the renal threshold may increase with renal insufficiency. Other agents will be ineffective or will result in hyperkalemia. No late distal tubular agents should be used in combination, because hyperkalemia will undoubtedly result.

Vasodilator Therapy.[2,3,11] Vasodilators, since their introduction in the 1970s, have offered impressive hemodynamic and clinical benefit to patients with heart failure and high systemic vascular resistance. Vasodilators lower systemic mean and systolic pressure. This decrease in end-systolic pressure without alteration of early systolic pressure effectively increases the stroke volume and therefore the cardiac output. The lowered systolic pressure reduces left ventricular stroke work demands. The commonly used vasodilators, their dose, and the frequency of administration are listed in Table 2.2–7. Vasodilators fall into three general categories: direct-acting, neurohumoral, and calcium-channel blocking agents.

Direct-acting Vasodilators. The oldest vasodilator is nitroglycerin. Nitrates attach at the nitrate receptor and result in venous, more than arterial, vasodilation. This decreases preload and has little effect on systemic resistance or blood pressure. Oral agents are deactivated in the liver on first pass from the intestine and therefore must be given in high doses. Cutaneous therapy likely results in nitrate receptor down-regulation and subsequent tachyphylaxis. Hydralazine directly affects arterial smooth muscle and is a potent arterial vasodilator. Although short-term hemodynamic studies demonstrate a 40 to 50 percent increase in cardiac output with hydralazine, long-term studies suggest much less sustained improvement, if any at all. Doses of hydralazine below 50 mg every 6 hours do not offer a vasodilating effect in most patients. Hydralazine and nitroglycerin together offer a more effective combination with proved long-term efficacy.

Neurohumoral Agents. Prazosin is a potent vasodilator because of its effect on blocking postsympathetic alpha-adrenergic receptors and inhibition of phosphodiesterase. Prazosin dilates both the arterial and the venous systems. The long-term efficacy of prazosin

TABLE 2.2-7. COMMONLY USED VASODILATORS

Category	Agent	Mechanism of Action	Usual Oral Dose (mg)	Frequency of Administration (hr)	Long-Term Efficacy
Direct vasodilators	Nitrates	Nitrate receptor	40	q4–6	+
	Hydralazine	Arterial smooth-muscle dilator	50	q6	±
	Nitrates + Hydralazine	Arterial and venous smooth muscle	Same	q6	+ +
Neurohumoral	Prazosin	α_1-Adrenergic receptor blockade	1–5	q6–8	±
	Captopril	Blocks angiotensin I conversion to angiotensin II	6.25–25	q8	+ + +
Ca^{++} blocker	Nifedipine	Ca^{++} flux—smooth-muscle dilation	10–20	q6–8	+

remains unproved, with conflicting results in prospective trials. Captopril prevents the conversion of angiotensin I to angiotensin II and blocks the degradation of bradykinin—both of which result in vasodilation of the arterial and venous systems. Long-term, prospective randomized trials have proved the efficacy of captopril in improving hemodynamics and exercise capacity. Side effects include thrombocytopenia, rash, and proteinuria. Enalapril, a captopril congener, may have fewer side effects. As angiotensin-converting enzyme inhibitors reduce aldosterone, potassium loss may become less profound despite continued diuretic use, and the aldosterone antagonist diuretic spironolactone may become less effective.

Many neurohumoral agents display a first-dose response. Marked hypotension may occur with the first administration of prazosin or captopril but is not apparent subsequently. The initial dose of each drug should therefore be small (0.5 to 1 mg prazosin, 6.25 mg captopril), and the drug should be administered at night so that the patient will be supine when the maximal effect occurs.

Calcium-Channel Antagonists. The blockade of calcium channels diminishes smooth-muscle tone and dilates both arteries and veins. Only nifedipine is suitable in patients with dilated cardiomyopathy,

because verapamil has too great a negative inotropic effect. The vasodilating properties of nifedipine are usually greater than its modest negative inotropic effect as long as doses less than 20 mg every 6 hours are used. Very few long-term studies have been performed with nifedipine in congestive heart failure, although it appears to maintain its initial hemodynamic effect in the long term. Nifedipine may cause some flushing, lower extremity fluid retention, and gastrointestinal distress.

There is no perfect vasodilator yet available. The use of one class of vasodilators may result in a rebound increase in other compensatory mechanisms, often reducing or negating the initial benefit of the drug used. Before a drug is abandoned, it is important to ascertain that the appropriate initial agent was chosen, that the dose was appropriate, and that minor adjustments in diuretic therapy will not improve the patient's condition.

Inotropic Agents. The only inotropic agent available for oral use is digitalis. Digitalis interferes with sodium-potassium adenosine triphosphatase, causing an increase in intracellular sodium levels. A sodium-calcium exchange results in an increased concentration of intracellular calcium. Increased intracellular calcium results in greater actin-myosin interaction and increased contractility.

The cellular mechanism controlling inotropism is demonstrated simplistically in Figure 2.2–6. Ultimately, contractility relates to the availability of calcium to the interactive proteins actin and myosin and the level of intracellular cyclic adenosine monophosphate (AMP). The availability of intracellular calcium to actin and myosin is controlled by troponin and other regulatory cellular proteins. There are as yet no clinically available agents to control the troponin avidity for calcium uptake; however, mechanisms that increase intracellular calcium increase contractility. Agents that increase membrane-bound adenylate cyclase will increase not only cyclic AMP but also protein kinases, which subsequently increase calcium influx. Adenylate cyclase may be stimulated by G regulatory proteins, which are enhanced by adrenergic stimulation. Of the clinically available adrenergic agents, norepinephrine displays excessive vasoconstriction, and epinephrine excessive chronotropic properties for clinical use. Dopamine and dobutamine are intravenously administered sympathomimetic agents used for patients with advanced and severe heart failure in whom all alternative therapy has failed. Because cyclic AMP is deconjugated by phosphodiesterase, agents that inhibit phosphodiesterase (amrinone, milrinone) will increase cyclic AMP and contractility. Several new inotropic agents are under active investigation. Currently available inotropes, including digitalis, may improve contractility and reduce symptoms but may also promote ventricular irritability and shorten life span.

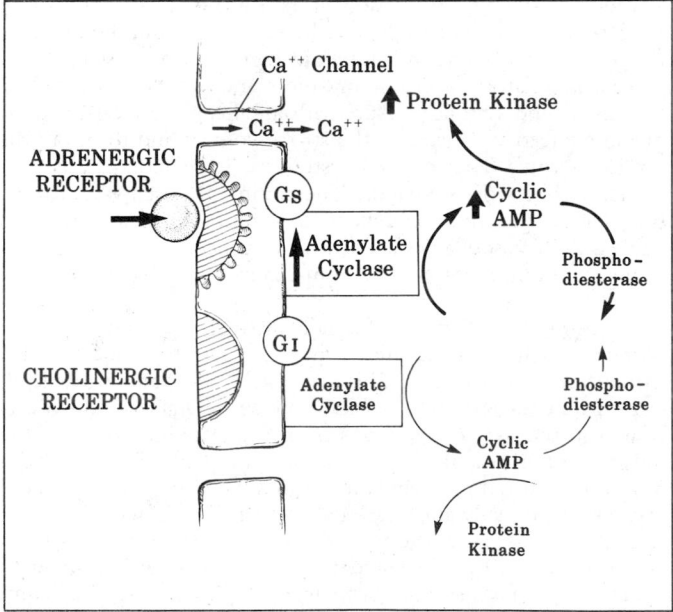

Figure 2.2–6. Cellular modulation of contractility. Increased cyclic AMP or intracellular Ca^{++} results in increased contractility. Stimulation of the adrenergic receptor results in an increase in the G regulatory protein and a subsequent increase in membrane-bound adenylate cyclase. Adenylate cyclase elevation results in an increase in cyclic AMP. Cyclic AMP may increase intracellular protein kinases, which increase calcium transport into the cell. G$_S$ = G-stimulating protein; G$_I$ = G-inhibitory protein; AMP = Adenosine monophosphate.

CARDIAC TRANSPLANTATION

Heart transplantation is no longer "experimental" and is now accepted as a standard part of the armamentarium in the treatment of heart failure. Only heart failure patients with an anticipated survival of 6 months to 1 year should be considered. One-year posttransplant survival rates of 85 percent and 5-year survival rates of 60 to 70 percent have been achieved with the recent advances in

immunosuppressive therapy. Nevertheless (1) the results are less rewarding in children and in patients over 60 years of age, (2) patients must have demonstrated compliance with treatment and have supportive families, and (3) transplantation cannot be considered in patients with systemic disease states that would result in recurrence of cardiac deterioration (e.g., amyloidosis or sarcoidosis). Additionally, cardiac transplantation entails tremendous short- and long-term costs. Transplantation replaces a life-threatening cardiac illness with a multitude of controllable medical problems requiring careful, life-long surveillance. These problems include immunosuppressive drug toxicity, infection, rejection, and accelerated coronary atherosclerosis due to drug-induced cholesterol abnormalities, hypertension, and rejection-mediated endothelial damage. Nonetheless the increase in longevity and the improvement in life-style are truly rewarding in appropriately chosen candidates.

REFERENCES

1. Abelmann WH: Myocarditis. N Engl J Med 275:832, 1966
2. Captopril Multicenter Research Group: A placebo-controlled trial of captopril in refractory chronic congestive heart failure. J Am Coll Cardiol 2:755, 1983
3. Franciosa JA, Dunkman WB, Leddy CL: Hemodynamic effects of vasodilators and long-term response in heart failure. J Am Coll Cardiol 3:1521, 1984
4. Fuster V, Gersh BJ, et al: The natural history of idiopathic dilated cardiomyopathy. Am J Cardiol 47:525, 1981
5. Goodwin JF, Oakley CM: The cardiomyopathies. Br Heart J 34:545, 1972
6. Johnson RA: Heart failure. In Johnson RA, Haber E, Austen WG (eds): The Practice of Cardiology. Boston, Little, Brown, 1980, p. 31
7. Johnson RA, Palacios I: Dilated cardiomyopathies of the adult. N Engl J Med 307:1051, 1119, 1982
8. Kannel WB, Castelli WP, et al: Role of blood pressure in the development of congestive heart failure. N Engl J Med 287:781, 1972
9. Lee DC-S, Johnson RA, et al: Heart failure in outpatients: A randomized trial of digoxin vs. placebo. N Engl J Med 306:699, 1982
10. Maron BJ, Epstein SE: Hypertrophic cardiomyopathy: A discussion of nomenclature. Am J Cardiol 43:1242, 1979
11. Packer M, LeJentel TH: Physiologic and pharmacologic determinants of vasodilator response: A conceptual framework for rational drug therapy for chronic heart failure. Prog Cardiovasc Dis 24:275, 1982
12. Regan TJ: Alcoholic cardiomyopathy. Prog Cardiovasc Dis 27:141, 1984

CHAPTER 2.3

Cardiac Murmurs and Other Manifestations of Valvular Heart Disease[14]

Nicholas J. Fortuin, Stephen C. Achuff, and Richard S. Ross

The diagnosis of cardiovascular disease depends on the synthesis of all the available clinical information, but some objective finding must be taken as the focal point about which the differential diagnosis is developed. Heart murmurs, which are subject to precise description with regard to timing and location of maximum audibility, frequently form such a starting point.

In this chapter, cardiac murmurs are used as a basis for a consideration of the physical findings and laboratory abnormalities associated with valvular lesions and acyanotic congenital abnormalities. Later sections deal with the cause, pathophysiology, evaluation, and management of each of these lesions. Since surgical management plays such an important role in this type of cardiac disease, a portion of the chapter is devoted to general considerations of cardiac surgery and problems related to the use of prosthetic heart valves.

THE DIFFERENTIAL DIAGNOSIS OF MURMURS

The other aspects of the cardiovascular and general physical examination (Chapter 2.1) are essential in the differential diagnosis of murmurs. The remainder of this chapter is based on a primary classification of murmurs by usual timing and point of maximum intensity, as described in Figure 2.1–3, and is organized around a series of tables listing other physical findings and laboratory tests that are helpful in reaching a diagnosis. Not all murmurs will behave in the prototypical manner described in the tables. For example, in some patients with aortic stenosis, the murmur will be heard best at the apex of the heart, and in some with mitral regurgitation the murmur will radiate to the base. The cardiac abbreviations used in the tables are explained in Chapter 2.1.

SYSTOLIC MURMURS

Left Second Interspace

The most common murmur is the early-systolic murmur heard best in the left second interspace. It is usually a crescendo-decrescendo or ejection murmur. The six most common possibilities are listed in Table 2.3–1. Differentiation is difficult because these murmurs arise in the main pulmonary artery, right ventricular outflow tract, or proximal aorta. These structures are close to the chest wall in the region of the left second interspace; the closer the apposition, the more prominent are the auscultatory phenomena.

The innocent murmur of a normal heart with a normal flow is usually short, not very loud, and not widely transmitted. It may be more difficult to hear during inspiration or in the sitting position. The murmur cannot be heard in the back or over the neck vessels. The absence of symptoms and other abnormal physical findings may be all that is necessary to establish this diagnosis, but if uncertainty persists, then a chest roentgenogram, an ECG, and an echocardiogram may provide support for or against this diagnosis.

The innocent murmur may be longer and louder in the presence of an abnormality of shape of the thorax, such as pectus excavatum or a small anteroposterior diameter, as seen in the "straight back syndrome." Wide splitting of the second sound, palpable systolic activity parasternally, rSr' in lead V₁ of the ECG, and a large cardiac silhouette on the posteroanterior chest roentgenogram may be seen in these patients and may contribute to the suspicion of a left-to-right shunt at the atrial level. The echocardiogram, which shows normal right ventricular size, is usually adequate to distinguish between these two conditions.

The physiologic murmurs of high flow due to fever, thyrotoxicosis, pregnancy, and anemia are louder and longer than the inno-

TABLE 2.3–1. SYSTOLIC MURMURS—LEFT SECOND INTERSPACE

Diagnosis	Auscultation	Other Physical Examination	Radiograph	ECG	Cardiovascular Laboratory Findings	Echocardiogram
Innocent murmur	Murmur variable with respiration	Likely in normal thin chest, straight spine, or pectus excavatum	Normal or pectus deformity Straight dorsal spine	Normal	Normal	Normal
Physiologic murmurs	Disappears with treatment of primary condition	Signs of thyrotoxicosis, anemia, fever, pregnancy, etc.	Normal	Normal	Increased cardiac output	Active LV wall motion
Atrial septal defect	S_2—wide, fixed split Middiastolic rumble LLSB	RV lift PA lift	Prominent RV Vascular lungs	Incomplete RBBB	Left-to-right shunt into RA	Dilated RV, paradoxic septal motion
Pulmonary stenosis	EC expiration S_2 split, P_2 soft or absent	Thrill Venous *a* wave prominent	Prominent RV outflow Poststenotic dilation PA	RVH—tall RV, Right axis deviation—peaked P waves	Pressure gradient RV-PA	Normal or RVH
Idiopathic dilation of pulmonary artery	EC	PA lift	Large PA	Normal	Negative except for large PA on angiography	Normal
Small ventricular septal defect	Pansystolic plateau murmur S_2 split	Thrill	Normal	Normal	Small left-to-right shunt into RV	Normal, may detect shunt with Doppler flow mapping

Note: The cardiac abbreviations used in this table are explained in Chapter 2.1.

cent murmur but are still crescendo-decrescendo murmurs and end about two thirds of the way through systole, well before the second sound. These murmurs may have a scratchy or harsh quality that may diminish when the patient sits up and takes a deep breath. The chest roentgenogram, ECG, and echocardiogram are normal unless the high flow has been present for a long time, as in a patient with sickle cell anemia in whom cardiac chamber enlargement has developed.

Increased flow through the right ventricle and pulmonary artery is also the cause of the systolic murmur in the left second interspace of a patient with a left-to-right shunt through an atrial septal defect or anomalous pulmonary venous return to the right atrium. Other physical findings are helpful in making this diagnosis. Wide splitting of the second heart sound is usually present, and the degree of splitting either does not vary or varies only slightly with respiration. Hyperactivity or even a heave may be felt in the left parasternal region. A middiastolic murmur may be heard at the lower sternal border. The simple laboratory studies provide diagnostic information; the ECG almost always shows incomplete or complete right bundle-branch block, the roentgenogram cardiomegaly with prominence of the central and peripheral pulmonary vasculature, and the echocardiogram an enlarged right ventricle with paradoxical motion of the ventricular septum.

A loud and long murmur suggests pulmonary stenosis. This murmur may extend upward to the aortic component of the second sound; the pulmonic component may be diminished or absent but, when present, is delayed. Both the intensity and duration of the murmur are directly related to the severity of the stenosis. The murmur is widely transmitted over the precordium and is often heard in the back and even over the neck vessels. The pressure in the right ventricle is high, but it is unusual to feel a parasternal heave. A systolic thrill in the left second interspace, however, is generally present. The ejection click, which is heard in valvular pulmonic stenosis but not infundibular obstruction, may disappear during inspiration. Right ventricular hypertrophy is present on the ECG when obstruction is severe. The chest roentgenogram will show prominence of the main pulmonary artery and the proximal portion of the left pulmonary artery and normal peripheral vasculature.

Clinical evaluation is sufficient for accurate diagnosis in the vast majority of patients with a systolic murmur in the left second interspace; cardiac catheterization and angiography are rarely necessary. However, cardiac catheterization and angiography may be indicated to establish the severity and exact form of the disorder in anticipation of surgical correction in those patients with organic heart disease.

Right Second Interspace

The ejection systolic murmur that is loudest in the right second interspace is related to turbulence of flow in the outflow tract of the left ventricle, at the aortic valve, or in the aorta. Aortic stenosis is the most important organic lesion associated with this murmur but may be simulated by the other conditions listed in Table 2.3–2.

The murmur of aortic stenosis is characteristically crescendo-decrescendo or ejection in type; if the lesion is severe, the murmur is loud, long, and associated with a systolic thrill in the right second interspace and over the carotid arteries. The murmur is often well heard at the apex, where it may have a musical quality. The carotid pulse is slow in rising, and the pulse pressure is small. Although the systolic murmur is always heard, the other auscultatory signs depend on the type of lesion present. The second aortic sound is often absent when the valve is calcified and rigid, but in a young person it may be loud and clear if there is congenital aortic stenosis with a flexible, mobile, diaphragm type of valve. A loud early-systolic ejection click also is heard when the valve is flexible, not when it is rigid. Mobile and flexible valves become rigid and calcified with the passage of years.

When aortic regurgitation is severe, the systolic stroke output increases and a short, but very loud, early systolic murmur may be generated in the aortic root from the increased flow, even though no obstruction exists. The systolic murmur may even be associated with a thrill, but the true nature of the murmur can be recognized by the cardiac and peripheral signs of aortic regurgitation.

Murmurs of mitral regurgitation may be transmitted to the base of the heart and heard in the right second interspace. This unusual transmission is probably related to impingement of the systolic regurgitant jet on the atrial wall at its point of contact with the aorta. This murmur can be differentiated from that of aortic stenosis by its holosystolic character, the absence of peripheral signs of aortic stenosis, and the typical murmur of mitral regurgitation at the apex. Of course, aortic and mitral valve disease commonly coexist in rheumatic heart disease.

The murmur of pulmonary stenosis occasionally is heard well to the right of the sternum, but only with transposition of the great vessels is it louder on the right than on the left side. Trans-

TABLE 2.3–2. SYSTOLIC MURMURS—RIGHT SECOND INTERSPACE

Diagnosis	Auscultation	Other Physical Examination	Radiograph	ECG	Cardiovascular Laboratory Findings	Echocardiogram
Aortic stenosis calcific (age >40 yr)	Systolic murmur transmitted to neck and apex Diminished or absent EC and A$_2$ S$_4$ gallop	LV heave Slow-rising pulse Narrow pulse pressure Systolic thrill	Calcified Ao valve LV enlargement Dilated ascending Ao	LVH	Pressure gradient between LV and Ao	Calcification Ao valve. Thick LV wall. High-velocity jet on Doppler.
Aortic stenosis congenital (child and young adult)	Systolic murmur transmitted to neck and apex Loud EC and A$_2$ S$_4$ gallop	LV heave Slow-rising pulse Narrow pulse pressure Systolic thrill	LV enlargement Dilated ascending Ao	LVH	Pressure gradient between LV and Ao	Eccentric Ao valve closure
Aortic regurgitation	Decrescendo diastolic murmur Early-systolic murmur Middiastolic and presystolic murmur at apex (Austin Flint)	Wide pulse pressure Quick-rising pulse LV heave	Dilated Ao LV enlargement	LVH	No pressure gradient at Ao valve Aortic regurgitation on angiocardiography	Fluttering MV, dilated LV, LA Regurgitant flow on Doppler
Mitral regurgitation	Holosystolic murmur, not transmitted to neck, heard better at apex and axilla	LV heave	Calcium at MV Big LA	LVH Broad P waves AF	No pressure gradient at MV Mitral regurgitation on angiocardiography	Mitral prolapse, thick leaflets, dilated LV, regurgitant flow on Doppler
Aortic sclerosis	Short systolic murmur	Age usually >50 yr Evidence of atherosclerosis	Calcium in aortic arch	Normal	No pressure gradient	Thick aortic leaflets with normal opening
Bicuspid aortic valve	Short systolic murmur Early decrescendo diastolic murmur EC	Common in youth May be associated with coarctation	Usually normal	Normal	Aortic regurgitation: none, mild, or very rarely severe	Eccentric Ao valve closure
Aortic dilation or aneurysm	Short systolic murmur Diastolic murmur may be present Tambour S$_2$ Lift in right second interspace	Signs of syphilis or Marfan syndrome	Dilated Ao Calcium in ascending Ao in syphilis	Normal	Dilated Ao	Dilated proximal Ao
Hypertension	Short systolic murmur Loud A$_2$S$_1$ may be present	Hypertension	LV enlargement	LVH	LV pressure elevated	Thick LV walls

Note: The abbreviations used in this table are explained in Chapter 2.1.

mission of the murmur to the neck vessels is not proof of aortic origin, since loud murmurs due to pulmonary stenosis can be heard there.

Ejection systolic murmurs in the right second interspace are often heard in elderly patients with aortic atherosclerosis. Many of these patients have sclerotic changes in the leaflets of the aortic valve, but only a few will have hemodynamically significant obstruction. Assessment of the carotid upstrokes, valve orifice on echocardiography, and flow velocity across the valve by Doppler echo will distinguish the lesion from aortic stenosis.

Radiologic examination of the heart is helpful. Dilation of the ascending aorta and enlargement of the left ventricle are seen in both aortic stenosis and regurgitation. The finding of calcification in the aortic valve area on chest roentgenogram, fluoroscopy, or echocardiography provides confirmatory evidence for the diagnosis of calcific aortic stenosis. The absence of aortic valve calcification in an older patient with a systolic murmur is evidence against the presence of significant aortic stenosis. In the patient with aortic regurgitation, echocardiography will help to differentiate lesions of the aortic valve from those of the aortic root and, by measurement of left ventricular chamber size, will provide some quantitative assessment of the severity of the volume load.

Apex and Left Lower Sternal Border

The conditions responsible for a systolic murmur at the apex or along the lower left sternal border are listed in Table 2.3–3.

The organic murmurs of mitral and tricuspid regurgitation and of ventricular septal defect are heard at the apex or between the apex and the left lower sternal border and typically are holosystolic. They begin with the onset of ventricular systole, and hence S$_1$, and usually extend throughout systole, ending with S$_2$ or slightly later, when the ventricular pressure falls below atrial pressure. Only the murmur of mitral regurgitation is loudest at the apex and transmitted into the axilla. That of the small ventricular septal defect, referred to as Roger's murmur, is heard best along the lower left sternal border but may be audible at the apex. The murmur of tricuspid regurgitation typically is loudest at the sternal border or even to the right of the sternum, but frequently it is loud at the apex. The increase in intensity of the murmur during inspiration, the prominent v waves in the jugular veins, the systolic pulsation of the liver, and signs of right ventricular hypertension support the diagnosis of tricuspid regurgitation. In doubtful cases, Doppler echocardiography with flow mapping can be used to locate the regurgitant jet or left-to-right shunt with a ventricular septal defect.

TABLE 2.3–3. SYSTOLIC MURMURS—APEX AND LEFT LOWER STERNAL BORDER (LLSB)

Diagnosis	Auscultation	Other Physical Examination	Radiograph	ECG	Cardiovascular Laboratory Findings	Echocardiogram
Mitral regurgitation						
• Chronic	Holosystolic usually radiating to axilla S_1 soft S_3 common	LV heave	Big LA and LV MV calcification	Broad, bifid P waves AF common	LA pressure elevated, big v waves Mitral regurgitation by angiography	MV prolapse, leaflet thickening, dilated LV, LA
• Acute	Crescendo-decrescendo murmur, holosystolic or ending before S_2, radiation to base or axilla, S_4	Signs of PH	Minimal LV and LA enlargement Pulmonary congestion	Normal	Large LA v waves Mitral regurgitation by angiography	Flail mitral leaflet, vegetations. Normal or slightly dilated LV, LA with active wall motion
Hypertrophic cardiomyopathy (IHSS)	Crescendo-decrescendo murmur, S_4 Modified by squatting and Valsalva maneuver	Rapid, bifid carotid, LV heave	Normal or LVH	LVH Large P wave WPW syndrome	Small LV systolic volume Gradient LV cavity to outflow tract	Asymmetric septal hypertrophy, systolic anterior motion of MV
Ventricular septal defect (small)	Holosystolic LLSB, high-pitched, harsh	Thrill LLSB	Heart small	Normal	Left-to-right shunt Normal pressures	Normal
Tricuspid regurgitation	Holosystolic maximum toward sternum, increase with inspiration, not transmitted to axilla	v Waves in JVP Pulsating liver Signs of RV hypertension and congestive failure	Big RA and VC Large heart	Right axis deviation	Elevated v waves RA	Dilated RV, paradoxical septal motion
Aortic stenosis (transmitted)	Ejection—early-systolic murmur—also heard right second interspace	Thrill—right second interspace	LV large Aortic-valve calcification	LAD and LVH	Pressure gradient aortic valve	Calcified Ao valve
Mitral-valve prolapse	Mid- to late-systolic murmur, may be preceded by click or clicks	Pectus excavatum	Normal	Abnormal T waves	Prolapse of leaflets of MV by angiography midsystole with subsequent regurgitation	Prolapse of MV leaflets
Papillary muscle dysfunction	Mid, late, or pansystolic murmur S_4 gallop		Normal or mild LVH	MI or abnormal ST-T waves	Regurgitation by angiography	Often normal, LV wall motion abnormality

WPW = Wolff-Parkinson-White; JVP = jugular venous pressure; LAD = left axis deviation. Note: The other abbreviations used in this table are explained in Chapter 2.1

When mitral regurgitation occurs abruptly, as with rupture of chordae tendineae or severe papillary muscle dysfunction, the blowing, pansystolic murmur typical of chronic mitral regurgitation may not be heard. In acute mitral regurgitation, the murmur may be of the crescendo-decrescendo type, and harsh and rasping in character. The murmur can radiate well to the upper sternal areas. A fourth heart sound and signs of pulmonary hypertension are usually present. In this situation the chest roentgenogram and echocardiogram will show the left atrium and ventricle to be only minimally enlarged, but there are prominent signs of pulmonary congestion.

The murmur associated with mitral valve prolapse is typically late systolic in timing and is usually introduced by one or more midsystolic clicks. The murmur and clicks may be highly variable in intensity and timing.[7,8] The late systolic timing of the murmur is explained by the fact that the mitral valve is competent early in systole but gives way or falls back into the atrium later in systole. As the mitral regurgitation becomes more severe, it will be present throughout systole, and at this time the murmur becomes holosystolic. This change in the murmur is often associated with the onset of symptoms and enlargement of the heart. When the murmur is late in onset, it indicates that the regurgitation is not severe, and this condition is compatible with a long period of normal cardiac function. Rupture of the chordae tendineae and infective endocarditis are common explanations of the rapid progression of mild to severe regurgitation in some of these patients.

Murmurs due to alteration in function of the papillary muscles are common in patients with ischemic heart disease. Most fre-

quently the murmur is low in intensity, diamond shaped, and well localized to the apex. Such murmurs and those confined to late systole do not signify hemodynamically significant mitral regurgitation. Papillary muscle dysfunction or localized rupture may cause more severe mitral regurgitation, but in this situation the murmur is usually pansystolic and the associated findings are similar to those seen in patients with acute mitral regurgitation due to other causes. The severity of the mitral regurgitation associated with papillary muscle ischemia may vary remarkably; at times the patient may be comfortable and the murmur faint, and at other times the patient may be in severe respiratory distress with a loud, long apical systolic murmur.

In patients with hypertrophic cardiomyopathy (IHSS), the cardiac murmur is midsystolic in timing and has a crescendo-decrescendo shape. This murmur may simulate aortic stenosis at the left sternal edge but may sound more like mitral regurgitation at the apex. This auscultatory quandary should immediately suggest hypertrophic cardiomyopathy. A characteristic feature of the murmur of hypertrophic cardiomyopathy is modification of the murmur by certain maneuvers. In some patients the murmur will be intensified by the Valsalva maneuver and decreased when the patient assumes the squatting posture. Associated findings of a rapid, bifid carotid pulse and the characteristic echocardiographic findings of extreme septal hypertrophy and systolic anterior motion of the mitral valve also help to establish the diagnosis.

The murmur of a ventricular septal defect may be heard all over the precordium, including the apex, but is always loudest along the left sternal border. It is typically more harsh than that of

mitral or tricuspid regurgitation. If the defect is small, the murmur may be the only abnormality detectable on physical examination. Larger defects may be associated with a palpable thrill and a middiastolic murmur at the apex caused by the increased flow across the mitral valve in diastole. Ventricular septal defects with a large left-to-right shunt are rare in adults.

Valvular aortic stenosis must be considered among the common causes of apical systolic murmurs, because the high-frequency, musical components of the aortic stenosis murmur may be transmitted down the long axis of the left ventricle to the apex. In this situation the murmur may be heard poorly in areas between the apex and the base. Its origin can be determined by the presence of other signs of aortic stenosis, such as abnormal carotid pulses and transmission of the murmur to the neck vessels, and by the absence of signs of significant mitral regurgitation such as left atrial enlargement.

DIASTOLIC MURMURS

Apex

A diastolic murmur at the apex is typically due to stenosis of an atrioventricular valve, but other conditions may be responsible (Table 2.3–4).

Mitral stenosis is the most important cause. The characteristic murmur is rumbling, low pitched, heard best at the apex, and occasionally audible only in a very small area—usually directly over the apical impulse. Exercise sometimes is necessary to bring it out, and it is also more prominent with the patient in the left lateral decubitus position. Presystolic accentuation of intensity and frequency is an important characteristic of this murmur. It may be difficult to hear, especially when there is a low cardiac output or severe pulmonary congestion. Its presence can be suspected on the basis of other signs, such as a snapping, loud first heart sound at the apex and an opening snap of the mitral valve, which gives a characteristic cadence. Silent mitral stenosis should be suspected in

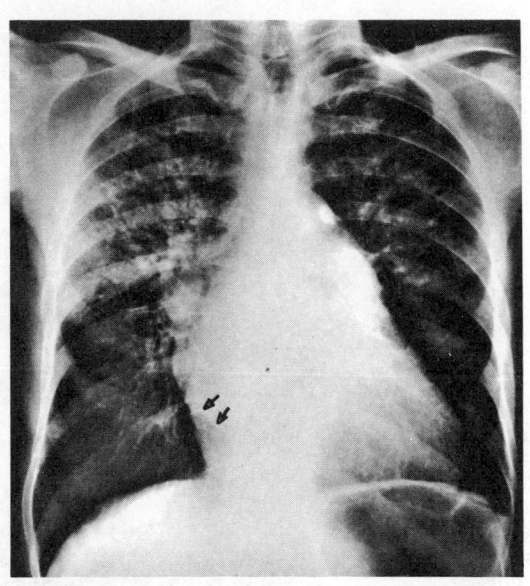

Figure 2.3–1. Chest radiograph of patient with mitral stenosis, showing double density at lower right border of heart, which represents lower border of enlarged left atrium (*arrows*). Right ventricular outflow tract and pulmonary artery are also enlarged.

every patient with signs and symptoms of pulmonary hypertension with pulmonary congestion without another obvious cause, with atrial fibrillation, or with systemic embolization. Support for the diagnosis of mitral stenosis may be provided by the radiologic examination, which may reveal a double density along the border of the right side of the heart, indicating that the left atrium is enlarged (Fig. 2.3–1). Kerley B lines at the lung bases are also char-

TABLE 2.3–4. DIASTOLIC MURMURS—APEX

Diagnosis	Auscultation	Other Physical Examination	Radiograph	ECG	Cardiovascular Laboratory Findings	Echocardiogram
Mitral stenosis	S_1 snapping OS present Middiastolic rumble Presystolic murmur	RV lift	Big LA MV calcification Kerley B lines	RAD Broad notched P waves	Mitral diastolic pressure gradient	Thick MV leaflets with flat diastolic closure Dilated LA
Mitral regurgitation (diastolic flow murmur)	S_1 soft or absent S_3 present Middiastolic murmur Systolic murmur of mitral regurgitation	LV lift	LA large LV large	LAD LVH	Gross mitral regurgitation	Normal diastolic MV motion
Flow murmur secondary to increased pulmonary blood flow, e.g., ASD, VSD, or PDA	S_1 normal S_2 fixed split in ASD Murmurs of primary lesion		Hypervascular lung fields		Proof of primary lesion	Normal diastolic MV motion Active LV wall motion
Tricuspid stenosis	Diastolic murmur heard best near sternum Increased by inspiration	Big *a* waves in JVP	Big RA and VC		Tricuspid diastolic pressure gradient	Thickened TV leaflets Gradient on Doppler
Aortic regurgitation (transmitted)	Decrescendo diastolic murmur LLSB Onset with S_2	Signs of aortic regurgitation LV lift	Large LV	LAD LVH	Signs of aortic regurgitation	Fluttering MV
Aortic regurgitation (Austin Flint)	S_1 normal or soft OS absent Middiastolic rumble Presystolic rumble	Peripheral signs of aortic regurgitation LV lift	Large LV	LAD LVH	Signs of aortic regurgitation	Fluttering MV with rapid diastolic closure

RAD = Right axis deviation; LAD = left axis deviation; JVP = jugular venous pressure. The other abbreviations used in this table are explained in Chapter 2.1.

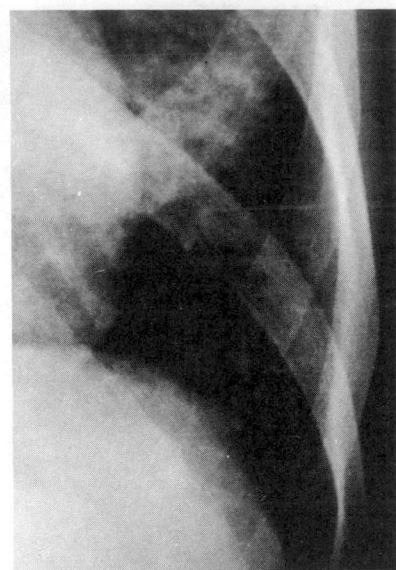

Figure 2.3–2. Left costophrenic angle from chest radiograph of patient with mitral stenosis showing linear streaks of increased density known as Kerley B lines.

acteristic of mitral stenosis (Fig. 2.3–2). The ECG may show broad, notched P waves or atrial fibrillation. The echocardiogram provides the most reliable noninvasive laboratory information about the presence or absence of mitral stenosis; abnormal motion of the anterior and posterior leaflets, increased number of echoes from the leaflets, slow filling of the left ventricle, and enlargement of the left atrium may all be recognized.

Diastolic murmurs at the apex may also be heard in other conditions. Rarely, the tricuspid valve is involved in rheumatic heart disease and may become stenotic. The murmur usually is loudest at the lower left sternal border and may increase in intensity during inspiration. Marked distension of the jugular veins is present and the *a* wave is prominent if the patient is in sinus rhythm.

The middiastolic part of the murmur of aortic regurgitation is occasionally transmitted to the apex and may lead to the incorrect diagnosis of associated mitral stenosis. This error can be avoided by carefully tracing the transmission of the diastolic murmur from the left sternal border to the apex.

A second source of diagnostic error in the same setting is the Austin Flint murmur. The timing of this murmur is middiastolic or presystolic, or both and has the same rumbling character as the murmur of mitral stenosis. It originates at the mitral valve and is probably related to flow through the mitral valve, which is turbulent because of rapid and early mitral valve closure as a consequence of the regurgitant stream and rising diastolic pressures in the left ventricle.[10] The Austin Flint murmur is best differentiated from that of mitral stenosis by the absence of a snapping first heart sound and an opening snap. If the blood pressure is elevated by a vasopressor drug or handgrip exercise, the Austin Flint murmur will increase in intensity because the aortic regurgitation is increased, whereas the murmur of mitral stenosis will be unchanged. However, if the cause is rheumatic, both valves may, of course, be involved. The echocardiogram provides valuable information to help distinguish the Austin Flint murmur from the rumble of mitral stenosis.

Increased flow through a nonstenotic atrioventricular valve can produce a diastolic murmur that simulates the murmur, but not the other auscultatory signs, of mitral stenosis. In the patient with mitral regurgitation the inflow into the left ventricle during diastole is increased and may be double or triple the normal flow. This gives rise to a diastolic murmur even in the presence of pure mitral regurgitation. This murmur usually follows a very loud third heart sound gallop.

Increased flow through the atrioventricular valves secondary to increased pulmonary blood flow can also cause murmurs resembling those of mitral stenosis. The high-flow circuit includes the tricuspid but not the mitral valve in patients with a defect in the atrial septum. In cases of ventricular septal defect and persistent ductus arteriosus, the increased flow passes through the mitral but not through the tricuspid valve. Diastolic murmurs of similar character also are heard in sickle cell and other anemias and may lead to an incorrect diagnosis of mitral stenosis.

Second and Third Left Interspace

Diastolic murmurs at the base of the heart usually represent regurgitation at one of the semilunar valves (Table 2.3–5). These murmurs characteristically occur in early diastole and are decrescendo in type, with the maximum intensity immediately after the second heart sound. The murmurs of both aortic and pulmonary regurgitation are best heard along the left sternal border in the third and fourth interspaces, but the aortic murmur also is heard at the right of the sternum in the second interspace. The pulmonary diastolic murmur usually is not audible to the right of the sternum. When an aortic diastolic murmur is heard better on the right side, aortic root disease should be suspected as the cause of the aortic regurgitation. Syphilis, dissecting aneurysm, or rupture of a sinus of Valsalva must be given special consideration in these situations.

One must decide whether a decrescendo diastolic murmur at the base of the heart is due to aortic regurgitation or to pulmonary regurgitation resulting from pulmonary hypertension. This problem arises frequently in patients with mitral stenosis who might reasonably be expected to have either or both of these lesions. If the murmur is that of pulmonary regurgitation, simple mitral valvotomy is the treatment of choice, whereas if there is significant aortic regurgitation, it may be an incorrect course of action. Doppler echocardiography with flow mapping can be used to make this distinction, but the following clinical observations may be helpful in bedside differentiation. Peripheral signs of aortic regurgitation—wide pulse pressures and so on—are the best evidence that the murmur arises at the aortic valve. Evidence of left ventricular hypertrophy favors an aortic origin. Finally, on statistical grounds a basilar diastolic murmur in a patient with rheumatic heart disease is most likely to be of aortic origin, even in the presence of pulmonary hypertension.

Isolated pulmonary regurgitation attributed to disease of the valve rather than to pulmonary hypertension occurs rarely. In this entity the diastolic murmur is low pitched and not of the decrescendo type.

Diastolic murmurs at the base of the heart may be transmitted from other areas. The diastolic component of the continuous murmur of a persistent ductus arteriosus is heard here occasionally, but the more typical, continuous nature can be appreciated on auscultation under the left clavicle. The diastolic component of other continuous murmurs, especially that of coronary arteriovenous fistula, may be confused with the murmur of aortic insufficiency.

CONTINUOUS MURMURS

A continuous murmur is one heard throughout both phases of the cardiac cycle. The intensity may vary, but there is persistent sound throughout both parts of the cycle. It is sometimes difficult to distinguish such a murmur from prolonged systolic and diastolic murmurs of severe aortic valve disease, but there is usually an identifiable pause separating the systolic and diastolic components in the latter. The most characteristic feature of a continuous murmur is the fact that it runs over or past the S_2. The essential physiologic requirement for the generation of a continuous murmur is continuous flow through an abnormal communication during all phases of the cardiac cycle. Thus a pressure gradient must be present during both systole and diastole. Communication may exist between the aorta and the pulmonary artery (persistent ductus), between the aorta and the chambers of the right side of the heart (ruptured sinus of Valsalva aneurysm), or between an artery and a vein.

TABLE 2.3–5. DIASTOLIC MURMURS—SECOND INTERSPACE, RIGHT AND LEFT (BASE)

Diagnosis	Auscultation	Other Physical Examination	Radiograph	ECG	Cardiovascular Laboratory Findings	Echocardiogram
Aortic regurgitation	Murmur decrescendo heard right second interspace and third left interspace S_2 may be of decreased intensity, but normal S_2 does not exclude severe AR	LV lift Peripheral signs of wide pulse pressure	Large LV	LVH LAD	Aortic regurgitation by angiocardiography	Fluttering MV, dilated LV Aortic regurgitation by Doppler flow mapping
Pulmonary regurgitation	S_2 (P_2) loud if PR secondary to PH Murmur left second interspace, not to right of sternum In absence of PH P_2 normal. Murmur rough and scratchy crescendo-decrescendo	RV lift Peripheral signs of AR absent	Avascular lung fields if PH present	RAD RVH	Aortic valve competent	Dilated RV, paradoxical septal motion Pulmonary regurgitation by Doppler flow mapping
Diastolic component of continuous murmur (transmitted)	Characteristic continuous murmur heard elsewhere (e.g., under left clavicle or over neck)					Normal or dilated LV, LA

LAD = Left axis deviation; RAD = right axis deviation. The other abbreviations used in this table are explained in Chapter 2.1.

The murmur of persistent ductus arteriosus resembles the sound of machinery, with maximum intensity in systole at or near the second sound. Both phases are best heard under the left clavicle, but sometimes one of the components will be audible in the left second interspace and will lead to the incorrect diagnosis of semilunar valve disease. Additional signs are a wide pulse pressure, evidence of left ventricular overload, and, occasionally, a middiastolic flow murmur at the apex, mimicking mitral stenosis. On a chest radiograph the pulmonary arteries are seen to be enlarged and the lung fields vascular.

An arteriovenous malformation of the coronary circulation is another cause of continuous murmur. The point of maximal intensity is usually over the left sternal border. Communication of a dilated coronary artery directly with one of the chambers of the right side of the heart or with the coronary sinus produces a continuous murmur that may be confused with that of a persistent ductus arteriosus. However, the murmur differs from that of persistent ductus in usually being loudest over the lower end of the sternum or between the sternum and the apex and in having a peak intensity that does not occur in association with the second heart sound.

A communication between the aorta and a chamber of the right side of the heart may be formed by rupture of an aneurysm of the sinus of Valsalva. It is usually the right sinus of Valsalva that ruptures into either the right ventricle or the right atrium. The continuous murmur is often of grade 5 or 6 in intensity and accompanied by a thrill. The point of maximal intensity varies with the specific anatomy of an individual case but is usually best heard along the lower left sternal border. The diastolic component is louder than the systolic, which may help in its differentiation from persistent ductus arteriosus. Patients with this condition usually give a history of sudden onset of congestive heart failure, sometimes associated with a feeling of tearing or breaking within the chest.

A systemic arteriovenous fistula in the chest wall or neck may produce a continuous murmur. Such a fistulous communication may develop between the internal mammary artery and vein, as a result of a penetrating wound, or between the carotid or vertebral artery and a jugular vein, as a result of central venous pressure line insertion. Pulmonary arteriovenous fistulas must also be considered and are associated with faint, continuous murmurs over the part of the lung that contains them.

Other causes of continuous murmurs are congenital aortopulmonary communication, ventricular septal defect with aortic regurgitation, and two surgically created types of anastomosis: one between the subclavian artery and the pulmonary artery (Blalock-Taussig operation) and the other between the aorta and the pulmonary artery (Potts operation).

The diagnosis of the typical persistent ductus arteriosus usually can be made easily without catheterization, but the differential diagnosis of the other causes of continuous murmurs requires the use of the laboratory. Right- and left-sided heart catheterization, indicator dilution studies, and contrast radiography are often necessary to locate the points of origin and termination of the shunt.

Venous "hums" may be confused with continuous murmurs of organic origin. If a venous hum is suspected, the diagnosis can be established by a few simple maneuvers. First, the sound is louder in the neck than over the chest. Second, it may be altered when a patient turns his head or breathes and usually disappears entirely with pressure over the jugular vein just above the clavicle. Such a murmur is usually rough, harsh, and irregular in character. It is loudest in diastole and is diminished or absent with the patient in the recumbent position.

A stenotic area in a carotid artery or another branch of the aortic arch may be the source of a bruit heard over the chest. If the stenosis is of such degree that a pressure gradient (and hence flow) persists throughout diastole, the murmur will be continuous. If it arises in the innominate artery or one of its branches, it is heard better under the right clavicle and in the neck than over the heart. Abnormality of peripheral pulses or a difference between the blood pressure in the two arms may be present. A similar mechanism explains the continuous murmur heard in the presence of multiple areas of stenosis in the peripheral pulmonary arteries.

In pregnancy and the early postpartum period, one may hear over the upper part of the chest a continuous murmur that has been called a mammary souffle. This murmur may be confined to systole but may extend beyond the second sound into diastole. Characteristically, it can be obliterated by firm pressure with the bell of the stethoscope.

SPECIFIC VALVE ABNORMALITIES

AORTIC STENOSIS[12,15]

Obstruction to left ventricular outflow can occur above (supravalvular) or below (subvalvular) the aortic valve but is most common at the aortic valve itself. Subvalvular aortic stenosis is a congenital

lesion in which a discrete fibrous membrane or tunnel causes obstruction. In patients with hypertrophic cardiomyopathy (IHSS), a gradient may be recorded between the body of the left ventricle and the area just beneath the aortic valve, but this results from rapid and complete emptying of the ventricle, rather than from left ventricular outflow obstruction. Supravalvular aortic stenosis is also a congenital lesion and practically always associated with a peculiar abnormal physiognomy with elfin facies. Whereas rheumatic fever may damage the aortic valve and produce changes leading to aortic stenosis, isolated aortic stenosis without associated mitral involvement rarely is caused by rheumatic fever but is usually due to a congenital abnormality of the aortic valve or calcification of a normal valve.[22]

Congenital aortic valve disease producing left ventricular outflow obstruction is seen at two different age periods. Patients with valves that are stenotic from birth usually come to the attention of the physician in childhood or early adulthood because of the presence of a heart murmur or symptoms related to left ventricular outflow obstruction. Such congenitally stenotic valves may show signs of progressive narrowing with age as a consequence of abnormal hemodynamic stress and valve calcification. A second and larger group of patients with congenitally malformed valves does not develop aortic stenosis until the sixth or seventh decade, when valve calcification occurs and is responsible for progressive obstruction. These patients often have a history of a cardiac murmur from early adulthood, but signs and symptoms of left ventricular outflow obstruction are not seen until the congenitally abnormal valve, which is usually bicuspid, becomes calcified. In elderly patients, calcification of a normal aortic valve may cause obstruction.

Patients tolerate severe degrees of aortic obstruction for long periods without symptoms. The left ventricle is able to compensate for the abnormal pressure-work that it must perform because of its ability to hypertrophy. Ultimately, however, even this compensatory mechanism proves inadequate, or the hypertrophy may alter the diastolic function of the heart so that pulmonary congestion develops. Thus some patients with aortic stenosis may initially have symptoms of left ventricular failure. Angina pectoris is also a frequent symptom even in the absence of left ventricular failure or coronary atherosclerosis because left ventricular stroke work and muscle mass are increased while coronary perfusion pressure may progressively diminish with increasing valve obstruction. The third cardinal symptom of aortic stenosis is syncope, usually exertional. The mechanism underlying this symptom may be inability to augment cardiac output because of fixed outflow obstruction or even a reflex-induced fall in cardiac output. In some cases, cardiac arrhythmias are the cause of the syncopal episodes; heart block is especially common in patients with calcific aortic stenosis. Once any of these symptoms develop, their progression is usually rapid, or the patient may die suddenly. Sudden death is unlikely to occur before the appearance of other symptoms, however. The appearance of any symptom in the patient with suspected aortic stenosis demands prompt investigation.

The severity of aortic obstruction may be accurately assessed at the bedside. The key to the evaluation is the character of the arterial pulse. In severe disease the carotid pulse is retarded in upstroke and small in volume, and the systolic blood pressure and the pulse pressure are reduced. In older patients with coexistent sclerosis of large vessels, these arterial signs may not be present. The intensity of the systolic murmur does not necessarily correlate with the severity of the lesion, but the peak intensity will occur progressively later with increasing obstruction. With severe stenosis the murmur is long and extends almost to the end of left ventricular systole, which may actually be after P_2 (paradoxic splitting of S_2). Left ventricular hypertrophy will usually be obvious by palpation, ECG, echocardiography, or chest roentgenogram. In older patients, significant aortic stenosis is unlikely if valve calcification is not demonstrated at fluoroscopy or echocardiography. Quantitative application of Doppler techniques with the use of maximal velocity of flow across a diseased aortic valve gives sufficiently reliable estimates of the gradient that cardiac catheterization is seldom

necessary simply to assess the severity of aortic stenosis. Catheterization should be performed, however, in preparation for surgical intervention to determine whether significant coronary atherosclerosis is present and concomitant coronary artery bypass grafting is thus required.

There is little justification for medical therapy for the symptomatic patient with aortic stenosis. Symptoms indicate that the left ventricular outflow obstruction is severe and that surgical therapy is indicated. In younger patients with mobile, noncalcified valves, commissurotomy may effectively relieve obstruction, but this is rarely possible when the valve is calcified, and in this situation the valve must be replaced with a prosthesis. The reduction in cardiac work that occurs after successful aortic replacement will improve symptoms even in patients with coronary atherosclerosis or left ventricular dysfunction, although the immediate postsurgery mortality rate will be higher among these patients. Bypass of significantly obstructed coronary arteries is usually performed at the time of aortic valve replacement. Recently the technique of balloon valvuloplasty has been applied successfully to patients with critical aortic stenosis who, because of advanced age, prohibitive surgical risk, or refusal to undergo operation, have no other options. Short-term symptomatic relief is seen in the majority of these patients, but the duration and extent of palliation are currently unknown.[6]

AORTIC REGURGITATION[16,26]

Aortic regurgitation may result from disease processes affecting the aortic valve leaflet (rheumatic heart disease), supporting structures in the aortic root above the valve (dissecting aneurysm), or supporting structure below the valve, as in the case of a ventricular septal defect located high in the septum. The most common causes of these abnormalities are listed in Table 2.3–6.

An understanding of the pathophysiology of aortic reflux allows an accurate assessment of the severity of the lesion at the bedside. The left ventricle dilates in order to increase stroke volume, which is necessary to maintain an adequate forward flow and accommodate the volume of blood that refluxes backward. The size of the left ventricle, determined by palpation, chest roentgenogram, or echocardiography, is a rough guide to the severity of the volume load. Systolic pressure increases because of the excess stroke volume. Aortic diastolic pressure falls in proportion to the severity of the backward diastolic leak, and therefore the pulse pressure is wide. In most cases of severe aortic regurgitation, systolic pressure exceeds 140 mm Hg and diastolic pressure is less than 60 mm Hg. In many cases, accurate determination of diastolic pressure by sphygmomanometer is not possible, Korotkoff sounds being heard all the way to zero pressure. Peripheral resistance de-

TABLE 2.3–6. ETIOLOGY OF AORTIC REGURGITATION

Disease of aortic valve
  Rheumatic
  Congenital deformity
  Infective endocarditis
  Rupture, spontaneous or traumatic

Disease of aortic root
  Syphilis
  Dissecting aneurysm
  Cystic medial necrosis with dilation
  Inflammatory disease
    Rheumatoid spondylitis
    Reiter syndrome
    Relapsing polychondritis
    Giant cell aortitis

Disease of subvalvular structure
  Aneurysm of sinus of Valsalva
  High ventricular septal defect
  Subaortic fibrous stenosis

creases to promote forward blood flow; this, in conjunction with the increased stroke volume, imparts the characteristic hyperkinetic circulatory signs recognized in the carotid pulse, which is quick, at full volume, and often bifid, and in peripheral arteries, where palpation reveals a collapsing (water-hammer) pulse. Although the distensibility or compliance of a ventricle chronically exposed to a volume load such as aortic regurgitation increases, eventually left ventricular diastolic pressure rises as the severity of the volume load progresses; the left ventricular diastolic pressure may be very high (50 to 60 mm Hg) and may actually support the aortic diastolic pressure. A very high ventricular diastolic pressure is also likely when the aortic regurgitation develops abruptly, as in acute aortic dissection or acute infective endocarditis with valve rupture. In this situation, left ventricular stiffness and compliance are normal and dilation has not had a chance to develop. In addition, if the peripheral flow is reduced, reflex vasoconstriction develops. This high diastolic blood pressure in the aorta and the peripheral vasoconstriction may mask the classic peripheral signs of severe aortic regurgitation. Because the ventricular diastolic pressure rises so high and equals the aortic diastolic pressure in about middiastole, the diastolic murmur may be short. Further the high ventricular diastolic pressure closes the mitral valve in middiastole; thus the first heart sound is absent at the onset of systole. The echocardiogram is invaluable in this setting and demonstrates fluttering of the anterior leaflet of the mitral valve and premature diastolic closure of the mitral valve.

The intensity of the aortic diastolic murmur does not correlate with the severity of reflux, but the presence of an Austin Flint murmur indicates that aortic regurgitation is severe.[10] In the patient with clinically severe aortic regurgitation, cardiac catheterization is usually not needed to assess the need for or type of surgical intervention. Sufficient morphologic information about the aortic valve and aortic root, as well as accurate assessment of left ventricular function and possible other valve involvement, can generally be obtained with two-dimensional echocardiography. In the setting of acute infective endocarditis, catheterization may even be unduly hazardous because of the potential for dislodging vegetations.

Patients may tolerate even severe degrees of aortic regurgitation for long periods with preservation of excellent effort tolerance. Symptoms of congestive heart failure or angina do not occur until the left ventricle is unable to maintain an adequate forward stroke volume. In patients with chronic aortic regurgitation, this is usually due to the development of left ventricular dysfunction, a result, perhaps, of chronic excessive stretching and tearing of sarcomeres (see Chapter 2.2) or intrinsic disease of the left ventricular myocardium. As with aortic stenosis, once symptoms appear, the progression to more severe symptoms and death is usually rapid and little affected by medical therapy. Aortic valve replacement should therefore be recommended for patients with symptoms of aortic regurgitation. Unfortunately, even successful valve replacement at this time, although important to interrupt the progression of symptoms, may leave the patient with a dilated ventricle that is abnormal in its function. The dilemma of when to recommend surgery for the asymptomatic patient with evidence of severe aortic regurgitation is one of the most difficult in clinical cardiology.[3] A prospective study of patients with rheumatic aortic regurgitation indicated that in asymptomatic patients with any of the following, there is high likelihood that symptoms will develop or death will occur in 3 to 6 years: (1) systolic blood pressure over 140 mm Hg and diastolic pressure less than 40 mm Hg; (2) cardiomegaly as indicated by chest roentgenogram (cardiothoracic ratio >55 percent); or (3) left ventricular hypertrophy with strain as determined by ECG.[27] Strong consideration should be given to surgery in this group of patients before onset of symptoms or in asymptomatic patients who show evidence of progressive cardiac enlargement.[2] Surgery is also advisable before symptoms appear when aortic root disease is responsible for aortic reflux. Patients with Marfan syndrome, inflammatory aortitis, or dissecting aneurysm may die as a result of aortic rupture due to progressive aortic dilatation. Echocardiography permits identification and follow-up of such patients.

Elective replacement of the aortic root and valve is recommended if the diameter of the aorta exceeds 5.5 to 6.0 cm when the diameter is increasing.

MITRAL STENOSIS[25,28]

In the adult, mitral stenosis is almost always the result of rheumatic heart disease. In spite of this, only half the patients can recall an attack of acute rheumatic fever in childhood. Mitral obstruction occurs in the years after the initial insult to the valve, sometimes as a result of continuous low-grade rheumatic activity but more commonly because of long-standing hemodynamic stress to a diseased valve. Mitral stenosis may therefore be progressive in the adult in spite of adequate prophylaxis against recurrent streptococcal infection. As the mitral orifice narrows, left atrial pressure rises so that an adequate cardiac output can be maintained, and a pressure gradient is produced between the left atrium and the left ventricle. The resultant increase in left atrial pressure is reflected backward to pulmonary veins, capillaries, and arteries and is responsible for the most common symptom of mitral stenosis—dyspnea on exertion. Patients may not notice breathlessness until unusual circulatory needs are called for, as with pregnancy or excessive physical activity or when a bout of rapid atrial fibrillation occurs. The result may be abrupt and severe elevation of left atrial pressure, leading to pulmonary edema or extravasation of blood into the alveoli, producing hemoptysis. More commonly, the dyspnea is insidious in onset and slowly progressive. When mitral obstruction becomes more severe, cardiac output cannot increase in response to demands, giving rise to the symptom of fatigue. This universal complaint may occur so gradually that the patient does not realize that his activities are restricted, and sometimes only in retrospect, after surgical correction, does he recognize the severity of his effort incapacity. Long-standing left atrial hypertension causes enlargement of the left atrium, which is responsible for atrial arrhythmias, particularly atrial fibrillation, which produces further impairment of cardiac output. The enlarged fibrillating atrium is a site for the formation of a clot, which may be dislodged as a systemic embolus. In some patients, marked left atrial enlargement does not occur, left atrial hypertension is more severe, and pulmonary arteries constrict to produce "reactive" pulmonary hypertension. Such patients may show predominant signs and symptoms of right-sided heart failure early in their course. Some patients respond to elevated pulmonary venous pressure with bronchospasm so that asthmatic features may dominate the presentation. Patients with mitral stenosis are more prone to bronchopulmonary infection. In older patients this may be responsible for the development of chronic bronchitis and emphysema. Cough, especially at night, is a frequent early symptom.

Clinical evaluation of the severity of mitral stenosis should begin with the understanding that the principal manifestations of the lesion will be predominantly in the lungs and right side of the heart. Symptoms, generally a good guide to the severity of the valvular disease, may be misleading in mitral stenosis. Occasionally, patients with mild obstruction may develop severe pulmonary congestion during stress or a paroxysm of rapid atrial fibrillation, whereas some patients with severe "reactive" pulmonary hypertension may be relatively protected from pulmonary congestion and have few complaints. Signs of pulmonary hypertension on physical examination or radiography, or signs of right ventricular hypertrophy by ECG, always indicate that the mitral stenosis is severe. The chest roentgenogram is invaluable in assessing the severity of obstruction. With elevation of left atrial pressure there is a redistribution of blood flow from the lower part of the lungs to the upper part. This produces prominence of the vasculature in the upper lung fields and a reduction of vasculature in the lower lung fields in the upright chest roentgenogram. This finding, in association with evidence of left atrial enlargement, strongly suggests the diagnosis of mitral stenosis. The presence of Kerley B lines (Fig. 2.3–2) usually indicates that mean left atrial pressure

is 25 mm Hg or higher. Lesser degrees of pulmonary congestion are seen with less severe disease. Because the mitral valve opens earlier with increasing left atrial pressure, the degree of narrowing of the S_2–opening snap interval will be a general index of the severity of obstruction.

In the young patient the diagnosis of mitral stenosis can usually be made with confidence on the basis of symptoms, physical findings, and changes on chest roentgenogram. In older patients the characteristic physical signs may be altered because of valve calcification, obesity, emphysema, pulmonary hypertension, or reduced cardiac output. However, truly "silent" mitral stenosis is distinctly uncommon. Clues to the presence of the lesion are usually apparent to the careful observer. The presence of mitral stenosis should be diligently searched for and the diagnosis suspected in any of the following clinical situations: (1) unexplained pulmonary hypertension, (2) recurrent atrial fibrillation, (3) systemic embolization, (4) asthma with atypical features, (5) chronic obstructive pulmonary disease where dyspnea is out of proportion to the objective evidence of lung disease, and (6) unexplained congestive heart failure. It is also important to recognize that the clinical findings of mitral stenosis may be mimicked closely by other conditions—for example, atrial myxoma and atrial septal defect, the latter particularly in middle-aged or older patients. The diagnosis of mitral stenosis can be confirmed or established confidently in nearly all cases by echocardiography (see Chapter 2.1).

There are two surgical procedures available to treat the patient with mitral stenosis: mitral commissurotomy and valve replacement with a prosthetic device. In the former operation the surgeon attempts to split the fused commissures of the mitral valve by hand or with a mechanical dilator (closed commissurotomy) or under direct inspection with a scalpel (open commissurotomy). This procedure is highly effective in properly selected cases and may restore the mitral orifice to nearly normal dimensions. Many patients will continue to be free of severe mitral obstruction even 20 years after operation. The operative mortality rate should be 1 percent or less in well-selected patients operated on by experienced surgeons.[1] The disadvantages of the procedure are that (1) it cannot be performed if mitral regurgitation is present, (2) significant mitral regurgitation may be produced if the valve is fibrotic and calcified, (3) the valve orifice may be only temporarily stretched and not actually increased in size, and (4) mitral restenosis may occur. In spite of these considerations, mitral commissurotomy should always be performed when feasible in the patient with mitral stenosis who requires surgery. Unfortunately, in not all instances is it possible to achieve successful mitral commissurotomy. With increasing thickness of the valve, fibrosis and fusion of subvalvular structures, and valve calcification, commissurotomy becomes more difficult. These factors are more likely to be found in older patients and those with a long history of symptomatic disease. These complicating factors are also more common in male patients. Therefore most patients over the age of 40 years, particularly men, will require mitral valve replacement. The mortality rate with this procedure is slightly higher than that associated with commissurotomy, and the risk of subsequent embolization, although low, is significant even with anticoagulant therapy. Valve obstruction, however, will be effectively relieved.

The decision as to when to intervene surgically in the course of mitral stenosis will vary with the type of operative procedure anticipated. Thus, if one can confidently expect to achieve success with mitral commissurotomy, patients with early and mild (New York Heart Association [NYHA] class II) symptoms may be referred for surgery. Early operation in these patients can be expected to improve symptoms and retard the development of pulmonary vascular disease. The ideal patient will be a woman in her late twenties or thirties with modest effort intolerance and physical signs suggesting a pliable mitral valve, such as a loud and snappy S_1, a loud opening snap, and prominent presystolic rumble. When mitral valve replacement is the likely procedure, surgery should be delayed until the development of more-severe symptoms (NYHA class III or IV). An exception to this general rule is the presence of

pulmonary hypertension that, when confirmed by catheterization, represents an indication for commissurotomy or valve replacement even in the absence of severe symptoms.

In the past, mitral valve surgery was recommended for all patients with mitral stenosis whose presentation included systemic embolization, but this is no longer thought to be necessary. Surgery should be carried out in patients who also have moderate or severe hemodynamic abnormalities, but those with milder disease can be effectively managed with long-term anticoagulation.

Cardiac catheterization should be performed in most patients in whom surgery is considered, particularly those over the age of 40 years, those with return of symptoms after previous mitral surgery, those with suspected pulmonary hypertension, and those with other valvular lesions. The younger patient (in whom coronary artery disease is unlikely) with obvious findings of mitral stenosis and confirmatory evidence of significant obstruction on echocardiography can be sent to surgery without the need for catheterization.

As noted in the discussion of aortic stenosis, certain patients with severely symptomatic mitral stenosis will not be candidates for surgery but may benefit from balloon valvuloplasty. Long-term data are lacking, but several studies have documented good short-term results.[19]

MITRAL REGURGITATION[11,23,24]

Effective closure of the mitral valve requires the interaction of various components of the complex mitral apparatus, consisting of valve leaflets, chordae tendineae, papillary muscles, valve annulus, and left ventricular myocardium. Disease processes affecting any of these structures may result in mitral regurgitation. The more common causes of mitral regurgitation are listed in Table 2.3–7.

Contrary to widely held opinion, rheumatic heart disease accounts for only a small percentage of patients with pure mitral regurgitation (less than 5 percent). Most patients with severe mitral regurgitation will show myxomatous change in the valve leaflets. This lesion, which also is called mitral valve prolapse, Barlow syndrome, or floppy mitral valve, may be a manifestation of an inherited connective tissue disorder, such as Marfan syndrome, but it occurs most commonly as an isolated abnormality. The mitral regurgitation associated with this lesion is usually mild, but examples of more severe disease due to this abnormality are encountered with increasing frequency, suggesting that some of these patients are prone to progression of the lesion, usually as a result of progressive dilation of the mitral annulus. Rupture of chordae tendineae occurs more frequently in patients with myxomatous disease of the valve and may also occur without obvious cause or as a result of infective endocarditis or chest trauma. Dysfunction or rupture of a papillary muscle is usually a manifestation of ischemic heart disease and may occur during the evolution of acute myocardial infarction or develop insidiously in patients with chronic ischemic heart disease. Some degree of mitral regurgitation is frequent in patients with primary myocardial disease and is due to left ventricular dilation, which causes malalignment of papillary muscles or myopathic involvement of the papillary muscles themselves.

TABLE 2.3–7. ETIOLOGY OF MITRAL REGURGITATION

Rheumatic heart disease

Congenital heart disease
  Endocardial cushion defect
  Corrected transposition of the great vessels

Mitral prolapse (myxomatous degeneration, "floppy" valves)

Ruptured chordae tendineae

Valve perforation or loss of substance (infective endocarditis)

Papillary muscle rupture or dysfunction

Calcification of the mitral annulus

Primary myocardial disease

Of all valvular lesions, chronic mitral regurgitation is the best tolerated because the left ventricle ejects the extra volume load into a low-resistance chamber, the left atrium. The extra work the left ventricle must bear will be much less in this situation than when the total stroke volume must be ejected into a high-resistance circuit, as in aortic regurgitation, so that excellent compensation can be maintained for many years in spite of a severe valvular leak. The left atrium enlarges gradually to accommodate the regurgitant volume; because of its distensibility, left atrial pressure may remain normal even though the volume of mitral regurgitation is large. Because the posterior left atrial wall is in direct continuity with the posterior mitral valve leaflet, progressive left atrial enlargement causes further separation of mitral leaflets and increasing incompetence of the valve. Patients with chronic mitral regurgitation have a slowly progressive disease course in which symptoms of fatigue and mild breathlessness wax and wane over many years. Signs and symptoms of severe pulmonary congestion do not appear until the regurgitant volume becomes very large and the left ventricle is unable to maintain an effective forward output. Clinical guidelines to the severity of the lesion will be reflected best in the size of the left ventricle, as determined by palpation, echocardiography, or chest roentgenogram, and in the severity of pulmonary venous congestion.

When mitral regurgitation occurs acutely, as with rupture of chordae tendineae or papillary muscle, the left atrium has little time to accommodate to the extra volume load, and left atrial pressure may rise precipitously to very high levels, even though the regurgitant volume may not be large. These patients will usually have an abrupt onset of symptoms related to pulmonary congestion. The heart size may be normal or only slightly enlarged, but the lungs will show signs of pulmonary congestion. Occasionally, papillary muscle dysfunction may be responsible for intermittent acute mitral regurgitation, which may present a confusing picture of episodic pulmonary edema followed by relatively symptom-free intervals. The cardiac murmur may be absent or soft in this situation and the diagnosis of mitral valve dysfunction difficult to establish. Figure 2.3–3 shows the roentgenographic appearance associated with acute and chronic mitral regurgitation. The major factor responsible for the difference in presentation is the distensibility of the left atrium.

Cardiac catheterization is indicated in the symptomatic patient with mitral regurgitation to determine the level of pulmonary artery and left atrial pressure, assess severity of the mitral leak by cineangiography, and determine the presence or absence of coronary atherosclerosis. As with other valve lesions discussed earlier, two-dimensional echocardiography with Doppler flow mapping will obviate the need for more extensive catheterization studies in many patients with mitral regurgitation. On occasion it may be difficult to distinguish between the patient with primary myocardial disease with associated mitral regurgitation and the patient with severe organic valvular disease with associated ventricular dilation. Echocardiography is helpful in this situation as well. The patient with primary mitral regurgitation shows increased wall movement, whereas the patient with cardiomyopathy shows impaired motion.

Repair or replacement of the mitral valve with a prosthetic device should be recommended for patients with severe symptoms (NYHA class III or IV) of mitral regurgitation. Some surgeons prefer plastic repair of the mitral valve apparatus in carefully selected patients with mitral regurgitation.[5] When technically feasible, repair of ruptured chordae, resection and plication of redundant myxomatous leaflets, and mitral annuloplasty are as effective, from a hemodynamic standpoint, as prosthetic replacement and additionally avoid the potential for long-term complications of an implanted device. The operative mortality rate in mitral valve replacement is 5 percent or less at most centers. The improvement in long-term survival rates and the interruption of progression of symptoms by such surgery have been amply documented. It should be recognized that delay of surgery until class III or IV symptoms appear will leave the patient with an enlarged heart that does not function normally even after successful surgery.[4] However, the course of mitral regurgitation may be so prolonged and benign before severe symptoms occur that it hardly seems justifiable to recommend operation earlier.

MEDICAL AND SURGICAL MANAGEMENT OF THE PATIENT WITH VALVULAR HEART DISEASE[20,21]

The management of a patient with valvular heart disease must be based on a thorough understanding of the natural history of the disease. The physician must recognize that mild valvular lesions are well tolerated and may be compatible with a normal, active life. The remarkable ability of the heart to compensate for extra loads imposed by valve dysfunction makes it possible for patients with major valve disease to live active, productive lives for many years. The good physician realizes that patients with even minor valvular abnormalities are justifiably frightened by their conditions and that part of his job is to lessen this psychologic burden. It is reassuring to emphasize to the patient that he may carry on most normal activities and even exercise vigorously.

Most disease processes affecting valvular structures produce their effects gradually over many years, and therefore the natural history of most valvular lesions evolves slowly. First priority must be given to the prevention of events that will accelerate the evolution of the disease process, such as a recurrence of acute rheumatic fever or an attack of bacterial endocarditis. Recurrences of rheu-

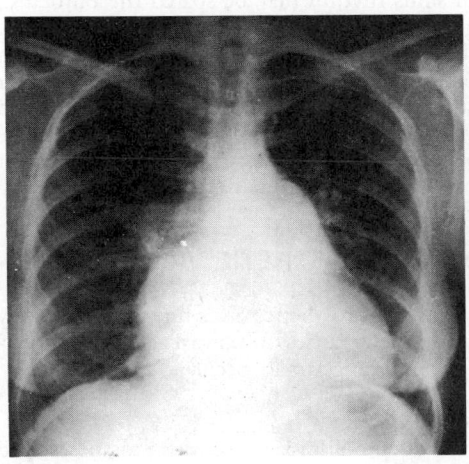

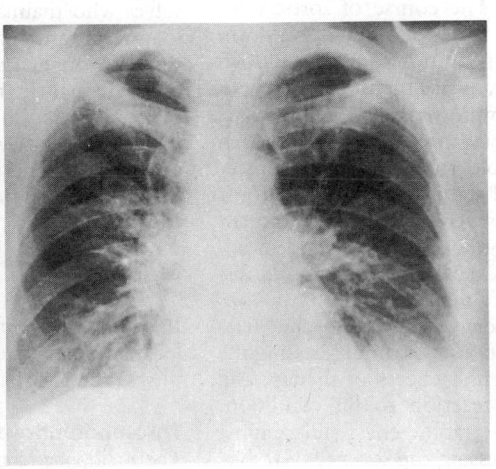

Figure 2.3–3. A. Chronic rheumatic heart disease with long-standing severe mitral regurgitation. Left atrium and left ventricle are markedly enlarged, but lung fields show few signs of pulmonary congestion. **B.** Acute mitral regurgitation due to ruptured chordae tendineae. Heart size is normal, but there is marked pulmonary congestion.

A   B

matic fever are prevented by the administration of daily penicillin or sulfa drugs to protect against streptococcal infection, at least until age 40 years. All patients with valvular lesions, whether rheumatic or congenital, should receive prophylaxis against bacterial endocarditis in the form of penicillin or other appropriate antibiotic at the time of dental or surgical procedures. Medical therapy may help to improve compensation and ensure slow progression, thereby deferring surgical intervention. Digitalis preparations are beneficial because of their inotropic action on the left ventricle and their action in slowing the ventricular response in atrial fibrillation. Diuretics may alleviate pulmonary or systemic congestion. Atrial systole plays an important role in maintaining forward stroke volume in patients with mitral and aortic stenosis, and therefore the onset of atrial fibrillation may herald symptomatic deterioration. Reestablishing normal sinus rhythm by electrical or pharmacologic cardioversion and maintenance of sinus rhythm with antiarrhythmic drugs may allow the patient to live many years with minimal symptoms. The enlarged, fibrillating left atrium of patients with mitral valve disease is a potential source of embolic material, and anticoagulant therapy is indicated to prevent systemic emboli if there are no major contraindications. Patients with valvular heart disease may have disease processes that affect other parts of the heart and are responsible for worsening symptoms. For example, myocardial disease is common in patients with rheumatic heart disease, and this may limit compensation. Coronary artery disease may coexist in older patients and may be less well tolerated because of the extra cardiac work the valvular lesion entails.

Repair or replacement of cardiac valves has had a major effect in improving the natural history of valvular heart disease.[17,18,26] Durable prosthetic devices of excellent hemodynamic design are available for valve replacement, and the operation can be done in many centers with an operative mortality rate of less than 5 percent. However, prosthetic valves all have a finite life span and their own complications, and the operation itself continues to carry a certain unavoidable minimal rate of morbidity and mortality. Many postoperative problems relate to the fact that long-term anticoagulation is usually necessary. Timing is all-important in making the recommendation for valve replacement. The physician must understand the natural history of the unoperated valvular lesion so that he will not intervene too early (and thereby deny the patient years of prosthesis-free living) or too late (after irreversible damage has occurred to the left ventricular myocardium or pulmonary vasculature).

It is true, in general, that mechanical problems, such as valvular lesions, that are responsible for symptoms should be treated by mechanical means (i.e., valve repair or replacement). In most instances the patient tells the physician when valve surgery is needed, not directly, but in the form of symptoms. In general, it is a mistake to treat major symptoms for too long with medication or reassurance. In aortic valve disease the presence of even mild symptoms such as angina pectoris or breathlessness is an indication for consideration of surgical therapy. The course of aortic valve disease moves rapidly once symptoms develop. The interval from onset of symptoms to major decompensation or even sudden death may be brief. The appearance of adverse manifestations with mitral disease is less rapid. Because symptoms may wax and wane for many years, the physician can adopt a more leisurely approach to surgical intervention. It is advisable to recommend surgery when symptoms reach NYHA class III status—and earlier in some patients. When clinical signs point to severe valvular involvement or pulmonary hypertension, valve surgery may be advised in advance of symptomatic deterioration. Coexistence of valvular disease with myocardial or coronary artery disease may prompt consideration of intervention before severe symptoms occur. It is useful to observe the patient at several points in time, assessing the rate of progression of the disease and the effects of therapy and determining the patient's emotional reaction to his condition. Laboratory studies such as electrocardiography, chest radiography, and echocardiography are useful in assessing the severity of the lesion and its effect on the left ventricle. Progressive evidence of cardiac enlargement or left ventricular hypertrophy may precede a change in the patient's symptomatic status and provide early warning that the time for surgical treatment is near. When clinical signs indicate acute valve destruction, as in infective endocarditis, valve replacement must be performed urgently and may be lifesaving, even though active infection persists.[9]

The patient's general medical and emotional status must be carefully assessed as part of the evaluation for surgery. If severe disease of other organ systems exists, the physician may elect a conservative approach to therapy for the valvular lesion. The physician must determine whether the patient's other disease can be effectively managed before recommending valve replacement. Advanced age is not a contraindication to valve surgery if the patient does not have other debilitating medical illness. Many patients over the age of 80 years have had successful valve replacement.[13] Coronary artery disease that coexists with valvular disease can often be treated with bypass surgery at the time of valve replacement. Symptomatic or asymptomatic extracranial cerebrovascular disease should be thoroughly evaluated, because some carotid lesions can be corrected at the time of, or before, the valve operation.

The information provided by cardiac catheterization may be helpful in deciding on surgical therapy, but this procedure is not necessary for all patients undergoing operation. It should be emphasized that the decision to operate on a valve is made from clinical information obtained by history, physical examination, and careful follow-up of the patient, and not from catheterization studies. In most cases the experienced clinician can easily determine the severity of the primary valve lesion. Catheterization is used to assess the function of the other valves, determine whether coronary artery disease is present, evaluate left ventricular function, measure the level of pulmonary artery pressure, and confirm the severity of the primary valve lesion. Some patients, particularly younger ones, may be referred for valve operation without catheterization when clinical findings are obvious and there is no suspicion of complicating circumstances. In some cases catheterization may be dangerous, as in active infective endocarditis, and in some the information provided may be misleading, as in assessing the severity of mitral stenosis in older patients who have a great deal of subvalvular disease.

The physician should play an active role with the cardiac surgeon in deciding what type of operative procedure or valve prosthesis is to be used. Repair of a valve (i.e., mitral commissurotomy or repair of certain mitral regurgitation lesions), when feasible, is always the preferred procedure because the patient is left with his own native valve, which may function effectively for many years. Prosthetic valves have remained implanted for more than 20 years, and therefore there is good information on the natural history of these devices. The experience with heterograft tissue valves is much shorter, but these devices, usually employing porcine valves, have the advantage of physiologic hemodynamic design and are less prone to produce thromboemboli. Thus patients receiving tissue valves who maintain sinus rhythm may be spared the burden of long-term anticoagulation. The shortcoming of bioprosthetic valves is longevity, because degenerative changes and calcification occur frequently, making reoperation necessary within 10 years for many patients. Prosthetic valves, which are made from plastics and metals, have shown continued design improvement and can be expected to function effectively for 20 years or more. The major drawback is the necessity of long-term anticoagulant therapy.

COMPLICATIONS OF PROSTHETIC VALVES

In the majority of instances, prosthetic valves function effectively for many years and the patient carries on normal activities. Nevertheless the following complications may occur.

Thromboembolism
The incidence of thromboembolism is lower with prostheses used since 1970, but this complication has not been eliminated. Emboli

usually occur because the patient has not achieved an adequate level of anticoagulation (two to three times the control level). The addition of a platelet-inhibiting agent such as dipyridamole to warfarin may lower the incidence of this dread complication.

Infection

A foreign body within the circulation is a natural repository for blood-borne infection. For this reason, patients should be given prophylactic antibiotics, preferably by the parenteral route, during dental or other minor surgical procedures and at the earliest signs of any infection. Infective endocarditis on a prosthetic valve is a dread complication that carries a mortality rate in excess of 25 percent. Infections acquired in the early postoperative period are caused by organisms such as *Staphylococcus aureus* and *S. epidermidis*, *Candida*, and gram-negative bacteria and are difficult to eradicate by antibiotic therapy alone. Because the mortality rate is in excess of 50 percent for this group of patients, reoperation should be considered early in the course of the infection. Prosthetic valve endocarditis occurring after 3 months postoperatively can be cured with antibiotic therapy alone, but the occurrence of heart failure, systemic emboli, conduction disturbance, evidence of valve dehiscence, or persisting fever or bacteremia during the course of treatment demands consideration of prompt surgical intervention.

Prosthesis Malfunction

Prosthesis malfunction may occur as a consequence of thrombus formation, alteration in the structure of the moving ball or disk by wear and tear or swelling, sticking of the ball or disk in the cage, improper seating of the prosthesis, or improper size of the prosthesis. The latter two problems will usually be evident in the early postoperative period as a refractory low-output state or intractable pulmonary congestion. The other manifestations usually develop insidiously several years after successful valve replacement. Prosthesis malfunction is notoriously difficult to detect even with the aid of catheterization and angiography, although recently Doppler echocardiography has proved extremely useful in assessing prosthesis-related obstruction or regurgitation, with both mechanical and tissue valves. It should be suspected in the patient with a prosthetic valve who shows any of the following:

1. Alteration of the timing or quality of opening and closing sounds
2. Development of a new regurgitant murmur
3. Embolization
4. Increased severity of intravascular hemolysis
5. Development of heart failure or angina after a period of improvement
6. Occurrence of syncope

Paravalvular Leak

Regurgitation of blood between the prosthetic valve ring and the heart valve annulus usually results from tearing of suture material either spontaneously or after damage of heart tissue by infection. If the regurgitation is minimal, the course is stable, but severe regurgitation requires further surgery. It has been reported that severe paravalvular leak may be present in the absence of a significant regurgitant murmur, especially around valves inserted in the mitral area.

Hemolytic Anemia

The red blood cell's survival time is shortened in all patients with prosthetic valves, probably because of battering and destruction of cells by the intravascular foreign body. Fragments of red cells and schizocytes may be seen in the peripheral blood smear. The amount of hemolysis is usually mild and easily compensated for by increased reticulocytosis. Rarely hemolysis may be severe enough to produce anemia. This usually occurs in association with prosthesis dysfunction or a regurgitant leak. Chronic intravascular hemolysis results in the loss of iron in the urine in the form of hemosiderin, and iron deficiency may be produced after several years.

REFERENCES

1. Bonchek LI: Current status of mitral commissurotomy: Indications, techniques, and results. Am J Cardiol 52:411, 1983
2. Bonow RO, Picone AL, et al: Survival and functional results after valve replacement for aortic regurgitation from 1976 to 1983: Impact of preoperative left ventricular function. Circulation 72:1244, 1985
3. Bonow RO, Rosing DR, et al: The natural history of asymptomatic patients with aortic regurgitation and normal left ventricular function. Circulation 68:509, 1983
4. Borow K, Green LH, et al: End-systolic volume as a predictor of postoperative left ventricular performance in volume overload from valvular regurgitation. Am J Med 68:655, 1980
5. Cosgrove DM, Chavez AM, et al: Results of mitral valve reconstruction. Circulation 74 (Suppl 1):I-82, 1986
6. Cribier A, Savin T, et al: Percutaneous transluminal balloon valvuloplasty of adult aortic stenosis: Report of 92 cases. J Am Coll Cardiol 9:381, 1987
7. Criley JM, Heger J: Prolapsed mitral leaflet syndrome. Cardiovasc Clin 10:213, 1979
8. Devereux RB, Perloff JK, et al: Mitral valve prolapse. Circulation 54:3, 1976
9. Dinubile MJ: Surgery in active endocarditis. Ann Intern Med 96:650, 1982
10. Fortuin NJ, Craige E: On the mechanism of the Austin Flint murmur. Circulation 45:558, 1972
11. Hammermeister KE, Fisher L, et al: Prediction of late survival in patients with mitral valve disease from clinical, hemodynamic, and quantitative angiographic variables. Circulation 57:341, 1978
12. Hossack KF, Neutle JM, et al: Congenital valvular aortic stenosis. Natural history and assessment for operation. Br Heart J 43:561, 1980
13. Jamieson WRE, Dooner J, et al: Cardiac valve replacement in the elderly: A review of 320 consecutive cases. Circulation 64 (Suppl 2):II-177, 1981
14. Leatham A: Auscultation of the heart and phono-cardiography. Edinburgh, Churchill Livingstone, 1975
15. Lombard JT, Selzer A: Valvular aortic stenosis. A clinical and hemodynamic profile of patients. Ann Intern Med 106:292, 1987
16. Morganroth J, Perloff JK, et al: Acute severe aortic regurgitation. Ann Intern Med 87:223, 1977
17. Munzor S, Gallardo J, et al: Influence of surgery on the natural history of rheumatic mitral and aortic valve disease. Am J Cardiol 35:234, 1975
18. Murphy ES, Kloster FE: Late results of valve replacement surgery. Mod Concepts Cardiovasc Dis 48:30, 1979
19. Palacios I, Block PC, et al: Percutaneous balloon valvotomy for patients with severe mitral stenosis. Circulation 75:778, 1987
20. Rahimtoola SH: Valvular heart disease: A perspective. J Am Coll Cardiol 1:199, 1983
21. Rapaport E: Natural history of aortic and mitral valve disease. Am J Cardiol 35:221, 1975
22. Roberts WC: Anatomically isolated aortic valve disease: A case against its being of rheumatic etiology. Am J Med 49:151, 1970
23. Roberts WC, Perloff JK: Mitral valvular disease. A clinico-pathologic survey of the conditions causing the mitral valve to function abnormally. Ann Intern Med 77:939, 1972
24. Selzer A: Nonrheumatic mitral regurgitation. Mod Concepts Cardiovasc Dis 48:25, 1979
25. Selzer A, Cohn KE: Natural history of mitral stenosis. Circulation 45:878, 1972
26. Smith HJ, Neutze JM, et al: The natural history of rheumatic aortic regurgitation and the indications for surgery. Br Heart J 38:147, 1976
27. Spagnuolo M, Kloth H, et al: Natural history of rheumatic aortic regurgitation. Criteria predictive of death, congestive heart failure and angina in young patients. Circulation 44:368, 1971
28. Wood P: An appreciation of mitral stenosis. Br Med J 1:1051, 1113, 1954

CHAPTER 2.4
Pericarditis

Stephen C. Achuff

Pericardial disease[3,6,15] merits discussion separate from other disorders of the cardiovascular system even though it is encountered relatively infrequently in general medical practice. Its importance lies in the fact that it may mimic more common cardiac conditions, and serious, even life-threatening errors of diagnosis and treatment may be committed. Alternatively, timely consideration of a pericardial process may lead to a completely different and ultimately successful course of therapy, for example, pericardiectomy for occult constrictive pericarditis in a patient with hitherto refractory congestive heart failure. Moreover, the types of pericardial disease encountered currently differ substantially from those of an earlier era, as evidenced by the increased prevalence of such diseases as radiation- and drug-induced pericarditis, postpericardiotomy syndrome, and infectious pericarditis in immunosuppressed patients. This chapter discusses the widely varying clinical manifestations of pericardial disease and an approach to managing the specific problems presented by each of the most common forms.

ACUTE PERICARDITIS

CLINICAL FEATURES (Table 2.4–1)

Chest pain is the presenting symptom in the majority of patients with acute pericarditis. The pain may be either sharp or dull and oppressive. It is typically retrosternal, with radiation to the left trapezius ridge. It is usually exacerbated by deep breathing or lying supine and is relieved by sitting up and leaning forward. Pain is not an invariable complaint, and some patients with significant pericardial effusion have dyspnea and signs of right-sided heart failure. The extreme form of this presentation is cardiac tamponade with hypotension or shock. Fever is associated with most types of acute pericarditis. In certain settings, such as after open heart surgery or in immunosuppressed patients, fever is the first abnormality that prompts consideration of a pericardial disease process.

The hallmark physical finding of acute pericarditis is the triphasic friction rub, the three components corresponding to ventricular systole, early diastolic ventricular filling, and late diastolic atrial systole. One or more components are heard in over 90 percent of patients with acute pericarditis, regardless of the amount of pericardial effusion. The rub is heard best just to the left of the sternum in the third or fourth intercostal space and is often variable with respiration and body position. The character of the typical rub is leathery, scratchy, or grating, and it has a more superficial quality than the first and second heart sounds or most cardiac murmurs. Because many patients will have associated left pleural inflammation, the chest should be auscultated both during normal breathing and with held respiration. Care must also be taken to ensure firm and uniform contact of the stethoscope with the chest wall, because closely spaced ribs or the movement of chest hair may create sounds that simulate a pericardial friction rub.

LABORATORY FINDINGS

A standard 12-lead ECG is the most useful single laboratory test for a patient with suspected acute pericarditis. Although the pericardium itself is electrically silent, involvement of the subepicardial myocardium produces characteristic PR segment, ST segment, and T-wave changes without alteration of QRS morphologic features

(Fig. 2.4–1).[14] PR segment depression is a specific but not invariable ECG finding in acute pericarditis. Most precordial and limb leads will show ST segment elevation. The only lead that often shows ST depression is aV_R, but there is no "reciprocal" depression (as in acute myocardial infarction) in leads opposite the injured area of myocardium. Serial tracings will generally allow the clinician to distinguish between pericarditis and infarction because each condition produces typical evolutionary patterns. The only other situation where widespread ST segment elevations may simulate the changes of pericarditis is the juvenile or early repolarization variant seen in some healthy young and middle-aged people. In this condition the PR segments are normal, and there is little or no change in the ST segments on serial ECGs.

Blood studies are usually not helpful in the diagnosis of acute pericarditis. The erythrocyte sedimentation rate and white blood cell count are often, but not invariably, elevated. When abnormal they are more useful in following the course of the disease and the response to therapy, and later in suspected recurrences. Specific blood tests may be ordered when one is considering the various causes of acute pericarditis (see below), for example, LE cell, serum complement, and antinuclear factor determinations in cases of possible systemic lupus erythematosus (SLE). Likewise, the chest radiograph offers no finding specific for acute pericarditis but should be obtained to exclude other conditions that enter into the differential diagnosis. Echocardiography should be performed when the cardiac silhouette is enlarged clinically or radiographically but need not be done in every patient with typical and uncomplicated acute pericarditis. However, an echocardiogram is mandatory if pericardiocentesis is to be undertaken for other than emergency indications.

DIFFERENTIAL DIAGNOSIS

The patient with the sudden onset of chest pain who is found to have a pericardial friction rub and ST segment elevations on an ECG is readily recognized as having acute pericarditis. The differential diagnosis in less classic presentations is much the same as outlined in the section on acute myocardial infarction (see Chapter 2.8). In questioning the patient about pain, the clinician should focus on the quality and exact location and radiation of the chest pain, the relation to breathing and body position, and any associated symptoms, such as cough with blood or sputum production,

TABLE 2.4–1. CLINICAL MANIFESTATIONS OF ACUTE PERICARDITIS

History	Chest pain: Varies with respiration and body position
Physical examination	Friction rub: Three components Fever
ECG	ST segment elevation in multiple leads without reciprocal depression PR segment depression T-wave inversion
Chest radiograph	Normal Enlarged with pericardial effusion Left pleural effusion
Blood studies	Elevated sedimentation rate Leukocytosis

dyspnea, or vomiting. Other diagnoses, such as acute myocardial infarction, aortic dissection, pulmonary embolism, pneumonia, pneumothorax, cholecystitis, or pancreatitis, should be entertained if the history is appropriate. Physical examination may narrow the list of possibilities, but in most instances the clinician should obtain chest radiographs and a 12-lead ECG. Special studies such as arterial blood gas determinations, ventilation perfusion lung scan, aortography, and abdominal ultrasonography, are reserved for evaluating specific conditions that may be confused with pericarditis. The condition most frequently mistaken for acute pericarditis is myocardial infarction, and hospitalization with serial observation, ECGs, and serum enzyme studies is warranted to make this distinction.

ETIOLOGY

Table 2.4–2 lists the various causes of acute pericarditis most likely to be encountered in the present era. Still the most common is acute idiopathic or nonspecific pericarditis. This is seen primarily in adolescents and young adults, who will often have a history of a preceding viral infection days or weeks before the onset of chest pain and fever. Presumably the pericarditis is a delayed hypersensitivity response to the virus, but the attempt to identify a specific agent is seldom successful. Direct infection of the pericardium (and sometimes the myocardium as well) has been reported in outbreaks of Coxsackie B virus, echovirus, adenovirus, mumps, and infectious mononucleosis. Purulent pericarditis, caused by bacteria, fungi, or protozoa, is uncommon but increasing in frequency because of the large number of patients undergoing open heart surgery, patients receiving chronic immunosuppressive therapy, and users of illicit drugs.[12] Occasionally, infection will spread to the pericardial space from a contiguous pleuropulmonary focus or from infective endocarditis. Acute tuberculous pericarditis is rare in the US

TABLE 2.4–2. CAUSES OF ACUTE PERICARDITIS

Idiopathic (nonspecific)

Infectious
- *Viral:* Coxsackie virus, echo virus, adenovirus
- *Bacterial:* Staphylococcus, Pneumococcus, Haemophilus
- *Fungal: Candida, Aspergillus, Nocardia, Histoplasma*
- *Mycobacterial: Mycobacterium tuberculosis*

Connective tissue disease
- Systemic lupus erythematosus, rheumatoid arthritis, scleroderma

Radiation-induced disease

Neoplastic disease
- Metastatic lymphoma, lung and breast cancer

Drug-induced disease
- Procainamide, hydralazine, phenytoin, minoxidil

Delayed myocardial injury
- Postmyocardial infarction (Dressler syndrome)
- Postpericardiotomy syndrome
- Postcardiac trauma

Metabolic
- Uremia
- Myxedema
- Cholesterol pericarditis

Miscellaneous
- Type A aortic dissection, sarcoidosis, pancreatitis

today but is still the underlying cause of some cases of chronic constrictive pericarditis. Among connective tissue diseases, SLE is the most common cause of acute pericarditis. Pericarditis in SLE is usually part of a more widespread polyserositis with renal involvement, although pericardial effusions and pericardial thickening are fre-

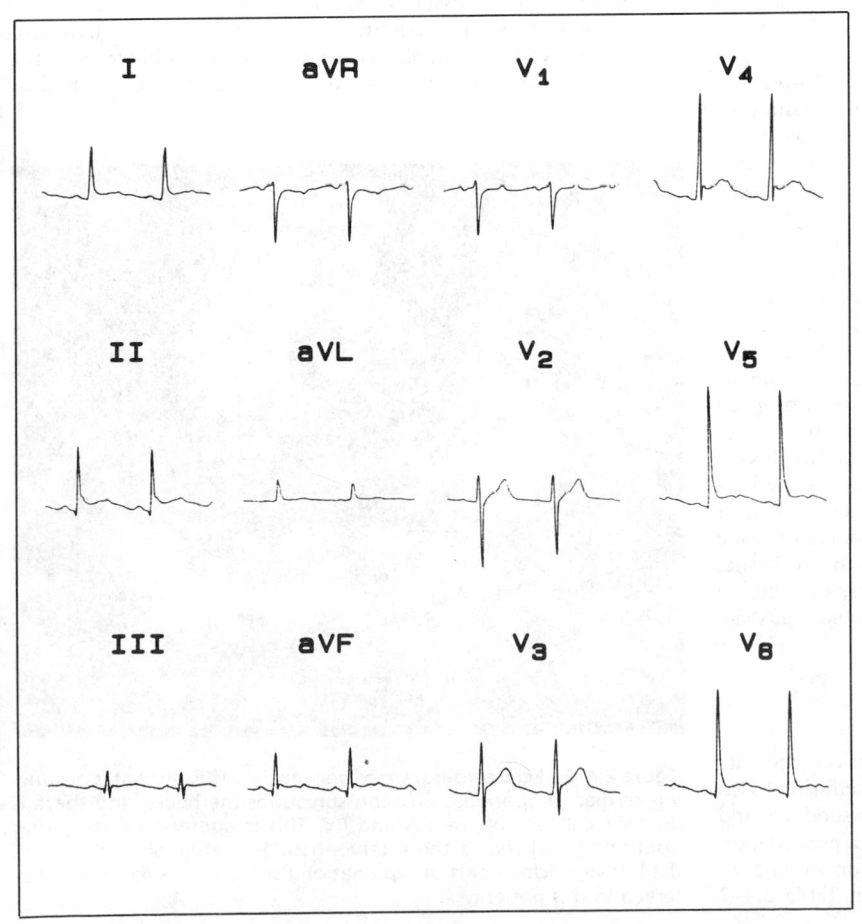

Figure 2.4–1. ECG in acute pericarditis. ST segments are elevated in multiple limb and precordial leads. There are no reciprocal ST segment depressions as in acute myocardial infarction. Note PR segment depression in leads V$_4$ to V$_6$.

quent findings in rheumatoid arthritis. Radiation-induced pericarditis is an important and not infrequent complication of therapy for neoplastic disease. High-dose mediastinal radiotherapy for lymphoma and for lung and breast cancer may cause an acute pericarditis, pericardial effusion with tamponade, or chronic constrictive pericarditis—the latter not becoming clinically apparent for 5 to 10 years or more after treatment. Direct pericardial involvement with tumor is also an increasingly common cause of acute pericarditis and does not necessarily signal a terminal phase of the disease. A number of drugs have been associated with acute pericarditis, most notably procainamide and hydralazine, probably because of their propensity to induce or unmask a form of lupus erythematosus. Pericarditis, a frequent early accompaniment of acute myocardial infarction, cardiac surgery, and blunt or penetrating trauma, is due to epicardial injury or inflammation. Weeks or months later, however, patients may have chest pain, fever, and signs of pericarditis, pleuritis, or both, often with large effusions. These problems are thought to result from an immunologic reaction, either autoimmune or in response to a previous viral infection, because antiheart and antiviral antibodies have been demonstrated in patients with this syndrome. Uremia is the most common metabolic abnormality associated with pericarditis.[9] It is seen often in hemodialysis units and may remit with an increase in the frequency of dialysis treatments. In other patients it is more likely due to a concurrent or reactivated viral infection of the pericardium. Patients with type A aortic dissections (see Chapter 2.11) often have a concomitant pericarditis due to leakage of blood into the pericardial sac. The clinician must be aware of this association and not focus on the pericarditis to the extent of overlooking the primary problem of dissection.

TREATMENT

Acute idiopathic pericarditis is typically a benign and self-limited disorder requiring only symptomatic treatment. Pain relief is provided by analgesics and nonsteroidal anti-inflammatory drugs such as aspirin, indomethacin, or ibuprofen. Usually a 1-week course of therapy is sufficient for a symptomatic response, as well as return of the sedimentation rate and white blood cell count to normal. All these agents may be associated with gastrointestinal upset, so that antacids and sometimes an H_2 blocker such as ranitidine should be given concurrently. At least one recurrence may be expected within a few months of the original episode in approximately 15 percent of patients. In this event, a longer course of anti-inflammatory therapy is undertaken. The temptation to prescribe corticosteroids should be resisted as long as possible, not only because of the greater incidence and severity of side effects but also because some patients will become steroid-dependent and may never be completely weaned. Truly refractory cases do occur, however, with multiple recurrences over a period of 5 to 10 years or more.[4] Corticosteroids should be reserved for this type of patient, and if withdrawal becomes difficult, consideration should be given to surgical removal of the pericardium. Treatment of most other causes of pericarditis involves primary therapy for the underlying condition, for example, more intensive dialysis in uremic pericarditis; radiotherapy or chemotherapy in neoplastic pericarditis; or corticosteroid or immunosuppressive therapy in connective tissue diseases. Purulent pericarditis is seldom cured with antibiotics alone, with the exception of tuberculous pericarditis, and surgical drainage should be instituted promptly after a microbiologic diagnosis has been established.

COMPLICATIONS[5,11]

Apart from recurrent episodes of pain and inflammation, the only significant complication of pericarditis is pericardial effusion. This is particularly important when the fluid accumulates suddenly and produces cardiac tamponade. Sometimes this mode of presentation of acute pericarditis obscures the other signs of the underlying inflammatory process. Any of the conditions listed in Table 2.4–2

may be associated with effusion, and whether or not tamponade ensues depends on the rapidity with which effusion develops. As little as 200 ml of fluid accumulating in minutes or hours may cause tamponade and shock, whereas subacute and chronic effusions as great as 2 L may be well tolerated. The diagnosis of important pericardial effusion can usually be made at the bedside. Elevation of the jugular venous pressure is the most reliable sign, and the neck veins should be inspected frequently in any patient with acute pericarditis. Tachycardia, dyspnea, peripheral pallor or cyanosis, and muffled heart sounds indicate significantly compromised cardiac function. In this situation a pulsus paradoxus should be apparent (i.e., greater than 10 mm Hg inspiratory fall in the systolic blood pressure, as determined by careful sphygmomanometry).[2] Chest radiography will show an increased cardiac silhouette, and the ECG will show generalized low-voltage and sometimes complete electrical alternans, a decrease in size of the entire P-QRS-T complex with alternate beats. The simplest and most reliable laboratory technique for demonstrating pericardial effusion is echocardiography (Fig. 2.4–2). With large effusions the heart may be seen to swing in the pericardial space corresponding to electrical alternans on the ECG. In cardiac tamponade the right atrium and right ventricle often show late diastolic collapse. During inspiration the right ventricular diameter increases because there is abnormal septal motion toward the left ventricle and a resultant decrease in diameter of this latter chamber. These relative changes in ventricular size during inspiration account in part for the pulsus paradoxus seen with cardiac tamponade.

PERICARDIOCENTESIS[8]

The diagnosis of cardiac tamponade demands prompt therapeutic action; usually this means percutaneous needle or catheter aspiration of the effusion. Because of the inherent risks the procedure should be done by an experienced and skilled operator, preferably in the catheterization laboratory or intensive care unit, where reliable ECG and hemodynamic monitoring are available. Atropine should be given as premedication to prevent vasovagal hypotension. It is usually desirable to thread a short catheter over the needle after entry into the pericardial space has been confirmed by

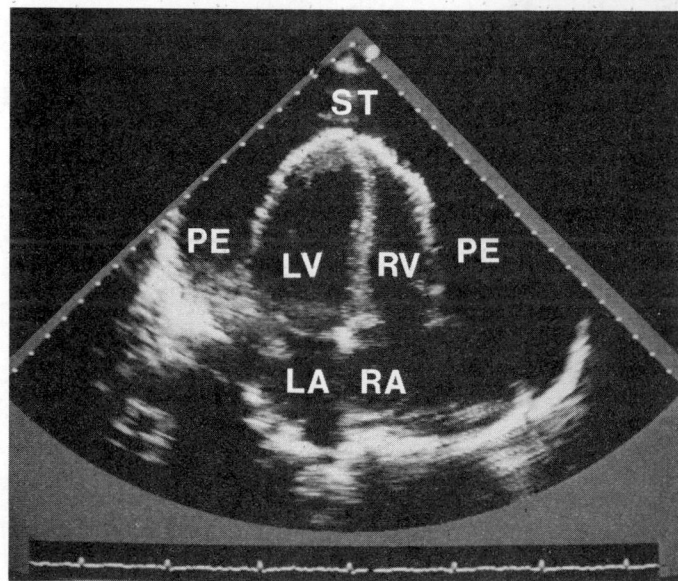

Figure 2.4–2. Echocardiogram of pericardial effusion that is producing cardiac tamponade. Effusion surrounds the heart, and there is diastolic collapse of the RA and RV. This image was taken during inspiration and shows the interventricular septum shifted toward the left ventricle, a partial explanation for the pulsus paradoxus observed in this patient.

TABLE 2.4–3. PERICARDIAL COMPRESSIVE SYNDROMES

• Cardiac tamponade
• Effusive-constrictive pericarditis
• Chronic constrictive pericarditis

TABLE 2.4–4. CLINICAL MANIFESTATIONS OF CONSTRICTIVE PERICARDITIS

History	Edema, ascites, dyspnea
Physical examination	Elevated jugular venous pressure Kussmaul sign Early diastolic knock Edema, hepatomegaly, ascites
ECG	Low voltage Nonspecific ST segment and T-wave changes Atrial fibrillation
Radiography	Heart size usually enlarged Chest radiograph may show calcium in pericardium Chest CT scan or MRI shows thickened pericardium
Catheterization	Early diastolic dip followed by diastolic plateau in ventricular pressure Equalization of diastolic pressures in all chambers

aspiration of fluid. This allows easy removal of large amounts of effusion; the catheter may also be left in place for drainage, over hours or days, and for instillation of chemotherapeutic agents in selected cases of purulent or malignant pericarditis. In elective cases, when the procedure is being done for diagnostic purposes, pericardiocentesis should always be preceded by echocardiography. Before the introduction of echocardiography, pericardiocentesis had a higher morbidity rate than at present, probably because it was attempted in patients with cardiomegaly and little, if any, actual effusion. The diagnostic yield of pericardiocentesis will be greatest in patients with pericarditis related to neoplastic, infectious, and connective tissue disease. Results of fluid analysis are nonspecific in pericarditis related to idiopathic, radiation-induced, and frequently even tuberculous disease.

SUBACUTE AND CHRONIC PERICARDITIS[1]

Any of the various types of acute pericarditis discussed earlier may evolve into the pericardial compressive syndromes listed in Table 2.4–3. The main differentiating feature is the time course involved, since they share the same causes, pathophysiology, and principles of management. Although cardiac tamponade is a dramatic and acutely life-threatening condition, the effusive-constrictive and chronic constrictive syndromes develop insidiously and may not be discovered until a prolonged period of disability and unsuccessful treatment has passed. The original inflammatory insult to the pericardium may have gone unrecognized or been long forgotten, making correct diagnosis all the more difficult.

CLINICAL FEATURES

The fundamental pathophysiologic problem in the pericardial compressive syndromes is impaired inflow of blood into the right side of the heart. The symptoms and signs are therefore those of systemic venous congestion with progressively deteriorating cardiac output due to underfilling of the ventricles. Sometimes the constrictive process is particularly severe around the left atrium, resulting in pulmonary vascular congestion. In addition, if the fibrosis extends into the epicardium, systemic and pulmonary venous congestion is due to a combination of pericardial and myocardial involvement. Table 2.4–4 lists the principal clinical and laboratory features of constrictive pericarditis. Edema, ascites, and dyspnea are the common presenting signs. The protean clinical manifestations of constrictive pericarditis often lead to erroneous diagnoses.

The combination of cachexia, hepatic enlargement, hypoalbuminemia, and ascites may suggest cirrhosis of the liver, or prominent albuminuria may result in the mistaken diagnosis of nephrosis. A number of incorrect cardiac diagnoses may also arise from misinterpretation of physical findings. Probably the most common error relates to the interpretation of the pericardial knock, which may be mistaken for a gallop sound and may lead to the diagnosis of cardiomyopathy or be considered an opening snap, leading to the incorrect diagnosis of mitral stenosis.

A high jugular venous pressure is often the key to diagnosis, but the pressure may be abnormal only after exercise or volume loading. One feature of constrictive pericarditis is the rapid Y descent of the jugular venous pulse. This finding of a collapsing pulse in the neck veins mirrors the changes in intracardiac pressure illustrated in Figure 2.4–3. Pulsus paradoxus and even a pericardial friction rub may be present in effusive-constrictive pericarditis, whereas Kussmaul sign (inspiratory increase in the jugular venous pressure) is typical of predominantly constrictive disease. Murmurs are usually absent, but a characteristic early diastolic knocking sound is sometimes heard. This sound corresponds to the period of maximal ventricular filling and is attributed to the abrupt cessation of filling by the fibrotic, noncompliant pericardium. Hepatomegaly, edema, and ascites may be of massive proportions.

LABORATORY FINDINGS

The ECG is almost always abnormal, usually showing low voltage, ST segment and T-wave changes, and not infrequently atrial fibrillation. The chest radiograph generally shows an enlarged cardiac

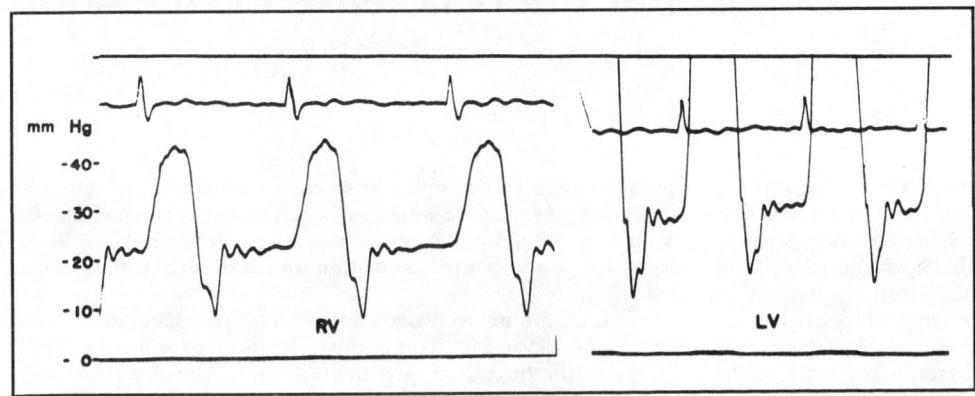

Figure 2.4–3. Intraventricular pressures from a patient with constrictive pericarditis and atrial fibrillation. The pressure does not continue to rise throughout diastole because all the filling occurs early. RV and LV diastolic pressures are shown at a higher level of amplification. Note that pressures in right and left ventricles have similar contour and reach approximately the same level at the end of diastole.

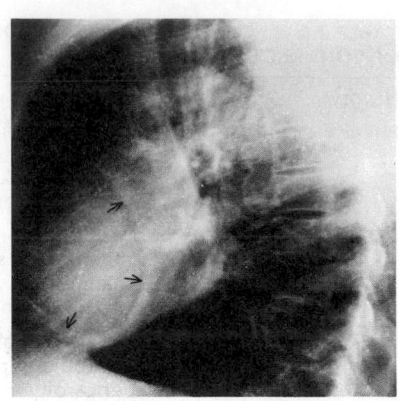

Figure 2.4–4. Lateral roentgenogram in constrictive pericarditis demonstrating pericardial calcification. The calcium is most likely to appear in the region of the atrioventricular groove and on the diaphragmatic surface of the heart. Fluoroscopy is often helpful in differentiating pericardial from pulmonary calcification.

the catheterization laboratory to determine whether hemodynamic compromise persists after removal of the fluid.

TREATMENT

Once the diagnosis of a pericardial compressive syndrome has been established, the only definitive treatment is removal of fluid, pericardium, or both. Occasional patients with primarily an effusive process, particularly those whose disease is radiation-induced or secondary to a connective tissue disease or uremia, will be managed successfully with pericardiocentesis and systemic or instilled corticosteroids. Once constriction is well established, however, there is no effective temporizing therapy, and operative removal of the visceral and parietal pericardium should be undertaken promptly. Deferring pericardiectomy may cause irreversible myocardial changes and result in suboptimal long-term improvement.

silhouette, although not to the degree expected, given the magnitude of hemodynamic compromise. The finding of calcific deposits in the pericardium on radiography or fluoroscopy gives an important clue to the diagnosis (Fig. 2.4–4). In effusive-constrictive disease the echocardiogram shows evidence of pericardial fluid or, in some cases, of pericardial thickening, but it does not show specific signs of the constrictive process. Chest CT scan and MRI are promising newer techniques for defining more accurately the degree and extent of pericardial thickening.[7,13]

The cardiovascular diagnostic laboratory may provide confirmation of the diagnosis by demonstration of a characteristic pressure tracing of arrested filling (Fig. 2.4–3). Ventricular filling is limited to the first part of diastole. Atrial pressure is high, and as the tricuspid valve opens, blood quickly fills the ventricle to capacity. There is no further filling during the remainder of diastole, and pressure and volume in the heart remain constant. The rapid inflow results in the dramatic drop in venous pressure observed in the neck veins as the collapsing pulse. The steep Y descent is responsible for the characteristic pressure contour in the cardiac chambers, which has been referred to as the square root sign ($\sqrt{\ }$). In constrictive pericarditis, the filling of both sides of the heart is limited by the pericardium, and therefore the end-diastolic pressures in the right and left ventricles tend to be identical ("equalized"). A similar hemodynamic and clinical picture may be manifested by patients with restrictive cardiomyopathy due to infiltrative diseases of the myocardium such as amyloidosis, hemochromatosis, or sarcoidosis (see Chapter 2.2).[10] Endomyocardial biopsy may have to be performed to differentiate these conditions from constrictive pericarditis. When effusive-constrictive pericarditis is suspected, it may be useful to perform pericardiocentesis in

REFERENCES

1. Cameron J, Oesterle SN, et al: The etiologic spectrum of constrictive pericarditis. Am Heart J 113:354, 1987
2. Fowler NO: Physiology of cardiac tamponade and pulsus paradoxus. Mod Concepts Cardiovasc Dis 47:109, 1978
3. Fowler NO: The pericardium in health and disease. Mount Kisco, NY, Futura Publishing, 1985
4. Fowler NO, Harbin AD: Recurrent acute pericarditis: Follow-up study of 31 patients. J Am Coll Cardiol 7:300, 1986
5. Guberman BA, Fowler NO, et al: Cardiac tamponade in medical patients. Circulation 64:633, 1981
6. Hancock EW: Management of pericardial disease. Mod Concepts Cardiovasc Dis 48:1, 1979
7. Isner JM, Carter BL, et al: Computed tomography in the diagnosis of pericardial heart disease. Ann Intern Med 97:473, 1982
8. Krikorian TG, Hancock EW: Pericardiocentesis. Am J Med 65:808, 1978
9. Kumar S, Lesch M: Pericarditis in renal disease. Prog Cardiovas Dis 22:357, 1980
10. Meaney S, Shabetai R, et al: Cardiac amyloidosis, constrictive pericarditis and restrictive cardiomyopathy. Am J Cardiol 38:547, 1976
11. Press OW, Livingston R: Management of malignant pericardial effusion and tamponade. JAMA 257:1088, 1987
12. Rubin RH, Moellering RC: Clinical, microbiologic and therapeutic aspects of purulent pericarditis. Am J Med 59:68, 1975
13. Soulen RL, Stark DD, Higgins CB: Magnetic resonance imaging of constrictive pericardial disease. Am J Cardiol 55:480, 1985
14. Spodick DH: Acute pericarditis: ECG changes. Primary Cardiol 8:78, 1982
15. Spodick DH: The normal and diseased pericardium: Current concepts of pericardial physiology, diagnosis and treatment. J Am Coll Cardiol 1:240, 1983

CHAPTER 2.5
Congenital Heart Disease in the Adult

Thomas A. Traill

Adult patients with congenital heart disease usually have medical evaluation for a symptomless heart murmur or an abnormal chest radiograph. The number of patients with symptoms of breathlessness, fluid retention, or cyanosis is small. Since the majority of potentially serious defects are detected and treated surgically in childhood, the range of malformations seen in adult practice is not representative of congenital heart disease as a whole. Patients include many with mild lesions who need treatment, some whose

heart disease is too complex or severe for surgical correction, and only a few who require surgical repair. The last group includes patients with atrial septal defect, coarctation of the aorta, aortic stenosis, and a number of less common defects such as tetralogy of Fallot.

It is traditional to divide congenital heart diseases into "acyanotic" and "cyanotic" conditions. The former are usually simple "holes in the heart" or valve abnormalities, which do not cause

arterial desaturation. The latter are more complex defects, in which a communication between the systemic and pulmonary circulations, such as a ventricular septal defect (VSD), is combined with circumstances that cause venous blood to bypass the pulmonary circuit and cross directly through the defect into the systemic circulation. For this right-to-left shunting to be clinically obvious, there must be severe obstruction to flow through the pulmonary artery. Except in a few rare diseases, obstruction to pulmonary blood flow occurs either at the level of the pulmonary valve or in the form of obstructive pulmonary vascular disease.

ACYANOTIC LESIONS

VENTRICULAR SEPTAL DEFECT

When a VSD is large (approximately the size of a dime in an infant or a quarter in an adult), the defect itself offers no resistance to flow, and the right ventricular pressure is equal to the left ventricular pressure. With equal pressures in the two ventricles, the direction and volume of shunting across the defect are determined by the relative vascular resistance in the pulmonary and systemic circuits. At birth the pulmonary vascular resistance (see Chapter 2.6) is very high, so that even with severely increased pressure supplying the pulmonary artery, the volume of pulmonary blood flow is not greatly increased. At this stage there is no murmur, and heart disease is not suspected. During the first 2 or 3 days after birth, however, as the pulmonary vascular resistance falls to as little as 10 percent of the systemic resistance, a large left-to-right shunt develops; thus the pulmonary blood flow may be several times the cardiac output. The result is severe pulmonary congestion: the infant is breathless, cannot feed, and fails to gain weight.

In the next few months, either the defect may be closed surgically (in times past when infant surgery was more risky, a physiologic means of palliation was to place a constricting band around the main pulmonary artery), the defect may reduce spontaneously, or the pulmonary vascular resistance may rise in reaction to the high flow and pressure. The initial result of an increase in pulmonary vascular resistance is reduction in the excessive pulmonary blood flow with improvement in symptoms. As the reactive vascular changes progress, however, they eventually limit pulmonary blood flow until the left-to-right shunt is replaced by right-to-left shunting and cyanosis develops. This situation, referred to as the Eisenmenger syndrome, can occur in response to any type of lesion capable of permitting a large left-to-right shunt.

In adult patients, simple VSD is much less common than in children. Many or most small defects (less than 3 mm) close in infancy or childhood, and those seen in adult life are the lesions of intermediate size, neither very large nor small enough to have closed spontaneously. Patients are typically asymptomatic and normally developed, and the only abnormal physical finding is a loud pansystolic murmur at the lower left sternal border. The intensity of the murmur is no indication of the size of the defect; indeed, a "pinhole" defect in the muscular (trabecular) portion of the ventricular septum may produce a palpable thrill. A clue to such a small muscular defect may be a rapid decrescendo murmur in late systole as the hole is pinched off by the contracting myocardium.

Adults with VSD rarely develop any serious hemodynamic disturbance. Very occasionally the flow across the defect and the resultant volume load on the left ventricle are sufficient to cause cardiac dilation and a gradual deterioration in left ventricular function. This situation is analogous to chronic mitral regurgitation of moderate severity and represents an unusual indication for surgical repair. More commonly, the indications for surgery are recurrent infective endocarditis or the development of aortic regurgitation. The latter occurs as a complication of defects of the septum immediately beneath the right coronary cusp of the aortic valve. The valve leaflet may then herniate down into the right ventricle, and if aortic regurgitation is allowed to persist until it becomes hemo-

dynamically significant, irreparable damage to the valve is likely and replacement will be required.

LEFT-TO-RIGHT SHUNTS AT ATRIAL LEVEL

Defects of the atrial septum and anomalies of pulmonary venous return, including scimitar syndrome and sinus venosus defect, all have similar pathophysiologic and clinical effects, related to high flow through the right ventricle and pulmonary artery. Young adults with atrial septal defect (ASD) are usually asymptomatic, and they are referred for evaluation because of a heart murmur or an abnormal chest radiograph. A few complain of mild exertional dyspnea. Physical examination reveals a healthy, normally developed young person. The *a* wave in the jugular pulse is prominent, and there may be a right ventricular lift. Auscultation reveals characteristic wide, fixed splitting of the second heart sound. There is usually an ejection systolic murmur due to increased flow through the right ventricular outflow tract, and there may be an additional diastolic rumble, reflecting increased flow through the tricuspid valve. In patients with ostium secundum ASD, the ECG typically shows partial or complete right bundle-branch block. The presence of left axis deviation (a superior vector) on the ECG usually indicates an ostium primum defect, the simplest expression of an atrioventricular canal defect (or endocardial cushion defect). This type of defect is associated with abnormalities of the atrioventricular valve ring; the mitral valve is displaced forward and toward the apex, as may be shown by echocardiography or angiography, and the leaflets may be cleft or dysplastic and allow mitral regurgitation.

The volume of left-to-right shunting through the pulmonary circulation may be inferred from the chest radiograph (Fig. 2.5–1) or the echocardiogram (Fig. 2.5–2). The latter shows enlargement of the right ventricle and pulmonary artery, with flattening of the septum. The shunt is quantified at catheterization as the ratio of pulmonary flow to systemic flow, typically between 1.5:1 and 4:1. Such estimates are always approximate, and it is dangerous to set a particular value of shunt size below which surgical correction is unnecessary.

The natural history of ASD dictates that the majority of patients should be referred for surgical repair. Although symptoms are rarely present in the young, there is no natural tendency toward closure, and in patients over the age of 40 years the lesion eventu-

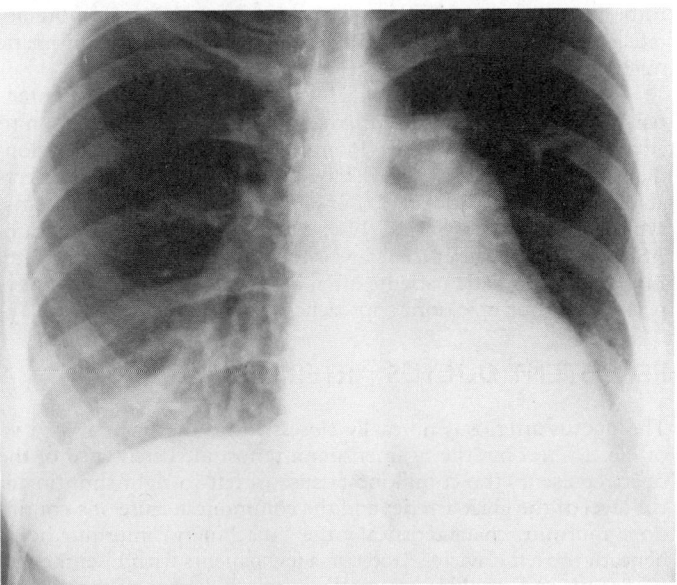

Figure 2.5–1. Chest radiograph of a patient with atrial septal defect, showing enlarged pulmonary arteries and increased pulmonary vascularity.

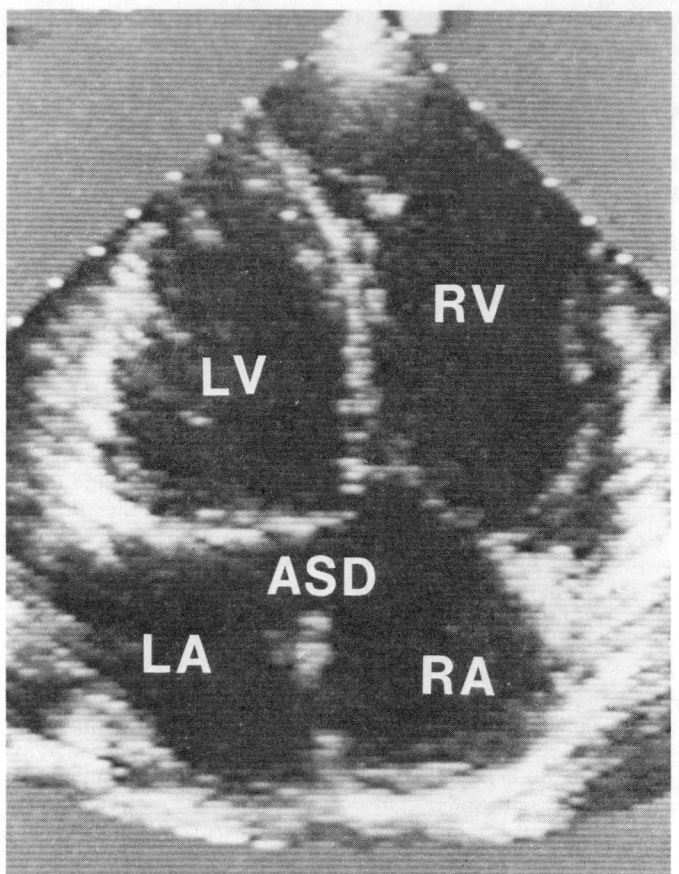

Figure 2.5–2. Echocardiogram (apical view) showing an atrial septal defect (ASD) with enlargement of the right ventricle (RV). RA = right atrium; LA = left atrium; LV = left ventricle.

ally causes fluid retention, atrial arrhythmias, cardiomegaly, and dyspnea. In elderly symptomatic patients, symptoms may mimic the clinical presentation of chronic mitral stenosis, which is easily excluded by echocardiography, or cor pulmonale, which may be a difficult source of confusion. Although such patients often appear to be unpromising candidates for surgery, the operative mortality rate is low, and the benefit of repair, even in the symptomatic stage, is remarkable.

Other aspects of the natural history of ASD include the potential for paradoxical embolism, which represents another reason to advocate surgical closure. Endocarditis, however, is rare. Development of pulmonary vascular disease is not as common as in defects at ventricular or aortic level, nor is it as rapid. In a few patients, typically in their twenties, Eisenmenger syndrome complicates ASD. Surgical repair at this stage is too dangerous to contemplate. Elderly symptomatic patients often have moderate pulmonary hypertension, but it seldom approaches the systemic level.

PERSISTENT DUCTUS ARTERIOSUS

The ductus arteriosus normally closes within the first day or two of life, to become the ligamentum arteriosum. Persistence of the duct represents the commonest cause of left-to-right shunting at the level of the great arteries and the commonest cause of a continuous murmur, characteristically the "machinery" murmur heard beneath the left clavicle. Except in a few patients with Eisenmenger syndrome and in elderly patients, surgical closure of the duct is recommended even in the absence of hemodynamic upset, since the operation is straightforward and the natural history includes a significant risk of bacterial endocarditis.

LEFT-SIDED OBSTRUCTIVE LESIONS

Congenital obstructive lesions of the left side of the heart include coarctation of the aorta (discussed in Chapter 2.10) and various anomalies of the aortic valve, mitral valve, and left atrium. Their physiologic effects are the same as those of their acquired counterparts.

Aortic stenosis (AS) may be valvular, typically with unicuspid or bicuspid valve, or it may occur above the valve (supravalvular AS) or below it (subaortic stenosis). Fixed subaortic lesions represent a spectrum from a discrete fibrous rim or diaphragm immediately beneath the aortic valve to a tubular fibromuscular constriction extending into the left ventricular cavity. These lesions should not be confused with IHSS or hypertrophic cardiomyopathy (HCM). The term "idiopathic hypertrophic subaortic stenosis" was coined when "functional" obstruction to left ventricular ejection was postulated on the basis of a pressure gradient demonstrable in many cases between the apex of the ventricle and the subaortic region at the end of the ejection phase. However, it has since been recognized that this pressure gradient is neither a constant finding in this disease nor a significant pathophysiologic mechanism, and the condition should be thought of as a cardiomyopathy, characterized by impaired diastolic function, rather than as a form of subaortic stenosis (see Chapter 2.2).

Congenital mitral stenosis may resemble its acquired counterpart with commissural fusion. Other varieties include parachute mitral valve, in which both mitral leaflets are supported by a single papillary muscle, and supravalvular mitral stenosis, or cor triatriatum, in which a membrane, often perforated by only a tiny hole, is situated above the mitral valve in the left atrium.

RIGHT-SIDED OBSTRUCTIVE LESIONS

The physiology of right-sided obstructive lesions differs in some respects from the corresponding abnormalities on the left side, because the structure of the right ventricle differs markedly from that of the left and because the foramen ovale exists as a potential valve allowing right-to-left shunting between the atria when normal flow through the right heart is impeded.

Right Ventricular Outflow Obstruction

The most common kind of pulmonary stenosis is congenital valvular stenosis. The pulmonary valve commissures are fused so that during ejection the structure forms a dome, with a jet of blood leaving through the small central orifice. The valve is mobile and usually creates a characteristic ejection sound as it assumes this shape, preceding a loud ejection systolic murmur. The pulmonary closure sound is typically soft and delayed, in proportion to the severity of obstruction. A dysplastic valve, consisting of a thick, immobile fibrous rim, is typical of pulmonary stenosis in Noonan syndrome. Neither this variety nor obstruction below the level of the valve due to congenital infundibular stenosis creates an ejection sound. Infundibular obstruction with VSD, referred to as tetralogy of Fallot (discussed below), is the commonest congenital cause of cyanosis in adults.

The natural history of severe, isolated, right ventricular outflow obstruction is generally predictable from the gradient between the right ventricle and pulmonary artery. When this exceeds about 40 mm Hg, there may be an increase in right ventricular hypertrophy, and right atrial hypertension, fluid retention, and in some cases syncope may occur. Surgical relief of the obstruction is therefore indicated, by valvotomy, balloon dilation, or resection of the lesion. When the gradient is less, progression is unusual, and the natural history is benign. Although definitive assessment often requires catheterization, the ECG is a useful indicator of the severity and progression of right ventricular hypertrophy. A monophasic R wave in lead V_1 is a sure indication that right ventricular pressure is similar to the systemic pressure. A chest radiograph shows normal peripheral pulmonary vasculature unless there is an associated

shunt. In the case of valvular stenosis, poststenotic dilation causes widening of the main pulmonary artery shadow.

Obstruction of the right side of the heart that occurs within the body of the right ventricle is a secondary phenomenon when right ventricular hypertrophy causes enlargement of the trabecular system and development of an anomalous right ventricular muscle bundle separating the outlet of the ventricle from the inlet region.

Ebstein Anomaly

Ebstein anomaly is the commonest congenital lesion of the right ventricle and the tricuspid valve. A portion of the valve, usually part of the anteromedial leaflet, is attached in the body of the right ventricle and results in functional obstruction to right ventricular filling, often with tricuspid regurgitation. Ebstein anomaly and other, rarer congenital abnormalities of the right ventricle, including Uhl anomaly, may all be associated with cyanosis when a patent foramen ovale allows right-to-left shunting across the atrial septum.

The clinical severity of Ebstein anomaly is variable. Sometimes the lesion causes severe cyanosis and requires surgical treatment in infancy. In this situation the prognosis is poor. By contrast, many adult patients are virtually asymptomatic. They may have a considerable degree of cardiomegaly, mainly due to right atrial enlargement, but cyanosis is often mild and may fluctuate in severity over the years. Physical examination reveals a quiet cardiac impulse and the characteristic auscultatory feature of a loud, delayed tricuspid closure sound, often referred to as the "sail sound." In addition, there may be a nondescript systolic murmur at the base. The ECG is often bizarre, with a wide pattern of right bundle-branch block, and arrhythmias are common. The echocardiogram is characteristic, showing dilation of the right side of the heart with a large, displaced tricuspid valve.

CYANOTIC CONDITIONS

MECHANISMS OF CYANOSIS

Congenital heart anomalies that result in cyanosis all consist of complex combinations of abnormalities, which together cause venous blood to reach the systemic output—that is, right-to-left shunting. Three underlying mechanisms are responsible. Most patients have obstructed pulmonary blood flow, due either to pulmonary stenosis or to increased pulmonary vascular resistance; this obstruction is combined with a communication between the two sides of the heart, across which right-to-left shunting occurs. In this first group are patients with tetralogy of Fallot, which consists of a VSD and pulmonary stenosis at the level of the infundibulum.

The second mechanism is typified by transposition of the great arteries, in which the aorta arises from the right ventricle and the pulmonary artery from the left ventricle. In this and certain related conditions, the two circulations are effectively parallel, so that oxygenated blood circulates continuously in the pulmonary circuit, mixing with the systemic circulation only across an ASD and through the persistent ductus arteriosus.

The third way for venous blood to reach the systemic circulation is found in the condition known as single ventricle, in which all of the blood entering the atria is mixed together in one chamber before being ejected into the aorta and the pulmonary artery. The resulting degree of cyanosis depends on the relative contributions of pulmonary venous blood and systemic venous return to the final mixture. This ratio is determined by the volume of pulmonary blood flow in comparison with the cardiac output. If there is no resistance to ejection into the pulmonary circuit, the pulmonary blood flow is high and the resulting mixture is largely oxygenated blood; cyanosis is therefore scarcely detectable. Such a patient is likely eventually to develop Eisenmenger syndrome. When there is severe pulmonary stenosis, the physiology is more like that of tetralogy of Fallot. The pulmonary pressure and flow are low, and cyanosis is obvious. These considerations apply whatever the level of the "central mixing" and whatever other defects may be present. For example, in tricuspid atresia, the pathophysiology is determined not by the absence of the right atrioventricular orifice but by the presence of a functional single ventricle, with a degree of pulmonary stenosis that varies from patient to patient.

APPROACH TO THE PATIENT

Two fundamental questions should be asked when one is planning the diagnostic evaluation of a patient with cyanotic congenital heart disease:

1. Is pulmonary blood flow reduced because of Eisenmenger syndrome, or because of stenosis at the level of the pulmonary valve?
2. Does the heart contain a complete "set of parts"—two atrioventricular valves, two ventricles, and two great arteries?

The two answers will determine long-term treatment strategy. If the patient's cyanosis is caused by pulmonary vascular disease, the only immediately available treatment is supportive, and further diagnostic studies are not required. On the other hand, if the patient has a low pulmonary arterial resistance and two ventricles, each with an atrioventricular valve, complete surgical correction may prove to be possible, and the anatomy and function of the heart should be investigated in detail.

PULMONARY VASCULAR DISEASE

Pulmonary vascular obstructive disease is discussed in Chapter 2.6. The clinical diagnosis of Eisenmenger syndrome is usually straightforward. In many cases, although not all, the history is consistent with the presence of a left-to-right shunt in childhood, followed by the insidious development of cyanosis; this sign is often noticed before any serious impairment of exercise capacity occurs. In addition to cyanosis and clubbing of the fingers, there is right ventricular hypertrophy and a palpable tap at the upper left sternal border, corresponding to a very loud pulmonary valve closure sound. The chest radiograph is characteristic, with enlargement (frequently massive) of the central pulmonary arteries and peripheral "pruning" of the smaller vessels. In contrast, the patient whose obstruction to pulmonary blood flow is at the level of the pulmonary valve has a soft, delayed, or absent pulmonary closure sound, and the chest radiograph shows a pulmonary artery that is more likely to be reduced in size than enlarged. The history will include cyanosis beginning soon after birth, and the patient may even have had previous palliative surgery in the form of a shunt procedure.

TWO VENTRICLES OR ONE?

After it has been established that the patient has a low pulmonary artery pressure, and therefore that surgical treatment may be possible, the next step is to determine whether there are two ventricles. Physical signs alone cannot provide the answer. The ECG may offer clues, but the echocardiogram provides the most direct approach, showing unequivocally whether there is a septum separating two atrioventricular orifices. In patients with one ventricle, who often have a rudimentary anterior chamber that is remote from the inlet portion of the heart, the echocardiogram demonstrates the number and positions of the atrioventricular valves, thus distinguishing cases of "double inlet ventricle" (single ventricle) from tricuspid atresia. In patients who have two ventricles and may thus be candidates for complete surgical correction, catheterization and angiography are necessary to complete the detailed information required before operation can be advised.

TETRALOGY OF FALLOT

The commonest cyanotic condition in the adult, tetralogy of Fallot, is a complex lesion characterized by stenosis of the right ventricular infundibulum in association with a VSD straddled by the aorta. The four elements of the "tetralogy" thus consist of (1) VSD, (2) pulmonary stenosis, (3) aortic override, and (4) right ventricular hypertrophy. Because the muscular narrowing of the infundibulum increases as the right ventricle hypertrophies, the obstruction to pulmonary blood flow tends to increase with the years. The typical patient is not overtly cyanotic at birth or even in the first months of life, but he gradually becomes so during the first few years. When infundibular stenosis is severe, "cyanotic spells" may ensue, during which spasm of the hypertrophied infundibulum acutely obstructs pulmonary blood flow. Propranolol, with its negative inotropic effect, is used for palliation of this situation, but prompt surgery is essential. "Squatting," a maneuver by which the child abruptly increases venous return, temporarily dilating the right ventricle and the right ventricular outflow tract, is also a feature of severe right ventricular outflow obstruction. The patient who survives to adult life without corrective or palliative surgery has clubbing of the fingers, polycythemia, often rather pronounced acne, and exercise impairment due to fatigue and dyspnea. Fluid retention and syncope are late manifestations.

Examination of the heart reveals right ventricular hypertrophy, an easily detectable aortic closure sound (because it arises closer than normal to the chest wall), and a soft delayed or absent pulmonary valve closure sound. In the typical case there is a loud ejection systolic murmur with no ejection click.

The chest radiograph indicates pulmonary oligemia, and the ECG shows right ventricular hypertrophy, confirmed by echocardiography. The latter documents the presence of two ventricles separated by a normally formed septum. If the great arteries are in their normal spatial relationship, then the differential diagnosis includes tetralogy of Fallot, pulmonary atresia with VSD, double-outlet right ventricle, and pulmonary stenosis with right-to-left shunting at the atrial level. A quiet heart with a continuous murmur from congenital systemic to pulmonary collateral vessels favors the diagnosis of pulmonary atresia.

Similar ventricular architecture is found in a group of conditions in which the spatial position and ventricular connections of the great arteries are reversed. The simplest case, transposition of the great arteries, is not seen in adults, but certain variants are compatible with long-term survival. "Corrected transposition" refers, not to a state after surgery, but to congenital correction by virtue of ventricular inversion (discordant atrioventricular connec-

tion) with transposition (discordant ventriculoarterial connection). Usually the aortic valve is in an anterior left-sided position.

MANAGEMENT

The principles of surgical management of cyanotic lesions follow naturally from the pathophysiology. When cyanosis is the result of inadequate perfusion of the lungs, the first aim of therapy is to increase pulmonary flow. Ideally this can be achieved by total surgical correction; however, a systemic-to-pulmonary shunt should be created when the lesion is too complex, when there is a single ventricle, or when the pulmonary arteries are absent or hypoplastic and thus inadequate to allow the right ventricle to pump the entire systemic flow. The Blalock-Taussig operation connects one of the subclavian arteries to the ipsilateral pulmonary artery. Other, less frequently used shunts include the Waterston-Cooley shunt, in which the ascending aorta is connected to the right pulmonary artery; the Potts procedure, in which the descending aorta is connected to the left pulmonary artery; and the Glenn operation, in which the superior vena cava is joined to the right pulmonary artery. The Glenn operation was a natural predecessor to the Fontan operation for tricuspid atresia, in which the entire systemic venous return bypasses the absent right ventricle through a direct connection between the right atrium and the pulmonary artery. This approach has proved remarkably successful and raises obvious physiologic questions about the real function of the normal right ventricle.

Cyanosis results in polycythemia; when successful surgical correction of the cardiac lesion is impossible, an elevated hematocrit is an important cause of morbidity and death, with complications including intravascular thrombosis and brain abscess. Routine venesection, with clear fluid replacement to maintain blood volume if necessary, is advocated to keep the hematocrit at less than 60 to 65 percent.

REFERENCES

1. Adams FH, Emmanouilides GC: Heart Disease in Infants, Children and Adolescents, 3d ed. Baltimore, Williams & Wilkins, 1983
2. Becker AE, Anderson RH: Pathology of Congenital Heart Disease. London, Butterworths, 1981
3. Roberts WC (ed): Adult Congenital Heart Disease. Philadelphia, Davis, 1987
4. Wood P: The Eisenmenger syndrome: Or pulmonary hypertension with reversed central shunt. Br Med J 2:701, 755, 1958

CHAPTER 2.6
Pulmonary Hypertension

Thomas A. Traill and John R. Michael

A number of different diseases lead to an increase in pulmonary artery pressure, or pulmonary hypertension. They are discussed together in this chapter because their clinical presentations overlap, and they demand a common diagnostic strategy. Table 2.6–1 lists the most frequent causes of pulmonary hypertension grouped according to the site and cause of obstruction in the pulmonary circuit. The pulmonary capillary wedge pressure obtained by right-sided heart catheterization provides a close estimate of the pulmonary venous pressure and can thus be used to separate causes of pulmonary hypertension into those due to downstream obstruction in the left side of the heart and pulmonary veins and those in which the abnormality begins in the pulmonary arteries and arteri-

oles. It is important to distinguish between elevation of the pulmonary artery pressure and elevation of the pulmonary vascular resistance. The former can occur because of downstream obstruction or because of a high pulmonary blood flow, even in the presence of normal pulmonary vessels. An elevated pulmonary vascular resistance implies functional (potentially reversible) or structural abnormality of the arteries or arterioles, often referred to as "pulmonary vascular disease." Such elevation of the resistance in the pulmonary circuit may be "primary" (idiopathic), but it more commonly occurs as a result of an identifiable stimulus to reactive changes in the small vessels.

The normal systolic pulmonary artery pressure is 15 to 28

TABLE 2.6–1. CAUSES OF PULMONARY HYPERTENSION

Downstream obstruction
- Raised left ventricular filling pressure
- Mitral stenosis
- Left atrial myxoma
- Cor triatriatum
- Congenital pulmonary vein anomalies
- Pulmonary veno-occlusive disease

} Wedge pressure high

Communication between systemic and pulmonary circulation
- With left-to-right shunt (low resistance) } Plexogenic pulmonary
- Eisenmenger syndrome   } arteriopathy

Primary pulmonary hypertension

Thromboembolic pulmonary hypertension

Cor pulmonale
- Chronic respiratory failure
    - Chronic obstructive lung disease
    - Sleep apnea
    - Kyphoscoliosis
    - Muscular dystrophy
- Obliterative parenchymal disease
    - Fibrosing alveolitis
    - Cystic fibrosis

} Wedge pressure normal

Miscellaneous
- High altitude
- Schistosomiasis
- Hepatic cirrhosis (Banti syndrome)

mm Hg. The diastolic pressure, which is usually similar to the pulmonary capillary wedge pressure, is 5 to 15 mm Hg, and the mean pulmonary artery pressure is 10 to 22 mm Hg. The pressure gradient across the pulmonary vascular bed is thus much less than in the systemic circuit, so that the pulmonary vascular resistance is normally 10 percent of the systemic vascular resistance. Metabolic changes, in particular hypoxia, may cause reversible increases in pulmonary vascular resistance. A permanent increase indicates the presence of pulmonary vascular disease. In primary pulmonary hypertension or Eisenmenger syndrome the pulmonary vascular resistance may equal or exceed the systemic vascular resistance. In some such patients, pharmacologic effects are still demonstrable, and vasodilator drugs or an increase in inspired oxygen may cause a temporary fall in resistance. This is usually manifested not as a decrease in pressure but as an increase in pulmonary blood flow.

CLINICAL FEATURES IN PULMONARY HYPERTENSION

In patients with mild pulmonary hypertension, features of the primary disease usually determine the clinical picture, and the only clues to pulmonary hypertension may be an accentuated pulmonary closure sound (P_2) and subtle evidence of right ventricular hypertrophy. As pulmonary vascular disease becomes severe, however, manifestations of pulmonary hypertension and right-sided heart failure predominate, so that irrespective of the initiating cause, most patients with severe pulmonary vascular disease have similar signs and symptoms.

The earliest symptom is fatigue. Exertional dyspnea begins gradually and is seldom severe until a late stage of the disease. Ankle swelling, abdominal discomfort, and an increase in girth reflect fluid retention and passive hepatic and splanchnic congestion. With further progression of the disease, anorexia, weight loss, angina caused by right ventricular ischemia, and syncope develop. Small hemoptyses are common, particularly in association with respiratory infections. Occasionally, massive hemoptysis occurs.

Physical examination reveals a chronically ill patient who is often tired and breathless when crossing a room. Mild cyanosis may be present because of right-to-left shunting across the foramen ovale. Severe central cyanosis with finger clubbing usually indicates that the patient has Eisenmenger syndrome. Peripheral pulses are of small volume. The jugular venous pressure is elevated, often with a systolic wave of tricuspid regurgitation. The precordial impulse includes a prominent right ventricular lift and palpable bulge in the second left intercostal space over the pulmonary outflow tract. On auscultation, the P_2 is accentuated, audible even at the apex, and often preceded by a systolic murmur and ejection click. In advanced cases, the Graham Steell murmur of acquired pulmonary valve regurgitation may be present. The roentgenographically demonstrated heart size depends on the initiating cause but is seldom large. The proximal pulmonary artery segment is prominent, and the distal pulmonary vessels are "pruned" (Fig. 2.6–1). The echocardiogram demonstrates right ventricular hypertrophy with increased cavity size. The short-axis cross section shows flattening of the septum and, in extreme cases, bulging of the septum into the left ventricular cavity. The most important aspect of the echocardiographic examination is to identify or exclude primary left-sided heart disease, in particular mitral stenosis or other, rarer causes of left atrial obstruction. It is essential not to overlook such treatable causes of pulmonary hypertension, and before echocardiography was widely available, it was often necessary to perform cardiac catheterization to exclude occult mitral disease. In a few such cases the only other clue to left-sided heart disease is the presence of both left atrial and right ventricular hypertrophy on the ECG.

SPECIAL CLINICAL TYPES OF PULMONARY HYPERTENSION

PULMONARY HYPERTENSION IN LEFT-SIDED HEART DISEASE

Pulmonary artery pressure automatically increases in response to a rise in pulmonary venous pressure. The change in pulmonary artery pressure is usually commensurate; thus, in common forms of left-sided heart disease, mild pulmonary hypertension forms only

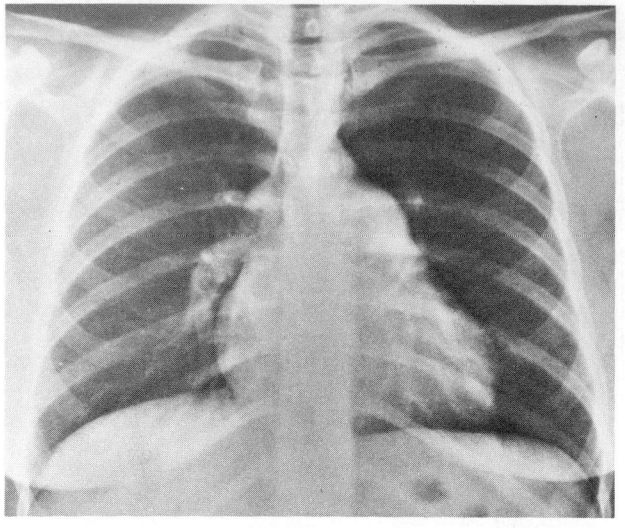

A

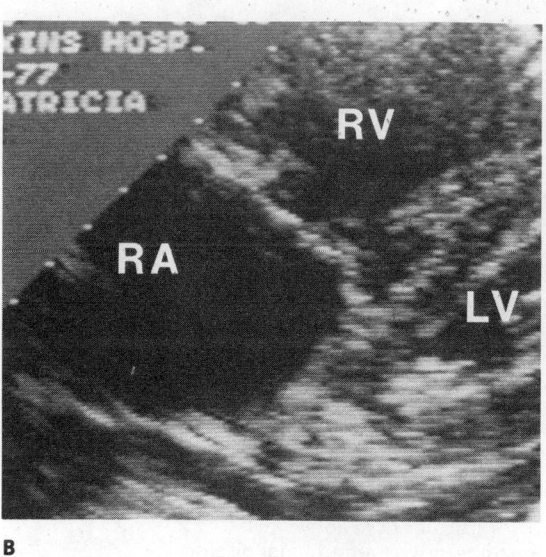

B

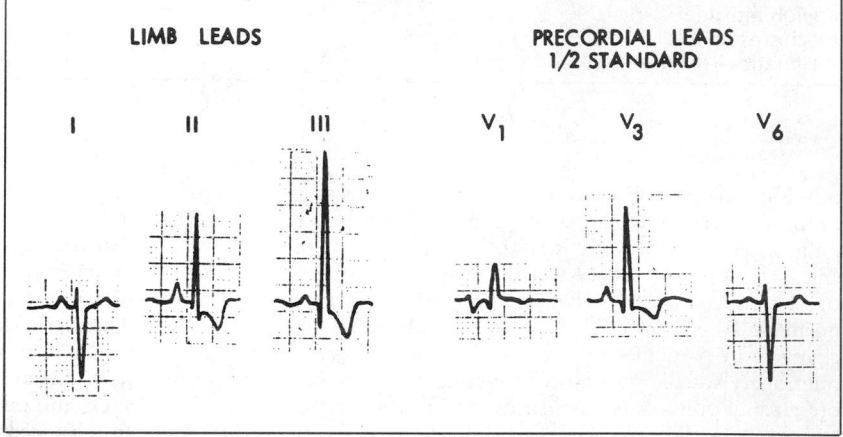

C

Figure 2.6–1. A. Chest radiograph in primary pulmonary hypertension, showing increased size of the main and proximal pulmonary arteries with "pruning" of peripheral vessels. **B.** Echocardiogram in short axis view showing enlargement of the right ventricle (RV) and atrium (RA) with compression and distortion of the left ventricle (LV). **C.** ECG shows right axis deviation, right atrial enlargement, and right ventricular hypertrophy.

a minor aspect of the clinical picture. In a few patients, however, particularly those with obstruction at the left atrial level as a result of mitral stenosis, "reactive" pulmonary hypertension may develop. In the early stages this represents an increase in pulmonary artery pressure that is disproportionate to the rise in pulmonary venous pressure but is still reversible after corrective surgery. With the passage of time, however, fixed pulmonary vascular changes develop; thus in a few patients with mitral stenosis, severe pulmonary hypertension develops and may dominate the clinical presentation.

PRIMARY PULMONARY HYPERTENSION[2]

Several causes of pulmonary vascular disease are associated with identical morphologic changes in the pulmonary arterioles and small pulmonary arteries, best referred to as "plexogenic pulmonary arteriopathy."[6] "Primary pulmonary hypertension" is used to describe the idiopathic form of this kind of vascular disease, in which the disease originates in, and is confined to, the small pulmonary arteries. In the earlier stages there is pronounced hypertrophy of the pulmonary arteriolar media, with an "onionskin" type of intimal fibrosis and, in advancing cases, fibrinoid necrosis and a characteristic "plexiform" lesion. These changes may be

complicated by intravascular thrombosis and may lead to widespread obliteration of small pulmonary vessels.

The pathogenesis of primary pulmonary hypertension is not understood, but it is widely suspected that the initiating event is intense pulmonary arteriolar spasm. Consistent with this view is the association with Raynaud phenomenon, either in the patient or in the patient's family, and with systemic sclerosis and the "CREST" syndrome (calcinosis, Raynaud phenomenon, esophageal dysfunction, sclerodactyly, and telangiectasia) (see Chapter 8.5).[5] Although it might be supposed that pulmonary hypertension complicating systemic sclerosis is merely a result of pulmonary fibrosis (see below), plexogenic pulmonary arteriopathy may occur in systemic sclerosis independent of the degree of fibrosis in the parenchyma.

Most patients are young, typically presenting in their early twenties, with an overall age range from childhood to late middle life. There is a pronounced female preponderance of 4:1 or 5:1, and there are occasional familial occurrences. The disease is presumed to have a presymptomatic phase during which pulmonary hypertension develops. At the time of presentation, patients often have pulmonary artery resistance and pressure similar to those in the systemic circulation, with fixed or reduced cardiac output, right ventricular dilation, and increased right ventricular filling pressure.

The prognosis for patients with primary pulmonary hyperten-

sion is poor. The majority of patients live no more than 5 years from the time of first diagnosis. Treatment with vasodilators, in particular the calcium-channel blocker nifedipine, is helpful in only a small proportion (10 to 15 percent) of patients. Many physicians advise anticoagulation, both because of the possibility that the patient has chronic thromboembolic disease and because in situ thrombosis may accelerate the progression of the idiopathic condition. However, the benefits of anticoagulation are not established. Currently the only definitive therapy appears to be transplantation of the heart and lungs. This has been performed in a number of centers with encouraging results.

CHRONIC THROMBOEMBOLIC PULMONARY HYPERTENSION

A small number of patients with a clinical presentation identical to that of the idiopathic form of primary pulmonary hypertension prove to have chronic thromboembolic disease[1] (see Chapter 3.8). In some cases this is related to the use of the contraceptive pill, but only a few patients have clinical evidence of systemic venous disease or venous thrombosis. The diagnosis is often difficult to make at the bedside, but ventilation-perfusion scans usually reveal multiple perfusion defects. Pulmonary arteriography is hazardous and has its chief value in acute or subacute massive pulmonary embolism when thrombolytic or surgical treatment is under consideration. When patients with chronic thromboembolic pulmonary vascular disease have persistently high pulmonary artery pressure, the prognosis is poor, as in primary pulmonary hypertension.

PULMONARY VENO-OCCLUSIVE DISEASE

Obstruction at the pulmonary venous level is a rare cause of pulmonary hypertension. In babies, congenital anomalies of pulmonary venous return may occur with or without an obstructive component. In either case, early correction is required. In a few adults with acquired pulmonary hypertension the diagnosis turns out to be a variant of pulmonary vascular disease known as pulmonary veno-occlusive disease, a fibrosing condition affecting small pulmonary veins and venules.[1] The clinical clue to this condition is a presentation with established pulmonary hypertension and a history of episodic pulmonary edema. Right-sided heart catheterization reveals variable wedge pressures, depending on whether the wedged position communicates with an obstructed or still patent segment of the pulmonary venous system.

EISENMENGER SYNDROME

Eisenmenger syndrome may be defined as a congenital cardiac defect complicated by irreversible pulmonary vascular disease with a resistance so high that the shunt is bidirectional or reversed. Any of the congenital systemic-to-pulmonary communications normally associated with left-to-right shunting may be complicated by Eisenmenger syndrome[3]—for example, ventricular septal defect, persistent ductus arteriosus, atrial septal defect, or more complex lesions that cannot be surgically corrected in infancy, such as single ventricle. When pulmonary vascular disease complicates congenital heart disease, the abnormality resembles plexogenic pulmonary arteriopathy of primary pulmonary hypertension, and it seems likely that they have a common pathogenesis involving vasospasm.

One might imagine that modern pediatric and surgical expertise would make Eisenmenger syndrome a disease of the past and that children with cardiac defects carrying the potential for pulmonary vascular disease would be detected and treated early in life. However, a number of patients with congenital heart disease continue to be seen by a physician for the first time at ages from 5 to 25 years with established and inoperable pulmonary vascular disease. They come from families at all socioeconomic levels, and it must be assumed that many have been expertly examined as infants or young children. Thus a proportion of patients develop the Eisenmenger reaction without going through the stage of having a large and clinically apparent left-to-right shunt. One presumes that vasospasm occurs from birth and that the high pulmonary vascular resistance that is normal during intrauterine life does not fall after delivery (see Chapter 2.5).

COR PULMONALE

To the pathologist the term "cor pulmonale" means right ventricular enlargement caused by disease of the respiratory system with pulmonary hypertension. In clinical practice the expression implies also that there is evidence of right ventricular failure. We may distinguish two general mechanisms by which lung disease causes pulmonary hypertension. In a few patients, such as those with fibrosing alveolitis, pulmonary vascular obstruction is a result of obliteration of the pulmonary vascular bed as part of the underlying disease. Simple destruction of the pulmonary vasculature, however, has to be extensive to cause pulmonary hypertension; for example, pneumonectomy does not, of itself, cause a rise in pressure in the remaining pulmonary artery. In the majority of patients with cor pulmonale the primary mechanism is pulmonary artery vasoconstriction due to chronic arterial hypoxemia. This, rather than destruction of lung tissue, is the cause of pulmonary hypertension and cor pulmonale in patients with chronic respiratory failure due, for example, to emphysema, chronic bronchitis, sleep apnea, kyphoscoliosis, cystic fibrosis, or muscular dystrophy.

In patients with cor pulmonale the cardiac complications of their pulmonary disease usually develop late in the course of a long-standing respiratory disorder. Typically, fluid retention develops, and there are signs of right ventricular enlargement with a rise in jugular venous pressure and development of tricuspid regurgitation. The cardiac signs in these patients may be difficult to appreciate clinically, because of the chronic changes in the lungs. Echocardiography, when it is possible, demonstrates right ventricular enlargement and flattening of the septum. On the chest radiograph an enlargement of the main pulmonary artery or the right descending pulmonary artery to 16 mm or more suggests the presence of pulmonary hypertension. Patients in whom pulmonary hypertension develops because of fibrosing alveolitis generally have a vital capacity and a diffusing capacity for carbon monoxide less than 40 percent of the predicted values. In patients with emphysema and chronic bronchitis the development of pulmonary hypertension usually results in Pa_{O_2} values of less than 60 mm Hg and forced expiratory volume at 1 second (FEV_1) of less than 1 L.

Chronic respiratory disease is common in the population and can accompany pulmonary hypertension without being its cause. Thus, before one diagnoses a condition as cor pulmonale, it is important to be alert for primary cardiac disease—in particular, mitral stenosis or atrial septal defect. Elderly patients with primary cardiac conditions and severe fluid retention frequently appear to be poor candidates for surgical correction and yet may obtain spectacular benefit when an underlying cardiac cause is correctly diagnosed and treated.

Management of cor pulmonale consists of treating the underlying condition and optimizing the patient's oxygenation and fluid balance. Since fluid retention is due both to elevated pressures in the right side of the heart and to the renal effects of combined hypoxemia and hypercapnia, treatment directed at reversing the abnormal blood gas values is preferable to overreliance on diuretics. The patients are sensitive to underfilling of the right side of the heart, and zealous efforts to achieve a normal jugular venous pressure may result in a low cardiac output state and azotemia. The use of digitalis has little to contribute and may be hazardous in chronic hypoxemic states. The only exceptions may be patients with biventricular failure or with supraventricular tachycardia. Treatment with oxygen has little effect in patients whose pulmonary hypertension is due to obliteration of the pulmonary vascular

bed, but it can be effective in those who have a high degree of pulmonary vascular resistance because of chronic hypoxemia. Patients with chronic lung disease who have a Pa$_{O_2}$ less than 60 mm Hg should be treated with low-flow oxygen.[4] In these patients the continuous use of oxygen selectively vasodilates the pulmonary circulation and lowers pulmonary arterial pressure, thereby improving survival, exercise performance, and quality of life.

REFERENCES

1. Edwards WD, Edwards JE: Clinical primary pulmonary hypertension: Three pathologic types. Circulation 56:884, 1977

2. Haworth SG: Primary pulmonary hypertension. Br Heart J 49:517, 1983
3. Haworth SG, Sauer V, et al: Development of the pulmonary circulation in ventricular septal defect: A quantitative structural study. Am J Cardiol 40:781, 1977
4. Nocturnal Oxygen Therapy Trial Group: Continuous or nocturnal oxygen in hypoxemic chronic obstructive lung disease. Ann Intern Med 93:391, 1980
5. Salerni R, Rodnan GP, et al: Pulmonary hypertension in the CREST syndrome variant of progressive systemic sclerosis (scleroderma). Ann Intern Med 86:394, 1977
6. Wagenvoort CA, Wagenvoort N: Primary pulmonary hypertension: A pathologic study of the lung vessels in 156 clinically diagnosed cases. Circulation 42:1163, 1970

CHAPTER 2.7

Thoracic Pain and Angina Pectoris

Nicholas J. Fortuin and Gary D. Walford

Thoracic pain may have its origin in the various tissues of the chest wall, the neck, the intrathoracic structures, or areas below the diaphragm. When the pain arises in the skin or superficial structures, it usually can be localized accurately by the patient. When it arises in deeper structures, it may be diffuse and difficult to localize, or it may radiate in such a pattern as to mislead both patient and physician into believing that the abnormality lies beyond the limits of the thorax. This apparent lack of relationship between the location of the pain and the site of the lesion is explained by the fact that many thoracic structures, including the heart, the aorta, the pleura, and the esophagus, are supplied by sensory fibers from the same segments of the spinal cord. The afferent fibers from the heart and pericardium are carried principally in the sympathetic nerves, but some reach the central nervous system by way of the vagal and phrenic nerves. The phrenic nerve also carries the pain fibers from the pericardium, diaphragm, and diaphragmatic pleura, and this pathway accounts for the referral of pericardial pain to the trapezius region and to the shoulder.

The cause of cardiac pain is not known with certainty. The myocardium and the pericardium can be the source of cardiac pain, but pain probably does not originate in the coronary arteries. Available evidence indicates that the myocardium itself gives rise to pain when coronary blood flow is inadequate. Inadequate coronary blood flow may be the consequence of fixed or transient obstructive disease in coronary arteries or of the imposition of an extreme demand on the myocardium in the presence of normal vessels, as in the case of aortic valve disease, hypertrophic cardiomyopathy, or systemic hypertension.

PATHOPHYSIOLOGY OF MYOCARDIAL ISCHEMIA[14]

When the oxygen requirements of the myocardium exceed the supply of oxygen derived from coronary blood flow, the myocardium becomes hypoxic. The factors determining myocardial oxygen demand and oxygen supply are shown in Figure 2.7–1 and the consequences of ischemia are listed at the bottom. This diagram can be used to explain the way various factors precipitate angina and how various therapeutic measures bring about relief.

The major factors determining oxygen demand are heart rate, left ventricular wall stress, and the contractile state of the myocardium. Heart rate is increased during exercise, with excitement, and as a response to catecholamine stimulation. Wall stress is directly proportional to ventricular volume and arterial blood pressure, and it is inversely proportional to the thickness of the ventricular wall. The larger the left ventricular volume or pressure, the higher the oxygen cost per unit of work. As a result, therapeutic measures that allow the ventricle to operate at a smaller volume or lower pressure are beneficial. The contractile state of the myocardium is most commonly altered by catecholamines or sympathetic stimulation, both of which shift the heart to a steeper function curve, increase the rate of tension development in the myocardium, and hence increase the oxygen cost.

The factors influencing supply are coronary blood flow and the oxygen-carrying capacity of the blood. In most situations the oxygen content is not important, and the most important factors in supply are coronary blood flow, which is determined by aortic pressure, and coronary vascular resistance. For this reason any disease such as atherosclerosis that alters coronary vascular resistance is important.

In addition, spasm of large epicardial coronary arteries may cause transient increases in resistance and thus severely restrict coronary blood flow. Both the distribution of flow and the total amount of flow are of importance in providing oxygen to the myocardium. The inner subendocardial regions of the ventricle are especially susceptible to ischemia. Catecholamine stimulation, by increasing the rate of tension development, decreases the flow to the endocardium.

Pain and electrocardiographic changes are the common clinical manifestations of myocardial ischemia. The impairment of ventricular function is of importance because it initiates positive feedback loops that may tend to perpetuate the ischemic condition. The poorly functioning ventricle may dilate, and this increases wall stress and oxygen consumption, which tend to aggravate the ischemic condition. The rise in end-diastolic pressure that accompanies left ventricular dysfunction is due to an acute alteration in ventricular relaxation and compliance. This may also reduce subendocardial blood flow in diastole. Ventricular dysfunction may also lead to decreased arterial pressure and hence lower coronary perfusion pressure. The metabolic consequences of ischemia are many, but the most thoroughly studied is the shift from aerobic to anaerobic metabolism. The metabolic products of anaerobic metabolism may be important in the production of the pain of myocardial ischemia and are an important stimulus to coronary vasodilation.

Obstruction of one of the major extramural coronary arteries by an atherosclerotic plaque is responsible for myocardial ischemia in most patients with angina pectoris. Usually several coronary arteries are involved, with narrowings obstructing 75 percent or

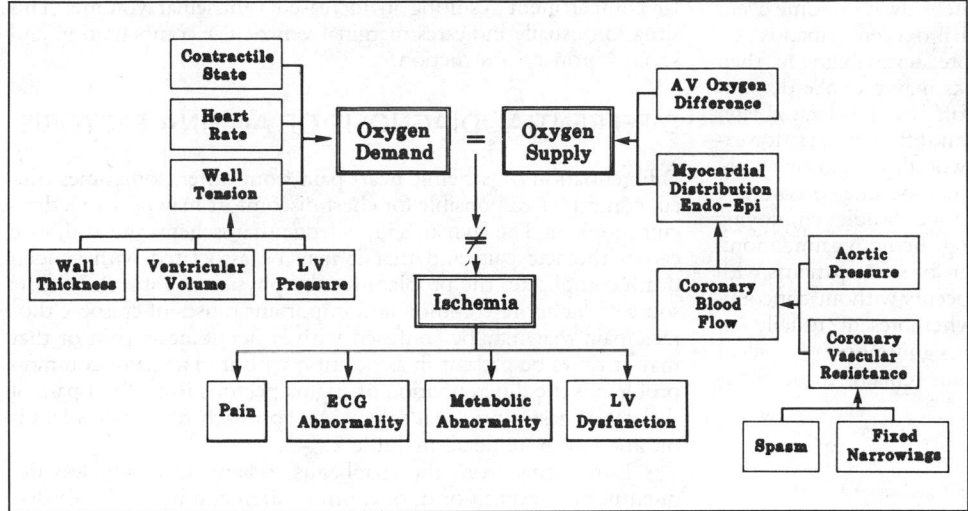

Figure 2.7–1. The pathophysiology of myocardial ischemia. The factors contributing to myocardial oxygen requirement are listed at the left. The factors regulating myocardial blood flow are listed at the right and the consequences of myocardial ischemia at the bottom of the figure.

more of the vessel lumen at single or multiple sites serially distributed. Proximal narrowing of a single vessel is the cause in a minority of patients, and a small percentage will show no definite evidence of atherosclerosis as detected by coronary angiography. Disease of the small intramural coronary arteries of the myocardium may be the cause of myocardial ischemia in some of these patients. Arteriographic studies of the coronary arteries have documented the occurrence of reversible coronary artery spasm as a cause for some instances of myocardial ischemia. Spasm may occur in normal arteries or at the site of an atherosclerotic plaque. The cause of coronary spasm remains unknown. Humoral mechanisms, such as thromboxane A_2 and histamine, have been suggested by experimental studies, but there has been scanty evidence to support their role in human coronary spasm. The focal nature of coronary spasm suggests that local endothelial factors promoting increased vascular reactivity may be important. In addition to localized spasm causing coronary obstruction, recent evidence suggests that coronary arteries may show active vasomotion, which may be responsible for changes in coronary vascular resistance. Other causes of fixed coronary artery obstruction include embolic disease, which is particularly likely in the presence of mitral valve disease; ostial aneurysm; Takayasu arteritis and other large-vessel arteritides, including polyarteritis and giant cell arteritis; congenital abnormalities of the coronary arteries; and Kawasaki disease, which may produce aneurysms of the coronary arteries.

ANGINA PECTORIS

Typical angina pectoris can be recognized easily. It is substernal in location and almost never inframammary or strictly precordial. Radiation into the left shoulder and down the inner aspect of the left arm into the ring and little fingers is frequent but not universally present. The character of the discomfort is often "visceral" in quality and will be described by the patient as squeezing, constrictive, oppressive, or similarly vague in nature and usually is not described as a "pain." It may also be characterized as stabbing, sharp, burning, or even tingling. "Numbness" is another word sometimes used by the patient. Sometimes the patient is not aware of discomfort but complains of dyspnea, a symptom that frequently accompanies angina. The right arm, neck, jaw, and throat may be occasional sites of radiation. Rarely, the pain is felt in these areas alone, and the chest is not involved. The discomfort usually persists for 1 to 5 minutes. Sharp, shooting pain lasting for only a few seconds or aching discomfort of several hours' duration is unlikely to be due to myocardial ischemia.

The distribution and character of the pain are far less specific in establishing the diagnosis than its relationship to exertion, which is the most important feature of angina pectoris. The patient experiences pain on exertion that subsides or disappears, usually within 5 minutes, when he rests. The amount of exertion required to produce the pain varies from day to day, but the relationship is qualitatively the same. The patient usually will say that its appearance makes him stop what he is doing. If the pain subsides while exercise continues at the same rate, it is unlikely to be angina. Distress may be provoked sooner and by less activity in cold weather, or it may occur more readily after eating or during emotional upset. The patient with typical angina pectoris cannot continue exertion at the same rate after the pain appears but sometimes can do more work after a brief period of rest.

Relief of the pain by rest is an important characteristic of angina pectoris, but the response to nitroglycerin also is important. Most patients who benefit are relieved in 3 to 4 minutes after placing the tablet under the tongue, and in many instances, relief comes after only 20 or 30 seconds. Equivocal relief or relief that comes only after 10 or more minutes makes it unlikely that myocardial ischemia is responsible for the pain. The diagnosis of myocardial infarction must be considered if pain characteristic of myocardial ischemia persists for 20 minutes to an hour.

The physician must remember that the failure of nitroglycerin to relieve pain can be due to deterioration of the preparation as a result of age and exposure to heat, light, or moisture. This should be suspected if the patient reports that the side effects (headache, throbbing in the throat, and flushing) previously associated with the administration of the drug are now absent. The response to nitroglycerin can be helpful in establishing the diagnosis of angina pectoris, but it should never be the principal evidence on which the diagnosis is based. Relief of chest discomfort by nitroglycerin is not specific for myocardial ischemia, because this drug may relieve other types of chest pain such as that due to esophageal spasm.

STABLE ANGINA PECTORIS

Patients with angina pectoris can be categorized into stable and unstable groups. Stable angina indicates that the pain has been present for some time (months to years), occurs predictably with exertion, and is alleviated rapidly by rest and nitroglycerin. In such patients there may be times when angina occurs more frequently, such as during emotional stress, or times when angina occurs infrequently. Patients with stable angina may experience pain without physical exertion, for example, after a heavy meal, during emo-

tional upset, or during a nightmare, but there always is some event that is responsible for increasing myocardial oxygen demands.

Patients with stable angina may note a variability in their threshold for pain. Sometimes minor tasks may provoke discomfort in the morning hours, but major effort is well tolerated later in the day. Patients may note variability on different days; for example, pain may occur more readily on workdays than on weekends. This variable threshold to angina may be due to coronary spasm or changes in coronary vasomotor tone. Studies employing ambulatory ECG monitoring, stress testing, hemodynamic monitoring, and radionuclides have shown that for some patients with angina, evidence of myocardial ischemia occurs without concomitant chest symptoms. Chest discomfort, when present, usually follows other evidence of ischemia. The significance of "silent ischemia" in patients with stable symptoms remains to be determined.

UNSTABLE ANGINA PECTORIS[13]

When ischemic cardiac pain occurs at rest without obvious provoking factors, with minimal effort, or for prolonged periods, the patient is said to suffer from unstable angina pectoris, a syndrome that stands in an intermediate position between stable angina pectoris and acute myocardial infarction. Other terms for this syndrome include preinfarction angina, crescendo angina, intermediate coronary syndrome, and acute coronary insufficiency. The unstable angina syndrome includes a variety of clinical presentations. Patients may experience angina for the first time with exertion and then note a crescendo pattern of increasing angina with less and less effort. Other patients with stable angina may note an increase in the frequency of pain and a decrease in the amount of effort required to bring on pain. Angina may occur at rest or may be of increased duration and severity, requiring more nitroglycerin for relief. Other patients with the syndrome have prolonged episodes of ischemic pain that resemble acute myocardial infarction but without subsequent laboratory confirmation of muscle necrosis. Such episodes may occur repeatedly. Common to each presentation is the occurrence of myocardial ischemia with minimal or no obvious increase in myocardial oxygen demands. This implies a recent change in the coronary circulation's ability to deliver oxygen in the absence of clinical evidence of myocardial infarction. Thrombus formation on a preexisting area of atherosclerosis, hemorrhage into an atherosclerotic plaque, or coronary spasm all may play some role in the etiology of this syndrome.

Variant (Prinzmetal) Angina[13]

Patients with an unusual form of unstable angina, variant (Prinzmetal) angina, experience recurrent episodes of typical anginal pain at rest, often despite well-preserved effort tolerance. The causal role of myocardial ischemia in the patient's pain may be difficult to establish unless an ECG is recorded during an episode of pain. In contrast to patients with chronic stable angina who demonstrate ST segment depression with myocardial ischemia, patients with variant angina show ST segment elevation, often of a striking degree and resembling acute infarction, which disappears with relief of the anginal attack. Coronary spasm may play an important role in the production of this syndrome. One third of patients show no evidence of coronary atherosclerosis, and the remainder have major proximal obstruction lesions. Reversible spasm of both diseased and normal coronary arteries in association with the clinical manifestations of the syndrome has been observed by coronary angiography during spontaneous attacks, or it may be provoked by vasospastic agents such as ergot alkaloids.[8]

Angina Decubitus

Some patients may awake with angina not associated with dreaming after they have spent several hours in the recumbent position. This is termed "angina decubitus." This clinical presentation is analogous to paroxysmal nocturnal dyspnea and is due to the increased oxygen demands that occur with fluid shifts into the vascular compartment resulting in increased ventricular volume. This situation usually indicates marginal ventricular compensation and severe coronary obstruction.

DIFFERENTIAL DIAGNOSIS OF ANGINA PECTORIS

Differentiation of ischemic heart pain from other, sometimes trivial, conditions responsible for chest discomfort may present a difficult problem. The layman's knowledge that ischemic heart disease causes thoracic pain and that it may be associated with sudden death complicates the problem for the physician. Table 2.7–1 lists some of the more common and important causes of episodic thoracic pain that may be confused with ischemic heart pain or that may at times be present in association with it. The most common problem is the differentiation of angina pectoris from chest pain of skeletal or gastrointestinal origin. An approach to this problem is outlined in more detail in Table 2.7–2.

Pain arising from the esophagus, biliary tract, and less frequently the stomach or duodenum is often confused with cardiac pain because the character and location of the pain may be similar. The relation to exertion is the major differentiating feature. The pain of reflux esophagitis is not usually accentuated by exertion or relieved promptly by rest. Eructation may ameliorate reflux pain and may also be beneficial to some patients with angina. Antacids may provide relief in gastrointestinal disease but do not affect cardiac pain. The response of ischemic cardiac pain to nitroglycerin is not specific because esophageal spasm, which often accompanies reflux esophagitis, may be relieved by this drug. Passage of a gallstone or acute cholecystitis and esophageal spasm may produce episodic retrosternal pain, which is easily confused with the acute cardiac pain of prolonged ischemia or infarction.

The differentiation of these conditions is made more difficult because ECG changes may accompany the gastrointestinal disorders and because disease in the gastrointestinal tract may serve as a trigger for acute cardiac events.

Musculoskeletal Pain

The skeletal system may be the source of pain that can be mistaken for angina pectoris. Such pains may originate from arthritis or lesions in the cervical spine, or from intercostal neuritis or myositis. Skeletal pains frequently are brought on or aggravated by exertion. Walking or working with the hands, with the associated motion of the thoracic skeleton, results in pain. The hyperventilation of walking is associated with an increase in the intensity of the pain originating in the chest wall or diaphragm. In contrast to angina pectoris, skeletal pains usually are slow to subside and persist for several hours at a low level of intensity after a bout of activity. Skeletal pain may be present when the patient awakens and before he has gotten out of bed. Angina pectoris appears often while he is washing, shaving, and dressing.

A common cause of chest pain is muscle or ligament strain frequently brought on by unaccustomed exercise and located in the costochondral or chondrosternal junction or chest wall muscles. Localized tenderness is usually present, and the pain is often clearly related to movements involving the painful site. Deep breathing, turning, or twisting, and movements of the shoulder girdle and arm, often will elicit the pain. The discomfort may be brief, lasting for only a few seconds, or it may last for several hours. Therefore it is often possible to distinguish it clearly from angina, which has a duration intermediate between the two extremes. Musculoskeletal pain is often sharp and sticking in the affected site but may extend upward to the shoulder and into the neck. It is aggravated by rotation of the head or forceful downward traction of the shoulder, and there may be associated circulatory disturbances in the arm.

EVALUATION OF THE PATIENT WITH CHEST PAIN

A careful history by an experienced physician is the most important diagnostic test for the patient with chest pain. Information about

TABLE 2.7–1. EPISODIC THORACIC PAIN

Presenting Condition	Symptom
Angina pectoris	Substernal visceral discomfort or distress, provoked by effort, emotion, eating, and, occasionally, by lying down. Relieved by rest and nitroglycerin
Pleural pain	Precipitated by breathing or coughing: usually described as sharp. Associated physical and radiographic findings of pleurisy
Esophageal pain	Burning and substernal, with occasional radiation to the shoulder. Nocturnal occurrence (when lying flat). Relief with food or antacids or sometimes nitroglycerin
Peptic ulcer	Nearly always infradiaphragmatic and epigastric. Nocturnal occurrence and daytime attacks relieved by food. Not worsened by activity
Biliary disease	Usually under right scapula, prolonged in duration. Biliary disease is more important as triggering mechanism for angina than as a mimic
Cervical disc	History of injury is common; may be provoked by activity. Persists after activity is discontinued. Local palpation and movement may produce pain
Arthritis-bursitis	Usually of long (hours) duration. Local tenderness or pain with movement
Hyperventilation	Tingling in circumoral area or hands; anxiety. Usually marked complaints of breathlessness without evidence of lung disease
Chest wall (musculoskeletal)	Provoked by movement, especially twisting, bending, etc. Usually long-lasting and often associated with local tenderness
Psychoneurosis	Virtually always after anxiety; poorly described complaints; inframammary location of pain

the location, character, radiation, duration, and precipitating and alleviating factors of the pain will establish the diagnosis in the majority of patients. There is no correlation between either the duration or the severity of the complaint and the cause of the pain. Although many physicians continue to put great emphasis on the radiation of pain into the left arm or shoulder, this is of limited value in the differential diagnosis, because conditions other than angina pectoris produce such radiation. The physician must not forget that pain provoked by activity and relieved by rest may be caused by shoulder and neck movements during exercise.

Patients with chest pain as a manifestation of an emotional disorder are particularly difficult to evaluate. In depressive reactions and anxiety states, chest pain that may have many features of angina may be a prominent symptom. The physician must be especially careful to establish the proper diagnosis based on objective findings in these patients because the erroneous diagnosis of cardiac disease serves to heighten anxiety, creating a cycle leading to severe cardiac neurosis, worsening depression, and job disability. Early recognition of the functional nature of the pain and appropriate reassurance can alleviate the symptom and improve the

TABLE 2.7–2. DIFFERENTIAL DIAGNOSIS OF ANGINA PECTORIS

	Angina Pectoris	Skeletal Pain	Gastrointestinal Pain
General Features			
Family history	Premature death in male relatives		
Past history	Cigarette smoking, hypertension, hypercholesterolemia, and diabetes	Trauma to neck or back	Indigestion
Onset of illness	Usually certain of month of onset, if not specific day	Uncertain of date of onset	Uncertain of date of onset
Duration of illness	Usually not more than 5 years without objective manifestations (i.e., ECG changes)	May have been present for many years	May have been present for many years and seasonal in occurrence
Individual Attack			
Precipitation	Effort is prime precipitator. Also may come with emotion, food, and, occasionally, on lying down	Skeletal motion or hyperventilation—associated with effort rather than work, per se	Nervous tension and food Relation to effort is vague or absent
Duration	Until effort stops. Disappears in 1–3 min. Patient cannot continue. Must stop	May last many minutes to hours after rest. Patient can continue effort	Variable Up to several hours
Relief	By cessation of effort. Administration of nitroglycerin often, but not always, successful	Change in position, heat, and aspirin	Change in position, eructation, milk, or bowel movement. Nitroglycerin may be effective
Nocturnal attacks	May be awakened from sound sleep. Relief by sitting up Rare in absence of angina of effort	Trouble falling asleep	Early morning hours. Relief by antacid. May never occur in daytime or on exertion
Time of day	More likely soon after arising, shaving, washing. Effort after meals	Worse in evening, especially after day of physical exertion	Anytime. Related to food, recumbency, tension
Season and weather	Less exertion will bring on in cold weather	Worse in winter and damp weather	No relation

emotional state. The occurrence of syndromes such as vasoregulatory asthenia or mitral valve prolapse (Barlow syndrome) with great frequency in anxious patients with cardiac complaints adds to the diagnostic difficulty because electrocardiographic changes at rest or with exercise, cardiac arrhythmias, or abnormal physical findings are frequent in these syndromes and may lend credence to the diagnosis of organic cardiac disease.

Even when ischemic heart disease is present, a second disease process often can be identified to explain certain features of the syndrome that do not fit the diagnosis of angina pectoris. Gastrointestinal disease (especially esophagitis), musculoskeletal disease, and emotional disorders frequently are present in patients who have true angina pectoris.

Physical Examination

Careful observation of the patient during the physical examination may provide information regarding the lability of his cardiovascular system and general emotional status. The deep breathing required for auscultation of the lungs may provoke vague chest complaints. Chest pain due to inflammation of the muscles of respiration can also be provoked by the maneuver and can be clearly differentiated from chest pain of cardiac origin. Variability in blood pressure during the examination indicates lability of cardiovascular control, as does undue cardiac acceleration with a change of position.

Findings of a physical examination of the patient with angina pectoris are usually normal when the patient is free of pain. Hypertension, diabetes, tobacco stains, or obesity, when present, suggests proneness to coronary artery disease. If, during examination, the patient is experiencing an attack of chest pain, cardiac auscultation should be carried out immediately and an ECG obtained. A fourth heart sound, reflecting the altered diastolic compliance of the ventricle, may be present. Systolic murmurs due to papillary muscle dysfunction and a precordial bulge due to localized ventricular dysfunction may appear transiently.

An important point is the reproduction of the pain under observation. This may be accomplished by simple maneuvers during the examination, thereby satisfying both physician and patient that the cause of the pain is known and, in some instances, not serious. Manipulation of the neck and percussion of the spine may reproduce pain of skeletal origin. Palpation of the surface of the thorax also may provide evidence of arthritis or cervical disc disease, myalgia, or costochondritis (Tietze syndrome); on rare occasions it may locate tenderness resulting from neoplastic disease of the ribs. Hyperventilation for 1 to 2 minutes may reproduce chest pain in some anxiety-prone patients. When reproduction of the pain by simple means is not possible, reasonable efforts to provoke it by special procedure, such as exercise stress testing and esophageal perfusion, may be undertaken.

Special Testing in the Evaluation of Chest Pain[15]

The Electrocardiogram with Pain.
An ECG taken during an episode of spontaneous pain provides diagnostic information. The finding of peaked or inverted T waves or ST segment depression or elevation during an episode of pain, followed by the disappearance of these changes after the episode, is evidence for myocardial ischemia. An episode of spontaneous pain at rest with ST segment elevation is presumptive evidence of spasm, whether the vessel is normal or narrowed by atherosclerotic plaque. Conversely, a normal or unaltered ECG obtained during an episode of pain is evidence against the cardiac origin of the pain but does not exclude it.

Exercise Stress Testing.[12]
Exercise stress testing may provide important insights into the cause of chest pain. The study allows the physician to observe the patient under conditions that may reproduce the pain. If the patient reacts casually to the pain or continues to exercise with pain, angina is unlikely because most patients are frightened by anginal discomfort and instinctively stop exercise. The patient may develop severe dyspnea with pain, which may be a clue to advanced coronary disease. The ECG or radioisotope

studies may show objective changes suggesting transient myocardial ischemia (see Chapter 2.1). The absence of such abnormalities may be evidence against a cardiac cause of the pain and may reassure both the patient and the physician. The stress test may provide evidence about the severity of coronary artery disease. Severe coronary obstruction in multiple arteries is suggested by the appearance of chest pain or ECG change at a low work load or heart rate, a fall in blood pressure during exercise, severe ST segment depression (>2 mm), or the appearance of multiple areas of decreased perfusion on thallium testing. Conversely, well-maintained exercise capacity, even in association with anginal pain or ECG changes, indicates a favorable prognosis.

Stress testing is performed frequently in asymptomatic patients as a means of detecting early evidence of coronary artery disease. Although in some cases an abnormal test result may be due to painless myocardial ischemia, in many the ECG abnormalities represent a false-positive response. Before the physician concludes that the patient has coronary artery disease, other confirmatory tests such as a stress test with thallium or even coronary arteriography should be performed.

Coronary Arteriography.
Coronary arteriography is valuable in the study of patients with angina and has a low morbidity rate (2 percent) and mortality rate (about 0.1 percent in adults, and directly related to the severity of the patient's disease and age).

The indications for coronary arteriography vary widely in different centers, depending on the importance put on knowing "the anatomy" (i.e., the number of vessels involved with atherosclerosis and the severity of the narrowings) to determine prognosis and on the enthusiasm for surgery and percutaneous transluminal coronary angioplasty. When the diagnosis of angina pectoris is secure based on historical or electrocardiographic information, when symptoms are stable while the patient is on a good medical regimen, and if performance on an exercise test is good, then medical therapy seems most appropriate; there is little to be gained by arteriographic definition of arterial lesions. On the other hand, even stable symptoms can be "disabling" to active patients, and the gratifying early success in relieving symptoms now being achieved with percutaneous transluminal coronary angioplasty has liberalized the traditional indications for catheterization.

When the cause of chest pain cannot be determined, arteriography may be important either to exclude coronary artery disease in the patient who is being treated for it with insufficient evidence or to establish the diagnosis in the patient with atypical angina. In some patients with established coronary artery disease, particularly those who are very young or those with demanding employment, the need for prognostic information based on arteriographic findings may be an indication for study. Arteriography must be performed in all patients being evaluated for coronary artery bypass surgery.

Current techniques permit good radiologic visualization of both coronary arteries by the selective injection of radiopaque material. Atherosclerotic narrowings and obstructions can be seen and the patterns of epicardial blood flow identified. If narrowings are present, the diagnosis of atherosclerotic coronary artery disease is established. False-positive arteriograms occur rarely, if at all, and may be due to spasm caused by the catheter in an otherwise normal vessel or to inadequate injection of the radiopaque dye, causing areas of underfilling to give the false appearance of a lesion. False-negative arteriograms are possible because a lesion may be located at a site that is not well visualized, such as at the origin of the vessel when the catheter tip might actually be beyond the lesion or at an area where several vessels overlap. In appropriate patients whose coronary arteries initially appear normal, provocative tests for coronary artery spasm may be performed.[8]

The clinical importance of arteriographic findings is sometimes difficult to assess and must be based on a clear understanding that the demonstration of atherosclerotic narrowing does not prove that the patient's symptoms can be attributed to myocardial ischemia. If the arteriographic findings are clearly those of severe

disease, the information is of great value. One can then be certain about the existence of ischemic heart disease and safely attribute the chest pain or electrocardiographic abnormalities to this condition. If the arteriogram reveals only minor or no atherosclerotic changes, the physician must be cautious in his interpretation. Ischemic heart disease is not likely to be present if the arteriogram is normal. However, the method provides adequate visualization of only the large coronary arteries, and the possibility that disease may be present in small vessels cannot be excluded. Small-vessel disease may be the cause of angina in that small group of patients with typical angina pectoris who have an abnormal exercise test result and normal coronary arteries on arteriography. This test must therefore be evaluated along with other clinical and laboratory evidence. Other cardiac causes of the patient's symptoms must be sought if the arteriogram is normal, for example, coronary artery spasm, cardiomyopathy (especially of the hypertrophic form), myocardial bridging, or mitral valve prolapse. Regardless, it should be reassuring that the finding of normal coronary arteries in the patient with angina who does not have spasm is associated with a good prognosis.[9] Unfortunately, some patients are not reassured by a finding of "no cardiac disease" by laboratory tests but continue to be disabled by their chest pain.

Echocardiography. Echocardiography in combination with Doppler ultrasound is useful as an adjunct to the history and physical examination in diagnosing other cardiac conditions that may account for chest pain, such as valvular, pericardial, cardiomyopathic, or congenital abnormalities. It should be emphasized that the presence of these conditions does not preclude the coexistence of coronary artery disease. Their presence may confound the interpretation of an exercise test and may even increase the risks associated with performing it.

Ambulatory ECG Monitoring. It is good practice to obtain an ECG during any episode of pain that occurs while the patient is accessible, such as in the physician's office or on the hospital ward. The fortuitous occurrence of pain in the physician's office is not to be expected. Holter monitoring may be useful in the evaluation of patients with recurrent chest pain that is not reproducibly induced by exertion, namely that due to coronary artery spasm, or in the evaluation of patients with coronary artery disease who have no angina but have come to the physician's attention because of other symptoms, such as syncope, that may be due to ischemia-induced arrhythmias.

AN APPROACH TO EVALUATION AND MANAGEMENT OF PATIENT WITH CHEST PAIN

If the patient has angina pectoris with symptoms during rest or minimal exertion, or if the angina is prolonged, his condition is considered unstable. Medication is therefore begun immediately, and hospitalization may be justified before proceeding. Most patients can be evaluated as outpatients. On the basis of a detailed history, careful physical examination, chest radiograph, and resting ECG, the physician should establish a working diagnosis and categorize the patient's chest pain into one of four general diagnostic groups: (1) angina pectoris, (2) noncardiac pain, (3) cardiac pain related to other cardiac conditions (e.g., mitral valve prolapse, aortic stenosis, hypertrophic cardiomyopathy, pericarditis, or pulmonary hypertension), and (4) chest pain of uncertain cause. Only in a minority of patients will classification be in the last category.

Certain special tests, as discussed earlier, may be of aid in diagnosis, but they should be used judiciously and may not be needed at all. For example, if the patient is elderly and the history is clearly that of angina, it may not be necessary to do any further testing, and therapy can be started immediately. If the pain is noncardiac, tests such as exercise testing may not be helpful and could be misleading if a false-positive result is obtained. When the cause of pain is not readily apparent by initial clinical evaluation, special testing

is useful. If noninvasive testing is not informative, coronary angiography may be needed to determine whether coronary artery disease is present or not. The finding of other cardiac abnormalities does not establish a causal relationship between the abnormality and the symptom of chest pain. For example, mitral valve prolapse is common in the population as is chest pain. The coexistence of the two does not implicate the prolapse as a cause of the chest pain. Epidemiologic studies have established that chest symptoms are no more common in patients with prolapse than in those without this abnormality. Patients who have nonischemic chest pains and evidence of mitral prolapse should not be told that they have a cardiac disorder that is the cause of their chest complaints. This only heightens the patient's anxiety about his symptom.

THERAPY FOR ANGINA PECTORIS

GENERAL THERAPEUTIC MEASURES

The goals of therapy are to improve the quality and duration of life for a patient with a chronic disease. Before the physician considers specific therapy, it is important to emphasize the need for a strong patient-physician relationship, the benefit of modifying risk factors to improve the long-term prognosis, and the possible role of noncardiac disease in exacerbating angina pectoris.

The patient with angina pectoris needs a physician who will see him repeatedly and help him adjust to his disease. A single visit with an abbreviated diagnostic and prognostic summary is inadequate and may do great harm. The physician must be sure of his diagnosis and must not convey to the patient any doubts he may have. If the diagnosis is in doubt, further study is indicated. Other causes of thoracic pain must be excluded as primary or contributing causes. The patient must be taught to recognize the pains that are of cardiac origin and to realize that not every chest pain he may experience is the result of cardiac disease. Sometimes the majority of the pains experienced by a patient with proved angina pectoris are caused by musculoskeletal factors or esophagitis, and simple measures directed at these conditions may reduce the number of attacks.

The physician must emphasize that the prognosis is not necessarily poor, especially considering recent advances in medical therapy, coupled with a growing understanding of when it is most appropriate to use invasive therapy.

The ideal treatment for angina pectoris is one that would bring about the regression of the atheromatous lesions or the elimination of coronary artery spasm. The basic cause of atherosclerosis and spasm are unknown, but a number of factors are known to increase the risk of development and progression of ischemic heart disease and can be modified (see Chapter 2.8). These include high concentrations of serum cholesterol, hypertension, sedentary lifestyle, type A personality, and cigarette smoking. The patient must be taught that he can have an impact on the long-term course of his disease through modification of risk factors.

There is now evidence that reduction of hyperlipidema,[10] cessation of smoking, and control of hypertension improve prognosis. It is therefore essential that the patient give up cigarette smoking, and the physician should not equivocate on this recommendation. Weight reduction is beneficial but often difficult to achieve in middle-aged, sedentary individuals. Weight reduction in combination with a diet and drug therapy, when appropriate for the underlying lipid disorder, will help to reduce blood lipids. Control of blood pressure by weight loss, dietary sodium restriction, or drugs may reduce the frequency of anginal attacks and may retard progression of atherosclerosis. Most physicians believe that the relationship between the risk factors and disease is so strong that every reasonable effort should be made to eliminate risk factors whenever possible. Correction is therefore recommended when it can be effected by measures that are not hazardous. The patient with angina pectoris should be encouraged to engage in moderate exercise,

such as regular walking. As his tolerance increases, he may be permitted to engage in a sport that does not produce pain or to pursue light jogging, swimming, or cycling.

Effort capacity may improve as a result of regular exercise, and the patient's general state of well-being and confidence will also increase. Generalizations cannot be made about management, and each patient should be encouraged to establish, within his limitations, a program of activity that is as nearly normal as possible. To help the intelligent patient avoid attacks, an explanation of myocardial blood flow in terms of supply and demand will be useful; for others, simpler explanations must be provided. In any event, patients must learn that effort provokes and rest relieves the pain of angina pectoris; that effort in the cold or after eating is often less well tolerated; that more work can be tolerated if it is undertaken slowly; and that he must avoid situations that require that he hurry. Other important measures include reduction in work involvement, avoidance of fatigue, and allowance of increased time for rest and pleasurable, relaxing activities.

SPECIFIC MEASURES IN THE TREATMENT OF ANGINA PECTORIS

Faced with a patient with recent-onset angina or one who shows a changing pattern of pain, the physician should be alert to precipitating factors that may be responsible for increasing myocardial oxygen needs or decreasing supply (see p. 88). For example, hyperthyroidism or the administration of thyroid hormone to patients with myxedema may be responsible for worsening anginal pain. In diabetic patients who are taking insulin, hypoglycemic episodes may precipitate angina attacks, particularly at night. The production of angina by paroxysmal arrhythmias may mask other symptoms (e.g., palpitations) that would more directly lead to the diagnosis of the arrhythmia itself. Worsening angina may reflect increasing left ventricular dilation consequent to left ventricular failure, as in some cases of angina decubitus. Cardiomegaly may be a clue to such a mechanism. Such patients often improve with digitalization and diuretic therapy. It is not often appreciated that the balance between oxygen supply and demand in the myocardium may be so tenuous that a small reduction in the blood hemoglobin level (i.e., reduction of hematocrit by 5 or 6 points) may account for worsening angina. Such a change may be a clue to occult gastrointestinal blood loss, often from a large-bowel carcinoma. Erythrocytosis, of even modest degree, also may aggravate ischemia if the increased viscosity causes decreased blood flow.

In addition to correcting abnormalities extrinsic to the heart, therapy is initiated to minimize the adverse effects of the intrinsic coronary artery abnormality—coronary spasm or fixed atherosclerotic disease—by means of medical therapy, percutaneous transluminal coronary angioplasty (PTCA), and coronary artery bypass surgery (CABS). The goals of therapy to relieve symptoms and prolong life, must be kept in mind as decisions regarding therapy are made. Each therapy has certain benefits and carries certain risks that must be understood to make rational decisions, and these benefits and risks will be discussed specifically in the following sections of this chapter. However, the first step in choosing the most appropriate long-term therapy for a given patient is to use the clinical and anatomic information, as described above and in Table 2.7–3, to establish the patient's prognosis in general terms.[15] This is important because there is evidence to indicate that for some groups of patients with angina, prognosis can be improved by surgical treatment whether symptoms are severe or not. The major factor adversely affecting prognosis is the degree of impairment of left ventricular function. This can be assessed clinically by looking for evidence of previous myocardial infarction by ECG, for evidence of cardiomegaly by radiographic or physical examination, for poor exercise capacity, or, in advanced stages, for evidence of pulmonary congestion. More specific evidence may be obtained by assessing the function of the left ventricle by echocardiography,

TABLE 2.7–3. FACTORS ADVERSELY AFFECTING PROGNOSIS IN CORONARY ARTERY DISEASE

Severity of left ventricular dysfunction
- Previous myocardial infarction
- Cardiomegaly
- Poor treadmill performance
- Congestive heart failure
- Poor LV function on ventriculography

Severity of ischemia
- Easily provoked, severe, or prolonged symptoms
- Dyspnea associated with angina
- Resting ECG changes
- Exercise test: Low work load, low heart rate hypotension, severe ST segment depression or elevation
- Multiple, large, or long-lasting perfusion defects on radionuclide study with exercise
- Left main coronary artery disease
- Multiple vessel disease
- Proximal left anterior descending coronary artery disease

Associated noncardiac problems
- Advancing age
- Hypertension
- Diabetes
- Uncontrolled hyperlipidema or continued cigarette smoking

radionuclide angiography, or contrast ventriculography. If left ventricular function is normal, the prognosis is generally good. A second important determinant of prognosis, which is independent of ventricular function, is the severity of myocardial ischemia. This may be manifested by frequent or prolonged ischemic symptoms or ECG changes at rest. During stress testing, short duration of exercise, a low heart rate at onset of symptoms, a fall in blood pressure, and severe ST segment depression are indicative of severe ischemia. Coronary angiography provides more precise anatomic information about the extent of disease responsible for ischemia. Patients with involvement of the left main coronary artery, obstructive disease in all major arteries, or disease in the proximal anterior descending artery have a worsened outlook. In addition, noncardiac factors (e.g., increased age) and associated medical problems (e.g., hypertension or diabetes) affect prognosis adversely. For most patients, prognosis can be adequately determined on the basis of clinical findings and stress test results, with the addition of coronary arteriography allowing more precise definition.

The decision to recommend surgical therapy is based primarily on two major questions: First, can surgery prolong life expectancy over that with medications alone? Second, is the patient incapacitated by his symptoms despite maximally tolerated medical therapy? Regarding the first question, randomized studies, to date, have shown that regardless of symptoms, CABS is superior to medical therapy for prolonging life in patients with left main coronary artery stenosis of 50 percent or greater and in patients with three-vessel coronary artery disease who have abnormal left ventricular function. The role of PTCA will be discussed below, but it may be thought of as an alternative to surgical therapy for some patients who have had an inadequate response to medical therapy. No randomized trial has yet been done to determine the efficacy of PTCA on long-term prognosis. Patients with mild to moderate angina, with single-, double-, or triple-vessel CAD, or with normal left ventricular function have not shown improved survival time as a result of surgery. Furthermore no randomized study has shown that bypass surgery prevents myocardial infarction in these patients. Many patients live long and fruitful lives after the onset of angina pectoris on medical therapy alone. Patients with angina who have a normal ECG at rest and normal blood pressure have shown an expected yearly mortality rate of 1.6 percent, which is only slightly different from that of healthy age-matched control subjects.

MEDICAL THERAPY

The discussion presented above clearly shows the importance of an adequate trial of medical therapy in most patients. This can only be accomplished if the physician has knowledge about the specific medications to be used. They include three groups: nitrates, beta blockers, and calcium-channel antagonists.

The goal of medical therapy for angina pectoris can be appreciated by a review of Figure 2.7–1. The balance between myocardial oxygen demand and supply by means of coronary artery blood flow can be improved by either decreasing demand or increasing supply. Table 2.7–4 summarizes the effects of medical therapy on the factors that affect supply and demand. The medications in common use act primarily by decreasing demand, although calcium-channel blocking agents and nitrates can increase supply in situations where there is coronary artery spasm and are therefore the treatment of choice for this problem.[3] Ideally, therapy should be directed at the prevention of myocardial ischemia and not just at the relief of pain. As previously discussed in this chapter, not all ischemia is manifested as symptoms. The patient may be rendered asymptomatic by any of several programs, but the absence of symptoms alone does not mean that the probability of death or myocardial infarction will be reduced by the therapeutic measures, because ischemia may be still occurring. Thus it may be beneficial to determine objectively the efficacy of therapy in preventing or minimizing ischemia by using exercise testing or ambulatory monitoring.

Nitrates

Nitroglycerin. It is probable that the most important action of nitroglycerin is reduction of the work of the heart by diminishing ventricular wall stress. Left ventricular volume is reduced as a result of peripheral venous dilation and, to a lesser extent, by a drop in arterial pressure.

Patients with angina pectoris usually learn to control the number of attacks by modifying the amount and speed of physical exertion and avoiding tension-inducing experiences. When attacks cannot be avoided in this way, nitroglycerin is recommended. Patients should be encouraged to use it freely and not avoid its use; it does no harm to take the drug unnecessarily for an attack that would have passed without it. Occasionally, mild attacks that might have been aborted by the use of nitroglycerin become severe.

Nitroglycerin taken prophylactically may permit greater effort without angina. For example, it may be taken before facing a stressful business situation, before physical exertion, or before sexual intercourse. The effect may be maintained for 20 to 30 minutes.

The effective dose of nitroglycerin must be determined by experiment, since there is variability from patient to patient and in the same patient from time to time. The usual dose is 0.4 mg taken sublingually, but some physicians prefer to start with a smaller dose to avoid the unpleasant side effects at the beginning of therapy. The dose should be adjusted upward if pain is not relieved and there are no adverse effects, such as a significant drop in blood pressure or headache. It may be advisable to have the patient seated during the initial trial of the drug. The hemodynamic, and hence the therapeutic, actions of the drug are dependent on the effect of

gravity; the medication will therefore have less effect if the patient lies down. If the initial dose (0.4 mg) results in uncomfortable headaches and flushing, it should be adjusted downward because a smaller dose may be just as effective in relieving pain. Some patients will not get relief with 0.4 mg, and a regular dose of 0.6 mg may be required. Contrary to what patients often fear, the drug usually does not lose effectiveness with frequent use. When a dose that formerly relieved attacks suddenly becomes ineffective, it is likely that the drug has deteriorated. To ensure potency, patients should be advised to carry at least a daily supply and to replace unused tablets every few weeks from a bottle that is kept in a cool, dark place. A slight tingling under the tongue usually accompanies the use of a tablet that is still potent. A recently released aerosol formulation is available that will deliver the equivalent of a 0.4-mg-tablet dose by being sprayed under the tongue. Clinical experience will determine whether it is a viable alternative to the tablet.

Occasionally, even potent nitroglycerin in adequate amounts fails to relieve what the patient interprets as an attack of angina pectoris. He should be warned that if chest pain is not relieved by two or three tablets within a 15-minute period, his chest pain may be due to a myocardial infarction and he should seek his physician's advice before taking more medication. Rarely, the drug not only fails to relieve pain but actually seems to make it worse. This paradoxical effect is probably due to exaggerated splanchnic pooling or to an exaggerated fall in systemic blood pressure and may be circumvented if the patient lies down before taking the medication.

Long-acting Nitrates.[16] Nitroglycerin may be administered as a 2 percent ointment that is applied to the skin. Absorption through the skin is slower than through the mucous membranes, and the therapeutic action may persist for up to 6 hours. The dose must be determined by trial and error in each patient and is measured in inches of ointment squeezed from a tube. Nitroglycerin ointment is especially useful in the management of nocturnal angina. An application at bedtime may make it possible for the patient to sleep throughout the night. The patient should apply the ointment gently, because vigorous rubbing may lead to intense headache and a shortened duration of action. Other topical nitrate preparations use a membrane that permits continuous absorption through the skin over a 24-hour period. These patch formulations have the advantage of convenience, but their sustained efficacy at this interval at the present dose is under question. Furthermore, all long-acting nitrates, used continuously, may produce tolerance that decreases the clinical efficacy after the first few hours of use.

Long-acting effects of other nitrates, such as erythrityl tetranitrate or isosorbide dinitrate, occur when the drugs are administered in chewable or sublingual form so that absorption through the buccal mucosa may occur. More prolonged action may follow oral administration in patients who require large doses of the drugs because of metabolism by the liver. The therapeutic effects are maximal in 20 to 30 minutes and may persist beyond 2 to 3 hours. Although some patients may find benefit from routine administration of the drug every 4 to 6 hours, others will achieve maximal efficacy by taking the drug in anticipation of activities and repeat-

TABLE 2.7–4. EFFECTS OF MEDICATIONS ON MYOCARDIAL OXYGEN SUPPLY AND DEMAND

| | Nitrates | Beta Blockers | Ca Antagonists | | |
			Nifedipine	Diltiazem	Verapamil
Demand					
Contractile state	—	↓	↑	↓	↓↓
Heart rate	↑	↓	↑	↓	↓↓
Wall stress	↓	↓	↓↓	↓	↓
Supply					
General coronary artery tone	↓	↑	↓↓	↓	↓
Focal coronary artery spasm	↓	↑	↓↓	↓	↓

ing the dosage every 2 hours if increased activity levels persist. In patients with unstable angina, it is effective to combine 2-hourly administrations of a chewable or sublingual nitrate with the use of nitroglycerin ointment.

Beta-blocking Agents[4]

The physiologic effect of catecholamines is mediated through two types of cell-surface adrenergic receptors, alpha and beta, which are distinguished by their relative affinities for the different types of catecholamines. Alpha-adrenergic receptors have more affinity for epinephrine and norepinephrine than for isoproterenol; the affinity is opposite in the case of beta-adrenergic receptors. The alpha-adrenergic receptor is found mostly in vascular smooth muscle, where it initiates vasoconstriction. The beta-adrenergic receptor has two subtypes, beta-1, and beta-2. The ventricular myocardium receptors are almost exclusively beta-1 and initiate increases in heart rate and contractility, whereas beta-2 receptors are found as part of the atrial receptors and exclusively in bronchial and vascular smooth muscle, where stimulation initiates bronchodilation and vasodilation, respectively.

Beta blockers bind to the cell surface beta-adrenergic receptors, where they inhibit the binding, and therefore the action, of catecholamines. Thus their therapeutic action is to reduce myocardial oxygen demands primarily by decreasing heart rate and ventricular contractility, particularly during exercise, when catechol levels rise, by the competitive inhibition of beta-adrenergic receptor sites in the ventricular myocardium. Beta blockers also lower blood pressure through an uncertain mechanism that may include a combination of lowered cardiac output, the inhibition of renin release, and a direct central nervous system effect in lowering sympathetic nerve discharge to the peripheral vasculature. Thus exercise performance improves after the use of beta-adrenergic blocking drugs because the response of the combination of factors that increase oxygen demand (heart rate, contractility, and systolic pressure) to any given level of exercise is reduced. The result is a delay in the appearance of the critical level of oxygen demand at which angina appears. The beta-adrenergic blocking drugs are usually used in combination with nitrates and calcium-channel antagonists. Most patients will show dramatic improvement in angina after beta-ad-

renergic receptor in initiating vasoconstriction in peripheral vessels. able to resume nearly normal activities while remaining free of pain. All available formulations have equivalent antianginal effects but different pharmacologic properties regarding pharmacokinetics, receptor cardioselectivity, intrinsic sympathetic activity, and membrane-stabilizing activity that yields a quinidine-like antiarrhythmic activity. These properties offer different dosing strategies in patients who are more likely to suffer side effects from a given formulation. These properties are discussed below and outlined in Table 2.7–5.

Pharmacokinetics are determined by whether the beta-blocking drug is more lipid or more water soluble. Solubility in lipids is exhibited by propranolol, pindolol, and metoprolol. These preparations are metabolized rapidly (short-acting), cross the blood-brain barrier poorly (fewer central nervous system effects), and are excreted mostly by the kidney.

"Cardioselectivity" means that the particular drug blocks primarily the beta-adrenergic receptor of the heart, the beta-1 receptor. This characteristic is relative, however, rather than absolute. Thus the cardioselective, or beta-1 selective, drugs (atenolol and metoprolol) are less likely to cause bronchoconstriction or peripheral vasoconstriction than are nonselective (i.e., beta-1 and beta-2) blocking drugs. In patients with asthma, however, even the relatively cardioselective agents can cause enough inhibition of the bronchodilatory effects of the beta-2 receptor to "induce" bronchospasm. Similarly, in the peripheral vasculature, beta-1 blocking drugs may be better than drugs that block both beta-1 and beta-2 receptors but may still cause enough inhibition of the beta-2 vasodilatory effect to leave unopposed the effect of the alpha-adrenergic receptor in initiating vasoconstriction in peripheral vessels. This may not be a problem in patients when antianginal therapy includes other drugs that are vasodilators (e.g., nifedipine). A recently available preparation, labetalol, combines beta blockade with alpha blockade and has an obvious advantage in patients unable to tolerate beta blockade alone.

"Intrinsic sympathomimetic activity" means that the drug initiates some stimulation of the receptor to which it is binding. Beta blockers with this characteristic simulate the effect of catecholamines at rest but exhibit beta-blocking properties during exercise.

TABLE 2.7–5. PHARMACOLOGIC PROPERTIES OF BETA BLOCKERS

Name	Usual Total Daily Dosage (mg)	No. of Doses Per Day	Half-Life (hr)	Excretion	Lipophilicity[a]	Cardioselectivity
Propranolol[b] (Inderal)	80–360	1–4	1–6[c]	Hepatic	High	No
Metoprolol (Lopressor)	50–200	1–2	2–4[c]	Hepatic	Moderate	Yes
Atenolol (Tenormin)	25–200	1–2	6–9	Renal	Low	Yes
Nadolol (Corgard)	20–320	1	16–24	Renal	Low	No
Timolol (Blocadren)	10–40	2	4–6	Hepatic and renal	Low	No
Pindolol[d] (Visken)	7.5–22.5	3	3–4	Renal and hepatic	Moderate	No
Acebutolol[d] (Sectral)	400–1200	2–4	3	Hepatic and renal	Moderate	Yes
Labetalol[d,e] (Normodyne or Trandate)	300–1200	3	6–8	Renal and hepatic	Low	No

[a]Determined on the basis of relative solubility in lipid relative to water.
[b]Membrane-stabilizing activity.
[c]Longer-acting preparation available.
[d]Intrinsic sympathomimetic activity.
[e]Alpha-adrenergic receptor blockade.

This characteristic may be useful in patients who have resting brady-cardia or marginal ventricular function—and who therefore may benefit from a faster resting heart rate or the effect of adrenergic stimulation on contractility at rest—but in whom exertion induces ischemia, which causes cardiac function to deteriorate.

The role of membrane stabilization is unclear and probably is not achieved by clinically applied doses.

The side effects of beta blockade are predictable because of the blunting of the effects of catecholamines: lassitude and depression in patients with a predisposition to the side effect; bronchocon-striction; vasoconstriction (vasospastic angina if it affects the coro-nary artery and Raynaud phenomenon or exacerbation of periph-eral vascular disease if it affects the peripheral vasculature); impotence; "masking" or worsening of insulin-induced hypogly-cemic episodes; and worsening heart failure and heart block. The drugs must be used cautiously, if at all, when these conditions are anticipated, and certain precautions, such as the use of a pacemaker in a patient with bradyarrhythmia or digitalis and diuretics in the patient with poor ventricular function, should be considered. The condition of some such patients with congestive heart failure and severe angina may improve if small doses of beta-blocking drugs are combined with digitalis and diuretics because the positive effects of relieving ischemia are greater than the negative effects on contrac-tility in maintaining overall cardiac function. An additional "side effect" has to do with reports of severe myocardial ischemia after abrupt withdrawal of beta blockers; withdrawal should therefore be gradual or closely supervised.

Calcium-Channel Blocking Drugs[3]
Intracellular calcium plays a key role in initiating vasoconstriction, increases in heart rate, and increases in cardiac contractility. Cal-cium enters the cells of vascular smooth muscle, cardiac conduc-tion pathways, and contractile tissue through membrane channels. These channels, which are controlled by electrical activity (action potentials), other ions (sodium and perhaps potassium), and neurotransmitters (catecholamines, acetylcholine), can be blocked and intracellular calcium levels lowered by the calcium-channel blocking drugs. A decrease in calcium levels, in turn, results in vasodilation, slowed heart rate, and reduced contractility. In addi-tion, by an unknown mechanism, these drugs decrease oxygen de-mand on the heart for a given work load at a given heart rate. Thus a higher work load is possible before angina occurs, and in this respect, they act much like beta-blocking drugs in benefiting the exercising patient through an "oxygen sparing" effect.

Nifedipine, verapamil, and diltiazem are presently available calcium-channel blockers, but new formulations are being evalu-ated. At clinically tolerated oral doses of 10 to 30 mg three or four times a day, nifedipine is the most potent dilator of systemic and coronary arteries; verapamil, 80 to 120 mg given orally three or four times a day, is the most potent at slowing heart rate and de-creasing oxygen demand. Diltiazem, given at doses of 30 to 90 mg orally three or four times a day, can be viewed as a compromise, yielding less vasodilation than nifedipine but more than verapamil and less heart rate slowing and oxygen sparing than verapamil but more than nifedipine. The side effects of nifedipine relate to vaso-dilation: headache, flushing, hypotension, peripheral edema. Hy-potension is exacerbated by nitrates and is most pronounced in the dehydrated patient. The worst side effect of verapamil is conduc-tion block, especially of the atrioventricular node, and verapamil should be avoided or its use monitored carefully in patients with conduction abnormalities. Verapamil and, to a lesser and variable extent, diltiazem increase serum digoxin concentration by lower-ing renal clearance. Thus digoxin dosage should be lowered by about 50 percent and levels monitored when given with verapamil or diltiazem. Diltiazem has similar but less severe side effects than verapamil and, along with verapamil, may cause constipation. All three drugs are negatively inotropic, but this effect is least notice-able for nifedipine, where the decrease in blood pressure provides an afterload reduction that permits maintenance of cardiac output.

The differing clinical effects offer a rationale for combining nifedipine with either diltiazem or verapamil. The latter two drugs have effects similar to beta blockers and, in fact, have been com-pared favorably to beta blockers as single agents in the treatment of angina pectoris.[6]

Other Pharmacologic Agents
Inspection of Figure 2.7–1 will aid understanding of the mecha-nism of action of cardiac glycosides and diuretics in the treatment of angina. Left ventricular dysfunction may be improved by cardiac glycosides and the ventricular volume and wall stress decreased. Diuretics operate by decreasing plasma volume, ventricular vol-ume, and wall stress. Diuretics may have an additional beneficial effect by lowering elevated blood pressure, thus reducing oxygen consumption. Cardiac glycosides and diuretics are especially useful in patients with nocturnal angina. Additional measures that may be helpful in this particular type of angina are salt restriction and sleeping with the head of the bed elevated. Digitalis is also useful in slowing the ventricular rate in atrial fibrillation and preventing supraventricular tachycardia. Aspirin inhibits platelet-mediated vasoconstriction and coagulation and thus has a rationale in man-agement of angina as an adjunct to other regimens. Further study is required before its use in stable angina is established.

PERCUTANEOUS TRANSLUMINAL CORONARY ANGIOPLASTY[5]

In those patients in whom there is no clear indication that CABS will prolong life (see discussion above), PTCA has been employed to relieve symptoms when medical therapy is unsatisfactory.

PTCA is accomplished by engaging the coronary artery ostium with a catheter, called a guiding catheter, by means of a technique similar to that used for routine arteriography. The site of the lesion is identified by injection of radiopaque contrast solution, and then a small, flexible, balloon-tipped catheter is inserted through the guiding catheter and down into the diseased vessel to bridge the site of stenosis with the balloon. The balloon is inflated to com-press the material within the lesion, fracture the atherosclerotic plaque, and stretch the artery. The ideal candidate for successful PTCA is a patient with symptoms of recent onset (6 months) that are refractory to medical therapy and that are caused by a single, proximal, noncalcified lesion. Success at significantly reducing the lesion in these patients is close to 90 percent; however, 20 to 30 percent will return to their predilation severity of stenosis in the first year and require a second procedure. The complication rate includes a fraction of a percent for mortality (0.2 in the first 2000 patients done by the originator of the technique, Dr. Andreas Gruentzig) and 1 to 2 percent for acute infarction requiring emer-gency bypass surgery. The importance of surgical backup in the overall safety of the patient cannot be overstated when it is consid-ered that another 4 to 5 percent may require urgent surgery when angioplasty results in worsening of the lesion without total occlu-sion. Patients are treated with antiplatelet agents and calcium-channel antagonists after the procedure and followed up with either repeat angiography or exercise testing. Long-term patency is being evaluated and appears to be maintained in most patients. PTCA may be employed in selected patients with multivessel dis-ease or occlusions in bypass grafts. For example, in a patient who has had an inferior infarction as a result of right coronary artery occlusion, dilation of a lesion in the left anterior descending coro-nary artery may alleviate postinfarction angina. The precise indica-tion for PTCA will be better understood after randomized clinical trials are done.

CORONARY ARTERY BYPASS SURGERY[1,2]

Most patients undergo coronary bypass surgery for relief of symp-toms, usually after medical therapy has been tried but has not been successful or well tolerated by the patient. Some patients without severe symptoms but with disease of the left main artery or severe

disease in multiple vessels undergo surgery to improve prognosis, particularly if there has been previous damage to the left ventricle.

Bypass is accomplished by using segments of saphenous vein to connect the aorta to the distal coronary artery beyond the stenosis or by creating an anastomosis between the distal end of the internal mammary artery and the coronary artery beyond the stenosis. The operative mortality rate approaches 1 percent in centers with wide experience with the procedure. Enhanced myocardial blood flow is the mechanism of improvement in a large proportion of patients, but other mechanisms, such as intraoperative infarction of ischemic myocardium or denervation, may be responsible, in part, in some patients.

Patients with diffuse atheromatous disease extending to the distal coronary arteries or patients with small vessels, apparently an important factor in the poorer results for women, are less likely to have a successful operation. Older subjects also have poorer results. Recent studies indicate that anginal symptoms may return in 5 percent of patients a year after successful bypass surgery, and that the rate of disease progression in the grafts is accelerated with time, so that at 10 years more than 50 percent will be severely diseased.[1] This indicates that for many, and perhaps all, this form of therapy represents a useful but temporary palliation of myocardial ischemia in the natural history of a lifelong disorder. Graft patency is improved by using the internal mammary artery when feasible (90 percent patency at 10 years) and by the use of antiplatelet agents, aspirin and dipyridamole.

It should be emphasized that most studies comparing medical and surgical therapy have focused on the ability of each to prolong life. The quality of life is also an important factor, and frequently medical therapy fails in this regard. CABS has been repeatedly shown to improve the quality of life in those patients in whom medical therapy failed. However, it should not be undertaken with the assumption that risk-factor modification can be neglected or that CABS ensures a long-term solution or cure. The risk of myocardial infarction remains unchanged by CABS, but there is some evidence that the infarction may be smaller if it does occur.

When stenosis develops in functioning bypass grafts, angioplasty may be an effective means of reestablishing patency. Repeat operations are possible, but the success rate declines and the mortality rate increases with each additional operation.

MANAGEMENT OF UNSTABLE ANGINA PECTORIS[7,11,13]

Patients with unstable angina should be treated in a hospital with close monitoring. In many instances, hospitalization and rest alone will restore stability because the patient is removed from a stressful home or work situation. Other patients will require intensive triple drug therapy with nitrates, calcium-channel antagonists, and beta blockers, which may be instituted rapidly, depending on the clinical need. Intravenous nitrates and heparin may be helpful. Nitrates are particularly important because they reduce myocardial oxygen demands and also may prevent coronary artery spasm, which may play an important role in producing pain in this syndrome. Aspirin may also be beneficial. In most cases, intensive medical therapy

will be effective in controlling the attacks. Because the short-term prognosis for such patients is excellent, emergency arteriography or surgery is not indicated, although most patients should have arteriography at some point. In patients whose condition is refractory to these measures, intraaortic balloon counterpulsation will provide relief of pain and allow arteriography to be performed safely. If symptoms do not abate with medical treatment that can be given on an ambulatory basis, or if angina becomes incapacitating with resumption of activity, coronary arteriography is indicated to determine whether coronary artery obstructions are amenable to PTCA or CABS.

REFERENCES

1. Bonow RO, Epstein SE: Indications for coronary artery bypass surgery in patients with chronic angina pectoris: Implications of the multicenter randomized trials. Circulation 72(suppl 5):23, 1985
2. Bourassa MG, Fisher LD, et al: Long-term fate of bypass grafts: The Coronary Artery Surgery Study (CASS) and Montreal Heart Institute experiences. Circulation 72(suppl 5):71, 1985
3. Conti CR, Pepine CJ, et al: Calcium antagonists. Cardiology 72:297, 1985
4. Frishman WH: Clinical differences between beta-adrenergic blocking agents: Implications for therapeutic substitution. Am Heart J 113:1190, 1987
5. Gruentzig AR, King SB III, et al: Long-term follow-up after percutaneous transluminal coronary angioplasty: The early Zurich experience. N Engl J Med 316:1127, 1987
6. Humen DP, O'Brien P, et al: Effort angina with adequate beta-receptor blockade: Comparison with diltiazem alone and in combination. J Am Coll Cardiol 7:329, 1986
7. Kaplan K, Davison R, et al: Intravenous nitroglycerin for the treatment of angina at rest unresponsive to standard nitrate therapy. Am J Cardiol 51:694, 1983
8. Kaski JC, Crea F, et al: Local coronary supersensitivity to diverse vasoconstrictive stimuli in patients with variant angina. Circulation 74:1255, 1986
9. Kemp HG, Kronmal RA, et al: Seven-year survival of patients with normal or near normal coronary arteriograms: A CASS Registry Study. J Am Coll Cardiol 71:479, 1986
10. The Lipid Research Clinics Coronary Primary Prevention Trial Results. II. The relationship of reduction in incidence of coronary heart disease to cholesterol lowering. JAMA 251:36, 1984
11. Luchi RJ, Scott SM, et al: Comparison of medical and surgical treatment for unstable angina pectoris: Results of a Veterans Administration cooperative study. N Engl J Med 316:977, 1987
12. McNeer JF, Margolis JR, et al: The role of the exercise test in the evaluation of patients with ischemic heart disease. Circulation 57:64, 1978
13. Rahimtoola SH: Unstable angina: Current status. Mod Concepts Cardiovasc Dis 54:19, 1985
14. Ross RS: Pathophysiology of the coronary circulation. The Sir Thomas Lewis Lecture. Br Heart J 33:173, 1971
15. Silverman KJ, Grossman W: Angina pectoris: Natural history and strategies for evaluation and management. N Engl J Med 310:1712, 1984
16. Thadani U, Fung JL, et al: Oral isosorbide dinitrate in angina pectoris: Comparison of duration of action and dose-response relation during acute and sustained therapy. Am J Cardiol 49:411, 1982

Acute Myocardial Infarction
Alan D. Guerci and Myron L. Weisfeldt

As many as 1 million acute myocardial infarctions (MIs) occur annually in the United States. Approximately one third of these are fatal, with the majority of deaths occurring before the patient reaches a hospital. Acute MI is the most common cause of death in the United States.

PATHOGENESIS

ATHEROSCLEROSIS AND THROMBOSIS

Thrombotic occlusion of atherosclerotic lesions of coronary arteries is the proximate pathogenetic event in nearly all acute transmural MIs.[7] Spasm of coronary arteries and coronary artery embolism also account for some infarcts,[21] and an even smaller number are the result of congenital anomalies of the coronary circulation. Thrombosis superimposed on inflammatory or proliferative arteritides, as in certain connective tissue diseases or in secondary syphilis, is a rare cause of acute MI.

Coronary atherosclerosis is primarily a disease of the proximal and mid-portions of the large epicardial vessels. Coronary angiograms obtained in the first 4 hours after the onset of transmural infarction demonstrate total occlusion of the infarct-related artery by thrombus in approximately 85 percent of cases and subtotal occlusions in most of the remaining 15 percent.[7] When thrombolytic therapy is successful in dissolving the infarct-related thrombus, a tight coronary stenosis, with 70 to 99 percent reduction in luminal diameter, generally persists. Thus MI usually occurs when an atherosclerotic narrowing is already advanced. Finally, acute MI is a marker for multivessel coronary artery disease. The majority of survivors of a first MI have a >50 percent stenosis in one or both of the remaining two large epicardial coronary arteries.[29,32]

The factors that promote thrombosis of coronary atheromas are not fully characterized. Ulceration or rupture of plaques, with exposure of collagen and other thrombogenic tissue factors, is known to occur; and it is likely that the turbulent flow and stasis distal to tight coronary stenoses are conducive to platelet aggregation and fibrin deposition.[9]

PATHOPHYSIOLOGY

The consequences of acute MI are dependent on the size and location of an infarct. Infarct size, in turn, is determined by the size of the ischemic region and the intensity and duration of the ischemia. Thus it is appropriate to review the anatomy of the coronary vessels and those factors which govern myocellular viability.

CORONARY ARTERY ANATOMY

The left main coronary artery ordinarily supplies blood to about 70 percent of the left ventricle. Clinicopathologic correlations indicate that an acute MI involving more than 40 percent of the left ventricle causes intolerable mechanical dysfunction, with cardiogenic shock and death in the majority of cases. Thus, in the absence of extensive collateral flow from the right coronary artery, acute occlusion of the left main coronary artery has immediate and devastating effects on contractility. Death may occur within seconds.

The left anterior descending coronary artery is usually the largest of the three coronary arteries. It carries blood to the anterior free wall, the anterior half (or more) of the septum, and variable amounts of the lateral wall (Fig. 2.8–1). Thus the left anterior descending artery typically perfuses 40 to 50 percent of the left ventricle, and proximal anterior descending occlusions are often lethal. The left anterior descending artery also perfuses the bundle of His and the initial portions of the right and left bundles as they traverse the high part of the septum. In addition to pump failure, intraventricular conduction disturbances and complete heart block (resulting from block beyond the atrioventricular [A-V] node) commonly result from proximal occlusions of the left anterior descending artery.

The circumflex coronary artery, which also arises from the left main coronary artery, carries blood to the posterior wall, variable amounts of the lateral wall, and variable amounts of the inferior wall. In general, the circumflex artery is not a large vessel, and circumflex occlusions are usually well tolerated. Involvement of the posterior papillary muscle may cause severe mitral regurgitation, however, and in occasional patients in whom the circumflex perfuses most or all of the inferior wall (so-called left dominant circulation), circumflex occlusion may cause severe pump failure.

The right coronary artery supplies the right ventricle; variable amounts of the inferior septum, inferior free wall, and posterolateral wall; and, in approximately 90 percent of persons, the A-V node. As in the case of the circumflex coronary artery, the right coronary artery usually perfuses a less than critical amount of left ventricular myocardium, and right coronary occlusions do not ordinarily result in severe left ventricular dysfunction. Right coronary occlusions more commonly cause heart block or extensive right ventricular dysfunction.

ISCHEMIA AND NECROSIS

The heart possesses only a limited capacity to withstand ischemia. Animal studies and more limited data from human subjects indicate that necrosis consequent to total occlusion of a coronary artery is usually complete in 4 to 6 hours. Animal models also suggest that perfusion must remain above approximately 40 percent of preocclusion levels for the ischemic tissue to survive.[27]

An important variable in determining whether ischemic tissue undergoes necrosis is collateral flow. Collateral flow is highly variable but may be sufficient to prevent a large infarction. Patients with total occlusion of a coronary artery and abundant collateral perfusion with preserved regional ventricular function are the exception, however, and not the rule. Furthermore such patients seldom have acute MI. Thus, ipso facto, most patients with acute MI have inadequate collateral flow. Unfortunately, there are no simple clinical or laboratory means by which patients with negligible collateral perfusion can be distinguished from those whose collateral flow is greater and might be manipulated to the patient's benefit.

SUBENDOCARDIAL INFARCTION

Whereas thrombotic occlusion of large epicardial coronary arteries accounts for the overwhelming majority of transmural MIs, the pathogenesis of nontransmural or subendocardial infarctions is less well understood. Left ventricular wall stress and myocardial oxygen

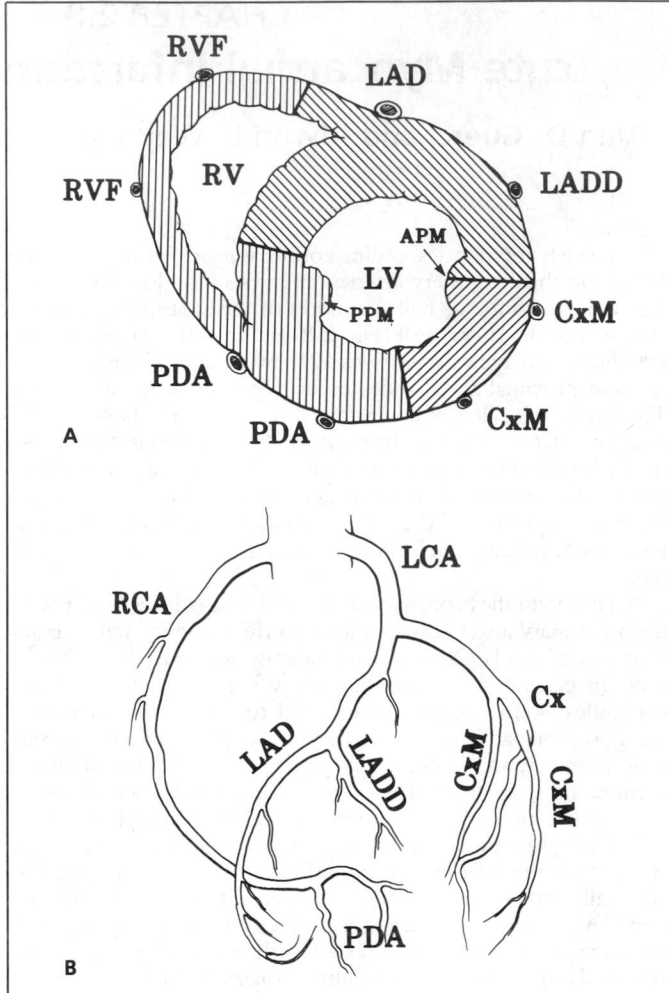

Figure 2.8–1. Representative human coronary artery anatomy. **A.** Vascular territories at midventricular level. LV = left ventricle; RV = right ventricle; LAD = left anterior descending coronary artery; LADD = diagonal branch of the LAD; CxM = circumflex marginal coronary artery; RVF = right ventricular free wall branch; APM = anterior papillary muscle; PPM = posterior papillary muscle. **B.** Left anterior oblique view. Posterior descending arteries move from plane of diagram toward reader's eye and are foreshortened. RCA = right coronary artery; LCA = left coronary artery; Cx = circumflex; PDA = posterior descending artery.

demand are greatest in the subendocardium, and subendocardial blood flow is more readily decreased than blood flow to subepicardial layers by the compressive effects of elevated left ventricular end-diastolic pressure. Thus, in regard to both oxygen supply and demand, the subendocardium is at greater risk of ischemia than is the subepicardium. The combination of increased myocardial oxygen demand, resulting from increased heart rate or blood pressure, and fixed blood supply due to a critical coronary stenosis, undoubtedly accounts for some subendocardial infarcts. This is particularly likely during exposure to uncontrollable stresses, such as severe hypertension, general anesthesia, postoperative recovery, and hypovolemia due to hemorrhage. Many subendocardial infarctions, however, occur in patients who have neither tachycardia, hypertension, nor hypotension. Thus subendocardial infarction results from a diverse set of processes, including (1) transient total or subtotal occlusion of large epicardial coronary arteries, due either to thrombosis with spontaneous thrombolysis or to spasm; (2) total occlusion of secondary coronary arteries (e.g., diagonal branches of the left anterior descending coronary artery or the pos-

terior descending branches of the right coronary artery); (3) total occlusion of large epicardial coronary arteries with sufficient collateral flow to preserve subepicardial but not subendocardial tissue; and (4) prolonged ischemia caused by a tight coronary stenosis in the presence of increased oxygen demand.[8]

CLINICAL FEATURES

INITIAL PRESENTATION

Patients with acute MI usually have squeezing or crushing retrosternal pain that frequently radiates to the neck, jaw, or left arm. Radiation to the right arm or back is less common. The majority of patients have had similar, although milder, discomfort in the preceding hours or days, and those with chronic angina typically experience a worsening of their symptoms for several days before an infarction.

Whereas completely asymptomatic MIs are unusual, unrecognized infarctions are not. Not all patients find the discomfort of acute MI so intolerable as to require immediate medical attention. In some the pain is epigastric and mistaken for indigestion. In others, the arm or neck discomfort overshadows the chest pain and the cardiac origin is not obvious. Still other patients have accompanying complications, such as shortness of breath or some combination of malaise, weakness, and anxiety. These latter symptoms may be the only conscious manifestations of a reduction in cardiac output and a secondary increase in adrenergic tone. Serial ECGs from longitudinal studies of large employee groups suggest that as many as 10 to 15 percent of patients with infarcts do not seek medical attention. An additional 10 to 15 percent die suddenly, usually from ventricular fibrillation before hospital admission.

PHYSICAL EXAMINATION

Just as the symptoms of MI are diverse, a wide range of physical findings may be encountered. No physical findings are specific, and the most common abnormalities in the initial stages of MI are those associated with pain. Anxiety and diaphoresis occur in the majority of patients, and mild shortness of breath is also frequently observed.

For a number of reasons, abnormalities that are actually manifestations of myocardial ischemia and infarction, rather than errors in diagnosis or treatment, are referred to as "complications." This custom prevails partly because abnormalities demonstrable by physical examination often develop hours or even days after the patient is admitted to the hospital. In addition, these abnormalities usually dictate treatment and prognosis. Because of the delayed expression of many of the clinical findings of acute MI, and because of the natural connection between physiologic derangements common to acute MI and treatment, other abnormalities, particularly those of heart rate, breathing, and heart sounds, are described in the section on complications, presented later in this chapter. Attention will first be focused on laboratory studies and considerations of differential diagnosis appropriate to the patient's presentation.

LABORATORY STUDIES

Electrocardiography
The ECG is the single most important laboratory test in the diagnosis of the initial phase of acute MI. ST segment elevation is the hallmark of acute transmural ischemia, whereas ST segment depressions, T-wave inversions, or both are typical of ischemia confined to the subendocardial half of the left ventricle.

The ECG is by no means infallible in the diagnosis of acute MI. The early stages of transmural infarcts may be manifested by relatively nonspecific ECG features, such as ST segment elevation

of less than 0.1 mV, or unusually tall, peaked T waves. Rarely, patients with acute transmural infarcts have normal ECGs at the time of presentation. These problems of sensitivity and specificity are even more common in the diagnosis of subendocardial infarcts. Minor nonspecific ST-T wave changes may be the only ECG evidence of a subendocardial infarct.

Nevertheless, the ECG remains a vital diagnostic tool that offers insight into the stage, location, and extent of an infarct (Figs. 2.8–2A and 2.8–3A).

The ST segment elevations of transmural MI usually subside within a few days; as this takes place, T waves commonly invert. R-wave amplitude begins to decline within hours, and R-wave loss, to whatever extent it is destined to occur, is usually complete in a day or two. The evolution of Q waves parallels the loss of R-wave amplitude: Q waves begin to appear in a few hours and ordinarily reach their full development in 24 to 48 hours (Figs. 2.8–2B and 2.8–3B).

The ST-T segment changes of subendocardial infarction may persist indefinitely or resolve after a few days. Subtle loss of R-wave amplitude, with or without permanent T-wave inversion, may be the only sustained evidence of a subendocardial infarct.

The term "transmural," as commonly used, is an oversimplification. ST segment elevation does not necessarily connote ischemia involving the full thickness of a region of the left ventricle, and neither the evolution of 40 msec Q waves nor even the loss of all R waves is absolutely specific for transmural infarction. For this reason, some authorities have proposed that the terms "Q wave" and "non-Q wave" infarction replace "transmural" and "subendocardial" in the interpretation of ECGs.

Serologic Tests

With the loss of membrane integrity characteristic of necrosis, myocardial enzymes leak into the serum. Measurement of creatine kinase (CK), aspartate aminotransferase (AST) (formerly serum glutamic-oxaloacetic transaminase [SGOT]), and lactate dehydro-

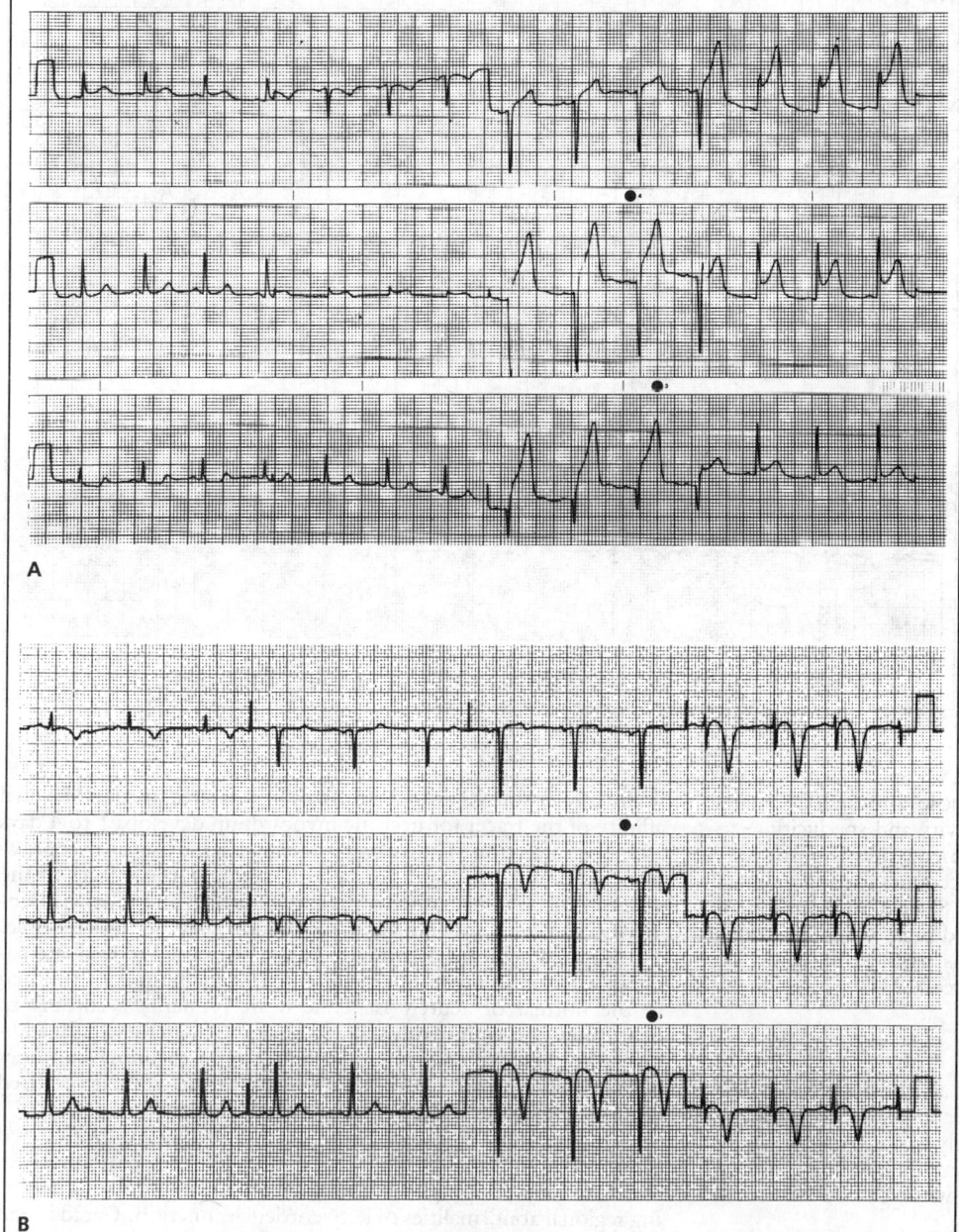

Figure 2.8–2. ECG in anterior myocardial infarction. **A.** Acute phase is indicated by ST segment elevations in leads I, aV$_L$, and V$_1$ to V$_6$. Tall, peaked T waves, so-called hyperacute T waves, are also present in leads V$_2$ to V$_5$. **B.** Late phase, recorded 2 weeks later. Loss of R-wave amplitude and T-wave inversions are evident in leads in which ST segments were elevated, and QS complexes have developed in leads aV$_L$, V$_2$, and V$_3$. Persistent ST segment elevations in leads V$_2$ to V$_5$ suggest dyskinesis of anterior wall.

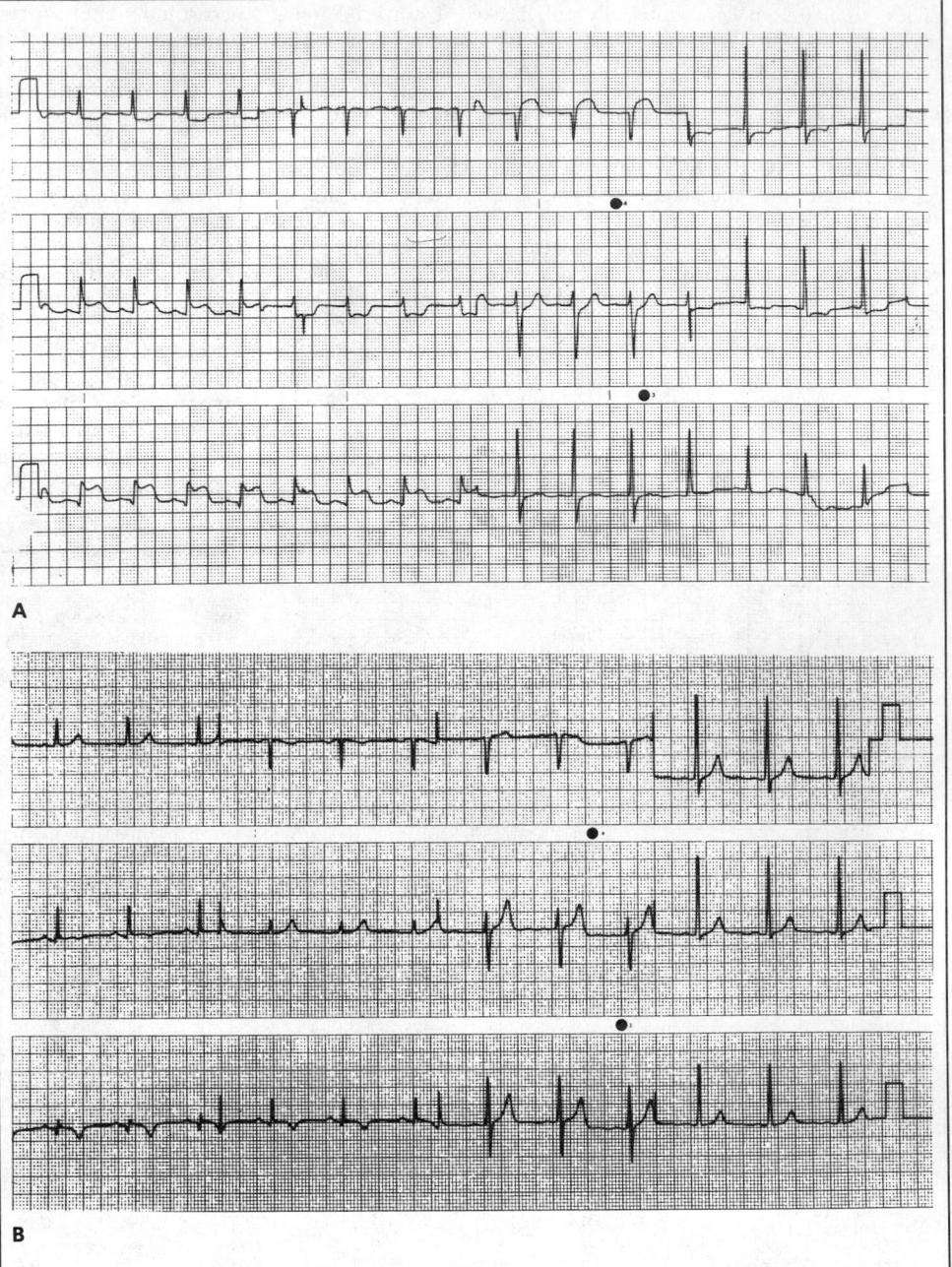

Figure 2.8–3. ECG in inferior MI. **A.** Acute phase is evidenced by ST segment elevations in leads II, III, and aV_F. ST segment depressions in anterior leads, most noticeably I and aV_L, were not accompanied by abnormalities of perfusion or motion in anterior wall; hence these are benign, ''reciprocal'' ST segment depressions. **B.** Late phase. R-wave loss is most prominent in lead III, where there is also a pathologic Q wave. T waves here inverted in leads II, III, and aV_F, and reciprocal ST segment depressions have resolved.

genase (LDH) has been used for this purpose, although CK analysis is preferred because of its relative sensitivity and specificity.

The time course of release of these enzymes is portrayed in Figure 2.8–4. The CK-MB isoenzyme accounts for approximately 15 percent of myocardial creatine kinase. Skeletal muscle ordinarily contains less than 3 percent CK-MB, and brain tissue has none of the MB isoenzyme. Thus CK elevations with more than 3 or 4 percent MB isoenzyme generally indicate an MI.

Radionuclide Imaging

Several techniques involving intravenous administration of radioactive tracers have been developed in order to assess myocardial perfusion, the presence or absence of recently infarcted tissue, and left ventricular function. Although these examinations are not performed routinely, they may be of value when clinical features of a particular case are inconsistent.

The most specific of these tests uses pyrophosphate labeled with technetium-99, which localizes in infarcted tissue. Maximal affinity of the tracer for necrotic myocardium develops 1 to 4 days after the infarction. Difficulties associated with use of pyrophosphate scanning are its uptake by bone, so that the images of the sternum and ribs may obscure the cardiac image, and relative insensitivity, so that a subendocardial infarction may be undetectable. Thallium-201 chloride scanning has also been used to evaluate patients with acute myocardial ischemia, but thallium is distributed in the normal or acutely ischemic heart primarily according to blood flow and is not truly a measure of the infarct itself. In addition, the presence of a perfusion defect on a thallium scan does not, by itself, provide information regarding the time it occurred (i.e., old defects and new defects look the same).

Technetium-99 gated blood pool scanning, in which red blood cells are labeled with the tracer, provides a noninvasive means of measuring right and left ventricular function and detecting regional abnormalities of left ventricular function. Gated blood pool scanning cannot distinguish between old and new infarction.

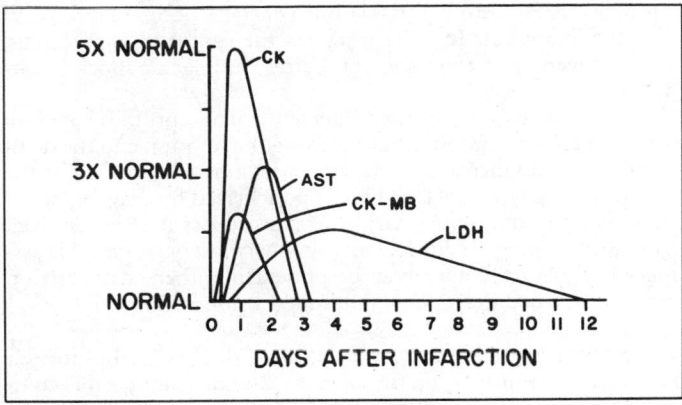

Figure 2.8–4. Time course of serum enzyme concentration after typical MI. CK = creatine kinase; AST = aspartate aminotransferase; CK-MB = isoenzyme of CK, which is found mainly in myocardium and is therefore more specific for myocardial damage. LDH = lactate dehydrogenase.

DIFFERENTIAL DIAGNOSIS

Several other diagnoses must be borne in mind in the evaluation of symptoms thought to be due to myocardial ischemia. Inasmuch as several of these diseases are in themselves life threatening, a thorough workup of the patient may require invasive and somewhat risky procedures in a patient who, in fact, has an acute MI and nothing else.

Unstable Angina

The character, location, and radiation of anginal pain may be so similar to that of an acute MI as to obscure the diagnosis. Although chest pain lasting more than 20 to 30 minutes is usually thought to indicate an infarction, the pain of unstable angina may wax and wane so that it is impossible to determine its total duration. Serial ECGs and CK determinations usually suffice to establish the correct diagnosis. Patients in whom evidence for an infarct is ultimately lacking are best classified as having unstable angina (see Chapter 2.7).

Aortic Dissection

Dissecting hematomas of the thoracic aorta, generally referred to by the misnomer "dissecting aortic aneurysm," ordinarily produce severe chest pain that may be indistinguishable from that of an acute MI. Indeed, if the dissection extends into the aortic root, it may actually occlude one of the coronary ostia and cause an infarction.

Several clinical features of aortic dissection help differentiate dissection from infarction. The pain is often described as tearing in quality, it frequently radiates to the back, and, from the clinician's point of view, it often seems worse than the pain of an infarction. Dissection of the aortic root may cause aortic regurgitation, and dissection of the brachiocephalic or left subclavian artery will result in differences in blood pressure in the right and left arms.

Aortic dissection does not, by itself, produce ECG changes characteristic of acute MI. Thus the ECG may be helpful in ruling out an MI in patients with aortic dissection alone. On the other hand, among patients with abnormal baseline ECGs or patients with an MI resulting from a dissection, the ECG may be of no value. The finding of a widened superior mediastinal shadow on a routine chest radiograph suggests the diagnosis of dissection. Echocardiography, CT scanning, and MRI are other noninvasive means that may establish the diagnosis. When these means fail, aortography becomes necessary.

Pulmonary Embolism

Chest pain, shortness of breath, and nonspecific ST-T wave abnormalities may accompany acute pulmonary embolism. The development of pleuritic chest pain, a pleural friction rub, infiltrates on a chest radiograph, and the frequent nonspecificity of the ECG changes may be useful differentiating features. The latter point cannot be overemphasized. Pulmonary embolism and MI may both cause chest pain, shortness of breath, lung infiltrates, and hypotension. However, pulmonary embolism does not, by itself, cause ST segment elevations, and even massive pulmonary embolism may be associated with only minor and nonspecific ST-T wave changes. As a rule, hypotension and respiratory distress due to acute MI are accompanied by gross ECG abnormalities, such as clear-cut ST segment elevations, widespread ST segment depressions, or widespread and deep T-wave inversions. These latter changes may occur in pulmonary embolism, but hemodynamic instability in the absence of such changes, as sometimes occurs in pulmonary embolism, should always raise suspicion of a cause other than MI.

Other diseases of the lungs and thoracic cavity may mimic acute MI. These include pneumonia, pneumothorax, and pneumomediastinum. Chest radiography and careful physical examination are usually sufficient to establish the correct diagnosis.

Pericarditis

The pain of pericarditis can usually be distinguished from the pain of MI on the basis of the history alone. Pericardial pain is typically made worse by lying in the supine position and better by sitting up and leaning forward. Pericardial pain also has a pleuritic component in most cases (i.e., it is made worse by deep breathing). A pericardial friction rub helps to establish the diagnosis.

In some cases, serial ECGs and CK determinations are required to establish the diagnosis. The CK level is usually normal in pericarditis, and the ST segment elevations characteristic of pericarditis have an upward concave contour. In addition, the ST segment elevations of pericarditis are commonly widespread, often occurring in the distribution of more than one coronary artery.

Other Conditions

Esophageal spasm may cause pain that is indistinguishable from that of acute MI, but esophageal spasm does not cause ECG changes or CK elevations. Pancreatitis and biliary tract disease may cause low retrosternal and epigastric pain similar to that of an MI and sometimes may cause T-wave inversions and minor ST segment elevations. As in the case of esophageal spasm, typical evolutionary ECG changes and CK elevations do not occur.

Chest wall abnormalities such as rib fractures or herpes zoster radiculitis may also cause pain similar to that of an MI, but these conditions usually cause chest wall tenderness and can be diagnosed correctly on the basis of careful clinical examination.

HOSPITAL COURSE

The patient's hospital course is characterized by clinical events that can be termed either manifestations or complications. The distinction between the two terms is somewhat arbitrary. For example, every patient who has a myocardial infarction has some impairment of myocardial function because myocardial cells are ischemic or necrotic. The magnitude of the effect depends on the number of cells damaged. In the majority of patients with a first myocardial infarction, there is no clinical manifestation of left ventricular dysfunction initially, and therefore when clinical evidence of dysfunction develops, often later in the course, it is termed a complication. The same is true of arrhythmias, with occasional premature beats being a common manifestation and an indication of some electrical instability. On the other hand, it is the risk of ventricular fibrillation that necessitates electrocardiographic monitoring.

Treatment is focused on analgesia and bed rest during the first day, with resumption of a normal diet, ambulation, and observa-

tion for complications in the days that follow. Patients with an MI that remains uncomplicated can be discharged 5 to 10 days after admission.

COMPLICATIONS

Acute MI can be complicated in a variety of life-threatening ways. In most cases, abnormalities arise as a consequence of the size and location of the infarct. These complications include mechanical, electrical, ischemia-related, and miscellaneous complications. In each instance, detection and appropriate therapy require meticulous serial examinations.

Mechanical Complications

Congestive Heart Failure. The most common mechanical complication of acute MI is congestive heart failure, which may range from symptomless basilar lung congestion to cardiogenic shock. An inverse relationship exists between the size of an infarct and residual left ventricular function. Among previously normal persons, persistent evidence of heart failure at rest usually indicates at least an intermediate-sized infarct. When left ventricular function is already impaired, a small infarct may precipitate heart failure.

Left-sided heart failure due to MI is generally similar in its clinical expression to heart failure from other causes. Shortness of breath, rales, radiographic evidence of lung congestion, and hypoxemia are the most common manifestations. A heaving or paradoxical left ventricular impulse may be present in more severe cases, particularly in patients with anterior infarcts. An S_3 gallop correlates closely with elevated filling pressures. Sinus tachycardia is also an important sign of heart failure; indeed, suspicion of ventricular failure should be aroused whenever an afebrile and pain-free patient's heart rate is persistently above 90 beats/min.

The earliest stages of cardiogenic shock may be relatively subtle. There are two reasons. First, cardiovascular reflexes have evolved to maintain blood pressures in the face of declining contractility by increasing the heart rate and the peripheral resistance. Second, diaphoresis and cool, clammy skin can be a nonspecific response to pain. Together with sinus tachycardia, however, diaphoresis and cool, clammy skin in pain-free patients are ominous signs, even in the absence of obvious respiratory insufficiency or hypotension. In more extreme cases, severe lung congestion, livedo reticularis, metabolic acidosis, oliguria, and hypotension supervene.

Not all of the hypotension that accompanies acute MI is due to severe left ventricular dysfunction. Hypotension in association with bradycardia is not unusual and is seen most often in inferior infarction. Hypotension may also be seen in patients with either relative (i.e., vasodilator induced) or absolute intravascular volume depletion or in patients with right ventricular infarction (see below).

Mitral Regurgitation. Mitral regurgitation occasionally complicates MI and is most often due to ischemia of the posterior papillary muscle or surrounding areas of the inferior wall. Rupture of a papillary muscle occurs infrequently and is a catastrophic event, producing immediate and overwhelming pulmonary edema with hypotension and cardiogenic shock.

The murmur of acute papillary muscle dysfunction is typically located at the apex with radiation to the axilla, but it may be loudest along the left parasternal area with radiation to the base. More important, the murmur often has a decrescendo quality, because the left atrium has not had time to dilate and a relatively small regurgitant volume may suffice to bring left ventricular and left atrial pressures into equilibrium. This accounts for the observation that severe acute ischemic mitral regurgitation may be associated with a murmur that is only grade I or II in intensity. In such cases the presence of tall V waves in a wedged pulmonary artery catheter pressure tracing confirms the diagnosis.

Ventricular Septal Defect. Rupture of the interventricular septum occasionally complicates anterior and inferior infarctions. The tim-

ing of septal rupture is variable but generally occurs 3 to 7 days after the infarction. In most instances the rupture is devastating, causing severe lung congestion and often cardiogenic shock or cardiac arrest.

The diagnosis of ruptured interventricular septum is based on development of a systolic murmur along the sternum and the demonstration of an increase in oxygen content in venous blood at the level of the right ventricle. This can be achieved by drawing blood gas samples from a pulmonary artery catheter as it is passed from right atrium to right ventricle to pulmonary artery. A palpable systolic thrill over the apex may be present in either postinfarction ventricular septal defect or severe mitral regurgitation.

Ventricular Free-Wall Rupture. Rupture of the free wall of the left ventricle is an unusual and, in most cases, immediately lethal complication of transmural infarction. Like rupture of the interventricular septum, it tends to occur 3 to 7 days after infarction.

In rare cases, pericardial adhesions adjacent to the infarct confine the hemopericardium to a small area. This condition is known as left ventricular pseudoaneurysm and urgently requires surgical correction.

Right Ventricular Infarction. The right ventricle is perfused by the right coronary artery. In about one third of inferior infarcts, the right coronary artery occlusion is sufficiently proximal to cause extensive right ventricular necrosis.

The primary clinical manifestation of right ventricular infarction is a low output state (e.g., tachycardia, hypotension) that is out of proportion to left ventricular failure. Some lung congestion may coexist with this condition because of infarction of the inferior wall of the left ventricle, but this is ordinarily not severe. In more extreme cases the compensatory increase in right ventricular end-diastolic volume and pressure is so great that a tamponade-like condition is established. The distended right ventricle competes with the left ventricle for space within the pericardium, and equalization of filling pressures occurs.

Although demonstration of ST segment elevation in lead V_4R (an electrode placed in the right fifth intercostal space, at the midclavicular line) has been used to identify patients with right ventricular infarction,[12] the diagnosis is usually made on clinical grounds. Jugular venous distension or demonstration of elevation of right ventricular end-diastolic pressure equal to the wedged pulmonary artery pressure is usually sufficient to establish the diagnosis.

Electrical Complications

Acute MI is associated with a wide variety of arrhythmias, both ventricular and supraventricular.[16] Only the most common and most important will be discussed.

Sinus bradycardia is observed frequently in patients with inferior infarcts. It may be the result of ischemia of the sinoatrial node or of activation of negative chronotropic and vasodepressor reflexes induced by ischemia of the basilar portion of the inferior wall. In the latter case, hypotension usually accompanies the bradycardia.

Sinus tachycardia, premature atrial contractions, and atrial fibrillation are also common in MI. In the majority of cases they share a common cause: atrial distension due to ventricular failure. Because these rhythms may be the only clinical manifestations of heart failure, they demand serious attention. Alternatively, premature atrial beats and atrial fibrillation may result from postinfarct pericarditis that extends to the atrial surface. True atrial infarcts are uncommon and lack specific clinical features.

Premature ventricular depolarizations occur in the majority of acute MIs, and nonsustained ventricular tachycardia is present in as many as 30 percent of cases. Sustained ventricular tachycardia occurs less frequently.

Primary ventricular fibrillation (i.e., ventricular fibrillation in the absence of severe congestive heart failure) occurs in 5 to 10 percent of acute MIs. As in the case of ventricular premature beats, most primary ventricular fibrillation occurs early in the course of acute MI, with 80 percent of cases developing within 12 hours of symptom onset.

Primary ventricular fibrillation is more common in patients with large infarcts than in patients with small infarcts. Several other life-threatening arrhythmias, particularly asystole and electromechanical dissociation, are also usually confined to patients with large infarcts.

Heart Block. Of the several conduction disturbances common to acute MI, A-V nodal block is the most serious. The A-V node is perfused by the right coronary artery in about 90 percent of persons. Thus inferior infarcts may be accompanied by ischemia of the A-V node. Mobitz I heart block usually precedes complete heart block, and subsidiary pacemaker tissue low in the node or the bundle of His often emerges to maintain ventricular contraction. Even when complete heart block does occur in inferior infarction, the ischemic A-V nodal dysfunction generally resolves after a few days and conduction returns spontaneously.

In contrast, the A-V block that sometimes complicates anterior infarcts tends to be devastating. Such block implies extensive necrosis of the septum and anterior wall. Subsidiary pacemaker tissue is not reliable because the left anterior descending coronary artery supplies the distal portion of the bundle of His and the proximal portions of the right bundle and left anterior fascicle as they course through the high part of the septum.

The complete heart block of anterior infarcts is often heralded by intraventricular conduction disturbances, or Mobitz II block. When complete right or left bundle-branch block occurs in the course of an infarction, the risk of progression to complete heart block is in the range of 15 percent. For either right bundle-branch block with left anterior hemiblock or right bundle-branch block with left posterior hemiblock, the risk of progression to complete heart block approaches 30 percent; when right bundle-branch block alternates with left bundle-branch block, the risk exceeds 40 percent.[14]

Whereas isolated first-degree A-V block does not carry a high risk of progression to complete heart block, first-degree A-V block in association with left or right bundle-branch block progresses to complete heart block in about 20 percent of cases.[14]

Ischemia-related Complications

Postinfarction Angina. Angina that occurs at rest or with minimal exertion in the first few days after an MI is a serious problem, with 1-year mortality rates as high as 50 percent.[30] The risk is greatest when the ischemia occurs in a vascular territory other than that of the infarct or when a subendocardial infarction is due to a high-grade stenosis without permanent total occlusion in a large epicardial artery. In the former situation, usually accompanied by ST segment depressions in leads remote from the infarct, a second transmural infarction may occur, whereas in the latter case, characterized by ST segment elevation in leads in the region of infarction, the subendocardial infarct may become transmural. Small extensions along the margins of an infarct tend to be less threatening.

The acute phase of transmural infarction may be accompanied by ST segment depression in ECG leads facing regions of the ventricle remote from the infarct. ST segment depressions signify true ischemia in less than 50 percent of cases, and in the remaining patients the ST segment depressions are a benign reciprocal change. Chest pain or left ventricular failure out of proportion to the apparent size of the infarct suggest true ischemia. This suspicion can be confirmed by the demonstration of ventricular wall motion or perfusion defects in the region of the ST segment depressions.[33]

Miscellaneous Complications

Pericarditis frequently occurs 1 to 4 days after transmural infarction. The clinical features are similar to pericarditis from other causes: pleuropericardial pain, a pericardial rub, fever, and ST segment elevations.

Low-grade fever and leukocytosis are expected in the first few days after infarction, particularly in patients with large infarcts. The fever of MI does not ordinarily exceed 38.9C (102F), and the white blood cell count usually remains below 15,000.

Pulmonary or systemic emboli occur in 5 to 10 percent of MIs unless specific precautions are taken to reduce their incidence. The risk of pulmonary embolism in MI is primarily attributable to bed rest. Systemic emboli, on the other hand, usually originate from left ventricular mural thrombi. Left ventricular mural thrombus formation is primarily dependent on extensive wall motion abnormalities. Most cases are a consequence of large anterior infarcts.

A number of poorly understood complications of acute MI were encountered years ago but are rarely seen today. Dressler syndrome, for example, is an apparently autoimmune pericarditis that occurs weeks to months after the infarction. The shoulder-hand syndrome is a reflex neurologic dystrophy, with pain and stiffness in the shoulder and pain and vasomotor instability in the forearm and hand. Analgesics and aggressive physical therapy are urgently required for effective treatment of this condition.

TREATMENT

An all-inclusive review of the treatment of MI is beyond the scope of this text. This section will discuss general measures applicable to all MIs, the treatment and prevention of complications, salvage of acutely ischemic myocardium, and long-term care.

GENERAL MEASURES

Patient comfort is of paramount concern, particularly in the first few hours of an MI. Opiates are usually required for analgesia, although they may aggravate the bradycardia caused by inferior infarcts and the hypotension resulting from any infarct. Despite these potential problems, 2 to 4 mg of morphine sulfate can be given intravenously at 5-minute intervals until the patient is comfortable. Sedation, usually with a benzodiazepine, may also be advisable. Diazepam, 5 or 10 mg given orally at 6- to 12-hour intervals, is one of many benzodiazepines suitable for this purpose.

Bed rest and a clear liquid diet are usually indicated for the first hospital day. Patients with an uncomplicated infarct can spend time in a chair and progress to solid foods on the second hospital day and should be encouraged to walk by the third or fourth hospital day. This progression of activity must proceed more slowly in patients with complications. Because bed rest and low-bulk foods given in the first few days after an MI may cause constipation, it is generally advisable to prescribe a stool softener.

Removal of unnecessary tubing (e.g., intravenous lines, oxygen) is also good for patient morale. Lidocaine and oxygen may be discontinued as early as the second hospital day in patients with uncomplicated infarcts.

Primary ventricular fibrillation develops in 5 to 10 percent of acute MIs. Although less common, sustained ventricular tachycardia and complete heart block are not rare. Because these rhythms usually occur without premonitory symptoms, ECG monitoring is advisable for at least 24 hours. Indeed, this need for ECG monitoring constitutes the principal reason for the existence of coronary care units.

Mild to moderate hypoxemia is not uncommon in acute MI and is generally the result of ventilation-perfusion mismatch in the lungs, which responds to low flow oxygen (2 to 4 L/min by nasal cannula or mask). Because hypoxemia of this magnitude may develop without warning in the first 24 hours of an infarction and may contribute to recurrent ischemia or arrhythmias, routine administration of oxygen for the first 24 to 48 hours of acute MI is indicated. This approach is preferable to the routine determination of arterial blood gas levels.

MECHANICAL COMPLICATIONS

Congestive Heart Failure

The most common mechanical complication of acute MI is congestive heart failure. Mild heart failure can be treated with diuretics.

Digitalis preparations are usually withheld for several days until sinoatrial and atrioventricular nodal function stabilizes.

Patients with more severe left ventricular failure, that is, those with moderate lung congestion or even pulmonary edema, often benefit from vasodilator therapy in addition to diuretics (Table 2.8–1). Intravenous nitroglycerin has a greater dilatory effect on systemic veins than systemic arteries. As a consequence, nitroglycerin reduces preload more than it reduces afterload, and it tends to relieve lung congestion more than it increases cardiac output. Coronary vasodilation and short duration of action are additional advantages of intravenous nitroglycerin. The usual starting dose is 5 μg/min. Infusion rates in excess of 400 μg/min do not ordinarily provide additional benefit.

When afterload reduction is a primary goal of therapy, as in severe mitral regurgitation or ventricular septal defect, nitroprusside is the drug of choice. As with nitroglycerin, the usual starting dose is 5 μg/min, and the dose is increased until the desired endpoint is reached or hypotension prevents the use of more of the drug. Thiocyanate toxicity, manifested by slurred speech, muscle twitching, and restlessness, may be encountered in patients with renal insufficiency or after prolonged administration of high doses.

Hypotension is a common problem in patients with acute MI. Arrhythmias, activation of vasodepressor reflexes, intravascular volume deficits, concomitant therapy with vasodilators, and right or left ventricular failure account for nearly all cases. Whereas the first of these causes is usually self-evident, the others may not be.

If a hypotensive patient with no bradycardia is breathing comfortably and the lungs are not congested, it is appropriate to administer 200 to 500 ml of normal saline solution over 3 to 5 minutes and then to reevaluate the patient. If, on the other hand, there is evidence of respiratory compromise, or if more than 1 to 2 L has been delivered intravenously and the patient remains hypotensive with uncertain intravascular volume status, it is appropriate to initiate invasive hemodynamic monitoring with pulmonary and

systemic arterial catheters (Fig. 2.8–5). Pulmonary artery catheterization may also be useful in patients with persistent pulmonary edema. There are several justifications for this approach. First, there is no consistent relationship between central venous and left ventricular filling pressures in patients with acute MI. As a consequence, the level of the jugular venous pulse does not provide a reliable estimate of left ventricular preload. Second, in patients with normal pulmonary capillary permeability, pulmonary congestion begins to develop at approximately the same hydrostatic pressure that maximizes or nearly maximizes left ventricular function: 15 to 20 mm Hg. Thus, in patients with hypotension and low filling pressures, the pulmonary "wedge" pressure can usually be raised to 15 to 20 mm Hg by fluid administration without compromising lung function. Alternatively, in patients with severe lung congestion, it is often possible to reduce the wedge pressure to 15 or 20 mm Hg with diuretics and vasodilators without a precipitous decline in cardiac output or blood pressure.

Patients with cardiogenic shock require support with inotropic drugs more potent than digitalis. Vasoconstriction is also often needed. Dopamine is in most cases the drug of choice for this purpose. Its positive inotropic effects overshadow its vasoconstrictive properties at low and intermediate doses (2 to 10 μg/kg/min), and it is usually only a weakly positive chronotrope.

Norepinephrine and dobutamine may also be valuable in the treatment of cardiogenic shock. Norepinephrine is a potent vasoconstrictor, however, and may stimulate excessive renal and mesenteric vasoconstriction. In contrast, dobutamine is a fairly potent vasodilator, and blood pressure may fall despite its positive inotropic actions.

Blood pressure permitting, the addition of a vasodilator to dopamine or norepinephrine may be beneficial in cardiogenic shock, particularly when pulmonary artery pressures are thereby reduced.[10]

Intra-aortic balloon counterpulsation is generally to be avoided in patients with cardiogenic shock. Whereas aortic balloon

TABLE 2.8–1. TREATMENT OF HEART FAILURE IN ACUTE MYOCARDIAL INFARCTION

Killip Class[a]	Clinical Findings	CVP	PCW	Cardiac Output	Approximate Hospital Mortality Rate	Treatment[b]
I	No evidence of heart failure	N	N	N	<5%	None necessary
II	Mild to moderate CHF: bibasilar rales and/or S$_3$ gallop	N	↑	N	10%	Diuretics; consider vasodilators or digitalis
III	Severe CHF: rales above tip of scapula, S$_3$ gallop, sinus tachycardia, frank pulmonary edema	N	↑	↓	30%	Diuretics and nitrates; if response inadequate, consider catecholamines (e.g., dobutamine or dopamine), if evidence of ongoing ischemia, consider IABC, coronary angiography
IV	Cardiogenic shock: BP <90 and signs of systemic hypoperfusion (e.g., cool, clammy skin; oliguria; metabolic acidosis)					
	Specific subsets: Hypovolemia	↓	↓	↓		Intravascular volume expansion
	Right ventricular infarction	↑	N	↓		Intravascular volume expansion; consider dopamine
	Rupture of papillary muscle or VSD	N or ↑	↑	↓		Vasodilator therapy (especially nitroprusside); catecholamines (e.g., dopamine and IABC if necessary); urgent angiography and surgery advisable
	Left ventricular pump failure	N	↑	↓	80%–90%	Dopamine, vasodilators if tolerated; IABC to be avoided unless there is evidence of ongoing ischemia

[a]Reference 18.
[b]See reference 10 for detailed discussion of this subject.
CVP = central venous pressure; PCW = pulmonary capillary wedge pressure; N = normal; CHF = congestive heart failure; IABC = intraaortic balloon counterpulsation; BP = blood pressure; VSD = ventricular septal defect.

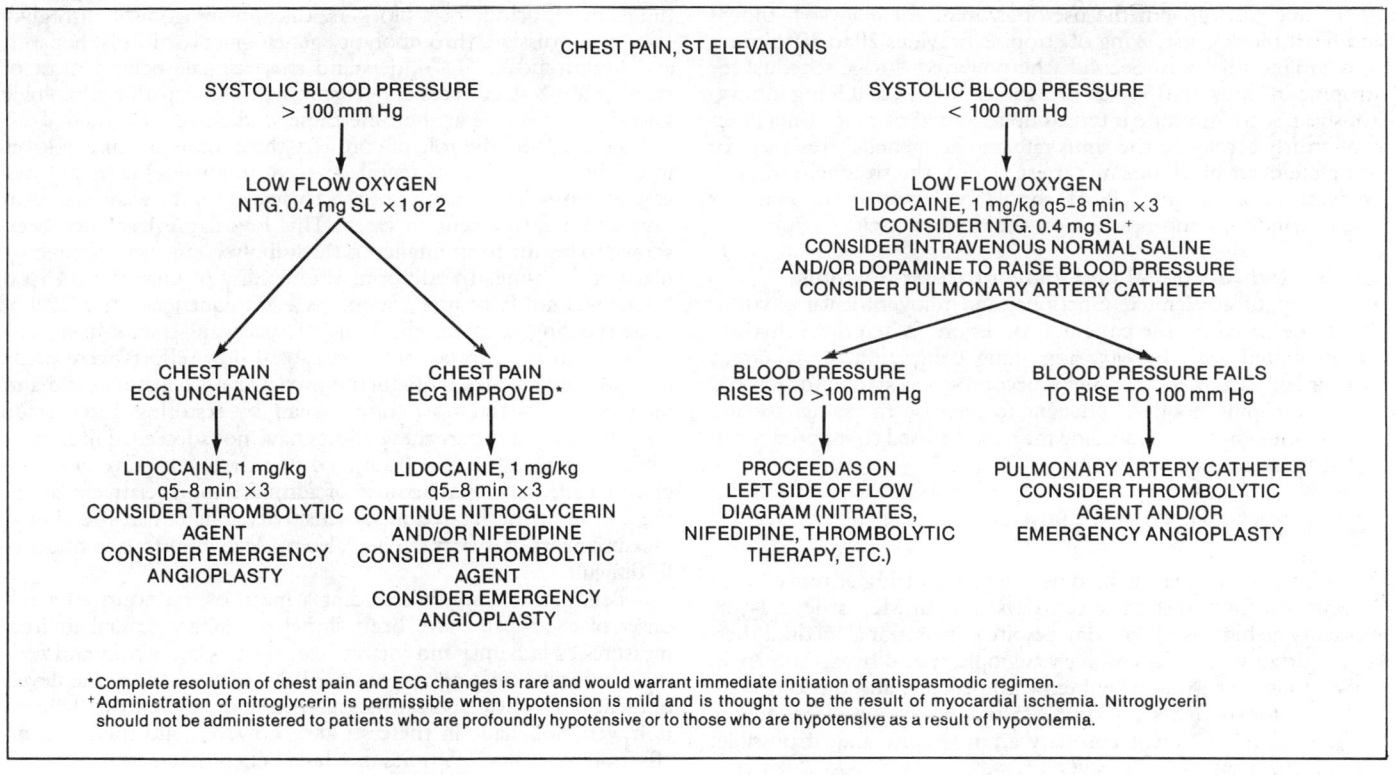

Figure 2.8–5. Treatment options for early phases of acute MI. These treatment decisions should be made within 15 (left side of flow diagram) to 60 minutes (right side) of presentation.

counterpulsation is of great value in patients with ventricular septal defect, mitral regurgitation, or recurrent ischemia, it has not been shown to reduce the size of the index infarct or the mortality rate in cardiogenic shock. Aortic balloon counterpulsation may dramatically improve the patient's condition, but it places the patient, family, and physician in the difficult position of artificially supporting a nonviable patient. The mortality rate for MI complicated by cardiogenic shock remains in excess of 80 percent.

In addition to hemodynamic support, patients with infarct-induced severe mitral regurgitation or ventricular septal defect urgently require coronary arteriography, left ventriculography, and, if possible, corrective surgery.

Right Ventricular Infarction
Right ventricular infarction presents a number of special problems. As a rule, the administration of large volumes of normal saline solution (as much as several liters) will raise right ventricular preload by a sufficient amount that cardiac output and blood pressure are restored to normal or nearly normal levels. Monitoring of central venous and pulmonary arterial pressures is often a useful guide to fluid therapy in these cases. In cases of extreme right ventricular dysfunction, fluid loading may so dilate the right ventricle that the filling of other chambers is impaired by a lack of space within the pericardium. The treatment of such patients is empiric, relying on careful observation of the relationship of right- and left-sided filling pressures, cardiac output, and systemic arterial pressure. With careful hemodynamic monitoring and inotropic support, the condition of some of these patients will stabilize as right ventricular function improves or the pericardium stretches.

ARRHYTHMIAS

Ventricular Fibrillation
Primary ventricular fibrillation (i.e., fibrillation in hemodynamically stable patients) occurs in 5 to 10 percent of patients with

acute MI and can usually be prevented by the administration of lidocaine (2 to 3 mg/kg over 20 minutes, followed by continuous intravenous infusion at 10 to 40 μg/kg/min).[20] Eighty percent of cases occur in the first 12 hours after the onset of chest pain, and warning arrhythmias are neither sufficiently specific nor sensitive to guide therapy. It is appropriate, therefore, to treat all patients in the initial stages of documented acute MI with lidocaine for 12 to 24 hours. Patients with ongoing ventricular ectopy, particularly those with ventricular tachycardia or fibrillation while receiving lidocaine, often require longer therapy, the addition of other antiarrhythmic agents, or both.

Bradyarrhythmias and Heart Block
In patients with inferior MI, sinus bradycardia, Mobitz I second-degree A-V block, and even complete heart block usually respond to atropine. Alternatively, the Mobitz II block and complete heart block, which sometimes complicate anterior infarction, do not reliably respond to atropine. Temporary transvenous pacemakers are recommended in these situations. Temporary pacemakers are also recommended by most cardiologists for right or left bundle-branch block and first-degree A-V block, bifascicular block, and alternating right and left bundle-branch block.[14] Routine prophylactic temporary pacing for isolated new right or left bundle-branch block is controversial. The decision is perhaps best made by assessment of the overall clinical situation. The development of right or left bundle-branch block in the setting of an anterior infarction, in which case the emergence of subsidiary pacemaking tissue cannot be relied on, favors the insertion of a temporary pacemaker.

Patients in whom temporary transvenous pacemakers are inserted prophylactically but are not used (i.e., in whom complete heart block does not develop) do not ordinarily require permanent pacemakers. In contrast, patients with anterior infarcts who develop complete heart block and subsequently regain conduction do need permanent pacemakers. As many as two thirds of such patients will develop high-grade atrioventricular block over the next year.[14]

Three rules govern the use of atropine for bradyarrhythmias and heart block. First, 2 mg of atropine provides 20 to 30 minutes of complete vagolysis. Second, the preferred dosage schedule for atropine in sinus bradycardia or Mobitz I block is 0.5 mg intravenously at 3- to 5-minute intervals up to a total of 2 mg; 1 mg doses may greatly accelerate the sinus rate and are generally reserved for complete heart block or sinus arrest. Third, the treatment of sinus bradycardia or Mobitz I block should be based on the patient's overall condition and not just on the rhythm itself.

Accelerated Junctional and Idioventricular Rhythms

Treatment of accelerated junctional and idioventricular rhythms should be based on the patient's condition. When these rhythms are associated with hypotension, lung congestion, or recurrent myocardial ischemia, treatment becomes necessary. Administration of atropine is often sufficient to increase the sinus rate and restore sinus rhythm. Lidocaine may also be used to suppress accelerated idioventricular rhythms.

POSTINFARCTION ANGINA

Postinfarction angina, defined as angina occurring at rest or with minimal exertion in the first few days after an MI, carries a 1-year mortality as high as 50 percent despite conventional medical therapy. Mortality rates for coronary angioplasty and bypass surgery in this setting are substantially below 10 percent, and the long-term prognosis for survivors is good.[2,6] Postinfarction angina is therefore an indication for urgent coronary arteriography and, if possible, revascularization.

MISCELLANEOUS PROBLEMS IN THERAPY

Anticoagulation

The risk of pulmonary embolism is approximately 6 percent in patients with acute MI. The risk of systemic embolization, principally stroke, is almost as high. These risks can be reduced by approximately 70 percent with full-dose heparinization followed by anticoagulation with warfarin or one of its congeners.[34]

Since intermittent subcutaneous administration of "low dose" heparin is effective in preventing deep vein thrombosis and pulmonary embolism, an important question is which patients are in jeopardy of systemic embolization. It is apparent that patients with large infarcts and, in particular, large anterior infarcts, are at greatest risk of mural thrombus formation and subsequent embolization. It seems appropriate to induce anticoagulation in such patients for at least 1 month. The value of prolonged anticoagulation in patients with anterior infarction is uncertain, although one study suggests that anticoagulation should be maintained indefinitely.[26] In the remaining patients, that is, those with subendocardial infarcts and nonanterior infarcts, anticoagulation can be discontinued when the patients are fully ambulatory.

Pericarditis

The pericarditis that occurs several days after transmural MI does not ordinarily respond to salicylates. Indomethacin, 50 mg given orally three to four times a day, usually provides relief within a few hours. Treatment is ordinarily continued for a week.

When gastrointestinal upset or acute renal failure requires termination of therapy with indomethacin, a short course of high-dose therapy with glucocorticoids (e.g., prednisone, 40 mg daily for 3 to 5 days) is also effective. If at all possible, however, glucocorticoids are to be avoided in the first few weeks after acute MI, for they delay scar formation, promote infarct expansion, and increase the risk of myocardial rupture.

MYOCARDIAL SALVAGE

In the past 20 years, a wide variety of agents have been employed in an attempt to prevent the necrosis of acutely ischemic myocardium; these include beta blockers, calcium antagonists, nitroglycerin, nitroprusside, thrombolytic agents, glucocorticoids, heparin, and hyaluronidase. To understand the rationale behind most of these studies, it is necessary to summarize the pathophysiologic knowledge available at the time these studies were initiated.

Before 1980 the role of coronary thrombosis in acute MI was in doubt. Autopsy data revealed severe multivessel coronary disease in most fatal infarcts, but occlusive thrombi were found in only about 50 percent of cases. This low figure has since been shown to be due to spontaneous thrombolysis, an event not recognized at the time. In addition, the rapidity of infarction (4 to 6 hours) was not fully appreciated. As a consequence of this level of understanding, and on the basis of successful results in experimental animals with abundant collateral flow, efforts were made to reduce infarct size by reducing myocardial oxygen demand and increasing collateral flow, rather than by restoring anterograde flow. For the most part these efforts have not succeeded in human subjects, although it may be argued that the agents have not been given an adequate trial because of administration relatively late in the course of the infarction. Insensitivity inherent in the clinical measurements of infarct size has also made demonstration of benefit difficult.

Beta blockers administered at a mean of 3.4 hours after the onset of chest pain have been shown to reduce several indirect measures of ischemia and infarct size, such as chest pain and ventricular fibrillation, and to preserve R waves and reduce the development of Q waves. Direct measurements of left ventricular function were not made in these studies, however, and there was no effect on mortality.[15] Studies in which beta blockers were administered at means of 8 to 11 hours after the onset of chest pain have detected no effect on infarct size or mortality.[28] These results, together with the fact that beta blockade is hazardous in patients with the greatest need for myocardial salvage—those with large infarcts—do not permit an unqualified endorsement of beta blockade for acute MI.

Although individual trials of intravenous nitroglycerin have produced conflicting data with regard to infarct size and mortality, pooled data from these studies show a 20 percent reduction in mortality associated with nitroglycerin administration.[36] Nifedipine, verapamil, nitroprusside, and hyaluronidase have failed to reduce infarct size or mortality when administered a mean of 6 to 12 hours after the onset of chest pain.

In contrast, intravenous administration of 1.5 million U of the thrombolytic agent streptokinase over 1 hour has been shown to reduce infarct size and mortality by a small but highly significant amount statistically when administered within 6 hours of the onset of chest pain.[13] This benefit is concentrated in patients with anterior infarcts and those who are treated within 1 hour of the onset of chest pain. Intracoronary streptokinase and emergency coronary angioplasty have also been found to preserve left ventricular function and reduce mortality.[17,25,31] Although these approaches are associated with higher recanalization rates and lesser degrees of residual stenosis in the infarct-related coronary artery than intravenous streptokinase, they are not widely applicable. Many hospitals lack the facilities for catheterization and angioplasty. Even among hospitals that can perform these procedures, the delays associated with emergency cardiac catheterization may negate the benefit of intracoronary therapy.[1]

As experience with streptokinase has accumulated, it has become apparent that thrombolytic therapy is limited in several ways. Intravenous streptokinase dissolves the infarct-related thrombus in 60 to 90 minutes in only about half the patients, and because of the high-grade residual stenoses that typically persist after successful thrombolytic therapy, reocclusion and reinfarction rates are as high as 20 percent.[35] In the years ahead, it is likely that tissue plasminogen activator will replace streptokinase. Tissue plasminogen activator, a natural human thrombolytic agent, is nonantigenic and relatively clot-specific. Allergic reactions have not been reported with its use, and it is faster and more effective than streptokinase.[35] Strategies for identification of patients at risk of reocclusion are

still evolving, but current practice includes catheterization of all patients in whom thrombolytic therapy is thought to have successfully lysed the infarct-related clot. It is also generally agreed that patients with greater than 70 percent stenoses need some form of urgent revascularization procedure, either angioplasty or coronary bypass surgery. Optimal timing for revascularization has not yet been defined.

Blood pressure permitting, it is appropriate to initiate therapy for all acute MIs with one or two 0.4 mg sublingual nitroglycerin tablets (Fig. 2.8–5). Nitroglycerin is a potent coronary vasodilator and occasionally provides dramatic improvement or aborts the infarct completely. Although such improvement is unusual, the ease and rapidity with which nitroglycerin can be administered and the fact that its administration does not interfere with other measures that may subsequently become necessary seem to justify this approach. If the patient's condition and the ECG have not improved within 5 to 10 minutes of drug administration, it is appropriate to shift the focus of therapy to other agents, particularly thrombolytics.

LONG-TERM CARE

A wide variety of approaches have been employed to minimize the incidence of sudden cardiac death or recurrent MI among survivors of MI. This section will focus on the major determinants of survival after infarction, risk stratification, treatment with beta-adrenergic blocking drugs or aspirin, and general rehabilitative measures.

General Considerations
Death rates among infarct survivors are approximately 10 percent during the first year and 3 to 5 percent annually for each of the next several years. The single most important determinant of survival is residual left ventricular function. One study, for example, found an almost exponential increase in death rates as ejection fraction fell below 40 percent. Whereas patients with ejection fractions of 60 percent or greater had 1-year mortality rates of approximately 2 percent and those with ejection fractions of 40 percent to 59 percent had only a small additional risk, nearly half of the patients with ejection fractions less than 20 percent had died in the first year after their infarctions.[23]

The number and severity of coronary artery stenoses and high-grade ventricular ectopy have also been identified as risk factors for death in the years after a MI.[23,29] Because these problems are treatable in a way that poor left ventricular function is not (treatment of congestive heart failure is aimed at symptoms and does little for the left ventricle itself), their detection is an important part of postinfarction care. Indeed, many authorities have incorporated screening for myocardial ischemia and ventricular ectopy into a predischarge routine.[5]

Low-Level Stress Testing
Several studies have shown that patients in whom myocardial ischemia is provoked by a low-level stress test (e.g., target heart rate 70 percent of age-predicted maximum) performed 1 to 3 weeks after an acute MI have a 20 percent risk of recurrent infarction or death over the next year, whereas those without ischemia have a mortality risk of 2 to 5 percent.[19] On the basis of these studies, it is common practice to perform coronary arteriography and, if appropriate, coronary angioplasty or bypass surgery on patients with ischemic responses. However, it is not known whether such patients can be treated as safely with aggressive antianginal therapy followed by angioplasty or surgery in the event of failure of medical therapy.

Ambulatory Electrocardiographic Monitoring
The detection of frequent premature ventricular beats or nonsustained ventricular tachycardia with 24 hours of ambulatory ECG (Holter) monitoring obtained 1 to 2 weeks after MI is associated

with an increased risk of sudden cardiac death.[22,23] The occurrence of high-grade ventricular ectopy is also closely correlated with severe left ventricular dysfunction, however, and it is not completely established that the ventricular ectopy is truly an independent risk factor. Likewise, it has not been demonstrated that prophylactic antiarrhythmic therapy can prevent the sudden deaths that are associated with ventricular ectopy.

Beta Blockade
The long-term administration of beta blockers, initiated 1 to 4 weeks after infarction, has been shown repeatedly to reduce mortality rates among selected infarct survivors by approximately one third.[3,11,24] This reduction in mortality appears to persist for at least 3 years and is primarily due to a reduction in sudden cardiac death among patients with arrhythmias or mild congestive heart failure during the in-hospital phase of their infarction.[11,24]

Aspirin
Several large studies have tested the hypothesis that antiplatelet therapy with aspirin can reduce the incidence of recurrent infarction and death. Although these studies have provided conflicting results, a recent analysis of pooled data from these trials concluded that aspirin use is associated with a 10 percent reduction in mortality.[4,34]

General Rehabilitative Measures
General rehabilitative measures should be aimed at the restoration of physical and social function and, where possible, the elimination of risk factors for atherosclerosis.

Most patients can begin walking on the third or fourth hospital day and can be discharged 1 to 2 weeks after the infarction. Low-level, predischarge exercise testing is especially useful in this setting, because apart from long-term prognostic information, it provides specific guidelines about safe or unsafe physical activity.

Because a period of 6 or more weeks is required before transmurally infarcted myocardium is completely replaced by scar tissue, patients are usually advised to avoid strenuous exercise and, in particular, isometric exercise during this period. Stretching exercises, walking, and light household chores can be performed during this time. Sexual activity is permitted, but some restraint is advised. The cardiovascular demands of sexual intercourse between married partners are equivalent to walking at a brisk pace or climbing two flights of stairs.

Depending on the size of the infarct and the nature of the patient's work, most patients can return to work 1 to 3 months after an MI. Patients with large infarcts and poor left ventricular function should not resume strenuous physical labor. Selected patients may benefit from supervised exercise in formal rehabilitation programs. The major advantages of these programs are that they can be effective in building confidence and that they acquaint patients with the discipline and invigoration of regular exercise. Regular exercise may also stimulate collateral coronary artery blood flow.

Risk factor modification is a worthy goal. Control of hypertension, cessation of smoking, and reduction of cholesterol levels are all associated with reduction of cardiovascular morbidity and mortality after MI.

In addition to anxiety about the safety of daily activities, depression and denial are common problems after MI. Most patients respond to a sympathetic and frank appraisal of their physical limitations and prognosis. Those who do not respond usually react favorably to professional counseling. Every effort should be made to return the patient to a normal social and economic life.

REFERENCES

1. Anderson JL, Marshall HW, et al: A randomized trial of intravenous and intracoronary streptokinase in patients with acute myocardial infarction. Circulation 70:606, 1984

2. Baumgartner WA, Borkon AM, et al: Operative intervention for post-infarction angina. Ann Thorac Surg 38:265, 1984
3. Beta-Blocker Heart Attack Trial Research Group: A randomized trial of propranolol in patients with acute myocardial infarction. JAMA 247:1701, 1982
4. Canner PL: Aspirin in coronary heart disease: Comparison of six clinical trials. Isr J Med Sci 19:413, 1983
5. DeBusk RF, Blomqvist CG, et al: Identification and treatment of low risk patients after acute myocardial infarction and coronary artery bypass graft surgery. N Engl J Med 314:161, 1986
6. DeFeyter PJ, Serruys PW, et al: Coronary angioplasty for early post-infarction unstable angina. Circulation 74:1365, 1986
7. DeWood MA, Spores J, et al: Prevalence of total coronary occlusion during the early hours of acute myocardial infarction. N Engl J Med 303:897, 1980
8. DeWood MA, Stifter WF, et al: Coronary arteriographic findings soon after non-Q-wave myocardial infarction. N Engl J Med 303:417, 1986
9. Folts JD, Crowell EB, Rowe GG: Platelet aggregation in partially ob-structed vessels and its elimination with aspirin. Circulation 54:365, 1976
10. Forrester JS, Diamond G, et al: Medical therapy of acute myocardial infarction by application of hemodynamic subsets. N Engl J Med 295:1356, 1404, 1976
11. Furburg CD, Hawkins CM, Lichstein E: Effect of propranolol in post-infarction patients with mechanical or electrical complications. Circula-tion 69:761, 1984
12. Geft PL, Shah PK, et al: ST elevation in leads V_1 to V_5 may be caused by right coronary occlusion and acute right ventricular infarction. Am J Cardiol 53:991, 1984
13. Gruppo Italiano per lo Studio della Streptochinasi Nell' Infarto Miocar-dico (GISSI): Effectiveness of intravenous thrombolytic treatment in acute myocardial infarction. Lancet 1:397, 1986
14. Hindman MC, Wagner GS, et al: The clinical significance of bundle branch block complicating acute myocardial infarction. 2. Indications for temporary and permanent pacemaker insertion. Circulation 58:689, 1978
15. International Collaborative Study Group: Reduction of infarct size with the early use of timolol in acute myocardial infarction. N Engl J Med 310:9, 1984
16. Julian DG, Valentine PA, Miller GG: Disturbances of rate, rhythm, and conduction in acute myocardial infarction. Am J Med 37:915, 1964
17. Kennedy JW, Ritchie JL, et al: The western Washington randomized trial of intracoronary streptokinase in acute myocardial infarction: A 12-month follow-up report. N Engl J Med 312:1073, 1985
18. Killip T, Kimball JT: Treatment of myocardial infarction in a coronary care unit: A two-year experience with 250 patients. Am J Cardiol 201:457, 1967
19. Krone RJ, Gillespie JA, et al: Low level exercise testing after myocardial infarction: Usefulness in enhancing clinical risk stratification. Circula-tion 71:80–89, 1985
20. Lie KI, Wellens HJ, et al: Lidocaine in the prevention of primary ven-tricular fibrillation. N Engl J Med 291:1324, 1974
21. Maseri A, L'Abbate A, et al: Coronary vasospasm as a possible cause of myocardial infarction: A conclusion derived from the study of "pre-infarction angina." N Engl J Med 299:1271, 1978
22. Moss AJ, David HT, et al: Ventricular ectopic beats and their relation to sudden and non-sudden cardiac death after myocardial infarction. Circulation 60:998, 1979
23. Multicenter Postinfarction Research Group: Risk stratification and sur-vival after myocardial infarction. N Engl J Med 309:331, 1983
24. Norwegian Multicenter Study Group: Timolol induced reduction in mortality and reinfarction in patients surviving acute myocardial infarc-tion. N Engl J Med 304:802, 1981
25. O'Neill W, Timmis GC, et al: A prospective randomized clinical trial of intracoronary streptokinase versus coronary angioplasty for acute myocardial infarction. N Engl J Med 314:812, 1986
26. Report of the Sixty Plus Reinfarction Study Research Group: A double-blind trial to assess long-term or anticoagulant therapy in elderly pa-tients after myocardial infarction. Lancet 2:889, 1980
27. Rivas F, Cobb FR, et al: Relationship between blood flow to ischemic regions and extent of myocardial infarction. Circ Res 39:439, 1976
28. Roberts R, Croft C, et al: Effect of propranolol on myocardial infarct size in a randomized blinded multicenter trial. N Engl J Med 311:218, 1984
29. Sanz G, Castañer, et al: Determinants of prognosis in survivors of myo-cardial infarction. N Engl J Med 306:1065, 1982
30. Schuster EH, Bulkley BH: Early post-infarction angina: Ischemia at a distance and ischemia in the infarct zone. N Engl J Med 305:1101, 1981
31. Simoons ML, Serruys PW, et al: Improved survival after early throm-bolysis in acute myocardial infarction. Lancet 2:578, 1985
32. Turner JD, Rogers WJ, et al: Coronary angiography soon after myocar-dial infarction. Chest 77:58, 1980
33. Vatner SF: Correlation between acute reductions in myocardial blood flow and function in conscious dogs. Circ Res 47:201, 1980
34. Veterans Administration Cooperative Trial: Anticoagulants in acute myocardial infarction. JAMA 225:724, 1973
35. Williams DO, Borer J, et al: Intravenous recombinant tissue type plas-minogen activator in patients with acute myocardial infarction: A re-port from the NHLBI Thrombolysis in Myocardial Infarction Trial. Circulation 73:338, 1986
36. Yusuf S, Collins R: IV nitroglycerin and nitroprusside therapy in acute myocardial infarction reduces mortality: Evidence of randomized con-trolled trials (abstr). Circulation 72 (suppl 3):224, 1985

CHAPTER 2.9
Cardiac Arrhythmias

Thomas Guarnieri and Lawrence S.C. Griffith

The normal excitation of the human heart initiates contraction in an orderly and synchronous fashion, thereby producing an effec-tive cardiac output. Excitation begins in the sinus node, which, by virtue of its inherent automatic behavior, is the primary cardiac pacemaker. Impulses generated in the sinus node result in atrial contraction and, through an extensive conduction system, ventric-ular contraction. A cardiac arrhythmia is said to exist when the normal order of excitation is perturbed, through changes in either automaticity, conduction, or both.

ANATOMY AND PHYSIOLOGY

The sinus node is the primary pacemaker of the heart. It surrounds the sinus node artery at the junction of the superior vena cava and the right atrium. Atrial pathways from the sinus node to the A-V node (internodal pathways) have been described, but their role in conduction is unclear.

The atria and the ventricles are electrically linked in a complex area known as the A-V junction (Fig. 2.9–1). The proximal por-tion of the junction is made up of the intersection of the atrial fibers and the A-V node, found at the base of the atrial septum. The vascular supply of the A-V node comes from the A-V nodal artery, originating in 90 percent of individuals from the distal right coronary artery.

The bundle of His, enveloped by connective tissue, emerges from the A-V node at the central fibrous body and courses to the muscular septum. The branching portion of the His bundle exits from the central fibrous body and cascades down the septum in the form of the left bundle and the right bundle (Fig. 2.9–1). The

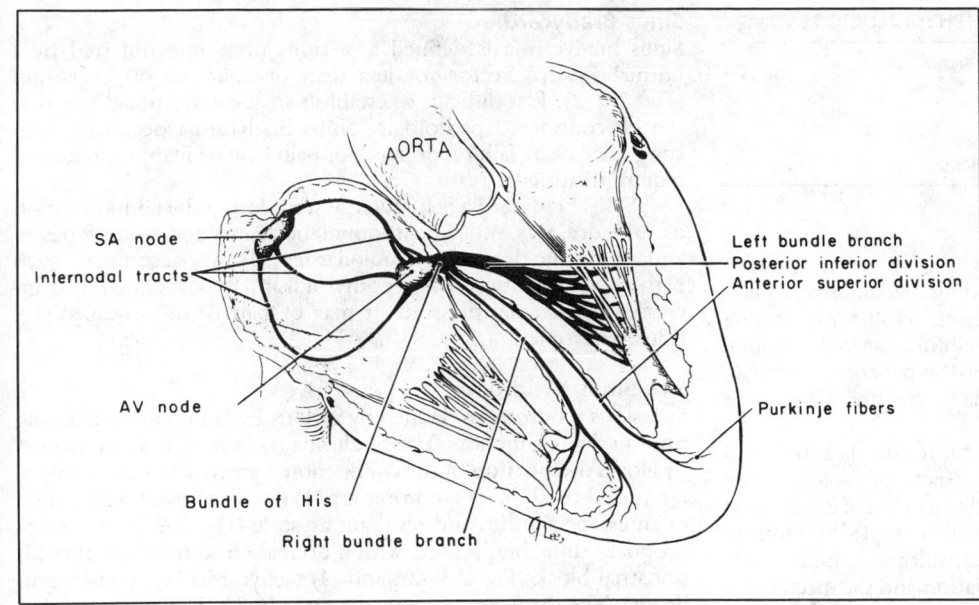

Figure 2.9-1. Anatomy of impulse conduction.

left bundle has been classified electrocardiographically as having two major fascicles, the left anterior and the left posterior, although this anatomic division may not be distinct. The right bundle is a more discrete fiber, coursing down the septum and arborizing in the right ventricle. The blood supply to the His bundle and the bundle branches is complex and variable. The common His bundle and the first third of the right bundle are generally supplied by the A-V nodal artery, whereas the distal right bundle, common left bundle, and left anterior fascicle are supplied by the left anterior descending coronary artery. The posterior fascicle receives blood from both the left anterior descending artery and the A-V nodal artery. Knowledge of these vascular relationships is helpful in understanding the occurrence of various types of conduction abnormalities in ischemic heart disease.

The conduction system of the heart is richly innervated by both the sympathetic and the parasympathetic nervous systems. Stimulation of the cardiac sympathetic fibers enhances automaticity and conduction velocity throughout the heart. Conversely, the parasympathetic nervous system exerts its effect primarily above the bundle of His. Parasympathetic (vagal) stimulation decreases automaticity and conduction through both the sinoatrial node and the A-V node but does speed atrial conduction.

DIAGNOSIS OF ARRHYTHMIAS

The first principle in the approach to the patient with a cardiac arrhythmia is to achieve the correct diagnosis. In many cases this will require a careful analysis of the history and the physical examination, and a repeated review of the ECG. In some individuals the correct diagnosis may require several ECGs or the use of specialized devices, including ambulatory monitors or intracardiac recordings.

After diagnosis, the arrhythmia must be viewed in context. For example, premature ventricular contractions occur in many young and healthy individuals, and their presence is harmless. Conversely, frequent premature ventricular contractions in a patient with an acute myocardial infarction may portend a life-threatening arrhythmia. In some cases a cardiac arrhythmia reflects the subject's physiologic state. For example, the bradycardia seen in trained distance runners represents a conditioning effect and is not an arrhythmia per se. On the contrary, some rhythm disorders are distinct entities. The A-V reciprocating tachycardia (paroxysmal supraventricular tachycardia) seen in individuals with the Wolff-Parkinson-White syndrome is based on the alterations in the anatomy and physiologic characteristics of the conduction system and is a problem unto itself.

Cardiac arrhythmias must also be viewed in relation to the hemodynamic alterations they cause. Bradycardia alters cardiac output by producing a low mean blood pressure because of the prolonged time the heart is in diastole, whereas tachycardia produces low output because of incomplete filling of the ventricles and, in some cases, disturbed patterns of contraction. Additionally, in those rhythms where A-V synchrony is interrupted, the contribution of atrial contraction to the cardiac output may be lost.

DETECTION OF CARDIAC ARRHYTHMIAS

Occasionally the patient's history may be sufficient for diagnosis. Some patients with paroxysmal atrial fibrillation can "tap out" an irregularly irregular rhythm. In general, though, a history of palpitations is not reliable for the diagnosis of arrhythmias. Some individuals with serious arrhythmias (e.g., ventricular tachycardia) may have asymptomatic but nonsustained periods of arrhythmias, which are an important warning sign. On the other hand, rhythm disorders that produce acute changes in cardiac output and loss of consciousness, whether from a slow heart rate or a rapid heart rate, are not well reported.

The physical examination during an episode of cardiac arrhythmia is an important and often overlooked part of the diagnostic evaluation. Of particular help is the evaluation of the jugular venous waveform. The presence of flutter waves is an important clue to the diagnosis of atrial flutter. The presence of cannon waves suggests junctional or ventricular tachycardia with ventriculoatrial dissociation. If the cardiac rhythm is regular, the varying intensity of the first heart sound suggests A-V dissociation.

The standard for the diagnosis of cardiac arrhythmias remains the ECG. It cannot be overemphasized that the recording of a 12-lead ECG during cardiac arrhythmia (as opposed to a rhythm strip only) is an important factor in the diagnosis of the arrhythmia. Careful examination of the tracing from each lead of the 12-lead ECG is mandatory in determining the exact relationship between the atria and the ventricles. The ECG's accuracy can often be augmented by the use of specialized lead systems (Lewis leads or esophageal leads), which attempt to record atrial activity more accurately.

Many cardiac rhythm disorders are paroxysmal, and the physi-

TABLE 2.9–1. INDICATIONS FOR ELECTROPHYSIOLOGIC TESTING

• Diagnosis of wide QRS complex tachycardia
• Pharmacologic control of arrhythmias
• Arrhythmia mapping
• Testing efficacy of antitachycardia devices

cian does not have the benefit of a recording made during an episode of cardiac arrhythmia. In these cases, Holter monitoring or transtelephonic monitoring is very helpful. Especially helpful with the Holter monitor is the ability of the patient to correlate the presence of symptoms and arrhythmia by the use of a diary or a signal button attached to the device.

The most specialized method for both the diagnosis and provocation of cardiac arrhythmias is the electrophysiology study (Table 2.9–1). The electrophysiology study enables the intracardiac electrograms to be recorded. It was originally designed to measure the His potential but has evolved into a multiple-catheter study that can accurately measure both the initiation and the mechanism of many cardiac arrhythmias. It has been especially helpful in the diagnosis of arrhythmias of uncertain mechanism (the wide QRS complex tachycardia) and has been used of late for guiding therapy in the treatment of ventricular tachycardia. The electrophysiology study is mandatory if surgical treatment of an arrhythmia is planned.

CLASSIFICATION OF ARRHYTHMIAS

BRADYCARDIA

The term "bradycardia" is applied when the heart rate is less than or equal to 60 beats/min. Bradycardia is not necessarily pathologic, because it can be present in conditioned athletes or in anyone during sleep. Bradycardia becomes pathologic when the heart rate is too slow to sustain cardiac output and thereby produces symptoms. Bradycardia of various types is common in elderly persons, and as such its presence is not sufficient in many cases to explain symptoms. Symptoms must be clearly correlated with the presence of the rhythm disorder. Bradycardia or asystole may be transient in individuals with severe conduction system disease. In many of these individuals, multiple recordings are necessary to document the presence of severe bradycardia occurring with symptoms.

Sinus Bradycardia

Sinus bradycardia is defined as a sinus node rate (inferred by a normal P-wave vector) of less than or equal to 60 beats/min (Fig. 2.9–2). It is difficult to establish an absolute cut-off rate that can be considered pathologic. Sinus bradycardia occurring with congestive heart failure, exercise, or pain may be inappropriate and require treatment.

Sinus bradycardia is frequently seen during the administration of such drugs as antisympathomimetic agents and some types of antiarrhythmic drugs (e.g., amiodarone). It may accompany such pathologic conditions as hypothyroidism, hypothermia, and increased intracranial pressure. It may be part of the so-called sick sinus syndrome.

Sick Sinus Syndrome

Sick sinus syndrome is defined by various ECG findings suggesting sinus node dysfunction. The syndrome is commonly accompanied by global dysfunction of the conduction system. The main components of the sick sinus syndrome are (1) sinoatrial arrest with failure of an escape rhythm and resultant asystole (Fig. 2.9–2), (2) inappropriate sinus bradycardia with a decrease in cardiac output, (3) sinoatrial block (Fig. 2.9–2), and (4) tachycardia-bradycardia syndrome. The third component, sinoatrial block, may be recognized by a periodic failure of the P wave to appear or from a decrease in the P-P intervals before the P wave. It is important to examine the ECG for evidence of an atrial premature contraction that is not conducted through the A-V node and thus mimics sinus block. The fourth component of the sick sinus syndrome, known as tachycardia-bradycardia syndrome, is a common variant of the sick sinus syndrome. It is characterized by a pause after a period of tachycardia, generally atrial fibrillation—hence the name "tachycardia-bradycardia syndrome." Occasionally, atrial fibrillation with a slow ventricular response rate is called the sick sinus syndrome because cardioversion of this rhythm may result in asystole. The cause of sick sinus syndrome is not clear, but the abnormality is generally characterized by a diffuse fibrosis of the conduction system.

Sinoatrial block is an uncommon finding but is seen in the presence of structural disease of the atrium or drug toxicity. Digitalis, quinidine, and other type I agents can precipitate sinoatrial block. Although vagal stimulation can also precipitate sinoatrial block, in general there is an underlying cause, such as ischemia or a degenerative process.

Junctional Rhythm (Junctional Escape)

Junctional rhythm, so called because it arises in the A-V junction, represents an escape mechanism when there is failure of impulse

Figure 2.9–2. A. Sinus bradycardia. Atrial and ventricular rate of 37 beats/min with constant P-R interval of 0.14 second. Chronic 2 to 1 sinoatrial block is alternative explanation for this form of bradycardia. **B.** Sinoatrial block, 2 to 1. Interval between third and fourth P wave is exactly twice the normal interval, as seen between the first, second, and third P waves. Left bundle-branch block pattern is also present. **C.** Sinus arrest. After three normal-appearing P-QRS-T complexes, there is no evidence of impulse formation or transmission for 1.5 seconds. At that time a QRS complex appears as a result of impulse that was probably generated in the A-V junction. This is an escape junctional beat. Before second escape junctional beat is generated, sequential activation of the atrium, A-V node, and ventricle is resumed from sinoatrial node.

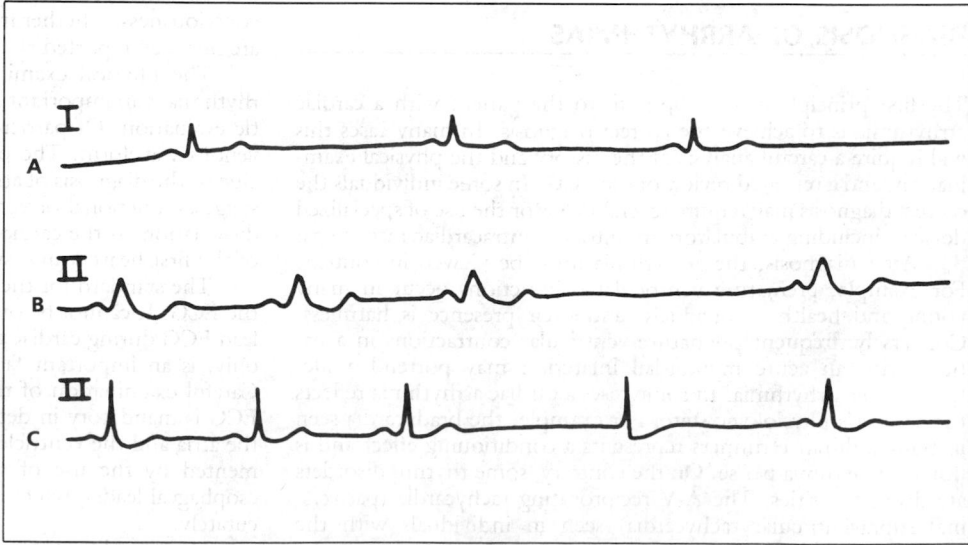

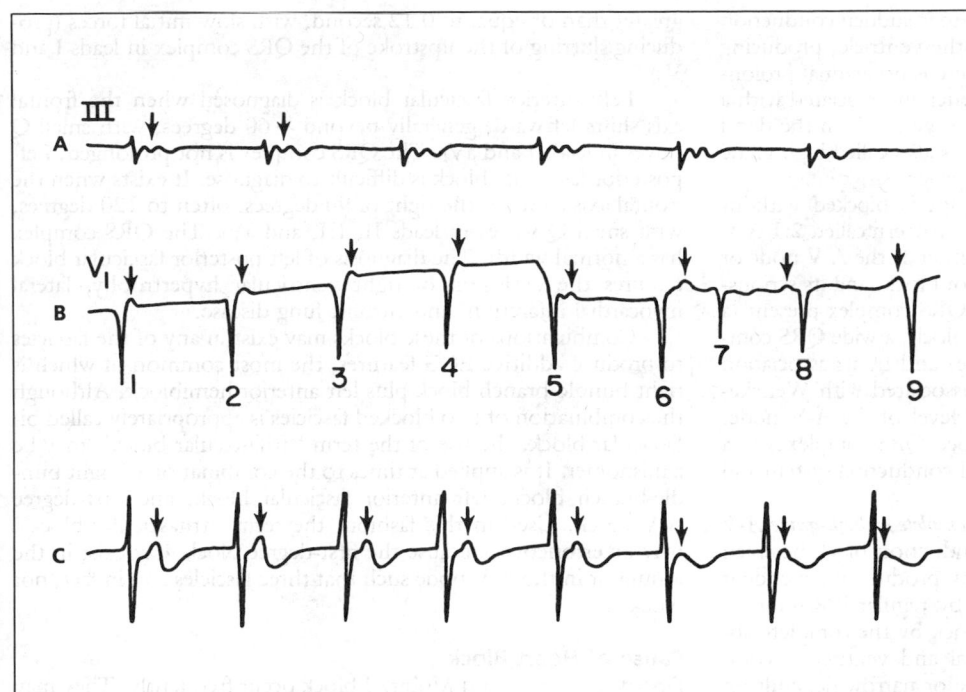

Figure 2.9–3. A. Junctional bradycardia with retrograde activation of atrium. P wave follows each QRS complex. Inverted P wave in this lead and lead II and upright P wave in lead aV$_R$ result from retrograde depolarization of atrium. B. Junctional rhythm with capture beats, also known as A-V dissociation. In this strip, QRS complexes numbered 1 to 6 are result of impulses generated in the A-V junction. However, atrium continues to be depolarized from impulse generated in sinoatrial node at a rate slightly slower than rate of impulse generation in A-V junction. Fourth and fifth P waves follow QRS complex at a time when A-V node is still totally refractory and thus are not transmitted to ventricle. Sixth P wave occurs during relative refractory period, however, and is conducted with prolonged PR interval. C. Junctional rhythm with isorhythmic dissociation. Rates of impulse formation in sinoatrial node and A-V junction are very similar, and P waves are in close association with QRS complexes, but sequential activation of atrium, A-V node, and ventricle is not present.

formation or conduction (Fig. 2.9–3). The rate and form of the rhythm depend on its origin. Rhythms arising in the proximal A-V node result in a narrow QRS complex and a rate of 40 to 60 beats/min, whereas those arising in the His, Purkinje, or distal conducting system have a wide QRS complex with a rate of 20 to 40 beats/min. It is not infrequent for junctional rhythms arising in the proximal A-V node to have retrograde capture of the atrium or to be dissociated from the atrial rhythm altogether.

The most common causes of junctional rhythms are intoxication from digitalis or other A-V node–blocking drugs. This rhythm is also common during acute inferior myocardial infarction.

Atrioventricular Block

A-V block exists when the atrial impulse to the ventricles is delayed or blocked in the A-V junction, the distal conducting system, or both. The impairment of the conduction is said to be fixed (independent of rate) or functional (rate dependent).

Historically, ECG findings have been used to categorize A-V block as either first-degree, second-degree (Mobitz type I, or Wenckebach, and Mobitz type II), or third-degree block. In general, the progression from first-degree through third-degree block

represents a continuum of physiologic and pathologic severity, with third-degree block being the most severe. Just as essential as determination of the type of heart block present is characterization of the escape pacemaker, since it is the escape pacemaker that is ultimately important in maintaining cardiac output.

First-degree heart block is characterized by a P-R interval greater than 0.20 second. Usually the delay occurs in the A-V node, although with diffuse conduction-system disease the delay can exist at multiple levels of the conduction system.

Second-degree A-V block is divided into Mobitz I, or Wenckebach block and Mobitz II block. In Mobitz I block the QRS complex is typically normal and the block is characterized by a progressive prolongation of the P-R interval until a QRS complex fails to follow a P wave (Fig. 2.9–4). The amount of increase in the P-R prolongation with each beat progressively lessens, thereby shortening the R-R interval. The pattern produced on the ECG is one of "grouped" beating. The ratio of the number of QRS complexes to the number of P waves characterizes the Wenckebach phenomenon (3:2 means three P waves to two QRS complexes). The ratio of the number of P waves to QRS complexes may vary from sequence to sequence, giving a variety of ECG patterns. Mobitz I A-V block is generally localized to the A-V node and may, in fact, be a transient phenomenon.

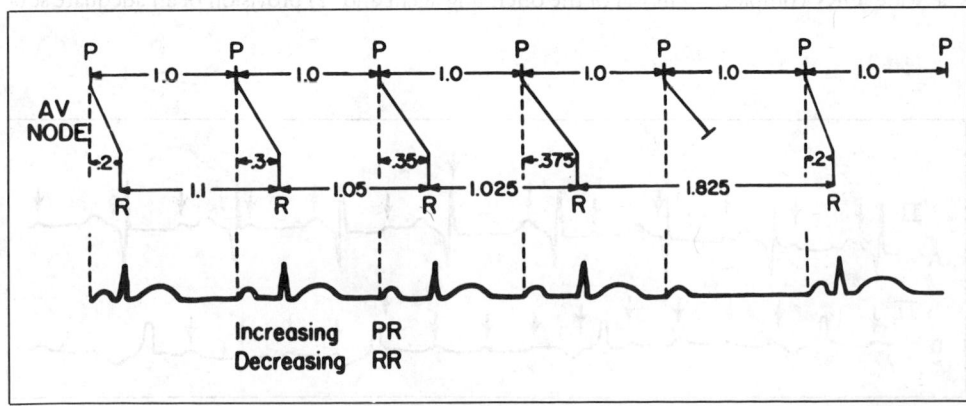

Figure 2.9–4. Schematic representation of Wenckebach phenomenon, in which P-P interval remains constant but P-R interval becomes progressively longer while R-R interval becomes shorter. Note that fifth P wave is not conducted to ventricle and results in dropped beat, which allows A-V node to rest and thus conduct sixth P wave with short P-R interval.

Mobitz II A-V block exists when there is sudden conduction failure of one or more atrial impulses to the ventricle, producing an "all or none" conduction pattern. There is no gradual prolongation of the P-R interval. Mobitz II is generally associated with a wide QRS complex, and the site of block is generally in the distal part of the conducting system. Mobitz II is also called high-grade A-V block because it carries an ominous prognosis.

Occasionally every other QRS complex is blocked without changing P-R or P-P intervals, producing a pattern called 2:1 A-V block. The level of 2:1 block may occur either at the A-V node or in the distal conduction system. The site of block (and its seriousness) can be judged both by the type of QRS complex present (a narrow QRS complex suggests A-V node block; a wide QRS complex suggests block below the His bundle) and by its association with other forms of A-V block. When associated with Wenckebach block, the block is generally at the level of the A-V node. When fixed or associated with two dropped QRS complexes in a row, it is probably at the level of the distal conduction system and should be regarded as Mobitz II.

Third-degree A-V block (also called *complete or high-grade A-V block*) exists when there is a complete conduction block between the atrial impulse and the ventricles that produce independent rhythms (Fig. 2.9–5). It is characterized by regular R-R intervals on the ECG. It differs from Mobitz II block by the complete absence of a relationship between the atrial and ventricular complexes. Whether the QRS complex is wide or narrow depends on the area of block, although in advanced forms of heart disease it is almost always wide. In congenital heart block or after surgically induced heart block, the QRS complex may be narrow. With advanced conduction-system disease, the rate of the subsidiary pacemaker may be slow and may indicate an ominous prognosis. In third-degree heart block, the regularity of the R-R interval may be disturbed by shifts in the site of the escape pacemaker, premature ventricular contractions, or temporary or partial reinstitution of conduction.

Bundle-Branch Block. Delay or block of impulse conduction in one of the three conducting fascicles produces a characteristic ECG pattern that is termed right bundle-branch block, left bundle-branch block, left anterior fascicular block, or left posterior fascicular block (Fig. 2.9–6). In some cases the block may occur in the various components of the bundle-branch system; a frequent combination, for example, is left anterior fascicular block and right bundle-branch block. Some of the combinations are dictated by a common compromise of the vascular supply of the conduction system.

Right bundle-branch block produces a wide QRS complex, greater than or equal to 0.12 second, with slow terminal forces (producing a slurred S wave in lead I and lead V_6). The initial forces are sharp, because the interventricular septum of the heart continues to be depolarized in the normal left-to-right fashion. So-called incomplete right bundle-branch block can be identified by a QRS complex that is between 0.10 and 0.12 second in duration but that is similar in appearance to right bundle-branch block.

Left bundle-branch block produces a wide QRS complex, greater than or equal to 0.12 second, with slow initial forces (producing slurring of the upstroke of the QRS complex in leads I and V_6).

Left anterior fascicular block is diagnosed when the frontal axis shifts leftward, generally beyond −60 degrees, with small Q waves in leads I and aV_L. The QRS complex is not prolonged. Left posterior fascicular block is difficult to diagnose. It exists when the frontal axis shifts to the right of 90 degrees, often to 120 degrees, with small Q waves in leads II, III, and aV_F. The QRS complex has a normal width. The diagnosis of left posterior fascicular block requires the exclusion of right ventricular hypertrophy, lateral myocardial infarction, and chronic lung disease.

Combinations of these blocks may exist in any of the fascicles to produce additive ECG features, the most common of which is right bundle-branch block plus left anterior hemiblock. Although the combination of two blocked fascicles is appropriately called bifascicular block, the use of the term "trifascicular block" may be a misnomer. It is applied at times to the combination of right bundle-branch block, left anterior fascicular block, and first-degree A-V block. Used in this fashion, the term "trifascicular block" may be erroneous, because the first-degree block may exist in the atrium or in the A-V node such that three fascicles are, in fact, not blocked.

Cause of Heart Block

First-degree block and Mobitz I block occur frequently. They may be seen in acute rheumatic fever or other infectious processes of the myocardium, including acute myocarditis. Many drugs cause first-degree or Mobitz I block, including digitalis, beta blockers, calcium-channel blockers, and amiodarone. Other common causes are invasion of the conduction system by granulomatous disease, surgical and catheterization trauma, and congenital abnormalities of the conduction system. Mobitz II block and third-degree A-V block occur after myocardial infarction and in patients with a fibrotic or degenerative process of the conduction system. As noted, high-grade A-V block signals an ominous form of conduction system disease because of slow and unpredictable escape pacemakers. All degrees of heart block may occur in acute myocardial infarction or in chronic ischemic disease. Notably, most episodes of heart block occurring in the acute phase of inferior myocardial infarction are reversible. Forms of heart block or bundle-branch block during an anterior myocardial infarction signify a poor prognosis, not necessarily on the basis of conduction, but because of the amount of myocardium destroyed.

Clinical Manifestations

Generally Mobitz I block and first-degree heart block are asymptomatic. Episodic Mobitz II block and episodic complete heart block can produce grave problems. When associated with a slow escape pacemaker or with asystole, they may produce syncope, low cardiac output, congestive heart failure, or death.

Treatment of Heart Block

The treatment of heart block is based on two principles: (1) removal of the offending agent and (2) provision of an adequate sub-

Figure 2.9–5. A. Complete heart block—junctional pacemaker. Narrow QRS complex and relatively rapid rate of 70 beats/min indicate that ventricular pacemaker is relatively high in A-V junctional tissue. P waves are indicated by arrows. **B.** Complete heart block—idioventricular pacemaker. Wide QRS complex and very slow rate indicate that pacemaker is located in ventricle, usually in distal part of the Purkinje system.

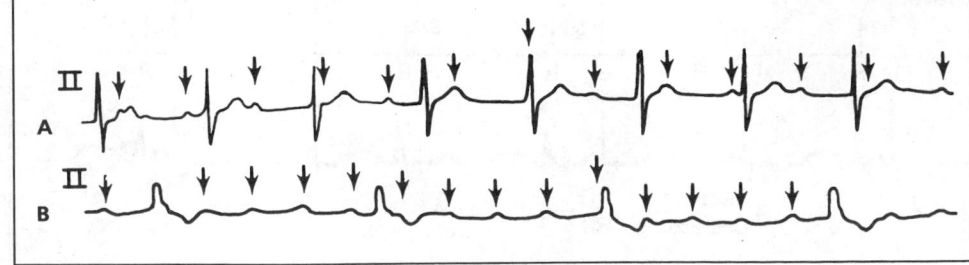

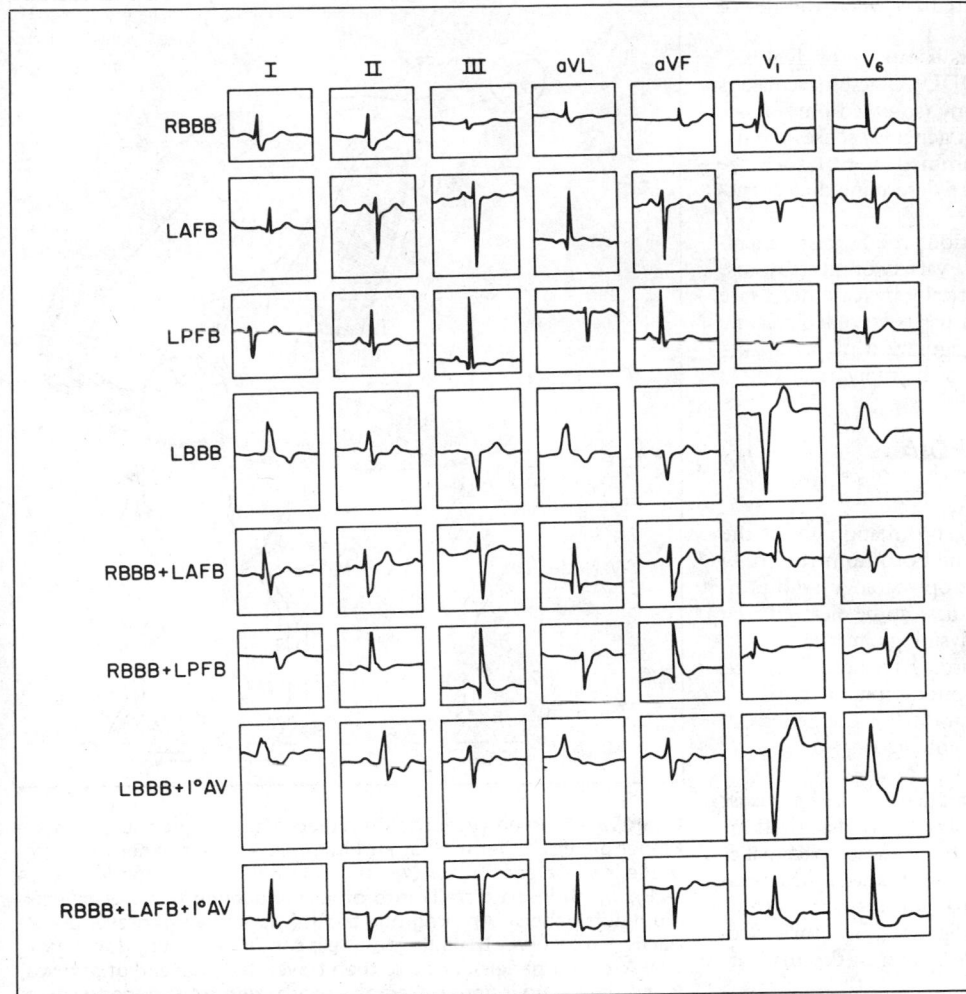

Figure 2.9–6. Electrocardiographic patterns associated with fascicular blocks. RBBB = right bundle-branch block; LAFB = left anterior fascicular block; LPFB = left posterior fascicular block; LBBB = left bundle-branch block; 1°AV = first degree of A-V block. Top three patterns (RBBB, LAFB, LPFB) represent unifascicular block; next three patterns (LBBB, RBBB plus LAFB, and RBBB plus LPFB) represent bifascicular blocks; and bottom two patterns (LBBB plus 1°AV, and RBBB and LAFB and 1°AV) represent two forms of trifascicular block.

sidiary pacemaker. Drugs that produce heart block must be removed, or if indispensable, they must be accompanied by the use of a pacemaker. In acute situations, 1 mg of atropine given intravenously may transiently improve A-V conduction in blocks located in the A-V node but rarely is effective for more serious forms of A-V block, particularly those seen with anterior myocardial infarction.

As noted earlier, it is rare for first-degree block or Mobitz type I second-degree block to require treatment other than removal of the causative factor. In episodes that are drug induced and occur at the A-V node, atropine may transiently improve conduction.

High-grade A-V block, whether established or transient, requires artificial pacing. Exceptions to this rule are seen in patients with inferior myocardial infarction and transient heart block and in patients with congenital heart block or surgically induced heart block whose escape pacemaker is adequate to maintain blood pressure and cardiac output.

In most patients, high-grade A-V block is not improved by atropine. Intravenously administered isoproterenol or epinephrine may increase the rate of junctional or ventricular pacemakers. However, caution must be exerted in using these agents in the face of acute myocardial infarction. Artificial pacing is the treatment of choice.

Pacemakers. Since the first pacemakers were implanted in 1950, there has been a revolution in the type and variety of pacemakers useful for the treatment of intractable bradycardia or heart block. With the advance in the technology of pacemakers has come controversy over the indications for permanent pacing. In general,

pacemakers are indicated for symptomatic bradycardia or heart block (Table 2.9–2).

Pacemaker systems now include complex generators that are programmable for rate, sensitivity, energy, and chamber or chambers paced and sensed. Because of these complexities a nomenclature for pacing has been established to identify pacer function (Table 2.9–2). The simplest code identifies the chamber(s) paced and sensed and the method (response mode) of sensing—either inhibition or triggering or both. An example is a dual-chamber pacemaker configured in the DVI mode. This means that both the atria and the ventricles are paced (D); the pacemaker senses the ventricle

TABLE 2.9–2. PACEMAKERS: INDICATIONS AND CODES

Indications for Permanent Pacing

- Complete or advanced A-V block
- Sick sinus syndrome and "tachycardia-bradycardia syndrome"
- Symptomatic sinus bradycardia
- Mobitz II A-V block
- Hypersensitive carotid sinus syndrome (see Chapter 15.5)

Pacemaker Codes

Chamber paced: *Dual,*[a] *Ventricular, Atrial*

Chamber sensed: *Dual, Ventricular, Atrial*

Response mode: *Dual, Inhibited, Triggered*

[a]"Dual" means that both chambers are sensed or paced, or that the pacemaker is both inhibited and triggered by the different signals it senses.

(V); and the pacemaker output is inhibited (I) when the device senses an adequate ventricular rate.

The current generation of pacemakers is capable of dual pacing, dual sensing, and a dual response (DDD). These pacemakers thus restore cardiac rate and A-V synchrony (so-called physiologic pacing). In the DDD mode the pacemaker generally senses the native atrial depolarization and, after a programmed interval, paces the ventricle. This allows the native atrial rate to determine the ventricular pacing rate.

In patients with sinus node dysfunction, the newest generation of pacemakers can "sense," through a variety of mechanisms, when exercise has begun and can automatically increase heart rate to satisfy exercise demands. This function has been called *adaptive pacing*. The type and programmable configuration of pacemaker function can be complex, and therapy must be individualized.

ECTOPIC BEATS AND TACHYCARDIA

Mechanisms
Over the past two decades a great deal of information about the mechanism of cardiac arrhythmias has come both from the study of isolated tissue and from invasive electrophysiology studies in man.[9] In many cases, therapy for tachycardias can be dictated by a precise understanding of the disturbed physiologic mechanism.

Classically, the mechanisms of tachycardia have been discussed in terms of alterations in automaticity, conduction, or both. In the last 10 years, another potential mechanism for the genesis of cardiac arrhythmias, called triggering, has emerged.

Abnormal Automaticity. Abnormal automaticity is said to exist when a subsidiary pacemaker usurps control of the cardiac rhythm. This is differentiated from the emergence of an escape pacemaker when conduction is blocked or normal automaticity has been aborted. There are many causes of abnormal automaticity, including drugs (especially catecholamines and digitalis), ischemia, electrolyte disturbances, or even abnormal stretching of the myocardium.

Reentry. The three conditions required for reentry are a closed-loop circuit for the reentrant mechanism, unidirectional block in one part of the circuit, and slow conduction in the other part of the circuit. There is now substantial evidence documenting reentry as a common mechanism for cardiac arrhythmias in man (particularly the Wolff-Parkinson-White syndrome) (Fig. 2.9–7). Many data suggest but do not prove that reentry is a cause of ventricular tachycardia and atrial flutter. Conditions known to lead to reentry may be produced by drugs, ischemia, or infarction.

Triggering. Recently a new mechanism for cardiac arrhythmias has been proposed. In digitalis intoxication arrhythmias, it is postulated that tachycardia emerges from calcium-overloaded cells on the basis of reexcitation during the action potential. This mechanism depends on the conditions set by the previous beat—hence the term "triggering." Much speculation has centered on the role of triggered arrhythmias as a cause of ventricular tachycardia.

Premature Beats
Ectopic Beats. "Ectopic beats" is an old ECG term, meaning "beats coming from out of place." The term is not helpful, because it offers no explanation either for diagnosis or for treatment.

Premature Atrial Contractions. Premature atrial contractions (PACs) arise anywhere in the atria (Fig. 2.9–8). They are a normal finding in most persons but are important because they may initiate episodes of tachycardia in the atrium (particularly atrial fibrillation) or in the A-V node. They are frequently seen when the atria are distended. They may be caused by drugs (catecholamines, theophyllines) or may be associated with anxiety, stress, or caffeine

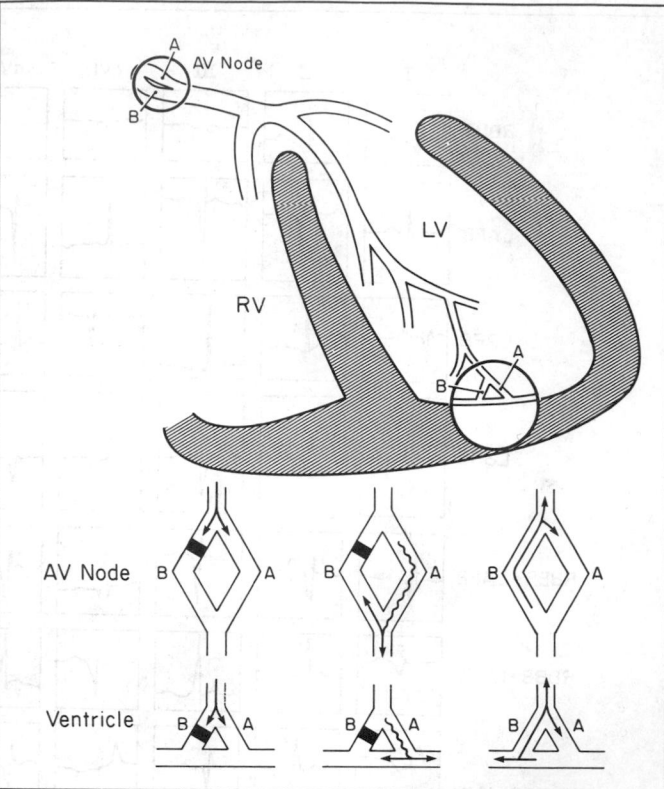

Figure 2.9–7. Reentry mechanisms diagrammed for either A-V node (upper panels) or ventricular Purkinje fibers (lower panels). Antero-grade impulse encounters two separate pathways of conduction (A + B), which insert distally into other conducting tissue or myocardium (left panels). Anterograde block (stippled area) prevents conduction in pathway B, while impulse is conducted slowly down pathway A (center panels). Impulse then travels to distal end of pathway B and finds it no longer refractory, conducting retrograde to site of origin of impulse and again anterograde down pathway A (right panels). Repetitive impulses can be produced by continued circular activation of conducting loop. RV = right ventricle; LV = left ventricle.

use. They are seen frequently with pericarditis and myocarditis and after myocardial infarction.

PACs are recognized as premature beats with P waves that may differ significantly from the sinus P wave. They may fail to conduct through the A-V node because of physiologic refractoriness and are referred to as blocked PACs. They may also penetrate and reset the sinus node, causing pauses on the ECG. If the PAC comes early enough in the cardiac cycle, it may encounter refractoriness in the distal conducting system and be conducted as an aberrant, or wide, QRS complex beat.

Premature Junctional Beat. Premature junctional beats arise anywhere in the A-V junction and, as a result of retrograde conduction, cause atrial depolarization (Fig. 2.9–8). On the ECG they usually result in narrow QRS complexes, either without preceding P waves or with retrograde P waves. As with PACs, they may enter the refractory period of the distal conducting system and be conducted aberrantly. Premature junctional beats are seen with digitalis excess, after myocardial infarction (especially inferior), or with catecholamine or theophylline use.

Premature Ventricular Beat. Premature ventricular beats are one of the most common cardiac arrhythmias in patients with or without heart disease (Fig. 2.9–8). They are wide, bizarre beats (generally

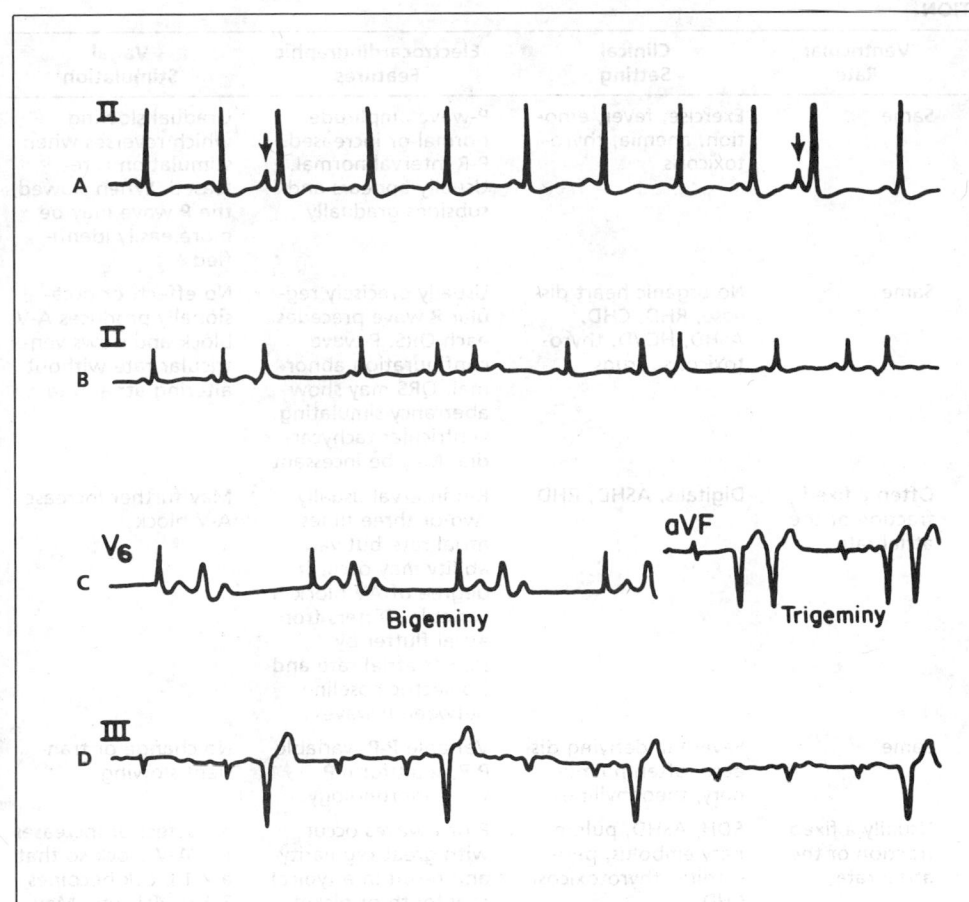

Figure 2.9–8. Premature contractions. A. Premature atrial contraction. P wave associated with atrial premature contraction (third complex) appears different in configuration from other P waves. This atrial premature beat is followed by normal QRS pattern, but such premature beats need not be conducted to ventricle or may be conducted in aberrant fashion, simulating right bundle-branch block. **B.** Premature junctional contraction. In this case, premature impulse was conducted not only to ventricles but also to atria in retrograde fashion, resulting in inverted P wave. Retrograde conduction is not necessarily part of junctional premature contractions. **C.** Premature ventricular contraction. Lead V_6—Premature ventricular contractions are represented by wide, bizarre QRS complexes, each of which follows normally conducted beat. This relationship is termed bigeminy. Lead aV_F—Every normally conducted beat is followed by two premature beats of ventricular origin in this ECG, demonstrating trigeminy. Less serious type of trigeminy is characterized by repetitively occurring sequences containing two normally conducted beats and premature ventricular beat. **D.** Premature ventricular contractions. In this patient with atrial fibrillation, interval between conducted and premature, or ectopic, beat is same on each occasion. This fixed relation of ectopic to conducted beat is termed fixed coupling.

greater than 0.12 second). Retrograde conduction to the sinus node causes resetting, or the beats may be blocked in the A-V node and occur with a compensatory pause.

The importance of premature ventricular beats must be assayed in context. When they occur in otherwise healthy individuals, they are harmless. In patients with heart disease, particularly with acute myocardial infarction, they may foretell the onset of ventricular tachycardia or fibrillation. One of the major difficulties in treating patients with premature ventricular beats and serious heart disease is to determine in which individuals the premature ventricular beats, occurring either singly or in short salvos, portend future and serious cardiac arrhythmias. To date, there is no satisfactory understanding of which patients will go on to have serious ventricular tachycardia, although most clinicians regard frequent or complex premature ventricular contractions occurring after myocardial infarction as ominous.

Premature ventricular beats may be seen in response to various types of medications (catecholamines, caffeine, theophyllines, digitalis). They may be observed in any form of acute heart disease, including ischemic heart disease, myocarditis, or rheumatic fever. In the presence of digitalis or acute ischemic heart disease, hypokalemia may be an important exacerbating factor.

TACHYCARDIA (Table 2.9–3)

General Assessment

The importance of accurate diagnosis of tachycardia before intervention is related to the hemodynamic consequences of the arrhythmia. Patients with cardiac arrest, acute myocardial ischemia, or pulmonary edema should be given emergency cardioversion and cardiopulmonary resuscitation. When the clinical situation is not an emergency, important information from the history and physical examination should be sought. It is vital that a 12-lead ECG (not just a rhythm strip) be obtained.

The Problem of the Wide QRS Complex Tachycardia[10]

The clinician is confronted frequently with a regular tachycardia that is made up entirely of wide QRS complexes with no readily discernible atrial activity (Table 2.9–4).[10] It must be decided which is present: ventricular tachycardia or supraventricular tachycardia conducting with bundle-branch block (so-called supraventricular tachycardia with aberrancy).

There are several clues that help differentiate ventricular tachycardia from supraventricular tachycardia with aberrancy. An effort should be made to determine the A-V relationship during the tachycardia, because a wide QRS complex tachycardia with A-V dissociation is almost always ventricular tachycardia. The presence of cannon waves or varying first heart sounds suggests A-V dissociation. Multiple leads on the ECG (with Lewis or esophageal leads) should be examined to ascertain the atrial and ventricular relationship. If the patient has an underlying normal QRS complex, it is rare for aberrantly conducted SVT to have a QRS complex greater than 0.14 second. Occasionally the shape of the QRS complex in lead V_1 is helpful for making the differential diagnosis. Last, the response of the tachycardia to vagal stimulation (carotid sinus massage) should be noted. The easiest maneuver for stimulating the vagus is carotid sinus massage.

Carotid Sinus Massage. Before carotid sinus massage is attempted, the carotid artery should be carefully auscultated for a bruit, which may indicate atherosclerotic disease and as such would be a contra-

TABLE 2.9–3. TACHYCARDIA CLASSIFICATION

Diagnosis	Atrial Rate (beats/min)	Ventricular Rate	Clinical Setting	Electrocardiographic Features	Vagal Stimulation
Sinus tachycardia	100–180 (in children may be above 200)	Same	Exercise, fever, emotion, anemia, thyrotoxicosis	P-wave amplitude normal or increased. P-R interval normal. Usually appears and subsides gradually	Gradual slowing which reverses when stimulation is released. When slowed, the P wave may be more easily identified
Ectopic atrial tachycardia	110–200 (faster in children)	Same	No organic heart disease, RHD, CHD, ASHD, HCVD, thyrotoxicosis, drugs	Usually precisely regular P wave precedes each QRS. P-wave configuration abnormal. QRS may show aberrancy simulating ventricular tachycardia. May be incessant	No effect, or occasionally produces A-V block and slows ventricular rate without altering atrial rate
Ectopic atrial tachycardia with A-V block	120–220	Often a fixed fraction of the atrial rate	Digitalis, ASHD, RHD	R-R interval usually two or three times atrial rate but variability may occur if degree of AV block is variable. Differs from atrial flutter by slower atrial rate and isoelectric baseline between P waves	May further increase A-V block
Multifocal atrial tachycardia	>100	Same	Severe underlying disease, often pulmonary; theophylline	Variable P-P, variable P-R, multiform P wave morphology	No change or transient slowing
Atrial flutter	220–320	Usually a fixed fraction of the atrial rate	RDH, ASHD, pulmonary embolus, pericarditis, thyrotoxicosis, CHD	P or f waves occur with great regularity and result in a typical saw-tooth or picket fence undulation in leads 2, 3, aV$_F$, V$_1$ and V$_2$	No effect or increases the A-V block so that a 2:1 block becomes 3:1 or 4:1, etc. May rarely terminate the flutter
Atrial fibrillation	Not discernible	40–300	RHD, ASHD, pericarditis, thyrotoxicosis, CHD, pulmonary embolus	Totally irregular R-R interval; baseline may have fine or coarse fibrillatory waves; in some instances, no evidence of atrial activity discernible and diagnosis rests on grossly irregular ventricular response	Increase in degree of A-V block and slowing of ventricular rate
Supraventricular tachycardia (PSVT; formerly paroxysmal atrial tachycardia [PAT])	120–220	120–220	No organic heart disease; ASHD, RHD, CHD	Regular R-wave interval; P waves may occur before, with, or after the QRS; QRS as in sinus or with aberrancy	May have no effect or may terminate tachycardia abruptly
Nonparoxysmal (accelerated) junctional tachycardia	70–120	70–120	Digitalis intoxication; inferior MI	Same as above except slower rate; QRS as in normal sinus rhythm, may have A-V dissociation	No effect or minimal slowing
Wolff-Parkinson-White syndrome A-V reciprocating tachycardia	140–220	140–220	No organic heart disease, CHD, RHD	Regular R waves; retrograde P waves after QRS	No effect or terminate spontaneously, with resumption of preexcitation
Atrial fibrillation	Not discernible	40–300		Bizarre, irregular QRS, with no discernible P wave; ventricular rates may approach 300	No effect unless conduction is over A-V node

(continued)

TABLE 2.9–3. TACHYCARDIA CLASSIFICATION (Continued)

Diagnosis	Atrial Rate (beats/min)	Ventricular Rate	Clinical Setting	Electrocardiographic Features	Vagal Stimulation
Accelerated idioventricular rhythm (AIVR)	80–130	80–130	Acute inferior infarction; amiodarone	Rate often very close to sinus rate; wide QRS complexes similar to VPBs; A-V dissociation common	No effect
Ventricular tachycardia	60–140	140–280	Acute myocardial ischemia or infarction, anoxia, electric shock, digitalis, trauma; no organic heart disease	Broad, bizarre, slightly irregular QRS complexes; independent and slower P wave rate sometimes determined; fusion beats may appear	No effect or may very rarely convert to sinus rhythm
Ventricular flutter and fibrillation		300 or greater	Acute myocardial ischemia or infarction, anoxia, electric shock, digitalis, trauma, quinidine	Disorganized, grossly irregular wave pattern	No effect

CHD = congenital heart disease; RHD = rheumatic heart disease; ASHD = arteriosclerotic heart disease; HCVD = hypertensive heart disease; VPB = Ventricular premature beats.

indication to massage. The massage should be performed at the bifurcation of the carotid artery, below the angle of the jaw. Massage should at first be gentle, because the presence of a hypersensitive reflex may result in asystole. The duration should never exceed 4 or 5 seconds and should always be unilateral. The ECG should be recorded during the carotid massage.

Sinus Tachycardia (Table 2.9–3)
Sinus tachycardia in the adult is a regular, narrow-complex tachycardia at a rate greater than 100 beats/min, generally less than 180 to 190 beats/min. A normal P wave precedes each QRS complex, and onset and decline are gradual. Sinus tachycardia represents a normal response to exercise, stress, anxiety, and fear, but it may be a significant compensatory mechanism in congestive heart failure or volume depletion. It may accompany fever, hyperthyroidism, or the use of vagolytic drugs, particularly atropine-like agents. It is generally slowed but not terminated by carotid sinus massage.

Sinus heart must be distinguished from sinus node reentry, a rare form of reentrant tachycardia, and from sinus arrhythmia, which is probably a normal variant of sinus rhythm. Sinus node reentry is a paroxysmal arrhythmia with a rate between 120 and 150 beats/min and is characterized by a normal P wave preceding a normal QRS complex. It resembles sinus tachycardia because the reentry is within the sinus node itself. Sinus arrhythmia occurs frequently and represents a physiologic response in sinus rate to sympathetic or parasympathetic stimulation. It is frequently seen in normal respiratory cycles but may be exaggerated in serious forms of heart disease.

Ectopic Atrial Tachycardia (Table 2.9–3)
There are three forms of ectopic atrial tachycardia encountered in clinical practice: ectopic atrial tachycardia; multifocal atrial tachycardia; and digitalis-induced atrial tachycardia, sometimes called paroxysmal atrial tachycardia with or without A-V block.

In ectopic atrial tachycardia the heart rate is between 110 and 200 beats/min, and the tachycardia may be incessant. The cause is unknown, but this form of tachycardia is frequently seen as a sequela to myocarditis or rheumatic fever, being more frequent in children than in adults.

Ectopic atrial tachycardia is characterized by an abnormal P wave preceding a normal QRS complex. The abnormal P wave is consistent with the ectopic site of the tachycardia. In some cases there may be varying degrees of A-V block because of physiologic refractoriness. Carotid massage may result in increased A-V refractoriness and a decrease in the ventricular rate but generally has little effect on the rate of the tachycardia.

Multifocal atrial tachycardia is a chaotic form of atrial tachycardia, with a rate greater than 100 beats/min, and is characterized by at least three or four forms of P waves, varying P-R intervals, and varying R-R intervals. It is differentiated from atrial flutter or atrial fibrillation by the presence of discrete P waves. Multifocal atrial tachycardia is commonly seen in patients with advanced forms of heart disease and particularly in severe forms of underlying obstructive lung disease. Some investigators have suggested that it may be caused by digitalis excess. Recent data suggest that high levels of theophylline may cause multifocal atrial tachycardia.

Digitalis excess can cause ectopic atrial tachycardia (Fig. 2.9–9) with or without an abnormal P-wave. Because of the digitalis excess, there is frequent block of the atrial impulses in the A-V node—hence the term "paroxysmal atrial tachycardia" with block. This term is a poor one because this form of tachycardia is not paroxysmal and should not be confused with A-V node reentrant tachycardia.

Atrial Flutter (Table 2.9–3)
Atrial flutter is characterized by rapid but organized beating of the atria at a rate between 220 and 360 beats/min, with the ventricular rate dependent on the refractoriness of the A-V node

TABLE 2.9–4. DIFFERENTIATION OF SUPRAVENTRICULAR TACHYCARDIA WITH ABERRANCY FROM VENTRICULAR TACHYCARDIA

Favors SVT	Favors VT
QRS duration ≤0.14 sec	QRS duration >0.14 sec
Right bundle-branch block pattern	Left bundle-branch block pattern
Triphasic RSR in lead V_1	Monophasic or biphasic QRS complex in lead V_1
Normal axis	Left axis deviation Fusion beats A-V dissociation

SVT = supraventricular tachycardia; VT = ventricular tachycardia.

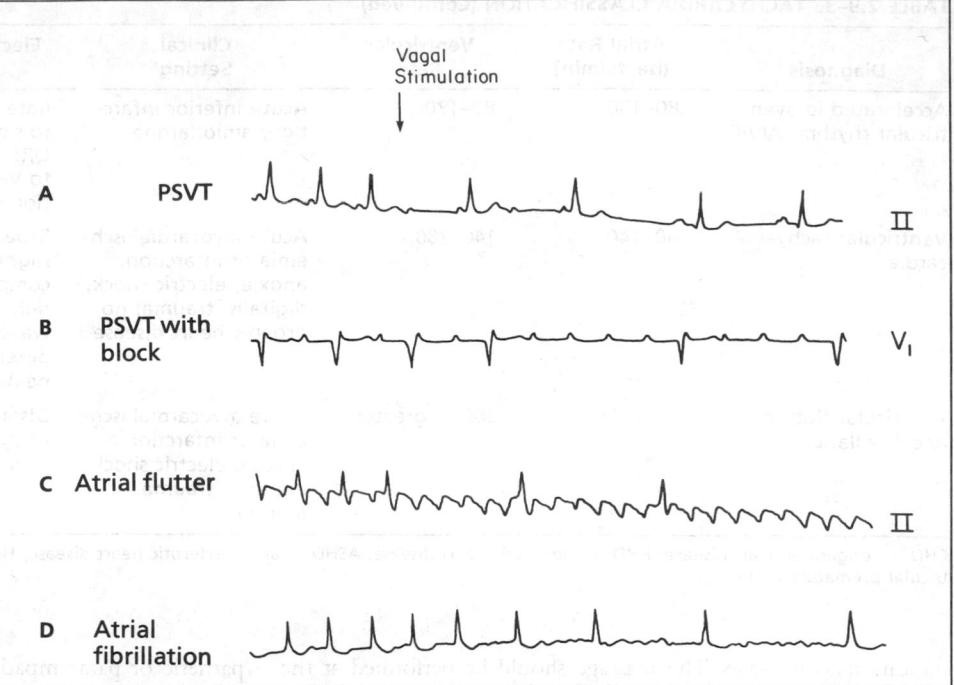

Figure 2.9–9. Common supraventricular tachycardias. Response to vagal stimulation is illustrated in right-hand two thirds of each tracing. **A.** PSVT—paroxysmal supraventricular tachycardia. Vagal stimulation either will have little detectable effect on rhythm or will convert it to normal sinus rhythm. **B.** Atrial tachycardia with block. Anterograde block is increased, but normal sinus rhythm rarely ensues. **C.** Atrial flutter. A-V block is increased, making flutter waves easier to identify, but conversion to normal sinus rhythm does not occur. **D.** Atrial fibrillation. A-V block is increased, making atrial fibrillation waves easier to identify, but atrial fibrillation persists.

(Fig. 2.9–9). The lower rate of the tachycardia (to differentiate it from atrial tachycardia) is not well defined and may vary with various types of antiarrhythmic drugs, particularly the type I agents or amiodarone.

Electrocardiographically, atrial flutter produces a characteristic undulating, or flutter, baseline that is best seen in the inferior leads (II, III, or aV$_F$). Carotid sinus massage frequently produces a decrease in the ventricular response rate because of increasing A-V node refractoriness. The response rate of the ventricle to the atrial flutter is variable (2:1, 3:1, or varying patterns). A 1:1 pattern is rare unless preexcitation is present or the patient has been treated with a quinidine-like agent without digitalization.

Atrial flutter is generally associated with some form of organic heart disease, myocarditis, or coronary artery disease, but it may also be seen in healthy young individuals. It is a common rhythm after open heart surgery and after correction of complex congenital heart disease.

Atrial Fibrillation (Table 2.9–3)
Atrial fibrillation is probably the most common of all atrial arrhythmias (Fig. 2.9–9). Although it is not uncommon in individuals without heart disease (lone atrial fibrillation, or "holiday heart"), it is most frequently associated with organic heart disease. It is a common rhythm in persons with a distended atrium resulting from valvular heart disease (especially mitral valve disease), ischemic heart disease, post-myocardial infarction, pericarditis, and chronic obstructive lung disease. Long-standing hypertension is often a cause of atrial fibrillation. Atrial fibrillation is sometimes seen in acutely ill persons with systemic illnesses, especially thyrotoxicosis or septicemia.

Atrial fibrillation is characterized by random, indiscrete, and disorganized atrial activity, the frequency of which is difficult to distinguish on the ECG. The ventricular response rate is classically "irregularly irregular" (variable R-R intervals), consistent with concealed conduction of the atrial impulses through the A-V node. The concealed conduction is also responsible for the intermittent aberration of the conducted beats, called Ashman phenomenon, recognized as ventricular complexes with "right bundle-branch block" morphologic features that follow a long-short R-R sequence. This aberration is frequently confused with premature ventricular beats. It is known that the refractoriness of the

His-Purkinje system, especially the right bundle, is directly proportional to the duration of the preceding R-R interval. Therefore a long R-R cycle may increase the refractory period of the right bundle, and thus the next conducted beat may be aberrant. This phenomenon represents a normal increase in refractoriness of the His-Purkinje system.

Besides the hemodynamic consequences of a rapid ventricular response, the rhythm itself may pose another risk to the patient: embolic stroke. Data from the long-term Framingham study suggest that chronic atrial fibrillation is a serious risk factor for stroke. Although not proved, the theory is that when atrial fibrillation is associated with significant cardiomegaly, this risk factor is probably increased.

Paroxysmal Supraventricular Tachycardia
Paroxysmal supraventricular tachycardia (PSVT) (Fig. 2.9–9) as it is most properly called, is also called paroxysmal atrial tachycardia, paroxysmal nodal tachycardia, A-V node circus movement tachycardia, paroxysmal A-V junctional tachycardia, or junctional tachycardia. The term "paroxysmal atrial tachycardia" is both an anachronism and a misnomer—it was originally believed that the tachycardia arose in the atrium. It is clear that the mechanism of PSVT is either reentry within the A-V node (about 75 percent of all PSVT) or reentry using a concealed accessory A-V pathway (approximately 15 percent of cases; see the discussion of Wolff-Parkinson-White syndrome, below). Both mechanisms produce a paroxysmal narrow QRS complex tachycardia.

The ECG shows a regular narrow QRS complex tachycardia at a rate between 120 and 220 beats/min. P waves are retrograde and either are not visible on a standard surface ECG or are seen superimposed in the T wave or in middiastole. PSVT stops and starts suddenly, most often initiated by a premature atrial or ventricular contraction. Conduction may be aberrant, giving the impression of ventricular tachycardia (see the discussion of wide QRS complex tachycardia, above). The classic response of PSVT to carotid massage or to Valsalva maneuver is sudden cessation; this is consistent with the increase of the refractoriness of the A-V node and with termination of the reentrant arrhythmia.

PSVT is a common arrhythmia seen in otherwise healthy persons. It may complicate or be unmasked by other forms of heart disease, including acute MI, myocarditis, or rheumatic fever. Sys-

temic illness of any sort may also precipitate PSVT, as may exercise, stress, caffeine, or emotion.

Nonparoxysmal Junctional Tachycardia

Nonparoxysmal A-V nodal tachycardia (accelerated A-V junctional rhythm) is an automatic rhythm originating within the A-V junction. The rhythm is recognized as a narrow QRS complex rhythm that is considerably slower than PSVT (between 70 and 120/min). There may be retrograde capture of the atrium, or in many cases A-V dissociation may be present. Depending on the site of automaticity, conduction of the QRS complex may also be aberrant, producing a wide QRS complex rhythm. Unlike PSVT, nonparoxysmal junctional tachycardia is not perturbed by carotid sinus massage, a feature consistent with its automatic behavior.

Nonparoxysmal junctional tachycardia is commonly seen in digitalis intoxication or with inferior MI. It can also be seen after the administration of atropine or catecholamines.

Wolff-Parkinson-White Syndrome (Preexcitation)

The Wolff-Parkinson-White syndrome is the most common member of the family of preexcitation syndromes (so-called because the ventricle is "preexcited" through an accessory pathway that bypasses part or all of the normal A-V node His-Purkinje system (Fig. 2.9–10).[5] The bypass tract has two important consequences: (1) it sets up a pathway for A-V reentrant tachycardia (PSVT), and (2) it provides a pathway from the atrium to the ventricle that bypasses the physiologic refractoriness of the A-V node, thus allowing the potential for extraordinarily rapid conduction of atrial impulses to the ventricle. Wolff-Parkinson-White syndrome produces a characteristic ECG with a short P-R interval and a slurred QRS complex (the delta wave). The short P-R interval and the slurring of the initial forces of the QRS complex represent the bypass of the A-V node with preexcitation of the ventricle.

It should be noted that the diagnosis of the Wolff-Parkinson-White abnormality is based on electrocardiographic evidence. This diagnosis does not suggest a specific arrhythmia, and individuals with Wolff-Parkinson-White syndrome may have other forms of arrhythmia not related to the accessory pathway. In fact, most individuals with the Wolff-Parkinson-White abnormality are probably asymptomatic.

There are two common arrhythmias seen with the Wolff-Parkinson-White syndrome. The first is A-V reciprocating tachycardia. In this tachycardia, there is anterograde conduction over the A-V node His-Purkinje system and retrograde reentry over the accessory pathway. During the tachycardia, the ECG may be indistinguishable from A-V node reentrant tachycardia (PSVT).

The second arrhythmia that patients with the Wolff-Parkinson-White syndrome may experience is atrial fibrillation. In these individuals there may be rapid conduction of the atrial impulses over the accessory pathway, which produces a wide and bizarre

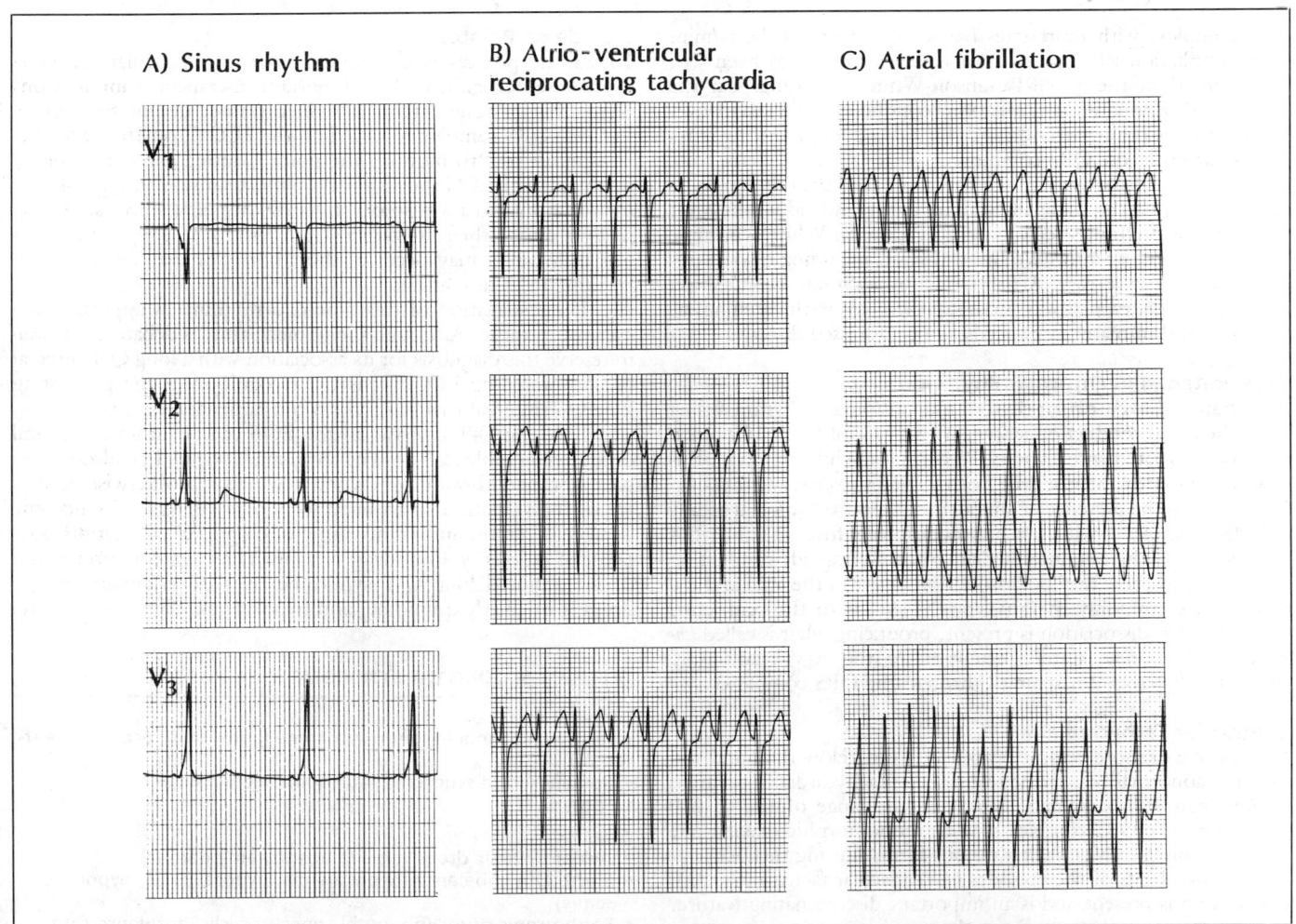

Figure 2.9–10. Electrocardiographic evidence of Wolff-Parkinson-White syndrome in leads V_1, V_2, and V_3 (same patient). **A.** Sinus rhythm with preexcited QRS complexes. Note short P-R interval and broad QRS complex. **B.** A-V reciprocating tachycardia. QRS complex is now normal; anterograde conduction is over normal conduction system. **C.** Atrial fibrillation. Wide bizarre QRS complexes result from conduction over accessory pathway.

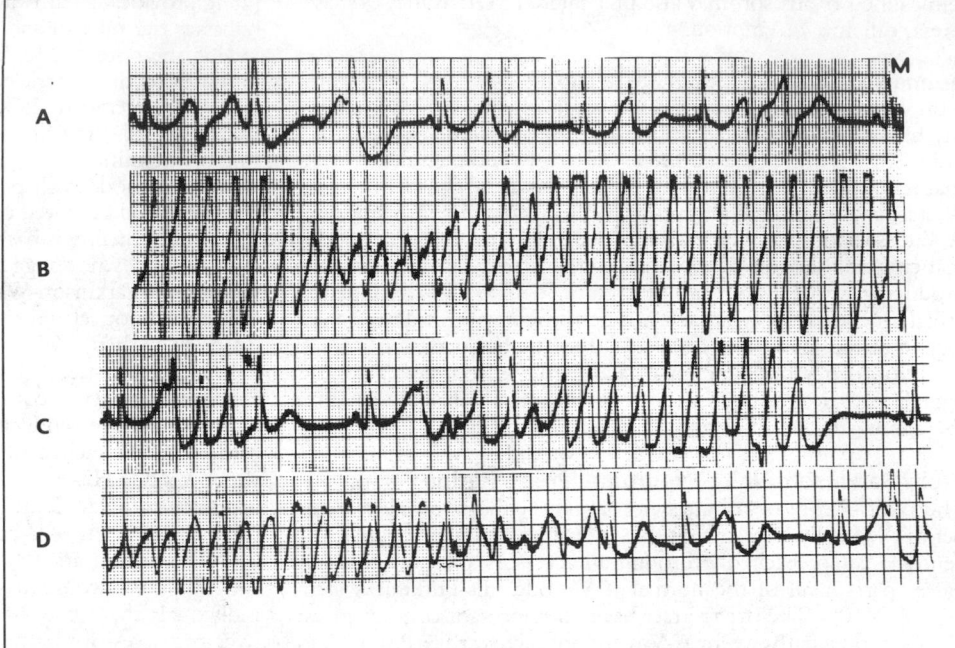

Figure 2.9–11. Torsade de pointes. **A.** Multifocal premature ventricular beats in patient with prolongation of Q-T interval. **B, C, and D.** Typical torsade de pointes ventricular tachycardia with undulation of ventricular depolarization about electrocardiographic baseline.

QRS complex, with heart rates between 200 or 300 beats/min. Atrial fibrillation leading to ventricular fibrillation has been well documented in the Wolff-Parkinson-White syndrome. On the other hand, during atrial fibrillation, conduction may occur over both the accessory connection and the A-V node, producing striking variations of the QRS complex.

The Wolff-Parkinson-White syndrome (and the other preexcitation syndromes) are generally seen in healthy individuals. As with PSVT, the arrhythmias seen in Wolff-Parkinson-White syndrome may complicate other forms of heart disease, including myocarditis or ischemic heart disease. Atrial fibrillation with rapid conduction over the accessory pathway may represent a life-threatening arrhythmia and in many cases needs to be addressed directly.

Accelerated Idioventricular Rhythm
Accelerated idioventricular rhythm is an automatic rhythm arising from the distal conduction system with a rate of 60 to 100 beats/min and associated with a wide QRS complex. This rhythm is commonly seen with inferior MI, with digitalis excess and hypokalemia, and in the presence of amiodarone. Electrocardiographically the QRS complex is wide but may occasionally fuse with the sinus complex to produce an intermediate form. Retrograde conduction may occur, or there may be dissociation between the atria and the ventricles. Commonly the atrial rate is similar to the ventricular rate, although dissociation is present, producing what is called *isorhythmic dissociation*. Careful attention to the A-V relationship shows the P waves "marching" through the QRS complexes.

Ventricular Tachycardia
When three or more ectopic beats arise from below the bundle of His, the abnormality is termed ventricular tachycardia. The rate is greater than 100 beats/min, usually in the range of 130 to 210 beats/min. The QRS complex may be monomorphic (having one form) or polymorphic (having various forms) during the tachycardia. In two thirds of the episodes of ventricular tachycardia, A-V dissociation is present and is an important discriminating feature.

Ventricular tachycardia is usually associated with organic heart disease, particularly ischemic heart disease or cardiomyopathy. It may be seen with rheumatic heart disease, digitalis excess, or hypertensive or valvular heart disease. An occasional patient with ventricular tachycardia may seem to have no primary organic heart disease.

Torsade de Pointes
Torsade de pointes is a particular type of ventricular tachycardia whose recognition has important therapeutic implications (Fig. 2.9–11).[8] The rhythm is termed torsade de pointes because the wide QRS complex recorded on the ECG during the tachycardia appears to "turn about the point" during the course of arrhythmia. The ECG shows a wide, almost sinusoidal, type of ventricular tachycardia whose axis shifts 180 degrees ("turns about the point") during the tachycardia (Fig. 2.9–11). This type of ventricular tachycardia may occur as short bursts or may be sustained, resulting in cardiac arrest.

The recognition of this type of arrhythmia is important because of its cause. Although the nomenclature is debated, it is well to reserve this diagnosis for its association with a long Q-T interval on the preceding ECG.[2] It is the recognition of the preexisting long Q-T interval that has serious consequences for therapy.

The long Q-T interval on the ECG can be either congenital or acquired (Table 2.9–5). The congenital long Q-T syndromes are seen with or without deafness and may occur in otherwise healthy young individuals. The acquired form of the long Q-T syndrome is more common and is increasingly recognized as a serious side effect of various types of drug therapy. The most common causes of the acquired long Q-T syndrome are type Ia antiarrhythmic drugs (particularly quinidine) and hypokalemia. Simultaneous hy-

TABLE 2.9–5. LONG Q-T SYNDROME

Congenital
- Jervell and Lange–Nielsen syndrome (autosomal recessive, deafness)
- Romano-Ward syndrome (autosomal dominant)
- Sporadic

Acquired
- Antiarrhythmic drugs (type Ia agents, amiodarone)
- Electrolyte imbalance (hypokalemia, hypocalcemia, hypomagnesemia)
- Psychotropic drugs (phenothiazines, tricyclic, antidepressant agents, lithium)
- CNS abnormalities (subarachnoid hemorrhage, tumor)
- Organophosphorus poisoning
- Miscellaneous (myocardial infarction, myocarditis, mitral valve prolapse)

pokalemia and administration of a type I antiarrhythmic agent (Tables 2.9–6 and 2.9–7) is a common combination. Other drugs such as the phenothiazines and the tricyclic antidepressants have been implicated. It is important to recognize the long Q-T interval in association with this rhythm, because treatment is directed primarily at removing the offending agent.

Ventricular Fibrillation

Ventricular fibrillation is disorganized, chaotic activity of the QRS complex on the surface ECG. It is differentiated from ventricular tachycardia because of its disorganization. It produces no effective cardiac output and without immediate cardioversion results in death. It is generally recognized as a terminal arrhythmia, although there have been cases of "primary" ventricular fibrillation.

TREATMENT OF TACHYCARDIA

The treatment of tachycardia is dictated both by the nature of the arrhythmia and by the context in which it occurs. In some cases no treatment is necessary, whereas in others rapid cardioversion is the treatment of choice. Before initiating pharmacologic treatment of a tachycardia, particularly when it is paroxysmal or recurrent, one should always ask two questions: Is treatment necessary? If so, what is the safest and most effective method of treatment? The answers to these questions are important, because most antiarrhythmic drugs have a narrow therapeutic/toxic ratio.

All too often, nonpharmacologic treatment of tachycardia is overlooked. Particularly important in the treatment of ventricular tachycardia in patients with ischemic heart disease is the maintenance of a stable serum potassium concentration. Prevention of myocardial ischemia or decreasing heart size may be beneficial in many types of atrial or ventricular arrhythmia. Alterations in lifestyle—including a decrease in stress, an aerobic conditioning program, and avoidance of caffeine and alcohol—may all prove useful in the initial treatment of cardiac arrhythmias.

Antiarrhythmic Drugs

The development of newer antiarrhythmic drugs has progressed greatly in recent years. The Vaughan-Williams classification of antiarrhythmic drugs has been a useful though limited scheme (Table 2.9–6). Antiarrhythmic drugs are classified on the basis of their effects on isolated cardiac tissue. Within each class, several agents are grouped because of a common effect on the cardiac membrane. Within each class, however, the drugs may be remarkably different in pharmacokinetics and in toxicity.

Type Ia Agents. Quinidine, procainamide, and disopyramide are classified as type Ia agents because they are classic membrane anesthetics and increase conduction time and refractoriness in cardiac muscle (Table 2.9–6). The agents (particularly quinidine) may cause increased conduction through the A-V node because of a centrally mediated vagolytic action. This is important to remember when treating atrial flutter or atrial fibrillation, because the agents may cause a paradoxical increase in the ventricular response rate resulting from a decrease in the refractoriness of the A-V node. In the treatment of atrial flutter-fibrillation, therefore, drugs that increase A-V node refractoriness are given before administration of the type Ia agent is started.

Type Ia drugs are useful for atrial flutter-fibrillation, ectopic atrial tachycardia, and ventricular arrhythmias. The drugs should not be used in individuals with a prolonged Q-T interval because of their tendency to increase this Q-T interval. These drugs may also slow conduction in the His-Purkinje system and should be used cautiously in patients with preexisting heart block.

Although these agents have similar electrophysiologic effects, their side effects and pharmacokinetics differ markedly. Quinidine, for example, may produce intolerable gastrointestinal side effects (nausea, vomiting, and diarrhea) in up to 20 percent of patients. Use of procainamide, on the other hand, may be limited by allergic side effects, including the induction of a systemic lupus erythematosus syndrome, which develops in 15 to 20 percent of patients who take the drug for longer than 1 year. Disopyramide produces urinary retention and has remarkable negative inotropic properties.

Type Ib Agents. Lidocaine, tocainide, phenytoin (diphenylhydantoin), and mexiletine are type Ib agents, because they have little effect on the effective refractory period of normal myocardial tissue. Lidocaine is the primary antiarrhythmic agent for acute ventricular arrhythmias in myocardial infarction. It is always used parenterally. Oral lidocaine-like drugs—tocainide and mexiletine—have recently been developed.[1]

Phenytoin has electrophysiologic properties similar to those of lidocaine but with a long half-life. Its use has not received broad support because its efficacy has been disappointing. Some clinicians have found it useful for the treatment of ectopic atrial tachycardias.

The primary toxicity of lidocaine and tocainide is CNS related. Tremors, confusion, and seizures are the side effects most commonly seen with lidocaine. Lidocaine is dependent on hepatic blood flow for its elimination; conditions that reduce hepatic blood flow (e.g., congestive heart failure with decreased cardiac output) may cause a remarkable reduction in lidocaine clearance, with possible toxic effects.

TABLE 2.9–6. ANTIARRHYTHMIC AGENT CLASSIFICATION

	Ia	Ib	Ic	II	III	IV
	Quinidine Procainamide Disopyramide	Tocainide Lidocaine Phenytoin Mexiletine	Flecainide Encainide	Propranolol Nadolol Timolol Metoprolol Pindolol Atenolol	Amiodarone Bretylium	Verapamil Nifedipine Diltiazem
Atrial						
CT	↑	→	→ ↑	→ ↑	→ ↑	→
ERP	↑	→	→ ↑	→ ↑	↑	→
A-V node						
CT	↑ → ↑	→ ↓	↑	↑	→ ↑	↑
ERP	↑ → ↑	→	↑	↑	↑	↑
H-P-VM						
CT		→ ↑	↑	→	→ ↑	
ERP	↑	→	↑	→	→	
Automaticity	↑	↓	→ ↓	↓	→ ↓	→

CT = conduction time; ERP = effective refractory period; H-P-VM = His-Purkinje-ventricular muscle; ↑ = increase; ↓ = decrease.

TABLE 2.9–7. FEATURES OF COMMONLY USED ANTIARRHYTHMIC AGENTS

Agent	Route	Dose	Interval (hr)	Peak Levels (hr)	Elimination Metabolism	$t_{1/2}$ ± SD
Quinidine sulfate	PO	800–3000 mg/day	4–6	$\frac{1}{2}$	>90% liver	7 ± 3 hr
	IM	800–3000 mg/day	4–6	$\frac{1}{2}$		
Procainamide	PO	1000–4000 mg/day	3–4	1–1$\frac{1}{2}$	50% liver	3–4 hr
	IM	1000–4000 mg/day	3–4	$\frac{1}{2}$	50% kidney	
	IV bolus	100–200 mg q 5 min		Immediate		
	Infusion	20–50 µg/kg/min				
Disopyramide	PO	400–800 mg/day	6	1$\frac{1}{2}$	50% liver	7 ± 4 hr
					50% kidney	
Phenytoin	PO	200–600 mg/day	12	2–6	>90% liver	22 ± 8 hr
	IV load	700–1000 mg		Immediate		
	Maintenance	200–600 mg/day	12			
Lidocaine	IV bolus	0.5–2.0 mg/kg	—	—	>95% liver	1–2 hr
	Infusion	10–50 µg/kg/min				
Tocainide	PO	200–800 mg/day	8	1–2	30% kidney	14 ± 3 hr
					>70% liver	
Flecainide	PO	100–200 mg/day	8–12	1–4	>80% liver	12–27 hr
Encainide	PO	75–200 mg/day	8	1–4	50% liver	6–10 hr
					50% kidney	
Amiodarone	PO	200–600 mg/day	24	?	?	? 3–6 wk
Bretylium	IV	5–10 mg/kg	—	Immediate[a]	80% kidney	6–8 hr
	IM	Infusion 1–2 mg/min (up to 30 mg/kg/min)				

[a]Onset of action may require several minutes.
$t_{1/2}$ = half-life; GI = gastrointestinal; PVCs = premature ventricular contractions; VTs = ventricular tachycardia; VF = ventricular fibrillation.

Type Ic Agents. Flecainide and encainide are type Ic antiarrhythmic agents recently released for use.[3] They share the common theme of type I agents in being membrane anesthetics. They tend to increase refractoriness in atrial and myocardial cells, although to a lesser extent than do type Ia agents. They also increase refractoriness of the A-V node and the His-Purkinje system, unlike type Ia and Ib agents. They are also differentiated from type Ia agents because they have little effect on the Q-T interval per se, as seen on the surface ECG.

Flecainide has proved to be an effective agent in the treatment of ventricular arrhythmias. It is a well-tolerated oral agent with a reasonably long half-life. Visual disturbances and gastrointestinal upset are the primary side effects associated with flecainide. Its usefulness in the long-term management of patients with serious ventricular arrhythmias remains to be documented.

Type II Agents. Within the past few years, several new beta-blocking agents have appeared (Tables 2.9–6 and 2.9–7). Now available are nonspecific beta blockers, cardioselective beta blockers, and beta blockers with partial agonist or intrinsic sympathomimetic ac-

tivity. Dose range for these drugs depends on the pharmacokinetics dictating administration from once to four times daily. The mechanism of action of this group of antiarrhythmic drugs is competive antagonism of beta-1 receptors. These agents are particularly useful in treating tachycardias that use the A-V node (atrial fibrillation or PSVT), because they cause increased refractoriness of the A-V node and can either stop reentrant tachycardia or slow atrial conduction through the A-V node. It is also clear that these agents may have an effect on ventricular arrhythmias that is mediated by the sympathetic nervous system—particularly those arrhythmias that may be related to ischemia. Clinical trials have documented that low doses of beta blockers can reduce the incidence of sudden cardiac arrest after myocardial infarction.

The side effects of these agents depend largely on their pharmacokinetics and selectivity (Table 2.9–8). Agents that are more selective for beta-1 receptors have less effect on the blockade of bronchial or peripheral smooth muscle, permitting their use in reactive airway disease. None of these agents, however, is pure or specific, and with increased dose they may have beta-2 antagonism. These agents may produce significant extracardiac side effects, in-

Therapeutic Serum Level (μg/ml)	Active Metabolite	Extracardiac Side Effects	Indications
2–5	No	GI symptoms (20–30%) Cinchonism Thrombocytenia Hemolytic anemia Skin rash Fever	Atrial arrhythmias Preexcitation syndromes PVCs, VT
4–8	N-acetylprocainamide	Hypotension (IV) Skin rash Fever Lupus erythematosus syndrome (40%)	See quinidine
2–5	No	Blurred vision Dry mouth Constipation Urinary retention	See quinidine
10–20	No	Ataxia Nystagmus Gingival hyperplasia Fever Hepatitis Skin rash Macrocytic anemia	PVCs (digitalis toxicity)
2–6 (plasma)	Yes	Seizures Apnea Hallucinations	VT
3–8	?	Thrombocytopenia Drowsiness Paresthesias	PVCs, VT
0.2	No	GI symptoms Headache Drowsiness	PVCs, VT
?	O-desethylencainide	GI symptoms Headaches Blurred vision	PVCs, VT
?	Desethylamiodarone	Photosensitivity Hepatitis Corneal opacities Hypothyroidism Hyperthyroidism Pulmonary fibrosis Peripheral neuropathy	VT/VF
?	No	Hypertension Hypotension Tachycardia Nausea and vomiting	VT or VF

cluding depression, impotence, or cognitive dysfunction in elderly persons. In combination with other agents (particularly calcium-channel blockers, digitalis, or amiodarone), they may produce significant bradycardia and hypotension.

Type III Agents. Amiodarone and bretylium are dissimilar compounds that share the common feature of prolonging the action potential duration. Bretylium is a potent sympathetic ganglionic blocker that inhibits norepinephrine release. These ganglionic blocking properties do not define its antiarrhythmic properties, and the basis for the antiarrhythmic properties of bretylium remains in question. Amiodarone is a benzofuran derivative with a chemical structure resembling that of thyroxine.[11] The drug's antiarrhythmic mechanism of action also remains unclear, although recent evidence suggests that a combination of sodium-channel blockade, antisympathetic activity, and a primary and undefined effect combine to prolong the duration of the drug's period of action.

Bretylium is given intravenously. Its most remarkable side effect is an initial transient hypertension (discharge of norepinephrine) followed by hypotension resulting from ganglionic blockade.

Amiodarone's pharmacologic and chemical properties make it a unique but potentially toxic agent.[11] It is administered orally. Amiodarone or its metabolites are deposited in many organs, including the lung, liver, myelin sheaths, and fatty tissues. The half-life of the drug has not been well established but is on the order of several weeks or months.

Amiodarone may cause either hypothyroidism or hyperthyroidism. The drug causes corneal microdeposits, which are present in almost all individuals who take the drug. These deposits generally do not interfere with vision. The drug may also cause serious pulmonary insufficiency, peripheral neuropathies, and hepatitis.

Both bretylium and amiodarone are reserved for the treatment of serious and refractory ventricular tachycardia. The toxic/therapeutic ratios of both drugs do not make them, as yet, first-line drugs for the treatment of ventricular tachycardia.

Class IV Agents. The calcium antagonists represent one of the most significant advances in the treatment of supraventricular arrhythmias. The drugs act by competitive antagonism of calcium entry through the slow channels, particularly in the A-V and sino-atrial nodes (Table 2.9–9). Additionally, because of the block of

TABLE 2.9–8. CLASSIFICATION OF BETA BLOCKERS

	Oral Daily Dose (mg)	Systemic Absorption (%)	Major Elimination	Half-Life (hr)	Protein Binding (%)	Selectivity	ISA
Atenolol	50–200	50	Kidney	7	10	Beta 1	0
Metoprolol	100–400	50[a]	Liver	3	12	Beta 1	0
Nadolol	40–640	30	Kidney	24	30	Beta 1 and 2	0
Pindolol	20–60	95	Kidney (50%) Liver (50%)	8	40	Beta 1 and 2	+
Propranolol	40–640	20[a]	Liver	4	80	Beta 1 and 2	0
Timolol	20–60	50[a]	Kidney	4	10	Beta 1 and 2	0

[a]Good gastrointestinal absorption, but first pass through liver reduces systemic delivery.
ISA = intrinsic sympathomimetic.

calcium entry, they have negative inotropic effects on working myocardium, dilating smooth muscles both in the coronary arteries and in other arterial beds. The calcium antagonists, especially verapamil, are highly effective means of managing arrhythmias involving reentry through the A-V node or of controlling the ventricular response rate during atrial fibrillation or atrial flutter. Intravenous verapamil is effective in terminating PSVT in approximately 70 to 80 percent of cases. It has thus become the pharmacologic treatment of choice for the termination of acute intermittent PSVT. Intravenous verapamil will also convert atrial flutter or atrial fibrillation in a much smaller percentage of cases, perhaps 10 to 20 percent.

The calcium antagonists appear to undergo extensive hepatic metabolism before elimination. Verapamil has a large hepatic first-pass effect, which may explain why it is less effective given orally than intravenously.

The calcium antagonists have a generally good therapeutic index and are well tolerated. Intravenous verapamil, however, can cause hypotension and bradycardia. The drug should be carefully administered to those patients with depressed cardiac function or advanced conduction disturbance.

Management of Acute Tachycardia

The management of an episode of acute tachycardia differs from the prevention of tachycardia. The aggressiveness with which an acute episode of tachycardia should be treated depends on the context in which the arrhythmia occurs and its hemodynamic consequences. The management of the acute episode, when hemodynamic compromise is not present, can be divided into four stages: (1) sedation or removal of the offending stimuli, (2) vagal stimulation where appropriate, (3) pharmacologic therapy, and (4) cardioversion.

Stage 1: Sedation and Removal of Offending Stimuli. In episodes of recurrent arrhythmia (particularly PSVT), sedation or removal of stimulating agents is the safest way to treat the arrhythmia. Sedation is a convenient way to decrease the sympathetic tone on which many of these arrhythmias thrive. Abstinence from caffeine or other agents may be helpful. It is clear that withdrawal from alcohol (the "holiday heart") may also be a significant factor in the initiation of these arrhythmias.

Stage 2: Vagal Stimulation. In persons with recurrent arrhythmias using the A-V node, vagal stimulation can be important for terminating the arrhythmia. Many patients learn variations of Valsalva maneuver on their own. The patient should always be instructed to be recumbent during this maneuver. They should also be instructed that if carotid sinus massage is attempted, it should be done only for a few seconds and only unilaterally.

Stage 3: Pharmacologic Therapy. The choice for pharmacologic therapy in each arrhythmia is a complex one (see Tables 2.9–6 and 2.9–9). For the short-term treatment of PSVT, intravenous verapamil has become the drug of choice. In the treatment of acute ventricular tachycardia (nonhemodynamically compromising), the drug of choice remains lidocaine.

Stage 4: Cardioversion. Electrical cardioversion remains the treatment of choice in patients whose tachycardia is poorly tolerated. It is not reserved for ventricular tachycardia alone but should be considered in the management of any rapid tachycardia (with the exception of sinus tachycardia) that is hemodynamically compromising. Specifically, cardioversion remains an important mainstay in the management of both acute and chronic atrial fibrillation (Table 2.9–10).

With some notable exceptions, cardioversion has a long history of safety and efficacy. In the vast majority of patients, cardioversion can be carried out uneventfully when simple precautions are taken. (See the discussion of contraindications to cardioversion, below.)

In certain arrhythmias, particularly atrial flutter and PSVT, cardioversion will occur with lower energies, on the order of 25 to 50 watt-seconds. It is desirable to use as low an energy level as possible during cardioversion. On the other hand, cardioversion of ventricular tachycardia or ventricular fibrillation should begin at 200 watt-seconds.

Contraindications to Cardioversion. There are few absolute contraindications to cardioversion. It was once held that patients taking

TABLE 2.9–9. CALCIUM ANTAGONISTS

	Dose (mg)		Relative Effects[a]		
	IV	Oral	Cardiac Contractility	A-V Conduction	Peripheral Resistance
Diltiazem	5–20	30–90 qid	↓ ↑	↓ ↓	↓ ↓
Nifedipine	—	10–30 qid	↓	↓	↓ ↓ ↓
Verapamil	5–20	80–120 tid or qid	↓ ↓	↓ ↓ ↓ ↓	↓ ↓

[a]All effects tend to be decreased; the relative magnitude of decrease is expressed as the number of signs.

TABLE 2.9–10. REVERSION OF ATRIAL FLUTTER AND FIBRILLATION

I. Purpose
   A. To restore control of the rate to the sinus node
   B. To restore synchronous atrial and ventricular activity
   C. To reduce the incidence of systemic and pulmonary emboli

II. Reversion is particularly indicated when atrial flutter or fibrillation:
   A. Appears as a result of a nonrecurrent stimulus such as cardiac catheterization or surgery
   B. Is of recent onset (If cardiac surgery is anticipated, reversion may be postponed until after operation.)
   C. Is associated wtih hyperthyroidism (Reversion should follow control of metabolic state.)
   D. Appears after cardiac surgery
   E. Is symptomatic (Palpitations and easy fatigue develop after mild exercise.)
   F. Is associated with a history of recent embolism (Anticoagulants should usually be administered for 4 to 6 weeks before reversion is attempted.)

III. Reversion is unlikely to be sustained with:
   A. Long-standing arrhythmia—especially in association with a large heart and a large left atrium
   B. History of previous reversion with relapse while receiving antiarrhythmic drugs (not applicable in patients with paroxysmal arrhythmias)
   C. Unrelieved mitral valve disease or a dilated left atrium (Occasionally reversion is worthwhile even though sinus rhythm persists for only a short period.)

IV. Reversion is dangerous with:
   A. Evidence of digitalis intoxication
   B. Known left-atrial thrombus
   C. High-degree A-V block
   D. Sinus node disease

digitalis should have the drug withheld for 24 to 36 hours before cardioversion. Recent data suggest that as long as patients do not have digitalis toxic effects, cardioversion may be undertaken safely. Cardioversion should not be employed in patients with atrial fibrillation and a very slow response rate or in those with clear evidence of sick sinus syndrome or subsidiary pacemaker dysfunction. In these patients, cardioversion may result in asystole. Cardioversion should also be withheld in patients with a recent embolic stroke. Patients with atrial fibrillation of longer than 1 week, especially with mitral valve disease, should have 4 to 6 weeks of warfarin therapy before elective cardioversion.

Nonpharmacologic Treatment of Arrhythmias, Including Electrical Devices and Surgery

A number of arrhythmias have proved to be remarkably difficult to control with drug therapy alone, and several other modes of nonpharmacologic therapy have been developed.

Surgery. Surgical treatment of cardiac arrhythmias has evolved considerably in the last 10 years.[4] Surgical division of the accessory pathway is a remarkably effective means of treating the arrhythmias of the Wolff-Parkinson-White syndrome. Many clinicians now refer healthy young individuals who have had life-threatening atrial fibrillation for this elective procedure, rather than imposing a lifelong commitment to a variety of pharmacologic agents. In patients whose intractable ventricular tachycardia is associated with ventricular aneurysms or ischemic heart disease, several surgical procedures have been devised to "ablate the arrhythmic focus."[6] These procedures are predicated on the principle that the site of the arrhythmia can be electrically isolated; they have been reserved for patients with intractable ventricular tachycardia.

Pacers and Cardioverters. Many forms of reentrant tachycardia can be eliminated by patient-activated or automatic pacemakers. These devices can sense the presence of tachycardia and deliver rapid atrial or ventricular pacing in a specified algorithm; this pacing is capable of terminating the tachycardia. Additionally, external and implantable cardioverters and defibrillators have recently been introduced and approved.[7] These appliances are capable of out-of-hospital cardioversion and defibrillation. They are an important adjunct for the patient with serious and recurrent ventricular tachycardia and fibrillation that have not been well controlled with pharmacologic therapy.

REFERENCES

1. Alpert JS, Haffajee CI, et al: Chemistry, pharmacology, antiarrhythmic efficacy and adverse effects of tocainide hydrochloride: An orally active structured analogue of lidocaine. Pharmacol Ther 3:316, 1983
2. Bhandari AK, Scheinman M: The long QT syndrome. Mod Concepts Cardiovasc Dis 54:45, 1985
3. Bigger JT: Symposium on flecainide acetate. Am J Cardiol 53:1B, 1984
4. Cox JL: The status of surgery for cardiac arrhythmias. Circulation 71:413, 1985
5. Gallagher JJ, Pritchett ELC, et al: The preexcitation syndromes. Prog Cardiovasc Dis 20:285, 1978
6. Josephson ME, Harken AH, Horowitz LN: Endocardial excision. A new surgical technique for the treatment of recurrent ventricular tachycardia. Circulation 60:1430, 1979
7. Mirowski M, Reid PR, et al: The termination of malignant ventricular arrhythmias with implanted automatic defibrillator in human beings. N Engl J Med 303:322, 1980
8. Smith WM, Gallagher JG: Les torsades de pointes: An unusual ventricular arrhythmia. Ann Intern Med 93:578, 1980
9. Spear JF, Moore EN: Mechanisms of cardiac arrhythmias. Ann Rev Physiol 44:485, 1982
10. Wellens HJJ, Bar FWHM, Lie KI: The value of the electrocardiogram in the differential diagnosis of a tachycardia with a widened QRS complex. Am J Med 64:27, 1978
11. Zipes DP, Prystowsky EN, et al: Amiodarone: Electrophysiological actions, pharmocokinetics and clinical effects. J Am Coll Cardiol 3:1059, 1984

CHAPTER 2.10
Systemic Hypertension

Paul K. Whelton
and R. Patterson Russell

MEASUREMENT OF BLOOD PRESSURE

An elevated blood pressure, like an elevated body temperature, may be due to a variety of underlying causes. If the elevation is sustained, cardiovascular complications are likely to result. High blood pressure is one of the most serious and potentially avoidable public health hazards in the developed world. Although many questions remain unresolved, the natural history and the value of treatment are better defined for persons with high blood pressure than for those with most other disease processes.

In clinical practice, repeated measurements of a patient's systolic or diastolic blood pressure often provide estimates that vary by more than 20 to 30 mm Hg. This is particularly the case when observers are unaware of the results of previous blood pressure measurements. Such variability is usually unnecessary and may lead

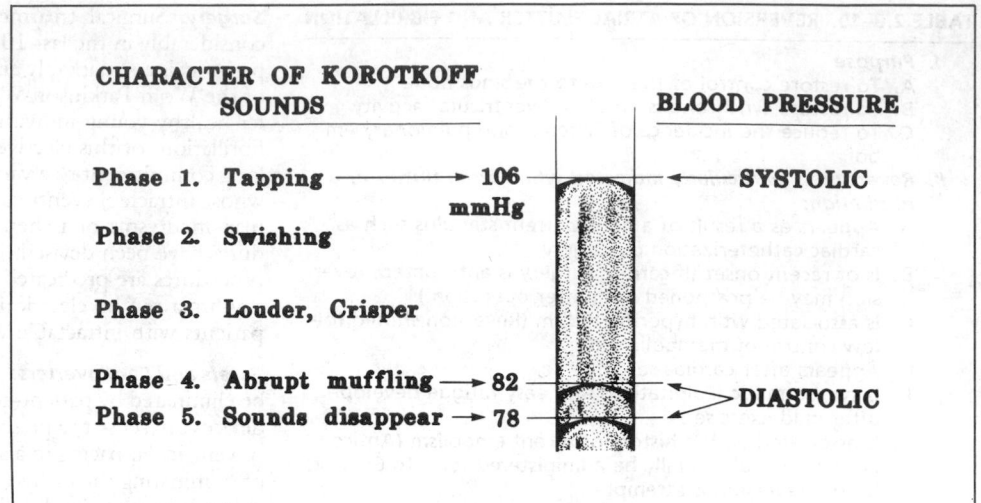

CHARACTER OF KOROTKOFF
SOUNDS   **BLOOD PRESSURE**

Phase 1. Tapping ──────→ 106 ◄─── SYSTOLIC
                              mmHg

Phase 2. Swishing

Phase 3. Louder, Crisper

Phase 4. Abrupt muffling ─→ 82 ┐
Phase 5. Sounds disappear ─→ 78 ┘──── DIASTOLIC

Figure 2.10–1. Graphic representation of the relationship of Korotkoff sounds to blood pressure measurement.

to serious errors in management. Differences between blood pressure measurements generally result from a mixture of random biologic variation in the patient's own level of blood pressure and systematic differences in observer technique and criteria. In an individual patient, the effects of random variation in blood pressure can be substantially reduced by the use of an average of serial blood pressure determinations. Systematic differences are mostly observational in nature, but some result from a patient's own response to the circumstances of their measurements. Much of the well-documented placebo effect of antihypertensive therapy results from a gradual reduction in the within-subject response to blood pressure determinations as patients become accustomed to the personnel, the procedure, and their surroundings. Systematic errors are not diminished by the use of an average blood pressure, but they can be reduced to an acceptably low level by standardizing the circumstances, criteria, and technique of blood pressure measurement.

For many years the American Heart Association has provided recommendations to meet the basic requirements of standardization.[8] In brief, a patient is comfortably seated in a quiet room with the forearm supported, at heart level, on a smooth surface. Tight arm clothing is removed and the sphygmomanometer cuff positioned just above the antecubital space so that the center of the cuff bladder is over the brachial artery. The bladder should nearly encircle the patient's arm and be approximately 20 percent wider than arm diameter. Cuff pressure is raised rapidly to about 30 mm Hg above the point at which the patient's radial pulse disappears. The observer's eyes should be level with the manometer from which the applied pressure is being read. With the stethoscope applied firmly but gently over the patient's brachial artery, cuff pressure is slowly reduced at a rate of 2 to 3 mm Hg per second while the observer records the systolic and diastolic blood pressures.

Systolic blood pressure is recorded as the pressure at which Korotkoff sounds appear (phase 1) (Fig. 2.10–1). In patients whose blood pressure is difficult to record, Korotkoff sounds may be augmented by raising the patient's arm before cuff inflation, increasing the rate of inflation, and instructing the patient to open and close the fist several times just before measurement.

Diastolic blood pressure is normally recorded as the pressure at which Korotkoff sounds become muffled (phase 4) or disappear (phase 5). Virtually all epidemiologic and clinical trial information is based on phase 5 measurements. In addition, disappearance of Korotkoff sounds is a better indicator of intra-arterial diastolic blood pressure than is muffling. On occasion, phase 5 is either absent or occurs at a very low level of blood pressure; in such instances, phase 4 recordings provide the only reliable estimate of diastolic blood pressure. This is particularly the case in hyperdy-

namic states such as aortic regurgitation, pregnancy, and thyrotoxicosis. Both phase 4 and phase 5 of diastolic blood pressure should always be recorded when they are separated by more than 4 to 6 mm Hg.

DETECTION AND CLASSIFICATION OF THE HYPERTENSIVE PATIENT

The use of blood pressure levels to categorize individuals as hypertensive or normotensive is of doubtful biologic validity. Nevertheless, such categorization proves useful as an operational means of case definition and therapeutic decision making. Hypertension may be detected by community-wide, occupational-health, or self-measurement screening techniques. An additional and highly effective strategy in many developed countries is to measure the blood pressure of all patients who seek health care for other reasons. Individuals should be informed clearly that a single elevated blood pressure reading does not identify the presence of hypertension but indicates the need for further observation. It must be emphasized that blood pressure screening can be effective only if adequate arrangements are made for follow-up. In addition to the basic recommendations for hypertension detection (Table 2.10–1), certain subsidiary classifications are often helpful. Patients with blood

TABLE 2.10–1. RECOMMENDATIONS FOR FOLLOW-UP OF AN INITIAL BLOOD PRESSURE MEASUREMENT AND FOR FINAL CLASSIFICATION OF HYPERTENSIVE STATUS IN U.S. ADULTS

Average Blood Pressure (mm Hg)		Initial Follow-up	Final Classification[a]
Systolic	Diastolic		
>240	>115	Immediately evaluate or refer to source of care	Severe hypertension
200–239	105–114	Evaluate or refer within 2 wk	Moderate hypertension
160–199	90–104	Confirm and evaluate within 2 mo	Mild hypertension
140–159	85–89	Recheck within 1 yr	Borderline high pressure
<140	<85	Recheck within 2 yr	Normal pressure

[a]Based on average of two or more measurements on at least two subsequent visits. Final classification should be based on highest grade of either systolic or diastolic blood pressure.

pressures that fluctuate across the arbitrary line dividing normotension from hypertension are often said to have labile hypertension. The term "accelerated hypertension" is applied to patients who exhibit a rapid and progressive rise in blood pressure over the course of several months. Isolated systolic hypertension describes patients with an average systolic blood pressure greater than 160 mm Hg who have a diastolic blood pressure less than 90 mm Hg. Malignant hypertension is a clinical diagnosis based on the presence of hypertensive papilledema.

Hypertension may also be classified as primary or secondary, depending on the presence or absence of a recognizable underlying cause. Hypertension is primary or essential in more than 90 percent of patients. Secondary hypertension may be further classified on the basis of therapeutic response. Some causes of secondary hypertension are amenable to correction and must be carefully considered in every hypertensive patient. In the remainder, the underlying cause cannot be corrected, but its recognition may be helpful in the choice of optimal antihypertensive drug therapy.

PREVALENCE AND CAUSES OF HYPERTENSION

Table 2.10–2 provides some estimates of the prevalence of high blood pressure in the United States according to age, race, and sex.[10] Although the prevalence rates provided are based on a single measurement, which tends to overestimate an individual's average blood pressure, they do provide a rough approximation of the situation in the community. As is readily apparent, hypertension is a pervasive disease that is particularly common in the black population. In most societies there is a tendency for blood pressure to rise with age. In females, systolic blood pressure rises at a more or less constant rate throughout life, whereas in males the rate of rise during adolescence is faster but is subsequently less than in females. In both sexes, diastolic blood pressure rises more gradually with aging; consequently, pulse pressures are wider in elderly persons. The statement that "average blood pressure rises with age" conceals a wide range of individual trends. Persons fortunate enough to start life with relatively low levels of blood pressure show the least tendency for blood pressure to rise with aging, whereas those whose initial blood pressure is relatively high are most likely to become hypertensive. In the United States, there is little difference between average blood pressure in black infants and white infants, but black adults tend to have blood pressures that are 5 to 10 mm Hg higher than their white counterparts. Many studies have demonstrated that hypertension is more common in lower socioeconomic groups.

Because hypertension often runs in families, clinicians have long suspected a genetic influence. Population studies have confirmed a familial resemblance across the entire spectrum of blood pressure levels, and even more convincing evidence of a genetic

influence comes from twin and adoptive studies. However, environmental factors appear to play the dominant role in most persons with hypertension. Of the many environmental factors that may be important in the genesis of hypertension, excessive calories and salt intake have received the greatest attention. A close association exists between blood pressure and body weight, especially during adolescence and middle age. In addition, weight loss often results in a reduction of blood pressure in obese persons. Interpopulation studies suggest the presence of a relationship between salt intake and the presence of hypertension. Experimentally, blood pressure can be modulated by administering a diet that is either extremely high or low in salt content. It has been difficult, however, to demonstrate convincingly a relationship between salt intake and blood pressure in most Western societies. Some investigators have argued that salt intake merely represents a marker of the civilizing process and plays no active role in the genesis of hypertension. In recent years, increasing interest has centered on the possibility that high blood pressure may result from a chronic deficiency of potassium or calcium intake. Magnesium deficiency and heavy metal exposure have also been suggested as etiologic possibilities. Their role is more controversial. Emotional stress undoubtedly leads to an acute rise in blood pressure, but it has been more difficult to document the role of stress in sustained elevations of blood pressure. Finally, the presence of a relationship between excess alcohol intake and high blood pressure has been well demonstrated. This in itself, however, cannot account for the majority of instances in which hypertension occurs. In summary, many etiologic possibilities have been advanced but none has been conclusively demonstrated as the principal underlying cause of essential hypertension. Indeed, it seems likely that the cause of hypertension is multifactorial in most patients.

RISKS OF HYPERTENSION

Epidemiologic studies have repeatedly demonstrated the presence of a strong relationship between blood pressure and cardiovascular risk.[1,6] Risk increases in a curvilinear fashion with progressively higher levels of blood pressure, and the risk applies equally to elevations of systolic and diastolic blood pressure. In the classic 1959 Build and Blood Pressure insurance industry report, the blood pressure that appeared to be optimal for longevity was less than 110/70 mm Hg.[1] On an individual basis, patients with moderate or severe hypertension are at much greater risk than their counterparts with mild hypertension. Mild hypertension is so common, however, that it is responsible for most of the cardiovascular complications that can be attributed to the effects of sustained hypertension in the general community.[14]

The main causes of sickness and death in hypertensive patients are cardiovascular, cerebrovascular, peripheral vascular, and renal disease. The relationship between hypertension and stroke is very striking. For instance, in the Framingham study, hypertension (blood pressure >160/95 mm Hg) was associated with a 5- to 30-fold increase in the risk of stroke, depending on the age and sex of the group being studied.[6] The relative likelihood of developing congestive heart failure or a dissecting aneurysm of the aorta is also closely related to an individual's level of blood pressure. At every age and at every level of severity, however, the main hazard facing the hypertensive patient is from coronary artery disease. This is true in both sexes, but the absolute risk of coronary artery disease is considerably higher in men than women. Although hypertension is an important predictor of coronary artery disease, the likelihood of myocardial infarction is dramatically influenced by other cardiovascular risk factors. The extent of this variability is well illustrated by the Framingham study results shown in Table 2.10–3. The table identifies an enormous degree of variation in the probability of the development of cardiovascular disease at four levels of systolic blood pressure, depending on the presence or absence of six cardiovascular risk factors. The therapeutic implications of this

TABLE 2.10–2. PREVALENCE OF ADULT U.S. POPULATION WITH A SYSTOLIC BLOOD PRESSURE > 160 mm Hg OR DIASTOLIC BLOOD PRESSURE > 95 mm Hg ON A SINGLE MEASUREMENT[a]

Age (yr)	White		Black	
	Male	Female	Male	Female
18–24	5	1	5	5
25–34	8	4	18	10
35–44	17	10	38	28
45–54	26	19	37	51
55–64	31	32	50	54
65–74	35	42	50	59

[a]Adapted from Table 40 of Health and Nutrition Examination Survey, Vital and Health Statistics. Series 11, No. 203. Washington, DC, US Department of Health, Education, and Welfare, 1977.

TABLE 2.10–3. PROBABILITY PER 1000 OF DEVELOPMENT OF CARDIOVASCULAR DISEASE DURING 8-YEAR FOLLOW-UP OF U.S. MALES AND FEMALES WITHOUT OR WITH OTHER RISK FACTORS[a]

Systolic BP (mm Hg)	Males				Females			
	Age 35 yr		Age 55 yr		Age 35 yr		Age 55 yr	
	Without[b]	With[c]	Without[b]	With[c]	Without[b]	With[c]	Without[b]	With[c]
105	6	269	55	563	4	62	34	248
135	9	371	85	674	6	92	52	337
165	14	486	130	768	9	136	78	439
195	23	602	193	841	13	195	115	547

[a]"Cardiovascular disease" refers to new onset of coronary heart disease, cerebrovascular accident, congestive heart failure, or intermittent claudication.
[b]Nonsmoker with no LVH or ECG, no glucose intolerance, and a serum cholesterol level of 185 mg/dl.
[c]Smoker with LVH on ECG, glucose intolerance, and a serum cholesterol level of 385 mg/dl.
Adapted from Framingham Study, Section 28, 1973.

variability in risk are twofold. First, the management of hypertensive patients should be multifactorial. Too often, patients with high blood pressure are treated exclusively with hypotensive medications, and little or no attempt is made to alter other cardiovascular risk factors. Second, the decision to institute antihypertensive therapy should probably be influenced by the presence or absence of other cardiovascular risk factors.

EVALUATION OF THE HYPERTENSIVE PATIENT

Once the presence of hypertension is confirmed, the next steps are to (1) determine whether the elevation is primary or secondary, (2) identify and, where possible, treat any other cardiovascular risk factors, and (3) ascertain the degree of vascular disease present in such target organs as the central nervous system, eyes, heart, and kidneys. A complete history and physical examination supplemented by selective laboratory studies will provide this information. In the history taking, inquiry should be made regarding the family history of hypertension and cardiovascular complications; the presence or absence of central nervous system, cardiac, and genitourinary symptoms; dietary habits; and, in women, the history of previous hypertension associated with pregnancies or the use of oral contraceptives. Physical examination enables the physician to assess the degree of target organ involvement through careful evaluation of the ocular fundi, heart, and central nervous system. In addition, signs of specific correctable conditions such as coarctation of the aorta, Cushing syndrome, and renovascular hypertension may be detected. Initial laboratory studies should include the following:

1. Urinalysis and serum creatinine determination
2. Serum potassium and uric acid determinations
3. Fasting blood sugar and lipid-lipoprotein profile
4. Complete blood cell count
5. ECG
6. Chest radiograph
7. Echocardiogram (optional)

Additional studies may be desirable, depending on the drug(s) selected for therapy and the patient's blood pressure response. However, if a patient's blood pressure is responsive to a simple medical regimen, elaborate search for a correctable cause is not indicated.

CLINICAL PRESENTATION

The four common clinical presentations of patients with primary or essential hypertension are outlined in Table 2.10–4. Most hypertensive patients initially have an asymptomatic elevation of blood pressure and have no additional physical signs or laboratory abnormalities. In those who are symptomatic, common complaints include headaches, vertigo, tinnitus, nosebleeds, nervousness, and palpitations. Such symptoms may result from the anxiety associated with disease labeling of asymptomatic individuals. Alternatively, they may represent the first manifestation of vascular damage after prolonged exposure to high blood pressure. Funduscopic evidence of arteriolar narrowing is often the earliest finding of hypertensive damage on the physical examination (see Chapter 17.6). A slight ventricular heave, ST-T wave changes on the ECG, and trace proteinuria may also be present.

Less frequently, patients have more obvious complications because of the effects of sustained high blood pressure on the heart, cerebral circulation, and kidneys. Left ventricular hypertrophy is more closely related to severity than duration of hypertension and is manifested clinically by the appearance of a left ventricular heave, a prominent fourth heart sound, and electrocardiographic evidence of left ventricular hypertrophy. Cardiac dysfunction culminates in symptoms and signs of left- and right-sided congestive heart failure. Occasionally, patients with essential hypertension come to medical attention for the first time during an attack of acute pulmonary edema, angina pectoris, or myocardial infarction.

The most common symptom attributable to the effects of hypertension on the cerebral circulation is headache. The classic headache of hypertension is a throbbing, occipital pain that is worst on awakening and gradually improves with activity. In general, the higher the pressure, the more severe is the headache. The importance of performing an adequate funduscopic examination cannot be overemphasized. Arteriolar tortuosity and arteriovenous compression are common manifestations of hypertensive vascular damage in the retina. Flame-shaped hemorrhages and soft, ill-defined "cotton-wool" exudates suggest the presence of severe hypertension and should alert the treating physician to the necessity for a rapid reduction in the patient's blood pressure.

A decrease in renal blood flow and tubular function are the first signs of hypertensive renal disease. Renal insufficiency and proteinuria are more commonly noted in patients with long-standing, severe, or malignant hypertension and in those with underlying renal parenchymal disease.

Patients who enter the *malignant phase* of hypertension are almost always symptomatic and generally die within a 6- to 12-month period if untreated. Most patients with malignant hypertension have very high blood pressures, but the diagnosis is based on the presence of hypertensive papilledema rather than the absolute level of blood pressure. "Hypertensive encephalopathy" is a term used to denote the occurrence of cerebral episodes in severely hypertensive patients. Many such patients have malignant hypertension, and virtually all have intensely constricted retinal arteries. These episodes are characterized by violent headaches, vomiting, visual impairment, drowsiness, and transient neurologic features,

TABLE 2.10–4. PRIMARY OR ESSENTIAL HYPERTENSION: MODE OF PRESENTATION

Presentation	Possible Symptoms	Common Physical Signs	Laboratory Abnormalities
Symptomless	None	Elevated blood pressure alone	None
Symptomatic but no major complication	Headache, vertigo, tinnitus, nosebleeds, nervousness, palpitations	Narrowing of retinal arterioles Slight ventricular heave	*ECG:* ±ST-T wave changes *Urine:* ±urinary protein
Symptomatic with: Cardiac complications	Dyspnea, orthopnea Angina pectoris	$S_4 \pm S_3$ Enlarged heart Ankle edema	*ECG:* Left ventricular hypertrophy or ST-T wave changes *Radiograph:* Left ventricular dilation
Central nervous system complications	Occipital headaches Dizziness, vertigo Deterioration of vision or mental function	Narrowed, tortuous retinal arteries that compress and "nick" the retinal veins Transient or permanent neurologic changes	±Bloody cerebrospinal fluid
Renal complications	Nocturia or polyuria		*Urine:* 1–2+ proteinuria, decreased specific gravity, or both *Blood:* Increased serum creatinine level
Malignant phase	Severe headaches Visual impairment Weight loss ± symptoms of hypertensive encephalopathy	Any of the above, plus papilledema and retinal hemorrhages, or exudates	Any or all of the above, plus microscopic or gross hematuria, heavy proteinuria, and hemolytic anemia

and they usually culminate in catastrophic central nervous system complications if untreated. Hypertensive encephalopathy represents the most positive indication for immediate hospitalization and reduction in blood pressure.

SECONDARY CAUSES OF HYPERTENSION

In recent years it has been repeatedly demonstrated that a thorough evaluation of all hypertensive patients to search for secondary causes of hypertension is economically and scientifically unsupportable. A brief evaluation, including a careful history and physical examination, is mandatory, however, in every patient because even by the most conservative estimates, between 0.5 and 1.5 million hypertensive persons in the United States have potentially correctable forms of the disease. The search for an underlying cause of hypertension becomes particularly relevant in patients who fail to respond satisfactorily to antihypertensive drug therapy. Figure 2.10–2 outlines a general approach to the detection, evaluation, and treatment of hypertensive patients. The principal clinical and laboratory features of the secondary forms of hypertension are summarized in Table 2.10–5.

Secondary hypertension usually results from underlying renal or endocrine disease. Several forms of secondary hypertension can be directly linked to derangements of the renin-angiotensin-aldosterone system, and a disorder of this system may also play a role in the pathogenesis of essential hypertension. A schematic outline of factors that influence renin secretion and metabolism is provided in Figure 2.10–3. Briefly, the proteolytic enzyme renin is secreted by juxtaglomerular cells within the kidney. Renin hydrolyzes the hepatic glycoprotein renin substrate to form the decapeptide angiotensin I. Principally under the influence of a pulmonary converting enzyme, this peptide is further reduced to form the octapeptide and biologically active metabolite angiotensin II. Angiotensin II, the most potent pressor known to man, influences blood pressure directly by causing arteriolar vasoconstriction and indirectly by increasing secretion of the salt-retaining adrenal mineralocorticoid, aldosterone.

Normally, renin is secreted in response to a depletion of extracellular fluid volume and a reduction in renal perfusion pressure. Activation of the renin-angiotensin-aldosterone system serves as a valuable homeostatic mechanism to prevent a threatened fall in blood pressure. However, inappropriate stimulation of the system can result in systemic hypertension. For example, in many patients with constriction of the renal artery, renal hypoperfusion leads to excessive renin production and angiotensin II–mediated hypertension. Likewise, primary aldosteronism produces a volume expansion–mediated form of hypertension. Antihypertensive drugs have important effects on the renin-angiotensin-aldosterone system. Hyperreninemia is common during vasodilator and diuretic therapy, whereas adrenergic inhibitors such as methyldopa, clonidine, and beta blockers tend to reduce renin secretion. The converting enzyme inhibitors enalapril and captopril block conversion of angiotensin I to its active metabolite angiotensin II. Finally, the potassium-sparing agent spironolatone is a competitive inhibitor of the effect of aldosterone at sodium-potassium exchange sites in the distal tubule of the kidney.

RENAL PARENCHYMAL DISEASE

Hypertension is one of the most frequent complications of renal failure.[11] It is usually no more than a transient phenomenon in acute renal failure but constitutes a more serious complication in patients with chronic renal failure, because many of these patients ultimately die from vascular complications. Treatment of hypertension provides an effective way of delaying the progression to end-stage renal disease. In general, the hypertension results from an excessive retention of salt and water. In this instance, adequate diuresis should be the initial goal of therapy. In approximately 5 to 10 percent of patients, the hypertension is renin-angiotensin mediated, and administration of a converting enzyme inhibitor or a beta blocker is more important. Nephrectomy, although effective in lowering blood pressure in this latter group of patients, is best reserved for those who are functionally anephric and who have not benefited from an adequate trial of therapy with a converting enzyme inhibitor.

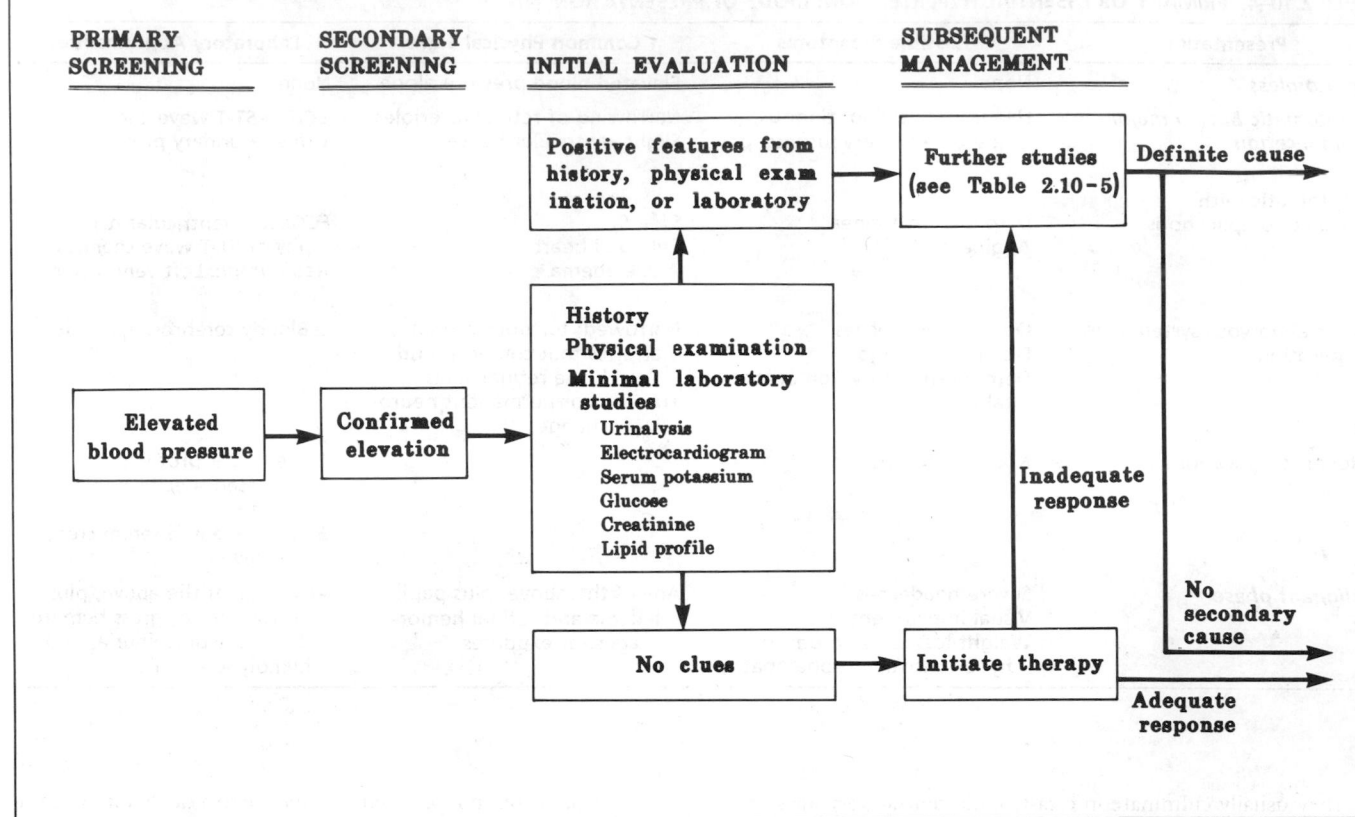

RENOVASCULAR HYPERTENSION

Hypertension results from underlying renal ischemia in less than 1 percent to more than 5 percent of hypertensive patients, depending on whether the physician is operating in an unselected or a referral practice. The specific types of vascular, parenchymal, and capsular involvement that may produce renal ischemia include the following:

I. Large-vessel disease
    A. Atherosclerotic vascular disease
    B. Fibrous dysplasia or fibromuscular disease
    C. Arteritis
    D. Other
II. Parenchymal lesions
    A. Unilateral pyelonephritis
    B. Juxtaglomerular cell tumors
    C. Wilms tumors
III. Capsular lesions
    A. Hematoma

Typically, renovascular hypertension results from deposition of an atherosclerotic plaque close to the ostium of the main renal artery or a fibrous-fibromuscular narrowing in the mid- to distal portion of the right renal artery. Since only a small percentage of the hypertensive population has underlying renal ischemia, it is unreasonable to embark on an expensive and time-consuming search for renovascular disease in all such patients. If the patient is not a suitable candidate for percutaneous transluminal angioplasty or surgical intervention, special investigational procedures are generally unwarranted.

History and Physical Examination

The fibromuscular form of renovascular hypertension is most frequently identified in young white women, whereas the atheroscle-rotic form is typically a disorder of older men and women. Furthermore the disease is more common in patients with severe hypertension and in those whose blood pressure is difficult to manage or abruptly rises after previously satisfactory control. A bruit that lateralizes to the side of the abdomen is strongly suggestive of renal artery stenosis. Careful abdominal auscultation in a quiet room will facilitate detection of the distinctive high-pitched, usually continuous, bruit in about 30 percent of patients with renovascular hypertension.

In many patients the decision to perform renal arteriography is strongly influenced by the results of ancillary laboratory studies. In general, screening laboratory studies should be obtained in all patients who have untreated diastolic blood pressures >110 mm Hg or in those who present management problems and are under the age of 50 years.

Screening Laboratory Studies

Pyelography is one of the simplest and most accurate screening tests available in the average hospital. Early films from a rapid-sequence "hypertensive" pyelogram provide the most sensitive indication of renal vascular disease, namely a discrepancy (delay on the involved side) in appearance time of contrast medium in the kidneys of 1 minute or more. Other suggestive findings are hyperconcentration of dye in the late films and a difference in size between the kidneys of at least 1.5 cm. Pyelography may also reveal the presence of renal parenchymal disease. Although less specific, isotope renography can be used as an initial screening test in patients who are allergic to pyelographic dye. Elevated levels of peripheral plasma renin activity (PRA) in relation to the patient's posture and 24-hour urinary sodium excretion are helpful when present. Many patients, however, have normal levels.

Renal Arteriography

In general, renal arteriography should be performed in the following groups of patients:

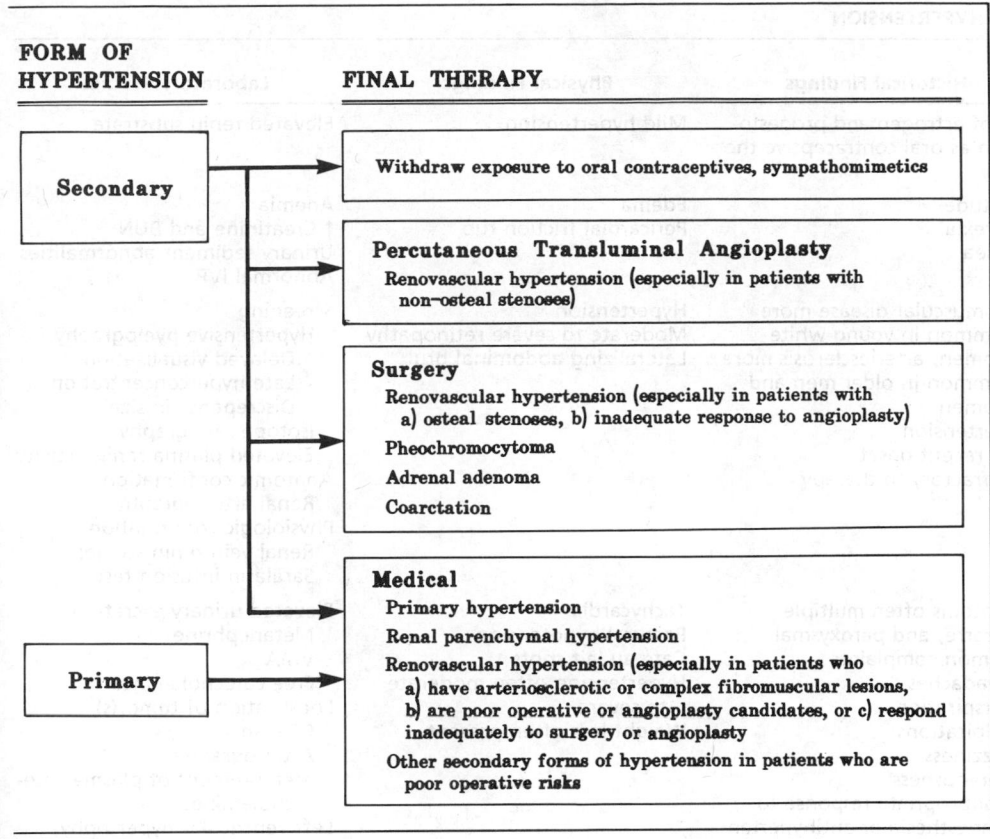

FORM OF HYPERTENSION	FINAL THERAPY

Secondary

Withdraw exposure to oral contraceptives, sympathomimetics

Percutaneous Transluminal Angioplasty
Renovascular hypertension (especially in patients with non-osteal stenoses)

Surgery
Renovascular hypertension (especially in patients with
  a) osteal stenoses, b) inadequate response to angioplasty)
Pheochromocytoma
Adrenal adenoma
Coarctation

Medical
Primary hypertension
Renal parenchymal hypertension
Renovascular hypertension (especially in patients who
  a) have arteriosclerotic or complex fibromuscular lesions,
  b) are poor operative or angioplasty candidates, or c) respond
  inadequately to surgery or angioplasty
Other secondary forms of hypertension in patients who are
  poor operative risks

Primary

Figure 2.10–2. Flow diagram depicting the sequential evaluation of a hypertensive patient from first detection to final therapy.

1. White women less than 50 years old with an untreated average diastolic blood pressure of >110 mm Hg
2. Patients with a lateralizing abdominal bruit
3. Patients with a positive result on a laboratory screening procedure
4. Patients whose treatment is problematic

Angiography not only allows assessment of the technical feasibility of an angioplastic or surgical procedure but, when combined with the available clinical information, usually permits accurate prediction of the underlying vascular abnormality.

Physiologic Studies

The mere demonstration of an arteriographic or pyelographic abnormality in a hypertensive patient is not sufficient indication for an angioplastic or surgical intervention. One must be reasonably certain that the demonstrated lesion is responsible for the hypertension and that its repair will be followed by a return of blood pressure toward, if not completely to, normal. Many studies have demonstrated the usefulness of comparing renal vein renin activity (RVRA). Most often this comparison is expressed as a ratio of involved to uninvolved RVRA, and ischemia is diagnosed when the ratio is 1.5 or greater. Additional criteria, however, including the absolute difference in RVRA between the two renal veins and the presence or absence of contralateral RVRA suppression, permit a more accurate diagnosis.[12,15] Standardized tests based on blood pressure or renin response to infusion of the angiotensin II receptor blocker saralasin acetate have proved equally useful as a means of quantitating the physiologic importance of renovascular lesions in hypertensive patients.

Treatment

In most patients the initial approach should be medical. Administration of a drug regimen that includes a converting enzyme inhibitor will often reduce blood pressure successfully. Renal function should be assessed carefully, however, because functional hypoperfusion of the kidneys with resultant renal failure is not uncommon in patients with bilateral renovascular disease. Once blood pressure has been successfully controlled, serious consideration should be given to an attempt to revascularize the ischemic kidney by percutaneous transluminal angioplasty or surgical revascularization. This is particularly the case in patients with fibromuscular disease, because most patients derive a long-term cure after successful revascularization. Percutaneous transluminal angioplasty provides a less invasive therapeutic option and is probably as effective as surgery, provided it is possible to dilate the stenotic area satisfactorily. Although it is often possible to dilate ostial arteriosclerotic lesions, the resultant benefit may be transient, because the stenotic lesion frequently returns to its former position after the dilating cathetic has been withdrawn. Surgery provides an alternative therapeutic option for patients in whom angioplasty has been unsuccessful or is technically not feasible. When surgery is undertaken, all possible efforts should be made to preserve renal mass, although the final decision as to whether a renovascularization procedure, segmental resection, or nephrectomy will be performed can be made only at the time of operation. In patients who are being managed with a long-term medical regimen, one must be certain that blood pressure is adequately controlled and renal function is stable. If not, the need for angioplasty or surgery should be carefully reconsidered.

PHEOCHROMOCYTOMA

Pheochromocytoma, which results from excessive catecholamine production, is a rare but well-characterized cause of hypertension.[9] Important end products of catecholamine biosynthesis are normally found in the brain (dopamine), autonomic nervous system (norepinephrine), and adrenal medulla (norepinephrine and epinephrine). After release from the autonomic nervous system and

TABLE 2.10–5. SECONDARY FORMS OF HYPERTENSION

Condition and Probable Prevalence (%)	Historical Findings	Physical Findings	Laboratory Studies
"Oral contraceptive" hypertension (<5)	Use of estrogen and progestogen as oral contraceptive therapy	Mild hypertension	Elevated renin substrate
Parenchymal renal disease (<5)	Lassitude Anorexia Nausea	Edema Pericardial friction rub	Anemia ↑ Creatinine and BUN Urinary sediment abnormalities Abnormal IVP

Renovascular hypertension (<5)	Fibromuscular disease more common in young white women; arteriosclerosis more common in older men and women
	Hypertension
	  Of recent onset
	  Refractory to therapy
		Hypertension
		Moderate to severe retinopathy
		Lateralizing abdominal bruit
			Screening
			  Hypertensive pyelography
			    Delayed visualization
			    Late hyperconcentration
			    Discrepancy in size
			  Isotope renography
			    Elevated plasma renin activity
			Anatomic confirmation
			  Renal arteriography
			Physiologic confirmation
			  Renal vein renin studies
			  Saralasin infusion test

Pheochromocytoma (<1)	Symptoms often multiple, bizarre, and paroxysmal
	Common complaints
	  Headaches
	  Perspiration
	  Palpitations
	  Dizziness
	  Nervousness
	  Inappropriate response to anesthesia or antihypertensive drugs
		Tachycardia
		Postural hypotension
		Café au lait spots
		Hypertension often moderate to severe
		Weight loss often present
			Elevated urinary excretion
			  Metanephrine
			  VMA
			  Free catecholamines
			Localization of tumor(s)
			  CT scan
			  Arteriography
			  Measurement of plasma catecholamines
			Left ventricular hypertophy, hyperglycemia, and proteinuria common

Primary aldosteronism (<1)	Weakness
	Muscle cramps
	Paresthesias
	Tetany
	Polyuria, polydipsia
		Mild hypertension
		Chvostek or Trousseau sign
			Before treatment
			  Hypokalemia, kaliuresis
			  Alkalosis
			  ↓ Plasma renin activity on low sodium intake
			  ↑ Plasma aldosterone on high sodium intake
			Localization studies
			  CT scan
			  Venography
			  Adrenal vein steroid determinations

Cushing syndrome (<1)	Sexual dysfunction
	Weakness
	Backache
		Plethora
		Central obesity
		Hirsutism
		Purple striae
		Ecchymoses
			Polycythemia
			Hyperglycemia
			Osteoporosis
			Increased urinary levels
			  17-Ketosteroids
			  11-Oxysteroids

Coarctation of aorta (<1)	Asymptomatic hypertension in childhood
	Intermittent claudication
		Changes in legs versus arms
		  Lower blood pressure
		  Diminished or delayed pulses, or both
		Precordial murmur
		Intercostal pulsations
			Chest radiograph changes
			  Rib notching
			  Numeral "3" sign
			Left ventricular hypertrophy

BUN = blood, urea, nitrogen; IVP = intravenous pyelogram; VMA = vanillylmandelic acid.

adrenal medulla, 90 percent of epinephrine and norepinephrine is reabsorbed unchanged. The remaining 10 percent is metabolized by catechol-o-methyltransferase (COMT) to metanephrine-normetanephrine and by monoaminoxidase to vanillylmandelic acid (VMA).

The diagnosis of pheochromocytoma may be accurately confirmed by biochemical analysis of the urinary catecholamines epinephrine and norepinephrine or the metabolites metanephrine, normetanephrine, and VMA. With the development of more sensitive and accurate biochemical tests, pharmacologic interventions such as histamine stimulation and phenotolamine blockade have come to play a very limited role in the diagnosis of pheochromocytoma. Depending on the biochemical screening test used, there are a number of reasons why one might obtain a false-positive or false-negative result. Some of these are outlined in Table 2.10–6. Patients may be asymptomatic and normotensive at the time of presentation to the physician, but more frequently they complain of headaches, excessive perspiration, palpitations, nervousness, nausea, vomiting, and weight loss. Their hypertension is often severe and is frequently accompanied by evidence of left ventricular hy-

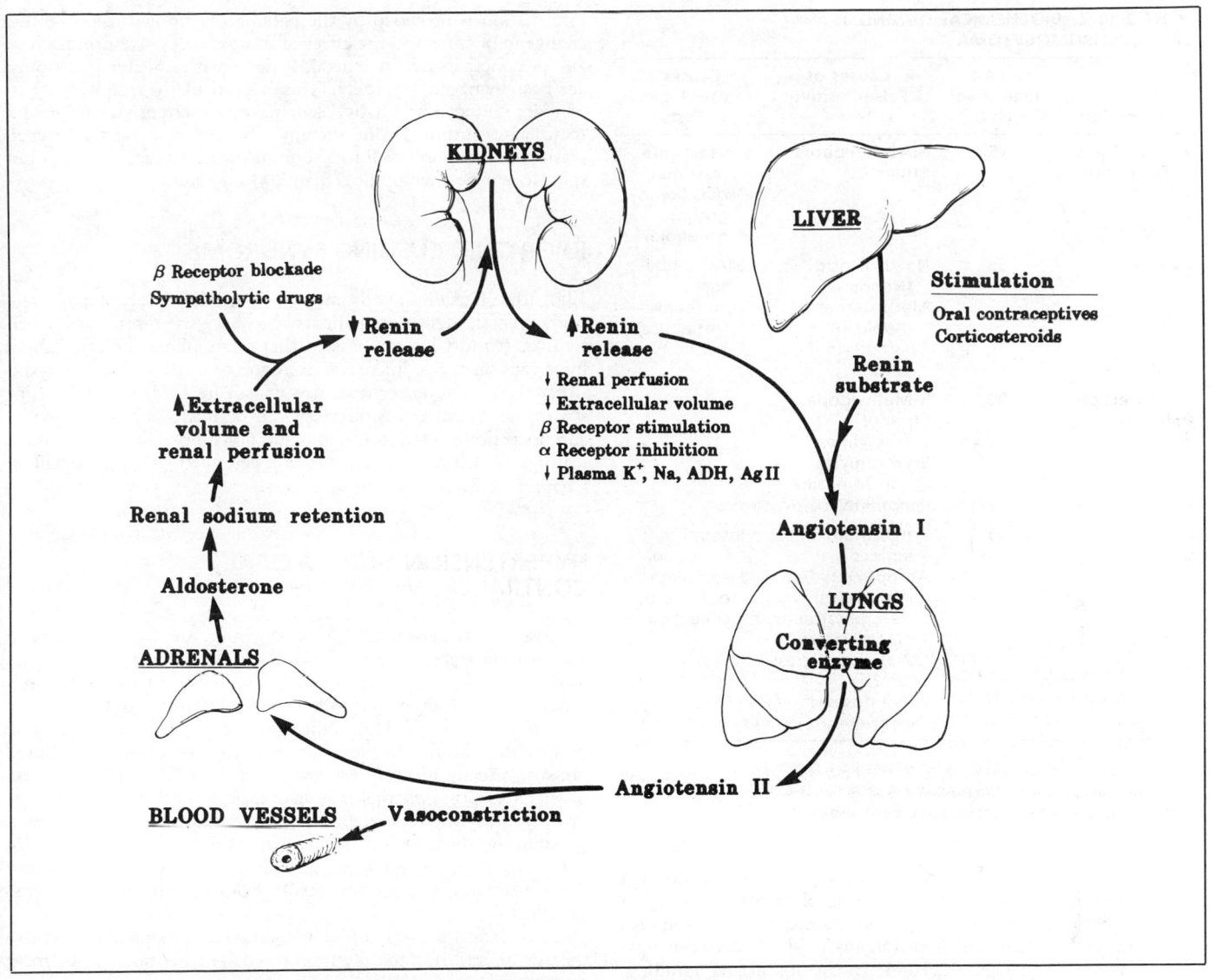

Figure 2.10–3. Schematic outline of factors that influence homeostasis of the renin-angiotensin-aldosterone system. Under normal circumstances, the system helps to prevent hypotension. Excessive production of angiotensin or aldosterone is pathophysiologic mechanism responsible for several of most common forms of secondary hypertension. ADH = antidiuretic hormone.

pertrophy, retinopathy, and proteinuria. In addition, tachycardia is common and hyperglycemia is seen in approximately 60 percent of patients. As with renovascular hypertension, it is not reasonable to screen the entire hypertensive population for the possibility of pheochromocytoma. However, this form of hypertension should be considered in any patient with severe hypertension, paroxysmal symptoms, excessive headaches or sweating, tachycardia, hyperglycemia, hypermetabolism without hyperthyroidism, or a paradoxical response to hypotensive or anesthetic agents.

More than 90 percent of pheochromocytoma patients have solitary benign adrenal adenomas, but some tumors are multiple, ectopic, or malignant. These tumors occur with greater frequency in younger patients and in those with familial tumors. Some of the latter will have medullary carcinoma of the thyroid and parathyroid tumors (multiple endocrine adenomatosis, Sipple syndrome type II). In addition, a wide variety of disease entities have been associated with pheochromocytoma, including cholelithiasis, neurofibromatosis, congenital cyanotic heart disease, polycythemia, and renovascular hypertension.

Pheochromocytomas can usually be localized with an abdominal CT scan. More invasive tests, such as abdominal-thoracic arte-

riography and vena cava catecholamine sampling, are best reserved for patients in whom recurrent, ectopic, or multiple tumors are thought likely. These invasive tests should be performed only under carefully monitored conditions, because administration of contrast medium and catheter manipulation almost invariably activate the tumor. Once the diagnosis is established, patients can be treated either medically or surgically. Since the perioperative mortality rate is generally less than 3 percent and the postoperative results are usually excellent, surgery is indicated in most patients. Medical therapy is usually reserved for preoperative management, poor surgical candidates, and patients with malignant tumors. It includes hydration, alpha- or beta-receptor blockers or both, and, on occasion, the tyrosine hydroxylase inhibitor α-methyl-p-tyrosine.

PRIMARY ALDOSTERONISM

Primary aldosteronism is present in less than 1 percent of the hypertensive population. Although malignant hypertension is unusual, there are no other historical or physical features that help to

TABLE 2.10–6. BIOCHEMICAL DIAGNOSIS OF PHEOCHROMOCYTOMA

Urinary Test	Patients Identified (%)	Causes of False-Positive Tests[a]	Causes of False-Negative Tests
Metanephrines and normeta-nephrines	95	MAO inhibitors Ethanol	Certain contrast materials (Renografin) Propranolol
VMA	95	Nalidixic acid (Negram)[b] Methocarbamol (Robaxin) Guaifenesin (Robitussin)	MAO inhibitors Disulfiram (Antabuse) Ethanol
Free catecholamines	90	α-Methyldopa Ethanol Tetracyclines Erythromycin Chlorpromazine Quinidine	
All of the above	99	Sympathomimetic amines Abrupt clonidine withdrawal Severe physical or mental stress Other neural crest tumors Large doses of L-dopa	Intermittent secretion Incomplete or incorrect collection

MAO = monoamine oxidase.
[a]Adapted in part from Manger WM, Gifford RW: Pheochromocytoma. New York, Springer-Verlag, 1977 (Table 6.14).
[b]Common trade names identified in parentheses.

identify these patients. The cardinal manifestations of the disorder are hypertension, kaliuresis in the setting of hypokalemia, and a deranged pattern of renin-angiotensin-aldosterone secretion. An algorithm for evaluation of hypokalemia in the hypertensive patient is presented in Figure 2.10–4. In the absence of vomiting, diarrhea, excessive licorice intake, or the use of diuretics or laxatives, hypokalemia in a hypertensive patient should be carefully evaluated. Patients who develop hypokalemia during administration of thiazide diuretics deserve evaluation if their hypokalemia cannot be easily corrected after discontinuation of the diuretic agent.

Urinary potassium excretion is best quantitated by obtaining a 24-hour urine specimen while the patient still has hypokalemia and a liberal salt intake but is not taking diuretics. In this setting, most patients with aldosteronism excrete more than 30 mEq of potassium per day. The diagnosis of primary aldosteronism can subsequently be confirmed by the demonstration of low, nonstimulable plasma renin activity and elevated, nonsuppressible plasma aldosterone concentration. The renin-angiotensin-aldosterone system is usually stimulated by ambulation and either short-term administration of a loop diuretic or a 3 to 5 day diet with a sodium content of 20 mEq/day. In contrast, the system is usually suppressed by volume expansion and overnight assumption of the supine position. Because hypokalemia that occurs for any reason may influence renin activity and aldosterone production, blood samples for these assays should be obtained after potassium repletion.

The diagnosis of primary aldosteronism can usually be established with some certainty. It is equally important, however, to determine whether the disease resulted from a unilateral adrenal adenoma or from bilateral adrenal hyperplasia, because only the former is surgically correctable. The two conditions may be differentiated by abdominal computed axial tomography, adrenal venography, and hormonal sampling from the adrenal veins. Additional information is provided by the patient's hormonal response to a change in posture and the effect of short courses of spironolactone and dexamethasone. In general, patients with unilateral adenomas are best managed surgically. This is particularly true of patients who are young, severely hypokalemic or hypertensive, and unable to tolerate spironolactone therapy. Patients with bilateral hyperplasia often respond well to a sodium-restricted diet and low-dose spironolactone therapy (less than 200 mg/day).

IDIOPATHIC CUSHING SYNDROME

Idiopathic Cushing syndrome is an unusual cause of hypertension, even though most patients who have the disease are hypertensive. It must be emphasized that many obese subjects exhibit hypertension and an increased excretion of urinary 17-hydroxycorticosteroids. The latter does not constitute evidence of Cushing syndrome, because this diagnosis can be made only when hyperadrenocorticalism is autonomous and nonsuppressible. The clinical features of Cushing syndrome are described in more detail in Chapter 14.3.

HYPERTENSION DURING ORAL CONTRACEPTIVE THERAPY

An association between oral contraceptive use and hypertension was first suggested in 1967, and it is now abundantly clear that most patients taking oral contraceptives have systolic blood pressure elevated by about 5 to 6 mm Hg and diastolic blood pressure by about 1 to 3 mm Hg. Although severe hypertension is a rare occurrence, the rise in blood pressure may be impressive. Blood pressure usually reverts back to its previous level after cessation of therapy, although this may take as long as 3 months. Several investigators have reported that oral contraceptives increase renin substrate production, but the precise mechanisms of this form of hypertension are as yet unclear. Likewise, it is not clear whether the increase in blood pressure results from an estrogen or a progestin effect.

The blood pressure of all women receiving oral contraceptive therapy should be carefully monitored. Furthermore, since most women receiving oral contraceptive therapy experience a rise in blood pressure, the criteria for selection of patients and the need for subsequent close observation are most critical in those who have other cardiovascular risk factors.

COARCTATION OF THE AORTA

Coarctation should be considered in young patients with long-standing mild hypertension. Commonly, these patients are asymptomatic, but some complain of headaches or experience intermittent claudication. Physical examination reveals arterial hypertension in the upper extremities, with the pressure in the right arm often exceeding that in the left. Demonstration of a palpable pulse in the femoral artery does not exclude the diagnosis of coarctation, but the femoral pulse is reduced in amplitude and delayed in onset, and the pressure in the legs is less than that in the arms. There may be a systolic murmur over the precordium and sometimes over the back in the region of the narrowed aortic segment. Radiographic clues include rib notching, characteristically seen at the lower border of the outer third of the ribs, and the "3" sign contour of the left upper border of the heart. Thoracic aortography is helpful in defining the length and precise location of the narrowed segment.

Potential complications of untreated coarctation include aortic dissection or rupture, infective endocarditis, subarachnoid hemorrhage due to associated berry aneurysms, and congestive heart failure. Surgical results are excellent and the perioperative mortality rate is low if surgery is performed early in life.

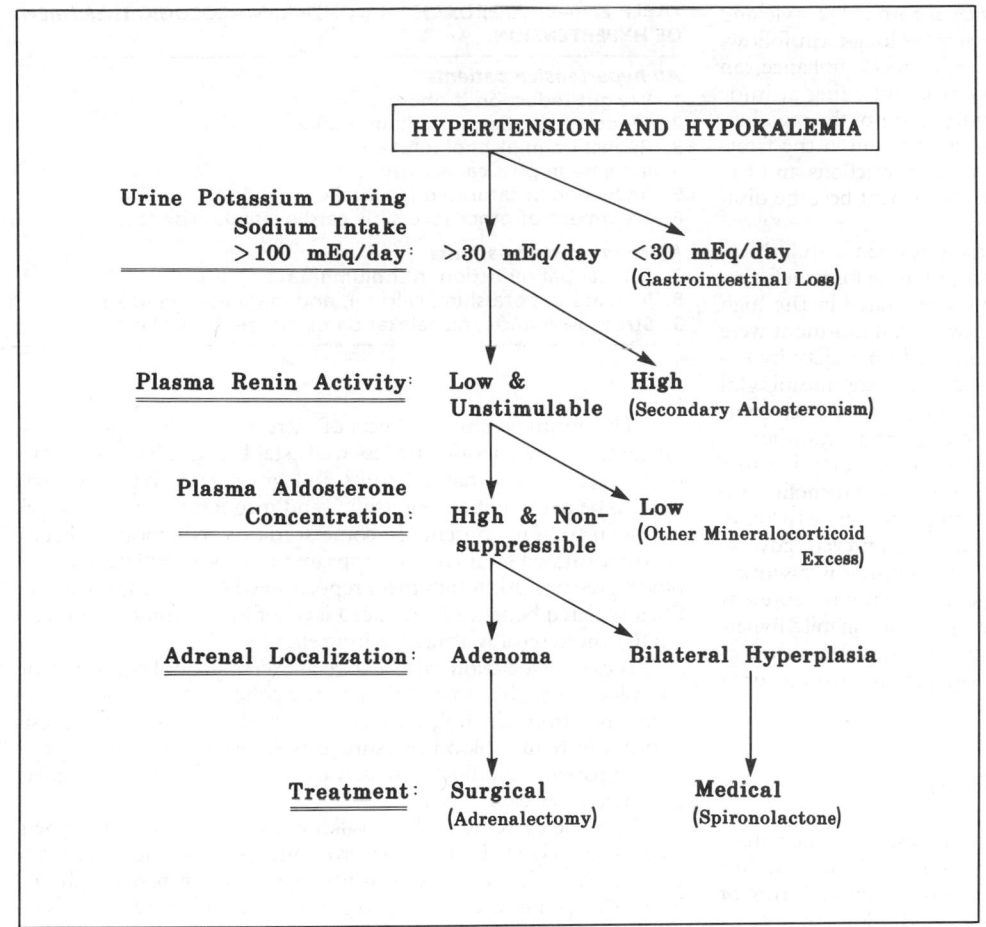

HYPERTENSION AND HYPOKALEMIA

Urine Potassium During
Sodium Intake
>100 mEq/day: >30 mEq/day   <30 mEq/day
(Gastrointestinal Loss)

Plasma Renin Activity: Low &   High
Unstimulable   (Secondary Aldosteronism)

Plasma Aldosterone
Concentration: High & Non-   Low
suppressible   (Other Mineralocorticoid
Excess)

Adrenal Localization: Adenoma   Bilateral Hyperplasia

Treatment: Surgical   Medical
(Adrenalectomy)   (Spironolactone)

Figure 2.10–4. Approach to evaluation of hypokalemia in hypertensive patients.

OTHER CAUSES OF SECONDARY HYPERTENSION

In many diseases, hypertension is an important if not a primary manifestation. Systolic hypertension is often noted in patients with thyrotoxicosis. In such patients, lid lag, hand tremor, tachycardia, and thyroid enlargement or nodularity should suggest the appropriate diagnosis. Blood pressure returns to its previous level once a euthyroid state is reached, and the patient rarely requires more specific therapy. Hypertension may occur in patients with tumors of the brain, infections of the brain stem, and lesions of the autonomic nervous system, such as spinal cord injury or acute porphyria. Although these disorders of the central nervous system frequently produce striking hypertension, the blood pressure usually reverts toward normal after the acute episode has subsided.

Hypertension is also a prominent feature of toxemia of pregnancy. Most patients with toxemia have mild hypertension, but some progress to the malignant phase, which may result in convulsions and permanent renal damage. In general, toxemia presents a greater threat to the fetus than to the mother. Levels of blood pressure that would not merit treatment under ordinary circumstances should be carefully evaluated if they develop during the first trimester of pregnancy.

APPROACH TO TREATMENT OF ESSENTIAL HYPERTENSION

GENERAL RECOMMENDATIONS

General guidelines for the treatment of patients with essential hypertension are provided in Table 2.10–7 and specific recommendations with respect to nonpharmacologic and pharmacologic ther-

apy in Tables 2.10–8 and 2.10–9, respectively. Treatment should be initiated only after a careful assessment of the patient's blood pressure, his cardiovascular risk status, and the presence or absence of other complicating factors that might influence the patient's response to a given treatment. In a chronic condition such as essential hypertension, it is important that the patient become an active partner in the treatment process. Patients should understand (1) the rationale for initiating treatment, (2) the usual inadequacy of symptoms as a reliable indicator of blood pressure control, (3) the

TABLE 2.10–7. GENERAL GUIDELINES FOR TREATMENT OF HIGH BLOOD PRESSURE

Hypertensive Category	Recommended Action[a]
Malignant	Immediate hospitalization and antihypertensive drug treatment
Moderate or severe (systolic BP ≥200 or diastolic BP ≥105 mm Hg)	If elevation confirmed at second visit, begin drug and nondrug treatment
Mild (systolic 160–199 or diastolic 90–104 mm Hg)	If elevation confirmed at three visits, attempt lowering of blood pressure by nondrug or nondrug and drug treatment. Antihypertensive drug therapy frequently required for those with highest pressures
Borderline high (systolic 140–159 or diastolic 85–89 mm Hg)	Provide follow-up. Consider nonpharmacologic treatment

[a]Treat other reversible cardiovascular risk factors in all patients.

compatibility of long-term treatment with a normal life-style and an excellent prognosis, and (4) the necessity for long-term follow-up and compliance with the treatment regimen. Compliance can be maximized by demonstrating a responsive and caring attitude on the part of the health care team, simplification of the regimen, and involvement of a family member or close friend in the treatment process. Unnecessary dietary and other restrictions and frequent office visits should be avoided lest the patient become disillusioned, noncompliant, or semi-invalid.

Risk information presents the treating physician with a therapeutic dilemma. Patients with the greatest potential for benefitting from antihypertensive drug therapy are concentrated in the high end of the blood pressure distribution. However, if treatment were confined to such patients, the burden imposed on society by hypertension could not be substantially reduced. Any meaningful attempt to decrease the brunt of blood pressure–related complications mandates treatment of the much larger number of asymptomatic individuals with mild hypertension. In this situation, one is treating many to save a few, and the risk/benefit ratio is more precarious than when one is treating patients with more severe hypertension. Special care to recognize and prevent adverse effects resulting from therapy for mild hypertension is essential. For obvious reasons, nonpharmacologic interventions represent the most appealing form of antihypertensive therapy in mild hypertension. Unfortunately, such recommendations are often either ignored or incompletely effective, and most patients require drug therapy to normalize their blood pressure.

NONPHARMACOLOGIC TREATMENT

In recent years there has been increasing interest in the nonpharmacologic approach to treatment of hypertension.[5,7] In part this reflects the fact that patients with progressively milder forms of hypertension are being considered as candidates for long-term therapy. Nondrug treatment is variously recommended as the initial therapeutic approach, as an adjunct to long-term drug therapy and as a means to gradually reduce the requirement for drugs once a satisfactory degree of blood pressure control and rapport with the patient have been established. In each setting, favorable reports have been published, but results from long-term, rigorously performed trials are scarce.

Table 2.10–8 identifies nine nonpharmacologic hypertension treatment approaches that have been ordered according to the presumed benefit of each intervention. The most substantial evidence in favor of an antihypertensive effect from nondrug therapy comes from trials of weight reduction in obese patients with hypertension. Many patients find it difficult to achieve and maintain their ideal body weight. This should not be a deterrent, however, because useful reductions in blood pressure can result even when the degree of calorie restriction and associated weight loss is limited. Less consistent results have been reported with modest restrictions in sodium intake. However, the normal intake of salt in Western countries is excessive, and at least some individuals appear to benefit from this advice. Thus a trial of moderate sodium restriction seems appropriate in most patients. Such advice is particularly sensible in patients receiving concurrent diuretic treatment, because reduced sodium intake will blunt the degree of diuretic-induced urinary potassium wasting. Patients and any other party responsible for the preparation of their food should be instructed to read the labels of all canned and packaged goods carefully, because sodium is commonly used to flavor or preserve processed foods. Provided the patient is prudent in his or her choice of food and avoids the use of table salt, sodium intake can be reduced from the usual level of 140 to 200 mEq/day to approximately 70 to 100 mEq/day. For more enthusiastic patients, sodium intake can be reduced even further and the probability of a reduction in blood pressure increased. This mandates very careful attention to dietary practices, however, and can be disruptive to home life.

TABLE 2.10–8. APPROACH TO NONPHARMACOLOGIC TREATMENT OF HYPERTENSION

All hypertensive patients
1. Weight reduction if obese
2. Modest reduction in sodium intake
3. Reduction in alcohol intake
4. Increase in physical activity
5. Reduction in saturated fat intake
6. Treatment of other reversible cardiovascular risk factors

More interested patients
7. Substantial reduction in sodium intake
8. Increase in potassium, calcium, and magnesium intake
9. Stress avoidance and relaxation or biofeedback therapy

The antihypertensive effects of increased levels of potassium, calcium, and magnesium are less well established. However, a diet that is generous in natural fruits and green leafy vegetables will tend to be high in fiber, potassium, and magnesium intake, as well as low in sodium content. In some studies a reduction in dietary polyunsaturated fat intake has appeared to result in lower levels of blood pressure. Although these reports need further confirmation, the associated benefit of a reduced level of low-density lipoprotein (LDL) cholesterol is attractive in itself.

A close association exists between excess alcohol consumption and blood pressure. In addition to the other potential benefits of abstinence from alcohol, an increasing body of evidence suggests that it will reduce blood pressure as well. At a minimum, hypertensive patients should be advised to consume less than 2 ounces of ethanol per day.

Isotonic exercises such as walking, jogging or swimming help to reduce weight, LDL cholesterol, and possibly blood pressure levels as well. For all these reasons, hypertensive patients should be encouraged to exercise on a regular basis, under the supervision of an appropriate professional.

A variety of relaxation and biofeedback therapies have been advocated for the treatment of hypertension. Although such approaches have rarely been evaluated in a rigorous fashion, they may be useful in treating selected patients with mild hypertension. As with all forms of nonpharmacologic treatment, the individual patient's response should be monitored carefully; when the response is inadequate, antihypertensive drug therapy should be considered as an alternative or concurrent form of treatment.

ANTIHYPERTENSIVE DRUG THERAPY

Value of Drug Treatment

Although useful, the knowledge that a given drug can lower blood pressure successfully is an inadequate basis for initiating such treatment. One must have more substantial evidence of a benefit from the therapy before recommending a lifelong course of treatment. Epidemiologic studies suggest that the recent widespread use of antihypertensive drugs in the community may be responsible for an impressive decrease in the frequency of malignant hypertension and an acceleration in the decline of the mortality from stroke.[13] Controlled clinical trials, however, provide the best evidence in favor of a beneficial role for antihypertensive drug therapy.

Because the outcome was almost uniformly unfavorable in untreated patients, it was relatively easy to demonstrate the value of drug therapy in malignant and nonmalignant but severe hypertension. Much larger and more rigorous trials were required to establish the value of antihypertensive drug treatment with milder forms of hypertension. During the past two decades, a variety of trials have been designed to test the hypothesis that antihypertensive drug treatment is beneficial in patients with mild to moderate hypertension. The results of nine such trials are presented in Figure 2.10–5. For each trial, the relative benefits of antihypertensive drug treatment and the confidence that can be ascribed to

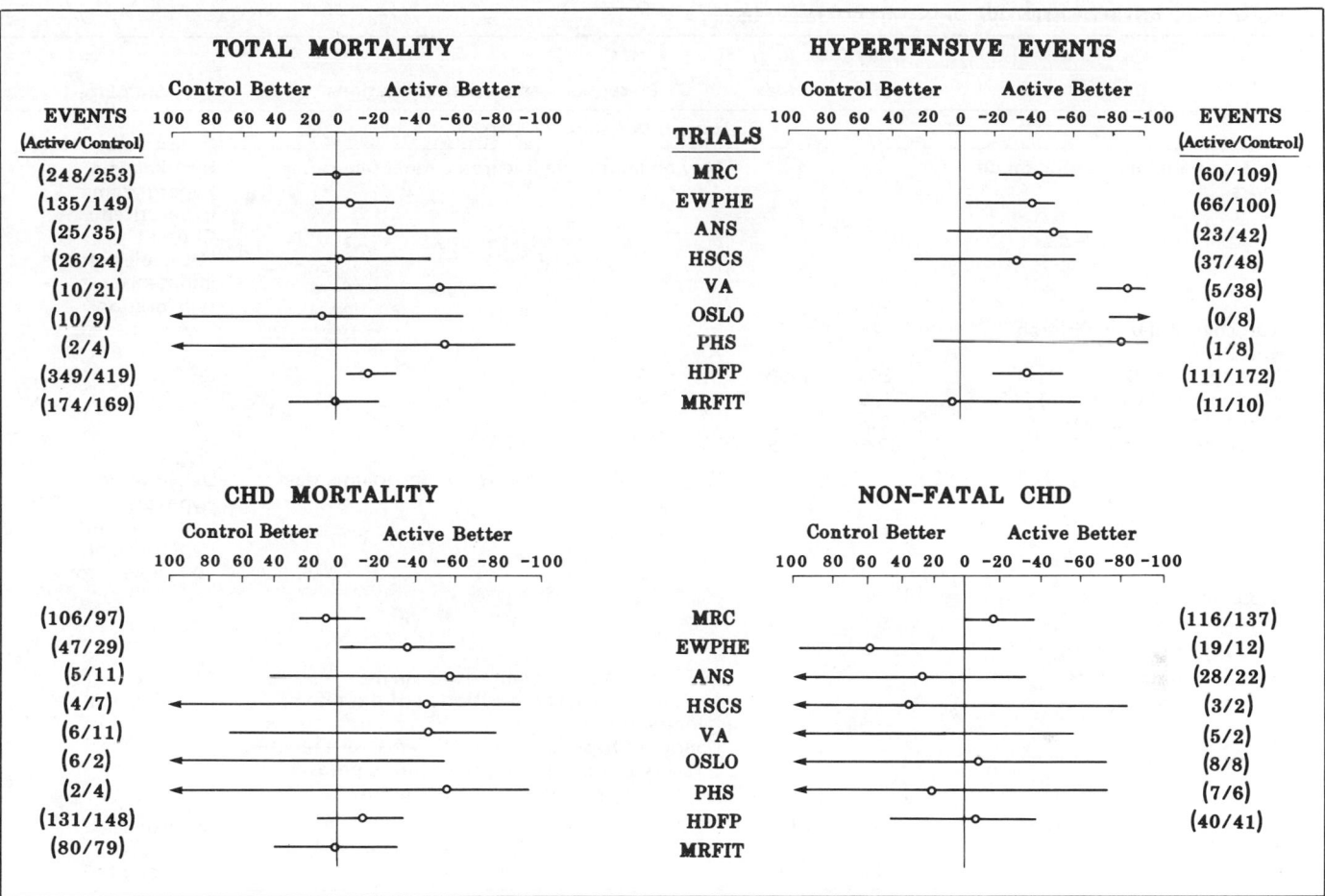

Figure 2.10-5. Value of antihypertensive drug therapy in mild to moderate essential hypertension. Point estimate and 95% confidence interval for relative difference (%) between active and control treatment in nine published trials (MRC = Medical Research Council Study; EWPHE = European Working Party on Hypertension in the Elderly Study; ANS = Australian National Study; HSCS = Hypertension Stroke Cooperative Study; VA = Veterans Administration Study; OSLO = Olso Study; PHS = Public Health Service Study; HDFP = Hypertension Detection and Follow-up Program; MRFIT = Multiple Risk Factor Intervention Trial).

these findings are displayed for the following four major outcomes: (1) total mortality rate, (2) hypertensive events (fatal and nonfatal strokes and congestive heart failure), (3) coronary artery disease mortality rate, and (4) nonfatal coronary artery disease. In addition, the number of events on which the results are based is identified. In eight of the nine trials, there was a substantial reduction in the relative frequency of hypertensive events among subjects in the active treatment group. In addition, the incidence of left ventricular hypertrophy and progression to more severe levels of hypertension was almost uniformly lower in those receiving active treatment. Most of the trials provided suggestive, albeit nonsignificant, evidence that drug treatment reduces mortality among persons with coronary artery disease. In one trial, the Hypertension Detection and Follow-up Program,[4] the reduction was both substantial (20 percent) and significant even in participants with mild hypertension. The latter group also experienced a 20.3 percent reduction in all-cause mortality.

In summary, the results of these nine trials leave little doubt that antihypertensive drug treatment of patients with mild to moderate hypertension results in an overall benefit. However, one must be careful in generalizing this group experience to the individual patient, and controversy remains as to whether every patient with mild hypertension should receive antihypertensive drug therapy if nonpharmacologic measures fail to provide adequate blood pressure control. The possibility that adverse effects during long-term drug therapy might counterbalance or outweigh the benefits of treatment are of greatest concern in the management of "low risk," mild hypertension in which average diastolic blood presure is between 90 and 94 mm Hg. This is especially the case in patients who have no end-organ damage and few, if any, associated cardiovascular risk factors. Some physicians prefer to withhold antihypertensive drug therapy in such patients. However, at a minimum they should be treated with a nonpharmacologic approach. Likewise, they should be followed up carefully, because in many the blood pressure will increase to levels at which the need for drug treatment is more clearly established.

Drug Categories

Table 2.10-9 groups antihypertensive drugs by the frequency of their use in treating patients with uncomplicated essential hypertension. Thus group I is composed of diuretics; group II, adrenergic inhibitors; group III, angiotensin-converting enzyme inhibitors; group IV, calcium-channel blockers; and group V, direct vasodilators.

TABLE 2.10–9. ANTIHYPERTENSIVE DRUGS IN COMMON USE

Drugs[a]	Daily Dose (mg)		Precautions and Contraindications	Side Effects
	Min	*Max*		
Group I: Diuretics				
Thiazides and related sulfonamide diuretics			May be ineffective in chronic renal failure	Hypokalemia Hyperglycemia Hyperuricemia GI upset LDL cholesterol Impotence Dehydration
Hydrochlorothiazide (Esidrix; HydroDIURIL)	25	100		
Chlorothiazide (Diuril)	250	1000		
Chlorthalidone (Hygroton)	25	50		
Metolazone (Zaroxolyn)	2.5	5		
Indapamide (Lozol)	2.5	5		
Loop diuretics			Excessive diuresis may precipitate volume depletion	Dehydration Hypokalemia Hyperglycemia Hyperuricemia LDL cholesterol
Furosemide (Lasix)	40	480		
Bumetanide (Bumex)	0.5	10		
Ethacrynic acid (Edecrin)	25	200		
Potassium-sparing agents			Ineffective as antihypertensive agents Must be used in combination with thiazide or loop diuretics Danger of hyperkalemia in patients with renal failure or receiving supplementary potassium or other drugs that spare potassium	GI upset Hyperkalemia
Spironolactone (Aldactone)	25	100		Gynecomastia
Amiloride (Midamor)	5	10		
Triamterene (Dyrenium)	50	100		Renal stones
Group II: Adrenergic Inhibitors				
Beta-adrenergic inhibitors			Contraindicated in sick sinus syndrome, heart block, asthma, chronic obstructive pulmonary disease, and congestive heart failure Use with caution in patients with diabetes mellitus or peripheral vascular disease	GI upset Bradycardia Fatigue Insomnia Vivid dreams Impotence Bronchospasm Cold extremities Heart block ↓ HDL cholesterol Hypertriglyceridemia
Nonselective beta blockers				
Propranolol (Inderal)	40	480		
Nadolol (Corgard)	40	320		
Timolol (Blocadren)	20	60		
Relatively cardioselective beta blockers				Extracardiac side effects less common at low doses
Atenolol (Tenormin)	50	200		
Metoprolol (Lopressor)	100	400		
Beta blockers with intrinsic sympathomimetic activity				Side effects may be less common than with nonselective beta blockers
Pindolol (Visken)	10	60		
Acebutolol (Sectral)	400	1200		
Combined alpha and beta blockers				
Labetalol (Normodyne; Trandate)	200	1200		Nausea Dizziness Headache
Centrally acting adrenergic inhibitors				
Clonidine (Catapres)	0.2	2.4	Rebound hypertension may occur with abrupt discontinuation of clonidine or guanabenz	
Guanabenz (Wytensin)	8	32		
Methyldopa (Aldomet)	250	2000		Hepatitis Hemolytic anemia
Alpha-1 adrenergic blockers				
Prazosin (Minipress)	1	40	Orthostatic hypotension, especially in elderly patients or insulin-dependent diabetics	First dose "syncope" Dizziness Palpitations Headaches
Terazosin (Hytrin)	1	20		

(continued)

TABLE 2.10–9. ANTIHYPERTENSIVE DRUGS IN COMMON USE (Continued)

Drugs[a]	Daily Dose (mg)		Precautions and Contraindications	Side Effects
	Min	Max		
Group II: Adrenergic Inhibitors (Cont.)				
Peripheral-acting adrenergic inhibitors				
Reserpine (Serpasil)	0.1	0.25	Depression, peptic ulcer, ulcerative colitis	Nasal congestion Depression Increased appetite Weight gain
Guanethidine (Ismelin)	10	300	Pheochromocytoma, nonhypertensive congestive heart failure Use of monoamine oxidase inhibitors	Postural and exercise hypotension Diarrhea Impotence Retrograde ejaculation
Group III: Angiotensin-Converting Enzyme Inhibitors				
Captopril (Capoten)	25	150		Rash Dysgeusia Hyperkalemia Reversible acute renal failure in patients with bilateral renal artery stenosis Neutropenia, especially in patients with renal or collagen vascular disease Proteinuria (rare at recommended doses)
Enalapril (Vasotec)	5.0	40		Headache Dizziness Fatigue
Group IV: Calcium Channel Blockers				
Nifedipine (Procardia)	30	180		Dizziness, headaches, hypotension
Verapamil (Calan, Isoptin)	240	480	Use with caution in patients with congestive heart failure or heart block	Edema, flushing, constipation
Diltiazem (Cardizem)	120	360		Nausea
Group V: Direct Vasodilators				
			May precipitate angina in patients with coronary heart disease	Tachycardia, fluid retention
Hydralazine (Apresoline)	50	300	Hypersensitivity	Headaches and myalgia Lupus erythematosus-like syndrome (rare at recommended doses)
Minoxidil (Loniten)	5.0	100		Hypertrichosis Pericarditis (rare)

[a]Generic name is given in parentheses.

Hemodynamic Effects

Diuretics facilitate sodium excretion by the kidney, which initially reduces plasma volume and cardiac output. With continued use, cardiac output returns toward normal but peripheral resistance falls, and this is the major factor responsible for their long-term antihypertensive effects. Some adrenergic inhibitors, such as the beta blockers, appear to lower blood pressure by effecting a reduction in cardiac output. Others, such as methyldopa, clonidine, prazosin, and reserpine, work primarily by decreasing peripheral vascular resistance. Direct vasodilators, such as hydralazine and minoxidil, have an even more potent effect on peripheral vascular resistance. However, fluid retention and an increase in plasma volume are common occurrences during the administration of these agents. Such fluid retention limits the antihypertensive efficacy of direct vasodilators and to a lesser extent adrenergic inhibitors when they are used as first-step therapy. The predominant hemodynamic effect of angiotensin-converting enzyme inhibitors such as captopril and enalapril is to lower peripheral vascular resistance by decreasing angiotensin II production and bradykinin degradation. They can also induce diuresis and thus reduce plasma volume, however, by inhibiting the production of aldosterone. Calcium-channel blockers such as nifedipine, diltiazem, and verapamil have similar hemodynamic effects, although their site of action differs. The adrenergic inhibitor guanethidine is unique in that it lowers both cardiac output and peripheral vascular resistance.

Specific Drug Regimens

Many schemes for antihypertensive drug therapy have been proposed over the past 20 years, but none is perfect. Obviously, therapy should be tailored to meet the needs of the individual patient.

The choice of drugs should be influenced not only by the severity of a patient's hypertension and the presence or absence of end-organ damage but also by such widely diverse factors as the patient's financial resources and the familiarity of the physician with the drug and its side effects.

Currently, most authorities recommend a stepped-care approach to drug administration.[5] Although diuretics and beta blockers are frequently recommended as the first-step drugs of choice,[5] angiotensin-converting enzyme inhibitors, calcium-channel blockers, or other adrenergic inhibitors provide an alternative option (step 1: group I, II, III, or IV agent). Diuretics and calcium-channel blockers appear to be most effective in older and black patients, whereas beta blockers and converting enzyme inhibitors are generally more effective in younger and white patients. Substitution of an alternative drug from group I, II, III, or IV or combination therapy with a diuretic and a group II, III, or IV agent (step 2: group I plus group II, III, or IV agent) should be considered for patients in whom initial monotherapy produces an inadequate blood pressure response. If step 2 combination therapy proves ineffective, triple therapy with a diuretic, adrenergic inhibitor, and direct or indirect vasodilator (step 3: group I and group II agents plus group III, IV, or V agent) is appropriate. Provided there are no contraindications, beta blockers are the adrenergic inhibitors of choice in such combinations. If a patient continues to have hypertension on this triple-therapy regimen, careful consideration should be given to the possibility of dietary or drug noncompliance or the presence of an underlying correctable cause for the hypertension. If these possibilities can be excluded, various combinations of drugs from groups II, III, and IV should be added to a group I loop diuretic and the more potent group V vasodilator minoxidil (step 4).

Follow-up and Goals

Generally, antihypertensive drug therapy can be started on an outpatient basis. The primary goal of treatment is to achieve and maintain a systolic blood pressure <160 mm Hg and a diastolic blood pressure <90 mm Hg with minimal side effects. Initially, patients should be seen at 2- to 4-week intervals, but once their blood pressure is well controlled, they usually need to return no more often than every 3 to 6 months. Between office visits, blood pressure control may be monitored by means of blood pressure recordings in the home or workplace. Complicated regimens should be avoided, and combinations of drugs with different sites of action are preferred to combinations of several drugs with similar sites of action.

Individual Drugs

Diuretics are the most frequently used antihypertensive drugs.[2] They are effective as sole agents in the treatment of mild hypertension and in this setting will decrease systolic blood pressure by approximately 10 to 20 mm Hg and diastolic blood pressure by 5 to 10 mm Hg. Diuretics are especially effective in the treatment of black and elderly patients. In more severe hypertension, diuretics potentiate and complement the actions of adrenergic inhibitors, angiotensin-coverting enzyme inhibitors, calcium-channel blocking agents, and vasodilators. Of the many diuretics available, thiazide and thiazide-like agents are the most frequently used to treat hypertensive patients. Chlorothiazide and hydrochlorothiazide are often administered twice daily, whereas longer-acting thiazide-like agents such as chlorthalidone and metolazone are given once daily. Furosemide is the preferred diuretic in patients with renal insufficiency and in regimens that include the potent vasodilator minoxidil. All thiazide and thiazide-like agents may induce hypokalemia, hyperglycemia, hyperuricemia, and hyperlipidemia. The physician should measure serum potassium, glucose, LDL and high-density lipoprotein (HDL) cholesterol, triglyceride, and uric acid levels before initiating therapy and should monitor them periodically thereafter. Serum potassium levels should be checked at 6- to 12-month intervals. Hypokalemia should be prevented in all patients receiving digitalis or steroid therapy and treated in those who become symptomatic, have underlying coronary artery disease, or have an average serum potassium level <3.0 mEq/L.

The necessity for treating apparently healthy asymptomatic patients with an average serum potassium level between 3.0 and 3.5 mEq/L is controversial.[16,17] Treatment can be accomplished in one of three ways. Restricting dietary salt intake may decrease renal potassium wasting and often corrects milder forms of hypokalemia. Supplemental potassium may be provided by dietary changes or in the form of potassium chloride tablets or elixirs. Of these, the latter is best, since dietary changes are often unreliable and potassium chloride tablets occasionally lead to small-bowel ulceration or obstruction. In many patients the addition of a potassium-sparing agent, such as amiloride or triamterene, is the most acceptable and effective form of therapy. Hyperkalemia, the most dangerous side effect of such treatment, is principally noted in patients with renal insufficiency or those in whom the agent is used in conjunction with potassium supplementation, converting enzyme inhibitor therapy, or a nonsteroidal anti-inflammatory agent.

Beta blockers, the combined alpha- and beta-adrenergic blocker labetalol and methyldopa, clonidine, guanabenz, prazosin, reserpine, and guanethidine are all effective adrenergic inhibitors. Beta blockers should be avoided in patients with a history of bronchospasm, asthma, or congestive heart failure, and they should be used cautiously in those with cardiac conduction defects, diabetes mellitus, or peripheral vascular disease. In most other patients they are well tolerated and are particularly valuable in the treatment of patients with hyperdynamic circulatory states, renin-angiotensin–dependent hypertension, coronary insufficiency, arrhythmias, or a high risk of acute myocardial infarction. Methyldopa, clonidine, guanabenz, and reserpine have similarities, in both their mode of action and their side effects. All four appear to act primarily on the central nervous system, even though each has additional effects on the peripheral autonomic system. Potential side effects during methyldopa, clonidine, and guanabenz therapy include sedation, dry mouth, and dizziness, whereas nasal congestion, lethargy, and increased appetite are more common with reserpine. Each of the four may, on occasion, induce more serious adverse effects, such as hepatitis and hemolytic anemia with methyldopa; depression and aggravation of peptic ulcer disease with reserpine; and rebound hypertension after abrupt withdrawal of clonidine or guanabenz. In addition to a standard oral tablet, clonidine is available as a 7-day patch preparation. The patch is particularly useful in noncompliant patients and for treatment during the perioperative period. Prazosin and terazosine differ from all other adrenergic inhibitors in that they appear to work primarily as alpha-1 receptor blockers. In addition to lowering blood pressure, they may increase HDL cholesterol and lower LDL cholesterol. The most important side effect that can be encountered during prazosin treatment is that of hypotension after initiation of therapy (first-dose phenomenon). This is uncommon if therapy is initiated at a dose of 1 mg twice daily and the patient is instructed to take the first capsule at bedtime while supine. Patients should, however, be warned of the possibility of initial dizziness, and the drug is best avoided in elderly arteriosclerotic patients with impaired autonomic responses. Guanethidine is a long-acting and very potent peripherally active adrenergic inhibitor. However, because of its side effects, which include postural and exertional hypotension, retrograde ejaculation, impotence, and diarrhea, guanethidine is usually reserved for use in patients with exceptionally resistant hypertension. Guanethidine should be administered with extreme caution in patients who have coronary, cerebral, or renal insufficiency.

Converting enzyme inhibitors, such as enalapril and captopril, are particularly useful in patients with unilateral renovascular hypertension or high renin essential hypertension. They are, however, well tolerated and often effective in patients with other forms of essential hypertension as well. Captopril-induced side effects include skin rashes, dysgeusia, and, more rarely, proteinuria or leukopenia. Either agent can precipitate hyperkalemia in patients with renal insufficiency or a poorly functioning renin-angiotensin-aldosterone axis. Likewise, either can induce or worsen renal failure in patients with bilateral renovascular disease. However, preliminary data suggest that converting enzyme inhibition may slow the progression of renal disease in certain patients with renal insufficiency.[3]

Calcium-channel blocking drugs such as nifedipine, diltiazem, and verapamil are effective in lowering blood pressure when given alone or in combination with a diuretic. As with beta blockers, these agents are especially valuable in the treatment of patients with hypertension and angina. They also appear to work well in elderly and black patients. Verapamil is the drug of choice for hypertensive patients with supraventricular tachyarrhythmias. However, calcium-channel blockers should be used with caution in patients with congestive heart failure or heart block. Major side effects include flushing, headaches, dizziness, constipation, and edema.

Since increased peripheral vascular resistance appears to be the primary physiologic defect in most patients with established essential hypertension, the use of direct vasodilators has for many years generated a great deal of interest. Hydralazine and minoxidil are the only direct vasodilators approved for oral use in the United States. Both are effective vasodilators, but sodium retention and reflex tachycardia usually complicate their use. This complication mandates the concomitant use of a diuretic and an adrenergic inhibitor such as a beta blocker. Hydralazine may induce a peripheral neuropathy and a reversible lupus erythematosus–like syndrome, especially when it is used in doses greater than 300 to 400 mg per day. For this reason, antinuclear antibody titers should be monitored every 6 months.

Minoxidil is more potent than hydralazine. Its use is, however, uniformly associated with the occurrence of resting tachycardia, an increase in cardiac output, weight gain, and edema. In addition, hypertrichosis is common and pericardial effusion has been reported in some patients. Minoxidil should be considered as a substitute for hydralazine when full-dose conventional triple therapy has failed in a compliant patient. When minoxidil is given in combination with a beta blocker and a loop diuretic, normalization of blood pressure is usually possible even in patients with the most resistant forms of hypertension.

HYPERTENSIVE URGENCIES AND EMERGENCIES

Moderate or severe elevations of blood pressure sometimes place a person at imminent risk of a hypertensive complication unless the blood pressure is promptly lowered. The rapidity with which blood pressure should be lowered depends not only on the patient's blood pressure level but also on the presence or absence of other findings that influence the likelihood of an acute hypertensive complication. Situations in which blood pressure must be lowered within 1 hour are often termed "hypertensive emergencies."

Most patients with a hypertensive emergency have symptoms and signs of central nervous system or cardiovascular disease, including alteration in mental status, papilledema, focal neurologic deficits, angina pectoris, dyspnea, rales, and acute changes on the ECG. Classic examples of hypertensive emergencies include (1) hypertensive encephalopathy, (2) hypertension-induced angina pectoris, intracranial hemorrhage, acute left ventricular failure with pulmonary edema, type B aortic dissection (see Chapter 2.11), and (3) severe hypertension associated with acute myocardial infarction, toxemia of pregnancy, or extensive burns or head trauma.

TABLE 2.10–10. COMMON DRUG REGIMENS FOR TREATMENT OF HYPERTENSIVE URGENCIES AND EMERGENCIES

Drug Name[a]	Route of Administration	Usual Dose	Usual Time of Onset	Side Effects
Sodium nitroprusside (Nipride)	Intravenous	Titrated infusion of 50–100 mg/L Dextrose in water solution (0.005–0.01 mg/kg/min)	Immediate	Hypotension GI upset Tachycardia Sweating Edema Rash Thiocyanate toxic effects Methemoglobinemia
Phentolamine[b] (Regitine)	Intravenous	5–10 mg (rapid injection)	Immediate	Hypotension Tachycardia Flushing
Diazoxide (Hyperstat)	Intravenous	50–100 mg minibolus every 5–15 min	3–5 min	Hypotension GI upset Local pain Tachycardia Sweating Angina ↑ Uric acid ↑ Blood sugar
Nitroglycerin (Tridil)	Intravenous	5–10 μg/min	2–5 min	Hypotension Bradycardia Tachycardia GI upset Flushing Methemoglobinemia
Labetalol (Normodyne; Trandate)	Intravenous	20–30 mg every 10–15 min (maximum 300 mg)	5–10 min	Hypotension GI upset Local pain Scalp tingling Burning sensation in throat and groin
Nifedipine (Procardia; Adelat)	Oral or sublingual	10 mg every 15–30 min (maximum 60 mg)	5–20 min	Hypotension GI upset Tachycardia Headache
Clonidine (Catapres)	Oral	0.1 mg every hr (maximum 0.5–1.0 mg)	1–3 hr	Hypotension Sedation Dry mouth

[a]Proprietary names are given in parentheses.
[b]Indicated only for patients with pheochromocytoma crisis.

Situations that are less dramatic but nevertheless mandate control of blood pressure within a 24-hour period are commonly referred to as "hypertensive urgencies." These include accelerated or malignant hypertension in a patient without evidence of an impending complication and moderate or severe hypertension in the perioperative period or in patients requiring emergency surgery. It is not always possible to make a clear distinction between hypertensive urgency and hypertensive emergency.

A variety of drug regimens have been proposed for the treatment of patients with a hypertensive urgency or emergency. Elements of the most frequently used regimens are presented in Table 2.10-10. Perhaps the most reliable and predictable approach is to use one of the intravenously administered direct vasodilators: sodium nitroprusside or diazoxide.

Sodium nitroprusside lowers blood pressure within seconds, and its effect can be reversed within an equally short period of time. Constant, careful blood pressure monitoring is essential during the administration of this agent. Effective in every form of hypertension, it is the drug of choice for patients with hypertension-related acute pulmonary edema, coronary insufficiency, and aortic dissection. Sodium nitroprusside dilates venous as well as arterial smooth muscle and often decreases cardiac output, even though reflex tachycardia is a uniform occurrence. Sodium nitroprusside is partly metabolized to sodium thiocyanate, but this does not usually constitute a problem unless the drug is administered in high dosage or for a prolonged period to a patient with renal insufficiency.

Although less potent than sodium nitroprusside, diazoxide usually begins to lower blood pressure within minutes of administration, and its effects last for a minimum of 4 to 6 hours. Diazoxide should be administered rapidly in 50 to 100 mg doses every 5 to 15 min until the desired fall in blood pressure is achieved. Afterward, blood pressure should be checked every 15 to 30 min and additional 50 to 100 mg doses given when necessary.

Phentolamine is the drug of choice in pheochromocytoma crisis, but sodium nitroprusside is also effective. Alternative means of rapidly lowering blood pressure include intravenous administration of labetalol or nitroglycerin, oral or sublingual nifedipine administration, and rapid oral clonidine loading. Whichever method is chosen, blood pressure must be monitored carefully and the dangers of an overly aggressive approach to blood pressure reduction must be balanced against the risks of the high blood pressure itself. Likewise, once initial control of blood pressure has been established, patients should be rapidly switched to an oral antihypertensive drug regimen.

REFERENCES

1. Build and Blood Pressure Study. Chicago, Society of Actuaries, 1959
2. Cloher TP, Whelton PK: Physician approach to the recognition and initial management of hypertension: Results of a statewide survey of Maryland physicians. Arch Intern Med 146:529, 1986
3. Hollenberg NK: Advances in therapeutics: Converting enzyme inhibition and the kidney. Am J Med 79(Suppl 3C):1, 1985
4. Hypertension Detection and Follow-up Program Cooperative Group: Five year findings of the Hypertension Detection and Follow-up Program. JAMA 242:2562, 1979
5. The Joint National Committee on Detection, Evaluation, and Treatment of High Blood Pressure: Their 1984 Report. Arch Intern Med 144:1045, 1984
6. Kannel WB: Role of blood pressure in cardiovascular morbidity and mortality. Prog Cardiovasc Dis 17:5, 1974
7. Kaplan NM: Non-drug treatment of hypertension. Ann Intern Med 102:359, 1985
8. Kirkendall WM, Feinleib M, et al: Recommendations for human blood pressure determination by sphygmomanometers. Subcommittee of American Heart Association Postgraduate Education Committee. Circulation 62:1146A, 1980
9. Manger WM, Gifford RW: Pheochromocytoma. New York, Springer-Verlag, 1977
10. Roberts J, Maurer K: Blood pressure levels of persons 6–74 years: United States 1971–1974. Series 11, No. 203. Washington, DC, National Center for Health Statistics, 1982
11. Russell RP, Whelton PK: Hypertension in chronic renal failure: Clinical presentation, prognosis, pathophysiology and treatment. Am J Nephrol 3:185, 1983
12. Vaughn ED, Buhler FR, et al: Renovascular hypertension: Renin measurements to indicate renal plasma flow and sore for surgical curability. Am J Med 55:402, 1973
13. Whelton PK: Declining mortality from hypertension and stroke. South Med J 75:33, 1982
14. Whelton PK: Essential hypertension: Therapeutic implications of epidemiologic risk estimation. Hypertens 2(Suppl 2):3, 1984
15. Whelton PK, Harrington DP, et al: Renal vein renin activity: A prospective study of sampling techniques and methods of interpretation. Johns Hopkins Med J 141:112, 1977
16. Whelton PK, Watson AJ: Diuretic-induced hypokalemia and cardiac arrhythmias. Am J Cardiol 58:5A, 1986
17. Whelton PK, Whelton A, Walker WG (eds): Potassium in Cardiovascular and Renal Medicine. New York, Marcel Dekker, 1986

CHAPTER 2.11
Diseases of the Aorta

A. Michael Borkon and Vincent L. Gott

The term "aneurysm" is derived from the Greek *aneurysma,* meaning a widening. An aneurysm refers to any dilated blood-containing sac involving an artery, a vein, or the heart. Aortic aneurysms most commonly arise as a consequence of arteriosclerosis, aging, or hypertension. True aneurysms of the aorta may be fusiform or saccular. The fusiform variety, which involves the entire circumference of the aorta, is the most common form of arteriosclerotic aortic aneurysm. Saccular aneurysms involve only a portion of the aortic wall and appear as an outpouching from the lateral wall of the blood vessel. Saccular aneurysms, although rare now, were once usually due to syphilis.[4] Unlike true aneurysms, which involve all or a portion of the vessel wall layers, a false aneurysm is confined by only a fibrous capsule, usually the result of arterial trauma or a contained rupture of a true aneurysm. Bacterial or fungal infections may result in mycotic aneurysms. Aneurysms may rupture, compress adjacent structures, form arteriovenous fistulas, produce distal embolization, or become infected.[8]

THORACIC ARTERIOSCLEROTIC ANEURYSMS

The most common cause of thoracic aortic aneurysms is arteriosclerosis. The most prevalent locations for arteriosclerotic aneurysm formation are, in decreasing order, the infrarenal abdominal aorta, descending thoracic aorta, popliteal artery, ascending aorta,

and aortic arch. Most arteriosclerotic aneurysms occurring in the descending aorta are fusiform and are seen in patients over 60 years of age. Men are affected more than women, and often there is a history of hypertension. Aneurysms may be found concomitantly in multiple sites, and evidence of occlusive arteriosclerotic vascular disease may be present as well. Arteriosclerotic aneurysms of the ascending aorta begin above the aortic root and are usually limited to the ascending aorta. Occasionally the aortic arch may be involved. Aneurysms involving the descending aorta begin at the base of the left subclavian artery and taper down at the level of the diaphragm. The arteriosclerotic aneurysmal process may extend to involve the suprarenal abdominal aorta.

SIGNS AND SYMPTOMS

Many thoracic arteriosclerotic aortic aneurysms are asymptomatic, being recognized on routine chest radiograph as a mediastinal mass (Fig. 2.11–1A). Thus an aortic aneurysm should be considered in the differential diagnosis of any asymptomatic mediastinal mass. Ascending aortic aneurysms usually display signs, whereas those of the arch frequently are associated with symptoms, most commonly acute or chronic chest pain. Chronic chest pain, arising from erosion or compression of adjacent structures, may radiate into the neck, shoulder, or back. Acute pain is usually a sign of sudden expansion, rupture, or dissection. Respiratory symptoms, shortness of breath, dyspnea on exertion, hemoptysis, and cough may be due to compression of the left main-stem bronchus or the trachea. Compression of the left recurrent laryngeal nerve may produce hoarseness, and esophageal compression can result in dysphagia. Aortic regurgitation is unusual in ascending arteriosclerotic aortic aneurysms but common with annuloaortic ectasia or dissec-

tions. In such cases, a diastolic murmur and peripheral signs of aortic regurgitation can often be elicited. Thrombus formation develops along the inner wall of the aneurysm, and distal emboli may produce a cerebrovascular accident; an acute abdomen due to emboli of the celiac, mesenteric, or renal vessels; or limb or digit ischemia. The signs and symptoms of a thoracic aortic aneurysm depend on its size and location.

EVALUATION

Evaluation of the patient with a thoracic aneurysm begins with a comprehensive history and physical examination. Evidence of an aneurysm may not be apparent, but other manifestations of arteriosclerosis may be found, including carotid and femoral bruits, an abdominal aortic aneurysm, or hypertension. Concomitant aneurysms of the abdominal aorta and the femoral and popliteal arteries are common. A murmur of aortic regurgitation is unusual. The posteroanterior chest radiograph will frequently demonstrate the presence of a mediastinal mass suggestive of an aneurysm. Further investigation should include a CT scan of the chest (Fig. 2.11–1B), which may facilitate diagnosis as well as demonstrate the aneurysm's location and size. If an operation is indicated, an arteriogram may further delineate the anatomic relationships of the aneurysm. Progressive layering of thrombus occurs within the dilated aorta, resulting in a channel of blood flow that tends to maintain a relatively normal dimension. Since an arteriogram shows only intraluminal dimensions, however, aneurysm size may be underestimated. The CT scan will demonstrate the true diameter of the aneurysm and can be used to detect changes in size. The recent development of MRI may supplant the use of CT and arteriography in evaluation of aortic aneurysms.

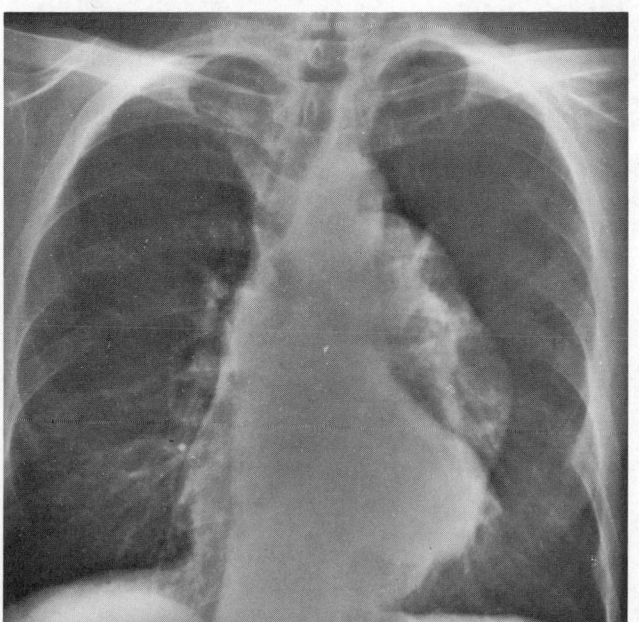
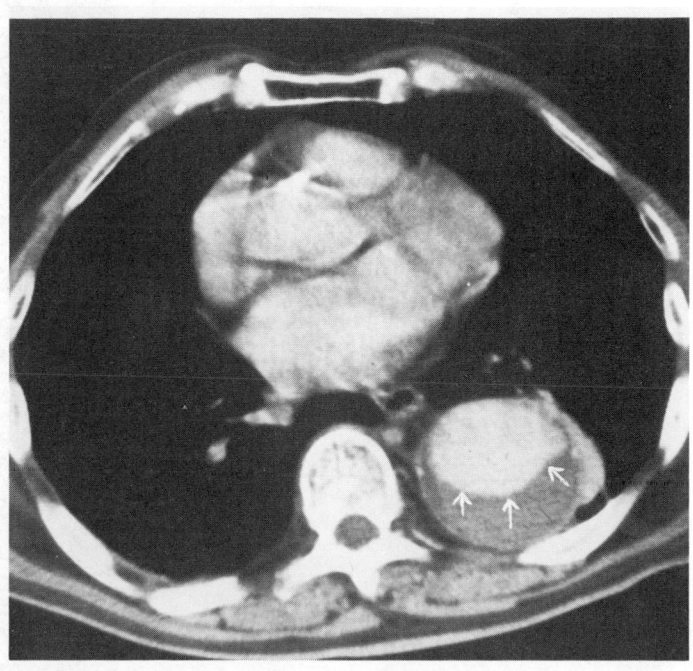

A

B

Figure 2.11–1. A. Chronic arteriosclerotic descending thoracic aortic aneurysm presenting as asymptomatic posterior mediastinal mass. **B.** Chest CT scan of same patient, showing aneurysm. Note small lumen (arrows), enhanced by contrast medium, and adjacent thrombus.

MANAGEMENT

Management of patients with these aneurysms depends on the size and location of the aneurysm, the clinical setting, and the relative risk of rupture versus operative repair. Because frequent complications after aneurysm repair include myocardial infarction, stroke, and respiratory and renal failure, preoperative assessment of these systems will enable one to predict operative risk. The greatest risk posed by an aneurysm is rupture, and a direct relationship exists between aneurysm size and the risk of rupture. Patients with aneurysms greater than 6 cm who have a low operative risk should be considered for elective repair. For other patients, CT scans should be obtained at 6- or 12-month intervals to assess aneurysm growth. These patients include asymptomatic patients with stable aneurysms less than 6 cm in diameter and high-risk patients with large thoracic aneurysms. Since thoracic aortic aneurysms frequently expand without symptoms, once- or twice-yearly monitoring by CT or MRI scan is important. If the aneurysm increases in size, the patient should be referred for operation. Symptoms of pain or compression of adjacent structures should also prompt urgent consideration of operative intervention.

Syphilitic aneurysms are more prone to rupture than arteriosclerotic aneurysms. Aneurysms of the descending thoracic aortic may expand or rupture rapidly, producing acute chest and back pain. Exclusion of myocardial infarction and pulmonary embolus is important; however, unnecessarily delayed treatment of an acute expanded aneurysm will ultimately lead to death from rupture and exsanguination. Ascending aortic aneurysms may have a similar presentation, and because of their intrapericardial location, they may have features of cardiac tamponade.

Aneurysms are repaired by replacing the dilated segment of aorta with a Dacron graft. Partial circulatory support of the lower extremity and visceral vessels is frequently used for repair of descending thoracic aneurysm. Full cardiopulmonary bypass, occasionally with deep hypothermia and circulatory arrest, is required for repair of ascending and arch aortic aneurysms. A ruptured thoracic aortic aneurysm carries an exceedingly high mortality rate, whereas elective repair in a low-risk patient can be carried out safely with a less than 10 percent chance of death.

THORACIC AORTIC DISSECTION[1,5,9]

The term "dissecting thoracic aortic aneurysm" is a misnomer and should be discarded in favor of "thoracic aortic dissection." An aortic dissection is characterized by an intimal tear that allows blood to be propelled by the force of systemic blood pressure through the aortic media in a course parallel to that of the blood flow. A transverse intimal tear can be identified in the majority of dissections. It arises in the ascending aorta in about 70 percent of patients. The tear will be found in the aortic arch in about 10 percent of patients, in the proximal descending thoracic aorta in about 20 percent, and infrequently in the abdominal aorta. The dissection process usually does not involve the entire circumference of the aorta but, rather, spirals along the greater curvature of the aorta (Fig. 2.11–2). Because the dissection occurs in the outer half of the medial layer of the aorta, the outer covering of the false channel is exceedingly thin and prone to rupture. Occasionally, the false channel will reenter into the true lumen in a distal location. Most aortic dissections occur in patients between 40 and 60 years of age; men are afflicted three times as commonly as women. Hypertension, trauma, and cystic medial necrosis may be contributing factors. Occasionally, an ulcerative plaque may be the site of intimal disruption, but frequently no underlying abnormality of the aorta can be identified. Figure 2.11–3 illustrates the classification of aortic dissection. The traditional DeBakey classes I and II[2] now signify simply ascending, or type A, aneurysms, whereas DeBakey class III refers to descending, or type B, aneurysms.[6] Acute life-threatening complications of aortic dissection are rupture with exsanguination, development of cardiac tamponade, and aortic

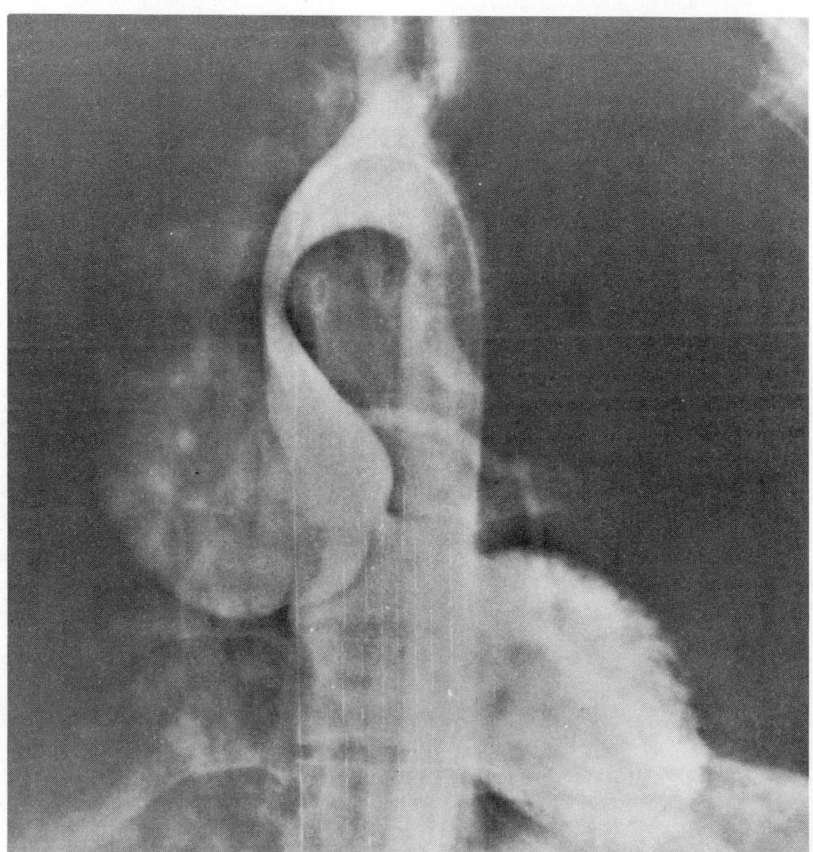

Figure 2.11–2. Aortogram of ascending aortic (type A) dissection, revealing spiraling of dissection plane into false lumen around greater curvature of ascending aorta and arch. In addition, aortic regurgitation is present, filling left ventricle with contrast medium.

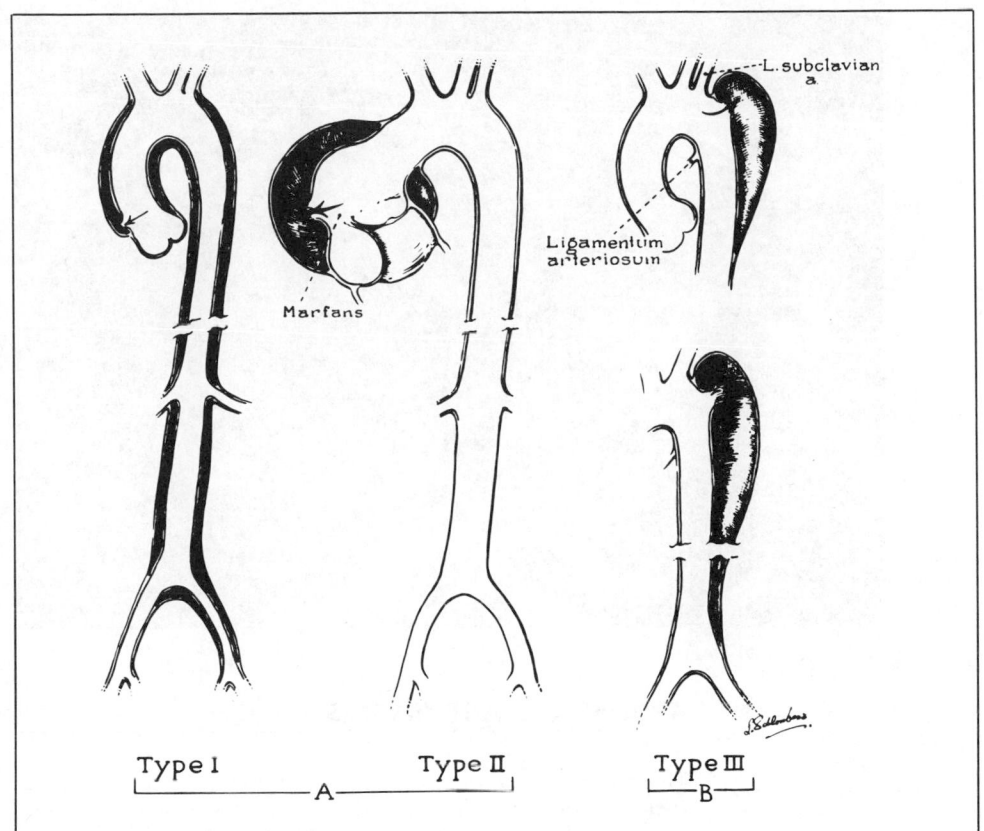

Figure 2.11–3. Classification of aortic dissection. DeBakey types I and II are equivalent to type A, or ascending aortic dissection; type III and type B are synonymous for dissections beginning distal to left subclavian artery in descending thoracic aorta.

regurgitation due to loss of suspension of aortic valve leaflets. Myocardial infarction may result from occlusion of the right coronary artery, which is frequently compressed during the dissection process. Late consequences of aortic dissection are chronic aneurysm formation, aortic regurgitation, and visceral or limb vessel ischemia.

SIGNS AND SYMPTOMS[10]

The most common presentation of an acute aortic dissection is severe chest pain, either substernal or interscapular, that is crushing or tearing and often radiates from front to back. Syncope and hypotension may accompany the onset of pain. Major arterial vessels can be occluded in the process of dissection, resulting in cerebral, spinal cord, limb, or visceral vessel ischemia. The presentation of an acute aortic dissection must be differentiated from that of myocardial infarction, pulmonary embolus, acute abdomen, and acute visceral or limb ischemia.

Physical examination often reveals a clammy, pale, acutely ill patient. Although most patients with aortic dissection have a hypertensive history, this finding may not be observed in the acute setting. Neurologic deficit or a pulse discrepancy between the arms may indicate head or arm vessel compromise. Similarly, acute abdominal pain or diminished femoral pulse may suggest visceral vessel or lower limb compromise. A diastolic murmur of aortic regurgitation strongly suggests an ascending aortic dissection.

EVALUATION

The diagnosis of an acute aortic dissection is suspected by the clinical presentation and confirmed by chest CT or aortography. Frequently, upper mediastinal widening may be detected on the posteroanterior radiograph, suggesting an aortic dissection. An intimal flap or a false lumen (Fig. 2.11–4) can be identified by CT scan. An aortogram will help delineate the extent of dissection and may be helpful in identifying associated compromise of visceral or extremity vessels.

MANAGEMENT

Initial management of patients with suspected acute aortic dissection is control of hypertension with vasodilators and beta blockers to diminish the possibility of further dissection or rupture, followed by expedient laboratory evaluation.[12] Aneurysms involving the ascending aorta (type A) are associated with improved survival rates if managed by operative repair. To prevent the frequent occurrence of intrapericardial rupture, the surgeon interrupts the dissection process by dividing the ascending aorta and oversewing the proximal and distal dissection planes. Aortic continuity is reestablished by insertion of a Dacron graft. In the presence of aortic regurgitation, the leaflets may be resuspended, rendering the valve competent. The distal dissection plane, which may extend into the descending thoracic or abdominal aorta, often becomes obliterated; continued regular examination of the distal aorta with a plain radiograph or CT scan is required because of possible late aneurysm formation. Acute descending (type B) thoracic aortic dissections are best managed nonoperatively unless there is evidence of continued chest pain, development of a pleural effusion, neurologic symptoms, or visceral limb vessel ischemia—in which case operation should be performed. Patients with a chronic descending thoracic aortic dissection should be carefully followed up with chest radiographs and CT scans, because the condition may require repair if the aorta begins to expand.

MARFAN SYNDROME (CYSTIC NECROSIS)

The most frequent cause of death in patients with Marfan syndrome is cardiovascular disease. Ruptured aortic aneurysm or aortic dissection is common.[7] Fusiform or saccular aneurysms may de-

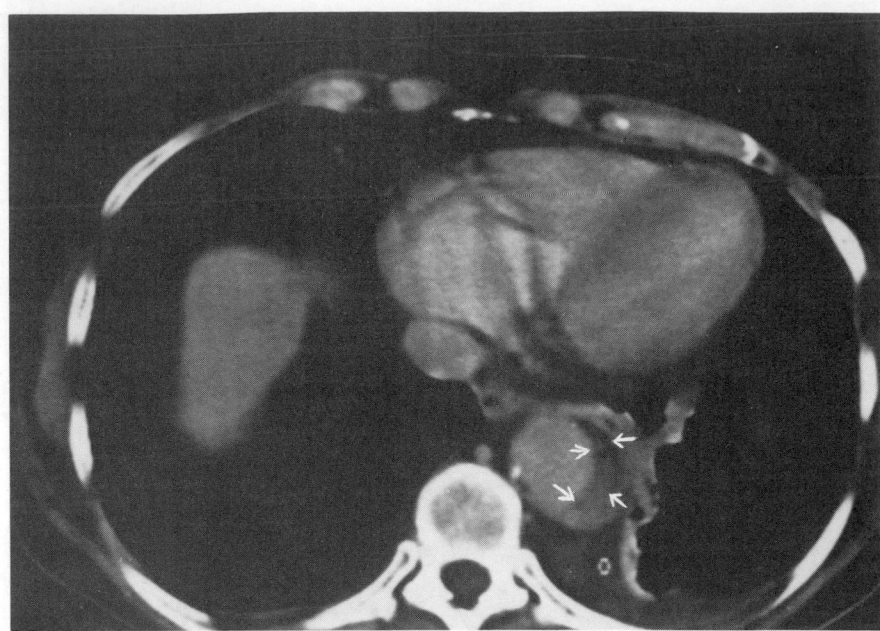

Figure 2.11–4. CT scan of patient with descending thoracic aortic dissection. False lumen (arrows) is present in descending thoracic aorta.

velop in the ascending aorta, increase to a significant size before symptoms develop, and then suddenly rupture. Concomitant aortic regurgitation is often present. Typically these aneurysms are found within the aortic root, but multiple sites are also common. Figure 2.11–5 shows the typical "gourdlike" or "pear-shaped" arteriographic appearance of an ascending aortic root aneurysm found in patients with Marfan syndrome. Because of the risk of ascending aortic rupture or dissection, patients with Marfan syndrome should be screened by echocardiography to determine the presence of aortic root enlargement. Elective repair, replacing the aortic valve and the ascending aorta with a valved Dacron graft and reimplanting the coronary arteries, may be carried out with a low risk of operative death. As in nonmarfanoid patients, operation should be considered once echocardiography shows that the aortic root diameter has exceeded 6 cm, a size at which the risk of rupture has been found to increase.[3]

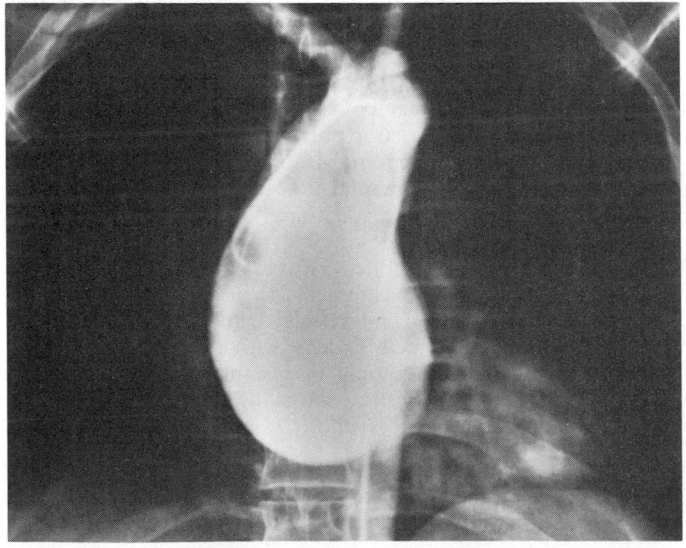

Figure 2.11–5. Ascending aortogram of patient with Marfan syndrome, revealing characteristic pear-shaped aneurysm of ascending aorta and root.

ABDOMINAL ANEURYSMS

The infrarenal abdominal aorta is the most frequent site of arterial aneurysm formation. The majority of these aneurysms are arteriosclerotic and fusiform, and most are discovered on routine physical examination or during evaluation for back discomfort. A palpable, expansile, and occasionally tender mass can be felt above the umbilicus and below the xiphoid process. Ultrasound examination is the most practical test to determine the presence and size of the aneurysm. Complications of untreated abdominal aortic aneurysms include rupture, distal embolization, infection, aortoenteric fistula, aortocaval or renal vein fistula, and left colon ischemia.

The rate of expansion of infrarenal abdominal aortic aneurysms is unpredictable, and rupture frequently occurs if they remain untreated. Although the risk of rupture is related to size, even small aneurysms can give way without warning. Accepted indications for operation include diameter greater than 6 cm, concomitant symptoms, or evidence of expansion.[11] The operative mortality rate is less than 4 percent and related to complications of a cardiopulmonary nature. As a consequence, preoperative evaluation should include investigation of possible coronary artery disease and of lung and renal function.

REFERENCES

1. Cooke JP, Safford RE: Progress in the diagnosis and management of aortic dissection. Mayo Clin Proc 61:147, 1986
2. DeBakey ME, Cooley DA, Creech O Jr: Surgical considerations of dissecting aneurysm of the aorta. Ann Surg 142:586, 1955
3. Gott VL, Pyeritz RE, et al: Surgical treatment of aneurysms of the ascending aorta in the Marfan syndrome. N Engl J Med 314:1070, 1986
4. Heggtveit HA: Syphilitic aortitis: A clinicopathologic autopsy of 100 cases: 1950–1960. Circulation 29:346, 1964
5. Miller DC: Acute dissection of the aorta: Continuing need for earlier diagnosis and treatment. Mod Concepts Cardiovasc Dis 54:51, 1985
6. Miller DC, Stinson EB, et al: Operative treatment of aortic dissections. J Thorac Cardiovasc Surg 78:365, 1979
7. Murdoch JL, Walker BA, et al: Life expectancy and causes of death in the Marfan syndrome. N Engl J Med 286:804, 1972
8. Roberts WC: The Aorta: Its Acquired Diseases and Their Consequences as Viewed from a Morphologic Perspective. New York, Grune & Stratton, 1979

9. Roberts WC: Aortic dissection: Anatomy, consequences, and causes. Heart J 101:195, 1981
10. Slater EE, DeSanctis RW: The clinical recognition of dissecting aortic aneurysm. Am J Med 60:625, 1976
11. Szilagyl DE, Smith RF, et al: Contribution of abdominal aortic aneurysmectomy to prolongation of life. Ann Surg 164:678, 1966
12. Wheat MW Jr, Haris PD, et al: Acute dissecting aneurysms of the aorta. J Thorac Cardiovasc Surg 58:344, 1969

CHAPTER 2.12

Peripheral Vascular Disease[9]

G. Melville Williams

Vascular abnormalities involving the extremities increase in frequency with age and are a major cause of disability in the United States. The challenge in managing patients with "peripheral vascular disorders" comes from the realization that although peripheral manifestations are frequently symptoms of a generalized, systemic disease, the peripheral problem itself demands solution for the well-being of the patient. Reconstructing an occluded femoral artery will not cure atherosclerosis, but it may mitigate a major problem for the patient. The specificity of symptoms and the availability of extremities for examination enable the physician to make a diagnosis of the extent and severity of the disease reliably and to plan therapy rationally.

PATHOPHYSIOLOGIC CONSIDERATIONS

Blood flow to an extremity is determined by the difference between the arterial and venous pressure divided by a complex set of resistances and capacitances. Figure 2.12–1 illustrates these relationships. Extremity circulation is depicted as an arterial segment composed of relatively noncompliant (low capacitance) vessels and a distal or arteriolar resistance. The venous side is more complicated and is shown as a group of vessels with a large capacitance and a proximal resistance. This resistance is caused by constrictions at joints and at the diaphragm. Flow in the all-important capillary bed is increased by an increase in arterial pressure, and it is diminished by an increase in resistance proximal to the capillary bed. The effects of pressure changes on the veins are far more complex because of the very large capacitance of the veins. Thus the increase in venous pressure at the ankle produced by taking a sudden upright posture is not reflected immediately by diminished capillary flow, because blood fills the compliant veins (Fig. 2.12–2). The capacitance of the veins is 18 times greater than that of the arteries, permitting blood to flow through capillaries during intermittent periods of high venous pressure.

An atherosclerotic plaque that occludes the lumen of an artery 70 percent or less is frequently unaccompanied by reduced flow and pressure under resting conditions. However, when the distal resistance is reduced by exercise, the plaque becomes significant and restricts flow, resulting in muscle ischemia, which is appreciated as a crampy pain. Sclerotic plaques that reduce the lumen 90 percent or more will reduce flow and pressure at rest and cause much more dramatic ischemia and pain during exercise (Fig. 2.12–3). Very large aneurysms increase the compliance of the arterial tree, diminishing peak systolic pressure and flow through the capillary bed. However, this rarely leads to symptoms.

The pathogenesis of venous insufficiency in the legs is far more complex and requires greater elaboration. The venous system has been likened to a ladder. The saphenous veins constitute one vertical strut and the deep veins situated between muscles represent the other. The rungs of the ladder are made of multiple "perforating" veins, so called because they penetrate the fascia to drain blood from the superficial extrafascial veins to those within the muscle compartment. All major veins possess valves that permit centripetal flow only. When muscle contraction occurs, the veins are compressed and blood, prevented from flowing distally by valves, is propelled up the leg. When relaxation occurs, the pressure in the deep venous system becomes lower than that in the superficial system and flow is established from superficial to deep veins through the perforating veins, or rungs of the ladder.

Impaired venous return in the upright position occurs when there has been destruction of deep venous valves after thrombosis and recanalization. Patients with paralysis, severe arthritis, or other pain syndromes also develop postural venous insufficiency because muscle contraction is essential for prograde venous flow against gravity.

DIAGNOSTIC SYMPTOMS AND SIGNS

ARTERIAL INSUFFICIENCY

The signs and symptoms of peripheral arterial disease are determined by the location and degree of vascular obstruction, the rapidity with which this obstruction develops, and the presence or absence of collateral channels. The initial symptom of arterial disease is the pain of muscle ischemia or claudication. Characteristically, this is a sensation of fatigue, dull aching, or crampiness felt in the muscle. It is induced by a constant degree of exercise and completely relieved by 5 to 10 minutes of rest. Patients with musculoskeletal disease or venous insufficiency also commonly complain of pain produced by exercise and relieved by rest. Careful questioning of the patient will, however, disclose clear-cut differences in most cases. The patient with arterial insufficiency acquires pain during exercise; his exercise tolerance is reasonably stable, dependent only on the rapidity and duration of exercise; and the relief of pain occurs rapidly. By contrast, the pain associated with musculoskeletal disorders,[7] as well as with venous insufficiency, may begin during exercise or several hours after a period of exercise; there are fluctuations in exercise tolerance; and the pain is relieved by rest, but relief may be delayed for several hours or days (Table 2.12–1).

The location of ischemic pain is determined by the sites of arterial obstruction. If pain is felt in the calf muscles, the major obstruction is probably in the superficial femoral artery. Pain in the thigh occurs with disease of the common femoral or external iliac artery. If pain is experienced in the buttock, there is obstruction in either the common iliac artery or the distal aorta. Impotence is another sign that may reflect distal aortic disease; impotence and bilateral buttock and thigh claudication together constitute Leriche syndrome.

Constant pain in a resting extremity raises the possibility of acute arterial occlusion. Patients without any preceding history of claudication who seek medical attention for a painful extremity most likely have had an arterial embolus. Excruciating pain is an early prominent feature after complete occlusion of a large, normal artery. With the passage of time, however, severe pain is frequently replaced by paresthesias, providing the patient with false optimism.

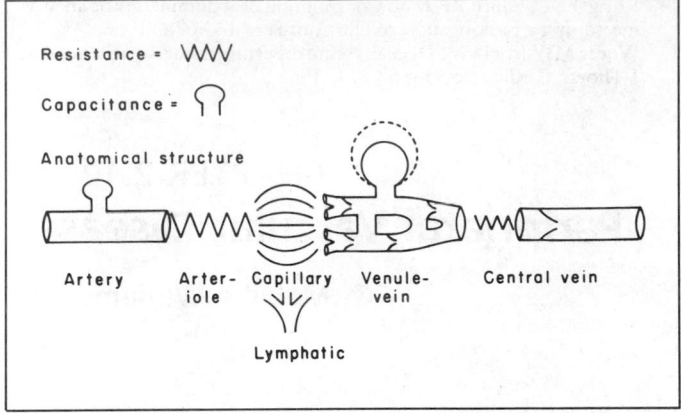

Figure 2.12–1. Diagram of peripheral circulation.

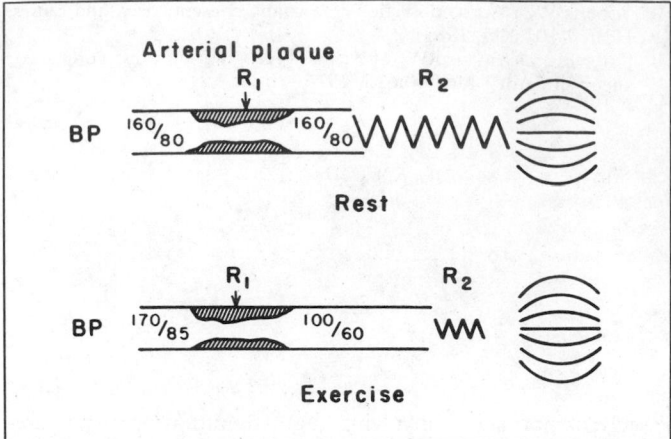

Figure 2.12–3. Mechanism of blood pressure (BP) reduction distal to partial occlusion produced by exercise. When vascular resistance falls in exercising muscle, plaque becomes significant, and it is detected by measuring pressure before (R_1) and after (R_2) exercise.

The physician who examines such a patient will find the extremity pale and pulseless below the site of occlusion. Thus there are four adjectives all starting with the letter *p,* that describe the signs and symptoms of acute arterial occlusion—painful, paresthetic, pale, and pulseless. The site of the occlusion can frequently be deduced from the level of change of skin temperature: ankle and foot, popliteal occlusion; lower leg, superficial femoral occlusion; midthigh, iliac artery occlusion; inguinal ligament, aortic occlusion.

The patient with a preceding history of claudication who has chronic extremity pain while at rest, ulceration, or both will most often have multiple and extensive arterial stenoses or occlusions. Palpation of brachial, radial, carotid, aortic, femoral, popliteal, and pedal pulses provides important information. These pulses are graded from 0 to 4+, and considerable time is required even by

experienced examiners to decide whether a pulse is absent. If the examiner cannot feel a pulse well enough to count it, the score is 0. Equivocation is a poor practice.

An especially valuable sign of chronic arterial ischemia is extreme pallor of the forefoot on elevation and rubor on dependency. The test is performed by elevating the extremity while the patient lies supine. The degree of blanching is noted. The extremity is then lowered by having the patient sit on the edge of the bed or examining table, and the time required for maximal "blushing" to occur is recorded. In the normal or hyperemic individual, the foot becomes only slightly pale on elevation and maximal color is present as soon as the leg is made dependent. In patients with ischemia, there is a delay of at least 20 seconds and sometimes as much as 2 minutes before the capillary blush becomes maximal. If a patient has this sign, called dependent rubor, severe ischemia is present. An existing skin lesion or even a clean incision carried through this area of rubor will not heal. Evaluation in patients with dark skin is more difficult, but it can still be done by noting the color of the plantar surface of the foot and ankle. Dependent rubor indicates maximal small vessel vasodilation caused by tissue ischemia.

Trophic changes in the skin are less reliable indices of ischemia. It is not uncommon to find patients with advanced ischemia, particularly if acute, with normal nail and hair growth, whereas abnormal skin appendages and skin texture are seen in a variety of nonvascular disorders.

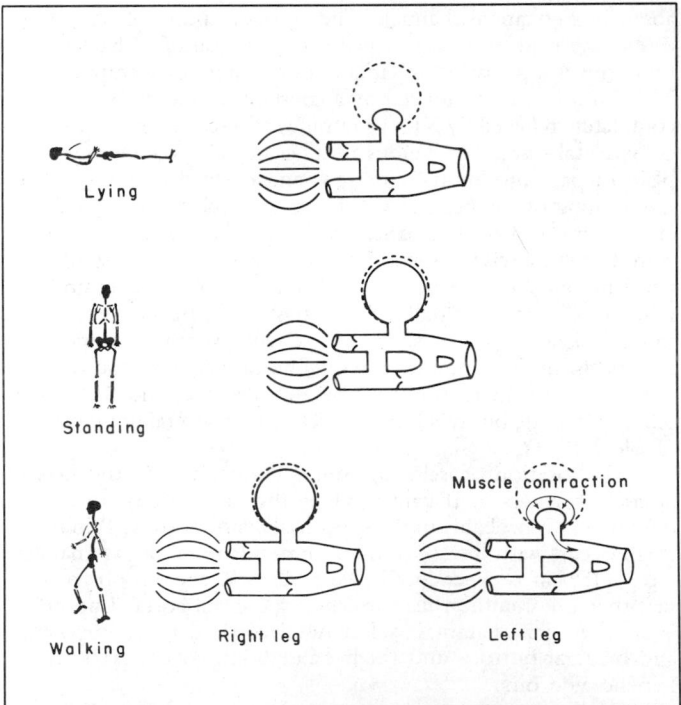

Figure 2.12–2. Diagrammatic schema illustrating value of venous capacitance. When a person stands, the effect of gravitation pressure is to cause pooling of blood in capacitance veins. There will be no increase in pressure in capillary bed until capacitance is full. When a person walks or runs, capacitance modulates venous return; as one leg fills on relaxation, the other empties on pushing off.

TABLE 2.12–1. DIFFERENTIAL DIAGNOSIS OF LEG PAIN: SIGNS AND SYMPTOMS

Disease Entity	Exercise Related	Site	Pulses	Other Findings
Ischemia	4+	Muscle	↓↓ to 0	Pallor → rubor
Compression of cauda equina	3+	Sacral nerve roots	±	↓ Reflexes
Arteritis	2+	Joints, lateral thigh, shin	±	Joint effusions
Venous insufficiency	2+	Calf, foot	±	Edema, stasis dermatitis
Neuropathy	0	Glove, stocking	±	↓ Sensation

VENOUS INSUFFICIENCY

The symptoms and signs of venous insufficiency depend in large measure on whether the processes are acute or chronic, and localized or generalized. Acute venous insufficiency may be caused by thrombophlebitis, trauma, or external venous compression. Steady pain, swelling, superficial venous distension, muscle compartment tenderness, and a dusky, cyanotic skin color are the major signs and symptoms. Extreme degrees of acute venous obstruction induce arterial vasoconstriction, which further reduces capillary flow. Gangrene may result. Such extremities will be massively swollen and cyanotic, giving rise to the term "phlegmasia cerulea dolens."

Patients with chronic venous insufficiency will complain of aching pain in the lower leg after periods of standing or sitting. As insufficiency progresses, the skin becomes thickened and brown. Secondary varicosities, pruritus, and ulceration are late manifestations. Although patients frequently attribute an ulcer to trauma, ulcers caused by venous hypertension occur in predictable locations. The area of skin anterior and superior to the medial malleolus is drained by branches of the long saphenous vein and is the most common site of ulceration, probably because the greatest focus of high venous pressure will occur when valves are disrupted in this system. It has been stated that the malleoli divide arterial and venous ulcerations, with the former occurring inferior and the latter superior to the malleoli.

The patient with chronic venous disease should be examined in the standing and supine positions. Edema is the primary finding in most patients. Standing may disclose the presence of dilated superficial veins. The pressure in these veins is generally high when the legs are dependent. Simple palpation before and after the patient stands on his toes ten times will rapidly differentiate patients with trivial varicosities from those whose varicosities are the result of deep venous pathologic changes. In the presence of a competent deep system, the pressure falls appreciably with exercise. In the presence of an incompetent deep venous system, the pressure will remain high despite exercise.

An attempt should be made to determine the presence and magnitude of venous valvular insufficiency. This is done by placing the patient in the supine position, elevating the extremity to empty the veins, and applying a rubber tourniquet above the knee. When the patient stands, the presence or absence of filling of the dilated superficial veins is noted while the tourniquet is in place and immediately after it is removed. If very marked increase in filling occurs with removal of the tourniquet, the major source of filling of these superficial veins is reflux down an incompetent saphenous vein. If the veins dilate very rapidly while the tourniquet is in place, they are clearly filling by means of incompetent perforators situated below the tourniquet. It is frequently possible to palpate dilated perforator veins by feeling "holes," or defects, 0.5 to 1 cm in size in the fascia of the lower leg. Thus, on physical examination alone, it is possible to judge the extensiveness of the venous problem and to determine whether or not surgical resection of a few or many incompetent, valveless veins is likely to aid the patient.

LABORATORY AIDS IN DIAGNOSIS OF VASCULAR DISEASE

Doppler Flow Probe

Of the special diagnostic aids, the Doppler flow probe has assumed the most important role in the evaluation of patients with vascular disease. The available models are all extraordinarily sensitive detectors of flow. Thus flow may be detected by the Doppler probe in pedal vessels even in cases of severe ischemia. If one is to avoid overestimating circulatory adequacy, pressure measurements are mandatory.

The measurement of segmental limb pressures is easily done with the Doppler flow probe. Pressure in the thigh can be determined by applying a large cuff to the thigh and determining the pressure at which flow is extinguished in the popliteal or tibial artery as monitored by the Doppler probe. By placing the cuff around the calf, measurements of calf pressures can be obtained as the examiner determines which pressure is associated with the loss of pedal flow. Calf and thigh pressures are compared with each other and with the brachial artery pressure to provide an objective assessment of the degree of arterial disease. If resting calf pressures are one fifth of those recorded in the brachial artery, severe ischemia is present and limb loss is imminent. If calf pressure is one half of the brachial artery pressure, claudication is the expected symptom. If the pressure is 80 percent or greater of the brachial artery pressure, some explanation other than arterial insufficiency must be found for the patient's symptoms, particularly if the pressure is sustained after exercise. If thigh pressure is normal and calf pressure low, the occlusion is in the distal femoral or popliteal system. If thigh pressures are also low, significant iliac or aortic disease is present. Occasionally, flow cannot be eliminated by cuff pressures greater than 200 mm Hg. This finding suggests the presence of extensively calcified vessels and invalidates the test.

Plethysmography

A number of sensitive instruments are available that measure changes in the volume of a part. Some of them record the changes in volume associated with cardiac ejection (e.g., pulse volume recorders). Other instruments make use of the normally compliant venous system to measure inflow. In these tests a tourniquet is inflated to 60 mm Hg pressure to occlude venous return, and the change in volume with time during the first 10 to 20 seconds is recorded as flow. For example, the flow to a finger can be estimated by suddenly inflating a proximal tourniquet and measuring the acute increase in volume of the finger.

Deductions can also be made about the presence or absence of venous obstruction with the use of the principles of plethysmography. If a tourniquet applied to the thigh is inflated to occlude venous return, the volume in the calf increases. If, however, an occlusion is present, the increase in volume is less than expected because the capacitance is full. Further, release of the tourniquet is followed by a slower-than-normal return of blood volume to resting levels. Sufficient data have been generated with the use of these principles of diminished filled volume and delayed emptying to state that plethysmography will detect significant thrombi in the femoral and iliac venous systems. Plethysmographic techniques are much less accurate below the knee, where the veins form a parallel rather than a series circuit and thrombi are far less apt to cause physiologic obstruction.

Angiography

Angiography remains the reference method for assessing the cause and severity of peripheral vascular disease. The technique, employing videotape and subtraction of background (digital subtraction angiography), allows visualization of most arteries and veins after the intravenous injection of contrast.[3] Thereby the risks of arterial puncture are obviated. The ease of performance of this procedure may lead to its overuse, for seldom is arteriography required to make practical decisions in the management of patients with peripheral vascular disease. Rather, its major application is in the evaluation of cerebral, renal, and visceral vessels when other tests are less able to predict patency. Standard arteriography is required in individuals requiring surgery for the relief of intractable symptoms. Properly performed, it provides the surgeon with the information he needs to make judgments about the type of surgery to be performed and the likelihood of success.

Venography is indisputably the most accurate method for the detection of venous thrombi. The procedure must be carried out by skilled personnel to avoid problems associated with extravasation of contrast material and to be certain that the deep veins are adequately filled. Concern is still expressed about the toxicity of contrast material. However, the clinical incidence of important

complications is low, and venography is indicated to establish the diagnosis of phlebitis in most patients.

ISCHEMIC PERIPHERAL VASCULAR DISEASE ENTITIES

RHEOLOGIC ABNORMALITIES

Ischemia may be caused by rheologic problems, as well as by structural narrowing of the blood vessel wall. Every patient with ischemic manifestations should therefore be evaluated with this thought in mind, particularly if the symptoms involve the digits and if multiple extremities are affected. The most common rheologic disorders are sickle-cell anemia, polycythemia vera, macroglobulinemia, and the presence of cold agglutinins. The effect of these various disorders is to render the blood more viscous, thereby deterring flow through the capillary bed. Raynaud disease, which is an unusually severe vasoconstrictive response to cold, may well be a rheologic problem in some patients, for it has recently been reported that periodic plasmapheresis successfully ameliorates symptoms.

ARTERIAL EMBOLISM

An arterial embolus should be suspected in any individual who experiences the sudden loss of circulation to an extremity. Although most emboli can be easily removed by modern surgical techniques, the mortality rate remains high and surprisingly constant at 15 to 30 percent. Thus the problem in a significant number of patients is not so much the ischemic limb but the underlying problem, such as heart failure or an unresolved nidus of thrombus providing the source for secondary emboli to important visceral and cerebral arteries.

Emboli may originate from the left atrial appendage in patients with atrial fibrillation. Others originate in the left ventricle when the endocardium is damaged and the left ventricle contracts poorly. An intracardiac tumor may be the source of emboli. Recent studies suggest that 90 percent of patients with arterial emboli have heart disease, but the heart may not be the source in all. Emboli may come from the venous side of the circulation, passing through a patent foramen ovale. Finally, a thrombus may form in the aorta itself and be shed distally. Of these various sources, recent evidence suggests that paradoxic emboli originating from the venous circulation and mural aortic thrombi are more frequent causes of acute circulatory failure than previously suspected.

It is obvious that to reduce the risk of complications and death, the physician must search for the source and cause of an embolus and correct the primary cause whenever possible. The successful management of patients with arterial emboli depends on the collaboration of physician, surgeon, and diagnostic laboratories. The first practical decision to be made is whether or not the patient can withstand angiography and general anesthesia. If the patient has had a recent myocardial infarction and is in low-output failure or is having ventricular arrythmias, treatment of these problems assumes priority. However, simultaneous attempts should be made to restore peripheral circulation, because continued ischemia causes pain, anxiety, and the release of toxic metabolic products.

For a hemodynamically unstable patient, nonoperative therapy seems attractive. High-dose heparin therapy (50,000 to 100,000 units per day) is designed to inhibit coagulation completely, allowing the patient's own fibrinolytic system to lyse the occluding clot. More recently, enzymatic lysis of the embolus has been advocated. For prevention of systemic fibrinolysis that may partially lyse the primary source of the embolus (e.g., left ventricular mural thrombus), the enzyme is delivered through an intra-arterial catheter placed at the proximal extent of the clot. Locally active tissue plasminogen activators will probably become the enzymes of the future. At present, high-dose urokinase or streptoki-

nase infusions are given and clot lysis is studied at 1 to 3 hours by repeat arteriography; successful lysis has been reported to occur in 75 to 85 percent of patients.

Attempts to lyse an embolus enzymatically have several serious limitations. Enzymatic lysis requires time and is not suitable for patients with paralyzed limbs. Furthermore, the logistics of transporting the patient with complicated monitoring equipment and caring for him during the process of arteriography and infusion are cumbersome. Finally, high-dose, short-term enzyme therapy may be only partially successful, and the necessarily protracted infusion of the enzymes may lead to continuing ischemia. Consequently, although surgery seems to be drastic therapy for these patients, it is frequently less stressful, particularly when there are emboli in the extremities, which can be removed in the majority of cases under local anesthesia.

The sudden loss of circulation in an otherwise stable patient with no acute complicating cardiovascular condition is a less severe problem, but delay should be avoided. Evaluation should be thorough but expeditiously completed. Special attention should be directed to symptoms of preceding ischemia of the involved limb or of cardiac arrhythmias. An ECG and an echocardiogram should be obtained. Noninvasive tests of venous patency of the legs should be done. Scanning with the use of radioactive indium–labeled platelets offers promise of localizing areas of active thrombus and should be done in conjunction with angiography after the patient has been hydrated well. In cases of upper extremity emboli, the aortic arch and the origin of the involved vessel must be visualized. In the case of lower extremity embolization, biplane views of the abdominal aorta are indicated, along with views of the site of occlusion. Enzymatic lysis of the embolus or thrombus should be considered.

There is also an intermediate category of patients: those who have had a recent myocardial infarction but are stable at the time of the embolic event. More experience is needed to document the relative frequency of embolic sources in this group of patients before one can proceed with rational therapy. In our recent experience, however, the extraction of one embolus is likely to be followed by the presence of a second unless the cause is eradicated. Thus we currently favor an aggressive approach to detect the source of embolization before proceeding with therapy. An alternative approach is to reserve aggressive diagnostic procedures for those patients who experience recurrent emboli.

ARTERIOSCLEROSIS

Occlusive arteriosclerosis may be localized to a single area. Only a minority of patients have coexisting symptomatic carotid, coronary, aortic, iliac, and femoral artery occlusive disease. In terms of the practical management of the patient, more is to be gained by considering the process localized and amenable to treatment than is to be gained by an overly pessimistic view of the intractable nature of this disease.[4]

Abundant evidence supports the concept that much more is to be gained by medical rather than surgical management of patients with nondisabling calf claudication.[5] Medical management consists of the following: (1) cessation of all smoking, (2) control of hypertension, (3) weight reduction, (4) dietary management of hyperlipidemia, (5) exercise (principally walking to the point of claudication three times a day), and (6) proper care of the feet to prevent infection and cold exposure. The physician may expect the development of collateral circulation to take 6 months. This process can be followed by noting changes in work tolerance and in segmental limb pressures. As a general rule, surgery for the relief of claudication alone should not be undertaken when this symptom has been present for less than 6 months unless the work tolerance is clearly lessening rapidly. Vasodilator drugs have not proved effective. There may be a role for agents that inhibit platelet aggregation such as aspirin or dipyridamole, and a trial of pentoxifylline (Trental) is indicated in the active patient. This agent decreases

blood viscosity by altering the membrane of the red blood cell, a process requiring 6 weeks of therapy. Clinically, it is the only agent known to increase exercise tolerance. Significant improvement is rarely achieved, however. Most patients report no effect or, at most, a 10 to 30 percent increase in exercise tolerance.

Balloon dilation is assuming a greater therapeutic role in patients with symptomatic atherosclerotic disease.[6] If the femoral pulses are diminished, indicating iliac stenosis, angiography is indicated. Short areas of stenosis can be dilated with success in 90 percent. In a significant proportion, the iliac plaques, partially dislodged by the dilating balloon, are resculptured, giving the arterial lumen a smooth appearance on an angiogram. Results of balloon dilation of the femoral arteries depend on runoff from the popliteal artery. Excellent symptomatic relief is achieved when short occlusions or stenoses are dilated and the distal runoff is good.

Surgery remains the treatment of choice in most patients with disabling claudication, pain during rest, or gangrene. Overall, the patient with bilateral hip and thigh claudication who has absent femoral pulses has an 85 percent chance at 5 years and an 80 percent chance at 10 years of complete symptomatic relief by surgery. A patient with significant calf claudication, rest pain in the foot, or both, who has femoral but no popliteal pulses, has a 70 percent chance of complete symptomatic relief by surgery at 5 years. A patient with calf claudication and rest pain in the foot but with a popliteal pulse has a nearly equal chance of long-term symptomatic relief. In every instance of lower extremity occlusive disease, the chances for successful surgery outweigh those of failure.

Surgical reconstruction should be considered in all patients with intractable claudication, but fewer and fewer meet this criterion. Intractability judged by the individual's need to perform a certain amount of work with his legs; the judgment must be made in the context of his overall health and by means of objective measurements of segmental pressures that have failed to improve or have worsened. The patient should be informed about, and willing to accept, a surgical procedure that has a 5 percent chance of making his circulation acutely worse, necessitating amputation.

Diabetic patients have three discrete problems leading to difficulties with their extremities. First, they have an increased frequency of arteriosclerosis, which also occurs at an earlier age and in small arteries. Second, they have a high frequency of neuropathy, which results in anesthetic joint disease in the feet. Third, they have an increased susceptibility to infection. These problems render the management of the diabetic patient with a foot lesion especially complicated.

The so-called trophic foot ulcer of the diabetic patient is characterized by its location on the plantar aspect of the foot directly beneath a joint, most commonly the metatarsophalangeal joint. Callus surrounds the ulcer, which is rarely, if ever, painful. The pathogenesis is best explained by chronic, unappreciated trauma causing deterioration and rupture of the capsule of the anesthetic joint. Fragments of the cartilage are extruded, eventually eroding the skin from within. Proper management depends on the reduction of trauma to the joint involved, and to this end there is no substitute for special shoes. At times surgery is indicated, but the procedure should never be less than the excision of the involved joint.

THROMBOANGIITIS OBLITERANS

Thromboangiitis obliterans, a disease entity initially described by Buerger, was thought to be extremely rare 10 years ago, but at present virtually all physicians caring for patients with vascular disease agree that this is a distinct and not infrequent pathophysiologic entity. It is characterized by (1) necrosis of the digits of both hands and feet, (2) occurrence before the age of 40 years in patients who are predominantly male, Jewish, and heavy cigarette smokers, (3) occlusion of small- and medium-sized arteries below the elbow and below the knee, and (4) the frequent coexistence of thrombophlebitis, which may be either superficial or deep (Table 2.12–2).

TABLE 2.12–2. MANIFESTATIONS OF ATHEROSCLEROSIS, THROMBOANGIITIS OBLITERANS, AND RAYNAUD DISEASE

	Athero-sclerosis	Thrombo-angiitis Obliterans	Raynaud Disease
Age of onset (yr)	>40	<40	<40
Intermittent digital pallor	Absent	Absent	Hallmark
Persistent pain, cyanosis, and necrosis of fingers	Absent	Present	Rare and late in course
Cold sensitivity	Present	Present	Extreme
Claudication in palms and soles	Absent	May be present	Absent
Claudication in calves and thighs	Present	Late in course	Absent
Occlusion of arteries distal to elbow and knee	Rare	Present	Absent
Occlusion of arteries above elbow and knee	Present	Rare and late in course	Absent
History of phlebitis	Rare	Frequent	Rare

Patients with Buerger disease generally have severe pain in one or more digits. A few have claudication in the hand while writing or in the sole of the foot while walking. Virtually no other disease entity produces this type of claudication. If the physical examination demonstrates the loss of one or more tibial arteries or the loss of either the radial or ulnar artery, the diagnosis is virtually established.

Allen sign is useful for demonstrating occlusion of the ulnar or radial artery or of the palmar arch vessels that connect the two. The test is performed by elevating the hand and closing the fist while the examiner compresses both the radial and ulnar arteries. The hand is then opened and closed until pallor is noted. After a minute, pressure on the ulnar artery is released while the examiner notes the color of the hand and fingers while maintaining pressure on the radial artery. If the ulnar artery and palmar arch are patent, the hand will assume a normal pink color immediately. If the ulnar artery is occluded, the hand will remain blanched. If the palmar arch is incomplete, the fifth or fourth finger will assume a normal color while the first three fingers remain blanched. Patency of the radial artery can be demonstrated in the same way by compressing the ulnar instead of the radial artery. Similar information can be obtained by use of the Doppler flow probe.

Withdrawal from tobacco is the most important part of treatment. This is more easily said than done, for the extent of addiction is severe in the majority of these patients. The value of platelet antagonists, anticoagulation with warfarin, and steroids remains unproved. Some patients benefit from sympathectomy.

VASOCONSTRICTIVE DISORDERS

Vasoconstriction of the hands and feet is a normal sympathetic response to cold that preserves core body temperature. This reflex is exaggerated in a variety of systemic diseases, causing patients to complain of pain and pallor in one or more fingers or toes after exposure to cold or even during emotional upsets (Table 2.12–2). When this symptom complex exists singly, it is called Raynaud disease; when it exists as one manifestation of a collagen vascular disorder or a rheologic disorder, it is termed Raynaud phenomenon. The diagnostic study of patients with exaggerated cold pressor responses includes assays of complement levels, rheumatoid factor, antinuclear factor, and sedimentation rate. In addition, patients with structural occlusion have increased cold sensitivity, and thorough vascular examination should be done.

In the case of Raynaud disease, where no structural changes exist early in the course of the disease, treatment is predicated by common sense. Patients are reassured if a thorough examination demonstrates the absence of structural damage to important arteries of the involved extremities. Simple measures, such as wearing gloves inside of mittens in the wintertime and using the elbow to test for the temperature of water, should be explained by the physician. If symptoms persist or become worse despite commonsense measures, a trial of agents blocking alpha-adrenergic responses or calcium-channel blocking agents may be undertaken. Nifedipine (10–20 mg, three or four times daily) has the greatest potency and it should be recommended to patients whose employment depends on cold exposure of their extremities. Surgery, consisting of sympathectomy, is reserved for patients who have tissue loss and is rarely necessary. Although early results are generally good, recurrent symptoms develop in the upper extremities in most patients after 5 years. It must be stressed, therefore, that the foremost aim of the physician in treating patients with Raynaud disease or phenomenon is to alter habits of cold exposure, just as his aim in the patient with Buerger disease is to have this patient eliminate smoking.

ANEURYSMS OF THE ILIAC, FEMORAL, AND POPLITEAL ARTERIES

Arteriosclerotic aneurysms of the femoral and popliteal arteries are likely to shed emboli and finally thrombose rather than rupture. The typical history is one of recurrent episodes of pain, principally in the foot but at times in the calf musculature. Examination at this stage of the disease will disclose the presence of the pulsating mass in the groin or behind the knee and irregular red-blue patches of skin on the foot. Continued embolization, thrombosis, and loss of the extremity are almost inevitable in untreated patients. Reconstruction of arterial circulation after thrombosis of a popliteal aneurysm is not nearly as successful as primary resection before thrombosis. Thus all patients with an extremity aneurysm should undergo resection and graft replacement when the aneurysm is found.

Many instances of rupture of an iliac artery aneurysm have been reported. However, iliac aneurysms are not detected on physical examination or routine radiographs, and the incidence of rupture remains unknown. In the otherwise healthy patient, surgery is the preferred method of treatment, but one could not argue with the choice of sonography or CT scanning for patients with cardiopulmonary disease, which increases surgical risk.

DISORDERS OF THE VENOUS SYSTEM

ACUTE THROMBOPHLEBITIS

The principal signs and symptoms of acute thrombophlebitis are calf pain and aching, edema, and muscle tenderness (see the discussion of chronic venous insufficiency, below). The majority of hospitalized patients with deep venous thrombosis will have no symptoms, and only 50 percent of those thought to have phlebitis clinically demonstrate it on venography. Thus it is hard to escape the view that reliance must be placed on the laboratory for the diagnosis of thrombophlebitis.

Venous stasis and hypercoagulability are the two major causes of thrombophlebitis. Superficial phlebitis may be a manifestation of an underlying malignancy but may also occur in venous varicosities or for no known reason. Of itself, the process has little risk of embolizing or contributing to venous stasis. It is appropriate to treat the isolated superficial phlebitis symptomatically with heat and rest. Should other superficial veins become involved, the process must be taken more seriously and consideration given to systemic anticoagulation. Such patients should be hospitalized and should undergo venography and other tests in a search for an occult malignancy.

The patient with calf pain and ankle edema of acute onset should undergo an initial noninvasive assessment of venous patency. If the test result is positive, treatment with heparin is begun immediately. It is still wise to confirm the diagnosis by venography or digital subtraction angiography, which can be done several hours or even a day later. In cases where the noninvasive test discloses no venous obstruction, heparinization may be safely deferred until a venogram can be performed. Note that irrespective of the results of the noninvasive test, venography is recommended, because neither the disease process nor the means of treatment is trivial, and it is essential to apply the reference method (i.e., venography) to establish this diagnosis. The management of patients with deep venous thrombosis may vary in its details, but there is general agreement that patients should be anticoagulated with intravenous heparin and switched to long-term therapy with warfarin after 5 to 7 days.

CHRONIC VENOUS INSUFFICIENCY

The management of a patient with chronic venous insufficiency and a stasis ulcer may be gratifying, because all ulcers can be healed.[8] One needs only to put the extremity higher than the heart to correct the underlying cause of venous hypertension and treat secondary problems of infection and skin loss appropriately. The patient with a large infected ulcer should be admitted to the hospital and placed on a regimen of bed rest, antibiotics, and topical care of the ulcer. In a matter of 3 to 5 days the ulcer will improve to such a degree that the patient may be discharged after application of Unna paste boot, or may undergo skin grafting if the ulcer is greater than 3 cm in diameter. The use of Unna boot is the best way to achieve compression of incompetent veins, allowing healing to progress while the patient is ambulatory.

Once the ulcer has healed, the patient must wear custom-made elastic stockings to limit the increase in venous pressure that caused the problem. Surgery is reserved for those who cannot or will not wear these stockings and have recurrent ulcers. The very elderly patient may not be capable of putting these stockings on and may have to wear Unna boots permanently.

REFERENCES

1. Brewster DC, LaSalle AJ, et al: Factors affecting patency of femoropopliteal bypass grafts. Surg Gynecol Obstet 157:437, 1983
2. Collen D, Lijnen HR: New approaches to thrombolytic therapy. Arteriosclerosis 4:579, 1984
3. Crummy AB, Strother CM, et al: Computerized fluoroscopy: Digital subtraction for intravenous angiocardiography and arteriography. Am J Roentgenol 135:1131, 1980
4. DeBakey ME, Lowrie GM, Glaeser DH: Patterns of atherosclerosis and their surgical significance. Ann Surg 201:115, 1985
5. Imparato AM, Kim G, et al: Intermittent claudication: Its natural course. Surgery 78:795, 1975
6. Kadir S, Kaufman SL, et al: Angioplasty. In Selected Techniques in Interventional Radiology. Philadelphia, Saunders, 1982
7. Karayannacos PE, Yahson D, Vasko JS: Narrow lumbar spinal canal with "vascular" syndromes. Arch Surg 111:803, 1976
8. Linton RR: The post-thrombotic ulceration of the lower extremity: Its etiology and surgical treatment. Ann Surg 138:415, 1953
9. Rutherford RB (ed): Vascular Surgery. Philadelphia, Saunders, 1977
10. Szilagyi DE, Elliott JP, et al: A 30-year survey of the reconstructive surgical treatment of aorto-iliac occlusive disease. J Vasc Surg 3:421, 1986
11. Szilagyi DE, Smith RF, et al: Contribution of abdominal aortic aneurysmectomy to prolongation of life. Ann Surg 164:678, 1966

CHAPTER 3.1
An Introduction to Respiratory Diseases

Peter B. Terry, Wilmot C. Ball, Jr.,
and Stephen P. Peters

The cardinal manifestations of pulmonary diseases are symptoms of cough, dyspnea, and chest pain; signs of sputum production, hemoptysis, fever, wheezing or labored breathing, rales, cyanosis; radiologic findings of infiltration or mass lesion; and respiratory functional changes of airway obstruction, diminished lung volumes, hypoxemia, and hypercapnia. Whereas acute respiratory diseases are usually symptomatic and associated with physical findings, chronic respiratory diseases are more likely detected, particularly in their earliest stages, only by careful assessment of radiographs, pulmonary function tests, and special studies.

The diagnosis of pulmonary diseases rests principally on a careful history and physical examination, a thorough inspection of high-quality radiographs, spirometry, selected additional tests of respiratory and nonrespiratory lung function, and special procedures such as bronchoscopy, thoracentesis, tissue biopsy, and scintigraphy. This chapter summarizes the clinical manifestations of pulmonary diseases caused by abnormalities of the respiratory and nonrespiratory functions of the lung and presents diagnostic approaches to patients so afflicted.

EVALUATION OF COUGH AND SPUTUM

HISTORY AND DIFFERENTIAL DIAGNOSIS

Cough is part of the normal defense mechanism for cleansing the tracheobronchial tree. It is a reflex act usually arising from stimulation of the bronchial mucosa at some point between the larynx and second order bronchi or from sources as distant as the alveoli and tympanic membranes. The stimulus may be provided by inhaled particulate matter, by mucus secreted by cells lining the tracheobronchial tree, by inflammatory exudate originating in the pulmonary parenchyma or the conducting airways, by the presence of a benign or malignant tumor within the bronchus, or by pressure on the outer wall of the bronchus. Cough may occasionally be produced by conditions involving the pleural surfaces or from stimulation of the external auditory canal, as by impacted cerumen.

Dry or nonproductive cough of acute onset is the typical response to inhalation or aspiration of a foreign body or irritant; is a common early symptom of acute bronchitis, asthma, or pneumonia (especially of viral origin); and may be a prominent manifestation of pulmonary embolization. Chronic, nonproductive cough suggests an endobronchial tumor, extrinsic pressure on the trachea or on a bronchus, one of the diffuse forms of pulmonary infiltration or fibrosis, pulmonary congestion due to early heart failure, or recurrent aspiration of food or gastric contents.

Sputum is not produced by healthy persons, and its presence is a sign of disease. A productive cough of acute onset is generally indicative of a viral or bacterial infection in the tracheobronchial tree. A chronic productive cough suggests bronchitis or bronchiectasis.

GROSS EXAMINATION OF SPUTUM

Yellow or green sputum suggests a bacterial infection in the tracheobronchial tree or lung parenchyma. A large number of eosinophils associated with an allergic condition may also produce yellow sputum. A rust-colored sputum, which is produced by blood evenly dispersed in yellow pus, is most commonly seen in pneumococcal pneumonia. Sputum in *Klebsiella* pneumonia also frequently contains blood but is often bright red and more translucent and viscid. Purulent sputum with a foul odor is usually indicative of anaerobic infection, commonly due to streptococci or bacteroides in a lung abscess. Sputum that is mucoid in character is least helpful diagnostically and may result from any form of long-standing bronchial irritation.

INTERPRETATION OF BLOOD IN THE SPUTUM

Blood-streaked sputum is most commonly caused by acute bronchitis, pneumonia, and other forms of bronchopulmonary suppuration. When not readily attributable to one of these conditions, or when bleeding is persistent or recurrent, full investigation, including bronchoscopy, is warranted. Slight but persistent bleeding is most suggestive of bronchial carcinoma, while recurrent episodes of minor hemoptysis are more common in bronchiectasis, endobronchial tuberculosis, and mitral stenosis. Production of larger amounts of blood suggests pulmonary infarction, bleeding within a tuberculous cavity, or upper-lobe (dry) bronchiectasis. Expectoration of clots may be seen with pulmonary infarction. Care must be taken in evaluating the history of hemoptysis to be certain that the point of bleeding is not in the nose or the nasopharynx, with secondary aspiration of blood.

EVALUATION OF DYSPNEA

Shortness of breath, either during exercise or rest, is a common manifestation of many forms of pulmonary and cardiovascular disease. It denotes the patient's awareness of respiratory effort that is excessive for his level of physical activity. The neural pathways involved in the production of dyspnea are not completely understood, and a single mechanism has not yet been proposed to account satisfactorily for all the clinical situations in which dyspnea may be experienced.

In patients with pulmonary disease the presence of dyspnea is closely related to abnormalities in the mechanics of breathing. There is a good correlation between the level of inspiratory work and dyspnea. Increased inspiratory work and dyspnea are found in conditions in which the lungs or thorax are stiffer than normal, such as pulmonary fibrosis, because the inspiratory muscles have to develop greater tension to produce the same tidal volume (Chapter 3.5). When the thoracic volume is abnormally large, as in emphysema and acute asthma, greater inspiratory muscle tension is

required to produce the tidal volume (see Chapters 3.6 and 3.7). Resistance to airflow is so high at normal lung volumes that the patient breathes near total lung capacity and uses accessory inspiratory muscles. In the acute asthmatic attack, the presence of dyspnea is highly correlated with the retraction of the sternocleidomastoid muscles. In emphysema, loss of elastic recoil results in a large lung volume so that accessory muscles are used during breathing at rest.

The neural pathway by which dyspnea is sensed may begin in the respiratory muscles themselves. It has been suggested that whenever the length-tension relations of the respiratory muscles are inappropriate for the task required, neural traffic reaching the central nervous system from muscle spindles results in the sensation of dyspnea.[4]

Neural receptors within the lungs also are likely to be of great importance in dyspnea. J receptors are vagal nerve endings in the interstitial space between pulmonary capillaries and alveoli. When stimulated, they cause hyperpnea and a number of somatic and visceral reflex effects that decrease muscular activity during exercise. They are inactive during normal breathing but are stimulated by pulmonary congestion and edema. It is believed that the J receptors are stimulated by the presence of pulmonary capillary hypertension and interstitial edema and that this mechanism is of paramount importance in the sensation of dyspnea associated with left ventricular failure. A similar mechanism explains orthopnea, in which these receptors are activated by the increased congestion of the lungs that occurs in the supine posture. The J receptors are also stimulated by pulmonary emboli and inflammation. Some of the dyspnea in restrictive pulmonary disease associated with stiff lungs may well be related to excessive stimulation of nerve endings within the interstitial spaces.

Abnormalities of blood gases do not appear to be directly related to the sensation of dyspnea. The blood gases, however, do affect the level of ventilation and are thus indirectly of great importance. The limitation of muscular exercise in the normal person at high altitude is certainly in part related to the greater ventilatory stimulus from hypoxia, for maximal exercise at any altitude is reached at an approximately equivalent level of ventilation. Muscular exercise in the patient with serious pulmonary insufficiency is likely to be limited by the sensation of dyspnea that results from an inappropriately high degree of respiratory work. Prevention of the ventilatory stimulus from a decrease in arterial oxygen tension by increasing the level of inspired oxygen concentration therefore allows the patient to perform a greater degree of muscular exercise at the same minute ventilation.

Dyspnea can be viewed as an imbalance between the ventilatory stimulus and the capacity to respond to the stimulus. In the patient with pure left ventricular failure, the prime cause of the dyspnea is the increased neural stimulus from the congestion, although the congestion does cause some increase in stiffening of the lungs. The decrease in dyspnea on assuming the upright posture is probably related to the decrease in the stimulus. In the patient with asthma or emphysema, the dyspnea is primarily related to the reduced capacity to respond to the ventilatory stimulus. The dyspnea can be decreased by improving mechanical function, for example, bronchodilators, or decreasing the ventilatory stimulus, for example, improving the level of oxygenation.

EVALUATION OF PAIN

Inflammation of the parietal pleura is the most common cause of pain associated with respiration. A complaint of respiration-related pain may also be elicited from patients with intercostal nerve damage, rib fractures, muscle injury, or costochondral junction separation. A history of factors that precipitate and relieve the pain, as well as palpation or movement of the involved area, is helpful in determining the cause. Unremitting, unilateral pain of weeks to months duration in the absence of infection, trauma, or psychiatric disease suggests a neoplastic origin.

EVALUATION OF PHYSICAL SIGNS

Inspection, palpation, percussion, and auscultation are used to gain information about both anatomic and physiologic abnormalities of the lungs. Physical findings may provide information that cannot be deduced from radiographic study. Examples are wheezing as a sign of airways obstruction, late inspiratory crackles as a manifestation of congestive heart failure, and a pleural friction rub as a sign of pleural disease.

INSPECTION

Inspection during quiet breathing and forced expiration permits recognition of tachypnea, hyperpnea, labored respiration, suprasternal or intercostal retractions, hyperinflation, asymmetry of expansion, and discoordination of the respiratory muscles. Restrictive and obstructive ventilatory abnormalities can also be detected by inspection.

PERCUSSION

Impaired resonance (dullness to percussion) results whenever something more dense than air-filled lung lies directly beneath the chest wall. Common causes are fluid in the pleural space, fibrous thickening of the pleura, consolidation or atelectasis of the lung, and a large peripherally located mass in the lung. A truly flat percussion note at one lung base usually signifies a large pleural effusion or elevation of the diaphragm. Increased resonance may be generalized when the lungs are hyperinflated (as in emphysema) and may be localized to one side over a pneumothorax or a large bullous lesion.

BREATH SOUNDS

Normal inspiratory breath sounds are produced by turbulent flow within large and medium-sized airways including subsegmental bronchi and may be heard at the open mouth as random noise that covers a wide frequency spectrum. These sounds vary in intensity with rate of airflow and are abnormally loud when medium-sized airways are narrowed, as in asthma and bronchitis. As the sounds are transmitted through normal lung to the chest wall, most of the high-frequency components are attenuated; the resulting sound heard through the stethoscope is termed vesicular breathing. When lung parenchyma and chest wall are normal, differences in intensity of vesicular sounds at the chest wall reflect regional differences in ventilation. A local decrease in intensity may also result from impaired transmission of sound. Pleural effusion, pleural thickening, and pneumothorax are examples of this and result in distant or absent breath sounds. An abnormal increase in intensity of breath sounds is always accompanied by a change in their character, which may range from a slight harshness of quality to fully developed bronchial breathing. These changes are due to increased transmission of the higher-frequency components of breath sounds originating in the larger airways. Bronchial breathing may be heard over consolidated, atelectatic, or compressed lung, provided the airway to this portion of the lung remains patent. Similar changes may be heard over extensively damaged lung in tuberculosis, bronchiectasis, and various forms of chronic pulomonary fibrosis.

VOICE SOUNDS

Transmission of spoken or whispered voice sounds to the chest wall may also be altered by the presence of disease. In many instances changes in voice sounds may be more readily appreciated than the corresponding alterations in breath sounds, especially when the latter are difficult to hear because of obesity, a noisy environment, or other factors. Distant or inaudible sounds may be

produced by a large pleural effusion, pneumothorax, or bronchial occlusion. Increased transmission of voice sounds is associated with a change in their character so that they assume a higher pitched, less muffled quality than normal and often permit distinct recognition of the words spoken. This is called "bronchophony" and is heard over areas of consolidation, infarction, atelectasis, or compression of lung. In its extreme form (egophony) the spoken words assume a nasal or bleating quality and the sound *ee* is heard through the stethoscope as *ay*. This sound is most common when solidified lung and pleural fluid are both present but may be heard over an uncomplicated lobar pneumonia or pulmonary infarction. Transmission of whispered voice sounds with abnormal clarity (whispered pectoriloquy) has the same significance as bronchophony.

ADVENTITIOUS SOUNDS

Much confusion in the reporting and interpretation of physical findings has resulted from the multiplicity of terms used to describe adventitious lung sounds. It is now recommended that all the common abnormal lung sounds be referred to as either *crackles* or *wheezes*.

Crackles
Crackles are nonmusical individual clicking sounds previously referred to as "rales" or "crepitations." Each explosive sound is produced by the opening of a medium or small airway in an abnormally deflated area of lung. When coarse crackles occur only during the first half of inspiration, they are generally a manifestation of severe obstructive pulmonary disease. Fine crackling heard entirely or predominantly during late inspiration is characteristic of diffuse interstitial disease, areas of lung contracted by fibrosis or atelectasis, and lung stiffened by pneumonia or the effects of interstitial congestion due to heart failure. In any generalized process the less-distended dependent lung is most likely to produce crackles, which are therefore heard at the bases when the patient is erect. A few basilar end-inspiratory crackles are normally present after prolonged shallow breathing but are abolished by a few deep breaths. A pleural friction rub, although classified as crackling, is usually recognizable as a sequence of evenly spaced sounds, in late inspiration and early expiration, localized low in the axilla or over the lung base posteriorly. Low-pitched discontinuous sounds may be produced by exudate within the large airways; these sounds show considerable variation from breath to breath and are often abolished by coughing.

Wheezes
Wheezing refers to musical sounds heard either at the mouth or through the stethoscope. When low-pitched, they are sometimes called "rhonchi." These sounds are generated by the vibratory motion of airway walls, not by the vibration of an air column, and only medium and large airways can produce these sounds. Multiple high-pitched wheezing sounds are the result of an increase in bronchomotor tone, as in asthma.

EVALUATION OF LABORATORY STUDIES

MICROSCOPIC SPUTUM EXAMINATION

For microscopic examination, sputum is collected in a container to facilitate the selection of a drop-sized sample of optically dense material.[6] This is smeared on a glass slide, covered and examined immediately. The presence of alveolar macrophages under low power is evidence that the material arose from deep within the lung. The presence of greater than ten squamous epithelial cells per low-power field suggests contamination with saliva and indicates an inadequate specimen. In patients with asthma, low-power examination may reveal the laminated whorls called "Curschmann spirals," or "Charcot-Leyden crystals," which are thought to represent the coalescence of eosinophilic granules. Cellular detail is best appreciated by use of the oil immersion lens.

The sputum in patients with asthma shows a predominance of eosinophils. In contrast, sputum composed predominantly of neutrophils correlates with the presence of bacterial infection, with 85 percent of such specimens showing pathogenic organisms on culture. A specimen containing a predominance of neutrophils should be Gram stained for identification of bacteria. Predominance of a specific organism may be used as a generally reliable guide for the selection of antibiotics in patients suspected of having pneumonia. On rare occasions the discovery of macrophages filled with large globules of fat in a patient with an unexplained infiltrate gives the only clue to the diagnosis of lipid pneumonia and may obviate the need for thoracotomy. The presence of lipid is confirmed by Sudan III stain of the sputum. When carcinoma of the bronchus is present, cytologic study with special stains will reveal malignant cells in the majority of cases.

EVALUATION OF CHEST ROENTGENOGRAPHY

Chest roentgenograms serve to record the presence or absence of disease on the date of the examination, and serial examinations serve to document change. It is possible to make a presumptive etiologic diagnosis in a number of conditions on the basis of chest roentgenograms alone, while in other instances the nature of a lesion can be determined only by bacteriologic or cytologic studies. A negative radiographic examination does not necessarily imply that disease is absent; a lesion may be too small to be recognized radiographically. For example, a solitary pulmonary nodule must be 4 to 5 mm in diameter, and a pleural effusion must measure 200 to 300 ml before it can be identified.

Interpretation of chest roentgenograms requires knowledge of the normal roentgen anatomy of the thorax and an ability to recognize and analyze deviations from the normal. This ability is developed through experience gained by the orderly and detailed study of many normal and abnormal films. It is important to recognize the limitations imposed by technically suboptimal films and to repeat the examination whenever necessary. If standard views of good quality do not provide an adequate definition of the gross anatomy of an abnormal finding, additional views or special examinations may be useful.

The objective of the examination of chest films is the localization and description of abnormal lung findings and, when possible, the recognition of specific morphologic change. This exercise should not be preceded by attempts to arrive at a specific diagnosis or even a differential diagnosis. Recognition of the fact that a certain density is the result of loss of volume (atelectasis), infiltration, or accumulation of pleural fluid will be of considerable help in defining the etiology or specific disease entity. However, pulmonary lesions should first be classified in reference to their location, contour, configuration, number, and size.

The examination of a chest film with intrathoracic disease should begin with an attempt to determine the anatomic location of each lesion. The classification by location can be subdivided into lobar or segmental abnormalities or into diffusely scattered lesions. The topographic arrangement of the pulmonary lobes and segments on posteroanterior and lateral films must be known for precise description of localized lung lesions. Displacement of the trachea or esophagus and bone involvement, such as erosion of dorsal vertebral bodies, ribs, or the sternum are ancillary observations to define the extent of a disease process.

Localization is of importance not only for descriptive purposes but also for differential diagnosis and management. For example, a density on the chest radiograph does not necessarily represent a pulmonary lesion but may instead be part of the pleura or mediastinum. Localization is also helpful with less well-defined lesions. For instance, pulmonary disease localized to the lung bases is frequently observed in infections secondary to bronchiectasis, aspiration, collagen vascular diseases, or idiopathic pulmonary fi-

brosis. Diseases such as bronchopneumonia and fungus infection may occur anywhere in the lung parenchyma. A lobar or segmental pattern suggests pneumonia, endobronchial disease, or infarction.

The physician's ability to localize lesions is aided greatly by a number of special radiographic signs. Two that are extremely reliable in localizing pulmonary infiltrates and mass lesions are the silhouette sign and the air bronchogram. The silhouette sign occurs when the normally sharp borders between mediastinal structures or the diaphragm and the lung become blurred (Fig. 3.1–1). Normally the contours of the heart and great vessels are sharply delineated against the surrounding lung. This contrast in density between lung tissue and other thoracic structures is the result of the differential x-ray absorption of the air-containing lung and these other organs. Thus, whenever lung tissue in contact with the cardiac contour is not aerated, this absorption differential does not exist and the heart border will be blurred. Since the heart is located in the anterior compartment of the thoracic cavity, a disease process blurring the heart border must also be located anteriorly. Masses or infiltrates located posteriorly in the lung will not affect the sharpness of the cardiac silhouette because the heart is still surrounded by aerated lung tissue.

The air bronchogram is helpful in distinguishing intrapulmonary lesions from lesions in the mediastinum or the pleural space. Under normal conditions the bronchi contain air and, hence, are not visible if surrounded by aerated lung. If surrounded by pulmonary infiltrate, the bronchi will be seen as linear air shadows and, hence, prove the intrapulmonary location of a disease process. Air bronchograms can be observed in pneumonia, pulmonary infarction, bronchiectasis, and pulmonary edema. An air bronchogram can also be observed in a partially collapsed lung where bronchi are crowded together. Whenever bronchi within consolidated lung contain inspissated mucus, inflammatory debris, or tumor, they will not be visible.

Rounded lesions are called "nodules," or, if larger, "masses" (Chapter 3.3). Linear lesions may be called "strands," or "bands," depending upon their size. Streaky or linear densities in the lung may represent pulmonary vessels, fibrosis, or atelectasis. Short horizontal lines in the lower lung fields are frequently the result of discoid atelectasis and represent incomplete aeration or a small pulmonary infarct. When linear lesions appear to form a network, they are said to be reticular. In general, acute and subacute inflammatory lesions have an ill-defined border and are said to be infiltrates. Chronic inflammation and neoplasms are usually well demarcated. Large pulmonary infiltrates involving an entire lobe are referred to as a "lobar consolidation." They may increase the lung volume and displace the pleural fissures. Decrease in lung volume is usually due to tissue necrosis or atelectasis.

OBLIQUE VIEWS

The oblique views are sometimes helpful in localizing a lesion and in separating a parenchymal density from overlying structures. They are also used in evaluating heart chamber size, heart valve calcification, and in separating vascular structures from mediastinal or parenchymal masses. Minimal oblique views are frequently more helpful than the standard 45-degree oblique films.

LATERAL DECUBITUS (RECUMBENT) VIEWS

Lateral decubitus views are used to demonstrate the presence of small pleural effusions and to determine if pleural fluid is loculated. On a decubitus film, free fluid runs up the dependent chest wall or layers along the mediastinum. Loculated accumulations may change shape but do not change position. Free fluid in the lower hemithorax frequently shifts so that the underlying lung and pleura previously obscured by the fluid can be visualized, allowing the differentiation of effusions secondary to parenchymal infiltrates (parapneumonic effusions) from primary pleural disease. Decubitus views may aid in outlining the confines of a cavity, demonstrating air-fluid levels within cavities and differentiating pyopneumothorax from large lung abscesses.

LORDOTIC VIEW

The lordotic view projects the clavicles and first ribs above the lung, allowing the apices to be viewed more clearly. Anterior lesions are projected upward and posterior lesions downward, making this view useful in localizing lesions seen poorly on the lateral or oblique views.

Figure 3.1–1. Silhouette sign. **A.** Posteroanterior view of right middle lobe infiltrate. Note blurring of adjacent right heart border—*silhouette sign.* **B.** Lateral view of same patient. In contrast, note sharp borders of infiltrate with minor and major fissures. Other commonly silhouetted structures are diaphragms by lower lobe infiltrates and left heart border by lingular infiltrates.

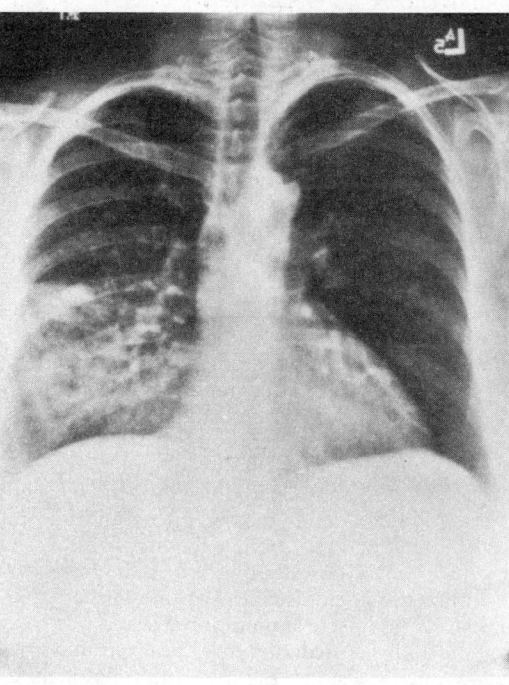

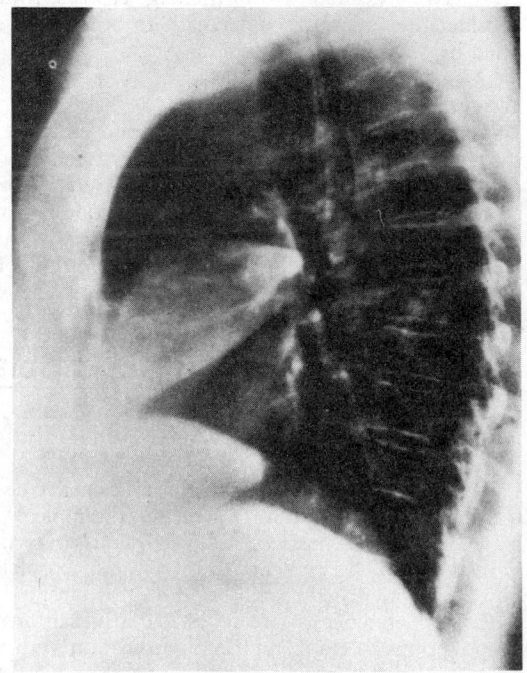

A

B

EXPIRATORY FILM

A small pneumothorax is frequently seen only on a film taken during full expiration. Superimposed inspiratory and expiratory films may be used to evaluate lack of diaphragmatic movements, such as that which occurs with air trapping in emphysema or with neuromuscular disease. Unilateral hyperinflation secondary to the ball-valve effect of an endobronchial tumor or aspirated foreign body can be detected by inspiratory and expiratory films. The mediastinum shifts away from the side of the lesion because the affected lung cannot empty during expiration.

COMPUTED TOMOGRAPHY (CT)

CT examinations of the chest should not be requested indiscriminately but should be used to resolve specific problems that are not clarified by routine examinations.[14] Since CT can identify pulmonary nodules with greater sensitivity than regular radiographs, it is useful when the likelihood of small tumor metastases is high, such as in the patient with melanoma or the patient with an apparently single nodule and a known primary tumor elsewhere. This sensitivity is not without its hazards. The CT may lead to the discovery of unexpected nodules interpreted as metastatic lesions that in fact represent granulomatous lesions. CT does, however, permit the quantitative measurement of the radio-density of small nodules, allowing high-density nodules to be recognized as inflammation even when calcification is not visible.[15] Extremely low density may indicate fat or a fluid-filled lesion. Mediastinal masses can often be seen with clarity in axial sections and can readily be distinguished from vascular structures if CT examination is performed after intravenous injection of contrast material.

The staging of lung cancer may be approached more rationally with the demonstration of hilar, paratracheal, or subcarinal lymph nodes by CT. Main and lobar bronchi can be visualized, allowing for the demonstration of intrinsic lesions or secretions, extrinsic compression, and the patency of airways within dense infiltrates.

Pleural disease is more reliably distinguished from parenchymal disease by CT, which has proven useful in patients with pneumonia in which complicating pleural effusion or empyema is suspected. Emphysema, blebs, and bullous lesions not seen on routine chest films can be readily recognized with CT scanning.

FLUOROSCOPY

Chest fluoroscopy delivers considerably more radiation than is required for exposure of films and should be used only when necessary. It is the best method for demonstrating immobility or paralysis of a diaphragm. During a rapid inspiratory sniff, the chest wall is fixed and the normal diaphragm descends; a paralyzed diaphragm will move upward because of the increased intra-abdominal pressure caused by descent of the diaphragm on the other side. Fluoroscopic examination with the application of a metallic marker is often helpful in choosing the proper location for withdrawal of fluid from a loculated pleural effusion or empyema.

RADIOISOTOPE STUDIES

Detection of regional abnormalities in the distribution of pulmonary blood flow and ventilation can be accomplished by radioisotope scanning of the lungs.[1] Perfusion scans are usually made with a gamma camera after intravenous injection of Tc-99m-labeled microspheres; anterior, posterior, and both lateral and oblique views should be obtained and interpreted in conjunction with a Xe-133 posterior ventilation scan and a chest radiograph taken at the same time.

Multiple segmental or lobar defects unaccompanied by corresponding ventilation defects or infiltrate on the chest film strongly suggest pulmonary embolism.[2] If underlying pulmonary parenchy-

mal disease, such as emphysema, is responsible for the perfusion defect, a ventilation scan will show a filling defect in the same area. The distribution of inhaled Xe-133 during a single breath and the time required to wash the Xe-133 out of the lung are important in assessing parenchymal or airway disease. When widespread parenchymal disease is present, the absence of characteristic changes on ventilation and perfusion scans does not exclude pulmonary embolism. In addition, nonsegmental patchy filling defects may be produced by pulmonary emboli, and pulmonary arteriography may be required for confirmation of the diagnosis. Serial lung scans are useful in following the patient with pulmonary embolism. This problem is discussed further in Chapter 3.8.

Perfusion scans are useful in the evaluation of resectability of bronchogenic carcinoma. A large area of reduced blood flow on the affected side indicates that involvement of the hilar vessels is likely, and when the entire lung is unperfused, the chance of a successful resection is small.

In the patient with impaired pulmonary function who requires thoracotomy and resection of lung tissue, scans permit prediction of the effect of operation on pulmonary function, and may be critical in establishing operability.[10]

Gallium scans of the lung may be helpful in assessing the abundance of inflammatory cells in diffuse parenchymal disease.[7] Detection of these inflammatory cells occurs with active inflammation and is absent with arrested fibrosis. Knowledge of disease activity is particularly helpful in determining the role of steroid therapy in idiopathic pulmonary fibrosis or sarcoidosis.

ULTRASOUND

Echo studies appear to have their greatest usefulness in localizing small areas of effusion or empyema for thoracentesis. They are not entirely reliable in distinguishing solid from liquid subpleural material, and they will not detect lesions separated from the chest wall by aerated lung.

EVALUATION OF RESPIRATORY FUNCTION

Diseases that produce significant anatomic alterations in the pulmonary parenchyma or disturbances in the mechanical operation of the chest wall or diaphragm result in abnormalities of pulmonary function. Laboratory measurements of these derangements are clinically useful both in the diagnosis and management of chest disease.[3]

The most useful pulmonary function tests include measurements of forced expiration (spirometry), diffusing capacity, and arterial blood gases. Measurements of alveolar ventilation, dead space, airway resistance, forced inspiratory flows, elastic recoil pressure, percent right-to-left shunt, respiratory muscle strength, and pulmonary artery pressure may be helpful in selected cases. Exercise tolerance tests with or without supplemental oxygen are useful in the evaluation of disability and in assessing the need for ambulatory oxygen therapy. Table 3.1–1 shows examples of the application of physiologic testing in specific clinical problems.

SPIROMETRY

Abnormalities of pulmonary mechanics are commonly evaluated by means of spirometry, that is, vital capacity and one or more parameters of airflow during forced expiration. Vital capacity is defined as the largest volume of air that the patient can exhale voluntarily, beginning with the lungs fully inflated. Weakness, pain on deep breathing, poor comprehension, or lack of cooperation on the part of the patient may result in an underestimate of the vital capacity. The result is compared either with previous measurements made on the same patient or with average normal values

TABLE 3.1–1. EXAMPLES OF APPLICATION OF PULMONARY FUNCTION TESTING

Clinical Problem	Suggested Studies	Results and Comments
Wheezing or other evidence of airway obstruction	Spirometry	Indices of expiratory flow reduced. Confirms and quantifies severity of obstruction. Immediate improvement after bronchodilator is typically seen with asthma
	Lung volumes (He or N_2)	Increased in emphysema and asthma. May be normal in chronic bronchitis and reduced in bronchiectasis. Markedly elevated residual volume suggestive of pulmonary emphysema
	Diffusing capacity	Normal in asthma, normal or slightly reduced in bronchitis, low in emphysema
	Airway resistance	High in most forms of obstructive pulmonary disease, but may be normal in emphysema
	Elastic recoil pressure	Low in uncomplicated emphysema, normal in bronchitis, asthma
Severe obstructive airway disease; suspected respiratory failure	Arterial blood	High P_{CO_2} indicates hypoventilation. O_2 saturation below 80% indicates need for oxygen therapy. Rising P_{CO_2} may indicate need for respirator.
Status asthmaticus	Arterial blood	P_{CO_2} >50 mm Hg usually indicates very severe impairment and need for intensive supervision
	Peak expiratory flow	Excellent method for following course of attack
Evaluation of operative risk	Spirometry	Severity of obstruction related to operative risk
	Arterial blood	Elevated P_{CO_2} means high anesthesia risk
	Exercise ability	Inability to perform mild exercise usually correlates with high risk
Unexplained coma	Arterial blood	High P_{CO_2} may explain coma. Normal P_{CO_2} rules out hypoventilation as cause of coma
Diffuse pulmonary infiltration or fibrosis	Spirometry	Reduced vital capacity suggests stiff lung, provides baseline for evaluation of course or treatment
	Diffusing capacity	Degree of reduction indicates extent of damage to lung. Baseline for treatment
	Arterial blood	P_{O_2} may be minimally abnormal early and markedly abnormal in severe fibrosis
Pulmonary hypertension	Spirometry	Usually little loss of vital capacity in multiple emboli or primary pulmonary hypertension, marked loss in diffuse fibrosis
	Diffusing capacity	Low in diffuse fibrosis; normal or only slightly reduced value suggests pulmonary vascular disease
	Arterial blood	Recurrent small to medium sized pulmonary emboli unlikely with normal arterial oxygen tension
Polycythemia	Arterial blood	Low P_{O_2} and saturation suggest secondary polycythemia
Mitral stenosis	Diffusing capacity	Severe reduction suggests irreversible damage to lung
	Postexercise vital capacity	Useful in following course of disease
Suspected scleroderma with normal x-ray	Spirometry	Early restrictive ventilatory defect
	Diffusing capacity, compliance	Low values support diagnosis
High serum bicarbonate levels	Arterial blood	Normal P_{CO_2} with high pH and bicarbonate indicates metabolic alkalosis P_{CO_2} >55 indicates compensated respiratory acidosis unless pH very high
Dyspnea without clinical signs of heart or lung disease	Spirometry and diffusing capacity	Lung disease as cause of dyspnea unlikely with normal spirograms and diffusing capacity
	Arterial blood	May be normal with significant disease. Abnormality suggests underlying pathology

based on sex, age, and height. Because of normal variation, an isolated measurement of vital capacity can be considered abnormal only when it is less than 85 percent of the predicted value.

Reduction in vital capacity is common in association with airway obstruction of any cause. In the absence of obstruction a small vital capacity usually indicates that the total lung capacity is also reduced and that a restrictive ventilatory defect is present. The restriction may be secondary to interstitial fibrosis, pleural or parenchymal space-occupying lesions, chest wall deformity, neuromuscular disease, or heart failure.

Spirometer tracings made during forced expiration (forced expirograms) are the most convenient indirect method of assessing the presence and severity of an obstructive ventilatory defect. The 1-second forced expiratory volume (FEV_1), expressed in liters or in percent of the measured vital capacity (FEV_1 percent), is the most convenient and useful measurement for evaluating prolonged expiration. Airways obstruction is the characteristic physiologic abnormality in asthma, chronic bronchitis, and emphysema. The mechanisms and clinical manifestations of airways obstruction are discussed in Chapters 3.6 and 3.7.

DIFFUSING CAPACITY

The diffusing capacity (DL_{CO}) is measured with carbon monoxide as the test gas and is expressed in milliliter uptake per minute per millimeter of mercury partial pressure difference across the alveolocapillary membrane. Perhaps the greatest clinical usefulness of diffusion measurements is in the group of diffuse parenchymal diseases that produce more profound abnormalities in gas exchange than in pulmonary mechanics (see Chapter 3.5). Interstitial fibrosis even in the presence of minimal radiographic abnormality is commonly associated with a reduction in diffusing capacity. Diffusion measurements are also useful in the differentiation of emphysema from bronchitis and asthma. Pure chronic bronchitis and asthma cause little or no reduction in diffusing capacity, whereas emphysema is characterized by a significant decrease in DL_{CO} (see Chapter 3.7). The presence of pulmonary hypertension and cor pulmonale correlates well with gross reduction in the diffusing capacity in both emphysema and in diffuse interstitial disease. The diffusing capacity for carbon monoxide may remain nearly normal in pulmonary vascular lesions, such as multiple pulmonary emboli, and may therefore occasionally be useful in differential diagnosis.

In the interpretation of diffusion measurements it is important to bear in mind that a low diffusing capacity almost always results from loss of functioning alveolocapillary surface area rather than from thickening of alveolar walls. While a severe reduction in the diffusing capacity is a potential cause of hypoxemia, the low arterial PO_2 at rest in patients with diffuse lung disease is more likely to be due to ventilation to perfusion ($\dot{V}/\dot{Q}$) abnormality (see next section).

ARTERIAL BLOOD GAS STUDIES

Measurements of O_2 tension, CO_2 tension, and pH of arterial blood have proven to be of great usefulness in the diagnosis and therapy of a wide variety of clinical conditions. From these measurements approximate values of bicarbonate and oxygen saturation can be calculated. A single arterial blood study affords a complete picture of the acid–base status of the patient and is useful in a variety of renal and metabolic problems.

The partial pressure of carbon dioxide in arterial blood (Pa_{CO_2}), which does not differ substantially from the partial pressure of carbon dioxide in alveolar gas (PA_{CO_2}), is determined by the balance between delivery of carbon dioxide to the alveoli and its removal by ventilation. Maintenance of a normal arterial carbon dioxide tension requires that alveolar ventilation be kept proportional to metabolic carbon dioxide production. A sustained arterial PCO_2 of 80 mm Hg, for example, indicates that the level of alveolar ventilation is half of normal, that is, half that which would be appropriate for the existing rate of metabolic carbon dioxide production.

Hypercapnia is thus the result of inadequate alveolar ventilation and may be observed in patients whose control of breathing is impaired (sedative or narcotic overdose, central nervous system [CNS] lesion, primary hypoventilation syndrome) or who are unable to meet ventilatory demands because of respiratory muscle paralysis. Chronic CO_2 retention is most common in patients with severe obstructive pulmonary disease, especially chronic bronchitis, and usually when the 1-second forced expiratory volume has fallen to 1 L or less. A normal or slightly low arterial PCO_2 is maintained in most patients with a restrictive ventilatory abnormality. However, Pa_{CO_2} may rise acutely in patients very severely ill with pneumonia, pulmonary edema, or even extensive fibrosing alveolitis. Since the presence of an increased dead space may cause a marked discrepancy between alveolar ventilation and minute ventilation, the adequacy of alveolar ventilation cannot always be predicted by bedside observation. Sampling of arterial blood for measurement of Pa_{CO_2} is therefore indicated whenever alveolar hypoventilation is suspected.

As alveolar ventilation falls and arterial PCO_2 rises, there is a reciprocal fall in alveolar O_2 tension that may lead to hypoxemia.

The oxygen tension of alveolar gas may be estimated from a simplification of the alveolar air equation:

$$PA_{O_2} = PI_{O_2} - \frac{Pa_{CO_2}}{R}$$

where PA_{O_2} = alveolar O_2 tension, PI_{O_2} = inspired O_2 tension (150 mm Hg for room air at sea level), Pa_{CO_2} = arterial PCO_2, which is assumed to equal alveolar PCO_2, and R = respiratory exchange ratio. The respiratory exchange ratio, defined as ratio of CO_2 output to O_2 uptake by the lungs, is equal to the respiratory quotient in the steady state, and has a numerical value of about 0.8. R may be measured by analysis of expired air or may be estimated under non-steady-state conditions. Although the simplified equation presented here is inaccurate when inspired O_2 is above 50 percent, it provides a convenient clinical method for predicting alveolar PO_2 in a patient receiving supplemental oxygen.

Hypoxemia may result from three separate mechanisms:

1. Low alveolar oxygen tension (hypoventilation, breathing low-oxygen mixtures, high altitude)
2. Failure to achieve equilibrium between alveolar and capillary oxygen tensions (diffusion defect)
3. Effective shunting of blood from the venous to the arterial side (direct anatomic shunt, perfusion of poorly ventilated alveoli)

Arterial PO_2 is normally slightly less than end-capillary PO_2 because of the admixture of venous blood. Most of this is due to the effect of uneven ventilation to perfusion ($\dot{V}/\dot{Q}$) ratios in the normal lung, which results in overperfusion of portions of lung relative to their ventilation. The total shunt effect in a young normal individual is less than the equivalent of 6 percent of cardiac output and results in an O_2 tension difference between alveolar gas and arterial blood (A − a O_2 difference) of up to 15 mm Hg.

A slightly larger A − a O_2 difference leading to mild hypoxemia is common in bronchitis, bronchiectasis, emphysema, atelectasis, pneumonia, the early stages of many diffuse pulmonary lesions, and a host of other conditions in which the V/Q ratio is not uniform throughout the lung.

When severe hypoxemia occurs as a manifestation of lung disease, the predominant mechanism may be admixture of venous blood through unventilated lung regions (true shunt), as in the adult respiratory distress syndrome. Increasing the inspired oxygen concentration in this situation has only a small effect on arterial PO_2.

Hypoxemia produces important physiologic changes, especially in cerebral and cardiac function. Chronic mild hypoxemia may result only in a sense of fatigue, a subtle impairment of judgment, and a slight tachycardia, with increase in cardiac output. A more abrupt and severe reduction in arterial oxygen tension may produce gross disturbances in behavior or loss of consciousness and may give rise to a fatal cardiac arrhythmia. Although disturbances of consciousness resulting from carbon dioxide retention are generally promptly and fully reversible, even a brief period of severe cerebral hypoxia may result in irreversible damage to the brain or may produce an altered state of consciousness from which recovery requires hours or days.

LUNG VOLUMES

Functional residual capacity (FRC) may be measured by equilibration of air in the lungs with an insoluble gas such as helium, or by measuring the total amount of nitrogen washed out of the lungs during the breathing of pure oxygen. Total lung capacity (TLC) is the total volume of air in the lungs at full inflation, and residual volume (RV) is the volume of air remaining in the lungs after a complete expiration. Measurements using these methods are not reliable in the presence of severe airway obstruction and abnormal

distribution of inspired air, since they may underestimate true lung volume. A more accurate way of determining FRC is by plethysmography. An increase in RV is seen with airway obstruction of any cause but is most marked in emphysema or during an acute attack of asthma. Reductions in TLC are seen with pulmonary fibrosis resulting from sarcoidosis, scleroderma or fibrosing alveolitis, neuromuscular disease, skeletal deformities, and space-occupying lesions within the chest.

PHYSIOLOGIC DEAD SPACE AND VENOUS-ADMIXTURE-LIKE EFFECT ($\dot{V}/\dot{Q}$ ABNORMALITIES)

When arterial blood samples are drawn in conjunction with the collection and analysis of expired air, physiologic dead space and venous-admixture-like effect may be calculated. Physiologic dead space is the portion of each inspiration that fails to take part in gas exchange in the lung. It includes the anatomic dead space (volume of the conducting airways) and a portion of the inspired air that ventilates underperfused or nonperfused alveoli (high $\dot{V}/\dot{Q}$ ratio). Abnormally large values may be found in any disease characterized by nonuniform involvement of the lung, especially those in which vascular occlusion or obliteration is a feature. Venous-admixture-like effect is the portion of cardiac output that is effectively shunted from right to left because of blood flow through poorly ventilated areas of lung (low $\dot{V}/\dot{Q}$ ratio). It is abnormally increased in a variety of lung diseases and therefore has little value in differential diagnosis.

COMPLIANCE AND AIRWAY RESISTANCE

More direct methods than those discussed are available for measuring the mechanical properties of the lungs. Pulmonary compliance, defined as the number of liters change in static lung volume produced by a 1 cm H_2O change in transpulmonary (alveolar minus intrapleural) pressure, is a measure of the distensibility of the lungs. The measurement of transpulmonary (elastic recoil) pressure at functional residual capacity and at full lung inflation may be useful in the diagnosis of several diseases. For example, there is a loss of recoil in emphysema and an increase in recoil in interstitial fibrosis.

Airway resistance is the pressure difference in centimeters of water between alveoli and mouth required to produce an inspiratory or expiratory flow rate of 1 L/sec. These studies are technically much more complex than spirometry and are seldom available on a routine basis but are valuable investigative tools and are occasionally helpful in an individual clinical problem.

FLOW VOLUME LOOPS

These measurements of airflow allow one to determine whether the limitation of airflow is during inspiration, expiration, or both. Inspiratory flow patterns are predominantly affected by extrathoracic (upper) airway obstruction as seen in laryngeal cancer or paralyzed vocal cords.[9]

EXERCISE TESTING

Measurement of ventilation parameters and gas exchange during exercise can help to define the contributions of lung and heart disease in patients with combined disabilities. Determination of arterial blood gases during exercise can also show whether significant arterial hemoglobin desaturation is occurring, indicating the need for supplemental oxygen.[18]

MUSCLE STRENGTH MEASUREMENTS

Respiratory muscle strength may be reduced in neurologic or neuromuscular disease.[5] Diminished strength, fatigue, or poor mechanical advantage can contribute, however, to reduced pulmonary performance in patients with increased respiratory loads, such as pulmonary emphysema and pulmonary fibrosis, or reduced muscle mass, such as with malnutrition. On occasion acute isometric measurements may not reveal inspiratory or expiratory muscle weakness in the presence of muscle fatigue from inadequate energy stores or sustained loads. Inspiratory muscle strength is most frequently measured by performing a maximal static inspiratory effort from resting or residual lung volume against an obstructed mouthpiece with a small leak to minimize oral pressure artifacts. Expiratory force may similarly be measured from total lung capacity for an overview of muscle strength. Detection of muscle fatigue often requires repetitive measurements over some period of time.

SLEEP STUDIES

Sleep-related breathing disorders may be diagnosed by measuring airflow at the mouth and nose simultaneously with thoracic cage and abdominal movements in the sleeping patient. Absence of airflow with continuing respiratory efforts suggests upper airway obstruction, while absence of airflow and respiratory efforts suggests a central respiratory disorder (see Chapter 3.7).[12]

NONRESPIRATORY FUNCTIONS OF THE LUNG

The respiratory system, like the integument and the gastrointestinal system, provides an interface between the organism and the environment. Although the primary role of the respiratory tract is gas exchange, it also performs a number of important nonrespiratory functions: air filtration and conditioning; synthesis of important proteins, lipids, and inflammatory and modulatory molecules; metabolism of drugs, hormones, and other natural products; and maintenance of the integrity of the organism from the external environment. These processes are finely regulated, and it appears that upset of this balance in the direction of either deficiency or excess can be harmful.

AIR FILTRATION AND CONDITIONING

Under normal conditions at rest, the nasal mucosa and nasopharynx perform the major part of filtering and conditioning inspired air. Because the nasal cavity narrows in the region of the turbinates, the airstream is accelerated and flow becomes turbulent. These forces cause most particles above 10 μm in diameter to deposit on the nasal mucosa. At the same time, the nasal mucosa conditions and humidifies the inspired air so that air delivered to the lower bronchi and alveoli is at body temperature and fully saturated with water. At rest, such conditioning occurs in the nasopharynx and the first few generations of airways. If an individual breaths in frigid air ($-17C$) while exercising and increases his total ventilation from a resting value of 7.5 to 60 L/min, conditioning of inspired air is incomplete so that at the sixth or seventh generation airways, the inspired air temperature is approximately $27C$.[2] The consequences of heating and humidifying inspired air appear important in the pathogenesis of exercise-induced asthma.

Particles of respirable size (0.5 to 3 μm) remain suspended until they reach the terminal and respiratory bronchioles, where they are deposited on the airway surface because of gravitational forces. This and other physical factors play an important role in determining the pattern of injury by various inhaled substances. Particulate material, such as organic dusts (silica), allergens, and infectious agents, deposit largely according to size as described previously. The degree of penetration to lower bronchial generations, however, depends on many factors such as the concentration of agent, the pattern of breathing (nose or mouth), and velocity (inspiratory flow rate) and amount (minute ventilation) of air inspired. The design of inhaled therapeutic agents must also take

these factors into consideration. Agents whose target are the bronchial tree (e.g., most bronchodilators) should be between 3 and 10 μm, while agents must be between 0.5 and 3 μm to have any hope of reaching terminal bronchioles, and perhaps alveolar structures.

STRUCTURAL ELEMENTS

Supporting structures of lung parenchyma include collagen (60 to 70 percent), elastin (25 to 30 percent), glycosaminoglycans (<1 percent), and fibronectin (0.5 percent). Although the major structural element is collagen, elastin is responsible for the characteristic pressure-volume changes associated with lung inflation (see following discussion). Collagen performs a restraining function at high lung volumes. Exposure of lung tissue to elastase(s), such as that found in polymorphonuclear leukocytes, results in a destruction of elastin and a loss of lung elastic recoil. The destructive effect of such elastases may be amplified in patients with a genetic or acquired deficiency of the major elastase protease inhibitor, α-1-antitrypsin or α-1-antiprotease. The normal α-1-antiprotease phenotype is MM, while the most common phenotype associated with a deficiency of this inhibitor is termed "ZZ" and is associated both with premature emphysema and with juvenile cirrhosis in some patients.

Lung glycosaminoglycans come in two forms: hyaluronate and sulfated moieties. Although these molecules make up only a small portion of lung extracellular matrix and are usually very stable, they appear to play an important role in the synthetic and restructuring process that follows lung injury. Fibronectin, a serum protein synthesized by fibroblasts, endothelial cells, and macrophages, also appears important in the parenchymal response to lung injury. Fibronectin, termed a "competence" factor, appears to be important in the functioning of the extracellular cytoskeleton and to play a permissive role in fibroblast replication. Uncontrolled action of "competence" and "progression" factors such as alveolar macrophage derived growth factor (AMDGF), can result in fibroblast accumulation, such as that seen in granulomatous lung disorders.

The lung is lined with a surface active material important in maintaining alveolar stability at low lung volumes. This material, termed "surfactant," is primarily phospholipid, although protein components have also been identified. Surfactant is synthesized by type II pneumocytes. The major clinical condition associated with a deficiency of surfactant is the respiratory distress syndrome of the newborn.

The tracheobronchial tree is also lined with a mixture of other secretions. These segregate microscopically into a sol phase, which is adjacent to the surface of epithelial cells, and a gel phase, which is more superficial. These secretions are 2 to 5 μm thick and line the airways from alveoli to the trachea. Cilia beat in the aqueous sol phase. Protein components of these secretions include immunoglobulins (IgA, IgE, and IgG), albumin, α-1-antiprotease, α-1-antichymotrypsin, other protease inhibitors, α-2-macroglobulin, haptoglobulin, ceruloplasmin, transferrin, lysozyme, amylase, lactic dehydrogenase, kallikrein, peroxidase, β_{1c}-globulin, lactoferrin, hydroperoxidase, and mucous glycoproteins.

Mucous glycoproteins are a heterogeneous group of glycoproteins with O-linked glycosides attached to a protein core. This mucus layer is thought to provide an important protective function for the airways by physically and chemically preventing invasion of the airways by foreign agents, by providing a favorable environment for the action of immunoglobulins and cilia, and by providing an effective transport system for aspirated materials (with the mucociliary apparatus). Kartagener syndrome, characterized by situs inversus, paranasal sinusitis, and bronchiectasis, is associated with ciliary dysmotility and impaired mucociliary transport because of a disordered microtubular arrangement and an absence of normal dynein arms in the cilia. This disorder appears to be associated with a more generalized dysfunction of cilia and often includes sterility in men and chronic bronchitis and otitis media; it has been referred to as the "immotile cilia syndrome."

METABOLIC FUNCTIONS

The lung is involved in the generation and metabolism of a wide variety of locally active substances such as hormones, which are known as "autacoids."

A wide variety of normal lung cells produce biologically active substances, including biogenic amines such as histamine; peptides such as bradykinin; lipids derived from arachidonic acid such as prostaglandin $F_{2\alpha}$, thromboxane A_2, leukotrienes C_4, D_4, and E_4 (slow reacting substance of anaphylaxis), proinflammatory compounds with spasmogenic properties; leukotriene B_4, which is chemotactic for polymorphonuclear leukocytes; prostaglandin E_2 and prostacyclin, which are vasodilators and can cause smooth muscle relaxation; phospholipids including the phospholipid components of surfactant and platelet activating factor; and immunoregulatory molecules including interferon and interleukins. Pulmonary tumors may secrete a wide variety of hormones including adrenocorticotropic hormone, antidiuretic hormone (arginine vasopressin), parathyroid hormone, gonadotropins, calcitonin, growth hormone, vasoactive intestinal peptide, glucagon- and insulin-like peptides, prolactin, serotonin, and prostaglandins.

The lung also metabolizes certain biologically active substances. Although it can rapidly transform angiotension I to angiotension II by means of a converting enzyme, the lung more commonly inactivates biologically active compounds. The lung rapidly clears or inactivates bradykinin, serotonin, prostaglandins E_2 and $F_{2\alpha}$, some leukotrienes, some steroids (e.g., testosterone), adenosine triphosphate, and adenosine diphosphate. While these metabolic functions serve to regulate the immediate environment of the lung, they also have the potential to prevent potentially harmful compounds from entering the systemic circulation.

PULMONARY DEFENSE MECHANISMS INCLUDING INFLAMMATION AND REPAIR

Defense mechanisms of the lung include barrier and clearance properties provided by respiratory mucus and the mucociliary escalator; phagocytic, metabolic, and digestive functions provided by alveolar macrophages and recruited polymorphonuclear leukocytes; and specific immunologic defenses provided by antigen processing cells and lymphocytes.

Alveolar macrophages play a central role in pulmonary defense mechanisms. These cells isolate invading organisms and material by phagocytosis; transport ingested materials; destroy ingested materials by oxidation, proteolysis, and hydrolysis; and prepare antigen for presentation to T lymphocytes. In addition, they appear to coordinate the resolution of the inflammatory process, including the process of repair. Such processes appear to be finely regulated, and this regulation of the pulmonary immune process seems to differ from the systemic immune response. For example, cellular immune responses of the lung appear blunted when compared to systemic (i.e., splenic) responses. Teleologically, such a system is beneficial to the host in avoidance of infection as well as the consequences of uncontrolled pulmonary inflammation.

Uncontrolled pulmonary inflammation is probably important in the pathogenesis of a number of interstitial lung diseases. This view is supported by studies that have used the technique of bronchoalveolar lavage. The pattern of cells obtained in lavage fluid appears to represent or mark particular classes of disease processes. These include the systemic granulomatous disease; sarcoidosis, in which increased numbers of T lymphocytes have been observed in lung lavage fluid from patients with active disease; and idiopathic (i.e., cause unknown) pulmonary fibrosis, in which increased numbers of polymorphonuclear leukocytes have been observed. The finding of a particular pattern of cells cannot, in general, estab-

lish a particular diagnosis (an exception may be histiocytosis X); however, it can provide important supportive evidence.

EVALUATION OF NONRESPIRATORY FUNCTIONS OF THE LUNG

Derangement of the nonrespiratory processes of the lung often leads to disease, as examples cited earlier have shown. Disorders of "nonrespiratory" lung function, however, often come to light because of their impact on gas exchange properties of the lung. The lung, like most organs, responds to insult or injury in a limited number of ways. For example, the airways react to insult via two major mechanisms: mucus hypersecretion (chronic bronchitis) or narrowing (obstructive lung disease). Obstructive lung diseases lead to hyperinflation of the lungs and can be due to smooth-muscle hypertrophy and contraction (bronchial asthma) or to destruction of elastic elements of the lung (emphysema). Numerous agents attack the interstitial components of the lung. These may be infectious (as in a viral pneumonia), toxic (as in exposure to various dusts), or immunologic (as in connective tissue diseases), and may be associated with either lymphocytic (e.g., sarcoidosis) or neutrophilic (e.g., idiopathic pulmonary fibrosis) alveolitis. Interstitial lung diseases lead to a restrictive function and difficulty with gas exchange, often manifested by a decrease in the diffusing capacity.

Table 3.1–2 lists a number of useful tests for the differential diagnosis of pulmonary disease. While several disorders listed require special tests to confirm a suspected diagnosis, other diagnoses are a byproduct of the physical examination and routine laboratory studies (e.g., Kartagener syndrome with situs inversus). A number of other readily available, standard tests include detailed serological evaluation for patients with a suspected connective tissue disease, an L/S ratio on amniotic fluid for fetuses at high risk for

premature birth, and sweat chloride test for patients suspected of having cystic fibrosis. The diagnosis of α-1-antitrypsin (α-1-antiprotease) deficiency can be suspected on clinical grounds (premature emphysema, often of the lower lobes), and confirmed by serum protein electrophoresis showing a flat α-globulin region. This protein is an acute phase reactant and can increase, particularly in heterozygotes, during times of stress. More definitive information can be obtained with a quantitative measurement of the protein or, preferably, a protease inhibitor (Pi) typing.

Many immunodeficiency states can be diagnosed in part by quantitative measurement of immunoglobulins. These include disorders associated with an increased quantity of immunoglobulin, such as the hyperimmunoglobulin E state. Lymphocytes subtyping, particularly in patients with helper (T_4) and suppressor (T_8), phenotypes, is available in most medical centers now that the deficiency of helper T lymphocytes in patients with the acquired immune deficiency syndrome has been recognized. Skin testing to determine in vivo response to various antigens often provides information that cannot be obtained from in vitro methods. The presence of immediate skin test reactivity has been a valuable tool in the diagnosis and treatment of airborne allergic disease; the immediate skin test response to *Aspergillus* spp. is positive in over 95 percent of patients with allergic bronchopulmonary aspergillosis. Results of delayed skin testing may also be useful; however, they rarely provide more than supporting data.

Almost all asthmatics show an increase in nonspecific bronchial responsiveness to nonspecific agents such as histamine and methacholine. Although the diagnosis of bronchial asthma is made clinically, inhalation challenge testing may confirm an impression of bronchial hyperresponsiveness or aid in exploring possible precipitants such as exercise, cold air, and environmental or occupational agents.

Bronchoalveolar lavage is a useful adjunct to bronchoscopy in several clinical settings, including the diagnosis of infections in

TABLE 3.1–2. EVALUATION OF "NONRESPIRATORY" FUNCTIONS OF THE LUNG

Test	Disease
History	
Physical examination	
Routine laboratory examination	
• Hematology	
• Chemistries	
• ECG	
• Chest roentgenograph	Situs inversus (Kartagener syndrome)
• Routine pulmonary function testing	
Serological evaluation (ANA, C_3, C_4, CH_{50}, rheumatoid factor)	Connective tissues disorders
Lecithin/Sphingomyelin (L/S) ratio	Respiratory distress syndrome of the newborn
Sweat chloride	Cystic fibrosis
Serum protein electrophoresis	Alpha-1-antitrypsin deficiency
• Alpha-1-antiprotease quantitation	Alpha-1-antitrypsin deficiency
• Protease inhibitor (Pi) typing	Alpha-1-antitrypsin deficiency
Quantitative immunoglobulin determination	Immunodeficiency states, dysgammaglobulinemias
Lymphocyte subtyping	Acquired immunodeficiency syndrome and related disorders
Skin testing	
• Immediate	Atopic status, allergic bronchopulmonary aspergillosis
• Delayed	Sarcoidosis (anergy)
Special pulmonary function tests	
• Inhalation challenge (histamine, methacholine, antigen, exercise, cold air, occupational agents)	Bronchial asthma, particulary with unusual precipitants
Bronchoalveolar lavage	Infections (special stains, culture), interstitial lung diseases (cell count and differential), foreign matter (particles as with asbestos exposure), research tool
Biopsy	Infections, pulmonary alveolar proteinosis, ciliary dysfunction syndromes (ciliary structure by electron microscopy)

immunocompromised hosts. Its use to obtain cells to diagnose an ongoing "alveolitis" or to document exposure to an occupational agent (such as asbestos) is primarily a research tool, as are techniques to measure alveolar macrophage production of factors such as interleukins and fibronectin. Such procedures are safe, however, and relatively noninvasive and promise to provide important information concerning the pathogenesis of numerous diseases of the lungs. Finally, special handling of biopsy specimens, such as electron microscopic study of cilia, may be useful in selected cases.

EVALUATION OF TISSUE AND CELLS

THORACENTESIS

This technique is used in the evaluation of pleural effusion. Indications and interpretation of results are discussed in Chapter 3.4. It should be noted that thoracentesis involves some risk of lung injury or induction of pneumothorax and should be performed with close attention to proper technique.

BRONCHOSCOPY

The development of the flexible fiberoptic bronchoscope has greatly enhanced the capability of bronchoscopy and has broadened the diagnostic and therapeutic indications for its use[8] (Table 3.1-3). The conventional rigid bronchoscope is excellent for removal of foreign bodies or tenacious secretions. The fiberop-

TABLE 3.1-3. INDICATIONS FOR BRONCHOSCOPY

Indication	Comments
Diagnostic	
Hemoptysis	Best performed when bleeding has almost stopped
Chronic unexplained cough	May be early manifestation of endobronchial tumor
Undiagnosed mass	Transbronchial biopsy may be performed
Delayed resolution of pneumonia	Excludes bronchial obstruction as cause
Localized atelectasis	Identify cause of bronchial obstruction if present
Evaluate operability in lung cancer	Extent of proximal endobronchial spread or peribronchial compression or fixation can be assessed
Positive sputum cytology with negative x-ray	Fiberoptic scope will permit localization of nearly all occult lung cancer
Lung abscess	Exclude bronchial obstruction, obtain material for culture
Tracheal extubation	Evaluate trauma to airway resulting from intubation
Therapeutic	
Control of hemorrhage	Endobronchial lesion may occasionally be cauterized
Removal of foreign body	Rigid bronchoscope preferred
Lobar atelectasis in patient on respirator	Aspiration of secretions through bronchoscope permits reexpansion
Lung abscess which drains poorly	Repeated endoscopy may promote drainage

tic bronchoscope permits visualization of bronchial orifices beyond the level of subsegmental bronchi. The optical system produces magnification of the image so that excellent detail is visible even in very small airways. The flexible shaft makes it ideally suited for patients with cervical spine abnormalities or displacement of the trachea. A number of brushes, curettes, and microbiopsy forceps devised for use with the fiberoptic bronchoscope have extended the range over which diagnostic information can be obtained. Under fluoroscopic guidance these devices can be placed into a small lesion in the periphery of the lung.

The lowest risk is achieved when bronchoscopy is performed under topical anesthesia, which is satisfactory for most procedures. In anxious or uncooperative patients, or when a very lengthy procedure is required, general anesthesia is more satisfactory.

BRONCHOALVEOLAR LAVAGE

Cells and proteins found in the small airways and alveolar structures may be sampled by instilling, aspirating, and then examining sterile saline solutions introduced via a fiberoptic bronchoscope.[13] Changes in the normal percentages of cells may suggest both the type and activity of diseases, such as sarcoidosis, idiopathic interstitial fibrosis, or hypersensitivity pneumonitis. Lavage is also helpful in diagnosing opportunistic infections in immune compromised hosts.

BIOPSY PROCEDURES

When a definitive diagnosis cannot be established by simpler means, it is often necessary to obtain tissue for microscopic examination. A wide variety of biopsy procedures are potentially useful in obtaining suitable tissue from the lung, bronchi, pleura, or mediastinum, and it is important to select the procedure with the lowest risk and greatest likelihood of recovering material that will be diagnostic. Table 3.1-4 provides information regarding the selection of a specific biopsy procedure depending on the nature and location of the lesion.

Bronchial Biopsies
During the course of diagnostic bronchoscopy with either rigid or fiberoptic instruments, any visible endobronchial lesion or abnormal-appearing area of bronchial mucosa will be biopsied. Various types of biopsy forceps are available for this purpose, and the biopsy may be performed under direct vision. Larger fragments of tissue can be obtained through the rigid bronchoscope, but various-sized microforceps and curettes suitable for use with the fiberoptic instrument often yield satisfactory tissue specimens.[11] Biopsy of normal-appearing bronchial mucosa will sometimes provide histologic confirmation of the diagnosis of pulmonary sarcoidosis. Biopsy of spurs proximal to the origin of a peripheral carcinoma is useful in establishing the presence or absence of mucosal and submucosal spread of the tumor.

Brush Biopsy
This procedure, either under direct vision through the bronchoscope or under fluoroscopic guidance, is a very valuable technique because of the low incidence of complications. Tissue fragments adhering to the stiff nylon brush may provide a specific diagnosis of infection, by smear or culture, or may permit a diagnosis of tumor on cytologic or histologic examination. If a localized lesion can be adequately seen in two projections under the fluoroscope, a brush biopsy can be obtained even when the lesion is too peripheral to be seen directly with fiberoptic bronchoscopy. The diagnostic yield from such biopsies is approximately 85 percent in bronchogenic carcinoma; a diagnosis of Hodgkin disease, *Pneumocystis* pneumonia, tuberculosis, or fungus infection can also be made by this technique.

TABLE 3.1–4. NONTHORACOTOMY BIOPSY TECHNIQUES

Type of Lung Disease	Procedures	Indications
Diffuse parenchymal	Transcatheter bronchial brush biopsy	Most helpful in acute infections
	Bronchoscopy, open tubed or fiberoptic (FOB) with brushing, washing and biopsy	Best procedure with least risk for acute or chronic disease
	Needle biopsy (cutting)	Ability to tolerate pneumothorax. No pulmonary hypertension.
	Mediastinoscopy	With hilar adenopathy
Localized	Pleural biopsy	With pleural effusion
Peripheral	Transcatheter bronchial brush biopsy or FOB with brushing and biopsy	Ability to visualize lesion in two planes on fluoroscopy. Excellent for cancer. Good for infectious infiltrates.
	Aspiration needle biopsy, cutting if aspiration unproductive	Obstructed bronchus preventing endoscopic diagnosis (common with larger lesions). Ability to visualize lesion in two planes. Denser lesions yield larger specimens.
Midlung	FOB with brushing, washing, and biopsy	Fluoroscope usually not necessary with FOB
	Mediastinoscopy	With lesions ≥3 cm in diameter or questionable hilar node involvement, or when tumor is known to be large cell undifferentiated carcinoma
Central	Rigid bronchoscopy, FOB on standby	Should yield diagnosis in almost all cases of epidermoid carcinoma
	Mediastinoscopy	Necessary for staging and determination of operability in all cases
	Transbronchial needle aspiration	For staging and determination of operability of cancer

Transbronchial Lung Biopsy

Tissue may be obtained through the bronchoscope by wedging a small biopsy forceps into the lung parenchyma. In diffuse disease, lung tissue can be recovered in most instances and is usually sufficient to provide a tissue diagnosis (see Chapter 3.5). In the case of a localized lesion in the periphery of the lung, fluoroscopic guidance will be required. Complications such as hemoptysis and pneumothorax are infrequent but occur more commonly with this technique than with simple bronchial brushing. The yield is substantially higher with transbronchial biopsy in most types of diffuse disease.

Transbronchial Needle Aspiration

Recently a needle has been developed for use with the fiberoptic bronchoscope to puncture the walls of the trachea or a major bronchus.[17] This allows for sampling of mediastinal, hilar, and subcarinal lymph nodes in the staging of lung cancer (see Chapter 3.3).

Pleural Biopsy

Percutaneous needle biopsy of the pleura is a simple and safe procedure in the presence of pleural effusion and is indicated whenever the etiology of an exudative effusion is not proven. This procedure is discussed further in Chapter 3.4. Pleuroscopy, or open biopsy of the pleura by means of a limited thoracotomy, will provide specimens of pleura when needle biopsy has failed and an etiologic diagnosis is mandatory.

Percutaneous Lung Biopsy

Biopsy through the chest wall under local anesthesia may be the procedure of choice for localized lesions near the pleural surface and in some patients with diffuse lung disease.[3] A plain needle for aspiration of tissue and a cutting needle have both been used for this purpose. In general, the aspiration technique should be tried for solid lesions and the cutting needle used only if aspiration is not successful. The cutting needle will be necessary in patients with diffuse disease. An experienced operator may achieve a high percentage of definitive diagnoses in patients with malignancy or inflammatory disease. The chief complication is pneumothorax, which occurs in 20 percent of cases but requires insertion of a chest tube in only about 10 percent. Hemoptysis is common but is rarely serious, and intrapleural bleeding is rare.

MEDIASTINOSCOPY

Endoscopic examination of the mediastinum is performed under general anesthesia through a small skin incision at the suprasternal notch.[3] Visualization and biopsy of abnormal tissue in the area around the trachea, carina, and proximal right mainstem bronchus can be carried out. The left lower paratracheal and left mainstem bronchus area cannot be visualized by this technique. Risk of the procedure is little more than the risk associated with general anesthesia.

Mediastinoscopy is most useful in the evaluation of resectability in the patient with lung cancer (see Chapter 3.9). Positive nodes along the trachea or on the side opposite the primary lesion preclude resection for cure. In the case of positive lower mediastinal hilar nodes on the side of the primary, some surgeons will attempt resection if the lesion is a squamous carcinoma. Bronchogenic carcinoma presenting as a centrally located mass will show mediastinal node involvement in nearly half of all cases. Small cell carcinoma has an even higher rate of spread to mediastinal nodes, and mediastinoscopy is often required to establish a diagnosis. Since small cell carcinoma is usually not a resectable lesion, mediastinoscopy is not indicated for staging when the cell type is already known. Peripherally located squamous and adenocarcinomas are less likely to involve mediastinal nodes than are centrally located primary tumors. Mediastinal involvement with large cell carcinoma is common, regardless of the location of the primary.

Mediastinoscopy is also useful in the diagnosis of sarcoidosis, tuberculosis, histoplasmosis, and Hodgkin disease, since these conditions commonly involve mediastinal lymph nodes. This procedure has a high yield in sarcoidosis and should be considered when no skin lesions are present and peripheral lymph nodes appear uninvolved.

Previous mediastinoscopy is one of the few firm contraindications to mediastinoscopy, since adhesions make an adequate dissection difficult or impossible. Superior vena cava obstruction is not a contraindication but requires particular care in the initial incision and subcutaneous dissection.

DIAGNOSTIC THORACOTOMY

Transbronchial or percutaneous lung biopsy may be unsuccessful or contraindicated in a significant number of patients with an undi-

agnosed pulmonary lesion. In this and certain other specific situations, open thoracotomy may be required for diagnosis.

The solitary peripheral nodule may present such a situation (see Chapter 3.3). When old and recent radiographic findings seem to indicate tumor presence, excisional biopsy is usually called for. This is especially true when the abnormality is too small or poorly seen for needle biopsy under fluoroscopy. A full posterolateral thoracotomy is usually performed and the area in question examined under direct vision. Biopsies may be taken for frozen section; the extent of the disease can be accurately evaluated, and, if appropriate, definitive resection may be undertaken.

When a solitary nodule appears unlikely to represent a tumor, every effort should be made to establish a diagnosis short of thoracotomy. Percutaneous needle biopsy or transbronchial biopsy may succeed in proving such a lesion to be inflammatory.

Another common indication for open-lung biopsy is in the patient with diffuse parenchymal lung disease that is progressive and symptomatic. Although transbronchial or percutaneous biopsies are frequently positive, they are subject to considerable sampling error and may not provide a specimen that is fully representative of the disease process. When the process is acute and generalized, a lingular biopsy through a small anterior thoracotomy is a satisfactory procedure and offers the advantages of low risk and minimal postthoracotomy discomfort. When there are multiple areas of involvement that appear by radiograph to differ in age or structure, the thoracotomy should permit inspection of a whole lung as well as biopsy of areas representing the most recently involved and the most severely involved and areas appearing relatively normal.

A third situation in which open-lung biopsy is preferred is in the patient with leukemia, lymphoma, or other systemic disease who develops an acute pulmonary infiltrate while taking high-dose steroids and cytotoxic chemotherapeutic agents. In many of these patients it is essential that a definitive diagnosis be established without delay so that appropriate therapy may be instituted. Transbronchial or needle biopsy techniques occasionally provide too little tissue for frozen sections and may be found to be inadequate after the delay required for permanent sections. Many such patients will be found to have two or more complicating infections at the same time, and under these circumstances small biopsy samples may be seriously misleading. Because of simplicity and low morbidity, however, transbronchial lung biopsy is usually attempted before diagnostic thoracotomy in the majority of immune compromised patients developing acute diffuse lung disease.

REFERENCES

1. Alderson PO: The roles of radionuclide studies in the diagnosis of pulmonary disease. In Siegelman SS (ed): Pulmonary System: Practical Approaches to Pulmonary Diagnosis. New York, Grune & Stratton, 1979
2. Alderson PO, Ruyanavech N, Secker-Walker RH: The role of ^{133}Xe ventilation studies in the scintigraphic detection of pulmonary embolism. Radiology 120:633, 1976
3. Baker RR, Stitik FP, Summer WR: Preoperative evaluation of patients with suspected bronchogenic carcinoma. Curr Probl Surg 1, December 1974
4. Campbell EJM, Agostoni E, Davis JN (eds): The Respiratory Muscles: Mechanics and Neural Control. Philadelphia, Saunders, 1970
5. Derenne J, Macklem PT, Russos C: The respiratory muscles: Mechanics, control, and pathophysiology. Am Rev Respir Dis 118:119, 1978
6. Epstein RL: Constituents of sputum: A simple method. Ann Intern Med 77:259, 1972
7. Line BR, Fulmer JD, et al: Gallium-67 citrate scanning in the staging of idiopathic pulmonary fibrosis: Correlation with physiologic and morphologic features and bronchoalveolar lavage. Am Rev Respir Dis 118:355, 1978
8. Marici FN: The flexible fiberoptic bronchoscope. In Johnston RF (ed): Pulmonary Care. New York, Grune & Stratton, 1973
9. Miller RD, Hyatt RE: Obstructive lesions of the larynx and trachea: Clinical and physiologic characteristics. Mayo Clin Proc 44:145, 1969
10. Olsen GN, Block AJ, et al: Pulmonary function evaluation of the lung resection candidate: A prospective study. Am Rev Respir Dis 111:379, 1975
11. Parks RD: Bronchial brushing and transbronchial biopsy. In Johnston RF (ed): Pulmonary Care. New York, Grune & Stratton, 1973
12. Phillipson EA: Control of breathing during sleep. Am Rev Respir Dis 118:909, 1978
13. Reynolds HY, Newball HH: Analysis of proteins and respiratory cells obtained from human lungs by bronchial lavage. J Lab Clin Med 84:559, 1974
14. Siegelman SS: Computed tomography. In Siegelman SS (ed): Pulmonary System: Practical Approaches to Pulmonary Diagnosis. New York, Grune & Stratton, 1979
15. Siegelman SS, Zerhouni EA, et al: CT of the solitary pulmonary nodule. Am J Roentgenol 135:1, 1980
16. Turino GM: The lung parenchyma—A dynamic matrix. J Burns Amberson lecture. Am Rev Respir Dis 132:1324, 1985
17. Wang KP, Marsh BR, et al: Transbronchial needle aspiration for diagnosis of lung cancer. Chest 80:48, 1981
18. Wasserman K, Whipp BS: Exercise physiology in health and disease. Am Rev Respir Dis 112:321, 1975
19. West JB: Pulmonary Pathophysiology—The Essentials. Baltimore, Williams & Wilkins, 1977

CHAPTER 3.2
Localized Pulmonary Infiltration

E. James Britt, Robert A. Wise, and J.T. Sylvester

Localized pulmonary infiltrates are defined as radiodensities within the lung parenchyma that involve only a portion of the lung and that cannot be classified as mass lesions. The distinction between localized infiltrate and mass lesion is sometimes difficult and is based upon the more distinct borders and quasispherical shape of the latter. The causes of mass lesions (see Chapter 3.3) should always be kept in mind when evaluating the etiology of an apparent localized pulmonary infiltrate. Orientation of this and many of the succeeding chapters of this section around roentgenographic findings rather than a symptom or a physical finding emphasizes the importance of the chest radiograph in the management of lung diseases. The chest radiograph may be obtained because of a symptom or physical finding or as a primary screening examination. The history and physical examination often must be interpreted in light of the chest radiograph, rather than the other way around. The general approach to interpretation of the chest radiograph is discussed in Chapter 3.1.

Lung infiltrates may be classified as alveolar, interstitial, or cavitary. Alveolar infiltrates are homogeneous. Sometimes multiple rosettes several millimeters in diameter are seen at the border of these infiltrates. The presence of such rosettes, thought to represent acinar shadows, is pathognomonic for alveolar disease. Air bronchograms are frequently present. Alveolar infiltrates are found in diseases in which alveoli are filled with edema fluid, cells, blood,

or other foreign material. Common causes of alveolar infiltrates are pulmonary edema, bacterial pneumonia, and pulmonary infarction.

An interstitial infiltrate appears as fine lines (reticular) or dots less than 3 mm in diameter (nodular) or both lines and dots (reticulonodular). This type of infiltrate is associated with diseases in which the predominant pathologic process is in the interstitium of the lung. Localized interstitial infiltrates are commonly caused by viral, mycobacterial, and fungal infections. Lymphangitic carcinomatosis, sarcoidosis, pneumoconiosis, interstitial pneumonitis, and hypersensitivity reactions usually cause diffuse interstitial infiltrates, but they may present with localized densities.

A cavity appears as an air density within an infiltrate. Cavitary infiltrates occur when a necrotizing process has caused sloughing of lung parenchyma, which is then expectorated, leaving a hole within the lung. Incomplete drainage of such a cavity may appear

as a linear air-fluid level that will change its orientation in decubitus views. Lucencies within an infiltrate do not always imply cavitation. For example, irregular resolution of a pneumonia or an infiltrate superimposed on pulmonary emphysema may produce multiple small radiolucencies that mimic a cavitary infiltrate. A list of causes of cavitary infiltrates is given in Table 3.2–1.

Localized infiltrates frequently produce a change in the volume of the lung previously occupied by air. A change in volume is shown by appropriate shifts of the fissures, diaphragms, mediastinum, or hila from their normal location. Decreases in volume are often seen in airway obstruction, pulmonary embolism, and in the healing stages of parenchymal inflammation. An increase in the volume of the lung associated with the infiltrate, classically seen in *Klebsiella pneumoniae* infection, is also commonly seen with the staphylococcal, mixed anaerobic, and type III *Streptococcus pneumo-*

TABLE 3.2–1. CAUSES OF PULMONARY CAVITATION

Condition	Radiologic Appearance	Characteristic Features
Specific Infection		
Primary lung abscess	Thick-walled cavity with surrounding infiltrate and air fluid level; frequently located in dependent lung zones	Copious foul sputum. Predisposing conditions: alcoholism, neurologic disease, or esophageal disease
Tuberculosis	Usually upper lobes. May be multiple. Wall usually 2–5 mm thick, contour smooth or irregular. Fibrosis and calcification common	Sputum almost invariably positive in untreated cases. Positive tuberculin skin test
Atypical mycobacteriosis	Indistinguishable from tuberculosis	Identification of atypical mycobacteria on culture. Common in AIDS population
Amebic abscess	Right lower lobe. Pleural effusions, empyema, or pleural adhesions may be present	Extension from hepatic abscess. Amebas may be present in stool and sputum
Fungal Diseases		
Coccidioidomycosis	Usually thin-walled cavity or no evidence of disease in surrounding lung. May be thick-walled, multiple, with fluid level and with extensive parenchymal disease	Occasional cough and hemoptysis, often asymptomatic. Sputum culture positive for *Coccidioides immitis*
Histoplasmosis	Simulates tuberculosis. Chronic fibrocavitary disease in apical or subapical regions	Elevated complement fixation titer. Positive sputum cultures for *Histoplasma capsulatum*
Aspergillosis	Intracavitary fungus ball (mycetoma)	Positive sputum culture for *Aspergillus*. Positive precipitins for *Aspergillus*. Secondary invasion of pre-existing cavity or cyst
Actinomycosis	Suppurative abscesses with widespread intrapulmonary consolidation. Most commonly involves lower lobes. Pleural involvement common	Chest wall sinuses, common. Cultures of sputum or sinus drainage positive. Sulfur granules in sputum
Cavitary Neoplasm		
Bronchogenic carcinoma	Irregular inner wall of cavity, eccentric cavitation	Cigarette smoking male over 40. Cough and hemoptysis. Sputum cytology positive
Metastatic carcinoma	Often multiple	Primary disease elsewhere may be evident. Usually squamous type
Lymphoma	Often multiple. May be associated with hilar node enlargement	Peripheral adenopathy usually present
Miscellaneous		
Silicosis or pneumoconiosis	Conglomerate masses with cavitation. Associated diffuse changes	Occupational history
Pulmonary infarction	Peripheral density, often with atelectasis	Secondary infection by contamination from bronchial tree or septic pulmonary embolism
Infected bronchogenic cyst	Usually single. May be close to carina or in peripheral lung field	Asymptomatic until infected. Symptoms usually chronic
Polyarteritis nodosa and Wegener granulomatosis	Often multiple nodules which cavitate	Evidence of extrapulmonary disease
Rheumatoid lung nodules with cavitation		Associated joint manifestations. Positive serologic test for rheumatoid disease
Caplan syndrome (rheumatoid arthritis) with pneumoconiosis of coal miners	Commonly occurs in lower lobes	Occupational history. Associated joint manifestations. Positive serologic test for rheumatoid disease
Sarcoidosis	Fibrotic infiltrate and hilar adenopathy	

niae infections. All of these infections may lead eventually to cavitation, which then heals with volume loss.

Thoracic adenopathy may occur in the hilar, anterior mediastinal, paratracheal, or subcarinal regions. Causes of thoracic adenopathy are listed in Table 3.2–2.

The presence of a *pleural effusion* associated with a localized infiltrate is found with neoplasia, bacterial infection, or pulmonary infarction. While radiographically nonspecific, pleural fluid is an important source of diagnostic material and therefore should carefully be sought, with additional decubitus views, if necessary.

CLINICAL EVALUATION

The clinical history should be directed toward identification of associated underlying conditions and environmental exposures and should attempt to identify the onset of the illness, its course, and the current state of the patient.

A history of associated conditions or exposures is important. Alcoholics frequently develop tuberculosis, lung abscess, aspiration pneumonia, and pneumonia due to the pneumococcus or *Klebsiella pneumoniae*. Diabetics are predisposed to bacterial pneumonia, tuberculosis, and fungal infections. Immunodeficiency due to neoplasm, steroid therapy, or chemotherapy is commonly complicated by infection with opportunistic organisms such as fungi, *Pneumocystis carinii*, and viruses. Homosexuals, drug addicts, and hemophiliacs have been recognized to be prone to the development of the acquired immunodeficiency syndrome (AIDS) and a resultant high incidence of *Pneumocystis carinii* pneumonia and *Mycobacterium avium-intracellulase* and cytomegalovirus infections, as well as other conditions associated with defects in cell-mediated immunity.[4,6] The patient with a bleeding disorder may develop spontaneous pulmonary hemorrhage with localized consolidation in the face of little or no hemoptysis. Aspiration pneumonia commonly occurs after loss of consciousness or cardiac arrest. A history of travel to an endemic area may suggest a specific diagnosis, such as coccidioidomycosis after travel in the southwestern United States. Exposure to parrots or parakeets may suggest psittacosis, while exposure to forest animals may suggest tularemia or pneumonic plague.

Constitutional symptoms are nonspecific but help to date the onset and progression of the illness. Fever suggests infection, but it may also be seen with neoplasms, sarcoidosis, and hypersensitivity pneumonitis. An illness of acute onset suggests bacterial pneumonia or pulmonary embolism, while an insidious onset suggests malignancy or mycobacterial infection.

Cough or a change in a chronic cough pattern may also help to date the onset of the illness. The character of the sputum may suggest a diagnosis. Malodorous sputum is typical of anaerobic infection. Hemoptysis commonly accompanies bronchogenic carcinoma, tuberculosis, bronchiectasis, bacterial infections, and pulmonary infarction.

Physical examination of the chest is not as helpful as the chest radiograph in the diagnosis of localized infiltrates. There are exceptions to this rule. Crackles may be heard early in pneumonia or pulmonary edema when the chest radiograph is normal. At times, using the chest radiograph, it may be difficult to differentiate a consolidated pneumonia from a localized pleural effusion. Increased sound transmission over an area of dullness is found with consolidation of lung, while decreased sound transmission over an area of dullness is characteristic of a localized pleural effusion.

The general physical examination may prove helpful in assessing the functional status of the patient as well as the cause of the infiltrate. The presence of cyanosis and the use of accessory muscles of respiration are clues that the disease process is seriously impairing respiration. Cachexia, adenopathy, poor dental hygiene, the absence of pharyngeal reflexes, and signs of cardiac disease and venous insufficiency are helpful findings that should be sought in every patient with a localized pulmonary infiltration.

DIFFERENTIAL DIAGNOSIS

Once the roentgenographic picture, history, physical examination, and clinical setting are assessed, the differential diagnosis of the pulmonary infiltrate may be approached by routinely considering a number of etiologic possibilities (Table 3.2–3). The pace of the evaluation will be determined in part by the condition of the patient. Individuals who are critically ill require that a firm diagnosis be established within hours. Presumptive diagnoses may be made and treatment begun before definitive confirmation is obtained. The immunosuppressed patient represents a special class of patient—extensive and rapid evaluation is necessary. In the stable, less critically ill patient, there may be ample time to obtain old radiographs and to await the results of specialized laboratory testing.

INFECTION

The first consideration is whether the infiltrate is caused by infection. Productive cough, purulent sputum, fever, rales, signs of

TABLE 3.2–2. CAUSES OF THORACIC ADENOPATHY

Disease	Comments
Sarcoidosis	Most common cause of bilateral hilar adenopathy. Paratracheal adenopathy common
Lymphoma	Frequently asymmetrical and involves the anterior mediastinum. One third of cases have associated pleural effusion
Bronchogenic carcinoma	Unilateral adenopathy is the presenting radiographic finding in 12%–35% of cases. Adenopathy in the radiographic absence of a primary lesion suggests small cell carcinoma
Acquired immuno-deficiency syndrome (AIDS)	Up to 8% of susceptible individuals symptomatic with *Pneumocystis* may present with adenopathy only
Primary tuberculosis	Adenopathy is virtually always present in children and frequent in adults. When present, it is usually asymmetrical
Histoplasmosis	Commonly occurs with primary infection in children and heals with calcification. Commonly asymmetrical
Tularemia	Hilar adenopathy, usually ipsilateral, occurs in approximately one third of pneumonic cases
Mycoplasma pneumoniae infection	Hilar adenopathy occurs in one fourth of childhood cases and uncommonly in adults
Pneumoconiosis	Hilar adenopathy common in silicosis, and uncommon in asbestosis and simple coal workers' pneumoconiosis
Idiopathic inflammatory lymphadenitis	Uncommon. Characteristic histopathology
Infectious mononucleosis	Uncommon
Erythema nodosum	This may be a *forme fruste* of sarcoidosis
Angioimmunoblastic lymphadenopathy	Generalized lymphadenopathy. Associated interstitial pneumonitis
Cystic fibrosis	Prominent cystic bronchiectasis

TABLE 3.2–3. DIFFERENTIAL DIAGNOSIS OF A LOCALIZED PULMONARY INFILTRATE

	Radiologic Appearance	Clinical Findings	Note
Malignancy			
Bronchogenic carcinoma	May present as pneumonia or infiltrate distal to a proximal obstructing lesion	Weight loss, anorexia, cough, hemoptysis in a smoker, paraneoplastic syndromes may provide a clue (see text)	Sputum cytology may be positive with proximal lesions
Bronchoalveolar cell carcinoma	Indolent segmental or lobar pneumonia	Copious thin mucoid sputum	
Hodgkin lymphoma	Parenchymal infiltrates occur only as a direct extension of mediastinal disease except in treated cases. Recurrent disease may occur as a solitary infiltrate usually outside of prior radiation fields	Painless, progressive enlargement of lymph nodes, splenomegaly, fever, weakness, pruritis	Reed–Sternberg cells have occasionally been identified in the sputum
Mechanical Obstruction			
Atelectasis	Linear or plate-like densities in dependent portions of lung	Common in postoperative and in other immobilized patients. Predisposing factors include hypoventilation, anesthesia, sedation, and analgesics	
Bronchopulmonary aspergillosis	Migratory infiltrates, evidence for mucoid impaction	Progressive or recurrent attacks of asthma in an individual with a longstanding history; fever and expectoration of brown mucus plugs	Positive skin test and precipitins against Aspergillus species. Elevated IgE level
Foreign body	Variable; hyperinflation with check valve phenomenon, atelectasis and collapse with complete obstruction	History of object in mouth, dental visit, poor dentition, etc. Right side most common because of straight right mainstem bronchus	Nonmetallic objects may not be radiopaque
Right middle lobe syndrome	Recurrent right middle lobe infiltrates	Historically, tuberculosis is most common; endobronchial tumor or foreign body must be ruled out[a]	Abnormal collateral ventilation may play a role (see text)
Bronchial adenoma	Localized infiltrate with atelectasis though chest film is often normal	Recurrent cough, hemoptysis, fever in a young adult	
Inhalation			
Aspiration pneumonia	Alveolar infiltrate with dependent zones or diffuse alveolar infiltrates	See text	See text
Suppurative lung abscess	Dense homogenous infiltrate progressing to cavitation with an air fluid level. Most commonly involves the superior segment of the right lower lobe	History of unconsciousness, alcoholism, seizure disorder, oropharyngeal suppuration, or copious foul sputum. Fever, weight loss and anemia	Anaerobic organisms cultured from transtracheal aspirate
Lipoid pneumonia	Chronic progressive lower lobe infiltrates may simulate lung mass	History of mineral oil use	Lipid-laden macrophages in sputum
Other materials Hydrocarbons Milk Near drowning	Either localized or diffuse alveolar infiltrates	Usually acute event with specific history	
Blood	Usually lower lobe infiltrates	Epistaxis, hematemesis or hemoptysis from any cause	Clears in 3–4 days
Embolic			
Pulmonary embolism	Segmental basal homogenous infiltrate which abuts the pleural surface	Sudden onset of dyspnea and pleuritic pain in an immobilized or predisposed patient	Subtle and variable presentations make a high index of suspicion necessary
Fat embolism	Diffuse infiltrates	Skeletal trauma, petechiae, mental confusion and respiratory distress	Fat globules in the urine have been described
Septic emboli	Multiple small infiltrates which cavitate	Suspect in intravenous drug abuse, pelvic inflammatory diseases, and in right-sided subacute infective endocarditis	Common staphylococcal etiology

(continued)

TABLE 3.2–3. DIFFERENTIAL DIAGNOSIS OF A LOCALIZED PULMONARY INFILTRATE (Continued)

	Radiologic Appearance	Clinical Findings	Note
Immunologic			
Systemic lupus erythematosus	Recurrent or migratory infiltrates	Negative sputum and blood cultures; other clinical evidence for active systemic lupus erythematosus	Caution: infection is still the most common cause of infiltrates in these patients
Rheumatoid arthritis	Predominantly affects lung bases	Middle-aged men more than women	High titer of rheumatoid factor
Dermatomyositis	Bibasilar infiltrates	Muscle weakness and skin rash	Hypoventilation and atelectasis, secondary to muscle weakness, aspiration, secondary to dysphagia and alveolitis all must be considered
Scleroderma	Bibasilar infiltrates		Aspiration must be considered because of esophageal involvement
Ankylosing spondylitis	Hyperinflation and upper lobe fibrotic and bullous disease	Clinically evident in young males more than females; chronic low back pain; spontaneous pneumothorax occurs	HLA-B27 associated
Goodpasture syndrome	Diffuse interstitial infiltrates	Dyspnea, hemoptysis, and hematuria in a young adult male	Antiglomerular basement membrane antibodies found
Idiopathic pulmonary hemosiderosis	Diffuse interstitial infiltrates	Iron deficiency, cough and dyspnea in children 10–12 yr old	No renal involvement
Wegener granulomatosis	Multiple round infiltrates with cavitation common	Sinusitis, hemoptysis, pleuritic chest pain, hematuria, and skin rash, 5th decade	A localized or limited form occurs
Other			
Radiation pneumonitis	Geometric infiltrate corresponding to radiation portal	Dry cough and dyspnea occurring days to 6 mo following treatment	Diagnostic change in sputum cytopathology has been described
Congenital: Bronchopulmonary sequestration	Cystic infiltrate in posterior segment of left lower lobe more than right lower lobe	History of prior abnormal chest film helpful	
Trauma	Focal infiltrate not always in area of trauma may be delayed 4–12 hr	History of blunt trauma to thorax	Progressive hypoxemia from 4–24 hr after insult
Pulmonary infiltrates with eosinophilia: Löffler syndrome	Transient migratory infiltrates		Ascariasis common, other parasites possible
Chronic eosinophilic pneumonia	Chronic peripheral infiltrates	Atopic individual: fever, malaise, cough, dyspnea for 1–2 mo	
Drug allergy	Patchy infiltrates	Nitrofurantoin, para-amino salicylic acid, tricyclic antidepressants, hydrochlorothiazide	

[a]Recurrent infiltrates in the same location suggest a proximal obstructing lesion. However, recurrent pneumonia, secondary to predisposing conditions, is most common.

consolidation, and leukocytosis increase the likelihood of infection. The Gram stain of the sputum may provide presumptive bacteriologic information. Cultures of the sputum and blood often provide confirmatory information. When pneumonia is evident clinically and cultures fail to provide a specific diagnosis, the primary atypical and more unusual causes of pneumonia must be considered. These include pneumonias caused by mycoplasma and organisms in the legionella group, chlamydia and rickettsial groups, and viruses. In some cases, recognition of these atypical causes will lead to a specific form of treatment. Occasionally, special culture and staining techniques and serologic studies and lung biopsy may be required. The diagnosis and treatment of pneumonia is fully discussed in Chapter 9.6.

MALIGNANCY

Next, consider malignancy. Bronchogenic carcinoma (see Chapter 6.22), the most common lung neoplasm, usually arises in the segmental bronchi. As a result, the radiologic manifestation of bronchogenic carcinoma may not be the mass itself but rather obstructive pneumonitis or atelectasis. A history of weight loss, malaise, anorexia, and progressive dyspnea in a patient who smokes suggests bronchogenic carcinoma. Recurrent small amounts of hemoptysis may also be evident. With a central lesion obstructing a bronchus, sputum cytology is likely to reveal malignant cells. Paraneoplastic syndromes, such as pulmonary osteoarthropathy, Cushing syndrome, and the syndrome of inappropriate ADH secretion, and

hypercalcemia also suggest carcinoma, as do neurologic signs of a cranial space-occupying lesion due to early metastasis.

Bronchoalveolar cell carcinoma is a well-differentiated adenocarcinoma originating from epithelial cells in the alveoli or terminal airways.[11] It accounts for 1 to 10 percent of all primary lung cancers and presents commonly as a persistent or poorly resolving solitary pulmonary infiltrate resembling a segmental or lobar pneumonia. It may also present as a well-circumscribed mass, single or multiple nodules, or in a diffuse form. Pleural effusion is found in 10 percent of cases. Cavitation is also described. One half of patients are asymptomatic when the lesion is first noticed. Chest pain, cough, dyspnea, and weight loss are common complaints in the remainder. The production of mucoid sputum in large quantities is suggestive of bronchoalveolar cell carcinoma. This symptom, however, is seen infrequently and only with extensive disease. Diffuse rales are striking on physical examination. Diagnosis, which is often delayed until other more common causes of localized infiltrates are excluded, is made by lung biopsy. Histologically, the tumor must be distinguished from metastatic adenocarcinoma.

Hodgkin disease may present as a localized pulmonary infiltrate, although the most common roentgenographic finding is hilar and mediastinal adenopathy. Pulmonary infiltration usually occurs as a direct extension of mediastinal involvement. After radiotherapy, this lymphoma may recur as a pulmonary infiltrate in the absence of adenopathy and is usually located in areas of lung not previously irradiated. Lung parenchymal involvement by non-Hodgkin lymphoma is present only when there is widespread systemic involvement. The disease is usually manifested as masses or nodules. Primary pulmonary lymphoma is uncommon.

BRONCHIAL OBSTRUCTION

Mechanical obstruction of a bronchus frequently causes loss of volume. The affected lung may appear as a localized area of increased radiodensity because of the crowding and consolidation of the normally translucent alveolar structures. Localized obstruction may result from a mucous plug, tumor, or foreign body.

Postoperative patients are subject to atelectasis secondary to mucous plugs. Impaired clearance of secretions and hypoventilation due to pain, anesthesia, and sedative and analgesic drugs are contributing factors. Dependent portions of the lung are most susceptible. Treatment of atelectasis should include suctioning, postural drainage, and encouragement to cough and inspire deeply.

Atelectasis secondary to mucous plugs may also occur in asthmatic individuals. Progressive or recurrent attacks of asthma in an individual with atopic history, accompanied by expectoration of brownish sputum and an occasional bronchial cast suggests *bronchopulmonary aspergillosis*. Migratory pulmonary infiltrates are common. Even the upper lobes may become atelectatic. Fever and eosinophilia are common. The diagnosis is established by the appropriate clinical picture, a positive *Aspergillus* skin test and serum precipitins, an elevated IgE level, and isolation of the organism from the sputum.

Bronchial adenoma is a tumor that frequently causes mechanical obstruction.[9] It is slow growing and has a low-grade malignant potential. It arises from the alveolar lining cells and is more common in women than in men and in individuals under age 40. The majority of patients present with symptoms of cough and hemoptysis. Treatment is surgical.

Foreign-body aspiration may also present as a localized infiltrate. Patients with obtundation, poor dentition, recent dental procedures, and seizure disorders are prone to aspiration. Bronchoscopy is both diagnostic and therapeutic.

Mechanical obstruction is a common cause of recurrent infiltrates in the same location. The "middle lobe syndrome" is recurrent middle lobe infiltrates or atelectasis, or both, thought to result from extrinsic compression of the middle lobe bronchus by peribronchial lymph nodes. In the past, tuberculosis was a common cause. Bronchogenic carcinoma is more common today. Surpris-

ingly, at bronchoscopy the middle lobe bronchus is patent in many cases. Recent observations suggest that collateral ventilation to the middle lobe is poor, rendering it more susceptible to collapse than other areas of lung.[8] Recurrent infiltrates may appear in the absence of obstruction, such as the recurrent pneumonias that occur in patients with alcoholism, diabetes, chronic sinusitis, congestive heart failure, bronchiectasis, and aspiration.[13]

EMBOLISM

Pulmonary thromboembolism may produce a pulmonary infiltrate and consolidation. The infiltrate may represent hemorrhage, edema, or tissue necrosis and is characteristically basilar and wedge-shaped, with its base against the pleural surface. *Fat embolism* must be considered in individuals suffering from skeletal trauma, who develop mental confusion, respiratory distress, severe hypoxia, and petechial hemorrhage in the skin.

ASPIRATION

Pathogenesis
Aspiration of foreign material into the lung also may cause localized pulmonary infiltrates. An example is aspiration of gastric contents.[1,2,14] The bronchial tree is normally protected from gastric aspiration by a series of barriers. The lower esophageal sphincter prevents reflux from the stomach. The height of the esophagus in the upright position serves as a hydrostatic barrier to reflux. The coordinated swallowing mechanism closes the epiglottis while clearing the oropharynx. Laryngeal reflexes cause glottic closure following mechanical or chemical irritation. An intact cough reflex clears the material from the tracheobronchial tree.

Any disruption of these barriers favors the aspiration of gastric or oropharyngeal contents. The most common disruption is sleep. Nearly half of normal subjects have been found to aspirate pharyngeal contents during sleep. Although this aspiration is apparently of little clinical consequence in healthy persons, it may be a significant threat to persons with underlying cardiac or pulmonary disease. Risk factors that predispose to aspiration are listed in Table 3.2–4.

When aspiration occurs, the major deposition occurs in the dependent zones of the lungs. For example, in the supine position, the superior segments of the lower lobes and the posterior segments of the upper lobes will be dependent. In the prone position the anterior segments of the upper lobes and the middle lobes will be at risk. In general, aspirated material is more likely to be deposited on the right side than the left.

Clinical Features
The clinical episode of aspiration is frequently not observed, and the patient may present with a catastrophic illness characterized by dyspnea, hypoxemia, hypotension, and alveolar pulmonary infiltrates that may be difficult to distinguish from acute myocardial infarction, pulmonary embolism, or overwhelming sepsis. Alternatively, the patient may present with unexplained fever, an infiltrate localized to the dependent lung zones, superimposed bacterial pneumonia, or unexplained deterioration in arterial oxygenation. Silent aspiration of gastric or oropharyngeal contents may be the most common cause of hospital-acquired pneumonia.

Historical features that suggest the possibility of aspiration include a history of prolonged or violent coughing spells following a meal or an episode of vomiting, but this history is often lacking. The diagnosis can be established with confidence if particulate matter is suctioned from the tracheobronchial tree. Although gastric acid is rapidly neutralized by tracheobronchial secretions and tissue, the finding of acidic fluid in the tracheal secretions supports the diagnosis. In addition, the bronchoscopic finding of diffuse bronchial mucosal erythema and edema extending to the subsegmental bronchi is compatible with the diagnosis of aspiration of

TABLE 3.2–4. RISK FACTORS FOR ASPIRATION

Impairment of Consciousness
  Anesthesia
  Alcoholism
  Seizure disorder
  Stroke
  Heroin addiction
  Coma
  Cardiac arrest

Impairment of Esophageal Function
  Esophageal stricture, benign or malignant
  Hiatus hernia, incompetent esophageal sphincter
  Achalasia
  Tracheoesophageal fistula
  Zenker diverticulum
  Nasogastric intubation

Impairment of Swallowing Mechanism
  Pseudobulbar palsy
  Tracheostomy
  Laryngeal carcinoma

Impairment of Cough Mechanism
  Neuromuscular weakness
  Local intratracheal anesthesia

Increased Bacterial Inoculum
  Periodontitis
  Tonsillar abscess
  Dental abscess
  Sinusitis

gastric contents. One should always keep in mind that illness, such as cerebrovascular insufficiency, acute myocardial infarction, and pulmonary embolism, can precede and induce aspiration of gastric contents.

Prognosis

The prognosis of aspiration pneumonia is variable. Some patients will succumb rapidly either from asphyxiation due to occlusion of the trachea or from acute overwhelming pulmonary edema, hypoxemia, and circulatory collapse. A second group of patients will develop lung infiltrates, which gradually clear over several weeks. A third group of patients shows initial improvement after the acute episode but succumbs to secondary infection. The mortality of aspiration pneumonia depends upon the type and quantity of aspirated material as well as the premorbid state.

Treatment

The initial therapy of aspiration of gastric contents should be directed toward securing patency of the airway with suctioning, intubation, and, if necessary, bronchoscopy. Supplemental oxygen should be administered to combat hypoxemia. If necessary, positive pressure ventilation should be applied. Positive end-expiratory pressure may be necessary to overcome hypoxemia and allow the use of nontoxic concentrations of inspired oxygen. Hemodynamic parameters should be closely monitored. Intravenous fluids should be administered to combat hypovolemia and hypotension.

Bacterial superinfection is common because of impairment of local pulmonary defense mechanisms. Infection acquired outside the hospital is commonly due to mixed aerobic and anaerobic organisms similar to those residing in the host's oropharynx. Infection acquired within the hospital frequently is caused by aerobic Gram-negative bacteria as well as mixed aerobic–anaerobic infections.[10] The diagnosis of superinfection is difficult because acid aspiration per se will cause a clinical picture similar to bacterial pneumonia. Antibiotic therapy should be guided by the results of sputum smears and cultures. Transtracheal aspiration is helpful in selected cases to obtain sputum for cultures uncontaminated by oropharyngeal flora. In general, antibiotics should be reserved for patients in whom aspiration is followed by progressive lung infiltrates, pu-

rulent sputum, or fever. Corticosteroids in pharmacologic doses have been long thought to be of benefit for acid aspiration, particularly if given early; however, the efficacy of such treatment is unproven.

Aspiration of gastric contents is frequently a preventable disease. Preventive measures include proper administration of tube feedings, maintenance of nasogastric tube patency, having susceptible patients sit upright during and after feeding, proper inflation of tracheostomy balloons, careful clearance of vomitus and pharyngeal secretions in patients with impaired consciousness during transport and hospitalization, positioning of unconscious or vomiting patients in the lateral decubitus or prone position, and meticulous anesthetic technique.

The lung is also vulnerable to aspiration of a variety of other foreign materials. *Lipoid pneumonia* is a chronic, slowly progressive infiltrate in the dependent lung zones caused by aspiration of mineral oil used as a stool softener or as a vehicle for nose drops. Hydrocarbon aspiration occurs commonly following ingestion of these substances and causes an acute diffuse alveolitis with pulmonary hemorrhage and edema. Hydrocarbons should not, in general, be lavaged from the stomach because of the risk of aspiration during the procedure. When aspirated into the trachea, food particles cause a granulomatous alveolitis with a subacute course over several days. Milk, commonly aspirated by children, causes an acute chemical bronchitis and pneumonitis. Near drowning may involve aspiration of gastric contents as well as water, and the clinical sequelae of the episode depend upon whether the water was contaminated, the duration of the submersion, and temperature of the water.

AUTOIMMUNE DISORDERS

Localized pulmonary infiltrates are seen in several *autoimmune disorders*.[7] While infection is still the most common cause of a pulmonary infiltrate in systemic lupus erythematosus, recurrent or migratory infiltrates or atelectasis are also characteristic of lung involvement in lupus. Dyspnea, high fever, and cough associated with hemoptysis and a bilateral alveolar filling process, and negative sputum and blood cultures suggest acute lupus pneumonitis. Apical pleural thickening and fibrosis may mimic the early infiltrate of tuberculosis in patients with ankylosing spondylitis. Pathologically, interstitial fibrosis is found. The presence of proximal muscle weakness or tenderness and erythematous rash should suggest polymyositis or dermatomyositis as a cause of bibasilar infiltrates. These infiltrates may result from a fibrosing alveolitis or from recurrent aspiration secondary to swallowing abnormalities associated with the disorder.

Goodpasture syndrome is characterized by pulmonary hemorrhage and renal failure. It occurs most commonly in young adult males. Diffuse infiltrates are more common than localized infiltrates. Antibodies directed against glomerular basement membrane can be found. Idiopathic pulmonary hemosiderosis appears to be a separate entity, more common in children under 10 years of age. Extensive alveolar infiltration may occur without clinically apparent hemoptysis. *Wegener granulomatosis* is a granulomatous vasculitis that presents most commonly in middle age. The chest radiograph will reveal rounded single or multiple infiltrates, which may be cystic or cavitary, although single nodules or localized infiltrates are reported. The illness presents with malaise and weakness, sinusitis, hemoptysis and pleuritic chest pain, skin rash, and hematuria. A limited form of the illness is also described. Therapy with cyclophosphamide has resulted in an improved prognosis for these patients.

OTHER

Bronchopulmonary sequestration is a *congenital malformation* in which a portion of a lobe fails to communicate with the normal

bronchial tree and receives its blood supply from a major systemic artery, usually the descending thoracic aorta. Bronchopulmonary sequestration is usually recognized as the result of pneumonia presenting radiographically, commonly as a cystic infiltrate in the posterior basilar bronchopulmonary segment of the left lower lobe, or less often in the corresponding location on the right. The diagnosis must be confirmed by identifying the blood supply to this segment by aortography. The importance of recognizing the abnormal blood supply derives from the intraoperative hazard of surgical resection when the abnormal blood supply is not appreciated.

Localized infiltrates in patients undergoing radiation therapy suggest *radiation pneumonitis*.[5] The infiltrate may appear 2 to 3 months following exposure, or as early as several days or as late as 6 months following treatment. The etiology is suggested by the sharp borders of the infiltrate, which correspond to the outline of the radiation port. Patients have nonproductive cough and dyspnea. Lung biopsy will reveal a pneumonitis showing endothelial damage, interstitial and alveolar edema, swelling and nuclear damage in the epithelial cells, polymorphonuclear infiltration, and vascular thrombosis. Eventually, most patients will develop evidence of fibrosis in the area of pneumonitis.

The combination of *pulmonary infiltrates* and *peripheral blood eosinophilia* can occur in several disorders.[12] Löffler syndrome and chronic eosinophilic pneumonia are diseases of unknown etiology in which patients may be found to have nonsegmental areas of infiltration radiographically, with blood eosinophilia. In Löffler syndrome, the infiltrates are fleeting. Chronic eosinophilic pneumonia is a prolonged illness with fever, malaise, anorexia, weight loss, and dyspnea. The symptomatic and roentgenographic pictures are dramatically and promptly reversed with steroid therapy.

A growing number of therapeutic agents have been recognized as causes of the syndrome of pulmonary infiltrates and eosinophilia (Table 3.2–5). The hypersensitivity reaction may be accompanied by dyspnea, cough, and fever. Pleural effusion may also be found. When an acute reaction goes unrecognized, chronic intermittent exposure may lead to loss of lung volume and roentgenographic evidence of fibrosis.

Diagnosis may be difficult because of the nonspecific nature of the findings, the inability to attribute the reaction to a specific drug in patients receiving multiple drug regimens, and the possibility that an underlying disease may account for the reaction.

Illicit use of therapeutic agents, such as the habit of "mainlining" (intravenous injection) crushed tablets, can produce striking dyspnea, infiltrates, and eosinophilia in which the reaction is attributed not to the drug itself but to the materials used in the matrix of the tablet.

Parasites whose life cycle involves transit through the lungs, such as ascariasis, strongyloidiasis, and ancylostomiasis, pulmonary larva migrans, and schistosomiasis, may cause the syndrome. Tropical eosinophilia, a disease seen in individuals who live or travel in the tropics, causes an asthmatic illness or an illness consisting of malaise, weight loss, fever, cough, and dyspnea. Roentgenographic abnormalities include a diffuse micronodular infiltrate and hilar adenopathy. High levels of antibody to filarial antigen are found, and patients will demonstrate improvement on treatment with antifilarial chemotherapy.

TABLE 3.2–5. COMMON DRUGS CAUSING HYPERSENSITIVITY LUNG DISEASE[3]

- Nitrofurantoin
- Sulfonamides
- Diphenylhydantoin
- Carbamazepine
- Chlorpropamide
- Imipramine
- Isoniazid
- Others

REFERENCES

1. Bartlett JG, Gorbach SL: The triple threat of aspiration pneumonia. Chest 68:560, 1975
2. Bynum LJ, Pierce AK: Pulmonary aspiration of gastric contents. Am Rev Respir Dis 114:1129, 1976
3. Cooper JAD, White DA, Matthay RA: Drug induced pulmonary disease. Am Rev Respir Dis 133:321 and 488, 1986
4. Curran JW, Evatt BL, Dale HL: Acquired immunodeficiency syndrome: The past as prologue. Ann Intern Med 93:401, 1983
5. Gross NJ: Pulmonary effects of radiation therapy. Ann Intern Med 86:81, 1977
6. Hopewell PC, Luce JM: Pulmonary involvement in the acquired immune deficiency syndrome. Chest 87:104, 1985
7. Hunninghake GW, Fauci AS: Pulmonary involvement in the collagen vascular diseases. Am Rev Respir Dis 119:471, 1979
8. Inners CR, Terry PB, et al: Collateral ventilation and the middle lobe syndrome. Am Rev Respir Dis 118:305, 1975
9. Lawson RN, Ramanathan L, et al: Bronchial adenoma: Review of an 18-year experience at the Brompton Hospital. Thorax 31:245, 1976
10. Lorber B, Swenson P: Bacteriology of aspiration pneumonia: A prospective study of community and hospital acquired cases. Ann Intern Med 81:329, 1974
11. Mario M, Galy P: Bronchioalveolar cell carcinoma. Clinicopathologic relationships, natural history and prognosis in 29 cases. Am Rev Respir Dis 107:621, 1973
12. Ottesen EA: Eosinophilia in the lung. In Kirkpatric CH, Reynolds HY (eds): Immunologic and Infectious Reactions in the Lung. New York, Marcel Dekker, 1976
13. Winterbauer RH, Bedon GA, Ball WC Jr: Recurrent pneumonia, predisposing illness and clinical patterns in 158 patients. Ann Intern Med 70:689, 1969
14. Wynne JW, Wodell H: Respiratory aspiration of stomach contents. Ann Intern Med 87:466, 1977

CHAPTER 3.3
Mass Lesions and Pulmonary Nodules

Stephen R. Selinger, Peter B. Terry, and Ko-Pen Wang

Spherical or oval lesions within the lung parenchyma or the mediastinum are termed "nodules" and "masses." They require careful and expeditious investigation because they may represent a treatable infection or a resectable tumor.

Many such nodules and masses present without symptoms, while others cause chest pain, cough, or hemoptysis. The symptoms produced depend in large part upon the extent of disease and location of the lesion. These features also determine the diagnostic approach to the problem. It is, therefore, most convenient to approach mass lesions within the chest in terms of their anatomic location (as shown in Figure 3.3–1 and Table 3.3–3) and radiographic presentation.

MEDIASTINAL MASSES

The mediastinum is the extrapleural space bounded by the sternum anteriorly, the vertebral column posteriorly, and the two pleural cavities on the left and right; it extends from the diaphragm to the thoracic inlet.[4,7,8,12] The mediastinum is arbitrarily divided into four compartments (Fig. 3.3–1). The normal structures of the mediastinum and embryonic rests can give rise to tumors and mass lesions. Neoplasms originating outside the mediastinum, infections, and multisystem diseases such as sarcoidosis can involve the mediastinum.

CLINICAL MANIFESTATIONS

Symptoms associated with mediastinal masses usually arise from the local effects of the mass and thus vary with the location, size, compressibility, rate of growth, and invasiveness of the lesion. Any large mass, especially a malignant tumor, may invade or erode into normal structures, causing characteristic symptoms and signs. An estimated 35 to 44 percent of patients with primary tumors of the mediastinum are asymptomatic when found on chest films.[3,10,12,14,15] In symptomatic patients, the most common complaints are cough, chest pain, and dyspnea. In some instances the principal clinical findings are remote from the mediastinum. These may be simply the general systemic effects of infection or malignancy—fever, asthenia, anorexia, weight loss, and anemia—or para-

neoplastic syndromes associated with a specific type of mediastinal lesion. An example is the thymoma, which may be associated with myasthenia gravis, erythroid hypoplasia, Cushing syndrome, dermatomyositis, Whipple disease, or agammaglobulinemia.

DIAGNOSIS AND MANAGEMENT

Determination of the exact location of a mediastinal mass is of considerable value in differential diagnosis. The diagnosis of a mass found in a mediastinal compartment is generally a reflection of the normal structures found in that location; embryonic rests of tissue; infections, tumors, or multisystem diseases that may involve that location. For example, thymoma is the most common anterior mediastinal tumor. Posterior mediastinal tumors are most often of neural origin. Middle mediastinal masses are most commonly caused by lymph node enlargement from sarcoidosis, tumor, or chronic granulomatous infection. The sites of some of the commonly occurring lesions and their clinical manifestations are outlined in Table 3.3–1 and Figure 3.3–1.

Noninvasive Studies

Posteroanterior, lateral, and oblique radiographs of the chest are essential guides to the location and character of the mass. Careful study of changes in density suggesting fat, cystic changes, calcification, or bone erosion is important. Computed tomography (CT) has changed the noninvasive evaluation of abnormal mediastinal radiographs. Anatomic locations can be precisely defined, and the character and density of lesions can furnish valuable clues as to etiology. Contrast enhancement may suggest or rule out a vascular lesion. CT has largely supplanted the need for conventional tomography or ultrasound evaluation. On occasion, fluoroscopy may be useful in the assessment of diaphragmatic and mediastinal mobility and will demonstrate movement of the mass in relation to swallowing, respiration, and cardiac pulsation. Movement of the vocal cords can also be observed by contrast radiography. Fluoroscopy may also detect the expansile pulsation of an aneurysm, but errors of interpretation caused by transmitted pulsations are frequent. Examinations with radiopaque materials in the esophagus, tracheobronchial tree, or blood vessels may be definitive. Isotope scanning procedures are useful in identifying thyroid masses and in demonstrating abnormal distribution of blood flow to the lungs.

Invasive Studies

Despite the excellent imaging afforded by CT, a histologic diagnosis is required in the majority of mediastinal lesions. The invasive study chosen to make a histologic diagnosis depends upon the anatomic location of the mass and should always be the procedure that imparts least risk to the patient. In addition, the potential information to be gained from the chosen procedure should always have some impact upon the management of the patient. Often the information gained will make a more invasive, risky procedure unnecessary. For example, the identification of mediastinal involvement often indicates that a bronchogenic carcinoma is unresectable.

Mediastinoscopy allows biopsy of lesions in the anterior and middle mediastinum that are adjacent to the trachea.[1] The subcarinal and hilar regions cannot be accessed by this technique. Transbronchial needle aspiration performed during fiberoptic bronchoscopy has allowed access to right and left paratracheal, subcarinal, and hilar regions.[13] This has eliminated the need for thoracotomy in some instances. Many anterior and middle mediastinal tumors not adjacent to the tracheobronchial tree still require thoracotomy for diagnosis. The proximity of vascular structures to these regions has limited the usefulness of percutaneous needle aspiration and biopsy.

Open thoracotomy is the most direct method of establishing an etiologic diagnosis when simpler procedures have failed. Although the risk of elective thoracotomy is low, the therapeutic im-

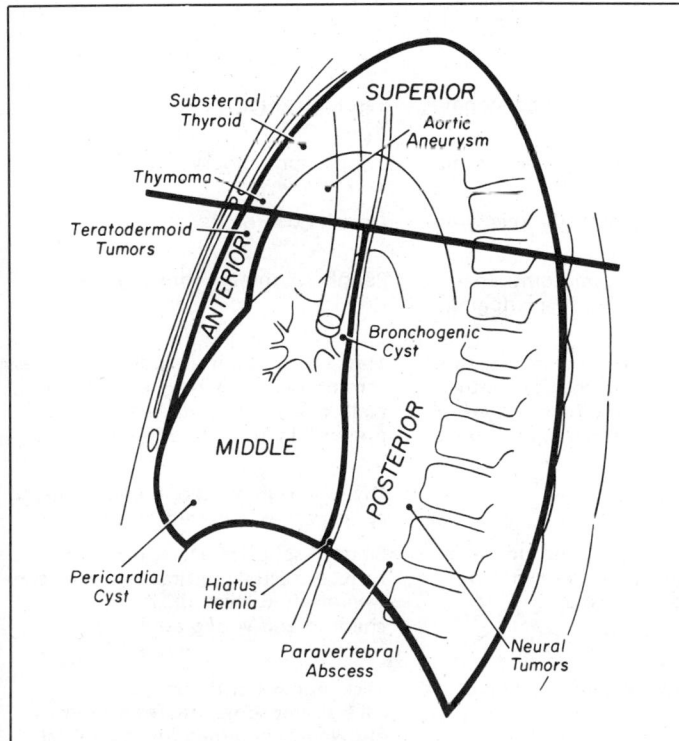

Figure 3.3–1. Diagram illustrating mediastinum and site of common primary lesions. Customary subdivisions are shown. Important structures in these subdivisions are as follows: Superior mediastinum—aortic arch and major branches; superior vena cava and innominate veins; thymus; trachea, esophagus, thoracic duct; vagus, phrenic, sympathetic nerves; left recurrent laryngeal nerve; lymph nodes. Anterior mediastinum—lymph nodes, fibroareolar tissue. Middle mediastinum—heart, pericardium, ascending aorta; proximal pulmonary vessels; phrenic nerves; tracheal bifurcation; lymph nodes. Posterior mediastinum—descending aorta and branches; azygos and hemiazygos veins; esophagus, thoracic duct; vagus and sympathetic nerves; lymph nodes.

TABLE 3.3–1. MEDIASTINAL MASSES

Mass and Incidence[a]	Other Locations	Clinical Manifestations	Diagnostic Aids
Anterior Mediastinum			
Thymoma (18%)	Malignant thymoma can spread to posterior mediastinum	Associated with myasthenia gravis, erythroid hypoplasia, Cushing syndrome, dermatomyositis; 30% are malignant	Tensilon test, bone marrow aspiration, 17-KS, 17-OHCS, plasma cortisol, antithymic and antimuscle antibodies
Lymphoma (12%)	Middle posterior (hilar adenopathy)	Pressure on surrounding structures; lymph node enlargement elsewhere; systemic manifestations (anemia, fever, etc.)	May be lobulated, bilateral but asymmetrical; biopsy of other nodes, bone marrow biopsy
Germ cell tumors (12%)		Pressure on surrounding structures; may rupture into bronchus or pleural cavity; bulging anterior chest wall; clubbing; 20% are malignant	Often large; teeth, bone, fatty layer may be visible on radiograph; most common in young adults
Substernal thyroid (6%)	Middle	Pressure on recurrent laryngeal nerve, trachea blood vessels; hyperthyroidism	May be palpable in neck; moves with swallowing; may be visualized on I-131 scan
Lipoma (<1%)	Middle	Usually asymptomatic	Smooth margins; fat density on CT
Middle Mediastinum			
Lymph nodes			
Bronchogenic carcinoma (esp. small cell); carcinoma of upper GI tract, prostate, kidney		Cough, hemoptysis, dyspnea, weight loss	Sputum cytology, bronchoscopy, mediastinoscopy
Sarcoidosis		Often asymptomatic; other clinical evidence of sarcoidosis—erythema nodosum uveitis, parotitis, CNS involvement, arthritis	Commonly bilateral hilar and right paratracheal; hyperglobulinemia; hypercalcemia, decreased pulmonary compliance and DLCO despite clear lungs in CXR; positive Kveim test
Chronic infections • Tuberculosis • Histoplasmosis	Anterior	Evidence of systemic infection; symptoms of pulmonary infection, bronchial compression; erosion into a bronchus	Cultures, skin test, history of exposure
Acute infections • Infectious mononucleosis		Sore throat, rash, cervical adenopathy	Serologic tests
Hodgkin disease	Anterior	Other involved nodes; systemic symptoms	Lymph node biopsy
Non-Hodgkin lymphoma		Other involved nodes; systemic symptoms	Lymph node biopsy
Leukemia	Anterior	Systemic signs and symptoms; anemia, thrombocytopenia, splenomegaly	Peripheral smear, bone marrow
Aortic aneurysm	Superior, posterior	Pressure on all surrounding structures including bone; may leak or rupture into adjacent viscera; Marfan syndrome; history of trauma, atherosclerosis, syphilis	Mass shows expansile pulsation unless thrombosed; may have calcification in wall; tracheal tug, different blood pressure in arms, arteriography
Pericardial cyst (6%)	Anterior	Not symptomatic	Often at right cardiophrenic angle; cystic nature apparent on CT
Bronchogenic cyst (8%)	Anterior	Tracheal compression; secondary infection; material may be expectorated through bronchial communication	Smooth spherical mass, often adjacent to tracheal bifurcation; may contain air fluid level; most common in children and young adults
Posterior Mediastinum			
Neurofibroma, neurosarcoma (10%)		Pressure on spinal cord and nerve roots	Recklinghausen disease with café-au-lait spots, neurofibromas elsewhere, enlarged intervertebral foramina, erosion of vertebral pedicles; myelogram
Ganglioneuroma (5%)		Compressed trachea, esophagus, great vessels; Horner syndrome	High urinary vanillylmandelic acid; gait abnormalities from extension into spinal canal; most common in young adult
Neurolemmoma (4%)		Involves bone and encroaches on spinal canal	Myelogram
Neuroblastoma (2%)		Nonproductive cough and wheeze; often extends into spinal canal and produces gait abnormalities	Most common in children

(continued)

TABLE 3.3–1. MEDIASTINAL MASSES (Continued)

Mass and Incidence[a]	Other Locations	Clinical Manifestations	Diagnostic Aids
Posterior Mediastinum (Cont.)			
Pheochromocytoma (1%)		Hypertension	Elevated urinary catecholamines
Paravertebral abscess		Back pain, fever, evidence of tuberculosis elsewhere	Fusiform mass; bone changes on radiograph; cultures for tuberculosis, fungi, and staphylococcus
Esophageal Lesions			
Diverticulum		Regurgitation, repeated aspiration	Barium swallow; mass may show air fluid level
Hiatus hernia			

[a]Incidence in 1252 cases taken from 11 series, 1952–1972. Refers only to primary tumors of the mediastinum.[3,12]
DLCO = diffusing capacity; CXR = chest radiogram; CT = computed tomography.

plications of the anticipated findings must be weighed against the operative risk in each case.

EVALUATION OF MEDIASTINAL LYMPHADENOPATHY

Lymph nodes are present in every division of the mediastinum, but the largest number appears in the superior and middle mediastinum, in close proximity to the trachea and its bifurcation. Their enlargement may be produced by infections, including primary tuberculosis, histoplasmosis, coccidioidomycosis, actinomycosis, and other fungus diseases. Acute lymphadenopathy may be seen occasionally with pneumococcal pneumonia or lung abscess, with pertussis and tularemia, and with infectious mononucleosis. A number of cancers may present with mediastinal lymph node metastases; these are discussed in Chapter 6.22.

There are many causes of lymph node enlargement that would not justify thoracotomy for diagnosis. Mediastinal lymphadenopathy is best approached diagnostically by mediastinoscopy, transbronchial needle aspiration, or parasternal incision. In sarcoidosis, a common cause of bilateral hilar adenopathy, transbronchial biopsy of the lung parenchyma, has a high yield (80 to 90 percent) even when the lungs appear normal roentgenographically.

SOLITARY PULMONARY NODULES

The solitary pulmonary nodule, often referred to as a "coin lesion," is a common abnormal roentgenographic finding. It is defined as a single rounded or oval lesion of less than 6 cm in diameter, lying within the lung parenchyma with aerated lung around it. It is a frequent incidental finding on a routine radiograph in an asymptomatic patient. The immediate problem is to determine the likelihood of primary malignancy and the need for thoracotomy. Although most lesions are benign granulomas, as many as 40 percent of solitary nodules referred for resection are malignant tumors.[5,6,11] Resectability of pulmonary neoplasms is clearly related to early diagnosis, reaching 75 percent in small (less than 6 cm), asymptomatic lesions, in contrast to 30 percent resectability when all types of bronchogenic carcinoma are included. Furthermore the smaller the lesion at the time of resection, the better the survival rate. Forty to fifty percent of patients survive for at least 5 years after resection of a malignant coin lesion compared with less than 10 percent overall survival in bronchogenic carcinoma. Therefore aggressive management is justified in many of these patients, especially if they are at risk for bronchogenic carcinoma and are potential surgical candidates.

CLINICAL FEATURES

Table 3.3–2 summarizes features helping to differentiate benign from malignant nodules.[2]

Table 3.3–3 summarizes the clinical and radiologic features of the common and uncommon types of pulmonary nodules. Symptoms related directly to the presence of the nodule are commonly absent. Many nodules are noted incidentally on chest radiographs performed for another purpose. A pulmonary nodule, however, can be associated with symptoms related to an underlying multisystem disease, a paraneoplastic syndrome, or distant metastases. Historical features suggestive of malignancy include heavy smoking, hemoptysis, age over 40, and known previous malignancy elsewhere. Residence in an area endemic for fungi may suggest chronic granulomatous infection, especially in a young, nonsmoking patient.

The nodule itself can seldom be detected by examination of the chest. Careful search should be made for evidence of primary or metastatic tumor elsewhere. The presence of rheumatoid arthritis suggests the possibility of a rheumatoid nodule in the lung, especially if superficial nodules are present. Bloody nasal discharge or destructive lesions in the nasal passages suggest Wegener granulomatosis. Cutaneous and mucosal telangiectases or a bruit over the chest wall may be present if the lesion is a pulmonary arteriovenous fistula.

In the absence of extrapulmonary symptoms and signs a primary malignancy elsewhere presenting in the lungs as a solitary metastasis is most unlikely. Extensive roentgenographic surveys of the urinary tract and skeletal and digestive systems are not justified until the pulmonary lesion has been diagnosed as malignant. For a solitary nodule, the yield is small from expensive radiographic surveys; where multiple nodules are concerned, the yield may be higher but biopsy of the lung nodules would be necessary to confirm the presence of metastases. When a known primary neoplasm of the gastrointestinal or urogenital system is present, the likelihood of a solitary metastasis is increased.

TABLE 3.3–2. DIFFERENTIATION OF BENIGN AND MALIGNANT NODULES

Probably Malignant
- Serial film show recent origin or rapid growth
- Umbilication or notching of the margin of the nodule
- Eccentric cavitation with irregular wall thickness
- Noncalcified fuzzy lesion in a male smoker over age 40
- Positive sputum cytology

Probably Benign
- Lesion with sharp margins in patient under age 35
- Radiograph stability for 2 years
- Radiograph appearance characteristic of lesion associated with proven systemic disease
- High density on CT

Almost Surely Benign
- Solid or laminated calcification
- Radiograph stability for 5 years
- Lesion with sharp margins in patient under age 30 with positive tuberculin skin test
- Serial films show evolution characteristic of inflammatory lesion

TABLE 3.3–3. DIFFERENTIAL DIAGNOSIS OF PULMONARY NODULES

Type and Incidence	Radiologic Appearance	Characteristic Features
Neoplasms		
Bronchogenic carcinoma (10–25%)	Fuzzy borders, often umbilicated margin; progressive enlargement over weeks or months; calcification rare (<1%); cavitation, if present, is often eccentric	Highest incidence in cigarette smokers; often asymptomatic; occasionally hemoptysis; cytology occasionally positive; most common in men over 40
Bronchial adenoma (2% that of carcinoma)	Sharply demarcated; calcification rare; predilection for right upper lobe, middle lobe, and lingula	Cough and hemoptysis in one third of cases; often visible at bronchoscopy; 10% develop distant metastases; occurs equally in men and women; younger age group than bronchogenic carcinoma
Metastatic lesions (5–15%)	Uncalcified; spherical; sharp or fuzzy margins; often multiple	Symptoms almost always absent; primary malignant tumor elsewhere; bronchoscopy and cytology usually negative
Bronchiolar-alveolar carcinoma (rare)	Air bronchogram; frequently slow growing	Symptoms often absent; cytology may be positive
Benign Pulmonary Tumors		
Hamartoma (5–10%)	Round or oval; majority well demarcated and lobulated; 30% calcified; slow growth is characteristic	Symptoms usually absent
Granulomas		
Tuberculosis, histoplasmosis, coccidioidomycosis, rarely brucellosis, and mineral oil aspiration (60%)	Two thirds show calcification; laminar or solid calcification pathognomonic; sharply defined margins; occasionally linear strands to hilus or pleural surface; satellite lesions common in tuberculosis; may be multiple	Symptoms usually absent; exposure by contact or endemic area; skin tests positive; sputum cultures usually negative
Uncommon Pulmonary Nodules		
Bronchogenic cyst (2%)	Central or lower lobe location with sharp margins; occasional fluid level	Asymptomatic until communication with bronchus established
Hydatid cyst (rare)	Ovoid, sharply circumscribed; may be lobulated; fluid level may be present; meniscus of air at apex of cyst may be visible on tomogram	Association with sheepherding dogs; palpable or calcified hepatic cyst; echinococcal hooklets in sputum
Pulmonary infarct (rare as solitary nodule)	Fairly rapid resolution on serial films; small pleural effusion	Pleuritic pain and pleural rub; elevated serum lactic dehydrogenase; lung scan may show segmental defects in other areas
Round Atelectasis	Associated with pleural plaques	History of asbestos exposure
Rheumatoid granuloma (rare)	Well circumscribed and uniformly dense; may be calcified; may have associated diffuse basal fibrosis; pleural effusion often present	Rheumatoid arthritis; lesion resolves rapidly on steroid therapy; rheumatoid factor present
Pulmonary arteriovenous fistula (rare)	Spherical and usually well circumscribed; rarely calcified; vessels leading to hilus visible on tomogram	Cutaneous and mucosal telangiectases may be present; cyanosis and polycythemia; audible bruit over lesion; angiography diagnostic
Intrapulmonary hematoma (rare)	Dense, circumscribed; progressive shrinkage on serial films	History of thoracic trauma or recent wedge resection
Chronic focal pneumonitis (rare)	Rapid resolution with antibiotics	Recent episode of pneumonia
Bronchopulmonary sequestration (uncommon)	Usually left lower lobe; may contain air-fluid level	Asymptomatic unless infected; complications rare
Hematogenous abscesses (uncommon)	Usually multiple; more numerous in lower lobes	Patient very ill; gram-negative organisms often responsible; blood cultures frequently positive
Wegener granulomatosis (rare)	Usually multiple; nodules of varying size; cavitation frequent	Sinus, nasal, renal or other organ involvement

A number of radiographic features suggest whether a pulmonary nodule is benign or malignant (Table 3.3–2). Granulomas are usually subpleural in location, with sharp margins. Solid or laminated calcification occurs only in granulomas and excludes bronchogenic carcinoma. In contrast, primary lung carcinomas often have indistinct borders. Granulomatous disease is uncommon in the anterior segments of the upper lobes; the presence of a nodule in one of these regions strongly suggests carcinoma. Apart from the presence of solid or laminated calcification, however, no combination of radiographic features on a single examination will safely exclude malignancy.

Previous radiographs can furnish valuable information regarding the growth characteristics of a lesion in question and suggest that a nodule is benign. Radiograph stability for at least 5 years or

TABLE 3.3–4. MULTIPLE NODULES

Neoplastic	Developmental	Infectious	Immunologic
Lymphosarcoma	Pulmonary arteriovenous fistulas	Bacterial abscesses	Lymphomatoid granulomatosis
Hematogenous metastasis		*Coccidioides immitis*	Wegener granulomatosis
Multiple myeloma		*Paragonimus westermani*	Rheumatoid necrobiotic nodules
Papilloma			

shrinkage suggestive of an inflammatory lesion may be accepted as evidence that a nodule is benign. The growth rate of a primary lung malignancy may appear slow, however. The doubling time of a bronchogenic carcinoma varies from 30 (small cell) to 460 days (median, 120 days). Because the volume of a spherical lesion varies with the cube of the radius, in one doubling time a 1 cm lesion will grow to 1.25 cm. This apparently slow growth rate dictates that great care must be taken in comparing radiographs and that one must use sufficiently old films for comparison. A doubling time of less than 30 days (rapid growth rate) suggests that one is dealing with an inflammatory process.

Some lesions may be clearly localized and characterized from posteroanterior and lateral chest films alone, but localization is commonly aided by the use of apical lordotic or oblique views. CT is usually required to obtain precise information about the character of the borders and the presence or absence of calcification, and may reveal multiple nodules where only a single lesion is visible on standard radiographs. In addition, the densities of pulmonary nodules may be determined with computed tomography.[9] High-density lesions have been associated with a benign diagnosis, while low-density readings are found in both benign and malignant diseases.

Extrapulmonary lesions, such as interlobar pleural effusions, pleural plaques and tumors, chest wall tumors, and skin tumors, must be excluded. Application of a metallic marker to the nipples or cutaneous nodules removes all doubt about whether they are responsible for the roentgenographic shadow in question. *Every effort must be made to obtain all previous chest films* to determine the stability and duration of the lesion.

DIAGNOSTIC STUDIES

Although a positive skin test does not establish the diagnosis, negative tests with tuberculin, histoplasmin, and coccidioidin make malignancy more likely. In such instances, immediate thoracotomy generally may be indicated, even in a person under 35 years of age. A strongly positive tuberculin test does not exclude malignancy.

Percutaneous needle biopsy is covered thoroughly in Chapter 3.1 and is effective about 80 percent of the time in obtaining sufficient tissue for diagnosis. It is nearly always indicated to have tissue confirmation of malignancy before beginning therapy. In a patient too ill to undergo general anesthesia and thoracotomy, needle biopsy offers a simple method of obtaining a tissue diagnosis with acceptably low morbidity.

The greatest value of bronchoscopic and percutaneous biopsy procedures is in proving the diagnosis of a malignant neoplasm. This information will sometimes justify thoracotomy in a poor-risk patient or will assist in persuading a patient that operation is essential. These procedures are less satisfactory in proving that a nodule is benign, since recovery of a small fragment of inflammatory tissue does not exclude tumor.

When less invasive studies are nondiagnostic, thoracotomy is necessary for the proper diagnosis and management of all lesions thought to be probable or possible primary malignancies without apparent spread. Thoracotomy is required to establish a diagnosis of benign tumor as well. Thus diagnostic thoracotomy is indicated except in those few patients showing strong evidence of a benign lesion, that is, stability of the lesion for 5 years or characteristic laminar or solid calcification. Other factors deterring one from tho-

racotomy include significant obstructive airway disease and serious arteriosclerotic cardiovascular disease. In uncomplicated cases the mortality and morbidity of this procedure is generally low.

MULTIPLE NODULES

Multiple pulmonary nodules may represent developmental lesions, infections, neoplasms, or immunologic diseases (Table 3.3–4). The differential diagnosis and diagnostic approach are governed by the clinical setting and radiograph characteristics. Diagnostic thoracotomy is rarely indicated if malignancy is suspected because curative resection is extremely rare. Consequently, tissue diagnosis is sought with bronchoscopic or percutaneous needle biopsy.

PULMONARY MASSES

Solitary lesions larger than 6 cm in diameter are termed "masses." Virtually all the entities that may be responsible for solitary nodules may also produce larger masses. Additional diagnostic possibilities include masses resulting from conglomerate silicosis, mucoid impaction in asthmatics, and an intrapulmonary sequestration cyst.

REFERENCES

1. American Thoracic Society: Diagnostic mediastinoscopy. Am Rev Respir Dis 105:487, 1972
2. Baetson EM: An analysis of 155 solitary lung lesions illustrating the differential diagnosis of mixed tumors of the lung. Clin Radiol 16:51, 1965
3. Benjamin SP, McCormack LJ, et al: Primary tumors of the mediastinum. Chest 62:297, 1972
4. Crowe JK, Brown LR, Muhm JR: Computed tomography of the mediastinum. Radiology 128:75, 1978
5. Cummings SR, Lillington GA, Richard RJ: Managing solitary pulmonary nodules. Am Rev Respir Dis 134:453, 1986
6. Gracey DR, Byrd RB, Cugell DB: The dilemma of the asymptomatic pulmonary nodule in the young and not-so-young adult. Chest 60:479, 1971
7. Hyson EA, Ravin CE: Radiographic features of mediastinal anatomy. Chest 75:609, 1979
8. Leigh TF, Weens HS: The Mediastinum. Springfield, Ill, Thomas, 1959
9. Proto AV, Thomas SR: Pulmonary nodules studied by computed tomography. Radiology 156:149, 1985
10. Rubush JI, Gardner IR, et al: Mediastinal tumors. J Thorac Cardiovasc Surg 65:216, 1973
11. Siegelman SS, Stitik FP, Summer WR: Management of the patient with a localized pulmonary lesion. In Siegelman SS, Stitik FP, Summer WR (eds): Pulmonary System. Practical Approaches to Pulmonary Diagnosis. New York, Grune & Stratton, 1979
12. Silverman NA, Sabiston DC Jr: Primary tumors and cysts of the mediastinum. In Hickey RC, Clark RL (eds): Current Problems in Cancer. Chicago, Year Book Medical Publishers, 1977
13. Wang KP, Marsh BR, et al: Transbronchial needle aspiration for diagnosis of lung cancer. Chest 80:48, 1981
14. Wychulis AR, Payne WS, et al: Surgical treatment of mediastinal tumors. J Thorac Cardiovasc Surg 62:379, 1971
15. Young R, Pochaczevsky R, et al: Cervicomediastinal thymic cysts. Am J Roentgenol 117:855, 1973

CLINICAL MANIFESTATIONS

SYMPTOMS

Pleural effusion may be associated with symptoms caused by inflammation of the parietal pleura or compression of the lung. When the volume of fluid is small, pleural pain (pleurisy) is often present. A small inflammatory effusion is often accompanied by pleurisy and a friction rub. Pleurisy is commonly characterized as a sharp, stabbing sensation absent or minimal during quiet respiration but intensified during full inflation of the lungs. It must be differentiated from other types of pain accentuated by inspiration. These include the pain associated with rib fracture or costochondritis, nerve root compression, herpes zoster, acute bronchitis, and various cardiovascular and esophageal lesions. When there is direct involvement of the parietal pleura by tumor or by infection, as in empyema, constant dull aching pain independent of respiration may result.

Large or bilateral pleural effusions may lead to dyspnea. Orthopnea is uncommon in the absence of congestive heart failure. The accumulation of pleural fluid in patients with severe heart disease or with chronic obstructive pulmonary disease may result in dyspnea that seems disproportionate to the volume of fluid present. In this group of patients, removal of even small amounts of fluid may produce marked improvement in symptoms. The accumulation of significant volumes of pleural fluid sometimes does not cause symptoms, and the presence of pleural effusion can only be recognized on routine radiographs of the chest.

PHYSICAL SIGNS

Accumulation of fluid usually occurs first at the bases of the lung, and the earliest physical signs are localized to this area. When the volume of pleural fluid is small, differentiation from elevation of the diaphragm, atelectasis, and consolidation may be difficult. It is usual to find a dull to flat percussion note over the area of fluid, together with reduced or absent breath sounds in this area. An area of bronchial breathing, accompanied by an alteration of the quality of voice sounds or frank egophony, is sometimes heard over the adjacent compressed lung. When the amount of fluid is large, the volume of the involved hemithorax may appear to be increased, and expansion during inspiration may be reduced. Unless the mediastinum has become fixed in position by invasion with tumor, or portions of lung on the affected side have become completely atelectatic, the mediastinum is usually shifted away from the side of a large effusion.

RADIOGRAPHIC APPEARANCE

When there are no adhesions between the visceral and parietal pleura, the earliest sign of fluid in the pleural space that can be appreciated on plain films of the chest is blunting of the costophrenic angle on the posteroanterior view and loss of sharp demarcation of the posterior portion of the diaphragm in the lateral view. With the accumulation of larger volumes of fluid, the outline of the diaphragm in the lateral view is completely lost, and the posteroanterior view shows an area of opacificaton at the lung base, often tapering up the lateral chest wall in the form of a meniscus. When a major portion of the hemithorax is radiopaque, air-filled bronchi in the compressed and atelectatic lung may be crowded together and displaced into the upper lung field. The heart and other mediastinal structures are characteristically shifted toward the uninvolved side.

When less than 300 ml of pleural fluid is present, the posteroanterior roentgenogram may show no abnormality. Furthermore, blunting of the costophrenic angle may be caused by old inflammatory adhesions. Lateral decubitus films may be very helpful in these situations, since as little as 15 ml of free pleural fluid may be recognized as a layer of density along the inner margin of the dependent chest wall. Examination of the thorax by computed tomography (CT) is also a sensitive method for identifying free pleural fluid. CT may also be useful when parenchymal and pleural densities are difficult to separate on plain films.

If previous inflammatory disease has caused adhesions between visceral and parietal pleura, the fluid may be loculated rather than free in the pleural cavity. When it is confined to the region between the lower lobe and the diaphragm (infrapulmonary effusion), it may resemble an elevated diaphragm. The effusion may lie within a fissure (interlobar effusion), most commonly the major fissure on the right. The posteroanterior film in such cases may show a shadow that resembles an intrapulmonary tumor. A loculated pleural effusion may also produce a shadow that lies flat against the pleural surface and bulges into the lung field in one or more locations. The simultaneous presence of fluid and air within the pleural space produces a sharply demarcated horizontal line in an upright film and can usually be readily identified. Placement of a radiopaque marker during fluoroscopy or diagnostic ultrasound may be used for more accurate localization of loculated fluid to assist in achieving complete removal by thoracentesis.

MECHANISMS OF PLEURAL EFFUSION

The pleural cavity normally contains a small volume of thin serous fluid formed for the most part by transudation from the parietal pleural surface.[2] Recent evidence suggests that fluid, including particulate matter and cellular debris, is removed through lymphatic channels that arise from lacunae on the parietal pleural surface.[5] The visceral pleural surface in man is supplied by the bronchial circulation, but with drainage into the pulmonary vein. The normal balance between formation and removal of fluid may be compromised by a partial or complete obstruction of the lymphatic circulation, by a rise in either the pulmonary venous or the systemic venous pressures, or by a decrease in the colloid oncotic pressure of plasma. In the presence of pulmonary venous hypertension, fluid may enter the pleural space from the lung surface. Since a significant portion of the lymphatic drainage from the abdomen passes by way of the diaphragm, especially on the right, a variety of inflammatory conditions within the abdomen or the presence of ascites may be accompanied by accumulations of pleural fluid on the right. Small perforations or defects in the diaphragm itself sometimes allow bulk flow of ascitic fluid from the abdominal cavity into the chest. Accumulation of noninflammatory pleural fluid may therefore occur in any condition that results in ascites, in obstruction to the venous or lymphatic drainage of the lung, or in either isolated left-sided or isolated right-sided congestive heart failure. The pleural effusion of heart failure occurs most commonly in the presence of combined ventricular failure. A severe reduction

in the level of plasma protein concentration may contribute to the accumulation of noninflammatory pleural fluid.

Inflammatory effusions result from inflammation of structures adjacent to the pleural space, usually just beneath the visceral pleura within the lung, but occasionally from lesions within the mediastinum, diaphragm, or chest wall. Removal of this fluid by the normal clearing mechanisms may be considerably retarded by the presence of inflammatory obstruction of the lymphatic channels draining the thorax, and secondary inflammation of larger areas of pleural surface may result in the very rapid outpouring of fluid.

The simultaneous presence of air and fluid within the pleural cavity, unless air has been introduced during thoracentesis or surgery, almost always implies the presence of a bronchopleural fistula, resulting most commonly from tuberculosis, pyogenic pneumonia, lung abscess, or malignant tumor.

When the thoracic duct is lacerated or interrupted by trauma or obstructed by tumor, lymph may accumulate in the pleural space. This condition is termed "chylothorax" and is identified by the milky appearance of the fluid, fat droplets on staining with Sudan III, and a total neutral-fat content greater than 0.5 g/dl.

DIAGNOSTIC MEASURES

Unless the etiology has been clearly established, the mere presence of fluid within the pleural cavity constitutes an indication for thoracentesis. This simultaneously serves the purpose of providing fluid for examination, permitting better radiographic visualization of the lung following the removal of fluid, and relieving symptoms. The gross appearance of the fluid should be carefully noted and specimens obtained for various laboratory examinations. A minimum examination would consist of the measurement of total protein and lactic dehydrogenase (LDH) content, the determination of total and differential cell counts, and examination of the spun sediment with Wright stain. When the etiology of the effusion is not firmly established, the fluid should be subjected to appropriate bacteriologic study for pyogenic organisms, fungi, and *Mycobacterium tuberculosis,* and to cytologic examination for the presence of malignant cells. Under certain circumstances (see following discussion), it may be useful to analyze the fluid for glucose and amylase and to determine its pH. If a milky appearance of the fluid suggests chylothorax, determination of total neutral fat should be obtained and the fluid examined for fat droplets by staining with Sudan III.

In many situations in which an inflammatory effusion is known to be present or suspected, needle biopsy of the parietal pleura with an Abrams or a Cope biopsy instrument may be performed at the time of initial thoracentesis.[3] These biopsies have shown a 60 to 75 percent positive yield in patients with tuberculous or malignant pleural effusions and may provide a diagnosis in cases where bacteriologic or cytologic examination of the fluid is unrewarding.[4] When biopsy is indicated, it is best performed while free fluid is still present within the pleural cavity, since this protects the lung from injury by the biopsy instrument. When a diagnosis has not been established despite one or more needle biopsies, thoracoscopy with biopsy of the pleura under direct vision is often successful.

DIFFERENTIAL DIAGNOSIS

In determining the etiology of a pleural effusion it is useful to establish whether the fluid is a transudate or an exudate. Transudative effusions are caused by elevated systemic or pulmonary venous pressure or by decreased plasma oncotic pressure; the pleural surfaces are not directly involved by the primary pathologic process. In contrast, an exudative effusion results from inflammation or other disease of the pleural surface, or from lymphatic obstruction.

Table 3.4–1 lists the principal causes of transudative and exudative effusions and also shows a number of less common causes of pleural effusion. Most transudative effusions have protein concentrations of less than 3 g/dl. Exudative effusions usually contain more than 3 g protein per deciliter; those due to tuberculosis or pyogenic infection frequently show a protein concentration above 5 g/dl. More reliable separation may be made by measuring the LDH concentration of pleural fluid and serum and by comparing pleural fluid and serum protein concentrations. An LDH concentration greater than two thirds of the normal serum level, a pleural fluid-to-serum LDH ratio greater than 0.6, or a pleural fluid-to-serum protein ratio greater than 0.5 establishes the presence of an exudative effusion with high reliability.

The presence of gross blood in the pleural fluid is most common when the effusion is due to trauma, tumor, or pulmonary infarction. It may also result from bleeding induced at the time of a previous thoracentesis and is occasionally seen in effusions due to tuberculosis and pneumonia. Blood-tinged fluid with fewer than 10,000 RBC/μl is commonly found in an inflammatory effusion of any cause and is therefore of little diagnostic aid. Noninflammatory effusions usually contain only small numbers of white blood cells, predominantly lymphocytes, while total counts above 2500 are usually seen in inflammatory exudates. The majority of these cells may be polymorphonuclear leukocytes early in the course of a bacterial or tuberculous infection or following pulmonary infarction, but later in the course of the disease mononuclear cells generally predominate. In an occasional case the pleural fluid may contain an exceptionally high percentage of eosinophils, even in the absence of blood eosinophilia. This is a relatively nonspecific finding but may be associated with pneumothorax or may be induced by multiple thoracenteses or intrapleural bleeding. Eosinophilia is unusual in effusions due to tuberculosis and malignancy. Wright stain of the centrifuged sediment will allow identification of mesothelial cells, which are large cells with basophilic cytoplasm, a large nucleus with finely stippled chromatin, and one to three bright blue nucleoli. Tuberculous effusions rarely show more than 1 percent of these cells, whereas most nontuberculous effusions contain over 5 percent mesothelial cells.

Chemical analysis of pleural fluid may provide additional clues to diagnosis. Pleural fluid glucose is only occasionally significantly lower than serum glucose when the effusion is caused by tuberculosis or tumor, but is usually very low (0 to 16 mg/dl) in effusions due to rheumatoid arthritis or in empyema fluid. The pH of pleural fluid is usually 7.30 or greater; lower values are occasionally seen in tuberculous and malignant effusions.[1] A value below 7.20 in a parapneumonic effusion commonly is associated with the development of an empyema and results from excessive production of carbon dioxide by leukocytes in the fluid. Moderate elevation of pleural fluid amylase is occasionally seen in malignant effusions, but markedly elevated amylase levels indicate either pancreatic disease or rupture of the esophagus with leakage of salivary amylase into the pleural space.

TREATMENT

Effective management requires that the etiology of the effusion be established and that specific treatment be applied where possible. In the case of noninflammatory effusions, correction of the underlying abnormality, perhaps accompanied by thoracentesis for removal of the bulk of the fluid, will usually result in rapid clearing of the effusion. When pleural inflammation is present, reabsorption of pleural fluid may be slow, and repeated thoracentesis may be required to keep the pleural cavity dry even after institution of specific therapy. It is important in these cases that reasonable effort be made to keep the pleural cavity free of fluid to prevent the development of fibrosis in the pleural space, with subsequent loss of pulmonary function. If this is not done, subsequent surgical decortication may be required. In tuberculous effusions, once ef-

TABLE 3.4–1. CAUSES OF PLEURAL EFFUSION

Common Causes of Transudative Effusion

Congestive heart failure	Usually chronic biventricular failure Usually bilateral Pleuritic pain and friction rub uncommon
Cirrhosis	In presence of ascites Effusion usually confined to or larger on the right Serum proteins often low
Nephrotic syndrome	Associated with hypoproteinemia and generalized edema and ascites

Common Causes of Exudative Effusion

Tuberculosis	Effusion usually unilateral, may be asymptomatic Often no parenchymal lesion on x-ray
Bronchogenic carcinoma	Effusion often bloody and large, may recur rapidly after removal Parenchymal or hilar lesion usually visible on x-ray after thoracentesis
Bacterial pneumonia	Sterile effusion must be differentiated from empyema Fluid frequently becomes loculated
Viral and mycoplasma pneumonia	Pleurisy and bilateral effusion common
Pulmonary infarction	Pleural pain commonly present Effusion usually small in amount but often bloody
Lymphoma	Most common in Hodgkin disease Often associated with mediastinal node or parenchymal involvement
Metastatic tumor	Effusion often bilateral Parenchymal lesions usually apparent
Trauma	Associated with intrapleural bleeding
Abdominal surgery	Small effusions common but usually resolve in 48 hr

Less Common Disorders in Which Effusion Occurs Frequently

Pleural mesothelioma (malignant)	Fluid may be high or low in protein content Effusion chronic and recurrent, may be bilateral and involve pericardium Irregular thickening of the pleura usually present History of asbestos exposure
Asbestos pleural effusion	Recurrent exudative effusion in absence of mesothelioma Fluid may contain many eosinophils
Meigs syndrome	Benign ovarian tumor with ascites and hydrothorax Fluid protein concentration usually low
Pancreatitis	Effusion more common on left side Fluid may have amylase higher than in blood
Postcardiotomy syndrome	Associated with fever and pericarditis
Systemic lupus erythematosus	Usually associated with pleuritic pain, often with areas of plate-like atelectasis on x-ray

Disorders Only Occasionally Accompanied by Effusion

Rheumatoid arthritis	Pleural fluid glucose commonly below 12 mg/dl LDH usually very high
Other collagen diseases (polyarteritis, scleroderma, Wegener granulomatosis)	Usually associated with activity of the underlying disease
Fungus infections (actinomycosis, histoplasmosis, coccidioidomycosis)	Effusion or empyema occasionally complicates chronic pulmonary infection
Hypothyroidism	Low-protein effusion may occur in absence of congestive failure
Sarcoidosis	Extreme rarity of pleural effusion is useful in differentiating from tuberculosis

fective antituberculous chemotherapy has been instituted, it may be advisable to administer corticosteroids in an effort to hasten resolution of the effusion and prevent pleural fibrosis. When pleural effusion due to malignant disease recurs rapidly, requiring repeated thoracentesis, reaccumulation may be retarded by insertion of a chest tube and instillation of a sclerosing agent such as tetracycline.

EMPYEMA

Accumulation of pus within the pleural space (empyema) is an occasional complication of bacterial pneumonia or lung abscess and should be distinguished from the more common sterile inflammatory effusion. The fluid usually is thick and has the turbid appearance of frank pus, containing over 30,000 WBC/μl and often showing the etiologic bacterial agent on Gram stain and in culture. Empyema fluid caused by anaerobic organisms, especially *Bacteroides* or streptococci, often has a foul odor. A chronic empyema in a patient already treated with antibiotics may pose a problem in identification, since the fluid may have become thinner and the culture may be sterile. The leukocyte count of the fluid under these circumstances is probably the most reliable distinguishing feature. In addition, pleural fluid with a pH below 7.20 should strongly suggest empyema.

The presence of an empyema should be suspected whenever a patient with bacterial pneumonia shows either persistence or re-

currence of fever after appropriate antibiotic treatment. Evidence of even a small amount of pleural fluid in this setting requires thoracentesis for diagnosis. Although empyemas usually arise by extension of bacterial infection through the visceral pleura from the lung, they may also result from perforation of the esophagus, subphrenic abscess, or as a complication of surgery.

Successful management of the patient with empyema requires both the administration of appropriate antibiotics and the maintenance of effective drainage. Prompt recognition and institution of drainage provide the greatest likelihood that the empyema space will close without becoming chronic. When a small empyema is discovered early in the course of infection, attempts to close the space by repeated thoracentesis may be justified. This is seldom successful, however, and the prompt insertion of a chest tube with connection to water-seal drainage is the usual treatment. After several days without adequate drainage, most empyemas become loculated so that a tube is no longer effective, and in this situation

thoracotomy with removal of the empyema sac and decortication of the lung results in a more rapid recovery.

REFERENCES

1. Good JT Jr, Taryle DA, Sahn SA: The pathogenesis of low glucose, low pH malignant effusion. Am Rev Respir Dis 131:737, 1985
2. Light RW: Pleural Diseases. Philadelphia, Lea & Febiger, 1983
3. Poe RH, Israel RH, et al: Sensitivity, specificity and predictive values of closed pleural biopsy. Arch Intern Med 144:325, 1984
4. Prakash UBS, Reiman HM: Comparison of needle biopsy with cytologic analysis for the evaluation of pleual effusion. Analysis of 414 cases. Mayo Clin Proc 60:158, 1985
5. Albertine KH, Wiener-Kronish JP, Staub NC: The structure of the parietal pleura and its relationship to pleural liquid dynamics in sheep. Anat Res 208:401, 1984

CHAPTER 3.5
Diffuse Pulmonary Infiltration and Fibrosis

Carol J. Johns and Sandra M. Walden

This chapter discusses a variety of conditions that produce abnormal radiographic images widely distributed throughout both lungs.[7] The clinical manifestations associated with these radiographic abnormalities may be minimal or incapacitating, depending on the nature and extent of the condition. Some patients are asymptomatic, presenting because of an abnormal routine chest radiograph, while others present with cough, dyspnea, decreased exercise tolerance, cyanosis, cor pulmonale, or heart failure—all the result of impaired lung function. Systemic manifestations of illness such as fever, fatigability, anorexia, and weight loss predominate in some disorders. In these the physical examination may be normal or may reveal related systemic findings, lung restriction, inspiratory lung crackles, airway obstruction, clubbing, or evidence of cor pulmonale. In certain multisystem diseases, such as progressive systemic sclerosis (scleroderma), rheumatoid arthritis, uremia, and the lymphomas, the pulmonary manifestations may be only incidental findings. Diffuse disease may also exist without radiographic changes, especially in early *Pneumocystis carinii* pneumonia and occasionally in sarcoidosis and idiopathic pulmonary fibrosis. Rapid changes are unusual except in pulmonary edema or rapidly progressive infections.

RADIOGRAPHIC FEATURES

The abnormal chest roentgenogram conveys specific information useful in guiding the clinical investigation of the patient with diffuse lung disease. The radiographic abnormalities can usually be described either as alveolar, or as interstitial with nodular, reticular, and noduloreticular patterns. These patterns are presented in Chapter 3.1. Computed tomography may provide additional information about the presence and location of enlarged lymph nodes and details of the pattern of infiltration or anatomic change. For example, subpleural infiltrates are characteristic of early sarcoidosis with active inflammation.

Radiographic changes may be evident without symptoms, and rapid change is unusual except with pulmonary edema and intrapulmonary hemorrhage. Certain radiographic changes imply chronicity of disease. In inflammatory disorders, cystic dilation of distal air spaces (bronchiolectasis) may occur, producing a coarse reticular

pattern with air spaces 5 to 6 mm in diameter. When extensive, this pattern is referred to as "honeycomb lung" and may be seen in any diffuse *fibrosing alveolitis*. Subpleural clusters of rounded lucencies are especially well seen at the lung bases. Proliferation of fibrous tissue may produce thick linear shadows and gross shrinkage and distortion of the lung parenchyma.

Many diseases have both alveolar and interstitial components, and it is often impossible to distinguish these pathologic processes by radiographic studies. Making a diagnosis from the radiographic pattern alone has serious limitations, but a series of films can be diagnostically useful, yielding important information about the time course of a disease. Sometimes radiographic abnormalities associated with the parenchymal densities are of great help in identifying the underlying process. Examples of this are bilateral diaphragmatic pleural calcification, which is nearly always caused by asbestos exposure, and eggshell calcification of hilar nodes, which is rare except in patients with silicosis.

PULMONARY FUNCTION TESTING AND PHYSIOLOGIC ABNORMALITIES

Diseases characterized by filling of the alveoli or infiltration of the interstitial tissues of the lung usually cause abnormalities in pulmonary mechanics and gas exchange. The characteristic pattern in most of these diseases is a reduction in lung volumes (restrictive ventilatory defect), usually without airway obstruction; alveolar hyperventilation (low arterial PCO_2) with a reduced arterial PO_2 due largely to abnormal ventilation-perfusion ratios; and a variable but often severe reduction in diffusing capacity. The deposition of any abnormal material results in stiffening of the lungs and reduction in the volume normally occupied by air. This is manifest by a decreased compliance of the lungs and restriction with a reduction in vital capacity, total lung capacity, and residual volume.

Since the airways are only indirectly affected by processes confined to the interstitial spaces, airway obstruction is often conspicuously absent in this group of diseases. Distortion or narrowing of airways, with resulting obstruction to the flow of air, may occur in complicated cases or in late stages of the chronic diffuse fibrosis, including sarcoidosis, however. Reversible airway obstruc-

tion indicates increased airways reactivity, as is noted in hypersensitivity pneumonitis and sarcoidosis. These physiologic abnormalities and methods for the clinical evaluation of pulmonary function are discussed more generally in Chapter 3.1.

TABLE 3.5–1. RADIOGRAPHIC PATTERNS[7]

Alveolar (Air Space Filling)
Fluid
- Pulmonary edema—congestive failure
- Heroin overdose
- Uremia
- Inhaled fumes
- Aspiration

Blood
- Vasculitis
- Goodpasture syndrome
- Idiopathic pulmonary hemorrhage
- Invasive aspergillosis in immunosuppressed host
- Bleeding diatheses

Cells
- Pneumonia (bacterial, fungal, tuberculous, viral)
- Debris (pulmonary alveolar proteinosis)
- Pneumocystis carinii
- Eosinophilic pneumonias
- Alveolar cell carcinoma

Interstitial
Edema
- Lymphatic obstruction (Kerley B lines)
- Leukemia
- Chronic congestion
- Capillary leak (arabinoside-C)

Cellular Infiltrates
- Interstitial pneumonitis
- Sarcoidosis
- Drug effects
- Leukemia
- Lymphangitic spread of tumor (breast, stomach, pancreas, lung, biliary tract)
- Hypersensitivity pneumonitis
- Radiation pneumonitis

Fibrosis
- Idiopathic pulmonary fibrosis
- Sarcoidosis
- Pneumoconioses
- Scleroderma

Iron Deposits
- Siderosis
- Hemosiderosis

Cystic Spaces
- Emphysema
- Sarcoidosis
- Eosinophilic granuloma
- Cystic fibrosis
- Familial fibrocystic dysplasia
- Chronic fibrocystic inflammatory disease

Diseases Characteristically Involving Upper Lobes
- Tuberculosis
- Sarcoidosis
- Silicosis
- Coal workers' pneumoconiosis
- Eosinophilic granuloma
- Cystic fibrosis

Diseases Characteristically Involving Lower Lobes
- Alveolar proteinosis
- Asbestosis
- Aspiration
- Berylliosis
- Scleroderma
- Bronchiectasis

APPROACH TO DIAGNOSIS

Diffuse roentgenographic abnormalities are produced by a wide variety of underlying diseases, but it is clearly important to make a definitive diagnosis whenever possible. The most practical approach is to narrow the differential diagnosis as much as possible using the appearance of the chest roentgenogram together with information from the history and physical examination. From the radiograph one can determine some anatomic characteristics of the lesion. Table 3.5–1 presents a systematic approach to radiographic patterns. The duration of symptoms, together with a review of previous films (if available), will indicate whether the process is acute, chronic, or static. The history permits evaluation of the possibility of a familial disorder or a disease caused by aspiration or inhalation of a foreign substance. In addition, the importance of

TABLE 3.5–2. DIAGNOSTIC FEATURES OF DIFFUSE PULMONARY INFILTRATION

Often Asymptomatic
- Sarcoidosis
- Siderosis (arc welders), early pneumoconiosis
- Carcinoma of thyroid with diffuse pulmonary metastases
- Eosinophilic granuloma (histiocytosis X)
- Löffler pneumonia, lipoid pneumonia
- Alveolar proteinosis (minimal infiltrates)

Fever
- Infections, collagen diseases, leukemia, lymphoma
- Hypersensitivity pneumonitis
- Sarcoidosis (erythema nodosum or active hepatic disease)
- Drug reactions

Hemoptysis
- Advanced fibrocystic disease with superimposed bacterial or fungal infection or mycetoma (esp. sarcoidosis and tuberculosis)
- Bronchiectasis
- Idiopathic pulmonary hemosiderosis
- Cavitary disease—tuberculosis, fungal disease, Wegener granulomatosis
- Vasculitis—Wegener granulomatosis, Goodpasture syndrome, polyarteritis
- Invasive aspergillosis
- Blood dyscrasia or anticoagulant overdose
- Trauma—contusion
- Pulmonary emboli with infarction

Bronchial Obstruction or Wheezing
- Asthma, allergic bronchopulmonary aspergillosis
- Hypersensitivity pneumonitis—infrequently
- Tropical eosinophilia
- Eosinophilic granuloma (histiocytosis X)
- Bronchiolitis obliterans[5]

Mediastinal Adenopathy
- Sarcoidosis—usually symmetrical bilateral hilar and often with right paratracheal adenopathy
- Lymphoma—often asymmetrical
- Granulomatous infections—tuberculosis, histoplasmosis, usually asymmetrical and often calcified when old
- Fungal infections
- Wegener granulomatosis—uncommon
- Silicosis—eggshell or ring calcification (seen also in sarcoidosis and postirradiation Hodgkin disease)

Pleural Disease
- Tuberculosis and acute pneumonias—effusion or empyema
- Collagen vascular diseases—effusion
- Asbestosis—calcification, especially diaphragmatic pleura
- Neoplasms, effusion—often bloody
- Pulmonary emboli with or without infarction—effusion
- Congestive failure—transudative effusion
- Sarcoidosis—effusion rare and usually small

possible environmental and occupational exposures requires a lifetime job history. Together, the history and physical examination provide clues to the presence of associated systemic disease. Priority in thinking should be given to any specific disorders suggested by the information so obtained; to those diseases, for example, infections, for which specific treatment exists; and to common rather than rare diseases. A few specific clinical findings that are often helpful are shown in Table 3.5–2. Finally, it is useful to refer to a comprehensive list of disease categories (Table 3.5–3) to be certain that no important diagnostic possibility is being overlooked.

DIAGNOSTIC PROCEDURES

The roentgenographic and clinical features often strongly suggest a diagnosis that can be confirmed by conventional means. For example, appropriate cultures may prove the diagnosis of infection; biopsy of a characteristic skin lesion, lymph node, or liver may support the diagnosis of sarcoidosis; and the demonstration of a malignant tumor outside the thorax may account for diffuse metastases throughout the lungs. Seeking all readily accessible clues often obviates the need for major invasive procedures.

SPUTUM EXAMINATION

This subject is discussed in detail in Chapter 3.1. In patients with bacterial or fungal infections or with *Pneumocystis carinii* pneumonia, appropriate smears and cultures may establish a diagnosis. Periodic acid-Schiff (PAS) stain of formalin-fixed sputum may show the characteristic alveolar material present in alveolar proteinosis. Cytologic study may reveal tumor cells. Large numbers of eosinophils in the sputum suggest a hypersensitivity disorder involving the lung. Oil droplets within macrophages support the diagnosis of lipoid pneumonia. Hemoptysis is often diagnostically helpful (see Table 3.5–2).

LYMPH NODE BIOPSY

Palpable superficial lymph nodes may be biopsied with little discomfort and risk to the patient. Such a biopsy is often useful in the diagnosis of sarcoidosis, tuberculosis, Hodgkin disease and other lymphomas, and metastatic carcinoma. A granulomatous reaction is nonspecific, however, and may occur as a response to hypersensitivity, fungal or bacterial infection, parasitic infestation, the deposition of foreign chemical substances, tuberculosis, or sarcoidosis. Careful bacterial cultures of biopsy material are always important.

Mediastinoscopy with node biopsy is a safe and useful procedure in staging tumors or when lymphoma is suspected. It has a high yield in sarcoidosis but is rarely necessary to make the diagnosis.

BRONCHOSCOPY AND LUNG BIOPSY

Biopsy procedures are discussed in detail in Chapter 3.1. Transbronchial lung biopsy is especially useful with multilobar disease, for example, in suspected sarcoidosis, metastatic neoplasm, or opportunistic infection in immunocompromised hosts. Four adequate specimens containing alveoli should be obtained. This is the procedure of choice in sarcoidosis when other features or more superficial abnormalities do not establish a diagnosis.[2] Findings of nonspecific pneumonitis do not exclude a potentially treatable disorder but do reduce the likelihood of a granulomatous pneumonitis.

Lung brushings dependably produce organisms in *P. carinii* pneumonia in immuncompromised hosts. Needle aspiration or biopsy of paratracheal or subcarinal nodes may provide useful cytologic material revealing tumor or granulomas.

Open-lung biopsy carries a low risk, especially in young patients without complicating heart disease, and provides a tissue specimen of adequate size. Open-lung biopsy is necessary occasionally to verify diffuse lung disease, such as bronchiolar carcinoma, eosinophilic granuloma (histiocytosis X), pulmonary alveolar proteinosis, berylliosis, desquamative interstitial pneumonia, drug reactions, and idiopathic pulmonary fibrosis. In this last disease, determination of the presence of an active inflammatory process and the degree of fibrosis is useful in predicting the response to corticosteroids.[3] The value of open biopsy in seriously immunosuppressed patients is unclear, since broad coverage of all suspected infections usually must be initiated immediately when diffuse infiltrates or symptoms appear.[1,13]

Answers to three questions may aid in the decision regarding the need for open lung biopsy: (1) Does the patient have a lesion amenable to treatment? (2) Are there sufficient indications for treatment if the suspected diagnosis proves correct? (3) Is it important to know of an occupational exposure or a specific environmental agent present in the lungs?

Lung tissue should be subjected not only to histologic study but also to a careful search for fungi and tubercle bacilli, using all appropriate staining and cultural techniques. Chemical and spectrographic analysis may be indicated to identify such substances as silicon and beryllium.

Percutaneous lung biopsy is useful when peripheral discrete or general confluent masses are present. Biopsy with a no. 18 needle provides a larger specimen than transbronchial lung biopsy and is especially useful with peripheral lesions. Tumor, fungi, and amyloid usually are readily identified. Severe obstructive airway disease and bullous lesions are relative contraindications.

MANAGEMENT

Specific treatment obviously requires a definitive diagnosis. Although many of the diseases discussed in this chapter are not responsive to therapy, it is important that all treatable possibilities be given special consideration. Table 3.5–4 lists a number of diseases amenable to treatment.

ASSESSMENT OF DISEASE ACTIVITY

First, it is essential to determine activity or progression by symptoms, previous radiographs, and measurements of pulmonary function. The degree and course of impairment are crucial factors in long-range management decisions, especially in sarcoidosis.[2] The importance of diligently seeking previous radiographs also cannot be overestimated. Furthermore, active disease can be measured retrospectively by demonstrating reversibility in response to treatment.

Gallium-67 lung scans have been used to assess the presence of an active inflammatory component with affinity for gallium. The nonspecificity and varying sensitivity as well as the radiation burden are significant limiting factors in its usefulness.

Bronchoalveolar lavage[4,12] with study of the cellular elements and chemical mediators of inflammation and fibrosis can give information about the activity and nature of the alveolitis. In sarcoidosis the increased numbers of T-helper lymphocytes and activated T lymphocytes are thought to correlate with disease liable to progression. With idiopathic pulmonary fibrosis, increased numbers of polymorphonuclear leukocytes (PMNs) are noted. There is

TABLE 3.5-3. CLASSIFICATION OF DIFFUSE INFILTRATIONS AND CHARACTERISTIC FEATURES

Disease	Special Features
I. Familial or Congenital	
Familial fibrocystic dysplasia	Early clubbing; multiple tiny cysts
Cystic fibrosis	Children and young adults affected; viscous tracheobronchial secretions; chronic and recurrent pyogenic infections; microabscesses; positive sweat test
Alveolar microlithiasis	Asymptomatic fine nodular alveolar calcification
Familiar dysautonomia	Autonomic nervous system dysfunction; aspiration pneumonitis
II. Infections	
Bacterial	Fever, cough, sputum
Mycobacterial (tuberculosis)	Gradual onset, fever, positive tuberculin skin test, cough, weight loss, miliary disease may be indolent
Fungal	Localized or diffuse lesions; often superimposed on underlying disease
Parasitic (schistosomiasis, ascariasis)	Bronchial asthma, eosinophilia, precipitins and complement fixing antibodies
Pneumocystis carinii	Immunosuppressed or debilitated patients, especially with AIDS
Viral	Cough, dyspnea, fever, myalgia; patchy infiltrates or diffuse changes
III. Inhaled Irritants	
Chemical Fumes	
Nitrogen dioxide	Silo-filler's disease; disabling dyspnea, exposure-related
Chlorine, phosgene	Exposure history; abrupt onset of cough and dyspnea
Cadmium	Exposure history; steroids may be lifesaving
Metal fume fever (brass and zinc)	Occupational history (galvanizing); fever and chill on exposure
Trimellitic anhydride	Exposure: rubber industries, metal refining, polyurethane plastic resins; pulmonary disease anemia syndrome; hypersensitivity pneumonitis; delayed onset asthma, rhinitis, cough, myalgia; hemorrhagic pneumonitis
Polyvinyl chloride	Exposure: plastics industry; interstitial pulmonary fibrosis with granulomatous reactions
Polymerizing chemicals such as diisocyanates	Exposure to polyurethane foam, rubber, plastics, or resins; worse beginning of work week; minor patchy, soft opacities
Mineral Dusts	
Asbestosis	Exposure history (insulation construction, shipyard work, etc.); long latent period; interstitial disease progressing to diffuse, coarse fibrosis and honeycomb pattern, most often bibasilar; shaggy heart border; calcified pleural plaques, often diaphragmatic and pericardial surfaces; pleural effusions; associated with lung cancer and pleural mesothelioma
Berylliosis	Exposure history (aircraft manufacturing, metallurgy, rocket fuels, radiographic casings); granulomatous changes may resemble sarcoidosis
Coal workers pneumoconiosis	Coal dust exposure; occasional progressive massive fibrosis
Silicosis (see Fig. 3.5-1)	Exposure history (sandblasting, quarrying, mining, foundry glass, and ceramics work); associated mycobacterial disease; nodular silica deposits and progressive fibrosis and retraction; eggshell calcification of hilar nodes
Siderosis (iron oxide)	Exposure history (arc welding); no symptoms or disability; simple nodular pattern on radiograph; iron-laden macrophages without fibrosis
Talcosis	Exposure history; micronodule patterns; intravenous narcotics with crushed tablets
Organic Dusts[6,11]	
Extrinsic asthma	Inhaled antigens; mucous plugs or impactions (status asthmaticus); eosinophilia and eosinophils in sputum
Allergic bronchopulmonary aspergillosis[9]	Clinical asthma: eosinophilia; multiple and varying infiltrates with rounded visible shadows of fungal plugs; mycelia of *Aspergillus* cultured in sputum; *Aspergillus* precipitins in serum; increased IgE; responds to corticosteroids
Hypersensitivity pneumonitis[6] (extrinsic allergic alveolitis)	Exposure history essential; cough and dyspnea; may remit with removal from exposure; responds to corticosteroids
Farmers' lung	Exposure to moldy hay; serum precipitins for spores of *Micropolyspora faeni, Thermoactinomyces vulgaris*
Humidifier/air conditioner lung	Thermophilic actinomycetes in ventilation systems at home or at work
Bird fanciers' lung	Exposure to avian proteins, pigeon breeders
Pituitary snuff users' lung	Bovine and porcine proteins
Bagassosis	Moldy sugar cane exposure; serum precipitins for *Thermoactinomyces*
Byssinosis	Exposure history (raw cotton, flax, or hemp); reversible airway obstruction; chronic bronchitis and emphysema; radiographic changes usually minimal
Isocyanates	Paint catalyst, exposure in paint workers, porcelain finishers

(continued)

TABLE 3.5–3. CLASSIFICATION OF DIFFUSE INFILTRATIONS AND CHARACTERISTIC FEATURES (Continued)

Disease	Special Features
IV. Neoplastic	
Bronchiolar (alveolar cell) carcinoma	Cough, sputum, weight loss; alveolar pattern, (localized or diffuse); may present as solitary nodules
Hematogenous metastases	Melanoma, breast, testis, chorioepithelioma, thyroid, pancreas, kidney
Lymphangitic carcinomatosis	Breast, stomach, pancreas, lung, biliary tract
Leukemia (lymphatic more common)	Fever; leukostasis with WBC 200,000/mm³; blood and bone marrow changes; diffuse perihilar pattern; mediastinal nodes common
Lymphoma	Parenchymal nodules, especially nodular sclerosing Hodgkin; mediastinal nodes
V. Metabolic	
Uremia	Renal failure; pulmonary edema pattern
VI. Aspiration	
Aspiration pneumonitis	Disturbed consciousness or disorders of swallowing; local anesthesia of the pharynx; drowning; basal or posterior patchy pneumonitis
Lipoid pneumonia	Intranasal oily drops; mineral oil laxative in elderly
Kerosene pneumonia	Kerosene ingestion
VII. Drug Reactions[3]	
Cytotoxic Drug Reactions	
Most common: bleomycin[a], nitrosourea *Uncommon:* cyclophosphamide[a] (Cytoxan), methotrexate[a], azathioprine (Imuran), chlorambucil (Leukeran), busulfan (Myleran) *Rare:* procarbazine HCl[a]	See Table 3.5–4; fever without chills; onset 2–6 mo after initiation of therapy; may not resolve with drug withdrawal; worsened by combined cytotoxic agents; gradual progression of alveolar interstitial infiltrate and decreased diffusing capacity, bizarre alveolar nuclei on biopsy. Bleomycin may generate oxygen radicals that produce lung injury; oxygen administration accelerates bleomycin toxicity; cytotoxic lung injury may predispose to infection
Noncytotoxic Drug Reactions	Fever less often than with cytotoxic drug reactions; severity may be dose-related; dyspnea resolves with discontinuation of drug, improves with steroids
• Chemotherapeutic agents[12] Methotrexate[a] most common	Produces a noncytotoxic reaction; fever, cough, dyspnea
Cytosine arabinoside (Ara-c)	Intense pulmonary edema, both noncardiogenic and cardiogenic; usually fatal
• Antiarrhythmics Amiodarone	Dyspnea, leukocytosis, elevated erythrocyte sedimentation rate (ESR); diffuse interstitial or alveolar pattern resolves with discontinuation of drug; corticosteroid therapy may improve
Procainamide	Drug-induced lupus syndrome
• Antibiotic agents Nitrofurantoin	*Acute:* severe dyspnea, fever, cough, eosinophilia, resolves with discontinuation. *Chronic:* interstitial fibrosis
Amphotericin	Diffuse interstitital infiltrate, hemoptysis, hypoxemia
Sulfasalazine	Dyspnea, cough, eosinophilia; diffuse interstitial infiltrate with rare fibrosing alveolitis; usually resolves with discontinuation
• Opiates Heroin, methadone, propoxyphene	Transient noncardiac pulmonary edema; talcosis due to impurities in preparation; associated with midline granulomatosis
• Antihypertensives Hydralazine	Hypersensitivity pneumonitis; lupuslike syndrome; clears slowly with withdrawal of drug
Hydrochlorothiazide (uncommon)	Reversible noncardiogenic pulmonary edema; clears with withdrawal
• Miscellaneous Gold salts	Interstitial pneumonitis, fibrosis, anaphylactoid reactions
D-penicillamine	Goodpasture syndrome, allergic alveolitis, interstitial pneumonitis
Cocaine	Talcosis; inhaled forms (free-base) may induce pulmonary edema, acute respiratory distress syndrome, or permanent interstitial fibrosis
Oxygen toxicity	Usually occurs with >60% Fio_2 >24 hr; exudative and proliferative phases; diffuse hemorrhagic capillary damage
VIII. Physical Agents	
Postirradiation fibrosis[8]	Sharp borders reflecting the port used, 6–12 wk after radiation treatment begun; can be diffuse or localized; occurrence and severity related to volume and dose of lung irradiation; worsened by concomitant chemotherapy or steroid withdrawal; improves with high-dose corticosteroids started immediately with onset of pneumonitis; may progress gradually to fibrosis over 6–12 mo

(continued)

TABLE 3.5–3. CLASSIFICATION OF DIFFUSE INFILTRATIONS AND CHARACTERISTIC FEATURES (Continued)

Disease	Special Features
IX. Circulatory	
Hemodynamic: mitral stenosis or chronic left ventricular failure	Pulmonary edema; Kerley B lines, hemosiderosis, lower lobe fibrosis
Thromboembolic: multiple pulmonary emboli	Episodic dyspnea, atelectatic streaks, pulmonary hypertension, positive lung scan
Fat embolism	Recent fracture; localized changes or diffuse pulmonary edema
Lymphangiography	Recent lymphangiogram: ground glass appearance
X. Connective Tissue Diseases[9]	
Scleroderma	Systemic manifestations of sclerosis (skin changes, gastrointestinal tract and joint symptoms); cystic changes at lung bases
Polyarteritis nodosa	Subacute febrile systemic disease; variable manifestations of pneumonia, asthma, hemoptysis
Wegener granulomatosis	Necrotizing granulomatous lesions of upper airways, lung, and kidneys; may be limited to lungs; multiple nodular masses that may cavitate
Systemic lupus erythematosus	Small atelectatic streaks with occasional patchy pneumonitis; pleural effusion common; antinuclear factor; pulmonary disease more common in procainamide-induced disease
Rheumatoid lung disease	Rheumatoid pulmonary nodules and endarteritis; pleural effusion common
Caplan syndrome[11] (rheumatoid pneumoconiosis)	Coal workers' pneumoconiosis; clinical signs of rheumatoid arthritis; rheumatoid factor; occasional progressive massive fibrosis
Idiopathic pulmonary fibrosis[4] (synonyms—see text)	Dyspnea, clubbing; diffuse fine fibrosis Cor pulmonale; possible multiple agents or factors elicit this; some respond to corticosteroids; immunologic mechanisms possible
XI. Eosinophilic Pneumonias	
Löffler syndrome	Fever, eosinophilia, asthma; minimal or no pulmonary symptoms; recovery usually within a month; transitory and migratory alveolar infiltrations
Prolonged pulmonary eosinophilia	Chronic patchy infiltrations
Tropical eosinophilia	Asthmatic attacks; biologic false-positive serologic test for syphilis; complement fixation positive for filarial antigens; may respond to diethylcarbamazine
XII. Miscellaneous	
Sarcoidosis[2,10]	Granulomatous involvement of lungs, lymph nodes, eyes, skin, liver, spleen, salivary glands, muscle, etc.; variable symptoms; hilar adenopathy frequent; tuberculin anergy; increase in gamma globulins; elevation of serum angiotensin-converting enzyme; responds to corticosteroids
Pulmonary alveolar proteinosis	PAS-staining material occasionally in sputum; pulmonary lavage with saline produces clearing; chronic alveolar infiltration; often perihilar distribution; cellular debris fills alveoli without interstitial change; nocardiosis may develop
Eosinophilic granuloma (histiocytosis X)	Begins in childhood with slow progression; airway obstruction common; may have diabetes insipidus; pneumothorax common; associated bone lesions common; honeycomb cystic lung in later stages; no hilar adenopathy; cytotoxic agents recommended
Goodpasture syndrome[9]	Hemoptysis, anemia, and renal failure; acute hemorrhagic pneumonitis and nephritis; patchy infiltrates; linear irregular thickening of glomerular and alveolar basement membrane on electron microscopy; cytotoxic specific anti-glomerular basement membrane antibody
Idiopathic pulmonary hemosiderosis	Recurrent hemoptysis, anemia, hemosiderin-laden macrophages in sputum; fine reticular shadows with interstitial fibrosis; varying infiltrates with blood; mechanism uncertain
Rejection phenomenon in homotransplantation	Circulating antibody against donor cells; acute vasculitis; destruction of grafted organ; cytotoxic tissue-specific antibody–type II immunologic reaction
Lymphomatoid granulomatosis	Varied patterns; unknown cause; fever, skin, kidney, and marrow involvement; corticosteroids and cyclophosphamide
XIII. Secondary Pulmonary Fibrosis	
Bronchiectasis	Cough and purulent sputum of long standing
Bronchitis and obstructive pulmonary disease	Impaired forced expiratory flow; hyperinflation; increased linear markings

[a]These drugs can cause both cytotoxic and noncytotoxic reactions.

TABLE 3.5–4. THERAPY OF DIFFUSE PULMONARY LESIONS[1,6,14]

I. **Specific chemotherapy for infections**
  - Timely use of broad-spectrum antibiotics is essential in immunosuppressed hosts; withdrawal of immunosuppressive agents may be necessary, especially with cytomegalovirus
II. **Removal from exposure for occupation pulmonary diseases**
III. **Corticosteroid treatment**
  - Sarcoidosis
  - Incapacitating or progressive disease; persistent disease, with functional impairment without evidence of spontaneous remission for more than 1 yr
  - Hypersensitivity pneumonitis if symptomatic and not responding to simple environmental removal of the offending antigen
  - Pulmonary vasculitis
    Polyarteritis nodosa, systemic lupus erythematosus, Wegener granulomatosis
  - Eosinophilic granuloma (histiocytosis X)
    Effect uncertain
  - Therapeutic trial in idiopathic fibrosing alveolitis
    More likely helpful with more inflammatory picture and less fibrosis; "desquamative" features, rather than "mural" changes may suggest a more favorable response or milder disease
IV. **Immunosuppressive or cytotoxic agents**
  - Neoplastic disease: lymphomas, leukemia, carcinoma of breast, metastatic seminomas, etc.
  - Wegener and lymphomatoid granulomatosis (cyclophosphamide often combined with corticosteroids)
  - Eosinophilic granuloma (histiocytosis X)
  - Lupus erythematosus
  - Rheumatoid arthritis
V. **Pulmonary lavage for alveolar proteinosis**
VI. **Hormone therapy for some neoplasms, e.g., carcinoma of the breast**

no doubt that bronchoalveolar lavage provides an important research tool for better understanding of disease mechanisms, but it has limited usefulness in guiding treatment. Results are variable and methods are not standardized, with no clearly identifiable markers to direct therapy.

Elevations of serum angiotension converting enzyme[10] are thought to reflect the presence of active granulomatous inflammation and have been observed with 75 percent of patients with active untreated sarcoidosis, but the finding is variable and has much less specificity than originally hoped. It is not reliable in predicting the need for further corticosteroid treatment.[2,4,10,14]

The vigor of the diagnostic approach will be determined by the severity of disease. Objective evidence of change assists in the assessment of response to treatment (radiographic changes and serial measurements of pulmonary function, as well as changes in symptoms and other clinical findings). These points are particularly pertinent in patients treated with corticosteroids but apply as well to patients with infections treated with antimicrobials.

CORTICOSTEROID THERAPY

Steroid therapy appears to help many patients with sarcoidosis, fibrosing alveolitis, connective tissue disease involving the lung, and certain other disorders of an immunologic type.[2,5,14]

Furthermore, in some instances of progressive or seriously incapacitating disease, a therapeutic trial of steroids is indicated even when a specific diagnosis has not been made. Open-lung biopsy may occasionally be deemed inadvisable or not likely to reveal a specific diagnostic picture, but transbronchial lung biopsy can almost always be performed. The risks and potential value of steroid use must be weighed and the effects objectively assessed. Careful prior exclusion of infectious disease is important in deciding on a trial of corticosteroid therapy.

IMMUNOSUPPRESSIVE AGENTS

The role of these agents in diffuse lung disease remains relatively uncertain except in lymphomas and leukemia. Benefit from cyclophosphamide combined with prednisone therapy has been demonstrated in Wegener granulomatosis and lymphomatoid granulomatosis.[9,14] These agents have an anti-inflammatory action as well as a specific inhibitory effect on immunologic reactions. Their use is indicated in patients with vasculitis, usually in combination with corticosteroids.

SUPPORTIVE TREATMENT

Supportive treatment is important not only in conjunction with specific therapy: It may also be initiated when other treatment is not available or indicated. Symptomatic remedies for troublesome cough, limitation of physical activity, treatment of congestive failure, and measures to combat secondary bacterial infection may be of great therapeutic value. Oxygen administration may occasionally be needed to relieve hypoxia. Since airway obstruction with alveolar hypoventilation is an unusual and late feature, oxygen usually can be administered safely with little risk of depressing respiration and retaining carbon dioxide.

SPECIFIC PROBLEMS IN DIAGNOSIS AND MANAGEMENT

TUBERCULOUS AND FUNGAL INFECTIONS

The importance of promptly identifying potentially treatable infections, such as tuberculosis, cannot be overemphasized. Treatable infectious agents must always be sought, especially in patients with altered host defenses. The development of tuberculosis may be the first clue to the immunosuppression associated with human immune virus (HIV) infection, before AIDS is identified. The presence of fine miliary micronodular lesions should always suggest the possibility of *miliary tuberculosis*.

The urgency of beginning appropriate chemotherapy may not be recognized, as symptoms may vary from mild illness to severe dyspnea and prostration. The presence of fever and rapidly progressive disease favors tuberculosis rather than sarcoidosis, which can produce a similar roentgenographic appearance. The tuberculin skin test is usually positive but may be negative in the presence of overwhelming disease or in older patients whose skin reactivity is not normal. Liver biopsy is positive in over 90 percent of cases, and acid-fast tissue stains commonly show tubercle bacilli. The use of at least two or three effective antituberculous drugs is essential in tuberculosis to prevent the emergence of drug resistance. Treatment must be continued for a sufficient period of time to eradicate the disease, usually 9 months if isoniazid and rifampin are included in the regimen. Pyrazinamide and streptomycin often are added to this regimen for the first 2 months to strengthen the regimen and shorten the overall treatment to 9 months. When poor compliance is anticipated, supervised chemotherapy may allow a shorter treatment period of 6 months. Daily treatment for 2 months followed by 4 months of twice weekly isoniazid and rifampin can be effective.

Failure of primary treatment may indicate the presence of drug resistance. Drug resistance should be suspected in foreign-born patients from developing countries, and treatment should be initiated with three drugs. If the patient has been treated before, it is important to include drugs to which the organisms probably are sensitive. Rifampin is an excellent mycobactericidal drug, but *neither rifampin nor any single drug should ever be added to a failed or failing regimen*. Sensitivity studies and a careful history of drugs previously administered are essential when drug resistance is suspected.

Communication with the appropriate health department is

valuable for investigating case contacts and for managing the disease. Recognition and management of tuberculosis is outlined in Chapter 9.6. Other nontuberculous mycobacteria, such as *M. kansasii* and *M. avium-intracellulare,* can cause pulmonary disease. The latter is frequently noted in AIDS patients.

Fungal infections must be differentiated from tuberculosis and appropriately treated. It is important to recognize saprophytic fungi (i.e., *Aspergillus fumigatus* in sarcoidosis), which are frequently present in intracystic or intracavitary mycetomas but which may not be responsible for any invasive disease. *Aspergillus* can produce extensive necrotizing disease and hemorrhage in seriously immunocompromised hosts.

ENVIRONMENTAL AND OCCUPATIONAL DISEASE[11]

The exposure to a variety of inhaled irritants at home and in the workplace produces a group of diffuse lung disorders that are being encountered with increasing frequency. Taking a careful lifelong work and symptom history is essential to establish suspicion of an exposure-related illness, especially since these diseases may present with chronic nonspecific complaints. Knowledge of the hazards related to specific occupations may also permit a presumptive diagnosis of these disorders. This section will consider a few examples of the occupationally related lung diseases (see Table 3.5–3).

Mineral Dusts

The pneumoconioses are frequent causes of diffuse nodular or reticular lesions in the lung. In the United States, asbestosis, coal workers' pneumoconiosis, and silicosis are the most common types.

Asbestos. Asbestos consists of a number of naturally occurring fibrous hydrated silicates that resist all forms of destruction. This substance has been commonly used in the construction industry to strengthen materials such as cements, pipes, insulation, fillers, paints, and brake materials. Although those most at risk have been workers directly handling these materials, such as those employed in shipyards and construction, significant exposure has been recognized through atmospheric pollution at school and in the home. Not all workers exposed to asbestos develop asbestosis. The severity and duration of exposure appear to be important, but the precise associations have not been delineated. Exposure is also associated with an increased incidence of mesothelioma and lung cancer, with the latter particularly in cigarette smokers. Even with regular exposure to asbestos, these findings develop only after a latent period of 10 to 20 years in most cases and may progress in severity even with removal from contact with asbestos. Radiographic features are shown in Table 3.5–3. Pulmonary function tests may reflect the progression of restrictive disease.

Silicosis. Silicosis develops after exposure to dust containing high concentrations of silicon dioxide. Particles 3 to 5 mm in diameter are most likely to produce disease. The more common occupations in which significant silica exposure may occur include mining and quarrying of sandstone, granite or quartz, stonecutting, masonry, sandblasting, glass and ceramics manufacturing, enameling, and foundry work (see Table 3.5–3). The diagnosis of silicosis (Fig. 3.5–1) is based on characteristic radiographic findings in patients with the appropriate exposure history. Many patients who are asymptomatic when first seen for their "abnormal chest radiograph" eventually develop progressively worsening dyspnea on exertion and chronic productive cough. Pulmonary hypertension and resultant cor pulmonale may occur in advanced cases despite removal from dust exposure years earlier. Silicosis predisposes to tuberculous infections, which often accelerate progressive massive fibrosis. Atypical infections with *M. avium-intracellulare* and *M. kansasii* as well as other opportunistic organisms also occur with

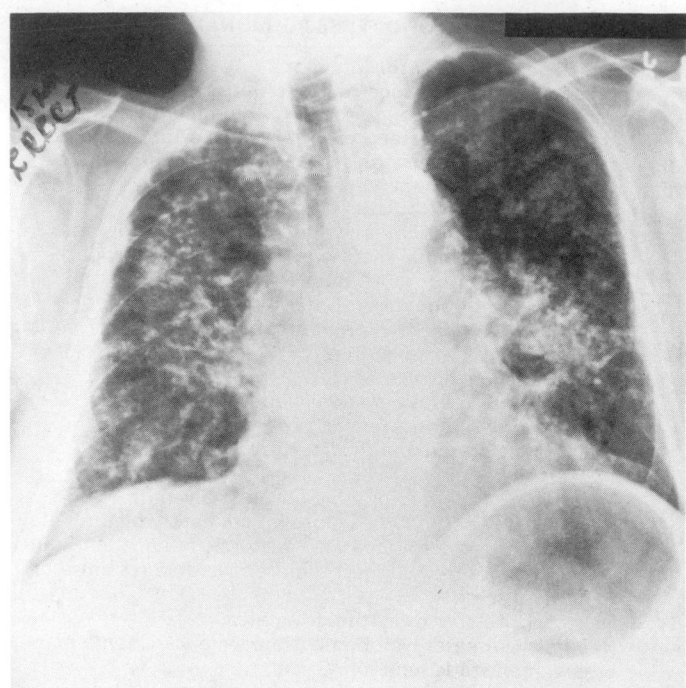

Figure 3.5–1. Silicosis in a 70-year-old man with 35 years of silica exposure as a ceramics worker.

increased frequency in these patients. Radiographic features of silicosis are described in Table 3.5–3.

Coal Workers' Pneumoconiosis. Coal workers' pneumoconiosis (CWP) develops in coal miners, carbon electrode workers, and graphite workers who inhale carbon dust. Normal mucociliary mechanisms are overwhelmed, and the dust is retained in the respiratory bronchioles and alveoli, causing a tissue reaction and the development of *coal macules* with areas of focal emphysema. With "simple" CWP, workers are typically asymptomatic except for a mild cough productive of blackish sputum. Unlike patients with silicosis, disease in them does not progress after they are removed from exposure. Obstructive defects detected on pulmonary function testing are usually due to concomitant cigarette abuse. Radiologic findings of simple CWP consist of diffuse, small (1 to 5 mm in diameter) nodular infiltrates, predominantly in the upper lung fields.

In "complicated" pneumoconiosis, or progressive massive fibrosis (PMF), opacities in the upper lung fields are at least 1 cm in diameter but may progress to encompass an entire lobe. Cavitation can occur due to ischemic necrosis or tuberculosis. *Caplan syndrome,* or rheumatoid pneumoconiosis, is associated with rheumatoid arthritis. This syndrome is similar to PMF, although the pulmonary lesions begin more peripherally and are more rapidly progressive than in PMF. Caplan syndrome can be seen in workers exposed to coal dust, silica, or asbestos. Treatment with immunosuppressive agents such as D-penicillamine has been promising.

Beryllium. Beryllium is a rare element used commercially as beryllium aluminum silicate. Beryllium poisoning may occur in acute or chronic form, although the intense exposures producing acute reactions of fulminant pulmonary edema rarely occur nowadays. A more benign form of the acute disease presents as a dry, nonproductive cough with substernal chest pain, dyspnea on exertion, anorexia, fatigue, and weight loss several weeks to months after exposure begins. *Chronic berylliosis* develops insidiously after a latent period as long as 15 years after exposure has ceased, presenting

with progressive dyspnea on exertion and mild cough, fatigue, weight loss, and arthralgia. Severe interstitial fibrosis may occur.

Inhalation of radiopaque dusts such as iron, tin, and barium generally produce benign nonspecific pneumoconioses in which these inorganic particles are retained in the lungs but do not cause toxic, allergenic, or inflammatory lung reactions (see Table 3.5–3). Although the roentgenographic effects are dramatic, little associated clinical disability occurs unless these agents are inhaled as mixed dusts that include fibrogenic agents such as silica.

Organic Dusts

The inhalation of organic particles or gases may lead to a number of pulmonary diseases, most commonly acute and chronic asthmatic responses. *Hypersensitivity pneumonitis*, also known as *extrinsic allergic alveolitis*, results from the sensitization and recurrent exposure to a specific antigenic substance. An increasing number of organic dusts (Table 3.5–3) are being recognized as causative agents.

Hypersensitivity pneumonitis should be suspected in patients with repeated bouts of influenza-like pneumonitis, active interstitial lung disease, or an appropriate exposure history. Disease is thought to result from a combination of type III and type IV immunologic reactions to the sensitizing antigen (see following discussion). The clinical onset may be acute or insidious. The *acute* form usually occurs with intermittent intense exposure to the agent to which the person is sensitized. Symptoms usually begin abruptly between 4 and 6 hours after exposure, with fever, chills, malaise, dyspnea, and nonproductive cough, which gradually subside over several hours to days. Occasionally, there is an immediate bronchospastic response as well. Removal from further exposure and treatment with corticosteroids accelerate resolution.

A *chronic* form of hypersensitivity pneumonitis results from a less intense but continuous exposure, such as with humidifier or air conditioner or bird fanciers' pneumonitis. Fever and chills may be absent, and patients present with progressive dyspnea on exertion, cough productive of mucoid sputum, fatigability, anorexia, and weight loss. The disease may progress to severe disability from pulmonary interstitial fibrosis despite withdrawal from exposure. A key to management lies in the recognition and termination of exposure to the offending antigen as early as possible. Corticosteroids may help accelerate remission if given early enough. The chest radiograph shows a diffuse interstitial infiltrate, which may progress to parenchymal retraction or honeycombing, or both.

IMMUNOLOGIC PULMONARY REACTIONS[6,9,14]

Four basic immunopathologic processes have been defined. Complex interrelationships exist in immunologic reactions, however, and often more than one type of response is involved in a clinical immunologic syndrome.

Type I: Immediate Hypersensitivity

In this type of immune reaction exposure to a specific antigen causes the production of a specific antibody (IgE). On a subsequent exposure the IgE combines with the allergen to initiate a sequence of biochemical reactions resulting in the release and synthesis of chemical mediators such as histamine, prostaglandins, and leukotrienes. The response may be systemic (anaphylaxis) or confined to specific organ systems such as the skin (urticaria), airways (allergic asthma), or, less commonly, lung parenchyma (interstitial or alveolar edema). These reactions are discussed in detail in Chapters 3.7: (Obstructive Lung Disease) and 7.1: (Immunologic Diseases).

Type II: Cytotoxic Tissue-specific Reactions

These reactions involve cytotoxic tissue-specific IgG and IgM antibodies, which react with an intrinsic antigenic constituent of the target organ cell, or an intrinsic cellular component similar to an extrinsic antigen. An example is *Goodpasture syndrome*.

Type III: Immune Complex Reactions

Immune-complex reactions result in deposition of antigen-antibody complexes along alveolar-capillary membranes in response to inhalation of specific antigens. This mechanism is involved in *hypersensitivity pneumonitis* (extrinsic allergic alveolitis) as described earlier. *Pulmonary vasculitis* as seen in *polyarteritis nodosa, Wegener granulomatosis,* and *lymphomatoid granulomatosis* also involve immune complex deposition. Response to steroids and immunosuppressive treatment has been encouraging.

Type IV: Cell-mediated Delayed Hypersensitivity

Delayed hypersensitivity is mediated by the interactions of sensitized lymphocytes with antigen, resulting in the release of substances that produce a maximal inflammatory immunologic response at 48 to 72 hours. These reactions are exemplified by the production of granulomatous nodules in tuberculosis and are also thought to be involved in chronic berylliosis.

SARCOIDOSIS[2,4,10,14]

Sarcoidosis is a granulomatous disease of unknown etiology that requires more detailed description because of its frequency as a cause of diffuse pulmonary infiltrations and its protean and variable manifestations. The most common pulmonary manifestation is hilar adenopathy, which is often associated with right paratracheal adenopathy. This is termed "type I sarcoidosis" without evident pulmonary infiltration, and spontaneous remission is frequent. If nodes persist when pulmonary infiltrations are visible, it is termed "type II." Infiltrations without adenopathy are labeled "type III A." Type III B indicates the presence of coarse fibrosis. Natural progression of the disease is pictured in Figure 3.5–2. The pulmonary lesions vary from those roentgenographically invisble through small nodular lesions of 2 to 3 mm to large confluent masses several centimeters in diameter. Soft infiltrates of a ground glass or "alveolar" type may also be observed. A reticulonodular pattern is frequent, with some fine interstitial infiltrates or fibrosis, or both, and the disease may progress to severe diffuse fibrocystic changes. In the absence of known environmental hazardous exposure, sarcoid is the most common cause of diffuse infiltration, and it is particularly likely when symptoms and degree of illness seem mild in relation to the extent of the radiographic changes. The clinical presentation can vary, however, from the incidental radiographic finding to debilitating febrile systemic illness or severe cough and dyspnea. The disease occurs most frequently in young adults and is more common and severe in black patients. Peripheral lymphadenopathy, hepatosplenomegaly, uveitis, and skin lesions are often present. Parotid and lacrimal gland enlargement and nervous system and myocardial disease with arrhythmias may be observed. Such clinical findings as depression of delayed hypersensitivity reactions (tuberculin, mumps, *Candida*), increased serum globulin, elevated alkaline phosphatase, hypercalciuria, and hypercalcemia also suggest the presence of sarcoid.

The diagnosis of sarcoidosis depends on the compatible clinical and radiologic picture and on granulomas on tissue biopsy (with reasonable exclusion of other causes of granulomatous disease). Biopsy information is sought from the most accessible tissue that seems abnormal. Transbronchial lung biopsy is especially useful, but characteristic histologic lesions may also be demonstrated in lymph nodes, skin lesions, liver, minor salivary glands in lip biopsy, or conjunctiva. The latter has a low yield except when the conjunctiva appears nodular.

Spontaneous remission is common in many patients with mild sarcoidosis, and no treatment will be required. In the absence of severe incapacitating disease, patients should be observed for several months without treatment to assess the likelihood of a spontaneous remission. Relapses are uncommon following spontaneous remissions. If the disease progresses or if significant disease persists in 6 to 12 months, most clinicians agree that corticosteroid

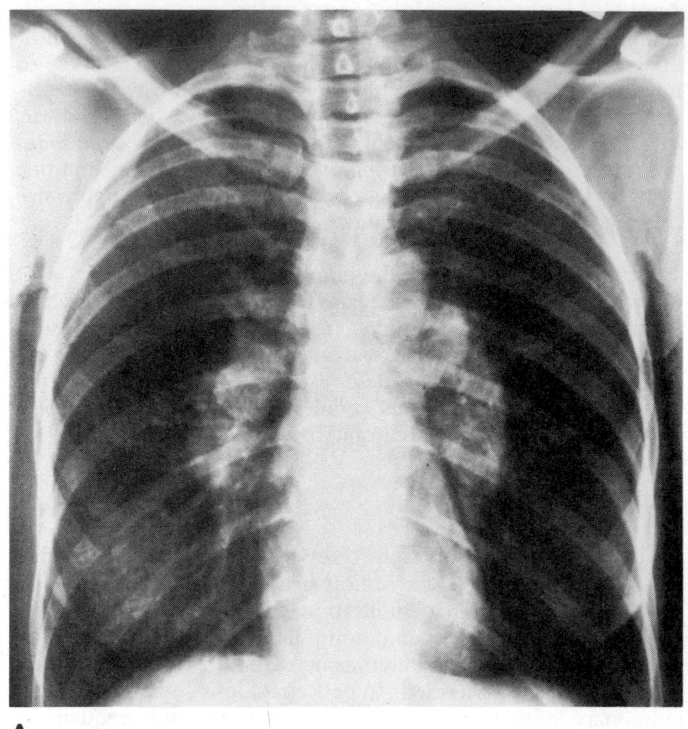

A

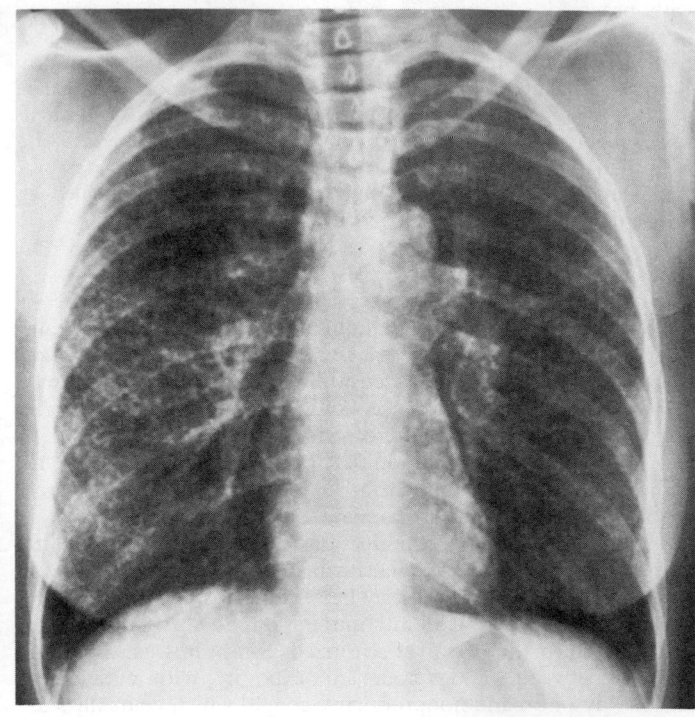

B

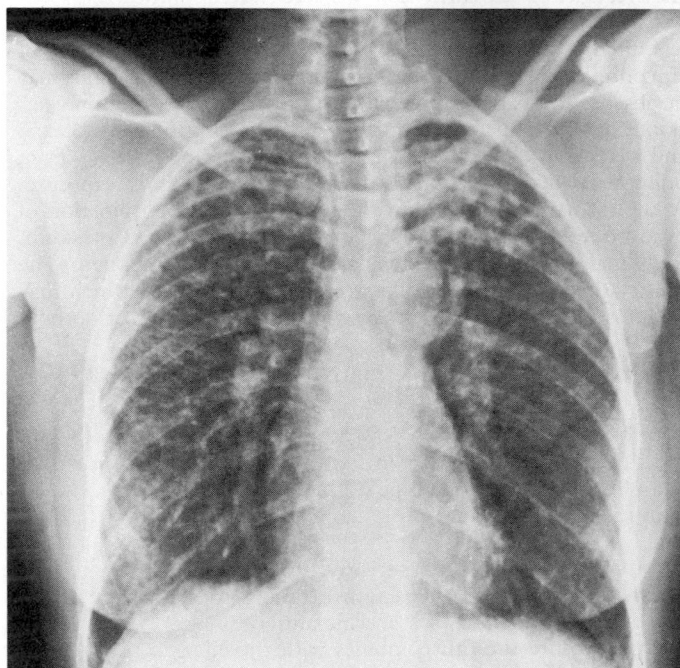

C

Figure 3.5–2. Sarcoidosis in a 43-year-old black woman. **A.** Type I: Bilateral hilar adenopathy (1/7/83). **B.** Type III: Reticulonodular infiltrates, one year later; nodes have regressed (3/16/84). **C.** Coalescent infiltrates with early fibrocystic changes, 2 years later (4/25/86).

treatment should be initiated. Mediastinal or hilar or peripheral lymphadenopathy alone is usually not sufficient indication for systemic treatment. Treatment should be initiated in seriously ill patients as soon as histologic support of the diagnosis is obtained and other causes of granulomatous disease reasonably excluded.

Corticosteroids often produce a dramatic therapeutic effect in sarcoidosis. Dyspnea and pulmonary function may improve within 2 to 4 weeks, and radiographs may also document significant improvement. Treatment should be withdrawn if such objective im-

provement is not clearly documented in 2 months. Treatment is initiated with 40 mg prednisone daily for 2 weeks, 30 mg daily for 2 weeks (using divided doses for the first 4 weeks), then single daily 8 AM doses of 25 mg for 2 weeks, followed by 20 or 15 mg daily for at least 4 more months. Alternate-day therapy for maintenance treatment is recommended by some physicians, but daily treatment facilitates compliance. Low doses of 10 to 15 mg daily rarely cause problems and are effective in controlling the inflammatory process. Tapering of drugs should be gradual and cautious, since

relapse may occur. Monthly evaluations should be made, especially at the end of the treatment and in the first 3 months thereafter. If symptoms, function tests, and chest radiographs worsen, treatment can often be reinstituted at the dose previously known to maintain stability. Some patients may require lifetime low-dose maintenance therapy.

Chloroquine has proven helpful in chronic indolent mucocutaneous sarcoidosis (500 mg daily for 2 weeks, then 250 mg daily for several months) but has not seemed effective in pulmonary sarcoidosis. Because of the potential of retinal and corneal damage, chloroquine is usually given for no longer than 6 months. Courses of treatment for skin lesions, nasal obstruction, and sinusitis can be repeated at 6-month intervals.

IDIOPATHIC PULMONARY FIBROSIS[4,14]

A group of similar inflammatory disorders that appear to involve predominantly the alveolar walls is referred to by the term "fibrosing alveolitis" and results in *idiopathic pulmonary fibrosis*. These disorders are characterized by varying degrees of interstitial cellular infiltration, desquamation of cells into the alveolar spaces, and deposition of fibrous tissue. The terms "interstitial pneumonitis" and "diffuse interstitial fibrosis" refer to the same group of disorders, which include the condition refered to as "Hamman–Rich syndrome" and "muscular cirrhosis of the lung." In some instances this may represent a hypersensitivity penumonitis with an unknown offending agent. Bronchoalveolar lavage may be useful in distinguishing the predominance of neutrophils in this condition from the increased lymphocytes observed in sarcoidosis.

Prednisone therapy is generally started with a dose of 60 mg per day and reduced gradually over a period of weeks until a plateau of improvement is reached, as judged by symptoms, radiographic changes, and repeated pulmonary function tests. A maintenance dose of 15 to 30 mg per day is often required to prevent relapse.

DIFFUSE INFILTRATIVE DISEASE IN IMMUNOSUPPRESSED PATIENTS

Patients with impaired immune defense systems often present with diffuse pulmonary infiltration. Susceptible hosts include patients with: (1) AIDS; (2) organ transplants; (3) malignant disease: leukemia, lymphoma, widely metastatic carcinoma; (4) granulocytopenia; (5) any systemic disease causing immunosuppression or requiring immunosuppressive drug therapy; (6) chronic renal or liver insufficiency. In these patients, common infections can produce totally uncharacteristic roentgenographic patterns, and agents that are not usually pathogenic may cause rapidly progressive pulmonary infections. *Pneumocystis carinii* pneumonia in AIDS patients is an example of this (Fig. 3.5–3). Table 3.5–5 summarizes the possibilities that must be considered for immunosuppressed hosts.[13] The main problem is to differentiate superimposed infection from extension of the underlying disease and reactions to drugs or irradiation used for treatment. Other common noninfectious pulmonary complications in these hosts include diffuse pulmonary hemorrhage, pulmonary emboli, and pulmonary edema (both cardiogenic and noncardiogenic). Sputum studies, bronchoalveolar lavage, or transbronchial lung biopsy often provide the diagnosis.[16] An aggressive therapeutic approach is often warranted, since many of these reactions are rapidly fatal if untreated. Broad-spectrum antibiotics can often be used for bacterial, fungal, and viral infections until further information becomes available.[1]

Open-lung biopsy is rarely useful in the diagnosis of acute infectious processes. This procedure may be very helpful, however, in the diagnosis of noninfectious processes such as drug reactions, lymphoma, or lymphangitic spread of metastatic carcinoma.

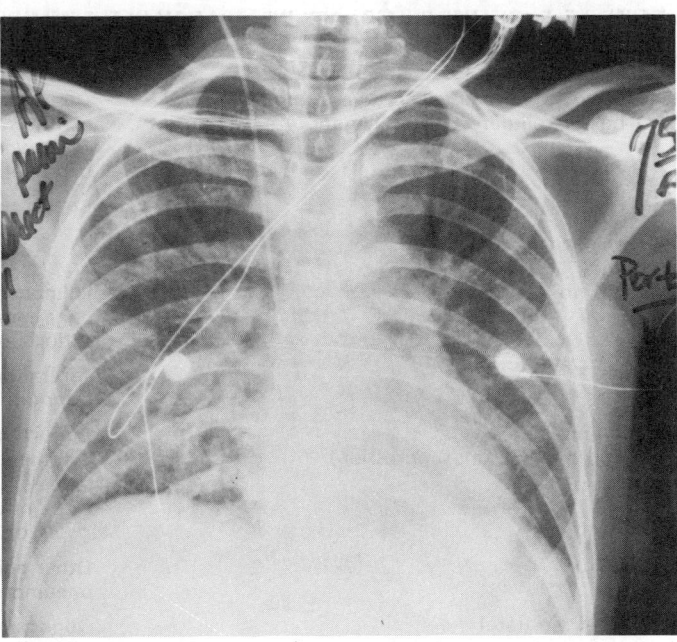

Figure 3.5–3. *Pneumocystis carinii* pneumonia in a 32-year-old heroin addict with AIDS. The homogeneous acinar pattern is a result of alveolar filling.

REFERENCES

1. Armstrong D, Gold JWM, et al: Treatment of infections in patients with the acquired immunodeficiency syndrome. Ann Intern Med 103:738, 1985
2. Bascom R, Johns CJ: The natural history and management of sarcoidosis. Adv Intern Med 31:213, 1986
3. Cooper JAD Jr, White DA, Matthay R: Drug-induced pulmonary disease. Am Rev Respir Dis 133:321 (Part I), 133:488 (Part II), 1986
4. Crystal RG, Bitterman PB, et al: Interstitial lung disease of unknown cause: Disorders characterized by chronic inflammation of the lower respiratory tract. N Engl J Med 310:154, 235, 1984
5. Epler GR, Colby TV, et al: Bronchiolitis obliterans organizing pneumonia. N Engl J Med 312:152, 1985
6. Fink JN: Hypersensitivity pneumonitis. J Allergy Clin Immunol 74:1, 1984
7. Fraser RG, Pare JAP (eds): Diagnosis of Diseases of the Chest, 2d ed. vol I–IV, Philadelphia, WB Saunders, 1977
8. Gross NJ: Pulmonary effects of radiation therapy. Ann Intern Med 86:81, 1977
9. Harmon EM: Immunologic lung disease. Med Clin North Am 69:705, 1985
10. James DG, Jones-Williams W: Sarcoidosis and other granulomatous disorders. In Smith LH (ed): Major Problems in Internal Medicine, vol 24, Philadelphia, WB Saunders, 1985
11. Keith WKC, Seaton A (eds): Occupational Lung Diseases, 2d ed, Philadelphia, WB Saunders, 1984
12. Reynolds HY: Bronchoalveolar lavage: State of art. Am Rev Respir Dis 135:250, 1987
13. Rosenow EC III, Wilson WR, Cockerill FR III: Pulmonary disease in the immunocompromised host. Mayo Clin Proc 60:473 (Part I), 60:610 (Part II), 1985
14. Schwartz MI (ed): Interstitial lung diseases: 28th Annual Aspen Lung Conference. Chest 89(Suppl):107S, 1986
15. Weiner RS, Bortin MM, et al: Interstitial pneumonitis after bone marrow transplantation. Ann Intern Med 104:168, 1986
16. Williams D, Yungbluth M, et al: The role of fiberoptic bronchoscopy in the evaluation of immunocompromised hosts with diffuse pulmonary infiltrates. Am Rev Respir Dis 131:880, 1985

TABLE 3.5–5. DIFFUSE PULMONARY INFILTRATION IN THE IMMUNOSUPPRESSED HOST[13]

Disease	Features
Acquired Immunodeficiency Syndrome (AIDS) T-helper cell defect and B lymphocyte dysfunction	**Opportunistic infections:** often multiple and fatal despite aggressive treatment; *Pneumocystis carinii* most common, (Fig. 3.5–3) mycobacteria (especially *M. avium-intracellulare*), *Cryptococcus neoformans,* cytomegalovirus (CMV) (alone or often in combination with the above agents)
	Kaposi sarcoma may spread to the lungs
Organ Transplantation Kidney <1 mo	**Pulmonary edema** with fluid overload or decreased organ function and **pulmonary embolism** (first 2 to 3 wk) account for one-third of all pulmonary complications, with cardiomegaly and pleural effusion in two-thirds
	Aspiration pneumonia infections: bacteremia from infected wound or intravascular line
1–4 mo (maximal immunosuppression)	**Opportunistic infections** most common during this period Cytomegalovirus most frequent, with bilateral symmetric diffuse interstitial process; usually not severe and self-limited; respiratory failure uncommon; may cause neutropenia and be associated with **superinfection** with *P. carinii, Aspergillus,* or *Cryptococcus,* with severe, progressive, life-threatening disease
	Other primary infections: *P. carinii;* varicella zoster causes life-threatening pneumonia; *Nocardia, mycobacteria, adenovirus*
>3–4 mo (late)	**Opportunistic infections:** *C. neoformans, P. carinii, Legionella, Mycoplasma,* other fungal infections
Bone marrow <30 days	*Pseudomonas aeruginosa* from wound or intravascular line
30–100 days	**Opportunistic infections:** as with kidney transplants; cytomegalovirus most common cause of interstitial pneumonitis
	Interstitial pneumonitis[15] begins within 50–75 days; occurs in 20%–30%, and fatal in half; often idiopathic
	Drug-induced pulmonary disease[3] (cyclophosphamide and methotrexate) may play a role in interstitial pneumonitis
>100 days	**Graft-versus-host disease (CBH):** major factor contributing to death; **chronic GVH:** begins within 100–400 days with cough, obstructive lung disease, bronchospasm; lymphocytic bronchitis and necrotizing bronchiolitis obliterans may be fatal[5]
	Late infections: Varicella zoster, *Staphylococcus aureus, Streptococcus pneumoniae* **Relapse** of the **basic underlying disease** such as leukemia
Heart–lung	Cardiac pulmonary edema with rejection; *P. carinii* common
Liver	Similar to kidney transplant
Malignant Tumors Carcinoma and sarcoma	**Hematogenous or lymphangitic spread;** usually no fever; insidious onset; diagnosed by sputum cytology or biopsy (transbronchial or transthoracic) in 50%–90% of cases
Lymphoma	Local or diffuse infiltrates; **disease recurrence or extension** often requires mediastinoscopy or thoracotomy; fever frequent; nodules may cavitate; pleural effusion in one-third; mediastinal and hilar nodes common unless prior irradiation; most frequent in nodular sclerosing Hodgkin disease; nodes less frequent in lymphocyte depleted non-Hodgkin lymphoma
	Drug reaction due to cytotoxic therapy
	Infections due to corticosteroids and immunosuppressive agents or granulocytopenia (see below)
Leukemia	Pulmonary infiltrate in 60%–80%
Untreated	**Infections** in 70% and proportional to degree of neutropenia
	Intact T-cell and B-cell populations make opportunistic infections less common; **bacterial pneumonia** most common; **hemorrhage** occurs with platelets below 15,000/mm³ and often without hemoptysis
	Leukemic infiltrates may occur, usually diffuse; most common in **acute** nonlymphocytic leukemia with high percentage of blasts in blood, or in **chronic** lymphocytic leukemia
	Leukostasis with WBC >200,000/mm³ produces dyspnea, although chest roentgenogram may be normal; hypoxemia out of proportion to pulmonary function studies; may produce infarction and become infected; **hairy-cell leukemia** predisposed to granulomatous infection; **pleural effusion** from leukemic pleural infiltrates in chronic myelogenous leukemia; **lymphadenopathy** with lymphatic leukemia

(continued)

TABLE 3.5–5. DIFFUSE PULMONARY INFILTRATION IN THE IMMUNOSUPPRESSED HOST[13] (Continued)

Disease	Features
Granulocytopenia (Neutrophils <500/mm³) secondary to myelosuppressive therapy	**Infections:** 90% frequency; fever >38C best predictor of presence of infection; minor lesions commonly cause life-threatening infections; can occur any time in the course of granulocytopenia; **initial infections:** 50% gram-negative sepsis with adult respiratory distress syndrome (ARDS) most common; *S. aureus* common; **secondary infections** occur within 10–14 days of initial antibiotic therapy: **Fungal infections** most common secondary infection: candidiasis, aspergillosis, often with hemoptysis **Viral infections:** CMV, herpes simplex, herpes zoster **Bacterial:** *Staphylococcus epidermidis* increasing frequency
Drug-Induced Pulmonary Disease Bleomycin (occurs in 10% of all patients treated with *bleomycin;* more if over age 70 and if cumulative total dose >450 U)	See Table 3.5–3; mimics other diseases such as infections, underlying diseases, i.e., lymphoma, leukemia, or metastatic lymphangitic carcinoma; generally diagnosed by exclusion; diffuse changes but not always uniform; symptoms and abnormal gallium-67 scan may precede roentgenographic changes; small pleural effusion in 10%
Cytosine Arabinoside (Ara-c)	See Table 3.5–3
Chronically Immunosuppressed Hosts (dose-related effects of chronic corticosteroid therapy, alkylating agents, or antimetabolites; impaired antibody, cellular, and inflammatory responses)	Gram-negative pneumonia with ARDS most common; *Staphylococcus aureus,* *Streptococcus pneumoniae,* atypical pneumonias (*Legionella, Mycoplasma*), fungal and viral infections also common; *P. carinii* pneumonitis may become manifest as corticosteroids are tapered
Chronic renal insufficiency (impaired granulocyte and T cell function with altered tumor surveillance)	Increased susceptibility to **infections; metastatic pulmonary calcification** in half of the patients on dialysis
Connective tissue disease (immunocompromised with corticosteroids or immunosuppressive agents or both)	**Infections; drug effects; disease recurrence:** Goodpasture syndrome; acute lupus erythematosus
New "Unrelated" Pulmonary Disease	Cardiac pulmonary edema, pulmonary emboli, oxygen toxicity, noncardiac edema from leukoagglutinating reaction, new or second unrelated malignant neoplasm, infection, aspiration pneumonia, ARDS, hemorrhage into the lung, emboli related to lymphangiography, radiation reaction

CHAPTER 3.6
Asthma

Eugene R. Bleecker
and Martin D. Valentine

Asthma is a clinical syndrome characterized by increased responsiveness of the airways to a variety of diverse stimuli that cause widespread narrowing of the intrapulmonary airways resulting in intermittent dyspnea and wheezing. The major features of asthma are reversible airflow obstruction, symptom-free periods between attacks, and increased bronchomotor responsiveness. While it is estimated that 3 percent of the population in the United States has asthma, other individuals with chronic obstructive pulmonary disease (COPD) may develop intermittent, reversible airflow obstruction that clinically resembles asthma. Furthermore, in some asthmatics, airflow obstruction may be progressive, leading to the development of chronic irreversible airways disease. The interrelationships between reversible (asthma) and fixed (COPD) airflow obstruction make understanding the pathogenesis and therapy of asthma important (Fig. 3.6–1).

HYPERREACTIVITY OF THE AIRWAYS

Asthma is characterized by an exaggerated bronchoconstrictor response to various physical, chemical, and pharmacologic stimuli.[4]

Clinically, asthmatic subjects may develop wheezing or coughing and may be aware of dyspnea or other symptoms of airflow obstruction following exposure to inhaled dusts, vapors, cold air, or exercise. When patients with asthma inhale biochemical mediators such as histamine, cholinergic agents such as methacholine, or irritants such as citric acid, dust, or cigarette smoke, they respond with a greater degree of bronchoconstriction than do normal subjects.[7] Airways reactivity testing can be used to diagnose asthma when this disorder is suspected but is not obvious from the clinical presentation. In patients with well-characterized asthma the degree of increased nonspecific airways reactivity is thought to correlate with the severity of asthmatic symptoms and individual therapeutic requirements. Airways reactivity may represent an important risk factor that can predict more rapid loss of pulmonary function in individuals with COPD.[5] Thus the presence of increased levels of airways reactivity in asthma and COPD suggests that common factors may be important in the pathogenesis of both these disorders (Fig. 3.6–1).

The fundamental mechanisms responsible for airways hyperreactivity are the subject of intense investigation.[4] Some proposed mechanisms emphasize the role of alterations in airway smooth

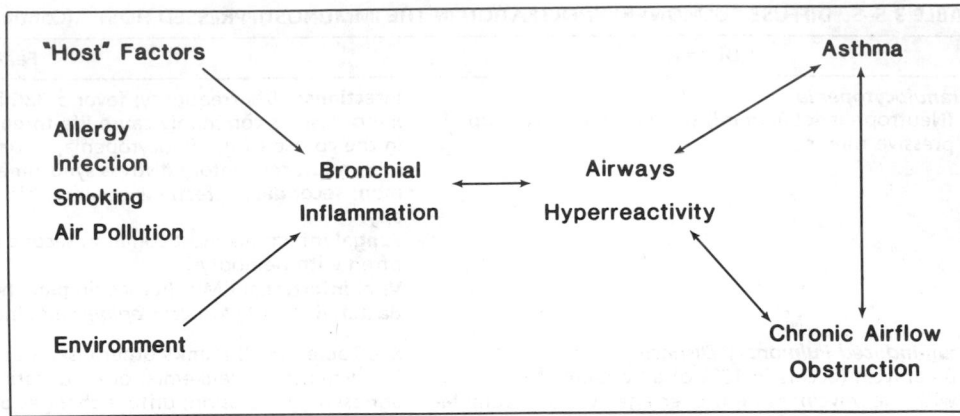

Figure 3.6–1. Pathogenesis of asthma and relationship to chronic obstructive lung disease. Host and environmental risk factors may lead to the development of bronchial inflammation and airway hyperreactivity. In some individuals typical asthma develops while in others there are combinations of asthma and chronic airflow obstruction.

muscle tone and the effects of airflow obstruction on particle deposition. In theory, when there is bronchoconstriction, inhaled substances or irritants are preferentially deposited in the larger airways. This increased concentration on the surface of the central airways could contribute to the heightened bronchial responsiveness found in asthmatics. Other studies indicate that hyperreactivity may be related to an abnormality of the regulation of airway smooth muscle and bronchial secretions by the autonomic nervous system.[2] Examples of these neural mechanisms are as follows: (1) increased sensitivity of cholinergic airway receptors could produce bronchoconstriction through activation of reflex pathways carried in the vagus nerves; (2) insensitivity of beta-adrenergic receptors on bronchial smooth muscle may be caused by an intrinsic defect in beta-receptor function in asthmatics or by prolonged therapy with sympathomimetic agonists; (3) a defect in neural airway control by the nonadrenergic, noncholinergic nervous system that normally serves to inhibit bronchial smooth muscle contraction; or (4) abnormal release from sensory nerve ending of neuropeptides that can trigger inflammatory mediator release and bronchoconstriction.[2]

While each of these potential mechanisms may play a role in the development of airways hyperresponsiveness, there is evidence to suggest that bronchial inflammation may be a common factor that contributes to the development of increased airways reactivity in both asthma and COPD (Fig. 3.6–1).[13] It is possible that the initial trigger is the release of mediators from bronchial mast cells, macrophages, and epithelial lining cells. These substances cause the migration of inflammatory cells that include neutrophils, eosinophils, and platelets into the airways. The activation of neu-

trophils and platelets results in the release of other mediators that include proteases and oxygen free radicals. While the eosinophil has functions that serve to control and inhibit inflammation, for example, the release of histaminases, phosopholipases, and arylsulfatases, it can also produce other substances including leukotrienes, platelet-aggregating factor, and granule-derived mediators such as major basic protein, peroxidases, and a neurotoxin. These substances can cause local injury in the airways. Once initiated, this sequence of inflammatory events could cause all the pathophysiologic changes found in asthma, including alterations in epithelial integrity, abnormalities in the autonomic neural control of airway tone, changes in mucociliary function, and increased responsiveness of bronchial smooth muscle (Fig. 3.6–2).

CATEGORIES OF ASTHMA

The causes of hyperreactivity of the airways relate to the pathogenesis of asthma, and they also provide a basis for dividing asthma into diagnostic categories. It should be emphasized that these different categories represent points on a clinical spectrum and that there is considerable overlap in the majority of patients.

EXTRINSIC ALLERGIC ASTHMA

In some asthmatic patients, environmental exposure to the pollens of grasses, ragweed, or other specific allergens such as animal dan-

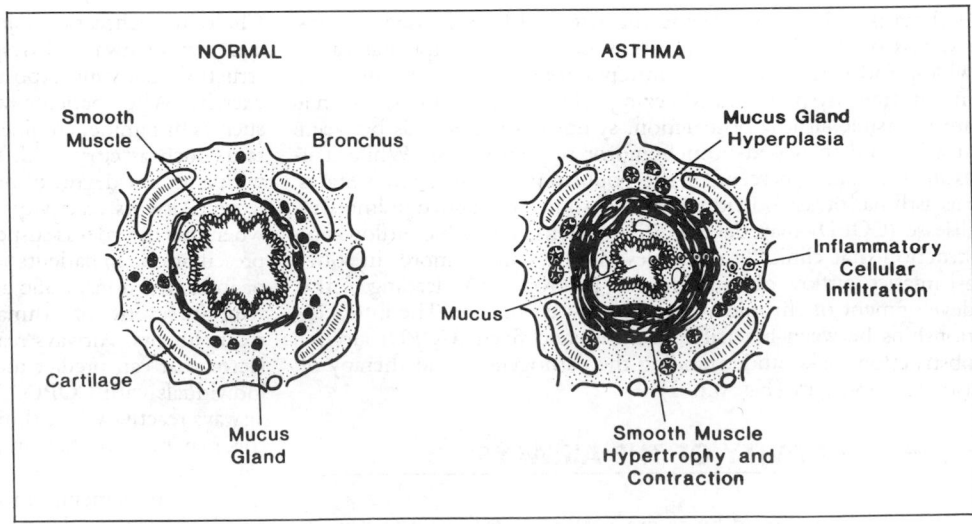

Figure 3.6–2. Schematic representation of the morphology of normal airways and the pathologic changes found in asthma.

der, dust, or some occupational agents produces an asthmatic attack. These allergic asthmatics usually note the onset of symptoms during childhood or adolescence and frequently have other allergic diseases including allergic rhinitis, eczema, and urticaria. Hereditary factors seem important in the etiology of asthma in these allergic individuals, since they often have relatives with asthma and other allergic diseases. In addition, they display increased nonspecific airways reactivity, since asthmatic attacks are also triggered by numerous nonallergic causes. The clinical course of allergic asthma is characterized by intermittent episodes of bronchospasm with relatively symptom-free periods between attacks. Often this disease symptomatically improves as these individuals enter adulthood, but in some, asthma may persist or recur during middle or old age.

In allergic asthmatics, reactions producing acute attacks of airway obstruction are caused by IgE-mediated immediate hypersensitivity reactions closely associated with the development of bronchial inflammation.[1] A specific antigen in these allergic patients will cause a wheal and flare reaction when injected intradermally and airflow obstruction when inhaled. These physiologic events are attributable to the biologic activities of a group of chemical mediators immunologically released from appropriate target cells (Table 3.6–1). Exposure to an antigen in susceptible individuals causes the production of specific reaginic antibody (IgE), which fixes to basophils and mast cells. Repeat exposure to the antigen initiates a sequence of reactions resulting in the formation, release, and synthesis of mediators. Some of these mediators such as histamine and high-molecular-weight eosinophil and neutrophil chemotactic factors are stored within basophils and mast cells (Table 3.6–1). Other mediators are formed from membrane phospholipid stores by metabolism of arachidonic acid through two biochemical pathways (Fig. 3.6–3). The cyclooxygenase pathway results in the formation of prostaglandins and thromboxanes, while the lypoxygenase pathway results in the production of leukotrienes. These mediators can produce numerous physiologic and cellular events including contraction of bronchial smooth muscle, alterations in vascular smooth muscle tone, aggregation and degranulation of platelets, increased membrane permeability, and attraction of inflammatory cells (Table 3.6–1).[1] Thus, an antigenic stimulus that can produce acute bronchospasm also causes inflammatory changes in the airways through a series of immunologic and biochemical reactions. In man, mediator release is depen-

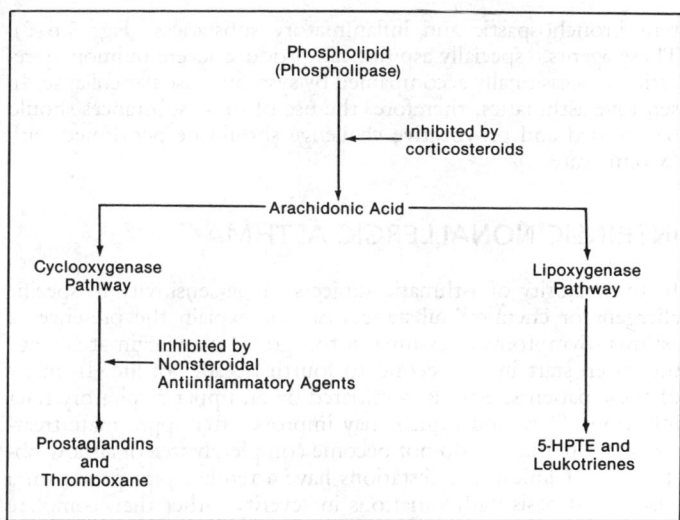

Figure 3.6–3. Arachidonic acid metabolic pathways showing the breakdown of membrane phospholipids and metabolism of arachidonic acid to prostaglandins (cyclooxygenase pathway) and leukotrienes (lipoxygenase pathway).

dent on these complex interactions; in addition, they are modulated directly by the local levels of mediators (histamine and prostaglandins), by endogenous levels of hormones, and perhaps by autonomic neural reflex pathways. Some of these interactions serve as a basis for the pharmacologic therapy of allergic asthma. For example, circulating beta-adrenergic catecholamines, histamine, and prostaglandin E_2 can increase intracellular levels of cyclic AMP and thus inhibit mast cell mediator release. In contrast, alpha-adrenergic agonists facilitate mediator release by decreasing cellular cyclic AMP levels. Cholinergic agents may enhance mediator release by affecting a different cell-receptor site associated with an increase in cyclic GMP. Corticosteroids may affect membrane phospholipid metabolism, preventing formation of arachidonic acid and thus altering the development of these inflammatory processes (Fig. 3.6–3).

NONALLERGIC EXTRINSIC ASTHMA

This category includes asthma that occurs after exposure to various chemical agents that do not seem to provoke a classic IgE immunologic reaction. Many of these triggers are found in occupational and industrial settings.[6] For example, exposure to toluene-2-4-diisocyanate (TDI) or phthalic anhydride, chemicals used in the manufacture of plastics, can produce an asthmatic syndrome in some workers. Other examples include exposure to metal fumes and salts (chromium, nickel, ammonium); wood particles (oak and western red cedar); vegetable, grain ("baker's asthma"), and coffee bean dusts; industrial chemicals (epoxy resins, soldering fluxes); pyrolysis products of plastics ("meat wrapper's asthma"), enzymes (*Bacillus subtilis* in detergents); and pharmaceutical agents (penicillin, pancreatic enzymes).[6] Individuals who have asthma related to these occupational or industrial exposures frequently display increased levels of nonspecific airways reactivity that appear to reflect the frequency of exposure and the severity of their disease.

Other agents, such as aspirin, nonsteroidal anti-inflammatory drugs (indomethacin, phenylbutazone), and tartrazine (yellow food dye No. 5), may also precipitate or worsen bronchial asthma. It is interesting that nonsteroidal anti-inflammatory agents prevent the synthesis of prostaglandins from arachidonic acid in cell membranes. This may facilitate the production of other products of arachidonic metabolism that include leukotrienes, which are po-

TABLE 3.6–1. INFLAMMATORY MEDIATORS RELEASED DURING IMMEDIATE HYPERSENSITIVITY REACTIONS

Mediator	Function
Histamine	Airway smooth muscle contraction, increased vascular permeability, vasodilation, chemotactic properties
Eosinophil and neutrophil chemotactic factors	Attraction of neutrophils and eosinophils
Platelet aggregating factor	Platelet aggregation and release of mediators (serotonin) from platelets
Prostaglandins	
PGD$_2$	Airway smooth muscle constriction, chemotaxis, vasodilation
PGF$_{2a}$	Airway and vascular smooth muscle constriction
PGE$_1$ and PGE$_2$	Airway and vascular smooth muscle dilation
Leukotrienes	
LTC$_4$, LTD$_4$, LTE$_4$	Airway smooth muscle constriction, increased vascular permeability
LTB$_4$	Chemotaxis of neutrophils and eosinophils

tent bronchospastic and inflammatory substances (Fig. 3.6–3). These agents, especially aspirin, can produce severe pulmonary reactions, occasionally accompanied by systemic vascular collapse. In sensitive asthmatics, therefore, the use of these substances should be avoided and provocative challenge should be performed with extreme care.

INTRINSIC NONALLERGIC ASTHMA

In the majority of asthmatic subjects, hypersensitivity to specific allergens or chemical substances cannot explain the presence of asthma. Symptoms of asthma in this group may begin at any age but often start in the second to fourth decades of life. In many of these patients, asthma is initiated by an upper respiratory tract infection. These individuals may improve after appropriate treatment but frequently do not become completely free of airflow obstruction. Clinical manifestations have a tendency to persist on a year-round basis with variations in severity rather than complete symptomatic remissions. Some of these patients have a history of cigarette smoking and chronic bronchitis that either precipitates or complicates their asthma. Others who initially have intermittent episodes of bronchospasm develop a clinical course complicated by progressive and irreversible airflow obstruction as is found in patients with COPD (Fig. 3.6–1).

Patients with "nonallergic" or "intrinsic" asthma have an as yet undefined abnormality that makes their airways hyperreactive to a multitude of stimuli including inhaled irritants, exercise, and psychologic factors. Airways reactivity and asthmatic symptoms may worsen after various environmental exposures (cigarette smoke, air pollutants) or during upper respiratory infections—responses associated with the development of bronchial inflammation.[13] While evidence of specific allergy to inhaled and ingested antigens is lacking, serum IgE levels are often normal, and allergic skin testing is negative; these nonallergic or intrinsic asthmatics do have increased numbers of eosinophils in their circulation and bronchial secretions.

EXERCISE-INDUCED ASTHMA

In a large percentage of subjects with asthma, exercise can produce wheezing and dyspnea that occur shortly after completing exercise. This response to exercise is one example of bronchial hyperreactivity characteristic of all types of asthma.[3] In some mild asthmatics, however, exercise-induced bronchospasm may be the dominant clinical manifestation of their disease. It is related to the effects of hyperventilation during exercise when cool, relatively dry air is rapidly inspired.[11] It can be reproduced by hyperventilation with cold, dry air, which is thought to cause heat loss in the airways and changes in the osmolarity of bronchial secretions.

Exercise-induced asthma may be precipitated by outdoor activities during the winter in cold climates, while swimming in an indoor pool is less likely to produce bronchospasm, since the ambient temperature and humidity of inspired air is higher and airway cooling does not occur. It can be prevented by treatment before exercise with either an inhaled sympathomimetic agent or drugs that effect the release of inflammatory mediators such as chromolyn.

CLINICAL FEATURES

Dyspnea, cough, and wheezing are the most common clinical features associated with asthma. In most patients, acute asthmatic attacks lasting for hours or days are separated by remissions during which symptoms are reduced or absent. Even when an asthmatic is subjectively improved, there may be considerable impairment of respiratory function that is not fully appreciated by routine clinical assessment.[12]

During a mild attack the patient notes wheezing and cough but can perform ordinary tasks without difficulty. Physical examination reveals inspiratory or expiratory wheezing, or both, accentuated by a forced expiration. With increasingly severe attacks, dyspnea is present during mild exertion and eventually persists even at rest. Coughing becomes more pronounced, but it may be difficult for the asthmatic to raise sputum. The lungs become hyperinflated, and breath sounds become distant with high-pitched inspiratory and expiratory wheezes.[15] The term "status asthmaticus" describes a severe prolonged asthmatic attack refractory to the usual modes of therapy (see Chapter 4.6). Patients experiencing severe asthmatic attacks are extremely dyspneic and use accessory muscles of respiration to be able to breathe at high lung volumes.[15] Objective pulmonary function tests, such as serial spirometry and blood gases, should be employed to assess the severity of an asthmatic attack and to monitor therapy.

Although many cardiorespiratory diseases are characterized by wheezing, dyspnea, and cough, the differential diagnosis of an acute asthmatic attack can usually be made with little difficulty on the basis of an adequate medical history and physical examination. The major entities that must be excluded include acute left ventricular failure, an aspirated foreign body, pulmonary thromboembolism, an endobronchial tumor, and other forms of chronic obstructive airway disease. Occasionally there may be confusion between upper and lower airway obstruction. For example, extrathoracic airway obstruction caused by a tracheal or laryngeal tumor may give rise to a clinical presentation simulating asthma. Patients with large airway obstruction, however, usually present with inspiratory stridor loudest in the region of the obstruction. In differentiating upper and lower airways obstruction, a comparison of maximum inspiratory and expiratory flow rates is useful. With lesions in the upper airways, inspiratory flow rates are reduced because of extrathoracic airway collapse during inspiration. Indirect laryngoscopy or direct nasopharyngoscopy with a bronchoscope can be used to visualize and diagnose an anatomic abnormality in the upper airway.

PATHOPHYSIOLOGY OF AN ACUTE ASTHMATIC ATTACK

Increases in airflow resistance alone do not explain all the clinical and physiologic findings characteristic of asthma. During an asthmatic attack, airways tend to close, and the asthmatic must breathe at high lung volumes to keep airways open and permit gas exchange.[15] The work of breathing increases, and accessory muscles of respiration (sternocleidomastoid muscles) must be used to maintain this level of hyperinflation. In fact the use of accessory muscles of respiration correlates better than dyspnea and wheezing with a severe impairment of pulmonary function during an acute asthmatic attack.[12] Severity should be objectively measured by two simple parameters of forced expiration. The forced expiratory volume in 1 second (FEV_1) reflects expiratory airflow obstruction, while the reduction in forced vital capacity (FVC) correlates with the increased tendency for airway closure and hyperinflation of the lung. Severe attacks associated with significant hypoxemia and increases in arterial CO_2 levels occur where the FEV_1 falls below 25 percent of predicted or approximately 1 L.

During a severe asthmatic attack, hypoxemia and hyperinflation of the lung increase pulmonary vascular resistance and lead to pulmonary hypertension, manifested electrocardiographically by acute right axis deviation, "p" pulmonale, and right ventricular strain.[15] The negative pleural pressures needed to inflate the lungs produce an increased afterload on the left ventricle. Changes in left ventricular function are clinically evident when a significant pulsus paradoxus develops during severe asthmatic attacks.

LABORATORY FINDINGS

Pulmonary function tests reveal the characteristic signs of bronchial obstruction including a reduction in the FEV_1 and vital capacity.[12] When the FEV_1 falls below 1 L, significant abnormalities in arterial blood gas tensions frequently occur. Spirometry should be used to monitor the severity of the attack and the response to bronchodilator therapy. To distinguish patients with asthma from those with emphysema, measurement of the single breath diffusing capacity for carbon monoxide can be helpful. The diffusing capacity is typically low in emphysema but normal in asthma. Arterial hypoxemia commonly develops during acute attacks of asthma because of abnormalities in the matching of ventilation and perfusion caused by bronchospasm, occlusion of airways with mucus, and regional alterations in pulmonary blood flow. During mild to moderate asthmatic attacks there is alveolar hyperventilation, and arterial CO_2 tension is reduced. With a severe asthmatic attack alveolar hypoventilation occurs and the arterial PCO_2 rises. Therefore, an increase in arterial PCO_2 during the course of an acute asthma attack to levels greater than 40 mm Hg should be viewed with alarm.

A chest roentgenogram should be obtained in any severe attack that does not respond to appropriate therapy or when there is a clinical suspicion of pulmonary infection. The characteristic radiographic abnormality during an acute attack is hyperinflation of the lungs with an increase in the anteroposterior diameter of the chest, lowering and flattening of the diaphragm, and increased radiolucency of the lung fields. In contrast to emphysema, hyperinflation is reversed during remission. The chest roentgenogram should be carefully examined for the presence of pneumonia, atelectasis secondary to mucus plugging, pneumomediastinum, and pneumothorax. If there is a history of headaches or nasal congestion, sinus films should be obtained.

Sputum should be examined and cultured when there is a clinical suspicion that a bacterial infection has either triggered or complicated an asthmatic attack. A complete blood count with a differential will be useful to document the presence of eosinophilia as well as to evaluate an infectious process.

MANAGEMENT OF ASTHMA

The successful management of asthma requires measures designed to avoid precipitating factors, while simultaneously treating the clinical manifestations and preventing the complications of the disease. Therapy will be ineffective and serious errors may result if any one of these factors is neglected.

GENERAL MEASURES

In some asthmatics, triggers of an attack can be easily recognized and controlled, while in others precipitating factors are less well defined and more difficult to determine. In general, patients with asthma should avoid exposure to irritating fumes, dusts, aerosol sprays, and air pollutants. Asthmatics should not smoke and should not be exposed to cigarette smoke in poorly ventilated spaces. Passive exposure to cigarette smoke can result in worsening of respiratory function in individuals with hyperreactive airways. It may also be necessary to control environmental temperature and humidity with an air conditioner whose filter should be changed regularly to avoid accumulation of airborne molds and fungi. In rare circumstances removal to a more favorable climate may be indicated.

Attacks of asthma can be precipitated by emotional factors.[2] This may present difficult therapeutic problems, since asthma can be a chronic, debilitating disease that may prove psychologically traumatic to both the patient and family. In a severe attack, while sedation may be helpful in relieving emotional stress, the relief of

anxiety resulting from the patient's confidence in his physician and nurses as well as treatment with the appropriate regimen is often of greater importance. Sedatives and tranquilizers administered during acute asthmatic attacks may worsen respiratory muscle fatigue and precipitate respiratory failure.

INFECTION

Upper respiratory infections can increase airways reactivity and precipitate bronchospasm in asthmatics.[4] Even in normal individuals, upper respiratory infections can produce transient episodes of bronchial hyperreactivity that may be associated with a persistent, dry cough and mild bronchospasm. These individuals respond better to therapy with a bronchodilator than with a cough suppressent.

Although infection is not a part of every asthmatic attack, its presence should be looked for carefully by evaluating the clinical course and the results of a chest roentgenogram and sputum examination. Occasionally an asthmatic's sputum may appear to be grossly purulent because of the presence of eosinophils; therefore, microscopic sputum examination and culture are indicated when treatment of a respiratory tract infection is considered. The antibiotic of choice is either tetracycline or ampicillin administered for 7 to 10 days, unless the results of a sputum culture or drug hypersensitivity dictate the use of another antibiotic.

ALLERGY TO SPECIFIC INHALED, INGESTED, OR INJECTED SUBSTANCES

Allergy to specific inhaled, ingested, and injected substances may be detected by obtaining a complete medical history, by skin testing, and by evaluating the effects of exposure to the suspected allergens. Desensitization is more effective in individuals with a limited number of allergies that appear to trigger asthmatic symptoms. For example, those individuals with animal dander sensitivies who cannot avoid exposure to this antigen often respond to immunotherapy. In contrast, desensitization is less effective in adult asthmatics with skin test reactivity to multiple allergens that are poorly related to their clinical disease. In these individuals, avoidance of a specific allergen may be preferable to immmunotherapy.[10]

PHARMACOLOGIC THERAPY

Five different groups of drugs are available for the treatment of asthma: (1) sympathomimetics, (2) methylxanthines, (3) anticholinergic agents, (4) antiallergic agents, and (5) corticosteroids.

Sympathomimetic Agents

These drugs may be divided into agents that have predominantly alpha-adrenergic activity or beta$_1$- and beta$_2$-sympathomimetic selective actions.[16] The desirable therapeutic effects are due to the beta$_2$-sympathomimetic actions of these drugs. Stimulation of beta$_2$-receptors increases cyclic AMP levels in mast cells, basophils, and bronchial smooth muscle, thereby inhibiting mediator release and directly dilating airway smooth muscle. The undesirable side effects of sympathomimetics are due to their beta$_1$-activity, which stimulates the cardiovascular system and may cause tachycardia and arrhythmias.

These agents are effective bronchodilators that should be administered initially as aerosols, since they will produce local bronchial smooth muscle dilation with fewer systemic side effects.[8] The more selective and prolonged actions of the newer beta$_2$-agonists are preferred over older, less selective drugs (Table 3.6–2). Oral preparations of these agents are associated with more frequent side effects that include systemic circulatory effects, anxiety, and skeletal muscle tremor.[16] Parenteral administration of sympathomimetic

TABLE 3.6–2. INHALED BETA-SYMPATHOMIMETIC AGONISTS

Generic Name	Beta Selectivity	Onset of Action (min)	Peak Effect (min)	Duration of Effect (hr)
Isoproterenol	B₂ = B₁	1–5	5–15	1–2
Isoetharine	B₂ > B₁	5	5–15	2–3
Metaproterenol	B₂ > > > B₁	1–5	30–60	2–5
Terbutaline	B₂ > > > B₁	1–5	30–60	2–5
Bitolterol	B₂ > > > B₁	3–5	30–60	4–8
Albuterol	B₂ > > > > B₁	5–15	30–60	3–6

agents should be reserved for the treatment of acute asthmatic attacks that do not respond to aerosol therapy.[8]

Methylxanthines

Theophylline derivatives are effective bronchodilators that may also improve respiratory muscle strength and endurance. They are available in a variety of preparations that differ in their bioavailability and duration of action.[17] The physician should become familiar with two or three of these prepartions such as an inexpensive, short-acting preparation (generic aminophylline) and a long-acting theophylline preparation. They can be used in combination with sympathomimetic agonists, since they have different modes of action. Individualization of drug dosage frequently requires the determination of plamsa theophylline levels. Plasma levels between 10 and 20 μg/ml are considered therapeutic, but even at these recommended levels side effects may occur in some individuals.[14] At plasma levels higher than 20 μg/ml serious side effects such as nausea, vomiting, central nervous system irritability, and tachyarrhythmias are likely to occur. Peak plasma levels usually occur 1 to 2 hours after oral administration, so blood specimens should be drawn during this period when evaluating for toxicity.

Intravenous aminophylline is initially administered with a loading dose of 5 to 6 mg/kg followed by a continuous infusion of 0.9 mg/kg/hr. In individuals with conditions known to interfere with theophylline metabolism by the liver (congestive heart failure, cirrhosis, respiratory failure, drugs) the maintenance doses should be reduced by 50 percent, and plasma theophylline levels should be carefully monitored. In obese individuals, theophylline dosage should be calculated based on ideal body weight, since the drug is less well distributed in adipose tissue. In children and in heavy smokers, theophylline may be metabolized more rapidly, and there may be increased drug requirements.

For oral therapy with a short-acting preparation, the recommended starting dose is 200 mg three or four times daily, but as much as 1200 to 1600 mg may be required by some patients. The dose can be increased every 2 to 5 days while the patient is observed for therapeutic and toxic side effects. Minor side effects that include nervousness, nausea, and headache occur with initial use of oral theophylline but frequently resolve with continued therapy. The use of long-acting preparations administered once or twice a day may appear to improve patient compliance, but the absorption of many of these long-acting agents may be affected by the relationship to food intake as well as the fat content of the meal. The prescribing physician must therefore have specific knowledge of the pharmacology of the individual theophylline drug preparations.[17]

Anticholinergic Agents

These agents were used earlier in this century but lost favor because of potential local and systemic side effects that could result in the drying of respiratory secretions, blurred vision, and cardiac and central nervous system stimulation.[2] Atropine is the most potent anticholinergic agent available, but its inhalation results in varying degrees of systemic absorption in different individuals. These agents are contraindicated in patients with narrow angle glaucoma or bladder neck obstruction due to prostatic hypertrophy. Although atropine may be effective in treating bronchospasm, it is not officially approved for use as a bronchodilator by the Food and Drug Administration. A newer drug (ipratroprium) with no systemic absorption and minimal effects on mucociliary function has been in use for some time in other countries and has recently been approved in the United States. The onset of action of ipratroprium, when inhaled, is more delayed than that of aerosolized sympathomimetics (Table 3.6–2). Its peak effect occurs within 30 to 60 minutes, and its duration of action is 3 to 6 hours. This drug appears to be a more effective bronchodilator in patients with chronic bronchitis and airflow obstruction than in asthmatics. Some patients with asthma respond with significant and prolonged bronchodilation, however, and a therapeutic trial with ipratropium coupled with objective testing with spirometry may be useful in their treatment.

Antiallergic Drugs

Cromolyn is not a bronchodilator, and its exact mechanism of action is not fully understood. It is thought to stabilize mast cells and basophils, thereby preventing the release of inflammatory mediators. It is available as a nebulized solution and a metered-dose inhaler. Cromolyn is used as a prophylactic agent in allergic asthmatics; it may also be effective in some nonallergic intrinsic asthmatics, especially children and adolescents. Therapeutic responses should be reviewed after 1 month of treatment by evaluating symptoms, frequency of asthmatic attacks, and the results of spirometry. Patients should realize that this drug is a prophylactic agent, not intended for the treatment of acute asthmatic attacks. The one exception is its use in preventing the development of exercise-induced bronchospasm, when acute administration just before exercise usually reduces or blocks the development of postexertional bronchospasm.

Corticosteroids

Corticosteroids and anti-inflammatory agents that are useful in the treatment of bronchospastic diseases. Steroids may act synergistically with bronchodilators, making asthmatic airways more responsive to these agents. The mechanisms of action of corticosteroids are not fully understood but may be related to their effects on arachidonic acid metabolism and other cellular anti-inflammatory properties (Fig. 3.6–3). When used to treat acute asthma, their onset of therapeutic effects is delayed for as long as 6 to 12 hours.[9] They may be administered orally, intravenously, and as aerosols. Because of the serious side effects from long-term systemic steroid therapy, its use should be reserved for severe asthmatics whose disease is not controlled with standard bronchodilators and for the treatment of status asthmaticus. When steroid therapy is undertaken in the ambulatory patient, pulmonary function tests should be used to evaluate their effectiveness objectively. Alternate-day therapy should be attempted, and the lowest effective dose should be employed. Intermittent or "burst" therapy for periods of 7 to 10 days using high doses (40 to 60 mg of prednisone) may be started and tapered rapidly in the treatment of severe exacerbations of bronchospasm. This approach will not produce clinically significant changes in adrenal function but may cause transient steroid-induced abnormalities in glucose metabolism. Inhaled corticosteroid preparations with minimal systemic absorption may be used to reduce or eliminate the requirement for systemic corticosteroids or as primary therapy for asthma. Steroid aerosols are frequently administered in combination with other bronchodilators.

APPROACH TO THE PHARMACOLOGIC THERAPY OF ASTHMA

The therapeutic regimen in the treatment of asthma must be individualized for each patient. During a remission, occasional use of an aerosolized sympathomimetic agent may be all that is required

to treat intermittent episodes of bronchospasm. In asthmatics who require continuous bronchodilator treatment, one can prescribe either an aerosolized selective beta$_2$-sympathomimetic or a theophylline preparation. Nebulized bronchodilators can be used to control acute mild exacerbations and as prophylactic agents before undertaking activities known to cause bronchospasm. Cromolyn provides effective prophylactic therapy for allergic and exercise-induced asthma and may be useful in the treatment of other forms of asthma. When additional therapy is indicated, asthmatics should be treated with both aminophylline and beta$_2$-agonists, as these agents have different mechanisms of action and have additive effects as bronchodilators when used in combination. The role of anticholinergic agents still needs to be determined, but some patients, especially those with asthmatic bronchitis, have excellent bronchodilator responses to inhaled ipratroprium. Traditionally, initial therapy in asthma has employed bronchodilators, and the use of corticosteroids has been reserved for severe asthmatics or acute exacerbations of asthma. In view of the importance of bronchial inflammation in the pathogenesis of this disorder, inhaled cortiscosteroids may be useful in the therapy of less severe asthmatics to prevent the development of inflammatory events and to reduce airways reactivity (Fig. 3.6–1). Systemic corticosteroids should be reserved for status asthmaticus and for severe asthma unresponsive to standard therapy.[9] Whenever possible, aerosolized corticosteroids should be used to reduce the dose of systemic steroids when they are administered for prolonged periods.

Acute asthmatic attacks are best treated with aerosolized or subcutaneous injections of a sympathomimetic agonist.[8] Aminophylline is not as potent or rapid in relieving bronchospasm, but it should be used during severe asthma that does not respond to sympathomimetic agents alone. During severe attacks, acute high-dose therapy with corticosteroids may be necessary.[9]

COMPLICATIONS

The course of asthma may be changed drastically by the development of medical complications, and the goal of management is, first, their prevention, if possible, and, second, their treatment when necessary.

In acute asthma, bronchodilators may cause a transient small decrease in arterial PO_2 (5 to 10 mm Hg), but this is easily treated with supplemental oxygen. In very rare instances the propellants used in commercial metered-dose inhalers produce irritation and bronchospasm. This paradoxical response can be evaluated in the pulmonary function laboratory by performing serial spirometry before and after the administration of the specific bronchodilator preparation and can often be treated by switching to a different agent.

Sympathomimetics and theophylline preparations may cause cardiac arrhythmias in susceptible patients.[14] It should be noted that bronchospasm with resultant hypoxemia can also trigger cardiac arrhythmias, and in these situations the administration of bronchodilators often improves the arrhythmia.

Mucus impaction and bronchospasm can cause microatelecta-

sis and even lobar collapse. Usually atelectasis improves after treatment with bronchodilators, hydration, and physical therapy. Bronchoscopy is rarely needed and may be harmful because it can worsen bronchospasm in asthmatics and provides only temporary relief of atelectasis.

While infectious processes often precipitate asthmatic exacerbations, bronchitis and pneumonia can develop during acute asthma. Development of purulent respiratory secretions during an asthmatic attack requires reevaluation for superimposed infection.

Allergic bronchopulmonary aspergillosis may complicate asthma. This syndrome is characterized by febrile episodes, cough productive of purulent sputum with dark brown plugs and bronchial casts, eosinophilic pulmonary infiltrates, and focal proximal bronchiectasis. When it occurs, patients have serum precipitins and an immediate or delayed skin reaction to the aspergillus antigen. Therapy with corticosteroids may improve bronchospasm and prevent the development of bronchiectasis.

REFERENCES

1. Austen KF, Orange RP: Bronchial asthma: The possible role of the chemical mediators of immediate hypersensitivity in the pathogenesis of subacute chronic disease. Am Rev Respir Dis 112:423, 1975
2. Bleecker ER: Cholinergic and neurogenic mechanisms in obstructive airways disease. Am J Med 8(5A):93, 1986
3. Bleecker ER: Exercise-induced asthma. Physiologic and clinical considerations. Clin Chest Med 5:109, 1984
4. Boushey HA, Holtzman MJ, Sheller JA: Bronchial hyperreactivity. Am Rev Respir Dis 121:389, 1980
5. Britt EV, Cohen B, et al: Airways reactivity and functional deterioration in relatives of COPD patients. Chest 77:260, 1980
6. Brooks SM: Bronchial asthma of occupational origin. Scand J Works Environ Health 3:53, 1977
7. Chatham M, Bleecker ER, et al: A comparison of histamine, methacholine and exercise airways reactivity in normal and asthmatic subjects. Am Rev Respir Dis 126:235, 1982
8. Fanta CH, Rossing TH, McFadden ER Jr: Emergency room treatment of asthma. Am J Med 72:416, 1984
9. Fanta CH, Rossing TH, McFadden ER Jr: Glucocorticoids in acute asthma. A critical controlled trial. Am J Med 74:845, 1983
10. Lichtenstein LM: An evaluation of the role of immunotherapy in asthma. Am Rev Respir Dis 117:191, 1973
11. McFadden ER: Respiratory heat and water exchange: Physiological and clinical implications. J Appl Physiol 54:331, 1983
12. McFadden ER, Kiser R, DeGroot WJ: Acute bronchial asthma: Relations between clinical and physiologic manifestations. N Engl J Med 288:2221, 1973
13. Nadel JA: Inflammation and asthma. J Allergy Clin Immunol 73:651, 1984
14. Nicklas RA, Whitehurst VE, et al: Concomitant use of beta-adrenergic agonists and methylxanthines. J Allergy Clin Immunol 73:20, 1984
15. Rebuck AS, Read J: Assessment and management of severe asthma. Am J Med 51:788, 1971
16. Webb-Johnson DC, Andrews JL: Bronchodilator therapy (2 parts). N Engl J Med 297:476, 1977
17. Weinberger M: The pharmacology and therapeutic use of theophylline. J Allergy Clin Immunol 73:525, 1984

Chronic Obstructive Pulmonary Disease and Sleep Apnea Syndromes

Gail G. Weinmann, Phillip L. Smith, and Harold A. Menkes

CLINICAL TYPES

Chronic obstructive pulmonary disease (COPD) is a nonspecific term referring to a group of diseases characterized by cough, chronic sputum production, dyspnea, and irreversible expiratory air flow obstruction. In the United States the vast majority of COPD is related to smoking and results from chronic bronchitis and emphysema, but with improved medical therapy an increasing number of patients with bronchiectasis from cystic fibrosis and immotile cilia syndrome survive and present with airway obstruction in adulthood. With antibiotics and immunizations, bronchiectasis from pneumonitis is becoming a less frequent cause of COPD.

The hallmark of COPD is irreversible obstruction of expiratory air flow. After a full inspiration, normal subjects are able to forcibly exhale at least 75 percent of their total vital capacity within 1 second as measured with a spirometer. Thus the ratio of their forced expiratory volume in 1 second to forced vital capacity (FVC) is 75 percent or greater. Patients with airway obstruction either from asthma or COPD have decreased FEV_1 and FEV_1/FVC. In asthma this fall is due to hyperresponsive airways and is reversible with therapy, but in COPD it is due to permanent changes and is not reversible. Reversible and irreversible components may coexist, leading to terms such as "asthmatic bronchitis."

CHRONIC BRONCHITIS

Chronic bronchitis is a condition characterized primarily by excessive mucous secretion and cough. Airway obstruction may be absent in some patients or may appear only with superimposed acute infection. Morphologic changes are limited to the bronchial walls, which show loss of cilia and increases in size and number of mucous glands. Glands have dilated ducts and extend further into the peripheral airways than normal. A chronic inflammatory infiltrate is present in the mucosa, and there is often occlusion of the peripheral airways with secretions. Chronic or recurrent bacterial infections are common. Classically, the patient with pure chronic bronchitis has been called the "blue-bloater." Dyspnea may be mild or moderate and cough prominent, and the patient may have hypercapnia, hypoxia, secondary erythrocytosis, pulmonary hypertension, an enlarged heart, and episodes of right-sided heart failure.

EMPHYSEMA

Emphysema is characterized by alveolar wall destruction, which leads to loss of elastic recoil and compliant, collapsible airways. Although it is technically a diagnosis that can be made only by the pathologist, certain clinical and radiographic characteristics distinguish this condition during life. In addition to the dyspnea and airway obstruction, patients with emphysema have low diffusing capacities, increased residual voumes and total lung capacities, and hyperlucent lung fields on chest radiograph. These clinical findings correlate with destruction of alveolar ducts and alveolar walls.

Centrilobular emphysema starts in the center of the lobule and bears a well-documented relationship to cigarette smoking and antecedent chronic bronchitis. It localizes primarily to nondependent or apical lung. Panlobular emphysema, which involves the whole lobule uniformly, is far less common. It may be associated with hereditary α_1-antitrypsin deficiency and tends to occur in dependent or basilar lung regions. With advanced disease it is difficult to distinguish centrilobular from panlobular emphysema, and patients dying with advanced disease usually have elements of both. Classically, the patient with pure emphysema has been called the "pink puffer." Unlike the "blue bloater," this patient's dyspnea is prominent, but the cough is trivial and the arterial blood gases are relatively normal at rest. This patient is thin and has a small heart.

While chronic bronchitis and emphysema are described here as separate entities, it is important to note that many patients have elements of both diseases.

ASTHMATIC BRONCHITIS

A subset of patients who present with a typical picture of COPD have airways obstruction partially reversible with bronchodilators. They may also have bronchial hyperreactivity and complain of episodes of increased dyspnea and wheezing typical of asthma without a history of atopy. Yet because of an irreversible component these patients are not just asthmatic. The term "asthmatic bronchitis" has evolved to convey the idea of coexisting reversible and irreversible airway obstruction. This concept may have important therapeutic implications, as patients may benefit from aggressive bronchodilator therapy in both the short and the long run.

OTHER OBSTRUCTIVE LUNG DISEASES

Bronchiectasis refers to destroyed bronchi and has much in common with chronic bronchitis. It differs, however, because it is caused by recurrent infections that lead to copious secretions and, later, development of obstructive lung disease. In the normal host, bronchiectasis is caused by recurrent or prolonged pneumonia of either bacterial origin (especially pertussis) or viral origin (especially measles or influenza). It can also occur when inherited or acquired defects interfere with normal defense mechanisms in the lung (e.g., in cystic fibrosis, immotile cilia syndrome, agammaglobulinemia). In the past these diseases have been in the domain of the pediatrician, but with improved survival and improved recognition of milder forms, they are now coming to the attention of the internist.

Cystic fibrosis (mucoviscidosis) is an inherited autosomal recessive disease of the exocrine glands that results in inspissated secretions, pancreatic insufficiency, and bronchiectasis. The pediatric patient often presents with failure to thrive, heat stroke, or recurrent infections, but the older patient with a milder disease may present with COPD. Diagnosis is confirmed by the finding of elevated chloride concentration in the sweat. Immotile cilia syndrome is caused by abnormal cilia and ciliary function and results in recurrent infections of the sinuses and respiratory tract. Patients with agammaglobulinemia also have recurrent infections of the sinuses and respiratory tract. Early therapy in all of these diseases is directed at prevention and control of infections. When airway obstruction develops, the clinical manifestations and therapeutic principles are the same as in COPD. Rarely, bronchiectasis is sufficiently localized to be amenable to surgical excision.

RISK FACTORS

Pulmonary function as measured by the FEV_1 decreases with age in normal nonsmoking adults at the rate of 15 to 30 ml/yr. Thus age is a major determinent of ventilatory function. But this "normal" loss of function does not lead to symptomatic disease. The single most important risk factor for the development of COPD is cigarette smoking; approximately 80 percent of COPD can be attributed to this.[3] Despite the clear association between smoking and COPD, however, less than 20 percent of people who regularly smoke develop significant airway obstruction. This suggests that other host or environmental factors are important. In 1963 investigators described early-onset familial emphysema in patients with very low levels of α_1-antiprotease in their serum.[5] This rarely encountered condition is a genetically determined abnormality that increases the risk for COPD at least tenfold. Large epidemiologic studies have shown that when controlling for age and smoking history, other factors—including low socioeconomic status (perhaps because of increased exposure to urban and industrial pollutants), a first-degree relative with COPD, type A blood, and male gender—are also associated with an increased risk for COPD.

Smoking nevertheless remains the most important treatable factor in the development of COPD. Smoking leads to increased numbers of macrophages and neutrophils, which release protease in the lungs; reduces the function of antiproteases; and interferes with repair processes in the lungs. In addition to smoking, which affects metabolic rate and weight as well, dietary factors also may increase the risk for developing smoking-related lung disease and mucus hypersecretion.[14]

The role of passive smoking is being investigated.[3] Recent evidence has shown that parental smoking, especially maternal smoking, may increase respiratory illness and symptoms in children. Whether this will result in disease in later life is unknown.

Asthma is characterized by hyperresponsiveness of airways to a variety of stimuli. The relationship between airway hyperreactivity and risk for COPD has been debated for years. Some investigators argue that the reversible obstruction that occurs in asthmatics is unrelated to COPD, while others believe that the presence of hyperreactivity is an important risk factor for COPD. Recent studies support the latter hypothesis. Approximately half the patients with COPD have hyperreactive airways when challenged with bronchoconstrictors such as histamine or methacholine. Furthermore, COPD patients who are hyperreactive lose lung function at a faster rate than those who are not. Thus airway hyperreactivity may predispose an individual to the development of COPD. If so, exposure to environmental contaminants known to increase airway reactivity, such as influenza viruses, sulfur dioxide, and ozone, may potentiate the risk for COPD.

While certain occupational exposures are clearly related to the development of chronic lung disease, their role in the development of COPD is not clear. Coal dust exposure has an effect that is separable from cigarette smoking, but the prevalence of significant ventilatory obstruction may be as low as 1 to 5 percent with high exposure. Cotton and grain dust exposure produce occupational asthma, but chronic airway obstruction has been observed in up to one quarter of nonsmoking grain workers.

CLINICAL MANIFESTATIONS

Dyspnea is usually the chief complaint of a patient with COPD who is presenting for the first time. The presence of associated symptoms such as cough, chronic sputum production, ankle edema, weight loss, or paroxysmal nocturnal dyspnea will depend on the severity of disease and whether emphysema or chronic bronchitis predominates. In the majority of patients with chronic airway obstruction, both conditions are present when the patient seeks medical attention. There is almost always a history of smoking. Although the patient may say that the symptoms are of recent onset, careful questioning usually reveals that episodes of cough and sputum and decreasing exercise tolerance developed over a period of years. The onset of symptoms is so insidious that the patient often attributes his declining exercise tolerance to age or deconditioning and does not seek medical attention until symptoms are debilitating or a complication has supervened. Severe airway obstruction may be encountered as an incidental finding in a preoperative evaluation. The sensation of shortness of breath is frequently aggravated by dampness, cold, dust, or upper respiratory tract infections, which progress to produce acute purulent bronchitis. The onset of symptoms may be dated to a cold that "settled in the chest" and never resolved.

Early in COPD the physical examination may be normal. As the disease progresses, an increasing number of physical signs become apparent. The chest may appear barrel-shaped, and scattered wheezes or crackles may be heard. Evidence of airway obstruction may be absent but, if present, is best observed during maximal forced expiration. For this purpose the physician auscultates the chest while the patient first inhales fully and then exhales as rapidly as possible through an open mouth. Even when wheezing is not heard, prolongation of forced expiration beyond 4 to 5 seconds indicates airway obstruction. In more advanced disease, scattered wheezing may be heard during tidal breathing, particularly in the patient with chronic bronchitis during an exacerbation. The diffuse melodious wheezes heard in asthma are atypical, however. The patient with chronic bronchitis and little emphysema may present with recurrent purulent bronchitis and respiratory failure accompanied by signs of right-sided heart failure. In contrast, the patient with emphysema and little bronchitis presents with physical signs of lung hyperinflation such as increased anterior posterior chest diameter, widened intercostal spaces, hyperresonant percussion note, obliteration of the area of cardiac dullness, low diaphragm, and diminished breath sounds. The patient with predominantly emphysema usually has carbon dioxide retention and right-sided heart failure only as a terminal event, when adequate alveolar ventilation is a mechanical impossibility. These findings are subject to large observer error, correlate poorly with severity of obstruction, and are not dependable for distinguishing among asthma, bronchitis, and emphysema.

Late in their disease or during an acute decompensation, both types of patients have tachycardia, tachypnea with a prolonged expiratory phase, and pulsus paradoxus. They use their accessory muscles of respiration and purse their lips to control expiratory flow and to maintain airway caliber. The clinical presentation in the most severely ill patients may be dominated by manifestations of hypoxia and hypercapnia (such as altered consciousness ranging from drowsiness to frank psychosis or coma, cyanosis, and cardiac irritability). Rarely, carbon dioxide retention is sufficient to produce increases in intracranial pressure and papilledema.

Patients with bronchiectasis often seek medical attention before marked obstruction is present because of copious sputum production (up to a cup per day) or because of recurrent bouts of infection. The patient's breath may have a foul odor from pulmonary or sinus infections. Clubbing, atypical for other forms of COPD, may be present. Late in the disease, right-sided heart failure occurs.

LABORATORY FINDINGS

The hallmark laboratory finding in COPD is a decreased forced expiratory flow rate measured by spirometry. The vital capacity may be normal or low, but the FEV_1, peak expiratory flow rates, and other assessments of expiratory flow are reduced. The FEV_1 is used to estimate the degree of obstruction. It is unusual to see a patient with an FEV_1 above 2 L who experiences dyspnea during normal physical activity. An FEV_1 of less than 1 L, however, is usually associated with dyspnea on level walking or climbing one flight of stairs. Carbon dioxide retention of cor pulmonale is usually associated with an FEV_1 of less than 1 L.

Lung volumes measured with helium dilution are abnormal in COPD. Residual volume is elevated in airway obstruction from any cause, since small airways tend to close and trap gas behind them. In emphysema, functional residual capacity and total lung capacity are also elevated because of a loss of elastic recoil. In contrast to bronchitic patients, the patient with emphysema has a low diffusing capacity due to loss of alveolar surface area. Elastic recoil pressure measured with an esophageal balloon is also decreased because of the destruction of elastin in alveolar walls. The decrease in diffusing capacity and loss of elastic recoil measured during life correlate with the extent of emphysema seen microscopically.

Arterial blood gas determinations are necessary in the evaluation and management of patients with obstructive disease to determine the adequacy of alveolar ventilation and oxygenation. Arterial blood gases, however, correlate only roughly with the degree of obstruction as measured by spirometry. The patient with emphysema who has a strong drive to breathe will maintain normal arterial blood gases or show only slight hypoxia at rest despite complaints of dyspnea. By contrast, the patient with bronchitis may have no complaints of dyspnea while having a PO_2 less than 65 mm Hg. Prolonged, significant hypoxia results in erythrocytosis. Hypercarbia results in compensatory retention of bicarbonate. If significant hyperinflation is present, the ECG shows low voltage and, if pulmonary hypertension is present, signs of right ventricular strain.

RADIOGRAPHIC FINDINGS

As much as 50 percent of patients with significant chronic airway obstruction have normal or near-normal chest radiographs. Others show a variety of findings that are nonspecific and of limited value in identifying or differentiating the common forms of obstructive pulmonary diseases. Nevertheless, radiographic assessment in all patients with COPD is essential to excluding other associated pulmonary disease such as pneumonia or cancer.

Common findings on chest radiograph in patients with COPD from emphysema are increased radiolucency of the lung, a flat diaphragm, a large retrosternal airspace, and an angle of greater than 90 degrees between the diaphragm and sternum on lateral films. These findings indicate hyperinflation and should not be considered diagnostic of a specific type of lung disease. A more diagnostic finding in emphysema is regional or generalized loss of vascularity with rapid tapering of the proximal branches of the pulmonary artery. This finding, which is frequently subtle on plain radiographs, is more easily appreciated with CT of the chest. Similarly a CT scan may reveal striking bullae in the upper lobes that are missed on a plain radiograph. Bullous lesions in the lower lobes, particularly in a patient less than 40 years of age, should alert the physician to a diagnosis of α_1-antitrypsin deficiency.

Patients with chronic bronchitis show less hyperinflation but may have subtle increases in lung markings, suggestive of thickening of the bronchi. In bronchiectasis the increase in markings is occasionally sufficient to produce the "railroad track" sign of two parallel thickened bronchial walls. In cystic fibrosis, unlike other conditions, bronchiectasis and scarring are predominantly in the upper lobes.

DIFFERENTIAL DIAGNOSIS

When a patient presents with complaints of dyspnea on exertion, cough, paroxysmal nocturnal dyspnea, orthopnea, and a history of smoking, COPD and left ventricular dysfunction are the two primary diagnostic considerations. It is noteworthy that smoking is a major risk factor for cardiac as well as lung disease and that cardiac complications of smoking are more common than pulmonary complications. Since similar symptoms occur in both heart and lung disease, they may not be helpful in distinguishing between

the two. Crackles are heard in COPD as well as left-sided heart failure, and bronchial wall edema in congestive heart failure (CHF) may produce wheezes. Signs of right-sided heart failure such as ankle edema, jugular venous distension, or a hepatojugular reflex are caused by COPD as well as left-sided heart failure. The presence of an S_3, cephalization of blood flow on chest radiograph, and the presence of hypertension in a patient known to be normotensive, however, point toward the diagnosis of left ventricular failure. The heart sounds may be difficult to hear or the chest radiograph hard to interpret for blood flow pattern in COPD.

Perhaps the simplest and most definitive differentiation between a patient with COPD and a patient with CHF is based on a spirogram. In CHF the FVC falls, but it is unusual for the FEV_1 as a percentage of FVC to fall below 70. In contrast the patient with COPD may have a reduced FVC, but the characteristic abnormality is a marked reduction in the FEV_1/FVC ratio. In some cases it may be necessary to perform a cardiopulmonary exercise test or an echocardiogram to assess left ventricular function. If a trial of diuretic therapy is considered too dangerous, measurement of pulmonary capillary wedge pressure as an indicator of left atrial pressure will distinguish between the two. Since left ventricular failure is not uncommon in patients with COPD, it is often necessary to treat both.

Other causes of dyspnea can be distinguished from COPD on the basis of history, physical examination, and spirometric evaluation. In asthma the history of dyspnea is episodic and the obstruction reversible with bronchodilators. Early interstitial pulmonary fibrosis may mimic chronic bronchitis by chest radiograph but will produce a restrictive ventilatory defect apparent with spirometry. Primary pulmonary hypertension may mimic emphysema because of a paucity of peripheral vasculature and a low diffusing capacity. It tends to be a disease of young women; no hyperinflation occurs, and there is minimal airway obstruction as measured by spirometry, however.

It is usually not critical to distinguish among the chronic obstructive airway diseases, since therapy is directed toward reversing the pathophysiologic sequelae of disease (e.g., dyspnea, hypoxia). The exception to this rule is the identification of the patient with bronchiectasis because of cystic fibrosis. A long history, upper lobe involvement, and symptoms of malabsorption or heat intolerance easily identify the patient with severe disease. Milder forms should be sought in anyone with bronchiectasis, especially in a patient who grows mucoid *Pseudomonas* on sputum culture. The diagnosis alerts the physician to watch for pancreatic insufficiency and to provide genetic counseling.

MANAGEMENT

Since debilitation develops as a result of airways obstruction, any mode of intervention that reduces the decline in pulmonary function should be implemented. The most important intervention available is cessation of smoking. A smoker who quits will not regain lung function, but the rate of loss will revert to that of a nonsmoker (Fig. 3.7–1). Indeed, even individuals at highest risk (e.g., homozygote PiZ with low α_1-antitrypsin levels) show a dramatic reduction in the rate of lung function decline when they stop smoking. Two thirds of patients with chronic bronchitis note improvement in cough and sputum production within weeks after stopping, and many report improved exercise tolerance. Whether the recent trend to switch to smoking cigarettes with less tar and nicotine will have any effect on rate of lung function loss is not yet known.[3]

Other modes of therapy are directed at improving lung function and general well-being and preventing or treating complications. The most effective method of improving lung function is bronchodilator therapy. To decrease dyspnea and improve exercise tolerance, exercise programs directed at increasing respiratory muscle strength have been tried.[6] An exercise program may improve

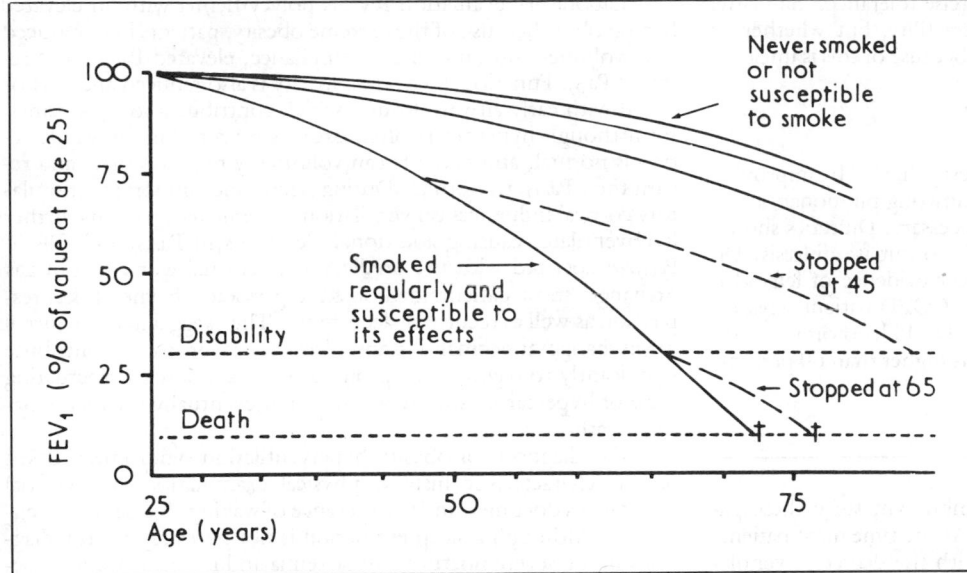

Figure 3.7–1. Effect of age and smoking on FEV_1. Normals and smokers who are not susceptible to the effects of smoking lose lung function slowly (15 to 30 ml/yr) throughout adult life, as shown by the upper curve. A susceptible smoker will lose lung function at an accelerated rate as shown by the lower curve. The rate of loss will depend on susceptibility. If smoking is stopped, the rate of loss will revert to that of a nonsmoker. (*From Fletcher C, Peto R: The natural history of chronic airflow obstruction. Br Med J 1:1645, 1977.*)

cardiovascular fitness and a sense of well-being. Complications such as pneumonia are best prevented with antipneumoccocal vaccination and yearly vaccination against influenza. Complications such as pulmonary hypertension secondary to hypoxia must be treated with oxygen.

PHARMACOTHERAPY

The general approach, mechanisms of action, and complications of bronchodilator therapy are outlined in detail in the chapter on asthma (Chapter 3.6) and can be applied to patients with COPD. The discussion here will be confined to aspects that relate particularly to COPD.

All patients with COPD should be tested for response to inhaled bronchodilators as part of their initial evaluation. If the spirogram obtained 15 to 30 minutes after an inhaled bronchodilator shows a 15 percent or greater increase in either the FEV_1 or FVC compared to before bronchodilators, then some benefit from chronic bronchodilator therapy is assured. If their response is poor, it does not preclude a better response with prolonged treatment. The evaluation should be repeated after 1 to 2 months of bronchodilator therapy. Although sympathomimetic drugs and theophyllines remain the cornerstone of therapy in both asthma and COPD, there is evidence that atropine and its congeners will produce bronchodilation in patients with COPD.[4] Theophyllines, although used primarily for their bronchodilatory effect, may provide additional benefit in COPD because they improve mucociliary clearance and diaphragmatic contractility.[1] Cromolyn is not useful in COPD unless there is a coexistent allergic component.

Improvement with corticosteroids can be predicted if the patient responds promptly to inhaled sympathomimetic bronchodilators.[8] Steroids should not be used if adequate exercise tolerance can be achieved with other agents. If exercise tolerance is still severely impaired after using other modes of therapy, a trial of prednisone (20 to 40 mg per day) is warranted. The trial should be preceded by spirometric assessments of lung function, repeated 2 to 4 weeks later. If no objective improvement is demonstrated, steroids should be discontinued.

OXYGEN

Continuous low-flow oxygen (1 to 4 L by nasal cannula) is indicated for the patient with a resting PO_2 of 55 mm Hg or less. Pa-

tients with exercise-induced dyspnea whose PO_2 is 65 mm Hg or less at rest should be evaluated with a cardiopulmonary exercise tolerance test to see if the PO_2 falls with exercise. If the PO_2 falls significantly during exercise and oxygen improves exercise performance, supplemental oxygen should be provided for routine activities. The major complication of oxygen therapy in some patients is depression of ventilatory drive and hypercapnia. Small elevations of PCO_2 are acceptable and well tolerated, but patients must be monitored closely and the lowest possible concentration of oxygen given.

Oxygen therapy improves cognitive function, exercise tolerance, and pulmonary hemodynamics. Long-term studies show that it also improves survival.[7,9] A major conclusion from these data is that oxygen supplementation is beneficial and should be given continuously for maximum benefit.

INFECTION CONTROL

Patients with COPD have impaired pulmonary defense mechanisms and thus are more susceptible to serious sequelae of viral infections. Vaccination for pneumococcus and influenza has been shown to decrease the complication rate in these patients. Bouts of acute purulent bronchitis are usually due to an overgrowth of normal mouth flora such as *Haemophilus influenzae* or *Streptococcus pneumoniae*. When the sputum changes color in patients with bronchitis, they should be treated with a broad-spectrum antibiotic that covers these pathogens, such as ampicillin, trimethoprim-sulfamethoxazole, tetracycline, or erythromycin. Patients with bronchiectasis have impaired mucociliary clearance and often benefit from a regular program of postural drainage and assisted coughing. Mucolytic agents have been proposed for patients with highly viscous sputum found in bronchiectasis. Their use, however, is controversial, and they may induce bronchospasm in some patients with COPD.

RESPIRATORY MUSCLE TRAINING

A current area of active research focuses on exercise training to improve the strength of the respiratory muscles. There is evidence that respiratory muscles can be strengthened through exercise such as breathing through resistors, and this increased strength may result in increased maximum minute ventilation. Whether this is of clinical benefit is unclear, however, since psychologic and motiva-

tional factors play important roles in exercise tolerance.[6] Similarly, aminophylline increases diaphragm contractility, but whether its use results in symptomatic improvement because of this is unclear.[2]

OTHER

Treatment of right-sided heart failure is best achieved by improving arterial PO_2 to at least 55 mm Hg by maximizing pulmonary function and using supplemental oxygen if necessary. Diuretics should be added if correction of hypoxemia fails to initiate diuresis. Digoxin should be used only if there is clear evidence of left-sided heart failure, since hypoxia may make the COPD patient sensitive to the arrhythmogenic potential of digitalis. Phlebotomy is indicated for erythrocytosis if the hematocrit is higher than 60 percent.

COURSE AND PROGNOSIS

The natural history of early COPD is unknown, since these patients do not come to medical attention. At the time most patients seek medical advice, survival correlates with the degree of ventilatory impairment. An FEV_1 of less than 0.750 L is associated with a reduction in 5-year survival to one third of normal. Survival from the onset of breathlessness in emphysema is likely to be shorter than in patients with bronchitis.

SLEEP APNEA SYNDROMES

The highly complex rhythmic control of ventilation depends on both cortical and brainstem control mechanisms, which are modulated by afferent sensory input from both chemical (CO_2 and O_2) and reflex neural stimulation. The synchronized output of the brainstem controller results in the phasic activation of the respiratory muscles including the diaphragm, intercostal muscles, and the oropharyngeal muscles, which are responsible for maintaining upper airway patency. Dysfunction of the brainstem, the chemical sensors, or the muscles of respiration may result in the failure to initiate or maintain adequate alveolar ventilation.[10,11]

OBESITY HYPOVENTILATION SYNDROME

The obesity hypoventilation syndrome is a relatively rare clinical syndrome characterized by morbid obesity, alveolar hypoventilation with hypoxemia, hypersomnolence, polycythemia, and cor pulmonale. Because of the excessive appetite and similar appearance of patients to the fat boy in Dickens' *Pickwick Papers,* these individuals have been referred to as "pickwickian." At present, it is unclear why certain morbidly obese individuals develop CO_2 retention, but it appears that the pathogenesis of this disorder results from either a suppression of the neural output of the central nervous system or a mechanical inability to respond to normal afferent ventilatory stimuli. Regardless of the primary defect, once carbon dioxide retention is established, patients are at marked risk for developing progressive daytime and nocturnal hypoxemia, which in turn produces pulmonary hypertension, cor pulmonale, and sudden death.

These patients complain of a lifelong history of severe obesity, although they generally present with an additional acute weight gain with the onset of cor pulmonale. Dyspnea on exertion and morning headaches are common, but the most striking feature of this syndrome is hypersomnolence manifested by inappropriate sleep, often while eating or talking. In the extreme, patients spend the majority of their existence sleeping. On physical examination they are morbidly obese with noticeable cyanosis, pedal edema, and sometimes engorged neck veins. An increased second heart sound and hepatic enlargement may be present.

Laboratory evaluation reveals polycythemia with an elevated hemoglobin. Because of the extreme obesity, patients have reduced lung volumes and pulmonary compliance, elevated Pa_{CO_2}, and reduced Pa_{O_2}. Functional residual capacity is also reduced and is associated with early airway closure, which contributes to hypoxemia. Even though hypercarbia often exceeds 50 mm Hg, airway function is normal, and patients can voluntarily hyperventilate and return their Pa_{CO_2} to normal. During sleep, since important stimulatory cortical influences on ventilation are removed, patients further hypoventilate, causing additional elevations in Pa_{CO_2} and falls in Pa_{O_2}. Associated with the predictable nocturnal worsening of gas exchange, most patients demonstrate periodic Cheyne-Stokes respiration as well as recurrent sleep apnea. The exaggerated nocturnal gas-exchange abnormalities and sleep apnea probably contribute significantly to daytime symptoms as well as to a self-perpetuating cycle of hypercarbia and hypoxemia that eventually causes premature death.

The diagnosis of obesity hyperventilation syndrome is based on the characteristic history, physical examination, and arterial blood gases documenting the presence of waking alveolar hypoventilation. Although a sleep evaluation is not necessary for the diagnosis of the severe nocturnal hypoxemia and hypercarbia, it is useful in the management for periodic breathing and sleep apnea. The ideal therapy for obesity hypoventilation is weight reduction, which decreases the mechanical load and reverses the hypercarbia and hypoxemia. Alternatively, respiratory stimulants such as progesterone and supplemental oxygen will significantly improve gas exchange and relieve the cor pulmonale. In general, tracheostomy has not been needed as a primary form of therapy.

SLEEP APNEA

The sleep apnea syndrome represents a primary failure in the regulation of respiration during sleep. The ultimate result of the syndrome is clinical symptoms while the patient is awake.[11] Original descriptions of sleep apnea were made in morbidly obese patients with obesity hypoventilation; however, it is now recognized that the majority of patients are mildly to moderately overweight and do not hypoventilate. Patients with sleep apnea who are not overweight generally have coexisting central nervous system illness or anatomic alterations in the upper airway. The hallmark of this disorder is recurrent apnea associated with hypoxemia, arousal from sleep, and loud snoring.

The pathogenesis of sleep apnea is unclear; however, it appears that there is either an alteration in the metabolic control that initiates respiration or an increased relaxation of the upper airway muscles leading to obstruction of the oropharynx. Characteristically, two major types of breathing pattern result: *central* apnea, which is characterized by an absence of neural respiratory output and thus inactivity of the respiratory muscles; or *obstructive* apnea, which is characterized by occlusion of the upper airway despite continued respiratory muscle activity. In a true sense, all apneas are "central" in origin, since most aspects of the phasic regulation of respiration are modulated by the central nervous system.

The major clinical feature of this disorder is the recognizable intermittent sleep-associated apnea accompanied by disruptive snoring. Since patients are usually unaware of their breathing pattern, bed partners are often the major source of accurate historical detail. Initially, the recurrent apneas are infrequent and not associated with significant hypoxemia; therefore, daytime hypersomnolence begins insidiously and may be ignored. As the severity of apnea progresses, disabling hypersomnolence develops, usually in the absence of overt signs of cor pulmonale. Additional symptoms include cognitive dysfunction, manifested as memory loss or inability to concentrate, and loss of libido. In contrast to those with the obesity hypoventilation syndrome, patients with apnea usually do not have morning headaches and do not complain of dyspnea on exertion.

The typical patient on physical examination is male, middle-aged, mildly to moderately overweight, and hypertensive. Patients should be carefully examined for clinically apparent hypothyroidism because of the frequent association with obstructive sleep apnea. Infrequently, there are associated upper-airway structural abnormalities such as adenotonsillar hypertrophy, microagnathia, and enlarged tongue associated with acromegaly.

While overweight hypersomnolent patients who snore should be suspected of having sleep apnea, the diagnosis can be confirmed only by a complete physiologic monitoring of sleep. These recordings should include electroencephalographic (EEG) descriptions of nonrapid eye movement and rapid eye movement (non-REM and REM) sleep, measurements of respiration to define the type of apnea, ear oximetry to determine the level of hypoxemia, and ECG monitoring to note any associated life-threatening arrhythmias. Patients with clinically significant apnea demonstrate frequent periodic central or obstructive apneas occurring at a frequency of 30 to 40 episodes per hour.

The therapy for patients with sleep apnea depends both on the type and severity of the apnea. In general, all patients should avoid respiratory depressants such as sedatives, hypnotics, and alcohol, since frequency of apnea and associated hypoxemia is worsened. Minimal weight reduction in patients with predominantly obstructive apnea markedly improves oxygenation, reduces the frequency of apnea, and improves daytime hypersomnolence.[12] Correction of anatomic narrowing by removal of tonsillar or adenoidal hypertrophy may be useful in some patients. Newer forms of reconstruction of the upper airway have been partially sucessful; increasing upper-airway size seldom eliminates obstructive sleep apnea. Pharmacologic management of obstructive apnea with tricyclic antidepressants, respiratory stimulants, and oxygen have proven useful in selected patients. Patients with severe obstructive apnea benefit from either tracheostomy that bypasses the area of obstruction or constant pressure applied to the nose, which prevents collapse of the upper airway.[13] Treatment of central apnea, on the other hand, has been less successful. Supplemental nasal oxygen consistently reduces the severity of apnea and hypoxemia, but other pharmacologic medications such as progesterone and theophylline produce variable results.

REFERENCES

1. Aubier M, DeTroyer A, et al: Aminophylline improves diaphragmatic contractility. N Engl J Med 305:249, 1981
2. Belman M, Sieck G, Mazar A: Aminophylline and its influence on ventilatory endurance in humans. Am Rev Respir Dis 131:226, 1985
3. Fielding B: Smoking: Health effects and control. N Engl J Med 313:491, 555, 561, 1985
4. Gross NJ Skorodin MS: The role of parasympathetic system in airway obstruction due to emphysema. N Engl J Med 311:421, 1984
5. Laurell C-B, Ericksson S: The electrophoretic alpha$_1$-globulin pattern of serum in alpha$_1$-antitrypsin deficiency. Scand J Clin Lab Invest 15:132, 1963
6. Levine S, Weiser P, Gillen J: Evaluation of a ventilatory muscle endurance training program in the rehabilitation of patients with chronic obstructive pulmonary disease. Am Rev Respir Dis 133:400, 1986
7. Medical Research Council Working Party: Long-term domiciliary oxygen therapy in chronic hypoxic cor pulmonale complicating chronic bronchitic and emphysema. Lancet 1:681, 1981
8. Mendella LA, Mangrede J, et al: Steroid responsiveness in stable chronic obstructive pulmonary disease. Ann Intern Med 96:17, 1982
9. Nocturnal Oxygen Therapy Trial Group: Continuous or nocturnal oxygen therapy in hypoxemic chronic obstructive lung disease: A clinical trial. Ann Intern Med 93:391, 1980
10. Philipson EA, Bowers G: Sleep disorders. In Fishman AP (ed): Update: Pulmonary Diseases and Disorders. New York, McGraw-Hill, 1982, p. 256
11. Sleep Apnea Disorders. Med Clin North Am 69(6), 1985
12. Smith PL, Gold AR, et al: Weight loss in mild to moderately obese patients with obstructive sleep apnea. Ann Intern Med 103:850, 1985
13. Sullivan CS, Issa FG, Berthan-Jones M: Reversal of obstructive sleep apnea by continuous positive airway pressure applied through the nares. Lancet 2:862, 1981
14. Tockman M, Khoury M, Cohen B: The epidemiology of COPD. In Petty TL (ed): Chronic Obstructive Pulmonary Disease, 2d ed. New York, Marcel Dekker, 1985, p. 43

CHAPTER 3.8
Pulmonary Thromboembolism

William R. Bell

Although pulmonary thromboembolism has been recognized for centuries, it remains one of the most common and difficult problems in the clinical practice of medicine. It is a disease that crosses all traditional specialities and subspecialties of medical practice. There are numerous reasons why this disease is difficult to manage, but the major source of distress to the physician is the difficulty encountered in establishing the diagnosis. Pulmonary embolism has no typical, specific, or uniform mode of presentation. In general the patient feels very ill and has complaints referable to the thorax. Pulmonary emboli most commonly occur in patients who are at greatest risk. Autopsy studies indicate that pulmonary thromboembolism is the most frequently missed diagnosis directly responsible for patient mortality. In 40 to 60 percent of patients who die of pulmonary emboli, the diagnosis and treatment were incorrect.[5,7]

In the United States, the annual incidence of symptomatic pulmonary emboli is estimated to be 650,000, and for approximately 38 percent of these the experience is fatal. The mortality is fivefold to sixfold greater in a group of patients in which the diagnosis is not established. Since less than 10 percent of these patients have associated incurable disease, most of them can be saved if there is an early, accurate diagnosis and immediate treatment.

PATHOPHYSIOLOGY

Pulmonary thromboembolism is defined as impaction of thrombus or other foreign material in the pulmonary arteries. With rare exception, the embolus originates at a distant site (distal to the right atrium) and travels to the lungs via the venous circulation. The most common source of thrombi is thought to be the venous vasculature of the lower extremities. Almost all pulmonary emboli consist of thrombotic material (fibrin, red cells, white cells, and platelets) but, on rare occasions, nonthrombotic materials, such as fat, bone marrow, air, amniotic fluid ("squams"), tumor, and a wide variety of exogenous foreign bodies may embolize into the lungs.

The embolic material in the pulmonary vasculature produces complete or partial obstruction of right heart blood flow to the distal alveolar-capillary sites of gas exchange, and this initiates physiologic reactions in the heart and lungs. The hemodynamic consequences of the reduction in vascular cross-sectional areas are an increase in pulmonary vascular resistance and pulmonary artery pressure and distention of the pulmonary artery. When severe, the pulmonary hypertension can result in right heart failure with reduced cardiac output. Although these hemodynamic alterations are well documented in man their precise mechanism has not been established. Theoretically, the enormous pulmonary arteriocapillary reserve capacity should provide more than adequate compensation for the areas obstructed by embolic material. In this disease, however, pulmonary hypertension has been documented when less than 50 percent of the vascular bed is obstructed. Neural reflexes or vasobronchoconstriction by humoral mediators, such as serotonin, bradykinin, fibrinopeptides A and B, and prostaglandin, may be responsible.

As a result of embolic obstruction, a portion of the lung may be ventilated, but not perfused with blood. This results in a respiratory microunit that is not capable of physiologic gas exchange. In response to this alteration, there is constriction of the alveolar spaces and bronchial airways to the affected area. If the vascular obstruction is complete, vessel breakdown distal to the site of obstruction may occur with hemorrhage producing damage to the ventilatory space. Portions of the lung will be without perfusion and ventilation, and when numerous alveolar units are severely damaged, focal infarction may develop. The rarity of this event is probably related to the dual blood supply of the lungs. The lungs receive blood from the bronchial arteries as well as from the pulmonary arteries and the bronchial circulation continues to function in spite of pulmonary artery obstruction. Regardless of the location and size of vessel obstructed, pulmonary infarction spreads to a pleural interlobar or visceral surface. The size of the clot(s) and vessel obstructed are not determining factors in the development of infarction. This is more likely due to the development of tissue necrosis, hemorrhage into interstitial and alveolar areas, and associated pleuritis, with resultant atelectasis and hypoventilation in the adjacent pulmonary parenchyma.[3] In approximately 40 percent of patients with pulmonary infarction associated with pulmonary emboli, there is an associated pleural effusion that may be serous, but usually is serosanguineous.

THROMBOGENESIS

The inciting event for pulmonary emboli is the formation of venous thrombosis. Although it has been known for over 100 years that damage to the vessel wall intima, stasis, and aberrations in the coagulation-fibrinolytic mechanisms are critical factors in the development of a thrombus, the precise inciting trigger has not been identified. Direct damage to vessel wall intima from any cause induces thrombus formation. Stasis, the relative slowing of blood flow, facilitates interaction between coagulation factors, platelets, and vessel surface and also impedes the clearance of "activated" coagulation factors and thus provides optimal conditions for thrombus formation. Venous stasis is most commonly associated with the development of deep vein thrombosis in man. Although extensive studies have been performed on the blood coagulation system, no acceptable mechanism has been identified to explain the "hypercoagulable state." The pocket above the venous valves of the leg veins is probably the site of origin of most pulmonary emboli. The relative frequency with which pulmonary emboli originate in the leg veins, as compared with the veins of the pelvis, abdominal cavity, inferior vena cava, upper extremities, and right heart chambers, has not been established. Within the legs, the area above the knee is the most frequent source of emboli.

COEXISTING RISK FACTORS

Pulmonary thromboembolism occurs with increasing frequency in patients with certain underlying diseases.[1,4,6,8,9] The most common coexisting condition is immobilization resulting from a disabling illness. This is followed closely in frequency by peripheral venous disease, including thrombophlebitis, venous varicosities, with accompanying insufficiency and stasis, cardiopulmonary disease, the use of oral contraceptives, recent surgery, and obesity. Less common coexisting illnesses include endocrine and metabolic disease, pelvic disease, hypertension, the postpartum period, and malignant neoplasms. Approximately 5 percent of patients with pulmonary emboli have no recognizable concurrent or prior illness.

CLINICAL FEATURES[1,4,6]

Regardless of the clinical setting or associated symptoms or signs, pulmonary thromboembolism usually presents abruptly. Nearly all patients experience chest pain, which is more commonly pleuritic than nonpleuritic, and dyspnea. These symptoms are so common that the absence of dyspnea, chest pain, or tachypnea makes the diagnosis of pulmonary emboli unlikely. Other common symptoms include diaphoresis, cough and hemoptysis, and apprehension. In some patients, leg cramps, palpitations, syncope, nausea, vomiting, chills, and angina-like chest pain occur. Many of these symptoms are noted transiently for several days before the diagnosis is established.

Physical examination commonly reveals tachypnea, fever, and tachycardia. Hypotension leading to shock may occur in some patients and is almost always associated with massive (greater than two lobar arteries occluded) emboli. The combination of rales, rhonchi, wheezes (most likely secondary to bronchospasm), and a pleural friction rub are present in the majority of patients. Cardiac signs, which may call attention to right heart involvement, include accentuated pulmonic component of S_2, right ventricular lift, S_4 gallop, ejection murmur at left sternal edge, or signs of systemic venous congestion. It is unusual to find clinically evident thrombophlebitis of the lower extremities at the time of diagnosis. Unilateral leg swelling, determined visually or by circumferential measurements at defined positions above and below the knee, when present, suggests the presence of deep vein thrombosis. More commonly observed are signs of chronic venous disease, such as tortuous varicosities, mild edema, and skin changes of stasis.

None of the above-mentioned signs or symptoms are specific for pulmonary emboli. They are present in many other diseases, including congestive heart failure, pneumonia, chronic lung disease, and myocardial infarction. It is difficult to establish the diagnosis of pulmonary emboli from clinical findings alone. The physician must first think of it when the patient presents with these nonspecific symptoms in an appropriate setting. He may then call upon laboratory aids to confirm or often deny his clinical suspicion.

LABORATORY STUDIES[8,9]

ELECTROCARDIOGRAM

In more than one third of the patients the ECG is normal, while in others there are nonspecific abnormalities that are not helpful in making the diagnosis. The changes observed in the ECG do not correlate with the size of the emboli, location, or hemodynamic alterations. The most frequent ECG abnormalities are changes in the ST segment and T wave in right precordial leads. The time-honored alterations of P pulmonale, peaking of P wave, right axis deviation, $S_1Q_3T_3$ pattern, atrial fibrillation, and changes of right

ventricular hypertrophy are observed only occasionally. Almost all of the ECG abnormalities are transient, lasting only a few hours or days. Although the ECG may not provide specific diagnostic information, abnormalities noted here may provide a clue that an acute cardiopulmonary event has occurred. The ECG is useful in excluding myocardial infarction.

CHEST ROENTGENOGRAM

Intravascular thrombi have the same radiodensity as the blood and surrounding tissues and cannot be visualized with plain radiographs. The most frequently observed abnormalities are the secondary pulmonary parenchymal changes of consolidation and atelectasis often with unilateral diaphragmatic elevation. Pleural effusion occurs in about one third of the patients and may be bilateral. In 60 percent of patients the effusion contains red blood cells. Increase in major vessel and cardiac chamber size may occur, but is rare. Infrequently, changes compatible with pulmonary parenchymal infarction (pleural based, triangular, wedge-shaped density), abrupt vessel cutoff, and large areas of radiolucency secondary to oligemia are seen. Changes of parenchymal infarction, when present, usually occur 18 to 36 hours following the embolic event. The chest roentgenogram is normal in approximately half of the patients with documented pulmonary thromboembolic disease.

The chest radiograph is most helpful in a patient suspected of having emboli when it is normal. The combination of a normal chest radiograph and an abnormal lung isotope perfusion scan should heighten the suspicion of the diagnosis.

HEMATOLOGY AND COAGULATION STUDIES

The erythrocyte sedimentation rate and white blood cell count may be minimally elevated. Infrequently, the white blood cell count (with a normal differential distribution) may increase to 15,000 to 20,000/mm³. The platelet count and the plasma fibrinogen concentration are either normal or moderately elevated. Fibrinogen-fibrin degradation products may be elevated at some time in the course of the illness, but are not elevated at the time of the acute event, and, therefore, are not helpful in making the diagnosis or making the decision to institute therapy.

CHEMISTRY STUDIES

Measurement of serum enzymes or isoenzymes offers little diagnostic help in patients with pulmonary emboli. Although minimal ele-

vations in bilirubin, alkaline phosphatase, LDH, SGOT, and SGPT can be detected, they are transient and do not occur with any predictability. Presently, there is no biochemical test that has been proven to be efficacious in making or supporting the diagnosis of pulmonary thromboembolism.

ARTERIAL BLOOD GASES

Although approximately 80 percent of the patients with pulmonary emboli have a reduced Pa_{O_2} on room air, this test has several limitations as a diagnostic test. At least 15 percent of the patients with even massive emboli have Pa_{O_2} levels of 90 mm Hg or greater. In diseases such as acute and chronic lung disease and cardiac disease where pulmonary embolism is common, the Pa_{O_2} level may be reduced prior to the embolic event. If a recent, normal set of arterial blood gas determinations is available for comparison, repeat study at the time of symptoms suggestive of emboli may provide evidence favoring the diagnosis.

ISOTOPE LUNG SCANNING[1,10]

Pulmonary isotopic perfusion lung scanning is a valuable technique in the investigation of a patient with suspected pulmonary emboli. This technique is sensitive and provides accurate information about blood flow in pulmonary vessels as small as 15 μm in diameter. It is performed by injecting isotopically labeled denatured protein particles (microspheres) into a peripheral vein. When the microspheres reach the lung, they are held up transiently in capillaries, allowing external gamma detectors to image the distribution pattern of radioactivity in the lung. Currently, the detectors image six different views of the lungs: anterior, posterior, right and left lateral, and right and left oblique (Fig. 3.8–1). This technique can be performed easily and quickly, without discomfort or morbidity to the most seriously ill patient. The diagnostic utility of this technique is severely limited because of its lack of specificity. Anything that alters blood flow, such as infectious processes, congestive heart failure, infiltrative neoplasms, or asthma, as well as intraluminal vascular obstruction, can yield an abnormal distribution pattern of radioactivity in the lungs. If a properly performed lung scan (six views) reveals bilateral segmental defects, at best this can strongly suggest, but does not confirm, the diagnosis of pulmonary emboli. The greatest utility of the lung perfusion scan is in excluding the diagnosis of pulmonary emboli. Because of its sensitivity, a normal perfusion scan effectively excludes the diagnosis of pulmonary emboli. An inconclusive, abnormal scan is helpful at

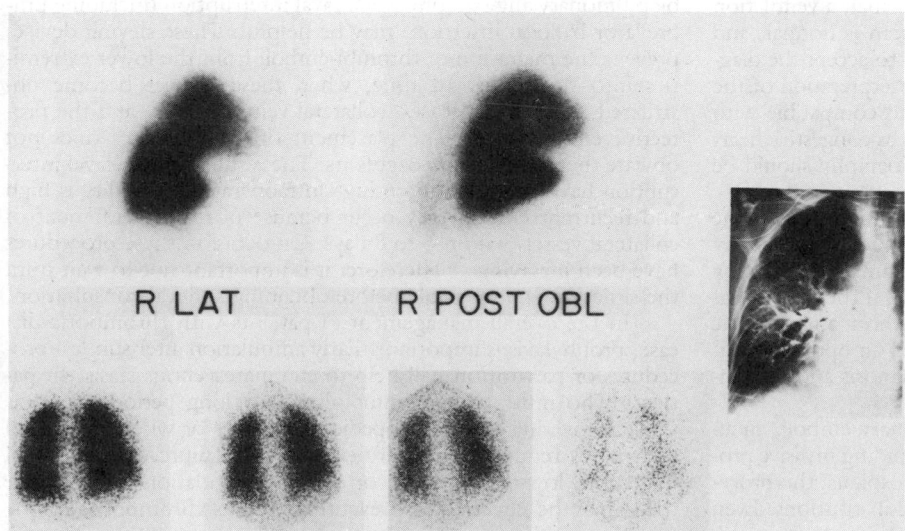

Figure 3.8–1 Ventilation and perfusion scans shown in conjunction with selective right lower lobe pulmonary arteriogram in patient with pulmonary embolism. Segmental perfusion defect in right mid-lung field seen in right lateral and right posterior oblique views of perfusion scan (top). Ventilation scan (bottom) is normal. Arteriogram (right) demonstrates emboli in artery to right mid-lung field.

R LAT   R POST OBL

the time of angiography, to direct the angiographer to look closely at areas suspected of having emboli.

The inhalation of radioactive gas (xenon) can be used to examine the function of the ventilatory compartments of the lung, and is often performed after the perfusion scan to determine whether ventilatory abnormalities are responsible for perfusion defects. Theoretically, if there is intraluminal obstruction due to thrombi, the perfusion scan will be abnormal, but the ventilation scan will be normal. In a patient with pulmonary emboli, the defects seen on perfusion scan will not be matched by defects on the ventilation scan. Unfortunately, this ideal situation is not always present. If the blood vessels are damaged by extensive embolic obstruction, the adjacent ventilatory compartments may be deranged. The defect seen on perfusion scan may be matched by a similar defect on ventilation scan; such a combination may be interpreted erroneously as pulmonary parenchymal disease, and not thromboembolism. Whether the combination of perfusion and ventilation lung scanning will improve the accuracy of the perfusion scan alone in supporting the diagnosis of pulmonary embolism remains to be established.

PULMONARY ANGIOGRAPHY

The pulmonary angiogram is the best available technique to establish the presence of pulmonary emboli. Although this technique is not infallible, recent studies have demonstrated that the occurrence of false negatives or false positives is rare. The discomfort to the patient, the personnel, expense of equipment, and time required limit the routine use of this technique but do not negate its usefulness. The morbidity and mortality are less than 1 percent.

Recent angiographic studies have documented that emboli are commonly bilateral. Infrequently (10 to 15 percent), the emboli are confined to one lung and these are usually multiple. In some patients, resolution of thrombi may occur as early as 15 to 20 days following the embolic event. The combination of angiographic and lung perfusion scanning studies has demonstrated that nearly two thirds of the patients have residual vascular defects one year following the diagnosis. CT and MRI scans are not useful, given currently available techniques.

DIAGNOSTIC APPROACH

If the history and the physical examination are suggestive of emboli, the patient should receive a lung perfusion scan directly. An arterial blood gas determination may be helpful. If the lung perfusion scan is normal, the investigations can cease; pulmonary emboli are excluded. If the lung perfusion scan is abnormal, a ventilation scan should be performed. If the ventilation scan is normal, and clinical features are appropriate, it is reasonable to accept the diagnosis of emboli and institute therapy. If the interpretation of the prefusion and ventilation scans is abnormal and compatible with emboli, but there are additional problems, such as congestive heart failure, chronic lung disease, and asthma, angiography should be performed to settle the issue.

There are other clinical situations where confirmation of the diagnosis by angiography is important. These include a past history of bleeding or untoward reaction to anticoagulants, prior to any surgical procedure, including umbrella insertion, if the patient has a past history of recurrent pulmonary emboli without angiographic documentation, or if the patient has been placed on optimal medical management without substantiating the diagnosis and his condition deteriorates.

Given the difficulty of recognizing pulmonary emboli, an algorithm is useful in facilitating diagnosis and avoiding invasive procedures. Angiography is not available at many hospitals; this procedure is available on a limited basis only at some institutions. Even when angiography is available, it is not possible to perform this study in every patient suspected of venous-thromboembolic disease. The combination of ventilation-perfusion lung scanning along with Doppler ultrasound and impedance plethysmography performed on the lower extremities provides evidence for an accurate diagnosis in 80 to 89 percent of patients. An arterial PO_2 of greater than 85 mm Hg plus a low-probability lung ventilation–perfusion scan has a negative predictive value of 98 percent. One must recognize that movement from test to test along a "decision tree" (Fig. 3.8–2) is predicated upon probability and predictability rather than on the relative degree of certitude provided by angiographic techniques. A decision tree is of greatest help when angiographic techniques are not available.

MANAGEMENT

The most important initial step in treatment is administration of adequate fluid volume to increase the venous pressure in order to promote maximal blood return to the right heart. Anticoagulant or thrombolytic therapy should be instituted promptly, as soon as the diagnosis is made. In addition, supportive measures such as oxygen and, if indicated, minimal effective doses of analgesics, aminophyline for bronchospasm, digitalis for heart failure, and/or vasopressors for hypotension should be administered (see Chapter 2.2). For patients with uncomplicated pulmonary emboli the initial agent of choice is intravenous heparin, which should be administered for 10 to 14 days. Before discontinuation of heparin, oral anticoagulants should be instituted and continued for 6 weeks to 6 months or longer. The duration of oral anticoagulation must be guided by the status of the patient. In those patients with risk factors such as obesity, congestive heart failure, venous disease of the lower extremities, or a history of recurrent thrombotic disease, oral anticoagulation may be continued indefinitely. In patients who are temporarily immobilized, oral anticoagulant therapy should continue until the patient is fully ambulatory.

In those patients with massive or submassive emboli who experience cardiopulmonary compromise, prompt restoration of blood flow is needed to return the cardiac index to normal. Thrombolytic agents, streptokinase or urokinase, infused for 12 to 24 hours, can induce clot dissolution and return cardiopulmonary hemodynamics toward normal within hours, which does not occur with heparin therapy (see Chapter 6.24).[1,2] In these situations available data indicate thrombolytic agents to be the initial treatment of choice. Surgical embolectomy should be considered in the patient who is receiving optimal medical therapy but shows clinical deterioration or persisting hypotension. If anticoagulation is ineffective in preventing recurrent embolic episodes, as documented by pulmonary angiography, vena caval interruption (including umbrella or balloon insertion) may be helpful. These sieving devices prevent the migration of thrombi-emboli from the lower extremities into the lungs. In time, when these devices become obstructed, blood flow ceases, collateral veins develop, and the protective effect is lost. The placement of these devices does not obviate the need for anticoagulants. The results of vena caval interruption have been disappointing—intraoperative mortality is high and recurrent emboli may occur because of the development of collateral vessels within 6 to 8 days. On occasion these procedures have been lifesaving.[11] Therefore, it is important not to wait until the situation is irreversible before obtaining surgical consultation.

In the overall management of patients with thrombotic disease, prophylaxis is important. Early ambulation after surgical procedures or parturition will help to eliminate venous stasis. In patients who must remain immobilized for long periods, such as those recovering from orthopedic procedures or when prolonged bed rest is required for treatment of heart failure or myocardial infarction, low-dose heparin or oral anticoagulation (see Chapter 6.24) may be effective in preventing venous thrombosis. Elastic support stockings may promote venous flow in the legs as may leg muscle contraction against resistance.

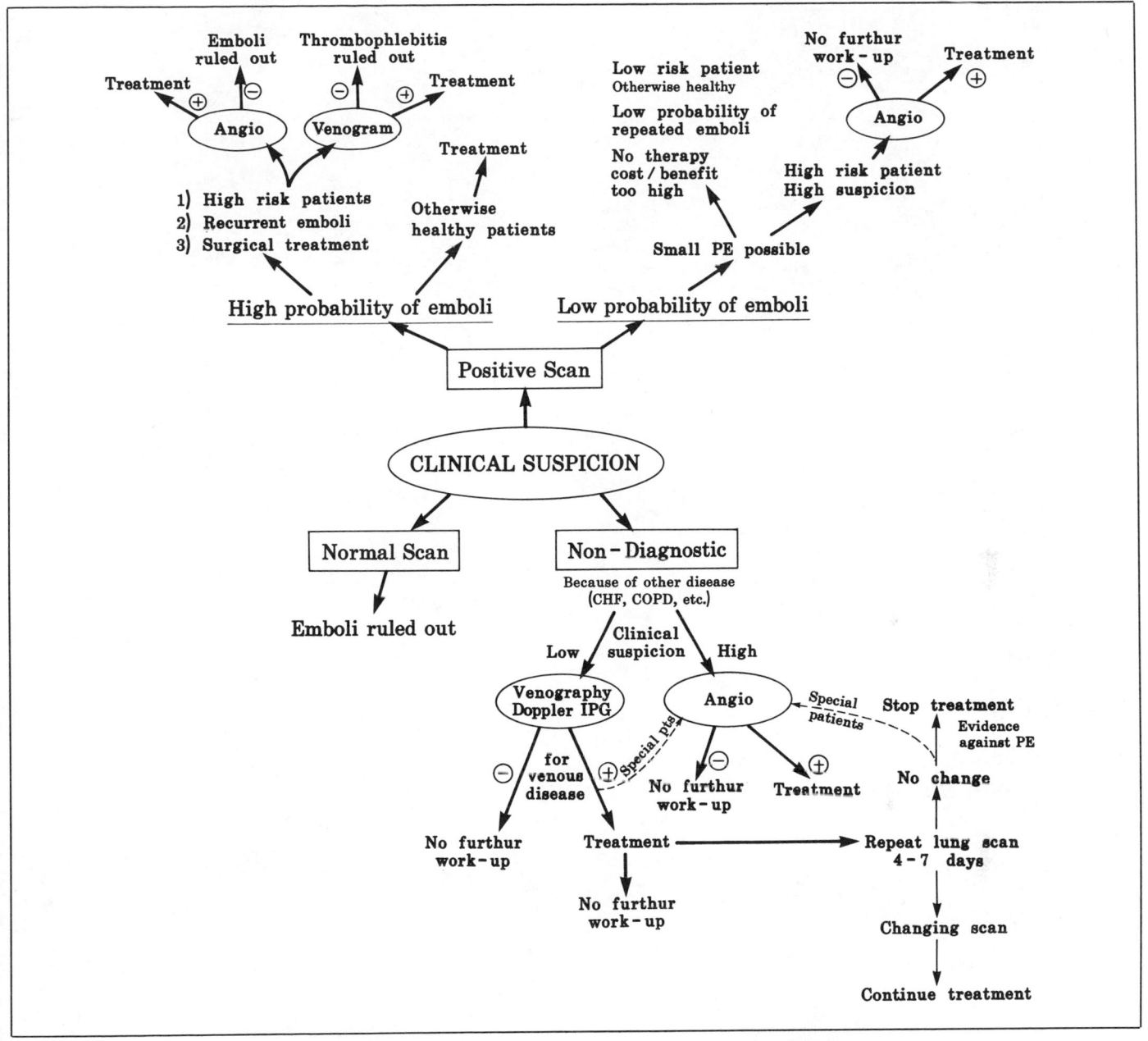

Figure 3.8–2. Decision tree for diagnosis of pulmonary emboli.

REFERENCES

1. Bell WR, Bartholomew JR: Pulmonary thromboembolic disease. In O'Rourke RA (ed): Current Problems in Cardiology, Chicago, Year Book Medical Publishers, 1985, p. 1
2. Bell WR, Meek AJ: Guidelines for the use of thrombolytic agents. N Engl J Med 301:1266, 1979
3. Bell WR, Simon TL: Current status of pulmonary thromboembolic disease: Pathophysiology, diagnosis, prevention and treatment. Am Heart J 103:239, 1982
4. Bell WR, Simon TL, DeMets DL: The clinical features of submassive and massive pulmonary emboli. Am J Med 62:355, 1977
5. Freiman DG, Suyemoto J, Wessler S: Frequency of pulmonary thromboembolism in man. N Engl J Med 272:1278, 1965
6. Goldhaber SZ (ed): Pulmonary Embolism and Deep Venous Thrombosis. Philadelphia, WB Saunders, 1985, p 1
7. Gorham LW: A study of pulmonary embolism. Arch Intern Med 108:8, 418, 1961
8. A National Cooperative Study: The urokinase-streptokinase pulmonary embolism trial. JAMA 229:1606, 1974
9. A National Cooperative Study: The urokinase pulmonary embolism trial. Circulation 47(Suppl 11):1, 1973
10. Robin ED: Overdiagnosis and overtreatment of pulmonary embolism. Ann Intern Med 87:775, 1977
11. Silver D, Sabiston DC: The role of vena caval interruption in the management of pulmonary embolism. Surgery 7:1, 1975

CHAPTER 4.1

Circulatory and Ventilatory Management of the Critically Ill Patient: General Aspects

Peter Rock, William R. Furman,
and J.T. Sylvester

This chapter presents general aspects of circulatory and ventilatory management of critically ill patients. Subsequent chapters deal with management of specific disorders.

EVALUATION OF CIRCULATION

Assessment of cardiovascular function is central to the management of the critically ill patient. Noninvasive methods subject the patient to little or no risk but provide only indirect assessment of perfusion adequacy. Invasive methods provide more exact information at the cost of greater risk. Before resorting to invasive methods, the physician should carefully consider potential risks and benefits. In general, as much information as possible should be obtained by noninvasive means before invasive methods are used.

NONINVASIVE METHODS

When the sphygmomanometric technique is used to measure arterial blood pressure, attention must be paid to the size and placement of the pressure cuff. A cuff that is too small or too loosely applied will cause an artificially high reading. Auscultation of the blood pressure may be difficult when pressure is very low or in patients with peripheral vasoconstriction. In these cases, ultrasonic Doppler flow detectors should be substituted for the stethoscope. When frequent blood pressure determinations are necessary, it may be advisable to use an automated sphygmomanometer. Because blood pressure is a function of cardiac output and systemic vascular resistance, it cannot be used to assess the adequacy of cardiac output. Many organs, notably the kidneys and the brain, autoregulate their flow over a wide range of perfusion pressures; however, renal blood flow will decrease when mean arterial blood pressure falls below 80 mm Hg, and cerebral blood flow will decrease when mean arterial blood falls below 60 mm Hg.

Sinus tachycardia is often an early indication of intravascular volume depletion. Cool, clammy skin develops as the body redirects blood flow from the periphery to essential organs; however, patients with septic shock or hyperthermia may have preserved peripheral flow (so-called warm shock). Cyanosis may reflect inadequate tissue perfusion or pulmonary dysfunction. The rapidity of skin capillary refill provides another index of peripheral blood flow. Delirium or stupor are early signs of inadequate brain perfusion. A urine output greater than 0.5 ml/kg/hr suggests that renal perfusion is adequate.

Electrocardiography is used to detect disturbances of heart rate, rhythm, and electrical conduction. Echocardiography permits assessment of ventricular ejection fraction, valvular function, and global or regional abnormalities in myocardial wall motion. Radionuclide cardiac imaging performed with portable cameras can also provide information about ejection fraction and myocardial wall motion in critically ill patients.

INVASIVE METHODS

Arterial Catheters
Indications and Risks. An arterial catheter allows continuous monitoring of blood pressure and repeated blood sampling for determination of blood gas values and other variables. In most critically ill patients, the benefits of arterial catheters outweigh the risks, which include infection, thrombosis, and unintentional arterial injection. To prevent infection, the connecting tubing and flushing solution should be changed daily. The catheter should be removed after 3 days unless infection is obvious, in which case it should be removed immediately. If reinsertion at a new site is unlikely to be successful, the physician must decide whether the benefits of continued catheterization outweigh the risks of infection, thrombosis, or management without the catheter. Thrombosis and subsequent distal ischemia are more likely in patients who are hypotensive or who are being treated with vasoconstrictor agents. Catheter removal is indicated in the presence of signs of distal ischemia such as pallor, decreased temperature, or pain. Distal ischemia and necrosis may also result from unintentional arterial injection. Substances injected forcefully into a radial artery can reach the head by retrograde arterial flow. To avoid arterial injection, the arterial line and its connecting tubing should be clearly labeled.

Insertion. Arterial catheters are usually inserted into the radial artery, but the femoral, dorsalis pedis, and axillary arteries can also be used. The femoral artery is useful when other pulses are impalpable; however, femoral catheters may be more subject to infection and thrombosis. The brachial artery should not be used because collateral circulation around the elbow may be inadequate. Before cannulating the radial artery, adequacy of the collateral circulation should be assessed with the Allen test.

Percutaneous cannulation is preferred to surgical "cut-down" because the incidence of infection is less. To cannulate an artery percutaneously, the site is made sterile, the artery is located by palpation, and the overlying skin is infiltrated with lidocaine and then nicked with a surgical blade at the insertion site. The needle over which the catheter is mounted is advanced through the skin nick toward the heart at a 45-degree angle to the artery until the artery is punctured, as indicated by a surge of blood into the catheter. The catheter is then advanced into the artery over the stationary needle. Successful cannulation of the artery is signaled by easy insertion of the catheter and free-flowing blood return. If resistance is met during catheter insertion, the needle should be removed and the catheter gradually withdrawn. The appearance of blood flow indicates that the catheter tip is in the arterial lumen

and the catheter should be readvanced. Under no circumstances should the catheter be withdrawn over the needle while the needle and catheter are still in the patient. Such a maneuver may shear off the catheter tip.

Alternatively, arterial cannulation can be achieved by the Seldinger technique. The artery is entered with a thin-walled needle and a flexible guide-wire inserted through the needle. The needle is then removed, and the wire is left in the artery. The catheter is inserted into the artery over the wire and the wire removed. This technique should be used to cannulate the axillary and femoral arteries. It may also be used to cannulate the radial artery.

After the catheter has been inserted, it should be secured with a skin suture and covered with a sterile dressing. The tubing from the catheter must be connected with a locking connector to avoid accidental disconnection.

Pressure Monitoring. To measure blood pressure, the catheter is connected to a pressure transducer by means of fluid-filled, low-compliance tubing. Increasing the length of this tubing lowers the resonant frequency of the system and increases the likelihood of artifacts. Bubbles or kinks in the tubing can damp the tracing and artificially lower recorded blood pressure. Transducers should be calibrated by exposing them to a known pressure. Automated electronic calibration systems should be used only if routinely verified by direct pressure calibration. The level of the right atrium should be used as the hydrostatic zero reference point. In a supine patient this is approximated by the midaxillary line. The transducer must be placed at this level when making measurements.

Central Venous and Pulmonay Artery Catheters

Indications and Risks. A central venous catheter permits determination of central venous blood pressure, facilitates venous blood sampling, and provides a route for intravenous administration of medications, fluids, and blood products. These catheters are employed in critically ill patients when hemodynamic instability or administration of large volumes of fluids is present or anticipated. A triple-lumen, thermistor- and balloon tipped pulmonary artery catheter permits sampling of mixed venous blood and measurement of central venous pressure, pulmonary arterial and wedge pressures, and cardiac output. Pulmonary artery catheters are also available with electrodes that allow pacing of the atrium or ventricle, alone or in combination. Pulmonary artery catheters are used in patients with life-threatening hemodynamic instability or severe respiratory failure. In selected stable patients these catheters may be placed electively for diagnostic purposes or to assess the patient's response to therapeutic interventions.

Unlike arterial catheters, central venous or pulmonary artery catheters (Table 4.1-1) can present life-threatening risks. To avoid air embolism during insertion, the patient should be maintained in a supine, head down position. The catheter or its connecting tubing should never be opened to air. Resuscitative drugs, including lidocaine, should be readily available to treat insertion-related arrhythmias. Unintentional arterial puncture, which occurs in 2 to 10 percent of cases, can cause cerebral ischemia in patients with atherosclerotic carotid disease and compromise the tracheal lumen. Pressure should be applied directly to the punctured artery for several minutes to ensure hemostasis. Perforation of the myocardium by the guide wire or catheter can cause pericardial tamponade. Laceration of the thoracic duct may occur when the catheter is inserted from the left side of the neck. A chest radiograph should be obtained after insertion, not only to verify the catheter's position but also to identify a pneumothorax if present. Since pulmonary artery catheters are longer and more frequently manipulated, they have greater potential for infection and venous thrombosis. Obviously infected catheters should be removed immediately and all other catheters removed after 3 days. Reinsertion, if necessary, should be performed at a new site. Other complications include endocarditis, pulmonary infarct, pulmonary artery rupture and hemorrhage, intravascular knotting of the catheter, and air embolism secondary to balloon rupture. Ventricular ectopy commonly

TABLE 4.1–1. COMPLICATIONS OF PULMONARY ARTERY CATHETERIZATION

Insertion	Pneumothorax, hemothorax, hydrothorax, chylothorax, arterial puncture, mediastinal hematoma, nerve injury, cardiac value injury
Thrombosis	Pulmonary emboli, pulmonary infarction, venous or endocardial thrombosis
Hemorrhage	Myocardial or vascular perforation, pulmonary artery rupture
Arrhythmias	Premature ventricular contractions, ventricular tachycardia or fibrillation, right bundle branch block
Infection	Intravascular infection, endocarditis, sepsis

occurs as the catheter is advanced through the heart. Because transient right bundle branch block may also develop, pulmonary artery catheterization should be attempted with great caution in patients with preexisting left bundle branch block. The physician should consider prophylactic placement of a transvenous pacemaker to treat complete heart block, should it occur.

Insertion. As insertion sites the antecubital, femoral, and external jugular veins provide low risk of arterial puncture and pneumothorax and permit control of bleeding in patients with a defect in coagulation. On the other hand, it may be difficult to reach the central circulation from these sites because of tortuosity of the vessels or the presence of valves. Nevertheless, the external jugular vein should be used in a first attempt to enter the central venous system unless the patient is in extremis and no delay can be tolerated. The antecubital site may be useful in patients with a coagulopathy or in whom a pneumothorax would be particularly hazardous.

Greater success in central venous catheterization can be achieved by insertion through the internal jugular or subclavian veins. The subclavian route of cannulation is associated with a higher rate of pneumothorax. Moreover, if unintentional arterial puncture occurs with the subclavian approach, it will not be possible to tamponade the site of bleeding. The internal jugular route is therefore preferred. When appropriate, the patient should receive sedation before insertion. The patient's heart rate and rhythm, blood pressure, and respiratory rate and pattern should be monitored, preferably by an assistant. It may be advisable to administer oxygen in certain patients.

The patient should be positioned so that the site of insertion is below the level of the heart. This decreases the possibility of air embolism and distends the vein, facilitating cannulation. After sterile preparation, the site of insertion should be infiltrated with lidocaine. Two insertion sites have proved useful for internal jugular catherization.

The *paracarotid approach* takes advantage of the position of the internal jugular vein immediately lateral to the carotid artery in the midportion of the neck. The patient's head should be turned slightly to the opposite side and the carotid artery located at the level of the thyroid cartilage by palpation. One or two fingers should be placed directly over the artery to identify its location. Excess pressure should be avoided because it may slow the heart or compress the vein. After anesthetizing the skin 0.5 cm lateral to the palpating fingers, a 22-gauge "finder" needle on a 10-ml syringe containing local anesthetic is inserted lateral to the palpating fingers, directed perpendicular to the bed and slightly laterally, and quickly advanced a few millimeters. The presence of the needle within the vein should then be tested by gently aspirating the syringe. Excessive suction may cause the vein to collapse and make identification difficult. If the needle is not within the vein, it should be advanced in increments of several millimeters to a maximum depth of 3 to 5 cm, aspirating after each increment. If the

vein is not identified, the needle should be withdrawn, removed, and redirected slightly more medially. The needle should not be redirected while deeply inserted, as the tip of the needle may lacerate vital structures. The direction of the needle should not carry it under the palpating fingers. When the vein is identified, the direction and depth of the finder needle are noted and used to guide insertion of a thin-wall 16-gauge needle capable of taking a flexible guide-wire. If there is resistance to guide-wire insertion, the wire should be removed and the syringe reattached to check for the free flow of blood. Insertion of an excessive length of wire should be avoided because of the risk of atrial or ventricular arrhythmias and myocardial perforation. The catheter is next inserted over the wire. A small skin nick at the site the wire enters the skin may facilitate entry.

The *anterior approach* requires identification of the insertion site at the apex of the triangle formed by the medial and lateral heads of the sternocleidomastoid muscle and the clavicle. After identifying the carotid artery by palpation, the finder needle should be inserted at a 45-degree angle to the skin toward the ipsilateral nipple. If the vein is not encountered, the needle should be withdrawn to the skin surface and redirected in a slightly more medial direction. When the internal jugular vein is found, it is cannulated using the guide-wire technique previously described.

With either approach, great care must be taken to avoid catheterization of the carotid artery. Arterial blood will ordinarily be redder than venous blood and pulse out of the needle; however, these signs can be unreliable in hypoxic patients with high venous pressure. If the placement of the needle or catheter is questionable, location should be determined by connecting the device to a pressure transducer and inspecting the measured pressure waveform. Under no circumstances should catheterization proceed if there is doubt as to the venous nature of the blood. This is particularly important for catheterization of the pulmonary artery, which requires placement of a large introducer.

The most commonly used pulmonary artery catheter has three lumens. The distal lumen opens at the tip of the catheter and is located in a pulmonary artery when the catheter is correctly placed. The proximal lumen opens at a side hole 30 cm from the catheter tip and is usually in the right atrium. The third lumen allows inflation of the balloon at the catheter tip. The inflated balloon carries the catheter into the pulmonary artery by acting as a

"sail" in the wind of blood flow. A thermistor at the tip permits the determination of cardiac output by thermodilution. Before insertion, the proximal and distal lumens must be filled with heparinized saline and the balloon checked for leaks.

Because of its large diameter, the pulmonary artery catheter must be inserted through a special sheath, which is usually inserted into a central vein over a guide-wire previously placed through a central venous catheter. The sheath has a diaphragm that prevents blood from flowing out when the catheter is in place and a sidearm for the administration of fluids. Once the sheath has been inserted, it should be secured with a skin suture. The pulmonary artery catheter is then introduced into the sheath for approximately 20 cm. The central venous position of the catheter is confirmed by inspection of the pressure waveform (Fig. 4.1–1). The balloon is then inflated with 1.5 ml of air and the catheter advanced while the pressure waveform is observed. The right ventricular waveform is characterized by a diastolic pressure that is close to central venous pressure. Advancement into the pulmonary artery is signaled by the development of a diastolic pressure greater than central venous pressure. The catheter is then advanced until it wedges, as indicated by a sudden fall in pressure and the appearance of a left atrial waveform. Normally the right ventricle is 50 cm from insertion sites in the neck. Failure to reach the ventricle with 65 cm of catheter suggests that the catheter is in the inferior vena cava or coiling in the right side of the heart. In this case the catheter should be withdrawn. Whenever the catheter is withdrawn, the balloon should be deflated. When the catheter is correctly positioned, a protective plastic sheath is pushed over the catheter and connected to the introducer sheath. This keeps the catheter sterile, allowing further manipulation if necessary. The pressure waveform must be continuously displayed to permit recognition of migration into the wedge position or the right ventricle. Migration into the wedge position could lead to a pulmonary infarct; migration into the ventricle could cause ventricular arrhythmias. Occasionally, successful insertion of a pulmonary artery catheter requires bedside fluoroscopy. Stiffening the catheter by injecting cold saline, turning the patient, or advancing the catheter while the patient takes a big breath may facilitate passage into the pulmonary artery.

Pressure Monitoring. Central venous pressure is usually measured intermittently with a fluid-filled manometer; however, a trans-

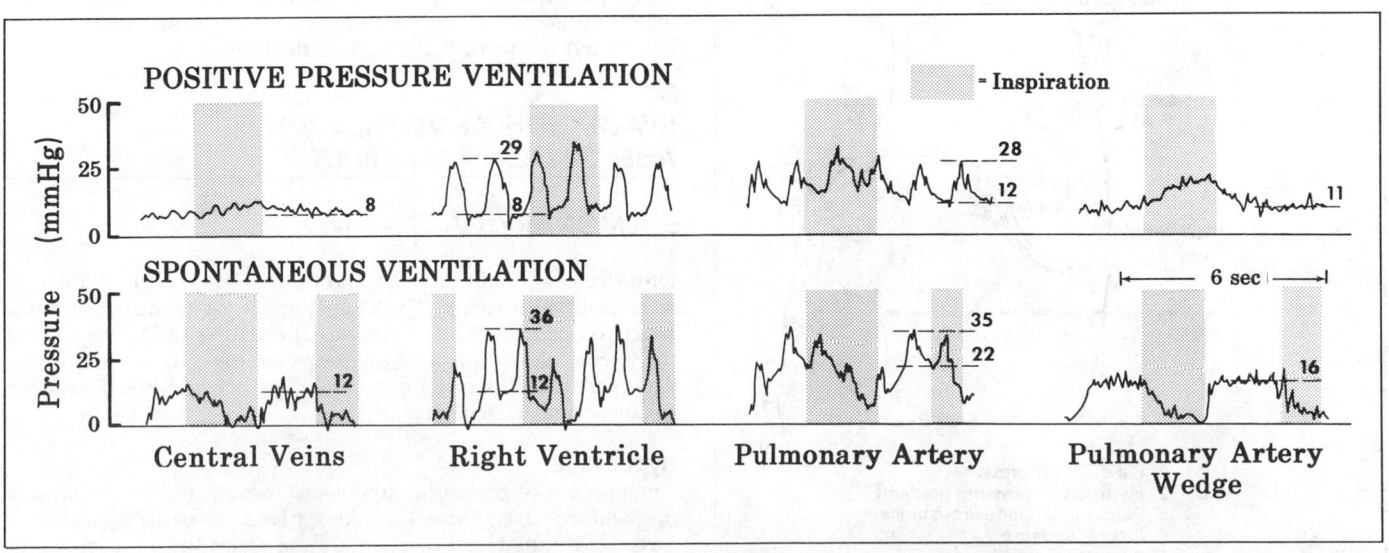

Figure 4.1–1. Recordings of central venous, right ventricular, pulmonary arterial, and pulmonary artery wedge pressures from a Swan–Ganz catheter in a patient breathing spontaneously and a paralyzed patient on a positive-pressure ventilator. Note that inspiration causes a negative deflection of the tracing with spontaneous ventilation, and a positive deflection with positive-pressure ventilation. In both cases, measurements are made at end-expiration.

ducer can be used if continuous monitoring is necessary or it is desired to inspect the pressure waveform. Pulmonary artery pressures are routinely measured with transducers. It is particularly important to place the transducer at the correct zero hydrostatic reference level (the level of the right atrium) because errors of only a few millimeters of mercury can be significant in these ordinarily low pressures.

Before using central venous and pulmonary artery wedge pressures to estimate the filling pressures of the right and left ventricles, the physician must evaluate the influence of numerous artifacts. Ventricular filling pressure is the difference between the pressures inside and outside the ventricle (i.e., the transmural pressure) at end diastole. Because central venous and pulmonary arterial wedge pressures are measured relative to atmospheric pressure, they will not accurately reflect filling pressures if the pressure surrounding the heart and intrathoracic vessels is significantly different from atmospheric pressure. For this reason, measurements should be performed at end-expiration, when intrapleural pressure is usually close to atmospheric pressure. In patients treated with positive end-expiratory pressure (PEEP), however, the positive pressure applied to the airways can be transmitted to the pleural space and intrathoracic vessels, artifactually elevating central venous or pulmonary arterial pressures. When uncertainty exists, pleural pressure can be measured with an esophageal balloon.

If pleural pressure artifacts can be eliminated, central venous pressure can be assumed to equal intraluminal right atrial pressure; however, it can sometimes be unwise to assume that pulmonary artery wedge pressure equals intraluminal left atrial pressure (Fig. 4.1–2). A catheter in the wedge position occludes a pulmonary artery, creating a static column of fluid between the catheter tip and the junction of pulmonary veins draining the occluded and nonoccluded lung regions. Interruption of this column (capillary compression secondary to hyperinflation or vascular kinking secondary to atelectasis), increased pulmonary venous resistance (pulmonary vasospasm), or increased flow through nonoccluded lung may therefore cause wedge pressure to depart significantly from intraluminal left atrial pressure. Finally, stenosis of the mitral or right atrioventricular valve can cause atrial (and therefore central venous or wedge) pressures to exceed ventricular filling pressures.

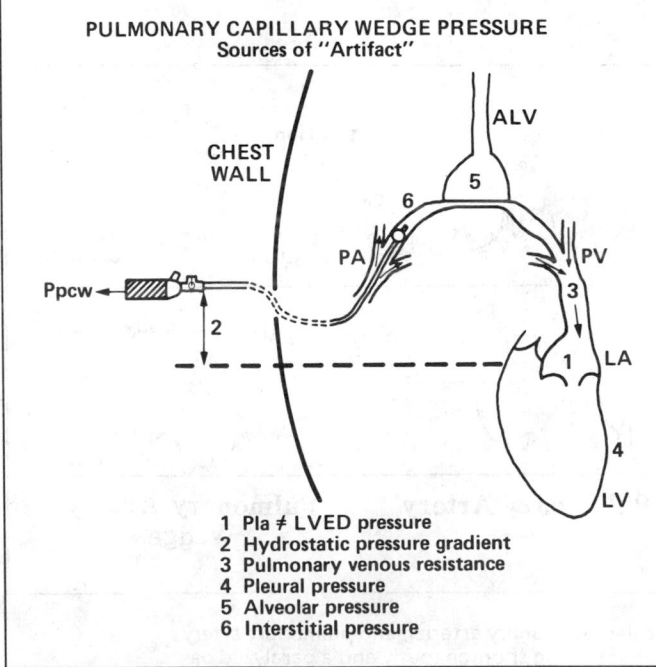

Figure 4.1–2. Sources of artifact in measurment of pulmonary capillary wedge pressure (Ppcw) when used as an index of left ventricular end-diastolic (LVED) pressure.

TABLE 4.1–2. FORMULAS AND NORMAL VALUES FOR HEMODYNAMIC INDICES

Cardiac index (CI)	$= \dfrac{\text{Cardiac output}}{\text{Body surface area}}$	2.2–4.0 L/min/m²
Stroke volume (SV)	$= \dfrac{\text{Cardiac output}}{\text{Heart rate}}$	1 ml/kg
Systemic vascular resistance (SVR)	$= \dfrac{\text{MAP} - \text{RAP}}{\text{Cardiac output}}$	11–15 mm Hg min/L
Pulmonary vascular resistance (PVR)	$= \dfrac{\text{MPAP} - \text{PCWP}}{\text{Cardiac output}}$	1–1.5 mm Hg min/L
Left ventricular stroke work index (LVSWI)	$= \dfrac{(\text{MAP} - \text{PCWP})\,(\text{CI})}{\text{Heart rate}}$	3.7 mm Hg L/m²

Measurement of Cardiac Output. The pulmonary artery catheter permits repeated measurements of cardiac output by thermodilution. In this technique, 10 ml of cold 5 percent dextrose is rapidly injected into the right atrium through the proximal lumen while pulmonary artery temperature is measured continuously from the thermistor at the catheter tip. To obtain cardiac output, a computer divides the product of injectate volume and the difference between body and injectate temperature by the concentration-time integral of the difference between body and pulmonary artery temperature after taking into account the specific heats of 5 percent dextrose and blood and loss of "cold" from the system. Ice-cold injectate gives a better signal-to-noise ratio and is therefore preferred to room temperature injectate in patients with large fluctuations in baseline pulmonary artery temperature. The technique has few complications. Excessive use in patients with poor renal function could cause fluid overload. Infection or sepsis is possible. Rarely, the cold injectate can cause sinus pause, sinus arrest, or other bradycardias. The most serious complication is inappropriate management deriving from errors in measurement. Measurements should therefore be performed in triplicate, and the thermodilution curve recorded to detect unacceptable levels of noise and rule out artifacts due to poor injection technique.

As shown in Table 4.1–2, several hemodynamic indices can be derived from measurements of systemic, pulmonary artery, and wedge pressures, cardiac output, and heart rate. These include estimations of resistance to flow in the systemic and pulmonary circulations and the work performed by the heart.

EVALUATION OF VENTILATION AND OXYGEN TRANSPORT

PULMONARY GAS EXCHANGE

Disturbances of pulmonary O_2 and CO_2 exchange occur frequently in critically ill patients. The evaluation of gas exchange depends largely on measurement of the partial pressures of O_2 and CO_2 in the arterial blood (Pa$_{O_2}$, Pa$_{CO_2}$). Impaired oxygenation and disorders of CO_2 elimination often occur together, but it is instructive to consider them separately.

Hypoxemia

An approach to the pathophysiologic assessment of hypoxemia is diagrammed in Figure 4.1–3. At sea level, arterial PO_2 normally exceeds 90 mm Hg. Lower values can result from a decrease in inspired O_2 tension, hypoventilation, right-to-left shunt, or ventilation-perfusion mismatch. The first is a problem only at high altitude. Hypoventilation, indicated by elevation of arterial CO_2 tension, always contributes to hypoxemia. The magnitude of contribution can be assessed by calculating the alveolar-arterial PO_2 difference (P[A − a]$_{O_2}$):

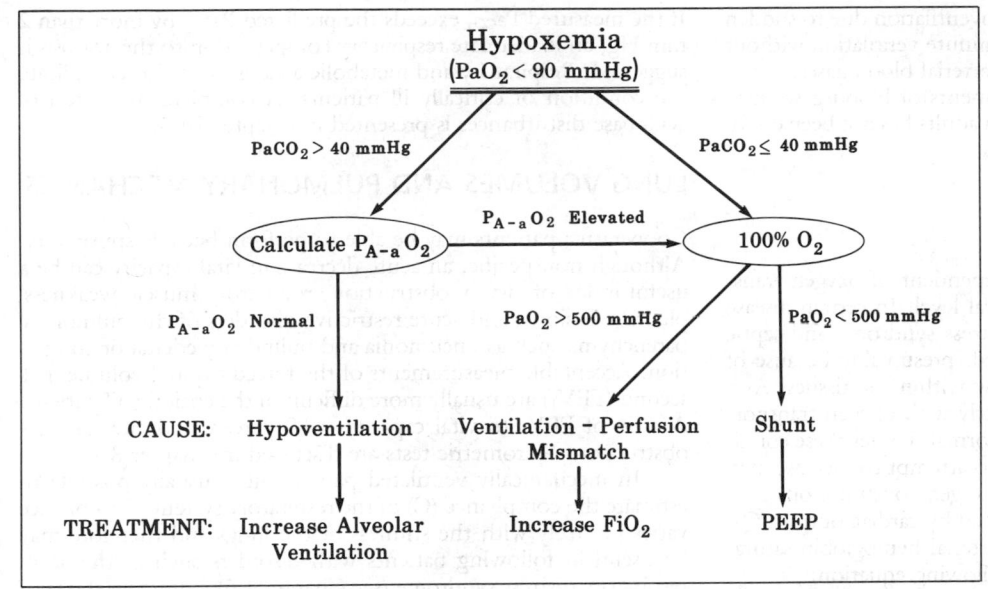

Figure 4.1–3. Pathophysiologic assessment of hypoxemia.

$$P(A - a) O_2 = FI_{O_2} (PB - Pw) - Pa_{CO_2}/R - Pa_{O_2}$$

where FI_{O_2} is the fractional inspired O_2 concentration, PB is barometric pressure (760 mm Hg at sea level), Pw is the vapor pressure of water at the patient's temperature (47 mm Hg at 37C), and R is the ratio of CO_2 production to O_2 consumption (usually 0.8). $P(A - a)O_2$ expresses the efficiency with which a lung exchanges O_2. In a perfect lung the $P(A - a)O_2$ would be zero; however, slight shunting and imperfect ventilation-perfusion matching cause the $P(A - a)O_2$ to be <10 mm Hg in healthy young patients breathing room air and <20 mm Hg in healthy old patients. The normal value of $P(A - a)O_2$ increases with FI_{O_2}; therefore initial assessment should be performed with the patient breathing room air. In an individual patient, changes in the efficiency of pulmonary O_2 exchange can be evaluated by measuring $P(A - a)O_2$ at the same FI_{O_2}. A normal $P(A - a)O_2$ in a hypoxemic, hypercapnic patient indicates that hypoventilation is the sole cause of the hypoxemia. If $P(A - a)O_2$ is elevated, shunt or ventilation-perfusion mismatch also contribute.

Ventilation-perfusion mismatch can be distinguished from shunt by measuring Pa_{O_2} while the patient breathes 100 percent O_2; however, this should not be done in patients who may hypoventilate in response to oxygen (see Chapter 4.7). When Pa_{O_2} exceeds 500 mm Hg under these conditions, the major cause of hypoxemia is ventilation-perfusion mismatch. When Pa_{O_2} is significantly less than 500 mm Hg, the major cause is shunt. If desired, the shunt fraction ($\dot{Q}s/\dot{Q}t$) can be quantified as follows:

$$\dot{Q}s/\dot{Q}t = (Cc - Ca)/(Cc - C\bar{v})$$

where Cc, Ca, and C$\bar{v}$ refer to the content of oxygen in end-pulmonary capillary, arterial, and mixed venous blood, respectively, while the patient breathes 100 percent O_2. Ca and C$\bar{v}$ can be measured directly, or Ca can be measured and C$\bar{v}$ calculated, assuming an arterial-venous O_2 content difference of 4 ml/dl. Assuming complete saturation of hemoglobin and an end-capillary P_{O_2} equal to alveolar P_{O_2} ($PA_{O_2} = PI_{O_2} - Pa_{CO_2}$ on 100 percent O_2) Cc can be calculated as follows:

$$Cc = 1.39 \, Hb + 0.003 \, PA_{O_2}$$

where Hb is hemoglobin concentration, 1.39 is the O_2 carrying capacity of hemoglobin in milliliters per gram, and 0.003 is the plasma solubility of O_2 at 37C in milliliters per deciliter per millimeter of mercury. As a rough guide the physician can remember

that a Pa_{O_2} of 50 mm Hg on 100 percent O_2 indicates a shunt fraction of about 50 percent.

As shown in Figure 4.1–3, determining the pathophysiologic cause of hypoxemia has important therapeutic implications. Hypoventilation is usually treated by increasing alveolar ventilation. Ventilation-perfusion mismatch is treated by increasing FI_{O_2}. Positive end-expiratory pressure may be indicated when right-to-left shunting is due to alveolar filling or collapse is present.

Hypercapnia
Arterial P_{CO_2} is determined by the rate of CO_2 production ($\dot{V}_{CO_2}$) and alveolar ventilation ($\dot{V}A$) according to the following equation:

$$Pa_{CO_2} = K\dot{V}_{CO_2}/\dot{V}A = K\dot{V}_{CO_2}/\dot{V}_E - \dot{V}_D$$

where K is a constant equal to 8.63, $\dot{V}_E$ is minute ventilation, and $\dot{V}_D$ is dead-space ventilation. This equation reveals that Pa_{CO_2} increases whenever alveolar ventilation decreases relative to CO_2 production. Thus, alveolar hypoventilation is defined by an increase in Pa_{CO_2} above its normal value of 35 to 45 mm Hg. Conversely, alveolar hyperventilation is defined by a decrease in Pa_{CO_2}. Hypoventilation can result from a decrease in minute ventilation, as in barbiturate overdose and respiratory muscle weakness, or an increase in dead-space ventilation, as in pulmonary emphysema. Minute ventilation can be measured directly. Dead-space ventilation can be calculated as follows:

$$\dot{V}_D = \dot{V}_E (Pa_{CO_2} - PE_{CO_2})/Pa_{CO_2}$$

where PE_{CO_2} is mixed expired CO_2 tension. The causes and management of hypoventilation are discussed in Chapter 4.7.

Noninvasive Assessment of Pulmonary Gas Exchange
Arterial oxygen saturation can be monitored continuously by ear or finger oximeters. These devices can be used to detect decreases in saturation that result from untoward events such as ventilator disconnection, mucus plugging of airways, pulmonary emboli, pulmonary edema, and bronchospasm. A disadvantage is their insensitivity to the effects of changes in Pa_{O_2} occurring at saturations >90 percent. The noninvasive and continuous nature of the measurement, however, is a strong recommendation for their use in appropriate patients.

Carbon dioxide concentration in exhaled gas can be measured breath by breath with infrared or mass spectrometry. End-tidal CO_2 concentration can be considered an estimate of alveolar or arterial P_{CO_2} and used to guide ventilator settings and weaning at-

tempts and to detect quickly acute hypoventilation due to sudden increases in dead space or decreases in minute ventilation without resorting to frequent measurements of arterial blood gases.

Although transcutaneous measurements of blood gases may be helpful in children, their usefulness in adults has not been established.

OXYGEN TRANSPORT

Normally, oxygen consumption is independent of oxygen transport unless transport falls below a critical level. In certain disease states, such as the adult respiratory distress syndrome and septic shock, this critical level can be increased, presumably because of defects in the distribution of blood flow within the tissues. As a result, oxygen consumption varies directly with oxygen transport even when the quantity of transport is normal. Under these conditions, it is reasonable for the physician to attempt to increase oxygen transport until it no longer limits oxygen consumption.

Oxygen transport ($\dot{Q}_{O_2}$) is determined by cardiac output ($\dot{Q}$), hemoglobin concentration (Hb), and arterial hemoglobin saturation with O_2 (Sa_{O_2}) according to the following equation:

$$\dot{Q}_{O_2} = 13.9 \; \dot{Q} \; \text{Hb} \; Sa_{O_2}$$

where 13.9 is the product of the capacity of hemoglobin to combine with O_2 in milliliters per gram and a correction factor to convert deciliters to liters. Maximizing Sa_{O_2} by increasing inspired O_2 concentration, instituting mechanical ventilation, and administering positive end-expiratory pressure is important, but therapeutic manipulations of cardiac output and hemoglobin concentration are frequently easier to accomplish and must not be ignored. Oxygen transport can be measured directly if a thermistor-type pulmonary artery catheter is in place. The effects of changes in $\dot{Q}_{O_2}$ or O_2 consumption ($\dot{V}_{O_2}$) can be assessed by calculating $\dot{V}_{O_2}$ as:

$$\dot{V}_{O_2} = (Ca - C\bar{v})\dot{Q}$$

Alternatively, $\dot{V}_{O_2}$ can be calculated from ventilatory variables:

$$\dot{V}_{O_2} = \dot{V}_E \frac{1 - F_{E_{O_2}} - F_{E_{CO_2}}}{1 - F_{I_{O_2}}} - F_{E_{O_2}}$$

where $F_{E_{O_2}}$ and $F_{E_{CO_2}}$ are the mixed expired concentrations of O_2 and CO_2 and $F_{I_{O_2}} < 1.0$.

ACID-BASE IMBALANCE

Changes in Pa_{CO_2} alter acid–base balance according to the Henderson–Hasselbalch equation:

$$pH = 6.1 + \log [HCO_3]/0.03 \, Pa_{CO_2}$$

The increase in Pa_{CO_2} caused by hypoventilation will therefore decrease arterial pH, resulting in respiratory acidosis. Acute hypoventilation in a previously normal patient will decrease pH by 0.008 U for every 1 mm Hg increase in Pa_{CO_2}. A pH change less than this suggests that hypoventilation has been present long enough (about 3 days) to allow a compensatory increase in [HCO_3] by renal mechanisms. Metabolic acidosis occurs commonly in critically ill patients, particularly as lactic acidosis secondary to inadequate O_2 transport. Metabolic acidosis stimulates ventilation, but complete respiratory compensation may take hours because the pH of the cerebrospinal fluid (CSF) bathing the chemoreceptors changes only slowly. Empiric relations have been established that relate the expected change in Pa_{CO_2} to the change in [HCO_3] during metabolic acidosis. One such relation is

$$\text{Predicted } Pa_{CO_2} = 1.5 \, [HCO_3] + 8$$

If the measured Pa_{CO_2} exceeds the predicted Pa_{CO_2} by more than 2 mm Hg, an inadequate respiratory compensation to the acidosis is suggested. Respiratory and metabolic alkalosis can also complicate the condition of critically ill patients. A complete discussion of acid–base disturbances is presented in Chapter 10.3.

LUNG VOLUMES AND PULMONARY MECHANICS

Cooperative patients may be able to perform bedside spirometry. Although nonspecific, an acute decrease in vital capacity can be a useful index of airway obstruction, respiratory muscle weakness, pleural effusions, and acute restrictive disorders of the pulmonary parenchyma such as pneumonia and pulmonary edema or congestion. Acceptable measurements of the forced expired volume in 1 second (FEV_1) are usually more difficult in the critically ill patient. A ratio of FEV_1 to vital capacity <80 percent indicates airways obstruction. Spirometric tests are discussed in Chapter 3.1.

In mechanically ventilated patients, it is usually possible to estimate the compliance (C) of the respiratory system. Compliance varies inversely with the stiffness of the lungs and therefore may be useful in following patients with disorders such as the adult respiratory distress syndrome (see Chapter 4.5), adjusting the level of positive end-expiratory pressure, and in assessing the potential for weaning from mechanical ventilation. Compliance can be calculated as follows:

$$C = V_T/(P_{plat}-P_{ee})$$

where V_T is tidal volume, P_{plat} is the plateau reached by airway pressure during an inspiratory pause, and P_{ee} is end-expiratory pressure. Normally, C is about 100 ml/cm H_2O. It should be remembered that C is affected by the stiffness of the lung and the chest wall. To use C to assess changes in the former, it is necessary to assume constancy of the latter. This is reasonable only if the patient is completely relaxed during the measurement.

RESPIRATORY MUSCLE FUNCTION

Respiratory muscle weakness and fatigue are major causes of respiratory failure in critically ill patients. On physical examination, clues to the development of respiratory muscle fatigue include a progressively increasing respiratory rate and alterations of breathing pattern. Normally, the chest wall and abdomen move outward in concert during inspiration because of the elevation of the thoracic cage and downward movement of the diaphragm. With fatigue the pattern becomes paradoxical, as if the patient were resting the diaphragm while breathing with the chest wall muscles or vice versa; for example, outward movement of the chest wall is accompanied by inward movement of the abdomen, or conversely, outward movement of the abdomen is accompanied by inward movement of the chest wall. With marked fatigue there is a decrease in alveolar ventilation and an increase in Pa_{CO_2}.

As described previously, the vital capacity may be used to quantify respiratory muscle weakness. Ventilatory failure usually occurs when vital capacity falls below 10 ml/kg. Alternatively, the physician can measure the maximum inspiratory pressure by having the patient exert a maximal inspiratory effort against a closed airway with his lungs at residual volume. Normally, values more negative than -100 cm H_2O can be generated. Values ≥ -20 cm H_2O are frequently associated with ventilatory failure.

RESPIRATORY THERAPY

ADMINISTRATION OF OXYGEN

In the spontaneously breathing patient, O_2 can be administered by nasal cannula or face mask. The nasal cannula allows the patient to eat and drink without interrupting O_2 administration. It is well

tolerated by most patients except at flows >3 to 4 L/min, which dry and irritate the nasal mucosa. This method, however, results in a variable, unpredictable FI_{O_2} that depends on the flow rate of oxygen, the magnitude and pattern of minute ventilation, the presence of nasal obstruction, and whether the patient breathes through his nose or mouth. Furthermore, in hypoxemic patients who hypoventilate when Pa_{O_2} is increased, the fixed flow of O_2 delivered by nasal cannula will become less diluted by the patient's ventilation, further increasing FI_{O_2} and Pa_{O_2} and possibly worsening hypoventilation. Thus the nasal cannula should not be used in the initial management of critically ill patients. Various types of face masks are available. Oxygen concentrations are controlled by adjustment of air and O_2 flows at the wall outlet or by Venturi valves incorporated in the masks, which use a fixed flow of O_2 but entrain varying amounts of room air. These masks can provide O_2 concentrations between 24 and 40 percent and are particularly useful in hypoventilating patients who may hypoventilate further in response to an increase in Pa_{O_2}. A tight-fitting face mask with a reservoir bag and a nonrebreathing valve allows O_2 concentrations greater than 50 percent to be achieved, but even with this technique it can be difficult to exceed 70 percent because of the entrainment of air through leaks. This is particularly likely to occur in patients with high minute ventilations. In general, if an FI_{O_2} >50 percent is required, tracheal intubation should be considered.

Whatever the method of administration, the physician should use the lowest concentration of O_2 that produces an arterial O_2 saturation of 90 percent. When pH, Pa_{CO_2}, temperature, and 2,3-DPG levels are normal, this corresponds to a Pa_{O_2} of 60 mm Hg. With decreased pH or increased Pa_{CO_2}, temperature, or 2,3-DPG levels, the Pa_{O_2} at 90 percent saturation is increased because of a shift in the oxyhemoglobin dissociation curve to higher partial pressures. Under these circumstances the therapeutic goal should be a Pa_{O_2} of 70 to 80 mm Hg. Alternatively, the arterial O_2 saturation could be measured directly.

Except for purposes of quantifying the shunt fraction, 100 percent O_2 should be avoided. This concentration can increase the probability of O_2 toxicity and the shunt fraction. The latter occurs because perfused, poorly ventilated lung units that contain only CO_2, O_2, and water vapor are predisposed to absorption atelectasis. In patients with severe hypoxemia due largely to shunt, FI_{O_2} can usually be lowered from 100 to 75 percent without a significant decrement in Pa_{O_2}. In all patients the physician should attempt to keep FI_{O_2} below 50 percent to avoid O_2 toxicity.

TRACHEAL INTUBATION

Indications for tracheal intubation include apnea, hypoxemia requiring FI_{O_2} >50 percent, and acute hypercapnic respiratory failure unresponsive to conservative measures. Intubation may also be used to prevent pulmonary aspiration of gastric contents in patients acutely predisposed by disorders such as stroke or drug overdose and to permit hyperventilation of patients with increased intracranial pressure.

Complications of tracheal intubation are related to tube insertion or the duration of intubation (Table 4.1–3). Esophageal intubation and aspiration of gastric contents are common serious complications of insertion. The former can lead to upper airway obstruction and gastric distension and rupture. Esophageal intubation can usually be detected by careful, postinsertion auscultation over the chest and stomach as air is injected through the tube. When intubation is elective, local anesthesia of the upper airway may prevent gagging, vomiting, and aspiration. Awake patients may become hypertensive and tachycardic during laryngoscopy and intubation. Nasopharyngeal and tracheal structures may be injured. Tracheal penetration, for example, can lead to pneumomediastinum, pneumothorax, and mediastinitis. Overinflation of the cuff can compress the tube, obstruct its tip, or cause ischemia of the tracheal wall. To avoid this, the physician should inflate the

TABLE 4.1–3. COMPLICATIONS OF TRACHEAL INTUBATION

Related to insertion
- Esophageal intubation
- Aspiration
- Hypertension, tachycardia
- Injury to airway structures (broken or dislodged teeth; lacerations of lips, gums, vocal cords; tracheal penetration)
- Overinflation of cuff (tube obstruction, tracheal ischemia)
- Malpositioning of tube (obstruction of main-stem bronchus, nonocclusive cuff)

Related to duration
- Necrosis and injury of airway structures (vocal cord damage, tracheoesophageal fistula, bronchial stenosis)
- Infection (sinusitis, retropharyngeal abscess, nosocomial pneumonia)

cuffs to the minimum pressure necessary to achieve occlusion (usually <20 mm Hg). Inability to occlude indicates that the tube is too small or positioned too low, usually in the right main-stem bronchus. This can obstruct the contralateral lung, cause atelectasis, and worsen hypoxemia. To avoid malpositioning, radiopaque endotracheal tubes should be used and the position checked by chest radiography immediately after insertion and thereafter on a daily basis or whenever malpositioning is suspected.

The longer the duration of intubation, the more likely are complications such as vocal cord damage, tracheoesophageal fistula, tracheal stenosis, sinusitis, retropharyngeal abscess, and pulmonary infection. If intubation exceeds 2 to 3 weeks, the physician should consider tracheostomy, which bypasses the upper airway and thus avoids complications associated with those structures. Tracheostomy, however, shares all of the other complications and, in addition, has some of its own, such as hemorrhage, subcutaneous emphysema, and cellulitis of the neck. The patient is particularly vulnerable 1 to 2 days after tracheostomy, when edema and distortion of structures at the tracheostomy site can make reinsertion after inadvertent extubation difficult.

Before performing intubation the physician should confirm the availability of suction, oxygen, a selection of endotracheal tubes, a stylet to stiffen the tube if necessary, a hand bag ventilation system, and face masks in a variety of sizes. Appropriate resuscitative drugs, including atropine, lidocaine, epinephrine, and calcium, should also be immediately available. Oral intubation requires a laryngoscope, which consists of a handle and a detachable blade. A straight blade (Miller type) allows visualization of the vocal cords by lifting the epiglottis directly but may be difficult for the inexperienced operator to use because it crowds the oropharynx. The curved blade (MacIntosh type) is preferable because it permits the tongue to be swept aside, providing more room in the oral cavity for manipulation of the endotracheal tube. To intubate with this blade, the patient is placed supine and his head thrust forward and extended slightly to facilitate exposure of the cords. The mouth is opened widely with the fingers of the right hand. With laryngoscope held in the left hand, the blade tip is placed at the junction of the base of the epiglottis and the valleculae. Lifting the handle at a 45-degree angle to the floor without using the teeth as a fulcrum will elevate the epiglottis and expose the cords. The endotracheal tube is advanced through the laryngeal opening until the cuff is just past the vocal cords (usually 21 to 23 cm from the incisors in adults). It is important not to advance the tube further, because this can result in bronchial intubation. The cuff is then inflated until the air leak around the tube is eliminated. Correct placement of the tube should be immediately confirmed. On physical examination, outward movement of the chest during inspiration, fogging of the tube's internal wall during expiration, the presence of breath sounds bilaterally over the chest, and the absence of inspiratory sounds over the stomach indicate correct placement. Final confirmation by chest radiography should be obtained as

soon as possible. The endotracheal tube tip should be positioned several centimeters above the carina. When correctly positioned, the tube should be taped securely in place along with a rigid oral airway, which facilitates removal of oropharyngeal secretions and prevents the patient from biting the tube.

Experienced physicians can accomplish tracheal intubation by the nasal route; however, this route is contraindicated in patients with basilar skull fractures, in whom the risk of intracranial penetration is increased.

MECHANICAL VENTILATION

The indications for mechanical ventilation are the same as those listed for tracheal intubation. The ventilator most frequently used in medical intensive care units is volume-cycled and pressure-limited. This type of ventilator delivers a preset tidal volume unless an adjustable upper limit for airway pressure is reached. Pressure-cycled ventilators, which stop inspiration when a preset pressure is reached, and time-cycled ventilators, which stop inspiration after a preset time, are less useful. High frequency and jet ventilators deliver very small tidal volumes (usually < 100 ml) at very high frequencies (5 to 50 Hz). Their efficacy remains unknown and their use experimental.

When the physician decides to institute mechanical ventilation, he must select the mode of ventilation, tidal volume, frequency, the ratio of inspiratory to expiratory time (I:E ratio), FI_{O_2}, and level of positive end-expiratory pressure. The mode of ventilation should be assist-control or intermittent mandatory ventilation (IMV). In the former, the patient receives a breath whenever inspiratory muscle contraction generates an airway pressure sufficiently negative to trigger the ventilator. The threshold of the trigger is adjustable. If the patient does not make inspiratory efforts, the ventilator will deliver breaths at a specified tidal volume and frequency. The assist-control mode is commonly used to rest inspiratory muscles, because theoretically the only work the patient has to do is to activate the trigger. Hyperventilation, which occurs commonly in the assist-control mode, can usually be managed by decreasing tidal volume. IMV, which is used more often, delivers breaths at a specified tidal volume and frequency, usually in response to a triggering inspiratory effort (synchronous IMV, or SIMV). Between these breaths, the patient is allowed to breathe spontaneously. IMV is usually more effective than assist-control in patients with an irregular breathing pattern. Some authorities believe that IMV preserves respiratory muscle function in patients without preexisting respiratory muscle fatigue and weakness. IMV may also limit susceptibility to the decrease in cardiac output that can accompany positive-pressure ventilation and positive end-expiratory pressure (PEEP). With IMV the increases in pleural pressure due to the ventilator and PEEP, which tend to compress the right atrium and great veins and thereby decrease venous return, may be offset by the decreases in pleural pressure due to spontaneous inspiration.

A tidal volume of 10 to 12 ml/kg and a frequency of 10 to 12 breaths per minute are reasonable initial settings. Subsequent adjustments should be made as necessary to maintain adequate alveolar ventilation, as indicated by the Pa_{CO_2}. Upward adjustment of tidal volume is limited by the increasing risk of barotrauma at higher transpulmonary pressures, particularly in patients with destructive disorders of the pulmonary parenchyma such as emphysema. When frequency is increased, the time for passive expiration decreases, and alveolar pressure may not fall to the level of airway opening pressure before the next breath is delivered. Thus, breaths may "stack," leading to an increase in end-expiratory lung volume. This phenomenon of "auto-PEEP" is particularly likely to occur in patients with obstructive airways disease. Its presence can be detected by shutting off the ventilator and occluding the expiratory airway just before the ventilator's next breath. In a relaxed patient, the rise in airway pressure above the set end-expiratory pressure measures the magnitude of auto-PEEP. Auto-PEEP can

be relieved by decreasing respiratory frequency or the I:E ratio. The latter is accomplished by increasing the inspiratory flow rate. Normally, I:E is about 1:2. With obstructive airways disease, a value of 1:4 is more reasonable.

PEEP is employed to increase transpulmonary pressure and lung volume at end-expiration in order to inflate atelectatic or unventilated alveoli and airways, reduce right-to-left intrapulmonary shunt, and relieve hypoxemia. Although usually given by ventilator, in some patients PEEP can be administered by a tightly fitting face mask, in which case it is termed "continuous positive airway pressure" (CPAP). The indication for PEEP is severe hypoxemia refractory to increases in FI_{O_2} and associated with an acute, diffuse process in the lungs, such as pulmonary edema secondary to left ventricular failure or the adult respiratory distress syndrome. PEEP is contraindicated in patients with hyperinflated lungs and is not likely to be helpful when the pulmonary process is focal. The use and complications of PEEP are discussed in Chapter 4.5.

Before removing mechanical ventilation, the physician should correct factors that may prevent spontaneous ventilation such as malnourishment, fluid and electrolyte imbalance, cardiac failure, depressed mental status, fever, and pain. A vital capacity greater than 10 ml/kg, a maximum inspiratory pressure more negative than -20 cm H_2O, an FI_{O_2} less than 0.5, and V_D/V_E less than 0.6 are associated with successful weaning. Patients who chronically hypoventilate should have an arterial CO_2 tension near their baseline level, a normal pH, and an O_2 tension of 60 to 70 mm Hg before weaning is attempted.

Two approaches to weaning are commonly employed. In the first, mechanical ventilation is discontinued for 15 to 30 minutes while the physician monitors minute ventilation, respiratory rate, and pattern of breathing and other vital signs. A pulse or ear oximeter is also useful to monitor arterial oxygen saturation. Untoward events such as desaturation, hypotension, or respiratory muscle fatigue, indicate that mechanical ventilation should be reinstituted. If possible, an arterial blood sample should be drawn before reinstitution to quantify hypoxemia and hypoventilation, if present. If this initial trial is uncomplicated, the ventilator should be periodically withdrawn on a regular schedule, gradually increasing the frequency and duration of withdrawal. The pace of weaning will be dictated by the patient's response. The longer the patient has received mechanical ventilation, the slower the weaning process is likely to be. Between periods of withdrawal, the parameters of mechanical ventilation should be set to allow the respiratory muscles to be adequately rested. The other approach is to decrease gradually the frequency of breaths delivered by the ventilator in the IMV mode. In both approaches, it is frequently appropriate to maintain normal mechanical ventilation at night to permit sleep. When weaning has been achieved, it is advisable to observe the patient for an additional 12 to 24 hours before removing the endotracheal tube. Extubation should be performed by a physician skilled in intubation, especially in patients who may have developed upper airway obstruction secondary to prolonged intubation. Patients should not be fed for several hours after extubation because impaired swallowing may cause aspiration.

REFERENCES

1. Connors AF, McCaffree DR, et al: Evaluation of right-heart catheterization in the critically ill patient without acute myocardial infarction. N Engl J Med 308:263, 1983
2. Goldenheim PD, Kazemi H: Cardiopulmonary monitoring of critically ill patients. N Engl J Med 311:717, 776, 1984
3. Moser KM, Spragg RG: Use of the balloon-tipped pulmonary artery catheter in pulmonary disease. Ann Intern Med 98:53, 1983
4. O'Quin R, Marini JJ: Pulmonary artery occlusion pressure: Clinical physiology, measurement, and interpretation. Am Rev Respir Dis 128:319, 1983
5. West JB: Pulmonary Pathophysiology—The Essentials. Baltimore, Williams and Wilkins, 1982
6. Wiedemann HP, Matthay MA, et al: Cardiovascular-pulmonary monitoring in the intensive care unit. Chest 85:537, 657, 1984

CHAPTER 4.2
Cardiorespiratory Arrest

Nisha Chibber Chandra

Cardiorespiratory arrest—the sudden, unexpected cessation of effective cardiac and respiratory function—can result from diverse causes, particularly cardiac tachyarrhythmias or asystole.

Regardless of the underlying cause, treatment should initially be directed at restoring tissue oxygenation by the simple maneuver of chest compression and artificial ventilation. More definitive measures can then be directed toward the underlying cardiac problem. Because cardiopulmonary arrest is unexpected and because the underlying disorder is often reversible, all persons participating in patient care—indeed most people—should be familiar with basic life support techniques. Furthermore, because of the urgent nature of the situation and the large number of persons usually involved in the resuscitative effort, an organized approach is vital, and one person should assume primary responsibility.

Respiratory arrest, which shares many of the features of cardiorespiratory arrest, is most often due to acute airway blockage. It requires special, although simple, management. A discussion of respiratory arrest will be followed by a review of the management of cardiorespiratory arrest based on current information of the mechanism of blood flow in cardiopulmonary resuscitation (CPR).

MANAGEMENT OF ACUTE RESPIRATORY ARREST

Respiratory arrest is the sudden cessation of effective respiratory effort and is commonly caused by airway obstruction due to a foreign body such as a food mass. (The tongue is most often the cause of airway obstruction in the unconscious patient.) The patient rapidly becomes cyanotic, although cardiac function and ineffective ventilatory efforts may be maintained for several minutes. Opening of the airway or artificial respiration alone may result in the successful resuscitation of such a patient.

Maneuvers recommended by the American Heart Association for foreign body obstruction include the following[14]:

1. *Heimlich maneuver:* This consists of a series of sharp thrusts delivered with clenched fists over the upper abdomen of the patient by a rescuer standing behind the victim with his arms encircling the victim's upper abdomen and lower thorax. Although the technique has been criticized because it can lead to visceral injury,[11] when properly administered it is safe and effective. It can also be used on an unconscious supine patient with the force delivered by the rescuer's palm directed inward and cephalad from a position straddling the victim's thighs.
2. *Manual removal:* The victim's mouth should be opened and attempts made to dislodge any obvious foreign body. This maneuver should not be attempted while a respiratory arrest victim remains conscious and continues to attempt to clear his own airway.
3. *Back blows:* Three or four sharp blows high on the spine between the scapulae can often successfully dislodge foreign bodies.

MANAGEMENT OF ACUTE CARDIORESPIRATORY ARREST

In 1960, rhythmic chest compression was shown to generate blood flow and support vital organ perfusion during cardiac arrest until more definitive therapy could be provided.[9,10] These observations form the basis for cardiopulmonary resuscitation as it is practiced today. As a result, CPR is now administered by a network of laypersons, paramedics, nurses, and physicians, each capable of providing effective and increasingly sophisticated support to cardiac arrest victims.

MECHANISM OF BLOOD FLOW DURING CPR

Following the development of external chest compression it was assumed that blood flow during CPR was due to direct compression of the heart between the sternum and vertebral column. Central to the direct cardiac compression mechanism for blood flow was the concept that pressure gradients are established across the heart during chest compression and that blood flow occurs in proportion to these pressure gradients. In recent years a number of observations cast doubt on this hypothesis.

First, rapid, vigorous coughing (a maneuver that increases intrathoracic pressure) was shown to maintain consciousness during ventricular fibrillation for up to 45 seconds.[6] Second, animal experiments revealed virtual equivalence of pressure fluctuations in the right atrium, pulmonary artery, left ventricle, aorta, esophagus, and lateral pleural space during chest compression.[2]

Figure 4.2–1 displays respresentative intrathoracic pressures in experimental animals during CPR. Pressures in the heart and other intrathoracic structures rise by a similar amount during chest compression. Aortic pressure is transmitted efficiently to the carotid arteries, but retrograde transmission of intrathoracic pressure to the jugular veins is prevented by valves at the thoracic inlet. Thus, a peripheral arteriovenous pressure gradient is established during chest compression, with blood flow occurring as a result of this gradient.[12] When chest compression is released, intrathoracic pressures fall toward zero, and the return of systemic venous blood is unimpeded. Retrograde flow from extrathoracic arteries into the aorta is limited by its relative nondistensibility. In the system diagrammed (Fig. 4.2–1) the heart is a conduit, not a pump.

It follows that maneuvers that increase intrathoracic pressure during CPR will be accompanied by increased arterial blood pressure and flow. Indeed, this has been demonstrated in experimental animals and humans.[3,4] Epinephrine also substantially increases myocardial and cerebral flow during CPR by mechanisms related to its alpha-adrenergic effects, including increased arterial vascular tone resulting in higher aortic pressure during the release phase of chest compression, selective vasoconstriction with shunting of blood from nonessential tissues to the heart and brain, and prevention of carotid collapse, thus ensuring efficient transmission of intrathoracic arterial pressures to the brain.

Increased intrathoracic pressure is not the only mechanism by which blood flows during CPR. In some animal studies, intrathoracic vascular pressures exceed pleural pressure during chest compression. This suggests that cardiac compression sometimes occurs. The hemodynamics of CPR are less clearly characterized in humans. Although several lines of evidence favor the intrathoracic pressure model of blood flow,[3] direct cardiac compression sometimes occurs, as evidenced by unequal intrathoracic vascular and pleural pressures.

Animal data also suggest that during conventional CPR, three parameters of chest compression (chest compression force, duration, and rate) can be manipulated to optimize myocardial and cerebral flow. Increasing chest compression force and chest com-

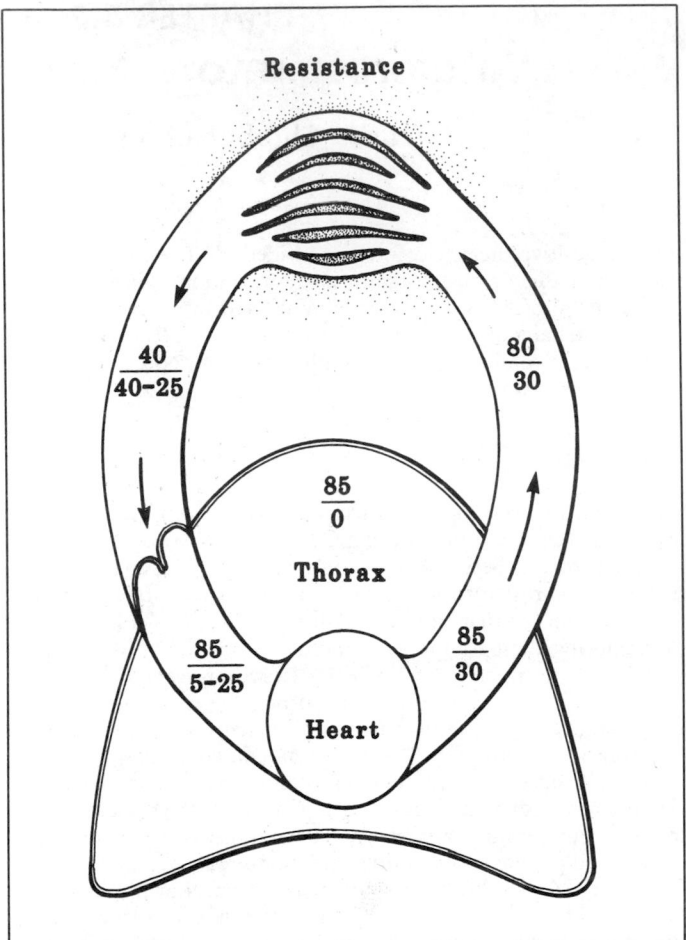

Figure 4.2–1. Representative pressures as recorded in experimental animals during conventional CPR. Systolic pressures indicate pressures recorded during chest compression, and diastolic, those recorded during the release phase of chest compression. Intrathoracic pressures were calculated from esophageal pressures. During chest compression the extrathoracic arterial pressure is similar to intrathoracic aortic pressure; however, extrathoracic venous pressure is markedly lower than intrathoracic venous (right atrial) pressure because of functioning venous valves at thoracic inlet. As a result there is an extrathoracic-arteriovenous pressure gradient and hence forward blood flow. In this model the heart serves only as a passive conduit during chest compression.

pression duration (to 45 to 50 percent of each compression-release cycle) will increase vital organ perfusion if blood flow during CPR is due to manipulation of intrathoracic pressure. In such cases, increasing the rate of chest compression will *not* increase vital organ perfusion. If, however, blood flow during CPR is a result of direct cardiac compression, as in open-chest cardiac massage, vital organ perfusion will increase with increasing chest compression force and rate but will *not* be affected by changes in chest compression duration.[8] But at higher chest compression rates (80 to 100/min), the time for each chest compression-release cycle decreases and prolongation of compression duration is easily achieved. Thus, irrespective of the primary mechanism of blood flow during CPR, higher chest compression rates probably optimize vital organ perfusion during resuscitation.

Based on these data, the new American Heart Association recommendations for chest compression incorporate an increase in chest compression rate from 60/min to 80 to 100/min.[14]

TIMING OF CPR

Cardiac arrest is the sudden cessation of effective mechanical function of the heart. Prompt recognition is essential: the success of resuscitative measures depends on the speed with which they are initiated following arrest. Permanent cerebral anoxic injury is likely to occur if total circulatory arrest lasts more than 4 to 6 minutes.

Cardiac arrest should be considered in the differential diagnosis of sudden collapse; its diagnosis rests on unresponsiveness, pulseless major vessels, and absent heart sounds. Respirations may continue for a few minutes following arrest, but they rapidly become inadequate. It is imperative to initiate CPR as soon as the clinical diagnosis is made and not to wait for respiration to cease. In the management of a patient in cardiac arrest the "ABC rule" must be remembered: A, airway (establishment of a patent); B, breathing (ventilation); and C, circulation.

VENTILATION DURING CPR

Ventilation, a critical component of CPR, should be initiated as soon as the need for CPR is recognized. It is important to clear the airway of loose foreign material and dentures. Next the head should be positioned to eliminate upper airway obstruction by the base of the tongue. The two techniques now employed are comparable in efficacy:

1. *Head tilt–chin lift method:* In this maneuver, the head of the victim is tilted back by gentle pressure on the forehead, and the chin lifted forward, with the jaw supported by the other hand.
2. *Head tilt–neck lift method:* This method is similar, but the neck, instead of the jaw, is gently lifted anteriorly while the head is tilted back. This technique is not recommended if cervical spine injury is suspected.

If no spontaneous respirations are present or if existing respiratory efforts are feeble, mouth-to-mouth ventilation should be initiated immediately, with adequacy of ventilation gauged by a rise and fall of the patient's chest with each delivered breath.

The bag-and-mask technique of oxygen delivery is commonly used by the equipped rescuer in conjunction with a mechanical airway device. The curved plastic "airway" is the simplest of such devices, is easily positioned, and facilitates maintenance of an unobstructed airway by moving the tongue anteriorly. However, during prolonged CPR, adequate ventilation may be difficult to maintain with the bag-and-mask technique, and gastric distention and aspiration may occur.

The esophageal obturator airway has been shown to be a useful and effective technique for emergency ventilation. With this device, gastric distention and aspiration are prevented by balloon obstruction of the esophagus, and ventilation is achieved through proximal openings in the pharyngeal portion of the esophageal obturator tube. Patients may, however, aspirate when the esophageal balloon is deflated. In the newer esophageal obturator airway devices, a nasogastric tube can be inserted through the esophageal obturator to drain the stomach. Risk of aspiration is thereby minimized. Other complications include esophageal rupture and inadvertent insertion into the trachea, with resultant cerebral hypoxia.

The ideal device for establishing and maintaining a patent airway is an endotracheal tube. Endotracheal intubation enables a rescuer to hyperventilate an arrest victim and thereby lower arterial PCO_2, thus compensating for the metabolic acidosis of cardiac arrest.[2,5] Endotracheal intubation requires considerable skill. Ventilation (by mouth-to-mouth or bag-and-mask methods) and chest compression should not be discontinued for prolonged periods while attempting to intubate arrest victims. Proper tube position in the trachea must be confirmed by noting breath sounds over both lung fields, the absence of air sounds over the stomach, and the rise and fall of the patient's chest with each ventilation.

CHEST COMPRESSION DURING CPR

Once adequate ventilation is achieved, manual chest compression should be initiated. The heel of the hand should be placed over the lower third of the sternum and the chest compressed 3.5 to 5 cm at a rate of 80 to 100/min. Chest compression should be maintained for 50 percent of each chest compression-release cycle. A prolonged compression duration is achieved at this high compression rate without having to consciously pause at peak chest compression (see above discussion: Mechanism of Blood Flow During CPR). During chest compression a major arterial blood vessel should be palpated. With each chest compression, an arterial pulse should be felt. A diminished or absent pulse indicates inadequate chest compression force, hypovolemia, pericardial tamponade, or tension pneumothorax. If two trained rescuers are performing CPR, every fifth chest compression should be followed by ventilation. Lay rescuers should perform *only* one-person CPR, in which situation every 15th chest compression should be followed by two slow ventilatory breaths (1 to 1½ sec each).[14]

The American Heart Association has approved the use of pneumatic chest compression devices for CPR.[14] These devices are as effective as manual CPR and have no greater incidence of side effects or complications. Mechanical devices have the advantage of providing constant and adequate chest compression without operator fatigue. They also facilitate transport of patients undergoing resuscitation, and chest compression does not have to be interrupted during defibrillation.

DEFINITIVE THERAPY OF CARDIAC ARREST

Definitive therapy of cardiac arrest is based on ECG assessment of cardiac activity. In general, rhythms associated with cardiac arrest fall into one of the following categories: ventricular tachycardia or fibrillation, asystole or complete heart block, and electromechanical dissociation.

If a defibrillator is available before an ECG can be obtained and cardiac arrest has been established, a 200-joule countershock should be administered without delay. This approach is based on two facts: First, ventricular tachyarrhythmias account for most cardiac arrests. Second, direct-current countershock is not likely to worsen the situation in cases of asystole, complete heart block, or electromechanical dissociation.

Ventricular Tachycardia or Fibrillation (Fig. 4.2–2)

Once ventricular fibrillation or tachycardia is identified, electrical defibrillation should be performed as soon as possible (Fig. 4.2–2). Direct current defibrillation is employed with one electrode paddle placed at the right upper sternal edge and the other placed to the left of the cardiac apex. The paddles should be well coated with electrode paste and held firmly against the chest in order to decrease the transthoracic impedance. The anteroposterior paddle position is occasionally used and presents certain theoretical advantages over the more conventional anterolateral placement; however, the anteroposterior approach is somewhat awkward and no study has shown it to be superior to the anterolateral position.

The current American Heart Association recommendations call for one and, if necessary, a second 200- to 300-J countershock and, if fibrillation persists, a third 360-J countershock in the initial treatment of ventricular fibrillation. These three shocks should be delivered in rapid succession. Earlier recommendations called for higher energy defibrillation and suggested that heavier patients be defibrillated with even higher energy levels. However, 85 to 90 percent of patients weighing up to 90 kg can be successfully defibrillated by using 175 to 200 J.[15] Furthermore, repeated high-energy defibrillation may result in myocardial injury.

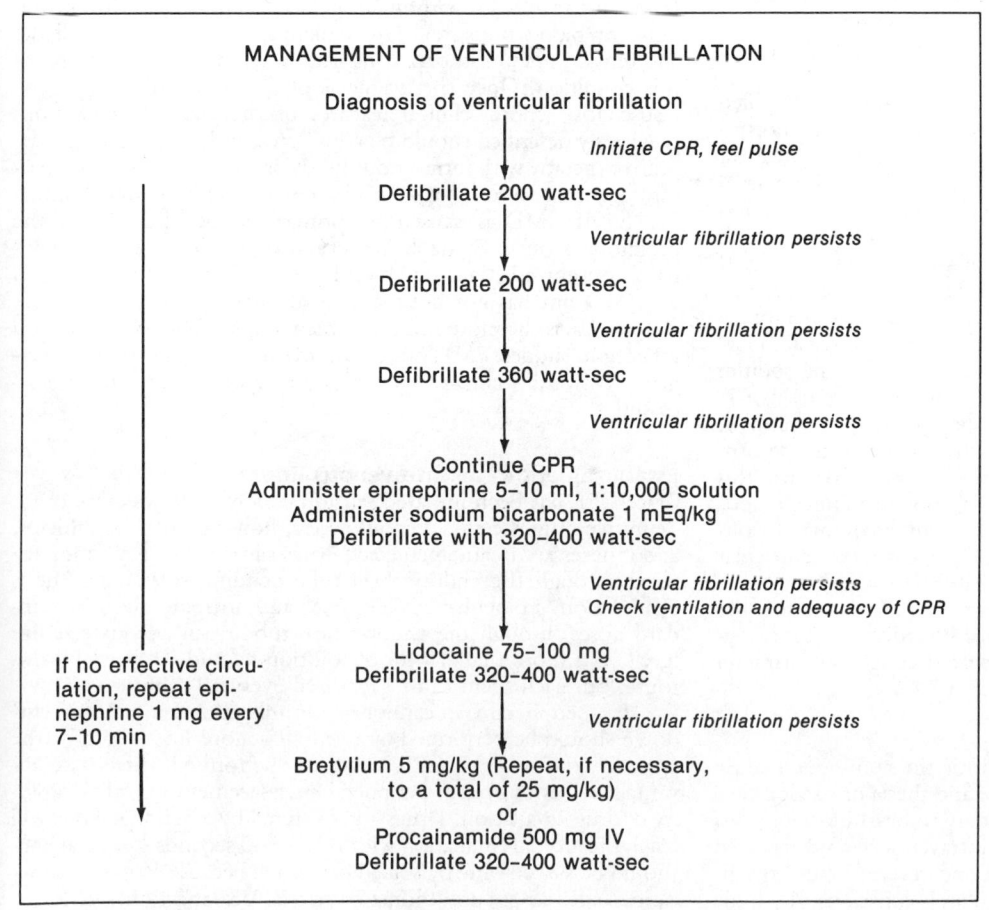

Figure 4.2–2. Flow chart for management of ventricular fibrillation.

If the ECG shows fine fibrillation, or if the three initial defibrillation attempts are unsuccessful, epinephrine (5 to 10 ml of 1:10,000) should be administered intravenously and CPR should be continued. Epinephrine makes ventricular fibrillation more responsive to defibrillation, probably by improving coronary flow during CPR. If repeated attempts at defibrillation fail, it is likely that myocardial ischemia and systemic acidosis or hypoxia are severe. CPR should be continued, with epinephrine administration every 5 to 10 minutes. Sodium bicarbonate should also be administered at this time (1 mEq/kg IV). Supplemental oxygen at the highest available concentration should always be given the victim of cardiac arrest. Hyperventilation to compensate for metabolic acidosis may also be helpful. Repeated attempts at defibrillation should be performed with 320 to 400 J.

If ventricular fibrillation persists despite these measures, lidocaine is the antiarrhythmic agent of choice. It should be given intravenously in a dose of 1 mg/kg every 3 to 5 minutes up to a total of 3 mg/kg.

If ventricular fibrillation is not abolished by lidocaine, epinephrine, and repeated countershocks, bretylium tosylate should be administered intravenously in a dose of 5 mg/kg. Direct current countershock should be repeated. Additional bretylium, in doses of 10 mg/kg, should be given at 10- to 15-minute intervals up to a total of 25 mg/kg. Procainamide is an acceptable alternative and is given as a 500-mg loading dose intravenously over 5 minutes and repeated after 5 minutes if necessary. If a hemodynamically stable rhythm is established but the patient again develops ventricular fibrillation, especially with acute myocardial infarction, propranolol may be used. It should be given only if the previously described drug therapy fails. Appropriate dosage is 1 to 2 mg by slow intravenous injection over 3 to 4 minutes. A total of 5 to 10 mg may be needed. After successful cardioversion an intravenous infusion of lidocaine, bretylium, or procainamide should be maintained for at least 24 hours. Bretylium and procainamide can produce significant hypotension, which usually lessens when the drug infusion is discontinued. Factors perpetuating ectopy, for example, ischemia, hypokalemia, and hypoxemia, should be treated appropriately if present.

Hyperkalemia, a cause of ventricular fibrillation, is identified on the ECG by the presence of tall peaked T waves with a normal QT interval or a "sine-wave" ventricular tachycardia on prearrest tracings. Hyperkalemia can cause atrioventricular block, intra-atrial or intraventricular conduction delays, ventricular fibrillation, and rarely, asystole. Life-threatening hyperkalemia is best treated with an intravenous infusion of 10 to 30 ml of a 10 percent solution of calcium gluconate, with ECG monitoring. Calcium counteracts the adverse effects of potassium on the neuromuscular membrane by competitive inhibition but does not alter plasma potassium levels. Hyperkalemia should be subsequently treated using sodium bicarbonate, glucose-insulin infusions, or ion exchange resins.

The "precordial thump" was once popular for the treatment of ventricular standstill.[13] Ventricular tachycardia can also be converted to sinus rhythm with precordial percussion. Because this technique may precipitate ventricular fibrillation in an unconscious patient who is not in cardiac arrest, current recommendations specify its use only in situations of ECG-confirmed ventricular tachycardia or fibrillation before a defibrillator is available.

Cough has been shown in rare instances to convert ventricular tachycardia to a supraventricular rhythm. If cardiac arrest is recognized before consciousness is lost,[6] repeated cough can maintain consciousness by raising the intrathoracic pressure.

Asystole of Heart Block

Asystole due to excess vagal stimulation is the commonest cause of cardiac arrest during the induction of anesthesia or surgical procedures. Asystole may also occur secondary to heart block or sinus node disease. Atropine (1 mg), given intravenously and repeated in 5 minutes, can successfully prevent and reverse bradyarrhythmias in such situations. Again, if the patient is conscious, rhythmic forceful coughing can maintain adequate vital organ perfusion until

definitive treatment can be initiated. In out-of-hospital or spontaneous cardiac arrest, studies show that success of resuscitation can be gauged by the initial rhythm. Asystole carries the worst long-term prognosis, probably because many of these patients are discovered after a long period of cardiac arrest. If asystole is diagnosed, vigorous precordial blows may restart the heart. Rhythmic precordial percussion can be continued as needed for profound bradycardia or asystole while a major arterial pulse is palpated, until other definitive treatment becomes available. If chest blows fail, CPR should be immediately initiated and intravenous epinephrine (5 to 10 ml of 1:10,000 solution) administered. Acidosis and hypoxemia should be corrected by inducing hyperventilation and administering sodium bicarbonate if appropriate (see following discussion). Resuscitative measures may sometimes result in the return of a slow ventricular rhythm with a pulse that can subsequently be supported with atropine (1 to 2 mg IV) or isoproterenol until a temporary pacemaker can be placed. Attempts at external pacing are occasionally effective. Infrequently, very fine ventricular fibrillation may appear like a straight line on a single-lead ECG and thus be mistaken for asystole. In such instances, where the diagnosis of asystole is in question, it is suggested that a perpendicular ECG lead be analyzed. This can be rapidly performed, if "quick-look" paddles are being used, by simply changing paddle position by 90 degrees. If fine ventricular fibrillation is present, a more typical ECG fibrillation pattern will become apparent on monitoring a perpendicular lead, whereas in true asystole a straight line will persist in all ECG leads. If ventricular fibrillation is diagnosed, a 200-J countershock should be immediately delivered. Successful cardioversion of "asystole" has been reported in some patients who likely had fine ventricular fibrillation that was initially misinterpreted.

Electromechanical Dissociation

Electromechanical dissociation (EMD) is defined as organized electrical cardiac activity without evidence of effective perfusion (no pulse or blood pressure). Hypovolemia, pericardial tamponade, and tension pneumothorax constitute the most treatable causes of this condition. Once the diagnosis of EMD is made during any resuscitative effort, clinical features of the treatable conditions previously described should be considered and, if appropriate, definitive therapy with intravenous fluids or blood replacement, pericardiocentesis, or chest tube placement should be initiated immediately. If EMD is caused by primary myocardial failure, the prognosis is grave. Epinephrine should be administered and ventilation optimized. Calcium chloride (5 to 7 mg/kg) has been used for EMD but has not been shown to improve survival rates. Its routine use is therefore not recommended. With acute myocardial infarction, sudden EMD often indicates myocardial rupture; emergency pericardiocentesis followed by surgical repair is rarely successful.

Establishment of an Intravenous Route

Once CPR has been initiated, an intravenous line is necessary for definitive drug therapy. Venous access, however, may be difficult, and if necessary in an emergency, drugs can be effectively administered through the endotracheal tube pending successful venous cannulation. Epinephrine, lidocaine, and atropine given in standard doses through the endotracheal tube reach adequate serum levels. No more than 10 ml of solution should be given by this route, but each agent can be repeated every 10 minutes.

If a peripheral vein cannot be cannulated, a femoral vein cutdown should be performed or a central venous line placed by the percutaneous route. If CPR is properly performed, there is no advantage to central versus peripheral line placement regarding rapidity of drug circulation. Drugs administered by a peripheral line will reach the arterial circulation within 15 to 30 seconds.[1] Central lines should be placed only by skilled personnel because serious complications such as pneumothorax or arterial laceration can occur. Intracardiac injections may produce coronary lacerations and should

be used only if venous or endotracheal access is unobtainable or CPR is ineffective in generating a pulse.

Termination of CPR

Despite aggressive resuscitative efforts, patients in cardiac arrest may not regain spontaneous circulation. The decision to terminate resuscitative efforts is difficult and should be based on the physician's assessment of the underlying cause of the arrest and the cerebral, cardiovascular, and general status of the patient. Absence of organized ECG activity after 15 to 20 minutes of adequate CPR and appropriate definitive therapy is likely to be associated with a poor outcome. Persistent deep unconsciousness with absence of respiration and reflexes suggests profound cerebral ischemia, and prolonged resuscitative efforts are usually unsuccessful. These broad guidelines must, however, be altered in patients in whom hypothermia, barbiturate overdose, or electrocution is suspected, as recovery with return of good cerebral function has been documented hours after beginning resuscitation.

Postarrest Care

Following successful resuscitation, patients should be monitored in an intensive care unit because cardiac arrhythmias and hemodynamic and ventilatory instability are common. Respiratory support may be necessary initially, and frequent arterial blood gas determinations should be made in order to treat the hypoxemia and acidosis that often occur after arrest. To manage fluid status correctly and optimize cardiac function, pulmonary artery catheterization may be required.

The treatment of postarrest encephalopathy consists of prevention of recurrent hypoxia or hypotension; maintenance of normal serum glucose, electrolytes, and osmolality; and reduction of cerebral edema. Although widely used, glucocorticoids and barbiturates have not been shown to reduce postarrest cerebral edema. Hyperventilation and consequent hypocapnia-induced cerebral vasoconstriction may be beneficial in this regard. Prognosis of patients with ischemic encephalopathy is related to the depth and duration of cerebral dysfunction. Failure to recover neurologic function within 24 hours of resuscitation is an ominous sign. If recovery does occur, postarrest amnesia, behavioral disturbances, or neurologic deficits may be manifest. Renal and hepatic failure, pneumonia, bowel ischemia, and sepsis are other frequent postresuscitation complications that require early and aggressive management.

MAJOR DRUGS USED DURING CPR

Drugs used for the treatment of specific arrhythmias are reviewed in Chapter 2.9.

Because it promotes myocardial and cerebral perfusion, epinephrine should be administered whenever CPR is needed to support the circulation. In addition, its positive inotropic and chronotropic properties make it useful for asystole, heart block, and EMD. It should be administered intravenously or endotracheally in a dose of 0.5 to 1 mg every 5 to 10 minutes.

Norepinephrine

Norepinephrine (Levophed) is a potent vasoconstrictor and inotropic agent and, like epinephrine, should increase blood pressure and cerebral and myocardial perfusion during CPR. Less experience has been accumulated with norepinephrine, however, and the potency of its renal and mesenteric vasoconstrictive effect presents a theoretical drawback. Subcutaneous extravasation also causes severe tissue necrosis. This agent is most useful in the treatment of profound hypotension, as its chronotropic effects are significantly less than those of epinephrine. *Dopamine* (a chemical precursor of norepinephrine) and *dobutamine* (a synthetic catecholamine) have little use during CPR but are preferred over epinephrine for use as inotropic agents after successful resuscitation because of their lesser chronotropic and vasoconstrictive effects.

Isoproterenol

Isoproterenol is a synthetic catecholamine with almost pure beta-agonist effect. It can therefore lower arterial pressure during CPR and decrease vital organ perfusion. *Its use should be strongly discouraged if CPR is in progress.* Isoproterenol is useful in the treatment of bradycardia due to heart block in the presence of adequate blood pressure, that is, in the post-resuscitative period, until temporary pacing can be established.

Sodium Bicarbonate

Sodium bicarbonate is used during arrest to correct metabolic acidosis.[5] The latest American Heart Association recommendations have deemphasized the role of bicarbonate therapy because the primary treatment of the metabolic acidosis of cardiac arrest is adequate alveolar ventilation and reduction of arterial PCO_2. Sodium bicarbonate (1 mEq/kg) should be administered only *after* 10 minutes have elapsed, that is, following the initiation of CPR initial definitive pharmacologic and electrical therapy. Half the dosage of bicarbonate may be repeated after 15 minutes if necessary. The administration of bicarbonate in the absence of adequate ventilation can result in rising levels of PCO_2. For most clinical situations encountered during CPR, bicarbonate should not be regarded as a "first line" drug. Ideally, the dose of bicarbonate should be gauged by calculating the base deficit. Excessive administration of sodium bicarbonate can result in metabolic alkalosis, hypernatremia, and hyperosmolality. Bicarbonate is most useful and required in large doses during the early post-resuscitative period, when profound metabolic acidosis can occur.

Calcium Chloride

Calcium chloride (5 to 7 mg/kg) is used to enhance the contractile state of the heart and is indicated in severe hypotension or hyperkalemia. It is no longer recommended for use in EMD or asystole during CPR.

OUTCOME OF RESUSCITATION

Since 1961 the rate for successful out-of-hospital resuscitation with a paramedic response system has improved from 24 to almost 40 percent. Factors favorably affecting successful out-of-hospital resuscitation include time from collapse to beginning of CPR (less than 4 minutes), total duration of CPR (less than 7 minutes), and time to successful delivery of definitive care (less than 10 minutes). In a community with extensive training of citizens in CPR and a nearly ideal emergency medical system, 31 percent of all out-of-hospital arrests were successfully resuscitated, 19 percent discharged from the hospital, with most of the discharged patients (250 out of 276) able to return home; more than 66 percent of those patients who were working before the arrest returned to gainful employment.[7] The outcome of resuscitation could be further improved with better training of laypersons in CPR and the widespread use of paramedical response systems.

REFERENCES

1. Bishop RL, Weisfeldt ML: Sodium bicarbonate administration during cardiac arrest. Effect on arterial pH, PCO_2 and osmolality. JAMA 235:506, 1976
2. Chandra N, Guerci A, et al: Contrasts between intrathoracic pressures during external chest compression and cardiac massage. Crit Care Med 9:789, 1981
3. Chandra N, Rudikoff M, Weisfeldt ML: Simultaneous chest compression ventilation at high airway pressure during cardiopulmonary resuscitation. Lancet 1:175, 1980
4. Chandra N, Weisfeldt ML, et al: Augmentation of carotid flow during cardiopulmonary resuscitation in dogs by ventilation at high airway pressures simultaneous with chest compression. Am J Cardiol 48:1053, 1981

5. Chazan JA, Stenson R, Kurland GS: The acidosis of cardiac arrest. N Engl J Med 278:360, 1968
6. Criley JM, Blaufuss AH, Kissel GL: Cough-induced cardiac compression: Self-administered form of cardiopulmonary resuscitation. JAMA 236:1246, 1976
7. Eisenberg MS, Hallstrom A, Bergner L: Long term survival after out-of-hospital cardiac arrest. N Engl J Med 306:1340, 1982
8. Halperin HR, Tsitlik JE, et al: The determinants of vital organ flow during cardiac arrest in dogs. Circulation 73:539, 1986
9. Jude JR, Kouwenhoven WB, Knickerbocker GG: Cardiac arrest: Report of application of external cardiac massage in 118 patients. JAMA 178:1063, 1961
10. Kouwenhoven WB, Jude JR, Knickerbocker GG: Closed-chest cardiac massage. JAMA 173:1064, 1960
11. Redding JS: The choking controversy: Critique and evidence on the Heimlich maneuver. Crit Care Med 7:475, 1979
12. Rudikoff MT, Maughan WL, et al: Mechanisms of blood flow during cardiopulmonary resuscitation. Circulation 61:345, 1980
13. Scherf S, Bornemann C: Thumping of the precordium in ventricular standstill. Am J Cardiol 5:30, 1960
14. Standards and guidelines for cardiopulmonary resuscitation (CPR) and emergency cardiac care (ECC): JAMA 255:2905, 1986
15. Weaver WD, Cobb LA, et al: Ventricular defibrillation: A comparative trial using 175-J and 320-J shocks. N Engl J Med 307:1101, 1982

CHAPTER 4.3
Shock

Roy G. Brower, Peter Rock, W. Lowell Maughan, and J.T. Sylvester

Shock is a syndrome caused by inadequate tissue perfusion. Typically, an initial insult such as hemorrhage or septicemia is followed by compensatory cardiovascular responses, including vasoconstriction and tachycardia. If the insult continues, compensation eventually fails and the clinical picture progresses from anxiety, pallor, diaphoresis, and oliguria to coma, anuria, circulatory collapse, and death. In previously healthy patients, shock is usually obvious when systolic blood pressure falls below 90 mm Hg; however, in patients with chronic hypertension, shock can occur when blood pressure is normal. If shock is severe or prolonged, it may become irreversible; therefore, it is important to recognize and treat shock as soon as possible.

PATHOPHYSIOLOGIC CLASSIFICATION

Shock states can be classified according to the magnitude of cardiac output. When cardiac output is normal or high (high-output shock), inadequate tissue perfusion results from maldistribution of flow among or within organs. This can occur when decreased systemic vascular resistance causes arterial blood pressure to fall below levels necessary to maintain normal perfusion to all organs, as in spinal cord injury; when local humoral or reflex control of arterial caliber is abrogated by the release of vasoactive mediators, as in endotoxic or anaphylactic shock; or when nutrient microvessels are blocked, as in disseminated intravascular coagulation.

Inadequate tissue perfusion caused by low cardiac output (low-output shock) can be caused by dysfunction of the heart or the vasculature. Cardiac dysfunction can be assessed from the cardiac output, or Frank-Starling, curve in which cardiac output is plotted against cardiac filling pressure (Fig. 4.3-1). This relationship reveals that cardiac output increases toward a maximum as filling pressure increases. An improvement in cardiac function, manifested by an upward shift in the curve (higher cardiac output at the same filling pressure), occurs when myocardial contractility increases or afterload decreases. Cardiac dysfunction, manifested by a downward shift (lower cardiac output at the same filling pressure), occurs with decreased contractility, increased afterload, dysrhythmia, or acute valvular dysfunction.

The heart's filling pressure is also the back pressure to blood flow from the systemic vasculature to the heart, the venous return. The relationship between filling pressure and venous return (the venous return curve) characterizes the function of the vasculature (Fig. 4.3-1). This relationship shows that venous return decreases as cardiac filling pressure increases. The flow-axis intercept of the venous return curve is the mean systemic pressure, the pressure that drives blood back to the heart from the periphery. Mean systemic pressure varies directly with the volume of blood distending the vasculature and inversely with vascular compliance. It should not be confused with the mean arterial pressure of the systemic circulation. An improvement in vascular function, manifested by a shift of the venous return curve to the right (higher venous return at the same cardiac filling pressure), occurs when blood volume increases or vascular compliance decreases. Vascular dysfunction, manifested by a shift to the left (lower venous return at the same cardiac filling pressure), occurs when blood volume decreases or vascular compliance increases. It is also possible for the slope of the venous return curve to change; for example, it becomes shallower when the resistance to venous return is increased, as in polycythemia or compression of the great veins.

In a steady state, cardiac output is equal to venous return.[2,17] If the cardiac output and venous return curves are plotted on the same axes (Fig. 4.3-2), they intersect at only one point (the equilibrium point). This defines the only cardiac output–venous return and filling pressure possible for a given set of curves. Thus, the decrease in cardiac output characteristic of low-output shock can result from a leftward shift of the venous return curve (low vascular volume, high vascular compliance, high resistance to venous return) or a downward shift of the cardiac output curve (low contractility, valvular dysfunction, dysrhythmia).

Which mechanism predominates in a patient can be determined by measuring cardiac output and estimating the filling pressures of the right and left sides of the heart from central venous and pulmonary artery wedge pressures, respectively (see Chapter 4.1). In high-output shock, cardiac output is high and filling pressures are normal. Low-output shock can be cardiogenic or vascular. In cardiogenic low-output shock, a low cardiac output is associated with elevation of filling pressures. In vascular low-output shock, both cardiac output and filling pressures are low. Classification of shock in this manner is important because it guides management.

SPECIFIC SHOCK SYNDROMES

Characteristic clinical and pathophysiologic features of several commonly encountered shock syndromes are described in the following sections. When appropriate, specific aspects of management are

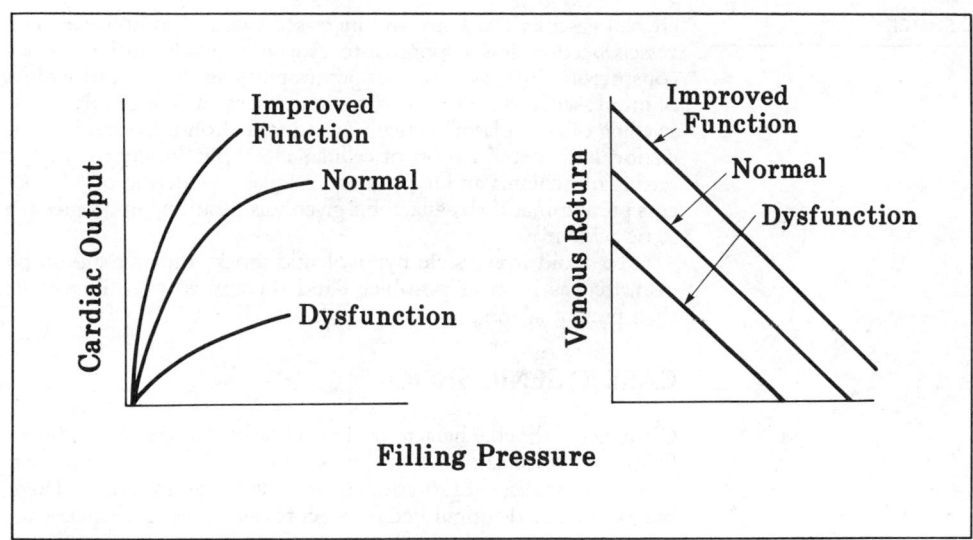

Figure 4.3–1. Cardiac output (Frank-Starling) curve (*left*) and venous return curve (*right*).

also discussed. General aspects of management are discussed in the following section.

HYPOVOLEMIC SHOCK

Patients with hypovolemic shock present with low cardiac output and low filling pressures caused by the loss of fluid from the intravascular space. This type of shock is frequently the result of severe gastrointestinal hemorrhage from peptic ulcers, esophageal varices, or colonic diverticula. In the setting of trauma, hemorrhage is usually apparent, but large amounts of blood or plasma can also sequester in the extravascular space of soft tissues (hematoma) or third spaces (hemoperitoneum, hemothorax). Severe gastrointestinal illnesses such as cholera can result in hypovolemic shock if the rate of fluid lost from the bowel exceeds the rate at which fluids can be ingested and absorbed. In the very old and the very young, relatively mild gastroenteritis can result in marked dehydration and shock. Burn patients have massive losses of fluid and protein, and adequate replenishment is a key element in survival. Similarly, patients with pancreatitis or a perforated viscus frequently require large amounts of fluid to maintain an adequate intravascu-

lar volume. Other causes of hypovolemic shock are listed in Table 4.3–1.

Much of our knowledge about hypovolemic shock was obtained from experiments in animals following withdrawal of blood.[3,4] Hemorrhage decreases the volume of blood distending the capacitance vessels of the circulation, thereby decreasing mean systemic pressure, venous return, and cardiac output. Within minutes, however, compensatory responses occur. Intense sympathoadrenal discharge results in peripheral vasoconstriction, increased peripheral vascular resistance, redistribution of cardiac output to essential organs such as the heart and the brain, reduced vascular compliance, and restoration of the pressure gradient for venous return. Activation of the renin angiotensin-aldosterone system further increases vascular tone and causes renal sparing of fluids and electrolytes. Increased circulating levels of antidiuretic hormone contribute to the maintenance of intravascular volume.

If the loss of intravascular volume is mild, shock may not occur and recovery is likely with little or no intervention. If the volume loss is severe, however, shock will develop. Two phases of hypovolemic shock have been recognized. During the early reversible phase, cardiac output and arterial blood pressure can be returned to normal and the likelihood of survival enhanced by

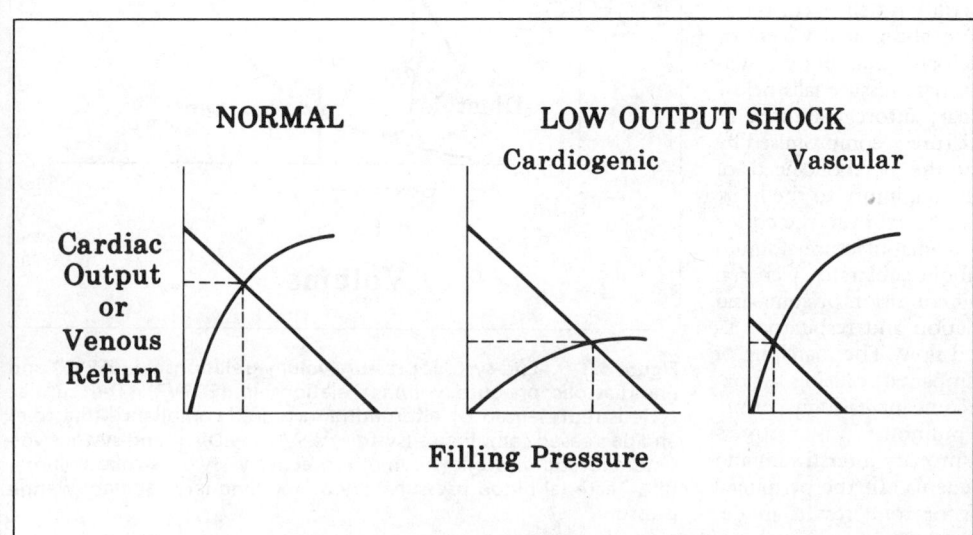

Figure 4.3–2. Cardiac output and venous return relationships plotted on the same axes. The intersection of these relationships determine the steady-state level of cardiac output/venous return. Depressed cardiac output may be caused by cardiogenic or vascular dysfunction.

TABLE 4.3–1. CAUSES OF HYPOVOLEMIC SHOCK

Bleeding
Gastrointestinal
- Peptic ulcer
- Diverticuli
- Esophageal varices
- Mallory-Weiss tear

Trauma
- External bleeding
- Internal sequestration of blood
  Hemoperitoneum
    Splenic rupture
  Hemothorax
    Aortic rupture or dissection
    Laceration of pulmonary vessel
    Laceration of intercostal vessel
  Hematoma

Dehydration
Gastrointestinal fluid losses
- Viral enteritis
- Bacterial enteritis
  Cholera
  Shigella

Renal fluid losses
- Diabetes mellitus
- Diabetes insipidus
- Excessive diuretics

Cutaneous fluid losses
- Burns
- Perspiration

Internal fluid sequestration
- Ascites
  Peritonitis
  Cirrhosis
  Nephrosis
- Intestinal obstruction
  Carcinoma
  Volvulus
  Adhesions

administration of adequate amounts of suitable fluids. In the canine hemorrhage model, this phase lasts approximately 90 minutes after 40 percent of the blood is rapidly removed. If fluid resuscitation does not occur or is inadequate, shock becomes irreversible and subsequent interventions result in only minor or transient improvements.

The irreversible phase is characterized by functional deterioration in several organs. Myocardial contractility is depressed, possibly by a circulating peptide released from abdominal viscera or skeletal muscle (myocardial depressant factor).[3] In addition, myocardial perfusion may be inadequate if arterial pressure falls below 50 to 60 mm Hg, the usual limit of coronary autoregulation. This effect is potentiated if the coronary vasculature is compromised by atherosclerosis. With inadequate perfusion the metabolic needs of the myocardium cannot be met, and ischemic injury to the heart occurs. In the kidney, blood flow is redistributed from the cortex to the medulla. The liver loses its ability to manufacture albumin and to metabolize lactate and other metabolic substrates. Cerebral blood flow may be compromised, causing confusion or coma and alterations in EEG activity. Hyperventilation and respiratory alkalosis can further decrease cerebral blood flow. The matching of ventilation and perfusion in the lung is impaired, causing hypoxemia. The pulmonary vasculature may become increasingly permeable. With fluid resuscitation, the rise in pulmonary vascular pressures may cause fluid to leak into the pulmonary interstitium and alveolar spaces, resulting in pulmonary edema. In the peripheral circulation, loss of spontaneous vasomotor tone results in de-

creased vascular resistance and increased vascular compliance. The vessels become less responsive to exogenously administered vasoconstrictors. Increased vascular permeability results in a further loss of intravascular fluid to the interstitial spaces. At the cellular level, swelling of endoplasmic reticulum and mitochondria occur in association with deterioration of cellular metabolic functions. In the setting of ischemia and hypoxemia, cellular production of ATP occurs predominantly by anaerobic glycolysis, resulting in progressive lactic acidemia.

To avoid irreversible hypovolemic shock, therapy should be instituted as soon as possible. Fluid therapy is more important than pressor agents.

CARDIOGENIC SHOCK

Cardiogenic shock, characterized by a low cardiac output and high filling pressures, can be caused by systolic or diastolic dysfunction of cardiac muscle, dysrhythmia, or valvular dysfunction. These causes must be distinguished from acute right ventricular overload, as occurs with massive pulmonary embolism.

Dysfunction of Cardiac Muscle
A decrease in systolic function of the heart secondary to a decrease in myocardial contractility causes a downward shift in the cardiac output curve (Fig. 4.3–1). This shift, however, can also result from deterioration of diastolic function or increased ventricular afterload and is not specific for decreased contractility. To distinguish among these possibilities, it is useful to consider the heart as a muscular chamber that changes from a relatively compliant state during diastole to a relatively noncompliant state during systole.[11] The end-diastolic pressure-volume relationship (EDPVR) and the end-systolic pressure-volume relationship (ESPVR) of the heart are illustrated in Figure 4.3–3. The heart begins its contraction on its EDPVR and ends its contraction on its ESPVR. These two rela-

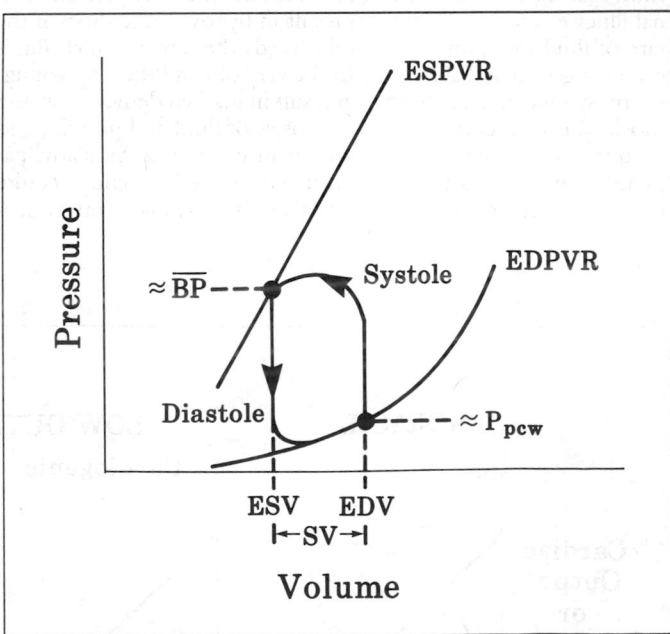

Figure 4.3–3. End-systolic pressure volume relationship (ESPVR) and end-diastolic pressure volume relationship (EDPVR). The cardiac cycle is represented by alternating increased compliance (diastole) and decreased compliance (systole). ESV and EDV = end-systolic volume and end-diastolic volume, respectively. SV = stroke volume. BP = arterial blood pressure. Ppcw = pulmonary capillary wedge pressure.

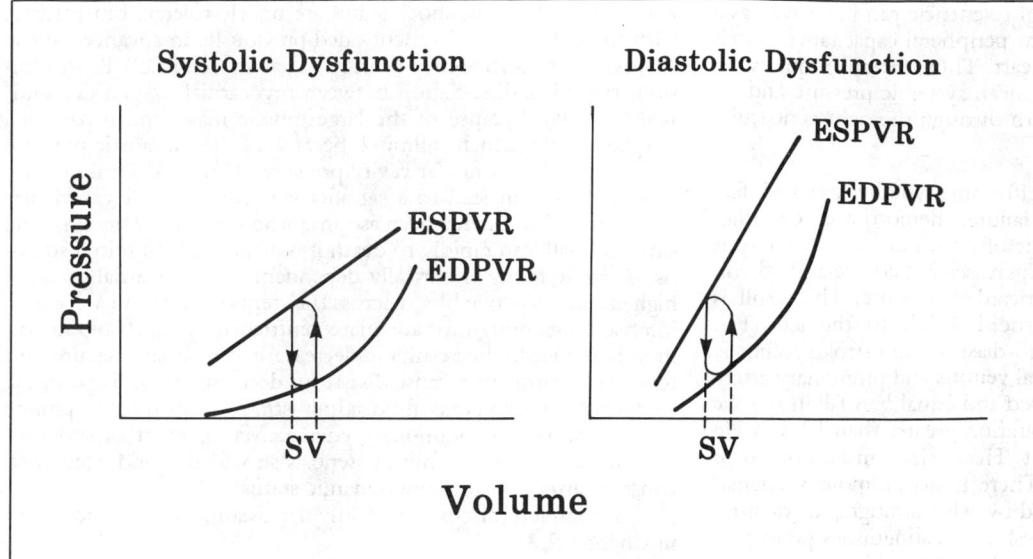

Figure 4.3–4. Stroke volume (SV) may be decreased by systolic dysfunction, indicated by the decreased slope of the end-systolic pressure volume relationship (ESPVR), or diastolic dysfunction, indicated by the increased slope of the end-diastolic pressure volume relationship (EDPVR).

tionships determine the limit of cardiac performance under any given contractile state of the ventricle.

An increase in the contractile state of the ventricle causes a shift in the ESPVR to the left, whereas a decrease in contractility shifts the ESPVR to the right (Fig. 4.3–4). A steeper ESPVR means that at any given end-systolic volume, the end-systolic pressure developed by the ventricle will be greater. A shallow ESPVR indicates systolic dysfunction: end-systolic pressure will be less at any given end-systolic volume. A change in the stiffness of the ventricle during diastole changes the EDPVR (Fig. 4.3–4). Increased stiffness causes diastolic dysfunction by shifting the EDPVR to the left and decreasing the diastolic filling that occurs at a given end-diastolic pressure. As shown in Figure 4.3–4, deterioration in either systolic or diastolic function will decrease stroke volume if end-diastolic filling pressure is unchanged. With severe dysfunction, stroke volume is likely to remain low even if end-diastolic filling pressures are increased by compensatory reflexes or the administration of fluids or pressors. Although a deficit in stroke volume can be offset by an increase in heart rate, this mechanism is limited because the time for diastolic filling decreases as heart rate increases. If the stroke volume deficit is not overcome by increased heart rate, cardiac output will fall.

The pressure-volume analysis can be used clinically if stroke volume (SV) is known and left ventricular end-systolic and end-diastolic pressures are estimated from mean arterial and pulmonary artery wedge pressures, respectively. It is usually possible to classify end-systolic and diastolic volumes (ESV, EDV) as normal or increased from the stroke volume and the heart size estimated from a posteroanterior chest film. Alternatively, they can be calculated directly if left ventricular ejection fraction (EF) is known (EDV = SV/EF, and ESV = EDV − SV). Such calculations allow the physician to determine whether cardiogenic shock (low cardiac output, high filling pressures) is due to impaired systolic function (low end-systolic pressure relative to end-systolic volume) or impaired diastolic function (high end-diastolic pressure relative to end-diastolic volume). Normal values for end-systolic and end-diastolic pressures and volumes are shown in Figure 4.3–5.

Systolic Dysfunction. The most common form of systolic dysfunction leading to shock is acute myocardial infarction, discussed in Chapter 2.8. Other causes of systolic myocardial dysfunction that can lead to shock are coronary insufficiency (see Chapter 2.7) and

myocarditis (see Chapter 2.2). In addition, systolic dysfunction is a frequent complication of shock from other causes. Factors contributing to myocardial depression under these conditions include myocardial ischemia secondary to low coronary perfusion pressure, hypoxia, acidosis, and elaboration of myocardial depressant factors.

Right ventricular infarction deserves emphasis, because unlike left ventricular infarction the shock it causes can usually be reversed if recognized and managed properly. The history is frequently suggestive of myocardial infarction. The ECG is consistent with infarction of the inferior myocardium. Cardiac output is low, and central venous pressure is equal to or greater than pulmonary artery wedge

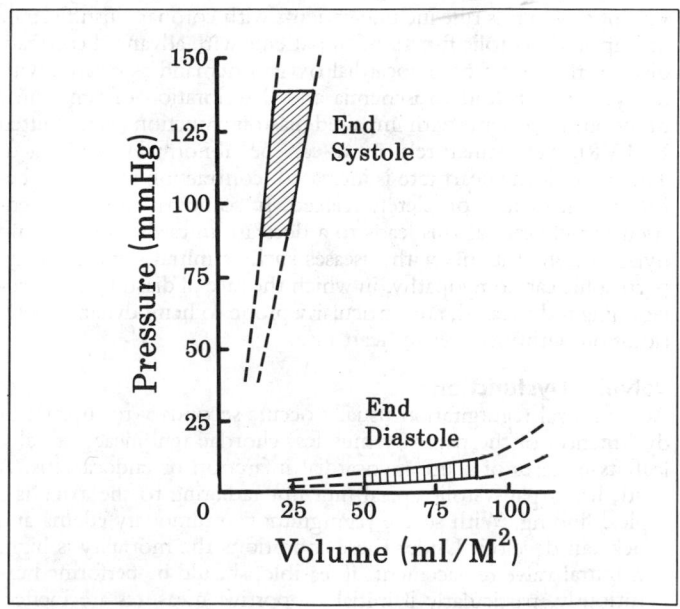

Figure 4.3–5. Normal ranges for left ventricular end-systolic and end-diastolic pressure–volume relationships are shown (*shaded portions*). Ranges of pressure and volume are shown (*dotted lines*) that could occur in shock conditions when left ventricular function is normal.

pressure. In this condition, the right ventricle can be viewed as a passive conduit leading blood from peripheral capacitance vessels to the pulmonary circuit and left heart. Thus, therapy requires the administration of fluids to elevate mean systemic pressure and increase the gradient for venous return through the right ventricular conduit.

Diastolic Dysfunction. Pericardial effusions, whether due to infection, malignancy, chronic renal failure, hemorrhage, or other causes, can progress until the limit of pericardial distensibility is reached. Beyond this point, small increases in pericardial fluid volume lead to large increases in pericardial pressure. The result is cardiac compression, a shift of the EDPVR to the left (Fig. 4.3–4), and markedly decreased end-diastolic and stroke volumes. With pericardial tamponade, central venous and pulmonary artery wedge pressures are typically elevated and equal.[13] A fall in systolic arterial blood pressure during inspiration greater than 10 mm Hg (pulsus paradoxus) may be present. Heart size can be normal or enlarged on a chest radiograph. There is no pulmonary edema. Definitive diagnosis is accomplished by echocardiographic demonstration of pericardial fluid. This test also distinguishes pericardial tamponade from right ventricular infarction, which can present with similar hemodynamic findings. Although definitive therapy may require prolonged treatment of an underlying condition, acute removal of even small amounts of pericardial fluid with an electrocardiographically guided, percutaneous needle can be life saving.

In advanced states of ventricular hypertrophy, as occurs with aortic stenosis, the end-diastolic pressure-volume relationship can be shifted to the left because of increased muscle mass. When there is a need for increased cardiac output, therefore, the heart may be unable to respond without the development of very high end-diastolic pressures. This can lead to pulmonary edema and hypoxemia.

Dysrhythmia

Ventricular fibrillation, severe bradycardia, or tachycardia can cause low-output shock. These disorders are discussed in Chapter 2.9. It is important to realize that tachycardia, even if severe, can be a result rather than a cause of shock. In this case, treatment should be directed at the underlying cause rather than the tachycardia. Exceptions to this rule include patients with coronary insufficiency or impaired diastolic function. In patients with advanced coronary disease, the increased myocardial oxygen demand associated with tachycardia can lead to ischemia and deterioration of ventricular function. In patients with impaired diastolic function (a left-shifted EDPVR), ventricular relaxation can be abnormally prolonged. Therefore, if the heart rate is increased, contraction may begin before the heart has completely relaxed. In some patients with ventricular tachycardia, this leads to a decrease in cardiac output and hypotension. Patients with diseases such as mitral stenosis or hypertrophic cardiomyopathy, in which the rate of diastolic ventricular filling is decreased, are particularly prone to hemodynamic deterioration with increases in heart rate.

Valvular Dysfunction

Acute mitral regurgitation usually occurs secondary to rupture or dysfunction of the papillary muscles, chordae tendineae, or valve leaflets in cases of acute myocardial infarction or endocarditis. A loud, harsh pansystolic apical murmur radiating to the axilla is a typical finding. With severe regurgitation, pulmonary edema and shock can develop. Under these conditions the mortality is high, and mitral valve replacement, if feasible, should be performed expeditiously, particularly if initial supportive measures are ineffectual. Acute aortic regurgitation can occur with dissecting aortic aneurysms, endocarditis, trauma, or dysfunctional prosthetic valves. Coronary artery disease can be a difficult problem in this situation because high wall tension in the dilated ventricle during systole and the rapid decline of aortic pressure during diastole decreases diastolic coronary flow. Again, valve replacement is indicated.

Although stenosis of the aortic or mitral valve is rarely a pri-

mary cause of shock, shock states are poorly tolerated in patients with these disorders. As mentioned previously, in advanced aortic stenosis the hypertrophied heart has a left-shifted EDPVR. In addition, there is a dissociation between myocardial oxygen demand, which is high because of the large muscle mass, and myocardial oxygen supply, which is limited because of the low aortic pressure relative to left ventricular cavity pressure. Thus, a decrease in systolic pressure can lead to a significant decrease in left ventricular function and a further decrease in aortic pressure. This unstable situation will lead rapidly to death if not reversed. In mitral stenosis, diastolic filling is critically dependent on a left atrial pressure high enough to drive blood across the stenotic valve and a diastolic interval long enough for adequate ventricular filling. If blood volume is reduced, the resultant decrease in left atrial pressure and reflex tachycardia may cause disastrous decreases in cardiac output. Conversely, overzealous fluid administration can quickly plunge these patients into pulmonary edema. Management of shock in patients with aortic or mitral stenosis should be conducted with constant attention to hemodynamic status.

A complete discussion of valvular dysfunction can be found in Chapter 2.3.

SEPTIC SHOCK

Septic shock occurs in the presence of microbial pathogens or their toxins in the blood or tissues. In the United States, approximately 300,000 patients per year are affected. With a mortality rate of 50 to 75 percent, septic shock is a major cause of hospital deaths. This disorder is more likely to develop in a compromised host. Alcoholics, patients receiving steroids or other immunosuppressive drugs, victims of the acquired immunodeficiency syndrome (AIDS), malnourished individuals, patients at the extremes of age, patients suffering from hypothermia or hyperthermia, and patients with end-stage organ failure are at particular risk.

The most common cause of septic shock is gram-negative bacteremia, but the syndrome also occurs with gram-positive bacteremia and with fungal, rickettsial, or viral infections. The pathogenesis is incompletely understood but probably involves activation of the complement, coagulation, and kinin systems of the blood by microbial components or toxins. Endotoxin, a lipopolysaccharide component found in the cell walls of all gram-negative bacteria, is one such substance. Secondary events include adherence and aggregation of polymorphonuclear leukocytes and platelets to endothelium, endothelial damage and capillary leakage, vasodilation, disseminated intravascular coagulation, and myocardial depression.

Clinically, sepsis may be heralded by fever and shaking chills or hypothermia. Altered mental status, decreased urine output, and hyperventilation often occur before the development of frank shock. Hypotension is initially associated with high cardiac output, possibly due to increased perfusion of dilated low-resistance vascular beds. Perfusion of the skin persists; the skin remains warm, hence the label "warm shock." If therapy is not instituted in a timely fashion or if the infection is severe, cardiac output eventually falls. This may be caused by hypovolemia secondary to fluid extravasation from damaged capillaries or loss of systemic vascular tone. This causes a further fall in blood pressure; anuria; and cold, clammy skin (so-called cold shock). Approximately 10 percent of septic patients develop the adult respiratory distress syndrome (see Chapter 4.5), manifested by severe dyspnea, diffuse pulmonary infiltrates, and refractory hypoxemia.

Treatment of septic shock requires fluid resuscitation and the administration of pressors, but these measures are frequently unsuccessful. Naloxone, an opiate and endorphin antagonist, was found to be effective in the therapy of a variety of shock states in animals, including endotoxic shock. Clinical trials, however, have failed to confirm the effectiveness of this agent in human septic shock.[9] High doses of corticosteroids have been advocated by some. Typically, methylprednisolone is administered in a single dose of 30 mg/kg, which may be repeated in 4 hours if shock persists. In a recent controlled trial, corticosteroids decreased the mor-

tality from septic shock during the earlier stages of illness, but the mortality rate was ultimately the same in control and treated patients.[15] In another recent study, antiserum directed against endotoxin improved survival in patients with gram-negative sepsis.[19] Although this therapy is promising, its ultimate utility remains to be determined.

The most important therapeutic step in septic shock is identification and treatment of the underlying infection. The lungs, urinary tract, and gastrointestinal tract are the most common sources. If a source of infection is not immediately identified, a careful search must be instituted. Particular attention should be given to the possibilities of abdominal, pelvic, or thoracic abscesses and infections of the joints or paranasal sinuses. All possible cultures should be obtained and appropriate broad-spectrum antibiotic coverage instituted as soon as possible. More specific antibiotic treatment may be possible when the results of cultures and antibiotic sensitivities become available. A short delay in therapy can result in death of the patient.

MASSIVE PULMONARY EMBOLISM

Massive pulmonary embolism causes an acute severe increase in pulmonary vascular resistance secondary to mechanical obstruction of the vessels and pulmonary vasospasm from release of vasoactive mediators. The resultant increase in right ventricular afterload can rapidly lead to right ventricular failure, elevation of central venous pressure, decreased venous return, shock, and death. Patients who survive long enough to receive the attention of a physician are usually hypoxic, tachypneic, and tachycardic. Some patients will wheeze, suggesting the incorrect diagnosis of asthma. The neck veins are usually distended, indicating increased central venous pressure. A right ventricular heave and gallop rhythm may be present. The ECG may reveal atrial or ventricular arrhythmias, as well as signs of right ventricular strain. Cardiac enlargement may be present on the chest radiograph. Insertion of a pulmonary artery catheter may be difficult because of right ventricular enlargement, increased propensity for arrhythmias, or the presence of obstructing thrombi in large pulmonary arteries. Pulmonary artery pressure is characteristically elevated, but a mean pressure >40 mm Hg is rarely seen except in patients with preexisting cardiopulmonary disease. The pulmonary artery wedge pressure can be normal or elevated. Remarkable symptomatic and objective improvement may occur when thrombi fragment and move peripherally in the lung.

The diagnosis should be suspected whenever sudden hemodynamic deterioration occurs in a predisposed patient or in a patient not known to have preexisting heart disease. Definitive diagnosis can be difficult and may require selective pulmonary angiography if radioisotopic perfusion and ventilation scans of the lung are indeterminant.

Initial therapy consists of the aggressive administration of fluids to expand vascular volume and increase the pressure gradient for venous return. Oxygen by face mask or nasal cannula is usually necessary. Pressor agents may be required to raise arterial pressure. Occasional patients with severe, refractory hypoxemia may benefit from intubation and artificial ventilation. Because recurrent embolization can be fatal, anticoagulation with heparin should be instituted as soon as possible. Thrombolytic agents such as urokinase and streptokinase speed reversal of shock and may be life saving. Surgical removal of pulmonary thrombi is rarely successful and should be considered only when all other measures have failed. A detailed discussion of the management of pulmonary embolism can be found in Chapter 3.8.

OTHER SHOCK SYNDROMES

Tension Pneumothorax
If air enters the pleural space in sufficient volume, pleural pressure may rise above atmospheric pressure. This may occur as a result of trauma such as a knife wound to the chest or of barotrauma from

mechanical ventilation. Clinical manifestations include respiratory distress, tachypnea, cyanosis, tachycardia, shift of the trachea away from the side of the pneumothorax, and hyperresonance and decreased breath sounds on the affected side. The chest radiograph reveals a collapsed lung with shift of the mediastinum to the contralateral side. Shock is thought to result from compression of the great veins and heart and blockade of venous return. Hypoxemia may occur from shunting through the collapsed lung. Acidosis may result from ventilatory compromise or lactic acidemia due to low cardiac output. Tension pneumothorax requires immediate thoracostomy and evacuation of the air through a chest tube.

Anaphylactic Shock
Anaphylactic shock is the life-threatening manifestation of an immediate hypersensitivity reaction. Exposure of sensitized individuals to certain antigens (penicillin and other drugs, insect venoms) results in massive release of mediators such as histamine, eosinophil chemotactic factor, and proteolytic enzymes from mast cells. The physiologic consequences include increased vascular permeability, bronchospasm, upper airway compromise due to soft-tissue swelling, pulmonary hypertension, platelet aggregation, and systemic hypotension. Shock is thought to result from (1) decreased venous return due to dilation of systemic capacitance vessels and hypovolemia and (2) right ventricular failure secondary to severe pulmonary hypertension. Patients may present with wheezing, itching, swelling of the tongue, nausea, vomiting, abdominal pain, altered mental state, or loss of consciousness. Treatment includes removal of the inciting substance, oxygen supplementation, prompt and aggressive fluid resuscitation, administration of epinephrine, theophylline, corticosteroids, and histamine receptor blockers such as diphenhydramine. Attention must be paid to maintaining the airway. Endotracheal intubation or tracheostomy may be required. Individuals who have suffered an anaphylactic reaction should wear a bracelet that identifies the reaction and the antigen.

Aortic Dissection
Aortic dissection exists when the aortic intima is disrupted and blood enters the wall of the aorta. Signs and symptoms vary with the location of dissection. Ascending aortic dissections may produce shock from (1) occlusion of the origins of the main coronary arteries, (2) acute aortic valve regurgitation, (3) bleeding into the pericardial sac with consequent pericardial tamponade, or (3) bleeding into the pleural space or other cavities with consequent hypovolemic shock. Descending aortic dissections may produce shock from bleeding. Causes of aortic dissection include hypertension, Marfan syndrome, and trauma. Patients may present with severe acute chest pain in the case of an ascending dissection, whereas acute onset of back pain suggests descending aortic dissection. Absent or diminished peripheral pulses may be due to obstruction of vessels leading to the limbs as well as hypotension. Neurologic signs and symptoms may result from obstruction of the carotid or spinal arteries. Diagnosis is made by computerized tomography and angiography. Ascending dissections require surgical intervention; descending dissections may be managed medically, although these may ultimately require surgery as well. In both types of dissection, therapy that lowers systemic blood pressure (assuming the patient is not yet in shock) and decreases myocardial contractility may be helpful in limiting the progression of the dissection.

MANAGEMENT

GENERAL APPROACH

To manage shock effectively, the physician must make the diagnosis, institute initial management, identify pathogenetic and pathophysiologic causes, and institute specific therapy.

The complete shock syndrome is generally easily recognized; however, the early stages of shock may be manifested only by anxiety and hyperventilation. Heart rate and blood pressure can be

normal when the patient is recumbent. Orthostatic tachycardia and hypotension indicate that homeostatic mechanisms are approaching the limit of compensatory capacity. It is of paramount importance to make the diagnosis as early as possible so that therapy can be instituted before shock becomes irreversible.

Once shock is recognized, the patient should be kept warm and placed in the supine or head down position, unless this is precluded by orthopnea. The history, physical examination, and initial laboratory studies should be directed toward revealing the source of shock and assessing its severity. Vital signs should be monitored closely. The history may indicate trauma or anaphylaxis. Fever suggests sepsis and should prompt culturing of possible sources of infection. The ECG may suggest cardiogenic shock. A fluid challenge, such as 100 ml of Ringer lactate given intravenously over 10 to 15 minutes, may help to determine if hypotension is due to inadequate vascular volume. Initial therapy should include oxygen, especially if arterial blood gas measurements reveal hypoxemia, hyperventilation, and metabolic acidosis. A central venous catheter allows assessment of central venous pressure, serves as a conduit for the administration of fluids and medications, and provides a route for later insertion of a pulmonary artery catheter, if necessary. The adequacy of perfusion can be assessed by measuring hourly urine output with a urinary catheter. A nasogastric tube may reveal a previously unsuspected upper gastrointestinal hemorrhage. Radiographs of the chest and abdomen may suggest left ventricular failure (enlarged cardiac silhoutte, perihilar alveolar infiltrates) or a perforated viscus (subdiaphragmatic air).

The cause of shock is usually apparent after the initial evaluation, and specific therapy can then be instituted. Whether or not a specific diagnosis is made, many patients with supine hypotension will require a pressor agent to maintain coronary and cerebral perfusion. The rates and amounts of pressors and fluids administered will be dictated by the patient's response. In some cases, the patient's condition can be quickly stabilized. In others, a positive response to initial therapy may be minimal or absent, indicating that more aggressive managment is necessary.

Measurement of cardiac output and filling pressures with a pulmonary artery catheter (see Chapter 4.1) allows shock to be classified pathophysiologically and is useful for monitoring the therapeutic response. In *vascular low-output shock* (low cardiac output and filling pressure), fluids and vasoconstrictor agents are given until filling pressures are stable at normal values. Filling pressures should be monitored carefully to avoid iatrogenic pulmonary edema. *Cardiogenic low-output shock* (low cardiac output and high filling pressures) is most often the result of left ventricular ischemia or infarction, but other conditions can produce a similar hemodynamic picture. An elevation of central venous pressure to a level equal to or greater than pulmonary artery wedge pressure suggests right ventricular infarction, massive pulmonary embolism, or pericardial tamponade. The electrocardiogram and echocardiogram will help distinguish among these possibilities. Volume administration is a key initial therapeutic maneuver in right ventricular infarction and massive pulmonary embolism, but pericardial tamponade requires pericardiocentesis as soon as possible. When pulmonary artery wedge pressure exceeds 20 mm Hg, fluids should be administered with great caution, if at all. Rather, therapy should be directed toward improving the ionotropic state of the myocardium, eliminating the dysrhythmia, or correcting valvular dysfunction. If the patient has tension pneumothorax or is being ventilated with positive end-expiratory pressure, filling pressures may be elevated because of increased pleural pressure. In these cases, shock may be vascular (decreased venous return) rather than cardiogenic, and fluid administration is indicated. *High-output shock* (normal or high cardiac output and filling pressure) is almost always caused by septicemia. Therapy should include fluid administration, pressors, and rapid detection and treatment of the underlying infection.

FLUID RESUSCITATION

When fluids are indicated, the physician must choose the quantity and type of fluid to be infused.

Types of Fluid

Blood. Blood is an excellent fluid for vascular volume expansion, because the cellular elements remain in the vascular space, and the oncotic pressure of the plasma protein helps to retain water in the vascular space as well. Blood transfusion is therefore an effective means of increasing mean systemic pressure and venous return. Moreover, by increasing hemoglobin concentration, blood transfusion increases arterial oxygen content and systemic oxygen transport, the product of cardiac output and arterial oxygen content. These properties make blood transfusion an obvious choice in the treatment of hemorrhagic shock and other forms of shock associated with moderate or severe anemia. On the other hand, blood is expensive and requires special skills and equipment to procure, process, store, and dispense. Moreover, transfusion reactions may occur, and there is a small but significant risk of the transmission of infectious agents such as hepatitis virus, cytomegalovirus, and human immunodeficiency virus (HIV). Blood is usually given in the form of type-specific and cross-matched packed red blood cells (PRBCs), a unit of which contains the red blood cells from one unit of blood separated from the other cellular elements and most of the plasma.

Colloid Solutions. Albumin, human plasma protein fraction, and hetastarch[8] are excellent intravascular volume expanders and are especially useful when it is necessary to raise cardiac output and arterial pressure quickly. The oncotic pressure provided by the protein or starch molecules retains water in the vascular space and draws additional water into the circulation from the extravascular space. Colloid solutions are more easily stored and handled than blood, but they are expensive. Also, if too much colloid solution is inadvertently given, the vascular congestion that ensues may be difficult to reverse quickly. Dextran solutions are no longer recommended for volume expansion because they can induce antigenic reactions and coagulation abnormalities. Hetastarch, when given in large amounts, has also been associated with abnormal bleeding tendency. Hypotension has occasionally been observed in patients given plasma protein fraction. This may be due to the presence of vasoactive peptides, amines, or sodium acetate.

Crystalloid Solutions. Crystalloid solutions have no oncotic pressure and move quickly into the extravascular space, thus only a fraction of the volume administered ultimately remains in the intravascular space. This may be advantageous, because many patients in shock have decreased interstitial and intracellular, as well as intravascular, water. Moreover, the risk of vascular congestion from overzealous crystalloid administration is less than with colloid solutions or blood. Normal saline contains modestly high concentrations of sodium and chloride, but if renal function is not impaired these excesses are easily handled. Lactated Ringer solution is a more physiologically balanced electrolyte solution, containing calcium and potassium ions. Bicarbonate ion is unstable in these solutions, but the lactate in Ringer solution is metabolized to bicarbonate unless hepatic function is impaired. There is a theoretical objection to the administration of lactate to shock patients, many of whom are in moderate-to-severe lactic acidosis due in part to hepatic dysfunction.

Approach to Fluid Resuscitation

Fluid resuscitation usually begins with administration of crystalloids. The patient may fail to respond initially if the total body fluid deficit is large or if there is continuing rapid depletion of intravascular volume. When shock is due to hemorrhage, it is frequently necessary to use blood to ensure adequate oxygen carrying capacity and oxygen delivery. The amount needed depends on the amount of blood lost and the normal intravascular volume of the patient. As a general rule, it is advisable to infuse PRBCs to maintain hemoglobin concentration no less than 10 g/dl. Patients in hemorrhagic shock should also receive crystalloid solutions, which help to fill the depleted intravascular space, raise the gradient for venous return, and repair the deficit in extravascular fluid commonly associated with hypovolemic shock. The utility of crystal-

loid solutions in hemorrhagic shock has been convincingly demonstrated in animal studies. Dogs that received crystalloid infusions in addition to blood fared substantially better than those that received blood alone.[10] Indeed, effective fluid resuscitation from hemorrhagic shock can frequently be accomplished with crystalloid solutions alone, as long as the resulting anemia can be tolerated. If only crystalloid solutions are used in resuscitation from hemorrhage, it may be necessary to administer three to five times as much volume as that lost from the intravascular space.

Except when hepatic function is impaired, endogenous replacement of albumin lost by hemorrhage is usually rapid; however, colloid solutions are useful in the most extreme cases of hypovolemic shock, when intravascular volume must be raised quickly. In this case, crystalloid solutions and PRBCs are usually administered as well.

In hypovolemic shock without blood loss as well as in septic shock, it is frequently necessary to expand both the intravascular and extravascular spaces. Crystalloid solutions in large quantities are generally used for this purpose. Colloid solutions are used if serum albumin concentration is less than 2 g/dl. PRBCs are indicated if anemia is also present or if there is marked endothelial damage and extravasation of fluid.

SYMPATHOMIMETIC AMINES

Sympathomimetic amines are administered to increase systemic vascular resistance, decrease systemic vascular compliance, increase myocardial contractility, or increase heart rate. As shown in Table 4.3–2, the available agents vary markedly in their ability to produce these effects. This variability depends largely on the extent to which the agents interact with the various adrenergic receptors (Table 4.3–3). In addition, effects may vary with dose, depending on the affinity of the agent for a particular type of receptor. The physician must use the agent that most closely satisfies the needs of his patient and that exacts a minimal cost in terms of adverse effects.

Because sympathomimetic amines have a short half-life, they must be administered by continuous intravenous infusion. The short half-life is an advantage, allowing the infusion rate to be rapidly titrated to the appropriate level. Ideally, these agents should be administered through a central venous catheter with a constant infusion pump and with continuous monitoring of arterial pressure with an intra-arterial catheter. The optimal dose is the lowest capable of achieving the desired effect. Duration of therapy should be minimized. Sympathomimetic amines are a temporary measure used to support the patient until the underlying disorder can be corrected.

Specific Drugs

Dopamine. Dopamine is a metabolic precursor of norepinephrine and is the most commonly used pressor in the management of

TABLE 4.3–2. EFFECTS OF VASOACTIVE AGENTS ON HEMODYNAMIC VARIABLES

Drug	SVR	Myocardial Contractility	Heart Rate	Cardiac Output
Dopamine 0–5 μg/kg/min	0	+	0	0
Dopamine 5–10 μg/kg/min	+	+ +	+	+
Dopamine >10 μg/kg/min	+ +	+ +	+ +	+ +
Dobutamine	0/−	+ + +	0	+ +
Epinephrine	0/+ +	+ + +	+ +	+ +
Norepinephrine	+ +	+ +	0/+	+/−

SVR = systemic vascular resistance; 0 = no effect; + = modest effect; + + = intermediate effect; + + + = marked effect; − = decrease.

TABLE 4.3–3. EFFECTS OF VASOACTIVE AGENTS ON RECEPTORS

Drug	Receptors			
	Dopaminergic	*Alpha*	*Beta-1*	*Beta-2*
Dopamine 0–5 μg/kg/min	+ + +	0	0	0
Dopamine 5–10 μg/kg/min	+ + +	+	+ + +	+ +
Dopamine >10 μg/kg/min	+ + +	+ + +	+ + +	+ +
Dobutamine	0	+	+ + +	+
Epinephrine	0	+ + +	+ + + +	+ +
Norepinephrine	0	+ + + +	+ + +	+
Isoproterenol	0	0	+ + +	+ + + +

0 = no effect; + = modest effect; + + = intermediate effect; + + + = strong effect; + + + + = very strong effect.

shock. At doses up to 5 μg/kg/min, dopamine causes vasodilation of the renal and splanchnic beds by stimulating dopaminergic and beta-2 receptors. Urine output may increase secondary to increased renal blood flow, but cardiac output, heart rate, and blood pressure are usually unaffected. At 5 to 20 μg/kg/min, myocardial contractility and heart rate increase because of beta-1 stimulation. Despite progressive vasoconstriction due to alpha stimulation, systemic vascular resistance may not change, possibly because of offsetting vasodilation in the kidneys, gut, and skeletal muscle. Cardiac output, heart rate, and blood pressure are usually increased. At doses greater than 20 μg/kg/min, alpha-mediated vasoconstriction begins to dominate in most vascular beds. Systemic vascular resistance increases, and blood flow is redistributed to the brain and heart.

Norepinephrine. Norepinephrine is a potent stimulator of alpha and beta-1 receptors but has little effect on beta-2 receptors. It increases systolic, diastolic, and pulse pressures. If hypertension occurs, reflex vagal discharge may cause bradycardia. Resistance to blood flow increases in most circulatory beds, including the skin, splanchnic system, muscle, kidney, and liver. Coronary blood flow is relatively well preserved. Norepinephrine is commonly employed in situations where blood pressure must be quickly restored above critical levels to avoid myocardial or cerebral ischemia. Because it can increase arterial pressure so effectively, norepinephrine may increase renal blood flow and urine output despite renal vasoconstriction. The dose of norepinephrine can vary widely: 4 to 5 μg/min may be effective in some patients, whereas 30 to 40 μg/min may be required in others. Lack of response to high doses of norepinephrine is usually a grave prognostic sign.

Epinephrine. As a potent stimulant of alpha and beta receptors, epinephrine increases heart rate and myocardial contractility and causes vasoconstriction in most vascular beds. Beta-2 stimulation, responsible for vasodilation in the coronary and skeletal muscle vasculature, can limit the pressor effects of lower doses (10 to 30 μg/min) and redistribute blood flow away from the splanchnic bed. In high doses it is the pressor of choice during cardiac arrest (see Chapter 4.2) or anaphylactic shock.

Dobutamine. Dobutamine increases myocardial contractility with little or no effect on heart rate. It causes less systemic vasoconstriction than dopamine because it is less potent as an alpha agonist. Dobutamine may thus be preferable to dopamine when decreased myocardial contractility plays a major pathogenetic role. However, dobutamine can cause hypotension if its effects on cardiac output do not overcome the vasodilation secondary to stimulation of beta-2 receptors. The use of dobutamine should probably be limited to patients who are normotensive or only minimally hypotensive.

Isoproterenol. Isoproterenol is a powerful beta agonist with virtually no alpha effects. It increases heart rate and contractility, causes vasodilation in skeletal muscle, and increases cardiac output. Despite the rise in cardiac output, blood pressure usually falls. Isoproterenol markedly increases myocardial oxygen requirements while reducing coronary perfusion pressure. Tachyarrhythmias and ventricular fibrillation are common adverse side effects. Its use should be limited to the emergency treatment of severe heart block in acute myocardial infarction after atropine has proved ineffective and before artificial pacing has been established (see Chapter 2.9).

Principles Underlying Choice and Use

It is frequently necessary to initiate vasopressor therapy before the cause of shock is known. Dopamine is commonly selected in this situation. One advantage of this drug is that at lower doses it increases flow to the kidneys. At higher doses this salutary effect is gradually outweighed by alpha-receptor stimulation. Dopamine has alpha and beta receptor effects and thus may increase cardiac contractility and systemic vascular resistance.

If the cause of the shock condition is known, it may be possible to select a pressor agent to specifically counteract the pathophysiologic defect. For example, because dobutamine is primarily an inotrope, it may be useful when myocardial function is depressed. In contrast, norepinephrine may be most useful when systemic vascular resistance is low and cardiac function is acceptable, as in septic shock. Epinephrine, like dopamine, has alpha and beta affects and therefore may be used in many of the same situations as dopamine. Epinephrine, however, is more potent than dopamine, and it is therefore more difficult to titrate the dose of epinephrine to obtain the desired effect. Epinephrine is generally reserved for situations in which dopamine is not effective. One exception to this is anaphylactic shock, in which epinephrine is usually the vasopressor of choice. Isoproterenol markedly increases myocardial oxygen requirements but does not increase myocardial oxygen supply; it therefore may precipitate myocardial ischemia. Moreover, isoproterenol does not raise blood pressure and is therefore not suited for use in shock.

HYPOXEMIA AND ACIDOSIS

Arterial blood gas analysis should be performed to assess oxygenation and acid–base state. Hypoxemia, if present, should be corrected (see Chapter 4.1). Metabolic acidosis may be due to accumulation of lactate, ketones, or organic acids of endogenous (chronic renal failure) or exogenous (poisoning) origin. Severe acidosis may depress myocardial function; therefore intravenous bicarbonate injection is often used to reverse acidosis. Recently, however, the use of bicarbonate in this setting has been questioned.[16] Mechanically ventilated patients may not be able to eliminate the excess CO_2 produced during buffering of exogenously administered bicarbonate; therefore, it may be necessary to adjust ventilator settings to provide increased alveolar ventilation. Use of bicarbonate does not eliminate the need to identify and vigorously correct the underlying disease.

MECHANICAL DEVICES USED TO TREAT SHOCK

The *intra-aortic balloon* may be used in patients with cardiogenic shock (see Chapter 2.8).[12,14] Inserted percutaneously or by surgical cut-down of the femoral artery, this device reduces left ventricular afterload by deflating during systole and improves coronary artery perfusion by inflating during diastole. The balloon pump is useful in the management of temporary myocardial dysfunction, as occurs after coronary artery bypass surgery,[12] or in patients awaiting cardiac surgery (valvular replacement, correction of a ventricular septal defect, or cardiac transplantation). It should not be used in patients with irreversible cardiac failure. Military antishock trousers (MAST) are used to treat hypovolemic shock, particularly in the initial management of the trauma victim.[1,7] This inflatable garment encloses the lower extremities and abdomen. When inflated, it increases venous return by squeezing on venous capacitance vessels and increases systemic vascular resistance by compressing arterial vessels. Although rarely used in the intensive care unit, MAST may be employed to test the response of the patient to a volume challenge ("autotransfusion") without actually administering fluids.[5] Rapid deflation of MAST should be avoided, as hypotension may ensue.

REFERENCES

1. Gaffney FA, Thal ER, et al: Hemodynamic effects of medical anti-shock trousers (MAST garment). J Trauma 21:931, 1981
2. Guyton A, Jones C, Coleman T: Circulatory Physiology: Cardiac Output and Its Regulation. Philadelphia, WB Saunders, 1973
3. Hess ML, Warren M, Okabe E: Hemorrhagic shock. In Burton MA, Lefer AM (eds): Handbook of Shock and Trauma. Vol 1: Basic Science. New York, Raven Press, 1983, p 393
4. Hinshaw L: Overview of hemorrhagic shock. In Cowley RA, Trump BF (eds): Pathophysiology of Shock, Anoxia, and Ischemia. Baltimore, Williams & Wilkins, 1982, p 203
5. Jastremski MS, Beney KM: Military antishock trouser (MAST). Application as reversible fluid challenge in patients on high PEEP. Chest 85:595, 1984
6. Kennedy JW, Baxley WA, et al: Qualitative angiocardiography. I. The normal left ventricle in man. Circulation 34:272, 1966
7. McSwain N: Pneumatic trousers and the management of shock. J Trauma 17:719, 1977
8. Puri VK, Padipaty B, White L: Hydroxyethyl starch for resuscitation in patients with hypovolemia and shock. Crit Care Med 9:833, 1981
9. Rock P, Silverman H, et al: Efficacy and safety of naloxone in septic shock. Crit Care Med 13:28, 1985
10. Rush BF: Volume replacement: When, what, and how much. In Schumen WM, Nyhus LM (eds): Treatment of shock: Principles and Practice. Philadelphia, Lea & Febiger, 1974, p 23
11. Sagawa K: The end-systolic pressure-volume relation of the ventricle: Definition, modifications, and use. Circulation 63:1223, 1981
12. Scheidt S, Wilner G, et al: Intra-aortic balloon counter-pulsation in cardiogenic shock. N Engl J Med 288:979, 1973
13. Shabetai R: Cardiac tamponade. In: The Pericardium. New York, Grune & Stratton, 1981, p 224
14. Sobel BE: Cardiac and noncardiac forms of acute circulatory failure (shock). In Braunwald E (ed): Heart Disease. Philadelphia, WB Saunders, 1984, p 578
15. Sprung CL, Caralis PV, et al: The effects of high-dose corticosteroids in patients with septic shock. A prospective, controlled study. N Engl J Med 311(18):1137, 1984
16. Stacpoole PW: Lactic acidosis: The case against bicarbonate therapy for organic acidosis: The case for its continued use. Ann Intern Med 106:615, 1987
17. Sylvester JT, Goldberg HS, Permutt S: The role of the vasculature in the regulation of cardiac output. Clin Chest Med 4(2):111, 1983
18. Yang SS, Bentivoglio LG, et al: From Cardiac Catheterization Data to Hemodynamic Parameters. Philadelphia, FA Davis, 1978
19. Ziegler EJ, McCutchan JA, et al: Treatment of gram-negative bacteremia and shock with human antiserum to a mutant *Escherichia coli*. N Engl J Med 307(20):1225, 1982

Pulmonary Edema

Alan D. Guerci and John R. Michael

Most pulmonary edema develops because of an increase in microvascular pressure or an increase in the permeability of the pulmonary vessels to protein and solute. This chapter focuses on the pathophysiology, diagnosis, and therapy of pulmonary edema caused by an increase in microvascular pressure. The pathophysiology and management of pulmonary edema caused by an increase in the permeability of the pulmonary vessels is discussed in Chapter 4.5.

PATHOPHYSIOLOGY

Movement of fluid across the pulmonary vessels is determined by the hydrostatic pressure difference between microvascular pressure and the interstitial pressure that surrounds the vessel, by the oncotic pressure gradient between the oncotic pressure of plasma and interstitial fluid, and by the permeability of the microvascular membrane to solute and protein.[16] Because the pressure in the pulmonary microvessels exceeds the pressure in the interstitium of the lung, a hydrostatic pressure gradient normally promotes the movement of fluid out of the pulmonary vessels into the lung interstitium. A protein oncotic pressure gradient opposes the hydrostatic pressure gradient because the protein concentration is greater in plasma than in the interstitial fluid. Under normal conditions, these two opposing forces result in a net movement of fluid out of the vessels into the interstitium. The lymphatics remove this fluid, thereby preventing pulmonary edema.

If pulmonary microvascular pressure rises, the hydrostatic gradient increases, promoting fluid movement into the lung interstitium. The increased interstitial fluid is returned to the systematic circulation by the lymphatics. Because fluid removal through the lymphatics can increase dramatically, an increase in lung water does not occur until the capacity of the lymphatics has been exceeded. Excess fluid accumulates first in the lung interstitium rather than in the alveolar spaces. If, however, extra fluid continues to enter the lung interstitium, alveolar flooding will eventually occur.[16] Experimentally, pulmonary edema or an increase in lung weight does not occur in the presence of normal protein oncotic pressure until pulmonary microvascular pressure exceeds 20 to 25 mm Hg.[8] Although a decrease in plasma protein oncotic pressure alone will not produce pulmonary edema, it will increase at least transiently the amount of fluid that moves out of the pulmonary vessels at a given microvascular pressure.[4,8,12] Consequently, patients who have a low serum protein concentration may develop pulmonary edema at microvascular pressures less than 20 to 25 mm Hg.

Pulmonary microvascular pressure or pulmonary venous pressure may increase as a result of an extra work load placed on the heart, a decrease in myocardial contractility, restriction to ventricular filling, or a combination of these factors.

DIAGNOSIS

The diagnosis of pulmonary edema is generally straightforward. Patients typically present with the sudden onset of severe respiratory distress. The patient is terrified, feels as if he were drowning, and sits bolt upright gasping for breath. In most patients this presentation coupled with a history of prior heart disease and diffuse rales

makes the diagnosis apparent. The most common mistake in the emergency situation is to make an erroneous diagnosis of pulmonary edema in elderly patients with respiratory failure due to chronic bronchitis, asthma, or emphysema. Conversely, elderly patients with pulmonary edema may be mistakenly thought to have respiratory failure due to chronic bronchitis. Such mistakes may result in inappropriate and potentially dangerous therapy, for example, using epinephrine for a patient with pulmonary edema or morphine for a patient with respiratory failure caused by chronic bronchitis or emphysema. Diagnostic confusion may occur because patients with both diseases can present with extreme dyspnea, wheezing, pulsus paradoxus, hypoxemia, and hypercapnia. This error can be avoided by obtaining information about the patient's prior medical history and medications and by obtaining a chest radiograph.

The history may provide important clues about precipitating factors, including increased salt intake, noncompliance with medications, infection, tachycardia, bradycardia, myocardial ischemia, thyroid disease, pulmonary embolism, severe anemia, or the recent use of drugs that depress myocardial contractility or cause salt retention.

On physical examination the patients are markedly agitated, tachypneic, and diaphoretic. They may also be cyanotic with cold, ashen skin, indicating a low cardiac output and increased peripheral vascular resistance from activation of the sympathetic nervous system. As a consequence of the increased sympathetic activity, most patients at presentation will have an elevated blood pressure. The presence of hypertensive changes in the retinal vessels helps to distinguish patients with chronic hypertension from patients with acute hypertension.

Arterial blood gas determinations generally document hypoxemia, hypercapnia, and acidosis. The hypercapnia has three causes: inadequate alveolar ventilation due to alveolar flooding; airway narrowing by peribronchial edema; and respiratory muscle fatigue secondary to the increased work of breathing and inadequate oxygen delivery to the diaphragm and other respiratory muscles. The acidosis is usually mixed metabolic and respiratory.[1] The chest radiograph generally shows bilateral alveolar infiltrates and an enlarged heart. The presence of a normal-sized heart on the chest radiograph of a patient with pulmonary edema should suggest the possibility of mitral stenosis, a left atrial myxoma, noncardiogenic pulmonary edema, or a recent myocardial infarction with a stiff left ventricle that has not had time to dilate.

Cardiogenic pulmonary edema can often be distinguished from noncardiogenic pulmonary edema based on the clinical picture alone. Prospective studies indicate, however, that perhaps 15 to 20 percent of patients may be initially misclassified.[5] Characteristics that help to separate the two groups are the clinical setting in which the pulmonary edema develops, the chest radiograph pattern, the pulmonary microvascular pressure as estimated by the pulmonary capillary wedge pressure, and the ratio of albumin or total protein in the alveolar fluid to that in the plasma.

Certain conditions predispose patients to the development of noncardiogenic pulmonary edema (see Chapter 4.5). These conditions include sepsis, fracture of the long bones, rapid transfusion of 5 to 10 units of blood, neurologic lesions that increase intracranial pressure, aspiration of gastric contents, or inhalation of smoke or toxic chemicals. The history in such cases differs markedly from the usual sequence of events in patients with cardiogenic pulmonary edema.

Patients with cardiogenic pulmonary edema usually have an enlarged heart that is revealed by a chest radiograph, whereas patients with noncardiogenic pulmonary edema often have a normal-sized heart. In cardiogenic pulmonary edema the pulmonary capillary wedge pressure usually exceeds 18 to 25 mm Hg. In contrast, patients with noncardiogenic pulmonary edema typically have a wedge pressure less than 10 to 15 mm Hg. Patients with noncardiogenic pulmonary edema have an increase in the vascular permeability to protein—and, consequently, a higher concentration of albumin or total protein in the alveolar fluid than in patients with cardiogenic pulmonary edema. Although not measured routinely, the ratio of alveolar to plasma protein concentration can help to distinguish these two types of pulmonary edema. In cardiogenic pulmonary edema the ratio is generally 0.4 to 0.5, whereas in noncardiogenic pulmonary edema it is typically between 0.7 and 1.0.[6]

Some patients develop pulmonary edema because of an increase in both microvascular pressure and permeability. This may occur in patients with noncardiogenic pulmonary edema who become volume-overloaded or have coexistent cardiac disease. Clinical studies suggest that a combined defect may be more common than is generally realized. Studies in experimental animals, for example, indicate that severe myocardial ischemia may increase pulmonary vascular permeability.[15]

TREATMENT

In patients with pulmonary edema it is important to assess the problem quickly to determine whether special conditions exist that alter the approach to therapy (Table 4.4–1).

The treatment goals are to reduce pulmonary venous pressure, identify precipitating factors, and determine the underlying cardiac disorder (Table 4.4–2). Pulmonary venous pressure can be reduced by having the patient sit upright and by the administration of oxygen, morphine sulfate, nitrates, and diuretics. Morphine dilates systemic veins, thereby reducing venous return and decreasing pulmonary venous pressure. In addition, the anxiety-reducing effects of morphine decrease circulating catecholamines, leading to a fall in systemic vascular resistance. This in turn lowers afterload on the left ventricle, thereby augmenting cardiac output. Morphine sulfate should be given intravenously in 2- to 6-mg increments. Doses can be repeated at 5- to 10-minute intervals, up to a total dose of 16 mg. The amount and frequency of each dose is determined by the patient's blood pressure, level of consciousness, and respiratory status. Morphine should not be given to patients with a systolic blood pressure less than 90 mm Hg, with a depressed level of consciousness, or with depressed respirations. Morphine antagonists should always be available.

Most nitrates predominantly dilate systemic veins. Nitroprusside is the major exception because it dilates arteries and veins equally. Sublingual nitroglycerin (0.4-mg tablets) offers the advantages of easy, immediate delivery and rapid onset of action. Since intravenous nitroglycerin requires careful titration, sublingual nitroglycerin generally establishes a therapeutic level more rapidly than does intravenous infusion. Sublingual nitrates are thus preferred in the initial management of patients with pulmonary edema

TABLE 4.4–1. RAPID ASSESSMENT OF PATIENT WITH PULMONARY EDEMA

- Respiratory status
- Level of consciousness
- Blood pressure
- Evidence of myocardial ischemia
- Arrhythmia
- Valvular heart disease
- Prosthetic valve
- Renal failure

TABLE 4.4–2. TREATMENT OF PULMONARY EDEMA

	Dosage	Monitor
Oxygen	100%	Arterial blood gas analysis
Patient upright		
Morphine	2–6 mg IV, repeat q5–10min up to maximal of 16 mg	Blood pressure Level of consciousness Respiratory status
Nitrates	Sublingual 0.4 mg every q2–5min Avoid topical nitrates Use IV nitrates in patients with shock	Blood pressure
Diuretics	Furosemide 40 mg IV Bumetanide 1 mg IV	Blood pressure Volume status Potassium
Miscellaneous		
Rotating tourniquets	Do not block arterial inflow Use on only three extremities Rotate q15–20min	Generally unnecessary
Phlebotomy	Remove 250–500 ml	Only if other measures fail
Aminophylline	Generally unnecessary 6 mg/kg load over 30 min; 0.5 mg/kg/hr maintenance	Heart rate Avoid with myocardial ischemia
Sodium bicarbonate	Avoid	

who are not hypotensive. Intravenous nitrates should be used in hypotensive patients. Large amounts of sublingual nitrates are often required: 0.4 mg may be given every 2 to 5 minutes. Care must be taken to ensure that the tablets dissolve under the patient's tongue. Sublingual absorption can be increased by keeping the mouth moist, using water-soaked pads if necessary. As with morphine, nitroglycerin should not be given routinely to patients with severe hypotension (systolic blood pressure less than 90 mm Hg). Topical nitrate preparations should not be used in patients with pulmonary edema, because the peripheral vasoconstriction makes cutaneous drug absorption unreliable.

Potent, rapidly acting diuretics are the third class of drugs used to lower pulmonary venous pressure. Furosemide (Lasix) and bumetanide (Bumex) are the drugs of choice. Furosemide dilates systemic veins even before diuresis occurs, thus lowering pulmonary venous pressure. For most patients, 40 mg intravenously is an adequate initial dose. For patients already receiving larger oral doses of furosemide, an intravenous dose equivalent to twice the patient's regular dose is usually effective. One milligram of bumetanide is generally equivalent to 40 mg of furosemide. Often 20 to 30 minutes are required before these drugs induce diuresis. If urine output has not improved after 30 minutes, the diuretic may be repeated at double the previous dosage. As with morphine and nitrates, furosemide and bumetanide should not be given to hypotensive patients. Because these diuretics can cause life-threatening kaliuresis, serum electrolytes should be measured frequently.

OTHER MEASURES

Several other forms of therapy are occasionally helpful. Rotating tourniquets are generally unnecessary and ineffective. They may, however, decrease venous return sufficiently to benefit some patients and should always be applied when the patient is in extremis. Tourniquets should be placed on only three extremities and ro-

tated every 15 to 20 minutes. They should not be applied so tightly that they obstruct arterial inflow. The removal of 250 to 500 ml of blood by phlebotmy may also reduce pulmonary vascular congestion but should be tried only when other measures fail.

Although aminophylline is sometimes recommended for the treatment of pulmonary edema, it is not a first-line drug. Wheezing is generally due to airway narrowing caused by fluid in the sheaths that surround the airways. This wheezing responds promptly to the usual therapy for elevated pulmonary venous pressure, and aminophylline is usually unnecessary. Furthermore, aminophylline may result in tachycardia, which should be avoided in patients with myocardial ischemia.

Dialysis may be required in patients with moderate renal insufficiency and is generally necessary in anuric patients. Morphine, nitrates, and phlebotomy are useful temporizing measures until dialysis can be arranged. In addition to volume overload, uremia can also depress myocardial contractility. Dialysis improves both abnormalities.[10]

ASSOCIATED PROBLEMS

Intubation
Although a fixed rule is difficult to establish concerning intubation, patients with severe respiratory acidosis (pH <7.10, Pa_{CO_2} >70 mm Hg), severe hypoxemia (Pa_{O_2} <50 mm Hg) despite oxygen therapy or altered consciousness should be intubated. One should not hesitate to intubate patients with pulmonary edema who develop respiratory failure and CO_2 retention, since once the edema clears, they are usually easily extubated.

Once intubated, the patient should be initially given 100 percent oxygen. Oxygenation may be improved further by 5 to 15 cm H_2O of positive end-expiratory pressure. The patient should be hyperventilated to correct respiratory acidosis or compensate for metabolic acidosis. Mechanical ventilation, in addition to correcting acidosis and hypoxemia, also reduces the work of breathing and, consequently, the percentage of cardiac output that goes to the diaphragm and other respiratory muscles. Furthermore, the increase in alveolar pressure caused by mechanical ventilation, especially when augmented with positive end-expiratory pressure, decreases venous return, shifts fluid out of alveoli,[9] and reduces the afterload on the failing left ventricle.[13]

The administration of sodium bicarbonate should be avoided in the treatment of pulmonary edema. Although the acidosis is a mixed respiratory and metabolic acidosis, the respiratory acidosis predominates and quickly resolves as gas exchange improves. The metabolic acidosis also rapidly reverses with standard therapy. In addition, an ampule of sodium bicarbonate provides a large sodium load and may significantly increase serum osmolality. Finally, the administration of a standard ampule of bicarbonate in a patient with concomitant respiratory acidosis can transiently increase Pa_{CO_2} by 10 to 20 mm Hg.[2] Because carbon dioxide rapidly diffuses into the myocardium, sodium bicarbonate can paradoxically worsen intracellular acidosis and ventricular function. The primary role of digitalis in the treatment of acute pulmonary edema is to slow the ventricular rate in patients with atrial fibrillation or other supraventricular tachycardias. Except for rate control, digitalis has a limited role in the management of acute pulmonary edema.

The majority of patients with pulmonary edema do not require catheterization of the right side of the heart and measurement of pulmonary arterial and capillary wedge pressures. Catheterization of the right side of the heart, however, may be necessary in patients who do not respond as expected during the first few hours of therapy and is generally indicated for patients requiring therapy with vasopressors or high doses of intravenous nitrates.[3,5]

Shock
The combination of pulmonary edema, severe hypotension (systolic blood pressure usually <90 mm Hg), and inadequate tissue perfusion (livedo reticularis, altered mental status, oliguria, and metabolic acidosis) necessitates treatment with inotropic drugs and the withholding of vasodilators and diuretics until blood pressure and tissue perfusion increase. Dopamine, dobutamine, and norepinephrine (Levophed) are all potent and have a serum half-life of less than 3 minutes. Important differences in their actions may be exploited to a particular patient's benefit. Dopamine improves mesenteric and renal blood flow at low and intermediate doses (1 to 10 µg/kg/min), thus facilitating diuresis. At higher doses of dopamine (10 to 20 µg/kg/min), generalized vasoconstriction tends to predominate. The usual starting dose is 5 to 10 µg/kg/min, depending on the severity of the hypotension. Dobutamine, a synthetic catecholamine, is used in the same dose range (2 to 20 µg/kg/min). As a rule, these two drugs produce similar increases in stroke volume and cardiac output. Dobutamine, however, can be a potent vasodilator and may aggravate hypotension unless cardiac output increases enough to compensate for the decrease in systemic vascular resistance. Norepinephrine produces more potent vasoconstriction and less of an increase in heart rate than does dopamine. The initial dose of norepinephrine is usually 25 to 50 µg/min, and this can be increased every 3 to 5 minutes until the desired blood pressure is obtained.

Once blood pressure and tissue perfusion are adequate, diuretics and nitrates can be given to reduce pulmonary venous pressure. Nitrates also increase cardiac output and may augment the renal response to diuretics. In hypotensive patients, nitrates should be given intravenously. In general, nitroglycerin and nitroprusside are both effective. Nitroprusside is a more potent arterial dilator, but at high doses it may produce cyanide toxicity (manifested by nausea, vomiting, confusion, and muscle spasms).[14] Starting doses for both drugs are the same (0.1 µg/kg/min), and 50 to 200 µg/min is commonly required. Dosage may be increased by 5 to 25 µg/min every 5 to 20 minutes. Hypotension, the most common adverse effect, is usually short-lived and can be treated by reducing the nitrate dose.

Although it is difficult to generalize, several guidelines should be followed in the care of patients with pulmonary edema and severe hypotension. First, continuous monitoring of pulmonary and systemic arterial pressures is necessary for effective treatment.[3] Second, vital organ perfusion is usually inadequate at systolic blood pressures below 90 mm Hg and usually adequate at pressures above 100 mm Hg. Therefore, catecholamine and vasodilator dosages should be adjusted accordingly. Third, pulmonary edema develops at pulmonary venous pressures above 20 mm Hg. Blood pressure permitting, a wedge pressure less than 20 mm Hg should be the goal of vasodilator and diuretic therapy. Finally, to the greatest extent possible, intravascular overload should be treated with diuretics rather than ever increasing doses of nitrates.

SPECIAL SITUATIONS

The management of pulmonary edema varies from the standard approach in certain situations.

Myocardial Ischemia
When acute myocardial ischemia precipitates pulmonary edema, the vascular congestion results from the sudden redistribution of volume into the lung, and intravascular volume may be normal. Morphine and especially nitroglycerin are preferred over diuretics because these medicines obviate the risk of diuretic-induced volume depletion and hypotension.

The acute onset of pulmonary edema following a recent myocardial infarction should suggest a ventricular septal defect from rupture through the ventricular septum or mitral regurgitation from papillary muscle rupture or dysfunction.[7]

Arrhythmias
Heart block and ventricular or supraventricular arrhythmias may precipitate pulmonary edema, particularly in patients with preex-

isting heart disease. Therapy in these situations should focus on controlling the arrhythmia (see Chapter 2.9). Patients with pulmonary edema due to supraventricular or ventricular tachycardias may need direct current cardioversion. Conscious patients should always be sedated before cardioversion.

Valvular Heart Disease

Two forms of valvular disease frequently cause pulmonary edema requiring specific modifications of therapy: regurgitant lesions and mitral stenosis. Aortic regurgitation, mitral regurgitation, and acquired left-to-right shunts such as a ventricular septal defect secondary to myocardial infarction or a ruptured sinus of Valsalva aneurysm can produce fulminant pulmonary edema. Although emergency surgery is usually required for lesions severe enough to cause pulmonary edema, afterload reduction with nitroprusside reduces the regurgitant flow and is the cornerstone of medical efforts to stabilize these patients.

Mitral stenosis poses special problems. First, the auscultatory hallmarks of mitral stenosis—a loud first heart sound, an opening snap, and a diastolic rumble—may be difficult to appreciate in the noisy and frenetic atmosphere that usually surrounds the emergency treatment of pulmonary edema. Nevertheless, several findings point to the correct diagnosis. First, the diagnosis should always be considered in patients with pulmonary edema and a normal cardiothoracic ratio on chest radiograph. Second, atrial fibrillation with a rapid ventricular response and pulmonary edema in a young or middle-aged person should suggest the possibility of mitral stenosis or a left atrial myxoma.

The correct diagnosis is of vital importance in patients with mitral stenosis, for not only does the focus of therapy differ from that in routine cases of pulmonary edema, but standard therapy with venodilators and diuretics can be fatal because the decrease in venous return and intravascular volume can dramatically reduce left ventricular filling, cardiac output, and arterial blood pressure. Medical therapy cannot affect the fundamental problem in mitral stenosis, which is decreased orifice size. Nevertheless the major physiologic problem in mitral stenosis, the transvalvular pressure gradient, can be lessened by measures that slow the heart rate and increase diastolic filling time. This lowers left atrial (and pulmonary venous) pressure while increasing left ventricular filling, cardiac output, and systemic arterial pressure. For this purpose verapamil is the drug of choice. Five milligrams can be given intravenously in 1 or 2 minutes and repeated at 5-minute intervals until a heart rate of 60 to 80 is obtained or until a total of 15 mg has been administered. Verapamil should not be given to patients with severe hypotension unless the clinician is confident that the hypotension is caused by the tachycardia. Otherwise, cardioversion is indicated. If verapamil does not control heart rate, digoxin, 0.25 mg, can be given intravenously and repeated in 1 hour and then at 4-hour intervals up to a total dosage of 1 to 1.5 mg. If these efforts fail to reduce the ventricular rate and improve pulmonary edema, propranolol (0.1 mg/kg IV) can be administered slowly and cautiously (over 5 to 20 minutes). Propranolol is contraindicated in patients who are hypotensive or have severely depressed myocardial contractility. If a patient with pulmonary edema from mitral stenosis fails to respond to medical therapy, emergency balloon dilation or surgery may be life saving.[11]

Patients with Prosthetic Valves

Dysfunction of aortic or mitral valve prostheses can cause pulmonary edema. Careful auscultation and echocardiography may establish the correct diagnosis. It is well to remember that echocardiography usually provides only indirect evidence of the prosthesis dysfunction. Conventional echocardiography is not sensitive in the detection of occlusive thrombi or regurgitant flow, and the sonoreflective characteristics of prosthetic devices may even obscure a Doppler image of regurgitant flow. On the other hand, good left-ventricular function and coexisting pulmonary edema would suggest a regurgitant lesion, whereas normal contraction of a small, slowly filling left ventricle and dilation of the left atrium, right ventricle, or both, would suggest thrombosis of a mitral prosthesis. In the absence of a clear explanation for persistent pulmonary edema in a patient with a prosthetic valve, cardiac catheterization is generally advisable. Indeed, thorough cardiologic evaluation, including echocardiography, magnetic resonance imaging,[17] and/or cardiac catheterization should be considered in every patient with unexplained refractory pulmonary edema.

REFERENCES

1. Aberman A, Fulop M: The metabolic and respiratory acidosis of acute pulmonary edema. Ann Intern Med 76:173, 1972
2. Bishop RL, Weisfeldt ML: Sodium bicarbonate administration during cardiac arrest. JAMA 235:506, 1976
3. Connors AF Jr, McCaffree DR, Gray BA: Evaluation of right heart catheterization in the critically ill patient without acute myocardial infarction. N Engl J Med 308:263, 1983
4. Dodek PM, Rice TW, et al: Effects of plasmapheresis and of hypoproteinemia on lung liquid conductance in awake sheep. Circ Res 58:269, 1986
5. Fein AM, Goldberg SK, et al: Is pulmonary artery catheterization necessary for the diagnosis of pulmonary edema? Am Rev Respir Dis 129:1006, 1984
6. Fein A, Grossman RF, et al: The value of edema fluid protein measurement in patients with pulmonary edema. Am J Med 67:32, 1979
7. Feneley MP, Change VP, O'Rourke MF: Myocardial rupture after acute myocardial infarction. Ten-year review. Br Heart J 49:550, 1983
8. Guyton AC, Lindsey AW: Effect of elevated left atrial pressure and decreased plasma protein concentration on the development of pulmonary edema. Circ Res 7:649, 1959
9. Malo J, Ali J, Wood LDH: How does positive end-expiratory pressure reduce intrapulmonary shunt in canine pulmonary edema? J Appl Physiol 57:1002, 1984
10. Nixon JV, Mitchell JH, et al: Effect of hemodialysis on left ventricular function. J Clin Invest 71:377, 1983
11. Palacios IF, Lock JE, et al: Percutaneous transvenous balloon valvotomy in a patient with severe calcific mitral stenosis. J Am Coll Cardiol 7:1416, 1986
12. Parker RE, Wickersham NE, et al: Effects of hypoproteinemia on lung microvascular protein sieving and lung lymph flow. J Appl Physiol 60:1293, 1986
13. Pinsky MR, Summer WR, et al: Augmentation of cardiac function by elevation of intrathoracic pressure. J Appl Physiol 54:950, 1983
14. Schulz V: Clinical pharmacokinetics of nitroprusside, cyanide, thiosulphate, and thiocyanate. Clin Pharmacokinet 9:239, 1984
15. Slutsky RA, Peck WW, Higgins CB: Pulmonary edema formation with myocardial infarction and left atrial hypertension: Intravascular and extravascular pulmonary fluid volumes. Circulation 68:164, 1983
16. Staub NC, Nagano H, Pearce ML: Pulmonary edema in dogs, especially the sequence of fluid accumulation in lungs. J Appl Physiol 22:227, 1967
17. Westcott JL, Steiner RM: Clinical applications of magnetic resonance imaging (MRI) of the heart. Cardiovasc Clin 17:323, 1986

CHAPTER 4.5
Hypoxic Respiratory Failure:
~~Ad~~ult Respiratory Distress Syndrome

David B. Pearse, E. James Britt,
and J.T. Sylvester

INTRODUCTION AND CLINICAL FEATURES

The adult respiratory distress syndrome (ARDS) is a clinical description of severe lung injury characterized by increased permeability of alveolar-capillary membranes and the development of protein-rich pulmonary edema. The syndrome is defined by severe dyspnea, diffuse alveolar infiltration on the chest radiograph, marked hypoxemia refractory to increases in inspired O_2 concentration, and the absence of left ventricular failure. ARDS is associated with a diverse group of disorders (Table 4.5–1). When a single predisposing condition is present, the risk of developing ARDS is variable, with an overall risk of 6 percent. Gastric aspiration and pneumonia caused by gram-negative bacilli are associated with the

TABLE 4.5–1. DISORDERS ASSOCIATED WITH ADULT RESPIRATORY DISTRESS SYNDROME

Aspiration
- Gastric contents
- Fresh and salt water
- Hydrocarbons

Central Nervous System
- Trauma
- Anoxia
- Increased intracranial pressure

Drug Overdose
- Acetylsalicylic acid
- Heroin
- Methadone
- Propoxyphene
- Barbiturate

Hematologic Alterations
- Disseminated intravascular coagulation
- Massive blood transfusion
- Postcardiopulmonary bypass

Infection
- Sepsis (gram-positive or -negative)
- Diffuse pneumonia
- Tuberculosis
- Peritonitis

Inhalation of Toxins
- Oxygen (high concentrations >60%)
- Smoke
- Corrosive chemicals (NO_2, Cl_2, NH_3, phosgene, cadmium)

Metabolic Disorders
- Pancreatitis
- Uremia

Shock
- Any etiology (rare in cardiogenic)

Trauma
- Fracture (large bone)
- Lung contusion
- Nonthoracic
- Burn

highest incidence rates (36 and 12 percent, respectively). Patients with multiple predispositions have an overall risk of 25 percent.[4]

Most patients who develop ARDS are already hospitalized for associated disorders. Occasionally, patients will present with ARDS without an identifiable cause. Early in the evolution of ARDS there is often a latent period when patients are stable, without respiratory signs or symptoms. Gradual tachypnea may develop with hypocapnia and mild hypoxemia. The onset of ARDS is heralded by acute respiratory distress, pink to red frothy sputum, diffuse chest rales upon examination, and widespread infiltrates on the chest radiograph. Although it is presently not possible to predict if a predisposed patient will develop ARDS, it is known that 90 percent of patients who develop the syndrome require mechanical ventilation within 3 days of the initiating insult.[4]

Pulmonary edema due to left ventricular failure must be ruled out. Sometimes this can be accomplished by history, physical examination, ECG, and echocardiography. Standard chest radiography may also be helpful. Pulmonary edema due to left ventricular failure is characterized by cardiomegaly, an inverted blood flow distribution, peribronchial cuffs, an even distribution of alveolar infiltrates, and pleural effusions. In ARDS the heart size and blood flow distribution are usually normal, whereas peribronchial cuffs and pleural effusions are uncommon. There is a peripheral distribution of infiltrates, and air bronchograms are frequently observed.[7] In many patients, however, the distinction between ARDS and left ventricular failure will not be clear, and pulmonary artery catheterization will be required.

Approximately 150,000 new cases occur each year in the United States. With advances in respiratory care, few patients now die from respiratory insufficiency; however, the mortality remains at 60 to 70 percent. One third of deaths occur within 72 hours as a direct result of the underlying illness. Most of the remainder occur within 2 weeks from infection or multiple organ system failure.[1] The prognosis for survivors appears good. Few are symptomatic, and residual pulmonary function abnormalities, if present, are usually mild.[3]

PATHOGENESIS AND PATHOPHYSIOLOGY

The pathogenesis of ARDS is unknown. The diversity of associated clinical conditions suggests that many mechanisms of injury may exist. Some conditions (e.g., lung contusion and aspiration of gastric acid) cause direct injury to the lung parenchyma. Others (e.g., sepsis, shock, and nonthoracic trauma) activate indirect mechanisms that may involve cellular and humoral mediators.

Many of the disorders associated with ARDS are thought to activate complement products such as C5a, which may cause polymorphonuclear neutrophils (PMN) to aggregate and adhere to pulmonary endothelium. Other humoral substances, possibly from alveolar macrophages, may play a role in this process. The activated PMNs are thought to migrate into the pulmonary interstitium and release toxic products that damage the alveolar-capillary membrane.[11] These include oxygen radicals (superoxide anion, hydrogen peroxide, hydroxyl radical), proteolytic enzymes (elastase, collagenase), and metabolites of arachidonic acid (prostaglandins,

thromboxanes, leukotrienes). In support of this sequence of events, large numbers of PMNs are seen in lung biopsy specimens from patients with ARDS; moreover, PMNs chemoattractants and PMN-derived proteolytic enzymes have been found in bronchoalveolar lavage fluid. Some experimental models of ARDS demonstrate an injurious role for the PMN. On the other hand, some animal models of lung injury appear to be PMN-independent or to show extensive pulmonary sequestration of activated PMNs with only transient pulmonary dysfunction. In addition, ARDS has occurred in patients rendered neutropenic by treatment for hematologic malignancy. These observations suggest that pathways of injury other than the PMN must exist.

The common occurrence of disseminated intravascular coagulation, thrombocytopenia, and platelet-fibrin emboli in patients with ARDS prompted investigation of a possible link between disordered coagulation and lung injury.[9] Although fibrin degradation products caused increased pulmonary endothelial permeability when infused into animals, it is unknown if these products cause human lung injury. Platelets sequester in the lungs of ARDS patients; however, it has not been established that platelets contribute to lung injury.

Despite the diversity of associated conditions, the pathologic appearance of the lungs is uniform. Grossly, the lungs are airless, heavy, red, and indurated. In the acute phase, light microscopy reveals proteinaceous fluid in the interstitium, and erythrocytes, leukocytes, cellular debris, and fibrin in the alveoli. Hyaline membranes occur in some alveoli, and platelet-fibrin thrombi are seen in vessels. On electron microscopy, type 1 alveolar epithelial cells exhibit swelling, vacuolization, necrosis, and sloughing. Less severe changes are seen in capillary endothelial cells. The acute phase of the syndrome is followed by a chronic phase, characterized by proliferation of type 2 alveolar epithelial cells, influx of plasma cells, histiocytes, and lymphocytes, and the formation of interstitial and intra-alveolar fibrin. In some patients, this reparative process leads to resolution. In others, a fibrosing alveolitis ensues, resulting in interstitial fibrosis.

Most of the acute pathophysiologic abnormalities are caused by formation of pulmonary edema. Edema formation is governed by the hydrostatic and colloid osmotic pressure gradients between the vascular space and interstitium, the area and permeability of the vascular-interstitial interface to water and protein, and the rate of lymph flow from the lung. In ARDS the permeability of the endothelial membrane is increased. The intravascular hydrostatic pressure may also be increased because of pulmonary vasoconstriction. As a result, fluid enters the interstitium at an increased rate. If the capacity of the lymphatics to remove fluid is exceeded, fluid collects in the interstitial spaces around vessels and airways. When the capacity of the interstitium to store fluid is exceeded, fluid overflows into the alveoli.

Alveolar flooding and collapse lead to profound gas exchange abnormalities. Right-to-left shunts caused by perfused but unventilated alveoli produce severe hypoxemia refractory to increases in inspired oxygen concentration. Interstitial edema, intraluminal fluid, and bronchospasm narrow small airways, decreasing regional ventilation. These underventilated units can collapse and worsen the shunt or remain open and contribute to hypoxemia through ventilation-perfusion mismatch. Despite the marked pathologic changes of alveolar-capillary membranes, diffusion impairment is thought not to contribute to hypoxemia. Neither does hypoventilation, because arterial PCO_2 is characteristically low.

As edema fluid collects in the interstitium and alveoli, the lung becomes smaller and stiffer. Surface tension forces increase because of dilution and alteration of surfactant. Inspissated fluid, peribronchial edema, and bronchospasm increase airways resistance. With pulmonary compliance and lung volume reduced and airways resistance increased, the patient must work harder to maintain an adequate functional residual capacity and minute ventilation. The increased work of breathing can lead to respiratory muscle fatigue, further decreases in lung volume, and worsening gas exchange.

MANAGEMENT

Except when a treatable cause of ARDS can be identified, therapy can only be supportive. The goals of supportive management are to maintain O_2 transport, limit pulmonary edema, and avoid complications. The physician must not be so distracted by the patient's considerable immediate needs that he fails to identify and treat the underlying condition. Because of the severity of the gas exchange defect, these patients are almost always initially hospitalized in the intensive care unit.

All patients will require oxygen. Treatment with oxygen begins when the patient can no longer maintain an arterial oxygen saturation >90 percent breathing room air. This usually occurs when the arterial PO_2 falls below 60 mm Hg; however, if acidosis and fever are present, the oxyhemoglobin dissociation curve can be shifted to the right, increasing the O_2 tension required to achieve 90 percent saturation. To avoid toxicity, the inspired O_2 concentration should be kept as low as possible. Oxygen toxicity is thought to occur when cellular antioxidant systems are overwhelmed by increased production of toxic O_2 products such as the superoxide anion, hydrogen peroxide, and the hydroxyl radical. These highly reactive species attack lipids and proteins, causing disruption of membranes and inactivation of enzymes. Although inspired O_2 concentrations <50 percent do not adversely affect pulmonary function acutely in healthy human subjects, this may not be true in ARDS patients, whose lungs may have already sustained considerable oxidative injury. Currently it is unknown what concentration of O_2 is safe in patients with ARDS. Moreover, there is no proven treatment for O_2 toxicity.

As the work of breathing increases and respiratory muscle fatigue develops, the patient fails to maintain adequate lung volume. Progressive atelectasis, right-to-left shunting, and hypoxemia develop despite increased inspired O_2 concentrations. At this point, the physician usually resorts to tracheal intubation and mechanical ventilation to reverse atelectasis and relieve the work of breathing. Occasionally, this can be accomplished simply by ventilating the patient at a tidal volume of 12 to 15 ml/kg and a frequency sufficient to maintain a normal arterial CO_2 tension. More often, however, it is necessary to administer PEEP.[6] PEEP acts by increasing transpulmonary pressure and lung volume, thereby opening closed airways, inflating collapsed alveoli, reducing right-to-left shunt, and improving arterial oxygenation. PEEP can also increase lung compliance and thereby decrease the work of breathing. PEEP does not decrease extravascular lung water. Rather, experimental evidence suggests that PEEP augments edema formation. This may occur because the increase in lung volume lowers interstitial pressure, thereby increasing the transvascular hydrostatic pressure gradient. Early use of PEEP in patients at risk for ARDS does not decrease the subsequent incidence of the syndrome.

PEEP is usually begun at 3 to 5 cm H_2O and increased by increments of 3 to 5 cm H_2O until oxygenation improves or 20 cm H_2O is reached. During these maneuvers, inspired O_2 concentration should be held constant. Lack of improvement may indicate that the patient is preventing increases in transpulmonary pressure by contraction of the expiratory muscles. In this case, paralytic agents may be helpful. When oxygenation improves, it is frequently possible to reduce PEEP by 5 cm H_2O, because the transpulmonary pressure necessary to open collapsed alveoli is usually greater than that required to keep them open. When oxygenation is adequate, inspired O_2 concentration should be reduced to as low a level as possible, preferably <50 percent. Occasionally, PEEP can be administered by a tightly fitting face mask. Usually, however, this is not well tolerated. Furthermore, if the patient vomits, the risk of aspiration is increased.

To avoid adverse side effects, it is important to use the lowest level of PEEP necessary to achieve adequate oxygenation. The adverse effects of PEEP are several. Barotrauma (pneumothorax, pneumomediastinum) can occur at all levels of PEEP. A PEEP-induced increase in pleural pressure can compress the right atrium

and great veins, thereby decreasing venous return and cardiac output. A decrease in cardiac output can result in a lower mixed venous O_2 tension and thus a lower arterial O_2 tension for any degree of shunt. Cardiac output is usually not affected by levels of PEEP under 15 cm H_2O if adequate vascular volume is maintained. A fall in cardiac output can be reversed by careful administration of intravenous fluid. PEEP may decrease blood flow to ventilated alveoli resulting from capillary compression, causing an increase in dead space. When minute ventilation and CO_2 production are constant, a decreased alveolar ventilation and increased arterial PCO_2 could result. This problem can be corrected by increasing minute ventilation. If PEEP is used in the presence of a focal pulmonary process such as lobar pneumonia, diversion of blood flow from ventilated alveoli can increase shunt fraction and worsen hypoxemia. PEEP is therefore not indicated for treatment of hypoxemia resulting from focal lung disease.

Because of these adverse effects, the physician must carefully reassess the patient at each level of PEEP. The influence of PEEP on gas exchange and cardiac output cannot be predicted, which emphasizes the importance of a controlled, incremental approach. PEEP should never be interrupted for vascular pressure measurements. This practice can result in profound hypoxemia. An optimal level of PEEP is that which allows adequate arterial oxygen saturation without significant reduction in cardiac output at an inspired oxygen concentration below 50 percent. In most ARDS patients this can be achieved with levels of PEEP between 10 and 20 cm H_2O.[10]

The elimination of hypoxemia may be of no benefit if accomplished at the expense of cardiac output. It is the transport of oxygen from the lung to the tissues that must be maximized. Oxygen transport is the product of arterial oxygen content and cardiac output. Thus, decreased cardiac output should be avoided and an adequate arterial O_2 tension maintained. In addition, hemoglobin concentration should be kept in the normal range. Even slight degrees of anemia cannot be tolerated in these patients.

Careful hemodynamic management is essential and usually requires catheterization of the pulmonary artery with a thermistor-tipped, balloon-flotation catheter capable of providing measurements of cardiac output by thermodilution (see Chapter 4.1). When the permeability of the lung is increased by injury, small changes in intravascular pressure lead to large changes in fluid filtration. Thus, pulmonary artery and wedge pressures should be kept as low as possible by careful fluid management and judicious use of diuretics while avoiding decreases in cardiac output. Pulmonary vasodilators have been effective in animal models of ARDS, but experience in patients is limited. Left ventricular failure should be avoided. When renal failure complicates the picture, dialysis should be performed without delay if indicated. A pulmonary artery catheter also allows measurement of O_2 transport and mixed venous oxygen content. The latter is needed to calculate shunt fraction. When O_2 consumption is constant or increasing, an increase in mixed venous O_2 content may indicate increased effectiveness of tissue perfusion.

Multiple organ system failure and secondary infection such as gram-negative pneumonia are major causes of death in ARDS.[8] Prolonged illness and hospitalization are associated with colonization of the oropharynx by gram-negative bacteria. Antacids used to lower the risk of gastrointestinal bleeding have been incriminated as potentiators of gram-negative bacterial growth in the stomach. Altered mental status may predispose to aspiration. Host resistance may be compromised by poor nutrition. Endotracheal tubes, which prevent coughing and provide a convenient portal of entry for organisms contaminating ventilators and respiratory therapy equipment, should be removed as soon as possible. The same is true of intravascular and bladder catheters, which potentiate the risk of sepsis. Early diagnosis and judicious use of antibiotics may prevent the development of resistant organisms and improve survival. Aerosolized antibiotics have been advocated by some to prevent secondary pneumonias, but their efficacy remains uncertain.

Upper gastrointestinal hemorrhage, usually from peptic ulcers, is a common complication. Bleeding may be potentiated by disseminated intravascular coagulation and thrombocytopenia. The mortality rate is higher and hospital stay is longer among patients with bleeding. Administration of antacids frequently and in sufficient quantity to maintain gastric pH >4.0 will reduce the likelihood of upper gastrointestinal hemorrhage. Cimetidine has been less effective. There is little rationale to support administration of both agents.

Specific treatments for ARDS are being sought. Corticosteroids have received considerable attention because they stabilize cell and lysosomal membranes and inhibit a variety of granulocyte functions; however, preliminary results of a recent multicenter trial of corticosteroid therapy in ARDS suggest that these agents had no effect on mortality.[2] More encouraging results have been obtained with prostaglandin E_1, a pulmonary vasodilator that also inhibits platelet aggregation, macrophage activation, and neutrophil function. A recent placebo-controlled, prospective trial found that prostaglandin E_1 significantly improved 30-day survival in patients with ARDS.[5] This result awaits confirmation.

REFERENCES

1. Bell RC, Coalson JJ, et al: Multiple organ system failure and infection in adult respiratory distress syndrome. Ann Intern Med 99:293, 1983
2. Bernard GR, Luce JM, et al: High-dose corticosteroids in patients with the adult respiratory distress syndrome. N Engl J Med 317:1565, 1987
3. Elliott CG, Morris AH, Cengiz M: Pulmonary function and exercise gas exchange in survivors of adult respiratory distress syndrome. Am Rev Respir Dis 123:492, 1981
4. Fowler AA, Hamman RF, et al: Adult respiratory distress syndrome: Risk with common predispositions. Ann Intern Med 98:593, 1983
5. Holcroft JW, Vassar MJ, Weber CJ: Prostaglandin E_1 and survival in patients with the adult respiratory distress syndrome: A prospective trial. Ann Surg 203(4):371, 1986
6. Loyd JE, Newman JH, Brigham KL: Permeability pulmonary edema: Diagnosis and management. Arch Intern Med 144:143, 1984
7. Milne ENC, Pistolesi M, et al: The radiologic distinction of cardiogenic and noncardiogenic edema. Am J Radiol 144:879, 1985
8. Montgomery AB, Stager MA, et al: Causes of mortality in patients with the adult respiratory distress syndrome. Am Rev Respir Dis 132:485, 1985
9. Rinaldo JE, Rogers RM: Adult respiratory distress syndrome: Changing concepts of lung injury and repair. N Engl J Med 306(15):900, 1982
10. Shapiro BA, Cane RD, Harrison RA: Positive end-expiratory pressure in acute lung injury. Chest 83(3):558, 1983
11. Tate RM, Repine JE: Neutrophils and the adult respiratory distress syndrome. Am Rev Resp Dis 128:552, 1983

CHAPTER 4.6
Status Asthmaticus

Gail G. Weinmann, Eugene R. Bleecker,
and John R. Michael

Status asthmaticus refers to a severe asthma attack that is refactory to the usual forms of therapy. It is a life-threatening medical emergency that requires immediate hospitalization for intensive treatment. The incidence of status asthmaticus is difficult to determine because of the lack of a consistent definition, but each year in the United States severe asthma accounts for 130,000 hospitalizations and 2000 to 4000 deaths.

CLINICAL PRESENTATION

The patient with status asthmaticus presents with the typical clinical features of a severe asthma attack. Similarly, the physiologic findings in status asthmaticus represent the most severe end of the spectrum (see Chapter 3.6).

The primary complaint is extreme shortness of breath, often associated with chest tightness and severe anxiety. The dyspnea may have developed suddenly, but more typically the patient gives a history of dyspnea and increasing use of medication over several days to a week. The patient appears to be in severe respiratory distress and may be able to talk only in single syllables between breaths. The patient usually presents with tachycardia, tachypnea, and hypertension from anxiety, dyspnea, and hypoxemia. The respiratory rate is variable and may be misleadingly low (20 to 30 breaths per minute) for the severity of the attack. Flow through narrowed airways produces wheezing. In severe asthma, air flow may be so diminished that wheezes are not heard.

The major pathophysiologic findings are decreased expiratory flow rates, abnormalities of gas exchange, air trapping, mucous plugging of airways, decreased forced vital capacity, and elevated static lung volumes (Fig. 4.6–1). Because of air trapping and an unconscious effort to breathe at high lung volumes, the asthmatic patient develops a negative pleural pressure. The negative pleural pressure markedly increases the work of breathing, adding to the sensation of dyspnea and increasing the afterload on the left ventricle, which contributes to the development of pulsus paradoxicus.

To gauge the severity of an asthma attack one should evaluate a number of objective and subjective criteria because no single factor is totally reliable (Table 4.6–1). A history of previous intubation for asthma or recent emergency room visits should signal the physician that the patient is likely to have severe asthma. Tachycardia greater than 130 beats per minute, pulsus paradoxus greater than 20 mm Hg, or diminished breath sounds are commonly used indicators of severity. Arterial blood gas studies usually reveal hypoxemia with hypocapnia and a respiratory alkalosis. A normal or elevated $PaCO_2$ indicates alveolar hypoventilation and severe mismatching of ventilation and perfusion. Occasionally, the work of breathing is extreme enough to produce a metabolic acidosis. An FEV_1 less than 1 L, a peak expiratory flow rate (PEFR) less than 100 L/min, or the inability to perform any pulmonary function test point to a severe asthma attack. The chest radiograph generally shows hyperinflation because of air trapping. If the hyperinflation is severe, the diaphragrms may become inverted. The electrocardiogram usually reveals sinus tachycardia but may also show signs of right-sided heart strain such as right axis deviation and P pulmonale. Cyanosis, an abnormal mental status, the appearance of fatigue, respiratory acidosis, metabolic acidosis, secondary electrolyte abnormalities, an infiltrate or pneumothorax on chest radiograph, or lack of response to therapy are signs of a potentially fatal asthma attack.

TREATMENT

The primary objective is to prevent complications of hypoxemia such as arrhythmias or cardiopulmonary arrest. All patients should receive supplemental oxygen by face mask or nasal cannula. Oxygen therapy rarely suppresses ventilatory drive in patients with uncomplicated asthma, unlike the response in patients with acute respiratory failure caused by chronic bronchitis or emphysema. Relief of hypoxemia with supplemental oxygen therapy will reduce the likelihood of cerebral anoxia, ventricular arrhythmias, respiratory muscle fatigue, pulmonary hypertension, or impaired myocardial contractility.

The second objective is to reverse the asthma attack (Table 4.6–2).[10,11] (See Chapter 3.6 for mechanisms, untoward effects, and contraindications of specific agents used in asthma.) A flow sheet that includes physiologic data (vital signs, blood gases, spirometry readings) and drugs administered is helpful in evaluating response and anticipating complications. Sympathomimetic drugs are the first choice in acute asthma because of their rapid onset of action and efficacy.[9] As in the treatment of all types of asthma,

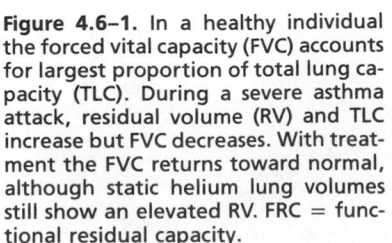

Figure 4.6–1. In a healthy individual the forced vital capacity (FVC) accounts for largest proportion of total lung capacity (TLC). During a severe asthma attack, residual volume (RV) and TLC increase but FVC decreases. With treatment the FVC returns toward normal, although static helium lung volumes still show an elevated RV. FRC = functional residual capacity.

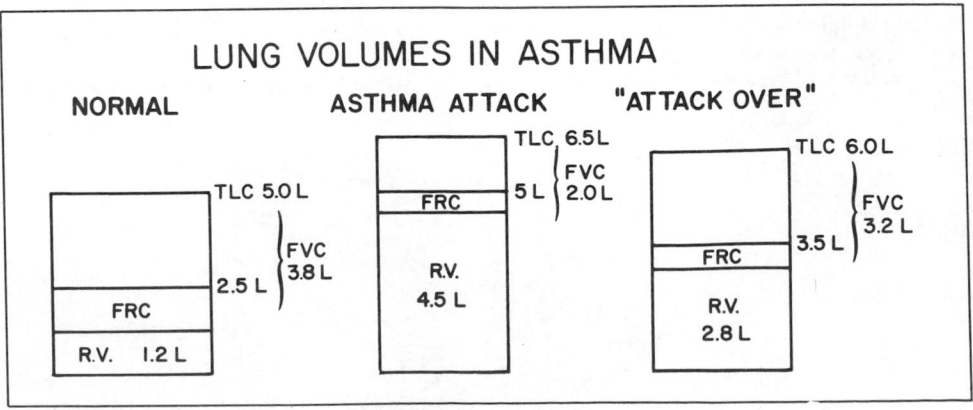

TABLE 4.6–1. SIGNS INDICATING ASTHMATIC CRISIS

History
- Previous intubation(s)
- Recent hospital admissions or emergency room visits

Physical Examination
- Tachycardia >130/min
- Pulsus paradoxus >20 mm Hg
- Accessory muscle use
- Diminished breath sounds
- Absence of wheezes
- Inability to cooperate with tests
- Altered consciousness
- Cyanosis

Laboratory Signs
- Arrhythmias
- Normal or elevated $Paco_2$
- Hypoxia <60 mm Hg
- Metabolic acidosis
- FEV_1 <1 L, PEFR <100–120 L/min

inhalation is the preferred route of administration because it has a lower incidence of side effects. Although patients with status asthmaticus are usually treated by nebulization, epinephrine or other sympathomimetics can also be given subcutaneously. Subcutaneous injection of these drugs is generally safe in children or young adults because these patients are at lower risk for developing severe hypertension or arrhythmias than are older adults, who may have occult cardiac disease. The initial timing of bronchodilator therapy is the same, whether given as an aerosol or as an injection: up to three doses in the first hour (see Table 4.6–2).[3,9] Intravenous isoproterenol (0.5 to 5 μg/min) is rarely used and should be reserved only for those patients who fail to respond to the usual forms of therapy. Intravenous isoproterenol can induce fatal arrhythmias even in young children with normal hearts.

Many patients may be initially unresponsive to sympathomimetic therapy. It is unclear whether this is due to tachyphylaxis of

TABLE 4.6–2. PHARMACOLOGIC THERAPY OF STATUS ASTHMATICUS

Route	Drug	Dose
Sympathomimetics		
Inhalation	Isoproterenol	0.5 ml 1:200 in 2.5 ml saline q20min × 3, then q2–4h
	Metaproterenol	0.3 ml in 2.5 ml saline q20min × 3, then q3–6h
	Isoethrane	0.5 ml in 2.5 ml saline q20min × 3, then q3–6h
	Atropine	1–3 mg in 2.5 ml saline q6–8h
Subcutaneous	Epinephrine	0.3 ml 1:1000 q20min × 3
	Terbutaline	0.25 mg q30min × 2
Theophylline		
Intravenous	Aminophylline	Load with 5.6 mg/kg over 30 min if not taking theophylline; then start infusion of 0.3–0.9 mg/kg/hr. If taking a theophylline preparation, start infusion without a loading dose
Steroid		
Intravenous	Methylprednisolone	40–125 mg q6h
	Hydrocortisone	100–400 mg q6h

the beta-adrenergic receptors or whether beta-adrenergic receptor insensitivity is part of the underlying defect in asthma. Despite the reduced response to beta-adrenergic stimulation, such therapy should be continued unless significant side effects develop, because eventually beta-adrenergic sensitivity will be restored.

Theophylline is an effective bronchodilator and should be used in anyone requiring hospital admission for asthma (see Table 4.6–2). In many patients with severe asthma, therapeutic theophylline levels appear to provide an additional bronchodilator effect in addition to that produced by other drugs. In the patient with a severe asthma attack, theophylline should be started immediately in case the patient is resistant to sympathomimetic therapy. In status asthmaticus, theophylline should be given intravenously rather than orally to avoid any question about absorption. The plasma half-life of theophylline varies greatly among individuals; plasma levels should be followed to provide maximum efficacy with minimum toxicity (see Chapter 4.7, Table 4.7–9). Older patients with liver disease or congestive heart failure may need one-third to one-half the dose necessary to produce a therapeutic level in a young, otherwise healthy patient (see Chapter 4.7, Table 4.7–9). In patients who have been taking theophylline, it is wise to obtain a serum level before beginning therapy and then start a constant infusion without giving a loading dose. If the initial serum level is subtherapeutic, the patient should be given one-half the usual loading dose of theophylline and continued on the maintenance infusion.

Corticosteroids are unquestionably effective in the treatment of asthma. Early treatment with steroids reduces the severity of an acute attack and increases the rate of recovery. How steroids work is unclear, but restoring beta-receptor activity may be one important mechanism.[8] Like theophylline, steroids should be given intravenously, but specific preparations and doses over a certain level (40 mg of methylprednisolone or 250 mg of hydrocortisone every 6 hours) do not appear to produce different outcomes.[4,6] Steroid therapy should be given early, continued for at least 48 hours, and not tapered too rapidly. Patients who were not taking steroids before admission can usually have the dose tapered over 1 to 4 weeks. In other patients, tapering of steroids may require weeks to months. Since inhaled steroids may cause bronchospasm, they are generally not used in the treatment of status asthmaticus.

Although atropine or related agents seem to be valuable for certain chronic asthmatics, their role in status asthmaticus is less clear. The concern over their potential to increase sputum viscosity has probably been excessive; thus a trial of aerosolized atropine is probably warranted in the refractory patient who responds poorly to sympathomimetics and theophylline.[1,7] Atropinelike drugs are contraindicated in patients with narrow-angle glaucoma or bladder-neck obstruction.

Many patients with status asthmaticus may be volume-depleted because of diaphoresis, tachypnea, and poor oral intake for several days. Fluid management should restore euvolemia over 24 to 48 hours. This may help mobilize secretions. Most infections that trigger an asthma attack are viral rather than bacterial. Because studies have shown that recovery from a routine asthma attack is unaffected by antibiotic administration,[5] antibiotics should be reserved for the patient who has overt signs of bacterial infection such as a chest radiographic infiltrate, leukocytosis, fever, or purulent sputum with numerous neutrophils and organisms. Use of mucolytic agents has been advocated and is tempting given the tenacity of the sputum. Although mucolytic agents may reduce sputum viscosity, there is no evidence that they improve outcome. Because these agents may cause bronchospasm in some patients, they are not generally used.

A few patients will not improve despite maximal pharmacologic therapy and will require intubation and artificial ventilation to prevent life-threatening hypoxemia. Clear-cut indications for intubation include an altered level of consciousness, development of a severe metabolic acidosis, a superimposed pneumothorax, and persistent hypoxemia. In less clear-cut cases, the most important factor is whether the patient is beginning to tire.

In previous decades the mortality rate for patients with severe asthma who required mechanical ventilation ranged from 15 to 30 percent.[2] The majority of deaths occurred because of barotrauma from the high airway pressures required to ventilate these patients adequately. The high airway pressure develops because of airway narrowing, obstruction of airways with mucus, air trapping, and the tendency of the anxious patient to "fight" the ventilator. The high mortality rates led to a change in ventilator management in these patients.

Now the primary goal of mechanical ventilation in severe asthma is to provide adequate oxygenation. This is usually easily accomplished with high concentrations of supplemental oxygen. In these patients it is crucial to keep the airway pressure below 60 cm H_2O. Techniques that keep the airway pressure below this limit include reducing the inspiratory flow rate and the ventilator rate while maintaining a long expiratory time to avoid air trapping. Most patients after intubation are so agitated they cannot relax and breathe with the ventilator. If the patient cannot cooperate and the airway pressure consistently exceeds 60 cm H_2O, the patient may need to be sedated and paralyzed to suppress spontaneous respiratory movements in order to reduce airway pressure and achieve effective ventilatation. By using these manuevers, the patient can generally be adequately ventilated and a Pa_{CO_2} in the range of 40 to 50 mm Hg and an airway pressure less than 60 cm H_2O can be achieved. Occasionally, keeping the airway pressure less than 60 cm H_2O will lead to an elevated Pa_{CO_2}. This is acceptable as long as the patient is well oxygenated, hemodynamically stable, and not severely acidotic (pH <7.20). This approach has dramatically reduced the mortality rate in patients with status asthmaticus who require mechanical ventilation.[2]

In severe asthma, unlike other types of respiratory failure, diazepam (1 to 5 mg) is the preferred drug for sedation because it does not have the histamine-releasing properties of morphine. For the same reason, pancuronium rather than succinylcholine is preferred for achieving paralysis of the respiratory muscles. If all else fails, general anesthesia with halothane has been reported to reduce airway resistance.

Sedatives are absolutely contraindicated in anyone with severe asthma unless ventilation is controlled. The agitation that accompanies asthma is secondary to the increased work of breathing and can be considered protective. The most effective way to relieve the agitation is to improve the asthma. Although some physicians advocate bicarbonate therapy for an extremely low pH to restore maximum medication efficacy, if the respiratory failure is not improved the infused bicarbonate will be converted to carbon dioxide which adds to the respiratory acidosis.[10,11] If a patient has severe respiratory or metabolic acidosis, the best way to minimize acid and CO_2 production and increase CO_2 elimination is to begin mechanical ventilation.

REFERENCES

1. Bryant DH: Nebulized ipratropium bromide in the treatment of acute asthma. Chest 88:24, 1985
2. Darioli R, Perret C: Mechanical controlled hypoventilation in status asthmaticus. Am Rev Respir Dis 129:385, 1984
3. Fanta CH, Rossing TH, McFadden ER Jr: Emergency room treatment of asthma. Am J Med 72:416, 1982
4. Fanta CH, Rossing TH, McFadden ER Jr: Glucocorticoids in acute asthma: Clinical controlled trial. Am J Med 74:845, 1983
5. Graham VAL, Milton AF, et al: Routine antibiotics in hospital management of acute asthma. Lancet 1:418, 1982
6. Haskell RJ, Wong BM, Hensen JE: Double-blind, randomized clinical trial of methylprednisolone in status asthmaticus. Arch Intern Med 143:1324, 1983
7. Karpel JP, Appel D, et al: A comparison of atropine sulfate and metaproterenol sulfate in the emergency treatment of asthma. Am Rev Respir Dis 133:727, 1986
8. Morris HG: Mechanism of action and therapeutic role of corticosteroids in asthma. J All Clin Immunol 75:1, 1985
9. Rossing TH, Fanta CH, et al: Emergency therapy of asthma: Comparison of the acute effects of parenteral and inhaled sympathomimetics and infused aminophylline. Am Rev Respir Dis 122:365, 1980
10. Summer WR: Status asthmaticus. Chest 87 (Suppl 1):875, 1985
11. Sybert A, Weiss EB: Status asthmaticus. In Weiss EB (ed): Bronchial Asthma, 2d ed. Boston, Little, Brown, 1985, p 808

CHAPTER 4.7
Hypercapnic Respiratory Failure

Stephen R. Selinger, E. James Britt, and John R. Michael

DEFINITION

The normal range for Pa_{CO_2} is 35 to 45 mm Hg. A Pa_{CO_2} greater than 48 mm Hg indicates hypercapnic respiratory failure, which may be acute or chronic. The patient's history and an analysis of the relationship between pH and Pa_{CO_2} help to distinguish between acute and chronic hypercapnic respiratory failure. The arterial P_{CO_2} reflects the balance between the body's production of CO_2 and the lung's elimination of CO_2, a balance determined by alveolar ventilation (Table 4.7-1). Although unusual conditions such as severe hyperthermia or status epilepticus can result in a transient marked increase in the body's production of CO_2, an increase in CO_2 production by itself rarely causes a sustained increase in arterial P_{CO_2}. The most common reason for an elevated Pa_{CO_2} is inadequate alveolar ventilation. Alveolar ventilation refers to that portion of the total ventilation that reaches the alveoli and results

Patients with respiratory failure can be divided into two groups: those whose primary defect is inadequate oxygenation of the blood (hypoxic respiratory failure) and those whose basic problem is inadequate elimination of carbon dioxide because of alveolar hypoventilation (hypercapnic respiratory failure). The arterial blood gases in a patient with hypoxic respiratory failure reveal a normal Pa_{CO_2} and profound hypoxemia, which is refractory to high concentrations of oxygen because of intrapulmonary shunting of blood past nonventilated alveoli. In contrast, the hallmark of hypercapnic respiratory failure is an elevated Pa_{CO_2}. These patients will also generally have a reduced Pa_{O_2} while breathing room air because of alveolar hypoventilation and, if there is underlying lung disease, because areas of the lung have a ventilation-to-perfusion ratio of less than 1. Hypoxic respiratory failure occurs predominantly in patients with pulmonary edema due to ARDS or congestive heart failure. The diagnosis and management of these diseases are discussed in Chapters 4.4 and 4.5.

TABLE 4.7–1. ALVEOLAR VENTILATION EQUATION

$$Pa_{CO_2} = Constant \times \frac{Carbon\ dioxide\ production\ by\ the\ body}{Alveolar\ ventilation}$$

$$\frac{Total\ minute}{ventilation} = \frac{Alveolar}{ventilation} + \frac{Dead\text{-}space}{ventilation}$$

in gas exchange with the pulmonary capillary blood. Total ventilation can be effective (alveolar ventilation) or ineffective (dead-space ventilation) (Table 4.7–1). Dead-space ventilation refers to ventilation of areas of the lung that are not perfused or are underperfused for the amount of ventilation (areas with a ratio of ventilation to perfusion greater than 1). The excess ventilation is wasted because it does not contribute to gas exchange with the pulmonary capillary blood. A decrease in alveolar ventilation may occur because of a decrease in total ventilation, an increase in the percentage of total ventilation that is wasted (increased dead-space ventilation), or a combination of these two mechanisms. Patients who develop hypercapnic respiratory failure despite having normal lungs do so primarily because of a decrease in total minute ventilation; whereas patients with lung disease retain CO_2 primarily because of an increase in wasted ventilation. In patients with lung disease who develop hypercapnic respiratory failure, total minute ventilation may be increased, normal, or decreased.

GENERAL MANAGEMENT

In the management of patients with hypercapnic respiratory failure, three critical questions should be answered.

What is the Reason for Alveolar Hypoventilation?
The major categories of disorders that produce hypercapnic respiratory failure are listed in Table 4.7–2. In approaching a patient it is helpful to consider the possible contribution of an abnormality at each level of the respiratory system.

Are Lungs Normal or Abnormal?
Hypercapnic respiratory failure may develop in patients with normal or abnormal lungs. Many processes can cause alveolar hypoventilation without producing lung disease. For example, patients with depressed respiratory drive from a sedative drug overdose or patients with weak respiratory muscles from neuromuscular disease may hypoventilate and thus develop hypercapnic respiratory failure. The underlying disorder in these patients, however, increases their risk for developing pneumonia or aspirating gastric contents. In these patients the development of lung disease as a complication of the underlying illness increases the likelihood that they will develop respiratory failure.

One may quickly determine whether the lungs are normal or abnormal from the past medical history, chest radiograph, and calculation of the alveolar-arterial oxygen gradient (Table 4.7–3). Patients with normal lungs will generally have only a slight increase in the normal alveolar-arterial oxygen tension gradient of 10 to

TABLE 4.7–2. CAUSES OF HYPERCAPNIC RESPIRATORY FAILURE

- Central nervous system (CNS) disorders
- Spinal cord lesions
- Neuromuscular disease
- Chest wall disease
- Upper airway obstruction
- Lower airway disease

TABLE 4.7–3. CALCULATING THE ALVEOLAR–ARTERIAL O_2 GRADIENT

Alveolar P_{O_2} = [(Barometric pressure − Water vapor pressure) × Fraction of inspired oxygen] − (Pa_{CO_2}/Respiratory quotient)

Example: In a patient breathing room air with a barometric pressure of 747 mm Hg, water vapor pressure of 47 mm Hg, Pa_{CO_2} of 40 mm Hg, and respiratory quotient of 0.8,

$$Alveolar\ P_{O_2} = (747 - 47) \times 0.21 - 40/0.8$$
$$= 147 - 50$$
$$= 97\ mm\ Hg$$

While the patient is breathing room air, the alveolar oxygen tension is normally 10 to 15 mm Hg higher than the arterial oxygen tension.

15 mm Hg while breathing room air. In contrast, patients with abnormal lungs will have a widened alveolar-arterial O_2 gradient.

Is Respiratory Failure Acute or Chronic?
This question can be answered by analyzing the relationship between the arterial Pa_{CO_2} and the pH (Table 4.7–4).[3,13] Because many patients may have a chronically elevated Pa_{CO_2}, these calculations are more useful in a patient if baseline arterial blood gas values are available.

DIAGNOSIS

Acute hypoxemia or hypercapnia can produce nonspecific but dramatic changes in central nervous system (CNS) function. Depending on the magnitude of the change in Pa_{CO_2} or Pa_{O_2}, apprehension, confusion, obtundation, or even coma may occur. Consequently, the possibility of acute hypercapnic respiratory failure should be considered in any patient who demonstrates a change in his level of consciousness. In contrast to the often dramatic manifestations of acute hypercapnia or hypoxemia, the chronic effects may be difficult to detect. Chronic hypercapnia produces minimal CNS or cardiovascular effects (including cerebral vasodilation,

TABLE 4.7–4. ACUTE OR CHRONIC HYPERCAPNIA

Acute Hypercapnia
$$\Delta pH = 0.008 \times \Delta Pa_{CO_2}$$

Example: Patient presents with pH 7.32 and Pa_{CO_2} 50 mm Hg. Assuming a baseline pH of 7.40 and Pa_{CO_2} of 40 mm Hg, the change in Pa_{CO_2} is 10 mm Hg and the change in pH is 0.08. These changes suggest acute hypercapnia, which has caused acute respiratory acidosis.

Chronic Hypercapnia
$$\Delta pH = 0.003 \times \Delta Pa_{CO_2}$$

Example: A patient with long-standing COPD presents with a gradual worsening of his shortness of breath over the past week, pH of 7.37, and Pa_{CO_2} of 50 mm Hg. Assuming a baseline pH of 7.40 and Pa_{CO_2} of 40 mm Hg, the change in Pa_{CO_2} is 10 mm Hg and the change in pH is 0.03. These changes suggest chronic hypercapnia, which has caused a chronic respiratory acidosis.

Mixed Acute and Chronic Hypercapnia
Example: A patient with chronic obstructive lung disease presents with worsening shortness of breath and a pH of 7.29 and Pa_{CO_2} of 60 mm Hg. Baseline arterial blood gases indicate chronic respiratory failure with a pH of 7.37 and Pa_{CO_2} of 50 mm Hg. The recent change in Pa_{CO_2} is 10, and the change in pH from baseline is 0.08. These results indicate acute hypercapnia superimposed on chronic hypercapnia.

which may cause headaches), whereas chronic hypoxemia impairs judgment and motor function. Because these changes are nonspecific, the clinical suspicion of hypercapnic respiratory failure depends on the patient's complaint of respiratory distress, physical findings that suggest respiratory failure, or the presence of a disorder that leads to alveolar hypoventilation.

Patients with hypercapnic respiratory failure due to upper airway obstruction, lower airway disease, or chest wall disease will generally complain of difficulty breathing. Patients with alveolar hypoventilation due to CNS disorders or neuromuscular disease may or may not complain of dyspnea. Physical findings that suggest the possibility of alveolar hypoventilation are an abnormally slow respiratory rate in an obtunded patient, paradoxical movement of a segment of the chest wall during inspiration, or discoordinated movement of the respiratory muscles. Normally the chest and abdomen move in concert: outward together during inspiration and inward together during expiration. If the chest and abdomen are moving in the opposite direction, this indicates respiratory muscle weakness, and the physician should suspect alveolar hypoventilation and hypercapnic respiratory failure. Confirmation of the diagnosis requires the measurement of arterial blood gases.

CAUSES OF ALVEOLAR HYPOVENTILATION

CENTRAL NERVOUS SYSTEM DISORDERS

Alveolar hypoventilation caused by a decrease in the neural output from the pontine-medullary centers that control respiration most commonly results from sedative drug overdose or an increase in intracranial pressure following CNS injury. CNS abnormalities do not decrease respiratory drive unless the lesion directly involves the respiratory center or is extensive enough to cause an increase in intracranial pressure with compression of the center. Typically, such patients are comatose and have gross neurologic findings and a poor prognosis. Thus the development of respiratory depression in a patient with a cerebral hemorrhage, tumor, stroke, or head injury is an ominous sign.

The respiratory rate may serve as a useful clinical guide for monitoring the degree of respiratory depression because most sedative or narcotic drugs reduce ventilation by decreasing the respiratory rate rather than the tidal volume. The barbiturates are an exception to this rule, depressing primarily the tidal volume. Respiratory arrest in sedative drug overdoses is the result of progressively decreasing respiration over time rather than the sudden development of apnea, the exception being glutethimide, which may cause sudden apnea.

In patients with a sedative overdose, the need to intubate is usually apparent from the clinical status. Patients who are comatose or who have convulsions, an absent gag reflex, or an elevated Pa_{CO_2} should be intubated to protect their airway and reduce the likelihood of complications such as aspiration of gastric contents.

SPINAL CORD LESIONS

Injury to the upper cervical cord is the most common spinal cord lesion leading to respiratory failure. The innervation of the diaphragm, the major respiratory muscle, arises from the third through the fifth nerve roots. The following rhyme serves as a useful mnemonic for this anatomy: "C three, four, and five keep you alive." Injury to the cord at or above this level causes paralysis of both hemidiaphragms, whereas injury below this level does not generally affect diaphragmatic function. When there is spinal cord edema, the degree of respiratory muscle paralysis following injury may be greater in the first few days and the patient may temporarily need support with mechanical ventilation.

Occasionally paralysis of one or both of the hemidiaphragms develops from injury involving the phrenic nerves. Paralysis of one hemidiaphragm usually causes only mild disability; paralysis of

both hemidiaphragms produces severe disability.[5] Patients with bilateral paralysis generally present with dyspnea. One clue to this diagnosis is the complaint that dyspnea worsens when lying down.

NEUROMUSCULAR CAUSES

The most common neuromuscular disorders that cause alveolar hypoventilation and hypercapnic respiratory failure are myasthenia gravis, the Guillain-Barré syndrome (acute polyneuritis), muscular dystrophy, and demyelinating diseases such as amyotrophic lateral sclerosis. The symptoms and respiratory parameters that should be followed in patients with neuromuscular disease are indicated in Table 4.7–5. Deciding whether to intubate these patients is difficult. Some patients may not complain of shortness of breath and may deny distress despite progressive weakness. Thus the physician cannot always count on the patient's symptoms as an early warning of trouble. Particularly worrisome signs are the inability to swallow saliva or cough effectively. A patient who must be suctioned to remove saliva that he cannot swallow is at extreme risk because he can no longer protect his airway.

Serial monitoring of forced vital capacity (FVC) and the forced expiratory volume in 1 second (FEV_1) can be helpful. The FVC and FEV_1 should fall in parallel. A fall in FEV_1 disproportionate to the fall in the FVC suggests airway obstruction with secretions and the need for intubation. Especially worrisome is a decreasing FVC coupled with an increasing respiratory rate. A FVC less than 1 L or a maximum inspiratory force less than −20 cm H_2O indicates severe weakness of the respiratory muscles. Arterial blood gases are not a sensitive index of the need for intubation; that is, patients who are tiring or having difficulty handling secretions may not initially have an elevated Pa_{CO_2}. The decision to intubate is difficult because one does not want to do so needlessly. Conversely, failing to intubate the patient with progressive weakness who is no longer able to protect his airway or take an adequate tidal volume can result in his death. The clinical axiom in monitoring patients with neuromuscular disease is, "If the patient has started to retain CO_2, you have waited too long to intubate." It is important to consider and discuss with the patient and the family the advisability of intubation in patients with an untreatable progressive neuromuscular disease.

CHEST WALL ABNORMALITIES

Kyphoscoliosis is the most common chronic chest wall disorder leading to CO_2 retention. Mild degrees of kyphoscoliosis do not cause respiratory difficulty, but patients with severe kyphoscoliosis often have a chronically elevated Pa_{CO_2} and a long history of dyspnea on exertion. The presentation and management of these patients is similar to that of patients with chronic obstructive lung disease. Hypercapnic respiratory failure develops because of the increased work of breathing caused by the stiff chest wall, the mechanical disadvantage that the deformed chest imposes on the respiratory muscles, and the mismatching of ventilation and perfusion, which increases wasted ventilation.

TABLE 4.7–5. PARAMETERS TO BE FOLLOWED IN PATIENTS WITH NEUROMUSCULAR DISEASE

Worrisome Signs
- Difficulty in handling secretions
- Difficulty swallowing
- Ineffective cough
- Increasing respiratory rate

Worrisome Measurements
- FVC <1 L or 15 ml/kg
- Maximum inspiratory force < −20 cm H_2O
- Elevated Pa_{CO_2}

Multiple rib fractures or fractures on both sides of the sternum may produce an unstable segment of the thorax ("flail chest"). A flail chest occurs most commonly after accidents but may develop following cardiopulmonary resuscitation. During inspiration, the unstable segment of the chest wall moves in when the rest of the chest wall is moving out. This paradoxical motion reduces the efficiency of ventilation with decreasing alveolar ventilation. Respiratory failure develops not only because paradoxical motion and chest pain limit ventilation, but because these patients often have an underlying contusion of the lung that further impairs gas exchange. Patients who have respiratory distress in association with a flail chest should be intubated and treated with PEEP. Initially the patient should be slightly hyperventilated in order to suppress spontaneous respirations. The increased lung volume caused by PEEP will prevent atelectasis, and PEEP and mechanical ventilation will tend to minimize inward movement of the unstable chest wall segment, thus helping to stabilize the injured chest wall.

UPPER AIRWAY OBSTRUCTION

Upper airway obstruction is a suprisingly common problem. The major causes are listed in Table 4.7–6. Patients generally present with fatigue and severe dyspnea. Patients with extrathoracic obstruction, that is, obstruction of the nasopharynx, larynx, and extrathoracic trachea, typically have stridor (a harsh, high-pitched sound that becomes more pronounced during inspiration). Hoarseness, in contrast, indicates involvement of the vocal cords.

Patients with tracheostomy tubes require special consideration. A tracheostomy tube is a foreign body, so when these patients present with acute respiratory failure they may have an obstructed tube. Obstruction may be present even though it is possible to pass a suction catheter through the tube. These tubes may be blocked by dry, caked secretions despite a narrow, open channel through the middle. Thus, an initial step in the management of acute respiratory failure in a patient with a tracheostomy tube is to replace the tube.

Adults who develop infectious epiglottitis usually present with chills, fever, dysphagia, a sore throat, and difficulty handling their saliva. They prefer to sit forward to facilitate breathing. Hoarseness is uncommon. A swollen epiglottis will usually be seen on soft tissue radiographs of the neck (lateral view). Upper airway obstruction in the adult due to croup is uncommon, and when obstructive symptoms develop in this situation, there may be the possibility of a previously unrecognized pathologic laryngeal condition.

Unilateral vocal cord paralysis is usually well tolerated, but bilateral paralysis generally produces significant symptoms. An enlarged thyroid may compress the trachea, causing respiratory distress. An intrathoracic goiter is often not palpable in the neck but will generally be visible on the chest radiograph. Inhalation of smoke or noxious chemicals frequently injures the upper airway, causing edema and obstruction. Patients with moderate to large surface area burns who undergo rapid fluid replacement are at extreme risk for developing laryngeal edema. When burn patients are evaluated, the presence of soot about the face or in the nares or mouth should suggest the possibility of upper airway injury.

TABLE 4.7–6. CAUSES OF UPPER AIRWAY OBSTRUCTION

- Foreign body
- Anaphylaxis
- Infection
- Tumor
- Trauma
- Vocal cord paralysis
- Goiter
- Chemical injury
- Smoke inhalation

The presence of dyspnea in patients with upper airway disease indicates severe obstruction. The normal diameter of the trachea is 20 mm. In healthy subjects the diameter may be reduced to 6 mm before dyspnea occurs, but a further increase in obstruction can lead to fatigue and hypercapnic respiratory failure.

The primary goal of therapy is to maintain an open airway. In a patient with acute upper airway obstruction who is not in extremis, the upper airway should be examined by the most experienced person available, even if it results in a slight delay in treatment. Patients with acute epiglottitis should ideally be examined in the operating room because of the possibility of acute spasm and closure of the airway. In patients who are in extremis, intubation should be performed immediately. If time allows, the patient should be intubated by an experienced anesthesiologist with facilities ready to perform an emergency tracheostomy. Once a patent airway is ensured, respiratory distress is usually eliminated and attention can turn to diagnosis and definitive therapy.

LOWER AIRWAY DISEASE

The major diseases of the lower airways that cause hypercapnic respiratory failure are asthma, chronic bronchitis, emphysema, and cystic fibrosis. The pathophysiology of asthma is discussed in Chapter 3.6 and the management of status asthmaticus in Chapter 4.6. The pathophysiology, diagnosis, and outpatient therapy of chronic bronchitis and emphysema are discussed in Chapter 3.7. This chapter will discuss the therapy of acute respiratory failure caused by chronic bronchitis and emphysema.

Patients with acute respiratory failure due to chronic bronchitis, emphysema, or both frequently have a long history of smoking and of increasing problems with cough, sputum production, and shortness of breath. The forced vital capacity is usually less than 1 L. When these patients develop acute exacerbations, they generally give a history of gradually progressive shortness of breath over several days. The family may also note impaired judgment and agitation. On physical examination, these patients are usually in obvious respiratory distress with an increased respiratory rate, labored breathing, and use of accessory muscles. They also have the characteristic physical findings that suggest chronic obstructive pulmonary disease (COPD): hyperresonance, decreased breath sounds, and prolonged expiration. There may be evidence of right ventricular failure as indicated by edema, a pulsatile liver, a parasternal lift, and the murmur of tricuspid regurgitation. They are generally confused but conscious. Altered consciousness is produced by the combined effects of acidosis, hypoxemia, and hypercapnia. Some patients become lethargic, whereas others are agitated and combative. Semicoma or coma is not usually present unless the Pa_{CO_2} exceeds 75 mm Hg and the Pa_{O_2} is less than 35 mm Hg.

MANAGEMENT OF ACUTE RESPIRATORY FAILURE IN PATIENTS WITH COPD (Table 4.7–7)

If time permits, it is helpful to obtain arterial blood gas analysis before beginning therapy in order to assess the degree of ventilatory impairment. Oxygen therapy should then be started. Although these patients are acidotic and have an elevated Pa_{CO_2}, the initial therapy is oxygen because the major risk is hypoxemia. In patients with chronic bronchitis or emphysema, oxygen may be delivered through a Venturi mask or by nasal prongs. A Venturi mask allows control of the inspired oxygen concentration because it maintains the oxygen concentration constant over a wide range of oxygen flow rates. In contrast, with nasal prongs the inspired oxygen concentration can vary widely, depending on the minute ventilation and whether breathing is through the mouth or nose. The concentration of inspired oxygen given by nasal prongs also depends on the oxygen flow rate. The gauges that regulate oxygen flow rate, however, are often imprecise at flow rates less than 3 L,

TABLE 4.7–7. MANAGEMENT OF ACUTE RESPIRATORY FAILURE IN COPD

- Low-flow oxygen (24% by Venturi mask)
- Search for treatable precipitating conditions
- Nebulized bronchodilators
- Intravenous aminophylline
- Intravenous fluid
- Consider antibiotics
- Corticosteroids
- Replete potassium, phosphate, and magnesium

and an increase in oxygen flow rate can drastically increase the inspired oxygen concentration, leading to depression of respiratory drive. In the initial management of these patients it is therefore preferable to deliver oxygen through a Venturi mask. The only exception is the patient who will not keep a face mask on or in whom the mask interferes with the ability to bring up secretions.

Although high concentrations of oxygen can suppress ventilatory drive in patients with COPD and acute hypercapnic respiratory failure, only a rare patient will have a significant decrease in minute ventilation when treated with 24 percent oxygen by Venturi mask. Part of the increase in Pa_{CO_2} produced by oxygen therapy is not due to a decrease in respiratory drive and minute ventilation but to the effect that increasing PO_2 has on the binding of CO_2 to hemoglobin (Haldane effect). At low oxygen tensions, more carbon dioxide binds to hemoglobin than at higher oxygen tensions. Thus an increase in PO_2 with oxygen therapy reduces the amount of CO_2 bound to hemoglobin, thereby increasing the amount dissolved in plasma. This leads to an increase in measured Pa_{CO_2} of approximately 3 to 5 mm Hg. More important than the absolute change in Pa_{CO_2} caused by oxygen therapy is evidence of CO_2 narcosis or increase in acidosis. An increase in Pa_{CO_2} without clinical evidence of deterioration or substantial decline of the pH is not worrisome.

A common mistake is to suddenly stop oxygen therapy because of concern about an elevated Pa_{CO_2} and the possibility of suppressed hypoxic ventilatory drive.[4,10] If ventilatory drive has been suppressed by oxygen therapy, removing oxygen will not be helpful because it will cause the arterial PO_2 to fall much more rapidly than the rate of return of the stimulus to breathe. Consequently, removing oxygen in this situation exposes the patient to a hazardous combination: depressed alveolar ventilation without supplemental oxygen.

The best way to avoid this situation is to begin with low concentrations of oxygen, for example, 24 percent, and gradually increase the concentration—depending upon the patient's clinical condition, Pa_{O_2}, Pa_{CO_2}, and pH. If clinical deterioration has occurred despite therapy with a low concentration of oxygen and if ventilation appears to be depressed, the appropriate therapy is not to stop oxygen therapy in the hope that this will stimulate respirations but to make arrangements for intubation.

After beginning oxygen therapy, the next step is to identify as quickly as possible any precipitating conditions that require special therapy. Table 4.7–8 lists the most common events that precipitate acute respiratory failure in patients with obstructive lung disease. There may not be, however, a readily apparent precipitating cause.

TABLE 4.7–8. PRECIPITATING CONDITIONS FOR ACUTE RESPIRATORY FAILURE

- Respiratory tract infections
- Systemic infection
- Congestive heart failure
- Pulmonary emboli
- Pneumothorax
- Sedatives
- Gastrointestinal bleeding

Because these patients have generally developed respiratory failure over a period of 2 to 7 days, they are often volume-depleted and need intravenous fluid.

Initial drug therapy should include nebulized bronchodilators and intravenous aminophylline. Nebulized bronchodilators should be used initially every 1 to 2 hours depending on the patient's condition. They have a rapid onset of action, and the effect lasts for several hours. Fewer systemic side effects are seen than with parenteral bronchodilators, and they are effective even in patients who have already been using sympathomimetic drugs.

In the patient who has not been taking a theophylline preparation, a loading dose of aminophylline of 5.6 mg/kg can be given and a maintenance infusion started (Table 4.7–9). In the patient who has been using theophylline, a serum concentration should be determined. Generally a loading dose of aminophylline is not given to these patients; instead, a constant infusion of aminophylline is begun. If the initial serum concentration is less than 5 μg/ml, a loading dose should be administered and the maintenance dose continued. The clearance rate of aminophylline varies widely, depending on genetic factors, smoking history, the presence of liver disease, and concurrent medications. Consequently, it is important to measure serum theophylline levels and adjust the maintenance infusion appropriately.[7] The desirable range for serum theophylline is between 10 and 15 μg/ml. The beneficial effects of greater concentrations do not justify the increased risk of untoward reactions such as multifocal atrial tachycardia, ventricular arrhythmias, and seizures. There are several reasons to use theophylline in this setting: it is not only a bronchodilator but also a vasodilator that may reduce pulmonary arterial pressure and the work load on the right ventricle. Theophylline also appears to prevent diaphragmatic fatigue and speed the recovery of an already fatigued diaphragm.[12]

During episodes of acute respiratory failure, these patients frequently develop multifocal atrial tachycardia. This arrhythmia is often a sign of theophylline toxicity, hypokalemia, or hypomagnesia.[8] Correcting these abnormalities often slows the rate substantially and may restore normal sinus rhythm. If the abnormal rhythm persists and the rapid rate leads to difficulty, verapamil or a beta blocker will often control the ventricular rate.[9] Digitalis is generally ineffective in treating multifocal atrial tachycardia and should be avoided.

Bronchitis or pneumonia may precipitate an episode of respiratory failure. The most commonly encountered organisms are *Streptococcus pneumoniae*, *Haemophilus influenzae*, and *Pneumophila legionella*. Patients who have been recently hospitalized, live in nursing homes, or are taking corticosteroids are at increased risk for developing gram-negative pulmonary infections. Antibiotics are generally used in patients who have clinical evidence of bronchitis such as increased sputum production or a change in the character of the sputum. These patients frequently do not have a fever or leukocytosis. An appropriate broad-spectrum antibiotic should be chosen based on the results of a Gram stain of the sputum.

TABLE 4.7–9. AMINOPHYLLINE DOSAGE

Group	Maintenance Dose[a,b] (mg/kg/hr)
Young adult smokers	0.8 (0.7)
Otherwise healthy nonsmoking adults	0.5 (0.43)
Older patients and patients with cor pulmonale	0.3 (0.26)
Patients with congestive heart failure, liver disease	0.1–.2 (0.1)

[a]Based on estimated lean (ideal) body weight.
[b]Equivalent anhydrous theophylline dose indicated in parentheses.
Adapted from FDA Drug Bulletin, Feb. 1980.

Corticosteroid therapy in these patients speeds the rate of improvement in vital capacity.[1] A commonly used dose is the equivalent of 40 to 60 mg of prednisone a day given intravenously for the first few days. Once the patient has clearly improved, the daily amount should be slowly tapered. Because corticosteroids can contribute to the development of hypokalemic metabolic alkalosis, it is important to use a preparation such as dexamethasone or methylprednisolone, which have minimal mineralocorticoid effects.

Patients with chronic obstructive lung disease may have low body stores of phosphate or magnesium. Profoundly depressed serum phosphate or magnesium levels may decrease the contractility of the respiratory muscles and thus contribute to the development of acute respiratory failure.[2] In most patients with respiratory failure, however, the serum levels of phosphate and magnesium are only moderately reduced. Although slightly reduced levels are unlikely to affect muscle function significantly, it is prudent to correct any abnormalities.

Diuretics play a limited role in the treatment of these patients. The retention of fluid results primarily from the combined renal effects of hypoxemia and hypercapnia.[6] Correction of the arterial blood gases with appropriate therapy will generally initiate diuresis. Diuretic use without appropriate potassium supplementation may result in hypokalemia, predisposing the patient to multifocal atrial tachycardia or ventricular arrhythmias. Diuretic use may also lead to metabolic alkalosis, decreased respiratory drive, and further elevation of Pa_{CO_2}. Diuretics should thus generally be reserved for those patients who have persistent edema despite improvement in their arterial blood gas values. Digitalis is of limited value except in patients with rapid supraventricular arrhythmias or with biventricular heart failure.[11]

Occasionally, despite appropriate therapy, patients will deteriorate and require intubation. Ideally, the question of intubation for a patient with severe obstructive lung disease should be discussed with the patient and family while the patient's condition is stable. Patients who have been intubated have a 3-year survival rate ranging between 35 and 50 percent, and almost all patients with chronic obstructive lung disease who require intubation can be extubated before leaving the hospital; therefore patients should not be denied intubation solely because of the concern that they cannot be extubated.

The need for intubation is determined primarily by the clinical status of the patient rather than by the arterial blood gases. The patient who is comatose or obtunded needs intubation. Patients who are unable to cooperate with therapy because of combative behavior or lethargy should be intubated also, as should patients who appear to be tiring. If the patient's condition is deteriorating, it is preferable to intubate electively rather than to wait until the patient has a respiratory arrest. It is desirable to intubate the patient with the largest possible endotracheal tube to facilitate the removal of secretions and minimize the airway resistance produced by the endotracheal tube. The endotracheal tube should have a high-compliance, low-pressure balloon that will reduce the chance of tracheal injury secondary to pressure necrosis.

Beginning mechanical ventilation in a patient with chronic bronchitis and emphysema may be followed by hypotension. Because of the increased lung compliance in patients with emphysema, most of the increase in intrathoracic pressure produced by positive-pressure ventilation will be transmitted to the pleural space, increasing pleural pressure. The resulting increase in pressure around the heart will in turn increase right atrial pressure, thus reducing venous return and cardiac output. The airway obstruction and loss of lung elastic recoil will impair emptying of air from certain areas of the lung, leading to air trapping. This trapped air will further increase intrathoracic pressure and reduce venous return. Any degree of volume depletion will amplify the fall in venous return produced by the increase in intrathoracic pressure. Thus if a patient with chronic bronchitis or emphysema who is placed on a ventilator becomes hypotensive, the most likely explanation is a decrease in venous return. This can be corrected by increasing intravascular volume.

In patients with severe hypercapnia who are placed on mechanical ventilation, the elevated Pa_{CO_2} should be slowly reduced to a level that produces an arterial pH in the range of 7.30 to 7.40. As a result, the Pa_{CO_2} will often remain above 45 to 50 mm Hg. Overaggressive hyperventilation can result in acute alkalosis, which predisposes the patient to seizures and ventricular arrhythmias.[14]

REFERENCES

1. Albert RK, Martin TR, et al: Controlled clinical trial of methylprednisolone in patients with chronic bronchitis and acute respiratory insufficiency. Ann Intern Med 92:753, 1980
2. Aubier M, Murciano D, et al: Effect of hypophosphatemia on diaphragmatic contractility in patients with acute respiratory failure. N Engl J Med 313:420, 1985
3. Bear RA, Gribile M: Assessing acid–base imbalances through laboratory parameters. Hosp Pract (11):157, 1974
4. Campbell EJM: Respiratory failure, the relation between oxygen concentration of inspired air and arterial blood. Lancet 2:10, 1960
5. Derenne JP, Machlem PT, et al: The respiratory muscles: Mechanics, control, and pathophysiology. Am Rev Respir Dis 118:119, 581, 1978
6. Heinemann HO: Right-sided heart failure and the use of diuretics. Am J Med 64:367, 1978
7. Intravenous dosage guidelines for theophylline products. FDA Drug Bull. Feb:4, 1980
8. Levine J, Michael JR, et al: Multifocal atrial tachycardia: A theophylline-induced rhythm. Lancet 1:12, 1985
9. Levine J, Michael JR, et al: Treatment of multifocal tachycardia with verapamil. N Engl J Med 312:21, 1985
10. Massaro DJ, Katz S, et al: Effect of various modes of oxygen administration on the arterial gas values in patients with respiratory acidosis. Br Med J 2:627, 1962
11. Mathur PN, Powles ACP, et al: Effect of digoxin on right ventricular function in severe chronic airflow obstruction: A controlled clinical trial. Ann Intern Med 95:283, 1981
12. Murciano D, Aubier M, et al: Effects of theophylline on diaphragmatic strength and fatigue in patients with chronic obstructive pulmonary disease. N Engl J Med 311:349, 1984
13. Narins RG, Emmett M: Simple and mixed acid–base disorders: A practical approach. Medicine 59:161, 1980
14. Zwillich CW, Pierson DJ, et al: Complications of assisted ventilation. Am J Med 57:161, 1974

Status Epilepticus

Allan Krumholz and Robert S. Fisher

Status epilepticus is the most severe and dangerous form of epilepsy. Any type of seizure may present as status epilepticus, but generalized convulsive or tonic-clonic status epilepticus poses the greatest danger. Status epilepticus may be precipitated by serious underlying brain disease[1] and can cause neuronal cell damage, permanent neurologic impairment, and death.[7,9,10] Because prompt, appropriate therapy prevents many of these complications, status epilepticus should be considered a medical emergency.

The term "status epilepticus" designates epileptic seizures of any type that are protracted or repeated without recovery of consciousness so as to create an enduring epileptic state.[4] The seizure duration required for a designation of "status" has varied from 10 minutes to several hours, but 30 minutes is a common and reasonable criterion.[7]

EPIDEMIOLOGY

Like epilepsy, status epilepticus is a relatively common disorder. It is estimated that 4 percent of all seizure patients develop status epilepticus, and approximately 5 percent of all seizure visits to hospital emergency departments are for this disorder.

The proper treatment and ultimate prognosis of status epilepticus is highly dependent on its underlying cause. Among patients with prior known epilepsy the prognosis for status epilepticus is generally good; the mortality rate is below 3 percent, and seizures usually respond well to initial therapy.[1,7] For those patients whose status epilepticus is symptomatic of a serious brain or systemic disorder other than epilepsy, however, survival rates and outcomes are poorer, with a mortality rate of about 15 percent.[1] Status epilepticus may be the first evidence of a disorder such as a brain tumor, stroke, or encephalitis. Systemic metabolic disorders, including hypoglycemia, hyponatremia, hypoxia, or uremia may also cause status epilepticus, and these seizures can be particularly difficult to control until the underlying systemic disorders are corrected.[7] Still, regardless of cause, status epilepticus should be promptly treated and controlled because status of long duration is associated with poorer outcomes.[1]

CLASSIFICATION

Appropriate therapy of status epilepticus requires proper diagnosis and classification. Prolonged generalized convulsive or grand mal seizures have adverse systemic consequences and need to be stopped quickly. Less severe or more limited forms of status epilepticus, such as partial motor and nonconvulsive absence status epilepticus, are less damaging and may not demand as aggressive therapy.[7,11] With these therapeutic considerations in mind, status epilepticus is best classified into those seizures with convulsive motor symptoms, so called "convulsive status," and those without motor convulsions, "nonconvulsive status" (Table 4.8–1).

Convulsive seizures account for about 80 to 90 percent of all status epilepticus and consist of several seizure types (Table 4.8–1).[7] Generalized convulsive seizures, as occur in grand mal or tonic-clonic status epilepticus, may be generalized from their onset, but they may also have a partial onset and only later or secondarily generalize. Myoclonic status epilepticus is characterized by rapid, often asynchronous and irregular muscle jerks. This type of status epilepticus, without impaired consciousness, is generally associated with primary generalized epilepsy and has a good prognosis. When myoclonic status epilepticus is associated with coma or metabolic disorders, for example, following cardiopulmonary arrest, the prognosis for survival or recovery is poor.[7] Partial motor seizures, even though convulsive, do not have the severe systemic consequences and poor prognosis of generalized convulsive seizures unless they secondarily generalize. Partial seizures do, however, suggest the possibility of focal structural brain disease.

Nonconvulsive status epilepticus may account for 10 to 20 percent of all instances of status epilepticus. The two major forms are absence status epilepticus and complex partial status epilepticus (Table 4.8–1).[7] Compared to convulsive status epilepticus, nonconvulsive status epilepticus is rare and its manifestations subtle, so diagnosis is often delayed. Presenting manifestations include confusion, speech arrest, automatic behavior, and amnesia.

Characteristically, absence status epilepticus presents suddenly as a dreamlike confusional state, with varying degrees of responsiveness and awareness, reactive automatisms, eye blinking, and facial movements.[11] The diagnosis, once suspected, is best confirmed by electroencephalography (EEG), which demonstrates characteristic diffuse or generalized irregular spike and wave discharges. Absence status epilepticus has been reported to go on for days without serious consequences, so therapy, although similar to that for convulsive status epilepticus, need not be as aggressive.[11] Although absence or petit mal status epilepticus is the most common form of nonconvulsive status epilepticus, complex partial status epilepticus may occur more frequently than previously suspected.[2]

Complex partial status epilepticus is defined as repeated complex partial or psychomotor seizures without recovery of consciousness between the seizures. The confusional state is therefore marked by symptoms characteristic of repeated individual complex partial seizures: staring, mutism, nonreactive automatisms, stereotyped movements, chewing, lip-smacking, and picking movements.[2,5] This form of status epilepticus is also confirmed by EEG, which typically demonstrates focal temporal sharp or paroxysmal activity coinciding with clinical symptomatology.[2] Although the adverse systemic consequences of complex partial status epilepticus are not as severe as those of generalized convulsive status epilepticus, persistent neurologic deficits, particularly cognitive deficits and memory loss, are reported, so prompt control of complex partial status epilepticus is advised.[5]

TABLE 4.8–1. CLASSIFICATION OF STATUS EPILEPTICUS

Convulsive
Generalized
- Tonic-clonic or grand mal
- Tonic
- Myoclonic
- Secondarily generalized, with partial onset

Partial
- Partial motor (epilepsia partialis continua)

Nonconvulsive
Generalized
- Absence or petit mal

Partial
- Complex partial or psychomotor

RISK OF STATUS EPILEPTICUS

Severe uncontrolled generalized convulsive seizures have been demonstrated to result in permanent brain damage in experimental models and in human studies. The risk is greatest when seizures go on for over 60 minutes and cause adverse systemic and metabolic disturbances, which may secondarily damage brain tissue (Table 4.8–2).[9,10]

Furthermore, sustained cerebral seizure activity itself, even without the influence of secondary metabolic derangements (Table 4.8–2), has been demonstrated to alter cerebral neuronal functions such as protein metabolism and to result in brain injury.[4,9] Cerebral injury following status epilepticus principally involves the hippocampal cortex, cerebellum, and neocortex. The more severe effects on the brain are substantially diminished by eliminating or reducing the adverse systemic influences of convulsive status epilepticus (Table 4.8–2). Consequently, to prevent cerebral injury associated with status epilepticus, it is important to bring generalized convulsive seizures under control promptly.[4,9]

DIAGNOSTIC EVALUATION

The diagnostic evaluation of status epilepticus should be individualized and guided by historic data and clinical and laboratory findings. Although status epilepticus is a medical emergency, a careful and systematic evaluation of the patient is necessary before initiating anticonvulsant therapy. While the patient is being stabilized, a concise but well-directed history and physical examination can be performed and screening metabolic studies obtained. A history of previous seizures, drug or alcohol abuse, or systemic metabolic illness such as diabetes or uremia could alter management. In addition, the presence of focal neurologic signs, evidence of significant head trauma, or fever and nuchal rigidity should alert the clinician to the need for urgent diagnostic studies or specific forms of therapy other than anticonvulsants. The neurodiagnostic studies that are most useful after stabilization of the patient include computed tomography (CT), lumbar puncture, and EEG. CT scanning is the most effective method for diagnosing structural brain lesions such as tumors, abscesses, or hematomas. Cerebrospinal fluid (CSF) analysis detects associated nervous system infections or inflammatory disorders. Although mild CSF pleocytosis has been noted in some patients with convulsive status epilepticus, caution is advised before attributing cells in the spinal fluid to seizures because of the frequent association of status epilepticus with serious infections or inflammatory conditions.[1] The EEG confirms the presence of status epilepticus and may be particularly valuable in situations when the presence, nature, or persistence of seizures is in doubt. This would include conditions such as nonconvulsive status, suspected psychogenic or pseudoseizures, and paralysis due to neuromuscular blocking agents.

TABLE 4.8–2. POTENTIAL ADVERSE SYSTEMIC CONSEQUENCES OF GENERALIZED CONVULSIVE STATUS LASTING MORE THAN 60 MINUTES

- Hyperthermia
- Hypotension
- Hypoxia (aspiration)
- Decreased cerebral perfusion
- Autonomic instability (cardiac arrhythmias)
- Hypoglycemia
- Hyperkalemia
- Lactic acidosis
- Myoglobinuria

TREATMENT

Therapeutic efforts in status epilepticus should not be limited solely to stopping seizures but must also recognize the importance of stabilizing and maintaining vital functions during status epilepticus (Table 4.8–3). Initially, attention should be directed to securing an airway, maintaining blood pressure, and supporting cardiovascular function. An intravenous line should be placed. Before parenteral drugs are administered, however, blood should be drawn to monitor glucose, electrolytes, urea, and, when appropriate, anticonvulsant levels. The ECG should be monitored, oxygen administered, and arterial blood gas levels determined. While these measures are being taken, a brief history can be obtained and a screening physical and neurologic examination performed. Glucose, 50 ml of a 50 percent solution, should be administered intravenously. In possible alcohol abusers its administration should be preceded by 100 mg of thiamine because of the risk of precipitating Wernick syndrome.[4] Parenteral therapy with primary or first-line anticonvulsants for status epilepticus is considered if seizures persist after the patient's condition has been stabilized. The choice of drugs for use in status epilepticus is limited to those available for parenteral administration and includes benzodiazepines, phenytoin, and barbiturates.

Benzodiazepines are the drugs of choice for the rapid termination of all forms of status epilepticus and should be given when a seizure does not stop spontaneously within a reasonable time (e.g., 2 to 4 minutes in the case of tonic-clonic seizures). Diazapam 10 to 20 mg or lorazepam 4 to 8 mg is given intravenously with careful monitoring of respirations and blood pressure. Lorazepam is thought to have some potential advantages over diazepam, including longer duration of action and lower risk for causing apnea.[4] Preliminary studies, however, have failed to demonstrate a definite therapeutic advantage for lorazepam.[8] A reasonable rate for intravenous administration of diazepam and lorazepam is 2 mg/min. Because the anticonvulsant effects of the benzodiazepines subside within 15 to 45 minutes, a longer-acting agent, such as phenytoin, should usually be administered after successful benzodiazepine therapy.

Phenytoin has proven to be a mainstay in the control of status epilepticus.[4] The current protocol is a loading dose of 18 mg/kg of phenytoin administered intravenously at a rate not to exceed 50 mg/min. ECGs and blood pressure should be monitored, as particular care is required when administering phenytoin to patients with cardiac disease. Hypotension can occur and is best corrected

TABLE 4.8–3. THERAPY OF GENERALIZED CONVULSIVE STATUS EPILEPTICUS

Stabilize the Patient (0–10 min)
- Maintain airway O_2, sustain blood pressure and
- monitor ECG, intravenous and 50% glucose-thiamine

Stop the Seizures
Primary anticonvulsants (5–15 min)
- Diazepam (10–20 mg IV)
- Lorazepam (4–8 mg IV)
- Phenytoin (18 mg/kg IV)

Secondary anticonvulsants (30–60 min)
- Phenobarbital (20 mg/kg IV)
- Diazepam as a continuous infusion (100 mg, in 500 ml of 5% glucose, at 40 ml/hr)

Tertiary anticonvulsants and therapy (after 60 min)
- General anesthesia
  Halothane
  Short-acting barbiturate (pentobarbital)
  Neuromuscular paralysis
- Paraldehyde (4% solution in normal saline IV)
- Lidocaine (1–3 mg/kg IV at <50 mg/min)

by decreasing the rate of intravenous infusion or stopping infusion and increasing fluid volume before resuming infusion. Phenytoin alone has been used successfully as the initial form of therapy in status epilepticus and may be especially useful when it is necessary to avoid depression of consciousness. Because it may take 20 or 30 minutes to build up effective levels, phenytoin has become less popular than benzodiazepines for initial therapy of status epilepticus. Outpatients already receiving phenytoin for seizure control may be given additional phenytoin if benzodiazepines do not stop their seizures. With status epilepticus, administration of phenytoin may proceed before anticonvulsant serum levels return, because status epilepticus rarely occurs in the presence of therapeutic levels and transient toxicity is more acceptable than continued status epilepticus. The combination of diazepam and phenytoin will terminate status epilepticus in 80 to 90 percent of cases.[1,4] Generally, once seizures stop, phenytoin may be given in a maintenance dose of approximately 5 mg/kg daily, and drug levels should be monitored.

If seizures persist or recur after the above-mentioned measures have been taken, second-line anticonvulsants, such as phenobarbital or diazepam, as a continuous infusion should be considered.[1,4] Furthermore the patient will probably need intubation and monitoring in an intensive care unit. Phenobarbital is administered intravenously at a rate not to exceed 100 mg/min until the seizures stop or a total dose of 20 mg/kg is reached.[6] Diazepam, 100 mg diluted in 500 ml of 5 percent dextrose solution and infused at a rate of approximately 40 ml/hr, should maintain diazepam blood levels of 0.2 to 0.8 μg/ml.[4] By the time these secondary anticonvulsants have been administered, 60 minutes or more have usually passed, a time span that seems to be associated with systemic and metabolic problems that may complicate management and lead to further brain injury. Consequently it is important to attend to these complicating factors (Table 4.8–2) while proceeding with tertiary treatment for intractable status epilepticus (Table 4.8–3).

When seizures persist despite appropriate primary and secondary therapy (Table 4.8–3), the likelihood of a good outcome is substantially reduced. Nevertheless, control of seizures should still be aggressively pursued in the next stage of therapy using anesthetic doses of drugs and neuromuscular blockade. Inhalation anesthetics, such as halothane, or short-acting barbiturates, such as pentobarbital, can usually arrest clinical and electroencephalographic seizures, but these drugs have considerable potential toxicity.[4,6] For example, pentobarbital has serious cardiovascular side effects and can cause direct myocardial depression.[6] The use of these anesthetic agents is best directed by an experienced anesthesiologist or intensive care specialist in a carefully monitored and well-supervised intensive care unit. Neuromuscular blocking agents paralyze and reduce metabolic demands and muscle breakdown, but they do not influence the abnormal brain electrical activity associated with status epilepticus. For paralyzed individuals and others, EEG monitoring may be helpful to determine the continued presence of subclinical seizures. Various other anticonvulsant agents, including paraldehyde and lidocaine, have been advocated for use in status epilepticus, but their efficacy has been less thoroughly documented.

Paraldehyde may be administered intravenously as a 4 percent infusion in normal saline. The rate of infusion is titrated to control seizures. Maximal dosages for paraldehyde are not well established, but caution is advised as a total daily dose of 15 g is approached. Paraldehyde has been reported to cause hypotension and pulmonary edema, particularly when administered in high concentrations or by rapid infusion. Because paraldehyde in high concentrations may decompose plastic, it should be transferred by glass syringes and stored in glass bottles. Paraldehyde may also decompose into potentially toxic products with age or exposure to light, so it should be used only when fresh and protected from light.[3]

Lidocaine has been reported to control status epilepticus in some patients refractory to other therapy. A test dose of 1 to 3 mg/kg IV may be given at a rate not to exceed 50 mg/min. Seizures are reported to stop within minutes. If this initial treatment is successful but seizures recur, a maintenance infusion of 1 to 4 mg/kg/hr may be continued, but a total hourly lidocaine dose of greater than 200 to 300 mg may be hazardous. Lidocaine may cause hypotension and cardiovascular complications, so ECG and blood pressure should be carefully monitored.[3]

If general anesthesia with drugs such as halothane, pentobarbital, or paraldehyde is used, the goal should be to maintain anesthesia at a level that will prevent seizures without endangering the patient. Therapy is continued until seizures no longer recur, and EEG monitoring may be used to evaluate therapy and determine when the dosage of these medications may be tapered. Usually, tapering can be started within 4 to 6 hours of anesthetic induction, but if seizures recur, anesthesia may need to be reinduced. It is important to distinguish conditions that are not true status epilepticus and are unlikely to benefit from aggressive seizure treatment, such as severe encephalopathies with associated epileptiform EEG changes or sporadic focal muscular or myoclonic contractions.

Finally, one must weigh the need for continued aggressive therapy of status epilepticus against the potential risks on an individual basis. During the entire course of therapy for refractory status epilepticus, careful management of systemic metabolic problems (Table 4.8–2) should be emphasized. Furthermore, attempts to control seizures should be coordinated with appropriate diagnostic studies to define the cause of status epilepticus, with special emphasis on treatable disorders that may be preventing control of seizures and contributing to morbidity.

REFERENCES

1. Aminoff MJ, Simon RP: Status epilepticus. Am J Med 69:657, 1980
2. Ballenger CE, King DW, Gallagher BB: Partial complex status epilepticus. Neurology 33:1545, 1983
3. Browne TR: Paraldehyde, chlormethiazole, and lidocaine for treatment of status epilepticus. In Delgado-Esqueta AV, Wasterlain C, Treiman DM, Porter RJ (eds): Status Epilepticus, Mechanisms of Brain Damage and Treatment. New York, Raven Press, 1983, p 509
4. Delgado-Esqueta AV, Wasterlain C, et al: Management of status epilepticus. N Engl J Med 306:1337, 1982
5. Engel JE, Ludwig BI, Fetell M: Prolonged partial complex status epilepticus: EEG and behavioral observations. Neurology 28:863, 1978
6. Goldberg MA, McIntyre HB: Barbiturates in the treatment of status epilepticus. In Delgado-Esqueta AV, Wasterlain C, Treiman DM, Porter RJ (eds): Status Epilepticus, Mechanisms of Brain Damage and Treatment. New York, Raven Press, 1983, p 499
7. Hauser WA: Status epilepticus: Frequency, etiology, and neurological sequelae. In Delgado-Esqueta AV, Wasterlain C, Treiman DM, Porter RJ (eds): Status Epilepticus, Mechanisms of Brain Damage and Treatment. New York, Raven Press, 1983, p 3
8. Leppik IE, Derivan AT, et al: Double-blind study of lorazepam and diazepam in status epilepticus. JAMA 249:1452, 1983
9. Meldrum BS, Brierley JB: Prolonged epileptic seizures in primates: Ischemic cell change and its relation to ictal physiological events. Arch Neurol 28:10, 1973
10. Meldrum BS, Horton RW: Physiology of status epilepticus in primates. Arch Neurol 28:1, 1973
11. Porter RJ, Penry JK: Petit mal status. In Delgado-Esqueta AV, Wasterlain C, Treiman DM, Porter RJ (eds): Status Epilepticus, Mechanisms of Brain Damage and Treatment. New York, Raven Press, 1983, p 61

CHAPTER 4.9
Elevated Intracranial Pressure

Daniel F. Hanley, Henry Brem, Hamilton Moses III, and Mark C. Rogers

NORMAL ANATOMY AND PHYSIOLOGY OF THE CRANIAL VAULT

The skull is a rigid barrier that protects the CNS from physical forces applied externally. The skull also limits the expansion of intracranial contents by fixing the volume within the cranial vault. Normal intracranial pressure (ICP) involves a balance between three separately regulated compartments: the brain tissue volume (1400 ml, 90 percent), the cerebral blood volume (75 ml or 5 percent), and CSF volume (75 ml or 5 percent). The brain tissue volume is protected by the blood-brain barrier. Diseases often disrupt this regulating mechanism and lead to increases in brain tissue volume. Cerebral blood volume varies with the regulation of blood flow to brain tissues, which is impaired by severe head trauma and sustained hypoxia or ischemia. Factors that increase and decrease blood volume include cerebral activity, PO_2, PCO_2, venous return, and vasoactive drugs. CSF volume is the most dynamic of these intracranial compartments. Choroid plexus tissue located in the lateral third and fourth ventricles produces CSF, which flows out around the brain stem and is reabsorbed into the sagittal sinus and the sleeves of the spinal nerve roots. When brain or cerebral blood volume increases, CSF volume normally compensates by decreasing. Two mechanisms are responsible for this compensation: (1) movement of CSF from the cranial space to the spinal space and (2) increased absorption of CSF. Increased production of CSF occurs rarely and does not ordinarily account for disorders of intracranial pressure. Diseases such as hydrocephalus develop when CSF volume is increased because flow is obstructed or absorptive mechanisms are not functioning.

Intracranial pressure normally ranges between 0 and 15 mm Hg. Changes in volume in any individual compartment are usually matched with opposite changes in the other compartments. When compensation for increased volume does not occur, intracranial pressure rises. As is typical of incompressible fluids in rigid containers, small increases in volume produce large rises in pressure (Fig. 4.9–1).

PATHOPHYSIOLOGY

The pathophysiologic consequences of severe elevations of intracranial pressure are uniformly similar despite multiple causes (Table 4.9–1). At high intracranial pressures, cerebral perfusion is impaired, resulting in ischemic damage. Asymmetrically increasing volumes (i.e., mass lesions) lead to intracranial shifts, which usually cause direct tissue damage. These compartmental shifts are described in detail in Chapter 15.10 (see Table 15.10–3). The rate at which intracranial pressure rises is often indicative of the seriousness of the process. Rapidly expanding masses often lead to complications such as brain herniations and ischemic damage, whereas slower processes often are better tolerated (e.g., the expansion over many years of a meningioma). Lesions expanding over minutes and hours are thus more likely to present as global cerebral dysfunction and more slowly progressive lesions as focal deficits.

CLINICAL PRESENTATION

It may be difficult to differentiate common, benign complaints from those reflecting an emergent situation requiring rapid diagnosis and prompt therapy. The importance of understanding cranial vault physiology lies not only in adjusting treatments to decrease elevated pressure but also in recognizing the *clinical imperative* of a patient whose neurologic condition is deteriorating from intracranial hypertension. Here, timely and effective decisions must be made. In eliciting a history the clinician must be sensitive to groups of symptoms likely to be associated with acute ICP elevations. The clustering of historical indicators into consistent symptom complexes makes the diagnosis of acute intracranial pressure syndrome likely. This syndrome should be evaluated immediately and not confused with complaints best managed at a later date.

GENERAL SYMPTOMS

Headache
The headache associated with increased intracranial pressure or intracranial masses is important to distinguish from the headaches of many other causes (see Chapter 15.9). There are certain features that should warn the physician that a headache may be associated with increased intracranial pressure or an intracranial mass:

- Nocturnal headaches or headaches present on arising
- Headaches in a patient of middle age who previously has not had headaches or has had a different type of headache
- The evolution of the headache to a dull ache, present continually, and made worse by coughing and straining
- Headaches associated with altered mental state and/or nausea
- Headache in a child under age 10, unless there is a strong family history of headaches

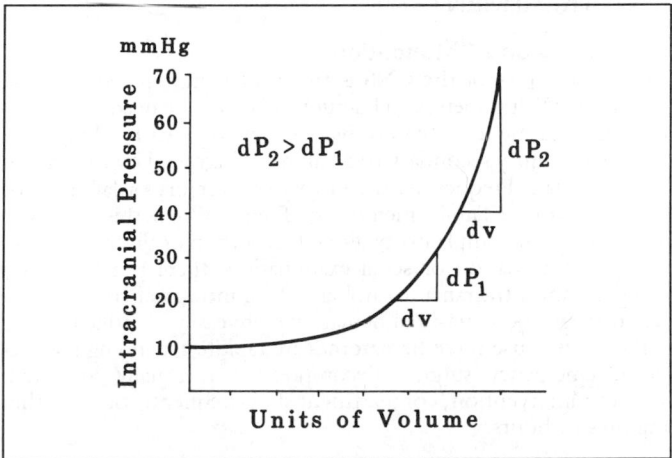

Figure 4.9–1. Relationship of intracranial pressure to volume. Theoretical intracranial volume-pressure curve. As intracranial volume and pressure (ICP) rise, uniform increments of volume (dV) cause larger and larger rises in intracranial pressure (dP). Intracranial elastance (dP/dV) thus increases in parallel with the intracranial pressure during progressive addition to the volume of the intracranial contents. Intracranial compliance is defined as dV/dP, and it changes in reciprocal fashion. Note that dV/dP_2 is less than dV/dP_1. Thus the intracranial compliance falls as the intracranial pressure is elevated. See text. (*From Miller JD, Leach P: J Neurosurg 42:274, 1975.*)[6]

TABLE 4.9–1. MECHANISMS OF INTRACRANIAL PRESSURE ELEVATION

Compartment	Pathophysiology	Clinical Example
Brain volume		
Edema	Cytotoxic or vaso-genic	Anoxia or head trauma
Mass effect		
Acute	Vessel wall dys-function	Parenchymal hema-toma
Chronic	Tumor growth, edema	Meningioma, glioma
Blood volume		
Intravascular	Vasodilation	Hypoxia, hypercapnia, vasodilators
Extravascular	Hemorrhage with mass effect	Epidural hematoma
CSF volume	Obstruction of fo-ramen of Monro	Hemispheric tumor (glioma)
	Obstruction of aqueduct and outlet of fourth ventricle	Posterior fossa tumor
	Obstruction of subarachnoid space	Chronic meningitis, carcinomatosis
	Overproduction of CSF	Choroid plexus papil-loma

Mental Status

The changes in mental state are also distinctive. The early changes may be subtle and consist of lethargy, slowness of action or decision, irritability, and some loss of normal social behavior. These symptoms may be falsely attributed to depression or the effects of chronic headache. In later stages, more significant disorders of consciousness occur. Patients may require stimulation and time to arouse but then show acceptable behavior. Subsequently, they return to somnolence if not stimulated. This is followed by the development of stupor and finally coma. Some patients may go through a stage of irrational hyperactivity before coma.

ACUTE SYNDROMES: URGENT DIAGNOSIS AND TREATMENT

Head Injury and Obtundation

Traumatic injury of the CNS is the most common serious brain condition.[5] With open skull fracture and coma the need for evaluation and treatment is obvious; however, mild direct head injury or concussive injury secondary to a fall may be ignored by the patient and physician. Frequently, the history of an injury or fall must be obtained from a family member or friend. When this history is associated with complaints of altered sensorium or findings of progressive obtundation or serial examination, there is a likelihood of significant intracranial pathology. Both intra-axial contusion or hemorrhage and extra-axial hematomas are easily identified with a CT scan. Because these hematomas are rapidly expanding mass lesions, emergency surgical decompression is usually indicated. Without intervention, compartment shifts frequently occur within minutes to hours.

Syncope, Headache, and Meningismus

Ruptured cerebral arterial aneurysms and other vascular lesions frequently present with *abrupt onset* of severe headache, associated syncope, or near syncope and are followed by milder but persistent head discomfort. The description of severe pain with an onset over seconds and associated altered consciousness accompanied by a faint, fall, or tonic extensor posturing can frequently be elicited in the history. Chronic headache is more prevalent by at least a factor of 100 to 1; thus it is not uncommon to find a patient with syncope or unremitting head pain of several days duration and an un-

usually abrupt onset grouped with patients awaiting elective evaluation for migraine and tension headache. A careful history often avoids this error. Physical examination should include particularly careful attention to the presence of meningismus, retinal hemorrhages, cranial nerve palsies, and other focal neurologic deficits. Any doubts regarding the diagnosis should be resolved immediately by a CT scan. If the scan does not show a focal mass or shift, a lumbar puncture should be performed to determine the presence of subarachnoid blood and to measure spinal fluid pressure. Hydrocephalus or elevated pressure usually requires prompt intervention. A second episode of acute hemorrhage or the more gradual onset of obstructive hydrocephalus commonly occurs and can lead to further deterioration in function as a consequence of the additional increase in intracranial pressure.

Focal Deficit, Obtundation

Brain tumors or any other space-occupying mass lesion can be associated with an initial deficit that increases in severity because of edema formation or hemorrhage, with subsequent loss of homeostasis in cranial vault pressure and a compartment shift and obstructive hydrocephalus. Onset of compartment shift and obstructive hydrocephalus usually takes place over several hours, but both can progress in minutes once the patient is obtunded. The physician usually confronts this situation in the hospital setting as the family or hospital staff observes that the patient is "not himself," is slow to arouse, or is frequently sleeping. Recognition of these symptoms requires a repeated neurologic examination and funduscopic examination. A precise anatomic definition of the process usually requires a prompt CT scan.

Seizures

The onset of seizures (generalized or focal) may be associated with intracranial hypertension caused by an occult mass. Individuals presenting with seizures should have a careful examination for papilledema and focal deficits. A CT scan is best performed with the initial evaluation if a mass lesion is to be definitely ruled out. Status epilepticus is particularly dangerous in this situation, as cerebral volume regulating systems frequently decompensate. The results are compartmental shifts and uncontrolled intracranial hypertension.

CRITICAL CARE TECHNIQUES

The optimal management of intracranial hypertension requires prompt identification of high-risk patients and diagnostic monitoring of intracranial pressure.[7] A patient is at high risk for cerebral injury from ICP when he presents with an acute syndrome, as described earlier, or when he has neurologic deficits from known head injury, acute hydrocephalus, Reye syndrome, or parenchymal brain hemorrhage. The presence of intracranial hypertension is suggested by obtundation, presence of a Cushing response (bradycardia and hypertension), physical findings of a herniation syndrome, or a CT image revealing compartment shift or hydrocephalus. Patients with these findings can be grouped together for purposes of initial management. The absence of these findings does not prove that ICP is normal.

MEASUREMENT

High-risk patients should undergo immediate direct assessment of intracranial pressure. Lumbar puncture is dangerous for these individuals, as herniation syndromes can be provoked. Critical interventions are best made with information derived from direct measurement of intracranial pressure, frequent CT images of the injured area, or both. Pressure measurement is achieved by placing an ICP monitoring device through a burr hole into the vault of the skull. Intracranial pressure monitoring is an emergency procedure that should be undertaken with the assistance of a neurosurgical consultant. There are three types of devices: intraventricular cathe-

ters, subarachnoid screws, and extradural sensors. The intraventricular device is a flexible Silastic catheter that is directed into the lateral ventricle. It measures the pressure of the ventricular CSF by providing an external fluid pathway to a bedside pressure transducer. Its use is indicated when emergency monitoring of obstructive hydrocephalus is planned, and it allows for the rapid and continuous drainage of CSF. Its greatest disadvantage is the risk of ventricular bacterial infection, which occurs in 1 to 5 percent of the patients catheterized.

The subarachnoid screw is a hollow device that provides a fluid pathway from the superficial cortical area (subarachnoid space) to an external pressure transducer. These devices are less difficult to place, do not require manipulation of brain tissue, and are accompanied by a lower infection rate than intraventricular catheters. Subarachnoid screws are particularly helpful in monitoring the ICP of head injury victims who have small or collapsed cerebral ventricles. Their disadvantages include the inability to withdraw CSF. These devices are also less accurate in measuring ICP because surface cortical measurements do not always reflect changes in the intraventricular pressure. These inaccuracies are more evident at pressures greater than 30 mm Hg; thus the sensitivity and usefulness of these devices is not impaired greatly by this limitation.

Epidural devices are disposable transducers placed in the epidural space. The transduction of pressure force takes place at the dura. These devices have essentially the same limitations as the subarachnoid screw. They are commonly used for postoperative monitoring of neurosurgical patients because of the ease of placement at the time of surgery. The device should be compatible with the critical care unit display system so that the ICP may be displayed for continuous observation. Audible alarms and parameter trending devices are useful formatting options for ICP measurements; they are common to the display systems in many critical care units.

Not infrequently a high-risk patient is identified in an outpatient setting without easy access to critical care and CT technology. Such patients are best managed by transfer to the appropriate critical care environment and given concurrent empiric treatment for elevations of ICP. For the obtunded patient without focal neurologic deficits, however, a diagnosis of bacterial meningitis should be entertained. An outpatient lumbar puncture and administration of intravenous antibiotics should be initiated before transfer in this situation.

TREATMENT

Respiratory Measures
CNS diseases often produce mechanical respiratory failure and impaired airway reflexes. Either of these neurologic deficits may accelerate a worsening ICP. Optimal care of patients with intracranial hypertension requires protection of the airway with an endotracheal tube and maintenance of a normal Pa_{O_2} and Pa_{CO_2}. Both hypoxia and hypercapnia produce cerebral vasodilation and are accompanied by rises in ICP. For the compromised cranial vault with poor compliance, these rises in pressure will have serious consequences. Conversely, mechanical hyperventilation lowers Pa_{CO_2} significantly and produces cerebral vasoconstriction. This maneuver can be quickly performed and is effective in lowering ICP rapidly over a few minutes. Mechanical ventilation and PEEP are often required to maintain a Pa_{O_2} of 80 to 100 mm Hg. This level of oxygenation produces a greater than 90 percent hemoglobin saturation, adequate to prevent Po_2-mediated cerebral vasodilation and maintain systemic oxygen consumption. Both mechanical ventilation and PEEP are associated with elevated intrathoracic pressures, which are sometimes transmitted to the intracranial space through veins and CSF pathways. These pressure elevations can be minimized by reducing chest wall resistance with neuromuscular blocking agents and sedatives.

Pharmacologic Measures
Osmotic diuretics act by producing an osmolar gradient that favors the passage of water from the brain into the systemic circulation.[3]

Mannitol and glycerol both function through this mechanism. Mannitol also produces an increased urine output, as it is not transported across the kidney collecting tubules. It is frequently used to decrease the brain volume compartment. Its beneficial effects on ICP will last for several hours, but repeat doses are almost always required.[6] Care must be taken not to produce a hyperosmolar state (i.e., in excess of 315 mosm). Loop diuretics also produce a negative free water balance that is partly accounted for by decreased brain water content. They are best used in combination with mannitol, when their synergistic action improves ICP control. Corticosteroids are thought to stabilize the blood-brain barrier. Clear demonstrations of their ability to reduce brain swelling and improve neurologic symptoms for patients with brain tumors have led to their use in many clinical situations. Their mechanism of action differs from that of diuretics, and they often produce long-lasting effects. Their benefits in nonneoplastic diseases are not well demonstrated.

Circulatory Measures
Adequate cerebral perfusion is a major goal of treating elevated ICP. A good estimate of the cerebral perfusion pressure (CPP) may be produced by subtracting ICP from mean arterial pressure (MAP), thus, $CPP = MAP - ICP$. Maintaining a CPP greater than 60 mm Hg minimizes the possibility of ischemia-induced cerebral damage. In many patients an adequate CPP can be maintained only by simultaneous efforts to increase MAP and decrease ICP. Mean arterial pressure elevation usually requires a pressor to increase systemic vascular resistance and an ionotrophic agent to increase cardiac output.

General Medical Measures
Elevated body temperature produces increased metabolic requirements for oxygen delivery, including an increased cerebral metabolic rate for oxygen ($CMRo_2$). These requirements are associated with increased ICP. Antipyretics and topical cooling measures should be applied to minimize $CMRo_2$. Similarly, seizures represent a situation of markedly increased brain work and $CMRo_2$ and are often accompanied by serious elevations of ICP. Seizures should be terminated with a rapid-acting barbiturate or benzodiazepine. Subsequent seizures are best prevented with a long-acting anticonvulsant such as phenytoin or phenobarbital. For most brain diseases, seizures are a likely complication; thus, it is best to administer anticonvulsants prophylactically when treating elevated ICP. Head position can also be associated with increased ICP. Both "head down" and "head sideways" positions are associated with increased cerebral venous volumes and elevated ICP. These positions are best avoided, even though they do not always produce ICP changes. Continuous monitoring of ICP is helpful in allowing for optimal positioning of the patient.

Surgical Measures
When the primary problem is a mass that can be removed without great risk, definitive surgical therapy should be undertaken at the earliest possible time. In this situation medical therapies should be looked on as vital temporizing maneuvers. External ventricular drainage is a surgical maneuver that permits removal of CSF in substantial quantities. It is a bedside procedure that often is highly effective in controlling elevated ICP. In some severe global cerebral injuries the removal of damaged brain substance allows for improved ICP management. In selected patients the removal of normal temporal or frontal lobe tissue can prevent compartment shifts and ICP elevations.

ORGANIZING THERAPY FOR ACUTELY ELEVATED ICP

The first step in treating acute intracranial hypertension is to identify its cause. For any condition recognized as a neurologic emergency, the general sequence of diagnostic and therapeutic maneuvers is similar: (1) rapid, complete neurologic and general medical

examination; (2) appropriate respiratory and circulatory support; and (3) emergency CT scan to define the value of emergency surgical decompression of the cranial vault. If surgery is not contemplated, the patient should be sent to a hospital where serial neurologic evaluations can be reliably performed and interpreted. Changes in the patient's status should be followed by timely changes in therapy. For patients who cannot be aroused and who have an abnormal motor response to pain, intracranial pressure must be monitored.

When ICP is not elevated, the patient can be observed continuously for transient elevation of pressure. Repeat neurologic assessment should be performed frequently by physicians and nurses. The most commonly used assessment regimen involves the Glasgow Coma Scale and the British Medical Research Council Strength Scale for each limb (Table 4.9–2). When ICP is elevated, immediate efforts to reduce it below 20 mm Hg should be made. The most rapidly effective treatment is hyperventilation. This requires elective endotracheal intubation usually performed with local airway anesthetics, sedatives, and muscle relaxants. This sequence blocks Valsalva and other airway-mediated elevations of ICP. Hyperventilation alone usually controls ICP within minutes, but if it is ineffective, an osmotic agent such as mannitol should be used. Corticosteroids are usually added at this time for long-term control of ICP, particularly when it is due to cerebral edema of a neoplastic origin. For patients with poorly controlled ICP, surgical removal of brain tissue, parenchymal hematomas, or necrotic lesions should be considered. If the intracranial pressure remains elevated (i.e., >30 mm Hg), many experienced clinicians would add barbiturates in anesthetic doses (Table 4.9–3).

The most common complications contributing to persistently elevated ICP are hypoxia, hyperthermia, elevated airway pressures, and seizures. These abnormalities should be treated simultaneously if ICP is to be controlled rapidly. Pentobarbital provides the additional benefits of peripheral vasodilation (cooling) and strong anticonvulsant properties. It is an excellent adjunct to other traditional treatments for seizures (see Chapter 15.5). When the patient's condition is clearly deteriorating in the opinion of his physician or nurse observer, initial medical intervention should not wait for measurement of intracranial pressure or CT scanning. Similarly, emergency ventricular drainage can be effectively performed in the ICU or emergency ward if the situation demands it.

TABLE 4.9–2. NEUROLOGIC ASSESSMENTS TO DISCOVER TRANSIENT ELEVATION OF ICP

Glasgow Coma Scale

Eye opening	Spontaneous	4
	To speech	3
	To pain	2
	None	1
Best motor response	Obeys	6
	Localizes	5
	Withdraws	4
	Abnormal flexion	3
	Extensor response	2
	None	1
Verbal response	Oriented	5
	Confused conversation	4
	Inappropriate words	3
	Incomprehensible sounds	2
	None	1
		15

British Medical Research Council Strength Scale

Normal power	5
Active movement against gravity and resistance	4
Active movement against gravity	3
Active movement gravity eliminated	2
Flicker or trace contraction	1
No contraction	0

PROGNOSIS

Head Injury

Intracranial hypertension is a life-threatening situation. Elevation of ICP to the level of mean arterial pressure for any period of minutes is dangerous and, when it lasts for hours, is associated with poor outcome or death. Patients presenting with head injury and serious neurologic impairment nevertheless have a good prognosis if ICP can be adequately controlled in an emergent manner (50 to 75 percent survival; 25 to 50 percent with good to complete functional recovery).[5] In a smaller number of patients, prognosis is more directly related to the degree and extent of the primary injury and not to control of ICP.

Acute Obstructive Hydrocephalus

The short-term prognosis for acute obstructive hydrocephalus is excellent, but the long-term outcome depends on the underlying cause. For neoplasms the histology of the tumor is the best overall indicator (see Chapter 15.10). For aneurysmal hemorrhage with CSF obstruction, the location of the aneurysm, condition of the patient, and timing of surgery all seem to influence outcome. Some form of shunting is required in about one third of all patients with aneurysmal hemorrhage. The overall morbidity with acute aneurysms is 30 percent, and the mortality is 30 percent as well.

Reye Syndrome and Other Forms of Hepatic Encephalopathy

Reye syndrome is seen predominantly in children, with 90 percent of the cases reported in children less than 15 years of age. Elevation of ICP in these patients correlates strongly with poor outcome. When ICP is well controlled (15 to 20 mm Hg) in the setting of good supportive care, 80 percent of patients regain normal function. In adult patients the causes of hepatic encephalopathy are more diverse, and coma with severe intracranial hypertension is less common. A role for acute ICP management has recently been suggested. Outcome appears to depend on the cause of the hepatic failure and general supportive care.

Parenchymal Hemorrhage

Hypertensive hemorrhage is a common cause of stroke in adults. It produces herniation syndromes and acute obstructive hydrocephalus. Elevation of ICP has been treated successfully with ventricular drainage and surgical hematoma evacuation. The location of the hematoma correlates closely with the neurologic deficits. As in other disorders prolonged ICP elevation is a bad prognostic indicator. The importance and timing of medical and surgical treatment for ICP elevation in this disease remains controversial.

SUBACUTE ELEVATION OF ICP

Headache

Slowly expanding mass lesions are most often associated with focal neurologic deficits, but the associated disabilities may be minor or are inappropriately ignored. Long-standing, mild headache is described as an early and apparently benign complaint by many individuals; however, a more severe headache is often brought out by Valsalva or related maneuvers, coughing, straining, or sneezing. Further diagnostic evaluation may reveal a mass in the fourth ventricular region or a posterior fossa mass with obstructive hydrocephalus.

Confusion, Incontinence, and Abnormal Gait

Confusion, incontinence, and abnormal gait—unusual triad—often present in older adults, appearing gradually over several months. The inability to function at home or at work is the dominant complaint of the patient's family members. There may be incontinence or urgency. The gait is characterized by instability and a hesitancy to pick up the feet on stepping. These symptoms are reversible with CSF shunting if the triad is recognized early.

TABLE 4.9–3. MANAGEMENT OF INCREASED INTRACRANIAL PRESSURE

	Primary Maneuver	How Much	How Long Before an Effect	Time Action	Comments
Airway	Endotracheal intubation				Concurrent continous arterial pressure monitoring with frequent sampling of arterial gases recommended
	Hyperventilation	Pa_{CO_2} 20–25	1–5 min	6–24 hr	May require prolonged muscle relaxants
	Oxygenation	FI_{O_2}, PEEP	1–5 min	Long-term	
Pharmacotherapy	Mannitol	0.5–2 g/kg (IV)	15–60 min	4–6 hr	Serum osm should not exceed 315 mosm Discontinuation may be associated with elevated ICP
	Dexamethasone	≥10 mg (IV) bolus	Hours–days	6–48 hr	Higher doses indicated in patients with beneficial response
		Four q 6 hr maintenance			
Surgical Interventions Craniotomy	Removal of hematoma or brain		Immediate	Long-term	Best performed early Associated deficits may be severe
Ventricular catheterization	Cranial bur hole and sterile catheter insertion	Drain CSF to normal pressure	Immediate	Long-term	Negative pressure should not be used Antibiotic prophylaxis Infection rate after 72 hr
Anesthetic Interventions	Pentobarbital	20–35 mg/kg bolus			Requires cardiovascular monitoring and skilled cardiopulmonary support
		3–5 mg/kg/hr infusion	30–60 min	Dependent on level of anesthesia	

Asymptomatic Conditions

A number of conditions associated with diffuse increases in intracranial pressure often present with papilledema but with no global signs until late in their course (Table 4.9–4).

Large Head

The presence of an abnormally large (98th percentile) head circumference in an infant or child should suggest chronic intracranial

TABLE 4.9–4. INCREASED INTRACRANIAL PRESSURE WITHOUT LOCALIZING SIGNS

- Cerebral edema
    Vasogenic (increased permeability of blood vessels)
        Tumors in "silent" area, e.g., frontal lobe
        Toxins, e.g., lead
    Cytotoxic (increased uptake of fluid by cells)
        Anoxia
        Water intoxication
- Hypertensive encephalopathy
- Chronic obstructive lung disease with hypercapnia
- Chronic meningitis, e.g., tuberculous, fungal
- Pseudotumor cerebri
    Corticosteroid withdrawal
    Vitamin A intoxication
    Tetracycline (in children)
    Addison disease
- Posterior fossa tumors
- Choroid plexus papilloma
- Communicating hydrocephalus, e.g., post-meningitis, subarachnoid hemorrhage

hypertension. This finding is most frequently associated with hydrocephalus, although brain tumors may also be responsible. Less common findings include failure of the fontanels to close or, in adults, subcutaneous collections of CSF when the cranial vault has been breached.

THERAPIES FOR SPECIFIC SUBACUTE ELEVATIONS OF ICP

Pseudotumor Cerebri

Pseudotumor cerebri has multiple causes, such as otitis, endocrine disturbances, and drug intoxications[4] (Table 4.9–4). Withdrawing the causative agent, performing several lumbar punctures, or both are frequently associated with remission. Surgical intervention with a low-pressure CSF shunt is indicated for persistently elevated CSF pressures, long-standing headache, progressive loss of visual fields, or decreased visual acuity.[1] The use of steroids for this condition remains controversial.

Chronic Meningitis

Chronic meningitis is diagnosed by multiple examinations of CSF for bacteria, fungi, acid-fast bacilli, and neoplastic cells. A subcutaneous reservoir and an indwelling ventricular catheter may be required to administer antibiotics or chemotherapy.

Hydrocephalus

Elevations of ICP may be sustained (as in communicating and obstructive hydrocephalus) or intermittent (as in the syndrome of "normal pressure" hydrocephalus). In either situation it is best to obtain clear-cut evidence of intracranial hypertension from CT

scans before beginning treatment. This helps the surgeon match the pressure characteristics of the shunt to the hydrodynamic problem. More important, it ensures that the diagnosis is accurate before an artificial device is implanted; these devices have a low but significant failure rate (approximately 2 percent per year) and a higher rate of surgical complications (from 10 to 30 percent). The prognosis for idiopathic communicating hydrocephalus or congenitally acquired obstructive hydrocephalus is excellent, as ventriculoatrial and ventriculoperitoneal shunts are effective solutions for this problem. Occasional revision of the shunt may be required because of poor hydrodynamics or infection. For the syndrome of normal-pressure hydrocephalus, some improvement in gait and mentation can be expected in at least 50 percent of the patients treated.

COMMON PITFALLS IN DIAGNOSIS

Certain errors in the recognition of increased intracranial pressure occur with sufficient frequency to deserve special comment.

In elderly patients, mental and neurologic symptoms may be ascribed to senility or strokes. Papilledema, although present, is often not appreciated. Subdural hematomas may easily go unrecognized in this setting. This is particularly true for individuals receiving anticoagulants.

In alcoholics, manifestations of subdural and epidural hematomas may be mistakenly attributed to alcoholic intoxication, delirium tremens, ataxia, or peripheral neuropathies.

In the absence of focal signs, gradual changes in mental status are often attributed to depression, agitation, or other nonorganic mental illness. This is most common when the mass produces bizarre behavior rather than stupor (e.g., a frontal lobe mass). The administration of sedative, tranquilizing, or stimulant drugs often further obscures the clinical problem.

Abrupt changes in clinical status are often taken as evidence that the cause is a vascular lesion rather than a mass; however, such changes can be caused by neoplastic and nonneoplastic masses or other nonvascular lesions, usually because of local hemorrhage. When such a sudden change in status occurs, the outcome depends on the rapid diagnosis of its cause.

The absence of a history of trauma may be erroneously used to exclude subdural hematoma. More than half the patients with proven chronic subdural hematoma have no recollection of any preceding head trauma.

Similarly, the absence of fever or of leukocytosis does not exclude the possibility of a brain abscess. A well-encapsulated abscess may present solely as a mass lesion without any systemic manifestation of infection.

REFERENCES

1. Boddie HG, Banna M, Bradley WG: ''Benign'' intracranial hypertension. A survey of the clinical and radiological features and long-term prognosis. Brain 97:313, 1974
2. Cottrell JE, Turndrof H: Anesthesia and Neurosurgery. St. Louis, CV Mosby, 1980
3. Fishman R: Cerebrospinal Fluid—Disease of the Nervous System. Philadelphia, WB Saunders, 1980, p 63
4. Foley J: Benign forms of intracranial hypertension—''toxic'' and ''otitic'' hydrocephalus. Brain 78:1, 1965
5. Jennett B, Teasdale G: Management of Head Injuries. Philadelphia, FA Davis, 1981
6. Miller JD, Leach P: Effects of mannitol and steroid therapy on intracranial volume-pressure relationship in patients. J Neurosurg 42:274, 1975
7. Rogers MC, Traystman RJ (eds): Symposium on neurologic intensive care. In Critical Care Clinics. Philadelphia, WB Saunders, 1985

CHAPTER 4.10
Poisoning, Bites, and Stings

James J. Lipsky

POISONING

DIAGNOSIS AND MANAGEMENT

Exposure to any chemical substance that can cause injury or death constitutes a poisoning. The many problems associated with poisoning cut across all boundaries of medicine. Although the consequences of this fact may complicate the management of a poisoning, a logical systematic approach to all poisoned patients can still be undertaken. The management of the poisoned patient includes the general measures of supportive care as well as measures particular to the poison involved. In addition to medical problems, the poisoned patient may also have psychologic problems that must not be neglected. Measures undertaken in the management of the poisoned patient are listed in Table 4.10–1.

Consider the Possibility
Failure to consider the possibility of poisoning is a common error. For example, in a study of acetylsalicylic acid ingestion, a common poisoning, it was found that in 20 of 73 ingestions the diagnosis was initially missed.[2] The undiagnosed cases involved patients who initially gave no history of acetylsalicylic acid ingestion. Because

this group of patients had an increased mortality, arriving at the diagnosis quickly is important. Poisoning should be considered even when a history of such is not obtained.[9]

Maintain Vital Signs
The cornerstone of management of the poisoned patient is intensive supportive care to maintain vital functions.

Maintain Respiration
A patent airway must be established and maintained. The unconscious patient should be placed on his side to avoid aspiration. A cuffed endotracheal tube will assure a clear airway as well as prevent aspiration of gastric contents. If respiration is inadequate, mechanical assistance of ventilation is indicated.

Treat Shock
Maintenance of an adequate level of blood pressure may prove difficult. In general, shock should be treated initially with fluid replacement and, if possible, by elevation of the legs. If these simple measures fail to maintain tissue perfusion and urinary output, vasopressors are indicated (see Chapter 4.3).

TABLE 4.10–1. MEASURES IN THE MANAGEMENT OF THE POISONED PATIENT

- Consider the possibility
- Maintain vital signs
- Identify the poison
- Prevent continued absorption of the poison
- Hasten elimination of the poison
- Correct or prevent toxic effects of the poison

Watch the Temperature

The temperature of the severely poisoned patient should be carefully monitored and, if abnormal, corrected. Hypothermia may be present with overdoses of CNS depressants such as barbiturates. Hyperthermia may be associated with amphetamine or atropine poisoning.

Consider Cardiac Arrhythmias

The identification and treatment of cardiac arrhythmias is discussed in Chapter 2.9.

Identify the Poison

Although supportive care alone is often adequate management, it is important to identify those poisons for which specific antidotes exist. In identifying the poison or poisons, history, physical examination, and laboratory tests may all be helpful.

In obtaining the history it is always important to consider its reliability. Patients or those with them are often incorrect concerning the number of pills ingested. Pill containers should be obtained if possible. Often the pharmacist who filled the prescription can give helpful information. Remember that an empty pill container may not have contained the medication described on the label. Furthermore, the possibility of multiple poisonings should be considered. For example, alcohol may accompany ingestion of other agents such as barbiturates.

Identification of the poison by the physical examination is usually difficult since most poisons do not produce pathognomonic signs. Certain constellations of physical signs, however, may be associated with certain poisons (Table 4.10–2).

The laboratory is helpful in the identification of many substances. Blood, urine, and gastric contents can all be used. Many

TABLE 4.10–2. COMMON POISONS AND PHYSICAL SIGNS OF INGESTION

Poisons	Manifestations
Atropine-like agents Atropine, scopolamine, LSD, STP	Agitation, hallucinations, dilated pupils, beet-red color, dry skin, and fever
Amphetamines	Excessive activity, argumentativeness, tremors, headache, diarrhea, dry mouth with foul odor, sweating, tachycardia, arrhythmia, dilated pupils
Opiates	Slow respirations, pin-point pupils, euphoria, or coma
Organic phosphates or mushrooms (*Amanita muscaria*)	Salivation, lacrimation, urination, defecation, miosis, and pulmonary congestion
Barbiturates	Sleepy, slurred speech, nystagmus, staggering gait (ataxia) without alcohol odor to breath
Phenothiazines	Torsion head and neck syndrome, oculogyric crisis, and ataxia
Salicylates	Vomiting, hyperpnea, and fever

From Mofenson HC, Greensher J: Pediatrics 54:336, 1974.[9]

laboratories perform "toxicologic screens." The physician must know what is tested in these screens. A laboratory report of a negative toxicologic screen does not necessarily mean that the patient is not poisoned. It may only mean that the poison was not on the screen.

Although identification of the poison may be helpful, quantification is usually unnecessary. In most cases of poisoning, treatment would not be altered by knowledge of the blood level of the poison. Exceptions to this statement are few and include acetaminophen and acetylsalicylic acid. With these, a patient's initial physical examination may not indicate the severity of the poisoning, and proper therapy may be unnecessarily delayed. In the case of acetaminophen, antidotes administered in time may interdict the toxic effects of the drug but are ineffective if administered 8 to 10 hours after the poison has been ingested.

Prevent Continued Absorption

Emesis is an effective and rapid method to remove ingested poisons from the stomach. In the alert patient, emesis can be used in most poisonings with the exception of caustic alkali or small amounts of petroleum distallates. Emesis can be rapidly induced in some patients by mechanical stimulation of the oropharynx. Less rapid emesis can be induced pharmacologically by an emetic such as ipecac. A myopathy secondary to the frequent use of ipecac has been reported in some patients with eating disorders; however, this adverse effect is not a problem when ipecac is used as a single dose in the treatment of poisoning.[12] Apomorphine has also been used; however, this drug produces undesirable CNS depression.[6] Although emesis is generally considered to be the most effective way to empty the stomach, it does not always guarantee complete gastric emptying.[7]

Gastric lavage may also be employed to empty the stomach; however, a wide-bore orogastric tube is necessary if tablets and large particulate matter are to be aspirated. Most tablets cannot be aspirated through nasogastric tubes. If the patient is unconscious, gastric lavage may still be done. In this situation, a cuffed endotracheal tube should first be placed to prevent aspiration.

The sooner lavage is performed after an ingestion, the greater the benefit; however, because some poisons (such as acetylsalicylic acid) may cause pylorospasm and opioids (such as codeine) may cause ileus, lavage may still be worthwhile hours after the ingestion. In the case of acetylsalicylic acid, which does not rapidly leave the stomach, lavage should always be done. Lavage, like emesis, is not indicated for ingestion of caustic alkali or small amounts of petroleum products.

Following lavage or emesis, activated charcoal may be administered. Although activated charcoal adsorbs a wide range of poisons, it is not effective for all substances, for example, paraquat.

Following lavage or emesis, cathartics such as magnesium citrate may be given if ileus is not present.

Hasten Elimination of the Poison

Current methods for hastening elimination of some poisons are forced diuresis, dialysis, and charcoal or other hemoperfusion columns.[16] Before any of these procedures are undertaken, the physician should carefully consider whether they are indicated. The routine use of forced diuresis on poisoned patients is not recommended because this may result in the physician's having to treat fluid and electrolyte problems as well as the poisoning.

Drugs whose elimination may be hastened by a forced alkaline diuresis include lithium, salicylates, and long-acting barbiturates such as phenobarbital. Forced acid diuresis is helpful in the elimination of amphetamine. The use of peritoneal or hemodialysis may be useful in poisonings such as alcohol, phenobarbital, bromide, lithium, chloral hydrate, and salicylates. The clinical course of the patient, such as the maintenance of vital signs, should be the major factor in deciding if dialysis is to be used. The use of hemoperfusion columns may be useful for the treatment of ethchlorvynol or phenytoin poisonings.[14]

Correct or Prevent Toxic Effects of the Poison

In some poisonings, administration of a specific antidote is indicated (Table 4.10–3). Because it is difficult to be knowledgeable about every type of poisoning, one should not hesitate to seek sources of information on poisonings. Poison control centers are often helpful in providing information rapidly. Useful publications are listed in the references. The following sections in this chapter deal with some of the more common poisonings in adults.

SALICYLATES

Salicylate intoxication is common. Severe poisoning may be caused by acute ingestion as well as by chronic administration. The latter form of poisoning can result from accumulation of salicylates due to saturation of some of the metabolic processes in salicylate elimination. The severity of salicylate intoxication may initially be difficult to assess on clinical grounds. Patients can appear to be quite well or to have mild hyperventilation and tinnitus. Hyperpyrexia, nausea, and vomiting may also be present. Coma may not be an initial manifestation even in a heavy ingestion; however, in the absence of other causes, an altered state of consciousness indicates severe poisoning. The plasma salicylate level is the best way to assess severity. A nomogram devised by Done[3] indicates the severity of an ingestion based on the serum level and time after ingestion. Any level greater than 50 mg/dl at 4 hours after the ingestion indicates a potentially serious ingestion. The nomogram should not be applied to chronic ingestions, in which the severity of the poisoning is not always related to the salicylate level. In adults, salicylate poisoning may produce respiratory alkalosis with metabolic acidosis, whereas young children usually present with metabolic acidosis. Dehydration, hypokalemia, and hypoglycemia may also be present.

Treatment is directed at the removal of salicylate and the correction of the metabolic abnormalities. The gastric contents should be removed by emesis or lavage. Lavage may be effective as late as 4 hours after ingestion. Remember, "Don't procrastinate; it is never too late to aspirate salicylate." Alkalinization of the urine can enhance elimination of salicylate; however, in severe poisoning it may be difficult, if not impossible, to achieve an alkaline urine, particularly if hypokalemia is present. Therefore, one should not use the urinary pH to "titrate" the amount of bicarbonate administered. In cases of severe poisoning with profound acidosis, dialysis should be employed to remove the salicylates. Hypokalemia should be corrected with potassium administration and glucose given to correct hypoglycemia. In severe poisonings, glucose administration should be considered even in the presence of a normal blood sugar because experiments in animals have demonstrated decreased brain glucose under these conditions.[5]

ACETAMINOPHEN

Hepatic necrosis and subsequent death from liver failure are the most significant clinical problems following a large overdose of acetaminophen. The hepatic necrosis is the result of a toxic metabolite that is produced in increased amounts when large quantities of acetaminophen are ingested. The amount of acetaminophen necessary to produce liver damage is usually over 10 g in adults. Subsequent liver damage can be better predicted by determination of the level of acetaminophen in the serum. Levels greater than 200 μg/ml at 4 hours after the ingestion may indicate eventual liver damage, and levels greater than 350 μg/ml may be associated with very severe liver necrosis and possible death. Nomograms for assessing the severity of an acetaminophen ingestion based on the serum level and the time following the ingestion have been published.[20]

Treatment of acetaminophen ingestion is directed at inactivating the toxic metabolite or at preventing its production. Although the exact mechanism of action of cysteamine, methionine, and N-acetylcysteine has not been proved, these compounds have been shown to prevent or lessen liver damage if they are given less than 10 hours after the ingestion. Their administration more than 10 hours after ingestion does not appear to be efficacious.

Thus, antidotes should be given as soon as possible, even before the acetaminophen level is known. Both methionine and N-acetylcysteine are commercially available and have no significant undesirable side effects. Measures such as dialysis and forced diuresis are ineffective in acetaminophen ingestion.

LITHIUM

Lithium intoxication is usually associated with blood levels above 1.5 mEq/L. Lithium intoxication may result from acute ingestion as well as from chronic administration. Decreased tubular reabsorption of sodium leads to increased reabsorption of lithium. Consequently, elderly patients who are on salt-restricted diets or taking sodium-wasting diuretics are more susceptible to the development of toxicity from chronic administration. In mild cases of toxicity, there may be nausea and vomiting, polydipsia, and fine tremor of the hands as well as mental confusion. In more severe poisonings there is increased tremor, coma, and seizures. The ECG may show T-wave flattening or inversion. Treatment is directed toward removal of lithium from the body; this may be accomplished by forced alkaline diuresis with careful monitoring of fluid and electrolyte status. If necessary, peritoneal dialysis or hemodialysis can be used; however, forced diuresis may be as effective as either form of dialysis.

OPIOIDS

The syndrome associated with opioid overdoses comprises coma, flaccid paralysis, miosis, and respiratory depression. Pulmonary edema may occur several hours after the first symptoms. In narcotic overdose patients, other causes of coma, such as trauma, must be considered. If narcotic overdose is suspected, then the

TABLE 4.10–3. ANTIDOTES

Acetaminophen	N-Acetylcysteine 150 mg/kg IV over 15 min followed by 50 mg/kg IV over 4 hr and then by 100 mg/kg IV over 16 hr[15] N-Acetylcysteine may also be given orally *or* Methionine 2.5 g orally stat and q4h × 3
Anticholinesterases (organophosphate insecticides)	Atropine 2.0 mg IV repeated as needed Pralidoxime 1 g IV repeated as needed
Cyanide	Sodium nitrate 3%, 10 ml IV followed by sodium thiosulfate 25%, 50 ml IV
Ferrous sulfate	Deferoxamine 1 g IM initially followed by continuous intravenous infusion at a rate no more than 15 mg/kg/hr not to exceed 80 mg/kg/24 hr
Opioids (heroin, morphine, codeine, propoxyphene)	Naloxone 0.4–2 mg IV as initial dose; repeat as needed
Phenothiazines	Benztropine 2 mg IV or diphenhydramine 25–50 mg IV
Tricyclic antidepressants (amitriptyline, doxepin, imipramine)	Physostigmine salicylate 1–2 mg IV

specific narcotic antagonist, naloxone, should be administered immediately. The response to naloxone is both diagnostic and therapeutic. Because naloxone is a competitive antagonist of opioids, large doses may be required to reverse the effects of a large overdose of an opioid. Although the initial dose recommended is usually 0.4 mg IV, much larger doses may be needed. A total parenteral dose of 24 mg in a 70-kg patient has been given without adverse effect.[8] Because the effects of naloxone may last for only a few hours, one should carefully monitor the patient and readminister the antagonist if respiration and CNS depression redevelop. If pulmonary edema develops, it can be treated with oxygen and positive pressure ventilation.

TRICYCLIC ANTIDEPRESSANTS

Ingestion of excessive tricyclic antidepressants (amitriptyline, desipramine, doxepin, and imipramine) may result in CNS depression, anticholinergic manifestations, and cardiac arrhythmias. Although respiratory depression may be severe, patients are usually still responsive to painful stimuli. Cardiac arrhythmias may be life threatening, and prolongation of the QRS complex greater than 100 msec has been associated with serious intoxications.[19] Treatment of tricyclic poisoning is directed at reversing the anticholinergic manifestations. Physostigmine given intravenously may reverse the CNS effects. The reversal may be brief; thus careful monitoring of the patient should continue. Whether physostigmine is able to reverse the cardiac arrhythmias is debatable. Because physostigmine may itself be associated with toxicity, the administration of this antidote should be reserved for those cases in which supportive care alone is inadequate. The use of physostigmine by continuous intravenous infusion may lead to a greater chance of cholinergic toxicity. If hypotension is present, it may respond to volume expansion. Forced diuresis, hemodialysis, and charcoal perfusion are not effective measures in treating overdose of tricyclic antidepressants. Supportive care with physostigmine is usually sufficient.

ORGANOPHOSPHATES

Serious poisoning by organophosphates may be caused by exposure to commercial concentrates of insecticides. Exposure may occur through the skin, mucous membranes, respiratory tract, or gastrointestinal tract. The clinical features result from inhibition of acetylcholinesterase leading to excess acetylcholine. The clinical signs and symptoms of organophosphate poisoning are classified into muscarinic (including increased sweating, salivation, lacrimation, nausea, vomiting, increased bronchial secretion, and bronchoconstriction), nicotinic (including fasciculations, paralysis, and tachycardia), and CNS effects (including coma and respiratory depression). Low red cell or whole blood cholinesterase activity confirms the diagnosis.

Treatment of organophosphate poisoning involves several measures. Prevent continued exposure to the agent by washing the affected areas if necessary. Reverse muscarinic manifestations by administration of intravenous atropine in doses of 1 to 2 mg, repeating as often as necessary to maintain a mild degree of atropinization (dry mouth and mydriasis). Administer large amounts of atropine, even in excess of 100 mg/24 hr, to accomplish this. Because atropine does not reverse nicotinic effects such as muscular weakness leading to respiratory paralysis, pralidoxime in a dose of 30 mg/kg IV should also be administered. This agent reactivates acetylcholinesterase in many types of organophosphate poisoning and may also reverse the CNS effects of the poisoning.[10] Repeat administration every 30 minutes and assist ventilation mechanically if necessary. Use measurements of FEV_1 and vital capacity as a guide to the degree of respiratory insufficiency. In cases of severe poisonings, administration of antidotes for several days or longer may be required.

BARBITURATES

The most serious effects of an overdose of a barbiturate are respiratory depression, coma, shock, and hypothermia. The degree of severity of the intoxication is best assessed by the clinical state of the patient rather than the blood level of the barbiturate. The cornerstone of management of barbiturate overdose is intensive supportive care. There are no specific antidotes, and neuroleptic agents have no place in management. Respiration may have to be supported by mechanical ventilation. Shock associated with barbiturate ingestion appears to be due either to vasodilation or a relative decrease in intravascular volume.[18] Shock may therefore be initially treated with plasma expanders and elevation of the feet. Vasopressors may be required when volume expansion might precipitate heart failure or is ineffective. Hypothermia should not be overlooked. Efforts to hasten the elimination of barbiturates are of limited value except for the long-acting drugs, such as phenobarbital, for which forced alkaline diuresis may be effective. Hemodialysis may remove significant amounts of long-acting barbiturates but not the shorter-acting ones; however, dialysis is needed only in severely poisoned patients with a deteriorating clinical status.

CARBON MONOXIDE

Although exposure to carbon monoxide is usually associated with obvious sources such as exhaust fumes from automobiles without emission control devices, it may occur in less evident situations such as inadequately ventilated indoor charcoal fires or space heaters. Furthermore, the cherry-red flush of the skin associated with carbon monoxide poisoning is not a common clinical occurrence. When the diagnosis is made, the patient should be immediately removed from the source of carbon monoxide and 100 percent oxygen administered. Administration of oxygen will usually reduce carboxyhemoglobin to safe levels by 4 hours. Five percent carbon dioxide should *not* be used as a respiratory stimulant, because hypoxia is the major problem and respiration can be supported by mechanical ventilation if necessary. After therapy is initiated, attention should be directed to the possible effects of hypoxic tissue damage. Cerebral edema must be vigorously treated with hypothermia or corticosteroids. Myocardial ischemia or infarction or both may occur even in young adults; therefore the ECG should be monitored for several days after severe intoxication.

PHENOTHIAZINES

Phenothiazine overdose may produce coma, respiratory depression, and shock as well as extrapyramidal manifestations such as muscle rigidity and torticollis. Respiratory depression and shock are relatively uncommon, although when present, shock is profound. Cardiac arrhythmias that respond poorly to treatment may also be present. Shock should be treated with volume expansion and, if necessary, a vasopressor. Extrapyramidal effects can be abolished with the administration of diphenhydramine or benztropine. Forced diuresis or dialysis does not enhance the elimination of phenothiazines.

METHANOL AND ETHYLENE GLYCOL

Methanol and ethylene glycol are sometimes ingested as an ethyl alcohol substitute. Both produce toxicity because they are metabolized to toxic compounds. Methanol is metabolized to formaldehyde and then to formic acid. Ethylene glycol is metabolized to glycolate and subsequently to oxalate and other acids.[4] Toxicity from both of these substances may be delayed because of the time needed for metabolism. Coma and a profound metabolic acidosis may be a consequence of the ingestion of either of these substances. Chemical analysis of the blood is useful in distinguishing between the two

substances. Additionally, methanol may be associated with dilation of the pupils. Oxalate crystals may sometimes be found in the urine if ethylene glycol is ingested. Bicarbonate administration is used to correct the metabolic acidosis.

Hemodialysis is effective in the removal of both methanol and ethylene glycol, as well as their toxic metabolites. In methanol intoxication a serum concentration of 50 mg/dl methanol or, perhaps more important, 20 mg/dl formate indicates the need for dialysis.[11] In any clinically severe ethylene glycol poisoning, dialysis should be instituted. With either poisoning it is urgent that treatment prevent the formation of toxic metabolites. The initial metabolic pathway for these alcohols involves the enzyme alcohol dehydrogenase. Because ethanol is a more avid substrate for this enzyme than either methanol or ethylene glycol, ethanol administration is able to block the metabolism of these alcohols. An ethanol level of 100 mg/dl should be maintained; this level is achieved by a loading dose of 0.6 g/kg ethanol followed by approximately 100 mg/kg/hr by continuous intravenous infusion. Ethanol should be infused until the blood is cleared of methanol or ethylene glycol.

BITES AND STINGS

ARACHNID BITES

Only a few species of spiders have toxic bites that cause problems for humans. Unless the bite is observed or the spider found, the diagnosis may be difficult to make. The most common spider bite of medical consequence in the United States is that of the black widow, *Latrodectus* genus, which inhabits dry and dark places. The venom of *Latrodectus* contains neurotoxins that cause the release of acetylcholine. The clinical picture includes painful muscle rigidity along with increased cholinergic manifestations such as perspiration and salivation. Treatment includes supportive care. Muscle rigidity may respond to infusion of 10 percent calcium gluconate or intravenous diazepam. In cases of severe symptoms, antivenin may be used after the lack of sensitivity to horse serum has been determined.

The brown recluse spider, *Loxosceles reclusa*, which is found indoors as well as outside, has a cytotoxic multicomponent venom. Although most bites by this spider may be innocuous, severe tissue necrosis can occur at the site of the bite, and more rarely, a systemic reaction may occur from intravascular hemolysis and coagulation. Treatment of this spider bite is controversial; the use of steroids or local excision of the wound has been advocated. Although neither therapy has been definitely proved effective, steroids have been suggested for the treatment of systemic reactions.[1]

Reports of stings by scorpions are rare in the United States. Most bites occur on the hand. Toxicity is manifested by increased cholinergic as well as adrenergic activity. Treatment is supportive care, although propranolol may be used for countering hypertension and tachycardia.

SNAKE BITES

The poisonous snakes of the United States are in the pit-viper family (such as rattlesnakes, copperheads, and cottonmouths) and the coral snakes. Snake venoms are complex mixtures of substances that can produce various combinations of neurologic and cytotoxic effects. It is important to realize that not all snake bites lead to envenomation. The failure to develop edema at the site of the bite within an hour may indicate that envenomation has not occurred. The cornerstone in the management of snake bites is the rapid administration of antivenin—within 2 hours after the bite. Prior to the administration of antivenin, local incision and suction may be helpful if performed within the first 15 minutes. There does not appear to be any role for fasciotomies in the treatment of snake bite.[17]

STINGS

The most important toxicity associated with stings of the Hymenoptera (bees, hornets, yellow jackets, and wasps) is that of anaphylaxis. Various systemic reactions occur in response to Hymenoptera venom in about 0.5 percent of the population. Such reactions vary in severity from urticaria and pruritus to laryngeal edema, bronchospasm, and shock. Although there may be cross reactivity to antigens in the venom of yellow jackets and hornets, the venom of honeybees appears to be antigenically distinct. Anaphylaxis may also result from the sting of the ant (*Solenopsis* genus). Treatment of anaphylaxis to stings involves the careful removal of the stinger so as not to cause further injection of venom, and the administration of aqueous epinephrine, 1:1000, 0.2 to 0.5 ml, subcutaneously. For stings on an extremity, 0.1 to 0.2 ml of the epinephrine should be injected into the site of the sting and a tourniquet applied to prevent venous and lymphatic drainage from the site. In the presence of shock, 1.0 ml of 1:10,000 epinephrine may be given slowly intravenously. This dose may need to be repeated every 15 minutes. Endotracheal intubation may be needed for laryngeal edema. Persistence of shock may require treatment with fluids and vasopressors. If bronchial constriction has not responded to epinephrine, intravenous aminophylline may be useful.[13] Steroids are not an effective treatment for acute anaphylaxis. For those who have suffered systemic reactions to stings it is advisable to carry epinephrine autoinjectors that allow emergency self-treatment. Desensitization to venom may also be useful although the need for booster injections in some may be life-long.

REFERENCES

1. Anderson PC: Necrotizing spider bites. Am Family Practice 26:198, 1982
2. Anderson RJ, Potts DE, et al: Unrecognized adult salicylate intoxication. Ann Intern Med 85:745, 1976
3. Done AK: Salicylate intoxication: Significance of measurements of salicylate in blood in cases of acute ingestion. Pediatrics 26:800, 1960
4. Gabow PA, Clay K, et al: Organic acids in ethylene glycol intoxication. Ann Intern Med 105:16, 1986
5. Hill JB: Salicylate intoxication. N Engl J Med 288:1110, 1973
6. MacLean WC: A comparison of ipecac syrup and apomorphine in the immediate treatment of ingestion of poisons. J Pediatr 82:121, 1973
7. Matthew H: Gastric aspiration and lavage. Clin Toxicol 3:179, 1970
8. Matthew H, Lawson AAN: Opium alkaloids and morphine derivatives. In Treatment of Common Acute Poisonings, 3d ed. Edinburgh, Churchill Livingstone, 1975, p 138
9. Mofenson HC, Greensher J: The unknown poison. Pediatrics 54:336, 1974
10. Nambia T, Nolte C, et al: Poisonings due to organophosphate insecticides. Am J Med 50:475, 1971
11. Osterloh JD, Pond SM, et al: Serum formate concentrations in methanol intoxication as a criterion for hemodialysis. Ann Intern Med 104:200, 1986
12. Palmer EP, Guay AT: Reversible myopathy secondary to abuse of ipecac in patients with major eating disorders. N Engl J Med 313:1457, 1985
13. Patterson R, Valentine M: Anaphylaxis and related allergic emergencies including reactions due to insect stings. JAMA 248:2632, 1982
14. Pond S, Rosenberg J, et al: Pharmacokinetics of haemoperfusion for drug overdose. Clin Pharmacol 4:329, 1979
15. Prescott LF, Illingworth RN, et al: Intravenous N-acetylcysteine: The treatment of choice for paracetamol poisoning. Br Med J 2:1097, 1979
16. Rosenbaum JL (ed): Clinical aspects of hemoperfusion for intoxication. Clin Toxicol 17:493, 1980
17. Russell FE: Rattlesnake bite. JAMA 245:1579, 1981
18. Shubin H, Weil MN: The mechanism of shock following suicidal doses of barbiturates, narcotics, and tranquilizer drugs, with observations on the effects of treatment. Am J Med 38:853, 1965
19. Spiker DG, Weiss AN, et al: Tricyclic antidepressant overdose: Clinical presentation of plasma levels. Clin Pharmacol Ther 18:539, 1975
20. Symposium on paracetamol and the liver. J Int Med Res 4 (Suppl 4): 1976

Hypothermia and Hyperthermia

Keith T. Sivertson

BODY TEMPERATURE REGULATION

The ability of human beings to live anywhere in the world depends on their ability to regulate body temperature. Under temperate conditions, body temperature reflects the balance between heat production and heat loss. When subjected to thermal stress, emergency measures such as shivering and sweating are employed. If these emergency measures are overwhelmed, body temperature is altered outside the optimum range for physiologic function, and the performance of organ systems deteriorates.

Temperature regulation is centered in the brain, with two distinct control systems operating. The first, a perceptual-behavioral system, relies on cognitive manipulation of information provided by skin thermoreceptors. Thermal stress is then avoided by seeking shelter or adjusting clothing. The second control system is centered in the anterior hypothalamus. Central blood temperature receptors in the hypothalamus and peripheral skin thermoreceptors provide information about the temperature of the "core" (i.e., the temperature of the blood exiting the heart and flowing to the brain and other viscera), and the "shell" (i.e., the temperature of the skin and superficial blood in the trunk and extremities). The hypothalamus responds to maintain core temperature.

The anterior hypothalamus acts as the main "thermostat" in humans. Sensitivity of central thermoreceptors in the hypothalamus is about ±0.2C. The "set-point" of this hypothalamic thermostat can be affected by CNS disease or pyrogens. When affected by pyrogens, the hypothalamus defends a new set-point in the same way it defends normal temperature.

Efferent output from the hypothalamus is delivered by direct neural pathways or catecholamine release by the adrenal medulla. Vasomotor responses can alter skin blood flow 20-fold or more, adjusting the temperature at the air-skin interface. Thus the skin and extremities (the "shell") are the route of primary heat exchange. Vasodilation, panting, and, with more intense heat stress, sweating are adjustments to improve heat loss. With cold stress, peripheral vasoconstriction is the primary conservative response. Heat production may be increased by "nonshivering thermogenesis," an increase in metabolic rate mediated by norepinephrine release. In severe cold stress, shivering can for short periods increase heat production by an amount similar to that produced by maximum exercise. Shivering results from alternating contractions of opposing striated muscle groups producing no gross movement. Shivering is controlled by the hypothalamus and also involves a spinal reflex.

Heat exchange at the air-skin interface involves several physical mechanisms:

Radiation may contribute to heat gain or loss depending on the temperature of the environment and the presence of radiant heat sources. Radiation of heat to a relatively cooler environment accounts for 65 percent of heat loss. The presence of large radiant heat loads (e.g., sun, blast furnaces, large engines) may result in heat gain.

Convection by cooling air currents accounts for 15 percent of heat loss but can result in heat gain in very hot conditions (e.g., in a desert with high air movement).

Conduction by contact with a warmer or cooler object usually produces little heat exchange. Conduction may be the principal route of heat exchange in a person immersed in a fluid.

Evaporation such as sweating or "insensible" water loss from the skin and lungs may contribute to 20 percent of cooling at rest.

Sweating and evaporation account for the majority of heat loss when ambient temperatures are 95F (35C) and above. Humidity profoundly reduces the body's ability to cool itself by sweating. At a relative humidity above 75 percent, evaporation decreases; above 90 percent, evaporation virtually ceases. Sweat that does not evaporate but that simply drips from the skin contributes insignificantly to heat loss.

Inadequacy of thermoregulatory responses and the perceptual-behavior control system precipitates elevation or depression of core temperature, causing dysfunction of other organs, manifested as the clinical syndromes of hypothermia and hyperthermia.

HYPOTHERMIA

Hypothermia is arbitrarily defined as a core temperature of less than 35C (95.5F). Severe hypothermia is a core body temperature below 32C (90F). Changes with mild hypothermia (32 to 35 degrees) are a result of the body's physiologic attempt to maintain a normal temperature. Below 32C, however, abnormalities occur, resulting from the effects of cooling on body functions.[1,5] The numerous causes of hypothermia are listed in Table 4.11–1. The most common type is that of "urban hypothermia," which refers to chronic cooling in a debilitated person who is exposed to the weather. Alcohol and drug intoxication, stroke, extremes of age, and injury are frequent predisposing factors.

DIAGNOSIS

Recognition of hypothermia is theoretically simple, requiring only the use of a low-reading thermometer or thermistor. Because the patient with hypothermia can present with a broad spectrum of symptoms (Table 4.11–2), however, the possibility of hypothermia may be easily overlooked in the patient who is confused, hypotensive, bradycardic, or in ventricular fibrillation. Standard glass thermometers do not detect temperatures below 95.5F, require minutes to equilibrate, and must be shaken down between readings. Although special low-reading glass thermometers exist, the most practical method for following core temperature is an electronic thermistor placed 15 cm into the rectum. Although rectal temperatures typically lag 1 to 2 degrees behind midesophageal temperatures during cooling and rewarming, measuring rectal temperature is more practical than measuring esophageal temperature. Recognition of hypothermia depends on clinical suspicion and realization that hypothermia can occur with ambient air temperatures as high as 50F or even warmer if the patient is immobile, wet, or has other predisposing factors.

TREATMENT

Successful treatment of the hypothermic patient depends on accurate measurement of the patient's core temperature and determination of the circumstances of the cold exposure. The patient whose core temperature has been lowered over hours is likely to have exhausted compensatory mechanisms that maintain body temperature and is likely to be hypoglycemic, volume depleted, and acidotic.

As body core temperature falls, myocardial contractility, heart rate, and cardiac output decline faster than do the metabolic needs

TABLE 4.11–1. HYPOTHERMIA: CLINICAL SETTINGS[6]

Controlled (Induced)
- Treatment of hypermetabolic states
- Deep hypothermia for surgery

Accidental
- Environmental exposure
- Cold water immersion

Metabolic
- Hypothyroidism
- Hypoglycemia
- Hypopituitarism
- Hypoadrenalism

Hypothalamic and CNS Dysfunction
- Anorexia nervosa
- Shapiro syndrome (agenesis of corpus callosum)
- Spontaneous periodic hypothermia
- Tumor
- Wernicke encephalopathy
- Cerebrovascular disease
- Head trauma
- Spinal cord transection

Drug-induced
- Ethanol
- Barbiturates
- Phenothiazines
- General anesthetics

Dermal Dysfunction
- Erythrodermas
- Burns

Sepsis

Protein-calorie Malnutrition

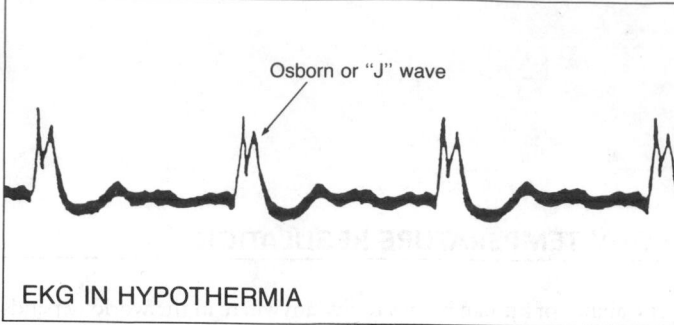

EKG IN HYPOTHERMIA

Figure 4.11–1. Electrocardiogram showing the J wave of hypothermia.

of the peripheral tissues. Respiratory rate decreases as well. Acidosis is thus frequently both respiratory and metabolic in origin. Myocardial electrical conduction is slowed before or at the same time as a myocardial contractility decreases. Electrocardiographic abnormalities include prolongation of PR and QT intervals and the QRS complex. The T-wave vector may be shifted and the terminal vector of the QRS complex altered, producing the J or Osborn wave[4] (Fig. 4.11–1). The Osborn wave typically appears at core temperatures of 32C to 33C, and its amplitude increases at temperatures below 30C. The exact cause of the Osborn wave is unknown, although it has been variously interpreted as reflecting anoxia, acidosis, or injury current. The Osborn wave is highly suggestive of hypothermia, although it may appear in subarachnoid hemorrhage without hypothermia.[4] Profoundly hypothermic patients typically have marked myocardial irritability. Because many therapeutic interventions have been reported to precipitate ventricular fibrillation, the patient should be manipulated as little as possible while receiving supportive care during rewarming.

The basic tenets of initial care are to avoid precipitating ventricular fibrillation, prevent further cooling, begin volume expansion, and treat hypoglycemia (if present). Active rewarming of the hypothermic patient should not be started in the field, except in the rapidly cooled and mildly hypothermic patient (core temper-

TABLE 4.11–2. CLINICAL FINDINGS IN HYPOTHERMIA

Confusion	32C
Pupils dilate	30C
Increased myocardial irritability	<30C
Coma	28C
EEG flat	20C
Asystole	15C

ature >32C), so as to avoid the danger of peripheral vasodilation caused by warming the extremities before warming the core. These dangers include rewarming shock and after-drop. Rewarming shock develops because of inadequate volume replacement combined with declining peripheral vascular resistance. After-drop refers to a continued fall in the core temperautre when cool blood from the extremities returns to the core. Concomitantly frostbitten extremities should not be rewarmed in the field. Tissue loss from thawing and refreezing is greater than from prolonged freezing alone.

Profoundly hypothermic patients may appear dead yet may have complete neurologic recovery if managed properly. Chest compression (see Chapter 4.2) should be begun in patients with ventricular fibrillation, asystole, or bradycardia without a palpable carotid pulse. Although chest compression may trigger ventricular fibrillation in a bradycardic patient, CPR must be started if a pulse is not felt.

On arrival in the hospital emergency department, appropriate supportive care must be rapidly undertaken (Table 4.11–3). Endotracheal intubation is indicated in those patients who are not breathing or do not have a gag reflex. Ventilation with oxygen before intubation prevents hypoxemia and reduces the risk of ventricular fibrillation during intubation. Arterial blood gas (ABG) values must be corrected for the effect of temperature (Table 4.11–4). The avoidance of respiratory or metabolic alkalosis appears to be important in preventing ventricular fibrillation. Fifty percent dextrose in water (50 to 100 ml IV) and thiamine (100 mg IV) should be routinely given because of the possibility of hypoglycemia or thiamine deficiency. Naloxone (2 mg IV) should be administered to the confused or unconscious patient to rule out concomitant narcotic overdose. Other drug therapy, especially in the patient with a core temperature of less than 30C, should be avoided. Insulin and antiarrhythmic drugs are typically ineffective in patients with a core temperature less than 30C. As the patient rewarms, insulin may become active and cause hypoglycemia. Antiarrhythmic drugs are unlikely to be effective below 30C, and the primary therapy of ventricular tachycardia or fibrillation is core rewarming and synchronized cardioversion or defibrillation.[1]

For the mildly hypothermic patient (>32C), passive rewarming may be adequate and attention should be directed to identifying associated illnesses or injuries. For the profoundly hypothermic patient, active rewarming is critical to survival. After supportive measures have begun, active rewarming measures should be started (Table 4.11–5). All patients should receive warmed (45C) humidified oxygen at a concentration of 50 percent or greater. All intravenous fluids should be warmed to 45C. Additional rewarming measures should be chosen based on the patient's temperature, other clinical factors (ventricular fibrillation, asystole), and the ability of the method to deliver heat to the patient (Table 4.11–6).

Emergency cardiopulmonary bypass through femoral arterial and venous cannulae is perhaps the method of choice for warming a patient with a nonperfusing cardiac rhythm or asystole.[2] Dual peritoneal dialysis catheters allow the exchange each hour of 4 to

TABLE 4.11-3. MANAGEMENT OF SEVERE HYPOTHERMIA: HOSPITAL CARE

1. Examine for and treat:
   - Airway obstruction
   - Bleeding
   - Head and neck trauma
2. Remove clothes
3. Vital signs, rectal temperature, and cardiac monitor
4. At least two large-bore IV
   - Administer: $D_{50}W$ (50–100 ml), thiamine (100 mg), naloxone (2 mg)
     IV fluid at 45C (titrate rate to vital signs and urine output)
   - Draw blood for: CBC, electrolytes, BUN, glucose
     Arterial blood gases corrected for temperature
5. Warm humidified O_2 (45C) 50–100% by face mask at 4 L/min
   Endotracheal intubation if necessary
   Do not overventilate
6. 12-lead ECG followed by continuous monitoring of the rhythm
7. Insert Foley catheter
8. Begin active core rewarming of the torso
9. Sodium bicarbonate should be used only for pH ≤ 7.2 (0.5–1.0 mEq/kg IV over 30–60 min).
10. Insulin should be given only if blood glucose is consistently over 400 mg/dl and temperature ≥30C
11. Chest radiograph, CPK, liver function tests, amylase, thyroid function tests, urine and blood for toxicology, lumbar puncture if indicated
12. Repeat arterial blood gas monitoring, glucose, and K^+ with each rise of 2C–3C
13. If extremities are frozen on arrival, keep them frozen until torso is warmed; then warm them rapidly
14. Continue cardiac and temperature monitoring for at least 24 hr after achieving normothermia
15. Follow-up chest radiograph

TABLE 4.11-5. REWARMING METHODS FOR HYPOTHERMIA

Passive Rewarming
- Removal from environmental exposure
- Insulating material (e.g., blankets)

Active External Rewarming
- Specially designed devices for trunk rewarming (circulated water jacket)
- Electric blankets
- Immersion in heated water

Active Core Rewarming
- Inhalation rewarming
- Warmed IV fluids
- Extracorporeal blood rewarming
- Hemodialysis
- Peritoneal dialysis
- Bladder irrigation
- Intragastric balloon
- Colonic irrigation
- Mediastinal irrigation via thoracotomy

a penicillinase-resistant penicillin or vancomycin, combined with an aminoglycoside, such as gentamycin, tobramycin or amikacin, and if anaerobes are suspected, clindamycin or metronidazole.

Patients with concomitant frostbite to the extremities should have their core rewarmed first before allowing the frostbitten extremities to thaw.[1] After the core temperature is above 32C to 34C, the frostbitten area should be rapidly warmed using a water bath with the temperature 42C to 44.4C to minimize pain during rewarming.[9]

Cardiopulmonary resuscitation must not be terminated too quickly. Case reports exist of full neurologic recovery following profound hypothermia and cardiac arrest requiring over 2 hours of CPR.[2] These cases suggest that heroic efforts are justifiable in the otherwise salvageable patient.

HYPERTHERMIA

Preventing an abnormal elevation in body temperature depends on maintaining a balance between heat dissipation and generation.

6 L of fluid heated to 45C. This provides a reasonable alternative to cardiopulmonary bypass and allows control of fluid balance and electrolytes. Gastric lavage with 45C fluid through an intragastric balloon, colonic lavage, or bladder irrigation through a three-way Foley catheter are all effective alternatives. The use of additional rewarming techniques will depend on what facilities are available.

Active external rewarming can be an acceptable alternative if the trunk is preferentially warmed using a device (circulated water jacket) designed for this purpose. This method of rewarming is preferable to total immersion of an unstable patient into a tub of hot water. Total immersion is potentially dangerous because of the limited access to the patient.

Underlying complications must be sought. Hypothermic patients frequently develop pneumonia, and hypothermic patients with underlying sepsis may have the worst prognosis of any subgroup.[6] Appropriate cultures should be obtained. If sepsis is suspected, antibiotic therapy should be initiated and should include

TABLE 4.11-4. CORRECTION OF ARTERIAL BLOOD GASES FOR BODY TEMPERATURE

	↑1C[a]	↓1C[a]
pH	↓0.015	↑0.015
P_{CO_2} (mm Hg)	↑4.4%[b]	↓4.4%[b]
P_{O_2} (mm Hg)	↑7.2%	↓7.2%

[a]Change with reference to 37C.
[b]Percent change of the value measured at standard 37C.

TABLE 4.11-6. ESTIMATED HEAT GAIN FROM ENDOGENOUS AND EXOGENOUS SOURCES

Heat Source	Calories Provided at Core Temp. of 28C[a]
Normal metabolic rate	70 kcal/hr
Maximal shivering	350 kcal/hr
Humidified O_2 at 20 L/min (45C)	30 kcal/hr
IV fluid (45C)	17 kcal/L
Peritoneal dialysis (45C) 1 L/hr	17 kcal/hr
4 L/hr	68 kcal/hr
Cardiopulmonary bypass (45C) 1 L/hr	17 kcal/hr
28 L/hr	476 kcal/hr
Trunk immersion in hot water (45C) Vasoconstriction present	600 kcal/hr
Vasodilation present	2400 kcal/hr

[a]A 70-kg human requires a gain of 60 kcal of heat to increase body temperature 1C.
From Myers RA, Britten JS, Cowley RA: JACEP 8:523, 1979.[5]

Clothing, ventilation, exercise, and water and salt repletion affect the heat load and the ability of the body to regulate body temperature. Heavy exercise should be avoided or modified in hot, humid weather. Salt and, more important, water repletion should be routine and occur before symptoms of heat illness occur. The very young, the very old, or persons with underlying diseases, particularly cardiovascular disease, are at special risk for illness from heat stress.

The clinical consequences of heat stress represent a continuum. The three most severe syndromes will be reviewed (Table 4.11–7).

HEAT CRAMPS

Heat cramps occur in large, heavily used muscle groups (i.e., calves), typically after long-term heat exposure. The cramping muscle can be relieved by passive stretching. Though the cause is not well defined, inadequate water and relative salt depletion are most commonly implicated. Water and mild salt supplementation appear to be effective prophylaxis in groups at risk (steel mill workers, football players). For the patient presenting with cramps, oral hydration with 0.1 percent NaCl solution or the intravenous infusion of 0.9 percent NaCl solution is effective therapy.

HEAT EXHAUSTION

Patients with heat exhaustion have more severe symptoms than do patients with heat cramps. The syndrome typically develops over days as compensatory mechanisms to maintain normothermia are taxed. Symptoms frequently include headache, irritability, anorexia, malaise, thirst, and muscle cramps. Orthostatic hypotension and syncope may occur. Tachycardia and tachypnea are frequent. Body temperature may be normal or only moderately elevated, typically to no more than 100F. Dehydration is common. Impairment of CNS function is minimal and nonspecific.

Diagnosis relies on a history of heat exposure, the symptoms described above, and an absence of concomitant disease. Treatment consists of rest in a cool environment and either oral rehydration with 0.1 percent salt solution or an intravenous infusion of 5 percent dextrose in 0.45 percent sodium chloride solution. Young, healthy patients with significant dehydration as indicated by either an elevated blood urea nitrogen, hematocrit, or orthostasis may require as much as 4 L of fluid over 6 to 8 hours. Older patients will require more judicious rehydration and should probably be hospitalized.

HEAT STROKE

Heat stroke represents a true medical emergency. The patient typically has an antecedent history of heat exposure, an elevated body temperature, and severe CNS dysfunction (i.e., delirium, coma, or seizures). The severity of the CNS dysfunction distinguishes heat stroke from heat exhaustion. Brain damage is common in severe cases.

There are two typical presentations of heat stroke. Classic heat stroke is most frequently seen in the elderly, the debilitated, or the very young. It tends to develop over a period of days, during a heat wave, and in persons who are unable to seek a cooler environment and maintain an adequate fluid intake. Exertional heat stroke typically occurs in young healthy persons working or exercising in an excessively hot and humid environment. The onset is rapid, and dehydration is typically less severe than in patients with classic heat stroke.

The symptoms of heat stroke result from diffuse cellular metabolic derangement and cell death. Creatine kinase, aspartate aminotransferase (AST), and lactic dehydrogenase serum enzyme levels may initially be strikingly elevated and may continue to increase for 7 to 10 days. Rhabdomyolysis results in myoglobinuria, which may lead to acute renal failure. Coagulation times are often abnormally prolonged, and disseminated intravascular coagulopathy is not uncommon. Despite an increase in cardiac output, hypotension may develop because of severe peripheral vasodilation and volume depletion. Systemic vascular resistance is low, secondary to profound cutaneous vasodilation. At temperatures above 40C, cardiac contractility decreases, and fluid therapy must be carefully monitored in the hypotensive patient.[7]

The search for concurrent disease is secondary in the initial treatment of heat stroke. Therapy to cool the patient must begin in the field and should not await precise determination of the cause of the hyperthermia. If the temperature is refractory to cooling efforts or if the patient remains comatose, other diagnostic procedures are immediately warranted. Lumbar puncture is necessary to exclude meningitis or encephalitis. Sepsis, head trauma, cerebrovascular accident, and thyroid storm should also be considered.

Rapid and immediate cooling is the primary therapy of heat stroke. Although there is much debate regarding the best method of cooling, it is generally accepted that the severity and duration of hyperthermia profoundly influences morbidity and mortality.[8] General supportive care is fundamental. Endotracheal intubation is advised for the patient with inadequate ventilation or an absent gag reflex. Supplemental oxygen; two large-bore intravenous lines; and continuous monitoring of ECG, central venous pressure, blood pressure, and urinary output (with a Foley catheter) should be standard components of management.

Cooling by immersion in a tub of ice water, like immersion for hypothermia, can be technically difficult when caring for an unstable patient. Increasing evaporation is technically simpler and probably equally effective. The patient is undressed and sprayed with cool water while fans blow room temperature air over the patient. This technique may produce cooling rates of 0.31C/min, a result similar or superior to the rate of cooling with ice bath immersion.[8] This technique allows easy access to the patient, intravenous lines, and monitoring devices.

Active cooling should be stopped when the body temperature reaches 39C to prevent overcooling. Hyperthermia may, however, recur in 4 to 6 hours and the patient's thermoregulatory mechanisms may be unstable for several weeks following heat stroke.[3] Fluid therapy must be carefully evaluated as hypotension may improve with cooling alone. Maintenance of an adequate urine output appears to decrease the risk of severe acute renal failure. Vasopressors should be used only as a last resort. Shivering, which

TABLE 4.11–7. CHARACTERISTICS OF HEAT ILLNESS

Syndrome	Symptoms/Signs	Treatment
Heat cramps	Onset after working in heat, cramps in heavily used muscle groups, temperature normal	Cool environment, oral hydration, mild salt supplementation with salt tablets
Heat exhaustion	Slow onset (days), headache, irritability, temperature normal to slightly elevated (100F)	Cool environment, oral and/or IV hydration
Heat stroke (classic, exertional)	Slow or rapid onset, delirium, coma, seizures, temperature markedly elevated (>104F)	Rapid cooling, intensive, supportive care

increases heat production, may be precipitated by cooling. Shivering, if it becomes a severe problem, will generally be suppressed by chlorpromazine, 25 to 50 mg IV. Chlorpromazine, however, lowers the seizure threshold and may cause hypotension. Pharmacologic treatment of seizures may include diazepam (up to 10 mg given slowly intravenously), phenytoin (15 mg/kg given intravenously in normal saline at no faster than 50 mg/min) or phenobarbital (120 to 240 mg given slowly intravenously every 20 to 30 min to a total of 400 to 600 mg). Some case reports have questioned the efficacy of phenytoin given alone.[8] Severe acidosis (pH <7.2) should be corrected with sodium bicarbonate (0.5 to 1.0 mEq/kg IV over 30 to 60 minutes), remembering that arterial blood gas results must be corrected for temperature (Table 4.11–4). Total body base deficit should be calculated and half of the deficit corrected with intravenous administration of 1 mEq/ml sodium bicarbonate.

The heat stroke patient will require intensive monitoring for 48 to 72 hours even if cooling is rapidly achieved and mental status improves. Jaundice, rhabdomyolysis, and acute renal failure may occur as late sequelae. Poor prognostic signs include coma for more than 10 hours, a markedly prolonged prothrombin time, or an AST level greater than 1000 IU/L.[8]

REFERENCES

1. Bangs CC: Hypothermia and frostbite. Emergency Med Clin North Am 2:485, 1984
2. Bangs CC, Hamlet MP: Hypothermia and cold injuries. In Auerbach PS, Green E (eds): Management of wilderness and environmental emergencies, 1st ed. New York, Macmillan, 1983, p 126
3. Clowes GHA Jr, O'Donnell TF Jr: Heat stroke. N Engl J Med 291:564, 1974
4. Gould L, Gopalaswamy G, et al: The Osborn wave in hypothermia. Angiology J Vasc Dis 36:125, 1985
5. Myers RA, Britten JS, Cowley RA: Hypothermia: Quantitative aspects of therapy. JACEP 8:523, 1979
6. Reuler JB: Hypothermia: Pathophysiology, clinical settings and management. Ann Intern Med 89:519, 1978
7. Schrier RA, Hano J, et al: Renal, metabolic and circulatory responses to heat and exercise. Studies in military recruits during summer training, with implications for acute renal failure. Ann Intern Med 73:213, 1970
8. Shibolet S, Lancaster M, Danon Y: Heat stroke, a review. Aviat Space Environ Med 47:280, 1976
9. TB MED 81, NAVMED P-5052-29, AFP161-11: Cold injury. Washington, DC, Departments of the Army, Navy and the Air Force Publications, 1976

Medical genetics is concerned with genetic disorders and with the role of genetic factors in all disease. *Clinical genetics* is that part of medical genetics concerned directly with the care of patients afflicted with genetic disorders and their families.

As a generalist and an adviser to prospective parents, the physician who cares for adult patients must be conversant, at least in a general way, with all genetic disorders. Genetic disorders are by no means the exclusive concern of the pediatrician. Increasingly, because of improved care, patients with grave genetic disorders are surviving to adulthood, and mild forms compatible with such survival are being recognized. Cystic fibrosis of the pancreas provides an example of both features. Many diseases that were first delineated on the basis of the most severe (and, as was thought, "textbook") cases are being recognized in adult patients. Furthermore, those genetic disorders that first manifest in adolescence or later are a significant segment of medical practice. Finally, the role the internist often fills as family physician offers the opportunity and responsibility to observe and respond appropriately to the particular genetic characteristics of patients and their families, and to use the information in the diagnosis and management of their health problems.

This section on medical genetics discusses an etiologic category of disease. After a discussion of general principles, including a review of the anatomy of the human genome, each of three main classes of genetic diseases is discussed: chromosomal aberrations, mendelian disorders, and multifactorial disorders. Pharmacogenetics and immunogenetics are accorded separate chapters because although these areas are important to medicine, they do not primarily represent disorders, as do the other three main topics. Of the several catagories of genetic disease, mendelian disorders are discussed most extensively. Principles of diagnosis, prognosis (genetic counseling), treatment, and prevention are presented. The number of mendelian disorders is large,[2] but they become more manageable in clinical practice when the basic principles underlying all of them are familiar to the physician. Also, mendelian disorders tend to fall into one of a few major groups according to pathogenetic mechanisms, such as inborn errors of metabolism ("enzymopathies"), transport disorders, receptor defects, and lysosomal disorders. Consequently, after the discussion of principles, major pathogenetic categories of mendelian disorders are illustrated. The contributions of molecular genetics, which have brought about a veritable revolution in clinical genetics ("the new genetics"), will be emphasized throughout the section.[43]

CHAPTER 5.1
General Considerations

Victor A. McKusick

GENETIC FACTORS IN DISEASE

Genetic factors play some role in most diseases[41] and, similarly, environmental factors play a role. Most diseases fall somewhere on a scale where genetic factors predominate on one end, and environmental factors predominate on the other. For example, phenylketonuria and galactosemia are near the "genetic end" but are not at the very end because diet, an environmental factor, influences these diseases. Similarly, tuberculosis is near the "environmental end," although again it is not at the extreme end because genetic constitution is shown by twin and ethnologic studies to play a significant role. Hypertension, peptic ulcer, diabetes, and many other disorders fall in a middle ground. Useful as this simplistic model is for conceptualizing the *relative* roles of genetic makeup and exogenous factors, few diseases can be positioned on such a scale with mathematical precision. Favism is, however, an example of a disease in which the relative roles of the two influences can be precisely stated. It would be placed in the very center of the scale; this disease has an absolute requirement for both deficiency of red blood cell glucose 6-phosphate dehydrogenase (G6PD) (an X-chromosomally determined defect) and for exposure to the fava bean (an exogenous agent). Both factors are necessary, but neither alone is sufficient to cause favism. An exogenous factor (thiamine deficiency) and an endogenous factor (mutation in transketolase) collaborate in "causing" the Wernicke-Korsakoff syndrome.[3,35]

Because of the influence of environmental factors in most genetic diseases, manipulation of the environment is an approach to their treatment. Furthermore, environmentally induced disorders or malformations often closely mimic genetic disorders. Thus the medical geneticist must keep environmental factors also prominently in mind.

Genetic diseases tend to fall into one of three categories: (1) "chromosomal aberrations,"[9] although usually not inherited in the usual sense of that word (they may be heritable), involve the genetic material and therefore are one form of genetic disease. (2) By typical pedigree patterns and other characteristics, many disorders reveal themselves to be the result primarily of mutation at a single genetic locus. These are called "mendelian disorders." (See McKusick's *Mendelian Inheritance in Man*[32] for a comprehensive listing of all known mendelian disorders.) The specific chromosome or even part of the chromosome carrying the specific causative gene is becoming known for an increasing number of disorders.[33] (3) Many common disorders, such as hypertension and cardiac malformations, are termed "multifactorial" because both genetic and nongenetic factors, often multiple in each case, collaborate in causation. ("Polygenic" describes multiple genetic background.) The "new genetics" is important for diagnosing, understanding, treating, and preventing all three categories of disease.[36,43]

This three-way classification is, like many classifications, to some extent arbitrary. As indicated earlier, environmental factors influence even "single-gene" disorders, as does the rest of the genetic makeup of the patient. Thus all are, in this context, multifactorial. Even in multifactorial disorders the operation of individual loci has been identified in an increasing number of instances. In chromosomal aberrations many genes are present in excess or are deficient; hence these might be termed polygenic or multifactorial. With improved methods for studying chromosomes ("high-resolution cytogenetics"), small chromosomal aberrations have been

found in certain mendelian disorders. But despite its arbitrariness, the classification is useful because the clinical approach to the three types of disease is different.

In addition to the three categories of genetic disease just discussed, a fourth large category, "somatic cell genetic disease," deserves mention. Findings of specific chromosome changes such as translocations or deletions in specific forms of neoplasia, discovery of oncogenes, and demonstration of a relationship between the chromosomal changes and oncogenes (see Chapter 6.12) show that neoplasms are fundamentally genetic diseases. In most instances the change is acquired in a given cell line and is not inherited; yet neoplasms have a change in the genetic material that is etiopathogenetically causative and therefore represent one category of genetic disease. Furthermore, evidence suggests that some sporadic congenital malformations are the result of somatic cell mutation; that is, they represent a form of somatic cell genetic disease, and most autoimmune diseases are probably in this category.

The four aspects of clinical medicine—diagnosis, prognosis, treatment, and prevention (see Editors' Note)—are as significant to clinical genetics as to all other parts of clinical medicine. Each category of genetic disease, particularly mendelian disorders, can conveniently be discussed under these four headings.

The methods of clinical genetics include pedigree construction; cytologic techniques, particularly study of the chromosomes in dividing somatic cells such as lymphocytes (p. 275ff), and study of biochemical characteristics of cultured skin fibroblasts; special biochemical tests of blood and urine for the diagnosis of inborn errors of metabolism; screening of neonates for genetic diseases such as phenylketonuria and testing for heterozygous carriers of genetic disease; amniocentesis, chorionic villus sampling, ultrasound, and other methods for prenatal diagnosis; genetic counseling; and special approaches (e.g., dietary) for treatment of inborn errors of metabolism. New methods of diagnosis[43] involve analysis of the genes themselves with recombinant DNA (deoxyribonucleic acid) probes and restriction enzymes ("Southern blotting" and related methods). Family linkage studies using DNA markers (restriction fragment length polymorphisms [RFLPs], also known as "riflips") have enabled prenatal diagnosis of disorders such as hemophilia, preclinical diagnosis of conditions such as adult polycystic kidney disease and Huntington disease, and carrier detection in disorders such as Duchenne muscular dystrophy. (See discussion on gene diagnosis, on p. 286.)

THE ANATOMY OF HUMAN GENOME

As stated earlier, this section on medical genetics is concerned with an etiologic class of disease, but it is also concerned, as are many of the other sections, with the disorders of a particular organ system—in this case, the human genome. As Berg[2] put it: "Just as our present practice of medicine relies on the sophisticated knowledge of human anatomy, physiology, and biochemistry, so will dealing with genetic disease in the future demand a detailed understanding of the molecular anatomy, physiology, and biochemistry of the human genome. We shall have to have physicians who are as conversant with the molecular anatomy and physiology of the chromosomes and genes as the cardiac surgeon is with the structure and workings of the heart and circulatory tree."

The chromosomes of normal diploid body cells number 46: 22 pairs of autosomes (nonsex chromosomes) and a pair of sex chromosomes, XX in the female, XY in the male. Existing techniques permit the demonstration of a distinctively banded staining pattern for each of the 24 different chromosomes, the 22 autosomes, the X, and the Y. In the lymphocytes of peripheral blood, stimulated to mitosis with phytohemagglutinin, chromosomes in metaphase have the appearance shown in Figure 5.1–1. In all, about 450 bands are discernible. By special methods (high-resolution cytogenetics), chromosomes at an earlier, more extended stage (prophase or prometaphase) can be stained, allowing definition of

850 or more bands. With banding methods the "lesion" has been specified in many previously incompletely (and sometimes incorrectly) delineated chromosomal aberrations, such as the Philadelphia chromosome of chronic myeloid leukemia; "new chromosomal syndromes" have been described by recognition of characteristic phenotypes of cytogenetically "pure culture" groups of cases, such as the trisomy 8 syndrome,[9] and small aberrations have been found to be the basis of previously etiologically obscure neoplasms, such as retinoblastoma, or congenital syndromes, such as the Prader-Willi syndrome.

Banding techniques have also provided the necessary anatomic detail for mapping genes to specific chromosomes or regions of chromosomes by the method of interspecies somatic cell hybridization and in situ hybridization. By these and other approaches such as family linkage study with DNA markers (see later discussion), the genic anatomy of the chromosomes has been determined in some detail. Figure 5.1–2 presents, in abridged form, some of that information. Note the location of the genes for the Rh and ABO blood groups (on chromosomes 1 and 9, respectively); for adrenocorticotropic hormone (ACTH) (proopiomelanocortin) [POMC] on 2), insulin (on 11), prolactin (on 6), and growth hormone and placental lactogen (on 17); for the heavy, kappa light, and lambda light chains of immunoglobulins (on 14, 2, and 22, respectively); for interferons (on 9 and 12); for the major histocompatibility complex, including HLA (on 6); for the globins of hemoglobins (on 11 and 16); and so on. The morbid anatomy of the human genome, that is, the chromosomal location of mutations responsible for various mendelian disorders, is presented later (see Fig. 5.3–10).

NORMAL MEIOSIS AND GAMETOGENESIS

As stated earlier, the nucleus of each somatic cell of humans contains 22 pairs of nonsex chromosomes (autosomes) and a pair of sex chromosomes (Fig. 5.1–1). (Some cells, such as megakaryocytes, are polyploid; their chromosome counts are multiples of the basic diploid number of 46.) In the fertilized ovum, the zygote, 23 of the chromosomes, one of each pair, are derived from the father via the sperm and 23 from the mother. In the process of mitosis, which occurs in somatic cells undergoing division, each chromosome is reduplicated so that each daughter cell receives the full complement of 46 chromosomes identical to those in the original zygote. By contrast the process of meiosis (etymologically this is the same word as *miosis*, which by usage refers exclusively to a reduction in pupil size) results in a reduction in chromosome number from the diploid number (23 pairs) found in somatic cells to the haploid number (23 unique chromosomes, one from each pair) characteristic of the gametes: eggs and sperm.

Meiosis (Fig. 5.1–3) occurs during the production of gametes in the ovary or testis. The process consists of two cell divisions, with chromosome reduplication occurring only once, early in the process. In the first meiotic division the reduplicated twin-stranded pairs of homologous chromosomes (e.g., the two chromosomes No. 1) come to lie side by side, attached at their centromeres, in a process called "synapsis." One of each pair goes to each pole, and the cell divides. The passage of one of a pair of homologous chromosomes into one daughter cell and its homologue into the other daughter cell is the basis of Mendel's first law, that of the segregation of alleles (alternative genes at the same locus on homologous chromosomes). In the case of one pair of chromosomes, if the maternally derived chromosome (or at least the chromosome with the maternally derived centromere) passes into cell 1, the paternally derived chromosome of the pair passes into cell 2. Completely independent of this is the matter of which daughter cell receives the paternal or maternal chromosome of another pair. Thus the events of the first stage of meiosis also constitute the basis of Mendel's second law, that of independent assortment of genes on separate (nonhomologous) chromosomes.

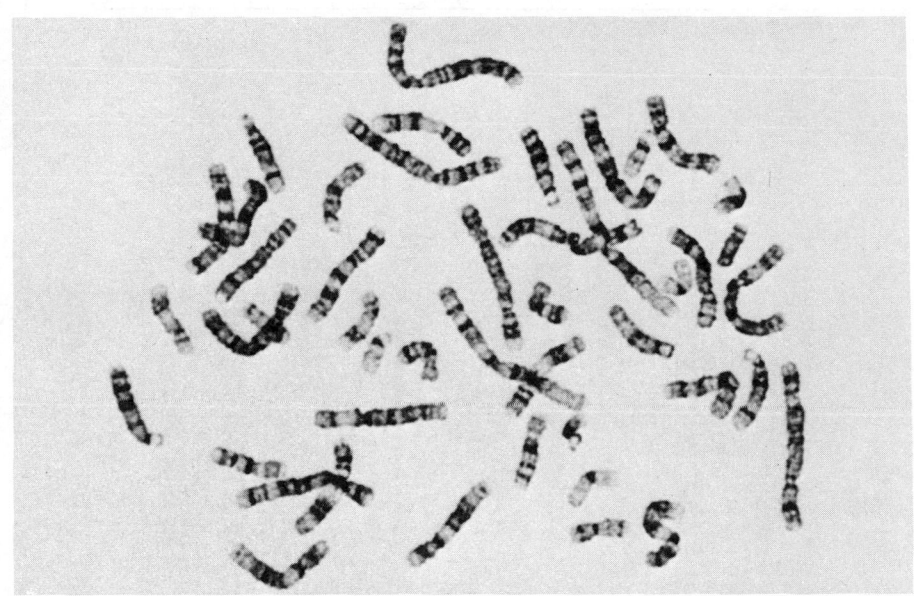

A

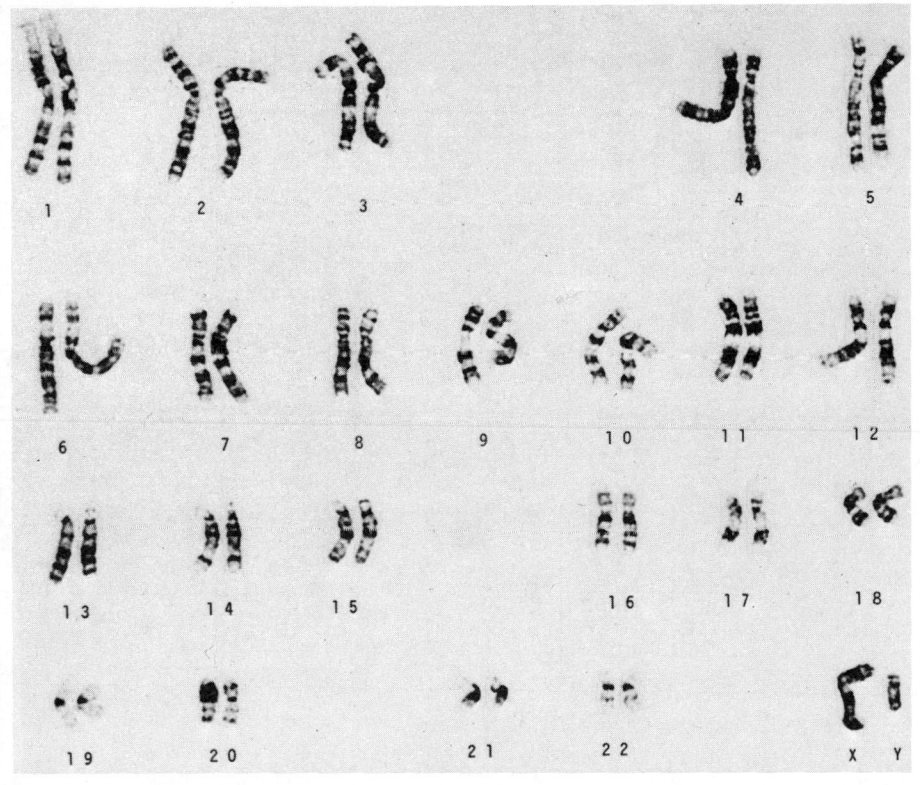

B

Figure 5.1–1. A. Chromosomes (in metaphase) of single lymphocyte from normal male, prepared and stained by trypsin-Giemsa banding technique. (Approximate magnification ×5000.) **B.** Same, arranged in karyotype. (*Courtesy Dr. Uta Francke.*)

In the second stage of meiosis (the equational division) the daughter cells, each of which contains half the number of chromosomes found in somatic cells and the primordial germ cells, undergo a mitosislike division. As a result the gametes have half the somatic number of chromosomes.

Another event fundamental to genetics occurs during meiosis, namely, crossing over, or recombination. Early in meiosis, at the stage when each chromosome has reduplicated and when the two chromosomes of each pair have undergone synapsis (the "four-strand stage"), homologous chromosomes exchange segments, so that a segment of the chromosome 1 originally derived, let us say, from the father may end up on the chromosome 1 with the cen-

tromere derived from the mother. An important consequence of the second stage of meiosis is separation of the products of crossing over. Independent assortment of the chromosomes in the first stage of meiosis results in great diversity of the gametes—2^{23} different gametes are produced with equal likelihood. The diversity of the gametes is further increased to a vast extent by crossing over. Thus a "shuffling of the genes" occurs in meiosis.

Because of crossing over, genes at different loci, that is, nonalleles, may show assortment, even if they are on the same chromosome. Indeed, if they are far apart on the same chromosome, the assortment may be completely independent, as though the genes were on separate chromosomes. If the genes are close together, the

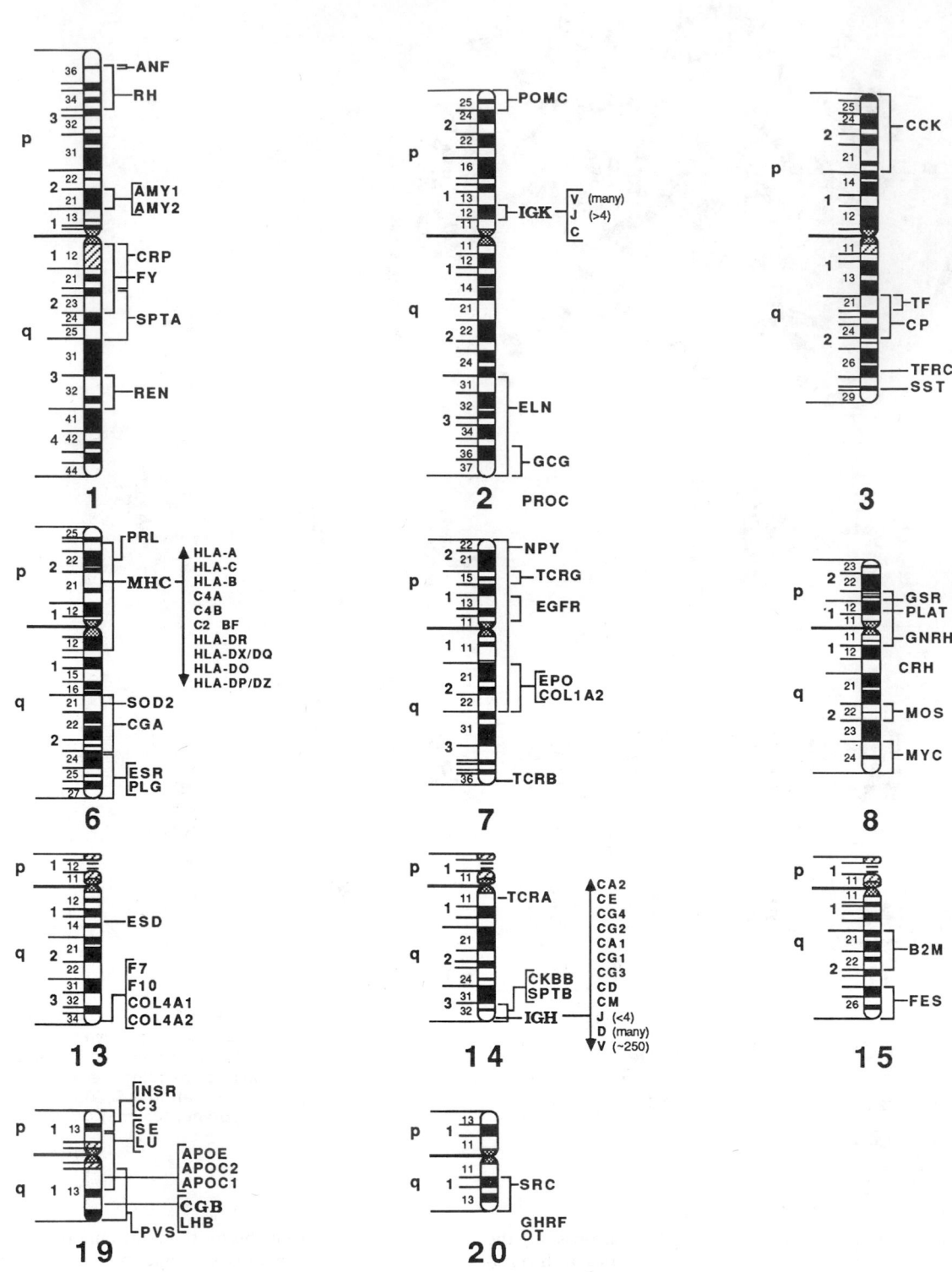

Figure 5.1–2. ''Genic anatomy'' of human chromosomes (abridged version). The detailed map and descriptions of methods of chromosome mapping are given elsewhere.[32,33] (*See Key to Figure 5.1–2 on p. 274.*)

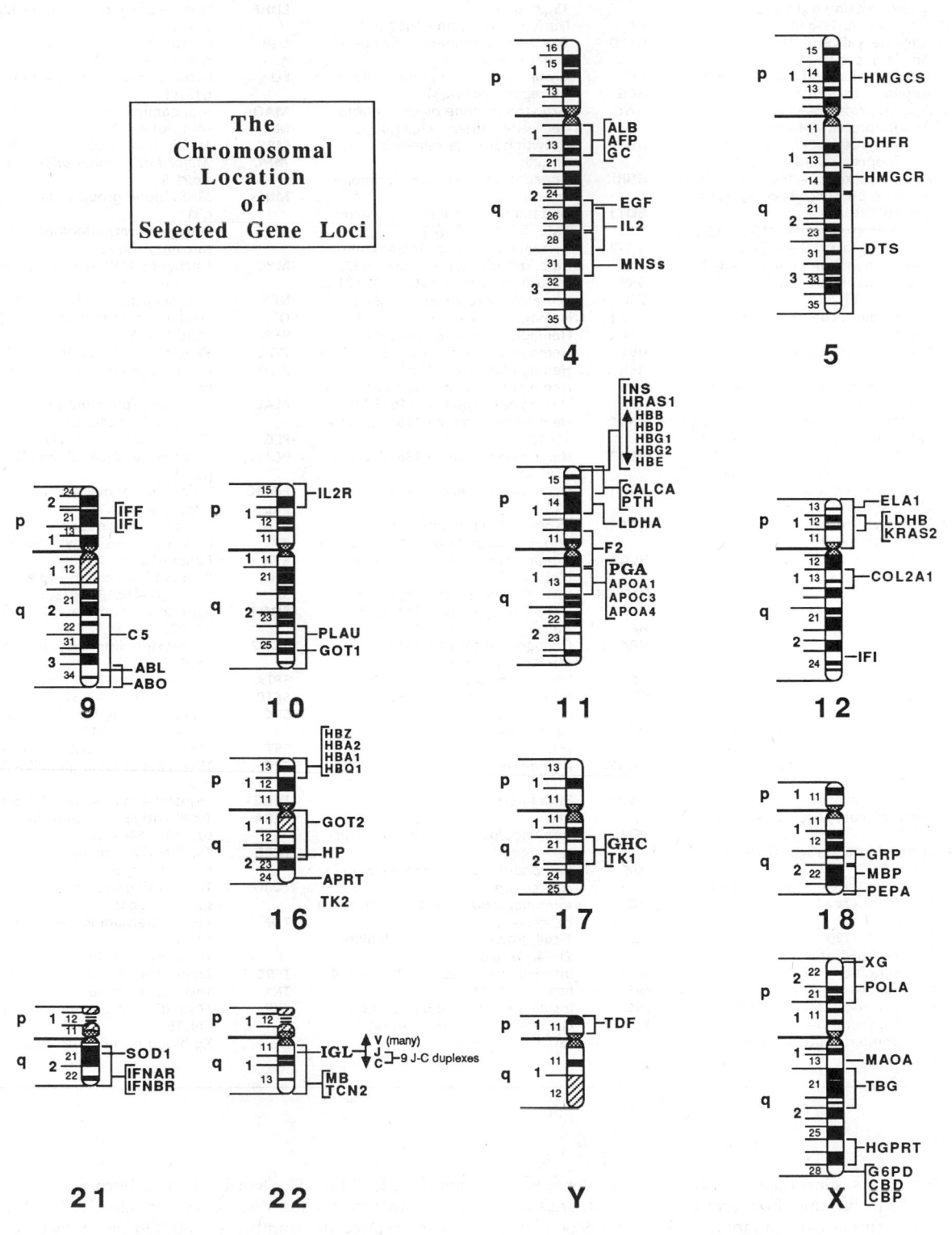

The
Chromosomal
Location
of
Selected Gene Loci

KEY TO FIGURE 5.1–2: Symbols in italic refer to gene clusters.

ABL	Oncogene ABL (Abelson)—9q34.1	F7	Clotting factor VII—13q34	LDHA	Lactate dehydrogenase A—11p15-p14
ABO	ABO blood group—9q34	FES	Oncogene FES (feline sarcoma)—15q25-q26	LDHB	Lactate dehydrogenase B—12p12.2-p12.1
AFP	α-fetoprotein—4q11-q13	FY	Duffy blood group—1q12-q21	LHB	Luteinizing hormone, beta-chain—19q13.32
ALB	Albumin—4q11-q13	G6PD	Glucose-6-phosphate dehydro-genase—Xq28	LU	Lutheran blood group—19p13.1-q13.11
AMY1	Amylase, salivary—1p21	GC	Group-specific component—4q12	MAOA	Monoamine oxidase A—Xq13
AMY2	Amylase, pancreatic—1p21	GCG	Glucagon—2q36-q37	MB	Myoglobin—22q11.2-q13
ANF	Atrial natriuretic factor—1p36.2	*GHC*	*Growth hormone/placental lacto-gen gene cluster—17q21.0-q22.0*	MBP	Myelin basic protein—18q22-qter
APOA1	Apolipoprotein A-I—11q13			*MHC*	*Major histocompatibility complex—6p21.3*
APOA4	Apolipoprotein A-IV—11q13	GHRF	Growth hormone releasing factor—Chr.20	MNSs	MNSs blood group system—4q28-q31
APOC1	Apolipoprotein C-I—19q13.1	GNRH	Gonadotropin releasing hormone—8p21-q11.2	MOS	Oncogene MOS (Moloney murine sarcoma)—8q22
APOC2	Apolipoprotein C-II—19q13.3	GOT1	Glutamate oxaloacetate transami-nase, soluble—10q25.3	MYC	Oncogene MYC (avian myelocyto-matosis)—8q24
APOC3	Apolipoprotein C-III—11q13	GOT2	Glutamate oxaloacetic transami-nase, mitochondrial—16cen-q22	NPY	Neuropeptide Y—7pter-q22
APOE	Apolipoprotein E—19q13.1	GRP	Gastrin releasing peptide—18q21	OT	Oxytocin-neurophysin I—Chr.20
APRT	Adenine phosphoribosyltransfer-ase—16q24	GSR	Glutathione reductase—8p21.1	PEPA	Peptidase A—18q23
B2M	Beta-2-microglobulin—15q21-q22	HBA1	Hemoglobin α₁—16p13.33-p13.11	*PGA*	*Pepsinogen A cluster—11q13*
BF	Properdin factor B—6p21.3	HBA2	Hemoglobin α₂—16p13.33-p13.11	PLAT	Plasminogen activator, tissue type—8p12
C2	Complement component-2—6p21.3	HBZ	Hemoglobin zeta—16p13.33-p13.11	PLAU	Urokinase (plasminogen activator, urinary)—10q24-qter
C3	Complement component-3—19p13.3-p13.2	HBB	Hemoglobin beta—11p15.5	PLG	Plasminogen—6q26-q27
C4A	Complement component-4S—9q22-q34	HBD	Hemoglobin delta—11p15.5	POLA	Polymerase, DNA, alpha—Xp22.3-p21.1
C4B	Complement component-4F—6p21.3	HBE	Hemoglobin epsilon—11p15.5	POMC	Proopiomelanocortin—2p25
C5	Complement component 5—9q22-q34	HBG1	Hemoglobin gamma 136 alanine—11p15.5	PRL	Prolactin—Chr.12
CA1	Carbonic anhydrase I—8q13-q22	HBG2	Hemoglobin gamma 136 glycine—11p15.5	PTH	Parathyroid hormone—11p15
CA2	Carbonic anhydrase II—8q13-q22	HBQ1	Hemoglobin theta-1—16p13.33-p13.11	PVS	Polio virus sensitivity—19q13-qter
CALCA	Calcitonin—11p15.4-p15.1			REN	Renin—1q32
CBD	Deutan color blindness—Xq28	HGPRT	Hypoxanthine-guanine phos-phoribosyltransferase—Xq26-q27.2	RH	Rhesus blood group—1p36.2-p34
CBP	Protan color blindness—Xq28	HLA	Human leukocyte antigen (multi-ple)—6p21.3	SE	Secretor—19p13.1-q13.11
CCK	Cholecystokinin—3pter-p21	HMGCR	HMG CoA reductase—5q13.3-q14	SOD1	Superoxide dismutase, soluble—21q22.1
CD	D constant region, IgH—14q32.33	HMGCS	HMG CoA synthase—5p14-p13	SOD2	Superoxide dismutase, mitochon-drial—6q21
CE	E constant region, IgH—13q32.33	HP	Haptoglobin—16q22.1	SPTA	Alpha-spectrin—1q22-q25
CG1-4	Gamma 1-4 constant region genes, IgH—14q32.33	HRAS1	Oncogene HRAS1 (Harvey rat sarcoma-1)—11p15.5	SPTB	Beta-spectrin—14q32
CGA	Chorionic gonadotropin, α-chain—6q21.1-q23	IFF	Fibroblast interferon—9p21	SRC	Protooncogene SRC (Rous sar-coma)—20q12-q13
CGB	*Chorionic gonadotropin, beta-chain—19q13.32*	IFI	Interferon, gamma or immune type—12q24.1	SST	Somatostatin—3q28
CKBB	Creatine kinase, brain type—14q32	*IFL*	*Leudocyte interferon cluster (alpha-interferon)—9p21*	TBG	Thyroxine-binding globulin—Xq21-q22
CM	Mu constant region, IgH—14q32.33	IFNAR	Alpha-interferon receptor—21q21-qter	TCN2	Transcobalmin II—22q11.2-qter
COL1A2	Collagen I, α₂-chain—7q21.3-q22.1	IFNBR	Beta-interferon receptor—21q21-qter	TCRA	T-cell antigen receptor, alpha subunit—14q11.2
COL2A1	Collagen II, α₁-chain—12q13.1-q13.3	*IGH*	*Immunoglobulin heavy chain clus-ter—14q32.33*	TCRB	T-cell antigen receptor, beta subunit—7q35
COL4A1	Collagen IV, α₁-chain—13q34	*IGK*	*Immunoglobulin kappa light chain cluster—2p12*	TCRG	T-cell antigen receptor, gamma subunit—7p15
CP	Ceruloplasmin—3q21-q24	*IGL*	*Immunoglobulin lambda light chain cluster—22q11.12*	TDF	Testis determining factor—Ypter-p11.2
CRH	Corticotropin releasing hormone—8q13	IL2	T-cell growth factor (interleukin-2)—4q26-q28	TF	Transferrin—3q21
CRP	C-reactive protein—1q12-q23	IL2R	Interleukin-2 receptor—10p15-p14	TFRC	Transferrin receptor—3q26.2
DHFR	Dihydrofolate reductase—5q11.1-q13.2	INS	Insulin—11p15.5	TK1	Thymidine kinase-1—17q21.0-q22.0
DTS	Diphtheria toxin sensitivity—5q15-qter	INSR	Insulin receptor—19p13.3-p13.2	TK2	Thymidine kinase, mitochondrial—Chr.16
EGF	Epidermal growth factor—4q25-q27	KRAS2	Oncogene Kras-2 (Kirsten rat sarcoma)—12p12.1	XG	Xg blood group—Xpter-p22.32
EGFR	Epidermal growth factor receptor—7p13-p11				
ELA1	Elastase-1—12p				
ELN	Elastin—2q31-qter				
EPO	Erythropoietin—7q21-q22				
ESD	Esterase D—13q14.11				
ESR	Estrogen receptor—6q24-q27				
F10	Clotting factor X—13q34				
F2	Prothrombin (clotting factor II)—11p11-q12				

assortment that occurs is less than completely independent. Studies of genetic linkage examine the extent to which traits are transmitted together in families, quantitate the degree of independence of assortment, provide a measure of the distance between genetic loci on the chromosome, and, when correlated with anomalous chromosomes in the family, indicate the precise chromosomal localization of genes—mapping the chromosomes of humans.[33]

The time course of meiosis, and of gametogenesis in general, is different in males and females. In the human female, germ cells multiply rapidly during early fetal life. Oogonia (the primordial germ cells of the female) cease to propagate after the fifth or sixth month of fetal life. The female infant is born with a full stock of oocytes that must last for her entire reproductive life. Estimates of this stock place the number at 750,000 per individual newborn female; however, many of these oocytes degenerate at various stages of oogenesis and at various times in the life of the female.

By the time of birth, the oocytes have completed most of the prophase of the first meiotic division and then regress into a long interphase-like dictyotene ("thick-thread") stage during which the nuclear membrane remains intact and the chromosomes are visible as threadlike or netlike structures. The dictyotene stage lasts for at least 12 years and even as long as 50 years. During this stage the

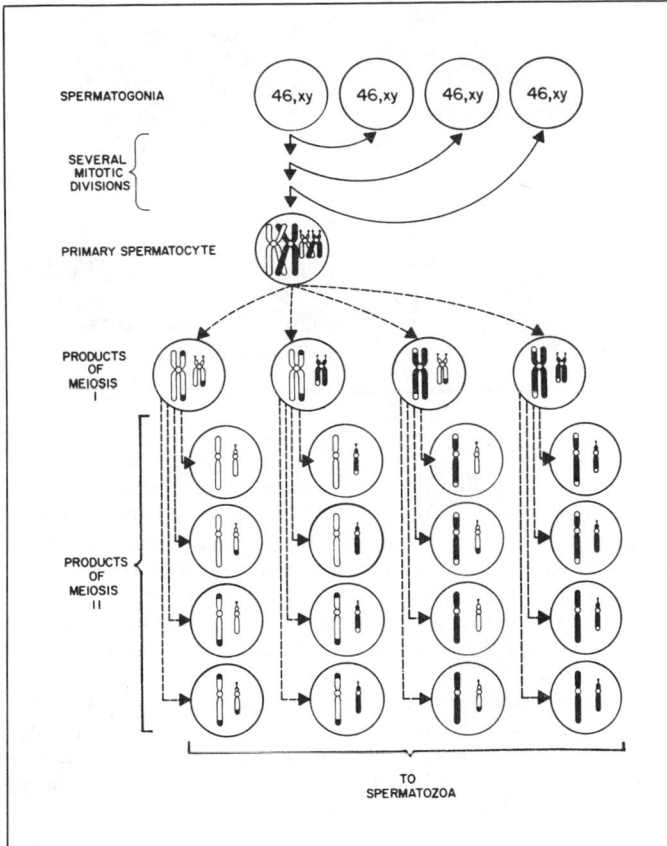

Figure 5.1–3. *Spermatogenesis,* showing normal meiosis. Only two pairs of chromosomes are shown. Crossing over, that is, exchange of segments between chromosomes, occurs in tetrad stage in primary spermatocyte. Diversifying effect of crossing over is indicated. Whereas in spermatogenesis, as diagrammed here, four gametes are produced from each primordial germ cell that enters meiosis, parallel process in the female, oogenesis, produces only one ovum, since in each stage of meiosis one of two daughter cells is cast off as a polar body. Diagram also indicates basis for increasing frequency of mutations with age in the male—"paternal age effect"; opportunity for occurrence and accumulation of mutations in initial mitotic diversions is illustrated.

DNA content is tetraploid (i.e., has twice as much chromosomal material as the normal diploid body cells), since each chromosome has replicated and no cell division has taken place.

Meiosis in the oocyte is resumed about the time of ovulation, and the first meiotic, or reduction, division is completed at that time. Pituitary gonadotropin stimulates this resumption of meiosis. The second, or equational, division of meiosis is usually completed only after the entry of the sperm into the ovum. In the female a polar body is extruded and lost as one product of each meiotic division. The chromosomes of the male and female pronuclei undergo a round of DNA synthesis and are therefore double, that is, have two chromatids, at the time they became commingled in the first mitotic division. With the completion of fertilization, the ovum becomes a zygote. The process of fertilization usually takes place in the ampulla of the fallopian tube. Uterine implantation of the human embryo occurs 6 to 7 days after ovulation.

Spermatogenesis differs from oogenesis in several important respects. The production of sperm is exceedingly abundant, and the total number produced in the lifetime of a male is astronomical. Proliferation of spermatogonia does not begin until puberty but thereafter may continue for the lifetime of the male; oogenesis through most of the first stage of meiosis is confined to intrauterine life. Four spermatids (and no polar bodies) are produced from each spermatogonium. The time for completion of the full cycle of spermatogenesis is about 64 days, in contrast to the 12 to 50 years of oogenesis.

This difference in the schedule of gametogenesis in males and females is responsible for the phenomena of maternal age effect in certain chromosomal aberrations (e.g., the frequency of Down syndrome [mongolism] is higher in offspring of older mothers) and paternal age effect in new mutations (e.g., the average age of fathers of new mutation cases of Marfan syndrome is about 7 years above the average, or said differently, older fathers have an increased risk of having children affected with a new mutation for some dominantly inherited disorder such as Marfan syndrome) (Fig. 5.1–3).

Mutations can also occur in early stages of development, such as in the round of DNA synthesis in the male and female pronuclei of the fertilized ovum. These, and mutations in somatic cells at a somewhat later stage, lead to a mosaic or sectorial state. If the mutation is dominant and if the germ cells are involved ("germinal mosaicism"), unaffected parents can have two or more affected children—an apparent exception to the usual pedigree pattern of dominant inheritance.

CHAPTER 5.2
Chromosomal Aberrations

Victor A. McKusick

ABNORMALITIES IN MEIOSIS AND GAMETOGENESIS

Normally, half the sperm contain 22 autosomes and a Y chromosome each, and half of them contain 22 autosomes and an X chromosome each. As a result, half of the fertilized eggs, or zygotes, will be XY (males) and half will be XX (females). So-called nondisjunction (Fig. 5.2–1) of a chromosomal pair during the process of meiosis may result in both members of a chromosomal pair being included in a germ cell, giving rise to a disorder such as the XXY (Klinefelter) syndrome, or in neither being present in a germ cell, giving rise to a condition such as the XO (Turner) syndrome. Missegregation of chromosomes, loss of one member of a pair, and

other accidents of cell division can also occur in an early cleavage stage of the zygote. Mosaicism may result from such accidents. For example, an XXX/XO mosaic might result from nondisjunction at an early cleavage of an XX zygote. (Some mosaicism is the result of loss of the extra chromosome from some cells in a developing zygote that was initially trisomic; e.g., mosaic XXX/XX.)

A point mutation, which is detected by the presence of a simply inherited disorder or trait in subsequent generations, can occur in the germ cells of either the male or the female. Mutation also occurs in somatic cells, where it does not differ in principle from that in the germ cells. Theoretically, if somatic mutations occurred in the zygote or at an early postzygotic stage, the individual might be affected with the given disorder. Furthermore, if a somatic mutation occurs at an appropriate postzygotic stage early in embryo-

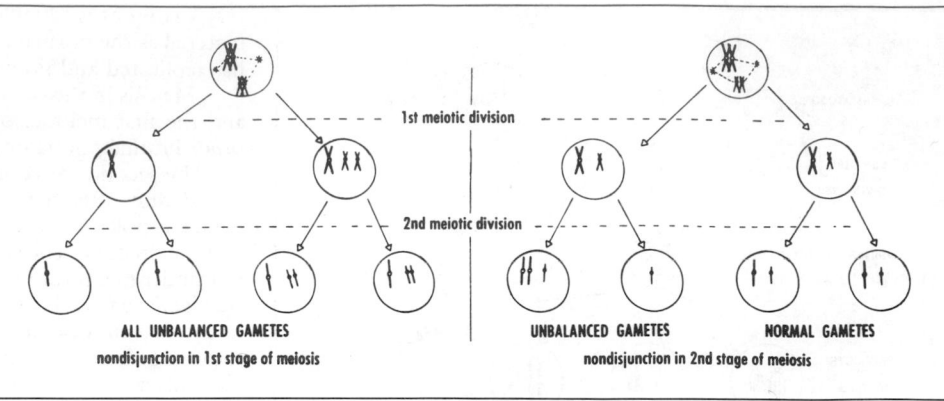

Figure 5.2–1. Abnormal meiosis, nondisjunction. Failure of homologous chromosomes to disjoin normally in the first meiotic division (*left*) and of two chromatids to separate and pass into separate cells in the second stage of meiosis (*right*) is illustrated. Nondisjunction and related accidents in segregation of chromosomes can also occur in mitosis, such as in early stages of the zygote.

genesis and if action of the mutant gene is locally manifest, a sectorial, or mosaic, situation might result. For example, if the normal allele of the gene for von Recklinghausen neurofibromatosis underwent mutation early in embryogenesis, one might observe a sector in which skin tumors and pigmented spots occur. An individual with such a condition would not transmit the disorder unless gonadal tissue was also involved. When a gonadal anlage cell suffers mutation, the situation is referred to as "gonadal mosaicism." An individual with this condition, although not showing signs of the disorder, may, if the condition is dominant, have more than one affected child. (Note the difference between mosaicism and chimerism. "Mosaicism" is the presence of two [or more] classes of cells representing variations on a single genome, e.g., somatic mutation mentioned earlier. "Chimerism" is a mixture of cells of different genomes, e.g., sometimes a dizygotic twin is found to have a minor cell line derived from the cotwin through early cross-transfusion in utero.)

As outlined for the sex chromosomes, missegregation of autosomes can occur in meiosis or in early mitotic stages, resulting in the presence of three of a particular chromosome rather than the normal two, a condition called "trisomy." This is what happens with chromosome 21 to result in Down syndrome (mongolism, or trisomy 21). Or only one of a particular autosome may end up in the zygote, a situation called "monosomy." Although monosomy of the X chromosome (Turner syndrome) is relatively well tolerated, monosomy of the autosomes leads to early embryonic death as a rule; trisomy of any except chromosomes 13, 18, and 21 is rarely found in liveborn infants. In rare instances patients have been found to have as many as five X chromosomes, presumably arising through nondisjunction in both the first and the second stages of meiosis. Such XXXXX individuals (and those who are XXXY, XXXX, and XXXXY) are severely retarded and have serious somatic malformations and abnormal sexual development. That they survive is related to the special mechanism by which X chromosomes in excess of one are rendered genetically inactive, at least in part or after a certain stage in embryogenesis. This special mechanism is responsible for normal dosage compensation in the female, in whom the excess of genetic material (two X chromosomes as compared to the one X chromosome of the normal male) would otherwise be disruptive. The one-inactive-X hypothesis (the Lyon hypothesis) concerns this mechanism of dosage compensation (Fig. 5.2–2).

Other chromosomal aberrations can occur during meiosis, not through missegregation but through chromosome breakage. A single break may lead to loss of that segment of the chromosome without a centromere. For example, the distal part of the short arm of chromosome 5 may be lost (5p−), leading to the clinical picture called the cri-du-chat syndrome. If two breaks occur in the same chromosome, an inversion may occur when the chromosome heals. If the two breaks are on the same side of the centromere, that is, in the same chromosome arm, it is termed a paracentric inversion. If the two breaks are on opposite sides of the centro-

mere, it is termed a pericentric inversion. If two breaks occur in separate chromosomes, pieces may be exchanged between them, so-called reciprocal translocation. Or two breaks occurring at the end of the certain chromosome may lead to a fusion chromosome (robertsonian translocation). The last is most frequently observed as occurring between chromosomes 21 and 14, which have their centromeres near the ends (they are so-called acrocentric chromosomes).

The individual who develops from a gamete carrying an inversion or a reciprocal translocation usually shows no abnormality but is likely to produce abnormal offspring because of the unbalanced gametes (with an excess or deficiency of genetic material, or both) that may be produced by such persons during meiosis.

DIAGNOSIS OF CHROMOSOMAL ABERRATIONS

Clinically, the chromosomes are most conveniently studied in circulating lymphocytes stimulated to mitosis with phytohemagglutinin. This mitogen is added to a small sample of blood in short-term culture. Colchicine is also added to arrest cell division and to

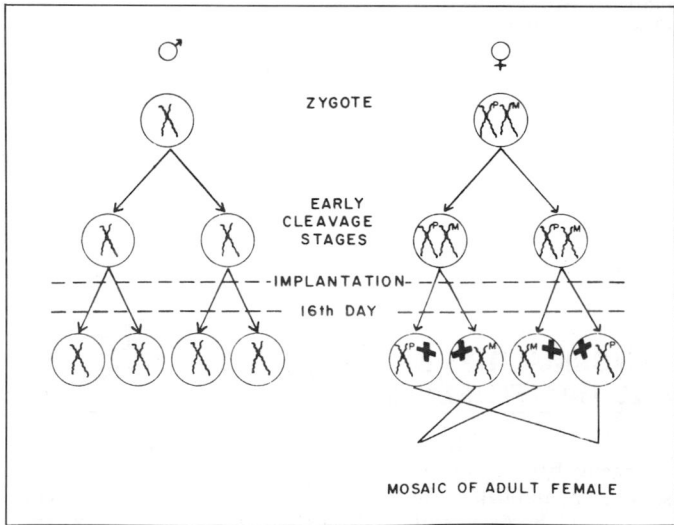

Figure 5.2–2. The Lyon principle. Some time between implantation and the 16th day in the normal female embryo, one X chromosome in each cell (*left*) becomes genetically relatively inactive and forms the Barr body, or sex chromatin. It is randomly determined whether the X chromosome contributed by the mother or father is the inactivated one in a given cell, but once decision is made in a given cell, all descendants of that cell have the same X chromosome inactive.

cause an accumulation of cells in metaphase, a stage of mitosis optional for study of the chromosomes. Treatment with hypotonic saline produces swelling of the nuclei and spreading of the chromosomes, so that they are more easily examined individually. Special treatment of various types have been developed, relating for example to pH, as well as special stains, to produce a banding pattern of the chromosomes. Each of the human 24 chromosomes (22 autosomes plus X and Y) has a unique and distinctive banding pattern (see Fig. 5.1–1). After short-term culture and treatment along the lines just indicated, the cells are spread, fixed, and stained for light microscopy at high magnification. (Electron microscopy has thus far yielded little clinically useful information.)

The metaphase chromosomes of a single lymphocyte have the appearance shown in Figure 5.1–1A. The photographic image of each chromosome is cut out, and the chromosomes are arranged in pairs; are identified by their relative lengths, ratio of arms, and specific banding patterns; and are laid out in a so-called karyotype, as shown in Figure 5.1–1B. (The schematic representation is called an ideogram.) Each of the metaphase chromosomes is double, that is, consists of two chromatids united at the centromere. Each chromosome has replicated in preparation for cell division, and each chromatid of a particular chromosome is destined to be that chromosome in one of the two daughter cells. (The separate chromatids of each chromosome are evident in preparations made by nonbinding methods. In banded preparations such as those shown in Figures 5.1–1 and 5.2–4, the chromatids are in close apposition.)

A now little-used method for diagnosing abnormalities in sex chromosome number is the buccal smear. The Barr body, demonstrable subjacent to the nuclear membrane in stained buccal mucosal cells, represents the one inactive X chromosome of the normal 46,XX female (Fig. 5.2–3). It is absent in the 46,XY male and present in double or triplicate in persons with the XXX or XXXX sex chromosome constitutions. Fluorescent Y chromatin is also demonstrable in specially stained mucosal cells and is a marker for the Y chromosome. It is absent in the XO (Turner) syndrome and double in XYY males. It may also be absent in the rare normal XY male who has a small Y chromosome missing the fluorescent part of its long arm. These methods have been largely superseded by chromosome studies (karyotyping).

Abnormalities of the chromosomes have been related causally to disorders in at least six categories (Table 5.2–1). In addition, increased chromosomal breakage is an integral feature of some mendelian syndromes, such as Fanconi anemia. Figure 5.2–4 is a composite of the karyotypic findings associated with some leading chromosomal abnormalities.

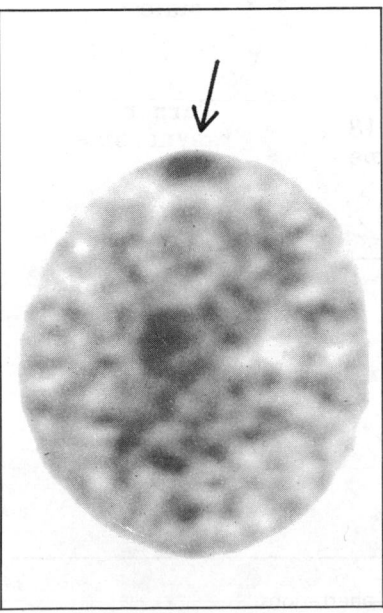

Figure 5.2–3. X chromatin (Barr body) in nucleus of female buccal mucosal cell.

TABLE 5.2–1. PHENOTYPES TO WHICH CHROMOSOMAL CHANGES HAVE BEEN CAUSALLY RELATED

- Sex abnormalities, such as XO Turner syndrome, XXY (Klinefelter) syndrome
- Mental retardation, such as trisomy 21 in Down syndrome, deleted short arm of chromosome 5 in cri-du-chat syndrome, fragile-X syndrome
- Complex malformation syndrome, such as D_1 trisomy (trisomy 13, or Patau syndrome)
- Behavioral abnormalities, such as XYY male
- Abortion—in one fifth to one half of spontaneous abortions in the first trimester, major chromosomal abnormalities are demonstrable in the conceptus
- Neoplasia, such as Philadelphia chromosome (9;22 translocation) in CML[39]

SEX ANOMALIES RESULTING FROM ABERRATION OF THE SEX CHROMOSOMES

Primary amenorrhea and male infertility are leading presenting complaints in adults with anomalies of the sex chromosomes. In the female with primary amenorrhea, clinical features may indicate either Turner syndrome or the testicular feminization syndrome; male infertility may indicate Klinefelter syndrome.

The buccal smear for determination of the X chromatin can be a first step in the laboratory confirmation of these diagnoses (Fig. 5.2–3). In a majority of instances, females with Turner syndrome are X-chromatin negative, like the normal male, and males with Klinefelter syndrome are X-chromatin positive, like the normal female. Apparent females with the testicular feminization syndrome are in fact males and are X-chromatin negative. Usually, and certainly in case of doubt, such as patients with Turner syndrome who are chromatin positive, direct studies of the chromosomes are indicated. In conventional cases of these three syndromes—Turner syndrome, Klinefelter syndrome, and testicular feminization—the sex chromosome findings are, respectively, XO, XXY, and normal XY. These are described in more detail below, and some of the more complicated related conditions are discussed.

TURNER SYNDROME

Short stature, primary amenorrhea, and lack of development of secondary sex characteristics are the cardinal features of Turner syndrome.[9] Other less consistent features are a webbed neck, lowset ears, a low posterior hairline, numerous pigmented nevi, a broad, shieldlike chest with widely spaced nipples, and brachydactyly, with particular shortening of some metacarpals, especially the fourth. Coarctation of the aorta, hypertension (without coarctation and probably secondary to vascular anomaly of the kidney), and angiomata of the bowel, leading to gastrointestinal bleeding, are features of a small but significant number of cases. On laparotomy the internal sex organs are found to be of female type, but the uterus is infantile and the ovaries are represented merely by fibrous streaks. Turner syndrome occurs about once in every 2500 female births.

About 80 percent of cases of the syndrome are X-chromatin negative and show 45 chromosomes, there being but a single sex chromosome, an X. The second sex chromosome, either an X or a Y, is missing. Turner syndrome is called the XO (read "X-oh") syndrome or the 45,X syndrome.

Most cases of Turner syndrome that are X-chromatin positive are found by chromosome study to fall into one of the following situations:

1. Some have 46 chromosomes, including one X chromosome and another large chromosome that is made up of

two long arms of an X chromosome, a so-called isochromosome X. Thus these individuals have three X-chromosome long arms and only one X-chromosome short arm. The deficiency of the short arm of the X chromosome is critical to the short stature that is part of Turner syndrome. The Barr body and the "drumstick" of the polymorphonuclear leukocytes (which is the equivalent of the Barr body) is unusually large in these isochromosome-X cases; other evidence indicates that the Barr body in each cell of these cases is formed by the anomalous large chromosome, the isochromosome. The anomalous X chromosome is the inactive one in most or all cells. Inactivation of the isochromosome with two long arms prevents ill effects of an extra dose of long-arm genetic material.

2. Some of the chromatin-positive cases are mosaics of XO cells and other cells such as normal XX. This situation arises as a result of an accident of mitosis in an early division of the zygote.

Noonan syndrome has somatic features like those of Turner syndrome, but the chromosomes are normal. It appears to be an autosomal dominant disorder. Both males and females are affected (previously called male Turner syndrome and female pseudo-Turner syndrome, respectively). In females sexual development is usually normal, whereas males usually have hypogonadism. Short stature, lowset ears, and webbed neck occur as in Turner syndrome. The sternum is often characteristically misshapen, having a sharp angulation at the angle of Louis (junction of the manubrium and corpus sterni) so there is pectus carinatum ("pigeon breast") above and pectus excavatum ("hollow chest") below.

OTHER X-CHROMOSOME ANOMALIES WITH FEMALE PHENOTYPE

The XXX (triple-X) female is the most frequent of the X-chromosome anomalies with the female phenotype, occurring probably about once in each 800 female births. The triple-X state is, however, less well known than many of the other X-chromosome anomalies, mainly because no characteristic disorder is produced. Although triple-X females often are mentally retarded and may have a schizophrenia-like condition, somatic abnormalities do not occur consistently. Menstruation may be normal. One would expect that half the ova of such women would carry two X chromosomes rather than one and that on fertilization an XXY or another XXX individual would be formed. This is a rarity, however; most offspring have been karyotypically normal.

As stated earlier, quadruple-X and even penta-X cases have been identified, but these are rare.

MALE INFERTILITY AND KLINEFELTER SYNDROME

Small testes and infertility are consistent features of Klinefelter syndrome. Gynecomastia is present in many, and the habitus is sometimes eunuchoidal, that is, the legs are disproportionately long and the fat distribution is feminine in type, with concentration about the hips. The beard and body hair are sparse, and normal male recession of the hairline does not occur. In older persons with the syndrome the face tends to be unusually wrinkled. Intelligence is on the average reduced, but mental retardation is rarely severe, and

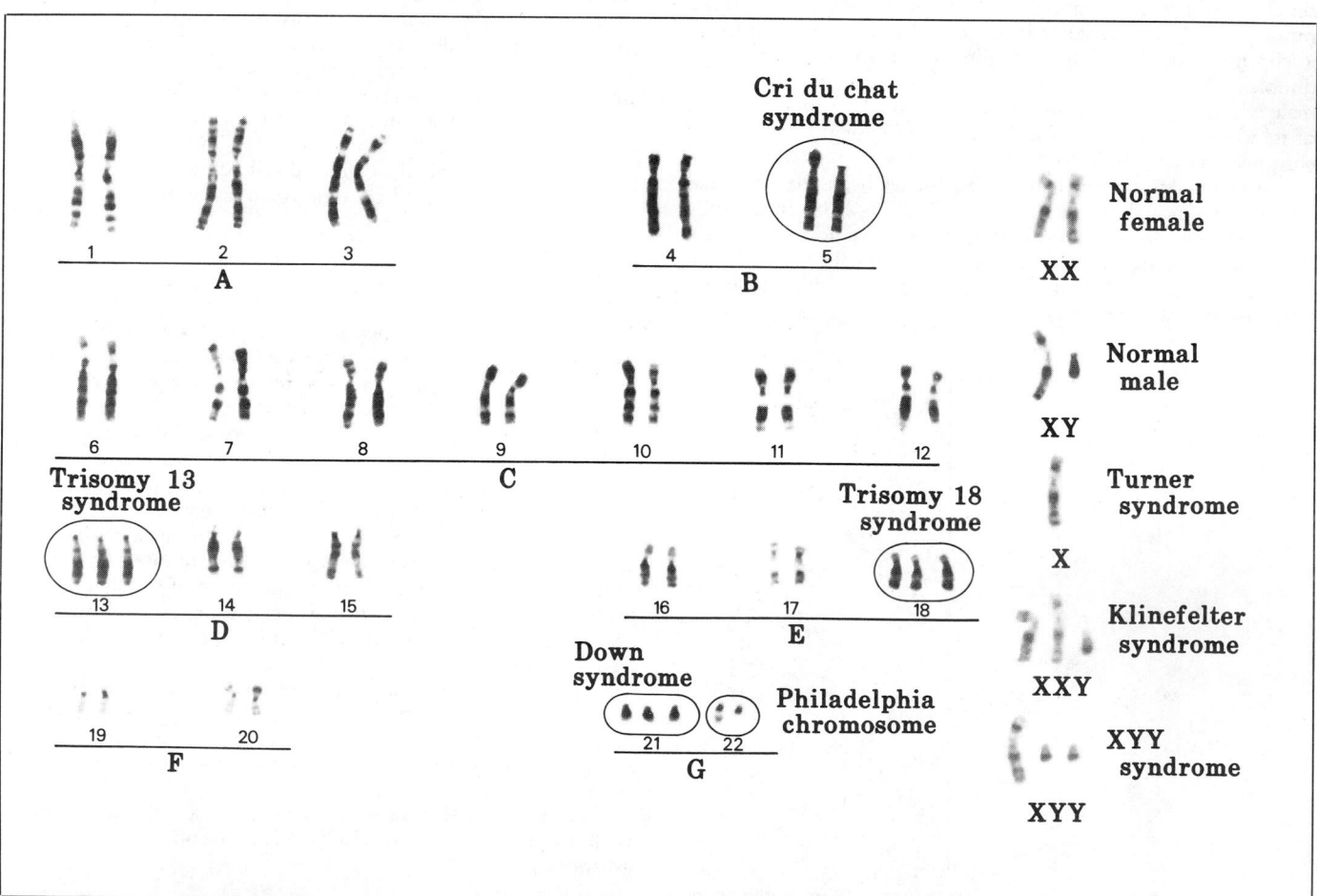

Figure 5.2–4. Composite karyotype showing selected major chromosomal aberrations.

some affected persons are quite intelligent. Congenital malformations are not associated with Klinefelter syndrome. About 1 in every 500 newborn males has this syndrome.

Typically, the patient is positive for both X and Y chromatin. High levels of pituitary gonadotropin (follicle-stimulating hormone) characterize the urinary hormone excretion. The histologic changes in the testes in postpubertal cases (ghostlike sclerosed tubules and Leydig cell hyperplasia) are also characteristic. In the prepubertal cases these changes are not present, and the main finding is absence or striking paucity of germ cells. The postpubertal changes are caused by the high concentration of circulating pituitary gonadotropins.

Other sex chromosome anomalies with the male phenotype include the XXXY (triple X-Y) syndrome and the XXXXY (quadruple X-Y) syndrome. In general, the features in the genitalia, habitus, and breasts are the same as in the XXY Klinefelter syndrome. A difference is the occurrence of severe mental retardation and some congenital malformations, such as radioulnar synostosis, in the XXXY and XXXXY states.

Missegregation of the Y chromosome in the second stage of meiosis can lead to sperm carrying two Ys and an individual who is karyotypically XYY. On the average, XYY males are taller and more liable to antisocial behavior than are their XY brothers.

The study of sex chromosome anomalies has taught us much about normal sex determination. With rare exception (and these instances are themselves instructive) testes develop if a Y chromosome is present and testes do not develop if the Y chromosome is absent. To be sure, the testis may not be normally functional (e.g., in the XXY [Klinefelter] syndrome). Furthermore, only part of the Y chromosome, in the mid or proximal part of the short arm, is critical to differentiation of the indifferent embryonic gonad into a testis. With the use of DNA markers, many XX males have been found to have genetic material from the short arm of the Y chromosome translocated onto the end of the short arm of the X chromosome. This exchange occurred during meiosis in the father and must have included the gene(s) for testis-determining factor.

MALFORMATION SYNDROMES DUE TO CHROMOSOMAL ABERRATIONS

The malformations in which microscopically identifiable chromosomal abnormality can be convincingly demonstrated are without exception complex anomalies (malformation syndromes). A prototype is Down syndrome. Excessive chromosome 21 material is a consistent karyotypic finding. In addition to mental retardation, leading features include a round small head, typical facies (epicanthus, Brushfield spots of the iris, a large furrowed tongue, cheilosis), short stature, a transverse palmar crease, brachydactyly with an incurved fifth finger, alopecia areata, cardiac malformation (atrioventricular canal defect), and progressive cataracts. Acute leukemia occurs with increased frequency in persons with Down syndrome.

Most cases of Down syndrome show three separate chromosomes 21 rather than the normal two. Meiotic nondisjunction with incorporation of both chromosomes 21 into the gamete is responsible. This accident occurs more often in older mothers. The overall frequency of Down syndrome is about 1 in 800 live births, but the frequency becomes as high as 1 in 80 in the offspring of mothers over 40.

Some cases of Down syndrome are found to be mosaics: some cells are trisomy 21, whereas others are of normal karyotype. Mosaic Down syndrome originates in an accident in an early cleavage stage. It may occur at a sufficiently late stage that only a small proportion of all cells are trisomic, and the individual shows few or no stigmata. However, if the gonad participates in the trisomy, such a person can give birth to trisomic offspring. (It is biologically possible for a female with Down syndrome to be the mother of a Nobel laureate! Females with nonmosaic trisomy 21 apparently conceive trisomy 21 and normal offspring in equal proportions. Because of fetal loss of trisomy 21, karyotypically normal offspring predominate among the children of women with Down syndrome.)

Other cases of Down syndrome are of one of the so-called translocation types. In many of these, a chromosomal rearrangement occurred in an earlier generation and multiple cases of mongolism occur in the family. A frequent type of translocation involves a union between a chromosome 21 and a chromosome of the 13 to 15 group. Carriers of a 14;21 translocation chromosome have a total of 45 separate chromosomes but are phenotypically normal because they neither lack a significant amount of chromosomal material nor carry an excess. In such individuals, however, accidents in meiosis are likely to occur. A ''balanced gamete'' is formed if the translocation chromosome goes into it without any other chromosome 14 or 21. But if both the translocation chromosome and the independent chromosome 21 get into the same gamete, a state trisomic for chromosome 21 is created in the zygote (after fertilization of the anomalous gamete by a normal 21-bearing gamete). The proportions of various types of offspring—normal, balanced carriers, and Down syndrome—are not as precise as are the genetic ratios observed with ''mendelizing'' traits. In part, this is because many of the aneuploid embryos die in utero. The proportion of children of 14;21 translocation carrier women who have Down syndrome is about 11 percent. Among the children of carrier males about 5 percent have Down syndrome.

When a parent is a translocation carrier, parental age is not a factor in the occurrence of mongolism. Translocation Down syndrome constitutes, however, less than 5 percent of all cases. Even in women of young maternal age, an isolated (i.e., nonfamilial) case of Down syndrome is more likely to be of conventional trisomy 21 type. For more precise prognostication, the chromosomes should be studied in any instance of more than one case of Down syndrome in a family. Even in families with two or more cases of Down syndrome, conventional trisomy 21 is frequently found. Some maintain that the karyotype should be determined in all cases of established or suspected Down syndrome.

Two other main types of chromosomal aberrations that have been related to specific malformation syndromes are trisomy 13 and trisomy 18 (formerly known as D_1 or Patau syndrome and E_1 or Edwards syndrome, respectively). Since chromosomes 13 and 18 are larger than chromosome 21 and presumably carry more genetic information, and features are more drastic in these disorders. Unlike persons with Down syndrome, no one with these aberrations has been known to survive.

Deletion of part of the short arm of one chromosome 5 produces a characteristic disorder called the cri-du-chat (cat-cry) syndrome because of the characteristic sound made by affected infants. This aberration is characterized by microcephaly and severe mental retardation. Patients with this disorder are common, especially since they survive to adulthood.

Banding techniques and high-resolution cytogenetics have permitted the phenotypic-karyotypic correlations necessary for delineation of some new chromosomal syndromes. The phenotype could be analyzed in a group of cases carrying precisely the same chromosomal abnormality. One of these syndromes is trisomy 8,[9] which bears similarities to Marfan syndrome.[19]

Although arachnodactyly, chest deformity, and gangly habitus suggest Marfan syndrome, trisomy 8 patients do not have the ocular and cardiovascular abnormalities of Marfan syndrome and show mental retardation, wide spacing between the first and second toes, and unusual creases of the palms and soles—all non-Marfan features. Most if not all are mosaics; that only a portion of their cells are trisomic for this relatively large chromosome may explain why the effects are not more drastic than they are.

The Prader-Willi syndrome is a congenital disorder characterized by morbid obesity with small hands and feet and usually mental retardation. A small abnormality in the long arm of chromosome 15 subjacent to the centromere has been found by high-resolution cytogenetics.[25]

Another important chromosomal abnormality associated with disease is the "fragile X," a break or gap toward the end of the long arm of the X chromosome. The fragile-X syndrome comprises mental retardation and large testes, with less striking or specific features such as prominent ears and jaw. This disorder is at the borderline between mendelism and chromosomal aberration; it is transmitted as an X-linked recessive trait with partial and variable expression in the heterozygous carrier females.[32] The chromosomal change is "brought out" by a culture medium deficient in folate. It is a relatively frequent cause of mental retardation, occurring in about 1 in 2000 males.

NEOPLASIA DUE TO CHROMOSOMAL ABERRATIONS

Since Boveri early in this century, genetic change in a clone of cells has been considered as the basis for malignancy—the "cause" of cancer. An increasing number of firmly established examples are now known in humans. In cases of chronic myeloid leukemia (CML) a distal part of the long arm of one chromosome 22 is translocated to another chromosome, most often to the end of the long arm of a chromosome 9.[39] The abnormal (partially deleted) chromosome is called the Philadelphia chromosome, having been discovered by Nowell and Hungerford of that city. Only blood cells show the abnormality. The chromosomal change is acquired, not congenital. Exposure to ionizing radiation (such as x-ray treatment used in the past for ankylosing spondylitis) is responsible in some cases for the chromosomal breakage that led to the oncogenic chromosomal rearrangement. Viral or chemical damage to the chromosomes is suspected in others.

It is now known that the 9;22 translocation (Philadelphia chromosome) of CML is reciprocal and that an "oncogene" symbolized ABL (for Abelson, the retrovirus it resembles in the DNA sequence), normally situated on the end of the long arm of chromosome 9, is translocated to 22. Oncogenes are normal constituents of the human genome that serve important functions in the control of cell proliferation. In CML the translocation brings the ABL oncogene into the proximity of a DNA sequence on chromosome 22 (called BCR1 for "breakpoint cluster region"). A fusion gene, consisting in part of the ABL gene and in part of BCR1, is implicated in the initiation of malignancy in this form of leukemia.

The Philadelphia chromosome can be of diagnostic value in patients who present atypically, for example, with the clinical picture of myelofibrosis. It also has prognostic significance. The Philadelphia chromosome is probably found in all CML cases, usually in the characteristic 9;22 translocation but sometimes in a different rearrangement that creates the ABL-BCR1 fusion gene. Those patients who appear to have CML but lack the Philadelphia chromosome or its equivalent must be considered to suffer from a fundamentally distinct entity. They tend to show a more rapid course and respond less favorably to therapy.[13]

When the Philadelphia chromosome is being tested for in samples of peripheral blood, phytohemagglutinin is omitted from the preparative procedure. In CML the circulating myeloid leukocytes usually include enough mitotic cells for study; phytohemagglutinin stimulates the unaffected lymphocytes.

Characteristic translocations of acquired nature occur in association with other forms of hematologic malignancy: such as 2;8 or 8;14 or 8;22 translocation with Burkitt lymphoma[22]; 15;17 translocation with acute promyelocytic leukemia. The MYC oncogene on chromosome 8 and the FES oncogene on chromosome 15 appear to be involved, respectively, in these two malignancies.

Solid tumors often show a deletion, either acquired or congenital. Congenital deletion of a band on the long arm of chromosome 13 (13q14) is associated with retinoblastoma. Congenital deletion of a band on the short arm of chromosome 11 (11p13) is associated with Wilms tumor (with or without other features of the WAGR syndrome: Wilms tumor/aniridia/gonadoblastoma/mental retardation). Acquired deletion of part of 3p occurs in small-cell cancer of the lung.

IN WHAT CASES SHOULD CHROMOSOME STUDIES BE DONE?

A chromosome analysis is time consuming and therefore expensive. Consequently, there must be careful selection of the cases to be studied. In X-chromosome abnormalities, a buccal smear combined with informed clinical observation often suffices. For example, in a teenage boy with gynecomastia, Klinefelter syndrome can be excluded with confidence if the testes are of normal or near-normal size; normal male findings on a buccal smear clinch the alternative diagnosis of adolescent gynecomastia.

Substantiation of the diagnosis of Down syndrome may be helpful in making arrangements for the care of the infant. Thus in suspected but uncertain cases, chromosome studies are indicated. In young parents of a child with Down syndrome, chromosome analysis can improve the precision with which the risk of subsequent children being affected is estimated. If one parent is a translocation carrier, the risk of another child's being affected is considerable.

In the differentiation of CML from leukemoid states, such as myeloid metaplasia, finding the Philadelphia chromosome (9;22 translocation) is as specific as finding *Mycobacterium tuberculosis* in the sputum of a patient with a pulmonary lesion.

As indicated earlier, some other hematologic malignancies are accompanied by specific chromosomal changes and information on the karyotype is useful in diagnosis, prognosis, and management.

Cases of congenital malformations in which chromosome abnormalities might be sought are so numerous that decisions must be made as to what types of cases are likely to "pay off." Complex, multiple-system malformations are the ones in which discernible chromosomal abnormalities are most likely to be found. Malformations with mendelian patterns of inheritance, such as the Ellis–van Creveld syndrome,[32] an autosomal recessive trait (see Table 5.3–7), are not likely to show chromosomal abnormalities.

In Fanconi anemia, Bloom syndrome, and ataxia-telangiectasia (all autosomal recessive disorders) increased chromosomal breakage and other abnormalities are found. The proclivity to leukemia and other malignancies shown by each of these conditions may be related to this chromosomal breakage. Study of the chromosomes can provide information corroborating the diagnosis.

Mendelian Disorders

Victor A. McKusick

Principles of diagnosis, prognosis (genetic counseling), treatment, and prevention will be presented in this chapter. Thereafter these principles will be illustrated with a discussion of eight special categories of mendelian disease: hemoglobinopathies; inborn errors of metabolism, including vitamin-responsive forms; lysosomal diseases; receptor disorders; defects in transmembrane transport; heritable disorders of connective tissue; mendelian malformations; and mendelian neoplasms. Pharmacogenetics and immunogenetics will also be discussed.

There is a large number of mendelian disorders, so that even though many of them are individually rare, in the aggregate they represent a significant aspect of clinical practice. Table 5.3–6 gives the numbers of firmly and provisionally identified mendelian traits, most of them "diseases," "disorders," or "defects," that have been identified in successive editions of *Mendelian Inheritance in Man*.[32] The steadily increasing numbers reflect advances in genetic nosology (meaning classification of genetic diseases, or, better, delineation of genetic diseases). The numbers become less formidable when the information concerning all the individual conditions is systematized on the basis of advances in fundamental knowledge in the last few decades. The discussion of the characteristics of eight categories of mendelian disorders will indicate the sort of systemization that is possible.

DIAGNOSIS

Basic to both diagnosis and prognosis is the genetic family history as incorporated in the pedigree. Three further principles of fundamental importance to the accurate diagnosis of mendelian disorders are genetic heterogeneity, pleiotropism, and variability. The laboratory diagnosis of mendelian disorders has some special aspects, particularly with regard to the identification of the basic "lesion" in DNA. "Gene diagnosis" by direct study of the gene or by the linkage principle is now feasible for an ever-increasing number of entities. These approaches are useful in prenatal diagnosis (e.g., of the thalassemias), in premorbid diagnosis (e.g., of Huntington disease[29]), and in carrier detection (e.g., of hemophilia).

THE FAMILY HISTORY

The family history carefully taken is a major tool of clinical genetics. In eliciting and recording a patient's complete history there is much to recommend obtaining the family history last. The description of the presenting problem and the past history concerning health and illness are valuable guides to the nature of the questions to be asked in taking the family history. For example, the questions to be asked of a 35-year-old man with chest pain compatible with angina pectoris are different from those to be asked of a 35-year-old man with failing vision and skin changes about the neck compatible with pseudoxanthoma elasticum.[31]

The past history and the methodical review of systems may suggest multiple-system involvement or may give evidence of long-standing minor stigmata of the disorder that brings the patient to the physician. Thus further background for the family history is provided. Frequently the complaint that brings the patient to medical attention is relatively trivial. This is especially true in genetic disorders, because the patient may have become accustomed to the condition through its presence from an early age or because of its slow development. Its grave potentialities may not be known to the patient unless there are other similar cases in the family.

In obtaining the family history, at least four general questions should be asked:

1. Has anyone in your family had a condition similar to yours?
2. Is there any condition that seems to "run in your family?"
3. Are your parents related by blood?
4. What was the ethnic origin of your parents?

The question about consanguinity is particularly important in the case of rare recessively inherited disorders. Since it is generally held that consanguinity is "bad" and since specific regulations with regard to the marriage of relatives are laid down by some religions and by some states, patients may be embarrassed by the question, but usually the physician thinks the question will be more embarrassing than it actually proves to be.

The rarer the recessive disorder, the more frequently the parents of affected persons are found to be consanguineous. Tay-Sachs disease is relatively frequent in Ashkenazi Jews, and the frequency of first-cousin marriages among parents of cases is relatively low, although higher than in the general population. In non-Jews the disorder is much less frequent, but a higher proportion of the parents are first cousins or related in some other manner. In families with cystic fibrosis, a relatively frequent disorder in persons of Northern European extraction, little increased parental consanguinity is expected, and little or none is found. When both parents are foreign born, even if the patient does not know them to be related, the presumption of consanguinity is strong if they came from the same village. The same is true if the parents came from the same rural area of the United States, where the forebears had lived for several generations.

Ethnic background is frequently of value in the appraisal of diagnostic possibilities. Anemia in a person of Mediterranean stock brings to mind possibilities different from those suggested by anemia in one of Swedish origin. Some rare recessive diseases are much more frequent in certain ethnic groups, for example, thalassemia[6,43] and G6PD deficiency in persons of Mediterranean origin, familial Mediterranean fever in Armenians and Sephardic Jews, and acatalasia in Japanese. Other diseases are notably rare in certain groups, for example, cystic fibrosis in blacks and phenylketonuria in Jews.

If the disorder in question is a recognized autosomal dominant trait and if the affected person is a sporadic case, the diagnosis may be "shored up" by finding advanced paternal age. Advanced paternal age points to new dominant mutation in the same manner as parental consanguinity suggests autosomal recessive inheritance.

After the general questions of the family history, a systematic inquiry should be made into the status, living or dead, and the state of health of all immediate relatives, particularly first-degree relatives (parents, sibs, and offspring). Whether the inquiry is carried further depends on the nature of the ailment and the results of the earlier questioning. Usually each close relative should be asked about individually, beginning with the parents. In questioning about the sibs, it is best to ask about each pregnancy of the mother in order, so that stillbirths, miscarriages, and infant deaths are not overlooked. If the patient is married and has children, the health of the spouse and all pregnancies resulting from the marital union are reviewed.

Organization of the family history is facilitated by a sketch of the family tree. The individual in a family who brings that family

to study—the patient in the usual clinical situation—is referred to in pedigree studies as the proband (or as the propositus or proposita). The proband is indicated in pedigree charts by an arrow. Males and females are most often represented by squares and circles, respectively. Consanguineous matings are indicated by a double marital line. If the mating is consanguineous, it is useful to complete the pedigree sufficiently to indicate how the parents are related. Individuals affected with a given disorder can be indicated by blacked-in symbols. If several characteristics are present in the family, various special methods can be used for indicating which are present in any given individual. There are conventions for indicating twins, monozygotic and dizygotic, and for abortions. Each individual in the pedigree is indicated by a number. The generations are numbered with Roman numerals, and the persons in each generation are numbered consecutively with Arabic numerals. Thus III-6 refers to the sixth person in the third generation of the family. These conventions are illustrated in Figures 5.3–1 to 5.3–6.

PEDIGREE PATTERNS OF MENDELIAN INHERITANCE

Based on the mechanics of the chromosomes in meiosis, genes are distributed in families in predictable patterns. Depending on whether the gene is located on an autosome or on an X chromosome and depending on whether the gene in single dose (heterozygous state) or only in double dose (homozygous state) results in the given phenotype, characteristic familial patterns of inheritance are demonstrated by simply inherited disorders.

When a gene in single dose causes a given effect, the phenotype is said to be dominant. When the effect is observed only in the homozygote (i.e., with the mutant gene in double dose), the phenotype is said to be recessive. In general, disorders resulting from defects in enzyme systems—such as all the inborn errors of metabolism—behave as recessives. Because of the margin of safety provided in most enzyme systems, phenotypic abnormality is evident only when all of a given enzyme is mutant (and deficient). On the other hand, disorders resulting from a change in the amino acid sequence of a structural or other nonenzymic protein are usually dominant. Consequences of the alteration in the physical and chemical properties of the particular protein are observable in the heterozygote even though only a portion of that protein is of the mutant type. Several of the heritable disorders of connective tissue are dominant. For example, the loose jointedness, cutaneous fragility, bruisability, and stretchability associated with the classic Ehlers-Danlos syndrome, which is inherited as a dominant, are thought to result from alteration in collagen. The differences in the nature of the defect in the dominant and recessive forms of methemoglobinemia and of the Ehlers-Danlos syndromes (p. 298) illustrate this principle. Some of the porphyrias are notable "excep-

tions that prove the rule"; although they are "caused" by an enzyme deficiency, they show autosomal dominant inheritance.

Dominance and recessiveness are attributes of the phenotype, not of the gene. In population genetics, for convenience, geneticists speak of dominant genes and recessive genes, but in clinical genetics confusion is avoided if the adjectives are used only in connection with specifically defined traits.

The pedigree patterns of *rare* simply inherited traits are characteristic for autosomal dominant, autosomal recessive, X-linked recessive, and X-linked dominant inheritance.

The characteristics of the pedigree of *rare autosomal dominant disorders* are outlined in Table 5.3–1.

The characteristics of the pedigree of *rare autosomal recessive disorders* are outlined in Table 5.3–2. In contrast to dominant diseases, which are transmitted to the offspring from one parent, each parent, although usually phenotypically normal, contributes a mutant gene to the affected offspring. *Recessive inheritance is inheritance from both parents.* On the average, of the children of two heterozygous parents, one fourth (homozygotes) will be affected, one half (heterozygotes) will carry a single mutant gene, and the remaining fourth will be normal (Fig. 5.3–2).

X-Linked Inheritance

Diseases or traits that result from genes located on the X chromosome are said to be "sex linked" or, more precisely, "X linked." If the condition is dominant, that is, is manifest when the gene is

TABLE 5.3–1. PEDIGREE CHARACTERISTICS OF UNCOMMON AUTOSOMAL DOMINANT DISORDERS

- Each affected individual has an affected parent, unless the condition arose by fresh mutation in the given individual. (Because of wide variability in severity of dominant traits, the parent may be too mildly affected to be recognized as a case.)
- An affected individual and a normal mate will have, on the average, affected and normal children in equal proportions.
- Normal children of an affected person will have all normal offspring.
- Males and females are affected in equal proportions.
- Affected males and females are equally likely to transmit the condition to male and female offspring. Specifically, male-to-male transmission occurs.
- Homozygotes may be born if two affected persons (heterozygotes) marry. Homozygotes are usually more severely affected than heterozygotes.
- On the average, the age of fathers of sporadic (new mutation) cases is elevated.
- The more severely the disorder interferes with reproduction, the larger is the proportion of cases that are sporadic ("new mutations").

TABLE 5.3–2. PEDIGREE CHARACTERISTICS OF UNCOMMON AUTOSOMAL RECESSIVE DISORDERS

- The parents are usually clinically normal.
- The larger the family, the more often will more than one child be affected.
- The rarer the mutant gene in the population, the more often will the parents be related.
- In marriages between individuals, each with the same recessive disease, all their offspring will be affected.
- Affected individuals who marry normal individuals have only normal offspring (unless the normal spouse is a carrier).
- The sexes are affected in equal proportions.
- If an affected individual marries a heterozygote, as is more likely to occur with consanguineous marriage, half the children would be affected, and a pedigree pattern simulating dominant inheritance would result.

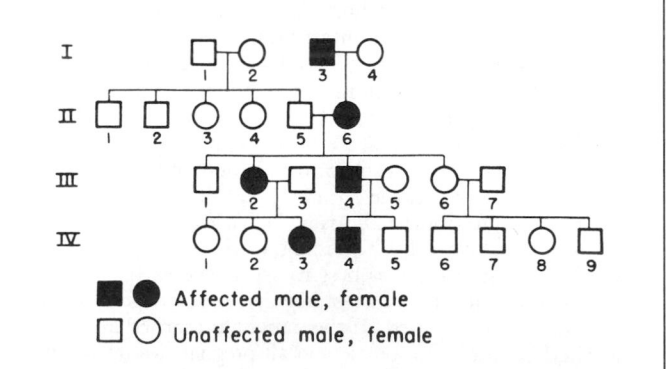

Figure 5.3–1. Autosomal dominant pedigree pattern (idealized).

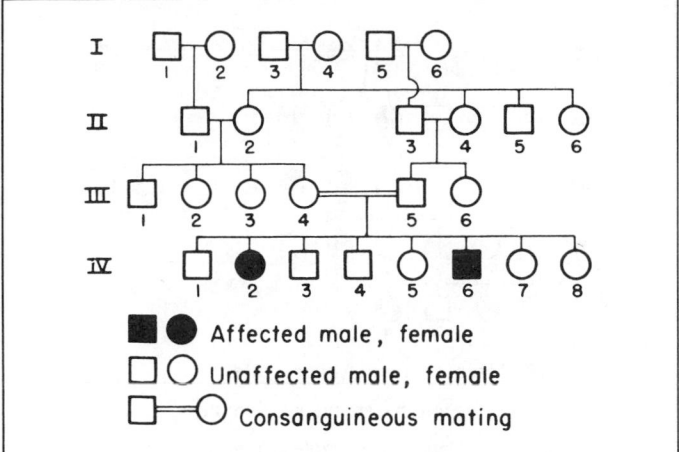

Figure 5.3–2. Autosomal recessive pedigree pattern (idealized). Parents are first cousins.

present in the heterozygous state in the female, either sex may be affected. If the condition is recessive and rare, females will seldom be affected, since homozygosity, or a double dose of the gene, is required. In males with only one X chromosome an X-linked gene is always expressed, regardless of whether the condition is dominant or recessive in the female. Since the male cannot inherit his X chromosome from his father, male-to-male (father-to-son) inheritance rules out sex-linked inheritance. The characteristic features of *X-linked recessive inheritance* are outlined in Table 5.3–3. (See Fig. 5.3–3.)

Some X-linked traits behave as dominants, that is, are expressed in the heterozygous female. The features are outlined in Table 5.3–4. Hereditary hypophosphatemia ("vitamin D–resistant rickets") is a good example (Figs. 5.3–4 and 5.3–5).

When an X-linked disorder is dominant but is lethal in utero to the hemizygous affected male, a characteristic pedigree pattern, schematized in Figure 5.3–6 and described in Table 5.3–5, results. Examples are one form of incontinentia pigmenti, focal dermal hypoplasia, and orofaciodigital (OFD) syndrome. The first two have, in association with congenital malformations, skin lesions whose spotty distribution may be a manifestation of the Lyon principle (Fig. 5.2–2). The only male cases of the OFD syndrome have been found either to have a closely simulating autosomal recessive disorder (OFD II) or to be instances of the XXY (Klinefelter) syndrome and are thus not true exceptions to this mode of inheritance.

Disorders with dominant inheritance and those with recessive inheritance were contrasted earlier with respect to the usual nature of the basic defects. They can also be contrasted with respect to

TABLE 5.3–3. PEDIGREE CHARACTERISTICS OF UNCOMMON SEX-LINKED (X-LINKED) RECESSIVE DISORDERS

When the disorder is such that affected males do not reproduce (e.g., Duchenne muscular dystrophy, testicular feminization syndrome):
- Only males are affected.
- According to theoretic expectations, about two thirds of cases have a carrier mother from whom the mutant gene is inherited; about one third of cases arise by new mutation in the X chromosome from the mother.
- In the inherited form, affected males may have affected brothers and affected maternal uncles. The new mutation cases are sporadic, that is, isolated cases.
- The sisters of inherited cases have a 50 percent chance of being carriers for the gene.
- A carrier sister transmits the gene to half her sons, who are affected, and to half her daughters, who are carriers.
- Unaffected males do not transmit the disorder.

When the disorder is such that affected males may reproduce (e.g., hemophilias A and B, G6PD deficiency):
- The proportion of cases that are inherited rises further above two thirds, the less is the reduction of average number of children produced by affected males.
- Affected males transmit the gene to *all* their daughters and to *none* of their sons.
- All phenotypically normal daughters of affected males are carriers.
- If married to a carrier female, affected males will have daughters, half of whom are homozygous and affected, half of whom are normal but carriers.
- Rare heterozygous females may be affected ("manifesting heterozygotes"), because of chances of lyonization.

variability and clinical severity. Dominant disorders tend to be more variable and also less severe than recessive ones. Because a dominant disorder may be so mild in a given individual, "skipped generations" may be observed in pedigrees. Reduced penetrance is mainly a feature of dominant traits. Reduced penetrance means that the expressivity (severity) of the trait is below the level of recognition.

All simply inherited genetic disorders arose by gene mutation at some time in the past. A given case may be the result of a new dominant mutation occurring in the germ cells of one or the other of the parents. Such cases will be sporadic, and there will not be the characteristic pedigree pattern shown in Figure 5.3–1. If, on the average, patients with a given dominant disorder have only half as many children as do unaffected persons in the general population and one assumes genetic equilibrium, then half the probands in any large series will be new mutations. An example is von Recklinghausen neurofibromatosis. In the case of some autosomal dominant disorders whose victims very rarely reproduce, almost all

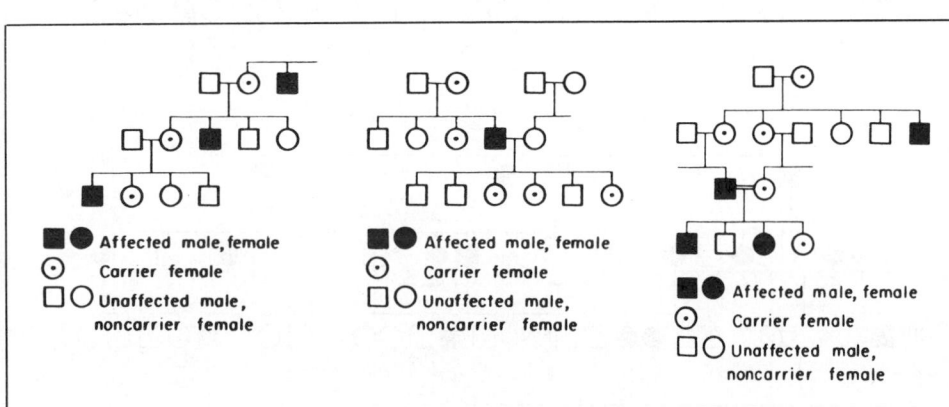

Figure 5.3–3. X-linked recessive pedigree pattern. **Left:** Oblique pattern of affected males and carrier females. **Center:** All daughters of affected male are carriers; all sons are unaffected. **Right:** Daughter of affected male married to carrier female may be homozygous and affected. The fact that a son is affected is not an exception to the rule of no male-to-male transmission, since mutant X chromosome came to affected son from carrier mother.

TABLE 5.3–4. PEDIGREE CHARACTERISTICS OF UNCOMMON X-LINKED DOMINANT DISORDERS

- Both males and females are affected, but females tend to be affected about twice as often as males.
- An affected female transmits the disorder to half her sons and half her daughters, on the average.
- An affected male transmits the disorder to *all* his daughters and to *none* of his sons.
- On the average, the heterozygous affected female tends to be less severely affected than the hemizygous male, and the disorder is more variable in heterozygous females.

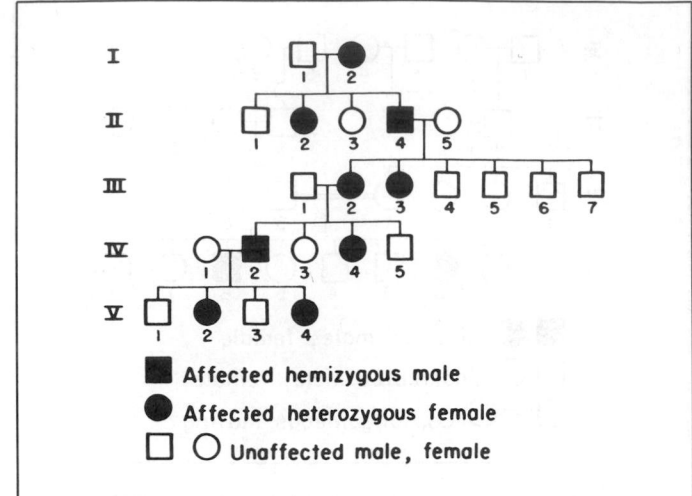

Figure 5.3–4. X-linked dominant pedigree pattern (idealized).

cases are the consequence of new mutation and are said to be sporadic. Fibrodysplasia ossificans progressiva, Apert syndrome, and perhaps progeria are examples. (For most such conditions the increased average age of fathers of new mutation cases is demonstrable.) It can be shown that with an X-linked recessive condition like Duchenne muscular dystrophy, in which no affected males reproduce, one third of cases arise by new mutation in the X chromosome carried by the mother's ovum, and in two thirds of cases the disorder is inherited from a carrier mother, the mutation having occurred in an earlier generation. At least such is the theoretic expectation.

GENETIC HETEROGENEITY[30]

It is axiomatic that the phenotype ("clinical picture") is not a necessary indication of the genotype (the genetic constitution) of the patient. This is the same as saying that any one of two or more different mutations can result in one and the same disorder. "Look alikes" should be distinguished because the mode of inheritance may be quite different, requiring different genetic counseling, and the clinical prognosis and appropriate management may differ. Indeed, the "look alike" may not be mendelian, but rather environmentally produced—a so-called phenocopy. (Genetic "look alikes" are called genocopies, or genetic mimics.) A major theme of clinical genetics in the last two decades has been identification of genetic heterogeneity in conditions previously thought to be single entities. Examples are the Ehlers-Danlos syndromes, the mucopolysac-

charidoses, and nonspherocytic hemolytic anemias, and the several forms of intestinal polyposis and multiple endocrine neoplasia. As reflected by the numbers given in Table 5.3–6, a rapid increase in the number of known mendelian disorders has occurred in the last two decades. This has resulted not so much from identification of new phenotypes as from discovery that one phenotype encompasses several separate genetic disorders.[30]

Genetic heterogeneity, the existence of separate entities, is discerned by (1) phenotypic differences, (2) biochemical differences, (3) genetic differences, and (4) physiologic differences.

Phenotypic Differences

The presence or absence of corneal clouding is one clinical feature distinguishing two forms of mucopolysaccharidosis,[34] the autosomal recessive type described by Hurler and the X-linked recessive form described by Hunter. The association of soft tissue and osseous tumors[32] distinguishes the colonic polyposis of Gardner syndrome from familial polyposis of the colon.

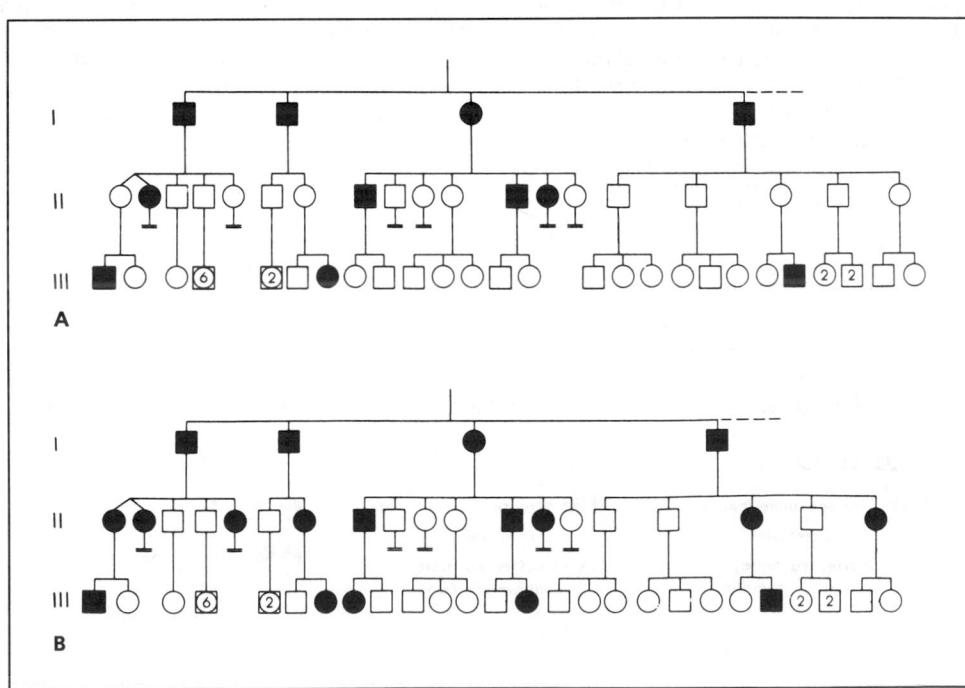

Figure 5.3–5. Hypophosphatemic (vitamin D–resistant) rickets. **A.** Skeletal signs of rickets were used as phenomissed by this method of study. **B.** Low serum phosphorus level was phenotype studied. With this phenotype the pedigree pattern is completely consistent with X-linked dominant inheritance.

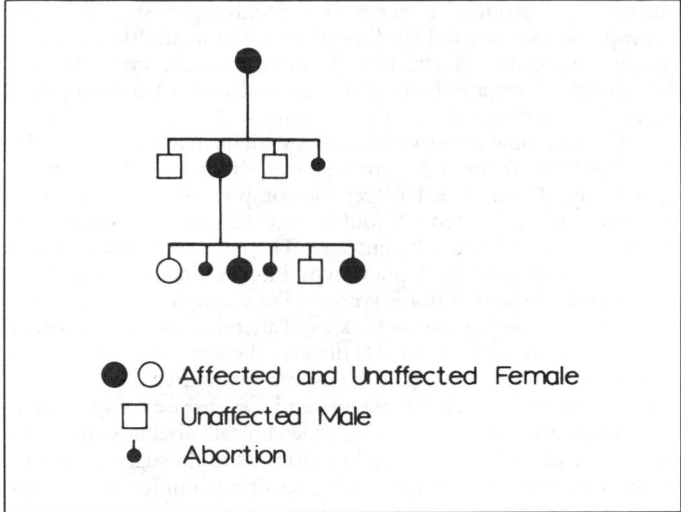

Figure 5.3–6. Pedigree pattern of X-linked dominant lethal in hemizygous affected male (idealized).

- Only females are affected (affected males are lost as abortions).
- An affected female transmits the disorder to half her daughters.
- There is a deficiency of sons of affected females.
- Affected females show an increased frequency of spontaneous abortion, these being hemizygous affected males.

two forms of elliptocytosis not linked to Rh are due to mutation in either alpha-spectrin or beta-spectrin.[33]

In many instances, congenital deafness (deaf-mutism) can be shown to be inherited as a simple autosomal recessive. Assortative (i.e., nonrandom) mating is often practiced by deaf-mutes; deaf persons marry other deaf persons much more often than would occur on a random basis. All children of two deaf persons, each from a family with a recessive pattern of inheritance, are deaf if the two parents are homozygous at the same locus. Families fulfilling this expectation have been observed. In other families, however, two parents, both affected by phenotypically identical recessively inherited deafness, have children who are all normal. The explanation is that the deaf parents are homozygous at different loci and suffer from genetically distinct forms of deafness.

Somatic cell genetics provides an elegant way to identify genetic heterogeneity. Fusion of cells from patients with what appear to be the same disorder (with deficiency of the same enzyme) may show complementation, with restitution of normal enzyme function. The explanation may be that the enzyme involved is made up of two different polypeptide chains and the cases involved have mutation in different chains. Or in one case it may be a regulator mutation, whereas the other has a structural mutation.

Biochemical Differences

Marfan syndrome and homocystinuria, despite phenotypic overlap (subluxation of lenses and skeletal abnormalities), are distinguished by biochemical identification of homocystine in the urine. Often when a biochemical "handle" is identified, phenotypic differences are then appreciated, permitting clinical differentiation. Such is, for example, now usually possible for Marfan syndrome and homocystinuria.[31]

Genetic Differences

Differences in mode of inheritance can distinguish entities. Spastic paraplegia, retinitis pigmentosa, and Charcot-Marie-Tooth peroneal muscular atrophy arc three disorders that arc inherited as autosomal dominants in some families, as autosomal recessives in others, and as X-linked recessives in yet other rare instances. Usually in conditions with three different modes of inheritance, the autosomal recessive form is clinically most severe, the dominant form least severe, and the X-linked form intermediate in severity.

At least two distinct forms of elliptocytosis (ovalocytosis), both inherited as dominants, were identified on the basis of linkage relationship, although no phenotypic differences were discernible. Linkage studies indicated that one form is determined by a gene at a locus close to that occupied by the Rh blood-group genes (now known to be chromosome 1), whereas a second form of elliptocytosis is determined by a gene (or genes) at some locus far removed from the Rh locus. Subsequently, it was found that the form of elliptocytosis linked to Rh is "caused" by a defect in protein 4.1 of the skeleton of the red blood cell membrane, whereas

Physiologic Differences

This approach to identification of genetic heterogeneity is nicely demonstrated by the hemophilias. Before about 1950, all sex-linked hemophilia was assumed to be one disease, although the possibility of multiple allelism had been suggested to explain the occurrence of mild and severe forms. It was then discovered that the blood from some hemophilic subjects would correct the clotting defect in others. The explanation is that the location of the defect in the chain of clotting reactions is different, so that bloods from two hemophilic persons complement each other, each providing an essential clotting factor missing in the other. Thus hemophilia A (classic hemophilia) and hemophilia B (Christmas disease) were distinguished. The protein clotting factors, antihemophilic globulin (factor VIII) and plasma thromboplastin antecedent (factor IX) are chemically distinct. Although both are determined by genes on the X chromosome, the genes are known to be on different parts of the chromosome. Linkage studies indicate that the hemophilia A gene is fairly close to the color-blindness locus and the G6PD locus (now known to be near the end of the long arm

TABLE 5.3–6. NUMBERS OF LOCI AS IDENTIFIED MAINLY BY MENDELIZING PHENOTYPES[a]

	McKusick's *Mendelian Inheritance in Man*[32]							
Phenotype	*1966*	*1968*	*1971*	*1975*	*1978*	*1983*	*1986*	*1988*
Autosomal dominant	269 (+568)	344 (+449)	415 (+528)	583 (+635)	736 (+753)	934 (+893)	1172 (+1029)	1446 (+1116)
Autosomal recessive	237 (+294)	280 (+349)	365 (+418)	466 (+481)	521 (+596)	588 (+710)	610 (+810)	627 (+851)
X linked	68 (+51)	68 (+55)	86 (+64)	93 (+78)	107 (+98)	115 (+128)	124 (+162)	139 (+171)
Total	574 (+913)	692 (+853)	866 (+1010)	1142 (+1194)	1364 (+1447)	1637 (+1731)	1906 (+2001)	2212 (+2138)

[a]Numbers in parentheses refer to those not yet fully established. Increasingly loci are identified by parasexual methods or methods of molecular genetics even though no mendelizing phenotypes (including disorders) have yet been related to the locus.

of the X), whereas the Christmas disease gene is far removed from these loci. Thus evidence from genetic linkage corroborates the conclusion from physiologic studies.

PLEIOTROPISM

Whereas genetic heterogeneity means that one (or almost the same) phenotype can result from any one of several genotypes, pleiotropism ("multiple effects") means that several phenotypic features can result from one gene. We have in clinical genetics many syndromes (meaning literally a "running together") based on the pleiotropism of individual genes; certain phenotypic features tend to occur together predictably. Sometimes there is an evident or at least plausible reason for the association. For example, in Marfan syndrome, association of lens dislocation and weakness of the aortic media are explicable on the basis of a connective tissue defect, even though the precise nature of that defect is not yet known. In other cases, the reason for syndromal association is not clear. For example, why should jejunal polyps and melanin spots of the buccal mucosa, lips, and digits be associated in the Peutz-Jeghers syndrome?[32]

Syndromal association in mendelian disorders is always based on pleiotropism, not on genetic linkage. Two genes at separate loci, even though closely situated on the same chromosome, become separated through the process of crossing over (p. 271). The closer the genes are, the longer the time (in generations) that is required for their separation. Genetic linkage does not cause a permanent association of genetic traits, nor does it account for mendelian syndromes. (Close linkage of loci with insufficient time for separation of specific alleles at these loci, so-called linkage disequilibrium, is probably responsible for certain HLA-and-disease associations [p. 302].)

The importance of pleiotropism to clinical genetics is in diagnosis. Some of the pleiotropic features are useful external clues to the presence of serious internal abnormalities. Table 5.3–7 lists examples.

VARIABILITY

Not only are there many mendelian disorders, but also each may vary rather widely in affected persons, even members of the same family. This is particularly true of autosomal dominant disorders. This variability is due in part to differences in the environment, intrauterine and extrauterine, in which the individual develops and lives, and due in part to differences in the rest of the genetic makeup of the affected persons.

Variability, probably due mainly to difference in genetic background, is illustrated by two brothers with Marfan syndrome, which was inherited from their father. One had ectopia lentis, striking arachnodactyly, severe scoliosis, and marked mitral regurgitation. The second brother in his teens had no ocular or recognizable cardiac abnormality, and only rather unspecific skeletal changes that alone would not have sufficed for a firm diagnosis of Marfan syndrome (for which there is not yet a laboratory test). That he, indeed, had Marfan syndrome was unhappily proved by his subsequent development of a dissecting aneurysm of the aorta. On the average, brothers share half their genes in common. Influence of differences in genetic background on the expression of mendelian syndromes is known in mice and other experimental animals. Usually one aspect of the syndrome, such as ectopia lentis in the example above, fails to be expressed.

Different mutations can occur in a given gene—allelic mutations—and although each may cause abnormality in a particular function controlled by that gene, the resulting abnormality may be quantitatively and even qualitatively different. Many examples are now known of allelic series as the basis of variation in genetic disease. Some enzymopathies occur in both vitamin-responsive and nonresponsive forms (see later discussion of homocystinuria), the former usually being clinically less severe. Deficiency of acid

maltase may produce a severe form of glycogen storage disease (Pompe disease) or a milder disorder manifest in adulthood as progressive myopathy. Cystinuria, Gaucher disease, cystic fibrosis, G6PD deficiency, and hemophilia are probably other examples of mendelian disorders with allelic variants.

In autosomal recessive diseases a patient may have a "double dose" of mutant genes at a given locus, but they are different mutant alleles. This is called a "genetic compound" or "compound heterozygote"; the term "double heterozygote" is reserved for heterozygosity at two different loci. The genetic compound usually is accompanied by a phenotype intermediate in severity between that of the two homozygotes. For example, among the hemoglobinopathies SS disease (sickle cell anemia) is a severe disorder, whereas CC disease is mild; SC disease, the genetic compound, is of intermediate severity (and has some qualitative clinical differences from both sickle cell anemia and CC disease). Especially in the case of autosomal recessives, wide clinical variability in a series of cases, with little intrafamilial variation, should suggest the existence of two or more mutant alleles, resulting in different homozygous states and genetic compounds.

GENE DIAGNOSIS

Molecular diagnosis of mendelian disorders ("gene diagnosis"[14,43] or "DNA diagnosis") can be performed for prenatal diagnosis (on DNA obtained by chorion villus sampling [CVS] or amniocentesis), for preclinical diagnosis (as in Huntington disease[29]; on DNA of circulating leukocytes), and for carrier detection (as in hemophilia). DNA diagnosis can take two forms: diagnosis by the linkage principle or direct demonstration of a lesion—for example, deletion or single nucleotide substitution—in the gene itself. When a given gene is known to be closely linked to a DNA marker, such as a restriction fragment length polymorphism (RFLP; "riflip") identified by Southern blot analysis, the disease gene can be identified by the company it keeps. This identification usually requires information about other members of the family and is impossible if the marker locus is invariant in the given family, that is, if relevant persons are not heterozygous. In the case of the β-thalassemias the identification of several closely linked RFLPs, constituting a "haplotype," increases the likelihood of finding informative families.

Oligonucleotide probes have been synthesized, matching a segment of the normal gene and a segment of the mutant gene containing a nucleotide substitution. In the case of the Hb S gene the nucleotide change is GAG to GTG as the sixth codon of the β-globin gene. Only the Hb S oligonucleotide probe hybridizes with the DNA of a person with sickle cell anemia; both the Hb S and the Hb A probes hybridize with the DNA from a person with sickle cell trait (SA).[8]

In some cases, deletion of the gene can be demonstrated by the fact that the cloned gene does not hybridize in southern blot analysis with the patient's DNA. In cases of an autosomal recessive form of growth hormone deficiency, the cloned gene probe fails to hybridize with the patient's DNA, indicating absence (deletion) of the gene.

PROGNOSIS

In genetic disease the question "What will be the outcome?" (see Foreword) has additional implications; it may apply to unborn offspring of the person seeking advice. Of course, prognosis in the usual sense of the implications of the disease for the length and quality of life is also important in clinical genetics. In addition, the question often asked by patients with genetic disease or by their families is "What will be the outcome of later pregnancies?" "I have such-and-such (or, such-and-such is in my family). Will I transmit it to my children?" or "My wife and I and our families do not have anything of this sort, but we have a child with such-

TABLE 5.3–7. SOME HEREDITARY SYNDROMES IN WHICH EXTERNAL MANIFESTATIONS AID IN THE DIAGNOSIS OF GRAVE INTERNAL DISORDERS[a]

Syndrome	External Clues	Internal Disorder(s) of Importance	Mode of Inheritance	Basic Defect
von Hippel-Lindau syndrome	Retinal angioma(s)	Cerebellar hemangioblastoma Pheochromocytoma Hypernephroma Polycythemia	Autosomal dominant	Unknown (structural defect)
Wilson disease (hepatolenticular degeneration)[7]	Kayser-Fleischer ring of cornea	Hepatic cirrhosis Basal ganglion degeneration	Autosomal recessive	Disorder of copper metabolism (low serum ceruloplasmin)
Pseudoxanthoma elasticum (Grönblad-Standberg syndrome)[31]	Characteristic changes in skin of neck, axillas, and flexural areas	Gastrointestinal hemorrhage Occlusive peripheral and coronary arterial disease	Autosomal recessive	Degeneration of elastic fibers
Hereditary hemorrhagic telangiectasia (Rendu-Osler-Weber disease)	Cutaneous and mucosal telangiectasia	Gastrointestinal hemorrhage Pulmonary arteriovenous fistulas Hepatic cirrhosis	Autosomal dominant	Structural anomaly of small arteries and veins
Marfan syndrome[31]	Ectopia lentis Long extremities	Aneurysm of aorta	Autosomal dominant	Connective tissue abnormality, exact nature unknown
Holt-Oram syndrome[38,42]	Absent or anomalous thumbs	Atrial septal defect	Autosomal dominant	Unknown
von Recklinghausen neurofibromatosis	Café-au-lait spots and fibromas of skin	Pheochromocytoma Meningioma Acoustic neuroma Hypoglycemia (with intraperitoneal fibroma)	Autosomal dominant	Unknown
Gardner syndrome	Osteomas of mandible and skull Sebaceous cysts	Premalignant polyps of colon and stomach	Autosomal dominant	Unknown
Peutz-Jeghers syndrome	Melanin spots of buccal mucosa, lips, and digits	Polyps of jejunum (and other portions of GI tract) producing intussusception, bleeding; rarely malignant	Autosomal dominant	Unknown
Ellis–van Creveld syndrome	Polydactyly and dwarfism	Single atrium	Autosomal recessive	Unknown
Albright hereditary osteodystrophy (pseudo- and pseudo-pseudohypoparathyroidism) (two or more forms)	Short metacarpals and metatarsals Round facies Subcutaneous calcification	Hypocalcemic tetany Mental retardation	Autosomal dominant	G protein, stimulatory, alpha subunit[4,26a]
Fabry diffuse angiokeratoma	Characteristic angiokeratomatous lesions of skin	Episodic abdominal pain Renal failure	X-linked dominant (or intermediate, since heterozygous females are more mildly affected)	Deficiency of α-galactosidase (ceramide trihexosidase)
Nail-patella syndrome	Dysplastic nails, hypoplastic or absent patellas, limitation of pronation and supination of elbows	Renal failure	Autosomal dominant Linked to ABO blood group locus	Unknown (structural defect)

[a]See McKusick's *Mendelian Inheritance in Man*[32] for references to specific entities.

and-such. Will our later born children have this condition also?'' Providing the answers to such questions is called genetic counseling. The following principles can be given:

1. Diagnosis is of the essence. Because of genetic heterogeneity, disorders of different modes of inheritance (or not hereditary at all) may appear similar and be given the same label. Familiarity with the world's experience with the familial occurrence of a given disorder or class of disorders (as recorded in *Mendelian Inheritance in Man*[32]) is essential.

A sign of competence is the ability to come to a correct diagnosis even though the physician has not seen the disease before. In clinical genetics the clinician is put to particular test because of the large number (Table 5.3–7) and individual rarity of genetic disorders.

2. In the case of autosomal dominant disorders, a sporadic case in a family may represent a new mutation. If the father is in his 40s or 50s, this possibility is given increased weight. The hazard to subsequently born children is negligible, although the affected person can transmit the disor-

der to descendants. Sporadicity may be only apparent however; one parent may, in fact, have the disorder in very mild form.

In some autosomal dominant disorders, a majority of affected persons have a fresh mutation. This is the case in 70 to 80 percent of cases of achondroplasia and an even higher proportion of cases of other conditions such as Apert syndrome (acrocephalosyndactyly). When experience teaches that the given disorder is fully penetrant (as it is in the two specific examples given), then fresh mutations can be concluded with relative confidence when both parents are unaffected. An equilibrium exists between addition of mutant genes to, and their removal from, the gene pool, that is, a balance between new mutations on the one hand and negative selection on the other. In Marfan syndrome, about 15 percent of cases are new mutants, and reproductive fitness is reduced by about 15 percent below the population average through death of affected persons before reaching or completing the reproductive age.

3. Once a couple has given birth to a child with a well-delineated autosomal recessive disorder, such as phenylketonuria, cystic fibrosis, and many others, the risk to subsequently born children can be stated precisely as 1 in 4. Even if three, four, or any number of affected children have been born, the risk is still 1 in 4 for *each* later born child—chance has no memory. It is useful to use the coin-tossing analogy. Regardless of the number of heads—or tails—thrown in a row, the chance of a head—or a tail—on the subsequent toss is always 50 percent. Otherwise, parents may think that they have had their one affected child in four and can expect to have three more children who will be normal.

4. For X-linked disorders such as hemophilia and Duchenne muscular dystrophy, the problems of genetic counseling are somewhat different. For example, what is the risk that a sister of the affected boy is a carrier and therefore liable to have affected sons? If the affected brother inherited his disorder from a carrier mother, the risk is different from that if the brother's disease arose by new mutation in the X chromosome contributed by his mother. If there are affected maternal uncles, then the chance of the sister's being a carrier is 1 in 2, the chance of her having a son (rather than a daughter) is 1 in 2, and the chance of her transmitting the hemophilia gene rather than the normal allele to her son is 1 in 2, giving a joint risk of 1 in 8 for a hemophilic son. If she already has had some normal sons, the risk of her being a carrier is reduced according to Bayes theorem.

5. Obviously, the ability to detect the heterozygous carrier state for recessive disorders is useful to genetic counseling. This is less the case in most rare autosomal recessives, because even if the person is a carrier (and the chances of this are 2 in 3 for the normal sib of a person with an autosomal recessive disorder), children will be affected only if the person marries another carrier. Among unrelated persons from whom a spouse is chosen, the frequency of heterozygotes ranges from 1 in 50 to 1 in 150 for most rare recessives. The risk is, of course, much higher if the person marries a first cousin; 1 in 4 is the chance of the first cousin's being a carrier.

On the other hand, to be able to detect female carriers of X-linked traits is of great value, because they can have affected sons regardless of the genotype of the husband. A low ratio of factor VIII procoagulant activity to factor VIII antigen is useful in detecting carriers for hemophilia A. Increased levels of creatine kinase are useful, although sensitivity and specificity of the test are imperfect, in detecting females carrying the gene for Duchenne muscular dystrophy.

6. In multifactorial conditions (see p. 303), for example, common congenital malformations such as cleft lip, cleft palate, and congenital heart disease, genetic risks can be estimated only in empirical terms. For example, in a collection of families with a single case of cleft lip, a frequency of 4 percent of cleft lip among offspring born subsequent to the affected child may have been found. If one parent is also affected, the risk is increased, and so on. Empirical risk figures undoubtedly exaggerate the risk in some families and underestimate it in others. In this situation, as in so many others of medical genetics, the likelihood of heterogeneity must also be kept in mind. One must look for objective features that may make it possible to arrive at a more precise estimate of genetic risk. As an example, one form of cleft palate is associated with a characteristic structural peculiarity of the lower lip, namely mucous pits or mucoceles. The lip anomaly behaves as a typical autosomal dominant condition. In only a certain proportion of persons with this lip anomaly does cleft palate also occur. One can at least assure those family members without the lip anomaly that the risk of having a child with a cleft palate is not increased.

7. Prenatal diagnosis by amniocentesis[17,43] or chorionic villus sampling[43] is a technique of preventive genetics. It has added a new dimension to genetic counseling. In the first of these methods, amniotic fluid is withdrawn percutaneously at about the 16th week of gestation. The amniocytes, cells in the amniotic fluid, which are fetal in origin, are studied for their chromosomal constitution or for levels of specific enzymes. Chromosomal aberrations can be detected. Indeed, screening for Down syndrome in the fetus of mothers over 35 years of age is a main indication for amniocentesis. If the conceptus is known to be at risk for a disorder for which an enzyme deficiency is known and if the enzyme is normally expressed in amniocytes (Tay-Sachs disease, galactosemia, and many other conditions are examples), then prenatal diagnosis by amniocentesis can be helpful. The objective is to help couples achieve a healthy family through selective abortion.

Other approaches have been developed for those genetic disorders with no chromosomal abnormality and those in which the biochemical defect is not discernible in amniotic cells. Some structural abnormalities can be visualized by ultrasonography or radiography or directly by fetoscopy. These include spina bifida cystica, anencephaly, the polydactyly of the Ellis–van Creveld syndrome, and hydrocephalus.

A newer method for obtaining fetal cells for prenatal diagnosis is chorionic villus sampling (CVS) through the cervix. CVS has the advantage that it can be done as early as 10 weeks of gestation. Gene diagnosis (p. 286) can be performed on the DNA of either amniocytes or chorionic villus cells.[43] Direct detection of DNA changes specific to disorders such as the thalassemias and sickle cell anemia[8] is possible.

Since by definition mendelian disorders are characterized by a change in the DNA, all should be amenable to gene diagnosis. In addition to use in prenatal diagnosis, the approach will have usefulness in diagnosis of doubtful cases, in premorbid diagnosis (i.e., before development of clinical manifestations, as in hereditary polyposis coli and Huntington disease), and in detection of heterozygous carriers of recessive disease.

8. In addition to a thorough knowledge of genetic principles and of the literature on the particular condition (both its genetics and its natural history), the genetic counselor should have common sense, good judgment, a sense of proportion, and empathy. The bald risk figures are not the whole or even the most important part of the information to be transmitted. The total "cost" must be considered. Cost can be thought of as the product of the recurrence risk and the burden (in terms of emotional and financial

TABLE 5.3–8. PERSPECTIVE IN GENETIC COUNSELING[a]

Defect	Recurrence	Burden
Anencephaly	Low	Low
Color blindness	High	Low
Congenital heart malformation	Low	High
Duchenne muscular dystrophy	High	High

[a]From E.A. Murphy.

stress). As indicated in Table 5.3–8, a condition such as Duchenne muscular dystrophy, with both high recurrence risk and high burden, carries the highest cost.

9. Genetic counseling should always be given in such a way as not to incite or aggravate anguish, although the advice should never depart from the truth. Often genetic counseling can give great relief. The counselee frequently has an exaggerated notion of the risk involved. For example, the nonhemophilic brother of a hemophilic cannot transmit hemophilia to his descendants, but he may not know that. That the normally statured offspring of two achondroplasts cannot transmit the disorders is another example.

TREATMENT

Therapy is not the "long suit" of clinical genetics. However, mendelian disorders are not as therapeutically hopeless as they might seem. There is, of course, a difference between treatment and cure. It is true that cure is not now possible unless the surgical correction of genetically determined abnormalities can be so considered. Opportunities for treatment in genetic disease arise from the fact that, at least to some extent, almost all genetic diseases are the result of the action of environmental as well as genetic etiologic factors.

The following are forms of therapy in genetic disease: elimination diets, dietary supplementation, avoidance of certain drugs, elimination from the body of affected tissue or toxic material, replacement of a missing gene product, enzyme induction, cofactor (vitamin) supplementation, replacement of defective tissue, and other forms of surgical therapy. Somatic cell gene therapy is a realistic possibility within the foreseeable future.

SPECIFICALLY RESTRICTED DIETS

In galactosemia and phenylketonuria, galactose and phenylalanine, respectively, cannot be metabolized properly, and pathologic effects result from the accumulation of these substances or their metabolic products. Elimination of galactose and phenylalanine from the diet at an early stage can prevent irreversible damage. Restriction of dietary phytanic acid has great benefit in Refsum disease.

AVOIDANCE OF DRUGS

Barbiturates and some other agents precipitate acute attacks of porphyria in the rare genetically susceptible person. Certain antimalarial and other drugs and also the fava bean precipitate hemolysis in persons with the X-linked genetic deficiency of erythrocyte G6PD (p. 300). Clearly preventive treatment consists of avoiding the offending agents.

ELIMINATION FROM THE BODY

Hemochromatosis is effectively treated by repeated venesection. The removal of the excess copper from the body in Wilson disease (hepatolenticular degeneration) by means of penicillamine,

which binds it and carries it out in the urine, is another case in point.

REPLACEMENT OF A MISSING GENE PRODUCT

The replacement of a missing gene product is illustrated by the administration of antihemophilic globulin in hemophilia A, of gamma globulin in agammaglobulinemia, of thyroid hormone in the several genetic defects of thyroid hormone synthesis, and of cortisone in cases of genetic defects in adrenal hormone synthesis. Administration of hematin,[24] the product of the pathway in which the enzyme defect of porphyria is sited, can benefit acute intermittent porphyria by feedback inhibition of the pathway.

Enzyme replacement is more difficult than is replacement of the nonenzymic substance just mentioned. Transfusion in patients with severe combined immunodeficiency due to lack of adenosine deaminase (ADA) has some benefit because of the ADA contained in the red blood cells.[20] Plasma transfusion in some lysosomal diseases (p. 293) has detectable but clinically insignificant effects. A more effective way to replace enzyme is by transplantation of tissue, such as bone marrow.

ENZYME INDUCTION

At least one example of enzyme induction by pharmacologic means is known. The Arias type of hyperbilirubinemia is mainly of cosmetic significance. Jaundice is lifelong. Phenobarbital in a dosage that is not objectionably sedative results in dramatic clearing of the icterus. The mechanism of benefit of "impeded" androgens in hereditary angioedema[16] may fall into this class.

COFACTOR (VITAMIN) SUPPLEMENTATION

In the case of so-called vitamin-dependent, or, better, vitamin-responsive, inborn errors of metabolism, administration of the vitamin cofactor in amounts 100 times or more greater than the minimal requirement "cures" the disease. B_6-responsive homocystinuria (p. 295) is one of the best examples.

REPLACEMENT OF DEFECTIVE TISSUE

Bone marrow transplantation has been successfully accomplished in Fanconi anemia for replacement of hematopoietic tissue, in osteopetrosis to replace the defective osteoclasts, and in certain genetic immunodeficiency states to reconstitute the immune system. Kidney transplantation has been performed in cases of hereditary cystic disease, cystinosis, Fabry disease, and the amyloid kidney of familial Mediterranean fever. Liver transplantation has been done in cases of cirrhosis due to α_1-antitrypsin deficiency.

OTHER FORMS OF SURGICAL THERAPY

Removal of the spleen in hereditary spherocytosis corrects the anemia, which is the main manifestation. In the Peutz-Jeghers syndrome simple removal of the intestinal polyps (which are usually not premalignant) cures this part—the only significant one—of the syndrome. Enucleation of the affected eye cures retinoblastoma, susceptibility to which is transmitted as an autosomal dominant trait in some families, if metastasis has not occurred. (In the familial form, however, retinoblastoma may occur in the contralateral eye, and the person who inherits the retinoblastoma gene has an increased risk of developing osteosarcoma.)

SOMATIC CELL GENE THERAPY

Methods for incorporating genes into somatic cells will permit, in the foreseeable future, correction of the molecular defect in disor-

ders such as thalassemia. Reimplantation of the patient's own bone marrow after extracorporeal gene therapy is an example of this approach.

PREVENTION

The most important and contributory service function of clinical genetics is preventive medicine. Primary prevention, avoidance of the occurrence of disease, is the objective of genetic counseling. Secondary prevention, avoidance, or amelioration of the effects of the disease, particularly through early detection and initiation of therapy, is a significant part of clinical genetics.

Genetic preventive measures include neonatal screening for inborn errors of metabolism, family screening for disorders such as colonic polyposis and Wilson disease, amniocentesis for prenatal diagnosis of chromosomal aberrations and inborn errors of metabolism, and population screening for heterozygous carriers of recessive disease.

Neonatal screening becomes important for any disorder that can be treated effectively. Phenylketonuria and galactosemia are cases in point. Early institution of therapy is essential before irreversible damage is done.

Any mendelian disorder for which there is useful therapy should be sought in other members of the family whenever an index case (proband) is detected. Examples include colonic polyposis, Wilson disease, hemochromatosis, Marfan syndrome, the porphyrias, and G6PD deficiency (Table 5.3–9). In some of these conditions, such as Wilson disease, a single testing is adequate to identify the presence of the disease. In others, such as colonic polyposis, periodic examination of persons at high risk is necessary.

This is "health maintenance" practiced at the family level. The mode of inheritance is important in deciding which relatives should be screened. Ordinarily, in the case of Wilson disease, a recessive, it is sufficient to screen sibs. In polyposis coli and acute intermittent porphyria, dominant disorders, it is essential to screen all first-degree relatives (parents, sibs, and offspring) and perhaps go further afield in the pedigree, depending on the findings in first-degree relatives.

Preclinical disease can be detected in sibs of persons with Wilson disease[7] and hemochromatosis,[10] and measures to reduce body stores of copper and iron, respectively, can prevent the development of cirrhosis and other pathologic changes. In the porphyrias and in G6PD deficiency, identification of affected relatives is important so that they may be warned against agents known to precipitate abnormality.

In addition to neonates and family members, the fetus is now also subject to screening for chromosomal abnormalities, specific inborn errors of metabolism, and some other abnormalities. Cells for study are obtained by amniocentesis[17] performed percutaneously in the second trimester of gestation or by CVS performed through the vagina in the first trimester of pregnancy. The chromosomes can be studied by the usual methods (p. 270). Karyotyping the fetus is the objective of amniocentesis when one of the parents carries a balanced chromosomal rearrangement, such as the fusion 14;21 chromosome that predisposes to Down syndrome in the offspring. The fetal karyotype can also be determined in the case of older mothers, because of their relatively high risk of bearing offspring with Down syndrome. It is strongly indicated in any mother over 40 and some recommend it for any mother over 35.

When parents are known to be heterozygous carriers of a particular autosomal recessive disorder (usually because of the birth of an affected child), the fetus can be tested for the disorder. Study of

TABLE 5.3–9. PRACTICE OF PREVENTIVE MEDICINE IN THE FAMILY[a]

Disease	Type of Inheritance	Detection of Defect	Treatment
Angioedema, hereditary	Autosomal dominant	C1 esterase inhibitor assay	"Impeded" androgen[16]
Coproporphyria	Autosomal dominant	Assay of coproporphyrinogen oxidase in white cells, fibroblasts	As for porphyria, acute intermittent (below)
Gardner syndrome	Autosomal dominant	Examination for bony and soft tissue tumors, colonic polyps	Colectomy
G6PD deficiency	X-linked recessive	RBC G6PD assay	Avoidance of hemolysis-inducing drugs
Hereditary spherocytosis	Autosomal dominant	Osmotic fragility of RBC	Splenectomy
Hemochromatosis[10]	Autosomal recessive	Measures of iron metabolism; HLA typing in families	Venesection
Homocystinuria, B₆ responsive[31]	Autosomal recessive	Homocystine in urine	Vitamin B₆
Marfan syndrome[31]	Autosomal dominant	Echography of ascending aorta	Propranolol
Malignant hyperthermia	Autosomal dominant	Blood CPK	Avoidance of anesthesia
Polyposis coli	Autosomal dominant	Colonoscopy	? Colectomy
Porphyria, acute intermittent	Autosomal dominant	Assay of uroporphyrinogen-1 synthetase in red cells	Avoidance of barbiturates, etc.; glucose, hematin for acute attacks[24]
Prolonged QT syndrome	Autosomal dominant	ECG	Antiarrhythmia drugs
Prolonged QT-deafness syndrome	Autosomal recessive	ECG	Antiarrhythmia drugs
Pseudocholinesterase deficiency (succinylcholine sensitivity)	Autosomal recessive	Assay of plasma pseudocholinesterase	Care in use of muscle relaxants in anesthesia
Porphyria cutanea tarda	Autosomal dominant	Assay of uroporphyrinogen decarboxylase in RBCs	Phlebotomy
Wilson disease[7]	Autosomal recessive	Ceruloplasmin, serum	Penicillamine

[a] This is a partial list for purposes of illustration. See McKusick's *Mendelian Inheritance in Man*[32] for additional references concerning specific disorders.

cultured skin fibroblasts has become a leading technique in clinical genetics. The fibroblast turns out to have, fortunate for clinical genetics, a wide enzymatic repertoire, a feature shared by amniotic cells and chorionic villus cells. Theoretically any disorder for which an enzyme deficiency has been identified in skin fibroblasts—and there are over 200 such disorders, almost all recessive, either autosomal or X linked—can be diagnosed antenatally by the enzymatic study of amniotic and chorionic cells. Notable exceptions to the rule that cultured skin fibroblasts can be used for diagnosis by enzyme assay are phenylketonuria and type 1 glycogen storage disease; phenylalanine hydroxylase and glucose 6-phosphatase are not found in cultured normal fibroblasts.

Gene diagnosis (p. 286), applied to the DNA of fetal cells, is the answer to many problems of prenatal diagnosis.[43] It has the advantage that the gene need not be functional in the tissue studied. DNA diagnosis is therefore applicable in hemoglobinopathies,[6] hemophilia, and the inborn errors of metabolism, phenylketonuria and type I glycogen storage disease, mentioned earlier.

Other methods of prenatal diagnosis include fetoscopy for direct observation of malformations and for fetal blood sampling. Ultrasonic visualization of some malformations is possible. α-Fetoprotein, the fetal equivalent of serum albumin, is elevated in the maternal plasma (and the amniotic fluid) when the fetus has anencephaly or spina bifida.

Screening for heterozygous carriers of recessive disease at a population level is worthwhile when heterozygotes are as frequent as 1 in 30 or higher and when the information can be put to the useful service of the persons found to be heterozygous. Tay-Sachs disease is a nearly ideal example. The frequency of Tay-Sachs disease (a progressive neurologic disorder of infants, leading to death in the first decade) is about 1 in 3600 in Ashkenazi Jews. The frequency of the Tay-Sachs gene is therefore about 1 in 60, and the frequency of heterozygotes about 1 in 30. (These estimates follow from the Hardy-Weinberg equilibrium, $p^2 + 2pq + q^2$, in which q is the frequency of the Tay-Sachs gene, q^2 is the frequency of Tay-Sachs homozygotes, and $2pq$ is the frequency of heterozygotes.) A test for heterozygotes—level of β-hexosaminidase A (hex A) in the blood is available. Furthermore, the homozygous affected fetus can be identified by measurement of hex A in cultured amniotic cells. Thus Tay-Sachs disease theoretically can be eliminated, if couples, both heterozygous, are identified by screening and their pregnancies are monitored by amniocentesis.

SPECIFIC CATEGORIES OF MENDELIAN DISEASE

Many of the principles outlined previously, as well as special considerations, are illustrated by the seven classes of simply inherited disorders discussed in this section (see also Table 5.3–9).

THE HEMOGLOBINOPATHIES

The hemoglobinopathies[6] are prime examples of molecular disease. Indeed, the molecular abnormality of hemoglobin in sickle cell anemia, demonstrated by electrophoresis, was the original basis for Linus Pauling's seminal concept. Many principles of biology and clinical genetics have been learned from the study of hemoglobinopathies or are illustrated by them. These include the nature of mutation at the DNA level; gene duplication as a mechanism of evolution; "switching off" of some genes and "switching on" of others during ontogeny; allelism and nonallelism among the various hemoglobin variants; pleiotropism (e.g., the manifold features of sickle cell anemia); genetic heterogeneity (e.g., the many different mutations that can lead to anemia, methemoglobinemia, or polycythemia); pharmacogenetics (e.g., drug-sensitive hemoglobinopathies such as Hb Zurich); selection by malaria to account for the high frequency of Hb, S, C, and E and the thalassemias; prenatal diagnosis by restriction enzyme analysis; and many more.

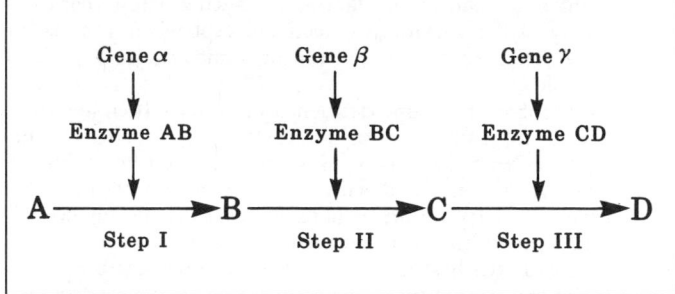

Figure 5.3–7. Genetic control of chain of reactions in metabolic pathway.

INBORN ERRORS OF METABOLISM

In inborn errors of metabolism,[40] the mutation has occurred in a gene that codes for an enzyme controlling a step in intermediary metabolism or in a synthetic pathway. Because of deficient activity of the enzyme, a block occurs in the chain of reactions, as diagrammed in Figure 5.3–7. Clinical abnormality results from toxic effects of metabolites that accumulate proximal to the block, or from deficiency of products of the metabolic or synthetic pathway. Alkaptonuria (p. 292) is an example of the former, and genetic defects in thyroid or adrenal hormone synthesis illustrate the latter mechanism. In some disorders, such as homocystinuria, both pathogenetic mechanisms may be operative. In some disorders a defect in feedback inhibition occurs because of deficiency of a product of the pathway, and some of the pathologic effects are produced or aggravated through excessive production of metabolites (Fig. 5.3–8). This happens in the porphyrias. Administration of hematin, the deficient product of the pathway, has therapeutic value.[24] The Lesch-Nyhan syndrome illustrates the same phenomenon.

Similar pathogenetic mechanisms operate in genetic defects of cortisol and aldosterone synthesis by the adrenal cortex. The two steroid hormones are synthesized from cholesterol through intermeshed synthetic pathways. Impairment of cortisol production results, through cybernetic mechanisms, in a compensatory increase in ACTH secretion by the anterior pituitary. Impairment of mineralocorticoid production results in a comparable compensatory increase in renin-angiotensin production. These compensatory mechanisms may return cortisol or aldosterone production to normal or near normal, but at the expense of excessive production of products and by-products that have undesirable hormonal effects, such as masculinization of the female.

Some inborn errors of metabolism are vitamin responsive, that is, are alleviated by specific vitamins in a pharmacologic dosage. The vitamin in each such case is a normal cofactor for the

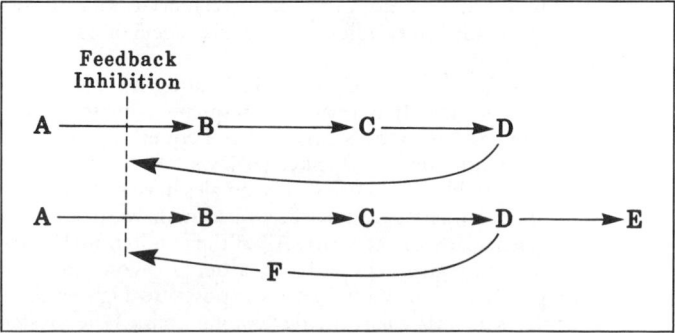

Figure 5.3–8. Control of gene action through feedback inhibition.

enzyme involved, and the mutation is of such a nature that catalytic activity of the enzyme is defective except when it is loaded with the vitamin cofactor. One form of homocystinuria (p. 295) is an example.

The number of enzyme deficiencies that have been identified now exceeds 200. Almost all of the resulting inborn errors of metabolism are inherited as recessives, either autosomal or X linked. Most enzymes are endowed with sufficient margin of safety that the partial deficiency found in heterozygotes has no phenotypic effects. Exceptions to this rule of thumb are four enzymopathies in the hematin synthesis pathway: acute intermittent porphyria, protoporphyria, porphyria cutanea tarda, and coproporphyria. (Congenital erythropoietic porphyria due to an enzyme deficiency in the same pathway is autosomal recessive.) In part the excessive function of δ-aminolevulinic acid synthetase because of reduced feedback inhibition by hematin[24] is probably the reason for disease even in the heterozygote. Furthermore the pathway may be stressed, leading to intermittent attacks or clinical exacerbation. Hereditary angioedema (Table 5.3–9) and antithrombin III deficiency ("thrombophilia") are two other dominantly inherited enzymopathies.

Dominantly inherited disorders usually involve a nonenzymic protein of structural or other function, such as collagen or hemoglobin. The methemoglobinemias illustrate this principle of the basic defect of dominants versus recessives. They all have the same phenotype, cyanosis (sometimes leading to confusion with congenital heart disease), but some are dominant and some recessive. Recessive methemoglobinemia is caused by deficiency of the enzyme methemoglobin reductase. Dominant methemoglobinemia is caused by one or another of the hemoglobins M.

The principles of pathogenesis, diagnosis, and treatment of inborn errors of metabolism will be further illustrated with phenylketonuria, alkaptonuria, and the Lesch-Nyhan syndrome.

Phenylketonuria

Phenylketonuria (PKU) is an autosomal recessive inborn error in the metabolism of the amino acid phenylalanine. The deficiency involves the enzyme phenylalanine hydroxylase, which catalyzes the addition of a hydroxyl group to phenylalanine to make tyrosine. Phenylalanine ingested in the form of dietary protein accumulates, and the products of alternative metabolic pathways, phenylketone substances, are excreted in the urine, giving the condition its name.

Severe mental retardation is the most consistent manifestation. Patients with this disorder tend to have light complexions. Relative deficiency of tyrosine, from which melanin is produced, or inhibition of melanin synthesis by phenylalanine or by a metabolic product are possible mechanisms of the light coloration. The patient is often noted to have a characteristic odor, referred to as "mousy." Neurologic features and behavioral peculiarities, such as unusual posturing and spasticity, are frequently present. Chemical tests for identifying PKU in the newborn period are now available. The Guthrie test makes use of phenylalanine-requiring bacteria for a bioassay of phenylalanine in blood. A low-phenylalanine diet prevents development of retardation. If the dietary regimen is initiated early, normal development can be achieved. That restriction of phenylalanine can be safely relaxed after age 5 or 6 is hoped but not yet proved.

Like many other rare recessives, PKU varies in frequency in different ethnic groups. It is relatively frequent in persons from northern Ireland and western Scotland, less frequent in American blacks, and very infrequent in Ashkenazi Jews.

Some untreated PKU homozygous females have had children; these have all been mentally retarded, and some have shown malformations, particularly of the heart. All of the children are heterozygotes, unless, of course, the father is a heterozygote. In utero the offspring of a woman with PKU is exposed to high levels of phenylalanine, which damages the developing brain. When tested after birth, the children may show no clue to the cause of the

mental retardation. Theirs is an unusual form of genetic disease—one based on the genotype of the mother, not their own.[23,27]

Alkaptonuria

Alkaptonuria (and the abnormal phenotype that accompanies it, ochronosis) is an inborn error in the degradation of homogentisic acid, a derivative of tyrosine (that is in turn derived from phenylalanine, as noted above). Homogentisic acid oxidase is deficient. By oxidation, which is favored in alkaline urine, homogentisic acid is converted to a black alkapton. Black diapers are often the first sign of the disease.

Arthritis of the spine becomes evident when the affected person reaches adulthood (20s or 30s). Calcification of the spinous ligaments or intervertebral discs produces a characteristic radiographic appearance. In vivo tanning of collagen is thought to be the mechanism of the damage to connective tissues. Sclerotic and calcific changes in the aortic valve are frequent. Black discoloration of the scleras and ear cartilages are clinically evident, and the costal cartilages are found at thoracic surgery or autopsy to be deeply pigmented. The pinnae become stiff and calcified; radiographs may even demonstrate ossification, as indicated by the presence of miniature marrow cavities. Black radiopaque prostatic stones are another feature of ochronosis.

The Lesch-Nyhan Syndrome

This syndrome is an X-linked recessive inborn error in purine metabolism. Hypoxanthine-guanine phosphoribosyl-transferase (HGPRT) is the enzyme deficient. This enzyme normally catalyzes the conversion of guanine to guanylic acid and of hypoxanthine to inosinic acid. Since guanylic acid no longer exercises its normal inhibitory effect on PRPP synthetase (Fig. 5.3–9), at the first and rate-limiting step on uric acid synthesis, hyperuricemia results. In addition to renal stones from hyperuricemia, the patients are mentally retarded, have choreoathetosis, and display compulsive self-mutilation, especially biting of fingers and lips. The pathogenesis of the neurologic features is not well understood.

Rare allelic forms of HGPRT deficiency have been found in which neurologic features are minimal or absent, and the patients are young adult males with gout as the only clinical abnormality. (Yet other patients with gout and urolithiasis are found to have a

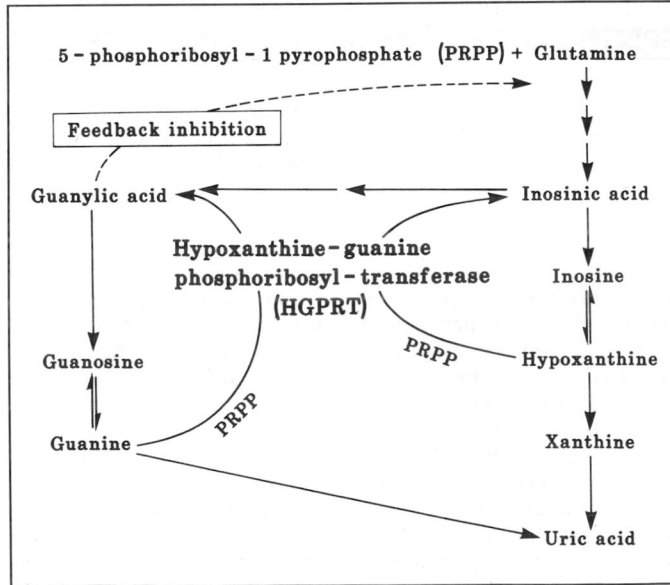

Figure 5.3–9. Schematic representation of purine metabolism with particular reference to uric acid synthesis. Basic defect in Lesch-Nyhan syndrome is deficient activity of HGPRT.

mutation of the enzyme PRPP synthetase such that it is not inhibited by guanylic acid. This disorder is also X-linked recessive.) These forms of hereditary hyperuricemia constitute only a small portion of any series of gouty patients.

Among the cultured skin fibroblasts of heterozygous females, the X linkage of the HGPRT locus is proved by demonstration of two classes of cells: one class with normal HGPRT and one with deficient HGPRT as in affected males. This finding is predicted by the Lyon hypothesis. Studies of mouse-human somatic cell hybrids confirm the X linkage and provide further information that the HGPRT locus is on the distal end of the long arm of the X.

Another significant genetic feature of individuals with the Lesch-Nyhan syndrome is that the great majority of their mothers are heterozygous carriers, which is much more than the anticipated two thirds. Those heterozygous women who do not have heterozygous mothers, that is, carry a new mutation, have older fathers on the average, which is the same finding as in new dominant mutations (p. 275). Mutation may be more frequent in the males than in females in Lesch-Nyhan syndrome and in other X-linked disorders.

LYSOSOMAL DISEASES

Lysosomes constitute the disposal and reclamation system of the cell. They are membrane-bound sacs that maintain a low pH and contain more than 60 acid hydrolases involved in degradation of nucleic acids, proteins, lipids, mucopolysaccharides, glycogen, and other macromolecules. Deficiency of specific acid hydrolases leads to specific disorders, including Fabry angiokeratoma, Tay-Sachs disease, type II glycogen storage disease (Pompe disease), Gaucher disease, and at least 10 enzymatically distinct mucopolysaccharidoses (of which Hurler syndrome, MPS I H, is the prototype). The characteristics of lysosomal diseases are listed in Table 5.3–10. The mucopolysaccharidoses and Fabry disease illustrate these characteristics.

The mucolipidoses and cystinosis are instructive variations on the theme of lysosomal disease. In I-cell disease, a mucolipidosis, multiple lysosomal enzymes fail to get into lysosomes because of mutation in the gene coding for an enzyme that adds a moiety necessary for their passage across the lysosomal membrane. In cystinosis the mutation involves the mechanism by which the substrate cystine is transported out of lysosomes.[15]

The Mucopolysaccharidoses
As indicated by Table 5.3–11, the mucopolysaccharidoses include a rather large number of conditions that earlier in their nosology were considered to be one entity, Hurler syndrome, and in individual cases can be confused with Hurler syndrome, at least at some stage in their clinical evolution. The Sanfilippo syndrome provides a striking example of this genetic heterogeneity. Four phenotypically virtually identical forms of the disorder (progressive and severe mental retardation with relatively mild changes in liver, joints, and bones and no corneal clouding) show deficiency of different acid hydrolases, each of which is normally involved in the cleavage of heparan sulfate.

Allelic variants are also evident in this category of genetic disease. Hurler and Scheie syndromes are "caused" by deficiency in

the same enzyme, α-L-iduronidase (which is now known to be coded by chromosome 22). Yet Hurler syndrome is a severe disorder, leading to death almost always before age 10, whereas Scheie syndrome (although characterized by corneal clouding and stiff joints, e.g., claw hands, as in Hurler syndrome) is accompanied by normal intelligence and long survival. Intermediate phenotypes may represent the expected genetic compound, or a compound heterozygote (the Hurler-Scheie syndrome), although parental consanguinity in some of these cases suggests that homozygosity for yet another allele at the α-L-iduronidase locus is the genetic basis.

Fabry Disease
Fabry disease is an X-linked recessive lysosomal disorder resulting from deficiency of ceramide trihexosidase (α-galactosidase A). Clinical features include crises of pain in the abdomen and limbs; characteristic skin lesions, which give rise to the synonym "diffuse angiokeratoma" and occur particularly around the umbilicus and in the bathing trunk area; a whorl-like corneal clouding; and progressive renal failure. Both affected males and heterozygous females show a whorl-like dystrophy of the cornea on slit-lamp examination. Heterozygous females rarely have skin lesions but late in life may develop renal failure. Variation, presumably allelic, is represented by families in which affected males have renal failure without angiokeratoma.

RECEPTOR DISORDERS

Familial hypercholesterolemia and the testicular feminization syndrome are genetic defects in, or deficiency of, specific receptors.

The defect in *familial hypercholesterolemia* involves the cell membrane receptor for low-density lipoprotein (LDL). On transport into the cell, LDL normally inhibits 3-hydroxy-3-methylglutaryl coenzyme A reductase (HMG CoA reductase), the enzyme catalyzing the rate-limiting step in cholesterol synthesis. Heterozygotes for the receptor defect have levels of plasma cholesterol in the range of 300 to 500 mg/dl. These individuals sometimes show xanthomas of tendons and have an increased risk of coronary occlusion and other complications of atherosclerosis. Homozygotes have plasma cholesterol levels is excess of 500 mg/dl, regularly have xanthomas, including a type called "xanthoma plana of the palmar creases," and usually succumb to coronary occlusion before age 20.

The defect in familial hypercholesterolemia was found by study of cultured fibroblasts from patients homozygous for the defect.[5] Again, heterogeneity is found. Some homozygotes have no receptor, whereas others have a functionally defective receptor. Rare homozygotes have a defective receptor that combines normally with LDL but cannot effect "internalization" of LDL. Yet another type of mutation leads to a form of an LDL receptor molecule that is not incorporated into the cell membrane. All these mutations are allelic, and genetic compounds have been observed.

Familial hypercholesterolemia in its heterozygous form is one of the most frequent genetic diseases, occurring in about 1 in 500 persons.

In the *testicular feminization syndrome* (better called "androgen insensitivity"), a defect occurs in a receptor that is situated in the cytoplasm and normally combines with dihydrotestosterone (DHT). The DHT-receptor complex is translocated into the nucleus where it acts on specific chromosomal sites to induce the action of specific genes controlling male secondary sex characteristics. Again, cultured skin fibroblasts were vital in the elucidation of the defect, and again genetic heterogeneity was found. Some cases appear to have a DHT receptor, but it is functionally ineffective, perhaps because that part of the molecule which interacts with DNA is defective.[32]

Clinically, testicular feminization is a form of male pseudohermaphroditism. Patients are karyotypically normal XY males but ap-

---

TABLE 5.3–10. CHARACTERISTICS OF LYSOSOMAL DISEASES

- Storage diseases
- Deposits in cells are membrane bound
- Clinical course is progressive
- Multiple organs and tissues are involved
- Stored material is chemically heterogeneous
- Treatment by providing missing enzymes potentially feasible

TABLE 5.3–11. THE MUCOPOLYSACCHARIDOSES[34]

Number[a]	Eponym	Clinical	Genetics	Urinary MPS	Enzyme Deficient
MPS I H (25280)	Hurler	Clouding of cornea, grave manifestations, death usually before age 10	Homozygous for MPS I H gene	Dermatan sulfate, heparan sulfate	α-L-Iduronidase
MPS I S	Scheie	Stiff joints, cloudy cornea, aortic valve disease, normal intelligence and (?) life span	Homozygosity for MPS I S gene	Dermatan sulfate, heparan sulfate	α-L-Iduronidase
MPS I H/S	Hurler-Scheie	Intermediate phenotype	Genetic compound of MPS I H and MPS I S genes (?)	Dermatan sulfate, heparan sulfate	α-L-Iduronidase
MPS II, severe (30990)	Hunter, severe	No corneal clouding, milder course than in MPS I H, death before 15 years	Hemizygous for X-linked gene	Dermatan sulfate, heparan sulfate	Iduronate sulfatase
MPS II, mild	Hunter, mild	Survival to 30s to 60s, fair intelligence	Hemizygous for X-linked allele	Dermatan sulfate, heparan sulfate	Iduronate sulfatase
MPS III A (25290)	Sanfilippo A		Homozygous for Sanfilippo A gene	Heparan sulfate	Heparan N-sulfatase (sulfamidase)
MPS III B (25292)	Sanfilippo B	Indistinguishable phenotype: mild somatic, severe central nervous system effects	Homozygous for Sanfilippo B gene	Heparan sulfate	N-acetyl-α-D-glucosaminidase
MPS III C (25293)	Sanfilippo C		Homozygous for Sanfilippo C gene	Heparan sulfate	Acetyl-CoA:α-glucosaminide N-acetyltransferase
MPS III D (25294)	Sanfilippo D		Homozygous for Sanfilippo D gene	Heparan sulfate	N-acetylglucosamine-6-sulfate sulfatase
MPS IV A (25300)	Morquio A	Severe, distinctive bone changes, cloudy cornea, aortic regurgitation	Homozygous for Morquio A gene	Keratan sulfate	Galactosamine-6-sulfate sulfatase
MPS IV B (25301)	Morquio B	Mild bone changes, cloudy cornea, hypoplastic odontoid	Homozygous for Morquio B gene	Keratan sulfate	β-Galactosidase
MPS V	—	—	—	—	—
MPS VI, severe (25320)	Maroteaux-Lamy, classic severe	Severe osseous and corneal changes, valvular heart disease, striking WBC inclusions, normal intellect, survival to 20s	Homozygous for Maroteaux-Lamy gene	Dermatan sulfate	Arylsulfatase B (N-acetylgalactosamine 4-sulfatase)
MPS VI, intermediate	Maroteaux-Lamy, intermediate	Moderately severe changes	Homozygous for allele at Maroteaux-Lamy locus or genetic compound	Dermatan sulfate	Arylsulfatase B (N-acetylgalactosamine 4-sulfatase)
MPS VI, mild	Maroteaux-Lamy, mild	Mild osseous and corneal changes, normal intellect, aortic stenosis	Homozygous for allele at Maroteaux-Lamy locus	Dermatan sulfate	Arylsulfatase B (N-acetylgalactosamine 4-sulfatase)
MPS VII (25322)	Sly	Hepatosplenomegaly, dysostosis multiplex, mental retardation variable, WBC inclusions	Homozygous for mutant gene at β-glucuronidase locus	Dermatan sulfate, heparan sulfate	β-Glucuronidase

[a]The five-digit number refers to entry in *Mendelian Inheritance in Man*.[32]

pear to be normal females in terms of development of secondary sexual characteristics such as breasts and external genitalia; however, they have primary amenorrhea, the vagina ends blindly, and they have testes in the inguinal canals, which often bring the "girls" to surgical attention for presumed hernia.

Although the term "testicular feminization" is perhaps too deeply imbedded in our medical vocabulary to be eliminated, in clinical practice "androgen insensitivity" is a designation much more acceptable to patients and their families. In complete androgen insensitivity, the patients are women who have female external genitalia and fully developed secondary female sexual characteristics (except that pubic hair is usually absent) but are infertile. The testes must be removed to avoid malignancy.

Testicular feminization shows the pedigree pattern of an X-linked recessive. Since affected males are infertile, however, the pattern cannot be distinguished from that of an autosomal dominant trait that is not expressed in heterozygous females (who are, as it were, already feminized). Cloning studies of cultured skin fibroblasts from heterozygous mothers of patients with testicular feminization proved X-linked recessive inheritance by demonstrating two classes of cells: One class has a deficient DHT receptor, just as in affected males, whereas the second cell line has a normal DHT receptor. This is the finding predicted for an X-linked trait by the Lyon hypothesis (p. 276; see Fig. 5.2–2).

Incomplete androgen insensitivity, due to a mutation presumably allelic to that responsible for testicular feminization, is the

basis of Reifenstein syndrome. The patients are almost always recognized as male. They may have normal or nearly normal male external genitalia and secondary sexual characteristics. Hypospadias, gynecomastia, and infertility were the features initially describing this syndrome, however.

DISORDERS OF TRANSMEMBRANE TRANSPORT: CYSTINURIA

Cystinuria was one of the four disorders that Garrod spoke of as inborn errors of metabolism in his famous lectures in 1908. Although the other three—alkaptonuria, albinism, and pentosuria—are indeed the result of enzyme blocks, cystinuria is a defect in an active transport mechanism in the renal tubule. Because of the mutation-determined defect, four basic amino acids—cystine, lysine, arginine, and ornithine—are imperfectly reabsorbed from the glomerular filtrate. Of these amino acids, cystine is relatively insoluble in urine, particularly acid urine, so that cystine stones form in the urinary tract. These stones are radiopaque by virtue of their high sulfur content. The diagnosis of cystinuria is made by finding the characteristic hexagonal, plate-like cystine crystals in the urine, and by a positive cyanide nitroprusside test on the urine. (Homocystine also gives a positive test; the two amino acids are distinguished by other methods such as high-voltage paper chromatography. Homocystinuria[31] is not accompanied by urolithiasis, because homocystine is more soluble in urine than cystine and is excreted in lower amounts.) The defect in cystinuria and in some other renal tubular transport defects can be demonstrated in the intestinal mucosa as well.

Heterogeneity in cystinuria is demonstrated by the fact that in some families only homozygotes have an abnormal secretion of amino acids. In these families cystinuria is recessive. In other families, heterozygotes (e.g., both parents of affected persons as well as half the sibs and offspring) excrete cystine and lysine (but usually not the other two amino acids) in intermediate amounts, and some heterozygotes develop cystine urinary stones. Evidence indicates that the genes responsible for these two forms of cystinuria are alleles, that is, are at the same genetic locus, and genetic compounds have been observed.

The treatment of cystine urolithiasis consists of maintenance of large urine volumes and alkaline pH. Penicillamine has also been used, on the rationale of the solubility of the mixed disulfide, cysteine-penicillamine.

Other genetic defects in transport mechanisms concern phosphate (hereditary hypophosphatemia, or vitamin D–resistant rickets), glucose (renal glycosuria), and hydrogen ion (renal tubular acidosis). Defects in transport across intracellular membranes appear to underlie some genetic disorders, for example, of glucose-6-phosphate into the endoplasmic reticulum in glycogen storage disease Ib, of cystine across the lysosomal membrane in cystinosis, and of cobalamin across the mitochondrial membrane in one form of methylmalonicaciduria. The precise nature of the transport defect in these several conditions is diverse.

HERITABLE DISORDERS OF CONNECTIVE TISSUE

The mucopolysaccharidoses, discussed earlier as lysosomal diseases, are one class among the heritable disorders of connective tissue,[31] since they concern one of the important elements of connective tissue, mucopolysaccharides. The fibrous elements of connective tissue—collagens and elastic fibers—are involved in Marfan syndrome, the Ehlers-Danlos syndrome, cutis laxa, osteogenesis imperfecta, and pseudoxanthoma elasticum. Collagen is damaged by accumulating metabolites in homocystinuria (to produce a clinical picture simulating Marfan syndrome in many ways) and in alkaptonuria (to produce a characteristic arthropathy).

Marfan Syndrome
Although the basic defect (apparently collagen) is just now being elucidated, it has been clear that it is a unitary one because Marfan syndrome is mendelian, specifically autosomal dominant. Abnormalities occur in three domains: (1) Ectopia lentis is the hallmark of ocular involvement but is found in only about three fourths of cases. Myopia and retinal detachment are other ocular features. (2) The skeletal features include long thin limbs, giving excessive height, an abnormally low ratio of upper segment to lower segment, arm span greater than height, and "spider fingers" (arachnodactyly). The joints are often abnormally loose, and scoliosis is severe in many. (3) Weakness of the aortic media is the most frequent life-imperiling cardiovascular feature, but "floppy mitral valve" (the Barlow or click-murmur syndrome) is frequent, and some patients have profound mitral regurgitation.

Largely because the basic defect is not known, there is no specific laboratory test for the diagnosis of Marfan syndrome. It remains a clinical diagnosis. Detection of ectopia lentis can help confirm the suspected diagnosis, but as noted earlier it is not always present; furthermore, ectopia lentis occurs with other conditions, such as homocystinuria (see later discussion) and the Weill-Marchesani syndrome (short stature and stiff joints with lens subluxation, an autosomal recessive). Enlargement of the aortic root by echography also supports the diagnosis of Marfan syndrome, but this finding may not be present at an early stage of the patient's disease. Family study, which should be done also for the practice of preventive medicine, can confirm the diagnosis if a history of dissecting aneurysm is obtained or if a relative is found with ectopia lentis or other clear signs of Marfan syndrome.

The aorta in Marfan syndrome is prone to dilation at the root and in the ascending portion, and dissection with rupture can occur. As a rule the first part to undergo progressive dilation is that within the radiographic silhouette of the heart. Hence, because of involvement of the sinuses of Valsalva, appreciable aortic regurgitation may precede aortic dilation of a degree evident to ordinary radiographic study. Echography is a useful noninvasive means of detecting this dilation. Dissecting aneurysm rarely, it seems, develops "out of the blue," but rather in an aorta that has already undergone dilation. Dissections are most often of the Debakey type II (limited to the ascending aorta) but DeBakey type I (extending throughout the length of the aorta) and DeBakey type III (involving the aorta distal to the left subclavian) have been encountered.

Propranolol, atenolol, and other beta-adrenergic blockers may be useful in staying the progress of aortic dilation and averting dissection. The rationale is reduction in the abruptness and force of ventricular ejection. Surgical replacement of the ascending aorta and aortic valve is performed in patients with advanced changes in the aorta.[19]

Patients with Marfan syndrome require lifelong periodic evaluation. In prepubertal girls induction of puberty with estrogen-progesterone to limit height and shorten the period of maximal risk of scoliosis may be indicated. The state of the aorta should be evaluated annually by echography in patients of all ages. The ocular features require regular check.

Homocystinuria
Homocystinuria is a garrodian inborn error of metabolism and secondarily a heritable disorder of connective tissue. The diagnosis is made by demonstration of homocystine in the urine and confirmed by demonstration of the specific enzyme deficiency in cultured skin fibroblasts. The enzyme involved is cystathionine synthase (or synthetase), which catalyzes the condensation of homocysteine and serine to form cystathionine.

As in Marfan syndrome, ectopia lentis is a leading feature. Whereas the lenses usually are displaced upward in Marfan syndrome, they are characteristically dislocated downward in homocystinuria. Also, whereas ectopia lentis is present at birth in Marfan syndrome (and may progress later), the ectopia lentis of homocystinuria is acquired, usually in the first years of life, but sometimes not until the 20s or later. Myopia is an ocular feature of homocystinuria that usually develops before ectopia lentis.

Skeletal features of homocystinuria include excessive height

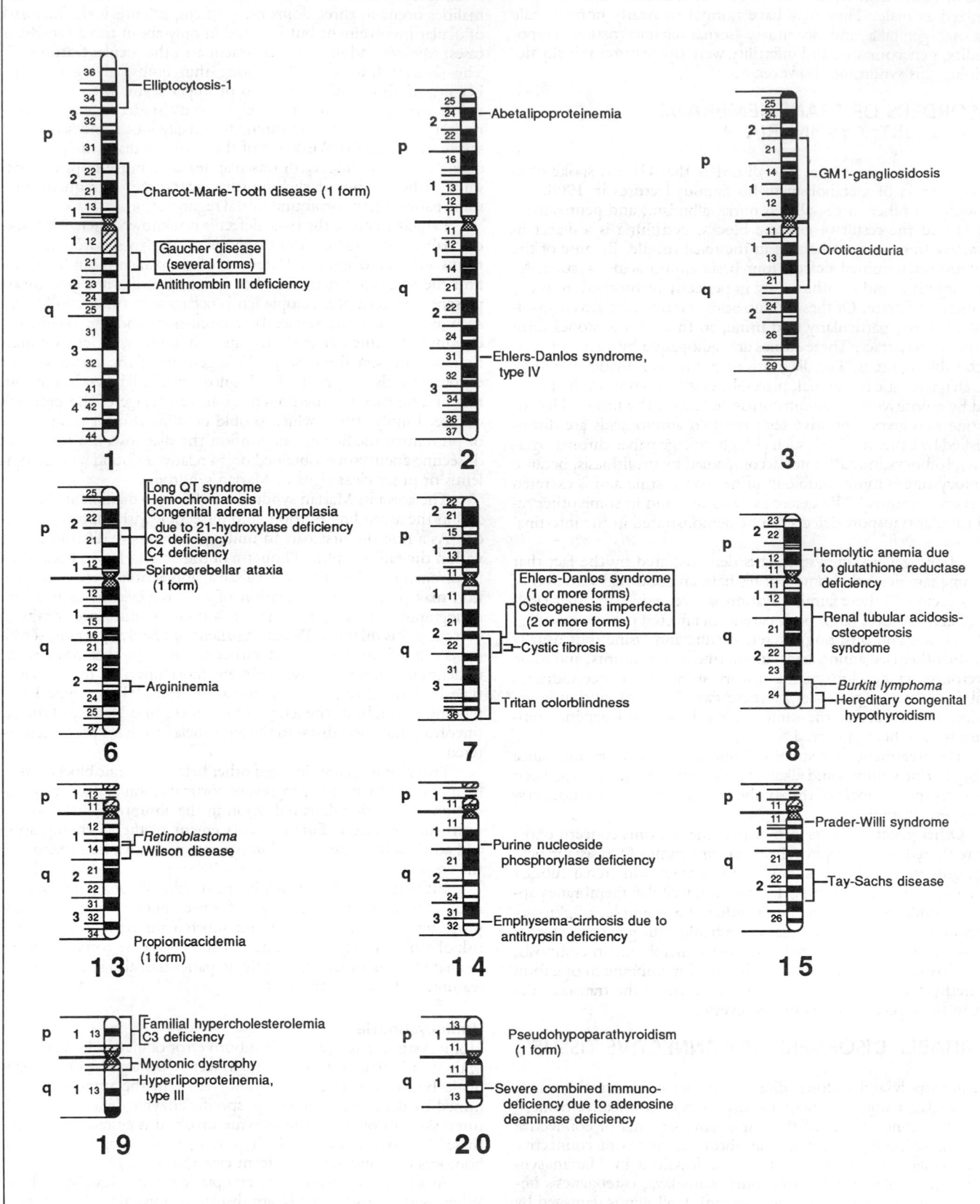

Figure 5.3–10. Morbid anatomy of human genome (abridged version). Locale of mutation underlying various diseases is indicated by chromosome by which name of disease appears. Regional location on given chromosome is known for some of these genes and indicated by lines to appropriate band(s). Disorders enclosed in box are produced by mutations at same locus, that is are

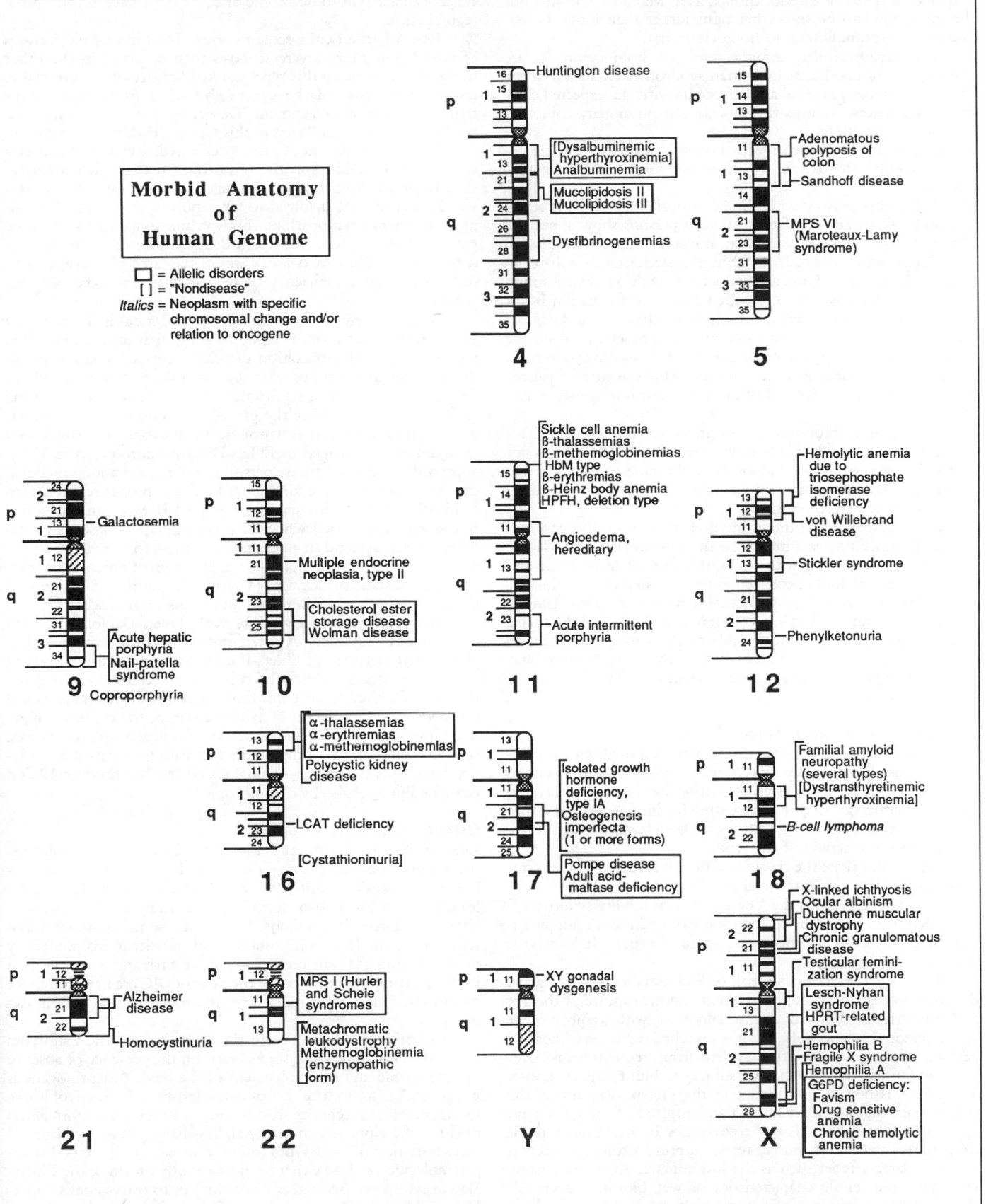

Morbid Anatomy of Human Genome

☐ = Allelic disorders
[ ] = "Nondisease"
Italics = Neoplasm with specific chromosomal change and/or relation to oncogene

4
- Huntington disease
- [Dysalbuminemic hyperthyroxinemia] / Analbuminemia
- Mucolipidosis II / Mucolipidosis III
- Dysfibrinogenemias

5
- Adenomatous polyposis of colon
- Sandhoff disease
- MPS VI (Maroteaux-Lamy syndrome)

9
- Galactosemia
- Acute hepatic porphyria
- Nail-patella syndrome
- Coproporphyria

10
- Multiple endocrine neoplasia, type II
- Cholesterol ester storage disease / Wolman disease

11
- Sickle cell anemia
- β-thalassemias
- β-methemoglobinemias HbM type
- β-erythremias
- β-Heinz body anemia
- HPFH, deletion type
- Angioedema, hereditary
- Acute intermittent porphyria

12
- Hemolytic anemia due to triosephosphate isomerase deficiency
- von Willebrand disease
- Stickler syndrome
- Phenylketonuria

16
- α-thalassemias
- α-erythremias
- α-methemoglobinemias
- Polycystic kidney disease
- LCAT deficiency
- [Cystathioninuria]

17
- Isolated growth hormone deficiency, type IA
- Osteogenesis imperfecta (1 or more forms)
- Pompe disease / Adult acid-maltase deficiency

18
- Familial amyloid neuropathy (several types)
- [Dystransthyretinemic hyperthyroxinemia]
- *B-cell lymphoma*

21
- Alzheimer disease
- Homocystinuria

22
- MPS I (Hurler and Scheie syndromes)
- Metachromatic leukodystrophy
- Methemoglobinemia (enzymopathic form)

Y
- XY gonadal dysgenesis

X
- X-linked ichthyosis
- Ocular albinism
- Duchenne muscular dystrophy
- Chronic granulomatous disease
- Testicular feminization syndrome
- Lesch-Nyhan syndrome / HPRT-related gout
- Hemophilia B
- Fragile X syndrome
- Hemophilia A
- G6PD deficiency: Favism / Drug sensitive anemia / Chronic hemolytic anemia

allelic disorders, even though clinical picture may be quite different. Conditions enclosed in brackets are "nondiseases"; that is, no clinical abnormality has been related with certainty to enzyme deficiency or other biochemical phenotype. See reference 33 for detailed information and description of mapping methods.

and deformity of the anterior thorax, as in Marfan syndrome, but the joints tend to be somewhat tight rather than loose. Osteoporosis is a feature limited to homocystinuria.

The cardiovascular complications of homocystinuria are thrombotic, not aortic, as in Marfan syndrome. Occlusion of the coronary, cerebral, or renal arteries occurs with the expected clinical consequences. Venous thrombosis and pulmonary embolism are also complications.

About half the patients with homocystinuria have some degree of mental retardation, a feature not found in Marfan syndrome.

As a group, persons with homocystinuria vary widely in severity, although within one family affected persons show about the same severity. This group variation, unusual for a recessive, is due to different, presumably allelic, forms of cystathionine synthase deficiency. In one form some residual activity of the enzyme is found in cultured fibroblasts and the patients respond to vitamin B_6 (or pyridoxine, a cofactor for cystathionine synthase), in a dosage of 100 mg a day or more, with clearing of homocystine from the urine, cessation of thrombotic accidents, and avoidance of ectopia lentis (if it has not already developed). This category of patient tends to be at the milder end of the spectrum; intelligence is usually normal.

Patients in a second group are more severely affected, have no detectable enzyme activity in cultured fibroblasts, and do not respond to pyridoxine. Restriction of methionine intake in the diet is the mainstay of therapy, supplemented by platelet-suppressing agents to prevent thrombosis.

Homocysteine and other sulfhydryl compounds that accumulate in homocystinuria interfere with cross-linking of collagen, probably by combining with the aldols formed from lysine and hydroxylysine residues in collagen as the first step in cross-linkage. Homocysteine has a close structural similarity to penicillamine, which has a similar effect on collagen cross-linkage. Endothelial denudation may underlie the thrombotic propensity of the disease. The mental defect of some individuals with homocystinuria may be related to a deficiency of brain cystathionine, as well as to intracranial thromboses.

The Ehlers-Danlos Syndromes

This group of disorders,[31] once thought to be a single entity, comprises at least 10, probably more, separate disorders. In several of them a basic defect in collagen formation has been identified. In each of them laxity of joints and stretchability, bruisability, and fragility of skin tend to be features, although some of these are inconspicuous in certain of the types.

Types I and II are the classic varieties, in severe and mild form, respectively. They are autosomal dominant.

Type III, also called the "benign hypermobility syndrome," is characterized mainly by striking loosejointedness. A floppy mitral valve may occur in this form, as in all others. It likewise is autosomal dominant.

Type IV (ecchymotic, arterial, or Sack-Barabas type) is a grave disorder because of proneness to spontaneous rupture of the gut and large arteries. The skin is unusually thin, with readily evident subcutaneous blood vessels, and it is stretched tightly over the face, ears, and fingers. Its fragility is evident from frequent breaks over the shins and other areas that are subject to blunt trauma. Loosejointedness is not striking except in the fingers. Rupture of the spleen from minor impact trauma and rupture of the gut for no apparent reason occur. Large ecchymoses or hematomas result from minor trauma or muscle tears. Rupture without dissection occurs in large arteries such as the innominate. At surgery, tissue may have the tensile characteristics of wet blotting paper. Although there is evidence of heterogeneity from mode of inheritance (both autosomal dominant and autosomal recessive forms are established), from electron microscopy and biochemical studies, and to some extent from clinical features, all seem to share a deficiency in production of type III collagen.

Type V is an X-linked recessive with the features of classic Ehlers-Danlos syndrome. Some affected boys have severe mitral regurgitation.

Type VI (the ocular-scoliotic form) has the cardinal features of type I plus more severe scoliosis than observed in the other forms and (unique to this type) marked fragility of the eye globe, leading to rupture of the cornea and sclera from minor blunt trauma and retinal detachment. Dissecting aneurysm of the aorta has been observed. Collagen in this type is deficient in hydroxylysine, because of deficiency of the specific hydroxylase that converts selected lysine residues in the protocollagen chain to hydroxylysine. Defective cross-linking of collagen results because hydroxylysine is, with lysine, involved in formation of cross-links. Like almost all other enzymopathies, this is an autosomal recessive. Some patients derive benefit from high doses of vitamin C, which is a cofactor for lysyl hydroxylase. Cases of the same phenotype without demonstrable deficiency of lysyl hydroxylase have been reported.

Type VII (arthrochalasis multiplex congenita) is characterized by profound joint laxity (leading to congenital dislocation of the hips and repeated subluxation of other joints such as the shoulders), stretchable and bruisable skin, and short stature. The basic defect in Ehlers-Danlos syndrome, type VII, is in cleavage of the extra piece off one end of the procollagen molecule at the time it is excreted from the cell of synthesis, the fibroblast. Intermolecular cross-linking of collagen in Ehlers-Danlos syndrome, type VII is apparently defective because persistence of the extra-long procollagen does not permit stacking of molecules in proper register. Two forms of Ehlers-Danlos syndrome, type VII exist: an autosomal recessive form with deficiency of a procollagen peptidase, that catalyzes the cleavage and an autosomal dominant form with an amino acid substitution in the $alpha_1$- or $alpha_2$-chain of procollagen, rendering it resistant to cleavage. (This may be another illustration of the basic difference of dominant and recessive disorders.)

There remain other families with Ehlers-Danlos syndrome that cannot be satisfactorily fitted into any of the above types. The genetic heterogeneity of Ehlers-Danlos syndrome is not surprising in light of the large size of the collagen molecules (and the genes that code for them), the considerable number of posttranslational processes in the formation of mature collagen, the existence of genetically and chemically distinct classes of collagen, and, in the case of type I collagen, heteromeric structure with two of its three polypeptide chains (the $alpha_1$-chains) coded by chromosome 17 and one (the $alpha_2$-chain) by chromosome 7.

Osteogenesis Imperfecta

Like Marfan syndrome and the Ehlers-Danlos syndromes, osteogenesis imperfecta is a major form of a heritable fibrous connective tissue disorder. "Brittle bones," blue sclerae, and deafness are leading features of a classic form known in the past as osteogenesis imperfecta tarda. It is inherited as an autosomal dominant. Osteogenesis imperfecta congenita (OIC) is classically manifested by many fractures that are already present at birth and is usually fatal in the neonatal period. Most of the cases of OIC are new dominant mutations, although a much rarer autosomal recessive form also exists.

In both the congenita and the tarda forms clinical subtypes have led to classification systems based on the presence or absence of blue sclerae and of involvement of the teeth ("dentinogenesis imperfecta"), as well as other characteristics. In each of these forms, molecular genetics studies show a variety of abnormalities of either the $alpha_1$-chain or the $alpha_2$-chain of type I collagen.[33] Thus mutation of some types and in some parts of the type I collagen molecule can lead either to one or another form of the Ehlers-Danlos syndrome (see earlier discussion) or to osteogenesis imperfecta and to a variety of different forms of one or the other of these. A similar phenomenon occurs in the case of the alpha-globin locus (on chromosome 16) and the beta-globin locus (on chromosome 11). Mutations in either locus can lead to thalassemia, methemoglobinemia, anemia due to unstable hemoglobin, or polycythemia.[33]

MENDELIAN MALFORMATION SYNDROMES

Although the common solitary malformations such as cleft palate, cardiac malformations, and spina bifida are multifactorial, some malformation syndromes are mendelian.[18] Autosomal dominant examples are Apert syndrome (acrocephalosyndactyly) and the Holt-Oram syndrome (Table 5.3–7). Autosomal recessive examples are the Ellis–van Creveld syndrome, cartilage-hair hypoplasia, and Kartagener syndrome. An X-linked recessive example is aqueductal stenosis (leading to hydrocephalus) with adducted thumbs.

The molecular basis of few mendelian malformation syndromes is known. In the future, study of this aspect is likely to be as contributory to normal developmental biology as study of genetic defects has been to the understanding of normal physiology and biochemistry, for example, of coagulation, intermediary metabolism, protein synthesis, transmembrane transport, lysosomes, cell surface receptors, and the like. Some mendelian defects in sexual development are now understood: (1) testicular feminization (p. 293), (2) the masculinized external genitalia of females with the several adrenal hyperplasia syndromes, and (3) the female phenotype in males with a defect or absence of the gene(s) that normally control differentiation of the testes.

The molecular defect in Kartagener syndrome is likewise known. This autosomal recessive malformation syndrome comprises dextrocardia (situs inversus viscerum), bronchiectasis, sinusitis, and male infertility.[11] Bronchial cilia and sperm show, by electron microscopy, a morphologic defect in dynein, which is essential to the motor function of cilia and the sperm tail. Thus bronchiectasis, sinusitis, and male infertility have ready explanations. Ciliated endothelium (or at least microtubules) may be involved in rotation of cardiovascular anlagen in early development. The dextrocardia may be lacking in as many as half of cases of the immobile cilia syndrome. A normal function of the mechanism defective in Kartagener syndrome may be determination of levorotation of the heart; when the mechanism is not operative, the rotation is to the right or to the left in equal proportions.

MENDELIAN NEOPLASMS

All cancers are genetic disorders inasmuch as a change in the genetic material underlies them. Some neoplasms are demonstrably mendelian, for example, familial polyposis coli, retinoblastoma, and the three forms of multiple endocrine neoplasia. Others, such as breast cancer and ovarian cancer, show a strong familial tendency, suggesting the operation of a "major gene" in some families.

The theory of Knutson proposes that many cancers, particularly childhood cancers such as retinoblastoma, which occur both on an inherited and a sporadic basis, may have two mutations as their "cause." The inherited cases have one mutation already and occurrence of a second leads to neoplasm. The inherited cases are likely to be bilateral and multifocal and to occur at an earlier age than the sporadic cases. This is evident in retinoblastoma, acoustic neuroma, and pheochromocytoma, for example. In the cases of retinoblastoma, the Knutson hypothesis has been confirmed at the DNA level. It is clear that retinoblastoma is recessive; the locus on

chromosome 13 must be a homozygous mutant for neoplasia to occur. Retinoblastoma, hereditary acoustic neuroma, and hereditary pheochromocytoma are considered autosomal dominant disorders because they are transmitted through successive generations. The recent molecular studies show that in fact they are recessive; the susceptibility is dominant.

MORBID ANATOMY OF HUMAN GENOME

Figure 5.3–10 is presented by way of summary of the foregoing discussion. It reflects the rapid progress in understanding of the genic anatomy of the human chromosomes that has occurred in recent years and will be, as Berg[2] indicated (p. 270), important to physicians concerned with genetic diseases in the future.

The disorders that are indicated here include

1. *Inborn errors of metabolism,* such as galactosemia (on chromosome 9)
2. *Lysosomal storage diseases,* such as Tay-Sachs disease (on 15) and Hurler syndrome (on 22)
3. *Heritable disorders of connective tissue,* such as the form of osteogenesis imperfecta due to mutation in the gene for the alpha$_2$-chain of type I collagen (on 7)
4. *Hemoglobinopathies,* including the thalassemias (on 11 and 16)
5. *Hereditary nonspherocytic hemolytic anemias,* such as that due to deficiency of glutathione reductase (on 8)
6. *Immunologic disorders,* such as deficiencies of C2 and C4 (on 6) and C3 (on 19), and severe combined immunodeficiency due to deficiency of adenosine deaminase (on 20)
7. *Disorders of coagulation,* such as antithrombin III deficiency (on 1) and hemophilia A (on Xq28)
8. *Neurologic disorders* of unknown biochemical defect, such as Charcot-Marie-Tooth disease (on 1), one form of spinocerebellar ataxia (on 6), myotonic dystrophy (on 19), and Duchenne muscular dystrophy (on Xp21)
9. *Receptor diseases,* such as testicular feminization (on the X chromosome near the centromere)
10. *Endocrine disorders,* such as congenital adrenal hyperplasia due to 21-hydroxylase deficiency (on 6) and one form of isolated growth hormone deficiency (on 17)
11. *Malformation syndromes,* such as the Prader-Willi syndrome (on 15)
12. *Miscellaneous disorders,* such as hemochromatosis (on 6) and postanesthetic apnea due to pseudocholinesterase deficiency (on 3)

The chromosomal locale of gene derangements that lead to neoplasms is indicated by deletion of specific chromosomal segments and by reciprocal translocations between chromosomes at specific breakpoints. In many of these, specific "oncogenes" (normal genetic components that probably serve a fundamental role in control of cell proliferation) have been identified at or near the site of deletion or chromosomal break. Examples cited earlier were the MYC gene and Burkitt lymphoma[22] and the ABL gene and chronic myeloid leukemia.[39]

Pharmacogenetics

Victor A. McKusick

Pharmacogenetics is concerned with the relationship between genetic constitution and the handling and effects of drugs. Particularly clear examples are the gene-determined differences[12] in the metabolism of isonicotinoyl hydrazide (isoniazid, or INH), the hemolytic anemia induced by primaquine and other drugs in persons with a defect in red cell G6PD, and hemolytic anemia induced by sulfonamides and other drugs in patients with hemoglobin Zurich.[32] The intolerance for certain substances demonstrated by patients with porphyria is an example of gene-drug interaction. Two examples from anesthesiology are succinylcholine apnea (pseudocholinesterase deficiency causing prolonged muscle paralysis) and malignant hyperpyrexia, often fatal, precipitated by a variety of anesthetic agents.

Differences in the rate of metabolism of the adrenergic beta-blocker metoprolol[26] and of the antiepileptic mephenytoin[21] are based on genetic polymorphism of separate cytochrome P450 enzymes involved in their metabolism. The consequence is that blood levels vary widely from person to person after the same oral dose. Nortriptyline, the mood elevator, also shows a variable rate of degradation based on the same polymorphism as that involved with metoprolol—known as "debrisoquin polymorphism"—having been first described in England on the basis of studies of that antihypertensive agent,[28] which is not used in the United States.

All of these examples have mendelian differences as their basis. They are, however, the exceptions. Most differences in the way drugs are handled and most differences in reactions to drugs are graded chracteristics and are probably multifactorial.

GENETIC DIFFERENCES IN THE METABOLISM OF INH

A number of pharmacologic agents, of which INH, a drug used in the treatment of tuberculosis, was the first to be studied from this point of view, are acetylated by a mechanism that shows genetic polymorphism.[12] About one half of all whites are rapid acetylators, and one half are slow acetylators. Slow acetylation is autosomal recessive. These phenotypes are sometimes referred to as rapid and slow inactivation, because the acetylated form of INH is chemotherapeutically ineffective.

Rapid acetylators get less adequate treatment of their tuberculosis from a given dosage of INH. On the other hand, slow acetylators are most likely to develop peripheral neuropathy because of high concentration of free INH. In practice, the genetic difference in rate of INH inactivation is usually not determined in the patient who is to receive antituberculous therapy with this agent, because INH is administered in adequate dosage to treat a tuberculous infection even in a rapid inactivator, and pyridoxine (vitamin B$_6$) is administered concurrently to prevent neuropathy.

GLUCOSE 6-PHOSPHATE DEHYDROGENASE DEFICIENCY

A defect of G6PD is present in the erythrocytes of many Americans of African and Mediterranean origin. This disorder is inherited as an X-linked recessive, its frequency being about 10 percent in American black males and about 1 percent in black females.

The red cell enzyme defect is no apparent impediment to the patient unless some exogenous factor is superimposed. The disorder was detected in Mediterranean peoples because of the widespread consumption of fava beans and in American blacks when primaquine was given for antimalarial prophylaxis during military service. The clinical picture is that of acute hemolytic anemia following ingestion of the agent by persons with the enzyme deficiency. Hemoglobinuria, anemia, jaundice, fever, leukocytosis, and renal failure can all result, and the acute episode may be fatal.

Young erythrocytes of G6PD-deficient persons have near-normal concentrations of G6PD, but as the red cells age, the enzyme decreases more rapidly than is normal and disappears relatively early in the red cell life span.

The long list of agents incriminated as factors precipitating hemolytic anemia includes such common medicaments as aspirin. Viral infections may also precipitate hemolytic crises, although the evidence is not conclusive, since antipyretic and other agents are usually administered in such cases. In the newborn infant who is G6PD deficient, hemolysis may be induced by the administration of some vitamin K preparations, by some agent taken by the mother before delivery, or by chemicals reaching the baby through the mother's milk.

In many populations of Africa, Sardinia, Sicily, and Greece, as well as among Sephardic and Iraqi Jews, its high frequency qualifies G6PD deficiency as a genetic polymorphism. Like the sickle gene, the G6PD deficiency gene probably owes its high frequency to protection against malaria that it bestows on either the hemizygous male or the heterozygous female or both.

G6PD deficiency provides yet another example of heterogeneity in genetic disease. The disease affecting Africans differs from that affecting Mediterranean peoples in that enzyme concentrations in the erythrocytes are not as low, and decreased G6PD activity in the leukocytes and some other tissues does not occur as it does in the Mediterranean form of the disease. Furthermore, the enzyme deficiency in blacks is accompanied by an electrophoretic peculiarity of the enzyme protein.

Some rare mutations in the G6PD molecule cause chronic nonspherocytic hemolytic anemia independent of drug exposure. About 200 mutant variants of G6PD have been identified by electrophoretic and other means. G6PD rivals hemoglobin as a demonstration of the biochemical diversity of humans.

CHAPTER 5.5
Immunogenetics

Victor A. McKusick

BLOOD GROUPS

The blood groups share with the hemoglobins the distinction of having contributed greatly to the formulation of principles of human genetics and of genetics in general.[37] Furthermore, blood groups are of great significance in medicine. The success of major surgery, the saving of life from exsanguinating disease or trauma, and the prevention of congenital abnormalities or fetal loss resulting from maternofetal incompatibility illustrate their important practical role.

Most of the blood groups are genetically determined variations in certain components of the red cell membrane. The Lewis system antigens are adsorbed on the surface of the erythrocyte, however. At least 12 different blood group systems, each determined by a separate locus, have been identified.

The different antigens on the red cells are identified by means of antibodies, proteins in serum that combine with the antigens and produce such effects as agglutination of the red cells. Some of the antibodies occur "naturally," for example, in the ABO blood group system: group A persons have in their serum antibody against group B cells; group B persons have antibody against group A cells, and group O persons have antibody against both group A and group B cells. These "natural" antibodies are probably the result of immunization by A-like or B-like antigens that are widely distributed in nature, such as in foods of plant origin. Because of natural antibodies, Landsteiner in 1900 was able to demonstrate the ABO blood types simply by mixing the serum and red cells of different persons.

To demonstrate the antigens of other blood groups, it is necessary to obtain the corresponding antibody by one of two main methods. In the case of MN blood groups, the antibody was produced in another species, the rabbit, by injecting human red blood cells. Rabbits injected with cells from persons of the MM genotype produced anti-M serum; cells from persons of the NN genotype stimulated production of anti-N serum. Cells from persons of the MN genotype, that is, heterozygotes, were agglutinated by either anti-M or anti-N rabbit serum.

The other method by which antibodies demonstrating blood groups are formed is the accidental development of antibody by a pregnant woman or a transfused patient. If the mother lacks a red cell antigen that is present in the fetus (who inherited it from the father), the mother may develop antibodies against the antigen when fetal cells leak over into the mother's circulation. Most of the Rh blood groups, as well as several of the other blood group systems, were discovered in the study of cases of maternofetal incompatibility. The same situation occurs in principle when the patients are tranfused with red cells containing antigens they do not possess and they develop serum antibodies against the antigens. The X-linked blood group Xg[a] was discovered in this way.

The blood groups are inherited as codominant traits; in the heterozygote, such as the AB person, both blood types are demonstrable. In many instances—in fact, so often that it is now considered a general principle—an antibody is eventually discovered for both antigens present in the heterozygote. Thus in the Kell system an antiserum was first discovered that agglutinated the red cells from persons of the genotype KK or Kk but not of persons of the genotype kk. Later an antiserum was found that agglutinated the red cells from persons of the genotype Kk or kk, but not KK.

The Rhesus (Rh) system is among the most complex identified in humans. A transatlantic controversy raged over whether multiple allelism or close linkage accounts for certain aspects of the diversity.[37] Specifically, Fisher and Race in England suggested that three closely linked loci are responsible for the Rh specificities that they call D, C, and E (in the order of their postulated order on the chromosome). On the other hand, Wiener in this country was of the view that a single, complex locus with many alleles is involved.

The Rh blood group system has been extensively studied, mainly because the Rh_o (D) antigen is the most antigenic outside the ABO system and hence is of great clinical significance.

MATERNOFETAL INCOMPATIBILITY

Maternofetal incompatibility[37] for the ABO blood groups may lead to early fetal death and abortion. It has been estimated that as many as 5 percent of conceptions are lost through ABO incompatibility. This phenomenon is not surprising, since the type O mother, for example, has natural antibody against type A and B antigens of fetal red cells and other tissues, including, perhaps, the placenta, which is largely of fetal genotype.

In the Rh system, unlike the ABO blood group system, the mother does not naturally carry antibodies against the Rh antigens that she does not possess. Trouble develops only if the mother becomes sensitized to what for her is a foreign antigen entering her system in the form of red cells from a fetus that contains a different Rh antigen through inheritance from the father. Sensitization of the mother is accomplished by actual bleeding from the fetus into the mother. Sensitive methods based on the demonstration of red cells containing fetal hemoglobin can detect the presence of very small amounts of fetal blood distributed in the mother's circulation. In subsequent pregnancies, if the fetus is again incompatible, the mother's titer of anti-Rh antibody may rise briskly, maternal antibody may cross the placenta to the fetus and the damaging effect on the infant may result in the characteristic clinical picture of hemolytic disease of the newborn (HDN), which can take the form of erythroblastosis fetalis, hydrops fetalis, or icterus neonatorum.

About 15 percent of whites are Rh negative. HDN would be much more frequent than it is if no other factors were involved. One factor is undoubtedly the low frequency of occurrence of sufficiently large fetomaternal bleeds; many Rh-incompatible pregnancies pass without their occurrence. Another important factor protecting against Rh sensitization is accompanying ABO incompatibility. If the red blood cells that bleed from the fetus to the mother are of an ABO blood type different from the mother's, the natural antibody of the mother is likely to destroy them before they can incite sensitization.

The main offender in the Rh type of HDN has been D. It has much greater antigenic propensities than the antigens C and E and the greatest of any blood group other than the ABO groups. Furthermore, the frequencies of the different Rh groups allow greater opportunity for this strong antigen to cause clinical disease. Obviously, once HDN has occurred, the risk that future children of an Rh-negative mother and an Rh-positive father will develop erythroblastosis is 100 percent if the father is DD, but is only 50 percent if he is Dd. Since in various populations some CDE combinations are more frequent than others, an estimate of whether the father is DD or Dd can be obtained from the reactions with anti-C, anti-c, anti-E, and anti-e antisera. (Unfortunately no anti-d antiserum is available.) For example, if the father is English and

reacts to anti-C, anti-D, and anti-e, but not to anti-c and anti-E, he must have CDe on one chromosome. The other chromosome may carry either CDe or Cde. Since in English populations CDe is about 41 times more common than Cde, it is likely that the man is homozygous DD (i.e., CDe/CDe).

The Rh-incompatible pregnancies most likely to lead to sensitization of the mother—those in which fetal bleeds occur into the maternal circulation—are identifiable by the demonstration of red cells containing fetal hemoglobin in the mother's blood. Fetal bleeds are most likely to occur in late pregnancy, especially with trauma to the placenta, such as occurs with forceps delivery. These observations, taken together with the natural protection afforded by ABO incompatibility, suggested that immunologic inactivation of the fetal Rh-positive red cells that leak into the mother's circulation by giving Rh antibody ("Rho-Gam") at the proper time and in the proper dosage would be a useful therapeutic approach. The approach is now fully validated and is routinely used.

HISTOCOMPATIBILITY

In addition to the ABO locus, the important histocompatibility locus in humans is HLA (so called because it is studied in human lymphocytes; A means it was the first human leukocyte locus to be designated). The HLA "locus" is in fact a region (on the short arm of chromosome 6) containing several separate but closely linked loci referred to collectively as the major histocompatibility complex (MHC). The best studied of these loci are HLA-A, HLA-B, HLA-C, and HLA-D/DR. The HLA antigens on the cell surface coded by these loci fall into class I (HLA-A, -B, and -C) and class II (HLA-D and -DR, a complex of several loci, including neighboring loci such as HLA-SB). Class III proteins coded by the MHC region include C2 and C4 (the second and fourth components of complement) and Bf (factor B of the properdin or alternate pathway). This complex of genes is situated on the short arm of chromosome 6 (see Fig. 5.1–2). (The locus for the 21-hydroxylase deficiency type of congenital adrenal hyperplasia is close to the HLA-B locus and the hemochromatosis locus is close to the HLA-A locus.)

The class I antigens occur on virtually all cells. They are tested for by means of antisera discovered in multiparous women or multitransfused patients (as in the case of blood group systems) or by specifically prepared monoclonal antibodies. The class II antigens are limited largely to lymphocytes. The HLA-D antigens are tested for by cellular techniques such as MLR (response in mixed lymphocyte culture). The HLA-DR ("D-related") antigens are tested for by serologic techniques. The chemical structure of all these antigens and of the genes that code them is now being defined.

Any one person has at least eight HLA alleles, two at each of the major loci mentioned: HLA-A, -B, -C, and -D/DR. The set of alleles on one chromosome is referred to as a "haplotype." A frequent haplotype in whites is, for example, A1-B8-Cw7-DR3. The diversity of MHC is enormous. Over 20 HLA-A alleles, 30 HLA-B alleles, 8 HLA-C alleles, 12 HLA-D alleles, 10 HLA-DR alleles, and 7 HLA-SB alleles are known. The number of possible combinations is therefore almost astronomical.

In a single family, because of the large number of different haplotypes in the population, the parents are likely to have, between them, four different ones—let us call them E, F, G, and H—the father being EF and the mother GH. The offspring will be of four different types: EG, EH, FG, and FH. The chance of two sibs being of identical HLA constitution is 25 percent. The parent and child can be of identical HLA constitution only if the two parents happen to have at least one haplotype in common. For this reason, sib-sib renal transplants are more frequently successful than parent-child transplants. (Actually more than four HLA constitutions may be found among sibs because although the HLA-A, -B, -C, and -D loci are closely linked they are still subject to low-frequency recombination through crossing over during meiosis in the parents.)

HLA typing is useful in kidney transplantation. Kidneys from HLA identical sibs enjoy almost 100 percent survival; kidneys from sibs that share only one haplotype fare less well; and kidneys from a sib with two different HLA haplotypes fare least well.

In the United States, kidneys from HLA identical but unrelated donors fare little better than do HLA-unlike cadaver kidneys. In the experience in Europe, appropriate HLA match does correlate with survival of the transplanted kidney. The discrepancy between intrafamilial usefulness of HLA match and the populational experience may be explained by the existence of other significant histocompatibility loci in the HLA region or elsewhere in the genome. Possibly greater homogeneity of European populations is responsible for the differences in American and European results.

MARKER AND DISEASE ASSOCIATION

Blood group and disease associations were identified in the 1950s. Persons of blood type O have an increased risk of peptic ulcer of the duodenum (about 1.5 times the risk of non-O persons) and persons who are also secretor negative (do not secrete ABO blood group substance into the saliva) have a risk almost 2.5 times that of non-O-secretor persons. The basis of this (and other) blood group and disease association is not genetic linkage. The non-O-secretor association with peptic ulcer has been observed in all ethnic groups. Genetic linkage produces no permanent association of traits in a population. Genetic linkage cannot account for either syndromes or marker-disease association. Rather, blood group and disease associations have their basis in the pleiotropic effect of particular alleles. (See discussion of linkage disequilibrium as an alternative mechanism for association, especially in the HLA system.)

An intimate association between a particular Duffy blood type and resistance to tertian malaria is now known. In the past when fever therapy, specifically malaria therapy, was used for central nervous system syphilis it was known that tertian malaria usually did not "take" in blacks; quartan malaria was used instead. The reason for the resistance to tertian malaria is now known to be the almost 100 percent frequency of the Duffy-null (Fy°) gene in West Africans and a high frequency in American blacks. The Duffy *a* or Duffy *b* allele determines a cell-surface component that is essential for the *Plasmodium vivax* organism to penetrate red blood cells.[33] Duffy-null cells lack this component. The Duffy-null blood type achieved high frequency in West Africa because of the protection it afforded against vivax malaria.

Examples of association of disease with specific HLA types are now known. The most striking are those between narcolepsy and HLA-DRZ and between HLA-B27 and ankylosing spondylitis. Almost all cases of ankylosing spondylitis are found to be B27; conversely, any B27 male has about a 20 percent risk of developing ankylosing spondylitis of some degree. The finding suggests a central pathogenetic role of B27 in this disease; possibly the cell surface component of this specific antigenic characteristic is a specific receptor for an etiologic agent such as a virus.

Other less strong HLA-disease associations have been found. Several diseases that appear from other evidence to have important immunologic aspects to their pathogenesis, such as diabetes and myasthenia gravis, show strongest association with specific HLA-DR alleles. These associations are of particular interest because of homology of the genes for class II antigens to the well-studied immune response (Ir) genes in the H2 complex in the mouse (the MHC equivalent of HLA in that species).

Some HLA and disease associations are thought to result from linkage disequilibrium, not from pleiotropism. The association of HLA-A3 and hemochromatosis is an example. Linkage disequilibrium means that the hemochromatosis locus is close to the HLA-A locus (a fact demonstrated by family linkage studies), that the specific mutation which causes hemochromatosis arose relatively recently in a chromosome that was carrying the HLA-A3 allele, and that a sufficient number of generations have not passed for equilibration with A3 and non-A3 alleles to occur through crossing-over. Any selective advantage to having the A3 and hemo-

chromatosis genes together would tend to maintain the linkage disequilibrium.

GENETIC IMMUNODEFICIENCIES

Another large aspect of immunogenetics concerns heritable defects in the immune mechanism: defects in immunoglobulins, cellular immunity, complement, interferon, and polymorphonuclear and macrophage function. Some of these are discussed elsewhere. An enzyme deficiency has been identified in some instances, such as severe combined immunodeficiency due to adenosine deaminase deficiency. The chromosomal location of some of the normal genes involved in the immune process is shown in Figure 5.1–2 and of the mutations underlying some of the immunodeficiencies in Figure 5.3–10.

CHAPTER 5.6

Multifactorial Disorders: The Genetics of Common Diseases

Victor A. McKusick

As indicated earlier, all disease is multifactorial. In all disorders, multiple genetic and nongenetic factors play some role even though nongenetic factors are small ones in some mendelian disorders and vice versa. Many common diseases, such as hypertension, atherosclerosis, cardiac malformations, emphysema, and peptic ulcer, "run in families" and in particular ethnic groups. A genetic background is indicated also by twin studies (comparisons of rate of concordance in monozygotic twins with that in like-sex dizygotic twins). Yet these conditions do not display simple mendelian pedigree patterns indicative of a monogenic basis. The genetic component of causation appears to be polygenic, that is, multiple genes each contribute to the development of the disorder.

In the case of some disorders that have a quantifiable feature, such as hypertension and hypercholesterolemia, the multifactorial and possibly polygenic nature of the trait is indicated by the fact that the distribution of the variable, blood pressure and serum cholesterol, is unimodal. Measured in a population, the values show no separation into two or more classes. Where on the distribution curve for blood pressure or cholesterol an individual falls depends on the particular assortment of genes inherited from the parents and the environment in which those genes function.

In connection with congenital malformations a threshold model is conceptually useful. Accumulation of a sufficient number of genetic and environmental risk factors takes the individual above a threshold, with resultant development of malformation.

Multifactorial or polygenic inheritance must not be confused with genetic heterogeneity. Diabetes, hypercholesterolemia, and hyperuricemia behave as multifactorial traits when viewed at the population level. At the family level, however, it is sometimes possible to identify a single gene locus that is mainly responsible for the disease in that family. Examples include MODY (maturity-onset diabetes of the young[1]), an autosomal dominant, familial hypercholesterolemia (p. 293), and gout due to HGPRT deficiency (p. 292). α_1-Antitrypsin deficiency is responsible for some of the familial occurrence of emphysema. Hyperpepsinogenemic peptic ulcer is an autosomal dominant form of that disorder. Malformations of the heart include some mendelian forms, although usually the simply inherited forms are malformation syndromes in which other pleiotropic effects of the gene reveal its unique nature. Examples are the Holt-Oram syndrome and the Ellis–van Creveld syndrome (see Table 5.3–7).

In due course one can anticipate that the specific biochemical function of each gene contributing to polygenic inheritance will be defined. The non-O-secretor association with peptic ulcer indicates two loci that each make a small contribution to causation of the disease. Ankylosing spondylitis, a common disorder, is an illuminating case. It was at one time thought to be a male-influenced autosomal dominant. Then multifactorial inheritance seemed more likely. With the discovery of the HLA-B27 association we came full circle. It can be viewed as a monogenic disease, or with equal or greater validity as a multifactorial disease. There are probably genetic factors in addition to HLA type; the reduced penetrance in females suggests this. Defects in the LDL receptor (p. 293) and in apolipoproteins such as apoA-1 and apoE are examples of single gene–determined components in the multifactorial causation of atherosclerosis. Gene-determined differences in membrane Na-K transport, as revealed by studies in red cells, may contribute to essential hypertension.[44,45] The identification of specific genes contributing to the cause of multifactorial disorders will probably be aided by mapping studies, using RFLPs as markers, for example.

In genetic counseling of common disorders, recognition of a mendelian subtype is obviously important. Lacking that, one must rely on empiric figures for predicting risk of recurrence. To answer the question, for example, "What chance is there that our next child will have cleft palate like our first child?", it is necessary to have information on a large series of the same situation. In such a series, what is the proportion of affected children born after an index case, given that the parents and other close relatives are unaffected? For most congenital malformations, the answer to this question is a few percent (1 to 4 percent).

The empirical risk estimate is a sliding one. Whereas if three children with an autosomal recessive disorder have been born from normal parents, the risk to a fourth-born child is still one in four; the risk increases for later born children in the case of more than one affected child with a common type of congenital malformation. If more than one sib is affected, the parents carry particular constellations of genes that are likely to cause the malformation. For many malformations, empirical figures are now available for the recurrence risk, depending on whether a single sib, a parent and child, two sibs, and so on, have been affected in the family.

REFERENCES

1. Bell JI, Wainscoat JS, et al: Maturity onset diabetes of the young is not linked to the insulin gene. Br Med J 286:590, 1983
2. Berg P: Nobel lecture: Dissections and reconstructions of genes and chromosomes. Science 213:296, 1981
3. Blass JP, Gibson GE: Abnormality of a thiamine-requiring enzyme in patients with Wernicke-Korsakoff syndrome. N Engl J Med 297:1367, 1977
4. Bourne HR, Kaslow HR, et al: Fibroblast defect in pseudohypoparathyroidism, type I: Reduced activity of receptor-cyclase coupling protein. J Clin Endocrinol Metab 53:636, 1981
5. Brown MS, Goldstein JL: A receptor-mediated pathway for cholesterol metabolism. Science 232:34, 1986
6. Bunn HF, Forget BG: Human Hemoglobins. Philadelphia, WB Saunders, 1985
7. Cartwright GE: Diagnosis of treatable Wilson's disease. N Engl J Med 298:1347, 1978
8. Chang JC, Kan YW: A sensitive new prenatal test for sickle cell anemia. N Engl J Med 307:30, 1982

9. de Grouchy J, Turleau C: Clinical Atlas of Human Chromosomes, 2d ed. New York, Wiley, 1984

10. Edwards CQ, Carroll M, et al: Hereditary hemochromatosis: Diagnosis in siblings and children. N Engl J Med 297:7, 1977

11. Eliasson R, Mossberg B, et al: The immobile-cilia syndrome: A congenital ciliary abnormality as an etiologic factor in chronic airway infections and male sterility. N Engl J Med 297:1, 1977

12. Evans, DAP, McKusick VA, Manley KA: The genetic control of isoniazid metabolism in man. Br Med J 2:485, 1960

13. Ezdinli EZ, Sokal JE, et al: Philadelphia-chromosome-positive and -negative chronic myelocytic leukemia. Ann Intern Med 72:175, 1970

14. Francomano CA, Kazazian HH: DNA analysis in genetic disorders. Ann Rev Med 37:377, 1986

15. Gahl WA, Bashan N, et al: Lysosomal cystine transport is defective in cystinosis. Science 217:1263, 1982

16. Gelfand JA, Sherins RJ, et al: Treatment of hereditary angioedema with Danazol: Reversal of clinical and biochemical abnormalities. N Engl J Med 295:1444, 1978

17. Golbus MS, Loughman WD, et al: Prenatal genetic diagnosis in 3000 amniocenteses. N Engl J Med 300:157, 1979

18. Goodman RM, Gorlin RJ: The Malformed Infant and Child: An Illustrated Guide. New York, Oxford University Press, 1983

19. Gott VL, Pyeritz RE, et al: Surgical treatment of aneurysms of the ascending aorta in the Marfan syndrome: Results of composite-graft repair in 50 patients. N Engl J Med 314:1070, 1986

20. Hirschhorn R, Papageorgiou PS, et al: Amelioration of neurologic abnormalities after enzyme replacement in adenosine deaminase deficiency. N Engl J Med 303:377, 1980

21. Kalow, W: The genetic defect of mephenytoin hydroxylation deficiency. Xenobiotica 16:379, 1986

22. Kirsch IR, Morton CC, et al: Human immunoglobulin heavy chain genes map to a region frequently involved in chromosomal translocations in malignant B-lymphocytes. Science 216:301, 1982

23. Komrower GM, Sardharwalla IB, et al: Management of maternal phenylketonuria: An emerging clinical problem. Br Med J 1:1383, 1979

24. Lamon JM, Frykholm BC, et al: Prevention of acute porphyric attacks by intravenous haematin. Lancet 2:492, 1978

25. Ledbetter DH, Mascarello JT, et al: Chromosome 15 abnormalities and the Prader-Willi syndrome: A follow-up report of 40 cases. Am J Hum Genet 34:278, 1982

26. Lennard MS, Silas JH, et al: Oxidation phenotype—a major determinant of metoprolol metabolism and response. N Engl J Med 307:1558, 1982

27. Mabry CC, Denniston JC, et al: Maternal phenylketonuria: A cause of mental retardation in children without the metabolic defect. N Engl J Med 269:1404, 1963

28. Mahgoub A, Idle JR, et al: Polymorphic hydroxylation of debrisoquin in man. Lancet 2:584, 1977

29. Martin JB, Gusella JF: Huntington's disease: Pathogenesis and management. N Engl J Med 315:1267, 1986

30. McKusick VA: On lumpers and splitters, or the nosology of genetic disease. Perspect Biol Med 12:298, 1969

31. McKusick VA: Heritable Disorders of Connective Tissue, 4th ed. St. Louis, CV Mosby, 1972

32. McKusick VA: Mendelian Inheritance in Man. Catalogs of Autosomal Dominant, Autosomal Recessive and X-linked Phenotypes, 7th ed. Baltimore, Johns Hopkins University Press, 1986

33. McKusick VA: The morbid anatomy of the human genome: The role of gene mapping in clinical medicine. Medicine 65:1, 1986; 66:1, 1987; 66:237, 1987; 67:1, 1988

34. McKusick VA, Neufeld, EF: The mucopolysaccharide storage diseases. In Stanbury JB, Wyngaarden JB, Fredrickson DS, et al (eds): The Metabolic Basis of Inherited Diseases, 5th ed. New York, McGraw-Hill, 1983

35. Nixon PF, Kaczmarek MJ, et al: An erythrocyte transketolase isoenzyme pattern associated with the Wernicke-Korsakoff syndrome. Eur J Clin Invest 14:278, 1984

36. Orkin SH: Reverse genetics and human disease. Cell 47:845, 1986

37. Race RR, Sanger R: Blood Groups in Man, 6th ed. London, Blackwell, 1975

38. Smith AT, Sack GH Jr, Taylor GJ: Holt-Oram syndrome. J Pediatr 95:538, 1979

39. Stam K, Heisterkamp N, et al: Evidence of a new chimeric bcr/c-abl mRNA in patients with chronic myelocytic leukemia and the Philadelphia chromosome. N Engl J Med 313:1429, 1985

40. Stanbury JB, Wyngaarden JB, et al (eds): The Metabolic Basis of Inherited Diseases, 5th ed. New York, McGraw-Hill, 1983

41. Thompson JS, Thompson MW: Genetics in Medicine, 4th ed. Philadelphia, WB Saunders, 1986

42. Van Regemorter N, Haumont D, et al: Holt-Oram syndrome mistaken for thalidomide embryopathy—embryological considerations. Eur J Pediatr 138:77, 1982

43. Weatherall, DJ: The New Genetics and Clinical Practice, 2d ed. Oxford, Oxford University Press, 1985

44. Weder AB: Red-cell lithium-sodium countertransport and renal lithium clearance in hypertension. N Engl J Med 314:198, 1986

45. Woods JW, Parker JC, Watson BS: Perturbation of sodium-lithium countertransport in red cells. N Engl J Med 308:1258, 1983

CHAPTER 6.1
Hematopoiesis

Lyle L. Sensenbrenner

Hematopoiesis encompasses the structure, function, and proliferation kinetics of the entire hematopoietic as well as the lymphoid (immune) system. In order to fully understand hematopoiesis, one must consider it as a part of this greater lympho-hematopoietic system. It is important to appreciate the common source and intricate structure-function relationships between the various elements of that system and the role each of these elements plays in regulating proliferation, maturation, and activity of the system as a whole. In the adult the mature system is composed of a series of organs (bone marrow, lymph nodes, thymus, spleen, and Peyer patches) and the various cellular elements which they produce, as well as the "channels" (lymphatic and vascular) which traverse and carry those elements to every tissue of the body.

PEDIGREE OF THE LYMPHO-HEMATOPOIETIC SYSTEM (Fig. 6.1–1)

PROGENITOR CELLS[4,5,8]

Using light microscopy one can recognize in the tissues of the hematopoietic system cells of each of the major hematopoietic lineages—erythrocytic, granulocytic, monocytic, lymphocytic, and megakaryocytic (Table 6.1–1). Various stages of cell maturation can be identified, including the earliest recognizable precursor, a primitive blast cell most commonly found in the bone marrow. Studies indicate that these recognizable precursors all give rise to more mature cells either with or without concomitant cell division. When precursor cells divide they do so by producing daughter cells, both of which are more mature than the parent cell from which they arose. The precursor pool is capable of expanding the total number of cells of a given lineage but only at the expense of increasing maturation. There is no true self-renewal of precursor cells. Thus, the pool of early precursor cells cannot sustain itself and would become exhausted if no earlier pool of cells existed to replenish it. Each recognizable precursor can be thought of as the source of a clone of cells produced by a series of divisions. The earlier the precursor, the larger its clone will be. At each division maturation occurs until the stage of differentiation is reached where division can no longer take place (orthochromatic monoblast, metamyelocyte and 64N megakaryocyte). The clone then ceases to expand, and terminal differentiation occurs.

In order to replenish the precursor pool there must exist an even more primitive "progenitor" cell, morphologically unrecognizable, which gives rise to the recognizable precursors. The first evidence of this was the demonstration in murine systems that small quantities of normal murine bone marrow injected intravenously into mice whose bone marrow had been totally destroyed by radiation would repopulate the entire lympho-hemotopoietic system with cells of donor origin. Further proof of the existence of such "stem cells" occurred when it was shown that lethally irradiated mice given small quantities of bone marrow intrave-

nously developed "colonies" of hematopoietic cells visible on the spleen surface. Studies showed that these colonies each arose from a single cell, which came from the donor marrow, and that approximately one of every thousand bone marrow cells injected was capable of producing such a colony. The cell giving rise to these colonies was termed the "colony-forming unit," or CFU. Since it developed in the spleen, it was called the CFU-spleen or CFU-S. These cells have no morphologically recognizable features and can be identified only after the fact, by observing their progeny in the recipient animal. Studies showed that single colonies frequently contained cells of several lineages (red blood cells, granulocytes, and monocytes), indicating that the CFU-S was truly a multipotent hematopoietic progenitor cell (Fig. 6.1–1).

Evidence now clearly demonstrates that the CFU-S progenitor pool is maintained by the proliferation of even earlier totipotent lympho-hematopoietic progenitor cells. In murine systems there is a small pool of totipotent hematopoietic progenitors that give rise to both lymphoid and hematopoietic cell lines (Fig. 6.1–1). These totipotent cells (the earliest stem cell) are the ultimate source in the adult of all multipotent and committed lymphoid and hematopoietic progenitors. The totipotent stem cell appears to be able to maintain itself throughout adult life but cannot be replenished if destroyed except by bone marrow transplantation. Most of the cells in the stem cell pool are not in cell cycle and divide infrequently. When they do divide, they appear to produce one totipotent daughter cell identical to the mother stem cell (a process called "self-renewal") and one daughter cell that goes on to proliferate more rapidly and form multipotent progenitors. The progeny of these multipotent progenitors become more firmly committed to the various cell lineages, finally producing recognizable precursors and ultimately mature cells. Thus, it is possible for daughter cells of the totipotent progenitor cell to produce billions of mature progeny in every lympho-hematopoietic lineage.

Every cell of the lympho-hematopoietic system is a progeny of the totipotent stem cell, including all lymphoid elements that migrate from their origin in the bone marrow either to the thymus, lymph nodes, spleen, and Peyer patches or into the tissues, where maturation, commitment, and the development of functional competence take place. The osteoclast, the cell that produces the marrow spaces in the originally solid bones, is also the progeny of the hematopoietic stem cell.

At given stages of maturation progenitor cells develop a series of "marker" proteins on their surface specific for particular lineages and degrees of differentiation. When injected into other species of animals these proteins elicit an immune response allowing the formation of monoclonal antibodies. Utilizing these antibodies, one can identify specific populations of cells of similar kind and at a similar state in their development. Many of these markers are very lineage-specific, while others are found at a particular stage of development in several lineages. Some, such as the lymphoid markers, are clearly associated with a particular cell function. It is believed that many of the markers are actually specific receptors that develop on the surface of the cell at a given time in its differen-

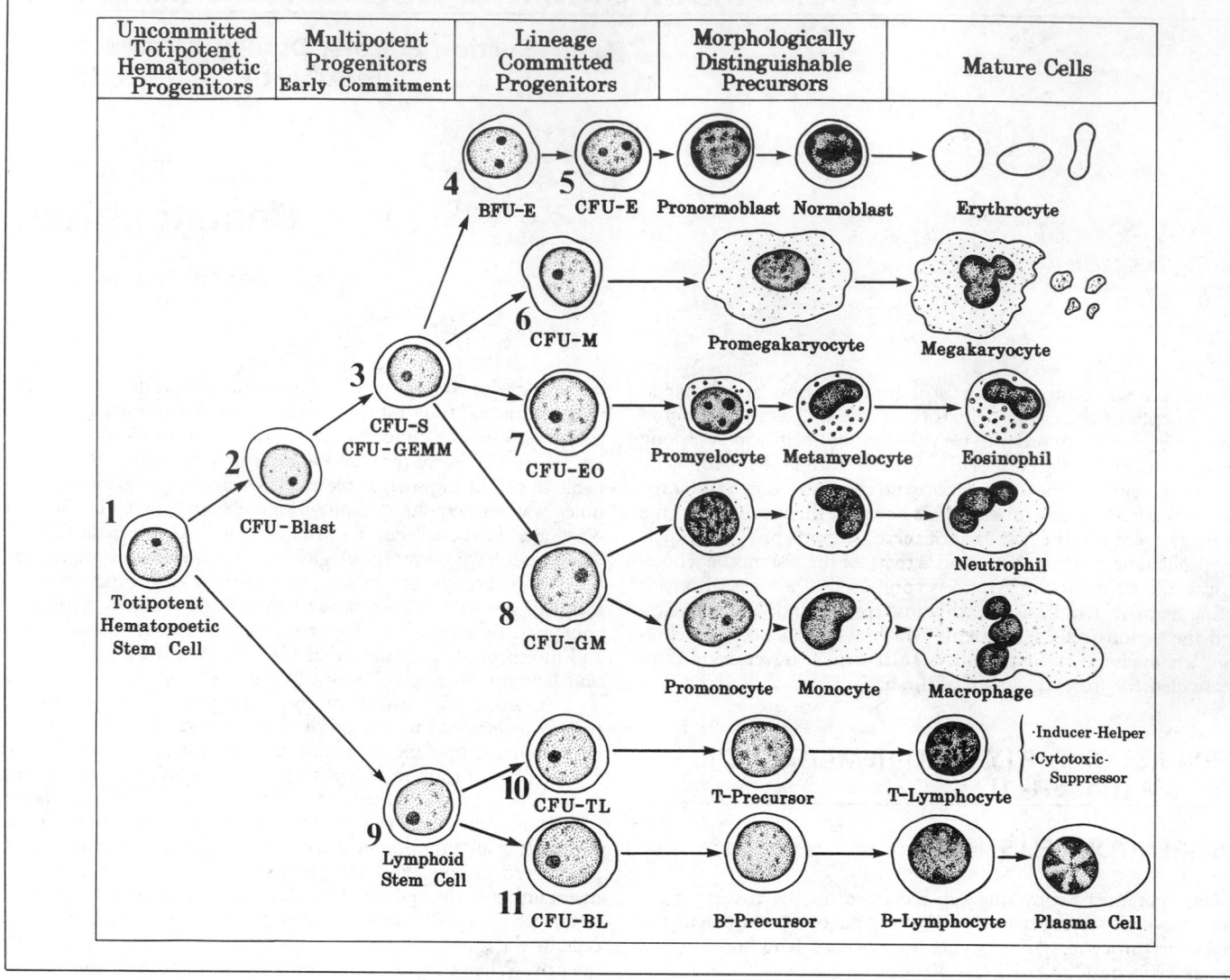

Figure 6.1–1. Cytogenealogy of blood cells.

TABLE 6.1–1. CLASSIFICATION OF HEMATOPOIETIC PROGENITOR CELLS

Progenitor Cell	Method of Identification	Associated Clonal Disorders of Hematopoiesis
Totipotent hematopoietic stem cell	Chromosomal markers Isoenzyme markers Allogeneic bone marrow reconstitution studies	Chronic myelogenous leukemia Idiopathic refractory sideroblastic anemia
Multipotent hematopoietic stem cell	Chromosomal markers Isoenzyme markers In vivo clonal assay (CFU-S) In vitro clonal assay (CFU-Blast, CFU-GEMM)	Polycythemia vera Idiopathic myelofibrosis Essential thrombocytopenia Paroxysmal nocturnal hemoglobinuria Acute leukemia Aplastic anemia
Granulocyte-macrophage progenitor cell	In vitro clonal assays (CFU-G, CFU-GM, CFU-M) (CFC-Eso, CFU-Bas)	Acute leukemia
Erythroid progenitor cell	In vitro clonal assays (BFU-E, CFU-E)	Pure red cell aplasia Acute leukemia
Megakaryocytic progenitor cell	In vitro clonal assays (CFU-Meg)	Acute leukemia

tiation process. Thus, by determining which particular receptors (markers) are present on a given cell, one can frequently determine both its lineage and stage of maturation.[3,4,7]

A genetic alteration of the stem cell pool will be carried by all subsequent progeny. The alteration will be manifested at the stage of development in which the affected gene is expressed. Thus a gene for an abnormal hemoglobin will be expressed only in those progeny committed to the erythroid line at the stage of hemoglobin production. A lethal defect expressed at the multipotent hematopoietic stem cell level will result in a failure of all hematopoietic progeny, and aplastic anemia will result while the lymphoid cell lineages may show little or no defect. Paroxysmal nocturnal hemoglobinuria represents a defect expressed in a multipotential hematopoietic progenitor that then appears to produce an unlimited number of multilineage progeny in a clonal fashion, all of which carry the same defect for increased susceptibility to complement lysis.

In the normal individual the lympho-hematopoietic system is in a dynamic state of equilibrium, constantly replenishing the multipotent and lineage-specific progenitor cells from a pool of totipotent stem cells. In the murine system, these multipotent progenitors and totipotent stem cells can be demonstrated to exist throughout much of the lympho-hematopoietic system including the peripheral blood and spleen as well as the bone marrow. Studies of patients undergoing bone marrow transplantation and the clonal nature of a variety of human disorders (chronic granulocytic leukemia, paroxysmal nocturnal hemoglobinuria) tend to indicate that a similar series of progenitor cells exists in humans.

The process by which a given multipotent progenitor is driven to commitment along a particular lineage is not clear. The evidence to date is somewhat conflicting. Some data support the idea that the microenvironment in which the stem cell lies plays a major role in bringing it into cycle and determining the differentiation pathway along which its progeny will develop. However, there is other evidence to support the concept that the onset of cell cycling and the route of differentiation is totally stochastic.

PROGENITOR CELL ASSAYS[4-6]

Since the various hematopoietic progenitor cells are not morphologically readily identifiable, numerous attempts have been made to "culture" these cells in vitro and to verify their presence by observing their progeny. Studies have defined the culture conditions under which a particular population of progenitors proliferate and differentiate, leading to a clearer description of their pedigree and some of their characteristics. By modifying these culture conditions various progenitors are identified. Clonal growth of progenitor cells was achieved utilizing a semisolid medium (agar, methylcellulose, or clotted plasma) in which anchorage-independent cells grow but have restricted migration capabilities. By providing lineage-specific "growth factors" produced in "conditioned media" or other cellular extracts, multiple progenitors were identified by their clonal growth characteristics and the histology of the mature cells in those clones. An early progenitor, designated the CFU-Blast, has been identified in vitro from the bone marrow and umbilical cord blood of humans. These cells are capable of producing colonies of undifferentiated primitive cells that on subculture can produce secondary colonies of hematopoietic cells of all lineages including other colonies of blasts. The CFU-GEMM also gives rise to colonies containing cells of multiple lineages (granulocytes, erythrocytes, megakaryocytes, and monocytes). Thus the CFU-GEMM is also a multipotent progenitor. BFU-E (burstforming unit—erythroid) in the presence of large quantities of erythropoietin gives rise to large late-developing colonies of erythroid cells, while the more mature CFU-E (erythroid) produces smaller, more rapidly developing colonies requiring less erythropoietin to induce differentiation. The CFU-GM (granulocyte, monocyte) give rise to both granulocyte and monocyte colonies. Lineage-specific progenitors producing pure colonies of eosinophils, granulocytes, macrophages, or megakaryocytes have also been identified (Fig. 6.1–1).

The use of in vitro colony-forming cell assays permits the study of the impact of disease processes on the proliferation and maturation of cells other than recognizable terminally differentiating hematopoietic cells. This gives one the ability to determine the target cell for a variety of human disease processes as well as insight into the mechanisms by which many of the complications seen are produced. In vitro clonal assays have a wide variety of clinical applications as well. For example, since the composition of the culture constituents utilized can be varied, it is possible to study the influence of defined chemical agents and cellular and humoral factors in the pathogenesis of hematopoietic disorders. An example is that of acquired immune neutropenia where one can predict the influence of agents such as corticosteroids.[1] In vitro culture of erythroid precursors is now widely employed to determine the mechanism involved in pure red blood cell aplasia. Clonal assays of leukemic cells permit the study of the cells' response to chemotherapeutic agents and to those agents used to promote cell differentiation. Identification of immunologically mediated mechanisms of aplastic anemia is made possible by the application of in vitro clonal assays to the study of patients' bone marrow and peripheral blood. The recently described in vitro assay for the very primitive human hematopoietic progenitor, CFU-Blast, will allow even further insights into normal and abnormal hematopoiesis.[8]

ANATOMY OF THE LYMPHO-HEMATOPOIETIC SYSTEM

BLOOD

Blood is the main distribution system for the cellular and humoral products of the lympho-hematopoietic system. It is a liquid tissue, a suspension of formed elements in a fluid plasma that circulates within the vascular space. Blood is a unique organ, having its own diverse cellular structure, multiple functions, and specific developmental history. The cellular contents of all lympho-hematopoietic organs including the blood are the product of the one small pool of totipotent lympho-hematopoietic stem cells. The cells in the blood are heterogeneous. Although most of the cells are end-stage, mature cells, some retain the capability of further differentiation and even multiple divisions. A red blood cell will travel approximately 175 miles during its 120-day life span, and the total mass of red cells constitutes a surface area of 3000 square miles. The functions of the cellular elements of the blood are to provide oxygen to the tissues (red blood cells), to prevent invasion of microorganisms or other foreign substances (white blood cells), to carry out immune surveillance (lymphocytes), and to promote hemostasis (platelets).

Since the blood extends throughout every tissue of the body and maintains to a great degree the hemostasis of the whole organism, it is not infrequent that a primary blood disorder may first be manifested by an apparent although secondary dysfunction of one of these other organs. It is just as likely that since the blood perfuses the microvasculature of every organ, thus coming into intimate contact with all parts of the body, a disease process originating in a particular nonhematopoietic organ may first be manifested by signs or symptoms of abnormalities of the blood. Thus, it is not uncommon that a patient may present with signs and symptoms of anemia while the primary problem is renal failure, or what appears to be primary heart failure may be secondary to the severe anemia of pure red blood cell aplasia.

Because of this very intimate relationship between the blood and all other body organs, a careful examination of the whole patient (history, physical examination, and examination of the elements of the peripheral blood) is an essential part of the evaluation of all disorders in which an abnormality in the hematopoietic system is suspected. Because of its accessibility, blood is the easiest

tissue to obtain for careful study. Examination of the cellular elements of the blood is as much a part of the physical examination as taking the blood pressure, auscultating the heart, or palpating the abdomen. Indeed, the physical examination is incomplete without a determination of the hemoglobin, hematocrit, red and white blood cell counts, differential count, platelet count, and a description of the blood cell morphology as seen in the blood smear.

BONE MARROW

When examined under light microscopy, the bone marrow is noted to consist of a heterogeneous population of cells of different origins in different stages of maturation randomly dispersed about the spicules. However, inspection by electron microscopy of a carefully prepared specimen shows that the bone marrow has a well-defined architecture that appears to be designed specifically for cell-cell interactions.[10]

The proliferative capacity of the bone marrow is equaled only by that of the skin and intestinal mucosa. In the normal healthy adult, approximately two million new red blood cells and platelets and nearly three quarters of a million granulocytes are produced every second.

Since in mammals hematopoiesis normally occurs only in extravascular sites, the mechanism for their delivery, when mature, to the blood stream requires that they traverse the endothelium lining the marrow sinuses. Migration is transcellular rather than between adjacent endothelial cells.

In the case of megakaryocytes, large pseudopod-like cytoplasmic processes extend into the blood stream, and the platelets are shed from them. The degree to which the sinus endothelial cells exert selectivity with respect to cell release, the direction of cellular traffic, and the acquisition of nutrients, regulatory macromolecules, and other agents is to a great extent unknown.

LYMPHOID SYSTEM

The lymphocytes and their related organs are an integral part of the lympho-hematopoietic system. The lymphoid system includes the thymus, lymph nodes, spleen, Peyer patches, and the various lymphatic channels that connect the lymphoid organs to the bloodstream and to each other. As noted in Fig. 6.1–1, the cells of the lymphoid system are derived from the same bone marrow totipotent hematopoietic stem cell as is the rest of the hematopoietic system. Commitment to lymphoid lineage appears to take place early, after which most of the cells migrate from the marrow through the blood stream to one of the lymphoid organs where further proliferation, commitment, and maturation take place.

FETAL HEMATOPOIESIS

The earliest identifiable hematopoietic cells appear as islands in the yolk sac during the first month of embryogenesis. Later these cells disappear, their fate unclear, and concomitant with the onset of fetal circulation hematopoiesis is initiated first in the liver and then in the spleen. Only in the later stages of fetal development do bones form. The bones are originally solid cores which are "invaded" by osteoclasts which dissolve the bone and leave behind the spaces into which the marrow will develop. It is of interest that the osteoclast is also a progeny of the hematopoietic stem cell. During embryogenesis, foci of hematopoiesis occur in a variety of tissues in addition to the liver, spleen, and marrow. These foci mimic the sites of hematopoiesis in lower organisms. The earliest identifiable cells to appear are erythroblasts, followed shortly by megakaryocytes, then granulocytes, lymphocytes, and finally monocytes.

Following birth there are changes in both the location of he-

matopoiesis and the overall mass of hematopoietic tissues. During fetal life, the cranium and vertebral bodies are major sites of blood formation. After birth, there is a gradual redistribution of the marrow to the developing bony skeleton, especially the ribs, pelvis, and sternum. Eventually the bone marrow volume exceeds blood cell production requirements, and fatty tissue gradually fills the unutilized space, especially in the bones of the limbs. Bone marrow and blood formation is then concentrated in the axial skeleton. In the adult, bone marrow comprises about 5 percent of the body weight, a mass comparable to that of the liver, reflecting the importance of blood in the body's economy.

In addition to anatomic distribution and cell mass, fetal hematopoiesis differs from adult hematopoiesis in a number of other aspects (Table 6.1–2). In the fetus, the predominant hemoglobins that appear in a sequential fashion as blood production shifts from the yolk sac to the liver and spleen are the embryonic hemoglobins and fetal hemoglobin, while in the adult, fetal hemoglobin constitutes 1 percent or less of total hemoglobin production and adult hemoglobin makes up the rest. After birth, erythropoiesis is dependent on the hormone erythropoietin, a glycoprotein synthesized predominantly in the kidneys.

IDENTIFIABLE CELLS IN THE BONE MARROW

ERYTHROPOIESIS[9]

In addition to the well-defined architecture of the marrow there is a clear organization of the recognizable cells contained within the bone marrow into small but distinct pools depending on their lineage, degree of maturation, and proliferative potential. Morphologically recognizable myeloid and erythroid precursors can be divided into proliferating (mitotic) and nonproliferating (nonmitotic) pools. Within the erythroid series the pronormoblast (rubriblast), basophilic normoblast (prorubricyte), and polychromatophilic normoblast constitute the mitotic pool while the orthochromatic normoblast (metarubricyte), which has lost the ability to synthesize DNA, and the reticulocyte compose the nonmitotic erythroid pools. The normal transit time for a red cell from the pronormoblast stage until its exit from the marrow is approximately 7 days, a short interval considering that the life span of a red cell is between 100 and 120 days. When there is a demand for red cells, marrow transit time is shortened, and reticulocytes are released prematurely into the circulation. These reticulocytes can be recognized in Wright-stained smears by their large size and polychromatophilic hue. Recognition of mature reticulocytes requires supravital staining with new methylene blue.

Mature red cells lack the capacity to synthesize proteins, and as a consequence are unable to replace enzymes and structural proteins that deteriorate as the cells age. Old red cells characteristically have reduced glycolytic activity; alterations in intracellular cation content; diminished surface area, surface charge, and cell size; and increased membrane rigidity, cell density, and fragility. They are

TABLE 6.1–2. COMPARISON OF FETAL AND ADULT HEMATOPOIESIS

Fetus	Adult
Extramedullary hematopoiesis in liver and spleen	Hematopoiesis only in the bone marrow
Erythropoiesis antedates renal development	
Erythropoiesis is dependent on the liver	Erythropoiesis is dependent on the kidneys
100% fetal hemoglobin	1% fetal hemoglobin
Erythropoietin is present	Erythropoietin is present

removed from the circulation by the reticuloendothelial system. Once ingested by macrophages, red cells are catabolized with the release of their iron for either reutilization by newly formed cells or storage, and the conversion of their heme content to carbon monoxide and bilirubin. The relationship of plasma-unconjugated bilirubin to bilirubin production is such that even if bilirubin production were to increase tenfold, as may occur in certain hemolytic disorders, plasma-unconjugated bilirubin seldom rises higher than 4.0 mg.

MYELOPOIESIS[2]

Among the morphologically recognizable precursors of the myeloid lineage there is also a mitotic pool composed of the myeloblast, promyelocyte, and myelocyte, and the nonmitotic pool containing the metamyelocyte, the band, and the segmented neutrophil. The normal transit time for a neutrophil from the myeloblast stage to the blood is 7 days. Of that time 4 to 5 days are spent in the nonmitotic pool. Given the short intravascular life span of the circulating neutrophil (14 hours) and its inability to recirculate having once left the blood stream, the nonmitotic neutrophil pool serves as a reserve for the continuous maintenance of an adequate blood neutrophil level and also an immediate source of neutrophils readily available to combat microbial invasion without the lag period required for the production of new cells. When the nonmitotic neutrophil pool is depleted, the host is at greater risk of infection. The nonmitotic reserve pool of the marrow is usually adequate if at least 25 percent of the neutrophils are at the band and segmented stages.

Neutrophils within the blood stream are divided into two approximately equal pools, a circulating pool and a marginated pool. Peripheral blood leukocyte counts provide a measure of only the circulating neutrophil pool; neutrophils marginated along postcapillary venules are not normally represented, but it is the release of these cells into the circulation that accounts for the leukocytosis associated with strenuous exercise, convulsions, paroxysmal tachycardia, and the administration of ether or epinephrine. Segregation of neutrophils between the circulating and marginating neutrophil pools is not always orderly, and this may account for the absence of the expected leukocytosis in some patients with infection. For this reason, the number of circulating band forms provides a better reflection of marrow neutrophil response than the total blood neutrophil count. Since delivery of neutrophils to the site of infection is the desired result, examination of the appropriate exudates for the presence of neutrophils is the best measurement of the adequacy of the host response.

In contrast to the neutrophil, little is known of the kinetics of the monocyte. Monocytes and their precursors constitute less than 1 percent of the marrow cell population and under normal circumstances are difficult to identify in the marrow with certainty. Compared to the neutrophil, there is no analogous monocyte reserve pool. These cells migrate from the marrow randomly and conduct their most important replicative activities in the tissues where they serve as the source of alveolar macrophages; Kupffer cells; and peritoneal, pleural, and reticuloendothelial macrophages.

MEGAKARYOCYTOPOIESIS

The least common of the hematopoietic cells is the megakaryocyte, a cell unique among mammalian cells for its polyploid DNA content. Megakaryocytes comprise less than 0.5 percent of the marrow cell population. Depending on its ploidy, each megakaryocyte produces between 4000 and 8000 platelets. Platelet release occurs by the extension of segments of megakaryocyte cytoplasm into the lumen of the marrow sinus. These cytoplasmic segments called proplatelets, fragment along demarcation membranes into platelets. Occasionally a megakaryocyte will pass into the circulation intact and become trapped within the pulmonary vascular bed where

it releases its platelets. In order of decreasing frequency the distribution of megakaryocyte ploidy within the marrow is 8N, 16N, and 32N. Megakaryocyte size, maturation, and ploidy appear to be linked, but ploidy and nuclear lobulation are not. The majority of the 8N megakaryocytes are immature and 95 percent of platelet-shedding megakaryocytes are 16N and 32N. When there is a demand for platelets megakaryocyte size, ploidy, and maturation rate increase; an increase in the number of megakaryocytes is a later event. Once released, at least 30 percent of circulating platelets are sequestered within the spleen and other extravascular sites. They can be released from these sites by epinephrine, exercise, or acute blood loss. Platelet life span is approximately 9 days. Unlike neutrophils, however, there is no substantial marrow reserve pool to compensate for a sudden reduction in the circulating platelet mass.

HEMATOPOIETIC GROWTH FACTORS[6]

The factors regulating hematopoiesis in the normal individual are complex. They include cellular as well as humoral influences that make up the microenvironment in which the hematopoietic cells proliferate and differentiate. Several humoral factors that directly influence hematopoietic cell growth and differentiation in vitro have been identified. Some of these have been shown to have significant effects in vivo as well.

ERYTHROPOIETIN[9]

Erythropoietin is a glycoprotein produced in the kidney and to a lesser extent in the liver. Renal hypoxia stimulates erythropoietin production; a surfeit of oxygen suppresses it. Extrarenal erythropoietin production is insensitive to hypoxia. Factors which decrease eythropoietin production include endotoxin, protein deprivation, and hypercapnea. Androgens and thyroid hormone on the other hand enhance it.

Under normal circumstances only minute quantities of erythropoietin (0.3 ng/ml) are in the plasma and only a fraction of that amount is excreted in the urine. With the recent availability of recombinant erythropoietin, sufficient amounts of the purified material are now available, and clinical studies of its usefulness in human disease states are being carried out.

Erythropoietin increases the number of cells differentiating into mature erythrocytes and augments their hemoglobin synthesis. It also facilitates the release of reticulocytes from the marrow.[9] A major target cell for erythropoietin appears to be the CFU-E and to a lesser extent the BFU-E.

GRANULOCYTE- AND MONOCYTE-STIMULATING FACTORS[6]

Recently several other humoral factors have been identified as granulocyte and monocyte growth regulators. These have now been purified, the specific DNA isolated and inserted into cells, and the recombinant hematopoietic growth regulators produced. These factors include recombinant granulocyte colony-stimulating factor (G-CSF) and the human recombinant granulocyte-monocyte colony-stimulating factor (GM-CSF). In vitro it has been shown that each of these factors can stimulate the clonal proliferation and maturation of progenitor cells. Human recombinant GM-CSF has a profound stimulating effect on the more mature granulocyte macrophage progenitor, CFU-GM (Fig. 6.1–1), and very little effect on the BFU-E or earlier progenitors. In vitro studies of G-CSF show it to have its major effect by stimulating the proliferation and maturation of those late progenitors committed to forming clones of granulocytes, and CFU-G. Although there is no absolute evidence at present that any of these factors play an important role in the regulation of hematopoiesis in vivo in the normal situation, recent studies indicate that "pharmacologic" doses of the materials

(GM-CSF) given to animals following lethal whole-body radiation and autologous bone marrow infusion markedly enhanced the recovery in the peripheral blood of granulocytes and platelets. Clinical studies are now underway to determine whether GM-CSF enhances the recovery of bone marrow function in patients with either aplastic anemia or severe bone marrow damage after suppressive chemoradiotherapy.

MULTILINEAGE-STIMULATING FACTOR

A factor shown to stimulate several cell lineages in vitro has been demonstrated in both murine and human cell systems. The material (multi-CSF or interleukin-3) has been isolated from a variety of cell sources, including stimulated normal lymphocytes. In vitro, it has been shown to stimulate the proliferation and differentiation of cells of the erythroid line (BFU-E), the granulocyte and monocyte line (CFU-GM), and the earlier multilineage progenitor CFU-GEMM. Its role in the regulation of hematopoiesis in vivo in the normal situation is unclear.

The use of growth factors as therapeutic tools for patients with bone marrow failure of a variety of etiologies is presently being evaluated. Growth factors may soon provide valuable adjuncts to our present modes of therapy.

REFERENCES

1. Bagby GC, Lawrence HJ, Neenhout RC: T-lymphocyte mediated granulopoietic failure: In vitro identification of prednisone-responsive patients. N Engl J Med 309:1073, 1983
2. Dancey JT, Deubelbeiss KA, et al: Neutrophil kinetics in man. J Clin Invest 58:705, 1976
3. Foon KA, Todd RF III: Immunologic classification of leukemia and lymphoma. Blood 68:1, 1986
4. Greaves MF, Chan LC, et al: Lineage promiscuity in hematopoietic differentiation and leukemia. Blood 67:1, 1986
5. Griffin JD, Lowenberg B: Clonogenic cells in acute myeloblastic leukemia. Blood 68:1185, 1986
6. Metcalf D: The molecular biology and functions of the granulocyte-macrophage colony-stimulation factors. Blood 67:257, 1986
7. Minden MD, Mak TW: The structure of the T-cell antigen receptor genes in normal and malignant T-cells. Blood 68:327, 1986
8. Rowley SD, Sharkis SJ, et al: Culture from human bone marrow of blast progenitor cells with an extensive proliferation capacity. Blood 69:804, 1987
9. Spivak JL, Graber SE: Erythropoietin and the regulation of erythropoiesis. Johns Hopkins Med J 146:311, 1980
10. Weiss L: The hematopoietic microenvironment of the bone marrow: An ultrastructural study of the stroma in rats. Anat Rev 186:161, 1976

CHAPTER 6.2
The Anemic Patient

Jerry L. Spivak

Under normal circumstances the circulating red cell mass is maintained at a constant level in a given individual, but among persons of the same age and sex that level may vary by more than 10 percent (Table 6.2–1). Furthermore, differences in red cell mass are also observed between children and adults, and, in adults, between men and women. Ambient oxygen tension also influences the red cell mass and altitude of residence must be considered when comparing the value for a particular individual with the expected norm. After adolescence, age alone does not influence the red cell mass and should never be invoked as a cause for impaired red cell production.

Two factors determine the circulating red cell mass—the life span of the red cells and the rate of effective red cell production. Red cell life span in humans is finite, normally 120 days. Consequently, in order to maintain a constant red cell mass, 0.8 percent of the circulating red cells (20 ml) must be replenished each day. Red cell production is regulated by the hormone erythropoietin and is dependent on an adequate supply of nutrients of which

iron, folic acid, and vitamin B_{12} are the most important. The difference in circulating red cell mass between men and women is probably a consequence of androgen production in men. Androgens enhance both the size of the erythropoietin-responsive cell pool in the marrow and the production of erythropoietin by the kidneys.

DEFINITION OF ANEMIA

Anemia can be defined quantitatively as a reduction in the circulating red cell mass below that considered to be normal for individuals of the same sex and age. Such a definition, however, provides no information about the ability of the circulating red cells to provide oxygen to the tissues. Thus an individual with a high carboxyhemoglobin level would be functionally anemic even though the circulating red cell mass was normal or elevated. Conversely, with a low-oxygen-affinity hemoglobin, tissue oxygenation might be adequate even though the circulating red cell mass was less than normal. However, since there is no simple method for evaluating tissue oxygenation and since a mild reduction in red cell mass unassociated with tissue hypoxia is often the first clue to the presence of a serious underlying disease, quantitative measurements are routinely employed to identify anemia. Unfortunately, in spite of the development of well-established norms (Table 6.2–1), physicians frequently fail to heed documentation of a reduced red cell mass until the level is well below the accepted normal range.[4]

Anemia develops when the demand for red cells exceeds the capacity of marrow to produce them. This may be due to excessive destruction of red cells, their loss by hemorrhage, impaired red cell production, or a combination of these. Acquired anemia is always a consequence of another disorder that must be identified. Treatment of the anemia alone by transfusion or hematinic agents is unacceptable.

TABLE 6.2–1. NORMAL RED CELL VALUES FOR ADULTS

	Males	Females
Hematocrit (%)	47 ±7	42 ±5
Hemoglobin (g/dl)	16 ±2	14 ±2
Red cell count ($10^6/\mu l$)	5.4±0.8	4.8±0.6
MCV (fl)	90 ±8	90 ±8
MCH (pg/cell)	29 ±2	29 ±2
MCHC (g/dl)	33.5±2	33.5±2

CLINICAL CONSEQUENCES OF ANEMIA

There is no correlation between the severity of an anemia and the nature of its underlying cause. The symptoms and signs associated with anemia depend on the cause of the anemia, its extent, the rapidity of onset, and the presence of other disorders that compromise the patient's health. Because the principal function of red cells is to carry oxygen to the tissues, fatigue, headache, and exertional dyspnea are common symptoms. The progression of anemia, however, may be so insidious that a profound reduction in red cell mass is tolerated with few symptoms. This is frequently the situation in pernicious anemia. Indeed, subjective complaints in this disorder may be sufficiently nonspecific that the nature of the underlying blood disorder is not recognized. In chronic, compensated hemolytic anemia, a state of ill health is often appreciated only in retrospect after the hemolytic process has been corrected.

A number of mechanisms are available to compensate for the decrease in oxygen transport associated with anemia. They include a reduction in hemoglobin-oxygen affinity, an increase in cardiac output, a reduction in peripheral vascular resistance and blood viscosity, a decrease in circulation time, an increase in oxygen extraction, and a redistribution of blood flow. The elevated cardiac output is due mainly to an increase in stroke volume; tachycardia is frequently not present. Usually the cardiac output does not increase until the hemoglobin level falls to 7 g/dl or less. There is no correlation, however, between the severity of the anemia and the cardiac output.[5] In sickle cell anemia, the cardiac output may be elevated when the hemoglobin level is 9 g/dl, while in the elderly, severe anemia may be associated with little change in the cardiac output. Even in the absence of cardiac disease, however, anemia can produce circulatory congestion and fluid retention.[9]

EVALUATION OF ANEMIA

HISTORY

Because of the intimate relationship between the blood and the other body organs, determination of the cause of anemia requires a logical approach to avoid misuse of the laboratory and inappropriate therapy. A careful history is the first step toward diagnosis. Knowledge of previous hematologic studies or blood donations will help date the onset of anemia. Inquiry concerning environmental or occupational exposures, travel, and drug and ethanol use is mandatory. Patients do not usually volunteer information concerning the use of nonprescription drugs, and occasionally a visit to the patient's medicine cabinet will be necessary. Investigation of gustatory behavior with respect to pica or exotic or irrational diets may be rewarding, as may questions concerning jaundice or dark urine. Given the central importance of the blood to the body's economy, scrutiny of all organ systems is obligatory. Hypothyroidism presenting with a mild normochromic, normocytic anemia is frequently missed because of failure to comply with this mandate. The family history is, of course, of great importance in determining whether a blood disorder is hereditary or if a genetic predisposition to certain autoimmune diseases exists. Frequently, relatives or close associates are better observers than the patient and may be able to provide important disease-related milestones with respect to the onset of pallor, jaundice, or constitutional symptoms, drug use, or toxic exposures.

PHYSICAL EXAMINATION

On physical examination jaundice, telangiectases, petechiae, ecchymoses, papillary atrophy of the tongue, lymphadenopathy, sternal or other bony tenderness, splenomegaly, hepatomegaly, leg ulcers, and neurologic abnormalities are important findings. Pallor is best evaluated from the mucous membranes, as alterations in blood flow, variations in pigmentation, and the presence of other disorders make the determination of pallor from skin examination unreliable. As a rough guide, however, pallor of the palmar creases is not usually observed until the hemoglobin level is 7 g/dl or less. As mentioned above, tachycardia is not usually observed unless the anemia is acute. Other evidence of hyperkinetic circulatory activity, however, such as a widened pulse pressure, accentuation of the first and second heart sounds, systolic flow murmurs, and a cervical venous hum, may be present.

The history and physical examination, together with a urinalysis, and examination of the stool for occult blood, an examination of a well-stained peripheral blood smear, a hemoglobin or red cell count, a mean corpuscular volume (MCV), and a corrected reticulocyte count, form the basis for the evaluation of an anemia. Positive findings obtained from the history or physical examination serve to focus attention on certain diagnostic possibilities and the need for immediate therapeutic intervention. Most often, however, the peripheral blood smear, the MCV, and reticulocyte count provide the information on which further diagnostic studies are based.

LABORATORY STUDIES

Red Cell Count, Hemoglobin Concentration, and Hematocrit

Three measurements are used interchangeably to quantify the concentration of circulating red cells—the red cell count, the blood hemoglobin concentration, and the volume of packed red cells (hematocrit). Once performed manually, these measurements are now routinely made with greater accuracy by electronic particle counters. The red cell count and hemoglobin concentration are measured directly; the hematocrit is derived from the mean red cell volume and the red cell count. A hematocrit determined in this fashion will always be lower than one determined directly by centrifugation of whole blood in a hematocrit tube, since trapped plasma increases the apparent hematocrit in the latter instance. In both iron deficiency anemia and megaloblastic anemia due to deficiency of vitamin B_{12} or folic acid, the difference between the two techniques is even greater because in these situations the red cells are more rigid than normal and more plasma is trapped.

The red cell count, the blood hemoglobin concentration, and the spun hematocrit are influenced by the plasma volume. Thus, they do not faithfully reflect the circulating red cell mass, but for routine purposes the ease with which these measurements are obtained outweighs this disadvantage. In certain clinical situations, however, such as erythrocytosis, a direct determination of circulating red cell mass by isotope dilution will be necessary to distinguish an absolute increase in red cell mass from a reduction in plasma volume.

Reticulocyte Count

The red cell count, the blood hemoglobin concentration, and the hematocrit are, of course, static measurements and reflect only the balance between production and destruction of red cells. For an estimate of effective red cell production both the presence of polychromatophilic red cells in the blood and the number of circulating reticulocytes can be used. Polychromatophilic red cells are reticulocytes that have been prematurely released into the blood stream before completion of hemoglobin synthesis.[8] Normally less than 0.1 percent of circulating red cells are polychromatophilic as identified by Wright-stained blood smears. With stimulation of the marrow by erythropoietin, the number of polychromatophilic cells increases exponentially and in the absence of intrinsic disease of the marrow can be used as an indicator of increased effective erythropoietic activity. Mature reticulocytes released into the blood can only be identified with supravital stains, but the reticulocyte count provides a simple means of quantitating blood production and identifying anemias due to impaired production of red cells. Since reticulocytes are enumerated as a function of red cell number, ane-

mia produces an apparent increase in the reticulocyte count. Furthermore, when anemia is severe, reticulocytes are released prematurely and spend a longer time in the circulation. As a consequence, the daily reticulocyte count may not faithfully reflect the actual rate of new blood production. To compensate for these effects and obtain a meaningful index of blood production, the raw reticulocyte count is corrected first for the degree of anemia:

$$\text{Reticulocyte count} \times \frac{\text{Observed hematocrit}}{\text{Normal hematocrit for sex and age}} = \text{Corrected reticulocyte count}$$

If the hematocrit is 25 percent or less, the corrected reticulocyte count should be divided by 2 to adjust for the prolonged maturation of the reticulocytes in the circulation. The corrected value can be employed as an index of effective erythropoiesis in comparison to normal.[6]

Red Cell Indices

Electronic particle counters also determine the MCV, the mean corpuscular hemoglobin (MCH), and the mean corpuscular hemoglobin concentration (MCHC) of red cells. These measurements have traditionally been used to characterize deviations from the mean in size and hemoglobin content of circulating red cells. However, of the three only the MCV is directly measured and of important discriminant value in patients with anemia; the MCH and MCHC are derived quantities and usually provide little additional information. The MCV is useful in screening for disorders producing macrocytosis or microcytosis. Since the MCV indicates only a central tendency and is subject to distortion by red cell fragmentation or agglutination, it must be coupled with examination of a carefully prepared blood smear. MCV values far outside the normal range are generally a consequence of advanced disease. Since different disorders can produce similar alterations in the MCV, the peripheral blood smear is useful in distinguishing between them. Furthermore, the peripheral blood smear provides the only

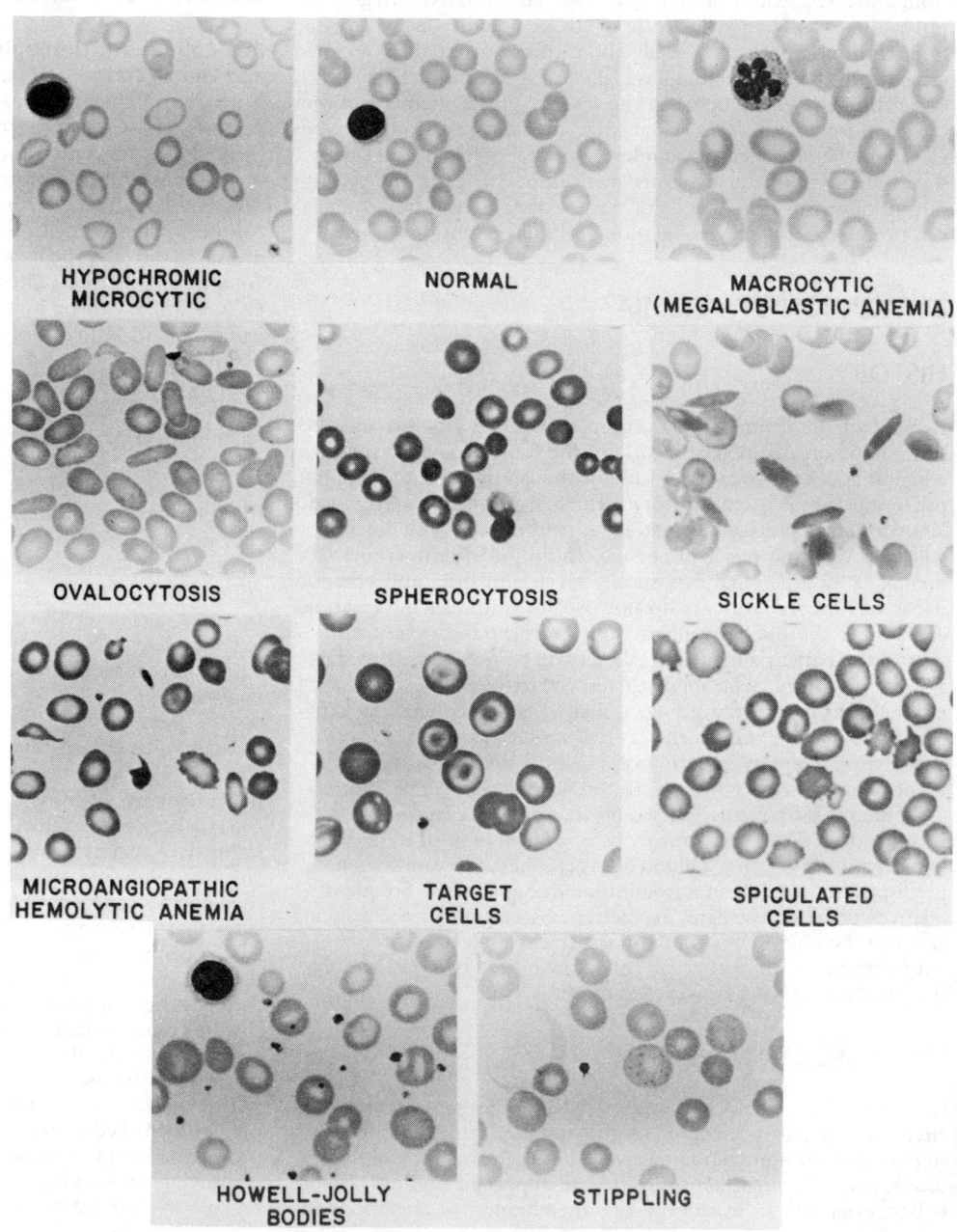

Figure 6.2–1. Normal and abnormal red cell morphology.

means for detecting red cell inclusions or abnormalities restricted to a portion of the circulating red cell population and corroborating results obtained by the particle counter. Indeed, the information obtained from the electronic particle counter and the peripheral blood smear complement each other and accurate interpretation of data derived from the electronic counter is not possible without reference to a well-prepared blood smear.

In addition to the MCV, MCH, and MCHC, electronic particle counters often provide a measurement of anisocytosis, the coefficient of variation of red cell volume (RBC CV), or red cell distribution width (RDW). Normally the distribution of red cell volume is Gaussian. Excessive heterogeneity of red cell volume (anisocytosis) is an early feature of disturbed erythropoiesis and is reflected by an increase in the RBC CV or RDW.[2] This measurement can be also used to distinguish between thalassemia trait and iron deficiency anemia. In thalassemia trait the RBC CV or RDW is normal; in iron deficiency, it is increased.[1] An increase in RBC CV can also occur when there is a bimodal distribution of red cell volumes. In this instance the MCV would not provide an accurate reflection of red cell volume.

Blood Smear

Figure 6.2–1 illustrates the type of diagnostic information that can be obtained from the peripheral blood smear that would not be provided by electronic particle counters. Thus, hypersegmented neutrophils and macroovalocytes suggest the presence of megaloblastic hematopoiesis. Howell–Jolly bodies are also seen in megaloblastic hematopoiesis; they are a feature of the postsplenectomy state and of hyposplenism as well. Red cell stipping may be due to a hemoglobinopathy, a sideroblastic process, or lead poisoning, while spiculated red cells may be seen in hypothyroidism, liver disease, and starvation. Abnormalities of red cell shape and size are a hallmark of hemolytic processes, and the type of morphologic abnormality may suggest the underlying cause of the hemolysis. Red cell fragmentation suggests mechanical intravascular destruction, which may be due to a vasculitis, a cardiac valvular abnormality, a metastatic tumor, or a consumption coagulopathy. Sickled erythrocytes are a pathognomonic feature of hemoglobin S, while ovalocytosis or spherocytosis suggest underlying abnormalities of the red cell cytoskeletal proteins. Spherocytes may also be the consequence of antibody-mediated red cell membrane loss. Other blood abnormalities not illustrated include red cell agglutination, which is seen with cold agglutinins; rouleaux formation, which occurs with hyperglobulinemia; and "blister-cells," which can develop in glucose-6-phosphate dehydrogenase (G6PD) deficient red cells.

To be of value the blood smear must be carefully made, since the risk of inducing misleading artifacts during preparation is great. Furthermore, not only must an oil-immersion lens be used for careful scrutiny of many areas of the smear, but to obtain maximal information, experience is required as well. Nevertheless, the peripheral blood smear represents an immediate tissue biopsy of great potential importance and should always be examined by the physician responsible for the patient.

CLASSIFICATION OF ANEMIA

Once the presence of anemia is established, the reticulocyte count and peripheral blood smear are used to distinguish hemolytic anemias or anemia due to blood loss in which the marrow is responding from anemias in which the primary defect is impaired red cell production. Hemolytic anemias are discussed in Chapter 6.6. Table 6.2–2 lists the many causes for hypoproliferative anemias. This group of anemias can be further subdivided for diagnostic purposes by using the MCV (Table 6.2–3). This morphologic classification provides a logical basis for further laboratory studies.

TABLE 6.2–2. CAUSES OF HYPOPROLIFERATIVE ANEMIA

- Impairment of renal function
- Impairment of pituitary or thyroid function
- Infection
- Inflammation
- Neoplasms, hematopoietic and nonhematopoietic
- Starvation
- Drugs, toxins
- Aplastic anemia
- Pure red cell aplasia
- Myelofibrosis
- Deficiency of iron, vitamin B_{12}, or folic acid
- Sideroblastic anemia

BONE MARROW ASPIRATION

Not only can a variety of different disorders cause similar changes in red cell size, but in many instances there are no discernible alterations of red cell size (Table 6.2–3). For these reasons examination of a bone marrow aspiration is often needed to determine the nature of the disorder causing anemia. A marrow aspirate is also necessary in the evaluation of leukopenia or thrombocytopenia. The stained marrow aspirate permits assessment of the composition of the marrow precursor cell populations and the presence of maturation or morphologic abnormalities of these cells. A marrow aspirate is useful in the evaluation of storage cell disorders and in the evaluation of neoplastic involvement of the marrow. It is the only reliable means for assessing marrow iron stores and provides a source of tissue for karyotypic analysis of hematopoietic cells.

BONE MARROW BIOPSY

In the event that marrow cannot be aspirated, a bone marrow biopsy should be performed. Marrow biopsy provides the only reliable method for evaluating marrow cellularity and architecture. The diagnosis of aplastic anemia can be established only by marrow biopsy and the procedure should be performed in every patient with pancytopenia, since in this situation the marrow aspirate can be misleading. Marrow biopsy is useful in staging Hodgkin disease and non-Hodgkin lymphomas and carcinoma of the lung. Bilateral

TABLE 6.2–3. MORPHOLOGIC CLASSIFICATION OF HYPOPROLIFERATIVE ANEMIAS

Normocytic Anemia
- Infection
- Inflammation
- Neoplasms
- Renal disease
- Pituitary or thyroid failure
- Starvation
- Aplastic anemia
- Pure red cell aplasia
- Myelofibrosis

Microcytic Anemia
- Iron deficiency
- Thalassemia
- Anemia associated with systemic disease
- Sideroblastic anemia[a]

Macrocytic Anemia
- Folic acid deficiency
- Vitamin B_{12} deficiency
- Thyroid disease
- Liver disease
- Sideroblastic anemia[a]
- Myelodysplasia
- Drugs

[a]May be dimorphic.

biopsies increase the yield of positive results by approximately 15 percent.[3] In disorders such as tuberculosis or sarcoidosis, the incidence of biopsies containing granulomas varies between 15 and 30 percent.[7]

In special situations sophisticated studies of red cell production and destruction such as ferrokinetics, red cell survival, sequestration, and clonal proliferation as well as tests of red cell structure and function may be necessary to identify the defect causing an anemia. The situations in which such tests are employed are discussed in the chapters that follow.

REFERENCES

1. Bessman JD, Feinstein DI: Quantitative anisocytosis as a discriminant between iron deficiency and thalassemia minor. Blood 53:288, 1979

2. Bessman JD, Johnson RK: Erythrocyte volume distribution in normal and abnormal subjects. Blood 46:369, 1975
3. Brunning RD, Bloomfield CD, et al: Bilateral trephine bone marrow biopsies in lymphoma and other neoplastic diseases. Ann Intern Med 82:365, 1975
4. Carmel R, Denson TA, Mussell B: Anemia: Textbook vs practice. JAMA 242:2295, 1979
5. Duke J, Abelmann WH: The hemodynamic response to chronic anemia. Circulation 39:503, 1969
6. Hillman RS, Finch CA: The misused reticulocyte. Br J Haematol 17:313, 1969
7. Munt PW: Miliary tuberculosis in the chemotherapy era: With a clinical review in 69 American adults. Medicine 51:139, 1971
8. Perrotta AL, Finch CA: The polychromatophilic erythrocyte. Am J Clin Pathol 57:171, 1972
9. Varat MA, Adolph RJ, Fowler NO: Cardiovascular effects of anemia. Am Heart J 83:415, 1972

Iron Deficiency Anemia

Jerry L. Spivak

Iron is the most important and abundant metal in the body. Both the abundance and importance of iron derive from its essential role in oxygen transport, cell respiration, and cell proliferation. As a consequence of the fundamental requirement of iron in energy metabolism, the body has a mechanism for enhancing intestinal iron absorption but lacks a mechanism for iron excretion. Although minute amounts of iron (1 mg/day) are lost by desquamation of epithelial cells and in the sweat, urine, and bile, these deficits are easily replenished by the diet. Consequently, iron deficiency in the adult is usually the result of blood loss for which the cause should be sought diligently. Since iron deficiency is always caused by some other disorder, blind therapy with iron is never justified, and in Western societies inadequate dietary intake should never be accepted as a cause of the deficiency state in an adult.

IRON ABSORPTION

The distribution of iron within the body for normal men and women is shown in Table 6.3–1. The bulk of the iron required daily for hemoglobin synthesis is provided by catabolism of senescent red cells while tissue iron stores provide a reserve to maintain hemoglobin synthesis when blood loss occurs or there is a sudden demand for red cells. Dietary iron serves to replenish ordinary daily losses. The iron content of the diet is linked to caloric intake; each 1000 calories ingested contains approximately 7 mg of iron.[8] Not all of this iron, however, is available for absorption. Dietary iron occurs in two forms, heme iron and nonheme iron, each of which is absorbed by a different mechanism. Heme compounds are absorbed intact with high efficiency in the upper small bowel. Once absorbed, iron is released from heme within the mucosal cells by heme oxygenase. In contrast to heme iron, the bioavailability of nonheme iron is poor. This is due in part to the manner in which the iron is complexed in particular foodstuffs such as spinach or rice, and in part to the adverse effect of other constituents of the diet on absorption of nonheme iron. Egg yolk, bran, tannates (tea and coffee), antacids, and antibiotics (tetracyclines) inhibit nonheme iron absorption; meat, fish, and ascorbic acid enhance it.

In addition to the quantity and quality of the diet, iron absorption is affected by the gastrointestinal environment. Nonheme food iron is generally in the oxidized ferric $(3+)$ form. Ferric iron is insoluble at the alkaline pH characteristic of the upper small bowel where iron absorption takes place. Chelation of ferric iron by sugars, amino acids, and ascorbic acid in the acid environment of the stomach renders it soluble and absorbable in the small bowel.[15] Thus, achlorhydria or loss of the gastric reservoir as well as motility disorders or damage to the bowel wall will impair nonheme iron absorption.

Regulation of the amount of iron absorbed daily occurs at the level of the mucosal cell through mechanisms which are not well understood. The mucosa serves as a barrier to the absorption of excessive quantities of iron which would prove toxic but is also capable of enhancing iron absorption up to five-fold to offset increases in daily iron requirements. The most important factors that influence iron absorption are body iron stores and the rate of red cell production, whether effective as in polycythemia vera or ineffective as in sideroblastic anemia or thalassemia.[5] Hemochromatosis represents a unique situation characterized by increased iron absorption in the absence of any physiologic stimulus.

TABLE 6.3–1. IRON BALANCE

	Adult Male (hemoglobin 16 g/dl)	Adult Female (hemoglobin 14 g/dl)
Hemoglobin iron (mg)	2500	1900
Storage iron (mg)	1000	500
Iron intake (mg/day)	10–15	10–15
Iron absorbed (mg/day)	1.0	1–2.5
Iron loss (mg/day)	1.0	1–2.5[a] (1.0–1.5 from menstrual loss)

[a]This increase in menstruating females is corrected by increased efficiency of absorption; however, the menstruating female whose iron loss increases further will become iron deficient.

IRON TRANSPORT

Once absorbed, iron enters the circulation bound to transferrin, an α-globulin with a molecular weight of 80,000 produced by the liver. Since free iron is toxic and forms insoluble precipitates at the pH of extracellular fluids, transferrin has an essential role in iron transport. It contains two binding sites for iron which, while not biochemically equivalent, appear to function in the same fashion with respect to the delivery of iron to cells. Transferrin binds only ferric iron, and thus ferrous iron being released from cells must first undergo oxidation. This process is catalyzed by ceruloplasmin.[14] The ferroxidase activity of ceruloplasmin may explain in part the hypochromic anemia associated with severe copper deficiency.

Normally, the binding sites of transferrin are only one third saturated. Iron is released from the protein only at specific cell receptors, after which the transferrin is freed to repeat its cycle of iron uptake and delivery. The number of specific receptors for transferrin determines the extent of iron delivery to a particular tissue.[8] Because of the high density of transferrin receptors on immature erythroid precursors, they receive the bulk of transferrin iron. However, when transferrin saturation falls below 16 percent, iron delivery to developing red cells is impaired. Conversely, when transferrin saturation exceeds 80 percent, iron loading of other tissues, particularly the liver, occurs. The liver, however, appears to be a passive recipient of iron, since it releases iron to the plasma when the plasma iron level falls.

Tissue macrophages, in contrast to erythroid precursors or hepatocytes, are unable to acquire iron from transferrin. Macrophage iron is obtained from the catabolism of senescent red cells. Approximately 75 percent of this iron is returned to the plasma for transport to erythroid precursors by transferrin. Since the bulk of the daily red cell iron requirement is provided by macrophages, these cells can have a profound influence on erythropoiesis. In the presence of inflammation or infection, release of iron from macrophages is retarded, plasma iron and transferrin saturation decline, and red cell production is diminished. The major pathways involved in iron transport are illustrated in Figure 6.3–1.

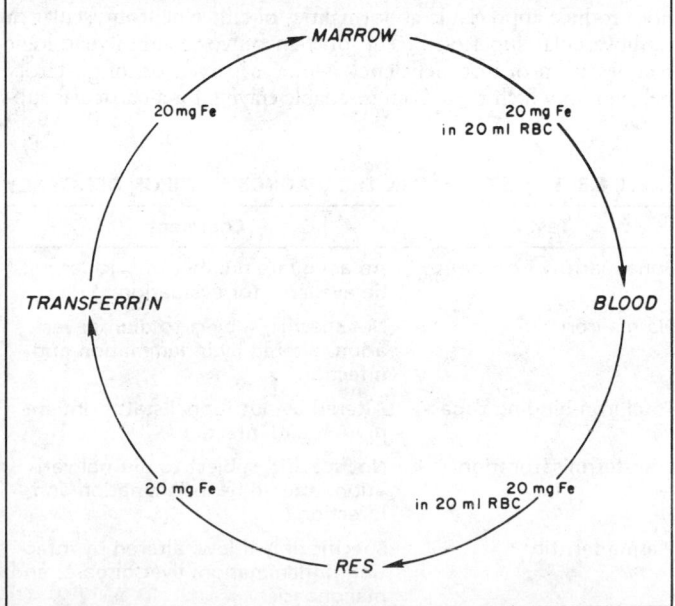

Figure 6.3–1. Schematic representation of daily exchange of iron in the adult. Daily losses and offsetting gastrointestinal iron absorption are not illustrated. RES = Reticuloendothelial system.

IRON STORAGE

Iron in excess of requirements for essential functions is stored either in ferritin or hemosiderin. Ferritin, a large and ubiquitous protein, the synthesis of which is stimulated by iron, can hold up to 4500 iron atoms.[1] Iron stored in the spherical ferritin molecule is readily mobilizable but also packaged in a manner that facilitates its excretion by the cell. In addition to its intracellular role in iron storage, ferritin also circulates in the plasma. Plasma ferritin, however, in contrast to the intracellular form, is virtually iron free and does not function as a transport protein.

Hemosiderin is an insoluble, paracrystalline aggregate of denatured ferritin molecules and other cell constituents most likely formed within lysosomes. The iron to protein ratio of hemosiderin is higher than that of ferritin, and when iron stores increase, it accumulates progressively within hemosiderin, not ferritin. Iron contained within hemosiderin is mobilized more slowly than soluble ferritin iron and represents the stable iron reserve which can be visualized by light microscopy using the Prussian blue stain.

IRON DEFICIENCY

When demands for iron for erythropoiesis exceed the capacity for iron absorption, a predictable sequence of events occurs which if iron stores are not replenished terminates in iron deficiency anemia (Fig. 6.3–2). The earliest sign of iron deficiency is depletion of marrow iron stores as determined by the Prussian blue stain. This is reflected by a decrease in plasma ferritin and subsequently an increase in plasma transferrin. When the amount of iron available for erythropoiesis falls below the minimal required level, plasma iron and transferrin saturation fall and there is an increase in free erythrocyte protoporphyrin. Initially, as anemia ensues erythropoiesis is normocytic, but microcytic red cells begin to appear in the circulation, producing an increase in the red cell distribution width (RDW; quantitative anisocytosis) which precedes a reduction in MCV. If iron deficiency persists, there is a further decline in red cell production and the red cells become progressively more microcytic and hypochromic. Iron deficient red cells are more rigid than normal red cells, and therefore severe iron deficiency anemia has a hemolytic component.

The causes of iron deficiency are many (Table 6.3–2) and not always evident. Women frequently underestimate the extent of menstrual blood loss, and occult gastrointestinal blood loss can be difficult to document. Even if gastrointestinal bleeding cannot be demonstrated, iron deficient men and postmenopausal women should have endoscopy or gastrointestinal radiographic contrast studies, or both, because occult blood loss can be the earliest sign of an intestinal carcinoma. Not infrequently, repeated examination of the stool for occult blood and sophisticated endoscopic and radiologic techniques are required to localize the site of gastrointestinal bleeding. If gastrointestinal evaluation is unrewarding, the urine should be examined as a possible site of iron loss.

DIFFERENTIAL DIAGNOSIS OF IRON DEFICIENCY

Microcytic, hypochromic erythropoiesis is not specific for iron deficiency. Other causes include thalassemia, sideroblastic anemia, the anemia associated with systemic disease, and copper deficiency. The tests useful in detecting iron deficiency along with the factors that can distort them are listed in Table 6.3–3. The most reliable test for demonstrating iron deficiency is a bone marrow iron stain provided an adequate aspirate is obtained and carefully scrutinized. A therapeutic trial of iron is, of course, the most conclusive evidence that iron lack is the cause of anemia, but such a trial must not be allowed to compromise a search for the cause of the iron deficiency. For routine purposes, the plasma ferritin is the best sin-

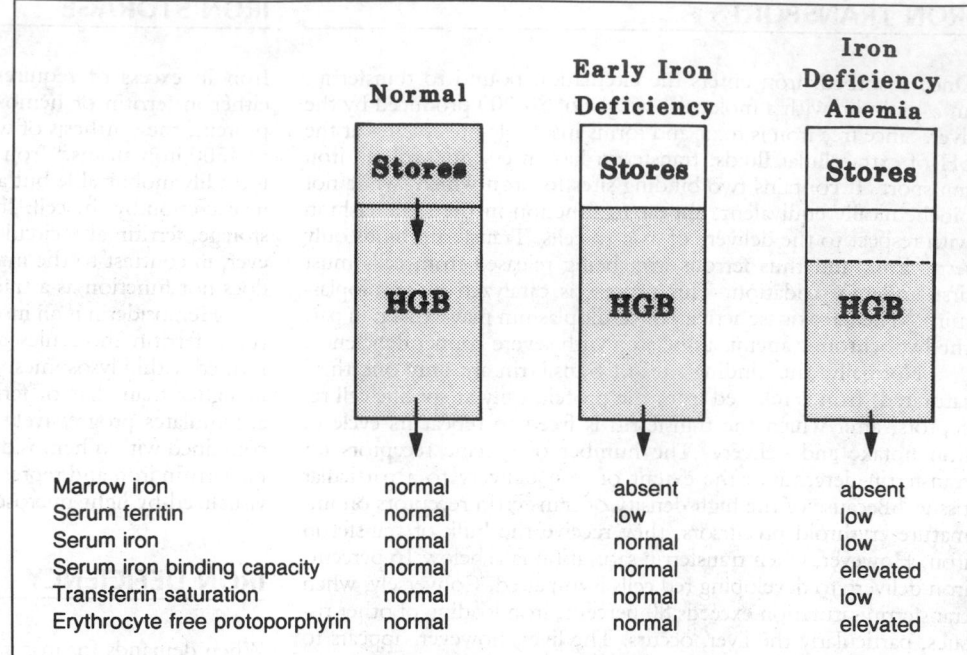

	Normal	Early Iron Deficiency	Iron Deficiency Anemia
Marrow iron	normal	absent	absent
Serum ferritin	normal	low	low
Serum iron	normal	normal	low
Serum iron binding capacity	normal	normal	elevated
Transferrin saturation	normal	normal	low
Erythrocyte free protoporphyrin	normal	normal	elevated

Figure 6.3–2. Sequence of changes associated in the development of iron deficiency.

gle screening test for iron deficiency since it more closely reflects body iron stores than the transferrin level.[11] A ferritin level less than 12 ng/ml is diagnostic of iron deficiency; in the presence of inflammation or infection, a ferritin level of 50 ng/ml or less suggests the presence of iron deficiency. The plasma iron level is not a sensitive test and even when low is not specific for iron deficiency. A transferrin saturation below 16 percent, while also not specific for iron deficiency, does indicate that the quantity of iron available for erythropoiesis is inadequate.[2] Thrombocytosis, for unknown reasons, may develop with iron deficiency and regress with iron therapy. Thrombocytosis is not, however, an invariable event and is also associated with other disorders (inflammation, infection) which themselves depress the plasma iron and transferrin saturation in the presence of adequate iron stores. A peripheral blood smear should, of course, always be examined. Basophilic stippling and red cell fragmentation suggest that microcytosis is due to thalassemia, while the presence of hypersegmented neutrophils with either normocytic or microcytic red cells suggests a combined deficiency state of iron and folic acid or vitamin B_{12}. The blood smear is also the only method for detecting the dimorphic red cell population of sideroblastic anemia and is an inexpensive method for evaluating the platelet count. Representative values for the laboratory studies described above in the various microcytic and hypochromic anemias are illustrated in Table 6.3–4.

TABLE 6.3–2. CAUSES OF IRON DEFICIENCY

Impaired Absorption
- Gastric surgery
- Achlorhydria
- Malabsorption syndromes
- Ingestion of clay or dirt

Increased Iron Loss
- Gastrointestinal hemorrhage
- Hookworm infestation
- Menstrual bleeding
- Pregnancy; lactation
- Phlebotomies
- Paroxysmal nocturnal hemoglobinuria
- Traumatic intravascular hemolysis
- Idiopathic pulmonary hemosiderosis

CLINICAL FEATURES OF IRON DEFICIENCY

In view of the essential role of iron in oxygen transport processes, it might be expected that iron deficiency would produce substantial systemic signs and symptoms. However, aside from the adverse effects associated with anemia and the underlying disease that produced the iron deficiency, few specific complaints can be attributed to iron lack in the adult. Abnormalities of epithelial surfaces such as glossitis, papillary atrophy, dysphagia, and spooning of the nails (koilonychia) are written about more frequently than they are observed. Certainly, the dysphagia-postcricoid esophageal web syndrome (Plummer–Vinson, Paterson–Kelly syndrome) is rarely seen now and may not have any relationship to iron lack. In contrast to experimental studies in animals, iron deficiency in humans does not produce appreciable abnormalities of either neuromuscular or cardiovascular function.[13] The one unequivocal nonhematologic manifestation of iron deficiency is pica, a perversion of gustatory behavior in which there is an insatiable craving for a particular sub-

TABLE 6.3–3. TESTS USED IN THE DIAGNOSIS OF IRON DEFICIENCY

Test	Comment
Bone marrow iron stain	An adequate number of spicules must be available for evaluation
Plasma iron	Not specific, subject to diurnal variation; altered by inflammation and infection
Total iron-binding capacity	Altered by nutritional status, inflammation and infection
Transferrin saturation	Not specific, subject to diurnal variation; altered by inflammation and infection
Plasma ferritin	Specific only if low; altered by infection, inflammation, liver disease, and malignancies
Erythrocyte-free protoporphyrin	Not specific; altered by lead poisoning, inflammation and infection
Red cell indices	Only the MCV is useful but is neither a specific or sensitive test

TABLE 6.3–4. REPRESENTATIVE LABORATORY ABNORMALITIES IN MICROCYTIC AND HYPOCHROMIC ANEMIAS

Test	Normal Range	Iron Deficiency	Anemia Associated with Systemic Disease	Thalassemia Trait	Sideroblastic Anemia
MCV (fl)	(80–99)	<80	<80	<80	80–>100
Plasma iron (μg/dl)	(65–175)	<30	<30	65–175	>200
Iron-binding capacity (μg/dl)	(300–360)	400	200	300–360	300–360
Transferrin saturation (%)	(25–50)	<16	<16	25–50	>80
Plasma ferritin (μg/l)	(20–250)	<12	20–1000	20–250	1000
Erythrocyte-free protoporphyrin (μg/dl)	(27–61)	180	180	27–61	180
Basophilic stippling	Absent	Absent	Absent	Usually present	Present
Marrow iron stores	Present	Absent	Present	Present	Increased

stance or food.[6] Compulsive ice ingestion (pagophagia) is a common form of pica, but the perversion may take more exotic forms. Patients rarely volunteer information about their dietary behavior, either because they are embarrassed by it or because they fail to recognize it as abnormal. In view of its diagnostic importance, evidence of pica should always be sought. As a corollary, dietary habits such as clay ingestion may lead to iron deficiency. Starch ingestion is not uncommonly associated with iron deficiency but starch itself does not inhibit iron absorption.

TREATMENT OF IRON DEFICIENCY ANEMIA

The treatment of iron deficiency anemia encompasses both the disorder causing the iron deficiency and correction of the iron deficit. When the source of iron loss cannot be identified, iron replacement sufficient to restore the circulating red cell mass without replenishing body iron stores permits early recognition of recurrent bleeding by a fall in the hematocrit. Based on the mechanism for absorption of nonheme iron, iron should be given in the ferrous form; chelators such as ascorbic acid are unnecessary and timed-release preparations should be avoided. In patients with a reduced gastric reservoir due to gastric resection, a liquid iron preparation (taken through a straw to avoid dental stains) should be employed. Otherwise 200 mg of elemental iron should be given each day on an empty stomach. Three tablets of ferrous sulfate provide the requisite quantity of elemental iron; with ferrous gluconate twice as many tablets are required because of its lower iron content. Inorganic iron can cause gastrointestinal disturbances and will discolor the stool. Increasing the dose gradually and administering iron with meals reduces discomfort. Antacids and antibiotics should not be taken simultaneously with iron. In the noncompliant patient, when large amounts of iron are required or when there is malabsorption or inflammatory bowel disease, iron can be given parenterally in the form of iron dextran. Regardless of the technique employed, intramuscular iron stains tissues. Intravenous administration of iron dextran should be reserved for situations in which there is insufficient muscle mass for intramuscular injections.[9] Iron dextran can cause fever, urticaria, arthralgias, lymphadenopathy, and anaphylaxis. Reactions, while unpredictable, are most common with large doses of iron dextran and in patients with inflammatory disorders such as rheumatoid arthritis or lupus erythematosus.

With iron therapy, a reticulocyte response is usually observed within 7 days. The rate of rise of the hemoglobin level varies with the degree of anemia. In general a 50 percent increment in the hemoglobin level occurs within a month and restoration of the hemoglobin level is not more rapid with parenteral iron than oral iron. Once the circulating red cell mass is restored to normal, several more months of therapy are required to replenish body iron

stores. The plasma ferritin level is a convenient guide for this, since it will remain low until iron stores are repleted.[16]

SIDEROBLASTIC ANEMIA

Iron not used in the synthesis of hemoglobin is sequestered in the red cell cytoplasm in ferritin. Normally aggregates for ferritin can be identified with the Prussian blue stain in 30 to 50 percent of developing red cells in the bone marrow. Nucleated cells containing Prussian blue stained granules are called sideroblasts; siderocytes are nonnucleated erythroid cells containing similar inclusions. The number of sideroblasts and siderocytes is markedly reduced with iron deficiency. Intracellular aggregates of iron increase red cell rigidity and are normally removed during passage through the spleen. Consequently, siderocytes are only present in the peripheral blood when the spleen is absent or nonfunctioning, when there is hemolysis with an increased delivery of reticulocytes containing siderotic granules to the circulation, or when there is a sideroblastic anemia.[3]

Under normal circumstances iron does not accumulate within mitochondria. In certain diseases, however, mitochondrial iron accumulation does occur (Table 6.3–4). Since red cell mitochondria are arranged in a perinuclear distribution, when loaded with iron they appear as a ring of granules around the nucleus with Prussian blue staining. This appearance has given rise to the term "ringed sideroblast." In addition to these cells, sideroblastic anemias are usually characterized by an increase in body iron stores, hyperferremia, increased transferrin saturation, and marrow erythroid hyperplasia, occasionally with megaloblastic features. Circulating red cells can be normocytic, macrocytic, or microcytic, and hypochromic. Hypochromia and microcytosis may be generalized or limited only to a portion of the red cell population, giving rise to a dimorphic pattern. Basophilic stippling may be prominent in the hypochromic cells and represents siderotic granules, not ribosomal RNA. Neutropenia, monocytosis, and alterations in the platelet count may be observed.

Chronic ethanol abuse is the commonest cause of sideroblastic anemia in a hospital setting. Ethanol-induced sideroblastic anemia is a reversible disorder and usually develops in a setting of folic acid deficiency and megaloblastic anemia.[7] Sideroblastic changes are also a feature of preleukemic disorders, and when such changes develop during alkylating agent therapy it may indicate the onset of leukemic transformation. In elderly patients, sideroblastic anemia often develops in the absence of any associated illness. This type of sideroblastic anemia has been designated idiopathic refractory sideroblastic anemia (IRSA).[10] Studies employing isoenzymes of G6PD suggest that IRSA is a clonal disorder of the pluripotent hematopoietic stem cell.[12] IRSA is usually refractory to pyrodoxine, which is beneficial in hereditary sideroblastic anemia, but less than

10 percent of patients with IRSA develop acute leukemia as part of their illness. Those who are predisposed to develop acute leukemia have severe anemia, a low reticulocyte count, a high transfusion requirement, and thrombocytopenia.[10] The development of hemoglobin H synthesis may also be a leukemic marker. For the most part the clinical course of idiopathic refractory sideroblastic anemia is dictated by the patient's transfusion requirement and the development of iron overload and myocardial failure.

REFERENCES

1. Aisen P, Listowsky I: Iron transport and storage proteins. Ann Rev Biochem 49:357, 1980
2. Bainton DF, Finch CA: The diagnosis of iron deficiency anemia. Am J Med 37:62, 1964
3. Cartwright GE, Deiss A: Sideroblasts, siderocytes and sideroblastic anemia. N Engl J Med 292:185, 1975
4. Cheng DS, Kirshner JP, Wintrobe MM: Idiopathic refractory sideroblastic anemia. Cancer 44:724, 1979
5. Conrad ME, Barton JC: Factors affecting iron balance. Am J Hematol 10:199, 1981
6. Crosby WH: Pica: a compulsion caused by iron deficiency. Br J Haematol 34:341, 1976
7. Eichner ER: The hematologic disorders of alcoholism. Am J Med 54:621, 1973
8. Finch CA, Huebers H: Perspectives in iron metabolism. N Engl J Med 306:1520, 1982
9. Hamstra RD, Block MH, Schocket AL: Intravenous iron dextran in clinical medicine. JAMA 243:1726, 1980
10. Kushner JP, Lee GR, et al: Idiopathic refractory sideroblastic anemia. Clinical and laboratory investigation of 17 patients and review of the literature. Medicine 50:139, 1971
11. Lipschitz DA, Cook JD, Finch CA: A clinical evaluation of serum ferritin as an index of iron stores. N Engl J Med 290:1213, 1974
12. Prchal JT, Throckmorton DW, et al: A common progenitor for human myeloid and lymphoid cells. Nature 274:590, 1978
13. Rector WG, Fortuin NJ, Conley CL: Non-hematologic effects of chronic iron deficiency. Medicine 61:382, 1982
14. Roeser HP, Lee GR, et al: The role of ceruloplasmin in iron metabolism. J Clin Invest 49:2408, 1970
15. Schade SG, Cohen RJ, Conrad ME: Effect of hydrochloric acid on iron absorption. N Engl J Med 279:672, 1968
16. Wheby MS: Effect of iron therapy on serum ferritin levels in iron-deficiency anemia. Blood 56:138, 1980

CHAPTER 6.4
Megaloblastic Anemia

Jerry L. Spivak

Megaloblastic anemia is produced by disorders that impair DNA synthesis (Table 6.4–1). Although the effects of many of these disorders are global, they are most marked in tissues with a high rate of cell turnover, particularly the blood. The characteristic morphologic, biochemical, and proliferative abnormalities associated with impaired DNA synthesis indicate the mechanism for anemia but not its etiology. Most often, megaloblastic anemia is due to a deficiency of either vitamin B_{12} or folic acid. Mammalian cells require both vitamins for DNA synthesis but lack the capacity to manufacture either. Therefore, when confronted with a patient with a megaloblastic anemia, it is the physician's obligation to determine if a vitamin deficiency state exists and, if so, its cause. Once these correctable forms of megaloblastic anemia are excluded, other etiologies can be considered.

FOLIC ACID

Folic acid (pteroylglutamic acid) is a water-soluble, heat-labile vitamin found in green leafy vegetables, liver, kidney, yeast, and certain fruits. It exists in food conjugated with varying numbers of glutamic acid residues. These are removed during absorption by mucosal γ-glutamyl peptidase. Absorption of folic acid takes place in the proximal third of the small intestine. The minimum daily folate requirement is 50 μg, and total body stores of folic acid are approximately 7 mg[11], a small quantity with respect to its turnover rate. Folic acid functions as a coenzyme in certain reactions involving a one carbon transfer. Reactions include the interconversion of serine and glycine, the conversion of deoxyuridylate to thymidylate, methionine synthesis, histidine catabolism, and the de novo synthesis of purines. For these reactions folic acid must first be reduced to tetrahydrofolic acid, a reaction catalyzed by the intracellular enzyme dehydrofolate reductase. Once reduced, the molecule can accept the methyl, formyl, and methylene groups involved in its various reactions. Folic acid circulates in the serum as N^5-methyl tetrahydrofolic acid. A serum protein binder exists but appears to have no important role in folate transport. Intracellular folate is converted to the polyglutamate form, a process that requires vitamin B_{12}. Under normal circumstances, body stores of folic acid provide a 4 to 5 month supply of the vitamin if intake is interrupted.[11] Folic acid deficiency can, however, occur more acutely in

TABLE 6.4–1. CAUSES OF MEGALOBLASTIC HEMATOPOIESIS

- Folic acid deficiency
- Vitamin B_{12} deficiency
- Acute leukemia and myelodysplastic syndromes
- Nitrous oxide inhalation
- Arsenic poisoning
- Chemotherapy

TABLE 6.4–2. CAUSES OF FOLIC ACID DEFICIENCY

Inadequate Intake

Defective Absorption
- Intrinsic bowel disease
- Blind loop syndrome

Impaired Utilization
- Ethanol
- Vitamin B_{12} deficiency
- Folic acid antagonists (dihydrofolate reductase inhibitors)

Increased Requirements
- Pregnancy
- Hemolytic anemia
- Myeloproliferative disorders
- Exfoliative dermatitis
- Hyperthyroidism
- Chronic hemodialysis

the setting of chronic alcoholism or increased demands for the vitamin.[7] The causes of folic acid deficiency are listed in Table 6.4–2.

VITAMIN B$_{12}$

Vitamin B$_{12}$ is a complex molecule consisting of a corrin ring containing a cobalt atom, both of which are linked to a single ribonucleotide moiety. This basic unit is known as a cobalamin. The function activity of cobalamins is determined by the nature of the ligand attached to the cobalt atom within the corrin ring. In humans, the principal forms of vitamin B$_{12}$ are deoxyadenosylcobalamin, which predominates in the tissues, and methylcobalamin, which predominates in the plasma.[13] Other cobalamins are present in the body but have no known biologic role.

Vitamin B$_{12}$ is a product of microbial metabolism and occurs in the diet only in foods of animal origin. Liver, kidney, eggs, and milk are rich sources of the vitamin. Absorption of vitamin B$_{12}$ requires the participation of intrinsic factor, a glycoprotein produced by gastric parietal cells. Vitamin B$_{12}$ extracted from food binds in the acid environment of the stomach to B$_{12}$ binders known as "R" proteins because of their rapid mobility during electrophoresis. The R protein-vitamin B$_{12}$ complex is degraded in the alkaline environment of the upper small intestine by pancreatic proteases and the free vitamin B$_{12}$ is bound by intrinsic factor.[12] The intrinsic factor-B$_{12}$ complex attaches to specific receptors in the ileum where, in the presence of calcium and a pH greater than 6.0, the complex is internalized. Once absorbed and released from intrinsic factor, vitamin B$_{12}$ binds to its carrier protein transcobalamin II, on which it is totally dependent for transport and delivery to cells. Unlike transferrin, transcobalamin II, after delivering vitamin B$_{12}$ to an intracellular location, is degraded by lysosomes and not recycled.[10] Other vitamin B$_{12}$ binding proteins, differing chemically from transcobalamin II and belonging to the R group of proteins, are present in the plasma.[9] These proteins, transcobalamin I and III, bind the bulk of plasma vitamin B$_{12}$ but have no known biologic function. Even in the presence of tissue vitamin B$_{12}$ deficiency, these binders do not release the vitamin. The concentration of the various vitamin B$_{12}$ binding proteins varies in certain disease states and may be of diagnostic significance (Table 6.4–3).

The minimal daily requirement for vitamin B$_{12}$ is 1 μg. Body stores are large with respect to its turnover rate, and the vitamin is efficiently conserved during its enterohepatic recirculation. Thus, in contrast to folic acid deficiency, deficiency of vitamin B$_{12}$ in the adult takes years to develop once absorption is interrupted. The disorders causing vitamin B$_{12}$ deficiency are listed in Table 6.4–4. As the table indicates, vitamin B$_{12}$ deficiency is essentially a consequence of malabsorption. While adults who ingest irrational diets that exclude all animal products develop low serum vitamin B$_{12}$ levels, most evidence suggests that even these individuals do not develop vitamin B$_{12}$ deficiency unless they acquire an absorptive defect.[2]

TABLE 6.4–3. DISEASE-INDUCED ALTERATIONS OF VITAMN B$_{12}$ BINDING PROTEINS

Disease	Elevated Binder
Chronic myelogenous leukemia	TC I
Leukemoid reaction	TC I
Polycythemia vera	TC III
Gaucher disease	TC II
Acute hepatitis	TC I

TC = Transcobalamin.

TABLE 6.4–4. CAUSES OF VITAMIN B$_{12}$ DEFICIENCY

Inadequate Intake

Impaired Absorption
- Gastric abnormalities
  Pernicious anemia
  Total gastrectomy
  Lye ingestion
  Congenital absence of intrinsic factor
  Biologically inert intrinsic factor
- Intestinal abnormalities
  Ileal resection or irradiation
  Granulomatous bowel disease
  Diverticulosis
  Congenital defect (Imerslund syndrome)
  Blind loop syndrome
  Fish tapeworm
  Drugs (PAS)
- Pancreatic insufficiency
- Congenital absence of transcobalamin II

INTERRELATIONSHIP OF VITAMIN B$_{12}$ AND FOLIC ACID

Vitamin B$_{12}$ is known to participate in only two metabolic processes in mammalian cells.[6] Deoxyadenosyl cobalamin serves as a coenzyme for the conversion of methylmalonyl coenzyme A to succinyl coenzyme A, which accounts for the methylmalonic aciduria associated with vitamin B$_{12}$ deficiency. The other and more important process clinically is the conversion of homocysteine to methionine, for which methylcobalamin serves as the coenzyme. It is this reaction that links vitamin B$_{12}$ and folic acid because the reaction is catalyzed by the enzyme 5-methyltetrahydrofolate-homocysteine transmethylase (Fig. 6.4–1). During this reaction, 5-methyltetrahydrofolate is converted to tetrahydrofolate. Tetrahydrofolate is the immediate precursor of N^5-N^{10} methylene tetrahydrofolate, which is required for the conversion of deoxyuridylate to thymidylate. Since thymidylate is required for DNA synthesis, deficiency of either vitamin B$_{12}$ or folic acid impairs DNA synthesis and leads to megaloblastic anemia. Essentially, vitamin B$_{12}$ deficiency creates a "folate deficient" state within the cell while N^5-methyltetrahydrofolate accumulates in the blood. This accounts for the identical morphologic manifestations of vitamin B$_{12}$ and folic acid deficiency as well as the ability of large doses of folic acid to correct the megaloblastic abnormalities due to vitamin B$_{12}$ deficiency. On the other hand, as would be expected, vitamin B$_{12}$ cannot correct a folate deficient state. In spite of the ability of folic acid to initially correct the anemia of vitamin B$_{12}$ deficiency, macrocytosis persists, and eventually marrow hypoplasia ensues.

SUBACUTE COMBINED DEGENERATION

An important difference between megaloblastic anemia caused by folic acid deficiency and that due to vitamin B$_{12}$ deficiency concerns the neurologic abnormality known as subacute combined degeneration, which is associated only with vitamin B$_{12}$ deficiency and is uncorrectable with folic acid.[17] Subacute combined degeneration is a process of myelin degeneration that involves the white matter of the dorsal and lateral columns of the spinal cord, and the peripheral nerves. Its earliest manifestations are paresthesias in a stocking-glove distribution, and loss of fine touch and vibratory sensation. As the disorder progresses clumsiness, ataxia, weakness, and spasticity ensue. The degree of recovery depends on the duration and severity of the neurologic abnormalities. By masking the anemia associated with vitamin B$_{12}$ deficiency, folic acid therapy permits

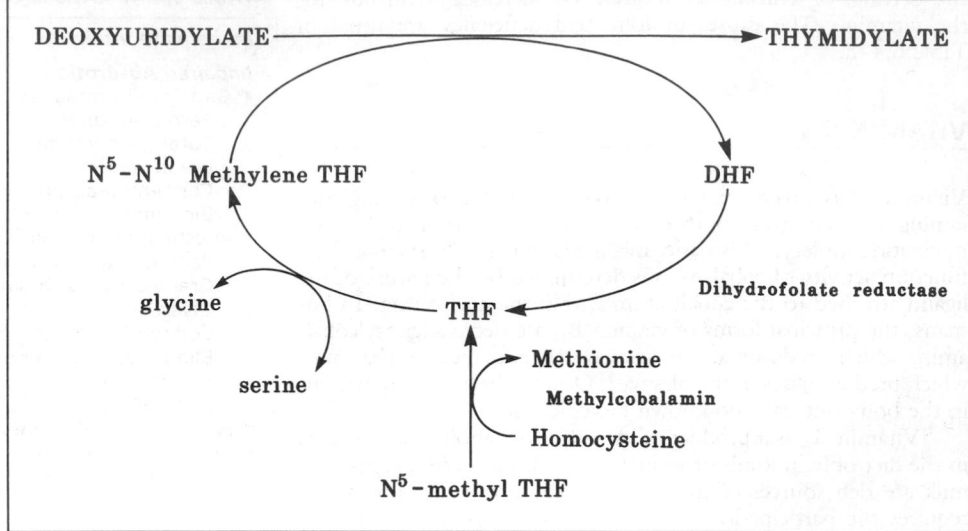

Figure 6.4–1. Metabolic interrelationship of vitamin B$_{12}$ and folic acid.

the neurologic abnormalities to progress because their cause remains unrecognized.

The biochemical basis for the neurologic abnormalities due to vitamin B$_{12}$ deficiency are not completely understood. Formerly, impairment of proprionate metabolism due to failure of isomerization of methylmalonyl coenzyme A to succinyl coenzyme A was thought to be involved. It has recently been suggested, however, that neurologic disease in patients with vitamin B$_{12}$ deficiency may be the consequence of a relative deficiency of methionine. According to this theory, when conversion of homocysteine to methionine is impaired, because of lack of vitamin B$_{12}$, intracellular folate levels fall and cells respond by diverting their available folate stores away from DNA synthesis to methionine synthesis.[15] A reduction in DNA synthesis also reduces the need for methionine further protecting the cell. When additional folate is provided in these circumstances, DNA synthesis is enhanced out of proportion to methionine synthesis, protein synthesis and protein methylation are compromised due to lack of the essential amino acid, and damage to myelin occurs.

PERNICIOUS ANEMIA

The classical and most common cause of vitamin B$_{12}$ deficiency is pernicious anemia, a hereditary disorder of gastric function with autoimmune features in which there is malabsorption of the vitamin. The fundamental lesion in pernicious anemia is gastric atrophy with achlorhydria and failure to secrete intrinsic factor. The major manifestations of the disease, therefore, are due to vitamin B$_{12}$ deficiency. Because pernicious anemia is also an autoimmune disorder these patients may develop other abnormalities such as

Hashimoto thyroiditis, hyperthyroidism, or vitiligo.[8] Pernicious anemia is also associated with Addison disease and hypoparathyroidism. Patients with adult-onset immunoglobulin deficiency or selective IgA deficiency also develop the disorder. Antibodies to parietal cells are found in approximately 80 percent of patients, while intrinsic factor antibodies are found in 50 percent. Both types of antibodies are present in gastric juice as well as the serum. Thyroid antibodies, lymphocytotoxins, and rheumatoid factor are also observed with an increased frequency. Racial differences exist with respect to both the age of onset and the incidence of antibodies. In black females, the disease occurs at an earlier age and with a higher frequency of intrinsic factor antibodies.[4] Patients with pernicious anemia have a higher incidence of gastric polyps and carcinoma than the general population. Because of this and because of its insidious onset as well as the risk of irreversible neurologic damage and the high incidence of associated endocrinologic disorders, pernicious anemia is a disorder of substantial importance to the physician. Fortunately, modern diagnostic techniques can facilitate its recognition if properly employed.

LABORATORY EVALUATION OF MEGALOBLASTIC ANEMIA

Macrocytosis is a hallmark of megaloblastic anemia due to vitamin B$_{12}$ or folic acid and may be the earliest clue to the disorder preceding anemia and other manifestations of the vitamin deficiency state by up to a year.[3] Unfortunately, it is a clue that is frequently ignored. Furthermore, macrocytosis is also a consequence of a variety of disorders in which there is no deficiency of vitamin B$_{12}$ or

TABLE 6.4–5. CAUSES OF MACROCYTOSIS

- Folic acid deficiency
- Vitamin B$_{12}$ deficiency
- Liver disease
- Alcoholism
- Sideroblastic anemia
- Aplastic or hypoplastic anemia
- Hypothyroidism
- Neoplasms
- Hemolytic anemia
- Drugs (azathioprine, methotrexate)

TABLE 6.4–6. FEATURES OF MEGALOBLASTIC HEMATOPOIESIS

Peripheral Blood
- Macrocytosis (oval macrocytes)
- Anisocytosis and poikilocytosis
- Howell–Jolly bodies
- Neutrophil hypersegmentation

Bone Marrow
- Hypercellularity
- Erythroid hyperplasia
- Megaloblastic erythropoiesis
- Neutrophil hypersegmentation
- Giant metamyelocytes

TABLE 6.4–7. FACTORS INFLUENCING THE SERUM FOLATE LEVEL

Falsely Low
- Recent low dietary intake
- Contamination of serum with radioisotopes (gallium 67, technetium 99m)

Falsely Normal or High
- Recent increase in dietary intake
- Hemolysis of sample
- Coexisting B_{12} deficiency

TABLE 6.4–9. FACTORS INFLUENCING SERUM VITAMIN B_{12} LEVEL

Falsely Low
- Folic acid deficiency (30–50%)
- Pregnancy (20%)
- Vegetarian diet
- Transcobalamin I deficiency
- Contamination of serum with radioisotopes (technetium 99m or gallium 67)

Falsely Normal or High
- Recent parenteral administration of vitamin B_{12}
- Radioassay artifact
- Chronic myelogenous leukemia, polycythemia vera
- Transcobalamin II deficiency
- Nitrous oxide inhalation

folic acid (Table 6.4–5). The degree of macrocytosis cannot be used to discriminate among these disorders, as can other features associated with megaloblastic hematopoiesis (Table 6.4–6). Careful scrutiny of a peripheral blood smear is of particular importance for several reasons. First, the macrocytes of folic acid or vitamin B_{12} deficiency differ from the macrocytes of other disorders because of their oval shape and lack of central pallor. Second, in megaloblastic anemia, there is striking red cell anisocytosis and poikilocytosis with microcytes, fragmented forms, and tear-drop cells, features not seen in other macrocytic disorders. Third, the peripheral blood smear is the only method for identifying the Howell–Jolly body, a DNA remnant found in red cells in megaloblastic anemia or when there is hypofunction or absence of the spleen. Fourth, the peripheral blood smear is the only method for identifying neutrophil hypersegmentation, an abnormality that is pathognomonic for megaloblastic maturation. Only severe neutropenia or a marked left shift of the granulocytes will mask hypersegmentation, which usually reappears once these abnormalities have been corrected. Neutrophil hypersegmentation persists for several weeks after therapy with folic acid or vitamin B_{12} has been initiated and is a valuable clue to the nature of the underlying anemia when therapy has been initiated blindly.[14] Hypersegmentation may also be the only clue to the presence of vitamin B_{12} or folic acid deficiency in the presence of iron deficiency, thalassemia trait, or renal disease.

Examination of a bone marrow aspirate serves to establish the presence of megaloblastic hematopoiesis in the patient with macrocytosis but is not diagnostic for a vitamin deficiency state since other disorders can produce megaloblastic maturation (Table 6.4–1). Most important, when iron deficiency is present, megaloblastic maturation can be masked, and the marrow aspirate may appear leukemic.[16] Therefore, a number of tests have been developed to establish whether a deficiency of either folic acid or vitamin B_{12} is present. None of these is totally sensitive or specific; all are subject to technical artifact and must be interpreted with caution.[1]

For the reasons listed in Table 6.4–7, the serum folate level is the least useful of all the tests and has no role in the diagnosis of megaloblastic anemia. As illustrated in Tables 6.4–8 and 6.4–9, the assays for red cell folate and serum vitamin B_{12} are not without their problems, including a consistent but undefined element of technical inaccuracy.[5] Furthermore, a deficiency of one vitamin often influences the level of the other. In view of these problems, an isolated assay for either red cell folate or serum vitamin B_{12} is not useful when a deficiency of either vitamin is suspected. Measurements for both must be obtained. A low red cell folate level in the presence of a normal serum vitamin B_{12} level indicates tissue folate deficiency; a normal red cell folate level in the presence of a low serum vitamin B_{12} level suggests vitamin B_{12} deficiency. When the levels of both are low, a Schilling test will be necessary to determine the nature of the vitamin deficiency state (Table 6.4–10).

Because vitamin B_{12} deficiency is almost always due to malabsorption, a Schilling test is not only useful for identifying megaloblastic anemia due to vitamin B_{12} deficiency but also for determining the mechanism for the malabsorption. Since megaloblastic anemia due to vitamin B_{12} deficiency responds to therapy with folic acid, the Schilling test is of particular value in patients who have been treated in a blind or "shotgun" fashion. It is important to remember that treatment with vitamin B_{12} will not correct malabsorption of the vitamin or impair performance of the Schilling test as long as vitamin B_{12} therapy is withheld during the period in which the test is performed. The type of information that can be obtained from the Schilling test is illustrated in Table 6.4–11. As shown in Table 6.4–12, performance of the Schilling test, like the other tests for vitamin B_{12} or folic acid deficiency, is not without its pitfalls.

TREATMENT OF VITAMIN B_{12} OR FOLIC ACID DEFICIENCY

The management of patients with vitamin B_{12} or folic acid deficiency consists of replenishing body stores of the vitamin and correcting the cause of the vitamin deficiency. In view of the insidious onset of vitamin B_{12} deficiency, profound levels of anemia are well-tolerated even by individuals of the advanced age at which pernicious anemia is usually manifest. Much of the symptomatology of vitamin B_{12} deficiency such as anorexia, irritability, confusion, glossitis, fever, or orthostatic hypotension is alleviated rapidly with vitamin replacement. In patients accustomed to anemia, transfusions may precipitate pulmonary edema and should be limited to cases of coronary artery insufficiency, gastrointestinal blood loss, fever, or infection. For correction of vitamin B_{12} deficiency, hydroxycobalamin (a precursor of the active forms of mammalian cobalamins) should be administered intramuscularly (or intrave-

TABLE 6.4–8. FACTORS INFLUENCING RED CELL FOLATE LEVEL

Falsely Low
- Vitamin B_{12} deficiency

Falsely Normal or High
- Early folate deficiency
- Blood transfusion
- Reticulocytosis

TABLE 6.4–10. THE SCHILLING TEST

- Oral administration of tracer dose of radioactive vitamin B_{12}[a]
- Saturation of binding sites by parenteral injection of 1 mg unlabeled vitamin B_{12}
- Collection of urine for 24 hours on 2 successive days for radioactivity measurements
- Normally, greater than 9% of administered dose is excreted in first 24 hr

[a]The simultaneous administration of two different isotopes of vitamin B_{12}, one of which is combined with intrinsic factor is not recommended because of the risk of an inaccurate and misleading result.

TABLE 6.4–11. CLINICAL USEFULNESS OF SCHILLING TEST

Cause of Vitamin B₁₂ Deficiency	Intestinal Vitamin B₁₂ Absorption		
	Without Intrinsic Factor	With Intrinsic Factor	After Antibiotic Therapy
Dietary deficiency	Normal	Normal	—
Lack of intrinsic factor	Low	Normal	—
Ileal disorder	Low	Low	Low
Bacterial over-growth	Low	Low	Normal

nously if there is thrombocytopenia) at a dose of 100 μg per day for 7 days. Thereafter 100 μg of the vitamin can be given weekly for 5 weeks to replenish body stores. As with other forms of anemia, the rate of response varies with the initial hematocrit; full recovery usually occurs within 2 months in the absence of complications such as iron deficiency or infection. Neurologic manifestations may take 6 months or longer to resolve if they are reversible. Patients who malabsorb vitamin B₁₂ are dependent on a parenteral source of the vitamin and must receive maintenance therapy at a dose of 100 μg per month for life.

Folic acid as a monoglutamate is well absorbed and most folate deficient patients will respond to 1 mg of the vitamin admin-

TABLE 6.4–12. FACTORS INFLUENCING SCHILLING TEST RESULTS

Falsely Normal
• Contamination of urine with other radioisotopes (technetium 99m or gallium 67)
• Treatment with corticosteroids

Falsely Low
• Incomplete urine collection
• Renal failure
• Inappropriate injection of vitamin B₁₂
• Drug ingestion (PAS, colchicine, neomycin, phenformin, anticonvulsants, KCl, ethanol)
• Folic acid deficiency
• Defective intrinsic factor preparation
• Gastric antibodies to intrinsic factor

istered daily. Replenishment of body stores may take several weeks. The duration of therapy will depend on the nature of the problem causing the deficiency. In certain situations where the patient is initially ill and the cause of the underlying vitamin deficiency is unclear, both folic acid and vitamin B₁₂ should be administered after the appropriate tests have been obtained. Combination therapy will not be harmful and valuable time will be saved by instituting therapy. Subsequently, depending on the results of initial studies, definitive tests can be performed to determine the nature of the vitamin deficiency.

REFERENCES

1. Carmel R: The laboratory diagnosis of megaloblastic anemias. West J Med 128:294, 1978
2. Carmel R: Nutritional vitamin B₁₂ deficiency. Ann Intern Med 88:647, 1978
3. Carmel R: Macrocytosis, mild anemia and delay in the diagnosis of pernicious anemia. Arch Intern Med 139:47, 1979
4. Carmel R, Johnson CS: Racial patterns in pernicious anemia. N Engl J Med 298:647, 1978
5. Cohen KL, Donaldson RM Jr: Unreliability of radiodilution assays as screening tests for cobalamin (vitamin B₁₂) deficiency. JAMA 244:1942, 1980
6. Das KC, Herbert V: Vitamin B₁₂-folate interrelations. Clin Haematol 5:697, 1976
7. Eichner ER, Pierce HI, Hillman RS: Folate balance in dietary-induced megaloblastic anemia. N Engl J Med 284:933, 1971
8. Goldberg LS, Fudenberg HH: The autoimmune aspects of pernicious anemia. Am J Med 46:489, 1969
9. Hall CA: Transcobalamins I and II as natural transport proteins of vitamin B₁₂. J Clin Invest 56:1125, 1975
10. Hall CA: The transport of vitamin B₁₂ from food to use within the cells. J Lab Clin Med 984:811, 1979
11. Herbert V: Experimental nutritional folate deficiency in man. Trans Assoc Am Physicians 75:307, 1962
12. Marcoulles G, Parmentier Y, et al: Cobalamin malabsorption due to nondegradation of R proteins in the human intestine. J Clin Invest 66:430, 1980
13. Matthews DM, Finnell JC: Vitamin B₁₂: An area of darkness. Br Med J 2:533, 1979
14. Nath BJ, Lindenbaum J: Persistence of neutrophil hypersegmentation during recovery from megaloblastic granulopoiesis. Ann Intern Med 90:757, 1979
15. Scott JM, Weir DG: The methyl folate trap. Lancet 2:337, 1981
16. Spivak JL: Masked megaloblastic anemia. Arch Intern Med 142:2111, 1982
17. Victor M, Lear AA: Subacute combined degeneration of the spinal cord. Am J Med 20:896, 1956

CHAPTER 6.5

The Hemoglobinopathies: Inherited Disorders of Hemoglobin Synthesis

Samuel Charache

MOLECULAR BIOLOGY

Human hemoglobin is composed of two pairs of polypeptide chains; in normal adults, alpha chains combine with beta, delta, or gamma chains to form hemoglobin A ($\alpha_2\beta_2$), A₂ ($\alpha_2\delta_2$), or F (fetal hemoglobin, $\alpha_2\gamma_2$). Structure and function of the hemoglobin A tetramer are known in exquisite detail[3]; among proteins it is remarkable for its stability, its ability to bind and release oxygen at physiologic oxygen pressures, and the modulation of its oxygen

affinity by allosteric effectors such as 2,3-diphosphoglycerate (2,3-DPG), H^+ ion, and CO_2. The gamma chains of fetal hemoglobin lack a binding site for 2,3-DPG, and as a result, fetal red cells have higher oxygen affinity than adult cells, an advantage in transporting oxygen across the placenta. The pair of genes that govern alpha-chain synthesis are on chromosome 16; those that govern beta-, delta-, and gamma-chain synthesis are clustered together on chromosome 11. Abnormalities of these genes can be produced by point mutations (i.e., substitution of one base for another) or by

unequal crossing over of DNA from one member of a pair to another (typically producing a deletion, or rarely an insertion, of genetic material). Either type of abnormality can affect hemoglobin structure, function, or synthesis.[1] A few examples are listed in Table 6.5–1, but many others have been described in recent years. Particularly in the thalassemia syndromes, differing mutations can have identical phenotypic expression.

In general, inherited disorders of hemoglobin synthesis are rare conditions, but a few occur in high frequency in certain population groups. These genetic polymorphisms (Table 6.5–2) are thought to exist because they convey an advantage to heterozygotes; evidence that such is actually the case is most plausible for hemoglobin S, which appears to protect heterozygous children from death due to falciparum malaria. β-Thalassemia syndromes may convey a similar advantage. Homozygotes for both the β^s or thalassemia genes are at a severe disadvantage, and initially did not survive to adult life in areas of endemic malaria.

In the United States today, the most common hemoglobinopathies are those associated with the sickle cell gene, and the most serious are the β-thalassemia syndromes. Only those two groups of disorders will be discussed here. There are only about 60,000 patients with sickle cell disease and less than 1000 with clinically significant thalassemia syndromes in this country. The intense interest that has been manifested in these disorders stems not only from the much larger numbers of patients in other countries, but because they are the most clearly understood of all "molecular" diseases.

SICKLE CELL DISEASE

Included under the designation of sickle cell disease are all the conditions that cause clinically significant illness due to sickling of red cells (Table 6.5–3). In the United States, it usually is taken to include sickle cell anemia, hemoglobin SC disease, and sickle/β-thalassemia. The pathogenesis is the same in the three disorders. However, the incidence and severity of most complications is greater in sickle cell anemia, because the red cells there contain a higher concentration of hemoglobin S. Patients with SC disease and sickle/β-thalassemia may have a normal lifespan and may be diagnosed as late as age 60 or 70. The same occasionally happens for patients with sickle cell anemia, but not very often.

PATHOGENESIS

Molecules of deoxygenated hemoglobin S align themselves into linear polymers; as the polymer fraction within the red cell rises, it loses deformability and eventually is deformed into a crescentic or holly-leaf shape. At the same time, or perhaps after multiple cycles of sickling and unsickling, the cell membrane is damaged, permitting loss of water and potassium ions. This causes intracellular hemoglobin S concentration to rise and thereby increases the likelihood that the cell will sickle at a given PO_2. Hemoglobin S may also denature into hemichromes, insoluble precipitates that adhere to the inner surface of the cell membrane and exaggerate its physical and functional abnormalities. Some abnormal hemoglobins seem to be able to "replace" molecules of hemoglobin S in the polymers, while others cannot; the severity of clinical illness in such compound heterozygotes depends on the likelihood that such replacement can occur, as well as on the intraerythrocytic concentration of hemoglobin S.[5] Sickle cell trait produces virtually no clinical manifestations because hemoglobin in AS cells does not polymerize at the PO_2 found in most organs of persons living at low altitudes. The renal medulla, probably because of its high osmolarity, is an exception to this rule: loss of water from red cells can raise the intracellular hemoglobin S concentration enough so that even AS red cells sickle. As a result, microinfarctions, hematuria, and even renal papillary necrosis can be seen in sickle cell trait.

TABLE 6.5–1. EXAMPLES OF MUTATIONS LEADING TO HEMOGLOBINOPATHIES

Type of Mutation	Disorder	Structural Alteration	Function	Synthesis
Point mutation				
Codon β6 GAG → GTG	Sickle cell anemia	β6 Glu → Val	Polymerizes when deoxygenated	Impaired dimer association
Codon β145 TAT → TAC	Hb Osler (polycythemia)	β145 Tyr → Asp	Increased oxygen affinity	Normal
Codon 42 TTT → TCT	Hb Hammersmith	β42 Phe → Ser	Unstable	Normal
Nucleotide −28 A → C[a]	β^+-Thalassemia	Normal	Normal	Transcription defect due to change in "TATA box" → decreased β-chain synthesis
Nucleotide 1 in β IVS-1 G → A[b]	β°-Thalassemia	—	—	Splicing defect in IVS-1 → no β-chain synthesis
α Terminator codon TAA → TAG	Hb Constant Spring	α chain elongated by 31 amino acids	?	Decreased α-chain synthesis
Unequal crossover				
Insert three codons between α118 and α119	Hb Grady	O → Glu-Phe-Thr	Increased oxygen affinity	Normal in vivo
Exchange between β and δ gene	Hb Lepore	N terminus δ chain C terminus β chain	Normal	Decreased β-chain synthesis
Delete five codons between β91 and β95	Hb Gun Hill (hemolytic anemia)	Lue-His-Cys-Asp-Lys → O	Unstable	Normal
Delete β-, δ-chain genes	Hereditary persistence of fetal hemoglobin (African type)	—	—	No β or δ chain synthesis. Increased γ chain synthesis
Delete α-chain gene	α Thalassemia	—	—	Decreased α chain synthesis

[a]Nucleotide 28 bases before the "methyl cap site" of the β globin gene.
[b]First nucleotide in the first intervening sequence of the β globin gene.

TABLE 6.5–2. GENETIC POLYMORPHISMS

Hemoglobinopathy	Ethnic Group	Homozygous Condition
Hb S	West Africa	Sickle cell anemia
Hb C	West Africa	Hb C disease
Hb E	Southeast Asia	Hb E disease
β-Thalassemia	Greece, Italy, Asia	Thalassemia major (see text)
α-Thalassemia	Asia, Greece, Italy	Hb H disease (see text)

Decreased deformability of sickle cells leads to occlusion of small blood vessels, with ischemia and infarction (the painful crises of sickle cell disease). Membrane damage leads to hemolytic anemia, with the usual consequences of that process. Anemia is severe in sickle cell anemia (hemoglobin concentration 5 to 8 g/dl) and limits the exercise capacity of patients. It is recurrent vasoocclusive episodes that produce major disability and bring patients to the physician, however.

DIAGNOSIS

Hemolysates prepared from blood of patients with sickle cell anemia contain only hemoglobins S, F, and A_2 after electrophoresis on cellulose acetate (pH 8.6) or agar (pH 6.0), but not all patients with that phenotype have sickle cell anemia (Table 6.5–4). In sickle cell anemia the solubility test or sickle cell preparation is positive; the MCV is normal or somewhat increased, and sickled forms, polychromasia, and nucleated red cells are seen on blood smears. In adults the smear shows evidence of loss of splenic function.

CLINICAL MANIFESTATIONS AND THEIR MANAGEMENT

Painful Crises

Pain starts suddenly, often in bones or joints, but at times in the abdomen or chest. Patients say that attacks are more common in rainy or cold weather, and sometimes occur after physical exertion or emotional stress. Those relationships, however, are imprecise. Infection, pregnancy, and trauma may precipitate problems, and crises themselves seem to make subsequent crises more likely. Efforts to connect some acute phase reactant in blood to the onset of crises have been unsuccessful, but altered properties of vascular endothelium could conceivably be involved in such events.

Sites of pain are often tender, and there may be local or sys-

TABLE 6.5–3. SICKLING DISORDERS

Sickle Cell Disease	% Hb S in Red Cells	Clinical Severity
Sickle cell anemia	90–97	Severe
S/D Punjab	50	Severe
S/O Arab	50	Severe
S/β-Thalassemia	70	Mild/moderate
S/C	50	Mild/moderate
Other Sickling Disorders		
S/HPFH[a]	70	No disease
Sickle cell trait	35	No disease

[a]African variety of hereditary persistence of fetal hemoglobin.

temic signs of inflammation (swelling, heat, fever), but none of these need be present. Similarly, increased leukocytosis may be seen—but there is no invariable clinical or laboratory concomitant of a painful crisis. Since much more treatable conditions—particularly infections—can present in exactly the same fashion, "vasoocclusive crisis" is a diagnosis of exclusion. A patient with sickle cell anemia who complains of bone pain may have bone marrow infarction or osteomyelitis. The physician must use all his skills and laboratory aids; at times no specific information is forthcoming. In the final analysis, the patient's statement of pain must be accepted.

After more treatable conditions are excluded, analgesics and other supportive measures are used.[7] Oral narcotics are preferable to parenteral ones, but patients in severe pain may not accept them. Oral hydration is preferable to intravenous fluid therapy. Patients will often drink carbonated beverages or water if they can reach them from their bed and if they are encouraged to do so. Oxygen therapy is unnecessary, unless the patient is hypoxemic. If he or she is, treatment should be vigorous (see below).

Usually patients with sickle cell disease will not visit the hospital emergency room unless their symptoms compel them to do so. Some visits can be forestalled by providing patients with a *small* supply of oral narcotic for home use. On the other hand, any patient with fever should be seen by a physician, and efforts should be made to ensure that patients have thermometers at home and know how to read them.

Acute Chest Syndrome

Special attention must be paid when patients present with chest pain, fever, and abnormal shadows on chest radiographs because any interference with oxygenation of the blood may have dire consequences. In children, who may have overwhelming infection and die abruptly, antibiotics should be used promptly. The physician has more leeway with adults, from whom pathogenic organisms often cannot be isolated. Most lesions in adults are probably pulmonary infarctions, caused by emboli of necrotic bone marrow or aggregates of sickled cells. A decision to use antibiotics should be made on the patient's overall condition, realizing that improvement may occur spontaneously.

Every patient with a pulmonary infiltrate should have his or her arterial PO_2 measured, as a guide to prognosis and therapy. Patients whose PO_2 is below 75 mm Hg should receive oxygen, and PO_2 should be measured again to be sure it rises. If it does not, pulmonary function is severely compromised, and partial exchange transfusion should be considered. Increased numbers of polymers begin to form within sickle cells as PO_2 falls, and reduction of the proportion of sickle cells may prevent further vascular occlusions.

Surgery

As noted above, trauma may precipitate crises, and major surgery can be followed by a series of events that are perplexing and dangerous. In addition, there is always some risk of cardiorespiratory arrest during general anesthesia, and the likelihood of resuscitation is probably quite small if there is "total body sickling" during a period of anoxia. For these reasons, *and without convincing proof that it is necessary,* some authorities recommend partial exchange transfusion before general anesthesia. No such rule is inflexible, but careful dialogue between internist, surgeon, and anesthesiologist *is* essential before all such procedures.

Gallbladder Disease

As with any chronic hemolytic anemia, gallstones are common. The risks of surgery, and the fact that the stones are often asymptomatic, must be balanced against the risk of a dangerous attack of acute cholecystitis. Not every patient with stones should be operated on, but all those with symptoms of fatty food intolerance or recurrent right upper quadrant pain should be referred to a surgeon.

TABLE 6.5–4. GENOTYPES THAT PRODUCE THE SFA$_2$ PHENOTYPE

| Patient's MCV | First-Degree Relatives with Sickle Cell Trait | First-Degree Relatives | | | Probable Genotype |
		Hb A$_2$	Hb F	MCV	
Normal	All	Normal	Normal	Normal	S/S
Low	Some	Increased in some	Normal or low	Low in some, but iron stores normal	S/β°-Thalassemia
Low	All; low % S in some	Normal	Normal	Low in some, but iron stores normal	S/S plus α-thalassemia
Normal	Some	Low in some	20% in some	Normal	S/HPFH
Low	Some	Low in some	20% in some	Low in some	S/$\delta\beta$-Thalassemia

Pregnancy

There are data to support *prophylactic* transfusion of pregnant women with sickle cell disease in order to improve both maternal and fetal outcome. Experts debate, however, whether transfusions should be given before there is suggestion of impending trouble, as the transfusions themselves carry some risk. A small controlled study suggests that transfusions should not be given unless the pregnant patient exhibits acceleration of the pace of her sickle cell disease, but more data are needed.

Women often worry, and sometimes ask, about the risk of becoming pregnant. With careful management, if pregnancy is desired, the risk (in experienced hands) is acceptable. Unwanted pregnancies represent a failure of medical management, and the internist or pediatrician should begin to discuss contraception in early adolescence. Oral contraceptives are preferable to abortion, and should not be dismissed as an alternative.

Genetic counseling is important but can be difficult to accomplish. Every patient should understand how he or she comes to have the disease as well as the risk (or lack of risk) of transmitting it to his or her children.[7] It must be stressed that the risk of one in four for an SS child in an AS/AS mating is true for each pregnancy; having one affected child does not mean that the next three will be AA or AS. Explanation of compound heterozygous states (SC, S β-thalassemia) is very difficult, and for worried parents, brief "one-time" explanations are often useless. Therefore, the services of a skilled counselor should be obtained, if necessary. Prenatal diagnosis is now a definite option for couples at risk.[2] Most major medical centers can provide the necessary information for referral.

Stroke

Cerebral vascular accidents cause serious disability in a few patients. In children, chronic transfusion for several years is generally accepted as therapy, but no data are available as to efficacy of such management for prevention of second strokes in adults.

Chronic Organ Damage

Repeated small infarctions eventually lead to organ dysfunction: bone, retina, liver, kidney, and heart are frequent sites of difficulty in older patients. The spine and long bones of middle-aged adults often show scars of previous damage; aseptic necrosis of the femoral or humeral head, or recurrent joint pain and effusion, can produce significant morbidity. Some patients obtain significant relief from insertion of prostheses; others do not. Secondary gout is another common cause of joint pain: allopurinol is a logical form of therapy, but hepatotoxicity tempers enthusiasm for its use. Retinal vascular proliferation is more common in hemoglobin-SC disease than in sickle cell anemia. It is not clear, however, that photocoagulation of early lesions (before they bleed) is advantageous. Older patients (>45) may be less able to tolerate anemia than young ones, and occasional small transfusions may significantly improve their exercise capacity.

Transfusion

Transfusion is used not only to increase the oxygen-carrying capacity of the blood, but also to improve its rheologic properties. Two opposing factors are evident when one measures the behavior of mixtures of normal and sickle cells: the greater the proportion of normal cells, the better, and the higher the hematocrit, the worse. In situations in which one is trying to improve flow (rather than oxygen-carrying capacity of the blood) the goal of transfusion should be at least 50 percent normal red cells without too much elevation of hematocrit. If a patient is severely anemic (hemoglobin 5.5 g/dl or less) this end can be achieved by careful administration of red cell concentrates, often with a potent diuretic to avoid circulatory overload. In patients with less severe anemia, prior phlebotomy is required; "recipes" for partial exchange transfusion have been devised, but expert advice on details is usually necessary.[4]

THALASSEMIA SYNDROMES[8]

Clinically, the thalassemia syndromes can be readily classified on the basis of transfusion requirements, survival, the presence of bony abnormalities (produced by excess erythropoiesis) and hemochromatosis. "Cooley anemia," or homozygous β-thalassemia, is the archetype, but many degrees of lesser clinical severity can be observed (Table 6.5–5). The inheritance of these conditions is difficult to ascertain, for there are many thalassemia syndromes of varying severity. Recently, it has become easier to recognize the different thalassemia genes through analysis of DNA, and a more satisfactory classification may soon emerge.[1]

PATHOGENESIS

The basic defect of all thalassemia genes is decreased production of a specific globin chain—alpha chains in α-thalassemia, and so forth. Production may be diminished or completely absent; clinically the distinction is most evident in conjunction with the presence of a gene for an abnormal hemoglobin. β°-Thalassemia genes produce total absence of beta-chain synthesis; an S/β° compound heterozygote produces only β^s globin chains. β^+-Thalassemia genes can produce some hemoglobin A; S/β^+ compound heterozygotes may have 10 to 30 percent hemoglobin A in their red cells, depending upon the severity of the β^+-thalassemia genes. Blacks homozygous for mild β^+-thalassemia may have only mild anemia while homozygosity for the Mediterranean type of β^+-thalassemia produces a very serious illness (Table 6.5–5). α-Thalassemias are classified somewhat differently from β-thalassemias because there are two alpha globin genes per chromosome; each of the total of four may be functional, hypoactive, or deleted. The α° haplotype $(- -)$ has no normal gene, the α^+ haplotype has one $(-\alpha)$, and homo-

TABLE 6.5–5. CLINICAL CLASSIFICATION OF THALASSEMIA SYNDROMES

β-*Thalassemia*
- Severe transfusion-dependent ("Cooley anemia")
  Homozygous β^+- or β^0-thalassemia
  Homozygous Hb Lepore (some cases)
  Compound heterozygous (β^+/β^0)
  Compound heterozygous (β^+ or β^0/Lepore) (some cases)
- Thalassemia intermedia (moderate anemia; may require transfusions occasionally)
  Homozygous mild β^+-thalassemia (type found in blacks)
  Compound heterozygous (mild β^+-/severe β^+)
  Compound heterozygous (β^+/hereditary persistence of fetal hemoglobin)
  Compound heterozygous (β^+/Lepore) (some cases)
  Homozygous $\delta\beta$-thalassemia
  "Severe" heterozygous β-thalassemia
- Thalassemia minor (mild microcytic anemia)
  Heterozygous β^+ or β^0
  Heterozygous $\delta\beta$ thalassemia
  Heterozygous Hb Lepore

α-*Thalassemia*
- Hydrops fetalis (death in utero)
  Homozygous α^0 thalassemia (no normal genes)
- Hemoglobin H disease (moderate anemia; hemolysis)
  Compound heterozygote (α^0/α^+) (one normal gene)
  Compound heterozygote (α^0/Hb Constant Spring) (one normal gene)
- Mild microcytic anemia
  Homozygous α^+ (two normal genes)
  Heterozygous α^0 (two normal genes)
  Compound heterozygous (α^+/Hb Constant Spring) (two normal genes)
- Minimal disease
  Heterozygous α^+ (three normal genes)

zygous α^+-thalassemia ($-\alpha/-\alpha$) is more or less clinically equivalent to heterozygous α^0-thalassemia ($--/\alpha\alpha$).

Some of the mechanisms of decreased globin synthesis in thalassemia are outlined in Table 6.5–1; many of them involve deletion of genes, or abnormal processing of DNA. A few abnormal hemoglobins are thalassemia-like; hemoglobins Constant Spring and Lepore produce α- and β-thalassemia, respectively. A few unstable hemoglobins are so very unstable that although globin production is normal, the product denatures so quickly that the final effect is thalassemia-like.[3]

Anemia is produced by the patient's inability to synthesize hemoglobin, and by hemolysis. The severity of anemia in β-thalassemia is governed in part by the activity of gamma-chain genes. If beta-chain synthesis is absent, and gamma-chain synthesis almost compensates for the deficit, the anemia may be mild. The severity of anemia is also governed by the presence of excess globin chains. In β-thalassemia, for instance, uncombined alpha chains accumulate ("unbalanced globin synthesis"); they are unstable, precipitate, and cause hemolytic anemia.

α-Thalassemia differs from β-thalassemia in two significant ways. First, alpha chains are necessary for formation of fetal hemoglobin ($\alpha_2\gamma_2$). A fetus who could not make alpha chains would be severely compromised, and probably would die in utero (hydrops fetalis). Second, beta and gamma chains are more stable than alpha chains, and the excess globin does not precipitate as quickly. Tetramers of beta chains (β_4, Hb H) and gamma chains (γ_4, hemoglobin Barts) are found in the red cells of patients with α-thalassemia. These hemoglobins are functionally useless, because of their very high oxygen affinity.

DIAGNOSIS

β-Thalassemia can occur in patients of any ethnic background, and "Mediterranean" anemia is common in many non-Mediterranean

peoples, including Asians and blacks. Malfunction of a single alpha gene ($\alpha-$) is common in blacks, but the two abnormal genes ($--$) seen in Mediterranean, Middle Eastern and Asian peoples are not. As a result, hemoglobin H disease ($\alpha-/--$) is rare in blacks and hydrops fetalis due to loss of all four normal alpha globin genes is almost unheard of.

If they have not been hypertransfused, patients with β-thalassemia major are pale and may be jaundiced (from intramedullary or extramedullary hemolysis) or pigmented (from iron overload). Bone marrow expansion is evident in the bones of the skull and face, and perhaps by bony deformity elsewhere; extra medullary hematopoiesis is reflected in hepatosplenomegaly. Anemia is marked with striking microcytosis, poikilocytosis, and erythroblastosis. Fetal hemoglobin is increased, sometimes markedly; hemoglobin A_2 may be low, normal, or increased. Both parents and any children should have microcytic red cells in the absence of iron deficiency, and elevated levels of hemoglobin A_2; hemoglobin F may be increased. Patients with thalassemia intermedia show lesser changes in the red cells, variable A_2 levels, and increased fetal hemoglobin.

Relatives of patients with β-thalassemia should have elevated proportions of hemoglobin A_2. If they do not, but do have increased fetal hemoglobin, $\delta\beta$-thalassemia—absence or malfunction of both the beta chain gene and the neighboring delta chain gene, needed for synthesis of hemoglobin A_2 ($\alpha_2\delta_2$)—should be suspected. An abnormal hemoglobin migrating like S at pH 8.6, but like A on agar, comprising 10 to 15 percent of a hemolysate and associated with microcytosis, is probably hemoglobin Lepore and has the same clinical significance as a β-thalassemia gene.

There is no easy way to diagnose α-thalassemia. One considers the possibility when a member of a high-risk group (blacks, Asians, and Caucasians from the Mediterranean area or Near East) has unexplained microcytosis, mild anemia, normal iron stores, and a normal hemoglobin A_2 level. Hemoglobin H disease is usually a mild hemolytic anemia, but since hemoglobin H is unstable, oxidant drugs can precipitate hemolytic crises similar to those seen in G-6-PD deficiency. Hemoglobin H can be demonstrated by electrophoresis or by tests for unstable hemoglobins. Loss of the four alpha genes ($--/--$) causes fetal death in utero, and α-thalassemia should be considered in the differential diagnosis of hydrops fetalis in persons from an appropriate population group.

CLINICAL MANIFESTATIONS AND THEIR MANAGEMENT

In contrast to sickle cell anemia, the overwhelming problem in thalassemia is the need for more hemoglobin. Transfusion requirements and the consequences of iron overload (hemochromatosis produced, in part, by those transfusions) dominate the clinical picture. Children who are not transfused show retarded sexual maturation.

Congestive heart failure may occur at hemoglobin concentrations tolerated well in other chronic anemias, probably because of cardiac hemochromatosis. Arrhythmias are common in older transfused patients, and may be an immediate cause of death. Other manifestations of hemochromatosis include hepatic cirrhosis and rarely diabetes. Joint symptoms may be related to bone disease as well as synovial iron deposits. As in any hemolytic anemia, folic acid deficiency may make anemia more severe, and increased bilirubin production can lead to gallstones and cholecystitis. Hypersplenism can also exaggerate the hematologic problem, and some patients profit from splenectomy.

Bone abnormalities produced by expansion of marrow activity, and retarded growth and development, can be prevented if children are maintained at near normal hemoglobin concentrations. Soft bones, due to replacement of bone by marrow, produce dental and orthopedic problems. Exuberant marrow growth may produce intrathoracic (paraspinal) masses of marrow that can be confused with neoplasms.

GENETIC COUNSELING

Counseling is more difficult than in sickle cell disease, for recognition of carriers and distinction of homozygotes from heterozygotes is much less accurate. Careful study of the patient's family, including measurement of red cell indices, blood counts, and hemoglobins A_2 and F, usually permit a reasonable guess of his or her genotype. Similar family studies of a prospective spouse's family may be necessary if he or she has either a slightly abnormal blood count or a positive family history. Prenatal diagnosis requires a sample of fetal blood in many instances and is less satisfactory than in sickle cell anemia.[2]

TREATMENT

Therapy is aimed at maintaining oxygen transport but avoiding or postponing iron overload, causing increased iron excretion. Infusion of "neocytes," young red cells separated from donor blood by differential centrifugation, has been suggested, but the high cost of preparing such cells militates against their general use.

Iron chelation therapy, once considered difficult or impossible, can now produce negative iron balance and prevent accumulation of iron. Prolonged subcutaneous or intravenous infusions of desferrioxamine are needed, week after week, to accomplish that end, and many patients are unwilling to adhere to such a regimen. Liver iron stores can be reduced, progression of cirrhosis arrested, and cardiac disease prevented, but there is no evidence that chelation therapy can reverse cardiac hemochromatosis once it becomes manifest.[9] New orally effective chelators are being sought; early use of such drugs could profoundly alter the course of many patients.

REFERENCES

1. Antonarakis SE, Kazazian HH Jr, Orkin SH: DNA polymerization and molecular pathology of the human globin gene clusters. Hum Genet 69:1, 1985
2. Boehm C, Kazazian HH Jr: Prenatal diagnosis of hemoglobinopathies—1983. Semin Perinatol 7:175, 1983
3. Bunn HF, Forget BG: Hemoglobin: Molecular, Genetic and Clinical Aspects. Philadelphia, WB Saunders, 1986
4. Charache S: Treatment of sickle cell anemia. Ann Rev Med 32:195, 1981
5. Charache S, Dover GJ, et al: Hydroxyurea-induced augmentation of fetal hemoglobin production in patients with sickle cell anemia. Blood 69:109, 1987
6. Serjeant GR: Sickle Cell Disease. Oxford, Oxford University Press, 1985
7. Vichinsky EP, Johnson R, Lubin BH: Multidisciplinary approach to pain management in sickle cell disease. Am J Pediatr Hematol Oncol 4:328, 1982
8. Weatherall DJ, Clegg JB: The Thalassaemia Syndromes. 3d ed. Oxford, Blackwell Scientific Publications, 1981
9. Wolfe L, Olivieri N, et al: Prevention of cardiac disease by subcutaneous deferexamine in patients with thalassemia major. N Engl J Med 312:1600, 1985

CHAPTER 6.6
The Hemolytic Anemias
Thomas S. Kickler

The hemolytic anemias are characterized by a shortened red cell life span. The red cell has evolved to a simple design whose main function is the delivery of oxygen to the tissues. It accomplishes this function efficiently with few basic elements—the red cell membrane, hemoglobin, and enzyme systems that maintain the integrity of the membrane and the labile hemoglobin molecule. Derangements in these red cell elements account for the intracellular hemolytic anemias. In contrast, the extracellular hemolytic anemias arise when various factors act upon the red cell to shorten its survival. These broad categories of *intracellular* and *extracellular* defects form the basis of the classification of the hemolytic anemias (Table 6.6–1). The following sections will describe the general approach to the diagnosis of a hemolytic disorder and the major hemolytic anemias. (See Chapter 6.5 for the disorders of hemoglobin.)

DIAGNOSIS OF HEMOLYTIC DISORDERS

A systematic analysis of clinical information, peripheral smear, and the measurement of the reticulocyte count is required when evaluating any type of anemia. Hemolysis is suggested when anemia occurs in the absence of bleeding and in the presence of increased erythroid production estimated by the reticulocyte count. Clinical signs and symptoms (Table 6.6–2) and blood smear abnormalities (Table 6.6–3) provide the initial clues to the mechanism of the hemolysis. Further specific tests will establish the diagnosis.

CLINICAL EVALUATION

Anemia since childhood, accompanied by a positive family history, suggests an intracellular defect. The recent onset of hemolysis suggests an acquired (extracellular) hemolytic condition. Concomitant illnesses such as systemic lupus erythematosus or a lymphoprolif-

TABLE 6.6–1. CLASSIFICATION OF HEMOLYTIC ANEMIAS

I. Inherited intracellular defects
  A. Membrane abnormalities
    1. Hereditary spherocytosis
    2. Hereditary elliptocytosis
    3. Hereditary stomatocytosis
    4. Hereditary pyropoikilocytosis
  B. Enzyme abnormalities
    1. Deficiency of erythrocyte glycolytic enzymes
    2. Deficiency of enzymes in the pentose-phosphate pathway and glutathione metabolism
  C. Hemoglobinopathies (see Chapter 6.5)
II. Acquired intracellular defects
  A. Paroxysmal nocturnal hemoglobinuria
III. Extracellular defects
  A. Immune hemolytic anemias
  B. Traumatic (microangiopathic) hemoyltic anemias
  C. Infectious agents
  D. Chemical and physical agents

TABLE 6.6–2. CLUES TO THE ETIOLOGY OF HEMOLYTIC ANEMIA

Clinical Setting	Cause of Hemolysis
A. Childhood onset with familial tendency	Intracellular abnormality
B. Concomitant illness	
1. Collagen vascular disease, lymphoproliferative disorders	Immune hemolysis
2. Malignant hypertension, disseminated intravascular coagulation, prosthetic heart valve, vasculitis, disseminated carcinoma	Microangiopathic hemolysis
3. Infection	Clostridia, malaria, pneumococcus, *Escherichia coli, Bartonella*
4. Hepatocellular disease	Spur cell anemia
C. Drug administration	Enzyme deficiency, unstable hemoglobin, immune hemolysis
D. Recent transfusion	Red cell alloantibody-induced hemolysis

TABLE 6.6–4. LABORATORY EVALUATION OF HEMOLYSIS

Laboratory Test	Results
General Tests	
• Reticulocyte count	Elevated in hemolysis (also in the presence of hemorrhage or bone marrow recovery from a nutritional deficiency or toxin)
• Haptoglobin, hemopexin	Reduced in intra- or extravascular hemolysis
• Plasma hemoglobin and urine hemosiderin	Present in intravascular hemolysis
• Chromium 51 red cell survival	Reduced
• Miscellaneous	
Bilirubin	Elevated unconjugated fraction
Lactic dehydrogenase	Elevated
Specific Tests	
• Osmotic fragility	Increased with spherocytosis, hereditary or acquired
• Direct antiglobulin test	Positive in immune hemolysis
• Enzyme assays	Reduced activity
G6PD	
Pyruvate kinase	
• Ham or sugar water test	Positive in PNH

See Chapter 6.5 for evaluation of hemoglobinopathies.

erative disorder are frequently associated with immune-mediated hemolysis. The recent administration of a drug to an individual of Mediterranean or African origin may suggest an intracellular defect (G6PD deficiency, for example). Hemolysis may develop in hospitalized patients with infections, on drugs, or with transfusion.

INITIAL LABORATORY EVALUATION[8]

Peripheral Smear Morphology
Hemolysis is suggested by the presence of polychromatophilic macrocytes on a Wright-stained smear. These blue-orange staining cells represent reticulocytes. When hemolysis is severe, greater marrow stress develops and younger reticulocytes appear, known as "shift reticulocytes." These cells have fine basophilic stippling. In severe hemolysis, nucleated red cells are readily found. The particular morphology of the red cells may suggest a specific disorder (Table 6.6–3).

Bone Marrow
In hemolytic anemias the bone marrow predictability shows erythroid hyperplasia. Since the bone marrow infrequently provides additional useful information, a marrow aspirate is generally not indicated in the evaluation of a patient with hemolysis, unless an associated disease is suspected.

TABLE 6.6–3. PERIPHERAL SMEAR MORPHOLOGY IN HEMOLYTIC ANEMIAS

Morphologic Abnormality	Disease
Spherocytes	Hereditary spherocytosis Immune hemolysis Extensive burns Clostridial sepsis Hb C disease
Schistocytes	Red cell fragmentation syndromes
"Blister" cells	G6PD deficiency
Target cells	Hemoglobinopathy
Spiculated cells	Pyruvate kinase deficiency Liver disease
Agglutination	Immune hemolysis

Laboratory Tests (Table 6.6–4)
The reticulocyte count is the most useful and most readily available test to assess the functional capacity of effective erythroid production. As described in Chapter 6.2 the reticulocyte count must be corrected for the degree of anemia. The degree of reticulocytosis will increase with the severity of the anemia, provided adequate iron, folate, and vitamin B_{12} are available. At times other laboratory tests may be useful in evaluating a hemolytic disorder. The most direct and precise measure of red cell survival is isotopic labeling of the patients' cells with Chromium 51. This costly and time-consuming test is rarely required except on occasions when investigating obscure reasons for hemolysis or when the presence of hemolysis is equivocal. The sites of red cell destruction, such as spleen and liver, can also be detected with this technique.[10]

If hemolysis is occurring intravascularly, plasma hemoglobin may be increased. This is usually accompanied by hemoglobinuria. With chronic intravascular hemolysis, a Prussian blue stain of the urine sediment will show hemosiderin present in renal tubular cells. Typically, patients with hemolysis caused by a prosthetic heart valve, immune transfusion reactions, or paroxysmal nocturnal hemoglobinuria will have hemosiderinuria. In severe cases loss of iron through the urine can lead to iron deficiency anemia.

A variety of chemical determinations are useful in establishing the presence of hemolysis. Bilirubin, being an oxidative metabolite of heme, is increased in hemolytic disorders. Specifically, the unconjugated or "indirect" form of bilirubin is elevated. The serum level of "direct" or conjugated bilirubin is normal unless hepatic or biliary disease are present. A second indicator of hemolysis is reduced or absent haptoglobin levels. This protein specifically binds free hemoglobin and the complex is cleared. Thus, patients with significant hemolysis, either intra- or extravascular, have low or absent haptoglobin levels.[11]

HEMOLYTIC ANEMIAS DUE TO HERITABLE INTRACELLULAR DEFECTS

MEMBRANE DEFECTS[12]

Viscoelastic properties of the red cell membrane contribute to the deformability of the cell so that it can survive turbulent flow yet be able to pass narrow capillaries. The red cell membrane cytoskele-

ton is composed of a network of intrinsic proteins. Spectrin, actin-like proteins, and ankyrin are the proteins that structurally determine the red cell shape and deformability. Abnormalities in the molecular structure of these proteins appear to be associated with the pathogenesis of hereditary spherocytosis, elliptocytosis and stomatocytosis.

Hereditary Spherocytosis

Clinical Features. Hereditary spherocytosis[17] is an autosomal dominant inherited defect of the red cell membrane characterized by anemia, splenomegaly, spherocytosis, and increased red cell osmotic fragility. With an incidence of approximately 200 per million, it is one of the most common hereditary hemolytic anemias in the United States. There is a wide spectrum of severity in the anemia. Some patients are incidentally diagnosed while others have severe hemolytic anemia. The symptoms of hereditary spherocytosis are those characteristic of chronic hemolytic disorders. The disorder is typically first noticed in childhood although the disease may be so mild that it goes unrecognized until adulthood. Biliary tract symptoms may be the presenting feature. Cholelithiasis has been found in over 40 percent of patients. Chronic leg ulcers may also complicate the disorder.

The course of the disease may be complicated by episodes of "aplastic crisis," where erythropoiesis is suppressed yet the hemolytic process continues. These episodes of life-threatening anemia develop, usually in association with infection, and are accompanied by leukopenia and thrombocytopenia. The crisis may last from 7 to 14 days.

Laboratory Findings. Patients with hereditary spherocytosis will have spherocytes and polychromatophilia on their blood smear. The mean cell volume is normal, but the mean cell hemoglobin concentration may be elevated (37 to 39 g/dl). The osmotic fragility test is useful in diagnosing the disorder. Because the red cells have a decreased surface-to-volume ratio they have an increased susceptibility to lysis by hypotonic saline. In the osmotic fragility test the lysis of test cells is compared to normal red cells using different concentrations of sodium chloride solution. At higher osmolalities spherocytic cells are more susceptible to lysis than the control cells. In those patients with only a small population of spherocytic cells, incubating the blood for 24 hours at 37C will enhance the abnormality. There is no correlation between the degree of anemia and the fragility of the red cells. It should be noted that in any condition in which spherocytes are present, for example, warm autoimmune hemolytic anemia, the osmotic fragility will be increased.

Management. The hemolysis in hereditary spherocytosis is relieved by splenectomy. Splenectomy should be suggested in any patient who has moderate or severe hereditary spherocytosis to avert the complications of the disorder, aplastic crisis, cholelithiasis, and chronic leg ulcers. The mortality and morbidity from splenectomy in hereditary spherocytosis are low. Delaying splenectomy to age 4 or 5 may reduce the risk of postsplenectomy sepsis.[14]

ENZYME DEFECTS

The glycolytic pathway, together with the oxidative hexosemonophosphate shunt and its dependent glutathione metabolism, provide the red cell with energy and protect the cell's constituents from oxidant injury. Any enzyme abnormality that leads to deficient energy generation or a reduction in a cell's capability to reduce oxidizing agents leads to hemolysis. Through the glycolytic pathway adenosine triphosphate (ATP) is generated. ATP is required for the maintenance of cell shape and membrane transport systems. The constant regeneration of glutathione provides protection from such oxidative stresses as drugs or infection. Glucose-6-phosphate dehydrogenase is the critical enzyme in the complex enzymatic process that recycles glutathione.

Glucose 6-Phosphate Dehydrogenase Deficiency (G6PD)[1]

G6PD deficiency is an X-linked disorder. At the molecular level several variants of G6PD have been described. Males being hemizygotes may be markedly deficient in enzyme activity. The majority of female heterozygotes show enzyme levels intermediate between normal and deficient activity. Although a spectrum of activity may be seen among females, few are as deficient as males with the disorder. This phenomenon relates to the degree of X-chromosome inactivation in females.

In patients of Mediterranean origin with G6PD deficiency, enzyme activity is typically less than 1 percent. These individuals are extremely sensitive to oxidant stresses. An African variant of the enzyme is found in 10 percent of black males. These individuals have G6PD activities about 15 percent of normal.

Clinical Features. The typical black individual with G6PD deficiency does not have any evidence of hemolysis unless challenged by oxidant drugs, infection, or noxious agents (fava beans). These hemolytic episodes are self-limited. Some variants may have chronic hemolysis characterized by episodes of accelerated hemolysis. In the acute event, hemolysis occurs intravascularly, and abdominal or back pain may occur in association with hemoglobinuria. In some cases, hemolysis is so severe that acute renal failure may develop. Drugs implicated as producing hemolysis are listed in Table 6.6–5.

Laboratory Findings. The peripheral smear is nondiagnostic. Frequently cells with displaced hemoglobin, "blister cells," are evident. A quantitative determination of G6PD establishes the diagnosis. If the enzyme activity in the red cells is determined at the time of acute hemolysis and reticulocytosis, normal to low normal activity may be found. A low normal value of G6PD in the presence of reticulocytosis may suggest the disorder. In these cases, the enzyme activity should be repeated after the hemolytic episode is over.

Treatment. G6PD deficient individuals should avoid drugs that may induce severe hemolysis. If hemolysis results in severe anemia, transfusions may be life-saving. Splenectomy is not beneficial in hemolytic anemia due to G6PD deficiency.

HEMOLYTIC ANEMIAS DUE TO ACQUIRED INTRACELLULAR DEFECTS

PAROXYSMAL NOCTURNAL HEMOGLOBINURIA

Paroxysmal nocturnal hemoglobinuria (PNH) is an acquired hematopoietic stem cell disorder that results in an intrinsic abnormality of red cells, platelets, and granulocyte membranes. An unexplained susceptibility to complement lysis leads to intravascular hemolysis. The etiology of the stem cell disorder is unknown. Chronic hemolysis dominates the clinical picture.[6]

The most serious complications of PNH include thrombosis and marrow aplasia with bleeding or infections. Thrombosis of large intra-abdominal veins, especially hepatic veins, are common.[7]

TABLE 6.6–5. AGENTS IMPLICATED IN PRODUCTION OF HEMOLYSIS IN G6PD DEFICIENCY

Acetanilid	Pentaquine
Nalidixic acid	Primaquine
Naphthalene	Sulfacetamide
Niridazole	Sulfamethoxale
Nitrofurantoin	Sulfanilamide
Pamaquine	Sulfapyridine

Since the hemolysis is intravascular, iron deficiency may develop in patients with protracted hemolysis. Renal abnormalities may complicate PNH either as a result of thrombosis or of chronic hemoglobinuria and hemosiderinuria. Aplastic anemia may be the predominant presenting finding in patients with PNH. Occasionally, some patients will present with isolated thrombocytopenia. Therefore, in any patient presenting with cytopenias of obscure etiology, the diagnosis of PNH should be considered.

The peripheral blood shows no diagnostic features. The bone marrow characteristically shows erythroid hyperplasia with absent iron stores. When there is pancytopenia, a hypoplastic marrow may be seen. The increased susceptibility to complement lysis forms the basis of the tests used in diagnosing PNH. Incubating red cells with sucrose (sugar water test), resulting in hemolysis of red cells with PNH membrane defect, is a sensitive screening test.[5] The acidified-serum lysis test (Ham test) should be done to confirm the diagnosis. PNH is discussed in more detail in Chapter 6.12.

ABNORMALITIES IN THE GLYCOLYTIC METABOLIC PATHWAY[16]

Pyruvate Kinase Deficiency

Pyruvate kinase deficiency is the most common deficiency in the glycolytic pathway, the others being rare. The inheritance is autosomal recessive. This hemolytic anemia arises because of impaired production of ATP. Most patients have a mild to moderate chronic hemolytic anemia and splenomegaly. The blood smear shows polychromatophilia and occasionally echinocytes. The diagnosis is confirmed by assay of the enzyme activity.

HEMOLYTIC ANEMIAS DUE TO ACQUIRED EXTRACELLULAR DEFECTS

IMMUNE HEMOLYTIC ANEMIAS

Immune hemolytic anemia is an acquired hemolytic condition caused by the product of autoantibodies against the patient's red cells. The immune hemolytic anemias are classified in Table 6.6–6. The characteristics of the hemolytic antibody and the presence or absence of an underlying illness form the basis of the classification. Warm autoimmune hemolytic anemia (AIHA) is characterized by autoantibodies that react at 37C. Cold AIHA is characterized by antibodies that have maximal reactivity at 4C. With the history and laboratory findings of an acquired hemolytic anemia, an immune mechanism should be evaluated. As discussed below, the hallmark of an immune hemolytic anemia is a positive direct Coombs test.

Warm Autoimmune Hemolytic Anemia[3,13]

This type of immune hemolysis is most common, accounting for approximately 70 percent of cases. Patients of all ages are affected,

TABLE 6.6–6. CLASSIFICATION OF AUTOIMMUNE HEMOLYTIC ANEMIAS

A. Warm Autoimmune Type
1. Primary warm autoimmune hemolytic anemia
2. Secondary warm autoimmune hemolytic anemia
   a. Collagen vascular diseases
   b. Lymphoproliferative disorders

B. Cold Autoimmune Type
1. Primary cold agglutinin syndrome
2. Secondary cold agglutinin syndrome
   a. Mycoplasma infections and infectious mononucleosis
   b. Lymphoproliferative disorders
3. Paroxysmal cold hemoglobinuria

C. Drug-Induced Anemias

but with a higher incidence occurring in females. Neoplasms of the reticuloendothelial system, collagen vascular diseases, inherited and acquired immunodeficiency states, and ulcerative colitis are diseases frequently associated with warm AIHA. The combination of warm AIHA and autoimmune thrombocytopenia is known as Evans syndrome.

Pathophysiology. IgG antibodies lead to shortened red cell survival principally by extravascular destruction in the reticuloendothelial system. The mononuclear phagocytes in these tissues possess Fc receptors for the immunoglobulin G (IgG) coating the red cells. If present, complement factors coating the red cells also facilitate the phagocytosis by the macrophage. In the process of phagocytosis, small portions of the red cell are ingested by the macrophage. If the ingestion is incomplete, the released red cell after resealing of its membrane will lose its typical convex appearance and appear spherical. The principal site of red cell destruction is the spleen, unlike in cold agglutinin disease, where the liver plays a predominant role.

Presenting Signs and Symptoms. The onset of anemia may be insidious or fulminant. In many patients, symptoms from the associated underlying illness will predominate. Jaundice, hemoglobinuria, and fever are infrequent clinical findings. Splenomegaly is present in about 50 percent of patients with warm AIHA, with hepatomegaly being present in one third of patients.

Laboratory Findings. The hemoglobin concentration is variable, but it is not uncommon to have values less than 7 g/dl. The blood smear shows spherocytes, polychromatophilia, and autoagglutination. Bilirubin values are normal in over half of patients. The reticulocyte count is typically elevated, but a reticulocytopenic form of the disorder can occur as well. In this case life-threatening anemia develops.

The hallmark of the disorder is a positive direct antiglobulin test (Coombs test). This fundamental immunologic test is used to detect increased levels of IgG or complement (specifically C3d) on the surface of the red cell. The test consists of adding goat or rabbit antihuman IgG or C3d or both to the patient's red cells to detect in vivo sensitization. Reactivity is determined by the presence of agglutination after incubation and centrifugation. This technique is also used to detect serum antibody by testing the patient's serum against normal red cells (the indirect Coombs test). In rare instances, the direct Coombs test may be negative due to the sensitivity of the standard direct Coombs test. In this situation, the diagnosis of Coombs-negative immune hemolytic anemia may be confirmed by more sensitive immunologic techniques such as radioimmunoassay. In warm AIHA IgG is found alone or in combination with C3. Because IgG and C3 potentiate each other's opsonic function, more severe hemolytic anemia is typical of patients whose red cells demonstrate both IgG and C3.

Therapy. Initial therapy for warm AIHA is the administration of corticosteroids. A therapeutic effect, with reduction of hemolysis, will be achieved in 80 percent of patients. This improvement will frequently be preceded by a significant rise in the reticulocyte count. If this does not occur, other associated conditions such as iron, folate, or B$_{12}$ deficiency should be sought. Once the anemia improves gradual reduction in the dose of corticosteroids is warranted, because of the tendency for clinical relapse. For the patient unable to tolerate long-term steroids or relapsing anemia after discontinuation of drug treatment, splenectomy is recommended. Before the introduction of corticosteroid therapy, splenectomy alone was helpful in 50 percent of patients. Splenectomy should not be undertaken lightly in this disorder because even with skilled surgeons, the morbidity and mortality are significant. Transfusion of red cells will have shortened survival paralleling the patient's autologous red cell destruction rate. Nonetheless, if transfusion therapy is considered lifesaving, red cells should not be withheld because of fear of a hemolytic reaction. The blood bank should be

consulted to assure that a clinically significant red cell alloantibody is not masked by the autoantibody.

Cold Agglutinin Disease (CAD)

In contrast to warm AIHA, cold autoimmune hemolysis involves IgM antibodies. More commonly, the patients are middle-aged or elderly. The cold agglutinin syndrome is less frequent than warm AIH, accounting for approximately 15 percent of the immune hemolytic anemias. Cold agglutinin disease may be associated with neoplasms, especially chronic lymphocytic leukemia, Waldenström macroglobulinemia, and lymphoma. In addition, it is associated with mycoplasma and Epstein–Barr virus infections.

Patients usually have less severe anemia than in warm AIHA. Nonetheless, the most frequent presenting symptoms are referable to the anemia. Upon exposure to cold temperatures, patients may develop hemoglobinuria. Associated with cold exposure and resultant autoagglutination in small capillaries, symptoms of acrocyanosis may occur.

Pathophysiology. As blood circulates through acral body areas where ambient temperatures are low, the IgM autoantibodies can bind to the patient's red cells. The hemolysis that follows is precipitated by the fixation of complement to the red cell surface. Hepatic macrophages are the primary effector cell in removing red cells coated with C3 in the form of C3b. Red cell destruction does not go unchecked since a plasma inactivator (factor I) cleaves C3b, converting it to C3d. These C3d cells are resistant to destruction and circulate normally.

Laboratory Findings. A characteristic finding is autoagglutination of the patient's red cells following phlebotomy. This finding can readily be observed upon making a blood smear. Other characteristic blood smear findings include mild spherocytosis and polychromatophilia. The characteristic serologic results include a positive direct antiglobulin test with complement sensitization. The presence of IgG on the patient's red cells is not characteristic of CAD. The responsible IgM antibodies are not detectable because they eluate off the red cell during in vitro testing procedures. Cold-reactive IgM autoagglutinins asssociated with immune hemolysis are present at titers greater than 1000 when tested at 4C. If the testing is carried out at progressively higher temperatures, the titers decrease. Pathologic IgM autoagglutinins typically react to temperatures of 30C. In chronic CAD, the IgM antibody is usually a monoclonal protein of the kappa light chain type. Polyclonal IgM immunoglobulins (with both kappa and lambda light-chain distribution) are found in the form of the disease that is associated with mycoplasmal or Epstein–Barr virus infections.

Therapy. Therapy is principally preventive in nature. Exposure to cold should be avoided. Wearing gloves, hats, and warm clothing when outdoor activities cannot be avoided should be recommended. Steroids and splenectomy are ineffective. Alkylating agents have been tried in patients with severe hemolysis and anemia. It is unclear whether this maneuver has provided any long-term benefit. If transfusions of red cells are required, administration of the blood through a blood warmer is prudent.

Paroxysmal Cold Hemoglobinuria[9]

Paroxysmal cold hemoglobinuria (PCH) is a unique autoimmune hemolytic disorder, caused by an IgG autoantibody. The antibody has reactivity against red cell P antigens. The disorder is characterized by acute onset of fulminant hemolysis associated with fever, chills, and abdominal pain. Hemoglobinuria always occurs. PCH frequently develops after a viral illness; in the past it was associated with syphilis. The antibody that mediates the disorder is an IgG antibody that binds to the red cell upon exposure to the cold. With warming, complement activation lyses the red cells intravascularly. The disorder is diagnosed by the Donath–Landsteiner test. This serologic test involves incubating the patient's serum with cells at 4C then warming the cells to allow complement activation to proceed. If this type of autoantibody is present, hemolysis of the cells will occur. PCH is usually a self-limited disorder and resolves spontaneously in a few days to weeks. Blood transfusion support, with warmed blood, may be required.

Drug-induced Immune Hemolytic Anemia[4]

Drug administration can lead to immune destruction of red cells by various mechanisms (Table 6.6–7). This type of immune hemolytic anemia accounts for approximately 10 percent of patients with immune hemolysis. Numerous drugs have been incriminated as inducing immune hemolytic anemia. However, the most frequently involved drugs are methyldopa, penicillin, and quinidine. The usual mode of onset of the anemia is gradual, although with drugs that can induce an immune complex type mechanism, the hemolysis may be acute and severe. The direct Coombs test will show IgG and/or complement sensitization of the red cells (Table 6.6–7). Methyldopa administration will frequently also lead to serum antibody (positive indirect test), unlike any of the other drugs. The management of these disorders is discontinuation of the drug.

RED CELL FRAGMENTATION SYNDROMES

Physical trauma may be sufficient to cause intravascular hemolysis with hemoglobinuria and hemoglobinemia. The surviving red cells take the form of schistocytes (fragments, helmets, or crescents), which readily distinguish red cell fragmentation syndromes from other acquired anemias.

TRAUMATIC CARDIAC HEMOLYSIS[15]

Hemolysis may develop following placement of a prosthetic heart valve or after an ostium primum repair of the atrium with an intracardiac patch. Rarely does intrinsic valve disease lead to hemolysis. Aortic prosthetic valves are more frequently associated with hemo-

TABLE 6.6–7. CLINICAL AND LABORATORY FEATURES OF DRUG-INDUCED IMMUNE HEMOLYSIS

Mechanism	Drug Example	Clinical Findings	Antibody Studies Direct Antiglobulin Test Findings	Antibody Properties
Possible alteration in suppressor lymphocyte populations	Methyldopa	10% of patients will have positive direct Coombs test; hemolysis is rare	IgG	IgG autoantibody
Immune complex	Quinidine	Acute hemolysis; renal insufficiency	Complement C3d	IgM or IgG
Drug absorption to red cells	Penicillin	History of high dose administration	IgG	IgG antibody that reacts only with drug-coated cells

lysis because of the greater turbulence in flow. The hemolysis accompanying nonsurgically corrected valvular disease is rarely severe. When hemolysis and hemosideruria have been prolonged, iron deficiency may develop. Daily iron supplementation should be instituted if significant hemolysis is present. Reoperation may be necessary for some patients with severe hemolysis.

MICROANGIOPATHIC HEMOLYTIC ANEMIAS

Red cell fragmentation occurring in association with small vessel disease may occur.[2] This type of hemolytic disorder is termed microangiopathic. The deposition of fibrin within the microvasculature or severe hypertension provide the conditions for fragmentation. A variety of clinical syndromes are associated with microangiopathic hemolytic anemia (Table 6.6–8). One of the most serious disorders is thrombotic thrombocytopenic purpura, discussed in Chapter 6.9.

Microangiopathic hemolytic anemia may be a prominent feature of disorders associated with vasculitis. These include polyarteritis nodosa, systemic lupus erythematosus, and acute glomerulonephritis. Associated with the vasculitis is fibrin disposition, which leads to red cell fragmentation. The peripheral smear of patients with disseminated intravascular coagulation (DIC) frequently shows red cell fragmentation. DIC may be the result of a variety of disorders such as sepsis, abruptio placenta, or disseminated carcinoma. In these conditions, the red cell fragmentation is due to fibrin deposition within the microvasculature. The hemolysis is rarely severe, and as the underlying disease is controlled, fragmentation ceases.

REFERENCES

1. Beutler E: Glucose-6-phosphate dehydrogenase deficiency and nonspherocytic hemolytic anemia. Semin Hematol 2:91, 1965
2. Brain MC: Microangiopathic hemolytic anemia. The possible role of vascular lesions in pathogenesis. Br J Haematol 8:358, 1962
3. Frank MM, Schreiber AD, Atkinson JP: Pathophysiology of immune hemolytic anemias. Ann Intern Med 87:210, 1977
4. Garratty G, Petz LD: Drug induced immune hemolytic anemia. Am J Med 58:398, 1975
5. Hartman RC, Jenkins DE: The sugar water test for paroxysmal nocturnal hemoglobinuria. N Engl J Med 275:155, 1966
6. Hartman RC, Jenkins DE, et al: Paroxysmal nocturnal hemoglobinuria: Clinical and laboratory studies relating to iron metabolism and therapy with androgen and iron. Medicine 45:331, 1966
7. Hartman RC, Luther AB, et al: Fulminant hepatic venous thrombosis in paroxysmal nocturnal hemoglobinuria. Definition of a medical emergency. Johns Hopkins Med J 146:247, 1980
8. Hillman RS: Characteristics of marrow production and reticulocyte maturation in normal man in response to anemia. J Clin Invest 48:443, 1969
9. Johnsen HE, Brostrøm K, Madsen M: Paroxysmal cold hemoglobinuria in children. Scand J Haematol 20:413, 1978
10. Najean Y, Cacchione R, et al: Methods of evaluating the sequestration site of red cells labeled with ^{51}Cr: A review of 96 cases. Br J Haematol 29:495, 1975
11. Nyman M: Serum haptoglobin. Methodological and clinical studies. Scand J Clin Lab Invest (suppl 39) 11, 1959
12. Palek J, Lux SE: Red cell membrane skeletal defects in hereditary and acquired hemolytic anemias. Semin Hematol 20:189, 1983
13. Petz LD, Garratty G: Acquired immune hemolytic anemias. New York, Churchill-Livingstone, 1980
14. Schwartz SI, Bernard RP, et al: Splenectomy for hematologic disorders. Arch Surg 101:338, 1970
15. Sears DA, Crosby WH: Intravascular hemolysis due to intracardiac prosthetic devices. Am J Med 39:341, 1965
16. Tanaka KR, Valentine WN, Miva S: Pyruvate kinase deficiency hereditary nonspherocytic hemolytic anemia. Blood 19:267, 1962
17. Weed RI: Hereditary spherocytosis. Arch Intern Med 135:1316, 1975

TABLE 6.6–8. CAUSES OF RED CELL FRAGMENTATION

Cardiac Abnormalities
• Cardiac prosthesis
• Unoperated valvular disease
• Valve homografts
• Coarctation of the aorta

Small Vessel Disease (Microangiopathic Hemolytic Anemia)
• Thrombotic thrombocytopenic purpura
• Vasculitis in collagen vascular diseases
• Hemolytic uremic syndrome
• Malignant hypertension
• Eclampsia
• Disseminated carcinoma
• Giant hemangiomas

CHAPTER 6.7
Anemia Associated with Systemic Disease

Jerry L. Spivak

Because of the central role of the blood in the body's economy and its intimate relationship with the other body organs, systemic disease or dysfunction of a particular organ can have a profound influence on blood production. Hypoproliferative anemia resulting from a systemic illness or organ dysfunction is the commonest type of anemia encountered in hospitalized patients.[23] Since its causes are many (see Table 6.2–2) and often correctable and since it is unresponsive to blind therapy with hematinics, the diagnostic approach must be thorough. When erythropoiesis is impaired by organ failure or a systemic disease, the red cells are usually normocytic and normochromic and provide little information concerning the nature of the underlying disorder. Examination of a bone marrow aspirate or biopsy is often required to distinguish the nonspecific anemia associated with inflammation, infection, or neoplasia from anemia due to intrinsic diseases of the marrow such as aplastic anemia, leukemia, myeloproliferative disorders, and myeloma. The marrow aspirate may also reveal maturation defects due to folic acid or vitamin deficiency that are masked in the peripheral blood due to thalassemia trait, simultaneous iron deficiency, or renal disease. Examination of the marrow is also the only means for establishing the presence of red cell aplasia and for evaluating iron stores in the presence of inflammation, infection, malignancy, or liver disease. Even a normal marrow aspirate is helpful in evaluating patients with a normocytic anemia, since it reduces the number of diagnostic possibilities. When marrow cellularity, morphology, and iron stores are normal, a hypoproliferative anemia is usually due to one of two causes: a reduction in erythropoietin production or end organ unresponsiveness to the hormone.

ANEMIAS DUE PRIMARILY TO ORGAN FAILURE

RENAL DISEASE

In the adult, the kidney is the major site of erythropoietin production; small amounts of erythropoietin are made in extrarenal sites such as the liver but are insufficient to sustain an adequate level of erythropoiesis.[13] With significant renal parenchymal damage, erythropoietin production is diminished but the characteristics of the anemia associated with renal disease also reflect the etiology of the renal disease. In acute renal failure, the anemia is usually a consequence of the disorder causing the renal disease (thrombotic thrombocytopenic purpura, hemolytic–uremic syndrome, malignant hypertension, renal cortical necrosis, hemolytic transfusion reaction, bacterial sepsis) with microangiopathic red cell abnormalities and an elevated reticulocyte count. In chronic renal failure due to intrinsic renal disease, the red cells are normocytic with a minor degree of poikilocytosis due to burr cells; red cell survival is modestly decreased, the proportion of erythroid precursors in the marrow is diminished and the reticulocyte count is low. The quality of the anemia may of course be modified by complications of the renal failure (inanition, bleeding, infection, and myelofibrosis due to secondary hyperparathyroidism) or its treatment (dialysis toxins such as aluminum, blood loss during dialysis, dialysis of folic acid, dialysis hypersplenism, and overtransfusion). Although much attention has been directed towards a role for uremic toxins in the anemia of chronic renal disease, with the exception of aluminum,[27] evidence supporting such a role is meager.[27] Plasma levels of both polyamines and parathyroid hormone are elevated in uremic patients. Both substances inhibit erythropoiesis under experimental conditions in vitro. However, neither has a central role in the anemia of uremia since the anemia can be corrected in humans by continuous peritoneal dialysis, which does not effectively remove either substance,[33] and experimentally in uremic animals by administration of erythropoietin.[12] The amelioration of anemia in renal dialysis patients who contract hepatitis[28] and the development of erythrocytosis associated with renal cyst formation in chronically dialyzed patients[26] as well as the lack of anemia in a uremic patient with polycythemia vera[29] also support the contention that insufficient erythropoietin production and not the presence of uremic toxins is the primary defect in the anemia associated with chronic renal disease.

Anemia is a major clinical problem in uremic patients, because of the expense of transfusions and their attendant hazards both to patients and their contacts. Numerous studies have demonstrated that parenteral administration of androgens can enhance red cell production and reduce or abolish transfusion requirements.[14,21] However, androgen therapy also poses a number of hazards, and the untoward effects of long-term therapy with these agents is unknown. They are also unlikely to be effective in anephric patients or in those with a high transfusion requirement.

Since erythropoietin lack is the principal cause for anemia in patients with end-stage renal disease, erythropoietin replacement would be the logical treatment. Human erythropoietin has been purified and molecularly cloned, and the recombinant product has been tested in humans. Recently, in two separate phase I and II clinical trials, it was demonstrated conclusively that recombinant erythropoietin corrects the anemia of end-stage renal disease and abolishes the need for transfusions in anephric patients.[11,32] When available, recombinant erythropoietin should prove to be the treatment of choice for the anemia of end-stage renal disease.

ENDOCRINE DISEASE

Erythropoietin is the only hormone obligatory for red cell proliferation and differentiation, but these processes may be modified directly or indirectly by other growth and developmental hormones.

Androgens enhance erythropoiesis directly by increasing the number of erythropoietin-responsive progenitor cells and indirectly by increasing renal erythropoietin production. Clinically, androgens are responsible for the difference in red cell mass between men and women after puberty, and lack of androgens accounts for the equalization that occurs with castration. Erythrocytosis is a complication of androgen therapy and may be a feature of virilizing tumors. Corticosteroids, growth hormone, and thyroid hormones appear to affect erythropoiesis indirectly through their influence on body metabolism and oxygen consumption. Thyroid hormones may also influence the metabolism of the red cell directly by altering its response to adrenergic agents.[24] Anemia is an uncommon complication of hyperparathyroidism, seen most often in the secondary form of the disease in patients on chronic hemodialysis as a consequence of myelofibrosis.[31] The anemia associated with endocrine disorders is nondescript and usually puzzling unless the intimate relationship of the blood to the body's economy is kept in mind.

THYROID DISEASE

Anemia is a feature of both primary and secondary hypothyroidism.[16] The anemia is generally mild, in part because of a simultaneous reduction in plasma volume as a consequence of the hypothyroid state. The red cells are usually normocytic, but acanthocytes may be prominent. Macrocytosis unassociated with folic acid or vitamin B_{12} deficiency and corrected by thyroxine therapy occurs in a small proportion of patients. Hypothyroidism may be a complication of pernicious anemia, and the two diseases can occur simultaneously. The link between them appears to be one of autoimmunity. Approximately 55 percent of patients with pernicious anemia have antithyroid antibodies, while 32 percent of patients with myxedema have antiparietal cell antibodies.[7]

Iron deficiency is a complication of hypothyroidism. In women, menorrhagia may be the cause. Whether malabsorption of iron has a role is unclear. Many patients have a reduced serum iron and transferrin saturation in the absence of iron deficiency, which responds to the administration of thyroxine alone.[16] In the patient with an uncomplicated disorder, correction of the anemia requires 6 months or more following initiation of thyroid hormone therapy.

POLYENDOCRINOPATHY SYNDROME

As a consequence of autoimmune disease, endocrine disorders may be associated with anemia independent of a link through body metabolism. The association between hypothyroidism and pernicious anemia has been mentioned. The incidence of pernicious anemia is also increased in patients with hyperthyroidism, adrenal insufficiency, or hypoparathyroidism.[7] Often multiple glandular abnormalities are present in the same patient, and in these patients pernicious anemia develops at an earlier age than is usual in individuals without endocrine abnormalities.

LIVER DISEASE

Anemia is a common complication of liver disease and can be produced by a number of mechanisms depending on the nature of the underlying hepatic disorder.[17] Blood loss leading to iron deficiency can occur as a consequence of esophageal varices, gastritis, or peptic ulceration. Malnutrition and ethanol abuse lead to folic acid deficiency. Portal hypertension is associated with an increase in plasma volume, which exaggerates the degree of anemia, and with splenomegaly, which can lead to red cell sequestration.

Abnormalities of red cell shape occur in liver disease in part because of failure of cholesterol esterification.[8] Red cell membrane cholesterol is in equilibrium with that in the plasma, and an in-

crease in plasma-unesterified cholesterol leads to an increase in red cell membrane cholesterol. This results in redundancy of the red cell membrane and the characteristic thin macrocytes and target cells associated with liver disease. In advanced alcoholic liver disease and rarely in fulminant viral hepatitis, acanthocytes (spur cells) and echinocytes (spiculated cells) are observed. The mechanisms responsible for these red cell changes are not entirely defined, but a recent study suggests that echinocyte formation in patients with liver disease is due to red cell binding of abnormal high density lipoproteins.[22] The role of these changes in the shape of the erythrocyte in the anemia of liver disease is unknown.

In addition to specific causes for anemia, there also appears to be a nonspecific depression of red cell production in liver disease. The affinity of hemoglobin for oxygen is reduced, and the hemoglobin-oxygen dissociation curve is shifted to the right.[4] Thus, at any given hemoglobin level more oxygen should be available to the tissues than expected under normal circumstances, and the need for a normal red cell mass may not be necessary. The fact that erythrocytosis develops in some patients with cirrhosis who have arteriovenous shunts suggests that the functional capacity of the marrow remains intact.

ANEMIAS DUE TO IMPAIRED MARROW FUNCTION

PURE RED CELL APLASIA

The syndrome of pure red cell aplasia (PRCA) is characterized by a normocytic, normochromic anemia, absence of reticulocytes, normal leukocyte and platelet counts, and a virtual absence of erythroblasts in the marrow with normal myelopoiesis and megakaryocytopoiesis.[18] Occasionally an increase in marrow lymphocytes and eosinophils is observed. PRCA may be congenital or acquired, and acquired PRCA can be primary or secondary (Table 6.7–1). In primary PRCA, no underlying disease, drug, or toxic exposure can be identified. Some patients with primary PRCA have circulating IgG which is cytotoxic to erythroid precursors; in others no cause for the PRCA is ever evident. In addition to antibodies cytotoxic to erythroblasts, other immunologic abnormalities have been observed in patients with primary PRCA. They include hypogammaglobulinemia, monoclonal gammopathy, and antinuclear antibodies and autoantibodies against red cells or platelets.

A striking feature of acquired PRCA is its close association with thymoma.[15] Fifty percent of patients with acquired PRCA have a thymoma, while approximately 5 percent of patients with

TABLE 6.7–1. CAUSES OF PURE RED CELL APLASIA

Congenital
• Diamond–Blackfan syndrome

Acquired
Primary
• Antibody-mediated
• Idiopathic

Secondary
• Thymoma
• Infections
• Renal failure
• Starvation
• Neoplasms (chronic lymphocytic leukemia, chronic myelogenous leukemia, Hodgkin disease, lymphoma, multiple myeloma, lung carcinoma, gastric carcinoma)
• Hemolytic anemia
• Systemic lupus erythematosus
• Drugs (phenytoin, isoniazid, chlorpropamide, tolbutamide, phenylbutazone, azathioprine, halothane, gold, sulfonamides, chloramphenicol, penicillin, phenobarbital)

a thymoma have PRCA. Most patients with a thymoma and PRCA are women, generally over the age of 50. PRCA never precedes the thymoma but can occur many years after the thymoma appears as well as after its resection. Thymomas are associated with other autoimmune disorders, and patients with thymoma and PRCA have developed systemic lupus erythematosus or myasthenia gravis.[19] There is no correlation between the histology of the thymoma and the development of PRCA or the other autoimmune syndromes.

The diagnosis of PRCA is established from a marrow aspirate. If the cellularity of the aspirate is inadequate, a biopsy must be performed. Because the marrow cellularity is normal in primary PRCA, the diagnosis is not infrequently overlooked. When there is an associated disorder such as myelofibrosis, chronic lymphocytic leukemia, or chronic myelocytic leukemia, the absence of erythroid precursors is even more likely to be missed.

Once a diagnosis of PRCA is established, it is necessary to determine its etiology. When due to a drug or infection, the disorder is self-limited. When present as a complication of an autoimmune disease or neoplasm, treatment of the underlying disease is required to obtain remission of the red cell aplasia. When PRCA is associated with a thymoma, thymectomy is usually required since other forms of therapy are ineffective in the presence of the tumor. Rarely irradiation has been effective in relieving PRCA when the thymoma is unresectable.

If no cause is apparent after an observation period of several months or thymectomy is ineffective, treatment with corticosteroids should be initiated. If no effect is seen within 2 months, immunosuppressive therapy with either cyclophosphamide or azathioprine should be tried. Immunosuppressive agents appear to be effective even if erythroblast antibodies are not detectable. Plasmapheresis has been beneficial in a few patients; splenectomy has been employed when immunosuppressive agents have failed. Spontaneous remissions occur in PRCA, as do relapses following remission induction with drugs.

PROTEIN-CALORIE MALNUTRITION

Starvation produces anemia, but the magnitude of the anemia may be obscured by changes in the plasma volume that are associated with the starved state. The principal defect appears to be a reduction in erythropoietin production.[1] While this in part reflects reduced metabolic demands with a decreased requirement for oxygen, synthesis of the hormone in response to hypoxia is also impaired. The latter may be a consequence of either protein lack or caloric deprivation. Caloric deprivation reduces the level of triiodothyronine (T_3), a hormone required for erythropoietin production.[5] The marrow response to erythropoietin appears to be intact unless the state of malnourishment is extreme. Anemia associated with protein-calorie malnutrition is usually normocytic, but acanthocytes may be prominent due to lack of serum betalipoprotein.[20] There is usually a reduction in marrow cellularity as well as the development of serous fat atrophy. The latter is manifested by the presence of amorphous, gelatinous, pink-staining material in the marrow aspirate. While described as a characteristic feature of anorexia nervosa, serous fat atrophy can be seen in starvation due to other causes.[9] In addition, in anorexia nervosa, as well as other forms of starvation, marrow necrosis occurs.[20] Thus, several factors are involved in the anemia associated with starvation. Leukopenia is also a feature of the starved state and involves lymphocytes, monocytes, and granulocytes, but the marrow granulocyte reserve appears to be normal.[3]

INFILTRATIVE DISEASE OF THE MARROW

Direct involvement of the marrow with suppression of normal hematopoiesis occurs in a variety of disorders in addition to hematologic neoplasms. They include Hodgkin disease, non-Hodgkin lymphomas, myeloma, malignant histiocytosis, malignancies of

other organs, particularly the lung, prostate, stomach, breast, and thyroid, disseminated infection with atypical mycobacteria, and Gaucher disease. Myelofibrosis or infiltration of the marrow by tumor or granulomas may stimulate extramedullary hematopoiesis with the appearance of nucleated erythroid and myeloid precursors and misshapen red cells (tear-drop forms) in the circulation. The term "leukoerythroblastic reaction" has been used to describe these abnormalities, which are not specific for invasion of the bone marrow by tumor but may be seen in a variety of nonmalignant disorders such as hemorrhage, hemolysis, megaloblastic anemia, drug reactions, and infections.[25] The absence of peripheral blood abnormalities, however, does not exclude the presence of tumor within the marrow. The degree of anemia associated with infiltrative disease of the marrow depends on the nature of the underlying disease and its duration. The extent of marrow involvement by tumor or reactive fibrosis is often not sufficient to account for the observed suppression of hematopoiesis. Other factors involved include inanition, marrow necrosis, and inhibition of hematopoietic cell proliferation by tumor products.

Pancytopenia or a leukoerythroblastic reaction without a discernible cause are indications for a bone marrow biopsy. Aplastic anemia cannot be differentiated from other causes of pancytopenia without a biopsy because this is the only technique for evaluating marrow cellularity. A biopsy is also necessary for establishing the presence of fibrosis within the marrow. Marrow fibrosis is a reactive phenomenon that is associated with acute and chronic myeloproliferative disorders, metastatic tumor, or certain metabolic abnormalities such as hyperparathyroidism. While tumor cells can be identified in marrow aspirates, the frequency with which metastatic tumor is identified is increased severalfold when a biopsy is obtained. Overall, the frequency of positive marrow biopsies in patients with malignant disease is approximately 30 to 40 percent, depending on the type of tumor. Performing bilateral biopsies can increase the yield 20 to 50 percent. In granulomatous disorders such as tuberculosis or sarcoidosis, bone marrow biopsy has a much lower diagnostic yield (15 to 30 percent) than either liver, lung, or lymph node biopsy.

INFECTION

Infections can produce anemia by a variety of mechanisms, depending on the type of infection and the characteristics of the host (Table 6.7–2).[2] Hookworm infection leads to iron deficiency and fish tapeworm infection to vitamin B_{12} deficiency if the parasite load is large. Hemolysis can be induced by direct infection of red cells (malaria, Bartonellosis), by toxin secretion (clostridia), or by immune mechanisms (mycoplasma, malaria, syphilis, infectious mononucleosis, and other viral infections). In patients with preexisting hemolysis, viral or bacterial infections accelerate red cell destruction by enhancing reticuloendothelial system activity. A predisposition to infection with certain organisms such as *Salmonella* also exists in hemolytic states because of involvement of the reticuloendothelial system in erythrophagocytosis. In sickle cell anemia, this relative reticuloendothelial cell blockade is magnified by splenic atrophy, increasing the risk of overwhelming infections with encapsulated organisms such as the pneumococcus. In individuals with red cell G6PD deficiency, viral or bacterial infections induce hemolysis probably as a consequence of oxidant injury to the red cells by hydrogen peroxide generated in activated leukocytes.

Suppression of hematopoiesis as well as increased cell destruction occurs as a consequence of certain infections. Aplastic anemia is a complication of viral hepatitis and, rarely, infectious mononucleosis. Bacterial and fungal infections can produce bone marrow necrosis. Patients with chronic hemolytic anemias also develop transient aplastic crises with viral infections. Although white cells and platelets as well as red cells may be involved, most often the transient aplastic crisis is manifested by the rapid development of profound anemia. While there is reason to believe that a similar transient depression of hematopoiesis occurs with viral infections in normal individuals, it only becomes clinically evident when there is a marked reduction in red cell life span. Consequently, when patients with chronic hemolytic anemia develop fever, the reticulocyte count should be monitored to detect the development of a transient aplastic crisis. Another clue is the lessening of jaundice in these habitually icteric individuals.

ANEMIA ASSOCIATED WITH SYSTEMIC DISEASE

Although infection, inflammation, and neoplasms can cause anemia by a variety of well-defined mechanisms, more commonly the anemia observed in these conditions is of a nonspecific nature and not distinguishable on the basis of the underlying illness.[6] The anemia is generally mild (hemoglobin levels of 10 to 11 g/dl), and the red cells are normocytic and normochromic, although microcytosis and hypochromia can be observed. The corrected reticulocyte count is low for the degree of anemia, and the bilirubin level is not elevated. Red cell life span is modestly reduced, but the marrow is unable to compensate even though its cellularity is normal and there is no evidence of maturation abnormalities. Serum iron and transferrin saturation are reduced, but in contrast to iron deficiency anemia, serum transferrin is low while serum ferritin levels are elevated and marrow iron stores are normal or increased. Erythropoietin levels are not appropriately elevated for the degree of anemia, but this is not invariable. Since chronic illness is often associated with a low serum T_3 level, the reduction in erythropoietin may only reflect a decrease in tissue oxygen demands.[30] Ferrokinetic studies have revealed a block in the release of reticuloendothelial iron to the plasma. This may be the most important abnormality in the anemia associated with systemic disease.[10] In certain situations, however, such as when there is tumor in the marrow, erythropoiesis may be ineffective, with resultant intramedullary cell death. The role of agents such as endotoxin, interleukin-2, interferon, and prostaglandins as well as cell-cell interactions involving lymphocytes, macrophages, and hematopoietic progenitor cells remains undefined. Not to be overlooked, however, is the contribution to the anemia provided by repeated phlebotomies for diagnostic purposes in a setting of limited marrow proliferative activity.

The anemia associated with systemic disease is, of course, a diagnosis of exclusion, and because it may in part mimic iron deficiency anemia, bone marrow aspiration may be required to establish the correct diagnosis. The anemia usually remits with alleviation of the underlying disease. Indeed, a gradual improvement in the hematocrit is a good indicator of successful therapy and is a

TABLE 6.7–2. INFECTION AND ANEMIA

Infection Deficiency Anemia
- Hookworm

Megaloblastic Anemia
- Fish tapeworm

Hemolytic Anemia
- Nonimmune
   Malaria
   Bartonellosis
   Clostridia
   Viral hepatitis
- Immune
   Malaria
   Syphilis
   Infectious mononucleosis
   Mycoplasma pneumoniae

Hypoproliferative or Aplastic Anemia
- Viral hepatitis
- Infectious mononucleosis
- Parvovirus

useful guide when treating patients with disorders such as bacterial endocarditis.

REFERENCES

1. Anagnostou A, Schade S, et al: Effect of protein deprivation on erythropoiesis. Blood 50:1093, 1977
2. Barrett-Connor E: Anemia and infection. Am J Med 52:242, 1972
3. Bowers TK, Eckert E: Leukopenia in anorexia nervosa. Arch Intern Med 138:1520, 1978
4. Caldwell PRB, Fritts HW, Cournand A: Oxyhemoglobin dissociation curve in liver disease. J Appl Physiol 20:316, 1965
5. Caro J, Silver R, et al: Erythropoietin production in fasted rats. J Lab Clin Med 98:860, 1981
6. Cartwright GE: The anemia of chronic disorders. Semin Hematol 3:351, 1966
7. Chanarin I: The Megaloblastic Anemias. Oxford, Blackwell Scientific, 1979, p 332
8. Cooper RA: Abnormalities of cell membrane fluidity in the pathogenesis of disease. N Engl J Med 297:371, 1977
9. Cornbleet PJ, Moir RC, Wolf PL: A histochemical study of bone marrow hypoplasia in anorexia nervosa. Virchows Arch A Path Anat Histol 374:239, 1977
10. Douglas SW, Adamson JW: The anemia of chronic disorders: Studies of marrow regulation and iron metabolism. Blood 45:55, 1975
11. Eschbach JW, Egrie JC, et al: Correction of the anemia of end-stage renal disease with recombinant human erythropoietin: Result of a phase I and II clinical trial. N Engl J Med 316:73, 1987
12. Eschbach JW, Mladenovic J: The anemia of chronic renal failure in sheep, response to erythropoietin-rich plasma in vivo. J Clin Invest 74:434, 1984
13. Fried W: Erythropoietin and the kidney. Nephron 15:327, 1975
14. Hendler ED, Goffinet JA, et al: Controlled study of androgen therapy in anemia of patients on maintenance hemodialysis. N Engl J Med 291:1046, 1974
15. Hirst E, Robertson TI: The syndrome of thymoma and erythroblastopenic anemia. Medicine 46:225, 1967
16. Horton L, Coburn RJ, et al: The haematology of hypothyroidism. Q J Med 45:101, 1976
17. Kimber C, Deller DJ, et al: The mechanism of anaemia in chronic liver disease. Q J Med 34:33, 1965
18. Krantz SB: Diagnosis and treatment of pure red cell aplasia. Med Clin N Am 60:945, 1976
19. Mackechnie H-LN, Squires AH, et al: Thymoma, myasthenia gravis, erythroblastopenic anemia, and systemic lupus erythematosus in one patient. Can Med Assoc J 109:733, 1973
20. Mant MJ, Faragher BS: The haematology of anorexia nervosa. Br J Haematol 23:737, 1972
21. Neff MS, Goldberg J, et al: A comparison of androgens for anemia in patients on hemodialysis. N Engl J Med 304:871, 1981
22. Owen JS, Brown DJC, et al: Erythrocyte echinocytosis in liver disease. Role of abnormal plasma high density lipoproteins. J Clin Invest 76:2275, 1985
23. Paine CJ, Polk A, Eichner ER: Analysis of anemia in medical inpatients. Am J Med Sci 268:37, 1974
24. Popovic WJ, Brown JE, Adamson JW: The influence of thyroid hormones on in vitro erythropoiesis. J Clin Invest 60:907, 1977
25. Retief FP: Leuco-erythroblastosis in the adult. Lancet 1:639, 1964
26. Shalhoub RJ, Rajan U, et al: Erythrocytosis in patients on long-term hemodialysis. Ann Intern Med 97:686, 1982
27. Short AIK, Winney RT, et al: Reversible microcytic hypochromic anemia in dialysis patients due to aluminum intoxication. Proc EDTA 17:226, 1980
28. Simon P, Meyrier A, et al: Improvement of anaemia in hemodialyzed patients after viral or toxic hepatic cytolysis. Br Med J 280:892, 1980
29. Spivak JL, Cooke CR: Polycythemia vera in an anephric man. Am J Med Sci 272:339, 1976
30. Utiger RD: Decreased extrathyroidal triiodothyronine production in nonthyroidal illness: Benefit or harm? Am J Med 69:807, 1980
31. Weinberg SG, Lubin A, et al: Myelofibrosis and renal osteodystrophy. Am J Med 63:755, 1977
32. Winearls GC, Oliver DO, et al: Effect of human erythropoietin derived from recombinant DNA on the anemia of patients maintained by chronic haemodialysis. Lancet 2:1175, 1986
33. Zappacosta AR, Caro J, Erslev A: Normalization of hematocrit in patients with end-stage renal disease on continuous ambulatory peritoneal dialysis. Am J Med 72:53, 1982

Bleeding: Hemostasis, Approach to Patient, and Vascular Defects

William R. Bell and Dudley P. Jackson

Humans are dependent for survival on the capacity of blood to remain fluid within the circulatory system and to effect hemostasis promptly following injury to blood vessels. Patients with bleeding are encountered frequently in the practice of medicine. Blood loss is minimized by (1) vascular integrity and the soft tissue support of small vessels, (2) circulating blood platelets, and (3) plasma proteins that are responsible for the coagulation process. A rational approach to the patient with bleeding requires an understanding of normal hemostasis.

HEMOSTASIS[3,9,11-13]

Normal hemostasis depends upon a complex series of interrelated reactions involving blood vessels, platelets, and coagulation. These mechanisms become operative immediately following disruption of the blood vessel wall.[7]

BLOOD VESSELS

The first change appreciated is contraction of the vessel wall mediated by nerve stimuli acting on smooth muscle. This vasoconstriction impedes blood flow to the site of disruption and is followed almost instantly by formation of a hemostatic plug consisting of masses of adherent and aggregated platelets that become meshed between strands of fibrin. Vasoactive substances liberated from platelets may enhance vasoconstriction.

PLATELETS

Disruption of the blood vessel wall also initiates changes in blood platelets involving a series of reactions designated as adhesion, release, and aggregation. Loss of vascular integrity and distortion of endothelial cells results in exposure of blood to collagen and connective tissue fibers, and platelets migrate and adhere to the dam-

aged site. This platelet adhesion is the initial event in formation of the platelet plug. The surface of the platelet consisting of the trilaminar plasma membrane covered with acid mucopolysaccharides and glycoproteins permits adhesion to the damaged endothelial cell in the presence of calcium, fibrinogen-fibrin, and von Willebrand factor (vWF). This interaction between platelet membrane and endothelial cell initiates transmission of stimuli to the internal milieu of the platelet resulting in the appearance of two phospholipase enzymes that initiate the metabolism of arachidonic acid. The free arachidonic acid is converted to a prostaglandin compound, endoperoxide PGG_2, by a cyclooxygenase enzyme. PGG_2 spontaneously converts to PGH_2, which subsequently is converted by thromboxane synthetase to thromboxane A_2. Formation of this compound and its secretion out of the platelet is the result of the platelet undergoing the release reaction. Thromboxane A_2 is unstable and directly induces the release reaction in surrounding platelets primarily by reduction of cyclic adenosine monophosphate (AMP) concentration and activity, thereby promoting the release reaction. This reaction results from the interaction of distinct components in the platelet cytoplasm that include granules, mitochondria, glycogen-containing particles, and a Golgi apparatus. Three types of granules of particular importance in the release reaction have been identified, and each contains components that mediate the aggregation of platelets. The alpha granules contain fibrinogen, platelet factor 4, β-thromboglobulin, platelet derived growth factor, fibronectin, and vWF; delta granules (dense bodies) contain calcium, adenosine diphosphate (ADP), potassium, serotonin, and catecholamines; and lambda granules (lysosomal granules) contain cathepsin, histone, β-glucuronidase and phosphatase. In response to stimuli initiated by the interaction of platelet and endothelial cell membranes these granules secrete and release their contents, which amplify the message of aggregation of additional platelets in the initiation of thrombus formation. The central component in amplification of this message is ADP. Exposure of the platelet membrane to ADP prepares and facilitates the glycoprotein IIb-IIIa receptor to bind fibrinogen to the platelet membrane. The bound fibrinogen (from the plasma or from the alpha granule) in the presence of calcium is the essential mediator of the aggregation reaction. The release reaction is inhibited or modulated by substances that increase the concentration of or prevent the degradation of cyclic AMP in the platelet internal milieu. The most important of these agents is prostacyclin (designated PGI_2) which is synthesized by vascular endothelial cells. PGI_2 enhances the activity and production of adenylate cyclase. This agent is the most potent inhibitor of platelet aggregation and platelet plug formation that has been identified in the human body.

COAGULATION

Platelets also participate in a facilitory manner in the interaction of coagulation proteins leading to formation of fibrin (see Chapter 6.10). Platelets provide a lipoprotein reaction surface upon which procoagulant enzymes and their respective substrates interact. A receptor site for factor Xa is exposed on activated platelets—i.e., platelets undergoing aggregation and the release reaction. Upon binding to the platelet membrane lipoprotein, factor Xa, along with factor Va, converts prothrombin (factor II) to thrombin, a potent serine protease. The thrombin initiates fibrin polymer formation from fibrinogen, which is intimately in place, thereby stabilizing and providing the network support structure of the hemostatic plug. The initiation of this localized process of solidification results from the release of four peptides from the dimeric fibrinogen molecule (two fibrinopeptides from the alpha chain and two fibrinopeptides from the beta chain) by the enzymatic cleavage activity of thrombin. Release of these peptides through sequential stages yields the lengthy fibrin polymer. This compound is connected by end-to-end and end-to-side anastomotic bonding and although stable can be reversibly solubilized in solutions of urea

and monochlor acetic acid. In the final stage of fibrin polymer formation the solid lattice support structure of fibrin becomes irreversibly insolubilized through the process of transamidation by factor XIII, a transglutaminase cross-linking enzyme that covalently links glutamyl and lysyl amino acid residues, in the presence of calcium, on carboxyl termini of adjacent lambda chains and approximated alpha chains. The resultant fibrin polymer is irreversibly insoluble and depending on the degree of cross-linking is resistant to the digestive degradation of plasmin. Retraction of the fibrin clot occurs, requires viable platelets, and is mediated by the contractile protein thrombasthenin. When this entire process is unchecked, as in certain pathologic states, it is the beginning of thrombus formation and vascular obstruction.

FIBRINOLYSIS

As blood vessels are repaired following injury, it is necessary that fibrin clots be broken down and removed in order to reestablish and maintain normal blood flow. The lysis of fibrin clots is accomplished by a proteolytic enzyme, plasmin. The active enzyme is derived from an inactive precursor, plasminogen, by the action of various substances present in plasma and tissues. One plasminogen activator, urokinase, has been purified from human urine; and another, streptokinase, has been purified from extracts of β-hemolytic streptococci. The circulating plasma usually contains potent inhibitors of fibrinolysis, and it is presumed that various components of the fibrinolytic system are adsorbed into the fibrin clot, thereby avoiding inactivation before the formation of active plasmin.

AN APPROACH TO THE BLEEDING PATIENT[1,3,9,11-13]

Bleeding may result from a defect in any stage of normal hemostasis, and in some instances multiple defects may be operative. Determination of the cause(s) of bleeding is aided by an etiologic classification (Table 6.8–1). The mode of presentation of the bleeding problem dictates the approach taken by the clinician during evaluation of the patient. The procedure most likely to identify the nature of the hemorrhage is a detailed personal and family history.[1] A careful physical examination is a necessity. Laboratory testing is essential for precise identification of disorders of blood platelets and coagulation but often is unnecessary in the evaluation of patients with vascular defects.

The first consideration is to decide whether the bleeding is secondary to vascular defects including mechanical manipulation or is resulting from endogenous pathology (i.e., disorder of platelets or coagulation). Bleeding associated with an anatomically identifiable focal lesion usually is the result of a mechanical problem inducing vessel disruption. Local bleeding disproportional to the degree of injury suggests an underlying hemostatic defect. Generalized, spontaneous bleeding usually is due to an underlying hemostatic defect that may be congenital or acquired. Congenitally inherited abnormalities of the platelet system, the coagulation system, or the fibrinolytic system usually are single defects, with rare exceptions confined to one of those three systems. In contrast, acquired hemostatic defects more commonly result from combined disturbances in those three systems.

PERSONAL HISTORY

The patient must be questioned as to whether the problem of bleeding has been lifelong thereby suggesting a congenital disorder, or is of recent onset suggesting an acquired disorder. Is the bleeding spontaneous or is trauma required for the bleeding to begin? Spontaneous bleeding without associated trauma suggests a hem-

TABLE 6.8–1. CAUSES OF BLEEDING

Vascular Defects
Mechanical
- Trauma
  Injuries and lacerations
  Factitious
  Abuse by others
- Erosions and ulcerations of vessels
- Orthostasis

Structural
- Congenital
  Hereditary hemorrhagic telangiectasia (Osler–Weber–Rendu disease)
  Cavernous hemangioma (Kasabach–Merritt syndrome)
  Angiokeratoma corporis diffusum (Fabry disease)
  Connective tissue disorders
    Ehlers–Danlos syndrome
    Marfan syndrome
    Pseudoxanthoma elasticum
    Osteogenesis imperfecta
- Acquired
  Senile purpura
  Excessive corticosteroids (steroid purpura)
  Scurvy
  Angiodysplasia of the gastrointestinal vessels
  Amyloidosis
  Kaposi sarcoma and other vascular tumors

Hypersensitivity States
- Vasculitis
- Henoch–Schönlein syndrome

Infections
- Bacterial
- Viral
- Parasites

Miscellaneous
- Purpura simplex
- Autoerythrocyte sensitization (? psychogenic purpura)
- Purpura associated with various dermatologic disorders

Disorders of Blood Platelets (see Chapter 6.9)
Quantitative Disorders
- Thrombocytopenia
  Congenital
  Acquired (the most common hematologic cause of bleeding)
- Thrombocytosis
  Primary
  Secondary

Qualitative Disorders
- Congenital
- Acquired

Disorders of Blood Coagulation (see Chapter 6.10)
Congenital
- Deficient synthesis of specific coagulation factor(s)
- Synthesis of functionally defective coagulation factor(s)

Acquired
- Accelerated utilization of coagulation factors (disseminated intravascular coagulation)
- Deficient or defective coagulation factor(s)
- Inhibitors of coagulation (anticoagulants)
  Spontaneous
  Therapeutic (see Chapter 6.25)

orrhagic disorder. The patient's response to surgery (including severing the umbilical cord at birth, circumcision, dental extractions, tonsillectomy, etc.) and major or minor trauma should be evaluated. Excessive bleeding following minimal trauma suggests a hemorrhagic disorder. The degree of trauma may be difficult to assess, and it should be recalled that certain types of surgery (e.g., tonsillectomy and adenoidectomy) are more likely to result in bleeding than are others (e.g., herniorrhaphy) even in normal individuals.

Bleeding resulting from vascular defects or platelet disorders usually occurs immediately after an exciting event such as trauma or surgery; in contrast, bleeding usually is delayed by several hours or days in patients with congenital disorders of coagulation. Has the patient required transfusion of blood resulting from substantial blood loss, and if so, did the bleeding cease, or did it continue despite transfusion? It is important to determine whether the bleeding was generalized or local. Was it confined to the area of trauma or surgery? Is the same site recurrently involved, or is the bleeding widespread and migratory? The time required for the bleeding to cease and the ecchymoses or purpura to clear without intervention, and the occurrence of delayed bleeding, are helpful in identifying the problem. The site and type of bleeding (i.e., skin, mucous membrane, articular, periarticular, subcutaneous soft tissue, gastrointestinal, genitourinary, central nervous system, etc.) must be ascertained. Cutaneous petechiae and spontaneous mucous membrane bleeding suggest a vascular or platelet disorder. Hemarthroses are common in congenital disorders of blood coagulation (e.g., hemophilia), but are not seen in disorders of platelets. Simultaneous bleeding from multiple nonadjacent sites is most consistent with concomitant disorders of coagulation proteins, platelets, and vascular integrity such as are seen in disseminated intravascular coagulation (DIC) or thrombotic thrombocytopenic purpura (TTP).

The history must be complete and extend beyond a discussion focused only on bleeding manifestations. Most acquired hemostatic defects are associated with underlying systemic illness. Symptoms suggestive of disorders of the liver, kidneys, collagen vascular system, and immune system should be sought. Abnormal bleeding may be a feature of neoplasia, infections, malabsorption, shock, and complications of obstetrics. Particular attention should be directed at a detailed history of drug intake. A variety of drugs may adversely affect vascular integrity, platelets, and coagulation proteins. Direct questioning regarding use of over-the-counter compounds containing aspirin is important. Certain antibiotics may alter platelet function and adversely affect coagulation proteins. Bleeding due to surreptitious use of anticoagulants has been well described, most often in individuals working in medically related fields.

FAMILY HISTORY

A detailed family history often is helpful in facilitating the correct diagnosis. At times, it confirms the diagnosis suggested by personal history and laboratory data. In pursuing the family history it is essential that the persons designated by the patient are, in fact, the true biologic mother, father, sibling, and so on, and not related by adoption or some other means. All available blood relatives should be questioned, their sex correctly identified, and then studied.

When taking a family history, knowledge of the inheritance patterns of the known hemostatic defects is essential. The most common inherited coagulation factor deficiency states are factors VIII and IX. Factor VIII deficiency is found in two distinctly different disorders: (1) hemophilia A, or classic hemophilia, and (2) von Willebrand disease. Factor IX deficiency is also known as hemophilia B, or Christmas disease. Of all known congenital coagulation deficiency states only hemophilia A and hemophilia B are X-linked recessively inherited. Von Willebrand disease (three different types) is inherited in an autosomal dominant pattern. Deficiencies of factors I, II, V, VII, X, XI, XII, prekallikrein, and high-molecular-weight kininogen are inherited in an autosomal recessive fashion. Classically, carriers and relatives of affected individuals possess a level of approximately 35 to 50 percent of normal of the deficient factor. An autosomal dominant pattern is observed in hereditary hemorrhagic telangiectasia, some qualitative platelet defects, and dysfibrinogenemia. Congenital multiple factor deficiency states usually are inherited in an autosomal dominant pattern. A negative family history does not eliminate the possibility of a congenital factor deficiency state because approximately 20 to 30 per-

cent of newly recognized factor deficiency states appear to result from spontaneous mutations.

PHYSICAL EXAMINATION

Particular attention should be given to the site and type of bleeding present. Cutaneous and mucous membrane bleeding in the form of petechiae and purpuric lesions is characteristic of thrombocytopenia, platelet dysfunction, and sometimes vascular defects. Ecchymoses (i.e., bruises) may be associated with any defect of hemostasis, but hematoma formation of cutaneous, subcutaneous, or deeper body tissues or organs is more characteristic of disorders of coagulation, especially coagulation factor deficiency states. The diagnosis of hereditary hemorrhagic telangiectasia and cavernous hemangioma often can be made when telangiectatic or localized endotheliomatous hemangiomatous lesions are identified. One must not confuse telangiectatic lesions, which blanch on pressure, and petechiae, which do not blanch. Signs of spontaneous hemarthroses are virtually diagnostic of congenital deficiency of a coagulation factor (i.e., factor VIII or IX).

The physical examination must extend beyond the bleeding lesions. A detailed examination of the skin and the presence of lymphadenopathy, splenomegaly, ascites, or other features of hepatic or renal disorders may provide useful clues. Stigmata suggestive of disorders of circulation, connective tissue, collagen vascular disease, neoplasia, and so forth, are important. In sum, proper evaluation of the patient with bleeding requires not only a detailed history but also a complete physical examination.

LABORATORY STUDIES

Although the history and physical examinations are the most helpful and reproducibly reliable screening techniques for hemorrhagic diseases, there are situations where some laboratory tests are indicated in the comprehensive approach to identify a patient at risk to bleed.[2,5,6,8] This problem arises in a patient who must experience a surgical procedure. The consequences of even routine and simple surgical procedures in the patient with an underlying hemorrhagic disorder may be disastrous and even fatal. Today because of the degree of subspecialization some physicians are not familiar with the appropriate questions or do not take the time to obtain an adequate personal and family history. Sometimes the patient cannot give a reliable history, and occasionally the patient cannot given any history because of an underlying disease process, i.e., seizures, coma, and so forth. Some patients with bleeding disorders are asymptomatic with a negative past history because they have never experienced trauma or a surgical procedure. Not all surgical procedures uncover a bleeding disorder, and some patients asymptomatically acquire a hemorrhagic disease following the last surgical procedure. Patients with various neoplastic diseases frequently have associated problems with bleeding.[10] Bleeding in the cancer patient may result from the primary disease process, the non-specificity of the therapy they must receive to treat the neoplasm, or from associated diseases, infection, metabolic disorders, and nutritional deficiency that are common in the patient with neoplasm. For these reasons and for patients who are in these categories, laboratory screening tests have a role in optimal patient management.

With an understanding of the various aspects of hemostasis one can thoughtfully select those laboratory studies that monitor the functional integrity of the different components and phases of the platelet function, coagulation factor, and fibrinolytic systems. The initial assessment of a bleeding disorder should include the following screening tests:

1. Platelet count and examination of peripheral blood film prepared with blood obtained from finger puncture to verify the platelet count and also to evaluate RBC and WBC morphology

2. Bleeding time—performed in a standardized manner by an experienced person—to provide information regarding platelets and blood vessels, as does a tourniquet test
3. Prothrombin time (PT)—to examine factors II, V, VII, and X
4. Partial thromboplastin time (activated [APTT] or nonactivated [PTT] technique)—to provide information on the intactness of all the coagulation proteins and their interaction (except factors VII and XIII). The test is most sensitive for factors VIII, IX, XI, and XII.[5]
5. If either the PT or APTT/PTT are prolonged, testing for the presence of a circulating anticoagulant must be performed
6. Thrombin clotting time (TT)—to provide information on the interaction of thrombin and fibrinogen and allow quantitation of the amount of fibrinogen present

If the above mentioned studies do not allow precise identification of the problem, individual specific coagulation factor assays and additional special studies may be required. Hemophilia A and hemophilia B can be separated from each other only by laboratory testing,[4] and this separation is crucial since the appropriate therapeutic modalities are different.

VASCULAR DEFECTS[3,9,11-13]

Bleeding due to defects of blood vessels (Table 6.8–1) are common and may be acquired or congenital. The cause of the defect may be obvious, but in many patients a detailed history and physical examination are required to recognize the cause and avoid unnecessary laboratory studies. Platelet numbers and function as well as the coagulation proteins usually are normal except as noted.

MECHANICAL DEFECTS

Trauma

Injuries and Lacerations. The most common cause of bleeding is injury to blood vessels. The causes of bleeding are easily recognized when the injuries occur in association with major trauma or surgery. In some instances, the injury may be less obvious. For example, a large subgaleal hemorrhage may be seen following a wrestling match in which prolonged or severe constriction and pressure have been applied to the head and neck. Petechiae or ecchymoses resulting from suction of the skin ("love bites") are well known. They are elliptical or round lesions of the skin that may appear after love making. The term "cyclops purpura" has been used to describe a rounded or circular lesion on the skin—often the forehead—of children following application of sucker toys.

Factitious. Factitial purpura is relatively common and may be difficult to diagnose. It is the result of self-flagellation with various objects or sucking of the skin including sucking of air from a glass or bag placed over the face. The lesions occur on the accessible areas of the body and may be quite bizarre depending upon the nature of the trauma. The term "Munchausen syndrome" has been used to describe individuals who simulate a bleeding state by self-induced hemorrhage. Hematuria due either to self-injury or addition of blood from another source to urine is a particularly common finding in this syndrome. Serious bleeding due to coagulation disorders may be induced by self-administration of anticoagulant agents. Patients usually deny self-inflicting trauma or surreptitious ingestion of drugs.

Abuse by Others. Bleeding due to this distressing cause is well described. The initial history may be misleading because of denial. Multiple lesions usually are present, often of different ages. The nature of the lesions depends on the type of trauma inflicted. The term "battered child" has been used to describe young children

with this disorder, and the presence of multiple injuries including recent or old fractures has been emphasized. Abuse by others can occur at any age and is being recognized with increasing frequency in the elderly.

Erosions and Ulcerations of Vessels

These lesions usually are the result of inflammation, infection, pressure, or mass lesions (i.e., tumors). Such lesions of cutaneous vessels are easily recognized. Diagnostic problems arise when the lesions occur in other sites—especially the respiratory, gastrointestinal, and genitourinary systems. Bleeding, especially severe bleeding, may be difficult to localize. Proper identification of the bleeding site often requires other diagnostic tests including invasive procedures.

Orthostasis

Purpura occurs most often at the site of maximum venous pressure in capillaries, usually the lower extremities. Purpura may be increased by constricting garments such as garters or arm bands. Purpura of the face, head, or neck may occur as the result of increased capillary pressure associated with the Valsalva maneuver, coughing, vomiting and retching, strangling, superior vena caval obstruction, or the current practice of hanging by one's feet for relief of back pain.

STRUCTURAL DEFECTS

Congenital Defects (see also Chapter 5.3)

Hereditary Hemorrhagic Telangiectasia (Osler–Weber–Rendu Disease). This disorder is transmitted as an autosomal dominant and is characterized by structural anomaly of arteries and veins—i.e., telangiectases—on the skin and mucosa. The visible telangiectases occur most often on the lips, tongue, palate, face, hands, and feet. The diagnosis usually is made on the basis of the history and physical examination, especially if the typical lesions are found on multiple members of the family. Bleeding occurs from the telangiectases most commonly in the form of epistaxes and gastrointestinal bleeding. The cutaneous lesions will bleed if traumatized, and hematuria may occur. Pulmonary arteriovenous fistula with polycythemia and hepatic cirrhosis have been described. Tests of blood platelets and coagulation are normal except for the rare patient with coexistent hemophilia or von Willebrand disease. Local measures may be helpful in treating active bleeding, but surgery rarely is indicated because of the likelihood of bleeding from other lesions. Chronic blood loss often results in iron deficiency anemia, which should be treated with oral iron therapy often on a continuing basis.

Cavernous Hemangioma (Kasabach–Merritt Syndrome). The lesions are cavernous ("strawberry"), soft vascular malformations often noted early in life. The lesions occur in the skin and various organs, especially the liver and spleen. The lesions frequently expand and can become quite large. Thrombocytopenia may be noted, and some of these patients develop findings of DIC.

Angiokeratoma Corporis Diffusum (Fabry Disease). This disorder is transmitted as X-linked dominant or intermediate. It is due to the absence of the enzyme trihexosylceramide galactosyl hydrolase from skin fibroblasts and is characterized by telangiectases that do not blanch completely on pressure and are often clustered on the abdomen, hips, scrotum, and thighs. Vasomotor disturbances, corneal opacities, and renal failure may be seen.

Connective Tissue Disorders. Platelet morphology and aggregation may be abnormal in certain heritable disorders of connective tissue, but the bleeding results from abnormalities of smaller blood vessels and associated connective tissue. Defective fibronectin has been considered to play a role in the platelet dysfunction and hyperextensibility of the joints. *Ehlers–Danlos syndrome* represents a group of disorders of collagen characterized by laxity and hyperextensibility of skin and joints, fragility of skin, and bleeding. The bleeding is most prominent in type IV, which may be inherited as autosomal dominant or autosomal recessive. Ecchymoses and subcutaneous hematomas are common, but bleeding may occur from multiple sites including following rupture of vessels. Elective surgery should be avoided because of the risk of bleeding and poor wound healing. *Marfan syndrome* is an autosomal dominant disorder due to a defect of collagen and characterized by excessive height, long thin extremities, weakness of the aortic media, ectopia lentis, and bleeding (ecchymoses and operative bleeding). *Pseudoxanthoma elasticum* is an autosomal recessive disorder of elastic fibers characterized by lax skin often with telangiectases and ecchymoses. Bleeding may occur from multiple organ systems. *Osteogenesis imperfecta* is an autosomal dominant disorder of collagen which results in defective bone matrix and brittle bones and may be associated with purpura, epistaxis, hemoptysis, and intracranial bleeding.

Acquired Defects

Senile Purpura. As the name implies, this disorder is seen in older individuals. It is characterized by intracutaneous hemorrhagic lesions occurring most commonly on the dorsum of the hands and the extensor surfaces of the wrists and forearms, but any area of the body may be involved. The overlying skin is thin and has a characteristic appearance resembling parchment paper due to loss of support tissue and collagen, which is thought to be the cause. The lesions are well demarcated, have a red-purple color, and move with the skin. Darkly pigmented areas may remain as the lesions resolve. This disorder usually can be identified on the basis of the history and physical examination. Care should be taken after venipuncture since this procedure may be followed by new lesions, but surgery carries no increased risk of bleeding. This disorder is of only cosmetic importance and is not associated with a hemorrhagic diathesis.

Steroid Purpura. Excessive corticosteroids, either endogenous (Cushing syndrome) or exogenous (long-term therapy), often result in cutaneous lesions indistinguishable from those seen in senile purpura and presumably due to increased catabolism of collagen. The presence of purple striae and other clues provided by the history and physical examination should result in the correct diagnosis.

Scurvy. Scorbutic bleeding (scurvy) characteristically presents with perifollicular petechiae and ecchymoses occurring most commonly on the legs. Gingival bleeding is common. Subperiosteal bleeding is seen in children. Subcutaneous hematoma and hemarthroses have been described, and sudden death may occur. The bleeding is attributable to decreased or defective collagen, which is attributable to defective hydroxyproline synthesis in the absence of vitamin C (ascorbic acid). Other features of scurvy including anemia and follicular hyperkeratosis may provide clues, and tests of capillary resistance (i.e., tourniquet test) are invariably abnormal. The bleeding manifestations (and abnormal tourniquet test) respond promptly to administration of vitamin C, which should be initiated promptly.

Angiodysplasia of the Gastrointestinal Vessels. This disorder or syndrome has not been fully characterized, but is being recognized with increasing frequency, especially with the use of new endoscopic techniques. Multiple arteriovenous malformations usually are present, and bleeding may occur from any level of the gastrointestinal tract. The lesions appear to be more common in older individuals and may be associated with valvular heart disease, renal disease, and possibly myelodysplastic syndromes. An inheritance pattern has not been defined, and possible overlap with congenital defects of small vessels (especially hereditary hemorrhagic telangiectasia) awaits further study. Therapy is difficult because bleeding may occur from various sites at different times, and visualization of the lesions per se does not establish them as the site of bleeding.

Amyloidosis. Purpura in patients with amyloidosis, in contrast to most other disorders, usually is manifest in the upper portions of the body. Periorbital ecchymoses are common. Large ecchymoses on the forehead, face, neck, and chest may occur spontaneously or with minimal trauma ("pinch purpura"). Bleeding from the gastrointestinal and urinary tracts may be seen. Infiltration of the blood vessel wall by amyloid causes the purpura. In addition to the loss of vessel wall integrity produced by the amyloidosis, some patients have an associated deficiency of coagulation factors X and IX (rarely factor VII). These disorders of coagulation appear to be due to binding of the factors to amyloid and in some instances loss into the urine (factor X) when there is renal glomerular involvement.

Kaposi Sarcoma and Other Vascular Tumors. Bleeding in Kaposi sarcoma results from the proliferation of vessels in the tumor. Dilated dermal vessels and proliferation of capillaries with local hemorrhage and hemosiderin deposition give rise to the early nodular lesions of the skin. An adequate biopsy is essential for the diagnosis. The relation of this disorder and the acquired immunodeficiency syndrome (AIDS) is discussed elsewhere (see Chapter 9.15).

HYPERSENSITIVITY STATES

Vasculitis
Purpura may result from direct vascular damage caused by drugs, toxins, chemicals, and infections. A relatively frequent cause of nonthrombocytopenic purpura secondary to loss of vessel wall integrity is vasculitis. The characteristic skin lesions occur in a symmetrical distribution most prominently on the extremities. A periungual distribution on fingers and toes is common. The buttocks often are involved, but the trunk and face usually are spared. Urticaria may precede the purpura, which often is palpable (macular, papular). The lesions may become necrotic. Hypersensitivity reactions often are the cause, and reactions to drugs are common. Numerous drugs have been incriminated,[3,9,11-13] including especially antibiotics, barbiturates and other sedatives, phenothiazines, and thiazide diuretics. Cutaneous vasculitis may be seen in the primary arteritides and connective tissue disorders including systemic lupus erythematosus, polyarteritis nodosa, rheumatoid arthritis, and Wegener granulomatosis. Vasculitis may be associated with paraproteinemic and dysproteinemic states often in association with neoplasms and hemoproliferative states (multiple myeloma and lymphoproliferative disorders). Waldenström macroglobulinemia and cryoglobulinemia may be associated with purpura, easy bruising, and epistaxis—and such patients may have associated abnormalities of platelets and coagulation. Cryoglobulinemic purpura, which is aggravated by exposure to cold, may exist in the absence of hematologic malignancies and may be seen in association with collagen vascular disorders and various infections. Cryofibrinogenemia, which is most commoly seen in association with malignancy, may be associated with cold-induced purpura.

Henoch-Schönlein Syndrome
This syndrome is most common in children but can be seen at any age. It is an acute vasculitis involving the gastrointestinal tract, kidneys, and joints as well as the skin. Cutaneous manifestations are similar to those seen in vasculitis of other causes. The skin lesions usually are well circumscribed, symmetrical, and prominent on the lower extremities. The lesions tend to coalesce with an advancing border. Gastrointestinal symptoms may include abdominal pain, vomiting, diarrhea, bleeding, and in children intussusception. Polyarthralgias are common, but frank arthritis is unusual. Glomerulonephritis and the nephrotic syndrome may be seen, and progressive renal failure may occasionally occur. The etiology is unknown, but formation of immune complexes and deposits of IgA in the vessel wall may play a role. Most patients recover completely in 4 to 6 weeks, but relapses may occur. Symptomatic treatment

is used, and occasionally corticosteroids have been employed but evaluation of the effect of therapy is difficult.

INFECTIONS

Bacterial, viral, and parasitic infections can cause abnormal bleeding, which may be severe. Multiple mechanisms have been identified, and more than one may be operative in the same patient. Direct damage to vessels may be produced by the infecting agent as demonstrated by finding the organism in the purpuric lesions associated with such infections as meningococcemia and various rickettsial diseases. Direct vessel damage may be produced by toxins, particularly endotoxins that damage the endothelium. Formation of immune complexes also may result in endothelial damage and vasculitis. Isolated thrombocytopenia may occur in association with many infections, including gram-negative and gram-positive bacterial infections—especially with sepsis, a variety of viral infections that can be serious (smallpox, yellow fever) or more common (rubella, chicken pox), and malaria. Thrombocytopenia with infections may be due to a direct effect of the infecting agent on platelets and the endothelium, but there is increasing evidence that immune mechanisms often are involved. Finally, bacterial infections may result in DIC, which can be severe and life-threatening.

MISCELLANEOUS

Purpura Simplex
This disorder, also known as simple easy bruising, is seen most often in women. The patients complain of easy bruising, especially on the hips and legs, often without recalled trauma. The lesions may exacerbate at the time of menses. Examination reveals small ecchymoses without induration or hematoma and no petechiae. In some cases there is a history of similar lesions in other female but not male members of the family, suggesting a hereditary familial disorder. It has been suggested that some cases represent mild forms of disorders of platelet function or von Willebrand disease. Tests of platelet function and coagulation rarely are indicated and when performed results are normal and there is no hemorrhagic diathesis. The disorder is only of cosmetic importance.

Autoerythrocyte Sensitization
This uncommon, acquired disorder of unknown etiology is seen almost exclusively in women. The patients may have a history of surgery or physical injury several weeks or months before the onset of bleeding. The patients then develop repeated episodes of swelling and bruising on the extremities, usually preceded or accompanied by pain or paresthesias at the site of bruising. Tests of platelet function and coagulation are normal. The characteristic painful lesions may be produced by intracutaneous injection of washed red cells or erythrocyte stroma from the patient's blood, suggesting autoerythrocyte sensitization during the preceding surgery or trauma. Psychiatric evaluations have demonstrated deep emotional disturbances with the suggestion that the disorder be designated "psychogenic purpura." The relation of this order to factitious purpura is uncertain.

Dermatologic Disorders
Purpura may be associated with a variety of dermatologic disorders and syndromes, which are discussed elsewhere (see Chapter 17.7).

REFERENCES

1. Bachmann F: Diagnostic approach to bleeding disorders. Semin Hematol 17:292, 1980
2. Barber A, Green D, et al: The bleeding time as a preoperative screening test. Am J Med 78:761, 1985

3. Colman RW, Hirsh J, et al (eds): Hemostasis and Thrombosis: Basic Principles and Clinical Practice, 2d ed. Philadelphia, JB Lippincott, 1987

4. Fareed J, Bick RL, et al: Molecular markers of hemostatic disorders: Implications in the diagnosis and therapeutic management of thrombotic and bleeding disorders. Clin Chem 29:1641, 1983

5. Giddings JC, Peake IR: Laboratory support in the diagnosis of coagulation disorders. Clin Haematol 14:571, 1985

6. Kaplan EB, Sheiner LB, et al: Usefulness of preoperative laboratory screening. JAMA 253:3576, 1985

7. Natelson EA: Human blood coagulation: Clinical and laboratory correlation. Clin Physiol Biochem 1:214, 1983

8. Rapaport SI: Preoperative hemostatic evaluation: Which tests, if any? Blood 61:229, 1983

9. Ratnoff OD, Forbes CD (eds): Disorders of Hemostasis. Orlando, Grune and Stratton, 1984

10. Seifter EJ, Bell WR (eds): Coagulation Disorders in the Cancer Patient. Mt Kisco, NY, Futura Publishing, 1984

11. Thorup OA Jr (ed): Leavell and Thorup's Fundamentals of Clinical Hematology, 5th ed. Philadelphia, WB Saunders, 1987

12. Williams WJ, Beutler E, et al (eds): Hematology, 3d ed. New York, McGraw-Hill, 1983

13. Wintrobe MM, Lee GR, et al (eds): Clinical Hematology, 8th ed. Philadelphia, Lea & Febiger, 1981

CHAPTER 6.9

Disorders of Blood Platelets

Dudley P. Jackson and William R. Bell

Blood platelets originate as fragments demarcated from the cytoplasm of megakaryocytes in the bone marrow and are released into the circulation. The intramedullary development of megakaryocytes and the production and release of platelets from the marrow is controlled, in part, by thrombopoietin. Circulating blood platelets are anucleate structures 2 to 3 μm in diameter, with a volume of 7.5 to 11.5 fl, that display many metabolic activities[8] upon which their physiologic functions are dependent. Platelets normally have a circulating life span of 10 ± 1.5 days, and at any given time two thirds of the total functioning platelets are in the circulating blood with one third in the spleen. The normal platelet count in humans is 150,000 to 400,000/μl. Bleeding may result from either quantitative or qualitative abnormalities of platelets (see Table 6.8–1).

THROMBOCYTOPENIA

Thrombocytopenia is defined as a platelet count of less than 100,000/μl. The hemorrhagic diathesis attributable to thrombocytopenia is designated thrombocytopenic purpura, which is the most common hematologic cause of abnormal bleeding. Petechiae on the skin and mucous membranes and cutaneous ecchymoses often are the initial manifestations. More serious forms of bleeding include epistaxes, gingival bleeding, genitourinary and gastrointestinal bleeding, and most seriously intracranial bleeding. Spontaneous hemarthroses do not occur. The bleeding often is intermittent and correlates only approximately with the platelet count. When the platelet count declines below 50,000/μl, one must be concerned about hemorrhage, especially if there is associated trauma. Spontaneous bleeding may occur with a platelet count less than 20,000/μl and is common when there are less than 10,000 platelets per microliter.

The approach to patients with thrombocytopenia requires an understanding of its cause(s), which can be classified on the basis of the mechanism(s) involved (Table 6.9–1). Management of the patient depends upon the degree of bleeding and the cause of the thrombocytopenia, which is determined by a detailed history, physical examination, and appropriate laboratory tests.[6] In all cases, a reduced platelet count should be verified by examination of an appropriately stained peripheral blood smear prepared directly from blood obtained by finger puncture without the use of an anticoagulant. Examination of smears of aspirated bone marrow or sections of marrow obtained by biopsy is essential. The selection of other laboratory tests depends upon the clinical presentation.

IMPAIRED PRODUCTION OF PLATELETS

Thrombocytopenia due to impaired production may be the result of decreased thrombopoiesis caused by a reduction of megakaryocytes in the marrow or by ineffective thrombopoiesis by megakaryocytes in the marrow (Table 6.9–1). Congenital forms have been described, but impaired production most often is an acquired disorder.

TABLE 6.9–1. CLASSIFICATION OF THROMBOCYTOPENIA

Impaired Production of Platelets
Decreased Thrombopoiesis (Megakaryocytes Decreased)
- Congenital—intrauterine infections, rare hereditary disorders, etc.
- Marrow injury—drugs, chemicls, irradiation, infection, aplastic anemia, etc.
- Marrow invasion—neoplasms, leukemia, fibrosis, etc.

Ineffective Thrombopoiesis (Megakaryocytes Normal or Increased)
- Congenital—associated with uncommon congenital disorders
- Deficiency of vitamin B_{12} or folic acid (megaloblastic megakaryocytes)
- Drugs (thiazide diuretics, alcohol, etc.)

Decreased Survival of Platelets
Immune-mediated
- Autoantibodies
  Idiopathic (immune) thrombocytopenic purpura (ITP)
  Systemic lupus erythematosus
  Drugs (quinine, quinidine, etc.)
  Neoplasms
- Alloantibodies
  Post-transfusion purpura
  Isoimmune neonatal thrombocytopenia

Nonimmune
- Disseminated intravascular coagulation (DIC)
- Thrombotic thrombocytopenic purpura (TTP)
- Hemolytic uremic syndrome (HUS)
- Sepsis
- Endothelial hemangioma
- Foreign surfaces (mechanical heart valves, circulating bypass pumps, etc.)
- Drugs (e.g., ristocetin)

Sequestration of Platelets
- Splenomegaly and hypersplenism

Dilution of Platelets
- Massive transfusions

Decreased thrombopoiesis due to marrow injury or invasion is relatively common. Treatment is directed at the underlying cause including removal of offending drugs or chemicals, supportive therapy, and efforts to restore normal bone marrow function. Some malignancies that invade marrow (e.g., leukemia) are treated with drugs that further decrease thrombopoiesis before improvement occurs. The major form of supportive therapy for control of hemorrhage is the use of platelet transfusions (see Chapter 6.24), which can be used prophylactically or therapeutically.[4,6] Restoration of bone marrow may be achieved in some cases of aplastic anemia and leukemia by use of immunosuppressive agents or bone marrow transplantation.

Recognition of ineffective thrombopoiesis is particularly important because of the availability of effective therapy in many cases. Thrombocytopenia due to deficiency of vitamin B_{12} or folic acid responds promptly (i.e., within 4 to 10 days) to administration of the appropriate vitamin. In some cases, alcohol produces ineffective thrombopoiesis, and in such cases withdrawal of alcohol results in disappearance of thrombocytopenia within a few days.

DECREASED SURVIVAL OF PLATELETS[1,6,9,12]

Platelets may be released normally from the bone marrow but be damaged and removed prematurely from the circulation. Most commonly this results from antibody-mediated platelet injury. Autoantibodies capable of destroying platelets may appear spontaneously (idiopathic thrombocytopenic purpura [ITP]) or in association with other disorders (systemic lupus erythematosus, neoplasms) or with the use of drugs (quinine, quinidine, etc.).

Immune-Mediated Thrombocytopenia

Drugs. Thrombocytopenia produced by drugs may be the result of direct damage to either the marrow megakaryocytes (e.g., myelosuppressive agents) or the circulating platelets (e.g., ristocetin). Commonly, however, immunologic mechanisms are involved in drug-induced thrombocytopenia. Agents such as quinine, quinidine, sulfonamides, and thiazides are common offenders, but any drug may be involved.

Whenever petechiae and purpuric lesions of the skin and mucous membranes are encountered and the platelet count is low, the patient and companions must be questioned exhaustively about the use of medications. The petechial and purpuric lesions are usually macular, nontender, nonpruritic, and without erythematous borders, in contrast to allergic reactions. This is important since some drugs can induce purpura without associated thrombocytopenia. The immunologic reaction that decreases platelet survival may occur in several different ways. The drug or a metabolite may act as a hapten and form a plasma protein complex that is antigenic. The drug-carrier protein (antigen)-antibody complex may be absorbed nonspecifically on the platelet. The altered platelet surface results in prompt removal by the reticuloendothelial system. Laboratory tests to identify if a drug is responsible or which drug is the causative agent are difficult and seldom reliable.

Management of the problem mandates immediate discontinuation of all medications. If thrombocytopenia persists for more than 2 weeks in the absence of all medications, another etiology should be entertained. The recovery interval may be longer in the presence of hepatic and renal insufficiency or if the offending agent is normally excreted very slowly. Purposeful readministration of the suspicious agent to confirm the diagnosis is not advisable unless there is no possible alternative and the agent under suspicion is essential for life. When reinstituting a drug regimen, administering one agent at a time is the best way to identify the responsible drug. To avoid a recurrence of thrombocytopenia a suitable substitute drug should be found. Since the drug-induced antibody is specific, one needs to find an agent of similar therapeutic utility with a molecular structure that differs from that of the offending agent.

Idiopathic (Immune) Thrombocytopenic Purpura. ITP is an illness with immunologically mediated thrombocytopenia appearing in the absence of an identifiable disease or exposure to any exogenous agents. This disease, also called autoimmune thrombocytopenic purpura (ATP), occurs in two forms—acute and chronic.

Acute ITP. Acute ITP occurs most commonly in the pediatric age group, with equal frequency in females and males. Commonly there is an immediate antecedent upper respiratory viral, and occasionally bacterial, infection. The patient presents with the abrupt appearance of generalized skin and mucous membrane petechiae and purpura. Gastrointestinal and genitourinary bleeding are often associated. The peripheral blood film is essentially devoid of platelets with the count usually between 10,000 and 20,000/μl. Associated fever, eosinophilia, and mild lymphocytosis are observed frequently. In contrast to chronic ITP, the acute form of the disease is self-limited, with spontaneous remission occurring in 80 to 90 percent of patients within 2 to 6 weeks. Usually there is no association with other immune diseases. In a small proportion of patients remission will occur later than 2 months. Treatment of any type is seldom required. If frank hemorrhage accompanies a platelet count of <20,000/μl a short course of corticosteroids in doses of 1 to 2 mg/kg should be considered. If there is no response in 3 to 4 months, splenectomy should be considered. Considerable effort and thought must be exerted to avoid splenectomy since undesirable sequelae may occur after removal of this organ. In addition to subdiaphragmatic abscess formation immediately after splenectomy, fulminant fatal sepsis has been reported during the ensuing weeks and years. Platelet transfusions are not helpful, because transfused platelets are eliminated from the circulation in a very few minutes.

Chronic ITP. The onset of chronic ITP occurs at any age but more commonly in females (3:1 to 4:1 over males) between the ages of 20 and 45 years. Usually an asymptomatic individual observes the presence of petechial lesions in the distal portions of the extremities and seeks medical attention. Occasionally the diagnosis is first considered when an unexpected low platelet count is identified at the time of an annual medical check-up. The spleen is usually not enlarged, the platelet count is reduced to 25,000 to 75,000/μl, and marrow megakaryocytes are increased or normal in number. Occasionally in the adult, chronic ITP is a part of or coexists with other immune diseases such as lymphoproliferative disorders, systemic lupus erythematosus, thyroid disease and, autoimmune hemolytic anemia (Evans syndrome). The etiology of the thrombocytopenia in ITP is a spontaneously appearing antibody (ITP factor) that damages the platelets, causing them to be removed from the circulation by the reticuloendothelial system. The ITP factor is an IgG class (7S subclasses 3 and 1), is species specific, can be absorbed by normal platelets, and probably does not fix complement per se. (C3 may be present on some platelets in this illness, however.)

The diagnosis of chronic ITP is largely one of exclusion. Only after all possible etiologic agents and diseases have been excluded can the diagnosis be made with certainty. Bone marrow examination reveals a cellular marrow with increased or normal numbers of megakaryoctyes. The demonstration of antiplatelet IgG on the platelet surface may be helpful, but the assay techniques used are difficult. Recently these assays have been seriously questioned regarding specificity.

Treatment. The diagnosis of ITP per se is not an indication for treatment. Therapy should be focused on prevention and control of bleeding and not on the platelet count, which does provide a measure of response to treatment. The established forms of therapy are corticosteroids and splenectomy. The initial treatment of choice is administration of an adrenocorticosteroid. In adults the usual starting dose is 60 mg (40 to 80 mg) of prednisone daily (15 mg orally every 6 hours), but equivalent doses of other preparations of corticosteroids can be used. Subsequent dosage is determined by the patient's response, with the objective of reducing

dosage to the lowest level that controls bleeding and maintains remission. Splenectomy should be considered when there is no response to prednisone, the dose of prednisone required is associated with significant side effects, or prolonged maintenance therapy (i.e., more than 6 months) is required. Other forms of therapy, which usually are reserved for patients with continued bleeding despite treatment with corticosteroids and splenectomy, include immunosuppressive agents, danazol (an impeded androgen), colchicine, and intravenous infusions of high-dose gamma globulin. The precise role of these forms of therapy in the management of ITP awaits further study. In the menstruating female, anovulatory agents may be helpful in controlling menstrual blood loss. The treatment of ITP in pregnancy is controversial and difficult because treatment must be appropriate for the mother, the fetus, and the newborn.[7]

Isoimmune Neonatal Purpura. A rare disorder in the newborn is thrombocytopenic purpura secondary to fetal maternal incompatibility. The infant's thrombocytopenia, usually severe, is thought to be due to transplacental passage of isoantibodies produced by the mother and directed against PI^{A1} antigens on the infant's platelets. The process is self-limited, and recovery to normal in 4 to 6 weeks is the rule.

Posttransfusion Purpura. The immune-mediated thrombocytopenia observed in this disorder is etiologically related to a previous blood transfusion. Classically, from 5 to 10 days following one or more units of whole blood, the platelet count will plummet to less than $10,000/\mu l$ in a 24-hour period. This is seen most frequently in females who have developed an antibody to a platelet antigen, PI^{A1}, which is present in more than 98 percent of the general population. Although this is extremely rare, it is frightening when it occurs, as hemorrhage is frequent. Corticosteroids may be of some benefit, but the platelet count may return to normal in 2 to 3 weeks in untreated individuals. Platelet transfusions are ineffective.

Nonimmune Thrombocytopenia

Thrombocytopenia occurring in the absence of immune-mediated mechanisms is observed in association with several disorders in which direct damage to platelets appears to be responsible for their premature removal from the circulation. Increased utilization or "consumption" of platelets associated with DIC, sepsis, and endothelial hemangioma is discussed in Chapters 6.8 and 6.10.

Thrombotic Thrombocytopenic Purpura (TTP).[10] This frequently fatal disease process occurs abruptly in previously healthy people. Thrombotic thrombocytopenic purpura is characterized by the following features: (1) severe thrombocytopenia, (2) microangiopathic hemolytic anemia (MAHA), (3) fever, (4) central nervous system disturbances, and (5) renal disease. It occurs more frequently in females. There is no single feature or test that is diagnostic. The diagnosis is made only after identifiable causes have been eliminated. Most helpful in diagnosis is the peripheral blood smear that uniformly contains striking red cell fragmentation, marked polychromatophilia, normal white blood cells, and decrease of platelets. The Coombs test is negative. The characteristic histopathologic lesion is fibrinogen-laden hyaline thrombus formation, which occurs secondary to severe endothelial cell damage and obstructs arterioles and capillaries in many places throughout the body. The combined use of corticosteroids, plasmapheresis, and plasma infusion has yielded complete remission in some cases and led to long-term survival.

The hemolytic-uremic syndrome (HUS) occurs predominantly in children and is very similar to TTP seen in adults except that fever and neurologic disturbances may be less frequent. Carcinoma-associated HUS (C-HUS) complicating therapy with mitomycin is being recognized with increasing frequency.[2] Transfusions of blood products (i.e., red blood cells, platelets, or plasma) should be avoided in patients with C-HUS if possible because they often are followed by pulmonary edema and worsening of the HUS.

Corticosteroids and plasmapheresis rarely are of benefit, but some success has been noted with immunopheresis using columns of staphylococcal protein A.

Traumatic Platelet Destruction. Severe thrombocytopenia is frequently observed in the presence of generalized infection. This may result from marrow megakaryocyte suppression or from direct damage to the platelet membrane from exotoxins or endotoxins released from micro-organisms. Mechanical devices placed in the vascular system such as prosthetic heart valves, Teflon septal patches, or Dacron vascular bypass grafts can damage platelet membranes, resulting in platelet removal from the circulation.

SEQUESTRATION OF PLATELETS

Abnormal distribution of platelets within the body is seen with hypersplenism and enlarged spleen syndromes and frequently gives rise to a modest reduction in the peripheral blood platelet count in the range of 50,000 to $80,000/\mu l$. Usually modest leukopenia and anemia are present concomitantly. The usual 30 percent of platelets residing in the spleen is increased to 60 to 80 percent in this situation. The bone marrow is characteristically normal. Platelet survival is normal with a delayed splenic transit time. Hemorrhage, because of thrombocytopenia, is unusual. Surgery usually can be accomplished without necessitating platelet transfusions. Splenectomy can be followed by restoration of the platelet count to near-normal levels but rarely is indicated in this disorder.

DILUTION OF PLATELETS

Thrombocytopenia does not occur following acute hemorrhage, but does occur following rapid replacement with large quantities of stored blood. The degree of thrombocytopenia is directly related to the number of transfusions and occurs regularly in patients receiving >14 units (7000 ml) of stored blood within a 24-hour period. Thereafter the platelets return to normal within 3 to 5 days. Use of fresh (i.e., <12 hours from donation) whole blood prevents this type of thrombocytopenia, but it is not always available in an emergency situation. Administration of excessive volumes of fluid of any type—including blood components without platelets—may result in dilutional thrombocytopenia, with platelet counts reduced to approximately 50,000 μl. Frequently there are simultaneous reductions in serum electrolytes. Treatment consists of fluid restriction and gentle diuresis.

THROMBOCYTOSIS

Thrombocytosis—i.e., a platelet count greater than $400,000/\mu l$—is seen in association with a variety of conditions (Table 6.9–2).

TABLE 6.9–2. SOME CAUSES OF THROMBOCYTOSIS

Myeloproliferative Disorders (Chapter 6.18)
- Essential thrombocythemia
- Polycythemia vera
- Chronic myelocytic leukemia
- Agnogenic myeloid metaplasia

Asplenia (from any cause)

Neoplasms (particularly carcinomas)

Inflammatory and Infectious Disorders
- Rheumatoid arthritis and acute rheumatic fever
- Ulcerative colitis and regional enteritis
- Periarteritis nodosa
- Infections—acute and chronic

Miscellaneous
- Trauma, surgical procedures, acute hemorrhage, iron deficiency anemia, recovery ("rebound") from thrombocytopenia, etc.

Thrombocytosis associated with the myeloproliferative disorders is termed thrombocythemia or primary thrombocytosis, and when associated with other disorders is termed secondary or reactive thrombocytosis (see Table 6.8–1).

MYELOPROLIFERATIVE DISORDERS
(See also Chapter 6.18)

The platelet counts in untreated patients with polycythemia rubra vera (PRV) and chronic myelocytic leukemia (CML) often are elevated to the range of 400,000 to 800,000/μl. Other clinical and laboratory findings establish these diagnoses. Therapy is directed at the leukemia in CML and at control of the red cell mass in PRV and rarely is needed for control of the thrombocytosis.

The most striking elevations of platelet counts are seen in patients with essential thrombocythemia (ET) and in some patients with agnogenic myeloid metaplasia in whom counts from 1 to 5 million per microliter or even higher may be seen. Precise differentiation of these two disorders at times is difficult because of overlapping clinical and laboratory findings. Spontaneous bleeding may occur in essential (hemorrhagic) thrombocythemia and may be associated with digital or cerebral ischemia, but thrombosis (venous or arterial) is seldom seen.

The morphology of platelets in thrombocythemia is abnormal, especially in patients with ET and agnogenic myeloid metaplasia. The platelets on smears of peripheral blood are large (giant), at times being larger than the red blood cells, with prominent granulomeres and hyalomeres, and fragments of megakaryocytes may be seen. When the blood clots, pseudohyperkalemia and spurious increases in acid phosphotase, lactic acid dehydrogenase, calcium, inorganic phosphorus, and uric acid may be observed because of release of these substances from the markedly increased platelet mass during clotting. If blood clotting is prevented and these measurements are determined on plasma, these values will be normal. Abnormalities of various in vitro platelet functions have been described in thrombocythemia, but the clinical significance of these findings is unclear.[11]

Treatment of ET is symptomatic (see Chapter 6.18). Therapy usually is held until onset of symptoms. Reduction in the platelet count with hydroxyurea or bulsulfan (Myleran) may lessen bleeding. Platelet pheresis can be used to reduce platelets in emergency situations.

ASPLENIA

Thrombocytosis occurs in virtually all asplenic states but rarely produces symptoms or requires treatment. Moderate thrombocytosis occurs following major surgery or trauma but usually persists only for 7 to 14 days. Following splenectomy, platelet counts begin to increase within several days, usually reaching peak levels in 2 to 4 weeks. The counts may achieve levels of 1 million per microliter or more and are higher than can be explained by removal of a site (i.e., the spleen) of a physiologic platelet pool. The platelet count usually returns toward normal within several weeks or months after splenectomy but occasionally may remain elevated for years. Routine anticoagulation because of thrombocytosis following splenectomy is not recommended.

NEOPLASMS

Thrombocytosis may occur in association with various carcinomas (particularly breast and lung) and sarcomas in the presence or absence of metastatic disease. Its role, if any, in the occurrence of Trousseau syndrome in patients with neoplasms is unclear (see Chapter 6.10). Thrombocytosis also may occur in association with Hodgkin disease and other lymphoreticular neoplasms.

INFLAMMATORY AND INFECTIOUS DISORDERS

Inflammation produced in experimental animals results in thrombocytosis of unknown cause. Thrombocytosis is associated with a variety of inflammatory and infectious diseases (Table 6.9–2). It is especially common in various inflammatory disorders of the bowel and rheumatoid arthritis and may provide a sensitive indicator of the activity of the basic disease. Detection of thrombocytosis may alert the clinician to search for a previously unsuspected inflammatory disorder, infection, or neoplasm.

QUALITATIVE DISORDERS OF PLATELETS

Spontaneous bleeding may occur with a normal platelet count as the result of qualitative defects of platelet function which may be either congenital or acquired disorders (Table 6.9–3). Most of these functional defects are inherent within the platelet, and rarely does the defect result from an abnormality of an essential plasma component.

CONGENITAL DISORDERS

These rare disorders represent experiments of nature, the study of which has enhanced understanding of blood platelets. Platelets are involved in a series of reactions in normal hemostasis (see Chapter 6.8), including adhesion, aggregation, release, and coagulation. Congenital defects in each of these reactions have been identified (Table 6.9–3), and in some instances more than one reaction is involved. These disorders are characterized by a prolonged bleeding time and abnormalities of one or more tests of platelet function. Platelet counts usually are normal but in some cases thrombocytopenia may be noted.

Defects of Adhesion (Bernard–Soulier Syndrome)
This is an autosomal recessive disorder characterized by the presence of giant vacuolated platelets in the peripheral blood, an abnormal prothrombin consumption test, absence of ristocetin-induced platelet aggregation which is not corrected by vWF, and deficient platelet membrane glycoprotein (GP) Ib. Severe bleeding may occur. Platelet transfusions may provide temporary benefit.

TABLE 6.9–3. QUALITATIVE DISORDERS OF PLATELET FUNCTION

Congenital
Defects of adhesion
• Bernard–Soulier (giant platelet) syndrome

Defects of aggregation
• Glanzmann thrombasthenia

Defects of release (secretion)
• Storage pool disease
• Prostaglandin synthesis impairment

Defects of procoagulant activity
• Platelet factor 3 (PF3) deficiency

Associated with other congenital disorders, including:
• Chédiak–Higashi syndrome
• Hermansky–Pudlak syndrome (oculocutaneous albinism)
• Wiskott–Aldrich syndrome
• Various hereditary disorders of connective tissue

Acquired
Drugs—aspirin, nonsteroidal anti-inflammatory agents, antibiotics, etc.
Uremia
Myeloproliferative disorders
Dysproteinemic syndrome
Storage pool deficiency (e.g., postcardiopulmonary bypass)
Miscellaneous other disorders

Defects of Aggregation (Glanzmann Thrombasthenia)

This autosomal recessive disorder is characterized by abnormal or absent clot retraction; failure of platelets to aggregate in response to ADP, epinephrine, collagen, thrombin, and arachidonic acid; and deficiencies of GP IIb-IIIa. If local hemostatic measures fail to control bleeding, platelet transfusions may be necessary.

Defects of Release (Secretion)

The inheritance patterns of these disorders have not been well established, but in some cases of storage pool disease an autosomal dominant pattern has been reported. Platelets from patients with storage pool disease do not undergo the normal physiologic release reaction. This reaction does not take place either because the granules or bodies within platelet cytoplasm do not deliver their contents to the cytoplasmic milieu or the contents normally stored in these compartments are absent or abnormal (i.e., prostaglandin synthesis impairment). In the absence of a normal release reaction, the secondary wave of platelet aggregation is missing in vitro. Storage pool disorders occur in association with other congenital diseases including the Chédiak–Higashi, Hermansky–Pudlak and Wiskott–Aldrich syndromes.

ACQUIRED DISORDERS

Acquired defects of platelet function are much more common than are congenital dysfunctions and occur in association with a variety of illnesses and the use of certain drugs. In many instances the platelet dysfunction is complex and often associated with abnormalities of vessels or coagulation. As noted above, the various in vitro abnormalities reported in the myelodysplastic disorders are of uncertain clinical significance.

Drugs[3]

A large number of drugs are known to inhibit in vitro platelet function, but the clinical significance of these test results is not always obvious. Ingestion of aspirin results in irreversible acetylation and inactivation of the platelet cyclooxygenase enzyme, thereby leading to inhibition of endoperoxide and thromboxane synthesis. These changes result in inhibition of platelet aggregation by ADP, epinephrine, and collagen, and in some individuals the bleeding time is prolonged. However, there is no evidence that standard doses of aspirin induce significant bleeding in otherwise normal individuals except for the occurrence of occult gastrointestinal blood loss. In contrast, patients with underlying hemostatic defects (i.e., von Willebrand disease, hemophilia, etc.) should not ingest aspirin since they may experience significant increase in bleeding following its use. Various nonsteroidal anti-inflammatory agents (indomethacin, sulfinopyrazone, phenylbutazone, etc.) also inhibit the platelet cyclooxygenase enzyme, but their effects are reversible and short-lived. A number of penicillins (carbenicillin, ticarcillin, ampicillin, etc.) in high doses inhibit platelet aggregation and induce significant bleeding by unknown mechanisms. Cephalosporins also may inhibit platelet function. Infusions of dextrans (bacterial polysaccharides used as volume expanders) often result in prolongation of the bleeding time.

Uremia[5]

Significant bleeding that contributes to morbidity and mortality is well recognized in uremia. The cause of the bleeding is complex but is characterized by a prolonged bleeding time, suggesting platelet/vessel abnormalities. Abnormal platelet aggregation by ADP, collagen, and epinephrine occurs. Possible platelet defects include abnormal GP Ib or its binding to vWF, a storage pool defect, and elevated platelet calcium. Retention of uremic products (e.g., gua-

nidinosuccinic acid) that inhibit platelet function may contribute to the bleeding. The abnormal bleeding usually is controlled by dialysis, but the abnormalities of platelet function may persist. Infusions of cryoprecipitate or DDAVP (1-deamino-8-D-arginine-vasopressin) may provide temporary improvement of hemostasis.

Dysproteinemic Syndromes

Spontaneous bleeding frequently is associated with dysproteinemic states. In these diseases, platelet dysfunction probably is due to coating of the platelet membrane by the abnormal protein and is indicated by a prolonged bleeding time, impaired platelet adhesion and aggregation, and reduced platelet factor 3 (PF3) availability. Alterations in blood coagulation, hyperviscosity, and thrombocytopenia also are common. Bleeding is controlled by reducing the concentration of the abnormal protein by chemotherapy or by plasmapheresis in the acute situation with severe hemorrhage.

Storage Pool Deficiency

Acquired storage pool deficiency has been described in association with a number of disorders including SLE, ITP, TTP, and DIC, but in all of these disorders multiple other factors contribute to the bleeding. Depletion of platelet granule contents presumably from mechanical trauma has been noted in several conditions including cardiopulmonary bypass procedures, but again, multiple abnormalities often are present.

REFERENCES*

1. Aster RH: Thrombocytopenia due to enhanced platelet destruction. In Williams WJ, Beutler E, et al (eds): Hematology. 3d ed. New York, McGraw-Hill, 1983, p 1298
2. Cantrell JE, Phillips TM, et al: Carcinoma associated hemolytic uremic syndrome: A complication of mitomycin-C chemotherapy. J Clin Oncol 3:723, 1985
3. Carvalho ALA, Rao AK: Acquired qualitative platelet defects. In Colman RW, Hirsh J, et al (eds): Hemostasis and Thrombosis: Basic Principles and Clinical Practice. 2d ed. Philadelphia, JB Lippincott, 1987, p 750
4. Consensus Conference: Platelet transfusion therapy. JAMA 257:1777, 1987
5. Costaldi PA, Gorman DJ: Disordered platelet function in renal disease. In Colman RW, Hirsh J, et al (eds): Hemostasis and Thrombosis: Basic Principles and Clinical Practice. 2d ed. Philadelphia, JB Lippincott, 1987, p 960
6. Jackson DP: Management of thrombocytopenia. In Colman RW, Hirsh J, et al (eds): Hemostasis and Thrombosis: Basic Principles and Clinical Practice. 2d ed. Philadelphia, JB Lippincott, 1987, p 530
7. Martin JN, Morrison JC, et al: Autoimmune thrombocytopenic purpura: Current concepts and recommended practices. Am J Obstet Gynecol 150:86, 1984
8. Phillips DR, Shuman MA: Biochemistry of Platelets. Orlando, Academic Press, 1986
9. Pizzuto J, Ambriz R: Therapeutic experience on 934 adults with idiopathic thrombocytopenic purpura: Multicentric trial of the cooperative Latin American Group on hemostasis and thrombosis. Blood 64:1179, 1984
10. Ridolfi R, Bell WR: Thrombotic thrombocytopenic purpura: Report of 25 cases and review of the literature. Medicine 60:413, 1981
11. Schafer AI: Bleeding and thrombosis in the myeloproliferative disorders (review). Blood 64:1, 1984
12. Shulman NR, Jordan JV Jr: Platelet immunology. In Colman RW, Hirsh J, et al (eds): Hemostasis and Thrombosis: Basic Principles and Clinical Practice. 2d ed. Philadelphia, JB Lippincott, 1987, p 452

*References 3, 9, and 11 to 13 cited in Chapter 6.8 also provide detailed information relating to topics in this chapter.

Disorders of Blood Coagulation

William R. Bell and Dudley P. Jackson

The coagulation process involves interaction between many different proteins, proteases, phospholipids, and the divalent cation Ca^{+2} (Table 6.10–1, Fig. 6.10–1). The coagulation process can be activated and proceed via two sequential pathways—the intrinsic system (components present within circulating blood) and the extrinsic system (which includes components present in the extravascular compartment). Cooperative integration of these systems maintains vascular integrity and preserves hemostasis. The hemorrhagic diathesis in patients with coagulation disorders is due to an abnormality of one or more plasma proteins necessary for normal blood coagulation or by the development of a circulating anticoagulant (see Tables 6.8–1 and 6.10–1 and Fig. 6.10–1). Specific laboratory tests are required for precise identification of these disorders.

CONGENITAL DISORDERS

These disorders are the result of either deficient synthesis of specific coagulation factors or synthesis of functionally defective coagulation factors (see Table 6.8–1). Congenitally inherited abnormalities of coagulation usually involve a single factor, although familial multiple factor deficiencies have been described.

FACTOR I DEFICIENCY

Afibrinogenemia

Hereditary afibrinogenemia (deficiency of fibrinogen) is an extremely rare autosomal recessive disorder associated with a high degree of consanguinity. Its clinical features are usually manifested at birth with persistent hemorrhage from the umbilical cord or circumcision site. Thereafter, the affected individuals may experience easy bruisability, epistaxis, gingival bleeding, and excessive hemorrhage following trauma or surgery. Defective wound healing and abnormal scar formation have also been reported. Hemarthroses and difficulty with menstrual bleeding are rare.

Laboratory findings include a decreased sedimentation rate and prolonged bleeding time. Because the routine screening tests of coagulation—prothrombin time (PT), activated partial thromboplastin time (APTT), and thrombin time (TT)—depend on the presence of fibrinogen to form the fibrin clot endpoints, these tests are strikingly abnormal in this disorder. Although fibrinogen cannot be detected in assays that measure clottable protein, trace amounts may be identified in affected plasmas subjected to immunoelectrophoresis. This suggests that the basic defect in this disorder is one of impaired or inadequate hepatic synthesis. Platelet dysfunction is attributed to the absence of fibrinogen on the platelet membrane. Occasional individuals are hypofibrinogenemic, with levels of fibrinogen less than 100 mg/dl. This quantity of fibrinogen is usually adequate to produce normal clotting studies and few clinical symptoms. These patients may represent heterozygotes of afibrinogenemic patients or may have dysfibrinogenemia.

Treatment of afibrinogenemia may be indicated prophylactically before and during surgical procedures and therapeutically to terminate episodes of persistent hemorrhage. This can be achieved by infusions of plasma or cryoprecipitate that are enriched with fibrinogen. The use of fibrinogen concentrates has been associated with an unacceptable risk of hepatitis. Fibrinogen infused into afibrinogenemic patients has a near-normal half-life.

Dysfibrinogenemia

Dysfibrinogenemias are usually inherited in an autosomal dominant manner. Approximately 150 abnormal fibrinogens have been identified. The complexity of the fibrinogen molecule, however, provides many more potential sites for alterations in structure and physical properties. Specific structural abnormalities have been demonstrated only in fibrinogens Detroit, Munich, Metz, Petoskey, Lille, Rouen, Manchester, Sydney I and II, and New York. The majority of dysfibrinogenemias produce an asymptomatic clinical course and are discovered fortuitously. Several others have been associated with mild bleeding manifestations, thrombotic episodes (Baltimore, Vancouver, Paris II, and Wiesbaden), and defective scar formation (Paris I, Cleveland I, and Wiesbaden).

Patients with dysfibrinogenemia have defective conversion of fibrinogen to fibrin. The abnormal fibrinogen interferes with fibrinopeptide release by thrombin, inhibits fibrin monomer polymerization, or prevents effective crosslinking of fibrin monomers. These defects are reflected by prolongation of the PT, APTT, and TT. Purified procoagulant enzymes derived from snake venoms, e.g., ancrod and reptilase, can be substituted for thrombin in the TT and provide information concerning fibrinopeptide release from abnormal fibrinogens. Fibrinogen concentrations determined as thrombin clottable protein are decreased, but when measured immunologically or quantitatively as protein are normal or increased. Dysfibrinogens have been analyzed for their carbohydrate content and have been electrophoresed on polyacrylamide gels, with variable results.

Experience with replacement therapy in dysfibrinogenemic patients is limited by the rarity of its occurrence. Usually replace-

TABLE 6.10–1. FACTORS INVOLVED IN BLOOD COAGULATION

Factor	Synonym	Site of Synthesis	In Vivo Half-Life
I	Fibrinogen	Liver	3–4.5 days
II	Prothrombin[a]	Liver	2–5 days
III	Thromboplastin	All body tissues	
IV	Calcium (Ca^{2++})		
V	Proaccelerin	Liver	15–36 hours
VII	Proconvertin[a]	Liver	2–6 hours
VIII	Antihemophilic globulin (AHG)	? Endothelial cell	6–10 hours
IX	Christmas factor[a]	Liver	8–12 hours
X	Stuart–Prower factor[a]	Liver	32–48 hours
XI	Plasma thromboplastin antecedent (PTA)	Unknown	40–48 hours
XII	Hageman factor	? Liver	48–52 hours
XIII	Fibrin stabilizing factor (FSF)	Liver, megakaryocyte	5–12 days
	Protein C[a]	Unknown	?
	Protein S[a]	Unknown	?

[a] Vitamin K–dependent.

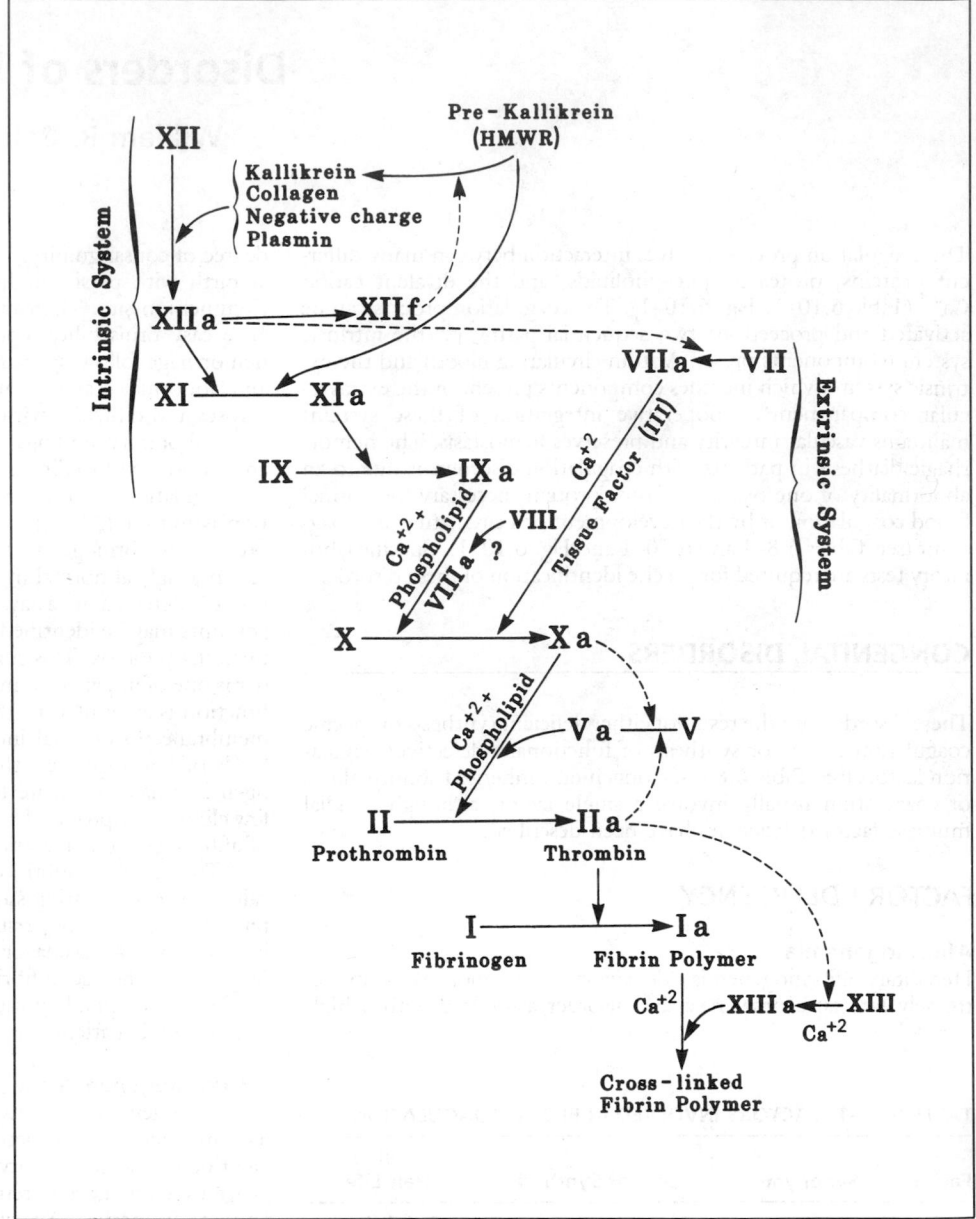

Figure 6.10–1. Diagram of the coagulation process showing components present in blood (intrinsic system) and those derived from extravascular sources (extrinsic system).

ment therapy is not necessary because adequate amounts of normal fibrinogen accompany the aberrant fibrinogen. If therapy is required, plasma infusions may be considered (Tables 6.10–2 and 6.10–3).

FACTOR II DEFICIENCY

Inherited in an autosomal recessive fashion, hypoprothrombinemia (deficiency of prothrombin) is the rarest of the hereditary coagulation disorders. Clinical bleeding is mild. Congenital dysprothrombinemias have also been reported; several have been characterized by reduced biologic prothrombin activity (15 to 50 percent of normal) but normal immunologic activity.

Prolonged PT, APTT, and variable clotting times are noted in laboratory specimens deficient in factor II. Bleeding times are usually normal. A two-stage prothrombin assay is necessary to confirm hypoprothrombinemia.

For those instances in which replacement therapy is needed in hypoprothrombinemia, plasma or purified prothrombin-complex concentrates can be used (Tables 6.10–2 and 6.10–3). The latter material is associated with a high frequency of hepatitis and may

be thrombogenic, particularly when administered to patients with preexisting hepatic dysfunction.

FACTOR III AND FACTOR IV

No reported congenital or acquired coagulopathies have been produced by deficiencies of factors III (thromboplastin) or IV (calcium). Thromboplastin is ubiquitous in most body tissues. Calcium ions are required only in trace amounts for coagulation. Before such a decreased level could be attained, other calcium-dependent body functions would fail and death would ensue.

FACTOR V DEFICIENCY

Hereditary proaccelerin deficiency is a rare autosomal recessive coagulopathy, which occasionally is associated with other congenital defects. Homozygotes possess factor V levels that are 9 to 10 percent of normal and demonstrate variable degrees of bleeding tendencies. Several instances of fatal hemorrhage resulting from tooth extractions and menses have been reported. Hemarthroses

TABLE 6.10–2. REPLACEMENT THERAPY FOR COAGULATION FACTOR DEFICIENCY

Source	Factors Present	Condition to be Treated	Risks
Plasma Fresh-frozen plasma Fresh whole blood	All known coagulation factors	Congenital and acquired deficiency states	Volume overload Hepatitis[a] AIDS
Cryoprecipitate	I, VIII, XIII	Hemophilia A von Willebrand disease Hypofibrinogenemia	Hepatitis[a] AIDS
Factor VIII concentrates	VIII, I, XIII	Hemophilia A Low-titer inhibitors against VIII	Hepatitis AIDS
Factor IX concentrates	II, VII, IX, X	Hemophilia B Hepatic failure	Hepatitis AIDS
Activated factor complexes	II, VII, IX, X	High-titer circulating inhibitors	DIC Shock Hepatitis AIDS

[a]Risk is very low.
AIDS = acquired immunodeficiency syndrome.

almost never occur. Heterozygotes generally have adequate levels of factor V to remain asymptomatic. Combined deficiencies of factors V and VIII have been identified more frequently than would be expected by chance alone.

Because factor V is involved in the common pathway of clotting, its deficiency produces an abnormal APTT and PT. The bleeding time is inexplicably prolonged in occasional affected individuals.

Replacement therapy in factor V deficiency (excluding disseminated intravascular coagulation) requires the use of fresh-frozen plasma. The characteristic lability and short plasma half-life (12 to

TABLE 6.10–3. QUANTITY OF REPLACEMENT THERAPY NEEDED IN FACTOR DEFICIENCY STATES

Indication For Replacement	Desired Factor Level to Control Hemorrhage[a] (% of Normal Activity)
Mild Hemorrhage • Acute hemarthrosis • Superficial soft tissue hematoma • Epistaxis, gingival bleeding • Unrelenting hematuria	15–25%
Major Hemorrhage • Extensive hemarthrosis and hematoma formation • Gastrointestinal hemorrhage • Retroperitoneal hemorrhage • Peripheral nerve deficit • Deep soft tissue hematoma formation • Presurgery prophylaxis	25–50%
Life-threatening Lesions • CNS hemorrhage • Pre-CNS surgery • Major extensive trauma	>50%

[a]This level is achieved by administration of the calculated dose required for the patient in need as follows: Units to be infused = [desired factor concentration − initial factor concentration] × plasma volume. By convention 1 ml normal plasma = 1 U of factor activity, 100% of normal activity = 1 factor U/ml plasma. Plasma volume = 5% × kg body weight.

36 hours) of factor V lead to a rapid loss of proaccelerin activity in stored plasma. Transfusions of normal platelets, which have factor V absorbed to their membranes, have also been used as replacement therapy (Tables 6.10–2 and 6.10–3).

FACTOR VII DEFICIENCY

Factor VII (serum prothrombin conversion accelerator, proconvertin) deficiency is an uncommon autosomal recessive coagulopathy associated with abnormal bleeding and thrombotic tendencies. Homozygotes usually have less than 10 percent of normal factor VII activity and experience mild to severe symptoms, including hemarthroses. Heterozygotes demonstrate decreased factor VII levels but are asymptomatic. Deep venous thrombosis and pulmonary emboli have been reported in several affected individuals. In addition, there is a high frequency of factor VII deficiency in patients with Dubin-Johnson syndrome.

Factor VII deficiency affects only the extrinsic system of clotting and is reflected by a prolonged PT with normal APTT and TT. Immunologic detection of factor VII antigen has been described in several patients with absent biologic activity. Replacement therapy can be accomplished by infusion of stored plasma. Factor VII is also contained in prothrombin-complex concentrates (Tables 6.10–2 and 6.10–3).

FACTOR VIII DEFICIENCY[4]

Factor VIII (antihemophilic factor, antihemophilic globulin) deficiency, classic hemophilia or hemophilia A, is inherited as a sex-linked recessive disorder. It is the most common severe congenital coagulopathy. Hemorrhagic complications may become obvious shortly after birth with circumcision and increase in severity and frequency with age and activity. The severity of bleeding symptoms appears related to the degree of factor VIII deficiency, so that severely affected individuals (factor VIII procoagulant activity less than 1 percent of normal) experience repeated and often spontaneous hemorrhagic episodes, most commonly hemarthroses. Repeated involvement of the joints ultimately produces crippling deformities and arthritides, which may require surgical intervention for synovectomy or joint replacement. The knees are most frequently involved, followed by the elbows and ankles, and, less commonly, the wrists, shoulders, and hips. Other hemorrhagic manifestations of severe hemophilia A include bleeding into subcutaneous and intramuscular compartments, hematuria, epistaxis, intracranial bleeding, gingival bleeding, hematemesis, melena, and "pseudotumor" formation. These may occur spontaneously or be provoked by minimal trauma. Soft-tissue hemorrhage into closed spaces may compromise sensory or motor function of nerves, dissect along fascial planes to compress vital structures (i.e., trachea, intestines), or form blood-filled loculations (pseudotumors), which may gradually increase in size and subsequently destroy adjacent soft tissue and bone. Retroperitoneal hemorrhage may mimic acute appendicitis or other causes of an acute abdomen. Hematuria is not uncommon, is usually microscopic and asymptomatic, and resolves spontaneously without treatment. Gastrointestinal bleeding (intraluminal and intramural) occurs occasionally but should not be attributed to the coagulopathy until the presence of an intrinsic lesion is ruled out. Intracranial hemorrhage is associated with a high mortality and requires prompt diagnosis and aggressive treatment.

Hemophiliacs with slightly less severe deficiencies of factor VIII activity (3 to 5 percent of normal) or mild deficiencies (5 to 25 percent of normal) rarely experience spontaneous hemorrhagic episodes but may become symptomatic following trauma or surgery. The degree of factor VIII deficiency remains constant throughout the life of the affected individual.

The presence of hemophilia A is determined by a prolonged

APTT, unless the factor VIII level is greater than 20 to 30 percent of normal. Whole blood clotting times are usually abnormal; PT, bleeding times, and TT are normal. Specific assay for factor VIII-procoagulant activity indicates a significantly reduced level, and the factor VIII-related antigen, as detected immunologically with heterologous antibody, is normal. Detection of related female carriers of hemophiliacs is based on obtaining factor VIII activities intermediate to normal values and values observed in the proband. This procoagulant activity serves as the numerator for a ratio constructed with the level of VIII antigen as the denominator. A result of less than 0.75 suggests the carrier state in family members of a congenitally deficient patient. Although hemophilia A can occur in the female offspring of a female carrier and affected male, this is an exceedingly rare event. The diagnosis of hemophilia A in a female requires exclusion of von Willebrand disease, a coagulopathy transmitted in an autosomal dominant manner.

The adequacy and promptness of replacement therapy in hemophilia A determine the subsequent morbidity and mortality of the disorder. For the majority of superficial soft-tissue injuries and hemarthroses, factor VIII levels should be raised to between 10 and 20 percent of normal. This can be accomplished with fresh-frozen plasma or cryoprecipitates of fresh plasma. When levels of factor VIII between 20 and 50 percent are required, as in major soft-tissue or visceral bleeds and in minor surgical procedures, use of cryoprecipitates or lyophilized concentrates is recommended. For major surgery and documented or clinically suspected central nervous system hemorrhage, factor VIII activities of 50 percent are considered adequate; however, because of the great risks of intracerebral bleeding, replacement to concentrations of 100 percent should be attempted. This is achieved most promptly and efficiently with lyophilized concentrates (Tables 6.10–2 and 6.10–3). Purified factor VIII (and factor IX) has been prepared by molecular biology cloning techniques and may provide an important advance in replacement therapy for hemophilia. An antifibrinolytic agent, ε-aminocaproic acid (EACA), may lessen bleeding following certain surgical procedures (dental extractions) but probably is contraindicated for control of hematuria because of the risk of formation of clots that may occlude the ureters or urethra.

VON WILLEBRAND DISEASE[2]

As originally recognized, von Willebrand disease (vWd) is inherited as an autosomal dominant disorder typically characterized by epistaxis, easy bruising, and mucosal and gastrointestinal hemorrhage. Menorrhagia is common in affected females. Spontaneous hemarthroses are rare. Posttraumatic bleeding often is prolonged. The degree of clinical symptomatology and laboratory abnormalities reflects heterozygous or homozygous inheritance patterns. A prolonged bleeding time is characteristic of the disease. In most cases the diagnosis is established in males and females who exhibit a mild or moderate bleeding disorder with prolonged bleeding times and abnormalities of other in vitro assays (Table 6.10–4). The family histories suggest that these are heterozygous defects. The homozygous disorder occurs much less commonly and is manifested by severe bleeding and very low levels of all assays (vWF:Ag< 1 percent, VIII:C< 5 percent, RCoF < 10 percent, for abbreviations see Table 6.10–4). This spectrum of disease activity is associated with varying but uniform reductions of all multimers that comprise the FVIII/vWF proteins and is designated type I vWd.

Recently, variants of vWd have been described (Table 6.10–4). The identification of these variants has been based on the relative decrease of some of the high-molecular-weight multimers of vWF:Ag in contrast to the lower-molecular-weight multimers. The differences in the vWF:Ag multimers is detectable on electroimmunoassay on sodium dodecal sulfate agarose or on crossed immunoelectrophoresis. Subdivision of these types depends on the hyperaggregability of platelets in the presence of suboptimal concentrations of ristocetin. Additional types of vWd are identified

TABLE 6.10–4. VARIANTS OF VON WILLEBRAND DISEASE

Type I	**Autosomal dominant** *VIII:C,vWF:Ag, and RCoF*—reduced in plasma *vWF:Ag*—multimeric structure qualitatively normal
Type II	**Plasma VIII:C > vWF:Ag or RCoF** *vWF:Ag*—abnormalities of multimeric structure
Type IIA	**Autosomal dominant** *vWF:Ag*—large and medium multimers absent in plasma and platelets *RIPA*—decreased
Type IIB	**Autosomal dominant** *vWF:Ag*—large multimers absent in plasma and normal in platelets *RIPA*—increased
Type IIC	**Autosomal recessive** *vWF:Ag*—large multimers absent in plasma and platelets *vWF:Ag*—multimers present are abnormal
Type III	**Autosomal recessive** *VIII:C*—markedly reduced *vWF:Ag, RIPA and RCoF*—absent
Pseudo-vWd (platelet-type vWd)	**Autosomal dominant** *VIII:c,vWF:Ag*—normal or decreased *vWF:Ag*—large multimers absent in plasma and present in platelets *RIPA*—increased and enhanced induction of thrombocytopenia
Acquired vWD	**Associated with an underlying disorder** Antibody directed against vWF:Ag or RCoF may be present

FVIII = factor VIII protein; VIII:C = factor VIII coagulant activity; VIII:Ag (VIIIC:Ag) = Factor VIII coagulant antigen, the antigenic expression of VIII:C; vWF(VIII/vWF) = von Willebrand factor protein; vWF: Ag(VIIIR:Ag) = von Willebrand factor antigen (FVIII-related antigen); vWd = von Willebrand disease; RIPA = ristocetin-induced platelet aggregation; RCoF = ristocetin cofactor assay, the ability of vWF to support RIPA.

because of the presence or absence of different size vWd:Ag multimers in circulating platelets versus plasma, the concentration of ristocetin cofactor RCoF, as well as the pattern of inheritance.

Infusions of normal fresh-frozen plasma or cryoprecipitate (prepared from normal plasma) correct the defects of vWd and should be administered for therapeutic and prophylactic purposes. They produce significantly higher and sustained levels of VIII:C activity than would be expected from the amount of factor VIII:C administered (Tables 6.10–2 and 6.10–3). Interestingly, infusion of plasma or cryoprecipitate prepared from plasma of patients with hemophilia A (factor VIII deficiency) also corrects the abnormalities in vWd but is not generally used for clinical situations. Factor VIII concentrates are not recommended in vWd because of their variable efficacy, which may be due to the inadvertent loss of high-molecular-weight multimers during processing. A synthetic analog of vasopressin, DDAVP (1-deamino-8-D-arginine-vasopressin) may increase VIII:C, vWF:Ag, and RCoF in some patients with vWd, perhaps by release of vWF from endothelial cells, thereby decreasing the need for transfusion. Patients with mild to moderate type I or type IIA vWd are the most likely to respond, but those with severe type I or type III rarely benefit. DDAVP should *not* be administered to patients with type IIB vWd and those with pseudo-vWd because of the risk of inducing thrombocytopenia. VWd variants accompanied by thrombocytopenia have been described, and in these cases platelet transfusions may be required.

FACTOR IX DEFICIENCY[4]

Congenital deficiency of factor IX (plasma thromboplastin component, Christmas factor) is known as Christmas disease or hemo-

philia B. It is clinically and genetically similar to hemophilia A but occurs less frequently. Homozygous females are rare, but symptoms may occur in females with X chromosome abnormalities such as Turner syndrome (XO). Combined deficiencies of factor VIII and IX have been described. Hemophilia B appears to be a heterogeneous group of disorders. The most common type is characterized by depressed levels of factor IX coagulant activity and normal factor IX antigen as detected by specific heterologous antibodies. Factor IX deficiency with absence of the factor IX antigen is associated with milder symptoms. A variant, designated hemophilia B^m, consists of an abnormal factor IX molecule that acts as a competitive inhibitor of factor VII. Plasma from B^m patients manifests a prolonged APTT and PT (using bovine brain as a source of thromboplastin) despite normal levels of all coagulation factors except IX.

Factor IX levels in homozygous hemophilia B are usually not as depressed as in hemophilia A. Thus, activity of less than 1 percent of normal is uncommon. Carriers are detected by their intermediate depressions of factor IX activity. Laboratory diagnosis for hemophilia B is characterized by a prolonged APTT and normal PT and TT. Bleeding times are usually normal. Specific factor IX assays reveal the deficiency.

Treatment of hemophilia B is similar to that for hemophilia A. Replacement is promptly and efficiently achieved with fresh-frozen plasma or prothrombin-complex concentrates (Tables 6.10–2 and 6.10–3). Circulating inhibitors may develop. Factor IX is not present in cryoprecipitate.

FACTOR X DEFICIENCY

Congenital factor X (Stuart-Prower factor) deficiency is a rare autosomal recessive disorder and clinically resembles factor VII deficiency. Several variants have been described, based on the presence or absence of factor X antigen as detected by a specific heterologous antibody. Acquired factor X deficiency occurs with vitamin K deficiency, hepatic disease, coumarin ingestion, and amyloidosis. Laboratory tests yield prolonged PT and APTT and normal TT and bleeding time. Specific factor X assay using Russell viper venom confirms the deficiency. Treatment is accomplished with fresh-frozen plasma (Tables 6.10–2 and 6.10–3).

FACTOR XI DEFICIENCY

Factor XI (plasma thromboplastin antecedent [PTA]) deficiency is a rare hereditary coagulopathy that has been reported to be transmitted both as an autosomal dominant and autosomal recessive trait. The disease occurs predominantly in Jewish individuals. The severity of the disease is variable and often remains asymptomatic until major trauma or surgery is encountered. Spontaneous hemorrhage and hemarthroses are rare. When bleeding does occur, its severity is not related to factor XI levels.

Laboratory work-up reveals prolonged APTT and whole blood clotting time. The PT is normal, and the bleeding time is rarely prolonged. The specific assay for factor XI and the APTT should be performed on fresh plasma collected in silicone-treated glassware, since factor XI is activated slightly by glass and by freezing. Replacement therapy can be accomplished with infusions of plasma (Tables 6.10–2 and 6.10–3).

FACTOR XII DEFICIENCY

Factor XII (Hageman factor) deficiency is usually inherited as an autosomal recessive trait. It is rarely associated with hemorrhagic complications, although mild bleeding and easy bruisability have been described in a few cases of severe deficiency. Affected individuals appear to have an increased tendency toward thromboembolic complications. The original proband, Mr. Hageman, died following deep leg vein thrombosis and massive pulmonary emboli. This may represent the incomplete or diminished intrinsic activation of plasminogen to plasmin by factor XII. Other investigators have suggested that factor XII inhibits platelet aggregation and that its deficiency promotes thrombogenesis through this mechanism.

As with deficiencies of factors XI, IX, and VIII, Hageman factor deficiency is associated with a prolonged APTT and a normal PT and TT. Whole blood clotting times performed in glass are also prolonged. The bleeding time is usually normal, although it was prolonged in the original proband. Specific assays for factor XII coagulation activity using established factor-deficient plasma indicate levels significantly below normal. No factor XII antigen has been demonstrated in affected patients.

Replacement therapy is theoretically unnecessary since clinical bleeding is rare; nevertheless, some hematologists recommend prophylactic infusions of plasma for factor XII deficient patients before surgery or following trauma (Tables 6.10–2 and 6.10–3).

FACTOR XIII DEFICIENCY

Congenital factor XIII (fibrin-stabilizing factor) deficiency is inherited as an autosomal recessive trait and in most cases becomes clinically apparent at birth with persistent umbilical bleeding. Although easy bruisability and hematoma formation are often prominent in deficient patients, spontaneous hemorrhage, mucous membrane bleeding, and hemarthroses are rare. Wound healing is defective, and dehiscence is common.

The diagnosis should be suspected when clinical bleeding begins 24 to 48 hours after the traumatic event in conjunction with normal screening tests of coagulation, e.g., PT, APTT, TT, bleeding time, whole blood clotting time, clot retraction, and specific assays for clotting factors. In each of these, the final fibrin clot appears friable and is soluble in urea (5 M) or in monochloracetic acid (1 percent). Only 1 percent factor XIII activity is necessary to crosslink fibrin clots normally and to render fibrin insoluble. Replacement therapy is achieved with administration of minimal quantities of plasma (Tables 6.10–2 and 6.10–3). The half-life of transfused factor XIII ranges between 95 and 125 hours.

DEFICIENCIES OF FLETCHER FACTOR; FITZGERALD, FLAUJEAC, WARREN, WILLIAMS, REID FACTOR; AND PASSOVOY FACTOR

Deficiencies of Fletcher factor (prekallikrein), Fitzgerald, Flaujeac, Warren, Williams, Reid factor (high-molecular-weight kininogen), and Passovoy factor have been recognized. They appear to be involved in the contact phase of the intrinsic pathway of coagulation. With the exception of Passovoy factor deficiency, they are asymptomatic. The hemorrhagic severity of Passovoy deficiency appears comparable to that seen in factor XI deficiency. Replacement therapy is accomplished with administration of fresh-frozen plasma. These deficiencies are characterized by a prolonged APTT and a normal PT and TT. In Fletcher factor deficiency, the APTT gradually shortens with incubation at 37C. Specific assays for prekallikrein and high-molecular-weight kininogen confirm the deficiencies. The abnormality present in the Passovoy defect has not been identified.

PROTEIN C AND PROTEIN C INHIBITOR[6]

A recently recognized component of plasma that interacts with procoagulant factors has been designated protein C. This glycoprotein-serine-protease zymogen has been isolated from human and bovine plasma. Protein C is a potent anticoagulant with species specificity. This molecule circulates in the blood inert in a precursor or proenzyme state. It becomes activated to protein Ca by thrombomodulin (a protein that resides on the surface of endothelial cells), with thrombin acting as cofactor. Protein C in its active form, protein Ca, plus a cofactor, protein S, selectively inactivates

factors V and VIII. In addition, protein Ca activates tissue plasminogen activator (tPA), which promotes the conversion of plasminogen to plasmin. Normal plasma contains a naturally occurring inactivator that modulates the activity of protein Ca and is designated protein C inhibitor. The biosynthesis of protein C, protein S, and protein Z (thought to act as a cofactor along with protein S) is dependent upon vitamin K, and they all contain several γ-carboxyglutamic acid residues. Similar in manner to other vitamin K–dependent procoagulant proteins (factors II, VII, IX, X), the synthesis of proteins C, S, and Z is altered in the presence of warfarin.

Two types of hereditary protein C deficiency have been recognized. In type I protein C deficiency there is a defect in one of the genes coding for protein C that will not permit translation. In these patients plasma protein C activity and antigen will be below the normal range, while the ratio of protein C activity and protein C antigen is within the normal range. In type II protein C deficiency, one of the genes coding for protein C has been modified, resulting in an abnormal gene product. In such patients the protein C antigen will be normal while protein C activity and the ratio of activity to antigen are below the normal range. Protein C deficient patients (heterozygotes and homozygotes) are at high risk for venous thromboembolism involving peripheral veins, lungs, cerebral veins, and the microcirculation of the subcutaneous tissue. Protein C deficiency has been reported as an isolated deficiency state and combined with a deficiency of factor V and factor VIII:C. Patients with isolated protein S deficiency suffering from recurrent venous thrombosis have been identified.

ANTITHROMBIN III

Antithrombin III (AT-III) is one of 10 naturally occurring plasma proteins that functions as an inhibitor in modulating the activity of the components of the procoagulant and fibrinolytic systems. This single-chain glycoprotein of 58,000 to 65,000 daltons circulates in the blood in the α_2-globulin region at a normal concentration of 18 to 30 mg/dl. It is synthesized in the liver and vascular endothelial cells. It functions predominantly as a cofactor that strikingly enhances the anticoagulant properties of heparin but exerts inhibitory activity against serine proteases factors IIa, IXa, Xa, XIa, XIIa, and plasmin. The congenital absence of AT-III occurs in an autosomal dominant pattern and is thought to be associated with an increased frequency of venous thrombosis. Three types of deficiency states have been described among several kindreds reported.

FAMILIAL MULTIPLE COAGULATION FACTOR DEFICIENCIES[10]

Two different types of multiple factor deficiencies have been identified. The first type is due to the coincidental concurrence of more than one hereditary single factor deficiency state. The second type is a single heritable disorder associated with deficiencies of two or more factors. Although these are very rare, the following combination of factor deficiencies have been identified in different families: V and VIII (secondary to protein C inhibitor deficiency); II, VII, IX, X (secondary to deficient γ-carboxylation of glutamic acid); VIII and IX; VII and VIII; VIII, IX, and XI; and IX and XI. Thorough evaluation of patients with unexplained prolonged prothrombin times and partial thromboplastin times (in the absence of circulating inhibitors) may lead to additional examples of multiple factor deficiencies in a single patient with familial inheritance.

THE FIBRINOLYTIC SYSTEM

The central component of the fibrinolytic system is plasminogen, which is synthesized in the liver and circulates in the blood as an inert precursor or proenzyme. Plasminogen is found in the euglob-

ulin fraction of the plasma in a concentration range of 12 to 15 mg/dl. The function of the plasminogen-plasmin proteolytic enzyme system is to bring about dissolution of excessive amounts of thrombus formation. This system can be activated by proteins found in different body tissues—plasma activator (vascular endothelial cells), tissue activator (uterus, ovary, neoplasms), and urinary activator (renal parenchymal cells). The degree of fibrinolytic activity by these endogenous activators is minimal and inadequate in pathologic states associated with thrombus formation. Two available agents, streptokinase (β-hemolytic streptococci) and urokinase (human urine or renal parenchymal cells), when exogenously administered activate the plasminogen system, generating plasmin that induces dissolution of pathologic thrombosis (pulmonary emboli, deep vein thrombosis, arterial thrombosis, etc.).

Within the recent past, extremely rare inherited disorders of the plasminogen system have been recognized. Defects in plasminogen or plasminogen activation have been observed to result in a propensity for recurrent thrombosis. Recurrent bleeding resulting from excessive fibrinolysis occurring because of congenital absence of one or more of the naturally present inhibitors of the plasminogen system (α_2-antiplasmin, α_2-antitrypsin, α_2-macroglobulin) has been recognized. These deficiency states are inherited as autosomal recessives and the treatment is fresh-frozen plasma replacement of these missing components.

ACQUIRED DISORDERS

Acquired disorders may result from deficient synthesis or synthesis of functionally defective coagulation factors or the presence of inhibitors of coagulation (see Table 6.8–1). Asparaginase may suppress synthesis of fibrinogen (factor I). Acquired dysfibrinogenemia has been reported in cases of hepatic disease, particularly hepatomas and hepatitis, and metastatic carcinomas. A deficiency of factor V, in association with other abnormalities, may be acquired during disseminated intravascular coagulation. Abnormalities of the vitamin K–dependent factors may accompany defective vitamin K metabolism. Factor IX deficiency may be seen in association with the nephrotic syndrome and proteinuria greater than 10 g per day. Combined factor IX and X deficiencies have been reported in amyloidosis (see Chapter 6.8). Acquired von Willebrand disease is a bleeding disorder that is seen in some patients who are afflicted with a variety of diseases including neoplasms, particularly lymphoma, leukemia, myeloproliferative disorders, connective tissue diseases, and dysglobulinemic states. The unique feature of some patients with this form of von Willebrand disease is the presence of an inhibitor directed against one or more of the properties of the factor VIII/vWF protein (Table 6.10–4). These individuals do not experience an incremental response in circulating levels of factor VIII following transfusion of cryoprecipitate or factor VIII concentrate.

DISSEMINATED INTRAVASCULAR COAGULATION[1,5,8]

Disseminated intravascular coagulation (DIC) is not a primary disease process, but a syndrome encountered in a wide variety of clinical situations (Table 6.10–5). It is characterized by the activation of the coagulation system with resultant "consumption" of a variety of coagulation proteins and platelets, which results in a hemorrhagic diathesis and, paradoxically, ischemic injury to various tissues, presumably due to vessel injury and thrombotic occlusion of small vessels. The fibrinolytic system is also activated, presumably as a homeostatic mechanism. The etiology of DIC is complex and not entirely understood. Factors known to be involved in its etiology are (1) entrance of extrinsic clot-promoting factors into the circulation (e.g., amniotic fluid embolism), (2) intravascular production of clot-promoting agents (e.g., acute intravascular hemolysis), and (3) vascular injury (e.g., infections). The clinical features

TABLE 6.10–5. SOME CAUSES OF DIC

Obstetrical Complications
- Premature separation of the placenta (abruptio placentae)
- Intrauterine retention of a dead fetus or placenta
- Amniotic fluid embolism
- Abortion: septic, or following instillation of hyperosmolar urea or hypertonic saline
- Toxemia

Infections
- Bacterial: sepsis with gram-negative and gram-positive organisms
- Viral
- Rickettsial
- Fungal
- Protozoal

Neoplasia
- Carcinoma: prostate, pancreas, breast, lung, etc.
- Acute promyelolytic leukemia, at presentation or during induction chemotherapy
- Sarcoma, including rhabdomyosarcoma and neuroblastoma

Trauma
- Shock, from whatever cause, including cardiopulmonary arrest
- Head injury
- Massive injuries, burns, and extensive surgery

Acute Intravascular Hemolysis
- Transfusion of incompatible blood
- Infusions of water: intravenously by error, by irrigation during surgery (TURP), submersion in fresh water

Miscellaneous
- Heat stroke
- Hypothermia
- Envenoming by poisonous snakes
- Autoinfusion of ascitic fluid

of DIC are bleeding and evidence of organ dysfunction. The severity of these features is variable and dependent upon the dynamics of the clinical setting. In acute forms of the syndrome, bleeding often is sudden in onset, with diffuse unprovoked bleeding from multiple locations, including recent venipunctures and the sites of indwelling catheters. Hemorrhage into any organ system may occur. Evidence of dysfunction of any organ system may be seen, and commonly involved areas are the skin, kidneys, lungs, liver, and central nervous system. In more chronic forms, recurrent bleeding of variable severity occurs often in association with frank evidence of thrombophlebitis (Trousseau syndrome). Laboratory studies characteristically reveal thrombocytopenia and a prolongation of the TT, PT, and APTT. Hypofibrinogenemia, or a decrease in fibrinogen from previously elevated levels, usually is noted. A rapid qualitative test, useful in an emergency for detection of hypofibrinogenemia, is the observation of an abnormal clot in glass tubes (the "clot observation" test). Tests for detection of fibrinogen-fibrin degradation products (FDP) are elevated. Tests of other coagulation factors may give variable results depending upon the assays used. Peripheral blood smears reveal microangiopathic changes in approximately 50 percent of patients.

Therapy mandates recognition and vigorous treatment of the underlying process. If this can be accomplished, the DIC is quickly brought under control and then disappears. For example, in patients with abruptio placentae, the level of fibrinogen rises rapidly following emptying of the uterus and reaches hemostatically effective levels within 6 to 12 hours. Patients with bleeding due to DIC require restoration of blood volume. Replacement with fibrinogen, while not harmful, rarely is necessary or effective unless or until the underlying disorder has been corrected. The use of heparin is controversial. Administration of heparin may result in increased bleeding before improvement in DIC occurs. In reported studies it has not reduced mortality, and generally its use is not recommended. The exception is DIC in Trousseau syndrome, in which

heparin often is useful. The use of EACA alone (i.e., without heparin) has been followed by serious and even fatal thromboembolism, and its use is not recommended except under unusual circumstances.

DISORDERS OF VITAMIN K–DEPENDENT COAGULATION FACTORS[6,7]

Vitamin K is the generic name for a group of naphthaquinones. It has long been recognized that synthesis of factors II, VII, IX, and X by the liver is regulated by vitamin K. More recently four additional vitamin K–dependent factors have been recognized and designated proteins C, S, M, and Z. Originally it was suggested that vitamin K deficiency resulted in decreased synthesis of these factors. More recently it has been demonstrated that vitamin K serves as a cofactor for a hepatic microsomal enzyme needed for post-translational completion of synthesis of the K-dependent factors. Thus deficiency of vitamin K results in synthesis of functionally defective (i.e., biologically inactive) proteins. Abnormalities of vitamin K metabolism are frequent causes of abnormal bleeding, which often include ecchymoses, epistaxis, gingival bleeding, gastrointestinal and genitourinary bleeding, and enhanced bleeding from esophageal varices. Laboratory diagnosis is relatively easy and includes a prolonged PT (due to deficiencies of factors II, VII, and X) and APTT (due to deficiency of factor IX) with confirmation by additional, more specific tests. Determination of the causes of these multiple deficiencies is enhanced by an understanding of the metabolism of vitamin K.

Vitamin K is not synthesized in humans. It is available from plant foods and is produced by intestinal bacteria. Hemorrhagic disease of the newborn is a preventable disorder attributable to vitamin K deficiency in the neonate before the diet and intestinal flora provide adequate amounts of the vitamin. Dietary inadequacy is an unusual cause of vitamin K deficiency in the adult, in part because of its availability from intestinal bacteria. The natural forms of vitamin K are lipid-soluble and require bile salts for absorption, which occurs chiefly in the small bowel. Thus, vitamin K deficiency can result from biliary obstruction (e.g., gallstones) from any cause as well as various malabsorption syndromes (e.g., sprue, celiac disease, inflammatory bowel diseases, short bowel syndrome, etc.). Parenchymal liver disease may lead to deficiency of the vitamin K–dependent coagulation factors, owing in part, to defective utilization of the vitamin for post-translational carboxylation of the factors. Cholestyramine, which is used to suppress itching caused by biliary tract obstruction and to reduce serum cholesterol, binds bile salts and may reduce absorption of vitamin K. Broad-spectrum antibiotics, which alter the intestinal flora, may limit availability of vitamin K from this important source and result in deficiency of vitamin K, especially if the patient's food intake is limited, as in the postoperative period. Broad-spectrum cephalosporin antibiotics (moxalactam, cefamandole) induce deficiency of vitamin K clotting factors and bleeding, blocking vitamin K–dependent peptide carboxylation by their N-methylthiotetrazole moiety. The effects of coumarin anticoagulants on the vitamin K–dependent coagulation proteins are discussed in Chapter 6.25. With the exception of patients with liver disease, all of these disorders are readily responsive to—and, most important, are preventable by—administration of appropriate preparations and doses of vitamin K.

INHIBITORS OF COAGULATION (ANTICOAGULANTS)

Spontaneous[3,4,9]
Acquired inhibitors of blood coagulation (circulating anticoagulants) develop in two clinical situations. They are encountered in individuals with congenital factor deficiencies (e.g., factor VIII or IX) who develop antibodies to the deficient factor following re-

peated exposure to sources of replacement therapy. The second situation involves the spontaneous development of inhibitors in individuals without preexisting coagulation abnormalities. These inhibitors specifically inactivate a previously activated clotting factor or interfere with the interaction of coagulation factors and platelets.

Approximately 10 to 15 percent of patients with classic hemophilia A (congenital deficiency of factor VIII) may eventually develop circulating inhibitors of factor VIII following factor VIII replacement therapy. The patient with such an inhibitor does not respond to subsequent replacement in the expected manner (Table 6.10–3), and if the inhibitor (anticoagulant) is present in high titer, does not respond at all. A low-titered inhibitor sometimes can be overcome by infusions of cryoprecipitate or factor VIII concentrate given in higher doses. When this maneuver fails (as in the presence of a high-titered inhibitor), other forms of therapy to be considered include the use of prothrombin-complex concentrates or activated factors, anti-inhibitor coagulant complexes containing a higher concentration of activated clotting factors (Autoplex or FEIBA), immunosuppressive agents, plasmapheresis, DDAVP, and factor VIII concentrates of bovine or porcine origin. The frequency of developing inhibitors in hemophilia B (congenital deficiency of factor IX) is approximately 2 to 3 percent, and the problems in therapy are similar to those in patients with hemophilia A and an inhibitor. Inhibitors of factor V have been reported in a few patients, but in most instances there was not clear evidence of preexisting congenital deficiency of factor V. Development of inhibitors in patients with congenital deficiency of other coagulation factors has rarely been reported.

Acquired inhibitors of coagulation factors usually are IgG immunoglobulins (IgG_4), although inhibitors of the IgM and IgA variety have been associated with abnormal paraproteinemias. Thus these antibodies may arise in patients with disorders such as multiple myeloma, macroglobulinemias, ulcerative colitis, and autoimmune diseases. An unexplained inhibitor of factor VIII develops rarely in the postpartum state and may be seen in elderly individuals without other associated disease. Severe bleeding may be seen, although hemarthroses are rare. Treatment often is difficult and is similar to that used in patients with congenital factor VIII deficiency (hemophilia A) and an inhibitor. Circulating anticoagulants have been related to the use of certain drugs, including antibiotics and phenytoin (Dilantin). Factor VIII inhibitors have been described with penicillin administration, and aminoglycosides have been implicated in the spontaneous development of factor V inhibitors. Antibodies against factor XIII have occurred with the use of isoniazid. In most instances inhibitors induced by drugs disappear eventually with termination of the medication.

A common interfering inhibitor occurs in systemic lupus erythematosus (5 to 10 percent of affected patients) and with few exceptions is directed toward the action of the prothrombin activator (a complex of factor Xa, factor V, phospholipid, and calcium). Other lupus anticoagulants have been identified infrequently against factor II activity and factors VIII, IX, XI, and XII. Recurrent deep venous thrombosis has been documented in several patients with lupus inhibitors against factors XI and XII. Acquired von Willebrand disease has been described in several patients with systemic lupus erythematosus. The inhibitor found in patients with systemic lupus erythematosus is commonly associated with a biologic false-positive test for syphilis. This inhibitor may be associated with an anticardiolipin antibody, which may correlate with recurrent miscarriage. Abnormal bleeding is uncommonly associated with the typical lupus anticoagulant. If low levels of factor II, thrombocytopenia, or uremia are also present, bleeding may occur. If acquired anticoagulants against factors VIII and IX exist in these patients, significant hemorrhage may occur and corticosteroid therapy should be instituted. Although the anticoagulant may not disappear immediately, its activity may decrease. Transfusions of fresh-frozen plasma are ineffective; treatment with immunosuppressive agents and factor concentrates have not been evaluated adequately.

Abnormalities of laboratory tests performed in the presence of a circulating anticoagulant depend on the site of action of the inhibitor. Characteristically, the abnormal test does not normalize when normal plasma is mixed with the sample containing the inhibitor. Incubation of the mixture at 37C for 1 hour may exaggerate the abnormality. In contrast, correction occurs when mixing experiments are performed in true coagulation factor deficiencies.

Therapeutic
The therapeutic use of various anticoagulants is discussed in Chapter 6.25.

REFERENCES*

1. Bell WR: Disseminated intravascular coagulation. Johns Hopkins Med J 146:289, 1980
2. Coller BS: Von Willebrand disease: In Colman RW, Hirsh J, et al (eds): Hemostasis and Thrombosis: Basic Principles and Clinical Practice. 2d ed. Philadelphia, JB Lippincott, 1987, p 60
3. Feinstein DI: Lupus anticoagulant, thrombosis, and fetal loss (editorial). N Engl J Med 313:1348, 1985
4. Lusher JM: Hemophilia: Current concepts of management and unresolved problems. Hematol Rev Commun 1:145, 1986
5. Marder VJ, Martin SE, et al: Consumptive thrombohemorrhagic disorders. In Colman RW, Hirsh J, et al (eds): Hemostasis and Thrombosis: Basic Principles and Clinical Practice, 2d ed. Philadelphia, JB Lippincott, 1987, p 975
6. Olson RE: Vitamin K. In Colman RW, Hirsh J, et al (eds): Hemostasis and Thrombosis: Basic Principles and Clinical Practice, 2d ed. Philadelphia, JB Lippincott, 1987, p 846
7. Ratnoff OD: Hemostatic defects in liver and biliary tract disease. In Ratnoff OD, Forbes CD (eds): Disorders of Hemostasis. Orlando, Grune and Stratton, 1984, p 451
8. Sach GH, Levin J, et al: Trousseau's syndrome and other manifestations of chronic disseminated coagulopathy in patients with neoplasms: Clinical, pathophysiologic and therapeutic features. Medicine 56:1, 1977
9. Shapiro SS: Hemorrhagic disorders associated with circulating inhibitors. In Ratnoff OD, Forbes CD, (eds): Disorders of Hemostasis. Orlando, Grune and Stratton, 1984, p 271
10. Soff GA, Levin J: Familial multiple coagulation factor deficiencies: I. Review of the literature: Differentiation of single hereditary disorders associated with multiple factor deficiencies from coincidental concurrence of single factor deficiency states. Semin Thromb Hemost 7:112, 1981

*References 3, 9, and 11 to 13 cited in Chapter 6.8 also provide detailed information relating to topics in this chapter.

Bone Marrow Failure

Lyle L. Sensenbrenner
and Albert H. Owens, Jr.

NORMAL HEMATOPOIESIS

Hematopoiesis in the normal state is an orderly process of cell proliferation and maturation that maintains the concentration of cellular elements in the peripheral blood and tissues necessary for good health (see Fig. 6.1–1).[4,5] This process is carefully controlled by a number of humoral and cellular mediators (Table 6.11–1).[3,4] For hematopoiesis to take place a favorable, delicately structured microenvironment is required.

The most primitive progenitors (pluripotent stem cells) of the lympho-hematopoietic systems may not be called upon to express their full functional potential during adult life. Their continued vitality and full range of biologic potential do become apparent, however, when bone marrow is transplanted from one individual to another and the recipient's entire lympho-hematopoietic cell system is fully reconstituted with donor-type cells. Following birth, the lymphoid system is usually sustained from the pool of lymphoid stem cells (see Chapter 7.1). Similarly, the other formed elements of the blood are maintained by the hematopoietic stem cell pool (see Chapter 6.1).

The most primitive hematopoietic stem cells are capable of some degree of self-renewal—perhaps even limitless self-renewal. They also produce progeny that are committed to differentiate along each of the specific cell lines. Thus, erythrocytes, granulocytic cells, and megakaryocytes are derived by a multistep process of proliferation, commitment, continuing differentiation, and maturation (see Fig. 6.1–1). It has been estimated that 25 to 35 cell divisions occur during the hematopoietic process, each with an additional degree of biologic commitment and differentiation.[1,5]

IMPAIRED HEMATOPOIESIS[5,6]

Impaired hematopoiesis results from defects in the stem cells per se or from disorders of the "physiologic environment" that regulates and normalizes blood cell self-renewal (Table 6.11–2). Hematopoietic stem cell defects may be congenital or acquired. At times it is possible to identify a specific nutritional deficiency (e.g., vitamin B_{12} or folic acid), toxin (e.g., chloramphenicol or benzene), or immunoglobulin (e.g., antibody against erythrocyte precursors or against erythropoietin) responsible for the defect. More often, however, the cause of the defective progenitor cell damage is not apparent.

The wide variety of morphologic abnormalities that result from hematopoietic stem cell defects can best be understood in terms of the biologic potential and commitment of the progenitor(s) primarily involved (see Fig. 6.1–1, Table 6.11–2). Further, the changes in cell morphology encountered during the course of disease can be understood in terms of disordered differentiation.

Defects in the more primitive hematopoietic stem cells (CFU-Blast, CFU-S, CFU-GEMM) may be expected to result in a failure of development of all subsequent hematopoietic elements in each of the various cell lines. A peripheral blood pancytopenia will ensue, and the bone marrow will appear hypoplastic. Similarly, disorders that primarily affect a committed progenitor will be manifested mainly in the cell line that develops from that progenitor. For example, the presence of an antibody directed against the early erythroid progenitor burst-forming unit–erythroid (BFU-E) will

result in a bone marrow devoid of any discernible red blood cell precursors, no red blood production, absence of reticulocytes in the peripheral blood and severe anemia, a condition known as pure red blood cell aplasia.

Stem cell disorders may lead to aplasia, dysplasia, or neoplasia (self-sustaining proliferation) of their subsequent hematopoietic elements depending on the nature and degree of the defect. Each of these morphologic abnormalities may result in a form of bone marrow failure (Table 6.11–3).

CLASSIFICATION[6]

Bone marrow failure results when the hematopoietic process is unable to produce sufficient numbers of properly functioning blood cells to sustain good health. Currently, bone marrow failure syndromes are classified according to the principal cellular abnormalities noted on routine cytologic examination of the peripheral blood and bone marrow (Table 6.11–4), and to the degree of severity of that abnormality. Although many congenital stem cell defects are apparent at birth or shortly thereafter, certain heritable disorders are not manifested until later in life.

Many bone marrow failure syndromes represent primary hematopoietic disease. However, more commonly blood cell development is impaired secondary to another systemic disease process such as infection, nutritional deficiencies, or renal failure (Table 6.11–4).

SIGNS AND SYMPTOMS

IMPAIRED CELL PRODUCTION

The clinical manifestations of bone marrow failure are determined in large measure by the cell line(s) involved, by the severity of the failure, and the rapidity of its onset (Table 6.11–5). Signs and symptoms of anemia are present if the erythrocytic series is compromised. Usually, the severity of the symptoms which the patient experiences is proportional to the rapidity of the onset of the anemia. Infections, especially with bacteria and fungi, result from the impaired production of normal granulocytes and monocytes. Bleeding and easy bruisability stem from a deficiency of platelets when megakaryocyte proliferation and differentiation is sufficiently impaired.

Patients with aplastic anemia develop all of these features to a varying degree since the basic defect in this disorder is located in the primitive hematopoietic stem cell. Patients with myelodysplastic disorders also demonstrate in varying degree signs and symptoms related to defects in all the cell lines. Although the bone marrow may appear to be cellular in many of the myelodysplastic disorders, hematopoiesis is often ineffective, resulting in selective cytopenias or blood cells that function poorly.

NEOPLASTIC CELL ACCUMULATION

In the myeloproliferative disorders, production of blood cells exceeds their destruction, resulting in excessive numbers of neoplastic cells that accumulate in the bone marrow and other tissue sites.

TABLE 6.11–1. PHYSIOLOGIC CONTROLS OF HEMATOPOIESIS

Site[a]	Mediator	Source	Action
(1) Uncommitted-earliest pluripotent stem cell	T-cell subset? Stochastic?	Thymus?	Regulates self-renewal (shown in mice)
(2) Multipotent hematopoietic + stem cells (CFU-Blast, CFU-S (3) CFU-GEMM)	Humoral activity; IL-3, GM-CSF (slight)	Stimulated T cells, monocytes	Stimulates cell division
(4) Burst-forming unit–erythroid (BFU-E)	IL-3, GM-CSF (slight)	Stimulated T cells, monocytes	Recruits erythropoietin-insensitive erythroid precursors to erythropoietin-sensitive state
(4) BFU-E and (5) colony-forming unit–erythroid (CFU-E)	Erythropoietin IL-3	Kidney and small amount extrarenal (liver)–stimulated lymphocytes	Stimulates development of erythrocytes from CFU-E and BFU-E
(6) Colony-forming unit–megakaryocyte (CFU-M)	Thrombopoietins (?) IL-3 (?)	Kidney (?)	Stimulates proliferation of megakaryocytes and release of platelets
(7) Colony-forming unit-eosinophil (CFU-Eo)	Eosinophil colony-stimulating factor	?	Stimulates proliferation of eosinophil precursors
(8) Colony-forming unit–granulocyte monocyte (CFU-GM)	GM-CSF	Monocytes, stimulated lymphocytes	Stimulates proliferation of granulocyte or monocyte precursors or both
	Granulocyte chalone	Mature granulocytes	Inhibits proliferation of CFU-GM; decreases granulocyte and monocyte production
	Prostaglandin IE	Macrophages	Inhibits production of granulocytes and macrophages
	Serum lipoproteins		Inhibits CFU-GM proliferation directly; inhibits GM colony-stimulating factor production
(9) Lymphoid stem cell and (10) colony-forming unit–T lymphocyte (CFU-TL)	IL-2, processed antigen	Macrophages that process antigen	Stimulates production of T-helper and suppressor cells and their lymphokines
(11) Colony-forming unit–B lymphocyte (CFU-BL) IL-4		Antigen-stimulated T-helper cells, macrophages	Stimulates maturation of B cells and antibody production

[a]Numbers refer to sites indicated in Figure 6.1–1, p. 306.

During this process, normal hematopoiesis is suppressed, and anemia, granulocytopenia, and thrombocytopenia develop. Furthermore, the accumulation of neoplastic cells in extramedullary sites leads to tumor formation and its attendant signs and symptoms. Intravascular plugs of blast cells may also impair circulation in the small vessels of the brain or the lungs. Thrombocythemia may also develop and lead to thrombosis of large vessels and bleeding disorders (see Chapter 6.8).

PARANEOPLASTIC MANIFESTATIONS

Neoplastic disorders often produce other signs and symptoms that are not directly due to the accumulation of excess tumor cells. For example, progranulocytic leukemia is associated with disseminated intravascular coagulation thought to be due to the release of a procoagulin from the neoplastic cells. Patients also develop fever, excessive uric acid production resulting in hyperuricemia, and sometimes uric acid renal stones. Hypercalcemia and hyperkalemia are among other physiologic abnormalities whose pathogenesis is not fully understood but which are often seen in neoplastic disorders.

MANIFESTATIONS OF ASSOCIATED DISEASE PROCESSES

Since bone marrow failure is frequently secondary to nonhematopoietic disorders, patients may also manifest a variety of signs and symptoms not related to the hematopoietic system. These symptoms would be characteristic of the nutritional deficiency, endo-

crinopathy, infectious disease, or intoxication that was also responsible for the impaired hematopoiesis (Table 6.11–5).

EVALUATION

When evaluating patients with bone marrow failure, the primary goal is to arrive at a rational management plan for each patient as expeditiously as possible. Several practical considerations should guide the physician to place special emphasis on certain aspects of the work-up:

1. What blood cell lines (types) are involved and how severe is the resulting functional deficit?
2. Are the functional defects due to impaired production of blood cells or to their increased destruction?
3. What is the cause of the hematopoietic failure?
   a. Is there evidence of a primary hematopoietic disorder?
   b. Is there evidence of an intoxication or a nutritional deficiency?
   c. Is the bone marrow failure due to a primary disease process outside of the hematopoietic system such as an infection or an endocrinopathy?
4. Will the process be self-limiting or progressive?
5. Is the process reversible? Are there indications for specific treatment?
6. Is the patient a candidate for allogeneic bone marrow transplantation?

TABLE 6.11–2. PATHOGENESIS OF BONE MARROW FAILURE SYNDROMES

Site[a]	Disorder	Blood and Marrow Morphology	Comments
(1) Pluripotent stem cell	Aplastic anemia (severe)	Severe reduction of all blood elements; severe marrow hypoplasia	Failure of all lymphoid and hematopoietic cell lines
(2) Multipotent hematopoietic + stem cell (CFU-Blast, CFU-S, (3) CFU-GEMM)	Aplastic anemia (severe), Fanconi anemia	Severe bone marrow hypoplasia; pancytopenia; lymphoid cell lines intact	Most common form of aplastic anemia; lymphoid elements normal. CFU-C, CFU-E, and BFU-E virtually absent
(4) Burst-forming unit–erythroid (BFU-E) and (5) colony forming unit–erythroid (CFU-E)	Pure red cell aplasia	Severe anemia, reticulocytopenia; red cell precursor virtually absent from marrow	Frequent association with thymoma; may be due to antibodies against red cell precursors or erythropoietin; CFU-E and BFU-E absent or sharply reduced
	Diamond–Blackfan syndrome	Severe anemia, reticulocytopenia; hypoplasia of red cell precursors in marrow	Congenital disorder; similar to pure red cell aplasia
(6) Colony-forming unit–megakaryocyte (CFU-M)	Congenital thrombocytopenias	Thrombocytopenia; marrow megakaryocytes decreased or absent	CFU-M essentially absent; intrauterine viral infection, drug reactions present similarly
(8) Colony-forming unit–granulocyte-monocyte (CFU-C, CFU-GM)	Congenital neutropenias, acquired neutropenias	Neutropenia, usually severe; granulocyte precursors absent from marrow	CFU-GM deficient; absence of stimulators in some instances; immune mechanisms involved in some cases
(9) Lymphoid stem cell, (10) colony-forming unit–T lymphocyte (CFU-TL) and (11) colony-forming unit–B lymphocyte (CFU-BL)	Immune deficiency disorders	Lymphopenia; hypocellularity of lymphoid organs; absence of plasma cells	Many congenital and acquired syndromes
T4 lymphocytes (helper cells)	AIDS	Normal or hypoplastic	Absence of T4 (helper) lymphocytes

[a]Numbers refer to sites of action in Figure 6.1–1, p. 306.

HISTORY AND PHYSICAL EXAMINATION

A careful family history will often aid in the identification of a heritable disorder. Ingenuity is often required in determining a patient's true biologic ancestry and the familial illnesses that may be related to hematopoietic failure.

An appropriate personal history will include the patient's occupation, potential exposure to drugs or chemical toxins, dietary habits, or evidence suggesting the origin of nutritional deficiencies. Seeking evidence of drug ingestion is especially important and should include items that might have been obtained "over the counter" as well as those prescribed by a physician. Chemical exposure is not always easy to identify, and several types of inquiry are often needed to determine the use of insecticides or organic solvents. For example, the potential exposures of farmers, chemical workers, automobile mechanics, or house painters are obvious compared to those associated with the pursuit of personal hobbies, casual automobile maintenance projects, or the many other facets of daily living.

The physical examination is likely to reveal evidence of significant anemia (pallor), granulocytopenia (infection), and thrombocytopenia (petechiae and ecchymoses). However, it is important that the examiner remain alert to evidence of neoplastic hematopoietic disorders (e.g., splenomegaly, lymphadenopathy, sternal tenderness, tissue infiltrates). Similarly, there may be stigmata of congenital disorders (e.g., the bone defects of Fanconi anemia or the skin abnormalities of dyskeratosis congenita) responsible for the bone marrow failure. On the other hand there may be evidence of nonhematopoietic disorders such as tuberculosis, renal failure, or hypothyroidism (Table 6.11–5), which can secondarily cause bone marrow failure.

TABLE 6.11–3. BLOOD DYSCRASIAS ASSOCIATED WITH IMPAIRED HEMATOPOIESIS[a]

Aplastic Syndromes
- Aplastic anemia
- Paroxysmal nocturnal hemoglobinuria
- Erythroid aplasia
- Hypoplastic neutropenia
- Amegakaryocytic thrombocytopenia

Dysplastic Syndromes
- Refractory anemia with excess blasts
- Refractory anemia with cytopenia
- Acquired idiopathic sideroblastic anemia
- Secondary myelodysplasias

Neoplastic Syndromes
- Acute myeloblastic leukemia
- Chronic myelocytic leukemia
- Polycythemia vera
- Myelofibrosis (megakaryocytic leukemia)
- "Smoldering leukemia"

[a]For further details see Chapters 6.12, 6.16, 6.17, 6.20, and 6.22.

PERIPHERAL BLOOD AND BONE MARROW ANALYSIS (Table 6.11–6)[6]

Careful examination of the peripheral blood will provide information about the concentration of its various cellular elements and their morphologic appearance. Thus, one will gain a precise appre-

TABLE 6.11–4. CLINICAL CHARACTERISTICS OF BONE MARROW FAILURE SYNDROMES

Line(s) Failing	Disease Syndromes	Manifestations	Diagnostic Considerations
All cell lines failing	Aplastic anemia	Pancytopenia. Bone marrow hypoplasia	Bone marrow biopsy confirms aplasia; plasma cells, mast cells, and lymphocytes common. Chromosome abnormalities may be present
	Reversible toxic suppression (radiation, drugs, toxins)	Pancytopenia. Bone marrow hypoplasia	Bone marrow biopsy confirms aplasia. Recovery evident with time
	Preleukemic states	Variable pancytopenia; abnormal cell types often present. Marrow likely cellular; all cell lines may be dysplastic	Bone marrow cellular; myelodyspoiesis prominent. Chromosomal abnormalities may foretell poor prognosis
	Paroxysmal nocturnal hemoglobinuria (PNH)	Hemoglobinuria, hemolysis; increased sensitivity of red blood cells to complement lysis. Pancytopenia. Aplastic anemia	Sugar water test, Ham test positive. Marrow may be cellular or hypoplastic. Acute leukemia may develop
	Myelophthisic states	Pancytopenia. Abnormal cells in peripheral blood	Bone marrow biopsy reveals infiltration of tumor or other abnormal cells
	Myelofibrosis	Anemia followed by pancytopenia. Hepatosplenomegaly common	Bone marrow biopsy shows fibrosis
	Vitamin deficiency	Macrocytic anemia followed by leukopenia, thrombocytopenia, and neurological defects	B_{12} absorption studies. B_{12} and folate levels. Red blood cell folate level. Bone marrow megaloblastic. Hypersegmentation of neutrophils
	Iron deficiency	Hypochromic anemia followed by leukopenia, thrombocytopenia	Sideropenia; iron stores low. Marrow usually cellular. Epithelial atrophy
Erythrocytes	Diamond–Blackfan syndrome	Congenital anemia, reticulocytopenia	Bone marrow shows few red blood cell precursors
	Transient erythroblastopenia of childhood	Anemia, reticulocytopenia, following viral infection	Bone marrow shows red cell aplasia. Recovery with time
	Pure red cell aplasia	Anemia, reticulocytopenia. Normal WBC and platelets	Bone marrow shows absent red blood cell progenitors. Circulating inhibitors of in vitro erythroid colony growth in some cases. Thymoma often present
	Anemia of renal failure	Anemia usually normochromic, normocytic; reticulocytopenia	Evidence of chronic renal failure. Bone marrow cellular, morphology normal
	Pituitary, thyroid, or adrenal cortical insufficiency	Usually normochromic anemia; rarely macrocytic or microcytic. Manifestation of endocrine insufficiency	Bone marrow normal. Thyroid function, other endocrine function studies abnormal
	Anemia of infection	Moderate anemia. Often microcytic	Low serum iron levels. Rapid iron turnover. Low iron binding capacity
	Anemia of cancer	Moderate normochromic anemia. Leukocytosis or thrombocytosis often present	Bone marrow may be normal or show metastatic tumor. Malnutrition and blood loss may complicate picture
	Starvation	Variable, slowly developing normochromic anemia due to vitamin, iron, other mineral, or true protein-calorie deprivation	Bone marrow may be fairly normal or show signs of specific vitamin or iron deficiency (e.g., macrocytosis, hypochromic red cells). Low serum albumin. Decrease in lymphocytes. Anthropometric studies showing starvation
Neutrophils	Cyclic neutropenia (congenital)	Congenital. Periodic infections at about 21-day intervals when granulocytes may be <100 per μl. Involves platelets and RBC as well, but only careful observation shows this	Serial bone marrows showing periodic proliferation of hematopoietic elements. Serial WBC show 21-day cyclic change in granulocytes from very low (<500) to normal
	Chédiak–Higashi syndrome (congenital)	Congenital. Mild to moderate neutropenia. Cutaneous and ocular hypopigmentation. Nystagmus. Frequent infections. Terminal lymphoma-like phase	Bone marrow aspiration hypercellular; vacuolization of granulocyte precursors. Large granules in mature granulocytic cells
	Chronic idiopathic neutropenia (congenital or acquired)	Monocytosis, neutropenia of many years duration. Infections, usually mild. Children may remit spontaneously	Bone marrow cellular; maturation arrest at myelocyte or metamyelocyte stage

(continued)

TABLE 6.11–4. CLINICAL CHARACTERISTICS OF BONE MARROW FAILURE SYNDROMES (Continued)

Line(s) Failing	Disease Syndromes	Manifestations	Diagnostic Considerations
	Drug-induced neutropenia 1. dose-dependent or idiosyncratic 2. immune-mediated	Transient agranulocytosis after drug ingestion	Bone marrow shows absence of granulocytic precursors, but normal number of progenitors
	Non-drug-induced immune neutropenia 1. isoimmune neonatal 2. autoimmune neutropenia	Neutropenia. Other cell lines normal	Bone marrow shows myelocytic hyperplasia, absence of mature neutrophils. Circulating antibodies to neutrophils. In vitro cultures reveal normal progenitors
	Felty syndrome	Neutropenia, splenomegaly. Rheumatoid arthritis	Bone marrow shows granulocytic hyperplasia. High rheumatoid factor titer. Positive ANA
Megakaryocytes	Congenital syndromes 1. May–Hegglin anomaly	Autosomal dominant. Thrombocytopenia. Good general health	Family studies. Giant platelets and neutrophils with Döhle bodies in blood
	2. Autosomal dominant thrombocytopenia	Thrombocytopenia; platelets normal. Mild bleeding	Family studies. Bone marrow shows small megakaryocytes. Platelet production ineffective
	3. Wiskott–Aldrich syndrome	Males. Thrombocytopenia. Immune defects; eczema. Lymphoproliferative disorders	Immune status studies. Marrow megakaryocytes appear normal
	4. Thrombocytopenia—absent radii syndrome	Autosomal recessive. Thrombocytopenia. Thumbs present but radii absent	Skeletal radiographs show absent radii. Family studies
	5. Intrauterine rubella infection	Thrombocytopenia, with or without bleeding Exposure to rubella during pregnancy	Bone marrow shows reduced or absent megakaryocytes
	6. Thiazide-induced thrombocytopenia	Thrombocytopenia, with or without bleeding. Exposure to rubella ing pregnancy	Bone marrow shows reduced or absent megakaryocytes
	Acquired syndromes 1. Postviral (rubella, varicella) thrombocytopenia	Thrombocytopenia, with or without bleeding. Recent viral infection or immunization with live vaccine (rubella, varicella)	Bone marrow shows vacuolated megakaryocytes, decreased numbers
	2. Drug-related (especially alcohol, thiazides)	Thrombocytopenia, with or without bleeding. History of ingestion	Marrow megakaryocytes absent or nearly so
	3. Ionizing radiation, cytotoxic drug-related	Thrombocytopenia, with or without bleeding. Usually being treated for neoplastic disease	Marrow hypocellular; megakaryocytes reduced or absent

ciation of the absolute and relative frequency of each cell type and be able to identify any abnormal cells present.

As aspiration and a needle biopsy of the bone marrow are required in order to evaluate fully the degree of cellularity and possible presence of tumor or other infiltrative disease processes. With care, a good quality needle biopsy can be safely obtained from the posterior iliac crest even from patients who are profoundly thrombocytopenic. A properly stained aspirate is useful in determining the relative proportion and maturation of each of the hematopoietic cell types in the marrow. A densely infiltrated or fibrotic marrow may lead to a "dry tap," a failure to obtain a specimen of bone marrow cells. Therefore, a biopsy is usually necessary to document profound aplasia as well as dense marrow infiltration or fibrosis.

IN VITRO CULTURE OF HEMATOPOIETIC PROGENITORS[5,6]

Current techniques permit the in vitro culture of many hematopoietic progenitor cells that cannot be distinguished on the routine morphologic studies of bone marrow (Table 6.11–7). At present, in vitro cultures may confirm the absence of a class of progenitors or suggest the possibility of a defect in an even more primitive stem cell.

Alternatively, cultural studies may show that progenitor cells are present in a patient's marrow and have full biologic potential but are not able to complete the normal processes of proliferation and differentiation in vivo because of a cellular or humoral defect in the bone marrow environment. For example, hematopoietic progenitors can be grown from even very hypocellular samples of bone marrow obtained from patients with severe aplastic anemia, severe neutropenia, or pure red blood cell aplasia. Perturbation of the culture conditions such as the addition of steroids, the removal of T lymphocytes or the addition of the patient's serum can often markedly enhance hematopoietic progenitor cell growth. These techniques may be used to define more precisely the pathogenesis of hematopoietic cell failure and predict the results of the application of similar techniques (therapy with adrenal corticosteroids or other immunosuppressive agents) to the clinical situation.

CHROMOSOMAL ABNORMALITIES[1]

The most frequent discrete, nonrandom chromosomal abnormalities associated with hematopoietic cell failure are those characteristic of the acute and chronic leukemias and certain of the non-Hodgkin lymphomas. Various chromosomal abnormalities are also present in about half of the patients with myelodysplastic syn-

TABLE 6.11–5. CLINICAL MANIFESTATIONS ASSOCIATED WITH BONE MARROW FAILURE

Due to Primary Blood Cell Production Failure

Erythrocytes	Pallor, weakness, easy fatigability Dyspnea, heart failure, renal and cerebral insufficiency, Roth spots in severe cases
Granulocytes	Infection, primarily bacterial Overwhelming sepsis due to bacteria and fungi in severe cases
Platelets	Easy bruisability Petechiae, ecchymoses, and hemorrhage in severe cases
All cell lines	Mixtures of the above manifestations

Due to Neoplasms of Hematopoietic Cells

Tumor formation	Splenomegaly, lymphadenopathy, soft tissue masses, bone infiltration
Small vessel plugging	Tumor cell accumulations, especially in brain, lung, and kidneys
Marrow infiltration	Sternal tenderness Hematopoietic cell failure

Paraneoplastic Syndromes

Progranulocytic leukemia	Disseminated intravascular coagulation
Several tumor types	Hyperuricemia, hypercalcemia, etc. (see Chapter 6.13 for details)

Features of Associated Systemic Diseases

Intoxications

Infections

Neoplasms (nonhematopoietic)

Nutritional disorders

Endocrinopathies and metabolic disorders

Diseases with disordered immunity

Renal insufficiency

Congenital abnormalities (e.g., skin, bone)

TABLE 6.11–6. EVALUATION OF BLOOD CELL LINES INVOLVED IN BONE MARROW FAILURE

Cell Line	Studies	Results and Interpretations
Erythrocytes	1. Reticulocyte concentration	1. Absence of reticulocytes implies impaired erythropoiesis. Presence of reticulocytes suggests increased destruction.
	2. Red blood cell, hemoglobin, and hematocrit determination	2. Decline in RBC count, Hgb, and Hct reflects degree and duration of bone marrow failure.
	3. Red blood cell size (MCV)	3. Macrocytosis suggests altered DNA synthesis (e.g., B_{12} and folate deficiency, folate antagonists).
	4. Hemoglobin concentration per RBC (MCHC)	4. Small, hemoglobin-deficient RBC suggest iron deficiency states, inability to utilize iron stores.
	5. Bone marrow morphology	5. Aspirate permits evaluation of number, morphology, and relative proportion of erythroid progenitors, their orderly progression to normal red blood cells, degree of hemoglobinization, cellular content and distribution of iron (sideroblasts), and iron stores in the marrow. Abnormal cell type may identify disease. Biopsy reveals evidence of infiltrative disease, confirms severe aplasia.
	6. Culture of bone marrow for BFU-E and CFU-E	6. Decrease or absence of BFU-E and CFU-E implies defect at progenitor stage or earlier. Growth in the presence of "erythroid aplasia" implies extrinsic inhibitor as in pure red blood cell aplasias.
Granulocytes	1. Total and differential WBC count	1. Reduction in granulocyte concentration proportional to degree of impairment provides no increased destruction.
	2. Bone marrow morphology	2. Precursors absent in hematopoietic failure: Megaloblastosis suggests altered DNA synthesis. Abnormal cell types may identify specific disease. Biopsy reveals infiltrative disease, severe aplasia.
	3. Culture of bone marrow CFU-GM with and without adrenal cortical steroid	3. Poor or absent CFU-GM growth implies defect at progenitor stage or earlier. Improved growth with steroid implies immune granulocytopenia.
	4. Test of peripheral blood cells as source of colony-stimulating activity	4. Low numbers of or defective monocytes will not provide colony-stimulating activity for normal GM colony growth.
Platelets	1. Platelet count	1. Counts must be confirmed by stained smear.
	2. Stained peripheral blood smear	2. Large platelet forms imply rapid platelet formation.
	3. Bone marrow morphology smear, and biopsy for evaluation of megakaryocyte number and morphology	3. Increased megakaryocytes in presence of thrombocytopenia implies increased platelet destruction. Absence of megakaryocytes implies defective progenitor. Abnormal cell types may identify specific disease. Biopsy may show infiltrative disease or severe aplasia.

TABLE 6.11–7. HEMATOPOIETIC PROGENITORS THAT CAN BE CULTURED FROM HUMAN BONE MARROW

Multipotent progenitors	Hematopoietic stem cell is reflected in the colony-forming unit–blast (CFU-Blast), the colony-forming unit-granulocyte, erythrocyte, monocyte, and megakaryocyte (CFU-GEMM), and the cells responsible for long-term marrow cultures
Bipotent progenitors	Colony-forming unit-granulocyte monocyte (CFU-GM)—this progenitor gives rise in vitro to colonies of granulocytes and monocyte-macrophages
Progenitors committed to single cell line differentiation	
Erythrocyte	Burst-forming unit-erythroid (BFU-E)—a progenitor committed to erythropoiesis that forms large erythrocyte colonies in vitro. Also present in peripheral blood
	Colony-forming unit-erythroid (CFU-E)—a later erythroid progenitor producing small erythrocyte colonies in vitro
Megakaryocyte	Colony-forming unit-megakaryocyte (CFU-M)—a progenitor committed to megakaryocytopoiesis, which gives rise to megakaryocyte colonies in vitro
Eosinophil	Colony-forming unit–eosinophil (CFU-Eo)—an eosinophil progenitor that produces eosinophil colonies in vitro

dromes. There is some indication that bone marrow failure patients with chromosomal abnormalities have a poorer prognosis and a greater propensity for developing acute leukemia than those who have 46 apparently normal chromosomes. As yet, no characteristic chromosomal abnormalities have been linked to aplastic anemia or paroxysmal noctural hemoglobinuria, although there has been a specific enzyme (acetylcholinesterase) deficiency detected in paroxysmal nocturnal hemoglobinuria. Pursuing studies of chromosomes has been difficult because of the profound hypocellularity of the bone marrow in many instances. However, more work in this general area is likely to be fruitful, especially utilizing the in vitro culture procedures, contemporary chromosomal banding methods, and the techniques of molecular biology.

MANAGEMENT

A management plan for each patient can usually be developed fairly promptly. The specific elements in the plan will reflect, in large measure, the answers to the questions posed in the preceding paragraphs.

SUPPORTIVE THERAPY

Blood component therapy provides appropriate support for many patients with severe impairments. Red blood cells can be transfused repeatedly over long periods (see Chapter 6.24). On the other hand, repeated transfusions of platelets frequently result in alloimmunization because of their contamination with white blood cells. This not only makes continued platelet support difficult or impossible but may preclude successful bone marrow transplantation at a later date (see Chapter 6.24). Recently techniques have been developed to remove more completely any contaminating white cells from platelet products, or render the nucleated cells nonimmunogenic by ultraviolet radiation which eliminates the dendritic cells. It is now fairly clear that it is the contaminating mononuclear cells that are responsible for initiating the alloimmunization to platelets. Granulocyte transfusions play a limited role, but they may be life-saving in profoundly granulocytopenic patients who have infections caused by antibiotic-resistant microorganisms.

SPECIFIC THERAPY

An examination of Tables 6.11–4 and 6.11–5 reveals a number of diseases possibly responsible for hematopoietic cell failure that require specific treatment, often with curative intent. It is important to continue to search for "treatable possibilities" during each patient's course.

Some patients with severe bone marrow failure are candidates for bone marrow transplantation (see Chapter 6.12). This is especially true for patients with severe asplastic anemia, the congenital immunodeficiency disorders, acute or chronic myelocytic leukemia, or high-risk acute lymphocytic leukemia. With improved techniques for clinical bone marrow transplantation, its application to other severe hematopoietic disorders such as thalassemia and myelofibrosis is being explored as well.

If a bone marrow transplant is to be carried out in a patient with aplastic anemia, it is best to do so as early in the course of the disease as feasible. This minimizes the likelihood of alloimmunization through repeated blood product transfusions and also avoids the need to carry out the transplantation procedure in an individual who has been compromised by multiple prior infections and bleeding episodes (Chapter 6.12).

Treatment is also available for patients with profound aplastic anemia who do not have an appropriate bone marrow donor available to them. Some success has been achieved by using adrenal corticosteroids in conjunction with antilymphocyte or antithymocyte globulin. Remissions have also been obtained following intensive treatment with cyclophosphamide with or without cyclosporine (see Chapter 6.12). Androgens occasionally ameliorate hematopoietic cell failure, but in most instances they are incapable of modifying severe degrees of impairment when used alone.

REFERENCES

1. Lajtha LF: The common ancestral cell. In Winthrobe MM (ed): Blood: Pure and Eloquent. New York, McGraw-Hill, 1980
2. Lichtman MA: The ultrastructure of the hematopoietic environment of the marrow: A review. Exp Hematol 9:391, 1981
3. Metcalf D: The molecular biology and functions of the granulocyte-macrophage colony stimulating factors. Blood 67:257, 1986
4. Ogawa M, Porter PN, Nakahata T: Renewal and commitment to differentiation of hematopoietic stem cells (an interpretive review). Blood 61:823, 1983
5. Quesenberry PJ: Concise review: Synergistic hematopoietic growth factors. Int J Cell Cloning 4:3, 1986
6. Williams WJ, Beutler E, et al (eds): Hematology, 3d ed. New York, McGraw-Hill, 1983

Aplastic Anemia and Paroxysmal Nocturnal Hemoglobinuria

Lyle L. Sensenbrenner
and Albert H. Owens, Jr.

Aplastic anemia and paroxysmal nocturnal hemoglobinuria (PNH) are considered together because they present differing clinical features that reflect a basic abnormality in the hematopoietic stem cell. The defect in both disorders causes a failure of hematopoiesis affecting all cell lines. Patients with aplastic anemia demonstrate a virtual absence of the early multipotent hematopoietic progenitor cell compartment (Fig. 6.12–1) and thus of all subsequent progenitors, precursors, and mature cells in all hematopoietic lines. The defect in PNH, on the other hand, results in the production of a clone of cells that are unusually sensitive to complement-mediated lysis, so that the marrow appears cellular, and all lineages are present. The resulting mature cells are rapidly destroyed, resulting in severe pancytopenia. Potentially both disorders are amenable to stem cell replacement therapy (allogeneic bone marrow transplantation). In the case of PNH, a disorder that appears to have a specific genetic defect, the disorder may potentially be curable some day by the insertion of a correct gene into the existing but defective multipotent hematopoietic stem cells. Elucidation of the pathogenetic mechanisms leading to these disorders and the circumstances responsible for their "spontaneous" resolution will enhance the potential for developing even more sophisticated forms of therapy.

APLASTIC ANEMIA

Aplastic anemia, an unexpected pancytopenia of the peripheral blood elements in the presence of a very hypoplastic bone marrow, results from a profound disorder in the proliferation, commitment, and maturation of the totipotent hematopoietic stem cell or its early progeny. This stem cell disorder leads to a marked reduction of all subsequent progeny, the functioning hematopoietic cell mass. This results in severe impairment of the production of mature, functionally competent erythrocytes, granulocytes, monocytes, megakaryocytes, and platelets (Chapter 6.1, Fig. 6.1–1). Routine morphologic studies of the peripheral blood reveal a pancytopenia expressed by decreased numbers of red blood cells (anemia), granulocytes (neutropenia), and platelets (thrombocytopenia). The number of lymphocytes is variable, frequently normal but occasionally severely depressed as well. The active hematopoietic elements in the bone marrow are replaced, to a large extent, by fatty tissue.[5]

Aplastic anemia results from either an intrinsic defect in the earliest stem cells, resulting in dysfunction or stem cell depletion, or from an alteration in the "physiologic microenvironment" of the bone marrow, rendering it nonsupportive of normal hematopoiesis. Evidence for each type of hematopoietic defect has been forthcoming from animal studies. It is difficult, however, to achieve analogous observations in humans.

The high frequency of successful allogeneic bone marrow transplantation in patients with aplastic anemia suggests that a structural microenvironmental defect sufficient to result in marrow aplasia either is infrequently the etiology of the disorder, or those patients who do have microenvironmental defects can have the defect corrected by the transplantation of cellular elements from normal bone marrow. Since hematopoietic progenitor colonies can be cultured in vitro from many patients with severely hypoplastic marrow, it seems likely that in a significant number of cases aplastic anemia may result from the presence of an inhibitor to normal hematopoiesis or from the lack of a necessary growth factor. The inability to culture hematopoietic colonies in vitro from marrow

cells obtained from other patients with similar clinical manifestations is compatible with the notion that the normal hematopoietic stem cells have been "exhausted" or severely damaged.

When the peripheral blood and bone marrow of patients with aplastic anemia is periodically subjected to routine morphologic analysis, some variation in hematopoietic function is usually noted. In part, this may be due to a spotty distribution of "hematopoietic islands" throughout an otherwise fatty marrow. True variations in cellular concentrations, however, will be encountered in the peripheral blood and marrow. Variable abnormalities in cell morphology will also be encountered. Both types of change are reflective of the disordered hematopoiesis that underlines this disease.

CLASSIFICATION[5]

Hematopoietic stem cell disorders capable of causing aplastic anemia may be either congenital or acquired through exposure to a variety of etiologic agents including drugs, ionizing radiation, or several chemicals, especially the organic solvents. Further, on rare occasions aplastic anemia has been shown to follow several systemic diseases, especially a group of viral illnesses including non-A, non-B hepatitis and infectious mononucleosis. Other preexisting disease states that sometimes lead to aplastic anemia are characterized by metabolic abnormalities such as panhypopituitarism or disordered immunity (Table 6.12–1). In many cases, however, the etiology of the aplastic anemia is unclear and classified as idiopathic because no specific causative factor is apparent.[1,5]

Heritable Aplastic Anemia (Table 6.12–2)
Fanconi anemia is perhaps the best characterized of these rare disorders. The diagnosis is usually suspected in those cases of aplastic anemia in which there is a definite family history of impaired hematopoiesis or the patient manifests the disorder in the first decade of life in association with developmental anomalies typical of Fanconi anemia in other organ systems. The disease may be present, however, with no manifestation other than a demonstrated increased fragility and decreased ability of chromosomes to be repaired when exposed to alkylating agents.

The mode of inheritance of many of the congenital aplastic anemia syndromes is less well characterized. When no familial pattern is obvious, it has been suggested that the hematopoietic stem cell disorder may have resulted from an in utero exposure to a bone marrow–damaging agent. A study of the chromosomes of bone marrow cells is frequently difficult to carry out because of the scarcity of cells suitable for cytogenetic study. However, evidence for chromosomal instability, chromated breaks, and various rearrangements has been reported in a few case studies. In Fanconi anemia, there is thought to be a significant defect in DNA repair. These same DNA abnormalities may well bear a relationship to the development of carcinomas and acute leukemia seen in some patients.

Acquired Aplastic Anemia
Acquired aplastic anemia occurs relatively rarely. In the United States, six to seven cases per million population are reported yearly. There is no clear age or sex preference for disease onset, although the incidence increases exponentially with age after 40, and the disease is slightly more common in males.[10]

A great many drugs frequently used in current clinical practice have been implicated in the pathogenesis of aplastic anemia. Several hundred drugs have been reported to the American Medical

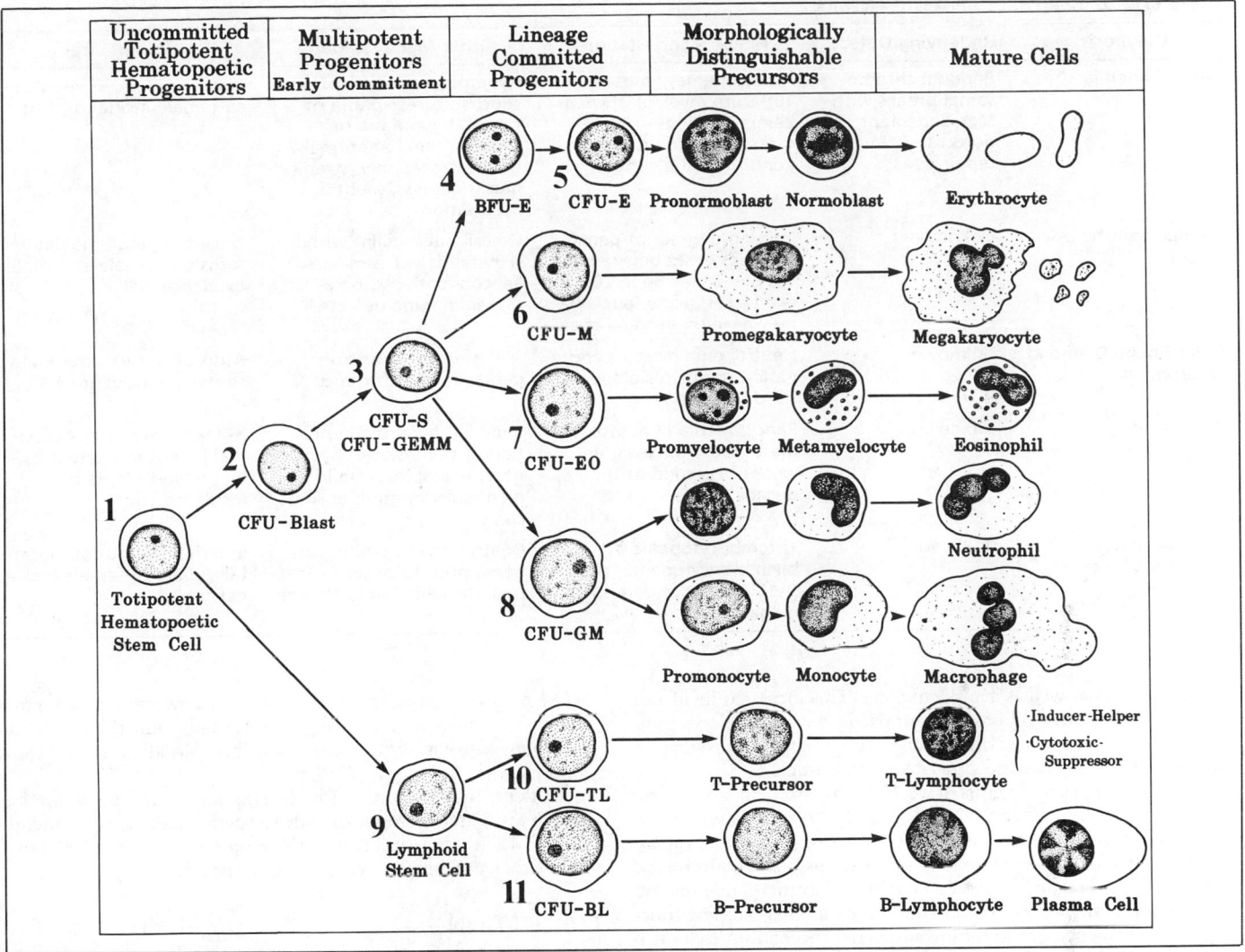

Figure 6.12–1. Cytogenealogy of blood cells.

Association registry because of the suspicion that they may have caused aplastic anemia (Table 6.12–3). The clear implication of a particular drug, however, is often difficult because of the rarity of aplastic anemia and the frequent use of a multiplicity of agents in treating a particular patient.

Perhaps the antibiotic chloramphenicol has received the widest attention as a cause of aplastic anemia over the past 30 years. On rare occasions chloramphenicol causes a severe, self-sustaining impairment of hematopietic stem cell function leading to severe aplastic anemia. This has been reported to occur approximately once in every 40,000 patients receiving the drug and has been reported following such minimal exposure as the use of chloramphenicol antibiotic eye drops. On the other hand, chloramphenicol-induced marrow hypoplasia can be a self-limiting disorder, and many patients have had the good fortune of recovering completely. Vacuolization of chromosomes can be observed following chlor-

amphenicol administration, and it is possible that DNA damage underlies the irreversible hematopoietic stem cell defects, leading to aplastic anemia and eventually the development of paroxysmal nocturnal hemoglobinuria and acute leukemia that has been reported following the use of the drug. Although chloramphenicol-induced DNA damage may be a random event, it is also possible that there is a genetically-determined susceptibility (not now recognized) that is responsible for this type of adverse drug reaction.

Benzene and many halogenated hydrocarbon chemicals are commonly used in industry and about the home. The etiologic relationship of benzene to aplastic anemia and other hematopoietic disorders including leukemia is clearer than is the case with many of the other compounds. Nonetheless, the potential for exposure to marrow-toxic chemicals is very high for many people who follow a normal life style in a modern industrialized society. The rarity of the disease in the presence of this high likelihood of exposure suggests the necessity in many cases of a second factor such as a genetic predisposition, alteration of the immune response, or accompanying viral illness in order to induce the disease.

Ionizing radiation damages hematopoietic precursor cells in proportion to the dose given. Erythroid progenitors seem most susceptible to damage followed by the granulocyte-monocyte cell series and the megakaryocytes. At lower doses (under 300 to 400 rads of whole body exposure) there is potential for hematopoietic recovery. Above this dose level, the marrow damage may be irreversible.

Continuous exposure of the bone marrow to low doses of irradiation has been associated with both an increased incidence of

TABLE 6.12–1. ETIOLOGY OF APLASTIC ANEMIA

- Heritable disorders
- Acquired disorders
    Ionizing radiation
    Chemicals
    Infections
    Metabolic abnormalities
    Immune disorders
    Myelodysplasias
- Idiopathic aplastic anemia

TABLE 6.12–2. HERITABLE APLASTIC ANEMIAS

Diagnosis	Underlying Defect	Hemic Manifestations	Other Manifestations	Inheritance
Fanconi anemia	Random chromosomal breaks with rearrangement; defect in DNA repair	Pancytopenia; onset age 5–10; acute myeloblastic leukemia develops in some cases; poor growth of progenitor cells in culture	Hyperpigmentation of skin; short stature; aplasia of radius, hypoplasia of thumbs; renal abnormalities; microcephaly, strabismus, deafness, mental retardation	Autosomal recessive. Male-to-female incidence, 1.5:1
Familial aplastic anemia	Unknown	Varying degrees of pancytopenia; onset before age 10; onset may be in 20s or even later; acute leukemia may develop in some cases	Occasional families with skeletal defects similar to Fanconi patients; occasional immune defects	Uncertain; multiple patterns seen; male-to-female incidence, 4:1
Shwachman–Diamond syndrome	Unknown	Neutropenia most severe; pancytopenia develops in third of cases	Metaphyseal dysostosis; pancreatic insufficiency	Autosomal recessive; male-to-female incidence 1:1
Dyskeratosis congenita	Unknown	Pancytopenia in approximately 50% of cases; develops in second or third decade of life	Reticular hyperpigmentation of skin, dystrophy of nails, leukoplakia; mild mental retardation in some cases	X-linked recessive; Autosomal inheritance also possible; male-to-female incidence, 10:1
Amegakaryocytic thrombocytopenia	Unknown	Thrombocytopenia at birth; pancytopenia, age 5–10; absent or very small megakaryocytes	Death from thrombocytopenia prior to onset of pancytopenia in most cases	Inheritance patterns uncertain; male-to-female incidence, 2:1

aplastic anemia as well as acute leukemia. This increased incidence of bone marrow disease has been noted in workers following radium and thorium ingestion as well as in patients given radiation therapy for spondylitis and other benign disorders.

Cases of aplastic anemia have been reported in association with many systemic diseases (Table 6.12–4). In most the underlying pathogenetic mechanisms by which the disease produces aplastic anemia have not been worked out. It seems possible, however, that viruses and related agents could damage normal gene function in hematopoietic progenitor cells and create a self-sustaining functional impairment. A commonly suspected mechanism by which several etiologic agents and systemic diseases produce aplastic anemia is that hematopoietic progenitor cells are continually damaged by an ongoing autoimmune reaction that results following initial damage by the drug, toxin, or infectious agent.[10]

CLINICAL MANIFESTATIONS

The onset of the symptoms and signs of aplastic anemia is frequently insidious. Those primarily due to hematopoietic cell failure are weakness and easy fatigability (anemia), fever and repeated infections (granulocytopenia), and easy bruisability and bleeding (thrombocytopenia). Symptoms are more pronounced when the disease progresses rapidly. The threshold for symptoms of anemia are lower in older individuals (Table 6.12–5), and these patients tend to present with symptoms when their blood counts are close to normal.

Patients may also present with signs and symptoms stemming from an associated systemic disorder underlying the aplastic anemia (Table 6.12–4). It is important to recognize these diseases, especially if they can be reversed by timely specific therapy.

EVALUATION

The general approach to evaluating patients with hematopoietic failure is set forth in Chapter 6.11.

Formal criteria for the diagnosis of severe aplastic anemia have been agreed to by several groups of clinical investigators (Table 6.12–6). The main objective criteria are derived from routine morphologic assessments of the peripheral blood and bone marrow.[4]

Pancytopenia is invariably present in aplastic anemia, but its severity is variable. Even when patients present with profound pancytopenia, it is well to question the diagnosis of aplastic anemia until it is clearly established.

Confirmation of the diagnosis of aplastic anemia requires aspi-

TABLE 6.12–3. CHEMICAL CAUSES OF APLASTIC ANEMIA

Drugs[a]	Insecticides	Solvents
Chloramphenicol	Chlordane	Benzene
Hydantoin	DDT	Carbon tetrachloride
Pyrazolones	Lindane	Stoddard solvent
Gold compounds	Parathione	Toluene
Phenothiazines	Arsenic compounds	
Sulfonamides	Pentachlorophenol	
Sulfonylureas		
Thiouracils		

[a]The American Medical Association maintains an extensive registry of drugs implicated in the induction of blood dyscrasias.

TABLE 6.12–4. SYSTEMIC DISORDERS ASSOCIATED WITH APLASTIC ANEMIA

Infections
- Hepatitis, mononucleosis, cytomegalovirus, disseminated tuberculosis

Myelodysplasias
- Paroxysmal nocturnal hemoglobinuria

Diseases with Disordered Immunity
- Collagen-vascular disease
- Diffuse eosinophilic fasciitis
- Graft-versus-host reactions

Endocrine-metabolic Disorders
- Pancreatic dysfunction
- Pregnancy

TABLE 6.12–5. CLINICAL MANIFESTATIONS OF APLASTIC ANEMIA

Signs and Symptoms	Threshold	Remarks
Anemia		
Weakness, pallor	Hematocrit <30	Slower onset results
Heart failure	Hematocrit <15	in lower symptomatic threshold
Thrombocytopenia		
Petechiae, ecchymoses	Platelets <40,000/μl	Chronic thrombocytopenia often well tolerated
Major bleeding	Platelets <10,000/μl	Platelet support given for bleeding
Granulocytopenia		
Regional tissue infection	Granulocytes <500/μl	Local signs minimal; little or no pus
Bacteremia organisms of high and low virulence	Granulocytes <100/μl	Infection progresses rapidly; fever, sepsis frequent

ration and biopsy of the bone marrow. By chance, a small focus of hypercellular marrow might be aspirated from a patient with aplastic anemia, giving the false impression of normal cellularity on smears of that aspirate. Further, a nonproductive aspirate might result from a marrow heavily infiltrated with neoplastic cells or from extensive myelofibrosis leading to an erroneous impression of hypoplasia. In either instance, a needle biopsy of the iliac crest will clarify the situation and demonstrate the degree of hematopoietic hypoplasia present.

The in vitro culture of bone marrow hematopoietic progenitor provides a means for exploring some of the pathogenic possibilities during the evaluation of aplastic anemia patients. The in vitro culture of bone marrow progenitors in the presence of subsets of lymphoid cells from aplastic anemia patients has shown marked inhibition of hematopoietic colony growth in some cases. In other instances, the serum from patients with aplastic anemia markedly inhibited the growth of normal progenitor cells. On the other hand, one can sometimes show that in vitro perturbation of the culture condition by the addition of antithymocyte globulin,

TABLE 6.12–6. DIAGNOSTIC CRITERIA FOR APLASTIC ANEMIA[a]

I. Severe Aplastic Anemia
  A. Peripheral pancytopenia (at least two must be present)
    1. Reticulocyte count <1% when corrected to a Hct of 40% (40,000/μl)
    2. Granulocyte count <500/μl
    3. Platelet count <20,000/μl
  B. Bone marrow hypoplasia (one of the following)
    1. Biopsy markedly hypocellular (<25% of normal)
    2. Biopsy mildly hypocellular (25%–50% of normal, with <50% of cells nonhematopoietic and nonneoplastic)
    3. Platelet count <100,000/μl

II. Moderate Aplastic Anemia
  A. Peripheral pancytopenia (at least two must be present)
    1. Reticulocyte count <1% (40,000/μl)
    2. Granulocyte count <1500/μl
  B. Bone marrow hypoplasia <30% normal number of hematopoietic cells in biopsy

III. Mild Aplastic Anemia
  A. Peripheral pancytopenia
    1. Hematocrit <38%
    2. Granulocyte count <1,800/μl
    3. Platelet count <140,000/μl
  B. At least one hypocellular bone marrow biopsy

[a]See reference 54.

methylprednisolone, or chloramphenicol or the removal of a subset of lymphoid cells occasionally results in marked enhancement of hematopoietic colony growth. This type of evidence lends credence to the concept that some cases of aplastic anemia result from severe stem cell damage, whereas others may be due to the lack of a necessary accessory growth factor or to the presence of a specific inhibitor of hematopoietic growth such as an immune reaction (cellular or humoral).

Hemostatic function studies are generally normal, except for those related to the degree of thrombocytopenia present. Ferrokinetic studies reflect the marked impairment of erythropoiesis. Plasma erythropoietin concentrations and erythropoietin excretion in the urine generally exceed normal values.

Grading the severity of aplastic anemia is important to the formulation of a management plan for each patient (Table 6.12–5). Many patients with mild aplastic anemia are symptomatic for months, but their prognosis for long-term survival and eventual recovery is fairly good. In marked contrast is the outlook for patients with severe aplastic anemia, who have an average life expectancy of 3 to 4 months. Rapid progression of signs and symptoms is also associated with a poor prognosis. In addition, males tend to do less well than females, and those presenting with prominent bleeding manifestations also have a poorer outlook.[3]

DIAGNOSTIC CONSIDERATIONS

Since a great many systemic disorders will impair hematopoiesis to a significant degree, leading to pancytopenia, the diagnostic evaluation of patients with suspected (idiopathic) aplastic anemia should be conducted carefully with this fact in mind (Table 6.12–7). In general, the main element leading to the discovery of these underlying diseases is alertness to their potential existence. The diagnostic methods are not particularly difficult per se.

MANAGEMENT

It is important to distinguish between patients with mild aplastic anemia and those with a severe impairment (Table 6.12–6). Patients with severe aplastic anemia require prompt and vigorous therapy because of their limited life expectancy (Table 6.12–8).

True remission of severe aplastic anemia in the absence of treatment is very rare. Death is usually related to the consequences of overwhelming infections due to antibiotic-resistance microorganisms. Bleeding complications also contribute significantly to morbidity and mortality, especially when patients become refractory to platelet transfusion because of alloimmunization.

Bone Marrow Transplantation

Allogeneic bone marrow transplantation has improved the outlook for patients with severe aplastic anemia to a remarkable degree. More than 50 percent of patients undergoing a bone marrow transplant for severe aplastic anemia remain alive and disease-free for more than 2 years (Table 6.12–9). Thus far very few relapses have been reported in patients after that time.[3,4,9]

Prime candidates for marrow transplantation are patients with severe aplastic anemia who are less than 50 years of age and have no other major organ system impairment. Further, the prospective recipient must not be immunized against the minor antigens on the potential donor's cells, as might be the case if there were many prior blood product transfusions or multiple pregnancies.

Suitable donors are usually siblings who are human lymphocyte antigen (HLA)–identical (genotypically identical) to the recipient and are emotionally and physically fit. It is now technically possible to transplant across major ABO blood group incompatibilities so that matching of red blood cell antigens is not required. Studies are being carried out in several centers in an attempt to extend the pool of prospective donors to include well-matched nonfamily members. A national registry of potential bone marrow donors and their HLA type is being developed for this purpose.

TABLE 6.12–7. DISORDERS TO BE DISTINGUISHED FROM APLASTIC ANEMIA

Disorder	Distinguishing Features	Comments
Paroxysmal nocturnal hemoglobinuria (PNH)	Presence of complement-sensitive red blood cells	PNH is a clonal disorder that may merge with aplastic anemia and acute leukemia
Preleukemia	Peripheral blood and marrow show dysplastic cells; chromosomal abnormalities	Myelodysplastic disorders merge with aplasias and neoplasms
Hematopoietic neoplasms	Peripheral blood and marrow show tumor cells; chromosomal abnormalities	Marrow aplasia may precede leukemia or occur during treatment
Marrow replacement	Marrow biopsy shows cancer, fibrosis, storage disease or osteopetrosis; splenomegaly frequent	Marrow aplasia may occur during cancer treatment
Infection	Culture, serology, and biopsy show viral infection, mycobacterial or fungal infection, parasitism	Marrow hypoplasia and pancytopenia may not be profound
Deficiency disorders	Hematopoietic cells usually show changes of B_{12}, folate, pyridoxine deficiency	

Lympholytic Therapies

More than half the patients with severe aplastic anemia do not have a suitable bone marrow donor available. Further, most patients are over age 50 or have some physiologic impairment that precludes bone marrow transplantation. In these instances, treatment with antilymphocyte globulin, antithymocyte globulin, cyclophosphamide, adrenal corticosteriods, or other immune suppressive agents should be considered.

Several types of experimental data indicate that thymocytes (and in certain situations, other lymphoid cells) have both a stimulating and inhibitory influence on hematopoiesis. Further, there are data that suggest that disordered immunity is responsible for some cases of severe marrow aplasia.

Therapeutic trials with antilymphocyte or antithymocyte globulin, cyclophosphamide, cyclosporine or adrenal corticosteroids have resulted in a significant improvement in the severe hematopoietic impairment of some patients. Estimating the frequency, extent, and duration of these remissions is a matter of current clinical investigation. Significant responses, however, are seen in about half of the patients. Relapses following treatment are common.[3]

Androgen Therapy

Androgens and etiocholanolone have been used in the treatment of aplastic anemia. Some degree of success has been encountered in a small proportion of patients with a mild impairment, usually after treatment courses in excess of 1 month. These agents are rarely, if ever, able to induce a significant improvement by themselves in patients with severe aplastic anemia.[4]

Supportive Therapy

Red blood cell transfusions are essential in the management of the anemia. Effective red cell transfusion therapy can in some cases be continued over prolonged periods (Chapter 6.24). However, iron overload with its consequent organ toxicities will eventually result if care is not taken to prevent it.

Platelet transfusions have been clearly shown to be effective in the management of bleeding due to severe thrombocytopenia. By maintaining a platelet count in these patients of greater than $20,000/\mu l$, one can be fairly certain that spontaneous bleeding will rarely occur except from previously existing lesions. In addition the judicious use of platelet transfusions can on occasion allow one to maintain a platelet count greater than $50,000\ \mu l$, a range in which even many major emergency surgical procedures can safely be done. Repeated platelet transfusions, however, often result in alloimmunization. Not only will alloimmunization make future platelet transfusions ineffective, but it also may preclude successful allogeneic bone marrow transplantation (Chapter 6.24). Adrenal corticosteroids appear to be of limited use in treating patients with thrombocytopenic bleeding. In women with severe thrombocytopenia, it may be wise to suppress ovulation with an appropriate hormonal agent such as norethynodrel or megestrol acetate.

Infections in patients with severe granulocytopenia are difficult to manage successfully. Properly chosen antibiotics promptly administered are the mainstay of effective treatment (Chapter 9.2). Granulocyte transfusions are of limited value and are most useful in supporting patients with severe infections due to antibiotic-resistant organisms. It is technically difficult, however, to harvest a large enough number of granulocytes for effective replacement therapy in adults. The incidence of severe side effects from granulocyte transfusion is very high, and support for longer than a few days is impractical. In addition, maintaining patients for prolonged periods in a relatively microbe-free "clean environment" (protective isolation with measures to reduce skin and gut microorganisms) for the purpose of preventing severe infection is usually impractical.

Patients with mild aplastic anemia should be encouraged to maintain normal daily activities insofar as possible. Patients and families who are properly informed about the nature of the disorder are generally prudent in avoiding the risks of trauma and infection. Simple procedures such as the use of antiseptic soap, the use of an electric razor rather than a blade, and the avoidance of intramuscular injections and other traumas are important for patients to follow in order to reduce morbidity as much as possible.

TABLE 6.12–8. PROGNOSIS IN APLASTIC ANEMIA

Category	Survival	Causes of Morbidity
Mild	75% live 3–4 mo ~50% live 1 yr ~20% live 5 yr	Iron overload (RBC transfusions), recurrent infections, anemia, progression to severe aplasia
Severe	50% live 3–4 mo ~30% live 1 yr ~20% live 5 yr	Infection, bleeding, anemia

PAROXYSMAL NOCTURNAL HEMOGLOBINURIA (MARCHIAFAVA–MICHELI SYNDROME)[2,8]

Paroxysmal nocturnal hemoglobinuria (PNH) is an acquired disorder, but its precise etiology is unknown. A consideration of PNH is included in this chapter because it is a hematopoietic stem cell disorder. Although the resulting erythrocyte defects are more prominent, it is clear that granulocytes and platelets are also af-

TABLE 6.12–9. TREATMENT OF APLASTIC ANEMIA

Therapy	Indications	Outcome
Allogeneic bone marrow transplantation	Severe aplasia Age < 50 HLA-identical sibling donor available	Early problems with severe aplasia, graft-versus-host disease; over 50% disease free survival at 2 yr; no relapses
Antithymocyte globulin Antilymphocyte globulin	Severe aplasia Not suitable for marrow transplantation No donor available	Early improvement in aplasia ~50% of cases; complete ~10%; relapses common
Cyclophosphamide (45 mg/kg/day × 4)	Severe aplasia Not suitable for marrow transplantation No donor available	Early problems with aplasia, CY toxicity; one course sufficient trial; response rate ~30%
Adrenal corticosteroids (methylprednisolone, 5–30 mg/kg/day)	Severe aplasia Not suitable for marrow transplantation	Toxicity problems; sustained or transient remissions in 2–4 weeks
Androgen (oxymethalone, 3–5 mg/kg/day)	Most effective in mild aplasias	Responses in ~5% of cases when androgen is given from 1 to 4 months; relapses common

fected. Studies in G-6-PD heterozygotes indicate that PNH cells constitute a clone of cells derived from what was probably a single hematopoietic stem cell. This would imply that the disorder results from the transformation and self-sustained proliferation of a single cell, much like a neoplasm.[2] Recently it has been shown that the hematopoietic cells of patients with PNH lack the enzyme acetylcholinesterase in their cell membrane. Whether or not this deficiency is the cause of the increased complement lysis seen in the cells of these patients is not clear.[8]

PNH is a rare disorder. Frequently it arises in the setting of an injured marrow. For example, many patients present initially with drug-induced or idiopathic aplastic anemia.[2] During the course of the disease, the cellular morphology of the marrow may change somewhat (myelodysplasia) and a "subclone" of complement-sensitive erythrocytes (PNH cells) may arise. Granulocytes and platelets in these patients also demonstrate a marked increased susceptibility to complement mediated lysis. Further, acute myeloblastic leukemia develops in a small proportion of cases. These facts seem consistent with the notion that PNH is a myelodysplastic disorder that arises from an underlying abnormality in a "transformed" hematopoietic cell.

CLINICAL MANIFESTATIONS

Traditionally, PNH has been considered as one of the hemolytic anemias because red cell destruction and hemoglobinuria are such prominent clinical features of the disorder. The hemoglobinuria is irregular in its occurrence, and contrary to what the name of the disease suggests, it is often not nocturnal, but seems to be more closely related to sleep at any time of the day or night. Increased hemoglobinuria seems to occur not only in relation to sleep, but also at the time of infection, surgery, and perhaps increased physical exertion. The precise reasons for the association of hemolysis with these factors is unknown.

The chronic hemolysis encountered in PNH is due to an erythrocyte membrane defect that renders these cells more sensitive to complement-mediated lysis than red cells normally are, and most of the diagnostic tests employed are based in this finding. Complement-mediated lysis of PNH erythrocytes can be activated by lowering pH (acid hemolysis, Ham test), by lowering ionic strength (sugar-water test), by increasing magnesium concentrations, and by antibodies. It is possible to grade the sensitivity to hemolysis of PNH erythrocytes by using graded concentrations of complement in in vitro tests, and one finds their distinct population of red blood cells based on their relative sensitivities. Most patients demonstrate only two of these populations in their peripheral blood, and some patients demonstrate all these. Only a rare patient has a pure population of only one PNH cell line.

Iron deficiency may develop in patients with protracted courses because significant amounts can be lost from the body as hemoglobin and hemosiderin in the urine. Various abnormalities of renal function may develop also. Some of the defects in tubular function are thought to be related to the persistent hemoglobinuria and hemosiderinuria.

Although chronic hemolysis and its consequences dominate the clinical picture, it is clear that granulocytes and platelets are defective also. Patients with PNH are usually granulocytopenic, which may in part explain their repeated infections. However, the infections are more likely attributable to the functional defects that these granulocytes demonstrate, including defective phagocytosis and decreased mobility and chemotaxis. Platelets also show a marked increase in complement-mediated lysis-releasing multiple factors that may in part be responsible for the thromboembolic phenomena seen in these patients. Hemorrhage is a frequent complication, especially in those patients undergoing an aplastic phase.

Thrombosis of large intraabdominal veins occurs frequently, especially involvement of the hepatic veins. This is associated with abdominal pain and rapid enlargement of the liver (Chapter 13.5) frequently leading to death. Major thrombosis of cerebral veins also occurs and may lead to death. Thrombosis of multiple small veins frequently occurs in the kidney and brain also. Although their occurrence may not cause prominent clinical symptoms, over time these thrombotic complications lead to significant impairment of renal and cerebral function.

DIAGNOSTIC CONSIDERATIONS

Hemoglobinuria is a prominent feature of this disease, and the presence of hemoglobin casts in the urine is commonly detected. However, there are times when hemoglobin is not easily demonstrable in the urine. Hemosiderinuria is a much more constant finding. In fact, one should question the diagnosis of PNH if excessive amounts of hemosiderin are not being excreted in the urine.

Pancytopenia is more prominent in PNH than in other hemolytic anemias, but the white blood cell counts and platelet counts vary within wide limits. The red blood cells are often macrocytic but may be hypochromic and microcytic, reflecting iron deficiency. The anemia is usually very severe. The leukocyte alkaline phosphatase may be low.

In most cases the bone marrow is very cellular and some degree of erythroid hyperplasia may be evident. The architecture of the hematopoietic cells is likely to be abnormal, however, and dysplastic-appearing cells may be seen. Varying degrees of ineffective hematopoiesis exist. At the time of an aplastic phase, the bone marrow will be quite hypoplastic in appearance.

The increased sensitivity of PNH red blood cells to complement-mediated hemolysis is best searched for by using the sucrose hemolysis (sugar-water) test. If this test is positive, a complete Ham acid hemolysis test will best confirm the diagnosis. During the course of PNH, the concentration of complement-sensitive erythrocytes in the circulating blood may be too low to detect by the sucrose hemolysis screening test, especially if there have been recent transfusions of red blood cells.

MANAGEMENT

Supportive therapy for patients with PNH requires repeated red blood cell transfusions because of anemia and replacement iron therapy when a deficiency has developed. Red cells used for transfusion purposes, however, must be washed free of plasma factors to prevent an exacerbation of hemolysis. Androgens (e.g., fluoxymesterone, 20 to 30 mg per day) and glucocorticoids (e.g., prednisone, 20 to 60 mg on alternate days) have shown mixed results. However, the long-term use of these drugs does not seem warranted unless there is clear evidence of continuing benefits at dose levels that do not produce troublesome side effects.

Anticoagulants, especially heparin, are used in the management of acute venous thromboses. No data suggest, however, that long-term anticoagulation has a beneficial effect on the ultimate course of the disease. Allogeneic bone marrow transplantation should be considered in the treatment of patients with severe PNH, especially since the disorder probably resides in the hematopoietic stem cell. The indications and related considerations are similar to those for patients with aplastic anemia. Experience with bone marrow transplantation in PNH, however, is quite limited.[9]

PNH may progress rapidly and result in death within a few months. Most patients, however, pursue a more chronic course during which the signs and symptoms of the disorder wax and wane. Occasionally, the disorder resolves spontaneously and all evidence of the PNH cellular clone disappears.

Most patients with active PNH eventually die of their disease. Death often follows a massive venous thrombosis of the hepatic or a cerebral vein. Occasionally the illness terminates with the development of acute myeloblastic leukemia.[7]

REFERENCES

1. Bennet JM, Catovsky D, et el: Proposals for the classification of the myelodysplastic syndromes. Br J Haematol 51:189, 1982
2. Beutler E: Paroxysmal nocturnal hemoglobinuria. In Williams WJ, Beutler E, et al (eds): Hematology, 3d ed. New York, McGraw-Hill, 1983
3. Camitta BM, Storb R, Thomas ED: Aplastic anemia. N Engl J Med 306:645, 712, 1982
4. Camitta BM, Thomas ED, et al: A prospective study of androgens and bone marrow transplantation for the treatment of severe aplastic anemia. Blood 53:504, 1979
5. Erslev AJ: Aplastic anemia. In Williams WJ, Beutler E, et al (eds): Hematology, 3d ed. New York, McGraw-Hill, 1983
6. Gerson WT, Fore DG, et al: Anticonvulsant-induced aplastic anemia: Increased susceptibility to toxic drug metabolites in vitro. Blood 61:889, 1983
7. Nowell PC: Preleukemias. Hum Pathol 12:522, 1982
8. Rosse WF: The control of complement activation by blood cells in paroxysmal nocturnal hemoglobinuria. Blood 67:268, 1986
9. Santos GW: History of bone marrow transplantation. Clin Haematol 12:611, 1983
10. Szklo M, Sensenbrenner L, et al: Incidence of aplastic anemia in metropolitan Baltimore: a population based study. Blood 66:115, 1985

CHAPTER 6.13
Biology of Human Neoplasia

Albert H. Owens, Jr.,
and Stephen B. Baylin

INTRODUCTION

Neoplastic disorders are the second most common cause of death in the United States. Extensive studies detail the morbid anatomy of neoplasia. A less extensive knowledge exists about the causative agents involved. Current clinical investigation is increasingly concerned with the biochemical and molecular abnormalities associated with tumors as well as with the proper evaluation of therapeutic results.

Physicians, who must base their therapeutic and preventive practices on existing knowledge, are faced with a bewildering array of reported facts. The following chapters are designed to orient students to the major concepts concerning human neoplasia and to direct them to the relevant literature.

This chapter considers the salient features of the biology of human tumors—causal factors, modes of clinical presentation, and expected course and survival. These features are introduced as physicians most commonly encounter them, and then their pathogenesis is explained.

Chapter 6.14 deals with the principles underlying the management of patients with neoplastic disorders. A general scheme of systematic patient evaluation is suggested, and the utility and limitations of presently available therapeutic modalities are discussed. Particular attention is paid to the biologic effects of irradiation and systemic therapy, as well as to their specific indications and therapeutic results, in order to provide a logical approach to management.

In Chapters 6.15 to 6.23 the leukemias and lymphomas and breast, bronchogenic, and bowel cancers are discussed to illustrate the several biologic and therapeutic principles previously presented.

CLINICAL MANIFESTATIONS

Neoplastic diseases are ubiquitous and protean in their manifestations. They are properly considered in virtually every differential diagnosis. Their prompt identification and rational treatment are derived from our current understanding of the circumstances of their origins, their anatomic extents, the associated physiologic abnormalities, and expected clinical courses.

Fundamentally, neoplastic diseases are defined by their biologic characteristics. In general, a neoplastic disease consists of an altered cell population that has become unresponsive to normal controls and to the organizing influences of adjacent tissues. Relatively unrestrained cell proliferation and growth are common to all neoplasms. In contrast to benign tumors, malignant neoplasms

exhibit the additional general properties of local tissue invasion and metastatic spread to distant anatomic sites.[2,3,15,20]

Experience in correlating the microscopic examination of tissue with the nature of clinical disease has allowed the identification of certain histologic abnormalities as being predictive of neoplastic biologic behavior. Among these histologic abnormalities are a high frequency of mitotic figures, derangements of nuclei and nucleoli, an alteration of normal tissue architecture, and evidence of the invasion of adjacent structures or distant metastatic spread.

Histologic examination of tissue specimens or exfoliated cell preparations is the main clinical diagnostic method. Characteristic histologic aberrations predict neoplastic diseases with a high degree of accuracy. Hence, common clinical parlance includes the phrase "proved by biopsy." However, this predictive relationship is not infallible. For example, lymph node abnormalities associated with insect bites, diphenylhydantoin administration, or systemic lupus erythematosus may be mistaken for malignant lymphoma. Conversely, the microscopic appearance of follicular carcinoma of the thyroid or chondrosarcoma may not reflect the malignant nature of these diseases.[2,10]

TUMOR CELL BIOLOGY

Cancers commonly arise in tissues with self-renewing cell systems. They may be viewed as a clonal expansion of cells that underwent malignant transformation at some stage of cell maturation prior to final differentiation. In many ways cancers are caricatures of normal cellular replication and maturation. In fact, the increasing biologic diversity that develops in tumor cell populations probably arises from imperfect attempts at maturation.[14,15]

Although clonal in origin, cancers are usually composed of heterogeneous cell populations. Genetic instability is a biologic property attributed to cancer cells that underlies the changing cellular morphology and behavior of individual tumors, e.g., an increased propensity to metastasize and the emergence of drug resistance. Gene amplifications and rearrangements occur more commonly in cancer cells and account for some of these alterations in cell function.

The main biologic properties displayed by tumor cells are not necessarily "malignant" but, rather, may reflect certain normal activities of the cells involved. Lymphocytes, granulocytes, and macrophages "invade" tissues and move to distant parts of the body as part of their normal functioning. Further, during embryogenesis various cells move to different sites, implant, and develop within new organs and tissues. Many of the phenotypic markers found on cancer cells (e.g., carcinoembryonic antigen, α-fetoprotein, fetal isozymes) are also present in immature normal cells. Thus, it appears that normal cells contain genetic information for cancerlike traits.

CYTOGENETIC OBSERVATIONS

One clue that both the genesis of cancers and their progression are linked to genetic changes is provided by the frequent chromosomal abnormalities observed. An ever-expanding list of tumor-specific karyotypic changes has resulted from the progressive improvement in chromosome banding techniques. Some of these changes have now been linked to molecular events that may be "causative" for specific cancers. Early on a foreshortened chromosome 22 (Philadelphia chromosome, Ph[1] chromosome) was found specifically related to chronic granulocytic leukemia, and more recently a characteristic translocation t(9q+; 22q−) was found in all myeloid cell lines and presumed present in the hematopoietic stem cell. It is now realized that this translocation places the c-abl oncogene from chromosome 9 into a region of chromosome 22, which results in an increased kinase activity for this gene.[9] Currently, several neoplastic disorders are characterized by specific karyotypic abnormalities, e.g., the monosomy 5 and 7 associated with acute leukemia

arising from myelodysplasia, the 22q− change associated with meningioma, the 3p− change linked to small cell cancer of the lung, the 8;21 translocation found with the M2 subgroup of acute granulocytic leukemia, and the translocations involving chromosome 8 found in Burkitt lymphoma. This latter change results in a translocation of the c-myc oncogene from chromosome 8 into promoter regions of immunoglobulin genes. This results in increased expression of the c-myc gene which plays a key role in cell proliferation. It is apparent that an increasing number of nonrandom abnormalities will be recognized from among the wide variations in chromosome number and appearance associated with most all types of neoplasia.[9,17]

ONCOGENES AND NEOPLASIA

The techniques of molecular biology have provided astounding recent insight into the potential mechanisms underlying the formation of human tumors. Much attention has been devoted to the potential role of "oncogenes" in the cause of cancers. At least 20 "oncogenes" have now been described, and each of these cellular DNA sequences has a high degree of homology to the known transforming sequences of retroviruses.[18] It is possible that these genes play a role in normal growth and development processes, although this remains to be shown. Arguments have been advanced that support qualitative or quantitative abnormalities of oncogene expression as key to the process of tumorigenesis. Quantitative changes can result from genetic changes such as the chromosome translocations discussed above—or from genetic events such as gene amplification that have particularly been associated with c-myc family genes. Qualitative changes, particularly associated with gene mutations, are increasingly being observed for the RAS family of oncogenes. In at least one group of tumors, the T-cell lymphoid neoplasms, the presence of a retroviral DNA sequence, the human T-cell virus (HTLV), in the genome, may be causative.[12] The next years will see an increasing list of tumor-specific gene alterations that could prove diagnostically and therapeutically important.[4,6,13,18]

FACTORS PREDISPOSING TO NEOPLASIA

Epidemiologic studies have identified environmental hazards, social practices, and heritable factors that seem responsible for variations in the incidence and clinical course of several cancers. These interrelationships are quite complex, and the discovery of the precise etiologic agents responsible for most cancers is thwarted further by the prolonged period of oncogenesis. Certain environmental factors and host (patient) characteristics, however, are of proven practical clinical utility.[10,15]

HERITABLE HUMAN NEOPLASMS

The increased incidence of neoplastic diseases within certain families has been noted frequently. A clearly defined pattern of inheritance has been established only rarely, however, and it is often difficult to assess the importance of environmental factors. Retinoblastoma, lipomatosis, colonic polyposis, and the other disorders listed in Table 6.13–1 may present in families with a pattern of dominant inheritance. In some families the association of pheochromocytoma and medullary carcinoma of the thyroid, cerebellocortical hemangioblastoma, or neurofibromatosis seems to be inherited as a dominant trait. The multiple endocrine neoplasm syndromes, I, II, and III, involving the pituitary, thyroid, and pancreatic islet cells, follow a dominant inheritance pattern in some cases, as does hereditary adenocarcinomatosis (adenocarcinomas of the colon, stomach, uterus, and ovary occurring in different members of the same family). In at least one tumor inherited on such a dominant basis, retinoblastoma, the causative gene may

TABLE 6.13–1. HERITABLE NEOPLASMS

Neoplasm	Clinical Manifestations
Skin and Subcutaneous Tissue	
Nevoid basal cell cancers	Dominant inheritance; onset from childhood to middle age; associated with multiple anomalies of skin, connective tissue and skeleton
Trichoepithelioma	Dominant inheritance; onset usually at puberty; basal cell cancers may be associated
Lipomatosis	Dominant inheritance; sarcomatous change occurs rarely
Gastrointestinal Tract	
Colonic polyposis	Dominant inheritance; malignant potential high
Nervous System	
Retinoblastoma	Dominant inheritance; incomplete penetrance; familial history in 5–10% of cases; bilateral tumors more likely than in sporadic cases
Chemodectoma	Dominant inheritance; carotid body tumors may be bilateral; may secrete catecholamines
Endocrine System	
Medullary thyroid cancer	May be associated with pheochromocytoma, parathyroid tumors and mucosal neuromas; may secrete calcitonin and other polypeptide hormones
Multiple endocrine adenomas	Onset in third to fifth decades; includes adenomas of pituitary, parathyroid, and pancreatic islet cells; various hormones secreted

TABLE 6.13–2. HERITABLE DISORDERS AND NEOPLASIA

Nonneoplastic Disorder	Neoplasm
Chromosomal Abnormalities	
Down syndrome (trisomy-21)	Acute leukemia (granulocytic)
Bloom syndrome	Acute leukemia
Fanconi anemia	Acute leukemia
Immunodeficiencies	
Ataxia telangiectasia, Wiskott–Aldrich	
Bruton agammaglobulinemia (X-linked)	Lymphoreticular neoplasia, possibly other tumor types
Late-onset deficiencies	
Chédiak–Higashi (lysosomal)	
Skin and Subcutaneous Tissue Abnormalities	
Albinism (pigmentation)	Squamous skin cancer
Xeroderma pigmentosa (DNA repair)	Squamous and basal cell skin cancers
Dyskeratosis congenita	Squamous cancer of skin and mucous membranes
Tylosis	Esophageal cancer
Café-au-lait pigmentation	Neurofibromatosis and related tumors. Sarcomas occur in 10% of cases
Mucocutaneous pigmentation (Peutz–Jeghers)	Intestinal polyposis (hamartomas); malignant potential low
Hamartoma Syndromes	
Retinal angiomas (von Hippel–Lindau disease)	Multiple angiomas of cerebellum
Tuberous sclerosis	Multiple cerebral gliomas
Multiple exostoses	Chondrosarcomas develop, 5–10% of cases

have been cloned. In this disease patients inherit a defective allele on chromosome 13. Subsequent abnormalities on the opposite allele occur in the retinal cells that form tumors. Other inherited tumors may result from such a series of genetic events.[13]

There are several relatively rare heritable nonneoplastic disorders and hamartomatous abnormalities that have been associated with malignant tumors with great frequency (Table 6.13–2). For the most part, the chromosomal instability syndromes and the immunodeficiency disorders are transmitted as autosomal recessive characteristics, as are albinism and xeroderma pigmentosa.[13]

The relative incidence of various neoplastic diseases with respect to age, sex, and other constitutional factors indicates that several additional host determinants exist. Acute (lymphocytic) leukemia is essentially a disease of childhood. Malignant melanoma is essentially a postpubertal phenomenon. Testicular tumors and Hodgkin disease are most frequently diseases of young adults. Breast cancer is far more common in women than in men. In both sexes the incidence of the chronic leukemias, myeloma, and the common cancers has been observed to increase progressively with advancing age.

ACQUIRED ANTECEDENT DISORDERS

Acquired nonneoplastic clinical disorders have been associated with an increased incidence of malignant tumors (Table 6.13–3). In general, these neoplasms have arisen from tissues undergoing prolonged regenerative activity. Perhaps the increased rate and extent of cellular proliferation enhances the development of true neoplasia. In any event, it is important that a physician observing patients with these nonneoplastic disorders be aware of their association with true neoplastic states. In some instances immediate

therapy is indicated, and in others careful serial observation is required to detect evolving tumors before they become extensive.[2,7,10]

There are additional disorders to be considered in this category because they too are significant with respect to the development of malignant neoplasms. For example, Bowen disease of the skin, regarded as a low-grade neoplasm by some, tends to evolve into a squamous cancer. In many cases, Bowen disease is also associated with cancers of the respiratory, gastrointestinal, or genitourinary tract.

Nonfamilial polyps (benign neoplasms) developing in the intestinal tract are regarded by many as "premalignant lesions." Colonic polyps are observed more frequently in older age groups, but there is a difference of opinion regarding the tendency of various types of polyps to develop into carcinoma. Their malignant potential is lower than that of the various familial polyposes. Similarly, chondromas of bone will occasionally develop into sarcomas.

Our knowledge of clinical disorders currently recognized as "premalignant" is largely limited to those occurring in sites accessible to serial examination. Pathologic studies strongly suggest that lesions with similar clinical significance also exist in more inaccessible sites. For example, squamous metaplasia of the bronchial epithelium has been correlated with an increased incidence of squamous cancer.

ENVIRONMENTAL CARCINOGENS

Chemical and Physical Agents

Specific etiologic agents have been identified and associated with several clinical neoplastic diseases. These external environmental

TABLE 6.13–3. ACQUIRED CLINICAL DISORDERS AND RELATED NEOPLASMS

Acquired Disorder	Neoplasm
Skin and Mucous Membranes	
Actinic dermatitis, keratoses	Squamous cancer of skin
Thermal burns	Chronic sunlight (ultraviolet) exposure of farmers, sailors, etc
Leukoplakia	Squamous cancer of mouth, vagina, bladder (leukoplakia is a term often loosely defined)
Paget disease of nipple	Adenocarcinoma of breast; associated intraductal cancer defines therapy of Paget lesions
Bowen disease	Cutaneous carcinoma in situ sometimes associated with arsenic ingestion or ionizing irradiation; often associated with respiratory, gastrointestinal, or genitourinary cancers
Hematopoietic Tissue	
Aplastic anemia	Acute leukemia
Paroxysmal nocturnal hemoglobinuria	Acute leukemia
Gastrointestinal Tract	
Sideropenic dysphagia	Squamous cancer of oropharynx and proximal esophagus (Plummer–Vinson, Patterson–Brown–Kelly syndrome)
Cirrhosis of liver	Hepatic cell adenocarcinoma with postnecrotic and alcoholic cirrhosis Deficient diet (protein), parasitism related in some geographic areas
Chronic ulcerative colitis	Adenocarcinoma of colon, multiple sites, developing in relation to pseudopolyp formation
Genital Tract	
Chronic cervicitis	Squamous cancer of cervix, especially with multiparity, lower socioeconomic status; rare in Jews
Chronic balanitis	Squamous cancer of penis; rare in men with neonatal circumcision
Skeletal System	
Paget disease of bone	Osteogenic sarcoma

factors are primarily chemical or involve ionizing or ultraviolet radiation. Table 6.13–4 lists the more common carcinogens and relates them to the resulting neoplasms. Comments concerning the populations usually at risk (by occupation), the nature of the exposure, and other clinical evidences of such contact are also included. In each instance, the chemical compound (or mixtures) or physical energy has been shown to be carcinogenic in laboratory animals. Studies of atom bomb survivors have also clearly shown an increased incidence of acute and chronic granulocytic leukemia as well as myelofibrosis with myeloid metaplasia. Further, fetal x-radiation markedly increases the risk of dying from a malignant disease before 10 years of age.[7,10]

In general, occupational cancers appear at the site of the most intense and prolonged exposure to the carcinogen. These sites, of course, vary with the type of exposure and the physiologic disposition of the carcinogens that are taken into the body. Usually there is a relatively long latent period (years) before the clinical emergence of the neoplasm. The characteristics of these tumors and their subsequent courses appear to differ little from their spontaneous counterparts.

Several epidemiologic surveys have linked cigarette smoking to an increased incidence of cancer, cardiovascular disease, chronic bronchitis, and pulmonary emphysema. Cigarette smokers have a substantially greater risk than nonsmokers of developing cancer of the bronchus, larynx, oral cavity, esophagus, and urinary bladder. Further, smoking compounds the carcinogenicity of other agents such as asbestos.

Our burgeoning technology is producing potential carcinogens at an ever-increasing rate, and the population is exposed to them through air, water, and food. Mycotoxins from various molds associated with foodstuffs are among the most potent tumor inducers in laboratory animals. The relative cancer-causing risks of artificial sweeteners, other food additives, pesticides, and so on are a matter of great public concern. Physicians must remain alert to the potential long-term effects produced by hormones or other therapeutic agents. The high incidence of uterine cancer in postmenopausal women treated with estrogens and the high incidence of vaginal cancer in children born to mothers who were given stilbestrol during pregnancy are cases in point.

Viruses

Viruses have been shown to be oncogenic in several animal species. At least 12 strains of human adenoviruses are capable of inducing tumors in newborn laboratory animals or causing neoplastic transformation in cells in vitro. The human wart virus is known to induce papillomas in man. The Epstein-Barr virus (EBV), the cause of infectious mononucleosis, is linked to the occurrence of Burkitt tumor in Africa and nasopharyngeal cancer in Asia. Herpes simplex type II virus has been associated with cancer of the uterine cervix. Recently a unique family of retroviruses capable of transforming eukaryotic human cells has been isolated from patients with T-cell leukemia-lymphoma. Thus, human T-cell leukemia virus (HTLV-I) appears in a subset of these tumors, as does the virus HTLV-II in hairy cell leukemia.[12,18]

Serologic studies have identified tumor-related antigens in patients with acute leukemia, osteogenic sarcoma, melanoma, and other soft tissue sarcomas. Similar antibodies have been found in family members. These observations are compatible with a virus or other infectious agent as the causative agent in these tumors producing unrecognized infections in normal individuals.

Cancer Prevention

Recognition of environmental oncogenic agents is of significance in terms of preventive medicine. Identification of industrial hazards has relieved workers of the risks of exposure. Cessation of cigarette smoking will reduce the incidence of bronchogenic cancer. However, the environmental surveillance and the behavioral modifications necessary for rational cancer prevention are difficult to achieve.

The oncogenic process is a prolonged one. This has enabled clinicians to detect dysplastic or early in situ neoplastic lesions in such sites as the uterine cervix by means of periodic cytologic studies. In laboratory systems, the transformation process can be inhibited or reversed by such compounds as β-carotene and cisretinoic acid analogs. Thus there is an experimental basis for considering chemoprophylaxis trials, especially in individuals at high risk of developing cancer.[7,19] It also may become increasingly possible to identify persons at high risk by demonstrating certain gene sequences in their DNA, showing an abnormality of carcinogen-metabolizing or DNA-repair enzymes, or by some other cytogenetic or biochemical technique. Whether or not a vaccination program could prevent virus-caused neoplasms requires further research.

TUMOR IMMUNITY

In animal models, tumor-specific transplantation antigens have been demonstrated clearly. Distinctive antigenicity has been shown in "spontaneous" tumors and in tumors caused by chemicals,

TABLE 6.13–4. ETIOLOGIC AGENTS IN HUMAN NEOPLASMS: ENVIRONMENTAL CARCINOGENS

Causal Factor	Neoplasm	Evidence of Exposure	Occupation and Type of Exposure
Chemical Agents			
Aromatic amines, especially β-naphthylamine	Papilloma and cancer of bladder, urinary tract	Compounds in urine	Cutaneous, respiratory exposure; chemical workers producing dye stuffs, rodenticides, laboratory reagents
Benzol	Leukemia, lymphoma	Anemia, bone marrow aplasia	Cutaneous, respiratory exposure; coal tar refiners, solvent manufacturers, painters, printers, mechanics using solvents
Coal tar, pitch, creosote, anthracene	Cancer of skin, larynx, bronchus	Chronic dermatitis, warts, photosensitivity of hands, face, exposed areas	Cutaneous, respiratory exposure; coke oven workers, coal tar distillers, lumber industry, chemical workers
Petroleum, shale and paraffin oils, waxes, tars	Cancer of skin	Chronic dermatitis, wax boils, warts in exposed areas	Cutaneous exposure; workers in oil refineries, wax and asphalt producers, mechanics
Isopropyl oil	Cancer of sinus, larynx, bronchus		Respiratory exposure; producers of isopropyl alcohol
Asbestos	Cancer of bronchus, mesothelioma	Pulmonary asbestosis, asbestos bodies in sputum, asbestos warts on fingers	Respiratory exposure generally, >2 years; asbestos miners, shippers, millers, pipe fitters, others; generalized pulmonary fibrosis (asbestosis) present
Chromium	Cancer of bronchus	Chronic dermatitis, chrome holes in skin, perforated nasal system	Respiratory (and cutaneous) exposure; workers engaged in chromate ore reduction
Nickel	Cancer of nasal cavity, sinus, bronchus	Nasal polyps, chronic bronchitis, dermatitis	Respiratory exposure; nickel miners, shippers, and refiners; nickel carbonyl responsible agent (?)
Arsenic	Cancer of skin, bronchus, bladder	Keratoses (especially palms and soles)	Smelters, pesticide manufacturers
Vinyl chloride	Hemangiosarcoma of liver		Chemical workers
Physical Agents			
Ionizing radiation	Cancer of skin, thyroid, tongue, tonsil, sinus, bronchus, osteogenic sarcoma, leukemia	Radiation dermatitis	Percutaneous or systemic exposure for therapeutic purposes (e.g., treatment of spondylitis, polycythemia), or by accident (radium-dial workers); respiratory exposure; pitch-blende miners
Ultraviolet radiation	Cancer of skin	Chronic active dermatitis, hyperkeratosis, exposed areas	Cutaneous exposure; farmers, watermen, other outdoor workers; rarely predisposing factors (e.g., xeroderma pigmentosa)

physical agents, or various viruses. The major antigens in chemically induced tumors seem specific for each tumor. Tumors caused by the same DNA virus usually have common neoantigens but lack virion antigens. Tumors caused by the same RNA virus usually share common transplantation-type antigens and virion antigens. Certain tumor-associated antigens seem to be specified by genetic information intrinsic to the host (in contrast to the genetic material added by an oncogenic virus) and may be expressed normally during an earlier stage of development (fetal or embryonic antigens). It is postulated that these fetal antigens reappear during oncogenesis either by means of gene derepression or as the result of expansion of immature cells in the tumor clone.

Observations in humans suggest that there are analogous tumor-related and fetal antigens associated with a variety of neoplasms. For example, distinctive antigenicity is associated with Burkitt lymphoma, nasopharyngeal cancer, melanoma, osteogenic sarcoma, several types of soft tissue sarcoma, and neuroblastoma. Fetal antigens have been demonstrated in cancers of the large bowel, pancreas, and lung (carcinoembryonic antigen), hepatoma and embryonal carcinoma (α-fetoprotein), and in a wider variety of benign and malignant tumors (γ-fetoprotein). Carcinoembryonic antigen is also present in the blood of pregnant women, heavy smokers, and some patients with hepatic cirrhosis, pulmonary emphysema, and ulcerative colitis.

Studies in animals have defined humoral and cell-mediated immune responses to tumor-related antigens. It has been shown also that sensitized lymphocytes can be prevented from acting against tumor cells by the presence of "blocking or enhancing antibodies." Immunologic responsiveness to tumor antigens may be thwarted by the presence of suppressor T cells, large amounts of tumor (immune paralysis), or tolerance due to the introduction of tumor antigen very early in life (e.g., vertical transmission of murine leukemia or mammary tumor agents). In one experimental system (the induction of squamous cell skin cancers in mice by ultraviolet light), there is a specific nonresponsiveness to the tumor in animals fully capable of expressing a wide range of other immune reactions.

Again, there is evidence for analogous situations in humans, but the data are less complete. In general, cancer patients with a greater degree of immunoresponsiveness have a better prognosis.

It also seems clear that patients are capable of responding to autochthonous tumor antigens and that a reasonable biologic basis exists for useful immunotherapy employing either antibody action directly against the tumor or the targeting of radiation or other therapeutic modalities to the cancer cells. "Spontaneous remissions" in human cancer are a rare but well documented phenomenon. Immune mechanisms are thought responsible in some cases, but direct and conclusive evidence is lacking.[10]

MODES OF CLINICAL PRESENTATION

The manner in which neoplastic diseases present themselves clinically is varied and inconstant. Whereas categorization and generalization are necessary, oversimplification is unwarranted in that it frequently leads to an undesirable lessening of clinical diagnostic awareness. Our current ability to define, detect, and quantitate the neoplastic state clinically is limited, and thoughtful clinical observers will often find themselves taxed to capacity.

The onset of the neoplastic state is difficult to date in humans. When there has been a known carcinogenic exposure (e.g., atom bomb casualties, thymic irradiation, and chromate exposure), a prolonged latent or induction period is likely before clinically detectable disease evolves.[4,16]

IN SITU LESIONS

Commonly, carcinoma in situ is cited as a premalignant lesion or as the earliest recognizable stage of clinical cancer. Although discussed most often in relation to the uterine cervix, such morphologic abnormalities have been observed at many tissue sites. However, current knowledge of their biologic consequences is imperfect. It is probable that a significant portion of such noninvasive lesions do not develop into clinical cancer. Frequently, the entire in situ abnormality is removed by the biopsy procedure. In many instances these tissue changes evolve in sites that are inaccessible to serial observation and therapeutic resection. As the diagnostic terminology implies, current therapeutic practice calls for the removal of these in situ lesions where practicable.

QUIESCENT NEOPLASMS

Malignant neoplastic diseases may exist in humans for months or years and produce few symptoms. Their presence may be detected by chance during the course of a routine medical survey related to cancer detection or for some unrelated purpose. Although every reasonable effort should be made to treat minimal and potentially curable lesions appropriately and to treat progressive neoplasms as effectively as possible, the detection of a malignant disease does not lead to an active therapeutic program in all cases. At autopsy (after death from any cause), cancer of the prostate is found in men with an increasing frequency related to their age, such that 15 percent of men over age 40 will have this pathologic diagnosis. However, only 2 to 3 percent of men will develop clinical illnesses caused by advancing prostate cancer. Similarly, chronic lymphocytic leukemia may exist for long periods with few symptoms. Hence, in the absence of effective curative therapy, treatment is begun for palliative purposes only.[7,11,20]

The varied clinical abnormalities produced by advancing neoplastic diseases may be grouped into two categories based on their presumed pathogenesis: (1) abnormalities that stem directly from the presence of a tumor and (2) physiologic derangements that are produced indirectly.

MASS LESIONS AND RELATED SYNDROMES

The clinical syndromes commonly associated with progressive nonleukemic neoplasms are related primarily to the growth of tumor masses and the consequent physical alterations produced in adjacent organ systems. The findings include the presence of an obvious tumor mass; the existence of an ulcerative lesion that does not heal satisfactorily; chronic bleeding and the consequences of blood loss; bone destruction and its sequelae; involvement of the central or peripheral nervous system, with attendant seizures, paralysis, and pain; acute or chronic obstruction of a hollow viscus and related findings; obstruction of mediastinal structures and its sequelae; and involvement of serous surfaces, with the consequent fluid accumulation. These syndromes are, of course, nonspecific and may be produced by noncarcinomatous mass lesions of other etiologies that alter the structure and function of organ systems in a similar manner.

A commonly encountered clinical problem derives from the initial presentation of a tumor at a site distant from its origin. The more frequent sites of presentation of metastatic neoplasms are the cervical and supraclavicular lymph nodes, lungs, liver, bones, and brain. These and other sites are listed in Table 6.13–5, together with the most probable primary source of the tumor.[3,20]

PHYSIOLOGIC ABNORMALITIES

There is an ever-increasing appreciation of the many physiologic functional abnormalities that are associated with neoplastic diseases but not primarily related to the physical consequences of their presence. Indeed, these functional derangements may constitute the presenting symptom complex that confronts the physician. They may determine the nature of the patient's morbidity and shape the design of the therapeutic program.[5,7]

Tumors may arise in organs that normally produce physiologically active substances, such as hormones. When such tumors produce excessive amounts of these substances unmodified by normal feedback control mechanisms, characteristic clinical illnesses ensue. Such are the consequences of functional adenomas of the pituitary, parathyroid, thyroid, islet cells of the pancreas, and adrenal cortex and medulla.

More commonly, tumors arise from organs that do not produce physiologically active substances currently recognized under normal conditions of health. Certain of these tumors appear to elaborate polypeptides with hormonal activity. Bronchogenic neoplasms, for example, may produce an ACTH-like substance that can induce hyperadrenocorticism or substances that induce hypercalcemia. Similarly, physiologically active secretions of bronchogenic tumors may be responsible for the inappropriate secretion of antidiuretic hormone, the disproportionate anorexia and wasting, or the hypertrophic pulmonary osteoarthropathy occasionally encountered.[5]

The underlying mechanisms for such tumor cell activity may involve derepression or activation of genes coding for the hormones involved. However, there is increasing evidence that tumor cells may be "differentiating" or "maturing" along lines similar to those of the cell populations from which they arose. Hence the observed changes in tumor cell morphology and biologic behavior may be reflections of the normal processes in self-renewing cell systems.

Ectopic hormone–producing tumors may be classified into two groups according to their morphologic features, histochemical properties, and the types of hormones they secrete. One group appears to arise from cells that have a neuroendocrine differentiation phenotype. These include small cell lung cancer, medullary thyroid cancer, thymoma, pancreatic islet cell tumors, and carcinoid tumors. Tumor cells of this type contain large neurosecretory granules and are capable of synthesizing biogenic amines. They may secrete calcitonin, ACTH, melanocyte-stimulating hormone (MSH), vasopressin, insulin, gastrin, secretin, glucagon, serotonin, and histamine or related compounds. The second group of tumors are endodermal or mesodermal in origin—cancers of the bronchus, gastrointestinal tract, and kidney; sarcomas of connective tissue and blood vessels; lymphoreticular neoplasms; non-

TABLE 6.13–5. COMMON SITES OF CLINICAL PRESENTATION OF OBSCURE PRIMARY TUMORS

Site	Primary Tumor	Commentary
Skin and subcutaneous tissue	Melanoma, breast, bronchus, stomach, kidney	Lesions are generally infiltrative and widespread; stomach, colon, and ovarian cancers may present with metastatic masses in the umbilical area
Cervical lymph nodes	Nasopharynx, pharynx, oral cavity, thyroid	More distant metastases rarely seen except when progression of local disease has been curbed
Supraclavicular lymph nodes	Bronchus, breast, stomach, esophagus, pancreas, colon, testis, ovary, uterine cervix	Nonpalpable scalene lymph nodes infrequently yield the diagnosis of metastatic cancer
Inguinal lymph nodes	Genitalia, rectum	Inflammatory disease frequently encountered
Lung	Breast, colon, kidney, testis, stomach, melanoma, thyroid	Radiographic patterns may vary from a solitary lesion (rare) to multiple nodules (most common) to that of lymphangitic or hematogenous spread
Liver	Colon, breast, bronchus, stomach, pancreas	Hepatomegaly, usually without hepatic insufficiency; metastases commonly cause disproportionate elevation of alkaline phosphatase (hepatic isozyme)
Ovary	Colon, stomach	Metastases to the ovary (Krukenberg tumors) may exceed the size of the primary by several-fold
Bones	Breast, bronchus, kidney, prostate, thyroid	Marrow-bearing bones involved most frequently; lesions usually lytic, at times sclerotic
Central nervous system	Bronchus, breast, colon, kidney	Metastases usually multiple (70% of cases)
Serous cavities	Bronchus, breast, ovary, lymphoma	Cytologic studies to be interpreted with caution

germ-cell gonadal tumors; and adrenal cortical tumors. They may secrete substances mimicking the effects of parathyroid hormone, erythropoietin, gonadotrophins, prolactin, growth hormone, renin, or thyrotrophin.

PARANEOPLASTIC SYNDROMES

The characteristics of the more commonly encountered physiologic derangements associated with neoplastic diseases are presented in Tables 6.13–6 to 6.13–13. These abnormalities are listed in relation to the organ systems that they primarily affect and the neoplasms with which they are most commonly associated. Some of these derangements may be visualized as consequent to the elaboration of excessive amounts of normal cell products, others as being caused by deficiencies. The pathogenesis of many of them, however, remains ill-defined.

SKIN AND MUCOUS MEMBRANES

The skin and mucous membranes react in various ways to the presence of a neoplasm (Table 6.13–6). In a strict sense, the mucous membrane pigmentation described by Peutz and Jeghers is not caused by intestinal polyposis but, rather, represents a closely associated heritable abnormality. The pathogenesis of the acquired hyperpigmentation characteristic of acanthosis nigricans is unknown. Similarly, the generalized pruritus seen most commonly with Hodgkin disease remains an enigma. The herpes zoster infections in patients with Hodgkin disease are probably related to deficiencies in immune responsiveness, especially since the process frequently becomes disseminated, the generalized cutaneous lesions being clinically similar to those of varicella.

Several of these clinical manifestations are related to disturbances of the cutaneous circulation. Carcinoid tumors are believed to contain an enzyme that activates a bradykinin-like polypeptide responsible for the vasodilatation and flush observed in patients having such tumors. This physiologically active polypeptide may also be responsible for the associated asthma (bronchoconstriction). After a protracted period, a thickened, violaceous change develops in the skin and over the face, neck, and upper anterior

thorax of many of these patients. Over similar periods of time, clinical evidences of pulmonary hypertension and tricuspid valve deformity may evolve.

Systemic mast cell disease is characterized primarily by urticaria pigmentosa, diarrhea, hepatosplenomegaly, and sclerotic bone lesions. Abnormal proliferation of mast cells is noted in several tissues, particularly the bone marrow. These cells are responsible for the excessive production of histamine that causes at least part of the symptomatology.

The pathogenesis of Raynaud phenomenon associated with neoplastic diseases is not known in every instance. At times the presence of cryoglobulins is responsible. Purpura may be associated with macroglobulinemia and the resultant increased serum viscosity. More commonly, it is associated with thrombocytopenia. The latter may be related to the underlying neoplasm (generally of the hematopoietic tissue) or may result from the bone marrow–suppressant effects of chemotherapeutic agents or ionizing radiation. Care should be taken to avoid overlooking the possibility that purpuric lesions are manifestations of a coexistent bacteremia.

The erythema multiforme, exfoliative dermatitis, bullous pemphigoid lesions, and dermatomyositis seen with leukemia, lymphoma, and a wide variety of cancers are spoken of as "allergic manifestations" of the underlying neoplasm or hypersensitivity states that somehow derive from the presence of the tumor. Erythema multiforme has been described, on occasion, in association with surgical manipulation of the tumor mass or with radiotherapeutic treatment. Bullous skin lesions, exfoliative dermatitis, and, probably, dermatomyositis are of diverse etiologies, but the clinician should be aware of the possible presence of an associated neoplastic disease.

HEMATOPOIETIC SYSTEM

The most commonly encountered hematologic abnormalities are presented in Table 6.13–7.[10]

Polycythemia, induced by erythropoietin, is a rare manifestation that has been reported in association with hypernephromas, hepatomas, benign uterine myomas, and vascular cerebellar tumors, as well as with renal cysts. On occasion a patient's rubor and suffused conjunctivae and mucous membranes, considered to-

TABLE 6.13–6. PHYSIOLOGIC ABNORMALITIES CAUSED BY NEOPLASIA: SKIN AND MUCOUS MEMBRANES

Manifestations	Mechanism	Neoplasm
Pigmentation Abnormalities		
Acanthosis nigricans		Carcinomas of gastrointestinal tract, other viscera
Diffuse hyperpigmentation	ACTH-MSH secretion	Small cell cancers of lung, thymoma, carcinoid, islet cell cancer of the pancreas
Mucocutaneous pigmentation (Peutz–Jeghers)	Autosomal dominant inheritance	Intestinal polyps (malignant potential low)
Café-au-lait pigmentation	Autosomal dominant inheritance	Neurofibromatosis
Xeroderma pigmentosa	Autosomal recessive inheritance	Squamous cancer of skin
Erythemas and Vascular Abnormalities		
Eythroderma and exfoliative dermatitis		Lymphoma, leukemia; many tumor types
Flushing, vasodilatation	Bradykinin-like polypeptide secretion	Carcinoid tumors; cancers of pancreas, bronchus, stomach, and other sites
Urticaria		
Urticaria pigmentosa	Histamine secretion	Mast cell tumor
Urticaria, transient		Several tumor types
Bullous Lesions		
Erythema multiforme		Leukemia, lymphoma, other tumors
Pemphigoid		Melanoma, cancers of bronchus, stomach, other sites
Purpura and Ecchymoses	Thrombocytopenia, macroglobulinemia, cryoglobulinemia, intravascular coagulation, fibrinolysin secretion	Leukemia, lymphoma, myeloma, other tumor types
Pruritus	May be associated with urticaria, erythema	Hodgkin disease, polycythemia vera
Benign Tumors		
Dermal inclusion cysts (Gartner)	Autosomal dominant inheritance	Colonic polyposis and brain tumors
Mucosal neuromas	Autosomal dominant inheritance	Medullary cancer of thyroid, pheochromocytoma
Dyskeratosis congenita		Cancer of esophagus
Varied Pathogenesis		
Pyoderma (various microorganisms)	Depressed granulocyte function, impaired immunity	Leukemia, lymphoma, myeloma
Virus infections, often disseminated (herpes zoster)	Impaired immunity	Hodgkin disease
Dermatomyositis	Cancer-associated in 5–50% of cases > age 40	Several tumor types
Lichen sclerosus et atrophicus		Several tumor types
Paget disease of the nipple		Intraductal breast cancer
Hypertrichosis	Virilizing hormones, ectopic ACTH, gonadotropin	Ovarian and adrenal tumors; lung cancer and other types

gether with an elevated hematocrit and with what is taken as a palpable spleen, have led to an incorrect diagnosis of polycythemia vera, the renal tumor palpable in the left upper quadrant being mistaken for an enlarged spleen.

Anemia is one of the more frequent accompaniments of neoplastic disease. Commonly, it results from prolonged blood loss, especially from the gastrointestinal tract, which results in iron deficiency. This chronic bleeding represents a direct consequence of erosion of the tumor surface. At times a normochromic anemia results from an increased rate of erythrocyte destruction with or without demonstrable erythrocyte autoantibodies and with or without demonstrable increased splenic sequestration of red cells. In contrast to normal individuals, those with disseminated neoplasia often are unable to compensate for this increased red blood cell destruction; their maximal erythropoietic response is a fraction of that normally expected.

A depression of all formed elements of the peripheral blood

is often seen in patients with disseminated neoplastic disease, particularly those with tumors of hematopoietic tissues. The older concepts of myelophthisis as a determinant of decreased bone marrow function are being modified. Massive replacement of marrow by tumor cells is an infrequent occurrence and an insufficient explanation for the majority of the pertinent clinical abnormalities encountered. Several other factors known to depress erythropoiesis are commonly identified in this clinical setting. They include active infection, renal insufficiency, cytotoxic drugs, hormonal agents, and ionizing radiation. An additional factor, ill-understood at present, is the existence of substances produced by the tumor that depress erythropoiesis. For example, this is presumed to explain the erythroid hypoplasia seen on occasion in patients with thymic tumors.

The precise agent responsible for the leukemoid reactions and the thrombocytosis associated with neoplastic diseases is unknown. These phenomena are encountered more commonly in

TABLE 6.13–7. PHYSIOLOGIC ABNORMALITIES CAUSED BY NEOPLASIA: HEMATOPOIETIC SYSTEM

Manifestation	Mechanism	Neoplasm
Abnormal Red Cell Mass		
Erythrocytosis	Erythropoietin secretion	Renal cancer, hepatoma uterine myoma, cerebellar hemangioma
Anemia	Eythrocyte destruction by antibody	Leukemia, lymphoma, ovarian cancer
Normochromic	Erythrocyte distortion and destruction caused by mechanical forces (microangiopathic hemolytic anemia)	Cancers of the stomach, prostate, breast, lung, pancreas, colon
	Deficient erythrocyte production (''pure red cell aplasia'') possibly caused by suppressor lymphocytes	Thymoma, chronic lymphocytic leukemia
	Decreased production and survival of erythrocytes (''anemia of cancer'')	Many tumor types
Hypochromic	Blood loss, sometimes occult (gastrointestinal tract)	Tumors of GI and GU tracts, and head and neck
Abnormal Circulating White Cell Mass		
Leukemoid reactions	Marrow invasion by tumor (granulopoietin secretion?)	Many tumor types
Leukopenia	Decreased production (marrow invasion); decreased survival (sepsis, antibody)	Leukemia, lymphoma, other tumors
Abnormal granulocyte function	Impaired chemotaxis, phagocytosis, or digestion	Acute leukemia, rarely other tumors
Abnormal Circulating Platelet Mass		
Thrombocytosis (often bizarre forms)	Marrow invasion by tumor (thrombopoietin secretion?)	Myeloproliferative disorders, lymphoma, bronchogenic cancer, other types
Thrombocytopenia	Decreased production (marrow invasion); decreased survival (sepsis, antibody)	Hematopoietic tumors, also other types
Abnormalities of Bleeding and Clotting		
Prolonged bleeding	Various clotting factor deficiencies (liver failure)	Many tumor types
	Fibrinolysin secretion	Prostate cancer
	Circulating anticoagulants (antibodies)	Plasma cell dyscrasias
Intravascular coagulation	Tumor produced ''thromboplastin''	Many tumor types

tumors that involve bone marrow. It is important to remember that leukemoid reactions are of diverse etiologies, some of which merit specific therapy—tuberculosis, for example.

INFECTIONS AND HOST RESISTANCE

Clinically significant infections with a variety of microorganisms are common accompaniments of neoplastic diseases (Table 6.13–8). Infectious diseases may cause the presenting manifestations of neoplastic disorders or may complicate their course or treatment. Frequently, it is difficult to distinguish between fever related to the neoplastic process and that stemming from a coexisting infection.

Commonly, the microorganisms responsible for infectious disorders in this setting are indigenous to the patient. These infections are frequently associated with an obstructed hollow viscus or they may be related to surface ulceration or perforation. For example, pneumonia, lung abscess, cholangitis, or pyelonephritis may result from obstruction of the bronchi or of the biliary or lower urinary tracts by tumor. Similarly, urinary tract infections may be associated with neoplastic erosion of the bladder mucosa, and abdominal abscesses or peritonitis may stem from perforation of the gastrointestinal tract.

Clinically significant characteristics of this type of infectious disease are slow resolution despite adequate antimicrobial therapy and recurrence in the same site. Hence, it is important for the

TABLE 6.13–8. PHYSIOLOGIC ABNORMALITIES CAUSED BY NEOPLASIA: INFECTIONS AND HOST RESISTANCE

Infection	Abnormality	Neoplasm
Localized infections caused by a variety of microorganisms	Hollow viscus obstruction, surface erosion, break in physical barriers	Several tumor types
Systemic infections due to variety of microorganisms, especially gram-negative, *Staphylococcus,* rare pathogens, fungi	Impaired granulocyte response (quantitative) and perhaps function (qualitative). Often associated with bleeding into tissues	Leukemia, lymphoma, myeloma, and a variety of tumor types
Bacterial infections especially pneumococcal and other ''extracellular'' microorganisms	Impaired antibody response, hypogammaglobulinemia	Myeloma, chronic lymphocytic leukemia
Salmonella bacteremia	Uncertain	Lymphoma, gastrointestinal neoplasms
Tuberculosis, fungal, and viral (herpes zoster) infections, often disseminated	Impaired cell-mediated immune responses	Hodgkin disease, other tumor types

physician encountering these phenomena to suspect the possibility of an underlying neoplasm.

In addition to the local tissue or structural factors that predispose patients with neoplasia to infectious diseases, factors of lessened host resistance, not fully characterized, seem operative. For example, *Pseudomonas* bacteremia, an uncommon clinical occurrence, is apt to be found in association with neoplastic diseases as well as in other debilitating states. Similarly, staphylococcal bacteremia or postoperative wound infection is commonly encountered in patients with neoplasms.

Hematopoietic or lymphoreticular neoplasms predispose patients to certain recurrent acute infections, indolent infections, or infections caused by uncommon microorganisms. Patients with acute leukemia are prone to develop staphylococcal infections as well as gram-negative bacteremias. Individuals with chronic lymphocytic leukemia and myeloma are subject to recurrent infections of the skin, lung, and urinary tract, caused by a variety of organisms, including the staphylococci, streptococci, pneumococci, and gram-negative bacilli. Pneumococcal meningitis without an associated infection at the portal of entry (e.g., sinus, middle ear, or lung) is particularly likely to occur in association with multiple myeloma. Perirectal abscess is often encountered in patients with monocytic leukemia.

The increased incidence of herpes zoster infections in association with Hodgkin disease and other lymphomas is well known. This is regarded as an activation of a latent varicella infection by many, although many cases occur shortly after exposure to children with chicken pox. Similarly, tuberculosis and infections due to *Listeria* and fungi are linked to Hodgkin disease and other hematopoietic neoplasms. In these patients, these infections are often widespread.

Several underlying abnormalities of host defense mechanisms have been identified (Table 6.13–8). In acute leukemia, deficient granulocyte response to stimulation has been noted in skin window studies. Acquired hypogammaglobulinemia and impaired responsiveness to a primary antigenic stimulus have been described in patients with lymphoid neoplasms. Anergy to tuberculin despite previously established hypersensitivity has been seen to develop in relation to relapsing Hodgkin disease. Impaired homograft rejection and other evidences of deficient cell-mediated immune responses have been noted in patients with Hodgkin disease and several disseminated cancers.

Myeloma is usually characterized by the presence of an increased serum concentration of an immunoglobulin of a single molecular species. These patients may be regarded as having a monoclonal gammopathy in that the synthesis of one type of immunoglobulin or immunoglobulin fragment increases to the virtual exclusion of all others. An impairment in normal humoral antibody responses seems to correlate most closely with the increased incidence of bacterial infections seen in these patients.

The increased frequency of infections in patients with neoplastic diseases is due to multiple factors. It seems clear that impairments of granulocyte response and function, humoral antibody responses, and cell-mediated immunity play a role. However, more needs to be learned about the importance of local tissue factors and a variety of circulating factors such as properdin, interferon, and perhaps other important determinants as yet unidentified. In addition, physicians must remain aware of the fact that antitumor treatments (irradiation, cytotoxic drugs, cortisone analogues) affect hematopoiesis, immune responsiveness, and the systemic dissemination of several microorganisms.

ENDOCRINE SYSTEM

The various endocrine abnormalities attributable to neoplastic diseases may be related to tumors of the endocrine organs or tissues not known to produce hormones normally. An experienced physician, when caring for a patient whose illness stems from hormonal overproduction, will search for an underlying tumor. Also, when caring for a cancer patient, the experienced physician will remain alert to the possible ectopic secretion of hormones.

Benign or malignant tumors of the various endocrine glands at times elaborate physiologically active hormones in supranormal amounts and are unresponsive to the normal feedback control mechanisms. On occasion, further growth and infarction of such a tumor may lead to an abrupt deficiency of the related hormone. Similarly, nonsecretory tumors or metastatic deposits have been responsible for the ablation of various endocrine glands, such as the anterior pituitary ablation caused by an expanding intracellar chromophobe adenoma or the addisonian syndrome caused by the bilateral replacement of the adrenal cortex with metastatic bronchogenic cancer.

There is a wide variety of paraneoplastic syndromes due to the secretion of hormonal substances by tumors of nonendocrine tissue (Table 6.13–9). These hormones may be similar to their "normal" counterparts or they may have a somewhat altered molecular configuration or metabolic effects. The hormone production processes, however, are not responsive to the normal physiologic controls.[5]

METABOLIC SYSTEM

Tumors are known to produce several types of physiologically active substances, including hormones, enzymes, immunoglobulins and immunoglobulin fragments, prostaglandins, bioactive aromatic amines, and vasoactive peptides. Because the pathogenesis of many systemic tumor-associated syndromes remains in doubt, it seems likely that additional physiologically active tumor secretions will be identified. For example, humoral substances may be responsible for the tissue wasting, certain hepatic dysfunctions, certain cerebral dysfunctions, hematopoietic disorders, coagulopathies, and neuropathies.

Hypercalcemia is a common cause of morbidity in patients with a wide variety of neoplasia (Table 6.13–10). The onset of symptoms is usually insidious and may occur shortly after the patient is immobilized for some reason. Somnolence, dementia, constipation, polyuria, and polydypsia are the usual manifestations. The hypercalcemia and hypercalciuria result from the breakdown of bone. This progressive demineralization may be due to the action of parathyroid-like hormone or tumor-secreted prostaglandins.

Hyponatremia and water retention have been associated with bronchogenic cancer for many years (Table 6.13–11). Similar phenomena occur in association with chronic pulmonary diseases (tuberculosis, lung abscess), central nervous system trauma (skull fracture, concussion), vascular compromise (hemorrhage and thrombosis), infection (meningitis, syphilis, encephalitis), and a variety of other diseases. Inappropriate vasopressin secretion is responsible for the abnormalities of many of these cases. More recently, it has been appreciated that hyponatremia and volume expansion can result from the action of vincristine, a metabolite of cyclophosphamide, and other drugs on the renal tubule.

Metabolic acidosis in cancer patients is usually due to progressive renal insufficiency. Metabolic acidosis may result, however, from renal tubular dysfunction caused by the excretion of immunoglobulin fragments (e.g., L-chains) or other proteins (e.g., lysozymes) in the urine of patients with leukemia, lymphoma, or myeloma. The pathogenesis of renal tubular defects in other instances is unclear. Certain anticancer agents, however, can cause similar renal tubular dysfunction, e.g., streptozotocin and isophosphamide.

One form of metabolic acidosis encountered in patients with acute leukemia and lymphoma is due to excessive production of lactate by tumor cells ("lactic acidosis"). Lactic acidosis is seen more often in association with the massive tissue anoxia that accompanies shock, and it has been suggested that tissue anoxia caused by leukemia cell-related blood hyperviscosity and sludging is responsible for lactate overproduction in some cases (Table 6.13–11).

TABLE 6.13–9. PHYSIOLOGIC ABNORMALITIES DUE TO NEOPLASIA: ENDOCRINE SYNDROMES CAUSED BY ECTOPIC HORMONE SECRETION

Manifestation	Mechanism	Neoplasm
Hyperadrenal corticism	Ectopic ACTH secretion "Corticotropin-releasing factor" secretion	Small cell cancer of the lung, thymoma, carcinoid tumors, cancers of breast, ovary, and prostate
Hyperthyroidism	Ectopic "TSH secretion" (may be caused by excessive HCG)	Choriocarcinoma, placental tumors, embryonal cancer of testis
Hyperglycemia	Excessive secretion of HGH, catecholamines, glucagon, adrenal steroids, estrogens; body-wasting	Many tumor types
Hypoglycemia	Ectopic insulin or insulin-like hormone (somatomedin) Impaired glycogenolysis Excess tumor consumption of glucose Under-alimentation	Many tumor types
Feminization—sexual precocity	Ectopic gonadotropin secretion	Teratomas, bronchogenic cancer, especially giant cell, breast cancer, melanoma
Virilization—sexual precocity	Ectopic gonadotropin or ACTH secretion	Hepatoblastoma, melanoma, cancers of the lung and breast
Hypertension	Ectopic ACTH secretion Pressor amine secretion Renin secretion	Lung, thymic cancers Neurogenic tumors Renal tumors

TSH = Thyroid-stimulating hormone; HCG = Human chorionic gonadotropin. HGH = Human growth hormone.

The overproduction of hypoxanthine, xanthine, and uric acid is a consequence of the excessive cellular proliferation and destruction that accompanies a variety of neoplasms. In neoplastic disorders of some chronicity, continued hyperuricemia is associated with gout in some cases (e.g., the myeloproliferative disorders). At times, drug-induced massive tumor lysis results in transient hyperuricemia and uricosuria, especially in patients with leukemia and lymphoma. Indeed, anuria may result from the precipitation of uric acid crystals in the renal tubules. This may be prevented by maintaining an alkaline urine, pH 7 or above, and a daily urine volume in excess of 2 liters. However, it is more effective to use allopurinol, a xanthine oxidase inhibitor, because it retards the conversion of the more soluble precursors to uric acid.

Transient hyperkalemia is another consequence of massive tumor lysis. At times this has complicated the management of patients with tumors that are very responsive to chemotherapy, e.g., leukemia and lymphoma. Proper anticipation and prompt recognition are keys to successful management with fluids, glucose, and insulin as needed (see Chapter 10.2).

GASTROINTESTINAL SYSTEM

A syndrome of intractable peptic ulcer, gastric hypersecretion, and diarrhea has been described in association with non-β, islet cell tumors of the pancreas (Table 6.13–12). About two thirds of the tumors are malignant and one third are benign adenomas. In about 25 percent of cases, the functioning islet cell tumor occurs in patients with familial polyendocrine adenomas (anterior pituitary, parathyroid, thyroid). A gastrin-like substance secreted by the islet cell tumor seems responsible for the gastric hypersecretion. In some cases, non-β, islet cell tumors are associated with a profound watery diarrhea and hypokalemia ("pancreatic cholera"). Achlorhydria is present also. It appears that these tumors produce vasoactive intestinal peptides, some of which are not fully characterized. These peptides markedly stimulate small bowel secretions.[5]

CONNECTIVE TISSUES

The connective tissue disorders occurring in association with neoplastic diseases are presented in Table 6.13–13. Critical evaluation of these associations is often difficult because of the lack of detailed clinical and pathologic study. Few fundamental observations have been made about their precise pathogenesis, particularly with respect to the articular abnormalities.

Metastatic tumor involvement of muscles, joints, or adjacent connective tissue structures is rare, although involvement of bony structures is common. At times, rheumatic or arthritic complaints are due to these underlying bony lesions and may occur before the

TABLE 6.13–10. PHYSIOLOGIC ABNORMALITIES CAUSED BY NEOPLASIA: METABOLIC DISTURBANCES

Manifestation	Mechanism	Neoplasm
Hypercalcemia	Ectopic PTH-like secretion Prostaglandin secretion "Vitamin D-like activity" Osteoclast-activating factor secretion	Cancer of the bronchus, breast, kidney, colon; many tumor types Myeloma, lymphoma
Hypocalcemia	Hypomagnesemia inhibits PTH secretion Hyperphosphatemia due to rapid tumor (DNA) lysis ?Blastic bone metastases	Several tumor types Lymphoma, Burkitt tumor
Osteomalacia with hypophosphatemia	Tumor-derived factor, possibly a vitamin D antagonist	Mesenchymal tumors
Hyperuricemia, gout	Rapid tumor cell proliferation and breakdown	Myeloproliferative disorders, lymphomas

PTH = parathyroid hormone.

TABLE 6.13–11. PHYSIOLOGIC ABNORMALITIES CAUSED BY NEOPLASIA: WATER AND ELECTROLYTE DISTURBANCES

Manifestation	Mechanism	Neoplasm
Hyponatremia (volume expansion)	Ectopic vasopressin secretion	Lung cancer, lymphoma, other tumor types
Hypernatremia (volume depletion)	Hypercalciuria, hypokalemia, dysproteinemia (L-chain) or fragment effect on renal tubule	Myeloma, lymphoma, many tumor types
Hypokalemia	Ectopic ACTH secretion, L-chain nephropathy, lysozymuria (renal tubular damage)	Lung cancer, myeloma, leukemia, other tumor types
Hyperkalemia	Massive tumor breakdown Lactic acidosis	Leukemia, lymphoma
Metabolic acidosis	Renal tubular defects Lactic acidosis	Hematopoietic tumors
Metabolic alkalosis	Ectopic ACTH secretion	Bronchogenic cancer, other types
Nephrotic syndrome	Amyloidosis Antigen–antibody complexes	Cancers of bronchus, kidney, ovary, lymphoma

bone has been destroyed sufficiently to permit the lesions to be detected by radiographic examination.

During the course of acute leukemia, especially in children, joint symptomatology is encountered frequently. The clinical picture may imitate that of acute rheumatic fever. Rarely, arthralgia has been reported to precede the diagnosis of leukemia by several months. Usually, however, ample evidence of the leukemic process exists in association with the arthropathy. Leukemic infiltration of the synovia and subperiosteal tissue associated with hemorrhage is responsible for the clinical manifestations.

Rheumatoid arthritis, systemic lupus erythematosus, and periarteritis nodosa have been reported in association with lymphoreticular neoplasms. These associations must be accepted cautiously, since the morphologic changes in the lymph nodes of patients with collagen-vascular disorders may mimic those of lymphoma. An unexpectedly frequent association between Sjögren syndrome and histiocytic lymphoma has been reported also.

Arthropathies resembling rheumatoid arthritis have been seen with a variety of tumors, although the pathogenesis is unclear. In a small series of cases, acute arthritis of the small joints of the hands and feet in patients with adenocarcinoma of the pancreas was related to fat necrosis of the synovium or adjacent tissue. In another small series of patients with carcinoma of the prostate and rheumatoid-like arthropathy involving the hands, feet, shoulders, and knees, significant improvement was reported 7 to 12 days after estrogen administration was begun.

Although hypertrophic pulmonary osteoarthropathy may occur in a high proportion of individuals with mesothelioma, it is most commonly encountered clinically in association with bronchogenic carcinoma. Rarely, it is seen with intrathoracic metastatic lesions. The symptomatology derives from the subperiosteal new bone formation, which occurs more frequently along the tibiae, radii, and phalanges. The ankles, knees, wrists, and fingers are the most commonly symptomatic points. At times the periarticular swelling and the presence of a joint effusion, especially of the knees, may simulate rheumatoid arthritis. In most instances the digits are clubbed. Not all the factors that cause hypertrophic pulmonary osteoarthropathy are known, but the inappropriate secretion of growth hormone (HGH) is responsible for some of the manifestations.

Remissions of this syndrome have been seen after resecting the underlying tumor or simply interrupting the vagus nerves above the lung root. Response to corticosteroids and salicylates is inconsistent.

Amyloidosis occurs in 5 to 15 percent of patients with myeloma and has been reported in persons with Hodgkin disease, renal cell cancer, and several nonneoplastic disorders. Patients with amyloidosis have frequent rheumatic complaints. An arthropathy involving the larger joints has been noted and ascribed to amyloid deposits in the synovium. Signs of inflammation are uncommon. Para-articular deposits of amyloid on occasion result in a chronic tenosynovitis or pain and numbness in the hand along the distribution of the median nerve (carpal tunnel syndrome).

The incidence of neoplasia in patients developing dermatomyositis after the age of 40 is high, ranging from 5 to 50 percent. Cancers of the bronchus and breast are most commonly associated with dermatomyositis, but many diverse tumor types have been reported. The precise pathogenesis of the dermatomyositis (which may occur without dermal lesions) is uncertain, although it is generally related to allergy or hypersensitivity to an unknown tumor component. Improvement in the dermatomyositis may take place following tumor resection.

Scleroderma has been reported in association with various tumors, but it is not clear that this association is statistically significant. In a few cases, sclerodermatous skin changes have been related to a secreting carcinoid tumor. Bronchiolar carcinoma has been reported as a terminal event in a few patients with the chronic lung disease of progressive systemic sclerosis.

NEUROMUSCULAR SYSTEM

The neurologic disorders that accompany neoplastic diseases are most commonly caused by the involvement of the central nervous system by primary or metastatic tumors. On occasion, neurologic

TABLE 6.13–12. PHYSIOLOGIC ABNORMALITIES CAUSED BY NEOPLASIA: GASTROINTESTINAL DISTURBANCES

Manifestation	Mechanism	Neoplasm
Peptic ulcer Gastric, pancreatic hypersecretion	Ectopic gastrin or secretin secretion	Pancreatic islet cell tumors, carcinoids, rarely other types
Diarrhea, abdominal cramps, asthma, flushing (carcinoid syndrome)	Secretion of serotonin, bradykinin-like peptides	Carcinoid tumors
Watery diarrhea syndrome	Secretion of "vasoactive-intestinal peptide" or related hormones	Pancreatic tumors, bronchogenic cancer, rarely other tumors

TABLE 6.13–13. PHYSIOLOGIC ABNORMALITIES CAUSED BY NEOPLASIA: CONNECTIVE TISSUE DISORDERS

Manifestation	Neoplasm
Arthropathy Signs, especially in children, imitate rheumatic fever Subperiosteal and synovial leukemic infiltrates and hemorrhage	Acute leukemia
Arthropathy similar to rheumatoid arthritis involving small and large joints Special incidence suggested with cancer of prostate and pancreas	Lymphoma, several cancers
Hypertrophic pulmonary osteoarthropathy generally seen with digital clubbing; linked to ectopic hGH secretion Subperiosteal new bone formed, tibiae, radii, phalanges Arthropathy similar to rheumatoid arthritis	Intrathoracic tumors, especially bronchogenic cancer
Amyloidosis Rheumatic complaints frequent Arthropathy of large joints probably due to amyloid deposits in synovium Inflammatory signs rare Para-articular deposits occur; chronic tenosynovitis, carpal tunnel syndrome	Myeloma
Gout Increased uric acid in concentrations, in serum and urine, and secondary gout, especially in myeloproliferative disorders and myeloma	Hematopoietic tumors, myeloma
Dermatomyositis or myopathy without skin changes with onset after 40 yr of age has 5–50% association with neoplasia Increased incidence of scleroderma with tumors uncertain	Several cancers, hematopoietic tumors

deficits are the initial clinical manifestations of illness, as, for example, in 3 or 4 percent of patients with bronchogenic carcinoma.[7]

Metastatic deposits commonly develop within the brain and rarely develop within the spinal cord. Metastases account for approximately 20 percent of all intracranial tumors. The brain and cord may be affected indirectly by metastases developing within their bony coverings, the skull, and the spine, with a consequent extension inward through the dura or with a compromise of vascular supply. Spinal cord compression associated with tumorous destruction of the adjacent vertebral body is a not-infrequent occurrence during the course of many neoplastic diseases.

Several reports note the prolonged survival of patients who have undergone resection of solitary cerebral metastases and the primary tumors and serve to remind physicians of the practical importance attached to the clinical demonstration of the solitary deposit. Cerebral metastases are multiple in at least 70 percent of cases, however, and in only a small minority of instances are the remaining organ systems free of obvious involvement.[20]

Diffuse metastatic involvement of the meninges, particularly about the base of the brain, occurs less frequently. In contrast to carcinomas, the leukemias and lymphomas spread to the meninges more often than to the substrate of the brain. "Tumor meningitis" may present a difficult diagnostic problem, particularly when there are no other clinical manifestations of the neoplastic process. The patient may present with headache, signs of increased intracranial pressure, cranial nerve palsies, or diabetes insipidus (rarely) or as a case of aseptic meningitis.

A practical problem results from the appearance of neurologic symptoms in patients with neoplasms, particularly those as responsive to therapy as the leukemias and lymphomas. At present the nerve cell degenerations and the demyelinating disorders are unresponsive to known therapy. On the other hand, tumor cell infiltrates of the meninges or mass lesions will yield satisfactorily to treatment. The physician must also remain mindful of the not-infrequent meningeal infections with *Cryptococcus, Listeria*, mycobacteria, and other microorganisms in these patients. Neurologic symptoms may also result from small vessel damage attendant on marked erythrocytosis or leukocytosis, intravascular clotting or the bleeding diatheses associated with thrombocytopenia, clotting-factor deficiencies, or the macroglobulinemic high serum viscosity state.

Certain neuromuscular disorders associated with neoplastic diseases cannot be attributed to actual involvement with tumor tissue, although their pathogenesis has not been clarified (Table 6.13–14). There is paucity of pathologic studies dealing with such disorders, particularly of the spinal cord and peripheral nerves. Additional interpretive problems arise because apparently identical abnormalities are seen as accompaniments of nonneoplastic disorders (sarcoid, tuberculosis, alcoholism) and because ionizing radiations can produce such a lesion as myelitis, vincristine may induce a peripheral neuropathy, and corticosteroids may cause myopathy.

"Carcinomatous encephalomyeloneuropathy" is a term that encompasses the overlapping clinical syndromes resulting from neural cell degeneration in the cerebellar cortex, the dorsal spinocerebellar tracts, the posterior columns, and the corticospinal tracts. Less frequently, neuronal damage is seen in the brainstem nuclei, dorsal root ganglia, and anterior horns of the spinal cord. The corresponding clinical syndromes may be primarily disorders of mentation or cerebellar function, syndromes of sensory or motor neuropathy, or mixed polyneuropathy. Overlapping of these syndromes is common. Carcinomas of the bronchus, ovary, and breast are the most frequently associated tumors, although a few cases associated with Hodgkin disease have been reported.

"Progressive multifocal leukoencephalopathy" is a term used

TABLE 6.13–14. PHYSIOLOGIC ABNORMALITIES CAUSED BY NEOPLASIA: NONMETASTATIC NEUROMUSCULAR DISORDERS

Manifestation	Neoplasm
Encephalomyeloneuropathy Degeneration of neural cells causes psychologic disorders (dementia, depression); cerebellar disorders (dysarthria, ataxia); sensory, motor, or mixed neuropathies; mixed syndromes	Several cancers, especially bronchogenic, ovary, breast
Multifocal Leukoencephalopathy Demyelinating lesions bilateral, asymmetrical, especially of cerebral hemispheres causing dementia, hemiparesis, speech defects, occasional cerebellar signs	Lymphoma, leukemia
Carcinomatous Myopathy Weakness and wasting especially of proximal limb and girdle muscles, with or without inflammation (polymyositis) or skin lesions (dermatomyositis)	Several cancers, especially bronchogenic
Myasthenic Syndrome Weakness of proximal limb muscles, rarely cranial muscles; transient improvement with repeated contractions; poor response to neostigmine; sensitive to curare	Bronchogenic cancer, especially small cell
Myasthenia Gravis Thymoma occurs in 15–30% of cases; improvement noted after resection	Thymoma

for the syndromes that result from the bilateral, asymmetrical demyelinating lesions most commonly observed in the cerebral hemispheres, cerebellum, brainstem, and, rarely, spinal cord. These result in dementia, visual impairment, hemiparesis, speech abnormalities, and, rarely, cerebellar dysfunction. These disorders are related more frequently to leukemia and lymphoma, although instances have been reported in patients with carcinoma of the bronchus and breast. In general the clinical course of this demyelinating disorder is more rapid than that associated with nerve cell degeneration. There is some evidence that a slow virus infection is involved.

Slowly progressive weakness and wasting, especially of proximal limb and girdle muscles, are common presenting complaints of carcinomatous myopathy. In general the onset is insidious, although there are reports of an abrupt onset following the administration of a muscle relaxant during anesthesia. This myopathy may occur in association with clinical or pathologic evidence of inflammation (polymyositis) or skin involvement (dermatomyositis). It may also occur in association with neurologic abnormalities (neuromyopathy), making precise clinical definition difficult. Of practical importance is the association of cancers of the bronchus, breast, and other sites with myopathy of late onset unaccompanied by other systemic abnormalities. Adrenal corticosteroids may induce remissions in this syndrome, particularly in those patients with dermatomyositis.

A consistent relationship between these degenerative changes, which affect the nerve cells, myelin, or muscles, and the associated neoplasm has not been demonstrated. The demyelinating disorders have been identified relatively late in the course of the neoplastic disease, but the encephalomyeloneuropathies and myopathies may precede or develop subsequent to the initial tumor diagnosis. Remissions of the last group of disorders have been related to the resection or successful treatment of the underlying neoplasm. Spontaneous remission and exacerbations have also been noted, however, making interpretation of these events difficult.

A few patients with tumors who complain of weakness exhibit additional features that suggest myasthenia. Proximal muscle weakness is common, but cranial muscle weakness is rare. Although increased fatigability follows repeated contraction of the involved muscles, a transient increase in strength is noted commonly. There is little or no increase in muscular strength after neostigmine or edrophonium administration. In some, symptoms have abated following the administration of guanidine. Thus far, the vast majority of patients with this myasthenic syndrome have had small cell cancer of the bronchus. However, the Eaton–Lambert syndrome has also been associated with breast cancer and other tumors and has been described in otherwise normal persons.

Among individuals with typical myasthenia gravis there is a 15 to 30 percent incidence of thymoma. There is not an unusual incidence of other neoplasms among them. The precise pathophysiologic relationship between the thymoma and myasthenia is not clear. Remission of the myasthenia, however, has been noted after resection or radiation of the thymic tumor.

Another poorly understood and rare clinical syndrome relates to the somatic pain induced by drinking alcohol in certain patients with Hodgkin disease. This is also seen occasionally with other neoplasms.

EXPECTED CLINICAL COURSE AND SURVIVAL

The prognosis for patients with neoplastic diseases is based on a complex series of biologic interactions between the tumor and the host. Certain factors have been related to a desirable or undesirable outcome in groups of patients, but good judgment must be shown in applying such data directly to an individual patient. The efficacy of various types of therapeutic intervention is an important prognostic factor also. However, even in the most "favorable" or "localized" lesions, which can be "excised completely" or

"ablated" by radiation therapy, it seems likely that the integrity of the patients' biologic defense mechanisms is a major determinant of the overall outcome.

TUMOR-RELATED FACTORS

In general, the major prognostic determinants that relate to the tumor are the site of origin, the histologic type and grade, and the extent of disease at diagnosis (clinical stage). In certain sites, such as the breast and prostate, hormone responsiveness is an important prognostic characteristic. In other neoplasms, the tumor cell's sensitivity to drugs or the emergence of drug resistance affects the course and survival significantly.[2,7,10]

The histologic pattern of tumors arising in the same site has been related to prognosis. Selected examples are shown in Table 6.13–15. The relationships between cell type and survival in breast cancer and bronchogenic cancer are shown in Chapters 6.21 and 6.22. Histologic criteria for the degree of malignancy of a tumor have been based primarily on the degree of cellular differentiation, the degree of cellular and nuclear pleomorphism, and the frequency of mitoses. For example, Broder's original studies divided squamous cell carcinomas into four grades of malignancy (grades I to IV). In general, grade I (differentiated) patterns were predictive of the least aggressive tumor growth and dissemination whereas grade IV (undifferentiated) patterns were associated with the most rapid rates of tumor growth and spread and the least favorable prognosis for life (e.g., Table 6.13–15).

Precise cancer grading as introduced by Broder is a time-consuming procedure and is not too helpful in predicting the biologic behavior of a tumor in an individual patient. Grading is applied mainly to squamous cancers and is useful in the analysis of groups of patients. In cancers of the thyroid, ovary, and testis, a clear definition of the cell type is more informative (Table 6.13–15).

Neoplasms arising in different sites have differing potentials for growth and spread. In this regard, cancers of the tongue, thyroid, and skin, which commonly spread to regional lymph nodes but rarely spread to distant parts of the body, may be contrasted with that of bronchogenic carcinoma and malignant melanoma, where death is often related to distant metastatic deposits.

The biologic behavior of an individual tumor and the morphologic appearance of its constituent cells may change over time. This process, termed tumor progression, seems to reflect the genetic instability of tumor cells and to some extent the selective pressures of various treatments. Thus, tumor cell populations are likely to be heterogeneous with respect to various biologic properties. For example, cell subpopulations may evolve with a greater proliferative capacity, a propensity to metastasize, or resistance to antitumor drugs.[1,14]

Patients who present with localized neoplasms have the best chances of survival, and their expected survival decreases in propor-

TABLE 6.13–15. SURVIVAL WITH COMMON NEOPLASMS RELATED TO HISTOLOGIC TYPE

Site	Morphology	Survival at 5 Yr (%)
Thyroid	Follicular and papillary	80–90
	Medullary	50–60
	Undifferentiated	10–12
Testis	Seminoma	80–90
	Embryonal carcinoma	50–60
	Choriocarcinoma	5–10
Salivary glands	Acinar cell	80–85
	Low-grade mucoepidermoid	80
	High-grade mucoepidermoid	20–25
	Mixed malignant	35–40
	Squamous	15–20

tion to the observed extensiveness of disease (Fig. 6.13–1). Although this generalization is supported by data from many sources, there are also individuals who present with localized tumors but succumb rapidly to metastatic disease despite optimal therapy. Conversely, a few with widespread tumors survive for prolonged periods, sometimes with no treatment. The extent of a patient's neoplastic disease at a given point in time is expressed as its clinical stage. The systems employed in various institutions differ somewhat; however, stage I usually indicates a neoplasm confined to its site of origin and stage IV distant metastatic spread, with stages II and III representing intermediate gradations. Similar schemes have been applied to the clinical classification of Hodgkin disease and other lymphomas. In this instance, stages I and II designate localized and more widespread regional involvement, respectively, and stages III and IV indicate more widespread involvement, often associated with systemic symptomatology (see Chapter 6.19).

Another system for describing the clinical extent of neoplastic disease has been devised by the International Union Against Cancer. The TNM system is a rather straightforward description: T meaning tumor, N meaning nodes, and M meaning distant metastases. Numerical modifers (1, 2, 3) indicate the degrees of involvement. For example, a patient with a breast cancer in excess of 5 cm with axillary node involvement but no evidence of more distant spread would be classified as $T_3N_2M_0$. It seems likely that this staging system will gain wider use in clinical practice.[10]

HOST-RELATED FACTORS

Several host-related characteristics affect the prognosis of patients with neoplastic disease, but many are ill-defined. Overall, the survival of female patients is greater than that of males, and this holds true when cancer outcomes are examined site by site. Pregnancy per se does not seem to alter the course of malignant diseases in a major way, although there are many reports that indicate that accelerated tumor growth occurred in the postpartum period. The patient's race also relates to prognosis. In most cancers, the prognosis is better for whites than blacks (Fig. 6.13–1).[8]

Clearly age is of major importance. Neoplasms occur more commonly in older individuals than in younger ones, as do various degenerative diseases, notably of the cardiovascular system. These nonneoplastic diseases also limit life expectancy, particularly if they are responsible for a significant functional insufficiency of one of the major organ systems, such as the heart, kidneys, or liver. The several major physiologic abnormalities produced by neoplasms themselves may also be life-limiting, and these are not necessarily expressions of extensive neoplasia. Examples are hemolytic anemia, thrombocytopenic bleeding, hypercalcemia, and infection. At least half of cancer patients die of physiologic abnormalities due to their cancers or associated degenerative disorders and not from the direct consequences of tumor mass, ulceration, or obstruction. Methods of defining host resistance to tumors are yet imperfect, and this assessment in patients is complicated by the use of cytotoxic and immunosuppressive treatments. However, it seems clear that impaired functioning of the reticuloendothelial system is related to oncogenesis and that progressively more severe deficiencies of immune reactivity are associated with advancing neoplastic diseases. Defects in cell-mediated responses are particularly notable in disseminated lymphoma and many other cancers.

On the other hand, it is quite clear that patients are capable of responding to (autochthonous) tumor antigens. In Burkitt tumor, patients developing a delayed-hypersensitivity response to tumor membrane extracts during treatment have a better prognosis than

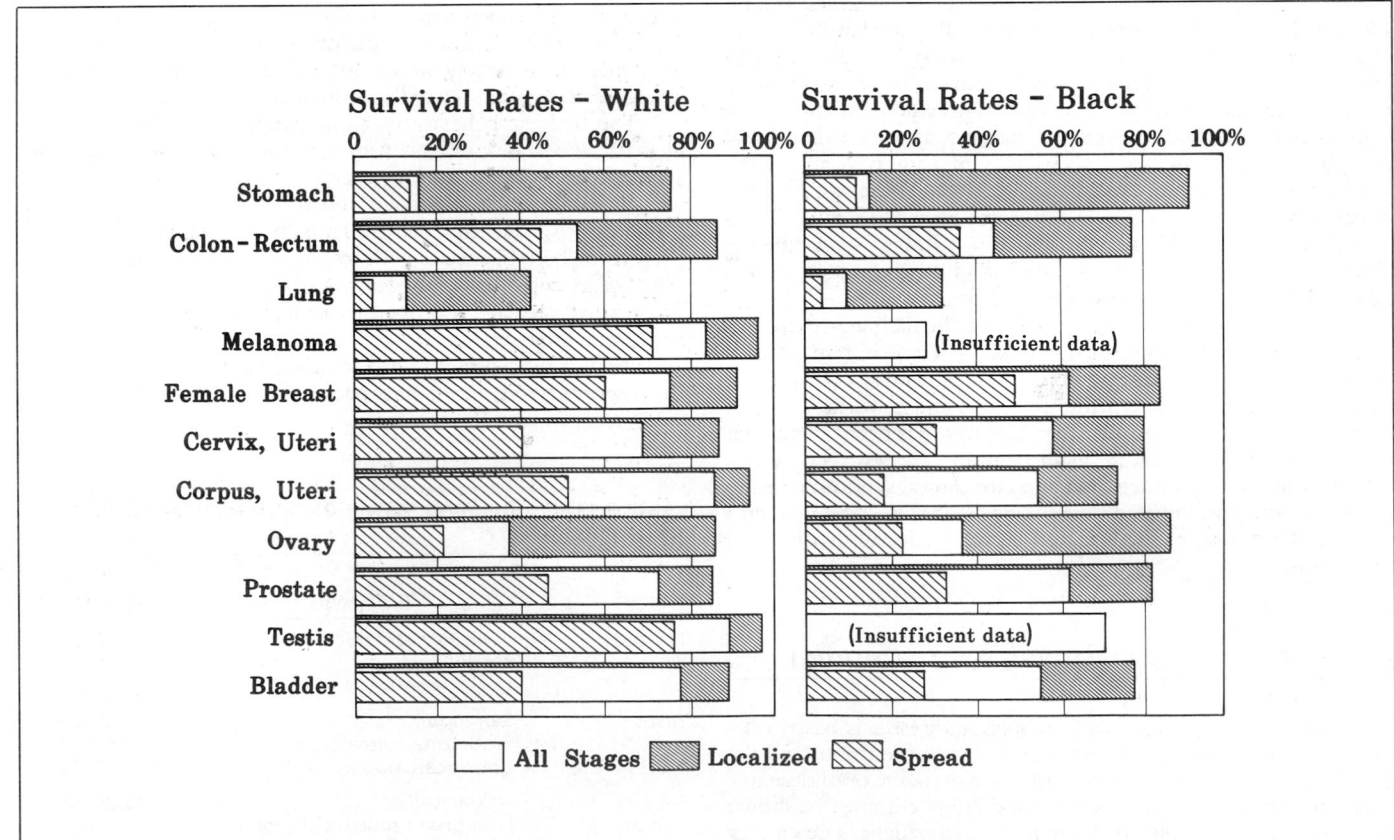

Figure 6.13–1. Five-year survival rates indicating that prognosis for patients with localized disease is better than outlook for patients with disseminated disease.

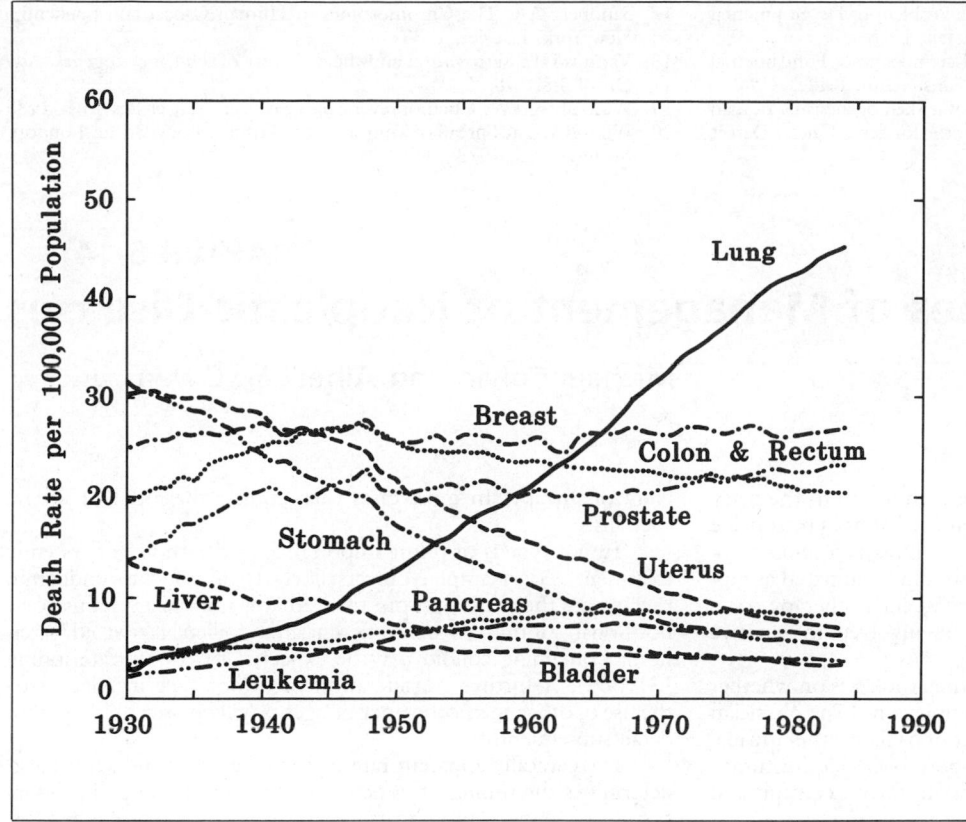

Figure 6.13–2. Cancer death rates standardized for age based on 1970 population statistics. Most notable is the steady increase due to bronchogenic cancer.

those who do not. Other studies indicate that the ability to develop (non-tumor-specific) cell-mediated immune responses correlates with a better prognosis following surgical resection of a wide variety of cancers. Thus, there is a beginning appreciation of host resistance factors important to prognosis.[10]

Clinicians often use the observed rate of tumor growth and spread as guides to management and prognosis in individual cases. In some instances where there is no potential for curative therapy, antitumor treatment may be withheld while the tumor remains indolent. A long interval between treatment of the primary tumor and recurrence usually signifies a better prognosis.

CHANGING CANCER SURVIVAL

Since there is no all-inclusive national repository of cancer statistics, estimates of incidence and survival are extrapolated from the experience recorded in several regional, population-based registries. Each year the American Cancer Society publishes a brief statistical resume and periodically the National Cancer Institute reports data from its SEER (Surveillance, Epidemiology, and End Results) program. Naturally there is a lag in reporting results, especially when 5-year survival figures are sought.[8]

An increasing number of cancer cases are encountered each year. During 1987, it is estimated that 965,000 cases were newly diagnosed, and 483,000 deaths will be recorded in the United States. In future years, it is expected that the number of new cases and the number of cancer deaths will continue to increase, especially in view of the "aging" of the population. Deaths due to bronchogenic cancer continue to increase at an alarming rate (Fig. 6.13–2).[8]

During recent years, the prognosis for survival in several cancer types has improved significantly. This is especially apparent in the younger age groups. Among the tumor types with an improved outlook are acute and chronic leukemia, Hodgkin disease and the lymphomas, myeloma, trophoblastic tumors, testis tu-

mors, cancers of the bladder, larynx, uterus, and thyroid, and several of the childhood tumors. The outlook for cancers of the colon, rectum, breast, and prostate improved for several years beginning in 1940, but there has been little change over the past 20 years. Unfortunately, the prognosis for cancers of the bronchus, pancreas, stomach, and certain other inaccessible sites has remained poor.

REFERENCES

1. Abeloff MD, Eggleston JC, et al: Changes in morphologic and biochemical characteristics of small cell carcinoma of the lung. Am J Med 66:757, 1979
2. Ackerman LV, del Regato JH: Cancer: Diagnosis, Treatment, and Prognosis, 6th ed. St Louis, CV Mosby, 1985
3. Atlas of Tumor Pathology, 2d series. Armed Forces Institute of Pathology. Washington, DC, beginning 1967
4. Barbacid M: Mutagens, oncogenes and cancer. Trends Genet 2:188, 1986
5. Baylin SB, Mendelsohn G: Ectopic (inappropriate) hormone production by tumors: Mechanisms involved and the biological and clinical implications. Endocr Rev 1:45, 1980
6. Bishop JM: Cancer genes come of age. Cell 32:1018, 1983
7. Calabresi P, Schein PS, Rosenberg SA (eds): Medical Oncology. New York, Macmillan, 1987
8. Cancer Facts and Figures 1987. New York, American Cancer Society, 1987
9. Croce CM: Chromosome translocations and human cancer. Cancer Res 46:6019, 1986
10. De Vita VT, Hellman S, Rosenberg SA (eds): Cancer, 2d ed. Philadelphia, JB Lippincott, 1985
11. Fer MF, Greco FA, Oldham RK (eds): Poorly differentiated neoplasms and tumors of unknown origin. Semin Oncol 9:40, 1982
12. Knudson AG Jr: Hereditary cancer, oncogenes and antioncogenes. Cancer Res 45:1437, 1985
13. Owens AH Jr, Coffey DS, Baylin SB (eds): Tumor Cell Heterogeneity: Origins and Implications. New York, Academic Press, 1982

14. Pierce GB, Shikes R, Fink LM: Cancer: A Problem of Developmental Biology. Englewood Cliffs, NJ, Prentice-Hall, 1978
15. Pullman B, Ts'o POP, Gelboin H (eds): Carcinogenesis: Fundamental Mechanisms and Environmental Effects. Amsterdam, Reidel, 1980
16. Ratner L, Sodroski JG, et al: Mechanism of leukemogenesis by human T-cell leukemia virus types I and II: role of the lor gene. Cancer Detect Prev 10:411, 1987

17. Sandberg AA: The Chromosomes in Human Cancer and Leukemia. New York, Elsevier, 1980
18. Varmus HE: Retroviruses and the discovery of cellular oncogenes. Adv Oncol 3:3, 1987
19. Wattenberg LW: Chemoprevention of cancer. Cancer Res 45:1, 1985
20. Willis RA: The Spread of Tumors in the Human Body, 3d ed. London, Butterworths, 1973

CHAPTER 6.14
Principles of Management of Neoplastic Diseases

Michael Colvin and Albert H. Owens, Jr.

The most important decision to be made with regard to the management of a cancer patient is whether that patient has a reasonable chance of cure. If curative antitumor therapy is possible and appropriate for the patient, then that therapy should be initiated as rapidly as possible. Surgery, radiation therapy, chemotherapy, or a combination of these modalities may be involved in curative therapy.

If curative therapy is not an option, then the decision whether to initiate antitumor therapy is a more complex one. The physician must decide whether the potential benefit of palliative therapy justifies the toxicity of such therapy. In addition to specific antitumor therapy, supportive therapy may be important for the comfort and well-being of the patient.

To establish the treatment options and to plan management it is critical that a systematic evaluation of the patient be carried out. Evaluation should include establishing a precise tumor diagnosis, delineating any associated physiologic abnormalities, and assessing any additional disease processes that may exist.

PATIENT EVALUATION

ANATOMIC DIAGNOSIS

A precise anatomic diagnostic formulation includes knowledge of the neoplasm's site of origin, tissue type, or both, as well as the anatomic extent of the disease process. The diagnosis is supported primarily by the microscopic examination of a tissue biopsy specimen or cell preparation considered in conjunction with the clinical disease state.[8]

A positive tissue diagnosis of the tumor is essential to avoid misdiagnosis and inappropriate treatment of nonneoplastic disease. Furthermore, it is important to determine the location of the neoplasm and the extent to which it has spread through the body, since these findings bear directly on the choice of a potentially curative or palliative therapeutic procedure.

The International Union Against Cancer has devised a systematic procedure for describing the extent of neoplastic disease that is being adopted widely as the basis for uniform diagnostic reporting and treatment planning (Chapter 6.13). This TNM classification applies to the clinical staging of patients not treated previously. The formulation describes the degree of involvement by the neoplastic process (numerals 1 to 3) as it relates to the *T*umor, the regional lymph *N*odes, and distant *M*etastases. Thus, a patient with a small epidermoid cancer of the uterine cervix confined to the primary site would be classified as $T_1N_0M_0$.[24]

The morphologic pattern (cell type and grade) of a tumor and its anatomic extent (clinical stage) are key data for treatment planning. All pertinent clinical data should be developed fully and all factors considered carefully when deciding on an individual program of therapy. In most cases this requires the input of several specialists.

Tumor type is of prime importance in the choice of systemic treatment. For example, cancers likely to respond to endocrine therapy are those arising from tissue that is normally responsive to hormonal stimuli. A well-differentiated follicular thyroid carcinoma containing colloid may be expected to concentrate iodine 131 (^{131}I). A further consideration of tumor type in relation to the use of other chemotherapeutic agents will be presented in more detail subsequently.

The clinically apparent rate of tumor growth and spread also determines the timing of noncurative therapy. In a small proportion of patients, tumors may remain indolent for prolonged periods and demand no therapeutic intervention.

PHYSIOLOGIC ABNORMALITIES

One of the spectrum of tumor-associated physiologic abnormalities (see Chapter 6.13) may be the primary determinants of the patient's prognosis and thus may demand primary therapeutic attention. Examples are massive hemorrhage from gastrointestinal tumor, a profound hemolytic process, hypercalcemia, and a major infectious process, such as pneumococcal meningitis.

The prime importance of logical physiologic therapy and thoughtful emotional support cannot be overemphasized. Often, in instances where the clinical application of potentially curative procedures is not appropriate or has failed, such supportive management provides far more comfort to the patient and the family than does the use of antitumor drugs.

ADDITIONAL DISEASE PROCESSES

Neoplastic diseases are most common in the older age groups. Therefore, patients with tumors may have coexisting disease processes, particularly of a degenerative nature. At times these nonneoplastic disorders are of prime clinical importance and determine the patient's prognosis. At other times the physiologic deficits produced by these disorders prohibit a major operative procedure or a potentially curative surgical resection. For example, a thoracotomy for the resection of a bronchogenic carcinoma would not be feasible in a patient with severe coronary artery disease, marked myocardial insufficiency, or marked respiratory insufficiency because of emphysema and bronchitis.

CURATIVE THERAPY

The optimal goal of an antitumor treatment regimen is complete eradication of all manifestations of the disease. With this in mind

the neoplastic cell has come to be regarded as the offending foreign organism or pathogenic parasite, and therapeutic efforts have been directed at removing or destroying the population of offensive cells.

SURGERY

The earliest successful treatment of neoplasms and the current main curative therapy is surgical excision. The major treatment benefits have accrued in cancers at accessible sites, where techniques of diagnostic surveillance are easily applied and excision can be carried out before the tumor has become extensive. The surgical approach is usually limited by the location and extent of the neoplasm rather than by the type of neoplastic cells or their metabolic characteristics.[8]

As the correlations of histologic characteristics with the natural history of tumors are established, however, the type of tumor may influence whether or not surgical therapy is appropriate. For example, the small cell histologic subtype of bronchogenic carcinoma is known to metastasize very early, and patients usually die of metastases rather than local recurrence of tumor. Therefore, initial "curative" resection of the primary tumor is not now the therapy of choice in patients with this type of bronchogenic carcinoma. Similarly, the increasing knowledge of the natural history of breast carcinoma has led to the use of less radical surgery and to more frequent use of adjuvant chemotherapy.[20]

As more successful techniques of radiotherapy and chemotherapy have been developed, surgery has been used in conjunction with these methods. For example, surgery designed to reduce tumor volume ("debulking") may enable their eradication by radiotherapy or chemotherapy. Also, patients with minimal residual testicular tumors following an otherwise complete response to combination chemotherapy have survived disease-free for many years after excision of the residual tumor.[10]

RADIATION THERAPY

Ionizing radiations of varying type and energy are employed to eradicate localized populations of neoplastic cells. As with surgical therapy, these procedures are limited chiefly by the location and anatomic extent of the lesion being treated. The greatest therapeutic successes are achieved with relatively small neoplasms that are detected before they have produced major organ system alterations or have spread beyond feasible treatment fields. Tumor cell eradication is limited by the lack of cytotoxic specificity of ionizing radiations. Thus, the tolerance of adjacent normal tissue limits the amount of radiation that can be directed at the tumor.[19,39]

Additional known biologic effects of irradiation must be considered when treating patients. At times, its effects on gonadal tissue are utilized in ablative therapy, but the possible mutagenic consequences of inadvertent nonlethal germ cell irradiation or unknown exposure of an early fetus must always be borne in mind. The carcinogenic potential of ionizing radiation has been clearly demonstrated in humans. In many therapeutic situations this delayed effect is of little practical consequence, but it should strongly militate against treating relatively young individuals for benign lesions or tumors that can be easily excised. Under certain circumstances (such as stage I cancer of the larynx), complete tumor cell ablation can be achieved by irradiation without the sacrifice of organ function (voice) that a curative surgical procedure might require.

SYSTEMIC THERAPY

There are compelling reasons to seek effective systemic treatments. Certain neoplastic disorders of hematopoiesis such as leukemia and multiple myeloma are disseminated widely in their earliest recognizable stage. Many neoplastic disorders of epithelial tissue are similarly disseminated. For example, apparently localized small cell cancer of the lung is in reality widely dispersed. By the same token, the emergence of distant metastases in patients who have had their limited stage breast cancer completely excised indicates that dissemination occurred prior to primary therapy.

Antineoplastic chemotherapy is considered curative in certain tumor types (e.g., trophoblastic tumors, testicular tumors, acute leukemia, Burkitt lymphoma, Hodgkin disease, non-Hodgkin lymphoma, childhood tumors) because of a significant frequency of disease-free remissions that extend for 5 years or more. In other circumstances, complete resolution of all clinically detectable disease can be achieved, but not for an indefinite period.[8,42]

All currently available antitumor drugs act on similar structures and metabolic pathways in normal and neoplastic cells. Consequently, their use is limited mainly by toxicity to normal tissues, notably the bone marrow, liver, kidneys, and nervous system. The emergence of drug resistance and the occasional location of tumors in the central nervous system or other anatomic sites inaccessible to drugs also limit their clinical utility. Many of the chemotherapeutic agents are mutagenic and carcinogenic, and these risks must be considered in their use.[6,14]

COMBINED OR ADJUVANT THERAPY

Therapeutic modalities have been combined in an effort to circumvent the limitations inherent in each. Radiation therapy is used preoperatively to reduce the tumor mass and render it resectable. A further goal is to prevent distant metastatic spread by devitalizing tumor cells prior to surgical manipulation. For example, preoperative irradiation is useful in the management of cancer of the body of the uterus, and there are some indications of its benefit in the treatment of patients with larger cancers of the head and neck and of the rectum. In many instances, however, the value of preoperative irradiation is disputed.[8]

Postoperative radiation therapy is used more widely. When tumors cannot be excised completely, as in the case of malignant brain tumors or large soft tissue sarcomas, postoperative irradiation can improve the outcome. Further, such a technique is used routinely and with good effect in the management of Wilms tumor.[8]

Chemotherapeutic agents have been used as adjuvants to radiation therapy with the thought of increasing the radioresponsiveness of the tumor and treating distant metastases that were not clinically apparent. Such a combined approach has proven advantageous in the treatment of retinoblastoma, Wilms tumor, head and neck cancers, Hodgkin disease and lymphoma among others. It appears that radiation therapy is most successful in dealing with large tumor masses, whereas chemotherapeutic agents can cope more effectively with smaller, widely disseminated deposits.

Chemotherapeutic agents have been used as adjuvants to surgery mainly to deal with clinically occult tumor dissemination. Most early trials failed to show any therapeutic advantage for this approach. In these trials however, low doses of drugs, and short periods of drug treatment were used. More recently, for example in breast cancer, it has been shown that the prolonged administration of cytotoxic drugs will delay or prevent tumor recurrence following surgery (see Chapter 6.21).[32,34]

SUPPORTIVE CARE

Extensive surgical procedures, intensive radiation therapy, and the vigorous use of chemotherapeutic agents have improved the results of cancer treatment. A favorable outcome, however, is often dependent on sustaining patients through limited periods of major physiologic impairment and readjustment. Intensive alimentation, reconstructive surgery, various restorative devices, blood component transfusion, and the control of infections are key considerations. Proper programs of rehabilitation and psychologic support

should be initiated with the beginning of antitumor treatment, especially in those cases where complete functional restoration is possible.

PALLIATIVE THERAPY

Patients with neoplastic disease that has progressed beyond hope of cure frequently have symptoms that are related to the presence of the tumor. Tumors may produce a wide variety of known biologically active substances, such as antidiuretic hormone, parathyroid hormone, gastrin, and serotonin, which will produce symptoms in the patient. There is also increasing evidence that many of the common systemic symptoms of tumors, such as cachexia or depression of immunity and bone marrow function, may be caused by as yet poorly characterized humoral substances produced either by the tumor or by inflammatory cells stimulated by the tumor.[3] Other symptoms may be related to mechanical effects of the tumor. Examples of mechanical effects of tumor masses include pain due to bony deposits, nerve root pressure, bleeding from a tumor surface, obstruction of viscera, healing ulceration, paralysis due to central nervous system or peripheral nerve compression, and serous cavity or subcutaneous fluid accumulation. Symptoms caused by the tumor constitute adequate indication for treatment, providing that there is a reasonable likelihood of achieving a good result.

In general symptoms caused by localized tumor masses are best treated by radiotherapy. The chronic leukemias, lymphomas, Wilms tumor, and neuroblastoma are radioresponsive tumors, whereas adenocarcinomas of the intestine, lung, kidney, and pancreas, and melanoma, osteogenic sarcoma, and fibrosarcomas are generally less responsive. Head and neck squamous tumors and cancers of the genitalia, bronchus, and esophagus are among those displaying an intermediate sensitivity. The use of ^{131}I offers satisfactory palliation to patients with colloid-forming carcinoma of the thyroid because of the selective uptake of iodine by this tumor.

On occasion a surgical procedure is most suitable, as in the relief of intestinal obstruction or the removal of an ulcerated breast lesion. At times a surgical procedure should be followed by a course of radiotherapy, as in acute spinal cord compression or extensive head and neck tumors. When the likelihood of a significant therapy induced remission is reasonable, it is important to support the patient in every way possible to permit completion of an adequate course of therapy. Many symptoms can be relieved by the judicious use of simple supportive measures.

Hormonal therapy, supplemental or ablative, can be very useful in the management of patients with tumors arising from endocrine-responsive tissues. The presence or absence of specific tumor cell hormone receptors provides a useful guide to therapy. Although tumor regrowth generally occurs after a period of time, "hormone responsiveness" usually indicates that subsequent endocrine manipulations will be beneficial.

BIOLOGIC EFFECTS OF ANTITUMOR THERAPY

A physician contemplating a specific therapeutic program must be thoroughly familiar with the varied biologic effects of available treatment modalities. The nature and basis of the effects of ionizing radiations, chemotherapeutic agents, and biological agents must be appreciated in order to prevent unintended discomfort to the individual being treated.

IONIZING RADIATION

The ionizing radiations employed therapeutically are of varying energies, but they produce qualitatively similar effects on exposed tissues. The sources of therapeutic ionizing radiations may be external to the patient, may be implanted in the tissues or body cavi-

ties, or may be given systemically in soluble chemical form such as $Na_2H^{32}P_2O_4$ and ^{131}I.

Whole-body irradiation is used infrequently in clinical practice. When used, therapy may be given from external sources, usually at a relatively low dose rate, or it may be given systemically in soluble isotopic form. Animals receiving high sublethal doses of whole-body irradiation quickly become listless and anorectic and may vomit. Similar effects are produced in patients who receive whole-body irradiation, 1000 rad at a dose rate of 5 rad per minute for purposes of immunosuppression prior to bone marrow transplantation.

Animals receiving lethal doses of whole-body irradiation usually die 7 to 14 days later as a consequence of bone marrow failure (marrow aplasia). The usual immediate causes of death are bleeding (thrombocytopenia) and infection (granulocytopenia). Animals receiving larger lethal doses die sooner because of gut damage or central nervous system derangement.

Most radiation therapy used clinically is directed toward specific anatomic sites or regions. The practical factors that limit the application of regional radiation therapy are the patient's systemic reaction and the effects produced on normal tissues within the field of treatment. Radiation sickness is characterized by general debility, anorexia, and vomiting. Symptoms that begin soon after the onset of treatment are related to dose and to volume and type of tissue treated and subside promptly on cessation of therapy or reduction in dosage.[19,39]

The normal tissues most commonly exposed in a treatment field include skin, mucous membrane, fat, connective tissue, muscle, bone, and cartilage. The intensity of the acute reaction observed in the skin or mucosa varies with the energy of the ionizing radiation and usually defines the tolerable dose when low energy radiation is being used. In many situations the acute or delayed changes produced in such tissues as the bone marrow, central nervous system, eyes, epiphyses, gonads, kidneys, and lungs are of great importance[8,39] (Table 6.14-1).

In general the early tissue effects of radiation (those produced in a matter of days) result from acute cell injury and death. At times this tissue necrosis is complicated by infection. Later (after a few weeks), tissue regeneration is completed but may be impaired by scarring and fibrosis. More severe late radiation effects (after months have elapsed) stem largely from vascular damage and include tissue atrophy or necrosis and ulceration, often in the skin. Vascular damage also determines the delayed development of impairments in other exposed organs—for example, radiation nephritis and radiation myelitis. Since ionizing radiations are carcinogenic, a rare delayed consequence is the development of another neoplastic disorder.

Ionizing radiations cause cell death, which may be defined as a loss of reproductive integrity. Exposed cells develop abnormalities of the nucleus, with visible chromosomal fragmentation and cross-linking. These result from the disruption of chemical bonds of the macromolecular cellular components, presumably through the intermediary of free radical formation. These changes may be modified by reparative mechanisms within the cell. The net damage to DNA seems to be of critical importance in determining the biologic expression of radiation effects.[19]

ANTITUMOR DRUGS

The antitumor drugs most commonly employed in current practice can be classified according to their presumed mechanisms of action (Table 6.14-2). Figures 6.14-1 and 6.14-2 are simplified schematic representations of the biochemical sites of action of cancer chemotherapeutic agents depicting the relationships of the agents to normal cellular metabolic processes.[6,14]

Tissue Proliferation and Drug Effects

By custom, the proliferative cycle that all types of dividing cells go through is divided into four phases—mitosis, G_1 (Gap$_1$), S (DNA

TABLE 6.14–1. BIOLOGIC EFFECTS OF IONIZING RADIATION: EXTERNAL SOURCE

Tissue Exposed	Clinical Manifestations
Skin and mucosa	Early erythema, desquamation followed by re-epithelialization, fibrosis (days) Later atrophy, telangiectasia develop Late necrosis, ulceration due to devascularization (mo) Still later, neoplasia
Hair	Epilation May recover in 5–12 mo depending on dose
Hematopoietic	Transient fall in reticulocytes, white cells, platelets, several days More marked when larger volume of marrow exposed during treatment of hematopoietic tumors May later result in marrow aplasia, fibrosis (mo)
Eye	Conjunctivitis, possible ulceration Sequence similar to mucosa Late cataract formation (mo to yr)
Lung	Acute radiation pneumonitis (days) related to lung volume exposed, perhaps related infection Late fibrosis (mo)
Heart	Acute and chronic pericarditis
Kidney	Delayed radiation nephritis (8–12 mo) due to vascular damage
Gonad	Sterility Mutational changes
Bone	Stops growth of ununited epiphyses; skeletal distortion results Late bone necrosis due to devascularization
Central nervous system	Delayed effects (mo) due to vascular damage, e.g., radiation myelitis More marked when larger volume of central nervous system exposed

synthesis), and G_2 (Gap$_2$). In most mammalian cells, S, the period of DNA synthesis, is of 6 to 8 hours duration and the G_2 phase lasts for approximately 2 hours. The G_1 phase is quite variable and it is during this period that cells perform many functions and increase their size. The G_0 phase has been added to describe cells that remain in G_1 for prolonged periods (nonproliferating).

Certain drugs such as mechlorethamine (HN2), 1,3-bis (2-chloroethyl)-1-nitrosourea (BCNU), and adriamycin react with cellular constituents irrespective of their proliferative activity (cell cycle–nonspecific agents). Other drugs are cycle-specific in their effect. For example, methotrexate, arabinosylcytosine, and hydroxyurea inhibit enzymes critical to DNA biosynthesis. Therefore, they are considered S-phase–specific agents.

Alkylating Agents

The cytotoxic actions of these drugs result from the covalent binding (alkylation) of the compound or a portion of it to a biologic target. Most of the alkylating agents in current use are nitrogen mustards, including cyclophosphamide, chlorambucil, melphalan, and mechlorethamine. Busulfan, long used in the therapy of chronic myelocytic leukemia, is a sulfonic acid ester. Other alkylating agents include the nitrosoureas (BCNU, CCNU), procarbazine, dacarbazine (DTIC), and hexamethylmelamine.

The toxicities common to alkylating agents include hematopoietic depression, gonadal dysgenesis, and nausea and vomiting. Most alkylating agents are immunosuppressive, with the exception of busulfan. Virtually all are mutagenic in model animal systems. Further, they are carcinogenic in humans, as shown by the occurrence of acute leukemia in a small percentage of patients treated extensively.

In addition to the undesirable effects that they share, many of the alkylating agents have unique toxicities. Hemorrhagic cystitis and alopecia are frequently caused by cyclophosphamide. High doses of this agent may produce cardiac damage and water retention caused by renal tubular dysfunction. Busulfan, when given for prolonged periods, can cause skin hyperpigmentation, pulmonary fibrosis, and a "pseudo-addisonian syndrome." Since procarbazine is an oxidant it may produce hemolytic anemia in susceptible individuals.

Alkylating agents react with a variety of biologic molecules, including amino acids, proteins, and nucleic acids. The reaction with DNA, however, appears to be the most important determi-

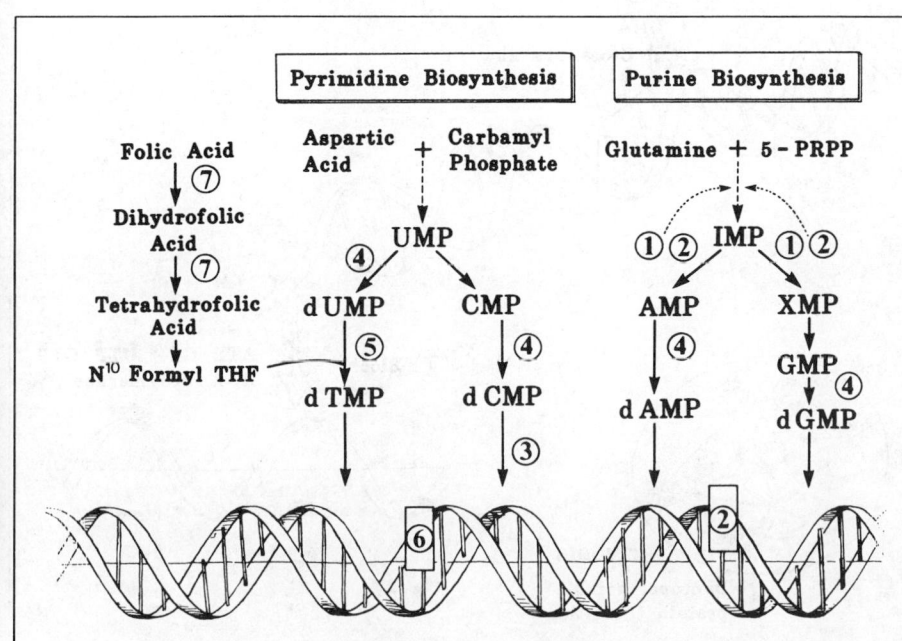

Figure 6.14–1. Major sites of action of antitumor drugs affecting DNA synthesis: 6-mercaptopurine ①, 6-thioguanine ②, arabinosylcytosine ③, hydroxyurea ④, 5-fluorouracil ⑤, 5-iodo-2′-deoxyuridine ⑥, methotrexate ⑦. Steps in purine biosynthesis: 5-phosphoribosyl 1-pyrophosphate (5-PRPP), inosinic monophosphate (IMP), xanthine monophosphate (XMP), guanosine monophosphate (GMP), deoxyguanosine monophosphate (dGMP), adenosine monophosphate (AMP), deoxyadenosine monophosphate (dAMP). Steps in pyrimidine biosynthesis: cytidine monophosphate (CMP), deoxycytidine monophosphate (dCMP), uridine monophosphate (UMP), deoxyuridine monophosphate (dUMP), deoxythymidine monophosphate (dTMP).

TABLE 6.14–2. CHARACTERISTICS OF COMMONLY USED ANTITUMOR DRUGS

Classification	Cell Cycle	Mechanism	Drug
Alkylating agents and platinum compounds	Cell cycle nonspecific React with biologic molecules irrespective of cell proliferation	Alkylation of nucleic acids, proteins, electron-rich molecules Probable critical target is DNA; covalent binding to purine and pyrimidine bases Cross-linking of DNA and/or DNA strand breaks	Mechlorethamine Cyclophosphamide Melphalan Chlorambucil Busulfan Carmustine Lomustine Semustine Procarbazine, DTIC Mitomycin-C Cis-platinum
Antimetabolites	Cell cycle specific Drug action may relate to specific phase of cell cycle S-phase most sensitive	Interfere with critical enzyme functions, especially those related to DNA biosynthesis Drugs are usually structural analogues of normal enzyme substrates	Methotrexate 6-Mercaptopurine 6-Thioguanine 5-Fluorouracil Ftorafur Cytosine arabinoside 5-Azacytidine Hydroxyurea
DNA intercalators	Cell cycle specific S-phase seems most sensitive Adriamycin; cycle nonspecific	Compounds of diverse structure that intercalate in the minor groove of DNA and interfere with transcription Drugs also cause breaks in DNA strands	Adriamycin Daunorubicin Bleomycin Actinomycin-D Mithramycin
Topoisomerase inhibitors	Cell cycle specific Exert maximal effects late in S or G2 and prevent cells from entering mitosis	Interacts with topoisomerase II to produce DNA strand breaks	Etoposide Amsacrine
Mitotic inhibitors	Cell cycle specific Metaphase arrest	Interactions with microtubular proteins prevent mitotic spindle formation and possibly other microtubular functions	Vinblastine Vincristine
Miscellaneous	Cell cycle nonspecific	Impairs 17-hydroxy-corticosteroid synthesis; damages adrenal cortex Asparagine-dependent tumor cells are susceptible to deprivation Produce DNA strand breaks	Mitotane L-Asparaginase Neocarzinostatin

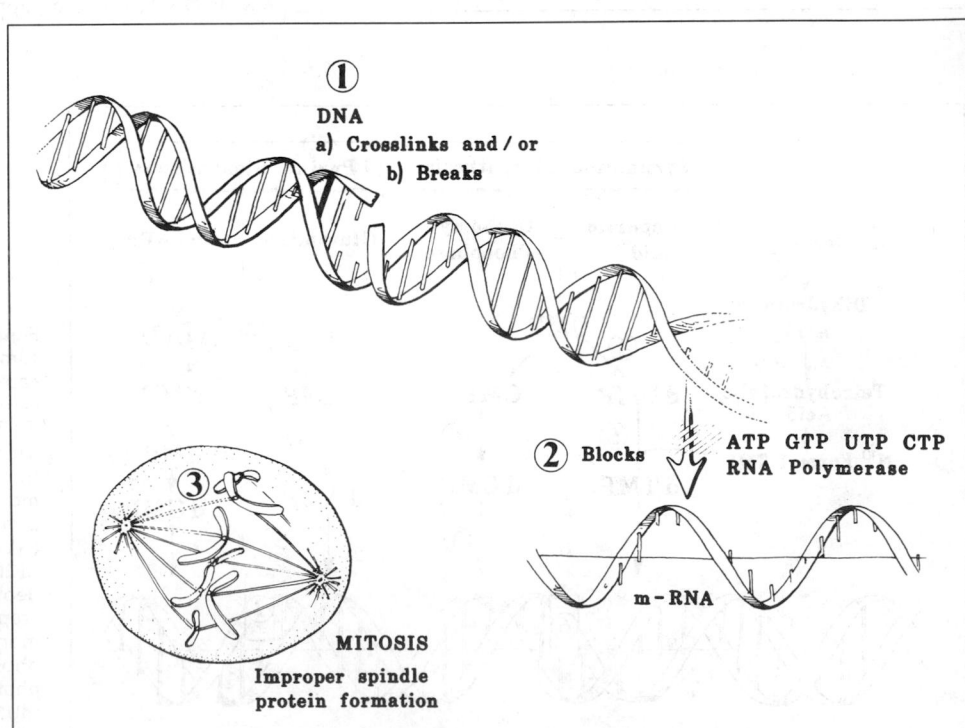

Figure 6.14–2. Major sites of action of antitumor drugs that interact with DNA or inhibit mitosis: alkylating agents ①, intercalators (dactinomycin, mithramycin, adriamycin, daunomycin) and topoisomerase inhibitors (etoposide, amsacrine) ②, vinca alkaloids ③.

① DNA
a) Crosslinks and/or
b) Breaks

② Blocks

ATP GTP UTP CTP
RNA Polymerase

m-RNA

③ MITOSIS
Improper spindle protein formation

nant of their antitumor effects. Agents with more than one alkylating group (polyfunctional) cross-link DNA strands and interfere with DNA replication. Monofunctional alkylating agents such as procarbazine and DTIC produce their DNA damage through single-strand breaks. The principal nucleotide target for the nitrogen mustards appears to be the *N-7* position of guanylic acid. The initial site of alkylation by the nitrosoureas may be the *O-6* position of guanylic acid.

Although it appears that the final chemical reactions with DNA are similar, the pharmacologic fates of these compounds, such as transport into the cell and chemical decomposition or metabolism to active or inactive species are quite different. These differences account for the unique clinical effects of these drugs. A tumor resistant to one alkylating agent, such as cyclophosphamide, may retain sensitivity to another, such as melphalan. Cyclophosphamide is relatively platelet-sparing. Rapid hematopoietic recovery is seen even after high doses of the drug, and repeated doses of cyclophosphamide do not result in cumulative bone marrow toxicity. In contrast, the nitrosoureas produce a delayed hematopoietic depression and cumulative bone marrow damage, making it difficult to administer repeated doses.

Platinum Compounds

A new class of antitumor agents that have assumed an important role in chemotherapy are the cis-platinum compounds. These compounds are coordination complexes of inorganic platinum that, like the alkylating agents, interact with DNA to produce interstrand and intrastrand DNA cross-links. These compounds have come to play an important role in the chemotherapy of testicular, ovarian, and head and neck cancer. The dose-limiting toxicity of the first member of this class was renal toxicity and, to a lesser extent, bone marrow suppression and hearing loss. Several newer platinum analogues have greatly reduced renal toxicity and ototoxicity, and their dose-limiting toxicity is bone marrow suppression.

Antimetabolites

Most antimetabolites in current use are purine or pyrimidine analogues or folic acid antagonists. Prior to producing their biologic effects, the purine and pyrimidine analogues must be converted in the target cell into nucleotides. The antimetabolites block DNA synthesis or cause defects in its structural integrity, and this occurs almost exclusively during the S-phase of the cell cycle (phase-specific). Their major toxic effects are observed in actively proliferating normal tissues, such as the bone marrow and intestinal epithelium. In addition, 6-mercaptopurine and methotrexate may cause hepatic cell damage.

Three purine analogues are employed widely. The administration of 6-mercaptopurine impairs several purine interconversions and inhibits de novo purine biosynthesis. Azathioprine (Imuran), a congener designed to protect the -SH group of 6-mercaptopurine from rapid metabolic breakdown, is used primarily as an immunosuppressant. Although 6-thioguanine interferes with purine biosynthesis and metabolic interconversions as much as 6-mercaptopurine, a significant amount of the analogue is incorporated into DNA. In some animal models the amount of DNA incorporation parallels therapeutic utility. In humans, the overall results of 6-thioguanine therapy are similar to those of 6-mercaptopurine.

When administered, the fluorinated pyrimidine analogues 5-fluorouracil and 5-fluoro-2'-deoxyuridine undergo a series of metabolic interconversions. In part, they are converted to 5-fluorodeoxyuridine monophosphate, which inhibits the enzyme thymidylate synthetase. This appears to be an important determinant of biologic effect. 5-Fluorouracil is also incorporated into RNA, and the drug may interfere with cellular function through this mechanism.

Arabinosylcytosine is an analogue of cytosine in which the ribose moiety is replaced by the sugar arabinose. The drug is converted to the nucleotide and as such interferes with DNA synthesis. Arabinosylcytosine nucleotide inhibits DNA polymerase and also produces chain termination after incorporation into the DNA strand.

Methotrexate and related compounds impair DNA synthesis by inhibition of dihydrofolate reductase, an enzyme essential for the synthesis of thymidylate. No congener has greater overall clinical utility than methotrexate. Citrovorum factor (tetrahydrofolic acid) administered shortly after (or before) methotrexate can prevent much of its toxicity, and the technique of "citrovorum factor rescue" has been used clinically to permit the administration of higher doses of methotrexate.

Hydroxyurea inhibits DNA synthesis without blocking RNA or protein synthesis. One of its main effects seems to be interference with the conversion of ribonucleosides to deoxyribonucleosides (inhibition of ribonucleoside diphosphate reductase).

Antibiotics

A great many antibiotics have been shown to have antitumor activity in various laboratory test systems. Of these, dactinomycin (actinomycin D), mithramycin, daunomycin, adriamycin, and bleomycin are in common clinical use.

Large doses of dactinomycin cause damage to proliferating tissues in the bone marrow, gastrointestinal tract, skin, and mucous membranes. These biologic effects are mainly due to the binding of dactinomycin to helical DNA and the consequent inhibition of DNA-dependent RNA synthesis. In greater concentration, the antibiotic will affect DNA synthesis and protein synthesis more directly. This selective action of dactinomycin has been used by molecular biologists as an investigative tool in clarifying many aspects of cell metabolism.

Mithramycin apparently has a very similar mechanism of action but may produce precipitous thrombocytopenia and fatal hemorrhage. Consequently, the drug is now rarely used as an antitumor agent. However, one of the effects of mithramycin is hypocalcemia, produced by the inhibition of the action of parathyroid hormone on bone. Since the hypocalcemic effect is seen at doses that rarely produce hemorrhagic toxicity, mithramycin is used to treat hypercalcemia and to control Paget disease of bone.

Daunomycin and adriamycin have similar chemical structures, but their mechanisms of action are not well understood. Both drugs intercalate with DNA and produce strand breaks, apparently through an oxidative mechanism. On the other hand, certain anthracycline antibiotics with antitumor activity do not enter the nucleus, thus indicating the existence of an important extranuclear site of action.

Daunomycin is used in the treatment of acute leukemia whereas adriamycin is used mainly in the management of lymphomas and several solid tumors. The usual treatment-limiting toxicity of both drugs is damage to the proliferating cells of the bone marrow, gastrointestinal tract, and skin and mucous membranes. Both antibiotics can cause serious damage to the heart that is cumulative. Therefore, total doses in excess of 500 mg/m^2 are not recommended.[6]

Bleomycin is a mixture of antibiotics that react with DNA, causing strand fission. Bleomycin also appears to inhibit some of the enzymes involved in DNA repair. Cells in the early S-phase seem most sensitive, and chromosomal fragmentation and mitotic arrest results. After administration, high concentrations of bleomycin remain in the skin, lungs, and responsive tumors. Damage to the skin and lungs usually limits clinical therapy.

Topoisomerase Inhibitors

Recently, several compounds have been found to exert cytotoxicity by interacting with the nuclear enzyme topoisomerase II to produce DNA strand breaks. Two such compounds, which are currently used clinically, are etoposide and amsacrine. Etoposide is an epipodophyllotoxin which is active against a number of tumors and is often used in the treatment of lung cancers and lymphomas. The principal toxicities of etoposide are leukopenia, hair loss, and nausea and vomiting. Amsacrine is an acridine derivative that is

useful in the treatment of acute nonlymphocytic leukemia. The dose-limiting toxicities of amsacrine are myelosuppression and gastrointestinal toxicity.

Mitotic Inhibitors

The vinca alkaloids, vinblastine, vincristine, and vindesine cause cells to arrest in metaphase by binding to microtubular proteins and preventing the assembly of the mitotic spindle. As might be expected, these agents are toxic to highly proliferative tissues. The dose-limiting toxicity of vinblastine is bone marrow suppression, whereas the dose-limiting effect of vincristine is neurotoxicity. The neurotoxicity of the vinca alkaloids is related to their interaction with neurotubules. However, the precise mechanism is poorly understood.

Mitotane (*o-p'*-DDD), used to treat adrenal cancer, came into clinical use because of its selective toxicity to adrenal cortical cells. Early degenerative lesions develop in the zona reticularis and the zona fasciculata and are accompanied by an impairment of 17-hydroxycorticosteroid synthesis. There is some evidence that mitotane inhibits enzymes important to steroid hormone production in the adrenal gland and enzymes responsible for the transformation of steroids in tissues as well. The clinical use of mitotane is limited primarily by skin eruptions, gastrointestinal intolerance, and mental derangements.

L-Asparaginase is an enzyme prepared from *E coli* or other microorganisms. Tumor cells lacking the capacity to synthesize asparagine are uniquely susceptible to this agent, which is used in the treatment of acute lymphocytic leukemia and lymphoma. The administration of L-asparaginase is limited by fever (endotoxin), chills, coagulation defects, hepatotoxicity, and pancreatitis.

STEROID HORMONES AND ANTIHORMONES

The steroid hormones of clinical importance in the treatment of neoplastic disease are androgens, estrogens, corticosteroids, and progestational agents. These hormones alter the morphology of responsive tumors, but the precise biochemical effect responsible for their tumor-controlling properties or their relatively tissue-specific action is not a matter of general agreement (Table 6.14–3).

During recent years, much has been learned about the sequence of events that relate to the binding of a steroid hormone to a target cell and the resultant biologic effects. For example, there are specific estrogen-binding proteins or estrogen receptors in estrogen-responsive cells. When the combined hormone and receptor protein enter the nucleus, specific stimulation of RNA polymerase and nucleic acid synthesis results. It is believed that similar mechanisms may be involved with other steroid hormones and their tissue responses.

Satisfactory oral and parenteral forms of these hormonal agents exist. To a large extent they are metabolized by the liver and the breakdown products eliminated in the urine and bile. Several of the listed tissue or metabolic effects of these hormones constitute their limiting toxicity clinically. On the other hand, certain of these effects, such as those of the corticosteroids on thrombocytopenic bleeding, hemolytic anemia, and calcium metabolism, are employed to advantage in the supportive care of patients.

Tamoxifen and nafoxidine have been introduced into clinical use because of their antiestrogenic properties. It appears that these compounds bind to estrogen receptors and block the effects of estrogens at the cellular level. These antiestrogens are particularly effective in the palliative therapy of postmenopausal patients with breast cancer, because a high percentage of the tumors in these patients will have estrogen receptors.

BIOLOGICAL THERAPY

IMMUNOTHERAPY

Animal studies indicate that a specific antitumor immune response is usually generated by the host. The reasons that tumors are able to escape this defense mechanism as they develop are not certain. In animal model systems, enhancement of the immune response by a variety of techniques has produced significant antitumor activity, including cures. It appears, however, that the number of malignant cells that can be eliminated by an immune mechanism is limited and that immunotherapy should be instituted when the least number of tumor cells is present.

Clinical trials have been carried out using a variety of methods to stimulate the immune response. These studies have used either immunization with irradiated autologous tumor cells or stimulation of the immune system with nonspecific adjuvants such as *Corynebacterium parvum*, BCG, and dinitrochlorobenzene (DNCB). Good results have been obtained with the DNCB treatment of

TABLE 6.14–3. BIOLOGIC EFFECTS OF STEROID HORMONES

Effects	Androgens	Estrogens	Progestin	Adrenocorticoids
Tissues	Stimulates growth of male sex tissues, body hair follicles, sebaceous glands, larynx, soft tissue and bones, erythropoietic tissue, closure of epiphyses	*Females:* Stimulates growth of breasts, nipples, uterus, pubic hair; proliferation of endometrium, myometrium, vaginal mucosa *Males:* Feminization of breasts, skin, hair, fat distribution; atrophy of genitalia	Maturation of breasts, endometrium, vaginal mucosa	Atrophy of thymus and lymphatic tissues and lympholysis; decrease in blood lymphocytes, eosinophils; increase in neutrophiles, platelets; increased liver glycogen; atrophy of muscles; osteoporosis
Metabolism	Increased RNA in target tissues; protein, calcium, and potassium anabolism; antagonizes estrogen action	Increased RNA in target tissues; protein and calcium anabolism; lowers blood lipids; antagonizes androgen action	Inhibits anabolic effects of androgens	Protein catabolism; enhances gluconeogenesis; increased secretion of gastric acid and pepsinogen; increased secretion of angiotensin, aldosterone; antagonizes insulin and HGH; stimulates erythropoiesis
Whole organism	Masculinization; growth spurt (prepubertal); increased tissue mass; sodium and water retention	Feminization; loss of libido (males); sodium and water retention Nausea	Sodium and water retention (large doses)	Sodium and water retention; hypertension; antiinflammatory; immunosuppression
Antitumor mechanisms	Directly on tumor cells; nuclear functions; anterior pituitary suppression Antiestrogenic effect	Direct effect on tumor cells; nuclear functions; anterior pituitary suppression	Effects on tumor unclear; anterior pituitary suppression	Effect on tumor cells; decreased glucose uptake

squamous cell and basal cell cancers of the skin. Also, useful and sometimes dramatic regressions of localized skin metastases of malignant melanoma and breast cancer have been obtained but with little effect on the visceral tumor.

With the development of techniques to produce monoclonal antibodies directed at specific antigens, the use of such antibodies for tumor therapy has become feasible. A major problem has been the failure to identify antigens that are specific to tumors. However, antibodies have been developed against tissue antigens that are present in high concentrations on certain tumors. For example, antibodies directed against idiotypic antigens have been shown to produce both partial and complete responses in patients with lymphomas,[25] but in most patients the responses have been partial and temporary. The use of monoclonal antibody therapy in solid tumors has been less successful. In order to enhance the antitumor activities of such antibodies, they have been coupled to radioisotopes or potent toxins, such as the ricin A chain. Such conjugates retain specificity to cells bearing the target antigen, yet do not depend on complement-dependent cytotoxicity to be effective against tumor cells. The initial clinical trials of antibody-conjugates have shown antitumor activity against both lymphomas and solid tumors.[7,27,35]

BIOLOGICAL RESPONSE MODIFIERS

A number of studies have evaluated the antitumor effects of peptides that are known to modulate cellular functions. The most thoroughly studied substances are the interferons, originally identified on the basis of their ability to render cells resistant to viral infection. Since large quantities of pure interferons have become available through recombinant DNA technology, these agents, especially α-interferon, have undergone extensive clinical trials. α-Interferon has been effective in the treatment of low-grade lymphomas, in which a 50 percent incidence of partial responses has been seen.[16] Particularly striking responses have also been seen in the treatment of hairy cell leukemia, a rare subtype of leukemia. In this disease the partial response rate has been approximately 70 percent, with good control of the symptoms.[16] The interferons have also shown some activity against solid tumors, in particular malignant melanoma and renal cell carcinoma. Other biologically active peptides, including tumor necrosis factor and interleukin 2, are currently undergoing clinical trial.

CELLULAR THERAPY

In 1985 Rosenberg and colleagues[31] reported the use of autologous lymphokine-activated killer (LAK) cells in the treatment of cancer patients. Mononuclear cells were harvested from these patients by leukopheresis, treated *in vitro* with interleukin 2, and then rein-

fused into the patients along with high doses of interleukin 2. Substantial responses were seen in patients with solid tumors, including renal cell carcinoma, melanoma, and colon carcinoma. Toxicity from the high doses of interleukin 2 is substantial, with severe fluid retention being the major problem. Because of the definite activity against solid tumors, this type of cellular therapy is now being extensively studied and compared to the administration of interleukin 2 alone.

SYSTEMIC THERAPY: SPECIFIC INDICATIONS

The general indications for the systemic treatment of neoplastic diseases have been discussed previously. Specific therapeutic indications are summarized here in relation to disease entities. Approximations of therapeutic usefulness are indicated by the frequency with which a neoplasm responds in relation to the cost in toxicity (Table 6.14–4).

A response is defined chiefly in terms of the objective clinical abnormalities that described the disease state at the beginning of therapy. For example, a complete response in acute leukemia implies a reversion to normal of the peripheral blood and marrow findings, as well as a resolution of all related symptomatology. In solid tumors, response implies a resolution of symptomatology and a decrease in tumor size or number by at least 50 percent without any evidence of disease progression. It must be pointed out, however, that the interpretation of clinical reports is difficult because of varied patient selection, response criteria, and other factors.

CHEMOTHERAPY

During the past few years it has become apparent that the use of cancer chemotherapeutic agents in combination may potentiate their effect on tumor cells. Drugs with differing mechanisms of action may be given simultaneously or in sequence with good effect. Combination chemotherapy is bearable because the adverse (toxic) effects of the drugs can, in some cases, be distributed over several tissues and not summate to severe intensity. Thus, the overall therapeutic outcome is much improved (Tables 6.14–5 and 6.14–6).

In many instances, more effective control of the tumor can be achieved by intermittent, intense courses of drug treatment spaced at intervals to permit recovery from toxicity. The success of this technique requires excellent supportive patient care.[26]

Leukemia
All types of acute leukemia are rapidly progressive and demand prompt treatment. Prolongation of useful life bears a direct rela-

TABLE 6.14–4. CLINICAL RESULTS OF SYSTEMIC CHEMOTHERAPY IN COMMON DISSEMINATED CANCERS

Potential Cure	Extended Survival	Useful Responses	Refractory
Acute lymphoblastic leukemia	Chronic granulocytic leukemia	Breast cancer	Bladder cancer
Acute myeloblastic leukemia	Lymphocytic lymphoma	Osteogenic sarcoma	Bronchogenic cancer
Hodgkin disease	Plasma cell dyscrasias	Colon cancer	Esophageal cancer
Histiocytic lymphoma	Chronic lymphocytic leukemia	Prostate cancer	Hepatic cancer
Burkitt tumor	Lung: small cell cancer	Endometrial cancer	Pancreatic cancer
Trophoblastic tumors	Ovarian cancer	Thyroid cancer	Stomach cancer
Testis tumors	Soft tissue sarcomas	Adrenal cortical cancer	Renal cancer
Ewing sarcoma	Neuroblastoma	Head and neck cancer	Uterine cervix cancer
Rhabdomyosarcoma	Thyroid: follicular cancer		Melanoma
Wilms tumor			
Retinoblastoma			

TABLE 6.14–5. EXPECTED RESULTS OF INITIAL CHEMOTHERAPY IN RESPONSIVE NEOPLASMS

Neoplasm	Drugs[a]	Expected Results	Comment
Leukemia			
Acute lymphoblastic	Prednisone Vincristine L-Asparaginase Daunorubicin	Complete remission in 90–95% of patients <age 15	"Prophylactic therapy" for meningeal leukemia "Maintenance therapy" for ~3 yr; 50% disease-free remissions >5 yr
Acute myeloblastic	Daunorubicin Arabinosylcytosine 6-Thioguanine	Complete remission in 50–60% of patients <age 65	Value of meningeal and maintenance therapy is uncertain Median disease-free remission ~2 yr
Chronic lymphocytic	Chlorambucil	Partial remission in 50–70% of cases	Disease often indolent Remissions maintained by continued therapy for 2–3 yr
Chronic granulocytic	Busulfan Hydroxyurea	Partial remission in >95% of cases	Remissions maintained by continued therapy for 3–5 yr
Lymphoma			
Hodgkin disease (stage III and IV)	Mechlorethamine Cyclophosphamide Vincristine Procarbazine Prednisone	Complete remission in 80% of cases	Radiation therapy to bulky tumors Continued therapy for 1 yr 30–60% disease-free remissions >5 yr
Low-grade non-Hodgkin lymphoma	Cyclophosphamide Vincristine Prednisone Interferon	Palliation of symptoms	Responsive to therapy, but sustained remissions are not seen
High grade non-Hodgkin lymphoma	Cyclophosphamide Vincristine Adriamycin Methotrexate Bleomycin Prednisone	Complete remissions in 50–70% of cases	Radiation therapy to bulky tumors 25–45% disease-free remissions >5 yr
Plasma Cell Dyscrasias			
Myeloma	Cyclophosphamide Melphalan Prednisone Adriamycin BCNU	Partial remission in 25–40% of cases	Remissions maintained by continued therapy for 1–2 yr Radiation therapy to mass lesions

[a]Drugs used in various combinations (see text).

tionship to the length of drug-induced disease remission (Table 6.14–5)[17,42]

Acute lymphocytic leukemia, predominantly a disease of childhood, will respond (complete response) to a number of drugs used singly—prednisone (55 percent), vincristine (50 percent), 6-mercaptopurine (35 percent), methotrexate (20 percent), arabinosylcytosine (20 percent), and cyclophosphamide (20 percent). More effective remission induction (>90 percent) can be achieved by using prednisone in combination with vincristine and L-asparaginase.[28]

At present, patients should be treated promptly on diagnosis with a multidrug "remission induction" regimen that includes prophylactic therapy for meningeal leukemia. Once a complete remission is achieved, prolonged "remission maintenance" or "consolidation" therapy is undertaken using multiple drugs intermittently in a planned sequence. It is to be expected that 50 percent or more of individuals on maintenance therapy will be alive at 5 years and free of evident leukemia.

Acute granulocytic leukemia, encountered most frequently in adults, is more refractory to treatment. The frequency of remission induction with single drugs is low—6-mercaptopurine (20 percent), arabinosylcytosine (20 to 30 percent), and methotrexate (10 percent). Cyclophosphamide is not effective at the usual dose levels but can induce complete remissions when given in high doses on an intermittent schedule.

Combination chemotherapy is clearly superior in inducing complete remissions in acute granulocytic leukemia. The drugs used in the most effective combinations include daunorubicin, arabinosylcytosine, and 6-thioguanine. Remission induction rates of 50 percent or more are to be expected in patients not previously treated. In contrast to acute lymphoblastic leukemia, median disease-free remission periods in excess of 2 years can be obtained without continued maintenance therapy.[28,41]

Preleukemia (see Chapter 6.16) represents a special case in that the disease process may remain static for prolonged periods (smoldering leukemia). The decision to begin multiagent chemotherapy is usually based on evidence of progressive marrow failure (especially thrombocytopenia and granulocytopenia) and progressive leukemia cell proliferation. The chronic leukemias, especially chronic lymphocytic leukemia, may pursue an indolent course for months or years. Because there is no evidence that prompt and aggressive therapy achieves superior long-term results, treatment is initiated only when the disease is progressing.

Busulfan will induce excellent and prolonged (years) partial remissions in nearly all patients (>95 percent) with chronic myelocytic leukemia. Splenic irradiation will achieve similar results, but it is generally more difficult to maintain satisfactory remission status without rather wide swings in disease activity. Hydroxyurea and 6-mercaptopurine may also be used to control disease manifestations.[29,42]

TABLE 6.14–6. EXPECTED RESULTS OF INITIAL CHEMOTHERAPY IN RESPONSIVE NEOPLASMS

Neoplasm	Drugs[a]	Expected Results	Comment
Lung cancer: small cell	Cyclophosphamide Adriamycin Vincristine Nitrosourea	Complete remission in 20–30% of cases	Radiation therapy to bulky tumors Median remission duration >2 yr
Breast cancer	Cyclophosphamide Methotrexate 5-Fluorouracil Adriamycin	Partial remission in 60–70% of cases	Radiation therapy to mass lesions Hormonal therapy useful in ER-positive tumors ER-negative tumors have higher growth fraction
Colon cancer	5-Fluorouracil Semustine Mitomycin C	Partial remission in 15–20% of cases	
Ovarian cancer	Cyclophosphamide Melphalan Adriamycin	Partial remission in 50–70% of cases	Surgery, radiotherapy for bulky tumor Some complete remissions obtained with combination chemotherapy
Trophoblastic tumors	Methotrexate Dactinomycin	Complete remission in >95% of cases	Nearly all cases remain disease-free >5 yr
Testis cancer	Cis-platinum Bleomycin Vinblastine	Complete remission in ~70% of cases	Remissions maintained by continued therapy for 1–2 yr Many disease-free remissions >5 yr
Wilms tumor	Dactinomycin Vincristine Adriamycin	Complete remission in 80–90% of cases	Surgery, radiotherapy for bulky tumor 60–80% cases disease-free >5 yr
Osteogenic sarcoma (localized)	Methotrexate Adriamycin	Surgery and chemotherapy yield ~50% disease-free survival >5 yr	Chemotherapy maintained ~2 yr Limb-preserving surgery possible
Ewing sarcoma	Cyclophosphamide Adriamycin Vincristine	Surgery and chemotherapy yield ~50% disease-free survival >5 yr	Chemotherapy maintained ~2yr
Rhabdomyosarcoma	Adriamycin Cyclophosphamide Vincristine	Surgery, radiotherapy, chemotherapy yield ~50% survival at 5 yr	Chemotherapy maintained 1–2 yr
Neuroblastoma	Cyclophosphamide Adriamycin Vincristine	Complete remission in 30–50% of cases	Surgery, radiotherapy for bulky tumor 20–25% of cases disease free at 5 yr

[a]Drugs used in various combinations (see text).

Chlorambucil, cyclophosphamide, and other alkylating agents can bring about prolonged partial remissions in 60 to 70 percent of patients with chronic lymphatic leukemia. Prednisone is also effective and is especially helpful in the management of hemolytic anemia, thrombopenic bleeding, and hypercalcemia. Combination chemotherapy to date has not yielded superior treatment results.[8,42]

Bone marrow transplantation for acute leukemia involves treatment of the patient with total body irradiation and very high doses of antitumor agents, followed by infusion of allogeneic bone marrow from a related or matched donor. Such therapy has not been effective in the treatment of patients who are in relapse. The use of allogeneic bone marrow transplantation in patients who have relapsed and then been retreated into a second or subsequent remission, however, results in a substantial percent of long-term remissions. The chance for a long-term remission in such patients with conventional chemotherapy is virtually nonexistent. If allogeneic bone marrow transplantation is performed in acute leukemia patients in first remission, 50 to 60 percent of these patients will then have long-term remissions or cures.[33] This number of long term remissions is higher than would be expected if the patients did not undergo the bone marrow transplantation, although some investigators believe that some of the newer and more intense induction regimens will produce a similar fraction of long-term first remissions. Allogeneic bone marrow transplantation has also resulted in a 50 to 70 percent rate of long-term remission in patients with chronic myelocytic leukemia. Recently, bone marrow trans-

plantation utilizing the patient's own marrow, which has been previously harvested and treated to eradicate residual tumor cells, has also resulted in a significant proportion of long-term remissions in patients with no hope of such results with conventional therapy.[43]

Lymphomas

Hodgkin Disease. In 1970 DeVita and colleagues reported that treatment of patients with advanced Hodgkin disease with a combination of nitrogen mustard (mechlorethamine), vincristine (Oncovin), procarbazine, and prednisolone (MOPP regimen) resulted in a high percentage of sustained complete remissions in these patients. A recent report summarized the results with this regimen at the National Cancer Institute after 14 years' experience. Eighty-four percent of the patients achieved a complete remission and 66 percent have remained disease-free for more than 10 years after treatment, confirming that MOPP is a highly effective therapy for Hodgkin disease.[23] Other investigators have reported that alternating MOPP therapy with courses of adriamycin, bleomycin, vinblastine, and dacarbazine (ABVD) is more effective than MOPP alone.[23] Subsequent studies, however, have not consistently confirmed that additional agents can improve on the results with MOPP.

Non-Hodgkin Lymphoma. A number of studies in recent years have demonstrated that low-grade lymphomas (well differentiated lymphocytic and nodular) respond initially to chemotherapy, but sustained remissions are not achieved.[30] Because of this finding and

the generally indolent nature of these neoplasms, patients with low-grade lymphomas are usually not treated unless their tumor is symptomatic, and intense treatment regimens are not usually administered. On the other hand, high-grade lymphomas (undifferentiated lymphocytic, diffuse histiocytic) have a high response rate to combination chemotherapy (50 to 70 percent complete responses) and about one half of these patients enter sustained complete remissions. The most commonly used regimen is a combination of cyclophosphamide, adriamycin (hydroxydaunorubicin), vincristine (Oncovin), and prednisone (CHOP regimen). Several reports have indicated that the addition of other agents, such as bleomycin, methotrexate, etoposide, procarbazine, and mechlorethamine, to the treatment resulted in a higher complete response rate.[12,21] Subsequent therapeutic trials, however, have failed to confirm the advantage of the more intense therapies, and the most appropriate combination therapy for high grade lymphomas is not certain.

A number of ongoing clinical trials have shown that very intense therapy and bone marrow rescue with either allogeneic or autologous bone marrow can result in long-term remissions in patients who have become refractory to conventional combination chemotherapy. The optimum induction therapy for such regimens and the role of in vitro treatment of the autologous bone marrow to eradicate residual tumor cells are not established.

Myeloma

Plasma cell myeloma often pursues an indolent course and may not require treatment. Cyclophosphamide, melphalan, and prednisone given as single drugs over an 8- to 12-week period will induce disease remissions in 20 to 30 percent of patients (Table 6.14–5). (The serum concentrations of myeloma protein provide an excellent guide to therapy.) These remissions generally are not as satisfactory as those achieved in the chronic leukemias. The combined use of prednisone and one of the alkylating agents produces a somewhat higher response rate than the alkylating agent alone. Higher doses of cyclophosphamide given intermittently are also effective.[8,42] Vincristine, BCNU, and adriamycin also are active against myeloma, and a recent comparative study found that the combination of vincristine, melphalan, cyclophosphamide, BCNU, adriamycin, and prednisone was superior to the combination of vincristine, cyclophosphamide, and prednisone.[9]

Trophoblastic and Germ Cell Tumors

Choriocarcinoma is a rapidly progressive disease and should be treated promptly. (Chorionic gonadotropin titers are a helpful guide to treatment.) Experience has shown that 90 percent or more of patients will respond to methotrexate or dactinomycin (Table 6.14–6). About half will remain disease-free for 5 years or longer and appear cured. The use of these drugs together or in sequence has increased the cure rate to about 75 percent. Refractory choriocarcinoma will respond to combination chemotherapy (e.g., methotrexate, dactinomycin, chlorambucil), and regressions have been reported following treatment with daunomycin, adriamycin, and bleomycin. Metastatic hydatidiform mole is a less aggressive disease and nearly all patients (95 percent) can be cured with methotrexate or dactinomycin.[8]

It is of some importance that complete disease control can be achieved without sacrificing the reproductive organs. Many posttreatment pregnancies have been carried to term successfully.

The treatment of disseminated testicular cancer has improved dramatically in the past decade. Cis-platinum, vinblastine, and bleomycin used in combination can induce complete remissions in 70 percent of patients. About one third of the patients who fail to obtain a complete drug-induced remission can be rendered disease-free by surgical removal of residual tumor masses. Of those who achieve a disease-free status, only 10 to 20 percent will relapse, most of them within the first year after therapy. Thus 60 to 70 percent of patients with disseminated testicular cancer appear to be curable.[8,10]

Adenocarcinoma of the ovary is responsive to alkylating agents and a number of other drugs, including cis-platinum, adria-

mycin, and hexamethylmelamine. Promising results with intensive combination chemotherapy have been reported. When compared to less toxic, single alkylating agent therapy, however, combination chemotherapy has not been shown to be consistently superior, especially in terms of survival.[4,44]

Childhood Tumors

Acute lymphocytic leukemia and lymphocytic lymphoma are among the most common neoplasms encountered in childhood. They are best managed with combination chemotherapy and with radiation therapy (see Chapters 6.16 and 6.19). Hodgkin disease is also managed similarly. It is important to begin treatment promptly in order to insure the best outcome. It may be expected that prolonged drug therapy will result in a retardation of linear growth.[42]

Brain tumors in children are managed primarily by surgery and radiation therapy according to their cell type. The role of chemotherapeutic agents in their treatment is under investigation. The intrathecal installation of antimetabolites such as methotrexate and arabinosylcytosine is useful in managing meningeal tumor and other superficial deposits. Vincristine, cis-platinum, and the nitrosoureas, given systematically, have produced regression of certain brain tumors. These leads are being explored, but it can be appreciated that the methodology for following the clinical effects of drugs on brain tumors is difficult.[6,8]

Over the past several years the prognosis for Wilms tumor has improved steadily (Table 6.14–6). In I and II patients presenting with localized disease, surgical excision of the tumor should be followed by radiation therapy to the region. III patients with more extensive local disease should be treated by surgery, followed by radiation therapy and chemotherapy with vincristine and dactinomycin. About 80 percent of such patients will be disease-free at 5 years. In patients presenting with metastatic disease or bilateral Wilms tumor, surgery and radiation therapy are the best means of managing the large tumor masses, and courses of dactinomycin, vincristine, and adriamycin are used to treat widespread disease. Complete remissions may be expected in two thirds of the cases or more, and about 40 percent will be alive and disease-free 2 years later.

Neuroblastoma presents usually as a disseminated disease. Surgical excision and radiation therapy are used to manage local tumor masses. (Neuroblastoma is very radioresponsive.) Vincristine, cyclophosphamide, dactinomycin, and adriamycin when employed as single agents have induced remissions in 30 to 50 percent of patients treated for disseminated disease. There is a body of opinion that suggests that surgical excision of apparently localized neuroblastoma (stages I, II, and III) should be followed by repeated courses of cyclophosphamide. More widely disseminated disease (stage IV) with bony metastases seems best managed with multiagent chemotherapy and radiation therapy.

The outlook for osteogenic sarcoma has improved greatly. Amputation is usually recommended when the tumor is resectable and when there are no evident pulmonary metastases. Intermittent courses of high-dose methotrexate followed by citrovorum factor have been given to patients following amputation. It would appear that such a combined approach has resulted in a 50 percent, 5-year, disease-free survival. High-dose methotrexate-citrovorum factor and adriamycin cause regressions in some patients with metastatic osteogenic sarcoma when given as single agents.

Ewing sarcoma may be difficult to distinguish from histiocytic lymphoma. It is a very radioresponsive tumor. The most successful plans of management employ radiation therapy to control the primary tumor mass and repeated courses of multiagent therapy to treat more widespread deposits (e.g., vincristine, adriamycin, and cyclophosphamide).

Similar therapeutic regimens have emerged for the soft-tissue sarcomas, especially rhabdomyosarcoma. Surgical excision and radiation therapy are the best means of managing bulky tumor masses. Combination chemotherapy (e.g., vincristine, adriamycin, and cyclophosphamide) can then be given in short courses over a

1- to 2-year period. With this approach, complete remissions have been achieved in 50 to 75 percent of patients who presented with metastatic disease, and most patients remain disease-free for over 1 year.

Solid Tumors in Adults

Although the overall results of drug treatment of the commonly occurring cancers of the breast, colon, bronchus, and other sites are not satisfactory, useful palliation can be obtained in many patients (Table 6.14–6). The nature of the possible tumor response must be balanced carefully against potential toxicity.

In breast cancer the use of combination chemotherapy following surgical resection appears to reduce the incidence of recurrent disease in women who have tumor involvement of axillary nodes (Chapter 6.21).[36] In patients with metastatic disease, multiagent chemotherapy has proven very useful, especially in managing individuals with progressive visceral organ involvement. For example, several large trials have revealed the efficacy of various drug combinations that include 5-fluorouracil (5-FU), methotrexate, vincristine, cyclophosphamide, and adriamycin given in short, intermittent courses over prolonged periods. Some 50 to 80 percent of cases respond with extensive tumor regression, and this status may be maintained for 8 to 10 months or more on the average. Thus, multiagent chemotherapy has replaced hormonal treatment as the initial modality in the management of rapidly progressive metastatic disease, especially in estrogen receptor–negative tumors.[8]

Best results in the treatment of metastatic cancer of the rectum and colon are achieved with 5-FU. Partial remissions of relatively short duration result in 15 to 20 percent of patients, especially those with less extensive tumor involvement of the parenchymal organs. Despite some encouraging early reports, the addition of a nitrosourea to 5-FU does not appear to increase the response rate in these tumors significantly. Therapy of metastatic gastric carcinoma with 5-FU, adriamycin, and mitomycin C (FAM regimen), however, has produced encouraging results, with a response rate of 25 to 30 percent.[13]

Metastatic adrenal cortical cancer will respond satisfactorily to several weeks of mitotane therapy in 30 to 35 percent of cases. Gastrointestinal intolerance, muscle aches, mental derangement, skin rashes, and the like make long-term treatment difficult.

The results achieved in small cell cancer of the lung have improved remarkably in recent years (see Chapter 6.22). Combination chemotherapy including such agents as adriamycin, cyclophosphamide, vincristine, a nitrosourea, and epipodophyllotoxin yields complete remissions in 20 to 30 percent of cases and partial responses in an additional 30 to 40 percent. At present the median period of disease-free remission is about 2 years.[1] Other types of bronchogenic cancer are much less sensitive to chemotherapy. Responses of short duration occur in 20 to 30 percent of cases; complete responses are rare.[15]

REGIONAL CHEMOTHERAPY

Topical applications of 5-FU or mechlorethamine have proven quite useful in the management of extensive squamous cell cancers of the skin and, in some instances, the lesions of mycosis fungoides. Alkylating agents instilled locally in high concentration are as efficacious as colloidal radioactive isotopes in the management of malignant effusions. The intrathecal administration of methotrexate or arabinosylcytosine can control meningeal leukemia, and prophylactic injections seem to prevent the clinical emergence of this complication in children with acute lymphocytic leukemia.

With the improvement of systemic chemotherapy for breast and bronchogenic cancer, meningeal involvement by these tumors is seen more frequently. The intrathecal administration of methotrexate and thiotepa is effective in this situation.[38] Regional perfusion or infusion therapy of a wide variety of tumors has been attempted, with variable results. The best outcomes have followed the perfusion of extremities bearing melanomas or sarcomas. Hepatic artery infusion of 5-fluorodeoxyuridine (5-FUdR) for the treatment of colorectal cancer metastatic to the liver has shown encouraging results.[11]

HORMONAL THERAPY

Hormonal therapy is used primarily for metastatic tumors of the breast and prostate that retain a degree of responsiveness to endocrine control. Progestins may cause remissions of endometrial cancer. Corticosteroids frequently induce remissions in acute lymphocytic leukemia and occasionally cause regressions of lymphomatous tumor masses and multiple myeloma. Thyroid hormone is used to suppress thyroid-stimulating hormone (TSH) secretion in patients following resection of their tumor, and hence reduce the likelihood of recurrent tumor growth.[8]

The clinical usefulness of hormonal agents and endocrine ablative procedures in selected neoplastic diseases is indicated in Table 6.14–7. The availability of clinically useful techniques for the measurement of estrogen receptors, progesterone receptors, and receptors for other steroidal hormones has provided a reliable basis for guiding hormonal therapy. This is especially true in breast cancer, where the presence or absence of estrogen receptors (ER) in each patient's tumor has become one of the prime determinants of the initial treatment prescribed for disseminated disease. For example, premenopausal patients with ER-positive cancers are likely to be treated with antiestrogens or with ovariectomy, and ER-positive, postmenopausal patients with an antiestrogen unless they have rapidly progressing disease with visceral organ involvement. There seems to be no value to "prophylactic castration" for the prevention of recurrence of breast cancer following primary curative resection (see Chapter 6.21).

TABLE 6.14–7. EXPECTED RESULTS OF HORMONAL THERAPY OF DISSEMINATED NEOPLASMS

Neoplasm	Therapy	Expected Result	Comment
Breast cancer (premenopausal, ER+)	Castration	Partial remission in 60–70% of cases	Estrogens will stimulate tumor growth
Breast cancer (postmenopausal, ER+)	Antiestrogen Androgen	Partial remission in 40–50% of cases Partial remission in 30–40% of cases	Adrenalectomy or hypophysectomy may yield a second remission in responsive patients
Breast cancer (ER–)		Rare response	Neither pre- nor postmenopausal patients are likely to respond
Prostate cancer	Estrogen	Symptomatic relief and some tumor regression ~60% of cases	Well-differentiated tumors (acid phosphatase +) likely responsive
Endometrial cancer	Progestin	Partial remission in 25–30% of cases	
Thyroid cancer	Thyroid hormone	Suppression of recurrent tumor growth (well-differentiated tumors)	Thyroid hormone continued indefinitely after surgery to suppress TSH

HYPERTHERMIA

A large body of laboratory investigation indicates that tumor cells are more damaged by transient temperature elevation (to about 43C) than are normal cells. At the present time, a variety of methods are used to produce localized heating of tumors. Regional hyperthermia is being evaluated when given alone or in combination with drugs or radiation therapy. The use of systemic hyperthermia for disseminated tumor has been associated with significant morbidity and has usually not resulted in tumor regression.[5]

DRUG SENSITIVITY TESTING

It would obviously be of benefit to be able to predict the sensitivity of a given tumor to drugs. Various techniques, most based on the inhibition of the uptake of radiolabeled DNA precursors, have been utilized with modest success in the past. Recently, a great deal of interest has been focused on drug sensitivity testing by examining the in vitro cloning ability of human tumor cells.[40] The main shortcoming with this technique has been the poor cloning and growth capability of human tumors in vitro.

A high percentage of human tumors do not show sufficient growth to permit sensitivity testing. If enough cells grow, however, drug resistance can be predicted with a high degree of reliability. It is likely that this technique will become more useful as better in vitro growth conditions are developed. Since the presence of a few resistant cells in several million are likely to be sufficient to prevent cure, however, this technique has obvious inherent limitations.

REFERENCES

1. Abeloff MD, Ettinger DS, et al: Intensive induction chemotherapy in 54 patients with small cell carcinoma of the lung. Cancer Treat Rep 65:639, 1981
2. American Joint Committee for Cancer Staging and End Results Reporting: Staging of Lung Cancer 1979, Chicago, 1979
3. Beutler B, Cerami A: Cachetin: More than tumor necrosis factor? N Engl J Med 316:379, 1987
4. Carmo-Pereira J, Costa FO, Henriques E: Cis-platinum, adriamycin, and hexamethylmelamine versus cyclophosphamide in advanced ovarian carcinoma. Cancer Chemother Pharmacol 10:100, 1983
5. Cavaliere R, Ciocatto E, et al: Selective heat sensitivity of cancer cells. Cancer 20:135, 1967
6. Chabner B: Pharmacologic principles of cancer treatment. Philadelphia, WB Saunders, 1982
7. DeNardo SJ, DeNardo GL, et al: Radioimmunotherapy of patients with B cell lymphoma using I-131 Lym-1MAb. J Nucl Med 27:903, 1986
8. De Vita VT, Hellman S, Rosenberg SA: Cancer: Principles and Practice of Oncology. Philadelphia, JB Lippincott, 1982
9. Durie BGM, Dixon DO, et al: Improved survival duration with combination chemotherapy induction for multiple myeloma: Southwest Oncology Group study. J Clin Oncol 4:1227, 1986
10. Einhorn LH, Williams SD, et al: Surgical resection in disseminated testicular cancer following chemotherapeutic cytoreduction. Cancer 48:904, 1981
11. Ensminger W, Niederhuber J, et al: Totally implanted drug delivery system for hepatic arterial chemotherapy. Cancer Treat Rep 65:393, 1981
12. Fisher RI, DeVita VT Jr, et al: Diffuse aggressive lymphomas: Increased survival after alternating flexible sequences of ProMACE and MOPP chemotherapy. Ann Intern Med 98:304, 1983
13. Gastrointestinal Tumor Study Group: A comparative clinical assessment of combination chemotherapy in the management of advanced gastric carcinoma. Cancer 49:1362, 1982
14. Gilman AG, Goodman LS, Gilman A: The Pharmacologic Basis of Therapeutics, 6th ed. New York, Macmillan, 1980
15. Golomb HM (ed): Non-small-cell lung cancer. Semin Oncol 10:1, 1983
16. Golomb HM: Interferons: Present and future use in cancer therapy. J Clin Oncol 4:123, 1986
17. Gunz FW, Henderson SS (eds): Leukemia, 4th ed. New York, Grune & Stratton, 1983
18. Gutterman JU, Fine S, et al: Recombinant leukocyte A interferon: Pharmacokinetics, single-dose tolerance, and biologic effects in cancer patients. Ann Intern Med 96:549, 1982
19. Hall EJ: Radiobiology for the Radiologist, 2d ed. Hagerstown, Harper & Row, 1978
20. Himel HN, Liberati A, et al: Adjuvant chemotherapy for breast cancer: A pooled estimate based on published randomized control trials. JAMA 256:1148, 1986
21. Klimo P, Connors JM: MACOP-B chemotherapy for the treatment of diffuse large-cell lymphoma. Ann Intern Med 102:596, 1985
22. Larkin JM, Edwards WS, et al: Systemic thermotherapy: Description of a method and physiologic tolerance in clinical subjects. Cancer 40:3155, 1977
23. Longo D, Young RC, et al: Twenty years of MOPP therapy for Hodgkin's disease. J Clin Oncol 4:295, 1986
24. Manual of Clinical Oncology: Edited under the auspices of the International Union Against Cancer. New York, Springer-Verlag, 1982
25. Miller RA, Maloney DG, et al. Treatment of B-cell lymphoma with monoclonal anti-idiotype antibody. N Engl J Med 306:517, 1982
26. Norton L, Simon R: Tumor size, sensitivity to therapy, and design of treatment schedules. Cancer Treat Rep 61:1307, 1977
27. Order SE, Stillwagon GB, et al: Iodine 131 antiferritin, a new treatment modality in hepatoma: A radiation therapy oncology group study. J Clin Oncol 3:1573, 1985
28. Powles R, McElwain T (eds): Leukemia I. Semin Hematol 19:3, 1982
29. Powles R, McElwain T (eds): Leukemia and Lymphoma II. Semin Hematol 19:4, 1982
30. Powles R, McElwain T (eds): Lymphoma III. Semin Hematol 20:1, 1983
31. Rosenberg SA, Lotze MT, et al: Observations on the systematic administration of autologous lymphokine-activated killer cells and recombinant interleukin-2 to patients with metastatic cancer. N Engl J Med 313:1485, 1985
32. Salmon SE, Jones SE (eds): Adjuvant Therapy of Cancer, III. New York, Grune & Stratton, 1981
33. Santos GW, Tutshcka PJ, et al: Marrow transplantation for acute nonlymphocytic leukemia after treatment with busulfan and cyclophosphamide. N Engl J Med 309:1347, 1983
34. Schabel FM: Concepts for systemic treatment of micrometastases. Cancer 35:15, 1975
35. Spitler LE, del Rio M, et al: Therapy of patients with malignant melanoma using a monoclonal antimelanoma antibody-ricin A chain immunotoxin. Cancer Res 47:1717, 1987
36. Tancini G. Bonadonna G, et al: Adjuvant CMF in breast cancer: Comparative 5-year results of 12 versus 6 cycles. J Clin Oncol 1:2, 1983
37. Terry WD, Rosenberg SA (eds): Immunotherapy of Human Cancer. New York, Elsevier, 1981
38. Trump DL, Grossman SA, et al: Treatment of neoplastic meningitis with intraventricular thiotepa and methotrexate. Cancer Treat Rep 66:1549, 1982
39. Vaeth JW (ed): Combined Effects of Chemotherapy and Radiotherapy on Normal Tissue Tolerance. New York, Karger, 1979
40. Van Hoff DD, Casper J, et al: Association between human tumor colony-forming assay results and response of an individual patient's tumor to chemotherapy. Am J Med 70:1027, 1981
41. Vaughan WP, Karp JE, Burke PJ: Long chemotherapy-free remissions after single-cycle timed sequential chemotherapy for acute myelocytic leukemia. Cancer 45:859, 1980
42. Williams WJ, Beutler E, et al (eds): Hematology, 3d ed. New York, McGraw Hill, 1983
43. Yeager AM, Kaizer H, et al: Autologous bone marrow transplantation in patients with acute nonlymphocytic leukemia, using ex vivo marrow treatment with 4-hydroperoxycyclophosphamide. N Engl J Med 315:141, 1986
44. Young RC, Chabner BA, et al: Advanced ovarian adenocarcinoma—A prospective clinical trial of melphalan versus combination chemotherapy. N Engl J Med 299:1261, 1978

CHAPTER 6.15
Disorders of White Blood Cells

Albert H. Owens, Jr.,
and Lyle L. Sensenbrenner

The major diagnostic classifications of white blood cell disorders continue to be based principally on the enumeration of the nucleated cells in the blood and the differential staining of leukocytes in the peripheral blood, bone marrow, lymphoid organs, and other tissues. It is important that physicians be familiar with the advantages and limitations of these simple morphologic techniques because they provide information vital to the solution of a wide variety of clinical problems.[2,6]

During recent times the characterization of white cells has been amplified by increasingly sophisticated technology. Electron microscopy has provided insights into the ultrastructure of white cells and the nature of their surfaces. Tissue transplantation studies, in vitro culture techniques, and the use of various specific biomarkers have provided evidence for the existence of a pluripotent hematopoietic stem cell that is capable of self-maintenance and differentiation along erythrocytic, granulocytic, megakaryocytic, and lymphoreticular lines. These same techniques have demonstrated the existence of a variety of humoral substances (colony-stimulating factors) that regulate and promote the growth of these cells. Recently, several of these factors have been purified, and the genes for their production identified and cloned. These purified growth factors are now available for clinical studies.[3] Modern marker techniques have permitted in vivo kinetic studies of the production, maturation, and tissue migration of leukocytes and a beginning appreciation of the factors that control and modulate these processes. Improved cell separation techniques together with sensitive and specific biochemical and histochemical methodology have increased our understanding of leukocyte composition and the mechanisms involved in motility, chemotaxis, phagocytosis, and lysosomal digestion. In addition, monoclonal antibodies have been used to detect and characterize several lineage-specific differentiation antigens that appear during normal leukocyte maturation. Some of this newer physiologic and biochemical knowledge has had an impact on clinical practice. For example, various qualitative defects in leukocyte phagocytosis and lysosomal digestion have been observed to be responsible for inadequate host defenses against invading microorganisms, and simple studies can be performed on peripheral blood leukocytes that will lead to their correct recognition.[6,7] The use of cell surface markers has allowed the classification of very undifferentiated tumor cell populations into myeloid or lymphoid types, a classification that influences significantly the type of therapy given and the ultimate results obtained.

In this chapter the white blood cells are identified briefly and their normal physiology and function outlined. The congenital and acquired qualitative defects of leukocyte function are considered together with the clinical syndromes they cause. Since the most common abnormalities in the number and tissue distribution of leukocytes are due to nonhematopoietic diseases, these several derangements are considered as diagnostic problems and the many potential underlying causes related to them. The primary proliferative abnormalities of white blood cells are also considered in sequence. Accounts of the leukemias and plasma cell dyscrasias are contained in Chapters 6.16, 6.17, and 6.20. Bone marrow failure is discussed in Chapter 6.11.

GENERAL CONSIDERATIONS

The total leukocyte count in the peripheral blood of normal adults ranges from 4000 to 10,000/μl. Of these, 55 to 65 percent are neutrophils, 1 to 3 percent eosinophils, 0 to 0.75 percent basophils, 25 to 35 percent lymphocytes, and 3 to 7 percent monocytes. In infants, especially newborns, white cell counts may be higher, even greater than 20,000/μl, and over 50 percent of the cells are lymphocytes.

In adults, significant fluctuations in the total leukocyte count can be seen during a short time (minutes to hours). This is usually associated with a rapid redistribution of granulocytes between the marginal and circulating pools in peripheral vessels and the ready reserve in the bone marrow. For example, strenuous exercise, pregnancy and labor, convulsions, paroxysmal tachycardia, and emotional panic frequently are accompanied by a neutrophilic leukocytosis because of rapid redistribution. A different type of variation in total granulocyte counts has been identified as well: cyclic changes with an amplitude of 2000 to 3000 granulocytes per microliter and a periodicity of about 20 days observed in normal individuals and attributed to variations in the rate of production of granulocytes mediated by humoral substances.

THE GRANULOCYTIC SERIES[4,6,7]

ORIGIN

The juvenile (band) and mature polymorphonuclear leukocytes (segmented cells) found in the peripheral blood are derived from granulocytic precursors located in the bone marrow. The myeloblast is the least differentiated identifiable form. As the cells mature they become smaller and their cytoplasm is less basophilic. In mature cells the nucleus is segmented and occupies proportionately less of the cell. Mature cells are described further as neutrophils, eosinophils, or basophils according to the staining characteristics of their prominent cytoplasmic granules (Table 6.15–1). Much evidence points to the existence of a stem cell population that remains largely in a nonproliferative state but is capable of differentiation into erythrocytic, megakaryocytic, and granulocytic cell types.

When considered in toto, the granulocytic cells compose a tissue of impressive size, approximating that of the liver (1300 to 1500 g). At any given time, less than 1 percent of the cells are circulating in the peripheral blood. The remainder are located, as developing and mature cells, in the marrow (about 800 to 900 g), in marginal intravascular (capillary) compartments, and in extravascular locations in all tissues, especially the lungs, liver, and spleen (about 500 to 600 g). The relatively large pools of mature granulocytes located in the bone marrow and aggregated along capillary walls serve as a ready reserve of motile phagocytic cells.

LIFE SPAN

The life span of the normal neutrophil is estimated to be between 10 and 15 days. Approximately 4 to 5 days are spent in the precursor pool in the marrow and an equal time in the marrow reserve. The time spent in the peripheral blood is less than 24 hours. The tissues in which most neutrophils are removed from the circulation are the lungs, liver, spleen, gastrointestinal tract, bone marrow, striated muscle, and kidney. Some granulocytes will survive an additional 4 to 5 days in extravascular sites.

Several factors are known to affect the concentration of circulating granulocytes (the size of the circulating pool). Rapid mobili-

TABLE 6.15–1. THE GRANULOCYTIC SERIES

Cell	Morphologic Features	Physiologic Function	Location
Myeloblast (15–20 μm)	Large nucleus, fine chromatin, usually two or more nucleoli Clear scant cytoplasms	Proliferation Marked DNA, RNA, protein synthesis	Confined to marrow except in disease
Myelocyte	Nuclear chromatin coarsens; nucleoli disappear Cytoplasm less basophilic, more abundant Prominent cytoplasmic granules develop	Progressive differentiation DNA, RNA, protein synthesis still prominent	Confined to marrow except in disease
Segmented cell (12–15 μm)	Band-shaped to multilobed nucleus; coarse chromatin Nuclear "drum stick" (Barr body) in 3% normal female cells Neutrophilic, eosinophilic, or basophilic cytoplasmic granules	Motility, chemotaxis, immune adherence, phagocytosis, and lysosomal digestion Glycolysis provides energy for phagocytosis Protein synthesis continues	Bone marrow Peripheral blood Tissues

zation of granulocytes from noncirculating pools in the bone marrow and along the margins of blood vessels can result from acute physiologic events such as violent exercise and emotional events, or the administration of pharmacologic agents such as endotoxin, adrenal corticosteroids, adrenalin, heparin, and etiocholanolone. The circulating leukocyte count may increase by a factor of 2 to 3, with children tending to be more reactive than adults.

Although there is much to suggest a positive feedback control of granulocyte production that operates on a stem cell precursor in a manner analogous to erythropoietin in erythropoiesis, the existence of "granulopoietin" has not been proven conclusively. There are substances in the serum of humans and other species that appear to stimulate and inhibit granulocyte proliferation (Chapter 6.11). A series of glycoproteins, "colony-stimulating factors," has been identified that appear to stimulate in vitro the proliferation of both "committed" progenitors and very early lineage-nonspecific cells that will mature into granulocytes and monocytes. These substances (interleukin-3, granulocyte-monocyte-stimulating factor, granulocyte-stimulating factor, and monocyte-macrophage-stimulating factor) have been identified, purified, their DNA cloned, and the recombinant material produced so that it is now available for clinical studies. Thus far serum levels of these growth factors have not been detected in humans, and their role as normal physiologic regulators of hematopoiesis is not clear. They may, however, eventually have therapeutic benefit in either specific or multilineage hematopoietic cell failure states. In addition, several investigators have claimed the existence of "chalone" and "antichalone" which inhibit the myelocyte (not the stem cell) or stimulate it to further proliferative activity (antichalone). Further work is needed to clarify these issues.

FUNCTION[5,6]

The mature granulocytes are concerned primarily with defending the body against invading microorganisms and other injurious agents. In order to achieve this purpose the granulocytes are motile, responsive to chemotactic stimuli, able to migrate through tissues, and capable of recognizing, phagocytizing, and digesting foreign objects.

Chemotactic factors cause the active, directional migration of granulocytes to involved tissue sites by a poorly understood series of events. Chemotactic factors are contained in necrotic tissue, bacterial lipopolysaccharides, complement components, and granulocytes themselves. Certain complement-dependent antigen-antibody interactions (opsonins) also stimulate the directional migration of granulocytes. Neutrophils and eosinophils are more responsive to these stimuli than are basophils.

The mechanism by which granulocytes recognize and bind to a foreign object are largely unknown. The energy required for phagocytosis is derived mainly from glycolysis. Phagocytic activity

seems to be increased in anemic individuals and those with fever. Phagocytosis is impaired in malnourished individuals and in the presence of high glucose concentrations. Many bacteria produce substances that inhibit phagocytosis—for example, somatic O antigens, capsular polysaccharides, exotoxins, and leukocidins.

Mature granulocytes contain two types of granules called by some "azurophilic" or primary, and "specific" or secondary. The azurophilic granules (membrane-bound lysosomes) are produced early in the maturation phase and contain a large complement of hydrolytic enzymes that are capable of digesting phagocytized material. There are enzymes capable of degrading nucleic acids, proteins, carbohydrates, and lipids. These granules also contain enzymes that attack collagen, glucuronides, and cell membranes (hemolysins). Other granule-associated materials are pyrogenic and thromboplastin-like, such as phagocytin, hyaluronic acid, and several mucopolysaccharides. The "specific" or secondary granules in mature cells are produced in myelocytes and metamyelocytes and contain alkaline phosphatase. During early stages of development the alkaline phosphatase activity is low or absent; later, it is variable. Myeloperoxidase, acid phosphatase, and arylsulfatase activity predominate in the early primary granule, while lysozyme, aminopeptidase, and collagenase are associated with the later specific granule.

Granulocytes also make a minor contribution to the body's defense mechanisms other than phagocytosis. In individuals with agranulocytosis, antibody production and the expression of immediate and delayed hypersensitivity are unimpaired. The mononuclear cell response to skin inflammation is delayed, however, suggesting that neutrophils enhance their migration to the injured site.

METABOLISM

Myeloblasts and myelocytes are capable of purine and pyrimidine biosynthesis and DNA and RNA synthesis as well. As granulocytes mature, their DNA and RNA content declines proportionately, and their nucleic acid synthetic capabilities are lost. Similarly, the tricarboxylic acid pathway enzymes decline in activity as the cells mature. Thus, glycolysis is the main energy-producing process in mature granulocytes, and it is important to the completion of locomotion and phagocytosis. Phagocytizing neutrophils are capable of converting oxygen to a series of compounds (including hydrogen peroxide) that have potent antimicrobial activity.

Granulocytes have a higher level of peroxidase, alkaline phosphatase, arginase, and arylsulfatase enzymes than do lymphocytes or other mononuclear cells found in hematopoietic tissue. Similarly, granulocytes contain more glycogen and vitamin B_{12} binding sites and their rates of glycolysis and respiration are greater. Eosinophils have higher levels of catalase and arylsulfatase activity than neutrophils. They contain only one type of large eosinophilic gran-

ule containing a myeloperoxidase, several cationic proteins, β-glucuronidase, acid β-glycerophosphatase, and arylsulfatase. Basophils are rich in acid mucopolysaccharides, heparin, histamine, and histidine decarboxylase. The full significance of all of these observations is unknown. Simple histochemical stains for myeloperoxidase aid in the clinical identification of myeloblasts, however, and stains for alkaline phosphatase help distinguish normal mature neutrophils.[2]

THE MONOCYTIC SERIES[1,3]

Monocytes in the peripheral blood are motile, phagocytic cells of varying size (16 to 30 μm). Large monocytes have a voluminous, kidney-shaped, or rounded, often folded, nucleus containing a fine chromatin network with small chromatin aggregates along the nuclear membrane. Their cytoplasm is abundant and stains gray-blue (Wright stain). It contains azurophilic granules. Small monocytes are often difficult to distinguish from large lymphocytes (15 to 20 μm). The nucleus of small monocytes is usually oval or rounded. The cytoplasm stains blue and contains new azurophilic granules. Monocytes give strong histochemical reactions for lysosomal enzymes (muramidase) and nonspecific esterases.

ORIGIN[4,6]

Monocytes and macrophages constitute a family of related phagocytic cells that are found in the blood, bone marrow, lymph nodes, spleen, liver, lungs, and a wide variety of tissues and body fluids. Monocytes and granulocytes develop from the same immediate bone marrow progenitor. Blood monocytes arise from precursors in the marrow. They are not fully mature cells, and they will divide and differentiate further in lymphoreticular tissues throughout the body. "Promonocytes" and "monoblasts" are difficult to distinguish with light microscopy. The kinetics of monocyte production as studied by current labeling techniques reveal them to be similar to granulocytes.

FUNCTION[1,3]

Monocytes are often found along the margins of small blood vessels. The ingestion of India ink particles and their propensity to adhere to surfaces have been used as an aid to the identification of monocytes.

Monocytes respond to chemotactic stimuli and foreign substances as do granulocytes. As they leave their marginal locations along small vessel walls and enter tissues, monocytes may be converted into large macrophages with increased phagocytic and digestive capacities. The life span of these macrophages may be pro-

longed in healthy tissue for many months. When monocytes and macrophages are mobilized to inflamed tissues they function in several ways. They produce glycoproteins (colony-stimulating factors) that stimulate granulopoiesis, monocytopoiesis, and lymphopoiesis.[3] They "process" antigen and induce lymphocytes into "blastic transformation." They interact with lymphocytes to produce "monocyte migration inhibition factor," which aids in the localization of more monocytes in antigen-containing areas. Further, monocytes and macrophages interact with antigen-antibody-complement complexes and elaborate chemotactic and opsonizing factors that promote phagocytosis. In the presence of *Mycobacterium tuberculosis* and similar stimuli, monocytes behave in a characteristic fashion by forming into epithelioid cells and multinucleated giant cells. They also ingest microorganisms and related particles.

Fixed-tissue macrophages, reticulum cells, and histiocytes have been thought to arise from the vascular endothelium, hence the term "reticuloendothelial system." It appears, however, that the stem cell for fixed-tissue macrophages as well as for motile monocytes is in the bone marrow. The main function of the mature reticuloendothelial cells (fixed-tissue macrophages), especially those located in the lungs, liver, spleen, and bone marrow, appears to be the trapping and cleaning of particulate matter from the blood stream by phagocytosis.

THE LYMPHOCYTIC–PLASMA CELL SERIES

Although lymphocytes are usually classified as small, medium, or large, it is more accurate to regard them as having a continuous spectrum of sizes that change in relation to their biologic function and degree of maturation. Small lymphocytes (4 to 10 μm) are the most numerous of these motile cells. The nucleus is large and stains a deep purple-blue, whereas the cytoplasm is scant and stains pale blue (Wright stain). Rarely, a few azurophilic granules may be present in the cytoplasm. Large lymphocytes (10 to 20 μm) contain larger nuclei, nucleoli, more abundant cytoplasm, and more ribosomes (Table 6.15–2).

The morphologic designation of "small lymphocyte" is rather ambiguous. Small lymphocytes may be quiescent for long periods, but they are not fully matured or end-stage cells. When stimulated by mitogens such as phytohemagglutinins they may "transform" into blast-like cells, initiate DNA, RNA, and protein synthesis, produce a variety of lymphokines, and divide or further differentiate. Lymphocytes also contain triglycerides, phospholipids, and lecithin. Further, they contain small amounts of glycogen and carry on both aerobic and anaerobic carbohydrate metabolism.

Lymphocytes have also been divided into long-lived and short-lived subpopulations based on the results of kinetic studies employing chemically labeled cells or cells containing x-ray–induced chromosomal abnormalities. The longer-lived cells are more

TABLE 6.15–2. THE LYMPHOCYTIC-PLASMA CELL SERIES

Cell	Morphologic Features	Physiologic Function	Location
Lymphoblast	Large nucleus, fine chromatin, usually a single nucleolus Clear cytoplasm	Proliferation	Germinal centers of lymph nodes, spleen, tonsils, gut, and other sites Not in blood
Lymphocyte	Small (4–10 μm) Rounded, deeply staining nucleus, masses of chromatin, no nucleoli Large (10–20 μm) Cytoplasm clear, deeply basophilic to light	Transformation to immunoblasts, plasma cells Cell-mediated immune responses Antibody synthesis	Lymphoid tissues Peripheral blood Bone marrow Tissues
Plasma cell	Large (10–20 μm) Eccentric oval nucleus Dense, coarse chromatin Basophilic cytoplasm, often vacuolated; perinuclear clear zone	Antibody synthesis	Lymph nodes Bone marrow Tissues Not in blood

plentiful (70 to 80 percent of the total) and have an estimated life expectancy greater then 100 to 200 days. These subpopulations cannot be distinguished accurately on morphologic grounds.

Further and now significant subsets of lymphocytes have been distinguished on the basis of the molecular configuration of their surface membranes, which are directly related to their function. Those derived from bone marrow (B lymphocytes, bursa-equivalent lymphocytes) are antibody-producing cells and contain various immunoglobulins or immunoglobulin fragments on their surface. On careful examination of the DNA in such B cells, one can detect rearrangements of the immunoglobulin gene, typical of antibody-producing cells, and an identifier that confirms that a cell population is of B-cell origin. These cells are located primarily in the germinal centers and medullary cords of lymphoid organs and are concerned principally with humoral immune responses. Thymic lymphocytes (T lymphocytes) represent between 60 and 80 percent of peripheral blood lymphoid cells and serve as both effectors and regulators of the vertebrate immune system. They contain one or more of a series of T or "theta" antigens on their surfaces. These antigenic determinates, which are presumed to be receptors on the cell surface, appear at various times during T-cell maturation and are associated with specific stages of development or cell function. T cells are capable of detecting perturbation on the surfaces of cells consequent upon invasion by viruses, bacteria, and intracellular parasites, or abnormalities produced by chemical or physical damage, or neoplastic transformation. They are found mostly around the germinal centers of lymph nodes and in the deep subcortical areas. T lymphocytes are the effector cells for cell-mediated immunity reactions and the cells that control humoral immune responses by B cells.

ORIGIN[6]

Transplantation studies indicate that the marrow contains pluripotential stem cells fully capable of reconstituting both the hematopoietic and lymphoreticular tissues. Labeling techniques show that lymphopoiesis in the marrow and thymus proceeds continuously and at a rapid rate. Marrow-derived cells migrate into the thymus in waves, where much of their differentiation takes place. Thymus-derived cells then enter the circulation. The thymus seems to be the main source of the long-lived lymphocytes that recirculate continuously through the body. The germinal centers of the various lymphoid organs are the principal sites of production of the short-lived lymphocytes generated in response to antigenic stimulation.

A variety of physiologic factors are thought to regulate the basal production and circulating levels of lymphocytes and their activation. Antigenic stimulation is known to be involved to a great extent as a promoter of lymphocyte production. The administration of ACTH and cortisone is followed by a transient lymphopenia and later lymphocytosis. Thyroid hormone stimulates lymphopoiesis. Growth hormone enhances the development of lymphoid tissues. In contrast, testosterone in large doses seems to prevent full lymphoid development.

FUNCTION

Lymphocytes are concerned primarily with responding to antigenic substances. During the early stages of a primary response, macrophages "process" antigen and interact with lymphocytes in a stimulatory fashion. The resulting immune responses are of two major types, cellular and humoral (antibody), and lymphocytes participate in both (see Chapter 7.1).

THE PLASMA CELL

Plasma cells develop from lymphoid precursors in germinal centers following antigenic stimulation. In addition, there is evidence that indicates that plasma cells are derived from lymphoid precursors in

the bone marrow and are thought to be the end-stage mature B lymphocyte. The earliest recognized plasma cell form is a large cell (20 to 30 μm) that may be difficult to distinguish from a blast cell. Mature plasma cells range in size from 4 to 20 μm. Their cytoplasm is basophilic and usually appears mottled. The nucleus contains dense clumps of chromatin (similar to a lymphocyte nucleus) that may be arranged to resemble the spokes of a wheel.

Normally plasma cells are seen in lymph nodes, bone marrow, and other tissues. They are not seen in the peripheral blood except in disease. The maturation time of the plasma cell is probably less than 12 hours, and their life span ranges from 2 to 4 days after the last mitosis. Rarely, plasma cells have been reported to be phagocytic; their chief function, however, appears to be antibody synthesis.

The plasmablast is seen in the peripheral blood and bone marrow only in multiple myeloma (see Chapter 6.20). It differs from the more mature plasma cell in having a large, eccentric nucleus with fine chromatin and one or more nucleoli. The cytoplasm is basophilic.

WHITE CELL DERANGEMENTS IN DISEASE

A frequently encountered clinical problem concerns the evaluation of abnormalities of the leukocytes in the peripheral blood. Such derangements may be reflected in the total white cell count, the proportion of the various (expected) cell types present, the appearance of grossly abnormal (unexpected) morphologic forms, or the presence of leukocytes unable to carry out their designated function because of congenital or acquired defects. The following text and tables consider the more commonly encountered derangements and their causes.

At times it is possible to detect enzyme defects in genetic disorders by examining the metabolic pathways, enzymatic reactions, or chemical constituents of circulating granulocytes.[5,6] Among these are glycogen-storage disease, galactosemia, maple-syrup-urine disease, orotic aciduria, acatalasia, and hypophosphatasia. There need not be obvious associated abnormalities of white cell number or morphology.

There are several distinctive morphologic abnormalities that can be encountered in circulating granulocytes and that provide important clues to the diagnosis of inherited or acquired systemic disorders (Table 6.15–3). Several distinctive heritable functional abnormalities of granulocytes have been discovered in children and adults who were troubled by serious repeated infections with a variety of microorganisms. These include defects in granulocyte mobility and chemotaxis ("lazy leukocyte" syndrome). Chronic granulomatous disease (chronic and recurrent infections) was described initially as a sex-linked disorder affecting male offspring of asymptomatic female carriers. The granulocytes of these patients are capable of phagocytosis but cannot digest certain microorganisms. Similar cases have been reported in females and appear to be inherited as an autosomal recessive defect. Affected individuals usually have repeated severe infections of the skin, mucous membranes, and airways with eventual systemic dissemination. Sporadic cases of similar granulocyte disorders have been reported as "variants" of chronic granulomatous disease. One autosomal recessive defect has been shown to result in myeloperoxidase deficiency and consequently clinical infections due to impaired granulocyte digestion of microorganisms.

It is a common event to be called upon to evaluate reports from routine peripheral blood examinations that indicate an abnormally high or low circulating white blood cell (granulocyte) count. It is critical to determine whether the circulating elements are the normal, mature cell types expected in the peripheral blood. Primary proliferative disorders of the hematopoietic system are usually identified by the preponderance of an abnormal cell type and evidences of organ enlargement and tissue infiltration.

Diurnal variations are observed regularly in the granulocyte

TABLE 6.15–3. CLINICALLY SIGNIFICANT MORPHOLOGIC ABNORMALITIES OF GRANULOCYTES

Abnormality	Significance
Döhle bodies Cyst-like cytoplasmic inclusions	*Acquired:* Infections, trauma, cancer, pregnancy, after cytotoxic drugs *Inherited:* May–Hegglin anomaly, with leukopenia, thrombocytopenia, giant platelets
Macropolycyte Large size (15–25 μm) with nuclear hypersegmentation	*Acquired:* Chronic infection, granulocytic leukemia after antimetabolites, folate, or B$_{12}$ deficiency *Inherited:* Autosomal dominant
Failure of nuclear lobe development (1–2 lobes only)	*Acquired:* Infections, leukemia, metastatic cancer, after drugs such as colchicine *Inherited:* Pelger–Huët anomaly autosomal dominant
Toxic granulations, vacuolization	*Acquired:* Infections (bacteremia)
Auer rods (malformed granules containing lysosomal enzymes)	*Acquired:* Acute granulocytic leukemia
Giant granules	*Inherited:* Disorders of polysaccharide metabolism, Alder–Reilly anomaly, with gargoylism
Large amorphous granulations, and inclusions	*Inherited:* Chédiak–Higashi syndrome (infections, albinism, neurologic defects, lymphoma) autosomal recessive

count, but the range is seldom greater than 2000 to 8000/μl. A neutrophil count as high as 15,000 to 20,000 may occasionally be encountered after strenuous exercise, maternal labor, or convulsions, and is often seen following acute hemorrhage or in the immediate postoperative period. A similar neutrophilia is noted following a transient granulocytopenia.

Growth factors, including human recombinant granulocyte-monocyte colony-stimulating factor, granulocyte colony-stimulating factor and interleukin 3 have been made available, and are at present undergoing initial clinical trials. Preliminary results indicate that these cloned growth regulatory factors may soon play a significant therapeutic role in a variety of disorders involving neutrophils and their production.

NEUTROPHILIA

Table 6.15–4 lists several common causes of significant neutrophilia. It can be seen that a frequent common denominator in

TABLE 6.15–4. CAUSES OF NEUTROPHILIA

Infections	Due to bacteria (especially pyogenic), mycobacteria, fungi, spirochetes, parasites May be localized or generalized
Metabolic disorders	Due to diverse causes resulting in uremia, diabetes, acidosis, gout, eclampsia
Neoplasms	Usually widely disseminated myeloproliferative disorders, lymphoma, metastatic carcinoma
Conditions causing cell necrosis or destruction	Infarction due to vascular disease (including polyarteritis) Intoxication due to drugs especially nephrotoxins and hepatotoxins Acute hemolysis, especially intravascular

these conditions is tissue inflammation, necrosis, or destruction. This neutrophilic leukocytosis is usually accompanied by an increase in the younger band or juvenile forms, and its magnitude is roughly proportional to the extent of the inflammatory or destructive process present. An orderly progression of younger and more mature morphologic forms is to be expected.

LEUKEMOID REACTIONS

Although its occurrence usually raises the fear of leukemia, a peripheral leukocyte count exceeding 50,000/μl may result from a variety of infections. For example, bacterial infections, such as pneumonia and meningococcal meningitis, may produce white cell aberrations mistaken for granulocytic leukemia. Similarly, pertussis and infectious mononucleosis may induce an abnormal lymphocytosis sometimes confused with lymphocytic leukemia. Disseminated tuberculosis can cause leukocyte changes that suggest the existence of all forms of lymphocytic, granulocytic, or monocytic leukemia. The fever, lymphadenopathy, and splenomegaly that attend some of these infections may further heighten the suspicion of leukemia.

Leukemoid reactions have been reported in association with various neoplastic diseases, particularly those involving the bone marrow. Other reports have related these white cell changes to drug reactions, hemorrhage, hemolysis, eclampsia, and severe burns. At times, a number of nucleated red cells and immature white cells appear in the peripheral blood in leukemoid reactions. Their clinical significance is discussed further in the section on leukoerythroblastosis.

When granulocyte constituents are released into tissues in large amounts because of cell breakdown, untoward consequences can result. Proteolytic enzymes can damage vascular membranes, glomeruli, collagen-elastic tissue, and so forth. Thromboplastin can lead to fibrin formation and eventual collagen deposition and scarring as in polyarteritis, glomerulitis, or arthritis. Problems can also be caused by other materials released from neutrophils such as the slow-reacting substance that causes smooth muscle contraction and increased vascular permeability (anaphylaxis), small cationic proteins that are vasoactive, and pyrogens which induce febrile reactions. Leukocytes that bind IgE, especially basophils, will release histamine on contact with antigen and initiate allergic reactions.

EOSINOPHILIA

The more common causes of a significant eosinophilia are listed in Table 6.15–5. Allergic disorders and hypersensitivity states associated with parasitic infestation or drug administration are the most frequently encountered etiologic entities. On occasion, eosinophilia has been reported as a familial anomaly, but in many such instances parasitic disease is responsible. Significant eosinophilia of unexplained pathogenesis is frequently seen in recipients of allogenic bone marrow transplants during the first 6 months to a year after engraftment.

BASOPHILIA

Basophilia is encountered infrequently. When noted, it is most frequently associated with one of the myeloproliferative disorders, especially chronic granulocytic leukemia. It has also been associated with Hodgkin disease, chronic hemolytic anemia, varicella infection, nephrosis, myxedema, contact dermatitis, allergic rhinitis, foreign-protein reaction, and graft rejections.

NEUTROPENIA

Neutropenia results from diverse causes. Although present knowledge of granulocyte kinetics in disease states is limited, it appears that a number of conditions produce neutropenia by virtue of im-

TABLE 6.15–5. CAUSES OF EOSINOPHILIA

Allergic states	Hay fever Asthma Exfoliative dermatitis Erythema multiforme Drug reactions
Parasitic diseases	Intestinal forms (hookworm, round worm) Tissue forms (toxicara, trichina, strongyloides, echinococcus)
Skin disorders	Pemphigus Dermatitis herpetiformis
Neoplasms	Myeloproliferative disorders Hodgkin disease Metastatic carcinomas T-cell leukemia or lymphoma
Other disorders	Scarlet fever Polyarteritis Eosinophilic granuloma Tropical eosinophilia Pernicious anemia Allogeneic bone marrow transplantation Hemodialysis or peritoneal dialysis Löffler syndrome

TABLE 6.15–6. CAUSES OF NEUTROPENIA

Infections	Acute viral (rubeola, hepatitis), rickettsial, bacterial (typhoid, brucella), or protozoan (malaria) All grave infections (bacteremia, miliary tuberculosis)
Marrow aplasia	Due to chemical or physical agents that regularly produce aplasia (e.g., antimetabolites, alkylating agents, benzol, ionizing radiation) or rarely produce aplasia (e.g., chloramphenicol, sulfonamides, thiouracil, amidopyrine) Due to unknown cause or related to myelophthisis (e.g., leukemia, neoplasia)
Nutritional deficits	Folic acid Vitamin B_{12}
Splenomegaly	Due to diverse causes (e.g., congestive, infiltrative)
Other disorders	Systemic lupus erythematosus Anaphylaxis, antileukocyte antibodies, immunodeficiencies, pancreatic exocrine deficiency, cyclic neutropenia (familial and sporadic)

paired granulocyte formation. For example, neutropenia may result from bone marrow damage due to chemical or physical agents and from maturation arrest related to dietary deficiencies, infectious diseases, and rarely autoimmune suppression or destruction of granulocyte precursors in the bone marrow. Neutropenia thought to be the result of an increased rate of destruction of granulocytes has tentatively been related to several disorders all resulting in splenomegaly. The precise role of leukoagglutinins in the etiology of neutropenia is not fully understood. In one instance, that of the neutropenia induced by amidopyrine, the presence of leukoagglutinins has been demonstrated, and they seem to be responsible for the agglutination of leukocytes and their rapid removal from the circulation. Another mechanism responsible for neutropenia is exemplified by the sequestration of granulocytes in the tissues, especially the gut, liver, spleen, and lungs, following anaphylactic shock. Some patients, especially those who have had a large number of blood product transfusions, will display severe neutropenia, and the presence of antineutrophil antibodies.

The more common causes of neutropenia are listed in Table 6.15–6. A more comprehensive discussion of agranulocytosis and related abnormalities may be found in Chapter 6.11.

THE MONONUCLEAR PHAGOCYTE

The mononuclear phagocytic cell system includes monocytes; fixed and mobile macrophages, as well as cells formed by the fusion of these cells; epithelioid cells; giant cells; and possibly osteoclasts. Monocyte-macrophage cell production takes place principally in the bone marrow where these cells share an immediate progenitor with granulocytic cells. The cells mature to the monocyte stage in the bone marrow and are then released into the peripheral blood. From the blood they migrate throughout the body tissues and come to populate tissues of several specific organs including lungs (alveolar macrophages), liver (Kupffer cells), peritoneum, and spleen. These monocyte-macrophages mature further in the peripheral organ, but retain their ability to divide. On occasion they will fuse to form multinucleated macrophages and are thought to be the origin of the epithelioid or giant cells found in some forms of inflammation. These cells are attracted to areas of inflammation by surface chemoreceptors, and when exposed to the product of cellular inflammation produce a variety of substances including mi-

gration-inhibition factor, which attracts and traps other monocytic cells in the area. These cells respond to various stimuli in a cooperative manner. The clinical and morphologic characteristics of this response vary according to the nature of the stimulus and the overall status of the host. The primary function of the monocytic cells is one of phagocytosis with the production of humoral regulatory factors an important secondary one. As part of the process, they have been shown to have an important function in the "processing" of antigens for lymphocytes, a primary step in the immune response.

MONOCYTOSIS

The most frequent causes of monocytosis are listed in Table 6.15–7. Since monocytes can frequently be confused with other cells (atypical lymphocytic myelocytes) it is important to verify all reports of monocytosis by carefully examining the peripheral smear of any patient reported to have this disorder. Monocytosis may be

TABLE 6.15–7. CAUSES OF MONOCYTOSIS

Infections	Bacterial: brucellosis, tuberculosis, subacute infective endocarditis, rarely typhoid fever Rickettsial: Rocky Mountain spotted fever, typhus Protozoan: malaria
Neoplasms	Monocytic leukemia Hodgkin disease and other lymphomas Myeloproliferative disorders Multiple myeloma Carcinomatosis
Connective tissue diseases	Rheumatoid arthritis Systemic lupus erythematosus
Other disorders	Chronic ulcerative colitis Regional enteritis Sarcoidosis Lipid-storage diseases Hemolytic anemia Hypochromic anemia Recovery from agranulocytosis

observed in relation to the increased myeloid activity induced by such common bacterial infections as pneumococcal pneumonia. It is seen frequently during the period of convalescence from such sepsis and also occurs during the recovery phase of marked neutropenia.

The special relationship of the monocyte to tuberculosis and tubercle formation has been cited. In disseminated tuberculosis, less mature monocytes (promonocytes) may be encountered in the peripheral blood. On occasion, failure to pursue a complete diagnostic evaluation has led to a mistaken diagnosis of leukemia.

The proliferative activity associated with responses of the monocyte-macrophage system may produce distressing results. Cell breakdown products may cause fever, tissue damage (proteolytic enzymes), gout (uric acid), and so forth. Organ enlargement and tissue destruction may result from "benign" disorders. For example, the continual proliferation of macrophages in Gaucher disease leads to destruction of liver, spleen, marrow, and bone and was once thought to be a malignant, neoplastic process. Impairments of hematopoietic function and immunoresponsiveness can also be encountered during violent reactions of the mononuclear phagocytic system, as can autoimmune hemolytic anemia and heightened reactivity to insect venoms and poison ivy.

MONOCYTOPENIA

A seldom noted and frequently insignificant finding is monocytopenia. It is frequently seen, however, as an accompaniment to bone marrow failure states and leukemic reticuloendotheliosis and following steroid therapy.

THE LYMPHOID SYSTEM

This system closely related to and sharing a common pluripotent stem cell pool with the hematopoietic system also functions primarily as a major host defense system. The major functions are to respond to antigenic stimuli by either immunoglobulin production (B cells) or reactive cell (T cells) infiltration. These reactives are closely integrated with the function of the monocytic-macrophage system, which "captures" and "processes" the antigen to which these cells respond. Disorders of lymphocytes are frequently manifested as a disordered immune system.

LYMPHOCYTOSIS

Acute viral infections and chronic granulomatous disorders are among the most frequent causes of lymphocytosis, being responsible for more than 35 percent of the cases (Table 6.15–8). A relative

lymphocytosis is present in most cases of neutropenia. The lymphocytosis associated with hyperthyroidism is also usually a relative one.

PLASMACYTOSIS

Plasma cells are not normally seen in the peripheral blood. Rarely, minimal peripheral plasmacytosis has been noted in association with the disorders listed in Table 6.15–9. Plasmacytosis above 10 percent has been reported in serum sickness, drug reactions, measles, scarlet fever, and the other disorders listed, but usually only an occasional plasma cell is seen. A more profound plasmacytosis or the presence of abnormal plasmablasts in the peripheral blood may be equated with the diagnosis of multiple myeloma (plasma cell leukemia).

Malignant plasma cell dyscrasias are characterized by the proliferation of a single clone of plasma cells, all producing a similar immune globulin. This can usually be detected by the presence of a monoclonal single peak on serum electrophoresis. In many B-cell disorders, however, no such peak (or spike) of protein can be detected. It has been shown, however, that B cells of a single clone all demonstrate the same B-cell immunoglobulin gene rearrangement, and malignant B-cell disorders can be identified by looking for this single common gene rearrangement on the B cells. Benign disorders of B cells tend to have a heterogeneous pattern of B-cell gene rearrangement.

Modest plasmacytosis is encountered more commonly in the bone marrow than in the peripheral blood. Mature plasma cells composing 5 to 15 percent (or more) of the observed nucleated cells may be related to the many disorders noted in Table 6.15–9. It is important in each instance to seek an explanation for bone marrow plasmacytosis. Several of the causative diseases are quite responsive to specific therapy. Others clearly carry grave prognoses.

LYMPHOPENIA

Severe depletion or near absence of lymphocytes and plasma cells has been reported in adults in connection with hypogammaglobulinemia and thymoma. In children a variable atrophy or virtual absence of these cells has been noted in several instances of congenital immunodeficiency syndromes (see Chapter 7.2). Selective depletion of a specific subset of lymphocytes (helper cells) is seen in AIDS. In that condition the antigenic marker on the helper T cell (T4 or CD4) appears to be a receptor to which the HIV virus binds

TABLE 6.15–8. CAUSES OF LYMPHOCYTOSIS

Acute infections	Infectious mononucleosis
	Infectious lymphocytosis
	Pertussis
	Mumps
	Rubella
	Infectious hepatitis
	Convalescent stage of many acute infections
Chronic infections	Tuberculosis, syphilis, brucellosis
Metabolic disorders	Thyrotoxicosis
	Adrenal cortical insufficiency
Neoplasms	Chronic lymphatic leukemia
	Lymphomas

TABLE 6.15–9. CAUSES OF BONE MARROW PLASMACYTOSIS

Acute infections	Rubella
	Rubeola
	Varicella
	Infectious hepatitis
	Infectious mononucleosis
	Scarlet fever
Chronic infections	Tuberculosis
	Syphilis
	Fungus
Allergic states	Serum sickness
	Drug reactions
Collagen-vascular disorders	Acute rheumatic fever
	Rheumatoid arthritis
	Systemic lupus erythematosus
Neoplasms	Disseminated carcinoma
	Hodgkin disease
	Multiple myeloma
Other	Cirrhosis of the liver

and is then internalized, thus allowing it to enter and selectively destroy all helper T-cells.

REFERENCES

1. Cline MJ, Lehrer RI, et al: Monocytes and macrophages: Functions and diseases. Ann Intern Med 88:78, 1978
2. Hayhoe FGJ, Flemans RJ: An Atlas of Hematological Cytology. New York, John Wiley, 1970
3. Metcalf D: The molecular biology and function of the granulocyte macrophage-colony-stimulating-factors. Blood 67:257, 1986
4. Quesenberry P, Levitt L: Hematopoetic stem cells. N Engl J Med 301:755, 1979
5. Tauber AI: Current news of neutrophil dysfunction. Am J Med 70:1237, 1981
6. Williams WJ, Beutler E, et al (eds): Hematology, 3d ed. New York, McGraw-Hill, 1983
7. Wintrobe MM (ed): Blood: Pure and Eloquent. New York, McGraw-Hill, 1980

CHAPTER 6.16
Neoplastic Diseases of Hematopoiesis

Philip J. Burke

Advances in the laboratory technology have forced a change in thinking about the origin and evolution of the myeloid malignancies. Evidence of clonal expansion involving most of the idiopathic abnormalities of the bone marrow suggests that all of these are stem cell neoplasms with varied growth advantages, rates of progression, and retained response to normal control mechanisms. For the sake of simplicity, the urge is to consider these apparently morphologically heterogeneous diseases in the spectrum of pluripotent stem cell failure that sometimes enters a malignant phase.

METHODOLOGIES

DNA hybridization technology has made possible critical observations that provide evidence for a multistep pathogenesis of hematopoietic neoplasms. Monoclonal antibodies and molecular probes now define phenotypic and genotypic lineages of malignant clonal hematopoietic cells and measure their expression of aberrant protein products.[4] With these methodologies, proto-oncogenes, cellular homologs of transforming sequences of retroviruses, have been incriminated in human leukemogenesis, and more than 20 proto-oncogenes have been mapped to chromosome breakpoint regions at specific chromosomal rearrangements in hematopoietic diseases. These oncogenes code for proteins with diverse functions including DNA binding, protein kinase, and cellular growth factor activities, factors involved in proliferation and differentiation of normal cells.[7]

New banding techniques define multiple complex chromosome changes that characterize most tumors, exhibit a high degree of nonrandomness, and impart a selective advantage to the cells in which they occur.[8] Incorporation of mutations in gene structure, or translocation of cellular oncogenes from one chromosome to another, are likely associated with malignant change and production of altered products. These chromosomal translocations may accomplish transformation by causing alterations in oncogene dosage or by activating normally quiescent oncogenes by bringing them into the transcriptional control of active genes. The latter event has been clinically demonstrated in B-cell neoplasms in which specific translocations transfer c-myc on chromosome 8 from its constitutive site to one next to immunoglobulin genes. In chronic myelocytic leukemia (CML), the oncogene c-abl is translocated from the distant long arm of chromosome 9 to the long arm of chromosome 22, resulting in the characteristic Philadelphia chromosome. As a consequence of this rearrangement, transcription of the fused c-abl and bcr gene on chromosome 22 results in a larger messenger RNA, and, therefore, expression of a larger and abnormal tyrosine kinase, one of the products of the four classes of oncogenes thus far determined (Table 6.16–1).

In addition, consistent abnormalities of chromosomes 5 and 7 are characteristic of leukemia secondary to previous cytotoxic antitumor therapy. Deletions on these chromosomes are in genes which influence growth factors or their receptors and which may lead to malignant transformation by loss of important humoral control mechanisms, such as the expression of a recessive gene on the analogous chromosome (Table 6.16–2).

A powerful new strategy for analysis of the clonal origin of

TABLE 6.16–1. ONCOGENES

Family	Properties	Genes	Location
Tyrosine kinases	EGF receptor	erbB1	7p 11–14
	CSA receptor	fms	5q 33
		abl	9q 34
		src	20q 12–13
		erbB2	17q 21
Serine-threonine kinases		mos	8q 22
		raf	7p 13
GTP-binding proteins		N-ras	1p 11–13
		HA-ras	11p 14–15
		Ki-ras-2	12p 12
Growth factor	PDGF	sis	22q 11-ter
Nuclear proteins		myc	8q 24
		fos	14q 21–31

PDGF = Platelet-derived growth factor; EGF = epidermal growth factor; CSA = colony stimulating activity.

TABLE 6.16–2. CHROMOSOMAL BREAKPOINTS LOCATED NEAR ONCOGENES OR REGULATORY GENES

Leukemia	Abnormality	Gene
AML-M2	t (8;21)	mos, Hu-ets2
AML-M4 EO	INV (16), t (16;16)	MT
AML-M5 a	t (9;11)	INF-α, INF-β, Hu-ets1
AML with increased basophils	t (6;9)	abl
AML with increased platelets	INV (3), t (3;3)	TF, TFR
MDS, t-AML	del (5)	CM-CSA, FMS
CML, ALL	t (9;22)	abl, bcr

ALL = acute lymphocytic leukemia; MDS = myelodysplastic syndrome; AML = acute myelocytic leukemia.

human cell populations also has been developed.[3] This technique involves the use of recombinant DNA probes to simultaneously detect restriction fragment length polymorphisms and methylation patterns on X-chromosome genes. With this technique, the coexistence of mature, clonal granulocytes with leukemic myeloblasts has been shown, proving that significant differentiation continues in these neoplasms, but that the relative proportion of divisions leading to duplication of stem cells rather than daughter cells is shifted. Clonal analysis of blood cells from patients in complete clinical remission of acute myelocytic leukemia (AML) confirm continued proliferation and differentiation of the neoplastic clone in a subset of patients. This terminal differentiation in some patients with acute leukemia and evidence of the clonal origin of the lineages of defined marrow elements supports the concept that the myeloproliferative diseases as a group are neoplasms arising from genetic or epigenetic changes effecting one cell and its progeny.

TABLE 6.16–3. DIAGNOSTIC CLASSIFICATION OF MYELOID NEOPLASMS

FAB (Classic)	Immunophenotype	Cytogenetics	Morphology
Myeloproliferative Disorders			
PRV (Polycythemia rubra vera)		+8	Hypercellular panmyelopathy
CML (Chronic myelocytic leukemia)	MY7, M78	t(9;22)	All marrow elements increased
MF (Myelofibrosis)			Leukoerythroblastosis, myelofibrosis, extramedullary hematopoiesis
ET (Essential thrombocythemia)			Platelet count $>100 \times 10^6/\mu l$, moderate increase all elements
Myelodysplastic Syndrome			
RA (Refractory anemia)		Normal	Anemia without blasts, cellular bone marrow, moderate dyserythropoiesis
RARS (Refractory anemia with ringed sideroblasts)		Normal	Anemia with <5% blasts; >15% nucleated cells are ringed sideroblasts
CMML (Chronic myelomonocytic leukemia)		Normal	RAEB plus monocytosis, immature granulopoiesis monocytosis $>1 \times 10^6/\mu l$
RAEB (Refractory anemia with excess blasts)		(−5/5q−), (−7/7q−), (20q−), (8+), (Y−)	Cytopenia of 2 or more elements, dyshematopoiesis, 5%–20% blasts
RAEB-t (Refractory anemia with excess blasts in transformation)		"	RAEB plus <20, <30% blasts in bone marrow, <5% blasts peripheral blood, Auer rods
Acute Myelocytic Leukemia			
M1 (Myelocytic, stem cell, undifferentiated)	Ia, MY7, MY9, MY10	Normal, INV(3), +8, t(9;22), 5q/−5, 7q/−7	90% undifferentiated blasts, <10% with granules, Auer rods
M2 (Myelocytic with maturation)	Ia, M7, MY9	Normal, t(8;21), +8, t(3;5), t(9;22), t(6;9)	Maturation to progranulocytes and beyond >10% with primary granules and Auer rods
M3a (Hypergranular, progranulocytic)	Ia,M7,MY9,VIM-2	t(15;17)	Hypergranular, primary granules, Auer rods, bizarre blasts, DIC
M3b (Microgranular, progranulocytic)			Progranulocytes with minimal granulation, bilobed nucleus, hyperleukocytosis, DIC
M4 (Myelomonocytic)	Ia,MY7,MY8,MY9, MO5, VIM-2	t(9;11), +8, t(6;9)	>20% monoblasts, >20% myeloblasts, monocytosis
M4 (Myelomonocytic, eosinophilia)		INV(16)	As above, with increased eosinophils
M5a (Monocytic)	VIM-2,MY9	t(9;11), t(11q23–25), +8, INV(16)	>80% monoblasts
M5b (Monocytic)			Monoblasts with >20% maturation
M6 (Erythrocytic)	Ia	Multiple	>50% nucleated erythroid cells, >10% bizarre erythroblasts, dyserythropoiesis, >30% myeloblasts, progranulocytes, may proceed to M2
M7 (megakaryocytic acute myelosclerosis)	Ia, Factor VIII, Ib, IIb/IIIa (EM-platelet peroxidase on nuclear membrane)	t(1;3), t27	Bizarre megakaryocytes with immature lobulation, increased platelets, myelofibrosis with heterogeneic peripheral blasts (confused with L1,L2,M1)
CML-BC (Chronic myelocytic in blast crisis)	Ia,MY7,MY9,VIM-2	t(9;22), −8, ISO 17 duplicated Ph[1]	M1,M2
AML (Secondary)	Ia,M7,M9,M10	5q−/7q−, 7q/−7 multiple	M1,M2,M7, can be bizarre with myelofibrosis
AML-ALL (Biphenotypic, hybrid)	Lymphoid and/or myeloid		Characteristics of varied myeloid and lymphoid lineage, may be hybrid or biphenotypic

PATHOGENESIS

Clonal hemopathies are phenotypically characterized by their origin in pluripotential stem cells, which are heterogeneous regarding their proliferative capacity, their response to regulation, and their physical properties. The varied clinical manifestations are consistent with the concept of clonal dominance and suppression. Suppression contributes to the lack of expansion of coexisting normal committed progenitor cells and their inability in a quiescent state to contribute to descendants. This lessened expression is in part the result of inhibition of the committed progenitor cell by tumor-elaborated substances, which do not affect the renewal potential of the pluripotent stem cell. Simultaneously, malignant clonal expansion and inherent instability lead to lack of differentiation and progression of uncontrolled growth and continued self-renewal of the selected, growth-favored clone. In addition, growth factors from the microenvironment of the bone marrow, which regulate stem cell growth and development, may also be aberrant in clonal neoplasia.

This concept contends that most hematopoietic neoplasms originate in a pluripotential stem cell and thereby confer abnormal morphology, cytogenetics, oncogene expression, and growth kinetics on all hematopoietic cells. In these myeloproliferative conditions, clonal expansion and progression end with death from the effects of either failure of all hematopoietic elements or transition to leukemia.

There is evidence for a multistep pathogenesis of hematopoietic myeloid malignancies. Some of the acute leukemias, the ultimate stage of the clonal hemopathies, are initially triggered by exposure to ionizing radiation, certain chemicals, and some chemotherapeutic drugs, especially alkylating agents, and certain genetic disorders. This process requires a sequence of steps. The chemical or environmental agent first interacts with functioning chromosomes, perhaps at a heritable fragile site. Subsequently, leukemogenesis may follow malfunction at the gene level following transposition of genetic material to promoter areas, etc. Amplification or modification of the gene product may then perpetuate leukemogenesis. These events may be subclinical and of long duration as in the prodromal stage of the myelodysplastic syndromes.[5]

TWO-STEP TREATMENT OF HEMOPATHIES

The duration of bone marrow failure and leukemic transformation is difficult to assess at initial clinical presentation. The onset is measured in years in some patients and in days in others. During this prodromal period, clonal cytopenias precede the eventual evolution to overt leukemia. The apparently normal cells are neoplastic, derived from a clone with proliferative advantage, but retain some integrity of normal differentiation programming. Ultimately, the phenotypically immature cells will predominate.[6]

Evidence of circulating tumor may be scanty. The bone marrow is generally hypercellular, with dyshematopoiesis in any residual normal-appearing cells, with or without the presence of myeloblasts. Normal numbers of stem cells reside in the marrow, their proliferation and maturation suppressed by the clonal neoplasm. These pluripotent cells, relatively resistant to the effects of cycle-active agents, will repopulate the marrow following the gross elimination of the neoplastic cells by cytotoxic drugs.

During this period, the effects of bone marrow failure and other altered host factors including an impaired immune system must be dealt with in a timely fashion. After effective chemotherapy reduces the cellular mass of the malignant clone, normal stem cells will randomly enter the cell cycle and repopulate the aplastic stroma. The desired antitumor effects of this aggressive approach must be balanced against the anticipated adverse effect of the drugs on normal bone marrow and other host tissues. The goal of therapy is the reduction of the clonal tumor mass, the recovery of a normal functioning bone marrow, and subsequent elimination of minimal residual tumor with intensive therapy.

CLASSIFICATION OF THE HEMATOPOIETIC MALIGNANCIES

The traditional classification of hematopoietic neoplasms by morphology has led to some phenotypically heterogeneous confusion. With better definition made possible by new technologies, these clonal neoplasms can be unified functionally as pluripotent stem cell disorders which display a wide spectrum of clinical and laboratory manifestations, but share a similar outcome.

The hematopoietic neoplasms are classified in the French-American-British (FAB) system by the morphology of the bone marrow elements and their histocompatible characteristics, with the subclasses ordered according to their rate of malignant transformation and growth.[2] All subtypes can be considered neoplastic on the basis of evidence of clonal expansion (Table 6.16–3).

The myeloproliferative disorders considered as a group include polycythemia rubra vera, chronic myelocytic leukemia, myelofibrosis, and essential thrombocythemia. The myelodysplastic syndrome is divided into five subgroups, and the aggressive, fulminant leukemias into M1 to M7, secondary, and the blast crisis of CML.[1]

The acute lymphocytic leukemias are classed according to morphology into L1 to L3 by the FAB method, and their virulence is determined more closely by their immunophenotype.[4]

REFERENCES

1. Bennet JM, Catovsky D, et al: Proposals for the classification of the myelodysplastic syndromes. Br J Haematol 51:189, 1982
2. Bennet JM, Catovsky D, et al: Proposed revised criteria for the classification of the acute myeloid leukemias: A report of the French-American-British cooperative group. Ann Intern Med 103:626, 1985
3. Fearon ER, Burke PJ, et al: Differentiation of leukemic cells to polymorphonuclear leukocytes in patients with acute nonlymphocytic leukemia. N Engl J Med 315:15, 1986
4. Foon KA, Gale RP, et al: Recent advances in the immunologic classification of leukemia. Semin Hematol 23:257, 1986
5. Galton DG: The myelodysplastic syndromes. Scand J Haematol 36:11, 1986
6. Koeffler HP: Myelodysplastic syndromes (Preleukemia). Semin Hematol 23:284, 1986
7. Lebowitz P: Oncogenic genes and their potential role in human malignancy. J Clin Oncol 1:657, 1983
8. Sandberg AA: The chromosomes in human leukemia. Semin Oncol 23:201, 1986

The Myeloid Neoplasms

Philip J. Burke

MYELOPROLIFERATIVE DISORDERS

POLYCYTHEMIA RUBRA VERA

Etiology and Pathogenesis

Polycythemia rubra vera (PRV) is a chronic proliferative disorder involving all bone marrow elements and is characterized by a plethoric, cyanotic appearance, splenomegaly, and an increased red cell mass. The etiology remains obscure. This disorder occurs principally during the middle years of life and is more common in men than in women.

Individuals with PRV may experience general debility and symptoms referable to multiple-organ systems. Many of the clinical manifestations may be related to the increased blood volume (increased red cell mass), increased blood viscosity, tendency to hemorrhagic and thromboembolic events, as well as to the underlying vascular disease (atherosclerosis and arteriosclerosis) commonly present in individuals of this age group.

Clinical Manifestations

The initial manifestations are variable. At times the diagnosis is made in asymptomatic individuals. Rarely, a massive gastrointestinal hemorrhage or thrombosis of a coronary or cerebral artery may be the first recognized sign of illness. More commonly, a variety of complaints, such as irritability, easy fatigability, headache, visual disturbances, tinnitus, abdominal fullness, and aching of the lower extremities, is noted. A peculiar pruritus is experienced by approximately half the patients, and it is often particularly severe after bathing. Other common presenting symptoms include dyspnea, angina, intermittent claudication, and dependent edema. Less commonly, gout is the initial clinical problem.

The physical findings include a ruddy cyanosis, especially about the face and ears. The florid complexion often appears weatherworn. Ecchymoses are common. The mucous membranes are quite reddened. The retinal veins are usually engorged. Hypertension is found in about half the cases. Peptic ulcer is encountered in 10 to 20 percent of instances and gouty arthropathy in 5 percent or fewer.

Splenomegaly is a cardinal feature of PRV, being present in 75 to 80 percent of cases on presentation. Early in the course of the disease the spleen may not have enlarged to palpable proportions. Later, a progressive increase in spleen size may herald increasing myeloid metaplasia with myelofibrosis or the onset of acute leukemia. Abdominal discomfort results from massive splenic enlargement, and this is periodically intensified by the occurrence of splenic infarcts. Modest hepatomegaly is observed in 30 to 50 percent of patients.

Before treatment, hematocrit values range between 55 and 80 percent. The white cell and platelet counts are elevated, the former usually ranging from $10 \times 10^9/L$ to $50 \times 10^9/L$ and the latter from $300 \times 10^9/L$ to $600 \times 10^9/L$. The red cells and white cells appear normal. There is a shift to the left in the granulocytic forms. Nucleated red cells and immature myelocytes are encountered occasionally. The granulocyte alkaline phosphatase concentration is high.

The bone marrow is usually quite cellular, and the elements present in normal relative proportions. The varying degrees of hyperplasia noted affect the granulocytic and megakaryocytic elements, as well as the erythroblastic elements, giving the impression of a panmyelopathy (Table 6.17–1). During the course of the disease, areas of myelofibrosis and osteosclerosis may be seen in the marrow and small foci of extramedullary hematopoiesis encountered, particularly in the liver and spleen.

The blood volume usually is increased, at times being nearly twice normal, principally because of an increase in the circulating red cell mass. Blood viscosity is increased in proportion to the hematocrit. Ferrokinetic studies reveal an increased plasma-iron turnover and erythrocyte production. Red cell life span is normal, as is arterial oxygen saturation. Radiographs of the bones generally reveal no abnormalities. The blood–uric acid concentration is high in a significant proportion of patients. Erythropoietin concentrations in serum or urine are usually lower than normal or undetectable. Serum vitamin B_{12} concentrations are usually increased.

Diagnosis

Plethora, ruddy cyanosis, splenomegaly, and hepatomegaly coupled with polycythemia in the absence of detectable cardiac or pulmonary disease leads promptly to the correct diagnosis in the majority of cases. A firm diagnosis is established with an increased red cell mass, normal arterial oxygen saturation, and splenomegaly. Thrombocytosis, leukocytosis, elevated granulocyte alkaline phosphatase activity, and increased serum vitamin B_{12} concentration are important secondary criteria.

Problems arise when individuals present solely with polycythemia or when the clinical features suggest an alternative myeloproliferative syndrome or an alternative cause for the hepatic and splenic enlargement. The polycythemic states (hematocrit >55 percent) result from increased erythropoiesis. In many instances of secondary polycythemia this increased red cell formation is mediated by erythropoietin. The increased erythropoietin secretion, in turn, may result from hypoxia or may reflect an inappropriate overproduction of this polypeptide by neoplasms or other lesions. Disorders productive of hypoxia or responsible for an inappropriate overproduction of erythropoietin as well as for hormonal and chemical agents must be excluded (Table 6.17–2).

When polycythemia is associated with increased white cell and platelet counts, the underlying illness is probably a myeloproliferative disorder. This probability is heightened by the coexistence of splenomegaly. The existence of an increased blood volume and increased blood viscosity may be seen in polycythemic states irrespective of their etiology.

At times, the physician is confronted by polycythemia without other evidence of myeloproliferation or any known causal condition. Stress erythrocytosis reported infrequently in anxious or hard-driving middle-aged individuals appears to be a relative polycythemia in that the red cell mass is normal but the plasma volume is decreased. Sometimes the basic diagnosis becomes clear only when additional findings develop.

Course and Management

Patients with PRV may be expected to survive for 10 to 20 years. The major medical problems encountered stem from the occurrence of vascular thromboses (and emboli) and hemorrhage. A peptic ulcer, which is common in these individuals, may be the site of gastrointestinal bleeding. Epistaxes, ecchymoses, and bleeding following dental extraction are more common. Intercurrent infections, particularly pulmonary, are a significant but lesser problem.

The immediate cause of death in this group of patients is principally the associated cardiovascular disease. Cerebral hemorrhage or thrombosis, myocardial infarction, and heart failure are the

TABLE 6.17–1. DIAGNOSTIC CLASSIFICATION OF THE MYELOPROLIFERATIVE DISORDERS

FAB (Classic)	Immuno-pheno-type	Cytoge-netics	Morphology
PRV (polycythemia rubra vera)	—	+8	Hypercellular pan-myelopathy
CML (Chronic mye-locytic leukemia)	MY7, M78	t(9;22)	All marrow elements increased
MF (Myelofibrosis)	—	—	Leukoerythroblas-tosis, myelofibrosis, extramedullary he-matopoiesis
ET (Essential throm-bocythemia)	—	—	Platelet count >100 × 10⁹/L; moderate increase all elements

most frequent terminal events. In 15 to 25 percent of the patients, the disease pattern changes and assumes the characteristics of granulocytic leukemia or myeloid metaplasia with myelofibrosis. At times, an acute granulocytic leukemia develops toward the end of the disease.

Management is directed toward maintaining the circulating red cell mass at a near-normal level by the use of venesection or myelosuppressive drugs. Functional deficits caused by coexisting vascular disease or other processes, for example, heart failure, angina, and peptic ulcer, require attention.

Venesection promptly reduces symptoms due to the increased blood volume. The repeated removal of 500 ml of whole blood every 2 to 3 days until the hematocrit approximates 55 percent may be followed by several months of remission. Symptomatic relief (and a normal red cell mass) often may be maintained by one or two similar venesections every 3 to 4 months. Erythropoiesis will not be limited until repeated phlebotomies have induced iron deficiency. Myelosuppressive therapy is required to control aggressive erythropoiesis, granulopoiesis, and thrombopoiesis.

Radioactive phosphorus, P-32, has been employed in the treatment of PRV for many years. Its use is discouraged because of the increased incidence of acute myelocytic leukemia in those

TABLE 6.17–2. CAUSES OF SECONDARY POLYCYTHEMIA

Associated with Hypoxia
• Cardiovascular disease, usually congenital, resulting in significant venous admixture
• Pulmonary disease resulting in
  Impaired gas diffusion
  Perfusion of poorly aerated lung
  Pulmonary arteriovenous fistulas
• High altitude residence
• Hypoventilation associated with obesity (Pickwickian syndrome)
• Hemoglobin variants with increased affinity for oxygen

Associated with Inappropriate Overproduction of Erythropoietin
• Tumors, benign and malignant, of the kidney, liver, central nervous system, uterus, ovary
• Renal cysts, rarely hydronephrosis

Associated with Adrenocortical Steroids or Androgens
• Adrenal hypercorticism, all types
• Virilizing tumors
• Therapeutic use of androgens (rarely corticoids)

Associated with Chronic Chemical Exposure
• Nitrites, sulfonamides, coal tar derivatives, and others producing methemoglobin and sulfhemoglobin
• Cobalt, various alcohols

treated patients. Hydroxyurea is presently the drug of choice, with doses of 1 to 2 g each day in intermittent courses controlling the evidence of panmyelopathy.[12]

CHRONIC MYELOCYTIC LEUKEMIA

Etiology and Pathogenesis
Chronic myelocytic leukemia (CML) is a myeloproliferative disorder that evolves through a number of biologic steps and clinical phases. Cytogenetic balanced translocations produce the characteristic Ph¹ chromosome, t(9;22); C-abl is consistently (90%) translocated from the distal long arm of chromosome 9 to the foreshortened long arm of chromosome 22. A probe of the hybrid gene composed of the breakpoint cluster region (bcr) and the activated c-abl oncogene demonstrates that all patients with CML have abnormal DNA alignments. As a consequence of this rearrangement, transcription of the fused c-abl and bcr on the genes of chromosome 22 results in a larger m-RNA and a larger protein with tyrosine kinase activity.[5]

There are several other mechanisms by which chromosomal abnormalities might influence the function of growth factors or their receptors and thus lead to malignant transformation. Loss of DNA may involve certain genes that regulate cell growth. Alternately, loss of genetic material may allow expression of a recessive mutant gene on the analogous chromosome. Ig gene rearrangement observed during the late aggressive phase confirms the clonal derivation of the neoplasm and its pluripotent stem cell origin.[8]

The initial step in genesis is likely exposure to chemical mutagens or radiation, an event that may result in clonal growth without a proliferative advantage until acquisition of the Ph¹-positive aberration, gene expression of an abnormal tyrosine kinase, and expansion of the myeloid stem cell compartment. Possibly involved in the intense myelofibrosis accompanying the cellular overgrowth is the activation of the c-sis oncogene, which is reciprocally translocated (t11;9) and produces platelet-derived growth factor (PDGF), a stimulator of collagen formation.

Classification
In the stable phase, which lasts for 2 to 6 years, the morphology of bone marrow cells is not unusual, although one or more elements may predominate in the hypercellular aspirate. With mutation and clonal evolution, 60 percent of patients will enter a myeloblast stage with myeloid antigen markers, while 30 percent will develop cells with a pre-B phenotype. At this time, the Ph¹ karyotype may persist, but additional abnormalities also will be evident (t9;22, +8, +9, isochrome 17, double Ph¹-positive, deletion Y).

CML may also present as acute myelocytic leukemia (AML) or more commonly as a Ph+ acute lymphocytic leukemia (ALL), which represents 20 percent of the ALL population and conveys a poor prognosis. Childhood Ph+ ALL is associated with a smaller tyrosine kinase than seen in the adult form of the disease. With remission, the bone marrow is free of the Ph¹-positive chromosome in one third of the cases, but remission duration is usually brief.

Clinical Manifestations
The onset of CML is insidious, as patients with this disorder may remain asymptomatic for many months. Common presenting complaints are weight loss, low-grade fever, weakness, dyspnea, palpitations, pallor, splenomegaly, and evidence of a generalized bleeding tendency. These manifestations may be attributed to the continued slow proliferation of long-lived granulocytes and progressive bone marrow failure. The abnormalities of granulocyte proliferation and survival often result in the accumulation of myeloid tissue five or ten times larger than the normal total mass. Aside from the symptoms due to tissue infiltration and mass lesions, patients with a large number of tumor cells may show signs of hypermetabolism or may develop gout due to prolonged hyperuricemia.

CML has been classified among the myeloproliferative disor-

ders because of its clinical similarity to PRV and myeloid metaplasia. The blood picture characteristically encountered early in the illness shows an orderly shift to the left with a rare myeloblast, more numerous myelocytes and metamyelocytes, and a preponderance of segmented forms. The leukocyte count may be as high as $1000 \times 10^9/L$. Anemia is often absent, and the platelet count may be higher than normal. Marrow smears reveal excessive numbers of myeloid cells similar to those found in the blood. Their alkaline phosphatase activity is lower than normal. The serum concentrations of vitamin B_{12} and its binding protein are characteristically increased.

CML must be distinguished from the other myeloproliferative disorders and the several conditions that may cause leukoerythroblastosis. A rapid diagnostic tool is now available that will detect with Southern blotting techniques the bcr in all cells without culture, and can therefore be used to screen patients with myeloid dysplasias for possible CML and its variants.

Course and Management

The course of CML is variable. Since the disease may remain relatively quiescent for prolonged periods, and since the goal of therapy is palliative, treatment is initiated when there is clear evidence of progression. The chief problems encountered in patients with progressive CML are related to the large spleen (and infarcts thereof), increasing anemia, hemorrhagic diathesis due to thrombocytopenia, increasing weight loss and debility, and, to a lesser extent, bone pain.

In the stable phase, all peripheral blood elements can fluctuate widely, but usually in a patient-specific cyclical manner. A stimulatory activity is present in the serum, acting in a reciprocal relation to the white blood count, but synchronous with the platelet count. There is little need in the adult to treat on the basis of these fluctuating counts unless the differential count includes a predominance of early forms, or is $>150 \times 10^9/L$. Intermittent therapy merely increases the amplitude of the rebound fluctuations. Children, however, tend to develop leukostasis at a lower white blood count and should be more carefully controlled.

Signs and symptoms of fatigue, bone pain, and hypermetabolism are easily controlled with daily oral hydroxyurea (Table 6.17–3). Hydroxyurea kills cells in cell cycle and is useful to rapidly reduce cell numbers when necessary. Long-term side effects are yet to be described. Reserved for the hydroxyurea refractory state, busulfan is an alkylating agent that is injurious to stem cells and produces a prolonged myelosuppression, pulmonary fibrosis, cataracts, and dryness of mucous membranes.

Since massive splenomegaly is a clinical problem during the terminal phases of CML, with platelet sequestration and pain, splenectomy may be entertained early. There is risk of postsplenectomy infection, and survival may not be prolonged.

Intensive therapy of CML, like that used in AML and aimed at complete remission with a Ph^1-negative state, has resulted in transient absence of Ph^1-positive cells in 25 percent of trials, but the duration of such mosiacism is brief. Whether such treatment prolongs survival is not yet known.[10]

Allogeneic bone marrow transplantation in young patients in stable phase with HLA-identical sibling donors has produced continuing long-term CML-free survival in 50 percent of patients treated. Results of similar trials with purged autologous bone marrow transplantation are too early to be evaluated. Apparently, significant complete remissions can be achieved with long-term therapy with α-interferon. The effect on overall survival is yet to be determined.

The terminal events of this illness are commonly related to the evolution of an acute phase characterized by the rapid proliferation of immature aneuploid myeloid cells, progressive anemia, thrombocytopenia, and an overall picture that resembles that of acute leukemia. Hemorrhage and infection are common causes of death. The disease in this phase is resistant to therapy. Treatment of the blast phase is unsatisfactory, with a median survival of 3 months. If the lymphoid variant is present, marked by terminal deoxynucleotyl transferase (TdT) and common acute lymphocytic leukemia antigen (CALLA) positivity, the majority of patients will achieve a complete remission of a few months duration with intensive treatment with prednisone, vincristine, and daunomycin.

Future Therapy. There is evidence in CML for persistence of normal hematopoietic precursors that are Ph^1 negative and are suppressed by clonal expansion of the abnormal cells with a proliferative advantage.[6] The urge in therapy is to reduce the number of abnormal and likely finite cells to allow functional recovery of the more differentiated committed precursor cells. Whether the Ph^1-negative cells that emerge after the annihilation of the leukemic cells are normal or merely neoplastic cells in a preleukemic phase is not clear. That malignant cells themselves can proliferate and differentiate in both CML and AML has been demonstrated by G-6-PD homozygosity, chromosome genetics, and molecular biologic studies using restriction fragment–length polymorphisms.[7] The prevalence of this maturation of leukemia is as yet unknown but indicates that drugs which force maturation rather than incur cytotoxicity will be of value in the treatment of this malignancy.

MYELOFIBROSIS

Many descriptive terms have been applied to the group of illnesses characterized by a leukoerythroblastic anemia, enlargement of the spleen and liver as the result of myeloid metaplasia, and a patchy or generalized fibrosis of the bone marrow. The etiology of this syndrome remains obscure. There is an increased incidence of myeloid metaplasia among atom bomb survivors and others exposed to ionizing radiation. One opinion relates this disorder to a neoplasm of reticuloendothelial cells involving principally the marrow, spleen, and liver. At present, many group this condition with the myeloproliferative disorders largely because of their overlapping clinical features and because of the occasional transition from one form to another.

A new subclass of AML based on the presence of platelet peroxidase on the blast cell using the electron microscope has been designated M7. This megakaryocytic leukemia is a fulminant disease that responds poorly to treatment and is associated with rapidly progressive fibrosis with increased amounts of circulating platelet–derived growth factor.

Clinical Manifestations

Myelofibrosis occurs in both sexes with equal frequency, generally after age 50. The primary complaints are weakness, easy fatigability, abdominal discomfort, and aching in the extremities, especially the legs. Less frequent symptoms are hemorrhage (skin and gastrointestinal tract), gout, and weight loss. Common physical abnormalities include pallor, ecchymoses or petechiae, striking splenomegaly, and more modest hepatomegaly. Icterus is present at times.

TABLE 6.17–3. TREATMENT OF CHRONIC MYELOCYTIC LEUKEMIA

Treatment	Median Survival From Treatment (mo)
None	30
Splenic irradiation	30
P-32	20
Splenectomy	40
Busulfan	40
Hydroxyurea	50
Intensive combination chemotherapy	55
Bone marrow transplantation	50% 5-year disease-free survival

Although a few patients may have a normal or even increased red blood cell mass early in their illness, one of the most characteristic features of this disorder is the leukoerythroblastic anemia. The red cells show marked anisocytosis and poikilocytosis. Nucleated red cells are often seen. The reticulocyte count is normal or moderately elevated.

The white cell count is usually elevated, and the differential shows a shift to the left. All types of immature granulocytes may be encountered in the peripheral blood, including an occasional myeloblast. The alkaline phosphatase stain shows high or normal amounts of enzyme; rarely, low values are obtained. In most cases the platelet count is elevated, and large, odd shapes are often encountered.

Attempts to secure marrow by aspiration may be unsuccessful. Biopsy techniques are more successful in providing the means of demonstrating the myelofibrosis and hypocellularity present. Osteosclerosis may be seen also. These marrow changes may be patchy early in the disorder; later they may be generalized. Indeed, it is not uncommon to encounter foci of hematopoietic cell hyperplasia. Biopsy or aspiration preparations from the spleen, the liver, and, rarely, the lymph nodes may show extensive extramedullary hematopoiesis (myeloid metaplasia).

Radiographs of the bones in 25 to 50 percent of cases show a patchy irregular osteosclerosis. The cortex of the long bones is often thickened. Osteoporosis has been noted also. The blood uric acid level is elevated in about 50 percent of instances, at times to twice normal levels.

Diagnosis

The hallmarks of myelofibrosis include a leukoerythroblastic anemia, marked splenomegaly and hepatomegaly with prominent myeloid metaplasia, and fibrosis or sclerosis of the bone marrow.

The diagnostic problems commonly confronted stem in part from the transition forms that exist between PRV, CML, and this disorder. In other instances, myelofibrosis must be distinguished from an aplastic or hypoplastic anemia. In addition, the physician must remain alert to the several possible causes of leukoerythroblastosis.

"Leukoerythroblastosis" is a term used to describe the presence of nucleated red cells and various immature myelocytic forms in the peripheral blood. When severe, this abnormality is striking, persistent, and usually accompanied by anemia. In its mildest forms there may be no anemia and only a few transiently circulating abnormal cells. Leukoerythroblastosis may result from myeloproliferative or from myelophthisic disorders (Table 6.17–4). Carcinomatosis and other myelophthisic processes are the most frequently encountered causes of marked leukoerythroblastosis.

Course and Management

The average prognosis for life ranges from 4 to 5 years, but with good supportive care many patients live much longer. The main continuing clinical problems are those stemming from the anemia, the markedly enlarged spleen, or the hemorrhagic episodes.

Symptoms resulting from severe anemia are relieved by transfusion. Not infrequently, a hemolytic anemia develops, and, rarely, the Coombs test may become positive. Splenectomy has been performed to relieve this hemolytic problem. Thrombocytopenia with bleeding also develops on occasion and may be relieved by splenectomy. Following splenectomy, however, the liver enlarges progressively (myeloid metaplasia), and the general course of the disease continues.

External radiation has been directed at the spleen to relieve local symptomatology or to combat hemolytic anemia or thrombocytopenia. The potential danger of irradiating the areas of extramedullary hematopoiesis has been stressed also. Busulfan has induced a decrease in spleen size in some patients and an improvement in their hematologic status, but it may have adverse effects on the remaining hematopoietic tissue. Hydroxyurea will likely relieve signs and symptoms of expanding disease when used judiciously.

The immediate causes of death relate to underlying cardiovascular disease affected adversely by anemia, thromboembolic events, or hemorrhage. A transition to chronic granulocytic or acute granulocytic leukemia may take place before death.

PRIMARY THROMBOCYTHEMIA

Primary thrombocythemia is a rare disease, primary in origin, characterized by a platelet count of $1000 \times 10^9/L$, hyperplasia of megakaryocytes, the absence of the Philadelphia chromosome, and no increase in red cell mass.[15] Like the other myeloproliferative disorders, it is a clonal disease, originating in a multipotential stem cell and occasionally interlinked with CML, PRV and myelofibrosis. Similarly, it is a disease of the patient over 50 and has an insidious onset. The majority of patients present with bleeding from the gastrointestinal tract, skin, or mucous membranes associated with a high platelet count in the peripheral blood. The bleeding can occur because of vascular thrombosis, infection, platelet function abnormalities, and consumption of coagulation factors. Both venous emboli and thromboses occur with gangrene and central venous and arterial occlusions may develop. Splenomegaly is present at diagnosis in ≥ 60 percent of patients. Laboratory features include a markedly elevated platelet count with platelet aggregates, giant platelets, cytoplasmic fragments, and abnormally shaped platelets. The bone marrow aspirate reveals megakaryocytic hyperplasia with a markedly hypercellular marrow. The megakaryocytes are large and abnormal. Because of chronic blood loss, most patients have iron deficiency anemia. There is an infrequent finding of an abnormality or deletion of the long arm of chromosome 21. As in the other myeloproliferative disorders, causes of secondary thrombocytosis must be ruled out, including PRV and CML.

Treatment of this disease is symptomatic. The use of alkylating agents and ^{32}P is not suggested because of the problem of late development of leukemia. Studies with acetylsalicylic acid have demonstrated a lack of effect. Prophylactic therapy with hydroxyurea is probably the treatment of choice if bleeding becomes a major problem. Otherwise therapy is held until necessary. Fifty percent or greater of the patients will survive longer than 5 years, with death caused by bleeding and thrombosis.

CONTRASTING CLINICAL FEATURES OF THE CHRONIC MYELOPROLIFERATIVE DISORDERS

Polycythemia rubra vera, myelofibrosis, and chronic myelocytic leukemia are considered together primarily because they manifest a chronic uncontrolled proliferation of hematopoietic stem cells and because their clinical features often overlap or change in an interrelating fashion with the passage of time. Although certain

---

TABLE 6.17–4. CAUSES OF LEUKOERYTHROBLASTOSIS

Abnormal Myeloproliferation Following:
- Blood loss or hemolysis
- Nutritional deficiency anemias

Myelophthisic Disorders
- Tuberculosis, especially disseminated
- Carcinomatosis (lung, breast, prostate)
- Xanthomatosis (Gaucher disease and others)
- Lymphoma
- Myeloma
- Myeloproliferative disorders

Severe Illness, Stress, Agonal States
- Infection
- Heart failure
- Uremia

basic morphologic resemblances are stressed, no implication with respect to etiology is intended. Continuing clinical experience serves to emphasize the diversity of findings manifested by different patients and by the same patient during the course of the disease. A patient with classic PRV may, after many months, develop an increasing anemia and progressive enlargement of the spleen and liver. Appropriate biopsies may reveal myelofibrosis and extramedullary hematopoiesis associated with a leukoerythroblastic anemia. Similarly, an individual with PRV may develop all the features of chronic granulocytic leukemia after the passage of months or years. The granulocyte alkaline phosphatase levels are usually elevated in these patients.

One percent or fewer of patients with PRV will develop acute myelocytic leukemia. This may evolve directly from the polycythemic status or may occur as a blast crisis in a person whose illness had previously become chronic granulocytic leukemia. The use of ^{32}P therapy or other forms of radiation therapy has been linked to a tenfold or greater increase in the incidence of acute leukemia.

Some patients with clear-cut myeloid metaplasia and myelofibrosis show transient polycythemia early in the course of their disease. The myeloid metaplasia syndrome seems unique among the myeloproliferative disorders because of the occasional associated occurrence of an autoimmune hemolytic anemia and the occasional associated development of thrombocytopenic purpura unrelated to therapy.

MYELODYSPLASTIC SYNDROME

During the prodromal period, before manifestations of overt leukemia, refractory cytopenias of varying duration and characterized by disordered hematopoiesis frequently occur. In these trilineage disorders in which the predominant cell may vary because of clonal progression and dominance over time, the classification is difficult.[1] To resolve this apparent heterogeneity, this constellation of marrow failure has been divided by morphologic criteria and histochemical stains into five subgroups (Table 6.17–5). Since all patients ultimately die of bone marrow failure or overt leukemia, it is clinically useful to consider these cytopenias from the beginning as neoplasms with a measurable preleukemic phase of variable length.

The term "preleukemic syndrome" is used to segregate those with signs of dyspoiesis in whom acute leukemia is imminent from those in whom the conversion is less certain.[14] For instance, those with refractory anemia with ringed sideroblasts (RARS), who also have hypercellular bone marrows with cytopenia, are less likely to undergo malignant transformation or progression prior to death. Unfortunately, overall survival in this group is not necessarily better than in those with an aggressive phase, as the patients succumb to the complications of bone marrow failure within several months.

The terms "myelodysplastic syndrome" (MDS), "smoldering leukemia," "preleukemia," and "refractory anemia with excess blasts in transformation (RAEB-t)" encompass a broad range of those patients presenting with a low percentage of leukemia cells and a protracted course to those with fulminant AML, with bone marrow replacement and a high percentage of blasts present at diagnosis. Overall, the group demonstrates a continuing progression of the same disease.

REFRACTORY ANEMIA

Refractory anemia (RA) usually occurs in patients over the age of 50 years with anemia as the main presenting symptom. The peripheral blood shows reticulocytopenia, variable dyserythropoiesis, and infrequently dysgranulopoiesis. Blast cells are not seen in the peripheral blood; when present they do not exceed 1 percent. The bone marrow is normal or hypercellular with erythroid hyperplasia and dyserythropoiesis. The granulocytic and megakaryocytic series almost always appear normal, and there are always fewer than 5 percent of blast cells. Rarely, patients with neutropenia and/or thrombocytopenia but no anemia can be included in this category.

Refractory Anemia with Ringed Sideroblasts
The main difference between RA and RARS is the presence of ringed sideroblasts accounting for more than 15 percent of all nucleated cells in the bone marrow. Ringed sideroblasts have several siderotic granules on the nuclear membrane arranged in a collar around the nucleus. Deficient hemoglobinization in some of the red cell precursors leads to a dimorphic picture in peripheral blood films.

Refractory Anemia with Excess Blasts
The age incidence in RAEB is similar to that of RA. There is always some degree of cytopenia affecting two or more of the bone marrow series. The peripheral blood shows conspicuous abnormalities in all three cell lines. In RAEB, in contrast to RA, dysgranulopoiesis is a common feature. There may be a small proportion of circulating blast cells (<5%). The bone marrow is hypercellular and shows varying degrees of either granulocytic or erythroid hyperplasia. There is always evidence of dysgranulopoiesis, dyserythropoiesis, or dysmegakaryocytopoiesis; ringed sideroblasts may be seen. The percentage of blasts (types I and II) in the bone marrow, by definition, is ≥5 percent up to 20 percent. There is almost always evidence of maturation in the granulocytic series to promyelocytes and beyond.

The percentage of blasts in the peripheral blood is less than 5 percent. The bone marrow resembles that of RAEB but may show a significant increase in monocyte precursors (promonocytes) often with fewer than 5 percent of blasts. In some patients with moderate monocytosis and bone marrow features identical to those of

TABLE 6.17–5. DIAGNOSTIC CLASSIFICATION OF THE MYELODYSPLASTIC SYNDROMES

FAB (Classic)	Cytogenetics	Morphology
RA (Refractory anemia)	Normal	Anemia without blasts, cellular bone marrow, moderate dyserythropoiesis
RARS (Refractory anemia with ringed sideroblasts)	Normal	Anemia with <5% blasts >15% nucleated cells are ringed sideroblasts
CMML (Chronic myelomonocytic leukemia)	Normal	RAEB plus monocytosis, immature granulopoiesis monocytosis >1 × 10^6/μl
RAEB (Refractory anemia with excess blasts)	(−5/5q−), (−7/7q−), (20q−), (8+), (Y−)	Cytopenia of 2 or more elements, dyshematopoiesis, 5–20% blasts
RAEB-t (Refractory anemia with excess blasts in transformation)	"	RAEB plus <20; <30% blasts in bone marrow, <5% blasts in peripheral blood, Auer rods

RAEB, the percentage of blasts may be higher than 5 percent and up to 20 percent.

Refractory Anemia with Excess Blasts in Transformation

This type includes cases of cytopenia in patients of any age, often with symptoms of brief duration, which do not strictly fit into either of the above categories or in any of the AML types (M1-M6). The hematological features are similar to those of RAEB but include 5 percent or more of blasts in the peripheral blood, more than 20 percent and up to 30 percent of blasts (types I and II) in the bone marrow, and presence of unequivocal Auer rods in granulocyte precursors. These patients with dyserythropoiesis may ultimately evolve from RA to RAEB or RAEB-t with eventual leukemia transformation if they have not succumbed to the effects of bone marrow failure.

CHRONIC MYELOMONOCYTIC LEUKEMIA

The defining feature of CMML is an absolute monocytosis (over $1 \times 10^9/L$). Often this is associated with an increase in mature granulocytes with or without evidence of dysgranulopoiesis (e.g., hypogranular and Pelger forms). It is a defined disease of the elderly, sometimes confused with CML because of a similar frequent high peripheral white blood count, a differential containing a progressive level of immature cells of the granulocytic series, hepatosplenomegaly, monocytosis, and a markedly hypercellular marrow. It terminates with an aggressive phase, consistent with a multistep evolution and clonal progression characterized by monocytosis with soft tissue invasion, bone pain, hypermetabolism, and leukostasis. In contrast to CML, however, chromosomal abnormalities are infrequent. Palliation can be achieved for variable periods in this fragile elderly population with blood product support and palliative drugs, the most effective being hydroxyurea. Evidence obtained by molecular biologic probes in some patients responding to therapy demonstrates mature granulocytes that are clonal, supporting trials of maturation agents as therapeutic tools to achieve terminal differentiation.

OTHER DISORDERS

5q MINUS SYNDROME

5q− syndrome is an entity distinct from those with multiple DNA deletions, which may include the loss of chromosome 5. The 5q− abnormality occurs with deletion of the long arm of chromosome 5, the site of the gene that encodes for both the GM-CSF and the CM-CSF receptors (see Table 6.16–2). Whether or not this relationship plays a causal role in the pathogenesis of the macrocytic anemia, hyponucleated megakaryocytes and elevated platelet counts observed in this syndrome is speculative. As a single DNA abnormality, the partial loss of chromosome 5 does not always predict for leukemia conversion, but the median survival is only 2 years nonetheless.[16]

CYTOGENETICS

As methods improve, the detectable incidence of chromosomal abnormalities in MDS increases (50 to 80 percent). They are those frequently seen in patients with AML secondary to treatment with antineoplastic drugs and ionizing irradiation and include deletions of chromosome 5 (−5,5q−), chromosome 7 (−7/7q−), chromosome 20 (20q−), an additional chromosome 8 (8+), and the loss of the Y chromosome. In MDS, as in secondary leukemia, the DNA abnormalities define neoplasia, leukemic conversion, and a poor prognosis. Response to treatment is low, the induced bone marrow failure prolonged, and the response brief. One factor mitigating a good response to cycle-active drugs is the consistently low tumor-growth fraction in MDS, quenching response to DNA-dependent drugs.

CLINICAL MANIFESTATIONS

MDS is characteristically a disease of the elderly (>70 years), with persistent cytopenias of a single or all lineages of the bone marrow elements in spite of a normal or hypercellularity of that organ, with ultimate conversion to leukemia or death from marrow failure likely within 2 years of diagnosis. MDS is neoplastic and lethal even without manifestations of overt leukemia.[9]

The signs and symptoms of MDS relate to the dominant cell line of the pluripotential clone most detectable at presentation. In half the cases, the cytopenia is discovered incidentally, with findings dependent on the extent of bone marrow failure and organ invasion. In others, infection, bleeding, marked weakness, and fatigue cause the patient to solicit help.

Virtually all patients have refractory anemia and many have pancytopenia, but isolated myeloid cytopenias are rare. The stained smear reveals abnormal red cells with macrocytosis and hypochromia, and circulating nucleated cells. There is neutropenia or thrombocytopenia in 50 percent of cases, with polymorphonuclear neutrophils (PMNs) $<2 \times 10^9/L$ characterized by hypogranulation and hyposegmentation in the neutrophils, and abnormal granule formation in the large platelets. The hypercellular marrow aspirate reveals abnormal growth and maturation of all elements, with erythroid hyperplasia, megaloblastosis, and marked dyserythropoiesis, sometimes with RARS. Other characteristic laboratory findings include increased serum and urine lysozyme (CMML), decreased PMN function, and a prolonged bleeding time.

With progression over time, and depending on the extent of the disease present when the patient was first found to have MDS, the picture may change from mild anemia to pancytopenia. In CMML a sudden increase in circulating monocytes and tissue invasion is a harbinger of the aggressive and terminal phase of the disease. In others, overt AML may signal the transformation to a fulminant leukemic phase.

TREATMENT

In this pluripotential stem cell disease, hope lies in new potential treatment areas: biomodulation with humoral factors to terminally differentiate leukemic cells and maturation of leukemia with cytotoxic agents. The advent of human-cloned colony-stimulating activities (CSA) suggests a role for growth stimulation of the pluripotential leukemic stem cell to drug sensitivity while forcing normal CFU-S to more rapid repopulation with normal marrow elements. These CSAs may also force maturation in the neoplastic cell.

ACUTE MYELOID LEUKEMIAS

DE NOVO ACUTE MYELOCYTIC LEUKEMIA

Classification

Acute myelocytic leukemia has recently been stratified on the basis of strict morphologic characteristics (Table 6.17–6). AML is characterized by aberrant cells with varying degrees of maturation, the majority in the myelocytic series, while some have monocytic characteristics and are associated with extramedullary infiltration. For example, M4 (myelomonocytic) leukemia occurs in one third of the patients and carries a high frequency of extramedullary disease and CNS invasion. M6 (erythroleukemia) is a rare variant that may ultimately progress to a myelocytic morphology. M7 (megakaryocytic leukemia), recently defined, is associated with bone marrow fibrosis and is diagnosed primarily by electron microscopic evi-

TABLE 6.17–6. DIAGNOSTIC CLASSIFICATION OF ACUTE MYELOCYTIC LEUKEMIA

FAB (Classic)	Immunophenotype	Cytogenetics	Morphology
M1 (Myelocytic, stem cell, undifferentiated)	Ia,MY7,MY9, MY10	Normal, INV(3), +8, t(9;22),5q/−5,7q/−7	90% undifferentiated blasts, <10% with granules, Auer rods
M2 (Myelocytic with maturation)	Ia,M7,MY9	Normal, t(8;21), +8, t(3;5),t(9;22),t(6;9)	Maturation to progranulocytes and beyond >10% with primary granules and Auer rods
M3a (Hypergranular progranulocytic)	Ia,M7,MY9,VIM-2	t(15;17)	Hypergranular, primary granules, Auer rods, bizarre blasts, DIC
M3b (Microgranular progranulocytic)	—	—	Progranulocytes with minimal granulation, bilobed nucleus, hyperleukocytosis, DIC
M4 (Myelomonocytic)	Ia,MY7,MY8,MY9, MO5, VIM-2	t(9;11), +8t, t(6;9)	>20% monoblasts, >20% myeloblasts, monocytosis
M4 (Myelomonocytic with eosinophilia)		INV(16)	As above, with increased eosinophils
M5a (Monocytic)	VIM-2,MY9	t(9;11),t(11q23–25), +8, INV(16)	>80% monoblasts
M5b (Monocytic)			Monoblasts with >20% maturation
M6 (Erythrocytic)	Ia	Multiple	>50% nucleated erythroid cells, >10% bizarre erythroblasts, dyserythropoiesis, >30% myeloblasts, progranulocytes, may proceed to M2
M7 (Megakaryocytic, acute myelosclcosis)	Ia, factor VIII, Ib, IIb/IIIa (EM-platelet peroxidase on nuclear membrane)	t(1;3),t27	Bizarre megakaryocytes with immature lobulation, increased platelets, myelofibrosis with heterogeneic peripheral heterogeneous blasts (confused with L1,L2,M1)
CML-BC (Chronic myelocytic in blast crisis)	Ia,MY7,MY9,VIM-2	t(9;22), −8,ISO 17 duplicated Ph[1]	M1, M2
AML (Secondary)	Ia,M7,M9,M10	5q−/7q−, 7q/−7 multiple	M1,M2,M7, can be bizarre with myelofibrosis
AML-ALL (Biphenotypic, hybrid)	Lymphoid, Myeloid		Characteristics of varied myeloid and lymphoid lineage, may be hybrid or biphenotypic

dence of platelet antibody on the nuclear membrane of cells. It can be confused with L1,L2 (lymphocytic) and M1 (myelocytic) leukemia.[2]

Cytogenetics and Immunophenotype

As prophase banding techniques improve, it is clear that a majority of patients with AML have at least one karyotypic abnormality with either a balanced translocation, deletion, or addition (Table 6.17–6). The most common chromosomal abnormality is a +8 or −7, a combination thereof, or a specific translocation, some with prognostic significance. For example, the t(8;21) occurs in 10 percent of patients with AML, predominantly the M1 and M2 subtypes; while M3 commonly has a translocation between chromosomes 15 and 17; and patients with M2 leukemia may have rearrangements within chromosome 16. In patients with leukemia apparently related to treatment of other malignancies, the 5/5q− and 7/7q− deletions are frequently seen.[16]

Immunophenotypes determined by specific monoclonal antibodies are subgrouped by panels of potent markers that accurately and rapidly separate lymphoid from myelocytic leukemia. Specific monoclonal antibodies, such as MY10, are associated with markedly primitive cells, a poor response to therapy, and a bad prognosis.

Combining morphology, histochemical stains, a battery of inclusive monoclonal antibodies, accurate karyotyping and cytogenetic analysis, and, when necessary, the electron microscope, the vast majority of patients with leukemia can be categorized and therapy begun.

Pathophysiology

The pathophysiology of acute leukemia is the consequence of bone marrow failure due to tumor-related suppression of normal hematopoiesis and the clinical expression of the malignant hematopoietic clone. The growth of blood cell precursors arrested at an immature stage of differentiation suppresses production of normal bone marrow elements, resulting in anemia, infection and bleeding, and the metabolic effects of increased cell turnover. Increased growth of leukemic cells and infiltration of virtually all organ systems completes the pathophysiologic complex. The signs and symptoms of bone marrow failure and infiltration of the central nervous system, liver, spleen, testes, ovary, lymph nodes, skin, and gastrointestinal tract, with varied degrees of failure of each organ, may contribute to the overall symptom complex at presentation.

The probability of achieving prolonged disease-free survival in acute leukemia has increased with the availability of active antitumor agents and enlightened scheduling of those agents.[17] Failure to obtain disease remission late in therapy involves either failure of support or tumor resistance, while early mortality relates to the pathophysiology of the tumor.

Although the combination of bone marrow failure and tumor invasion determines the clinical presenting features of acute leukemia, the aspects of clonal expression based on tumor mass, specific leukemia cell characteristics, and the rate of cell turnover determine the need for prompt intervention. Paradoxically, rapid cell kill with intensive drug treatment results in severe metabolic imbalances that are sometimes difficult to ameliorate. Survival also depends on the recognition of both disease- and treatment-related complica-

tions and the rational use of supportive measures that permit both disease eradication and treatment survival.

In some settings, immediate intervention is required. A scheme to rapidly decrease tumor mass safely entails awareness, rapid intervention, aggressive treatment, and critical care management in an emergency situation in all patients with hyperleukocytosis and large cell mass (Table 6.17–7).

In general, however, emergency therapy is not called for in patients presenting with AML. Unless there is a white blood count $>100 \times 10^9/L$, time can be taken to prepare the patient for systemic therapy after the appropriate diagnosis and clinical evaluation is made.

Treatment

Principles of treatment used in leukemia as a template disease remain applicable over time, while recipes of therapy change rapidly as new treatments are developed and new drugs are explored, with avenues now opened for biomodulation and maturation drugs. New tools to define successful therapy permit greater quantitation than the microscope, with detection of residual leukemia unsuspected on the pathology slides. Maximal reduction of tumor with the first treatment step can be achieved with noncompeting drug combinations, synergistic in time and action. Once remission is achieved, additional aggressive therapy is required to rid the patient of minimal residual disease and to produce a meaningful survival. The small amount of residual tumor exerts little proliferative suppression of normal tissue of the host, with the recovery of marrow, gut, and lung cells after treatment uninfluenced by products of the tumor itself. In this milieu, the tumor is less influenced by feedback mechanisms and is more responsive to normal hematopoietic and host factor regulation.

In complete remission, the patient is clinically prepared to withstand tissue toxicity and induced bone marrow failure. Now drugs can be used in a logical sequence timed to effect maximal pharmacokinetic results in a dose and schedule affording maximal cytokinetic advantage to the action of DNA-dependent, cell cycle–dependent, specific drugs such as cytosine arabinoside, daunomycin, avisacrine and eptopiside.

The rapid recognition and treatment of infection and the availability of intensive blood product support are essential to successful outcome of intensive antileukemic chemotherapy.[3] Prophylaxis against gastrointestinal-based infection with oral antibiotics

that act against aerobic bacteria, such as norfloxacin, will control endogenous host gram-negative organisms once the patient is rendered aplastic by disease or by cytotoxic drugs.[13] Surveillance cultures of the stool give advanced warning of impending overgrowth and systemic invasion. With the first fever during therapy (38.3C), immediate empiric antibiotics must be started and continued through therapy to prevent death by *Pseudomonas aeruginosa*.[3] Early use of amphotericin B controls fungal sepsis. Prophylactic platelet transfusions for platelet counts $<20 \times 10^9/L$ from random donors are effective in preventing bleeding during the initial induction course. With such cytotoxic and supportive therapy, reestablishment of a normal bone marrow (complete remission) can be anticipated in 65 percent of the patients treated. Twenty to 50 percent of patients will have a greater than 5-year survival without further therapy and may be cured.

As alternate second-phase therapy, once the patient under the age of 30 with an HLA-matched donor has achieved remission status, bone marrow transplantation should be considered. Although there are significant side effects of graft-versus-host disease (GVHD) and attendant chronic immunosuppression, the meaningful survival and cure rate in children is higher than that achievable with further courses of chemotherapy. Bone marrow transplantation, however, does not add significantly to survival greater than that achievable with chemotherapy in first remission in patients beyond the age of 30 and has no role in patients older than 50, because these patients fail to survive the ravages of GVHD.[4]

Unfortunately, chemotherapy of any kind is difficult to deliver to patients older than 60 years. In this population, which is more likely to experience MDS with leukemic progression or M4-M5 leukemias with poor prognosis, alternate therapy must be sought. With evidence that clonal maturation can be achieved after intensive therapy, noncytotoxic drugs may be found that will cause maturation. To date, retinoic acid, low-dose cytosine arabinoside, and vitamin D have had little success. However, with products of genetic engineering now available to the clinician, humoral regulators such as colony-stimulating activities hold the hope of the reestablishment of normal stimulation of proliferation and maturation. These noncytotoxic agents may biomodulate patients in remission to terminally mature their minimal residual tumor and allow the growth of normal polyclonal stem cell marrow recovery.[7]

Prognosis

As methods and therapy improve, the variables that predict the results of therapy change. Each new therapy, drug, and support system has altered the impact of infection, bleeding, and tumor mass effects, but high white count at presentation, obesity, and depressed functional status remain negative prognosticators (Table 6.17–8).

Cytogenetic banding techniques define some patients with certain chromosomal transformations such as (8;21) and (15;17) who fare better than those with deletions in their DNA content. For example, persistent abnormalities of the 5 or 7 chromosomes, apparently induced by mutagenic previous chemotherapy, portend a bad prognosis. The use of aggressive rational therapy has not yet been fully evaluated in this group. It is ironic that drugs that induce leukemia are used to attempt to eradicate it.

SECONDARY OR MUTAGEN-RELATED LEUKEMIA

In this variant of AML a prodrome occurs 1 to 7 years after exposure to a mutagen, usually chemotherapy or radiotherapy, in patients who were previously treated for another malignancy, such as Hodgkin disease, lymphoma, myeloma, or ovarian cancer. There is a direct relationship between the dose of scheduled chemotherapy and incidence of secondary AML, with a 20 percent chance of leukemia after long courses of alkylating agents. The preleukemic phase is characterized by ineffective erythropoiesis, dyspoiesis, and cytogenetic abnormalities. Pathognomonic for this disease is the loss of all or part of chromosome 5 and/or 7, abnormalities rarely

---

TABLE 6.17–7. MANAGEMENT OF HYPERLEUKOCYTOSIS AND TUMOR LYSIS SYNDROME

All Patients with Leukemia
- Institute allopurinol 600 mg PO stat, 300 mg PO qd × 5
- Institute aluminum hydroxide 30 ml PO stat and q4h
- Hydrate with 0.45 N NaCl without bicarbonate 150 ml/hr × 5 days
- Maintain urine output equal to hydration
  Furosemide IV as needed and effective
  Dopamine ≤3 µg/kg/min infusion
- Monitor K^+, PO_4, cr, sun, blood gases, q12h until stable
- Monitor PT, PTT, fibrinogen, FDP q12h until stable
- If positive tests develop, add heparin
- Dialyze early for increasing uric acid and/or renal failure
- Maintain platelet count $>20 \times 10^9/L$

Hyperleukocytosis
- Begin cell cycle–specific antileukemic therapy within 2 hr of admission
- Transfuse RBC only when WBC $<50 \times 10^9/L$, or when clinically imperative
- Maintain platelet count $>50 \times 10^9/L$

Coagulopathy—M3, Ongoing DIC
- Heparin 10 U/kg/hr by continuous infusion 6 hr prior to Rx or with treatment if hyperleukocytic
- Maintain platelet count $>50 \times 10^9/L$
- Monitor PT, PTT, fibrinogen, FDP q12h during drug infusion and until stable

TABLE 6.17–8. FAVORABLE INDICATIONS OF INDUCTION AND DURATION

Induction	Duration
Youth	Youth
De novo leukemia	De novo leukemia
Good performance status	
No extramedullary leukemia	
No bleeding	
No infection	
Low tumor mass	Low tumor mass
Low blast count ($<1 \times 10^9/\mu l$)	Low blast count
Residual normal marrow function	Complete remission
No disseminated intravascular coagulation	
No tumor lysis products	
No abnormal organ function	
FAB M1 to M4	FAB M1 to M3
Cytogenetics normal, t(8;21), INV 16, +8, +21, t(15;17)	Favorable genetics
Auer rods	
Rapid tumor reduction	Rapid tumor reduction
Good ARA-CTP uptake/retention	Good arabinocylcytodine triphosphate formation and retention
Increased growth of residual leukemia	Increased growth of residual leukemia
Minimal residual leukemia	Minimal residual leukemia
Poor growth in culture	Two courses of therapy

found in de novo AML (Table 6.17–6). The high incidence of a recognizable preleukemia phase compared to a 20 percent prodrome with de novo AML may relate to a proliferative disadvantage and slow cytokinetic rate because the tumor growth fraction is classically low. Additional chromosome abnormalities occur in the original abnormal clone in 75 percent of cases as the disease evolves to frank leukemia, but these are distinct from those associated with de novo AML. Although this syndrome is now more commonly attributed to chemotherapy, it is the type associated with benzene, chemical solvents, and other mutagens incriminated in leukemogenesis.[11] The preleukemia phase and ultimate poor response to chemotherapy places secondary leukemia functionally with the myelodysplastic syndrome because the majority of patients die within 2 years of either leukemia or the sequelae of pancytopenia.

Mutagen-related preleukemia evolves commonly to M2 or M4 leukemia with less than 1 year survival time. With appropriate aggressive therapy, survival time may be prolonged, but drug-induced bone marrow failure may be of long duration. Patients with preleukemia should be managed conservatively in the initial phase of the disease. Intensive combinations of chemotherapy or bone marrow transplantation may be used in the young, but only 50 percent of the patients will achieve remission, usually of brief duration.

REFERENCES

1. Bennet JM, Catovsky D, et al: Proposals for the classification of the myelodysplastic syndromes. Br J Haematol 51:189, 1982
2. Bennet JM, Catovsky D, et al: Proposed revised criteria for the classification of the acute myeloid leukemias: A report of the French-American-British cooperative group. Ann Intern Med 103:626, 1985
3. Burke PJ, Braine HG, et al: The clinical significance and management of fever in acute myelocytic leukemia. Johns Hopkins Med J 139:1, 1976
4. Champlin R, Gale R: Bone marrow transplantation for acute leukemia: Recent advances and comparison with alternative therapies. Semin Hematol 24:55, 1987
5. Collins SJ, Kubonishi I, et al: Altered transcription of the c-abl oncogene in K562 and other chronic myelogenous leukemia cells. Science 225:72, 1984
6. Dube ID, Gupta CM, et al: Cytogenetic studies of early myeloid progenitor compartments in Ph positive chronic myeloid leukemia. Br J Haematol 56:633, 1984
7. Fearon ER, Burke PJ, et al: Differentiation of leukemia cells to polymorphonuclear leukocytes in patients with acute nonlymphocytic leukemia. N Engl J Med 315:15, 1986
8. Foon KA, Gale RP, Todd RF III: Recent advances in the immunologic classification of leukemia. Semin Hematol 23:257, 1986
9. Galton DG: The myelodysplastic syndromes. Scand J Haematol 36:11, 1986
10. Griffin JD: Management of chronic myelogenous leukemia. Semin Hematol 23:20, 1986
11. Kantarjian HM, Keating MJ, et al: Therapy-related leukemia and myelodysplastic syndrome: Clinical, cytogenetic, and prognostic features. J Clin Oncol 4:1748, 1986
12. Kaplan ME, Mack K, et al: Long-term management of polycythemia vera with hydroxyurea: A progress report. Semin Hematol 23:167, 1986
13. Karp JE, Merz WG, et al: Oral norfloxacin for prevention of gram-negative bacterial infections in patients with acute leukemia and granulocytopenia. Ann Intern Med 106:1, 1987
14. Koeffler HP: Myelodysplastic syndromes (preleukemia). Semin Hematol 23:284, 1986
15. Murphy S, Harry I, et al: Essential thrombocythemia: An interim report from the polycythemia study group. Semin Hematol 23:177, 1986
16. Sandberg AA: The chromosomes in human leukemia. Semin Oncol 23:201, 1986
17. Vaughan WP, Karp JE, et al: Two-cycle timed-sequential chemotherapy for adult acute nonlymphocytic leukemia. Blood 64:975, 1984

CHAPTER 6.18
The Lymphoid Leukemias

Philip J. Burke

The lymphoid malignancies are a broad spectrum of bone marrow invasive diseases involving the cells of the immune system. At one end of the parabola is the fulminant, proliferative disease of children and adults, acute lymphocytic leukemia, and at the other, the terminally differentiated disease of the elderly, multiple myeloma. Between are a myriad of diseases that have defied classification by the pathologist and the light microscope. Now, new techniques, as in the myeloid malignancies, define the relationship of these diseases to each other and to normal cells. For example, neoplastic cells of B-lymphocyte lineage express surface light chain immunoglobulins that identify these tumors as clonal expansions.[3]

CHRONIC LYMPHOCYTIC LEUKEMIAS

Etiology and Pathogenesis
In contrast to CML, there is no evidence for involvement of carcinogens in the etiology of the chronic lymphocytic leukemias

(CLL). Chromosomal rearrangements occur in some, however, and are associated with translocation and activation of cellular oncogenes. In particular, in patients with T-cell and hairy cell leukemia and in a few patients with B-cell CLL, human retroviruses have been identified and may play a causative role.

Fundamental concepts have been defined in these malignancies. Specifically, in the acute T-cell leukemia of Asia, there is direct evidence of the integration of retroviral DNA into the genome of the patient with lymphoma. In Burkitt lymphoma, translocations between chromosomes 8 and 14 carry the myc oncogene to a promoter site on chromosome 14, with subsequent oncogene activation. DNA hybridization technology defines specific immunoglobulin gene configuration specific for each lymphoid clone and has defined homogeneous B-cell tumors. Combining monoclonal antibody recognition of surface and cytoplasmic markers, DNA technology, and the use of banding techniques to map chromosomal translocations and inversions in association with recognized oncogenes allows a clearer understanding of these lymphoid malignancies and their relationships to each other.

Classification

The chronic lymphoid malignancies can be divided into CLL, prolymphocytic leukemia, hairy cell leukemia, T-cell variants of all the above, non-Hodgkin lymphomas (see Chapter 6.19), and multiple myeloma (see Chapter 6.20).

Phenotypic and chromosomal markers are specific for a number of the subclassifications of the lymphoid malignancies (Table 6.18–1). B cells bear surface membrane immunoglobulins in virtually all cases. Those with chromosomal abnormalities involve 6, 12, 14, and 18, with trisomy 12 and 14q+ the most common. Its incidence of 3/100,000 people is equal to that of multiple myeloma and is in the same age group of 40 to 70 years. B-CLL accounts for 95 percent of cases in the West, while in Asia, T-cell variants are the more frequent form.[2]

B-CLL cells bind mouse erythrocytes and express membrane-bound immunoglobulins (SmIg). SmIg is an important marker of clonality for B-CLL, which expresses a single light chain. The batteries of monoclonal antibodies can now distinguish B-CLL from prolymphocytic leukemia and hairy cell leukemia and can demonstrate transformation to large cell lymphoma when cells are circulating or from the tumor biopsy. The most common membrane phenotypes of CLL are T1−, T3+, T4−, T6−, T8+, M1+, Leu7±. The rearrangement of the B chain or the T-cell receptor chain strongly supports the monoclonal nature of T-cell proliferation in T-CLL.[4]

In contrast to CML, the lymphocytic form frequently presents with painless, generalized lymphadenopathy. Splenomegaly is rarely of the magnitude encountered in the chronic granulocytic disorder. Anemia and bleeding tendencies are also seen. The clinical manifestations of CLL may be related to the proliferation and accumulation of long-lived, immunologically inert lymphocytes, progressive bone marrow failure, and increasing immunologic unresponsiveness (humoral immunity).

The clinical phenomenon of lymph node enlargement deserves special comment. Lymphoid tissue is responsive to many stimuli and participates in many regional or systemic diseases. Infections of all types, hypersensitivity states, collagen-vascular disorders, and thyrotoxicosis can produce regional or generalized lymphadenopathy. Some of these diseases can also produce transient abnormal blood lymphocytosis. Primary and metastatic neoplastic diseases also commonly involve the lymph nodes.

Neoplastic and nonneoplastic causes of lymph node enlargement are summarized in Table 6.18–2. It is often difficult to establish the cause of clinically significant lymphadenopathy, particularly at one point in time. The accurate pathologic interpretation of lymph node biopsy material demands an experienced pathologist and careful correlation with all available clinical data. A nonspecific clinical syndrome with nonspecific morphologic lymph node abnormalities may resolve completely or may develop into one of the lymphomatous neoplasms. On occasion, the neoplastic nature of the lymph node abnormality is appreciated correctly, but its precise classification is not possible. A patient with an undifferentiated malignant tumor may prove to have a lymphomatous disease on further study. Similarly, an abnormal cervical lymph node initially classified as lymphoma or histiocytic lymphoma may prove to be a metastatic deposit from an occult undifferentiated nasopharyngeal or bronchogenic primary neoplasm. Alternatively, the initial impression of neoplasia may prove incorrect and the lymph node alterations found to be part of a disorder such as systemic lupus erythematosus.

Clinically significant enlargement of the spleen also merits special attention. The spleen is part of the lymphoid organ of the body, and many of the comments made concerning the causes of lymph node enlargement are pertinent to splenomegaly. In contrast to the regional lymph nodes, the spleen is rarely involved with metastatic neoplasia. Involvement with primary lymphoid neoplasms is relatively common. The most frequent causes of splenomegaly are listed in Table 6.18–3.

The pathologic interpretation of altered splenic morphology may be difficult. On occasion, a spleen several times its normal size

TABLE 6.18–1. DIAGNOSTIC CLASSIFICATION OF THE LYMPHOID NEOPLASMS

FAB (Classic)	Immunophenotype	Cytogenetics	Morphology
Chronic Lymphocytic Leukemia (CLL)			
CLL (B-CLL)	Ia+,B1+,B2+,B4+,Leu1+, Smig+	+12,14q+, INV 14	Small lymphocytes
CLL (T-CLL)	Ia+, Leu1+, T	Normal	Small lymphocytes
CLL (Prolymphocytic)	Ia+,B4+,Smig+	t(6:12), DEL3	Prolymphocytes
CLL (Hairy cell)	Ia+, B1+,Leu M5,Leu14,Smig	Normal	Hairy cells (TRAP+)
CLL (Plasma cell)	PCA1+,B4+,Smig,CALLA+, LEU1−	Various	Plasma cells
CLL (Lymphosarcoma)	Ia+,B4+,B1+,Smig,CALLA+, Leu1−	Various	Cleaved lymphocytes
Acute Lymphocytic Leukemia (ALL)			
L1,L2 (Common)	CALLA+, tDt+,Ia+,B4+	t(4;22),t(9;22)	Small lymphocytes
L1,L2 (Pre-B)	CALLA+,tDt+,Ia+,CLG+,B4+	t(1;19),t(9;22)	Heterogeneous lymphocytes
L1 (T cell)	tDt, E receptor,Leu9, Leu1	t(11;14)	
L3 (B cell)	CALLA+,tDt−,B4+,SMIG+, HLA−DR	t(8;14)	Homogeneous large lymphoblasts with vacuoles and cleaved nuclei

TABLE 6.18–2. CAUSES OF LYMPH NODE ENLARGEMENT

Anatomic Site	Neoplastic	Nonneoplastic

Generalized enlargement	Leukemia
	  Chronic lymphocytic, acute, chronic granulocytic (acute phase)
	Lymphoreticular neoplasms
	  Hodgkin disease, lymphocytic and histiocytic lymphoma
		Acute infections
		  Bacterial, rickettsial, viral
		Chronic infections
		  Tuberculosis, syphilis, toxoplasmosis
		Hypersensitivity states
		  Serum sickness, drug reactions
		Collagen-vascular disorders
		  Systemic lupus erythematosus, rheumatoid arthritis
		Endocrine metabolic disorders: Hyperthyroidism, hypoadrenocorticism, hypopituitarism

Cervical nodes	Lymphoreticular neoplasms
	Metastatic neoplasms
	  Nasopharynx, oral cavity, pharynx, thyroid
		Acute infections (as above)
		Chronic infections
		  Tuberculosis, fungus
		Sarcoidosis

Supraclavicular nodes	Lymphoreticular neoplasms
	Metastatic neoplasms
	  Bronchus, breast, stomach, esophagus, pancreas, colon, genitalia
		Acute infections (as above)
		Chronic infections
		  Greater incidence reflecting intrathoracic tuberculosis, fungus diseases
		Sarcoidosis

Axillary nodes	Lymphoreticular neoplasms
	Metastatic neoplasms
	  Breast, rarely from bronchus
		Acute infections
		  Streptococcus, staphylococcus, P tularensis, cat-scratch disease

Mediastinal nodes	Lymphoreticular neoplasms
	Metastatic neoplasms
	  Bronchus, breast, stomach, pancreas, colon, genitalia
		Acute infections
		  Pneumonia, lung abscess, viscus perforation
		Sporotrichosis
		Chronic infections
		  Tuberculosis, fungus
		Sarcoidosis
		Erythema nodosum

Retroperitoneal nodes	Lymphoreticular neoplasms
	Metastatic neoplasms
	  Stomach, pancreas, colon, genitalia
	Retroperitoneal sarcoma
		Acute infections
		  Salmonella (other enteric fevers), viscus ulceration and/or perforation, abdominal abscess
		Chronic infections
		  Tuberculosis, fungus

Inguinal nodes	Lymphoreticular neoplasms
	Metastatic neoplasms
	  Genitalia, rectum
		Acute infections
		  Streptococcus, staphylococcus
		Venereal infections
		  Syphilis, lymphopathia venereum, granuloma inguinale

All sites	Congenital anomalies Lymphangioma, cystic hygroma	

fails to yield a pathognomonic histologic abnormality on comprehensive microscopic examination. Not infrequently, patients with classic manifestations of Hodgkin disease or lymphocytic lymphoma have had enlarged spleens removed earlier in their courses, with inconclusive pathologic descriptions after microscopic study. The appreciation of altered splenic morphology as it relates to the clinical evaluation of lymphoid neoplasms is limited by the infrequency or impossibility of serial studies.

Clinical Manifestations

CLL is the most frequent form of leukemia in elderly people and is usually diagnosed following routine blood examinations in otherwise healthy individuals or on the basis of widespread lymphadenopathy, fatigue, or weight loss. Usually the physical examination reveals no abnormalities, though in some cases generalized lymphadenopathy and splenomegaly are prominent findings. Persistent blood lymphocytosis over $15 \times 10^9/L$ without apparent cause, with lymphocytic infiltration of the bone marrow, is suggestive of the diagnosis of CLL. It is a neoplasm characterized by proliferation and accumulation of monoclonal small mature-appearing lymphocytes, usually B cell in origin.

Course and Management

CLL may remain indolent for months or years and require no particular therapeutic attention. When progressive, the major management problems stem from progressive increase in the size of lymph nodes and lymphoid tumor masses, a progressive anemia that may have a significant hemolytic component, a bleeding diathesis associated with thrombocytopenia, or infectious diseases attendant on hypogammaglobulinemia and other results of an acquired immunologic deficiency state. The most suitable therapeutic program will, therefore, combine pertinent elements of supportive and specific treatment.

Supportive Care. Systemic complications of CLL relate primarily to manifestations of the disease and not to its management, although tumor lysis and hyperuricemia can occur. The types of treatment used generally do not cause massive tumor kill immediately, nor is this necessary. True total complete remission or eradication of the disease has been rare in CLL, and attempts to treat aggressively have resulted in depression of normal marrow elements without clearing of the tumor. The systemic complications of CLL include hypogammaglobulinemia and recurrent infections,

TABLE 6.18–3. CAUSES OF SPLENOMEGALY

Neoplastic
- Primary lymphoreticular neoplasms
  Hodgkin disease, lymphosarcoma, reticulum cell sarcoma, chronic and acute lymphocytic leukemia, monocytic leukemia
- Primary hematopoietic neoplasms
  Acute myelocytic leukemia, myeloproliferative disorders (chronic myelocytic leukemia, myeloid metaplasia, polycythemia vera)
- Metastatic neoplasms (rare)
  Breast, melanoma, chorionepithelioma

Nonneoplastic
- Acute infections
  Bacterial, rickettsial, viral
- Chronic infections
  Bacterial (brucellosis, subacute bacterial endocarditis), tuberculosis, fungal, spirochetal, protozoan
- Sarcoidosis
- Hypersensitivity states
  Serum sickness, drug reaction
- Collagen vascular disorders
  Systemic lupus erythematosus, rheumatoid arthritis (Still disease, Felty syndrome)
- Endocrine-metabolic disorders
  Hyperthyroidism, lipoid storage disorders (Gaucher disease, Niemann-Pick disease)
- Hematologic disorders
  Pernicious anemia, Cooley anemia, iron deficiency anemia, congenital and acquired hemolytic anemias, thrombocytopenic purpura
- Congestive splenomegaly
  Portal or splenic vein thrombosis, cirrhosis of liver
- Cystic lesions
  Lymphangioma, hemangioma, post-traumatic

TABLE 6.18–4. STAGING OF CLL BASED ON SURVIVAL

Stage		Survival (Mo from Diagnosis)
0	Lymphocytosis >15 × 10^9/L μl Bone marrow infiltration >40%	150
I	Lymphadenopathy	100
II	Splenomegaly, hepatomegaly	70
III	Anemia (Hgb <11/g/dl or Hct <33%)	20
IV	Thrombocytopenia (platelets <100 × 10^9/L)	20

which rate a patient will progress. Some indications include high lymphocytosis, high white count, rapid tumor doubling, previous therapy, and poor response to initial therapy. Significant cytogenetic abnormalities are unknown.[8]

LARGE CELL LYMPHOMA

CLL can transform to new varieties of lymphoma, which include diffuse large cell lymphoma (Richter syndrome), a fulminant, debilitating, febrile, and, until recently, rapidly progressive disease. The development of large cell lymphoma occurs in at least 10 percent of patients and may be a new malignant clone with new genotype and phenotype. Also seen are prolymphoid transformation, lymphoblastic transformation, or even development of multiple myeloma.

HAIRY CELL LEUKEMIA

Hairy cell leukemia or leukemic reticuloendotheliosis, a chronic proliferative disease of older men with massive splenomegaly, cytopenia, and fibrotic bone marrow, was previously treated with splenectomy but now responds to interferon and deoxycoformycin with remarkably good results.

Diseases with lymphadenopathy and splenomegaly mimic many infectious, neoplastic, and immunologic diseases that are relatively benign in their manifestations and outcome. It is critical to rule out other causes of these findings (Table 6.18–2). With new hybridization techniques, it is less likely that a benign disease will be confused with a clonal neoplasm.

ACUTE LYMPHOCYTIC LEUKEMIAS

Primarily a disease of children, acute lymphocytic leukemia (ALL) constitutes 15 percent of adult acute leukemias, and is divided into three groups in the FAB classification. Most cases exhibit the common ALL antigen (CALLA) and B-cell gene rearrangement. ALL with T-cell phenotype is more common from 15 to 25 years of age, while acute undifferentiated or pre-B leukemia whose cells lack T or B characteristics and are CALLA-negative are seen more commonly in adults. B lymphocyte antigens are seen in approximately 5 percent of patients, T in 20 percent and neither in 75 percent. Virtually all patients with ALL have terminal deoxynucleotide transferase (TdT) (Table 6.18–1).

Clinical Manifestations
Like AML, clinical signs and symptoms are those of bone marrow failure, but there is higher frequency of lymphadenopathy, splenomegaly, mediastinal mass, and associated immunosuppression. This immunosuppression places the patient at risk for infections

which can be treated with γ-globulin and appropriate antibiotics. The immune-mediated anemia, thrombocytopenia, and neutropenia respond to prednisone and immunosuppressive agents, and occasionally to splenectomy and intravenous γ-globulin. Hyperviscosity syndrome has been seen with the IgM elaboration and treated as is multiple myeloma with plasmapheresis and chemotherapy. Hyperuricemia is rare, and hypercalcemia, except in the T-cell variant, is uncommon. If it occurs, it is treated primarily with hydration, diuretics, prednisone and calcitonin, and systemic chemotherapy.

Treatment. Alkylating agents (chlorambucil, cyclophosphamide) given for 4 to 8 weeks or more will induce good partial remission in 60 to 70 percent of the patients. Prednisone will show an antitumor effect in about 50 percent, and combination chemotherapy with drugs such as cyclophosphamide, vincristine, and prednisone may be superior. Adrenal corticosteroids are used frequently to suppress immune hemolysis, bleeding tendencies due to thrombocytopenia or hypercalcemia. Ionizing radiation may induce a marked resolution of lymphoid tumor masses. α-Interferon and deoxycoformycin may play a role in some of the B cell malignancies, but their efficacy is yet to be determined.

The course of CLL usually extends over a period of 5 years or longer. One third of cases are alive at 10 years after diagnosis. It is less common to observe a preterminal acute phase of this disorder than in chronic granulocytic leukemia. Death frequently results from an infectious disease, bleeding, the sequelae of severe anemia, an unrelated disease, or progression.

Prognosis
The introduction of a clinical staging system with prognostic significance has allowed comparison of therapeutic trials in patients with CLL (Table 6.18–4).[6] Nonetheless it is difficult to determine at

unique to the immunocompromised host. Nosocomial and parasitic infections, such as *Pneumocystis carinii* and atypical fungal organisms, in addition to those seen in the myeloid malignancies with granulocytopenia but intact immune responsiveness, must be suspected with each new fever. Since therapy is prolonged in ALL, consistent surveillance for pathogenic organisms is necessary even during remission after white blood cell recovery.

Course and Management

The preferred treatment varies with the phenotype. In all cases, combinations of drugs active against malignant lymphoblasts are required, together with treatment of the central nervous system for actual or potential leukemic cell infiltrates. The usual approach consists of a three-phase treatment of induction, CNS prophylaxis, and maintenance. Induction therapy includes prednisone, vincristine, L-asparaginase, and daunomycin. Optimal remission induction therapy in adult ALL is controversial. The use of vincristine and prednisone combined with L-asparaginase or an anthracycline produces remission rates of 85 percent. Consolidation or maintenance is commonly given with 6-mercaptopurine, methotrexate, cyclophosphamide, and prednisone in a cyclical fashion. Early consolidation and intensification therapy, particularly with a timed sequence including daunomycin, is effective in prolonging remission and preventing relapse, with a median remission duration of 50 months with up to 45 percent of patients remaining in continuous, complete remission beyond 5 years.

Unlike the disease in children the incidence of CNS leukemia in adult ALL is less than 10 percent in most series. Risk factors for CNS involvement include a high white cell count, T-cell phenotype, L3 Burkitt morphology. CNS relapse in childhood has been reduced from 50 to 5 percent with cranial irradiation and intrathecal methotrexate. Similar treatment reduces the incidence of CNS relapse in adults to about 10 percent. The current standard format calls for 60 months of treatment.[5]

Immunotherapy has not proven beneficial. Bone marrow transplantation has contributed somewhat, but only 30 percent of patients achieve a long survival. The host toxicity of bone marrow aplasia, immunosuppression, and graft-versus-host disease is high in patients >30 years of age.

Prognosis

Favorable prognostic features at diagnosis include young age, low white cell count, low number of circulating blasts, no mediastinal mass, no CNS involvement, L1 FAB classification, and karyotype of modal number >50.[1] Unlike the case in children, T-ALL is the most favorable subtype in adults. Remission rates usually exceed 80 percent and the remissions are long. Those with common ALL have an intermediate prognosis and those with null-ALL an inferior prognosis. Patients with hybrid leukemias and adults with B-ALL have the least favorable prognosis. Although there appears to be no difference in remission induction, most studies demonstrate that increasing age is associated with shorter remissions and decreased survival, with the breakpoint in age prognosis somewhere between 25 to 35 years. Also unfavorable is the remission induction duration of longer than 4 weeks, as is an abnormal karyotype with normal ploidy. Although rare at presentation, CNS leukemia is considered an adverse prognostic feature, especially when associated with L3 subtype. The presence of CNS involvement, however, has no significant influence on remission duration.[7]

REFERENCES

1. Crist W, Boyett J, et al: Clinical and biologic features predict a poor prognosis in acute lymphoid leukemias in children and adolescents. Med Pediatr Oncol 14:135, 1986
2. Croce CM, Nowell PC: Molecular basis of human B cell neoplasia. Blood 65:1, 1985
3. Foon KA, Gale RP, et al: Recent advances in the immunologic classification of leukemia. Semin Hematol 23:257, 1986
4. Gale R, Foon RA: Chronic lymphocytic leukemia: Recent advances in biology and treatment. Ann Intern Med 103:101, 1985
5. Hoelzer D, Gale RP: Acute lymphoblastic leukemia in adults: Recent progress, future directions. Semin Hematol 24:1, 1987
6. Rai KR, Sawitsky A, et al: Chronic lymphocytic leukemia. Med Clin North Am 68:697, 1984
7. Rivera GR, Mauer AM: Controversies in the management of childhood acute lymphoblastic leukemia: Treatment intensification, CNS leukemia, and prognostic factors. Semin Hematol 24:1, 1987
8. Sandberg AA: The chromosomes in human leukemia. Semin Oncol 23:201, 1986

CHAPTER 6.19
The Malignant Lymphomas

Albert H. Owens, Jr.

The malignant lymphomas are self-perpetuating proliferative disorders of the lymphoreticular cell system. As such they share a common cytogenealogy with the lymphocytic leukemias and with the plasma cell dyscrasias—disease processes that usually begin in the bone marrow (Table 6.19–1 and Figs. 6.19–1 and 6.19–2). Patients with malignant lymphomas are grouped together by clinicians, however, because of their distinctive presentations with a variety of extramedullary tumors, especially lymph node enlargement and splenomegaly.[4]

The incidence of malignant lymphomas appears to be increasing. During 1987, more than 7,000 cases of Hodgkin disease were newly diagnosed in the United States and about 28,000 cases of non-Hodgkin lymphoma as well.[3] Despite the eminent curability of many of these disorders, the malignant lymphomas are the seventh most common cause of cancer death.

ETIOLOGY AND PATHOGENESIS

Over the years several infectious agents have been considered as possible causes of Hodgkin disease and the other lymphomas. Early on *Mycobacterium tuberculosis* and related organisms were considered because of the common occurrence of tuberculosis in patients with Hodgkin disease. It appears, however, that the high frequency of mycobacterial and fungal infections in these patients is a consequence of an underlying defect in cellular immunity.[1]

Reports of the unusual occurrence of Hodgkin disease in "clusters" has provoked further consideration of infectious etiologies. Some epidemiologists have suggested, however, that the apparent "clusters" are chance phenomena. A few long-term follow-up studies have shown that patients who have had infectious

TABLE 6.19–1. NEOPLASTIC LYMPHORETICULAR PROLIFERATIVE DISORDERS

Disease State	Manifestations	
	Proliferative	*Immunologic*
Leukemia	Mild generalized adenopathy Splenomegaly	
Acute lymphocytic	Infiltration of blood, marrow, nodes, tissues with lymphoblasts	
Chronic lymphocytic	Infiltration of marrow, nodes, tissues with small lymphocytes	Progressive decrease in normal immunoglobulins and antibody response Decreased response of lymphocytes to mitogens
Lymphocytic lymphoma	Prominent generalized adenopathy Splenomegaly Mass lesions Infiltration of marrow common Variable small cell lymphocytosis	Autoimmune hemolytic anemia Rare monoclonal gammopathy
Plasma cell dyscrasias	Infiltration of marrow, tissues, blood with plasma cells Osteolytic bone lesions Rare adenopathy Rare splenomegaly	Overproduction of homogeneous immunoglobulin molecule or fragment (H-chain, L-chain) Progressive decrease in antibody response Low isoagglutinin titers
Histiocytic lymphoma	Regional or generalized adenopathy Splenomegaly Mass lesions Infiltration of marrow, nodes, tissue with abnormal histiocytic cells, also occasionally seen in blood	Rare monoclonal gammopathy
Hodgkin disease	Regional or generalized adenopathy Splenomegaly Mass lesions	Impaired cell-mediated immunity Decreased response of lymphocytes to mitogens Rare monoclonal gammopathy Autoimmune hemolytic anemia
Mycosis fungoides	Skin lesions predominate Lymph nodes, viscera are involved later Abnormal cells may be seen in blood and marrow	

mononucleosis have an increased risk of developing Hodgkin disease. Although the possible etiologic role of the Epstein-Barr virus (EBV) in Hodgkin disease has been explored in some detail, no conclusive causal relationship has been established. Similarly, the recently described human T-cell leukemia/lymphoma viruses (HTLV) have not been linked to Hodgkin disease as yet.

It is clear that both DNA and RNA viruses can cause malig-
nant lymphomas in cats, cows, rodents, and birds. In humans, the strong association between EBV infection and African Burkitt lymphoma is provocative. Similar findings are not forthcoming in other parts of the world, however. On the other hand, the evidence that a unique type-C RNA tumor virus can cause rather distinctive T-cell leukemias and lymphomas in adults is quite convincing.

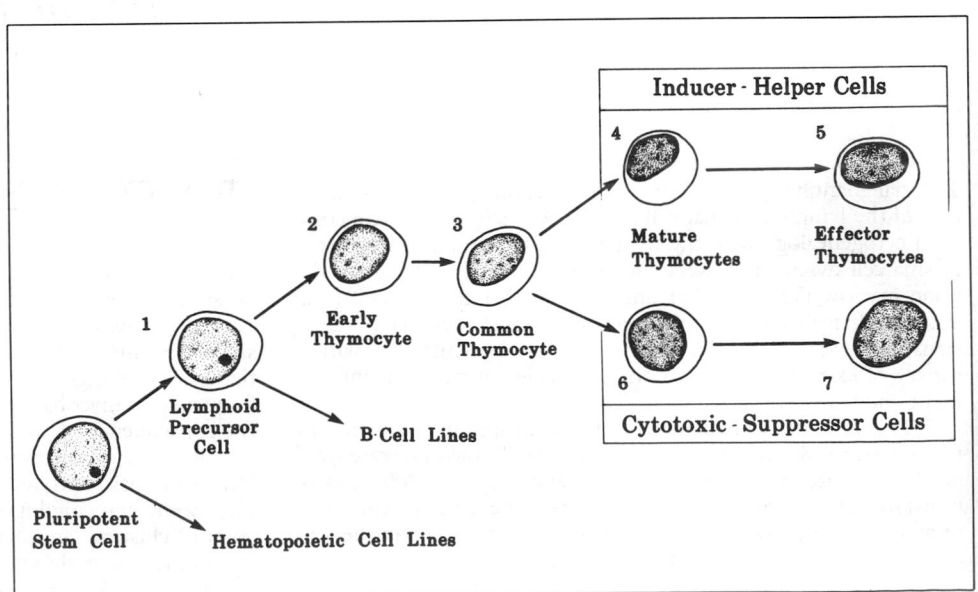

Figure 6.19–1. Cytogenealogy of T lymphocytes.

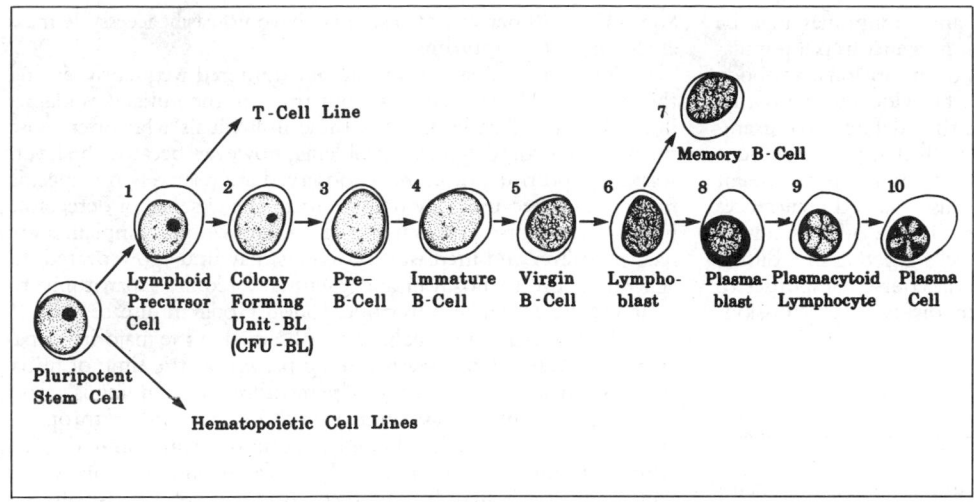

Figure 6.19–12. Cytogenealogy of B lymphocytes.

Recent research has been undertaken to evaluate the role of oncogenes, especially c-myc, in the pathogenesis of malignant lymphomas. It seems likely that retroviral oncogenes and their cellular counterparts that control the proliferation and differentiation processes do play an important role in the evolution of lymphomas, but the precise mechanisms are not yet clear. For example, cytogenetic studies in B-cell lymphomas (Burkitt) have shown a characteristic translocation of the c-myc oncogene from the short arm of chromosome 8 into the immunoglobulin heavy chain locus on the short arm of chromosome 14. Thus the translocated c-myc oncogene might come under the influence of a promoter region in the activated immunoglobulin gene and contribute to the neoplastic transformation of the cell.[12]

Ionizing radiation causes malignant lymphomas also. An increased incidence of lymphoma occurred in the atomic bomb survivors in Japan. Similarly, there was an unexpectedly high incidence of lymphoma in patients irradiated for ankylosing spondylitis.

Several clinical disorders have been linked with an increased risk of developing malignant lymphoma (Table 6.19–2). One feature most of them have in common is a major functional derangement of the immune system or exposure to cytotoxic and immunosuppressive therapy. Klinefelter syndrome has been related to the development of "reticulum cell sarcoma," but possible pathogenetic mechanisms are unclear. There is also an unexpectedly high frequency of histocompatibility antigen HLA-B12 in patients with malignant lymphoma, suggesting that constitutional factors predisposing to lymphoma development may exist.

CYTOGENEALOGY

The term malignant lymphoma emphasizes the rather characteristic types of tumor involvement that patients present with and the predictable patterns of spread that occur in the lymphoreticular tissues. Transition states between solid tumors (e.g., lymphocytic lymphoma) and leukemia (e.g., lymphocytic leukemia) are often seen, however. Further, it is possible to envision the patterns of tissue involvement and spread of neoplastic lymphoma cells in light of the "migration and homing" patterns of their normal counterparts. For example, follicular or nodular poorly differentiated lymphoma is a B-cell neoplasm that commonly spreads to involve the B-cell domains of the lymphoid tissues and bone marrow. In 85 percent of cases or more, the tumor is disseminated widely at the time of the initial clinical diagnosis. The transformed cell population probably arose from a migratory B cell and retained its ability to move about through the body and lodge in the usual B-cell areas.[7]

For the most part the malignant lymphomas are monoclonal neoplasms derived from the different developmental and functional subpopulations of lymphoreticular cells (Table 6.19–3). The conclusion that various of the lymphomas are monoclonal neoplasms is based on an analysis of cell surface markers (e.g., cell surface immunoglobulin, complement receptors, Ia antigens), cytogenetic abnormalities (e.g., the translocation 8q–:14q+), and DNA rearrangements (e.g., immunoglobulin gene rearrangements in B-cell lymphoma). Studies using a wide variety of monoclonal antibodies developed to human lymphocyte associated antigens also support the same conclusion.

TABLE 6.19–2. DISORDERS LINKED WITH MALIGNANT LYMPHOMA

Hereditary Disorders
- Ataxia telangiectasia
- Chédiak–Higashi syndrome
- Wiskott–Aldrich syndrome
- Swiss-type agammaglobulinemia
- Common variable immunodeficiency
- Klinefelter syndrome

Acquired Disorders
- Renal transplantation
- Sjögren syndrome
- Rheumatoid arthritis
- Systemic lupus erythematosus
- Acquired hypogammaglobulinemia

TABLE 6.19–3. CYTOGENEALOGY OF MALIGNANT LYMPHOMAS

Clinical Diagnosis	Cell of Origin
Hodgkin disease	Uncertain; likely macrophage/reticulum cell line
Non-Hodgkin lymphoma	
• Small lymphocytic	B cell; T cell (rarely)
• Intermediate lymphocytic	B cell
• Follicular lymphocytic	B cell
• Diffuse aggressive lymphocytic	B cell (65%); T cell (25%); histiocyte/reticulum cell (rarely)
• Burkitt lymphoma	B cell
• Lymphoblastic	B cell (10%); T cell (85%)
Mycosis fungoides	T cell

While the great majority of malignant lymphomas may be monoclonal neoplasms with apparently homogeneous cell populations as defined by histologic techniques or monoclonal antibody analysis, clinicians must remain alert to the wide variations that occur in the course of the disease entities thus defined. For example, B-cell lymphomas composed of small cells that produce nodular tumors may pursue an indolent course. Responses to treatment may be slow in coming, and repeated remissions and recurrences may extend over 5 to 10 years or longer. On the other hand, B-cell tumors composed of relatively large cells growing in a diffuse pattern usually pursue an aggressive clinical course. Responses to treatment may be dramatic.[13] Prolonged disease-free remissions may be achieved along with some cures.

HODGKIN DISEASE[4,10]

In 1832, Hodgkin described the autopsy findings in seven patients who died with generalized lymph node enlargement and splenomegaly. In 1856, Wilks graphically described Hodgkin disease as "characterized by a gradual progressive enlargement of the lymphatic glands beginning usually in the cervical region and spreading throughout lymphoid tissue of the body, forming nodular growths in the internal organs, resulting in anemia and usually a fatal cachexia." The pathologic characterization of this disorder relates mainly to the presence of a polycellular infiltrate composed of giant (Sternberg-Reed) cells, lymphocytes, plasma cells, monocytes, eosinophils, and neutrophils associated with a variable degree of fibrosis and necrosis.

Present evidence favors a macrophage-histiocyte origin for Hodgkin cells. Studies using T- and B-lymphocyte surface markers have produced conflicting results as to the cytogenealogy of these cells.

Chromosome analysis of Hodgkin disease tissue has usually revealed a mixture of normal and abnormal karyotypes. Although the 14q+ abnormality has been seen in a few cases, no consistent karyotypic abnormality has been found that is characteristic of the disease.

CLINICAL MANIFESTATIONS

Hodgkin disease is most commonly encountered in young people of all races. There is a bimodal incidence, with the first peak occurring between ages 15 and 35 and the second after age 50. Males are affected nearly twice as frequently as females.

The manifestations of Hodgkin disease are highly variable in nature and intensity. They may be systemic in character or may be referable primarily to one or more organ systems. It is convenient to group these features as they relate to the presence of solid tumor masses and associated hematologic, immunologic, or physiologic abnormalities.

The most common presenting complaints concern the painless, progressive, asymmetrical enlargement of cervical lymph nodes. Somewhat less frequent are the symptoms that stem from compression of various adjacent structures by expanding tumor masses. For example, cough, crowing dyspnea, dysphagia, and cervicofacial and upper-extremity edema may result from a mediastinal mass impinging on the tracheobronchial tree, superior vena cava, or esophagus. Similarly, low-back or abdominal discomfort, lower-extremity edema, or urinary or gastrointestinal dysfunction may result from retroperitoneal tumor, and left flank pain may result from an enlarged spleen.

There are nontender, rubbery, matted, or lobulated masses in the peripheral lymph node–bearing areas of 70 to 80 percent of affected persons. These masses usually are not attached to the overlying skin. Occasionally their size varies spontaneously over a period of several days. Palpable splenomegaly has been reported in 50 to 70 percent of cases. Radiographic examinations will identify a mass lesion in most of the patients without peripheral tumors. Some 10 to 20 percent of cases may have no easily accessible mass at the onset of symptoms.

Constitutional symptoms are encountered frequently during the course of Hodgkin disease, but they are the initial complaints in a minority of patients. It is these individuals who often pose the more difficult diagnostic problems, however, because the fever, weakness, pruritus, or cachexia observed are relatively nonspecific findings and because they may occur in the absence of detectable lymphoid tumors. For example, a patient whose complaints are recurrent fever and increasing weakness may undergo repeated diagnostic study to no avail and eventually require laparotomy to establish the existence of retroperitoneal Hodgkin disease.

Hematologic abnormalities are observed in the majority of patients with Hodgkin disease and are present at the time of initial diagnosis in about 30 percent. The most frequent finding is a normochromic anemia, most often a result of decreased erythropoiesis. At times, significant hemolysis can be demonstrated. The white cell count is often moderately increased, and a granulocytosis and monocytosis may be observed. An eosinophilia, usually less than 10 percent, may be seen in 10 to 20 percent of cases. Lymphopenia is common late in the disease. Thrombocytosis (platelet counts in excess of 400,000) is encountered at times and large bizarre forms may be observed. Sternberg-Reed cells are rarely identified in marrow aspirates but may be seen in 20 to 25 percent of patients if biopsy is employed.

A number of immunologic abnormalities have been associated with progressive Hodgkin disease. An unusual tendency toward viral, mycobacterial, and fungal infections has been noted. For example herpes zoster is encountered in 4 to 6 percent of cases. The incidence of active tuberculosis, is higher in patients with Hodgkin disease, than it is in the general population. In recent years, the frequency of fungus infections, especially cryptococcosis, appears to be increasing. The susceptibility to these infections has been related to the impaired ability to manifest delayed cutaneous hypersensitivity that is seen in more than half of the patients studied. Homograft rejection and lymphocyte responsiveness to mitogens are impaired also.[1]

Electrophoretic studies of serum proteins are often normal early in the course of the disease but may show a mild hypoalbuminemia and hyperglobulinemia (commonly α-2). Infrequently, a monoclonal gammopathy is encountered that is associated with bone marrow plasmacytosis. Antibody responsiveness generally remains unimpaired. Hypercalcemia and hyperuricemia occur occasionally. Low plasma zinc and elevated serum copper concentrations are associated with progressive Hodgkin disease.

DIAGNOSTIC CONSIDERATIONS

Since the majority of patients with Hodgkin disease present with readily accessible tumors, it is usually easy to establish a definitive diagnosis by the demonstration of the characteristic tissue morphology. The more common problems in diagnosis occur when (1) the patient presents with nonspecific constitutional symptoms, such as fever, in the absence of an identifiable tumor mass, (2) full consideration has not been given to the several possible causes of excessive lymphoreticular proliferation, (3) the morphologic pattern in the biopsy specimen is not characteristic enough to discriminate among the malignant lymphomas, (4) the report of a "positive biopsy" is accepted uncritically (e.g., biopsies from patients with disorders such as systemic lupus erythematosus or Whipple disease), or (5) the report of a "negative biopsy" (e.g., lymphoid hyperplasia) is accepted as eliminating the possibility of Hodgkin disease. At times, serial biopsies are required to establish a certain diagnosis.

COURSE AND MANAGEMENT[14]

The course of Hodgkin disease may vary greatly. Particularly in older patients, the illness may appear to be a rapidly progressive,

multicentric systemic disorder from the outset. More commonly, especially in younger individuals, Hodgkin disease begins as a localized disorder that spreads rather predictably to involve adjacent lymphatic tissue and is potentially curable. Since curative therapy requires that all existing disease be addressed, careful clinical staging is the cornerstone of proper patient management (Table 6.19–4).

It is difficult to detect all tissues involved with Hodgkin disease, especially in the abdomen. Retroperitoneal lymphography, as well as computed tomography and sonography, will reveal otherwise undetected disease in an impressive number of instances. Computed tomography is valuable in assessing intra-abdominal disease since it can detect areas of nodal involvement not usually visualized by lymphography. It is also useful in evaluating the extent of intrathoracic disease. Computed tomography does not replace lymphography, however, because it is not as sensitive a means of detecting minimal node involvement.

Laparotomy will reveal Hodgkin disease involvement of lymph nodes, spleen, and liver not detected by other means. In one series of patients with negative lymphograms, 25 percent of those without constitutional symptoms were found to have intra-abdominal Hodgkin disease at laparotomy, and 50 percent of those with symptoms had intra-abdominal disease. Nearly all clinically enlarged spleens prove to be involved, but 25 to 35 percent of normal-sized spleens are involved, too. Further, laparotomy has defined a small but definite proportion of "false-positive" lymphograms.

A proper staging laparotomy is a major surgical procedure. When coupled with a meticulous pathologic examination of all tissue samples removed, it can be a most informative undertaking. A staging laparotomy should not be completed routinely, however, especially because the procedure is associated with significant morbidity and mortality. It is essential that a complete staging laparotomy be performed when the outcome will determine the choice of therapy.

The currently used histologic classification of Hodgkin disease is based primarily on the observation of Lukes and associates (Table 6.19–5). The predominance of lymphocytic or histiocytic proliferation (or both) has been linked to localized disease and a better prognosis. In contrast, lymphocyte depletion is encountered more often in rapidly progressive disease and signifies a poor outlook for survival. Lukes interprets these patterns as representative of the patients' (immunologic) resistance and cites this as the most important determinant of the outcome of the disease.[8] Others have pointed out that splenic involvement and histopathologic evidence of vascular invasion carry a poorer prognosis.

The more widespread disease is associated with a poorer prognosis (Table 6.19–6). Further, the presence of constitutional symptoms is unfavorable. The prognosis for women seems consistently better than for men, irrespective of the stage of disease. Pregnancy has not been shown to have an adverse effect on survival, but it does present problems in the use of radiation therapy and cytotoxic drugs.

A sound treatment program for Hodgkin disease is based on an assessment of the diagnostic data, the anatomic extent of the disease and its rate of progress, the presence or absence of constitutional symptoms, and the possible existence of major physiologic abnormalities or intercurrent disorders that require more immediate therapy (e.g., bacterial infection, thrombocytopenia with bleeding, hemolytic anemia, hypercalcemia).

Truly localized Hodgkin disease (stages I and II) is managed best by radiation therapy (Table 6.19–6). Adequate tumoricidal doses (e.g., 4000 to 4500 rad in 4 to 5 weeks) must be delivered to the obviously involved areas and to adjacent lymphoreticular tissues using extended-field techniques (e.g., mantle and para-aortic fields). Because full doses are required to achieve curative results and because these dose levels are close to the tolerance of normal tissues, careful treatment planning and precise dose delivery are essential. A high proportion of stage II patients with systemic symptoms (stage IIB) or with mixed cellularity or lymphocyte-depleted histology relapse within 3 years. Many of these patients will have presented with large mediastinal masses. This has led to the use of combination chemotherapy as an adjunct to radiation therapy in these cases. With proper management, nearly 90 percent of stage I cases and about two thirds of stage II cases will be disease free at 5 years and may be presumed to be cured.

Patients with stage IIIA Hodgkin disease may be treated primarily with radiation therapy in centers where proper facilities exist (Table 6.19–6). There is a significant relapse rate, especially among patients with unfavorable histologic types. This has encouraged the adjunctive use of multiagent chemotherapy in these situations. In

TABLE 6.19–5. HODGKIN DISEASE: RELATIVE FREQUENCY OF HISTOPATHOLOGIC TYPE AND PROGNOSIS FOR SURVIVAL

Frequency (%)	Type	5-Year Survival (%)
10–15	Lymphocyte predominance	50–60
30–40	Nodular sclerosis[a]	45–55
20–40	Mixed cellularity	5–20
5–15	Lymphocyte depletion	0–10

[a]More common in younger age group.

TABLE 6.19–4. CLINICAL STAGING OF HODGKIN DISEASE (ANN ARBOR CLASSIFICATION)[a]

Stage	Description
I	Involvement of a single lymph node region (I) or of a single extralymphatic organ or site (I$_E$)
II	Involvement of two or more lymph node regions on the same side of the diaphragm (II) or localized involvement of an extralymphatic organ or site and/or one or more lymph node regions on the same side of the diaphragm (II$_E$)
III	Involvement of lymph node regions on both sides of the diaphragm (III), which may also be accompanied by localized involvement of an extralymphatic organ or site (III$_E$) or by involvement of the spleen (III$_S$) or both (III$_{ES}$)
IV	Diffuse or disseminated involvement of one or more lymphatic organs or tissues with or without associated lymph node enlargement

[a]Each stage is subclassified as A or B to indicate the absence (A) or presence (B) of systemic symptoms not otherwise explained: viz., weight loss greater than 10%; fever, and night sweats.

TABLE 6.19–6. HODGKIN DISEASE: CLINICAL STAGE, INITIAL THERAPY, AND EXPECTED SURVIVAL

Clinical Stage	Initial Therapy	Disease-Free Survival	
		2 Years (%)	5 Years (%)
I	Radiation therapy	85–90	85–90[b]
II	Radiation therapy[a]	85–90	60–70[b]
IIIA	Radiation therapy[a]	70–75	60–70
B	Combination chemotherapy[c]	60–80	40–45
IV	Combination chemotherapy[c]	60–70	30–40

[a]IIB and IIIA: add combination chemotherapy for mixed cellularity or lymphocyte depletion histology.
[b]Relapses more frequent with IIB staging and unfavorable histology.
[c]Add radiation therapy to manage bulky tumors.

most institutions, patients with stage III disease are managed primarily by means of combination chemotherapy.

Patients with stages IIIB and IV disease are best treated initially with multiagent chemotherapy (Table 6.19–6). Similar therapy is appropriate for patients who relapse following radiation therapy. A number of chemotherapeutic agents are useful in the management of Hodgkin disease, including the alkylating agents, the vinca alkaloids, procarbazine, the nitrosoureas, bleomycin, adriamycin, and the adrenal corticosteroids (see Chapter 6.14). A combination of antitumor agents with different mechanisms of action (e.g., mechlorethamine, vincristine, procarbazine, and prednisone) given concurrently and repeatedly over a 6-month period can induce a remission in nearly every patient treated. In fact, various complementary combinations of drugs seem to be equally effective in inducing long-term, disease-free remissions provided they are given in full doses and over a sufficiently prolonged period (6 months). Radiation therapy is employed often in an adjunctive role to eradicate bulky tumors. In many centers, the treatment of patients who appear to be in complete remission is stopped only after careful "restaging" fails to reveal evidence of persistent microscopic disease.

In general, about three quarters of previously untreated patients with advanced disease will remain in disease-free remission for 2 years. Over half of them may be expected to remain disease-free for 5 or more years and many are cured.

It is most important to an optimal long-term outcome to achieve maximal disease regression promptly during the initial course of treatment. The overall prognosis for patients with relapsing, previously treated Hodgkin disease is much less favorable. Because the desired outcome is achieved by applying combinations of treatments at dose levels that are near the biologic tolerance of most patients, it is important that all individuals under therapy be supervised closely and be given appropriate supportive care.

Common management problems in late-stage, relapsing Hodgkin disease result from progressive tumor growth (eventually resistant to therapy), anemia, bleeding, and other evidences of bone marrow failure, as well as from infections. Radiation therapy may be employed with profit to relieve abnormalities that result from persistent localized tumor masses. Infrequently, irradiation of an enlarged spleen will result in the resolution of constitutional manifestations and of distant tumor masses.

Adrenal corticosteroids may cause tumor lysis and a regression in systemic symptoms in a significant proportion of cases (about 25 percent). They are more useful in the management of such physiologic derangements as autoimmune hemolytic anemia, thrombocytopenia with bleeding, and hypercalcemia, however.

Rarely, acute leukemia and primary neoplasms of various types may develop in patients with long-term Hodgkin disease. These occurrences seem related to the carcinogenic properties of radiation therapy and chemotherapeutic agents. They also pose practical problems to physicians who manage these patients and who must remain alert to these eventualities.

NON-HODGKIN LYMPHOMAS[4,11,15,16]

Over the years, many types of malignant lymphomas have been described, most frequently on the basis of histopathologic features. In recent times, the terms giant follicle lymphoma, lymphosarcoma, and reticulum cell sarcoma have been replaced by the classification suggested by Rappaport and co-workers (Table 6.19–7). In general, clinicians have come to recognize that patients who have lymphomas with a nodular or follicular architecture (about one third of non-Hodgkin lymphomas) have a better outlook than those with a diffuse pattern. Pathologists and clinicians have employed the Rappaport system of classification (or closely related variants) under a wide variety of circumstances and it has proven to be very useful. Thus, even though many of the presumptions regarding cytogenealogy implicit in this system are incorrect, it must be regarded as the currently accepted standard in the United States.[7]

At present, clinicians tend to divide the malignant lymphomas into two groups: Hodgkin disease and the non-Hodgkin lymphomas. The latter is a more heterogeneous grouping that encompasses rather indolent disorders such as the nodular lymphocytic lymphomas as well as more aggressive neoplasms such as diffuse histiocytic lymphoma and Burkitt tumor (Tables 6.19–7 and 6.19–8).

Lukes and Collins (and others) have suggested a classification of non-Hodgkin lymphomas that is clinically relevant and based on the accumulating newer knowledge of the morphologic transformations associated with the normal functioning of the lymphoreticular cell system (Table 6.19–9). Their "functional classification" relates lymphoma cell morphology to the sequential stages in the histogenesis of normal T and B lymphocytes. Their morphologic observations are reinforced by the identification of T- or B-cell markers on the cell surfaces. Although clinically less useful from a practical point of view, the immunobiologic classifications provide a better conceptual framework for considering the various lymphoreticular proliferative disorders.

Immunobiologic observations indicate that the majority of non-Hodgkin lymphomas arise from the B-cell line (Table 6.19–9). Chronic lymphocytic leukemia and well-differentiated lymphocytic lymphoma appear to be closely related monoclonal neoplasms of B lymphocytes. On the other hand, lymphomas pre-

TABLE 6.19–7. HISTOPATHOLOGIC TYPES OF NON-HODGKIN LYMPHOMAS

Older Terms	Rappaport (1966)	Dorfman (1976)
Giant follicle lymphoma	Nodular lymphomas Lymphocytic, poorly differentiated Mixed lymphocytic and histiocytic Histiocytic	Follicular lymphomas[a] Small lymphoid Mixed small and large lymphoid Large lymphoid
Lymphosarcoma	Diffuse lymphomas Lymphocytic, well differentiated Lymphocytic, poorly differentiated	Diffuse lymphomas[a] Small lymphocytic[b] Atypical small lymphoid Lymphoblastic-convoluted and nonconvoluted
Reticulum cell sarcoma	Mixed lymphocytic and histiocytic Histiocytic, well differentiated Histiocytic, poorly differentiated Undifferentiated, pleomorphic	Mixed small and large lymphoid Histiocytic Large lymphoid[b] Undefined
Burkitt tumor	Undifferentiated, Burkitt type	Burkitt lymphoma

[a]Composite lymphomas comprised two well-defined cell types.
[b]Lymphomas showing plasmacytoid differentiated.

TABLE 6.19–8. NON-HODGKIN LYMPHOMAS: RELATIVE FREQUENCY OF HISTOPATHOLOGIC TYPE AND PROGNOSIS FOR SURVIVAL

Frequency (%)	Type	Survival 2 Yr (%)	5 Yr (%)
Nodular Lymphomas			
3	Lymphocytic, well differentiated	100	100
39	Lymphocytic, poorly differentiated	90	72
42	Mixed lymphocytic and histiocytic	93	60
16	Histiocytic	68	
Diffuse Lymphomas			
5	Lymphocytic, well differentiated	100	
19	Lymphocytic, poorly differentiated	48	32
19	Mixed lymphocytic and histiocytic	46	26
51	Histiocytic	30	18
6	Undifferentiated	35	

viously classified as histiocytic lymphoma or reticular cell sarcoma appear to have arisen from transformed lymphocytes of either the B- or T-cell type. A true histiocytic lymphoma seems to be a rare occurrence.

There are at present at least six different pathologic classifications for non-Hodgkin lymphoma in use throughout the world.[5,7,8] In order to facilitate international communication the National Cancer Institute sponsored a study by a representative group of experts that resulted in a unified Working Formulation for clinical use in the classification of non-Hodgkin lymphoma. This Working Formulation is compared to the Rappaport classification in Table 6.19–10.[9]

CLINICAL MANIFESTATIONS

The clinical manifestations of non-Hodgkin lymphoma are quite diverse, making short descriptions most difficult. The prognosis for survival is also quite variable. Table 6.19–8 presents the survival

TABLE 6.19–9. HISTOPATHOLOGIC TYPES OF NON-HODGKIN LYMPHOMAS: FUNCTIONAL CLASSIFICATION OF LUKES AND COLLINS (1974)

Type	Frequency (%)
U-cell (Undefined) Type	17
T-cell Types	15
Small lymphocyte	
Convoluted lymphocyte	
Sézary cell—mycosis fungoides	
Immunoblastic sarcoma	
B-cell Types	67
Small lymphocyte	
Plasmacytoid lymphocyte	
Follicular center cells	
Small cleaved	
Large cleaved	
Small transformed (noncleaved)	
Large transformed (noncleaved)	
Immunoblastic sarcoma	
Hairy cell leukemia	
Histiocytic Type	1

TABLE 6.19–10. COMPARISON OF WORKING FORMULATION AND RAPPAPORT CLASSIFICATION OF NON-HODGKIN LYMPHOMA

Working Formulation (1982)	Rappaport Classification (1966)
Low Grade	
Small lymphocytic	Diffuse, well-differentiated lymphocytic
Follicular, predominantly small cleaved cell	Nodular, poorly differentiated lymphocytic
Follicular, mixed small cleaved and large cells	Nodular, mixed lymphocytic and histiocytic
Intermediate Grade	
Follicular, predominantly large cell	Nodular histiocytic
Diffuse, small cleaved cell	Diffuse, poorly differentiated lymphocytic
Diffuse, mixed small cleaved and large cells	Diffuse, mixed lymphocytic-histiocytic
Diffuse large cell	Diffuse histiocytic
High Grade	
Large cell, immunoblastic	Diffuse histiocytic
Lymphoblastic, convoluted or nonconvoluted	Diffuse lymphoblastic
Small noncleaved cell Burkitt or non-Burkitt	Diffuse undifferentiated

outlook for patients with non-Hodgkin lymphoma classified according to the Rappaport system.[7] For convenience, selected clinical characteristics of these lymphomas and expected survival will be summarized using the Working Formulation terminology (Table 6.19–11).

Diffuse Well-Differentiated Lymphocytic Lymphoma (Malignant Lymphoma, Small Lymphocytic)

This disorder occurs most commonly in individuals over the age of 50 and is rarely seen in children and young adults. Males are affected nearly twice as often as females. Most tumors of this type are B-cell neoplasms. The less common well-differentiated T-cell tumors often affect younger individuals.

A majority of patients are asymptomatic when their disease is discovered. The usual presenting problems are connected with a painless, progressive, often symmetrical, generalized lymphadenopathy. The enlarged lymph nodes are rubbery, often discrete, and rarely adherent to the adjacent structures. Palpable splenomegaly is present in 20 to 25 percent of individuals on presentation. In 20 to 25 percent of cases, lymphoid tumor masses may present in the nasopharynx, oropharynx, or tonsillar areas. Furthermore, clinically detectable gastrointestinal tract involvement occurs in about 10 percent of cases. It is important to recognize extranodal lymphomas promptly because they require specific management.

Hematologic abnormalities are infrequent early in the course of lymphocytic lymphoma. As the disorder progresses, however, a normochromic anemia is commonly seen. Usually this relates to impaired erythropoiesis, but at times hemolysis is a major causal factor. In the more severe hemolytic states, the Coombs test is often positive. The platelet count generally is normal early in the disease but may be lower later on.

The relationship between well-differentiated lymphocytic lymphoma and chronic lymphatic leukemia (CLL) has been mentioned. These diagnostic entities likely represent different portions of the same basic disease spectrum, because transition states are often encountered. In one large series, lymphocytic lymphoma transformed into CLL in nearly 13 percent of the cases. Other observers have reported an absolute lymphocytosis in 15 to 30 percent of patients at some time during their course. At the time

TABLE 6.19-11. WORKING FORMULATION FOR THE CLASSIFICATION OF NON-HODGKIN LYMPHOMA

Subtype	Age at Onset (yr)	Sex Ratio (M:F)	Marrow Involvement (%)	Survival (%) 2 Yr	5 Yr
Small lymphocytic	26–79	1.2:1	70	80	60
Follicular, small cleaved cell	3–87	1.3:1	50	85	70
Follicular, mixed small cleaved and large cell	26–99	0.8:1	30	70	50
Follicular, large cell	16–82	1.8:1	34	62	44
Diffuse, small cleaved cell	10–91	2.0:1	32	62	35
Diffuse, mixed small cleaved and large cell	22–90	1.1:1	14	56	40
Diffuse large cell	10–88	1.0:1	10	48	34
Large cell, immunoblastic	10–81	1.5:1	12	40	30
Lymphoblastic	11–90	1.9:1	50	52	24
Small, noncleaved cell	3–90	2.6:1	14	32	23

of initial diagnosis, relatively arbitrary criteria are used to validate the terminology used. For example, patients presenting with a diffusely involved marrow who have a peripheral blood lymphocytosis in excess of 4000/mm³ are generally classified as having CLL.

As the disease progresses, patients may complain of increasing fatigue, lassitude, low-grade fever, night sweats and weight loss. The immunologic abnormalities that develop relatively late in the course of lymphocytic lymphoma are distinct from those that have been reported in Hodgkin disease. Bacterial infections are encountered with increasing frequency, and their occurrence may be correlated with a progressive decrease in γ-globulin concentration and an impairment in antibody response to specific antigen stimulation (e.g., pneumococcal polysaccharide).

Infrequently, macroglobulinemia (and its clinical consequences) is seen in association with lymphocytic lymphoma. Other monoclonal gammopathies have also been related to this disorder from time to time. Hypercalcemia may develop, too.

Nodular, Poorly Differentiated Lymphocytic Lymphoma (Malignant Lymphoma, Follicular, Small Cleaved Cell)

This subtype of non-Hodgkin lymphoma is most commonly encountered in adults and is rarely seen in children. Males and females are affected equally. Most tumors of this type are B-cell neoplasms.

At the outset, most patients are asymptomatic. They often tell of a painless, generalized lymphadenopathy which has waxed and waned over a period of several months or years prior to diagnosis. In general the course of the illness is rather indolent and the prognosis for survival is good (Tables 6.19–8 and 6.19–11).

The clinical manifestations of the nodular, poorly differentiated lymphocytic lymphoma are similar to those of the well-differentiated lymphoma. Spontaneous regressions occur more often in poorly differentiated lymphocytic lymphoma than any other subtype. Within 5 to 7 years of the initial diagnosis, about half of the patients will undergo a histologic transformation of their disease to a more aggressive subtype—generally a diffuse histiocytic (diffuse large cell) lymphoma.

Diffuse Histiocytic Lymphoma (Diffuse Large Cell Lymphoma)

Histiocytic lymphoma is encountered half as frequently as Hodgkin disease. It occurs in all age groups, but its peak incidence is between 40 and 60 years. The disorder is equally common in males and females.

Histiocytic lymphoma is characterized at first by the regional enlargement of lymph nodes or the development of prominent extranodal tumors and later by the generalized involvement of many organ systems. The invasive infiltrate characteristic of this disorder is composed predominantly of large mononuclear cells (15

to 35 μm) that contain delicate-appearing nuclear chromatin and often a single, prominent, dark-staining nucleolus. Recent studies indicate that histiocytic lymphomas in truth arise from transformed T- and B-lymphocyte precursors in nearly all instances. Although an authentic histiocytic lymphoma is a rarity, the term continues to be used in accordance with Rappaport's designation because of its clinical utility.

It is uncommon for individuals with histiocytic lymphoma to present with constitutional symptoms. The initial manifestations of this disorder most frequently are connected with a painless, asymmetrical regional lymph node enlargement, particularly in the cervical area. About one third of the patients may become symptomatic because of extranodal tumor masses, which are most apt to be encountered in the nasopharynx or oropharynx, tonsils, skin, gastrointestinal tract, or bones. Presenting complaints may also relate to enlarging mediastinal or retroperitoneal tumors.

On examination, the palpable peripheral masses are usually nontender, matted, and free of attachment to the overlying skin. A generalized lymphadenopathy is uncommon, and palpable splenomegaly is observed less frequently than in the other lymphomas (fewer than 20 percent of cases). Retroperitoneal lymph node involvement may be demonstrated in a high proportion of cases.

Hematologic abnormalities are uncommon in individuals with histiocytic lymphoma, especially during the early stages of the disease. Later, a normochromic anemia is seen commonly, and other evidences of progressive bone marrow failure may develop. On occasion, an autoimmune hemolytic process may be detected. Monocytosis has been reported with some frequency.

Histiocytic lymphoma at times develops into a leukemic disorder with the appearance of malignant histiocytes or monocytes in the peripheral blood and bone marrow. This outcome occurs in 3 to 5 percent of patients.

Immunologic abnormalities occur in patients with histiocytic lymphoma, but they have not been characterized as well as those of the other lymphomas. Viral infections (herpes zoster) and fungal infections (histoplasmosis, cryptococcosis) seem to occur with increased frequency in these patients. The serum concentration of gamma globulin usually is not altered. Monoclonal gammopathies have been reported in this setting, however, including the occasional occurrence of macroglobulinemia.

Large cell lymphomas of the immunoblastic subtype occur most often in the setting of immunodeficiency disorders, collagen-vascular diseases, or after renal transplantation. They pursue an aggressive clinical course, as do the other histiocytic (large cell) lymphomas.

The prognosis for patient survival has improved considerably with the advent of effective treatment. Unlike low-grade lymphomas in which cure is unlikely, patients with large cell lymphomas can look forward to complete eradication of their disease. The out-

look is especially good for individuals with localized disease (stages I and II).

Diffuse Lymphoblastic Lymphoma (Malignant Lymphoma, Lymphoblastic)

This convoluted T-cell lymphoma affects males twice as often as females and occurs more commonly in children and young adults. The cellular morphology of this lymphoma is similar to that found in many patients with T-cell acute lymphoblastic leukemia.

Patients frequently present with large mediastinal tumors, which may be responsible for a number of life-threatening problems (airway obstruction, superior vena cava obstruction, pleural and pericardial effusions). Presumably these lymphomatous tumors arise in the thymus. Although many patients with lymphoblastic lymphoma present with evident bone marrow involvement, they do not usually have a leukemic blood picture.

Untreated, lymphoblastic lymphoma will pursue a very rapid and fatal course. With appropriate therapy, however, it is among the most curable subtypes of non-Hodgkin lymphoma. The most effective therapy is based on the recognition that lymphoblastic lymphoma is most likely widely disseminated at the time of initial diagnosis, including CNS involvement. Therefore combination chemotherapy is the main treatment method. Radiation therapy is very effective in the management of large tumor masses.

Diffuse Undifferentiated Lymphoma (Diffuse Small Noncleaved Cell Lymphoma)

This B-cell lymphoma is a very aggressive tumor, which most commonly affects children and young adults. Both Burkitt and non-Burkitt types have been described, the latter encountered more often in adults.[2]

Burkitt tumor, which occurs most commonly in well-defined areas of tropical Africa, deserves brief mention because several of its characteristics suggest important implications for the types of lymphoma more commonly encountered in temperate climates. This lymphoma has a distinctive morphologic pattern. The neoplastic cells are rather uniform in appearance and appear to be derived from B-cell lymphoid precursors. The many large macrophages interspersed among the tumor cells often create a "starry sky" histologic pattern. Burkitt lymphoma presents primarily in children under 14 years of age, with a peak incidence in the 6th and 7th year. The manifestations of lymphoreticular proliferation are prominent, but leukemic transformation is rare. Particularly striking is the tumor involvement of the jaws and facial bones (about 50 percent of cases) and the intra-abdominal viscera. The disease is rapidly progressive, and most patients, if untreated, die within 1 year. Small numbers of similar cases have been reported in the United States and various other parts of the world.

In Africa, the epidemiologic characteristics of the disease are compatible with an infectious etiology and an arthropod vector. There may also be a relationship to endemic malaria. The Epstein–Barr virus (EBV) or a closely related agent has been identified as the possible cause of this lymphoma, and EBV antibodies have been found in the sera of all patients tested.

Burkitt tumor is highly responsive to combination chemotherapy. Nearly all treated patients improve promptly, and about half enter a prolonged complete remission. Indeed 50 percent or more of patients treated remain disease-free for over 2 years, and it seems likely that many are cured.

DIAGNOSTIC CONSIDERATIONS

The diagnosis of non-Hodgkin lymphoma presents few problems when an individual with little in the way of systemic symptoms manifests a painless, generalized lymphadenopathy. Biopsy is usually confirmatory.

Not infrequently, the physician must evaluate complaints caused by an enlarging tumor mass located in one of the lymph node–bearing areas, keeping in mind the multiple causes of lymph node enlargement. Similarly, the pressure of an extranodal mass (e.g., in the stomach, head and neck structures, mediastinum, or bones) leads to a consideration of the multiple pertinent possible causes. Again, tissue biopsy usually results in a definite diagnosis.

When patients present with fever and other constitutional symptoms or with derangements referable to one or more organ systems, the diagnostic problem is more complex. A majority of such individuals, however, have accessible tumor masses suitable for biopsy.

STAGING

The staging classification used for Hodgkin disease is generally applied to adult patients with non-Hodgkin lymphoma. Although there are several evident deficiencies to this method of staging patients, it is a useful guide to therapeutic decision making.

The same diagnostic procedures used in the evaluation of patients with Hodgkin disease are pertinent to the staging of individuals with non-Hodgkin lymphoma. Various histopathologic subtypes will require that special diagnostic attention be directed to specific anatomic sites, however. These sites include the lymphoid tissues of the nasopharynx, the gastrointestinal tract, mesenteric and retroperitoneal lymph nodes, the renal collecting system, the liver and spleen, the meninges, and the bone marrow.

Direct examination of the nasopharynx is indicated in most patients, followed by computed tomography to evaluate the extent of tumor involvement. Because mesenteric node involvement is common in non-Hodgkin lymphoma, computed tomography is recommended as well as bipedal lymphography. Abdominal ultrasonography is a very useful noninvasive method for repeatedly assessing possible lymphomatous obstruction of the renal collecting system. All patients should undergo needle biopsy of the bone marrow. Those with high-grade lymphoma should have a careful examination of their cerebrospinal fluid before beginning treatment.

Diagnostic laparotomy is usually not required in patients with non-Hodgkin lymphoma, because most are found to have stage III or IV disease before laparotomy is considered. An important subset of patients (about 10 percent), however, presents with extranodal lymphoma that is confined to the site of primary occurrence, especially the gastrointestinal tract, the head and neck, and the skeleton.

MANAGEMENT

As a group, patients with non-Hodgkin lymphoma have tumors that are very responsive to therapy. In fact, a significant proportion of patients can be cured.[13] Therefore, it is important to achieve a complete remission during the initial course of treatment and to continue therapy for a sufficiently prolonged period (e.g., 6 months) to maximize the possibility of achieving a curative result. Although they can achieve very useful results, subsequent treatment courses are not as successful in the long run.[6,11,16]

Although it is possible to set forth general guidelines for the treatment of patients with non-Hodgkin lymphoma (Table 6.19–12), such generalizations have limited utility. The optimal approach to a given patient is based on a thorough assessment of the histopathologic subtype of the lymphoma, the extent of the disease (stage), the functional impairments that exist, and the pace of the disease process. Low-grade lymphomas (Tables 6.19–10 and 6.19–11), which occur more commonly in older people, tend to follow an indolent course. The therapeutic approach to these patients is essentially palliative because cure seems beyond present treatment methods. On the other hand, the more aggressive tumors (intermediate and high-grade) pursue a more rapid course and demand prompt, vigorous therapeutic intervention, especially because many patients may be cured.

Chemotherapy is the main treatment method for patients with non-Hodgkin lymphoma. Single agents such as chlorambucil

TABLE 6.19–12. TREATMENT OF NON-HODGKIN LYMPHOMAS

Disease	Therapy
Low Grade	
Stages I and II	Radiation therapy–involved fields
Stages III and IV	Palliative radiation therapy, chemotherapy
Intermediate Grade	
Stages I and II	Radiation therapy[a]
Stages III and IV	Combination chemotherapy
High Grade	
All stages	Combination chemotherapy, CNS prophylaxis

[a]Add combination chemotherapy for large tumors, systemic symptoms.

and cyclophosphamide may control low-grade disease, stages III and IV, for months or even years (Tables 6.19–12 and 6.19–13). The treatment courses are relatively benign, and drug dosage can be managed easily in accordance with white blood cell and platelet counts. The duration of treatment is guided by the resolution of symptoms and tumor size since the therapeutic intent is palliation.

Generalized intermediate and high-grade disease (stages III and IV) is best treated by combinations of chemotherapeutic agents, each with different mechanisms of action (e.g., cyclophosphamide, vincristine, procarbazine, prednisone, doxorubicin,

TABLE 6.19–13. CHEMOTHERAPEUTIC REGIMENS FOR NON-HODGKIN LYMPHOMA

Low Grade	
Chlorambucil	6–12 mg PO daily or 30 mg/m² twice monthly
Cyclophosphamide	75–150 mg PO daily or 400 mg/m² for 3 days monthly
Intermediate and High Grade[a]	
M Mechlorethamine	6 mg/m² IV days 1 and 8
O Vincristine (Oncoin)	1.4 mg/m² IV days 1 and 8
P Procarbazine	100 mg/m² PO days 1 to 14
P Prednisone	40 mg/m² PO days 1 to 14
B Bleomycin	5 U/m² IV days 15 and 22
A Adriamycin	25/mg/m² IV days 1 and 8
C Cyclophosphamide	650 mg/m² IV days 1 and 8
O Vincristine (Oncoin)	1.4 mg/m² IV days 1 and 8
P Prednisone	60 mg/m² PO days 15 through 28
Pro Prednisone	60 mg/m² PO days 1 through 14
M Methotrexate	500 mg/m² IV day 15 with leucovorin
A Adriamycin	25 mg/m² IV days 1 and 8
C Cyclophosphamide	650 mg/m² IV days 1 and 8
E Etoposide	120 mg/m² IV days 1 and 8
C Cyclophosphamide	400 mg/m² IV day 1
O Vincristine (Oncoin)	1 mg/m² IV day 1
P Prednisone	40 mg/m² PO days 1 to 10
B Bleomycin	15 mg IV day 14
A Adriamycin	40 mg/m² IV day 1
M Procarbazine (Matulane)	100 mg/m² PO days 1 to 10

[a]Courses repeated every 3 to 4 weeks depending on patient tolerance. Therapy continued for 6 months or more depending on tumor response and toxicity.

bleomycin, methotrexate, etc.). Some treatment regimens use alternate courses of non-cross-resistant drugs to delay the emergence of drug-resistant tumor. Several multiagent combinations seem equally effective if given at full-dose levels for 6 months or more (Table 6.19–13). Radiation therapy is often employed in an adjunctive role to eradicate bulky tumors.

Although 80 percent or more of patients so treated may appear in complete remission, systematic restaging will reveal persistent lymphoma in about 20 percent. Therefore, careful restaging has become an important part of patient management in order to prevent premature cessation of treatment while there is a persistent tumor. Lymphomatous involvement of the CNS is a particular problem, especially in patients with high-grade disease. In fact, most contemporary treatment regimens call for CNS prophylaxis in these patients.

Depending on the histopathologic subtype, 25 to 50 percent or more of patients with non-Hodgkin lymphoma should be alive at 5 years, many of them disease-free and presumably cured (Tables 6.19–8 and 6.19–11). Bone marrow transplantation is being evaluated in this setting also as a possible means of increasing the cure rate.

Localized lymphomatous tumors (stages I and II and extranodal) respond readily to radiation therapy; usually doses of 4000 to 4500 rad are given over 4 to 5 weeks. Extended treatment fields (including total nodal irradiation) do not seem to offer a better prognosis. Perhaps this is not surprising in view of the fact that the vast majority of patients treated have widely disseminated, clinically occult disease at the time of their diagnosis. Nonetheless, between 50 and 60 percent of patients with localized lymphoma will remain disease free for 2 years or more following radiation therapy. The frequency of relapse, however, has led many to use combination chemotherapy given for 6 months or so after completion of radiation therapy in an attempt to eradicate all disease. This strategy is likely optimal for the management of patients with limited stage, intermediate-grade tumors (Table 6.19–12).

The major therapeutic problems encountered late in the course of patients with non-Hodgkin lymphoma are infections by bacteria, viruses, or fungi; anemia, at times hemolytic; progressively severe failure of all bone marrow elements; and the effects of enlarging tumor masses, eventually resistant to treatment. Radiation therapy applied to troublesome tumors can usually achieve useful palliation. Adrenal corticosteroids may induce tumor regression also. They are most helpful, however, in the alleviation of autoimmune hemolytic anemia, thrombocytopenic bleeding, and hypercalcemia.

MYCOSIS FUNGOIDES

Mycosis fungoides is a slowly progressive T-cell lymphomatous disorder that primarily involves the skin. A type-C retrovirus (HTLV) is the etiologic agent responsible. In its advanced stages, the disorder spreads to involve lymph nodes, spleen, bone marrow, blood, and various internal organs. The diagnosis is based on a characteristic histopathologic lesion, Pautrier abscesses, which contain a variety of normal and abnormal lymphoreticular cells infiltrating epidermal structures. In some cases, abnormal lymphoid cells with highly convoluted nucleus (Sézary cells) are found in the peripheral blood.

Men are afflicted twice as often as women. The earliest skin lesions are usually rather nonspecific in appearance. At times there is much erythema and pruritus. At this stage, a casual skin biopsy may be inconclusive, and biopsies of multiple sites may be required to establish a correct diagnosis. After several months or years, the plaquelike skin lesions may thicken into tumors. Lymph node involvement is usually manifest at this juncture and disease progression accelerates. Malignant lymphoreticular cell infiltrates next affect the liver, spleen, and a variety of internal organs. Although tumor infiltrates may compromise renal, cardiac, or CNS function,

death usually results from overwhelming bacterial, fungal, or viral infection.

Frequently, the earliest cutaneous lesions can be managed by ultraviolet radiation. The mechanisms responsible for this outcome are little understood. The more advanced plaquelike infiltrative lesions are managed best by electron beam therapy or the widespread topical application of mechlorethamine. More bulky tumor masses usually respond to radiation therapy, but the duration of these responses is quite variable. Disseminated lymph node and visceral disease is best managed by multiagent chemotherapy much like lymphocytic or histiocytic lymphoma.

REFERENCES

1. Aghai E: Hodgkin's disease: Malignancy, inflammation and abnormal immunity. Leuk Res 10:1267, 1986
2. Berger R, Bernheim A: Cytogenetics of Burkitt's lymphoma-leukaemia: A review. IARC Sci Publ 60:65, 1985
3. Cancer Facts and Figures. New York, American Cancer Society, 1987
4. De Vita VT, Jaffe ES, Hellman S: Hodgkin's disease and non-Hodgkin's lymphoma. In De Vita VT, Hellman S, Rosenberg SA (eds): Cancer, 2d ed. Philadelphia, JB Lippincott, 1985
5. Dorfman RF: Pathology of the non-Hodgkin's lymphomas: New classifications. Cancer Treat Rep 61:45, 1977
6. Gobbi PG, Cavalli C: Treatment of adult non-Hodgkin's lymphomas. Haematologica (Pavia) 71:321, 1986
7. Jaffe ES: Relationship of classification to biologic behavior of non-Hodgkin's lymphomas. Semin Oncol 13(suppl 5):3, 1986
8. Lukes RJ, Collins RD: Lukes-Collins classification and its significance. Cancer Treat Rep 61:971, 1977
9. National Cancer Institute Sponsored Study of Classifications of Non-Hodgkins' Lymphomas. Cancer 49:2112, 1982
10. Rosenberg SA: Hodgkin's disease. In Calabresi P, Schein PS, Rosenberg SA (eds): Medical Oncology. New York, Macmillan, 1985
11. Rosenberg SA: Non-Hodgkin's lymphoma. In Calabresi P, Schein PS, Rosenberg SA (eds): Medical Oncology. New York, Macmillan, 1985
12. Showe LC, Croce CM: Chromosome translocations in B and T cell neoplasias. Semin Hematol 23:237, 1986
13. Skarin AT: Diffuse aggressive lymphomas: A curable subset of non-Hodgkin's lymphomas. Semin Oncol 13(suppl 5):10, 1986
14. Straus DJ: Strategies in the treatment of Hodgkin's disease. Semin Oncol 13(suppl 5):26, 1986
15. Tubiana M, Carde P, et al: Non-Hodgkin's lymphoma. Cancer Surv 4:377, 1985
16. Yarbro JW (ed): Hematologic malignancies: Present status and future prospects. Semin Oncol 13(suppl 5), 1986

CHAPTER 6.20
The Plasma Cell Dyscrasias

Richard L. Humphrey
and Albert H. Owens, Jr.

Multiple myeloma and its variants, Waldenström macroglobulinemia, the heavy (H) chain diseases, primary amyloidosis, and related plasma cell dyscrasias, share two major features. The first is an uncontrolled proliferation of the lymphocyte-plasma cell series, and the second is the production of an excessive amount of homogeneous immunoglobulin (or subunit) by these cells. The type of protein produced serves as a convenient way to classify these disorders (e.g., IgG, IgA, IgD, or IgE myeloma). These disorders may overlap to some extent, however, and patients may display clinical features inconsistent with the disease process as suggested by the M component (e.g., IgM and skeletal lesions, IgG and hyperviscosity, and so on).

The homogeneity of the protein produced by any one patient, and its uniquely individual characteristics when compared with that from another patient, has led to the concept of a neoplastic transformation occurring within a single cell, leading to the proliferation of a clone of cells that may ultimately destroy the patient. Alternatively, if many cells are transformed simultaneously, one cell line may have a survival advantage so that when the disorder becomes evident clinically only one cell line is apparent. The infrequently observed biclonal or oligoclonal disorders might reflect the transformation of cells with equal proliferative capacity. In rare instances, the rule of "one cell–one antibody" seems to have broken down, with each cell making two or more immunoglobulins.

Patients with plasma cell dyscrasias are usually in their sixth decade or older. They may present with a variety of complaints, many rather nonspecific in nature. The abnormalities encountered most often are due to bone marrow failure, destruction of the skeletal system, progressive nephropathy, and susceptibility to infection.[12]

An increasingly large group of patients is discovered because they are found to have hyperglobulinemia when screened by a multichannel chemical analysis. Follow-up with serum protein electrophoresis or immunoglobulin quantitation or both reveals that the serum immunoglobulin concentration is elevated. At this juncture a critical distinction must be made as to whether the abnormality represents an exaggerated production of the otherwise normally heterogeneous immunoglobulins (polyclonal gammopathy) or the autonomous "neoplastic" production by a single clone of a homogeneous immunoglobulin (monoclonal gammopathy).[5,9]

HYPERGAMMAGLOBULINEMIA

POLYCLONAL GAMMOPATHY

Increased concentrations of serum immunoglobulins are seen in a variety of clinical disorders. For example, in acute and chronic infections, sarcoidosis, connective tissue disorders, and in many liver diseases, the concentrations of all or nearly all of the immunoglobulin classes are elevated (polyclonal gammopathy). This is an exaggeration of the normal situation in which antigen exposure is the driving force of the B cell transformation to plasma cells that results in immunoglobulin production (Fig. 6.20–1a,c). In recent years, very high levels of polyclonal immunoglobulin have been seen in some AIDS patients and, on occasion, to such an extent that hyperviscosity is of concern.

MONOCLONAL GAMMOPATHY

In the plasma cell dyscrasias and related disorders, there is a selective increase of a single molecular species of immunoglobulin (Fig. 6.20–1f). All molecules within this population are identical, being of one heavy (H) chain class and subclass, one type of light (L) chain, one genetic allotype, and so forth. With rare exceptions (e.g., H-chain diseases) these immunoglobulins are identical to normal antibodies with respect to their physical, chemical, structural, and antigenic characteristics. On occasion the monoclonal immunoglobulin has even been shown to have antibody-like activ-

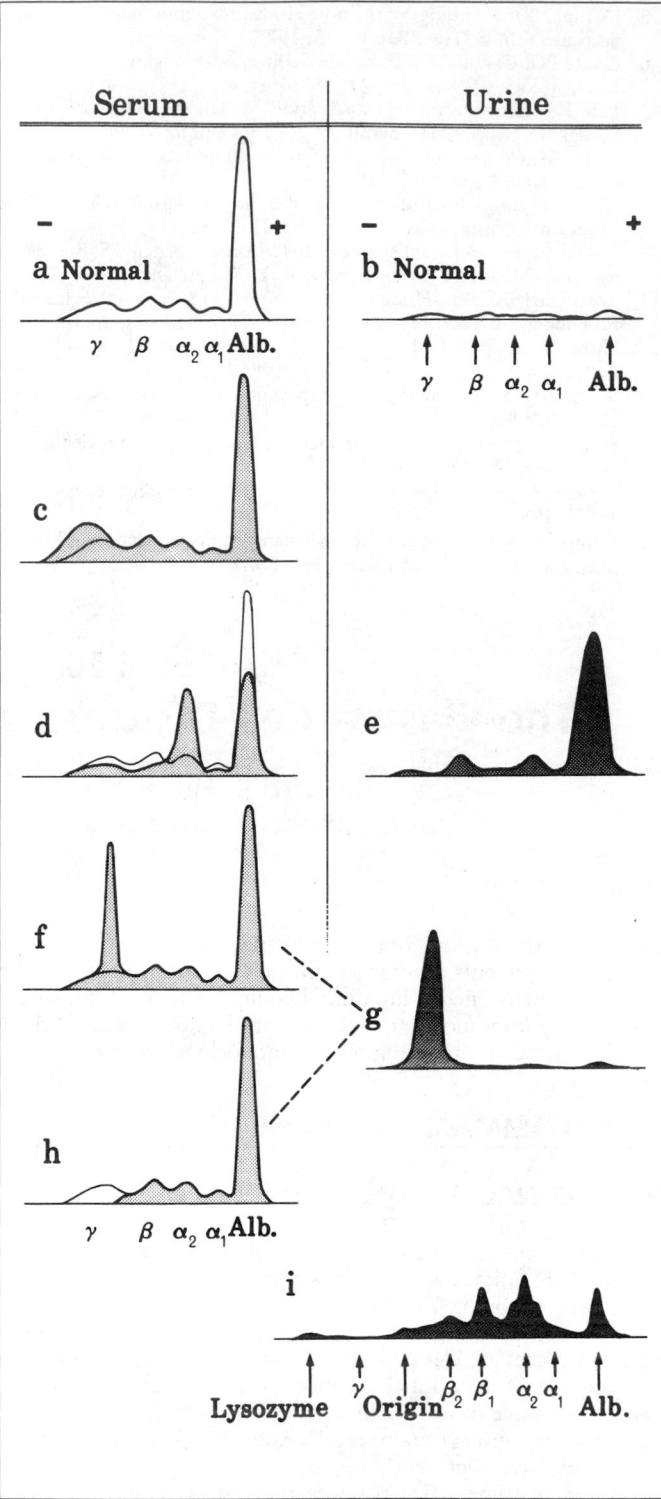

ity. These homogeneous proteins are often referred to as "M components," and the disorders characterized by their presence are called "monoclonal gammopathies" (Table 6.20–1).

In general the monoclonal immunoglobulins are composed of intact molecules, but occasionally only a part of the immunoglobulin structure is present. When excess L chain is synthesized it is readily filtered by the glomerulus, and if it exceeds the catabolic capacity of the renal tubular epithelium it will appear as a homogeneous protein in the urine (Fig. 6.20–1g). About half of these molecules display a peculiar thermal insolubility property (under acid conditions, precipitating at 40 to 60C and redissolving at 95C to 100C with repeat precipitation on cooling) and can properly be called Bence Jones protein. By extension, all free L chains (serum or urine) often are referred to as Bence Jones proteins whether or not they have this heat solubility property.[20]

There are a number of different clinical syndromes in which a protein is found related to the heavy polypeptide chain of either IgG, IgA, or IgM (γ, α, μ). Collectively, these have been called the "heavy-chain diseases."

The clinical circumstances in which such monoclonal immunoglobulins may be seen are diverse. The diseases most commonly associated with their presence, the plasma cell dyscrasias, are multiple myeloma and its variants, Waldenström macroglobulinemia, and primary amyloidosis (Table 6.20–2). Various lymphoreticular neoplasms (e.g., leukemias and lymphomas)[9] malignant tumors of epithelial structures (e.g., those of the lungs, gastrointestinal, and genitourinary tracts), and other diseases (e.g., polycythemia vera, renal tubular acidosis) may also be associated with a monoclonal immunoglobulin. Occasionally, the serum of an apparently normal individual will contain such a protein, particularly among the elderly.[5] Whether such individuals will develop other evidence of a progressive disorder or remain stable for years cannot be reliably predicted, and so these individuals should be followed at regular

TABLE 6.20–1. MONOCLONAL HYPERGAMMAGLOBULINEMIAS

I. Plasma Cell Dyscrasias
  A. Multiple myeloma (IgG, IgA, IgD, or IgE, ± free L chain; free L chain alone, rarely [<1%] no detectable immunoglobulin abnormality; very rarely bi- or oligoclonal)
  B. Macroglobulinemia (IgM ± free L chain)
  C. Heavy chain diseases (γ, α, or μ chain or fragment)
  D. Primary amyloidosis (IgG, IgA, IgM, or IgD, ± free L chain; free L chain alone, occasionally no detectable immunoglobulin abnormality)

II. Lymphoreticular Neoplasms
  Lymphoma, chronic lymphatic leukemia (often hypogammaglobulinemia; M component when present often IgM, occasionally IgG)

III. Nonlymphoreticular Neoplasms
  Cancer of colon, prostate, breast, stomach, and other sites (no consistent pattern of M components)

IV. Diseases with Autoimmune Features
  A. Mixed cryoglobulinemia (homogeneous IgM acting as anti-IgG) Cheltzer syndrome of Waldenström
  B. Hypergammaglobulinemic purpura (homogeneous IgG acting as anti-IgG)
  C. Cold agglutinin disease (IgM; κ predominantly)
  D. Sjögren disease (IgM)

V. Disorders of Varying and Unknown Etiology
  Chronic infections, parasitic diseases, cirrhosis of the liver, sarcoidosis, polycythemia vera, renal tubular acidosis (no consistent pattern of M components); Gaucher disease (IgG), pyoderma gangrenosum (IgA), lichen myxedematosus (IgG, λ predominantly)

VI. No Associated Disease
  "Benign" monoclonal gammopathy or monoclonal gammopathy of unknown significance (MGUS) (no consistent pattern of M components)

Figure 6.20–1. Diagrammatic representation of common serum and urine protein electrophoretic patterns. In each case normal (*heavy solid line*) is contrasted to abnormal (*shaded area*). **(a)** Normal serum. **(b)** Normal urine. **(c)** Chronic antigenic stimulation, resulting in broad-based increase in the γ region (polyclonal gammopathy). **(d)** Nephrotic syndrome, resulting in increase in α_2 region and decrease in other areas, especially albumin. **(e)** Glomerular proteinuria; pattern is dominated by albumin. **(f)** Monoclonal gammopathy, showing narrow-based "spike" in γ region. **(g)** Excess product proteinuria, showing narrow-based "spike" in β or γ region not corresponding to similar serum abnormality (Bence Jones protein). **(h)** Hypogammaglobulinemia, with virtual absence of protein in γ region. **(i)** Tubular proteinuria, in which globulins predominate. Multiple bands are present, including lysozyme.

TABLE 6.20–2. CLINICAL MANIFESTATIONS OF THE PLASMA CELL DYSCRASIAS

Manifestation	Myeloma	Macroglobulinemia	Primary Amyloidosis
Fever	Rare without infection	Frequent (unrelated to infection)	Rare without infection
Bacterial infection	>50% of cases	30% of cases	Uncommon
Amyloidosis	5–15% of cases	Infrequent (5%)	100%
Adenopathy, hepatosplenomegaly	Infrequent in absence of amyloidosis	Modest enlargement common	Adenopathy uncommon; hepatosplenomegaly common
Proteinuria	Bence Jones >50% of cases	Bence Jones 40% of cases	Nephrotic syndrome, 30% of cases
Azotemia	Common	Infrequent	Common in end stage
Osteolytic lesions	Solitary, 2–10% of cases. Multiple circumscribed lesions common	Uncommon (8%)	Rare
Osteoporosis	Common (60%). Without lytic lesions, 10% of cases	Frequent	Consistent with age
Neurologic	Root pain, cord compression. Rare peripheral polyneuropathy	Bizarre encephalopathy, myelitis, neuropathy frequent	Peripheral neuropathy, 30% of cases
Bleeding diathesis	30% of cases	50% of cases	Common
Blood and marrow	Marrow and sometimes blood and tissues infiltrated with plasma cells	Lymphocytoid–plasma cell infiltration of marrow, blood, nodes, and tissues	Low (5 to 10%) plasmacytosis in bone marrow
Monoclonal protein	IgG (~55%), IgA (~20%). Light chain alone (~25%). No serum or urine protein abnormality in <1%	IgM >3000 mg/dl	Common, especially λ light chain-related
Serum hyperviscosity	Rare	Common (75%) (50% symptomatic)	Rare unless IgM-related amyloidosis

intervals to observe for any evidence of progression. When stable over time this process has been called benign monoclonal gammopathy, or monoclonal gammopathy of unknown significance (MGUS). This latter term is preferable since the former presupposes knowledge about the future biologic behavior of the abnormal clone.

Monoclonal Immunoglobulin Identification

Zonal electrophoresis of the serum proteins on a supporting membrane (such as agarose or cellulose acetate) will be of great value if it reveals the very tall, symmetrical spike of an M component (Fig. 6.20–1f). M components can be stimulated on electrophoresis, however, by an extremely high concentration of polyclonal immunoglobulin (e.g., in AIDS), an increased α_2 macroglobulin (chronic inflammatory disease or the nephrotic syndrome; Fig. 6.20–1d), hemoglobin (hemolyzed sera), fibrinogen (plasma), increased lipoproteins, and a precipitate at the point of application of the serum to the strip. In addition, there are instances in which a monoclonal protein is electrophoretically heterogeneous (e.g., polymer formation or variable sialic acid content); hence the need for additional studies to add supporting information to that obtained by the serum protein electrophoretic pattern.

In the presence of an M component, immunoglobulin quantitation usually reveals a single class to be elevated, with a reduction in concentration in one or both of the other main classes. For example, IgG might be markedly increased while IgA and IgM are severely depressed. Immunofixation electrophoresis, in recent years, has largely replaced immunoelectrophoresis. This test will further reveal the monoclonal or polyclonal nature of the homogeneous band.

Demonstration of a single L-chain type (either all κ or all λ) is usually taken as confirmatory proof of the monoclonal nature of the protein. Other techniques, such as determination of molecular weight, carbohydrate content, L-chain typing after reductive cleavage of the molecule, and amino acid sequencing, may prove helpful in selected instances in establishing the molecular homogeneity of the immunoglobulin.

Immunoglobulin gene rearrangement studies are not as helpful in these diseases as they have proven to be in the diseases related to the earlier stages of B-cell maturation (e.g., lymphomas, leukemias). With these diseases, the demonstration of an immunoglobulin gene rearrangement may reveal the clonal nature of the disease process at a stage well before the cells have differentiated sufficiently to produce a detectable monoclonal immunoglobulin.[16]

Clinical Significance

The presence of a monoclonal immunoglobulin in high concentration in the serum has two major clinical implications. The first relates to its diagnostic significance (Table 6.20–1), with the final diagnosis depending on careful correlation of the laboratory tests with the clinical findings. The second concerns the physiologic abnormalities that the protein itself may cause. Such abnormalities occasionally result from high concentration of IgG or IgA immunoglobulins. About 70 percent of patients with a monoclonal IgM increase, however, will have symptoms attributable to the protein itself (e.g., hyperviscosity syndrome).

Occasionally, the monoclonal IgM (most frequently) or the IgG or IgA M component will have the property of gelling or precipitating at a temperature lower than body temperature (cryoglobulinemia).[16] Patients so affected may present with purpura, Raynaud's phenomenon, or even frank vascular obstruction with gangrene. Waldenström described a distinctive type of hypergammaglobulinemic purpura (not to be confused with his macroglobulinemia), primarily affecting young females.[9] Their latex fixation test is positive because of the small amounts of monoclonal IgG acting as an anti-IgG antibody. IgG-anti-IgG complexes are intermediate in size between the IgG and the IgM and can be resolved from the normal serum proteins by analytical ultracentrifugation. The complexes can also be detected by their reaction with the C1q component of complement, although serum complement levels are generally normal. The disease is usually benign and often spontaneous remission occurs. Therapy with corticosteroids is usually without demonstrable benefit (Table 6.20–1,IVB).

Meltzer et al[9] described another purpuric syndrome associated

with a monoclonal IgM that acts as an antibody against IgG. This disorder also primarily affects females, although it occurs at a somewhat older age. Occasionally, immune complexes are deposited on the glomerular membranes, resulting in progressive, fatal glomerulonephritis. Rarely, the amount of the monoclonal IgM may be so large as to cause hyperviscosity and require plasmapheresis. Treatment with alkylating agents, or other chemotherapeutic drugs, sulfhydryl reducing agents, splenectomy, or corticosteroids has been helpful in controlling symptoms and prolonging useful life in some instances (Table 6.20–1,IVA).

Another serious problem seen in patients with a monoclonal immunoglobulin relates to their severely disordered humoral immunity.[12] Patients with multiple myeloma, malignant lymphoma, and chronic lymphatic leukemia frequently develop an increased susceptibility to various infections, particularly bacterial infections. This acquired immunodeficiency (Fig. 6.20–1h) results from an impaired ability to synthesize specific antibody in response to antigenic challenge. This is due to the activation of phagocytic suppressor cells in the case of multiple myeloma and from suppressor T cells in chronic lymphatic leukemia. Replacement therapy with gammaglobulin preparations has not proven useful, nor has the prophylactic use of antibiotics. Febrile patients should be treated promptly with broad-spectrum antibiotics while awaiting specific identification of the causal organism and antibiotic sensitivity studies.

Amyloidosis of the kidneys, liver, heart, and gastrointestinal tract is also seen in association with plasma cell dyscrasias. Primary amyloidosis has been shown to be the variable end of light chains and consequently represents another way in which abnormalities of the metabolism of the immunoglobulins can result in disease.

MULTIPLE MYELOMA

Multiple myeloma, a plasma cell neoplasm with an incidence of approximately 3 per 100,000 is seen with increasing frequency in individuals over the age of 40. Mean and median age in most series approximates 60 years.[13] Its occurrence in men approximates that in women, but there is evidence that blacks are more susceptible and have an earlier age of onset. Although similarities exist between multiple myeloma and syndromes experimentally produced in laboratory animals (e.g., BALB/c mice), the pathogenesis of this disorder in humans largely remains unknown. Epidemiologic studies have revealed, however, that low-dose radiation exposure causes an increased incidence of myeloma.[10,19] No clear-cut role for chronic antigenic exposure has been demonstrated, although gallstones and liver disease are found with increased incidence in myeloma patients.

CLINICAL PRESENTATION

The onset and early course of multiple myeloma are usually insidious. Common complaints include weakness, anorexia, and weight loss and suggest a chronic progressive systemic illness. In more advanced cases, symptoms caused by bone involvement, anemia, renal insufficiency, neurologic deficits, and repeated bacterial infections may become increasingly prominent.

Skeletal Lesions
Bone pain of varying intensity is among the most frequent complaints of these patients. It is usually related to osteolytic lesions produced by focal accumulations of plasma cells. Although the lesions of myeloma are generally multiple, solitary skeletal defects are noted initially in 2 to 10 percent of cases. Their margins are sharply demarcated on radiologic examination; hence the common descriptive terms "punched out" and "soap bubble." They may be located in any part of the skeletal system but are identified most often in the red marrow–bearing areas of the skeleton such as the skull, spine, ribs, and pelvis. Soft tissue plasma cell tumors occur but are uncommon.

Diffuse demineralization of the bones is present in 60 percent or more of cases. Although it is most often associated with osteolytic defects, it may occur in their absence. The skeletal destruction has been related to the release of an osteoclast-activating factor (OAF) by the malignant plasma cells. Pathologic fractures and the collapse of demineralized vertebral bodies are frequent occurrences, producing nerve root or spinal cord compression. Hypercalcemia is frequently encountered in this setting but is rarely associated with tissue calcification or nephrolithiasis. Hypercalcemia can be a very severe and life-threatening problem and requires prompt treatment with saline hydration, and diuresis. Mithramycin, corticosteroids, and calcitonin have also been helpful.

About 15 to 20 percent of patients will have no demonstrable skeletal lesions at the time of their initial presentation. Failure to appreciate this fact at times obscures the diagnosis of multiple myeloma.

Nephropathy[18]
Over 50 percent of patients with multiple myeloma have free light chain (Bence Jones protein) demonstrable in their urine (Fig. 6.20–1g) at the time of their diagnosis, and 80 to 90 percent of patients develop some form of proteinuria during the course of their illness (Fig. 6.20–1e,g,i). The Bence Jones protein has the unique property of becoming insoluble at acid pH between 40 and 60C and redissolving at 95C. On occasion, the finding of proteinuria with this characteristic on routine urinalysis leads to the diagnosis of myeloma. The only certain way to determine the true nature of the proteinuria is to perform zonal electrophoresis (e.g., by cellulose acetate) followed by immunofixation electrophoresis with appropriate specific antisera. Many times, the amount of protein will be insufficient for electrophoresis, and concentrated samples (100 to 200×) will be required.

Light-chain proteinuria will often be missed if reliance is placed upon the screening tests using a dye-impregnated strip. The isoelectric point of the light chains is such that they often fail to induce a strong color reaction. A better screening test for the presence of proteinuria is the sulfosalicylic acid (SSA) precipitation test or the heat and acetic acid test, but these also may be negative if only small amounts of light chain are present. A positive SSA reaction in the presence of a negative dip stick test is presumptive evidence of Bence Jones proteinuria.[20]

Impairment of renal function can be either acute or chronic.[18] The acute form is almost always seen in patients with Bence Jones proteinuria whose illness is complicated by hypercalcemia and/or dehydration. These patients are candidates for aggressive support, including peritoneal dialysis or hemodialysis, because in many instances this acute renal failure is reversible. Acute renal failure has also been reported following intravenous pyelography, and this procedure should be avoided if possible in these patients or performed only after careful hydration.

Progressive renal insufficiency is a common occurrence and has been related to the presence of light chain proteinuria. Large numbers of eosinophilic lamellated casts are frequently present in the renal tubules, and the tubular cells themselves are markedly atrophic, often containing hyaline droplets and occasionally crystalline material. Glomeruli are usually normal for the age of the patient, but the loss of tubules is prominent, sometimes accompanied by interstitial fibrosis and a nonspecific cellular infiltration.

In the past, chronic impairment of renal function was attributed to renal tubular obstruction by these proteinaceous casts. It is now known that the kidney is the principal site for catabolism of free light chains and that toxic damage may be done to the renal tubular epithelium by the absorption and attempted catabolism of some of these Bence Jones proteins. Why some are nephrotoxic and others are not has been attributed to their isoelectric point, state of polymerization, and other physicochemical features, but a convincing molecular explanation has yet to be offered. Additional

factors contributing to renal insufficiency are amyloid deposits (seen in the blood vessels or glomeruli of 5 to 15 percent of cases), hypercalcemia (occasionally with nephrocalcinosis), and pyelonephritis.

A Fanconi-type renal tubular defect occurs infrequently in patients with multiple myeloma and results in glycosuria, aminoaciduria, renal tubular acidosis, hypokalemia, hypophosphatemia, and tubular proteinuria (Fig. 6.20–1i). Occasionally, this syndrome is incomplete, consisting only of the renal tubular acidosis.

The relative importance of these factors varies from case to case and must be considered together with the vascular lesions and possible prostatic obstructive uropathy common in this age group. Although discrete plasmacytomas or diffuse plasma cell infiltrates are occasionally encountered in the kidneys, they are rarely responsible for functional impairment.

Neuropathy

Neurologic signs and symptoms occur in about one third of patients with myeloma. Among the several factors responsible for the development of these often distressing abnormalities are nerve root or spinal cord compression because of skeletal fractures, vertebral collapse, or compression by a localized plasma cell mass. Amyloid can infiltrate peripheral nerves, and various poorly understood demyelinating syndromes can occur. These are often seen in conjunction with osteosclerotic skeletal change and are almost always seen with lambda as the light chain type. These different factors can result in various combinations of neurologic deficits, pain, weakness, and paresthesias according to the extent and location of the lesions in the nervous system.

Bacterial Infections

At times, patients with myeloma come to medical attention because of the repeated occurrence of pneumonia, meningitis, or urinary tract infections.[12] Their peculiar susceptibility to bacterial infections, especially pneumococcal, is related to their decreased ability to synthesize normal amounts of specific antibody following antigenic exposure (Fig. 6.20–1h). They should be thought of as functionally hypo- or agammaglobulinemic even though they may be chemically hypergammaglobulinemic because the M component does not provide normal antibody protection.

Hematologic Abnormalities

A normochromic normocytic anemia is an almost invariable accompaniment of multiple myeloma, and complaints related to anemia often bring patients to the physician. Rouleaux formation of the red cells complicates their proper enumeration, the preparation of blood smears, and blood typing and cross-matching procedures and results in a rapid erythrocyte sedimentation rate. Rouleaux formation and the elevated sedimentation rate may provide important early clues to the diagnosis of myeloma.

In addition to severe anemia, progressive plasma cell proliferation in the marrow may result in leukopenia and thrombocytopenia. Anemia may also result from hemolysis caused by warm or cold antibodies. Furthermore, renal insufficiency and blood loss may contribute to the anemia.

Occasional plasma cells are found in the peripheral blood of about 50 percent of cases, especially if buffy coat preparations are examined and, of course, are the means by which the tumor spreads. In 1 to 2 percent of individuals, plasma cells are sufficiently numerous (e.g., greater than $500/\mu l$) to suggest the term "plasma cell leukemia." Plasma cell leukemia may be the way in which the disorder presents, or it may be a late manifestation of an otherwise typical course for multiple myeloma. In either case, it seems to be extraordinarily resistant to chemotherapy and associated with a very short survival (median about 5 months).

Serum Protein Abnormalities

Hyperglobulinemia is observed in the majority of cases, and plasma cell dyscrasias are among the most common causes of serum globulin concentrations in excess of 5.0 g/dl. Excessive amounts of protein, homogeneous by electrophoretic (Fig. 6.20–1f,g) and immunochemical techniques, are found in the serum or urine of nearly all patients (M components). IgG or IgA M components and/or free light chains are encountered most often. In a few instances the identification of a serum or urinary protein abnormality of the myeloma type has preceded the appearance of other features of the plasma cell neoplasm by months or years. In general, the nature of the M component does not predict for survival or for response to therapy, but its physicochemical nature can lead to specific complications and symptoms.

Infrequently the IgG or IgA M components polymerize or physically associate in vivo and result in hyperviscosity. Because only about 40 percent of the IgG or IgA globulin is intravascular and the relationship between IgG or IgA concentration and viscosity is usually linear, plasmapheresis for the control of hyperviscosity in patients with multiple myeloma is much less effective than in Waldenström macroglobulinemia.

In other infrequent cases, cryoprecipitable globulins may result in Raynaud phenomenon or other vasoocclusive disturbances. Proteins that precipitate at 56C (pyroglobulins) have also been described but are of uncertain clinical significance. Certain myeloma proteins have also been observed to interact as antibodies with a variety of serum constituents with the resultant clinical and laboratory abnormalities dependent on the nature and type of this interaction.[16] For example, these proteins interacting with various clotting factors will behave as circulating anticoagulants and induce a bleeding diathesis.

DIAGNOSTIC CONSIDERATIONS

The common clinical manifestations of the plasma cell dyscrasias are compared and summarized in Table 6.20–2. The clinical diagnosis of multiple myeloma rests chiefly on the concurrent demonstration of compatible bone disease, characteristic monoclonal immunoglobulin in serum and/or urine, and typical plasma cell infiltration of the bone marrow or other tissue. Care must be taken, however, to exclude other causes of plasmacytosis such as hypersensitivity states, connective tissue disorders, cirrhosis of the liver, chronic infections, AIDS, and other neoplasms. Malignant plasma cells cannot be reliably distinguished from reactive ones on their light microscopic morphology, although various microscopic features (nuclear cytoplasmic asynchrony) have been described. No consistent or diagnostic chromosomal abnormalities have been described, but when present have been associated with more aggressive behavior of the tumor and poorer prognosis.

VARIANTS OF MULTIPLE MYELOMA

Light-Chain Disease (Bence Jones Proteinemia)[20]

In about 50 percent of the patients with IgG and IgA myeloma, the synthesis of the H and L chains appears to be well balanced and the serum immunoglobulin abnormality consists of an increased concentration of the monoclonal immunoglobulin and a reduction in the normal classes. In approximately 30 percent of the IgG and IgA myeloma cases, however, the immunoglobulin synthesis is more deranged and an excess of L chain is produced that fails to couple with H chain, escapes from the cell, and can be found in the serum by using sensitive techniques. Because of its small molecular weight (23,000 for the monomer), it is rapidly cleared from the serum through the glomerular membrane and is found in the urine (Fig. 6.20–1g). In about 25 percent of all patients with myeloma, normal cellular function is even more deranged, and L chain alone is synthesized. In these cases the serum abnormality is that of hypogammaglobulinemia (Fig. 6.20–1h). Overlooking this fact and not thinking of myeloma as a cause of hypogammaglobulinemia is a very common diagnostic error. An important clue, of course, is the presence of the Bence Jones protein in the urine.

With progressive renal deterioration and a failure to clear them from the serum, L chains will accumulate and may even reach a sufficiently high concentration to be visualized as a monoclonal band on electrophoresis. These cases (5 to 10 percent of all cases of multiple myeloma) have been designated as Bence Jones proteinemia. In some series, the patients synthesizing only L chains seem to have a somewhat more fulminant course with widespread bony disease, hypercalcemia, and relentless renal deterioration. This seems to be particularly true of those patients synthesizing the lambda type of L chains.

IgD Myeloma

Clinically, patients with IgD myeloma (about 1.5 percent of myeloma cases) are similar to those with IgG or IgA myeloma, but they seem to have a somewhat earlier age of onset and a more aggressive form of the disease. Most of the patients are male (two thirds to three fourths). It is of interest that some 93 percent of the reported cases have high concentrations of L chain in urine (versus 30 percent for IgG and IgA myeloma), with some 80 to 90 percent being of the lambda type (in contrast to about one third lambda in the other cases of myeloma). Serum concentrations of the IgD are often low, perhaps reflecting the short half-life of this molecule, and they may not appear as monoclonal spikes and hence be missed in routine zonal electrophoresis.

IgE Myeloma

Several cases of IgE myeloma have been recognized. Most of these patients had many circulating plasma cells (i.e., plasma cell leukemia) and did not have bony lesions, and almost all have had lambda light chains in their urine. Some of these patients have responded to melphalan or cyclophosphamide despite the poorer prognosis usually associated with plasma cell leukemia.

Nonsecretory Myeloma

Rarely (<1 percent), a plasma cell neoplasm will be observed that is not accompanied by an M component in either serum or urine. Some of these cases are marked by the cells' inability to secrete the M component after synthesis in the cytoplasm. Other cases seem to represent a total loss of the ability to synthesize an immunoglobulin molecule or fragment.

Extramedullary and Solitary Plasmacytomas

Patients with solitary plasmacytomas, especially if adequately treated (surgery, radiotherapy), may survive for many years. This is particularly true for those patients who have a soft-tissue plasmacytoma, many of whom are cured. It is usually observed that a solitary plasmacytoma in bone will eventually disseminate, but may take years to do so.

Amyloidosis

Extracellular proteinaceous fibrils can be found deposited in a variety of organs in 5 to 15 percent of individuals with multiple myeloma, particularly those producing L chains, especially of the lambda variety. These amyloid deposits are responsible for a variety of clinical findings depending on their extent and locations; for example, macroglossia, the carpal tunnel syndrome, restrictive cardiomyopathy, the nephrotic syndrome, postural hypotension, gastrointestinal bleeding, and various neuropathies.

COURSE AND PROGNOSIS

Untreated, median survival expectancy is approximately 12 months. Patients with several "risk factors," such as anemia (Hct <30 ml/dl), renal insufficiency (BUN >30 mg/dl), hypercalcemia (Ca^{++} >12 mg/dl), or being bedridden (poor performance status) have a median survival of only 6 to 8 months.

Other risk factors have been identified that also predict for shortened survival. These include hypoalbuminemia (<3 g/dl), thrombocytopenia (<20,000 μl), leukopenia (<1,000/μl), amy-

loidosis, plasma cell leukemia (>500 plasma cells/μl), failure to respond to treatment, or relapse after an initial response. Patients without these risk factors can have median survival expectancy of about 2 years, even without a response to treatment.

Another important determinant of survival is the tempo or pace of the disease. This is difficult to assess by the features of the disease at the time of presentation and often will be apparent only as the patient is followed. Although multiple myeloma advances with varying degrees of rapidity in different patients and may seem to remain static for prolonged periods, complete spontaneous remissions virtually never occur and progressive disease is always an indication for treatment. Response to treatment will significantly prolong survival and improve the quality of life.

MANAGEMENT

The major problems in the management of patients with myeloma are bone pain and structural defects of the skeleton, hypercalcemia, bone marrow failure with refractory anemia, leukopenia and thrombocytopenia, progressive renal insufficiency, and recurrent bacterial infections. Logical supportive treatment of these abnormalities is basic to optimal patient care. The maintenance of ambulation will help forestall bone demineralization and the development of hypercalcemia. In the management of renal insufficiency, the benefits of adequate hydration cannot be overstated. Depending on the status of the underlying disease, peritoneal dialysis or hemodialysis can be justified, and some patients have even been completely rehabilitated with cadaveric renal transplants.

In general, myelomatous tumors are moderately radiosensitive. Local radiation therapy used in conjunction with the appropriate orthopedic procedures, including internal fixation, often provides the best available palliation of local bone pain and permits rapid reambulation. Callus formation is commonly observed at the site of pathologic fractures, and recalcification may occur in osteolytic bone lesions following radiation.

A variety of agents and regimens have been studied and shown to induce partial remissions in 60 to 80 percent of patients.[3,4,8,13,15] Alkylating agents such as melphalan and cyclophosphamide are the mainstay of treatment programs that can also include BCNU, vincristine, adriamycin, and α-interferon. Such responses commonly are characterized by relief of symptoms, reduction in bone marrow plasmacytosis, decrease in L chain proteinuria, decrease in the serum M component, and improvement in hematocrit, white blood cell count, and platelets. Recovery of normal immunoglobulins and recalcification of bony lesions occur but are rare. Pulse doses of corticosteroids (e.g., prednisone) have been used in combination with alkylating agents and are clearly helpful in some patients, but their chronic use in patients with marked osteoporosis, renal insufficiency, and recurrent bacterial infections must be carefully considered because of their adverse effects on these conditions. There seems to be no relationship between the nature of the protein abnormality and the patient's response to systemic chemotherapy. Chemotherapeutic agents given at higher doses (e.g., cyclophosphamide)[15] or very intense regimens coupled with bone marrow transplantation are being investigated in the hope of improving survival or perhaps even establishing the possibility of cure. To date, combination chemotherapy has not provided any significant improvement over the results seen with the intermittent pulsing with melphalan and prednisone. Both γ- and α-interferon have been shown to be active with response rates in the 20 to 30 percent range.[4] Patients who achieve objective responses by any of these means have extended median survival expectancy, in some studies in the range of 4 or more years.

WALDENSTRÖM MACROGLOBULINEMIA

Macroglobulinemia[6] is a relatively rare disorder characterized by an uncontrolled proliferation of a single clone of lymphocytes, plasma

cells, or cells intermediate in morphology (lymphocytoid-plasma cells) that synthesize a homogeneous IgM. It is usually observed in individuals over the age of 50, with an incidence peaking in the sixth and seventh decades and of approximately twice the frequency in men than in women.

CLINICAL PRESENTATION

Macroglobulinemia may be a coincidental laboratory discovery before the onset of symptoms. The common complaints of weakness, lassitude, headache, weight loss, and mild exertional dyspnea are not distinctive and may be quite insidious in onset. As the disorder progresses, prominent features develop that mimic primary abnormalities of the cardiovascular, nervous, reticuloendothelial, or hematopoietic systems (Table 6.20–2). Many of the distinctive clinical features are related to serum hyperviscosity.

Cardiovascular System
Mild cardiac insufficiency accompanied by peripheral edema and pulmonary congestion is often encountered. Its severity is frequently related to the existing degree of serum hyperviscosity and the associated increase in plasma volume. Occasionally, low environmental temperature precipitates pain in the extremities, as in Raynaud syndrome, because of the cryoprecipitable properties of some of the Waldenström macroglobulins. Rarely, purpura, ulceration, and gangrene result from the occlusion of small blood vessels.

Nervous System
Neurologic symptoms and signs occur in about one quarter of the patients and comprise a variety of often bizarre patterns. Focal and diffuse encephalopathy, intracranial hemorrhage, myelitis, radiculitis, and peripheral neuropathy have been seen. Visual disturbances, often related to retinal hemorrhages, are common. Marked venous engorgement and segmentation of blood within the retinal vessels may be present (sausage veins). Examination of scleral conjunctival vessels with +40 diopter lens of the hand-held ophthalmoscope will often reveal dramatic intravascular sludging of the column of red blood cells ("box-car effect").

Reticuloendothelial and Hematopoietic Systems
Generalized lymphadenopathy is frequently observed but rarely is a prominent clinical feature. The liver and spleen are often slightly enlarged. An absolute lymphocytosis is seen infrequently in the peripheral blood, but more often leukopenia is encountered with a relative lymphocytosis. Abnormal circulating cells are often intermediate between lymphocytes and plasma cells in their morphology (lymphocytoid-plasma cells). Protein synthetic and immunofluorescent studies have demonstrated that these circulating cells synthesize the homogeneous IgM.

A normochromic anemia commonly accompanies macroglobulinemia. Hemolysis is demonstrated rarely, but when present may be accompanied by cold agglutinins. Many patients complain of a bleeding tendency, especially epistaxis and gingival oozing, and they may note cutaneous purpura. At times life-threatening gastrointestinal or intracranial hemorrhage occurs. The platelet count is often normal in these cases, with the coagulation abnormality related to the macroglobulin.

Other Systemic Effects
Bacterial infections are seen in about a third of the patients and account for many of the febrile episodes. Fever attributed to the disease itself is also seen, however, in contrast to myeloma, where this phenomenon is rare. Also in contrast to patients with myeloma, patients with Waldenström macroglobulinemia usually do not have bone lesions or skeletal pain, although osteoporosis is common. Hypercalcemia and renal insufficiency are also infrequent, although Bence Jones proteinuria has been reported in about 40 percent of cases.

DIAGNOSTIC CONSIDERATIONS

The diagnosis of Waldenström macroglobulinemia is based primarily on the coexistence of high serum concentrations of monoclonal IgM (defined as > 3000 mg/dl) associated with abnormal accumulations of lymphocytoid cells in the bone marrow and other tissues.[14] The predominant cells present may appear as typical plasma cells, cells intermediate between the lymphocyte and the plasma cell (most often), or nearly normal lymphocytes. Often, there is an associated increase in marrow basophils (tissue mast cells). Similar histopathologic findings may be noted in the lymph nodes, spleen, or in soft-tissue tumors. In some instances the biopsy may resemble lymphocytic lymphoma, histiocytic lymphoma, or, when scarring is prominent, Hodgkin disease. The liver (especially the portal areas) and the kidney may be infiltrated by these cells. PAS-positive staining, if present, is helpful but it is often not prominent. Amyloidosis has been associated with macroglobulinemia but is uncommon (< 5 percent of cases).

HYPERVISCOSITY SYNDROME

The IgM molecule is large and asymmetrical, having an axial ratio of about 10:1. As a consequence, it has a high intrinsic viscosity and significantly increases the viscosity of blood when it is present in high concentration. Levels of relative viscosity 10 to 15 times that of normal plasma may result. As a result of the interaction of the IgM with red cells, intravascular rouleaux formation (red cell clumping) may result in hypersequestration and shortened survival of circulating red cells, in addition to aggravating the blood viscosity. Coating of platelets interferes with their function in hemostasis. Blood flow in capillaries is compromised, and there may be anoxic damage and tissue hemorrhage. The work load on the heart is significantly increased.

The set of clinical features resulting from high blood viscosity has been termed the "hyperviscosity syndrome." This consists of a bleeding diathesis manifested as spontaneous bleeding from the mucous membranes into various tissues or at the sites of trauma. Visual disturbances result from intraocular hemorrhage and capillary stasis. A wide variety of neurologic symptoms, such as focal and diffuse brain syndromes, encephalopathy, and peripheral neuropathies, may also result from hemorrhage or capillary stasis. When severe, the hyperviscosity syndrome is life-threatening, leading to coma, convulsions, and fatal cerebrovascular accidents.

As a rule, hyperviscosity symptoms are not seen below a value of 3.0 (normal range of relative plasma viscosity is 1.5 to 1.9). The level of serum viscosity at which symptoms of the hyperviscosity syndrome arise, however, varies from individual to individual. The reasons for such variations are not fully understood, but the hematocrit level, the interaction of the IgM with red cells (rouleaux), and the presence of cardiovascular disease may make an individual less able to compensate for the circulatory derangements of increased blood viscosity and plasma volume. Whatever the factors are that cause this individual variation, the level of viscosity that will cause symptoms in a given individual is reasonably reproducible. This has been termed the "symptomatic threshold," and therapeutic measures (plasmapheresis or drug therapy) that maintain viscosity below this level will prevent the development of clinical symptoms.

This unique situation, in which the presence of the monoclonal IgM itself may account for significant symptomatology, has important therapeutic implications. Dramatic relief from neurologic symptoms, ocular disturbances, overt bleeding diathesis, and congestive heart failure may result from lowering plasma viscosity. Because most (about 80 percent) of the IgM is retained within the vascular space and since viscosity increases exponentially with increasing concentrations of IgM, plasmapheresis is an effective way of controlling this symptomatology. Because of this nonlinear relationship between viscosity and IgM concentration, modest re-

duction of IgM concentration will result in a clinically important reduction in blood viscosity.

COURSE AND PROGNOSIS

Waldenström macroglobulinemia may follow a relatively benign course for many years. Once major abnormalities develop, the usual prognosis for life is similar to that for patients with multiple myeloma. As the disorder progresses, its cellular proliferative aspects may become more prominent. An occasional patient may show a good response to therapy and be well controlled for several years, only to succumb to a disseminated proliferative phase indistinguishable from lymphocytic or histiocytic lymphoma. This can happen without an associated change in the concentration of the IgM as though a new clone has arisen that does not synthesize an immunoglobulin. In the usual situation, however, death is related to uncontrolled serum hyperviscosity, hemorrhage, or bacterial infection.

MANAGEMENT

The supportive care of individuals with macroglobulinemia is similar to that employed in multiple myeloma. In addition, plasmapheresis should be used to reduce plasma viscosity promptly and to correct the clotting defects caused by high serum concentrations of macroglobulin. Some patients can be managed for prolonged periods by plasmapheresis alone.

Alkylating agents, such as chlorambucil, cyclophosphamide, and melphalan, have been helpful in the longer term treatment of these patients. Useful responses may be expected in about 40 percent of patients who have been treated over a 3- to 4-month period with doses sufficient to produce mild leukopenia. These responses include a decrease in neoplastic tissue masses, a reduction of organomegaly, a lowering of serum macroglobulin concentration, reduced plasmapheresis requirement, an improvement in anemia, and a related improvement in the patient's symptoms. Responders have significantly longer average survival (49 months) than nonresponders (24 months). An occasional response has been produced by prednisone used alone, but it normally is given in combination with an alkylating agent.

THE AMYLOIDOSES

Amyloidosis[11] is a rare disorder encountered in fewer than 1 percent of autopsies at large general hospitals. It is characterized by the variable accumulation of an extracellular proteinaceous substance that may be found in nearly all tissues of the body. Amyloid is not starch, as the name implies, but rather a complex protein mixture dominated by a fibrillar component that can be visualized by electron microscopy.

DIAGNOSIS

The diagnosis is made histologically, although there may be certain clinical and laboratory features that strongly suggest the disorder. There are three ways to identify amyloid specifically. By light microscopy, using hematoxylin and eosin staining, there will be an amorphous, acellular, eosinophilic material infiltrating tissues and organs. More specific is the characteristic metachromatic reaction with stains such as crystal violet and fluorescence with stains like thioflavin-S. The amyloid material is identified most specifically, however, by its pink staining reaction with alkaline Congo red, which undergoes a brilliant yellow-orange to apple-green birefringence when examined with polarized light. This suggests an underlying ordered structure. Indeed, when examined by the electron microscope (the second method of identification), the amorphous material appears as a mat or web of fibrils of about 80 Å

diameter and unknown lengths (estimated in the thousands of Å). The third method, low-angle x-ray diffraction, reveals yet another level of organization in the amyloid fibril, that is, the polypeptide chains are largely arranged in an antiparallel β-pleated sheet. All of these methods give results that are largely without a counterpart in the normal individual and when taken together are highly specific for amyloid.

CLASSIFICATION

There have been many different attempts to subclassify this disorder based upon patterns of organ involvement, presence of associated disease or a positive family history, microscopic localization in tissue, ultrastructure of amyloid fibril, and so on. The problem with each of these has been the wide overlap of features exhibited by individual patients. A clinically useful and simple classification scheme is given in Table 6.20–3, and more extensive schemes are found in Glenner's two-part review.[11]

Amino acid sequence studies of the fibrillar component of amyloid from different patients have identified two major distinct biochemical forms. In the primary and myeloma-associated forms of amyloid, the fibrillar component was found to be the variable end of light chain or intact light chain. These forms of the disease, then, are truly forms of a plasma cell dyscrasia. In contrast, in the secondary and some of the hereditary forms (e.g., familial Mediterranean fever), the amyloid fibril is the same from patient to patient and is unrelated to immunoglobulin. A serum protein (SAA) is the precursor of this form of amyloid and, like C-reactive protein and other acute phase reactants, SAA is found to be elevated in chronic inflammatory states.

In most of the cases studied by these techniques, there has been no overlap between these two biochemical forms; however, in a few instances there is some evidence for the presence of both types of fibril or a discrepancy between the clinical and biochemical assignment. For the most part, however, the clinical and laboratory features fall into distinctive patterns. More recent information suggests that prohormones and an increasing list of other proteins[2] may be deposited in tissues in this structural form (Table 6.20–3).

Primary Amyloidosis

Since the demonstration of the immunoglobulin-like nature of the amyloid fibril, it is easier to understand why the symptoms and laboratory features of patients with primary amyloidosis resemble so closely those of patients with multiple myeloma-associated amyloidosis. In some cases it is hard to distinguish between these two possibilities, and often the arbitrary distinction for the diagnosis of myeloma is the existence of skeletal destruction and the degree of marrow replacement by plasma cells. Because the amyloid protein will differ from one patient to the next (variable end of L chain), there is some latitude for variation in the clinical expression of the disease (i.e., the organ predominantly involved, presence of serum or urinary M components, etc.). These variations are attributed to the physicochemical nature of that individual amyloid fibril, that is, its tissue or organ affinity, solubility, susceptibility to catabolism, and so on. Making allowances for these individual variations, a pattern emerges that is fairly characteristic.

The disease is rare before the age of 40. Peak incidence is in the middle 60s, with males outnumbering females. Symptoms are often nonspecific and insidious in onset, but fatigue, weight loss, and paresthesias are prominent. Depending upon the organ involvement, cardiac or renal insufficiency may dominate the clinical picture. Postural hypotension can occur and sometimes is very severe and difficult to manage. Carpal tunnel syndrome, nephrotic syndrome, and a sprue-like syndrome have also been noted. Physical findings include hepatomegaly, but splenomegaly and adenopathy are less common. Macroglossia with indentations on the tongue margins due to pressure of adjacent teeth is almost pathognomonic. Purpura is sometimes prominent, especially in areas subjected to trauma or increased hydrostatic pressure. Periorbital ec-

TABLE 6.20–3. CLINICAL CLASSIFICATION OF THE AMYLOIDOSES

Amyloid Classification	Associated Disease Process	Fibril Name	Parent Molecule	Distinguishing Features	Permanganate Treatment	Percent of Cases
Generalized or Systemic Forms						
Primary amyloidosis	No underlying or associated disease	AL	Immunoglobulin L chain or fragment (κ or λ)	No skeletal destruction Low (5–10%) bone marrow plasmacytosis	Resistant	50–60
Myeloma-associated	Multiple myeloma (5–15%) or Waldenström macroglobulinemia (<5%)	AL	L (κ or λ)	All other features of myeloma or Waldenström macroglobulinemia	Resistant	20–30
Secondary	Preexistent or coexistent chronic inflammatory or suppurative disease (e.g., rheumatoid arthritis)	AA	Serum amyloid A (SAA)	No M components in serum or urine No plasmacytosis	Sensitive	10
Hereditary or Familial Forms						
Familial Mediterranean fever	None	AA	Serum amyloid A (SAA)	Autosomal recessive inheritance Onset in childhood Recurrent serositis Nephrotic syndrome	Sensitive	Rare
Amyloidotic Polyneuropathy (FAP)	None	AF_p	Transthyretin (prealbumin) Chromosome 18	Autosomal dominant inheritance Adult onset Most of the various types are due to single base change (see Table 6.20–4)	Resistant	Rare
Localized or Limited Forms						
Senile Systemic Amyloid (SSA)						
Cardiac	None	AS_c		Age > 70, exclusively cardiopulmonary May be an autopsy finding and unimportant clinically	Resistant	5
Endocrine-Related						
Thyroid	None	AE_T	Calcitonin	Medullary carcinoma of thyroid	Unknown	Rare
Pancreatic islets	None	AE_P	Insulin	Insulinoma, diabetes		Rare
Respiratory Tract	None	AL	L (κ or λ)	Upper respiratory tract or lung	Resistant	Rare
Carpal Tunnel and Osteoarticular	Chronic hemodialysis	$AM\beta_{2m}$	β_2 microglobulin	Carpal tunnel and bone lesions	Sensitive	Increasingly seen in chronic dialysis patients
Nodular Cutaneous	None	AL	L (λ)	Some patients also have Sjögren syndrome	Resistant	Rare
Alzheimer disease (inherited form)	None	β protein	Larger unidentified protein expressed in brain, kidney, heart, etc.	Gene localized to chromosome 21 Autosomal dominant inheritance	Unknown	Rare
Down syndrome	None	β protein	Larger unidentified protein expressed in brain, kidney, heart, etc.	Gene localized to chromosome 21 Trisomy 21	Unknown	Rare
Hereditary cerebral hemorrhage	None	γ-trace protein	Urinary γ-trace basic protein (cystatin C)	Autosomal dominant inheritance Amyloid restricted to cerebral vessels leading to stroke	Unknown	Rare

chymosis from coughing, vomiting, or being placed in the inverted position (as for sigmoidoscopy) may be dramatic. The skin may be so fragile as to mimic epidermolysis bullosa or actually be infiltrated with nodules or plaques resembling xanthelasma. Laboratory findings may include proteinuria, sometimes in massive amounts, Bence Jones protein, serum M components, anemia, bone marrow plasmacytosis, and evidence of renal failure.

Albumin may be low and alkaline phosphatase elevated, but liver function, even with massive infiltration, usually is well preserved. In comparison with amyloidosis, in myeloma patients, in whom kappa light chain predominates (2/1; kappa/lambda), this ratio is reversed. Hence, lambda light chain seems to be more "amyloidogenic."

The diagnosis is established by histologic examination. Biopsy material is obtained more conveniently from the rectum (mucosa and submucosa), gingiva, tongue, or a clinically involved area of skin. Crosby capsule biopsy of the bowel and needle biopsy of the bone marrow, kidney, or liver may reveal the amyloid deposits. Endomyocardial biopsy via catheter has been of growing importance in establishing amyloid as the etiology in patients who present with otherwise unexplained restrictive cardiomyopathy. Bleeding can be a problem, and choice of biopsy site should partly be governed by the ease with which the complication of bleeding can be recognized and controlled.

Cardiac and renal failure are prominent causes of death, and median survival has been found to be about 15 months. Treatment to date has been largely supportive, but there are scattered reports of remissions induced with alkylating agents such as melphalan.[1] Steroids given alone do not seem to have contributed to the management of these patients. Chronic hemodialysis and peritoneal dialysis have been of help in selected patients, and a few patients have benefited from renal transplantation.

Myeloma-Associated Amyloidosis

Most of what was said above in relation to primary amyloidosis applies here. These patients, however, display skeletal destruction; more extensive bone marrow plasma cell infiltration; greater incidence and amounts of Bence Jones proteinuria and serum M components; and more anemia, hypercalcemia, and the like. In short, they not only seem to suffer the relentless damage due to the amyloid deposition but also are subject to all the difficulties of the progressive proliferation of the plasma cells themselves. Survival is accordingly less favorable than with either myeloma alone or primary amyloidosis, and median survival expectancy has been found to be about 5 months. Treatment should be pursued aggressively. The general principles of management are the same as for multiple myeloma.

Secondary Amyloidosis

This form of amyloidosis is seen in patients with coexistent chronic disease. In patients with long-standing suppurative disorders (osteomyelitis, bronchiectasis, pyelonephritis), lepromatous leprosy, paraplegia, tuberculosis, rheumatoid arthritis, or various malignancies, amyloid deposition was classically described as occurring predominantly in the liver, spleen, and lymph nodes (tissues rich in reticuloendothelial cells), as well as the kidneys and adrenal glands.

With the elucidation of the biochemical nature of the fibrillar component, it is clear that the vast majority of patients who have developed amyloidosis in this clinical setting are depositing a unique homogeneous protein (AA), which is the same from patient to patient. The hepatocyte synthesizes the serum precursor of this form of amyloid (AA) and is called SAA. There are several forms of SAA (genetic polymorphism). SAA behaves like other acute-phase reactants and is found in serum in increased amounts in inflammatory conditions. Animal studies have suggested that the clearance or catabolism of SAA is impaired in those individuals who subsequently develop amyloidosis. In large series of cases of amyloidosis, the secondary form accounts for 8 to 16 percent of the cases. In former years, tuberculosis led the list of associated diseases, but since this has come under control with effective antibiotic therapy, rheumatoid arthritis has become the most common associated disorder, with osteomyelitis second. The incidence among patients with rheumatoid arthritis ranges from 5 to 26 percent, and it should be suspected if unexplained proteinuria develops in such a patient. The clinical patterns seen in patients with secondary amyloidosis include the nephrotic syndrome, malabsorption, and neuropathy.

Management consists of adequate treatment and resolution of the underlying disease process. If this can be accomplished, there are a number of documented instances (as well as animal models) in which the amyloidosis resolves.

Familial or Hereditary Amyloidosis

There is a growing number of biochemically distinct varieties of hereditary amyloidosis, of both autosomal recessive and dominant modes of inheritance (Table 6.20–3).

With familial Mediterranean fever (FMF) there is biochemical information that reveals the amyloid in this situation to be AA in type. Its deposition is systemic, involving primarily the kidneys, liver, spleen, and adrenal glands. In this setting, proteinuria is often observed to progress to the nephrotic syndrome and eventually to increasing uremia, which results in death.

Recent studies have established the utility of colchicine therapy in reducing the frequency and severity of the febrile/peritoneal attacks of FMF, with clear evidence of prevention and delay of the deposition of amyloid and the extension of survival.

The application of the techniques of molecular genetics to the study of amyloidosis syndromes has begun to show evidence that a single amino acid substitution (mutation) in precise locations in a normal molecule is sufficient to lead to amyloid formation (Table 6.20–3). In some instances these studies have led to the ability to detect individuals who are carriers as well as those destined to develop the disease. Genetic and patient counseling are thereby enhanced. This is perhaps best exemplified in the group of disorders known as the familial amyloidotic polyneuropathies (FAP) (Table 6.20–4). To date there are at least four single amino acid substitutions in the transthyretin molecule (prealbumin) that result in somewhat different clinical expressions of amyloidosis. Other well-known kindreds remain to be studied. Exactly how a single amino acid substitution can result in clinically distinguishable syndromes also remains to be elucidated.

THE HEAVY CHAIN DISEASES

The heavy-chain diseases are rare lymphoproliferative disorders characterized by the presence in the serum and urine of immunoglobulin fragments related to the heavy (H) polypeptide chains. The H chains of the three major immunoglobulin classes (α, γ, μ) are involved with major deletions involving the V_H and C_{H1} regions.[16] The resulting polypeptide chains are only one half to three quarters the length of their normal counterparts. These fragments tend to have amino acid heterogeneity, electrophoretic heterogeneity, and a high carbohydrate content. They are often present in low concentration, resulting in a normal serum protein electrophoresis, or a low-level, broad-based band. No light chains are detected by immunofixation electrophoresis, and there are often only minimal or no abnormalities on urine protein electrophoresis. The clinical features of H-chain diseases overlap to some extent with other lymphoid neoplasms, but their unique biochemical features justify separate classification and a brief description (Table 6.20–5).

ALPHA (α) HEAVY-CHAIN DISEASE

To date several hundred cases of this disorder have been recognized, predominantly in young Arabs and non-Ashkenazi Jews residing in the Middle East. It is characterized by abdominal pain and severe malabsorption due to a malignant lymphoma ("Medi-

TABLE 6.20–4. FAMILIAL AMYLOIDOTIC POLYNEUROPATHIES (FAP)

Type	Amino Acid Substitution	Clinical Features
FAP Type 1 Androde (Portugal, Japan, Sweden, Greece, US)	Met substitutes for val at position 30	Especially lower limbs with severe autonomic dysfunction and cardiac myopathy Scalloped pupils Carpal tunnel syndrome
FAP Type II Rukavina (Indiana, Switzerland, Maryland)	Ser substitutes for ile at position 84	Upper limbs more affected than lower (may not be severe) Vitreous opacities Carpal tunnel syndrome Cardiomyopathy
FAP Type III (Iowa, Van Allen)	?	Upper and lower limbs affected Severe progressive nephropathy Peptic ulcer disease
FAP Type IV (Meretoja)	?	Corneal lattice dystrophy Cranial nerve palsies
FAP (Appalachia)	Ala substitutes for thr at position 60	Late onset (>60 yr) Cardiomyopathy Often lacks significant neuropathy and eye involvement
FAP (Jewish)	Gly substitutes for thr at position 49 and/or tle substitutes for phe at position 33	Possibly multiple variant alleles

terranean lymphoma") involving the small intestine and the mesenteric lymph nodes. The bowel wall and the lymph nodes are infiltrated by lymphocytes, reticulum cells, and numerous plasma cells. Bone marrow or other organ involvement does not usually occur. Children have been described with this protein abnormality in association with a pulmonary form of lymphoma.

On serum electrophoresis, some cases have had an abnormal band in the beta region. In all cases, characteristic abnormal alpha chains have been identified with no associated L chains. Free L-chain or Bence Jones protein has not been found in these cases. The abnormal alpha protein has not been found in the parotid saliva but is present in jejunal fluid associated with a secretory component.

Treatment has been with chemotherapy, chiefly alkylating agents or radiotherapy. About 10 percent of the patients have ex-perienced remissions with chemotherapy, but this has also occurred with antimicrobial therapy alone. This latter observation has suggested a possible premalignant phase related to chronic intestinal infection that undergoes malignant evolution.

GAMMA (γ) HEAVY-CHAIN DISEASE

This syndrome has been recognized in approximately 100 cases. The mode of onset is usually insidious, but may be rapid.

Clinically, the syndrome is characterized by fever; recurrent infections (particularly pneumonia); a peculiar (often transient) edema and erythema of the palate and uvula (attributed to lymphoid enlargement of Waldeyer ring); waxing and waning, general-

TABLE 6.20–5. CLASSIFICATION OF HEAVY CHAIN DISEASES

	Alpha	Gamma	Mu
Age at onset	10–30 yr	10–40 yr	>50 yr
Molecular weight	29,000–35,000 daltons	27,000–49,000 daltons	35,000–55,000 daltons
Presence of other M components	IgG	IgM, few IgG	IgA
Bence Jones protein	No	No	Yes
Amyloidosis	No	Yes	Yes
Hematologic findings	Anemia	Leukopenia (50%), atypical lymphocytosis, thrombocytopenia, eosinophilia, anemia (25%)	Resembles CLL
Organ involvement	Duodenum and jejunum, mesenteric lymph nodes, rarely respiratory tract	Bone marrow, lymph nodes, spleen, Waldeyer ring (85%)	Retroperitoneal nodes (often), bone marrow, skeletal destruction
Hepatosplenomegaly	Rare	Common	Yes
Lymphadenopathy	Rare	Often waxing and waning; sometimes painful	Rare
Histopathology	Massive infiltration of lamina propria and mesenteric lymph nodes	Plemorphic infiltrate; often nondiagnostic	Resembles CLL (60%) or non-Hodgkin lymphoma
Cytology	Lymphocytoid–plasma cells, occasionally immunoblasts	Lymphocytoid–plasma cells, eosinophils	Vacuolated lymphocytoid–plasma cells
Associated diseases	Chronic intestinal infection	Autoimmune disorders	Atypical CLL

ized lymphadenopathy, which is sometimes painful; and hepato-splenomegaly. (One patient has been described who had a clinical picture like alpha H-chain disease, but with gamma chain protein.)

Laboratory findings include a normochromic, normocytic anemia as well as frequent leukopenia, thrombocytopenia, and eosinophilia (sometimes marked). Many patients have had atypical lymphocytes or plasma cells in their blood, and a few cases have been diagnosed as plasma cell leukemia. Bone marrow plasmacytosis is common, as is hyperuricemia. Skeletal lesions have been uncommon.

Histologic examination of the bone marrow or lymph nodes often reveals a pleomorphic infiltration by plasma cells, reticulum cells, atypical lymphoid forms, and eosinophils. This tissue morphology has suggested the diagnosis of reactive hyperplasia, chronic inflammation, or Hodgkin disease, and sometimes repeated biopsies or autopsy is necessary to define the process as malignant lymphoma.

By definition, the feature common to all of these cases is the presence in serum and urine of a protein having the chemical and antigenic features of free gamma chains with no evidence of attachment to light chains. The concentration of the normal immunoglobulins is usually reduced.

Survival has ranged from just a few weeks to more than 5 years after the onset of symptoms. As the disease advances, recurrent bacterial infections and the progressive neoplastic growth present the main therapeutic problems. These patients require general supportive care similar to that for other lymphomas. Mechlorethamine, vincristine, procarbazine, and prednisone have been used with encouraging results. In several instances, splenic and nodal irradiation induced a partial regression in spleen size and temporary relief of systemic manifestations. Treatment of these patients with an alkylating agent (e.g., cyclophosphamide) alone has been disappointing.

Mu (μ) HEAVY-CHAIN DISEASE

An increased serum concentration of mu H chain has been demonstrated in a few cases of long-standing CLL or lymphocytic lymphoma. Clinically, these patients are unique in that they have retroperitoneal adenopathy and hepatosplenomegaly, but minimal peripheral adenopathy. In addition, the lymphocytoid-plasma cells are characterized by vacuolated cytoplasm.

Serum protein electrophoresis reveals hypogammaglobulinemia with no spike, and immunofixation electrophoresis is required to detect the abnormality. Many of these patients also have large amounts of free kappa chains (something not seen with alpha H-chain disease, and rare in gamma H-chain disease). In addition, bony lesions are seen (not present in alpha chain disease, and rare in gamma H-chain disease), as is amyloidosis (seen in only a few cases of gamma chain disease). The mu chain is not found in the urine because it tends to polymerize and is, therefore, too large to pass through the glomeruli. Fluorescent staining with specific antisera reveals that most of the cells make both the mu and kappa

chains. Their failure to be properly assembled into the whole molecule is related to a deletion in the mu chain. Many of these patients have responded to alkylating agent chemotherapy (e.g., chlorambucil) with good remissions lasting for several years.

REFERENCES

1. Camoriano JK, Greipp PR, et al: Resolution of acquired factor X deficiency and amyloidosis with melphalan and prednisone therapy. N Engl J Med 316:1133, 1987
2. Casey TT, Stone WJ, et al: Tumoral amyloidosis of bone of beta$_2$-microglobulin origin in association with long-term hemodialysis: A new type of amyloid disease. Hum Path 17:731, 1986
3. Cooper MR, McIntyre OR, et al: Single, sequential, and multiple alkylating agency therapy for multiple myeloma: A CALGB study. J Clin Oncol 4:1331, 1986
4. Cooper MR, Welander CE: Interferons in the treatment of multiple myeloma. Cancer 59:594, 1987
5. Crawford J, Eye MK, Cohen HJ: Evaluation of monoclonal gammopathies in the "well" elderly. Am J Med 82:39, 1987
6. Deuel TF, Davis P, Avioli LV: Waldenström's macroglobulinemia. Arch Intern Med 143:986, 1983
7. Durie BGM: Staging and kinetics of multiple myeloma. Semin Oncol 13:300, 1986
8. Durie BGM, Dixon DO, et al: Improved survival duration with combination chemotherapy induction for multiple myeloma: A southwest oncology group study. J Clin Oncol 4:1227, 1986
9. Farhangi M, Merlini G: The clinical implications of monoclonal immunoglobulins. Semin Oncol 13:366, 1986
10. Friedman GD: Multiple myeloma: Relation to propoxyphene and other drugs, radiation and occupation. Int J Epidemiol 15: 424, 1986
11. Glenner GG: Amyloid deposits and amyloidosis: The beta-fibrilloses. N Engl J Med 302:1283, 1333, 1980
12. Jacobson DR, Zolla-Pazner S: Immunosuppression and infection in multiple myeloma. Semin Oncol 13:282, 1986
13. Kyle RA: Diagnosis and management of multiple myeloma and related disorders. Prog Hematol 14:257, 1986
14. Kyle, RA, Garton JP: The spectrum of monoclonal gammopathy in CBO cases. Mayo Clinic Proc 62:719, 1987
15. Lenhard RE Jr, Oken MM, et al: High-dose cyclophosphamide. An effective treatment for advanced refractory multiple myeloma. Cancer 53:1456, 1984
16. Merlini G, Farhangi M, Osserman EF: Monoclonal immunoglobulins with antibody activity in myeloma, macroglobulinemia and related plasma cell dyscrasias. Semin Oncol 13:350, 1986
17. Rosen SM, Buxbaum JN, Frangione B: The structure of immunoglobulins and their genes, DNA rearrangement and B cell differentiation, molecular anomalies of some monoclonal immunoglobulins. Semin Oncol 13:260, 1986
18. Rota S, Mougenot B, et al: Multiple myeloma and severe renal failure: A clinicopathologic study of outcome and prognosis in 34 patients. Medicine 66:126, 1987
19. Shigematsu I, Kagan A: Cancer in atomic bomb survivors (GANN Monograph on Cancer Research No. 32). New York, Plenum/Japan Scientific Societies Press, 1986
20. Solomon A: Clinical implications of monoclonal light chains. Semin Oncol 13:341, 1986

CHAPTER 6.21
Breast Cancer

Martin D. Abeloff

Breast cancer is a rare occurrence in women under the age of 25, but it steadily increases in incidence throughout the years thereafter. Each year approximately 120,000 new cases of breast cancer are diagnosed in the United States and nearly half a million cases worldwide. Approximately 40,000 women in the United States die annually of metastatic breast cancer.

ETIOLOGY

Genetic factors appear to affect the incidence of breast cancer. Although detailed cytogenetic examination of breast cancer has lagged behind the study of hematopoietic neoplasms, available data

indicates that most breast cancers demonstrate chromosome alterations, usually hyperdiploidy with markers.[8] No clear association is known to exist between the currently recognized chromosome alterations in human breast cancer and specific cellular oncogenes.

Female relatives of breast cancer patients have a risk of developing breast cancer that is three to five times greater than the general population. When daughters of patients develop breast cancer it tends to occur at an earlier age. Asians are less susceptible to breast cancer than Caucasians. Although the incidence in Asians increases on migrating to the Western world, it is still lower than in Caucasian women.

Other factors that appear to relate to a higher risk of developing breast cancer include nulliparity, late first pregnancy, radiation, and benign proliferative disease. A recent study indicates that biopsy specimens lacking proliferative disease do not identify women at increased risk of cancer.[2] The numerical values for relative risk of cancer for patients with proliferative disease without cellular atypia and proliferative disease with atypia were 1.9 and 5.3, respectively. The risk of women with biopsy-proven atypia and a family history of breast cancer was 11 times that in women who had nonproliferative lesions without a family history of the disease.

The role of dietary fat content as a risk factor remains controversial. There is ample data from animal tumor models that a high-fat diet predisposes to breast cancer, but conflicting reports have appeared in regard to human breast cancer.[9] There is also recent evidence that the use of alcohol may increase the incidence of this neoplasm.[7]

PATHOGENESIS

The majority of breast cancers arise in the small mammary ducts. Noninvasive cancers (lobular carcinoma in situ and intraductal carcinoma) were considered to be rarities in the past, but incidence rates now appear to range from 1.4 to 10 percent. In patients with infiltrating cancer, several independent in situ lesions are often found on careful pathologic examination and may be present in the opposite breast also. Approximately 80 percent of breast cancers are classified as infiltrating ductal carcinoma (scirrhous adenocarcinoma). Infiltrating lobular carcinoma comprises 10 percent of cases. The less common histologic types (medullary, comedo, papillary, tubular, colloid, and adenocystic carcinomas) have a better prognosis than the more common infiltrating cancers.

It appears that breast cancer is a relatively slow-growing neoplastic process. Doubling times of breast cancer have been noted to vary widely, however, with averages of 40 to 300 days. Spread to the regional nodes is achieved via the draining lymphatics and to distant sites via the bloodstream.

CLINICAL MANIFESTATIONS

Fully 80 percent of women with breast cancer present with a painless lump that they found themselves. In 90 to 95 percent of cases, a firm breast mass is the major clinical finding. Retraction of the skin or nipple, patchy edema of the skin, or discharge from the nipple are likely to relate to an underlying cancer. On rare occasions, there are eczematoid changes or signs of tissue inflammation that are associated with a rapidly growing, aggressive cancer (inflammatory cancer).

It is rare for patients with breast cancer to present with systemic symptoms or with disseminated cancer. Breast cancer has been associated with various physiologic abnormalities that appear to be mediated by humoral substances (e.g., ectopic hormone secretion), but these syndromes are encountered less frequently than in other tumor types.

The extent of the disease at diagnosis is an important determinant of prognosis. Even in patients with distant metastases, the number of sites involved bears on longevity. The TNM clinical staging system is the one used most widely (see p. 382).

TABLE 6.21–1. RECURRENCE RATES IN BREAST CANCER PATIENTS WITH POSITIVE AXILLARY NODES

Axillary Lymph Nodal Status	Recurrence Rates (%) Following Radical Mastectomy		
	1.5 Yr	3 Yr	5 Yr
1–3 positive nodes	13	37	53
>4 positive nodes	52	68	80

Adapted from National Surgical Adjuvant Breast Program Studies; Fisher, B: Surgical adjuvant chemotherapy in cancer of the breast: Results of a decade of cooperative investigation. Ann Surg 168:337, 1968.

The important prognostic factor in patients with operable disease is the histologic status of the axillary lymph nodes (Table 6.21–1). The size of the primary tumor also has predictive importance. Nevertheless, although patients with stage I disease (small tumor size, histologically node-negative) comprise the best prognostic group, approximately 25 percent of these patients will experience a recurrence within 5 years of diagnosis. The presence or absence of estrogen and progesterone receptors in the primary tumor has been shown to have prognostic significance in stage I disease. Patients with histologically negative nodes and receptor-negative cancers will experience recurrence more quickly than patients with receptor-positive tumors. In addition, estimates of the tumor proliferative capacity by thymidine-labelling index studies or flow cytometry measurements of DNA content and ploidy may provide another means of prognosticating for relapse and survival (Table 6.21–2).[3] Studies are ongoing to assess the utility of growth factor receptors and oncogene expression of prognostic factors.

DIAGNOSIS

The diagnosis of breast cancer usually is not difficult. Certain benign lesions present as painless masses. These include adenofibromas, cystosarcoma phyllodes (rare cases are malignant), cystic disease, plasma cell mastitis, and fat necrosis. Intraductal papillomas may be appreciated as small masses, but there is generally a nipple discharge. Rarely do soft-tissue sarcomas, lipomas, and other connective tissue tumors present in the breast.

Surgical biopsy is the definitive diagnostic procedure, and this should not be delayed. In premenopausal women less than 20 percent of dominant masses in the breast will be malignant, but in postmenopausal women over 80 percent will be cancers.

COURSE AND MANAGEMENT

Breast cancer is one disease in which the utility of early detection has been demonstrated. It appears that regular breast self-examination and yearly mammography and physical examination carried out in asymptomatic women result in diagnosis of breast cancers at a more limited stage. A significant decrease in the case fatality rate (in women 50 years of age or older) has been demonstrated. Recent results from the Breast Cancer Detection Demonstration Project indicate comparable results in women under 40. The cur-

TABLE 6.21–2. PROGNOSTIC FACTORS INDICATING HIGH RISK OF RECURRENCE IN PATIENTS WITH PRIMARY BREAST CANCER

- Axillary lymph node involvement
- Larger tumor size
- Absence of estrogen and progesterone receptors
- High proliferative fraction indicated by thymidine-labeling index or DNA content studies

rent screening guidelines recommend performing mammography yearly in asymptomatic women aged 40 to 50 and older and following a similar routine in younger women with a personal or family history of breast cancer. It is estimated that currently only 15 percent of women aged 50 to 70 have annual mammography. If that percentage could be increased to 80 percent, mortality from breast cancer could be reduced by approximately 30 percent in the screened group.

LIMITED-STAGE CANCER

A careful and expeditious clinical staging evaluation is a necessary prerequisite to the decision for primary therapy. Key factors that are utilized in the decision-making process include menopausal status, pathologic size of primary tumor, histologic status of axillary lymph nodes, and estrogen and progesterone receptors. Therapeutic options for stages I and II lesions include mastectomy or excision of primary tumor accompanied by definitive radiation therapy without mastectomy. Axillary lymph node dissection or sampling should be performed to assess the need for systemic adjuvant therapy.

Operable stage III tumors can be treated initially with mastectomy followed by systemic therapy in conjunction with radiation therapy. Inoperable stage III disease and inflammatory breast cancer require vigorous multiagent chemotherapy to treat the primary tumor as well as occult distant metastases.[6] Radiation therapy can be employed to provide local control, and surgical management can be utilized in tumors rendered operable by the systemic therapy.

Although the majority of patients present with clinically localized disease, the prognosis is ultimately determined by the behavior of occult distant micrometastases present at the time of initial diagnosis. Once clinically detectable metastases are evident, cure is generally not achievable. One of the most important challenges in the management of breast cancer, therefore, is the eradication of occult micrometastases with systemic adjuvant therapy.

Significant advances have been made in adjuvant chemotherapy and hormonal therapy of breast cancer, but optimal therapy has not been defined for any subset of patients.[6] Based on the research data presented at the 1985 National Institutes of Health Consensus Development Conference,[5] a 12-member panel concluded that combination chemotherapy should be considered standard care for premenopausal patients with positive nodes regardless of hormone receptor status and that the antiestrogen tamoxifen is the treatment of choice for postmenopausal women with positive nodes and positive hormone receptor levels (Table 6.21–3). For postmenopausal women with positive nodes and negative receptor levels, chemotherapy may be considered but is not recommended

as standard practice. The efficacy of adjuvant therapy in patients with negative nodes has not been firmly established, but such therapy should be considered for high-risk patients in this group.

DISSEMINATED CANCER

Disseminated breast cancer is managed best with hormonal therapy or multiagent chemotherapy depending on the disease extent, the organ sites involved, the rate of progression of the disease, and the general medical condition of the patient (Table 6.21–3). The precise quantitation of estrogen receptor (ER) and progesterone receptor (PgR) in freshly excised tumor tissue is pivotal in constructing a rational treatment plan. In receptor-positive tumors, hormonal therapy will result in meaningful regressions in two thirds of the cases. In premenopausal patients with receptor-positive tumors, oophorectomy or antiestrogens (tamoxifen) are equally effective as first treatments. In postmenopausal patients, tamoxifen is generally preferred. Patients whose tumors are responsive to hormonal manipulations are likely to benefit from further endocrine therapy (aromatase inhibitors such as aminoglutethimide, estrogens, progestins, androgens) when their disease becomes progressive again.

The major indication for multiagent chemotherapy is disseminated disease that is rapidly progressive or involves major visceral organs.[1] Among the drugs used in current combinations are cyclophosphamide, methotrexate, 5-fluorouracil, and adriamycin. Meaningful partial remissions will be achieved in 50 to 70 percent of cases, but complete remissions are rare. The onset of antitumor response usually occurs within 4 to 8 weeks. When patients respond favorably, treatment is generally given over a protracted period, perhaps 12 to 24 months or until there is clear evidence of tumor progression. Radiation therapy is useful in the management of symptomatic tumor masses.

Chemotherapy is the most effective treatment for receptor-negative disseminated breast cancer or disease that is clinically refractory to endocrine therapy. (The likelihood of receptor-negative tumors responding to hormonal manipulations is quite small.) Although there is some evidence that ER-negative tumors have higher growth fractions, the clinical results to date are conflicting as to whether ER-positive or negative tumors are more responsive to multiagent chemotherapy.

SUPPORTIVE CARE

DIRECT EFFECTS OF TUMOR

The quality of life and in certain instances duration of survival of the patient with disseminated breast cancer can be significantly im-

TABLE 6.21–3. SYSTEMIC TREATMENT OF DISSEMINATED BREAST CANCER

| Patient Status | Tumor Characteristics | | Initial Treatment |
	Receptor	Metastatic Sites	
Clinically Occult Metastases			
Premenopausal	+ or −	Involved regional nodes	Adjuvant chemotherapy
Postmenopausal	+	Involved regional nodes	Antiestrogen therapy
Postmenopausal	−	Involved regional nodes	?Adjuvant chemotherapy
Clinically Obvious Metastases			
Premenopausal	+	Nodal, soft tissue, bones, pleura	Endocrine therapy: antiestrogen or bilateral oophorectomy
Postmenopausal	+	Nodal, soft tissue, bones, pleura	Antiestrogen
Premenopausal	+	Liver, lymphangitic lung	Combination chemotherapy ± endocrine therapy
Postmenopausal	+		
Premenopausal	−	Any site	Combination chemotherapy
Postmenopausal	−		

TABLE 6.21–4. COMMON COMPLICATIONS OF BREAST CANCER

- Chest wall recurrence
- Bony metastases
- Hypercalcemia
- Neurologic problems
    - Spinal cord compression
    - Intracranial metastases
    - Leptomeningeal metastases
- Malignant effusions—pleural, pericardial

proved by prompt diagnosis and therapy of the common major complications (Table 6.21–4).

Early detection of local-regional recurrence (chest wall, axillary, or internal mammary nodes) and prompt initiation of radiation therapy can prevent cosmetically disfiguring chest wall complications as well as neurologic impairment secondary to brachial plexus involvement. Likewise, the radiologic diagnosis of a focal osseous lesion as the cause of bony pain can enable the radiotherapist to relieve this pain and prevent a pathologic fracture. Elective orthopedic pinning should be considered when a painful lytic lesion disrupts the cortex of a weight-bearing bone.

The most common clinically significant metabolic complication of breast cancer is hypercalcemia. The symptoms of hypercalcemia (nausea, vomiting, constipation, polyuria, polydipsia, lethargy) can be mistakenly attributed to other effects of progressive cancer or side effects of narcotics and chemotherapy. A low index of suspicion for hypercalcemia is appropriate in non-ambulatory patients with extensive bony metastases. Hypercalcemia can be readily reversed with vigorous hydration, diuretics, and agents such as mithramycin and diphosphonates. Long-term control of hypercalcemia is dependent on successful therapy of the metastatic breast cancer.

Neurologic complications as a result of spinal cord compression, intracranial metastases, or leptomeningeal carcinomatosis represent a major cause of debilitation for the patient with advanced breast cancer. The key to effective therapy of epidural cord compression is establishing the diagnosis before significant neurologic impairment develops. Epidural spinal cord compression must be considered in the differential diagnosis of persistent back pain even without neurologic findings in a patient with breast cancer.

Respiratory and cardiac symptoms secondary to malignant effusions can be effectively managed by systemic therapy of breast cancer and by mechanical drainage procedures with installation of sclerosing agents. The selection of therapy is based on the distribution of other metastatic lesions, likelihood of response to chemotherapy or endocrine therapy, degree of physiologic compromise caused by the effusion, and rapidity of accumulation of the fluid.

COMPLICATIONS OF THERAPY

Skillful management of breast cancer not only requires understanding of the natural history of the disease process and the therapeutic options but also in-depth knowledge of the potential complications of the myriad surgical, radiotherapeutic, endocrine, and chemotherapeutic approaches. These complications of therapy can be particularly distressing to the patient in the adjuvant setting in which the patient begins treatment with few if any physical symptoms secondary to the cancer. Symptoms such as weight gain, alopecia, hot flashes, and other gynecologic effects secondary to artificially induced menopause can add further to the diminished self-image of a patient who has undergone surgical ablation of the breast. Considerable attention to psychosocial as well as medical supportive care is indicated in these situations.

REFERENCES

1. Consensus Conference: Adjuvant chemotherapy for breast cancer. JAMA 254:3461, 1985
2. Dupont WD, Page DL: Risk factors for breast cancer in women with proliferative breast disease. N Engl J Med 312:146, 1985
3. Hedley DW, Rugg CA, et al: Influence of cellular DNA content on disease-free survival of stage II breast cancer patients. Cancer Res 44:5395, 1984
4. Henderson IC: Chemotherapy for advanced disease. In Bonadonna G (ed): Breast Cancer, Diagnosis and Management, New York, Wiley, 1984
5. Proceedings of the NIH Consensus Development Conference on the Adjuvant Chemotherapy and Endocrine Therapy for Breast Cancer. In NCI Monograph No. 1, US Department of Health and Human Services, Bethesda, Md, 1986
6. Rouesse J, Friedman S, et al: Primary chemotherapy in the treatment of inflammatory breast carcinoma: a study of 230 cases from the Institute Gustave Roussy. J Clin Oncol 4:1765, 1986
7. Schatzkin A, Jones DY, et al: Alcohol consumption and breast cancer in the epidemiologic follow-up study of the First National Health and Nutrition Examination Survey. N Engl J Med 316:1169, 1987
8. Trent JM: Cytogenetic and molecular biologic alterations in human breast cancer: A review. Breast Cancer Res Treat 5:221, 1985
9. Willett WC, Stampsfer MJ, et al: Dietary fat and the risk of breast cancer. N Engl J Med 316:22, 1987

CHAPTER 6.22
Lung Cancer

Melvyn S. Tockman, Wilmot C. Ball, Jr., and Martin D. Abeloff

ETIOLOGY

Carcinoma of the lung (bronchogenic cancer) is the only malignant tumor whose incidence is increasing dramatically, and it is now the leading cause of cancer deaths in both men and women.[1] While there have been advances in methods for diagnosis and staging as well as treatment of lung cancer, almost 90 percent of those who develop lung cancer die of the disease. When a patient presents with symptoms, physical signs, or radiographic findings that suggest a diagnosis of lung cancer, it is the physician's responsibility to obtain histologic or cytologic proof of the diagnosis, to determine the cell type, and to stage the disease so that appropriate therapy can be chosen.

Bronchogenic cancers are thought to arise from the bronchial epithelium. Epithelial exposures to environmental agents have been causally associated with bronchogenic cancer. These agents include cigarette smoke, asbestos, chemicals (chromate, coke oven gases, bis-chloromethyl ether, nickel) and ionizing radiation (uranium ore).

Recent studies indicated the fundamental role of specific genetic factors in the carcinogenic process. For example, deletion in

the short arm of chromosome 3 (3p−) seems specifically related to small cell cancer.[10] According to the present understanding, DNA modification (somatic cell mutation) by activated carcinogens is the basic mechanism by which environmental agents "cause" pulmonary and probably all neoplasms. Genetic controls may regulate the concentrations of carcinogen-activating enzymes (aryl hydrocarbon hydroxylase) present in bronchial epithelial cells. In lung cancers, activation of members of several oncogene families have been described. The oncogene abnormalities can perhaps be explored as molecular probes in selecting patients for preventive therapy or as targets for specific anticancer treatments.[5]

Although the agents capable of causing bronchogenic cancer are diverse, none contributes as much to the increasing lung cancer incidence as does cigarette smoking. Lung cancer risk increases with the number of cigarettes smoked, the duration of smoking, and the tar content of the cigarettes. Recent evidence suggests that after controlling for cigarette smoking, the risk of lung cancer increases in proportion to the degree of airway obstruction, up to five-fold higher than among smokers without underlying pulmonary disease.[8] It has been postulated that the genetic substrate for development of chronic obstructive pulmonary disease is associated with that for the development of lung cancer. Of great importance is the fact that smoking cessation can greatly reduce the incidence of cancer in (former) cigarette smokers.

CLINICAL MANIFESTATIONS

Because of the absence of pain fibers in the lung parenchyma, a tumor arising in the lung often causes no symptoms unless it involves a bronchus, extends into adjacent structures, or produces distant metastases. In most cases, cough or chest pain is the initial complaint, but there is a wide spectrum of presenting clinical manifestations (Table 6.22–1). Patients with lung cancer often develop one or more of these manifestations as their disease progresses. Of special interest are the paraneoplastic syndromes (including weight loss) that in some instances may develop before the tumor itself is identifiable (Table 6.22–2). In about 10 percent of cases, lung cancer occurs in an asymptomatic individual and is first suspected because of a radiographic abnormality.

Manifestations unrelated to the primary tumor frequently are the first to become apparent clinically. For example, approximately one third of all bronchogenic cancers produce intracranial metastases, and 10 to 12 percent of these produce symptoms that precede those of the primary growth.

CELL TYPE

Although four major cell types are recognized (epidermoid or squamous cell carcinoma, adenocarcinoma, large cell carcinoma, and small cell carcinoma), there is good evidence that these cell types originate from a common tissue and represent clonal expansions of cells transformed at various stages of differentiation.[10] There is evidence too that the cancers themselves continue to "differentiate" and present mixed cell populations or altered cytomorphology at later points in the course of the disease. Cell type is associated with site of origin and rate of growth. Epidermoid and small cell cancers often arise centrally, while adenocarcinoma usually arises peripherally in the tracheobronchial tree. Epidermoid cancers are often preceded by multifocal dysplastic lesions or in situ cancers that are difficult to detect by ordinary clinical methods.

Small cell carcinoma is the most aggressive cell type, showing rapid growth and early metastasis to remote sites, and is usually treated with chemotherapy and radiation. The other cell types, collectively designated "non–small cell carcinoma," vary in their biological characteristics and clinical features. *Squamous carcinoma* typically arises within a large or medium bronchus, most frequently in an upper lobe, often spreads proximally within the mucosa, and

TABLE 6.22–1. CLINICAL MANIFESTATIONS OF LUNG CANCER

Location of Tumor	Symptoms and Signs
Primary Tumor	
Endobronchial tumor	Cough, hemoptysis, wheezing, dyspnea, lobar or segmental atelectasis, postobstructive pneumonia or abscess
Tumor extension to pleura	Chest pain, serous or bloody pleural effusion, dyspnea
Tumor in superior sulcus	Arm or shoulder pain (invasion of brachial plexus), Horner syndrome, vasomotor changes in hand
Mediastinal invasion	Pain in anterior chest, edema of arm and face (obstruction of superior vena cava), hoarseness (interruption of recurrent laryngeal nerve), paralysis of diaphragm (interruption of recurrent laryngeal nerve), paralysis of diaphragm (interruption of phrenic nerve), dysphagia, GI bleeding (invasion of esophagus), chylous pleural effusion (obstruction of thoracic duct), cardiac tamponade (pericardial effusion)
Distant Metastases	
Peripheral lymph nodes, skin, liver	Palpable tumor masses
Bone	Bone pain, pathologic fracture, signs of hypercalcemia
Nervous system	Paralysis, seizures, signs of increased intracranial pressure
Adrenal cortex	Adrenal insufficiency
Paraneoplastic Syndromes	See Table 6.22–2

commonly presents with cough, hemoptysis, wheezing, or postobstructive atelectasis or pneumonia. In only 20 percent is the primary lesion located in the periphery of the lung. Squamous carcinoma is the only cell type likely to be detected by sputum cytology before it produces a radiographic abnormality and may be multifocal in up to one fifth of cases. *Adenocarcinoma* nearly always arises as a nodule in the periphery of the lung. It may increase in size very slowly (up to 6 months to double in volume) but is more prone than squamous carcinoma to show lymphangitic spread in the lung, to produce pleural effusion, and to metastasize widely. Most "scar carcinomas" are adenocarcinomas. Bronchoalveolar carcinoma, a subtype of adenocarcinoma, has a tendency to spread via the airway, producing patchy, segmental, or even lobar infiltrates. Occasionally even a small tumor of this type is associated with copious sputum production. Multifocal and diffuse bilateral forms are sometimes seen. *Large cell carcinoma* is a poorly differentiated tumor characterized by rapid growth and early spread to mediastinal nodes. It usually begins as a peripheral nodule, which may become very large.

The spectrum of paraneoplastic syndromes (Table 6.22–2) also depends upon cell type. For example, Cushing syndrome and the syndrome of inappropriate antidiuretic hormone (ADH) release are seen almost exclusively in patients with small cell carcinoma, while hypercalcemia resulting from an ectopic parathormone-like substance is usually seen in squamous carcinoma.

Planning of both medical work-up and therapy depends upon the results of histologic or cytopathologic study of the tumor. For example, if needle biopsy of a lung nodule shows small cell carcinoma, a detailed search for metastases, including marrow biopsy,

TABLE 6.22–2. PARANEOPLASTIC SYNDROMES IN LUNG CANCER

Syndrome	Clinical Features	Associated Cell Type(s)
General		
Asthenia	Weakness, weight loss, anorexia	Any
Endocrine		
Cushing syndrome	Hypertension, hyperglycemia, hypokalemia	Small cell
Carcinoid syndrome	Diarrhea, flushing	Small cell
Hyperparathyroidism	Hypercalcemia	Squamous cell
Inappropriate ADH	Hyponatremia	Small cell
Ectopic gonadotropin	Gynecomastia	Any but mostly large cell
Ectopic insulin	Hypoglycemia	Squamous cell
Neuromuscular		
Cerebellar degeneration	Ataxia	
Peripheral neuropathy	Distal weakness, sensory loss	Any, but small cell most common, rarely adenocarcinoma
Multifocal leukoencepholopathy	Focal motor and sensory abnormalities	
Myopathy	Proximal muscle weakness and degeneration	
Eaton–Lambert (myasthenic) syndrome	Weakness improving on repeated stimulation	Small cell
Miscellaneous		
Hypertrophic pulmonary osteoarthropathy	Clubbing; bone pain in shins, ankles or hands	Usually squamous, never small cell
Migratory thrombophlebitis	May affect multiple sites or upper extremities	Any

TABLE 6.22–3. COMMON RADIOGRAPHIC PATTERNS IN CARCINOMA OF THE LUNG

Pattern	Characteristics	Associated Cell Type(s)
Solitary nodule	Borders indistinct if lesion small Low density by CT	Any, usually adenocarcinoma
Cavitary nodule	Irregular, thick cavity wall	Mostly squamous cell
Lobar atelectasis	Central mass often visible. Air bronchogram usually absent	Any, but mostly squamous cell
Segmental or lobar pneumonia	Pneumonia often chronic or poorly resolving usually associated with some loss of volume	Any
Hilar enlargement	From primary tumor: unilateral, discrete mass	Mostly squamous cell
	From node metastases: very large, sometimes bilateral	Typically small cell or large cell
Diffuse interstitial	Multinodular, reticular or linear pattern, Kerley B lines	Mostly adenocarcinoma
Diffuse bronchopneumonic	Alveolar densities in segmental or lobar distribution	Alveolar cell carcinoma

nign, but those greater than 1.5 cm have a high probability of containing tumor. Nodes of intermediate size must be evaluated by biopsy if the information is essential to staging (see below). When there is central, homogeneous, or "popcorn" calcification visible on plain films, or when a CT scan shows the representative density of the lesion to be greater than 175 Hounsfield units, it may be concluded that the nodule is benign. No other radiographic features are sufficiently reliable to allow the exclusion of lung cancer. Additional information on the differential diagnosis of mass lesions and pulmonary nodules can be found in Chapter 3.3 and Table 3.3–10.

is in order. A large peripheral lesion identified as large cell carcinoma might call for mediastinal exploration before resection, while this would be unnecessary for squamous carcinoma if no nodes are seen on computed tomographic (CT) scan.

RADIOGRAPHIC FEATURES

Findings on the radiograph of the chest are of major importance in the diagnosis of lung cancer. Although changes resulting from primary carcinoma of the lung cover a very wide spectrum, most cases show one of the features listed in Table 6.22–3 as the dominant abnormality. In a patient at high risk (e.g., a cigarette smoker over age 40), the finding of a lung nodule, an unexplained lobar atelectasis, a poorly resolving pneumonia or unilateral hilar enlargement should immediately initiate a work-up to prove or exclude the diagnosis of lung cancer. As shown in the table, some of the patterns suggest a specific cell type, and this is sometimes helpful in deciding how to proceed with the work-up.

When the abnormal finding is a solitary pulmonary nodule, it is very important to obtain previous chest radiographs for comparison, since the absence of change over a period of 2 years or longer suggests a benign lesion. CT is highly effective in characterizing the primary lesion, and is especially useful for centrally located tumors. It is also widely used to visualize the mediastinum. In general, mediastinal lymph nodes less than 1 cm in diameter are often be-

DIAGNOSIS AND STAGING

It has become standard practice to classify the extent of any non–small cell carcinoma using the TNM staging system, in which the primary tumor (T), node involvement (N), and distant metastases (M) are separately rated and combined into three stages (Table 6.22–4). Stage I includes cancers confined to the lung without spread to the mediastinum. Stage II comprises a small number of cases with large tumors and positive hilar nodes but without mediastinal involvement. Stage III includes cancers that extend outside the lung or have spread to the mediastinum or distant sites. Prognosis and choice of therapy are related to stage of disease in non–small cell carcinoma.

For small cell carcinoma a different scheme for staging is recommended since the TNM criteria do not correlate well with prognosis. "Limited" disease, defined by the absence of demonstrable tumor in the opposite lung and in remote sites, has a better outlook than "extensive" disease, even when there is lymphatic spread to the mediastinum and to supraclavicular lymph nodes. Staging of lung cancer, therefore, requires the gathering and interpretation of information concerning the location and extent of the primary lung tumor, the involvement of hilar and mediastinal lymph nodes, and the presence or absence of distant metastases.

In some cases the diagnosis of lung cancer, determination of

TABLE 6.22–4. STAGING IN LUNG CANCER

Non–Small Cell Carcinoma (TNM System)

Stage I	Primary tumor is entirely within the lung and more than 2 cm from the carina
	If there are hilar node metastases, primary is less than 3 cm in diameter
	There are no mediastinal or distant metastases
Stage II	Meets criteria for stage I except that primary tumor is greater than 3 cm in diameter and hilar node metastases are present
Stage III	Primary tumor extends into the chest wall, diaphragm or mediastinum *or*
	Primary tumor is less than 2 cm from the carina *or*
	There is atelectasis or pneumonia involving an entire lung *or*
	Malignant pleural effusion is present *or*
	There are metastases to the mediastinum or distant sites

Small Cell Carcinoma

Limited	Primary tumor is confined to one hemithorax
	Lymph node metastases are limited to the mediastinum, ipsilateral hilar nodes, and ipsilateral or contralateral supraclavicular nodes
	Pleural effusion may be present
Extensive	Primary tumor extends beyond the involved hemithorax *or*
	There are metastases in the contralateral lung or hilum *or*
	There are distant metastases

cell type, and accurate staging can be accomplished without invasive procedures. For example, if a patient with superior vena cava obstruction has right upper lobe atelectasis and a proximal mass and the sputum cytology is positive for squamous carcinoma, no additional procedure is required. In most cases, however, a biopsy or needle aspiration of the tumor or of involved nodes will be required to provide the needed information. Choice of a biopsy procedure will be dictated by consideration of risk to the patient, likelihood of a positive result, anticipated quality of the specimen to be obtained, and the possibility of ascertaining cell type and stage with a single procedure. Thus, biopsy of a superficially located lesion (skin, lymph node, bone) thought to be a metastasis is preferable to biopsy of the primary tumor because it is less invasive and if positive would also exclude surgery as a form of treatment.

Bronchoscopy is often the procedure of choice for diagnosis of lung cancer, especially when there are symptoms or signs of an endobronchial tumor (Table 6.22–1) or when the primary tumor is centrally located. In squamous cell carcinoma, a friable mass within the bronchial lumen can often be seen and biopsied under direct vision. Tumor involving a main bronchus less than 2 cm from the carina can be ascertained. If there is obstruction caused by extrinsic compression of a bronchus, as in small cell carcinomas a diagnosis is often possible by obtaining washing and brushings of the area for cytopathologic study. The most common complication of bronchoscopy in this setting is bleeding from the tumor.

When a suspected lung cancer is too peripheral to be reached by bronchoscopy, it may be approached through the chest wall if it is fluoroscopically visible. In experienced hands, percutaneous needle aspiration biopsy has a high diagnostic yield when the lesion is malignant. The main problems with this technique are that (1) pneumothorax is a common complication, especially when a large-bore needle is used, (2) the specimen obtained with a small-bore needle is suitable only for cytopathologic examination and may re-

sult in a less definitive diagnosis than a histologic specimen, and (3) the significance of a specimen that is negative for cancer is highly dependent upon the skill of the operator. There is, therefore, dispute about the need for needle aspiration biopsy in cases in which a lesion appears to represent a stage I lung cancer and the patient is a good operative risk.

When a decision regarding resectability rests upon the question of mediastinal node involvement and the results of CT are not definitive, direct examination and biopsy of these nodes is necessary, either by mediastinoscopy or parasternal exploration.[2] The dissection itself carries little risk, but general anesthesia is required. For this reason the patient is sometimes subjected to mediastinoscopy immediately followed by thoracotomy and resection if the mediastinal nodes are all negative on frozen section.

Patients with hematogenous metastases in other organs (stage III) will not profit from resection of the primary cancer. Early and occult metastatic spread in small cell carcinoma is so frequent that detailed study, including bone marrow biopsy, is required in order to determine the stage. In non–small cell carcinoma, however, extensive use of CT scans, contrast radiography, and radionuclide studies to search for clinically inapparent metastatic disease is not warranted. It is necessary only to pursue those clues provided by the history, physical examination, or basic laboratory work-up. Similarly, a solitary nodule in the lung does not justify a lengthy work-up for a primary tumor outside the lung, except in the patient who is at low risk for lung cancer, e.g., a young nonsmoker.

MANAGEMENT OF NON–SMALL CELL CANCER

The survival of patients with epidermoid or squamous cancer, large cell cancer, and adenocarcinoma can be related to the extent of disease (TNM stage) and the extent of physiologic impairment (activity status) at the time of diagnosis.

Patients with stage I or II disease at the time of diagnosis represent only about 25 percent of the population with non–small cell lung cancer, but they have a 40 to 50 percent survival rate following pulmonary resection.[6] For non–small cell lung cancer, therefore, surgery is the primary curative treatment. Non–small cell carcinoma is treated by complete surgical resection whenever possible. Because exploratory thoracotomy is associated with significant morbidity, it is important to identify the unresectable cases by careful preoperative staging. Patients who meet the criteria for TNM stages I or II are eligible for resection provided there are no coexisting medical problems that make the risk of operation unacceptable. There are three exceptions to the rule that stage III non–small cell carcinoma is not treated surgically. The first is the peripheral cancer that involves the chest wall but has not resulted in pleural effusion. Resection of these tumors along with a contiguous portion of the chest wall has resulted in about 20 percent long-term survival. The second is cancer arising in the apex (superior sulcus syndrome), which is treated with radiation therapy followed by surgical removal and carries a similar prognosis. Finally, there is controversy about the management of cases with mediastinal node metastases on the side of the lesion but not elsewhere. Some investigators recommend resection of the primary and radical mediastinal node dissection followed by irradiation of the mediastinum for such cases.

PREOPERATIVE EVALUATION

In patients with potentially resectable non–small cell lung cancer, the physician must assess the influence of any coexisting medical problems on the risk of operation. The likelihood of death from thoracotomy is increased by the presence of obstructive lung disease and coronary artery disease, both of which are common in the elderly patient who has been a smoker. The presence of angina, heart failure, poorly controlled arrhythmia, or recent myocardial infarction is usually regarded as a contraindication to surgery. In addition, obstructive lung disease increases the likelihood of post-

operative complications such as persistent air leak, atelectasis, pneumonia, and respiratory failure. In general, if spirograms show a forced expired volume in 1 second (FEV_1) of less than 1 liter, or if there is any degree of CO_2 retention or evidence of pulmonary hypertension, surgical treatment is inadvisable.

The patient's exercise tolerance should be evaluated preoperatively if there is any discrepancy between the degree of exertional dyspnea and the results of ventilatory studies. A rule-of-thumb evaluation of exercise tolerance can be carried out by climbing three flights of stairs with the patient. If the patient is able to hold a conversation without pausing for breath, his or her respiratory reserve is probably adequate to allow thoracotomy with lobectomy.

The effect of removal of functional lung tissue must also be considered. An estimate of this effect can be obtained by a quantitative partitioning of blood flow during perfusion scanning. For example, if 45 percent of the blood flow goes to the left lung, it can be estimated that 45 percent of the ventilatory function would be lost after a left pneumonectomy, and an anticipated postoperative FEV_1 can be calculated. If the calculated value is less than 1.0 L, pneumonectomy may result in chronic respiratory failure in those patients who survive. This method of estimating postoperative ventilatory status is quite reliable for pneumonectomy but tends to overestimate the loss from lobectomy.

NONOPERATIVE MANAGEMENT

In general, the course of bronchogenic carcinoma is distressingly short. The lymphatic and hematogenous dissemination of tumor cells occurs early in the natural history of the disease process. Death commonly results from distant metastases involving the liver, bones, and CNS.

Radiation therapy, the main palliative modality, is especially helpful in the management of hemoptysis, bronchial obstruction, compression of mediastinal structures, and pain. Radiation therapy is used also in the primary management of nonresectable, localized tumors, with good short-term success and a few long-term survivors. A recent controlled randomized study has shown no survival benefit for postoperative mediastinal radiation on completely resected stages II and III squamous carcinoma of the lung.[4] Such radiotherapy does protect against local recurrence of squamous carcinoma.

A number of cytotoxic agents can induce partial regressions in patients with distant metastases when given singly or in combination. The most effective regimens employ cisplatin, a vinca alkaloid (vincristine, vindesine), or a podophyllotoxin (etoposide). Objective response rates of 30 to 50 percent may occur particularly in patients with good ambulatory status. The potential benefits of such tumor shrinkage must be balanced against the toxicities of the cytotoxic regimens. In general, the chemotherapy of non–small cell lung cancer should be regarded as investigational.[7]

Certain patients with advanced stage adenocarcinoma and large cell cancer respond to systemic chemotherapy. Because of the poor prognosis of stages II and III adenocarcinomas and large cell carcinomas, however, investigations of chemotherapy as an adjuvant following surgical resection have been conducted.[3] A recent study has shown modest benefit of a combination of adjuvant cyclophosphamide, doxorubicin, and cisplatin in prolonging disease-free survival and overall survival in patients with stages II and III adenocarcinoma and large cell carcinoma. These results are encouraging but require confirmation before such therapy is accepted as standard care.

MANAGEMENT OF SMALL CELL CANCER

It is most important to identify small cell cancer promptly because this is generally a rapidly growing tumor and should be treated in an expeditious manner. Often tumor-secreted polypeptides (some of which are physiologically active) or other tumor products serve as effective biomarkers for the disorder, although distinctive markers initially present may be lost as the disease recurs and progresses.

Staging for patients with small cell lung cancer has different implications than for patients with other types of lung cancer because in general combination chemotherapy is the major treatment modality and surgical resection is not indicated. Determining the inital extent of disease is important, however, so that (1) the prognosis can be discussed with the patient and family, (2) the response to treatment can be adequately monitored, (3) the need for radiotherapy and, in highly selected cases, surgery can be assessed, and (4) in clinical investigations, uniform reporting and comparison of results can be accomplished.

Systemic combination chemotherapy is the major therapeutic modality. With current regimens employing drugs such as cyclophosphamide, doxorubicin, vincristine, etoposide, and cis-platin, approximately 10 to 15 percent of patients who present with localized disease (confined to one hemithorax) and 2 to 3 percent of patients with extensive disease will survive 2 or more years from the initiation of therapy.[9] A much larger percentage of patients will benefit from the antitumor therapy with relief of symptoms, improvement in quality of life, and frequently with extension of survival.

In patients with localized disease, radiation therapy directed to the primary tumor in conjunction with systemic chemotherapy decreases the local recurrence rate and may well improve survival. Elective cranial radiotherapy does reduce the frequency of clinical brain metastases in patients who have achieved complete remission with systemic therapy. Radiotherapy is the treatment of choice in patients with small cell cancer who have not responded adequately to chemotherapy.

Recently surgical excision of the primary tumor has been reinvestigated as an alternative to radiotherapy in the management of patients with localized small cell cancer. This appears to be beneficial in the small percentage of patients with small cell cancer who present with peripheral lesions and no hilar or mediastinal involvement.

MANAGEMENT OF SPECIFIC MANIFESTATIONS OF LUNG CANCER

As indicated in Table 6.22–1, the clinical manifestations of bronchogenic cancer can be categorized as (1) direct effects of the primary or metastatic tumor mass or (2) indirect or paraneoplastic effects of the cancer mediated by humoral factors or other tumor products. The most common manifestations of bronchogenic cancer requiring supportive care are listed in Table 6.22–5.

TABLE 6.22–5. SPECIFIC MANIFESTATIONS OF BRONCHOGENIC CARCINOMA REQUIRING SUPPORTIVE CARE

Direct Effects of Tumor
- Superior vena caval obstruction
- Bronchial obstruction
- Neurologic problems
    Spinal cord compression
    Intracranial metastases
    Leptomeningeal metastases
- Bony metastases
- Malignant effusions—pleural and pericardial

Indirect Effects (Paraneoplastic Syndromes)
- Endocrine syndromes
    Syndrome of inappropriate ADH secretion
    Ectopic ACTH production
- Neuromuscular disorders
    Encephalomyelitis
    Corticocerebellar degeneration
    Peripheral neuropathies
    Toxic effects of chemotherapy and radiotherapy

SUPERIOR VENA CAVAL SYNDROME

The obstruction of the superior vena cava by nodal involvement with cancer occurs most commonly in small cell carcinoma and squamous carcinoma of the lung. Metastases from other cancers can cause this syndrome, but benign causes (such as mediastinal fibrosis) are seen in less than 5 percent of the cases.

The physical findings (edema of face, neck, arms, and upper torso and prominent venous collaterals) are generally quite striking. These findings in a chronic smoker with a right lung mass on chest radiograph strongly suggests lung cancer. Diagnostic and other invasive procedures must be undertaken with caution because of the risk of hemorrhage secondary to injury to venous collaterals.

For patients with non–small cell cancer, radiation is the primary therapy. For patients with previously untreated small cell cancer, combination chemotherapy is the preferred treatment because it can provide control of the systemic neoplasm in addition to relief of the superior vena caval syndrome.

BRONCHIAL OBSTRUCTION

Major airway obstruction is commonly seen with lung cancer located centrally in the chest, particularly small cell carcinoma and squamous carcinoma. The same therapeutic principles that are applicable in management of superior vena caval syndrome apply in this situation. Postobstructive pneumonitis is a further complication of bronchial obstruction and can generally be relieved by radiation therapy.

NEUROLOGIC COMPLICATIONS

Myriad neurologic problems are found in patients with lung cancer, including mass lesions at varying levels of the neuraxis, paraneoplastic syndromes, and toxic effects of chemotherapy. Intracranial metastases are most commonly seen in small cell cancer and adenocarcinoma, while meningeal involvement is most frequently seen in small cell carcinoma.

A rare neurologic complication of cancer, intramedullary spinal metastasis, is worthy of note in that approximately 20 percent of reported cases have been in patients with small cell carcinoma of the lung. The signs and symptoms of intramedullary metastases can be indistinguishable from the more common epidural metastases and resultant cord compression that occurs secondary to all types of lung cancer. Brown–Séquard syndrome has also been reported in a number of cases. Since myelography can be interpreted as normal in cases of intramedullary lesions, a high level of suspicion is required.

Intracranial masses and spinal cord compression are best treated with radiation therapy. The paraneoplastic syndromes (such as limbic encephalopathy and cerebellar degeneration) that are most frequently associated with small cell lung cancer are not indications for radiation therapy but may respond to systemic therapy.

BONY METASTASES

Lytic and blastic osseous metastases often result in pain. Radiation therapy to the affected area is often effective in providing relief and may also prevent or delay the development of a pathologic fracture. Bony metastases are most common in small cell cancer. Hypercalcemia is commonly seen, however, in squamous carcinoma and rarely in small cell cancer. The hypercalcemia in squamous carcinoma of the lung appears to be secondary to the production of parathormone-like substance by this type of lung cancer.

ENDOCRINE SYNDROMES

In addition to the paraneoplastic syndrome of hypercalcemia, inappropriate secretion of ADH and ectopic production of ACTH constitute the most frequently occurring paraneoplastic syndromes in lung cancer. The latter two syndromes are generally seen in patients with small cell cancer.

These ectopic hormone syndromes are clinically important because (1) the endocrine abnormalities may themselves be a source of significant morbidity, (2) the initial clue to the diagnosis of bronchogenic cancer may be the hormone excess syndrome, and (3) the presence or reactivation of such a syndrome may provide an indication of the activity of the underlying tumor.

The optimal therapy of these syndromes is eradication or control of the cancer. Other measures are often required for symptom control such as water restriction and demeclocycline in management of the syndrome of inappropriate antidiuretic hormone (ADH) secretion, mithramycin in control of hypercalcemia, and drugs such as metyrapone, aminoglutethimide, and o,p'DDD in ectopic ACTH syndrome.

REFERENCES

1. Ginsberg RJ, Feld RD (eds): Fourth World Conference on Lung Cancer. Chest 89:199S, 1986
2. Haponik EF, Wang K: New methods for diagnosis and staging of mediastinal disease. In Aisner J (ed): Lung Cancer. New York, Churchill Livingstone, 1985
3. Holmes EC, Gail M: Surgical adjuvant therapy for stage II and stage III adenocarcinoma and large-cell undifferentiated carcinoma. J Clin Oncol 4:710, 1986
4. The Lung Cancer Study Groups: Effects of postoperative mediastinal radiation on completely resected stage II and stage III epidermoid cancer of the lung. N Engl J Med 315:1377, 1986
5. Minna JD, Ihde DC, Glatstein EJ: Lung cancer: Scalpels, beams, drugs, and probes. N Engl J Med 315:1410, 1986
6. Mountain CF: Therapy of stage I and II non-small cell lung cancer. Semin Oncol 10:71, 1983
7. Owens AH, Abeloff MD: Neoplasms of the lung. In Calabresi P, Schein PS, Rosenberg SA (eds): Medical Oncology—Basic Principles and Clinical Management of Cancer. New York, Macmillan, 1985
8. Tockman MS, Anthonisen NR, et al: Airways obstruction and the risk of lung cancer. Ann Intern Med 106:512, 1987
9. Vogelsang GB, Abeloff MD, et al: Long-term survivors of small cell carcinoma of the lung. Am J Med 79:49, 1985
10. Whang-Peng J, Kao-Shan CS, et al: Specific chromosome defect associated with small-cell lung cancer: Deletion 3p(14–23). Science 215:181, 1982

Colorectal Cancer

Gordon D. Luk

In the United States colorectal cancer[10] is associated with the second highest overall death rate for cancer of any site and accounts for about 20 percent of all deaths due to malignant disease, currently about 60,000 deaths annually. Colorectal cancer is also the second most frequent primary site of fatal cancer if both sexes are considered together. It will occur in approximately 5 percent of men and 6 percent of women in the United States. Incidence and death rates of this disease have not changed over the past 40 years. Fortunately, knowledge of the natural history and the biology of colorectal cancer has increased markedly, and this improved knowledge will undoubtedly lead to early identification of precursor lesions in high risk groups, which will permit careful screening and monitoring, and follow-up after surgical resection.

ETIOLOGY AND PATHOGENESIS

THE COLONIC EPITHELIUM

The available biologic evidence points to the adenomatous polyp in the colon as the precursor lesion to colorectal cancer. Available knowledge suggests that cancers may arise within the polyp, gradually destroy it by invasive growth, and proceed to penetrate into, around, and then through the bowel wall.

Studies of the colonic epithelium have shown fundamental differences between normal colonic epithelium and adenomatous epithelium. In normal colonic mucosa, cell proliferation is active but is restricted to the deepest third or half of the crypts of Lieberkühn. Cells produced by replication within the crypts migrate toward the colonic lumen and differentiate into two principal cell types, the goblet cells and the absorptive cells. Mitotic figures and uptake of tritiated thymidine predominate in the lower third to half of the crypts and decrease markedly when cells move from within the crypts to surface mucosa. One of the features of adenomas appears to be a loss of regulation of this dynamic process of cell proliferation, and exfoliation of cells from the surface epithelium appears to be poorly regulated. Cell proliferation, as evidenced by mitotic figures and thymidine uptake, takes place at all levels within the tissue. Both morphologically and dynamically, cells at the surface of an adenoma resemble the actively proliferating and minimally differentiated cells that normally constitute the lower third of the crypt (Fig. 6.23–1).

In summary a cardinal feature of adenomatous epithelium is the continuation of cell proliferation from within the crypt onto the epithelial surface. Exfoliation of cells cannot keep pace with tissue replication, and the accumulation of tissues that protrude into the bowel lumen then constitute the polypoid lesion. This failure of adenomatous epithelium to show normal regulation of cell proliferation may be the etiology of neoplastic growth.

ADENOMAS—MALIGNANT POTENTIAL

It is now widely accepted that the adenoma is the premalignant precursor lesion for colorectal cancer (Table 6.23–1). Direct evidence of this may never be available, as it would involve careful follow-up of unresected polypoid lesions. The presence of microscopic cancer foci cannot be excluded by simple biopsy of the polyp because of sampling error, so exact diagnosis requires complete excision of the polyp. Furthermore, current clinical wisdom suggests that all adenomas larger than 1 cm should be excised.[6]

Nevertheless, available evidence strongly supports the sequence of adenoma to colorectal cancer. When small cancers less than 0.5 to 1 cm are examined, residual adenomatous tissue is observed in up to 20 percent of specimens. Conversely, when adenomas are examined, they frequently contain areas of in situ or invasive malignancy, with incidence increasing with size. Adenomas smaller than 1 cm have about a 1 percent incidence of invasive malignancy; those between 1 and 2 cm have a 10 percent incidence, and those larger than 2 cm, about a 35 percent incidence. Furthermore, the risk of colorectal cancer has been shown to increase with the number of adenomas in the colon.

One of the most convincing arguments for the adenoma-to-cancer transition is the marked decrease in incidence of colorectal cancer when adenomas are routinely removed. This was shown in a large study of more than 20,000 individuals who underwent routine annual proctosigmoidoscopy and polypectomy when polyps were found. Twenty-five adenocarcinomas were detected on initial examination. Over the subsequent 90,000 patient-years of follow-up, however, only 13 of 90 (15 percent) of the expected number of additional cancers appeared (with expectation based on epidemiologic data). Moreover, the cancers were at an early stage of development, and all had an excellent chance for cure. Similar data have been obtained using fiberoptic colonoscopy and polypectomy in the follow-up of patients with colorectal cancer. Other biologic and pathologic laboratory evidence confirming the adenoma-to-cancer transition has also been put forth (Table 6.23–2).

HEREDITARY DISORDERS—POLYPS AND CANCER

Adenomatous Polyposis Coli (Familial Polyposis) Syndrome
In adenomatous polyposis coli (familial polyposis) syndrome the colon becomes covered by hundreds to thousands of adenomas, by age 15 to 25 years. Subsets of this disease involve variable expressions of extracolonic manifestations. In general, the disease is inherited as an autosomal dominant trait with virtually 100 percent penetrance. Unless colectomy or proctocolectomy is performed, over 50 percent of patients will have developed adenocarcinoma by age 37, and death from colon cancer approaches 100 percent by age 55.

Hereditary colorectal cancer, also described as hereditary nonpolyposis colorectal cancer (HNPCC), as well as Lynch syndrome I, is characterized by autosomal dominant inheritance with a low mean age (41 years) for the occurrence of colorectal cancer and a marked increase in proportion of tumors in the proximal colon. In this syndrome, a solitary adenoma or several adenomas may occur in a number of family members, although each affected member generally does not have more than 10 adenomas.

In some families, there is an increased risk of adenocarcinomas of all varieties, with a particular predominance of carcinoma of the colon, endometrium, and breast. Cancers tend to occur at an early age, and multiple primary malignant neoplasms are frequent. This pattern has also been termed the cancer family syndrome, or Lynch syndrome II.

Family History of Colorectal Cancer
Independent of polyposis syndromes and hereditary colorectal cancer, colorectal cancer has shown a modest familial aggregation, with certain families apparently at higher risk of having multiple family members who develop colorectal cancer. Using large pedigrees and the methods of genetic epidemiology, researchers have

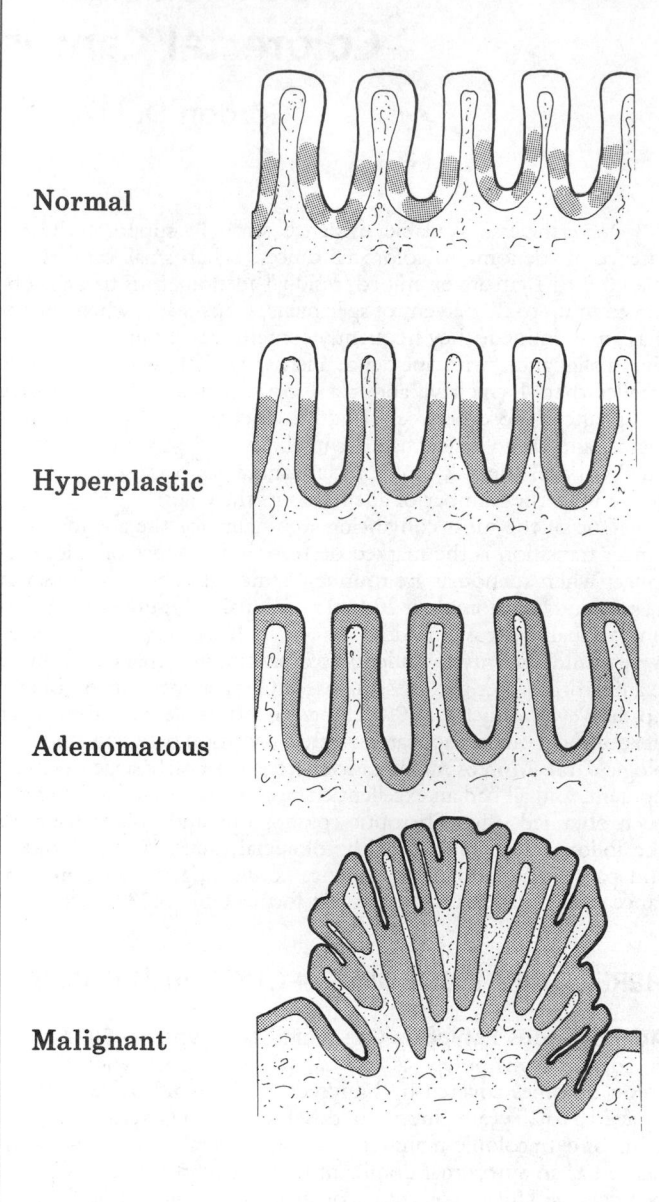

Figure 6.23–1. Epithelial replication in normal, hyperplastic, adenomatous, and malignant epithelium. Area of cell replication is indicated by shading. In contrast to normal mucosa and hyperplastic polyps, cell replication occurs in all regions of adenomatous and malignant epithelium. Loss of control of replication is characteristic of adenomatous and malignant epithelium.

TABLE 6.23–1. ADENOMAS: MALIGNANT POTENTIAL

Type (Alternate Names)	Incidence (%)	Invasive Malignancy (%)	Peak Age Incidence (%)
Adenomatous polyp (tubular adenoma, adenoma)	75	5	60
Villous polyp (villous adenoma)	10	40	65
Intermediate type polyp (tubulovillous adenoma)	15	20	60

TABLE 6.23–2. ARGUMENTS FOR THE EVOLUTION FROM ADENOMA TO COLORECTAL CANCER

- Patients kept adenoma free remain cancer free
- Increased incidence of cancer of greater size
- Increased incidence of cancer as the number of adenomas increases
- The peak age at which adenomas are diagnosed precedes that for cancer by about 5 years
- There is a similar distribution of adenomas and cancer within the large bowel
- The adenoma-to-cancer transition has been seen in familial polyposis

found subsets of colorectal cancers as well as colorectal adenomas that apparently occur in an autosomal dominant pattern, with incomplete penetrance.

Other Hereditary Polyposis Syndromes

In families with multiple juvenile polyps, the juvenile polyps could occur throughout the gastrointestinal tract, but colorectal cancer is generally uncommon. When present, it has apparently occurred in foci of adenomatous tissue and not in the juvenile polyp.

Similarly, in the Peutz–Jeghers syndrome, multiple hamartomatous polyps occur throughout the gastrointestinal tract and are associated with melanin pigmentation of the buccal mucosa, lips, and face. There is no good evidence for an increased risk of intestinal cancer, although an increased risk of cancers at other sites, occurring at an earlier age than in the general population, has recently been described.

RISK FACTORS FOR CANCER DEVELOPMENT[6]

A major risk factor for the development of colorectal cancer is the presence of adenomatous polyps. This risk is greatly increased in those with hereditary or multiple adenomatous polyps. A strong family history, as discussed above, is another risk factor (Table 6.23–3).

There is also an increased risk of colorectal cancer in patients with longstanding chronic ulcerative colitis for more than 10 years. In this disease, marked colonic mucosal dysplasia has been recognized as the precursor lesion for subsequent development of colorectal cancer.

Epidemiologic evidence suggests that dietary factors may play a role in ultimate cancer development.[7] Colorectal cancer is much more common in the developed Western world than in underdeveloped countries. This is thought to be related to the increased fiber and bulk in the diet in underdeveloped countries, which re-

TABLE 6.23–3. HIGH-RISK FACTORS FOR COLORECTAL CANCER

Age
- Over 40 years in asymptomatic men and women

Associated Disease
- Ulcerative colitis

Past History
- Colorectal cancer
- Colorectal adenoma
- Female genital cancer
- Female breast cancer

Family History
- Familial polyposis syndromes (including Gardner syndrome, Turcot syndrome, and Oldfield syndrome)
- Colorectal cancer
- Colorectal adenoma
- Cancer family syndrome

sults in a shortened transit time of fecal material with increased amount of unabsorbed fiber and increased stool bulk. Epidemiologic evidence also suggests that colorectal cancer is increased in areas with diets that are high in fat, particularly unsaturated fat and cholesterol. Supportive evidence includes the gradually increasing incidence of colorectal cancer in Japanese immigrants to the United States, who have adopted the American diet. Conversely, the high colorectal cancer incidence in United States citizens living in the industrial North seems to decrease upon migration to areas in the South with lower cancer incidence. Epidemiologic data also suggests that other dietary nutrients may play a role.[4] Internationally, geographic areas low in selenium in the soil show higher rates of colorectal cancer than areas with high selenium levels. Although the epidemiologic correlations are interesting and deserve further investigation, many other variables may account for these observations.

CARCINOGENESIS

Etiologic Agents

The process of carcinogenesis has been investigated in the rodent model. Many studies have demonstrated that the induction of colonic tumors in mice and rats by carcinogens might be enhanced by diets high in fat and cholesterol as well as diets low in selenium and in fiber. Furthermore, tumor induction is suppressed when selenium and fiber are returned to the diet. Other studies have demonstrated either no effect or the opposite effect, however. Nevertheless, use of the rodent carcinogenesis model has allowed further understanding of the biology and natural history of the carcinogenesis process. It also allows testing of potential chemopreventive agents.

Genetic and Chromosomal Changes

The oncogenes are homologs of retroviral sequences found in human cells and have been associated with higher incidence in tumor cells than in normal cells. It is now thought, however, that the oncogene might be expressed as a result of the increased cell proliferation rather than as a cause of the carcinogenesis process itself. In several experimental models, amplification (increased copy number of the particular gene sequence), mutation of the oncogene sequence, and increased expression of the messenger RNA coded by the oncogene sequence have been noted in higher incidence in colonic tumors than in normal colonic mucosa.

Genetic markers, such as chromosome abnormalities, have been non-uniform and not always demonstrable even in cancers. These genetic markers have not been useful in identifying the premalignant state. Recently, using molecular biology techniques including restriction fragment length polymorphism (RFLP) and in situ hybridization, the gene for familial polyposis has been localized to chromosome 5, most probably the long arm near bands 5q21–q22. These same investigations also found that at least 20 percent of sporadic human colon carcinomas demonstrate loss of a chromosome 5 allele. These results suggest that becoming recessive for the "familial polyposis gene" may be an important step in the development of colorectal cancers.

CLINICAL MANIFESTATIONS

Colorectal cancers generally do not extend far longitudinally along the bowel lumen, although circumferential tumors are not uncommon. Invasion through the bowel wall, with attachment to adjacent structures and organs, such as the genitourinary tract, abdominal wall, and small bowel, is frequent. Clinical manifestations and symptoms of colorectal cancer depend upon the location of the tumor in the colon (Table 6.23–4).

Right colonic lesions typically present with abdominal pain, unexplained iron deficiency anemia, and lower gastrointestinal (GI) tract bleeding. Occasionally, an asymptomatic abdominal

TABLE 6.23–4. COMPARISON OF THE FIVE MOST FREQUENT SYMPTOMS IN RECTAL, LEFT COLON, AND RIGHT COLON CANCER

Right Colon	Left Colon	Rectum and Rectosigmoid
Abdominal pain (75%)	Abdominal pain (75%)	Rectal bleeding (75%)
Weakness (25%)	Rectal bleeding (50%)	Constipation (50%)
Rectal bleeding (25%)	Constipation (50%)	Tenesmus (25%)
Nausea (25%)	Nausea (25%)	Diarrhea (25%)
Abdominal mass (25%)	Vomiting (25%)	Abdominal pain (25%)

mass may be noted by the patient or by the physician on physical examination. Rarely, the tumor obstructs the ileocecal valve, producing acute small bowel obstruction. Persistent, nagging lower abdominal pain is another complaint. Thus, any adult with unexplained iron deficiency anemia and GI tract bleeding should have an evaluation for carcinoma of the cecum and the right colon.

Tumors of the left colon, particularly of the sigmoid, usually present with abdominal pain and obstruction from circumferential "napkin-ring" growth. Gross blood per rectum is occasionally seen, but anemia is unusual.

Rectal tumors manifest with rectal pain, gross blood per rectum, tenesmus with a feeling of incomplete rectal evacuation, and, rarely, prolapse of tumor through the anus. In both sigmoid and rectal tumors, alternating diarrhea and constipation as well as decrease in caliber of stools is also occasionally seen.

Rectal lesions that have advanced beyond local lymph nodes may show perineural sheath invasion with consequent dull, boring pelvic pain. In villous adenoma of the rectum, profound electrolyte depletion, particularly of potassium, may be associated with the diarrhea.

Approximately one fourth of patients at the time of initial presentation have evidence of hematogenous distant metastases. The most common site is the liver, but lung metastases are also common. These can result in filling defects in the liver and pulmonary nodules.

DIAGNOSIS

CANCER SCREENING[3]

Cancer screening in the asymptomatic individual is recommended by The American Cancer Society. The current recommendations include routine annual digital rectal examinations for all persons aged 40 and over. A stool occult blood slide test should be added at age 50 on an annual basis, and sigmoidoscopy should be performed every 3 to 5 years after two initial negative sigmoidoscopies 1 year apart (Table 6.23–5).[9] Cancer screening should be particularly intensified in those special high-risk groups described earlier (Table 6.23–3), including those with hereditary syndromes, adenomatous polyps, history of adenocarcinoma, and ulcerative colitis and other high-risk factors.

In one study of close to 10,000 individuals aged 40 years and older, 1 percent of patients had at least one positive test for fecal occult blood. In these patients, neoplastic lesions were identified in 50 percent; these lesions were defined as polyps greater than 5 mm (38 percent) or cancers (12 percent). The other 50 percent of patients with fecal occult blood were found to have nonneoplastic lesions (including polyps smaller than 5 mm), diverticulosis, or no detectable abnormalities. Thus, the predictive value of occult blood testing appears to be on the order of 50 percent with a 0.5

TABLE 6.23–5. SUGGESTED SURVEILLANCE STRATEGIES FOR COLORECTAL CANCER

Risk Group	Strategy for Screening
Average risk: Persons over age 40	Yearly rectal exam and fecal occult blood testing beginning at age 40. Sigmoidoscopy every 3–5 years, or if rectal exam or fecal blood is positive. Air-contrast barium enema or colonoscopy if sigmoidoscopy is positive
Mildly increased risk: Persons with first-degree relatives with colorectal cancer; persons with history of cancer of genitourinary tract or breast	As above, but beginning 10 years prior to age of onset in relative; or when patient is found to have another cancer
Moderately increased risk: Persons with history of colorectal cancer or adenoma; persons with family history of the cancer family syndrome or colorectal cancer	Begin at time of diagnosis of colorectal cancer or adenoma, or at age 20 with family cancer history. Yearly rectal exam and fecal occult blood test. Air-contrast barium enema or colonoscopy every 1–3 years, of if rectal exam or fecal blood is positive
High risk: Persons with familial adenomatous polyposis syndromes or long-standing ulcerative colitis	Begin screening at age 10–14 in polyposis syndromes or after 7 years of pancolitis. Yearly sigmoidoscopy, with complete colonoscopy, every 1–3 years. Consider colectomy at the appearance of multiple polyps or at the time of confirmed diagnosis of dysplasia

percent false-positive rate. Nevertheless, only 12 cancers and 38 polyps were found after 10,000 patients were screened. This suggests that it will require 1000 occult blood examinations to discover one new case of colorectal cancer. For routine sigmoidoscopies, the yield could be even lower, requiring approximately 4000 examinations to discover one new case of colorectal cancer.

Colorectal cancer is one of the most common cancers, and the physician must be alert to clinical manifestations such as weight loss, blood in the stool, and change in bowel habits or stool characteristics. The potentially serious nature of these manifestations must be recognized and not attributed to hemorrhoids or other minor conditions until colorectal cancer has been definitely excluded. It must be stressed that colorectal cancer is curable if discovered early, and delay in diagnosis is a significant factor in poor prognosis.

MEDICAL HISTORY

A careful medical history is extremely important in the detection of possible manifestations of colorectal cancer. A positive family history or personal history of colorectal cancer, adenomas, and other malignancies (especially breast or endometrial) and a history of adenomas and ulcerative colitis should increase one's index of suspicion. Other symptoms should also be elicited, including general complaints of fatigue and weight loss as well as site-specific complaints, such as pneumaturia from a sigmoidovesical fistula.

PHYSICAL EXAMINATION

The physician should be careful to seek out external signs of internal malignancies, including dermatologic lesions. Abdominal masses may be felt, especially in right colonic cancer. Abdominal distension and hyperactive bowel sounds may suggest partial obstruction from a constricting lesion. The rectal examination must be a routine part of any physical examination, as about one fourth of all colorectal cancers may be detected by this procedure. One should be careful to search for a rectal mass, a rectal shelf, or a nodularity along the pelvic side wall. The presence of blood in the stool should also be excluded. In females, pelvic examination is important; the ovaries should be palpated to exclude ovarian metastases.

LABORATORY EXAMINATION

A microcytic hypochromic anemia may be indicative of iron deficiency anemia. An elevated alkaline phosphatase level may be the earliest sign of liver metastases.

DIAGNOSTIC TESTS

The sigmoidoscopic examination should be the first special diagnostic test performed. About one third of colorectal cancers may be seen with this instrument. A flexible fiberoptic sigmoidoscope can reach the splenic flexure and beyond, increase the extent of the large bowel visible, and detect up to two thirds of colorectal cancers. Any suspicious lesions should, of course, be biopsied.

If no lesions that could account for the clinical manifestations have been detected by sigmoidoscopy, the next examination should be either a barium enema or a colonoscopy. The choice often depends on the expertise of the specialist available. In general, a barium enema is preferable in the elderly; those with a known tortuous, long colon, and those with previous abdominal or pelvic operations. It must be stressed that an optimal barium enema depends on adequate and conscientious preparation to completely cleanse the colon. Cleansing is also very important for colonoscopy, although not as critical as for the barium enema, because the colonoscope is equipped with water jets that could be used to cleanse out particularly suspicious areas of the large bowel. For diagnosis of colorectal cancer and large polyps (>1 cm), a single-contrast barium enema is often adequate. A double-contrast barium enema should generally be reserved for those cases in which a search for minute and subtle changes of the mucosa and small polyps is required. The rationale and choice of the diagnostic procedure should be discussed beforehand with either the radiologist or the gastroenterologist-endoscopist.

METASTASES

Colorectal cancers generally spread by contiguous invasion or via regional lymph nodes, most commonly involving the liver and the lung. The search for metastases should include contiguous organs as well as the liver and lung. The sigmoidoscopy and barium enema should be reviewed to define the extent of the tumor if it is in the rectum. Cystoscopy and pelvic examination will help in determining local spread of the cancer.

For liver metastases, the alkaline phosphatase is of equal or greater usefulness than a liver scan. A routine chest film is done to exlude pulmonary lesions. The CT scan of the pelvic, abdominal, chest, and liver areas is probably the most sensitive test for detecting metastases.

BIOMARKERS[5]

The search for a serum biomarker or other biomarkers that can be obtained by noninvasive testing has been a laudable goal of facilitating the early diagnosis of colorectal cancer. No suitable marker is yet available, however. The carcino-embryonic antigen (CEA), one of the earliest and best known of tumor biomarkers, was once thought to be specific for colorectal cancer.[1] It has now been found

to be elevated with other cancers and benign inflammatory diseases of the bowel. Nevertheless, there is some suggestion that serial measurements of CEA levels both before and after surgery might provide a way of monitoring the adequacy of surgical resection and subsequent recurrence.

The search for new biomarkers for colorectal cancer is intense, with mucosal proliferation markers and carbohydrate markers being the current candidates under investigation. As described, abnormal increases in colonic mucosal cell proliferation have been interpreted as precursors of colorectal cancers. Thus, searches for mucosal cell proliferation markers or plasma markers of this increased mucosal cell proliferation is underway. The currently available antibodies raised against colonic cell surface carbohydrates and mucins have shed light on the biology of evolution from normal mucosa to adenocarcinoma, but they have not yet proved either sensitive or specific for colorectal cancer. Colonic mucosal cell proliferation markers may have potential diagnostic value, and may characterize those at high-risk for colorectal cancer. Furthermore, some of these markers, such as ornithine decarboxylase, may also provide a potential therapeutic target for suppression of the increased cell proliferation and, hence, for suppression of malignant transformation.

STAGING AND PROGNOSIS

DUKES CLASSIFICATION

The Dukes classification is widely accepted, although it has been changed and modified many times, and there is general confusion about the particular Dukes system that is being used. The Dukes classification system generally depends upon depth of anatomic spread and presence or absence of nodal metastases. The classifications offer a rough guide to prognosis but are limited by variations in both depth and anaplasia within a given tumor.

In general, one of the more widely used Dukes systems is the modification by Turnbull.

Stage A Tumor confinement within serosa
Stage B Tumor extension into pericolic fat
Stage C Tumor metastases to regional mesenteric lymph nodes but no evidence of distant spread
Stage D Tumor metastases to liver, lung, bone; seeding of tumor; tumor unresectable because of parietal invasion or adjacent organ invasion

This system clearly does not accurately separate the early primary tumor and lumps all lesions from the mucosa to muscularis propria into stage A. Also, the criteria for stage D classification is not completely defined. Nevertheless, the Dukes classification modifications are in wide use, and familiarity with the system is useful until other staging classifications are more universally accepted.

TNM CLASSIFICATION

The TNM staging system groups important prognostic variables concerning the size of the primary tumor (T), lymph node involvement (N), and distant metastases (M). Clearly, the TNM classification based on clinical evaluation alone prior to surgery will be different from classification after surgery or laparotomy (Table 6.23–6). The TNM classification is then divided into stage groupings in an attempt to stratify prognosis, which will be important in the research setting for studying the effect of treatment on prognosis (Table 6.23–7).

PROGNOSIS

For all patients with colorectal cancer combined, the 5-year survival rate and 5-year cure rate are both about 25 percent

TABLE 6.23–6. TUMOR (T), NODE (N), METASTASES (M) CLASSIFICATION OF COLORECTAL CANCER

T1	Mucosa or submucosa only
T2	Muscle or serosa
T3	Extension to contiguous structures, no fistula
T4	Extension to contiguous structures, with fistula
T5	Extension beyond contiguous structures
N0	No regional node involvement
N1	Regional node involvement
N4	Juxtaregional node involvement
M0	No distant metastases
M1	Distant metastases

(Table 6.23–8). The prognosis is clearly highly dependent on the stage at first diagnosis and the subsequent response to therapy. The prognosis is clearly much better for those patients whose diagnosis is made at an early stage.

Clinical features at first presentation also have an effect on prognosis. In general, prognosis is improved in those patients who are asymptomatic at first diagnosis or who first present with rectal hemorrhage, as well as those who present with a CEA of less than 5 ng/ml. Conversely, prognosis is worse when colorectal cancer is diagnosed in those at a young age, particularly those under 40. Prognosis is less favorable in those who present with obstruction, perforation, adjacent organ involvement, fistula formation, circumferential bowel tumor involvement, clinically fixed tumor, and tumor below the peritoneal reflection (Table 6.23–8).

Histologic grade also has an effect on prognosis. In general, the higher grade the tumor (the more poorly differentiated), the worse the prognosis.

The histopathology appears not to play a major factor in prognosis. The vast majority of colorectal cancers are adenocarcinomas, and to a much lesser degree, carcinoid tumors, leiomyosarcomas, and lymphomas.

THERAPY

LIMITED-STAGE DISEASE

Even though not properly classified as colorectal cancer, adenomatous polyps are an important consideration in therapy, as their removal markedly diminishes the subsequent occurrence of colorectal cancer. Generally, pedunculated polyps (those with a stalk) smaller than 2 cm can be easily removed via polypectomy with a cautery snare. For sessile polyps (without a stalk) and larger polyps, polypectomy carries a greater hazard of complication. In any case, it is important to consult closely with a pathologist, especially in reviewing the histopathology of the polypectomy margin. The presence of malignant cells could well dictate a laparotomy and resection of the colon to remove any remaining malignant cells.

TABLE 6.23–7. STAGE GROUPING FOR COLON CANCER

Stage I	T1	N0	M0
Stage Ib	T2	N0	M0
Stage II	T3, T4	N0	M0
Stage III	Any T	N1	M0
Stage IV	Any T	N4	M0
	Any T	Any N	M1

TABLE 6.23–8. PROGNOSTIC FEATURES OF PRIMARY COLORECTAL CANCER

Good Prognosis
- Diagnosis in asymptomatic patients
- Long duration of symptoms
- Hemorrhage as a presenting symptom
- Age >70 years
- Preoperative CEA <5 ng/ml

Poor Prognosis
- Young age
- Obstruction
- Free perforation
- Localized perforation with abscess formation
- Adjacent organ involvement
- Fistula formation
- Ulcerated primary tumor
- Rectal tumor
- Circumferential bowel lumen involvement
- Immobile tumor by rectal examination
- Perirectal lymphadenopathy by rectal examination
- Preoperative CEA >5 ng/ml

SURGERY

In general the first line of therapy for colorectal cancer is surgical. The general recommendation is for surgical resection of any resectable tumor, whether or not distant metastases have occurred. Leaving the colorectal cancer will most often result in subsequent complete bowel obstruction, which will then require emergency surgery, either resection or bypass of the obstruction.

In general, any resectable colorectal cancer should be removed by wide segmental resection of the colon and mesentery with intestinal anastomosis if the tumor is located above the peritoneal reflection, and abdominoperineal resection and permanent colostomy if the tumor is below the peritoneal reflection. If adjacent organs appear to be involved, they should be segmentally resected en bloc with the colon where possible. The operation of choice would clearly depend on the individual patient, and more important, on the skill, expertise, and experience of the surgeon. With good preoperative management and operative skill, up to 90 percent of all patients can receive curative or palliative surgical therapy with an operative mortality of less than 5 percent. The surgical mortality is higher for lesions in the rectosigmoid area and for tumors that have perforated or obstructed.

Although the removal of the regional mesenteric lymph nodes is important for staging purposes, radical extended lymph node dissections have not shown subsequent improved survival.

RADIOTHERAPY

Some surgeons prefer preoperative radiation therapy, but its efficacy in preventing metastatic disease has not been documented, and survival has not been convincingly improved. Nevertheless, low-dose radiotherapy appears to be as effective as moderate dose radiotherapy and has fewer complications. Postoperative abdominal radiation has also been done when the threat of intraperitoneal tumor seeding appears to be imminent. The choice of radiotherapy again depends on the availability, expertise, and experience of the radiotherapist, who must work closely with the surgeon and the medical oncologist.

CHEMOTHERAPY

Despite many reports that a variety of single-agent and multiagent protocols appear to be beneficial as adjuvant chemotherapy, the response rates in recurrent and metastatic cancers are very poor and of limited duration. A recent multicenter study has shown no significant improvement in survival with several adjuvant chemotherapy and radiotherapy protocols. Nevertheless, in the small subset of patients who show good to excellent response to 5-fluorouracil, there is some evidence of a prolonged median survival of 6 to 12 months.

Currently, chemotherapy, either as an adjuvant to surgery or as primary treatment in advanced or recurrent colorectal cancer, continues to remain an experimental maneuver. Progress in the treatment of patients can only be made by entrance of as many of these patients as possible into well-designed clinical trials.

Immunotherapy, either alone or in combination with chemotherapy, has been reported to show significant responses and improvement in survival in a very small number of patients. The particular immunotherapy modalities have included BCG, levamisole, as well as the more recently tested autologous cancer vaccines (vaccines made from the patient's own colon cancer cells) and the lymphokine-activated killer T cells (LAK) cell therapy. As in chemotherapy, progress in immunotherapy can be made only by entrance of an adequate number of appropriate patients into well-designed clinical studies.

DISSEMINATED AND RECURRENT DISEASE

Careful follow-up of colorectal cancer patients after the initial surgical resection is mandatory. A second primary colorectal cancer will occur in 3 to 16 percent of patients. In addition, these patients are also at increased risk for primary adenocarcinoma in other organs, especially breast and endometrial cancer. The incidence of second primaries and cancers in other organs is, of course, increased in those families characterized as having the cancer family syndrome, as described earlier. Careful follow-up can facilitate diagnosis of recurrent disease when it is still localized and amenable to further curative therapy. Systematic follow-up has resulted in cure in 5 to 10 percent of recurrent disease.

This careful follow-up can include history and physical examination every 3 to 4 months in the first year and every 6 months afterwards, together with barium enema or colonoscopy, and determination of alkaline phosphatase levels every 6 months to 1 year (Table 6.23–9).

TABLE 6.23–9. TESTS REQUIRED IN FOLLOW-UP OF COLORECTAL CANCER PATIENTS

Test	Year Postoperatively				
	1	*2*	*3*	*4*	*5*
History and physical examination[a]	3 monthly	3 monthly	3 monthly	6 monthly	6 monthly
Barium enema or total colonoscopy[b]	Yearly	Yearly	Yearly	Yearly	2 yearly
Suture line endoscopy	6 monthly	6 monthly	Yearly	—	—

[a]Breast check and cervical cytology yearly as well as alkaline phosphatase every 6 months.
[b]Barium enema or colonoscopy should be performed every 2–3 years for the remainder of the patient's life in order to detect possible metachronous colorectal cancers.

When recurrent disease is discovered, the primary mode of therapy is again surgical. If segmental resection is possible, it should be done whether or not lymph node metastasis or other dissemination of disease has occurred.

For patients who have an apparent complete resection of the primary colorectal cancer but limited hepatic metastases, resection of the tumor mass may result in a 20 to 30 percent chance of cure. Even in those patients who are not cured, the results suggest that survival may be prolonged.

Pulmonary metastases occur in approximately 15 percent of patients with colorectal cancer, and in 2 percent, these metastases are solitary. Resection of pulmonary metastases, when it is technically feasible, has resulted in improved survival to a 5-year survival rate of 30 to 35 percent.

Furthermore, in patients with a solitary pulmonary nodule in the setting of a coexisting or previous colorectal cancer, approximately half are due to metastatic disease and half are primary lung cancer. Thus, aggressive evaluation or resection of a solitary pulmonary nodule in the setting of colorectal cancer is imperative.

As described in the section on treatment for limited-stage disease, the optimal adjunctive therapy has not yet been clearly identified. Patients should be encouraged to enter well-designed experimental treatment protocols. If that is not possible, 5-fluorouracil as a single agent may offer some therapeutic efficacy with tolerable side effects.

SUMMARY

Colorectal cancer remains one of the most common malignancies in the United States for both men and women. The incidence rate of this tumor and survival following surgical resection have not improved in the last 40 years. As compared to the leukemias, the lymphomas, and other solid tumors, no effective chemotherapy regimens have been defined for colorectal cancer. Knowledge of the natural history, biology, and pathophysiology of colorectal cancer has increased markedly, however.

With this new knowledge, a strategy for the control of colorectal cancer is beginning to be formulated. The strategy includes:

1. Identification of colorectal carcinogens and protection from these substances, either by avoidance or by using chemoprotective and chemopreventive agents
2. Screening of the general population over the age of 40 years as well as high-risk populations
3. Identification of high-risk groups for careful follow-up
4. Adequate primary surgical resection combined with controlled clinical trials to test new adjuvant protocols
5. Careful follow-up and evaluation after primary surgical resection with aggressive therapy for localized recurrence and localized metastases
6. Continued aggressive and intensive search for effective therapeutic agents and biomarkers

With concerted effort, we should begin to improve our diagnosis, treatment, and prevention of this second most common cancer killer in the United States.

REFERENCES

1. Fletcher RH: Carcinoembryonic antigen. Ann Intern Med 104:66, 1986
2. Gastrointestinal Tumor Study Group: Adjuvant therapy of colon cancer: Results of a prospectively randomized trial. N Engl J Med 310:737, 1984
3. Gilbertsen V: Colon cancer screening: The Minnesota experience. Gastrointest Endosc 26:315, 1980
4. Kolonel LN, LeMarchand L: The epidemiology of colon cancer and dietary fat. Prog Clin Biol Res 222:69, 1986
5. Luke GD, Baylin SB: Ornithine deearboxylase as a biologic marker in familial colonic polyposis. N Engl J Med 311:80, 1984
6. Luk GD, Silverman AL, Giardiello FM: Biochemical markers in patients with familial colonic neoplasia. Semin Surg Oncol 3:126, 1987
7. Moore JR, Lamont JT: Colorectal cancer. Risk factors and screening strategies. Arch Intern Med 144:1819, 1987
8. Reddy BS: Nutritional aspects of colon cancer. Prog Food Nutr Sci 9:257, 1985
9. Simon JB: Occult blood screening for colorectal carcinoma. A critical review. Gastroenterology 88:820, 1985
10. Sugarbaker PH, Gunderson LL, Wittes RE: Colorectal cancer. In DeVita VT, Hellman S, Rosenberg SA (eds): Cancer, 2d ed. Philadelphia, JB Lippincott, 1985, p 795

CHAPTER 6.24
Transfusion Medicine

Thomas S. Kickler, Paul M. Ness, and Hayden G. Braine

Blood transfusion has four basic indications in clinical medicine. For patients with acute hemorrhage or other causes of hypovolemia, transfusions can be lifesaving by restoring the blood volume. For patients with chronic anemia refractory to other means of medical management, transfusions can restore the oxygen-carrying capacity. Many patients with acquired or congenital deficiency of platelets, leukocytes, or plasma proteins benefit by the use of blood products to replace these normal blood components. Finally, blood transfusion can be used as a means of removing toxic substances, as in exchange transfusions to remove bilirubin in hemolytic disease of the newborn.

As with any therapy, the potential benefit must be weighed against the potential risk before prescribing blood components. The physician can minimize the risks of isoimmunization and disease transmission by adherence to two basic transfusion principles. First, it is unnecessary to correct a deficiency to normal levels. Patients have normal hemostasis with platelet counts of $90,000/\mu l$ even though the lower limit of the normal range is $150,000/\mu l$, and the partial thromboplastin time is not prolonged with a 30 percent level of factor VIII even though the normal level is 100 percent. Physiologic levels should be restored, allowing the patient's homeostatic mechanisms to restore normality following acute replacement therapy.

The second basic transfusion principle is the use of specific blood components to correct a known deficiency rather than "nonspecific" therapy with whole blood for all indications. The modern blood bank can prepare several blood components from a single volunteer blood donation so that our limited national blood

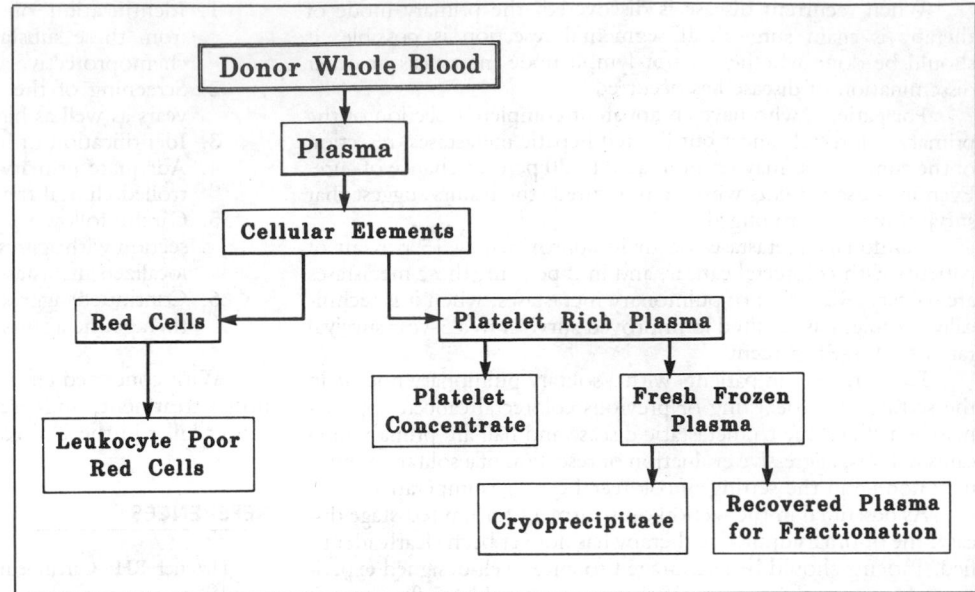

Figure 6.24–1. Donor whole blood.

supply can satisfy the increasing medical demands (Fig. 6.24–1). The routine use of blood components in medical practice is justified by the reasons and examples in Table 6.24–1.

RED BLOOD CELL PRODUCTS[2,15]

There are currently five different red cell products that meet various clinical indications for replacement of oxygen-carrying capacity and blood volume (Table 6.24–2).

RED CELL CONCENTRATES

Red cells are obtained from donor whole blood by removing plasma. The resultant unit of red cells has a hematocrit of 80 percent in a volume of approximately 300 ml. The red cell is the component of choice when restoration of oxygen-carrying capacity alone is required. It is the product of first choice for patients with chronic anemia or surgical hemorrhage where blood volume losses in adults are less than 1500 ml. Transfusions of red cells minimize volume expansion and maximally improve oxygen delivery.

RED CELL CONCENTRATES WITH ADDITIVE SOLUTIONS

Red cell concentrates are routinely collected in citrate phosphate dextrose with adenine allowing storage for 35 days (Table 6.24–3). Recently, new additive solutions have been introduced that permit 42-day storage. These solutions consist of an additional 100 ml of saline with dextrose, mannitol, and adenine, and are added after the removal of plasma from the unit of blood. The hematocrit of such units ranges between 50 and 60 percent. Since extra crystalloid solution is added, the red cells are less viscous, and predilution with saline to improve flow rates is not required.

WHOLE BLOOD

Massive hemorrhage is best treated with whole blood because red cells and volume are replaced simultaneously. Prompt correction

TABLE 6.24–1. BLOOD COMPONENT THERAPY

Justification	Transfusion Practice Example
1. Avoids circulatory overload	1. Red cells in chronic anemia avoids pulmonary edema
2. Limits harmful materials	2. Washed red cells eliminate K^+, NH_4^+, and H^+, which accumulate during storage and may be toxic in patients with renal or liver disease
3. Concentrates required material for effective levels	3. Cryoprecipitate or coagulation factor concentrates in hemophilia
4. Minimizes risk of disease transmission	4. Use of heat-treated clotting concentrates or albumin
5. Maximizes use of donated blood	5. One unit of donor blood can be used to provide red cells, platelet concentrate, cryoprecipitate, with residual plasma available for fractionation

TABLE 6.24–2. CLINICAL USE OF RED CELL COMPONENTS

Component	Indications
Red cells	Chronic anemia Surgical blood loss <1500 ml
Whole blood	Acute blood loss >1500 ml Exchange transfusion
Leukocyte-poor red cells	Febrile, non-hemolytic transfusion reactions
Washed red cells	Allergic reactions to plasma proteins (e.g., IgA) Removal of storage by-products for patients with severe renal or hepatic compromise
Frozen red cells	Rare blood preservation Autologous transfusion Febrile reactions refractory to leukocyte-poor blood

TABLE 6.24–3. PROPERTIES OF RED CELL CONCENTRATES STORED IN CPD-A

Parameter	Days of Storage		
	0	*28*	*35*
pH	7.55	—	6.71
Plasma K$^+$ (mEq/L)	4	76	78.5
Plasma Na$^+$ (mEq/L)	170	122	111
Red blood cell ATP (μmol/g Hgb)	3.84	2.46	1.9
Red blood cell 2,3-DPG (μmol/g Hgb)	13.5	0.53	0.35

Data from Moore GI, Peck CC, et al: Some properties of blood stored in CPD-A1 solution. A brief summary. Transfusion 21:135–137, 1981.[16]

of intravascular volume depletion is critical in the prevention of the sequelae of shock, that is, acidosis, renal failure, and disseminated intravascular coagulation. In the absence of whole blood, other red cell products can be combined with volume expanders (crystalloid or colloid) to treat massive hemorrhage, but whole blood use is a more efficient practice.

Whole blood is not a reliable source of platelets. Within 24 hours of collection and storage at routine blood bank 4C temperature, whole blood lacks viable platelets. In massively transfused patients, the use of platelet-free whole blood or red cells can result in dilution of the recipient's platelet count. Although the platelet count does not usually fall to levels associated with bleeding until 15 to 20 units of blood have been administered, coagulation monitoring and use of platelet concentrates for thrombocytopenic patients is recommended.

Whole blood use has been criticized as an inadequate source of coagulation factors. Factor VIII in stored whole blood falls rapidly to approximately 25 percent of normal, and factor V declines less rapidly to similar levels. The clinical significance of these deficiencies is minimal, however, since surgical hemostasis can be achieved with factor V and VIII levels that are 15 and 30 percent of normal, respectively. The other coagulation factors are stable in stored blood. Hence, in the absence of liver failure or DIC, whole blood can maintain adequate hemostatic levels.

LEUKOCYTE-POOR BLOOD

Patients receiving multiple transfusions or multiparous women may develop antibodies to leukocytes. When they are transfused with incompatible leukocytes, which contaminate red cell products, febrile nonhemolytic transfusion reactions may occur. These reactions can be prevented by the use of leukocyte-poor blood. A variety of techniques, including cell washing, filtration, and buffy coat removal, can remove at least 70 percent of leukocytes from blood products. Most patients will not experience febrile reactions with these products, but a few patients may require the additional leukocyte removal provided by frozen red cells.

WASHED RED CELLS

Red cells can be washed with isotonic saline to remove plasma. Patients who suffer repeated allergic reactions to plasma and patients with IgA deficiency should receive washed red cells.

FROZEN RED CELLS

Red cells can be frozen with a cryoprotective agent such as glycerol to extend the current 35-day liquid storage limitation to at least 3

years. Freezing red cells permits the accumulation of an inventory of red cells with defined antigen patterns for patients with complex antibody problems and patients requiring rare blood types. Autologous units can also be stored for future surgery or for patients with relapsing forms of anemia who are unlikely to have compatible blood available. The initial enthusiasm for frozen blood generated by the suggestions that hepatitis transmission and allograft rejection could be lessened by frozen red cell transfusion has not been justified by clinical trials. Frozen blood is used uncommonly, therefore, and the predicted growth for this product has not materialized.

FRESH-FROZEN PLASMA

Fresh-frozen plasma (FFP) is defined as the fluid portion of one unit of blood that has been centrifuged, separated, and frozen within 6 hours of collection. FFP contains the labile and stable components of the coagulation, fibrinolytic, and complement systems, as well as other plasma proteins that maintain oncotic pressure and immunity. Few specific indications for the use of FFP exist. These indications generally are limited to the treatment of congenital coagulation deficiencies in which specific factor concentrates are unavailable (see Chapter 6.10). In addition, for warfarin anticoagulated patients who are actively bleeding or require emergency surgery, FFP can be used to restore normal hemostasis.

FFP has become a popular volume replacement agent. Crystalloid and colloid solutions containing albumin or plasma protein fraction are preferable to FFP, however. Unlike FFP, these alternative therapies do not increase the risk of disease transmission. The practice of transfusing both packed cells and FFP to a patient massively bleeding not only doubles the disease transmission risk but also is more expensive. In these situations, whole blood would be more appropriate.

PLATELET COLLECTION AND TRANSFUSION

Prior to the use of platelet transfusion therapy, hemorrhage secondary to thrombocytopenia accounted for 50 percent of the mortality associated with bone marrow failure. With platelet transfusion support, this mortality has been reduced to less than 5 percent.[14] Thrombocytopenia alone, however, is not an absolute indication for platelet transfusion. Platelet transfusion is indicated only when thrombocytopenia results in hemorrhage or is highly likely to (Table 6.24–4). To develop a rational approach to platelet transfusion support, a thorough evaluation of the etiology of thrombocytopenia must be completed (Table 6.24–5).

ETIOLOGY OF THROMBOCYTOPENIA

Thrombocytopenia (peripheral blood platelet count less than 150,000/μl) may result from increased platelet consumption, platelet sequestration, decreased platelet production, or any combination of these factors. Platelet survival in the peripheral blood is normally 10 ± 1.5 days. A variety of conditions, including infection, trauma, vasculitis, arterial or venous thrombosis, and prosthetic heart valves, can decrease platelet survival by 50 percent or more, but thrombocytopenia usually does not result because bone marrow platelet production can normally be increased six- to eightfold. Platelet survival of less than 1 to 2 days generally cannot be compensated for by increased platelet production. Conditions capable of resulting in severely decreased platelet survival and thrombocytopenia include sepsis, disseminated intravascular coagulation, thrombotic thrombocytopenia purpura, the hemolytic uremic syndrome, and the immune thrombocytopenias.[9] It is important to identify the causes of increased platelet consumption in order to

TABLE 6.24–4. CURRENT INDICATIONS FOR PLATELET TRANSFUSION

Emergent:
- Platelet count <40,000/μl with clinical evidence of hemorrhage

Prophylactic:
- Platelet count <20,000/μl with severe bone marrow failure
- Prior to invasive procedures to maintain platelet count >80,000/μl for major surgery (laparotomy, thoracotomy, etc) to maintain platelet count >40,000/μl for minor procedures (spinal tap, endoscopy, etc)

Not Indicated:
- Disorders of increased platelet consumption

guide corrective therapy. Platelet transfusions alone are inadequate although they are of some use in controlling hemorrhage (Table 6.24–6).

Sequestration of platelets in the spleen may result in thrombocytopenia even though bone marrow platelet production and peripheral platelet survival are normal. Approximately one third of the peripheral platelet pool normally is sequestered in the spleen. Increased sequestration secondary to splenomegaly can result in mild to moderate thrombocytopenia. Thrombocytopenia less than 50,000 per μl is rarely caused by splenomegaly alone. Normally 10 to 20 percent of the peripheral platelet pool is sequestered in the liver. Increased hepatic platelet sequestration may result in thrombocytopenia such as that seen during severe hypothermia.

As thrombocytopenia secondary to splenic sequestration is not severe, platelet transfusion is usually not indicated. If significant splenic sequestration is present, platelet transfusion will result in less than the expected increment in circulating platelets, but those platelets that do circulate will have a normal survival. When platelet transfusion is used before splenectomy, the largest number of platelets should be transfused after the splenic artery is occluded in order to avoid sequestration of the transfused platelets.

Decreased bone marrow platelet production may be secondary to myelophthisis, developmental arrest, or hypoproliferative states. Infiltration of the bone marrow with cancer or fibrosis may result in an inadequate microenvironment to support thrombopoiesis.

TABLE 6.24–5. PATHOGENESIS OF SEVERE THROMBOCYTOPENIA

Consumption > Production	Decreased Production
Dilutional • Massive transfusion	*Congenital Disorders* • Fanconi anemia • Wiskott–Aldrich syndrome
Sequestration • Splenomegaly • Hypothermia	*Infection* • Rubella • Hepatitis • Cytomegalovirus
Immune Destruction • Autoimmune thrombocytopenia purpura • Drug-induced • Systemic lupus erythematosus • Evans syndrome	*Drugs and Toxins* • Cytotoxic drugs • Drug reactions • Hydrocarbons • Alcohol • Radiation
Nonimmune Destruction • Inflammation • Leukemia • Intravascular coagulopathy • Trauma • Arterial or venous thrombosis • Intravascular foreign body • Neoplasia • Hemangioma	*Vitamin Deficiency* • B₁₂ • Folate *Marrow Replacement* • Leukemia • Myeloproliferative disorder • Tumor • Osteopetrosis • Systemic histiocytosis • Gaucher disease • Amyloidosis

TABLE 6.24–6. CLINICAL EVALUATION OF SEVERE THROMBOYCTOPENIA

	Consumption >Production	Decreased Production
History	Massive transfusion Drug history Complicating medical problems Pregnancy	Recent viral infection Drug history Radiation exposure Exposure to toxins
Physical	Hepatosplenomegaly Purpura (DIC) Massive hemangioma Petechiae, ecchymoses Signs of complicating illness	Petechiae Evidence of tumor or leukemia Signs of vitamin deficiency or alcohol abuse
Peripheral blood	Evidence of increased marrow production: nucleated red cells, large platelets, immature granulocytes Evidence of increased destruction: damaged red cells, toxic granulation/vacuolization in leukocytes	Evidence of early cell release from marrow: nucleated red cells, large platelets Leukemic blasts or other evidence of tumor
Bone marrow	Hypercellular	Hypocellular or replaced with tumor Usually hypercellular in B₁₂ and folate deficiency Evidence of disordered myelopoiesis

Again, because of the great reserve capacity of normal bone marrow, such infiltration must be generalized in order to result in thrombocytopenia.

Thrombocytopenia secondary to deficient marrow production may also result from abnormal or impaired differentiation. In severe vitamin B₁₂ or folate deficiency, marrow megakaryocyte mass may be increased severalfold, but platelet production can be reduced to less than 10 percent of normal. Dysthrombopoiesis or impaired thrombopoiesis may also account for thrombocytopenia noted in leukemic or preleukemic conditions and paroxysmal nocturnal hemoglobinuria.

Thrombocytopenia due to decreased megakaryocyte numbers can occur as an isolated finding or in conjunction with deficits in erythroid or myeloid cell lines. In most instances an etiologic agent cannot be identified. In some cases chemical or radiation exposure, drug therapy, or viral infections can be incriminated. Cytotoxic drugs used as antineoplastic or immunosuppressive agents are commonly associated with pancytopenia. In most cases, such myelotoxicity is dose-related and reversible with cessation of therapy. Some agents, including the nitrosoureas, busulfan, L-phenylalanine mustard, and mitomycin-C, can produce prolonged periods of marrow hypoplasia.

Platelet transfusion therapy is most effective in thrombocytopenia secondary to bone marrow failure when there is an isolated defect in platelet production.[11]

THROMBOCYTOPENIA AND HEMORRHAGE

Platelet counts less than 100,000/μl are associated with a prolongation of the bleeding time, but spontaneous clinically significant hemorrhage is usually not observed unless the platelet count is less than 10,000/μl.[7] Petechiae and mucous membrane bleeding, the commonest physical signs of thrombocytopenia, usually do not develop until the platelet count is less than 40,000/μl (Table

TABLE 6.24–7. RELATIONSHIP BETWEEN PLATELET COUNT AND BLEEDING

Platelet Count	Clinical Findings
>100,000/μl	None
40,000–100,000/μl	Prolonged bleeding time Abnormal clot retraction No significant clinical abnormalities
10,000–40,000/μl	Petechiae, easy bruising, epistaxis
<10,000/μl	Major risk of bleeding, especially gastrointestinal and CNS

6.24–7). Patients with thrombocytopenia secondary to increased platelet destruction generally tolerate lower platelet counts with less evidence of bleeding than do patients with decreased platelet production. Hemorrhage is the greatest concern in the thrombocytopenic patient. Epistaxis, menorrhagia, and hematuria may be treated when detected. Intracranial hemorrhage, which may develop suddenly and be rapidly fatal, has been more difficult to manage. If the duration of thrombocytopenia is expected to be relatively short (less than 4 to 6 weeks) and the degree of thrombocytopenia severe (less than 10,000/μl), prophylactic platelet transfusion when the platelet count is less than 20,000/μl is usually employed. This transfusion strategy has been used in the treatment of acute leukemia. When thrombocytopenia is less severe and its duration indeterminate as in aplastic anemia, platelet transfusions are generally recommended only for documented bleeding or in preparation for invasive diagnostic or therapeutic procedures. Some authors feel that such a strategy may reduce the number of transfusions and thereby delay alloimmunization to platelet antigens.

PLATELET COLLECTION AND STORAGE

Single units containing 5 to 8 × 10^{10} platelets in a minimum of 50 ml of plasma are derived from whole blood during preparation of packed erythrocytes and plasma. These concentrates may be stored at room temperature (22C) for 5 to 7 days. To achieve a therapeutic dose, platelet concentrates are pooled and 3 to 6 U/m² are given. Platelet concentrates prepared from single units of whole blood usually are readily available, least expensive to prepare, may be stored up to 7 days, and involve negligible risk or discomfort for the blood donor. Bacterial contamination is an inherent risk of venipuncture, and storage greater than 5 days at room temperature of a contaminated concentrate may result in substantial morbidity and mortality to the transfused patient.

If HLA-matched platelets are required for an alloimmunized patient, 5 to 10 units of platelets must be obtained from a single HLA-matched donor by plateletpheresis. This is done either manually by serially collecting individual units of whole blood, separating the platelet fraction by centrifugation, and returning the erythrocytes and plasma to the donor, or by using one of several commercially available automated blood cell separators. While essential for the production of HLA-matched or CMV-negative platelet concentrates, plateletpheresis is more expensive and involves more donor risk because extracorporeal processing and reinfusion of blood and anticoagulant are required. Additionally, most automated cell separators require that many integral connections be made before use, thereby increasing the risk of bacterial contamination of the platelet product. For this reason the storage time for platelet concentrates prepared by plateletpheresis is usually restricted to 24 hours.

Whether obtained from whole blood donation or plateletpheresis, platelet concentrates should be ABO-compatible with the recipient. ABO compatibility does not significantly affect platelet survival, but infusion of large volumes of incompatible plasma may result in a hemolytic anemia. If ABO incompatible platelets must be used, washing and resuspension in saline will prevent hemolytic reactions.

Longer storage of platelets by freezing and cryopreservation at −90C to −196C would significantly improve platelet transfusion practice, particularly if inventories of HLA-typed platelets were available. Current techniques for platelet cryopreservation, however, incur a large platelet loss during freezing and thawing and result in a final product with poor posttransfusion survival. Consequently, cryopreserved platelets are not generally available.

EVALUATION OF TRANSFUSION OUTCOME

A successful platelet transfusion results in normal posttransfusion platelet recovery and survival. Platelet recovery is assessed by calculating the immediate (1 to 4 hours) posttransfusion increment in the recipient's platelet count:

$$\frac{\left(\begin{array}{c}\text{Posttransfusion} \\ \text{platelet count}\end{array} - \begin{array}{c}\text{Pretransfusion} \\ \text{platelet count}\end{array}\right) \times \left(\begin{array}{c}\text{Recipient} \\ \text{size in m}^2\end{array}\right)}{\text{Number of units transfused}}$$

$$= 10,000 \pm 5,000$$

where 1 unit = 5.5 × 10^{10} platelets.

A successful transfusion results in a corrected increment of 10,000 ± 5,000 (1 standard deviation). Patients without a functional spleen should have a corrected increment 30 percent higher. Patients with splenic sequestion will have lower corrected increments, but posttransfusion platelet survival will be normal.

With normal platelet survival, infusion of 3 to 6 units of platelets per square meter should result in a platelet count greater than 50,000/μl and adequate hemostasis for 3 to 5 days. In many clinical situations, however, normal platelet survival is not observed. Hemorrhage, fever, and infection, all frequently present in the patient with severe pancytopenia, may shorten platelet survival significantly. Consequently, critically ill patients may require more frequent platelet transfusions.

PLATELET TRANSFUSION FAILURE DUE TO IMMUNE DESTRUCTION

HLA antigens are expressed on circulating platelets. With transfusion, transplantation, or pregnancy, alloantibodies directed against this antigen system develop. Antigen exposure, concomitant cytotoxic or immunosuppressive therapy, and recipient genetic predisposition determine if an individual will become alloimmunized. While 40 to 80 percent of patients become alloimmunized after 1 to 2 months of transfusion support, a small population of patients are apparently resistant to sensitization to HLA antigens and never become alloimmunized.[6]

Studies indicate that serial platelet transfusions from one animal to another first result in shortened survival of tranfused platelets. With repeated sensitization, immediate posttransfusion platelet recovery is also reduced. The HLA specificity of posttransfusion alloantibodies is frequently quite broad. As few as three or four erythrocyte, platelet, or leukocyte transfusions can result in refractoriness to all but HLA-identical platelet concentrates.

Clinical identification of alloimmunization is difficult. If nonimmunologic causes of rapid platelet destruction and splenic sequestration are unlikely, a 1-hour posttransfusion platelet recovery less than 50 percent of expected is suggestive of immune platelet destruction. Over 80 percent of patients who develop alloimmunization to platelets also develop lymphocytotoxic antibodies. Screening patients requiring platelet transfusion support to detect the development of lymphocytotoxic antibodies is helpful in identifying those patients who will benefit from HLA-matched platelet transfusions. Several assays for the detection of antiplatelet antibodies have been proposed, but to date none have proved suffi-

ciently sensitive and specific to warrant general clinical use. Currently, an empiric trial of transfusion with HLA-matched platelets is the only definitive method to prove that platelet transfusion failure is mediated by anti-HLA alloimmunization.

HLA-A and -B loci antigens are the most important determinants of clinically significant alloimmune platelet transfusion failure.[21] Platelet concentrates obtained from donors identically matched at the HLA-A and -B loci with the recipient can result in normal posttransfusion platelet recovery and survival in patients absolutely refractory to HLA-mismatched platelets. Unfortunately the HLA-A and -B loci are highly pleomorphic. Over 16 A locus and 27 B locus antigen specificities have been identified. Thus, even for common phenotypes, the chance of identifying a four-antigen (A) match in a random population of blood donors is approximately 1 in 5000. In many donors only two or three antigens can be identified. As this usually reflects homozygosity at the A or B locus, such donors (BU match) are usually as effective as A matches. The majority of alloimmunized patients can also be successfully transfused with platelet products mismatched for one or two antigens (BX match) as long as the mismatched antigens are limited to those that are serologically similar to the recipient.[5] For example: HLA-A28 is serologically cross-reactive with HLA-A2 and frequently may be successfully substituted for HLA-A2. The ability to use BX matches successfully has increased the availability of suitable donors 150-fold, thereby making matched HLA platelets generally available. In situations when random donor HLA-matched platelets are not available, siblings of the patient and occasionally parents or children may be suitable matches, but should be used only after careful consideration of the fact that transfusions from such donors may sensitize the recipient to minor transplantation antigens and preclude subsequent bone marrow transplantation.

Non-HLA platelet antigens are apparently of minor importance in platelet transfusion. Five diallelic platelet antigen systems, designated PL^A, PL^E, Ko, BAIC, and PEN have been implicated as the cause of neonatal thrombocytopenia and posttransfusion purpura. The gene frequency of these antigens is sufficiently high that homozygotes lacking these antigens are uncommon and, therefore, they do not play a major role in posttransfusion alloimmunization.

All patients receiving platelet transfusion therapy should be carefully monitored for the development of alloimmunization. Screening for lymphocytotoxic antibodies should be performed prior to the start of therapy and weekly thereafter. Likewise the 1-hour posttransfusion-corrected platelet increment should be assessed frequently. When transfusion failures are detected, a trial of two HLA-matched (A or BU) transfusions are indicated. If transfusion with HLA-matched platelets gives a normal 1-hour posttransfusion increment, continued support with HLA-matched products is indicated. If matched platelets are not available, continued transfusion of nontyped products may result in increments (1000 to 4000 m^2/U) that are adequate to maintain platelet counts greater than 10,000/μl. In the most severe cases there may be no increment. Transfusing mismatched platelets in this setting will not prevent bleeding. Some clinicians, however, feel that in this situation 3 to 4 units of platelets given every 8 to 12 hours may improve survival (Table 6.24–8).

A number of patients experiencing platelet transfusion failure will not show an improved response to HLA-matched platelets. In some cases the cause of increased platelet consumption can be identified. Adequate treatment of the underlying disease (e.g., antibiotic therapy of bacteremia) may correct the problem. If splenomegaly can be incriminated, splenectomy may be considered if the patient's clinical situation permits. Every attempt should be made to eliminate drugs that impair platelet function, especially aspirin and high-dose therapy and penicillins. If uremia is present, dialysis may be considered. Frequent transfusions of small numbers of platelets may also be considered in this situation but their use is unproven, costly, and usually ineffective.

TABLE 6.24–8. CLINICAL EVALUATION OF PLATELET TRANSFUSION FAILURE

	Immune	Nonimmune
History	Multiple prior transfusion or pregnancies Drug hypersensitivity	Few or no transfusions or pregnancies
Physical	None	Splenomegaly Evidence of disorders leading to increased platelet destruction
Laboratory Lymphocytoxic antibody	Present in 85% of cases	Usually absent
Platelet-associated IgG	Direct test positive in ITP Indirect test positive in alloimmunization and some ITP	Usually absent

GRANULOCYTE TRANSFUSION

Infection secondary to granulocytopenia has become the leading cause of morbidity and mortality in patients with bone marrow failure (Table 6.24–9). Management of the severely neutropenic patient focuses on prevention of infection by markedly reducing the number of microorganisms in the gastrointestinal tract with oral nonabsorbable antibiotics, the use of reverse isolation techniques, and early empiric antibiotic therapy of suspected infection. In selected cases specific cell replacement therapy with granulocyte transfusion is an effective adjunct to overall infectious disease management.

GRANULOCYTE COLLECTION AND STORAGE

Preparation of granulocyte concentrates from normal donors became feasible with the development of centrifugal blood cell separators. Collection of adequate numbers of granulocytes from normal donors, however, has proved difficult. With current cell separators, 6 to 8 L of blood can be processed during a 2- to 3-hour donation. Granulocytes, however, cannot be separated from

TABLE 6.24–9. CAUSES OF SEVERE GRANULOCYTOPENIA

Increased Granulocyte Consumption	Decreased Granulocyte Production
Sequestration • Splenomegaly	**Congenital Disorders** • Fanconi anemia
Immune Destruction • Felty syndrome • Collagen vascular disorders	**Viral Infection**
Overwhelming Sepsis	**Drugs and Toxins** • Chloramphenicol • Propylthiouracil • Hydrocarbons • Cytotoxic drugs • Radiation
	Vitamin Deficiency • B$_{12}$ • Folate
	Marrow Replacement • Leukemia • Tumor • Myelofibrosis

erythrocytes unless the donor is treated with a compound that induces rouleauing of the erythrocytes. Hydroxyethylstarch or dextrans are usually used to achieve rouleauing. These agents also induce transient volume expansion and persist in the donor for variable periods of time. Donors may also be premedicated with steroids to mobilize the marginating granulocyte pool and marrow reserve, thereby inducing a leukocytosis and doubling the number of circulating granulocytes available for collection. With these steps yields of 1 to 3 $\times$ 10^{10} granulocytes can be collected from normal donors over a 2- to 3-hour period. Erythrocyte contamination, however, remains high and granulocyte concentrates must be ABO-compatible with the recipient. Lymphocyte contamination is also high and radiation of granulocyte concentrates to 1500 rad is usually recommended to prevent graft-versus-host disease from developing in patients who are severely immunodepressed.

Granulocyte concentrates may be stored at room temperature but should be used as soon as possible. Storage longer than 8 hours results in significant loss of granulocyte chemotaxis. Cryopreservation of granulocytes is currently not feasible.

INDICATIONS FOR GRANULOCYTE TRANSFUSION

In the early 1970s, gram-negative sepsis in the neutropenic leukemia patient was associated with a 60 to 80 percent mortality. The addition of four to eight daily granulocyte transfusions to standard antibiotic therapy reduced this mortality to less than 20 percent.[10] More recent studies have shown prophylactic granulocyte transfusions to be effective in reducing the incidence of bacteremia and local infections in neutropenic patients, but not effective in increasing overall survival.[20] Today improved supportive care without granulocyte transfusion has reduced the mortality of gram-negative sepsis to less than 10 percent. This has largely obviated the need for granulocyte transfusion. Granulocyte transfusion is now indicated only in the severely neutropenic patient (absolute granulocyte count $<100/\mu l$) with refractory sepsis due to multiple antibiotic resistant organisms and for neonatal sepsis.

The greatest difficulty in achieving effective granulocyte transfusion is obtaining an adequate cell dose. Normal adult granulocyte production approximates 1 $\times$ 10^{11} cells per day and is increased severalfold in response to infection. Even with the most efficient use of current technology, granulocyte concentrates prepared from normal donors contain only 1 to 3 $\times$ 10^{10} cells. This is an effective dose for neonates and small children, but is only marginally effective for adults.

ADVERSE EFFECTS

Chills and fever occur during 30 percent of granulocyte transfusions and frequently require premedication of the patient with steroids. Pulmonary infiltrates with associated dyspnea and wheezing have been noted in 10 to 15 percent of transfusions. Urticaria, generalized skin rashes, hypotension, and hypertension may also occur. Use of HLA-matched granulocyte concentrates may reduce the incidence of adverse reactions, but they are not generally available.

STEM-CELL TRANSPLANTATION

Human bone marrow contains totipotential stem cells capable of reconstituting normal lymphohematopoiesis following bone marrow ablative therapy. Transplantation of bone marrow has been employed to replace cellular deficits in lymphohematopoetic function in diseases such as aplastic anemia, congenital immune deficiency states, and thalassemia major. In addition it has been employed in conjunction with bone marrow ablative chemotherapy or radiotherapy in the treatment of cancer[13,19] (Table 6.24–10).

TABLE 6.24–10. CLINICAL MANAGEMENT OF ALLOGENEIC BONE MARROW TRANSPLANTATION

Pretransplant (Prior to Admission)
Evaluation of Recipient
- Disease status; stage and prognosis with transplant or alternate therapies
- Adequate organ function, especially cardiac, renal, hepatic, and pulmonary systems
- Psychosocial status
- Contraindications: infection, sensitization, etc.

Evaluation of Donor
- Contraindications of anesthesia
- Presence of normal marrow function
- Compatibility with recipient (HLA-A, -B, -D, and mixed leukocyte culture)

Preparative Regimen (Day −10 to 0)
- Immunosuppression: cyclophosphamide alone in nonsensitized patients; total body irradiation needed in sensitized patients
- Cytoreduction: cyclophosphamide, total body irradiation, busulfan, and other agents

Marrow Collection and Transfusion (Day 0)
- Collection under general anesthesia
- Sieving
- If major ABO incompatibility exists marrow may be depleted of red cells or recipient plasmapheresed to remove isoagglutinins

Severe Bone Marrow Aplasia (Day 0 to 21)
- Empiric management of fever and infection
- Platelet and red cell transfusion
- Hyperalimentation
- Fluid and electrolyte management

Postengraftment Problems (Day 21+)
- Acute graft-versus-host disease
- Interstitial pneumonitis
- Viral infections
- Chronic graft-versus-host disease
- Nutrition

DONOR SELECTION

The source of stem cells for transplantation may be from the patient for autologous reconstitution or from an HLA-identical donor for allogeneic transplantation. In cellular deficiency states autologous cells are obviously not available and an allogeneic donor must be used. In order to minimize the chance of rejection of the graft by the host or an immunologic attack on the host by the graft (graft-versus-host disease), the allogeneic marrow donor and recipient should be genotypically identical at the HLA-A and -B loci and nonreactive in the mixed lymphocyte culture (MLC). Bone marrow transplantation between siblings mismatched at a single HLA-A, -B, or -D locus due to recombination within the major histocompatibility complex has been performed successfully, but insufficient experience is available to recommend the routine use of such mismatches. Nonrelated HLA-A- and -B-locus identical and MLC nonreactive marrow donors also have been used successfully. The difficulty of identifying such nonrelated donors and the risk and discomfort of marrow donation limit the use of such donors.

For transplantation following marrow ablative therapy of cancer, allogeneic or autologous marrow can be used. When autologous marrow is employed it is preserved in liquid or frozen state until cytotoxic therapy is completed and then reinfused. Autologous bone marrow grafting has the advantage that the risks of graft rejection and graft-versus-host disease are minimal. Unfortunately, in many cases the autologous marrow may be contaminated with viable cancer cells, which may engraft with the normal stem cells. Techniques to remove tumor cells from marrow using in vitro treatment with drug or antibody are being investigated.

STEM CELL COLLECTION

Bone marrow is the most commonly used source of totipotent lymphohematopoietic stem cells in humans. After general anesthesia, multiple percutaneous aspirations of marrow are made along the anterior and posterior iliac crests of the donor. A volume of 500 to 1500 ml of a blood-marrow mixture anticoagulated with heparin and containing greater than 1×10^8 nucleated cells per kilogram of recipient weight is obtained. Adequate replacement of donor blood volume is essential during the collection.

PROCESSING, STORAGE, AND INFUSION

The aspirated marrow is filtered through graded sieves to remove particulate matter and create a single cell suspension. ABO blood group–compatible marrow may be infused through a vein without further processing. If there is an ABO blood group incompatibility between donor and recipient the large number of incompatible erythrocytes contained in the collected marrow would result in a hemolytic transfusion reaction. In such cases a leukocyte concentrate containing less than 25 ml of erythrocytes and 60 to 80 percent of the mononuclear cell fraction containing stem cells may be prepared by centrifugation and infused slowly.

Hematopoietic stem cells may be preserved in short-term (6- to 12-hour) liquid culture. Longer storage requires cryopreservation with cryoprotectant. Bone marrow preserved in liquid nitrogen ($-196C$) for over 3 years has been used successfully for transplantation. Although the minimum effective dose of stem cells is now known, most authors feel that more than 1×10^8 nucleated marrow cells per kilogram of recipient weight is desirable.

PRETRANSPLANT PREPARATIVE THERAPY

Syngeneic (identical twin) or autologous bone marrow can be transplanted without immunosuppression. To successfully engraft HLA-identical allogeneic marrow, treatment must be given before marrow infusion to eliminate residual recipient marrow and establish some degree of immunosuppression. If the recipient has not been sensitized by prior transfusion or pregnancy, pretreatment with cyclophosphamide alone is adequate. If the recipient has been sensitized, however, more intensive immunosuppressive regimens, usually employing total body irradiation, are used.

INDICATIONS FOR BONE MARROW TRANSPLANTATION

Allogeneic bone marrow transplantation is being investigated in a wide variety of malignant and nonmalignant diseases (Table 6.24–11). It has been shown to improve survival and is the treatment of choice for severe aplastic anemia. Bone marrow transplantation in acute leukemia in first or second remission results in a long-term disease-free remission in 30 to 60 percent of cases. Its overall superiority to conventional therapy, however, has not been proven. Bone marrow transplantation has been employed successfully in treatment of several congenital combined immune deficiency syndromes, thalassemia major, and Hunter syndrome. Its application in lymphoma, multiple myeloma, and other malignancies is being investigated.

Autologous bone marrow transplantation following intensive cytoreductive therapy has resulted in long-term remission and possibly cures in some leukemias and lymphomas refractory to conventional therapy.

RISKS IN BONE MARROW TRANSPLANTATION

Bone marrow transplantation involves many risks. Side effects of the pretransplantation preparative regimens vary according to the

TABLE 6.24–11. SPECIFIC DISORDERS TREATED BY BONE MARROW TRANSPLANTATION

Allogeneic
- Severe aplastic anemia (treatment of choice)
- Leukemia (reasonable alternative to other treatment)
  - Acute myelocytic and variants
  - Acute lymphocytic
  - Hairy cell leukemia
  - Chronic myelocytic
- Other neoplastic disorders (investigational)
  - Multiple myeloma
  - Breast cancer
  - Lymphoma
- Inherited metabolic disorders (investigational)
  - Adrenoleukodystrophy
  - Hurler syndrome
  - Gaucher disease
  - Maroteaux-Lamy syndrome
  - Metachromatic leukodystrophy
- Hemoglobinopathies (investigational)
  - Thalassemia major
- Severe combined immune deficiencies (treatment of choice)
- Osteopetrosis (treatment of choice)

Autologous
- Leukemia (investigational)
  - Acute lymphocytic
  - Acute myelocytic
- Other neoplastic disorders (investigational)
  - Lymphoma
  - Breast
  - Colon
  - Melanoma
  - Testicular carcinoma

agents used. All regimens, however, entail a period of 2 to 4 weeks of pancytopenia during engraftment. Platelet and red cell support and antibiotic treatment of infection are required routinely. Infections with herpesvirus and cytomegalovirus, as well as other opportunistic infections, are common, as is interstitial pneumonitis caused by the cytotoxicity of the preparative regimens or opportunistic infection. Of most concern is acute graft-versus-host disease encountered in 60 percent of allogeneic transplants and fatal in 10 percent of cases. This is manifested by a triad of generalized dermatitis, hepatitis, and enterocolitis. Treatment of graft-versus-host disease is difficult and usually involves use of prednisone, cyclosporine, and other immunosuppressive agents. A second syndrome with many features of autoimmune diseases, including dermatofibrosis and sclerosis, Sjögren syndrome, and progressive hepatitis, termed "chronic graft-versus-host disease," may be encountered weeks to years after bone marrow transplantation. This syndrome is more resistant to immunosuppressive therapy.

CLINICAL CONSIDERATIONS IN STORED BLOOD TRANSFUSION[3,12,16]

The preservation of blood in the liquid state is achieved by storage at 1 to 6C with anticoagulant preservatives that allow red cells to maintain adequate levels of adenosine triphosphate (ATP). The recent introduction of citrate phosphate dextrose with adenine (CPD-A1) has extended storage capability to 35 days. Liquid storage of red cells, however, leads to biochemical and functional changes that may affect the recipient. These changes are tabulated in Table 6.24–3 and should be recognized as potential causes of adverse effects in clinically compromised blood recipients.

HEMOGLOBIN FUNCTION

The pH of CPD-A1 blood falls during storage from accumulated hydrogen ions generated by the metabolism of glucose to lactate.

This pH fall decreases enzymatic activity in red cells with resultant decrease in 2,3-diphosphoglycerate (2,3-DPG) levels. This organic phosphate plays an important role in oxygen delivery to the tissues by stabilizing the deoxyhemoglobin conformation of hemoglobin favoring tissue oxygen delivery. In CPD-A1, 2,3-DPG is maintained for 12 to 14 days but then falls to low levels. This 2,3-DPG-depleted stored blood has increased oxygen affinity. The clinical importance of 2,3-DPG levels in transfused blood, however, is not resolved. In most recipients, transfused red cells regenerate 2,3-DPG levels within several hours so that hemoglobin oxygen affinity is corrected to normal within 24 hours. In the patient with adequate cardiac reserve, adequate oxygen delivery can be maintained by increasing cardiac output; in patients with compromised cardiac status, blood with normal 2,3-DPG is indicated for transfusion. Although the problems that may arise in patients with cardiopulmonary compromise due to 2,3-DPG depletion remain a concern, it is clear that the vast majority of patients are safely transfused with stored blood.

ACID LOAD

Stored blood demonstrates the biochemical changes of metabolic acidosis (plasma HCO_3-depletion) and respiratory acidosis (PCO_2 elevation). Patients can rapidly eliminate the excess CO_2 by pulmonary mechanisms, but the acid load has been a concern for massively transfused patients. The potential for acidosis is best handled by close monitoring of arterial blood gases in recipients of massive transfusions, rather than prophylactic administration of sodium bicarbonate.

POTASSIUM TOXICITY

Potassium accumulates because of leakage of intracellular potassium from red cells damaged during storage. Although the plasma potassium level of stored red cells may appear dangerously high, the total potassium load of a unit of packed red cells is usually small (>5.5 mEq). These levels are not harmful to most patients, and patients who may be harmed, such as neonates or patients with chronic renal failure, can be transfused with fresh or washed red cells.

CITRATE TOXICITY

CPD-A1 is a useful anticoagulant because the citrate component chelates calcium ions to prevent clotting. Transfusion of CPD-A1 blood can decrease the recipient's ionized calcium but is of concern only in massive transfusion or neonatal exchanges. Citrate toxicity has been difficult to document in adult patients, and calcium replacement therapy has been considered to have more risks than potential benefits.

ADVERSE EFFECTS OF TRANSFUSION
(Table 6.24–12)

TRANSFUSION REACTIONS[17,18]

Acute Hemolytic Transfusion Reactions
The signs and symptoms of an acute hemolytic transfusion reaction are triggered by the interaction of an antibody with transfused red cells, leading to complement activation and intravascular hemolysis. This type of hemolytic reaction most frequently occurs when ABO-incompatible blood is mistakenly transfused. The most serious sequelae of hemolytic transfusion reactions are acute renal failure and DIC. The DIC is most likely initiated by intravascular hemolysis and antigen-antibody complex activation of the coagulation process. The pathogenesis of the acute renal failure is

TABLE 6.24–12. RISKS OF TRANSFUSION THERAPY

Reaction	Examples
Disease transmission	Bacterial contamination of stored blood Viral—hepatitis B, non-A,non-B hepatitis, cytomegelavirus Protozoal—malaria, babesiosis Spirochete—syphilis Acquired immunodeficiency syndrome (AIDS)—HIV retrovirus
Alloimmunization	Red cell blood group antigen—hemolysis HLA antigens—febrile transfusion reactions, refractoriness to platelets Platelet antigens—posttransfusion purpura
Allergic reaction	Anaphylactic reactions to IgA in patients with IgA deficiency Urticaria
Circulatory overload	Whole blood transfusion to patients with cardiopulmonary compromise
Graft-versus-host disease	Viable lymphoid cells engrafted in immunocompromised transfusion recipients

postischemic in origin and is etiologically unrelated to hemoglobin toxicity. The decreased renal blood flow, particularly to the cortical area, may be related to release of vasoconstrictive substances that lead to increased stasis. DIC may play a role in inducing the renal failure from acute hemolytic reactions.

The most frequent signs of a hemolytic transfusion reaction are fever and chills. Vague symptoms of backache or flushing may be the only initial manifestations. In unconscious patients, hypotension and bleeding at surgical or venipuncture sites may be the initial clues. If sufficient amounts of incompatible red cells are transfused, hypotension and oliguria progressing to anuria can ensue.

When a hemolytic reaction is suspected, the transfusion must be stopped and samples sent to the blood bank for investigation. In general two simple tests are sufficient to confirm or exclude acute hemolysis: (1) visual inspection of the patient's serum for the pink coloration of hemoglobin, and (2) a direct Coombs test.

Initial treatment should not be delayed while awaiting laboratory confirmation. Aggressive treatment of hypotension and maintenance of adequate renal blood flow are the goals of the early therapy for hemolytic transfusion reactions. To promote urine output, 0.9 percent saline should be administered along with intravenous furosemide, which improves cortical blood flow. Mannitol, an osmotic diuretic, has been frequently recommended, but current debate exists concerning its usefulness. If anuria develops, the patient should be managed for acute renal failure, that is, fluid restriction, monitoring of electrolytes, and dialysis if required.

Delayed Hemolytic Transfusion Reactions
Delayed hemolysis results from an anamnestic antibody response to transfused red cell antigens in a previously immunized recipient. The alloantibody, usually an IgG immunoglobulin, typically is undetectable in pretransfusion testing. Upon rechallenge, the recipient produces increasing amounts of antibody, which can destroy the transfused cells by an extravascular mechanism. The most frequent presentation includes fever, an unexplained fall in hemoglobin, and jaundice. Renal failure is unusual. The direct Coombs test is positive until the transfused cells are destroyed. Serum alloantibody usually becomes easily detectable. Blood lacking the implicated antigens is required for future transfusions, even if the antibody again becomes undetectable.

Febrile Nonhemolytic Transfusion Reactions

Recipients who have been multiply transfused or pregnant are likely to experience febrile transfusion reactions. These reactions occur because patients become sensitized to granulocyte, lymphocyte, or platelet antigens. Commonly, the human histocompatibility antigens (HLA) are involved. The development of fever during transfusion is an indication to stop the transfusion because an acute hemolytic transfusion cannot be excluded without laboratory investigation. Febrile nonhemolytic transfusion reactions can be prevented by using leukocyte-poor red cells in patients with previous reactions.

Urticaria

Urticarial transfusion reactions most likely are caused by patient antibodies directed against donor plasma antigens. The severity of these reactions may be reduced by prophylactic antihistamines in susceptible patients. In patients requiring frequent transfusions who experience recurrent urticarial reactions or other allergic manifestations, washed red cells may be indicated.

Anaphylactic Transfusion Reactions

Although anaphylactic reactions to blood products are rare, they can occur in IgA-deficient patients who have antibodies to IgA. The incidence of IgA deficiency in blood donors is approximately 0.1 percent. To prevent reactions in sensitized patients, blood products free of IgA must be transfused. Extensively washed red cells may be used for red cell replacement. Plasma products must be obtained from IgA-deficient donors.

INFECTIOUS AGENTS TRANSMITTED BY TRANSFUSION[1,16]

Viral Hepatitis

Viral hepatitis remains a serious posttransfusion complication. Despite the elimination of paid blood donors and screening of donor blood for hepatitis B surface antigen, posttransfusion hepatitis still develops in as many as 10 percent of recipients. Many of these cases are anicteric and may be unsuspected clinically. Type B hepatitis accounts for only 10 percent of cases, with the remainder of the cases attributed to non-A,non-B hepatitis. The elimination of this type of hepatitis has been impeded by the lack of a serologic method for identification. Although the transmission pattern is similar to that of hepatitis B, non-A,non-B hepatitis is subclinical and anicteric in most cases. The mild nature of overt non-A,non-B hepatitis is misleading because hepatocellular necrosis has been seen in many cases, along with a propensity toward chronic hepatitis.

Acquired Immunodeficiency Syndrome (AIDS)

The transmission of AIDS by blood transfusion accounts for about 1 to 2 percent of known AIDS cases. AIDS has also occurred in hemophiliacs who have been treated with factor VIII concentrates. To prevent the risk of HTLV-III transmission, all blood and blood products are now tested for anti-HTLV-III. Furthermore, the use of a blood donor who may have been exposed to the virus is deferred. With these preventive measures, the risk of AIDS transmission by blood transfusion has been reduced. Because the incubation period of AIDS may be long, a detailed transfusion history covering the preceding 5 years should be obtained in any patient developing AIDS. If a transfusion-associated AIDS case is diagnosed, the blood bank should be notified to determine other patients at risk.

Cytomegalovirus

After the transfusion of blood, recipients may develop a mild febrile illness with splenomegaly; reactive lymphocytes may be seen in the peripheral blood. Cytomegalovirus (CMV) was originally described in cardiac surgery patients, accounting for the designation of postperfusion syndrome. It was subsequently observed that transfused blood could transmit CMV, leading to this syndrome.

Although CMV infection was initially attributed to fresh blood transfusions, it also occurs after the transfusion of stored blood. Patients who are immunosuppressed, such as renal or bone marrow transplant patients, are at greatest risk of CMV infection. CMV infection in neonates whose mothers lack antibody to CMV may be transmitted by blood products. To prevent CMV transmission to high-risk patients, blood products are used from donors who are negative for CMV antibodies.

Malaria

Malaria parasites can survive in stored blood and be transmitted to the recipient. Regulations eliminating prospective donors who have had malaria in the last 3 years or those who have traveled in endemic areas have made this adverse effect of transfusion rare. Nonetheless, the diagnosis of malaria should be considered in patients who have paroxysmal fever following transfusion.

Other Infections

Syphilis transmission has been reduced by using stored blood and serologic testing of donors. Other diseases transmitted by blood products include Chagas disease, toxoplasmosis, filariasis, and leishmaniasis.

DELAYED COMPLICATIONS OF BLOOD TRANSFUSIONS

Transfusion Hemosiderosis

Each unit of blood contains about 250 mg of iron. In those patients chronically transfused for congenital anemias or aplastic anemia, the iron load can become deleterious. Accumulation of iron in the heart, liver, and endocrine organs eventually leads to dysfunction. Iron chelation may help to maintain iron balance. The transfusion of reticulocytes and fractions of younger red cells (neocytes) may prolong the survival of transfused cells, decrease the required transfusion frequency, and lower the iron load.

Graft-Versus-Host Disease

Immunocompetent donor lymphocytes survive storage of red cell products and are present in large numbers in white cell or platelet products. These lymphoid cells can engraft in immunosuppressed recipients, leading to graft-versus-host disease. Irradiating blood products for recipients considered susceptible to graft-versus-host reactions eliminates the hazard. The typical radiation dose (1500 rad) has not been found to cause dysfunction of cellular or plasma elements in transfused blood.

RED BLOOD CELL TYPING

Blood groups are determined by the presence of antigenic substances on the red cell surface. These substances are either an integral part of the red cell membrane itself, such as Rh antigens, or are outward molecular extensions from the membrane, such as ABO antigens. The fact that these antigenic determinants are present on the red cells of some people and absent from the red cells of others is a result of genetic heterogeneity. Blood group inheritance follows Mendelian genetic laws.

Although the functions of blood group antigens remain speculative, their importance in clinical medicine cannot be questioned. The application of blood group serology is essential for the safety of blood transfusion practice as well as tissue transplantation. Blood groups are important markers in genetic and anthropologic studies. In addition, blood group identification is useful in paternity testing and forensic medicine.

THE ABO SYSTEM[15]

The ABO system was the first blood group recognized and remains preeminent in blood transfusion practice. In 1900, Landsteiner

tested red cells and sera obtained from his laboratory workers and noted that the sera from some workers agglutinated the cells of other workers but did not agglutinate their own cells. He divided individuals into three groups (A, B, and O) based on these experiments. In 1902, the fourth group, AB, was recognized. ABO classification is based on the detection of two antigens, A and B, on the red cells and two antibodies in the serum, anti-A and anti-B (Table 6.24–13). A reciprocal relationship exists whereby the presence of an antigen on the red cell prohibits the presence of an antibody against that antigen in the serum.

This reciprocal relationship is the basis of routine serologic practice in the blood bank. Two antisera, anti-A, and anti-B, are used to test the patient's red cells, a practice known as front typing or cell grouping. The patient's serum is also tested with cells of a known ABO group, known as back-typing or reverse grouping. These results are compared and are typically confirmatory; discrepant results can be an important clue to serologic difficulties and require further investigation in all cases.

The fact that patients routinely have anti-A, anti-B, or both in their serum if they lack the corresponding blood groups on their red cells explains the clinical importance of ABO blood group system recognition. The high density of ABO antigen sites on the red cell makes them ready targets for the IgM anti-A or anti-B isoagglutinins, and their interaction usually causes significant red cell destruction. ABO-incompatible blood, administered inadvertently, remains the most common cause of fatal transfusion reaction.

It is, therefore, highly desirable to transfuse patients with ABO-identical blood. Patients who are of the uncommon AB type have been considered as universal recipients in the past since they lack anti-A and anti-B; likewise, group O red cells (universal donor) are considered safe to administer to all patients. Blood supplies are generally adequate to avoid using universal donor blood except in cases of major trauma, where transfusion is mandated before blood grouping can be completed. Group O blood is administered as red cells in these occasions to avoid the potential problem of anti-A and anti B in the donor plasma.

The expression of ABO antigens on the red cell and in body fluids is the result of interactions of several genetic loci and the subsequent interaction of their gene products with precursor substances. ABO specificity on the red cell arises from glycosphingolipid molecules that are inserted into the red cell membrane. Expression of ABO antigens requires the presence of another gene, H. ABO antigens are expressed on glycoproteins that occur in body fluid secretions if the secretor gene Se is present. The Lewis gene, Le, also acts upon the oligosaccharide chain that determines A, B, and H activity. These genes are closely related and act on the same precursor substances but are not linked.

ABO expression requires the preliminary action of a transferase resulting from the presence of the H gene that conjugates a fucose molecule to the precursor chain. Patients who lack H are considered to be genotype hh and cannot add the fucose to product H substance. This fucose molecule is required for the action of specific ABO transferase; individuals who lack H, therefore, cannot produce ABO antigens. The hh genotype results in the rare Bombay phenotype. These patients lack H substance and ABO antigens on the red cells and produce antibodies against H, A, and B, permitting transfusion only with blood from donors with the Bombay phenotype.

ABO specificity is determined by the conjugation of sugar molecules to an oligosaccharide chain. The specific ABO gene product is an enzyme transferase that couples monosaccharides in a characteristic sequence to confer blood group specificity. H substance is the precursor molecule for the action of ABO gene products. If the A gene is present, a transferase is produced and attaches N-acetylgalactosamine (Gal NAc) to the H-substance–producing A antigen. In the presence of the B gene, a different transferase enzyme adds galactose to produce B substance. The third possible gene, O, is an amorph and produces no transferase so that the H substance remains unmodified. The A, B, and O genes are codominant.

THE Rh SYSTEM[15]

Awareness of the blood group system known as Rh began in 1939 with the detection of a case in which the mother of a stillborn baby had a transfusion reaction when given the husband's ABO-compatible blood. Her serum was found to react with her husband's red cells and approximately 80 percent of other ABO-compatible donors. These findings suggested that the mother's immune system had recognized and made antibody to a foreign antigen on the father's red cells and that the baby inherited the paternal antigen. In 1940, additional evidence was discovered that sera raised in rabbits and guinea pigs who had been injected with Rhesus monkey red cells would agglutinate Rhesus cells but also 80 percent of red cells from Caucasian blood donors—hence, the Rh designation. These findings led to the association of Rh incompatibility and erythroblastosis fetalis and were the discoveries that forecast the importance of the Rh blood group in routine transfusion practice.

Although the Rh blood group system has now been shown to contain at least 30 different specificities, the original specificity identified, Rho(D), remains the most important. Unlike the ABO system, antibodies to the D antigen arise only after stimulation from incompatible pregnancies or transfusions. The D antigen is clinically second to ABO because of its immunogenicity. It has been found that small aliquots of less than 1 ml of D-positive red cells can immunize Rh-negative recipients and that 50 to 75 percent of Rh-negative patients receiving Rh-positive blood will produce anti-D antibody. For these reasons, donor blood and patient's red cells are routinely typed for the D antigen. It is also routine that Rh-negative recipients receive Rh-negative blood products. The donor classification of Rh positive or negative is solely determined by the presence or absence of the D antigen on the red cells.

The highly immunogenic Rh blood group also plays an important role in the sensitization of mothers through fetomaternal hemorrhage, leading to hemolytic disease of the newborn. The likelihood of sensitization can be modified by the ability of passive immunity from injection of anti-D antibody to prevent the sensitization of Rh-negative mothers from the small amounts of blood

TABLE 6.24–13. ABO GROUPING

Cells Tested With:		Serum Tested With:		Interpretation	Frequency in US Population	
Anti-A	Anti-B	A Cells	B Cells	ABO Group	White	Black
0	0	+	+	O	45	49
+	0	0	+	A	40	27
0	+	+	0	B	11	20
+	+	0	0	AB	4	4

Data from Mourant AE, Kopec AC, Domaniewska-Sobczak K: The distribution of the human blood groups and other polymorphisms, 2d ed. London, Oxford University Press, 1976.

TABLE 6.24–14. RED CELL ANTIGENS AND DISEASE ASSOCIATIONS

Blood Group	Common Antigen	Disease Associations
Lewis	Le^a, Le^b	Renal transplantation antigen
P	P$_1$, P$_2$, p	Paroxysmal cold hemoglobinuria
I/i	I/i	Cold autoimmune hemolytic anemia Marrow stress or fetal erythropoiesis
Kell	K, k	Chronic granulomatous disease
Duffy	Fy^a, Fy^b	Malaria

passed from their Rh-positive babies at delivery. The routine administration of anti-D postpartum reduces the risk of sensitization from approximately 15 percent of mothers at risk to approximately 1 percent. This reduction in sensitization has decreased the incidence of hemolytic disease of the newborn due to anti-Rho(D) and thus has reduced fetal morbidity and mortality. Further reduction in Rh sensitization has been demonstrated by the antenatal injection of antibody at 28 weeks' gestation for all Rh-negative mothers.

OTHER BLOOD GROUPS

In addition to ABO and Rh, there are at least 300 blood group systems that can be detected on the surface of red blood cells. They can be considered in two groups: antigens whose absence commonly is accompanied by naturally occurring antibodies, and antigens in which alloantibodies are found only with previous sensitization. The former groups (Lewis, P, MNSs, I/i) are not commonly associated with transfusion problems, as the antibodies do not generally cause immune red cell destruction. The latter group can cause hemolysis and clinical problems but is less immunogenic than Rho(D). When these antibodies (Kell, Kidd, Duffy) are present, incompatible blood is avoided; however, no attempt is routinely made to administer donor blood that matches the patient's phenotype unless prior immunization has occurred. Occasionally, these blood groups or their antibodies accompany hematologic disease in noteworthy patterns or have important disease associations (Table 6.24–14).

REFERENCES

1. Aach RD, Kahn RA: Post-transfusion hepatitis: Current perspectives. Ann Intern Med 92:539, 1980
2. Chaplin H Jr: The proper use of previously frozen red blood cells for transfusion. Blood 59:1118, 1982
3. Counts RB, Maisch C, et al: Hemostasis in massively transfused trauma patients. Ann Surg 190:911, 1979
4. Curran JW, Lawrence DN, et al: Acquired immunodeficiency syndrome (AIDS) associated with transfusions. N Engl J Med 310:69, 1984
5. Duquesnoy RJ, Filip DJ, et al: Successful transfusion of platelets "mismatched" for HLA antigens to alloimmunized thrombocytopenic patients. Am J Hematol 2:219, 1977
6. Dutcher JP, Schiffer CA, et al: Long-term follow-up of patients with leukemia receiving platelet transfusions: Identification of a large group of patients who do not become alloimmunized. Blood 58:1007, 1981
7. Gaydos LA, Freireich EJ, Mantel N: The quantitative relation between platelet count and hemorrhage in patients with acute leukemia. N Engl J Med 266:905, 1962
8. Goldfinger D: Acute hemolytic transfusion reactions—A fresh look at pathogenesis and considerations regarding therapy. Transfusion 17:85, 1977
9. Harker LA, Slichter SJ: Platelet and fibrinogen consumption in man. N Engl J Med 287:999, 1972
10. Herzig RH, Herzig GP, et al: Successful granulocyte transfusion therapy for gram-negative septicemia. N Engl J Med 296:701, 1977
11. Higby DJ, Cohen E, et al: The prophylactic treatment of thrombocytopenic leukemic patients with platelets: A double blind study. Transfusion 14:440, 1974
12. Howland WS, Bellville JW, et al: Massive blood transfusion. V. Failure to demonstrate citrate intoxication. Surg Gyn Obstet 105:529, 1957
13. Johnson FL, Thomas ED, et al: A comparison of marrow transplantation with chemotherapy for children with acute lymphoblastic leukemia in second or subsequent remission. N Engl J Med 305:846, 1981
14. Levine AS, Schimpff SC, et al: Hematologic malignancies and other marrow failure states: Progress in the management of complicating infections. Semin Hematol 11:141, 1974
15. Mollison PL: Blood transfusion in clinical medicine, 4th ed. Oxford, Blackwell, 1979
16. Moore GL, Peck CC, et al: Some properties of blood stored in anticoagulant CPDA-1 solution. A brief summary. Transfusion 21:135, 1981
17. Perkins HA, Payne R, et al: Non-hemolytic febrile transfusion reactions. Quantitative effects of blood components with emphasis on isoantigenic incompatibility of leucocytes. Vox Sang 11:578, 1966
18. Pineda AA, Brzica SM, Taswell H: Hemolytic transfusion reactions. Mayo Clin Proc 53:378, 1978
19. Santos GW, Kaizer H: Bone marrow transplantation in acute leukemia. Semin Hematol 19:227, 1982
20. Strauss RG, Connett JE, et al: A controlled trial of prophylactic granulocyte transfusions during initial induction chemotherapy for acute myelogenous leukemia. N Engl J Med 305:597, 1981
21. Yankee RA, Graff KS, et al: Selection of unrelated compatible platelet donors by lymphocyte HL-A matching. N Engl J Med 288:760, 1973

CHAPTER 6.25
Anticoagulant and Thrombolytic Therapy

William R. Bell

Anticoagulants are substances that retard coagulation of the blood. The indications for their use in patients with pulmonary embolism, myocardial infarction, valvular heart disease, prosthetic heart valves, extracorporeal dialysis, and peripheral vascular disease are discussed in Chapters 2.3, 2.8, 2.12, 3.8, and 11.5, respectively.

There are two main categories of anticoagulants in common use: heparin and the coumarin-indanedione compounds.[13,16] The response of different individuals to the administration of both categories of anticoagulants is variable and, consequently, the dosage

must be adjusted in accordance with the response of the patient. Table 6.25–1 lists the usual dosage of some representative anticoagulants, but the precise dose and response of each patient must be determined. An adequate therapeutic level is selected on the basis of clinical experience as the level that reverses the abnormal process beng treated and provides the maximal depression of coagulation without increase in serious spontaneous hemorrhage. The clinician must be aware that deficiencies of coagulation factors and thrombocytopenia render the patient particularly sensitive to anticoagu-

TABLE 6.25–1. ANTICOAGULANTS: REPRESENTATIVE AGENTS

Class	Generic Name	Chemical	Trade Name	Routes of Adminis-tration	Usual Dose in Adults (Us)	Usual Onset of Peak Activity	Dosage Monitored by Measure-ment of	Antidote
Heparin	Heparin sodium[a]	Sulfate contain-ing mucopolysac-charide	Heparin sodium Liquaemin sodium Lipo-Hepin Panheprin	IV Continuous Intermittent	300–500/kg/24 hr 50–100/kg/q4 h	1–2 hr <30 min	Whole blood clotting time	Protamine sulfate

Class	Generic Name	Chemical	Trade Name	Routes of Adminis-tration	Initial (mg/24 hr)	Mainte-nance (mg/24 hr)		Dosage Monitored by Measure-ment of	Antidote
Coumarin	Bishydroxy-coumarin	3,3′-methylene-bis-(4-hydroxy-coumarin)	Dicumarol	PO	200–400	25–100	1.5–3 days	One-stage prothrombin time	2-methyl-3-phytyl-1, 4-naphthoqui-none(vitamin K₁)
	Warfarin sodium	3-(α-phenyl-β-acetyl-ethyl)-4-hydroxy-coumarin, sodium	Coumadin Panwarfin	PO or IV	25–50	2.5–10	1–2 days		and/or
Indanedione	Anisindione	2-phenyl-1, 3 indanedione	Miradon	PO	300	25–250	1–2 days		Transfusion of blood, or plasma fractions contain-ing the vitamin K–dependent clotting factors

[a] 1 mg of crystalline standard heparin sodium is equivalent to 100 USP units or 130 IU of heparin.

lants. In these instances, the usual doses may induce severe hemorrhage.

HEPARIN

Heparin, the most universally employed parenterally administered anticoagulant, is a sulfate containing heterogeneous mucopolysaccharide organic acid, with the highest anionic charge density recognized in living organisms. It interferes with coagulation at several steps—perhaps every step—in the coagulation scheme. It has been documented to inhibit the action of thrombin on fibrinogen; to inhibit many of the early stages of the cascade, including activation of factors VIII, IX, and X; and to interfere with the action of thrombin on platelets. The mechanism of the action of heparin is attributed to its ability to complex with an α_2-globulin (heparin-cofactor, antithrombin III) and in such combination augment the inhibitory capacity of this endogenous agent.[12] Heparin does not depress the production of any coagulation factor. In addition, heparin possesses anticomplement activity, is capable of releasing histaminase, and has lipemia-clearing activity resulting from the release of lipoprotein lipase. Heparin does not cross the placenta and is not secreted in breast milk.

MONITORING HEPARIN THERAPY

The quantity of heparin should be specified in units and not milligrams. Depending on the animal, anatomic source, and manufacturer, 1 mg of heparin may be equivalent to between 100 and 180 USP units (anticoagulating units) of heparin. The therapeutic antithrombotic dosage of heparin is best monitored by measurement of the whole blood clotting time. Clotting times can be measured by any of several rigidly standardized techniques, but the plain glass test tube technique (Lee-White), using venous blood, is the most reliable. In some centers, the recalcification time or the partial thromboplastin time (PTT) or the activated partial thromboplastin time (APTT) may be used to monitor heparin therapy. It must be recognized that some commercially available reagents

utilized in performing the PTT and APTT do not provide an accurate reflection of in vivo heparin anticoagulation. A Lee–White whole blood clotting time should be performed before escalating the dosage of heparin.

A control clotting time should be measured before the start of therapy. The dosage of heparin should be adjusted to maintain the clotting time at greater than 20 minutes, but not beyond 45 minutes. The ideal therapeutic range is thought to be between 25 and 35 minutes. Because the action of heparin can be altered by several drugs and heparin can disturb the action of several drugs, the clinician must be aware of these interrelationships.[5] Whenever heparin is employed, a flow sheet should be used to follow, on a daily basis, the patient's weight, date, hour of administration, agent (name, source, and type), dosage per 24 hours, whole blood clotting time or partial thromboplastin time (PTT), urine, and stool (for occult blood).

ADMINISTRATION

Aqueous heparin must be given parenterally. This agent is best administered via the intravenous route and may be given continuously or intermittently. Evenly sustained prolongation of the clotting time is most readily achieved by continuous intravenous infusion of heparin by a constant infusion pump and is the preferred manner of administration. The subcutaneous administration may cause erratic absorption, vessel puncture, bleeding, and discomfort, and is therefore a less desirable route of administration. The subcutaneous route can be used if careful monitoring of intravenous infusions is not available or if intravenous infusions interfere with ambulation. Because of the increased frequency of hemorrhage and erratic absorption, heparin should not be given intramuscularly.

Intravenous Route—Continuous Constant Infusion

A loading dose of 5000 units, given slowly in 10 to 20 ml diluent over 10 to 15 minutes, should be administered intravenously, and immediately following this, the constant infusion should be started (heparin, 200 to 350 U/kg of lean body mass in 250 to 500 ml of

5 percent dextrose to run 12 hours, or 300 to 500 U/kg in 1000 ml of 5 percent dextrose to run 24 hours). A whole blood clotting time should be checked 6 hours later. Depending on the whole blood clotting time at 6 hours, the dose, concentration of heparin, and rate of infusion should be adjusted and the whole blood clotting time or APTT rechecked *6 hours later*. This should be done until a satisfactory whole blood clotting time is obtained, at which time the appropriate dose of heparin should be continued via constant infusion and the whole blood clotting time determined every 12 hours for 2 to 3 days then every 24 hours for the duration of treatment.

Intravenous Route—Intermittent Infusion

The loading dose is given as in the case of continuous intravenous infusion. Following this, heparin, 50 to 100 U/kg of lean body mass should be given in 10 to 20 ml of 5 percent dextrose intravenously during a 10-minute period every 4 hours. During the first 24 hours of therapy, immediately before each 4-hour dose, the whole blood clotting time should be determined and recorded and the dose appropriately adjusted. Once the correct prolongation of the whole blood coagulation time is obtained, that dose of heparin should be given intravenously every 4 hours, with the whole blood coagulation time checked before the second and fourth dose each day for the duration of therapy.

Subcutaneous Route

When the subcutaneous route is used the approximate dosage schedule is 10,000 to 25,000 units every 6 to 12 hours. The clotting time should be measured 3 to 4 hours after the first dose and subsequent dosage adjusted to provide the desired prolongation. Thereafter, the clotting time should be measured every 12 hours or just prior to administration of the heparin to determine a possible cumulative effect. Heparin has been combined with agents such as gelatin, Pitkin menstruum, peanut oil, and beeswax, in an attempt to delay absorption and produce a more sustained effect. These preparations are not recommended because of varying rates of absorption, high frequentcy of local reactions, other undesirable side effects, and the difficulty of reversing the anticoagulant effect with specific antidotes.

The use of low-dose (5000 units subcutaneously every 8 hours) heparin for prophylactic therapy has been explored in several clinical areas.[2] Many studies employing low-dose heparin in prophylaxis of venous thrombosis have shown a reduction in the frequency of thrombosis. The low-dose heparin regimen has not been effective in major joint surgery, biliary tract surgery, and myocardial infarction. Because of a cumulative effect, some patients receiving low-dose heparin may become fully anticoagulated.

TOXICITY

The most common untoward reaction to heparin is bleeding and, although the true incidence is difficult to quantify, it may be as high as 25 to 35 percent, when all types of bleeding are considered. The problems of maintaining a constant rate of infusion during the administration of heparin are self-evident. Reactions to heparin, other than hemorrhage, are rare; the major ones are listed in Table 6.25–2. Hypersensitivity and anaphylactoid reactions have ranged from mild fever, urticaria, rhinitis, and conjunctivitis to sudden, severe hypertension, respiratory distress, and chest pain. Thrombocytopenia and transient alopecia may occur. Osteoporosis has been reported in some patients who received heparin for prolonged periods (more than 1 year).

ANTIDOTES

There are several antidotes that reverse the anticoagulant effect of heparin. These include protamine sulfate, hexadimethine bromide (polybrene), clupeine, polylysine, lysozyme, toluidine blue, fuchsin, and tryptophan.

TABLE 6.25–2. HEPARIN: UNTOWARD REACTIONS

- Hemorrhage
- Allergic reactions:
    Urticaria, fever
    Asthma
    Rhinitis, conjunctivitis
- Thrombocytopenia
- Alopecia
- Osteoporosis
- Arterial thrombosis
- Respiratory distress
- Hypotension
- Chest pain
- Dysesthesia pedis
- Hyponatremia
- Resistance

The antidote that is recommended and most commonly employed is protamine sulfate. The dose of protamine sulfate to be administered depends on the amount of heparin present. The amount of heparin present is dependent on the amount, the time, and route of the last dose of heparin given. The recommended dose is 1.0 mg for every 100 units (USP) heparin present in the body. It should be administered slowly, intravenously, and at a rate not greater than 5 mg per minute. No single injection of protamine sulfate should exceed 50 mg. The antiheparin effect lasts for approximately 2 hours. A clotting time should be checked approximately 15 minutes after the administration of protamine sulfate before an additional dose should be given. Some heparin effect may reappear after a single dose of protamine sulfate, especially if a large dose of heparin had been administered subcutaneously shortly before the injection of protamine.

Transfusions of blood, plasma, or other blood products are not antidotes against heparin, although they are of value in replacement therapy following hemorrhage.

COUMARIN-INDANEDIONE ANTICOAGULANTS

A large variety of coumarin-indanedione derivatives are commonly employed as anticoagulants.[13,16] These agents do not inhibit the rate of clotting when added to blood in vitro. When administered in vivo, they impair coagulation by altering the biologic function (clotting activity) of the end product of the vitamin K–mediated hepatic synthesis of factors II, VII, IX, and X. Normal levels (measured by immunologic techniques) of these factors are present during the administration of the coumarin-indanedione agents. Although the synthesis of factors II, VII, IX, and X is not depressed by these vitamin K antagonists, their functional properties are altered. The defect has been identified and is due to the absence of the second carboxyl group on the γ carbon of glutamic acid.[6]

The coumarin-indanedione anticoagulants have certain pharmacologic actions other than those related to coagulation. These include enhancement of uric acid excretion in the urine and a rise in serum transaminase and lactic dehydrogenase activity. Some patients who receive coumarin derivatives may excrete orange or reddish-colored urine, due to a metabolic breakdown product that gives this color in alkaline medium. This is not of clinical significance.

CONTROL OF DOSAGE

The one-stage prothrombin time test, devised by Quick, or one of its modifications is the most widely used test to monitor the effect of the coumarin anticoagulants. Following the administration of these agents, the coagulant activity of the vitamin K–dependent factors decreases in the following sequence: VII, IX, X, and II.

The order in which these disappear corresponds to the intravascular biologic half-life of these factors. The one-stage prothrombin time is influenced by changes in three of these factors (II, VII, and X), but there is close parallelism in the levels of factors VII and IX during therapy with the coumarin derivatives.[7] Thus, the one-stage prothrombin time is considered to be a reliable method for use in monitoring the effect and guiding the dosage of the coumarin anticoagulants.[7,13,16]

Because heparin can significantly affect the one-stage prothrombin time, the control prothrombin time should be obtained prior to the institution of heparin. It is desirable to adjust the coumarin anticoagulants to maintain the prothrombin time at a level of 15 to 25 percent of normal. This corresponds to a prolongation of the prothrombin time (in seconds) between 2 and 2.5 times the normal control (sometimes expressed as patient-to-control ratio).

ADMINISTRATION

The coumarin-indanedione derivatives are attractive because they can be administered orally. Some of these agents, for example, warfarin (Coumadin), can also be administered intravenously. The coumarin derivatives are preferred to the chemically similar indanedione derivatives because in clinical practice they produce fewer adverse side effects.[13] The approximate dosage schedules for bishydroxycoumarin, warfarin, and one of the indanedione derivatives are shown in Table 6.25–1.

There are two methods commonly utilized in the initiation of therapy with the oral anticoagulants. The older technique employs a "loading dose" of one of the coumarin derivatives (e.g., warfarin, 25 to 35 mg), after obtaining a control prothrombin time. Approximately 36 hours later, the prothrombin time is determined and a daily maintenance, usually 5 to 10 mg, is selected. The final single daily dose of anticoagulant is determined on the basis of daily measurement of the prothrombin time. The direction of change, as well as the absolute value of the prothrombin time, must be known in deciding the daily dosage.

The alternative technique is based on the observation that a "loading dose" produces a rapid fall in factor VII activity before other factor activities are depressed. Some investigators point out that even though there is prolongation of the prothrombin time, antithrombotic protection is not present until factor X activity is also reduced. Therefore, the recommendation has been made that smaller daily doses (warfarin, 10 to 15 mg) be given when therapy is initiated. The final daily dose is determined by observing the effect on the prothrombin time. Several days are often required to reach the desired therapeutic prolongation of the prothrombin time when the second method is employed. Regardless of which induction method of coumarin administration is selected, a reasonably stable maintenance dose can be achieved within 7 to 15 days. Once this has been achieved for several consecutive days, the prothrombin time can be checked at progressively longer intervals, from daily to twice weekly, then weekly while hospitalized. After discharge from the hospital, provided the patient's condition is stable and that a stable maintenance dose has been established, the prothrombin time determinations could be done at 2- to 3-week intervals. Clinical experience suggests that no longer than 3 weeks should pass without a prothrombin time check for the duration of therapy. If at any time during therapy with these agents the dose required increases to greater than 10 to 15 mg daily (warfarin), consultation with a coagulation specialist should be obtained.

Frequently, the oral anticoagulants are instituted near the end of a course of heparin therapy. Occasionally, therapy with the two agents may be initiated simultaneously. Because heparin can severely alter the prothrombin time, it is difficult to know when the coumarin-indanedione agents become effective. In most patients receiving continuous intravenous heparin, the prothrombin time can be reliably used as a measure of coumarin effect. In patients in whom heparin alters the prothrombin time it is possible to determine coumarin effect by using intermittent intravenous heparin therapy and determining the prothrombin time just before the next dose of heparin. In this way, the prothrombin time will be determined without significant influence by the presence of heparin.

A "rebound phenomenon" has been reported to occasionally follow the cessation of oral anticoagulant therapy. The precise nature of the rebound has not been defined. Some physicians feel that further thromboembolic episodes are more likely to occur at this time and recommend a gradual reduction in dosage over several days rather than abrupt discontinuation. The biologic half-life of these agents varies from 40 to 75 hours, however, and, with such a gradual disappearance from the body, additional efforts to taper the dose are unnecessary.

FACTORS INFLUENCING DOSAGE

A genetically determined hereditary (autosomal dominant) resistance to the anticoagulant effects of the coumarin-indanedione derivatives has been reported. To date, no heritable conditions associated with an increased sensitivity to these agents has been reported. Increased sensitivity to coumarin-indanedione derivatives may be produced by preexisting congenital or acquired hypoprothrombinemia, by disorders that interfere with the availability, absorption, or utilization of vitamin K, such as malnutrition, gastrointestinal disorders with decreased absorption of vitamin K (e.g., sprue, cystic fibrosis), oral antibiotics that alter intestinal bacterial flora, biliary obstruction, and liver disease. Hypermetabolic states, excessive intake of alcohol, and congestive heart failure may increase susceptibility of these anticoagulants. Females are more sensitive than males and dose requirements decrease with advancing age. Concomitant administration of many other drugs may either potentiate or decrease the response to the anticoagulant effects of these agents. A partial list is presented in Table 6.25–3. The prothrombin time of patients receiving the oral anticoagulants and any of these drugs must be monitored frequently. The simultaneous administration of other drugs may necessitate frequent alteration in the dose of the anticoagulant, either to maintain therapeutic effectiveness or to prevent potential disasters.[10,11]

TOXICITY OF ORAL ANTICOAGULANTS

The most common untoward reaction to the coumarin-indanedione anticoagulants is hemorrhage.[16] Other reactions, listed in Table 6.25–4, are rare.

ANTIDOTES

The anticoagulant effects of the coumarin-indanedione anticoagulants can be reversed by administration of vitamin K_1, which is a naturally occurring, oil-soluble, 3-phytyl derivative of 2-methyl-1, 4-naphthoquinone (vitamin K). Certain synthetic water-soluble vitamin K preparations, such as menadione and Hykinone, which are not 3-phytyl derivatives, are much less effective and should not be relied on as antagonists. The oil-soluble preparation of vitamin K_1 (Mephyton) should be administered intravenously at a rate not faster than 5 mg per minute. The water-soluble analogue of vitamin K_1 (Aqua Mephyton) is an effective antagonist and can be administered intravenously or orally, depending on the rapidity of effect that is desired. The subcutaneous and intramuscular routes can also be used but are less desirable because of variable absorption and local hematomas. The dose of vitamin K_1 depends on the amount and time of the last dose of anticoagulant and the urgency of the situation. In patients with life-threatening hemorrhage, if the dose of anticoagulant was not excessively large, 25 to 50 mg of vitamin K_1 given intravenously usually will produce a therapeutic effect within 4 hours, and within 12 to 24 hours the prothrombin time will have returned to control values. Such large doses of vita-

TABLE 6.25–3. SOME DRUGS THAT AFFECT THE RESPONSE TO COUMARIN-INDANEDIONE ANTICOAGULANTS

Anticoagulant Effects May Be Potentiated by:
- Pyrazolidine compounds
  - Phenylbutazone (Butazolidin)
  - Oxyphenbutazone (Tandearil)
- Antihyperlipidemic agents
  - Clofibrate (Atromid-s)
  - Dextrothyroxine (Choloxin)
- Anabolic steroids
  - Methandrostenolene (Dianabol)
  - Norethandrolone (Nilevar)
  - Oxymetholone (Adroyd)
  - Nandrolonedecanoate (Deca-Durabolin)
- Muscle relaxants
  - Phenyramidol (Analexin)
- Salicylates—in large doses
- Quinine, quinidine, cimetidine, amiodarone
- Sulfonamides and antibiotics (moxalactam)
- Disulfiram (Antabuse), mineral oil, glucagon

Anticoagulant Effects May Be Decreased by:
- Sedatives and hypnotics
  - Barbiturates
  - Glutethimide (Doriden)
  - Ethchlorvynol (Placidyl)
- Griseofulvin (Fulvicin, Grifulvin, Grisactin)
- Rifampin (Rimactane)
- Mercurial diuretics and some thiazides
- Multivitamins containing vitamin K
- Tranquilizers?
  - Meprobamate (Miltown, Equanil)
  - Haloperidol (Haldol)

Anticoagulant Effects Are Not Altered by:
- Diazepam (Valium)
- Chlordiazepoxide (Librium)
- Chlorothiazide (Diuril) in standard doses
- Flurazepam (Dalmane)

min K_1 may make the patient resistant to subsequent doses of anticoagulants for several days. Smaller doses (5 to 10 mg) of vitamin K_1 are given if the indications for its use are less urgent. The rise in serum transaminase and lactic dehydrogenase activity and the antithyroid activity produced by these agents are not reversed by any vitamin K preparation.

The clotting factors that are functionally altered by these anticoagulants are stable on storage and are present in acid-citrate-dextrose or citrate-phosphate-dextrose bank blood and fresh-frozen plasma. Transfusions of blood or plasma can act as antagonists to the coumarin-indanedione anticoagulants. A plasma fraction concentrate containing factors II, VII, IX, and X (Konyne, Proplex)

TABLE 6.25–4. COUMARIN-INDANEDIONE ANTICOAGULANTS: UNTOWARD REACTIONS

- Hemorrhage
- Skin lesions—rashes, necrosis, petechiae, purpura, exfoliation
- Syndrome of purple toes
- Nausea, vomiting, diarrhea
- Leukopenia
- Thrombocytopenia
- Agranulocytosis
- Eosinophilia
- Pyrexia
- Hepatic damage, hepatitis, jaundice
- Stomatitis, sore throat
- Nephropathy
- Alopecia
- Resistance

is an effective antagonist. Because of the significant recognized risk of hepatitis transmitted by these concentrates, however, their use is not recommended unless a life-threatening emergency is present.

HEMORRHAGE

Hemorrhage is the most commonly encountered complication of treatment with any of the anticoagulants. The incidence of serious hemorrhage is low and it is proportional to the intensity of the regimen employed. Fatalities have been reported, and moderate hemorrhage (that not requiring transfusion), such as hematuria, ecchymosis, hematomas, epistaxis, and melena, occurs in 10 to 35 percent of patients. Bleeding may involve any organ system, but certain types of hemorrhage deserve special mention. Hemopericardium occurs in some patients with myocardial infarction, and anticoagulant therapy may increase this tendency. Bleeding from the gastrointestinal tract may develop, and the term "anticoagulant ileus" has been used to describe obstructions of the small or large bowel due to hemorrhages into the abdominal wall, peritoneal cavity, mesentery, or wall of the bowel. Bleeding from the gastrointestinal, genitourinary, or respiratory tracts during anticoagulant therapy may indicate the presence of previously unrecognized lesions. Physicians should be especially alert to the possible development of subdural hematoma following head injury in patients receiving anticoagulants. Adrenal cortical insufficiency, due to bilateral adrenal hemorrhage, has been described. The occurrence of bleeding at the sites of intramuscular or subcutaneous injections of heparin has been mentioned. Patients receiving heparin should have daily physical examinations to detect abnormal bleeding and tests of urine and stool for occult blood.

Unusual care is required in performance of venipunctures and prolonged pressure should be applied to venipuncture sites. Invasive procedures should be avoided and, particularly in areas in which bleeding may be especially dangerous, are contraindicated. The introduction of needles or catheters into neck and subclavian veins must be avoided. Arterial punctures, lumbar punctures, thoracentesis, paracentesis, and subcutaneous and intramuscular injections should not be performed on patients receiving anticoagulants. In general, needles, cutting instruments of all varieties, and invasive procedures should be avoided during therapy with anticoagulants. An exception is the use of invasive procedures required for the management of the patient on anticoagulation, such as catheterization in pulmonary embolism, acute myocardial infarction (Swan–Ganz catheter), and unstable angina.

CONTRAINDICATIONS

Anticoagulants are contraindicated in patients with an active hemorrhagic diathesis and those who are allergic to these agents. Although heparin has been reported to be of possible benefit in patients with disseminated intravascular coagulopathy, a control study has not been performed, and the role of heparin in these clinical situations remains uncertain. Relative contraindications include intestinal ulceration, surgery of the CNS or eye, severe hypertension (diastolic over 130 mm Hg), a past history of cerebral hemorrhage, inadequate cooperation of the patient, or the absence of laboratory facilities. Anticoagulants must be used with utmost caution in pericarditis, diabetes mellitus, bacterial endocarditis, liver disease, steatorrhea, and malnutrition. Because they cross the placenta, the coumarin-indanedione agents are contraindicated during pregnancy and particularly at the time of delivery. These oral agents are secreted in breast milk and should not be given to nursing mothers.

THROMBOLYTIC AGENTS

Two thrombolytic agents, streptokinase (SK) and urokinase (UK), are currently available for the treatment of thromboembolic disease.[1,15] Indications for their use include massive and submassive emboli that have induced cardiopulmonary compromise; deep vein thrombosis, particularly when it extends into the thigh veins and inferior vena cava; arterial thrombo-occlusive disease; external A-V shunts; and acute myocardial infarction. Both agents must be given by continuous intravenous or arterial infusion. Their mechanism of action is to convert the inert proenzyme, plasminogen, to the potent proteolytic enzyme, plasmin. The latter exerts its therapeutic effect by attacking arginyl-lysyl bonds digesting fibrin clots. The biologic half-life of these agents in the blood is short, on the order of minutes in duration. For systemic therapy the usual dose of SK is 250,000 IU initially, given over 20 minutes, and 100,000 IU/hr for 24 to 72 hours. UK is given in a dose of 4000 IU/kg initially over 20 minutes, followed by 4000 IU/kg/hr for 12 or 24 hours. When a local perfusion technique is employed (infusing the thrombolytic agent via a catheter that has been passed adjacent to or into the substance of the thrombus) in a peripheral artery, vein, or graft the dose of SK is 7500 IU/hr by continuous infusion. The dose for infusion SK into the coronary ostia is a 20,000 IU loading dose, followed by 2000 IU/min for 60 to 90 minutes. For UK the intracoronary dose is 6000 IU/min for 120 minutes. As additional studies in patients with myocardial infarction are completed, the intracoronary route of administration is not commonly utilized. At present the most frequently utilized technique for employing thrombolytic therapy in acute myocardial infarction is a forearm vein infusion of SK 1 to 2 million IU over 15 to 60 minutes. Both agents can be administered in solutions of dextrose (5 percent), saline, or various combinations of these two excipients. The thrombin time is used to monitor therapy to ensure adequate but not excessive therapeutic activity of the fibrinolytic system. This test should be made preinfusion, 3 to 4 hours after initiation of the infusion to identify that activation of the fibrinolytic system has been achieved, and then every 12 hours for the duration of therapy. For therapeutic efficacy during infusion of the thrombolytic agents, the thrombin time should be 1.5 to 5 times prolonged over the preinfusion value. At the termination of thrombolytic therapy, the patient should be switched over to heparin and later to coumadin. When systemic thrombolytic therapy has been employed, heparin (without a loading dose) should be instituted when the thrombin time is less than twice the preinfusion value, usually a 2 to 3 hour interval. When a local perfusion technique is employed, heparin therapy should be instituted immediately upon cessation of the thrombolytic infusion, with a loading dose followed by a continuous intravenous infusion. In patients with myocardial infarction at the completion of thrombolytic therapy intravenous heparin is given. Where indicated, some patients are treated with angioplasty or surgical bypass, followed by an antiplatelet agent. During infusion with these thrombolytic agents, absolutely no invasive procedures of any type (save careful venipuncture) should be performed. Drugs that alter the coagulation system or interfere with platelet function are contraindicated. In the recommended therapeutic doses, both SK and UK are excreted in the form of inactive metabolites in the urine.

Undergoing clinical trial are a group of second generation thrombolytic agents. The design of these agents—recombinant tissue plasminogen activator (rt-PA), acylated-SK-plasminogen complex, and prourokinase—was intended to produce a product that would induce fibrinolysis only at the site of the thrombus formation. Studies to date indicate that all these agents induce a modest to mild degree of systemic fibrinogenolysis. One study with rt-PA suggests that it is more effective than SK in inducing coronary thrombolysis. A second study, essentially indicated to the aforementioned study, failed to show a significant difference between rt-PA and SK in establishing patency of the coronary arteries. The undesirable side effects of these agents, including hemorrhage, are not less frequent than seen with either SK or UK. Numerous studies of these agents in various types of thromboembolic diseases are in process.

Recently, a third thrombolytic agent has become commercially available. This is recombinant tissue plasminogen activator (rt-PA), for use in the treatment of acute myocardial infarction. The recommended route is intravenous in the following dose and schedule: 6 mg bolus followed by 54 mg, totaling 60 mg in the 1st hour, followed by 20 mg for 2 additional hours. Thus, the treatment time is 3 hours with a total dose not to exceed 100 mg.

ANTIFIBRINOLYTIC THERAPY

The degree of hemorrhage in many different disease processes is directly related to excessive activity of the plasminogen-plasmin proteolytic enzyme system. Control of this aspect of the pathogenesis of the disease problem is frequently therapeutically helpful in management of the underlying disease. In patients with congenital factor deficiency, particularly hemophilia-A, hemophilia-B, and von Willebrand disease, hemorrhage in the oropharynx is augmented by numerous proteases in the fluids of this anatomical compartment. In nonimmune and immune-mediated severe thrombocytopenia a significant percentage of blood lost from cutaneous and mucous membranes is promoted by the activity of the fibrinolytic system. Similar observations have been made in the bleeding associated with ulcerative colitis, genitourinary tract bleeding associated with prostatic surgery, and diseases or mechanical devices altering uterine endothelium.

Although there are several agents that can effectively inhibit the fibrinolytic system, two are currently commercially available; epsilon-aminocaproic acid (ε-ACA) and trans-p-aminoethyl-cyclohexane-carboxylic acid (AMCA). Both of these lysine analogs inhibit the plasminogen system by altering the configuration of the plasminogen molecule in a manner that prevents plasmin formation. Considerable clinical experience exists with the use of ε-ACA.[3] This agent may be given by mouth in tablet or elixir form and intravenously. The initial dose is given in the form of a 5-g loading dose followed by a maintenance dose of 1 to 2 g every 4 to 8 hours. A total dose of 30 g per day must not be exceeded.

When ε-ACA is used in the above-mentioned situations, controlled studies have demonstrated that patients with congenital factor deficiency require significantly less or no factor replacement therapy for dental procedures. Patients with severe thrombocytopenia may experience a reduction in bleeding despite no increase in the platelet count. In some instances uterine or urinary tract bleeding can be controlled with these agents.

A potential risk in using these agents is the induction of thrombus formation. Thus, before administration of either antifibrinolytic agent, one must demonstrate the absence of disseminated intravascular coagulation or Trousseau syndrome.

ANTIPLATELET AGENTS

Recent studies[4,15,17] have indicated possible efficacy of agents that inhibit platelet aggregation and release in the prophylactic treatment of thrombotic disease. The three agents that have been studied in large numbers of patients are aspirin (1.2 g), dipyridamole (200 to 400 mg), and sulfinpyrazone (600 to 800 mg). All of these agents are given orally, in divided doses over 24 hours. The clinical indications for the use of these agents are different for each drug. At present, the evidence suggests that aspirin may be helpful in prophylaxis against transient cerebral ischemic attacks; the other antiplatelet agents are not useful. Although some preliminary studies suggest that antiplatelet agents may be useful in ischemic heart disease and myocardial infarction,[8] their long-term value in reduc-

ing incidence or mortality rate remains unproved. Sulfinpyrazone may be useful in reducing the frequency of thrombotic occlusions in arteriovenous communications. Prevention of thromboembolism in patients with prosthetic devices, particularly heart valves, may be possible by combining one or more of the three antiplatelet agents with an orgal anticoagulant. The problems with drug interaction, however, require thoughtful consideration and careful monitoring. The value of the antiplatelet agents in the prevention of venous thrombosis is controversial. More negative than positive results with aspirin have been reported.

The beneficial effect of aspirin, in both transient ischemic attacks and reduction in venous thrombosis following hip surgery, was demonstrated in males but not in females.

Although some studies have demonstrated a favorable effect of the antiplatelet agents in some diseases, it is clear that additional studies are needed.

REFERENCES

1. Bell WR, Meek AG: Guidelines for the use of thrombolytic agents. N Engl J Med 301:1266, 1979
2. Clagett GP, Salzman EW: Prevention of thromboembolism in surgical patients. N Engl J Med 290:93, 1974
3. Gardner FH, Helmer RE: Aminocaproic acid: Use in control of hemorrhage in patients with amegakaryocytic thrombocytopenia. JAMA 243:35, 1980
4. Genton E, Gent M, et al: Platelet-inhibiting drugs in the prevention of clinical thrombotic disease. N Engl J Med 293:1174; 1236; 1296, 1975
5. Hansten PD: Drug Interactions: Clinical Significance of Drug-Drug Interactions and Drug Effects on Clinical Laboratory Results, 4th ed. Philadelphia, Lea and Febiger, 1979
6. Jackson CM, Suttie JW: Recent developments in understanding the mechanism of vitamin K and vitamin K-antagonist drug action and the consequences of vitamin K action in blood coagulation. In Brown EG (ed): Progress in Hematology. New York, Grune and Stratton, 1977, vol 10, p 333
7. Kazmier FJ, Spittell JA Jr, et al: Effect of oral anticoagulants on factors VII, IX, X, and II. Arch Intern Med 115:667, 1965
8. Klimt CR, Knatterud G, et al: Persantine-aspirin reinfarction study. Part II. Secondary coronary prevention with persantine and aspirin. J Am Coll Cardiol 7:251, 1986
9. Koch-Weser J: Coumarin necrosis. Ann Intern Med 68:1365, 1968
10. Koch-Weser J, Sellers EM: Drug interactions with coumarin anticoagulants. N Engl J Med 285:487, 547, 1971
11. O'Reilly RA, Aggeler PM: Determinants of the response to oral anticoagulant drugs in man. Pharmacol Rev 22:35, 1970
12. Rosenberg RD: Heparin action. Circulation 49:603, 1974
13. Sherry S (ed): Symposium: Thrombosis and anticoagulation. Am J Med 33:619, 1962
14. Verstraete M: Are agents affecting platelet functions clinically useful? Am J Med 61:897, 1976
15. Verstraete M: Biochemical and clinical aspects of thrombolysis. Semin Hematol 15:35, 1978
16. Vigran IM: Clinical Anticoagulant Therapy. Philadelphia, Lea and Febiger, 1965
17. Weiss HJ: Antiplatelet therapy. N Engl J Med 298:1344; 1403, 1978

CHAPTER 7.1
Adverse Immunologic Responses

Philip S. Norman, Elaine L. Alexander,
Marshall Plaut, and Richard L. Humphrey

PATHOGENETIC MECHANISMS

Immunologic reactions responsible for the pathogenesis of clinical disorders are qualitatively similar to normal responses and may be mediated by either the humoral or cellular arms of the immune system. Five main mechanisms are recognized: direct action of antibodies, cytotoxic reactions in which antibodies abetted by effector proteins damage cells, responses initiated by antigen combination with cytotropic antibodies on mediator-secreting cells such as mast cells and basophils (the classic allergic reactions), antigen-antibody complex formation resulting in activation of complement, and direct actions of lymphocytes without antibodies.

DIRECT ACTION OF ANTIBODIES

By their ability to combine with antigens that have biologic activity, antibodies are sometimes able to modify that activity without additional mediation of helper proteins or inflammatory cells. For instance, in hemophilia a total deficiency of factor VIII can leave the immune system capable of forming antibodies that inactivate transfused factor, thus complicating efforts at replacement.

Antibodies to cell surface receptors can modify cellular activity. In myasthenia gravis, antibodies to acetylcholine receptors lead to down-regulation of the number of available receptors and a reduced response to acetylcholine at the myoneural junction. In hyperthyroidism (Graves disease), antibodies to thyrotropin receptors are stimulatory and lead to excess thyroid hormone production because the antibody receptor complex is not readily degradable and the antibody is thus long acting. Antibodies to insulin receptors may lead to insulin resistance and antibodies to platelets may interfere with clotting and other platelet functions without destroying platelets.[1]

CYTOTOXIC ANTIBODY REACTIONS

When antibodies to cell constituents fix to their specific antigen and activate complement on the cell surface to accomplish cytolysis, they are referred to as "cytotoxic antibodies."[5] When the cells are foreign, the cytolysis is protective; when the cells are self, one type of autoimmune disease occurs. Examples of the latter include autoimmune hemolytic anemias, drug-related thrombocytopenias, and Goodpasture syndrome (see Chapters 6.7, 6.9, and 11.2). Antibodies to basement membrane in Goodpasture's syndrome result in pulmonary hemorrhage and glomerulonephritis without immune complex deposition in lung or glomeruli. Juvenile diabetes (see Chapter 14.7) may result from destruction of virus-infected pancreatic islet cells by this mechanism.

MEDIATOR RELEASE INDUCED BY CYTOTROPIC ANTIBODIES

Cytotropic antibodies fix to receptors on mediator-containing cells (mast cells and basophils), sensitizing those cells so that when subsequently exposed to antigen they rapidly secrete preformed or newly synthesized potent mediators of physiologic responses and inflammation. Physiologic mediators include histamine; leukotrienes C, D, and E; bradykinin-generating enzyme(s); and prostaglandin D_2, which initiate an immediate reaction characterized by smooth muscle contraction, itching, vasodilation, leakage of fluid from small blood vessels, edema, and hypersecretion of mucus (see Fig. 7.1–1). These phenomena tend to subside in minutes, but inflammatory mediators such as neutrophil, basophil, and eosinophil chemotactic factors and platelet-activating factor (acetyl-glyceryl-ether-phosphorylcholine) induce a local cellular response with eosinophils, neutrophils, and basophils, as well as mononuclear cells, which may last for several hours. This response is accompanied by a "late phase" of mediator release and a recrudescence of the early manifestations. The late phase may be responsible for a greater portion of the clinical manifestations of allergy than the immediate phase, since exposure often occurs over days or months. The early phase responds to mediator inhibitors such as antihistaminics, the late phase responds to anti-inflammatory drugs such as corticosteroids, and both phases respond to drugs inhibiting mediator release, such as cromolyn.[6]

In humans the only isotype of antibodies recognized as cytotropic is IgE. When the antigen is introduced rapidly by injection (drugs, diagnostic materials, insect stings) or ingestion (drugs, foods), the reaction may be rapid, generalized, and life threatening and is referred to as "anaphylaxis." Foods and additives may also cause a local reaction in the gastrointestinal tract consisting of nausea, vomiting, or diarrhea. When the antigen is introduced by inhalation, the reaction may be local and involve the nose if the particle is large (hay fever) or the lung if the particle is small (asthma). Usually the substance is otherwise innocuous and incites such reactions in a small proportion of individuals. The tendency to have IgE-mediated allergies is familial, partially explained by a recessive gene that confers elevated IgE levels in homozygotes, acting in conjunction with other genetic factors that govern recognition of antigenic determinants on environmental materials.

Mediator-containing cells are activated by stimuli other than an antigen-antibody union on their surface. Neural, chemical, and physical stimuli also induce mediator release, thus initiating symptoms that resemble allergic reactions even though no allergen exposure has occurred. These reactions can lead to late-phase reactions and may be important in rhinitis and asthma.

ANTIGEN-ANTIBODY COMPLEXES

Immune complexes produced by the interaction between antigen and antibody may circulate in the fluid phase in the bloodstream

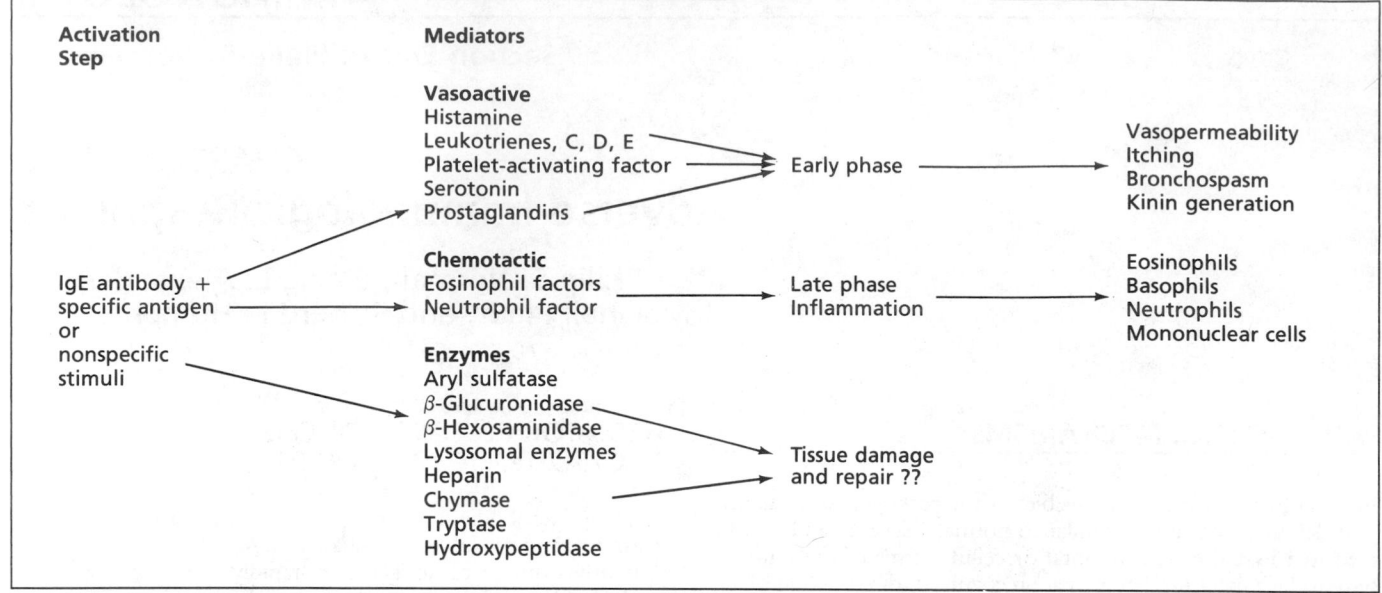

Figure 7.1–1. Mast cell events.

or lymph, or they may form in tissue from circulating or locally formed antibody interacting with a tissue-fixed antigen. Immune complexes can activate inflammatory mediators such as complement components, clotting factors, and proteolytic enzymes, which in turn initiate the influx of polymorphonuclear leukocytes. Although immune complexes are ordinarily cleared physiologically, if they are not cleared, they can lead to tissue damage and result in "immune complex disease." Factors such as the characteristics of the antigens and antibody, the ratio of antigen to antibody, charge, and the physical properties of the reaction medium determine the size (and pathogenicity) of an immune complex.

Complement modifies the structure and biologic activity of the complex by binding to the antigen-antibody complex. It is activated either by the "classical" pathway, initiated by the binding of C1 to antibodies (IgM or IgG) that have combined with corresponding antigens, or by the less selective "alternative" pathway, activated by particulate activators such as aggregated immunoglobulin or immune complexes. Normally activation of the classical pathway is followed by engagement of the alternative pathway, which binds a large number of C3b molecules to the complex. This process prevents the formation of large lattices and immune precipitation, maintaining complexes in solution and permitting diffusion of antigen-antibody complexes from their site of formation, thereby minimizing local inflammatory consequences. Immune complexes produced in the vasculature or cleared from tissue interact with receptors specific for C3b (CR1) on the surfaces of various types of cells, including erythrocytes, polymorphonuclear leukocytes, macrophages, B lymphocytes, some T lymphocytes, dendritic reticular cells in germinal centers, and glomerular podocytes.

Binding of opsonized immune complexes to CR1 on the surface of erythrocytes serves to prevent immune complex interactions with adjacent structures such as vascular endothelium and to carry immune complexes to the macrophage system of the liver, whereas immune complexes formed extravascularly are removed in the lymphocytic system. Immune complex formation is a normal host response to many biologic insults and routinely clears foreign antigens such as bacteria, viruses, and parasites. If the system fails, immune complex disease occurs.[7]

For instance, immune complex disease can be initiated by formation of *insoluble* or *precipitating* immune complexes in the presence of complement. The classic immune complex disease in hu-

mans is serum sickness, a clinical syndrome developing 8 to 12 days after the subcutaneous injection of horse serum, characterized by fever, lymphadenopathy, arthralgias, leukopenia, urticaria, and albuminuria.[1]

In patients with systemic lupus erythematosus (SLE), activation of complement at the site of immune precipitates leads to assembly of the complement membrane-attack complex (C5b-9) at the dermoepidermal junction of skin lesions and in glomeruli. Immune precipitates can be formed by passive depositions of circulating immune complexes into blood vessels or glomeruli or by in situ immune complex formation within tissue.[5,6]

Defects in one or more of the complex mechanisms that prevent the local accumulation of tissue immune complexes outside the fixed macrophage system may initiate or perpetuate immune complex diseases (Table 7.1–1). Patients with deficiencies of specific complement proteins (C1q, C1r, C1s, C4, C2, and C3) can develop immune complex diseases that resemble lupus erythematosus (lupus-like syndromes), suggesting that the classical complement pathway (C1 to C3) protects against immune complex disease. Presumably complement-dependent handling of immune complexes fails.

TABLE 7.1–1. HUMAN DISORDERS ASSOCIATED WITH CONGENITAL COMPLEMENT DEFICIENCIES

Component	Disease Association
Classical Pathway	
C1 to C4	Lupus-like syndrome characterized by glomerulonephritis, arthralgias/arthritis, vasculitis
C3	Recurrent, disseminated infections with pyogenic bacteria
Cytolytic Pathway	
C5 to C8	Disseminated neisserial infections, lupus-like syndrome, other rheumatic disorders
C9	None
CT inhibitor	Hereditary angioedema
C3b inhibitor	Recurrent infections with pyogenic bacteria

Failure to clear immune complexes may result from a receptor deficiency in many patients with SLE. A reduced number of erythrocyte CR1s limits the capacity of erythrocytes to carry and "buffer" immune complexes. Reduced binding of immune complexes to erythrocytes has also been observed in rheumatoid arthritis, cold agglutinin disease, and hematologic malignancies.[7]

Impaired physiologic clearance of immune complexes by the fixed macrophage system may contribute to immune complex disorders. The ability to clear immunoglobulin-coated erythrocytes is defective in patients with several immune diseases (including lupus erythematosus), correlates with the disease activity, and improves with therapy.

DELAYED AND LYMPHOCYTE-MEDIATED REACTIONS

Of the four distinct functional subsets of T lymphocytes—helper, suppressor, delayed hypersensitivity, and cytotoxic—delayed hypersensitivity T cells most often mediate adverse immunologic responses, although cytotoxic cells can also. T cells release soluble mediators, termed "lymphokines" (Table 7.1–2), which stimulate inflammatory reactions mediated by macrophages. Cytotoxic T cells also release a few lymphokines but in low concentrations; they lyse target cells but only at close range.[6]

Delayed Hypersensitivity

Delayed hypersensitivity represents the same events that occur when lymphocytes protect against intracellular bacteria such as *Mycobacterium tuberculosis* and *Listeria*, or fungi. Immune T cells recognize antigen, resulting in release of lymphokines that attract and activate macrophages, increase vascular permeability, and lyse cells. Recruitment of macrophages is delayed, peaking 24 to 48 hours after antigen exposure. A fully developed reaction shows cellular infiltration with macrophages, lymphocytes and other leukocytes, and fibrin deposition. Activated macrophages phagocytize and kill foreign organisms, release monokines (Table 7.1–3) that attract leukocytes and lymphocytes, and activate the complement and fibrin enzyme systems. While doing so, macrophages leak destructive enzymes, leading to the necrosis typical of delayed reactions.[8]

Delayed Hypersensitivity and Disease

Delayed hypersensitivity is part of the immune response to organisms such as *M. tuberculosis* and probably occurs in diseases characterized by mononuclear cell infiltrates, such as chronic active hepatitis, hypersensitivity pneumonitis, and sarcoidosis. Inhaled noninvasive organisms or antigens induce hypersensitivity pneumonitis, whereas the antigens of sarcoidosis are unknown.

In contact dermatitis, sensitized T lymphocytes react to chemicals (haptens) that combine with epidermal proteins to make complete antigens. These antigen-stimulated T cells recruit not only macrophages but also basophils; however, the pathophysiologic process of contact dermatitis is generally similar to that of delayed hypersensitivity. In contrast to the genetic predisposition required for immediate hypersensitivity, contact hypersensitivity to poison ivy can occur in the vast majority of normal persons.[8]

Cytotoxic T Cells

Cytotoxic T cells appear to be the primary protection against acute infections with viruses such as influenza. They usually do not recruit other cells or activate enzyme systems like complement or fibrin, hence are not inflammatory. Cytotoxic T cell lysis of large numbers of cells that bear an immunizing antigen may, however, be adverse. For example, when a virus infects many meningeal cells, cytotoxic T cells may virtually destroy the meninges.[1]

TABLE 7.1–2. LYMPHOKINES AND THEIR EFFECTS

Lymphokines	Effects
IL-2	*T cells:* growth *NK cells:* induction of activity
Interferon-g	*Macrophages:* activation, class II MHC expression, inhibition of migration; *NK cells:* induction of activity
IL-3	*Hematopoietic cells:* stimulation of differentiation (erythrocytes and myelocytes) *Mast cells:* growth, stimulation of histidine decarboxylase
IL-4 (BSF-1, BCGF-1)	*T cells:* growth *B cells:* growth/differentiation, secretion of IgE and other specific isotypes, class II MHC expression *Macrophages:* activation *Mast cells:* stimulation of growth
IL-5 (BCGF-2, TRF)	*B cells:* growth/differentiation, secretion of specific isotypes *Eosinophils:* growth/differentiation
Interferon-β2 (BCDF)	*B cells:* growth/terminal differentiation
GM-CSF	*T cells:* growth of some subsets *Hematopoietic cells:* stimulation of differentiation, especially of granulocytes and macrophages
Lymphotoxin	Cytolytic to (some) target cells
Leukocyte-inhibitory factor	Inhibit migration of granulocytes

Chemotactic factors for:
  Lymphocytes
  Monocytes/macrophages
  Neutrophils
  Fibroblasts
  Basophils	

Histamine-releasing factor(s)	Stimulate mast cell or basophil degranulation or both
Helper factor(s)	Stimulate immune response; both antigen-specific and nonspecific factors have been described
Suppressor factor(s)	Suppress immune response; both antigen-specific and nonspecific factors have been described
IgE-potentiating factor IgE-suppressor factor	IgE-binding factors that regulate IgE isotype response; similar factors regulate IgG and IgA
Glycosylation-enhancing factor Glycosylation-inhibiting factor	Regulate glycosylation of IgE-binding factors (and perhaps other factors) and thereby regulate isotype response

BSF = B-cell stimulatory factor; BCGF = B-cell growth factor; TRF = T-cell replacing factor; BCDF = B-cell differentiating factor; GM-CSF = granulocyte macrophage colony stimulating factor.

AUTOIMMUNE DISEASES

The diverse repertoire of specificities expressed by B and T lymphocyte populations include many that are directed to self-components. If there is a serious failure of complicated mechanisms by which the body distinguishes between self- and non-self-determinants (self-tolerance) and averts significant autoreactivity or autoimmunity, an autoimmune disorder may develop.

MacKay and Burnet[2] define autoimmune disease as "Any

TABLE 7.1–3. MONOKINES

- Lymphocyte-activating factors
  IL-1α
  IL-1β
  Others
- Interferon-α
- Tumor necrosis factor
- Chemotactic and activating factors for neutrophils
- Histamine-releasing factor(s)
- Arachidonic acid metabolites
- Reactive O$_2$ (O$_2$-, H$_2$O$_2$)
- Neutral proteases (e.g., plasminogen activator)
- Acid hydrolases
- Cytotoxic proteases
- Complement components

TABLE 7.1–4. ANTIGENS IN AUTOIMMUNE DISEASES

Disease	Autoantigen
Organ Specific	
Hashimoto thyroiditis	Thyroglobulin
Primary myxedema	Thyroid microsomes
Thyrotoxicosis (Graves disease)	
Pernicious anemia	Gastric parietal cells
Autoimmune atrophic gastritis	Intrinsic factor
Addison disease	Adrenal gland
Insulin-dependent diabetes	B-islet cell
Infertility	Testes
Postvasectomy syndrome	Sperm
Premature menopause	Ovary
Pemphigus vulgaris	Squamous epithelial cells
Bullous pemphigoid	Cutaneous basement membrane
Sympathetic ophthalmia	Uvea
Phacoantigenic uveitis	Lens capsule
Guillain-Barré syndrome	Peripheral nerve myelin
Chronic recurrent polyneuritis	?
Multiple sclerosis	?
Autoimmune hemolytic anemia	Erythrocyte surface antigens
Idiopathic thrombocytopenic purpura	Platelet
Idiopathic neutropenia	Neutrophil
Primary biliary cirrhosis	Smooth muscle
Chronic active hepatitis	Mitochondria
Cryptogenic cirrhosis	? Colon
Ulcerative colitis	
Goodpasture syndrome	Glomerular basement membrane
Interstitial nephritis	Tubulobasement membrane
Dermatopolymyositis	Transfer RNA synthetases
Rheumatoid arthritis	IgG (rheumatoid factor)
Scleroderma	SCL-70 centromere
Sjögren syndrome	Ro(SS-A/La(SS-B)
	IgG (rheumatoid factor)
	Antinuclear antibody
Non-Organ-Specific	
SLE	Antinuclear antibody
	Native DNA (double stranded)
	Single-stranded DNA
	Sm
	Small nuclear ribonucleoprotein (SmRNP)
	Ro(SS-A)
	La(SS-B)
	Cardiolipin
	Histone
	Ribosome

condition in which clinical symptoms or functional changes result from immunologic reactions of immunologically competent cells or antibodies, produced by the individual, with normal components of the body." Table 7.1–4 lists the heterogeneous autoimmune disorders with the antigens affected in rough order from organ specific to organ nonspecific.

Although information about the normal regulation of the immune response has greatly enhanced understanding of autoimmunity and autoimmune diseases, we still know relatively little about the mechanisms of tissue damage in human autoimmune disease.

Autoimmune disorders, except for those caused by cytotropic antibodies, mediate tissue damage by the immune processes already discussed. Not all autoantibodies, however, are pathogenic, and they may be found in apparently normal individuals or in some instances in preclinical disease.

Autoantibodies play a pathophysiologic role in hematologic disorders, antireceptor diseases, and bullous skin diseases, and they have been incriminated in several other autoimmune disorders in which their role has not been established directly.

Known autoantibodies against hematologic cells that induce cell damage and destruction (often utilizing the complement pathway) include antibodies that bind to erythrocyte surface determinants, resulting in the shortening of the erythrocyte life span and autoimmune hemolytic anemia; antibodies directed against platelet antigens, which can result in thrombocytopenia; and selective destruction of blood neutrophils by an immunologic mechanism. One or more of these autoimmune disorders may occur together, or in association with autoimmunity to other tissues.

Antireceptor antibodies cause a well-established group of autoimmune diseases by reacting with cell surface receptors involved in cell signaling. Myasthenia gravis (see Chapter 15.15) is caused by antibodies directed against the acetylcholine receptor at the neuromuscular junction. Graves disease (see Chapter 14.4), on the other hand, is caused by antibodies against the thyroid-stimulating hormone (TSH) receptor that bind on or near the TSH receptor on the thyroid cell and stimulate the thyroid cell to make excess thyroid hormone. In a small subset of diabetes mellitus patients, antibodies to the insulin receptor result in severe insulin resistance, which is usually associated with acanthosis nigricans (a rare skin disorder). The mechanism is more complicated than simple receptor blockade.[3,5]

Autoantibodies that cause antoimmune antireceptor disease have in common that they are IgG and must be bivalent to cause cross-linking of adjacent receptors on the cell surface. Clinical or laboratory evidence of other autoimmune disorders is common in antireceptor antibody disorders.

Several autoimmune cutaneous diseases are associated with tissue-specific autoantibodies. Pemphigus vulgaris (see Chapter 17.7) is characterized by a unique autoantibody that is specific for an epidermal cell surface antigen normally present in differentiating keratinocytes of squamous epithelia ("pemphigus autoantibod-

ies"). Bullous pemphigoid and its variant, herpes gestationis, also are highly specific autoimmune dermatologic disorders in which there are autoantibodies against antigens normally found within the cutaneous basement membrane zone ("pemphigoid autoantibodies").

Autoantibodies can bind to antigens and form immune complexes, which in turn induce disease such as SLE, as already discussed. In SLE antibodies are made into DNA (decyribonucleic acid) and are associated with disease activity. Immunocytochemical studies show that antibody and complement components, including the terminal activation pathway neoantigen C5b-9, are deposited in tissue lesions from skin and kidney. DNA has been eluted from immune complexes isolated from the kidney. Hence

immune complexes may circulate and be deposited in tissue or may be formed in situ and activate the complement cascade.

The development of lupus erythematosus skin lesions and congenital heart block in neonates has been linked to the transplacental passage of maternal IgG antibodies to Ro(SS-A) and La(SS-B) (small–molecular-weight ribonucleoproteins).[1]

Whether or not a specific autoantibody causes disease, it may be a valuable diagnostic marker for the presence of an autoimmune disorder (Table 7.1–5). Organ-specific autoantibodies such as antibodies to thyroglobulin and thyroid microsomes are seen in autoimmune thyroid diseases, and antibodies to gastric parietal cells and gastric intrinsic factor are observed in pernicious anemia with gastric atrophy (autoimmune-type gastritis) and associated autoimmune endocrine disorders. Autoantibodies are also made against pancreatic islet B cells, adrenocortical cells, ovaries and testicles (sperm). In addition, antibodies to glomerular basement membrane are seen in a subset of patients with glomerulonephritis (Goodpasture syndrome) and to tubular basement membrane in tubulointerstitial nephritis.[4]

Possible induction of autoimmune disorders by infectious agents is exemplified by carditis seen in rheumatic fever. A particular β-hemolytic streptococcal cell wall antigen has a molecular configuration similar to a sarcolemma antigen of heart muscle. During streptococcal infection, antibody produced against the streptococcal antigen is incidentally reactive with heart muscle (cross-reactive antibody).

In rheumatic diseases, organ *non*specific autoantibodies develop, such as antinuclear antibodies, antibodies to double- or single-stranded DNA, ribonucleoproteins [nRNP, Sm, Ro(SS-A), La(SS-b)], or IgG (i.e., rheumatoid factors). Some patients with autoimmune diseases make antibodies to subcellular organelles such as smooth muscle (primary biliary cirrhosis), metochondria (chronic active hepatitis), and centromere (scleroderma, CREST variant). In inflammatory muscle disease there are autoantibodies to various transfer RNA (ribonucleic acid) synthetases (histidyl, alanyl, and threonyl). Nevertheless the absence of serum autoantibodies does not exclude the presence of autoimmune diseases. With few exceptions, anti-antibodies are not "disease specific," and there is overlap between autoimmune disorders. In any event,

demonstration of serum autoantibodies often is a valuable adjunct in the evaluation of a suspected autoimmune disorder.[4]

T lymphocytes are not only present in affected tissues from patients with autoimmune disorders, but also are capable of inducing experimental autoimmune diseases. Helper T cells usually transfer disease either by directly causing tissue damage or inducing cytotoxic cells in the recipient. Although cytolytic–major histocompatibility complex (MHC) restricted T lymphocytes of the Lyt-2 phenotype from animals with thyroiditis have cytolytic activity against in vitro cultured thyroid cell monolayers, the direct demonstration of cytotoxic T lymphocytes in human autoimmune disease remains elusive. The role of natural killer (NK) cells and the participation of macrophages in autoimmune diseases are unknown.[1]

Establishing that the disorder is autoimmune is often difficult or impossible. Autoimmune disorders can be characterized by mechanism and organ specificity (Table 7.1–3). Some autoimmune disorders, however, affect multiple systems. One end of the spectrum is exemplified by Hashimoto thyroiditis, in which autoantibodies and invasive inflammatory lesions are directed against just one organ. Target organs affected in organ-specific disease include the thyroid, adrenal glands, stomach, pancreas, neuromuscular junction, and skin. The other end of the spectrum is typified by SLE, in which antibodies are directed to a variety of widely distributed antigens; hence the lesions are widely disseminated. Non-organ-specific diseases, which include rheumatologic disorders, involve the skin, kidney, serosa, joints, muscle, and nervous system.

Genetic control of the predisposition to autoimmune diseases is polygenic and multifactorial. Multiple cases of autoimmune disease can occur within members of the same family. In some instances, the same disease occurs in related individuals; more often, several autoimmune diseases are found. In some families organ-specific autoimmune diseases occur, whereas in others an increased frequency of systemic autoimmune diseases, multisystem immunopathies, and blood dyscrasias or cytopenias (non-organ-specific autoimmune disease) is the pattern.

Genetic markers associated with autoimmune diseases include products of the MHC, complement determinants, and the IgG heavy-chain marker. In particular, several class I and II cell surface antigens, products of the MHC, are associated. The haplotype HLA-D1,B8,DR3 occurs with particular frequency in the organ-specific diseases, except in chronic thyroiditis. This haplotype, the components of which are in linkage disequilibrium, also occurs in Sjögren syndrome, which is almost invariably associated with another class II molecule, HLA-DRw52. Rheumatoid arthritis, a non-organ-specific disorder, is associated with HLA-Dw4 and DR4. In insulin-dependent (type 1) diabetes mellitus, heterozygotes for HLA-DR3 and HLA-DR4 have a greatly increased risk of developing disease. DQ1/DQ2 heterozygosity appears to be associated with increased autoantibody production in autoimmune connective tissue disorders such as SLE and Sjögren syndrome.[8]

The consistently higher prevalence of autoimmune disease in women suggests that autoimmune disease expression may be under sex-linked genetic or hormonal influences.

EVALUATION OF IMMUNE FUNCTION

ENUMERATION OF T AND B CELLS AND T CELL SUBSETS

In a broad sense, T lymphocytes mediate cellular immune responses, whereas the B cells differentiate into lymphoid and plasma cells that synthesize antibodies and hence mediate humoral immune responses. Identification and enumeration of the circulating T and B cells can thus help in the diagnosis of autoimmune, lymphoproliferative, and immunodeficiency disease (e.g., acquired immunodeficiency syndrome [AIDS]) and may be of help in assessing

TABLE 7.1–5. COMPARISON OF ORGAN-SPECIFIC AND NON-ORGAN-SPECIFIC DISORDERS

	Organ-Specific	Non-Organ-Specific
Antigen	Localized to organ	Diffusely distributed
Lesions	Antigen in organ is target for immunologic attack	Immune complexes deposit systemically or in situ
Site of lesions	Endocrine organs	Skin, kidneys, joints, muscle
Examples:		
Thyroid	Hashimoto thyroiditis Primary myxedema Thyrotoxicosis	
Stomach	Pernicious anemia	
Adrenal glands	Addison disease	
Pancreas	Insulin-dependent diabetes	
Skin	SLE Scleroderma	
Kidneys	SLE	
Joints	Rheumatoid arthritis	
Muscle	Dermatopolymyositis	

the immune status of patients with cancer or those who are undergoing transplantation procedures.

T and B cells express different surface antigens that distinguish them from each other, as well as antigens and cell surface receptors that differ according to the stage of cell maturation (differentiation) (Figs. 7.1–2 and 7.1–3). These cell surface antigens provide a convenient way to detect and enumerate the different lymphoid cells, and techniques have been developed to use cells in suspension (e.g., in a blood sample or from a disrupted tissue) or in tissue secretion (frozen or fixed). For example, in the past T cells were enumerated by counting cells that would bind sheep red blood cells to their surface (rosette formation). More recently, cells labeled with fluorescent dye-labeled specific antibodies (usually monoclonal) that are directed against the cell surface markers of interest are counted under fluorescent microscopy or in a flow cytometer.[8]

Total T cells are recognized by monoclonal antibodies such as T3 and T11 (Fig. 7.1–2) and B cells by B1 (Fig. 7.1–3) and are expressed as a percentage of the peripheral lymphocytes. Normally T cells represent 50 to 80 percent of the blood lymphocytes, and B cells make up 5 to 20 percent.[8]

Subsets of T cells are recognized that mediate specific portions of the cellular immune response. T4 antibody identifies the helper/inducer cells, whereas T8 identifies the suppressor/cytotoxic lymphoid cells that control, modulate, and suppress B-cell activity. T4 cells represent 34 to 56 percent of the circulating lymphocytes, and T8 cells make up 18 to 32 percent. The ratio of T4 (helper) to T8 (suppressor) cells (T4/T8) is often calculated and may be clinically useful (normal range, 1.1/2.5). For example, ratios less that 1.1 may support an AIDS diagnosis, since T4 cells are usually severely depressed in this syndrome. Other more recently discovered subsets of lymphocytes can also be measured by fluorescent antibody assays or by functional assays. The NK cell is an example and may be found to be quite low in cancer patients, but increased after interferon therapy.

IMMUNOGLOBULIN LEVELS IN BLOOD AND BODY FLUIDS

The integrity of the humoral arm of the immune system is most often assessed by studying the total serum immunoglobulins,[8] but functional assays such as a specific antibody response to administered antigens (e.g., polyvalent pneumococcal vaccine) may also prove useful in selected instances. A battery of tests is required to screen adequately the serum immunoglobulins. These include a serum protein electrophoretic pattern that will permit quantitation of the (gamma) fraction (normal range, 0.7 to 1.7 g/dl), as well as a qualitative evaluation of the normal heterogeneity of the immunoglobulins (polyclonality).

Immunoglobulin quantitation can be accomplished with a number of techniques, such as laser nephelometry. Serum to be tested is diluted, a known amount of antibody specific for one of the major classes (e.g., anti-IgG or anti-IgM) is added, and the amount of light scattered by the resultant precipitate is measured and compared to standards. Immunoglobulin levels vary with age, but in an adult the normal range for IgG is 639 to 1349 mg/dl; for IgA, 70 to 312 mg/dl; and for IgM, 56 to 352 mg/dl. Deviations from these ranges may suggest a variety of disease states, but it should be emphasized that levels within these rather broad ranges do not prove normality or absence of illness.

Two final screening tests used to evaluate immunoglobulins are immunoelectrophoresis and immunofixation electrophoresis. These tests permit two-dimensional evaluation of immunoglobulins, determining their electrophoretic mobility and their normal heterogeneity, as well as their isotype (IgG, IgA, and IgM) and their light-chain type (kappa and lambda).

The other two immunoglobulin classes, IgD and IgE, are present in such low concentrations that more sensitive methods, such as radioimmunoassay, are required for their measurement. IgD has a normal range of 0 to 14 mg/dl and is rarely measured

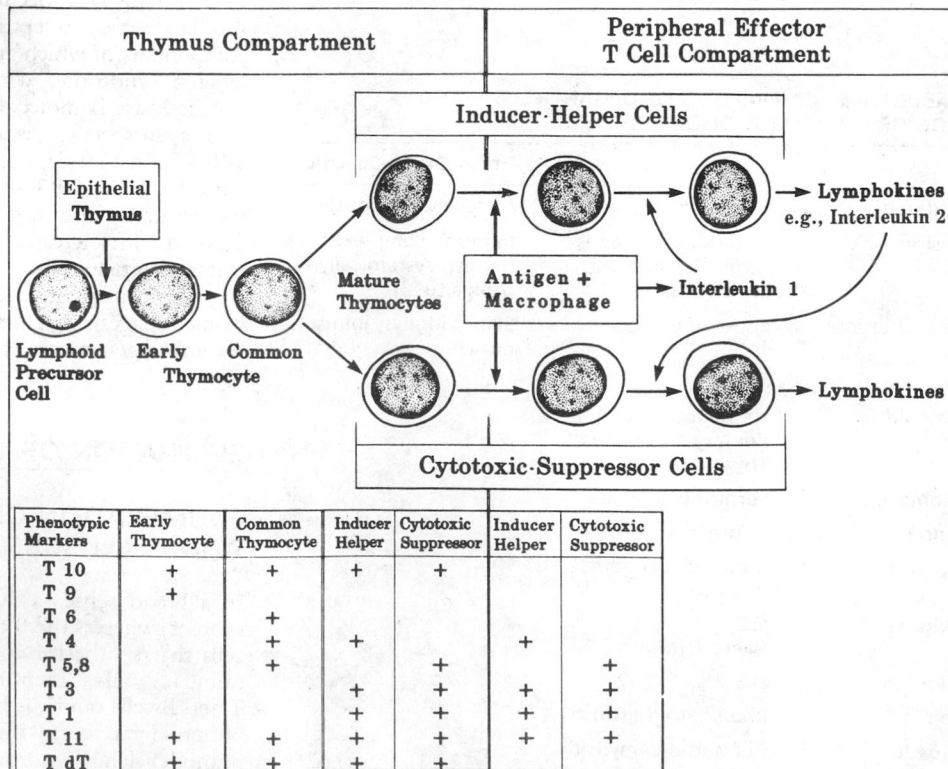

Figure 7.1–2. Schematic diagram illustrating major features of T cell ontogeny. Thymocytes can be discriminated by presence of T10 surface antigen and enzyme TdT (terminal deoxynucleotidyl transferase). Peripheral T cells can be recognized by presence of T1,3 markers. T11 recognizes thymocytes and peripheral T cells and is therefore a "pan" T marker. T4 recognizes the inducer-helper subset, and T5,8 aid in recognition of cytotoxic-suppressor cells.

Phenotypic Markers	Early Thymocyte	Common Thymocyte	Inducer Helper	Cytotoxic Suppressor	Inducer Helper	Cytotoxic Suppressor
T 10	+	+	+	+		
T 9	+					
T 6		+				
T 4		+	+		+	
T 5,8		+		+		+
T 3			+	+	+	+
T 1			+	+	+	+
T 11	+	+	+	+	+	+
T dT	+	+	+	+		

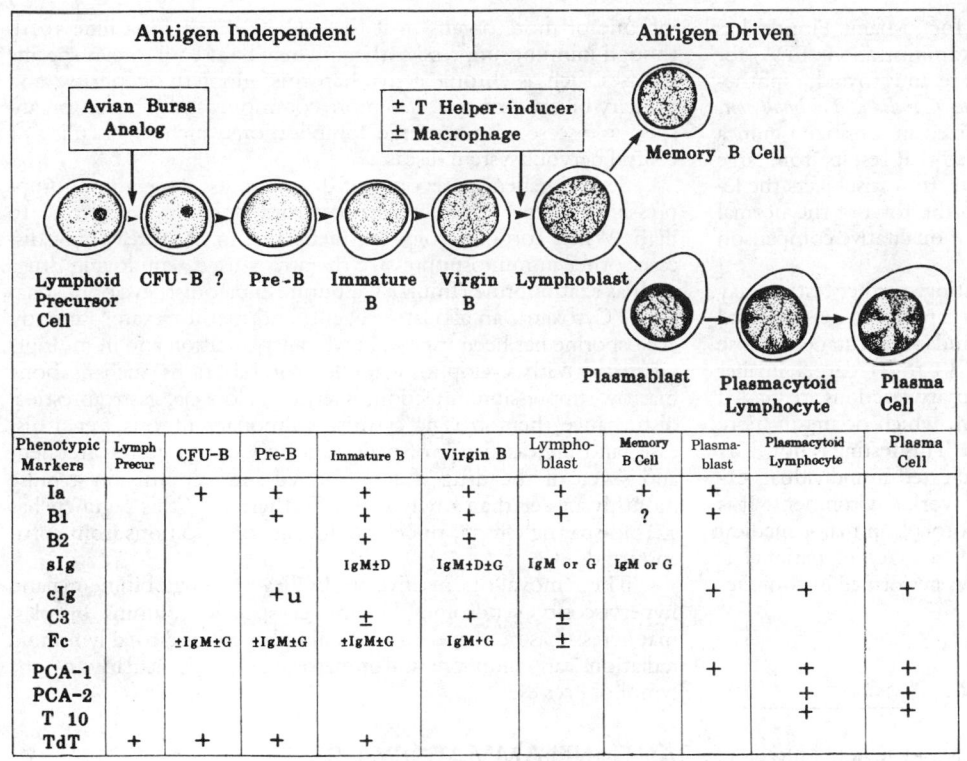

Phenotypic Markers	Lymph Precur	CFU-B	Pre-B	Immature B	Virgin B	Lympho-blast	Memory B Cell	Plasma-blast	Plasmacytoid Lymphocyte	Plasma Cell
Ia		+	+	+	+	+	+	+		
B1		+	+	+	+	+	?	+		
B2			+	+	+					
sIg				IgM±D	IgM±D±G	IgM or G	IgM or G			
cIg			+u					+	+	+
C3				±	+	±				
Fc		±IgM±G	±IgM±G	±IgM±G	IgM+G	±				
PCA-1								+	+	+
PCA-2									+	+
T 10									+	+
TdT	+	+	+	+						

Figure 7.1–3. Schematic diagram illustrating major features of B cell ontogeny. Ia and TdT are helpful in recognizing early B cell precursors. With some maturation B1 and B2 develop. Surface immunoglobulin (*SIG*) followed by cytoplasmic Ig (*CIG*) distinguishes B cells prepared to interact with antigen and ready to differentiate into plasma cells. Plasma cell associated (*PCA-1* and *2*) markers are not totally specific, but distinguish these cells when used together with T10 and secretion of immunoglobulin.

unless one suspects an IgD myeloma. Quantitation of IgE may sometimes be helpful in assessing allergic status, but it has a very broad normal range, extending from 5 to 472 ng/ml.

The determination of immunoglobulins by these and other assays in various body fluids may prove useful on occasion. For example, the presence of oligoclonal bands in ceribrospinal fluid with an increased level of IgG may add weight to the diagnosis of multiple sclerosis.

IMMUNE COMPLEX AND COMPLEMENT MEASUREMENTS

The sensitivity, specificity, and realiability of assays for the detection and measurement of circulating immune complexes in biologic fluids vary and virtually none are antigen specific.[4] Recognition of other molecules can result in false-positive results. No assay detects all immune complexes or distinguishes pathogenic from nonpathogenic immune complexes. Processing blood samples for serum modifies immune complex structure by complement action and releases immune complexes bound to CR1. Hence serum immune complex determinations are neither disease specific nor correlated with disease activity. Although immune complexes may play a major role in disease pathogenesis, the measurement of serum immune complex levels is not useful clinically.

On the other hand, the serum complement level is helpful, in that depression of serum complement is considered indicative of complement activation. Functional activation of the complement pathway is assessd by serum total hemolytic complement (CH$_{50}$), whereas individual complement components, most commonly C1q, C3, and C4, are measured by antigenic assays. A decrease in C1q or C4 indicates activation of the classical complement pathway, whereas an isolated decrease in C3 suggests selective activation of the alternative pathway. Decreases in C1q, C4, and C3 indicate activation of both pathways. Determination of complement component levels during disease activity is a static measurement of the dynamic process of complement activation, catabolism, and synthesis and does not always correlate with disease activity.

An increase in the serum SC5b-9 level, the attack complex of complement, provides definitive evidence for activation of the terminal components of complement, and research studies have been associated with active rheumatic or immunologically mediated neurologic disorders. When available, this sensitive assay should improve detection of complement activation. Immunocytochemical demonstration of immune complexes, complement, or membrane-bound C5b-9 tissue biopsy specimens of patients with autoimmune disorders may also establish activation of complement.

ANERGY TESTING

Individuals with deficient lymphocyte function have serious problems in resisting certain infectious agents (e.g., *M. tuberculosis* and other intracellular bacteria, fungi, protozoa, and viruses). One way to detect the deficiency is by anergy testing.[8] Anergy occurs in both congenital and acquired deficiency of T cell function and also in certain infectious diseases characterized either by unknown mechanisms, such as measles, or by those which overwhelm monocyte and macrophage defenses, such as miliary tuberculosis. A panel of antigens is injected intradermally and the diameter of induration is recorded at 24 and 48 hours. Positive reactions are defined arbitrarily as induration of greater than or equal to 5 mm. Nonreactive individuals are said to be anergic. Unfortunately, anergy testing was not standardized in the past, and anergy has at times been misdiagnosed as a result of either faulty antigens or a poor choice of antigens. For example, infants were called anergic simply for lack of exposure to bacterial or fungal antigens. Antigens commonly utilized include purified protein derivative of tuberculin and materials from streptococci, *Candida* and *Trichophyton* organisms, and mumps. The relevant antigen in these crude preparations has not been purified or identified to assist in standardizing the dose, however. The frequency of reactors to these antigens in the normal population depends on the batch of material, and varies from less than 50 percent, a frequency that would overdiagnose anergy, to 100 percent, which might underestimate anergy. Multitest cell me-

diated immunity from Merieux Institute, Inc., Miami, Florida, has been approved by the Food and Drug Administration (FDA) for testing and consists of puncture tests with tetanus toxoid, diphtheria toxoid, streptococcus, tuberculin, and *Candida, Trichophyton,* and *Proteus*. These antigens are standardized in sensitized guinea pigs and are tested in normal individuals so that results from large populations of normal subjects are known. In test subjects the lesion sizes are tabulated and compared to the total of the normal population, and a quantitative rather than qualitative comparison is made.[4]

If an individual is anergic by skin testing, further testing may be performed to establish the individual's capacity to be sensitized for lymphocyte reactivity by applying a standard epicutaneous dose of dinitrochlorobenzene (DNCB). After 14 to 21 days a smaller dose of DNCB is reapplied. Contact sensitivity reactions are graded on the basis of erythema and vesiculation, which occurs in more than 95 percent of the normal population. This testing is not FDA approved, and the procedure is contraindicated in individuals exposed to cross-reacting chemicals in their work environment. It is used most commonly in experimental protocols in major medical centers, where T lymphocyte functional activity of patients is changing over time. Anergy testing is often performed in conjunction with counting of T cell subsets.

THERAPEUTIC CONSIDERATIONS

Management of adverse immunologic reactions is only fully satisfactory if exposure to an external allergen can be terminated or an infectious agent eradicated before reactions to it do permanent damage. Nevertheless, a number of treatments and drugs have been developed that modify immunologic reactions, including immunization, immune suppression, anti-inflammatory drugs, antimediator drugs, and lymphokines.

Therapy in autoimmune disorders is multifaceted. In organ-specific disorders, the defect is often corrected by metabolic, biochemical, or pharmacologic means. For example, in hypothyroidism, thyroid hormone replacement is used, whereas in Graves disease (thyrotoxicosis) antithyroid drugs are normally prescribed. In autoimmune pernicious anemia, normal serum B_{12} levels are maintained by periodic injections of vitamin B_{12}. In myasthenia gravis, cholinesterase inhibitors are administered. When tissue damage is extreme and total function is lost (as in glomerulonephritis associated with lupus erythematosus or in severe deforming rheumatoid arthritis), kidney transplants, corrective surgery, or joint replacement may be necessary.

A simplified scheme of events with antibody-mediated and cellular reactions is shown in Figure 7.1–4, along with an indication of the site of action of these interventions.

IMMUNIZATION

Although immunization is the prime method of preventing infections, it is limited in modifying adverse reactions once they are initiated. Only in respiratory allergies and insect sting anaphylaxis does further parenteral immunization or immunotherapy seem to redirect adverse IgE antibody production to protective IgG antibody production (see Chapter 7.3).

IMMUNOSUPPRESSION

Another treatment approach for autoimmune disorders is to use anti-inflammatory agents and immunosuppressive drugs. Musculoskeletal symptoms of rheumatic disorders caused by inflammation are controlled by conventional anti-inflammatory drugs such as salicylates, nonsteroidal anti-inflammatory agents, and antimalarial drugs (e.g., hydroxychloroquine). Immunosuppressive drugs are used if there is evidence of progressive systemic disease involving one or more organs or if there is life-threatening illness. Although immunosuppressive therapy may be used in organ-specific diseases such as chronic active hepatitis, glomerulonephritis, and primary biliary cirrhosis, it is more commonly used in non-organ-specific disease with systemic complications, such as vasculitis or central nervous system disease.

Several general categories of drugs are used for immunosuppressive therapy. Usually corticosteroid doses are moderate to high. When corticosteroids are ineffective in life-threatening disease, other immunosuppressive therapy is used, employing drugs such as azathioprine (Imuran), a purine antagonist; cyclophosphamide (Cytoxan), an alkylating agent; and methotrexate. Recently cyclosporine has been used in renal transplantation and in multiple sclerosis. With cyclophosphamide, complications such as bone marrow suppression, infection, infertility, alopecia, gastrointestinal disturbance, hemorrhagic cystitis, pulmonary fibrosis, renal disease, and increased risk of malignancy appear to be less frequent and severe if the drug is administered intravenously in a pulse monthly rather than orally daily. Furthermore, this regimen has steroid-sparing effects, thereby reducing complications from corticosteroids.

The removal of causative antibodies in cryoglobulinemia and hyperviscosity syndromes by antigen-specific columns or plasmapheresis has been successful. Leukophoresis and total lymphoid radiation can eliminate inflammatory cells, particularly of the lymphoid series.

ANTI-INFLAMMATORY DRUGS

Anti-inflammatory drugs, both steroidal and nonsteroidal, interfere with leukocyte function in ways that reduce the intensity of inflammatory manifestions of disease.

ANTI-MEDIATOR DRUGS

These drugs block the effects of mediators generated by mast cells and basophils. Antihistamines, for instance, are blockers of the H1 effects of histamine and help relieve the symptoms of hay fever and urticaria. Their action is not exclusively antihistaminic and atropine-like effects may also be therapeutically useful. Drugs that raise intracellular adenosine 3':5'-cyclic phosphate (cyclic AMP), such as sympathomimetics or theophylline, have a dual action, both preventing mediator release and counteracting some mediator effects such as vasodilation and bronchospasm. Cromolyn sodium appears to block mast cell mediator release, at least in part. Drugs that block other mediators are in development.[8]

LYMPHOKINES

Lists of lymphokines and monokines are given in Table 7.1–2 and 7.1–3. Lymphokines act at very low concentrations, in the area of 10^{-12} M in some cases, and single lymphokines may have biologic effects on many different target cells, including T cells, B cells, macrophages, granulocytes, and mast cells. For example, although interferons were discovered by their antiviral activity, interferon-g also is a highly potent activator of macrophages and inhibitor of macrophage migration. Many lymphokines (first eight entries in Table 7.1–2) are purified and gene cloned; others are presently defined only by their functional activities. Lymphokines act on specific cell surface receptors. "Activating" stimuli for T cells, including antigens and mitogens, stimulate lymphokine secretion, and also stimulate expression of increased numbers of receptors for the lymphokines.

Several purified lymphokines are being used in experimental therapeutic trials in the treatment of cancer, immune deficiency, and autoimmune diseases. For instance, human mononuclear cells are cultured with interleukin 2 (IL-2) to generate lymphokine-activated killer (LAK) cells. Such LAK cells are potent cytotoxic cells,

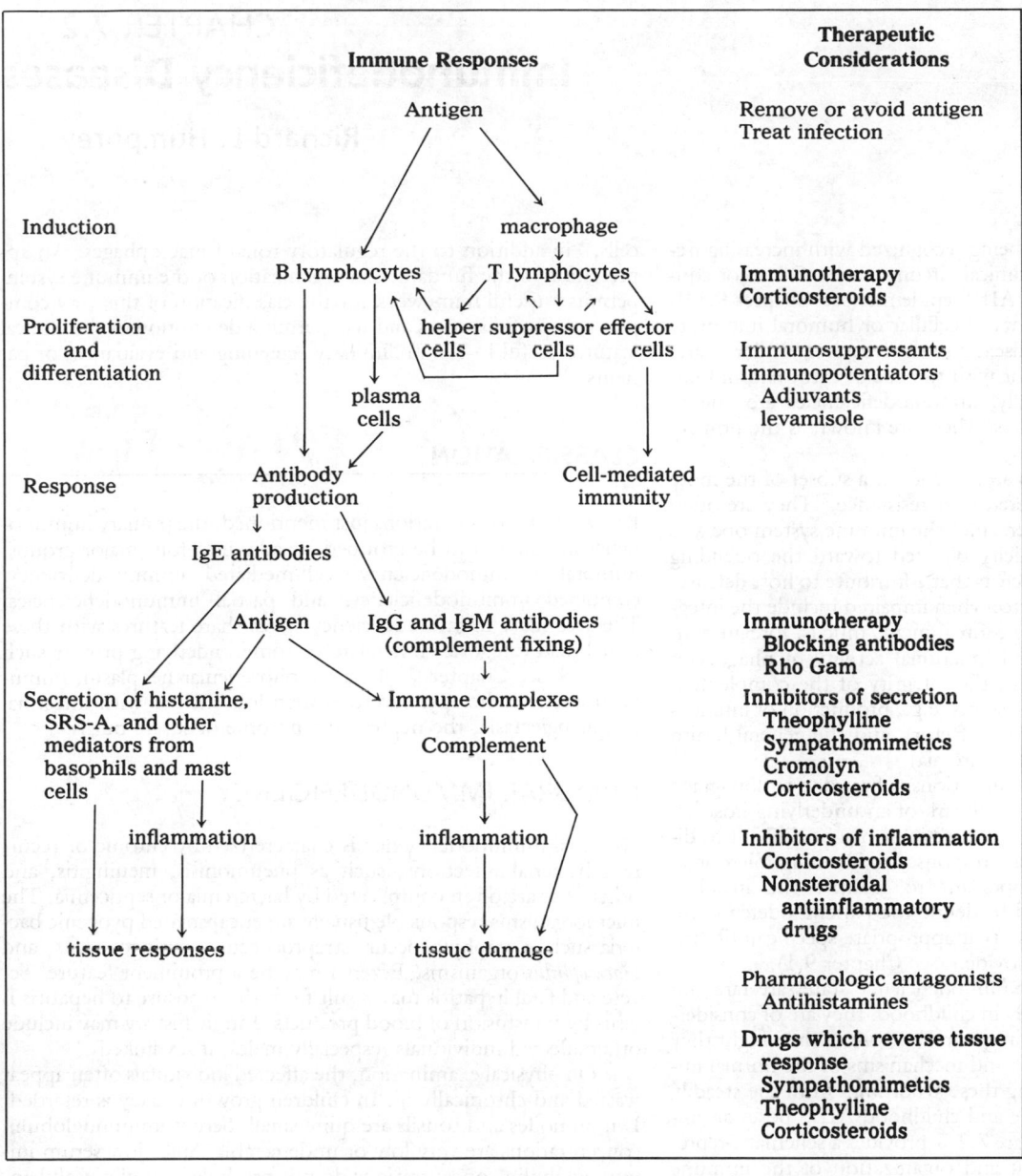

Figure 7.1–4. Therapeutic considerations in immunologic disorders.

which preferentially kill tumor cells. Preliminary results suggest that the combination of LAK cells and repeated injections of IL-2 has therapeutic benefits in some patients with certain types of cancer. Colony-stimulating factors or other factors that stimulate hematopoiesis are also being used in some cases of bone marrow failure.

REFERENCES

1. Dixon FJ, Fisher DW: The Biology of Immunologic Disease. Sunderland, Massachusetts, Hospital Practice, 1983.
2. MacKay JR, Burnet FM (eds): Autoimmune Diseases. Springfield, Ill, Charles C Thomas, 1963
3. Roitt IM, Brostoff J, Male DK (eds): Immunology. St. Louis, CV Mosby, 1985
4. Rose NR, Friedman H, Fahey JL (eds): Manual of Clinical Laboratory Immunology. Washington, DC, American Society for Microbiology, 1986
5. Rose NR, Mackay IR (eds): The Autoimmune Diseases. New York, Academic Press, 1985
6. Samter M (ed): Immunological Diseases, 3d ed. Boston, Little, Brown, 1978, vols 1 and 2
7. Schifferli JA, Ng YC, Peters DK: The role of complement and its receptor in the elimination of immune complexes. N Engl J Med 315:488, 1986
8. Stites DP, Stobo JD, Wells JV (eds): Basic and Clinical Immunology. Norwalk, Conn, Appleton & Lange, 1987

Immunodeficiency Diseases

Richard L. Humphrey

Deficiencies of immunity are being recognized with increasing frequency in a wide variety of clinical circumstances. Of major concern is the rapidly increasing AIDS epidemic (see Chapter 9.14). Apart from AIDS, impairments of cellular or humoral immunity are associated with acquired diseases of the lymphoreticular tissues (e.g., myeloma, lymphoma) or with the use of cytotoxic and immunosuppressive drugs. Rarely, immunodeficiencies are due to congenital or heritable disorders. These are known as the primary immunodeficiencies.[4]

Immunodeficiency states are, of course, a subset of the more general phenomenon of lowered host resistance.[7] They are often considered separately, however, since the immune system operates with a high degree of specificity directed toward the offending agent (e.g., antigen). Other factors that contribute to host defenses and result in decreased resistance when impaired include the integrity of mechanical barriers (e.g., integument, mucus, foreign bodies), the absolute number and functional activity of phagocytes (e.g., neutrophils, monocytes), the integrity of the complement cascade and other amplifying systems (e.g., production of interleukin 1 and 2, migration inhibition factor), and the general health status (e.g., starvation, diabetes, uremia).

Susceptibility to repeated infections, often due to low-grade or unusual pathogens, are the hallmark of an underlying host defense impairment. At times these infections may be difficult to diagnose because the classic tissue responses to invading microorganisms are lacking. It is important to identify the invading microorganism, however, and to define the patient's defense impairment as soon as possible so that appropriate specific antibiotic and supportive care can be provided (see Chapter 9.1).

Although the primary immunodeficiency states are rare and are recognized most commonly in childhood, they are of considerable importance for medicine in general because of the insight they give into the interrelationships and mechanisms of the normal immune response. Differentiating these syndromes from the steadily increasing problem of infantile and childhood AIDS poses an important clinical challenge. Figure 7.2–1 provides a schematic representation of the development and organization of the immune system. During embryonic development, hematopoietic and lymphoid precursor cells emerge in the yolk sac and migrate to the liver and later to primitive bone marrow. These lymphoid precursor cells come under the influence of two different organizing principles, the developing epithelial thymus and the avian bursa analogue.

The thymus, derived from epithelial outpouchings in the third and fourth pharyngeal pouches, induces differentiation of the thymus-dependent lymphocytes (T cells) that circulate to peripheral lymphoid tissue and mediate cellular immune reactions. These cellular immune reactions include delayed hypersensitivity skin reactions, homograft rejection, and graft versus host reactivity (see Chapter 7.1).

In birds the bursa of Fabricius (the bursa analogue in mammals is unknown; perhaps it is the bone marrow) induces differentiation of the bursa-dependent lymphocytes (B cells), which mediate humoral immunity. On encounter with an antigen (in some instances macrophage processing or helper T cell activity are required) B cells differentiate into plasma cells that secrete specific immunoglobulin (see Chapter 7.1). These two major divisions dominate the immune system: T cell–mediated cellular immunity and B cell–mediated humoral immunity. An additional set of complexities is introduced by the recognition of interactions between these divisions (Fig. 7.2–1): "helper T cells" and "suppressor T

cells," in addition to the regulatory role of macrophages. An appreciation of the fundamental organization of the immune system permits a useful framework for the classification of this very complex group of disorders and will permit a description of the clinical features useful in the preliminary screening and evaluation of patients.

CLASSIFICATION

Based on the considerations just mentioned, the primary immunodeficiency states can be grouped broadly into four major groups: humoral immunodeficiency, cell-mediated immunodeficiency, combined immunodeficiency, and partial immunodeficiencies. The secondary immunodeficiency states share features with these four broad categories but relate to some underlying process such as AIDS (see Chapter 9.14), a lymphoreticular neoplasm, immunosuppressive therapy, severe protein loss such as with intestinal lymphangiectasia, the nephrotic syndrome or severe burns.

HUMORAL IMMUNODEFICIENCY

Humoral immunodeficiency is characterized by chronic or recurrent bacterial infections, such as pneumonitis, meningitis, and otitis, that are often complicated by bacteremia or septicemia. The microorganisms responsible usually are encapsulated pyogenic bacteria such as staphylococcus, streptococcus, meningococcus, and *Haemophilus* organisms. Eczema may be a prominent feature. Severe and fatal hepatitis may result from the exposure to hepatitis B virus by transfusion of blood products. Family history may include other affected individuals (especially males, if sex linked).

On physical examination, the affected individuals often appear wasted and chronically ill. In children growth usually is retarded. Lymph nodes and tonsils are quite small. Serum immunoglobulin concentrations are very low or undetectable. Since low serum immunoglobulin concentrations do not preclude clinically useful antibody synthesis, responses to various antigens should be tested directly. The following tests are used because of their ready availability in most clinical settings: isohemagglutinin titers, Schick skin test (if abnormal, remains positive despite DPT [diphtheria-pertussis-tetanus] immunization), tetanus antitoxin titers, and absent response to pneumococcal (Pneumovax) or to typhoid-paratyphoid vaccination (febrile agglutinins). In addition, no plasma cells will be found on bone marrow aspiration or gut biopsy, and germinal centers and lymphoid follicles will be absent or poorly developed.

CELL-MEDIATED IMMUNODEFICIENCY

In contrast, cell-mediated immunodeficiency is characterized by a propensity for severe viral and fungal infections. The microorganisms responsible include cytomegalovirus, the herpes viruses, rubeola, rubella, *Candida* species, and *Histoplasma capsulatum*. If an individual is vaccinated against smallpox, disseminated vaccinia may result, and this is also true for vaccination with bacillus Calmette-Guérin (BCG) and other live attenuated organisms. In addition, the administration of live immunocompetent cells (e.g., blood or platelet transfusions) may result in graft-versus-host disease. The family history may be positive for similarly affected siblings or early infant deaths. On physical examination growth may

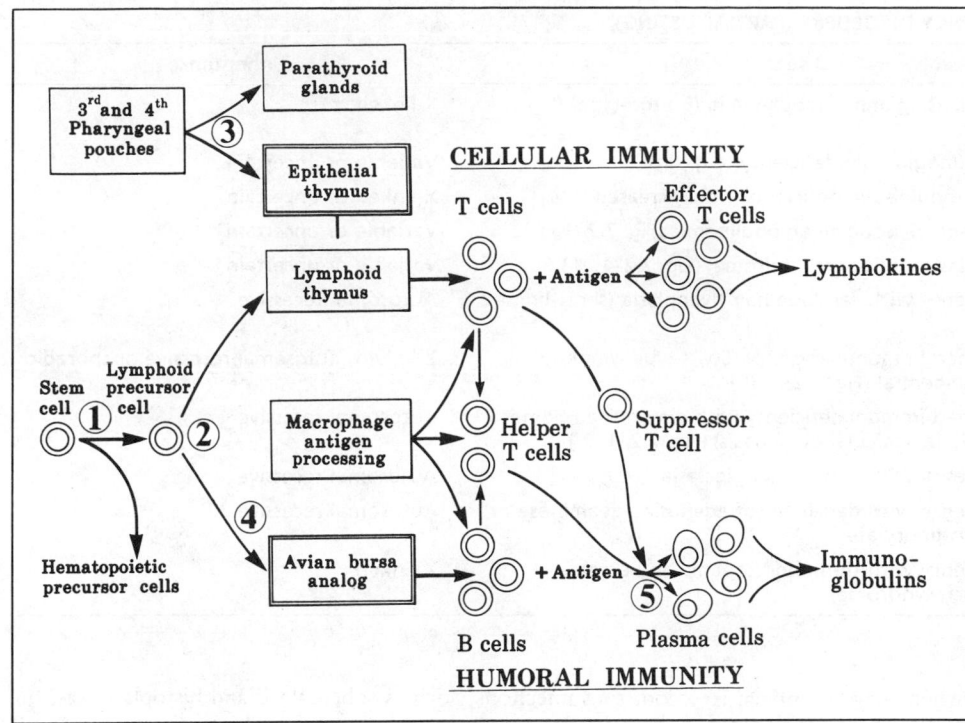

Figure 7.2–1. Development of the immune system is diagrammatically illustrated showing its separation into T cell-mediated cellular and B cell-mediated humoral components. Also illustrated are some interactions between various cell systems, including antigen processing by macrophage, helper T cell, and suppressor T cell-modulation of B cell activity. Postulated sites of defects giving rise to major (prototype) immunodeficiency syndromes are illustrated: (1) severe combined immunodeficiency with generalized hematopoietic hypoplasia (reticular dysgenesis); (2) severe combined immunodeficiency (Swiss-type lymphopenic agammaglobulinemia); (3) thymic hypoplasia (DiGeorge syndrome); (4) infantile X-linked agammaglobulinemia (Bruton-type); and (5) common variable immunodeficiency.

be retarded, lymph nodes and tonsils will be small, and the individuals may appear chronically ill. Routine laboratory studies reveal marked lymphopenia. The thymus usually is absent on lateral chext x-ray examination. Delayed hypersensitivity skin tests will demonstrate the marked impairment of cell-mediated immunity. (Normal adults have a median response of about three positive reactions to a battery that includes PPD, histoplasmin, *Trichophyton* species, *Candida* species, streptokinase/streptodornase, and mumps. In addition, more than 99 percent of normal individuals can be sensitized to DNCB.) Bone marrow aspiration shows reduced numbers of small lymphocytes, and tissue from a lymph node biopsy shows an absence of lymphocytes in the deep cortical areas and medullary cords.

Additional tests that have been used to define the impairment of these two parts of the immune system include measurement of the percentage of T and B cells among circulating lymphocytes, in vitro immunoglobulin production after stimulation with lipopolysaccharide or pokeweed mitogen, or in vitro response (e.g, tritiated thymidine incorporation) to phytohemagglutinin (PHA) or after incubation with allogeneic cells (mixed lymphocyte culture, or MLC). With the advent of highly specific monoclonal antisera (e.g., OKT series) and flow cytometry, the routine enumeration of both T and B cells and their subsets have become more readily available and precise. These laboratory tests are summarized in Table 7.2–2.

COMBINED AND PARTIAL IMMUNODEFICIENCY STATES

As implied in the title, these disorders combine in various ways the features of both the humoral and cell-mediated immunodeficiency states, or at the other extreme may be represented only by a minor defect in one or the other arm of the immune system. As will be discussed, severe combined immunodeficiency (Swiss-type lymphopenic agammaglobulinemia) represents a failure to develop both arms of the immune system, whereas the selective immunoglobulin deficiencies (e.g., isolated IgA deficiency) in many patients is not even associated with any clinical problems. The relationships between some of these deficiency states is diagram-

matically illustrated in Figure 7.2–1 with a partial listing in Table 7.2–1.

REPRESENTATIVE DISEASES

A few "classic" examples of the diseases that best typify and illustrate major features of the immunodeficiency syndromes will be discussed (Fig. 7.2–1, ④ and Tables 7.2–1 and 7.2–2). Several excellent comprehensive reviews are available for further study.[2,4–7]

Infantile X-Linked Agammaglobulinemia (Bruton-type)

Congenital sex-linked agammaglobulinemia always occurs in males, the recessive gene being carried by apparently normal women who are obligate heterozygote carriers of the defect. (Fig. 7.2–1, ④). Techniques are now available for demonstrating this carrier state.[3] When placentally transferred maternal antibodies disappear at about 6 to 9 months of age, a profound and lifelong deficiency of all types of circulating immunoglobulins becomes manifest. Although minute amounts of IgG and sometimes IgM are identifiable by sensitive immunochemical methods, functional levels of antibody are absent. Antigenic stimulation by bacterial or viral infections or by potent injected soluble or particulate antigens produces no demonstrable antibody response. These patients are capable of developing delayed or cellular hypersensitivity, however, and will display normal reactions to skin tests and can be sensitized with DNCB (Table 7.2–2). The lymph nodes, adenoids, and tonsils are small and hypoplastic and lack active germinal centers. Plasma cells are completely absent from lymph nodes, Peyer patches, appendix, and bone marrow. The thymus is histologically normal. Circulating B cells are markedly decreased or absent, and the defect seems to be a block in pre-B-cell differentiation to B cells. The carrier female (e.g., mother, sister), although immunologically normal, has B cells that are all of one active X chromosome type, suggesting a preferential loss of B cells that attempt to use the abnormal X (or inactivate the normal X) chromosome.[3] Clinically these patients are susceptible to repeated life-threatening pyogenic infections with organisms such as *Haemophilus*, *Streptococcus*, or *Staphylococcus*. Pneumonia, septicemia, meningitis, otitis, bronchitis, and sinusitis are recurrent problems. Viral and fungal

TABLE 7.2–1. PRIMARY IMMUNODEFICIENCY DISORDERS (PARTIAL LISTING)

Defect	Disease	Inheritance
B cells	Infantile X-linked agammaglobulinemia (Bruton-type) (Fig. 7.2–1,④)	X linked
	Selective immunoglobulin deficiency (e.g., IgA)	Variable or uncertain
	X-linked immunoglobulin deficiency with increased IgM	X linked or uncertain
	Common variable hypogammaglobulinemia (Fig. 7.2–1, ⑤)	Variable or uncertain
T cells	Thymic hypoplasia (DiGeorge syndrome) (Fig. 7.2–1, ③)	Variable or uncertain
	Immunodeficiency with cartilage-hair hypoplasia (short-limbed dwarfism)	Autosomal recessive
Combined B and T cells	Severe combined immunodeficiency (Swiss-type lymphopenic agammaglobulinemia) (Fig. 7.2–1, ①)	X linked, autosomal recessive or sporadic
	Severe combined immunodeficiency with generalized hematopoietic hypoplasia (reticular dysgenesis) (Fig. 7.2–1, ①)	Autosomal recessive
	Immunodeficiency with ataxia-telangiectasia	Autosomal recessive
	Immunodeficiency with deficiency of adenosine deaminase or nucleoside phosphorylase	Autosomal recessive
	Immunodeficiency with thrombocytopenia and eczema (Wiskott-Aldrich syndrome)	X linked

infections do not occur repeatedly, but when they do antigen is not cleared normally. For example, exposure to the hepatitis virus usually leads to fulminant hepatitis or chronic progressive hepatitis and is often fatal. Accordingly, transfusion with blood products should be avoided if at all possible.

Chronic gastrointestinal tract infection with rotavirus or *Giardia lamblia* may result in chronic diarrhea, spruelike malabsorption syndrome, and protein-losing enteropathy.

An unusual incidence of certain other conditions occurs with congenital sex-linked agammaglobulinemia. About one third develop clinically typical rheumatoid arthritis, including rheumatoid nodules. Histologically the lesions are also typical except for the absence of plasma cells. Tests for rheumatoid factor are invariably negative. This arthritis will subside with replacement gamma globulin therapy. Dermatomyositis or scleroderma has been recognized in other cases. In a few instances, progressive demyelination of the central nervous system has been observed, perhaps because of a chronic ECHO virus encephalitis.

Typical childhood eczema also occurs with increased frequency in patients with congenital sex-linked antibody deficiency. Skin tests to various allergens are negative, and the wheal and flare reaction is absent.

With an associated neutropenia, pneumonia caused by *Pneumocystis carinii* can occur, which is fatal in these patients unless treated promptly. There may be an increased incidence of granulomatous infections, such as tuberculosis and histoplasmosis, but these diseases respond to appropriate antibiotic therapy.

Treatment consists of prompt use of appropriate antimicrobials and long-term administration of gamma globulin. The prophylactic use of antibiotics is not likely to prevent many infections but only to select for antibiotic-resistant ones. Long-term results are fairly good, but these patients often develop chronic lung disease due to destruction of lung parenchyma by repeated infections. They are also prone to develop leukemia and lymphoma.

Thymic Hypoplasia (DiGeorge Syndrome)

Attention is drawn to infants with thymic hypoplasia (Fig. 7.2–1, ③) by the appearance of hypocalcemic tetany shortly after birth. This results from the failure of both the parathyroid gland and the thymus to be formed from the third and fourth pharyngeal pouches during embryonic development. A number of associated physical abnormalities often occur with thymic hypoplasia, including hypertelorism, antimongoloid slant of the eyes, low-set and notched ears, micrognathia, cardiac and aortic arch anomalies, and esophageal atresia.

The absence of the epithelial portion of the thymus results in a failure to develop T cells and cell-mediated immunity. To the extent that it is T cell independent, however, humoral-mediated immunity develops normally. The thymus is absent, and T lymphocytes are absent from blood and are not found in the

TABLE 7.2–2. LABORATORY EVALUATION OF IMMUNOCOMPETENCE

Humoral Immunity (B Cell Function)	Cellular Immunity (T Cell Function)
1. Immunoglobulin levels (IgG, IgA, IgM, IgE), serum protein electrophoresis, IgG subclass levels (1, 2, 3, 4)	1. Peripheral lymphocyte count and morphology
2. Isohemagglutinin titers (anti-A, anti-B)	2. Delayed hypersensitivity skin tests (e.g., PPD, histoplasmin, *Trichophyton* species, *Candida* species, mumps, streptokinase/streptodornase)
3. Tetanus antitoxin titers before and after immunization with tetanus toxoid or DPT	3. DNCB skin sensitization
4. Febrile agglutinins and specific antibody titers (before and after typhoid-paratyphoid immunization; Pneumovax, etc.)	4. Release of lymphokines (e.g., migratory inhibition factor [MIF], etc.)
5. In vitro immunoglobulin production following antigen or non-specific stimulation (e.g., pokeweed mitogen)	5. In vitro lymphocyte transformation by phytohemagglutinin or mixed lymphocyte culture
6. Biopsy bone marrow, lymph node, and gut and examine for plasma cells and germinal centers	6. Biopsy lymph node and examine for lymphocytes in thymus-dependent areas
7. Enumerate B cells in peripheral blood (e.g., surface Ig, flow cytometry; B1)	7. Enumerate and subclassify T cells in peripheral blood, e.g., flow cytometry using specific monoclonal antisera (e.g., OKT series, T3, 11; T4, T8)

thymus-dependent areas of the lymph nodes and spleen. These patients do not develop normal delayed hypersensitivity skin test reactions nor can they be sensitized with DNCB. These individuals are prone to develop infections with fungi, viruses, and opportunistic pathogens (e.g., *Pneumocystis*). Vaccination with live attenuated organisms leads to generalized disseminated fatal disease, and all such agents should be avoided. In addition, the transfer of live immunocompetent cells (blood, platelets, fresh plasma, or white cell transfusions) will lead to a rapidly fatal graft-versus-host disease. Thus these blood products should either be avoided or irradiated before use.

Correction in some instances has been achieved by means of early (14 weeks' gestational age) fetal thymus transplants with the beneficial effect perhaps mediated by the production of thymosin by the graft.

Severe Combined Immunodeficiency (Swiss-type Lymphopenic Agammaglobulinemia)

This disorder has several variants, with different modes of inheritance and somewhat different levels of severity (Fig. 7.2–1, ②).[2] Basically it can be thought of as a failure to develop lymphoid stem cells, resulting in an absence of both the cellular and the humoral components of the immune response. Exposure to live vaccines or blood products (hepatitis virus) may lead to serious infections. Recurrent severe infections of all types are the rule, and survival for more than a few months is unlikely. Successful treatment with correction of all of these abnormalities has been achieved using bone marrow transplantation from donors who are HLA histocompatible and also by using haploidentical bone marrow depleted of postthymic T cells.

Severe Combined Immunodeficiency with Generalized Hematopoietic Hypoplasia (Reticular Dysgenesis)

Immunodeficiency with generalized hematopoietic hypoplasia is characterized by a severe deficiency of both T cells and B cells, as well as a failure of development of granulocytes (Fig. 7.2–1, ①).[4,5] There have been only a few reported cases, all of whom have died with overwhelming infection within a few days to several weeks after birth. Marrow contains megakaryocytes and erythroid elements, but granulocyte precursors are absent. It is thought to be inherited as an autosomal recessive trait, but this has not been established with certainty. Bone marrow transplantation has been successful in providing complete correction.

Common Variable Immunodeficiency

This is a markedly heterogeneous group of disorders that will undoubtedly be more appropriately classified as further knowledge is developed (Fig. 7.2–1, ⑤).[4,5]

Altogether these patients represent the most common form of non-AIDS-related immunodeficiency. Often occurring in adults with a history of previous good health, the presumption is that their immune system was previously normal and so it is an "acquired" disorder. Sometimes an antecedent infection or other illness is recognized, but in most instances no "etiology" can be identified. Diagnostic and treatment implications are the same as discussed in the preceding sections, but when antibody deficiency is noted, particularly in the older age group, a search for underlying diseases such as chronic lymphocytic leukemia, lymphoma, and multiple myeloma is indicated.

Other conditions, such as collagen vascular disorders (rheumatoid arthritis, dermatomyositis), malabsorption, pernicious anemia, and the like, have been associated with or observed to develop in these patients. The malabsorption with steatorrhea is not accompanied by easily demonstrable changes in intestinal flora nor is it relieved by antibiotics. *Giardia lamblia* infestation should be considered and an intestinal biopsy performed to rule it out. There is also a high incidence of rheumatoid arthritis in the families of patients with hypogammaglobulinemia and in some families with SLE. Hemolytic anemia may occur, and several cases of megaloblastic anemia from vitamin B_{12} deficiency associated with defective absorption of vitamin B_{12} have been observed.

Frequent attacks of bronchitis and pneumonia lead to structural damage of the lungs, with lung abscess, empyema, diffuse fibrosis, or bronchiectasis. Also common are recurrent infections of the paranasal sinuses and middle ear. Repeated attacks of bacterial conjunctivitis may also occur. Episodes of acute pyoderma, meningitis, and urinary tract infections are noted with increased frequency but are less often a problem than sinopulmonary infections. Bacterial infections respond well to treatment with the appropriate antibiotic, and the course run by a single infection under treatment is not unusual. It is the high frequency of recurrence that constitutes the problem.

Recent studies indicate that in some of these patients the defect lies with overactive suppressor T cells, and these observations may lead to new ways to treat or control the disorder. In contrast, some patients lack B cells altogether, whereas other patients fail to produce or secrete immunoglobulin but have normal numbers of B cells. Autoantibodies to T and B cells have also been described.

Currently therapy consists of supportive care during the acute infection and prophylactic gamma globulin injections. Sometimes enough of the immune response remains so that anaphylaxis complicates the gamma globulin treatments; this requires very careful monitoring and observation during the injections. If this anaphylaxis develops, an occasional patient can still be helped if a single related donor can be used for plasma transfer or perhaps by the use of the newer intravenous gamma globulin preparations. Approximately 8 percent of these patients will develop malignancies, including leukemia, lymphomas, and epithelial tumors.

Selective Immunoglobulin Deficiencies

Selective immunoglobulin deficiencies occur in a variety of patterns and with varying degrees of completeness. The most common is the syndrome of isolated IgA deficiency. The incidence in the general population is about one case per 500 to 700. The mode of inheritance is uncertain or seems to vary among families. Fortunately most of these individuals are asymptomatic, but sinopulmonary infections are occasionally troublesome. Other syndromes have been recognized, and this deficiency has been related to allergies, autoimmune disorders, collagen vascular disorders, various malignancies, malabsorption, and mental retardation. The etiologic connection, if any, in most of these situations is obscure.

A serious difficulty for some of these patients is the presence of anti-IgA antibodies that can lead to gastrointestinal symptoms following milk ingestion. Another hazard that these patients face is with the administration of blood or plasma. They can develop antibodies to human IgA encountered in this fashion, and life-threatening anaphylaxis may result later when more blood or plasma is administered.

Sinopulmonary hygiene with specific antibiotic therapy is currently the only available treatment. No commercial source of IgA is available for administration; additionally, there would be serious reservations about its use (anaphylaxis), as well as probable lack of transport to the mucous membrane surface, and hence no effectiveness at the major deficient site.

The normal production and maturation of B cells destined to produce IgA depends heavily on helper T cell activity. Helper/suppressor ratios (and function?) are abnormal in bone marrow transplantation patients. Thus this class of immunoglobulin is low or absent for prolonged periods. This relationship also suggests that subtle abnormalities in T cell function may be responsible for the IgA deficiency in some instances.

IgG2 and IgG4 subclass deficiencies have been described in association with IgA deficiency and may be related to increased susceptibility to infection. IgE deficiency has also been seen in about half of the selective IgA deficient patients and is also recognized as an isolated defect.

Isolated IgG subclass deficiencies and selective failure to respond to certain whole classes of antigens have also been described.[1] It should therefore be realized that a normal level of IgG

may not rule out the presence of an immunodeficiency related to these more subtle defects.

Immunodeficiency with Deficiency of Adenosine Deaminase or Purine Nucleoside Phosphorylase

Combined T and B cell immunodeficiency results from the abnormality of purine metabolism created by deficiency of adenosine deaminase. In contrast, severely impaired T cell function with preserved B cell function is the result of purine necleoside phosphorylase deficiency. The selective toxicity for these enzyme deficiencies is seen in immune system functioning, which reveals a differential sensitivity on the part of the lymphoid cells to the accumulation of deoxyadenosine triphosphate and the blockage of the formation of S-adenosylmethionine (ADA deficiency) and to the accumulation of deoxyguanosine triphosphate (PNP deficiency).

In either case, the diagnosis is made by measuring the affected enzyme and finding very low or absent levels of activity in red blood cells, fibroblasts, or white blood cells. Carriers can be detected by finding half-normal levels.

Treatment has been accomplished most successfully by histocompatible bone marrow transplantation. If a suitable donor is not available, some patients have been helped by enzyme replacement (e.g., periodic red blood cell transfusions). This seems to work best when treatment can begin soon after recognition of the disorder.

REFERENCES

1. Ambrosina OM, Siber GR, et al: An immunodeficiency characterized by impaired antibody responses to polysaccharides. N Engl J Med 316:790, 1987
2. Buckley RH: Humoral immunodeficiency. Clin Immunol Immunopathol 40:13, 1986
3. Fearon ER, Winkelstein JA, et al: Carrier detection in X-linked agammaglobulinemia by analysis of X-chromosome inactivation. N Engl J Med 316:427, 1987
4. Rosen FS, Cooper MD, Wedgwood RJP: The primary immunodeficiencies. N Engl J Med 311:235; 300, 1984
5. Stiehm ER, Fulginiti VA (eds): Immunologic Disorders in Infants and Children, 2d ed. Philadelphia, WB Saunders, 1980
6. Twomey JJ (ed): The Pathophysiology of Human Immunologic Disorders. Baltimore, Urban & Schwarzenberg, 1982
7. Verhoef J, Peterson PK, Quie PG (eds): Infections in the Immunocompromised Host: Pathogenesis, Prevention, and Therapy. Amsterdam, Elsevier/North-Holland, 1980

CHAPTER 7.3
IgE (Anaphylactic) Reactions

Philip S. Norman

Most conditions regarded as allergic come about through an initial rapid release of locally active mediators from mast cells and basophils, usually triggered by a combination of IgE antibodies fixed to the cell surface and antigen (see Chapter 7.1). IgE antibodies, like other classes of antibodies, are synthesized and excreted in lymphoid organs, particularly those adjacent to the respiratory and gastrointestinal tracts, and circulate freely in body fluids.[3] Because specific receptors on mast cells and basophils recognize the Fc portion of the IgE molecules, however, most of the IgE formed resides on the surface of these cells and vanishingly small amounts are found in serum (5 to 500 ng/ml).

The ability to synthesize IgE antibody is not confined to allergic individuals; nearly everyone forms these antibodies, and they are greatly increased in the presence of parasitic infestations. A recessive gene appears to confer elevated serum IgE levels on homozygotes, but other factors, presumably immune response genes related to HLA types, appear to be necessary for the development of specific IgE antibodies. Thus some individuals with elevated IgE levels do not have a clinical allergy, and occasional individuals with normal IgE levels are allergic. There is a strong familial tendency to allergies. From 5 to 15 percent of individuals develop allergy to inhaled agents.

The disease caused by allergen exposure depends mainly on the site of entry. Inhaled allergens cause hay fever or allergic asthma (see Chapter 3.6); foods and food additives cause gastrointestinal allergy; injected materials (insect stings and drugs) and occasionally ingested foods and drugs cause anaphylaxis. The immediate reaction is often followed by a second phase, a recrudescence of symptoms hours later.

Mast cells, however, are triggered not only by IgE-mediated responses to allergens but also by other nonimmunologic stimuli. For example, changes in the osmolarity of their surroundings will initiate mediator release. Thus rapid injection of hypertonic substances such as radiographic contrast media may initiate anaphylaxis. Some people are unable to compensate for the drying effect of inhaling cold air and have rhinitis or asthma that is indistinguishable from an allergic reaction to an allergen. Cold air, which is also very dry air because it supports virtually no water vapor, causes rapid evaporation of water from the mucosal surface, leading to both cooling of the surface and a rise in local osmolarity. The early mediator release in such reactions may also be followed by a late phase.[3]

ANAPHYLAXIS

A systemic reaction occurs in the sensitized or susceptible individual within minutes after introduction of an agent capable of triggering mediator release and is manifested by collapse, profound hypotension, wheezing, and cyanosis. Autopsy may show almost no anatomic alterations but often reveals evidence of bronchoconstriction or edema of the upper airway to the point of closure.[2] Anaphylaxis is particularly likely to occur with injected agents, but its occurrence has been well documented after oral administration of foods and drugs. Anaphylactic sensitization to the venom of bees, yellow jackets, hornets, wasps, and fire ants occurs at times and may cause sudden death after one or more stings. Anaphylaxis not only occurs with serum or drugs given therapeutically but also after injected diagnostic reagents (Table 7.3–1). Intradermal skin testing of atopic individuals with pollen, inhalant, or food extracts carries a definite but small hazard of anaphylaxis. On rare occasions radiographic contrast media, sodium dehydrocholate, and local anesthetics also cause sudden shock and death after their administration. *These agents should never be injected into a patient without equipment for resuscitation, since the allergic reaction can be fatal.* Some anaphylactic reactions, such as those induced by contrast media or local anesthetics, do not appear to require prior sensitization and serve as examples of mediator release triggered by transient changes in osmolarity.

TABLE 7.3–1. AGENTS KNOWN TO CAUSE ANAPHYLAXIS

- Adrenocorticotropic hormone
- Allergenic extracts of pollens, molds, dusts, and foods
- Aminopyrine
- Amphotericin B
- Animal serums
- Chymotrypsin
- Heparin
- Human gamma globulin
- Indanedione derivatives
- Insect stings (bees, yellow jackets, wasps, hornets, and fire ants)
- Insulin
- Liver extract
- Local anesthetics
- Meprobamate
- Mercurial diuretics
- *p*-Aminosalicylic acid
- Penicillins
- Procainamide
- Radiographic contrast media
- Salicylates
- Sodium dehydrocholate
- Streptomycin
- Succinylcholine
- Sulfobromphthalein
- Sulfonamides

Anaphylaxis is best managed by prior detection of the tendency to react and avoidance of the offending agent. The detection of preexisting sensitivity to serums or drugs is difficult, however. Before serum or any drug known as an occasional cause of anaphylaxis is administered to a patient, careful inquiry about previous use and hypersensitivity to the agent should be made. If there is a history of hypersensitivity to a drug, an appropriate substitute should be sought. For animal sera, skin testing with a high dilution of serum is indicated. A wheal and erythema reaction indicates the need for caution in proceeding with antiserum therapy.

Skin testing for drugs, on the other hand, is highly unsatisfactory because *intracutaneous tests and patch tests with drugs are often negative when a patient has recently had a severe reaction to a drug.* In these cases the patient is probably sensitive not to the drug itself but to a protein conjugate or a metabolic product of the drug formed after administration.

In penicillin sensitivity, skin testing with both a "minor determinant mixture" (which contains penicillin) and penicilloyl polylysine will detect most anaphylactically sensitive individuals. A history of prior reaction to penicillin is a poor predictor of future reactions; 75 percent or more of patients with a suggestive history will have negative skin tests and can take penicillin safely.[1]

MANAGEMENT

Anaphylaxis requires emergency treatment to control circulation and respirations. Epinephrine hydrochloride, 0.3 to 0.5 ml of a 1:1000 solution, should be given subcutaneously or intramuscularly at once. If the patient is in shock with severe hypotension, additional epinephrine diluted to 1:100,000 may have to be given intravenously, along with additional fluids to restore circulating volume. The patient's head should be lowered. If there is evidence of airway obstruction, intubation or a tracheostomy is required. Antihistamines and corticosteroids are of no immediate value in treating anaphylaxis but may be required to control manifestations of a late-phase reaction.

When a patient has a prior history of anaphylaxis to a drug or a positive skin test but the drug is mandatory (e.g., penicillin or analogues in bacterial endocarditis or insulin in a diabetic) a desensitization regimen may be used. For penicillin a subcutaneous dose of 1000 U may be followed by a tenfold increase every 15 minutes until a full therapeutic dose is administered. For insulin, about one third the dose that caused previous systemic symptoms can be followed by a 5-U increase each time more insulin is indicated. With penicillin the IgE antibodies are undetectable while the drug is being given, but commonly return after the drug is discontinued. With insulin, developing IgG antibodies usually prevent later problems.

Immunization is the preferred approach for preventing anaphylaxis to insect stings in adults, since sensitivity is usually a straightforward IgE-mediated reaction to venom proteins. Intradermal skin tests with diluted venom from one or more of the Hymenoptera will produce a diagnostic wheal and erythema, and immunization with gradually increasing doses of the appropriate venom weekly will induce IgG antibodies and solid immunity. During seasons of high probability for stings, the patient should carry a kit containing injectable epinephrine until the immunity is established. The immunity must be maintained by booster injections every 8 weeks as long as annual tests indicate that IgE antibodies are still present. Insect-sting sensitivity in children, on the other hand, is often transient, and immunization is not needed unless the most recent anaphylactic reaction was unusually severe.[4]

HAY FEVER

Hay fever is characterized by recurrent, usually seasonal, rhinitis, with watery nasal discharge, sneezing, edema of the nasal mucous membranes, nasal obstruction, conjunctivitis, pharyngeal itching, and cough. These signs and symptoms result from exposure to otherwise innocuous agents.[6] The condition affects from 5 to 10 percent of the population.

INCITING AGENTS

The cause of hay fever in sensitized individuals is the inhalation of pollen from a relatively small number of plants.[5] These plants are widespread and propagate by producing large quantities of light, dry pollen that is easily blown about by the wind. Not all such pollens cause hay fever, however. Some do not contain antigens capable of inciting the disease. Pollens range in size from 10 to 100 mm, the size most suitable for entrapment on the moist surfaces of the turbinates. Pollen allergy characteristically produces nasal symptoms and occasionally causes asthma.

In the temperate zone of North America, there are three principal seasons in which pollen is spread: early spring (trees), early summer (grasses), and early fall (weeds). Ubiquitous outdoor molds, growing on decaying vegetation, also produce airborne spores in the fall. Local exposure to animal danders, housedust mites, insect detritus, and molds may cause symptoms like those of hay fever.

Ragweed is the most common cause of hay fever in the United States and may therefore be used as a general example. Ragweed plants are widespread, springing up as annual weeds wherever the ground is not under cultivation. The plants begin to produce pollen when they mature in August. A single plant can produce 2 billion grains of pollen, and an acre of ragweed has been estimated to produce 16 tons. Pollen is typically shed in the early morning hours. The grains are about 20 mm in diameter and are easily blown about by air currents; they have been found in the atmosphere 400 miles out to sea and at elevations of 14,000 feet. The concentration of pollen ranges up to several thousand grains per cubic meter of air on dry, windy days; on rainy days the air is often washed free of pollen. When the pollen grain is trapped in the nose of a sensitive individual, it releases its contents on the nasal mucosa. Of the proteins contained in the pollen, only a few act as sensitizing antigens. The major one of these, antigen E, has a molecular weight of 37,800 and represents only about 0.5 percent

of the extractable solids of pollen. A second antigen, "K," has a molecular weight of 38,200 and represents about 0.3 percent of the solids. Several smaller antigens are an occasional cause of sensitization.

PATHOGENESIS AND SYMPTOMS

The exposure of a sensitized person to pollen leads to the rapid development of hyperemia and edema of nasal mucosa, accompanied by hypersecretion of mucus, obstruction of the nasal airway, intense itching, and frequent sneezing.[6] The edema is at first unaccompanied by cellular infiltration, but after several hours the tissues become infiltrated with the eosinophils, basophils, and neutrophils of a late-phase reaction. At this point a second round of mediator release and symptoms may occur. Pollen can also be trapped in the eye and causes a reaction similar to that in the nose. *The severity of symptoms is closely related to the quantity of pollen inhaled,* as is shown by careful daily records of hay fever symptoms that correlate closely with pollen concentrations obtained by air sampling.

Secondary Factors
Nonspecific secondary factors may also influence the symptoms of allergies. During prolonged allergic reactions, such as continuous pollen exposure during a "season," the mucosa becomes "primed" for further reactions by the ongoing allergic inflammation, and less pollen is required to induce an intense reaction than when the mucosa had gone unchallenged. Priming is nonspecific; individuals are more sensitive after priming to allergens other than the priming allergen and to irritants such as smoke, chemical, or cooking odors. Atmospheric pollution in cities and days of high relative humidity may exacerbate symptoms. Emotional reactions involving disgust or hostility may increase the severity of symptoms. Exercise or excitement may temporarily lessen the manifestations of allergy followed by a rebound increase in symptoms. The manifestations of ordinary respiratory tract infections may be unusually severe during the hay fever season, although there is little evidence that seasonal allergy predisposes the sensitized individual to develop such infections.

DIAGNOSIS

The diagnosis of hay fever depends on *relating the symptoms to exposure to an inciting agent.*[6] A history of recurrent seasonal coryza and conjunctivitis strongly suggests allergy to pollen or hay fever caused by mold. Textbooks on allergy contain data for many localities on the average season of pollination of plants significant in hay fever. This information is obtained through air samples and the identification of pollens by their specific morphology. In addition, allergy clinics often perform air sampling as a guide to the current local situation. Correlation of such information with the patient's symptoms may provide the clue to the responsible agent. Environmental exposure to dusts, danders, molds, and so on must also be discussed closely with the patient; sometimes air in the home or place of work must be sampled.[1]

Skin Tests
The suspected sensitivity can be confirmed by skin testing with extracts of pollen or other allergens or by direct application of extracts to the membranes of the eye or nose. Very dilute solutions of the allergen must be employed to avoid inducing systemic reactions in allergic persons. A positive response is the rapid development of an allergic inflammation. Allergic individuals often have positive skin tests to a number of potential allergens that are unimportant in producing symptoms; thus *a positive skin test alone is not enough to make a causal diagnosis.* It is essential to correlate symptoms with exposure to allergens. In vitro tests for specific IgE antibodies by sensitive radioimmunoassays such as RAST (radioallergosorbent test) correlate well with skin tests and are useful in

diagnosing patients who have skin diseases that make skin testing impractical.

A thorough search for inciting agents by history and skin testing will fail to reveal a satisfactory allergic cause in many patients with typically allergic symptoms. Sinus radiographs may reveal structural abnormalities that will satisfactorily account for a few problems. But there remains a group of patients in whom the search for external causes of disease is not productive. They usually have nonseasonal perennial symptoms; some develop nasal polyps and have eosinophils in their nasal secretions. Whether these patients have allergic reactions to allergens that are as yet unrecognized, physically induced mediator release, chronic low-grade infections, physiologic disturbances (vasomotor rhinitis), or psychophysiologic reactions to environmental stress is not readily determined. The existence of such patients serves to emphasize that there is nothing specific about the symptoms usually associated with allergic reactions and that the same symptoms may arise from nonallergic causes.

TREATMENT

Avoidance
The first step in managing allergic rhinitis is to avoid the inciting agent. Local contamination with dusts, molds, insects, and so on should be eliminated by appropriate cleanliness or extermination. Many patients choose to go to areas free of pollens to which they are sensitive, either permanently or temporarily during the pollen season. Air conditioners or filters can clean the air in rooms or buildings. When the offending agent cannot be avoided, symptomatic relief can be achieved by a number of measures.

Drugs
Antihistamines taken orally (chlorpheniramine, 4 mg three or four times a day), vasoconstrictors applied locally (0.25 to 0.5 percent penylephrine) or taken systemically, and anticholinergics to dry secretions are all helpful measures.[6] A nonsedating antihistamine (terfenadine, 60 mg) needs to be taken only every 12 hours.

Immunotherapy
The only method of treatment that may alter the patient's basic reactivity is so-called desensitization, or more appropriately called "immunotherapy." Weekly or twice-weekly injections of gradually increasing amounts of extracts of the offending allergen are given before natural exposure is expected. In many cases, the patient's reactivity is sufficiently reduced for exposure to result in less severe symptoms. The application of graded concentrations of specific allergen to mucous membranes after desensitization shows that more allergen is now required for a reaction than before desensitization.

The mechanism by which the alteration is obtained involves several immunologic changes. Circulating antibodies of the IgG class, which can inhibit reactions in sensitized skin or histamine released by sensitized leukocytes, are increased by immunotherapy. Similar IgA and IgG antibodies in secretions are increased. The level of specific IgE antibodies also declines somewhat over several years of repeated injections, presumably because of stimulation of suppressor T cells. Cell sensitivity to histamine release by a specific antigen may be decreased also in patients with the most striking symptomatic response. IgG and IgA antibodies are immunologically specific for the antigen administered; decreases in cell sensitivity are not necessarily specific.

The degree of symptomatic relief is related to the dose of allergen administered, as shown in groups of patients under careful study. Better results are obtained with larger doses. Standardization of pollen extracts to express dosage in a universally applicable unitage, however, has been developed for only a few common allergens. When injections are discontinued, the IgG antibody level declines over several months, and during the next season of exposure the IgE antibody level rises sharply.

Immunotherapy may result in local or systemic allergic reactions, even anaphylaxis, as the dosage is increased. The amount of antigen needed to give adequate results is not predictable in the individual patient, and the dosage must be increased cautiously until a satisfactory result is achieved or until adverse reactions cause the procedure to be abandoned.

REFERENCES

1. Adkinson NF Jr: A guide to skin testing for penicillin allergy. Med Times 104:164, 1976

2. Austen KF: Systemic anaphylaxis in man. JAMA 192:116, 1965
3. Ishizaka K: Regulation of IgE synthesis. Annu Rev Immunol 2:159, 1984
4. Kagey-Sobotka A, Lichtenstein LM: The human immune response to insect stings. In Levine MI, Lockey RF (eds): Monographs in Allergy. Pittsburgh, Dave Lamber Associates, 1986
5. King TP, Norman PS: Antigens that cause atopic disease. In Samter M (ed): Immunological Diseases, 4th ed. Boston, Little, Brown, 1987
6. Norman PS, Lichtenstein LM: Allergic rhinitis. In Samter M (ed): Immunological Diseases, 4th ed. Boston, Little, Brown, 1987
7. Schleimer RP, Fox CC, et al: Role of human basophils and mast cells in the pathogenesis of allergic diseases. J Allergy Clin Immunol 76:369, 1985

Patients with rheumatic disorders seek specialized care for one of three reasons: (1) musculoskeletal pain or dysfunction, (2) a multisystem illness, or (3) the incidental discovery of a seroprotein abnormality.

Most common is the development of arthritis or "rheumatism," both of which rank high on the list of major health problems in terms of the prevalance of temporary, even permanent, disability. Classification is difficult for the spectrum of disorders, ranging from minor trauma to complex systemic illness, that may cause rheumatic symptoms. The "tentative" classification of the American Rheumatism Association[1] based on etiology and pathogenesis emphasizes the paucity of knowledge of disease mechanisms in this area of medicine. A practical and functional classification, although not encyclopedic, is presented in Table 8.1, which also guides the physician in the approach to the patient with rheumatic complaints.

No attempt is made to present clinical descriptions of all the disorders that may give rise to rheumatic symptoms. Initial consideration is given to the special features of history, physical examination, and laboratory data that are important in evaluating the patient with rheumatic manifestations. Subsequent chapters emphasize the diagnostic features and management of the more frequently encountered disorders. Finally, the differential diagnosis of multisystem disease and arthritis is discussed.

REFERENCES

1. McCarthy DJ (ed): Arthritis and Allied Conditions, 10th ed. Philadelphia, Lea & Febiger, 1984

TABLE 8.1. RHEUMATIC DISORDERS

Systemic Process
Systemic Features Dominant
- Systemic lupus erythematosus
- Systemic vasculitis
- Polymyositis
- Systemic sclerosis
- Sjögren syndrome
- Bacterial endocarditis
- Sarcoidosis
- Leukemias

Arthritis Dominant
- Adult rheumatoid arthritis

Arthritis with Extra-articular Lesions
- Ankylosing spondylitis
- Reiter syndrome
- Psoriatic arthritis
- "Colitic" arthropathy
- Gout
- Septic arthritis
- Hypertrophic osteoarthropathy

Arthropathy Alone
- Osteoarthritis
- Pseudogout
- Traumatic arthritis
- Tumors: bone, cartilage, synovium

Nonarticular Rheumatic Disease
- Bursitis, tendinitis
- Fasciitis
- Neuritis
- Nonorganic pain syndrome

CHAPTER 8.1
Evaluation of the Patient

Mary Betty Stevens

The essential and critical first step in evaluating the patient with rheumatic complaints is the comprehensive history and physical examination (Table 8.1–1). *Demographic features* are important (e.g., gouty arthritis in men and rheumatoid arthritis in women, Still disease in the young, and giant cell arteritis in the elderly). The significance of the *family history* in suggesting genetic factors (e.g., ankylosing spondylitis) and the *social history* in documenting exposures (e.g., arthritis of hepatitis) and relevant occupational or emotional trauma cannot be overemphasized.

Rheumatic problems must be localized to specific articular or periarticular structures and their *pattern and progression* precisely defined along with any *systemic features* that may be associated. The character, degree, and basis of disability must be carefully determined, because all too often a patient is "crippled" by a diagnostic label, not the disease process.

In the majority of instances, diagnosis can be made at this clinical level and will be supported by the judicious, selective use of ancillary studies. It should be emphasized that the laboratory data must be interpreted relative to the clinical situation and, with few exceptions (e.g., microcrystals in synovial fluid, organisms in fluids or tissue), the data are not absolutely diagnostic.

MUSCULOSKELETAL FEATURES

Because rheumatic complaints may result from disorders involving joints (arthropathy), periarticular soft tissues (bursitis, tendinitis), or tissue not directly related to joints (myositis, neuritis), the first step is to localize the site of involvement precisely. Pain caused by arthritis (i.e., joint inflammation) is usually confined to the joint or joints involved and is aggravated by joint movement. Symptoms of nonarticular rheumatism, such as tendinitis and bursitis, may mimic arthritic pain but can be distinguished on physical examination. Joint pain may occasionally be referred to other sites (e.g., in hip disease, pain may be primarily in the groin, anterior thigh, or knee); however, moving the involved joint will aggravate the pain and examination will elicit signs referable to the joint itself. Pain unrelated to joint motion or not localized to the joint or periarticular tissues argues against an organic rheumatic condition.

Patients who complain of arthralgia or myalgia unaccompanied by physical signs pose a difficult problem. Sometimes these symptoms are indicative of systemic disease (infectious, neoplastic, connective tissue disease, etc.); however, the most common causes

TABLE 8.1–1. APPROACH TO DIAGNOSIS

Clinical
- Host factors
- Musculoskeletal features
- Pattern of joint involvement
- Systemic manifestations

Laboratory
- Hematology
- Chemistries
- Serologic profile
- Synovial fluid analysis

Special Study
- Radiographs
- Other imaging techniques
- Tissue biopsy

of such rheumatic symptoms are simple fatigue, ill-defined pain syndromes, and psychologic disorders. The last are usually associated with a background of stress and emotional problems and, frequently, personal exposure to rheumatic disease; the persistence of complaints for prolonged periods without physical signs are characteristic of patients with psychologic disorders (sometimes termed "psychogenic rheumatism").

PATTERN OF JOINT INVOLVEMENT

The characterization of arthritis, *historically,* according to *onset* and *duration, intensity* of inflammation, *sites* and *progression* of joint involvement, is most valuable in establishing the diagnosis. A *history of prior episodes* (e.g., gout, Reiter disease) is helpful. A *migratory* pattern of arthritis, in which the arthritis leaves one joint as a new one is affected, is characteristic of acute rheumatic fever in contrast to the *additive* new joint involvement of rheumatoid arthritis. The *distribution* of the arthritis is of major diagnostic import. For example, the large joints are particularly involved in the arthritis of inflammatory bowel disease, whereas in rheumatoid arthritis the small joints are affected in a bilaterally symmetric fashion. Furthermore, processes commonly causing a *monarticular* arthritis (e.g., infection, trauma) differ from those presenting as a *polyarthritis.*

The *examination* of joints should include all the peripheral joints and axial skeleton. Each joint is evaluated for pain on motion, signs of inflammation, structural deformity, and dysfunction. Involvement of the joint itself is certain if there is an effusion or palpable *synovial hypertrophy;* both may be sufficient to produce a compressible distention of the joint capsule. The presence of a thickened synovium is a certain sign of chronic joint inflammation. Apparent joint enlargement may also be due to periarticular soft-tissue swelling or to marginal bony hypertrophy.

The differentiation between *inflammatory* and *noninflammatory* joint disease is key to successful management. In many cases the distinction is obvious on the basis of local signs of redness, heat, and exquisite tenderness, as in acute gout or pyogenic infection. More subtle evidences of inflammation usually accompany such chronic disorders as rheumatoid arthritis, in which an effusion and synovial membrane thickening may continue despite the absence of local heat or marked tenderness. Arthralgia alone and even joint tenderness, which are subjective manifestations, cannot be accepted as criteria of joint disease in the absence of additional signs of acute or chronic inflammation or structural changes.

The determination of *range of motion* should include an estimation of the degree of limitation and whether it is related to pain, soft-tissue swelling, contracture, or malalignment and bony deformity. *Crepitus* on motion usually is indicative of irregularity of the cartilaginous joint surfaces or bony contours. It may also arise from the soft tissues, for example, from an inflamed tendon moving through a thickened, irregular sheath. A greater-than-normal range of motion is important because it may not only suggest disruption of normal supporting structures but also predispose to trauma of joints and especially periarticular soft tissue. Furthermore, hyperextensibility may mask early structural changes that are disease related; this possibility reinforces the need for careful evaluation of involved and uninvolved companion joints.

Nonarticular rheumatic disorders most commonly include those of the periarticular soft tissues, such as tendonitis and bursitis. In these conditions, swelling and tenderness, when they occur, are confined to the affected periarticular structures. Pain can be elicited by direct pressure or by stretching or moving an involved tendon or muscle. Periarticular pain, muscle spasm, or tenderness may result from the unusual stress placed on these structures by altered joint posture and function, as well as from articular inflammation. When examination fails to demonstrate abnormalities of the joints or periarticular tissues, one should look for lesions of the bones or periosteum and for evidence of myopathic, neurogenic, or vascular disorders.

The presence of *structural change* or *deformity* may be helpful in characterizing the nature of the rheumatic processes. *Deformity* and *disability* are more likely to result from arthritis but can occasionally follow nonarticular processes (e.g., the contracted digits of reflex sympathetic dystrophy, swan-neck digital deformities of systemic lupus erythematosus, tendon contractures from disuse). Measurements of the degree of deformity are important in the overall assessment of the patient and in documenting progress. Recording the ranges of active and passive joint motion, noting fixed deformities, and assessing muscle strength are all helpful. Estimations of functional capacity can be made by asking the patient to perform a series of tasks that might be required in daily living, such as walking a measured distance or dressing; if these tasks are standardized and repeated at intervals, progress can be grossly estimated.

Deformity relates to structural alterations, and *disability* is a failure of the patient to function normally. A patient with rheumatic complaints may, therefore, be significantly disabled with or without an inflammatory or degenerative process affecting the articular structures and with little or no relationship to the degree of skeletal deformities. It is of therapeutic import to assess in every patient the deficit between normal function and performance and establish the basis for any disability.

SYSTEMIC MANIFESTATIONS[3,5]

The evaluation of patients with rheumatic complaints should include a survey of all organ systems. Arthralgia may be an early or presenting symptom of a multisystem disease, for example, systemic lupus erythematosus (SLE) or sarcoidosis. Muscle pain and especially weakness dominate the spectrum of polymyositis. A peripheral motor neuropathy frequently accompanies a systemic vasculitis. Furthermore, extra-articular manifestations of the arthritides that have diagnostic significance may be encountered (e.g., the subcutaneous nodules of rheumatoid arthritis, tophaceous deposits of gout, the multisystem manifestations of connective tissue disease) or therapeutic implications (e.g., the iritis in Still disease, the bowel lesion of Crohn disease).

IMAGING TECHNIQUES[7]

In general the changes noted on radiographic examination occur relatively late in the course of inflammatory joint disease; therefore, a normal radiograph by no means argues with the clinical diagnosis of arthritis. Radiographic examinations are of value, especially in patients with chronic joint disease, both in supporting

the clinical diagnosis and in evaluating the pattern and severity of articular changes. Early in the course of inflammatory joint disease, extra-articular radiographs are frequently of more diagnostic value than joint films (e.g., hilar nodes on chest radiograph or characteristic inflammatory changes in the small bowel).

Isotopic bone or joint scans are particularly helpful in patients with articular and periarticular pain but without clinical signs and radiographic abnormalities. Scans can detect occult synovitis and bony lesions (e.g., metastatic sites, ischemic bone necrosis).

HEMATOLOGY: BLOOD CHEMISTRY[2]

Hematologic abnormalities are generally nonspecific but can be critical in the differential diagnosis. For example, leukocytosis and thrombocytosis, features of systemic polyarteritis, argue against uncomplicated systemic lupus erythematosus in which leukopenia and thrombocytopenia are the expected abnormalities. Elevated levels of "acute-phase reactants" (erythrocyte sedimentation rate, C-reactive protein, serum glycoproteins) indicate the existence of an inflammatory condition. Although such elevations are of little differential diagnostic value, repeated determinations may be helpful in following the course of an inflammatory process.

Chemically, serum globulin elevations due to increased gamma globulin usually accompany a chronic inflammatory disorder, and they aid little in diagnosis unless marked in degree or monoclonal. Although hyperuricemia is not an absolute criterion for gout, an elevated serum uric acid is the general rule in acute gouty arthritis but must be interpreted in relation to the clinical setting. Similarly, in patients with muscle pain or weakness, serum elevations of enzymes localized in muscle may support the diagnosis of a polymyositis over an arteritis or neurogenic myopathy.

SEROLOGIC PROFILE[2,6]

The clinical specificities of circulating autoantibodies (Table 8.1–2) are not absolute; except for anti-Sm in systemic lupus, none is diagnostic of the disorder with which it is primarily associated. In addition to supporting the respective clinical diagnosis, however, some autoantibodies relate to clinical problems (e.g., Coombs and hemolysis, anti-ds DNA and nephritis), others mark risk factors in the underlying disease (e.g., anti-IgG and erosions in rheumatoid arthritis, anticoagulant and intravascular thrombosis or fetal loss in pregnancy), and still others identify disease variants of prognostic implications (e.g., antihistones and drug-induced lupus, anti-Ro(SSA) and subacute cutaneous lupus).

In addition to these markers of autoreactivity, the presence of specific antibodies (e.g., antistreptolysin O, antiviral) may confirm host response to infection.

SYNOVIAL FLUID ANALYSIS[9]

Synovial fluid should be analyzed whenever there is an accessible effusion. The hazards of aspiration are negligible, and the information gained may prove invaluable. In some instances, as in gout and infection, a diagnosis can be made from a few drops of fluid by the identification of crystals or organisms.

Synovial fluid analysis is particularly helpful in distinguishing the inflammatory from the noninflammatory causes of effusion (Table 8.1–3). Immediate indication of inflammation is obtained if the fluid is grossly turbid or purulent. Similarly, a bloody effusion suggests trauma, a bleeding disorder, or pigmented villonodular synovitis. Normally, synovial fluid is very viscid, but the *viscosity* is

TABLE 8.1–2. AUTOANTIBODIES

Antigen Specificity	Clinical Associations	
	Primary	*Miscellaneous*
IgG	RA	SBE, SLE, Sj, aging ($\geq$ 70 yr)
ANA (screen)	SLE	RA, CTD, discoid lupus, drug-induced lupus, miscellaneous inflammatory disorders
LE cell	SLE	RA, CTD, discoid lupus, drug-induced lupus, chronic hepatitis
ds-DNA	SLE	Lupus nephritis, rarely RA, CTD
Sm	SLE	SLE-specific
nRNP	SS	SLE, Sj
Histones	Drug-induced lupus	SLE
Ro(SSA)/La(SSB)	Sj	Subacute cutaneous lupus, SLE, vasculitis
Jo-1	PM	Pulmonary fibrosis in PM
BFP-STS, cardiolipin, anticoagulant	SLE	Interrelated. Risk markers for ___sis (rarely hem___ rhage) and pregnancy complications
RBC (Coombs), WBC platelet	SLE	Antibodies more frequent than ↓RBC, ↓WBC, ↓platelet

RA = rheumatoid arthritis; SLE = systemic lupus erythematosus; CTD = connective tissue diseases; Sj = Sjögren syndrome; SS = systemic sclerosis; ANA = antinuclear antibodies; PM = polymyositis.

reduced in many types of effusion, especially in severe inflammatory processes. Similarly, the firm *mucin clot* formed by normal and noninflammatory synovial fluid exposed to dilute acetic acid is, in contrast, friable or does not form at all when inflammation has depolymerized the protein-bound hyaluronate complexes.

The *white cell count* in synovial fluid is done as a blood white cell count, except that the usual diluents, which contain weak acids, may cause a mucin clot, trapping the cells and invalidating the count. Normal saline should therefore be used as a diluent. A small amount of methylene blue or another nuclear stain can be added if desired. The white cell count usually reflects the degree of inflammation, being under 2000 cells/μl in most noninflammatory effusions.

Synovial fluid analysis should also include the microscopic examination of a fresh smear for crystals or phagocytic inclusions, a bacterial smear and culture, and determination of glucose, protein, and complement content. Further discussion of the diagnostic significance of these procedures is contained in subsequent chapters.

SYNOVIAL BIOPSY[4,5,9]

Synovium, as a serous membrane, reacts in a limited way to insult. Most inflammatory disorders produce a nonspecific inflammatory response; however, a synovial biopsy can be diagnostic when granulomata, microcrystalline deposits, or neoplastic cells are present. Furthermore, the culture of synovial tissue may prove helpful even when synovial fluid is sterile.

TABLE 8.1–3. SYNOVIAL FLUID FINDINGS

Examination	Noninflammatory Effusions	Inflammatory Effusions	Diagnostic Features
Gross appearance	Clear yellow and viscid	Turbid with reduced viscosity	Grossly bloody effusions suggest trauma, bleeding disorders, pigmented villonodular synovitis, and, when fat droplets are present, a fracture communicating with the joint
White cell count (WBC)	<2000 cells/μl	>2000 cells/μl	>50,000 cells strongly suggests infection[a]
Glucose	Approximates blood glucose	May be reduced	Very low glucose strongly suggests infection[b]
Protein	2–3.5 g/dl	>3 g/dl	
Complement	Normal	Normal or high	Reduced in rheumatoid arthritis, especially relative to protein concentration
Microscopic crystals	None present except rarely cholesterol	Intracellular crystals in acute attacks	Urate crystals in gout; calcium pyrophosphate crystals in pseudogout
Cells	Predominantly mononuclear	Usually polymorphonuclear Phagocytic inclusions may be seen	Many phagocytic inclusions suggest rheumatoid arthritis (RA cells) Phagocytosis of leukocytes by macrophages in Reiter syndrome
Organisms	None	May be found in infection, intracellular or extracellular	Infection
Culture	Sterile	Sterile except in infection	Microorganism isolated

[a]But can occur in rheumatoid arthritis, Reiter syndrome, and microcrystalline arthritis.
[b]...found in 10% of rheumatoid effusions.

REFERENCES

1. Clinics in Rheumatic Disease, vols 1–12. Philadelphia, WB Saunders, 1975–1986
2. Cohen AS (ed): Laboratory Diagnostic Procedures in the Rheumatic Diseases. Boston, Little, Brown, 1967
3. Katz WA (ed): Rheumatic Diseases: Diagnosis and Management. Philadelphia, JB Lippincott, 1977
4. Kelley WN, Harris ED, et al (eds): Textbook of Rheumatology, 2d ed. Philadelphia, WB Saunders, 1985
5. McCarty DJ (ed): Arthritis and Allied Conditions, 10th ed. Philadelphia, Lea & Febiger, 1984
6. Parker CW (ed): Clinical Immunology. Philadelphia, WB Saunders, 1980
7. Resnick D, Niwayama G (eds): Diagnosis of Bone and Joint Disorders. Philadelphia, WB Saunders, 1981
8. Sheon RP, Moskowitz TW, Goldberg VM: Soft Tissue Rheumatic Pain: Recognition, Management, Prevention. Philadelphia, Lea & Febiger, 1982
9. Sokoloff L (ed): The Joints and Synovial Fluid. New York, Academic Press, 1978

CHAPTER 8.2
Systemic Lupus Erythematosus

Mary Betty Stevens

Systemic lupus erythematosus (SLE) is an immunologic disorder characterized clinically by inflammatory lesions in multiple organ systems and serologically by circulating autoantibodies and immune complexes. The clinical pattern and serologic profile vary greatly at onset and throughout the course of the disease; a reasonable question is whether SLE is truly a single disorder or a cluster of related syndromes varying in etiology or pathogenesis, or both.

Predisposing factors to SLE have been supported by clinical and experimental studies. *Genetically*,[2,10] the familial aggregation of SLE, the concordance of SLE in monozygotic twins, and the disease association with HLA-DR antigens (DR2 and/or DR3) are established. *Hormonal* factors have long been suggested by the dominance of women in all unselected series (approximately 8:1), with an increasing proportion of men in late-onset SLE in the older age group. Furthermore, in the experimental murine model of SLE (i.e., the NZB/W F1 hybrid mouse), maleness is associated with milder disease, slower in progression, and later in onset. Finally, the drug-induced subset of lupus and the photoactivation of cutaneous lesions suggest importance of *environmental* factors in some patients.

SLE can no longer be considered rare, especially in women. Blacks are affected more often than whites, but their reported increased severity of SLE has not yet been thoroughly analyzed in socioeconomic terms relative to medical care. Symptoms commonly begin between the ages of 15 and 40 years but can be noted at any age; neonatal lupus and the late-onset SLE in the elderly are unique subsets with expressions differing from those of typical adult SLE.

CLINICAL MANIFESTATIONS[4,8,12]

The type and severity of the initial manifestations of SLE vary greatly. Occasionally, patients present with a fulminant, febrile illness and functional deficit of many organ systems. There are also

those individuals without clinical symptoms who are detected through abnormal laboratory tests (e.g., biologic false-positive serologic test for syphilis). Most commonly, patients present with constitutional symptoms such as fever and malaise, as well as evidence of the involvement of several organ systems, especially the skin, joints, and serous membranes (Table 8.2–1).

The precise onset of SLE may be difficult to date. Frequently, over a period of months or years, a series of seemingly isolated illnesses may evolve into a pattern characteristic of SLE.

SYSTEMIC MANIFESTATIONS

Fever occurs in about 85 percent of patients durng periods of disease activity. Shaking chills are noted rarely and most often relate to a complicating infection or to antipyretic therapy. Malaise, easy fatigability, anorexia, and weight loss are also commonly encountered.

SKIN AND MUCOUS MEMBRANES[4,14]

A wide variety of skin and mucous membrane lesions have been noted in more than 75 percent of patients. The most characteristic dermal abnormality is butterfly erythema, which is distributed over the bridge of the nose and malar eminences in 40 percent of cases. Similar lesions, which at times become scaly and pruritic, may occur over the neck, upper chest, and extremities. Evanescent erythematous nodules on the digital pads and small, punctate, ulcerative lesions on the fingers and palms reflect an underlying vasculitis. Linear erythema along the margin of the eyelids is characteristic but infrequent. Ulcerative lesions may also be seen in the mucous membranes.

Many lesions occur that are less specifically related to SLE. Dermal atrophy, ulceration, and gangrene secondary to vascular insufficiency may develop in the setting of Raynaud phenomenon or arteritis. The occasional episodes of urticaria and angioneurotic edema are reminiscent of histamine-mediated responses. A third group of mucocutaneous lesions (purpura, petechiae, ecchymoses) reflects either an underlying hemorrhagic tendency or vasculitis.

The erythematous, scaling, disc-like plaques characteristic of discoid lupus erythematosus may occur in SLE. Involvement of the face and scalp is seen most often, with occasional extension to the trunk and extremities. Healing eventually occurs and results in atrophic, depigmented areas of skin. These discoid lesions may precede other systemic manifestations of SLE by months or years.

Photosensitive eruptions are noted in more than one third of cases. Frontal alopecia is frequent, especially in young women.

TABLE 8.2–1. INITIAL MANIFESTATIONS OF SLE (140 PATIENTS)

	Number of Patients
Arthritis or arthralgias	74
Skin rash	37
Fever	25
Pleurisy and/or pericarditis	16
Weight loss	9
Alopecia	6
Neuropsychiatric episode	5
Nephritis, thrombocytopenia, and BFP	3
Raynaud syndrome and anemia	2
Lymphadenopathy	1

Data from Johns Hopkins Rheumatic Disease Unit.

MUSCULOSKELETAL MANIFESTATIONS

Polyarthropathy is among the most commonly encountered manifestations of SLE, being present in 90 percent of individuals at some time during the course of their illnesses. Frequently, polyarthralgia is the dominant problem in the absence of objective joint abnormalities. Articular involvement is apparent as a presenting feature in three fourths of the cases.

An evanescent symmetric polyarthritis is observed most often. Any peripheral joint may be involved, especially interphalangeal and metacarpophalangeal. Mild deformities may develop in the digits, but the occurrence of contractures, ankylosis, and joint erosions on radiographs is unusual. As in rheumatoid arthritis, synovial (Baker) cysts can occur in the popliteal space and, with dissection or rupture, mimic thrombophlebitis.

Tenosynovitis occurs at times. A diffuse myopathy, especially one involving the pelvic and shoulder girdle musculature, is infrequent. Serum levels of muscle cell enzymes are elevated in those with myositis in contrast to patients with steroid-related myopathy or disuse wasting.

Ischemic bone necrosis of the femoral heads[21] is a common complication of SLE, especially in patients receiving corticosteroid therapy. Necrosis of humeral heads, knees, and carpal bones occurs less often.

OCULAR MANIFESTATIONS

The most characteristic ocular lesions are the cytoid bodies, which are found in 10 to 20 percent of patients. These small, oval, whitish opacities, occurring in the central portion of the fundus adjacent to blood vessels, represent foci of ischemic degeneration of the nerve-fiber layer of the retina. They may be difficult to distinguish from the lesions associated with diabetes mellitus, hypertension, bacteremia, and macroglobulinemia. Nonspecific conjunctivitis, retinal hemorrhages and exudates, and severe ocular lesions (e.g., retinitis, optic neuritis) leading to visual loss may also be encountered.

PLEUROPULMONARY MANIFESTATIONS[5,13]

Episodes of pleuritic pain are common and may occur without other detectable evidence of pleuritis or in association with a pleural rub or effusion.

An atelectasizing pneumonitis is a frequent pulmonary abnormality, especially in the older patient with late-onset SLE. Commonly, the development of pleural reaction and plate-like atelectasis at the lung bases are observed on serial chest films, unaccompanied by clinical findings. Widespread pulmonary lesions have been shown to impair alveolar-capillary diffusion, and marked respiratory insufficiency or the adult respiratory distress syndrome (ARDS) rarely develops. Recurrent pulmonary hemorrhage, also infrequent, is a poor prognostic sign.

CARDIOVASCULAR MANIFESTATIONS[12]

Cardiac lesions are observed in 50 percent of patients. Pericarditis is encountered most commonly. Although frequently sufficient to cause enlargement of the cardiac silhouette (on radiograph), pericardial effusions of large volume and tamponade are rare. Myocarditis, the most serious cardiac lesion, occurs in less than 10 percent of patients but is especially found in those with skeletal muscle inflammation.

Endocarditis is often present on pathologic examination. The characteristic vegetations (Libman-Sacks) are usually found under the mitral valve leaflets. Mitral stenosis has been observed as a consequence of lupus valvulitis; however, functional deficits ascribable to Libman-Sacks endocarditis are infrequent.

Hypertension in individuals with SLE usually relates to other renal involvement, steroid therapy, or both.

GASTROINTESTINAL MANIFESTATIONS[20]

Nearly 40 percent of patients with SLE complain of abdominal pain, which results from serositis or vasculitis. An acute abdominal condition, often difficult to interpret in the steroid-treated patient, may develop secondary to the disease (e.g., bowel perforation pancreatitis, peptic ulcer), its therapy, or an intercurrent process.

Dysphagia is an occasional symptom. Radiographic studies may reveal esophageal aperistalsis similar to that seen in systemic sclerosis. Similarly, segmental dilation may be noted in one or more regions of the small bowel.

Hepatomegaly is present in about one third of SLE cases. There is no distinctive hepatic functional abnormality or biopsy pattern characteristic of SLE. Severe functional impairment is rare.

RETICULOENDOTHELIAL MANIFESTATIONS

Palpable splenomegaly, observed in 15 to 20 percent of patients, is less common than local or generalized lymphadenopathy, which is especially prominent in children and young adults. Occasionally these abnormalities are sufficiently impressive to suggest lymphoma, but lymph node biopsy usually reveals a reticular hyperplasia.

NEUROLOGIC MANIFESTATIONS[6,11]

Mental or neurologic dysfunction is seen in 35 to 40 percent of patients with SLE. This usually relates to the central nervous system (CNS) rather than to peripheral nerves. Neuropsychiatric illness commonly occurs early in the course of SLE, especially within the first 2 years of illness.

A wide variety of behavioral disturbances, ranging from mild anxiety and minor memory defects to major psychoses, have been observed. Frequently, neuropsychiatric episodes of illness are not associated with cerebrospinal fluid abnormalities; however, evidence of disease activity in other organ systems is usually present.

Focal vascular lesions may result in seizures or frequently in multifocal neurologic deficits, and an "aseptic meningitis" may be seen in a small proportion of patients.

LUPUS NEPHRITIS[1,3,7,19]

Renal disease is present in most patients with SLE. Since progression to renal insufficiency and fatal outcome may occur, determining the presence or absence of renal involvement and its severity is important in prognosis and therapy.

Lupus nephritis commonly develops early in the course of SLE and infrequently after 2 or more years of disease activity. Rarely is nephritis the sole manifestation of the disease. Proteinuria and abnormalities of urinary sediment including hematuria, cylinduria, and pyuria are commonly found but may be minimal or transient early in the course of disease. At times, patients present with the nephrotic syndrome, but features of an acute glomerulonephritis are more common. In general, active nephropathy may be correlated with disease activity in other organ systems. In some cases the renal disease is not progressive and remains mild throughout the illness. Hypertension often develops in patients with advanced renal disease.

Percutaneous renal biopsy is valuable in assessing the renal status of the patient with SLE with respect to activity and severity of the nephritis. In some cases, renal biopsy may reveal involvement in patients with minimal or no abnormalities of their urinary sediments. In general, patients who have focal glomerulonephritis on biopsy have little functional impairment and a good prognosis.

More severe disease is typically associated with diffuse proliferative or membranoproliferative glomerulonephritis.

LABORATORY MANIFESTATIONS[12]

HEMATOLOGIC MANIFESTATIONS

A moderate normochromic anemia may be found in 80 percent of cases. A more severe anemia develops in relation to progressive renal insufficiency or superimposed infection. At times, an overt hemolytic anemia may develop; however, a positive Coombs test may be seen in individuals without evidence of shortened red cell survival. The red cell agglutinins usually are of the warm type and lack specificity for known blood group antigens.

A moderate leukopenia (2500 to 4000 WBC/μl) is seen in 50 percent of patients at some point in the course of their disease and is often associated with lymphopenia. A significant leukocytosis, rare in uncomplicated or untreated SLE, usually represents a response to corticosteroids or intercurrent infection.

Thrombocytopenia occurs in 30 percent of individuals with SLE but only occasionally produces a hemorrhagic diathesis. Thrombocytopenic purpura, however, can be the dominant disease manifestation. Circulating anticoagulants (antibodies to clotting factors) are more frequently associated with intravascular thrombosis, arterial and venous, than with bleeding.

The erythrocyte sedimentation rate and other acute-phase reactants are elevated in patients with active SLE and may remain slightly elevated during periods of apparent clinical remission.

IMMUNOLOGIC MANIFESTATIONS

Immunoglobulin abnormalities, many of which are relatively nonspecific, are present in most patients with SLE. Serum globulin concentrations in excess of 4.0 g/dl are seen in over 50 percent of cases. On electrophoresis, broad-based (polyclonal) gamma globulin elevations may be seen that contrast with the narrow peaks of the monoclonal dysproteinemias. Cryoproteins are sometimes present, especially in patients with active nephritis.

One of the hallmarks of SLE is serologic autoreactivity (see Table 8.1–2). The autoantibodies directed against red cells (Coombs test) may result in a hemolytic anemia, and autoantibodies that react with clotting factors (circulating anticoagulants) may cause intravascular clotting or a hemorrhagic diathesis. DNA or anti-DNA (native or double-stranded) immune complexes are responsible, in part, for induction of the glomerular lesions. Other immune complex systems have not been implicated in specific tissue injury, although patients with antibody to ribonucleoprotein (nRNP) have significantly more frequent sicca features and myositis. Anti-Ro(SSA), a predominantly cytoplasmic reactant, occurs in more than 25 percent of patients and also associates with the sicca complex in large part.

Most patients with SLE develop positive LE cell tests during their illness, but if they do not, the diagnosis is not excluded. The serum factor responsible for LE cell formation is an antibody capable of reacting with deoxyribonucleoprotein.

Several antinuclear and anticytoplasmic antibodies, generally neither species- nor organ-specific, have been identified in patients with SLE. Probably the most widely used method for detecting antinuclear factors employs immunofluorescence. The interpretation of antinuclear-antibody (ANA) titers varies according to the methodology and reagents used. The immunofluorescent assay for ANA detects multiple autoantibodies (including the LE cell factor) to nuclear constituents. In relation to the diagnosis of SLE, the test is more sensitive and therefore less specific than the LE cell phenomenon. Nearly all patients with active SLE are ANA positive. Because titers may vary according to the intensity of disease activity, serial ANA determinations may be of value in managing some patients.

TABLE 8.2–2. BIOPSY FINDINGS IN SYSTEMIC LUPUS ERYTHEMATOSUS

Skin
- Edema of the cutis, dilation of capillaries, liquefaction and degeneration of the basal layer, perivascular and subepidermal accumulation of cellular infiltrates with predominantly round cells
- Hyperkeratosis without parakeratosis
- Positive direct immunofluorescence for IgG immunoglobulin at dermal-epidermal junction (also in 60 percent of cases at uninvolved sites)
- Subcutaneous nodules histologically identical to the "rheumatoid" nodule

Lymph Node
- Reticulum and lymphoid cell hyperplasia
- Occasionally necrobiosis with cell degeneration, pyknosis, and formation of hematoxylin bodies

Muscle
- Nonspecific focal degeneration and perivascular round cell infiltration; histology indistinguishable from polymyositis may be found

Kidney
- Focal membranous, proliferative, and/or necrotizing glomerulonephritis
- Karyorrhexis and fibrinoid change often present with active disease
- Hematoxylin bodies rare, but diagnostic when present
- Diffuse membranous thickening with focal exaggeration (wire-loop lesions) is a fairly characteristic but late finding
- Positive direct immunofluorescence for IgG immunoglobulin in renal glomeruli and β1C globulin in nodular deposits beneath basement membrane. Complexes containing DNA can be eluted from the glomeruli

A persistent biologic false-positive (BFP) serologic test for syphilis may precede overt manifestations of SLE by months or years. Such reactions with cardiolipin antigen occur in individuals without histories of syphilitic infection. The chronic BFP and anticardiolipin antibody occurs in close association with circulating anticoagulants and thus can be related to intravascular events.

Serum complement is reduced in about three fourths of patients with active SLE. The observed reduction in complement levels may be correlated with the activity of the illness, especially in individuals with nephritis. Serum complement usually varies inversely with ANA titers. Because many disorders that simulate SLE, such as rheumatic fever, polyarteritis, and various infections, are usually characterized by a normal or elevated serum complement level, a low serum complement would favor the diagnosis of SLE. Reduced serum complement, however, may also be encountered in patients with serum sickness, acute glomerulonephritis, the nephrotic syndrome and, occasionally, other disorders. When hypocomplementemia is associated with ANA, especially in high titers, at least 85 percent of patients will have SLE.

Rheumatoid factors are present in almost 50 percent of patients at some time during the course of their disease. Unlike patients with rheumatoid arthritis, in SLE they are intermittently present and usually in low titer.

BIOPSY

Many of the tissue abnormalities encountered in biopsy specimens are relatively nonspecific (Table 8.2–2). Most characteristic of SLE are hematoxylin bodies (swollen cell nuclei devoid of cytoplasm and coated with globulin), but these are rarely found.

DIAGNOSIS[18]

The diagnosis of SLE is not a problem when the patient presents with several of the characteristic clinical and laboratory manifestations of a multisystem disorder. A febrile, young woman with a butterfly rash, arthritis, pleuritis, mild anemia, positive LE cell test, high ANA titer, and hypocomplementemia would be diagnosed promptly. Frequently, however, the course of the disease is chronic and evolves episodically over many years. In such cases, the relationship between seemingly isolated episodes of illness may not be appreciated. One must, therefore, interpret a patient's present complaint (e.g., arthritis) in the light of the past history. A prior attack of pleurisy or a skin eruption following sun exposure should give added meaning to the current complaint of arthritis.

Occasionally, the involvement of one organ system overshadows other features of SLE for prolonged periods. Because other clinical and laboratory features of the disorder may develop insidiously, they should be looked for repeatedly. Thus, idiopathic nephrosis, glomerulonephritis, hemolytic anemia, purpura, pleurisy, or pericarditis may eventually be recognized as components of a multisystem disorder.

There are no absolute criteria for the diagnosis of SLE, although revised criteria for its classification have been proposed recently by the American Rheumatism Association. Generally, definitive diagnosis rests on a combination of characteristic clinical and immunologic features, especially the LE cell and ANA tests. Although the presence of LE cells and ANA titers do not themselves establish the diagnosis, the absence of these immunologic abnormalities in symptomatic individuals casts some doubt on the presence of SLE. An ANA-negative patient with SLE with prominent photosensitive dermatitis in which renal and neuropsychiatric involvement is infrequent has recently been recognized, however; and in those patients with subacute cutaneous lupus (SCLE), anti-Ro(SSA) is present in the majority.

It is important to be aware of the various diseases that may produce symptoms similar to SLE, especially if specific therapy would alter their outcome (e.g., tuberculosis, subacute bacterial endocarditis, lymphoma). Furthermore, several manifestations of SLE overlap with those of the other collagen diseases, from which they should be distinguished (see Chapter 8.8).

COURSE AND PROGNOSIS[7,12]

In most instances the course of SLE is characterized by periods of remission and exacerbation, with the course protracted over many years, and the 10–year survival now approximates 90 percent. Rarely, the illness is fulminant, resulting in death in a few weeks.

Commonly, the various manifestations of SLE become evident sequentially over a period of years. Most recurrent episodes of disease activity are spontaneous, although in some instances intercurrent infection, drug administration, and severe emotional stress have been cited as precipitating factors. Remissions may occur spontaneously or in response to corticosteroid therapy and may last for months or even years.

There are no satisfactory data to describe the natural history of SLE. Recent survival rates at 5 (97 percent) and 10 (90 percent) years after diagnosis provide a basis for genuine optimism. Death results from renal failure, CNS involvement, acute abdominal catastrophes, or intercurrent infection. Severe disturbances, such as thrombocytopenia with bleeding, hemolytic anemia, fulminant arteritis, and lupus crises, are potentially fatal but frequently respond well to therapy.

Progressive nephritis with renal failure may continue despite satisfactory control of other disease manifestations. Individuals whose disease remains confined to the skin, joints, or serous surfaces or in whom immunologic abnormalities are present without vital organ involvement have good prognoses.

The effect of pregnancy on the course of SLE is variable and may be associated with exacerbations or remissions of the disease. Maternal ANAs and other antibodies have been shown to enter the fetal circulation, and SLE can affect the fetus (neonatal SLE), producing heart block and skin lesions when the mother is anti-

Ro(SSA) positive. Furthermore, fetal loss and placental vascular abnormalities have been associated with a maternal circulating anticoagulant and anticardiolipin antibody.

MANAGEMENT[15]

The therapeutic management of patients with SLE depends on the nature and severity of their disease manifestations. In addition to treatment designed to suppress inflammation and relieve symptoms, careful attention must be directed toward the general care of each patient. Furthermore, failure to recognize and deal with the personal needs of patients and their families can nullify an otherwise sound therapeutic program.

INTERCURRENT ILLNESS

It is important to remember that findings that develop during the course of SLE may be caused by intercurrent disorders. For example, infections caused by pyogenic bacteria, mycobacteria, or fungi may produce symptoms and signs that could be confused with those of SLE. Therefore, the pathogenesis of each new disease manifestation should be evaluated promptly in order to provide a firm basis for therapy.

PRECIPITATING EVENTS

At times, exacerbations of SLE seem to follow infections, drug administration, severe emotional turmoil, or surgical procedures. Similarly, exposure to the sun may result in worsening of dermal lesions. Such apparent precipitating events may be identified through the initial history or continued observation of each patient. It follows that sensible avoidance of these factors is in order. In general, nonessential surgical procedures and drug administration should be guarded against; however, care should be taken not to cripple patients with ritualistic prohibitions.

GENERAL THERAPY

Multiple therapeutic problems arise during the course of SLE, depending on the organ system involved and the related physiologic consequences. For example, lupus nephritis may result in progressive renal failure and hypertension. Furthermore, congestive heart failure may develop in this setting. Each of these abnormalities should receive the same basic supportive treatment accorded similar physiologic deficits due to other causes.

SUPPRESSIVE THERAPY

There is no known curative therapy for SLE. Nor is there evidence that suppressing minor manifestations of SLE early in its course will prevent the emergence of more serious multisystem involvement. Therefore, decisions concerning suppressive therapy are based on the nature and intensity of the disease manifestations. When needed, the safest antiinflammatory agents are employed in doses sufficient to allay clinical evidence of the disorder.

Thus, an asymptomatic individual with serum autoantibodies but without other abnormality requires no drug therapy. A patient with recurrent dermal lesions, myalgia, and arthralgia will benefit from salicylates or other nonsteroidal antiinflammatory drugs (NSAIDs) and antimalarials as well as from local therapy to the skin lesions. Patients with nephritis, myositis, or involvement of the myocardium or CNS usually require corticosteroids in high doses.

Salicylates and the NSAIDs

Salicylates are helpful in controlling musculoskeletal pain and should be prescribed so that adequate blood levels are maintained. In patients with polyarthritis the response is occasionally dramatic and may resemble that seen in rheumatic fever. Frequently, however, the response to salicylates is incomplete, and other agents are required. The choice of one NSAID over another can only be determined after specific drug trial and assessment of efficacy and tolerance.

Adrenal Corticosteroids

Corticosteroids are the most effective agents for suppressing inflammation. Steroids are reserved for those situations that will not yield to simpler measures. The prime indications for steroid therapy in SLE are active involvement of the kidneys, skeletal muscle and myocardium, central nervous system, hemolytic anemia, thrombocytopenia and in those with intravascular clotting, a complicated pregnancy associated with the lupus anticoagulant, and anticardiolipin antibody. At times, corticosteroids are needed to control progressive skin lesions, fever, and the other constitutional features of the illness.

The dosage level, schedule, and even route of administration of corticosteroids vary with the pattern and intensity of SLE activity. For individuals with minor manifestations, 20 mg of prednisone (or equivalent) in a single morning dose may be sufficient. Those with major organ involvement usually require therapy with 50 mg or more, occasionally 100 to 150 mg daily, initially. In the rare lupus crisis, an initial intravenous "pulse" of 1 g of methylprednisolone may be life-saving.

After successful suppression of disease activity for a few weeks, the dose of prednisone can be tapered slowly to levels of 20 to 30 mg daily. Below this level, reductions at a rate of 5 mg or less per month may be necessary to avoid exacerbation of the disease. In some instances, the drug can be withdrawn entirely. More often, prolonged maintenance at low-dose levels is required to prevent recurrence of symptoms.

Development of a Cushing habitus is common in patients treated with large doses of corticosteroids but can be controlled in large part with dietary restriction of calories. If renal function permits, a high-protein diet may be given to compensate partially for the protein-wasting effect of steroids. Diabetes occasionally occurs and may be modified by diet therapy and the use of oral hypoglycemic agents or insulin as needed. Fluid retention, rarely a problem when compounds producing little mineralocorticoid effect are used, can be managed by salt restriction or the use of diuretic agents. Hypertension usually requires control with antihypertensive drugs.

Peptic ulceration occurs and may cause significant bleeding or perforation. It should be remembered that corticosteroids may mask the clinical findings that usually result from a perforated ulcer.

Myopathy due to steroid administration is encountered infrequently. Fluorinated derivatives of prednisone are of special concern in this regard. The girdle musculature usually is affected most severely. Return of strength follows reduction of steroid dosage, coupled with a well-designed exercise program.

Posterior subcapsular cataracts are a late complication of steroid therapy encountered chiefly in individuals who have taken 15 mg or more of prednisone daily (or equivalent amounts of other congeners) for 2 years or more. Aseptic bone necrosis, especially in the heads of the femurs and humeri, is the most common cause of monarticular pain in treated SLE (25 percent). It should be remembered that pain may be present weeks, even months, before bone lesions are evident on radiographs.

Antimalarials

Hydroxychloroquine (Plaquenil) may control the discoid and other skin lesions as well as the rheumatic manifestations of SLE after several weeks of treatment. The drug is generally ineffective, however, in individuals with visceral involvement.

Gastrointestinal intolerance and dermatitis may occur in patients receiving an antimalarial. It should not be given to pregnant women because fetal abnormalities may result. Rarely, individuals who have taken hydroxychloroquine for several months, especially

those receiving more than 200 mg daily, may develop (pigmentary) retinal degeneration resulting in serious visual impairment. Deposits of the drug may also occur in the cornea.

Cytotoxic Agents

Azathioprine, cyclophosphamide, 6-mercaptopurine, and chlorambucil have been shown to suppress the manifestations of SLE. At present, there is insufficient evidence to compare long-term effectiveness and toxicity of these agents with corticosteroids. Generally, an immunosuppressive agent is added when corticosteroids fail to control the inflammatory process in major organ systems (i.e., kidney, CNS). Currently, any of these agents should be reserved for patients who are refractory to corticosteroids or who cannot tolerate the dosage level required.

SLE SUBSETS

Several syndromes sharing clinical or immunoreactive features with SLE should be differentiated from "typical" SLE. Drug-induced lupus and two cutaneous subsets—discoid lupus (DLE) and subacute cutaneous lupus (SCLE)—are especially important in view of differences in prognosis and required therapy. Infrequent are the SLE-like syndromes emerging in those at the extremes of age—neonatal lupus and late-onset SLE in the elderly.

Although ANA positivity can support the diagnosis of SLE, it is not diagnostic, and ANA negativity does not rule out SLE. Lupoid sclerosis, which is defined by ANA positivity coupled with clinical features of multiple sclerosis, is a rare and uncertain variant of SLE. Additional LE cell and ANA-positive disorders (e.g., other connective tissue diseases, rheumatoid arthritis, chronic active hepatitis) are readily recognized clinically.

DRUG-INDUCED SLE[9]

Adverse reactions to foreign protein and drugs of the serum-sickness type may closely mimic SLE clinically but seldom if ever are associated with ANA positivity. In contrast, there is a broad spectrum of chemically unrelated agents capable of activating SLE or unmasking a lupus diathesis or inducing a SLE-like syndrome de novo (Table 8.2–3). Prompt recognition of drug-associated lupus syndromes is the key to therapy because withdrawal of the agent usually causes the illness to subside and the serologic abnormalities to disappear.

The likelihood of a genetic predisposition to drug-induced lu-

TABLE 8.2–3. DRUG-INDUCED LUPUS: MAJOR AGENTS

Specific Generic Drug (Trade Name)	Risk
Hydralazine	+++
Procainamide	+++
D-penicillamine	+++
Isoniazid	++
Phenytoin (Dilantin)	++
Mephenytoin (Mesantoin)	++
Trimethadione	++
Ethosuximide	++
Propylthiouracil	+
Chlorpromazine and other phenothiazines	+
Methyldopa (Aldomet)	(+)
Quinidine	(+)

+++ = high; ++ = moderate; + = low; (+) = ANA-inducer, lupus uncertain.

pus is suggested by both the association with the slow-acetylator phenotype and, unlike SLE, by the enrichment of the HLA-DR4 alloantigen. The population is older than in idiopathic SLE and with less female dominance. The disease expression, similar to late-onset SLE, may thus be as host-modulated as drug-determined. Nonetheless the emergence of drug-induced lupus varies from one drug to another with respect to the required dose and duration of therapy. For example, high dosage and prolonged administration of hydralazine are the rule, whereas much smaller doses and briefer periods can be seen with procainamide or D-penicillamine.

The clinical features of drug-induced lupus are usually mild and include arthritis or arthralgia, myalgia, fever, and serositis. By definition, all patients are ANA-positive with antibodies to histones especially prominent; the anti-Sm and anti-ds DNA antibodies of idiopathic SLE are lacking in the drug-induced syndromes. LE cells (antideoxynucleoprotein) are usually demonstrated. Lymphadenopathy and renal and central nervous system involvement rarely, if ever, occur. In most patients the clinical and seroreactive complex subsides after withdrawal of the offending agent, but occasionally ANA positivity persists for prolonged periods.

Occasionally, patients have a history of features of SLE (i.e., an episode of arthritis or pleurisy, hyperglobulinemia) before drug administration; in some, added manifestations of SLE emerge after drug withdrawal. Such observations have suggested that an underlying lupus diathesis has been unmasked; however, the high prevalence of ANA positivity and a lupuslike syndrome, irrespective of age and sex, in those receiving procainamide supports the de novo induction of disease by this agent at least.

DISCOID LUPUS[4,14]

The typical skin lesions of discoid lupus are not common in patients with SLE, and they may recur or persist for many years in individuals who fail to develop evidences of a multisystem disorder. Perhaps 10 percent of patients presenting with discoid lesions will develop clinical and laboratory abnormalities characteristic of SLE during the later course of their illnesses. Because there are no features that identify these persons at the outset, it is wise to evaluate such patients thoroughly at periodic intervals. In some cases, joint pains, mild anemia, leukopenia, and even positive ANA may be encountered in the absence of other findings characteristic of SLE.

SUBACUTE CUTANEOUS LUPUS[12,17]

Subacute cutaneous lupus (SCLE), recently described, differs from discoid lupus in all respects (i.e., clinical, serologic, histologic) and has significantly less systemic involvement than typical SLE. Intense photosensitivity is the dominant manifestation. Polyarthritis is found in only a third, and less than 20 percent have serositis, neurologic involvement, nephritis, and hematologic abnormalities. The majority of patients are ANA-positive but otherwise are strikingly similar to the ANA-negative subset clinically and serologically with anti-Ro(SSA) positivity in approximately two thirds of both groups.

LATE-ONSET SLE[16]

Approximately 10 percent of adults with SLE are 50 years of age or older at the time of disease onset. The proportion of men is higher in the older age group. Skin lesions and arthritis, although common, are less prevalent than in the young adult, and lymphadenopathy and probably nephritis are also less frequent. More prevalent in the elderly are the pulmonary involvement (i.e., atelectasizing pneumonitis) and, immunologically, rheumatoid factor (anti-IgG) and anti-Ro(SSA). The late-onset subset, although not a unique syndrome, tends to have milder disease with a lower corticosteroid requirement, but the problem-oriented approach to therapy is the same in the elderly as in the young.

NEONATAL LUPUS[12,17]

Neonatal lupus is characterized primarily by the erythematous skin lesions, which are morphologically similar to those of SCLE in the adult. Less frequent is the complete heart block (≥ 35 percent), which can occur in the absence of cutaneous involvement and, in approximately 25 percent, may be associated with other congenital heart lesions. Occasionally, pneumonitis, lymphadenopathy, hepatosplenomegaly, and hematologic abnormalities are present.

At the time of pregnancy, approximately half the mothers of neonates with lupus are in apparently good health, whereas the other half have SLE or Sjögren syndrome, but anti-Ro(SSA)-positivity has been present in all. The data suggest that anti-Ro(SSA)-positive mothers with HLA-DR3 and antigens in linkage disequilibrium with -DR3 are at risk for infants with neonatal lupus, but the relative risk is yet to be quantified.

Maternal autoantibodies enter the fetal circulation and they, as well as the cutaneous lesions, disappear within weeks or months after birth. The cardiac involvement, if present, represents the only continuing problem, but emergence of typical SLE years later has been observed.

REFERENCES

1. Appel GP, Silva FG, et al: Renal involvement in systemic lupus erythematosus. Medicine 57:371, 1978
2. Arnett FC, Shulman LE: Studies in familial systemic lupus erythematosus. Medicine 55:313, 1976
3. Donadio JV, Burgess JH, Holey KE: Membranous lupus nephropathy: A clinicopathologic study. Medicine 56:527, 1977
4. Dubois EL: Lupus erythematosus. In Dubois EL (ed): A Review of the Current Status of Discoid and Systemic Lupus Erythematosus and Their Variants, rev. 2d ed. Los Angeles, USC Press, 1976
5. Eagen JW, Memoli VA, et al: Pulmonary hemorrhage in systemic lupus erythematosus. Medicine 57:545, 1978
6. Feinglass EJ, Arnett FC, et al: Neuropsychiatric manifestations of systemic lupus erythematosus: Diagnosis, clinical spectrum and relationship to other features of the disease. Medicine 55:323, 1976
7. Ginzler EM, Bollet AJ, Friedman MD: The natural history and response to therapy of lupus nephritis. Ann Rev Med 31:463, 1980
8. Harvey AM, Shulman LE, et al: Systemic lupus erythematosus: A review of the literature and clinical analysis of 138 cases. Medicine 33:291, 1954
9. Hess EV (ed): Kroc Foundation conference on drug-induced lupus. Arthritis Rheum 24:979, 1981
10. Hochberg MC, Boyd RE, et al: Systemic lupus erythematosus: A review of clinical laboratory features and immunogenetic markers in 150 patients, with emphasis on demographic subsets. Medicine 64:285, 1985
11. Johnson RT, Richardson EP: The neurological manifestations of systemic lupus erythematosus. Medicine 47:337, 1968
12. Lahita RG (ed): Systemic Lupus Erythematosus. New York, Wiley, 1987
13. Matthay RA, Schwartz MI, et al: Pulmonary manifestations of systemic lupus erythematosus. Medicine 54:397, 1975
14. Prystowsky SD, Herndon JH, Gilliam JH: Chronic cutaneous lupus erythematosus (DLE): A clinical and laboratory investigation of 80 patients. Medicine 55:183, 1976
15. Stevens MB, Hahn BH: Management of systemic lupus erythematosus. Bull Rheum Dis 32:35, 1982
16. Stevens MB: Connective tissue disease in the elderly. Clin Rheum Dis 12:11, 1986
17. Stevens MB: SLE: Clinical issues. Semin Immunopathol 9:251, 1986
18. Tan EM, Cohen JF, et al: The 1982 revised criteria for the classification of systemic lupus erythematosus. Arthritis Rheum 25:1271, 1982
19. Wagner L: Immunosuppressive agents in lupus nephritis: A critical analysis. Medicine 55:239, 1976
20. Zizic TM, Classen JN, Stevens MB: Acute abdominal complications of systemic lupus erythematosus and polyarteritis nodosa. Am J Med 73:525, 1982
21. Zizic TM, Hungerford DS, Stevens MB: Ischemic bone necrosis in systemic lupus erythematosus. Medicine 59:134, 1980

CHAPTER 8.3
Systemic Vasculitis

Mary Betty Stevens and Thomas M. Zizic

Systemic vasculitis encompasses varied disorders whose common denominator is necrotizing inflammation of blood vessel walls.[1,3] In most subsets, specific etiologic factors have not yet been identified. Studies in humans and experimental animals, however, support the role of large, soluble, circulating immune complexes capable of fixing complement in inducing vascular inflammation. Less certain are the additional possibilities of antibody-dependent direct vascular injury (i.e., antibodies to vessel wall antigens) and cell-mediated immunity. Immune mechanisms and induction of inflammation are detailed in Chapter 7.1.

Classification of the vasculitides is difficult and imperfect in view of their overlapping clinical and pathologic features. Table 8.3–1 proposes a basic approach to these patients and their special clinical problems. Among the disorders commonly associated with vasculitis are the other connective tissue diseases (especially SLE, dermatomyositis, and Sjögren syndrome), rheumatoid arthritis, systemic infections, and neoplasia.

POLYARTERITIS NODOSA[2,3,6]

Polyarteritis nodosa (PAN) is a disease of unknown etiology characterized by widespread segmental inflammation of medium-sized and small arteries, which usually results in a systemic illness with multisystem involvement. The clinical picture may vary considerably, depending on the organ or organs most critically damaged by the ischemia resulting from the vascular lesions.

Immune complex deposition in blood vessel walls has been implicated in the pathogenesis of PAN by immunohistology of involved vessels and on the basis of similarities to experimental immune complex disease as well as similarities of the clinical features to those with other immune complex disorders (e.g., serum sickness and SLE). Furthermore, the onset of symptoms may follow

TABLE 8.3–1. SYSTEMIC VASCULITIS

- Polyarteritis (nodosa)
- Granulomatous angiitis
  - Allergic granulomatosis (Churg-Strauss)
  - Wegener granulomatosis
  - Giant cell arteritis
  - Aortic arteritis (Takayasu disease)
  - Cranial arteritis
  - Lymphomatoid granulomatosis
- Hypersensitivity angiitis
- Vasculitis associated with other diseases

closely upon sensitivity reactions to such drugs as sulfonamides, iodides, penicillin, and thiouracil, or in association with hepatitis B antigen. Acute serous otitis media occasionally precedes necrotizing arteritis.

PAN is relatively uncommon, being less frequent, for example, than SLE or systemic sclerosis. In contrast to other disorders with immunologic features, it is two to three times more common in men than in women. It may occur at any age but is observed most frequently in the fourth through the sixth decades. There is no known racial or familial predisposition.

CLINICAL MANIFESTATIONS

Presenting Complaints
The initial manifestations of PAN are variable. Symptoms sometimes appear abruptly in a healthy individual, but often the process appears to follow a recent illness such as a respiratory infection or a drug reaction. Although disease of a single organ, such as nephritis or neuritis, may be the first manifestation of PAN, patients more often seem to be suffering from a subacute, febrile, systemic disease (Table 8.3–2). Fever, fatigability, myalgia, anorexia, and weight loss dominate the early symptomatology. The cumulative prevalence of clinical laboratory features of polyarteritis nodosa is found in Tables 8.3–3 and 8.3–4.

Skin and Mucous Membranes
Skin involvement occurs in more than 40 percent of patients. Small (0.5 to 1 cm) nodular lesions (arteritis) characteristically appear in the skin and subcutaneous tissues, occurring singly or in crops over any area of the body. Splinter hemorrhages in the nails and small periungual infarcts are characteristic although not invariably present. Nonspecific lesions (e.g., urticaria, petechiae, purpura, hemorrhagic bullae, and a variety of erythematous rashes) are encountered. Livedo reticularis and localized edema about the face, trunk, or extremities are occasional findings.

Ocular Manifestations
Four types of ocular manifestations are found in PAN:

1. Direct involvement of retinal vessels, with exudations, hemorrhage, "cytoid" bodies, arterial occlusion, papilledema, and optic atrophy
2. Exudative lesions of mesenchymal elements leading to episcleritis or iridocyclitis
3. Cerebral arterial disease with extraocular palsy, pupillomotor disturbance, and visual field defects
4. Hypertensive retinopathy associated with renal impairment

Cardiovascular Manifestations
Episodes of pericarditis with or without effusions may occur; a massive, bloody effusion with tamponade may result from a ruptured vessel. Patients may present with coronary insufficiency or

myocardial infarction caused by arteritis of the coronary vessels. Cardiac arrhythmias are occasionally encountered. Congestive heart failure may result from diffuse myocardial damage from arteritis or from hypertension secondary to renal arteritis.

Raynaud phenomenon is encountered infrequently. Rarely, lesions similar to thromboangiitis obliterans produce acrogangrene.

Gastrointestinal Manifestations[10]
Abdominal pain, nausea, vomiting, diarrhea, and intestinal bleeding are common manifestations of PAN. Depending on the extent and localization of vascular disease, almost any intra-abdominal disease may be mimicked. Hematomas (especially retroperitoneal) caused by the rupture of an arteritic lesion may present as a mass, often accompanied by pain and, when massive, by symptoms of acute blood loss. Catastrophic abdominal events occur in one fifth of patients. Bowel infarction is most frequent, followed by serious gastrointestinal bleeding and hepatic or splenic infarcts.

The liver is involved more frequently than has been recognized clinically. In those patients with PAN associated with hepatitis B antigen, liver involvement inevitably develops, although it may be late in appearance and mild in degree. A moderate degree of hepatomegaly is usually present. Pain over the liver and a friction rub may accompany hepatic infarction, and jaundice may develop if infarction is sufficiently extensive. Smaller, clinically silent infarc-

TABLE 8.3–3. CLINICAL FEATURES OF POLYARTERITIS (97 PATIENTS)[a]

Manifestations	Prevalence (%)
Renal	65
Hypertension	58
Fever	49
Pulmonary	42
Skin rash	41
Arthralgia/arthritis	40
Peripheral neuropathy	40
Peripheral vasculitis	35
Myalgias	33
Cardiac	30
Central nervous system	26
Hepatomegaly	22
Intestinal perforation	11

[a]From a series of angiographically or histologically proven polyarteritis.

TABLE 8.3–2. PRESENTING MANIFESTATIONS THAT SHOULD AROUSE SUSPICION OF POLYARTERITIS

- A nonspecific subacute or chronic febrile illness with loss of weight and leukocytosis
- An atypical abdominal illness, which may simulate a condition requiring laparotomy
- A primary renal disease frequently thought to be acute or subacute glomerulonephritis
- Polyneuropathy, sometimes in combination with myositis
- Bronchial asthma or focal pulmonary infiltrates suggesting infection
- Myocardial infarction or coronary insufficiency especially in association with any of the above
- Unexplained severe hypertension

TABLE 8.3–4. LABORATORY FEATURES OF POLYARTERITIS (97 PATIENTS)[a]

Manifestations	Prevalence (%)
Elevated ESR	89
Leukocytosis	78
Anemia	66
Thrombocytosis	58
Rheumatoid factor	37
Hepatitis-associated antigen	26
Cryoglobulinemia	25
Hypocomplementemia	21
Thrombocytopenia	18

[a]See footnote to Table 8.3–3.

tions may result in increased alkaline phosphatase and serum transaminases. Liver biopsy rarely yields a diagnosis of arteritis; in view of the risk of bleeding, imaging techniques (e.g., computed tomographic [CT] scan) have largely replaced invasive procedures.

Spleen and Lymph Nodes
Lymphadenopathy is not characteristic of PAN. Slight splenic enlargement is present in about 20 percent of the cases. Splenic infarction or perisplenic hemorrhage has been observed rarely.

Genitourinary Manifestations
Renal involvement is present in at least two thirds of patients. Occasionally, patients present with manifestations resembling those of acute, subacute, or chronic glomerulonephritis. More commonly, renal disease becomes evident later as systemic involvement progresses. Hypertension in PAN is generally secondary to renal disease. Hypertension may be mild and sustained; may fluctuate strikingly, suggesting pheochromocytoma; or may be severe, with a clinical picture of malignant hypertension.

There are two types of renal lesions, and they may occur simultaneously or independently: (1) a widespread focal or, occasionally, diffuse glomerulonephritis and (2) arteritis involving the renal artery and its branches. Renal arteritis may lead to renal infarction or to a perirenal or retroperitoneal hematoma.

The vessels of the bladder may be affected, producing hemorrhagic cystitis. Testicular infarction with severe pain and subsequent atrophy is more frequent in PAN than in any other single condition.

Musculoskeletal Manifestations
Myalgia and arthralgia are often prominent symptoms. Occasionally, trichinosis or primary myositis is suggested by the severity of the muscle pain. Later, profound weakness and atrophy may develop. Frank arthritis, present in approximately 40 percent of patients, occurs early in the course and most frequently involves the large joints (e.g., knees, ankles, wrists, elbows).

Neurologic Manifestations
The most common neurologic manifestation of PAN is a mononeuritis caused by arteritis of the nutrient vessels of major nerve trunks, such as the radial nerve, which causes wrist drop, and the peroneal nerve, which causes foot drop. Sensory and motor deficits, which may be symmetric, usually accompany this type of neuritis. Whereas the occurrence of peripheral neuritis in any obscure illness should always suggest the possibility of polyarteritis, involvement of several major nerve trunks (mononeuritis multiplex) is virtually diagnostic.

PAN may also affect other components of the nervous system in a variable and confusing pattern. Involvement of carotid, vertebral, meningeal, or deep cerebral vessels can lead to hemiplegia, transverse myelitis, convulsions, cerebellar dysfunction, extrapyramidal disorders, optic atrophy, or subarachnoid hemorrhage. Cranial nerve palsies are uncommon.

LABORATORY MANIFESTATIONS

Polyarteritis is usually associated with leukocytosis, often 15,000/μl or more. An increased platelet count (greater than 500,000/μl) is present in more than 50 percent of patients. Thrombocytopenia is present in 15 to 20 percent and has been associated with mesenteric arteritis. Anemia is usually mild and may be absent in the early phases. The erythrocyte sedimentation rate is almost always increased and generally reflects the intensity of disease activity. Proteinuria and, often, microscopic hematuria, pyuria, and casts are found in patients with glomerular disease. With renal arterial involvement, the urinalysis may be normal.

Rheumatoid factor is present in one third of patients and is more frequent in patients with mesenteric involvement. Hepatitis-associated antigenemia[8] and cryoglobulinemia are present in 25 percent of patients, and hypocomplementemia occurs in about one fifth, especially those with circulating complexes.

Biopsy
Typical lesions show segmental inflammation and necrosis of medium-sized or small arteries, usually extending throughout the vessel wall and disrupting the internal elastic lamina. Thrombosis, aneurysmal dilation, or rupture of the vessel and hemorrhage may be evident, as well as degeneration or infarction of the distal tissue. Lesions in all stages of development are encountered commonly.

If a skin nodule or tender muscle is apparent, a biopsy should be done. If not, selective biopsy of the deltoid muscle may be diagnostic, but the yield is low. In symptomatic patients, testicular or peripheral nerve biopsies may be more helpful.

A negative biopsy result does not exclude the diagnosis, and a positive biopsy result alone is not diagnostic for PAN. Similar vascular inflammation may occur in many disorders, even at the margin of suppurative bacterial lesions. The pathologic finding of arteritis must, therefore, be interpreted in relation to the clinical setting. This is especially true in patients with cutaneous vasculitis or when an isolated vasculitis is unexpectedly found in tissue (e.g., appendix or gallbladder) removed for another reason.

DIAGNOSIS

The diagnosis rests on a compatible clinical picture in conjunction with demonstration of arteritic lesions on biopsy or by imaging techniques. Leukocytosis and thrombocytosis are the most helpful laboratory features. The presence of fever, weight loss, and muscle or joint pain, combined with neural, cardiac, or renal lesions, is the most common clinical pattern suggesting the diagnosis of PAN. Although the coexistence of systemic symptoms and disorders in more than one organ system usually leads to the suspicion of polyarteritis, constitutional symptoms alone may dominate the early course of some patients. In others, an acute abdominal syndrome or abrupt onset of malignant hypertension may be presenting features (Table 8.3–2).

Arteriography[9] may be a useful diagnostic method, especially when biopsy material is negative for arteritis. In one series, 60 percent of patients with polyarteritis had aneurysms (usually multiple) demonstrated on angiography of hepatic, renal, and mesenteric circulations. CT scanning may demonstrate tissue infarcts (e.g., liver, spleen, kidney).

Differential Diagnosis
It is usually not difficult to distinguish PAN from other connective tissue disorders, even those in which arteritis is present, because of its clinical pattern, demographic features, and lack of serologic autoreactivity. The presence of HBsAg lends support to the diagnosis. In those instances when involvement of one organ system dominates the clinical picture for a time, polyarteritis may be confused with abnormalities of these organs (e.g., kidney, liver, peripheral or central nervous system) due to other causes. Similarly, when fever, weakness, and systemic symptoms are prominent, PAN must be separated from disorders capable of producing such symptoms (e.g., chronic infection, neoplasm, hyperthyroidism). Patients with cutaneous vasculitis may be febrile but may never develop visceral involvement. Angiographically, aneurysms may be demonstrated in fibromuscular dysplasia and pseudoxanthoma elasticum. These disorders can be differentiated on clinical grounds, and in contrast to PAN, a single aneurysm is the rule. Drug abusers and patients with atrial myxoma may have identical angiograms, but a careful drug history may establish the former and cardiac ultrasound, the latter.

COURSE AND PROGNOSIS[2]

The course of polyarteritis nodosa is variable, but in most cases the disease progresses at a varying rate over a period of months or years.

Spontaneous remissions and remissions induced by corticosteroid therapy have been reported.

Corticosteroid therapy has been reported to increase the 5-year survival rate from 12 percent in untreated patients to 50 percent in the steroid-treated group. Further improvement in the survival rate has been reported with the addition of cytotoxic drug therapy to steroids.[4,6] Nonetheless, the overall prognosis remains poor, and the disease is all too frequently fatal. Renal failure, massive retroperitoneal or gastrointestinal bleeding, perforation or infarction of the bowel, and CNS lesions are the major causes of death.

MANAGEMENT

The general principles of managing patients with PAN are similar to those described for managing patients with SLE (p. 498). Vigorous therapy with adrenal corticosteroids is required to control symptoms and to prevent disease progression. Prednisone or its equivalent is begun at a dose of 50 to 100 mg daily, and the patient is observed for evidence of disease regression (e.g., symptomatic improvement, lack of new lesions, and return of the erythrocyte sedimentation rate and platelet count to normal). Frequently, a higher dose may be required to control the disease. High dosage should be continued until stabilization has been achieved (in weeks or months). The dose is then gradually tapered if there is no recrudescence of the disease.

In addition to steroid therapy the early use of immunosuppressive drugs (especially cyclophosphamide and azathioprine) may be of significant benefit.[4,6] In one study the 5-year survival rate of 53 percent of patients treated with steroids alone increased to 80 percent, with median survival exceeding 12 years in patients receiving both steroids and immunosuppressives.

GRANULOMATOUS ANGIITIS

There is a spectrum of vasculitic syndromes ranging from the involvement of small vessels (arteriolar and venular) to inflammation of large arteries; a granulomatous reaction contributing to the inflammatory infiltrate occurs across this spectrum. Certain reasonably defined subsets have been identified with each having distinguishing features relative to the target population, the distribution and character of the vascular lesions, and the clinical dimensions of illness.

Allergic granulomatosis (Churg–Strauss syndrome)[3] is a rare variant of polyarteritis that differs clinically and pathologically. Pathologically, pulmonary involvement is dominant; small- and medium-sized arteries and veins are damaged by an intense inflammatory infiltrate that is granulomatous and eosinophilic. Middle-aged adults, slightly more men than women, are affected.

Clinically, allergic granulomatosis is universally associated with severe asthma; radiographically, pulmonary infiltrates are found in more than 90 percent of patients. The skin commonly has purpuric and nodular lesions that may evidence a granulomatous and eosinophilic vascular inflammation like that found in the lung or that may be a leukocytoclastic vasculitis. In more than 50 percent of patients a peripheral neuropathy indistinguishable from PAN (i.e., mononeuritis multiplex) occurs. Less frequent than in PAN are the cardiac, gastrointestinal, and renal manifestations. Hypertension is present in approximately 50 percent of patients.

Leukocytosis with a pronounced eosinophilia is the rule, and the sedimentation rate is usually elevated. Diagnosis is based on the association of asthma and peripheral eosinophilia with histologic evidence of a granulomatous vasculitis in the lung; it must be differentiated from PAN, Wegener granulomatosis, and other pulmonary syndromes with eosinophilia.

High-dose corticosteroid therapy, promptly instituted, has greatly improved the survival rate. The role of cytotoxic drug therapy, in addition, remains uncertain.

Wegener granulomatosis[3] is a disorder that targets primarily the upper respiratory tract, the lungs, and the kidney. An "incomplete Wegener" variant has been described in which the kidney is spared, but this may represent a stage in evolution rather than a discrete subset. The cardinal lesion—a necrotizing, granulomatous inflammation of small arteries and veins with giant cells—may be diffuse and widespread, but the diagnostic histopathology is found by lung biopsy. In contrast, the chronic inflammation of the upper respiratory tract and glomerulitis are less specific.

Young and middle-aged adults of both sexes are affected. The onset is usually insidious, with manifestations suggesting chronic sinus or other respiratory tract infection. Approximately two thirds of patients present with purulent rhinorrhea, antral pain, and epistaxis; in the other third, chronic cough, hemoptysis, or pleurisy are prominent at onset. As the disease progresses, mucosal ulceration and cartilaginous destruction of the nose may develop, as well as multiple pulmonary infiltrates or nodules. Eventually, generalized manifestations emerge, including fever, vasculitic skin lesions, musculoskeletal symptoms, peripheral neuropathy, and renal disease. Anemia, leukocytosis, and eosinophilia are present in the majority.

Corticosteroids alone have been ineffective, but steroids with cyclophosphamide, initiated early, have been shown to control the disease process. Other cytotoxic agents, although studied less extensively, seemingly produce more variable responses.

Giant-cell arteritis (GCA),[5] previously referred to as *temporal arteritis,* is a potent̶̶̶̶̶̶̶̶neralized, necrotizing granulomatous in̶̶̶̶̶̶ for thrombo- ̶̶̶̶̶ecting the elderly, infrequently seen before th̶̶amor-̶̶̶̶̶d typically found in women and Caucasians. Involvement of the temporal arteries is the rule, but disease of the ophthalmic and retinal vessels is common; there is overlap with the recently described *cranial arteritis* clinically, and with systemic arteritis.

The onset and course of GCA are variable; patients may initially consult their physician with cephalic or musculoskeletal symptoms or with systemic illness.

The cephalic phase of GCA is characterized most commonly by recurrent headache which, if bilateral, is usually more severe on one side. Jaw claudication may occur, and scalp tenderness as well as tenderness along the temporal arteries may be noted. The temporal arteries occasionally become prominent, even nodular; on palpation, asymmetry or loss of temporal artery pulsations is characteristic but not always present. Of most concern are the ocular complications in which vascular lesions affect the optic nerve and retina. Recurrent, transient visual loss (amaurosis fugax) can occur, and without prompt therapy, complete blindness may follow. Diplopia, also intermittent at first, and ophthalmoplegias are less common. Seldom do the ocular manifestations emerge in the absence of headache or other signs of temporal arteritis.

The musculoskeletal manifestations constitute the syndrome of *polymyalgia rheumatica (PMR),* which may or may not be associated with cephalic symptoms or detectable arteritis. Muscle pain and stiffness proximally in the shoulder and hip girdles are the dominant symptoms. When diagnosis is delayed and, as is all too often the case, symptoms persist for months without treatment, weakness and decreased range of motion of shoulders and hips can develop. The syndrome is characterized by an elevated sedimentation rate (usually greater than 50 mm/hr by the Westergren method) in almost all patients with active disease. In some patients with the PMR syndrome, diminished or absent pulsations in the temporal artery may be found in the absence of any cranial symptoms, and a temporal artery biopsy may reveal typical lesions of GCA.

Systemic features may occur at any time. Malaise and fatigability, anorexia with weight loss, and low-grade fever can be prominent. Among the generalized manifestations are cutaneous and visceral lesions, polyneuropathy, and an arthritis that particularly involves the central (e.g., sternoclavicular, achromioclavicular) and large joints. Mental confusion, seizures, hemiparesis, and coma have been noted.

The major complication of GCA is visual impairment, which can be prevented by early diagnosis and prompt administration of corticosteroids. The complete response of the muscle pain and stiffness within 24 to 48 hours after initiating steroid therapy is virtually diagnostic of the PMR-like component.

Aortic arch arteritis,[7] also referred to as "pulseless" disease and Takayasu disease, is characterized by a segmental panarteritis involving the elastic arteries originating from the aortic arch or thoracic aorta. It is seen almost exclusively in young women. An initial inflammatory phase, characterized by fever, night sweats, malaise, myalgia, and polyarthralgia, occurs in the majority. Months, even years, later the "pulseless" stage follows with symptoms of vascular occlusions. Occasionally, absent or variable pulses may be found on routine examination of the asymptomatic individual. Headache, syncope, reduced visual acuity, mental confusion, and convulsions may result from reduced cerebral blood flow. Symptoms may also include those of coronary insufficiency, heart failure, and arterial insufficiency of the upper extremities. These manifestations are often precipitated or accentuated by physical activity.

Pulses may be absent in the neck, head, and upper extremities, and the blood pressure may be unobtainable in the arms. There may be evidence of collateral circulation about the shoulders or elsewhere. A high-pitched systolic or continuous bruit may be noted over the upper chest. Anemia, leukocytosis, increased sedimentation rate, and hypergammaglobulinemia may be present.

Differential diagnosis involves aortic aneurysm, syphilitic aortitis, congenital anomalies of the aorta, and various tumors and infections of the mediastinum. Early diagnosis and prompt institution of corticosteroid therapy are essential, for many patients develop cerebral and cardiac insufficiency before the diagnosis has been suspected or established. The outlook is favorable with daily prednisone in moderate dosage (25 to 40 mg) initially; chronic low-dose (5 to 10 mg) maintenance therapy generally prevents late vascular complications and improves the survival rate.

RARE SUBSETS OF GRANULOMATOUS ANGIITIS

Recently, an *"isolated" arteritis of the CNS* has been emphasized. Cephalgia, altered mentation with impaired intellect, disorientation, and confusion are dominant presenting symptoms. Spinal cord vasculitis can occur. The histopathology and infrequently associated systemic manifestations (fever, arthralgias, myalgias) suggest an overlap with GCA in some. The existence of such an overlap is further supported by the predilection for the elderly of either sex. Diagnosis is difficult because laboratory study findings are normal except for occasional cerebrospinal fluid pleocytosis and protein elevation. Angiography is most helpful but not consistent with small artery narrowing and dilation in a "beaded" pattern. Corticosteroids appear to improve prognosis and prolong survival,

whereas the role of added cytotoxic drug therapy remains uncertain.

Lymphomatoid granulomatosis is as puzzling as it is rare, ranging from a "benign lymphocytic angiitis and granulomatosis" at one extreme to a frank lymphoma at the other. Fever and constitutional symptoms, respiratory manifestations, and central and peripheral neuropathy are cardinal features. Laboratory studies are not diagnostic; most helpful are the multiple nodular densities on chest radiograph. The histopathology is diagnostic; a bizarre, destructive, angiocentric inflammation involving small arteries and veins is the characteristic finding. The prognosis is poor, and the optimal therapeutic regimen is still undefined; however, corticosteroids appear to be beneficial. The value of cytotoxic drug therapy, in addition, is still undefined.

HYPERSENSITIVITY ANGIITIS

Hypersensitivity angiitis involves small vessels, both arteriolar and venular, especially in the skin, heart, and kidney. Polyarthritis is commonly present. The lesions are all the same age, suggesting a single precipitating event. Hypersensitivity vasculitis can follow exposure to foreign proteins, infectious agents, chemicals, and drugs. Often, a specific causative agent cannot be identified. Dramatic recovery follows withdrawal of the causative agent and the administration of adrenal corticosteroids.

REFERENCES

1. Christian CL, Sergent JS: Vasculitis syndromes: Clinical and experimental models. Am J Med 61:385, 1976
2. Cohen RD, Conn DL, Ilstrup DM: Clinical features, prognosis and response treatment in polyarteritis. Mayo Clin Proc 55:146, 1980
3. Cupps TR, Fauci AS: The vasculitides. In Thomas R, Fauci A (eds): Medicine, vol. 21. Philadelphia, Saunders, 1981
4. Fauci AS, Katz P, et al: Cyclophosphamide therapy of severe systemic necrotizing vasculitis. N Engl J Med 301:235, 1979
5. Hamilton CR Jr, Shelley WM, Tumulty PA: Giant cell arteritis including temporal arteritis and polymyalgia rheumatica. Medicine 50:1, 1971
6. Leib ES, Restivo C, Paulus HE: Immunosuppressive and corticosteroid therapy of polyarteritis nodosa. Am J Med 67:941, 1979
7. Schrire V, Asherson RA: Arteritis of the aorta and its major branches. QJ Med 33:439, 1964
8. Sergent JS, Lockshin MD, et al: Vasculitis and hepatitis B antigenemia. Medicine 55:1, 1976
9. Travers RL, Allison DJ, et al: Polyarteritis nodosa: A clinical and angiographic analysis of 17 cases. Semin Arthritis Rheum 8:184, 1979
10. Zizic TM, Classen JW, Stevens MB: Acute abdominal complications of systemic lupus erythematosus (SLE) and polyarteritis nodosa (PAN). Am J Med 73:525, 1982

CHAPTER 8.4
Polymyositis

Marc C. Hochberg

Polymyositis is a disorder of unknown etiology, characterized primarily by an inflammatory myopathy involving striated skeletal and, less commonly, cardiac muscle. Recent studies[5,11] support an autoimmune hypothesis, which considers tissue injury the consequence of cytotoxic lymphocytes specifically sensitized to antigens of skeletal muscle. A role for antecedent viral infection has been suggested by epidemiologic studies in children with dermatomyo-

sitis and supported by the development of viral-induced animal models of myositis. Moreover, a genetic predisposition has been suggested by the association of polymyositis with HLA-DR3 in Caucasians and HLA-DRw6 in blacks.[7] Fever, skin lesions (i.e., dermatomyositis), dysphagia, arthritis, vasomotor instability, and other visceral manifestations may occur, but weakness of limb girdle and proximal muscles is the dominant feature of the disease.

The major consideration in the patient with a polymyositis (Table 8.4–1) is whether the myopathy occurs alone, is associated with a neoplasm, or is one manifestation of a multisystem process (i.e., SLE, systemic sclerosis, Sjögren syndrome).

CLINICAL MANIFESTATIONS

PRESENTING COMPLAINTS

Polymyositis commonly begins insidiously. Patients with pelvic girdle involvement may note difficulty in rising from a reclining or sitting position or in climbing stairs. Weakness of the shoulder girdle usually begins with difficulty in raising and maintaining the arms overhead. Weakness of the neck flexors and pharyngeal weakness with dysphagia may also be early manifestations.

In some the onset is acute, and fever or skin rash (especially facial) may be associated with rapidly progressing muscle weakness, pain, tenderness, and even rhabdomyolysis.

SKIN AND MUCOUS MEMBRANES

Typical skin lesions occur in about 30 percent of cases (Table 8.4–1). Dusky, erythematous lesions appear on the face, neck, upper trunk, and proximal portions of the extremities. Periorbital edema often accompanies the facial rash. A characteristic lilac-colored or heliotrope rash over the eyelids is occasionally seen. In 20 percent of patients, patchy, erythematous, sometimes scaling maculopapular lesions are present over the knuckles (Gottron sign), knees, elbows, or medial malleoli. Erythema around the nail margins and erythema and atrophy of the finger pads may also occur. Cutaneous vasculitis (e.g., periungual infarcts, digital ulcers, tender dermal and subcutaneous nodules) occurs in 10 percent of patients.[6] Raynaud phenomenon occurs in 25 percent of patients overall but in about half of those with polymyositis associated with other connective tissue disease.

GASTROINTESTINAL MANIFESTATIONS

Dysphagia occurs in 40 percent of cases and may be associated with nasal regurgitation. Physiologic studies show impaired initiation of swallowing and diminished motor activity in the upper third of the esophagus (striated muscle). About 30 percent of patients with dysphagia show aperistalsis of the distal esophagus (smooth muscle), usually associated with Raynaud phenomenon. Motor dysfunction of the intestinal tract is rare. Abdominal pain and intestinal ulceration, perforation, and bleeding may be seen in childhood dermatomyositis (caused by vasculitis).[2]

MUSCULOSKELETAL MANIFESTATIONS

Weakness of the proximal limb girdle musculature is a cardinal feature of polymyositis. Although muscular pain and tenderness are common in the more acute cases, these features are often absent, especially when the onset is insidious.

Arthralgia or arthritis, especially of the fingers, wrists, and knees, occurs early in one third of cases, most often in those patients who have associated connective tissue disease. Muscular atrophy, contractures, and calcinosis are late features, occurring in a minority of patients but especially in children.

In the later stages of the disease the respiratory muscles may be severely weakened. Progressive respiratory insufficiency and pulmonary infection are frequently the causes of death. Such is particularly the case when there is associated cricopharyngeal involvement, with impairment of swallowing and consequent aspiration.

CARDIOPULMONARY MANIFESTATIONS

Cardiac involvement, consisting of ECG changes such as nonspecific ST-T wave changes, variable degrees of heart block and bundle branch block, atrial or ventricular arrhythmias, and congestive heart failure, may occur in up to one third of patients. Pulmonary involvement is usually manifested by interstitial fibrosis on chest

TABLE 8.4–1. DISTINGUISHING FEATURES OF TYPES OF POLYMYOSITIS

Type	Age and Sex Affected	Skin Lesions	Other Features
Polymyositis or dermatomyositis	Adults, especially fourth to sixth decades Female 3:1	Typical facial rash, extremity lesions, and cutaneous vasculitis in dermatomyositis	Insidious onset in those without skin lesions; occasional fever, muscle pain and tenderness Arthralgias or arthritis in 25% Raynaud in 15% Antibody to Jo-1 in 50% of polymyositis Usually steroid responsive
Childhood dermatomyositis	Usually age 5–14 No sex dominance	Typical facial and extremity lesions present	Contractures, calcinosis of muscles Vasculitic lesions prominent on biopsy Usually steroid responsive
Polymyositis or, more often, dermatomyositis with malignancy	Over age 45 No sex dominance	Typical facial lesions and Gottron sign in most	Acute or subacute onset; malignancy can be occult Raynaud not present Vasculitis clinically in 10% Seronegative Poor response to steroids but may improve with treatment of tumor
Polymyositis with connective tissue disorders	Age determined by associated disorder Females 8:1	Skin lesions of SLE, PSS, etc., dominant	Acute or subacute onset Major associations: SLE, SS, and Sjögren syndrome Clinicolaboratory features of associated disorder dominant Usually steroid responsive

roentgenogram (about 25 to 30 percent), or by restrictive ventilatory defect on pulmonary function testing, or by both. These abnormalities are comparable in type and extent to those seen in patients with systemic sclerosis but, in contrast, appear to respond to treatment with corticosteroids.

MALIGNANCIES[3,8]

The frequency of associated malignancy in adult-onset polymyositis varies from 7 to 24 percent with an average estimate of 13 percent based on ten series with approximately 600 patients. Solid tumors are found most often in these patients; carcinoma of the lung, prostate, and colon are commonly seen in men, and carcinoma of the breast, ovary, and lung are commonly seen in women. Those patients with malignancies are far less likely to have Raynaud phenomenon and other features of connective tissue disease, including autoantibodies. In contrast, patients with malignancies are more likely to have dermatomyositis than polymyositis, especially with superimposed cutaneous vasculitis. In addition, these patients tend to be older than those without malignancy; the frequency of associated malignancy was fivefold higher in myositis patients aged 45 years or more compared to those age 44 or below. Contrary to earlier impressions, this association does not appear limited to men but is nearly equal for both sexes. The majority of malignant lesions are diagnosed simultaneously or within 1 year after the diagnosis of myositis. Several authors have recommended that evaluations for malignancy be limited to those patients aged 45 and above with unexplained symptoms, abnormal physical or laboratory test findings, or a history of previous malignancy.[8]

LABORATORY MANIFESTATIONS

The laboratory findings that characterize polymyositis are shown in Table 8.4–2. Serum enzymes, such as serum aspartate amino transferace (AST), aldolase, lactic dehydrogenase (LDH), and creatine kinase (CK) are released from damaged muscle and elevated

TABLE 8.4–2. LABORATORY MANIFESTATIONS OF POLYMYOSITIS

Immunologic reactions
- ANA in some cases, especially those with associated CTD
- Antibody to Jo-1 frequent

Serum enzymes
- Elevated transaminases (AST and ALT), aldolase, creatine kinase, LDH, etc., during active stages of the disease

Electromyography
- Little or no reduction in total number of motor unit potentials on volitional contraction
- Individual potentials often of short duration, low amplitude, and polyphasic
- Spontaneous fibrillation and positive (sawtooth) potentials at rest
- Short bursts of rapidly repeating action potentials
- Abnormal intensity-duration curves

Muscle biopsy findings
- Focal or segmental degeneration of muscle fibers, sometimes with vacuolization
- Regeneration of damaged muscle fibers as evidenced by sarcoplasmal basophilia, large nuclei, and prominent nucleoli
- Necrosis of part of or whole muscle fiber with phagocytosis of its substance
- Infiltration of inflammatory cells most often in the perimysium near blood vessels, but sometimes diffusely
- Extreme variation in size of muscle fibers
- Interstitial fibrosis
- Vasculitis in childhood type

in the sera of almost all patients, reflecting to some degree the activity and severity of the myositis.

The electromyographic findings (Table 8.4–2) are not specific; however, characteristic small-amplitude, short-duration, polyphasic motor unit potentials are found in about 90 percent of patients. Increased membrane irritability at rest and bizarre high-frequency pseudomyotonic discharges also occur commonly.

The histologic pattern in various types of polymyositis (Tables 8.4–1, 8.4–2) is relatively uniform except where, for example, in childhood dermatomyatsitis vasculitis with endothelial proliferation, thrombosis, and infarction of muscle tissue is often prominent.[2] When seeking diagnostic material, one should take care to perform the muscle biopsy on an actively involved muscle, usually in the proximal groups.

Antinuclear antibodies are present overall in about 30 percent of cases, being most common in those with associated connective tissue diseases (especially systemic lupus erythematosus [SLE]) and rarely found in those with malignancies. A multiplicity of precipitating autoantibodies to extractable nuclear antigens have been found in myositis sera; the most sensitive is anti-Jo-1 antibody.[13] This is present in about 50 percent of patients with polymyositis and is associated with pulmonary fibrosis.[10]

DIAGNOSIS

The diagnosis of polymyositis is based chiefly on the occurrence of muscular weakness, especially of the girdle and proximal musculature, which is often associated with skin lesions, arthralgia or arthritis, and other features suggestive of connective tissue disorders (Table 8.4–1). The concentrations of one or more serum muscle enzymes are elevated in almost all patients with active polymyositis and, like electromyographic findings, help distinguish this disorder from other types of myopathy (Chapter 15.15). The histopathologic findings confirm the diagnosis.

COURSE AND PROGNOSIS

The natural course of polymyositis varies somewhat according to type (Table 8.4–1), but the prognosis has greatly improved in recent years. Factors associated with a poor prognosis are older age at diagnosis and cardiac involvement.[9] In the more chronic varieties, remissions and exacerbations may be seen, but without treatment the general trend is toward increasing impairment. The course of the myopathy can be altered beneficially by the administration of adrenal corticosteroids. Steroid-refractory patients may respond dramatically to the addition of an immunosuppressive agent, especially methotrexate.[1,4]

MANAGEMENT

The goals in the management of patients with polymyositis are to (1) suppress the inflammatory process in skeletal muscle and (2) minimize loss of muscle mass and strength. Early diagnosis and treatment are key to successful outcome.

General supportive care is important. Rest is helpful during disease activity, and measures such as passive exercises should be taken to preserve muscle strength and to prevent the development of contractures. All adult patients, especially over age 45, should be examined carefully for occult tumors. Occasionally the removal of a tumor has been associated with remission of the myositis. After the disease is controlled, physical therapy should be instituted to improve muscle strength. Nasogastric tube feeding or intravenous hyperalimentation may preclude the occurrence of aspiration in the patient with severe dysphagia. Antibiotics are used as needed in management of infectious complications.

Most patients with typical polymyositis or dermatomyositis

respond to adrenal corticosteroid therapy. Best results are obtained when treatment is instituted early. Although response to treatment is less dramatic in patients with advanced disease, all patients should nevertheless have a trial of corticosteroids. Such treatment is usually begun at high dose levels (60 to 80 mg of prednisone daily in adults and 1 mg/kg in children). When a maximal response has been achieved, the steroid dose should be reduced slowly (by about 10 percent of the daily dose every 2 to 4 weeks). Usually it is possible to reduce the dose to a small maintenance dose, and therapy may be discontinued in a few patients after several years. In patients refractory to steroid therapy or intolerant of the steroid dosage required for disease control, the addition of an immunosuppressive agent, especially methotrexate, has been beneficial.[1] Methotrexate is administered orally, each week, increasing the initial 7.5 mg dose to 15 to 25 mg as tolerated, until clinical and chemical remission is achieved.

REFERENCES

1. Arnett FC Jr, Whelton JC, et al: Methotrexate therapy in polymyositis. Ann Rheum Dis 32:536, 1973
2. Banker BQ, Victor M: Dermatomyositis (systemic angiopathy) of childhood. Medicine 48:261, 1968
3. Barnes BE: Dermatomyositis and malignancy. Ann Intern Med 34:68, 1976
4. Bohan A, Peter JB, et al: A computer-assisted analysis of 153 patients with polymyositis and dermatomyositis. Medicine 56:255, 1977
5. Currie S, Saunders M, et al: Immunologic aspects of polymyositis: The in vitro activity of lymphocytes on incubation with muscle antigen and with muscle cultures. QJ Med 157:63, 1971
6. Feldman D, Hochberg MC, et al: Cutaneous vasculitis in adult polymyositis/dermatomyositis. J Rheum 10:85, 1983
7. Hirsch TJ, Enlow RW, Bias WB: HLA-D related (DR) antigens in various kinds of myositis. Human Immunol 3:181, 1981
8. Hochberg MC: Polymyositis/dermatomyositis and malignancy. In Brooks P, York J (eds): Proceedings of the XVIth International Congress of Rheumatology. Amsterdam, Elsevier Science Publishers, 1985, p 279
9. Hochberg MC, Feldman D, Stevens MB: Adult-onset polymyositis/dermatomyositis: An analysis of clinical and laboratory features and survivorship in 76 patients with a review of the literature. Semin Arthritis Rheum 15:168, 1986
10. Hochberg MC, Feldman D, et al: Antibody to Jo-1 in polymyositis/dermatomyositis: Association with interstitial pulmonary disease. J Rheumatol 11:663, 1984
11. Johnson RL, Fink CW, Ziff M: Lymphotoxin formation by lymphocytes and muscle in polymyositis. J Clin Invest 51:2435, 1972
12. Reichlin M, Arnett FC: Multiplicity of antibodies in myositis sera. Arthritis Rheum 27:1150, 1984

CHAPTER 8.5
Systemic Sclerosis

Frederick M. Wigley

Systemic sclerosis (SS) is a chronic disease of unknown etiology characterized by sclerosis of the skin and subcutaneous tissue (scleroderma) and peripheral vascular instability (Raynaud phenomenon), as well as alteration in various internal organs, especially the lungs, heart, gastrointestinal tract, and kidneys.[7,10,11] Immunologic abnormalities are common but are generally nondiagnostic and clinically silent.[3]

Systemic sclerosis is not a rare disease, occurring somewhat less frequently than SLE but more commonly than polyarteritis or dermatomyositis. Women are affected twice as often as men, most commonly in the third to sixth decades of life.[4] Several possible associations of SS with genes of the major histocompatibility complex and an increasing number of familial cases have been reported, but no specific genetic factors have been identified.

CLINICAL MANIFESTATIONS

Raynaud phenomenon, present in 80 percent of patients with SS, is the most common presenting symptom, often preceding all other manifestations by years. Less frequently, patients may first note skin thickening and diffuse edema of the hands. Vague weakness, weight loss, fatigability, arthralgias, and musculoskeletal aching and stiffness are common early symptoms. Fever is uncommon and, when present, usually reflects an intercurrent process or overlap syndrome.

RAYNAUD PHENOMENON[9]

Raynaud phenomenon is characterized by reversible vasospasm of the digital vessels induced by cold exposure or emotional stress. Episodes are manifested by digital pallor and cyanosis associated with numbness and occasionally pain. The most common situation in which Raynaud phenomenon occurs is in primary Raynaud disease, in which no underlying cause or associated rheumatic disease can be defined. Local thickening of the skin and loss of the distal digital pad (sclerodactyly) is not specific for SS, but digital ischemia, ulceration and, rarely, gangrene are the most frequent complications of secondary forms of Raynaud phenomenon.[5] The complete picture of SS or another rheumatic disease may become evident following years of Raynaud phenomenon alone.

Raynaud phenomenon may be the peripheral manifestation of systemic vasospasm. It has been associated with migraine headache, atypical angina, and primary pulmonary hypertension. In patients with SS, studies have demonstrated that vasospasm likely occurs in the pulmonary, cardiac, and renal vessels.

SKIN AND MUCOUS MEMBRANES[7]

The skin and subcutaneous tissues are affected in most patients, although cases of systemic sclerosis without scleroderma are seen rarely.[8] Symmetric changes usually first appear in the distal portions of the extremities (especially the upper) and progress centrally. Initially, the skin is shiny and edematous. Later it becomes waxy, taut, and atrophic with diminished elasticity, sweating, and hair growth. The taut and thickened skin becomes bound to underlying structures, and contractures develop, which may limit skeletal movement. Facial involvement may result in a fixed expression with pursed lips, loss of normal wrinkling, and inability to close the eyelids tightly or fully open the mouth. A diffuse increase in skin pigmentation, as well as spotty areas of depigmentation, may characterize the involved sites. Telangiectases are common and often involve the mucous membranes of the mouth and lips as well as the skin of digits, nailfolds, palms, and trunk. Calcific deposits are sometimes present in subcutaneous tissue (calcinosis) but often escape detection except on radiographic examination.

The CREST syndrome (calcinosis, Raynaud phenomenon, esophageal dysfunction, sclerodactyly, telangiectasia) defines a variant of systemic sclerosis with limited skin involvement (fingers and face), fewer internal organ abnormalities, and a relatively benign course.

LUNGS

Pulmonary involvement is present in more than 70 percent of cases but is often asymptomatic, detected primarily by radiograph or pulmonary function tests.[2] When radiographic or severe pulmonary function abnormalities are present, the 5-year mortality rate approaches 50 percent. Episodic nonproductive cough is the earliest symptom; dyspnea is a late manifestation. Symptomatic pleurisy, effusion, or pneumothorax are rare. Bibasilar end-inspiratory rales due to pulmonary fibrosis are characteristic. The usual radiographic finding is a reticular or mottled infiltrate in the lower two thirds of the lung field.

A restrictive ventilatory defect with reduced lung volumes, or a low diffusing capacity, or both, is the most common abnormality seen with pulmonary function testing. A considerable variability in the course of pulmonary function exists; some cases improve, most slowly progress, and uncommonly rapid deterioration is seen. Severe Raynaud phenomenon, and a diffusing capacity of less than 40 percent of the predicted value have been associated with poor outcome.[2]

Pulmonary hypertension with cor pulmonale may exist as a result of extensive pulmonary fibrosis or secondary to direct involvement of the pulmonary vessels (Chapter 2.6). Obstructive airway disease, pulmonary infections, and respiratory failure secondary to myositis may also occur. The incidence of lung cancer is greater in patients with SS than in the general population.

CARDIAC MANIFESTATIONS

Primary cardiac involvement is present in up to 50 percent of patients at postmortem examination. Focal myocardial lesions, including contraction band necrosis and replacement fibrosis in the absence of changes in intramyocardial vessels, is characteristic. Congestive heart failure, cardiomegaly, arrhythmias, conduction defects, and sudden death can occur. Pericarditis is also common but is usually not apparent clinically. Right ventricular failure resulting from pulmonary hypertension is a major cause of mortality. Pathologic changes have been related to Raynaud phenomenon of myocardial vessels and subsequent tissue necrosis.

GASTROINTESTINAL MANIFESTATIONS

Although the gastrointestinal tract is almost always involved in SS, many patients are asymptomatic. Heartburn, dysphagia, and substernal or epigastric fullness are frequent complaints associated with esophageal dysmotility and gastroesophageal reflux. Esophagitis, peptic ulceration, and stricture formation are late complications. The characteristic physiologic changes found by manometric studies include diminution of peristaltic pressure in the distal two thirds of the esophagus and incompetence of the cardioesophageal sphincter. Delayed gastric emptying may also potentiate esophageal reflux. Dysmotility of the small and large intestine can present as abdominal discomfort, bloating, distention, or intermittent diarrhea alternating with constipation. Acute or chronic "pseudo-obstruction," true colonic impaction, or malabsorption secondary to bacterial overgrowth may occur. Radiographic studies may demonstrate dilation, delayed transient time, or large saccular dilations (pseudodiverticula). Rarely, in advanced intestinal disease, linear striates of gas within the bowel wall or pneumoperitoneum (pneumatosis cystoides intestinalis) occurs. Gastrointestinal involvement is a major cause of serious morbidity but an uncommon cause of death in systemic sclerosis.

The mechanism of motor abnormalities remains incompletely understood, but esophageal motility dysfunction has been closely linked to Raynaud phenomenon, which suggests a neurovascular defect. Impaired neuromuscular transmission and progressive atrophy of smooth muscle have been demonstrated as the major abnormalities of the bowel seen in systemic sclerosis.

KIDNEY MANIFESTATIONS[1]

Renal involvement, the major cause of death from SS, is evidenced by proteinuria, abnormalities of the urinary sediment, hypertension, and progressive renal failure. The scleroderma kidney is usually a late manifestation of SS, but in a few patients it occurs early with the abrupt onset of malignant hypertension. Sudden deterioration of renal function is usually associated with high renin levels. Biopsy reveals vascular lesions similar to those seen in malignant hypertension or allograft rejection. Occasionally, areas of cortical infarction are encountered. Renal involvement carries a grave prognosis.

MUSCULOSKELETAL MANIFESTATIONS

Polyarthralgia, stiffness, and occasionally a frank arthritis with inflammatory synovial fluid may occur, usually in the fingers, wrists, and knees.[7] Associated tenosynovitis gives rise to leathery friction rubs on motion.

Muscle weakness can occur secondary to loss of normal musculoskeletal use, malnutrition, or muscle atrophy and fibrosis. An inflammatory myositis can also be seen that is indistinguishable on muscle biopsy from polymyositis alone.

LABORATORY FINDINGS

Abnormal laboratory findings are often due to complications of visceral involvement. A mild normochromic, normocytic anemia may be present, or iron deficiency can develop secondary to esophagitis and upper gastrointestinal blood loss. Deficiency of vitamin B_{12}, or folate, or both, associated with malabsorption and bacterial overgrowth can accompany malnutrition. Proteinuria, azotemia, rapid renal failure, and angiopathic hemolytic anemia may occur as a manifestation of malignant hypertension.

A variety of immunologic abnormalities are found in systemic sclerosis. Hypergammaglobulinemia is present in about 50 percent of cases and has been reported in asymptomatic family members. Rheumatoid factor activity is present in 25 percent, and cryoglobulins can be found. Antinuclear antibodies are common, occurring in 40 to 90 percent of patients. Generally the titer is low, and antibodies may be directed against a variety of nuclear antigens that demonstrate a speckled pattern. Antibody directed against a nonhistone nuclear protein (SLC-70) has been found almost solely in patients with systemic sclerosis. Anticentromere antibody is found frequently in individuals with the CREST variant.

PATHOGENESIS

The cause of systemic sclerosis is unknown. The pathogenesis of the skin and internal organ involvement reflects collagen deposition and diffuse vascular abnormalities. An absolute increase in collagen with normal physical properties is found in the skin. Skin fibroblasts in culture synthesize more collagen than in controls and produce an immature collagen with a higher type III to type I collagen ratio. Cellular immunologic reactions have been postulated to trigger release of mediators that activate fibroblasts to produce excessive amounts of collagen. This theory is supported by the fact that patients with chronic graft-versus-host disease develop sclerodermatous skin and other features of systemic sclerosis. At

the same time, widespread vascular changes and the common occurrence of Raynaud phenomenon suggest that a primary vascular abnormality is present. Recent studies have implicated vasospasm as an initial event in the pathogenesis of renal hypertension, myocardial fibrosis, pulmonary hypertension, and esophageal dysmotility.

DIAGNOSIS

In the early stages of systemic sclerosis it may be difficult to make a specific diagnosis. Raynaud phenomenon may precede objective skin changes by years. Many manifestations of systemic sclerosis mimic other connective tissue disease, especially dermatomyositis, SLE, and rheumatoid arthritis. Overlap syndromes may further confuse the clinical diagnosis. Sclerodactyly, telangiectasia, esophageal dysmotility, and pulmonary fibrosis are not specific for systemic sclerosis; however, scleroderma proximal to the metacarpophalangeal joints, including face, neck, proximal extremities, or trunk, is diagnostic of systemic sclerosis.

Localized scleroderma presents with hardening of the skin similar to that seen in systemic sclerosis; however, Raynaud phenomenon, visceral involvement, and autoantibodies are usually absent. The *morphea* variant may occur as localized or diffuse patches. *Linear scleroderma* presents as streaks involving both skin and underlying structures, including muscle. The prognosis is excellent in these localized forms, but morbidity may be significant.

Eosinophilic fasciitis (Shulman syndrome) may mimic systemic sclerosis with pain, swelling, and induration of the skin and subcutaneous tissue.[12] Careful examination will show the skin to be delicate, overlying deeper masses of inflammatory tissue. Eosinophilia and hyperglobulinemia may be associated with this steroid responsive process. Several cases of aplastic anemia complicating the course have been reported. The diagnosis is established histologically.

Scleroderma must be differentiated from *scleredema,* which occurs commonly in children and young adults and may follow β hemolytic streptococcal infections. Scleredema may also occur in older adults with diabetes mellitus. The skin over the face, neck, and upper trunk usually appears brawny and does not pit. The arms and hands are involved in no more than 10 percent of cases, in contrast to scleroderma. Skin biopsy reveals an accumulation of mucopolysaccharide between the collagen fibers of the dermis. Resolution of the skin lesions begins in several weeks, and most cases clear completely in 18 to 24 months. Raynaud phenomenon does not occur.

Several other diseases may present with *"pseudoscleroderma"* and other features suggestive of systemic sclerosis, including carcinoid syndrome, chronic graft-versus-host disease, porphyria cutanea tarda, scleromyxedema, and exposure to bleomycin or polyvinyl chloride.

COURSE AND PROGNOSIS

Systemic sclerosis follows an extremely variable course. Patients may have persistent progressive disease or long periods of stability or improvement, even without treatment. The CREST variant lies within the spectrum of systemic sclerosis and generally follows a more benign course. Nonwhite females with systemic sclerosis have a higher mortality rate. Renal, cardiac, or pulmonary involvement is associated with a poor prognosis.

MANAGEMENT

No therapy has been proven to effectively alter the course of systemic sclerosis. Supportive measures that include physical therapy, avoidance of cold, the judicious use of sedatives and analgesics, and counseling of both patient and family are most important.

The many therapeutic problems that arise during the course of SS (e.g., heart failure, renal failure, hypertension, malabsorption) should receive the same basic therapy accorded similar physiologic deficits in other settings. For example, antibiotic treatment may dramatically improve intestinal malabsorption thus relieving nutritional anemia and allowing weight gain. The symptoms of reflux esophagitis have been improved by the addition of an H_2 blocker (cimetidine or ranitidine) to traditional methods of reflux treatment. Studies have demonstrated that Raynaud phenomenon may improve following the use of a calcium channel blocker (nifedipine or diltiazem). Sympathectomy and other vasodilators have not proven effective in the treatment of Raynaud phenomenon or the skin changes of SS. The use of the angiotensin-converting enzyme inhibitor, captopril, can reverse scleroderma renal crisis and malignant hypertension and provide sustained control.

Corticosteroids play a definite role only in the treatment of the myositis. They may also have transitory value in the early, edematous phase of scleroderma or in the treatment of rapidly progressive pulmonary disease. Nonsteroidal antiinflammatory drugs can be used to reduce articular symptoms. There is no solid evidence that other drugs (e.g., penicillamine, para-aminobenzoic acid, antimetabolites, or anticoagulants) will alter the course and eventual outcome.

REFERENCES

1. Cannon PJ, Hessar M, et al: The relationship of hypertension and renal failure in scleroderma (progressive systemic sclerosis) to structural and functional abnormalities of the renal cortical circulation. Medicine 53:1, 1974
2. Guttadauria M, Ellman H, et al: Pulmonary function in scleroderma. Arthritis Rheum 20:1072, 1977
3. Haynes DC, Gershwin ME: The immunopathology of progressive systemic sclerosis (PSS). Semin Arthritis Rheum 11:331, 1982
4. Medsger TA, Masi AT: Epidemiology of systemic scleroris. Ann Intern Med 74:714, 1971
5. Norton WL, Nardo JM: Vascular disease in progressive systemic sclerosis (scleroderma). Ann Intern Med 73:317, 1970
6. Peters-Golden M, Wise RA, et al: Clinical and demographic predictors of loss of pulmonary function in systemic sclerosis. Medicine 63:221, 1984
7. Rodnan GP, Fennell RN Jr: Progressive systemic sclerosis. Clin Rheum Dis 5:1, 1979
8. Rodnan GP, Fennell RN Jr: Progressive systemic sclerosis sine scleroderma. JAMA 180:665, 1962
9. Rodnan GP, Myerowitz RL, Justh GO: Morphologic changes in the digital arteries of patients with progressive systemic sclerosis (scleroderma) and Raynaud's phenomenon. Medicine 59:393, 1980
10. Siegel RC: Scleroderma. Med Clin North Am 61:283, 1977
11. Tufanelli DL, Windelmann RK: Systemic scleroderma: A clinical study of 727 cases. Arch Dermatol 84:359, 1961
12. Zuckner J: Eosinophilic fasciitis. Semin Arthritis Rheum 9:228, 1980

CHAPTER 8.6
Sjögren Syndrome
Mary Betty Stevens

The hallmark of Sjögren syndrome is an ocular and oral membrane dryness (the sicca syndrome), which results from an insufficiency of lacriminal, salivary, and mucous gland secretion. Equally characteristic is the variety of serum antibodies to autologous protein and cellular antigens.[2-4] The sicca syndrome may occur alone (primary Sjögren) or in association with rheumatoid arthritis or a connective tissue disorder (secondary Sjögren) such as SLE, SS, or polymyositis.

The sicca syndrome has been found in from 9 to 34 percent of patients with rheumatoid arthritis and seems more prevalent in those with severe and long-standing disease. Women, especially those in the fourth to sixth decades, are affected nine times more often than males. No familial or racial predisposition has been recognized.

CLINICAL MANIFESTATIONS[3,4]

SICCA MANIFESTATIONS

Patients may present with the primary sicca syndrome, or the ocular and oral involvement may develop during the course of rheumatoid arthritis or one of the connective tissue disorders. The eyes are involved in 80 to 90 percent of cases. Patients usually complain of a foreign body sensation or a feeling of grittiness but may also note burning and redness of the eyes or pain from corneal ulceration (keratoconjunctivitis sicca). Decrease in visual acuity is uncommon. The eyes may appear moist and without striking abnormality, even when deficiencies in tear formation are revealed by Schirmer test; slit-lamp examination reveals typical superficial filamentous erosions of the corneal epithelium and areas of punctate keratitis.

Dryness of the mouth (xerostomia) occurs in about 90 percent of cases. Recurrent salivary gland enlargement is characteristic but less common. Patients complain of soreness of the buccal lining, dry mouth, difficulty in eating dry foods, and excessive fluid intake because of impaired formation of saliva. Enlargement of the parotid glands (in 50 percent of cases) and submaxillary glands (in 20 percent) is usually bilaterally symmetric and painless.

Sicca manifestations are not always confined to the conjunctival and buccal membranes. Dryness and scaliness of the skin and decreased sweating may be noted. The entire respiratory tract may be involved, with dryness and crusting of the nose, dry throat, hoarseness, and a nonproductive cough as common symptoms. Gastrointestinal manifestations are uncommon, but achlorhydria is occasionally found and acute pancreatitis occurs rarely, with morphologic changes similar to those found in the salivary glands. Dryness of the vagina is common. Polyuria is frequent and is usually related to excessive fluid intake (to relieve the dry mouth). In a few patients, hyposthenuria unresponsive to water deprivation or vasopressin has been encountered.

SYSTEMIC MANIFESTATIONS

Although the systemic features of secondary Sjögren syndrome are predominantly those of the associated rheumatoid or connective tissue disease, patients with primary Sjögren syndrome may have extraglandular manifestations. Arthralgias and arthritis are common. A myopathy has been reported. Raynaud phenomenon oc-

curs in about 20 percent of cases and, like esophageal aperistalsis, may be encountered without the other features of systemic sclerosis. Vasculitis is common, especially in those patients with antibody to the cytoplasmic Ro(SSA) antigen.[1] Both vasculitis and lymphocytic infiltration can underlie cutaneous, nervous system, lung, and other organ lesions. Lymphadenopathy and organ lymphoid infiltrations can create the picture of pseudolymphoma,[5] usually late in the course of the disease. True lymphoma is an occasional disease outcome.

The association of maternal anti-Ro(SSA)-positive Sjögren syndrome with neonatal lupus supports the immunologic relationship with SLE.

LABORATORY MANIFESTATIONS

A mild anemia is found in about half the cases and leukopenia in up to one third. The erythrocyte sedimentation rate is often increased.

Hyperglobulinemia is noted in most cases. Rheumatoid factor is present in the majority, whether arthritis is observed or not. The sheep-cell agglutination test is positive less frequently than is the latex test using human F II gamma globulin.[3]

A variety of antibodies to tissue antigens that are not organ specific have been demonstrated. Antinuclear factors are present in about 60 percent (fluorescent technique) with LE cells usually found in those with rheumatoid arthritis or SLE. Antibodies to the Ro(SSA) and La(SSB) cytoplasmic antigens are frequent in primary and secondary Sjögren syndrome, especially in patients with vasculitis.[1] Antibodies to salivary or lacrimal gland extracts are not specific.

Isotopic scanning techniques may reveal sialadenitis and sialectasis in glands that are not clinically enlarged, but sicca symptoms are usually present before any radiographic changes are evident.

Salivary gland biopsy reveals normal acini replaced by an extensive lymphoid infiltration. Myoepithelial hyperplasia of the interlobular ducts is associated with proximal ductal dilation. Lip biopsy of minor salivary glands may reveal characteristic inflammatory and infiltrative changes and is a useful, low-risk diagnostic technique.

DIAGNOSIS

The diagnosis of Sjögren syndrome is based primarily on the association of xerophthalmia with xerostomia, often in association with rheumatoid arthritis or a connective tissue disorder.[4] Slit-lamp examination with rose bengal staining of the corneal erosions is necessary to confirm the presence of keratoconjunctivitis sicca. In some patients, especially those with asymmetric lacrimal or salivary gland enlargement, biopsy may be needed to distinguish Sjögren syndrome from sarcoidosis, lymphoma, and other tumors. Although autoantibodies are often present, there is no diagnostic pattern of seroreactivity, but anti-Ro(SSA) is highly associated with primary and secondary Sjögren syndrome and is less frequent in SLE.

COURSE AND PROGNOSIS

In patients with rheumatoid arthritis or one of the connective tissue disorders, the course and prognosis are determined by the underlying disease; the sicca symptoms usually remain mild. The ocular and oral involvement is usually more severe in individuals with the sicca syndrome alone; the late development of cryoglobulinemia, pseudolymphoma, and malignant lymphoma in these patients with primary Sjögren syndrome has been noted.

MANAGEMENT

Much can be accomplished with symptomatic measures to relieve ocular, oral, or mucous membrane dryness. Methylcellulose eye drops ("artificial tears") will relieve conjunctival dryness and prevent corneal erosions, and lozenges of glycerine or gelatin may alleviate oral dryness.

No specific treatment is known to alter the course of the sicca syndrome. Adrenal corticosteroids do not prevent progression of the disorder; their use and cytotoxic drug therapy are only justified in patients with otherwise unexplained (i.e., CNS) major organ involvement.

REFERENCES

1. Alexander EL, Hirsch TJ, et al: Ro(SSA) and La(SSB) antibodies in the clinical spectrum of Sjögren's syndrome. J Rheum 9:239, 1982
2. Anderson LG, Cummings NA, et al: Salivary gland immunoglobulin and rheumatoid factor synthesis in Sjögren's syndrome: Natural history and response to treatment. Am J Med 53:456, 1972
3. Block KJ, Buchanan WW, et al: Sjögren's syndrome, a clinical, pathological and serologic study of 62 cases. Medicine 44:187, 1965
4. Shearn MA: Sjögren's Syndrome. Philadelphia, WB Saunders, 1971
5. Talal N, Sokoloff L, Barth W: Extra-salivary lymphoid abnormalities in Sjögren's syndrome (reticulum cell sarcoma, "pseudolymphoma" macroglobulinemia). Am J Med 43:50, 1967

CHAPTER 8.7
Rheumatoid Arthritis

Thomas M. Zizic

Rheumatoid arthritis is a systemic disease characterized by a chronic proliferative and inflammatory reaction in the synovial membrane that eventually results in erosion and destruction of joint cartilage and supporting structures, giving rise to typical joint deformities and characteristic radiologic abnormalities. Synovial inflammation is accompanied by proliferation of the lining cells, many of which are rich in hydrolytic enzymes. Masses of the inflamed and hypertrophied tissue (pannus) extend into and erode the articular cartilages, especially at their margins, and weaken or destroy soft-tissue structures such as ligaments and tendons.

Another characteristic but less constant feature of rheumatoid arthritis is the rheumatoid granuloma, or rheumatoid nodule. This lesion is most frequently situated in the subcutaneous tissue adjacent to joints but may also occur in the synovial membrane and viscera.

CLINICAL MANIFESTATIONS

INCIDENCE

Rheumatoid arthritis has a world-wide distribution and affects approximately 1 percent of the adult population. The age of onset ranges from infancy to the ninth decade, with the peak being between the ages of 40 and 60. Females are affected twice as frequently as males. Over the age of 50 the sex incidence tends to equalize. Rheumatoid disease appears to be associated with HLA-DR4, suggesting possible hereditary predisposition to abnormal immunologic reactivity, which may be in response to an external etiologic agent as yet undefined. Because HLA-DR4 is associated only with seropositive RA and not seronegative RA, it is possible that these are different diseases.

ARTICULAR MANIFESTATIONS

The onset of rheumatoid arthritis is highly variable, ranging from the abrupt appearance of acute polyarthritis to the gradual development of stiffness and joint changes over a period of months or years. Symptoms may be intermittent, especially during the early course, but more often they are persistent and progressive.

Joint symptoms usually dominate the clinical course. Pain, stiffness, joint swelling, limitation of motion, and loss of function are present in variable degree. Another symptom is the so-called gel phenomenon, or stiffness after rest, which subsides after activity is resumed. Morning stiffness that persists for longer than 30 minutes after rising is often present. Eventually, displacement of normal alignment may result in severe loss of function.

The pattern of joint involvement is also highly variable. It may begin as a monarticular arthritis (usually in a knee) and remain so for months. More commonly, patients present with symmetric involvement of the small joints of the hands, wrists, and feet developing in an additive pattern. The elbows, shoulders, knees, hips, and ankles are also frequently involved, and the temporomandibular, sternoclavicular, and cricoarytenoid joints are occasionally affected, especially late in the course of the disease. Spine involvement is limited chiefly to the upper cervical segments. The symmetry of joint disease, in contrast to many other inflammatory joint disorders, is often complete and is one useful criterion for early diagnosis.

The pattern of rheumatoid arthritis in the hands is frequently characteristic, especially as the disease progresses. The distal interphalangeal (DIP) joints are usually spared but may be involved in children or those with disease onset over the age of 50. Swelling of the proximal interphalangeal (PIP) joints because of synovial and soft-tissue involvement frequently produces a fusiform enlargement of the fingers. Symmetric swelling of the metacarpophalangeal (MCP) joints (especially of the index and third fingers) and of the wrists is even more frequent than PIP involvement. Wrist involvement usually results in diffuse enlargement, soft-tissue swelling, and tenderness, particularly in the area of the ulnar styloids. A soft, boggy synovium with cyst-like prominences is often present over the dorsum of the hands and wrists due to a tenosynovitis of the extensor tendons. Frequently, synovial involvement at the wrist results in carpal tunnel entrapment of the median nerve, which can lead to digital pain, paresthesias, and loss of mus-

cle strength. Tinel sign is helpful in suggesting the diagnosis; it can be established with greater certainty by nerve conduction studies. Because of the limitation of motion in the MCP and PIP joints or both, the inability to make a tight fist is a common feature of rheumatoid hand involvement.

Because rheumatoid arthritis is both an inflammatory and proliferative process, the local tissue signs of acute inflammation are frequently minimal or absent. Thus the continued presence of a thickened synovial membrane or of pain on motion may be the only evidence of active synovitis. The absence of acute inflammatory signs does not mean that eventual joint destruction may not occur.

In most instances, deformity is produced by destruction of the supporting structures of the joint, imbalance of muscle action through atrophy, and tendon rupture or contracture. Ulnar deviation at the MCP joints is highly suggestive of rheumatoid disease. The extensor tendon may slip off the metacarpal head into the ulnar valley as the deformity develops, followed by subluxation of the proximal phalanx toward the palmar surface and to the ulnar side. Also common is hyperextension at the PIP joints with slight flexion at the DIP and MCP joints, the so-called swan-neck deformity. Another frequent alteration is flexion of the PIP joints and hyperextension at the DIP joints (boutonnière deformity). Thumb involvement often occurs at the MCP joint, resulting in flexion and inability to extend this joint. Rheumatoid disease of the foot commonly produces hallux valgus and cock-up toes, with upward displacement of the proximal phalanx at the metatarsophalangeal joint and flexion at the PIP joint of the toes. As a result, weight is borne distally entirely by the metatarsal heads, a frequent cause of pain on walking. Flexion contractures may follow involvement of the knees, hips, and elbows. Knee flexion markedly increases intra-articular pressure and predisposes to development of a popliteal (Baker) cyst. Its dissection mimics thrombophlebitis (i.e., pseudothrombophlebitis syndrome).[8]

EXTRA-ARTICULAR MANIFESTATIONS[3,11]

Rheumatoid arthritis is a systemic disease and may be accompanied by weight loss, low-grade fever, and anemia, as well as a variety of visceral lesions. In some patients these features are striking, but in most, articular disease dominates the clinical picture. Usually the number and severity of extra-articular features correlate with the severity and the duration of the arthritis.

The most characteristic extra-articular manifestation is the rheumatoid granuloma, or subcutaneous nodule. These nodules may be firmly attached to deeper structures or may be freely movable in the subcutaneous tissue. They are usually found over the extensor surfaces or the forearm along the ulnar ridge or in the ulnar bursa. They may be encountered over other pressure points, such as the ischial tuberosities or bony prominences of joints, and may develop along tendons or tendon sheaths. The rheumatoid nodule occurs in up to 35 percent of patients with rheumatoid arthritis and is almost pathognomonic. Nodules clinically and histologically identical to ''rheumatoid'' nodules can occur in systemic lupus erythematosus, and intracutaneous nodules that are histologically identical are found in granuloma annulare.

Lymphadenopathy is present in 25 percent of patients and extensive enough on occasion to suggest the diagnosis of lymphoma. Splenomegaly is present in 5 percent. Felty syndrome (vide infra) is occasionally associated with massive splenic enlargement.

Ocular involvement is not as common in adult rheumatoid arthritis as it is in the juvenile form. Dryness of the eyes accompanied by a foreign body sensation may result from keratitis sicca of secondary Sjögren syndrome (Chapter 8.6). Episcleritis has been observed in cases of rheumatoid arthritis in which necrotizing arteritis has developed. Rarely, granulomatous involvement of the sclera results in thinning and perforation of the eye and loss of vitreous (scleromalacia perforans).

One of the most frequent cardiac manifestations is pericarditis, present in about 25 percent of autopsied patients, but in the 5 percent with clinical manifestations, it may occasionally produce a large effusion and cardiac tamponade. Chronic constrictive pericarditis requiring surgical decortication of the heart is a rare complication.

Cardiac involvement with rheumatoid granulomas may occasionally give rise to arrhythmias. Because of the frequency of other types of cardiac disease in the same age group, certain diagnosis is not possible. Aortitis resulting from similar lesions is an uncommon cause of aortic regurgitation. Rarely unexplained left-sided heart failure may be the first sign of secondary amyloidosis.

Pleuritis occurs occasionally and may produce an effusion characterized by a low glucose content in the absence of any evidence of an infectious process. The complement titer is reduced in the rheumatoid effusion, suggesting immune complex fixation at the local membrane level.

Pulmonary involvement with rheumatoid granulomas is uncommon. Caplan described nodular pulmonary lesions in Welsh miners that in some instances preceded the onset of rheumatoid arthritis (Caplan syndrome); similar findings have also been described in other rheumatoid patients. Pulmonary insufficiency rarely results. Pulmonary fibrosis has been reported; the functional defect is impaired alveolar-capillary gas exchange and decreased diffusion capacity. The presence of laryngeal disease may be indicated by pain, hoarseness, and dysphagia as well as pulmonary function tests that show a reduced maximal breathing capacity, reduced peak inspiratory and expiratory flow rates, and extrathoracic obstruction on a flow volume loop.

Leg ulcers, especially over the malleoli, may develop in longstanding and severe disease. There are probably multiple factors involved in their formation, including inflammatory involvement of the small veins and arterioles.

Vasculitis or arteritis is recognized in approximately 5 to 10 percent of patients with rheumatoid disease and has been shown to be an early event in the development of rheumatoid nodules. The arteritis associated with rheumatoid arthritis may be necrotizing, disseminated, and indistinguishable from classic polyarteritis. More often it occurs in more isolated areas and tends to involve smaller vessels and to pursue a less progressive course. Endarteritis involving the digital vessels occasionally produces small areas of necrosis adjacent to nail margins. More commonly, vasculitis of the nutrient vessels to peripheral nerves may result in peripheral neuropathy, especially in the lower extremities. Occasionally, mesenteric vasculitis may lead to bowel infarction or perforation.

LABORATORY MANIFESTATIONS

HEMATOLOGIC MANIFESTATIONS

Mild anemia occurs in approximately 40 percent of cases. Typically it is the anemia of chronic disease, with a low serum iron and low serum iron-binding capacity. Iron deficiency itself is seen frequently, often as a result of gastrointestinal blood loss. Anemia caused by chronic folic acid deficiency has also been reported; thus, complete evaluation of any anemia is indicated, especially if the hematocrit is 30 percent or less.

Leukocytosis may occur and at times is striking. Leukopenia is also occasionally present—characteristically so in Felty syndrome, in which granulocytes are depleted. Most patients, however, have normal white cell counts. An elevated platelet count, which may accompany highly active disease, and eosinophilia are associated with increased extra-articular manifestations. The erythrocyte sedimentation rate and other acute-phase reactants (including the C-reactive protein) are elevated with active inflammation and are useful laboratory monitors of disease activity.

SEROLOGIC TESTS

Serologic tests for rheumatoid factor have proved helpful in clinical diagnosis and instrumental in the clinical separation of syndromes formerly considered as variants of rheumatoid arthritis. More than 50 percent of patients develop rheumatoid factor within 6 months and 75 percent within 10 months of disease onset. The test is based on the presence of gamma globulin (usually IgM) in rheumatoid serum, which reacts specifically as antibody to altered gamma globulin. Various particles or cells are used as carriers of the aggregated globulin (antigen) from human or animal sources, and the end point is agglutination.

The occurrence of rheumatoid factors is not limited to rheumatoid arthritis, although they occur most frequently and in highest titer in this disease. Rheumatoid factors are found in 5 to 10 percent of healthy individuals, depending on the test used; this incidence increases appreciably with age. Positive test results may also be seen in a variety of other diseases (Table 8.7–1). Titers are usually higher in rheumatoid arthritis than in these other disorders, but there is some overlap. Thus, a positive test is not diagnostic of rheumatoid arthritis and must be interpeted in the light of other clinical information. Despite its lesser sensitivity, the sheep-cell agglutination test (SCAT) is useful because of its greater specificity for rheumatoid arthritis. Rheumatoid factor tests are positive, with few exceptions, in patients with rheumatoid nodules, in those with variant syndromes (i.e., Felty, Sjögren, Caplan), and in most of those with extensive roentgenographic bony erosions. Twenty five to thirty percent of patients with definite rheumatoid arthritis have negative test results in the standard agglutination test systems, as neither high-affinity antibodies to IgG already complexed with IgG in serum nor bivalent antibodies (IgG and IgA) are detectable by agglutination reactions. Elevated levels of IgG rheumatoid factor are confined to patients with rheumatoid arthritis, but depending on the technique, the sensitivity may range from 50 to 85 percent of patients with rheumatoid arthritis, including positivity in more than 60 percent of patients with erosive rheumatoid arthritis who are seronegative for IgM rheumatoid factor.

Lupus erythematosus (LE) cell tests are positive in up to 25 percent of patients with rheumatoid arthritis. Typically, the number of LE cells seen in a preparation is less than in SLE. Antinuclear antibody (ANA) is also present in serum of 10 to 50 percent of patients with rheumatoid arthritis (depending on the technique used) but is also usually in low titer except in patients with severe and long-standing destructive rheumatoid disease or those with vasculitis and Felty and Sjögren syndromes.

Hypocomplementemia is an infrequent finding and has been associated with severe systemic disease and arteritis.[5]

SYNOVIAL FLUID (See Chapter 8.1)

Rheumatoid synovial fluid is characteristically turbid, with reduced viscosity, increased protein content, poor mucin clot, and slightly reduced glucose content. The white cell count is elevated (usually 5000 to 30,000/mm³), with predominantly a polymorphonuclear response at times of active disease. Phagocytes with cytoplasmic inclusions (the so-called RA cells) occur most frequently and abundantly in rheumatoid synovial fluid, although this finding is not specific. Cells with inclusions can be detected on examination of wet smears with high magnification in regular light, phase contrast microscopy, or with a supravital stain, such as 1 percent neutral red. The inclusions have been shown to contain fibrin, cell debris, and in some instances complexes of rheumatoid factor and gamma globulin. The detection of rheumatoid factor in eluates from washed, disrupted synovial fluid leukocytes has been reported. The complement level in rheumatoid synovial fluid is low compared to that in other types of inflammatory joint effusions, especially in relation to the total protein concentration. A low total hemolytic complement:protein ratio or C3 and C4 levels in the synovial fluid (less than 20 percent of serum levels) suggest an immune complex process in the synovium. When in addition the synovial fluid white count is more than 10,000/mm³ (which would be unusually high for SLE), rheumatoid arthritis is suggested as the cause of the immunologic process.

RADIOLOGIC ABNORMALITIES (Fig. 8.7–1)

Early in the course of rheumatoid arthritis no abnormality may be discerned radiographically other than soft-tissue swelling or the visualization of joint effusions. Periarticular osteoporosis is the earliest radiologic feature. The decrease in bone density is probably related to the remarkable increase in local blood flow in and around the inflamed joints and to disuse. In more advanced cases resorption of portions or even all of certain bones may occur. The carpal bones are particularly prone to undergo this change.

Juxta-articular erosions, sometimes having a punched-out appearance, result from replacement of bone at the margins of the articular cartilage by the synovial pannus. They may appear in any joint but are particularly prominent in the metacarpal heads, at the PIP joints, in the carpal bones, in the distal radius, radioulnar joint, and ulnar styloid. Large cystic erosions are sometimes seen in more advanced disease. As the inflammatory process continues, the entire articular cartilage is destroyed, especially in weight-bearing joints. The joint space becomes narrowed and may eventually disappear altogether. Subchondral sclerosis and bony proliferation or secondary degenerative arthritis eventually result. In the late stages of rheumatoid arthritis, the deformities noted grossly may also be observed radiographically.

BIOPSY[2]

The histopathologic changes in the rheumatoid nodule are characteristic but not absolutely diagnostic. Arteritis or vasculitis has been implicated in their production, but in the mature lesion vasculitis is seldom found. Generally, an area of central necrosis and fibrinoid degeneration is surrounded by epithelioid and chronic inflammatory cells in a palisading pattern, which in turn is enveloped by a collagenous capsule with perivascular collections of chronic inflammatory cells.

Muscle or sural nerve biopsy may demonstrate vasculitis. The presence of lymphorrhages in muscle and perivascular round cell infiltration are common in rheumatoid arthritis but are nonspecific findings and not indicative of arteritis. Lymph nodes usually show nonspecific hyperplasia of varying degree.

Synovial biopsy is seldom helpful, because the histologic picture is characteristic only in well-advanced cases. In the acute phase the synovial reaction consists of an inflammatory infiltration, an exudation of fibrin, and an intense proliferation of the superficial cell layers of the synovial membrane. Synovial hypertrophy may result in the formation of multiple villous projections. The lymphocytic and plasma cell infiltration of the deeper layers of the sy-

TABLE 8.7–1. PREVALENCE OF RHEUMATOID FACTOR

Diseases	Percent
Rheumatoid arthritis	80
Systemic lupus erythematosus	45
Systemic sclerosis	30
Subacute bacterial endocarditis	50
Interstitial pulmonary fibrosis	50
Liver disease	40
Waldenström macroglobulinemia	25
Tuberculosis, syphilis, leprosy	20
Sarcoidosis	20

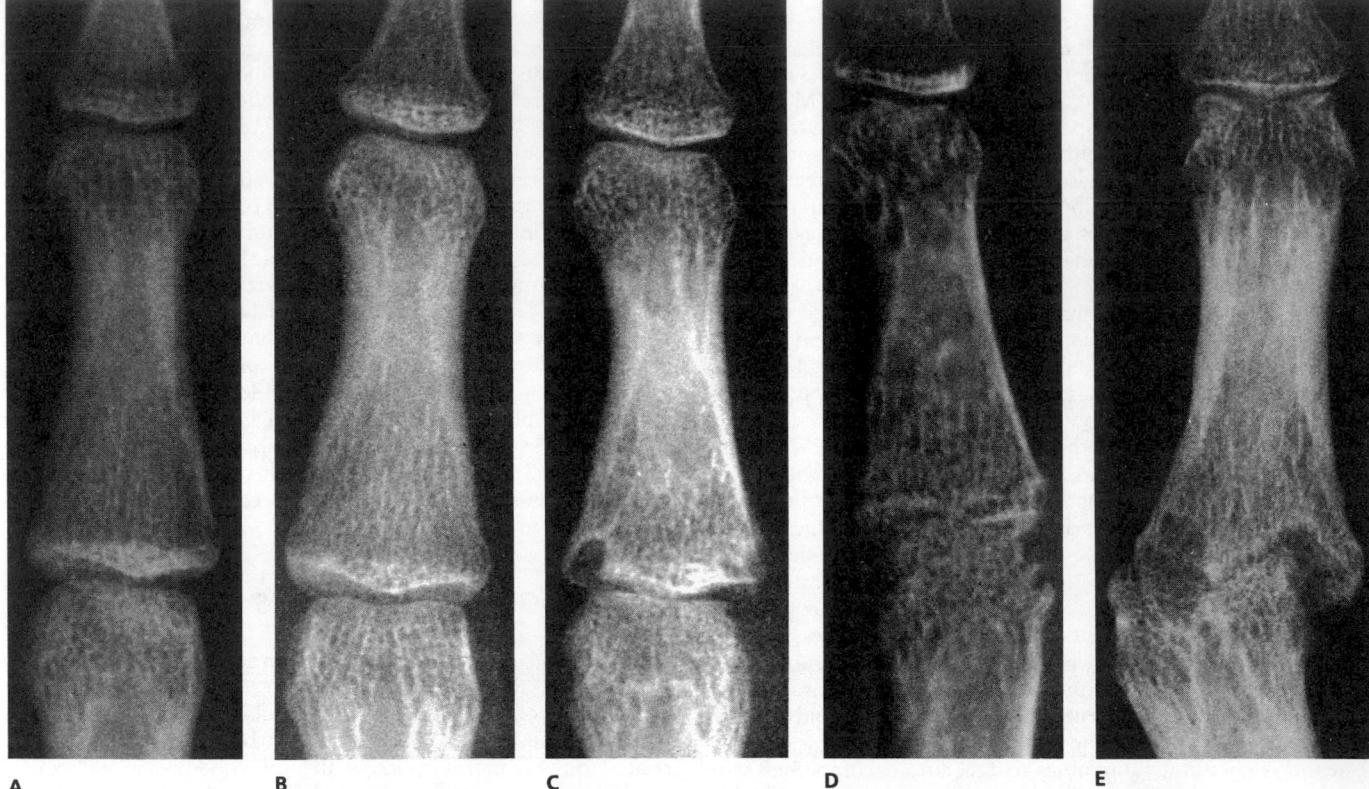

A   B   C   D   E

Figure 8.7–1. Radiologic progression of rheumatoid arthritis. **A.** A normal phalanx for comparison. **B.** Early rheumatoid involvement of a PIP joint in which soft-tissue swelling about the joint is the only abnormality. **C.** In a more advanced lesion there is soft-tissue swelling and periarticular osteoporosis. The joint space is narrowed, and there is a large "punched-out" erosion of the juxta-articular bone of the middle phalanx. In addition, several smaller irregular erosions are present at the articular margins on both sides of the PIP joint. **D.** Pronounced osteoporosis and marked narrowing of the joint space with ragged surface erosions on both sides of the PIP joint. **E.** Late stage shows destruction and erosion of both articular surfaces and underlying bone with subluxation at the PIP joint.

novium and in the regional lymph nodes has been related to the local production of rheumatoid factor.

DIAGNOSIS[7]

The diagnosis of rheumatoid arthritis depends on a combination of clinical, laboratory, and radiologic features that may require weeks, even months, to evolve. The pattern of the arthropathy is most helpful: an additive, symmetric, peripheral, inflammatory joint involvement. When subcutaneous nodules or erosive changes on the radiograph are added to the combination of a symmetric polyarthritis and rheumatoid factor positivity, the diagnosis of rheumatoid arthritis is certain. Rheumatoid factor positivity is a pivotal diagnostic issue, for it is not specific for rheumatoid arthritis and its absence does not rule out that diagnosis (Table 8.7–1). The serologic status must be thoughtfully interpreted in the light of the clinical setting. It is essential to recognize that time and continued observation may be necessary for diagnostic certainty. The diagnosis of rheumatoid arthritis can only be properly considered after 6 to 12 weeks of sustained, peripheral articular inflammation. An acute rheumatoid-like pattern of arthritis can occur with viral infections or associated with connective tissue disorders (e.g., SLE, systemic vasculitis, primary Sjögren syndrome) and, especially in the elderly, tumor syndromes. Thus, to be certain of the diagnosis of rheumatoid arthritis a period of follow-up may often be required, not only to see if the articular process of rheumatoid arthritis be-

comes established but also to allow extra-articular features of non-rheumatoid disorders, if present, to emerge.

COURSE AND PROGNOSIS[6,7]

The course of rheumatoid arthritis is variable, but approximately 60 percent of patients develop some degree of disability. At least a third have periods of remission lasting more than a year. Although the titer of rheumatoid factor does not closely reflect the course of the disease, patients with persistently positive tests (especially with high titers) early in the course of their disease have more severe disease. Patients with subcutaneous nodules and early radiologic signs of destruction have a poor prognosis. Patients with seronegativity and monarthritis or oligoarticular involvement generally do not develop destructive joint disease over an 8-year follow-up period.

Treatment will relieve the acute inflammatory manifestations of rheumatoid arthritis but cannot be considered curative. Because the prognosis for functional capacity and working ability is worse in rheumatoid arthritis than in the other inflammatory joint diseases, aggressive therapy is usually indicated. Fortunately, with aggressive therapy, major disability can be prevented in more than three fourths of patients. Because the course of rheumatoid arthritis is variable, the evaluation of therapeutic agents must be carefully controlled.

MANAGEMENT

The management of patients with rheumatoid arthritis is concerned mainly with suppressing the inflammatory aspects of the disease, preventing musculoskeletal deformity and dysfunction, correcting established deformities, and controlling the extra-articular features of the disease. Of equal importance is general medical care, prompt recognition and treatment of intercurrent illnesses (especially infections), and avoidance of circumstances likely to precipitate disease activity. Similarly, a sound patient-physician relationship is essential to an effective therapeutic program, as patients and their families often equate rheumatoid arthritis with hopeless invalidism and are in need of sensible emotional support and realistic optimism.

GENERAL MEASURES

A program of rest, exercise, and splinting is basic to the treatment of rheumatoid arthritis, irrespective of the drug therapy employed. Proper execution of such a program requires the continued cooperation of patient and physician at times in conjunction with the services of other skilled health professionals, especially orthopedists, physical and occupational therapists, and specialized nurses. Generally, such multidisciplinary services are most readily obtained at large treatment centers; it is important that they be made available early in the course of this disease in order to preserve maximum functional capacity.

Rest is important, especially during more active phases of the disorder; a proper balance of rest and therapeutic (not aimless) exercise is needed to maintain function.

Therapeutic exercises are designed to maintain and improve the range of joint motion and to promote muscular coordination and performance, thereby preventing fixed structural deformities. Both isotonic and isometric exercises are useful, the latter especially in maintaining muscle strength. The alleviation of pain and stiffness through the judicious use of heat and analgesic agents permits maximal participation in an exercise program.

Splinting is useful in managing highly inflamed joints and in preventing contractures and deformities; when these occur, serial casting may be corrective, especially if deformities are soft tissue in origin. Furthermore the use of orthopedic supports and other assistive devices may permit patients to compensate for functional impairments.

DRUG THERAPY

Current drug therapy (Table 8.7–2) cannot cure rheumatoid arthritis; however, when employed with appropriate adjunctive measures, drug treatment can suppress the inflammatory manifestations of the disorder and, in some cases, be associated with prolonged remissions (Table 8.7–1).

Nonsteroidal anti-inflammatory drugs (NSAIDs), a group of organic acid antagonists to prostaglandin synthetase, emerged following the discovery that a major action of aspirin was the inhibition of prostaglandin synthesis. Chemically they are derivatives of indole, enolic, or propionic acid (Table 8.7–2). They may substitute for salicylates when aspirin is not efficacious or not tolerated in adequate dosage. An advantage of the NSAIDs over aspirin is a lower incidence of gastrointestinal side effects. Most of these drugs compete with salicylates, so they are not administered simultaneously. Simultaneous administration also increases the frequency of gastrointestinal side effects. Prescribing drugs with a longer half-life or sustained-release (allowing dosage once or, at most, twice daily) may increase patient compliance.

When salicylates or a NSAID alone fail to control the disease, the next step is to add a *remittive agent* (i.e., an antimalarial, gold,

TABLE 8.7–2. DRUG THERAPY IN RHEUMATOID ARTHRITIS

Drug	Dosage (mg/day)
Antiinflammatory (NSAIDs)	
• *Salicylates*	
Acetylsalicylic acid (aspirin)	3.0–4.5 g
• *Indole Derivatives*	
Indomethacin (Indocin)	75–150
Sulindac (Clinoril)	300–400
Tolmetin sodium (Tolectin)	1200–1800
• *Propionic Acid Derivatives*	
Ibuprofen (Motrin)	1200–3200
Fenoprofen (Nalfon)	2400–3000
Naproxen (Naprosyn)	500–1000
• *Anthranilic Acid Derivatives*	
Meclofenamate sodium (Meclomen)	200–400
• *Enolic Acid Derivative*	
Piroxicam (Feldene)	20
Remittive	
Hydroxychloroquine (Plaquenil)	200
Gold	
Parenteral: Myochrysine, Solganal	[50]
Oral: auranofin	6
Penicillamine	250–750
Methotrexate	[5–15]
Sulfasalazine	500–2000
Corticosteroid	
Prednisone	5–15

[ ] = weekly dosage.

penicillamine, or methotrexate). With each, there is a lag time of several weeks before maximal response can be expected.

Hydroxychloroquine (Plaquenil), in conjunction with an NSAID, may alleviate the inflammation of rheumatoid arthritis, but 4 to 6 months of therapy are often required to achieve maximal benefit. When hydroxychloroquine is administered for prolonged periods (years), a few patients may develop retinal damage, but this is exceedingly rare. If adequate control is not achieved in 6 months, the drug should be discontinued.

Gold therapy (chrysotherapy) is used especially in early progressive rheumatoid disease. The use of *parenteral* gold is associated with improvement in more than half the patients with considerable and lasting improvement for 2 or more years in 20 percent. Several studies have shown less radiologic progression and erosions in patients who have responded clinically. Remission is seldom realized before a total administered dose of 500 mg, and 1.0 g or more may be required (i.e., 10 to 20 weeks of therapy). Maintenance of monthly doses of 50 mg may prolong a remission once obtained. *Oral* gold (auranofin), 3 mg twice daily, has recently been demonstrated to be clinically effective.

The major disadvantage of chrysotherapy is its potential toxicity. Patients should be closely watched, and a careful examination of skin and mucous membranes, urinalysis, and white blood cell count performed before each dose of drug. Most side effects with auranofin affect the lower gastrointestinal tract (abdominal cramps and diarrhea). Serious complications affecting the hematopoietic system and kidneys are less frequent than with intramuscular preparations.

D-penicillamine[4] is another slow-acting or disease-modifying drug approved for the treatment of rheumatoid arthritis. The majority of studies demonstrate the efficacy of penicillamine to be comparable to that of chrysotherapy but with slightly greater toxicity. Immunologic reactions (e.g., Goodpasture syndrome, polymyositis, myasthenia gravis, and lupus-like syndrome) may be induced. Greater caution should be used (i.e., more frequent

monitoring, lower dosages, and longer periods between dosage increments) if patients have a history of adverse reaction to gold, because proteinuria, rashes, and blood dyscrasias tend to recur, especially in HLA-DR3–positive patients with rheumatoid arthritis. Initial doses of 125 to 250 mg are increased by 125 mg bimonthly to a maximum of 750 mg per day.

Recently, there have been several well-controlled trials demonstrating the efficacy of *methotrexate*[12] in rheumatoid patients. There may be a significantly greater response in patients with the HLA-DR2 haplotype. Reasonable efficacy and low adverse reactions (<10 percent) are achieved by using a weekly, low dose of 7.5 to 10 mg per week. Methotrexate acts rapidly compared to gold and D-penicillamine in that at 6 weeks, the proportion of patients with improvement is comparable to that seen with auranofin or intramuscular gold at 6 months. Frequent side effects of methotrexate therapy are stomatitis, mild gastrointestinal irritation, and transiently elevated transaminase levels. Sustained elevation, or transaminase levels of more than twice normal, indicate the drug should be discontinued. Even though it is not oncogenic and is safer than other immunosuppressive drugs, methotrexate can cause unpredictable hepatic cirrhosis, pulmonary toxicity, and marrow toxicity. These effects are, fortunately, rare, but laboratory studies need monitoring at least every 2 to 4 weeks. Methotrexate has not yet been approved by the FDA for use in rheumatoid arthritis.

Recently, double-blind controlled studies comparing *sulfasalazine* with penicillamine and chrysotherapy have demonstrated significant clinical and laboratory improvements with all three drugs and support a disease-modifying action of sulfasalazine. The dose for sulfasalazine is 500 mg initially, increased by 500 mg at weekly intervals to a maintenance dose of 2 g daily. Improvement in clinical parameters generally occur within several months, with a slight lag in laboratory indices. The most frequent adverse effects are nausea, malaise, dyspepsia, and dizziness. Although patients with rheumatoid arthritis appear to tolerate sulfasalazine less well than patients with ulcerative colitis, side effects are frequent but seldom severe.

Adrenal corticosteroids are able to suppress the inflammatory aspects of rheumatoid disease more promptly than other agents now available; however, they are usually not used initially because of the undesirable side effects resulting from long-term administration. Steroid therapy may be considered early when salicylates and physical measures have failed to suppress intensely active and rapidly progressive disease, especially while remittive therapy is being established. Prednisone, in doses not exceeding 5 to 10 mg daily or even on alternate days, may provide necessary relief during this initial period of remittive-agent therapy before maximal benefit from these agents can be expected, after which their tapering to discontinuance is anticipated. Recently, there has been a greater use of a 3–day intravenous "pulse" of corticosteroid to immediately suppress inflammation until response to slow-acting agents takes place. When remission has been effected and maintained for a few weeks, the dose of prednisone should be tapered slowly and steadily until a minimal dose is achieved or the drug discontinued.

The injection of corticosteroids into joints has limited utility. Relief of symptoms may persist for several weeks and permit initiation of physical therapy, but reliance on repeated intra-articular corticosteroids is not advised. In some instances, pyogenic infections or deterioration of the joint have been observed following repeated intra-articular steroid injections.

Cyclophosphamide (Cytoxan) has been shown to be effective in rheumatoid disease, with regression of hypertrophic synovium and erosive changes. *Azathioprine* (Imuran) has also been reported to suppress the rheumatoid process, in some cases producing lasting remission. Nonetheless, these agents are strictly reserved for life-threatening systemic involvement (e.g., arteritis) or crippling articular disease that is refractory to conventional therapy. Only azathioprine has been approved by the FDA for use in rheumatoid arthritis.

ORTHOPEDIC SURGERY[10]

Two types of surgical procedures, synovectomy and joint reconstruction, may help patients with rheumatoid arthritis. Synovectomy appears at times to produce lasting improvement despite continued disease in other joints, but a recent 3-year study showed minimal clinical efficacy and no radiologic evidence of lasting benefit. Although synovectomy may be helpful in a single, refractory painful joint with invasive synovial proliferation and in wrists with threatened extensor tendon rupture, it would not appear to be of major value in general patient management. Recent advances in technique with total joint replacements have enhanced the usefulness of these reconstructive procedures. Relief of intractable pain and return to unassisted ambulation can now be expected from total hip and knee joint replacement.

RHEUMATOID VARIANTS

The variants of rheumatoid arthritis include juvenile rheumatoid arthritis and systemic forms of adult disease (i.e., rheumatoid arthritis with vasculitis and the syndromes of Felty, Sjögren, and Caplan). Only the frequently encountered juvenile-onset rheumatoid arthritis and Felty syndrome are discussed here. (See Chapter 8.6 for a discussion of Sjögren syndrome.)

JUVENILE RHEUMATOID ARTHRITIS[1]

Juvenile rheumatoid arthritis (JRA) is a chronic process with onset usually before the age of 16 and thought by most to be the childhood equivalent of adult rheumatoid arthritis. There are several basic similarities, and some patients continue to have active rheumatoid-like arthritis into adulthood.

Patients with JRA present in one of three ways: (1) a systemic illness, (2) a polyarthritis, or (3) involvement of one or at most very few (oligoarticular) inflamed joints. Those with onset of disease in early childhood commonly have the systemic form (Still disease). In this syndrome, joint symptoms are often overshadowed by a high, spiking fever (often double quotidian), erythematous rash, pleuropericarditis, splenomegaly, and generalized lymphadenopathy. The absence of renal disease, central nervous system involvement, and LE cells differentiate the disorder from SLE. Arthritis, which occurs in most cases, may be late to appear; thus the disease may present as an obscure febrile illness. The typical rash and the characteristic fever may suggest the correct diagnosis. Cervical spine involvement is common. Patients between the ages of 9 and 15 often present with polyarthritis and some deformity in the absence of marked systemic symptoms.

It is in the oligoarticular group that iridocyclitis occurs, which can result in visual loss. Ocular involvement does not necessarily coincide with active joint disease and is frequently associated with serum antinuclear antibody.

Some of those with disease onset in adolescence will have monarticular or oligoarticular arthritis. The significant association of HLA-B27 in boys with late-onset oligoarticular disease emphasizes the heterogeneity of juvenile chronic arthritis (see Chapter 8.9).

The overall prognosis in JRA is good, especially in those with monarticular involvement. Prolonged remissions are common; complete remission may occur, but in some, severely crippling deformities result. Amyloidosis is occasionally encountered, especially in Still disease.

Management is similar to that of adult rheumatoid arthritis. Salicylates alone or in combination with gold are the regimens of choice for most patients. Those with iridocyclitis should be promptly treated with corticosteroids to prevent blindness. The use of corticosteroids carries the additional hazard of altered normal growth in children. Preliminary studies with penicillamine sug-

gest that it may be of benefit in patients who do not benefit from treatment with gold. The slow-acting agents are reserved for children with an adult type of rheumatoid polyarthritis.

FELTY SYNDROME[7]

Rheumatoid arthritis, splenomegaly, and leukopenia (neutropenia) constitute the triad of Felty syndrome, which presents special problems.

Felty syndrome occurs equally in males and females. It usually begins after age 50 and is rare before age 35. Typical rheumatoid arthritis usually precedes splenomegaly and leukopenia by years. Arthritis is usually severe and associated with significant deformity but may be relatively inactive. The extra-articular manifestations of rheumatoid disease are frequently prominent in Felty syndrome. Severe weight loss and fever, sometimes episodic, may occur. Rheumatoid nodules occur more often than in uncomplicated rheumatoid arthritis. Leg ulcers and keratitis sicca are common. The spleen is usually only slightly enlarged but may be massive, suggesting lymphoma or chronic leukemia.

There is increased susceptibility to infection in Felty syndrome, but infections, when present, respond appropriately to antibiotics. Patients can mobilize granulocytes (although at a delayed rate) at local sites of infection despite their paucity in the circulation (fewer than 1500 WBC/mm³). In severe cases, mature granulocytes are virtually absent from the circulation and total white cell counts of fewer than 1000/mm³ are encountered. Anemia is moderate and rarely hemolytic. Thrombocytopenia may occur, although it is seldom severe enough to cause purpura. The bone marrow is cellular and shows a maturation arrest in the granulocytic series. Rheumatoid factor tests are invariably positive and occasionally in very high titer. Lupus erythematosus cells and antinuclear antibodies are also more common than in uncomplicated rheumatoid arthritis.

The basic management of patients with Felty syndrome is similar to that of patients with rheumatoid arthritis, with the frequent occurrence of infection in some posing an additional problem. Several reports have indicated striking improvement following splenectomy relative to reversal of the hematologic abnormalities, healing of ankle ulcers, and occasionally a cessation of infection. Such favorable results, however, if obtained, may be temporary. Recently, improvement in these features of Felty syndrome has been reported with chrysotherapy.

REFERENCES

1. Bujak JS, Aptekar RG, et al: Juvenile rheumatoid arthritis presenting in the adult as fever of unknown origin. Medicine 52:431, 1973
2. Goldenberg DL, Cohen AS: Synovial membrane histopathology in the differential diagnosis of rheumatoid arthritis. Medicine 57:239, 1978
3. Gordon DA, Stein JL, Broder I: The extra-articular features of rheumatoid arthritis. A systemic analysis of 127 cases. Am J Med 54:445, 1973
4. Hochberg MC: Auranofin or D-penicillamine in the treatment of rheumatoid arthritis. Ann Intern Med 105:528, 1986
5. Hunder GG, McDuffie FC: Hypocomplementemia in rheumatoid arthritis. Am J Med 54:461, 1973
6. Jacoby RK, Jayson MIV, Cosh JA: Onset, early stages and prognosis of rheumatoid arthritis: A clinical study of 100 patients with 11 year follow-up. Br Med J 2:96, 1973
7. Kaarela K: Prognostic factors and diagnostic criteria in early rheumatoid arthritis. Scan J Rheum 57(suppl):3, 1985
8. Katz RS, Zizic TM, et al: The pseudothrombophlebitis syndrome. Medicine 56:151, 1977
9. Mason DT, Morris JJ: The variable features of Felty's syndrome: Review of the literature and report of a case with massive splenomegaly. Am J Med 36:463, 1964
10. Mowat AG (ed): Surgical management of rheumatoid arthritis. Clin Rheum Dis 4, 1978
11. Vollertsen RS, Conn DL, et al: Rheumatoid vasculitis: Survival and associated risk factors. Medicine 65:365, 1986
12. Weinblatt ME, Coblyn JS, et al: Efficacy of low-dose methotrexate in rheumatoid arthritis. N Engl J Med 312:818, 1985

CHAPTER 8.8
Differential Diagnosis of Multisystem Disease

Mary Betty Stevens

The protean nature of the clinical manifestations of diseases with immunologic features results in their many varied presentations. The illness that appears at the onset may suggest that a single organ is principally involved, or there may be a confusing array of symptoms involving multiple organ systems. There are, however, certain patterns that occur repeatedly and that can alert the physician to the fact that one of these diseases is present. Certain clinical manifestations, occurring singly or in combination, signal the possibility that the patient may have a multisystem connective tissue disease (Table 8.8–1).

In evaluating the patient's presenting problem, one should keep in mind certain characteristic features of multisystem diseases with immunologic abnormalities, including:

1. Multiplicity of organ involvement
2. Chronicity of the illness combined with repeated failure to find a specific cause
3. Episodicity, with periods of activity interspersed with periods of spontaneous improvement
4. The tendency for some organs to be involved more than others and for this involvement to be the dominant feature of the disease for months or years

Additional problems are presented by the patient with a known connective tissue disease in whom an acute illness develops, a frequent event in the patient who is receiving one or more therapeutic agents. In such a circumstance the physician must ask several specific questions:

1. Is the acute illness the result of an exacerbation of the underlying disease, for example, SLE? If so, is it a spontaneous event? Is it a result of inadequate treatment? Was it precipitated by an infection or some other antigenic exposure, such as to a drug?
2. Is the present episode caused by the concurrent development of another type of "autoimmune" disease, for example, the appearance of Hashimoto disease in a patient with SLE or rheumatoid arthritis?
3. Is it a complication of concomitant treatment, for example, vertebral collapse, aseptic necrosis, or diabetes in a patient receiving high doses of an adrenal corticosteroid?

4. Is it a completely new and unrelated event? The connective tissue diseases may mimic many other diseases; it is easy to mistakenly attribute a new manifestation to the underlying chronic illness. For example, a patient with classic SLE who had been followed for many years developed jacksonian fits that were found to be caused by a meningioma, not by SLE. Similarly, a pleural effusion can be tuberculous or a joint septic rather than expressions of activity of underlying SLE or rheumatoid arthritis.

One of the most important principles in the consideration of the patient with multiple system manifestations is to rule out other diseases that may present in a similar fashion, particularly those that can be effectively treated. Only then can the diagnosis of a connective tissue disease be accepted. Some of the particular illnesses that must be considered in the study of this type of problem are listed in Table 8.8–2.

DIFFERENTIAL DIAGNOSIS AMONG DISEASES WITH IMMUNOLOGIC FEATURES

In the majority of cases, differential diagnosis can be made on the basis of the dominant clinical disease pattern. Most helpful is the presence or absence of manifestations, especially in certain combinations, that have a high degree of association with a particular clinical syndrome. For example, two young women are seen who have recently developed erythematous eruptions in a butterfly distribution, fever, diffuse muscle aching, and acute polyarthritis. In addition to these common symptoms, however, one patient has a history of several unexplained febrile episodes in the recent past with pleuritic pain, and laboratory investigations reveal microscopic hematuria, proteinuria, and antinuclear antibodies. With this combination of findings there can be little doubt that the diagnosis is SLE. In the other patient, weakness of the proximal muscle groups is demonstrated on examination, and serum transaminase concentrations are found to be increased. This clinical pattern is most compatible with dermatomyositis, rather than with SLE. SLE can be excluded with a greater degree of certainty in the absence of LE cells or of a high titer of antinuclear antibodies or hypocomplementemia. Thus, making a differential diagnosis of these disorders usually requires carefully assembling and analyzing clinical data, summarizing the features present, and adding significant negative information. A summary of some of the manifestations that may be useful in distinguishing these disorders is presented in Table 8.8–3.

TABLE 8.8–1. PRESENTING MANIFESTATIONS THAT MAY SUGGEST THE DIAGNOSIS OF A SYSTEMIC RHEUMATIC DISEASE

- Fever of unexplained origin
- Arthralgia or arthritis
- Myalgia or myositis
- Noninfectious pleuritis, pericarditis, or peritonitis
- Skin lesions, in particular erythema, nodules, purpura; membrane ulcerations
- Raynaud phenomenon or peripheral vasculitis
- Valvulitis or myocarditis
- Pneumonitis or pulmonary infiltration unresponsive to antibiotics
- Glomerulonephritis or nephrotic syndrome
- Peripheral neuropathy, especially mononeuritis multiplex
- Central nervous system manifestations, often localized and transient, which may mimic almost any neurologic syndrome
- Ocular involvement including keratitis, uveitis
- Lymphadenopathy and splenomegaly
- Acute hemolytic anemia, thrombocytopenia, leukopenia, eosinophilia
- Chronic false-positive serologic test for syphilis

TABLE 8.8–2. OTHER MULTISYSTEM DISEASES TO BE CONSIDERED IN THE DIFFERENTIAL DIAGNOSIS OF SYSTEMIC RHEUMATIC DISEASE

Infections
- Pyogenic with metastatic lesions
- Localized infection with multiple systemic manifestations
- Specific infection with multisystem involvement
  Tuberculosis
  Brucellosis
  Mycotic infections
  Syphilis
  Infectious mononucleosis
  Parasitic disease (e.g., trichinosis)
  Whipple disease

Granulomatous Diseases
- Sarcoidosis

Metabolic Diseases
- Porphyria
- Amyloidosis
- Chemical or drug toxicity or hypersensitivity (e.g., lead poisoning)

Neoplasms
- Metastatic neoplastic disease
- Tumors that produce a physiologically active polypeptide: carcinoma of the lung, carcinoid
- Benign atrial myxoma with tumor emboli
- Acute leukemia
- Hodgkin disease
- Lymphosarcoma
- Plasma cell disease, macroglobulinemia

Cardiovascular Disease
- Infective endocarditis with minimal systemic signs of infection
- Intramural thrombi with systemic embolization
- Multiple pulmonary embolization

TRANSITIONAL OR OVERLAP SYNDROMES[1,3,5]

Cases are being described with increasing frequency that have been designated as "transitional" or "overlap" syndromes involving features of SLE, rheumatoid arthritis, progressive systemic sclerosis, dermatomyositis, Sjögren syndrome, polyarteritis nodosa, and thrombotic thrombocytopenic purpura. In these cases the diagnosis of two or more of these diseases is suggested on the basis of the accumulated clinical, serologic, and histologic evidence. Some other patients with antibody to extractable nuclear antigens (ENA, especially RNP), have been diagnosed as having "mixed connective tissue disease," but most of these disorders evolve, with time, into systemic lupus or systemic sclerosis.[2,4]

These overlap syndromes involve many clinical, pathologic, and immunologic manifestations (Tables 8.8–4, 8.8–5, and 8.8–6). Moreover, these manifestations and the sequence in which they emerge present differing clinical problems, which may be of prognostic import.

1. *Manifestations common to more than one of the connective tissue diseases may be present without a characteristic pattern to establish the diagnosis of any single disorder.* Such is often the case early in the course of one of these disorders. For example, a young woman presented with clinical manifestations of Raynaud phenomenon, sclerodactyly, mild polyarthritis, anemia, increased sedimentation rate, and hyperglobulinemia. Latex fixation test results were positive in a titer of 1:640, but a sheep-cell agglutination test was negative. Antinuclear antibodies were demonstrated by the immunofluorescent technique in a titer of 1:80. Diagnoses of systemic sclerosis and SLE were suggested, but there was insufficient evidence to establish a definite diagnosis. Several months later this patient developed pleuritic pain, fever, skin lesions, and LE cells. She undoubtedly had SLE, but the same presenting manifestations

TABLE 8.8–3. SUMMARY OF MANIFESTATIONS THAT MAY BE HELPFUL IN DISTINGUISHING SYSTEMIC RHEUMATIC DISEASES

Disease	Clinical	Laboratory
Systemic lupus erythematosus	Females 8:1 Most common age at onset 15–40 yr Combinations of manifestations, e.g., fever (85%), skin lesions (85%) especially butterfly rash (30%), arthritis or arthralgias (90%), nephritis (60%), pleurisy and/or pericarditis (50%), central nervous system lesions (35%) especially psychosis	LE cells (65%–75%) Antinuclear antibodies (95%) usually in high titer especially anti-nDNA, anti-Sm antibodies Leukopenia (60%) Hemolytic anemia (10%) or positive Coombs test (25%), BFP reaction Low serum complement Basement membrane immunofluorescence on skin biopsy Hematoxylin bodies in lymph node or kidney biopsy (rare) Focal, proliferative or membranous glomerulonephritis on renal biopsy
Progressive systemic sclerosis	Females 2:1 Most common age at onset 20–50 yr Scleroderma present in almost all patients, Raynaud phenomenon (80%), altered intestinal motility, pulmonary fibrosis, myocardial failure, renal failure, occasional myositis and hypertension	Skin biopsy may show typical pattern of scleroderma Anti-Scl 70 and anti-centromere antibodies
Polymyositis (dermatomyositis)	Females 2:1 Most common age at onset 20–50 yr Proximal muscle weakness Heliotrope eruption on face or erythematous rash on extremities especially overlying joints (Gottron sign)	Elevated serum enzymes, such as SGPT, SGOT, CPK, aldolase Muscle biopsy showing inflammatory myopathy Electromyographic findings
Polyarteritis	Males 3:1 Most common age at onset 30–50 yr Combination of manifestations including fever, weight loss, arthralgia, myalgia, pulmonary lesions, nephritis, hypertension, focal infarction of heart, central nervous system, liver, bowel, etc. Peripheral neuropathy, especially mononeuritis multiplex	Leukocytosis Thrombocytosis Eosinophilia Necrotizing arteritis on biopsy
Rheumatoid arthritis	Females 2:1 Most common age at onset 30–50 yr Deforming, additive polyarthritis with radiographic changes, subcutaneous nodules Systemic features include arteritis with leg ulcers and peripheral neuropathy, pericarditis and pleurisy, pulmonary fibrosis, splenomegaly and Felty syndrome, sicca manifestations of Sjögren syndrome	Rheumatoid factors (70%) LE cells (20%) ANA positivity (30%) but usually in low titer Neutropenia (Felty syndrome) Thrombocytosis Hypocomplementemia (rare)
Sjögren syndrome (primary)	Females 4:1 Most common age ≥50 Xerophthalmia and/or xerostomia, salivary gland enlargement Extraglandular features include arthritis, vasculitis, pulmonary dysfunction, renal tubular acidosis, central and peripheral nervous system involvement	Anti-Ro(SSA)/La(SSB) precipitins Rheumatoid factors Antinuclear antibodies Minor salivary gland biopsy with lymphocytic infiltrates

could have been observed with SS. Only careful, continued observation and reevaluation will provide the final answer in such instances.

2. *In the presence of a definite connective tissue disorder, manifestations may develop that are far more characteristic of a second disease process.* The occurrence of a rheumatoid-like arthritis in association with several disorders has already been mentioned. Overlapping immunologic manifestations are the most frequently encountered. The hypothesis that autoantibodies are specific for a certain disease is not tenable (Table 8.8–6). For example, although the LE cell factor is more common in classic SLE, and rheumatoid factor more common in typical rheumatoid arthritis, these antibodies are found in other diseases with considerable frequency and even occasionally in supposedly normal individuals. Thus, an immunologic reaction commonly associated with one disorder does not necessarily alter the diagnosis when it is present in another.

Combinations of overlapping clinical, pathologic, or immunologic manifestations may also occur in patients without altering the basic diagnosis. Thus, the patient with classic rheumatoid arthritis and high-titered antinuclear antibody who develops leukopenia, anemia, and ankle ulcers would still be considered by most authorities to have rheumatoid arthritis, not SLE. Similarly, the diagnosis of systemic sclerosis rather than SLE would be made in the patient with typical scleroderma who has a pericardial effusion and antinuclear antibodies.

3. *Occasionally, one connective tissue disease tends to evolve into another or, less frequently, a complex illness emerges with features entirely characteristic of more than one disorder.* The coexistence of two disor-

TABLE 8.8–4. SOME OF THE OVERLAPPING CLINICAL MANIFESTATIONS OF SYSTEMIC RHEUMATIC DISEASES[a]

Disease	Fever	Erythematous Skin Eruption	Muscle Weakness	Polyarthritis	Sicca Syndrome	Pleurisy or Pericarditis	Pulmonary Fibrosis	Myocardial Disease	Hypertension	Raynaud Phenomenon	Altered Esophageal or Intestinal Motility	Nephritis	Focal Brain Involvement	Leukopenia	Hemolytic Anemia	Thrombocytosis
SLE	++	++	+	++	±	++	−	+	+	+	±	++	+	++	+	−
Polymyositis	+	++	++	±	±	±	±	±	−	±	±	−	−	−	−	±
Polyarteritis	++	±	+	+	±	±	−	+	+	±	−	++	+	−	−	++
Rheumatoid arthritis	±	−	+	++	+	+	±	−	−	±	±	−	−	−	±	+
Systemic sclerosis	−	−	+	±	±	+	+	+	+	++	++	+	−	−	±	±

[a]Estimations of approximate frequency: ++ = >50%; + = >10%; ± = <10%; − = not present.

TABLE 8.8–5. OVERLAPPING PATHOLOGIC MANIFESTATIONS OF SYSTEMIC RHEUMATIC DISEASES[a]

Disease	Myositis	Glomerulonephritis	Lymphocytic Infiltration of Solid Organs	Lymphoid Hyperplasia	Perivascular Inflammation	Vasculitis	Necrotizing Arteritis
SLE	+	++	+	++	+	+	+
Polymyositis	++	−	±	−	+	+	±
Polyarteritis	−	+	−	±	++	++	++
Rheumatoid arthritis	±	−	±	+	+	+	±
Systemic sclerosis	+	+	−	±	+	+	−

[a]Estimations of approximate frequency: ++ = >50%; + = >10%; ± = <10%; − = not present.

TABLE 8.8–6. OVERLAPPING SEROLOGIC MANIFESTATIONS OF SYSTEMIC RHEUMATIC DISEASES[a]

Disease	Hypergammaglobulinemia	LE Cells	ANA	anti-dsDNA	anti-ssDNA	anti-Sm	anti-nRNP	anti-Ro(SSA)[b]	Rheumatoid Factor	Positive Coombs Test	BFP Reaction	Reduced Serum Complement
SLE	++	++	++	++	++	+	+	+	++	+	+	++
Polymyositis	+	±	±	−	±	−	±	−	±	−	−	−
Polyarteritis	±	−	−	−	−	−	−	−	+	−	−	−
Rheumatoid arthritis	+	+	+	−	±	−	±	−	++	−	±	+
Systemic sclerosis	±	±	+	−	−	−	+	−	+	−	±	
Sjögren syndrome (primary)	++	+	+	−	±	−	±	++	+	−	−	−

[a]Estimation of approximate frequency: ++ = >50%; + = >10%; ± = <10%; − = not present.
[b]Especially in Sjögren syndrome (primary and secondary to SLE, RA, other).

ders in a single patient is not uncommon. For example, a patient initially had features of SLE, including fever, arthritis, Raynaud phenomenon, pleurisy, and LE cells. Then sclerodactylia, intestinal motor dysfunction, and pulmonary fibrosis subsequently became the dominant manifestations. This may be interpreted in several ways. The patient may be considered to have one disease (SLE) with overlapping manifestations of another (SS); both diagnoses may be considered applicable; or the diagnostic pattern is incomplete and the patient's disease should be in some intermediate category, such as an "overlap syndrome." The patients with anti-nRNP antibody and the combined features of SLE, scleroderma, and polymyositis are of special interest in this regard.

Another example of a high degree of overlap is the development of a generalized necrotizing arteritis indistinguishable from polyarteritis or of typical SLE, including nephritis, in a patient who has apparently had rheumatoid arthritis for many years.

SIGNIFICANCE OF OVERLAP IN DIAGNOSIS

Continued reevaluation of syndromes that are not clinically well defined is important, because in such situations the exclusion of disorders of known etiology is more difficult. In those patients who defy precise nosologic classification, broad descriptive terms (for example, "incomplete or atypical connective tissue disease

syndrome characterized by nondeforming polyarthritis, Raynaud phenomenon, and antinuclear antibody") or the use of multiple designations (for example, "rheumatoid arthritis and sclerodema") may be required.

Finally, it must be reemphasized that the therapeutic approach to the patient is not determined by a diagnostic label. Thus, in patients with overlap syndromes as in those with well-defined disease entities, management will depend on the type and the severity of clinical manifestations.

REFERENCES

1. Christian CL: Connective tissue disease: Overlap syndromes. In Cohen AS (ed): The Science and Practice of Clinical Medicine Rheumatology, New York, Grune and Stratton, 1979, p 154
2. LeRoy EC, Maricq HR, Kahaleh MB: Undifferentiated connective tissue syndromes (UCTS). Arthritis Rheum 23:341, 1980
3. Nimelstein SH, Brody S, et al: Mixed connective tissue disease: A subsequent evaluation of the original 25 patients. Medicine 59:239, 1980
4. Notman DD, Kirat N, Tan EM: Profiles of antinuclear antibodies in systemic rheumatic diseases. Ann Intern Med 83:464, 1975
5. Sharp GC, Irvin WS, et al: Mixed connective tissue disease—an apparently distinct rheumatic disease syndrome associated with a specific antibody to an extractable nuclear antigen (ENA). Am J Med 52:148, 1972

CHAPTER 8.9
Ankylosing Spondylitis and Related Disorders

Frank C. Arnett, Jr.

Ankylosing spondylitis, Reiter syndrome, and the arthropathies of psoriasis and inflammatory bowel disease share many overlapping clinical, radiographic, and genetic features. Spondylitis and sacroiliitis are prominent articular features in each. Rheumatoid factor and antinuclear antibodies are absent. Furthermore, the histocompatibility antigen HLA-B27 occurs with high frequency in all of these "spondyloarthropathies," lending support to their consideration as a disease group distinct from rheumatoid arthritis.[2,7,8]

ANKYLOSING SPONDYLITIS[10,13]

Ankylosing spondylitis (Marie–Strümpell arthritis) is primarily an inflammatory disease of the spine that produces bony fusion of articular and ligamentous structures. The disease primarily affects men (occurring three times as often as in women) and has its onset in young adult life. Familial clustering is common.

ARTICULAR MANIFESTATIONS

Typically, the onset of back symptoms is insidious. Pain often located in the lumbar or buttock areas may be severe but usually is not and may even be absent. Muscle spasm may be prominent, and tenderness over the sacroiliac joints is often encountered. Stiffness and limitation of motion develop gradually and spread to involve the entire spine in some patients. Characteristically there is a loss of lumbar lordosis; a dorsal kyphosis develops that may reach grotesque proportions. Involvement of the hips with the appearance of flexion contractures is also common. A convenient way to follow the progress of this deformity is to have the patient stand as straight as he can, with his heels to the wall, and to measure the distance from the wall to the occiput. Fusion of the costovertebral joints and the facet joints of the vertebrae limits expansion of the

chest. Because of this, breathing becomes largely diaphragmatic, but ventilatory function is usually not significantly impaired.

Peripheral joint involvement occurs most commonly in the hips and shoulders, with limitation of motion rather than pain. The manubriosternal joint may also be affected. Involvement of other peripheral joints is encountered occasionally, but many patients with such involvement are found to have psoriasis or Reiter syndrome.

EXTRA-ARTICULAR MANIFESTATIONS

Signs of systemic disease in ankylosing spondylitis are rare. An acute polyarthritis, resembling rheumatic fever or juvenile chronic arthritis, sometimes occurs several months or years before back symptoms appear. Iritis occurs in 15 to 25 percent of patients and may precede the development of back symptoms. Rheumatoid nodules do not occur. Fixation of the rib cage and dorsal kyphosis reduces the vital capacity. Rarely, apical fibrosis, with cavitary lesions resembling tuberculosis, is found. Occasionally, aortic regurgitation results from an inflammatory lesion that produces thickening of the aortic root and valvular cusps. Heart block may occur and is sometimes associated with aortic involvement.

LABORATORY FINDINGS

The sedimentation rate is usually elevated in the active phase of the disease, and a mild anemia may occur. Tests for rheumatoid factor are negative. The HLA-B27 histocompatibility antigen is found in 90 percent of patients compared to 8 percent of healthy individuals. Approximately 20 percent of B27-positive individuals develop signs of spondylitis.

RADIOLOGIC FEATURES

Marginal sclerosis, erosions, or fusion of the sacroiliac joints are constant findings and are usually the earliest abnormality detected. Spine involvement includes the facets and apophyseal joints. The disc spaces are well maintained. Marginal sclerosis, erosion, with "squaring" of vertebral bodies, and periosteal reaction are characteristic features. Fusion is accompanied by calcification in the anterior spinal ligament and actual bony bridging of all the vertebral segments, creating the appearance of a "bamboo" spine. Periosteal reaction due to inflammation of ligamentous insertions (enthesitis) also occurs in the pelvis, especially in the ischium, and results in striking radiologic abnormalities.

DIAGNOSIS

Ankylosing spondylitis is characterized primarily by pain, stiffness, and limitation of motion of the spine and by the associated radiologic abnormalities. Certain diagnosis may not be possible before bony ankylosis or typical radiographic findings develop. The occurrence of sacroiliitis in a young man or the association of back pain with iritis may suggest the diagnosis in this early phase. A summary of features helpful in differentiating ankylosing spondylitis from other arthritides of the spine is presented in Table 8.9–1.

COURSE

The disease progresses to spinal fusion in most instances. When fusion is complete, pain often subsides, and if functional position has been maintained, little disability results. Nerve root compression may occur but is rarely a serious problem. Subluxation or fracture of the upper cervical segments, with a consequent compression of the cord, is an unusual but potentially fatal event. Secondary amyloidosis has been reported in a few cases. Aortic regurgitation and complete heart block are also potentially serious but fortunately rare complications.

TABLE 8.9–1. DISTINGUISHING FEATURES OF ARTHRITIS OF THE SPINE

Disease	Age at Onset	Sex	Systemic Symptoms	Peripheral Arthritis	Area of Spine Involved	Radiographic Changes	Other Features
Ankylosing spondylitis	12–40	Males 3:1	±	Hips and shoulders	Entire spine	Obliteration of sacroiliac joints Sclerosis apophyseal joints Dorsal kyphosis Extensive fusion and ligamentous calcification	Negative rheumatoid factor Iritis (15%) HLA-B27 (90%)
Reiter syndrome	Young adults	Males 9:1	+ +	+ +	Sacroiliac joints Usually spotty, asymptomatic apophyseal joint disease	Extensive fusion uncommon except in sacroiliac joints	Eye disease Skin lesions Urethritis Negative rheumatoid factor HLA-B27 (75%)
Psoriatic arthropathy	20–60	Both sexes	+	+ +	Same as Reiter	Same as Reiter	Skin lesions Negative rheumatoid factor HLA-B27 (50%)
Colitic arthropathy	Children and young adults	Both sexes	+	+ +	Same as ankylosing spondylitis	Same as ankylosing spondylitis	Bowel involvement often subtle clinically Erythema nodosum Negative rheumatoid factor HLA-B27 (50%)
Rheumatoid arthritis	Any age	Females 2:1	+	+ +	Upper cervical segments	Erosion, fusion rare Subluxation, cervical spine, especially C1-C2	Rheumatoid factor Negative HLA-B27 Nodules
Osteoarthritis	Over 35	Both sexes	−	±	Cervical and lumbar segments No sacroiliitis	Sclerosis and spur formation Spondylosis	Nerve root compression
Tuberculosis	Usually young adults	Both sexes	+	−	Thoracic or lumbar segments	Destructive lesion in disc space with anterior collapse	Tuberculosis elsewhere
Ochronosis	Over 30	Both sexes	−	+	Diffuse	Disc degeneration and calcification. Secondary degenerative changes	Hereditary alkaptonuria
Other infections	Any age	Both sexes	+	±	Disc space Apophyseal joints Unilateral sacroiliac	No change, or destructive lesions of bone	All rare Brucellosis Syphilis Acute bacterial IV drug abuse

+ + = A frequent or characteristic manifestation; + = usually present but sometimes absent; ± = an occasional finding; − = no association.

MANAGEMENT

The prevention of deformity and the relief of pain are the major goals of therapy. Deformity can usually be prevented by physical therapy, a simple program of exercises or regular swimming, a firm mattress, and a low pillow. Salicylates may be helpful in relieving pain and merit initial trial; however, indomethacin or another NSAID is usually required for satisfactory results. The iritis may respond to topical corticosteroid but occasionally requires systemic administration for control.

REITER SYNDROME[1,3,6,10,11,12]

Reiter syndrome is the most frequent cause of arthritis in young men. Although often considered a venereal disease, venereal transmission has never been proved. Moreover, epidemic Reiter syndrome may follow acute bacillary dysentery or gastrointestinal infection with *Salmonella*, *Yersinia*, or *Campylobacter* species. Genetic factors also play a major role because HLA-B27 occurs in most patients.

CLINICAL MANIFESTATIONS

Although Reiter syndrome classically constitutes the triad of urethritis, arthritis, and conjunctivitis, a diagnosis is also possible without the ocular or urethral findings when characteristic skin lesions are present. These lesions, known as keratodermia blenorrhagica, appear on the palms of the hands and the soles of the feet and occasionally are present on the extremities or trunk. They appear first as erythematous macules and later become hyperkeratotic and indistinguishable from pustular psoriasis. Recent surveys of patients with gonococcal arthritis have failed to show any instances of keratodermia, and it is assumed that the older literature attributing this lesion to gonorrhea was inaccurate. Other skin lesions include circinate balanitis, painless superficial ulcers of the oral mucosa, and nail lesions. Ocular involvement may be only a conjunctivitis, but iritis may develop. Urethritis usually precedes the onset of arthritis by days or weeks and often fails to respond to antibiotic treatment. In some cases the urethral discharge may be overlooked unless examination is performed before urination in the morning. Usually, however, the discharge is quite evident and accompanied by dysuria. Identification of gonorrheal organisms in the urethral discharge does not indicate with certainty that the subsequent arthritis is due to gonorrhea unless the organism is also demonstrated in the joints and the arthritis responds promptly to penicillin.

The joint disease of Reiter syndrome is usually acute in onset and may be monarticular or polyarticular. The lower extremities are most often affected, especially the knees, ankles, and small joints of the feet. Affected digits have a "sausage" shape appearance. Pain in the heels is common and reflects inflammation at tendon insertions (enthesitis). The pattern of joint involvement is characteristically asymmetric. For example, a single PIP joint in one hand, one knee, and the opposite ankle may be affected. The arthritis usually persists for several months and then gradually subsides. Deformity may develop, with recurrent or residual chronic arthritis, but this is seldom as disabling as in rheumatoid arthritis. Chronic synovial thickening is less marked than in rheumatoid arthritis, and some deformity may result from periostitis and new bone formation rather than from joint destruction itself. Spinal involvement is spotty and asymmetric. The sacroiliac articulations are often affected. In contrast to ankylosing spondylitis, fusion and ligamentous calcification are uncommon.

Systemic signs are present to some degree in Reiter syndrome. Fever of 102F to 103F, persisting for days or weeks, may be seen in acute cases. Prolongation of the PR interval and, rarely, heart block may occur. Aortic regurgitation similar to that seen in ankylosing spondylitis has also been described in Reiter syndrome with spondylitis. Rarely, amyloidosis occurs.

LABORATORY STUDIES

Leukocytosis and elevation of sedimentation rate are common. Mild anemia also occurs. Tests for rheumatoid factor and antinuclear factor are negative. Synovial fluid is typically inflammatory, with cell counts up to 60,000/μl. Wright-Giemsa stain of synovial fluid cells may demonstrate a number of large macrophages containing one or more ingested polymorphonuclear leukocytes. More than half the patients will have the HLA-B27 histocompatibility antigen, especially those with chronic disease, iritis, and spondylitis.

RADIOLOGIC FINDINGS

No abnormalities may be noted early in the disease, but periarticular joint erosion closely resembling that of rheumatoid arthritis may develop subsequently. Periosteal reaction is often prominent and may be followed by new bone formation and bony fusion across joints. Periostitis of the os calcis with or without the formation of a calcaneal spur, apparent on lateral films of the foot, is sufficiently characteristic to be of some diagnostic value when present. Radiographic evidence of sacroiliitis and asymmetric spondylitis in association with peripheral arthritis should also suggest the diagnosis of Reiter syndrome.

COURSE

The acute episode usually subsides spontaneously after several weeks or months. Recurrences involving previously unaffected joints may occur at varying intervals, occasionally after a decade or more. Mild chronic symptoms may persist. A report on patients observed for many years suggests that recurrence and some degree of chronic symptoms may be the rule rather than the exception. The overall prognosis, however, is good, and extensive disability and deformity occur infrequently.

Although urethritis, ocular signs, skin lesions, and arthritis usually occur simultaneously in the initial episode, subsequent recurrence of these lesions may occur independently or in incomplete combinations.

MANAGEMENT

The major goal of treatment is the relief of inflammation. Splinting may be helpful. Indomethacin, tolmetin, or another NSAID can be used. Infrequently, moderate doses of adrenal corticosteroids are required. The iritis may respond to local application of steroids. The skin and nail lesions are resistant to therapy but eventually subside in most cases. Occasionally, lesions indistinguishable from psoriasis may persist.

PSORIATIC ARTHROPATHY[4,6,8,9]

Arthritis associated with psoriasis may take one of several clinical forms (see Table 8.9–2). Psoriasis may occur in a patient with typical rheumatoid arthritis with rheumatoid nodules and positive rheumatoid-factor tests. This association is infrequent and probably represents the coincidental occurrence of two rather common diseases.

An arthropathy directly related to psoriasis is now recognized. Psoriatic arthritis is characterized by asymmetric oligoarticular or polyarticular involvements with a predilection for the DIP joints. Distinctive punctate pitting of nails is almost always present. Nodules do not occur in these patients, and test results for rheumatoid factor are negative. The arthritis tends to be spotty in distribution and may be severely destructive or may be mild and minimally disabling. Spine involvement, especially sacroiliitis, is seen in 20 percent of cases.

TABLE 8.9–2. RELATIONSHIPS BETWEEN PSORIASIS AND ARTHRITIS

Clinical Patterns	Comment
Psoriatic arthritis	
• Asymmetric oligoarthritis (usual)	Affects 5–7% of patients with psoriasis
• Symmetric polyarthritis (less commonly)	Pathologic mechanisms probably intimately related
• DIP joint involvement	Severity of skin and joints not always parallel
• Nail pitting	
• "Sausage" digits	
• Sacroiliitis or spondylitis or both	
• Absence of nodules	
• Negative rheumatoid factor	
Rheumatoid arthritis	Coincidental occurrence of two common diseases
• Symmetric polyarthritis	
• Nodules	Each present in 2% of population
• Positive rheumatoid factor	
Gout	Frequency 4%
Hyperuricemia	Frequency 40%
	Probably reflects underlying defect in purine metabolism

Less commonly, psoriasis is associated with a mild rheumatoid-like symmetric arthritis. Patients with this type also do not have rheumatoid nodules or rheumatoid factor. There seems to be no definite correlation between the severity of the psoriasis and that of the arthritis. At times, psoriatic arthritis may be difficult to discriminate from Reiter syndrome.

Elevation of uric acid occurs in many patients with active psoriasis, and an association with gout has been reported.

The approach to the management of psoriatic arthropathy is similar to that employed in other spondyloarthropathies. If satisfactory results cannot be achieved with acetylsalicylic acid, indomethacin or another NSAID, adrenal corticosteroids may be used. Antimalarials, because of their tendency to exacerbate psoriasis, are not given to these patients. An antimetabolite such as methotrexate may control skin and joint symptoms but should be reserved for patients with severe disease.

COLITIC ARTHROPATHY[5,7,8,14]

The term colitic arthropathy has been applied to the arthritis associated with ulcerative colitis and Crohn disease. It is usually an acute process of mild to moderate intensity involving one or more joints. Its activity relates closely to that of the bowel disease. For example, after colectomy this type of arthritis goes into remission and does not recur unless the parent disease develops in the small bowel. Patients with this disorder do not usually develop chronic proliferative synovitis, so residual deformities are rare. Nodules and rheumatoid factors are absent. In childhood the arthritis may precede evidence of colitis. Erythema nodosum is an occasional extraarticular feature that, when present, is a useful aid in the diagnosis of arthritis with inflammatory bowel disease.

Finally, the association of sacroiliitis or spondylitis occurs in nearly 10 percent of patients with colitis, especially in those with HLA-B27 antigen. When these diseases are associated, their courses seem to be independent.

Because colitic arthropathy is usually a relatively mild disorder, it does not often present a difficult therapeutic problem. Salicylates are sufficient to control the symptoms in most cases. When the underlying bowel disease is brought under control, the arthropathy, except for spondylitis, usually subsides. Management of the spondylitis is the same as for ankylosing spondylitis.

JUVENILE CHRONIC ARTHRITIS (JCA)

Chronic arthritis in childhood has previously been termed juvenile rheumatoid arthritis (JRA), despite the broad variability in onset, clinical features, and course. Recent studies have shown that HLA-B27 is found in over one third of these children. The characteristics of this subset include late-childhood onset, male predominance, oligoarticular joint involvement, with subsequent development of sacroiliitis and spondylitis, and acute iritis. Rheumatoid factors and ANA are absent. Thus, this HLA-B27 group of children stands apart from those with JRA and relates more closely to children with ankylosing spondylitis or Reiter syndrome than to adult rheumatoid arthritis.

Therapy consists primarily of salicylates, possibly other NSAIDs, and physical therapy. Corticosteroids are rarely required and, when necessary, should be given on alternate days to minimize growth effects.

REFERENCES

1. Arnett FC, McClusky OE, et al: Incomplete Reiter's syndrome: Discriminating features and HLA-W27 in diagnosis. Ann Intern Med 84:8, 1976
2. Calin A (ed): The Spondyloarthropathies. Orlando, Fla, Grune & Stratton, 1984
3. Ford DK: Reiter's syndrome. Bull Rheum Dis 20:588, 1970
4. Gerber LH, Espinoza LR (eds): Psoriatic Arthritis. Orlando, Fla, Grune & Stratton, 1985
5. Haslock I, Wright V: The musculoskeletal complications of Crohn's disease. Medicine 52:217, 1973
6. McClusky OE, Lordon RE, Arnett FC Jr: HLA-27 in Reiter's syndrome and psoriatic arthritis. A genetic factor in disease susceptibility and expression. J Rheumatol 1:263, 1974
7. McEwen C, DiTata D, et al: Ankylosing spondylitis and spondylitis accompanying ulcerative colitis, regional enteritis, psoriasis and Reiter's disease. Arthritis Rheum 14:291, 1971
8. Moll JMH, Haslock I, et al: Associations between ankylosing spondylitis, psoriatic arthritis, Reiter's disease, and intestinal arthropathies and Behçet's syndrome. Medicine 53:343, 1974
9. Moll JMH, Wright V: Psoriatic arthritis. Semin Arthritis Rheum 3:55, 1973
10. Moller G (ed): Immunology of Reactive Arthritis and Ankylosing Spondylitis. Immunological Reviews, No. 86. Copenhagen, Munksgaard, 1985
11. Noer HR: An "experimental" epidemic of Reiter's syndrome. JAMA 198:693, 1966
12. Sairanen C, Paronen K, Mahonen H: Reiter's syndrome: A follow-up study. Acta Med Scand 185:57, 1969
13. Schlosstein L, Terasaki P, et al: High association of an HLA antigen, W27, with ankylosing spondylitis. N Engl J Med 288:704, 1973
14. Wright V, Watkinson G: The arthritis of ulcerative colitis. Medicine 37:243, 1959

Gout, Pseudogout, and Microcrystalline Synovitis

David S. Newcombe

Deposition of a variety of microcrystals in synovium frequently causes acute, and sometimes chronic, arthritis. The most common clinical disorders associated with microcrystalline synovitis are gout and pseudogout; a definitive diagnosis of these diseases depends on the identification of specific crystals in synovial fluid or, in gout, in tissue deposits (tophi). A self-limited episode of crystal-induced synovitis may follow the intra-articular injection of corticosteroid suspensions; rarely, the psychiatrically ill patient may induce factitious arthritis by injecting talc or face powder in the joints and periarticular tissues. Crystal size and solubility are key to inciting the cellular events.

Careful examination of synovial fluid is essential not only to distinguish specific crystals (Table 8.10–1) but also to differentiate these microcrystals from technical artifacts (e.g., anticoagulants, calcium oxalate, dust particles, and slide sealers) and other substances (e.g., collagen and fibrin fragments) that may mimic them.

MECHANISM OF MICROCRYSTALLINE SYNOVITIS

Acute crystal-induced synovitis results from complex interactions between synovium, factors regulating crystal formation and tissue-binding, phagocytes, and chemical mediators of inflammation.[8] The subsets of microcrystalline synovitis differ primarily with respect to the clinical setting and initial crystal-related event rather than the subsequent cellular process.

In gout, monosodium urate crystals may precipitate in synovium, cartilage, synovial fluid, and soft tissue, whereas in pseudogout, the shedding of crystalline calcium pyrophosphate dihydrate (CPPD) from cartilagenous deposits occurs initially. In both, the tissue macrophage may promote the fluid-phase inflammation through mediator-release after phagocytosis, which can stimulate the ingress of leukocytes into synovial fluid. Alternatively, microcrystals may be directly introduced into synovial fluid through dislodgement from articular deposits by physical trauma, by fluid and ionic shifts that alter their solubility, or by chemical changes in the cartilage matrix. The subsequent phagocytosis of free, insoluble crystals by leukocytes with their release of chemical mediators and lysosomal enzymes parallels the crescendo of the inflammatory reaction clinically. Still unexplained are the "shut-off" mechanisms that limit the acute attack.

GOUT

Gout is a derangement of purine metabolism that results in hyperuricemia, crystalline deposits of urate in tissues (tophi), and recurrent episodes of acute arthritis. There are two well-recognized forms of gout in which the acute arthritis is similar: primary gout, which is related to inborn metabolic errors, and secondary gout, in which hyperuricemia is produced by an increased breakdown of nucleic acids or interference with renal excretion of urate.

Primary gout is largely a disease of adult males. Onset before puberty is rare, and the incidence rises appreciably in early middle age. Primary gout and tophi are rare in women before menopause. In rare cases, primary gout is inherited as an X-linked recessive[2]; but in most cases, the familial occurrence suggests sex-influenced autosomal dominant or multifactorial inheritance.[11] A positive family history of gouty arthritis was obtained in slightly more than 50 percent of patients in one reported series, but in as few as 11 percent in another.[11]

CLINICAL MANIFESTATIONS

Acute Gouty Attack
The onset is abrupt and may follow trauma, surgery, fasting, dietary indiscretion or it may have no discernible stimulus. Intense inflammation develops with surprising rapidity. The patient may report being well on retiring and being unable to walk on arising. The metatarsophalangeal joint of the great toe is a typical site (podagra). Involvement of other joints is also common, especially the ankle, knee, wrist, elbow, and small joints of the hands or feet. Bursitis (especially olecranon) may occur with or without simultaneous joint involvement. The acute episode initially is generally monarticular but may affect several joints at once or in sequence.

Fever (101 to 103F) is often present. The joint involved becomes painful, tender, swollen, and red. Pain is so exquisite that the patient cannot move the affected joint or even bear the weight of bedclothes. The inflammatory process often extends above and below the joint, suggesting in some instances a cellulitis or superficial thrombophlebitis. Extensive effusions may occur in a large joint such as the knee. If no treatment is given, the acute episode will subside in a period of days, leaving no residual changes. Recurrence, however, is characteristic, and the history of repeated episodes of acute arthritis, especially when monarticular, and with symptom-free intervals between attacks, should always suggest the possibility of gout. Recurrent attacks frequently involve the same joint; once recurrence is established, there is wide variation in the frequency and severity of the acute attacks. During the interval between attacks (intercritical gout) patients may have no manifestations of the disease other than hyperuricemia.

Chronic Gouty Arthritis
Chronic gouty arthritis occurs primarily in patients who have tophaceous gout. These patients often have radiographic evidence of urate deposition in bone adjacent to the joints even in the absence of visible or palpable tophi.

Chronic gouty arthritis may cause morning stiffness and pain and swelling of multiple joints. Acute attacks of arthritis continue to occur and are commonly polyarticular. Effusions and synovial thickening may persist after the acute attack subsides. Deformity may result from the deposit of urate in soft tissue or bone. In its chronic and polyarticular form, gout may closely resemble rheumatoid arthritis; however, these disorders rarely occur together.

Extra-articular Features
The formation of soft-tissue deposits of sodium urate (tophi) increases with the severity of hyperuricemia and its duration. Topha-

TABLE 8.10–1. SYNOVIAL FLUID MICROSCOPY

Microcrystals	Birefringence
Calcium pyrophosphate dihydrate (CPPD)	+ weak
Calcium orthophosphate	+ strong
Monosodium urate	− strong
Cholesterol crystals	− strong
Hydroxyapatite aggregates	+/− (?)
Corticosteroid esters	+/− strong

ceous deposits are commonly found in bursae (especially olecranon and prepatellar), in the cartilage of the ear, in tendon sheaths, in articular cartilage and bone, and in soft tissue immediately adjacent to joints.

Tophi may be confused with rheumatoid nodules, especially when they occur on the extensor surface of the forearm in association with polyarticular gout. The gouty nodule is more gritty in consistency and irregular than the rheumatoid nodule, but biopsy may be required to differentiate them. Superficial deposits form hard, small, whitish plaques or nodules that may break through the overlying skin and discharge a chalklike mass of urate crystals.

Deposits of urate in tissue sites may result in damage or dysfunction. A tophus on a heart valve, causing a heart murmur, and in the vocal cord, producing hoarseness and obstruction, are examples of such rare clinical events.

Renal Calculi

About 10 to 20 percent of gouty patients eventually develop urate stones.[11] These are radiolucent unless mixed with calcium salts. Because asymptomatic hyperuricemia may precede acute gouty arthritis, urate stones may be the presenting manifestation of gout. Urate stones may also occur in patients with hyperuricemia who never develop arthritis. Urate renal calculi are more likely to occur in patients with the well-characterized genetic forms of primary gout (e.g., hypoxanthine-guanine phosphoribosyltransferase [HGPRT] deficiency, phosphoribosylpyrophosphate [PRPP] synthetase variants) and secondary gout because of their very high serum and urine concentrations of uric acid.[2,5,6] Following therapy for the primary disorder (e.g., leukemia), a massive precipitation of urate may occur and cause acute renal failure.

Renal Disease and Hypertension

Chronic renal disease may be associated with severe gout, but severe renal insufficiency rarely develops in the absence of hypertension. Multiple factors contribute to gouty nephropathy. The deposit of urates in the renal tubules may cause local obstruction and may predispose to infection. Hypertension and vascular disease may add to the tissue damage.

The relation of hypertension to the renal disease is complex. It is often not clear whether hypertension is a primary event or one secondary to the renal disease. There is a higher prevalence and earlier onset of hypertension in gouty subjects. The study of family members of patients with hyperuricemia and gout suggests that primary gout and hypertension are inherited by separate genetic factors. Aggressive management of hypertension is key, as hypertension is a major cause of morbidity and mortality in patients with gout.

LABORATORY MANIFESTATIONS

Hematologic Findings

Acute gout is usually accompanied by leukocytosis and elevation of the erythrocyte sedimentation rate and other acute-phase reactants. These findings are variable in chronic gouty arthritis.

Hyperuricemia

In the adult, clinically significant hyperuricemia exists when serum urate levels are ≥ 7 mg/dl, with the normal level in women ~ 1 mg/dl lower than in men. Although hyperuricemia is a cardinal feature of primary and secondary gout, it does not establish a diagnosis of gout and is often found in asymptomatic individuals, in those with renal insufficiency, and as a result of drug administration (Table 8.10–2), especially thiazide diuretics. It is also observed in other disorders that may cause joint symptoms, such as psoriasis and sarcoidosis. Asymptomatic hyperuricemia, established by elevated serum urate concentrations on repeated testing, is a common problem requiring careful evaluation to detect the underlying causal factors. In the majority, history and physical examination will identify the cause.

TABLE 8.10–2. DRUGS THAT AFFECT SERUM AND URINARY URIC ACID CONCENTRATIONS[a]

Drugs That May Increase Serum Uric Acid Concentrations
- Small doses of salicylate (< 2 g/24 hr)
- Thiazide diuretics
- Acetazolamide
- Pyrazinamide
- Ethambutol
- Cytotoxic drugs

Drugs That May Decrease Serum Uric Acid Concentrations
- Large doses of salicylates (4–6 g/24 hr)
- Phenylbutazone, oxyphenylbutazone
- Probenecid
- Sulfinpyrazone
- Allopurinol
- Corticosteroids and ACTH
- Coumarin compounds
- Estrogens
- Glyceryl quaiacolate or guaifenesin (Robitussin)
- Organic iodides (contrast dyes)

[a]Colchicine has no effect on serum uric acid.

Analysis of Synovial Fluid

The synovial fluid in acute gout is typical of inflammatory reactions, showing decreased viscosity, poor mucin clot, and polymorphonuclear leukocytosis (5000 to 50,000/μl).[4] Urate crystals can be identified in at least 90 percent of cases and provide the absolute diagnostic criterion. They are not as uniformly needlelike as in tissue tophi but can be identified within white cells or extracellularly by polarized light microscopy. Urates are highly refractile and stand out brightly when the Nicol prisms are crossed and the field is dark. Furthermore, with select filters, urate crystals demonstrate characteristic negative birefringence in compensated polarized light. Urate crystals are difficult to detect with regular light microscopy.

Biopsy

Identification of typical crystalline deposits may be made in a soft-tissue mass or synovial membrane removed by biopsy. The solubility of urates in aqueous solutions requires that absolute alcohol be used as a fixative for their preservation for histologic identification.

Radiologic Abnormalities

There are no radiographic findings in early gout except possible soft-tissue swelling. With continued urate deposition, punched-out, radiolucent areas of varying size develop in the bone adjacent to involved joints. The defects are often larger than those of rheumatoid arthritis and have overhanging margins (Fig. 8.10–1).

DIAGNOSIS

The diagnosis of gout is strongly suggested by the typical attack of acute arthritis, especially involving the great toe, and by the history of recurrent attacks with symptom-free intervals between episodes. A positive family history of primary gout and a history of renal calculi are also important diagnostic leads. The presence of tophi is diagnostic. In most patients the diagnosis rests on the clinical history and physical findings in conjunction with hyperuricemia and the presence of urate crystals in the synovial fluid or tissues.

PATHOGENESIS

Mechanisms of Hyperuricemia

Hyperuricemia represents an imbalance between endogenous production of uric acid (de novo biosynthesis or nucleic acid turnover), dietary intake, and renal or gastrointestinal urate excretion.[6]

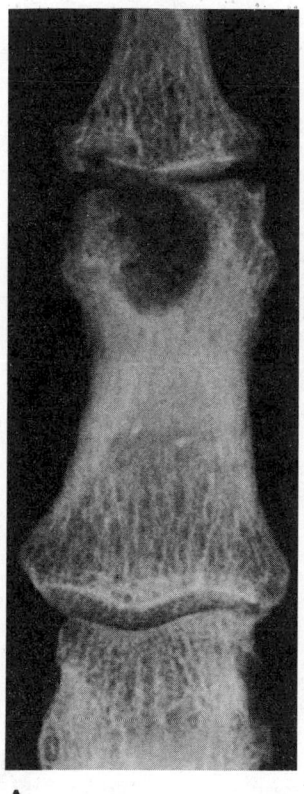
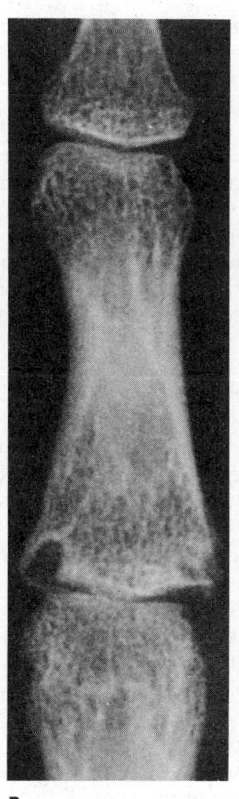
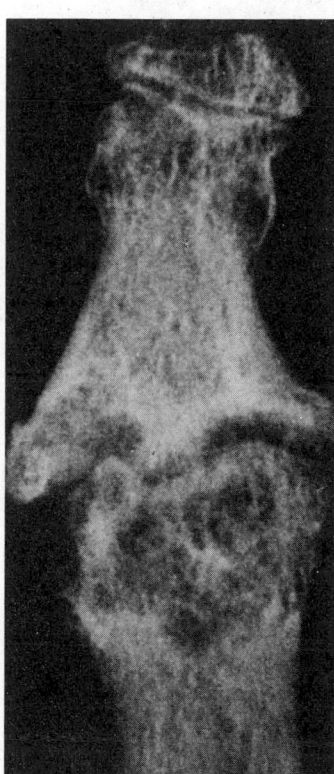

A   B   C

Figure 8.10–1. Comparison of punched-out lesions of gout, rheumatoid arthritis, and degenerative joint disease. **A.** Large punched-out lesion in the phalanx adjacent to and communicating with the distal interphalangeal joint (DIP) in a patient with tophaceous gout. There is no bony reaction around the defect or at the margin of the joint, no osteoporosis, and the joint space is not narrowed. A tophus exists in the adjacent soft tissue, accounting for the soft tissue enlargement. **B.** "Punched-out" erosion at the proximal interphalangeal (PIP) joint of a patient with rheumatoid arthritis. Note also the soft tissue swelling, osteoporosis, narrowing of the joint space, and smaller irregular erosions on both sides of the PIP joint. The DIP joint is not affected. **C.** Lesion of severe degenerative joint disease. There are many punched-out defects or pseudocysts in the bone adjacent to the PIP joint, with narrowing and irregular destruction of the joint space. There is also marked bony proliferation at both margins of the joint with overhanging edges. Soft tissue enlargement corresponds to the bony prominences. Note also similar involvement at the DIP joint.

In humans, only abnormalities of endogenous production or renal excretion are significant pathogenic factors. Primary gout is characterized, at least in a number of gouty subjects, by an overproduction of uric acid. A deficiency in a purine salvage enzyme, HGPRT, has been established as one mechanism of uric acid overproduction. An X-linked partial HGPRT deficiency has been associated with especially severe gouty arthritis of early onset.[2,5,6] Another specific enzyme defect, overactive PRPP synthetase, has been detected in several families.[6,11] This enzyme abnormality is also X-linked and is associated with severe gout and uric acid stones. A renal defect has been suggested in some gouty subjects who are normal or overproducers of uric acid. These examples illustrate that more than one mechanism accounts for the production of hyperuricemia in primary gout.[11,12]

In secondary gout the excessive uric acid is derived from the breakdown of purines or failure in renal excretion. Thus, secondary gout occurs with a variety of diseases associated with an overproduction and destruction of cells, especially blood cells (Table 8.10–3). Serum urate levels in patients with secondary gout are generally higher than in those with primary gout. Secondary gout more often arises as a result of the administration of drugs that interfere with the excretion of urate. It may occur in patients with chronic renal failure and in obese subjects on starvation diets. The hyperuricemia in the last situation may partly result from the competition of ketones and organic acids with urate in the tubular secretion of uric acid. The association of lead and gout has been known since the original description of the disease. Saturnine (lead-associated) gout is prevalent among patients drinking illicit lead-contaminated alcohol as well as those with heavy industrial exposure.[1]

The renal mechanism for the secretion of urate seems to be important in the pathogenesis of gout, as is the effect of various drugs on serum urate concentration. Normally, serum urate is completely filtered at the glomerulus and nearly completely reabsorbed in the proximal tubule.[4,12] An active secretory mechanism, and reabsorption in the distal tubule is responsible for the total urinary urate. This is also a site at which drugs may block urate secretion and promote the retention of urate in the serum. Drugs that are uricosuric act by blocking the reabsorption of urate in the proximal tubule. These drugs also often block tubular secretion but so overwhelm the reabsorption mechanism that the net effect is increased loss of uric acid in the urine. This accounts for the paradoxic effect of such drugs as salicylates, which may cause urate retention at low doses by blocking the tubular secretion mechanism and which are uricosuric at high doses because of their effect on reabsorption.

MANAGEMENT

At the outset, it must be emphasized that the pharmacotherapy of gout must be strictly compartmentalized relative to (1) the acute attack of gouty arthritis, (2) the intercritical period of persisting hyperuricemia, and (3) chronic, sometimes tophaceous, gout. In addition, special problems occur in the patient with asymptomatic hyperuricemia.

The Acute Attack

The aim of therapy for acute gouty arthritis is solely to suppress the acute inflammatory process. Synoviocentesis, essential for diagnosis, may also be of therapeutic benefit. Agents that reduce urate concentration (i.e., uricosuric drugs, allopurinol) should never be instituted during the acute attack or should continue without change in dosage if already being regularly administered when the acute episode occurs.

NSAIDS are the drugs of choice, especially phenylbutazone and indomethacin. Newer NSAIDs have been less well studied but are also efficacious (e.g., tolmetin sodium, ibuprofen, naproxen, piroxicam). Reliance on oral colchicine as the sole agent for treating acute gout has lost favor in view of its gastrointestinal toxicity, but the concomitant use of maintenance colchicine (i.e., 0.5 to 0.6 mg two or three times daily) may be of added benefit. With intolerance for NSAIDs, intra-articular or systemic corticosteroids transiently administered may interrupt the acute attack.

TABLE 8.10–3. HYPERURICEMIC DISORDERS[a]

Decreased Uric Acid Excretion
Renal
• Uremia
• Polycystic kidney
• Lead nephropathy
• Toxemia of pregnancy
• Bartter syndrome

Metabolic
• Hyperparathyroidism
• Hypothyroidism
• Acidosis
• Diabetes insipidus
• Paget disease

Miscellaneous
• Obesity
• Ethanol abuse
• Sarcoidosis
• Chronic berylliosis
• Down syndrome

Increased Uric Acid Production
Genetic
• HGPRTase deficiency
• PRPP synthetase overactivity
• Lesch-Nyhan syndrome
• Glycogen storage disease

Hematologic
• Myeloproliferative disorders
• Lymphoproliferative disorders
• Multiple myeloma
• Polycythemia
• Hemolytic anemia

Miscellaneous
• Obesity
• Ethanol abuse
• Psoriasis
• Solid tumors
• Tissue necrosis
• Convulsions
• Exercise

[a]For drugs, see Table 8.10–2.

After resolution of the acute attack, if it is the first attack, no continued treatment may be indicated. If there is a history of recurrent attacks, the chronic administration of colchicine (1.0 to 1.8 mg daily) may be necessary, especially if uricosuric drugs or allopurinol are to be instituted later. Recent clinical data have described a colchicine-induced myoneuropathy as a relatively common complication in gouty patients with diminished renal function taking modest doses of colchicine (1–1.5 mg/day). Clinical findings include proximal muscle weakness associated with a mild peripheral neuropathy. Laboratory findings demonstrate an increased serum creatinine (>1.6 mg/dl), elevated serum creatine kinase activity (>150 IV/L), and an abnormal electromyographic pattern. Muscle biopsy shows a distinctive lysosomal vacuolar myopathy. Reduction or discontinuance of colchicine results in a dramatic reversal of the muscle weakness that correlates with a return to normal creatine kinase activity.[12]

Intercritical Gout

General Measures. Diet is no longer severely restricted in patients with gout because of the difficulty in maintaining a truly low purine diet, the relatively small effect of normal dietary intake of purines on urate levels, and the greater efficacy of drug therapy in controlling the disease. Only foods very high in purines, such as glandular meats (i.e., liver, sweetbreads), should be limited.

It becomes important to avoid those drugs that promote hyperuricemia when possible. For example, salicylates should not be taken for minor analgesia and, in advance, acetaminophen (Tylenol) or propoxyphene HCl (Darvon) should be provided for such occurrences. The use of thiazide-like diuretics must be monitored in relation to urate levels.

In the obese patient, weight loss regimens should be devised to assure gradual and progressive reductions because of the adverse effects of starvation and the decreased renal urate secretion resulting from severe caloric restriction.

Caution relative to activities that traumatize the joints and periarticular structures should be exercised.

Prophylactic administration of colchicine should be instituted or continued in relation to surgical procedures. Again, analgesics other than aspirin should be provided for pain relief.

Measures to Reduce Urate Levels. Total body urate can be reduced either through enhanced renal excretion or through decreased uric acid production. Although the latter is more biochemically efficient and certain, the use of uricosuric agents has a long record of safety with efficacy over years, even decades, of observation.

Probenecid (0.5 to 1.0 g every 12 hours) is a well-established and safe uricosuric agent. As an alternative, sulfinpyrazone (Anturane) may be effective, but as a short-acting drug, it must be administered at 6-hour intervals with a total daily dose of 0.4 to 0.8 g. The institution of uricosuric drug therapy must be accompanied by forced fluids to prevent intrarenal urate precipitation and renal calculi. Serum uric acid levels must be monitored and the dosage of uricosuric agents adjusted to achieve the therapeutic objective of reducing the serum uric acid level to ≤ 6 mg/dl; and once initiated, uricosuric therapy should be continued indefinitely.

Allopurinol profoundly reduces serum urate by blocking the metabolic pathway of uric acid production through inhibition of xanthine oxidase. Because this agent does not produce its effect through the kidney and actually reduces the renal urate load, it is particularly useful in patients who have renal disease or renal calculi; however, renal stones composed of orotic acid, xanthine and oxipurinol occur (rarely) in patients treated with allopurinol. The initial dose of 100 mg allopurinol twice daily may be gradually increased to 400 to 600 mg daily to achieve the desired effect, but a maintenance dose of 300 mg daily is usually adequate.

The institution of agents to reduce urate levels must be undertaken in patients established on colchicine, 1.0 to 1.8 mg daily, to prevent acute gouty attacks that can otherwise occur with shifts in the urate pool.

Chronic Gouty Arthritis

In the patient with chronic gout, especially tophaceous gout, therapy must be directed against both the microcrystalline synovitis and the metabolic disorder. As in the acute attack, a nonsteroidal antiinflammatory drug and maintenance colchicine are established and then measures to lower urate levels added. Especially in severe tophaceous gout, allopurinol may be used in conjunction with uricosuric agents.

Surgery to remove large tophi that are draining or causing deformity or interfering with normal function is occasionally indicated.

It should be emphasized that chronic tophaceous gout is a preventable disorder in most patients maintained on an appropriate regimen. The most common cause of therapeutic failure in gout is inadequate follow-up and discontinuance of the maintenance drug program.

Asymptomatic Hyperuricemia

Asymptomatic hyperuricemia is a common problem differing from intercritical gout in that there is no evidence by history or examinations of any urate-related tissue damage. The higher the serum urate level, the more likely it is to be secondary to a definable underlying disorder of excretion or production, especially with serum uric acid levels consistently ≥ 13 mg/dl. The 24-hour urine uric acid level should be defined; under normal dietary conditions a

daily excretion of ≥ 1200 mg supports the need for therapy with allopurinol. In those with lower serum and uric acid levels, drug therapy to lower uric acid may be deferred, but patients should be regularly followed and their renal function monitored.

Any underlying disease (Table 8.10–3) should be treated appropriately whenever possible and, similarly, drugs increasing uric acid (Table 8.10–2) avoided. When disease-related therapy (e.g., cytotoxic drugs in malignancy) carries risk of a further increase in uric acid, transient prophylaxis with allopurinol and forced fluids may prevent uric acid calculi and nephropathy.

PSEUDOGOUT

Pseudogout is a microcrystalline synovitis induced by crystals of calcium pyrophosphate dihydrate and associated with calcification of hyaline and fibrocartilage (chondrocalcinosis).[9] More properly, this disorder is named calcium pyrophosphate dihydrate (CPPD) crystal deposition disease. Although the mechanism of cartilage calcification is poorly understood, the association of chondrocalcinosis and pseudogout with an array of disease processes suggests that multiple factors play a role. Although no cause-and-effect relationships have been established, certain genetic (e.g., hemochromatosis, Wilson disease, hypophosphatasia) and metabolic (e.g., hyperparathyroidism, acromegaly, hypothyroidism) disorders have been observed with unusual frequency.[9] Hereditary forms of CPPD disease have now been reported in many nationalities, with an autosomal dominant pattern of inheritance in some.

Pseudogout is rare before the fifth decade and increases in frequency with advancing age, which may help to explain an apparent association with degenerative osteoarthropathy.

CLINICAL MANIFESTATIONS

The term pseudogout was coined to emphasize the acute, episodic, gout-like attacks of synovial inflammation that are so characteristic of the disorder. Unlike gout, the large joints are preferentially involved in CPPD crystal deposition disease, especially the knee, which is the most frequent site of arthritis found in over half the cases. Involvement of the shoulder, hip, wrist, elbow, and MCP joints also occurs; acute inflammation of the first metatarsophalangeal (MTP) joint can mimic gouty podagra. Generally, episodes of pseudogout are less intense and more protracted than those of gout, but they may mimic gout in intensity, duration, and joint involvement. In both disorders, surgery, trauma, and medical stress are common precipitating events, but in pseudogout there are no drug or dietary risk factors. The only extra-articular feature of illness is the low-grade fever that frequently accompanies the acute attack.

In more than half the patients with chondrocalcinosis, multiple joints are involved with a chronic and progressive arthritis in some cases similar to rheumatoid arthritis and in others associated with articular changes indistinguishable from degenerative osteoarthropathy. Flexion contractures, especially of the knees, commonly develop. At least 20 percent of patients with CPPD are asymptomatic with radiographic evidence of chondrocalcinosis alone.

LABORATORY MANIFESTATIONS

Hematologic findings are nonspecific. The sedimentation rate is elevated during acute attacks, and a polymorphonuclear leukocytosis may occur. Serum findings are normal except as related to associated diseases. The finding of hyperuricemia (in ~ 20 percent) or, in the elderly, rheumatoid factor may confuse the picture and often delays diagnosis.

SYNOVIAL FLUID

The synovial fluid in acute pseudogout is typical of an inflammatory process except that a good mucin clot forms on exposure to dilute acetic acid in most instances, indicating a normal or nearly normal hyaluronate concentration. A leukocytosis (2000 to 50,000 cells/μl), predominantly polymorphonuclear, is present, the degree of white cell response relating to the duration and intensity of the acute attack. Intracellular and extracellular crystals of calcium pyrophosphate can be identified in more than 95 percent of effusions with careful examination. In ordinary light microscopy, the needle forms are difficult to distinguish from urate crystals, and even the more characteristic rodlike and rhomboid forms can be easily overlooked. With polarized light, calcium pyrophosphate crystals are not as highly refractive as urates, and, with select filters, calcium pyrophosphate crystals demonstrate weakly positive birefringence.[7]

As in gout, microcrystalline deposits are found in the synovial membrane.

RADIOLOGIC ABNORMALITIES

Chondrocalcinosis is the characteristic finding; linear, sometimes punctate or stippled, calcifications in the fibrocartilagenous menisci of the knees are most frequently seen. Additional common sites of calcification include the radioulnar joint, the symphysis pubis, the articular discs of the sternoclavicular joints, and, in the elbow, the articular cartilage of the humerus and radial head. Clinically, screening of chondrocalcinosis can be adequately realized with radiographs of the knees, pelvis, and wrists.

DIAGNOSIS

CPPD crystal deposition disease is suggested by the recurrent, episodic, intense attacks of arthritis so characteristic of microcrystalline synovitis, and the diagnosis is supported by the radiologic demonstration of chondrocalcinosis. The absolute criterion for diagnosis, however, is the demonstration of calcium pyrophosphate dihydrate crystals in the synovial fluid or synovial membrane of acutely inflamed joints. Diligent search for crystals with polarized light microscopy may be necessary when patients present in the late, subacute stage or with the chronic, polyarticular, rheumatoid-like picture. Diagnosis is especially difficult in those who have concomitant gout and pseudogout. It must be remembered that chondrocalcinosis is far more common in the elderly than the pseudogout syndrome, and synovial fluid analysis is also important to rule out other causes of joint inflammation (e.g., infection).

MANAGEMENT

General Measures
Bed rest is required during the acute episode. For several days thereafter, partial relief of weight bearing is usually necessary when the hip or knee is involved; analogous sparing of mechanical stress on upper extremity joints is essential with their involvement. Physical therapy can be beneficial after the acute attack has completely resolved, as it can maintain muscle strength, assure a maximal functional range of motion, and prevent contractures. Joint protection and avoidance of physical trauma are key in preventing recurrences.

The Acute Attack
As in gout, the aim of therapy is the suppression of the inflammatory synovial reaction; NSAIDs are the treatment of choice. Most experience has been with indomethacin (75 to 150 mg daily) and phenylbutazone (300 to 600 mg daily), either of which administered for several days is efficacious in most patients. The newer NSAIDs are likely to be of similar benefit. The synoviocentesis re-

quired for diagnosis may also reduce the inflammatory reaction; the judicious use of intra-articular corticosteroids is effective.

Chronic Pseudogout

Some patients with CPPD crystal deposition disease have frequently recurring attacks in a single joint or, more often, polyarticular attacks. Symptom-free intervals become less frequent and shorter in duration. Control of the chronic inflammation is attempted with NSAIDs, as in the acute attack. Response to maintenance levels of colchicine is variable and is best reserved for those with coexistent gout.

Asymptomatic Chondrocalcinosis

Because the fundamental defects in chondrocalcinosis are unknown, there is no preventive therapeutic program. Nonetheless, in the asymptomatic individual, as well as those with arthropathy, commonly associated diseases with CPPD should be sought and, if present, appropriately treated. Avoidance of physical trauma and transient NSAID prophylaxis in relation to surgery may prevent episodes of active synovitis.

OTHER MICROCRYSTALLINE DISORDERS

Microcrystalline-induced synovitis can occur with crystals other than monosodium urate and calcium pyrophosphate. The intra-articular injection of crystalline corticosteroid preparations is occasionally followed by a transient, acute arthritis. Even talc, self-administered by the psychiatrically ill patient (factitious arthritis), can evoke synovial inflammation. It would appear that the size and number rather than chemical structure of microcrystals are determinants of inflammation.

Recently recognized is an arthritis associated with hydroxyapatite crystals.[10,12] Although apatite has long been associated with periarticular inflammation and bursitis, these crystals, which are too small to be visualized by ordinary light microscopy, have now been demonstrated in synovial fluid cells and synovial membrane by electron microscopy. Light microscopy clues to the presence of apatite may be found when large clumps of crystals are present and appear as shiny cytoplasmic inclusions or, on Wright stained smears, purple inclusion bodies. In patients with an unexplained,

acute, microcrystalline arthritis, especially if monarticular and large joint, the possibility of hydroxyapatite-induced synovitis merits consideration. Management consists of rest and systemic anti-inflammatory agents or local intra-articular corticosteroids.

Calcium oxalate crystals have been identified in patients with chronic renal disease undergoing hemodialysis and are associated with synovitis of the knees.[3] Stiffness, moderate joint pain, and joint effusion with synovial fluid white cell counts always less than $2000/\mu l$ are characteristic. Serum oxalic acid levels are markedly elevated. No specific management program has been defined for this disorder, and the synovial effusions have been unresponsive to intra-articular steroids.

REFERENCES

1. Batman V, Maesaka JK, et al: The role of lead in gout nephropathy. N Engl J Med 304:520, 1981
2. Greene ML: Clinical features of patients with "partial" deficiency of the X-linked uricaciduria enzyme. Arch Intern Med 130:193, 1972
3. Hoffman GS, Schumacher HR, et al: Calcium oxalate microcrystalline associated arthritis in end-stage renal disease. Ann Intern Med 97:36, 1982
4. Kelley WN (ed): Crystal-induced arthropathies. Clin Rheum Dis vol 3(1), 1977
5. Kelley WN, Greene ML, et al: Hypoxanthine-guanine phosphoribosyltransferase deficiency in gout. Ann Intern Med 70:155, 1969
6. Kelley WN, Weiner IM: Uric Acid. Handbook of Experimental Pharmacology, vol. 51. Berlin, Springer-Verlag, 1978
7. Kohn NN, Hughes RE, et al: The significance of calcium phosphate crystals in the synovial fluid of arthritic patients. II. Identification of crystals. Ann Intern Med 56:738, 1962
8. Malawista SE, Duff GW, et al: Crystal-induced endogenous pyrogen production: A further look at gouty inflammation. Arthritis Rheum 28:1039, 1985
9. McCarty DJ, Silcox DC, et al: Diseases associated with calcium pyrophosphate dihydrate crystal deposition. A controlled study. Am J Med 56:704, 1974
10. Schumacher HR, Smolyo AP, et al: Arthritis associated with apatite crystals. Ann Intern Med 87:411, 1977
11. Wyngaarden JB, Kelley WN: Gout and Hyperuricemia. New York, Grune & Stratton, 1976
12. Twenty-fifth Rheumatism Review of Purine Metabolism, Gout, and Pseudogout. Arthritis Rheum 26:266, 1983

CHAPTER 8.11
Infectious Arthritis

Carol M. Ziminski

ACUTE BACTERIAL ARTHRITIS[3,5,8]

Bacterial infection of the joint usually presents as an acute febrile illness associated with monarticular or, less frequently, polyarticular arthritis. Large joints are primarily affected. Bacterial arthritis is usually acquired by the hematogenous route; the portal of entry is occasionally not evident. Important risk factors include an underlying chronic arthritis, a recent surgical procedure, joint trauma, and drug abuse. Most difficulty in diagnosis is encountered in those patients with an underlying chronic synovitis (e.g., rheumatoid arthritis) that predisposes to infection. In these patients, a superimposed septic joint may mimic a flare in the underlying disease. Furthermore, the underlying disease and its therapy may alter the presenting features of the infection. Factors commonly predisposing to septic arthritis are presented in Table 8.11–1.

Gonococcal Arthritis[7]

Infection with *Neisseria gonorrhoeae* is the leading cause of acute arthritis in young healthy adults, especially women. The incidence in men has been reduced by the use of antibiotics in the treatment of urethral infections, which are often more obvious in men than women. Because the primary infection in women may persist unrecognized and untreated, bacteremia with the seeding of joints is more likely to occur, often in association with menses or pregnancy. The acute attacks may subside in some patients without residual effects.

Migratory polyarthralgia is the common initial manifestation of disseminated gonococcal infection. Polyarthritis is present in approximately 50 percent of patients, but articular manifestations frequently settle in a single joint in which persistent infection is evident. Tenosynovitis, especially of the wrist, is also common, and soft-tissue inflammation may extend well beyond the limits of the

TABLE 8.11–1. PREDISPOSING FACTORS AND ORGANISMS IN SEPTIC ARTHRITIS

Predisposing Factors	Likely Organism
Host	
Children	*Haemophilus, Straphylococcus,* mumps, rubella
Young women (especially with menses, pregnancy)	Gonococcus
Homosexual men	Gonococcus, hepatitis B
Occupational	
Gardeners, florists, miners	Sporotrichosis
Medical personnel	Hepatitis B
Trauma, penetrating	*Staphylococcus*
Underlying Disease	
Rheumatoid arthritis	*Staphylococcus*
Prosthetic joint	*Staphylococcus, Streptococcus,* others
Focal infections (pneumonitis, sinusitis, peridontal sites, endocarditis, etc.)	*Staphylococcus, Streptococcus,* gram-negative (with urinary tract infections)
	Mycobacterium tuberculosis
Systemic disorders	
Systemic lupus	Gram-negative more often than gram-positive, fungal
Diabetes mellitus	Gram-negative, gram-positive, fungal
Myeloproliferative disorders and leukemias	Gram-negative
Multiple myeloma	Pneumococcus, others
Sickle cell disease	Pneumococcus, *Salmonella,* others
Therapy	
Cortiosteroids, cytotoxic and immunosuppressive regimens	Gram-positive, gram-negative, fungal

joint. Skin lesions are frequently observed and may be transient or may persist for several days. They appear most frequently on the forearms, thighs, or adjacent to joints as small macular or papular red spots that do not blanch on pressure. As they evolve, their centers may become vesicular or purulent. Biopsy of these lesions shows an inflammatory vasculitis; organisms are difficult to demonstrate but occasionally may be cultured. Perihepatitis or endocarditis may develop occasionally.

The diagnosis is established by isolating organisms from blood, joint fluid, or skin lesions or may be presumed from the demonstration of gonococci in cervical or urethral smears or cultures. Because of the fastidious growth requirements of the organisms, careful cultural techniques (including the inoculation of media at the bedside) may be required for their demonstration.

Staphyloccal Arthritis

Gram-positive organisms account for 80 to 90 percent of acute nongonococcal infectious arthritis, and staphylococci are responsible for the majority of those cases. Such infections especially occur in rheumatoid joints and in those patients receiving corticosteroids or with a prosthetic joint. Delay in treating a superficial infection adequately or failure to administer prophylaxis at the time of an invasive procedure imposes increased risk. Infrequently, infection may extend into the joint from an adjacent bony focus or may be introduced by penetrating trauma or surgical intervention.

Gram-positive bacterial arthritis is usually monarticular, except in patients with an underlying synovitis or with multiple joint prostheses and those who are immunosuppressed or severely debilitated. The knee is most frequently involved, with the shoulder, wrist, hip, and elbow also common sites. Periarticular inflammation is less common than in gonococcal arthritis.

Other Infectious Arthritis

Acute arthritis caused by streptococci and pneumococci is now relatively uncommon as a result of effective antibiotic treatment of the primary infection. Gram-negative bacilli have now emerged as an important cause of infectious arthritis. *Escherichia coli* is most frequently the causative organism, but *Pseudomonas aeruginosa* is especially prevalent in intravenous drug users. Involvement of sternoclavicular and sacroiliac joints has been noted particularly in these patients. *Haemophilus influenzae* is common in children from infancy to 8 years of age, but otherwise is a rare articular pathogen.

Neisseria meningitidis may also cause an acute polyarthritis. Pain is not often prominent, in contrast to other pyogenic infections. Joint symptoms commonly occur within a week after systemic signs or meningitis is evident. Arthritis may appear after antibiotics are given and at a time when other symptoms seem to be improving. Arthritis may also be a feature of chronic meningococcemia. In contrast to the prompt response of gonococcal arthritis, meningococcal arthritis does not subside rapidly with antibiotic therapy; however, residual joint damage is uncommon.

These types of bacterial arthritis, like staphylococcal types, are most likely to occur in the very young, the elderly, the chronically ill, and those with impaired host resistance.[6]

LABORATORY FINDINGS

Examination of synovial fluid is essential to the diagnosis of acute bacterial arthritis. Leukocytosis is present, with counts frequently exceeding $50,000/\mu l$. A high white cell count, however, may not be present early in the disease or if the disease's course is modified by therapy. The glucose level is usually low. Gram-stained smears of the joint fluid often reveal organisms, especially in pneumococcal, staphylococcal, and gram-negative bacillary infections. *Neisseria* organisms are seen infrequently on smear, except in a frankly suppurative arthritis, and they are difficult to culture. Bacteriologic culture of the needle used for synoviocentesis should be obtained even when synovial fluid cannot be aspirated. Blood cultures may confirm the presence of a bacteremia. Radiographs show few changes early in the disorder unless a focus of osteomyelitis is present. Later, joint destruction may become evident.

MANAGEMENT

Treatment is urgently required in infectious arthritis in order to prevent the destruction of cartilage and permanent joint damage. Joint fluid should be removed as completely as possible by repeated aspiration. If the arthritis is caused by a sensitive organism, such as the gonococcus or pneumococcus, aspiration and antibiotics begun early will assure an essentially complete recovery. If the organism is relatively resistant, such as the staphylococcus or a gram-negative bacillus, aspiration and antibiotics may be effective if started early. If, however, fever and arthritis (clinical signs and analysis of joint fluid) have not been substantially reduced in 48 to 72 hours, surgical drainage of the joint should be accomplished. If one is reasonably certain at the outset that the organism is resistant to antibiotics, immediate surgical drainage may decrease morbidity.

Septic arthritis responds to appropriate antibiotic treatment if the organism is sensitive and if the dosage employed is adequate. In gonococcal or pneumococcal arthritis, for example, parenteral procaine penicillin in a dose of 600,000 units every 6 hours is generally rapidly effective. Organisms resistant to penicillin were isolated from military personnel in Southeast Asia and are now being encountered in the United States. In patients with penicillin-resistant gonococcal arthritis or known allergy to penicillin, tetracycline, 500 mg every 6 hours, should be given. If a relatively resistant organism such as staphylococcus is suspected, larger doses of antibiotics should be employed (e.g., 12 million units of penicillin daily). The use of a penicillinase-resistant compound such as nafcil-

lin is advisable until sensitivities are known. The intrasynovial injection of antibiotics is not necessary in most infections. Of course, treatment of the primary focus of infection should not be neglected.

TUBERCULOUS ARTHRITIS[1,2]

The incidence of tuberculous arthritis has declined markedly with the availability of antituberculosis drugs and with improved early case-finding. Tuberculous joint disease is still seen, however, with some frequency, and early recognition is important because prompt treatment may prevent severe destruction of the involved joint.

CLINICAL MANIFESTATIONS

Tuberculous arthritis arises through hematogenous spread from an active focus of tuberculous activity elsewhere than in the joints. Some patients present with arthritic complaints, their primary tuberculous foci being quiescent, but the evidences of disseminated tuberculosis may dominate the clinical presentation.

The spinal joints are commonly affected, especially in children and young adults (Pott disease). Pain, tenderness, and muscle spasm are usually present in the area involved but may not be noticed in children until an abnormality of gait or posture develops. Progressive destruction of the disc space and vertebral body produces a kyphotic deformity. Adjacent soft-tissue abscesses often form and may impinge on nerve roots or cause cord compression.

In peripheral joints, the disease is generally monarticular, involving a large joint, especially the hip or knee. Pain, limitation of motion, and swelling are usually observed. The swelling is commonly unaccompanied by heat and is sometimes described as "doughy" because the synovial enlargement is accompanied by a relatively small effusion. A tenosynovitis at the wrist, especially on its volar aspect, may be encountered. Remissions and exacerbations of symptoms are not uncommon, and the course of the disorder may be surprisingly indolent.

LABORATORY FINDINGS

The synovial fluid white cell count is elevated, and the glucose content is markedly reduced. Organisms are occasionally found on smear, but culture of the fluid is more likely to yield positive results. Synovial biopsy should be performed if other tests have not confirmed the diagnosis.

Radiographs early in the course of the disease may be negative or may show only localized osteoporosis and soft-tissue swelling. As the lesion progresses, marginal erosions and decreased bone density are seen. Bone necrosis, producing radiodensities on either side of the joint, is a late finding. Eventually, extensive narrowing and destruction of the joint space and subchondral bone become evident. In the spine, the disc space is involved first, and the body of the vertebra soon after, causing partial collapse or erosion of the vertebra anteriorly.

MANAGEMENT

If begun early in the disease, prolonged treatment with antituberculosis drugs and immobilization of the involved joint may be sufficient therapy. Surgical intervention may be required to drain abscesses or remove necrotic debris. If the joint surface or bone has been extensively involved, fusion of the joint may be necessary. At times, when the diagnosis is strongly suspected, therapy may be initiated before bacteriologic confirmation to avoid joint destruction.

VIRAL ARTHRITIS[4]

Several viral infections, including hepatitis B, rubella, and mumps, may be associated with an acute polyarthritis. The course of viral arthritis is benign. Articular manifestations are prominent in approximately 20 percent of patients in the prodromal phase of hepatitis and may antedate the onset of clinical jaundice by days to weeks. Women may be at slightly greater risk for developing arthritis than men.

The polyarticular, often symmetric, arthritis usually begins abruptly, most commonly affecting the small joints of the hands, but any peripheral joint may be symptomatic. Skin involvement is frequently present in those with joint symptoms and often coincides with the onset of arthritis. Urticarial and maculopapular eruptions affecting primarily the lower extremities are most common, but purpura, petechiae, and angioneurotic edema may also be seen. Fever is present in half of those with arthritis; nausea, vomiting, and abdominal discomfort occur in a minority.

During the period of joint involvement, free HB_SAg is generally present in the serum, often at high titers, and liver function test results may also be mildly abnormal. Cryoglobulins have been reported in many patients. Joint fluid is typically inflammatory. Normal glucose levels help distinguish this effusion from bacterial arthritis.

Arthritis complicating naturally occurring rubella and following immunization with attenuated virus is most common in young adults, especially women. The synovitis is abrupt in onset, usually a few days after appearance of the morbilliform rash, but occasionally only after the rash has completely faded. Malaise, fever, and posterior cervical lymphadenopathy are often present. The most commonly affected joints are the small joints of the hands, wrists, knees, and ankles. The arthritis is typically migratory; joint effusions and tenosynovitis are common.

Leukopenia and inflammatory synovial fluid may be found. The latex test for rheumatoid factor is positive occasionally in naturally occurring but not in vaccine-induced disease. A rise in rubella titer in convalescent serum confirms the diagnosis.

No specific therapy is available for any of the virus-associated arthritides. In most cases the arthritis responds promptly and well to restriction of activity and nonsteroidal antiinflammatory drugs or simple analgesia. All manifestations usually subside within days to weeks without residual joint abnormality.

LYME DISEASE[9,10]

Lyme disease, first recognized in 1976, is caused by a spirochete (*Borrelia burgdorferi*), which is tick borne (*Ixodes dammini*).

The most common and distinctive feature is a cutaneous rash, erythema chronicum migrans, typically beginning as a red papule at the site of the tick bite and developing into a large annular lesion with central clearing. Systemic symptoms, including fever and chills, are often present. In 25 percent of patients, erythema chronicum migrans is not observed.

After 1 to 16 weeks, a relapsing monarticular or oligoarticular arthritis occurs. Knees, shoulders, elbows, ankles, and wrists, in that order, can be involved; temporomandibular arthritis may also occur. The duration is variable, lasting days to weeks, and recurrences are common. Joint destruction is unusual, but in 10 percent of patients, a chronic arthritis affecting one or both knees occurs.

Approximately 10 percent of patients present with neurologic involvement, predominantly aseptic meningoencephalitis, Bell palsy, or other radiculopathy. Cardiac involvement, usually manifested by conduction defects of ECG evidence of myopericarditis, is rare.

Laboratory study findings are generally not specific and are of limited value in establishing an early diagnosis, although specific antispirochetal antibodies will develop in most patients.

Early institution of antibiotic treatment (penicillin G or tetra-

cycline) results in more rapid resolution of skin lesions and decreased prevalence and severity of arthritis. The acute arthritis may respond to nonsteroidal anti-inflammatory drugs. Joint aspiration with occasional intra-articular corticosteroid injection may be helpful.

FUNGAL ARTHRITIS

Fungal arthritis is uncommon in healthy individuals. An acute sterile polyarthritis has been reported during the initial phase of infection with *Coccidioides immitis* and *Histoplasma capsulatum*. *Sporothrix schenckii* may infect a single joint or, less frequently, multiple joints near the inoculum site in gardeners, florists, and miners. Other fungi (especially *Cryptococcus, Candida, Coccidioides*) are usually found in patients who have serious underlying disease and are immunologically compromised by the illness or its therapy.

INFECTIOUS VERSUS REACTIVE ARTHRITIS

Microbial infections can cause acute inflammatory joint problems in two ways: direct septic arthritis or a postinfective reactive arthritis.

Acute infectious arthritis results most frequently from hematogenous dissemination but may also follow direct inoculation or local extension. Once a virulent organism establishes septic synovitis, joint destruction will generally occur unless the infection is eradicated early.

In contrast, a reactive arthritis that occurs 1 to 3 weeks after an extra-articular infection (e.g., upper respiratory tract) usually resolves spontaneously without cartilage or bone destruction. A chronic arthritis, however, may follow urogenital infections or bacterial dysentery and may represent a continuum with Reiter disease.

REFERENCES

1. Berney S, Goldstein M, Bishko F: Clinical and diagnostic features of tuberculous arthritis. Am J Med 53:36, 1972
2. Davidson PT, Horowitz I: Skeletal tuberculosis: A review with patient presentations and discussion. Am J Med 48:77, 1970
3. Goldenberg DL, Reed JI: Bacterial arthritis. N Engl J Med 312:764, 1985
4. Hyer FH, Gottlieb NL: Rheumatic disorders associated with viral infections. Semin Arthritis Rheum 8:17, 1978
5. Kelly PJ, Martin WJ, Coventry MB: Bacterial (suppurative) arthritis in the adult. J Bone Joint Surg 52A:1595, 1970
6. Morris JL, Zizic TM, Stevens MB: Proteus polyarthritis complicating systemic lupus erythematosus. Johns Hopkins Med J 133:262, 1973
7. O'Brien JP, Goldenberg DL, Rice PA: Disseminated gonococcal infection: A prospective analysis of 49 patients and a review of pathophysiology and immune mechanisms. Medicine 62:395, 1983
8. Rosenthal J, Bole GG, Robinson WD: Acute nongonococcal infectious arthritis. Arthritis Rheum 23:889, 1980
9. Steere AC, Green JG, et al: Successful parenteral penicillin therapy of established Lyme arthritis. N Engl J Med 312:869, 1985
10. Steere AC, Grodzicki RL, et al: The spirochetal etiology of Lyme disease. N Engl J Med 308:733, 1983

CHAPTER 8.12
Osteoarthritis

Marc C. Hochberg

Osteoarthritis, or degenerative joint disease, is a disorder in which joint cartilage and subchondral bone are primarily affected; the synovial membrane may be involved with changes secondary to local inflammation.[2-6,10] Biochemical changes in the proteoglycan matrix and increased hydration of cartilage associated with structural changes in the collagen framework lead to altered mechanical function of the cartilage. This change is followed by proliferation and remodeling of subchondral bone, which results in marginal spur formation. Destruction of superficial layers of the articular cartilage results in fragmentation, erosions of cartilage, and shedding of fibrils into the joint space. Inflammatory mediators, including prostaglandins, leukotrienes, histamine, superoxide radicals, interleukin-1, collagenases and metalloproteases derived from chondrocytes, synovial lining cells, and leukocytes are thought to play an important role in propagation of the original lesion. There are no systemic manifestations characteristic of this disease.

CLINICAL MANIFESTATIONS

EPIDEMIOLOGY[9]

Osteoarthritis is the most prevalent form of arthropathy; radiographic changes have been found in over one third of individuals, and the clinical diagnosis was made in 12 percent of persons examined in the United States Health and Nutrition Examination Survey, 1971 to 1975. Its prevalence increases with age, the majority of those over 60 being affected. Many individuals with radiographic changes are asymptomatic or nearly so. The onset and severity of the disorder have been related to several factors. The presence of Heberden nodes (marginal bony proliferation at the DIP joints) and Bouchard nodes (similar bony lesions at the PIP joints) follows a hereditary pattern with female preponderance. When related to trauma, metabolic and neuropathic disorders, or prior inflammatory arthritis, osteoarthritis is often referred to as secondary in type. When no precipitating factors save heredity can be identified, the disorder is called idiopathic (Table 8.12–1).

ARTICULAR MANIFESTATIONS[2,3]

The gradual onset of pain, stiffness, or aching in one or more joints is frequently first noted in middle life or beyond. Occasionally, minor trauma may precipitate symptoms. Pain in weight-bearing joints may be greatest after activity and may subside on rest. The mechanism of pain is multifactorial, from periosteal elevation at sites of bony remodeling, subchondral microfractures, capsular irritation from bony spurs, and biochemical mediators released from leukocytes and synovial living cells. In addition, periarticular muscle spasm is common. The stiffness after rest that is often noted is generally not so prolonged as it is in rheumatoid arthritis. Major disability rarely results, except when the knees or hips are involved.

On examination, signs of inflammation of the joint or surrounding soft tissues are rarely encountered. Swelling is minimal or absent, and effusions infrequently detected, except in the knees. Inflammation and effusion may be related to superimposed trauma, to the stress of continual weight-bearing, to loose bodies

TABLE 8.12–1. CLASSIFICATION OF OSTEOARTHRITIS

Idiopathic
- Localized (one joint or joint-group)
- Generalized osteoarthritis
- Erosive osteoarthritis
- Diffuse idiopathic skeletal hyperostosis (DISH)

Secondary
- Trauma
- Prior inflammatory joint disease (rheumatoid arthritis, infectious arthritis, others)
- Metabolic disorders (gout, CPPD, hemochromatosis, ochronosis, others)
- Neuropathic disorders
- Ischemic necrosis of bone
- Hemophiliac arthropathy
- Congenital disorders of cartilage or bone

within the joint, or to an intercurrent condition. Acute inflammatory "flares" in osteoarthritis may reflect shedding of calcium pyrophosphate dihydrate or hydroxyapatite crystals into the joint space. Deformities result largely from marginal bony overgrowth (osteophytes) and from the loss of articular cartilage, rather than from soft-tissue abnormalities. Crepitus is frequently felt.

The pattern of joint involvement is of some importance in differential diagnosis. Weight-bearing joints are the most common sites of symptoms. In the hands, involvement of the DIP joints (Heberden nodes) is commonly asymptomatic, whereas PIP involvement (Bouchard nodes) may cause stiffness. The MCP joints of the hands and wrists are rarely involved. Another common site is the first metatarsophalangeal joint, leading to lateral deviation of the great toe (hallux valgus) with pain on weight bearing.

Involvement of the knee joint may affect the patella also. Symptoms on walking or stair climbing result from the sliding of the uneven surface of the patella over the femur. Degeneration of cartilage on both sides of the tibiofemoral joint, especially on the medial aspect of the tibial plateau, produces some distortion of the joint space, so motion may be limited and lateral instability may result. New bone formation or a loose body occasionally produces a mechanical block to motion of the joint, limiting flexion more commonly than extension.

Involvement of the hip joint may result in pain that is referred to the thigh, knee, or groin and that is usually greatest upon bearing weight. Pain and limitation of motion of the hip (internal rotation, extension, or abduction) are frequent associated findings.

Involvement of the spine is asymptomatic in the vast majority of those with radiographic changes in cervical and lumbar segments. Associated degenerative disc disease may compound the problem of marginal spurring and foster nerve root compression. On examination, forced hyperextension may produce pain when lower cervical segments are involved, whereas forward flexion causes discomfort in upper cervical disease.

Primary generalized osteoarthritis is a syndrome to be differentiated from rheumatoid arthritis. Most patients are women, who are affected ten times as often as men, and who are of menopausal age. Involvement of the DIP and PIP joints and the carpal-metacarpal joints of the thumbs, as well as the knees, hips, and spine, is common. The polyarticular nature of the disorder, and the occasional occurrence of mild inflammatory changes in the joints, may be suggestive of rheumatoid arthritis. The presence of bony (not soft-tissue) enlargement of the finger joints, the sparing of MCP joints and wrists, the absence of systemic signs, and the radiologic findings permit ready differentiation of this disorder from the inflammatory arthritides.

Erosive osteoarthritis is a variant more difficult at times to distinguish from rheumatoid arthritis because of recurrent inflammatory episodes and a proliferative synovitis that leads to cartilage destruc-

tion and occasionally bony ankylosis. This process, affecting the DIP, PIP, and occasionally, MCP joints of middle-aged women, is felt to be distinct from either classic osteoarthritis or seronegative rheumatoid arthritis. The sedimentation rate is normal or only minimally elevated and tests for rheumatoid factor are negative. Radiographic examination is most helpful in supporting the diagnosis.

Diffuse idiopathic skeletal hyperostosis (DISH) is a variant with extraspinal manifestations. Hyperostosis of the spine characterized by large osteophytes leads to fusion of the anterior longitudinal ligament, especially in the thoracic spine. Extraspinal radiographic changes include bony spurs at sites of tendon attachment to bone as well as ligamentous calcification. Clinically, patients complain of stiffness and pain in the spine and peripheral joints but lack evidence of inflammatory involvement. This disorder must be distinguished from ankylosing spondylitis in which the apophyseal joint changes, not seen in DISH, are commonly present, and sacroiliitis is always seen.

LABORATORY AND RADIOLOGIC MANIFESTATIONS[6]

LABORATORY FINDINGS

There is no evidence of systemic disease. The synovial fluid is usually viscid, has few white cells, and has a good mucin clot. Cartilage fibrils may be found in the joint fluid, but their finding cannot be considered specific. Occasionally, however, especially with a superimposed crystal-induced synovitis, inflammatory fluid will be present.

RADIOLOGIC ABNORMALITIES

Narrowing of the joint space secondary to the loss of radiolucent cartilage occurs early. Subchondral sclerosis and marginal spur formation then develop and are the radiologic hallmarks of the disease. Osteoporosis is not a feature of degenerative joint disease. Erosions are also uncommon. Subchondral cysts are often seen and can be differentiated from erosions of rheumatoid arthritis, because the bony cortex overlying the cyst remains intact. In the spine, narrowing of the disc space is seen early, followed by bony proliferation at the anterior margins of the vertebral body. Spur formation also occurs posteriorly, tending to encroach on the neural foramina. Oblique views of the spine are helpful in demonstrating this latter finding and changes in the apophyseal joints.

DIAGNOSIS[1,7]

Osteoarthritis is characterized by its relatively noninflammatory nature and by the lack of systemic involvement. Symptomatic disease, which infrequently results in marked disability, is most likely to develop in weight-bearing joints. The typical physical and radiologic findings result from the degeneration of articular cartilage and overgrowth of subchondral bone.

A major problem in diagnosis results from the high prevalence of radiographic changes of osteoarthritis in older individuals, which is often asymptomatic. Thus, one must evaluate all joint complaints carefully to avoid the common error of ascribing them to easily demonstrable osteoarthritic lesions.

MANAGEMENT[7,8]

An important initial step in the management of symptomatic osteoarthritis is to reassure patients about the nature of the disorder,

its usual indolent course, and good prognosis. When weight-bearing joints are involved, rest from bearing weight is advisable. With spine involvement, immobilization may be helpful. Postural defects, obesity, occupational trauma, and other predisposing factors should be looked for and eliminated when possible. Muscle-strengthening exercises may enhance stability and minimize the likelihood of exacerbation by minor trauma.

Aspirin in moderate dosage is frequently beneficial. Other nonsteroidal antiinflammatory agents may be used when aspirin is ineffective or must be discontinued because of adverse reactions. Corticosteroids should not be administered systemically, but the injection of corticosteroid into a joint may provide relief. Repeated injections (more often than twice yearly) should be avoided.

Surgical measures are of benefit in lesions of the knee, hip, and spine. In severe lesions of the hip and knee, surgical procedures, including joint replacements, may provide relief of pain and improve ambulation. In spine disease, spontaneous fusion of the joint may occur and relieve symptoms. Operative fusion is employed in selected cases when symptoms persist despite conservative measures. Decompression of the spinal cord and nerve roots may be indicated in entrapment/compression syndromes.

REFERENCES

1. Altman R, Asch E, et al: Development of criteria for the classification and reporting of osteoarthritis: Classification of osteoarthritis of the knee. Arthritis Rheum 29:1039, 1986
2. Cooke TDV, Dwosh I (eds): Clinical pathologic osteoarthritis workshop: A synthesis of ideas, models, and research from an international viewpoint. J Rheumatol 10(suppl 9):1, 1983
3. Hochberg MC: Osteoarthritis: Pathophysiology, clinical features, management. Hosp Prac 19:41, 1984
4. Howell DS, Sapolsky AL, et al: The pathogenesis of osteoarthritis. Semin Arthritis Rheum 5:365, 1976
5. Howell DS, Talbott JE (eds): Osteoarthritis symposium. Semin Arthritis Rheum 11(suppl 1):1, 1981
6. Huskisson EC, Katona G (eds): New Trends in Osteoarthritis. Rheumatology: An Annual Review, vol. 17. Basel, S. Karger, 1982
7. Moskowitz RW, Howell DS, et al (eds): Osteoarthritis: Diagnosis and Management. Philadelphia, WB Saunders, 1984
8. Moskowitz RW: Management of osteoarthritis. Bull Rheum Dis 31:34, 1981
9. Scott JC, Hochberg MC: Osteoarthritis. I. Epidemiology. Md State Med J 33:712, 1984
10. Sokoloff L (ed): Osteoarthritis. Clin Rheum Dis 11:175ff, 1986

CHAPTER 8.13
Differential Diagnosis of Arthritis

Mary Betty Stevens

This chapter offers an approach to the diagnosis of the patient who presents with arthritis, emphasizing the clinical features pertinent to the differential diagnosis of the more common syndromes encountered. The character and pattern of articular involvement, especially whether one or multiple joints are affected by the disease process, is a primary diagnostic consideration. Although it must be emphasized that a monarthritis may represent the initial stage of a process that with time will involve multiple joints, there are certain disorders that remain predominantly monarticular and merit separate discussion.

POLYARTHRITIS

Patients with polyarthritis constitute a difficult group to diagnose properly, especially early in the course of disease. Despite differences in the underlying cause of the acute and chronic arthritides (Table 8.13–1), the patterns of arthritis and joint findings are often similar. In addition, arthritis is frequently but one aspect of some generalized disease process. Thus, one has to rely on a detailed analysis of historical data, careful physical examination, and selective laboratory studies to arrive at the correct diagnosis. Even so, in the early and acute phase, there are patients in whom the specific type of arthritis remains uncertain.

The clinical problems associated with acute and with chronic polyarthritis differ in several respects. Many of the disorders that produce an acute polyarthritis can be eliminated or given only minor consideration as possible causes of chronic arthritis, for example, pyogenic infections. Other disorders that do not present acutely must be considered when evaluating patients with chronic arthropathy—for example, osteoarthritis. Finally, those arthritides, such as rheumatoid arthritis and gout, which may present as acute or chronic disorders, offer different diagnostic problems, depending on the stage of disease when the patient seeks evaluation.

PERSONAL FACTORS

The age, sex, family, and social histories of the patient are important in considering the possible causes of polyarthritis. In the absence of rheumatic heart disease or a history of previous attacks, acute rheumatic fever is infrequent after the age of 21. Primary gout and ankylosing spondylitis are predominantly diseases of young men, and in both disorders a positive family history may be obtained. Reiter syndrome is almost exclusively a disease of men in the younger age groups, although the chronic arthritis of Reiter may extend into the fifth and sixth decades. Gonococcal arthritis is largely found in women. Chronic arthritis and tumor syndromes are more common in the older age groups. Osteoarthritis is unusual before the age of 35 unless there is some predisposing cause, and its incidence increases with advancing age.

Information about exposure to infections, antecedent procedures, and any history of drug or serum administration should be specifically sought in those with acute polyarthritis. Occupational demands and exposures are similarly important.

GENERAL MANIFESTATIONS

Most patients with acute polyarthritis have fever. In a child with polyarthritis a high fever (104F or higher) with marked diurnal peaks and especially a double quotidian pattern suggests juvenile rheumatoid arthritis (i.e., Still disease). Rheumatic fever is less likely to cause fever of this magnitude, and its fever shows less diurnal variation. Because bacteremia and viremia are mechanisms by which multiple joints are involved in an infectious process, the history of shaking chills and fever in a patient with acute polyarthritis should strongly suggest these possibilities. Shaking chills, however, may occasionally occur in the absence of infection, especially when salicylates have been administered to reduce fever.

Weight loss, fatigue, malaise, or myalgia that precedes the onset of polyarthritis suggests an underlying systemic disorder, such

TABLE 8.13–1. CAUSES OF POLYARTHRITIS

	Acute	Chronic
Infection	Acute bacterial, especially gonococcus and meningococcus Haverhill fever Subacute bacterial endocarditis Lyme arthritis Viral infection, rubella, other Syphilis (especially congenital)	 Viral infection, especially lymphogranuloma venereum Syphilis (especially congenital)
Sequel to infection	Acute rheumatic fever Whipple disease[7]	Jaccoud arthritis Whipple disease
Allergic or hypersensitivity disease	Drug reaction, serum sickness Henoch-Schönlein purpura Erythema nodosum Erythema multiforme	 Erythema nodosum
Connective tissue disease	Systemic lupus erythematosus Systemic vasculitis Systemic sclerosis Polymyositis/dermatomyositis Sjögren syndrome Relapsing polychondritis	Systemic lupus erythematosus Polyarteritis Systemic sclerosis Sjögren syndrome Relapsing polychondritis
Inflammatory joint disease, cause unknown	Rheumatoid arthritis Juvenile rheumatoid arthritis Reiter syndrome Behçet disease[2,10]	Rheumatoid arthritis Juvenile rheumatoid arthritis Agammaglobulinemia Reiter syndrome Psoriatic arthropathy Ankylosing spondylitis Behçet disease
Arthritis with disease of the intestinal tract	Ulcerative colitis Regional enteritis	 Regional enteritis
Metabolic disease	Gout	Gout Ochronosis[9] Type IV hyperlipoproteinemia[5]
Malignant disease	Multiple myeloma Lymphoma Leukemia	Multiple myeloma
Degenerative		Osteoarthritis Primary generalized osteoarthropathy
Miscellaneous	Hypertrophic pulmonary osteoarthropathy Sarcoidosis Pseudogout Amyloidosis Familial Mediterranean fever Sickle cell anemia	Hypertrophic pulmonary osteoarthropathy Sarcoidosis[6] Pseudogout Hemochromatosis[1] Acromegaly[8] Hemophilia Neurogenic Reticulohistiocytosis[3]

as one of the connective tissue disorders, infectious process such as subacute bacterial endocarditis, or tumor syndrome. Weight loss that is occasionally profound is evident in many patients during the course of rheumatoid arthritis. In contrast, osteoarthritis is characterized by the absence of any systemic signs.

ARTICULAR MANIFESTATIONS

The pattern of articular involvement is particularly valuable in differential diagnosis. It is essential to determine in detail, by history and physical examination, the character and distribution of joint symptoms, their intensity, and progression. For example, gout frequently involves the great toe, but in its polyarticular form it commonly does not affect that joint and instead involves knees, ankles, elbows, wrists, or small joints of the hands. Frequently, gonococcal arthritis begins as a polyarthritis and then settles predominantly in one or two joints. In both gout and gonococcal arthritis, tenosynovitis is common, which helps to distinguish them from rheu-

matoid arthritis or rheumatic fever. Furthermore, the intensity of joint inflammation in microcrystalline and septic arthritides is usually far greater than in other disorders, reflecting the phagocytic response to crystals and organisms in the synovial space.

The occurrence of similar attacks in the past is an important feature in the diagnosis of acute rheumatic fever, gout, Reiter syndrome, or systemic lupus erythematosus. In the majority of patients, rheumatoid arthritis is less episodic and, without therapy, is additive and progressive.

The symmetry of the joints affected in rheumatoid arthritis is also characteristic and contrasts with the usual pattern of psoriatic arthropathy and Reiter syndrome. On the hand the DIP joints are commonly spared in rheumatoid arthritis but are characteristically involved in the psoriatic and are also the sites of Heberden nodes. The PIP joints typically are involved in rheumatoid arthritis but also may be affected in osteoarthritis (Bouchard nodes). In contrast, the MCP joints are rarely affected in primary osteoarthritis, but are almost always involved in rheumatoid arthritis of the hands.

Reiter syndrome is most common in the lower extremities but may involve any joint. Hips and shoulders are the most frequently affected peripheral joints in ankylosing spondylitis. Other disorders that affect the lumbar spine and sacroiliac joints include psoriatic arthropathy, the arthritis of inflammatory bowel disease, and Reiter syndrome but not rheumatoid arthritis. When the axial skeleton is involved by the rheumatoid process, the upper cervical segments are affected, usually late in the course of the disease. Osteoarthritis is more likely to become symptomatic when present in weight-bearing joints; hence, complaints referable to knees or hips are most common.

Helpful in distinguishing osteoarthritis from inflammatory joint disease is the relationship between physical activity and joint symptoms. Stiffness after rest (gel phenomenon) that tends to subside with activity is commonly present in patients with polyarthritis, especially rheumatoid arthritis. In contrast, the pain and stiffness of osteoarthritis is intensified by activity and weight bearing. Thus, the early morning hours are the most difficult for patients with rheumatoid arthritis as compared to the end of the day for those with osteoarthropathy.

EXTRA-ARTICULAR MANIFESTATIONS

The extra-articular manifestations are often of more specific value in the differential diagnosis than the arthritis itself (Table 8.13–2). When certain of these manifestations occur concomitantly with arthritis, they may lead directly to the diagnosis; however, the arthritis may precede the obvious expression of the extra-articular abnormalities, and thus a continued search for them is required.

Since iritis may come and go independently of the arthritis, a history of iritis as well as the demonstration of synechiae or scars of an old process are also important. The uveitis of sarcoidosis that is granulomatous can usually be distinguished from other types. Sarcoidal lesions of the conjunctiva are commonly without symptomatic inflammation.

The type of skin involvement may be virtually diagnostic in some instances—for example, erythema marginatum in rheumatic fever, the typical butterfly rash of SLE, the circinate balanitis and keratodermia in Reiter syndrome, the transient rash of Still disease, and erythema chronicum migrans of Lyme arthritis. In psoriatic arthropathy, deep pitting of the nails is a common feature, leading one to suspect the correct diagnosis in patients whose skin lesions are quiescent or atypical. The diagnosis of serum sickness or a drug hypersensitivity reaction may be suggested by the presence of urticaria or erythema multiforme. Erythema nodosum may be associated with arthritis when there is no other evident systemic disorder; however, polyarthritis with erythema nodosum is often an early, sometimes presenting manifestation of sarcoidosis as well as a late manifestation of inflammatory bowel disease.

Pleurisy and pericarditis are common in SLE and Still disease and occur occasionally in adult rheumatoid arthritis. Moreover, serositis usually occurs early and may be an initial feature of SLE and juvenile rheumatoid arthritis, in contrast to the usual appearance late in the course of adult rheumatoid disease. Pulmonary hypertrophic osteoarthropathy is most often related to the presence of a pulmonary or pleural tumor and may be the initial manifestation of carcinoma of the lung. Clubbing of the fingers is invariably present in the patient with this condition.

The presence of a diastolic heart murmur in a young patient with acute polyarthritis immediately suggests acute rheumatic fever or subacute bacterial endocarditis (SBE). The presence of Libman-Sacks endocarditis in SLE correlates poorly with cardiac murmurs on physical examination.

In contrast to the usual sequence of events in ulcerative colitis and Crohn disease, the arthritis of Whipple disease may precede overt evidence of gastrointestinal involvement by months or even years. Reiter syndrome, in its epidemic form, has been described in association with acute bacillary dysentery, but the sporadic cases are more commonly associated with urethritis. The onset of gono-coccal arthritis in women frequently occurs in association with menses or pregnancy.

Evidence of nephritis in a patient with acute polyarthritis points toward the diagnosis of a multisystem disorder, especially SLE or polyarteritis. Careful search for infection (subacute infective endocarditis [SIE]) and detailed history of drug administration (serum sickness) are indicated in all patients with such a symptom complex, however.

LABORATORY FINDINGS

Routine blood counts are seldom of diagnostic value, although a modest degree of anemia is frequent in patients with rheumatoid arthritis, chronic infection (SIE), and the connective tissue disorders. When the anemia is hemolytic, especially Coombs test–positive, SLE is likely. Similarly, leukopenia and less frequently thrombocytopenia in patients with polyarthritis favor the diagnosis of SLE or rheumatoid disease.

Although acute-phase reactants lack diagnostic specificity, the sedimentation rate is almost always elevated in patients with active inflammatory joint diseases but rarely, if ever, in osteoarthritis. Similarly, serum globulin elevations are found in many disorders causing polyarthritis, but determination of specific antibody levels is more valuable than total globulin determinations.

Antinuclear antibodies (ANA), as demonstrated by the indirect immunofluorescent method, are present in all but 5 percent of patients with active SLE, usually in high titer, but may be found also in other disorders (e.g., rheumatoid arthritis and variants, progressive systemic sclerosis, chronic active hepatitis). A strongly positive LE cell test correlates more closely with the diagnosis of SLE but, even so, is not specific.

Rheumatoid factors (demonstrated by the latex fixation test) are present in most patients with adult rheumatoid arthritis and nearly all with the variants of Felty and Sjögren syndromes. In children with rheumatoid arthritis, rheumatoid factors are seldom found and they are characteristically absent in Reiter syndrome, psoriatic arthropathy, and ankylosing spondylitis. Rheumatoid factors, however, commonly occur in disorders other than rheumatoid disease, including approximately half the patients with SLE and SBE, and less frequently in other connective tissue disorders, sarcoidosis, chronic infections, and hepatocellular disease. Furthermore, circulating rheumatoid factors seem to represent a phenomenon of aging independent of disease and are detectable in almost half of healthy individuals over age 60.

Reduction of serum complement is characteristic of SLE, especially when concomitant with antinuclear antibodies in high titer. Hypocomplementemia also occurs in serum sickness (usually only a transient fall) and occasionally in SBE. When hypocomplementemia occurs in rheumatoid arthritis, it has been associated with the presence of peripheral vasculitis, circulating cryoprecipitable complexes, or other systemic features of rheumatoid disease.

Synovial fluid findings often provide the most useful information, especially in infection (high white blood count, low glucose, and organisms on culture or smear) and microcrystalline synovitis (urate crystals in gout, calcium pyrophosphate crystals in pseudogout). The presence of noncrystalline inclusions in phagocytes is a common finding in rheumatoid arthritis (protein complexes) and Reiter syndrome (white blood cells). Most helpful in rheumatoid arthritis and SLE is the demonstration of a reduced synovial fluid complement, especially relative to the protein concentration, which reflects intrasynovial utilization by immune complexes. The complement level is normal or elevated in most inflammatory synovial fluids, as in infection, gout, and Reiter syndrome. Even in the absence of such diagnostic findings as organisms or crystals, careful examination of synovial fluid is useful in discriminating between inflammatory and typically noninflammatory fluid of osteoarthritis. Of interest in this regard is the usual finding, difficult to explain, of a good mucin clot and marginal leukocytosis (< 5000 cells/μl) in SLE and rheumatic fever.

TABLE 8.13–2. EXTRA-ARTICULAR MANIFESTATIONS OF ACUTE AND CHRONIC POLYARTHRITIS

System	Manifestation	Disease Association
Ocular	Conjunctivitis	Reiter syndrome
	Episcleritis	Rheumatoid arthritis, polyarteritis
	Keratoconjunctivitis sicca	Sjögren syndrome
	Visual changes, band keratopathy	Juvenile rheumatoid arthritis
	Uveitis	Juvenile rheumatoid arthritis, Reiter syndrome, ulcerative colitis, regional enteritis, ankylosing spondylitis, sarcoidosis
Skin	Butterfly rash	Systemic lupus erythematosus
	Erythema marginatum	Rheumatic fever
	Urticaria, erythema multiforme	Drug reaction, systemic lupus erythematosus, serum sickness
	Keratodermia and circinate balanitis	Reiter syndrome
	Psoriatic lesions	Psoriatic arthropathy
	Transient red rash	Juvenile rheumatoid arthritis (Still disease)
	Small, red, nonblanching spots especially on upper extremities	Gonococcal arthritis, rubella, arthritis
	Erythema chronicum migrans	Lyme arthritis
	Petechiae and purpura	Henoch-Schönlein, systemic lupus erythematosus, subacute bacterial endocarditis
	Infiltrative lesions	Sarcoid, amyloid, reticulohistiocytosis
	Nail lesions	Psoriatic arthropathy, Reiter syndrome, systemic lupus erythematosus
Tendon	Tendonitis	Gonococcal arthritis, gout
	Tendon sheath effusions	Rheumatoid arthritis
Muscle	Myositis	Systemic lupus erythematosus, systemic sclerosis, polymyositis, Sjögren syndrome, sarcoidosis
	Nodules on extensor surfaces of forearms over joints, pressure points	Rheumatoid arthritis, rheumatic fever, gout (tophi), SLE
	Ulcers, especially ankles	Rheumatoid arthritis
Hematopoietic system	Lymphadenopathy, splenomegaly	Rheumatoid arthritis, Still disease, systemic lupus erythematosus, sarcoid, rubella, leukemia, lymphoma
	Bleeding disorders	Hemophilia, systemic lupus erythematosus
Pulmonary system	Pleuritis	Systemic lupus erythematosus, rheumatoid arthritis, juvenile rheumatoid arthritis
	Parenchymal infiltrates	Sarcoid, rheumatoid arthritis, polyarteritis, systemic lupus erythematosus
	Hilar adenopathy	Erythema nodosum, sarcoid, lymphoma
Cardiovascular system	Pericarditis	Rheumatic fever, systemic lupus erythematosus, Still disease, rare rheumatoid arthritis
	Myocarditis (including conduction defects)	Rheumatic fever, systemic lupus erythematosus, polymyositis
	Endocarditis (including murmurs)	Rheumatic fever, systemic lupus erythematosus, subacute bacterial endocarditis
	Aortitis (aortic regurgitation)	Ankylosing spondylitis, Reiter syndrome, rarely rheumatoid arthritis
	Raynaud phenomenon	Systemic sclerosis, systemic lupus erythematosus, rheumatoid arthritis
Gastrointestinal system	Malabsorption	Whipple disease (arthritis usually precedes gastrointestinal signs), systemic sclerosis
	Enteritis, colitis	Colitic arthropathy, arthritis with regional enteritis, Reiter syndrome, rheumatoid arthritis
Genitourinary system	Urethritis, prostatitis, vaginitis, cervicitis, pelvic inflammation	Gonococcal arthritis, Reiter syndrome
	Calculi, nephropathy	Gout
	Proteinuria, abnormal sediment	Polyarteritis, systemic lupus erythematosus, subacute bacterial endocarditis, serum sickness, systemic sclerosis
Neurologic system	Loss of proprioception, deep pain, e.g., tabes dorsalis, syringomyelia, diabetes mellitus	Neurogenic arthropathy

Joint radiographs are least helpful early in the course of polyarthritis except in the negative sense—to exclude such infrequent disorders as pulmonary osteoarthropathy, leukemia, or myeloma. Even with septic processes, it may require weeks, even months, for characteristic radiologic lesions to become evident. Occasionally, findings of gout or rheumatoid arthritis may be present early, but these are commonly absent until more chronic symptoms are evident. Radiographic findings of particular value are the periarticular osteoporosis and juxta-articular erosions characteristic of rheumatoid arthritis and the marginal sclerosis and bony spurs and bridges of osteoarthritis. Patients with chronic gout often have punched-out defects in bone adjacent to joints (urate deposits); the presence

of chondrocalcinosis, especially knees, wrists, or symphysis, alerts one to possible pseudogout. Destructive and asymmetric lesions in the distal phalangeal joints are characteristic of psoriatic arthropathy. Periostitis, so frequent in pulmonary osteoarthropathy, is also a feature of Reiter syndrome and the juvenile form of rheumatoid arthritis. Radiographs of the sacroiliac joints and lumbar spine are helpful early in those with low back syndromes (with or without peripheral arthritis) to distinguish the group of spondylitic disorders from degenerative joint and intervertebral disk disease.

Biopsy of the synovial membrane[4] is infrequently essential in acute and chronic polyarthritis. Although diagnostic synovial membrane features include the granulomata of tuberculosis and sarcoid, crystalline deposits, and abnormal cell types, these diagnoses can usually be established more readily on other grounds. Otherwise, the histology is seldom indicative of more than reactive synovium. In contrast, biopsy of the subcutaneous nodules or skin lesions may yield information of diagnostic value.

A summary of the distinguishing features of the major forms of acute and chronic polyarthritis is presented in Table 8.13-3.

COURSE

A significant number of patients with acute polyarthritis seen within the first 1 or 2 weeks of illness will have a self-limited process that subsides in a period of days or weeks, even without treatment. Many patients never have recurrences of arthritis. Some of these individuals may have unrecognized acute infections (possibly viral), and population surveys have shown that such single episodes of acute polyarthritis are rather common.

Recurrent episodes of arthritis suggest rheumatic fever, gout, Reiter syndrome, or a multisystem disease such as SLE. Similar bouts of synovitis with symptom-free intervals may be associated with inflammatory bowel disease, often in relationship to exacerbations of the intestinal lesions. Rheumatoid arthritis, psoriatic arthritis, and ankylosing spondylitis, after presenting acutely, usually persist and progress in the absence of therapeutic intervention. Finally, some patients with "undiagnosed polyarthritis" continue to have recurrent and unexplained synovitis. Even after months or years they fail to develop the articular features that allow further categorization or the extra-articular manifestations of the multisystem connective tissue disorders. Such patients require continued, long-term observation and anti-inflammatory therapy with constant reevaluation in search for specific cause.

It is important to recognize the development of residual joint damage with continued inflammation, whatever the cause. Infection, if not adequately treated in its early stages, may cause significant joint destruction within a few weeks. Residual changes are apt to follow closely the polyarticular onset of rheumatoid arthritis and are also common in Reiter syndrome, but fewer joints are usually affected in the latter.

DIAGNOSTIC VALUE OF THERAPEUTIC TRIALS

Information can be obtained occasionally in some types of acute polyarthritis. In cases of suspected gout, a prompt response following the administration of colchicine (especially intravenously) will help to confirm the diagnosis. In infectious arthritis, a rapid response may be obtained to appropriate antibiotics when a sensitive organism in involved. Careful collection of material for cultures is mandatory, of course, before a trial of antibiotics is undertaken.

Obviously, in conducting a therapeutic trial, only one agent should be administered. Placing a patient on salicylates and penicillin simultaneously, for example, may obscure a therapeutic response of some diagnostic value. Moreover, it must be remembered that spontaneous and rapid resolution of polyarthritis may occur in many patients placed on bed rest alone, so the results of therapeutic trials demand cautious interpretation.

MONARTICULAR ARTHRITIS

Processes capable of involving multiple joints may be encountered initially as monarthritides. Hence, many of the diseases discussed as causes of polyarthritis are listed again in relation to monarticular arthritis (Table 8.13–4). Several disorders, however, remain predominantly monarticular and are emphasized here. The most immediate concern of the physician dealing with the problem of acute monarthritis is to recognize septic arthritis and mechanical derangement of a joint, both of which can lead to unnecessary, sometimes permanent, disability if appropriate therapy is not promptly instituted.

ARTICULAR MANIFESTATIONS

The abrupt onset of monarticular arthritis, with intense local inflammation, fever, and peripheral and synovial fluid leukocytosis, should suggest infection or microcrystalline synovitis (gout, pseudogout) as the leading etiologic possibility. Because infection usually occurs through the bloodstream, a history of chills is common, and a focus from which the bacteremia originated may be evident (e.g., pneumococcal pneumonia, acute salpingitis, or soft-tissue abscess). Although large joints are most commonly involved in infection, one of the small joints of the hands or feet may occasionally be involved (especially with gonococci, meningococci, or SBE). An acute arthritis caused by gout or pseudogout may closely resemble infection, especially with regard to the intensity of articular inflammation. The metatarsophalangeal joint of the great toe (podagra) is frequently involved in acute gouty attacks early in the course of the disease and is seldom affected by other arthritides unrelated to trauma. Inflammation of the surrounding soft tissue resembling cellulitis or thrombophlebitis is common in acute gout. Trauma (e.g., a recent operation or local physical injury) often precedes an acute gouty attack.

Trauma is also a frequent precipitating factor in pseudogout. Pseudogout commonly affects the knees and, less frequently, elbows, hips, and wrists. Occasionally pseudogout is polyarticular. This syndrome of chondrocalcinosis and acute arthritis secondary to the presence of calcium pyrophosphate microcrystals in synovial fluid has been called pseudogout because of its clinical resemblance to gout, resulting from the fact that in both disorders, microcrystals are responsible for inducing inflammation.

Trauma may result directly in an acute painful swelling of a joint, especially when the injury involves rupture of a ligament or damage to cartilage. A history of significant trauma may be obtained in these patients, but not infrequently the injury may have been so minor an event that it is forgotten, or it may not be recalled for other reasons, such as alcoholism, seizures, or disorientation (especially in the elderly). Low-grade fever is sometimes associated with a traumatic effusion but rarely persists longer than 24 hours.

Acute painful swelling of a joint may be produced occasionally by a loose fragment of cartilage that is trapped or wedged between the articulating surfaces of a joint. Such loose bodies are common in osteoarthritis or osteochondromatosis and, especially in the knee, osteochondritis dissecans. A meniscus injury as well as a loose body may result in locking of the knee in addition to painful swelling.

Acute arthritis of colitic arthropathy is frequently a monarticular process. In most patients, active ulcerative colitis or regional enteritis is evident and the rheumatologic diagnosis is not difficult. In some, however, the bowel lesion is clinically silent. An added major consideration is acute infection secondary to a complication of inflammatory bowel disease.

Rheumatoid arthritis may remain localized to a single joint, especially the knee, for months and even years before other joints become involved. Rheumatoid arthritis with onset in the early teens may remain monarticular throughout its course. Intermit-

TABLE 8.13–3. IMPORTANT DIFFERENTIAL DIAGNOSTIC FEATURES OF ACUTE AND CHRONIC POLYARTHRITIS

Gonococcal Arthritis
- Young adults, especially females
- History of exposure
- Associated with menses or pregnancy
- After polyarticular onset, often settles in one or two joints; tenosynovitis prominent
- Association with skin lesions
- Frequent history of shaking chills, genitourinary symptoms (urethritis, salpingitis)
- Isolation of organism from genitourinary tract, blood joints, and skin lesions
- Response to penicillin

Viruses
- History of exposure, frequently during an epidemic
- Rise in serologic titer
- Leukopenia
- Spontaneous remission without sequelae in acute forms
- In lymphogranuloma venereum: chronic synovitis of large joints, hyperglobulinemia, positive Frei test

Acute Rheumatic Fever
- Child or young adult
- Evidence of recent beta streptococcal infection
- Migratory involvement of large joints; often previous attacks
- Association with carditis
- Response to aspirin

Serum Sickness or Drug Hypersensitivity
- History of drug administration, especially horse serum, penicillin, but also patent medicines
- Migratory involvement large and small joints
- Frequent association with rash (urticaria, erythema multiforme, others)
- Decreased serum complement level in serum sickness
- Response to drug withdrawal, antihistamines, or corticosteroid therapy

Connective Tissue Diseases
- Females predominate except in polyarteritis
- Joint involvement infrequently progresses to deformity
- Systemic signs and multisystem organ involvement, especially nephritis, in systemic lupus erythematosus and polyarteritis
- Serologic profile helpful, especially SLE

Rheumatoid Arthritis
- Women 2:1
- Initial frequent involvement hands (PIP, MCP joints) and wrist,
- Symmetric, additive involvement; chronically, all peripheral joints may be involved
- Morning stiffness prominent
- Subcutaneous nodules
- Tendon sheath effusions
- Characteristic deformities and erosive changes on radiograph in chronic stage
- Rheumatoid factor in up to 70% with time

Juvenile Rheumatoid Arthritis
- Onset before age 16
- Cervical spine involvement in 25%
- Growth-impairment variable, age-dependent
- Still disease associated with rash, serositis, lymphadenopathy, splenomegaly
- Subcutaneous nodules and rheumatoid factor uncommon
- Tends to remission at adolescence

Ankylosing Spondylitis
- Young men 9:1
- Spine disease with extensive fusion principal manifestation
- Hips and shoulders frequently involved
- Association with iritis, aortitis
- Subcutaneous nodules and rheumatoid factor not present

Reiter Syndrome
- Young men
- Genitourinary symptoms, signs (urethritis, prostatitis)
- Often asymmetric arthritis; most commonly lower extremities
- Tends to recur; knees, ankles, spine most often involved in chronic form
- Association with skin (keratodermia), membrane (oral, balanitis), and ocular lesions
- ECG changes may be present (heart block)

Psoriatic Arthropathy
- Typical skin lesions and nail involvement
- Asymmetric arthritis; frequent DIP joint involvement
- Spine disease, especially sacroiliitis
- Subcutaneous nodules and rheumatoid factor not present
- Hyperuricemia may be found

Arthritis of Inflammatory Bowel Disease
- Active ulcerative colitis, regional enteritis
- Large joints predominate
- Parallels course of intestinal disorder in most patients
- Negative rheumatoid factor tests

Erythema Nodosum
- Typical skin lesions
- Hilar adenopathy
- Arthritis usually lower extremities, especially ankles; usually evanescent
- May be associated with sarcoid, tuberculosis, regional enteritis, drug hypersensitivity, others

Sarcoidosis
- Arthritis usually occurs early in disease course, rarely progressive
- Hilar adenopathy and other systemic features
- Lesions demonstrable on biopsy of node or liver
- Hypergammaglobulinemia
- Elevated serum calcium or uric acid may occur

Gout
- Males or postmenopausal females
- Familial occurrence
- Podagra and prominent periarticular inflammation in acute attacks
- Precipitating factors (drugs, trauma, etc.)
- Tophi, clinically and radiographically, in chronic stage
- Increased serum uric acid and urate crystals in synovial fluid

Pseudogout (CPPD)
- Males predominate
- Mimics gout, with intense inflammation, especially knees
- Chondrocalcinosis on radiograph
- Calcium pyrophosphate crystals in synovial fluid

Hypertrophic Osteoarthropathy
- Clubbing of fingers
- Knees, wrists, ankles, fingers may be involved; rheumatoid-like
- Periostitis, especially at distal ends of long bones
- Association with pulmonary, mediastinal, other lesions—often malignant
- Course determined by underlying disease

Osteoarthritis
- Lower extremities predominate
- DIP (Heberden nodes) and PIP (Bouchard nodes) involvement
- Absence of MCP and wrist disease
- Pain after activity, improved with rest
- Absence of inflammatory signs
- Bony proliferation with spur formation

tent swelling of one or both knees, independently or simultaneously, in a young woman without marked articular symptoms or evident systemic features, suggests the diagnosis of intermittent hydrarthrosis. Exacerbation of joint swelling with menses is often observed with this condition.

Tuberculous arthritis is usually a subacute or chronic monarticular process. It may be produced by *Mycobacterium tuberculosis* and atypical chromogenic strains. Early recognition is imperative because specific therapy is available that will minimize otherwise inevitable joint destruction. The peripheral joint most frequently af-

TABLE 8.13–4. CAUSES OF MONARTICULAR ARTHRITIS[a]

Infection
- Acute bacterial (gonococcus, pneumococcus, streptococcus, staphylococcus, meningococcus, gram-negative)
- Tuberculosis
- Fungus

Inflammatory Joint Disease
- Rheumatoid arthritis (especially juvenile onset)
- Reiter syndrome
- Ulcerative colitis
- Regional enteritis

Metabolic
- Gout

Trauma
- Hemarthrosis
- Tear of ligament or cartilage

Osteoarthritis
- Primary
- Secondary (postinflammatory, posttrauma, neuropathic)

Neoplasms
- Pigmented villonodular synovitis (inflammatory granuloma or true neoplasm?)
- Primary (osteochondromatosis, lipoma, angioma, synovioma)
- Metastatic

Miscellaneous
- Intermittent hydrarthrosis
- Osteochondritis dissecans
- Bleeding disorders (hemophilia) with hemarthrosis

[a]Any form of polyarthritis may present initially with monarticular involvement.

TABLE 8.13–5. IMPORTANT DIFFERENTIAL DIAGNOSTIC FEATURES OF MONARTICULAR ARTHRITIS

Bacterial Infection
- Acute onset
- Focus of infection elsewhere
- Fever, occasionally chills
- Large joints primarily; intense inflammation
- Inflammatory synovial fluid with white blood cells often >50,000, low glucose, organisms on smear or culture
- Response to antibiotics

Tuberculous Arthritis
- Usually active tuberculosis elsewhere
- Tuberculin-positive
- Large joints (knee, hip) or tenosynovitis at wrist
- Cold inflammation clinically, but inflammatory synovial fluid
- Frequently bony involvement on radiograph
- Synovial biopsy characteristic
- Response to antituberculous therapy

Gout
- Acute onset
- Family history
- Men, postmenopausal women
- Often recurrent attacks in single joint, especially podagra
- Intense inflammation with uric acid crystals in synovial fluid
- Elevated serum uric acid
- Response to colchicine

Pseudogout (CPPD)
- Middle-aged, elderly men predominantly
- Mimics gout in acuteness and intensity of inflammation
- Calcium pyrophosphate crystals in synovial fluid
- Calcification joint cartilage knee, wrist, symphysis pubis

Trauma
- Abrupt onset
- Frequent history of significant direct trauma
- Lack of systemic signs
- Normal sedimentation rate
- Noninflammatory synovial fluid with red blood cells

Osteoarthritis
- Pain with weight bearing and exercise
- Minimal or absent inflammation
- Characteristic radiographic changes with subchondral sclerosis, marginal spur formation
- Chronic inflammation, recurrent trauma, and neuropathic (Charcot) joints predisposing factors

Osteochondritis Dissecans
- Acute and chronic symptoms
- Adolescents, young adults
- Knee joint predominantly involved
- Noninflammatory effusions related to extrusion of cartilage fragment into joint
- Radiograph characteristic with density or defect on articular surface of femoral condyle

Intermittent Hydrarthrosis
- Young women primarily
- One or both knees
- Effusion exacerbated with menses
- Synovial fluid nonspecific
- No systemic features
- Negative radiographs
- Rheumatoid arthritis develops subsequently in a few

Pigmented Villonodular Synovitis
- Knee joint primarily
- Recurrent bloody effusions and synovial hypertrophy
- Tumor versus granulomatous synovitis
- Characteristic biopsy
- Surgical removal necessary

fected in adults is the knee, in contrast to more common hip involvement in children. Spinal involvement (Pott diesase) is rarely associated with peripheral tuberculous arthritis.

Tumors involving joints are uncommon. The most frequently encountered tumor is benign osteochondroma, commonly multiple (multiple exostoses). Metastasis of tumors in the joint is rare, although extension to the joint of an adjacent bony tumor focus is occasionally seen.

The most common cause of chronic monarticular arthropathy is osteoarthritis. Knees or hips are the most frequently affected joints. Effusions may be encountered, especially in the knee, usually without evidence of significant inflammation.

Traumatic insult to a joint may produce recurrent or chronic symptoms that relate to the development of secondary degenerative change. Such may be the basis of neurogenic arthropathy, which is more often monarticular. Loss of proprioception in such disorders as tabes dorsalis, syringomyelia, and diabetes mellitus leads to repeated joint trauma, relaxation of supporting structures with marked instability and, finally, severe degenerative changes and bony proliferation. The knees are most frequently affected in tabes dorsalis, the shoulders and elbows in syringomyelia, and the ankles, tarsal, and metatarsal joints in diabetic neuropathy. Examination usually reveals an effusion, hypermobility of the joint, and remarkable bony overgrowth and crepitation in the advanced cases. Pain, when present, seems less in degree than the deformity and effusion should produce.

EXTRA-ARTICULAR FEATURES

The same concern for the patient's personal characteristics, environmental exposures, and general health status applies to those with monarticular arthritis as has been stressed for patients with multiple inflamed joints. Particularly important here is care in the documentation of exposure to infection and episodes of possible physical injury to the joint. It must be remembered that trauma, in addition to direct alteration of joint integrity, provides a frequent precipitating factor for acute microcrystalline synovitis. Similarly, a detailed history of drug administration may reveal agents (e.g., thiazides) that alter uric acid metabolism and favor gouty attacks. Septic arthritis is an increasing problem in drug abusers.

LABORATORY FINDINGS

Leukocytosis and elevation of the erythrocyte sedimentation rate are frequently found in acute infection, gout, and pseudogout but are usually absent in traumatic, degenerative, and neuropathic joint disease. Elevation of the serum uric acid favors the diagnosis of gout. A negative tuberculin skin test is substantial evidence against the diagnosis of tuberculosis.

Aspiration of synovial fluid is particularly useful in the diagnosis of monarticular arthritis. Mucin clot test findings are usually normal and the white cell count is usually less than 2000/µl in trauma, osteochondritis dissecans, neurogenic arthropathy, and osteoarthritis. Sanguinous effusions are characteristic of acute trauma but may also occur in pigmented villonodular synovitis, osteochondritis dissecans, and bleeding disorders. A white cell count higher than 50,000/µl and a low glucose level strongly implicate an acute bacterial infection, even though microorganisms may not be seen on smear or culture. A low synovial fluid glucose in a chronic monarthritis is highly suggestive of tuberculosis.

The recognition and identification of crystals in synovial fluid allow the diagnosis of gout or pseudogout to be made with certainty. The abundance of crystals varies with the time of synovial fluid examination relative to onset of the joint inflammation. During the first 12 hours or after the second day, crystals may be few and require careful search. In the acute inflammatory reaction they are predominantly intracellular, but in the interval or chronic phase they are extracellular.

Radiographic changes are helpful in distinguishing rheumatoid arthritis, gout, and osteoarthritis; however, it must be recalled that degenerative changes are commonly encountered and may be unrelated to the clinical problem. Chondrocalcinosis may be overlooked unless it is specifically considered. It usually occurs as a stippled, linear calcification of the meniscal or articular cartilage of the knee joint, in the wrist, hip, pubic symphysis, or intervertebral disks. Osteochondritis dissecans also presents a characteristic radiographic picture that is best seen in a tunnel view of the knee. The lesion is usually seen as a defect or density in the non-weight-bearing articular surface of the femoral condyle. Neurotrophic arthropathy is associated with an extreme degree of bony proliferation.

Acute infection has no radiologic manifestations unless it originates from a juxta-articular focus of osteomyelitis. Several weeks after an acute infection, a narrowing of the joint space may be evident because of the destruction of articular cartilage. Tuberculosis causes early narrowing of the joint space.

Biopsy of the synovium either opened by exploration or closed by needle techniques is of greatest usefulness in the patient with obscure monarticular arthritis. Confirmation of the diagnosis of tuberculous arthritis, sarcoidosis, pigmented villonodular synovitis and, occasionally, gout can be made on the basis of characteristic alteration of the synovial membrane.

A summary of the distinguishing features of various disorders producing monarthritis is presented in Table 8.13–5.

REFERENCES

1. Atkins CJ, McIvor J, et al: Chondrocalcinosis and arthropathy: Studies in haemochromatosis and in idiopathic chondrocalcinosis. QJ Med 39:71, 1970
2. Chajek T, Fainaru M: Behçet's disease: Report of 41 cases and a review of the literature. Medicine 54:179, 1975
3. Ehrlich GE, Young I, et al: Multicentric reticulohistiocytosis (lipoid dermatoarthritis): A multisystem disorder. Am J Med 52:830, 1972
4. Goldenberg DL, Cohen AS: Synovial membrane histopathology in the differential diagnosis of rheumatoid arthritis, gout, pseudogout, systemic lupus erythematosus, infectious arthritis, and degenerative joint disease. Medicine 57:239, 1978
5. Goldman JA, Glueck CJ, et al: Musculoskeletal disorders associated with Type IV hyperlipoproteinemia. Lancet 1:449, 1972
6. Gumpel JM, Johns CJ, Shulman LE: The joint disease of sarcoidosis. Ann Rheum Dis 26:194, 1967
7. Kelley JJ, Weisiger BB: The arthritis of Whipple's disease. Arthritis Rheum 6:615, 1963
8. Kellgren JH, Bau J, Tutton GR: The arthritis and other limb changes in acromegaly: A clinical and pathological study of 25 cases. QJ Med 21:405, 1952
9. O'Brien WM, LaDuc BN, Bunim JJ: Biochemical, pathologic and clinical aspects of alkaptonuria, ochronosis and ochronotic arthritis. Am J Med 34:813, 1963
10. Zizic TM, Stevens MG: The arthritis of Behçet's disease. Johns Hopkins Med J 136:243, 1975

CHAPTER 9.1
Clinical Management of Patients with Infectious Diseases

John G. Bartlett

Infectious diseases refer to pathologic processes resulting from microbes or microbial products. There has been a remarkable change in dealing with these conditions since the introduction of antimicrobial agents, initially with sulfonamides (Prontosil) in the mid-1930s and then with penicillin in the 1940s. Before these developments, infectious diseases accounted for more than half of all hospitalizations and were responsible for most fatalities.[9] At present, infectious diseases account for about 8 percent of all hospitalizations, and pneumonia, the leading cause of death due to infectious diseases, ranks sixth as a disease category responsible for fatality in the United States.[9] The discovery of antimicrobial agents has been described as the greatest lifesaving technologic development in the history of medicine, and it is credited with a 10-year extension in the average life expectancy. The impact of this curative revolution may be properly emphasized by noting that successful elimination of all deaths from cancer would result in only a 2-year extension in life expectancy. Further, use of these drugs is so simple that in 1960 Dr. Walsh McDermott wrote ''. . . with today's drugs it is possible to place in the hands of a barefoot, nonliterate villager more real power to affect the outcome of a child critically ill with, let us say, meningitis or pneumonia or tuberculosis, than could have been exerted by the most highly trained urban physician of 25 years ago.''[9]

Despite the progress, there has been a price to pay. Unbridled enthusiasm has led to extensive abuse with the consequence of selection and wide dissemination of antibiotic-resistant bacteria. Surveys in the United States indicate over 90 million prescriptions are written annually for antibiotics for ambulatory patients, and about one-fourth of all patients receive antibiotics during hospitalization. More important, retrospective surveys suggest that only about 40 percent of the antibiotic uses in the hospital are considered ''rational,''[11] and, according to one survey in the United States, nearly 60 percent of physicians use antibiotics in the management of the common cold.[17] The purpose of this chapter is to provide guidelines for the approach to the patient with a suspected infection. The major emphasis is on detection of the microbial agent and the judicious use of antibiotics with appropriate respect for statistical probabilities and precedent when empiric selections are necessary.

PATTERNS OF INFECTIONS

The microbes responsible for common infections are classified as bacteria, bacterialike (mycobacteria, mycoplasmas, chlamydiae, spirochetes and rickettsiae), fungi, viruses, and parasites (protozoa and worms). The types of infections and distribution of microbial pathogens within these categories primarily depend on the source of the patient population.

OFFICE AND CLINIC PRACTICE

Patients seen in offices or clinics account for about 600 million physician contacts annually in the United States. Surveys of practicing physicians indicate that the most frequent acute conditions leading to physician consultation are the common cold, influenza, and pharyngitis.[10,12] These are respiratory tract infections that are usually caused by viral agents, the etiology cannot be detected by the usual culture techniques, and they do not respond to specific forms of therapy. The most common treatable forms of infections seen in outpatients are bacterial infections, including streptococcal pharyngitis, otitis media, sinusitis, urinary tract infections, sexually transmitted diseases, and lower respiratory tract infections. The major pathogens in these cases include streptococci, *Streptococcus pneumoniae, Haemophilus influenzae, Escherichia coli, Neisseria gonorrhoeae,* and *Chlamydia.* The most frequently employed antimicrobial agents are penicillins, tetracyclines, erythromycins, and sulfonamides, which account for 80 percent of all outpatient prescriptions for antimicrobial agents.[13] These drugs are relatively cheap, show good bioavailability with oral administration, and have a long track record with extensive usage to establish both efficacy and relative safety.

HOSPITALIZED PATIENTS

Approximately 2.5 million patients are hospitalized annually in the United States for an infectious disease, accounting for approximately 10 percent of the total 281 million patient days in acute-care hospitals.[2] The most common forms of infections requiring hospital care are the urinary tract infections, which account for approximately one million hospitalizations per year, followed by lower respiratory tract infections, which account for approximately 600,000 (Table 9.1-1). The current estimate is that 93 percent of all community-acquired infections requiring hospitalization are caused by bacteria, and 6 percent are viral infections.[2] Drug utilization patterns within the hospital setting are far different because of the extensive use of parenteral agents, the most frequent in the United States being penicillins, cephalosporins, and aminoglycosides.[7]

HOSPITAL-ACQUIRED INFECTIONS

A ''nosocomial infection'' is defined as an infection that is acquired within the hospital setting that was not present or incubating at the time of admission. Extensive surveys indicate that 3.5 to 5 percent of all patients develop a nosocomial infection.[2,3,20] Approximately half of these infections are considered preventable, using the hospital infection control guidelines established by the Centers for Disease Control (CDC) and adopted by virtually all hospitals.[3] The most common infections are those involving the urinary tract, surgical wounds, and the lower respiratory tract (Table 9.1-1). The latter, hospital-acquired pneumonia, represents the most common lethal nosocomial infection, with mortality rates of about 20 percent. Bacteria are responsible for 90 percent of all nosocomial infections, with fungi accounting for most of the rest.[2] The bacteria encountered are unique in terms of species distribution and antibiotic sensitivity profiles compared to those encountered in community-acquired infections.[1] This presumably re-

TABLE 9.1–1. INFECTIONS IN U.S. HOSPITALS[a]

Type of Infection	Community Acquired (× 1000/yr)		Hospital Acquired (× 1000/yr)	
Genitourinary	1160	(38%)	830	(41%)
Lower respiratory tract	610	(20%)	240	(12%)
Upper respiratory tract	240	(08%)	10	(0.5%)
Enteric	80	(03%)	5	(0.2%)
Central nervous system	20	(0.7%)	5	(0.2%)
Disseminated and bacteremia	20	(0.7%)	190	(09%)
Other	890	(29%)	750	(37%)
Total	3030		2030	
Pathogens				
Bacteria	2820	(93%)	1830	(90%)
Viruses	180	(6%)	6	(0.2%)
Fungi	20	(0.7%)	200	(10%)
Parasites	10	(0.3%)	—	

[a]Data from the Communicable Disease Center based on the results of The Comprehensive Hospital Infections Project (CHIP) and the National Nosocomial Infections Study (NNIS). Surveys were performed in 89 U.S. hospitals during 1970–1976. Figures are for annual incidence × 1000 rounded to the nearest 10 or nearest significant number. Adapted from Dixon RE: Ann Intern Med 89:749, 1978.

flects clustering of highly vulnerable patients in a setting where there is extensive use of antibiotics. A similar situation is found in nursing homes.

The first clinically significant, serious consequences of antibiotic use within hospitals were penicillin-resistant strains of *Staphylococcus aureus* that were first noted in the early 1950s; these strains quickly became endemic in most hospitals throughout the world; and they became prevalent in the community about a decade later.[8] The usual determinants for this resistance were plasmids that encode for penicillinase production and are promoted by the widespread use of penicillins. In the early 1950s it was also noted that certain gram-negative organisms were naturally resistant to the antibiotics available at that time, and these gradually assumed greater importance. The gram-negative bacilli also became adaptive as new antibiotics became available, but their resistance patterns evolved in a particularly surreptitious fashion. Unlike *S. aureus*, the plasmids in these organisms encoded for resistance to several unrelated antibiotics, and transfer occurred not only between members of a single species, but also between different species and even between genera.[8] By the early 1970s, *Pseudomonas aeruginosa* was a well-established nosocomial pathogen, and by the mid-1970s there was a growing problem with aminoglycoside resistance in gram-negative bacilli. The plasmid-determined property of β-lactamase production then appeared in *H. influenzae*, *N. gonorrhoeae*, and *Bacteroides* species. In the early 1980s methicillin-resistant *S. aureus* became more widely disseminated, primarily in large, university-affiliated teaching hospitals.[14] This pattern of resistance, however, is somewhat different in that it appears to be chromosomal rather than transferred by plasmids.

The predominant organisms encountered in nosocomial infections in United States' hospitals are gram-negative bacilli, primarily *E. coli*, *P. aeruginosa*, *Klebsiella*, *Proteus*, *Enterobacter*, and *Serratia*.[2] The usual source of these bacteria is colonization of mucosal surfaces with resistant strains in hosts rendered susceptible by antibiotic treatment, debilitating conditions, and various medical procedures. Proof of the role of antibiotics in promoting the widespread dissemination of resistant strains is indirect but is supported by the fact that the highest rates of resistance are found in the hospitals

and in the agricultural industry, both settings where antibiotics are used extensively. The problem of antibiotic resistance is global in dimension, and certain characteristic plasmids also have been noted in widely separated geographic areas of the world.

Most authorities conclude that about half of nosocomial infections may be prevented by strict adherence to CDC guidelines.[21] The most important element of infection control is handwashing. Also important are barrier isolation techniques for resistant organisms in exudate or secretions. Another, based on 4 decades of experience, is restrained use of antibiotics.

INFECTIOUS DISEASES IN DEVELOPING COUNTRIES

As noted above, the most common infections encountered in office practice are viral infections, and the most frequent pathogens encountered in hospitalized patients in industrialized countries are bacteria, many or most of which originate from the normal flora of mucocutaneous surfaces. The experience in developing countries is quite different. Here, the most prevalent pathogens appear to be parasites and communicable agents that reflect crowding, poor sanitation, and limited health care resources (Table 9.1–2).[19] *Ascaris*, hookworm, and *Trichuris* are found in stools of a major portion of the three billion inhabitants of Africa, Asia, and Latin America.[18] These are worm infestations, the organisms usually do not replicate in the gastrointestinal tract, and symptoms reflect the total parasite load so that most patients remain asymptomatic. Other parasitic diseases that are highly prevalent in developing countries, but also cause substantial morbidity and mortality, are malaria and schistosomiasis. Agents of diarrheal disease, primarily rotavirus, cause repeated gastrointestinal infections in children and are responsible for about half of all childhood deaths. According to the World Health Organization, there are one billion episodes of diarrhea in children under 5 years, with five million deaths per year, or about 600 every hour. Diphtheria, measles, poliomyelitis, and tetanus are infections that have been largely controlled in industrialized nations, but continue to take a severe toll in the unimmunized and more vulnerable children from developing countries. The prevalence of serologic markers for hepatitis B is 70 to 90 percent in many of these countries, compared with 3 to 5 percent in the United States. Moreover, this infection is the most frequent cause of cirrhosis, and liver cancer associated with hepatitis B infection is

TABLE 9.1–2. MAJOR INFECTIOUS DISEASES OF AFRICA, ASIA, AND LATIN AMERICA (IN THOUSANDS PER YEAR): 1977–1978[a]

	No. with Infection	No. with Disease	No. of Deaths
Diarrhea	5,000,000	5,000,000	5–10,000
Malaria	800,000	150,000	1200
Schistosomiasis	200,000	20,000	500–1,000
Amebiasis	400,000	1,500	30
Hookworm	900,000	1,500	50–60
Trichiuriasis	500,000	100	low
Ascariasis	1,000,000	1,000	20
Filariasis	250,000	2–3,000	low
Giardiasis	200,000	500	very low
Dengue	3–4,000	1–2,000	0.1
Whooping cough	70,000	20,000	250–450
Measles	85,000	80,000	900
Typhoid	1,000	500	25
Tuberculosis	1,000,000	7,000	400

[a]Based on estimates from the World Health Organization. Adapted from Walsh JA, Warren KS: N Engl J Med 301:967, 1979.

the most common form of cancer in many parts of Africa and Asia. These data illustrate the unique geographic distribution of the pathogens, with major differences between industrialized countries and the developing world. This becomes an important consideration in any patient with a suspected infection who is a resident of Latin America, Asia or Africa, a refugee from these areas, or a recent traveler there.[18]

THE COMPROMISED HOST

The compromised host is defined as a person with a defect in the normal defense mechanisms that predisposes to infectious diseases.[16] The result may be unusually severe or recurrent infections with traditional pathogens, or they may involve certain "opportunistic" microbes, defined as organisms with minimal pathogenic potential that appear to cause disease almost exclusively in this population. The defects may be genetic, congenital, or acquired, and they may be primary or secondary to other disease processes or medications. There are five recognized categories:

1. Defects in B-cell function (humoral immunodeficiency), including hypogammaglobulinemia or a selective defect in IgA, IgM, or IgG.
2. Defects in T-cell function (defective cell-mediated immunity), including lymphoma, Hodgkin disease, cancer chemotherapy, corticosteroid administration, and the acquired immunodeficiency syndrome (AIDS).
3. Combined defects in T- and B-cell function (organ transplants).
4. Neutrophil defects with neutropenia, defective chemotaxis, or abnormal intracellular killing of bacteria (chronic granulomatous disease).
5. Complement defects (genetic defects of individual components, e.g., C_2 and C_3).

These conditions are discussed in more detail in Chapter 7.2, but three points are emphasized at this juncture:

1. The first point is that likely pathogens may be anticipated to some extent according to the nature of the defect (Table 9.1–3).[16] Patients with defects in humoral immunity, neutrophil function, or the complement system are prone to bacterial infections, usually with rather common bacterial pathogens. Unusual organisms are primarily found with defects in cell-mediated immunity (CMI). These include organisms that remain dormant in the body for extended periods without deleterious effects until the defect occurs, such as herpes simplex, herpes zoster, cytomegalovirus, and *Pneumocystis carinii*. Some organisms occasionally cause disease in otherwise healthy hosts but assume unusual pathogenic potential in the patient with defective CMI such as toxoplasmosis, cryptosporidia, *Strongyloides*, histoplasmosis, cryptococci, and mycobacteria, including atypical strains such as *Mycobacterium avium-intracellulare*. Still other organisms rarely cause any disease except in the compromised host such as phycomycetes (mucormycosis), invasive *Aspergillus*, disseminated or invasive candidiasis, *Listeria*, and *Nocardia*.
2. Clinical clues to the possibility of an immunodeficiency state are (1) the presence of an infection involving an opportunistic pathogen, (2) infections that are unusually serious, prolonged, or recurrent, (3) poor response to antibiotic treatment, or (4) clinical observations that are frequently associated with immunodeficiency states. The latter include chronic malabsorption, hematologic abnormalities, and autoimmune diseases.
3. Appropriate methods to document the defect depend on availability of tests and the type of defect suspected. The most frequently recommended screening tests are (1) a complete blood count to detect neutropenia, lymphopenia, or abnormal morphology of these cells, (2) measurement of levels of IgG, IgA, and IgM, (3) antibody levels to certain common infections or response to vaccines such as rubella, mumps, diphtheria, poliomyelitis, or tetanus as a functional assay of the humoral system, (4) an anergy

TABLE 9.1–3. PATHOGENS ASSOCIATED WITH IMMUNODEFICIENCY SYNDROMES

Humoral immunodeficiency	Pyogenic bacteria, *Giardia*, enteroviruses
Cell-mediated immunity	Bacteria—*Listeria, Salmonella, Nocardia* Viruses—H. simplex, H. zoster, CMV Protozoa—*Toxoplasma, P. carinii,* cryptosporidia Fungi—*Candida*, phycomycetes, *Aspergillus, Histoplasma, Cryptococcus* Parasites—*Strongyloides stercoralis* Mycobacteria—*M. tuberculosis*, atypical
Neutrophil deficit neutropenia	Enterobacteriaceae, *Pseudomonas, Aspergillus*
Defective chemotaxis	Bacterial infections
Intracellular killing	*S. aureus*, Enterobacteriaceae, *Pseudomonas Aspergillus, Nocardia*
Complement C2,3 deficiency	Streptococci, *H. influenzae*
C5 deficiency	Streptococci, *S. aureus*, Enterobacteriaceae
C6,7,8 deficiency	Disseminated *Neisseria* infection
Alternative pathway defect	*S. pneumoniae, H. influenzae, Salmonella*

screen to detect defects in CMI using several antigens such as *Candida*, tetanus, *Trichophyton*, mumps, and purified protein derivative (PPD), (5) T cell subset analysis to quantitate T cells by functional category, (6) assays of neutrophilic killing, and (7) evaluation of the complement system with total hemolytic complement (CH_{50}), and C_3 and C_4 levels.

PERSISTENT INFECTIONS

The natural history of most infections is characterized by microbial invasion followed by host response that is initially nonspecific and then antigen-antibody mediated. The end result is microbial elimination and recovery. There is increasing recognition of a group of microbial agents, primarily viruses, that violate this theme in that the putative organism is not eliminated because of various mechanisms that allow evasion of the immune system.[5] Persistent viral infections may cause persistent infection, they may remain latent and cause symptoms only when immune surveillance is compromised, they may cause autoimmune disease, and they may cause malignant transformation. Established associations are summarized in Table 9.1–4.

HOW TO USE THE MICROBIOLOGY LABORATORY

Infectious diseases are described as conditions caused by microbes or microbial products. Identification of the pathogen usually represents the foundation of a diagnosis and, to a large extent, dictates optimal treatment. This requires a basic understanding of diagnostic resources.

CLASSIFICATION

Microbial pathogens are classified according to selected properties as summarized in Table 9.1–5. There are major differences in the various categories in terms of growth requirements and the methods used to establish their role in disease. There are also major differences in size, which influence techniques used for direct observation in clinical specimens.

TABLE 9.1–4. VIRUSES THAT PRODUCE PERSISTENT INFECTIONS AND LATE SEQUELAE

Agent	Late Sequelae
Measles	Subacute sclerosing panencephalitis
Rubella	Congenital rubella
Herpesvirus	
Cytomegalovirus	Congenital CMV infection Mononucleosis-like syndrome, Pneumonitis, hepatitis, encephalitis
Herpes simplex	Recurrent genital or labial ulcers, disseminated infection
Varicella	Herpes zoster
Epstein-Barr virus	Nasopharyngeal carcinoma Burkitt lymphoma
Papovaviruses	
Polyomaviruses	JC virus—progressive multifocal leukoencephalopathy BK virus—nephritis
Papillomavirus	Laryngeal and genital warts Cervical carcinoma
Hepatitus B virus	Chronic hepatitis hepatic carcinoma
Agent(s) of non-A, non-B hepatitis	Chronic hepatitis
Retroviruses	
HTLV-I	Adult T-cell leukemia Tropical paraparesis
HTLV-II	Hairy-cell leukemia
HIV & HIV-2	AIDS and AIDS-related syndromes
Prions	
Kuru agent	Kuru
Creutzfeldt-Jakob agent	Creutzfeldt-Jakob disease

Bacteria

Bacteria of clinical significance can usually be recovered in microbiology laboratories using standard artificial (cell-free) media, including broth and solid agar supplemented with various nutrients. These media may be incubated in aerobic or anaerobic conditions, or in 5 to 10 percent CO_2, depending on the growth requirements for the suspected pathogens. The repertoire of media, incubation conditions, and methods of identification are usually stylized with relatively uniform policies in different laboratories depending on the type of specimen and the anticipated pathogens. Common clinical isolates (staphylococci, streptococci, *Neisseria*, *Enterobacteriaceae*, and *Pseudomonas*) generally show visible growth in 18 to 24 hours; identification may require an additional 2 to 24 hours; and sensitivity tests usually require 18 to 24 hours. Thus, the final report is usually available within 24 to 48 hours after initiation of bacteriologic processing. Specimens containing a mixed flora, anaerobes, or other relatively fastidious organisms may require longer periods.

Selected bacteria with special properties may be cultivated only by laboratories with special resources and then only by specific request. These include mycobacteria, anaerobic bacteria, spirochetes, *Mycoplasma*, and *Chlamydia*. Virtually all hospital laboratories offer mycobacterial cultures using specialized media that are held for 4 to 6 weeks, owing to relatively slow growth. Most mycobacteria have a replication time of about 20 hours compared to 20 to 30 minutes for "conventional" bacteria. Most hospital laboratories also offer anaerobic cultures, but the technical quality of the work is highly variable. Thus, some laboratories report isolation rates in as many as 40 percent in all specimens that are appropriate for anaerobic culture, whereas other microbiologists regard these organisms as rare isolates to be found only in unusual infections. Few clinical laboratories are able to cultivate *Mycoplasma*, *Chlamydia*, or spirochetes because of a lack of technical expertise and resources.

Fungi

Fungi generally are cultured on specific request utilizing selective media that inhibit bacteria. Recovery rates and interpretation of results are highly variable, depending on the specific fungus, specimen source, and clinical setting. Pathogenic fungi include *Histoplasma capsulatum*, *Coccidioides immitis*, *Blastomyces dermatitidis*, and *Cryptococcus neoformans*. Recovery of these organisms nearly always implies disease regardless of the specimen source. Opportunistic fungi include *Candida*, Phycomycetes, and *Aspergillus*. These organisms cause disease almost exclusively in patients with well-characterized defects in host defense mechanisms, and they commonly represent contaminants so that care must be exercised in attaching clinical significance to laboratory isolations. Dermatophytes cause infections that are confined to keratinized tissue including skin.

TABLE 9.1–5. PROPERTIES OF MICROBIAL PATHOGENS

	Bacteria and "Bacteria-like"					
	Conventional	*Spirochetes*	*Rickettsiae*	*Chlamydiae*	*Mycoplasmas*	*Mycobacteria*
Size (diameter)[a]	0.5–1 μm	0.2 μm	0.5 μm	0.3 μm	0.3 μm	0.5–1 μm
Visualization	Gram stain	Dark field exam	Gimenéz stain	Giemsa stain—elementary bodies Electron microscopy	Electron microscopy	Acid fast stain
Growth outside host cell	+	+	0	0	+	+
Laboratory media	Agar	Experimental animals	Tissue culture Embryonated eggs	Tissue culture Embryonated eggs	Hypertonic media	Agar
Normal flora	+	+	0	0	+ (not *M. pneumoniae*)	+ (not *M. tuberculosis*)
Usual method of disease detection	Culture	Serology Dark field exam	Serology	Culture Serology	Serology	Culture
Susceptibility to antibiotics	Virtually all	All (penicillin, tetracycline, etc)	All (tetracycline chloramphenicol)	All (tetracycline, erythromycin)	All (tetracycline, erythromycin)	Most

[a] Resolving power of naked eye is 100 μm; resolving power of light microscopy is 0.2 μm.

Viruses

Viruses usually cause infections that are self-limited. Relatively few of these infections may be treated, and attempts to make a specific etiologic diagnosis are usually not justified as practical or cost effective. The major methods of identifying a specific agent when appropriate are with viral cultures, serology, nucleic acid hybridization and antigen detection systems. Viruses are obligate intracellular parasites that cannot be grown on artificial media, so that tissue cultures are the usual method for cultivation. Most clinical microbiology laboratories do not offer this service. Even when these facilities are available there are notable limitations. For example, the virus of the common cold can be recovered from nasal secretions in only about 50 percent of patients with typical symptoms. The most common agents of viral gastroenteritis are rotavirus in children and the Norwalk agent in adults, neither of which can be readily grown even with optimal methods. Alternative methods are the enzyme-linked immunoabsorbant assay for rotavirus, or electron microscopy for detection of the Norwalk agent. None of the major causes of viral hepatitis (hepatitis A, hepatitis B virus, or the agents of non-A, non-B hepatitis) are recovered with tissue culture methods. Common viral agents that are most frequently recovered in clinical diagnostic virology laboratories are the herpesvirus group other than the Epstein–Barr virus (varicella-zoster, herpes simplex, and cytomegalovirus), adenovirus, enteroviruses (echo and coxsackie B), influenza (embryonated egg cultures preferred), parainfluenza, mumps, rubella, rubeola, and respiratory syncytial virus (extremely labile).

Parasites

Parasites are relatively large organisms with complicated life cycles. These organisms are rarely cultivated but are usually detected by direct smear to identify typical morphologic features, or with serologic studies.

THE NORMAL FLORA

Knowledge of the normal flora is a critical factor in the selection of specimens for culture and interpretation of results. It is also important in the understanding of the pathophysiology of many infections, since components of the "normal flora" are relatively common pathogens when they reach normally sterile sites.

Most mucocutaneous surfaces harbor a normal microflora

that include an imposing array of bacteria, some fungi, occasional viruses, and virtually no parasites.[6] The numerically dominant organisms are anaerobic bacteria, which represent the major form of life on humans. The complexity of the bacterial flora in some anatomic sites is awesome. For example, the normal tooth surface harbors approximately 70 different bacterial species, many of which cannot be readily recovered or taxonomically classified using current techniques. Other areas of the upper respiratory tract, referred to as ecologic niches, also harbor large concentrations of diverse populations of bacteria. Thus, the tooth surface, the pharynx, the buccal epithelial surface, and the tongue all harbor their own flora. Similarly, the gastrointestinal flora show major differences at various segments. Relatively low concentrations are noted in the stomach, where the major mechanism of population control is gastric acidity, and the organisms present are those washed down from the upper airways that survive the relatively hostile acid environment. In the small bowel, the major mechanism of population control is intestinal motility, which simply propels bacteria to more distant locations. The largest concentrations of bacteria are found in the colon, which is a relatively stagnant section of the intestinal tract. The colonic lumen harbors approximately $10^{11.7}$ bacteria per gram, there are estimates of as many as 400 microbial species, and these organisms constitute about 50 percent of the solid material in stool. The genital tract flora of women contains a complex array of organisms that are quite different during reproductive years, presumably reflecting major changes in the pH and cell type secondary to hormonal influence. All skin surfaces harbor a flora, although there are major differences between the types and concentrations of organisms according to temperature conditions and moisture content.

Most persons harbor yeast in the normal flora, especially *Candida* sp. These organisms have been recovered from up to 40 percent of all sputum cultures, 50 percent of stool specimens, and 30 percent of vaginal swabs, all in the absence of any pathology. Most healthy adults do not harbor or shed viruses from mucocutaneous surfaces, although viral cultures of stools from asymptomatic persons, especially children, may yield enterovirus or adenovirus. Members of the herpesvirus group (herpes simplex, varicella-zoster, cytomegalovirus, and Epstein–Barr virus) remain dormant within tissues of most persons for decades. Parasites are not considered normal flora, but they may be found in the absence of any detectable disease. This particularly applies to intestinal parasites such as *Trichuris, Giardia, Entamoeba histolytica, Ascaris,* and hookworm. None of these organisms are commonly found in stool of persons in industrialized countries, but they are sometimes found in travelers to developing countries and at least one type of intestinal parasite is found in stools of 30 to 80 percent of migrant farm workers or recent immigrants from those areas.[18] *P. carinii* and *Toxoplasma gondii* are examples of protozoa that remain dormant in tissue for decades in a fashion somewhat analogous to the herpesvirus group.

The data just summarized show that the predominant components of the normal flora are bacteria that populate mucocutaneous surfaces. The distribution of organisms is compartmentalized by anatomic sites (ecologic niches). The types and concentrations of microbes vary depending on a variety of factors, including the surface cell type, immunoglobulins, and environmental conditions such as oxygen concentration, redox potential, pH, and concentration of fatty acids. The flora becomes established shortly after birth and exposure to the external environment, and there are rapidly evolving changes during infancy, but once established, the flora of the skin, respiratory tract, and gastrointestinal tract usually remains relatively stable for extended periods. Some of these organisms are uniform within a species and constitute the autochthonous flora; other organisms are unique to the individual and represent a signature; whereas still others are only transiently present so that repeated cultures over extended periods in the same individual show some variations. There is little apparent benefit conferred by this commensal relationship to the host species, except for protection from intrusion by a virulent pathogen. Thus, rodents reared in germfree conditions appear to

Virus	Fungi	Parasites
0.02–0.3 μm	1–20 μm	10–50 μm
Electron microscopy	KOH	Light microscopy
0	+	Variable
Tissue culture	Agar	Rarely done
+ (Latent-herpes-virus group)	+ (especially *Candida* sp/)	+
Culture	Culture Serology	Visualization
Few	All (Amphotericin)	Most

TABLE 9.1–6. GUIDELINE FOR THE EXAMINATION OF SPECIMENS TO DETECT AGENTS OF INFECTIOUS DISEASES

Type of Infection	Specimen	Usual Stains[a]	Culture[b]	Other Tests	Comments
CNS infections Meningitis	CSF[c]	GS, India ink AFB	Aerobic bacteria Fungi Mycobacteria	Antigen detection tests for *S. pneumoniae, H. influenzae, N. meningitidis* Group B streptococci (pediatrics)	
Encephalitis	Brain biopsy[c]	FA for *H. simplex* GS, Giemsa, AFB	Aerobic and anaerobic bacteria, Fungi, *Nocardia* Mycobacteria		
Upper respiratory tract Pharyngitis	Pharyngeal swab	None	Aerobic bacteria	Monospot test Serology: EBV, toxoplasmosis, CMV	Usual pathogen sought is *S. pyogenes*, special processing and transport media required when gonococci suspected
Sinusitis	Sinus aspirate	GS	Aerobic and anaerobic bacteria		Sinus aspirates are usually done only by otolaryngologists; nasal swabs and nasal discharge are unreliable
Otitis media	Tympanocentesis[c]	GS	Aerobic bacteria		Tympanocentesis is not routinely performed; nasopharyngeal and throat cultures are unreliable
Epiglottitis	Blood only[c]	None	Routine		Swab of epiglottis contraindicated since this may cause acute respiratory obstruction
Thrush	Swab	GS or KOH prep	Fungi		Diagnosis is usually established by observing typical whitish patches plus yeast cells on direct smear
Dental	Aspirate	GS	Aerobic and anaerobic bacteria		
Pulmonary Pneumonia	Sputum, nasopharyngeal aspirates and tracheostomy aspirates	GS AFB KOH *Legionella* DFA	Aerobic bacteria Mycobacteria Fungi *Legionella*	Serology for mycoplasma (CF), *Legionella* (IFA), coccidioidomyces (CF), histoplasmosis (CF), influenza (CF), *Cryptococcus* (ID), *Chlamydia* (CF, IFA) etc.	Sputum cytology should be used to determine suitability for culture Quellung test to detect pneumococci
	Transtracheal or transthoracic aspirate[c]	Above	Above plus anaerobic bacteria		Invasive procedures requiring a skilled technician to be done when the anticipated yield justifies the risk
	Bronchoscopy specimens	GS AFB KOH	Aerobic bacteria Mycobacteria Fungi		Specimens include aspirates, brushings, washings, and biopsy. Use of protected brush and quantitative culture improves reliability for aerobic and anaerobic bacteria
	Lung biopsy[c]	H&E, AFB *Legionella* DFA Dieterle stain GMS	Aerobic bacteria Anaerobic bacteria Mycobacteria, Fungi *Legionella*, viral *Nocardia*		Usual methods are: (1) transbronchial biopsy, which provides smaller specimens subject to crush artifact; (2) open lung biopsy, which provides large specimens but requires general anesthesia and chest tube; or (3) transthoracic needle biopsy, which is seldom done

(continued)

TABLE 9.1–6. GUIDELINE FOR THE EXAMINATION OF SPECIMENS TO DETECT AGENTS OF INFECTIOUS DISEASES (Continued)

Type of Infection	Specimen	Usual Stains[a]	Culture[b]	Other Tests	Comments
Body fluids	Peritoneal fluid[c] Joint fluid[c] Pleural fluid[c] Blood[c]	GS KOH AFB GS (buffy coat)	Aerobic and anaerobic bacteria, fungi, *Mycobacteria* Aerobic and anaerobic bacteria, fungi	Antigen detection methods for *S. pneumoniae, H. influenzae, N. meningitidis,* group B streptococci, *Cryptococcus*	
Urinary tract Cystitis/pyelonephritis	Voided urine	MBS, GS AFB	Aerobic bacteria *Mycobacteria*	Antibody-coated bacteria, urinalysis	Usual diagnostic criterion is 10^5 bacteria/ml; culture should be repeated in asymptomatic women Concentration of 10^2 may be significant in women with dysuria-frequency syndrome
	Catheter	GS	Aerobic bacteria		Concentration 10^3 considered significant
	Suprapubic bladder asp.[c]	GS	Aerobic bacteria (Anaerobic bacteria)		Invasive diagnostic technique for children and adults with contaminated voided specimens Any bacteria are considered significant
	Partition urines	GS	Aerobic bacteria		Used primarily in patients with suspected chronic prostatitis: VB_1—1st voided specimen, VB_2—midstream; EPS—expressed prostatic secretions; VB_3—voided specimen immediately after massage
Genital tract Urethritis	Urethral discharge	GS FA stain for *Chlamydia*	Aerobic bacteria *Chlamydia*	Culture for *Chlamydia*	Expeditious processing or specialized transport required
Cervicitis	Cervical swab	GS FA stain for *Chlamydia*	Aerobic bacteria *Chlamydia*	Culture for *Chlamydia*	Inform lab of organisms sought—gonococcus (usual purpose), *S. aureus* (suspected toxic shock syndrome), group B streptococcus (parturition)
Genital ulcer	Swab/aspirate	GS Tzanck test (H. simplex) Darkfield (*T. pallidum*)	Aerobic bacteria	Serology for syphilis	Expeditious processing or specialized transport medium required for gonococcus
Pelvic inflammatory disease	Cervical swab	GS FA stain for *Chlamydia*	Aerobic bacteria (gonococci)		Expeditious processing or specialized transport medium required
	Culdocentesis laparoscopy[c]	GS	Aerobic and anaerobic bacteria		
Enteric diseases Diarrhea	Stool	MBS for leukocytes; O&P (preservative)	*Salmonella Shigella Campylobacter Yersinia V. cholerae V. parahaemolyticus*	Antigen detection methods for *C. difficile,* rotavirus, adenovirus; AFB for cryptosporidia Serology for enterovirus	Food poisoning—culture food for *Bacillus cereus, S. aureus, Clostridium perfringens* stool for *Bacillus cereus, C. perfringens* Traveler's—major agent is enterotoxigenic *E. coli* (ETEC), which cannot be detected by most laboratories; methylene blue stain used to distinguish inflammatory and secretory diarrheas

(continued)

TABLE 9.1–6. GUIDELINE FOR THE EXAMINATION OF SPECIMENS TO DETECT AGENTS OF INFECTIOUS DISEASES (Continued)

Type of Infection	Specimen	Usual Stains[a]	Culture[b]	Other Tests	Comments
Skin and soft tissues	Aspirates[b] Sinus drainage	GS KOH AFB	Aerobic and anaerobic bacteria, Fungi, mycobacteria	Intravenous lines should have quantitative culture (see Chapter 9.4)	Closed lesions (bullae, blebs, vesicles, abscesses, etc.) are valid for anaerobic culture; aspirates of cellulitis rarely yield bacteria
		Tzanck (H. simplex, varicella-zoster)			Tzanck stain and culture for H. simplex when indicated
	Biopsy	GS	Aerobic and anaerobic bacteria	Quantitative culture offered by some laboratories, especially for burns	

[a]Usual stains for exudate or tissue, abbreviations are GS = Gram stain, KOH = 10% potassium hydroxide, AFB = acid fast bacilli stain or modified acid fast stain, MBS = methylene blue stain, FA = fluorescent antibody, DFA = direct fluorescent antibody, GMS = Gomori methenamine silver, O&P = ova and parasites; H & E = hematoxylin and eosin.
[b]Appropriate types of cultures; many of these require a specific request.
[c]Indicates uncontaminated specimen.

thrive, grow larger, and live longer than their counterparts with a normal flora. Nevertheless, these animals fail to develop immunoglobulin levels against organisms that commonly colonize the intestinal tract, and they are unusually vulnerable to colonization and invasion by various microbial pathogens. The most common clinical example of an altered flora is in the patient receiving antibiotics, in which the changes reflect the dose, route of administration, pharmacokinetic properties, and the spectrum of the drug used. These patients are susceptible to colonization or "intrusion" with a variety of microorganisms, resulting in an altered "normal flora" that generally persists throughout treatment and for 2 to 3 weeks after antibiotics have been discontinued. On occasion, the consequence is an infection or "superinfection" by organisms that rarely cause disease in the absence of antibiotic exposure, such as candidiasis and *Clostridium difficile*-induced enteric disease. Additionally, antibiotic recipients within the hospital setting are uniquely susceptible to colonization by nosocomial pathogens, primarily gram-negative bacilli, which may become pathogens in the susceptible host or else serve as the source of plasmids in other colonizing bacteria.

SPECIMEN SELECTION

Most cultures are done to recover bacterial pathogens, and the usual specimens are exudate, body fluids, or tissue obtained from the site of the suspected infection. Patients with suspected bacteremia or "sepsis" should have cultures of blood and urine, but cultures of other sites in this setting should not be considered routine, and the common practice of culturing every orifice is ill-advised.

There are major differences in the quality of specimens for bacteria culture, depending largely on the distribution of the normal flora (Table 9.1–6). Specimens that virtually always contain colonizing bacteria include those from the lumen of the gastrointestinal tract, the mucosal surfaces of the upper airways, the genital tract, and the skin. Specimens are often collected from these sites in an attempt to find a specific pathogen. Thus, throat cultures are usually done to recover group A β-hemolytic streptococci, cervical cultures generally are processed only to detect *N. gonorrhoeae*, and stool is cultured only with selective media designed to recover certain enteric pathogens such as *Salmonella, Shigella,* and *Campylobacter.* Other specimens are not subject to contamination and are usually processed to detect a more encyclopedic array of bacteria, and interpretation of results is far simpler. These specimens include cultures of blood, body fluids (pleural fluid, joint fluid, bile, peritoneal fluid, and cerebrospinal fluid), aspirates of abscess contents, middle ear aspirates, transtracheal aspirates, culdocentesis aspirates, and biopsies of normally sterile organs.

As a general rule, the best specimens for the microbiology lab-oratory are liquid specimens. Swabs should be avoided whenever possible, since these tend to dry out and swab fibers may be deleterious to some bacteria. Exceptions are throat cultures utilizing a standard throat swab device with a fluid vial to prevent drying, and cervical swabs, which are processed immediately or placed in appropriate transport media.

The quality of specimens varies considerably, as noted, but there are some specimens that may be considered "precious" since they are obtained with invasive diagnostic techniques and yield unique microbial information that is not readily available from alternative sources. In my view, these should not be entrusted to the usual escort services of the hospital but should be hand-delivered for immediate processing. Specimens in this category include transtracheal aspirates, culdocentesis aspirates, suprapubic bladder aspirates, bone aspirates to detect osteomyelitis, and some specimens collected from the operating room. The physician who performs an invasive diagnostic technique will be well rewarded for effective communication with the microbiologist.

RAPID DIAGNOSTIC TECHNIQUES

The etiologic agent of most infections is detected by recovery of the pathogen from the infected site, an exercise that usually requires at least a day, often several days, and occasionally weeks. Rapid diagnostic techniques refer to more expeditious laboratory methods in which the time required for results is measured in minutes or hours. The most practical rapid tests are direct stains (Table 9.1–7).

Fluorescent-tagged antibody may be used to detect *Actinomyces,* herpes simplex, *Legionella,* pertussis, and parapertussis. Alternative antigen detection methods include latex particle agglutination, counterimmunoelectrophoresis, or enzyme-linked immunosorbent assays. Examples of organisms that may be detected with these techniques include *S. pneumoniae,* type B *H. influenzae,* group B streptococci, *N. gonorrhoeae, Neisseria meningitidis, Cryptococcus,* adenovirus, rotavirus, and sytomegalovirus. Another alternative to conventional culture that provides rapid diagnostic information is the nucleic acid probe. This technique uses the specificity of genetic sequences in chromosomes or plasmids to identify a species or strain; hybridization takes place only with a probe using complementary DNA or RNA nucleotide sequences. Most probes are radiolabeled and use roentgenography to produce an autoradiogram, or the probe is covalently linked to biotin or enzymes, and a protein marker is used that binds to the label. Nucleic acid probes are in the early stages of development but appear potentially useful in detecting virulence factors of bacteria (enterotoxigenic *E. coli* to detect LT and ST toxin), antibiotic resistance, specific microbes (*N. gonorrhoeae, Campylobacter, Chlamydia*), viruses (CMV, HIV), and parasites (*Plasmodium, Leishmania*).

TABLE 9.1–7. STAIN TECHNIQUES

Organism[a]	Usual Stain	Comment
Bacteria	Gram	Permits categorization as gram-positive or -negative and by morphology
Fungi	KOH/Gram	Gram—adequate for *Candida*. KOH preferred for most others; preferred tissue stains are methenamine silver, Giemsa and KOH
Mycobacteria	Acid-fast	Detects *M. tuberculosis*, atypical mycobacteria, *M. lepra;* modified acid-fast stain for *Nocardia*, *Legionella micdadei*, *Cryptosporidia*, and *Isospora*
Viruses	Tzanck test for inclusion bodies (herpesvirus group only)	All viruses are too small to visualize with light microscopy
Parasites	Direct exam of exudate; acid fast for *Cryptosporidia* and *Isospora*	Preferred tissue stains are Giemsa or methenamine silver
Chlamydiae	Cannot be visualized with light microscopy	Giemsa stain of tissue to detect elementary bodies

[a]Indirect fluorescent antibody stains and nucleic acid probes are alternative methods to visualize microbes that are usually species or strain specific.

INTERPRETATION OF CULTURE RESULTS

Interpretation of culture results depends on several interrelated variables:

1. The source of the culture, with distinction between specimens that are contaminated and those that are from normally sterile sites, is a fundamental issue in the interpretation of culture results. Some organisms represent pathogens almost any time they are recovered, regardless of the specimen source. Included in this group are: *Mycobacterium tuberculosis, Legionella sp.,* pathogenic fungi (*Blastomyces, Histoplasma,* and *Coccidioides*), *Mycoplasma pneumoniae, Chlamydia,* most enteric pathogens (*Salmonella, Shigella, Campylobacter, Yersinia, Vibrio cholerae*), and *Corynebacterium diphtheriae.* The second category of organisms includes relatively common bacterial pathogens that are readily interpreted as clinically significant when recovered in specimens that are collected from normally sterile sites, but also represent normal flora from mucocutaneous surfaces of healthy individuals. Organisms in this category include group A β-hemolytic streptococci, *S. pneumoniae, N. meningitidis, H. influenzae, S. aureus,* Enterobacteriaceae, *P. aeruginosa,* and many anaerobic bacteria (*Bacteroides* sp., fusobacteria, clostridia, and peptostreptococci). The third category of organisms are those that normally colonize the skin surface, have minimal pathogenic potential, and usually represent contaminants, unless they are repeatedly isolated from uncontaminated specimens and clinical correlations support their pathogenic role. Bacteria in this category include *Staphylococcus epidermidis,* diphtheroids, *Propionibacterium, Corynebacterium, Bacillus* sp., lactobacilli, *Streptococcus viridans,* and some anaerobes (*Veillionella,* eubacteria, bifidobacteria).

2. The pathogenic potential of the organism is another critical variable.
3. Interpretation must account for likely pathogens according to the host setting and the site of pathology.
4. Culture results should corroborate the results of direct stains. Discordance indicates a fastidious organism, improper culture techniques, misinterpretation or improper performance of the stain, the presence of nonviable organisms, the presence of contaminating organisms on the slide or stain, or previous treatment with antimicrobial agents that may preclude growth.
5. The concentration of organisms, particularly bacteria, is an important variable that is often overlooked. Quantitative cultures have been performed with specimens from a variety of sources including urine, bile, pulmonary secretions, abscess contents, and wounds. This work shows that bacterial infections are almost invariably associated with concentratons of at least 10^5/ml exudate or 10^5/g tissue.[15] The only specimen routinely cultured with quantitative techniques in most laboratories is urine, because this is easily accomplished with a quantitative loop. Most specimens, particularly exudate, pose a technical problem, since purulent secretions are tenacious and do not permit a uniform sampling size unless the specimen is liquefied. An occasional exception is that some clinical laboratories perform quantitative cultures on soft-tissue lesions that are biopsied, ground in a tissue grinder, and then serially diluted. This technique has been used to determine if wounds may be sutured with a primary closure, to determine the acceptability of a wound for skin grafting, and to predict burn wound sepsis. Although most specimens are not cultured quantitatively, comparable information may be obtained with semiquantitative analysis. The implication is that organisms in concentrations of 10^5 or more are generally recovered with "heavy" growth, or at least "moderate" growth. Organisms that are recovered in relatively small concentrations such as "light" growth on primary isolation plates or recovered only in broth media should be viewed with skepticism unless they are relatively fastidious, have unique pathogenic potential, or are consistently recovered from uncontaminated specimen sources.
6. Microbial therapy will rapidly modify the cultivable flora from infected sites. The culture that is obtained before the institution of treatment is the best one and should be viewed accordingly. This especially applies to specimens from potentially contaminated sites, since resistant organisms are to be anticipated. This usually represents "specimen superinfection," which must be distinguished from "patient superinfection."

TREATMENT GUIDELINES

GENERAL, SYMPTOMATIC, AND SUPPORTIVE CARE

The treatment of a patient with an infectious disease includes attempts to relieve patient suffering by means of "nonspecific" measures, an effort to prevent or treat pathophysiologic consequences of the infection using supportive measures, and a specific attack against the offending organism.

FEVER

Fever is a common manifestation of many infectious and noninfectious diseases and usually represents the final common pathway of an endogenous pyrogen. This is a valuable sign to assess the severity of the disease process and also the response to treatment. There

is also evidence that fever facilitates the host defense mechanisms against a microbial challenge by enhancement of phagocytosis, inhibition of occasional bacteria and viruses that are especially temperature labile, and promotion of interleukin activity.[4] The disadvantages of fever include (1) patient discomfort, (2) augmented metabolic demands, which may be particularly hazardous in patients with coronary insufficiency or congestive heart failure, (3) the consequences of hyperpyrexia with temperatures exceeding 106F, and (4) the possibility of inducing seizures, particularly in young children. The advisability of reducing fever is controversial, and the decision must be based on individual case information. Relevant issues are the magnitude of the fever, the consequences of increased metabolic demands as a result of associated conditions, patient discomfort, the security of the diagnosis, and the importance of utilizing fever to document therapeutic response. When the decision has been made to decrease temperature, the most frequently used antipyretics are acetaminophen and acetylsalicylic acid. The latter possesses anti-inflammatory action as well as antipyretic and analgesic action. Acetaminophen lacks the anti-inflammatory activity, which is rarely an advantage with infectious diseases, and it causes less toxicity so that many regard it as the antipyretic of choice. The usual dose in adults for either antipyretic is 0.6 to 0.9 g orally every 4 to 6 hours. It is recommended that this be given at regular intervals rather than for specific temperature elevations, since intermittent administration may result in wide fluctuations in the temperature profile that are often very uncomfortable for the patient.

PAIN

The relief of pain may be accomplished with antipyretics, but codeine and propoxyphene represent alternative agents for pain relief without affecting body temperature. Narcotics may be used for severe pain without altering fever, but these impose the hazard of addiction with prolonged courses.

SHOCK

The principles for managing septic shock are discussed in Chapter 4.3.

ASSOCIATED CONDITIONS

Patients with serious infections often have associated conditions that either increase the incidence or severity of the disease and require attention. These include correction of blood sugar in patients with diabetes, hydration for patients with fluid depletion, possible dialysis in patients with renal failure, reduction or elimination of chemotherapeutic agents that enhance susceptibility to infectious complications, and attempts to eliminate antibiotics when appropriate in order to prevent superinfections.

SURGERY

Surgery is often the most important facet of the treatment program. This particularly applies to patients with closed-space infections who require drainage and those with obstructing lesions with proximal infection. A commonly quoted adage is that all abscesses require drainage, but there are some notable exceptions. Most lung abscesses drain spontaneously and do not require surgical drainage. Approximately 70 percent of tubo-ovarian abscesses, most amebic liver abscesses, some pyogenic liver abscesses, and many cerebral abscesses respond to antibiotic treatment alone. Other abscesses, including intraabdominal abscesses, require some form of drainage either with surgery or with percutaneous techniques using ultra-sonic or computed tomographic guidance. Surgery is especially important in many soft-tissue infections that require debridement, drainage, or amputation.

FOREIGN BODIES

Infections associated with foreign bodies usually require removal of the foreign body, although there may be a trial of antibiotics when the necessary surgery is technically difficult or the device is particularly important. These guidelines apply to prosthetic heart valves, cerebrospinal shunts, LeVeen shunts, peritoneal dialysis devices, vascular grafts, joint prostheses, breast implants, intravenous catheters, and hemodialysis shunts.

SELECTION OF AN ANTIBIOTIC

The antibiotic revolution has been accomplished at considerable price in terms of abuse, unnecessary costs, serious side effects, and, perhaps most important, the problem of resistant bacteria. Thus, judicious use of these agents has become an essential component of both the art and science of medical practice. There are three fundamental questions in the patient with suspected infection. The first concerns the possibility that this represents a noninfectious process such as a collagen-vascular disease or tumor. These processes collectively actually outrank infections in causing fevers of unknown origin. The second question, assuming infection is present, concerns the likely etiologic agent on the basis of probabilities according to host setting, laboratory observations, and prior experience with similar infections. The final question concerns the advisability of treatment and the appropriate antibiotic regimen. There is a consensus that drug selection is clearly simplified if a pathogen is identified and susceptibility data are either predictable or available with in vitro testing. Nevertheless, many infections are treated, at least initially, with antibiotic regimens that are selected empirically. This approach is necessary because valid or uncontaminated cultures from the infected site are often not available, culture results are frequently not available at the time therapeutic decisions are required, and multiple published reports provide extensive information regarding regimens that are likely to be successful.

THERAPEUTIC RESPONSE

An important consideration in the treatment of infectious diseases is the anticipated response and the management plan for patients with treatable diseases who appear to have a suboptimal course. Included in the differential diagnosis are the following considerations:

1. Wrong diagnosis: This category includes noninfectious diseases and infections at alternative anatomical sites.
2. Wrong antimicrobial agent: This category applies to situations in which the microbial pathogen is resistant to the antibiotic, or the agent being given does not reach the inflammatory site. Data regarding the appropriate drug may be available with in vitro sensitivity tests or there may be need for empiric changes when valid cultures from the site of infection are not available.
3. Wrong regimen: The implication in this case is that the dosage or route of administration is inappropriate. The most common example is the aminoglycosides, which have a relatively close toxic-therapeutic ratio and are often given in subtherapeutic doses. Another concern is compliance, particularly in outpatients.
4. Need for surgery, drainage, or removal of a foreign body: Surgery often represents the mainstay of therapy, particularly in patients with closed-space infections, infections associated with obstructing lesions, or infections in the presence of foreign bodies.

5. Adverse drug reaction: Nearly all antibiotics and many other drugs may cause drug fever. Perhaps the most likely antimicrobial agents are sulfonamides, β-lactam agents (penicillins and cephalosporins), and amphotericin B. The fever pattern may be intermittent, spiking, or sustained, and eosinophilia is found in only about half of the cases. One useful clinical clue is that these patients often appear deceptively well despite the presence of fever. The appropriate management plan is to discontinue the drugs that are most likely to cause fever and use alternative agents from another pharmacologic class if continued treatment is necessary. Most patients respond within 48 to 72 hours. It should be noted that drug fever, per se, does not necessarily contraindicate the continued use of some agents that are essential for treatment.

6. Superinfection: Superinfections involve microorganisms that are resistant to the agents being given, are more likely to occur with broad spectrum regimens, and usually, but not invariably, involve the site of the original infection. The most common microbes are *S. aureus* (both methicillin-sensitive and resistant strains), *P. aeruginosa,* other resistant gram-negative bacilli, enterococci, and *Candida.* A characteristic feature of most superinfections is that the patient initially responds and then deteriorates. The usual method of detection is repeated cultures from potential sites of infection, but this is fraught with the hazard that sequential cultures subject to contamination by the normal flora are expected to yield bacteria that are resistant to the antibiotic given, and it is usually difficult to distinguish colonization from superinfection.

7. Inadequate host: This explanation is one of the most common reasons for the failure to respond, and it is also one of the most difficult to accept. A painful fact is that 20 to 30 percent of patients with pneumococcal pneumonia and bacteremia die despite treatment with penicillin, the mortality rate of gram-negative septicemia treated with appropriate drugs is 15 to 20 percent, and septic shock is associated with a 30 to 50 percent mortality rate despite the use of highly seasoned and widely accepted antibiotic regimens. These observations do not imply that other potential causes of failure to respond should not be sought. They do mean that host-defense mechanisms are critical, some infections are simply too far advanced at the time they are initially treated, and frequent changes in the antibiotic regimen without a sound scientific rationale are ill advised.

REFERENCES

1. Centers for Disease Control: National Nosocomial Infections Study Report, Annual Summary, 1979, issued March, 1982
2. Dixon RE: Effect of infections on hospital care. Ann Intern Med 89:749, 1978
3. Garner JS, Simmons BP: CDC guideline for isolation precautions in hospitals. Infection Control 4:249, 1983
4. Hanson DF, Murphy PA, et al: The effect of temperature on the activation of thymocytes by interleukins I and II. J Immunol 130:216, 1983
5. Haywood AM: Patterns of persistent viral infections. N Engl J Med 315:939, 1986
6. Kaiser MH, Cohen R, et al: Normal viral and bacterial flora of the human small and large intestine. N Engl J Med 274:500, 1966
7. Kennedy DL, Forbes MG, et al: Antibiotic use in U.S. hospitals in 1981. Am J Hosp Pharm 40:797, 1983
8. Lacey RW: Evolution of microorganisms and antibiotic resistance. Lancet 2:1022, 1984
9. McDermott W, Rogers DE: Social ramifications of control of microbial disease. Johns Hopkins Med J 151:302, 1982
10. McLemore T, Koch H: 1980 Summary: National Ambulatory Medical Care Survey. Vital and Health Statistics of the National Center for Health Statistics, No. 77, Feb 22, 1982
11. Moss F, McNicol MW, et al: Survey of antibiotic prescribing practice in a district general hospital. Lancet 2:349, 1981
12. National Center for Health Statistics: Physician visits: Volume and interval since last visit. Washington, D.C.: U.S. Government Printing Office. 1980 Summary, United States, Series 10, No. 144, 1980
13. National Center for Health Statistics: Drug utilization in office-based practice, a summary of findings. Washington, D.C.: U.S. Government Printing Office. National Ambulatory Medical Care Survey, United States, Series 13, No. 85, 1980
14. Peacock Jr. JE, Moorman DR, et al: Methicillin-resistant *Staphylococcus aureus:* Microbiologic characteristics, antimicrobial susceptibilities, and assessment of virulence of an epidemic strain. J Infect Dis 144:575, 1981
15. Robson MC, Krizek TJ, Heggers JP: Biology of surgical infections. In Current Problems in Surgery. Chicago, Year Book, 1973
16. Sen P, Kapila R, et al: Superinfection: Another look. Am J Med 73:706, 1982
17. Stolley PD, Becker MH, et al: Drug prescribing and use in an American community. Ann Intern Med 76:537, 1972
18. Ungar BLP, Iscoe E, et al: Intestinal parasites in a migrant farmworker population. Arch Intern Med 146:513, 1986
19. Walsh JA, Warren KS: Selective primary health care. An interim strategy for disease control in developing countries. N Engl J Med 301:967, 1979
20. Wenzel RP: Nosocomial infections, diagnosis-related groups, and study on the efficacy of nosocomial infection control. Am J Med 78:3, 1983
21. Williams WW: CDC guideline for infection control in hospital personnel. Infection Control 4:329, 1983

CHAPTER 9.2
Use and Misuse of Antimicrobial Agents

Paul S. Lietman

Several steps are required in the therapeutic approach to an infectious disease. After the initial decision as to the necessity of treatment is made, an antimicrobial agent is selected (Table 9.2–1), a therapeutic regimen is designed, and a plan for monitoring its effectiveness is formulated.

THE DECISION TO TREAT OR NOT TO TREAT

Although this decision is easy in the presence of a severe or life-threatening illness, it becomes more difficult with less severe or trivial infections and still more so when the therapy is aimed at preventing rather than curing an infectious disease.

Since infections by organisms such as pneumococci, which are highly sensitive to antimicrobial agents, may proceed rapidly toward life-threatening infection, one must begin treatment as early as possible. The manifest seriousness of some infections demands the immediate initiation of specific antimicrobial therapy without waiting for cultural proof of the specific organism involved and without knowing the sensitivities of that organism. Here the choice of an appropriate antimicrobial regimen depends on a sophisticated clinical estimate of the etiologic agent most likely to be involved as a base for the selection of the most logical antimicrobial

TABLE 9.2–1. ANTIMICROBIAL AGENTS IN CURRENT CLINICAL USE

	Mechanism of Action	Mechanism of Resistance	Serious Toxicity	Usual Daily Dose Range	Usual Dosage Interval (hr)
Penicillins monobactam, and thienamycin	Inhibition of bacterial cell wall synthesis by inhibiting the cross-linking reaction (transpeptidation)	Inactivation by β-lactamases Mutation in penicillin-binding proteins Impermeability	Anaphylactic shock Other allergic reactions Seizures Diarrhea		
Penicillin G				1.2–24 million	4–6
Procaine penicillin G				1–2 million U	12
Benzathine penicillin				1.2–2.4 million U	Monthly
Penicillin V				0.5–1 g	6
Ampicillin				1–12 g (R)	6
Amoxicillin				0.75–1.5 g (R)	6–8
Amoxicillin and clavulanate				0.75–1.5 g (R)	6–8
Carbenicillin			Bleeding Hypokalemia Sodium overload (4.7 mEq Na/g)	4–40 g (R)	3–6
Ticarcillin			Bleeding Hypokalemia Sodium overload (5.2 mEq Na/g)	2–20 g (R)	3–6
Ticarcillin and clavulanate			Bleeding Hypokalemia Sodium overload (5.2 mEq Na/g)	9–18 g (R)	4–6
Piperacillin			Bleeding Hypokalemia Sodium overload (1.85 mEq Na/g)	6–18 g (R)	4–6
Azlocillin			Bleeding Hypokalemia Sodium overload (2.17 mEq Na/g)	8–18 g (R)	4–6
Mezlocillin			Bleeding Hypokalemia Sodium overload (1.85 mEq Na/g)	6–18 g (R)	4–6
Methicillin		Inherent undefined resistance	Intersititial nephritis	6–12 g (R)	4–6
Nafcillin		Inherent undefined resistance	Neutropenia	3–6 g	4
Oxacillin		Inherent undefined resistance	Neutropenia	3–6 g (R)	4–6
Dicloxacillin		Inherent undefined resistance		1–4 g	6
Aztreonam				1–8 g (R)	6–12
Imipenem and cilastatin			Myoclonus Confusion Seizures Thrombophlebitis	1–4 g (R)	6–12
Cephalosporins	Same as penicillins	β-Lactamases of gram-negative organisms Inherent undefined resistance of staphylococci Impermeability	Anaphylactic shock Other allergic reactions Seizures Diarrhea Thrombophlebitis		
Cephalothin				2–6 g (R)	4–6
Cefazolin				1–12 g (R)	6
Cefadroxil				1–2 g (R)	12–24
Cephapirin				2–12 g (R)	4–6
Cephradine				2–8 g (R)	4–6
Cephalexin				1–4 g (R)	6–12
Cefuroxime				2.25–4.5 g (R)	8
Cefaclor				0.75–4 g	8
Cefamandole			Disulfiram-like reaction Hypoprothrombinemia	1.5–12 g (R)	4–8

(continued)

TABLE 9.2–1. ANTIMICROBIAL AGENTS IN CURRENT CLINICAL USE (Continued)

	Mechanism of Action	Mechanism of Resistance	Serious Toxicity	Usual Daily Dose Range	Usual Dosage Interval (hr)
Cephalosporins (*Cont.*)					
Cefoxitin				3–12 g (R)	4–8
Cefonicid				0.5–2 g (R)	12–24
Ceforanide				0.5–2 g (R)	12
Cefotetan				2–4 g (R)	12
Cefotaxime				2–12 g (R)	4–12
Cefoperazone			Disulfiram-like reaction Hypoprothrombinemia	2–12 g	6–12
Moxalactam			Disulfiram-like reaction Hypoprothrombinemia	2–12 g (R)	8–12
Ceftizoxime				2–12 g (R)	6–12
Ceftriaxone				1–4 g (R)	12–24
Ceftazidime				0.5–6 g (R)	8–12
Erythromycin	Inhibition of synthesis at translocation step	Decreased ribosomal binding	Hepatitis (with the estolate)	1–4 g (R,H)	6–12
Clindamycin	Inhibition of protein synthesis at peptidyl transferase step	Decreased ribosomal binding Impermeability	Colitis	0.5–1.5 g (R,H)	6–8
Chloramphenicol	Inhibition of protein synthesis at peptidyl transferase step	Acetylation by R factor–mediated enzyme	Aplastic anemia Transient bone marrow suppression Gray syndrome	2–6 g (H)	6
Tetracyclines	Inhibition of protein synthesis at initiation step	Impermeability due to defective transport	Diarrhea Superinfection Hepatitis		
Tetracycline				1–2 (R)	6
Oxytetracycline				1–2 g (R)	6
Minocycline			Vertigo	0.1–0.2 g (R)	6–12
Doxycycline				0.1–0.2 g	12–24
Aminoglycosides	Inhibition of protein synthesis at initiation step	Enzymatic modification by acetylation, adenylation, or phosphorylation	Neuromuscular paralysis Ototoxicity Nephrotoxicity		
Streptomycin				0.5–2 g (R)	12–24
Kanamycin				1 g (R)	6–12
Gentamicin				0.08–0.4 g (R)	8
Tobramycin				0.08–0.4 g (R)	8
Netilmicin				0.08–0.4 g (R)	8
Amikacin				1–1.5 g (R)	8
Polymyxins	Damage to membranes	Impermeability	Neuromuscular paralysis Nephrotoxicity Neurotoxicity		
Colistin				0.175–0.3 g (R)	6–12
Polymyxin B				1–1.75 million U (R)	12
Vancomycin	Inhibition of cell wall synthesis	Undefined mechanism	Fever Skin rash	2 g (R)	6–12
Rifampicin	Inhibition of RNA synthesis	Mutation in RNA polymerase	Hepatitis Induction of microsomal drug metabolizing enzymes	0.6 g	24
Sulfonamides	Inhibition of folic acid synthesis	Mutation in enzymes of folic acid synthesis	Fever Other allergic reactions Hemolysis with G6PD deficiency		
Sulfisoxazole				2–10 g (R)	6–8
Sulfamethoxazole				3 g (R)	8

(continued)

TABLE 9.2–1. ANTIMICROBIAL AGENTS IN CURRENT CLINICAL USE (Continued)

	Mechanism of Action	Mechanism of Resistance	Serious Toxicity	Usual Daily Dose Range	Usual Dosage Interval (hr)
Trimethoprim	Inhibition dihydro-folate reductase	Mutation in dihydro-folate reductase Alternate pathway	Transient hemato-poietic suppression Rash	0.2 g (R)	12–24
Trimethoprim–sulfamethox-azole	See both above	See both above	See both above	0.160 g trimethoprim (R) 0.8 g sulfamethoxa-zole	12
Nitrofurantoin	Undefined mecha-nism of action	Undefined resistance	Interstitial pneumoni-tis Pulmonary fibrosis Hemolysis with G6PD deficiency	0.2–1 g (R)	6
Nalidixic acid	Inhibition of DNA gyrase	Undefined resistance	CNS effects	2–4 g (R)	6
Norfloxacin	Inhibition of DNA gyrase	Undefined resistance	Nausea Headache Dizziness Fatigue	0.8 g (R)	12
Ciprofloxacin	Inhibition of DNA gyrase	Undefined resistance	Nausea Diarrhea Headache	0.5–1.5 g (R)	12
Metronidazole	Undefined mecha-nism of action	Undefined resistance	CNS effects Peripheral neurop-athy Disulfiram-like effect	0.75–2 g (H)	6–8
Isoniazid	Inhibition of my-colic acid syn-thesis	Mutation in mycotic acid synthesizing enzyme	Peripheral neurop-athy Hepatitis	0.3 g	24
Ethambutol	Undefined mecha-nism of action	Undefined resistance	Optic neuritis	1 g	24
Cycloserine	Inhibition of cell wall synthesis	Undefined resistance	CNS effects Allergic reactions	0.5–1 g	12
Amphotericin B	Interaction with ergosterol to damage mem-branes	Undefined resistance	Nephrotoxicity Fever and chills Phlebitis	0.015–0.1 g	24–48
Flucytosine	Inhibition of RNA synthesis	Impermeability Mutant conversion to fluorodeoxyuridine	Nephrotoxicity Transient bone mar-row suppression	0.35–1 g (R)	6
Ketoconazole	Inhibits synthesis of ergosterol	Undefined resistance	Hepatitis Effects on steroid syn-thesis	0.2–0.4 g	24
Miconazole	Inhibits synthesis of ergosterol	Undefined resistance	Phlebitis	0.6–3.6 g	8
Vidarabine	Inhibition of DNA replication	Undefined resistance	Fluid overload Transient bone mar-row suppression CNS effects	1 g	Over 12–24
Acyclovir	Inhibition of DNA replication	Mutation in herpes thymidine kinase or DNA polymerase	Phlebitis	1 g (R)	8
Zidovudine	Inhibition of viral reverse tran-scriptase	Undefined resistance	Anemia Leukopenia Nausea Headache	1.0 g	4
Amantadine	Inhibition of virus uncoating	Mutation in M pro-tein	Confusion Irritability Anxiety Ataxia Orthostatic hypo-tension	0.1–0.2 g (R)	12–24

(continued)

TABLE 9.2–1. ANTIMICROBIAL AGENTS IN CURRENT CLINICAL USE (Continued)

	Mechanism of Action	Mechanism of Resistance	Serious Toxicity	Usual Daily Dose Range	Usual Dosage Interval (hr)
Pentamidine	Unknown	Undefined resistance	Hypotension Hypoglycemia Arrhythmias Leukopenia Nephrotoxicity Hepatitis Skin rash	0.28 g (R)	24

(R) = Dosage adjustment needed in renal disease; (H) = dosage adjustment needed in hepatic disease.

agent or agents. This type of decision is essential with local infections judged to be proceeding toward septicemia, septicemia itself, most cases of meningitis, and many cases of pneumonitis.

More difficulty is encountered with less immediately serious infections. Here one is often justified in withholding treatment while collecting as much information as possible on which to base a rational decision. An example is the patient with a urinary tract infection who has an indwelling catheter in place or has a structural abnormality. In this situation one may first identify the organism and determine its sensitivities before initiating therapy, because any regimen selected is unlikely to successfully eradicate the organism. Faced with this knowledge, it may be best to refrain from subjecting the patient to the potential toxicity of the drug.

Perhaps the greatest misuse of antibiotics is in the treatment of viral or presumed viral illnesses. It has been stated that greater than 50 percent of common colds that are brought to the attention of a physician are treated with antibiotics. Although the argument is sometimes made that the antibiotic may prevent the occasional bacterial superinfection, this has not been documented. Clearly, this is a situation where even a remote chance of serious toxicity from the drug is unacceptable.

The use of antimicrobial agents to prevent infections is of proven value in only a few situations. These include the prevention of streptococcal infections in patients with rheumatic heart disease or past rheumatic fever (penicillin, a sulfonamide, or erythromycin), the prevention of meningococcal infection in close contacts of infected patients in epidemic situations (a sulfonamide if the meningococcus is sensitive, or minocycline or rifampin if not), the prevention of exacerbations of chronic bronchitis (ampicillin or tetracycline), the prevention of postoperative infections after vaginal hysterectomy, cesarean section, or abortion (cephalosporin), the prevention of postoperative infections after cardiovascular surgery (cephalosporin), the prevention of postoperative infections after clean-contaminated surgery of the head and neck or gastrointestinal tract (cephalosporin), the prevention of postoperative infections after major bowel surgery (oral neomycin and tetracycline), the prevention of tuberculous disease in tuberculin-positive patients receiving steroids (isoniazid), the prevention of influenza A (amantadine), and the prevention of a recrudescence of herpes simplex infection (acyclovir). Although of unproven value, the use of penicillin and an aminoglycoside is recommended by the American Heart Association for the prevention of infective endocarditis in patients with rheumatic or congenital heart disease who undergo dental manipulations or oral surgery. Similarly unproven is the widely advocated use of antibiotics in the presence of penetrating wounds, skull fractures, and other compound fractures.

THE CHOICE OF AN ANTIMICROBIAL AGENT

Without specific knowledge of the antimicrobial sensitivities of the organism involved in a particular infection, one must proceed on the basis of the usual sensitivities of similar organisms. With the emergence of resistance due to plasmid transfer between organisms of different species, one must be aware of the ecology of resistance in the particular population of patients being treated. Even within a single institution there may be wide divergences in the sensitivities of a group of organisms. A tabulation of drugs of choice and alternative drugs is presented in Table 9.2–2. One must emphasize, however, that the "drug of choice" may be determined on grounds other than clinical effectiveness. If several drugs are equally effective, selection of the "drug of choice" may be based on lower toxicity, lower cost, convenience of administration, or some combination of these factors. Individual considerations, including those presented below, may therefore alter one's "drug of choice" in a particular situation.[1-6]

BACTERIAL SENSITIVITIES

Sensitivity and resistance are relative terms based on the ability of a selected concentration of drug to inhibit bacterial growth (minimal inhibitory concentration or MIC) or to kill bacterial cells (minimum bactericidal concentration or MBC). The selected level separating sensitivity from resistance is somewhat arbitrarily chosen based on some relationship with the attainability of an effective plasma level. Several features of bacterial sensitivity testing should be kept in mind when evaluating the laboratory results and planning therapy. An organism may be "resistant," as defined by a lack of growth inhibition at concentrations achievable in plasma, and yet be quite "susceptible" to the higher concentrations of antibiotic achieved in urine. Conversely, an organism may be "sensitive" to the selected plasma level but "resistant" because the infection is in the meninges, where the concentration of the drug in question is less. It should also be noted that the MIC or MBC chosen is based on having that level of antibiotic constantly in contact with the bacterial cell over a 24- to 48-hour period. Consequently, one must consider the MIC or MBC as a minimal antibiotic concentration to be exceeded for all of or for at least a great proportion of each dosage interval.

The rate of killing of bacteria probably increases in some relation to the concentration of drug in the bacterium's environment. This is true for penicillin up to some plateau level, beyond which no further increase in killing rate occurs. For other antibiotics the plateau phenomenon does not appear to exist, and an increased rate of killing is associated with increasing concentrations of the antibiotic. Thus, for most antibiotics the dosage used for a serious infection is limited only by its toxicity and cost. One must always weigh the toxicity and cost of the antibiotic against the severity of the illness. It may be reasonable to risk some vestibular dysfunction or even hearing deficit as a result of gentamicin's ototoxicity to prevent death from a *Pseudomonas* septicemia. It may be reasonable to choose an expensive drug for a life-threatening infection but not for a trivial infection.

Finally, it should be recognized that the conditions under

TABLE 9.2–2. ANTIMICROBIAL SELECTION BASED ON ORGANISMS

	Drug of Choice	Alternative Drugs
Gram-positive Cocci		
Staphylococcus aureus		
• Nonpenicillinase producing	Penicillin G or V (oral)	Imipenem A cephalosporin Erythromycin Clindamycin Vancomycin
• Penicillinase producing	A penicillinase resistant penicillin	Amoxicillin and clavulanate Ticarcillin and clavulanate Imipenem A cephalosporin Erythromycin Clindamycin Chloramphenicol
• Methicillin resistant	Vancomycin	Trimethoprim-sulfamethoxazole
Streptococcus pyogenes		
• Groups A, C, G	Penicillin G or V (oral)	A cephalosporin Erythromycin Clindamycin Vancomycin
• Group B	Penicillin G or ampicillin	A cephalosporin Erythromycin Vancomycin
Streptococcus viridans	Penicillin G plus an aminoglycoside	A cephalosporin Erythromycin Vancomycin each plus an aminoglycoside
• *Streptococcus,* anaerobic	Penicillin G	Erythromycin Clindamycin Chloramphenicol A tetracycline
• *Enterococcus*	Ampicillin or amoxicillin or penicillin G plus an aminoglycoside	Erythromycin or vancomycin plus an aminoglycoside
• *Pneumococcus*	Penicillin G or V (oral)	A cephalosporin Erythromycin Clindamycin Chloramphenicol (meningitis) Vancomycin
Gram-negative Cocci		
Neisseria meningitidis		
• Meningitis or bacteremia	Penicillin G	Ampicillin Amoxicillin Cefuroxime Cefotaxime Ceftizoxime Ceftriaxone Chloramphenicol Trimethoprim-sulfamethoxazole
• Prophylaxis	Rifampin	Minocycline
Neisseria gonorrhoeae		
• Genital	Ceftriaxone or amoxicillin	Penicillin G Ampicillin Cefoxitin Spectinomycin Chloramphenicol Trimethoprim-sulfamethoxazole
• Extragenital	Penicillin G	A tetracycline
Gram-positive Bacilli		
Bacillus anthracis	Penicillin G	Erythromycin A tetracycline Chloramphenicol
Listeria monocytogenes	Ampicillin plus an aminoglycoside	Erythromycin A tetracycline Trimethoprim-sulfamethoxazole
Clostridium tetani	Penicillin G	A tetracycline
Clostridium perfringens	Penicillin G	Clindamycin Chloramphenicol A tetracycline Metronidazole
	Metronidazole	Vancomycin
Corynebacterium diptheriae	Penicillin G	Erythromycin

(continued)

TABLE 9.2–2. ANTIMICROBIAL SELECTION BASED ON ORGANISMS (Continued)

	Drug of Choice	Alternative Drugs
Gram-negative Bacilli (Cont.)		
Escherichia coli	Ampicillin	Amoxicillin Carbenicillin Ticarcillin Azlocillin Mezlocillin Piperacillin Aztreonam Imipenem A cephalosporin Chloramphenicol A tetracycline An aminoglycoside Trimethoprim-sulfamethoxazole Norfloxacin
Klebsiella pneumoniae	A cephalosporin	Amoxacillin and clavulanate Ticarcillin and clavulanate Mezlocillin Piperacillin Aztreonam Imipenem Chloramphenicol A tetracycline An aminoglycoside Trimethoprim-sulfamethoxazole Norfloxacin
Enterobacter	Cefotaxim, ceftriaxone, ceftizoxime	Carbenicillin Ticarcillin Azlocillin Mezlocillin Piperacillin Aztreonam Imipenem Chloramphenicol An aminoglycoside Trimethoprim-sulfamethoxazole Norfloxacin
Serratia	Cefotaxim, ceftriaxone, ceftizoxime	Carbenicillin Ticarcillin Azlocillin Mezlocillin Piperacillin Aztreonam Imipenem An aminoglycoside Trimethoprim-sulfamethoxazole Norfloxacin
Proteus mirabilis	Ampicillin	Carbenicillin Ticarcillin Azlocillin Mezlocillin Piperacillin Aztreonam Imipenem An aminoglycoside Trimethoprlm-sulfamethoxazole Norfloxacin
Proteus, indole-positive	Cefotaxime, ceftriaxone, ceftizoxime	Amoxicillin and clavulanate Carbenicillin Ticarcillin Azlocillin Mezlocillin Piperacillin Aztreonam Imipenem Chloramphenicol A tetracycline An aminoglycoside Trimethoprim-sulfamethoxazole Norfloxacin
Pseudomonas aeruginosa	Carbenicillin, or ticarcillin with an aminoglycoside (except streptomycin or kanamycin)	Azlocillin Mezlocillin Piperacillin

(continued)

TABLE 9.2–2. ANTIMICROBIAL SELECTION BASED ON ORGANISMS (Continued)

	Drug of Choice	Alternative Drugs
Gram-negative Bacilli (Cont.)		
Pseudomonas aeruginosa (Cont.)		Aztreonam Imipenem Ceftazadime Polymyxin Norfloxacin
Bacteroides • Respiratory	Penicillin G	Cefoxitin Cefotetan Clindamycin Chloramphenicol Metronidazole
• Gastrointestinal	Metronidazole	Ticarcillin Mezlocillin Piperacillin Cefoxitin Cefotetan Chloramphenicol
Salmonella	Chloramphenicol	Ampicillin Amoxicillin Trimethoprim-sulfamethoxazole
Shigella	Trimethoprim-sulfamethoxazole	Ampicillin A tetracycline Chloramphenicol
Haemophilus influenzae • Meningitis, epiglottitis	Chloramphenicol	Ampicillin Cefuroxime Cefotaxime Ceftriaxone
• Other infections	Ampicillin	Amoxicillin Cefaclor Cefamandole Cefotaxime Ceftizoxime Ceftriaxone A tetracycline Trimethoprim-sulfamethoxazole
Haemophilus ducreyi	Ceftriaxone	Erythromycin Trimethoprim-sulfamethoxazole
Bordetella pertussis	Erythromycin	Trimethoprim-sulfamethoxazole
Pseudomonas pseudomallei	Trimethoprim-sulfamethoxazole	A tetracycline
Pseudomonas cepacia	Trimethoprim-sulfamethoxazole	Imipenem Ceftazidime Chloramphenicol
Brucella	A tetracycline	Trimethoprim-sulfamethoxazole Chloramphenicol
Acinetobacter	Imipenem	Carbenicillin Ticarcillin Azlocillin Mezlocillin Piperacillin Minocycline Doxycycline An aminoglycoside Trimethoprim-sulfamethoxazole
Francisella tularensis	Streptomycin	A tetracycline Chloramphenicol
Yersinia pestis	Streptomycin	A tetracycline Chloramphenicol
Vibrio cholerae	A tetracycline	Trimethoprim-sulfamethoxazole
Fusobacterium nucleatum	Penicillin G	Metronidazole Clindamycin Chloramphenicol
Calymmatobacterium granulomatis	A tetracycline	Streptomycin
Spirochetes		
Treponema pallidum	Penicillin G	A tetracycline Erythromycin

(continued)

TABLE 9.2–2. ANTIMICROBIAL SELECTION BASED ON ORGANISMS (Continued)

	Drug of Choice	Alternative Drugs
Spirochetes (Cont.)		
Treponema pertenue	Penicillin G	A tetracycline Erythromycin
Leptospira	Penicillin G	A tetracycline
Borrelia recurrentis	A tetracycline	Penicillin G
Acid-fast Bacilli		
Mycobacterium tuberculosis	Isoniazid with rifampin	Streptomycin Kanamycin Para-aminosalicylic acid Ethambutol Pyrazinamide Cycloserine Capreomycin Ethionamide
Mycobacterium leprae	Dapsone	Rifampin Clofazimine
Mycobacterium avium-intracellulare	Isoniazid Rifampin Ethambutol Streptomycin	Clofazimine Capreomycin Ethionamide Imipenem Rifabutine Amikacin
Actinomycetes		
Actinomyces israelii	Penicillin G	A tetracycline
Nocardia	A sulfonamide	Trimethoprim-sulfamethoxazole Cycloserine
Fungi		
Candida albicans	Amphotericin B	Flucytosine Ketoconazole
Aspergillus	Amphotericin B	
Blastomyces dermatitidis	Amphotericin B	Ketoconazole
Chromomycosis	Flucytosine	Ketoconazole
Coccidioides immitis	Amphotericin B	Ketoconazole Miconazole
Cryptococcus neoformans	Amphotericin B	Flucytosine Ketoconazole

which the sensitivity is determined in vitro differ considerably from those existing at the site of infection. For example, protein binding is usually not considered in the determination of an MIC or MBC.

As a result of these considerations, the MIC or MBC should be viewed only as a rough guide to the likelihood of success or failure of treatment with the antibiotic tested against that particular organism. It is unlikely, however, that a systemic infection due to an organism shown to be resistant to a given agent in vitro will be effectively treated by that agent.

RESISTANCE PATTERNS

The ability of microorganisms to develop resistance to antibiotics and chemotherapeutic agents is truly remarkable, and the construction of a rational therapeutic regimen is greatly influenced by this phenomenon. For example, the mechanism of resistance that develops to erythromycin (an "induced resistance" in which low erythromycin levels encourage an increased resistance to the erythromycin) extends as well to clindamycin. Consequently, in treating an erythromycin-resistant organism one should not use clindamycin. Conversely, erythromycin would be poorly advised in an infection due to a clindamycin-resistant organism.

Resistance to the tetracyclines is usually on the basis of reduced permeability of an organism to the antibiotic. This resistance is shared by all of the numerous tetracycline derivatives and, conse-

quently, one should change categories of antibiotics if resistance to a tetracycline is seen.

Resistance to chloramphenicol often is mediated by an R factor, and simultaneously acquired resistance to multiple antibacterial agents is commonly seen. This acquired resistance to multiple drugs is due to the ability of the R factor DNA to carry into the bacterium information coding for several gene products capable of modifying several antibiotics. Thus, in addition to promoting the acetylation of chloramphenicol, the sulfonamides may be acetylated, kanamycin may be phosphorylated, gentamicin may be adenylylated, and the tetracyclines may be poorly transported into the bacterium. All of these resistances may be simultaneously conferred on a cell by the same R factor. As noted above, R factors may be transferred between bacterial species.

Resistance to the aminoglycosides (streptomycin, kanamycin, gentamicin, tobramycin, and amikacin) is usually by an R factor–mediated modification of the antibiotic. This modification may be by phosphorylation, adenylylation, or acetylation. The specificity of the R factor-mediated enzymes catalyzing these three modifications allows the modification of one of the aminoglycosides without necessarily conferring resistance simultaneously to the others. Thus, resistance to one aminoglycoside does not necessarily mean that resistance will be seen to the others. Individual sensitivities must be performed to each clinically useful aminoglycoside (currently gentamicin, kanamycin, tobramycin, and amikacin).

The β-lactamases inactivate penicillins and cephalosporins by

catalyzing hydrolysis of the β-lactam ring contained within these two antibiotic structures. A variety of β-lactamases differing in substrate specificity exist in both gram-positive and gram-negative organisms. In general, the staphylococcal β-lactamases are usually meant when the term *penicillinase* is used. These β-lactamases inactivate penicillin G, penicillin V, ampicillin, amoxicillin, carbenicillin, and ticarcillin, but fail to inactivate methicillin, nafcillin, oxacillin, cloxacillin, dicloxacillin, and the cephalosporins. A clever stratagem to circumvent these β-lactamases is the use of clavulanate, a β-lactamase inhibitor, concurrently with either amoxicillin or ticarcillin, thus converting drugs that are usually cleaved by these β-lactamases into useful antistaphylococcal drugs. Among the gram-negative organisms, the β-lactamase of *Pseudomonas* is capable of hydrolyzing penicillin, ampicillin, amoxicillin, and most of the cephalosporins but not carbenicillin or ticarcillin. The resistance of carbenicillin and ticarcillin to the *Pseudomonas* β-lactamase accounts in part for their usefulness in treating *Pseudomonas* infections.

The sulfonamides are inactivated by acetylation and this activity is often conferred by an R factor-mediated mechanism.

Resistance to trimethoprim is usually due to a mutation in the dihydrofolate reductase of the bacterium so that trimethoprim no longer binds to nor does it inhibit the mutant enzyme of the resistant species.

Resistance to acyclovir can be due to a mutation in the viral thymidine kinase, which activates the drug, or in the viral DNA polymerase, which is the site of action of the phosphorylated acyclovir.

THE SITE AND EXTENT OF INFECTION

Occasionally, the selection of a specific antimicrobial agent is based primarily on the site and extent of infection, and often the selection is influenced by it.

Urinary tract infections clearly can be eradicated by many chemotherapeutic agents that achieve adequate urinary levels but fail to achieve adequate plasma or tissue levels. From such observations one relates the effectiveness of therapy in urinary tract infections to the urinary levels of drugs and not to plasma or tissue levels. With some chemotherapeutic agents the urinary levels are adequate in spite of plasma and tissue levels that are never effective (such as nitrofurantoin, nalidixic acid, oxolinic acid, and Mandelamine). This approach also is useful in considering the appropriate dosage regimens of other drugs, such as penicillin, ampicillin, and carbenicillin, where even "resistant" organisms may succumb to the enormous levels achieved in the urine. The concentration of penicillins in the urine allows for the administration of much smaller doses than are required for systemic infections.

A second site of infection that often modifies the selection of an antibiotic is the cerebrospinal fluid (CSF) or meninges. Here the entry of the drug into the CSF becomes critically important, and several chemotherapeutic agents that are effective elsewhere are impotent in treating meningitis. Examples include cephalothin (and presumably other cephalosporins, with the exception of cefuroxime, cefotaxime, ceftriaxone, and moxalactam), clindamycin, erythromycin, and probably the highly protein-bound, semisynthetic, penicillinase-resistant penicillins such as nafcillin, oxacillin, cloxacillin, and dicloxacillin. Chloramphenicol assumes an increased importance in the treatment of meningitis because its levels in the CSF are one third to one half those in simultaneously measured plasma. Both trimethoprim and sulfamethoxazole enter the CSF as well.

The localization of bacteria within fibrin often requires the use of high doses of antibiotics to achieve penetration to the microorganism. This situation is seen with infective endocarditis.

An intracellular localization of organisms may require that the drug enter the cell. Chloramphenicol, rifampin, norfloxacin, ciprofloxacin, and trimethoprim are effectively distributed into cells while most of the others are not. In rare cases, such as in patients with chronic granulomatous disease where the cell's own bactericidal activity is impaired, the use of one of these drugs may be indicated in preference to a drug with greater in vitro sensitivity.

THE ADEQUACY OF HOST DEFENSE MECHANISMS

The selection of an antimicrobial agent is often influenced by the adequacy or inadequacy of the host defense mechanisms. Although this seems to be of documented value in relatively few situations, it is wise to consider host defense factors in choosing an appropriate drug.

In general, it is believed that "bactericidal" drugs should be used in preference to "bacteriostatic" drugs in patients with compromised host defense mechanisms including immune deficiencies, granulocytopenia, chronic granulomatous disease, patients after splenectomy, and patients who are immunosuppressed. Such "bactericidal" drugs include the penicillins, cephalosporins, and aminoglycosides, whereas erythromycin, the tetracyclines, chloramphenicol, and the sulfonamides are usually considered bacteriostatic. It should be recognized, however, that the terms "bactericidal" and "bacteriostatic" are not entirely clear in their meanings. Often, a drug is considered bacteriostatic at low concentrations and bactericidal at high concentrations, as claimed for clindamycin, chloramphenicol, and erythromycin. The bactericidal action of a drug is not usually a property of the drug itself but of the interaction between the drug, the microbe, and the environment. Penicillin, for example, is bactericidal if the microbe is in a hypotonic environment but not so if in a hypertonic milieu or in an abscess cavity. Trimethoprim is bacteriostatic if the organism is grown in a minimal medium but bactericidal if an exogenous supply of amino acids and purines is present. Chloramphenicol is bacteriostatic for *Escherichia coli*, but bactericidal for *Streptococcus pneumoniae, Neisseria meningitidis,* and *Haemophilus influenzae.* Thus the usefulness of these terms in clinical practice must not be overemphasized.

As previously cited, the penetration of a chemotherapeutic agent into host cells may be far more important than the categorization of the drug as "cidal" or "static."

THE PHARMACOKINETICS OF THE DRUG

Occasionally, the selection of an antimicrobial agent is based on the pharmacokinetics of the drug. For example, in patients with impaired renal function, most of the tetracyclines are retained with an enhanced risk of drug toxicity. Doxycycline, however, is excreted into the gut, and its kinetics do not change appreciably in the presence of diminished or changing renal function.

The individual kinetics of sulfamethoxazole and trimethoprim differ considerably in patients with severely compromised renal function, and the rational use of this fixed-dose combination then becomes difficult.

Most of the penicillins and cephalosporins are eliminated by glomerular filtration and active tubular secretion. Thus in renal disease the dose of most penicillins and cephalosporins should be reduced to minimize dose-related toxicities and cost.

In the presence of liver dysfunction, chloramphenicol cannot be efficiently detoxified by glucuronidation, and dose-related toxicity is seen more frequently, unless the plasma levels are followed to ensure a subtoxic concentration. Similarly, the plasma levels of gentamicin, kanamycin, tobramycin, and amikacin should be monitored in the patient with marked renal dysfunction to attain adequate levels with a minimum toxicity.

THE BENEFIT-TO-RISK RATIO OF THE DRUG

Both an estimation of benefit and an estimation of risk should be considered in the selection of any appropriate antimicrobial agent.

In general, greater risks are acceptable in the treatment of more severe infections, and no serious risks are acceptable in the treatment of minor infections. However, this axiom is violated frequently. For example, there is often concern about ototoxicity associated with the use of high doses of gentamicin even in the presence of a life-threatening *Pseudomonas* septicemia. Clearly, it is the proper choice to preserve life even at the expense of complete loss of vestibular function. Conversely, it has been estimated that about 50 percent of the use of clindamycin in a recent year was for self-limited upper respiratory tract infections. Yet clindamycin is occasionally associated with a pseudomembranous colitis, and at least two dozen deaths have been attributed to the colitis. Surely no mortality as a result of drug therapy is acceptable in the treatment of a trivial viral illness.

The proper estimation of a benefit-to-risk ratio requires accurate information quantifying the benefits attributable to the drug and accurate incidence figures with respect to the adverse reactions associated with it. Usually, neither of these is available in as firm a form as we would like. Consider, for example, the choice between ampicillin and chloramphenicol for the treatment of a serious *H. influenzae* infection. Usually, one would consider the two to provide about equal effectiveness and, consequently, the choice usually rests on the relative risks associated with the two drugs. Invariably, ampicillin has been chosen on grounds of lesser toxicity. But the available estimates of the incidence of fatal anaphylaxis associated with penicillin (1:10,000 to 1:100,000) and by inference also with ampicillin are in about the same range as the estimates of fatal aplastic anemia associated with chloramphenicol (1:15,000 to 1:60,000). Furthermore, the incidence of fatal thromboembolic phenomena associated with oral contraceptives is in the same range. Yet we find it acceptable to give oral contraceptives to normal women and we fear the administration of chloramphenicol even to the seriously ill.

COMBINATIONS OF ANTIMICROBIAL AGENTS

Often two or more antimicrobial agents are used simultaneously. Such combination chemotherapy is advantageous in several common clinical situations. The initial treatment of a serious infection in the absence of an identified bacteriologic agent constitutes the usual justification for the simultaneous use of two drugs. In this situation, one wishes to maximize one's chances of success by covering the most likely possibilities. In general, one assumes that the risk involved in the use of a second (or even third) drug is less than the risk associated with failure to appropriately attack the offending organism. One usually further assumes that the use of two or three "specific" antibiotics is preferable to the use of a single broad-spectrum antibiotic. Evidence for such an assumption is meager indeed. Nevertheless, this indication is reasonable on logical grounds and is clinically acceptable.

A second indication for combination chemotherapy takes advantage of the synergistic effect of some combinations on some bacteria or fungi. Although the situations with proven synergism are rare, they are of sufficient clinical importance to be considered. Perhaps the most commonly encountered example of synergism is in the combination of trimethoprim with sulfamethoxazole. In vitro synergism has been clearly demonstrated with this combination against a number of bacterial species. This synergism is based on the inhibition of two sequential steps in tetrahydrofolic acid biosynthesis by the two components. The combination of sulfamethoxazole with trimethoprim is also likely to be advantageous because of the rapid emergence of resistance that might be seen with trimethoprim alone and the diminution of this development with the simultaneous administration of a sulfonamide. Carbenicillin and gentamicin are synergistic against many strains (perhaps 30 percent of all strains) of *Pseudomonas aeruginosa*. About the same percentage of strains of *E. coli* are susceptible to a synergism between ampicillin and gentamicin. *Streptococcus viridans,* even though sensitive to penicillin, often shows synergism between penicillin

and an aminoglycoside. Some fungi are inhibited in a synergistic fashion by amphotericin B and flucytosine given concurrently.

A third rationale for the use of combinations of chemotherapeutic agents involves the simultaneous treatment of infections caused by multiple organisms. This may be considered particularly relevant in the treatment of contaminated gastrointestinal surgery after trauma or the rupture of a viscus. In this situation, there is experimental evidence for the effectiveness of clindamycin combined with an aminoglycoside to aim at both anaerobes and aerobic gram-negative bacilli.

A fourth indication for combination chemotherapy is an attempt to forestall the emergence of resistance to a single drug. This indication has been cited earlier with respect to the combination of trimethoprim with sulfamethoxazole. It also is frequently invoked in antituberculous chemotherapy in an effort to delay the emergence of resistance to isoniazid.

Although some significant advantages may accrue with the use of combinations of chemotherapeutic agents, some disadvantages are also apparent. The cost of therapy usually increases, the incidence of adverse reactions is compounded, a sense of security may be falsely engendered, and there may occasionally be antagonism between the components of the combination. Antagonism, although commonly considered, is rarely encountered at a clinical level. Two examples have been well documented. The combination of chlortetracycline with penicillin in the management of pneumococcal meningitis was associated with an increased mortality over that seen with the use of penicillin alone. No refutation of the conclusions of this study exists. However, the conclusions should not be extrapolated to other clinical infections, because no antagonism was seen with the simultaneous use of these two agents in the treatment of pneumococcal pneumonia.

The second situation of proven antagonism involves the inactivation of gentamicin and other aminoglycosides by high concentrations of carbenicillin and other penicillins. This inactivation has been clearly demonstrated in vitro, and the two drugs should not be added to the same intravenous bottle. The inactivation does not appear to occur in vivo in the usual case, but in the patient with markedly impaired renal function this inactivation may be realized.

DRUG INTERACTIONS

The selection of a chemotherapeutic agent is at times influenced by drug interactions. These interactions may be at many different levels ranging from direct chemical interactions, as noted previously for the inactivation of gentamicin by carbenicillin, through interactions affecting absorption, distribution, metabolism, and excretion. The absorption of the tetracyclines is impaired in the presence of iron salts, and the absorption of rifampicin is significantly diminished if para-aminosalicylic acid is concurrently administered. Both of these interactions are clinically significant. Many chemotherapeutic agents are tightly bound to plasma proteins, and the potential certainly exists for displacing these drugs by simultaneously administering other bound drugs. Conversely, the bound chemotherapeutic agent may displace other drugs, leading to elevated levels of the free drug. The metabolism of many drugs by way of microsomal drug-metabolizing enzymes is inhibited by chloramphenicol, and the metabolism of diphenylhydantoin is inhibited by isoniazid. The metabolism of theophyllin is inhibited by erythromycin. Conversely, the metabolism of many drugs is enhanced by inducers of microsomal enzymes, and rifampicin has been shown capable of such induction. This latter interaction has been shown to be clinically significant with respect to oral anticoagulants and to oral contraceptives as well. This type of interaction should be considered when selecting any chemotherapeutic agent that is significantly metabolized by the hepatic microsomal system. Drug interactions affecting excretion include the well-known effect of probenecid on the renal secretion of penicillins and the influence

of amphotericin-induced renal damage on the elimination of 5-fluorocytosine and the aminoglycosides.

THE RATIONAL ADMINISTRATION OF THE CHOSEN AGENT

Once the chemotherapeutic agent is chosen, the physician's next obligation is to provide the drug by way of an optimal regimen. Many of the considerations here are similar to those used in the selection of the drug. Several additional considerations are also important.

THE ROUTE OF ADMINISTRATION

Usually, if alternative routes of administration are available, the choice lies between oral, intramuscular, intravenous, and, occasionally, intrathecal routes.

Clearly, the oral route has many advantages and should be selected when possible for relatively minor infections. However, several disadvantages are also inherent in the oral administration of a drug. When patients will self-administer drugs, this is usually the only feasible route, but one should recognize that compliance is a major problem with any orally administered drug. Careful attention to compliance is in order in every patient since it is notoriously difficult to predict compliance or noncompliance. A second disadvantage is the unpredictability of absorption of many orally given drugs, although this problem may be overemphasized.

The intramuscular route obviates the need for a continuous intravenous line with its own propensity to serve as a nidus for infections. Furthermore, it is considerably less expensive considering the added cost of intravenous fluids. However, the seriously ill patient will usually have an intravenous line installed for other reasons, and its use for antimicrobial administration saves the patient from repeated intramuscular injections.

The intravenous route is frequently the route chosen in the seriously ill patient. In addition to the hygiene associated with an indwelling intravenous line, one has the additional problems of drug incompatibilities and drug stabilities. The list of incompatibilities is extensive and, as a generalization, one should attempt to deliver each drug singly and at its own time via the intravenous line. The delivery of drugs in an intermittent fashion allows this single drug administration and in addition attends to the problem of drug instability. The latter is particularly important with ampicillin and methicillin administration.

The intrathecal route is seldom used but is occasionally indicated in the treatment of difficult cases of meningitis. The problem arises here because of the severity of gram-negative meningitis and because of the inability of the aminoglycosides to enter the CSF. Although the usual method of delivery involves administration after a lumbar puncture, the flow of CSF prevents the antibiotic from entering the ventricles, and the intraventricular administration of the drug via a surgically placed reservoir has recently been advocated. Although this constitutes a major decision, the continuing high mortality associated with gram-negative meningitis demands that we continue our search for better treatment regimens.

THE RELATIONSHIP BETWEEN IN VIVO ANTIMICROBIAL LEVELS AND IN VITRO MINIMAL INHIBITORY CONCENTRATION (MIC)

The MIC has been described as it pertains to our selection of a therapeutic agent. Now we consider it again with regard to the relationship that should exist between the concentration of antimicrobial agent at the site of infection and the MIC of the organism. Because the MIC is performed by exposing the microbe to the drug continuously for the period of assay (usually 24 and sometimes 48 hours), a logical conclusion would be that this level of antimicrobial agent should be exceeded continuously. Exceptions can be immediately cited. For example, penicillin can be quite effective, even though the concentration falls to suboptimal levels for a part of each dosing interval. The same is certainly true of isoniazid. These exceptions may suggest that the above generalization applies less stringently to situations in which an irreversible interaction occurs between the drug and the organism. Nevertheless, even in these situations, it is advantageous to exceed the MIC for at least a large part of each dosing interval. The next decision is by how much to exceed the MIC. This question has been addressed in a formal manner for penicillin G, but far less information exists with other drugs. With increasing concentrations of penicillin G above the MIC, the bacteria are killed more rapidly and more effectively up to a point. Beyond this point the continued increase in concentration adds no more effectiveness to the system. Thus a plateau is reached beyond which more drug is of no advantage. This plateau is usually seen at a multiple of about 10 times the MIC of an organism. Other antimicrobials do not show this same plateau phenomenon, however, and increasing concentrations lead to increasing rates of bacterial killing. From this information one can tentatively suggest that the rate of bacterial growth inhibition or bacterial killing increases with increasing concentrations of an antimicrobial agent with the exception of the penicillins. In most cases, then, there should be no "optimal" multiple of the MIC that should be achieved. Instead, one should give as much of an antimicrobial agent as possible, at least in the seriously ill patient, without producing unacceptable toxicity and unacceptable cost.

DRUG DISTRIBUTION

The goal of chemotherapy is the eradication of the infection. To achieve that goal one must provide an adequate concentration of drug in the immediate environment of the organisms to be eradicated. It is difficult to assess the level of drug at the site of infection as access to compartments other than blood, urine, or CSF is difficult. One can use the available information on the penetration of drugs into urine, CSF, and models of interstitial fluid.

Most chemotherapeutic agents are eliminated in large part by the kidneys, and even with those drugs that are highly metabolized, a generous percentage of the administered dose is eliminated into the urine as the unmetabolized drug. Thus, urinary concentrations are often high and, if the drug is secreted into the urine (as are the penicillins and cephalosporins), may be enormous. Even a drug such as doxycycline, however, that may be eliminated largely by an extrarenal mechanism, provides adequate urinary concentrations for the treatment of many urinary tract infections. Thus the provision of adequate drug to the urine is rarely difficult.

Much more difficult is the provision of drug to the CSF. Although our understanding of antimicrobial penetration into the CSF is rudimentary, some information is available. Few antimicrobials enter the CSF with facility. One is usually faced with a choice between giving high levels of the drug intravenously in hope of driving enough into the CSF or giving the drug directly into the CSF via the lumbar route or the ventricular route. Direct instillation has received considerable recent support in the treatment of gram-negative meningitis with gentamicin. For most other drugs the alternative choice is usually made.

The distribution of antimicrobial agent into extravascular extracellular spaces has received renewed interest recently, but the guidelines remain scanty. In general, there is probably a reasonable correlation between plasma levels and interstitial fluid levels of most chemotherapeutic agents, although the kinetics of each compartment may vary. For this reason and because of the inability to directly measure the interstitial concentrations of an antimicrobial agent, one should strive for adequate plasma drug levels as an approximation of extracellular tissue levels. A unique site of drug distribution is prostatic fluid. Two chemotherapeutic agents (erythromycin and trimethoprim) are concentrated in this fluid.

INTERMITTENT VS. CONTINUOUS ADMINISTRATION

Although this issue has been debated for many years, no clear evidence in favor of intermittent or continuous administration has emerged. For practical reasons, an intermittent infusion is usually chosen. Care must be taken in using an intermittent regimen that the dosage interval is sufficiently short relative to the growth rate of the microorganism so that the microbes do not have a chance of recovering between doses. Perhaps one extreme example of this point is seen in the biweekly isoniazid regimens used in the treatment of tuberculosis. This is predicated upon the slow growth rate of the tubercle bacillus combined with the nearly irreversible interaction between isoniazid and the bacterium. A similar argument, although contracted in time, can be generated to explain the efficacy of penicillin given by intermittent dosing.

TOXICOLOGIC RESTRICTIONS

If the effectiveness of an antimicrobial agent increases with increasing concentration of the drug at the site of infection (as previously suggested), then adverse drug reactions that are dose related become important as restrictions on the amount of drug to be given. Examples of such dose-related toxicities include the neurotoxicity of penicillins, the nephrotoxicity of cephalosporins, aminoglycosides, polymyxin and amphotericin B, the ototoxicity of the aminoglycosides, the gray baby syndrome and possibly a similar adult syndrome with chloramphenicol, a transient bone marrow suppression with chloramphenicol, hepatotoxicity with the tetracyclines, sodium overload and bleeding with carbenicillin, ticarcillin, and ureidopenicillins, and diarrhea with most of the orally administered chemotherapeutic agents. As emphasized, however, in each individual situation one must carefully weigh the disadvantages of toxicity against the advantages anticipated from increased dosages.

MODIFICATIONS OF THERAPEUTIC REGIMENS

Modification of an otherwise optimal therapeutic regimen should be considered in the presence of renal or hepatic dysfunction.

Most antimicrobial agents are ultimately eliminated by the kidneys, and therefore any significant reduction of renal function should lead to a reappraisal of one's therapeutic regimen. Although an isolated impairment of tubular secretory capacity could theoretically lead to a change in the kinetics of elimination of the penicillins and cephalosporins, it is usually an impaired glomerular filtration that leads to a clinically important prolongation of the drug's residence in the host. Consequently, the dosage adjustments that are necessary usually correlate closely with the creatinine clearance or more roughly with the serum creatinine. In principle, a dosage adjustment should probably be made for nearly every chemotherapeutic agent in the face of moderate or marked glomerular dysfunction. Such adjustments are essential with a few drugs where dose-related toxicity occurs at drug levels near to those necessary for clinical effectiveness. The most common example is seen in the use of the aminoglycosides for major systemic infections. Because the margin of safety with these antibiotics is rather narrow, one is often bordering on the toxic level to achieve maximal effectiveness. A moderate change in glomerular filtration can then initiate a vicious cycle, with accumulation of the aminoglycoside, nephrotoxicity from the higher levels of drug, and greater accumulation of the aminoglycoside in a spiralling fashion. Nomograms and simple rules-of-thumb have been formulated to guide therapy in this situation, but the individual variation seen with each of the proposed guidelines makes a strong case for the monitoring of plasma aminoglycoside levels as a guide to dosage. Similar care should be taken with cephaloridine and other cephalosporins, vancomycin, polymyxin, the tetracyclines (with the exception of doxycycline, whose kinetics change little even with severe renal dysfunction), and 5-fluorocytosine.

Rational modification of antimicrobial dosage is much more difficult in the presence of hepatic dysfunction, for here the mechanisms of drug metabolism are variable and there is no commonality similar to the glomerular filtration of the kidney. Thus chloramphenicol is glucuronidated, clindamycin is demethylated and conjugated with sulfoxide, cephalothin is deacetylated, and the sulfonamides are acetylated. There is no commonly used "liver function test" that correlates well with any of these biochemical modifications. The best safeguard in the presence of liver dysfunction is to follow plasma levels if dose-related toxicity is a potential problem.

THERAPEUTIC MONITORING

To ensure a steady progression toward the eradication of an infection, it is essential that therapy be continually monitored after its initiation. This monitoring can be at a clinical, radiologic, microbiologic, or pharmacologic level and usually consists of some combination of these. Because the other modalities will receive consideration in the succeeding chapters on individual infectious diseases, only the pharmacologic level of monitoring is discussed here.

Two basically dissimilar approaches are available for antimicrobial monitoring. One can either measure the activity of a body fluid against a microorganism (and usually against the patient's own organism), or one can measure the concentration of the drug in an accessible fluid. Proponents of the former method (serum "cidal" levels) argue that the results are more indicative of the actual antimicrobial effectiveness because the determination measures the activity of the drug. Although the logic of this agreement seems persuasive, there is little evidence in support of this view. Equally unimpressive is the evidence that allows a measured "cidal" level to be considered inadequate, adequate, or optimal. Usually the level is considered adequate if the serum, plasma, or fluid can be diluted eightfold or more and still exhibit the inhibitory activity. It is also unclear when, in relation to a dose, one should seek such levels. Furthermore, it is apparent that once the serum, plasma, or other biologic fluid is diluted with a buffered salt solution, it no longer resembles the original fluid, and with increasing dilution the resemblence becomes even less. One of the consequences of the dilution of the fluid is the weakening of the plasma protein binding of some antibiotics. Thus highly bound antibiotics may appear increasingly active with dilution because of the availability of a greater percentage of the drug in the free or active state. Finally, the "cidal" level offers a composite answer in the presence of multiple antibiotics. Although this may be the desired measurement, it does not aid in the manipulation of each antimicrobial agent on an individual basis.

The alternative assay that is useful for antimicrobial monitoring is the measurement of absolute drug levels in the biologic fluid. Several new approaches, including enzymologic, radioimmunologic, and enzyme-linked immunoabsorbant assays have added to the ease with which a few chemotherapeutic agents can be quantified, and the more classical bioassay has been improved so as to provide greater rapidity and sensitivity. Although such antibiotic levels can be measured with ease, they provide only partial information and must be considered along with the tissue level of an antibiotic. The direct measurement of the concentration of the drug offers the additional advantages of providing individualized information about each drug and of allowing an assessment of the potential for dose-related toxicity.

It should be emphasized that the use of pharmacologic monitoring is of value primarily in the seriously ill patient or in the patient who has an underlying propensity to drug toxicity. Most infectious diseases can be adequately monitored at a clinical level and others with the addition of radiologic and bacteriologic assistance.

DURATION OF THERAPY

The decision to stop antimicrobial chemotherapy is usually based on a combination of empiricism, logic, and some scientific evidence.

Rarely is a regimen so standardized as to be nearly routine, but such is the case in the treatment of streptococcal pharyngitis, where a 10-day course of therapy is accepted by nearly all. Other rather standard durations of therapy include 4 weeks for infective endocarditis due to *S. viridans* and 6 weeks for some other endocarditides. Other clinical situations are less well defined and are based to a great extent on the course during therapeutic monitoring as previously noted. It is usually suggested that therapy continue for a few days after most evidence of infection has cleared. *Salmonella typhi* infections should be treated longer after the patient is afebrile; perhaps for an additional 14 days and *Shigella* infections for an additional 7 days. The duration of therapy in uncomplicated urinary tract infections is the subject of much debate.

REFERENCES

1. Gale EF, Cundliffe E, et al: The Molecular Basis of Antibiotic Action. New York, John Wiley and Sons, 1972
2. Garrod LP, Lambert HP, O'Grady F: Antibiotic and Chemotherapy. New York, Churchill Livingstone, 1981
3. Gilman AG, Goodman LS, Gilman A: The Pharmacological Basis of Therapeutics. New York, Macmillan, 1985
4. Mandell GL, Douglas RG, Bennett JE: Anti-infective Therapy. New York, John Wiley and Sons, 1985
5. The Medical Letter on Drugs and Therapeutics. Handbook of Antimicrobial Therapy, rev. ed. New Rochelle, NY, Medical Letter, 1986
6. Pratt WB, Fekety R: The Antimicrobial Drugs. New York, Oxford University Press, 1986

CHAPTER 9.3
Fevers of Obscure Origin

John J. Mann

Many patients who do not have localizing signs or symptoms will have fever as the dominant feature of their illness. The cause of fever may remain obscure despite appropriate microbiologic, radiologic, and serologic studies for the detection of specific infections. The problem is often confused by the premature use of therapeutic agents that alter the course of the illness, either by producing temporary defervescence or by inducing a febrile sensitivity reaction. The problem of the patient who has unexplained fever will serve to illustrate the principles outlined in the systematic approach to diagnosis and the necessity of constructing a careful plan for the management of a patient's illness (Chapter 1.4). The differential diagnosis in a patient who has obscure fever deserves special consideration as a common and often vexing challenge to the physician.

DEFINITION

Criteria for a diagnosis of fever of undetermined origin include illness of more than 3 weeks' duration, documented fever higher than 101F (38.2C) on several occasions, and failure of diagnosis after 1 week of study in the hospital.[11] Many common causes of fever are excluded by this definition, either because they can be readily diagnosed or because they are self-limited. The history, physical examination, blood counts, chest radiograph, and urinalysis and initial microbiologic evaluation are sufficient to establish a presumptive diagnosis in the majority of patients.

The causes of fever of undetermined origin are so varied and numerous that it is difficult to devise any fully practical classification of them. A simple and workable classification is presented in Table 9.3–1. Fever also may be noted in many other conditions not listed, such as in heat stroke and in congenital absence of the sweat glands. In these situations the cause of fever is usually obvious, and the abnormal temperature is not the important feature that calls for diagnostic study.

FEVER

It is important to recall that a low-grade fever does not always signify the presence of illness. The body temperature may rise above normal during exercise or excitement, particularly in a warm environment. A few individuals who are otherwise in perfect health persistently have a temperature of a degree or so above normal, a condition known as habitual hyperthermia. Psychogenic hyperthermia occurs in patients who become excessively preoccupied with minor temperature elevation due to anxiety.

The normal body temperature, as measured rectally, undergoes a diurnal variation from as low as 97.5F during the early morning hours to as high as 100.2F in the late afternoon or early evening. In most patients with fever, the temperature curve tends to follow the same pattern with higher levels occurring in the evening. The spikes of a widely swinging or hectic fever also usually occur in the evening. Rectal temperatures are about a degree higher than are oral readings, and axillary temperatures are about a degree lower than are oral temperatures. Rectal temperatures are preferred for patients who cannot cooperate sufficiently to obtain accurate oral readings.

Pattern and Degree of Fever

The heat-regulating mechanisms operating through the peripheral circulation and sweat glands usually prevent life-threatening elevations of body temperature, so that rectal temperatures exceeding 106F are unusual. Marked hyperthermia may be observed in patients with heat stroke or central nervous system lesions (meningitis, cerebrovascular accident, encephalitis, tumor of the hypothalamus, brain surgery, and trauma to the cervical cord). Other conditions sometimes causing elevations above 106F are lymphomas, acute yellow atrophy of the liver, thyroid crisis, fulminant pancreatitis, and drug reactions. Infections often associated with fevers above 105F are those of the urinary tract caused by gram-negative bacilli, meningococcemia, typhoid fever, brucellosis, tularemia, tuberculosis, malaria, relapsing fever, and leptospirosis. In contrast, some infections are characterized by low-grade or even no fever. Thus, not infrequently, disseminated fungal infections are associated with only mild elevation of temperature. Apart from these generalities, the height of the fever is not usually helpful in diagnosis. Thus, sensitivity to phenobarbital may produce as much fever as pneumococcal bacteremia.[3]

Occasionally, patients have recurrent febrile episodes over prolonged periods of time but enjoy relatively good health during the intervals. This is typical of Pel–Ebstein fever, which occurs in a small percentage of patients with Hodgkin disease. A number of other entities can be associated with this pattern, including malaria, relapsing fever, rat-bite fever, some forms of granulomatous pleuritis and pericarditis, drug reactions, inflammatory bowel dis-

TABLE 9.3–1. CAUSES OF FEVER OF UNKNOWN ORIGIN

Infections

Endovascular (streptococci, enterococci, staphylococci, and many others)

Extravascular focus

- Respiratory (lung abscess, empyema, bronchiectasis, pneumonia, sinusitis)
- Abdominal (appendiceal abscess, hepatic abscess, subdiaphragmatic abscess, psoas abscess, cholangitis)
- Genitourinary (renal carbuncle, perinephric abscess, kidney infection, prostatitis, pelvic abscess)
- Neurologic (brain abscess, epidural abscess, meningitis)
- Musculoskeletal (osteomyelitis, pyogenic arthritis, pyomyositis)

Specific infections

- Salmonellosis (typhoid, paratyphoid, other)
- Plague
- Parasitic infections (malaria, filariasis)
- Rickettsial infections
- Spirochetal infections (syphilis, leptospirosis)
- Listeriosis
- Viral infections
- Brucellosis
- Tularemia

Mycobacterial infections (tuberculosis, leprosy)
Fungal infections

Tumors (malignant or benign)

Hypernephroma
Carcinoma of gastrointestinal tract
Hepatic carcinoma (primary or metastatic)
Carcinoma of lung and pleura
Myxoma, simulating subacute bacterial endocarditis

Diseases of the Blood-Forming Organs

Leukemia
Hemolytic disorders
Pernicious anemia
Hodgkin disease and other lymphomas
Necrotizing lymphadenitis

Liver diseases

Hepatitis
Cirrhosis

Disorders Due to Toxins and Allergens

Allergenic drugs (sulfonamides, penicillin, iodides)
Foreign proteins (horse serum)
Products of tissue injury

- Myocardial infarction (including postmyocardial infarction syndrome)
- Pulmonary infarction
- Gangrene of extremities
- Tissue necrosis with remote sterile inflammation
- Accumulation of blood in body cavities or intestinal tract

Connective Tissue Disease

Still disease
Giant-cell arteritis
Systemic lupus erythematosus
Polyarteritis nodosa
Polymyositis
Rheumatic fever

Miscellaneous

Sarcoidosis
Inflammatory bowel disease

- Regional enteritis
- Ulcerative colitis
- Whipple disease

Metabolic

- Porphyria
- Gout
- Hyperthyroidism

Familial Mediterranean fever

Factitious Fever

ease, and familial Mediterranean fever. However, the search for less esoteric entities is often rewarding. Commonly, localized pyogenic infections of the biliary, genitourinary, gastrointestinal, or respiratory tracts are responsible for obscure intermittent febrile illnesses. Intermittent biliary obstruction (Charcot intermittent biliary fever), prostatitis, diverticulosis, or bronchiectasis are often overlooked yet readily treatable causes.

CHILLS

Although shaking chills occur most frequently in bacterial infections, especially when associated with bacteremia, they may also occur with drug reactions, neoplasms, collagen disorders, viral infections, and antipyretic treatment. Chills are therefore of limited help in distinguishing the cause of a febrile illness.

CAUSES OF FEVER OF UNKNOWN ORIGIN

Causes of fever of unknown origin (FUO) are categorized in Table 9.3–1. Differential diagnosis may be exceedingly difficult, because many diseases presenting an undiagnosed fever may have similar clinical manifestations. Thus, such frequent causes of FUO as chronic infections, neoplasms, collagen-vascular disorders, drug hypersensitivity states, and granulomatous diseases all may be associated with similar physical findings, including weight loss, chills, sweats, skin eruptions, arthritis, myositis, neuritis, and enlargement of the spleen, liver, and lymph nodes. These disorders also may present with only such nonspecific symptoms as irritability, malaise, easy fatigability, headache, and anorexia. Review of several large recent studies indicates that infections account for 36 percent of cases, neoplasms for 25 percent, autoimmune diseases for 10 percent, and miscellaneous diseases for 12 percent. Twelve percent of cases remain undiagnosed. The great majority of undiagnosed patients improved spontaneously, but some cases remained undiagnosed even after autopsy.[11] Petersdorf and associates repeated their study of unexplained fever 20 years after the original series.[9] They concluded that cancer had become the most common disease category, that abscesses represented a third of all infections, and that collagen diseases had become less frequent causes of unexplained fever.[9]

Commonly encountered causes of FUO will now be considered, with emphasis on the clues that may lead to the proper diagnosis.[4,6,11]

INFECTIONS

Bacteremia

Multiple blood cultures should be obtained in all cases of unexplained fever. Both aerobic and anaerobic techniques should be used, and the cultures should be held for more than 2 weeks to permit recognition of slow-growing organisms such as *Bacteroides*. In addition to obtaining blood cultures an hour before the daily temperature is expected, additional cultures spaced over the 24-hour period should be carried out because bacteremia may be intermittent. At least three cultures should be taken on the same day as well as on several subsequent days if there is a strong clinical suspicion of bacteremia.

Very often, septicemia begins without any apparent locus of origin. An insignificant skin puncture may be the starting point. It is always well to question a patient with septicemia about minor injuries, squeezing pimples, pulling hair, and so on. In women, the pelvic organs should always be a suspected source and examined carefully.

Antibiotic administration should be withheld until after the blood cultures have been obtained. Otherwise the correct diagnosis may never be made, and the successful management of the illness will be rendered more difficult, especially if improvement does

not occur. Once the cultures have been taken, appropriate antibiotics may be indicated if the patient is seriously ill. The initial treatment regimen can be appropriately altered when the causative organism is isolated and its antibiotic sensitivity is determined.

Localized Infections With or Without Abscess Formation

The observer should review systematically the possibility of a localized infection in the brain, meninges, pharynx, mediastinum, pericardium, endocardium, or thoracic cavity, below the diaphragm, in the liver or spleen, or in or about the kidneys, abdominal cavity, pelvis, perirectal area, prostate, bones and joints, or soft tissues. If such a systematic approach is not followed, with each possible locus considered in an orderly fashion, the cause of the patient's fever may well be overlooked. Certain localized infections deserve special mention here, although they are discussed more fully in other chapters.

Liver Abscess. Liver abscess often remains obscure clinically. Frequently, there is no obvious antecedent infection from which it could have originated such as colitis, ruptured appendix, and the like. The only manifestations may be fever, chills, anorexia, and malaise. The white blood cell count may be normal. The liver may be only slightly enlarged and not at all tender. The diaphragm may be high and fixed. A friction rub over the surface of the liver is only infrequently heard. Exploratory laparotomy may be the only means of discovering a liver abscess. Needle aspiration is helpful if it is positive, but it does not exclude abscess when negative. Moreover, it carries the danger of hemorrhage or irreversible shock if the contents of an abscess are spilled into the peritoneum. Radioisotopic scanning of the liver may reveal filling defects, but small abscesses (<2 cm) will be missed.[5]

Subdiaphragmatic Abscess. The subdiaphragmatic abscess can be as elusive as a liver abscess. The classic features of fixation and elevation of the diaphragm with secondary pleural reaction and ipsilateral tenderness in the shoulder muscles are not uniformly present. A subdiaphragmatic abscess may be found in patients whose histories reveal no obvious underlying cause. For example, several weeks after a seemingly uncomplicated operation, a patient developed a spiking fever, sweats, and malaise. Ultimately, a subdiaphragmatic abscess was found, and it was realized that the operation had been complicated by an infection, which had been masked by the postoperative administration of antibiotics.[1]

Cholangitis. Charcot fever produced by intermittent blockage of the biliary ducts is a common cause of periodic fever. Success in diagnosis depends on the detection of transient elevations of the serum bilirubin or alkaline phosphatase. For this reason these determinations should be made at the onset and the peaks of febrile episodes.

Appendicitis and Diverticulitis. In elderly persons or in those receiving adrenal steroids, acute appendicitis or diverticulitis may be overlooked or misjudged mainly because the usual manifestations of an acute inflammatory process may not be present. A ruptured viscus with abscess formation, sometimes associated with pylephlebitis, is not rare in these settings.

Perirectal Abscess. Perirectal abscess is a common cause of obscure fever in patients with diabetes or leukemia. It is readily diagnosed if a rectal examination is performed. Unfortunately, this is not always done. No febrile patient is too sick to have a rectal examination. Such abscesses may also complicate the course of regional enteritis, ulcerative colitis, diverticulitis, and granulomatous lesions involving the gut.

Perinephric Abscess. This infection is commonly mistaken for pyelonephritis or sepsis. Suggestive features are unilateral flank pain, dysuria, flank or abdominal mass, and lack of renal mobility on intravenous pyelogram. Organisms are usually aerobic, enteric, gram-negative bacilli, although gram-positive cocci can be responsible.

Prostatitis. The prostate can contain a reservoir of pathogenic bacteria and can be the focus for repeated febrile episodes. The history of febrile episodes occurring after long periods of riding or sitting should make one suspect the diagnosis.

Sinusitis. Sinusitis is a common disease that can cause fever. Normally the disease is clinically mild. However, in critically ill patients in association with endotracheal and nasogastric tubes, acute sinusitis may be responsible for prolonged unexplained fevers.[7]

Specific Infections

When the characteristic manifestations of a specific infection, such as typhoid fever, have reached their full development, the diagnosis is usually evident. It is in the early stages of the illness, when the only manifestations present are common to many infections, that problems of identification arise.

Salmonellosis. *Salmonella* infections are common and may follow typhoidal courses, with continual fever and chills for several weeks. Metastatic abscesses may be formed. There is an increased incidence of *Salmonella* infections in thalassemia, sickle-cell disease, leukemia, cirrhosis of the liver, neoplastic disease, and postsplenectomy. The organism can localize in neoplasms or hematomas, or in ulcerated plaques in the major arteries.

Malaria. Hundreds of millions of people live in areas where malaria still exacts a heavy toll. Physicians throughout the United States must consider malaria in the differential diagnosis of any febrile illness in patients who have traveled in endemic areas, particularly Southeast Asia. Even in patients who have never traveled to endemic areas, one should still consider the possibility of malaria acquired through artificial means such as blood transfusion or the sharing of common syringes; the latter possibility should particularly be considered in narcotic addicts.

Rickettsial Infections. A careful epidemiologic history, physical examination, and appropriate serologic studies usually serve to rapidly identify the rickettsial infections and remove them from the category of fevers of obscure origin.

Spirochetal Infections. Because of its protean manifestations syphilis must always be considered as a possible cause of fever (Chapter 9.15). Other spirochetes including *Leptospira* can cause prolonged febrile illnesses.

Viral Infections. Viral infections are not usually associated with fever of unknown origin. Most common viral illnesses are of short duration. Infectious mononucleosis, however, is a viral infection that is often overlooked. About 20 percent of patients have only fever, malaise, a refractory sore throat, and vague musculoskeletal complaints. The classic features of this illness may not be present. Although the febrile period usually lasts only 7 to 14 days, it may be prolonged for several weeks. The characteristic blood and serologic alterations may not make their appearance until late in the course, so that initially the correct diagnosis can be obscure.

In addition, an infectious mononucleosis-like illness has been described with cytomegalovirus, particularly after open-heart surgery and the use of the extracorporeal pump system. The heterophilic antibody test is negative, but diagnosis can be made by a rise in specific antibody in the serum and isolation of the organism from blood or urine. In patients with defective host defense mechanisms the cytomegalovirus can cause disseminated disease, with fever, hepatitis, lymphadenopathy, renal impairment, and pneumonia.

Prolonged fever with few localizing signs also may characterize

hepatitis. Although alterations in liver functions usually suggest the diagnosis, the occurrence of rashes and arthropathy may confuse the issue.

Granulomatous Infections. Not infrequently in the search for a diagnosis in a case of FUO, granulomas will be found in liver, lymph nodes, bone marrow, or other tissues. Although helpful, the presence of granulomas does not establish a diagnosis. Since the differential diagnosis includes many treatable conditions, it behooves the physician to make all efforts to establish a specific etiologic diagnosis. The following diseases have been associated with formation of granulomas in tissue: sarcoidosis, tuberculosis, fungal infections, brucellosis, tularemia, syphilis, leprosy, Hodgkin disease, drug reactions, and vasculitis. Recently, attention has been called to a group of patients with prolonged hectic fevers, marked constitutional symptoms, and usually only modest signs of disease. Biopsy of the liver shows multiple hepatic granulomas and there is a good response to corticosteroid therapy. Whether this entity of "granulomatous hepatitis" represents a separate disease is not yet clear. Tuberculosis and to a lesser extent disseminated fungal infections commonly present as fever of unknown origin and will be discussed in more detail.

Tuberculosis. Of all the chronic infections, tuberculosis is the one that most commonly presents as a fever of unexplained origin and is the one that is most commonly overlooked. This is a medical tragedy because it is so readily treated. Stead and others have contributed greatly to our understanding of the natural history of this complex disease.[14]

Primary Tuberculosis. Although the incidence of tuberculosis in the United States has decreased in the past 60 years, it is still a significant problem.[15] Early in this century, 80 percent of the population under age 20 had a positive tuberculin skin test. At present, less than 5 percent of young adults have a positive tuberculin skin test. However, in some urban centers half of the population over age 50 reacts to tuberculin.

Primary tuberculosis can be defined as the invasion of a nonimmune host by the tubercle bacillus. Most such individuals do not develop disease but show only a positive tuberculin skin test. The detection of these converters is extremely important since, if untreated, approximately 5 to 10 percent will develop significant clinical tuberculosis within 5 years, and an additional 2 to 5 percent will show recrudescence of their disease at a later time. When primary tuberculosis results in significant host injury, primary pulmonary tuberculosis results. Early in the disease the patient may be asymptomatic. With progression of the disease, weight loss, anorexia, fever, and mild respiratory symptoms appear. The chest radiograph shows patches of pneumonia almost always in the lower two thirds of the lung fields. Progression of the initial lesion may lead to pleurisy, pleural effusion, and cavitation with or without hemoptysis. Occasionally, the onset of primary pulmonary tuberculosis is more dramatic, with high fever, chills, marked respiratory symptoms, and leukocytosis; it also may masquerade as acute bacterial pneumonia.

Before the development of specific immunity, it is not unusual for the tubercle bacillus to disseminate widely throughout the body. Almost always this dissemination is silent, and lesions heal spontaneously with the development of immunity. Lesions tend to localize in areas characterized by high tissue oxygen tension (e.g., apex of the lung, kidney, brain, spine, and long bones). Uncommonly, disease will progress in these sites shortly after the initial infection. The results will be miliary tuberculosis or tuberculosis of extrapulmonary sites (e.g., meningitis, osteomyelitis) (Table 9.3–2). The prognosis then is ominous and prompt, and adequate treatment is necessary to prevent death.

Postprimary Tuberculosis. Postprimary tuberculosis can be defined as reappearance of active tuberculosis in a previously sensitized in-

dividual. In the past, this development was thought to be due to reinfection. At present, the evidence strongly indicates that postprimary tuberculosis develops not because of reinfection, but because of reactivation of dormant infection. This reactivation of the disease can occur a few months or many decades after the initial infection. It is more likely to occur when the host defense mechanisms are impaired by such things as steroid treatment, diabetes, cirrhosis, pneumoconiosis, neoplasms, and blood dyscrasias.

Postprimary Pulmonary Tuberculosis. Unlike in primary pulmonary tuberculosis, spontaneous healing in postprimary pulmonary tuberculosis is unusual, and tendencies to chronicity, liquefaction necrosis, and development of fibrosis are characteristic. Here again, the onset is usually insidious and extensive lung damage has usually occurred by the time the classic symptoms of fever, night sweats, weight loss, cough, and hemoptysis are noted. On chest film, lesions are usually located in the apices of the lungs and consist of fibronodular infiltrates, cavities, and fibrosis. Pneumothorax, pleurisy, and pleural effusions develop from extension of active tuberculous lesions to the pleura.

Postprimary Extrapulmonary Tuberculosis. As mentioned previously, seeding of tubercle bacilli throughout the body can occur during the primary phase of the disease. Table 9.3–2 lists the organs commonly involved in the recrudescence of active disease. Usually, symptoms will point to the specific organ involved. However, tuberculous peritonitis and tuberculosis of the genital tract often present with fever and nonspecific symptoms for prolonged periods of time. Diagnosis usually requires laparotomy.

Disseminated Tuberculosis. It may be particularly difficult to recognize tuberculosis in its disseminated form when there are no localized phenomena pointing to the diagnosis. Some patients can continue to work for a year or longer with active disseminated tuberculosis. The very mildness of the course may disarm and delude the physician into excluding this possibility because the patient does not appear sick enough. In addition, disseminated tuberculosis in the adult tends to be superimposed on a variety of illnesses that impair host defense mechanisms. In such cases the tuberculous infection may be completely overshadowed by the underlying disease.

Disseminated tuberculosis can occur with the primary or with the postprimary phase. It can be an acute illness, with high fever, chills, malaise, headache, and prostration. The fever is usually intermittent and well tolerated by the patient, who often is unaware of its presence despite peaks to 103F or 105F. Reversal of the normal diurnal variation or double quotidian fever patterns are sometimes seen. Pulmonary findings are usually unimpressive and sputum cultures are usually negative unless active pulmonary disease preceded the hematogenous spread. The chest film may show a miliary pattern that represents conglomeration of innumerable small miliary lesions. Hepatosplenomegaly, lymphadenopathy, and involvement of meninges, pericardium, pleura, peritoneum, eyes, and other organs may also develop. During acute miliary dissemination, polymorphonuclear leukocytosis is frequent and a leukemoid reaction with white blood counts as high as $100,000/\mu l$ may occur.

More commonly in the adult, disseminated tuberculosis follows a chronic course with low-grade fever and few or no pulmonary signs or symptoms. Other symptoms are nonspecific, and the physical alterations are common to a variety of disorders. Among the changes seen are hepatosplenomegaly, lymphadenopathy, muscle wasting, arthritis, chorioretinitis, hypergammaglobulinemia, hemolytic anemia or refractory anemia, leukopenia or leukocytosis, thrombopenia, or thrombocytosis. The tuberculin skin test may be negative. It is easy to understand why in these cases the diagnosis may be exceedingly difficult to establish. The most valuable diagnostic procedure is biopsy of the liver, which is indicated even in the absence of clinical liver involvement. Biopsy and culture of

TABLE 9.3–2. EXTRAPULMONARY TUBERCULOSIS

Site	Manifestations
Direct extension from pulmonary tuberculosis:	
Pleura	Dry pleurisy (fibrinous); pleuritic chest pain
	Wet pleurisy; effusion (often serosanguinous) with or without pulmonary involvement
	Empyema; complication of bronchopleural fistula
Larynx	Hoarseness, dysphagia
	Severe inflammation may endanger airway
	Formerly resulted in fibrosis and aphonia (now rare)
Bronchi and trachea	Cough, wheezing; bronchial obstruction (from granulation and ulceration) may lead to abscess formation or bronchiectasis
	Usually secondary to active pulmonary disease; occasionally results from rupture of caseous node into bronchus
	Responds well to chemotherapy; steroids may be dramatically beneficial
Alimentary tract	
• Buccal cavity, tongue	Painful ulcerations
	Usually late complication of chronic cavitary pulmonary disease
	Biopsy may aggravate
• Tonsil	Acquired from drinking infected milk (now virtually absent in U.S.)
• Esophagus and stomach	Rare; by extension from contiguous lymph nodes
• Intestine	Vague abdominal pain; constipation or diarrhea
	Usually secondary to swallowing heavily infected sputum in active pulmonary disease (contaminated milk is a source outside the U.S.)
	Ileocecal involvement commonest form
	May be confused with regional enteritis (Crohn disease)
	Fistula-in-ano and ischiorectal abscess formerly common with active pulmonary disease
Hematogenous and lymphogenous spread (or direct extension from nonpulmonary lesion):	
Disseminated hematogenous (miliary): acute	In childhood, follows soon after primary infection; in adults, may occur at any time in chronic active disease
	Abrupt onset of fever, chills, headache, malaise, prostration
	Leukocytosis up to 20,000 or leukemoid reaction
	Localization may involve one or more sites; lungs (dyspnea, sometimes scattered rales); miliary (millet seed) pulmonary radiograph lesions may be visible on chest film before acute symptoms, they proceed to conglomeration and cavitation
	Pleura (pleuritic pain, effusion)
	Meninges (meningitis develops in up to two thirds of untreated childhood cases)
	Eye (choroidal tubercles may be detected)
	Spleen (enlargement)
	Liver (hepatomegaly—increased alkaline phosphatase, bilirubin usually only minimally elevated; liver biopsy often positive for tubercles)
	Lymph nodes (enlargement)
	Peritoneum (with or without signs of peritonitis)
	Pericardium (pain, rub, tamponade)
Disseminated hematogenous (miliary): chronic	Dissemination occurs insidiously or in indolent intermittent episodes
	Signs and symptoms depend on organ sites predominantly involved
Nervous system	May not be acute in onset; irritability and listlessness in children
• Meningitis	Headache, and bizarre behavior in older children and adults
	Change of mental state, disorientation, and finally coma
	Stiff neck, cranial nerve signs
	Spinal fluid shows predominantly mononuclear pleocytosis (up to several hundred cells per mm^3), elevated protein, and low sugar
	Organism difficult to stain, though more often culturable
	Treatment must not await results of culture
	Untreated cases almost invariably fatal
	Without early treatment, permanent sequelae may include blindness, deafness, or mental deficiency

(continued)

TABLE 9.3–2. EXTRAPULMONARY TUBERCULOSIS (Continued)

Site	Manifestations
Hematogenous and lymphogenous spread (*Cont.*)	
Nervous system (Cont.)	
• Meningitis (*Cont.*)	Possible role of head trauma in localization of infection
	In addition to INH and rifampin, corticosteroids appear to ameliorate severe acute manifestations, relieve coma
	(Prevention of late sequelae is undocumented)
• Tuberculoma	Signs and symptoms of expanding intracranial mass
	Cannot easily be distinguished from neoplasm without surgical exploration
Lymph nodes	Pulmonary hilar involvement prominent in primary tuberculosis
	Mediastinal, tracheobronchial nodes may be source of spread to bronchi, pericardium, or elsewhere
	May cause cough and wheezing by pressure on bronchi
	Cervical lymphadenitis (scrofula)
	Painless swellings in the neck (single or multiple), nontender
	Tend to become matted
	May form cold abscess and chronic cutaneous sinus tracts
	Most often associated with pulmonary tuberculosis
	Some cases now caused by atypical mycobacteria
	Abdominal (mesenteric)
	May cause pain and fever or palpable abdominal masses
	Diagnosis usually requires laparotomy
Pericardium	Precordial pain, symptoms of cardiac tamponade, friction rub
	Ewart sign (posterior dullness and bronchial breath sounds due to lung compression by massive pericardial effusion)
	Usually arises by erosion of adjacent mediastinal node into pericardium
	Effusion may be predominantly a hypersensitivity reaction to tuberculoprotein
	Mycobacterium often not detectable by smear or culture
	Pericardiocentesis may aid diagnosis and treatment
	Late complication: constrictive pericarditis
Peritoneum	Acute onset with moderate abdominal pain, fever, distension from rapid accumulation of fluid
	Local abscess, adhesions, and loculations may produce doughy consistency
	Paracentesis may perforate bowel when significant adhesions are present
	May be insidious in onset
	Most often secondary to old abdominal focus
	Limited laparotomy for diagnosis and evacuation of fluid often indicated
	Response to chemotherapy is good
Kidney	Hematuria (microscopic or gross)
	Secondary bladder involvement may produce symptoms of cystitis; frequency, dysuria, pyuria
	Pyuria without bacteriuria on routine smear and culture always raises suspicion of renal tuberculosis
	Nephrectomy now rarely necessary because of good response to chemotherapy
Genital	
• Female	Salpingitis
	May be asymptomatic cause of sterility
	Menstrual irregularities may be present
	Pelvic peritonitis may be associated
	Adnexal mass usually detectable on pelvic examination
	Extension to ovaries or uterine endometrium may occur
	Endometrial curettage, leukorrheal discharge or menstruum may yield organism
	Surgical resection may be indicated after control of local peritonitis with chemotherapy
• Male	Epididymitis most frequently seen, though prostate and seminal vesicles often involved asymptomatically
	Acute swelling and tenderness or insidious appearance of slightly tender nodule
	Excision may be indicated to establish diagnosis

(continued)

TABLE 9.3–2. EXTRAPULMONARY TUBERCULOSIS (Continued)

Site	Manifestations
Hematogenous and lymphogenous spread (*Cont.*)	
Musculoskeletal system	Spine (tuberculous spondylitis or Pott disease)
	Starts as osteomyelitis of vertebral body
	Destruction with vertebral collapse followed by healing and ankylosis produces kyphosis (gibbus)
	Associated paravertebral cold abscess
	Treatment with decompression, curettage, and immobilization (external fusion of lateral spinous processes) plus chemotherapy
	Joints (large, weight-bearing joints; hip and knee, most common) pain, swelling
	Initial involvement usually in epiphysis of long bone or synovium
	Cartilage involvement is secondary; after destruction, ankylosis and immobilization may lead to healing
	Arthrodesis of large joints may not be required if early intensive chemotherapy is given

lymph nodes and bone marrow may yield similar information. The demonstration of acid-fast bacilli on stain or culture is diagnostic. As previously mentioned, the finding of granuloma without positive stains on culture is not diagnostic of active tuberculosis.

Fungal Infections. Fungal infections can present as febrile illnesses either during the acute primary pulmonary phase or more commonly when the disease has disseminated. Some of the features of the more common systemic mycotic infections are shown in Table 9.3–3.

Histoplasma capsulatum is a dimorphic fungus occurring both in yeast and mycelial forms. During human infection only the yeast form is produced. The vast majority of cases of histoplasmosis are asymptomatic. Skin test studies indicate rapid conversion to positivity during childhood in endemic areas. In some areas as many as 80 percent of children have a positive histoplasmin skin test by age 5. A certain number of asymptomatic infections result in pulmonary calcifications in the periphery of the lung parenchyma and in calcification of hilar nodes and spleen. This benign process represents over 99 percent of human infections.[13]

Acute Pulmonary Histoplasmosis. This benign and self-limited syndrome often occurs in small epidemics following exposure to contaminated chicken coops, caves, or freshly disturbed, shaded soil. The incubation period is 5 to 20 days, and the illness is characterized by fever, night sweats, chills, cough, chest pain, and less frequently, shortness of breath and hemoptysis. The severity of the symptoms varies from mild respiratory symptoms to severe prostration with high fever and cyanosis. The chest film usually shows bilateral disease with discrete or diffuse nodular pneumonic infiltrates with hilar lymphadenopathy. *Histoplasma capsulatum* may be cultured from sputum or gastric aspirates. Sometimes, even in these benign cases, the fungus can also be cultured from bone marrow or lymph node, indicating that the illness is not confined to the lungs. Usually the illness lasts from 2 weeks to 3 months, with spontaneous resolution. The prognosis is excellent, and treatment with amphotericin B is not required. The histoplasmin skin test is almost always positive, as is the serology.

Chronic Pulmonary Histoplasmosis. This illness, which occurs predominantly in adults, is entirely similar to chronic pulmonary tuberculosis. The symptoms are those of chronic pulmonary disease: cough, weight loss, dyspnea, recurrent fevers, hemoptysis, and chest pain.

The skin test is positive in 80 percent of cases, and the serology is positive in 90 percent of cases. Treatment with amphotericin B is effective.

Disseminated Histoplasmosis. Disseminated histoplasmosis has been observed at all ages but more commonly occurs at the extremes of life.[13] Symptoms and signs of pulmonary disease are absent in half of the patients. Ulcerative granulomatous lesions of the mouth, tongue, nose, pharynx, and larynx are suggestive of the diagnosis. Biopsy of these lesions will reveal the characteristic small intracellular yeast. The most commonly involved organs are the lungs, adrenal glands, liver, spleen, and lymph nodes. Clinically, hepatosplenomegaly is common, and in almost 20 percent of cases adrenal insufficiency will develop. Hematologic and liver function test abnormalities are common but nonspecific. The most helpful tool in diagnosis is culture of bone marrow. Positive results will be obtained in 75 percent of cases. The diagnosis cannot be ruled out by skin test (which is negative in 50 percent) or by serology (which is negative in 40 percent). The mortality of the untreated disease is well over 80 percent. Treatment with intravenous amphotericin B has reduced the mortality to 25 percent.

NEOPLASMS AND HEMATOLOGIC DISORDERS

Tumors are among the common causes of prolonged fever.[9] Although lymphomas and tumors of the kidney and liver are most likely to present with fever, any malignant tumor has the capacity to induce fever. Fever may be produced by tissue necrosis, involvement of the temperature regulating center, hemorrhage, secondary infection, or obstruction of the bronchus, ureter, or bile ducts. The temperature may be high and swinging, may be associated with chills, and may mimic the pattern followed in an infectious process.

Tumor as a cause of obscure fever may be overlooked for a variety of reasons. The frequency with which neoplasms present with fever may not be appreciated. There may be no historical or physical data pointing to the presence of a neoplasm, and laboratory changes are usually nonspecific. The tumor is often not detectable as a mass lesion even with the aid of special radiologic techniques. Its presence may be heralded by peripheral manifestations suggesting a different type of disease. Thus, bronchogenic tumor may present initially with severe joint pains (osteoarthropathy), which can be mistaken for those of rheumatoid arthritis. A lymphoma may be associated with a variety of skin eruptions, pancreatic carcinoma with polyphlebitis, carcinoma of the breast with peculiar neurologic alterations, and gastric cancer with a polymyositis. One must be familiar with these general disturbances produced by new growths (Chapter 6.13).

The fever associated with neoplasms of all sorts, including the leukemias, is often due not to the new growth itself but to some accompanying infection. Patients with neoplasms may have impaired immune responses, predisposing them to infection: once acquired, such infections may run rampant. For this reason the finding of a new growth in a patient with fever does not necessarily mean that the true cause of the fever has been located.

TABLE 9.3–3. COMMON SYSTEMIC MYCOTIC INFECTIONS

Disease	Source of Infection	Distinguishing Features
Histoplasmosis	Soil contaminated with bird droppings	High incidence of subclinical infections
	Worldwide, Mississippi Valley, Eastern and Central U.S.	Acute, subacute, or chronic pulmonary infection
	Airborne	Disseminated disease with hepatosplenomegaly, fever, anemia, skin and mucous membrane lesions
		Organism can be cultured from sputum, tissue, or bone marrow
		Reliable skin tests and serology except in disseminated disease (50 percent negative)
Cryptococcosis	Soil contaminated with pigeon droppings	Primary lesion, apparent or inapparent pulmonary lesion, coin lesion, or pneumonia
	Worldwide	Very high predilection for CNS infection mostly in patients with lymphoma, leukemia, or on steroids
	Airborne	Organisms frequently seen in CSF by India ink examination
		Can also involve bone, skin, mucous membranes, and kidneys
		Skin test not reliable
		Serology extremely useful: presence of cryptococcus polysaccharide antigen is diagnostic of active infection
Coccidioidomycosis	Dry desert soil, limited geographic distribution (Southwestern U.S.)	High incidence of subclinical infections
	Airborne	Acute, subacute, or chronic pulmonary infection
		Dissemination disease with involvement of skin, bones, viscera, and CNS
		Blacks and Filipinos particularly prone to disseminated disease
		Meningitis extremely chronic and prone to relapses
		Reliable skin tests for primary disease
		Serology extremely useful: Serum or CSF antibody complement fixation titer of 1:16 indicates serious illness
North American blastomycosis	Soil probably	Primary pulmonary infection usually inapparent
	North American continent, Southwestern U.S.	Disseminated disease with involvement of skin, lungs, bones, and urogenital tract
	Airborne	Characteristic verrucous or ulcerative skin lesions with central healing
		Skin test and serology not helpful
Sporotrichosis	Worldwide	Ulcerative skin lesion, usually on exposed surface, such as forearm, followed by lymphadenitis and lymphangitis with nodular ulcerations along lymphatics
	Often follows puncture wounds by rose or barberry thorns, splinters, or metal particles	May disseminate and produce widespread skin and mucosal lesions and less frequently bone, joint, and lung involvement
		Visceral lesions observed rarely
		Iodide therapy effective for skin involvement only
		Skin test and serology unreliable
Candidiasis	Normal inhabitant of man	Disseminated disease associated with debilitating illness, antibiotic or immunosuppressive treatment, indwelling intravenous or bladder catheters, gastrointestinal lesions, and diabetes mellitus
	Worldwide	Onset characterized by fever, chills, hypotension

(continued)

TABLE 9.3–3. COMMON SYSTEMIC MYCOTIC INFECTIONS (Continued)

Disease	Source of Infection	Distinguishing Features
Candidiasis (*Cont.*)		Organs involved are kidney, heart, lung, gastrointestinal tract, spleen, liver, skin, and mucous membranes
		Can present as endocarditis, meningitis, or endophthalmitis
		Skin test and serology unreliable
Phycomycosis (Mucormycosis)	Worldwide	Orbital cellulitis and necrosis in persons with acidosis (diabetic or renal)
	Common in animal feces and in decaying vegetable matter	Can also present a pulmonary or disseminated infection
	Possibly airborne	
Aspergillosis	Common saprophytes on decaying vegetable matter	Can present picture of asthma, allergic bronchopulmonary aspergillosis, fungus ball, necrotizing pneumonia, or disseminated aspergillosis
	Possibly airborne	The latter is characterized by tissue and vascular invasion with thrombosis and infarction in patients with lymphoreticular or hematopoietic malignancies

Benign tumors also may be the cause of fever. Patients with atrial myxoma may have a pattern of illness with fever and embolic manifestations simulating infective endocarditis.

Necrotizing lymphadenitis is well described in the Far East, where the entity was first observed. In this country it remains infrequently considered in the differential diagnosis of cervical lymphadenopathy and fever. There is a striking predominance in women. The course is benign but may be protracted and last for several months. Clinically this disease is often confused with lymphoma, systemic lupus erythematosus, or chronic infection. Diagnosis is made on the basis of distinctive histology and the clinical manifestations.[17]

LIVER DISEASE

Cirrhosis of the liver and hepatitis due to various agents may be associated with fever.[16] The laboratory findings associated with these disorders are often nonspecific. Even the presence of hepatitis viremia may not be related to illness (Chapter 13.3). Liver biopsy may be needed to distinguish granulomatous liver disease from neoplastic disorders or cirrhosis. Liver scans usually detect abscesses or tumor deposits.

DRUG FEVER

Drug reactions are an increasingly important cause of prolonged fever. The possibility of a drug reaction should always be an early consideration in dealing with puzzling fever.[3] Drug fever may be present with or without rash or eosinophilia.

Although certain drugs are more likely to cause fever than others are, it must be realized that any drug has the capacity to produce fever if it is given to a person who is hypersensitive to it.

A detailed drug history for each patient is essential. It should be explained to the patient that literally any drug or toxic agent is potentially capable of producing fever and that a detailed account of every medicine ingested and of all contact with toxic materials is desired. Patients (and some physicians) fail to appreciate that a drug well tolerated for many years may abruptly induce a reaction, including fever.

In the hospital it is a good practice to examine carefully the order sheets and nursing notes for the patient with unexplained fever. Drug hypersensitivity may produce clinical changes common to the collagen disorders, neoplasms, blood dyscrasias, and granulomatous infections and can be confused with such processes.

Often the problem can be clarified only by withdrawing all medications or by substituting drugs that the patient has never taken before.

CONNECTIVE TISSUE DISEASE

It is well known that the patient with systemic lupus erythematosus may not have the classic features of the disease in a readily recognizable pattern. The initial manifestations may be persistent fever that lasts for weeks before other significant abnormalities appear. Polyarteritis has also become increasingly familiar as a cause of obscure fever accompanied by weight loss and mild leukocytosis. Complicating infections and drug reactions are known to occur in this group of diseases, and it is important to rule out carefully such treatable illnesses as tuberculosis and other infections before accepting the diagnosis of a collagen disease when the classical manifestations of such a disease are not present.

Collagen vascular diseases are less likely to present as unexplained fever, according to recent reports, because of increased awareness and improved laboratory tests. However, Still disease and giant-cell arteritis remain two important considerations. Still disease, or adult juvenile rheumatoid arthritis, can present in young adults with high fever, rash, leukocytosis, and elevated erythrocyte sedimentation rate but without significant skeletal signs or symptoms and without positive specific laboratory studies. Management of this disease depends on the correct diagnosis. Diagnosis is made by the accurate interpretation of the various clinical features of the syndrome and exclusion of other possible diseases. Treatment of adult Still disease requires unusually high doses of aspirin or other nonsteroidal anti-inflammatory drugs, prednisone, or a combination of these drugs. Although many patients respond rapidly and dramatically, a significant number of patients have recurrent systemic attacks or may progress to deforming chronic arthritis.[8] Giant-cell arteritis must be suspected in older patients who have fever, anemia, and elevated sedimentation rate. At times, a trial with corticosteroids is the only way to settle the diagnosis.

MISCELLANEOUS

Among the causes of fever of obscure origin, sarcoidosis is important. This disorder may be characterized by little or no constitutional reaction or can be associated with marked wasting and a prolonged hectic fever. The distinction of this illness from tuberculosis or disseminated fungal infection is most difficult and is generally

made by exclusion after special stains of biopsy specimens and cultures fail to yield an etiologic agent.

Occult inflammatory diseases of the small and large bowel may be one of the most difficult and obscure causes of fever. Frequently symptoms that refer to the gastrointestinal tract are minimal and nonspecific. Contrast studies may be entirely negative, and only laparotomy will finally establish a diagnosis of Whipple disease or regional enteritis.

Occasionally, certain disorders of metabolism may primarily present with a fever, although more often than not they will declare themselves in a more familiar way. Hyperthyroidism, porphyria, and gout would be the main considerations, should this possibility arise.

Familial Mediterranean fever is a disease of unknown etiology that should be recognized on the basis of history. Characteristics of this disease are as follows: frequent positive family history, marked predilection for patients of Sephardic Jewish, Armenian, or Arab ancestry, predictable cycles of fever of abrupt onset and short duration associated with severe abdominal pain, polyserositis, and, less commonly, skin rash and arthritis. Colchicine has been found to be helpful in preventing attacks of familial Mediterranean fever.

FACTITIOUS FEVER

Fever is readily accepted as incontrovertible evidence of organic disease. However, factitious fever may be encountered when least expected. It is wise to give this possibility early consideration when dealing with puzzling fever.[12] It may be difficult, and at times almost impossible, to detect the manner in which the patient produced factitious fever. Such factitious fevers are most commonly seen in medical and paramedical personnel and members of their families. There are several points that may call attention to the possibility of factitious fever: failure of the temperature curve to follow the normal diurnal pattern, failure of the pulse to accelerate with sudden spikes of fever, rapid defervescence without sweating, and disparity between body and urine temperatures.

APPROACH TO THE PATIENT WITH FEVER OF UNKNOWN ORIGIN

Several general principles appear important: (1) No effort should be spared in the hunt for a specific diagnosis. (2) A well-organized systematic approach is required. (3) Once a significant abnormality has been uncovered, "go where the money is." (4) Most patients do not have rare diseases. They suffer from common diseases presenting in unusual fashions. (5) Time is usually not an important consideration—premature diagnostic or therapeutic interventions can further complicate a difficult problem. The mainstay of the clinical approach to the patient with fever of unknown origin remains an analysis of the data derived from an accurate, complete history and physical examination. In the history, particular attention should be paid to potential exposures, to the history of drug intake, to the details of the onset of the illness, and to the past history for clues to multisystem disease. Daily physical examination of the patient is important because changes in physical findings may give the clue to diagnosis. The following aspects of the physical examination are often neglected and yet many times prove to be rewarding: eye grounds, oral cavity, skin including palms and soles, diaphragmatic mobility, sternal tenderness, rectum, prostate, testes, pelvic organs in women, navel, auscultation of the liver, abdomen, and painful areas, and careful palpation for nodes, nodules, and areas of tenderness.

Routine laboratory studies should include a complete blood count, eosinophil count, erythrocyte sedimentation rate, urinalysis, blood chemistries, and examination of the stool smear. Blood cultures should always be obtained, and cultures of urine, sputum, stool, and cerebrospinal fluid are usually indicated. Screening studies for collagen vascular diseases may be helpful, but skin testing

and routine serologic studies are usually not useful. Routine radiologic studies should include radiographs of the chest and sinuses. Barium enema, upper gastrointestinal series, small bowel series, gallbladder study, and intravenous pyelography should be performed unless a specific clue points elsewhere. Despite the ready availability of many sophisticated, noninvasive diagnostic techniques, it is not clear which procedure or combination of procedures is most helpful. All such procedures have false-positive and false-negative rates of 10 to 33 percent. Radionuclide scans are best suited for screening and for evaluation of bones or liver. Ultrasound scans are useful in evaluating liver, kidneys, pancreas, and pelvis and in differentiating solid from liquid masses. Although computed tomography cannot serve for blind screening, it effectively delineates areas of possible pathology. Documentation of an abnormality by more than one technique decreases the incidence of false positive results but also decreases the sensitivity of the tests.[10]

The yield from bone marrow biopsy is low, but this procedure should be done routinely because it may be the only way to make the diagnosis of hematologic malignancies and certain infections such as histoplasmosis or tuberculosis. Liver biopsy should not be done in all patients since it has a low diagnostic yield. Liver biopsy is more likely to be helpful when hepatomegaly or abnormal liver function tests are present. One should proceed with biopsy of skin, muscle, temporal artery, lymph node, bone, lung, or gastrointestinal mucosa when there is a documented clinical abnormality. Rarely, a blind biopsy of muscle or temporal artery will lead to a specific diagnosis.

EXPLORATORY SURGERY

Not infrequently, in managing a patient with obscure fever, there comes a time when, despite one's best diagnostic effort, the cause of the patient's fever remains hidden. Then the difficult question has to be faced—should an exploratory laparotomy be performed? The answer to this question is extremely complex. Several guidelines have been offered and should be reviewed carefully in all cases.[1,2]

More recently ultrasonography and computed tomography have improved our ability to search for potential causes of fever of unknown origin, particularly within the abdominal cavity. As a result, exploratory laparotomy is used less frequently. However, false-positive and false-negative findings are sufficiently common[10] that the basic approach in making a decision to perform an exploratory laparotomy has not significantly changed. In general, an exploratory laparotomy is likely to be rewarding if there are symptoms or signs clearly pointing to some type of intraabdominal disease. Many disorders, although originating outside the abdominal cavity, may be accompanied by disturbances of bowel function, nausea, abdominal distension or pain, and mild derangement of liver function tests. On the other hand, exploratory laparotomy may be successful even in the absence of any suggestive symptoms or signs. In instances in which there is no clinical evidence whatever of intraabdominal disease, one should prolong the period of observation first and search the abdomen only if there is progressive deterioration of the patient's condition.

THERAPEUTIC TRIALS

As already stated, it is frequently difficult and sometimes impossible to detect on clinical grounds the specific cause of an illness presenting with fever, and the question of the wisdom and usefulness of a therapeutic trial often arises in such circumstances.

There are pros and cons to the use of a therapeutic trial in FUO. A therapeutic trial is no substitute for a thorough investigation of the patient's situation. Effective management of the patient's illness usually requires specific therapy, and suspicions or hunches are not sound bases for definitive therapy.

The trial usually entails the use of antibiotics, various steroids,

or antitumor agents, including radiation. All have potentially deleterious side effects that may complicate an already confused problem through the production of more fever, eruptions, jaundice, alterations in the blood, and so on. Not only may the patient's course be confused by the harmful side effects of such therapy, but any nonspecific beneficial effects that these agents produce may also mislead one into a false sense of achievement. Thus, a patient with a liver abscess may be symptomatically improved by being given corticosteroids, and hence valuable time is lost in bringing definitive therapy to bear.

A therapeutic trial may have a negative psychological effect on the patient and the family. Transient improvement may induce false hopes and dampen their willingness to embark upon some more difficult course, such as a longer period of observation or an exploratory operation, which may actually be the only avenue to recovery.

A therapeutic trial can become an undesirable delaying action when pushing ahead to definitive information by biopsy or exploratory laparotomy holds the single hope of recovery.

If clinical judgment indicates that none of the organ systems (heart, kidneys, etc.) is being seriously impaired by the underlying process, there is no reason for haste in beginning a therapeutic trial. Fever alone is no cause for hurry. Too often it becomes an alarm that results in actions that would never be employed after calm second thought. As a general rule, therefore, therapeutic trials in FUO are to be avoided except in very well-delineated circumstances.

On the other hand, rapidly advancing, life-threatening disease may indicate the use of a therapeutic trial, but even in this circumstance there is always time to secure material for important studies such as blood cultures.

If the decision is reached to attempt a therapeutic trial, several important considerations enter into the selection of an agent. First, it should be one to which the patient is least likely to have an adverse reaction. Second, to give the therapeutic trial differential diagnostic significance, the agent should be one of limited and, if possible, specific therapeutic effectiveness. Clearly, if an agent having a broad therapeutic potential is used, the patient's response to it will be of little diagnostic value. An obvious exception to this dictum is the critically ill patient, for whom adequacy of treatment must be assured from its very inception. In such instances, the desire to establish the specific diagnosis has to yield to the need to rescue the patient from the critical state. Therefore a broad therapeutic regimen must be devised, so that no treatable possibilities are overlooked. There may not be time for second attempts.

In addition to the most appropriate agent for the particular problem at hand being selected, it should be given in a dosage that will be effective and hence give a clear-cut, definite end point. Thus, if a patient is suspected of having systemic lupus erythematosus, it is an error to start a therapeutic trial with prednisone at a dosage level of only 20 mg, as this dosage is often inadequate. Enough of the drug must be given for the physician to be certain of its efficacy or lack of it. Clearly, it is also essential to continue the drug for a sufficient period of time.

REFERENCES

1. Altemeier WA, Culbertson WR, et al: Intraabdominal abscesses. Am J Surg 125:70, 1973
2. Baker RR, Tumulty PA, Shelley WM: The value of exploratory laparotomy in fever of undetermined etiology. Johns Hopkins Med J 125:159, 1969
3. Cluff LE, Johnson JE: Drug fever. Prog Allergy 8:149, 1964
4. Deller JJ Jr, Russell PK: An analysis of fevers of unknown origin in American soldiers in Vietnam. Ann Intern Med 66:1129, 1967
5. Grossman ZD, Wistow BW, et al: Radionuclide imaging, computer tomography, and gray-scale ultrasonography of the liver: A comparative study. J Nucl Med Allied Sci 18:327, 1977
6. Jacoby G, Swarz MN: Fever of undetermined origin. N Engl J Med 289:1407, 1974
7. Knodel AR, Beekman JF: Unexplained fevers in patients with nasotracheal intubation. JAMA 248:868, 1982
8. Larson EB: Adult Still's disease—Evolution of a clinical syndrome and diagnosis, treatment, and follow-up of 17 patients. Medicine 63:88, 1984
9. Larson EB, Featherston HJ, Petersdorf RG: Fever of undetermined origin: Diagnosis and follow-up of 105 cases, 1970–1982. Medicine 61:269, 1982
10. McNeil BJ, Sanders R, et al: A prospective study of computed tomography, ultrasound, and gallium imaging in patients with fever. Radiology 139:647, 1981
11. Petersdorf RG, Beeson PB: Fever of unexplained origin: Report of 100 cases. Medicine 40:1, 1961
12. Petersdorf RG, Bennett IL Jr: Factitious fever. Ann Intern Med 46:1039, 1957
13. Rubin H, Furcolow ML, et al: Seminar on mycotic infections: The course and prognosis of histoplasmosis. Am J Med 27:278, 1959
14. Stead WW: The pathogenesis of pulmonary tuberculosis among older persons. Am Rev Respir Dis 91:811, 1965
15. Stead WW, Kerby GR, et al: The clinical spectrum of primary tuberculosis in adults. Ann Intern Med 68:731, 1968
16. Tisdale WA, Klatskin G: The fever of Laennec's cirrhosis. Yale J Biol Med 33:94, 1960
17. Turner RR, Larkin J, Dorfman RF: Necrotizing lymphadenitis—A study of 30 cases. Am J Surg Pathol 7:115, 1983

CHAPTER 9.4

Bacterial Infections of the Skin, Muscle, and Bone

John G. Bartlett

PATHOPHYSIOLOGY OF INFECTIONS OF THE SKIN AND SOFT TISSUE

Skin consists of an outer ectodermal layer, the epidermis, which is firmly attached to the inner mesodermal layer, the dermis. The epidermis lacks a vascular supply and is relatively isolated from systemic host defenses. The dermis contains a lymphatic and vascular supply providing access to humoral or cellular defenses, but these structures also facilitate circumferential spread with lymphangitis or cellulitis. The skin is superimposed on subcutaneous tissue, the hypodermis, or tela subcutaneum. Skin appendages include sweat glands, hair follicles, sebaceous glands, apocrine glands, and nails that extend to the subcutaneous tissue, thus promoting spread to deeper structures. The deep fascia envelopes muscles and forms a barrier to the spread of superficial infections to muscular compartments. For this reason, most soft-tissue infections are restricted to the subcutaneous tissue and dermis.

The skin contains a resident and a transient microbial flora with concentrations that vary from 10^2 to 10^6 bacteria per cm^2,

depending on the anatomic site and sampling method. The lowest counts are found in dry, exposed, cool skin surfaces such as the extremities and face. Larger concentrations are noted in warm, moist areas such as the axillae, perineum, anterior nares, and toe webs. "Resident flora" refers to relatively stable bacterial populations in terms of microbial concentrations and specific species, the major components being diphtheroids, *Staphylococcus epidermidis*, and *Propionibacterium acnes*. These organisms rarely represent pathogens in skin and soft-tissue infections, but they are commonly recoverd in cultures as a result of surface contamination. The transient flora include organisms that are inconsistently present and presumably reflect acquisition from environmental sources. *Staphylococcus aureus* is frequently recovered in skin cultures but usually is a transient rather than true inhabitant. Aerobic streptococci are not part of the normal skin flora. Gram-negative bacilli are found primarily in warm, moist areas. Fungi, particularly species of *Candida* and dermatophytes, are also commonly found on normal skin. Viruses are rare in the absence of viral infections.

Electron microscopy shows bacteria normally inhabit the superficial two to three layers of desquamating cells of the epidermis. Deeper structures are protected by the anatomic barrier imposed by the intact dermis. Most infections result from direct entry of bacteria as a result of a breach in this mechanical barrier, by extension through the skin appendages, extension from deeper contiguous sites, or by hematogenous dissemination. Soft-tissue infections are difficult to produce with surface application or even direct microbial inoculation into subcutaneous tissue in the presence of normal defense mechanisms.[4] Contributing factors that are fundamental to the pathophysiology are (1) virulence of the microbe, (2) the inoculum size, (3) occlusive dressings, which prevent desquamation and provide a moist environment in which bacteria may proliferate, (4) significant disruption of the local area, (5) reduced vascular supply, (6) the presence of a foreign body, (7) compromise in systemic defense mechanisms, as with neutropenia, defective humoral defenses, and altered cellular immunity, and (8) disruption of lymphatic drainage or venous stasis. Clinical experience indicates that the site of infection usually reflects the virulence and concentrations of local bacteria superimposed on predisposing local conditions such as trauma, ischemia, lymphedema, venous stasis, and the location of certain appendages such as eccrine glands, sweat glands, or sebaceous glands.

Soft-tissue infections show considerable variation with respect to the responsible microbial pathogen, clinical presentation, therapeutic recommendations, and prognosis. The classification schemes used for tabular presentation here are primary soft-tissue infections that are common and usually superficial (Table 9.4–1), infections that are secondary to preexisting cutaneous lesions (Table 9.4–2), and deep or serious infections (Table 9.4–3). The

TABLE 9.4–1. PRIMARY PYODERMAS

Disorder	Organism	Usual Host/Site	Clinical Features	Treatment
Impetigo	*Strep. pyogenes* (*Staph. aureus;* streptococci, group B, C, or G)	Children May be epidemic Exposed areas	Vesicles with erythematous halos, then pustules and crusted lesions; lesions are painless	Careful and frequent cleansing; penicillin (erythromycin)
Bullous impetigo	*S. aureus*	Newborn and young children	Vesicles which progress to flaccid bullae	Penicillinase-resistant penicillin (erythromycin)
Erysipelas	*S. pyogenes* (streptococci, group B, C, or G; *S. aureus*)	Young children and older adults Areas of lymphatic obstruction or edema are predisposed	Painful erythematous, edematous, indurated, raised lesions with sharply demarcated margin; fever and leukocytosis are common	Penicillin (erythromycin)
Cellulitis	*S. pyogenes* *S. aureus* Others	Areas of prior trauma or ulceration	Painful, tender erythema with no elevation or sharp demarcation; systemic signs are variable	Penicillin, penicillinase-resistant penicillin or a cephalosporin
Lymphangitis	*S. pyogenes* (*S. aureus*)	Extremity	Erythematous streak with regional adenopathy	Penicillin; penicillinase-resistant penicillin; cephalothin or clindamycin
Folliculitis	*S. aureus* (*P. aeruginosa* Candida albicans)	Any area with hair follicles; areas exposed to swimming pool or whirlpool (*P. aeruginosa*)	Small erythematous papules with central pustule; no systemic signs	Saline compresses and topical antibiotics
Furuncles	*S. aureus*	Areas of friction, sweat and hair follicles—neck, face, axilla, and buttocks	Firm red nodule with progression to fluctuant painful mass and spontaneous drainage; fever and leukocytosis variable	Most heat application; antibiotics (usually penicillinase-resistant penicillin) for cases with extensive cellulitis, fever, or midface involvement; surgical drainage of large, fluctuant lesions
Carbuncle	*S. aureus*	Diabetics; usual areas are posterior neck, back, or thigh	Multiple abscesses that connect in subcutaneous tissue and drain along hair follicles	Incision and drainage; systemic antibiotics, usually penicillinase-resistant penicillin
Paronychia	*S. aureus* *S. pyogenes* *P. aeruginosa* Candida	Frequent hand immersion; nail fold	Periungual erythema and swelling with separation of nail fold from nail plate	

TABLE 9.4–2. INFECTIONS SECONDARY TO PREEXISTING CUTANEOUS LESIONS

Lesion or Setting	Major Microbial Pathogen	Preferred Antibiotic for Empiric Treatment[a]
Bites: Human 　　　Dog, cat	Oral anaerobes (*S. aureus*), *P. multocida* (*S. aureus*)	Penicillin (clindamycin) Penicillin (tetracycline or cephalosporin)
Burns	*P. aeruginosa*, other gram-neg. bacilli, *S. pyogenes* and other streptococci, *S. aureus*, *Candida*, *Aspergillus*	Aminoglycoside and penicillinase-resistant penicillin
Decubitus ulcer	Coliforms, *P. aeruginosa*, anaerobes including *B. fragilis* and clostridia, streptococci, *S. aureus* (usually polymicrobial)	Aminoglycoside and clindamycin, cefoxitin
Diabetic foot ulcer	Coliforms, *P. aeruginosa*, anaerobes, streptococci, *S. aureus* (usually polymicrobial)	Aminoglycoside and clindamycin, cefoxitin
Vascular gangrene	*S. aureus*, coliforms, anaerobes, streptococci	Aminoglycoside and clindamycin or cephalosporin
Sebaceous cysts	Anaerobic bacteria	
Pilonidal cysts	Anaerobic bacteria	
Dermatologic conditions with secondary infection: eczema, dermatophytes, acne, vesicular or bullous lesions	*S. pyogenes*, *S. aureus* (lesions in perineum, groin, and buttocks; colonic flora with coliforms and anaerobes)	Penicillinase-resistant penicillin or cephalosporin
Hidradenitis suppurativa	Anaerobes, coliforms, streptococci, *S. aureus*	
Intertrigo	*S. aureus*, coliforms, *Candida*	
Cutaneous surgical wound 　Clean surgery	*S. aureus*, *S. pyogenes*	Penicillinase-resistant penicillin or cephalosporin
Clean-contaminated or dirty 　　Colon	Anaerobes, coliforms, streptococci (usually polymicrobial)	Aminoglycoside and clindamycin
Pelvic	Anaerobes, coliforms, streptococci (usually polymicrobial)	Aminoglycoside and clindamycin
Biliary tract	Coliforms, clostridia, streptococci	Aminoglycoside and ampicillin
Gastroduodenal	Coliforms, streptococci	Cephalosporin
Trauma	*S. aureus*, *S. pyogenes*, clostridia	Penicillinase-resistant penicillin, cephalosporin
Intravenous infusion sites	*S. aureus*, coliforms, *P. aeruginosa*, *S. epidermidis*, *Candida*	Aminoglycoside and penicillinase-resistant penicillin or cephalosporin

[a]Guidelines provided for empiric choice with assumption that the clinical condition warrants systemic antibiotics and that there is no information from Gram stains or cultures to provide a more specific choice.

discussion is restricted to common and serious infections; the reader is referred to authoritative alternative sources for more extensive information.[11,13–15]

SUPERFICIAL SOFT-TISSUE INFECTIONS

IMPETIGO

Impetigo is a superficial infection of the skin, most common in children, which is usually caused by group A β-hemolytic streptococci. Epidemiologic studies indicate that the organism is acquired on normal skin approximately 10 days before the onset of detectable lesions. *S. aureus* is the primary pathogen in less than 10 percent of cases, although this organism is isolated commonly from lesions presumably reflecting secondary invasion. The infection is highly communicable, with spread being facilitated by crowding and poor hygiene. The initial lesions are small vesicles that pustulate and easily rupture. The purulent drainage dries to form a characteristic golden-yellow crust. Exposed areas are usually involved, and new lesions presumably reflect autoinoculation. The lesions are painless, remain superficial, heal without scarring, and are rarely accompanied by constitutional symptoms. The major concerns are

cosmetic considerations, communicability, secondary infection, and glomerulonephritis. Penicillin is regarded as the preferred antibiotic and is administered as a single intramuscular injection of benzathine penicillin (300,000 to 600,000 U for children or 1,200,000 U for adults) or orally (25,000 to 90,000 U/kg per day in four divided doses for 10 days). Erythromycin is the preferred alternative for penicillin-allergic patients and is administered in a 10-day oral regimen of 30 to 50 mg/kg per day for children or 250 to 500 mg four times daily for adults. There is no assurance that this treatment prevents pyoderma-associated nephritis. Bullous impetigo is a variant characterized by flaccid bullae that readily rupture. These lesions represent the cutaneous response to exfoliative toxin of *S. aureus* phage group II. The preferred drug for extensive disease is a penicillinase-resistant penicillin such as dicloxacillin (50 mg/kg per day in four divided doses for children) or erythromycin (30 to 50 mg/kg per day in four divided doses) for the penicillin-allergic patient.

ERYSIPELAS

Erysipelas is a superficial cellulitis of the skin with prominent lymphatic involvement, which is usually caused by group A streptococci, although occasional cases are produced by *S. aureus* or strep-

TABLE 9.4–3. DEEP AND SERIOUS SOFT-TISSUE INFECTIONS

	Clostridial Cellulitis	Synergistic Necrotizing Cellulitis	Gas Gangrene	Streptococcal Myonecrosis	Necrotizing Fasciitis	Infected Vascular Gangrene	Streptococcal Gangrene
Predisposing conditions	Trauma Surgical wound	Diabetes, prior local lesions, perirectal lesion	Trauma surgery	Trauma surgery	Diabetes, trauma surgery, perineal infection	Arterial insufficiency	Trauma, surgery
Incubation period	3 days	3–14 days	1–2 days	3–4 days	1–4 days	5 days	6 hr–2 days
Etiologic organism(s)	Clostridia	Mixed aerobic-anaerobic flora	Clostridia, esp. *C. perfringens*	Anaerobic streptococci	Mixed aerobic-anaerobic flora, esp. coliforms, *Bacteroides* and streptococci	Mixed aerobic-anaerobic flora	*S. pyogenes*
Systemic toxicity	Minimal	Moderate to severe	Severe	Minimal until late in course	Moderate to severe	Minimal	Severe
Course	Gradual	Acute	Acute	Subacute	Acute or subacute	Gradual	Acute
Wound findings							
Local pain	Minimal	Moderate to severe	Severe	Late only	Minimal to moderate	Minimal to moderate	Severe
Skin appearance	Swollen, minimal discoloration	Erythematous or gangrenous	Tense and blanched, yellow-bronze, necrosis with hemorrhagic bullae	Erythema or yellow bronze	Blanched, erythema necrosis with hemorrhagic bullae	Erythema or necrosis	Erythema, necrosis
Gas	Abundant	Variable	Usually present	Variable	Variable	Variable	No
Muscle involvement	No	Variable	Myonecrosis	Myonecrosis	No	Myonecrosis—limited to area of vascular insufficiency	No
Discharge							
Appearance	Thin dark	Dark pus or "dishwater"	Serosanguinous	Seropurulent	Seropurulent or dishwater	None	None or serosanguinous
Odor	Sweetish or foul	Putrid	Sweet or foul	Often putrid	Putrid	Putrid	No odor
Gram stain	PMNs and gram-pos. bacilli	PMNs, mixed flora	Sparse PMNs; gram-pos. bacilli	PMNs, gram-pos cocci	PMNs, mixed flora	PMNs, mixed flora	PMNs, gram-pos. cocci in chains
Surgical therapy	Debridement	Wide filleting incisions	Extensive excision, amputation	Excision of necrotic muscle	Wide filleting incisions	Amputation	Debridement on necrotic tissue

tococci, groups B (newborn infants), C, or G. About one third of patients have a preceding streptococcal respiratory tract infection. Other patients at increased risk are those with nephrosis, preexisting lymphatic obstruction, or edema. The lesion is bright red and indurated, and has an elevated border that is sharply demarcated from the adjacent uninvolved skin. The most common location is the butterfly area over the face, with involvement of the nose and cheeks. Fever and leukocytosis are common. The lesion usually remains confined to the dermis and lymphatics, although occasional patients develop cellulitis or bacteremia. The etiologic organism cannot be recovered from the skin surface and rarely can be isolated from the tissue with aspiration of the advanced edge. Penicillin is the preferred drug in doses ranging from intramuscular procaine penicillin (600,000 U every 8 to 12 hours) to aqueous penicillin G (3 million U intravenously every 4 hours). Patients who are allergic to penicillin should receive erythromycin orally in a dose of 500 mg four times daily for adults or, for more seriously ill patients, clindamycin in a dose of 600 mg intravenously every 8 hours. The preferred agent for patients with serious infections where both streptococci and *S. aureus* are possible etiologic agents is a penicillinase-resistant penicillin such as nafcillin in a dose of 1 to 2 g given intravenously every 4 to 6 hours. The preferred alternative agents for penicillin-allergic patients in this setting are intravenous vancomycin (1 to 2 g per day) or clindamycin (1.8 g per day).

LYMPHANGITIS

Lymphangitis implies inflammation of subcutaneous lymphatic channels and may be acute or chronic. With acute lymphangitis there are erythematous streaks that extend from an initial site of infection toward regional lymph nodes that are enlarged and tender. The course is typically rapid and, in fact, there may be systemic signs of infection before local signs other than pain are readily apparent. Cultures at the portal of entry or blood cultures will often yield the implicated organism. Cultures obtained by needle aspiration of the lymphangitic streak are generally negative. The most common pathogen is a group A *Streptococcus*, although occasional cases involve *S. aureus*. Patients may be treated with penicillin in regimens ranging from intramuscular procaine penicillin G (600,000 U once or twice daily) to aqueous penicillin G intravenously (500,000 to 2 million U every 4 to 6 hours). The preferred agent for seriously ill patients in the setting where *S. aureus* is an established or suspected pathogen is a penicillinase-resistant penicillin such as intravenous nafcillin (1 to 2 g every 4 to 6 hours), intravenous cephalothin (1 to 2 g every 4 to 6 hours), or intravenous clindamycin (600 mg every 8 hours). Other causes of acute lymphangitis include rat bite fever (*Spirillum minus*) or filariasis due to *Wuchereria bancrofti* or *Brugia malayi*. These should be considered in patients with a history of a rat bite or a geographic history with recent travel to Africa, Southeast Asia, or South America.

Chronic lymphangitis may be caused by *Sporothrix schenckii*, *Mycobacterium marinum*, *M. kansasii*, *W. bancrofti*, *B. malayi*, or *Nocardia brasiliensis*. The most common form in the United States is sporotrichosis, which is characterized by subcutaneous nodules occurring along the lymphatic channels. The responsible fungus, *S. schenckii*, is typically introduced at the site of trauma from a barberry bush or rose bush in a gardener. "Swimming pool granuloma" is caused by *M. marinum*, which often resides in swimming pools or fish tanks. This infection is usually a solitary nodular or ulcerative lesion at the site of prior injury, which serves as the portal of entry. However, patients occasionally have multiple nodules extending along lymphatics, as seen with sporotrichosis.

CELLULITIS

Cellulitis is an acute spreading infection involving the dermis and subcutaneous tissue. Common predisposing conditions include local trauma or an underlying skin infection such as a furuncle or a skin ulceration that becomes secondarily invaded. In some instances there is no apparent portal of entry, a finding that is most common in the lower extremity of patients with vascular insufficiency. The usual findings are local tenderness, pain, edema, warmth, or erythema. In contrast to erysipelas, the advanced edge is not sharply demarcated. There may be subcutaneous abscess formation, and the skin overlying the lesion may undergo necrosis with secondary ulceration. Systemic findings are variable, but patients with more serious infections may have fever, chills, leukocytosis, and bacteremia. Multiple organisms have been implicated, the most frequent being streptococci, and *S. aureau;* less common are *Haemophilus influenzae* (especially in children), *Streptococcus pneumoniae* and anaerobic bacteria.[15] Detection of the etiologic agent often proves difficult. Lesions associated with preceeding trauma, surgical incision, or skin ulceration often show a purulent discharge, but cultures of the exudate are subject to contamination by multiple bacteria from the skin flora and environmental sources. Aspiration of the leading edge of inflammation is often recommended, but these cultures are usually sterile. Full-thickness punch biopsies are more likely to yield positive cultures.[9] One well-known form of cellulitis that is particularly important to recognize is postoperative streptococcal cellulitis, a rampant infection that usually occurs 6 to 48 hours after surgery. This is earlier than most postoperative wound infections other than clostridial myonecrosis. It is characterized by a wound that becomes bright red, edematous, and painful, with a rapidly advancing discrete margin. Serous discharge expressed from the wound edge will show typical organisms on Gram stain, and cultures will yield group A β-hemolytic streptococci. Treatment consists of aqueous penicillin G in doses of 3 to 5 million units given intravenously every 4 hours.

ABSCESSES

Subcutaneous abscesses are most common in patients with folliculitis, cellulitis, or trauma. *S. aureus* is implicated in 25 to 50 percent of cases, is the major organism implicated in abscesses of the upper torso, and, when recovered, is usually present in pure culture. Contrary to popular teaching, most abscesses of the lower torso involve a polymicrobial flora with anaerobic bacteria, presumably of colonic origin, as the predominant pathogens.[12] This especially applies to abscesses in the perineal, inguinal, and buttock region. The usual finding is pain and swelling at the infected site. Additional associated findings often include induration, cellulitis, and regional adenopathy. Fluctuance may be difficult to detect, particularly with deep abscesses. When this diagnosis is considered, but not readily apparent, there should be a needle aspiration through sterilized skin. The actual size of the purulent collection is also often difficult to estimate on the basis of surface examination and, in most instances, is greatly underestimated. The preferred treatment is incision and drainage. Antibiotics are generally unnecessary with uncomplicated cases, except for patients who are clinically septic, patients who have abscesses in critical areas such as the central triangle of the face (which is drained by the emissary veins to the cavernous sinus), patients with severe compromise in host defense mechanisms, and infections associated with extensive cellulitis, lymphangitis, or regional adenopathy. The preferred agents for abscesses involving *S. aureus* are a penicillinase-resistant penicillin, a cephalosporin, erythromycin, or clindamycin. When anaerobes are involved, the preferred drugs are clindamycin or a penicillin.

HAIR FOLLICLE INFECTIONS

Folliculitis, furunculosis, and carbuncle are infections involving hair follicles that occur most frequently in areas subject to friction and perspiration, such as the neck, face, axillae, and buttocks. Folliculitis is restricted to hair follicles and appears as erythematous papules with or without a central pustule. Furunculosis refers to more extensive involvement of several hair follicles in a restricted area. The initial lesions are firm, painful, tender, red nodules that subsequently become fluctuant and may drain spontaneously. A carbuncle is a confluent infection in which there is penetration to the subcutaneous space with extensive undermining and deep abscess formation. The typical presentation is a painful, erythematous tender mass, with multiple draining sinuses in areas of thick inelastic tissue such as the posterior neck, back, or thighs. Factors that predispose to the incidence or severity of these infections include obesity, defects in neutrophil function, blood dyscrasias, poor hygiene, seborrhea, corticosteroid therapy, occlusive dressings, trauma such as hair plucking, and diabetes mellitus. Some patients with no clear predisposing conditions have repeated episodes of furunculosis over periods of years. *S. aureus* is responsible for most cases of folliculitis, furunculosis, and carbuncles. *Pseudomonas aeruginosa* has been implicated in folliculitis acquired from swimming pools or whirlpools. *Candida* occasionally causes folliculitis, but the lesions characteristically show typical satellite lesions and involve the intertriginous areas. Other organisms may be involved in the compromised host. *S. epidermidis* and diphtheroids are frequently present in sebum and often recovered in cultures, but seldom cause folliculitis. Treatment should include warm compresses and good hygiene with frequent use of antiseptic soaps. Patients with recurrent furuncles should wash frequently with soap to reduce *S. aureus* on the body surface; sheets and underclothing should be laundered at high temperatures and changed frequently, and draining lesions should be covered to prevent autoinoculation. The usual reservoir is the nose, but attempts to reduce nasal colonization are usually unsuccessful. Systemic antibiotics directed at *S. aureus* are advocated only for serious infections, including all patients with carbuncles, those with furuncles and extensive cellulitis or fever, or furuncles located in the mid-face region. Preferred agents for oral therapy are dicloxacillin (1 to 2 g per day), cephalexin (1 to 2 g per day), erythromycin (1 to 2 g per day), or clindamycin (1.2 g per day). More serious infections requiring parenteral therapy should be treated with a penicillinase-resistant penicillin such as nafcillin (4 to 8 g per day), cephalothin (4 to 8 g per day), vancomycin (1 to 2 g per day), or clindamycin (1.8 g per day). Incision and drainage is required for lesions characterized by fluctuant masses or confluent necrotic lesions.

INFECTIONS SECONDARY TO PREEXISTING LESIONS

ACNE

Acne vulgaris is a disease of sebaceous follicles characterized by comedones, papules, pustules, nodules, and cysts. The basic lesion is plugging of sebaceous follicles, particularly in persons who produce large amounts of sebum. Acne is not regarded as an infection per se, but *Propionibacterium acnes,* the dominant organism in the follicular flora, appears to play an important contributing role be-

cause of the production of a lipase, which breaks down fats in sebum to produce the free fatty acids implicated in evoking an inflammatory response. Long-term use of tetracycline (250 mg to 1 g orally per day) to reduce the fatty acid production by *P. acnes* is commonly advocated for severe cases. (Acne vulgaris is discussed in greater detail in Chapter 17.7.)

ECTHYMA

Ecthyma is similar to impetigo except that there is penetration through the epidermis resulting in a punched-out ulcer containing greenish-yellow crusts surrounded by a raised violaceous margin. The legs of children are the most frequently affected sites. These infections may occur de novo or they may represent bacterial invasion secondary to insect bites, minor trauma, eczema, pediculosis, and so on. The most frequent pathogen is group A β-hemolytic streptococcus. The lesions may resemble those produced by *P. aeruginosa* bacteremia in patients with severely compromised host defenses and bacteremia, but here the infection is limited to the soft tissue. Therapy should consist of removal of crust, warm compresses, and, with extensive lesions, systemic antibiotics such as penicillin or erythromycin using the same regimens advocated for impetigo.

BITES

Infected bites are similar to other soft-tissue infections associated with trauma except that the infecting pathogens commonly reflect the oral flora of the "donor" species. Another possibility is secondary invasion by the host's own cutaneous flora, the most frequent pathogen in this case being *S. aureus*. Infected human bites may occur as a result of a bite per se or a knuckle injury after a blow to the teeth ("clenched fist injury"). The major pathogens in these infections are oral anaerobic bacteria, such as anaerobic streptococci, *Bacteroides melaninogenicus*, fusobacteria, and spirochetes.[7] These lesions are often gangrenous, they may cause extensive tissue destruction, and most develop a putrid discharge. Oral antibiotics generally recommended for prophylaxis in outpatients with significant human bite injuries are penicillin G, penicillin V, ampicillin (250 to 500 mg, four times daily for 3 to 7 days), or ampicillin combined with clavulanic acid. More important, the wound should be thoroughly cleansed and debrided, and primary closure is avoided except for mutilating wounds, especially those involving the face. Patients with established infections often require debridement combined with parenteral administration of penicillin G (1 to 2 million U given intravenously every 4 to 6 hours) or clindamycin (600 mg intravenously every 8 hours).

Pasteurella multocida is a common pathogen in soft-tissue infections following animal bites. This is a small, gram-negative coccobacillus that is found in the upper respiratory tract of most cats, dogs, and many rodents. The usual lesion is erythematous and edematous, with a central ulceration and a seropurulent discharge. There may be rapidly spreading cellulitis, lymphangitis, lymphadenopathy, abscess formation, or osteomyelitis. Most patients with uncomplicated infections are afebrile, but they often have leukocytosis. This infection may be prevented with prophylactic penicillin (penicillin G, penicillin V, or ampicillin in oral doses of 250 to 500 mg four times daily for 5 to 7 days), or, for the penicillin-allergic patient, tetracycline in doses of 250 to 500 mg orally four times daily. Wound cleansing, debridement, avoidance of primary closure when feasible, rabies prophylaxis, and tetanus prophylaxis are additional important facets of management. Infections involving *Pasteurella multocida* may be treated with the same regimens advocated for prophylaxis if patients are not seriously ill. Patients with established infections requiring hospitalization should be treated with penicillin G in a dose of 400,000 to 2 million units every 4 hours or cephalothin in a dose of 1 to 2 g every 4 hours for 10 to 14 days.

Other considerations in the differential diagnosis of infections associated with animal bites are cat scratch disease and rat bite fever. *Cat scratch disease*, as the name implies, is most commonly associated with a cat scratch but may also be associated with a cat bite or simply a history of exposure to cats. The initial lesion is an erythematous papule followed 10 to 14 days later by tender regional adenopathy, which generally regresses within 6 weeks. The agent of this disease appears to be a fastidious gram-negative bacillus, but no antibiotic agent has established merit. *Rat bite fever* is an acute febrile illness caused by *Streptobacillus moniliformis* or *Spirillum minor* injected by the bite of a rat, mouse, or other rodent. *Streptobacillus moniliformis* is a pleomorphic gram-negative bacillus that may be recovered from blood, abscesses, or joint fluid. This causes a systemic illness with a relapsing fever pattern, an acute febrile systemic illness, and a generalized morbilliform or petechial rash after an incubation period of less than 10 days after rodent exposure. *S. minor* is a spirochete that may be detected by dark field examination of the infected site and, rarely, in peripheral blood smears. This agent also causes an acute relapsing febrile illness with a generalized rash, but the incubation period is 7 days to 3 weeks following exposure, and the bite site usually shows suppuration, ulceration, lymphangitis, and local adenopathy. Both organisms responsible for rat bite fever are susceptible to penicillin, which is regarded as the drug of choice.

INFECTED ULCERS

Secondary infections of decubitus ulcers, diabetic foot ulcers, and ischemic ulcers represent invasion of sites rendered susceptible by a decrease in local defense mechanisms including the loss of the formidable barrier of the intact skin. Cultures of purulent drainage, serous fluid expressed from the lesion edge, or biopsies of the ulcer bed usually yield a polymicrobial flora containing both aerobic and anaerobic bacteria. The most prevalent aerobic gram-negative bacillus is *Proteus*, and the most frequent anaerobic isolates are peptostreptococci, but almost any organism from the cutaneous or colonic flora may be found, including *S. aureus*. These same microbes may be recovered from cutaneous ulcers in patients with no overt evidence for infection. There is often direct extension to underlying bone with osteomyelitis. Both radiographs and scans (bone scan, indium-labeled white cell scan, and gallium scan), however, are often difficult to interpret. The main problem with the scans is that uptake in the adjacent soft-tissue infection renders these procedures sensitive but nonspecific. In many instances there is no way to resolve this diagnostic dilemma short of a bone biopsy. The most important facet of treatment for uncomplicated infections is good local care with debridement, avoidance of pressure, frequent cleansing, and avoidance of occlusive dressings that promote maceration of tissue. The need for vascular surgery should be carefully assessed by evaluating signs of ischemia, pulses, and Doppler measurements. The application of antiseptics or local antibiotics has no established benefit. Systemic antibiotics are reserved for cases in which there is extensive cellulitis, lymphangitis, tender adenopathy, extensive involvement of underlying soft tissue, osteomyelitis, signs of systemic infection, or bacteremia. The most frequent isolates in blood cultures are anaerobic bacteria, gram-negative bacilli, or *S. aureus*. Antibiotic recommendations for seriously ill patients are similar to those advocated for intra-abdominal sepsis because of similarities in the spectrum of bacteria involved. In septic patients an appropriate regimen before the availability of culture results is an aminoglycoside (gentamicin or tobramycin, 1.7 mg/kg every 8 hours) combined with clindamycin (600 mg every 8 hours) cefoxitin (2 g every 6 hours), or a single broad-spectrum agent such as cefoxitin (2 g every 6 hours), cefotetan (2 g every 8 to 12 hours), or imipenem (0.5 to 1 g every 6 hours).

BURNS

Sepsis is the major cause of mortality in patients with thermal injuries. Cutaneous burn-wound infection may be superficial, or it

may be severe, with "burn-wound sepsis," reflecting extensive invasion of viable tissue adjacent to the wound.[3] When accompanied by signs of sepsis, the mortality rate approaches 90 percent. The obvious cause is loss of intact skin as a microbiologic barrier. In full-thickness burns there is vascular occlusion that persists for 2 to 3 weeks before circulation is restored. The result is coagulation necrosis with large accumulations of nonviable tissue, the burn eschar, which provides an excellent culture medium. Susceptibility is enhanced by defects in polymorphonuclear chemotaxis and bactericidal activity. Organisms that colonize the surface are destroyed with the original injury, but the wound becomes colonized within 48 hours. Burn-wound isolates represent the patient's endogenous flora and the hospital flora. Major pathogens during the first 2 days are gram-positive bacteria, especially group A streptococci and, less commonly, *S. aureus.* By the third day, gram-negative bacteria appear. The major pathogens in late infections are *P. aeruginosa, Providencia stuartii, Enterobacter cloacae, Serratia marcescens,* and *Klebsiella* sp. These organisms proliferate in the eschar and are likely to invade the underlying subcutaneous tissue before the separation of the eschar with autografting by granulation tissue. Less common pathogens include fungi (*Candida, Aspergillus, Mucor,* and *Geotrichum*) and H. simplex. Management principles to prevent sepsis include early debridement of nonviable tissue, debridement of the eschar as it spontaneously separates, skin grafts for full thickness burns at 3 to 5 weeks, and topical antimicrobial agents such as mafenide acetate (sulfamylon) cream, silver nitrate (0.5%), or silver sulfadiazene (Silvadene).

Clinical signs of burn-wound sepsis appear late and there may be minimal findings in the wound. The most common presentation is systemic signs of sepsis with an altered mental status, tachycardia, tachypnea, fever or hypothermia, thrombocytopenia, leukocytosis or leukopenia, and hypotension. The major culture sources are blood cultures and biopsies of the burn wound, which are preferably done at regular 48-hour intervals using quantitative techniques. Empirical antibiotic regimens advocated should have a broad spectrum with activity against gram-negative bacilli and *S. aureus.* This often includes an aminoglycoside and a cephalosporin, or a penicillinase-resistant penicillin.

INFECTIONS RELATED TO INTRAVENOUS INFUSIONS

There are four types of infections associated with intravenous therapy:

1. The most common is cellulitis as indicated by induration, tenderness, and erythema, with or without a palpable cord, at the needle insertion site. These findings may also indicate mechanical or chemical irritation as well as infection.
2. Purulent thrombophlebitis with similar local findings, but there is suppuration within the vessel lumen or wall. Purulent exudate may be expressed, the patient may have persistent or refractory bacteremia, and surgical excision of the vein is often required.
3. Occult intravenous infusion site infections are characterized by positive blood cultures without local evidence of infection. This diagnosis is supported by recovering the same organism from the blood and intravenous cannula and the failure to detect an alternative portal of entry.
    The patient's skin flora is responsible for most of these three forms, and the dominant pathogens are gram-negative bacilli, *S. aureus,* and *S. epidermidis. Candida* sepsis is particularly common with intravenous hyperalimentation, and *S. epidermidis* is the most frequent pathogen with plastic lines such as Hickman catheters.
4. Another mechanism of infection is a contaminated infusate from the intravenous bottle, tubing, or various devices connected to the tubing. These infections may occur in

epidemics, and the usual pathogens are water-borne bacteria such as *Pseudomonas cepacia, Citrobacter freundii,* Enterobacter agglomerans, *Klebsiella,* and *Serratia.*

Factors that are associated with an increased risk for infection at intravenous infusion sites include prolonged duration of use, placement by cutdown rather than percutaneous puncture, and use of plastic catheters instead of needles. The latter is particularly important with lines that are left for extended periods. The current recommendation is that peripheral lines with plastic catheters or metal needles should be changed at 72-hour intervals. Arterial lines should be changed at 96 hours. Lines placed by tunneling through subcutaneous tissue do not require routine changes, but the entry site should receive meticulous wound care.

When line sepsis is suspected there should be cultures of blood using another peripheral vein, and any exudate that may be expressed from the needle puncture site should be Gram stained and cultured. Under ideal circumstances catheters with suspected or established line sepsis should be removed. The etiologic agent can usually be detected by direct Gram stain of the catheter for examination under oil immersion microscopy and by rolling a 5-cm segment onto culture media for quantitative culture.[2] The infusate also should be cultured if this is thought to be contaminated. Empirical antibiotic therapy for patients with suspected septicemia should include a regimen with activity versus staphylococci and gram-negative bacilli, such as an aminoglycoside combined with a cephalosporin, a penicillinase-resistant penicillin, or vancomycin. Any needle or line that can easily be replaced should be. Infections associated with lines placed by tunneling procedures are often considered critical; these may sometimes be treated without line removal, unless signs of sepsis or positive blood cultures persist with or recur after a course of antibiotics.

DEEP OR SERIOUS INFECTIONS OF SUBCUTANEOUS TISSUE, FASCIA, AND MUSCLE

These infections are generally classified according to etiologic agent, tissue plane involved, or selected characteristics in the clinical presentation (Table 9.4–3). This often gives the erroneous impression that these are distinct, easily differentiated entities, but in many instances there is significant overlap, and classification into precise categories may prove difficult or impossible. The most important factor in management concerns decisions regarding systemic antibiotics, diagnostic studies to differentiate certain syndromes as a guide to treatment and prognosis, and recognition of the critical role of surgery in treating many of these infections.

The classification scheme provided in Table 9.4–3 is the classic definition, but a much more practical approach (Table 9.4–4) recognizes two anatomic patterns with three groups of bacterial pathogens.

The anatomic patterns include infections involving the enveloping fascia that surrounds muscle groups, or "fasciitis." The sec-

TABLE 9.4–4. ANATOMIC PATTERNS OF BACTERIAL PATHOGENS

	Anatomic Pattern	
Bacteria	**Fasciitis**	**Compartment Infection**
Clostridia	Crepitant cellulitis	Gas gangrene
Streptococci	Streptococcal gangrene	Streptococcal myonecrosis
Mixed aerobic and anaerobic bacteria	Necrotizing fasciitis	Necrotizing synergistic cellulitis

ond is a deeper infection that involves the contents of the enveloping fascia and is referred to as "compartment infection" or "myositis." Fasciitis tends to extend along the fascia, sometimes with alarming rapidity despite seemingly appropriate antibiotic therapy. These lesions require surgical incision in the form of a fillet or removal of the fascia. When the compartment is involved there is inflammation within a closed space resulting in necrosis of the compartment contents. In this case, the necessary surgical procedure is debridement with excision of necrotic mucle or amputation. The most important role of the physician is to rapidly recognize these infections and proceed with early surgical intervention. Surgery is more easily accomplished with extremity involvement; it is often more mutilating and difficult when the abdominal wall or perirectal area is involved. With regard to diagnosis, the cardinal clinical features that should herald concern for the possibility of these infections are the following:

1. Severe pain that is spontaneous. The main differential is usually cellulitis that can be treated with antibiotics alone, but patients with cellulitis are more likely to show lesions that are tender and do not cause severe pain without manipulation. (Pain may be a deceptive feature by its absence in any soft-tissue infection in patients with neuropathies, especially diabetic patients.)
2. Bullous lesions may result from cutaneous necrosis after occlusion of deep vessels traversing the fascia or a compartment. Similar lesions also may be found with erysipelas, some forms of cellulitis (*P. aeruginosa, S. aureus*, streptococci), ischemic necrosis due to disseminated infection (meningococcemia, purpura fulminans, ecthyma gangrenosum, toxic shock syndrome, disseminated intravascular coagulation), toxins (brown recluse spider bites) or primary dermatologic diseases (bullous pemphigus).
3. Gas in the soft tissue may be detected by palpation, by radiograph, or by scans and often represents the production of volatile fatty acids by anaerobic bacteria. Again, the finding may be deceptive because of air introduced with irrigations.
4. Patients with systemic toxicity or deep soft-tissue infections are usually seriously ill, as indicated by high fever, high leukocyte counts, and delirium.
5. Deep infections, especially those involving the fascia, tend to spread rapidly, as indicated by sequential observation of marked borders.

Suspected deep infections require expeditious evaluation with early surgical intervention. Recommended diagnostic studies include radiographs, scans, needle aspiration, biopsy for frozen section, and exploration. Radiographs often show soft-tissue swelling that is nonspecific, or gas that is more worrisome. Computed tomography (CT) usually provides a fine anatomic description of the tissue plane involved and is highly recommended in suspect cases. Needle aspiration either blindly or under CT or ultrasound guidance will often yield important information, especially when the putrid, thin, gray "dishwater pus" characteristic of necrotizing cellulitis is found. This also may provide important specimens for bacteriologic studies when performed through intact skin. The problem is that there is little assurance that the proper anatomic site is sampled, so a negative aspirate is of limited value. An alternative is a full-thickness biopsy for frozen section that will provide a histologic description, defining the tissue plane involved. Despite all these recommendations, the most definitive diagnostic test is surgical exploration for direct visualization with the benefits of an anesthetized patient and use of optimal lighting in the operating room.

CLOSTRIDIAL INFECTIONS

Clostridia are relatively common isolates in various soft-tissue infections when proper cultures are performed, and they are particularly common in wound infections after intestinal surgery, traumatic injury, or ulcers located on the lower torso. These often represent simple contamination or colonization in which no pathogenic role can be readily discerned. Indeed, clostridia are recovered in 10 to 30 percent of all wounds among victims of serious civilian or battlefield injuries. The most prevalent species recovered is *Clostridium perfringens*, but a wide variety of other species may be found, including many that cannot be readily classified by most microbiology laboratories. The usual source is thought to be the colonic flora of the host, although another possible source is clostridial spores, which are almost universally present in soil samples. The important point to emphasize is that a diagnosis of clostridial infection must be based on clinical observations rather than on a bacteriology report.

Clostridial cellulitis is a soft-tissue infection involving *C. perfringens* or other clostridial species, often in association with additional aerobic and anaerobic bacteria. There may be extensive gas formation, with crepitation, leading to the frequent appellation "crepitant cellulitis." The major differential diagnosis is gas gangrene, although there are multiple other conditions that may be associated with gas in tissue. Unlike gas gangrene, clostridial crepitant cellulitis has a longer incubation period; a gradual evolution of symptoms; mild pain at the site of the infection; no skin discolorations, bullae, or necrotic surface lesions; and minimal systemic toxicity. Most important, there is no muscle involvement. If this is not found, only debridement of necrotic tissue is required, with drainage accompanied by penicillin given intravenously in doses of 6 to 20 million units daily. Mixed infections involving clostridia should be treated in an analogous fashion, using antibiotics based on results of Gram stains of exudate and cultures.

FASCIITIS

Necrotizing fasciitis refers to a deep infection that spreads within the fascial cleft between the subcutaneous tissue and the deep fascia with extensive undermining, sometimes complicated by skin gangrene as a result of vascular thrombosis. There is usually a break in the skin that provides a portal of entry such as a drug injection site, a decubitus ulcer, a diabetic foot ulcer, an enterostomy, an incised wound, or a perirectal abscess. More than half of cases occur in patients with diabetes. Earlier studies suggested streptococci and the term "streptococcal gangrene" was often applied. More recent studies indicate that most cases involve combinations of aerobic and anaerobic bacteria, the dominant isolates being coliforms, *Bacteroides* sp., peptostreptococci, and facultative streptococci. Gas in the soft tissue is common. The diagnosis may be established by passing a probe through the area of necrosis to demonstrate the extension along the fascial cleft. Other useful tests include a frozen section biopsy to demonstrate histologic changes and computed tomography to show the anatomic site of involvement. The most important therapeutic modality is surgery with a fillet combined with debridement of necrotic tissue. Antibiotics are directed against the infecting flora, generally requiring agents with activity against both coliforms and anaerobic bacteria. Penicillin is regarded as the preferred drug for cases in which streptococci or clostridia are predominant in Gram stains or cultures and should be given intravenously in doses of 3 to 4 million units every 4 hours. Infections involving a polymicrobial flora should be treated for both aerobic and anaerobic bacteria. Appropriate empirical regimens include an aminoglycoside (gentamicin or tobramycin, 1.7 mg/kg intravenously every 8 hours) combined with clindamycin (600 mg every 8 hours) or cefoxitin (2 g every 6 hours).

COMPARTMENT INFECTIONS

Clostridial Myonecrosis

Clostridial myonecrosis (gas gangrene) is a devastating infection characterized by myonecrosis and profound systemic toxicity. Most cases occur as complications of wounding from trauma or

surgery. The usual clinical settings are (1) traumatic injury or penetrating wounds, (2) surgery, especially intestinal or biliary tract operations, (3) uterine gas gangrene, which most frequently follows septic abortion, (4) soft tissue lesions associated with vascular insufficiency, (5) intestinal gas gangrene, which is usually found in compromised hosts, especially patients with leukemia, and (6) spontaneous gas gangrene, a rare form in which there is no readily identified predisposing condition. Critical interrelated factors in pathogenesis of the infection in most cases are wounding as a result of trauma or surgery, contamination with histotoxic clostridia and toxin elaboration promoted by a decreased oxidation-reduction potential at the site of injury. It is estimated that 30 to 80 percent of serious traumatic open wounds are contaminated with *C. perfringens* spores, although gas gangrene remains a relatively rare infection. These data emphasize the decisive role of local conditions that permit tissue hypoxia, such as vascular insufficiency, the presence of foreign bodies, necrosis, and concurrent infections involving other microbes. The usual incubation period from the time of wounding to the onset of symptoms is 2 to 4 days, with a range of 8 hours to several weeks. The first symptom is sudden and severe pain at the site of injury. At this time, observation of the wound typically shows tense edema and tenderness. Gas may be noted in the soft tissue according to palpation or radiographs, although this is not regularly found nor is it specific for the diagnosis. The skin is initially pale and then progresses to a magenta or bronze discoloration, often with cutaneous necrosis and hemorrhagic bullae. As the lesion evolves, there is a thin, serosanguinous discharge that often has a chrraracteristically sweet odor. The initial systemic findings include diaphoresis, low-grade fever, and tachycardia disproportionate to the temperature elevation. The tempo of the disease shows considerable variation, but in most instances there is rapid progression, with hemolytic anemia, hypotension, and renal failure. The patient typically remains alert despite profound systemic toxicity. The most frequent pathogen is *C. perfringens,* which is found in approximately 80 percent of cases with positive cultures. Other clostridial species implicated include *C. novyi, C. septicum, C. histolyticum, C. bifermentans,* and *C. fallax.* These species of clostridia produce over 20 exotoxins, including seven that are lethal to experimental animals. Perhaps the most important toxin of *C. perfringens* is the alpha toxin, which is a phospholipase that destroys cell membranes, alters capillary permeability, and causes severe hemolysis. *C. perfringens* is found in nearly all soil samples and is usually present as a component of the normal stool microflora of man. Thus, the agents of gas gangrene are ubiquitous, exposure is universal, and there is no necessity to isolate patients. The incidence of gas gangrene depends more on methods of wound management than exposure to the putative agent.

The diagnosis of gas gangrene is based on the constellation of clinical observations with supporting microbiologic studies. Gram stain of wound exudate or aspirates of bulla typically show large, gram-positive bacilli with blunt ends and a paucity of polymorphonuclear leukocytes. Approximately 15 percent of patients have clostridial bacteremia. It must be emphasized, however, that most patients with positive cultures, including blood cultures, for clostridia do not have gas gangrene. The definitive diagnostic procedure is surgical incision to expose muscle, which appears pale and edematous, beefy red, or, in advanced stages, black and friable.

Nonclostridial Myonecrosis
Nonclostridial myonecrosis includes diverse conditions classified by clinical setting and bacteriology as streptococcal gangrene, anaerobic streptococcal myonecrosis, synergistic necrotizing cellulitis, and infected vascular gangrene.

Myonecrosis involving streptococci resembles gas gangrene except that the tempo of the disease is less fulminant, local pain is not prominent in the early stages, soft-tissue gas is uncommon, and Gram stains of exudate show gram-positive cocci in chains as well as in polymorphonuclear cells. Treatment includes intravenous penicillin (3 to 4 million U intravenously every 4 hours) or clindamycin (600 to 900 mg intravenously every 6 to 8 hours) and surgical debridement.

The most common compartment infection involves a combination of aerobic and anaerobic bacteria and is often referred to by the somewhat deceptive term of "synergistic necrotizing cellulitis."[14] This is similar to necrotizing fasciitis, involving a mixed flora, except that the infection has extended beneath the fascia to involve the compartment. Most patients are diabetic, and they are often obese and have renal failure as well. The usual anatomic sites are the perirectal area or lower extremities. Common clinical features include bullous lesions, spontaneous pain, and gas. The diagnosis is based on characteristic clinical features, computed tomography showing myonecrosis with or without fasciitis, aspirates of the lesion, or surgical exploration. Aspirates show a characteristic "dishwater pus," a thin, grayish fluid with an extremely offensive putrid odor. Gram stains and culture of the exudate show a polymicrobial flora composed of coliforms, streptococci, and anaerobes. Blood cultures are positive in about 20 to 30 percent of cases, usually yielding coliforms such as *Escherichia coli* or anaerobes such as *Bacteroides* sp.[14] The mortality rate is 25 to 50 percent, and is highest in patients with perirectal lesions. This condition dramatically emphasizes the need for an expeditious diagnosis with rapid surgical intervention. Necrotic tissue must be debrided and many cases require reoperation almost daily to achieve adequate debridement. Antibiotic options include the intravenous regimens commonly used for intra-abdominal sepsis including an aminoglycoside, gentamicin, or tobramycin (1.7 mg/kg every 8 hours), combined with clindamycin (600 mg every 8 hours), metronidazole (500 mg every 6 hours), or cefoxitin (2 g every 6 hours). The muscle is nonviable, it fails to contract with stimulation, and the cut surface does not bleed. The most important therapeutic maneuver is extensive surgical debridement, with excision of involved muscles, amputation when an extremity is involved, or hysterectomy with uterine gas gangrene. The preferred antibiotics are aqueous penicillin G (10 to 20 million U daily for adults) or chloramphenicol (1 g intravenously every 6 hours). The therapeutic value of hyperbaric oxygen is debated, although there may be major problems in transferring critically ill patients to centers with this type of facility. Important supportive measures include fluid and electrolyte replacement, control of acidosis, transfusions for severe anemia, and appropriate management of renal failure. The overall mortality of gas gangrene in 116 reports summarizing over 1200 cases is 25 percent.

Pyomyositis
Pyomyositis is a primary bacterial infection of skeletal muscle that is usually due to *S. aureus.*[6] This is a rare infection in industrialized nations but is relatively common in the tropics, where it is referred to as "tropical pyomyositis." Blood cultures are usually negative, and muscle involvement is rarely noted in patients with disseminated staphylococcal infections. The usual presentation is an insidious onset of pain, swelling, and tenderness, usually involving a single muscle group of a lower extremity or trunk. Computed tomography will demonstrate the lesion, and needle aspirates yield purulent exudates that usually show *S. aureus* on Gram strain and culture. The treatment consists of incision and drainage combined with an antibiotic directed against *S. aureus* such as intravenous nafcillin (1 to 2 g every 4 to 6 hours) or cephalothin (2 to 4 g every 4 to 6 hours). Excision of the involved muscle is not necessary.

TETANUS

Tetanus is a neuroparalytic syndrome caused by the neurotoxin, tetanospasmin, produced by *C. tetani.* This disease requires a source of the organism, local tissue conditions that promote toxin production, and immunologic naïveté. The responsible organism has been recovered from 20 to 65 percent of soil samples. It is also commonly found in stool from a variety of animal sources, house dust, operating rooms, and contaminated heroin. In addition to wound contamination, important factors that contribute to the disorder are circumstances that promote reversion of spores to veg-

TABLE 9.4–5. TETANUS PROPHYLAXIS

Immunization Record	Wound[a]	Recommendation
Unimmunized, incomplete or unknown	Low risk	Toxoid[b] followed by complete immunization
	Tetanus prone	Toxoid plus TIG[c] 250–500 units using separate syringe and injection sites; complete active immunization
Primary immunization but no booster in 10 years	Low risk	Toxoid
	Tetanus prone	Toxoid, use of TIG is arbitrary
Primary immunization with booster within 10 years	Low risk	None
	Tetanus prone	Toxoid if 5 years since booster

[a]Tetanus prone wound indicates lesion which is severe, neglected, or over 24 hours old.
[b]Toxoid as DPT for children under 6 years, DT for person over 6 years.
[c]TIG indicates tetanus immune globulin.

etative forms with the production of neurotoxin. These are primarily local conditions such as tissue necrosis, suppuration, or the presence of a foreign body. The neurotoxin travels intra-axonally within membrane-bound vesicles at a rate of approximately 250 mm per day to the perikarya of motor neurons. After passage across the synaptic cleft it binds to a ganglioside and interferes with release of inhibitory transmitters, resulting in sustained contraction.

TYPES OF CLINICAL PRESENTATION

Recognized forms of tetanus include local, cephalic, generalized, and tetanus neonatorum. Generalized tetanus accounts for at least 80 percent of all cases. This may follow a trivial injury or may occur in association with a severe, contaminated crush injury. The usual incubation period between wounding and the onset of symptoms is 7 to 21 days, with a range of 1 to 60 days. The most common presenting symptom is trismus with tonic-clonic contractures of the face, neck, jaw, and abdomen. Additional features include irritability, restlessness, and dysphagia with hydrophobia. Persistent spasm of the back musculature results in opisthotonos. Tetanic seizures are characterized by sudden tonic contracture of the back musculature, flexion and adduction of the arms, clenched fists, and extension of lower extremities. Involvement of the autonomic nervous system may cause wide fluctuations in blood pressure, tachycardia, hyperthermia, cardiac arrhythmias, and diaphoresis. Complications include fractures from sustained contractions and convulsions, pulmonary emboli, involvement of the autonomic nervous system, coma, bacterial infections, and dehydration. The mortality rate in the United States is 25 to 30 percent. Poor prognostic factors are increased age, a rapid disease progression as measured by the time from wounding to the onset of symptoms, and a short period of onset, indicating the time from initial symptoms to generalized reflex spasms.

The most important therapeutic maneuver is to ensure airway patency and provide mechanical ventilation because of the tendency for respiratory arrest. Other therapeutic recommendations include (1) surgical debridement of the wound, (2) penicillin G given intravenously (1 to 2 million units every 4 to 6 hours for 10 days) or metronidazole given intravenously or orally (500 mg every 6 hours), or (3) tetanus immune globulin, preferably human hyperimmune globulin (500 to 6,000 units given intramuscularly), (4) cautious use of short-acting barbiturates, (5) chlorpromazine, meprobamate, or diazepam to control seizures, (6) reduced external stimuli that may precipitate spasms or convulsions, (7) tracheostomy, (8) maintenance of nutrition, hydration, and other

supporting measures, and (9) active immunization for all patients who recover, since natural infection does not produce detectable levels of circulating antibody.

Another form of the disease is *local tetanus*, in which the predominant involvement is in the extremity with the contaminated wound. This is a relatively unusual form, in which symptoms may persist for weeks or months, but the prognosis for recovery is excellent. Cephalic tetanus generally follows head injury or occurs in association with otitis media involving *Clostridium tetani*. Clinical symptoms are initially restricted to cranial motor nerve dysfunction, most frequently the seventh cranial nerve. The incubation period is only 1 to 2 days, and the prognosis is extremely grave. Tetanus neonatorum refers to generalized tetanus resulting from an infection of the umbilical stump with clinical expression at 3 to 10 days following birth. This form is found primarily in underdeveloped countries where a variety of contaminated materials are commonly used to either sever or dress the cord of newborn infants from unimmunized mothers. The mortality rate is generally reported at 70 percent or greater.

TETANUS PROPHYLAXIS

Tetanus is a preventable disease, with primary immunization followed by booster injections at 10-year intervals thereafter. Recommendations for wound management on the basis of the immunization history are summarized in Table 9.4–5.

OSTEOMYELITIS

Infections of bone are classified in three major categories: osteomyelitis following hematogenous spread of infection, bone infection secondary to a contiguous focus of infection, and osteomyelitis associated with vascular insufficiency[16,17] (Table 9.4–6). There are some unique bacteriologic patterns in selected clinical settings (Table 9.4–7).

HEMATOGENOUS SPREAD

Hematogenous osteomyelitis is classically described as a disease of children, with over 85 percent of cases in several large series involving patients of 16 years of age or less.[16] In this population the disease characteristically involves the metaphysis of long bones, especially the femur or tibia. The relatively high incidence during growth appears to reflect enhanced susceptibility of the vascular network of the metaphysis. At least one third of patients have a history of preceding blunt trauma to the area subsequently involved. The infection starts in the metaphyseal sinusoidal veins. It is contained by the epiphyseal growth plate and tends to spread laterally, with perforation of the cortex and a lifting of the loose periosteum.

Hematogenous osteomyelitis involving long bones is not only rare in adults, but different in its presentation. In these patients the growth cartilage has been resorbed so that the subarticular space is more vulnerable and the periosteum is firmly attached so that subperiosteal abscess formation is less common.

The most common form of hematogenous osteomyelitis in adults is vertebral osteomyelitis, especially in patients over 50 years of age.[17] The initial site of infection is the richly vascularized bone adjacent to cartilage. Eventually there is involvement of adjacent bone plates and the intervening intervertebral disc of the thoracolumbar, lumbar, or lumbosacral spine. This infection may extend longitudinally to involve other vertebrae, anteriorly to produce a paraspinal abscess, or posteriorly to form an epidural abscess. The latter is considered a serious complication because of possible cord compression with paraplegia or meningitis. A likely primary source for hematogenous dissemination in vertebral osteomyelitis can be found in about half of the cases. The most frequent sources are the genitourinary tract, skin, and respiratory tract.

S. aureus is implicated in 50 to 70 percent of cases of hema-

TABLE 9.4–6. TYPES OF OSTEOMYELITIS

	Hematogenous	Secondary to Contiguous Infection	Complication of Vascular Insufficiency
Overall incidence	20%	50%	30%
Age	1–16 yr >50 yr	>40 yr	>50 yr
Bones involved	Long bones (children) Vertebrae (adults)	Hip, femur, tibia	Feet
Predisposing causes	Trauma Bacteremia	Surgery Soft-tissue infection	Diabetes mellitus Vascular insufficiency
Major bacteria	*S. aureus* Gram-negative bacilli	Often polymicrobial *S. aureus*, gram-negative bacilli	Usually polymicrobial Gram-negative bacilli, anaerobes, streptococci, *S. aureus*
Presentation Initial episode	Fever, local pain, swelling, tenderness, limited movement	Fever, local pain, swelling, tenderness, limited movement	Ulceration drainage, ± pain
Recurrent	Sinus drainage ± pain	Sinus drainage ± pain	

togenous osteomyelitis. Enterobacteriaceae account for 20 to 30 percent of all cases and are more common in adults. A variety of other organisms also may be involved. *P. aeruginosa* is distinctly unusual except for osteomyelitis in drug addicts or following penetrating trauma of the foot (Table 9.4–6).

The classical presentation of acute hematogenous osteomyelitis is a precipitous onset of pain, swelling, chills, and fever. The usual symptoms with vertebral osteomyelitis are fever, back pain, and stiffness. Many patients have a more subacute form, with vague symptoms of 1 to 2 months' duration before presentation. In these cases there are few constitutional complaints, and local pain is the dominant symptom.

Patients with recurrent or chronic osteomyelitis often simply report increased drainage and pain following a prior episode involving the same anatomic site. One well-described variant is Brodie abscess, which is a subacute pyogenic osteomyelitis located in the metaphysis of long bone that is usually caused by *S. aureus*, with the major symptom of local pain and no fever.

CONTIGUOUS SPREAD

Osteomyelitis secondary to a contiguous focus of infection accounts for about 50 percent of all cases. The most common precip-

TABLE 9.4–7. BACTERIOLOGIC PATTERNS WITH OSTEOMYELITIS IN SELECTED CLINICAL SETTINGS

Clinical Setting	Major Pathogens	Major Sites
Prosthetic joint	*S. aureus*, *S. epidermidis*	Site of prosthesis
Parenteral drug abuse	*P. aeruginosa* *S. aureus*	Vertebral disc, pelvis
Sickle cell disease	*Salmonella*	Long bones; multiple bone involvement common
Puncture wound to foot	*P. aeruginosa*	Foot
Neonate	Group B streptococci *S. aureus*, *E. coli*	Long bones; joint involvement common, multiple bone involvement common
Chronic hemodialysis	*S. aureus*	Ribs, thoracic vertebra

itating factor is preceding surgery, especially open reduction of fractures involving the hip, femoral shaft, or tibial shaft. The next most common precipitating factor in this cateogry is a soft-tissue infection involving the digits of the hands or feet. Less common associated conditions include craniotomy, disc surgery, infected teeth, or radiation for malignant tumors, especially of the mandible. These infections usually become apparent within a month of the precipitating event, although many patients have chronic or recurrent infections that may be seen years or even decades later. The most common pathogen is *S. aureus*, followed by Enterobacteriaceae, *P. aeruginosa*, and streptococci. Many of these infections involve multiple bacteria, and this especially applies to cases that do not involve *S. aureus*. Infections associated with decubitus ulcers and diabetic foot ulcers usually involve a polymicrobial flora, including both coliforms and anaerobes.

VASCULAR INSUFFICIENCY

Osteomyelitis associated with vascular insufficiency accounts for about one third of all cases. Most patients are diabetic or have severe atherosclerosis, most are over 50 years of age, and the major site of infection is the toes or small bones of the feet. These infections usually involve multiple bacteria, including Enterobacteriaceae, *S. aureus*, anaerobic bacteria, and streptococci.

DIAGNOSIS

Diagnostic studies of major interest are radiographs or radionucleotide studies to demonstrate bone involvement, and cultures to identify the etiologic organism. Radiologic changes initially show lytic lesions, but these are not visible until 10 to 14 days after the onset. Further, new bone formation proceeds slowly so that it is not detected on radiograph for at least 1 month. Technetium and gallium scans are positive as early as 3 days after the onset of symptoms. These techniques do not differentiate cellulitis from osteomyelitis, and technetium scans performed after surgery or a fracture fail to distinguish bone repair and bone infection, as this test is a marker of osteoblastic activity.

Conclusive bacteriologic studies require isolation of the pathogen from either the bone lesion or blood cultures. Positive blood cultures are noted in approximately 50 percent of patients with acute untreated hematogenous osteomyelitis. Direct bone aspiration has a diagnostic yield of approximately 60 percent, and a surgical biopsy yields positive cultures in about 90 percent. Cultures from draining sinus tracts have shown poor correlation with cultures obtained directly from bone, especially when organisms other

than *S. aureus* are recovered.[10] These data indicate that bone biopsy or deep aspiration is clearly preferred and that cultures of wound drainage must be interpreted with caution.

TREATMENT

Treatment principles are quite different for acute and chronic forms of osteomyelitis. Antibiotics are the mainstay of treatment for acute cases, and the usual recommendation is parenteral drugs in high doses for 4 weeks. Limited data suggest that 2 weeks of intravenous therapy followed by 2 weeks of an orally effective antibiotic may be equally efficacious. The preferred initial regimen for acute staphylococcal osteomyelitis is a penicillinase-resistant penicillin such as nafcillin given intravenously in a dose of 1.5 to 2 g every 6 hours. Alternative agents are cephalothin (2 g every 6 hours) or clindamycin (600 mg every 8 hours). Antibiotic choices for osteomyelitis involving Enterobacteriaceae or *P. aeruginosa* should be based on in vitro sensitivity test results. The importance of bactericidal activity and the relative merits of drugs for bone penetration are debated but remain unresolved issues. Purulent collections sometimes require surgical drainage. Therapeutic guidelines for the management of chronic osteomyelitis are less precise, but here surgery appears to play a much more important role for removing sequestra and necrotic tissue. Microorganisms residing in dead bone may cause recurrent infections as late as 50 years after the initial episode.[18] Prolonged courses of antibiotics are given also. Most frequently they are begun by the parenteral route and then given by mouth for several weeks. The major goal of treatment is to prevent recurrent or chronic infection. Occasional complications noted in patients with chronic osteomyelitis are secondary amyloidosis, which has become extremely rare since the advent of antibiotics, and squamous cell carcinoma, which is detected in 0.2 to 1.5 percent of cases, with a mean delay of 34 years.[17] The prognosis in acute osteomyelitis is excellent, providing that appropriate antibiotic treatment is begun early in the course and continued for at least 3 weeks. The prognosis for chronic osteomyelitis is relatively poor since chronic or recurrent symptoms tend to be the rule regardless of management practices.

TUBERCULOUS OSTEOMYELITIS

Tuberculous osteomyelitis generally represents a complication of hematogenous dissemination from a primary infection in the lung. The most frequent sites of involvement are weight-bearing bones, including the spine, hip, knee, and ankles. About 50 percent of patients have tuberculous lesions in other anatomic sites.[5] Tuberculous spondylitis usually involves the lower thoracic or lumbar vertebrae. Skeletal involvement is insidious, and most patients have symptoms for months or even years before the diagnosis is established. Common presentations include local swelling and tenderness with long bone involvement, a chronic draining sinus, a painful or tender spine lesion, a kyphotic deformity, a neurologic deficit, or a lytic lesion discovered incidentally on radiograph. The best method to establish the diagnosis is often needle biopsy of bone lesions, sometimes with the assistance of guidance by computed tomography or fluoroscopy.

Treatment of spinal tuberculosis with two primary antituberculous drugs for 9 to 18 months appears to be as successful as surgical debridement or immobilization combined with chemotherapy.[1,8] Indications for surgery include progression of the disease during treatment, a paravertebral abscess, or an unstable lesion with threatened or established spinal cord compression.

REFERENCES

1. Bass JB, Farer LS, et al: Treatment of tuberculosis and tuberculosis infection in adults and children. Am Rev Resp Dis 134:355, 1986
2. Brun-Buisson MD, Abrouk F, et al: Diagnosis of central venous cather-related sepsis. Arch Intern Med 147:873, 1987
3. Curreri WP, Lutherman A, Braun DW: Burn injury. Analysis of survival and hospitalization time for 937 patients. Ann Surg 192:472, 1980
4. Duncan WC, McBride ME, Knox JM: Experimental production of infections in humans. J Invest Dermatol 54:319, 1970
5. Falk A: Results of long-term chemotherapy in spinal tuberculosis. XVII. A followup study of 235 patients. Am Rev Resp Dis 95:1, 1967
6. Gibson RK, Rosenthal SJ, Lukert BP: Pyomyositis. Increasing recognition in temperate climates. Am J Med 77:768, 1984
7. Goldstein EJC, Citron DM, Finegold SM: Role of anaerobic bacteria in bite-wound infections. Rev Infect Dis 6:S177, 1984
8. Gorse GJ, Pais MJ, et al: Tuberculous spondylitis. A report of six cases and a review of the literature. Medicine 62:178, 1983
9. Hook EW III, Hooton TM, et al: Microbiologic evaluation of cutaneous cellulitis in adults. Arch Intern Med 146:295, 1986
10. Mackowiak PA, Jones SR, Smith JW: Diagnostic value of sinus tract cultures in chronic osteomyelitis. JAMA 239:2772, 1978
11. MacLennan JD: The histotoxic clostridial infections of man. Bact Rev 26:177, 1962
12. Meislin HW, Lerner SA, et al: Cutaneous abscesses: Anaerobic and aerobic bacteriology and outpatient management. Ann Intern Med 87:145, 1977
13. Simmons RL, Ahrenholz DH: Infections of the skin and soft tissues. In Simmons RL, Howard RJ (eds): Surgical Infectious Diseases. New York, Appleton-Century-Crofts, 1982, p 507
14. Stone HH, Martin JD Jr: Synergistic necrotizing cellulitis. Ann Surg 175:702, 1972
15. Swartz MN: Skin and soft tissue infections. In Mandell GL, Douglas RG Jr, Bennett JE (eds): Principles and Practices of Infectious Diseases, 2d ed. New York, John Wiley & Sons, 1985, p 598
16. Waldvogel FA, Medoff G, Swartz MN: Osteomyelitis: A review of clinical features, therapeutic considerations and unusual aspects. N Engl J Med 282:198, 260, 316, 1970
17. Waldvogel FA, Vasey H: Osteomyelitis: The past decade. N Engl J Med 303:360, 1980
18. West WF, Kelly PJ, Martin WJ: Chronic osteomyelitis. I. Factors affecting the results of treatment in 186 patients. JAMA 213:1837, 1970

CHAPTER 9.5
Upper Respiratory Tract Infections

Patrick A. Murphy

Patients with upper respiratory tract infections often present vexing problems. Most of these infections are benign and self-limited, and many are caused by viruses for which we have no effective treatment. Some of them, however, are complicated by bacterial infection of the nasal sinuses or middle ear cavity, and if this is not recognized and treated, serious or lethal results, such as meningitis and septic thrombophlebitis, may follow. Some sore throats are caused by pathogens such as *Corynebacterium diphtheriae*, which may cause serious systemic complications, and others are secondary to illnesses such as agranulocytosis or acute leukemia. Diagnostic

facilities may be limited, because these patients are usually seen at home or in offices instead of in hospitals. Furthermore, there is no economic justification for expensive investigations for minor illnesses. The physician must therefore rely heavily on clinical features in reaching a diagnosis. Unfortunately, it is not possible to distinguish bacterial from viral infections on clinical grounds alone, because the manifestations may be the same. The physician must therefore be prepared to change the diagnosis and management as the patient's illness progresses and new information becomes available.

This chapter deals with management of the patient who has a cold, a sore throat, or tracheobronchitis. The common local complications such as sinusitis and otitis media are discussed, and the major bacterial infections of the pharynx, streptococcal and diphtheritic pharyngitis, are considered in more detail.

MANAGEMENT OF A COLD

When the major complaints are a runny nose, sneezing, and a dry cough with or without mild sore throat, viral infection can be diagnosed with reasonable confidence.[13] A large number of viruses may cause this syndrome, and as a rule their identification by culture or serologic tests is of no great importance. The only bacterial diseases causing primarily nasal symptoms are nasal diphtheria, which is rare, and infection by *Haemophilus influenzae* or meningococci. In these cases, the discharge is purulent from the onset. Viral infections are often associated with systemic symptoms such as headache, myalgias, and mild to moderate fever. The nasal discharge is clear mucus, and while tenderness over the sinuses is common, this is not severe, and spontaneous sinus pain is unusual. The eardrums are commonly retracted because of temporary eustachian tube blockage but are not inflamed. The cough, if present, is nonproductive, and the chest is clear to physical examination. Such a patient should be treated symptomatically. Recombinant human α interferon is now available, and intranasal administration of this material in large doses every 4 hours does improve the clinical symptoms of colds caused by rhinoviruses (but not other viruses). Large-scale use of this treatment seems impractical.

In most colds, after a few days the nasal discharge becomes mucopurulent, signaling that secondary bacterial infection has occurred. This in itself is not a cause for alarm and usually resolves spontaneously. However, bacteria may invade either the nasal sinuses or the middle ear, especially if mucosal swelling is severe enough to lead to obstruction of the sinus ostium or eustachian tube. Most cases of otitis media and purulent sinusitis will improve spontaneously, but this fact must not lull one into a false sense of security.

ACUTE SINUSITIS

The symptoms of acute sinusitis are sinus pain and tenderness, nasal blockage, and frankly purulent nasal discharge, with mild to moderate fever. Sometimes the inflammation is severe enough to cause nasal bleeding. The pain is usually moderate and due to absorption of air behind a blocked ostium; less often it is severe and due to the accumulation of pus under pressure (sinus empyema). Examination of the nose shows an inflamed, swollen mucosa and purulent discharge; if the nose is cleared by blowing, it may be possible to see reaccumulation of pus in a particular area, although commonly all the sinuses are involved to a greater or lesser degree.

The main principles of treatment are to establish drainage of the sinuses and to combat the infection with antibiotics. The inhalation of steam, whether medicated or not, is effective for temporarily clearing the nasal passages and promoting drainage. Oral "cold tablets" containing antihistamines and sympathomimetic drugs are entirely useless.[7] It is possible to achieve useful shrinkage of the nasal mucosa by nasal drops such as 0.5 percent ephedrine in saline, provided fairly large volumes (5 to 10 ml) are used and

the head is carefully positioned to ensure that the medication actually reaches the ostium of the sinus mainly affected. However, nasal sprays and drops as customarily used are without value. Modern endoscopes are so small and flexible that the ENT surgeon can insert one under the middle turbinate, inspect the orifices of all sinuses except the sphenoid, and cannulate them under vision for both diagnosis and therapy. This is the most efficient way to handle a severe case of acute sinusitis, but it obviously cannot be used for all cases.

The bacterial flora in acute sinusitis is varied, but most cases are due to pneumococci, streptococci, and *H. influenzae.* In addition, sinusitis may be caused by staphylococci, gram-negative rods, and anaerobic bacteria.[7,22] Gram-negative rods are especially common in the acute sinusitis of patients with indwelling nasogastric tubes.[4] The antibiotics commonly used for the treatment of acute sinusitis are amoxicillin, erythromycin, and trimethoprim-sulfamethoxazole, and in general they are effective.[7] Because drainage procedures are inadequate and no antibiotic can cover all possible organisms, treatment failure and the development of major complications are to be expected occasionally. Patients must be warned that treatment may not be effective and told to report back at once if deterioration or new symptoms occur, or if the symptoms continue unabated for a week. If antibiotics are clearly failing to control sinusitis, one should not hesitate to arrange for the most severely affected sinuses to be drained surgically.[5]

The major complications of sinusitis are due to erosion of bone and spread of the infection to adjacent structures. Obviously, the pathology will vary with the sinus affected, but the possibilities include orbital cellulitis, cavernous sinus thrombosis, meningitis, and brain abscess, usually in the frontal lobe. Severe local pain, headache, vomiting, high fever, shaking chills, and obvious systemic illness all suggest the onset of one of these complications. They urgently demand admission to hospital, accurate diagnosis, parenteral antibiotics in high dose, and surgical consultation. Computed tomography (CT) scans of the brain and pericranial structures have revolutionized the diagnosis of these conditions. As a rule, operative drainage of sinuses should be done after the acute infection has subsided, but there are exceptions. Some patients have bacterial sinusitis with every cold, and in them it is well to search for local abnormalities such as deviation of the nasal septum or nasal polyps. Surgical correction of these defects between acute attacks may lead to great improvement.

ACUTE OTITIS MEDIA

Infection of the middle ear cavity is easier to manage than acute sinusitis because one can see what is going on rather than having to infer it. The three cardinal symptoms are earache, discharge, and conductive deafness. Initially, pain may be due to lowered air pressure in the middle ear cleft, and the tympanic membrane is gray and retracted. In an established bacterial infection, the pain is due to accumulation of pus under pressure, and the tympanic membrane becomes red, loses its landmarks, and bulges. If it is perforated, pus can be induced to leak from the site of perforation by lowering the air pressure in the external auditory meatus.

The onset of discharge often is associated with a lessening of the pain, for obvious reasons. Deafness is not usually severe, and if it is severe it denotes an extensive infection. Abnormal bone conduction means that the infection has spread to the inner ear. Mild infections of the middle ear cavity may cause little pain and only moderate deafness, and examination shows only a few dilated vessels on the tympanic membrane and perhaps an accumulation of mucoid exudate behind the drum, with a fluid level.

The treatment of acute otitis media is antibiotics, sometimes with myringotomy in those cases in which there is severe pain and the drum is as yet intact. The responsible bacteria are usually pneumococci, streptococci, or *H. influenzae,* although almost any bacterium may be responsible on occasion, and in at least one third of cases, no bacteria can be grown from middle ear fluid.[2,6] If the

drum has perforated, or if myringotomy is done, then material for culture may be obtained that will guide antibiotic therapy; often, however, one must treat blindly. Because of the possible presence of *H. influenzae,* it is usual to recommend the use of amoxicillin for otitis media in children below the age of 8. In adults, penicillin is adequate. In penicillin-allergic patients, trimethoprim-sulfamethoxazole, erythromycin, or perhaps an oral cephalosporin may be tried. The important thing is to recognize that any antibiotic regimen is likely to fail on occasion. Vasoconstrictor nasal drops, and any sort of ear drops, are of dubious value.[3]

As in sinusitis, the chief dangers are obstruction of some narrow drainage pathway; accumulation of pus under pressure leading to necrosis of the mucoendosteum; osteomyelitis; and spread of the infection to surrounding structures. Infection of the middle ear cavity alone rarely leads to intracranial extension, probably because of spontaneous drainage through the eardrum. Infection of the mastoid antrum with occlusion of the aditus by swollen mucosa, however, is a classic source of septic thrombosis of the sigmoid sinus, extradural abscess, pyogenic meningitis, and brain abscess in either the temporal lobe or the cerebellum. Because most patients are treated with antibiotics, it is not usual nowadays for these complications to develop directly out of the acute otitis. Rather, the patient improves substantially, but persistent low fever, pain in the mastoid area, and continuing deafness signal continued infection, and if these warnings are neglected, disaster may ensue. If the patient is not returned completely to normal by a week of antibiotic treatment, an otologist should be consulted.

The actual onset of a major complication is marked by the symptoms previously discussed: headache, vomiting, fever, shaking chills, and systemic illness. Shaking chills particularly suggest septic thrombophlebitis. In addition, vertigo and nerve deafness may occur secondary to invasion of the inner ear, and there may be evidence of local abscess formation in the mastoid area. Rarely, one sees paralysis of the fifth or sixth cranial nerve due to osteitis of the petrous temporal bone. Urgent hospital admission, parenteral antibiotics, and surgical advice are appropriate.

Although intracranial complications of both sinusitis and otitis media may arise during the course of an acute respiratory infection in a person whose upper airway is basically normal, brain abscess, meningitis, and the like are actually more common as complications of chronic sinusitis or otitis media.[10]

MANAGEMENT OF A SORE THROAT

When the major complaint is sore throat, the cause may be either bacterial or viral, and the bacterial infections often demand specific treatment. Diagnosis from clinical features alone is possible in classic cases (Table 9.5–1), especially when it is known that an epidemic of sore throat due to a particular organism is in progress. Most sore throats are mild and present no distinguishing features on examination, however. One approach maintains that because of the danger of nephritis and rheumatic fever following streptococcal sore throat, all sore throats without exception must be cultured, and any with positive streptococcal cultures should be treated. Recent evidence suggests that for adults in this country, this approach involves an unreasonable investment of time and money (and risk of penicillin allergy) except under special circumstances.[16]

STREPTOCOCCAL PHARYNGITIS

Streptococcal pharyngitis is seen in its most classic form during epidemics in communities where people live in close physical proximity. Examples are schools, camps, and military training centers. Under these conditions, the introduction of a new streptococcal type may lead to rapid person-to-person transmission throughout the susceptible population. The organisms are well covered with protective M protein; inocula are large; clinical disease is severe;

and the incidence of sequelae is high. In the general population, many of the streptococcal carriers have established immunity to their own organism, which responds by losing much of its M protein and incidentally becoming less virulent. Disease due to these streptococci is milder, and the incidence of sequelae is much less. Under normal circumstances, about 5 percent of the asymptomatic general population and at least 10 percent of children carry group A, β-hemolytic streptococci in the pharynx. In the winter, families huddle together indoors, transmission occurs more frequently, organisms become more virulent, and both the carrier rate and the disease incidence are increased. It has been shown conclusively that infection is transmitted by respiratory droplets; dried streptococci in bed clothes, floor dust, and so on are incapable of causing disease.

Clinical Presentation

The classic symptoms are sore throat, dysphagia that may be so severe that only liquids can be swallowed, fever, and systemic upset. Cough, laryngitis, and coryza are rare, and their presence suggests some other diagnosis. On examination, the throat is intensely red and edematous, and if the tonsils are present there may be yellow flecks of exudate in the crypts that can easily be wiped away. Sometimes the exudate is confluent, but it remains yellow and easy to remove. The faucial pillars, the soft palate, and the uvula are swollen, and hypertrophy of lymphoid tissue under the posterior pharyngeal wall may produce a cobblestone appearance. The tonsillar lymph nodes are enlarged and tender, the temperature may range up to 104F or higher, and there is a neutrophil leukocytosis. Unfortunately, many proven streptococcal infections cause only mild symptoms, and a few are entirely asymptomatic.

The clinical diagnosis may be confirmed by a number of laboratory tests. The most important is culture of the throat, which in a typical case will demonstrate large numbers of mucoid colonies of β-hemolytic streptococci. Such streptococcal colonies are not necessarily group A, and this should be confirmed either by capillary precipitin or fluorescent antibody, which are specific tests, or by bacitracin sensitivity, which is easy and useful but has an error of about 5 percent in both directions. It is worth knowing that streptococci are delicate organisms that may easily die on cotton swabs if these cannot be plated immediately. A number of good transport media are available, and the organisms do survive well when dried on filter paper. The significance of small numbers of streptococci in the throat is less certain: many such cases are merely carriers of the organism, and the sore throat is due to concomitant viral infection.

Evidence of actual tissue invasion is provided by demonstrating significant (fourfold) rises in the serum levels of antibody to various streptococcal products. Antistreptolysin O is the classic antibody studied, and in throat infections significant rises are demonstrated in over 85 percent of cases. Other antigens, such as DNase B and NADase, may be useful as confirmatory tests in doubtful situations, although their main value is in the confirmation of streptococcal skin infections. Because streptococcal infections are universal, all normal human sera contain antibodies to streptococcal products; the mere presence of an antibody, no matter what the titer, does not prove that a current illness is due to streptococci. Serologic information, therefore, is only useful in retrospect.

The blood usually shows a neutrophil leukocytosis with white counts ranging up to about 20,000/μl in a severe infection. Higher values and gross shifts to the left would suggest some suppurative complication. Leukopenia is rare and would suggest either viral infection or perhaps the presence of some underlying condition that has lowered the blood neutrophil count and led to increased susceptibility to disease.

Therapy

Streptococcal pharyngitis is probably best treated by a single injection of 1.2 million units of benzathine penicillin G. This ensures that streptococci will be eradicated from the throat and that rheumatic fever will be prevented. Oral regimens must be continued

TABLE 9.5–1. DISTINGUISHING FEATURES OF INFECTIONS CAUSING PHARYNGITIS, TONSILLITIS, AND SORE THROAT

Etiology	Clinical Manifestations			Laboratory Findings		
	Symptoms	Local Appearance	Other Findings	Leukocyte Count	Culture	Other Findings
Group A β-hemolytic streptococci (streptococcal tonsillitis and pharyngitis)	Sudden onset, chills, headache, myalgia, vomiting; Painful swallowing	Fiery red edematous pharynx, tonsillar swelling; thin whitish yellow exudate restricted to tonsils; Cobblestone lymphoid hyperplasia of posterior pharynx	Fever up to 103–105°F; Patient looks ill; Tender cervical adenitis; Rash of scarlet fever (occasional)	10,000 to 15,000/μl	β-hemolytic streptococci on blood agar plates	Rising titer of antistreptolysin-O, antideoxyribonuclease B, and related antibodies
Corynebacterium diphtheriae (faucial diphtheria)	Gradual onset of chilliness, general malaise, mild sore throat; Swallowing is relatively painless; Laryngitis and airway obstruction may be present	Dull red injection, yellow-white adherent spots on tonsils; Dirty white or grayish yellow pseudomembrane; when stripped away a raw bleeding surface is exposed; Evidence of nasopharyngeal or laryngeal involvement may be noted	Moderate fever (101F–103F); May be few systemic manifestations until complications develop	Moderate leukocytosis, up to 15,000/μl	Throat swab onto Löffler, tellurite, and blood agar	Identification of typical organisms on stained smears of the lesion is occasionally helpful
Vincent angina (fusospirochetal pharyngitis)	Minimal save for local pain; Salivation	Superficial ulceration covered with a grayish white membrane that is easily removed; Foul odor	Minimal fever (up to 102F); Submaxillary node enlargement	May have slight leukocytosis	Not useful	Typical fusiform bacilli and spirochetes rapidly motile in wet preparations. Spirochetes stain poorly in fixed smears of exudate or necrotic tissue
Mycoplasma pneumoniae	Sore throat, cough	Nonspecific	Fever to 104F, Otitis media, pneumonia	Raised	M. pneumoniae	Complement fixation test positive; Cold agglutinins present
Candida (thrush)	Dysphagia, sore mouth and throat	Diffuse erythema, whitish mucoid exudate	May be none, but usually patient is already sick with some other disease and has been given antibiotics	No characteristic changes	Candida species	Stained smears of exudate show myriads of organisms in yeast form
Viruses Infectious mononucleosis	Gradual onset of malaise, headache, anorexia, sore throat	Edema, mild erythema; Tonsillar swelling and exudate; Pearly white membrane occurs which can be confused with diphtheria; May have coexistent streptococcal infection	Enlargement of nodes, especially posterior cervical, low-grade fever, splenomegaly, rashes, evidence of hepatitis; Illness may be prolonged	Leukopenia is common early, mild leukocytosis in second and third week; Lymphocytosis, especially with atypical cells	Negative for bacterial pathogens unless streptococcal infection coexists	Heterophile agglutinins; Stained smears of tonsillar exudate reveal myriads of atypical lymphocytes; EB virus antibody titer
Rhinoviruses (common cold)	Runny nose, sneezing	Clear, watery exudate	Low-grade fever	Normal		
Adenovirus	Sore throat; Cough; Conjunctivitis	Pharyngeal edema and erythema	Fever up to 102F	Normal	Adenovirus	
Coxsackie A (herpangina)	Sore throat	Vesicles on faucial pillars	Fever up to 102F	Normal	Coxsackie A16	
Herpes simplex (type I and II)	Sore throat and gums	Vesicles throughout mouth and on lips	Fever to 103F, gingivitis	Normal	Herpes simplex	Intranuclear inclusions in smears from vesicles. Fluorescent Ab positive.

for 10 days to achieve the same result; probably the best currently available is phenoxymethyl penicillin 250 mg four times daily. Patients who are genuinely allergic to penicillin should be treated with erythromycin 250 mg four times daily for 10 days. Culture of all family members makes little sense, because streptococci cannot be demonstrated in the throats of experimentally infected individuals until about 4 hours before symptoms of sore throat begin. Eradicative therapy for family members is indicated only when the strain of *Streptococcus* is known to be nephritogenic, and if this is the case, therapy should be given regardless of culture results because by the time symptoms and positive cultures develop it may be too late to prevent nephritis.

Complications

The complications of streptococcal pharyngitis are (1) spread of the infection in readily understandable ways, (2) scarlet fever (which is a systemic toxemia), and (3) glomerulonephritis, rheumatic fever, and other less common conditions, whose pathogenesis is not understood. Direct local spread of infection may produce peritonsillar abscess (quinsy), and abscesses may also develop in cervical lymph nodes or in lymphoid tissue of the posterior pharyngeal wall (retropharyngeal abscess). Acute streptococcal otitis media or sinusitis may occur, and, rarely, downward spread to the lungs produces streptococcal pneumonia. Streptococcal septicemia with secondary foci due to blood-borne spread is very uncommon except in debilitated people.

Scarlet Fever. Scarlet fever occurs when the streptococcus in the throat is lysogenized by a bacteriophage that codes for the production of the erythrogenic toxin. It is not agreed whether the toxin produces the rash directly or whether a state of hypersensitivity is responsible. The skin shows multiple, tiny erythematous papules that produce a generalized pink or red appearance from a distance. Circumoral pallor is classic. Later the rash becomes brownish, and extensive desquamation occurs. The tongue initially shows epithelial hypertrophy, leading to a thick gray coat, and subsequent desquamation leaves a red tongue with prominent fungiform papillae (the "strawberry tongue"). It is usually said that the presence or absence of scarlet fever does not affect the severity of either the suppurative or the nonsuppurative complications. This may be true now that antibiotic therapy is available, but it was not always so. The fact that small doses of purified toxin can kill rabbits and monkeys would suggest that its action extends beyond vasodilation in the skin.

A third group of complications appears not to require the presence of the organism in the lesions and includes rheumatic fever, acute glomerulonephritis, Sydenham chorea, and erythema nodosum. The clinical features of these illnesses are discussed elsewhere, and only their relationship to streptococcal sore throat is discussed here.

Rheumatic Fever. During epidemics of streptococcal infection, the peak incidence of rheumatic fever occurs about 3 weeks after the peak of pharyngitis, and this incubation period has been confirmed in military recruits and schoolchildren in whom the onset of infection could be timed precisely.[11] It does not shorten in second or subsequent attacks, even when these follow closely on a previous infection, and this long incubation period provides an opportunity for effective preventive therapy. Treatment with penicillin within 5 days of the onset of sore throat will completely prevent the subsequent onset of rheumatic fever, and treatment as late as 10 days after onset is of measurable value. Rheumatic fever may follow infection with many different streptococcal types, although some types are especially prone to cause the disease. During epidemics, rheumatic fever was found by Rammelkamp to follow 3 percent of proved cases of streptococcal pharyngitis. As mentioned earlier, however, the organisms are unusually virulent in these circumstances, and in the general population the figure is 0.3 percent and sometimes lower.

A different situation occurs in those who have been docu-mented as rheumatic with a previous attack of rheumatic fever. If a second streptococcal pharyngitis confirmed by culture and antibody rise is acquired within 6 months of an attack of rheumatic fever, the likelihood of recurrence is 50 percent. Over a 5-year period, the risk of recurrence following proved streptococcal pharyngitis slowly drops to about 10 percent and then appears to continue at that level indefinitely. The indefinite persistence of susceptibility to rheumatic fever is underlined by the fact that in Baltimore, 18 percent of all cases of rheumatic fever diagnosed between 1960 and 1964 occurred in adults and that the annual incidence in adults aged 20 to 39 was 3.1 per 100,000, or about 20 percent of the rate in children.[11]

Although rheumatic fever follows streptococcal infection, the exact pathogenesis is unknown, and, from the data just discussed, the occurrence of proved streptococcal infection with rises in serum antibody is not by itself enough even to guarantee a recurrence in subjects with known rheumatic tendencies. Clearly, there are associated factors, and what they may be is totally obscure. Genetic differences between rheumatic subjects and the general public have been suspected from family studies but the evidence is not conclusive. Racial and socioeconomic differences are not demonstrable if the rates are corrected for the degree of crowding. There is no evidence that rheumatic patients differ in their susceptibility to streptococcal infection: indeed, a comparative study between 164 families with at least one member with rheumatic tendencies and 179 normal families showed that the streptococcal isolation rates were identical for both adults and children.[12] Epidemiologic analysis suggests, in fact, that the only important determinant of the incidence of streptococcal infections is population crowding and that the rheumatic fever incidence is a simple function of the streptococcal attack rate.

There is abundant evidence that the antibody response to streptococcal infection is unusually intense in rheumatic subjects. This is a statistical phenomenon, there being extensive overlap with the normal at all ages; no level of antibody response to any antigen leads to a clear separation. There is evidence that streptococcal infections lead to the development of antibodies directed against cardiac muscle, and gamma globulin has been shown to be fixed to cardiac muscle in rheumatic subjects. However, similar antibodies occur also in normal people and after cardiac operations and myocardial infarctions. Furthermore, antibodies directed against vascular smooth muscle and skeletal muscle are also formed during streptococcal infections, but these tissues are not involved in rheumatic fever. In fairness, one must also add that antibodies directed against a glycoprotein in heart valves and against protoplasmic astrocytes have been discovered and are obviously of possible pathogenetic significance. Finally, lymphocytes sensitized against streptococcal antigens can kill beating heart muscle cultures, and it has been shown that patients with rheumatic fever have many more such lymphocytes than do normal subjects infected with streptococci. However, no one has yet integrated these immunologic observations into a coherent theory of pathogenesis.

How should we go about preventing rheumatic fever and rheumatic heart disease? There are two distinct questions here: the prevention of recurrent attacks of rheumatic fever in those who have already had one attack ("secondary prevention"), and the complete eradication of rheumatic fever ("primary prevention"). About secondary prevention there is no argument; it is known that the risk of recurrence is high and that continuous treatment with small doses of penicillin will reduce the risk to very low levels. What can be achieved was shown in a 10-year study in which patients were treated with 1.2 megaunits of benzathine penicillin G once monthly. No patient without cardiac damage at the outset developed it subsequently, and 70 percent of patients with established mitral incompetence at the outset lost their murmur.[18] Daily oral penicillin is less effective than monthly injections, as patients cannot be relied on to take it. No clinically important resistance of group A streptococci to penicillin G has occurred, and the incidence of allergic reactions seems to be low. Some cases of endocarditis due to *Streptococcus viridans* strains moderately resistant to pen-

icillin have been reported, but the incidence is low, and anyone who has had a clearly documented attack of rheumatic fever should be treated with intramuscular penicillin, probably for life. If the patient is allergic to penicillin, erythromycin is an acceptable substitute.

Primary prevention is a more thorny problem. Only about one third of cases of rheumatic fever occur after a sore throat for which the patient sought medical attention. In one third the symptoms are mild, and in one third there arc no symptoms at all. Considering the one third in whom prevention is possible, it is usually recommended that all patients complaining of sore throat should have a throat culture, and that if the culture is positive, they should be treated with penicillin. This general approach has been taken to its logical conclusion in Casper, Wyoming, where all children have monthly throat swabs, and any found to be harboring streptococci are treated. Another example of total prevention is in military camps, where epidemics are halted by treating the entire population of incoming recruits with prophylactic antibiotics.

An alternative viewpoint is gaining strength in Europe.[8] Death from a first attack of acute rheumatic fever is exceedingly uncommon, and chronic cardiac damage rarely results from a single attack. Sore throat is common; about 50 percent of the population has at least one sore throat per year. Only 20 percent of sore throats harbor streptococci, and only 3 percent are associated with a rise in ASO titer. Most people with positive streptococcal cultures do not have symptoms. Even if only patients with both a sore throat and a positive culture were treated, 20 percent of the entire population would receive a 10-day course of penicillin each year, and 20,000 cases of sore throat would have been diagnosed and treated to prevent one case of rheumatic fever. The mortality of penicillin treatment is uncertain but is thought to be of the order of 1 in 100,000 patients treated.[9] The conclusion is to reserve primary prevention for well-defined epidemic situations where streptococci are known to be prevalent and virulent, where most sore throats are streptococcal, and the risk of rheumatic fever is presumably about 3 percent. This is especially likely to be the case in Third World countries. Sore throats found under nonepidemic conditions in the general population of the United States should be managed symptomatically, with the time, effort, and money thus saved put into ensuring that those who have already had one attack of rheumatic fever do not get a second.[16]

Glomerulonephritis. Acute glomerulonephritis follows infection with only a few streptococcal types, and in the throat, this is usually type 12. The incidence of nephritis per proved type 12 streptococcal infection depends on how hard one looks. Obvious nephritis with edema, oliguria, and hematuria occurs in about 10 percent of cases, and if abnormal urine is accepted as the criterion, the incidence is above 20 percent. By renal biopsy, nephritis can be demonstrated in up to 50 percent of cases.

Acute poststreptococcal glomerulonephritis may occur at any age and is usually severe in adults. Why nephritis is so common after infection with particular streptococcal strains is unknown: electron micrographs show lumps of material underneath the glomerular epithelium that look like antigen-antibody complexes. In a few cases, streptococcal cell wall carbohydrates have been demonstrated in the lumps, along with antibody and complement components.

It is not at all certain that nephritis can be prevented by penicillin treatment of an established sore throat; in the only controlled trial of this question, no effect was demonstrable.[21] If there is protection, it is only partially effective. The patient should be treated mainly to prevent spread of the nephritogenic organisms to others, and there is a strong case for prophylactic treatment of close contacts, especially if they are adult. Once a patient has recovered from nephritis second attacks are uncommon, probably because of the persistence of type-specific protective antibody. Long-term penicillin therapy is therefore unnecessary.

Other Nonsuppurative Complications. Chorea usually occurs along with other manifestations of acute rheumatic fever, and long-term penicillin prophylaxis is indicated. What should be done in those cases where chorea is apparently an isolated manifestation is not altogether clear, because the etiology of such cases is obscure and they may not all be poststreptococcal. If there is serologic evidence of recent streptococcal infection, however, penicillin therapy would seem to be reasonable.

Erythema nodosum is sometimes due to streptococcal infection, and treatment with penicillin is then indicated. Long-term therapy is not required.

DIPHTHERIA

Diphtheria is a localized infection of the upper respiratory tract that may be associated with delayed systemic manifestations, chiefly myocarditis and peripheral neuropathy. The systemic manifestations are due to a toxin whose primary action is to block protein synthesis. Since the use of immunization on a large scale, diphtheria has become rare, but there was an epidemic in San Antonio in 1973 in a population in which immunization was not practiced. The penalty for missing the diagnosis for 24 hours may easily be the patient's life, so the disease must be recognized.[17]

Clinical Presentation

The patient has commonly been ill for a day or two with headache and malaise before developing a mild sore throat without much dysphagia and slight fever. He or she looks ill, with a gray pallor and a pulse rate raised out of proportion to the temperature. The tonsils are enlarged and the pharynx red and edematous. The membrane is dirty white in color and spreads not only over the tonsils but over the adjacent pillars of the fauces, the soft palate, and the uvula. This extratonsillar spread is pathognomonic. The membrane may spread downward to involve the larynx, and a common termination of untreated cases used to be death from laryngeal obstruction. The symptoms of laryngeal obstruction are hoarseness, stridor, and rib retraction on inspiration. The membrane is composed of necrotic epithelium, fibrin, and inflammatory cells, with the organism visible in the interstices. Because the epithelium is part of the membrane, it may be difficult to remove, and, when it is removed, a raw bleeding surface is left. Occasionally, no membrane is visible in the throat, and only the nasopharynx is involved. In this case the patient is usually less ill but has a blood-stained, purulent nasal discharge that may be unilateral.

The cervical lymph nodes enlarge early; this, combined with extensive edema of the tissues of the neck, may produce the classic bull neck appearance. In neglected cases, paralysis of the soft palate may lead to a nasal voice and the regurgitation of fluid through the nose. Usually by this time the membrane has partially sloughed and hangs in shreds from the pharyngeal wall.

Laboratory studies must demonstrate not only the organism but also that it is toxigenic. Smears of material from the edge of the membrane usually show gram-positive bacilli, but confirmation by culture is required because nonpathogenic corynebacteria may have similar morphology. Corynebacteria have simple growth requirements and will grow on most media, but because they may be overgrown by pneumococci and streptococci, it is best to plate swabs on blood or chocolate agar containing potassium tellurite. In the past, the colony morphology was thought to indicate whether or not the strain was toxigenic, but the correlations are only statistical and not useful in a particular case. Toxin formation is best demonstrated either by animal inoculation or by the Elek plate immunodiffusion procedure.

Therapy

The most important part of the therapy of diphtheria is to administer a large dose of antitoxin at the earliest possible moment. The aim is to provide enough to neutralize all the circulating toxin, to

neutralize any toxin that may be formed subsequently, and, hopefully, to neutralize toxin already bound to cells but not yet interiorized. The quantity given is 30,000 to 40,000 units in a moderately severe case, half being given intravenously and the rest intramuscularly. More is given if there is extensive involvement of the throat. The serum is prepared in horses, so the possibility of anaphylaxis should be borne in mind. Toxin already within cells is not accessible to antibody, and fatal myocarditis or severe neuropathy may still develop despite serum therapy. Cases treated on day 1 of the illness have a negligible mortality, whereas cases treated more than 4 days after the onset have the same mortality as controls.[17] There is therefore an obvious need for haste; serum should be given as soon as there is reasonable suspicion of the diagnosis without waiting for bacteriologic confirmation. If an adequate dose of antitoxin has been given at the outset, there is little point in giving more when paralysis or myocarditis later develops.

Antibiotics should also be given to eradicate the organism from the throat—both for the patient's sake and because convalescent carriers are a danger to others. It is usual to use penicillin, although there are indications that erythromycin might be even better.

Because of the dangers of laryngeal obstruction, myocarditis, and neurologic involvement, the patient should always be admitted to hospital and nursed in a unit capable of dealing with cardiac and respiratory crises if they should occur.

Complications

Complications are due to systemic absorption of diphtheria toxin produced in the throat. Toxigenic corynebacteria are lysogenized with β-prophage, and it can be shown that the phage carries the structural gene for the toxin. The mode of action of the toxin explains some of the clinical features and determines the approach to therapy. The toxin is a protein that is inactive until split into two chains by proteolytic enzymes at cell surfaces. One chain is required for the attachment to cell surfaces, the other is toxic if it can gain access to cell cytoplasm. The toxin action involves the enzymatic conversion of the translocation factor EF2 into an inactive form. Inactivation of all the EF2 molecules in a cell can be produced by only one molecule of toxin, but it is a process that requires many hours to complete. Once completed, protein synthesis is brought to a standstill. Functional damage will not be evident until the preformed supply of some critical protein has been exhausted.

Myocardiopathy. The most susceptible tissue is the heart, and some degree of myocarditis probably occurs in all cases. Clinical cardiac involvement occurs in about 10 percent of cases, especially when the throat disease is extensive. It is most commonly seen in the second week of illness, but may be earlier or later. Physical signs include sinus tachycardia, first-degree heart block, distant heart sounds, myocardial dilation, and low blood pressure. Severe myocarditis is indicated by congestive cardiac failure, second or third degree heart block, and ventricular tachycardias. Such patients have a bad prognosis and may die either from progressive congestive failure or suddenly from ventricular fibrillation or asystole. Treatment of the cardiac involvement with the usual regimens for congestive heart failure probably has little influence on the outcome. Pathologically, there is focal myocardial necrosis with edema, hyaline degeneration, and, sometimes, fatty change. The inflammatory response is usually minor. If recovery occurs, it is generally complete.

Neuropathy. Peripheral neuropathy is of two distinct types. Palatal paralysis is apparently caused by direct access of the toxin to the nerves, and a similar paralysis confined to the affected segment may be seen in wound diphtheria. As would be expected, it is usually the earliest neurologic symptom, appearing in the second or third week of illness. Other palsies are due to blood spread of the toxin and paralysis of accommodation is common in the third or fourth week. Subsequently, generalized polyneuritis may develop between the fifth and seventh week. It may produce death either by pharyngeal and laryngeal palsy, with aspiration pneumonia, or by paralysis of the diaphragm and intercostal muscles with respiratory failure. Treatment, thus, should include close observation of the patient's airway and vital capacity, with recourse to nursing with the patient in the prone position, endotracheal tubes, tracheostomy, and artificial ventilation as indicated. The lower limbs are generally more severely affected than the upper, and there may be extensive sensory involvement. The sphincters are almost always intact. If the patient survives, recovery may take many months but is usually complete.

VINCENT ANGINA

Vincent angina is synergic infection of the pharynx by two organisms, a spirochete and a fusiform gram-negative rod, which are normal inhabitants of the gingival crevices. Other bacteria, such as anaerobic streptococci and bacteroides species, also may be present in the lesions. The infection is usually found in persons with poor oral hygiene and is associated with more or less obvious gingivitis. It is especially common in malnourished, crowded populations and in patients with agranulocytosis or acute leukemia.

The major symptom is severe pain in the throat and gums, with dysphagia, dysarthria, and trismus. The breath is foul smelling, and the throat shows a gray-brown membrane that is easily wiped off. Fever is usually modest, and there is not much systemic disturbance unless the patient has an underlying condition. Motile spirochetes can be seen in wet preparations from the membrane, and several sorts of bacteria are usually demonstrable by culture under anaerobic conditions. The disease should be treated with 3 percent hydrogen peroxide mouthwashes and with systemic penicillin therapy. If a patient develops this infection despite previous good health and reasonable oral hygiene, a blood dyscrasia should be sought.

HAEMOPHILUS PHARYNGITIS

Until recently, *H. influenzae* infection was a rarity in adults because almost everyone had type-specific antibody in their serum as a result of infection in childhood. However, now a substantial number of adults do not carry protective antibody, whether because of the widespread use of antibiotics in children or because of better living conditions leading to a lower incidence of infection.[14]

The dominant clinical symptom is sore throat whose severity is out of all proportion to the visible change, coupled with dysphagia and hoarseness. The infection is commonly bacteremic, with high fever, neutrophilic leukocytosis, and positive blood cultures. Very soon, a dry, irritative cough and stridor are added, and the clinical condition deteriorates dramatically within a few hours. The patient becomes prostrated, with gross laryngeal obstruction and cyanosis, and may die within 24 hours of the onset.

The throat is red and swollen, but there are no ulcers or membranes, and nodes are not particularly prominent. A laryngeal mirror will show gross edema and redness of the epiglottis and aryepiglottic folds. All such patients should be admitted to the hospital, and if there is any evidence of respiratory obstruction, endotracheal intubation should be performed by an anesthetist in an operating room with a surgeon standing by to perform a tracheostomy if necessary. Normally the patient can be extubated after 48 hours. The best antibiotic is cefuroxime in doses of 1 g every 6 hours, because the same syndrome is sometimes caused by *Staphylococcus aureus*.

THRUSH

Candida albicans is part of the normal mouth flora and rarely causes trouble in healthy people. However, if the normal flora is altered

by antibiotic therapy, *Candida* may flourish and give rise to a characteristic syndrome. It is especially common when lozenges containing antibiotics have been prescribed, but it can also complicate systemic antibiotic therapy. In addition, it may be seen in sick people who have not been given antibiotics, particularly in those with leukemias or lymphomas.

The most common predisposing cause in adults at the present time is infection with HIV. Although thrush is not by itself sufficient for the diagnosis of AIDS, such patients also commonly have esophagitis, one diagnostic criterion. Even if the criteria for the diagnosis of AIDS are not satisfied when the patient is initially seen, it is common clinical experience that they will eventually emerge.

The throat is sore, but often the patient does not complain about it spontaneously. On examination there are pathognomonic patches of dead-white exudate on an erythematous background. Unlike food particles, they cannot be wiped away, and potassium hydroxide preparations show masses of yeasts and pseudohyphae. Thrush is usually merely a nuisance and responds well to mouthwashes with nystatin or to the old-fashioned painting with gentian violet. Occasionally, however, thrush spreads down the esophagus and causes esophagitis, which is characterized by severe pain on swallowing. This may be lethal if untreated and requires systemic chemotherapy with ketoconazole or amphotericin B. *Candida* esophagitis may occur in basically healthy people, but it is much more common in the immunosuppressed and is to be expected eventually in almost every case of AIDS. Therapy usually cures *Candida* esophagitis except in AIDS, when therapy must almost always be continued for life.

SYPHILIS AND GONORRHEA

Pharyngitis may occur in both syphilis and gonorrhea. Secondary syphilis is usually accompanied by a galaxy of physical signs—papular rash involving palms and soles, lymphadenopathy involving epitrochlear nodes, splenomegaly, arthritis, alopecia, conjunctivitis, condylomata, and so on. The pharyngitis is of gradual onset and is accompanied by mild to moderate fever. Inspection may show the classic snail track ulcers, and the lesions teem with spirochetes that can be seen on darkfield examination. Serologic tests for syphi-

lis are strongly positive. Gonococcal pharyngitis usually presents no distinguishing features on examination, and the cultural result is a surprise. Further details are contained in Chapter 9.14.

VIRAL PHARYNGITIS

In most viral upper respiratory infections, there is coryza or tracheobronchitis as well as sore throat. There may also be conjunctivitis, viral pneumonia, or gastrointestinal symptoms. Some groups of symptoms can be assigned with reasonable confidence to particular viruses (Table 9.5–2). Thus, acute respiratory disease in military recruits is characterized by high fever, headache, sore throat, and nonproductive cough. The throat is merely red, without exudate, and the causative agent is usually adenovirus type 4 or 7. Pharyngoconjunctival fever is the same infection, with more conjunctivitis and less bronchitis. Upper respiratory illness associated with nausea, vomiting, and diarrhea may be caused by ECHO viruses.

When sore throat is the principal complaint, adenovirus infection is most likely, followed by picornavirus infections. Herpangina is characterized by fever, sore throat, and a pathognomic vesicular eruption on the anterior pillars of the fauces. It is generally caused by coxsackie group A viruses. Primary herpetic gingivostomatitis usually occurs in children younger than the age of 5. However, it is occasionally seen in adults, and most such infections turn out to be due to herpes simplex type I rather than type II. The vesicles on the throat look like herpangina, but the gingivitis is diagnostic. Also, herpes simplex may recur in the pharynx of immunosuppressed people. Either form of herpetic infection can be diagnosed from the characteristic intranuclear inclusions, or by fluorescent monoclonal antibody, as well as by viral culture.

INFECTIOUS MONONUCLEOSIS

Infectious mononucleosis is a systemic illness, but sore throat may be the most prominent clinical feature. Usually the patient has been ill for a few days with fever and headache before the sore throat develops. The throat may be very sore, indeed, and examination then shows deep cut ulcers of the tonsils with a yellow slough at the base. Similar ulceration of the adenoids may cause a purulent postnasal discharge. In milder cases, the throat shows no

TABLE 9.5–2. COMMON RESPIRATORY INFECTION SYNDROMES

Infectious Agent	Rhinitis Coryza		Pharyngitis		Laryngitis		Tracheo-bronchitis		Pneumonia		Other Features
	Child	*Adult*	*Child*	*Adult*	*Child*	*Adult*	*Child*	*Adult*	*Child*	*Adult*	
Influenza virus	+	+	+	+	+	+	+	+	+	+	Severe myalgia, malaise, orbital headache
Adenoviruses	+	+	+	+	−	−	+	−	+	+	Keratoconjunctivitis; pleurodynia, orchitis, aseptic meningitis in recruits
Parainfluenza viruses	+	+	+	+	+	−	+	−	+	−	Croup
Coxsackie	+	+	+	+	−	−	−	−	−	−	Pleurodynia, orchitis, aseptic meningitis, pericarditis, herpangina
Respiratory syncytial virus	+	+	+	+	+	−	+	−	+	−	Little or no fever
Rhinoviruses	+	+	+	+	+	−	+	−	+	−	Little or no fever
Mycoplasma pneumoniae	+	+	+	+	+	+	+	+	+	+	Complement-fixation test positive; tetracyclines useful

specific features. Petechial hemorrhages at the posterior end of the hard palate may be seen but are not diagnostic.

Evidence of systemic illness may be provided by enlargement of cervical nodes other than the tonsillar group, generalized lymphadenopathy, splenomegaly, or hepatitis. The blood shows atypical lymphocytes, and these may also be found in smears from tonsils. The Paul-Bunnel test for heterophile red cell agglutinins becomes positive, as do tests for antibody to the Epstein-Barr (EB) virus. Even in cases with no clinical evidence of hepatitis, there are almost always elevated serum levels of enzymes, which normally are confined to liver cells.

Patients with infectious mononucleosis are usually slow to recover, and suffer from fatigue and low-grade sore throat for weeks. It is known that this virus persists for life, and some people have prolonged antibody responses to virus antigens that are expressed only early in virus replication. It has been suggested that there is a chronic form of EB virus infection, with clinical symptoms that may persist for years. Most observers are unable to distinguish this syndrome from chronic psychoneurosis, and it is not certain that it exists.

MYCOPLASMA INFECTIONS

Mycoplasma pneumoniae is the exception to the general rule that multiple organ involvement suggests viral infection that should be managed symptomatically. Most patients have upper respiratory symptoms, including sore throat, and only a minority actually develop pneumonia. The infections are insidious in onset and persistent once established. Often several members of a family are ill successively, and someone or other is ill for several months. People older than 40 are rarely affected; but characteristically, young adults are sicker than children. The disease responds fairly well to tetracycline or erythromycin therapy.

MANAGEMENT OF THE SORE THROAT

It is obvious that the initial management of all acute upper respiratory tract illnesses that include sore throat as one component should be symptomatic. As the disease progresses one should remember the possibility of secondary bacterial sinus or ear infections and the less likely possibility that the whole illness is due to *M. pneumoniae*. Whether to culture the throat for β-hemolytic streptococci is a question that each person must resolve for himself. It may be inevitable under present medicolegal conditions in this country, but it is by no means clear that it is totally rational.

When sore throat is the major complaint and especially when the patient is febrile and sick rather than merely inconvenienced, the probability of bacterial infection is higher. It is most important to exclude the rare but potentially lethal *C. diphtheriae* and *H. influenzae* infections, which are not hard to diagnose provided one thinks of them. In the presence of exudative tonsillitis of the classic streptococcal type, one can take a culture and give therapy immediately, preferably 1.2 million units of benzathine penicillin. Penicillin therapy does not measurably affect the duration of clinical symptoms, but suppurative complications do occur, and therapy is indicated when high fever and leukocytosis are present. When the sore throat shows no characteristic features and does not demand instant therapy, one can take a culture and institute penicillin therapy later if it is positive for streptococci. If a nephritogenic streptococcus is known to be about, therapy should be given immediately. If the culture shows only a few streptococci, it is likely that they are not the cause of the illness, and the need for therapy is moot. Many of these organisms are not group A, and those that are may be untypable because they have lost all or most of their M protein.

Whether antibiotics are given or not, the fever and general upset can be satisfactorily treated with acetaminophen, and various anesthetic lozenges may provide local analgesia. If the patient does not respond to treatment within a few days, infectious mononucleosis and blood dyscrasias should be considered.

MANAGEMENT OF TRACHEOBRONCHITIS

Most tracheobronchitis is caused by viruses, and recovery is rapid and spontaneous. Bacterial superinfection may occur, especially in patients with chronic obstructive pulmonary disease, asthma, bronchiectasis, and certain rare conditions such as cystic fibrosis. This may progress to severe and sometimes fatal bronchopneumonia, or may precipitate heart failure in a person with chronic cardiac disease. In addition, the viruses themselves may cause pneumonia, although this is ordinarily not severe and may only be diagnosed radiographically.

In adults, the commonest cause of tracheobronchitis without much coryza or sore throat is the influenza virus. Parainfluenza viruses, rhinoviruses, and the respiratory syncytial virus cause much less bronchitis in adults than they do in children. Exceptionally, Coxsackie and ECHO viruses may cause acute bronchitis in adults, and an occasional, but treatable, cause is *M. pneumoniae* infection.

The symptoms usually begin with headache, myalgia, and fever, with or without coryza or sore throat. The cough is commonly spasmodic and nonproductive, or there may be a small amount of whitish sputum. Dyspnea is not a feature if the lungs were previously normal, and the only pain is substernal soreness. There may be concomitant laryngitis with partial or total loss of voice. Stridor is almost unheard of in viral infections of adults and would suggest *Haemophilus* infection, or perhaps diphtheria.

Examination shows nothing specific. The patient has mild to moderate fever but is not usually very sick, and, in particular, is neither dyspneic nor cyanotic. The chest may show a few wheezes on auscultation, but there is no evidence of pulmonary consolidation.

In healthy people an annual bout of bronchitis is to be expected, and everyone has his or her own method of treating it. The physician's duty is limited to excluding pneumonia and signing whatever forms the patient may need to excuse him or her from work. Patients with chronic pulmonary disease deserve more attention, and there is solid evidence that they should be treated with antibiotics as soon as an attack of bronchitis develops. These patients carry pneumococci, streptococci, and *H. influenzae* in the tracheobronchial tree, and a viral infection that leads to lysis of ciliated epithelial cells may start a severe bronchopneumonia. Suitable drug regimens are tetracycline or ampicillin 500 mg every 6 hours. Antibiotics may also be given if a basically healthy person with acute bronchitis begins to cough up large quantities of purulent sputum. Bronchodilators may be required if there is much wheezing, especially in chronic bronchitis or asthma. Cough suppressants should be used judiciously, recognizing that cough is the best way of getting pus out of the airways and that respiratory depressants may precipitate respiratory failure in those with carbon dioxide retention. The cooperative patient will stop smoking until recovered. These simple measures suffice for the vast majority of cases. Laryngitis, if present, improves spontaneously along with bronchitis.

In elderly patients, patients already ill with some other disease, pregnant women, and postoperative patients, the bronchitis may progress to bronchopneumonia. Fever and general malaise become more pronounced, the cough becomes productive, with large amounts of purulent sputum, and dyspnea, tachypnea, and cyanosis appear. The chest now shows generalized coarse and medium crepitations, and there may be patches of dullness to percussion and bronchial breathing. Old people may become delirious. Such patients should be admitted to hospital and treated with oxygen, pulmonary toilet, and assisted ventilation, as necessary, combined with parenteral antibiotics. This is discussed more fully below. Bacterial infection of the sinuses or middle ear may also occur and is managed as discussed above.

INFLUENZA

The influenza viruses are the most important agents causing acute respiratory disease because although there is a relatively low case-fatality rate, enormous numbers of individuals are affected. During the influenza epidemic in the winter of 1962 to 1963 there were an estimated 80 million cases in the United States, and deaths from influenza and pneumonia increased by about 70,000. Because it is a well-studied epidemic viral disease, because of its prevalence and importance, and because it is a representative localized viral respiratory infection with prominent systemic manifestations, influenza is used here to illustrate certain general epidemiologic, clinical, and immunologic features of viral disease.

Epidemiology

Pandemics (worldwide epidemics) of influenza have been recorded at the rate of about four per century since 1610; the most severe pandemic occurred in 1917 to 1918, when an estimated 10 million persons died. In 1933, Smith, Laidlaw, and Andrews first isolated the virus, and serologic tests useful in diagnosis and in epidemiologic studies followed rapidly. By 1936 a practical method for the manufacture of a vaccine protective for animals had been found, and it was soon demonstrated that the vaccine offered some protection for humans. In 1947, however, there was an epidemic caused by the A-1 strain, and it became apparent that a new strain of the virus had appeared, against which the available vaccines offered little protection. In 1957 and in 1968, pandemics were caused by the Asian (A-2) and Hong Kong (A-3) strains.

The only important source of influenza virus is infected persons. The virus is readily found in respiratory secretions during the first few days of illness, but is rarely detectable for longer than the first week. Persistent carriers have not been demonstrated. There is evidence that inapparent or mild infections are more common than clinical disease; thus the viruses may persist in a population by causing sporadic mild illnesses resembling the common cold.

During nonepidemic periods, the viral antigens change slowly, and peptide mapping shows that successive single-base mutations leading to single amino acid substitutions are responsible for the changes (antigenic drift). The outbreak of a new pandemic is associated with a major change in the viral hemagglutinin to a completely new type (antigenic shift). The neuraminidase may or may not shift also. The mechanism for the shift(s) is probably that the virus has a segmented genome consisting of at least eight separate pieces of RNA. If two strains of influenza virus replicate in the same cell, then major recombination is possible. Perhaps the recombination occurs in an animal, rather than in humans. At any rate, a virus with a totally new hemagglutinin finds most of the world's population defenseless, with no preformed neutralizing antibody. A new neuraminidase is less dangerous because antibodies against this antigen have less influence on the outcome of infection.

The Asian strain of influenza virus was detected in China early in 1957 and possessed both a new hemagglutinin and a new neuraminidase. It was widely seeded throughout the United States by midsummer, but outbreaks of clinical disease occurred at that time only in camps, institutions, and communities in which schools were open. A substantial increase in cases occurred throughout the United States in September when schools reopened, but it was not until the onset of cold weather that the infection appeared in truly epidemic proportions. Thus widespread seeding of influenza virus may occur without epidemics being noted until other conditions are appropriate. This often leads to the simultaneous appearance of explosive outbreaks in widely distant areas. Wet weather, crowding, cold, stress, air pollution, and travel in closed vehicles are among the factors that have been proposed to explain this.[1]

Major influenza epidemics are caused only by type A strains. No part of the world escapes for long, widespread influenza recurring every 2 to 4 years. Nearly all epidemics reach their peak in the winter, with January and February the peak months in the northern hemisphere. Type B usually causes less severe epidemics, often localized to schools, military camps, and other closed populations, and occurring in 4- to 6-year cycles. Type C rarely causes epidemic disease.

Epidemics in any one locality tend to last only from 6 to 8 weeks. The short incubation period (2 to 3 days), the ease of transmission, the widespread seeding of the virus before the outbreak, and the high attack rates (50 to 75 percent when subclinical infections are included) may account for the short, explosive nature of the epidemics.

Clinical Presentation

The clinical manifestations of influenza vary from those of a mild upper respiratory illness to a severe pneumonia with involvement of many organs. There is little to distinguish the illness of isolated cases from that of disease caused by other common upper respiratory tract pathogens (Table 9.5–2), but a characteristic pattern is readily discernible when groups of patients are encountered, and the knowledge that influenza infection is prevalent is a most important clue to the diagnosis.

The incubation period is usually about 2 days. The patient characteristically has the sudden onset of prostration, myalgia, headache, retroorbital pain, and marked toxicity. Fever of 103F to 104F may ensue within a few hours. Bradycardia is common, but tachycardia is usually seen in the most severely ill. A flushed face and hot, dry skin are typical. Heliotrope cyanosis (reddish purple) suggests the diagnosis of influenzal pneumonia (pneumonia caused entirely by replication of influenza virus in the lung).

Systemic symptoms predominate during the first 24 to 48 hours of illness; as they subside, respiratory symptoms become prominent. Pharyngitis alone is distinctly unusual, but combinations with coryza, conjunctivitis, nasopharyngitis, tracheobronchitis, and bronchiolitis are common. Mucosal hyperemia is always present, and this may occasionally progress to hemorrhagic necrosis of the tracheobronchial mucosa. Scattered rhonchi or moist rales in the lungs are found in as many as a third of uncomplicated cases. Radiologic evidence of pulmonary involvement is also frequent. A dry, hacking cough and retrosternal burning are often most distressing parts of the illness. Secondary bacterial pulmonary infections are most frequent during the late stages of the illness and are heralded by the sudden return of high fever and prostration or by the appearance of dyspnea and cyanosis. Gastrointestinal manifestations are rare in influenza. Neurologic involvement, including meningoencephalitis, is not unusual in outbreaks. Myocarditis and pericarditis have also been reported; arrhythmias, hypotension, and cardiac failure are the usual manifestations.

Secondary bacterial infections of the ears, sinuses, bronchi, and lungs are frequent and important complications, and bacterial pneumonia is responsible for many of the fatalities. Bacterial infections occurring on the third to fifth day of influenza and influenzal pneumonia are particularly troublesome in patients with rheumatic heart disease, congestive heart failure or chronic pulmonary disease, and in pregnant women. Even in the absence of complications, the disease tends to be more severe in such patients. Influenzal pneumonia, which is usually diffuse and hemorrhagic, can sometimes be distinguished from secondary bacterial pneumonia in patients with influenza (Table 9.5–3).

In most patients, recovery takes place in a few days or, at most, a week, but delayed convalescence manifested by easy fatigability, persistent cough, recurrent myalgia, malaise, and depression may follow influenza. Subjective manifestations persisting beyond 3 weeks can be frequently related to a depression propensity of the patient.

Laboratory Findings

Leukopenia and lymphopenia are often seen early in influenza, but mild leukocytosis is more common. Brisk leukocytosis (more than 15,000/μl) suggests a secondary bacterial infection. Virus isolation in tissue culture or embryonated eggs is most readily accomplished with throat washings obtained before the sixth day of the illness. Hemagglutination-inhibition or complement-fixation tests are use-

TABLE 9.5–3. COMPARISON OF INFLUENZA VIRAL AND SECONDARY BACTERIAL PNEUMONIA

	Influenzal Pneumonia	Influenza with Bacterial Pneumonia
Onset	Seen early in illness, rapidly progressive	Several days after onset of influenza
Physical findings and chest x-ray	Diffuse infiltrates	Focal infiltrates Early pleural fluid (streptococci) Multiple cavities (staphylococci)
Sputum	Bloody, sparse bacteria and leukocytes	Purulent, many bacteria and leukocytes
White blood cell count	Often normal	Usually greater than 15,000/μl Polymorphonuclear leukocytosis
Erythrocyte sedimentation rate	Often normal	Usually increased
Prognosis	Mortality rate high, especially in patients with underlying disease (heart disease, chronic lung disease, pregnancy)	Responds to antibiotic therapy Greatest risk in patients with underlying cardiac or pulmonary disease

ful if both acute and convalescent sera are available. Virus isolation attempts are successful in only about 50 percent of the patients who develop serologic evidence of the illness.

Therapy

Most patients with influenza are given only supportive therapy. Several clinical studies show that amantadine in doses of 200 mg per day does lead to somewhat more rapid clinical improvement in persons infected with influenza A viruses. One study showed that 48 hours after treatment only 5 percent of college students treated with placebo were able to attend class, in contrast with 50 percent of those given amantadine. By 96 hours, however, over 90 percent of both groups were in class.[19] Amantadine is a mild reversible neurotoxin, and this is generally thought to outweigh its modest therapeutic effects for most patients. Elderly and debilitated patients, however, and those for whom quick return to health is important, should probably be treated with amantadine if it is known that the current epidemic strain belongs to group A. Amantadine is of no value for infections with influenza B. Codeine is particularly efficacious in alleviating myalgia, cough, and headache. Acetaminophen is useful but may make the patient more uncomfortable because of sweating and chilliness if it is given intermittently. Especially in children, aspirin should not be used because of the danger of Reye syndrome. Antibiotics are indicated when secondary bacterial complications develop, but do not influence the course of the viral illness and do not prevent bacterial complications. Sinusitis, otitis media, and purulent bronchitis are managed as discussed earlier. However, the onset of bronchopneumonia should be treated with a penicillinase-resistant semisynthetic penicillin, such as nafcillin, because many such cases are due to secondary staphylococcal infection. Cultures of the sputum and the blood should be done at the onset to determine the responsible organism, and therapy should be modified as appropriate. Such patients will of course need to be managed in the hospital, and until it is known that they are not coughing up *S. aureus*, they should be isolated. In addition to antibiotics, they will often require treatment for respiratory failure. Simple treatment is 24 or 28 percent oxygen by mask, humidification of the inspired air, nasotracheal suction, and postural drainage. Major crises may require tracheostomy and artificial ventilation.

Vaccination and Other Preventive Measures

It is easy to protect human volunteers against experimental challenge with influenza. Either formalinized whole virus vaccines or purified hemagglutinin (split virus) vaccines produce useful but not solid immunity. Split virus vaccines produce fewer side effects, especially in children, but are somewhat less effective stimuli of antibody production. Antibody responses are also influenced by previous experience with influenza infection; adults and older children usually require only one injection of vaccine, but children under 6

years usually need two. Provided that the vaccine virus is closely related to the epidemic strains, these vaccines also convey short-lived but useful immunity to wild-type influenza in the general population.

It is not practical to persuade the entire population every year to take a vaccine against an infection that is trivial in most people. Furthermore, in years in which the virus has a major antigenic shift, it probably would be impossible to make, test, distribute, and administer enough vaccine in time to abort the epidemic. Finally, the epidemic of Guillain-Barré syndrome following the swine flu immunization campaign of 1976 reminds us that no vaccine is free from side effects. For all these reasons, the current strategy is to vaccinate annually only that segment of the population likely to die of influenza. This includes persons older than 65 and people of any age who have chronic disease of the heart or lungs. Some physicians vaccinate all patients with any other chronic illness, but the evidence that this is useful is meager. Vaccination of healthcare workers also is recommended; it is hoped that they will remain available for work during an epidemic, and that they will not pass the virus to susceptible patients.

An adjunct in the control of influenza epidemics is the use of amantadine. There is clear evidence that this substance protects people against most influenza A strains if it is given before infection.[15] It can be given in a dose of 200 mg daily for 3 weeks after vaccination to provide protection while the antibody response is developing. Under epidemic circumstances, this can be very useful. Unfortunately, old people treated with amantadine have a fairly high incidence of (reversible) neurologic side effects.

Because the virus is widespread in a community during an epidemic, measures of isolation and quarantine are of little value. Crowding should be avoided, but measures that interfere with the normal activities of a community are not practical. Isolated populations may be protected during an epidemic by exclusion of visitors. During an epidemic, health authorities should give primary attention to minimizing complications in those who develop the disease.

REFERENCES

1. Asian Variant Influenza. Public Health Rep 73:99, 1958
2. Bluestone CD, Klein JO: Otitis media with effusion, atelectasis and eustachian tube dysfunction. In Bluestone CD, Stool SE (eds): Pediatric Otolaryngology. Philadelphia, WB Saunders, 1983, p 356
3. Cantekin EI, Mandell EM, Bluestone CD: Lack of efficacy of a decongestant-antihistamine combination for otitis media with effusion. N Engl J Med 308:297, 1983
4. Caplan ES, Hoyt NJ: Nosocomial sinusitis. JAMA 247:639, 1982
5. Evans FO Jr, Syndor JB, et al: Sinusitis of the maxillary antrum. N Engl J Med 293:735, 1975
6. Gwaltney JM: Virology of the middle ear. Ann Otol Rhinol Laryngol 80:365, 1971

7. Gwaltney JM, Syndor A, Sande MA: Etiology and antimicrobial treatment of acute sinusitis. Ann Otol Rhinol Laryngol 90:68, 1981
8. Haverkorn MJ, Valkenburg HA, Goslings WRO: Streptococcal pharyngitis in the general population. I. A controlled study of streptococcal pharyngitis and its complications in the Netherlands. II. The attack rate of rheumatic fever and acute glomerulonephritis in patients not treated with penicillin. J Infect Dis 124:339, 348, 1971
9. Idsoe O, Guthe T, et al: Nature and extent of penicillin side-reactions with particular reference to fatalities from anaphylactic shock. Bull WHO 38:159, 1968
10. Juselius H, Kaltiokallio K: Complications of acute and chronic otitis media in the antibiotic era. Acta Otolaryngol 74:445, 1972
11. Markowitz M, Gordis L: Rheumatic Fever, 2d ed. Philadelphia, WB Saunders, 1972
12. Matanoski GM, Price WH, Ferencz C: Epidemiology of streptococcal infections in rheumatic and non-rheumatic families. Am J Epidemiol 87:179, 1968
13. Monto AS, Ullman BM: Acute respiratory illness in an American community. JAMA 227:164, 1974
14. Norden CW, Callerance ML, Baum J: *Haemophilus influenzae* meningitis in an adult: A study of bactericidal antibodies. N Engl J Med 282:190, 1970
15. O'Donoghue JM, Ray CG, et al: Prevention of nosocomial influenza infection with amantidine. Am J Epidemiol 97:276, 1973
16. Pantell RH: Cost-effectiveness of pharyngitis management and prevention of rheumatic fever. Ann Intern Med 86:497, 1977
17. Russel WT: The epidemiology of diphtheria during the last 40 years. Medical Research Council: Special Report Series (London) 247:9, 1943
18. Tompkins DG, Boxerbau B, Liebman J: Long-term prognosis of rheumatic fever patients receiving regular intramuscular benzathine penicillin. Circulation 45:543, 1972
19. Van Voris LP, Belts RF, et al: Successful treatment of naturally occurring Influenza A/USSR/77 HINI. JAMA 245:1128, 1981
20. Wald ER, Milmoe GI, Bowen AD: Acute maxillary sinusitis in children. N Engl J Med 304:749, 1981
21. Weinstein L, LeFrock J: Does antimicrobial therapy of streptococcal pharyngitis or pyoderma alter the risk of glomerulonephritis? J Infect Dis 124:229, 1971

CHAPTER 9.6

Pneumonia

Patrick A. Murphy

Pneumonia poses some of the most fascinating diagnostic and therapeutic challenges in medicine. Acute inflammation in pulmonary tissue is usually caused by bacteria, and more than half of such cases are due to the pneumococcus. Even in patients presenting with pneumonia as the primary complaint, however, about half the cases are due to other organisms. Staphylococcal and gram-negative rod pneumonias carry a much worse prognosis than does pneumococcal pneumonia and require very different treatment. Furthermore, almost any bacterium can cause pneumonia on occasion; the list of exotic bacterial causes ranges from *Bacillus cereus* to *Pasteurella multocida*.

Pneumonia also may be caused by specialized bacteria, such as rickettsia and mycoplasmas, and in some circumstances by slow-growing organisms such as tubercle bacilli or *Nocardia*. Pneumonia due to viral infection is common; it seems likely that most cases are undiagnosed. Most pulmonary fungal infections are chronic, but there are exceptions. Even protozoa, such as *Pneumocystis carinii*, or helminths, such as *Ascaris lumbricoides*, may cause relatively acute pulmonary symptoms.

Finally, the clinical syndrome of fever and pulmonary infiltrate can also be due to a wide variety of noninfectious causes. Pulmonary embolism, allergic reactions to drugs or inhaled substances, aspiration pneumonia, and metastatic tumor are some of the possibilities.

Almost always, the available information is insufficient to make a precise diagnosis when the patient is first seen. Different organisms do tend to cause distinctive clinical syndromes, however, and a provisional diagnosis should be made on the basis of the clinical findings and rapidly obtainable laboratory results (Tables 9.6–1 and 9.6–2). Time must not be wasted in endless diagnostic maneuvers; unless bacterial pneumonia is thought to be improbable, the patient should be given antibiotics within an hour and a half of being seen. This chapter first deals with the various clinical patterns that may be seen in pneumonia and how to make an educated guess at the etiology. Second, it deals with the various techniques that can be used to firm up or alter the provisional diagnosis and how the common pneumonias should be managed.

PNEUMOCOCCAL PNEUMONIA

CLASSIC LOBAR PNEUMONIA

Lobar pneumonia is a localized disease; one lobe of one lung is consolidated, the remaining lobes are normal. It is true that sometimes more than one lobe is affected (double or triple pneumonia), but almost always there is one or more normal lobes. Most such cases are caused by the pneumococcus. The earliest manifestation is usually the abrupt onset of fever, with a shaking chill. Soon cough, purulent or rusty sputum, dyspnea, and pain in the side of the chest on inspiration or coughing supervene. Sometimes diaphragmatic pleurisy produces pain in the shoulder or in the upper abdomen.

On physical examination the patient appears acutely ill, febrile, often cyanotic, and has the characteristic physical signs of lobar consolidation. These include inspiratory lag and decreased respiratory excursions (splinting) of the involved hemithorax, with moderate percussion dullness, increased tactile fremitus, bronchial breath sounds, whispered pectoriloquy, and coarse inspiratory rales over the involved lobe. A pleural friction rub also may be heard over the area. Sometimes a sterile effusion develops along with the pneumonia; this will cause stony dullness to percussion and reduced-to-absent breath sounds. Frank empyema is unusual until the pneumonia has been established for a few days.

ATYPICAL PRESENTATIONS

Pneumococcal pneumonia is not always as easy to diagnose. Symptoms of fever, dyspnea, and pleuritic pain may precede physical or radiologic signs of pneumonia by as much as 24 hours. The earliest physical signs are fever and bronchial breathing; these suffice as the basis for a tentative diagnosis of pneumonia. In the elderly, pneumonia may cause little or no fever, and, especially in the presence of advanced emphysema, abnormal physical signs may be difficult to detect.[19] Often the most striking changes are delirium, stu-

TABLE 9.6–1. CLINICAL CLUES IN ETIOLOGIC DIAGNOSIS IN ACUTE PNEUMONIA

Etiologic Agent	Fever	Chills	Cough	Sputum	Other Features
Bacterial Pneumococcus (*Streptococcus pneumoniae*)	102–106F, usually sustained	Often single shaking chill at onset	Productive in 75% Pleuritic chest pain	Rusty, blood-streaked, mucopurulent	Preceding URI in many Herpes labialis frequent Lobar consolidation frequent
Staphylococcus aureus	Intermittent hectic, or sustained, 102–105F	Multiple	Pleuritic pain Often nonproductive when hematogenous in origin	Purulent, blood-streaked, occasionally gross hemoptysis	In infants, debilitated persons, or following influenza Lung abscess or pneumatocele
Group A β-hemolytic streptococci	Hectic, 104F or higher	Multiple	Productive Often with pleuritic pain	Purulent and bloody	Early pleural effusion and empyema common Often follows influenza or measles
Klebsiella pneumoniae (Friedländer bacillus)	Often remittent, 102–105F	Multiple	Productive Severe pleuritic pain	Thick, bloody, mucopurulent Gram stain very useful	Upper lobes; abscess Bulging fissure especially common in alcholics, diabetics
Haemophilus influenzae	Variable	Usually absent	Productive Wheezing common in children	Purulent Gram stain useful	Most common in alcholics or patients with chronic lung disease Lobar consolidation may occur
Bacteroides	101–104F	Multiple	Often not prominent	Gram-negative bacilli may be present on smear, fail to grow on aerobic media	1. Hematogenous pneumonia secondary to pelvic thrombophlebitis and bacteremia in young women Empyema not prominent 2. Aspiration pneumonia in older people Empyema often massive
Escherichia coli	100–103F	Multiple	Prominent	Thick, purulent, with gram-negative bacilli readily seen on smear	Usually associated with preexisting chronic debilitating illness Lower lobes almost always involved
Proteus	101–104F	Multiple	Prominent	Thick, purulent, with small gram-negative bacilli on smear	Usually superimposed on chronic lung disease Dense lobar consolidation, with multiple abscess formation
Pseudomonas	Reversal of diurnal temperature curve	Multiple	Prominent	Copious yellow or green sputum with gram-negative bacilli on smear	Usually diffuse bronchopneumonia in immunosuppressed patients
Francisella tularensis	102–105F, sustained	Variable	Often not prominent	Generally scanty Gram stain of little value	Previous exposure to rabbits, rodents, insect vectors Sometimes cutaneous ulcer Often severe toxicity
Legionella species	102–105F, sustained	Often	Dry early, productive later	Organisms sometimes visible with fluorescent antibody	Elderly men, common source epidemics, nosocomial. Delirium, diarrhea, shock

(continued)

TABLE 9.6–1. CLINICAL CLUES IN ETIOLOGIC DIAGNOSIS IN ACUTE PNEUMONIA (*Continued*)

Etiologic Agent	Fever	Chills	Cough	Sputum	Other Features
Mycoplasma *Mycoplasma pneumoniae* (Eaton agent)	101–104F	In less than 25%	Persistent, hacking nonproductive Pleurisy rare	Scant, mucoid	Physical findings often unimpressive Insidious onset Complement fixation test positive Tetracyclines and erythromycin effective
Chlamydiae *C. psittaci*	Variable, 101–105F	Shaking chills in one third	Dry, hacking, pleurisy rare	Small amount blood-streaked sputum	Acquired from birds Tetracyclines effective CF test positive
Rickettsiae *Coxiella burnetii* (Q fever)	Up to 105F	Common	Cough, and pleurisy late manifestations	Scant	Primarily a systemic illness Headache, myalgia CF test positive
Mycobacteria *Mycobacterium tuberculosis*	Usually under 102F, remittent or intermittent	May occur	Variable	Varies with stage of disease	History of exposure or previous tuberculous infection
Virus Influenza	Up to 105F	Suggestive of secondary bacterial infection	1. Dry cough 2. Productive cough	1. Scant or bloody 2. Purulent or bloody	1. True influenzal pneumonia, heliotrope, cyanosis, marked dyspnea 2. Secondary bacterial pneumonia, shaking chills, prostration
Varicella	Up to 105F	Rare	Usually harsh, dry cough, cyanosis	Scant (bloody)	Pulmonary involvement in 10% of adults with chickenpox Lesions may be miliary
Measles	Up to 105F	Rare	1. Dry 2. Productive	1. Scant 2. Copious, purulent	1. True measles giant cell pneumonia in persons with defective cell-mediated immunity 2. Secondary bacterial infection
Respiratory syncytial virus	Often mild	Rare	Dry	Scant	Children primarily, obstructive bronchiolitis
Adenovirus	Often mild	Rare	Variable	Scant	Most frequent in military recruits, often pharyngitis also
Fungi *Histoplasma capsulatum*	Variable	Rare	Usually nonproductive	Scant	Contact with bird droppings Culture and serologic evidence Self-limiting course
Coccidioides immitis	Variable	Common	Nonproductive, poorly localized chest pain	Scant	Often asymptomatic or flu-like Usually self-limited A wide range of pulmonary syndromes occur Erythema nodosum southwestern U.S.

(continued)

TABLE 9.6–1. CLINICAL CLUES IN ETIOLOGIC DIAGNOSIS IN ACUTE PNEUMONIA (*Continued*)

Etiologic Agent	Fever	Chills	Cough	Sputum	Other Features
Fungi (*Cont.*)					
Cryptococcus neo-formans	Usually low-grade	Rare	Often prominent	Scant	Pulmonary disease often silent, chronic, and not detected until meningitis appears Contact with pigeons
Aspergillus fumigatus	Up to 105F	Rare	Cough and pleurisy late manifestations	Scant, but smear shows diagnostic branching hyphae	Usually occurs in patients on steroid or immunosuppressive therapy (e.g., postrenal transplant)

por, congestive heart failure, or unexplained prostration. Unless pneumonia is actively sought in such patients, the diagnosis will be missed. Alcoholic patients may also present with fever and prostration out of proportion to the physical signs or with delirium tremens. One should remember that *Klebsiella pneumoniae* is not infrequently the cause of lobar pneumonia in alcoholics.

RECURRENT PNEUMOCOCCAL PNEUMONIA

Recurrent pneumonias often indicate underlying diseases, either local or systemic. Repeated bouts of pneumonia in the same area, and slow resolution of pneumonia, suggest bronchostenosis or bronchiectasis. In this circumstance, bronchoscopy should be done first, followed by a bronchogram if necessary. If bronchostenosis is found, determination of the etiology (by sputum cytology, culture for tubercle bacilli, bronchoscopic biopsy) is of greatest importance because the condition may be an early manifestation of a curable but potentially lethal disease (e.g., bronchogenic carcinoma, tuberculosis). Bronchiectasis should usually be managed by regular postural drainage with antibiotics as needed for exacerbations. Occasionally, segmental resection may be desirable.

Recurrent bouts of pneumonia in different sites should suggest systemic disease, such as systemic lupus erythematosus (SLE), or impaired immunologic defense mechanisms, as seen in patients with multiple myeloma. Early etiologic diagnosis and therapy are especially urgent when pneumonia occurs in association with such systemic disease. Whenever there is a question whether acute disease is due to acute bacterial infection or to underlying illness (e.g., SLE, polyarteritis), it is reasonable to manage the patient as though acute bacterial pneumonia were present.

PNEUMONIA DUE TO OTHER ORGANISMS

STAPHYLOCOCCAL PNEUMONIA[3]

Staphylococcal pneumonia is responsible for about one quarter of severe postinfluenzal pneumonia and occurs sporadically in individuals with impaired resistance to infection. It is relatively more common in old people than in the general population. Multiple chills and hectic fever are common, and the sputum is often bloody. Because the infection is necrotizing, abscesses occur early. In children, these abscesses may rupture into the pleura, producing the classic pyopneumothorax. Staphylococcal pneumonia may be hematogenous; the infiltrates being infected pulmonary emboli. The physical signs are less prominent than the radiographic findings, and there is usually an infected skin site that was the portal of entry. Often the patient is an intravenous drug abuser or has had an indwelling venous catheter for many days.

GROUP A STREPTOCOCCAL PNEUMONIA[2]

Group A streptococcal pneumonia was a common complication of influenza in the 1918 epidemic. It also occurs in a minute proportion of cases of streptococcal sore throat. There is early involvement of the lymphatic vessels, which become blocked by masses of organisms and inflammatory cells and are visible as streaks in the radiograph and as white cords at the autopsy table. Thin, bilateral pleural effusions accumulate very rapidly and usually contain streptococci. High fever, multiple chills, and severe bilateral pleural pain are characteristic.

KLEBSIELLA PNEUMONIA[7,15]

Klebsiella (Friedländer) pneumonia is classically a severe necrotizing upper lobar pneumonia seen most commonly in alcoholics. It may also affect diabetic people, old people, and persons with left heart failure, and often there is a great deal of bronchopneumonic as well as lobar involvement. The onset is usually fulminant with very viscid sputum, often grossly bloody. Sometimes there is a subacute course of days or weeks, and the illness may be mistaken for tuberculosis. The classic radiographic signs are bulging of the fissure and central cavitation, but they are not diagnostic. Healing is slow, and scarring is severe.

HAEMOPHILUS INFLUENZAE PNEUMONIA[4]

Haemophilus influenzae is the most common bacterium associated with acute respiratory failure in patients with chronic bronchitis. Many of the strains from these patients are noncapsulated, and it is uncertain that the bacteria in the sputum really cause the acute deterioration. There is no doubt that *H. influenzae* causes lobar or bronchopneumonia on occasion, because it has been isolated from the blood and/or empyemas in such patients. There are no distinguishing clinical features of this pneumonia.

PNEUMONIA DUE TO OTHER GRAM-NEGATIVE BACILLI[7,15]

Enterobacteria such as *Escherichia coli* or *Serratia marcescens* have caused an increasing proportion of nosocomial pneumonias during the last 2 decades. Most patients have had major operations or suffered from grave medical illnesses. Many were being artificially ventilated or had been given antibiotics. Similar cases may be caused by other gram-negative rods such as *Pseudomonas aeruginosa* or *Acinetobacter* species. These organisms are endemic in hospitals, are spread from one patient to another by the staff, are commonly

TABLE 9.6–2. LABORATORY STUDIES PERFORMED IN CASES OF PNEUMONIA

Etiologic Agent	Sputum Smear	Sputum Culture	Blood Culture	WBC	Chest Radiograph
Pneumococcus (*Streptococcus pneumoniae*)	Many gram-positive, lancet-shaped diplococci, often in sheets	Usually positive if sputum immediately plated on blood agar	Positive in over 20% of patients	Usually elevated (10,000–30,000/μl) but leukopenia may be present (alcoholics, overwhelming infections)	May be negative in early stages despite clear-cut clinical signs and symptoms of pneumonia. Infiltrates apt to be bronchopneumonic rather than lobar in unusually susceptible individuals
Staphylococcus aureus	Clusters of gram-positive cocci, often intracellular, usually present. May be absent if pneumonia is hematogenous	Usually positive	Frequently positive	Usually elevated (10,000–30,000/μl) but leukopenia may be present in overwhelming infections	Bronchopneumonic pattern with multiple infiltrates and early abscess formation. Pneumatoceles and pyopneumothorax common in children
Group A β-hemolytic *Streptococcus*	Of little value, since streptococci are abundantly present in normal flora	Usually positive	Often positive	Generally high (20,000–30,000/μl)	Extensive pleural effusions often present early. Frequent confluent involvement of two lobes
Klebsiella pneumoniae (Friedländer bacillus)	Gram stain of major value, showing gram-negative rods, often in pairs	Almost always positive	Positive in less than 20% of patients	Generally high (20,000–40,000/μl) but leukopenia may be present in overwhelming infections	Usually upper or right middle lobe involvement. Early abscess formation common
Haemophilus influenzae	Gram stain useful in showing small gram-negative coccobacilli, often in clumps, associated with gram-negative threadlike forms	Frequently positive if immediately plated on chocolate agar and incubated in CO_2 jar	Rarely positive in adults	Generally high (15,000–30,000/μl)	Frequently bronchopneumonic infiltrates, but may show lobar pattern
Legionella pneumophila	Gram stain usually negative for organisms. Many pus cells. Organisms may stain with fluorescent antibody	May be positive on charcoal yeast extract agar	Negative (almost always)	High (15,000–30,000/μl)	Alveolar infiltrates, initially patchy, becoming confluent
Bacteroides	Small, gram-negative bacilli usually seen	Negative unless anaerobic cultures carefully performed	Generally negative, except when pneumonia is associated with pelvic disease	Generally moderately elevated (15,000–20,000/μl)	In older people or alcoholics, pleural effusions early, often massive, generally obscure underlying bronchopneumonia
Escherichia coli	Gram stain of major value, consistently showing gram-negative bacilli	Almost always positive	Often positive	Generally high, with shift to left	Lower lobe bronchopneumonic infiltrates almost always present
Proteus	Predominance of small gram-negative bacilli	Almost always positive, persisting for days after appropriate antimicrobial therapy	Rarely positive	Generally high (15,000–30,000/μl)	Dense pneumonic infiltrates, generally with multiple abscesses
Pseudomonas	Gram-negative bacilli prominent	Uniformly positive, with organisms persisting during antimicrobial therapy	Initially negative. May be positive later in course of illness	Often normal early in illness, with later rise to 15,000–20,000/μl range	Diffuse bronchopneumonia with nodular infiltrates, frequently with multiple small abscesses

(continued)

TABLE 9.6–2. LABORATORY STUDIES PERFORMED IN CASES OF PNEUMONIA (*Continued*)

Etiologic Agent	Sputum Smear	Sputum Culture	Blood Culture	WBC	Chest Radiograph
Francisella (Pasteurella) tularensis	Generally not helpful	Positive if plated on cysteine-blood agar Cultural material hazardous to laboratory personnel	Almost always negative	Usually within normal limits, but marked leukocytosis (>20,000/μl) may occur	Perihilar infiltrate characteristic, often with enlarged hilar nodes
Mycoplasma pneumoniae	Not helpful	Positive in over 50% of cases if immediately plated on appropriate diphasic media, but not helpful in time to be of clinical value	Negative	Usually below 10,000, but up to 20,000/μl in 10% of clinical cases	Infiltrates may be perihilar or lobar Two or more lobes involved in one third of cases
Chlamydia psittaci Psittacosis Ornithosis	Not helpful	Not helpful	Negative	Usually within normal limits	Perihilar infiltrates most common
Coxiella burnetti (Q fever)	Negative	Not helpful	Not helpful	Variable	Patchy infiltrates, generally perihilar in distribution
Mycobacterium tuberculosis	Acid-fast stain positive with cavitary disease, but often negative with early pneumonia	Positive, but only after 4–6 weeks incubation	Negative	Often normal with acute pneumonia or with cavitary disease	Cavitary disease: upper lobe involvement may be confused with *Klebsiella pneumonia*
Influenza	Not helpful	Not helpful in time to be of clinical value	Negative	Moderate leukocytes (10,000–20,000/μl) may occur	Interstitial infiltrates, often in fine, widespread pattern
Varicella	Not helpful	Not helpful	Negative	Usually within normal limits	Same as influenza
Rubeola	Not helpful	Not helpful	Negative	Usually within normal limits	Same as influenza
Respiratory syncytial virus	Not helpful	Not helpful	Negative	Usually within normal limits	Same as influenza
Adenovirus	Not helpful	Not helpful	Negative	Usually within normal limits	Same as influenza
Histoplasma capsulatum	Intracellular organisms seen on PAS stain Also seen, less clearly, on Gram stain	Positive, often 4–8 days, on Sabouraud agar	Rarely positive	Variable, but generally within normal limits	Nonspecific, but often multiple, diffuse pulmonary infiltrates
Coccidioides immitis	Characteristic spherules with endospores after treatment with 20% potassium hydroxide	Positive on Sabourard agar but only after 5–10 days	Not helpful	Variable, but generally within normal limits	Multiple infiltrates and prominent hilar lymphadenopathy common Pleural effusions frequent
Cryptococcus neoformans	Often positive, with characteristic spherical yeast-forms (5–15μm) seen on India ink preparation	Positive on Sabouraud agar but only after 5–10 days	Often positive	Variable, but generally within normal limits	Nonspecific Usually dense, localized infiltration of basilar segments
Blastomyces dermatitidis	Often positive, with characteristic, thick-walled, single budding yeast cells of variable size (4–24μm)	Positive on blood or Sabourard agar, but only after 5–10 days	Negative	Variable, but generally within normal limits	Nonspecific Infiltration may be fine and diffuse, or well-localized and dense Thin-walled cavities may be present
Aspergillus fumigatus	May show segmented mycelia bearing small round spores, but frequently negative	Positive on Sabouraud agar, but of diagnostic value only if obtained directly from infected segment	Negative	Usually affects people with neutropenia	Initially multiple infiltrates, with later cavitation

resistant to antibiotics, and may be introduced directly down the trachea by ventilatory equipment. Cases of community acquired pneumonia due to these organisms also may occur in the elderly, in patients with chronic lung disease, in diabetics, and in alcholics. In the nosocomial cases, colonization of the throat or sputum by gram-negative rods usually precedes pneumonia by several days.

Previous colonization also may occur in chronic bronchitis or those with cystic fibrosis. In these cases, the pneumonia is generally caused by the organism(s) most prominent in sputum collected a day or two before the onset of pneumonia. The identity and antibiotic susceptibility pattern of the most probable organisms are, therefore, often available from the patient's chart. This is a much better guide than making guesses from the appearance of the sputum smear or the chest radiograph.

TULAREMIC PNEUMONIA[12]

In tularemic pneumonia there is usually a history of shooting and skinning rabbits in the patient's background. The disease is bacteremic, with high fever and severe systemic toxicity, and the pneumonia may be more evident on the radiograph than in the patient. Bilateral hilar adenopathy is suggestive.

LEGIONELLA PNEUMONIA[6,20]

Legionella pneumonia causes many different clinical pictures, and pneumonia is only one of them. As originally described, it was the cause of a severe pneumonia in middle aged and elderly males. Most of them smoked and drank heavily. The pneumonia was associated with widespread, patchy alveolar consolidation. Anoxia was severe, and mortality was high. The sputum contained pus cells, but few or no organisms. Patients frequently had evidence of extrapulmonary involvement: diarrhea and abdominal pain, delirium and stupor, jaundice, renal failure, and shock.

It is now possible to grow the organism and to identify cases by serologic means. By retrospective serologic surveys, it has been established that *Legionella* infection is a quite common cause of community-acquired pneumonia. In healthy people, the pneumonia is often mild. Several epidemics have involved acute febrile illness without pneumonia (Pontiac fever). Nosocomial epidemics affect primarily the patients, not the staff, and mortality may be high. The organism grows in water; epidemics may arise from point sources in cooling towers, air conditioners, or shower heads. There is general agreement that erythromycin is the most effective antibiotic in the treatment of this infection.

FUNGAL PNEUMONIA

The most common fungal pneumonia is acute primary infection with *Histoplasma capsulatum* or *Coccidioides immitis*. Other fungi, such as *Blastomyces dermatitidis,* may produce a similar picture. There may be a history of exposure, such as a visit to the San Joaquin Valley or cleaning out a chicken coop. In this case, several friends or family members are often affected also.

The dominant clinical feature is a spectacularly abnormal chest radiograph with generalized nodular and linear infiltrates and unilateral or bilateral hilar adenopathy. There may be the fungal equivalent of a primary (Ghon) complex. The patient is not usually particularly ill, although fever may be high. Cough is not prominent; there is little or no sputum, and dyspnea, cyanosis, and chest pain are uncommon. Many such patients never see a doctor and are diagnosed retrospectively by the presence of calcified nodules on the chest radiograph. In those with severe acute symptoms, the sputum often does not show fungi, and the diagnosis must be established serologically or by culture. Most people with acute fungal pneumonia recover uneventfully whether or not they are treated with amphotericin B.

Chronic fungal infections may follow the pattern of tuberculosis and may be complicated by bacterial pneumonias in the same way. The sputum smear usually does show fungi, spherules in coccidioidomycosis, small intracellular yeasts in histoplasmosis, and rather large yeasts showing the broad-based bud in blastomycosis. In immunosuppressed persons, many saprophytic or commensal fungi may cause pneumonia. As a rule, the sputum is unhelpful, and diagnosis requires the examination of lung tissue.

MYCOPLASMAL PNEUMONIA[13]

Mycoplasma pneumoniae is a common cause of pulmonary infections in children and young adults, especially in the age group of 5 to 35 years. These infections may occur sporadically or in epidemics that last months. Epidemics are especially common in school-aged children, within institutions, and within families. About 10 percent of infected patients have pneumonia, and 70 to 80 percent show evidence of tracheobronchitis, presumably reflecting a predilection of the organism for the respiratory mucosal cells. Characteristic features of mycoplasma pneumonia are fever, cough, malaise and a radiograph showing segmental bronchopneumonia in a lower lobe. The cough may be nonproductive or it may cause mucoid sputum that shows mononuclear cells and polymorphonuclear cells with no predominant likely pathogen on Gram stain. Most patients are not seriously ill and do not require hospitalization. Occasional complications include bullous myringitis, skin rashes (maculopapular, vesicular, erythema multiforme, erythema nodosum), intravascular hemolysis, neurologic complications (meningoencephalitis, Guillain-Barré syndrome, cerebellar ataxia, psychosis), myocarditis, and pericarditis. The organism can be recovered with special media, but few clinical laboratories offer this service. The cold agglutinin assay is usually positive with titers exceeding 1:128 in more severely ill individuals. The most specific serologic test is a complement fixation assay that shows a significant titer rise with sequentially collected specimens in up to 80 percent. The preferred treatment is with erythromycin or tetracycline; agents that are active against the cell walls of bacteria, such as penicillins and cephalosporins, are ineffective against *M. pneumoniae*.

PNEUMONIA IN SPECIAL CLINICAL SETTINGS

ASPIRATION PNEUMONIA[1,11]

In a sense, the vast majority of pneumonias are due to aspiration, as the pathogens are inhaled. The term is confined to the diseases resulting from aspiration of macroscopic quantities of material from the upper airway or of gastric contents. Two distinct syndromes occur. Gastric juice causes a chemical burn of the bronchial mucosa, which leads to leaky pulmonary capillaries and the loss of albuminous fluid from the plasma into the alveoli. Also, pulmonary surfactant is destroyed, and there is a progressive atelectasis. These processes are noninfective and are therefore unaffected by antibiotics. Aspiration of gastric juices carries a high mortality, despite expert respiratory support.

The second syndrome is due to infection; it may follow the first process if the patient survives, or it may occur independently. The upper airway normally contains large numbers of anaerobic bacteria that are of low pathogenicity. If grossly infected material is inhaled, however, these bacteria can cause a synergic necrotizing infection. The area of the lung affected is determined by the patient's position at the time the aspiration occurs. In the supine position, the most dependent areas are the apical segments of the lower lobes, and the posterior segments of the upper lobes. These are the areas most commonly involved. Right-sided involvement is more common than is left, allegedly because the right main bronchus is more or less a direct continuation of the trachea.

Aspiration pneumonia is uncommon in normal people except following anesthesia. Alcoholics and epileptics are classic victims,

as are those with neurologic diseases that impair swallowing and those with achalasia or other causes of esophageal obstruction. Patients without these predisposing features generally have grossly neglected teeth with extensive periodontal disease.

The aspiration may or may not be witnessed or remembered. The symptoms include fever, cough, sputum, dyspnea, and pleuritic pain. The course is subacute or even chronic, and the patient wastes rapidly. The sputum and breath have a characteristically foul smell. The chest shows evidence of segmental consolidation. It should be noted that an identical syndrome can follow bronchial obstruction from foreign body or tumor.

Sputum in these patients shows many pus cells, and a mixed bacterial flora. Sputum cultures are hard to interpret, because they generally show mixed respiratory flora. Cultures of transtracheal aspirates, however, confirm the presence in the lung of a mixed population of anaerobic and aerobic bacteria, and the same mixtures of organisms are recovered from pleural fluid. Treatment directed against the anaerobes generally leads to recovery. Transtracheal aspiration is a dangerous procedure in nonexpert hands, and patients are generally treated without a precise bacteriologic diagnosis.

PNEUMONIA IN PERSONS WITH CHRONIC LUNG DISEASE

Persons with chronic bronchitis, bronchiectasis, cystic fibrosis, and certain other chronic lung diseases start out with grossly impaired pulmonary function. They normally have productive cough and dyspnea, abnormal physical signs in the chest, and abnormal chest radiographs. Furthermore, relatively mild infections may throw these patients into acute respiratory failure, and because they have often been treated with antibiotics, they may be infected with resistant pathogens such as staphylococci or gram-negative rods. The most helpful symptoms and signs are fever, malaise, and new infiltrates on the chest radiograph.

PNEUMONIA IN IMMUNOCOMPROMISED HOSTS[18]

Persons with impaired host defense mechanisms include renal transplant recipients who are taking corticosteroids, cyclosporin A, or azathioprine, and those with neoplastic diseases who are taking various cytotoxic drugs, and often steroids as well. Such patients are prone to infection, and pulmonary infections form about one quarter of the total. Pneumonia in these patients shows many differences from pneumonia in normal people, and the management is totally different.

The organisms usually responsible for pneumonia are gram-negative rods and staphylococci. Why the pneumococcus is uncommon in these people is not clear. A sizable proportion of cases is due to viruses, but many are due to herpesviruses rather than influenza and adenoviruses. A numerically minor but very important group of cases is caused by *Pneumocystis carinii*. Fungal pneumonia is much more likely to be due to *Aspergillus* or *Candida* species than to the fungi pathogenic for normal people. These patients also may have pulmonary infiltrates secondary to infarction, tumor, or sensitivity to drugs.

The symptoms and signs of pneumonia are muted. Fever is almost constant, but cough and sputum are often absent. Dyspnea, tachypnea, and cyanosis are usually present, however. There may be little or no dullness to percussion, and on auscultation there may be only harsh breath sounds or minor degrees of bronchial breathing. Even the radiograph may be clear and may remain so. The reason for the dearth of symptoms and signs is probably that the patients have few or no inflammatory cells and cannot mount a local response. Lastly, bacterial pneumonia in these people progresses with appalling speed. The mortality in most large series treated in good hospitals is around 40 percent. Fungal and pneumocystis pneumonia are a little slower but are inevitably fatal without treatment. The logic of management is, therefore,

1. To culture blood, sputum, and pleural fluid if available
2. To put the patient on large doses of antibiotics covering both staphylococci and gram-negative rods
3. Unless there is clinical improvement within 48 hours, to add amphotericin B to the antibiotics and to pursue a tissue diagnosis of the infecting organism by whatever means is necessary

It is usual to escalate from transtracheal aspiration to endobronchial brushings and biopsy to open lung biopsy. Needle biopsy of the lung has largely been abandoned because of problems with inadequate samples, bleeding, and pneumothorax. There are, however, a number of centers that have obtained satisfactory results with transthoracic needle aspiration.

INTERSTITIAL PNEUMONIA[13,20]

Interstitial pneumonia results from infection of the alveolar walls and the spaces between them. In theory the alveoli do not contain exudate, but pathologic examination shows alveolar involvement in many cases thought by clinicians to be interstitial. It usually affects segments of the lung, but can affect a whole lobe and may be generalized. Often, consolidation occurs in one segment, clears there, and then affects another segment. Because the infiltrate is interstitial, there may be little or nothing abnormal on auscultation. The most common infectious causes are viruses, especially influenza and adenoviruses. *M. pneumoniae,* Q fever, and the bacillus of Legionnaires disease are all treatable causes of the syndrome, however. In immunosuppressed patients, interstitial pneumonia is suggestive of *P. carinii* infection. The most common radiographic finding here is "ground glass" infiltrates spreading from both hila.

Most patients with interstitial pneumonia due to infection give an acute history. Fever and cough either develop abruptly or are preceded by a few days of upper respiratory tract symptoms. Dyspnea and cyanosis are not usually marked, and pleural pain and effusion are uncommon, although not unknown. Typically, there is a distressing, hacking cough but little or no sputum. As a group, the patients are less ill than those with bacterial pneumonias.

In epidemic circumstances, the cause of the prevalent pneumonia may be known. Patients may give significant historical items, such as exposure to birds (*Chlamydia psittaci*) or cattle (*Coxiella burnetii*). Gram stains of the sputum show few or no leukocytes and no dominant bacteria. This is useful negative information, but a positive diagnosis can only be made by isolating the organism or by serologic means. Neither is immediately helpful, and the patient must be managed by clinical judgment.

LABORATORY STUDIES

All patients with pneumonia should have a Gram stain of the sputum, cultures of blood and sputum for bacteria, a white blood cell count (WBC) and differential, and a chest radiograph. If the patient does well some of these will prove superfluous, but they may be invaluable if the initial diagnosis was wrong. Usually, the specimens are taken, the radiograph is performed, and preliminary results such as Gram stains of sputum, WBC and differential counts are obtained before starting treatment. Clinical judgment will determine the process: If the patient is desperately ill, specimens can be taken immediately and examined after treatment has been started. The chest radiograph is a notorious cause of delay and can also be done later.

SPUTUM SMEAR

The specimen must be sputum; the physician should personally watch the patient cough and select a purulent sample for examina-

tion. Heat fixation of the slide is not usually necessary, and it impairs the assessment of cellular morphology. Several smears should be made and some unstained ones kept for later examination if necessary. The best indication that a specimen of sputum is authentic is the presence of alveolar macrophages; reasonable evidence is that it contains polymorphonuclear cells and a fairly uniform bacterial population. Mixed bacterial populations in genuine sputum suggest aspiration. The presence of epithelial cells and mixed bacteria means that the specimen is saliva.

In bacterial pneumonia, sheets of the responsible pathogen are usually seen, because organisms causing pneumonia are usually present in sputum at concentrations of about 10^8/ml (essentially never less than 10^6/ml). The smear is least useful for the diagnosis of pneumococcal pneumonia; this is because morphologically similar bacteria are common in the upper airway and because pneumococci disappear quickly from the sputum with antibiotic therapy. If sheets of extracellular diplococci are seen, pneumococcal pneumonia is probable, but their absence is uninterpretable. However, if polyvalent anticapsular pneumococcal antiserum is available ("Omniserum"), the diagnosis can be ruled in or out with better than 90 percent accuracy by doing a Quellung reaction on the sputum.

The real importance of performing a Gram stain of the sputum is to look for staphylococci and gram-negative rods. Staphylococci are characteristically round, occur in clumps, and are often seen inside the cytoplasm of leukocytes. Gram-negative rods are extracellular; short, fat rods suggest *Klebseilla;* long thin ones suggest pseudomonas, and coccobacilli suggest *H. influenzae.* However, it is unwise to rely on morphology to make a bacteriologic diagnosis; the patient should be treated for all the possibilities until cultures are available.

In pneumonia due to viruses and specialized bacteria such as mycoplasmas, the sputum shows few or no leukocytes and bacteria. As a rule, cells containing inclusion bodies or other obvious evidence of viral infection are also absent. Such cells may be demonstrable by the use of specific fluorescent antisera, however. Fluorescent antibody may also be used to demonstrate *Legionella* in sputum.

If sputum is not available, one must use clinical judgment about how far to pursue it. It would be absurd to do a transtracheal aspiration because a healthy young man with influenza has a segmental infiltrate. In an obtunded patient with bacterial pneumonia, it may be essential.

SPUTUM CULTURE

Sputum culture is usually positive in the more common bacterial pneumonias if proper cultural techniques are employed (Table 9.6–2). It must be realized, however, that sputum is collected through the mouth and is invariably contaminated with mouth flora, which may include many of the common causes of pneumonia. In addition, many patients with chronic bronchitis carry a resident population of bacteria in the tracheobronchial tree even when they are well. The mere presence of an organism in sputum cultures, even if the numbers are large, is not evidence of pneumonia caused by that organism.

In pneumococcal pneumonia, the sputum culture is often negative. The pneumococcus is a relatively fragile microorganism and may die if the specimen is allowed to sit for several hours before being streaked; it may also be overgrown by other organisms if the plate is not examined within 24 hours. It disappears irretrievably if even one dose of antibiotic has been given before the specimen was collected. Staphylococci and most gram-negative rods are less fastidious, and sputum cultures are usually positive. Special cultural techniques are required for *Francisella tularensis* and *Legionella pneumophila,* so the laboratory should be alerted if these organisms are suspected. Cultures of mycoplasma and of viral respiratory pathogens rarely yield positive results in time to be of therapeutic value. Likewise, fungus cultures seldom yield useful

diagnostic information in less than 4 or 5 days and are of little help in the early differential diagnosis of the pneumonia patient (Table 9.6–2).

BLOOD CULTURES

The advantage of blood culture is that if an organism grows from the blood (or from pleural fluid), there is no doubt about its pathogenicity. Up to 50 percent of pneumococcal pneumonias are bacteremic; in other bacterial pneumonias the figure is 20 percent or less. Blood culture is of no value in viral or rickettsial pneumonias.

LEUKOCYTE COUNT

Bacterial pneumonia is almost always accompanied by a brisk neutrophilic leukocytosis with a left shift. Low leukocyte counts occur in two circumstances: The patient may have none because of a disease or its treatment, or he or she may have such overwhelming infection that the marrow reserve of granulocytes has been exhausted. In the first case, the neutrophil count is simply low; in the second, the total count of neutrophils is low, but the proportion of immature forms is very high and the left shift very marked. The combination of low count and gross left shift is particularly likely to occur in alcoholics, elderly persons, and others whose bone marrow reserves of neutrophils are lower than normal. In the past it denoted a bad prognosis, but this is less true with antibiotic therapy.

Viral, rickettsial, and fungal pneumonias are usually associated with normal or low neutrophil counts, and there is no left shift. However, exceptions occur, and neutrophil counts in excess of 20,000 per μl with left shift have been seen in cases of pure influenzal bronchopneumonia. Traditionally, tuberculosis is associated with a normal neutrophil count, an elevated lymphocyte count if the prognosis is good, and an elevated monocyte count if the prognosis is bad.

THE CHEST RADIOGRAPH

The chest radiograph is an indispensable component of the evaluation for patients with suspected pneumonia. Virtually all patients show an infiltrate which is usually present at the time of initial evaluation and nearly always present within 24 hours after the onset of symptoms. Nevertheless, this examination shows considerable limitations in distinguishing between likely etiologic agents.[16]

The chest radiograph can suggest or confirm an etiologic diagnosis, but by itself it is insufficient to be more than suggestive. The features associated with bacterial pneumonia are, in descending order of reliability, cavitation, pleural effusion, lobar consolidation, bulging of the fissure, multiple small abscesses, segmental consolidation, and bilateral involvement. For viral pneumonia, the features are nodular infiltrates, diffuse involvement, reticular infiltrates, prominent bronchovascular structures, perihilar pneumonia, involvement of new areas, and hilar adenopathy.

Despite the overall variability in appearances, some bacteria do produce classical radiographic changes most of the time. Pneumococcal pneumonia usually shows a homogeneous lobar or segmented consolidation. Staphylococcal pneumonia is usually bilateral and basal, and abscesses usually form sooner or later. Streptococcal pneumonia is the only pneumonia in which early massive pleural effusions are common. *Klebsiella* pneumonia usually occurs in the upper lobes or the right middle lobe and is particularly likely to be associated with cavitation and the bulging fissure sign.

In viral, rickettsial, and mycoplasmal pneumonias, the appearances are generally similar, as described above. Two features most unsuggestive of a viral etiology are lobar consolidation and abscess formation. However, lobar consolidation is not uncommon in mycoplasmal pneumonia.

Apical cavitation is typical of chronic tuberculous and fungal infection.

CONDITIONS THAT MAY BE MISTAKEN FOR PNEUMONIA

A list of these conditions is given in Table 9.6–3, and a few are discussed below.

PULMONARY INFARCTION

Pulmonary infarction is very common and causes symptoms and signs that may be identical to those of bacterial pneumonia—fever, cough, bloody sputum, dyspnea, pleuritic pain, and basal consolidation. If the patient has recently had an operation or a baby or has a leg in a cast, the diagnosis may be easy. However, pulmonary infarctions may occur in young women in perfect health, especially if they use oral contraceptives.

The sputum may contain leukocytes but shows few or no bacteria. Cultures of blood and sputum are negative, although this is not immediately useful. There is usually no leukocytosis in pulmonary infarction, but this cannot be relied on. The chest radiograph may show basal segmental infiltrates with pleural effusions, but commonly the appearances cannot be distinguished from pneumonia.

The most useful investigations for differentiating pneumonia from infarction are the blood gases, the test for fibrin degradation products in the blood, and the pulmonary scan. Most patients with infarction have a low PO_2, often less than 60 mm Hg, and enough hyperventilation to produce a low PCO_2 as well. The plasma almost always contains fibrin degradation products. Segmental basal defects on the scan are associated with a high probability of pulmonary embolism. The definitive test is pulmonary angiography, but newer scans may make it of historical interest only. There are reports that gallium-67 citrate scans are positive in pneumonia and negative in infarction. Newer and more exciting scans use ^{11}CO or $^{15}CO_2$. Both these gases are very soluble in blood, and are normally rapidly removed from the lungs. In pulmonary infarction, the stagnant column of blood beyond the arterial block remains as a hot spot.

If there is real doubt as to the diagnosis, it may be safest to treat the patient for both conditions until the diagnosis is clear.

FRACTURED RIBS

Fractured ribs cause severe pain on inspiration but few or none of the other symptoms of pneumonia. Fractures may occur secondary to coughing or to metastases and may happen spontaneously in elderly people. They are easily detected by local tenderness and by exacerbation of the pain when one presses on the sternum; however, they may be difficult to see on radiographs.

TABLE 9.6–3. CAUSES OF PULMONARY INFILTRATES RESEMBLING PNEUMONIA CAUSED BY MICROORGANISMS

Condition	Distinguishing Features	
	Radiologic	*Other*
Pulmonary infarct	Wedge-shaped infiltrates, especially lower lobes Avascular areas	Sudden onset, sometimes hemoptysis, occasionally right heart strain
Atelectasis	Displacement of interlobar fissures, elevation of diaphragm, shift of mediastinum	Abdominal surgery, pleuritic pain, or other predisposing factor
Carcinoma, primary, or metastatic	Variable	Weight loss, signs of chronic illness Evidence of neoplasm elsewhere Cytology of sputum
Lymphoma	Variable Hilar and mediastinal adenopathy	Anemia, splenomegaly, lymphadenopathy
Chemical or lipoid pneumonia	Variable, not characteristic	History of ingestion or aspiration of oil, gasoline, kerosene
Irradiation pneumonitis	Variable	History of irradiation
Loeffler pneumonia	Migratory, patchy infiltrates, often multiple	Eosinophilia History of drug ingestion, helminthiasis
Pulmonary edema	Butterfly pattern of diffuse perihilar infiltrates, but localized infiltrates are not unusual	Cardiac disease, inhalation of noxious gases
Pulmonary alveolar proteinosis	Bilateral infiltrates radiating from hilum in butterfly fashion, especially lower lobes	Biopsy PAS-positive alveolar material
Idiopathic pulmonary hemosiderosis	Usually miliary mottling, with evanescent patchy infiltrates	Glomerulonephritis (Goodpasture syndrome), iron-deficiency anemia
Sarcoidosis	Hilar adenopathy, fine reticular parenchymal pattern	Other signs of sarcoidosis
Collagen-vascular diseases	Variable	Other evidence of the conditions
Uremic pneumonitis	Often butterfly pattern of diffuse perihilar infiltrates	Severe azotemia
Drug lung	Variable	History of drug ingestion

PULMONARY VASCULITIS

The list of conditions causing pulmonary vasculitis is very long, but only a few are likely to cause acute symptoms. They include SLE and the variants of polyarteritis. It is usually wise to treat for pneumonia initially if the diagnosis is in doubt.

SICKLE CELL DISEASE

Patients with hemoglobin SS disease often have attacks of fever, chest pain, and pulmonary infiltrate. Most of these episodes are probably noninfective, but antibiotics are, again, a wise precaution.

DRUG LUNG[10]

Most pulmonary reactions to drugs are chronic, but a few present acutely. Nitrofurantoin commonly does so. Drug-induced SLE is also worth remembering; the patients have antinuclear factor and may have any of the clinical features of spontaneous SLE. Hydralazine is a common cause. Some patients with pulmonary infiltrates have eosinophilia and would come under the general category of Löffler syndrome.

MANAGEMENT

The most important part of managing a patient with pneumonia is the selection of an appropriate antibiotic(s). One must also consider the patient's oxygenation and requirements for fluids and nutrition. Sometimes bacteria spread from the lung to other tissues; this must be recognized and treated. Later in the illness, it may become clear that the condition is not responding to treatment or that an initial improvement has been followed by deterioration.

ANTIBIOTIC TREATMENT

Antibiotic therapy has revolutionized the prognosis of pneumonia, but the disease remains a serious one. Pneumococcal pneumonia severe enough to require hospital admission still carries a mortality of 10 to 15 percent in most large series. Staphylococcal pneumonia mortality rates are of the order of 40 to 50 percent, and gram-negative rod pneumonias have mortalities in excess of 50 percent. Many factors are involved in these deaths, the most important being the type of patient who comes for treatment to university hospitals. They are often indigent, malnourished, or alcoholic, and frequently have other serious diseases, such as chronic lung disease or congestive heart failure. In addition, they present for treatment at an advanced stage. In all bacteremias, there is a point of no return, after which antibiotic therapy can no longer influence the outcome—this is seen particularly clearly in pneumococcal pneumonia, where most of the deaths occur in the first 24 hours. The second type of irretrievable situation that may be produced by delay is when the lung has become honeycombed with abscesses, when local spread has produced empyema or pericarditis, or when metastatic infections such as endocarditis, meningitis, or liver abscesses, have been established. Even if these are not immediately fatal, the patient faces a long, drawn-out illness, during which he or she will be liable to the illnesses of the bedridden—bedsores, pulmonary embolism, and bronchopneumonia.

In view of all this, it is important that delay is not compounded when the patient does reach the hospital. An abbreviated history covering the present illness, previous therapy, and other relevant information, such as drug allergies, can be completed in 15 minutes, and a physical examination in not much more. Chest radiograph, blood count, and blood and sputum cultures can be completed in another half hour, and treatment started. There is no excuse for the 5- or 6-hour delays that are common in most hospitals.

Pneumococcal Pneumonia
If the presumptive diagnosis is pneumococcal pneumonia, procaine penicillin is the drug of choice in a dose of 600,000 units twice daily intramuscularly. It is wise to give any sick patient a loading dose of 1 million units of crystalline penicillin intravenously, because procaine penicillin may not produce adequate blood levels for 2 or 3 hours. Pneumococci in the U.S. are almost invariably sensitive to these doses of penicillin, and the use of larger doses merely promotes colonization by staphylococci and gram-negative organisms, which may cause secondary pneumonia. In patients allergic to penicillin, erythromycin (2 g per day) is probably the best alternative. In some parts of the world, pneumococci resistant to penicillin and requiring treatment with vancomycin are common. Therapy should be continued for 1 week. As a rule, clinical improvement is noted within 24 hours, although sometimes the temperature may be elevated for 3 to 5 days. A patient who remains febrile after 1 week of treatment probably has undrained pus somewhere other than in the lung, as discussed below. The chest radiograph may remain abnormal for up to 3 months, however, and it is not necessary to continue therapy until the radiograph is normal. Resolution is normally complete.

Other Gram-positive Pneumonias
If clinical and laboratory features (Table 9.6–1 and 9.6–2) lead to the presumptive diagnosis of staphylococcal pneumonia, the best initial treatment is probably nafcillin in a daily dose of 6 to 9 g parenterally. If the staphylococcus turns out to be sensitive to penicillin G, this drug can be substituted in a dose of 4 to 6 million units daily. In patients said to be allergic to penicillin, skin testing should be done to confirm that anaphylactic sensitization exists. If the skin test is negative, there is no danger of death from anaphylaxis, although nafcillin therapy may later cause drug fever. If it does, cephalothin is usually tolerated. If the skin test is positive, neither penicillins nor cephalosporins should be used, and the best alternative is vancomycin 2 g daily parenterally. Vancomycin may also be required if the staphyloccocus is methicillin-resistant. Whatever antibiotic is selected should be continued for at least 3 weeks. The best treatment for hemolytic streptococcal pneumonia is penicillin G in a dose of 2 to 4 million units daily, parenterally.

Gram-negative Rod Pneumonias
In gram-negative rod pneumonias, treatment has hitherto been very unsatisfactory. Aminoglycosides have been the mainstay, but their therapeutic index is low, and even with monitoring of blood levels, renal failure and deafness were common. Furthermore, resolution of the pneumonia was often very slow, presumably because aminoglycosides do not diffuse readily, and are antagonized by pus. In my opinion, the availability of newer cephalosporins and penicillins should make it unnecessary to use aminoglycosides, except occasionally in hospital-acquired pneumonias.

Cefotaxime is essentially nontoxic, except for allergy, and it kills most gram-negative rods at concentrations of less than 0.1 μg/ml. It is not effective against most *Pseudomonas* sp, but these can be covered with piperacillin or ceftazidime. *Acinetobacter,* which is a rare cause of pneumonia, would still require the use of an aminoglycoside. One would not treat a patient with an aminoglycoside for gram-negative pneumonia unless he or she failed to respond to a third-generation penicillin or cephalosporin.

The antibiotics listed in Table 9.6–4 represent first guesses; in all cases the susceptibility of the infecting strain should be determined and therapy adjusted if necessary. Therapy in gram-negative rod pneumonias should be prolonged, especially for *Klebsiella* and *Pseudomonas* pneumonias. Tularemia is best treated with streptomycin, and the response to treatment is usually dramatic.

It is usually impossible to distinguish pneumonias due to mycoplasmas and rickettsiae from those due to viruses until serologic

TABLE 9.6–4. ANTIBIOTICS GENERALLY EFFECTIVE IN GRAM-NEGATIVE ROD PNEUMONIAS

Organism	Antibiotic
E. coli	Cefotaxime
Klebsiella	Cefotaxime
Proteus	Ticarcillin
H. influenzae	Ampicillin or chloramphenicol
Enterobacter	Cefotaxime
Serratia	Cefotaxime
Pseudomonas	Piperacillin or ceftazidime
Acinetobacter	Tobramycin

results become available. The treatable causes of the primary atypical pneumonia syndrome are M. pneumoniae, C. burnetii, Chlamydia psittaci, and Legionella species, especially L. pneumophila. Mycoplasma and the bacillus of Legionnaires disease respond best to erythromycin, 2 g per day. Because both these organisms are common causes of community-acquired pneumonia, and the other two are rare, it is recommended that all cases of atypical pneumonia be treated with erythromycin in the first instance. Tetracycline, however, is a much better drug for Q fever, psittacosis, and the newly described TWAR agent, which is a Chlamydia. If the patient's condition fails to improve, therefore, and if there is no evidence of infection with ordinary bacteria, a switch to tetracycline may be indicated.

Viral Pneumonia

Viral pneumonias used to be untreatable, but the beginnings of antiviral therapy are already with us. The most important instances are herpes simplex and varicella pneumonia, which can be treated with acyclovir (5 to 10 mg/kg intravenously every 8 hours). If a patient with obvious herpesvirus infection elsewhere develops a progressive pneumonia that does not seem to be caused by bacteria, it may be reasonable to proceed to acyclovir treatment, with or without a lung biopsy. Unfortunately, the most common herpesvirus causing pneumonia is cytomegalovirus, and for that no useful treatment is available. An acycloguanosine derivative was found to suppress viral replication but did not lead to decreased mortality. Herpesvirus pneumonias are rare in healthy people; they primarily affect the very young, the very old, and the severely immunosuppressed. In established influenzal pneumonia, amantadine is often given but it is dubious whether it affects the outcome.

Aspiration Pneumonia[1,11]

Aspiration pneumonia diagnosed soon after the aspiration of gastric juices is caused by chemical injury to lung tissue, which will not respond to antibiotics. Nonetheless, infection frequently develops, and there are differing opinions on what should be done. One school waits until infection develops, if it does, and then treats it. The school at the other extreme treats in-hospital aspiration prophylactically, with full antistaphylococcal and gram-negative coverage, because it is thought that these organisms cause a substantial proportion of nosocomial aspiration pneumonias. A middle school treats with low-dose penicillin or clindamycin to take care of the most common organisms, pneumococci and mouth anaerobes. There are no data supporting any of these positions, and the number and power of antibiotics given tend to be a function of the degree of illness of the patient. Although animal experiments suggest that steroids are useful if given before or within a few minutes after aspiration, it is generally impractical to give patients steroids this quickly, and they are not used.

Aspiration pneumonia presenting as an obvious infection, with fever, prostration, foul sputum, and cavitating pneumonia on

the chest radiograph, is best treated with clindamycin.[8] It should be remembered that patients may aspirate large objects such as pieces of food, teeth, and so forth. These will require diagnosis and removal by bronchoscopy before recovery is to be expected.

BLIND TREATMENT

Often the laboratory data gathered when the patient is admitted to the hospital provide no clue to etiologic diagnosis. In this setting, initial choice of antibiotics is influenced by the patient's clinical status. If the patient is young, previously healthy, and has fever, tachypnea, leukocytosis, and radiographic evidence of an infiltrate in one of the lower lobes, the presumptive diagnosis of pneumococcal pneumonia can be made and the patient treated with penicillin until the specific etiologic diagnosis is established. If, on the other hand, the patient has hypotension, cyanosis, confusion, and predominantly upper lobe or multilobar involvement, initial therapy should include drugs effective against Staphylococcus, Klebsiella and Legionnaires disease as well as the pneumococcus. Appropriate therapy in such a case might be cefotaxime 6 to 8 g per day plus erythromycin 2 to 4 g per day. The optimum antibiotic therapy would be determined by subsequent cultures and antibiotic sensitivity studies.

GENERAL MEASURES

Close Observation

Ideally, patients with pneumonia should be admitted to hospital for at least 48 hours, until it is clear that they are responding to treatment. This is not always possible, however, and it is clear that many cases of pneumococcal pneumonia can be adequately treated at home. A good person for outpatient management is one who is young, reasonably intelligent, has someone to care for him or her, and is not very sick. The patient should be made to understand that response to intramuscular penicillin is not guaranteed and that he or she should return to the hospital promptly if there is no improvement. Patients who are old, unreliable, anoxic, or suffer from other chronic diseases should always be admitted.

Rest and Hydration

In general, the patient should be allowed to undertake whatever activities he or she wishes, but it is wise to make sure that he or she is accompanied to the bathroom or elsewhere until clinical improvement occurs. Sick patients usually cannot drink enough to replace the several liters per day that they lose in sweating and through the respiratory tract. If dehydration is allowed to occur, bronchial secretions may become inspissated and may lead to atelectasis. It is therefore wise to use intravenous fluids for the first day or two.

Pleuritic Pain

If the pain is too severe to be managed with aspirin, it is probably better to induce local anesthesia by intercostal nerve block than to use codeine or stronger narcotics. This is because narcotics suppress the cough reflex. An agent like mepivicaine may provide anesthesia for 48 hours with only one injection, and a second may not be necessary.

Cough

Paroxysms of coughing may be very exhausting, especially to patients with heart disease. They may also seriously interfere with oxygenation. Moderate doses of codeine (32 mg) may suppress paroxysms, but it is unwise to use large doses because the cough reflex may be totally suppressed.

Cyanosis

There are three major mechanisms by which cyanosis may develop in pneumonia. In pneumococcal pneumonia, there may be exten-

sive blood flow through an airless consolidated lobe or lobes, so that a large fraction of the cardiac output is not oxygenated. Obviously, neither oxygen nor tracheobronchial suction is very effective for this condition, but it responds spontaneously in a day or two as the pneumonia improves. In bronchopneumonia, there are consolidated areas, but in addition, many airways are blocked by purulent secretions that add a component of ventilatory failure. Here, postural drainage, assisted coughing, and tracheobronchial suction can produce considerable improvement. Especially in exacerbations of chronic bronchitis, alveolar hypoventilation may rapidly become extreme, and severe carbon dioxide retention and hypoxemia develop. Such patients need antibiotics, bronchodilators, efficient physical therapy, tracheobronchial suction, and cautious 24 or 28 percent oxygen therapy. If these measures fail, endotracheal intubation and artificial ventilation may be necessary. Lastly, in extensive viral (influenzal) pneumonia there may be interstitial pulmonary edema, leading to a "diffusion block" type of respiratory failure with hypoxemia and hypocapnia. This state usually responds to oxygen therapy with positive end-expiratory pressure, although high concentrations may be required. If not, there is some evidence that forced dehydration with fluid restriction, and large doses of diuretics may be helpful.

Shock

When hypotension results from severe hypoxia, therapy is directed as discussed in the section on cyanosis. Gastric dilation and paralytic ileus are fairly common complications of pneumonia, especially with lower lobe involvement. They are readily detectable on physical examination and corrected by nasogastric intubation. When neither significant hypoxia nor gastric dilation is present, the hypotension may be the result of bacteremia, and treatment for bacteremic shock should be initiated.

COMPLICATIONS

Serious metastatic infections often occur in the patient with pneumonia despite appropriate antibiotic therapy. They include empyema, lung abscess, pericarditis, brain abscess, meningitis, pyarthrosis, and endocarditis.

Pleural Effusion

Despite penicillin therapy, pleural effusion occurs in about 5 percent of patients with pneumococcal pneumonia. It is seen in a much higher proportion of patients with streptococcal pneumonia, and it is almost invariably present in individuals with *Bacteroides* infections of the lung. When significant pleural effusion is present, fluid should always be removed by thoracentesis and examined for pyogenic and acid-fast organisms. If the effusion is thick, purulent, or foul smelling, it is best to drain it by means of an intercostal tube at the outset because multiple thoracenteses usually fail eventually, and by that time more extensive surgery may be necessary. Even when the fluid is thin, it is deemed wise to install a tube if it reaccumulates after a single thoracentesis. Laboratory criteria suggesting the need for chest tube drainage are visible organisms on Gram stain, a pH of less than 7.2, a glucose of less than 60, and a high lactic dehydrogenase (LDH) level.[9]

Lung Abscess

Abscess formation, always uncommon in pneumococcal pneumonia, is relatively common in *Staphylococcus, Klebsiella, Bacteroides, Proteus,* and *Pseudomonas* pneumonias. It is common in pneumonia secondary to aspiration of oral contents. Abscesses are treated by encouraging drainage by physical therapy and sometimes by endoscopic aspiration. Most of the pneumonias in which abscesses occur are already being treated with maximal doses of antibiotics, and there is no indication for a change in therapy unless it is shown that the organism is resistant to the drugs being used. A slow response to treatment of a necrotizing pneumonia is expected, and

antibiotic therapy should be continued longer than with a simple pneumonia. Lung abscess secondary to aspiration pneumonia responds well to fairly low doses of penicillin G, 2 to 4 million units per day. A controlled clinical trial has shown that clindamycin is significantly better, however, and a switch should be made if the patient fails to improve with penicillin.[8]

Pericarditis

Pericarditis usually causes precordial pain and a friction rub but may occur without either. It is especially common with empyema and should be considered in any patient who remains febrile and sick after his or her empyema has been drained. The chest radiograph may or may not be helpful, but echocardiography will demonstrate even small effusions. As with any other abscess, drainage is required. Needle aspiration is commonly done, but serious complications or death may result, and in a large institution it is best to drain the pericardium surgically.

Brain Abscess and Meningitis

Brain abscess is typically a complication of aspiration pneumonia, and the usual flora are *Bacteroides* and anaerobic streptococci. The condition may follow an obvious lung abscess or may occur after an episode of aspiration that was clinically minor. Brain abscess also occurs occasionally following staphylococcal pneumonia. Headache, vomiting, and unusual behavior are the most common symptoms; fever is slight and may be absent. The best diagnostic test for brain abscess is computerized axial tomography; if this is not available, brain scan is almost always positive. Lumbar puncture should not be done because of the danger of coning.

Meningitis is most common with pneumococcal pneumonia and requires therapy with large doses of penicillin. If it complicates gram-negative pneumonia, maximal doses of third-generation penicillins or cephalosporins will be required. If an aminoglycoside must be used, it should be given intrathecally and perhaps intraventricularly as well as systemically.

Pyarthrosis

The symptoms of a septic joint are severe local pain and inability to move the limb. On examination, the joint is hot, red, very tender to touch, and contains a purulent effusion. Usually, the organism is visible on Gram stains of the joint fluid. Antibiotics penetrate well into joints, and modification of dose is not usually required. Drainage is required, however, and if the fluid accumulates despite repeated taps, the joint should be opened surgically.

Persistent Bacteremia

When blood cultures remain positive 24 hours after therapy has started, infective endocarditis is a probable explanation. The patient may also have undrained pus in the pleural space or one of the other sites previously discussed. If there is no evidence of a septic focus elsewhere, the patient should be assumed to have endocarditis whether or not there is a murmur. Antibiotic treatment should be escalated until the serum bactericidal level is satisfactory (1:8 or better), and therapy should be continued for 3 to 6 weeks, depending on the organism.

Superinfection

Superinfection with organisms resistant to penicillin is unusual in pneumococcal pneumonia if the recommended dosage is employed. It is seen regularly with high doses, however, or when antibiotics with an unnecessarily broad spectrum are employed, and the secondary pneumonias are more lethal than the primary. Superinfection is common in *Klebsiella* pneumonia because of the combinations of broad-spectrum antibiotics that are usually used. If respiratory signs and symptoms fail to improve after 5 to 6 days of treatment, the sputum must be cultured again. If a new organism resistant to the antibiotics employed is found and no other complications of pneumonia are detected, the antibiotic regimen should be altered as indicated by sensitivity studies.

UNFAVORABLE COURSE AND ITS MANAGEMENT

Patients with unfavorable courses fall into two main groups. In the first, the pneumonia does not respond to treatment either clinically or radiologically. In the second group, the pneumonia resolves satisfactorily, but the patient remains febrile or becomes febrile again after the initial improvement.

Atelectasis

Atelectasis of all or part of a lobe may occur at any stage of acute pneumonia and usually results in increasing tachypnea and, if an entire lobe is involved, in severe dyspnea. Often the atelectatic area will clear with coughing, deep breathing, or forced expiration. If clearing is not observed in 2 to 3 hours after these respiratory maneuvers, bronchoscopic aspiration should be carried out, because the affected area may become fibrotic and functionless if the atelectasis persists.

Delirium

Delirium is a common complication of pneumonia, and because meningitis is a fairly common complication of bacteremia, lumbar puncture should always be done. If pyogenic meningitis is not adequately treated, all the signs of meningitis may be suppressed by the low doses of penicillin prescribed for the pneumonia, only to recur in fulminant form several days after cessation of treatment. Hypoxia is a frequent cause of delirium in the older pneumonia patient. Delirium tremens is commonly observed when alcoholics develop bacterial pneumonia. When it occurs (and meningitis and hypoxia have been excluded), it is treated with hydration and benzodiazepines.

Failure of Pneumonia to Resolve

If the patient is clinically well, afebrile, eating, and walking about without discomfort, the persistence of radiographic changes is no cause for alarm. It is not necessary to increase the dose of antibiotics, change the treatment, or continue for a longer time than usual.[5] Even pneumococcal pneumonia may take weeks to clear on the radiograph. Most other bacterial pneumonias are slower to resolve and may leave permanent scarring.

If the infiltrate persists and the patient remains sick, he or she should be completely reassessed, starting with a new physical examination. The first consideration is to rule out infection anywhere other than in the lung. It is essential to make sure that no part of the infiltrate represents infected pleural fluid, perhaps trapped in one of the fissures. The most useful diagnostic measures are computed tomographic (CT) scans or sonograms of the chest. The next most likely possibility is that the bacterial diagnosis is wrong and that the antimicrobial agent is inappropriate or is being used in dosages that are too small. If bacteria are isolated only from the sputum, they may be irrelevant to the illness. New cultures should be obtained and the treatment altered if necessary. If the evidence for bacterial etiology is good and the antibiotics are adequate as assessed in vitro, persistence or worsening of the infiltrate suggests inadequate drainage of pus. Staphylococcal and gram-negative rod pneumonias are characteristically necrotizing, causing multiple abscesses. A common explanation is bronchial obstruction, usually due to a tumor. Failure to resolve may also be a consequence of underlying tuberculous or fungal infection.

If the infiltrate persists but there is no unequivocal evidence of bacterial infection, other possibilities should be considered. The most important in normal people are the treatable causes of the primary atypical pneumonia syndrome. In immunosuppressed people, one should be most concerned about infection with saprophytic fungi and pneumocystis. Lastly, the whole illness may be noninfectious, and the patient should be assessed for the diseases listed in Table 9.6–3. Because these are many and various, one should only order tests when the diagnosis under consideration is clinically plausible.

Persistent Fever

Streptococcal, staphylococcal, and gram-negative rod pneumonias are characteristically slow to respond, and fever may persist up to 2 weeks in uncomplicated cases. If the patient is febrile but the chest symptoms and signs are improving and the radiograph shows initial clearing, then it is probable that the drugs used were appropriate and the doses adequate. In this case, nothing further need be done. If the patient is febrile and sick despite apparent improvement in the pneumonia, the likeliest explanation is an undrained focus of infection, either in the chest or elsewhere. A thorough search for empyema, pericarditis, and the other entities just discussed should be made. Sometimes, metastatic abscesses turn up in very unusual places, such as the vertebral column or the spleen, and in case of difficulty it is wise to investigate any area where the patient has even mild complaints.

Return of Fever

When fever returns after an initial improvement, the likeliest explanation is superinfection in the lung or some other site. Superinfection in the lung produces a return of respiratory symptoms and a deterioration in respiratory function.[17] If these are not present, the commonest sources of fever are the urine and intravenous catheter sites. Recurrent fever may also be due to a metastatic infection with the original organism. Drug allergy usually develops after 7 to 10 days of treatment, but it may be earlier in sensitized patients. It is often accompanied by eosinophilia, pruritus, and skin rashes. However, the neutrophil count is commonly normal. When the drug is withdrawn, the temperature usually falls to normal within 48 hours. Very occasionally, the original organism develops resistance to the antibiotics employed and causes a relapse. Obviously, a change of antibiotic is indicated.

MYCOBACTERIAL INFECTIONS

TUBERCULOSIS

Tuberculosis is now a disappearing disease in the United States. Except for pockets in large cities such as New York and Chicago, very few new infections are being established in young people. The rate of tuberculin positivity among people born in the United States is below 1 percent at the age of 21. This means that most clinical tuberculosis now is a reactivation in old people of disease acquired many years ago. There is a certain amount of tuberculosis in alcoholic and drug-dependent skid-row populations and in children exposed to them. An increasingly important source of new cases is immigrants.

Tuberculosis can present in a large number of ways. Children may have symptoms and signs of a primary complex—a small lung lesion and enlarged regional nodes. The nodes may be big enough to cause bronchial obstruction. Miliary disease and tuberculous meningitis are now rare. In immigrants, or in alcoholic adults, the classic cavitating upper lobe disease may be seen. The sputum smear is strongly positive for acid-fast bacilli. If the infection is relatively recent (less than 2 yr), one may see tuberculous pleural effusion. This is typically large and unilateral. It seems to be mostly a hypersensitivity phenomenon, and tubercle bacilli may be very few in the fluid, although they can often be cultured from it. Generally, the sputum is negative for tubercle bacilli.

In the context of an apparent pneumonia, tuberculosis may present in three main ways. A tuberculous focus in a node or in the lung may erode into a bronchus and result in widespread or lobar contamination with tuberculous pus. A rapid consolidation occurs, which is accompanied by high fever. Most of the changes are due to allergy to tuberculin and other bacterial products. Acid-fast bacilli may be scarce in the sputum, and substantial or complete resolution is common even in the absence of therapy (epitu-

berculosis). A more ominous illness is true tuberculous broncho-pneumonia. Here the course is relentlessly downhill, and the patient dies in a matter of weeks without therapy (galloping consumption). The sputum is strongly positive for tubercle bacilli. Lastly, pulmonary tuberculosis of the ordinary type may be complicated with a pneumococcal or other pneumonia. Sputum from cases of pneumonia should always be stained for acid-fast bacilli.

Elderly persons with reactivation disease may present with classic cavitating pulmonary tuberculosis, or with one of the pneumonic presentations previously discussed. Frequently they have lower lobe pneumonias without prominent apical changes. They also may develop caseation necrosis in lymph nodes, however, and the lungs may be clear on radiograph. Frequently the involved nodes are in the abdomen and are very hard to detect. Such patients may have fever of unknown origin for weeks or months. Often, the diagnosis is established by finding caseating granulomas in a liver biopsy. In some patients, however, the presence of miliary tuberculosis or tuberculous meningitis is recognized only at autopsy.

Spread of tubercle bacilli throughout the body occurs in essentially every primary tuberculous infection, and secondary foci are established in many different organs. If these subsequently break down, localized tuberculosis will result. Renal tuberculosis, bone and joint tuberculosis, Potts disease of the spine, pelvic tuberculosis in women (which presents as infertility) and tuberculous epididymitis or prostatitis in men are all still seen occasionally.

ATYPICAL MYCOBACTERIAL INFECTIONS

Because infection by human tubercle bacilli has become rare, infection by atypical mycobacteria has become relatively more common. Probably there has been no true increase in incidence for most of the population, although certain groups of immunosuppressed people are unquestionably prone to develop atypical mycobacterial infection. Atypical infection almost always involves just the chest, although miliary disease, meningitis, and other manifestations of generalized disease have been described. Generalized infection with *M. avium-intracellulare* is a common termination of the acquired immunodeficiency syndrome.[14] Cervical lymph node tuberculosis in children is frequently due to atypical organisms, but it has an excellent prognosis and probably does not need any treatment other than surgical drainage.

The typical adult patient with atypical mycobacterial infection is a middle-aged or elderly male with established chronic bronchitis, usually due to smoking. The mycobacterial disease may be of any degree of severity, but on the whole it is milder than that of true tuberculous infection. Many patients live in virtual symbiosis with their organisms for years. They do die faster than normal people of the same age, however, and some of these deaths are due to active pulmonary infection. In immunosuppressed patients, such as those with renal transplants or AIDS, infection typically progresses relentlessly to the death of the patient.

INFECTIVITY IN HOSPITALS

A common problem with tuberculosis is that the diagnosis is missed for a period because no one thinks of it. During this time the patient is in an open ward, and numerous hospital staff members are exposed to infection. When the tuberculosis is discovered, a large number of tuberculin tests, medical examinations, and chest radiographs become necessary. With atypical infections, these precautions are unnecessary because the organisms are of very low pathogenicity for normal people. All cases of tuberculosis, typical and atypical, should be reported to the State Health Department on the official form. Health department employees are generally the best people to trace contacts and examine family members.

MANAGEMENT

Human tuberculosis is now fairly easy to treat. The classic modes of treatment, worked out over many years and known to be effective, involve the use of two active drugs for 18 months to 2 years. If there are pulmonary cavities exceeding 2 cm in diameter, or large caseating masses elsewhere, there is sound evidence supporting the use of three drugs for the first 2 months of therapy. An example of such a regimen would be isoniazid (INH), 300 mg daily, plus ethambutol, 15 mg/kg daily for 18 months, supplemented by intramuscular injections of 1 g streptomycin three times weekly for the first 2 months. This regimen would be expected to cure at least 95 percent of cases, with most of the failures attributable to poor compliance. After treatment, the expected recurrence rate in the first 5 years should be 1 percent or less. If the organism is resistant to one or more primary drugs, it is generally possible to construct a satisfactory alternative using one or more of the following: rifampin, pyrazinamide, capreomycin, ethionamide, or para-aminosalicylic acid. Certain areas of the country have large numbers of tuberculous adults living on skid row who have been partially treated for tuberculosis on numerous occasions and have in their sputum multiple drug-resistant tubercle bacilli. Tuberculous children from such areas should initially be treated with three drugs to which resistance is not common in the local community.

Classic regimens make great demands on patient and physician because of the time involved. Shorter regimens are possible, provided that both INH and rifampin can be used simultaneously. This requires that the organisms are not resistant to either antibiotic, and that the patient does not develop significant hepatic toxicity. It is currently thought that INH plus rifampin for 9 months, with the addition of streptomycin in the first 2 months of therapy if there are cavities, is adequate treatment for all forms of tuberculosis. If the patient is unreliable, as much of the therapy as possible should be supervised.

For special purposes, larger numbers of drugs and even shorter times can be tried. Thus, in Hong Kong, a population of imprisoned drug addicts was treated with INH, rifampin, streptomycin, pyrazinamide, and ethambutol for only 4 months. Over 80 percent were quiescent 1 year after stopping treatment.

The treatment of atypical mycobacterial infections must be individualized. Not all patients need to be treated. If treatment is required, it may be difficult, because the organisms tend to be insensitive to most antibiotics. *M. kansasii* is generally only sensitive to INH at 10 μg/ml, rather than the 2 μg/ml required by most human tubercle bacilli. *M. avium-intracellulare* is pan-resistant. It is usual to use combinations of antibiotics in high doses for a long time. Often, one hears of patients being treated with five, six, or even seven drugs simultaneously. Isoniazid is generally given even if the organisms appear to be insensitive by laboratory tests. Because combinations of antibiotics are rarely tested, laboratory tests of susceptibility are not of much help in most patients, and the patients' response or failure must be assessed clinically. Uncontrollable atypical infection may sometimes necessitate old-fashioned surgical procedures such as thoracoplasty.

Patients being successfully treated for tuberculosis should develop an appetite, put on weight, feel better, stop coughing, show resolution of infiltrates on chest radiograph, raise their hematocrit, and lower their erythrocyte sedimentation rate. Positive sputum smears may be seen for months after the start of successful treatment. Most of these organisms are nonviable, and almost all are noninfectious. Even positive sputum cultures may be found several months into therapy; they may appear and disappear as tuberculous foci break down and drain into the bronchi. Again, most of these organisms appear to be noninfectious. This was established during the treatment of tuberculosis under grim slum conditions in Madras, India. No hospital beds were available, and strongly positive patients were given treatment and sent home. They lost the ability to infect their children within a week of starting treatment. Based on this, it is currently recommended that patients

with open tuberculosis be isolated for 2 weeks at the beginning of therapy; after that, isolation should be discontinued, without regard to sputum smears or cultures.

REFERENCES

1. Bartlett JG, Gorbach SL: The triple threat of aspiration pneumonia. Chest 68:560, 1975
2. Basiliere JC, Bistrong HW, Spence WF: Streptococcal pneumonia: Recent outbreaks in military recruit populations. Am J Med 44:580, 1968
3. Fisher AM, Trevor R, et al: Staphylococcal pneumonia: A review of 21 cases in adults. N Engl J Med 258:919, 1958
4. Hirschmann JV, Everett ED: *Haemophilus influenzae* infections in adults. Medicine 58:80, 1979
5. Jay SJ, Johansen WG, Pierce AK: The radiographic resolution of *Streptococcus pneumoniae* pneumonia. N Engl J Med 293:798, 1975
6. Kirby BD, Snyder KM, et al: Legionnaires disease: Report of sixty-five nosocomially acquired cases, and a review of the literature. Medicine 59:188, 1980
7. LaForce AM: Hospital acquired gram negative rod pneumonias. Am J Med 70:664, 1981
8. Levison ME, Mangura CT, et al: Clindamycin compared with penicillin for the treatment of anaerobic lung abscess. Ann Intern Med 98:466, 1983
9. Light RW: Management of parapneumonic effusions. Chest 70:325, 1976
10. Lippman M: Pulmonary reactions to drugs. Med Clin North Am 61:1353, 1977
11. Lorber B, Swenson RM: Bacteriology of aspiration pneumonia: A prospective study of hospital and community acquired cases. Ann Intern Med 87:329, 1974
12. Morgan HJ: Pleuropulmonary tularemia. Ann Intern Med 27:519, 1947
13. Murray HW, Masur H, et al: The protean manifestations of *Mycloplasma pneumoniae* infection in adults. Am J Med 58:229, 1975
14. Ogawa SK, Smith MA, et al: Tuberculous meningitis in an urban medical center. Medicine 66:317, 1987
15. Phair JP, Basseris HP, et al: Bacteremic pneumonia due to Gram-negative bacilli. Arch Int Med 103:2147, 1983
16. Tew J, Calenoff L, Berlin BS: Bacterial or non-bacterial pneumonia: Accuracy of radiological diagnosis. Radiology 124:607, 1977
17. Tillotson JR, Finland M: Bacterial colonization and clinical superinfection of the respiratory tract complicating antibiotic treatment of pneumonia. J Infect Dis 119:597, 1969
18. Williams DM, Krick JA, Remington JS: Pulmonary infection in the compromised host. Am Rev Respir Dis 114:359, 1976
19. Verghese A, Berk SL: Bacterial pneumonia in the elderly. Medicine 62:271, 1983
20. Yu VL, Kroboth FJ, et al: Legionnaires' disease: A new clinical perspective from a prospective pneumonia study. Am J Med 73:357, 1982

CHAPTER 9.7
Infective Endocarditis
John J. Mann

Infective endocarditis is caused by the implantation of microorganisms on the endocardium followed by tissue damage. Infective arteritis refers to the same process in extracardiac arterial structures. This localized infection is associated with prominent systemic manifestations and sometimes dramatic structural alterations. The systemic symptoms are often manifestations of bacteremia, emboli, metastatic abscesses, or immune phenomena. Structural alterations include destruction of valves or other cardiac structures with the frequent development of congestive heart failure. The aim of therapy must include not only the eradication of the infection but also the repair of the structural damage. Major recent changes in the treatment of endocarditis relate to the increasingly important role of surgery in the acute phase of the illness.[26]

PATHOGENESIS

Bacterial endocarditis occurs either in patients with preexisting endocardial damage or in patients with normal heart valves in whom the bloodstream has been invaded by virulent microorganisms (e.g., staphylococci, enterococci). Transient and asymptomatic bacteremia is the usual event inciting the endocardial infection. A careful historical review for conditions predisposing to bacteremia may furnish clues to the nature of the organism. The mouth is the usual portal of entry for α-streptococci. Dental procedures, poor dental hygiene, gingivitis, tonsillectomy, and viral upper respiratory tract infections have been implicated, because transient bacteremia has been demonstrated in association with these conditions. Enterococci are normal fecal inhabitants, and gastrointestinal and genitourinary factors, such as prostatitis, catheterization, urologic surgery and instrumentation, parturition, and septic abortion, frequently are responsible for transient enterococcal bacteremia. Cuta-

neous furuncles, cardiac surgery, infected wounds, and (occasionally) osteomyelitis are the usual sources of staphylococci. Addicts using narcotics intravenously are especially likely to develop staphylococcal endocarditis of the tricuspid valve, but may also develop α-streptococcal, enterococcal, or candidal infection of the left heart valves.[19] Candidal endocarditis should be suspected in patients with embolic complications involving larger vessels. Patients with pneumococcal pneumonia, bacteremia, and meningitis occasionally develop pneumococcal endocarditis of the aortic valve. In the preantibiotic era endocarditis afflicted mostly young adults with rheumatic heart disease. Currently the disease is most common in elderly patients with degenerative forms of cardiovascular disease or with no clinically obvious heart disease. Endocarditis occurs on atheromatous deposits, calcifications of the mitral annulus or aortic valve, thrombi overlying areas of myocardial infarction, and surgically altered endocardium.

Mitral valve prolapse presents an important dilemma in the genesis of bacterial endocarditis. This condition is an important precursor of infective endocarditis. The prevalence of mitral valve prolapse in the general population has been estimated to be 5 to 10 percent. This implies that the risk of endocarditis in mitral valve prolapse must be low. Current knowledge would favor restricting the use of prophylactic antibiotics in mitral valve prolapse to those patients with a clear-cut systolic murmur. Prophylaxis is probably not indicated in patients with an isolated click.[9]

Children who develop the disease usually have congenital heart disease. Interventricular septal defects, patent ductus arteriosus, coarctation of the aorta, bicuspid aortic valves, and the tetralogy of Fallot are the most important predisposing congenital lesions. Rheumatic, degenerative, and congenital heart diseases act similarly by producing an opportunity for deposition of platelets and fibrin on a heart valve. This results in the formation of a nonbacterial thrombotic endocarditis. Bacteremia by any of the mecha-

nisms described may transform this into bacterial endocarditis. Several investigations have demonstrated the repetitive production of bacterial endocarditis by intravenous injections of even nonvirulent bacteria in animals with catheter-induced nonbacterial thrombotic endocarditis.[5] In contrast, animals with normal heart valves do not develop bacterial endocarditis. A prospective autopsy study of 55 patients who had undergone pulmonary artery catheterization revealed endocardial lesions in 53 percent, sterile thrombus in 20 percent, and infective endocarditis in 7 percent.[20]

MICROBIOLOGY

Almost any microorganism may cause endocarditis; most bacteria and fungi, some viruses, and rickettsiae have been implicated as have *Legionella pneumophila* and chlamydial organisms. Over the past 75 years there have been fewer cases due to *Streptococcus viridans*, *Neisseria gonorrhoeae*, and *Streptococcus pneumoniae* and an increase in the incidence of staphylococci, enterococci, fungi, and unusual organisms.[22,25]

In association with cardiac surgery, immunosuppression, and narcotic addiction there has been an increased incidence of gram-negative bacteria causing infective endocarditis. In the past the incidence of gram-negative endocarditis was 1 to 3 percent. During the last decade the incidence has increased to 5 or 10 percent in normal valves and 15 percent in prosthetic valves. The organisms included *Haemophilus*, *Actinobacillus actinomycetemcomitans*, *Cardiobacterium hominis*, *Eikenella corrodens*, and others.[6] Currently, gram-positive cocci (streptococci and staphylococci) account for 55 percent of cases.

Streptococcus bovis deserves special mention because of its association with carcinoma of the colon.[12]

In 5 to 20 percent of cases cultures are sterile. Certain clinical settings tend to be associated with specific microorganisms. Subacute endocarditis in a young person with rheumatic mitral disease is usually associated with *Streptococcus viridans*. Staphylococci cause 50 percent of cases of acute endocarditis. Endocarditis that follows genitourinary manipulation is usually due to enterococci. Prosthetic valve infections are usually due to staphylococci, less commonly to streptococci, gram-negative bacteria, and fungi. Drug addicts are particularly prone to develop either right- or left-sided endocarditis secondary to staphylococci or pseudomonads. Severely compromised patients treated with intensive courses of antibiotics often develop fungal endocarditis, most commonly due to *Candida*, less commonly due to *Aspergillus*, *Histoplasma*, and others.

CLINICAL FEATURES

It has been traditional to label cases of endocarditis as subacute or acute. Subacute endocarditis usually occurs in patients with known underlying heart disease. The illness has been of long duration, slow progression with sterile emboli, and little change in cardiac status. The organism usually is *S. viridans*. Acute endocarditis often occurs without previous heart disease, with abrupt onset and prominent constitutional symptoms, early appearance of new murmurs, suppurative emboli, early anemia, and often marked leukocytosis. Congestive heart failure is commonly present. Obviously, the timing and choice of therapy will be influenced by the type of endocarditis.

PRESENTATION OF ENDOCARDITIS

Fever and Heart Murmur

Fever is the cardinal manifestation of infective endocarditis and the sign most frequently present. There is little that is characteristic about the fever. Generally, it is intermittent, irregular, mild, and not associated with shaking chills, but with more virulent organisms the course may be septic. Afebrile periods occur but are rarely prolonged, and fever is in all series the most frequent and reliable sign of endocarditis. Fever may be absent in cases complicated by severe congestive heart failure or uremia and during the administration of antimicrobial drugs.

The presence of a cardiac murmur is a common but not required feature. A murmur is absent initially in up to 50 percent of patients with right-sided endocarditis.[1] Murmurs are commonly absent during the early stage of acute endocarditis. Changing murmurs are present in the minority of cases. Even when present, murmurs may be unimpressive, particularly apical systolic murmurs. If needless deaths are to be prevented, infective endocarditis should be suspected in every patient with *fever and cardiac murmur* or *fever and anemia*, especially if the fever lasts more than a week. Familiarity with all the varied manifestations of the disease and a high index of suspicion make it even more likely that an early diagnosis will be made.

The unfortunately common practice of using antimicrobial drugs in treating undiagnosed febrile disease complicates the recognition of infective endocarditis. A patient with endocarditis given a short course of antibiotics may improve and become afebrile, even when the antibiotic was merely bacteriostatic. However, when antibiotics are discontinued, the illness will recur. Recurrent febrile disease because of inappropriate diagnosis and treatment is unfortunately often seen in patients with endocarditis. Attempts to establish the diagnosis by blood culture may be unsuccessful while the antibiotics are continued. For these reasons, recurrent febrile illness with short remission induced by antibiotic treatment and associated with negative blood cultures must be suspected of being infective endocarditis, particularly in the patient with valvular or congenital cardiac disease.

The onset of endocarditis is often vague and insidious, marked by anorexia, easy fatigability, weight loss, low-grade fever, malaise, myalgia, and arthralgia. Often, it is only after treatment has been effective that the patient becomes aware that he or she has not felt well for several months. Such presentations are characteristic of subacute infective endocarditis, in which *S. viridans* or group D streptococci are most frequently incriminated. Abundant serum antibodies to these relatively avirulent organisms are usually present at the time of clinical onset. Adverse effects of the interaction of antibody with bacterial antigens may account for some of the clinical manifestations. Purpura, clubbing arthralgias, nephritis, decreased serum complement, elevated gammaglobulins, positive rheumatoid factor, and positive antinuclear antibody test are immunologic features of endocarditis that can lead to confusion in diagnosis.

Emboli and Vascular Accidents

The manifestations of infective endocarditis are protean, because practically any organ can become involved. The most common localized manifestations of the disease are outlined in Table 9.7–1. Mycotic aneurysms, infarction, bleeding, and septic emboli account for most of the regional manifestations. Because friable, easily dislodged, valvular vegetations are almost invariably present in infective endocarditis, it is not surprising that embolic phenomena are seen so frequently. They may be the initial manifestation of the disease and are often fatal. Emboli can involve any organ but are most frequent in spleen, kidney, heart, brain, and, with right-sided endocarditis, lung. Suppurative pulmonary emboli are particularly common in narcotic addicts with staphylococcal infections of the tricuspid valve. It is particularly important to consider endocarditis in elderly patients with strokes. When the infective agent is the α-streptococci, it is rare for the embolic lesions to suppurate.

Splenomegaly

Whereas splenomegaly is seen in nearly half of patients with subacute infective endocarditis, clinically apparent splenomegaly occurs in less than a quarter of individuals with acute infective endocarditis.[13] The sudden appearance of splenomegaly with left upper

TABLE 9.7–1. MANIFESTATIONS OF INFECTIVE ENDOCARDITIS

General	Anorexia, weakness, malaise, fever, weight loss
Central nervous system	Emboli, mycotic aneurysms, brain abscess, meningitis, cerebrovascular accidents, paresis, diffuse encephalitis, coma, subarachnoid hemorrhage
Ocular	Roth spots
Cardiopulmonary	Progressive valvular damage, rupture of chordae tendinae, markedly changing murmurs Pulmonary emboli and infarction, hemoptysis Congestive heart failure Coronary embolism, myocarditis, myocardial valve ring abscess
Gastrointestinal	Splenomegaly, abdominal pain Splenic infarcts, mesenteric vascular occlusion Abnormal liver function tests
Genitourinary	Albuminuria, hematuria, embolic glomerulonephritis Flank pain, renal infarction Diffuse glomerulonephritis, uremia
Dermatologic	Petechiae, splinter hemorrhages, Osler nodes, Janeway lesions, pallor, icterus Pustular skin rashes
Extremities	Myalgia, arthralgia, arthritis, clubbing, osteomyelitis
Hematologic	Leukocytosis, anemia, elevated sedimentation, reduced serum complement, hyperglobulinemia, antigammaglobulin factor with positive Rose or latex fixation tests, positive antinuclear antibody test

quadrant pain and a friction rub in the region of the spleen suggests splenic infarction. The spleen is the most frequent site of recognized infarction, but renal infarcts are almost as common.

Nephritis and Uremia

Focal embolic glomerulitis with "flea-bitten" kidneys is frequent in endocarditis, and repeated search for hematuria and intermittent albuminuria is important in establishing the diagnosis. A diffuse proliferative glomerulonephritis, probably caused by circulating antigen-antibody complexes and occasionally producing uremia, is sometimes the outstanding feature of the illness, especially with staphylococcal or culture-negative endocarditis.[8] In this setting the illness can easily be mistaken for systemic lupus erythematosus.

Neurologic Manifestations

Neurologic complications occur in 40 percent of patients. Cerebral embolism, mycotic aneurysm, brain abscess, purulent meningitis, and aseptic meningitis are the most common manifestations.[18]

Cutaneous Manifestations

Since clubbing of the fingers and anemia are relatively late signs, they are not helpful in making an early diagnosis. Petechiae, especially those in the retina and with white centers (Roth spots), strongly suggest the diagnosis. Petechiae are most frequently seen in the oral mucosa, especially on the palate, in the retina and conjunctiva, over the upper anterior chest, and on the distal extremities. Nontender splinter hemorrhages are seen in the nail beds but are nonspecific. Erythematous macules and papules (Janeway lesions) occur on the palms and soles and may be especially prominent and early manifestations of acute infective endocarditis. Tender, raised, erythematous lesions encountered in the pads of

fingers and toes (Osler nodes) are of great diagnostic importance but occur in less than 25 percent of cases with subacute endocarditis and are very rarely seen in acute infective endocarditis.[13] Petechiae, splinter hemorrhages, Osler nodes, and emboli may continue to appear for several weeks during effective antibiotic therapy.

HEART FAILURE AND AORTIC INSUFFICIENCY

In the preantibiotic era, patients with endocarditis died usually from the bacterial infection. At present, congestive heart failure is the most common cause of death. The development of heart failure is associated with acute endocarditis, virulent microorganisms, and aortic insufficiency or, less commonly, mitral insufficiency.[6] Severe valvular damage with or without rapidly changing murmurs may occur in a few days, leading to the sudden onset of heart failure in a previously healthy person. The severity of aortic insufficiency may be difficult to assess clinically because of its rapid development. The classic signs of aortic insufficiency depend on the presence of a large pulse pressure. When aortic insufficiency develops rapidly, the left ventricular end diastolic pressure rises steeply, thus preventing a fall in diastolic pressure. In this setting wide-open aortic insufficiency can be present without the usual clinical findings.

LABORATORY DIAGNOSIS

Normocytic normochromic anemia is usually present. The rapid development of anemia indicates acute infection and the sedimentation rate is almost always elevated. These two parameters are useful in judging results of therapy.

Only slight leukocytosis is expected in subacute infective endocarditis, and even this is absent in about 50 percent of patients with subacute disease. Usually increased numbers of immature granulocytes are found in the blood. Leukocytosis greater than 15,000 is common with acute infective endocarditis. When, however, leukocytosis of this degree occurs in the course of subacute infective endocarditis, it suggests a complication such as an infarct. Demonstration of immature granulocytes may be helpful in patients suspected of having endocarditis despite sterile blood cultures.

Hyperglobulinemia and significant titers of rheumatoid factor are seen in about 50 percent of patients with subacute infective endocarditis. Microscopic hematuria is common; a few patients develop the full picture of glomerulonephritis with red blood cell casts, proteinuria, and low serum complement.[8]

With proper techniques, positive venous blood cultures can be obtained in almost all patients with infective endocarditis.[2,13] The frequency of positive cultures is equally great when the focus of infection is in the right side of the heart.[1] In most reported series, however, the blood has been sterile in about 15 percent of the cases. The bacteremia is characteristically continuous, and the usual pathogens can be readily isolated if both aerobic and anaerobic media are used and incubated for 3 weeks. Gram stains of all cultures should be made before they are discarded as negative. In many laboratories, cultures are discarded if they are negative after only 1 week's incubation. One pair of blood cultures should be incubated at room temperature. Prior antibiotic therapy may delay growth of the organism but does not necessarily preclude growth if the infection is still active. Four to six blood cultures should be obtained over the course of 12 to 72 hours. The time of day at which they are taken is of little importance. Arterial blood cultures are of no special value, but bone marrow cultures may be useful if unusual pathogens are suspected or when venous cultures remain sterile. If six cultures are negative, it is unlikely that additional blood cultures will be helpful. About 1 ml of blood should be used for each 10 ml of culture media, and penicillinase should be added if the patient has recently received penicillin or one of its analogs.

Careful in vitro sensitivity testing of recovered organisms is crucial. Tube dilution sensitivity studies should include determinations of minimum inhibitory concentration and minimum bactericidal concentration (MBC). After the antibiotic regimen has been started, the ability of the patient's serum to inhibit or kill the infecting organism should also be determined. It is traditional to recommend that a serum MBC of 1:8 or more be achieved to ensure successful therapeutic outcome. A recent multicenter collaborative study supported the finding that peak serum bactericidal titers of 1:64 or more and trough serum bactericidal titers of 1:32 or more predicted bacteriologic cure in all patients. The serum bactericidal test was a poor predictor of bacteriologic failure and clinical outcome.[23]

PATIENT MANAGEMENT

MEDICAL MANAGEMENT

Synergism between cell-wall active antibiotics, such as penicillin, and aminoglycoside antibiotics, such as streptomycin or gentamicin, has been well documented by in vitro experiments[10] and by studies on experimental endocarditis in animals.[3] This synergism is essential for the complete killing of even sensitive organisms such as *S. viridans*. It also has been demonstrated experimentally for more resistant streptococci and even staphylococci. A bactericidal regimen is essential if cure rather than mere suppression of infective endocarditis is to be achieved. Combinations of bactericidal and bacteriostatic drugs should be avoided in this disease, as the net effect may be bacteriostatic. The temptation to begin therapy before obtaining adequate blood cultures should be resisted, unless the diagnosis is obvious or the patient is very ill. Once adequately spaced blood cultures have been obtained, therapy may begin, directed toward the organism or organisms that appear on clinical grounds to be the most likely offenders. Standard regimens are indicated in Table 9.7–2. The recommendations are based on the concept that endocarditis is always fatal when untreated and extremely dangerous when undertreated. Modifications are made on the basis of the clinical response or on the basis of laboratory information such as final culture reports, sensitivity tests, and determination of serum activity. It is important to realize that clinical response is always the best indicator and should take precedence over the information received from the laboratory.

Streptococci that are killed by ≤ 0.1 μg/ml of penicillin are classified as penicillin-sensitive and are the most common cause of infective endocarditis. They include *S. viridans* and *S. bovis*. For patients not allergic to penicillin the three regimens used in Table 9.7–2 give equally excellent cure rates (>98 percent) and low relapse rates. The major advantage of the first regimen is the avoidance of the low risk of streptomycin-associated vestibular toxicity. This may be most important in older patients or in patients with impaired renal function. The major advantage of the 2-week regimen is that it is more cost effective than 4 weeks of hospitalization. Because it is a newer regimen, we may need additional studies to confirm its long-term effectiveness. Cephalothin, cefazolin, or vancomycin are acceptable alternatives for patients allergic to penicillin. Cephalosporins should be used cautiously in penicillin-allergic patients. In enterococcal endocarditis and endocarditis due to streptococci resistant to ≥ 0.1 μg/ml of penicillin, a combination of antibiotics as shown in Table 9.7–3 is necessary. Cephalosporins and penicillinase-resistant penicillins should not be used alone or in association with an aminoglycoside. The dose of the antibiotic and the choice of the aminoglycoside should be based on in vitro synergy studies. In patients allergic to penicillin, desensitization can be done if the skin test is negative. In patients with a positive penicillin skin test, the only alternative is to use vancomycin in association with an aminoglycoside.

The mortality of staphylococcal endocarditis remains high, and the course is usually complicated by heart failure, valve destruction, valve abscess, and suppurative emboli. The selection of an ideal regimen remains controversial because of the presence of antibiotic tolerance and resistance. The addition of an aminoglycoside to a cell-wall-active antibiotic, such as nafcillin, produces a synergistic effect in vitro and in experimental staphylococcal endocarditis in rabbits. This synergism has not been clearly demonstrated in humans, and combination regimens tend to cause greater toxicity. The decision to add an aminoglycoside to the regimen shown in Table 9.7–4 rests on such factors as severity of illness, in vitro studies for synergism, and response to treatment.[11] An aminoglycoside can be added for the initial 3 to 5 days of therapy, but a longer term should be reserved for unresponsive infections. In penicillin-allergic patients, vancomycin is the drug of choice, with cephalosporins and clindamycin as acceptable alternatives in selected patients. The treatment of endocarditis due to penicillin-resistant *Staphylococcus epidermidis* is particularly difficult and should be based on careful sensitivity studies. The combination of vancomycin, rifampin, and gentamicin is an appropriate initial regimen.

Treatment of the less common organisms responsible for endocarditis must be based on careful in vitro studies. Combinations of penicillin or ticarcillin and an aminoglycoside are usually required. Fungal endocarditis is usually treated with amphotericin B and 5-fluorocytosine. Surgical removal of the infected valve is often

TABLE 9.7–2. REGIMENS FOR PENICILLIN-SENSITIVE *STREPTOCOCCUS VIRIDANS*

Antibiotic	Dosage	Route	Duration (weeks)
Aqueous penicillin G	10–20 million U/day[a]	IV	4
Aqueous penicillin G	10–20 million U/day[a]	IV	4
or			
Procaine penicillin G	1–2 million U/6 hr	IM	4
plus			
Streptomycin	7.5 mg/kg (not to exceed 500 mg)/12 hr	IM	2
Aqueous penicillin G	10–20 million U/day[a]	IV	2
or			
Procaine penicillin G	1–2 million U/6 hr	IM	2
plus			
Streptomycin	7.5 mg/kg (not to exceed 500 mg)/12 hr	IM	2

[a]Either continuously or in equally divided doses every 4 hours.

TABLE 9.7–3. REGIMENS FOR *ENTEROCOCCUS* AND PENICILLIN-RESISTANT *STREPTOCOCCUS*

Antibiotic	Dosage	Route	Duration (weeks)
Aqueous penicillin	20–40 million U/day[a]	IV	4–6
or			
Ampicillin	12 g/day[a]	IV	4–6
plus			
Streptomycin	7.5 mg/kg (not to exceed 500 mg)/12 hr	IM	4–6
or			
Gentamicin	1.0 mg/kg (not to exceed 100 mg)/8 hr	IM or IV	4–6

[a]Either continuously or in equally divided doses every 4 hours.

TABLE 9.7–4. REGIMENS FOR *STAPHYLOCOCCUS AUREUS* OR *EPIDERMIDIS*

	Antibiotic	Dosage	Route	Duration (weeks)
Penicillin-sensitive	Aqueous penicillin G[a]	20 million U/day[b]	IV	4–6
Penicillin-resistant	Nafcillin[a] *or* oxacillin[a]	2 g/4 hr	IV	4–6
Methicillin-resistant	Vancomycin[a] *plus* rifampin	0.5 g/6 hr	IV	4–6
		300 mg/12 hr	Oral	4–6

[a]Gentamicin: 1 mg/kg every 8 hours may be added; see text.
[b]Either continuously or in equally divided doses every 4 hours.

required in fungal endocarditis and in endocarditis due to resistant bacterial organisms such as *Pseudomonas*.

SURGICAL MANAGEMENT

As previously indicated, eradication of the infection is only the first step in management. Often the structural damage must be repaired surgically. Recently it has become clear that early surgery is important in the management of heart failure developing in the course of endocarditis.[16] This is particularly true when aortic insufficiency is present. Sudden death is common in this setting. When heart failure is absent, medical therapy alone is effective. When heart failure is severe, that is, requiring more than digitalis, early surgery to correct the valvular incompetence is mandatory. When heart failure is mild, the decision is often difficult and must be based on an assessment of both the severity and progression of the valvular damage. This may require cardiac catheterization, because clinical signs may be misleading.[25]

In addition, echocardiography can provide a rapid, noninvasive diagnosis of bacterial vegetation in some patients. Two-dimensional echocardiography appears to be superior to M-mole echocardiography in diagnosing complications of endocarditis.[17] It also may identify patients with more severe diseases that are likely to require surgery.[21]

Other indications for surgery include the following: failure to sterilize the bloodstream infection; recurrent significant emboli, particularly cerebral and coronary emboli; prosthetic valve infection; cardiovascular accidents such as ruptured cusps, chordae, septum; mycotic aneurysms; and, possibly, progressive renal failure. Recent experience has indicated that surgery can be performed in the first few days of antibiotic treatment without significant increase in subsequent infection of the prosthetic valve.[7,26]

COMMON MANAGEMENT PROBLEMS

Prosthetic Valve Endocarditis (PVE)
Prosthetic valve endocarditis (PVE) is a serious complication of cardiac valve replacement and accounts for an increasing percentage of all cases of infective endocarditis.[24] Early-onset PVE occurs within 2 months of surgery and is usually due to microbial contamination occurring during surgery or soon after from postoperative infections. Late-onset PVE resembles native valve endocarditis and is thought to be due to transient bacteremias. Staphylococci account for almost half the cases of the early-onset PVE and one third of those of late-onset PVE. *S. epidermidis* is the single most common organism in both groups. Aerobic gram-negative bacilli are the second most frequent cause of early-onset PVE, whereas streptococci are more common in late-onset PVE. Fungi, particularly *Candida* and *Aspergillus,* are important causes of early-onset PVE and are seen less commonly with late-onset PVE. A wide variety of other bacterial and fungal species have been reported to cause PVE.

Clinically, patients with late-onset PVE resemble those with native valve endocarditis. In early-onset PVE the diagnosis is difficult because of the presence of other infectious complications such as pneumonia, urinary tract infection, mediastinitis, or wound infection. New murmur, hypotension, heart failure, new cardiac conduction abnormalities, splenomegaly, and leukocytosis are more prevalent in early-onset PVE. Peripheral manifestations are more common in late-onset PVE. Echocardiography, echophonocardiography, and cinefluoroscopy have generally not been helpful in making the diagnosis of PVE. Sustained bacteremia is the most important clue to the diagnosis of PVE, but particularly in the early postoperative period it may be difficult to separate PVE from bacteremia due to other postoperative infections.

The initial antibiotic regimen should include vancomycin and an aminoglycoside because of frequency of methicillin-resistant staphylococci and gram-negative bacilli. The regimen is then adjusted based on careful in vitro sensitivity studies. Despite intensive antimicrobial therapy the mortality remains high. Overall mortality is around 50 percent, 40 percent with early-onset PVE and 70 to 80 percent with late-onset PVE. Early surgical intervention is indicated particularly in cases of early-onset PVE associated with a nonstreptococcal agent, a new murmur, heart failure, repeated major emboli, valve prosthesis malfunction, persistent fever, fungal endocarditis, relapse of infection, or atrioventricular conduction disturbances.

Negative Blood Cultures in Suspected Subacute Infective Endocarditis
The incidence of sterile blood cultures in published series averages 5 to 20 percent. In most cases, sterile blood cultures result from prior antibiotic therapy, failure to obtain sufficient cultures, use of improper media, failure to observe the cultures for at least 3 weeks, or incorrect diagnosis. The so-called sterile phase of the disease is a distinctly unlikely explanation, especially early in the illness. Active rheumatic fever, drug fever, sterile embolization in association with congestive heart failure, rheumatic pneumonitis, the postcommissurotomy syndrome, and connective-tissue disorders are the most common conditions masquerading as endocarditis. Atrial fibrillation and congestive failure suggest sterile emboli and weigh against the diagnosis of endocarditis in such patients; anemia favors it. Atrial myxoma, tuberculosis, lymphoma, and occult neoplasm or abscess should also be considered.

It is common practice to begin therapy for infective endocarditis in such patients after six blood cultures have been obtained. Some recommend that therapy be directed against viridans streptococci; others believe the possibility of enterococci should be the determinant of therapy. There is no simple answer. Because the prognosis is less favorable in patients with sterile blood cultures, vigorous therapy appears to be indicated, with 20 million units of penicillin and 1 g of streptomycin per day for 6 weeks. Oxacillin or nafcillin may be added if the clinical picture suggests acute infective endocarditis. For suspected prosthetic valve endocarditis, vancomycin and an aminoglycoside should be used. If therapeutic re-

sponse is observed, a full course of antibiotics is indicated. Defervescence, a rising hematocrit and reticulocytosis, the return of the appetite and the leukocyte count to normal, and the appearance of a sense of well-being in the patient are helpful signs. If there is no response in 2 weeks, therapy should be discontinued and the patient reevaluated. Treatment of infective endocarditis is expensive, inconvenient, and potentially dangerous and should not be undertaken lightly. Whenever possible, a therapeutic trial should be avoided, since it is rarely helpful and is often confusing.

Recurrence of Fever During Treatment of Proved Endocarditis

When fever recurs in patients being treated for endocarditis, inadequate antibiotic therapy is usually suspected, but it is rarely the cause when appropriate, standard, bactericidal regimens are used (Table 9.7–2). This is not surprising when one realizes that many forms of antibiotic therapy that are incapable of curing endocarditis are capable of suppressing most of the manifestations of the infection. It is rare for the organisms to become resistant during therapy. Drug fever, intercurrent infections, sterile abscesses at injection sites, embolization, thrombophlebitis at the site of intravenous therapy, superinfection of the valve with a resistant strain, metastatic abscesses, bleeding mycotic aneurysms, and coexisting disease should be suspected. Ancillary evidence supporting these possibilities should be sought (eosinophilia, rash, new physical findings, and so on). Nonessential drugs that may cause fever, such as sedatives, should be discontinued. More blood cultures should be obtained, and penicillinase (8000 U/ml of blood) should be added to the cultures if any of the penicillin analogues are being used in treatment. Determination of the bactericidal activity of serum from the patient against the offending organism may be helpful. Some enterococcus strains may require 50 million to 100 million units of penicillin daily. If serum diluted 1:8 in broth is bactericidal, therapy is probably adequate, and there is little reason to increase the dose of antibiotics.

If drug fever is suspected and an alternative bactericidal regimen is available, it may be wise to discontinue the suspected antibiotics. If no other antibiotic regimen is suitable, the presumed allergic reaction may be treated with antihistamines, aspirin, or adrenal corticosteroids as needed.

Fever After Cardiac Surgery

When patients undergoing cardiac surgery develop fever in the postoperative period, a stitch abscess of the myocardium, of the great vessels, or at the site of a prosthesis is an all too frequent cause.[15] Blood cultures are almost always positive with this complication but may be sterile until antibiotics are discontinued. Other causes of fever should be considered; among them are drug fever, viral hepatitis, wound abscess not involving the heart, pneumonia, atelectasis, empyema, osteomyelitis, endarteritis at the site of femoral cannulation, urinary tract infection, postcardiotomy syndrome, and cytomegalovirus infection. Intracardiac infections are more frequent in poor-risk patients undergoing long and technically difficult operations and in patients in whom it was difficult to achieve hemostasis.

If an intracardiac infection seems likely, an intensive and prolonged course of antibiotic therapy should be given. This is very hazardous unless the microbial etiology has been established. Control of the infection prepares the patient for reoperation, which is usually necessary. It is practically impossible to cure the infection unless the prosthesis or infected suture is removed, but a few patients have been cured when infection caused by very sensitive organisms was treated intensively for prolonged periods with bactericidal therapy.

Prophylactic Antibiotics

Prophylactic antimicrobial drugs should be given to patients with congenital or acquired valvular heart disease at the time of diagnostic or therapeutic manipulations involving the teeth and the upper respiratory or urinary tracts.

The experimental endocarditis model suggests that oral penicillin, erythromycin, tetracycline, ampicillin, cephalothin, and many other single agents are not effective. In contrast, vancomycin or the combination of penicillin with an aminoglycoside is effective.[4] Prophylaxis for mitral valve prolapse was discussed earlier in this chapter. The American Heart Association recommendations have been revised, and follow-up doses are now limited to a single dose administered 6 hours after the procedure.

REFERENCES

1. Bain RC, Edwards JE, et al: Right-sided bacterial endocarditis and endarteritis: Clinical and pathologic study. Am J Med 24:98, 1958
2. Bennett IL Jr, Beeson PB: Bacteremia: A consideration of some experimental and clinical aspects. Yale J Biol Med 26:241, 1954
3. Durack DT, Pelleher L, Petersdorf RB: Chemotherapy of experimental streptococcal endocarditis. II. Synergism between penicillin and streptomycin against penicillin-sensitive streptococci. J Clin Invest 53:829, 1974
4. Durack DT, Petersdorf RG: Chemotherapy of experimental streptococcal endocarditis. I. Comparison of commonly recommended prophylactic regimens. J Clin Invest 52:592, 1973
5. Garvey GH, New HC: Infective endocarditis—An evolving disease. A review of endocarditis at the Columbia Presbyterian Medical Center 1968–1973. Medicine 57:105, 1978
6. Geraci JE, Wilson WR: Endocarditis due to gram-negative bacteria. Mayo Clinic Proc 57:145, 1982
7. Griffin FM Jr, Jones G, Gobbs CG: Aortic insufficiency in bacterial endocarditis. Ann Intern Med 76:23, 1972
8. Gutman RA, Striker GE, et al: The immune complex glomerulonephritis of bacterial endocarditis. Medicine 51:1, 1972
9. Hickey AJ, MacMahon SN, et al: Mitral valve prolapse endocarditis: When is antibiotic prophylaxis necessary? Am Heart J 109:431, 1985
10. Hunter TH: The treatment of some bacterial infections of the heart and pericardium. Bull NY Acad Med 28:213, 1952
11. Karchmer AN: Staphylococcal endocarditis—laboratory and clinical basis for antibiotic therapy. Am J Med 78(suppl 6B):116, 1985
12. Klein RS, Reuco RA, et al: Association of *Streptococcus bovis* with carcinoma of the colon. N Engl J Med 297:800, 1977
13. Lerner PI, Weinstein L: Infective endocarditis in the antibiotic era. N Engl J Med 274:199, 259, 288, 323, 1966
14. Lord JW, Imparato AM, et al: Endocarditis complicating open-heart surgery. Circulation 23:608, 1970
15. Medical Letter: Prevention of bacterial endocarditis. Med Lett Drug 26:3, 1984
16. Mills J, Utley J, Abbott J: Heart failure in infective endocarditis: Predisposing factors, course treatment. Chest 66:151, 1974
17. Mintz GS, Kotler MA, et al: Comparison of two-dimensional and M-mole echocardiography in the evaluation of patients with infective endocarditis. Am J Cardiol 43:738, 1979
18. Pruitt AA, Rubin RH, et al: Neurologic complications of bacterial endocarditis. Medicine 57:329, 1978
19. Ramsey RG, Gunnar RM, Tobin JR: Endocarditis in the drug addict. Am J Cardiol 25:608, 1970
20. Rowley KM, Clubb KS, et al: Right-sided infective endocarditis as a consequence of flow-directed pulmonary artery catheterization. N Engl J Med 311:1152, 1984
21. Wann LS, Dillon JC, et al: Echocardiography in bacterial endocarditis. N Engl J Med 295:135, 1976
22. Weinstein L, Rubin RH: Infective endocarditis. Prog Cardiovasc Dis 16:239, 1973
23. Weinstein MP, Stratton CW, et al: Multicenter collaborative evaluation of a standard serum bactericidal test as a prognostic factor in infective endocarditis. Am J Med 78:268, 1985
24. Wilson WR, Danielson GK, et al: Prosthetic valve endocarditis. Mayo Clin Proc 57:155, 1982
25. Wilson WR, Giuliani ER, et al: General considerations in the diagnosis and treatment of infective endocarditis. Mayo Clin Proc 57:81, 1982
26. Wise JR, Cleland WP, et al: Urgent aortic valve replacement for acute aortic regurgitation due to infective endocarditis. Lancet 2:115, 1971

Infections of Gastrointestinal Tract

Nathaniel F. Pierce and John G. Bartlett

Infections of the gastrointestinal tract are second in frequency only to those of the upper respiratory tract. They affect all ages but are most frequent among children. Cases may be sporadic, but epidemic spread can occur. In developing countries, acute gastrointestinal infections are a major cause of morbidity and mortality, especially among small children. Causative agents include viruses, bacteria, and protozoa. The most frequent symptoms of infection are vomiting and diarrhea. Evidence of mucosal damage, including bleeding, exudate formation, and perforation, also may occur.

This chapter concerns gastrointestinal infections that are transmitted by the fecal-oral route. Intestinal infections that are sexually transmitted are considered in Chapters 9.14 and 9.15.

THE INTESTINAL FLORA

Intestinal bacteria are most numerous in the distal ileum and colon, where bowel contents move slowly. The large and relatively stable populations at these sites (10^{11} bacteria per gram of colonic contents) reflect a balanced ecosystem that is sustained by interactions between the various bacterial species and by the host immune response at the mucosal surface. The proximal small intestine has far fewer bacteria, about 10^3 per ml of fluid.

The normal flora is relatively stable, but may be altered by a variety of events, including damage to the mucosa (irradiation or cytotoxic drug therapy), changes in intestinal motility (diarrhea, intestinal stasis, or the presence of "blind loops" of gut), interference with bacterial growth (antibiotic therapy), or the introduction of a new viral, bacterial, or protozoan agent. Colonization with new microbial agents is usually brief, ending in a few days or weeks as the host develops a specific mucosal immune response. Most episodes of transient colonization are asymptomatic. When the colonizing agent is a pathogen, however, symptoms may develop. Specific symptoms are determined by the portion of the bowel involved and the virulence mechanisms of the pathogen.

EPIDEMIOLOGY AND SUSCEPTIBILITY TO INFECTION

Some gastrointestinal infections are spread by direct fecal-oral contamination, for example, *Shigella* and rotavirus. Most, however, follow ingestion of fecally contaminated water or food. Thus, they are common in conditions of poor sanitation, especially when host susceptibility is high. The combination of poor sanitation and high host susceptibility permits epidemic spread, which can occur with almost any enteric pathogen. Spread of infection is also aided by the occurrence of numerous asymptomatic infections during which affected persons pass large numbers of pathogenic bacteria, viruses, or parasite cysts in their feces.

Host susceptibility is determined primarily by prior infection, which often provides some degree of immunity. Additional determinants include malnutrition, which may impair mucosal immune mechanisms, and impaired gastric acid production, which increases susceptibility to acid-sensitive bacteria, such as *Vibrio cholerae*. Because they lack acquired immunity, children are the most frequent victims of enteric infection. Adults who escape infection during childhood remain susceptible and are at high risk when traveling to areas of low sanitation. This explains the high incidence of travelers' diarrhea, often due to toxigenic *Escherichia coli*, among persons traveling from developed to underdeveloped countries.

Some enteric infections, especially viral ones, exhibit a seasonal pattern that is unexplained. Thus, enteroviruses cause disease primarily in the late summer and fall, whereas rotavirus infections occur mostly in winter months.

PATHOGENESIS OF INTESTINAL INFECTIONS

BACTERIAL INFECTIONS

Most enteric pathogens cause disease by one of three mechanisms: (1) the production of enterotoxins, (2) invasion and damage of the mucosa, or (3) mucosal invasion leading to bacteremia and extraintestinal foci of infection (Tables 9.8–1 and 9.8–2). With some, these mechanisms may be combined.[12]

Toxicogenic bacteria that colonize but do not invade the mucosa include *V. cholerae,* some *E. coli,* and possibly others. Colonization occurs in the small bowel, where the enterotoxin is produced and acts on the mucosa to cause secretion of an isotonic electrolyte solution, which leads to watery diarrhea. *V. cholerae,* serotype 01, and *E. coli* produce antigenically related protein enterotoxins that cause electrolyte secretion by stimulating adenylate cyclase activity and raising the level of cyclic adenosine monophosphate (cAMP) in mucosal epithelium.[8,11] Some *E. coli* produce an unrelated heat-stable enterotoxin that induces secretion by increasing levels of cyclic guanosine monophosphate (cGMP) in mucosal cells. Enterohemorrhagic *E. coli* causes bloody diarrhea ascribed to production of a toxin that is antigenically related to the enterotoxin produced by the Shiga bacillus.[8] A similar organism, or other enterotoxins, may be important in diarrhea caused by some strains of shigella, salmonella, aeromonas, *Vibrio parahaemolyticus,* and *V. cholerae* other than the 01 serotype. Additionally, some bacteria grow in contaminated food, ingestion of which causes vomiting or diarrhea without bacterial colonization of the intestine; the illness usually lasts less than 24 hours. These bacteria, which include *Clostridium perfringens* and toxigenic strains of *Staphylococcus aureus,* and *Bacillus cereus,* are the major causes of food poisoning. Finally, colonic overgrowth by *Clostridium difficile* may complicate antibiotic therapy, especially in patients who are chronically ill or recovering from surgery; the result is colitis with mucosal damage and diarrhea, probably mediated by cytotoxins of the offending organism.[1]

Invasive organisms include *Shigella, Salmonella,* enteroinvasive strains of *E. coli, Campylobacter jejuni,* and *Yersinia enterocolitica.* Invasion occurs in the distal ileum and colon. *Shigella* and invasive *E. coli* disrupt the mucosa, inducing a vigorous inflammatory response with signs of colonic irritation (tenesmus, abdominal pain) and the appearance of blood, mucus, and pus in the stool; infections with *C. jejuni* often cause a similar clinical picture.[2] Bacteremia with these organisms is unusual. In contrast, mucosal invasion by salmonellae causes little local inflammation but may be the first step leading to bacteremia and the syndrome of enteric fever. Diarrhea may also occur and is possibly mediated by an enterotoxin. It is uncertain how *Y. enterocolitica* causes diarrhea, but infection with this agent is often complicated by bacteremia and symptoms of systemic infection.

TABLE 9.8–1. BACTERIAL INFECTIONS OF THE INTESTINE

Mechanism	Major Symptoms	Fecal Leukocytes	Common Causative Organisms
Enterotoxin released in small bowel	Watery diarrhea, vomiting	No	Toxigenic *E. coli, V. cholerae, V. parahaemolyticus*
Food contaminated with toxin-producing organism	Vomiting, diarrhea	No	*S. aureus, C. perfringens, B. cereus*
Cytotoxicity by bacterial toxin	Diarrhea, often with colitis or pseudomembranous colitis	Variable	*C. difficile*
Mucosal invasion causing inflammation (also possible enterotoxin)	Dysentery, blood, or mucus in stool, fever, tenesmus, "toxicity"; may have watery diarrhea at onset	Yes	*Shigella*, invasive *E. coli*, some *Salmonella, V. parahaemolyticus, Y. enterocolitica, C. jejuni*
Mucosal invasion leading to bacteremia	"Enteric fever," some have watery diarrhea at onset	Yes	*Salmonella*, including *S. typhi*

VIRAL INFECTIONS

Acute gastroenteritis, with vomiting, diarrhea, and low-grade fever, also is caused by a variety of viral agents (Table 9.8–2).[3] The rotavirus is the major cause of acute dehydrating watery diarrhea in infants. Other viruses, including caliciviruses, parvoviruses, coronaviruses, and adenoviruses, also cause diarrhea in humans and in animals. The most commonly known cause of viral gastroenteritis in adults is the Norwalk agent. This organism may cause sporadic cases, but it also is responsible for large outbreaks.[3,7] Viruses replicate in the small-bowel mucosa, inducing mild inflammatory changes and transient flattening of the villi. Secretion of water and electrolytes occurs during mucosal repair, probably because of a transient predominance of immature mucosal cells. Malabsorption of dietary ingredients, especially lactose, also contributes to the diarrhea.

Other viral infections of the gut may produce no enteric symptoms, but lead to systemic spread with serious consequences, as occurs with poliomyelitis, other enterovirus infections, and infectious hepatitis.

PROTOZOAN INFECTIONS

Three protozoans, *Giardia lamblia, Cryptosporidium* sp and *Entamoeba histolytica*, are important causes of intestinal infection (Table 9.8–2). Each are acquired by ingestion of cysts from the feces of an infected individual. *G. lamblia* adheres to the mucosa of the jejunum and causes flattening of the villi. Flatulence, abdominal pain, malabsorption, and malodorous watery diarrhea are common symptoms, but the mechanism by which these are produced is uncertain. *E. histolytica* usually reside in the lumen of the colon, but occasionally penetrate colonic or ileal mucosa, producing characteristic ulcerative lesions and an inflammatory exudative response, frequently with bleeding; the clinical picture may resemble that caused by ulcerative colitis. In some instances *E. histolytica* migrate by the portal circulation to lodge in the liver or elsewhere and produce abscess formation. Cryptosporidia colonize the small bowel and cause watery diarrhea. In the immunocompetent host the disease is self-limited; in the immunodeficient patient, especially patients with AIDS, there may be chronic, debilitating diarrhea.[4]

CLINICAL CONSEQUENCES OF INTESTINAL INFECTION

The clinical conquences of intestinal infection are determined by the virulence mechanisms of the infective agent and the site of infection. They include water and electrolyte loss, intestinal malab-

sorption, blood and protein loss, systemic toxicity, and extraintestinal infection.

WATER AND ELECTROLYTE LOSS

The clinical effects of watery diarrhea are due entirely to the loss of water and electrolytes. Liquid stool is usually isosmotic with plasma, but its electrolyte composition is determined by the speed of passage through the gut and the presence of osmotically active derivatives of food. Electrolyte concentrations are highest when stool loss is rapid and there is no dietary intake (Table 9.8–3). When stool losses are combined with losses in urine, and losses by evaporation and vomiting, the usual net deficit is isotonic with plasma, that is, isotonic dehydration occurs. In some cases, water is lost in excess of sodium, giving hypertonic dehydration; this usually occurs when feeding of hypertonic fluids, such as undiluted cow's milk, is continued during diarrhea or when water intake is inadequate to replace evaporative losses.

The most important effect of watery diarrhea is the loss of isotonic saline. This causes extracellular volume depletion, which leads progressively to hypotension, shock, and eventually death. When this loss equals 10 percent of the body weight, death is near and the signs of saline depletion are obvious: poor skin turgor, cold cyanotic extremities, feeble or absent radial pulse, stupor, oliguria, and flat neck veins. On the other hand, loss of only half this amount, 5 percent of the body weight, may appear deceptively benign, the only signs being thirst, a feeling of fatigue, and possibly accentuated postural changes in pulse. It is important that patients with saline depletion be recognized and treated at this point, because symptoms and the risk of serious morbidity and mortality increase rapidly with further unreplaced fluid losses.

Bicarbonate loss during watery diarrhea causes metabolic acidosis, which may be severe; Kussmaul respirations develop as a compensatory mechanism. There is also a shift of blood volume into the pulmonary circulation, which may cause pulmonary edema if hypovolemia is corrected without concurrent correction of the acidosis (e.g., by giving normal saline).

Acute diarrhea also causes potassium depletion, but hypokalemia may not develop until the acidosis is corrected. Symptomatic hypokalemia is uncommon in adults unless there is preexisting potassium depletion. Signs of hypokalemia, including arrhythmias and paralytic ileus, are more common in children.

INTESTINAL DAMAGE AND MALABSORPTION

The most common manifestation of intestinal damage by enteritis is lactose intolerance due to loss of the brush border enzyme lactase. This enzyme splits lactose into absorbable glucose and galac-

TABLE 9.8–2. CAUSES OF ACUTE INFECTIOUS DIARRHEA

	Agent	Disease Form(s)	Comments
Viruses	Rotavirus and pararotavirus	Childhood diarrhea	Most common cause of childhood diarrhea in winter
	Norwalk agent, small rounded viruses	Acute diarrhea with cramps, vomiting, "intestinal flu"	Epidemics and sporadic cases, involving all ages
	Adenoviruses	Childhood diarrhea, especially types 40 and 41	Also occurs in bone marrow transplant recipients
	Calicivirus	Childhood viruses	Outbreaks and sporadic cases
Bacteria	Toxigenic *E. coli*	Watery diarrhea	Two types of toxin; important cause of traveler's diarrhea
	Invasive *E. coli*	Dysentery	Resembles shigellosis clinically
	Enteropathogenic *E. coli*	Watery diarrhea	Specific serotypes cause diarrhea
	Enterohemorrhagic *E. coli*	Bloody diarrhea	Usually caused by serotype 0157:H7
	V. cholerae, serotype 01	Severe watery diarrhea	Now present in South Asia, the Mideast, Africa, and U.S. Gulf Coast
	V. cholerae, other serotypes	Watery diarrhea	Especially in areas near salt water
	V parahaemolyticus	Watery diarrhea or dysentery	Poorly cooked shellfish are common source; may cause sepsis
	Aeromonas	Acute or chronic diarrhea	Untreated water
	C. jejuni	Watery or bloody diarrhea	Most common bacterial agent of diarrhea in developed world
	S. aureus	Vomiting and watery diarrhea; food poisoning	Preformed heat-stable enterotoxin in food; onset 2–4 hours after eating
	C. perfringens	Water diarrhea; food poisoning	Bacterial contamination of poorly cooked meat, poultry, or beans; onset 8–14 hours after eating
	B. cereus	Vomiting or diarrhea; food poisoning	Heat-stable enterotoxin; onset 2–14 hours after eating
	C. difficile	Diarrhea with colitis or pseudomembranous colitis	Caused by antiobiotic therapy, most commonly clindamycin, ampicillin, or cephalosporin
	Salmonella sp	Enteric fever, watery diarrhea, focal extraintestinal infections	Organisms (except *S. typhi*) in many processed foods; febrile enteritis is common form; gallbladder carriers for *S. typhi*
	Shigella sp	Watery diarrhea or dysentery; systemic complications with *S. dysenteriae* or *S. flexneri*	Person-to-person spread; infective inoculum may be very low
	Y. enterocolitica	Water diarrhea or dysentery	May also develop sepsis, arthritis, mesenteric lymphadenitis, erythema nodosum
Protozoa	*G. lamblia*	Watery diarrhea; chronic diarrhea with malabsorption	Spread by contaminated water
	E. histolytica	Dysentery or hepatic abscess	Often asymptomatic
	Cryptosporidium	Watery diarrhea	Prolonged diarrhea in immunosuppressed host, especially with AIDS

tose. When lactose hydrolysis fails, it is fermented by intestinal bacteria, producing acid, gas, and osmotically active fragments that draw more water into the intestine, thus aggravating the diarrhea. Lactose intolerance occurs, to some extent, with all forms of infectious enteritis that involve the small intestine; it may last for weeks, or even months, after the infection is terminated.

Other disaccharides, fats, and vitamins also may be malabsorbed during or shortly after diarrhea. This, combined with the common practice of withholding food during diarrhea, contributes to the cycle of diarrhea-malabsorption-malnutrition that occurs among the underprivileged throughout the world.

ENTERIC BLOOD AND PROTEIN LOSS

Anemia and hypoproteinemia, due to intestinal loss of blood and serum proteins, are serious complications of severe enteritis, such

TABLE 9.8–3. ELECTROLYTE CONTENT OF PLASMA AND STOOL DURING WATERY DIARRHEA (mEq or mmol/L)

	Plasma Normal	Watery Stool[a]	Plasma Severe Diarrhea[b]
Sodium	140	30–140	130–144
Potassium	4	10–30	3.5–5
Bicarbonate	25	10–50	7–15
Chloride	100	40–105	105–120

[a]Sodium and chloride content increase and potassium decreases with increasing rate of loss of stool. Bicarbonate declines with uncorrected acidosis or organic acids in stool, as occurs with lactase deficiency and continued milk intake.
[b]Typical values for isotonic dehydration.

as that caused by *Shigella* or *Clostridium difficile*. When this occurs in patients already malnourished or chronically ill, the risk of mortality is greatly increased.

FEVER, TOXICITY, AND SEPSIS

Patients with diarrhea caused by invasive bacteria often have fever, headache, myalgia, abdominal pain, malaise, tenesmus, and prostration. Children with shigellosis also may develop grand mal seizures. *Salmonella* bacteremia may cause localized infection (osteomyelitis, aortitis, abscesses), especially in compromised patients, such as those with sickle cell disease, immune deficiencies, or neoplastic disease. Enteric fever is a prolonged febrile bacteremic infection caused by *Salmonella typhi,* or sometimes other salmonella serotypes, in which diarrhea and localized systemic infections are not major features. Systemic infection with *Y. enterocolitica* may cause abdominal pain, mesenteric lymphadenitis, and a syndrome indistinguishable from acute appendicitis.

PATIENT MANAGEMENT

DIAGNOSIS

Determination of the cause of an episode of intestinal infection is important for two reasons: (1) to guide the use of antimicrobial therapy, and (2) to assist public health workers in their epidemiologic studies and control efforts. Unfortunately the etiologic agent for an acute episode of diarrhea often is unidentified despite a thorough diagnostic evaluation.

The patient should be questioned concerning important symptoms that characterize the illness, such as fever, vomiting, abdominal pain, tenesmus, blood or pus in the stool, and duration of illness. Other important data include information on recent travel (especially to areas of poor sanitation), similar symptoms among family members or other contacts, recent antibiotic therapy, recent ingestion of raw or poorly cooked seafood, and gastric surgery or the use of antacids. Physical findings that should be sought include evidence of saline depletion (decreased skin turgor, postural hypotension, or tachycardia), fever, and abdominal tenderness.

Diagnostic studies aimed at determining the etiologic agent are summarized in Table 9.8–4. Initial evaluation should include (1) the appearance of the stool (i.e., watery, mucoid, or bloody) and (2) tests for fecal blood and leukocytes. With these results it is usually possible to determine whether diarrhea is virus or toxin mediated (i.e., watery stool without blood or fecal leukocytes) or due to invasive or cytotoxin-producing bacteria (i.e., bloody, mucoid stool or stool with fecal leukocytes; see Table 9.8–1).[2,6] In most instances, stool and blood should also be cultured for pathogenic bacteria. For stool culture, both selective and nonselective media should be used, including specialized media or growth conditions for isolation of *C. jejuni, Y. enterocolitica,* and *Vibrio* sp (in areas near the sea). The choice of additional diagnostic studies should be guided by results of the initial evaluation. For example, evidence of colitis (e.g., fever, abdominal pain, tenesmus, and mu-

TABLE 9.8–4. TESTS FOR THE ETIOLOGY OF INTESTINAL INFECTION

Procedure	Comment
Stool Examination	
Appearance	Watery stool suggests enterotoxin or viral diarrhea; mucoid, bloody stool suggests invasive agent
Methylene blue stain for leukocytes	PMNs suggest mucosal invasion and damage; mononuclears suggest *S. typhi* (Table 9.8–1)
Tests for Specific Etiologic Agents	
Fresh, 37C wet preparation for amebas	Identification of pathogenic trophozoites requires experienced observer
Stool concentrate	For cysts of *E. histolytica, G. lamblia;* needs experienced observer
ELISA of stool for rotavirus or adenovirus	Especially for children <2 yr old
Stool acid-fast stain	For cryptosporidia
Test for cytotoxin of *C. difficile*	Tissue culture assay; requires a reference laboratory
Stool culture	Helpful for *Salmonella, Shigella, Vibrio, Aeromonas, Campylobacter,* and *Y. enterocolitica;* testing of *E. coli* for enterotoxin, invasiveness, and serotyping requires a reference laboratory
Blood, urine culture	Frequently positive in enteric fever due to *S. typhi* or other salmonellae; also may be positive for *Y. enterocolitica*
Other Tests	
Sigmoidoscopy	To diagnose inflammatory colitis (i.e., due to *C. difficile*) or amebiasis
Duodenal aspiration	For recovery of trophozoites of *G. lamblia;* jejunal biopsy may also be diagnostic
Serology	
Typhoid fever	Rise in antibody to O antigen (Widal test); not entirely specific
Cholera, toxigenic *E. coli*	Frequent rise in antibody to cholera toxin or heat-labile *E. coli* toxin; rise in bactericidal antibody to *V. cholerae;* requires reference laboratory
Viral diarrhea	Rise in antibody to specific virus; requires reference laboratory
Amebiasis	Elevated indirect hemagglutination titer

coid stool with blood and leukocytes) suggests a diagnosis of shigellosis but also may require that fresh stool be examined for cysts or trophozoites of E. histolytica and tested for the cytotoxin of C. difficile[1]; additionally, sigmoidoscopy may be required to confirm the diagnosis of colitis, to help distinguish between amebiasis, bacterial enterocolitis, and ulcerative colitis, and to obtain optimal samples for detection of amebae. On the other hand, acute watery diarrhea without fecal leukocytes, occurring in an infant, suggests a viral etiology, or possibly disease due to toxigenic E. coli; appropriate studies would include ELISA assays of stool for rotavirus, and testing of fecal E. coli for enterotoxin production. Unfortunately, some diagnostic studies, such as tests of E. coli for enterotoxin production, are available only in reference laboratories. Serologic studies usually are not helpful except in amebiasis.

TREATMENT

The major objectives of treatment are (1) prompt replacement of water and electrolyte losses and (2) termination of infection and control of toxicity. Additionally, nutritional maintenance is important for malnourished patients.

Water and Electrolyte Replacement

For patients with watery diarrhea, water and electrolyte replacement should begin promptly; when serious dehydration exists, the need is urgent. The goals are to correct existing water and electrolyte deficits and then replace ongoing stool losses until diarrhea stops. This can be done by two methods:

1. Oral replacement using a glucose- or sucrose-electrolyte solution.[10,13]
2. Intravenous infusion of electrolyte solutions.

Oral rehydration is convenient for all patients who can drink and are not seriously hypovolemic; it can be used in any treatment setting and is the most practical therapy where treatment facilities are limited, as is often the case in underdeveloped countries. Intravenous therapy is acceptable in modern hospitals and is essential to correct hypovolemia with shock.

The first step is estimation of the fluid deficit. A rule-of-thumb is that a 5 percent loss of body weight (mild dehydration) produces minimal signs (thirst, slight tachycardia, slightly diminished skin turgor), whereas a 10 percent deficit (severe dehydration) is nearly lethal (causing severe thirst, anuria, markedly decreased skin turgor, feeble or absent radial pulse, hypotension, and stupor). For rapid rehydration of severely dehydrated patients, an intravenous infusion must be quickly established. The replacement fluid should have an electrolyte content nearly isotonic with plasma and include appropriate electrolytes to correct serious existing deficits, including metabolic acidosis and potassium depletion. Ringer lactate is the best commercially available solution but requires potassium supplementation to a total of 15 mEq/L. Normal saline is the poorest electrolyte solution but is much improved when supplemented with bicarbonate (30 mEq/L) and potassium (15 mEq/L). In severely hypovolemic patients, at least half the estimated fluid deficit should be infused as rapidly as possible (e.g., 30 minutes), the rest being given over 2 to 4 hours.

For patients with moderate or mild dehydration, oral replacement therapy is usually ideal (see below). If intravenous therapy is used, however, replacement may be given over 6 to 8 hours. Any ongoing losses should also be replaced as they occur; when possible, stool should be measured and replaced volume-for-volume with the same intravenous fluid. Adequate "free" water, given as water by mouth or as a dextrose-water infusion, is needed to replace evaporative and urinary losses. Satisfactory volume replacement is indicated by a full peripheral pulse, adequate urine output, good skin turgor, and a stable posthydration body weight.

Oral therapy with a glucose- or sucrose-electrolyte solution (Table 9.8–5) is effective for acute dehydrating diarrhea of any eti-

TABLE 9.8–5. COMPOSITION OF ORAL GLUCOSE- OR SUCROSE–ELECTROLYTE SOLUTION

	Grams/L		mmol/L
NaCl	3.5	Na$^+$	90
NaHCO$_3$	2.5	K$^+$	20
KCl	1.5	Cl$^-$	80
Glucose or Sucrose	20 40	HCO$_3^-$	30
		Glucose or sucrose	110 110

ology in patients of all ages.[10,13] The glucose or sucrose is required to facilitate sodium and water absorption. The solution can be prepared as needed using table salt, baking soda, potassium chloride, and glucose or sucrose. It should not be heated and need not be sterile. Patients with severe dehydration, inability to drink, or paralytic ileus require initial intravenous rehydration (50 to 100 ml/kg), after which the oral solution can usually be used. Further intravenous fluids are not usually needed. Most patients will take, ad libitum, sufficient amounts of the oral solution to restore and maintain fluid and electrolyte balance. Patients with rapid continuing diarrhea may need encouragement to drink the needed amounts. Vomiting usually stops after initial intravenous rehydration of severely hypovolemic patients and seldom interferes seriously with oral therapy. When vomiting does persist, the amounts are usually small in relation to the volumes of stool and oral solution and can be replaced by additional oral solution. If vomiting is severe and there are signs of increasing dehydration, intravenous replacement must be used.

Antimicrobial Therapy

Antibiotics are useful in specific enteric infections (Table 9.8–6) but are never a substitute for adequate rehydration.[12] Oral tetracycline benefits cholera by reducing the volume of stool, the duration of diarrhea, and the duration of excretion of the pathogen. Antibiotics are also of benefit for shigellosis; however, knowledge of antibiotic sensitivity patterns in the area should be used to guide antibiotic selection. In contrast, antibiotic treatment of Salmonella gastroenteritis prolongs the convalescent carrier state and is contraindicated except when disease is severe or occurs among infants, the elderly, or debilitated persons. Systemic salmonella infections, such as typhoid fever, enteric fever, and focal extraintestinal infections, require specific therapy, however. Chloramphenicol (50 mg/kg/day) or ampicillin (100 mg/kg/day), each to be given in divided doses for at least 14 days, is usually effective, but the sensitivity of the organism should be confirmed. Antibiotics are of unproven value in treating diarrhea caused by C. jejuni or Y. enterocolitica, but they may eliminate fecal carriage of the pathogen and should be used for bacteremic infections. Oral vancomycin or metronidazole is effective for colitis due to C. difficile.[1] Antibiotics have no proven value in acute nonspecific diarrhea.

Treatment of infection with E. histolytica or G. lamblia also is summarized in Table 9.8–6. Because stool examination for giardial cysts may be negative during active disease, a trial of therapy is sometimes appropriate, especially in persons with a history of exposure and typical symptoms (i.e., foul watery flatulence, vague epigastric discomfort), and in whom duodenal intubation to search for trophozoites is not available.

Other Medications

Opiates and their derivatives (deodorized tincture of opium, Lomotil) relieve peristaltic cramping and diminish stool frequency during mild diarrhea. They are useless, however, in serious watery diarrhea and should be avoided in diarrhea due to invasive patho-

TABLE 9.8–6. ANTIMICROBIAL THERAPY OF ACUTE INTESTINAL INFECTIONS

Organism	Antimicrobial Therapy	Adult Dosage (Preferred Agent)	Comment
Shigella	Trimethoprim-sulfamethoxazole (ampicillin)[a]	2 tablets q12h for 5 days 1 tablet; T 80 mg, S 400 mg (500 mg q6h, for 5 days)	Confirm sensitivity in laboratory; ampicillin or tetracycline are suitable for sensitive strains
Salmonella	Ampicillin (chloramphenicol or trimethoprim-sulfamethoxazole)	1 g q4–6h for 3–5 days (500 mg q6h for 3–5 days; or 2 tablets q12h for 3–5 days)	Confirm sensitivity in laboratory; no antibiotics for uncomplicated enteritis; see text for treatment of enteric fever
C. jejuni	Erythromycin	250 mg qid for 5 days	Eliminates organism from stool and prevents relapses; no proven effect on illness
Aeromonas	Aminoglycoside (trimethoprim-sulfamethoxazole)	1.7 mg/kg IV q8h	
Y. enterocolitica	Gentamicin (third-generation cephalosporin; trimethoprim-sulfamethoxazole	Use dosage appropriate for systemic infection; give parenterally	Diarrhea and mesenteric adenitis subside spontaneously; treat bacteremia according to bacterial sensitivity
V. cholerae	Tetracycline (nitrofurantoin)	500 mg q6h for 2–3 days (100 mg q6h for 2–3 days)	
E. coli	Subsalicylate bismuth (trimethoprim-sulfamethoxazole, doxycycline)	60 ml qid for 5 days	Traveler diarrhea
C. difficile colitis	Vancomycin (metronidazole)	125–500 mg q6h for 10–14 days	Parenteral vancomycin is ineffective; metronidazole is preferred for less seriously ill patients to reduce cost
G. lamblia	Metronidazole or tinidazole (quinacrine hydrochloride)	250 mg tid for 5–7 days, 1.5 g once	Trial of therapy for typical, undiagnosed cases; relapses require treatment
E. histolytica	Metronidazole plus Iodoquinol (emetine hydrochloride)	750 mg tid for 5–10 days 650 mg tid for 21 days	For diarrhea or dysentery, with fecal trophozoites
Cryptosporidia	(No specific treatment)		

[a]Second-choice therapy is shown in parentheses; all medications are oral unless otherwise stated.

gens, such as *Shigella,* because systemic symptoms are worsened. Nonspecific absorbants such as kaolin, pectin, and charcoal have no proven value and can interfere with absorption of antibiotics.

Diet

Patients with diarrhea should not be starved. In uncomplicated cases, food intake should be guided by the patient's appetite. Foods containing lactose should be resumed slowly. Boullion, chicken soup, cereals, toast, and bananas are well tolerated. Special efforts should be made to maintain nutrient intake in malnourished patients.

PREVENTION

Safe water supply, effective sewage disposal, and careful food preparation have diminished enteric infections in developed nations. Enteric viral infections remain frequent, however, and salmonella species are widespread in processed foods. Lack of environmental sanitation in many developing nations makes control of enteric infections almost impossible.

IMMUNIZATION

Poliovaccine is the outstanding example of effective immunoprophylaxis of an enteric infection. The oral live vaccine has the apparent advantage of inducing mucosal immunity and thus preventing asymptomatic intestinal infection. A recently developed live oral typhoid vaccine, based on the avirulent *S. typhi* mutant, Ty21a, has also proved both safe and highly effective in field trials.[9] It appears to be more protective than the traditional parenteral typhoid vaccine. Parenteral cholera vaccine is ineffective in preventing

intestinal colonization with *V. cholerae* and only modestly protective against clinical cholera. Prospects are excellent for the development of effective vaccines against the newly described diarrheagenic viruses (e.g., rotavirus), and increasing knowledge of the mechanisms of intestinal immunity suggest that oral immunization against other enteric bacterial infections also may be possible.

AVOIDING ANTIBIOTIC ABUSE

Treatment with almost any type of antibiotic can predispose to the development of enterocolitis due to *C. difficile.* Reducing the incidence and severity of this disease requires that antibiotics be used judiciously and that patients be observed carefully during treatment. If possible, antibiotic therapy should be ended promptly for patients who develop diarrhea during treatment.

REFERENCES

1. Bartlett JG, Chang TW, Onderdonk AB: Colitis by *Clostridium difficile.* Rev Infect Dis 1:370, 1979
2. Blaser MJ, Wells JG, Feldman RA: Campylobacter enteritis in the United States. Ann Intern Med 98:360, 1983
3. Cukor G, Blacklow NR: Human viral gastroenteritis. Microbiol Rev 48:157, 1984
4. Current WL, Reese NC, Ernst JV: Human cryptosporidiosis in immunocompetent and immunodeficient persons. N Engl J Med 308:1252, 1983
5. Guerrant RL, Shields DS, et al: Evaluation and diagnosis of acute infectious diarrhea. Am J Med 78 (suppl 6B):91, 1985
6. Harris JC, Dupont HL, Hornick RB: Fecal leukocytes in diarrheal illness. Ann Intern Med 76:697, 1972

7. Kuritsky JN, Osterholm MT, Greenberg HB: Norwalk gastroenteritis: A community outbreak associated with bakery product consumption. Ann Intern Med 100:519, 1984

8. Levine MM: *Escherichia coli* that cause diarrhea: Enterotoxigenic, enteropathogenic, enteroinvasive, enterohemorrhagic, and enteroadherent. J Infect Dis 155:377, 1987

9. Levine MM, Kaper JB, et al: New knowledge on pathogenesis of bacterial enteric infections as applied to vaccine development. Microbiol Rev 47:510, 1983

10. Palmer DL, Koster FT, et al: Comparison of sucrose and glucose in the oral electrolyte therapy of cholera and other severe diarrheas. N Engl J Med 297:1107, 1977

11. Pierce NF, Greenough WB, Carpenter CCJ: *Vibrio cholerae* enterotoxin, and its mode of action. Bacteriol Rev 35:1, 1971

12. Quinn TC, Beuder BS, Bartlett JG: New developments in infectious diarrhea. Disease-a-Month 32:166, 1986

13. Santosham M, Daum RS, Dillman L: Oral rehydration therapy of infantile diarrhea. N Engl J Med 306:1070, 1982

CHAPTER 9.9
Intra-abdominal Sepsis

John G. Bartlett

Intra-abdominal sepsis refers to infections within the abdominal cavity and external to the lumen of the gastrointestinal tract. Included are a variety of disease processes involving the peritoneal surface and parenchymal organs such as the liver, spleen, and pancreas. Infections restricted to the intestinal mucosa usually involve enteric pathogens and are considered in Chapter 9.8.

PATHOGENESIS OF INTRA-ABDOMINAL INFECTIONS

As with most infections, intra-abdominal sepsis represents the consequences of the interaction between host defense mechanisms and a microbial challenge.[1] The peritoneal cavity is the largest preformed extravascular space in the body with a surface area that approximates the total cutaneous surface. There is usually less than 50 ml of peritoneal fluid that is clear and contains less than 250 cells per microliter with approximately 50 percent macrophages and 40 percent lymphocytes. The peritoneal fluid has minimal antibacterial activity, which is primarily complement-mediated.

MICROBIAL INOCULA

Most infections of the abdominal cavity involve bacteria that normally colonize the gastrointestinal tract. The usual mechanism for infections involving serosal surfaces (nonparenchyma organ infections) is a breach in the mucosal barrier as the result of an associated disease process such as peptic ulcer disease with perforation, appendicitis, diverticular disease, inflammatory bowel disease, penetrating trauma, and intestinal surgery. Both the types and concentrations of bacteria in the inoculum depend on the level of the gastrointestinal tract involved (Fig. 9.9–1). The stomach usually harbors a relatively sparse flora of penicillin-sensitive gram-positive bacteria, which originate in the oropharynx. The major mechanism of population control is gastric acidity so that the concentrations of bacteria are substantially larger in patients with gastric achlorhydria as a consequence of aging or ingestion of several commonly used medications. The small bowel also harbors a sparse number of bacteria, but here the major limiting factor is constant peristalsis, which simply propels the bacteria to the more distal segments. Patients with intestinal stasis lose this protective mechanism and often have overgrowth with a flora that is similar to that in the colon. The implication is that perforation of the stomach or small bowel under otherwise physiologic conditions results in contamination with relatively small numbers of bacteria. With strangulation obstruction, however, the inoculum of bacteria may be analogous to that with colonic perforation.

The largest microbial population in the human body is the relatively stagnant distal segment of the intestinal tract, the colon, where the concentrations of bacteria reach 10^{12}/g of intestinal contents. This approximates the geometric limits with which bacteria occupy space so that the dry weight of stool is almost entirely bacteria. Approximately 99 percent are anaerobic bacteria. Coliforms and *Bacteroides* species are virtually always present, and the total number of species represented in an individual patient is estimated at 400 to 500. These observations provide a rational explanation for the prevalence of colonic disease in association with intra-abdominal sepsis and the considerably greater threat posed by colon surgery compared to surgery on more proximal portions of the gastrointestinal tract.

CHEMICAL IRRITANTS

In addition to the microbial populations, it is important to note that there also may be chemical irritants or adjuvants included in inocula originating from the contents of the lumen. Chemical irritants include the pancreatic enzymes, bile, and gastric acid, which can initiate an inflammatory response independent of bacteria. Adjuvant substances include hemoglobin, the fiber content of stool, fibrin, necrotic tissue, barium sulfate, and bile salts.[1] Studies in experimental animals indicate that these promote the inflammatory process either by chemotaxic properties or by resisting phagocytosis. The importance of these adjuvants is emphasized as intra-abdominal sepsis appears to be far more complicated than a simple microbial insult. In experimental animals, intraperitoneal challenge with broth cultures of bacteria may result in acute septicemia, but there is minimal inflammation within the peritoneum causing peritonitis or abscesses. These latter effects, which are the common sequelae of intestinal perforation, are noted only when the bacterial challenge is accompanied with an appropriate adjuvant.[1,3]

LYMPHATIC DRAINAGE

The only portion of the peritoneal surface that may clear bacteria independently of an inflammatory reaction is the inferior surface of the diaphragm, which contains lacunae of the lymphatic system with stoma of 8 to 12 mm in diameter. These serve as channels for drainage from the peritoneal cavity to the anterior mediastinal lymphatics and then to the systemic circulation. The diaphragmatic clearance mechanism represents the first line of defense when bacteria are introduced into the abdominal cavity and it is facilitated by the negative pressure of diaphragmatic movements that favor bacterial migration to the subdiaphragmatic location. The potential advantage is rapid elimination of bacteria introduced into the peritoneal cavity, but the disadvantage is that the lymphatic clearance mechanism may be overwhelmed, resulting in bacteremia.

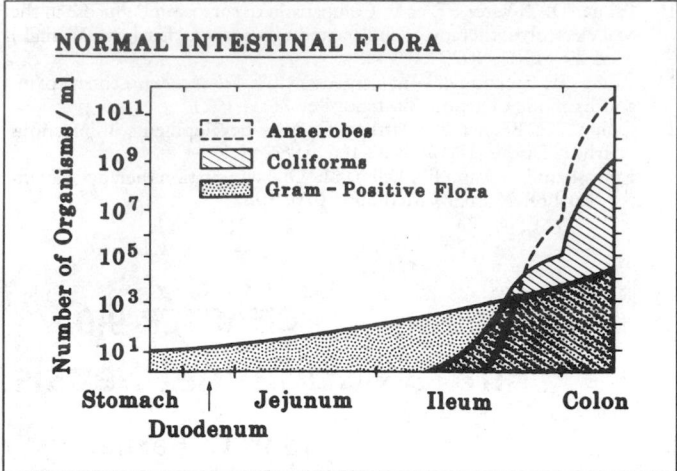

Figure 9.9–1. The microbial flora usually found at various levels of the gastrointestinal tract.

INFLAMMATORY RESPONSE

The second line of defense is the inflammatory response, which occurs within minutes. Initially, there is an influx of polymorphonuclear leukocytes. Bacteria activate the alternative complement system, opsonic (principally C3b) and chemotactic (principally C5a) factors are released, and opsonized bacteria are phagocytosed. Bacteria that are not eliminated successfully with the initial inflammatory response cause an aggregation of neutrophils, edema fluid, and viable bacteria that become entrapped as loculated collections or abscesses with a collagen wall. This response has the advantage of localizing the microbial insult. The disadvantage is that the microbes involved are relatively well protected from host defenses as well as systemically administered antibiotics. Neutrophils have a finite life of 2 to 5 days, so they break down within these loculated collections and release osmotically active products, causing the abscesses to increase in size with time.

CLINICAL MANIFESTATIONS

Clinical observations correlated with the data just summarized provide the rationale for considering intra-abdominal sepsis a "biphasic disease."[3] The initial insult may be free perforation of the intestine, with generalized peritonitis and the usual signs of an acute abdomen. Alternatively, the infection may be successfully restricted to its site of origin to form a "phlegmon," indicating localized peritonitis without the collagen wall of encapsulation found with abscesses. The phlegmon may be a much more subtle process than generalized peritonitis, and it often escapes clinical detection. The omentum facilitates the localization process by virtue of its mobility and high vascularity. With either localized or generalized peritonitis, a common sequelae is the second stage of the infection, which is characterized by intra-abdominal abscesses.

MONOMICROBIAL AND POLYMICROBIAL INFECTIONS

Infections of the abdominal cavity may be classified as monomicrobial or polymicrobial depending on the number of bacterial species located at the infected site. Common examples of monomicrobial infections are biliary tract infections, pancreatic infections (pancreatic abscess or infected pseudocysts), and spontaneous peritonitis. These are infections in which a single organism is usually involved, the predominant isolates being *Escherichia coli*, other col-

iforms, and streptococci. Most other infections of the abdominal cavity involve a complex mixture of aerobic and anaerobic bacteria derived from the normal intestinal flora (Fig. 9.9–1). The initial inoculum in cases associated with colonic disease presumably includes the 400 to 500 bacterial species noted previously so that the recovery of multiple organisms at the infected site is not surprising. Nevertheless this represents a distillate of the initial inoculum because only a small fraction of bacterial species survive. It is presumed that vagaries in the ability of various organisms to survive in a new environmental milieu or microbial virulence factors are involved in the selection process. The predominant isolates in exudate or blood cultures are coliform bacteria, principally *E. coli*, and *Bacteroides* species, especially *B. fragilis*[1] (Table 9.9–1). Intra-abdominal sepsis associated with diseases of the stomach and small bowel tend to involve the more simplified flora of the upper gastrointestinal tract with gram-positive aerobic bacteria comprising the dominant isolates.

PERITONITIS

Primary Peritonitis

Peritonitis may be considered primary or secondary, depending on associated conditions. Primary, or "spontaneous," peritonitis is an infection of the peritoneal cavity found in patients with ascites, usually adults with cirrhosis or children with nephrosis.[5] The suspected pathophysiologic mechanism is bacteremic seeding of a susceptible nidus, and the usual pathogens are coliform bacteria, especially *E. coli* or streptococci, including *S. pneumoniae*. The diagnosis is suspect in a patient with prior ascites, abdominal tenderness, fever, and peritoneal fluid containing over 300 leukocytes per microliter with a dominance of polymorphonuclear cells. This diagnosis is established with positive cultures of peritoneal fluid or blood in the typical setting.

Secondary Peritonitis

The most common form of peritonitis is the secondary form involving bacteria derived from the intestinal flora that contaminate the peritoneal cavity by direct extension as a result of a breach in mucosal integrity. The peritoneal surface serves as a semipermeable barrier to passive bidirectional flow of water and solutes. The acute inflammatory reaction with generalized peritonitis may result in a net flow of 300 to 500 ml of fluid per hour into the peritoneal

TABLE 9.9–1. BACTERIOLOGY OF PERITONITIS AND INTRA-ABDOMINAL ABSCESS[a]

	No.	(%)
Aerobic bacteria		
E. coli	235	(60)
Klebsiella-Enterobacter	101	(26)
Proteus	87	(22)
Pseudomonas	30	(08)
Enterococcus	66	(17)
Streptococci (other)	108	(28)
Anaerobic bacteria		
Bacteroides sp	288	(72)
B. fragilis	153	(38)
Eubacteria	94	(24)
Clostridia	67	(17)
Peptostreptococci	55	(14)
Peptococci	42	(11)

[a]Based on a study of 391 patients.
Adapted from Ahrenholz DH, Simmons RL: In Simmons RL, Howard RJ (eds): Surgical Infectious Diseases. New York: Appleton-Century-Crofts, 1982.[1]

cavity, so that the hemodynamic consequences may be comparable to those of a 50 percent body surface burn. The initial symptom is usually pain, frequently sudden, that may be localized or generalized and is aggravated by any movement. There is generalized tenderness, rebound tenderness, and voluntary muscular guarding when the parietal peritoneum becomes inflamed. Common associated findings are fever, leukocytosis, nausea, vomiting, ileus, abdominal distension with hyperresonance, and diminished or absent bowel sounds. The net fluid flux into the abdomen results in dehydration, a declining urinary output, and hypovolemic shock. These are the characteristic signs and symptoms associated with the classic acute abdomen.

Localized Peritonitis

Localized peritonitis refers to an inflammatory response restricted to the site of visceral inflammation, such as appendicitis or diverticulitis. These processes tend to be much more indolent in course and subtle in presentation. The initial symptom is often a vague pain, reflecting irritation of the visceral peritoneum, which produces minimal signs of localization. Subsequent involvement of the parietal peritoneum of the anterior abdominal wall permits the eventual appreciation of localized pain. This may never be apparent, however, with an inflammatory reaction in certain relatively inaccessible areas such as the subdiaphragmatic space or pelvis. Common associated findings include nonspecific findings of an inflammatory reaction such as fever and leukocytosis.

INTRA-ABDOMINAL ABSCESS

Intra-abdominal abscesses are purulent collections containing bacteria, neutrophils, and necrotic debris entrapped within a fibrous capsule. The most common predisposing causes are appendicitis, diverticulitis, prior intestinal surgery, trauma, and colonic carcinoma. Some patients have no obvious source of contamination.[1] The time interval between initial seeding of the peritoneal surface and clinical expression of an abscess is highly variable, ranging from days to years. Intra-abdominal abscesses may be distributed anywhere in the abdominal cavity, although there are certain preferential sites. A review of 540 cases of abdominal abscesses showed 36 percent involved the peritoneal surface, 38 percent were in the retroperitoneal space, and 26 percent were visceral[2] (Table 9.9–2). Intraperitoneal abscesses may occur adjacent to the area of initial inflammation, reflecting successful localization at the portal of entry, such as diverticular abscess or periappendiceal abscess. With free perforation the eventual location of abscesses reflects flow patterns of the intestinal contents that are governed by anatomic landmarks, gravity-favoring caudal spread, and intraperitoneal pressure gradients such as the diaphragmatic movement that favors cephalad spread. Thus flow tends to be upward, causing abscesses to localize in the subphrenic spaces, or downward, causing abscesses in the pericolic gutters and the pelvis.

Clinical Syndromes

Clinical manifestations are variable, with three recognized patterns: (1) the abscesses may follow immediately in the wake of generalized peritonitis; (2) there may be a biphasic clinical course in which the initial event apparently resolves, followed by an asymptomatic interlude that may last for days, months, or even years, which is in turn followed by the recurrence of symptoms involving microbes seeded at the time of the initial insult; and (3) there may be an insidious course with no obvious preceding event. The dominant complaints of the patient with an intra-abdominal abscess are also highly variable. Enteroparietal abscesses usually cause pain, tenderness, and a palpable mass. More difficult to detect are intraloop, intramesenteric, or subphrenic abscesses, because pain is often minimal or absent and there is usually no palpable mass. Pelvic abscesses may be palpated with rectal or vaginal examination, although the symptoms are often sufficiently vague that the appropriate examination is not performed.

Subphrenic abscesses are relatively common and are especially elusive to detect. The most common preceding conditions are prior surgery, perforated peptic ulcer disease, abdominal trauma, and acute appendicitis.[1] Most patients complain of abdominal pain that is diffuse and poorly localized. Respiratory symptoms, shoulder pain, chest pain, and weight loss are common associated complaints. Chest radiographs show pleural effusions, diaphragmatic elevation, or atelectasis in two thirds of cases. Retroperitoneal abscesses are usually associated with abdominal or flank pain, and about half of the patients show a flank mass or tenderness. The source of contamination is equally divided between a renal source (pyelonephritis or renal abscess) and intestinal source (appendicitis, diverticulitis, or pancreatitis). The patient may have a limp and often prefers to recline with flexion and abduction of the thigh to relax the psoas muscles. Pain may be elicited with extension of the thigh. Approximately one third of all intra-abdominal abscesses follow intestinal surgery. This causes the diagnostic problem imposed by the difficulty of interpreting pain in postoperative patients, the associated use of analgesics, and the paucity of meaningful findings with physical examination because of postoperative distension and tenderness.

Diagnostic Tests

Most patients with intra-abdominal abscesses have fever and leukocytosis. There also may be abnormal liver function tests, a pleural effusion, elevated diaphragm, or atelectasis on chest radiograph (subphrenic abscess), or positive blood cultures. *Bacteroides* bacteremia particularly suggests intra-abdominal sepsis. All of these findings are supportive but not diagnostic.

An important recent advance in the detection of intra-abdominal abscesses is the use of ultrasound, indium labeled neutrophil scans, or computed tomography. The preferred method is usually computed tomography, which appears to provide the optimal anatomic definition and shows sensitivity and specificity approaching 95 percent.[6,9] The results with ultrasound are somewhat less impressive. This procedure offers an advantage for seriously ill patients, however, because it can be done at the bedside, and it also avoids exposure to radiation. Gallium scans require 48 to 72 hours and fail to distinguish tumors from inflammatory masses. Gallium also is excreted into the bowel, confusing interpretation. Indium-labeled neutrophil scans obviate many of these disadvantages, but their main advantage is the ability to detect inflammatory lesions at extraintestinal sites. These scanning techniques have revolutionized the diagnostic evaluation of patients with suspected intra-abdominal sepsis. Intra-abdominal abscesses previously accounted for a significant portion of infections presenting as fever of un-

TABLE 9.9–2. LOCATION OF INTRA-ABDOMINAL ABSCESSES[a]

	No.	(%)	No.	(%)
Total cases			501	
Intraperitoneal			194	(36)
Right lower quadrant	84	(16)		
Left lower quadrant	28	(5)		
Pelvic	27	(5)		
Subphrenic	10	(2)		
Retroperitoneal			203	(38)
Visceral			143	(26)
Hepatic	69	(13)		
Pancreatic	34	(6)		
Tubo-ovarian	26	(5)		
Biliary tract	13	(2)		

[a]Reflects the experience of a general surgery service.
Adapted from Altemeier WA, Culbertson WR, Fullen WD, Shook CD: Am J Surg 125:70, 1973.[2]

TABLE 9.9–3. INTRA-ABDOMINAL SEPSIS: CLINICAL MANIFESTATIONS AND MANAGEMENT

Condition	Underlying or Associated Diseases	Bacteriology	Treatment [a]	Diagnostic Studies	Comment
Peritonitis Intestinal diseases	Perforated viscus, post-op intestinal surgery, diverticulitis, appendicitis, perforated peptic ulcer, inflammatory bowel disease, ruptured abscess	Coliforms *Bacteroides* sp Clostridia Streptococci	Supportive measures (see text) Antibiotics: Aminoglycoside + clindamycin, cefoxitin, metronidazole, or chloramphenicol ± penicillin or ampicillin; cefoxitin, cefotetan or imipenem may be used as single agents Surgery: to repair defect	Abdominal radiograph (ileus, free air) Contrast studies of gastrointestinal tract (may be contraindicated) CT scan or ultrasound Diagnostic paracentesis	May be generalized (generalized peritonitis) or localized (phlegmon) Extensive pre-operative studies are often not necessary or warranted with generalized peritonitis
Primary or "spontaneous"	Ascites usually secondary to cirrhosis (adults) or nephrosis (children)	Coliforms Streptococci	Antibiotics—Aminoglycoside + cephalosporin or ampicillin; second- or third-generation cephalosporin	Ascites fluid with >300 WBC/μl and a predominance of polymorphonuclear cells	Suspect in any patient with ascites and unexplained fever
Foreign body	Peritoneal dialysis	*S. aureus* *S. epidermidis* Coliforms *Candida*	Continuous dialysis to prevent loculations; removal of catheter if infection is recurrent or refractory or there is significant fall in dialysis capability Antibiotics based on cultures and Gram stain	Cloudy dialysate fluid Culture and gram stain of dialysate fluid or centrifuged fluid Hypoalbuminemia Rapid fall in dialysis capacity	Incidence of 0.3%–0.7% per dialysis Culture of dialysis fluid may be positive without clinical evidence of infection Culture is negative in 15%–35% of those with clinical evidence of infection; endotoxin in dialysate accounts for some aseptic cases
	Ventriculoperitoneal shunt	*S. epidermis* *S. aureus*	Antibiotics based on cultures using intravenous and intraventricular administration Shunt removal usually required	Shunt fluid with leukocytes and positive cultures	Incidence of 20%
Intra-Abdominal Abscess	Perforated viscus, post-op intestinal surgery, diverticulosis, appendicitis, inflammatory bowel disease, colonic carcinoma	*Bacteroides* sp Coliforms Clostridia Streptococci	Drainage: surgical drainage or percutaneous drainage with ultrasound or CT guidance Antibiotics: Aminoglycoside + clindamycin, cefoxitin, metronidazole or chloramphenicol ± penicillin or ampicillin; cefoxitin, cefotetan or imipenem may be used as single agent	Radiographs (chest, abdomen and contrast studies) variable depending on size, location and number of abscesses CT or ultrasound are preferred tests	May be solitary or multiple; favored locations are lower quadrants, pelvis subphrenic or subhepatic
Visceral Abscess Hepatic abscess Pyogenic	Biliary tract disease Intra-abdominal sepsis in portal drainage system Distant site of suppuration Cryptogenic (20–40%)	Coliforms Anaerobes Streptococci *S. aureus*	Antibiotics: Aminoglycoside + clindamycin, cefoxitin, metronidazole or chloramphenicol ± penicillin or ampicillin Drainage: Needle aspiration, percutaneous catheter drainage, surgical drainage	Lab: Increased WBC, bilirubin and alkaline phosphatase; decreased albumin Chest radiograph abnormal (50%)—atelectasis, elevated diaphragm, pleural effusion Radionucleotide scan, CT scan or ultrasound	Approximately 50% are solitary and 50% are multiple. Mortality rate is significantly worse for multiple abscesses (75% vs. 25%) Favored treatment for solitary abscess is surgical drainage combined with antibiotics

(continued)

TABLE 9.9–3. INTRA-ABDOMINAL SEPSIS: CLINICAL MANIFESTATIONS AND MANAGEMENT (*Continued*)

Condition	Underlying or Associated Diseases	Bacteriology	Treatment[a]	Diagnostic Studies	Comment
Visceral Abscess (Cont.)					
Amebic	Geographic history of exposure in Mexico or Southeast Asia	*E. histolytica*	Metronidazole (500–750 mg tid for 10 days) + diiodohydroxyquin Needle aspiration for large abscesses, dangerous location or failure to respond to medical treatment	*E. histolytica* serology: especially indirect hemagglutination assay with titer $\geq 1{:}128$, usually $>1{:}1028$ Liver function tests: Similar to pyogenic liver abscess Radionucleotide scan, CT or ultrasound (preferred methods)	Distinguish from pyogenic abscess with serology, needle aspiration, or therapeutic trial with metronidazole Alternative to metronidazole is chloroquine ± emetine Major complication is perforation into abdominal cavity (peritonitis), lung (lung abscess or empyema), or pericardium (pericarditis)
Splenic abscess	Endocarditis Distant site of suppuration Hemoglobinopathy Trauma	*S. aureus* Streptococci Coliforms Anaerobes *Salmonella*	Splenectomy Antibiotics: Aminoglycoside + cephalosporin or clindamycin	Chest radiograph—elevated diaphragm, effusion, atelectasis Radionucleotide scan, ultrasound, CT scan	
Pancreatic abscess or infected pseudocyst	Acute pancreatitis	Coliforms Streptococci	Drainage required Aminoglycoside + chloramphenicol or cephalosporin	Amylase increased in 30–70% Abdominal radiograph—displacement of gastric air, retroperitoneal gas, wide duodenal loop, or obliteration of psoas shadow CT scan or ultrasound, preferably with diagnostic aspiration	Suspect in patients with acute pancreatitis who have persistent sepsis (30%) or improve and then deteriorate after a 1–3 wk lull (30%) Main differential is pancreatic pseudocyst and edematous pancreas
Tubo-ovarian	Pelvic inflammatory disease	Anaerobes Streptococci Coliforms *N. gonorrhoeae* *Chlamydia* (?)	Antibiotics: Aminoglycoside + cefoxitin, clindamycin or metronidazole	Pelvic mass; ultrasound or CT scan	70% respond to antibiotics
Biliary Tract Infections					
Cholecystitis	Obstructed cystic duct; usually choledocholithiasis (95%) acalculus (5%) Increased incidence with diabetes, pancreatitis, cirrhosis, hemolytic anemia, inflammatory bowel disease	Coliforms Enterococci Clostridia	Antibiotics: Ampicillin or cephalosporin ± aminoglycoside Surgery: cholecystectomy early or late Cholecystostomy for emergency decompression	Lab: WBC $\leq 15{,}000/\mu l$; liver function tests variable Cholangiography—nonvisualization, gallstones, dilated common duct etc. Echo or radionucleotide (preferred methods of evaluation)	Relative merits of early surgery (within 1–2 wk of onset of symptoms) and late surgery (4–8 wk) are debated Bile cultures are positive in 50–70% of patients
Cholangitis	Biliary stasis—primarily choledocholithiasis or postoperative stricture	Coliforms Anaerobes	Antibiotics—Aminoglycoside + clindamycin, cefoxitin, metronidazole or chloramphenicol ± penicillin or ampicillin Surgery—exploration of common duct	Lab: elevated bilirubin alkaline phosphatase, transaminase Blood culture positive in ~50% Definitive diagnosis: percutaneous transhepatic cholangiogram	Suspect in patients with Charcot-triad: fever, abdominal pain, and jaundice Rare in patients <50 years except those of Chinese extraction
Emphysematous cholecystitis	Diabetes, males > females	Coliforms Clostridia	Antibiotics: Ampicillin or penicillin + aminoglycoside Early surgery mandatory	Radiograph showing gas in biliary radicles, gallbladder, or pericholecystic tissue	Tendency to perforation and gangrene; mortality rate high

(continued)

TABLE 9.9–3. INTRA-ABDOMINAL SEPSIS: CLINICAL MANIFESTATIONS AND MANAGEMENT (*Continued*)

Condition	Underlying or Associated Diseases	Bacteriology	Treatment [a]	Diagnostic Studies	Comment
Biliary Tract Infections (Cont.)					
Empyema	Complication of acute cholecystitis	Coliforms Enterococci Clostridia	Antibiotics: Ampicillin or cephalosporin + aminoglycoside Early surgical drainage mandatory	Mass in gallbladder	Purulent collection in gallbladder; patients usually severely ill; major complication is perforation; mortality rate high

[a] Treatment guidelines include recommended antimicrobial agents for empiric use assuming that no culture results or in vitro sensitivity test results are available. Doses for adults with normal renal function are: aminoglycoside–tobramycin *or* gentamicin (1.7 mg/kg q8h), amikacin (5.0 mg/kg q8h); clindamycin (600 mg q8h); cefoxitin (2 g q6h); chloramphenicol (1 g q6h); metronidazole (500 mg q6h); ampicillin (2 g q4–6h); cefotetan (1.5–2 g q8–12h); imipenem (0.5–1 g q6h).

known origin, and this observation led many authorities to advocate laparotomy when alternative diagnostic tests were unrewarding (see Chapter 9.3). It is now unusual for such abscesses to account for prolonged unexplained fevers, owing to the frequent use and diagnostic accuracy of these tests.

PATIENT MANAGEMENT

Major considerations in treatment strategies concern decisions regarding surgery and antibiotic options. Surgery frequently plays a decisive role for correction of the basic defect and for drainage of purulent collections. The selection of antibiotics is simplified if bacteriologic studies are available, but this is often unrealistic, because of limited access to the infected site for specimens, the delay in laboratory reporting, and the difficulty encountered in achieving a complete bacteriologic analysis of polymicrobial infections. Thus antibiotic regimens are usually selected empirically.

EMPIRIC ANTIMICROBIAL THERAPY

The empiric selection of antibiotic regimens should account for anticipated patterns of bacteria according to the site and type of infection (Table 9.9–3). The decision is complicated by the fact that most infections are polymicrobial, with involvement of multiple aerobic and anaerobic bacteria. Experimental animal studies of the septic complications that follow colonic perforation suggest that both coliform bacteria and anaerobes are pathogenic.[3] The major anaerobe of concern is *B. fragilis,* because of its high prevalence at the infected site; frequency as a cause of bacteremia; documented pathogenicity in experimental animals; and resistance to many commonly used antibiotics. The preferred antibiotics for *B. fragilis* are clindamycin, metronidazole, cefoxitin, cefotetan, ticarcillin-clavulanic acid, imipenem, and chloramphenicol. Aminoglycosides are usually advocated for coliforms such as *E. coli, Proteus, Klebsiella* or *Enterobacter*. These organisms also may be susceptible to cefoxitin, cefotetan, ticarcillin-clavulanic acid, or imipenem, permitting use of a single drug for all anticipated pathogens. The enterococcus often is present at the infected site as well, so that some authorities include ampicillin or add penicillin to regimens including an aminoglycoside.[1] The role of the enterococcus in intra-abdominal sepsis is controversial; therapy directed against this organism is best justified if it is recovered from blood cultures, is recovered from the infected site in pure culture, or the patient is not responding to a regimen inactive against it. Nearly all clinical trials show comparable results with various regimens, providing there is activity against coliforms and *B. fragilis*.[7,10,11] Nevertheless, a critical review of these trials[11] suggests suboptimal science and the need for better analytic methods.[7,10]

PHASES OF INFECTION AND ANTIBIOTIC CHOICE

The selection of antimicrobial agents and anticipated results are governed to a large extent by the phase of the infection in which the patient is treated. Experimental animal studies show that drug efficacy is substantially modified, with progressive delays in the institution of appropriate agents.[4] Treatment may be divided into three phases as a result of these observations:

1. *Before infection.* Prophylaxis is most realistic in patients undergoing surgery for conditions in which the incidence of postoperative infection is sufficiently high to justify preventive therapy. The most effective method of prophylaxis is to deliver drugs in a fashion that will provide serum levels at the time surgery is performed. An alternative approach with elective colon surgery is to use oral antibiotics such as erythromycin and neomycin before surgery in an attempt to reduce the colonic flora, which serves as the major source of pathogens in postoperative infections.[8]

2. *Early inflammatory phase.* This stage is associated with logarithmic bacterial growth and invasion at the infected site, such as generalized peritonitis or a phlegmon. This early phase of an established infection is the time antibiotics are most effective, and it is consequently considered the critical interval. Delays in the use of appropriate agents are likely to result in progressive deterioration or temporary improvement followed by the second phase of the biphasic disease characterized by abscesses. Virtually all antibiotics penetrate into the peritoneal cavity well to achieve relatively high levels within peritoneal fluid. Thus systemic administration is generally preferred and local application is not necessary.

3. *Abscess phase.* Drainage represents the most important facet of treatment once abscesses have formed. The traditional method is surgical drainage under direct visualization. An alternative method for solitary abscesses is percutaneous drainage using computed tomography or ultrasonic guidance.[6] The role of antibiotics once abscesses have formed is poorly defined. These drugs may be justified as an effort to prevent bacteremia or to limit local extension, but they generally fail to sterilize intra-abdominal abscesses and cannot be construed as a substitute for mechanical drainage. A potential problem in some patients is that antibiotics attenuate the clinical signs and symptoms, resulting in an unnecessary delay in establishing the diagnosis.

REFERENCES

1. Ahrenholz DH, Simmons RL: Peritonitis and other intra-abdominal infections. In Simmons RL, Howard RJ (eds): Surgical Infectious Diseases. New York, Appleton-Century-Crofts, 1982, p. 795

2. Altemeier WA, Culbertson WR, et al: Intra-abdominal abscesses. Am J Surg 125:70, 1973
3. Bartlett JG: Lessons from an animal model of intra-abdominal sepsis. Arch Surg 113:853, 1978
4. Bartlett JG, Dezfulian M, Joiner K: Relative efficacy and critical interval of antimicrobial agents in experimental infections involving *Bacteroides fragilis*. Arch Surg 118:181, 1983
5. Conn HO, Fessel JM: Spontaneous bacterial peritonitis in cirrhosis: Variations on a theme. Medicine 50:161, 1971
6. Gerzof SG, Robbins AH, et al: Percutaneous catheter drainage of abdominal abscesses. N Engl J Med 305:653, 1981
7. Harding GKM, Buckwold FJ, Ronald AR: Prospective randomized comparative study of clindamycin, chloramphenicol and ticarcillin, each in combination with gentamicin in therapy for intra-abdominal and female genital tract sepsis. J Infect Dis 142:384, 1980
8. Kaiser AB: Antimicrobial prophylaxis in surgery. N Engl J Med 315:1129, 1986
9. McNeil BJ, Sanders R, et al: A prospective study of computed tomography, ultrasound, and gallium imaging in patients with fever. Radiology 139:647, 1981
10. Nichols RL, Smith JW, et al: Risk of infection after penetrating abdominal trauma. N Engl J Med 311:1065, 1984
11. Solomkin JS, Meakins JL Jr, et al: Antibiotic trials in intra-abdominal infections. Ann Surg 200:29, 1984

CHAPTER 9.10
Infections of the Urinary Tract

Andrew R. Mayrer and B. Frank Polk

Symptomatic bacteriuria represents one of the most frequent infectious diseases encountered in the practice of medicine in developed countries. Certain populations are at particular risk for urinary tract infections, such as women of childbearing age, in whom the incidence is at least 10 percent. The associated morbidity and use of health care resources in this group alone may be judged by their 5 million annual visits to physicians' offices for treatment.[17] Other populations most susceptible to urinary tract infections and their consequences include children, pregnant women, the elderly, individuals with structural abnormalities of the urinary tract, and those whose urinary tracts are aided by instruments or that contain foreign bodies (indwelling catheters). Recurrent infections involving the renal parenchyma may cause chronic renal failure, especially in patients with obstructive lesions of the urinary tract. Infections of the urinary tract are the most common cause of gram-negative bacillary bacteremia, the complications of which may include metastatic abscess formation, septic shock, and death. These outcomes are particularly associated with hospital-acquired infection due to an indwelling bladder catheter or infection that occurs in the presence of urinary tract obstruction.

PATHOPHYSIOLOGY

Uropathogenic bacteria usually derive from a patient's fecal flora, which has colonized the vaginal introitus, perineum, or distal urethra. The most common route of infection is ascent from the urethra to the bladder and, frequently, through the ureter to the kidney (upper tract infection). Fewer than 10 percent of renal infections originate hematogenously, such as the renal carbuncle, which may develop during staphylococcal sepsis.

The microflora of the distal urethra normally contains skin commensals such as α-hemolytic streptococci, diphtheroids, and coagulase-negative staphylococci (*S. epidermidis* and *S. saprophyticus*). The perineal area in women, however, also is colonized with variable numbers of facultative gram-negative bacilli of the family Enterobacteriaceae (e.g., *Escherichia coli*), the origins of which are fecal. Urethral massage as well as periurethral trauma during sexual intercourse may permit periurethral gram-negative flora, as well as some skin commensals, to gain access to the bladder through the shorter female urethra.[2,3] The role of urethral trauma in the pathogenesis of symptomatic ascending urinary tract infections is more evident, in either sex, following one-time urethral catheterization (1 to 2 percent risk per catheterization) or the placement of an indwelling urethral catheter (greater than 50 percent risk by 30 days).

Normal host defenses in the urinary tract regularly prevent most introduced bacteria from colonizing and invading tissue. Specifically, the antegrade, unimpeded flow of adequate volumes of urine and its regular, complete evacuation from the bladder serve as effective clearance mechanisms. Any interference with these mechanisms results in increased susceptibility to infection. For example, prostatic hypertrophy or urinary tract nephrolithiasis may obstruct the outflow of urine or inhibit bladder evacuation. Consequent stasis of urine permits ascending bacteria to multiply, thereby amplifying the inoculum effect and the likelihood of tissue invasion. Once introduced into an obstructed urinary tract, bacteria also may proliferate at the site of obstruction, that is, in the periprostatic tissue or urinary tract stones themselves. Such foci frequently provide the basis for recurrent infections.

The composition of urine generally is regarded as an additional host-defense mechanism against ascending pathogens. Although urine may serve as a variable culture medium for gram-negative and gram-positive bacteria, its normally acid pH, high osmolality, and concentrations of urea are more likely to be inhibitory, rather than supportive, of bacterial growth. Urinary organic acids of dietary origins may provide suitable substrates for bacterial metabolism and growth, but a variety of other normal urinary proteins, such as secretory IgA and Tamm-Horsfall urinary glycoprotein (uromucoid or urinary slime), probably contribute to the inhibition or immobilization of ascending pathogens. Host defenses in the renal parenchyma include the high oxygen tension of the renal cortex and the hyperosmolar milieu of the medulla, although the latter may conversely reduce the effectiveness of polymorphonuclear phagocyte function or complement activation. Finally, tissue-based immune surveillance mechanisms such as macrophages and circulating humoral substances also contribute to the host's defense mechanisms.

A variety of phenotypic and genotypic characteristics of urinary tract bacterial isolates have been investigated as potential virulence factors. In general, the means by which such factors confer virulence include (1) greater access of bacteria to tissue, (2) increased resistance to host defenses, (3) enhanced growth of bacteria in vivo, and (4) increased tissue damage. Certain structural properties of uropathogens, such as flagella, provide the means of motile ascent that facilitates successful access to renal tissues. Other structures of *E. coli* known as fimbriae, or pili, produce hemagglutination of human erythrocytes and are capable of mediating bacterial attachment to uroepithelial cells in vitro. Most uropathic strains of *E. coli* possess the common type I fimbriae that bind to mannose-containing residues such as uromucoid.[19,20] Other bacterial fimbriae exhibit mannose-resistant hemagglutination (MRHA); these are significantly associated with symptomatic urinary tract infec-

tions.[10] One variety of *E. coli* MRHA fimbrial adhesion possesses P blood group-specific antigens (P-fimbriae), which bind to glyco-lipid receptors on uroepithelial cells.[13,15,19] P-fimbriae were present on more than 90 percent of urinary *E. coli* causing acute pyelo-nephritis in a pediatric population, as compared with less than 20 percent of *E. coli* strains causing cystitis and asymptomatic bacteri-uria.[13] The evidence that fimbrial-mediated adhesion is important in the pathogenesis of urinary tract infections has derived largely from patients with uncomplicated episodes of infection. In contrast, the role of this virulence factor is much less important in patients with recurrent or chronic infections, or in those with underlying struc-tural defects or vesicoureteral reflux.

Resistance to host defenses characterizes other putative viru-lence factors of uropathic bacteria. For example, *E. coli* strains that bear the polysaccharide capsular antigen K in high titers are more likely to be associated with urinary tract invasion than strains with lower titers of the K antigen.[12] In vitro studies with K antigens demonstrated their ability to inhibit phagocytosis as well as the complement-dependent bactericidal activity of serum, such as op-sonization.[9] Enhanced virulence by virtue of impaired host de-fenses also has been proposed as a mechanism by which urease-producing bacteria (e.g., *Proteus* species) may cause pyelonephritis. Specifically, the enzymatic degradation of urea by urea-splitting or-ganisms liberates ammonia, a toxic inhibitor of phagocytosis and complement-mediated bacterial cell lysis. Finally, nonimmune mechanisms of impaired host defenses may be induced by the local elaboration of gram-negative bacterial lipopolysaccharides with en-dotoxic properties. Among the many properties of such endotoxic substances are the inhibition of ureteral peristalsis and the elicita-tion of vasoconstriction in exposed tissues, both of which may contribute to tissue invasion.

Other characteristics of uropathogens have been associated with enhanced in vivo growth potential in the urinary tract. One of these, plasmid-mediated colicin V production, has been de-tected more frequently in invasive urinary tract bacterial strains than in noninvasive strains. The production of colicin V is closely linked to the genetic expression of iron sequestration which, in turn, confers growth and selection advantages to bacterial patho-gens. On a more macroscopic level, the catheterized urinary tract may be particularly susceptible to the elaboration of large amounts of fibrous exopolysaccharide glycocalyx by populations of gram-negative bacilli. Such a glycocalyx matrix provides a protective bio-film that may permit enhanced bacterial survival and multiplica-tion.[4]

Finally, virulence properties of uropathogens may relate to their enhanced ability to mediate tissue damage. One example may be hemolysin formation, which has also been demonstrated more frequently among uropathogens than nonpathogens.[11]

CLINICAL MANIFESTATIONS

The usual symptoms of a urinary tract infection are urinary fre-quency and dysuria that is sometimes accompanied by fever and flank pain. These findings are often nonspecific, however, and reli-able localization of infection within the urinary tract on the basis of signs and symptoms alone is frequently not possible. For example, urinary frequency, dysuria, suprapubic pain, and pyuria were found in similar frequencies in patients with acute urinary tract infections of proven renal or bladder origins.[5] The additional pres-ence of shaking chills, fever, flank pain, and costovertebral angle tenderness adds greater specificity to the localization diagnosis of acute pyelonephritis. The classic description of acute cystitis (low-grade fever, dysuria, urgency, frequency, suprapubic pain, and he-maturia) may be found, however, in patients with renal bacteriuria as well as in women with low colony count periurethritis (acute urethral syndrome).

Despite the varied and frequently overlapping acute urinary tract infection syndromes, the following classification scheme may

be helpful in approaching the management of patients with infec-tions of the urinary tract.

ASYMPTOMATIC BACTERIURIA

Asymptomatic bacteriuria is defined by the presence of $\geq 10^5$ colony-forming units (CFU) per milliliter of a single bacterial spe-cies in at least two consecutive clean-voided or catheterized urine specimens obtained from a patient without symptoms or signs re-ferable to the urinary tract. The prevalence of asymptomatic bacte-riuria is approximately 1 percent in young girls, and increases grad-ually throughout life; asymptomatic bacteriuria may be found in 3 to 5 percent of sexually active women of childbearing age and 10 to 20 percent of noncatheterized, healthy women 65 years of age or older. The prevalence of asymptomatic bacteriuria in young boys and men is considerably less than in age-matched females, and probably does not exceed 10 percent of noncatheterized, healthy men 65 years of age or older.

Asymptomatic bacteriuria, as defined above, usually is discov-ered during the investigation of unrelated complaints, or in the course of a routine screening. The vigor of urologic evaluation or treatment of patients with asymptomatic bacteriuria should be guided by certain epidemiologic associations. For example, patients with asymptomatic bacteriuria who are also pregnant or have known structural abnormalities of the urinary tract are more likely to develop an invasive infection and certain complications such as increased perinatal morbidity and mortality. Therefore, asymp-tomatic bacteriuria in these patients should be treated and followed carefully for associated recurrences or complications. Boys with asymptomatic bacteriuria detected during the first year of life fre-quently have underlying structural abnormalities of the urinary tract, which should be investigated and treated accordingly. The approach toward asymptomatic bacteriuria in other children should generally be guided by the clinical course after diagnosis. The development of one or more symptomatic urinary tract infec-tions or subtle manifestations of vesicoureteral reflux, such as per-sistent enuresis, frequently warrants invasive urologic study and chronic suppressive therapy. Recent long-term studies of school-girls with asymptomatic bacteriuria have demonstrated their in-creased risk of symptomatic infections and renal scarring,[8] but showed no clear-cut benefit from treatment.[18] Similarly, in the ab-sence of frequent symptomatic infections or abnormal urinary tracts, there is little evidence that empiric therapeutic intervention is of any benefit to asymptomatic bacteriuric adults or to the el-derly.[1]

ACUTE UNCOMPLICATED
URINARY TRACT INFECTION

Acute uncomplicated urinary tract infections occur predominantly in women and, although often associated with the trauma of sexual intercourse, are not associated with any apparent predisposing ana-tomic abnormality. As noted previously, fecal organisms such as antibiotic-sensitive strains of *E. coli* are usually etiologic. Uncom-plicated infections respond quickly to antimicrobial therapy, par-ticularly if they are localized to the bladder or to the urethra. Un-complicated infections with renal localization tend to respond less quickly to therapy and typically manifest relapses after single-dose or short-course therapeutic regimens.[22] In general, recurrent infec-tions in women are common and are classified as reinfection (infec-tion with a new organism) or relapse (infection with the same organism). The former recurrence pattern usually represents symp-tomatic bladder bacteriuria and is presumably a consequence of heavy perineal and introital colonization with facultative gram-neg-ative bacilli. Recurrent infections of the relapse variety, however, are more likely associated with a persistent renal focus of bacteriuria in men or women, or a chronic prostatic focus of infection in the lower urinary tract of men. The recognition and differentiation of these two types of recurrent urinary tract infection are important in

determining the scope of any urologic evaluation or antimicrobial management.

ACUTE COMPLICATED URINARY TRACT INFECTION

Acute complicated urinary tract infections represent urinary infections occurring in persons with urinary stasis due to a neuropathy or structural abnormalities of the urinary tract. Most frequently these occur in children with congenital abnormalities of the urinary tract, men with prostatic enlargement, and adults with nephrolithiasis or other structural abnormalities. Neurotrophic bladder dysfunction most commonly occurs in patients with spinal cord trauma and diabetes. The bacteriology and therapeutic outcome in these patients is much less predictable than in acute uncomplicated urinary tract infection. Eradication of infection as well as the avoidance of renal parenchymal damage are determined to a great extent by the early recognition and correction of the underlying lesion, when feasible, and avoidance of unnecessary urinary catheterization.

PERSISTENT BACTERIURIA

Patients of all ages may demonstrate alternating periods of symptomatic and asymptomatic bacteriuria. Frequently these patients are elderly and, if male, will likely have an underlying obstructive uropathy with a persisent focus of infection. Children with vesicoureteral reflux and women of child-bearing age with recurrent symptomatic infections commonly demonstrate persistent bacteriuria during asymptomatic intervals. Therapy in these patients is directed against symptomatic episodes or continuous suppression in an attempt to prevent symptomatic episodes or renal parenchymal damage. A careful search for a correctable anatomic focus of infection is warranted in most patients with persistent bacteriuria.

ACUTE URETHRAL SYNDROME

As a form of acute uncomplicated urinary tract infection, the acute urethral syndrome may account for 30 to 50 percent of episodes of dysuria, with frequency and pyuria in women. Typically, quantitative culture of voided urine reveals only 10^2 to 10^4 CFU/ml of a single gram-negative coliform pathogen. The dysuria and pyuria manifestations of the acute urethral syndrome must be distinguished from genital herpes simplex infection, vaginitis, or urethral infection with *Chlamydia trachomatis*.

CHRONIC PYELONEPHRITIS

Chronic pyelonephritis describes a clinicopathologic entity of chronic tubulointerstitial nephritis with scarring that occurs in usually bacteriuric patients. As such, chronic pyelonephritis causes 25 to 33 percent of end-stage renal failure. The frequently bacteriuric groups at greatest risk for this outcome include children and adolescents with unsuspected vesicoureteral reflux, adults with obstructive nephropathy, and possibly, patients who are chronically catheterized. Many patients with chronic pyelonephritis have no history of acute urinary tract infections or bacteriuria. Thus the role of continuing or recurrent urinary infection in the progression of this disease is uncertain, and a number of investigators have suggested immunopathogenic origins for chronic pyelonephritis.[16]

LABORATORY DIAGNOSIS

Microscopic examination of freshly voided, uncentrifuged, midstream urine for the presence of pus cells and bacteria is the simplest way to make a presumptive diagnosis of urinary tract infection. Specifically, the presence of bacteria at a concentration of one per high powered microscopic field (in stained or unstained preparations) indicates a bacterial count of $\geq 10^5$ CFU/ml. Similarly, the presence of polymorphonuclear leukocytes in an unspun preparation indicates a significant inflammatory response in the urinary tract. Alternatively, highly specific urine dip sticks are available for the detection of leukocyte esterase derived from urinary pus cells.

Quantitative bacterial culture of voided urine (or urine obtained by catheterization or suprapubic aspiration) remains the most valuable tool in the diagnosis of urinary tract infection. A urinary bacterial colony count of $> 10^5$ CFU/ml is, by definition, found in asymptomatic bacteriuria but is also invariably found in acute uncomplicated urinary tract infections that involve the kidneys or bladder. As described previously, the acute urethral syndrome is characterized by $< 10^5$ CFU/ml of urinary tract pathogens. Urine obtained by suprapubic aspiration should be sterile. Clean-voided specimens may contain scant numbers of contaminants, but in noninfected men and women should be $< 10^2$ and $< 10^3$ CFU/ml, respectively. Normal urine obtained by straight catheterization also should contain $< 10^2$ CFU/ml, whereas the urine from patients with indwelling bladder catheters (30 days or more) typically contain $\geq 10^5$ CFU/ml even in the absence of symptomatic infection.

Additional technical problems may limit the use of bacterial colony counts in urine specimens. For example, falsely elevated colony counts commonly occur from the use of inadequate periurethral cleansing before voiding. Delay in the prompt plating of a urine specimen may permit bacterial multiplication and spuriously elevated counts, but this may be obviated by storage at 4C for up to 24 hours before plating. Falsely low colony counts may result from administration of antibiotics to the patient or from contamination of the urine specimen by antiseptics or disinfectants.

BACTERIOLOGY

Facultative gram-negative bacilli of fecal origin that colonize the periurethral area represent the most frequent cause of urinary tract infections. *E. coli,* particularly of certain serotypes or strains that possess virulence factors described previously, is the most common uropathogen. Other organisms, such as *Enterobacter, Klebsiella, Proteus,* and *Pseudomonas,* are more commonly associated with complicated, persistent, or relapsing infections. Similarly, multiple antibiotic-resistant organisms are found in patients with complicated infections or infections associated with indwelling bladder catheters.

The most common gram-positive organism to cause urinary tract infection is *Streptococcus faecalis* (group D enterococci). Less frequently, staphylococci may cause urinary tract infections, and include *S. aureus* as a metastatic complication of hematogenous infection and *S. saprophyticus* as an invader by the usual ascending route. Urinary tract infections during pregnancy and the puerperium may be caused by group B *Streptococcus* in 5 to 10 percent of instances.

Anaerobic organisms are associated with fewer than 1 percent of urinary tract infections, but may produce infection in the presence of obstruction or suppurative infections such as periurethral or prostatic abscesses, or fistulous communication between the gastrointestinal and genitourinary tracts. Viruses have not been implicated as specific urinary tract pathogens in adults, although some may be detected during systemic infection (cytomegalovirus). Among the fungi, species of *Candida* may cause urinary tract infections, particularly in patients with compromised host defenses, diabetes mellitus, extensive antibiotic exposure, or indwelling bladder catheters. Tuberculous infections may involve the genitourinary tract, often occurring in conjunction with coliform bacteriuria, hematuria, and pyuria.

RADIOLOGIC EXAMINATION

Radiodiagnostic and urologic procedures (intravenous pyelogram, cystoscopy, voiding cystourethrogram or retrograde ureteric study,

renal ultrasound, renal CT scanning, and gallium scanning) have important roles in the detection of abnormalities that may cause infections or their complications. None of these studies is considered cost effective in most women with recurrent urinary tract infections.[17] Most patients with relapsing or persistent urinary tract infections should have a careful examination of the urinary tract, including cystoscopy and intravenous pyelography, to exclude obstructing or deforming lesions that may be surgically correctable. Renal ultrasound and CT scanning are also useful to detect obstruction as well as to detect infected renal cysts or complicating abscesses. Voiding cystourethrogram is the procedure of choice to demonstrate vesicoureteral reflux in children and young adults. Gallium and CT scans may identify the subset of pyelonephritis patients with nonsuppurative inflammatory infiltrate of the renal parenchyma (acute lobar nephronia), which frequently fails to respond to conventional antimicrobial therapy. The long-term prognosis of recurrent infections is excellent when radiologic examinations yield only normal findings.

LOCALIZATION OF INFECTIONS

The localization of infection to the upper and lower urinary tracts may be accomplished directly by the bladder washout technique of Fairley, bilateral ureteral catheterization, or direct renal biopsy, although these procedures are rarely necessary. A variety of indirect localization tests have been investigated that include antibody-coated bacteria in urine, maximal urinary concentrating ability, serum antibody titers to infecting bacteria, urinary "glitter cells," serum C-reactive protein, urinary enzyme excretion, and serum antibody to urinary Tamm-Horsfall protein. These lack the accuracy and cost-effectiveness required of a clinically useful test. The response to single-dose antimicrobial therapy has been used increasingly to distinguish uncomplicated, lower urinary tract infections and the acute urethral syndrome from upper urinary tract infections.

PATIENT MANAGEMENT

The therapy of acute uncomplicated urinary tract infections consists of appropriately selected antibacterial agents given parenterally or orally, depending on the seriousness of the infection. In addi-

tion, therapy of complicated urinary tract infections must include the relief of any obstructive lesion that may be present. In general, the pharmacokinetics of most commonly administered antibiotics (penicillins, cephalosporins, sulfonamides, and others) are such that achievable urinary antibiotic levels exceed by many times the simultaneously achievable serum levels. Therefore, it is rarely necessary to adjust urinary pH to maximize the bactericidal effects of particular antibiotics. Similarly, although adequate urinary volume is a useful host-defense mechanism, water intake is not especially critical during the management of most urinary tract infections with antibiotic agents. Sufficient water intake should be maintained when using sulfonamides to avoid renal tubular precipitation of sulfonamide crystals. Monitoring and adjustment of serum antibiotic levels is generally not necessary during the treatment of uncomplicated urinary tract infections but is appropriate when complicated infections are associated with sepsis or foci of renal parenchymal involvement.

Tables 9.10–1 and 9.10–2 provide guidelines for the duration and type of therapy for the most commonly encountered groups of patients with urinary tract infections. Such categorizations presume the prompt acquisition of an adequate patient history as well as the results of urinalysis and culture and any appropriate urologic evaluations, as discussed previously. As a general rule, antibiotic treatment of urinary tract infections should be restricted to patients who have symptoms ascribed to the infection and to asymptomatic infections in children and pregnant women.

ASYMPTOMATIC BACTERIURIA

Asymptomatic bacteriuria in nonpregnant women in the absence of prior urologic instrumentation, indwelling bladder catheterization, or obstruction generally does not warrant antimicrobial therapy. In contrast, pregnant women with asymptomatic bacteriuria are at increased risk for both acute pyelonephritis and perinatal mortality and morbidity and should be managed with a 7- to 14-day course of a sulfonamide (unless they are in the third trimester), ampicillin, or nitrofurantoin. Following therapy, pregnant patients should be monitored carefully with repeat urine cultures. Chronic antimicrobial prophylaxis of asymptomatic bacteriuria should be carefully considered for young children who may have vesicoureteral reflux or anatomic abnormalities, and in male patients who may have obstructive lesions of the urinary tract.

TABLE 9.10–1. MANAGEMENT GUIDELINES FOR URINARY TRACT INFECTIONS

Patient Profile	Anticipated Pathogen	Probability of Tissue Invasion	Treatment	Prognosis
Female with few prior episodes, reliable for follow-up, symptoms <3 days	Sensitive *E. coli*	Low	Single dose regimen	Excellent
Female with few prior episodes, poor follow-up anticipated, or prolonged symptoms prior to treatment	Sensitive *E. coli*	Variable	3–10 days, prophylaxis for closely spaced recurrences	Good
Female with many prior episodes, history of early recurrence, diabetes, renal transplant	Variable sensitivities	High	4–6 wk, prophylaxis for closely spaced recurrences	Fair
Males with recurrent infection, chronic prostatitis, or anatomic abnormality	Variable sensitivities	High	4–6 wk (12 wk for chronic prostatitis) Prophylaxis for closely spaced infections	Fair
Neurogenic bladder, large volume residual	Variable sensitivities	High	Treatment only for symptomatic episodes Intermittent catheterization for neurogenic bladder	Poor
Continuous drainage required	Variable sensitivities	Very high	Treatment only for sepsis	Poor

Adapted from Kunin CM: Am J Med 71:849, 1981.[14]

TABLE 9.10–2. ANTIBIOTIC REGIMENS FOR TREATMENT AND PREVENTION OF URINARY TRACT INFECTIONS

Single dose regimens

   Amoxicillin: 3 g orally

   Sulfisoxazole: 2 g orally

   Trimethoprim-sulfamethoxazole: 2 DS tablets orally

   Kanamycin: 500 mg IM

Conventional oral antimicrobial regimens (3–10 days or 4–6 weeks—see text)

   Ampicillin: 250–500 mg orally qid

   Tetracycline: 250–500 mg orally qid

   Sulfisoxazole: 0.5–1 g orally qid

   Trimethoprim-sulfamethoxazole: 1 DS tablet orally bid

   Cephalexin: 250–500 mg orally qid

   Nitrofurantoin: 50–100 mg orally qid

   Indanyl carbenicillin: 0.5–1 g orally qid

Parenteral regimens for empirical use in septic patients

   Aminoglycoside: gentamicin (1.7 mg/kg q8h), tobramycin (1.7 mg/kg q8h) or amikacin (5 mg/kg q8h) plus ampicillin (1–2 g q4–6h) or ticarcillin (3 g q4h)

   Cephalosporin ± aminoglycoside

Prophylactic regimens (usually given 6 mo to 1 yr)

   Trimethoprim-sulfamethoxazole: half a tablet orally daily or 3× per week

   Macrodantin: 50 mg orally daily

   Trimethoprim: 100 mg orally daily

   Ampicillin (250 mg), amoxicillin (250 mg), or trimethoprim-sulfamethoxazole (1 tablet) after intercourse for women with appropriate histories

ACUTE UNCOMPLICATED INFECTIONS

Antimicrobial therapy is fairly simple in these infections because of the susceptibility of the infecting pathogens and the limited extent of tissue invasion. Studies in recent years have repeatedly demonstrated that single-dose antimicrobial therapy is as effective as traditional 7- to 14-day courses.[6,22] Specifically, single-dose therapy is effective in approximately 85 percent of acute uncomplicated infections and is associated with significantly fewer antibiotic side effects and alterations in normal host flora as compared with conventional therapy. Follow-up cultures or urinalyses are not necessary in women with occasional acute uncomplicated infections. In contrast, women with two or three reinfections per year should be considered candidates for chronic antimicrobial prophylaxis after eradication of symptomatic bacteriuria by a single dose or short course (3 to 7 days) of appropriate therapy. A variety of such prophylactic regimens are available, such as a single-strength tablet of trimethoprim-sulfamethoxazole at bedtime 3 to 7 times weekly or 50 mg of nitrofurantoin at bedtime every night. Depending on the frequency of reinfection, chronic prophylaxis for 12 months or more should be considered.

ACUTE COMPLICATED INFECTIONS

Anatomic abnormalities or obstructive lesions should be identified and corrected accordingly. Single-dose antibiotic therapy is not appropriate for acute complicated infections; courses of 2 to 6 weeks' duration should be administered.[23] Because of the required duration of therapy to eliminate the foci of such infections, it is of critical importance to obtain pretreatment urine cultures and anti-

biotic sensitivities to select an appropriate antibiotic regimen. Trimethoprim-sulfamethoxazole is particularly useful in male patients with a prostatic source of infection. Frequent relapses with the same infecting organism also may be managed with chronic antimicrobial suppression, although the prevention of symptomatic bacteriuria in this predominantly male population is not as successful as that in women with frequent reinfections.

PERSISTENT BACTERIURIA

Bacteriuria with the same organism that persists despite appropriate antibiotic therapy is usually associated with a chronic focus of infection, that is, prostatitis, nephrolithiasis, or bladder diverticula. If the inability to eradicate bacteriuria is associated with an inability to remove the focus of infection, management options may be limited to the treatment of only those episodes that are associated with symptoms. Similarly, persistent bacteriuria that is associated with chronic indwelling bladder catheterization should be managed with therapy directed at symptomatic episodes only, and should not include chronic prophylaxis, because of the anticipated emergence of multiply resistant microorganisms.

ACUTE URETHRAL SYNDROME

Women with dysuria and pyuria in association with low-count bacteriuria generally harbor invasive strains of gram-negative bacilli, S. saprophyticus, or C. trachomatis.[24] Such women, in the absence of clinically evident genital herpes or vaginitis, should be managed with single-dose therapy as for acute uncomplicated infections. Failure to relieve symptoms in the several days after single-dose amoxicillin (3 g po) or trimethoprim-sulfamethoxazole (2 double-strength tablets po) should prompt a brief course of tetracycline or erythromycin for a presumptive chlamydial infection.

ACUTE PYELONEPHRITIS

The subset of patients with acute uncomplicated or complicated urinary tract infections who also manifest combinations of systemic toxicity, rigors, flank pain, and costovertebral angle tenderness should be managed more conventionally. Specifically, carefully obtained cultures of both blood and urine should be obtained, and empiric parenteral antibiotic agents should be administered. The presence of bacilli on stained or unstained preparations of urine should be broadly covered with an aminoglycoside agent (gentamicin, tobramycin, or amikacin), pending the final results of cultures. A penicillin, such as ampicillin, is frequently added to the empiric regimen of severely ill patients to provide adequate coverage against enterococci. In any event, the definitive therapeutic regimens should be selected on the basis of the final results of cultures and sensitivities and should be continued for a minimum of 10 to 14 days. Provided that an obstructive lesion is not present, and that a satisfactory response to parenteral therapy has occurred, suitable oral agents may be used for much of the 10 to 14 days of therapy.

FOLLOW-UP AND INTERIM EVALUATION

Follow-up cultures in the week after cessation of antibiotic therapy or urinary tract infections is indicated in any patients with complicated infections as well as in children, and in males. Such cultures should be considered optional in most women whose symptoms have resolved. As indicated previously, the inability to eradicate bacteriuria should alert the clinician to the possibilities of an unsuspected obstructive lesion, the use of inappropriate antimicrobials, or patient noncompliance.

SPECIAL PROBLEMS

THE URINARY CATHETER

In contrast to the low infection attack rate associated with one-time straight catheterization of the bladder (1 to 2 percent), an indwelling bladder catheter predisposes to infection at a cumulative rate of at least 50 percent by 30 days.[25] Catheter-associated urinary tract infections represent the most common form of nosocomial infection in hospitals as well as chronic care nursing facilities, and contributes to increased mortality.[21] This marked risk for infection may be minimized in several ways. First, chronic bladder catheterization should be avoided wherever possible. Second, chronic catheterization should be restricted to those patients requiring treatment of bladder outflow obstruction or those in whom an external drainage device, such as condom catheter systems in men or diaper appliances in women, are not feasible. Third, if a catheter is required, careful aseptic technique should be employed during insertion, and the catheter should be used for the shortest possible time. Patients with neurogenic or spastic bladders should receive optimal pharmacologic management before resorting to chronic indwelling bladder catheterization. Fourth, only closed drainage systems should be used to minimize the introduction of more virulent organisms into the urinary tract. Any obstructed catheter should be changed promptly. Fifth, systemic or oral antimicrobial prophylaxis should not be administered to patients with chronic indwelling catheters, nor should irrigants or antimicrobial solutions be instilled into the lumen or collection bag.

OTHER SYSTEMIC ILLNESSES

Patients with metabolic abnormalities, such as diabetes mellitus, and patients who are neutropenic from certain malignancies or cytotoxic therapies are particularly susceptible to the invasive complications of bacteriuria. Instrumentation and urologic manipulation should be avoided wherever possible, because, once colonized, these patients are particularly susceptible to persistent bacteriuria, acute pyelonephritis, and sepsis. Diabetic patients are also highly susceptible to renal parenchymal complications of urinary tract infections such as acute papillary necrosis, acute lobar nephronia, and renal abscess formation. They also are more likely to acquire nonbacterial forms of urinary tract infection such as pyelonephritis due to species of *Candida*.

REFERENCES

1. Boscia JA, Kobasa MS, et al: Therapy vs. no therapy for bacteriuria in elderly ambulatory nonhospitalized women. JAMA 257:1067, 1987
2. Bran JL, Levinson ME, Kaye D: Entrance of bacteria into the female urinary bladder. N Engl J Med 286:626, 1972
3. Buckley RM, McGuckin M, MacGregor RR: Urine bacterial counts after sexual intercourse. N Engl J Med 298:321, 1978
4. Costerton JW, Irvin RT, Cheng K-J: The bacterial glycocalyx in nature and disease. Annu Rev Microbiol 35:299, 1981
5. Fairley KF, Carson G, et al: Site of infection in acute urinary tract infection in general practice. Lancet 2:615, 1971
6. Fihn SO, Stamm WE: Interpretation and comparison of treatment studies for uncomplicated urinary tract infections in women. Rev Infect Dis 7:468, 1985
7. Fowler JE Jr, Pulaski ET: Excretory urography cystography and cystoscopy in the evaluation of women with urinary tract infection: A prospective study. N Engl J Med 304:462, 1981
8. Gillenwater JY, Harrison RB, Kunin CM: Natural history of bacteriuria in schoolgirls. N Engl J Med 301:396, 1979
9. Glynn AA, Howard CJ: The sensitivity to complement of strains of *Escherichia coli* related to their K antigens. Immunology 18:331, 1970
10. Green CP, Thoms VL: Hemagglutination of human type O erythrocytes, hemolysin production, and serogrouping of *Escherichia coli* isolates from patients with acute pyelonephritis, cystitis, and asymptomatic bacteriuria. Infect Immun 31:309, 1981
11. Hughes C, Hacker J, et al: Hemolysin production as a virulence marker in symptomatic and asymptomatic urinary tract infections caused by *Escherichia coli*. Infect Immun 39:546, 1983
12. Kaijser B: Immunology of *Escherichia coli*: K antigen and its relation to urinary-tract infection. J Infect Dis 127:670, 1973
13. Kallenius G, Mollby R, et al: Occurrence of P-fimbriated *Escherichia coli* in urinary tract infections. Lancet 2:1369, 1981
14. Kunin CM: Duration of treatment of urinary tract infections. Am J Med 71:849, 1981
15. Lefler H, Svanborg-Eden C: Glycolipid receptors for uropathogenic *Escherichia coli* binding to human erythrocytes and uroepithelial cells. Infect Immun 34:930, 1981
16. Mayrer AR, Miniter P, Andriole VT: The immunopathogenesis of chronic pyelonephritis. Am J Med 75:59, 1983
17. National Center for Health Statistics: Ambulatory medical care rendered in physicians' offices: United States, 1975. Adv Data 12:1, 1977
18. Newcastle Covert Bacteriuria Research Group: Covert bacteriuria in schoolgirls in Newcastle upon Tyne: A 5-year follow-up. Arch Dis Child 56:585, 1981
19. O'Hanley P, Lark D, et al: Molecular basis of *Escherichia coli* colonization of the upper urinary tract in BALB/c mice. J Clin Invest 75:347, 1985
20. Orskov I, Ferencz A, Orskov F: Tamm-Horsfall protein or urumucoid is the normal urinary slime that traps type I fimbriated *Escherichia coli*. Lancet 1:887, 1980
21. Platt R, Polk BF, et al: Mortality associated with nosocomial urinary tract infection. N Engl J Med 307:537, 1982
22. Souney P, Polk BF: Single-dose antimicrobial therapy for urinary tract infections in women. Rev Infect Dis 4:29, 1982
23. Stamm WE, McKevitt M, Counts GW: Acute renal infection in women: Treatment with trimethoprim-sulfamethoxazole or ampicillin for two or six weeks. Ann Intern Med 106:341, 1987
24. Stamm WE, Wagner KF, et al: Causes of the acute urethral syndrome in women. N Engl J Med 303:409, 1980
25. Warren JW, Platt R, et al: Antibiotic irrigation and catheter-associated urinary tract infections. N Engl J Med 299:570, 1978

CHAPTER 9.11
Infections of Central Nervous System

Diane E. Griffin

The central nervous system (CNS) is relatively protected from infection. It is protected from external invasion by the scalp, skull, and leptomeninges and from internal invasion by the blood-brain barrier. When infection occurs, it may be localized to the meninges (meningitis), occur diffusely in the parenchyma of the brain (encephalitis) or spinal cord (myelitis), focally (abscess), or in combinations of these locations (meningoencephalitis, encephalomyelitis, and others). CNS infections may be caused by parasites, fungi, mycobacteria, bacteria, rickettsia, mycoplasma, or viruses. Diseases may be mild and self-limited or rapidly fatal. Prompt treatment is

often effective for many of the more severe diseases and, for this reason, CNS infection must be recognized early and the probable infective agent determined rapidly.

SIGNS AND SYMPTOMS

Central nervous system infection initiates three processes that cause most of its manifestations: inflammation, increased intracranial pressure, and tissue necrosis. Each may result in headache. Inflammation of the meninges causes reflex paraspinous muscle spasm, which is reflected by an opisthotonic posture (particularly in children), nuchal rigidity, inability to straighten raised leg (Kernig sign), and flexion of the leg when the head is flexed (Brudzinski neck sign). Chronic meningeal inflammation also may involve the cranial nerves, resulting in cranial nerve palsies. Inflammation within the brain parenchyma may result in seizures, altered states of consciousness, or focal neurologic deficits. Tissue necrosis may result directly from the replication of the organism or from vascular thrombosis secondary to the inflammation. This, as well as increased intracranial pressure, also may result in altered states of consciousness, acute changes in personality or behavior, or focal neurologic deficits. Fever generally accompanies acute CNS infections but may be absent during chronic infections.

INITIAL EXAMINATION

The initial examination should include evaluation for cranial trauma, level of consciousness, cranial nerve palsies, focal deficits, meningismus, and increased intracranial pressure. If papilledema is present, a lumbar puncture may be contraindicated.

A search should be made for other foci of infection and for physical signs suggesting a specific microbial etiology. Physical findings may suggest the specific cause of CNS infection. Cutaneous petechiae and purpuric lesions strongly suggest meningococcal infection, although Rocky Mountain spotted fever and ECHO virus infection also are associated with a spotty exanthem. Meningitis in a patient with middle ear or sinus infection, cerebrospinal fluid (CSF) rhinorrhea, or pneumonia suggests a pneumococcal etiology, whereas mumps virus would be the likely cause of encephalitis in an individual with parotitis.

The evidences of CNS infection may be attributed to or masked by other disease processes. Fever may be attributed to a recognized infection elsewhere such as bacterial pneumonia, endocarditis, otitis, or sinusitis. Similarly, altered CNS function may be blamed on alcoholism, head trauma, stroke, brain tumor, subarachnoid hemorrhage, or senility. Treatable CNS infection, particularly bacterial meningitis, must be ruled out in such patients. This is usually done by lumbar puncture and careful CSF examination.

EXAMINATION OF CEREBROSPINAL FLUID

Cerebrospinal fluid is formed within the ventricular system by secretion from the choroid plexus and transudation of cerebral interstitial fluid. This fluid circulates through the ventricular foramina, down over the surface of the spinal cord and roots, and up through the basal cisterns to the sites of reabsorption over the surface of the brain. Normally the fluid is crystal clear, contains fewer than five mononuclear cells, has a protein content of 45 mg/dl or less, of which 14 percent or less is gamma globulin. The glucose concentration of CSF is greater than half the blood glucose, and CSF is under less than 180 mm H_2O pressure.

CNS infection usually produces changes in the CSF. These may include an increase in the number of cells (pleocytosis), increased protein concentration, and decreased glucose concentration (Table 9.11–1). Careful examination of this fluid is key to the diagnosis of many CNS infections. The cells should be counted and a differential performed (Table 9.11–2). Lymphocytes usually predominate in mycobacterial, fungal, rickettsial, and viral infections, whereas a predominance of polymorphonuclear leukocytes is the hallmark of bacterial and amebic infections. Uncentrifuged CSF with one polymorphonuclear leukocyte, or more than five mononuclear cells, is abnormal. In addition to identifying the nature of the cells present, the CSF should be examined for presence of the infecting agent. Mycobacteria, amebas, bacteria, or fungi may be seen by direct microscopic examination with a wet mount or the acid-fast, Gram or India ink stains. Microbial antigens also may be detected immunologically, that is, by countercurrent immunoelectrophoresis, radioimmunoassay, or enzyme immunoassay. CSF should be cultured for fungi, mycobacteria, bacteria, and viruses, because cultures may be positive when other detection

TABLE 9.11–1. SPINAL FLUID FINDINGS IN CNS INFECTIONS

	Cell Count (μl)	Cell Type	Glucose (mg/dl)	Protein (mg/dl)	Microscopic Examination	Culture
Normal	0–5	Mononuclear	40–80 or $\frac{1}{2}$ of serum level	10–45	Negative	Negative
Meningitis						
Viral	10–2,000	Early, mostly PMNs; late, mostly mononuclear cells	Normal	Normal to 100	Negative	Sometimes positive
Untreated bacterial	10–100,000	Predominantly PMNs	Low	Normal to 600, usually increased	90% positive	90% positive
Partially treated bacterial	10–10,000	Predominantly PMNs	Low or normal	Usually increased	Positive, or negative; bacteria may stain poorly	Frequently negative
Tuberculous	10–1,000	30–100% mononuclear	Low, may be normal early	Elevated, 100 to 500	Rarely positive	Usually positive
Fungal	5–1,000	Predominantly mononuclear	Low, occasionally normal	Normal to 500	India ink positive for cryptococci	Usually positive
Encephalitis	0–2,000	Early, mostly PMNs; late, mostly mononuclear	Normal	Normal to 120	Negative	Negative
Brain abscess	5–500	Mixture of PMNs and mononuclear	Normal	Normal to 500	Negative	Negative

TABLE 9.11–2. STEPS IN EVALUATION OF CELLS IN CEREBROSPINAL FLUID

I. Perform chamber count and differential
Count the number of cells in all 9 ruled squares (0.9 μl) of a hemocytometer filled with undiluted CSF. Multiply by 1.1 to obtain count per microliter. Identify each cell under high power.
  A. *If there are too many white cells*
    Dilute CSF 1 to 11 with Turck solution in WBC pipette. Count the number of cells in all 9 ruled squares (0.9 μl) of hemocytometer. Multiply by 10 to obtain count per microliter. Identify each cell or up to 100 cells under high power.
  B. *If there are too many red cells*
    1. Evaluate red cells by hematocrit
    2. Perform chamber count and differential after acid hemolysis. Dilute glacial (28%) acetic acid 1 to 11 with CSF in a WBC pipette. The acid hemolyzes the red cells without much dilution of the white cells.
    3. Count the number of cells in the 9 ruled squares (0.9 μl) of a hemocytometer. Multiply by 1.1 to obtain the number of cells per microliter. Identify each cell or up to 100 cells under high power.

II. If there are increased polymorphonuclear cells, obtain
  A. Cultures for bacteria (including warmed chocolate agar in carbon dioxide for meningococci), fungi, tubercle bacilli, and viruses
  B. Glucose and protein
  C. Gram stain of centrifuged sediment
  D. Acid-fast stain of centrifuged sediment

III. If there are increased mononuclear cells, obtain
  A. to D. as in II
  E. India ink preparation: Cover a drop of CSF (or spun sediment) containing the cells with a coverslip. Put a split drop of India ink at the edge of the coverslip. Look for a clear halo around the cell indicating the capsule of cryptococcus

IV. If there are bizarre or unidentified cells, obtain
  A. to D. as in II
  E. As in III
  F. Wright stain of sediment (lymphoma)
  G. Cytopathologic examination of sediment (tumor)

methods are negative and may provide a source of additional important information (speciation, antibiotic sensitivity, and so on). Because CNS infection is frequently a complication of systemic disease, other relevant body sites also should be cultured, such as blood, stool, throat, sputum, or urine, depending on the differential diagnosis.

The protein content of the CSF increases with most infections. The increase may be slight with viral infections but is usually greater with bacterial, fungal, or tuberculous infections. An increase in protein may be the only abnormality in brain abscess. CSF glucose is usually low in untreated bacterial meningitis and frequently low in fungal and tuberculous meningitis. CSF glucose also may be depressed in some viral encephalitides, CNS sarcoid, CNS tumors, and subarachnoid hemorrhage. Lowered CSF glucose is probably caused by altered glucose transport between blood and CSF.

PATHOPHYSIOLOGY

Organisms can enter the CNS directly, through the olfactory mucosa, by retrograde transport of peripheral nerves, or from the blood. Direct entry is a route used most frequently by bacteria and occasionally by fungi. Local infection of the soft tissues or skull may complicate wounds caused by trauma or surgery and result in direct extension of the infection to the CNS. The organisms involved in such infections are varied but frequently include staphylococci and gram-negative rods. Either abscess or meningitis may result. Skull fractures also may result in CSF rhinorrhea, which characteristically allows entry of the *Pneumococcus* into the CNS from the nasopharynx, resulting in meningitis.[9]

Infections of orifices adjacent to the CNS (the paranasal sinuses and the middle and external ear) may be complicated by invasion of the adjacent bone and subsequent spread of infection to the CNS. Meningitis may result, but brain abscess is more common. Brain abscesses after sinusitis are most frequently in the frontal lobe, whereas those complicating otitis media may be in the cerebellum (from mastoid air cells) or temporal lobe (from tegmen tympani). Bacteria most likely to cause acute sinusitis and otitis media are the *Pneumococcus*, unencapsulated strains of *Haemophilus influenzae*, mixed anaerobes, and *Staphylococcus aureus*. In diabetics a particularly malignant infection of the sinuses may be caused by fungi of the order Mucorales (*Absidia, Mucor,* and *Rhizopus*), which invade vessels and may spread rapidly to the CNS.[12] Diabetics also are particularly vulnerable to "malignant external otitis" caused by *Pseudomonas aeruginosa,* which may result in meningitis as well as cranial nerve palsies by direct invasion of these structures.[5] In the nondiabetic individual external otitis is not significantly associated with CNS infections.

Entry through the olfactory mucosa is possible because the olfactory nerve endings and meninges are exposed or in close approximation to the environment in the nasal mucosa. Occasionally bacteria and viruses infecting the upper respiratory tract may enter the CNS by this route. Only in meningitis caused by free-living amoebae (*Naegleria* or *Acanthamoeba*), acquired from swimming in freshwater lakes, does this appear to be a clinically important route of entry.[3]

Peripheral nerves, which have their cell bodies within or adjacent to the CNS, transport substances both to (retrograde) and from (anterograde) the cell body. Certain viruses, such as rabies, polio, herpes simplex, and herpes zoster, may be transported by these nerves and thus gain access to and spread within the CNS. The most striking example of this mode of entry is rabies virus, which enters exclusively by this mechanism.

By far the most frequent route of entry into the CNS for bacteria, mycobacteria, fungi, parasites, and most viruses is by the bloodstream. There are several vascular sites where organisms may enter: the meninges, the brain parenchyma, and the choroid plexus. Meningeal and cerebral capillary endothelial cells are linked by tight junctions and are, therefore, relatively impervious to organisms, unless previous damage has occurred. Some viruses are capable of replicating in endothelial cells and may use this property to their advantage for CNS invasion. Choroid plexus capillary endothelial cells, however, are fenestrated and may provide a greater opportunity for invasion of the CSF than the meningeal vessels themselves. The most important correlate for vascular entry of microbes into the CNS is the number of organisms per unit volume of blood. Characteristics of the invading organism (size and encapsulation) and of host defenses (antibody, complement, and phago-

cyte integrity) that affect clearance from the blood, therefore, are crucial in determining whether CNS infection will occur.

SPECIFIC CENTRAL NERVOUS SYSTEM INFECTIONS

VIRAL MENINGITIS

A number of viruses can cause meningitis (Table 9.11–3), a disease that occurs most frequently in children and young adults. The most likely etiologic agent varies with the season. In temperate climates the enteroviruses (ECHO, Coxsackie, and polio), which cause over half of viral meningitis, are most common in the summer and fall. Mumps is encountered most frequently in the spring of the year. The herpes viruses occur without seasonal variation.

Cerebrospinal fluid findings are shown in Table 9.11–2. Cell counts are usually between 100 and 500/μl. Early in the illness, polymorphonuclear cells may predominate, but there is a rapid conversion to mononuclear cells. The specific etiology is determined by isolation of the virus from the CSF or demonstration of a significant rise in virus-specific antibodies in the serum during the course of the illness. Isolation of the virus from the pharynx, stool,

or rectal swab suggests, but does not prove, that the agent caused the episode of meningitis. All of these methods of specific diagnosis take time. Early in the course of the disease, CNS infections that require specific therapy and have a poor prognosis if untreated must be seriously considered and ruled out before assuming a viral etiology. Repeat CSF examinations often are helpful in making this differentiation.

The disease is usually brief and requires no specific therapy. Headache and stiff neck are common complaints, but altered consciousness is not and may suggest another diagnosis or the presence of viral encephalitis in addition to meningitis. Patients are usually much improved in 1 to 3 days.

BACTERIAL MENINGITIS

The immediate differentiation of bacterial meningitis from other varieties of CNS infection depends on examination of the CSF (Table 9.11–2) and physical findings. Bacterial meningitis is strongly suggested by the finding of a predominantly polymorphonuclear pleocytosis with a total cell count ranging from 100 to many thousand per microliter and a co-existent low CSF glucose. The demonstration of bacteria on Gram stain of centrifuged CSF confirms the diagnosis and permits tentative identification of the

TABLE 9.11–3. CLINICAL FEATURES OF CNS INFECTIONS

Type of Meningitis	Site of Primary Infection	Special Clinical Features	Treatment	Comment
Viral				
Enteroviruses[a] ECHO Coxsackie Poliomyelitis	GI tract	Rashes common, pleuritis, pericarditis, paralysis (polio)	Supportive	Prevention by immunization (poliomyelitis); summer and fall
Mumps[a]	Salivary glands	Clinical mumps or orchitis may not occur	Supportive	CSF glucose may be low; Prevention by immunization; spring
Lymphocytic choriomeningitis	Possibly respiratory tract	Exposure to mice or hamsters	Supportive	CSF cells may be >2000/μl and glucose may be low
Herpesviruses				
Herpes simplex type 2	Genital tract	Vesicular skin eruption	Supportive or acyclovir	May be recurrent
Varicella zoster	Respiratory tract	Vesicular skin eruption	Supportive, adenine arabinoside or acyclovir	
Epstein–Barr	Oropharynx	May precede other signs or symptoms of infectious mononucleosis	Supportive	CSF may contain atypical lymphocytes
Mycoplasma	Respiratory tract	More common in children	Tetracycline	CSF may contain many PMNs early
Gram-Positive Bacteria				
S. pneumoniae[a]	Lung, ear, sinuses, nasopharynx	Antecedent infection common; pneumonia, endocarditis, sinusitis; previous head trauma	Penicillin; chloramphenicol is second choice	Search for focal infection (sinuses, ears) Most frequent in infants, the elderly, alcoholics
S. aureus	Endocarditis skin, sinuses, often no primary apparent	Usually associated with septicemia, brain abscess, epidural abscess, thrombosis of venous sinuses	Penicillinase-resistant penicillin	Abscess formation common
S. aureus	Foreign body	Associated primarily with ventricular shunts or reservoirs	Methicillin, local vancomycin	Removal of foreign body may be necessary
Other Streptococci	Skin, sinus, wound, septicemia	Usually associated with parameningeal focus	Penicillin; add gentamicin for group D streptococci	Group B infections common in newborn

(continued)

TABLE 9.11–3. CLINICAL FEATURES OF CNS INFECTIONS (Continued)

Type of Meningitis	Site of Primary Infection	Special Clinical Features	Treatment	Comment
Gram-Positive Bacteria (Cont.)				
Listeria	GI tract or possibly respiratory tract	Common in infants, elderly, alcoholics, malignancy, and immunocompromised states; subacute course in adults	Ampicillin or penicillin; gentamicin may also be necessary	May be confused with diphtheroids in culture; may occur in epidemics
Gram-Negative Bacteria				
N. meningitidis[a]	Nasopharynx	Petechial or purpuric skin rash, arthritis, shock, disseminated intravascular coagulation	Penicillin; chloramphenicol is second choice	May occur in epidemics; fulminant disease common; recurrent or familial disease associated with complement deficiencies; vaccine for types A and C available
H. influenzae[a]	Nasopharynx, respiratory tract	Croup, epiglottitis, subdural effusions common in infants	Cefotaxime or chloramphenicol and ampicillin until sensitivity is known	Uncommon after the age of 6 years; resistance to ampicillin increasing; vaccine available
Salmonellae	GI tract, gallbladder	Associated with septicemia	Ampicillin or chloramphenicol	Rare in uncomplicated enteritis
E. coli Klebsiella Proteus Pseudomonas	Wound, GI tract, urinary tract, bacteremia	Common in newborn. May follow neurosurgery or trauma	Cefotaxime, gentamicin or ampicillin; adjust therapy for sensitivity of organism	Intraventricular administration of aminoglycosides necessary to achieve adequate levels
Brucella	GI tract	Subacute or chronic picture. Fever often absent	Tetracycline plus rifampin	Mononuclear pleocytosis with elevated pressure Cultures positive
Spirochetes				
Syphilis	Genital	Wide spectrum of CNS changes	Penicillin	Follows inadequate treatment of primary disease
Leptospirosis	Possibly lung or GI	Hepatitis, conjunctivitis, extreme muscle tenderness	Penicillin	Exposure to urine of rodents, dogs, swine
Lyme disease	Tick bite	Cranial and peripheral nerve involvement common	Penicillin	Geographically restricted Erythema chronicum migrans Weeks to months before CNS disease or arthritis
Mycobacteria				
M. tuberculosis[a]	Lung, latent CNS tubercle	Focal neurologic signs common. Obvious pulmonary or disseminated TB often not present	INH and rifampin	Meningeal signs may be minimal, neurologic signs prominent
Fungi				
Cryptococcus[a] neoformans	Lung	Headache, waxing and waning symptoms common	Amphotericin and 5-fluorocytosine	Often associated with immunosuppressed state
Coccidioides immitis	Lung	Disseminated disease often present	Amphotericin (may need to be given intraventricularly)	History of travel or residence in American southwest
Histoplasma capsulatum	Lung	Complement-fixing antibody increased	Amphotericin	
Blastomyces dermatitidis	Lung	Skin lesions	Amphotericin	
Candida	Wound, IV site	Retinal lesions may be visible	Amphotericin (5-fluorocytosine may need to be added for C. tropicalis)	Associated with immunosuppression or hyperalimentation
Encephalitis Alphaviruses				
Western equine	Mosquito bite	More severe in children	Supportive	Avian reservoir; summer
Venezuelan equine	Mosquito bite	Illness usually mild	Supportive	Rodent reservoir; amplified in horses; summer

(continued)

TABLE 9.11–3. CLINICAL FEATURES OF CNS INFECTIONS (Continued)

Type of Meningitis	Site of Primary Infection	Special Clinical Features	Treatment	Comment
Fungi (Cont.)				
Alphaviruses (Cont.)				
Eastern equine	Mosquito bite	70% mortality	Supportive	Avian reservoir; eastern coast of U.S.; summer
Flaviviruses				
St. Louis	Mosquito bite	More severe in older individuals	Supportive	Avian reservoir; urban and rural epidemics; summer
Japanese	Mosquito bite	More severe in younger individuals	Supportive	Porcine reservoir; common throughout Asia; summer
Tick-borne	Tick bite	Strains differ in severity of illness	Supportive	Rodent reservoir; rare in U.S.; spring, summer
Herpesviruses				
Herpes simplex[a] type 1	Oropharynx or latent infection of ganglia	Signs of temporal lobe mass	Acyclovir	Brain biopsy for diagnosis
Varicella-zoster	Skin, ganglia	Cerebellar signs common, vasculitis may occur	Acyclovir	Unusual complication of chicken pox or shingles; may occur as skin lesions are clearing
Cytomegalovirus	Nasopharynx	Associated with CMV mononucleosis	Supportive	
Epstein–Barr	Nasopharynx	Cerebellar signs common	Supportive	Recovery usually complete; atypical lymphocytes in CSF
Other				
California (La Crosse)	Mosquito bite	Most common in children	Supportive	Midwestern & Western U.S.; summer
Mumps	Salivary gland	Hydrocephalus may occur as a late complication	Supportive	Vaccine available; spring
Rabies	Animal bite, inhaled bat excreta (caves)	Invariably fatal unless vaccine given before onset of clinical disease	Supportive	Immunization after exposure; study animal's brain for virus
Mycoplasma	Respiratory tract	Respiratory symptoms present in 50%	Tetracycline	Mortality and long-term morbidity significant
Bacteria				
Listeria	GI tract	Most common in patients with compromised cellular immunity; onset may be subacute	Ampicillin or penicillin; gentamicin may also be necessary	
Localized Intracranial Infection				
Anaerobes[a]				
Bacteroides Streptococci	Lung or pelvic abscess, or no focus found	Common in brain abscess, subdural empyema	Chloramphenicol or metronidazole	Examine smears for mixed flora; anaerobic culture
Staphylococci[a]	Parameningeal focus, endocarditis, neurosurgery	Common in subdural empyema, septic thrombophlebitis	Methicillin, drainage of empyema or abscess	Search for primary site
Streptococci	Sinusitis or otitis, bacteremia	Occur in subdural empyema, epidural abscess	Penicillin, drainage	Drain primary site in ear or sinuses
Enteric bacteria	Surgery, trauma, or bacteremia	Occur in brain abscess, subdural empyema, epidural abscess	Cefotaxime if sensitive, otherwise dependent on sensitivity pattern; drainage	More frequent in newborn and elderly
Nocardia	Lung	Occasional cause of brain abscess or subdural infection	Drainage; sulfonamide	More frequent in immunocompromised individuals
Cysticercosis	GI tract	Focal signs, seizures	Symptomatic	Multiple space-occupying lesions on brain CT; calcific densities on body radiographs; common in Mexico, Central and South America

[a]Indicates most common organisms.

infective agent by morphology and staining characteristics. Specific bacterial etiology is confirmed by culturing the organism from the CSF.

Bacterial meningitis may be caused by any of a number of bacteria. In the individual without a direct site of entry, a few organisms predominate.[7] These are *H. influenzae, Neisseria meningitidis,* and *Streptococcus pneumoniae,* all encapsulated organisms that usually enter the CNS by way of a high-grade bacteremia. *H. influenzae* infections occur largely in children under 6 years of age, a time of poor antibody response to the capsular polysacchride, but may also occur in the elderly.[1] *N. meningitidis* infections occur in the antibody-negative child and in young adults, often in association with a deficiency in one of the late complement components necessary for lysis of this organism.[16] *S. pneumoniae* is the most common cause of bacterial meningitis in adults. It occurs most frequently in infants, the elderly, and in persons of any age with a history of head trauma or functional asplenia. Pneumococcal infections also occur in association with sinusitis, pneumonia, endocarditis, myeloma, chronic lymphocytic leukemia, and alcoholism more often than other causes of bacterial meningitis.[2,9] *S. aureus* and the gram-negative enteric rods may produce meningitis in association with systemic infection, particularly in infants and the elderly, but also are frequently associated with cranial trauma or neurosurgery. *Staphylococcus epidermidis* CNS infections are particularly associated with implanted shunts or reservoirs.[18] *Listeria* meningitis occurs most often in neonates, the elderly, and in individuals with compromised cellular immune responses.[4,19] Physical examination of all patients with suspected meningitis should include a careful search for a focus of infection that may have given rise to bacterial meningitis by direct extension or by production of a bacteremia.

Differentiation of bacterial meningitis from other types of meningitis becomes more difficult after partially effective antibiotics have been administered for even a day or two. The CSF will usually remain abnormal, but the Gram stain of the CSF is less likely to be positive, and the organism may not grow on culture. Several days of therapy are required, however, to decrease the number of polymorphonuclear leukocytes and to reverse the high protein and low glucose levels in the CSF.[13] Such patients must be treated as having bacterial meningitis while the physician attempts to determine the true etiology of the CNS disease.

TUBERCULOUS MENINGITIS

Tuberculous meningitis occurs by hematogenous spread of the organisms during miliary disease, or by reactivation and rupture of a previously latent CNS tubercle. The disease progresses over a period of several days to several weeks with steadily increasing symptoms. The predominant clinical manifestations are headache, nuchal rigidity, lethargy, and progressive deterioration of mental function. The chronic and fibrosing nature of the meningitis may lead to cranial nerve palsies and obstructive hydrocephalus. Patients with miliary CNS disease (usually children) may have demonstrable tuberculosis involving other organs but negative purified protein derivative (PPD) skin tests. Patients with reactivated CNS disease frequently do not have demonstrable infection in other organs but usually have positive skin tests.[6] Cerebrospinal fluid findings in tuberculous meningitis are shown in Table 9.11–2. When examined early in the course of disease, the CSF findings may be similar to those in viral meningitis with a normal glucose, mononuclear pleocytosis, and elevated protein. Later the CSF glucose is usually low, an indication for the initiation of antituberculous therapy. Treatment usually must be begun without a definitive diagnosis, since the organisms are rarely seen on acid-fast stains of the CSF and therapy cannot be delayed until culture results become known. Optimal culture requires 5 to 10 ml of CSF.

FUNGAL MENINGITIS

The clinical picture of fungal meningitis varies widely and depends, in part, on the infecting agent[17] (Table 9.11–3). Cryptococcal meningitis may be acute, subacute, or chronic. Acute to subacute cryptococcal meningitis is seen primarily in individuals immunosuppressed either by their underlying disease or by chemotherapy.[11,17] In this setting initial CNS symptoms are often mild and nonspecific (headache, nausea, dizziness, irritability) gradually progressing to symptoms of clumsiness, somnolence, and visual blurring. Physical findings may include altered consciousness, stiff neck, cranial nerve deficits, and abnormal reflexes.

The chronic form of cryptococcal meningitis occurs most frequently in apparently otherwise healthy, elderly individuals. It should be considered in the diagnosis of mental disorders in the elderly. Symptoms of recurrent headache and difficulty with mentation may evolve slowly over many months and have a waxing and waning course. Fever and nuchal rigidity are usually absent. Papilledema is noted in about one third and cranial nerve palsies in about one fifth of the cases. Dementia may develop secondary to direct infection of the brain parenchyma or to the presence of hydrocephalus.[6]

Meningitis caused by *Coccidioides immitis* usually occurs within 6 months after the primary infection and involves primarily the basilar meninges. The most common symptom is headache, but fever, confusion, seizures, stiff neck, diplopia, ataxia, and focal neurologic deficits may occur. The diagnosis is made by culture or by demonstrating complement-fixating antibody in the CSF. The disease should be suspected in a patient with a compatible clinical picture and history of travel or residence in the American southwest. Early diagnosis is important, because early treatment appears to correlate with successful outcome. Meningitis may also be caused by *Histoplasma capsulatum.* As a manifestation of diseminated infection it may be associated with hepatosplenomegaly, fever, lymphadenopathy, weight loss, and an ulcerated or indurated lesion in the nasopharynx. Similarly, disseminated blastomycosis may present as a chronic meningitis.[6]

Cerebrospinal fluid findings in fungal meningitis are usually similar to those in tuberculous meningitis but in some cases of cryptococcal meningitis may be entirely normal (Table 9.11–2).[11] Direct examination of centrifuged spinal fluid with India ink is important for recognition of cryptococci in the acute form of the disease. The organisms can be differentiated from leukocytes by their large, clear capsule and budding morphology. Organisms are less likely to be seen in the chronic form of the disease, but the capsular antigen is detectable by immunologic methods, although it may be necessary to test several samples of CSF. Culture of the CSF remains the most sensitive diagnostic test for this disease.

OTHER TYPES OF MENINGITIS AND MENINGEAL SYNDROMES

Three spirochetal diseases—syphilis, Lyme disease, and leptospirosis—are associated with meningitis or meningoencephalitis. A syndrome similar to viral meningitis may be associated with secondary syphilis, whereas meningovascular syphilis is a tertiary complication of untreated syphilis. Prominent complaints of the latter include headache, intellectual impairment, and focal neurologic deficits that may include cranial nerve palsies and impairment of the pupillary light reflex. CSF shows a mononuclear pleocytosis with elevated protein and normal sugar. Serologic tests for syphilis are positive in serum and CSF.

Lyme disease is transmitted by ticks and characteristically begins with an annular skin lesion that may be followed, up to 6 weeks later, by meningitis with or without symptoms of encephalitis or arthritis. Neurologic signs often fluctuate, but cranial and peripheral nerve deficits are common. CSF findings are similar to those of viral meningitis. The diagnosis is usually made serologically.[15]

Leptospirosis may also include meningitis. Patients may have a variety of abnormalities associated with this infection, including fever, headache, conjunctivitis, impaired renal function, jaundice, and cough. The disease follows contact with infected animal urine. The disease may be mild and self-limited or rapidly fatal. CSF find-

ings are similar to those in viral meningitis. The diagnosis is usually made by culturing the organisms from the blood or by demonstrating a rise in the titer of complement-fixing antibody.

Free-living amebas, normally found in soil and in freshwater, may cause a severe, acute form of meningitis in individuals swimming in freshwater lakes. The most prominent complaint is severe frontal headache and fever. CSF findings are similar to those of bacterial meningitis (polymorphonuclear pleocytosis, low sugar, high protein) except that red cells are common, bacteria are absent, and motile amebas may be identified on a wet mount of CSF. The disease progresses rapidly, ending fatally in several days unless recognized.[8] Treatment with amphotericin has been reported to be successful if begun promptly.

A syndrome resembling viral meningitis also may be seen in association with *Mycoplasma pneumoniae* infections. Although death has been reported from associated encephalitis, the course is usually indistinguishable from viral meningitis.[14] Nuchal rigidity and pleocytosis also may be produced by a variety of processes that are not CNS infections, such as demyelinating and autoimmune diseases. These are commonly associated with CSF mononuclear cell counts of less than 200/μl, only light elevations in protein, and normal glucose concentrations. Another important cause of mononuclear pleocytosis is a parameningeal focus of infection such as sinusitis, mastoiditis, or vertebral osteomyelitis. Chemical meningitis may follow the intrathecal injection of contrast media, air, or anesthetic agents. Neoplastic diseases may seed the meninges, producing a pleocytosis, sometimes with decreased glucose. CSF cytology should reveal the nature of the cells.

VIRAL ENCEPHALITIS

The clinical picture of viral encephalitis varies from a mild, unrecognized infection to a rapidly lethal disease. Severity of disease is related to specific etiology and to the age of the patient (Table 9.11–3). Mild encephalitis (meningoencephalitis) also may be associated with some causes of viral meningitis such as mumps and enteroviruses.

Cytomegalovirus, Epstein-Barr virus, Western and Venezuelan equine, and St. Louis and California encephalitis are all relatively mild diseases in which fatalities are infrequent. Mortality is greater, and sequelae more severe, when the encephalitis is caused by herpes simplex type 1, Eastern equine, Japanese, or rabies virus infections.

The clinical picture provides little help in determining etiology, but a travel and contact history may be important. The arthropod-borne viruses, alphaviruses, flaviviruses, and bunyaviruses are present only during the seasons of their respective vectors (Table 9.11–3). Onset for all is typically abrupt, with severe headache and fever. If the meninges are also involved, nuchal rigidity may be present. Mental symptoms range from confusion and apathy to delirium, tremor, ataxia, and coma. Seizures are common, and cranial nerve palsies may be present. The hypothalamus and pituitary may be involved, causing severe hyperthermia or poikilothermia, diabetes insipidus, and inappropriate secretion of antidiuretic hormone. Herpes simplex encephalitis may present initially with symptoms of personality change, hallucinations, aphasia, and clinical and radiographic evidence of a temporal lobe mass lesion. Brain biopsy with pathology, culture, or fluorescent antibody staining is necessary for definitive diagnosis.[18]

LOCALIZED INTRACRANIAL INFECTION

Localized intracranial infection includes brain abscess, subdural empyema, epidural abscess, and septic thrombophlebitis of the major venous sinuses. Single brain abscesses most frequently develop from a contiguous source of infection such as the middle ear, mastoids, or paranasal sinuses. Abscesses of hematogenous origin are commonly multiple except right to left cardiovascular shunts.

Clinical signs may develop rapidly or slowly over a few weeks. Severe headache is often the earliest symptom. Evidence of increased intracranial pressure, focal neurologic deficits, seizures, and altered consciousness are often late features. Fever may be absent or low grade. The bacteria involved reflect the flora of the infected focus of origin. In abscesses the anaerobes (*Bacteroides* and streptococci) are common, but frequently more than one bacterial strain is present. Streptococci, enterobacteria, and staphylococci are frequent aerobic pathogens.

Infection of the subdural or epidural space almost always occurs as a complication of frontal sinusitis, craniotomy, or mastoiditis and suggests the presence of local osteomyelitis. Fever and focal headaches are the most common complaints and are often accompanied by an alteration in mental status and seizures. These processes may be preceded or accompanied by suppurative intracranial thrombophlebitis. Signs will depend on the veins involved. Cortical vein thrombosis may result in impaired consciousness, focal neurologic deficits, seizures, and increased intracranial pressure. Cavernous sinus thrombosis usually follows facial infection and results in the rapid appearance of proptosis and ophthalmoplegia. As with brain abscesses, the organisms present in these suppurative processes will reflect those present in the original site of infection.

Important diagnostic techniques to detect and differentiate these processes include careful neurologic examination, computed tomographic (CT) scanning (for brain abscesses and subdural empyema), and arteriography (for subdural empyema and thrombophlebitis). Skull films may demonstrate mastoiditis or sinusitis. Lumbar puncture is of limited value and may be dangerous. CSF pressure is often elevated and may contain increased protein or cells (Table 9.11–2), but these findings are not diagnostic. Bacteria are not present in the CSF unless the infection has extended to the meninges.

INFECTION IN IMMUNOCOMPROMISED HOST

Several types of CNS infections are seen in the host immunocompromised by underlying disease or chemotherapeutic regimens used for immunosuppression or treatment of malignancy. Patients with defects in clearance of organisms from the blood due to asplenia or humoral immune defects tend to have more frequent and more fulminant infections with common bacterial pathogens (*S. pneumoniae, N. meningitidis,* and others).[2,16] Patients with defects in cellular immunity have increased susceptibility to new infection by a variety of more unusual pathogens[8,11,17,19,22] and to reactivated infection of organisms previously contained by the immune response.[10,21] Opportunistic infections of the CNS are second only to pulmonary infections as a cause of morbidity and mortality in chronically immunosuppressed patients.

The organisms and the CNS diseases most commonly produced are listed in Table 9.11–4. Symptomatologies are as variable as the pathogens, but patients frequently have nonspecific complaints of recurrent headache and memory loss evolving over many weeks. Focal deficits may be present. The diagnosis of many of these diseases is difficult. CSF parameters may be normal or only slightly abnormal. Serology may not be helpful. *Cryptococcus, Candida,* and *Listeria* cause meningitis and may be cultured from the CSF, but brain biopsy or aspiration is required for the diagnosis of most of the other pathogens.

TREATMENT OF CENTRAL NERVOUS SYSTEM INFECTIONS

VIRAL INFECTIONS

With the exception of vidarabine or acyclovir for the treatment of herpes simplex[20] and varicella zoster virus infections, specific antiviral therapy is not currently available for viral meningoencephalitis.

TABLE 9.11–4. CNS INFECTIONS IN PATIENTS WITH DEFICIENCIES IN CELLULAR IMMUNITY

Organism	CNS Disease
Viruses	
Progressive multifocal leukoen-cephalopathy (JC)	Focal demyelination
Herpes simplex, types 1 and 2	Focal encephalitis
Cytomegalovirus	Diffuse cerebritis
Varicella zoster	Angiitis
Epstein–Barr	Primary lymphoma
Measles	Subacute encephalitis
Human immunodeficiency virus	Dementia
Bacteria	
Listeria monocytogenes	Meningitis, cerebritis
Nocardia	Abscess
Fungi	
Cryptococcus neoformans	Meningitis, cryptococcoma
Aspergillus	Vascular occlusion
Candida	Meningitis, microabscesses, vasculitis
Pseudallescheria boydii	Multiple abscesses
Parasites	
Toxoplasma gondii	Mass lesion

Patients in coma caused by encephalitis may make remarkable recoveries even after prolonged periods of unconsciousness. For this reason vigorous supportive treatment is indicated. Every effort should be made to avoid the complications of respiratory therapy, catheters, and intravenous lines, and complications should be treated vigorously if present. Blood glucose levels and electrolytes should be monitored closely. Seizures should be controlled, if they occur, with diphenylhydantoin or phenobarbital. Cerebral edema can be damaging and should be monitored in obtunded patients and controlled with removal of CSF, osmotic agents, or other means (see Chapter 4.9). Corticosteroids are of unproven value.

BACTERIAL INFECTIONS

Antibiotic treatment of bacterial infections of the CNS should begin as soon as possible. Antibiotics must be chosen for their ability to achieve therapeutic levels in the CNS without systemic toxicity as well as their bactericidal activity against the presumed pathogen. Dosages of antibiotics frequently used and effective for CNS infection are given in Table 9.11–5. In bacterial meningitis, treatment should begin after the initial examination of the patient, examination of the CSF, and obtaining necessary cultures, a process which should not require more than 30 minutes. If a bacterial etiology is not apparent at this point and the patient is not acutely ill, it may be wise to withhold therapy and repeat the lumbar puncture in 8 to 12 hours, at which time the CSF findings may be more diagnostic. In an acutely ill patient, it is often necessary to treat for the most likely bacterial pathogens even if evidence of a specific etiology is lacking.

Antibiotic treatments for specific causes of bacterial meningitis are summarized in Table 9.11–3. For *H. influenzae* meningitis, both chloramphenicol and ampicillin should be used for initial treatment, as organisms may be resistant to either. Cefotaxime has been proposed as single-drug initial therapy, but experience with this regimen is still limited. In patients allergic to penicillin, chloramphenicol also should be used to treat pneumococcal and menin-

gococcal infections. If the bacterial etiology is unknown, children should receive chloramphenicol and ampicillin, young adults should be given penicillin or chloramphenicol, and older adults penicillin or ampicillin and cefotaxime. If staphylococcal infection is suspected, initial therapy should include methicillin or nafcillin. Infections caused by enteric rods are treated with ampicillin or cefotaxime, depending on the sensitivity of the organism. Chloramphenicol is not bactericidal for most enteric gram-negative rods and, therefore, is not acceptable treatment for meningitis caused by these organisms. If the organism is sensitive only to aminoglycosides, therapy must be given intrathecally (8 mg gentamicin per day) using an intraventricular reservoir and intravenously (5 mg/kg per day) to achieve therapeutic levels throughout the ventricular and subarachnoid space. Ticarcillin or piperacillin given systemically may improve the efficacy of the aminoglycoside for certain organisms. CNS syphilis and Lyme disease should be treated with intravenous penicillin.

Therapy should be continued for 14 to 21 days. Longer courses may be required. The patient should be afebrile for at least 3 days before treatment is discontinued, and the CSF WBC should be $<30/\mu l$, none of which are polymorphonuclear. The CSF glucose should be normal, and the protein content only minimally elevated. Values exceeding this require a reevaluation of the adequacy of the therapy and a search for a loculated infection.

The prognosis in bacterial meningitis is determined by the causative organism and the condition of the patient when treatment is started. Factors contributing to a poor prognosis include meningitis caused by the *Pneumococcus* or *Staphylococcus,* severe neurologic deficit or coma at the onset of treatment, and underlying diseases of the host (malignancy, alcoholism, diabetes, or immunodeficiency). Mortality in pneumococcal meningitis remains between 25 and 30 percent, whereas in meningococcal or *H. influenzae* meningitis it is about 5 percent.

Treatment of localized CNS infections depends on the type of infection and the causative organisms. Intracranial abscesses should be treated initially with parenteral penicillin, a penicillinase-resistant penicillin, and chloramphenicol or metronidazole. If there is an otic source cefotaxime should be added. Treatment should begin as soon as the diagnosis is considered. Early surgical drainage is crucial in treatment of subdural empyema and, except for the early cerebritis stage, may be necessary for optimal management of brain abscess. Antibiotic therapy may be revised based on Gram stain and culture of abscess fluid but should be continued

TABLE 9.11–5. ANTIBIOTICS FOR BACTERIAL INFECTIONS OF CNS

Antibiotic	Age	Daily Dosage (IV)
Penicillin	Adult	$16–24 \times 10^6$ U
	Child	250,000 U/kg
	Neonate	100,000 U/kg
Ampicillin	Adult	12 g
	Child	300–400 mg/kg
	Neonate	100–200 mg/kg
Methicillin[a]	Adult	12–18 g
	Child	100–200 mg/kg
	Neonate	100–200 mg/kg
Chloramphenicol	Adult	4–6 g
	Child	75 mg/kg
	Neonate	25–50 mg/kg
Moxalactam *or* cefo-taxime	Adult	6–12 g
	Child	150–200 mg/kg
	Neonate	150–200 mg/kg

[a]Nafcillin or oxacillin also may be used. Dosage is two thirds of that for methicillin in adults and the same as methicillin in children and neonates.

for at least 3 weeks after drainage. If the origin of the infection, e.g., mastoid or sinus, yields other organisms on culture, the antibiotic therapy should be revised appropriately. Septic thrombophlebitis is treated by antibiotics alone; many episodes are caused by staphylococci and should be treated parenterally with methicillin or nafcillin in high dosage.

TUBERCULOUS INFECTIONS

Therapy for tuberculous meningitis usually employs a two-drug regimen (INH 400 mg daily and rifampin 600 mg daily). Ethambutol (25 mg/kg), pyrazinamide (2 g), and ethionamide (1 g) may be used as adjunctive therapy. Treatment should continue for at least 18 months. Short-term use of high-dosage adrenal corticosteroids may diminish cerebral edema and decrease the risk of herniation in persons with markedly elevated intracranial pressure. Response to treatment is slow; in fact the patient may continue to deteriorate for several days after treatment has begun. Most patients become afebrile in 1 to 4 weeks. CSF leukocyte count, glucose, and protein content may not become normal for several months. Tuberculous meningitis has the poorest prognosis in patients less than 2 years of age and in those with severely altered CNS function at the onset of treatment. Even with recovery from infection, permanent neurologic sequelae are common.

FUNGAL INFECTIONS

Intravenous amphotericin B (0.5 to 1.0 mg/kg per day) is the drug of choice for the most common forms of fungal CNS infections and infections caused by amebae. It is fungistatic rather than fungicidal and produces untoward side effects including fever, headache, nausea and vomiting, phlebitis, anemia, hypokalemia, and renal tubular dysfunction. For cryptococcal meningitis and *Candida* infections, the best results are achieved by the combined use of amphotericin B (0.3 mg/kg per day) and 5-fluorocytosine (150 mg/kg per day) for 6 weeks. During combined therapy, patients should be monitored frequently for bone marrow, as well as renal, toxicity. For coccidioidal meningitis, intrathecal amphotericin B therapy (0.5 mg per day) is necessary in addition to systemic therapy. Usually several months of therapy are necessary to achieve cure.

PREVENTION

Vaccines are available against certain viral CNS infections, including mumps, poliomyelitis, Japanese encephalitis, and rabies, and against the bacterial infections caused by group A and C *N. meningitidis* and *H. influenzae* type b. The meningococcal vaccine is used to prevent disease in closed populations (such as the military) or in epidemics but is not recommended for general use. The *Haemophilus* vaccine is recommended for children between 2 and 6 years of age who are exposed or have siblings who are exposed to groups of other children. A polyvalent pneumococcal vaccine is also available for use in persons with increased risk of pneumococcal infection.

Prevention of secondary cases of menigococcal and *H. influenzae* disease also is possible by antibiotic prophylaxis of close contacts. Rifampin, 600 mg a day for 4 days, is the drug of choice. Minocycline, 100 mg every 12 hours for 5 days, is also effective for meningococcal prophylaxis but may cause disturbing vestibular symptoms.

REFERENCES

1. Berke SL, McCabe WR: Meningitis caused by gram-negative bacilli. Ann Intern Med 93:253, 1980
2. Burman LA, Norrby R, Trollfors B: Invasive pneumococcal infections: Incidence, predisposing factors, and prognosis. Rev Infect Dis 7:133, 1985
3. Carter RF: Primary amoebic meningo-encephalitis: An appraisal of present knowledge. Trans R Soc Trop Med Hyg 66:193, 1972
4. Cherubin CE, Marr JS, et al: Listeria and gram-negative bacillary meningitis in New York City, 1972–1979: Frequent causes of meningitis in adults. Am J Med 71:199, 1981
5. Doroghazi RM, Nadol JB, et al: Invasive external otitis: Report of 21 cases and review of the literature. Am J Med 71:603, 1981
6. Ellner JJ, Bennett JE: Chronic meningitis. Medicine 55:341, 1976
7. Finland M, Barnes MW: Acute bacterial meningitis at Boston City Hospital during 12 selected years, 1935–1972. J Infect Dis 136:400, 1977
8. Frazier AR, Rosenow EC, Roberts GD: Nocardiosis: A review of 25 cases occurring during 24 months. Mayo Clin Proc 50:657, 1975
9. Hand WL, Sanford JP: Post-traumatic bacterial meningitis. Ann Intern Med 72:869, 1970
10. Jemsek J, Greenberg SB, et al: Herpes zoster-associated encephalitis: Clinicopathologic report of 12 cases and review of the literature. Medicine 62:81, 1983
11. Kovacs JA, Kovacs AA, et al: Cryptococcosis in the acquired immunodeficiency syndrome. Ann Intern Med 103:533, 1985
12. Lehrer RI, Howard DH, et al: Mucormycosis. Ann Intern Med 93:93, 1980
13. Mandal BK: The dilemma of partially treated bacterial meningitis. Scand J Infect Dis 8:185, 1976
14. Ponka A: Central nervous system manifestations associated with serologically verified mycoplasma pneumoniae infection. Scand J Infect Dis 12:175, 1980
15. Reik L, Steere AC, et al: Neurologic abnormalities of Lyme disease. Medicine 58:281, 1979
16. Ross SC, Densen P: Complement deficiency states and infection: Epidemiology, pathogenesis, and consequences of Neisserial and other infections in an immune deficiency. Medicine 63:243, 1984
17. Salaki JS, Louria DB, Chmel H: Fungal and yeast infections of the central nervous system: A clinical review. Medicine 63:108, 1984
18. Schoenbaum SC, Gardner P, Shillito J: Infections of cerebrospinal fluid shunts: Epidemiology, clinical manifestations, and therapy. J Infect Dis 131:543, 1975
19. Stamm AM, Dismukes WE, et al: Listerosis in renal transplant recipients: Report of an outbreak and review of 102 cases. Rev Infect Dis 4:665, 1982
20. Whitley RJ, Alford CA, et al: Vidarabine versus acyclovir therapy in herpes simplex encephalitis. N Engl J Med 314:144, 1986
21. Wong B: Parasitic diseases in immunocompromised hosts. Am J Med 76:479, 1984
22. Yoo D, Lee WHS, Kwon-Chung KJ: Brain abscesses due to *Pseudallescheria boydii* associated wth primary non-Hodgkin's lymphoma of the central nervous system—A case report and literature review. Rev Infect Dis 7:272, 1985

Systemic Viral Infections

John Modlin

INFECTIOUS MONONUCLEOSIS

Infectious mononucleosis is an acute illness resembling typhoid fever that occurs principally in adolescents and young adults. Approximately 80 percent of cases of infectious mononucleosis are serologically related to infection with the Epstein-Barr virus (EBV) by a positive heterophile reaction. About half of heterophile-negative cases of infectious mononucleosis are caused by the human cytomegalovirus (CMV), and the remainder are caused either by EBV or by other agents such as toxoplasmosis or rubella virus.

Infectious mononucleosis occurs principally in 15- to 25-year-old persons from the middle and upper socioeconomic strata who have escaped EBV infection earlier in life.[9] College students develop mononucleosis at an annual rate of 0.5 to 12 percent. Most cases occur sporadically as a result of intimate oral contact; asymptomatic persons shedding virus are expected to play a prominent role in transmission. Both CMV and EBV mononucleosis also can be transmitted by transfusion of fresh blood (postperfusion syndrome). Although EBV and CMV infection occurs at all ages, symptomatic illness occurs mostly in postpubertal adults, in whom approximately 50 percent of EBV infections and 5 percent of CMV infections among healthy adults produce the infectious mononucleosis syndrome.

After an incubation period of 30 to 50 days (shorter for transfusion-acquired cases) there is an abrupt onset of fever, malaise, and pharyngitis. Many patients also complain of chills, headache, photophobia, anorexia, dysphagia, myalgia, or a distaste for cigarettes. A physical examination often reveals periorbital edema, tonsillar enlargement with erythema and exudate, palatine petechiae, cervical adenopathy, and splenomegaly. Less common findings include jaundice and hepatomegaly. A maculopapular rash occurs in about 10 percent of patients unless they have been given ampicillin, which leads to generalized rash in about 90 percent of patients with acute infectious mononucleosis. A complete blood count drawn during the acute illness will show a peripheral blood WBC in the range of 12,000 to 50,000/μl with most of the increase caused by a rise in the number of lymphocytes. Eight to ten percent or more of the total WBC will be atypical lymphocytes. If liver function tests are obtained, a mild hepatitis can be demonstrated in more than 80 percent of cases. The clinical and laboratory features of illness caused by EBV and by CMV are nearly identical, except that CMV mononucleosis is not associated with an exudative pharyngitis or extensive lymphadenopathy.

In practice, the diagnosis of mononucleosis rests on the demonstration of (non-EBV-specific) heterophile antibodies in the patient's serum. The classic Paul-Bunnell-Davidsohn heterophile reaction is mediated by IgM antibodies that agglutinate sheep red blood cells (RBCs) after absorption of the test serum by guinea pig RBCs. Many clinical laboratories now employ slide or spot tests using horse or ox RBCs, which are more sensitive and more specific than tests based on sheep RBCs. Heterophile antibiodies are found in 75 percent of patients with EBV mononucleosis by the end of the first week of illness, and in 97 percent by the end of the third week.[10] They may persist for up to a year afterward. In unusual, atypical, or complicated cases, it may be desirable to test the patient's serum for antibodies directed against a variety of EBV-specific antigens, but these assays are not widely available. CMV mononucleosis is heterophile negative; diagnosis requires recovery of CMV from the blood, urine, or oropharynx, or demonstration of a rise in CMV-specific antibody titer.

The symptoms of infectious mononucleosis abate slowly, so that 50, 80, and 97 percent of patients are free of symptoms by 2, 3, and 4 weeks, respectively. Complications with protean manifestations are unusual but well described. They include hemolytic anemia, immune thrombocytopenia, pneumonia, myopericarditis, splenic rupture, severe hepatitis, and bacterial superinfection. Involvement of the central nervous system (CNS) occurs in less than 1 percent of cases; encephalitis, aseptic meningitis, transverse myelitis, hearing loss, and peripheral neuropathy (especially Guillain–Barré syndrome) are each associated with EBV mononucleosis.

Some individuals can have recurrent fever, malaise, pharyngitis, cervical adenopathy, or neuropsychiatric symptoms for months or years after onset of acute EBV mononucleosis.[23] In addition, a familial, X-linked immunodeficiency syndrome has been described in which affected males develop acquired agammaglobulinemia or lymphomas following EBV mononucleosis.[22] Except in these cases, mononucleosis related deaths are very rare, and are usually secondary to CNS disease, splenic rupture, or upper airway obstruction from severe tonsillitis.

Acutely ill patients should be advised to avoid strenuous exercise and contact sports, even though most will do so on their own. Steroids are sometimes useful in the management of airway obstruction or thrombocytopenia, but should generally be avoided otherwise, because they do not alter the natural history of the illness. Acyclovir, which has some activity against EBV in vitro, reduces the oropharyngeal shedding but does not affect the clinical course of disease or the development of latent infection.[1]

MEASLES

Measles (rubeola) is caused by a member of the *Morbillivirus* genus of the family Paramyxoviridae. The virus represents one of the most highly infectious agents known, and primary infection confers lifelong immunity to disease. Virtually all cases of measles occurred in young children before the deployment of measles vaccines in the 1960s; however, the widespread use of measles vaccine in developed countries has allowed many nonimmune persons to escape childhood exposure to measles and remain susceptible as adults. During 1986, nearly 30 percent of all measles cases reported to the Centers for Disease Control occurred in persons 15 years of age and older.[7] Outbreaks of measles now occur among adolescents and adults in colleges and other institutional settings.

Transmission occurs by the respiratory route. After an incubation period of 9 to 11 days, fever appears with signs of upper respiratory tract infection including cough, coryza, and conjunctivitis. Koplik spots are blue-white punctate lesions that appear on the buccal mucosa within 2 to 3 days of onset of symptoms in most cases of measles. The morbilliform rash begins on the face 3 to 4 days after onset of the fever and rapidly progresses distally to the trunk and extremities while becoming confluent on the face and neck. In uncomplicated infections, the fever and respiratory symptoms begin to abate rapidly after 4 or 5 days, and the rash fades, sometimes with desquamation.

Measles is generally mild in children, but can be severe in young infants and adults. Respiratory complications, including otitis media, croup, bronchitis, bronchiectasis, and pneumonia, are common. CNS complications are unusual, but serious. Postinfectious encephalitis, which affects 1 child in 1000 with measles, generally appears abruptly during convalescence from the rash ill-

ness. Recurrence of fever, diminution of consciousness, and generalized seizures are typical of measles encephalitis. The mortality rate is as high as 20 percent and about one third of survivors are left with significant neurologic impairment.[17]

Subacute sclerosing panencephalitis (SSPE) is an extremely rare (5 to 10 cases per 10^6 measles cases),[18] progressive, degenerative disease of the CNS. Measles virus has been isolated from brain tissue in some patients, and all have high titers of measles antibody in the CSF. Onset of CNS symptoms usually occurs years after natural measles infection (mean of 7 years). The majority of patients with SSPE give a history of measles at an early age.

The diagnosis of measles is most often a clinical diagnosis. When laboratory confirmation is desirable, determination of acute and convalescent measles hemagglutination inhibition antibody titers is the easiest and most reliable means. Antibody is usually detectable with the appearance of the rash and rapidly rises to peak levels in 3 to 4 weeks. A fourfold rise is diagnostic. Virus can be isolated from throat washings during the prodrome and the first 1 or 2 days of the rash. The Centers for Disease Control (CDC) now recommends that all suspected measles cases in the United States be confirmed by laboratory diagnosis.

Immune serum globulin (ISG) in a dose of 0.2 ml/kg will prevent or modify measles when given anytime during the incubation period. ISG is recommended for all susceptible measles contacts, especially infants 4 to 12 months of age. Live attenuated measles vaccine confers lifelong immunity in at least 95 percent of recipients. It is indicated for all immunocompetent persons over 15 months of age who have not previously received vaccine and who were born after 1957.[4]

RUBELLA

Rubella is a mild, exanthematous disease that naturally infects children, adolescents, and young adults. The illness caused by rubella is generally mild and rarely produces serious complications. The primary clinical and public health importance of rubella derives from infection of pregnant women and subsequent transplacental transmission to the fetus with resulting chronic infection and embryopathy. Once a universal disease in the United States, the incidence of rubella has fallen dramatically since the introduction of live, attenuated rubella virus vaccine in 1969. Before the availability of rubella vaccine, rubella was endemic at low levels with a marked seasonal variation. Cyclical epidemics of rubella occurred with a periodicity of 6 to 9 years, in which the incidence of reported disease increased from 3- to 10-fold over endemic levels. The last worldwide epidemic, the largest observed, occurred from 1963 to 1965. National reporting for rubella began in the late 1960s; 29 cases per 100,000 were reported in 1969, the year of vaccine licensure. The incidence of rubella declined sharply until 1974, when it remained level until 1979. Since, the incidence of reported disease has declined to extremely low levels, in part because of national immunization initiatives and the inclusion of rubella vaccine with measles vaccine (MMR). In 1985 a provisional total of 604 cases were reported in the United States or 0.25/100,000.[5] Serologic surveys carried out in several urban locations nationwide indicate that 15 to 25 percent of persons older than 15 years of age remain susceptible, a percentage that has not changed substantially since the introduction of vaccine.[3] In isolated, remote populations, the susceptibility of the population may be considerably higher.

Rubella virus is highly communicable. Infected persons may shed rubella virus in the upper respiratory tract from 1 week before to as long as 3 weeks after the onset of acute illness,[13] and transmission to susceptible persons occurs by the respiratory route. Approximately 50 percent of rubella infections are asymptomatic. In the remainder, onset of illness occurs after an incubation period of 14 to 18 days with simultaneous onset of rash, fever, and mild upper respiratory tract symptoms. The rash is typically a salmon-pink, macular pruritic exanthem that begins on the face and neck, spreads to the trunk and proximal extremities, and fades within 1 to 3 days of onset. Fever, when present, is generally low grade. Posterior cervical and occipital adenopathy is a hallmark of rubella, which may be present as the only symptom. Node enlargement, which is present as early as 7 days before the rash, peaks with onset of the rash. The occasional presence of generalized adenopathy and splenomegaly may lead to a mistaken diagnosis of infectious mononucleosis. Pharyngitis and conjunctivitis are common.

Many persons experience only mild illness, and virtually all recover within 3 to 4 days. The major complication is acute polyarthralgia involving the proximal interphalangeal joints, metacarpal phalangeal joints, wrists, elbows, or knees with tenosynovitis or the carpal tunnel syndrome. The latter occurs in 15 to 25 percent of rubella cases in postpubertal women and in a smaller number of children.[8] Joint symptoms usually begin during convalescence and persist for days to several weeks. The pathogenesis of the arthritis may involve immune complexes; rubella virus has been isolated from the joint fluid in cases of acute arthritis associated with live, attenuated rubella virus vaccine.[19] Rare complications include thrombocytopenic purpura, pancytopenia, orchitis, and postinfectious meningoencephalitis.

The diagnosis of rubella is usually based on the demonstration of a rise in specific humoral antibody titer. Serum antibody first appears within 1 to 3 days of the onset of the rash, and then peaks 2 to 6 weeks later. The hemagglutination inhibition (HI) test remains the gold standard for the diagnosis of acute rubella. Titers of less than 1:8 are considered negative, and seroconversion to positive, or a fourfold rise in antibody titer, indicates a diagnosis of recent rubella. Many immune persons may have a negative rubella HI titer, since the HI test is less sensitive than other, more recently developed serologic methods like enzyme-linked-immunosorbent assay (ELISA) and latex agglutination.[15] None of the newer methods are sufficiently standardized to allow a specific diagnosis of acute rubella, but they are widely used for serologic screening of pregnant women, hospital employees, and others.

IgM antibody appears first, peaks in 2 to 6 weeks, and declines to undetectable levels within 6 months. The presence of IgM antibody thus indicates recent rubella infection. Rubella-specific IgM serology is especially useful in the diagnosis of congenital rubella syndrome in the newborn. Both acquired and congenital rubella also can be diagnosed by recovery of rubella virus in cell culture, but the isolation procedure is lengthy and laborious and is not widely available.

The risk of fetal infection and the risk of congenital anomaly resulting from infection are both highest when maternal rubella occurs during the first month of gestation and declines thereafter.[8] Congenital anomalies are detected early in life in 60 percent of infants born to mothers experiencing rubella in the first month of pregnancy. Corresponding estimates for the second and third month are 25 to 40 percent and 10 to 30 percent, respectively. Although the risk of congenital anomalies is low when rubella occurs after the first trimester, as many as 60 percent of second- and third-trimester infections result in fetal infection and congenital abnormalities that are not detected until later in childhood.

The classic triad of congenital abnormalities due to rubella consists of cataracts, deafness, and congenital heart disease. Ocular defects and congenital heart disease result when maternal rubella occurs during the first 60 to 90 days of gestation, whereas hearing loss results from gestational rubella any time in the first 4 months. Other common findings of congenital rubella noted early in life include low birth weight, thrombocytopenia and purpura, organomegaly, hyperbilirubinemia, hemolytic anemia, osteitis of long bones, meningoencephalitis, and failure to thrive. Many of these phenomena resolve within the first few weeks of life. Pneumonitis is uncommon except with the late-onset type of congenital rubella.[24] Many anatomic and physiologic abnormalities are detected in some children with congenital rubella as they grow and develop. These include hearing loss, genitourinary tract abnormalities, diabetes mellitus and other endocrinopathies, hypogammaglobulin-

emia, and mental deficiency. An interesting, but tragic, progressive neurologic disorder that is clinically and pathologically similar to subacute sclerosing panencephalitis has been described in four adolescents with congenital rubella syndrome.[14] This rubella panencephalitis is thought to result from persistence of rubella virus in the CNS.

The RA27/3 virus is now the only rubella vaccine strain distributed in the United States. It produces seroconversion in 95 percent of seronegative susceptible persons, and successfully boosts the antibody titer in previously seropositive persons with low antibody titers.[2] RA27/3 vaccine causes fever and rash in 4 and 10 percent of seronegative recipients, respectively. The most important adverse effects of rubella vaccine are arthralgias and arthritis, which occur in nearly the same frequency as with natural rubella. The incidence of arthralgias after vaccination varies with rubella immune status, age, and sex. Immune recipients experience joint symptoms at a frequency that is no greater than controls. The highest risk of joint symptoms is among postpubertal women who have a 15 to 25 percent incidence of arthralgias and arthritis. Men (5 to 10 percent) and prepubertal children of both sexes (2 to 10 percent) have a lower incidence. Onset of joint symptoms is generally 7 to 21 days after vaccination. Symptoms most commonly involve the fingers, hands, wrists, and knees; most joint pains resolve within a week, although persistent and recurrent symptoms for up to 8 years is reported.

Rubella vaccine virus is shed in the nasopharynx of vaccinated persons in very low titers. Because studies in schools, institutions, and family settings have shown that susceptible contacts remain seronegative, however, there is no contraindication to immunizing contacts of pregnant women. Although rubella vaccine is contraindicated in pregnant women, there are data that indicate that the teratogenic potential of the vaccine virus is virtually nonexistent.[6]

Persons immune on the basis of both natural disease and as a result of vaccination are frequently reinfected with rubella after exposure to natural disease or administration of a booster dose of live vaccine virus. Reinfection is almost always asymptomatic and produces an anamnestic humoral antibody response with little or no rubella-specific IgM. There are at least 10 cases of reinfection reported to have occurred during pregnancy; interestingly, none have been in previously vaccinated women. The laboratory evidence supporting reinfection is questionable in several of these cases. Two women gave birth to affected infants. Despite these reports, the paucity of documented cases indicates that reinfection poses very little risk to the fetus.

VARICELLA

Varicella (chickenpox) is a common acute illness characterized by fever and vesicular exanthem that principally affects prepubertal children. Varicella is the manifestation of primary infection with varicella-zoster virus (VZV), a member of the human herpesvirus family. Reactivation of latent VZV infection later in life is the cause of herpes zoster (shingles), a painful vesicular eruption that is usually limited to the dermatome innervated by one sensory nerve. The clinical course of both varicella and zoster depends on the patient's age and the presence or absence of underlying cellular immunodeficiency.

Seroprevalence surveys indicate that 50 percent of children acquire antibody to VZV by 6 years of age in most urban areas, and more than 95 percent have antibody by 13 years of age. In the tropics and in some isolated areas, however, the proportion of adults who remain susceptible may range higher than 20 percent.[26] Infection confers lifelong immunity to varicella, although subclinical reinfections may occur commonly. Approximately 4 percent will subsequently develop herpes zoster sometime later in life.

VZV is highly contagious and person-to-person spread occurs readily among susceptible persons within households and institutional settings such as day-care centers, schools, and hospital wards. Persons shedding virus from 1 to 2 days before the onset of the varicella rash and persons with active herpes zoster are potential transmitters of VZV. Infectivity declines with drying and crusting of the skin lesions during either varicella or zoster. Transmission of VZV by the respiratory route is assumed; airborne spread is well documented in nosocomial settings.

As many as 10 to 20 percent of primary VZV infections are asymptomatic or mild enough to escape notice. Clinical disease follows an incubation period that is normally 11 to 21 days, but may be as long as 30 days in cases modified by administration of varicella zoster immune globulin (VZIG). In normal children the initial manifestation of low-grade fever is followed within 12 to 48 hours by onset of a generalized exanthem. Several crops of lesions may develop over a period of 1 to 5 days. The individual lesions appear at first as papules and rapidly evolve into 1 to 4 mm vesicles with a thin, erythematous base. Histologically the lesions are confined to the epidermis with some inflammatory cells extending into the dermis beneath. The vesicles evolve into small pustules with infiltration of polyps into the vesicular fluid, crust over within 2 to 5 days of their appearance, and rapidly heal without scarring. An enanthem consisting of shallow ulcerative lesions of the oral mucous membranes often parallels the appearance of the rash. The majority of varicella cases cause only mild discomfort and little limitation of normal activity. Secondary cases within the same household may be more severe than the index case.

Immunocompromised patients, especially those receiving chemotherapy or organ transplants, develop high fever and a more extensive exanthem during varicella. The individual lesions are larger, extend deeper into the dermis, and resolve more slowly. Thirty percent or more of immunocompromised children develop visceral involvement with varicella, including hepatitis, pneumonia, encephalitis, or myocarditis. Varicella pneumonia is a life-threatening complication, which may cause death in as many as 5 to 10 percent of immunocompromised children with unmodified varicella.[11]

Varicella in otherwise healthy adults also may be more severe than in normal children with a prodrome of fever, chills, and myalgias. Adults also experience a higher rate of complications and death. A study of varicella occurring in military personnel found that 16 percent had radiographic evidence of pneumonia, even though only 2 to 4 percent had symptoms suggestive of lower respiratory tract involvement.[25] Pregnancy may enhance the risk of varicella beyond that normally experienced by adult women.[20]

Secondary bacterial infections of the skin represent the most frequent complication of varicella in healthy children; cellulitis, impetigo, and erysipelas due to staphylococci or streptococci are most common. Acute cerebellitis (cerebellar ataxia) may occur 1 to 3 weeks after the rash. About 30 percent of affected patients will have a low-grade cerebrospinal fluid (CSF) leukocytosis, and most recover completely in days to weeks. Less common CNS complications include Reye syndrome, postinfectious encephalitis, aseptic meningitis, Guillain-Barré syndrome, and transverse myelitis. Arthritis, nephritis, nephrotic syndrome, and orchitis also are associated with acute varicella. Hematologic complications include thrombocytopenia and epistaxis. Hemorrhagic varicella is a dreaded form of the disease with a clinical picture of purpura fulminans and the pathologic picture of diffuse intravascular coagulation.

A syndrome of congenital malformations is an unusual but well-documented sequelae of varicella occurring during the first trimester of pregnancy.[27] Affected infants exhibit circumferential lesions of limbs, limb atrophy, eye defects, or cerebral atrophy. When maternal varicella occurs during the perinatal period, there may be a risk to the newborn infant of developing severe, fatal infection.[16]

The diagnosis is usually based on a history of exposure to varicella or herpes zoster and the finding of the typical vesicular exanthem. Demonstration of multinucleated cells and intranuclear inclusions by Giemsa stain of cells scraped from the base of one or more lesions (Tzanck prep) is a simple and rapid technique for di-

agnosis available to experienced clinicians. In addition, VZV may be recovered from vesicular fluid in cell culture, or acute infection can be demonstrated serologically by demonstration of a fourfold or greater rise in specific VZV antibody titer. Although many methods have been described, the fluorescent antimembrane antibody (FAMA) remains the standard method by which other serologic methods are compared.

Varicella in normal children requires no specific therapy other than symptomatic relief of the pruritus that often accompanies the rash. Similarly, adults with varicella are generally observed unless they develop signs of visceral disease. Varicella occurring in immunocompromised patients of any age is an indication for specific antiviral therapy. Intravenous acyclovir in a dose of 500 mg/m^2 every 8 hours has been proved to hasten recovery and reduce the risk and severity of visceral complications of varicella in children with various underlying conditions.[21] Acyclovir has several advantages over adenine arabinoside and α-interferon, which also have been demonstrated to be effective in controlled clinical trials.

Varicella also can be prevented by both passive and active immunization. Human varicella-zoster immune globulin (VZIG) will prevent or modify infection of susceptible immunocompromised patients when it is administered within 3 days of exposure. VZIG has no effect when given late in the incubation period or after the onset of symptoms. VZIG recipients will either remain seronegative, develop subclinical VZV infection with seroconversion, or develop mild varicella. Active immunization with an experimental live, attenuated varicella virus vaccine will prevent clinical varicella in about 80 percent of children with acute leukemia, and modify illness in the minority that develop symptoms after exposure.[12] VZV vaccine has also been widely tested in normal children and susceptible adults, but it has not yet been licensed in the United States.

REFERENCES

1. Andersson J, Britton S, et al: Effect of acyclovir on infectious mononucleosis: A double-blind, placebo-controlled study. J Infect Dis 153:283, 1986
2. Balfour HH, Balfour CC, et al: Evaluation of Wistar RA 27/3 rubella virus vaccine in children. Am J Dis Child 130:1089, 1976
3. Bart KJ, Orenstein WA, et al: Universal immunization to interrupt rubella. Rev Infect Dis 7(suppl):S177, 1985
4. Centers for Disease Control: Measles prevention. MMWR 31:217, 1982
5. Centers for Disease Control: Rubella and congenital rubella syndrome—United States, 1984–1985. MMWR 35:129, 1986
6. Centers for Disease Control: Rubella vaccination during pregnancy—United States, 1971–1985. MMWR 35:275, 1986
7. Centers for Disease Control: Measles—United States, 1986. MMWR 36:301, 1987
8. Cooper LZ, Krugman S: The Rubella Problem. New York, Year Book Medical Publishers, 1969
9. Evans AS, Niederman JC, McCollum RW: Seroepidemiologic studies of infectious mononucleosis with EB virus. N Engl J Med 279:1121, 1968
10. Evans AS, Niederman JC, et al: A prospective evaluation of heterophile and EBV-specific IgM antibody tests in clinical and subclinical infectious mononucleosis. Specificity and sensitivity of the tests and persistence of antibody. J Infect Dis 132:546, 1975
11. Feldman S, Hughes WT, Daniel CB: Varicella in children with cancer. Seventy-seven cases. Pediatrics 56:388, 1975
12. Gershon AA, Steinberg SP, et al: Live attenuated varicella virus. JAMA 252:355, 1984
13. Green RH, Balsamo MR, et al: Studies of the natural history and prevention of rubella. Am J Dis Child 110:348, 1965
14. Johnson RTL: Progressive rubella encephalitis (editorial). N Engl J Med 292:1023, 1975
15. Kleeman KT, Kiefer DJ, Halbert SP: Rubella antibodies detected by several commercial immunoassays in hemagglutination inhibition-negative sera. J Clin Micro 18:1131, 1983
16. Meyers JP: Congenital varicella in term infants: Risk reconsidered. J Infect Dis 129:215, 1974
17. Miller HG, Stanton JB, Gibbons JL: Para-infectious encephalomyelitis and related syndromes: A critical review of the neurological complications of certain specific fevers. Q J Med 25:427, 1956
18. Modlin JF, Jabbour JT, et al: Epidemiologic studies of measles, measles vaccine, and subacute sclerosing panencephalitis. Pediatrics 59:505, 1977
19. Ogra PL, Herd JK: Arthritis associated with induced rubella infection. J Immunol 107:810, 1971
20. Paryani SG, Arvin AM: Intrauterine infection with varicella-zoster virus after maternal varicella. N Engl J Med 314:1542, 1986
21. Prober CG, Kirk LE, Keeney RE: Acyclovir therapy of chickenpox in immunosuppressed children—A collaborative study. J Pediatr 101:622, 1982
22. Purtilo DT: Pathogenesis and phenotypes of an X-linked recessive immunoproliferative syndrome. Lancet 2:882, 1976
23. Straus SE, Tosato G, et al: Persisting illness and fatigue in adults with evidence of Epstein–Barr virus infection. Ann Intern Med 102:7, 1985
24. Tardieu M, Grospierre B, et al: Circulating immune complexes containing rubella antigens in late-onset congenital rubella syndrome. J Pediatr 97:370, 1980
25. Weber DM, Pellicchia JA: Varicella pneumonia. JAMA 192:572, 1965
26. Weller TH: Varicella and herpes zoster. N Engl J Med 309:1362, 1434, 1983
27. Williamson AP: Varicella-zoster virus in the etiology of severe congenital defects. Clin Pediatr 14:553, 1975

CHAPTER 9.13
Fungal Infections

John G. Bartlett

Fungi differ from bacteria in that they are eukaryotes, contain a discrete nucleus, and may reproduce sexually or asexually. Many are biphasic, having one form in nature and another at body temperature in the infected host. Infections caused by fungi are referred to as mycoses or mycotic infections. Fungi that invade only keratinized areas of the body including the skin, hair, and nails are dermatophytes and are reviewed in Chapter 17.7.

A large number of fungi cause diverse conditions in clinical medicine, but a convenient conceptual approach is to classify fungi as pathogenic and opportunistic (Table 9.13–1). Pathogenic fungi commonly infect the healthy host and include *Histoplasma capsulatum*, *Coccidioides immitis* and *Blastomyces dermatitidis*. Opportunistic is defined as "persons or parties (in this case fungi) that adapt themselves to make profitable use of the circumstances of the moment." Opportunistic fungi seldom cause infections, unless deranged host defenses provide the opportunity. The most frequent examples are *Candida* species, Phycomycetes, and *Aspergillus*. Contributing factors in most of these infections are antecedent antibiotic usage, reduced capacity to mount a polymorphonuclear response with neutropenia, or defective cell-mediated immunity resulting from acquired immunodeficiency syndrome (AIDS), corticosteroid treatment, lymphomas, or cancer chemotherapy.

TABLE 9.13–1. DISTINCTIVE FEATURES OF PATHOGENIC AND OPPORTUNISTIC INFECTIONS

	Pathogenic Fungi	Opportunistic Fungi
Examples	Histoplasmosis Blastomycosis Coccidioidomycosis	*Candida* Phycomycetes *Aspergillus*
Geographic distribution	Restricted to endemic areas	Ubiquitous
Host	Usually healthy	Usually compromised (neutropenia or defective cell-mediated immunity)
Diagnosis	Recovery of fungi or demonstration with stains of exudate or tissue	Demonstration of invasive disease with tissue biopsy usually required

Most fungi are found in nature, primarily soil and organic debris, although the major natural habitat for *Candida* species is the mucous membranes of the host. The pathogenic fungi tend to be found in specific geographic locations, whereas opportunistic fungi are ubiquitous. Virtually all healthy persons regularly encounter the opportunistic fungi, whereas contact with the pathogenic fungi is generally restricted to persons who reside in or travel to endemic areas.

The usual methods of detecting specific fungi are the common tools of microbiology including cultivation of the putative agent, detection of these organisms with appropriate stains of exudate or tissue, and occasionally, the use of serologic or skin tests. Interpretation of results is notably different for various fungi, however, based in part on their classification as pathogenic or opportunistic. When pathogenic fungi are encountered they are by definition implicated as agents of disease since these are not laboratory contaminants nor are they found in the normal flora. By contrast, the opportunistic fungi often represent contaminants in the laboratory or commensals that simply reside at uninfected sites. The implication is that opportunistic fungi may be considered pathogens only with the demonstration of invasive disease using biopsies, repeatedly positive cultures from normally sterile sites, or careful clinical correlations.

Cryptococcus neoformans does not obey these rules and is a rather common clinical isolate. It may be pathogenic to the healthy host but is also an opportunist in that many of the infected patients have the same defects noted previously. Pathogenic fungi, although most frequently found in the healthy host, tend to cause more serious problems such as disseminated disease in the compromised host.

HISTOPLASMOSIS

Histoplasma capsulatum is a biphasic fungus found in mycelia form in the environment and in yeast form at 37C in tissue. The organism is distributed worldwide, but is most prevalent in river valley areas in temperate and tropical zones. In the United States the endemic area includes the middle west, primarily the Mississippi and Ohio River valleys, and the river valley areas of the East. Eighty percent or more of persons residing in the Mississippi and Ohio River valleys have positive skin test to histoplasmin, indicating prior infection.

The *mechanism of infection* is inhalation of microconidia from the mycelia form in soil. Feces from birds or bats often carry large concentrations of histoplasma, and may be the source of epidemics such as in bat-infested caves (cave disease) or in old buildings infested with birds or bats. After inhalation of microconidia, the organism reproduces locally and then disseminates hematogenously.

The disease is often asymptomatic and recognized only with subsequent skin tests, a radiograph showing calcification of the pulmonary parenchyma and hilum (Ghon complex) or splenic calcifications indicating previous dissemination.

The *major clinical forms of histoplasmosis* are primary histoplasmosis, chronic pulmonary histoplasmosis, and disseminated histoplasmosis.[11] The initial infection is not recognized by the host or is simply ascribed to the flu in over 90 percent. Symptoms, when present, often include cough, fever, myalgias, and pleuritic chest pain. The severity of symptoms tends to correlate with inoculum size. Chest radiographs usually show infiltrates, hilar, or mediastinal lymph nodes. Less commonly there may be erythema nodosum, erythema multiforme, or arthralgias, all being most common in previously healthy young, adult women. These symptoms generally resolve without therapy. Reinfection may occur, but this also tends to be a benign, self-limited disease. Late sequelae include chronic or cavitary lung disease, mediastinal fibrosis, constrictive pericarditis, and disseminated disease. The most common is chronic pulmonary histoplasmosis associated with persistent symptoms, including cough, fever, and malaise. This is most common in men with chronic obstructive airways disease or emphysema. Again, most cases resolve spontaneously over 2 to 4 months, leaving residual pulmonary fibrosis. In approximately 25 percent there is progression to chronic cavitary disease with thick-walled cavities that may be complicated by bronchogenic spread to other sites in the lung.

Disseminated histoplasmosis indicates symptomatic, extrapulmonary histoplasmosis often representing reactivation of latent foci long after earlier dissemination at the time of immunosuppression.[8] Most patients have depressed cell-mediated immunity as with AIDS, organ transplantation, or corticosteroid administration. Alternatively, there may be dissemination with extrapulmonary symptomatology at the time of the original infection, a form most frequently seen in infants. Symptoms associated with disseminated disease include weight loss, fever, malaise, hepatosplenomegaly, lymphadenopathy, and bone marrow suppression.[8] As with most fungi (Table 9.13–2), *H. capsulatum* has favored anatomic sites for clinical expression with disseminated disease. The most frequent are the bone marrow and the oral mucosa. With bone marrow involvement there is anemia, leukopenia, or thrombocytopenia. The usual oral lesion is a painful ulceration in the oral cavity, pharynx, or larynx. Less common sites of dissemination include the gastrointestinal tract (primarily the ileocecal region), the adrenal glands resulting in adrenal insufficiency, or the central nervous system (CNS) with cerebritis or meningitis. There is also a focal chorioretinitis involving the macula that is ascribed to a hypersensitivity response to *H. capsulatum*, although the etiologic role of this fungus has not been clearly established.

The favored methods used to establish the *diagnosis* include cultivation of the organism from pulmonary secretions or from disseminated sites, tissue stains to detect typical morphologic forms, or antigen detection in urine or blood using a radioimmunoassay.[10] Sputum cultures rarely yield the organism in patients with self-limited pulmonary disease; cultures are positive with sputum from 50 to 70 percent of patients with chronic cavitary disease and from 50 to 90 percent of sites of dissemination. The organism is generally easily recognized as small (2 to 3 $\times$ 3 to 4 μm) ovoid yeast forms, usually within macrophages. Preferred stains are periodic acid-Schiff (PAS), Giemsa, or methenamine silver; the organism stains poorly with hematoxylin-eosin (H and E). A histoplasmin skin test is available, but its utility is limited by the frequency of positive results in patients from endemic areas and the significant rise in serologic titers that may result. As a consequence, the skin test is used primarily for epidemiologic studies and is not useful as a diagnostic tool. Serologic tests include complement fixation (CF) using mycelial or yeast form antigens that should show a single titer of at least 1:64 or, preferably, a fourfold rise in paired sera separated by 3 weeks. The immunodiffusion test detects antibodies to M and H bands, and is significant when both bands are demonstrated. These serologic tests are relatively insensitive in acute pul-

TABLE 9.13–2. CLINICAL FORMS OF MYCOTIC INFECTION

Infection	Usual Mechanism of Acquisition	Forms of Infection	Major Sites of Dissemination
Histoplasmosis	Inhalation	Primary pulmonary Chronic (progressive) pulmonary Disseminated	Marrow Oropharyngeal mucous membranes
Coccidioidomycosis	Inhalation	Primary pulmonary Chronic (progressive) pulmonary Disseminated	Skin and soft tissue Bones and joints Meninges
Blastomycosis	Inhalation	Primary pulmonary Chronic pulmonary Disseminated	Skin Bone and joints Male genitourinary tract
Cryptococcosis	Inhalation	Primary pulmonary Chronic pulmonary Disseminated	Meninges Skin Bone
Candidiasis	Endogenous	Mucocutaneous: oral esophageal, vaginal, paronychia, intertrigo, cystitis, or peritonitis Endocarditis Fungemia Disseminated	Renal Ocular Skin
Phycomyces	Inhalation	Rhinocerebral mucormycosis Pulmonary	
Aspergillosis	Inhalation	Aspergilloma Allergic bronchopulmonary Invasive pulmonary Localized: cutaneous, sinusitis, burn wounds, endophthalmitis Disseminated	Brain Liver Renal

monary histoplasmosis and in disseminated infection in the compromised host.

Treatment is generally restricted to patients with progressive pulmonary disease, chronic cavitary pulmonary histoplasmosis, and those with disseminated disease. For chronic cavitary disease the recommendation is for oral ketoconazole (400 mg per day for 6 to 12 months),[3] surgical resection of chronic, localized lesions, or amphotericin B (usually a total dose of 2 g). Immunocompetent patients with disseminated disease may be treated with oral ketoconazole, but immunosuppressed patients should receive amphotericin B.

COCCIDIOIDOMYCOSIS

Coccidioidis immitis is a diphasic fungus with a mycelia form in nature and large spherules (10 to 50 μm in diameter) containing endospores at 37C in tissue. The organism is found in semi-arid climates corresponding to the distribution of the lower Sonoran life zone, primarily southwestern United States (New Mexico, Arizona, Texas, and California), certain parts of South America, and Central America. The largest endemic area in the United States is the southern part of the San Joaquin valley, leading to the common reference as valley fever.

The *pathogenesis* of the disease involves inhalation of arthrospores; ensuing events are determined by host resistance and inoculum size. Disseminated disease is far more common in men, especially in Filipinos and Blacks, and in patients with compromised cell-mediated immunity.

The *clinical forms* correspond largely to those described for histoplasmosis as primary coccidioidomycosis, chronic progressive pulmonary coccidioidomycosis and disseminated coccidioidomycosis. Again, most infections are asymptomatic or regarded as a nonspecific respiratory illness. Symptoms, when present, usually include cough, fever, and pleuritic chest pain; occasionally patients develop erythema nodosum, erythema multiforme, and arthral-

gias, most commonly young adult, white women. Chest radiographs may show localized infiltrates, especially nodules that may be single or multiple, sometimes associated with hilar adenopathy or pleural effusion. Chronic progressive pulmonary coccidioidomycosis is a chronic disease associated with weight loss, fever, dyspnea, and chest pain. Late findings include cavitation or thin-walled cysts that may be detected on routine chest radiographs of asymptomatic patients. Extrapulmonary coccidioidomycosis reflects disseminated disease, either as a component of the original illness, or reactivation of latent foci, most frequently at a time of compromised cell-mediated immunity. The most common sites for disseminated disease are the skin and subcutaneous tissue, bones, joints, or meninges.

The *diagnosis* is made by recovery of the fungus from respiratory secretions or sites of dissemination, although the yield may be relatively low. Alternatively, typical spherules containing endospores may be demonstrated in exudates with a KOH wet mount or biopsies using H and E, PAS, Gridley, or methenamine silver stains. Skin tests are primarily useful for epidemiology studies; skin test conversion may be demonstrated with the initial infection, and skin test reversion (a positive test that becomes negative) supports the probability of disseminated disease. In contrast with histoplasmosis, the coccidioidin skin test does not alter serologic tests and is consequently more widely applied. Serologic tests are very helpful, because the titer tends to correlate directly with the severity of the disease. The complement fixation (CF) test usually becomes positive about the third week of illness, and persistent titers exceeding 1:32 strongly suggest disseminated disease. A positive CF test in CSF is considered diagnostic of meningitis.

Treatment is usually not advocated for patients with primary pulmonary coccidioidomycosis, because this usually resolves spontaneously. Some have suggested a 1-g course of amphotericin B for selected patients at risk for dissemination, such as black men, Filipinos, and patients with compromised cell-mediated immunity. Patients with progressive pulmonary coccidioidomycosis are often treated with ketoconazole (400 to 800 mg for 6 months or longer) or amphotericin B (1 to 2 g). Patients with disseminated disease

outside the CNS require amphotericin B (2 g or more). Coccidioidomycosis meningitis should be treated with intrathecal amphotericin B, often administered by an Ommaya reservoir in combination with intravenous amphotericin B.

BLASTOMYCOSIS

Blastomycosis dermatidis is a dimorphic fungus occurring as mycelia-bearing conidia in nature, and as large (8 to 15 μm diameter) encapsulated yeasts at 37C in the infected host. The endemic areas in the United States are the southeastern, south central, and midwestern states and regions adjacent to the Great Lakes. The natural habitat is not known, because the fungus is infrequently found in soil samples.

The organism is acquired by inhalation of conidiospores that cause a primary infection in the lung. This is usually asymptomatic, but some patients have flulike symptoms, pleuritic chest pain, arthralgias, or erythema nodosum. Complications include chronic pulmonary infections, cavity formation, pleural involvement, pulmonary fibrosis, and hematogenous dissemination. Chronic pulmonary infection may cause prolonged fever, weight loss, cough, pleuritic chest pain, or hemoptysis. Host factors responsible for maintaining control of blastomycosis are poorly understood, but dissemination is associated with defective cell-mediated immunity in at least some hosts. The major foci of dissemination are the skin and subcutaneous tissue, bones, joints, and the male genital tract.

The *diagnosis* of blastomycosis is usually made by KOH preparations of sputum or exudate from infected sites, recovery of the organism by culture, or the demonstration of typical forms in biopsy specimens. The organism appears characteristically as a large yeast with single budding daughter cells attached at a broad base. Preferred stains are methenamine silver or PAS. Histologic studies of pulmonary or skin lesions show noncaseating granulomas. There is no useful skin or serologic test.

Treatment is often not required for the acute pulmonary form, because most cases are self-limited and the diagnosis is rarely established. Nevertheless it is not possible to determine which individuals will develop progressive disease, so that many patients with acute pulmonary disease are treated. The preferred drugs are ketoconazole (400 mg per day for 6 months)[3] or amphotericin B in a total dose of 1.5 to 2.5 g.

CRYPTOCOCCOSIS

Cryptococcus neoformans is a spherical or ovoid yeast measuring 4 to 7 μm that is enveloped by a thick gelatinous polysaccharide capsule, sometimes with budding cells and a narrow attachment. The organism is widely distributed in nature and is found in exceptionally high concentrations in pigeon feces, although most patients with cryptococcosis have little or nothing to do with pigeons.

The usual mechanism of acquisition is by inhalation, and the *major recognized forms* of the disease are pulmonary or disseminated cryptococcosis. The pulmonary form may be associated with fever, cough, weight loss, and pleuritic pain, or it may be asymptomatic. Chest radiographs are variable in showing a single nodule, multiple nodules, infiltrates, a miliary pattern, cavitation, hilar adenopathy, or a pleural effusion.[6] In many cases the diagnosis is established when a thoracotomy is performed for a suspected neoplasm. Dissemination occurs primarily in patients who have defective cell-mediated immunity, especially patients with AIDS. Like most fungi, *C. neoformans* shows a propensity to disseminate to specific anatomic sites, and the primary target is the meninges, where it causes a basilar meningitis. Less common sites for disseminated disease are the skin, mucous membranes, and bone. Cryptococcal meningitis is suspect in any patient with chronic meningitis, and especially those with defective cell-mediated immunity who complain of headache, mentation changes, blurred vision, or meningismus.

The *diagnosis* of pulmonary infection may be made with cultures of sputum or bronchial washings using selective media, or India ink preparations of respiratory secretions, but the yield is relatively poor, and many cases are not established until a thoracotomy is performed for a suspected neoplasm on chest radiograph. The organism occasionally is recovered in blood cultures or urine cultures. In patients with meningitis, the diagnosis is usually readily established by detection of cryptococcal antigen with the latex agglutination test, which is positive in 95 percent of cases; alternative methods to establish the diagnosis include recovery of the organism in culture or demonstration of the typical encapsulated yeast forms with the India ink preparation. A general recommendation is that a lumbar puncture to detect cryptococcal meningitis should be performed when this organism is detected at any anatomic site.

Patients with pulmonary cryptococcosis generally do not receive treatment in the absence of meningitis. Sequential chest radiographs should be obtained to determine if the pulmonary lesion resolves spontaneously, stabilizes, or progresses.[6] Candidates for antifungal therapy include patients with progressive pulmonary infection, some compromised hosts with pulmonary disease, and all patients with disseminated disease. Cryptococcal meningitis is the only mycotic infection in which there is agreement regarding specific details of treatment, and even these are now becoming controversial as a result of AIDS. The specific recommendation is a 6-week course of amphotericin B (0.3 mg/kg per day) combined with flucytosine (150 mg/kg per day).[1] About half of patients receiving this regimen will show a toxic reaction, the most common being azotemia and marrow suppression.[9] Some patients will relapse and require a second course or a more ambitious regimen of amphotericin B. Patients with AIDS virtually always relapse and should continue to receive intermittent amphotericin B. An alternative strategy for patients who relapse or fail to improve is delivery of amphotericin B intrathecally, often with an Ommaya reservoir. One theoretical disadvantage of this approach is that cryptococcal meningitis, unlike coccidioidal meningitis, is usually an encephalitis as well as a meningitis.

CANDIDIASIS

There are numerous species of *Candida*, but the most commonly encountered in normal flora and at infected sites is *Candida albicans*. The organisms appear as egg-shaped budding yeasts, and in infected tissue or exudate they may appear as pseudohyphae. *Candida* species are the most frequent fungi recovered in clinical specimens and usually represent simple contaminants. Routine cultures of healthy individuals yield these organisms in 30 percent of respiratory tract specimens, 65 percent of stool specimens, and 50 percent of vaginal swabs.

The clinical features of candidiasis are highly variable depending to a large extent on the host. Most patients harbor the organism as a component of the normal flora, and most infections are thought to be endogenous. Both granulocytes and cell-mediated immunity appear to be important host defense factors.[2]

Clinical manifestations of candidiasis may be classified as mucocutaneous infections, fungemia, endocarditis, and disseminated candidiasis. Mucocutaneous infections are extremely common and associated with a variety of host settings. With oral candidiasis (thrush), vaginal candidiasis, *Candida* dermatitis, and cystitis there is no fungal invasion and the basement membrane is intact. *Candida* esophagitis, enteritis, and colitis reflect fungal invasion with disruption of the basement membrane and ulceration. A variety of associated conditions are thought to predispose to these. *Candida* overgrowth syndromes include diabetes, antibiotic use, pregnancy, and AIDS or other causes of defective cell-mediated immunity. Esophagitis is considered diagnostic of AIDS unless there is another explanation for defective cell-mediated immunity. Cutaneous forms include perianal infections, intertrigo, and paronychia. Chronic mucocutaneous candidiasis is a relatively rare disease asso-

ciated with limited defects in T-cell function characterized by persistent superficial *Candida* infection of the skin, nail, mucous membranes, and scalp.

C. albicans is the most common fungus recovered in blood cultures. Less common species in rank order are *C. tropicalis*, *C. parapsilosis*, *C. glabrata* (formerly *Torulopsis glabrata*) and *C. krusei*.[5] In many instances this appears to be a benign self-limited event that resolves spontaneously with removal of any indwelling vascular lines. Disseminated disease or endocarditis is to be suspected when blood cultures are persistently positive. *Candida* endocarditis occurs most frequently in the setting of a prosthetic valve, and less commonly among intravenous drug abusers. Disseminated candidiasis is a relatively common finding in autopsy series among patients with leukemia, lymphomas, and those receiving cancer chemotherapy. The most common sites of disseminated disease are the kidneys, eyes, and skin. Funduscopic examination often shows typical raised, white fundal lesions that are considered diagnostic of disseminated disease. Renal involvement may include renal abscesses with progressive renal insufficiency, but care must be exercised in the interpretation of urine cultures, because recovery of *Candida* from this source usually reflects cystitis of uncertain significance. The skin lesions are typically maculonodular with an erythematous base. The *diagnosis* of superficial *Candida* infections simply requires swabs or scrapings of infected sites for KOH wet mount, Gram stain, or culture. The diagnosis of disseminated disease may be especially difficult, because the recovery of *Candida* from most sites reflects surface involvement or contamination by the normal flora. The preferred method is to demonstrate typical organisms in tissue biopsies or recovery of the organism from an uncontaminated source on multiple occasions.

Mucocutaneous forms of candidiasis may receive treatment with topical agents such as nystatin or clotrimazole, or with orally administered ketoconazole.[2] Cystitis often may be eradicated by local bladder installations of amphotericin B, although the necessity to treat this condition is often controversial. Amphotericin B (1.5 to 2 g) with or without flucytosine must be used for disseminated disease. A common plan in patients with positive blood cultures is low-dose amphotericin B therapy (0.3 mg/kg for 10 days). Patients with endocarditis require valve replacement accompanied by the administration of amphotericin B with or without flucytosine.

PHYCOMYCOSIS (MUCORMYCOSIS)

Mycotic infections are caused by the genera *Mucor*, *Rhizopus*, *Absidia*, and *Cunninghamella*, which belong to the order Mucorales and appear morphologically identical with highly characteristic broad (usually 10 to 15 μm) nonseptate hyphae and right-angle branching. These organisms are distributed throughout the world in decaying matter and soil.

The organism may be acquired by inhalation, ingestion, or wound contamination with spores. The infection is characterized by invasion of blood vessels with thrombosis and infarction. Two types of hosts are susceptible, diabetics with ketoacidosis and patients with major defects in host defenses. The characteristic disease in diabetics is rhinocerebral mucormycosis, which occurs primarily in those with ketoacidosis but which also may develop in patients with hematologic malignancies complicated by neutropenia. The infection spreads through contiguous structures without respect for anatomic planes, resulting in orbit involvement with ophthalmoplegia; destruction of cranial nerves II, IV, V and VI; and extension to the carotid artery, cavernous sinuses, meninges, and brain. A second common form of the disease is pulmonary mucormycosis, which usually occurs in patients with hematologic malignancy or cancer chemotherapy complicated by neutropenia and often cell-mediated immunity as well. The clinical and radiographic findings frequently simulate those seen with pulmonary embolism and infarction, sometimes with cavitation. Disseminated disease is relatively uncommon.

The *diagnosis* of phycomycosis requires the demonstration of typical hyphal forms in tissue or with KOH preparations. Smears of sputum or wound exudate rarely show the fungus, and cultures of either these or tissue specimens infrequently yield the microbe. Even when it is recovered, there is often a question of plate contamination by airborne spores.

Amphotericin B should be given aggressively and as early as possible when this diagnosis is likely. There should be a rapid increase in dosage and a total dose of 2 to 3 g is generally advocated. For rhinocerebral mucormycosis in diabetics there should also be aggressive debridement of the lesion and prompt steps taken to control diabetic acidosis.

ASPERGILLOSIS

Aspergillus species occur in nature as hyphae with conidia, and in tissue and exudate as branched, septate hyphae measuring 2 to 5 μm in diameter with branching at about 45-degree angles. The organism is distributed throughout the world, most frequently in decaying vegetation.

Disease is usually acquired by inhalation of airborne conidiospores. Epidemics have occurred within hospitals among burn victims and immunosuppressed hosts, presumably because of inadequate filtration of hospital air.

Diseases caused by *Aspergillus* are highly variable, depending on the host. One of the more common forms is an aspergilloma or fungus ball composed of a tangled mass of hyphae within a pulmonary cavity caused by another disease process. This is usually a benign process unless there is severe hemoptysis. Another common pulmonary form is allergic bronchopulmonary aspergillosis resulting from hypersensitivity to the antigens of aspergillus colonizing the bronchial mucosa seen in patients with asthma.[7] This represents a common form of the pulmonary infiltrate with eosinophilia (PIE) syndrome. Invasive pulmonary aspergillosis is a serious complication found exclusively in the compromised host, primarily patients with leukemia or lymphomas, those receiving cancer chemotherapy and recipients of organ transplants when both neutropenia and defective cell-mediated immunity play contributing roles.[4] The usual finding is a bronchopneumonia or vascular invasion with thrombosis and infarction, sometimes with cavity formation. The invasive pulmonary form may be complicated by dissemination to the brain, kidneys, liver, and other organs.

Aspergillus is relatively difficult to cultivate from sputum with all forms of pulmonary aspergillosis, and it is difficult to recover from other potential sites of infection as well. More frequently, typical hyphal forms are seen with impression smears and biopsies using methenamine silver stains or PAS stains. *Aspergillus* precipitins in serum usually are present with aspergillomas and the allergic bronchopulmonary form, but they are not helpful with invasive or disseminated aspergillosis.

Therapeutic recommendations depend largely on the form of aspergillosis. Most aspergillomas do well without specific forms of therapy unless there is extensive hemoptysis, which is probably best treated with segmental resection. The allergic bronchopulmonary form of aspergillosis may respond to corticosteroids. Invasive forms of the disease require amphotericin B with rapid increases in daily dosage to 1 mg/kg per day and a minimum total dose of 2 g.

REFERENCES

1. Bennet JE, Dismukes WE, et al: A comparison of amphotericin B alone combined with flucytosine in the treatment of cryptococcal meningitis. N Engl J Med 301:126, 1979
2. Bodey GP: Candidiasis: A growing concern. Am J Med 77:1, 1984
3. Dismukes WE, Cloud G, et al: Treatment of blastomycosis and histoplasmosis with ketoconazole. Ann Intern Med 103:861, 1985
4. Gerson SL, Talbot GH, et al: Prolonged granulocytopenia: The major

risk factor for invasive pulmonary aspergillosis in patients with acute leukemia. Ann Intern Med 100:345, 1984

5. Horn R, Wong R, et al: Fungemia in a cancer hospital: Changing frequency, earlier onset, and results of therapy. Rev Infect Dis 7:646, 1985

6. Kerkering TM, Duma RJ, Shadomy S: The evolution of pulmonary cryptococcosis: Clinical implications from a study of 41 patients with or without compromising host factors. Ann Intern Med 94:611, 1981

7. Patterson R, Greenberger PA, et al: Allergic bronchopulmonary aspergillosis: Staging as an aid to management. Ann Intern Med 96:286, 1982

8. Sathapatayavongs B, Batteiger BE, et al: Clinical and laboratory features

of disseminated histoplasmosis during two large urban outbreaks. Medicine 62:263, 1983

9. Stamm AM, Diasio RB, et al: Toxicity of amphotericin B plus flucytosine in 194 patients with cryptococcal meningitis. Am J Med 83:236, 1987

10. Wheat LJ, Kohler RB, Tewari RP: Diagnosis of disseminated histoplasmosis by detection of *Histoplasma capsulatum* antigen in serum and urine specimens. N Engl J Med 314:83, 1986

11. Wheat LJ, Slama TG, et al: A large urban outbreak of histoplasmosis: Clinical features. Ann Intern Med 94:331, 1981

12. Young RC, Bennett JE, et al: Aspergillosis: The spectrum of the disease in 98 patients. Medicine 49:147, 1970

CHAPTER 9.14
Sexually Transmitted Diseases

Thomas C. Quinn and Bradley Bender

Sexually transmitted diseases (STDs) are a major and growing public health problem. The medical, social, and economic impact of these diseases far exceeds that previously attributed to the traditional venereal diseases—syphilis, gonorrhea, chancroid, lymphogranuloma venereum, and granuloma inguinale, which now account for only a fraction of STDs. Pathogens such as *Chlamydia trachomatis*, herpes simplex virus, hepatitis B, cytomegalovirus, *Trichomonas vaginalis,* and others are trasmitted primarily through sexual intercourse, and like gonorrhea have become epidemic in many countries. In addition, it has become more evident in the past decade that many of these infections are associated with a wide range of clinical complications that extend beyond the traditional sphere of venereology. Consequently the medical and public awareness of STDs and their associated complications have become more readily accepted, and an increasing emphasis has been placed on the training of physicians in this area.

Factors responsible for the metamorphosis of classical venereology to the study of the new generation of STDs are multifactorial. Among the factors responsible are changes in sexual behavior, advances in medical technology, and enhanced awareness of the complications of STDs by public health authorities, physicians, and the public.

First, there has been a marked increase in the incidence of several STDs, such as those due to *Neisseria gonorrhoeae,* herpes simplex virus, and *C. trachomatis.* This trend parallels the increment in the sexually active 18- to 30-year-old segment of our population, which is derived from the "baby boom" of the 1950s. Concomitantly, sexual behavior has changed, resulting in sexual activity at an earlier age and with an increased number of partners. For example, in one study the proportion of 17-year-old women who engage in premarital intercourse rose from 25 percent in 1971 to almost 50 percent in 1979; for age 19 the frequency increased from less than 50 to nearly 70 percent. The widespread use of non-barrier contraceptives has also contributed to the present epidemic of STDs.

A second major factor for the present epidemic is the improved recognition of STDs because of technologic advances in microbiology, improved clinical recognition of syndromes associated with STDs, and new epidemiologic information regarding their transmission. The recent development of cultures for herpes simplex virus and *Chlamydia* has enabled clinicians to diagnose these infections and their associated complications more readily. The recognition of hepatitis B and a wide range of enteric infections in homosexual men has affected the approach to the management of these disorders and related entities.

Lastly, the growing awareness of the consequences and com-

plications of STDs has motivated public health officials, medical institutions, and the public to support research and control programs in this area. The impact of STDs on pelvic inflammatory disease, infertility, ectopic pregnancy, and maternal, fetal, and infant infection has now been recognized and accepted throughout our society. The relationship of STDs to neoplasia, such as human papilloma virus and carcinoma of the vulva or cervix, and the role of sexually transmitted agents in the development of the highly fatal AIDS,[27] has emphasized the medical and social aspects of STDs throughout the world.

The purpose of this chapter is to review many of these STD pathogens (Table 9.14–1) and some of their associated clinical complications. An emphasis on diagnosis, treatment, and prevention is provided to develop a comprehensive approach to many of these common clinical problems.

GONORRHEA

Despite a slight decline in the incidence rate in the 1980s, there are still more than 1 million cases of gonorrhea reported annually in the United States, making this the most common reportable disease.[5] The causative organism is *N. gonorrhoeae,* a gram-negative diplococcus typically found within polymorphonuclear leukocytes present in discharge material from a variety of body sites such as the urethra or cervix. The organism is capable of infecting or colonizing a wide range of columnar or transitional epithelial mucous membranes. These include the urethra of men and women, a variety of genital glands such as Tyson or Cowper in men and Bartholin in women, the uterine cervical canal and fallopian tubes, epididymis, the anal canal, distal rectum, conjunctiva, and pharynx. Frequently, infection of the endocervix, anal canal, and pharynx have no specific or nonspecific symptoms. Aside from infections of the endocervix and urethra, the infectiousness and natural history of infections at other sites are not well understood.

Except in the neonate and in some young children, gonorrhea is virtually always transmitted sexually. Approximately 90 percent of women will acquire gonorrhea after genital intercourse with an infected man, while only one third of men will acquire gonorrhea after relations with an infected woman.[21] In addition to this preference for female sites, the complications of gonococcal infection are also more severe in the female. Local complications of pelvic inflammatory disease (PID), perihepatitis, infertility, and premature delivery are both more common and more severe than the rare epididymitis or urethral stricture that may occur in men.

TABLE 9.14–1. SEXUALLY TRANSMITTED DISEASES[a]

Pathogen	Disease	Complications	Diagnosis	Treatment[b]
Bacteria				
Neisseria gonorrhoeae	Urethritis, cervicitis, proctitis, pharyngitis, vaginitis, conjunctivitis	Pelvic inflammatory disease, urethral strictures, septic arthritis, endocarditis, epididymitis, prostatitis, infertility, ectopic pregnancy, prematurity, blindness	Gram stain showing gram-negative intracellular diplococci; growth on Thayer-Martin medium under 5% CO_2	See Tables 9.14–2, 9.14–3
Treponema pallidum	Syphilis	Tabes dorsalis, Charcot joints, meningovascular syphilis, dementia, aortitis, gummas, congenital syphilis	Darkfield examination of chancre, condyloma lata, or lymph node aspirate. Serologic tests for syphilis	*Early:* benzathine penicillin G 2,400,000 U IM *Late:* As above, once a week for 3 consecutive wk *Neurosyphilis:* Aqueous crystalline penicillin G, 3,000,000 U IV q4h × 10 days
Chlamydia trachomatis	Urethritis, cervicitis, proctitis, lymphogranuloma venereum (LGV)	Pelvic inflammatory disease, epididymitis, infertility, ectopic pregnancy, prematurity, neonatal pneumonia	Isolation in tissue culture Direct monoclonal Fluorescent antibody (ELISA)	Tetracycline or erythromycin 500 mg po qid × 7 days For LGV: as above for at least 2 wk, or until lesions are healed; also see Table 9.14–3
Ureaplasma urealyticum	Urethritis[c]	Prostatitis[c]		Tetracycline or erythromycin 500 mg po qid × 7 days
Mycoplasma hominis	Urethritis[c]	Pelvic inflammatory disease[c]		Tetracycline or erythromycin 500 mg po qid × 7 days
Haemophilus ducreyi	Chancroid	Spontaneous rupture of fluctuant nodes	Isolation on supplemented chocolate agar	Erythromycin 500 mg po qid × 7 days *or* TMP-SMX 160 mg po bid × 7 days or until lesions are healed; ceftriaxone 250 mg IM once is also effective
Calymmatobacterium granulomatis Mobiluncus sp.	Granuloma inguinale	Squamous cell carcinoma	Giemsa or Wright stain of scraping or biopsy showing coccobacilli in cytoplasm of mononuclear cells	Tetracycline 500 mg po qid until lesion is healed
Gardnerella vaginalis	Nonspecific vaginitis[c] (bacterial vaginosis)	Postpartum endometritis[b]	See Table 9.14–6	Metronidazole 500 mg po bid × 7 days or Ampicillin 500 mg po qid × 7 days
Group B streptococci	Asymptomatic carriage	Neonatal sepsis and meningitis	Isolation on blood agar	Aqueous penicillin G 50,000 U IM to neonates of mothers who are carriers
Fungi				
Candida albicans	Vaginitis		Fungal elements on 10% KOH preparation	Miconazole or clotrimazole 100 mg intravaginally daily × 7 days
Viruses				
Herpes simplex virus	Genital herpes, proctitis, pharyngitis	Recurrent attacks, disseminated disease, meningitis, neonatal herpes, autonomic dysfunction	1. Tzanck smear showing multinucleated giant cells 2. Tissue culture 3. Fourfold rise in complement fixing antibodies	Acyclovir 200 mg orally 5 × daily for 10–14 days or until healing of lesions Symptomatic therapy: Analgesics, sitz bath
Hepatitis A virus	Acute hepatitis		Serology—see Chapter 13.3	

(continued)

TABLE 9.14–1. SEXUALLY TRANSMITTED DISEASES [a] **(Continued)**

Pathogen	Disease	Complications	Diagnosis	Treatment[b]
Viruses (Cont.)				
Hepatitis B virus	Acute hepatitis	Chronic carriage, chronic hepatitis (active or persistent), periarteritis nodosa, glomerulonephritis, aplastic anemia, hepatoma	Serology—see Chapter 13.3	
Cytomegalovirus	Infectious mononucleosis syndrome	Congenital birth defects, prematurity, pneumonia (in immunocompromised) inflammatory colitis	1. Tissue culture 2. Serology	
Papilloma virus	Condyloma acuminatum	Cervical carcinoma[c] HPV 16, 18	Clinical appearance	Podophyllin 10–25% compound applied to lesions and washed off in 4 hr
Poxvirus	Molluscum contagiosum		Cytoplasmic inclusions on microscopy	Removal of caseous center
Human immunodeficiency virus (HIV), also known as HTLV-LAV	Acquired immunodeficiency syndrome	Kaposi sarcoma, *Pneumocystis carinii* pneumonia, and other opportunistic infections	See Chapter 9.15	See Chapter 9.15
Protozoa				
Trichomonas vaginalis	Vaginitis		Motile organisms on wet mount	Metronidazole 2 g po
Ectoparasite				
Sarcoptes scabiei var *hominis*	Scabies	Norwegian scabies in immunosuppressed	Characteristic burrows	Lindane 1% lotion or cream applied to body and washed off the next day
Pthirus pubis	Pubic lice		Combing of hair and microscopic examination	Lindane shampoo of infested area and wash in four minutes

[a]This table does not include infections associated with homosexual men, see Table 9.14–7.
[b]From Centers for Disease Control: Sexually transmitted disease treatment guidelines, 1985. MMWR 34:755, 1985.
[c]Suspected.

GONOCOCCAL INFECTIONS IN MEN

Urethritis, the most common manifestation of gonorrhea in men, is asymptomatic in 5 percent of newly infected patients. The usual incubation period is 2 to 5 days after sexual contact, but the disease infrequently occurs up to 2 to 3 weeks later. Symptoms are variable, changing from a thin, mucoid discharge to one that is grossly purulent. Meatal irritation, dysuria, and frequency are common associated complaints. If the symptoms are ignored or the infection is only partially treated, it can persist in an asymptomatic or mildly symptomatic state and can spread to produce epididymitis, prostatitis, and (rarely) disseminated gonococcal infection.

Homosexual men who participate in receptive anal intercourse are susceptible to anorectal gonococcal infections. Indeed, this is the most common cause of proctitis in homosexual men. The disease is asymptomatic in 20 to 50 percent of infected individuals and is typically mild in symptomatic men who may complain of pruritus, discomfort, tenesmus, and mucopurulent discharge.[26] Gonococcal pharyngitis occurs mostly in individuals who perform fellatio, but it is postulated that this infection can also occur after anilingus or cunnilingus with an infected partner. In symptomatic cases, the presentation is nonspecific with sore throat, erythema, pharyngeal exudate, and cervical adenopathy. The majority of pharyngeal infections are asymptomatic, however, emphasizing the importance of routine urethral, rectal, and throat cultures in high-risk individuals such as homosexual men.

GONOCOCCAL INFECTIONS IN WOMEN

Gonorrhea in women is manifested by urethritis, with frequency and dysuria, and by cervicitis, with a purulent cervical-vaginal discharge, dyspareunia, abnormal menstrual flow, and pelvic pain or discomfort. Anorectal involvement, which is usually asymptomatic, occurs in up to 50 percent of women with cervical gonorrhea.[39] Anorectal gonorrhea is frequently the result of rectal-vaginal contamination and does not necessarily imply that the patient has participated in rectal intercourse. Women who participate in anal intercourse or fellatio, however, are as susceptible to gonococcal proctitis or pharyngitis, respectively, as homosexual men who engage in these sexual practices. Anorectal symptoms are present in less than 10 percent of infected women. The most frequent complaints are anal itching, painful defecation, mucopurulent discharge, and constipation. Signs of anorectal infection include erythema and edema of the anal crypts, anal discharge, and, rarely, rectal bleeding from ulcerative proctitis.

One of the most serious complications of cervical gonorrhea is the development of pelvic inflammatory disease, which may occur in 10 to 20 percent of infected women. This complication is discussed later since it may involve multiple agents.

In prepubescent girls, the vaginal mucosa is susceptible to invasion by the gonococcus, the disease manifesting as a vulvovaginitis. Infection of prepubertal patients older than 1 year of age with gonorrhea is prima facie evidence of sexual molestation.

DISSEMINATED GONOCOCCAL INFECTION

Blood-borne dissemination of *N. gonorrhoeae* is rare, probably occurring overall in less than 1 percent of all gonococcal infections. Actual rates depend on the type of infecting strain and on host defense factors. Strains that are prone to disseminate tend to be nutritionally deficient auxotypes, which are less likely to cause symptomatic disease, such as a urethral discharge; are most resistant to the bactericidal action of normal human sera and complement; are more difficult to culture; and are more susceptible to antibiotics. For the last reason, disseminated gonorrhea is easy to treat, relative to other disseminated bacterial infections. The disease is characterized by fever, polyarthralgias, and a rash. The rash consists of one or two lesions present on distal extremities and is characterized as petechial, papular, hemorrhagic, or necrotic. Intracellular gram-negative diplococci representative of *N. gonorrhoeae* can be frequently demonstrated in scrapings of these lesions. The joints involved include the wrists, ankles, and knees; and in most cases tenosynovitis rather than frank arthritis is present. Septic arthritis can occur, however, and *N. gonorrhoeae* is the most common cause of infectious arthritis in young adults. Early in the arthritis-dermatitis gonococcal syndrome, blood cultures may be positive for *N. gonorrhoeae*. Joint fluid cultures are frequently negative for the pathogen until a frank arthritis has developed, however, at which time the joint effusions are culture positive and the blood cultures revert to negative.[20] Recurrent episodes of this syndrome are described in patients with defects in the terminal components of the complement cascade.[32]

DIAGNOSIS AND TREATMENT

Despite the development of a wide variety of new tests designed to detect *N. gonorrhoeae* in specimens from mucous membranes, a Gram stain smear and cultures that are directly inoculated onto selective media (e.g., Thayer-Martin, Martin-Lewis, and NYC) remain the best methods. A Gram stain smear of urethral exudate from infected men will demonstrate intracellular gram-negative diplococci in more than 90 percent of symptomatic males with gonococcal urethritis. In women, the Gram stain smear of cervical exudate will be positive in approximately 70 percent of those infected. The Gram stain is positive in only 30 to 50 percent of patients with rectal gonorrhea. Gram stains of pharyngeal exudate are not useful because of confusion with *Neisseria* species normally present in the pharynx. Although a negative Gram stain does not rule out the diagnosis of gonorrhea, a positive Gram stain for intracellular gram-negative diplococci taken from the urethra, cervix, or rectum is strongly supportive of gonococcal infection.

Regardless of the result of the Gram stain, cultures of the specimen and of multiple sites should be done in all cases in which there is a suspicion of gonococcal infection. The sensitivity (true positive) of a single culture swab is 90 to 98 percent in symptomatic men with urethritis and 80 to 90 percent in women with cervicitis. Rectal and pharyngeal cultures are slightly less reliable and repeated cultures may be necessary. Delay in plating, improper handling, failure to use selective media, or failure to incubate plates under high CO_2 tension may result in a false negative culture rate of 20 percent or more. Cultures of multiple sites are important to perform to confirm the results of the Gram stain as well as detect cases in which the Gram stain was negative. Additionally, isolates recovered in culture can be screened for penicillin resistance, which is especially important in high-risk individuals. The mechanism of penicillin resistance is usually by production of a β-lactamase, and these strains are referred to as penicillinase-producing *N. gonorrhoeae* (PPNG). PPNG originated in the Far East and presumably were imported to the United States by returning servicemen and refugees from Southeast Asia. Within the United States the number of PPNG cases has risen dramatically from 328 cases in 1979 to 4457 in 1986. Patients who have had sexual contact in Southeast Asia, who were exposed to patients with known PPNG infection, or who have a positive culture after completing therapy should all be screened for penicillin resistance. These individuals should be treated presumptively for PPNG, with spectinomycin. Penicillin-resistant gonococcal strains that do not produce penicillinase are referred to as "chromosomally-mediated resistant *N. gonorrhoeae*" (CMRNG).[8] These strains are also increasing in prevalence and require treatment protocols similar to those outlined for PPNG, with close follow-up for subsequent treatment failures.

The treatment regimens for various forms and complications of gonorrhea are outlined in Table 9.14–2. Additional management includes testing and treatment of sexual contacts, a serologic test for syphilis, and firm instructions to avoid sexual contact until a repeat culture of the infected site is taken about 1 week after completion of therapy for test of cure. In addition, all women and homosexual men treated for gonorrhea should have anal canal and pharyngeal cultures obtained routinely.

CHLAMYDIA TRACHOMATES

Chlamydia trachomatis is clearly one of the most common sexually transmitted pathogens in developed countries. There is an annual

TABLE 9.14–2. TREATMENT OF GONORRHEA[a]

	Penicillin Sensitive[b]	Penicillin Resistant[b]
Uncomplicated gonorrhea (urethritis, cervicitis, asymptomatic carrier, sexual contact)	Amoxicillin 3 g *or* Ampicillin 3.5 g PO *plus* probenecid 1 g PO *or* APPG[c] 4,800,000 U IM *plus* probenecid 1 g PO *or* Ceftriaxone 250 mg IM once	Spectinomycin 2 g IM *or* Ceftriaxone 250 mg IM once
Anorectal gonorrhea	APPG 4,800,000 U IM *plus* probenecid 1 g po	Spectinomycin 2 g IM *or* Ceftriaxone 250 mg IM
Pharyngeal gonorrhea	APPG 4,800,000 U IM *plus* probenecid 1 g po	Trimethoprim *or* sulfamethoxazole (80 mg and 400 mg repeated) nine tablets po daily for 5 days
Gonococcal ophthalmia	Aqueous crystalline penicillin G 10,000,000 U IV daily for 5 days	Cefoxitin 1 g IV qid for 5 days *or* Ceftriaxone 1 g IM daily for 5 days
Disseminated gonococcal infection	Aqueous crystalline penicillin G 10,000,000 U IV daily, followed by amoxicillin *or* ampicillin 500 mg po qid for 7 days	Cefoxitin 1 g IV qid for 7 days *or* Ceftriaxone 1 g IV daily for 7 days
Pelvic inflammatory disease	See Table 9.14–3	

[a]All regimens are single dose unless specified.
[b]From Centers for Disease Control: Sexually transmitted disease treatment guidelines, 1985. MMWR 34:755, 1985.
[c]Aqueous procaine penicillin G.

incidence of approximately four million infections in the United States as compared to the one million for gonococcal infections.[7] In general, the clinical manifestations and distribution of this organism are similar to those observed for gonococcal infections. There are also similar epidemiologic patterns for the two organisms, with the same high-risk groups (sexually active teenagers, particularly from economically disadvantaged groups). Indeed, the two infections often occur together. Approximately 20 percent of men with gonococcal urethritis have concomitant chlamydial infection, and approximately 40 percent of women with gonorrhea have chlamydial infections of the cervix. In most settings, other than STD clinics, chlamydial infections are more common than gonococcal infections. For example, routine screening of women attending family planning clinics found chlamydial infection rates to be 5 to 10 times that observed for gonococci. Thus, chlamydial infections are extremely common, and the clinical spectrum of these clinical infections is diverse.

C. trachomatis is a gram-negative, obligate, intracellular bacterium that for many years was thought to be a virus. The organism is now classified as a bacterium on the basis of cell wall analysis, susceptibility to antibiotics, and the presence of both DNA and RNA. The genus *Chlamydia* is divided into two species, *C. trachomatis* and *C. psittaci*. By immunofluorescence techniques, *C. trachomatis* can be divided into 15 different serovars.[7,18] Serovars A through C cause severe conjunctivitis, known as epidemic trachoma, in developing countries. Serovars D through K are sexually transmitted and cause urethritis, epididymitis, proctitis, cervicitis, salpingitis, and, in the neonate, conjunctivitis, otitis, and pneumonia. Serovars L1 through L3 are more virulent than the other serovars and cause lymphogranuloma venereum (LGV).

CHLAMYDIAL INFECTIONS IN MEN

C. trachomatis is a major cause of nongonococcal urethritis (NGU) and is found in up to 35 to 50 percent of cases. This condition usually occurs in young sexually active men who have a mucopurulent discharge following an incubation period of 1 to 3 weeks. It is usually milder than gonococcal urethritis. Other symptoms include dysuria and pruritus. Although the discharge is not as purulent as the typical case of gonococcal urethritis, there is sufficient overlap between the two syndromes to make them impossible to differentiate on clinical grounds. In general, when chlamydial diagnostic facilities are not available, the diagnosis of NGU is established by exclusion (failure to find gram-negative intracellular diplococci in Gram stain smear of the urethral discharge), and treatment with tetracyclines is instituted. When tissue culture facilities are available, cultures should be obtained by inserting a swab 1 to 2 cm within the urethra and promptly transporting it to the laboratory in special media.

Postgonococcal urethritis is a specific subset of NGU that occurs in men who have been treated successfully for gonorrhea but have a persistent urethral discharge. The great majority of these men had concomitant chlamydial infections. The penicillins used to treat gonococcal infection are inactive against chlamydiae.

The major complication of chlamydial urethritis is epididymitis. Approximately one third of epididymitis cases in young, sexually active men are due to gonococcal infection, with the other two thirds caused primarily by *C. trachomatis*. The organism may be recovered from urethra and epididymal aspirates.

In homosexual men an inflammatory proctitis can result from infection with *Chlamydia*.[33] Similar to gonococcal proctitis, most of these infections are asymptomatic or mild with major complaints of anorectal discharge, constipation, tenesmus, and pruritus. Erythema of the rectal mucosa and mucopurulent discharge are frequently present. Infection with the LGV serovars, however, may induce a more severe ulcerative proctitis, which clinically and histopathologically resembles granulomatous colitis or Crohn disease.

Another complication associated with chlamydial infection in men is the development of Reiter syndrome, characterized by urethritis, conjunctivitis, arthritis, and a dermatologic rash (see Chapter 8.9). Men with Reiter syndrome have *C. trachomatis* isolated from the urethra in 40 to 70 percent of cases.[25] It is not known whether chlamydiae are the direct cause of this syndrome or are associated with urethritis in these patients, however.

CHLAMYDIAL INFECTIONS IN WOMEN

Cervicitis is the most common manifestation of *C. trachomatis* infection in women, and it may be mild or asymptomatic. Patients may complain of a vaginal discharge and on examination the cervix is found to be red and friable, with a mucopurulent discharge from the os. Similar to urethritis in men, concomitant infections with *C. trachomatis* and *N. gonorrhoeae* frequently occur. Following treatment for gonorrhea, persistent symptoms of mucopurulent endocervicitis represent the female counterpart of postgonococcal urethritis in men.

The most important complication of chlamydial infection in the female is acute salpingitis. This organism is recognized in Sweden, where gonococcal infections have been more effectively controlled than in the United States, as a leading cause of acute salpingitis.[28] The chlamydial disease is clinically milder than salpingitis associated with gonococcal or anaerobic bacterial infection, but the ultimate prognosis in terms of fertility may be worse.

Another common condition in women is the acute urethral syndrome, which is characterized by dysuria and pyuria in association with a bacterial urine culture with bacterial counts $<10^5$/ml of urine. In one study *C. trachomatis* was the most common agent isolated in this infection.[38] This syndrome is discussed further in Chapter 9.10.

PERINATAL AND OCULAR INFECTIONS

A newborn infant exposed to cervical *C. trachomatis* infection during birth has approximately a 60 percent risk of acquiring a chlamydial infection. Approximately one third to one half of the exposed infants will develop conjunctivitis, and another 10 to 20 percent will develop pneumonia. In addition, otitis media in children under 1 year of age has been associated with chlamydial infection. Inclusion conjunctivitis of the newborn is an acute mucopurulent conjunctivitis with onset between 5 to 21 days of age. If untreated, the condition will usually resolve spontaneously after a course of several months. Chlamydial pneumonia of infants occurs between 2 to 12 weeks of age. The infants are afebrile, have a staccato cough, and are usually tachypneic. Radiographic findings include hyperexpansion of the lungs with a mild interstitial infiltrate. Immunoglobulins, particularly the IgM class, are elevated, and eosinophilia is frequently present.

LYMPHOGRANULOMA VENEREUM

The serovars L1, L2, and L3 cause lymphogranuloma venereum (LGV), which is a systemic sexually transmitted infection. In 1986, there were 396 reported civilian cases of LGV in the United States. The LGV serovars are more invasive than the other *C. trachomatis* strains, and the target organs typically involve lymphoid tissue. After an incubation period of 1 to 3 weeks, a small painless papule appears at the site of inoculation. This heals spontaneously within several days. Several weeks later, however, it is followed by prominent inguinal lymphadenopathy, especially in men. This adenopathy is unilateral in two thirds of the cases and bilateral in the remainder. In 20 percent of cases, enlargement of nodes above and below the inguinal ligament result in the "groove sign." The nodes progressively enlarge over the next month and become fluctuant; they are frequently referred to as bubos. If therapy is delayed, the overlying skin becomes inflamed, and draining fistulas may appear. Systemic symptoms of fever, myalgias, and malaise are

common. Late complications such as anorectal strictures or recto-vaginal fistulas may occur in neglected cases.

DIAGNOSIS AND TREATMENT

Chlamydial infections are difficult to diagnose for several reasons. First, they usually cause mild or asymptomatic infection, which can easily be overlooked. Second, coincident infections with gonorrhea occur, and this may lead the physician to overlook the possibility of chlamydial infection. Third, *C. trachomatis* is an obligate intracellular parasite that requires tissue culture facilities for cultivation that are not available to all physicians. Finally, serologic diagnosis of *Chlamydia* is useful in the diagnosis of LGV and pneumonia of the newborn, but of low utility in other infections with *Chlamydia*, in which high background prevalence rates render serodiagnosis less useful. Clinical suspicion therefore remains the key in the diagnostic evaluation of these clinical syndromes. Men with urethritis and a Gram stain showing polymorphonuclear leukocytes without intracellular diplococci should be treated empirically for NGU.[2] Women with cervicitis or salpingitis and negative Gram stain and culture for *N. gonorrhoeae* should be presumed to have *C. trachomatis* infection. Confirmatory cultures for *C. trachomatis* are indicated, but treatment should begin without delay.

More recently, two rapid methods of antigen detection have been developed that may be used if culture is not available or too expensive.[18] In one method, referred to as the direct-smear FA test, specimen material is obtained by swab and applied directly to a slide, which is fixed and then incubated with a fluorescein-conjugated monoclonal antibody before being examined under a fluorescent microscope. Elementary bodies of *C. trachomatis* stain a bright apple-green and are readily identified by a trained microscopist. The other rapid test measures antigen-antibody reaction in an enzyme-linked immunoabsorbent assay (ELISA) and can be used for processing large numbers of specimens. Both tests are rapid, inexpensive, and relatively sensitive (80 to 90 percent) and specific (92 to 97 percent) compared to culture.

Tetracycline is the treatment of choice for all chlamydial infections. The dose is 500 mg orally four times a day. Treatment should last for a minimum of 7 days. In LGV, treatment should continue for at least 2 to 3 weeks. In pregnant women and newborns, erythromycin 500 mg orally four times a day is recommended instead of tetracycline. Fluctuant bubos in LGV should be aspirated as needed to prevent spontaneous rupture. As with other STDs, examination and treatment of sexual partners is indicated.

HERPES SIMPLEX VIRUS

Herpes simplex virus (HSV, herpesvirus hominis) is a member of the herpesvirus group, which also includes varicella-zoster, cytomegalovirus, and Epstein-Barr virus. There are two types of herpesvirus, which were initially distinguished by clinical and epidemiologic behavior and classified as HSV-I and HSV-II. They can be identified now by serologic and microbiologic techniques. Both of these spherical viruses consist of an internal core of double-stranded DNA, surrounded by an icosohedral capsule and a lipoprotein envelope with an overall diameter of 150 to 200 nm. Replication occurs only within the host cell nucleus. The most distinguishing and clinically significant feature of HSV infection is the ability of the virus to establish a latent infection within sensory nerve ganglia of the spinal cord. Reactivation of the latent infection results in recurrences of viral lesions in the area of the original infection.

Approximately 90 percent of genital herpes in the United States is due to HSV-II, and 90 percent of oral labial herpes is due to HSV-I. Estimates of the incidence of new cases of genital herpes range from 200,000 to 1,000,000 a year, with the most likely figure in the neighborhood of 400,000 to 600,000. Further, it has been estimated that there was a tenfold increase in the number of office visits for genital herpes in the period 1966–1981, from 30,000 to 295,000.[5] Although these incidence figures are lower than those of gonorrhea and chlamydial infection, herpes infections are recurrent; thus, the prevalence of genital herpes (the number of existing cases of active infection at any time) is probably greater than for any other sexually transmitted disease. Serologic surveys indicate that about 20 percent of adult Americans have evidence of previous HSV-II infection, a large proportion of whom suffer from recurrences of genital herpes, and it is estimated that anywhere from 5 to 25 million Americans may be actively infected. The mode of transmission is through direct contact, with an average incubation period between 2 to 7 days. The virus initially replicates within the epithelial cells, resulting in cell lysis and stimulation of a local inflammatory response. The result is the characteristic thin-walled vesicle on an inflammatory base present on the skin and mucous membranes. The virus travels via sensory nerve pathways and establishes residence within trigeminal, sacral, or vagal ganglia. Reactivation can occur and is frequently associated with prodromal symptoms such as numbness and tingling in the area of subsequent vesicle formation. The exact factors responsible for reactivation are undetermined, but psychologic stress and menstruation are established risk factors.[19]

PRIMARY GENITAL HERPES

A high frequency of systemic symptoms characterizes primary or initial HSV infections.[9] Fever, malaise, headaches, and myalgias appear in the first 4 or 5 days and decrease over the next week. The local lesion begins as multiple painful vesicles that eventually ulcerate in 3 or 4 days. The lesions develop crusts and epithelialize over the next week. In severe cases, formation of new vesicles also can occur during this time. Tender, nonfluctuant inguinal lymphadenopathy is seen in most patients with genital HSV infection. Typically, HSV can be isolated from the lesions until reepithelialization has taken place. The lesions are most commonly seen on the glans and shaft of the penis in men and the labia, vagina, and cervix in women. Patients who participate in receptive anal intercourse can develop herpes proctitis.[17] The presenting complaints are fever, severe anorectal pain, constipation, difficulty in initiating urination, sacral dermatome paresthesias, and tenesmus. Perianal ulcers occur in 70 percent of cases, and inguinal lymphadenopathy is common. Sigmoidoscopic examination reveals mucosal friability and ulcers in the distal 5 to 10 cm of the rectum, and intranuclear inclusion bodies are found on rectal biopsy.

RECURRENT GENITAL HERPES

Recurrent HSV infections are generally milder than primary infections.[9] About one half of patients will have a prodrome characterized as a burning or tingling sensation in the subsequent area of vesicle development. Less than 10 percent of patients will have systemic symptoms. After a few hours to several days of the prodrome, about four to six small vesicles that are both painful and pruritic will appear. These ulcerate and form either multiple small ulcers or one or two large ones. Recurrent lesions last about 10 days. Recurrences are much more common in patients with primary genital herpes infected with HSV-II than with HSV-I.

COMPLICATIONS

The most important complication is the risk of transmission by an infected mother to her infant during delivery. The transmission occurs by direct contact of the infant with herpetic lesions during passage through the cervix and vagina. Neonatal herpes infections are frequently fatal or associated with significant neurologic sequelae. Cesarean section largely eliminates this risk, and it has become mandatory for women who come to term with active lesions or who are known to be shedding virus.

Other complications that are more common in women and occur mostly with primary infections include aseptic meningitis, seen in about 20 to 30 percent of patients, autonomic nervous system disorders (urinary retention, impotence, decreased rectal sphincter tone), sacral paresthesias, and myelitis. Autoinoculation can result in typical herpetic ulcers or herpes keratitis if a patient should touch a lesion and then touch another mucous membrane or his or her eye. If there are small breaks in the skin, local herpetic lesions can evolve. When the terminal phalanx is involved the condition is referred to as herpetic whitlow, a condition that occurs not infrequently among medical personnel. Disseminated HSV infections may occur in immunosuppressed patients, resulting in multisystem organ involvement. They are associated with a high mortality.

DIAGNOSIS AND TREATMENT

The clinical presentation of a patient with HSV infection usually suggests the diagnosis. The finding of multinucleated giant cells on scrapings of the ulcer base stained with methylene blue (Tzanck smear) is essentially diagnostic. A Papanicolaou smear of a cervical scraping in a woman with cervical herpes may yield the same information. The virus also can be cultured from the vesicle or ulcer in the majority of cases, but the special viral media is often not readily available. In primary HSV infections, a fourfold or greater increase in complement fixing serum antibodies is seen,[10] whereas in recurrent HSV infections serology is frequently nonspecific and nondiagnostic.

Acyclovir is the only drug that has been shown to be helpful for herpes. Administration of oral acyclovir 200 mg 5 times daily for primary HSV lesions decreases viral shedding, formation of new lesions, and pruritus.[4] It is ineffective in preventing the number or severity of recurrences, however. Patients with complications severe enough to require hospitalization should be given intravenous acyclovir 5 mg/kg every 8 hours for 5 to 7 days.

Treatment for recurrent episodes should be limited to those patients who typically have severe symptoms and who are able to begin therapy at the beginning of the prodrome or within 2 days of onset of lesions. Acyclovir 200 mg orally 5 times daily for 5 days may shorten the main clinical course by about 1 day. For frequent recurrences (6 or more per year) continuous treatment with acyclovir 200 mg orally 2 to 3 times daily will reduce the frequency of active disease by at least 75 percent.[14,40] After cessation of acyclovir clinical episodes may recur at the same frequency. The suppressive regimen is contraindicated in pregnant women.

Counseling is especially important in the management of this infection. Patients often feel extremely guilty about this disease and, despite the proliferation of public information on herpes, continue to be ignorant regarding many aspects of the infection. The high infectivity of the active lesion and the low transmissibility during remissions should be stressed. The marked variability of the course and its relationship to stress needs to be emphasized. Because of the association between genital herpes and carcinoma of the cervix, the importance of yearly Papanicolaou smears for women should be emphasized.

PELVIC INFLAMMATORY DISEASE

The term "pelvic inflammatory disease" (PID) refers to the clinical syndrome associated with ascending spread of microorganisms from the vagina and cervix to the endometrium, fallopian tubes, and contiguous structures. PID is one of the most significant complications of STDs in women, and is probably the most common serious infection in women of child-bearing age.[15] PID is the major cause of female infertility and ectopic pregnancy, each of which have tripled in incidence over the past decade. In the late 1970s, it was estimated that there were 850,000 cases of PID annually,

resulting in 2,500,000 physician visits, 250,000 hospitalizations, and 150,000 surgical procedures.[12] The total cost of the disease for 1979 was approximately $1.25 billion; if the long-term sequelae such as ectopic pregnancy and infertility are included, the cost estimate rose to over $2.7 billion. Other complications of PID include abscesses of the salpinx, ovary, or both, rupture of the abscess and, rarely, death. Chronic complications, though less severe, are more common. The risk of infertility is 18 percent following one episode of PID, 34 percent after two and 75 percent after three or more.[41] Chronic abdominal pain with dyspareunia can be particularly distressing. There is also a sevenfold to tenfold increase in ectopic pregnancies among women with a history of PID.[42]

Acute PID is almost exclusively a disease of sexually active women. The risk appears to be several times greater in sexually active teenagers who are 15 to 16 years of age and among women 20 to 24 years of age. Seventy-five percent of women with PID are less than 25 years of age and 75 percent are nulliparous. Reasons for the higher susceptibility of younger women to PID include a larger number of sexual partners, high frequency of anovulatory cycles, lower prevalence of immunity to STD pathogens, and possibly a delay in securing medical care. Other risk factors include a past history of gonorrhea or salpingitis, and use of an intrauterine device.

The etiology of PID is complex and polymicrobial. Two major groups of organisms are thought to be responsible for this syndrome—exogenous STD agents, which include N. gonorrhoeae, C. trachomatis, and Mycoplasma, and endogenous microorganisms, which are primarily facultative or strictly anaerobic organisms. STD agents account for 75 percent of PID cases in women below the age of 25. Consequently, PID is frequently classified as gonococcal or nongonococcal in origin. Gonococcal PID is defined by the recovery of N. gonorrhoeae from cervical culture. The percentage of cases of PID that are due to N. gonorrhoeae varies in different locations: in Sweden 10 to 20 percent; in Seattle 50 percent; in Los Angeles 65 percent; and in Dallas and Memphis 68 and 85 percent, respectively. When the peritoneum of these patients is sampled by culdocentesis, three patterns of infection emerge: (1) N. gonorrhoeae alone; (2) N. gonorrhoeae with mixed aerobic-anaerobic bacteria; and (3) mixed aerobic-anaerobic bacteria without the gonococcus. The aerobic organisms include gram-negative bacilli, streptococci, staphylococci, and Haemophilus species, whereas the anaerobic organisms include Bacteroides fragilis, other Bacteroides species, Clostridium species, peptococci, and peptostreptococci. The mycoplasmas of M. hominis and Urea urealyticum also have been isolated, but the role of these organisms in the pathogenesis of PID remains uncertain.

In nongonococcal PID, the above-mentioned organisms, along with Chlamydia trachomatis, have been recovered. In Sweden and other countries, it is believed that C. trachomatis alone or in conjunction with mixed aerobic-anaerobic organisms are responsible for a greater proportion of PID cases than is gonorrhea. The role of other organisms is controversial, though one study has shown significant change in antibody response to the capsular polysaccharide of B. fragilis in those women in whom this organism was recovered.[24] Other than as a complication of STDs, PID may arise following abortion, hysterosalpingography, insertion of an intrauterine contraceptive device (IUD), and dilation and curettage. These infections are also of polymicrobial origin, and most frequently involve mixed aerobic-anaerobic organisms.

The pathogenesis of gonococcal PID begins with cervical infection. Intracanalicular spread of the organism to the uterine cavity and the fallopian tubes occurs in certain susceptible individuals and an inflammatory response resulting in either endometritis or salpingitis develops. The presence of other organisms is thought to be due to secondary invasion.[15] In cases in which C. trachomatis is isolated, the same sequence of events probably occurs, except that Chlamydia produces a less intense inflammatory response, resulting in milder clinical findings. When peritoneal exudate from a salpingitis spreads to the right upper quadrant, perihepatitis may occur.

DIAGNOSIS AND TREATMENT

The clinical presentation of patients with PID is variable. In acute PID, patients typically complain of a history of abdominal pain or discomfort for 2 weeks or less. In gonococcal PID the symptoms may begin soon after menses, though in nongonococcal PID the disease may manifest itself at any time during the cycle. Complaints such as dysuria, vaginal discharge, abnormal vaginal bleeding, dyspareunia, pain on defecation, nausea, vomiting, fever, and chills are present to variable degrees. If perihepatitis is present, the woman also may complain of right upper quadrant pain that radiates to the right shoulder. Lower abdominal tenderness varies from mild to severe, with rebound tenderness frequently present. Vaginal speculum examination reveals a mucopurulent cervicitis in the majority of women with gonococcal or chlamydial PID. Cervical motion tenderness may be evident, as well as tenderness on palpation of the adnexal area on rectovaginal examination. Differential diagnosis should include acute appendicitis, ectopic pregnancy, endometriosis, ovarian cyst or tumor, and urinary tract disease. Sonography, laparoscopy, and culdocentesis are frequently used to confirm the diagnosis of PID and to rule out the above-mentioned conditions.

Unfortunately, no clinical or laboratory findings short of laparoscopy are diagnostic of PID, and there is reluctance to perform laparoscopy in all suspected cases. The following minimum criteria for the clinical diagnosis therefore have been suggested[36]:

1. Abdominal tenderness
2. Cervical motion tenderness
3. Adnexal tenderness with bimanual examination

In addition, at least one of the following five criteria should be present:

1. Temperature greater than 38C
2. A pelvic mass on examination or sonography
3. Intracellular gram-negative diplococci on Gram stain of cervical exudate
4. White blood count greater than or equal to 10,000/μl
5. Purulent material obtained by culdocentesis or laparoscopy

The decision regarding hospitalization for patients with PID is also controversial. Patients who fulfill the following criteria should definitely be considered for hospital admission and intravenous antibiotic therapy[36]:

1. Patients with diffuse rebound tenderness
2. Patients with a mass
3. Pregnant patients
4. Patients who fail outpatient therapy
5. Patients who cannot take oral therapy because of nausea or vomiting
6. Patients in whom the diagnosis is uncertain or surgical emergencies need to be excluded
7. Patients for whom outpatient follow-up cannot be arranged

Recommendations for inpatient and outpatient therapy are outlined in Table 9.14–3. It should be noted that these recommendations were drawn up on the basis of microorganisms identified in several studies and that they have not been validated by an extensive experience. Other measures important to good patient management include removal of the IUD if present, contraceptive counseling, bed rest, careful follow-up, and examination and treatment of sexual partners.

For those patients who fail to respond to the treatment, four possibilities should be considered. First, there may be resistant organisms present; these include PPNG, *C. trachomatis,* or anaer-

obes. Second, an abscess may have developed and may require surgical drainage. Third, if the patient has participated in sexual intercourse during or after therapy, reinfection is a possibility. Last, the diagnosis of PID may have been erroneous, and other conditions need to be excluded.

TABLE 9.14–3. TREATMENT OF PELVIC INFLAMMATORY DISEASE

Drug Regimens	Comments
Outpatient: Aqueous procaine penicillin G, 4,800,000 U IM *or* Cefoxitin 2 g IM *or* Ampicillin 3.5 g PO *or* Amoxicillin 3 g PO *Each combined with:* Probenecid 1 g PO *Each of the above combined with:* Doxycycline 100 mg PO bid for 10–14 days	Substitute spectinomycin 2 g IM in penicillin-allergic patients Effective against *N. gonorrhoeae* or *C. trachomatis*
Inpatient[a]: Cefoxitin 2 g IV qid *plus* Doxycycline 100 mg IV bid *followed by* Doxycycline 100 mg PO bid for 10–14 days	Effective against *N. gonorrhoeae, C. trachomatis,* anaerobes, and most gram-negative rods
or Gentamicin 2 mg/kg IV q8h *plus* clindamycin 600 mg IV q6h *followed by* Clindamycin 450 mg PO qid for 10–14 days	Optimal therapy against anaerobes and gram-negative rods Less effective against *N. gonorrhoeae* and *C. trachomatis*

[a]Inpatient regimens consist of a parenteral regimen to be given at least 4 days and until the patient is afebrile 48 hours. Oral agents may then be given to complete a total course of 10 to 14 days.
From Centers for Disease Control: Sexually transmitted disease treatment guidelines, 1985. MMWR 34:755, 1985.

SYPHILIS

Syphilis is a chronic, systemic infection due to *Treponema pallidum.* Osler referred to syphilis as the "great imitator," owing to the wide variety of clinical presentations, and stated, "he who knows syphilis, knows medicine." Though the number of new cases of other sexually transmitted diseases has risen dramatically in recent years, the incidence of syphilis has remained relatively stable over the past 2 decades at 10 per 100,000 population. In the United States there were 27,883 cases of primary and secondary syphilis and 68,125 cases of all stages of syphilis reported in 1986.[5] There has been a recent change in its epidemiology, however; infectious syphilis now is more common among male homosexuals or bisexuals who are prone to have multiple, anonymous, and transient liaisons. In addition, anal and oral chancres are frequently missed by medical examiners, and the diagnosis of syphilis in these cases is not frequently considered. Currently over half the reported cases of syphilis are in homosexual or bisexual men.

ACQUIRED SYPHILIS

T. pallidum is transmitted by intimate sexual contact, penetrating mucous membranes and apparently unbroken skin through minute abrasions. The disease is divided into different stages, as outlined in Table 9.14–4.

TABLE 9.14–4. SYPHILIS IN UNTREATED PATIENTS

Stage	Typical Findings	Onset After Exposure	Persistence	Serology % Reactive	
				VDRL	FTA-ABS
Primary	Chancre	21 days (10–90)	2–12 wk	72	91
Secondary	Rash, condyloma lata, mucous patches, fever, lymphadenopathy, patchy alopecia	6 wk to 6 mo	1–3 mo	100	100
Early latent	Relapses of secondary syphilis	<1 yr	Up to 1 yr	73	97
Late latent	Clinically silent	>1 yr	Lifelong unless tertiary syphilis appears	73	97
Tertiary	Neurosyphilis, cardiovascular syphilis, gummas	1 yr until death	Until death	77	99

Primary Stage

Following sexual contact with an infected partner, the organism penetrates the skin, replicates at the site of primary inoculation, and spreads systemically. The typical chancre appears 21 days later (range, 10 to 90 days) as a painless papule that evolves in a 2 to 20 mm diameter painless ulcer with an indurated edge. The lesion usually appears on the penis, labia, or cervix, but the anus or mouth can be involved if the patient participates in anal or oral intercourse. Firm, nontender inguinal adenopathy may occur with genital lesions. The chancre heals within 2 to 6 weeks, leaving no scar.

Secondary Stage

The primary stage may have been unrecognized. It may overlap in 25 percent of cases with the secondary stage, which develops approximately 6 weeks to 6 months after exposure. The characteristic finding in this stage is the appearance of a maculopapular rash. The lesions are erythematous and symmetrical and can involve any part of the body, although lesions on the palms and soles highly suggest secondary syphilis. It is important to remember that secondary syphilis is a systemic disease, and complaints such as weight loss, fever, and malaise are common. Generalized nontender lymphadenopathy also is found, and patchy alopecia in association with the rash is characteristic of this disease. Condyloma latum, a flat, wartlike lesion, may be found in intertriginous areas and around the anal canal. These must be differentiated from condyloma acuminatum, a fleshy genital wart (described later). Mucous patches are superficial, gray erosions of the mucous membranes that are present in about a third of the cases. All cutaneous lesions are infectious, particularly condyloma lata and mucous patches.

About 15 to 30 percent of patients will have an abnormal cerebrospinal fluid, although clinical meningitis is rare. Hepatitis, immune-complex nephropathy, arthritis, periostitis, uveitis, and proctitis occur, but are uncommon. One of these complications also may be the only manifestation of secondary syphilis. In untreated patients, the secondary stage will last from 1 to 3 months.

Latent Stage

After the secondary stage, patients enter into a clinically silent, that is, latent stage. This is divided into early (duration less than 1 year) and late (duration more than 1 year) latent syphilis. Patients can have relapses of secondary syphilis during this time. The majority of relapses occur in the first year and are typically milder than in the secondary stage of syphilis.

Tertiary Stage

Approximately 30 percent of patients in the preantibiotic era developed tertiary syphilis. This stage is rare today because of the wide availability of penicillin. The three forms of the disease are cardiovascular syphilis, neurosyphilis, and benign gummas.

Cardiovascular Syphilis. Cardiovascular syphilis is more common in men and in blacks, and occurs in about 10 to 20 percent of untreated cases. There is destruction of the elastic tissues due to endarteritis obliterans, causing aneurysmal dilation of the ascending aorta. This results in heart failure and coronary ostial obstruction. This complication may be even more prevalent than suspected, because autopsy studies have revealed evidence of aortitis in 30 to 50 percent of untreated syphilitics.

Neurosyphilis. Neurosyphilis occurs in 4 to 6 percent of untreated cases and has a variety of manifestations. Asymptomatic neurosyphilis applies to patients with no neurologic signs or symptoms but with a reactive blood serology and an abnormal cerebrospinal fluid. Meningovascular syphilis refers to a relatively acute presentation of delirium, seizures, headache, and neck stiffness. In tabes dorsalis there are signs of posterior column degeneration, with ataxia, areflexia, sensory deficits, "lightning pains" in the extremities, impotence, and urinary retention or incontinence. The sensory deficits can lead to trophic joint changes (Charcot joints). General paresis presents as dementia with an insidious onset of personality changes, irritability, insomnia, poor judgment, and declining mental capacity. The Argyll-Robertson pupil is seen in both general paresis and tabes dorsalis. This is a small, irregular pupil that can accommodate but fails to react to light.

Gummas. Gummas are late syphilitic lesions that consist microscopically of nonspecific granulomas. Essentially any organ can be involved, but the skin, skeletal system, liver, oral cavity, and upper respiratory tract are the most commonly affected.

SYPHILIS IN PREGNANCY

Women who acquire syphilis during pregnancy or become pregnant during the first year of the disease have an 80 to 90 percent chance of transmitting the disease to the fetus. Even though the risk decreases, an infected mother can still transmit syphilis to her fetus during late latent syphilis. Routine serologic screening of pregnant women, which results in therapy before the 19th week, will prevent congenital infection, and treatment thereafter can arrest further progression.

CONGENITAL SYPHILIS

Congenital syphilis results from transplacental spread of *T. pallidum* from the mother to the fetus. Transmission is rare before the fourth month of gestation, and early abortion is not seen. Untreated maternal infection may result in prematurity, stillbirth, neonatal death, and early or late congenital syphilis. Treatment of the mother during the first 4 months of pregnancy virtually eliminates the risk of congenital syphilis.

Clinical manifestations of early congenital syphilis are usually seen in the first 2 years of life. The affected child is usually healthy at birth, and the earliest symptom is a nasal discharge (snuffles) appearing between 2 to 8 weeks of age. This is followed by a variety of mucocutaneous lesions. In contrast to adults, the rash may be vesicular or even bullous. Pseudoparalysis resulting from painful osteochondritis, hepatosplenomegaly, lymphadenopathy, anemia, thrombocytopenia, and leukocytosis are commonly seen. Congenital rubella, cytomegalovirus, herpes simplex virus, and toxoplasmosis have similar clinical findings and must be differentiated from congenital syphilis.

Late congenital syphilis comprises those features that appear after 2 years. It is analogous to tertiary syphilis in the adult, except that cardiovascular disease is rare. Periostitis and osteochrondlitis result in frontal bossing, anterior bowing of the tibia ("saber shin"), and deafness due to cochlear degeneration. Dental abnormalities are characteristic: Hutchinson teeth (widely spaced, tapered incisors with a central notch) and mulberry molars (6 year molars with multiple, small cusps). Interstitial keratitis presents with photophobia, pain, tearing, and blurred vision. Interstitial keratitis, neural deafness, and the typical dentition form Hutchinson triad. Up to one third of infected children have asymtomatic neurosyphilis, with the symptomatic forms, such as general paresis, tabes dorsalis, and localized gummas, usually appearing in adolescence.

DIAGNOSIS AND TREATMENT

Knowledge of the biologic basis of the various serologic tests for syphilis is essential for their use in diagnosis. There are two basic types, a nonspecific reagin antibody and a specific antitreponemal antibody. The most common reagin antibody tests are the rapid plasma reagin (RPR) and the venereal disease research laboratory (VDRL) tests. The RPR and VDRL represent antibodies that are produced against a lipoprotein antigen resulting from the combination of the spirochete and host tissue. The tests have different sensitivities for each stage of the disease and are useful in screening because of their reliability, simplicity, and low cost. False-positive results are common and are seen acutely in various bacterial or viral infections, and chronically in persons with autoimmune diseases, in addicts, and in the elderly. They usually have a titer of less than 1:8.

A specific antitreponemal test must be performed for confirmation of the reagin test. The most widely used is the fluorescent treponemal antibody-absorption (FTA-ABS) test. This is an immunofluorescent test that is performed by first treating the patient's serum to remove nonspecific treponemal antibodies. The patient's absorbed serum is then placed on a slide containing *T. pallidum*. Fluorescein antihuman globulin is added and the slide is examined under a fluorescent microscope. Borderline tests are neither positive nor negative and need to be repeated. False positive tests can occur in patients with systemic lupus erythematosus and other autoimmune diseases. These are distinctive because of their beaded appearance under microscopy. Once a person has a positive FTA-ABS test, he or she generally remains positive for the rest of his or her life.

Darkfield examination of the chancre or the lesions of secondary or congenital syphilis also can be performed. The serous fluid from the lesion is placed on a slide, covered, and examined under phase microscopy. The presence of spirochetes is pathognomonic for syphilis. The test cannot be performed on oral or rectal lesions because of the large number of intestinal spirochetes that might cause a false positive test.

Penicillin is the treatment of choice for all stages of syphilis. Serum levels of 0.03 μg/ml are spirocheticidal. For syphilis of less than 1 year's duration, benzathine penicillin G, 2.4 million units, intramuscularly in one dose is adequate. In syphilis of more than 1 year's duration, except neurosyphilis, the same dose of penicillin should be given once a week for 3 consecutive weeks. For penicillin-allergic patients, tetracycline, 500 mg, by mouth, four times daily should be given for 15 days in early infections and 30 days in late infections.

Neurosyphilis is more difficult to treat because benzathine penicillin does not provide treponemicidal levels of penicillin in the CSF.[30] Therefore it is recommended that the patients be admitted to the hospital and treated with aqueous crystalline penicillin G, 12 to 24 million units, intravenously, daily for 10 days. Consultation with an infectious disease specialist is recommended for patients with penicillin allergy and neurosyphilis.

A common reaction following the treatment of syphilis consists of shaking chills, fever, myalgias, headache, tachycardia, and exacerbation of the inflammatory reaction at local sites of the disease. This is called the Jarisch-Herxheimer reaction and is seen in 50 percent of primary syphilis cases, 75 percent of secondary cases, and 30 percent of neurosyphilis cases. The massive release of treponemal lipopolysaccharides, which act as an endotoxin, is primarily responsible for this transient reaction.[16]

Follow-up of patients is especially important in this disease. Repeat quantitative VDRL titers at 1,3,6, and 12 months is recommended. The titer should revert to negative or decrease by fourfold dilutions and remain low. If this does not occur, the patient should be treated again with the above regimens. Penicillin-resistant treponemes do not exist.

CHANCROID

Chancroid is characterized by one or more genital ulcers caused by *Haemophilus ducreyi*, a facultative anaerobic gram-negative coccobacillus. Chancroid is endemic in tropical and subtropical countries; only 3,756 civilian cases occurred in the United States in 1986.[5] After an incubation period of 2 days to 2 weeks (median, 7 days), there appears a small, painful papule that ulcerates in 1 to 2 days. Lack of circumcision is an established risk factor in men. There are occasionally multiple "kissing" lesions due to autoinfection. In women, ulcers are more numerous, tend to be less painful, and cluster around the cervix. Unilateral, tender, fluctuant inguinal lymphadenopathy is common. Differential diagnosis includes herpes, primary syphilis, granuloma inguinale, and lymphogranuloma venereum.

Diagnosis is made by culturing the edge of the ulcer or lymph node aspirate on supplemented chocolate agar. Treatment is erythromycin 500 mg orally four times daily or trimethoprim-sulfamethoxazole, one double strength tablet twice daily for 10 days or until the ulcer and lymphadenopathy resolve. The susceptibility of *H. ducreyi* to these antimicrobial agents varies widely, and susceptibility patterns should influence selection of antibiotics. Other alternative treatment regimens include ceftriaxone 250 mg intramuscularly in a single dose, trimethoprim-sulfamethoxazole 640 mg and 3200 mg, respectively (4 double-dose tablets), orally in a single dose, or amoxicillin 500 mg plus clavulinic acid 125 mg 3 times daily for 7 days. Fluctuant nodes should be aspirated as needed to minimize the risk of spontaneous rupture.

CONDYLOMA ACUMINATUM

There has been a recent marked increase in the occurrence of anogenital warts. Office visits for genital warts have increased 459 percent for the period 1966–1981, from 169,000 to 946,000.[5] Anogenital warts (condyloma acuminata) are caused by human papillomaviruses (HPV). These double-stranded DNA viruses are transmitted through sexual intercourse, with an incubation period of 1 to 2 months. The disease appears as pink or brown cauliflower-like lesions on the glans penis, vulva, urethra, cervix, perineum, and anorectal regions. These lesions may be mildly pruritic, but are mainly cosmetically unappealing. The highly infectious condyloma lata of secondary syphilis need to be differentiated from these warts. This is usually done on the basis of their characteristic

appearance and by performing darkfield microscopy for spirochetes. Flat genital warts are most representative of condyloma lata.

Therapy varies according to the site of involvement. For external genital and perianal warts, application of podophyllin 10 to 25 percent in compound tincture of benzoin is advocated. The podophyllin should be applied to the wart, avoiding the normal surrounding tissue, and washed off in 4 hours. Treatment may be repeated weekly for four applications. For failures and treatment of cervical, vaginal, anorectal, or oral warts, cryotherapy, electrocauterization, or surgery is recommended. Because of the association of cervical warts, particularly with HPV 16 and 18, and with cervical neoplasms,[11,27] routine Papanicolaou smears of women with this lesion are advocated.

ECTOPARASITES

Ectoparasites are parasites that live on the integument of their hosts. The two most common, *Phthirus pubis* (pubic or crab louse) and *Sarcoptes scabiei* var *hominis* (scab mite), cause pediculosis pubis and scabies, respectively. These infections are transmitted by prolonged personal contact, including sexual intercourse.

The primary symptom of pediculosis is itching, primarily in the genital area, although any hairy part of the body can be involved. Close examination of the affected areas shows "nits" (actually these are eggs) attached one-half to 1 inch from the base of the hair shaft. The actual lice can also be seen on the skin: they are pinhead sized and yellow-gray. Frequently, reddish papules are present because of local irritation. Diagnosis can be made clinically or by examining hair combings under low-power microscopy.

Scabies is also characterized by pruritus that is typically worse at night. Typically the lesions are symmetric and consist of pathognomonic burrows due to the female mite. The burrow varies from 1 to 10 mm in length and is wavy and thready. The most common sites are the interdigital web spaces of the hand, flexor aspect of the wrist and elbow, belt line, the penis and scrotum in men, and around the nipples in women. In patients with immune deficiencies, thousands of mites can infest the individual in a condition known as Norwegian scabies.

The epidemiology of these diseases differs from most STDs: (1) there is an increased prevalence in heterosexuals as opposed to homosexuals[23]; (2) the act of simply sleeping together is more important than a brief sexual contact; and (3) fomites are important in their transmission since the parasites can live outside their host for brief periods.

Gamma benzene hexachloride (lindane) is the treatment of choice for both infections. For pediculosis (or scabies of the scalp), the medication is applied as a shampoo that should be washed off in 4 minutes. For scabies a 1 percent lotion or cream is applied to the body from the neck down and washed off the next day. A single application is usually effective for scabies, while a second application 1 week later may be necessary for pediculosis. Overuse may cause neurotoxicity (seizures), especially in children. Because of household transmission, all members of the household should be treated concurrently. Additionally, the bed linens and all clothing should be laundered on the day of therapy. The pruritus may persist for several weeks after treatment for scabies because of persistence of antigens in the skin.

GRANULOMA INGUINALE

Granuloma inguinale (donovanosis) is an STD due to *Calymmatobacterium granulomatis,* an encapsulated, short, gram-negative bacillus. It is the rarest of all STDs reported in the United States, with only 61 civilian cases in 1986.[6] Most of these infections were in homosexual men. Like chancroid, it is much more common in tropical and subtropical countries. The incubation period is 2 to 4 weeks, and the infection first appears as a painless, indurated papule. After 1 to 4 weeks, a beefy, granulomatous ulcer with elevated borders develops. Lymphadenopathy is uncommon, but the surrounding induration can extend into the inguinal region, resulting in a pseudobubo. The lesion resembles squamous cell carcinoma, which may also complicate long-standing cases, emphasizing the need for biopsy in uncertain cases.

Diagnosis is made by Wright or Giemsa stain of a scraping of the ulcer bed or of biopsied tissue. The presence of blue-black bipolar staining bacilli (Donovan bodies) in the cytoplasm of large mononuclear cells is pathognomonic. Contrary to its name, granulomas are not present.

The treatment is tetracycline 500 mg four times daily. This should be continued until the lesions have healed completely. For treatment failures, ampicillin 500 mg four times daily, streptomycin 0.5 to 1.0 g twice daily, gentamicin 1 mg/kg twice daily, and chloramphenicol 500 mg four times daily all have been advocated.

MOLLUSCUM CONTAGIOSUM

Molluscum contagiosum is a benign epidermal neoplasm due to a poxvirus. This DNA virus is difficult to grow in tissue cultures, and the disease has a long incubation period of up to 6 months. The lesion appears as a flesh-colored 2- to 5-mm papule, which then becomes umbilicated. A cheesy material can be expressed from the center of the lesion, and multiple lesions are common. Diagnosis is made by the clinical appearance, which is highly suggestive. Confirmation can be obtained by biopsy or examination of the expressed caseous material, which reveals molluscum bodies (basophilic cytoplasmic inclusions filled with the virion).

Treatment consists of removal of the caseous center by pressure after nicking the center with a scalpel or needle. Spontaneous resolution occurs in many cases. Podophyllin 20 percent compound or cryotherapy with liquid nitrogen can be employed in resistant cases.

APPROACH TO COMMON CLINICAL PROBLEMS

A POSITIVE SEROLOGIC TEST FOR SYPHILIS

A frequent clinical problem is the management of the patient with a positive serologic test for syphilis (STS). The biologic basis for these tests is explained in the previous section on syphilis. The challenge to the physician is to determine whether a positive VDRL or RPR result represents true disease or a biologic false positive (BFP). There are no hard and fast rules, but general guidelines can be given:

1. BFPs nearly always have a titer less than or equal to 1:8 Acute BFPs occur in infectious hepatitis, mononucleosis, pneumonia, malaria, chickenpox, measles, leprosy, and recent vaccinations. Chronic BFPs occur in autoimmune disorders, such as systemic lupus erythematosus and rheumatoid arthritis in the elderly and in intravenous drug abusers.
2. A patient with a positive VDRL and a negative FTA-ABS usually has a BFP. The exception occurs in early primary syphilis. In this case a chancre is usually present (or soon will be), and the titer is usually greater than 1:8. The test should be repeated in 1 month if no therapy is given.
3. Patients with a history of adequate treatment and low titers do not need further evaluation.
4. If an earlier VDRL is available, the results of the titer should be obtained. If the patient was treated between the two tests, there should be at least a fourfold fall in the titer. Otherwise the patient should be re-treated. A stable or increasing titer indicates the occurrence of reinfection or treatment failure.

TABLE 9.14–5. CLUES IN DIFFERENTIAL DIAGNOSIS OF GENITAL ULCER

	Herpes	Syphilis	Chancroid	LGV	Granuloma Inguinale
History	Recurrences	Homosexual/bisexual men	Overseas contact	Overseas contact, or homosexual/bisexual men	Overseas contact
Systemic symptoms	Present in 1st degree herpes	Present in 2nd degree syphilis	Absent	Gastrointestinal symptoms in some cases	Absent
Ulcer (number)	Multiple	1–2	1–3	1	1
Vesicles	+	—	—	—	—
Pain	+ +	—	+ +	+	—
Induration	—	+ +	—	—	+ +
Adenopathy	Tender	Firm, nontender	Tender, may suppurate	Tender, groove sign	Pseudobubo

— = Rare; + = occasional; + + = characteristic.

Examination of the CSF in these patients is another consideration. The problem arises because of failure of the standard three doses of benzathine penicillin to achieve detectable levels in the CSF and persistent CSF pleocytosis after this therapy.[27] Any patient with neurologic abnormalities therefore should have a lumbar puncture performed, and CSF syphilis serology obtained. For neurologically normal patients with syphilis of less than 1 year's duration, CSF examination is not needed, as the risk of neurosyphilis is very small. Similarly, elderly patients with no neurologic symptoms do not need a CSF examination since *asymptomatic* neurosyphilis is rare after syphilis of 30 years' duration.[22] Patients with CSF abnormalities such as a pleocytosis or positive CSF serology for syphilis should be considered to have neurosyphilis and treated as indicated in Table 9.14–1. Follow-up CSF examination after intravenous therapy is not indicated.

GENITAL ULCERS

The etiology of ulcerative genital lesions varies in different areas of the world. In the United States and other industrialized countries, 40 to 65 percent of the patients have genital herpes, 15 to 20 percent have syphilis, 1 to 2 perent have chancroid, and the remaining have nonvenereal lesions. Trauma, either direct or secondary to excoriation, is the most common cause of nonvenereal genital ulcers.

Clues in the diagnosis of a genital ulcer are given in Table 9.14–5. Despite the characteristic clinical picture in some patients, the clinical diagnosis should always be confirmed by laboratory testing. Further, the simultaneous occurrence of two or more pathogens in the same patient is not uncommon.

The following general guidelines are useful in patients with genital ulcers:

1. Since the consequences of untreated infection are so great, syphilis should always be excluded by dark-field examination and serology.
2. Typical painful ulcers, especially if accompanied by a history of recurrence and vesicle formation, strongly suggest the diagnosis of herpes.
3. If the patient has an ulcer that suggests syphilis, therapy should be initiated before the patient leaves the clinic.
4. Patients who are from Asia or Africa, or who have had a recent overseas sexual contact, should be evaluated for chancroid, LGV, and granuloma inguinale.
5. The inguinal region always should be examined. Characteristic adenopathy may be seen (Table 9.14–5).
6. Noninfectious etiologies should be considered only after serial observation and infectious causes have been ruled out.

7. Only when adequate diagnostic facilities are not available is empiric treatment warranted.

VAGINAL DISCHARGE

Not all cases of vaginal discharge are due to STDs, but because they are such a common problem among sexually active young women, these syndromes are included in this chapter.

Both vaginitis and cervicitis cause a vaginal discharge, and the two entities can be separated only by vaginal speculum examination. If the patient has cervicitis, a Gram stain should be done of the cervical discharge and treatment instituted for *N. gonorrhoeae, C. trachomatis,* or both as indicated by culture and Gram stain results as discussed. If the patient has a vaginal discharge further evaluation is indicated (Table 9.14–6). A normal physiologic discharge is characterized by a thin, clear, scanty mucous. It causes no symptoms and serves to protect the vaginal mucosa.

Yeast vaginitis is usually due to *Candida albicans,* although other related fungi can cause identical symptoms. These patients usually have intense pruritus associated with vulvovaginitis. Diabetes and use of systemic antibiotics are common risk factors. The discharge has a cottage-cheese consistency, and there may be adherent plaques on the vaginal wall. Diagnosis is made by mixing the discharge with 10 percent potassium hydroxide (KOH). KOH dissolves the secretions and under microscopy the characteristic fungal elements are easily seen. Treatment consists of local instillation of an antifungal agent. Recurrent vulvovaginal candidiasis is not uncommon. Superficial candidal dermatitis of the penis of the sex partner occasionally occurs. In this case the partner should be treated simultaneously with a topical antifungal agent. Next, intermittent administration of oral ketoconazole (400 mg per day) for 5 days after onset of menses may be beneficial.[35]

Trichomonas vaginalis is a small (7 × 10 μm), motile, pear-shaped protozoa. It causes a profuse vaginal discharge that is often frothy. About 50 percent of infections are asymptomatic. Examination of vaginal secretions mixed with an equal proportion of physiologic saline demonstrates the characteristic motile flagellate in at least three-quarters of cases. Metronidazole in a single 2 g oral dose is curative in greater than 90 percent of cases. Routine treatment of sexual partners is also advocated.

Nonspecific vaginitis, also referred to as bacterial vaginosis, is commonly seen in medical practice. Vaginal cultures reveal the presence of *Gardnerella vaginalis* (formerly known as *Haemophilus vaginalis* or *Corynebacterium vaginale*) in over 90 percent of cases and an increased concentration of anaerobic bacteria particularly *Mobilucas species.* The exact pathogenesis of the syndrome is uncertain, but it is believed that it is due to an interaction between certain anaerobic bacteria and *G. vaginalis.*[1,37] On microscopy, a character-

TABLE 9.14–6. DIAGNOSIS AND MANAGEMENT OF VAGINITIS

Etiology	Symptoms	Odor	Color	Consistency	Diagnosis	Therapy
Candida sp.	Pruritus, irritation	None	White	Thick, curdlike, scant	Presence of fungal elements on 10% KOH preparation	Miconazole *or* clotrimazole 100 mg intravaginal daily for 7 days
Trichomonas vaginalis	Profuse discharge, pruritus	Foul	Yellow, green	Frothy, profuse	Presence of motile trichomonads on wet mount	Metronidazole 2 g PO (single dose)
Nonspecific vaginitis	Vaginal odor	Fishy odor with 10% KOH preparation	Clear, white	Thin, homogeneous	1. Clue cells on wet mount 2. Vaginal pH above 4.5 3. Thin discharge 4. Fishy odor	Metronidazole 500 mg PO bid for 7 days

istic clue cell is seen on a saline preparation. The clue cell is an epithelial cell that has a granular appearance due to small gram-negative coccobacilli.

Diagnosis of nonspecific vaginitis is based on the exclusion of other causes of vaginitis, and the patient should have at least three of the following criteria[1]:

1. Vaginal pH above 4.5
2. Fishy odor of secretions with KOH treatment
3. A thin, homogeneous discharge
4. Clue cells on saline preparation

Treatment consists of metronidazole 500 mg, orally twice a day for 7 days. The use of an antibiotic effective only against anaerobes (and not *G. vaginalis*) serves to emphasize the importance of these organisms in this syndrome.

EPIDIDYMITIS

The epididymis is a thin tubular structure adjacent to the posterior surface of the testis. It serves to store spermatozoa until ejaculation occurs. Epididymitis presents with either sudden or gradual onset of pain in this region. On examination, the scrotum on the involved side is usually swollen and erythematous. Gentle palpation, however, reveals that the swelling is generally limited to the cord.

Epididymitis in sexually active men younger than age 35 is predominantly due to an STD, either *N. gonorrhoeae* or *C. trachomatis*.[3] Most patients also have a spontaneous or expressible urethral discharge. A Gram stain of the discharge will indicate the required therapy. Patients with gram-negative intracellular diplococci should be treated for gonorrhea (Table 9.14–2), followed by 10 days of oral doxycycline, and those without diplococci should be treated for *C. trachomatis* (Table 9.14–1).

Epididymitis in men older than age 35 is usually caused by a uropathogen. This age difference is apparently secondary to both the decreased incidence of STDs in older men and the increased incidence of acquired genitourinary tract abnormalities such as prostatic hypertrophy or calculi. These patients often have other symptoms of a urinary tract infection. Concurrent prostatitis is frequent. Treatment is guided by results of a midstream urine culture.

Tuberculosis was once a common cause of epididymitis. It is now rare in the United States. Most cases have concurrent involvement of the kidney, prostate, or seminal vesicles.

Two important diseases that can be confused with epididymitis are torsion of the testicle and testicular carcinoma. Torsion of the testicle is most frequent in adolescents. Patients have pain, and on examination the swelling involves the testis more than the epididymis. The testes also may be high in the scrotum. Pyuria and urethral discharge are typically absent. Surgical exploration is frequently indicated. The incidence of testicular carcinoma peaks in the 20s, the same age as most men with epididymitis. Even though most tumors are painless, the presence of pain does not rule out carcinoma. In difficult diagnostic cases or in those patients who fail to respond promptly to antimicrobials, urologic consultation should be obtained.

INTESTINAL INFECTIONS IN HOMOSEXUAL MEN

Because of sexual practices that involve fecal or rectal contact (anilingus, anal intercourse), homosexual men are susceptible to sexually transmitted gastrointestinal infections. The presenting symptoms include tenesmus, mucopurulent or bloody anal discharge, anal pain, constipation, diarrhea, abdominal cramps, and bloating. In one study, 80 percent of patients coming to an STD clinic with gastrointestinal symptoms were found to have an intestinal or rectal pathogen, with multiple pathogens identified in 22 percent of the cases. Additionally, 40 percent of homosexuals without gastrointestinal complaints were found to harbor pathogens.[34] The wide variety of organisms found in the evaluation of homosexual men is shown in Table 9.14–7. The initial evaluation of homosexual men should include a routine history and physical examination. Additionally, the patient should be questioned about his sexual practices including anilingus, fellatio, anal intercourse, and the number of different sexual partners. Careful inspection of the perianal area and anoscopy should be done. The presence or absence of ulcers, mucosal erythema, and friability should be noted, and a rectal swab should be obtained for Gram stain and gonorrhea culture. An RPR or VDRL serology should be obtained and a darkfield examination of suspicious external lesions should be performed. Frequently, an etiologic diagnosis can be made on the basis of these procedures. The presence of intracellular gram-negative diplococci indicates the diagnosis of gonorrhea. The combination of severe anorectal pain, multiple perianal or rectal ulcers, inguinal lymphadenopathy, urinary retention, and sacral paresthesias is distinctive enough to suggest a clinical diagnosis of herpes proctitis. Anorectal mass lesions suggest two possibilities. The first is syphilis (either primary or secondary), which can be confirmed by darkfield examination or a serologic test for syphilis. The second is carcinoma, which appears to be increased in patients who practice receptive anal intercourse.[13] Homosexual men also are subject to local traumatic injuries.[31]

Those patients with abnormal anoscopy in whom an immediate diagnosis cannot be made should undergo sigmoidoscopy. If the inflammation is limited to the distal 15 cm, the patient has proctitis; if it extends beyond the distal 15 cm, he has proctocolitis. Most of the patients with proctitis will have *N. gonorrhoeae*, HSV, non-LGV *C. trachomatis*, or *T. pallidum* identified as the putative agent, although other agents can cause this syndrome. Proc-

TABLE 9.14–7. GASTROINTESTINAL INFECTIONS ASSOCIATED WITH HOMOSEXUAL MEN

Syndrome	Pathogen	Treatment
Proctitis	*Neisseria gonorrhoeae*	Aqueous procaine penicillin G 4,800,000 U IM *plus* Probenecid 1.0 g PO
	Chlamydia trachomatis (non-LGV)	Tetracycline 500 mg PO qid for 7 days
	Herpes simplex virus	Stool softeners, analgesics, sitz baths Acyclovir 200 mg PO 5 times/day for 14 days
	Treponema pallidum	Benzathine penicillin G 2,400,000 U IM
Proctocolitis	*Entamoeba histolytica*	Metronidazole 750 mg PO tid for 10 days *plus* Diiodohydroxyquin 650 mg PO tid for 20 days
	Campylobacter sp.	Erythromycin 500 mg PO qid for 7 days (severe cases)
	Shigella sp.	Trimethoprim/sulfamethoxazole (160 mg/800 mg) PO bid for 7 days
	Chlamydia trachomatis (LGV)	Tetracycline 500 mg PO qid for 21 days
	Salmonella sp.	Chloramphenicol 500 mg IV qid for 10 days
Enteritis	*Giardia lamblia*	Metronidazole 250 mg PO tid for 7 days *or* Quinacrine hydrochloride 100 mg PO tid for 7 days
	Cryptosporidium sp.	Supportive, fluid therapy
Other	*Strongyloides stercoralis*	Thiabendazole 25 mg/kg PO bid for 2 days
	Enterobius vermicularis	Mebendazole 100 mg PO once; repeat at 2 weeks

tocolitis is usually caused by enteric pathogens that include *Campylobacter* sp, *Shigella* sp, *C. trachomatis* of the LGV serovars, and *Entamoeba histolytica*. Work-up should be directed toward the identification of these agents.

Patients with normal findings on anoscopy including absence of rectal leukocytes should be considered to have enteritis. These patients mainly complain of diarrhea, abdominal cramps, and bloating. The work-up should focus on enteric and protozoan infections, especially *Giardia lamblia*.

Asymptomatic homosexual men also need a complete evaluation because of asymptomatic carriage of many pathogens. Cultures for all of the potential pathogens would be prohibitively expensive, however. All of the patients should have a serologic test for syphilis, undergo anoscopy, and have a Gram stain of a smear of their rectal mucosa with a culture for *N. gonorrhoeae*. Those with abnormal rectal mucosa or rectal leukocytes need further evaluation, as 75 percent of these patients harbor an identifiable pathogen. In addition to *N. gonorrhoeae*, most of these pathogens are protozoa, so a stool evaluation for these patients is warranted. The practice of anilingus is significantly correlated with the acquisition of parasitic infestations[34] and history of this practice should also prompt a stool examination.

REFERENCES

1. Amsel R, Totten PA, et al: Nonspecific vaginitis. Am J Med 74:14, 1983
2. Arnold AJ, Kleris GS: The borderline smear in men with urethritis. JAMA 244:157, 1980
3. Berger RE, Alexander ER, et al: Etiology, manifestation and therapy of acute epididymitis: Prospective study of 50 cases. J Urol 121:750, 1979
4. Bryson YJ, Dillon M, et al: Treatment of first episodes of genital herpes simplex virus infection with oral acyclovir. A randomized double-blind controlled trial in normal subjects. N Engl J Med 308:916, 1983
5. Centers for Disease Control: Annual Summary 1986: Reported morbidity and mortality in the United States. MMWR 35:1, 1986
6. Centers for Disease Control: Chromosomally mediated resistant *Neisseria gonorrhoeae*–United States. MMWR 33:208, 1984
7. Centers for Disease Control: *Chlamydia trachomatis* infections. MMWR 34:53S, 1985
8. Centers for Disease Control: Sexually transmitted diseases treatment guidelines 1985. MMWR 34:755, 1985
9. Corey L, Adams HG, et al: Genital herpes simplex virus infections: Clinical manifestations, course, and complications. Ann Intern Med 98:958, 1983
10. Corey L, Holmes KK: Genital herpes simplex virus infections: Current concepts in diagnosis, therapy, and prevention. Ann Intern Med 98:973, 1983
11. Crum CP, Ikenberg H, et al: Human papillomavirus type 16 and early cervical neoplasia. N Engl J Med 310:880, 1984
12. Curran JW: Economic consequences of pelvic inflammatory disease in the United States. Am J Obstet Gynecol 138:848, 1980
13. Daling JR, Weiss NS, et al: Correlates of homosexual behavior and the incidence of anal cancer. JAMA 247:1988, 1982
14. Douglas JM, Critchlow C, et al: A double-blind study of oral acyclovir for suppression of recurrences of genital herpes simplex virus infection. N Engl J Med 310:1551, 1984
15. Eschenbach DA: New concepts of obstetric and gynecologic infection. Arch Intern Med 142:2039, 1982
16. Gelfand JA, Elin RJ, et al: Endotoxemia associated with the Jarisch–Herxheimer reaction. N Engl J Med 295:211, 1976
17. Goodell SE, Quinn TC, et al: Herpes simplex, proctitis in homosexual men. N Engl J Med 308:868, 1983
18. Grayston JT, Wang S: New knowledge of chlamydiae and the diseases they cause. J Infect Dis 132:87, 1975
19. Guinan ME, MacCalman J, et al: The course of untreated recurrent genital herpes simplex infection in 27 women. N Engl J Med 304:759, 1981
20. Holmes KK, Counts GW, et al: Disseminated gonococcal infection. Ann Intern Med 74:979, 1971
21. Hooper RR, Reynolds GH, et al: Cohort study of venereal disease. I: The risk of gonorrhea transmission from infected women to men. Am J Epidemiol 108:136, 1978
22. Jaffe HW, Kabins SA: Examination of the cerebrospinal fluid in patients with syphilis. Rev Infect Dis 4:S842, 1982
23. Judson FN, Renley KA, et al: Comparative prevalence rates of sexually transmitted diseases in heterosexual and homosexual men. Am J Epidemol 112:836, 1980
24. Kasper DL, Eschenbach DA, et al: Quantitative determination of the serum antibody response to the capsular polysaccharide of *Bacteroides fragilis* ss. *fragilis* in women with pelvic inflammatory disease. J Infect Dis 138:74, 1978
25. Kousa M, Saikku P, et al: Frequent association of chlamydial infection with Reiter's syndrome. Sex Trans Dis 5:57, 1978
26. Lebefeff DA, Hochman EB: Rectal gonorrhea in men: Diagnosis and treatment. Ann Intern Med 92:463, 1980
27. Ludwig ME, Lowell DM, Livolsi VA: Cervical condylomatous atypia and its relationship to cervical neoplasia. Am J Clin Pathol 76:255, 1981
28. Mardh P, Ripa T, et al: *Chlamydia trachomatis* infection in patients with acute salpingitis. N Engl J Med 296:1377, 1977
29. Masur H, Michelis MA, et al: An outbreak of community-acquired *Pneumocystis carinii* pneumonia: Initial manifestation of cellular immune dysfunction. N Engl J Med 305:1431, 1980
30. Mohr JA, Griffiths W, et al: Neurosyphilis and penicillin levels in cerebrospinal fluid. JAMA 236:2208, 1976
31. Owen WF: Sexually transmitted diseases and traumatic problems in homosexual men. Ann Intern Med 92:805, 1980
32. Petersen BH, Lee TJ, et al: *Neisseria meningitidis* and *Neisseria gonor-*

rhoeae bacteremia associated with C6, C7, C8 deficiency. Ann Intern Med 90:917, 1979

33. Quinn TC, Goodell SE, et al: *Chlamydia trachomatis* proctitis. N Engl J Med 305:195, 1981

34. Quinn TC, Goodell SE, et al: The polymicrobial etiology of intestinal infections in homosexual men. N Engl J Med 309:574, 1983

35. Sobel JD: Vulvovaginal candidiasis. What we do and do not know. Ann Intern Med 101:390, 1984

36. Spence MR: Pelvic inflammatory disease. Dermatologic Clinics 1:65, 1983

37. Spiegel CA, Amsel R, et al: Anaerobic bacteria in nonspecific vaginitis. N Engl J Med 303:601, 1980

38. Stamm WE, Wagner KF, et al: Causes of the acute urethral syndrome in women. N Engl J Med 303:409, 1980

39. Stansfield VA: Diagnosis and management of anorectal gonorrhoea in women. Br J Vener Dis 56:319, 1980

40. Straus SE, Tukiff HE, et al: Suppression of frequently recurring genital herpes: A placebo-controlled double-blind trial of oral acyclovir. N Engl J Med 310:1545, 1984

41. Westrom L: Effect of acute pelvic inflammatory disease on fertility. Am J Obstet Gynecol 121:707, 1975

42. Westrom L: Incidence, prevalence, and trends of acute pelvic inflammatory disease and its consequences in industrialized countries. Am J Obstet Gynecol 138:880, 1980

CHAPTER 9.15

Acquired Immunodeficiency Syndrome

Cheryl L. Newman and Thomas C. Quinn

The acquired immunodeficiency syndrome (AIDS) was first recognized as a distinct and newly expressed syndrome in the summer of 1981 when physicians reported five cases of *Pneumocystis carinii* pneumonia and 26 cases of Kaposi sarcoma in previously healthy men in New York and Los Angeles.[8] Since then, there has been an extraordinary increase in the number of reported cases of opportunistic infections and malignancies occurring in such immunocompromised individuals with AIDS. Within the relatively short span of 7 years, AIDS has become a global epidemic with estimates of over 100,000 cases of AIDS, 500,000 cases of AIDS-related conditions (ARC), and 5 to 10 million carriers of the AIDS virus, the latter responsible for the continued transmission of AIDS. In 1987, approximately 50,000 cases of AIDS were officially reported to the Centers for Disease Control, and approximately 1.5 million people had become infected with the AIDS virus.[5] From these statistics the U.S. Public Health Service estimates that by 1991 over 270,000 cases of AIDS will occur with over 54,000 deaths in that year alone from AIDS. In 1991 it is estimated that AIDS will become one of the leading causes of premature mortality, and over 8 to 10 billion dollars will be expended in providing for the health care of AIDS patients in that year alone.[6] With an 80 percent mortality rate 2 years from time of diagnosis and with the current lack of effective curative drugs or vaccines, AIDS clearly has become one of the most serious epidemics of this century.

VIRAL ETIOLOGY AND IMMUNOPATHOGENESIS

AIDS is characterized by the unusual occurrence of life-threatening opportunistic infections or malignancies in an individual who has severe depression of the cell-mediated immune system. This immunosuppression is caused by the loss of the T-helper (T4 or CD4) lymphocytes, which coordinate the cellular activities of the cell-mediated immune system. Intensive clinical, epidemiologic, immunologic, and virologic investigations over the past several years have firmly established that the causative agent of AIDS is a retrovirus that selectively infects the T4 lymphocyte and eventually causes the death of the cell. The AIDS virus has been previously referred to as the human T-lymphotrophic virus-3 (HTLV-III), lymphadenopathy associated virus (LAV), or AIDS related virus (ARV), but the currently accepted designation is the human immunodeficiency virus (HIV), because the above prototype viruses identified by individual scientists have been shown to be essentially the same virus. More recent studies in West Africa have discovered another closely related but distinct retrovirus in patients with AIDS,[23] but because of differences in the genomic structure of this virus, it is referred to as HIV-II, and the original virus is now referred to as HIV-I.

The AIDS virus is a retrovirus capable of replicating in a limited number of cells in the human body, including lymphocytes, macrophages, and cells of the central nervous system. Typical of retroviruses, HIV produces an enzyme, reverse transcriptase, which once inside the cytoplasm of the host cell, produces a DNA copy of its RNA genetic information. The DNA copy is then integrated into the genetic information of the host cell and remains integrated for the life of that cell, which may be as long as the life of the individual. When the host cell, in this case the T4 lymphocyte, is activated by exposure of various antigens, the virus replicates itself through activation of the *tat* viral gene. Eventually new viruses are released from the host cell, resulting in cellular lysis of the infected cell, and HIV invades other infected cells, continuing the cycle. These biologic factors, coupled with the lack of evidence of acquired immunity to HIV, have led to the recognition that once an individual is infected with HIV and develops detectable antibodies, that individual is potentially infected for life. Serologic screening assays, such as the enzyme-linked immunosorbent assay (ELISA), are used to detect the presence of antibodies to HIV as evidence of HIV infection (Table 9.15–1).[28] The pathogenesis of HIV is related to the suppression and eventual destruction of the T-helper (T4) lymphocytes that are critical in maintaining cell-mediated immunity. In addition, neurologic disease appears to be a direct result of HIV-induced destruction of brain cells.

VIRAL TRANSMISSION

The number of viral particles needed to initiate infection, the form in which they are transmitted, the relationship of cofactors, and the possible routes of entry are not known. These early events of the infectious process and the sites of replication of the virus in the body are not well defined. Some of the possibilities include direct entry of the virus into the blood with binding to T4 lymphocytes or invasion or phagocytosis by blood-borne or tissue macrophages that populate the epithelial cell linings of the vaginal, urogenital, or gastrointestinal tract. HIV is known to multiply in lymphocytes and macrophages, and the latter may be involved in dissemination of HIV to other organs, including the central nervous system.

HIV can be repeatedly recovered from AIDS patients and people found to have antibody to the virus. HIV has been isolated from a wide variety of bodily fluids from infected individuals, including blood, semen, vaginal fluid, tears, saliva, bone marrow, urine, cerebrospinal fluid, lymph nodes, and brain tissue. Epidemi-

TABLE 9.15–1. PREVALENCE OF ANTIBODY TO HIV IN VARIOUS U.S. POPULATION GROUPS (1986–1987)

Group	Percent Infected
Homosexual men	
• STD clinic (San Francisco)	72
• Random	33–70
IV drug users	
• New York City	59–87
• San Francisco	9
• Baltimore	41
Hemophiliacs (factor VIII therapy)	70–90
Female prostitutes	
• Seattle	5
• Miami	40
Women	
• Blood donors (Atlanta)	0.01
Men	
• Military applicants	0.15

ologic studies, however, have firmly established that only blood, semen, and vaginal secretions provide sufficient virus for transmission.[8] Consequently, infection has only been found to be transmitted by intimate sexual contact, injection of infected blood or blood products, and by birth to an infected mother. These modes of transmission are also well reflected in the epidemiologic characteristics of AIDS. Casual contact with an infected person, whether symptomatic or asymptomatic, has not been found to transmit HIV. This includes hand shaking, sharing of common drinking glasses, clothing, toilets, or residing in the same home. There has also been no documented evidence that insect vectors or vaccines are implicated in the transmission of HIV.

Sexual transmission, including both homosexual and heterosexual activities, appears to be the predominant mode of transmission of HIV (Table 9.15–2). Among homosexual men, receptive anal intercourse is a more effective means of transmission than either insertive anal intercourse or other types of oral-genital intercourse. Among heterosexuals, vaginal intercourse appears to be responsible for the transmission of the virus from men to women and from women to men.[18] Several studies in sexually transmitted disease clinics and among patients in Africa suggest that the presence of other sexually transmitted diseases including genital ulcerations may enhance transmissibility of the virus, particularly from women to men.[17,23] The exact risk of infection for a susceptible person having a single sexual encounter with an infected partner is unknown. Abstinence, a consistent monogamous relationship, or consistent use of condoms during intercourse appear to be protective in preventing the transmission of HIV.

Inoculation of HIV intravenously via blood transfusion, transfusion of infected blood products such as factor VIII or IX

TABLE 9.15–2. TRANSMISSION PATTERNS OF HIV[a]

Sexual	Homosexual activity
	Bisexual activity
	Heterosexual activity
Blood	Transfusion with infected blood or blood products (factor VIII or IX concentrate)
	Parenteral exposure to HIV-blood-contaminated needles or syringes (e.g., IV drug use)
Perinatal	In utero
	Parturition
	Postnatal

[a]No evidence of casual contact transmission

concentrates, or exposure to blood-contaminated needles and syringes commonly shared by intravenous drug users appear to be efficient means of transmission.[21] Large inoculations given in the form of transfused blood almost universally result in infection, whereas small inocula of blood on the end of a needle in the case of an accidental needlestick of a health care worker seldom results in infection. HIV infection via blood-borne transmission appears to be a function of the concentration of infectious virus in the blood, which is relatively low. Although the risk to health care workers of HIV infection from accidental needlestick or direct skin exposure to HIV-contaminated blood of a patient is low, HIV infection can occur in these circumstances, and the recommended safety precautions such as wearing gloves when in direct contact with infected blood must be followed to prevent transmission.[11]

Perinatal transmission represents the other major mode of transmission from infected mother to child. Perinatal transmission can apparently occur in utero, during parturition, or during the postpartum period, possibly from breastfeeding. The relative efficiency of perinatal transmission is not known, but it is estimated that approximately 50 percent of children born to an infected mother will become infected. These transmission rates may vary considerably depending on the immunologic competence of the mother, levels of neutralizing antibody, levels of circulating virus, and possibly other co-factors. The effect pregnancy may have on the natural history of HIV infection, and conversely, what effect HIV infection may have on the pregnancy, such as congenital defects, prematurity, or spontaneous abortion, is unknown. Presently, HIV-infected women of child-bearing age are advised to avoid pregnancy.[11]

NATURAL HISTORY OF HIV

Shortly after exposure to HIV, the individual may exhibit an infectious mononucleosis-like illness. The illness is characterized by a nonspecific viral illness with complaints of fever, malaise, weakness, rash, muscle pain, and headache.[7] Aseptic meningitis with recovery of the virus from the cerebrospinal fluid also has been reported during this acute phase. The illness lasts for approximately 2 to 3 weeks. Within 2 to 6 months after the acute infection, the infected individual may develop antibodies to HIV. The individual may then be asymptomatic for a period of several months to more than 7 years. However, as the virus continues to replicate and selectively destroy and deplete T-helper (T4) lymphocytes, cellular immunosuppression progresses, and the patient eventually develops symptoms. Presently, the mean incubation period from time of exposure to the development of AIDS-like symptoms is 6 years, illustrating the chronic nature of this viral infection. Nearly all patients illustrate some immunologic abnormalities after HIV infection, and the virus can be recovered from circulating lymphocytes during any given period after infection (Table 9.15–3).

The development of symptoms is highly variable. Approximately 50 to 60 percent of infected individuals will develop chronic lymphadenopathy, a diarrhea-wasting syndrome, local or diffuse neurologic problems, or other clinical-immunologic abnormalities within 3 to 5 years after exposure.[12,15] Two years after infection, approximately 5 percent of infected seropositive individuals develop life-threatening opportunistic infections or malignancies. An additional 5 percent of seropositive individuals then progress to AIDS each year, so that approximately 25 to 30 percent of infected individuals develop AIDS within 5 to 6 years after infection. Because these figures are cumulative, it is estimated that the majority of HIV-infected individuals will develop AIDS or a related encephalopathic illness within 10 to 15 years of exposure.

Natural history studies have examined a number of variables and cofactors that might influence progression of HIV infection. Cofactors, in general, may influence HIV infection at two different periods: cofactors that affect acquisition of infection, such as genital ulcerations or other sexually transmitted diseases, and cofactors

TABLE 9.15–3. REPORTED IMMUNOLOGIC ABNORMALITIES IN AIDS

Quantitative abnormalities of T lymphocytes
- Decreased numbers of T4 helper cells
- Variably altered numbers of T8 suppressor cells

Functional abnormalities of T lymphocytes
- Anergy
- Decreased proliferative responses in vitro
- Decreased cytotoxic lymphocyte function
- Decreased ability to provide help to B lymphocytes for immunoglobulin production
- Diminished lymphokine production
- Depressed clonal expansion of lymphocyte subsets

Functional abnormalities of natural killer cells
- Decreased in vitro cytotoxicity

Functional abnormalities of B lymphocytes
- Elevated serum immunoglobulin levels
- Circulating immune complexes
- Inability to mount a serologic response following de novo immunization
- Spontaneous proliferation
- Refractoriness to T-cell-dependent or independent mitogens signals in vitro

Functional abnormalities of monocytes and macrophages
- Diminished chemotaxis
- Decrease in vitro killing of parasites
- Spontaneously increased interleukin-1 secretion
- Spontaneously enhanced prostaglandin E_2 production

Serologic abnormalities
- Suppressor factors in sera
- T-cell-derived suppressor substances
- Possible antilymphocyte antibodies
- Elevated acid-labile α-interferon
- Elevations in β-2-microglobulin
- Elevations in α-1 thymosin
- Decreased serum thymulin levels

that affect disease progression once infection has occurred. It has been documented that those that have been infected the longest have the highest risk of developing AIDS. In prospective studies of seropositive individuals, a number of factors were found to influence progression to AIDS among the seropositive individuals.[15,22] In these studies a decreased number of T-helper lymphocytes ($<300/mm^3$), low level of antibody to HIV (particularly anti-p24), a high titer of antibody to cytomegalovirus, and a history of sex with someone in whom AIDS developed were independently associated with the subsequent development of AIDS. These variables may be markers rather than determinants of disease progression, however. A vigorous antibody response to HIV infection may confer at least temporary protection against the progression of immunodeficiency to AIDS, or a low level of antibody to HIV may reflect a later stage of infection. The increased risk associated with a history of having had sex with someone who had AIDS may indicate an earlier infection with a more virulent strain of HIV. Additional prospective studies of such individuals are required to further understand the natural progression of HIV, but these factors may be useful in counseling HIV seropositive persons and in designing studies of clinical intervention.

Isolated and unusual cases have been reported in which individuals remain seronegative for a long period of time, although their infections were proven by cultivation of the virus from the blood. This possibility has raised some concerns about the failure to detect infected individuals who wish to donate blood, although essentially 99 percent of infected individuals will have detectable antibodies to HIV. Recent development of an antigen assay may be of some usefulness in the detection of circulating antigen in antibody-negative individuals.

EPIDEMIOLOGY

After the identification of the first AIDS cases in the United States in 1981, the Centers for Disease Control formulated a case definition that was adopted by the World Health Organization (Table 9.15–4). Although this definition has undergone several modifications as more has been learned about the disease, it has essentially remained the same and has been quite useful in monitoring disease trends. Presently, an individual is identified as having AIDS if he or she is found to have a reliably diagnosed disease that is at least indicative of an underlying cellular immunodeficiency and has no known cause of immunosuppression other than infection with HIV. Infections that qualify for this definition are shown in Table 9.15–1. Malignancies that indicate AIDS primarily include Kaposi sarcoma and a variety of other lymphomas. Additional illnesses that strongly suggest but are not diagnostic of AIDS include the appearance of dementia or a myelopathy in the absence of a concurrent illness or condition other than HIV, a wasting syndrome with a profound involuntary weight loss of more than 10 percent of the baseline body weight, and either chronic diarrhea lasting for more than 1 month or chronic fever and weakness lasting for more than 1 month in the absence of any concurrent illness other than HIV.

Using this definition, 38,160 patients in the United States, including 37,635 adults and 525 children, meet the definition for patients with AIDS and have been reported to the Centers for Disease Control as of July 1987. Of these patients, 57 percent of the adults and 61 percent of the children are known to have died, including over 80 percent of those patients diagnosed 2 years previously. Since the initial reports of AIDS in early 1981, the number of cases reported for each 6-month period continues to increase. The increases are not exponential, however, as evidenced by the lengthening period of time required to double the number of

TABLE 9.15–4. CASE DEFINITION OF AIDS

Presence of a reliably diagnosed disease at least moderately suggestive of a cellular immunodeficiency, occurring in an individual with no known cause of underlying immunodeficiency other than infection with HIV.

Opportunistic Infections

Protozoa	*Pneumocystis carinii* pneumonia
	Toxoplasma gondii encephalitis or disseminated disease
	Cryptosporidia enteritis >1 mo
Fungi	Cryptococcal meningitis or disseminated infection
	Candida esophagitis
	Bronchial or pulmonary candidiasis
	Disseminated histoplasmosis
Bacteria	Disseminated *Mycobacterium avium-intracellulare*
	Disseminated *Mycobacterium kansasii*
Viral	Chronic mucocutaneous herpes simplex virus >1 mo
	Disseminated cytomegalovirus
	Progressive multifocal encephalopathy (JC papovavirus)

Cancers
- Kaposi sarcoma in HIV-positive patient
- Primary brain lymphoma
- Non-Hodgkin lymphoma (small noncleaved lymphoma, immunoblastic sarcoma of B cell, or unknown immunologic phenotype)

Chronic Lymphoid Interstitial Pneumonitis
- Children under 13 years of age if HIV-seropositive

Other Conditions
- Acceptable if serology or culture HIV-positive

cases. Cases have now been reported from all 50 states, the District of Columbia, four U.S. territories, and from 119 other countries of the world.

In the United States, *Pneumocystis carinii* pneumonia continues to be the most common opportunistic disease reported among AIDS patients. Sixty-six percent of the patients had *Pneumocystis carinii* pneumonia, 24 percent had other opportunistic infections without *Pneumocystis,* and 10 percent had Kaposi sarcoma alone. Ninety-five percent of the patients with Kaposi sarcoma were homosexual or bisexual men.

Among adult AIDS patients in the United States, 93 percent are men and 7 percent women. There has been no significant change over time in the distribution of male patients by age and race. Ninety percent of the men with AIDS are 20 to 49 years of age with a mean age of 36.8 years. Sixty-three percent are white, 22 percent are black, 14 percent are Hispanic, and 1 percent are of other race or ethnicity. Eighty-eight percent of the women reported with AIDS are also between 20 to 49 years of age with a mean age of 34.9 years. In contrast to the men, 27 percent are white, 52 percent are black, 20 percent are Hispanic, and 1 percent are of other race or ethnicity. Sixty-seven percent of the women had *Pneumocystis,* 31 percent had other opportunistic infections, and 2 percent had Kaposi sarcoma alone.

Nearly all adult AIDS patients can be placed in groups that suggest a possible means of disease acquisition (Table 9.15–5). The proportion of female AIDS cases who were heterosexual partners of persons with AIDS or at risk for AIDS increased significantly between 1982 and 1986 from 12 to 27 percent, a trend that may prove to be a good marker for following trends in heterosexual transmission.[18] Except for women with a coagulation disorder, the number of AIDS cases reported continues to increase in all patient groups.

The epidemiology of AIDS in other countries such as Canada and Europe is quite similar to that described for the United States with a male-to-female ratio of 13:1 and with the predominance of cases occurring among homosexual and bisexual men and intravenous drug users. In tropical countries such as in Africa and in the Caribbean, however, the male-to-female ratio is 1:1, and the majority of cases are identified in heterosexually active individuals. One of the primary risk factors for transmission of HIV in these countries is the heterosexual promiscuity that may exist among female prostitutes and men attending sexually transmitted disease clinics.[23] Prevalence rates of infection with HIV range from 20 to 80 percent among these promiscuous individuals. Exposure to infected blood transfusions and blood-contaminated needles used for medicinal purpose further amplifies the transmission of HIV among the general population of these tropical countries. With such high rates of infection among women of child-bearing age, a rapid rise in the number of cases among children is now occurring in these countries.

CLINICAL MANIFESTATIONS

The clinical manifestations of HIV are diverse and range from asymptomatic infection to overwhelming illness due to HIV-induced encephalopathy, multiple opportunistic infections, or malignancies. The CDC has developed a classification scheme for the various stages of HIV infection (Table 9.15–6). Clinical findings on physical examination thus depend on the clinical stage of the disease. Despite the wide range of agents responsible for the opportunistic infections and malignancies that characterize AIDS, however, there are some signs and symptoms peculiar to symptomatic ARC or AIDS that are summarized below.

HISTORY

In addition to documentation of a detailed sexual and medical history for information pertaining to a patient's risk group for acquisition of HIV infection, the medical history also should focus on clinical symptoms that suggest a chronic illness (Table 9.15–7). Subsequent to the development of overt AIDS, many patients have a prodrome characterized by progressive fatigue, anorexia, and unexplained fever. Weight loss of greater than 10 pounds (4.5 kg) during the preceding 3 months is often noted.

Nonproductive cough and progressive dyspnea are the most frequently mentioned cardiopulmonary symptoms and may reflect the insidious development of an opportunistic pneumonia. In addition to weight loss, anorexia, odynophagia, and dysphagia, gastrointestinal history often reveals symptoms of chronic or recurrent diarrhea and proctitis, abdominal pain, and occasional jaundice due to hepatosplenomegaly, cholecystis, or hepatitis-associated opportunistic infections or malignancies. Although diarrhea may be caused by the more common gastrointestinal pathogens, as seen in the "gay bowel syndrome," chronic diarrhea of several liters of watery stool per day more likely reflects diarrhea caused by an opportunistic pathogen such as *Cryptosporidium* or *Isospora.*

TABLE 9.15–5. AIDS CASES IN THE UNITED STATES BY TRANSMISSION CATEGORY AS OF JULY 1987

Transmission Category	Percent of Cases Reported		
	Male	*Female*	*Total*
Adults			
• Homosexual/bisexual	71	—	66
• IV drug user	14	50	16
• Both homosexual and IV drug user	8	—	8
• Hemophilia	1	0	1
• Heterosexual contact with AIDS patient or high-risk person	2	29	4
• Transfusion	1	11	2
• Undetermined	3	10	3
Total	100	100	100
Pediatric			
• Parent with AIDS or at risk for AIDS			78
• Transfusion			12
• Hemophilia			6
• Undetermined			4
Total			100

TABLE 9.15–6. CDC CLASSIFICATION SCHEME HIV INFECTION

Group	Description
I	Acute HIV infection
II	Asymptomatic seropositivity
III	Persistent generalized lymphadenopathy (PGL)
IV	Severe AIDS-related diseases
A	Constitutional disease (persistent fever, weight loss, or unexplained diarrhea)
B	Neurologic disease (dementia, myelopathy, or peripheral neuropathy)
C-1	Opportunistic infections of CDC surveillance definition (see Table 9.15–4)
C-2	Other recurrent infections (see text)
D	Opportunistic malignancies of CDC definition
E	Other serious conditions (including thrombocytopenia, Hodgkin disease)

TABLE 9.15–7. CLINICAL MANIFESTATIONS OF AIDS PERTINENT SIGNS AND SYMPTOMS

History
- Weight loss, fatigue, fevers, chills
- Visual changes, dysphagia, oral ulcers
- Dyspnea, cough, hemoptysis
- Diarrhea, abdominal pain, jaundice, anorexia, nausea, vomiting, rectal pain or ulcers
- Genital ulcers, impotence, dysuria, oliguria, hematuria
- Personality changes, sleep disorders, seizures, depression, weakness, numbness, difficulty with memory, headaches
- Changes in hair, skin, or nails

Physical Examination
- Cachexia, temporal wasting, eczema, chronic onychomycosis, Kaposi sarcoma lesions
- Thrush, oral ulcers, oral hairy leukoplakia
- Cotton wool spots, retinal hemorrhages, retinal detachment
- Tachypnea, tachycardia, rales, rhonchi, wheeze
- Jaundice, abdominal tenderness, hepatosplenomegaly, perirectal ulcers
- Genital ulcers
- Lymphadenopathy
- Hyperreflexia or hyporeflexia, gait abnormalities, abnormal mental status, diminished distal vibration or pinprick sensation, dystonia

A history of genital ulcerations, dysuria, incontinence, and sexual dysfunction may be present. Although uncommon, prostatitis and bladder and kidney infections may occur. Asymptomatic progressive focal and segmental glomerulosclerosis with and without nephrosis can develop, and the presence of hematuria, oliguria, and edema should be noted.

Neuropsychiatric symptoms include headaches, seizures, and confusion that may be caused by underlying encephalitis, meningitis, brain abscess, or tumor. Visual blurring, suggesting chorioretinitis, also may be present. Mild focal weakness caused by a myopathy or mononeuritis, or a more profound paralysis as seen in the AIDS-associated Guillian-Barre syndrome or viral myelopathy may be noted. Painful dysesthesias of the distal extremities often are reported. Before the development of overt AIDS encephalopathy, many patients note loss of libido, personality changes, impaired memory, sleep disorders, and a slowness of thinking. Other psychiatric symptoms include profound depression, paranoid psychosis, and severe anxiety disorders.

Symptoms of skin, hair, and nail disorders may reflect chronic immunodeficiency, hormonal abnormalities, or nutritional deficiencies associated with the HIV wasting syndromes. History of specific skin lesions suggesting Kaposi sarcoma or chronic fungal or herpetic infection should be sought.

PHYSICAL EXAMINATION

The general physical examination in full-blown AIDS may reveal overt cachexia (Table 9.15–7). Skin should be examined for the presence of purplish raised lesions of Kaposi sarcoma and other infectious lesions. Seborrheic dermatitis and the dermatomal vesicular eruption of herpes zoster are occasionally seen. Tattoos should be noted. Nails may reflect chronic onychomycosis. Peripheral or periorbital edema caused by protein losses from nephrosis or nutritional deficiencies may be seen.

Funduscopic examination may reveal cotton wool spots alone or exudative hemorrhagic lesions with or without retinal detachment as seen in cytomegalovirus or toxoplasmosis retinitis. Visual acuity may or may not be impaired, depending on the location of the retinal lesions. The presence of cotton wool spots in the retina without a definable opportunistic infection is common, and may represent immune complex deposition.

Oral examination in patients with ARC or AIDS typically reveals the white mucosal patches of oral candidiasis. Esophagoscopy in the patient with dysphagia may further reveal esophageal ulcers or plaques caused by *Candida*, herpes simplex, or CMV. Additionally, painful oral ulcers, particularly of the palate, can be seen. In some but not all cases, herpes simplex can be isolated from these lesions. Oral hairy leukoplakia, a hairy-appearing whitish plaque usually seen along the lateral border of the tongue, is occasionally present and is probably caused by an infection with one of the herpes viruses. Kaposi sarcoma lesions seen in the oral cavity may suggest gastrointestinal involvement.

The thoracic examination in the patient with pulmonary disease may reveal tachypnea, rales, wheezes, or rhonchi. Although cardiac lesions such as marantic endocarditis, pericarditis, and myocarditis have occasionally been reported as a complication of disseminated Kaposi sarcoma or other opportunistic infection, cardiac abnormalities are infrequent.

Abdominal examination may reveal hepatosplenomegaly, tenderness, or masses. Ascites or jaundice are rarely seen as primary manifestations of AIDS, but may occur as a consequence of the end stage of many of the AIDS-associated illnesses such as disseminated Kaposi sarcoma, lymphoma, or overwhelming opportunistic infection. Steatohepatitis, as a cause of significant hepatomegaly without other evidence of significant liver dysfunction, has been seen.

Chronic proctitis usually caused by herpes simplex is a frequent finding and is manifested by painful shallow erosions in the perirectal area. Proctitis secondary to other infections such as gonorrhea, giardiasis, amebiasis, or chlamydia can occur and be associated with the presence of blood, pus, or diarrhea. Inflammatory or malignant masses such as rectal lymphoma are occasionally found by rectal examination.

Nervous system manifestations of AIDS may result from opportunistic infections, malignancies, or HIV infection itself as seen in the subacute encephalitis syndrome. This is a progressive dementing syndrome in which the earliest signs may be minor impairments of cognitive functions such as calculation and memory skills. Personality changes and other psychiatric syndromes ranging from mild depression to overt psychosis also can be seen. With time, this syndrome relentlessly progresses, and the more usual signs of dementia become apparent. Dystonia, psychomotor retardation, and other Parkinson-like features can be seen. Eventually the patient becomes incontinent and unable to walk, talk, or maintain self-care. Other physical signs of neurologic dysfunction in AIDS depend on the location and type of lesion but can include delirium, dementia, focal or generalized seizures, motor and sensory deficits, abnormal movements such as clonus and dystonia, deep tendon reflex abnormalities, and gait disorders.

Although lymphadenopathy is one of the early hallmarks of HIV infection, especially during the prodromal stages before the development of ARC, it is well known that many patients with end-stage AIDS have minimal adenopathy. In fact, prominent lymphadenopathy during the later phases of illness may suggest the presence of lymphoma or the lymphadenopathic form of Kaposi sarcoma.

LABORATORY FINDINGS

Laboratory abnormalities associated with HIV infection, like clinical manifestations, depend on the stage of the disease. Seropositivity as determined by ELISA and Western blot analysis is the hallmark of infection. Most patients will have detectable virus by culture during some stage of the disease. With development of symptomatic ARC or overt AIDS, lymphopenia occurs and the ratio of T-helper cells to T-suppressor cells is generally depressed below 1.0. Most patients are anergic. Neutropenia and thrombocytopenia, which in some cases are immunologically mediated, can be seen. Most patients are anemic as well. Abnormalities of liver

and renal function and electrolytes may occur because of superimposed opportunistic diseases.

OPPORTUNISTIC INFECTIONS

Before the discovery of the viral etiology of AIDS, it was apparent that the major morbidity and mortality associated with the acquired immunosuppression was secondary to opportunistic infections. Despite our ability to treat many of the opportunistic pathogens effectively,[31,32] the occurrence of multiple infections in a single patient continues to complicate clinical care. As shown in Table 9.15–4, the case definition of AIDS depends on documentation of an opportunistic illness. Although the number and type of opportunistic diseases is large, the more common AIDS-associated infections and malignancies are discussed later.

FUNGAL INFECTIONS

Although not included in the case definition of AIDS, thrush or oral candidiasis is the most common infection occurring in AIDS patients and is often the earliest sign of immunodeficiency. When localized to the mouth, thrush is usually asymptomatic; with extension to the esophagus, dysphagia and odynophagia often occur. On esophagoscopy or barium swallow, mucosal ulceration can be seen. The characteristic whitish mucosal plaques can be easily scraped for gram stain or KOH wet preparation, which reveals budding yeast and pseudohyphae. Oral nystatin or topical clotrimazole is usually effective in controlling oral candidiasis. Treatment of esophageal candidiasis is more difficult; ketoconazole is sometimes effective, although severe esophagitis usually responds best to a short course of low-dose amphotericin B. Esophageal and mucocutaneous candidiasis are often chronic and recurrent; retreatment or suppressive therapy may be indicated in some patients. Disseminated candidiasis is not a usual complication of HIV-induced immunosuppression, although it may occur preterminally secondary to line sepsis or surgery.

Cryptococcal infection in AIDS usually starts as meningitis, although systemic disease due to *Cryptococcus neoformans* has been well documented and usually occurs as fungemia or pneumonia. Disseminated cryptococcosis involving the liver, lungs, spleen, bone marrow, lymph nodes, adrenals, as well as CNS has been noted on autopsy in some cases. The patient with cryptococcal meningitis usually has a history of chronic headache, fever, and mild confusion. Lumbar puncture may reveal elevated CSF pressure, slightly depressed CSF glucose concentrations, increased protein, and mild CSF pleocytosis. Although the Gram stain and India ink preparations are often positive, the cryptococcal latex agglutination test is the most rapid and reliable method of establishing the diagnosis. Occasionally patients with cryptococcal meningitis may have little or no alteration of the CSF glucose, protein, and cells; in these cases, detection of cryptococcal antigen in the CSF is especially useful. In disseminated cryptococodis, cultures of blood, urine, and sputum may be positive. Biopsy of infected tissue will reveal mucicarmine-positive yeast cells; this characteristic carminophilic pink capsule serves to distinguish this yeast from some of the other opportunistic yeasts such as *Blastomyces* or *Histoplasma*.

The mainstay of therapy for cryptococcal infection in AIDS is amphotericin B, preferably, in combination with flucytosine. Unfortunately, many patients may not tolerate this combination because of flucytosine-induced neutropenia, thrombocytopenia, and gastrointestinal toxicity. In those cases, monotherapy with full-dose amphotericin B (0.7 to 1 mg/kg per day) is indicated. CSF parameters should be followed periodically. Despite appropriate and prolonged treatment, many patients, though symptomatically improved, may have persistently positive cryptococcal antigen titers in the CSF. Titers in excess of 1:8 at the completion of a course of therapy are often associated with clinical and mycologic relapse.

Despite appropriate and successful initial therapy, over fifty percent of patients may experience relapse. Thus, some type of suppressive therapy is indicated in many patients; low-dose chronic or intermittent prophylactic amphotericin B administration is now advocated by many clinicians.

Disseminated histoplasma infection may develop in AIDS patients after inhalation of *H. capsulatum* spores from contaminated soil. Lymphohematogenous dissemination occurs, and the patient typically presents with unexplained fevers and hepatosplenomegaly with liver dysfunction, lymphadenopathy, and pancytopenia. Meningitis and chorioretinitis are also seen. Biopsy of infected tissues reveals PAS or methenamine silver-positive small budding yeasts often clustered in histiocytes. Unlike the more usual non–AIDS-associated histoplasma infections, granulomas are not usually seen. Although typically causing necrotizing lesions of the skin and bone, *Histoplasma duboisii*, a saprophytic soil fungus in Central and West Africa is associated with disseminated histoplasmosis in African AIDS patients.

Coccidioides immitis, a dimorphic fungus endemic in the southwestern United States may also cause disseminated disease in AIDS patients. Although *Aspergillus* infection has been typically associated with immunosuppression produced by cytotoxic drugs and steroids, disseminated aspergillosis is rare in AIDS patients, except preterminally. Serologic and skin tests, though helpful if positive, may be negative in the face of impaired cellular immunity, therefore the diagnosis of invasive fungal infections generally rests on biopsy and culture of involved tissues or body fluids. Initial therapy with amphotericin B is the treatment of choice. As with cryptococcosis, chronic suppressive therapy may be indicated. Some investigators suggest that ketoconazole may have a potential role for suppressive therapy, especially in histoplasmosis.

PROTOZOAL INFECTIONS IN AIDS

The most frequently identified opportunistic infection associated with AIDS is *Pneumocystis carinii* pneumonia (PCP), which is present in over 60 percent of adult AIDS patients. This ubiquitous protozoan parasite of the subphylum Sporozoa was originally described by Chagas in 1907 and was subsequently found to be a cause of opportunistic pneumonia in immunosuppressed patients, especially those undergoing therapy for malignant diseases or after organ transplantation.

Patients with PCP note the insidious onset of fever, chills, nonproductive cough, dyspnea, and malaise. These symptoms often precede the diagnosis by several weeks, although an occasional patient has an abrupt onset of respiratory failure. Early in the infection the chest examination and radiographs may be clear, and only mild hypoxia at rest is noted. At this stage, the gallium lung scan is often positive, and the lung diffusion capacity may be abnormal. With progression, diffuse reticulonodular bilateral interstitial infiltrates develop. As this organism cannot be readily cultured, diagnosis depends on demonstration of the parasite in lung tissue or pulmonary secretions. In some cases, pneumocysts can be recovered from expectorated sputum, though transbronchial biopsy with brushings and washings are usually needed for the recovery of the organism. Recently the use of the bronschoscope to perform a wedged bronchoalveolar lavage has obviated the need for a transbronchial or open lung biopsy. This less invasive procedure involves the instillation and rapid removal of a large volume of saline through a catheter wedged into a bronchial tributary, thereby sampling the distal alveoli. This technique is said to be as sensitive as open lung biopsy for the diagnosis of *Pneumocystis* infection.

Therapy of PCP involves appropriate ventilatory support and therapy with either pentamidine via intravenous or intramuscular injection, or intravenous trimethoprim-sulfamethoxazole. Thirty to fifty percent of people are unable to tolerate a complete course of the initial anti-*Pneumocystis* agent, requiring a switch to alternative therapy. Both pentamidine and trimethoprim-sulfamethoxa-

zole are associated with a 50 to 60 percent incidence of adverse reactions. Trimethoprim-sulfamethoxazole most frequently causes fever, rash, leukopenia, and abnormal liver function tests. Pentamidine may induce hypoglycemia, hyperglycemia, neutropenia, and renal dysfunction. Although hypotension may develop with overly rapid intravenous infusion, this method is often better tolerated than intramuscular pentamidine, which is associated with painful sterile abscess formation. When administered intravenously, pentamidine should be infused slowly, over 1 hour to obviate side effects. Either regimen results in a 60 to 80 percent response rate, even in recurrent disease. Because of the high incidence of adverse reactions and appreciable therapeutic failure rate of 20 to 40 percent, alternative therapies are being investigated.

Although dapsone, alone or in combination with trimethoprim, was effective in animal pneumocystosis, limited use in humans was associated with a nearly 60 percent rate of adverse reactions. Administration of aerosolized pentamidine directly into the bronchial tree has been successful in some patients and was associated with much fewer side effects than conventional parenteral therapy. Difluoromethylornithine (DFMO), an inhibitor of ornithine decarboxylase and polyamine biosynthesis, has been successfully used in the treatment of other protozoal infections such as trypanosomiasis. In limited compassionate protocol use in AIDS patients, DFMO has been effective in the treatment of PCP in patients who have failed conventional therapy. Randomized clinical trials to further evaluate this drug are pending. An additional alternative therapy for PCP is the combination of leucovorin and trimetrexate, a lipid soluble analogue of methotrexate. The addition of this antifolate compound to leucovorin ameliorates the myelosuppression and gastrointestinal toxicity of this potent antiparasitic compound. Encouraging results have been observed after use of this new drug combination in patients who either failed to respond or were intolerant of conventional therapy.

The recurrence rate for PCP in AIDS is approximately 20 to 40 percent, with the majority of recurrences occurring within the first year after the initial episode. Although controversial, chemoprophylaxis regimens including daily or biweekly trimethoprim-sulfamethoxazole, weekly dapsone or pyrimethamine-sulfadoxine (Fansidar), or monthly pentamidine have been recommended by some clinicians. The reported mortality of PCP is 10 to 30 percent. Despite appropriate therapy, less than 20 percent of patients requiring ventilatory support will survive.

Although long recognized as pathogens in the gay bowel syndrome, neither amebiasis nor giardiasis is diagnostic of AIDS. Two other gut parasitic infections occurring with much higher incidence in the AIDS population are *Cryptosporidium* and *Isospora*.

Cryptosporidium is a protozoal coccidian that historically has caused intestinal disease in a wide variety of animals. It became a recognized human pathogen in the 1970s and has been infrequently associated with self-limited traveler's diarrhea as well as diarrheal disease in children and some immunosuppressed adults. With the advent of AIDS, it became recognized as a cause of chronic, often severe, watery diarrhea. The parasite attaches to the epithelial surface of the small and large intestine causing an often massive efflux of fluid, occasionally up to 20 L per day. Although cryptosporidia can be seen in gut biopsy specimens, detection of the acid-fast oocysts in the stool using a modified Ziehl-Neelsen technique or fluorescent auramine stain of stool concentrates, is the usual method of diagnosis.

Isospora belli, like cryptosporidia, attaches to (and may invade) the small intestinal epithelium causing chronic profuse watery diarrhea. Diagnosis depends on detection of oocysts in iodine-stained specimens. Apart from fluid and nutritional support, therapy of *Cryptosporidium* with spiramycin or *Isospora* with trimethoprim-sulfamethoxazole has not been uniformly encouraging. Attempts to suppress the secretory diarrhea with a prostaglandin inhibitor such as indomethacin has occasionally resulted in a dramatic reduction in diarrheal fluid losses.

Toxoplasma gondii, an intracellular coccidian parasite, was first isolated from a rodent in 1908, although the cat is the definitive host. Despite the high frequency of human infection due to exposure to *Toxoplasma* oocysts, clinical illness is rare and organisms typically encyst and become latent within host tissues. In the setting of AIDS-induced immunosuppression, however, reactivation of latent infection may occur, usually resulting in *Toxoplasma* encephalitis or disseminated toxoplasmosis. Clinically, subacute or chronic encephalitis begins with fever, confusion, seizures, and headache. Focal neurologic findings and chorioretinitis may be found. Computed tomographic scans typically reveal single or multiple contrast-enhancing ring lesions, though other opportunistic CNS mass lesions may mimic these findings. Serologic tests are helpful if positive, although a negative IgM titer does not preclude the diagnosis in this setting. Although biopsy of the CNS lesions is often positive, revealing tachyzoites and cysts on Wright or Giemsa staining, definitive diagnosis may be difficult because of the inaccessibility of some lesions to biopsy and negative serologic studies. In these cases, presumptive diagnosis is often made, and therapy with the combination of pyrimethamine and a sulfonamide is begun. Alternative therapy with spiramycin, clindamycin, or trimetrexate-leucovorin has been proposed.

VIRAL INFECTIONS IN AIDS

Members of the herpes virus group are the most frequently identified viruses causing disease in the AIDS patient. In particular, cytomegalovirus (CMV) infection has contributed substantially to AIDS-associated morbidity and mortality. Although many HIV-infected patients harbor latent CMV, clinical disease usually takes the form of CMV retinitis, which may occur in the early stages of AIDS, or interstitial pneumonitis, which typically appears later. CMV retinochoroiditis may be asymptomatic initially but with progression typically causes loss of vision. Ophthalmologic examination often reveals perivascular exudative hemorrhagic lesions, occasionally associated with retinal detachment. CMV pneumonia produces a diffuse or focal interstitial and hemorrhagic pneumonitis that radiographically appears similar to most other forms of AIDS-associated opportunistic pneumonia. Gastrointestinal CMV involvement may cause profound diarrhea and mucosal ulceration with hemorrhage. Nervous system invasion by CMV has been associated with subacute encephalitis, peripheral neuropathy, and a Guillain-Barré-type syndrome. In the CNS, microglial nodules harboring cytomegalic cells predominantly in the gray matter can be seen at autopsy. Finally, disseminated disease and CMV wasting syndrome occur.

Definitive diagnosis of specific tissue invasion by CMV is best made by biopsy and demonstration of the typical cytomegalic cells containing intranuclear and intracytoplasmic inclusions. Experimentally, viral nucleic acid may be detected by Southern and in situ hybridization techniques. In cases of retinitis, the diagnosis can be made clinically by an experienced ophthalmologist. Serology is of little help in the diagnosis of invasive disease because most patients have preexisting titers to CMV. Viral cultures of blood or buffy coat, urine, and other body fluids may be positive although the incubation period may range from days to a few weeks before typical cytopathic changes are seen in the viral tissue culture line. Additionally, AIDS patients may chronically excrete CMV without having apparent clinical disease.

Until recently there has been no effective therapy for CMV infection. The new investigational drug, ganciclovir, is a guanosine analogue that has been shown to inhibit CMV proliferation in vitro. In clinical studies it has been most effective in the treatment of CMV retinitis; some, but not all, patients with pneumonia or gastrointestinal CMV infection have responded. As with most latent herpetic infections, however, cessation of therapy is associated with clinical and virologic relapse, and maintenance suppressive therapy is probably indicated.

Herpes simplex and varicella zoster virus also occur with increased frequency in AIDS patients. Chronic mucocutaneous her-

petic infections typically appear in the oral or anogenital regions; esophageal involvement mimicking *Candida* esophagitis is frequent. Acyclovir therapy effectively controls these infections, although recurrence is common. Localized herpes zoster is common in HIV-infected patients and infrequently disseminates. When it does, high-dose acyclovir therapy is generally efficacious.

Progressive multifocal leukoencephalopathy (PML), a demyelinating disorder of the CNS white matter caused by infection with a papovavirus, is said to occur in 1 to 4 percent of AIDS patients. Symptomatically, patients most frequently complain of gait disorders, visual loss, extremity weakness, and headaches. Confusion progressing to stupor may result. Computed tomographic scanning shows focal nonenhancing hypodense white matter lesions without mass effect, although magnetic resonance scanning is said to be more sensitive, especially at detection of subtle early lesions. CSF studies are normal or nondiagnostic. Definitive diagnosis by biopsy reveals demyelination and necrosis. Polyomavirus inclusions can be detected by immunologic methods; viral particles may be seen by electron microscopy. Currently there is no effective therapy for PML; the disease is inevitably fatal in most patients, although rare reports of spontaneous improvement or stabilization exist.

BACTERIAL INFECTIONS IN AIDS

Typical mycobacterial infections due to *Mycobacterium tuberculosis* have been recognized as a cause of disease in normal and immunocompromised hosts. In particular Haitian and African AIDS patients frequently have serious pulmonary or disseminated *M. tuberculosis* infections. The atypical mycobacteria, although ubiquitous, were infrequently identified as human pathogens until the advent of AIDS. Disseminated infection with *Mycobacterium avium-intracellulare* has been uniquely associated with AIDS in American and European patients. Disseminated *M. kansasii* has been infrequently reported as well. The patients with *Mycobacterium avium-intracellulare* infection present with prolonged fever, anemia, malaise, and wasting; many have coexisting opportunistic pathogens. Most are found to be bacteremic when special mycobacterial isolation media is used for culture. Aspirates of liver and bone marrow are also positive. Consistent with the heavy burden of mycobacteria in the blood are the striking number of organisms found invading the liver, spleen, and other organs at autopsy. True granulomas typical of usual granulomatous infections are generally not found. Diagnosis is made by culture of body fluids and tissues or acid-fast staining of biopsy specimens. Disseminated *M. avium-intracellulare* infections often fail to respond to antituberculous therapy. If instituted, treatment should include at least rifampin, ethambutol, and amikacin. Cycloserine and ethionamide or ansamycin or clofazamine may be added.

Bacteremias due to *Streptococcus pneumoniae*, *Haemophilus influenzae*, *Salmonella* sp, and *Listeria* have been occasionally reported in AIDS and ARC patients. *Nocardia* and *Legionella* pneumonias, and enteritis caused by *Salmonella*, *Shigella*, and *Campylobacter* may occur as well.

MALIGNANCIES AND AIDS

Although formerly known to cause chronic endemic disease in African and Mediterranean elderly men, Kaposi sarcoma is now the most common opportunistic neoplasm associated with AIDS. Cutaneous Kaposi sarcoma is usually indolent and appears as erythematous or violaceous nontender macular or papulonodular lesions. Visceral extension to involve the gut, lung, liver, spleen, and lymph nodes may occur. In rare patients an aggressive form of Kaposi sarcoma previously seen only in African children, the lymphadenopathic variety, occurs, often without cutaneous lesions. Management includes observation for localized cutaneous disease;

multiagent combination chemotherapy including vinblastine, VP16, α-interferon, and irradiation have been tried with modest success in some cases. Although there is currently no cure for Kaposi sarcoma, few patients actually succumb; rather, their ultimate course is determined by the coincidental development of opportunistic infections.

Apart from Kaposi sarcoma, non-Hodgkin lymphomas (including Burkitt lymphoma) are the most frequently identified opportunistic malignancies. These high grade B cell lymphomas often originate in extranodal sites, such as the CNS. Similar to the African Burkitt lymphomas and lymphomas in posttransplant patients, these neoplasms are frequently EBNA positive suggesting the possible role of persistent polyclonal B cell proliferation caused by Epstein-Barr virus in their pathogenesis.

Although not included in the CDC surveillance definition, Hodgkin disease has occurred in homosexual men who are HIV seropositive. Unique features of Hodgkin disease in these patients such as an increased prevalence of advanced-stage disease (mixed cellularity and lymphocyte depleted) and an unusual predilection for cutaneous and rectal involvement can be seen. Small cell carcinomas, particularly of the pancreas, rectosigmoid, and lung, and both oral and anal squamous cell malignancies have been reported as well.

THERAPY OF HIV INFECTION

Until recently, the management of HIV infection has focused predominantly on treatment of opportunistic infection and AIDS-associated malignancies. Specific antiviral therapy directed toward inhibition of replication of the AIDS retrovirus has resulted in the development of a variety of new therapeutic agents of which azidothymidine (AZT [Retrovir]) is the prototype. Additionally, agents that either stimulate immunologic cells, such as interferons, or replace the exhausted immune system, such as thymic transplantation, are being studied for their potential utility in combination with the newer antiretroviral drugs.

Knowledge of the molecular biology and understanding of the complicated life cycle of HIV has suggested multiple potential targets for therapeutic intervention (Table 9.15–8).[10,19] AZT is the most extensively studied of the reverse transcriptase inhibitors.[30] These agents are 2'3'-dideoxynucleosides and act by inhibiting the replication of the AIDS retrovirus by substitution of a thymidine analogue in which the usual 3' hydroxyl group is replaced by an azido group.[2,30] In a large placebo-controlled study of AZT a disproportionate rate of death occurred in the placebo group, and the study was discontinued prematurely. This and subsequent data suggest that AZT may prolong duration and quality of life in AIDS patients. The drug is currently available for use in patients with symptomatic HIV infection (AIDS or advanced ARC) who have either prior cytologically confirmed *Pneumocystis* pneumonia or an absolute T-helper lymphocyte count of less than 200 cells/mm³.

The recommended initial dose of AZT is 200 mg every 4 hours by mouth. AZT has good oral bioavailability and penetrates the blood brain barrier; thus it may be of benefit in the management of HIV dementia and other related neurologic syndromes. Unfortunately, substantial toxicity has been associated with its use. Anemia and granulocytopenia are the most frequently recognized serious side effects, and their development appears to be inversely correlated with the pretreatment hemoglobin level and leukocyte count and directly related to the duration of therapy. Other reported side effects include headache, anorexia, nausea, myalgia and insomnia. Biweekly hematologic monitoring is recommended, and side effects are managed by dose reduction or discontinuation of therapy.

Dideoxycytidine is another dideoxynucleoside which acts in a manner similar to AZT. As a cytosine analogue it becomes incorporated into the replicating viral DNA chain and thus inhibits reverse transcriptase activity. It is more potent and less marrow toxic than

TABLE 9.15–8. ANTIRETROVIRAL THERAPY

Agents	Proposed Mechanism of Action	Toxicities
AZT (azidothymidine [Retrovir])	Dideoxynucleoside reverse transcriptase inhibitor	Anemia, leukopenia, headache, myalgia
Dideoxycytidine	Dideoxynucleoside reverse transcriptase inhibitor	Potentially less marrow toxic and more potent than AZT
Suramin	Reverse transcriptase inhibitor	Adrenal insufficiency, proteinuria, neutropenia
Ribavirin	Guanosine analogue that inhibits 5' capping of mRNA	Anemia, liver enzyme elevations
Foscarnet (Phosphonoformate)	Reverse transcriptase inhibitor	Renal toxicity
HPA 23	Polyanion competitive inhibitor of reverse transcriptase	Thrombocytopenia, liver enzyme elevations
Peptide T	? Inhibits viral attachment	Minimal reported toxicity
AL721	? Inhibits viral attachment	Minimal reported toxicity
Rifabutine	Reverse transcriptase inhibitor	Minimal reported toxicity
Ampligen	Mismatched double-stranded RNA	Minimal reported toxicity

retrovir; clinical trials utilizing this agent in the treatment of AIDS are presently underway.

Suramin was the first antiretroviral agent and first reverse transcriptase inhibitor described. Response to therapy with suramin was variable in a small clinical trial with occasional clinical improvements, but with no immunologic improvements, being noted.[3] Side effects associated with its use include fever, proteinuria, neutropenia, and adrenal insufficiency. It is probably ineffective as a single agent for treatment of HIV infection but may be useful in combination with immunomodulator therapy.

Ribavirin, a guanosine analogue with known activity against a wide variety of DNA and RNA viruses, has recently been shown to inhibit HIV replication in vitro. This drug acts to inhibit HIV replication primarily through interference with the guanylation step required for 5' capping of viral mRNA. Early clinical trials demonstrated a virustatic effect and minor clinical benefit in the treatment of symptomatic ARC and AIDS patients. The most prominent toxicities were anemia and hepatic enzyme elevations. In vitro, ribavirin has been shown to inhibit the antiviral effect of AZT on HIV replication.[27] Results of a large placebo-controlled study of this agent are pending, and it is currently not licensed for use in HIV infection.

Phosphonoformate or foscarnet is a reverse transcriptase inhibitor with in vitro antiretroviral activity. Renal toxicity is the most serious associated toxicity. Clinical trials using this agent in the treatment of AIDS are underway.

HPA 23 is a polyanion-competitive inhibitor of reverse transcriptase that was shown to be virustatic and associated with clinical stabilization in a small uncontrolled clinical trial.[25] As with foscarnet, clinical trials are still underway to determine its ultimate utility in the management of HIV infection.

Peptide T is a synthetically produced eight-amino acid sequence peptide that corresponds to a portion of the binding epitope within the gp 120 viral envelope protein. As this epitope mediates binding of the virus to the T4 antigen on lymphocytes,

blockade of this site by peptide T may interfere with subsequent attachment of the virus, thereby blocking infectivity. Although further clinical trials are planned, preliminary use in a small group of AIDS patients with HIV dementia syndrome was associated with immunologic and neurologic improvement and overall clinical stabilization.[29]

AL-721 is a novel lipid compound that inhibits HIV replication in vitro, possibly by extracting cholesterol from the lymphocyte membrane or by altering the lipid-containing viral envelope.[26] Either mechanism could result in inhibition of viral attachment. Clinical trials are underway.

Rifabutine is an antimycobacterial agent with in vitro activity against HIV. In other settings, it is well absorbed orally and has little toxicity. Its activity in the management of HIV is yet to be determined.

Ampligen is a mismatched double-stranded RNA molecule with antiretroviral activity and immunomodulatory and lymphokine stimulatory properties. In limited clinical trials it partially restored immunologic function and improved the clinical status of patients with serious HIV infections.[4,20]

IMMUNOLOGIC MODIFIERS

α-Interferon is a leukocyte-derived immunomodulatory glycoprotein that suppresses HIV replication, possibly by interfering with viral assembly and release (Table 9.15–9). In a clinical trial of α-interferon in Kaposi sarcoma, partial tumor responses were noted.[16] Side effects associated with high-dose therapy included fatigue, headache, fever, chills, and myalgias. Although probably not useful as a single agent, it may be beneficial in combination with antiretroviral agents.

γ-Interferon, a lymphokine that stimulates the intracellular killing capacity of blood monocytes, is deficient in AIDS patients. Although in vitro monocyte oxidative capacity was restored after incubation with γ-interferon, in vivo administration actually resulted in suppressed monocyte function.[14] It therefore probably has little role in the treatment of AIDS.

Interleukin-2 (IL-2) is a T-cell-derived growth factor that controls natural killer cell responses and T- and B-cell growth and dif-

TABLE 9.15–9. IMMUNOMODULATOR THERAPY IN AIDS

	Proposed Mechanism	Comments/ Toxicities
Immunologic Modifiers		
α-interferon	Immunomodulator and antiretroviral activity (may inhibit viral assembly and release)	Some antitumor effect in Karposi sarcoma; fever, headache, chills, myalgia
γ-interferon	In vitro stimulates defective monocyte oxidative killing capacity	Minimal benefit with in vivo use
Interleukin-2	In vitro restores defective natural killer cell responses; promotes differentiation and proliferation of T and B cells	Partial virustatic and antitumor responses in killer cells with in vivo use
Transplantation		
Thymic and bone marrow transplantation	Replace immunologically active cells	May be of benefit if combined with antiretroviral therapy

ferentiation. As with α-interferon, minor antitumor responses were associated with its use in Kaposi sarcoma patients.[24] The overall utility of IL-2 in the management of AIDS is unknown.

Attempts to replace the devastated immune system of the AIDS patient by implantation of cultured thymic fragments or bone marrow transplantation have met with limited success, possibly because of failure to control continued HIV replication.[9] Use of these techniques in combination with antiretroviral therapy may be beneficial.

AIDS VACCINE

Most of the current approaches to the development of an AIDS vaccine involve the use of a subunit as the immunogen.[1,11,13] This subunit generally represents a portion of the virus, such as the HIV viral envelope protein, which is known to be immunoreactive. Multiple methods of synthesis of this subunit are currently under investigation. Some methods use genetically engineered mammalian cells to synthesize the viral envelope protein, whereas other methods chemically synthesize these subunit proteins. Alternatively, viral protein can be directly purified from whole virus or can be incorporated into a recombinant vaccinia vector. Antiidiotypic vaccines also are being studied as potential AIDS vaccines.

REFERENCES

1. Barnes D: Strategies for an AIDS vaccine. Science 233:1149, 1986
2. Broder S (ed): AIDS: Modern Concepts and Therapeutic Challenges. New York, Marcel Dekker, 1986, p. 335
3. Broder S, Yarchoan R, et al: Effects of suramin on HTLV-III/LAV infection presenting as Kaposi's sarcoma or AIDS-related complex: Clinical pharmacology and suppression of virus replication in vivo. Lancet 2:627, 1985
4. Carter WA, Strayer DR, et al: Clinical, immunological, and virological effects of ampligen, a mismatched double-stranded RNA in patients with AIDS or AIDS related complex. Lancet 2:1286, 1987
5. Centers for Disease Control: Update: Acquired immunodeficiency syndrome—United States. MMWR 35:757, 1986
6. Coolfont Report: A PHS plan for prevention and control of AIDS and the AIDS virus. Public Health Rep 101:341, 1986
7. Cooper DA, Gold J, et al: Acute AIDS retrovirus infection. Lancet 1:537, 1985
8. Curran JW, Morgan WM, et al: The epidemiology of AIDS: Current status and future prospects. Science 29:1352, 1985
9. Danner SA, Schuirman H, et al: Implantation of cultured thymic fragments in patients with acquired immunodeficiency syndrome. Arch Intern Med 146:1133, 1986
10. DeVita VT, Broder S, et al: Developmental therapeutics and the acquired immunodeficiency syndrome. Ann Intern Med 106:568, 1987
11. Francis DP, Chin J: The prevention of acquired immunodeficiency syndrome in the United States. JAMA 257:1357, 1987
12. Francis DP, Jaffe HW, et al: The natural history of infection with the lymphadenopathy-associated virus/human T-lymphotropic virus type III. Ann Intern Med 103:719, 1985
13. Francis DP, Petricciani JC: The prospects for and pathways toward a vaccine for AIDS. N Engl J Med 229:1352, 1985
14. Gelmann EP, Preble OT, et al: Human lymphoblastoid interferon treatment of Kaposi's sarcoma in the acquired immune deficiency syndrome. Am J Med 78:737, 1985
15. Goedert JJ, Biggar RJ, et al: Three-year incidence of AIDS in five cohorts of HTLV-III-infected risk group members. Science 231:992, 1986
16. Groopman JE, Gottlieb MS, et al: Recombinant alpha-2 interferon therapy for Kaposi's sarcoma associated with the acquired immunodeficiency syndrome. Ann Intern Med 100:671, 1984
17. Guinan ME, Hardy A: Epidemiology of AIDS in women in the United States. JAMA 257:2039, 1987
18. Heterosexual transmission of human T-lymphotropic virus type III/lymphadenopathy-associated virus. MMWR 34:561, 1985
19. Mitsuya H, Broder S: Strategies for antiviral therapy in AIDS. Nature 325:773, 1987
20. Montefiori DC, Mitchell WM: Antiviral activity of mismatched double-stranded RNA against human immunodeficiency virus in vitro. Proc Natl Acad Sci 84:2985, 1987
21. Peterman TA, Jaffe HW, et al: Transfusion-associated immunodeficiency syndrome in the United States. JAMA 254:2913, 1985
22. Polk BF, Fox R, et al: Predictors of the acquired immunodeficiency syndrome developing in a cohort of seropositive homosexual men. N Engl J Med 316:61, 1987
23. Quinn TC, Mann JM, et al: AIDS in Africa: An epidemiologic paradigm. Science 234:955, 1986
24. Rook AH, Masur H, et al: Interleukin-2 enhances the depressed natural killer and cytomegalovirus specific cytotoxic activities of lymphocytes from patients with the acquired immune deficiency syndrome. J Clin Invest 72:398, 1983
25. Rozenbaum W, Dormont D, et al: Antimoniotungstate (HPA 23) treatment of three patients with AIDS and one with prodrome. Lancet 1:450, 1985
26. Sarin PS, Gallo RC, et al: Effects of a novel compound (AL721) on HTLV-III infectivity in vitro. N Engl J Med 313:1289, 1985
27. Vogt MW, Hartshorn KL, et al: Ribavirin antagonizes the effect of azidothymidine on HIV replication. Science 235:1376, 1987
28. Weiss SH, Goedert JJ, et al: Screening test for HTLV-III (AIDS agent) antibodies: Specificity, sensitivity and applications. JAMA 253:221, 1985
29. Wetterberg L, Alexius B, et al: Peptide T in treatment of AIDS. Lancet 1:159, 1987
30. Yarchoan R, Weinhold KJ, et al: Administration of 3' Azido 3' deoxythymidine, an inhibitor of HTLV-III/LAV replication to patients with AIDS or AIDS-related complex. Lancet 1:575, 1986
31. Young LS: Management of opportunistic infections complicating the acquired immunodeficiency syndrome. In Cooney T, Ward T (eds): AIDS and other medical problems in the male homosexual. Med Clin North Am 70:677, 1986
32. Wood RW, Collier A: Acquired immunodeficiency syndrome. Infect Dis Clin North Am 1:145, 1987

CHAPTER 9.16
Geographic Medicine

R. Bradley Sack

Natural barriers that once served efficiently to limit diseases to certain geographic areas are gradually being eliminated in the process of world development. Time, mountains, and oceans are being surmounted by rapid and frequent movement of persons throughout the world. Meanwhile, disease patterns are changing, often for unknown reasons, and therefore some of the older "classic" literature in tropical and geographic medicine is now chiefly of historical interest. For these reasons it is quite probable that physicians in the United States will be coming in increasing contact with diseases that are largely unfamiliar to them.[7]

These "obscure" diseases are, however, of major importance to the health of most of the world's population, and they provide

TABLE 9.16–1. TREATMENT REGIMENS FOR SELECTED PARASITIC INFECTIONS

Disease	Pathogen	Drug of Choice	Alternatives
Blood and Tissue Protozoa			
Malaria	*Plasmodium falciparum, P. vivax, P. malariae, P. ovale*	Chloroquine phosphate (PO) 1 g stat, 0.5 g in 6 hr, then 0.5 g daily × 2 days (total 2500 mg)	
All *plasmodia* except chloroquine-resistant *P. falciparum*		Chloroquine hydrochloride (IV) *or* quinidine gluconate (drug and dose schedules available from CDC)	
Chloroquine-resistant *P. falciparum*	*P. falciparum*	Quinine sulfate (650 mg PO tid × 3 days) *plus* pyrimethamine (25 mg PO bid × 3 days) *plus* sulfadiazine (500 mg PO qid × 5 days) Quinine dihydrochloride (IV) *or* quinidine gluconate (as above)	
Prevention of relapse	*P. vivax* and *P. ovale* only	Primaquine phosphate 15 mg base (26.3 mg/day × 14 days)	
African trypanosomiasis			
Early stages	*Trypanosoma gambiense, T. rhodesiense*	Suramin[a] (IV)	Pentamidine
Late CNS stage		Melarsoprol[a]	Tryparsamide plus suramin
American trypanosomiasis	*T. cruzi*	Nifurtimox[a] (PO)	None
Amebic meningoencephalitis	*Naegleria* sp.	Amphotericin B (IV)	None
Blood and Tissue Helminths			
Visceral larva migrans	*Toxocara canis*	*For severe symptoms only:* Diethylcarbamazine *or* thiabendazole *plus* prednisone	Mebendazole
Trichinosis	*Trichinella spiralis*	*For severe symptoms only:* Thiabendazole *plus* prednisone	Mebendazole
Filariasis	*Wuchereria bancrofti, Brugia malayi, Loa loa, Acanthocheilonema perstans*	Diethylcarbamazine	None
Onchocerciasis	*Onchocerca volvulus*	Diethylcarbamiazine followed by samurin[a]	Mebendazole
Schistosomiasis	*S. mansoni*	Praziquantel	Oxamniquine
	S. hematobium	Praziquantel	None
	S. japonicum	Praziquantel	None
Echinococciasis	*Echinococcus granulosus* and other species	Surgical excision of cysts	Mebendazole
Cysticercosis	*Taenia solium*	Praziquantel	Surgery
Intestinal Protozoa			
Amebiasis, asymptomatic	*Entamoeba histolytica*	Diiodohydroxyquin (650 mg PO tid × 20 days)	Diloxanide furoate or paromomycin
Mild to moderate intestinal disease		Metronidazole (750 mg PO tid × 10 days) *plus* diiodohydroxyquin (650 mg PO tid × 20 days)	Paromomycin
Severe intestinal disease		Metronidazole (750 mg PO tid × 10 days) *plus* diiodohydroxyquin (650 mg PO tid × 20 days)	Dehydroemetine *plus* diiodohydroxyquin *or* emetine *plus* diiodohydroxyquin
Hepatic abscess		Metronidazole (750 mg PO tid × 10 days) *plus* diiodohydroxyquin (650 mg PO tid × 20 days)	Dehydroemetine followed by chloroquine phosphate plus diiodohydroxyquin
Giardiasis	*Giardia lamblia*	Quinacrine hydrochloride (100 mg PO tid × 5 days)	Metronidazole, Furazolidone
Intestinal Helminths			
Ascariasis	*Ascaris lumbricoides*	Pyrantel pamoate (single dose of 11 mg/kg PO—maximum 1g) *or* mebendazole (100 mg PO bid × 3 days)	Piperazine citrate

(continued)

TABLE 9.16–1. TREATMENT REGIMENS FOR SELECTED PARASITIC INFECTIONS (Continued)

Disease	Pathogen	Drug of Choice	Alternatives
Intestinal Helminths (Cont.)			
Trichuriasis	*Trichuris trichiura*	Mebendazole (100 mg PO bid × 3 days)	None
Hookworm	*Necator americanus, Ancyclostoma duodenale*	Mebendazole *or* pyrantel pamoate (same doses as above)	None
Strongyloidiasis	*Strongyloides stercoralis*	Thiabendazole (25 mg/kg PO bid × 2 days)	None
Tapeworm infections	*Taenia saginata, T. solium*	Niclosamide† (single PO dose, 2 g) *or* praziquantel (10–20 mg/kg, once)	Paromomycin

ᵃAvailable from Center for Disease Control, Atlanta, Georgia.
Abstracted from Medical Letter 28:9–18, 1986.

fundamental insights into basic host-parasite relationships and microbial mechanisms of pathogenesis. As these diseases are now being studied more intensively with modern scientific methodologies, new methods of diagnosis and treatment are being developed; unfortunately, much of this information is outside the scope of knowledge of most U.S.-trained physicians and, therefore, is unavailable to the U.S. population that might benefit from it.

This chapter is written primarily for physicians in the United States who will, on occasion, have need to diagnose and treat these geographically determined illnesses. Some of the changing aspects of global infectious diseases will be discussed, as well as possible means to their diagnosis and treatment. Since specific details of each illness can be found from other sources, the primary aim here will be to heighten the physician's awareniess for these diseases.

CHANGING PATTERNS OF GEOGRAPHIC ILLNESSES

Patterns of disease spread may be readily observed, although the causative factors may not be understood. Epidemics of *Shigella* dysentery and typhoid fever caused by strains of bacteria carrying plasmids that confer multiple-drug resistance (R factors) have appeared and disappeared over a several year period in Central America and Southeast Asia. Diseases usually controlled through the provision of safe water and sewage disposal can suddenly appear when these become inadequate. The recent occurrence of cholera in the United States exemplifies this. Malaria resistant to chloroquine is spreading geographically and is important to physicians first encountering patients with this disease. Drug resistant tuberculosis, now highly prevalent in certain areas of Southeast Asia, may be encountered in persons arriving from these areas. Probably the major change in worldwide disease patterns has been the elimination of smallpox through intensive circumscribed vaccination efforts.

As new bacteria and viruses are discovered to be etiologic agents of infectious diseases, our understanding of their geographic niche gradually becomes clear. Lassa fever, first thought to be a rare, highly lethal disease, is now known to be a common, mild febrile illness in most persons who are infected. Rotavirus-mediated diarrheal disease, first discovered as a major cause of infantile diarrhea in temperate climates, is now known to have a worldwide distribution, including the tropics. Most recently AIDS, originally found almost exclusively in a few high-risk populations in the United States, is now known to be widely distributed in other distant geographic areas, notably central Africa.

Geographic foci of unusual diseases also exist in North America, such as those for plague (southwest), coccidioidomycosis (San Joaquin Valley in California), Rocky Mountain spotted fever (the southeastern seaboard), and even echinococcus (Alaska).

CHANGES IN THERAPY FOR GEOGRAPHIC ILLNESSES

Improvements in therapy for many of these diseases continue to be made, but may not be known to most physicians in the United States. Effective means for treating cholera that were developed in cholera-endemic areas were not practiced during some of the recent outbreaks of cholera in Europe and Africa resulting in an unacceptably high mortality rate. Many of the drugs now known to be effective for some of these geographically determined diseases are not available in the United States (Table 9.16–1).

DIAGNOSIS AND TREATMENT OF GEOGRAPHIC ILLNESSES

How then does the physician develop an enlightened awareness of these diseases? Probably the first, most important consideration is the recognition of a history of travel by the patient: to be aware that modern transportation can virtually place someone in almost any geographic area within hours and may (1) lead to unusual exposures and (2) bring the person to the United States well within the incubation period of most infectious diseases. For physicians in the United States then, it is important to recognize disease in travelers returning to the United States or in persons immigrating either temporarily (as students) or permanently to this country.[2,6]

Once a possible history of exposure through travel can be established, it is important to inquire specifically about exposures: animals, rural areas, insects (if known), and presumed sanitation of consumed food and water.

Then, of course, it is necessary to know which diseases are endemic to the area and their seasons of transmission. Since this information is constantly changing, standard texts may be inadequate for this purpose. This up-to-date information is most readily available through two sources: the Centers for Disease Control *Morbidity and Mortality Weekly Report* and the *Weekly Epidemiologic Record of the World Health Organization*. Obviously, disease patterns do not conform to political units, the basis on which these reports are prepared, and it is necessary to realize the importance of broad ecologic regions, common because of their general aspects of geography and climate.[2] A summary of some of these diseases is given in Table 9.16–2. Fortunately, most diseases of travelers, because they are caused by viruses or enteric pathogens, are self-limited and may require no specific therapy.

Specific diagnosis of these diseases, once suspected through a history of travel or exposure, and a physical examination, which may be helpful (and can be diagnostic in some situations), can be made through (1) isolation and identification of the pathogen from

TABLE 9.16–2. INFECTIONS THAT MAY POSE A SERIOUS HEALTH HAZARD TO TRAVELERS OR PERSONS LIVING IN SELECTED GEOGRAPHIC REGIONS OR SUBJECT TO EXPOSURE IN CERTAIN ENVIRONMENTAL SITUATIONS

Disease	Pathogen	Usual Mode of Transmission	Incubation Period (days)	Laboratory Diagnosis	Primary Geographic Location
Viral, Chlamydial, and Rickettsial					
Lassa fever	Lassa fever virus	Not known	~14	Viral isolation, Ab titers	Africa
Yellow fever	Yellow fever virus	Vectors (mosquitoes)	3–6	Liver biopsy, viral isolation	Central Africa, South Africa
Hemorrhagic fever	Tickborne arboviruses, dengue virus, arenaviruses, Marburg agent, etc.	Vectors (ticks, mosquitoes), contact	Variable	Viral isolation, Ab titer, EM for Marburg agent	Worldwide; individual species often localized to select geographic areas
Viral encephalitis	Many arboviruses, herpesvirus, myxoviruses, enteroviruses, etc.	Vectors (mosquitoes), airborne, fecal, oral	3–10 or longer	Viral isolation, Ab titer	Worldwide; individual species often localized to select geographic areas
Rabies	Rabies virus	Contact (animal bites)	10 to much longer (months)	Viral isolation, Ab titer, brain biopsy	Worldwide
Hepatitis A	Hepatitis A virus	Fecal-oral	15–45	Liver biopsy, enzymes, Ab titer	Worldwide
Hepatitis B	Hepatitis B virus	Contact (blood)	45–180	Liver biopsy, antigen and Ab detection, enzymes	Worldwide
Typhus	*Rickettsia prowazekii*	Vectors (lice, fleas)	7–15	Ab titer (including Weil-Felix)	Worldwide
Spotted fever	*R. rickettsi*, etc	Vectors (ticks)	3–12	Ab titer (including Weil-Felix)	Eastern U.S.
Scrub typhus	*Rickettsia tsutsugamushi*	Vectors (mites)	6–12	Ab titer (including Weil-Felix)	Southeast Asia
Bacterial and Fungal					
Epidemic meningitis	*Neisseria meningitidis*	Airborne	Variable	CSF examination, culture	Africa, South America
Diphtheria	*Corynebacterium diphtheriae*	Airborne	1–7	Culture	Worldwide
Anthrax	*Bacillus anthracis*	Contact (animals, soil), airborne	1–7	Exudate, examination, culture	Worldwide
Plague	*Francisella pestis*	Vectors (fleas), airborne	1–12	Exudate, examination, culture	Worldwide, southwestern U.S., Southeast Asia
Cholera	*Vibrio cholerae*	Waterborne, foodborne	1–3	Culture, stool examination	Asia, Africa
Typhoid and paratyphoid	*Salmonella sp.*	Fecal-oral, waterborne	3–15 or longer	Culture, Ab titer	Worldwide, developing countries
Bacillary dysentery	*Shigella* sp.	Fecal-oral, waterborne	1–2	Culture	Worldwide, developing countries
Enterotoxic diarrhea	*Escherichia coli*, enterotoxigenic	Fecal-oral, foodborne	1–2	Culture	Worldwide, developing countries
Melioidosis	*Pseudomonas pseudomallei*	Contact (soil), airborne	2 or longer	Culture	Southeast Asia
Bartonellosis	*Bartonella bacilliformis*	Vectors (sandflies)	7–14	Culture, blood examination	Andes Mountains
Leptospirosis	*Leptospira* sp.	Waterborne, contact (animal urine)	2–20	Culture, Ab titer	Worldwide
Relapsing fever	*Borrelia* sp.	Vectors (lice, ticks)	4–18	Blood examination (Giemsa)	Africa, worldwide
Leprosy	*Mycobacterium leprae*	Contact (personal, soil?)	Variable but long (months)	Skin snip or blood examination	Worldwide
Tuberculosis	*M. tuberculosis*	Airborne, food (dairy products)	Variable	Sputum or exudate examination, culture, biopsy	Worldwide

(continued)

TABLE 9.16–2. INFECTIONS THAT MAY POSE A SERIOUS HEALTH HAZARD TO TRAVELERS OR PERSONS LIVING IN SELECTED GEOGRAPHIC REGIONS OR SUBJECT TO EXPOSURE IN CERTAIN ENVIRONMENTAL SITUATIONS (Continued)

Disease	Pathogen	Usual Mode of Transmission	Incubation Period (days)	Laboratory Diagnosis	Primary Geographic Location
Bacterial and Fungal (Cont.)					
Coccidiodomycosis	Coccidioides immitis	Airborne (soil)	Variable	Sputum examination (KOH), culture	Southwestern U.S.
Protozoan					
Falciparum malaria	Plasmodium falciparum	Vectors (anopheline mosquitoes)	10–14	Blood examination (Giemsa)	Tropics
Vivax malaria	P. vivax	Vectors (anopheline mosquitoes)	10–14	Blood examination (Giemsa)	Tropics
Quartan malaria	P. malariae	Vectors (anopheline mosquitoes)	18–42	Blood examination (Giemsa)	Tropics
Kala azar	Leishmania donovani	Vectors (sandflies)	60 to much longer (months)	Bone marrow and blood, splenic biopsy	Tropics
African sleeping sickness	Trypanosoma brucei	Vectors (tsetse flies)	14 or longer	Blood, LN, and CSF examination (Giemsa)	Tropical Africa
Chagas disease	Trypanosoma cruzi	Vectors (reduviid bugs)	Variable	Blood and marrow examinations (Giemsa) biopsy	South America
Amebiasis	Entamoeba histolytica	Waterborne, fecal-oral	Variable	Stool, exudate, or tissue examination	Worldwide
Giardiasis	Giardia lamblia	Waterborne, fecal-oral	Variable	Stool or duodenal aspirate examination	Worldwide
Cryptosporidiasis	Cryptosporidium	Waterborne, fecal-oral	Variable	Stool, stain	Worldwide
Helminthic					
Strongyloidiasis	Strongyloides stercoralis	Contact (soil)	Variable	Stool or duodenal aspirate examination	Worldwide
Eosinophilic meningitis	Angiostrongylus cantonensis, etc.	Food (snails, shrimp)	Variable	CSF examination	South Pacific
Filariasis	Wuchereria bancrofti, Brugia malayi, Onchocerca volvulus, Dipetalonema sp.	Vectors (mosquitoes, black-flies, etc.)	Variable but long (months)	Blood, urine, effusion, LN or skin snip examination	Tropics
Schistosomiasis	Schistosoma mansoni, S. haematobium, S. japonicum	Contact (water containing cercariae from snail host)	30–60	Stool or urine examination, rectal biopsy, Ab titer	Tropics
Paragonimiasis	Paragonimus westermani	Food (crabs, etc.)	Variable (months)	Sputum and stool examination biopsy	Far East
Echinococciasis	Echinococcus sp.	Fecal-oral (dog feces)	Variable (months)	Ab titer, fluid examination (surgically resected cyst, non aspirate)	Worldwide

body fluids or tissues and (2) specific immunologic responses to the pathogen. In some cases, it is necessary to treat on the suspicion of a specific diagnosis, since laboratory confirmation may not be available for many days. Such is the case with diphtheria or rickettsial diseases such as Rocky Mountain spotted fever or suspected drug-resistant malaria.

Laboratory tests are constantly being improved and current literature must be consulted for the most recent ones. Appropriate types of laboratory examinations for diagnosis are also listed in Table 9.16–2.

LABORATORY EXAMINATIONS

CULTURES AND MICROSCOPIC EXAMINATIONS

The most common presentations of patients who have recently been in the developing world are diarrhea, fever, skin lesions, or the report of eosinophilia on a routine laboratory report. The diagnosis of these relatively nonspecific syndromes will depend to a large degree on the clinical laboratory. The differential diagnosis will of ne-

cessity be based on the travel history and exposures; once this has been formulated, the appropriate laboratory examinations can be done.

Cultures for bacteria and fungi, and cell count and differential from body fluids, can often be diagnostic.[7] In addition, special examinations for larger parasitologic forms may be indicated. Sources of these diagnostic materials include:

Blood

Thick blood films, hemolyzed and stained by Giemsa or Fields methods, facilitate detection of malaria parasites, hemoflagellates, and microfilariae; identification can then be made in corresponding well-stained thin films. When malaria is suspected, multiple blood smears should be examined at 6- to 12-hour intervals, regardless of the fever pattern.

Bone Marrow

Culturing of bone marrow is the most sensitive technique for diagnosing typhoid fever and brucellosis.

Urine, Pleural, and Ascitic Fluids

Search of centrifuged sediment from body fluids may sometimes reveal filarial worms or their microfilariae.

Cerebrospinal Fluid

Certain amebae that are usually free living (members of the genera *Naegleria* and *Acanthamoeba*) may be isolated from the CSF of patients with primary amebic meningoencephalitis. Trypanosomes are present in the CSF during the later stages of African sleeping sickness. Subadult rat lungworms, *Angiostrongylus cantonensis,* may occasionally be aspirated from the subarachnoid space of human patients with eosinophilic meningitis caused by this parasite.

Tissue Aspirates and Biopsy Material

Skin snips, slits, or needle aspirates from the advancing margin of skin lesions, as in the diagnosis of leprosy, may be useful also in demonstrating the etiologic agents of cutaneous leishmaniasis, onchocerciasis, streptocerciasis, creeping eruption (due to canine hookworm larvae), scabies, and other cutaneous parasitic infections. Lymph node aspirates or biopsy may reveal trypanosomes or *Toxoplasma gondii;* adult filarial worms may be found on dissection or sectioning of lymph nodes from patients with bancroftian or Malayan filariasis. When searching for protozoal parasites in fresh biopsy material (lymph nodes, liver, bone marrow, lung, or other), stained tissue impressions greatly facilitate the examination and should be made in addition to the usual fixed tissue sections. Helminths are difficult to identify in tissue sections. Although an experienced parasitologist may easily recognize the higher taxonomic category to which the parasite belongs, the species may be impossible to determine. It is wise to preserve a portion of fresh tissue for crush preparations between glass slides or for tearing apart under a dissecting microscope in an effort to recover whole worms or identifiable large fragments. Biopsy of a rectal valve margin may be a useful maneuver in diagnosing schistosomal infections, especially *Schistosoma mansoni.*

Feces

Routine bacteriologic examination for *Shigella* and *Salmonella* may be rewarding, but the most common cause of travelers' diarrhea, enterotoxigenic *Escherichia coli,* cannot be identified except by special techniques not now routinely available. Other specific pathogens, such as riones, *Cryptosporidia,* and *Campylobacter,* require special media for their isolation.

Intestinal protozoa and helminths are usually detected by the presence of diagnostic stages in the stools. These include the motile trophozoites or thin walled cysts of protozoa and the eggs, larvae, or adult stages of helminths, the latter either entire or as detached segments (tapeworm proglottids). Because of the enormous disparity in size of these objects, varying from several meters for the larger tapeworms and about 30 cm for a mature ascarid worm to protozoa smaller than an erythrocyte, stool examination must be conducted at several levels of magnification. After careful gross inspection, fecal suspensions in saline are scanned methodically under low-power light microscopy and critical identification is then made under higher power (including the $100\times$ oil immersion lens for stained protozoa).

Loose, watery specimens that may contain actively motile amebic trophozoites containing ingested red blood cells should be examined promptly; specimens kept at room temperature longer than one-half hour will usually show only inactive, rounded-up precystic stages that are quite nondiagnostic. Fresh diarrheal specimens that cannot be examined immediately should be preserved in polyvinyl alcohol solution in vials and on slides prepared for permanent staining.

All specimens should be examined in warm saline coverslip preparations, supplemented by iodine- or methiolate-iodine-stained suspensions for identification of protozoal cysts.

Formed stool specimens, kept under refrigeration (not frozen) if examination is delayed more than a few hours, should also be examined by using one of the techniques for concentration of protozoal cysts and helminth eggs.

Even when concentration techniques are used to full advantage, detection of intestinal parasites is enhanced by examining a series of specimens (usually three or more) collected on different days from each individual patient. Examination of sigmoidoscopic curettings from suspected amebic ulcers aids in finding trophozoites of *Entamoeba histolytica;* material from the wall of abscesses in liver or other tissue, from the margin of abdominal or perineal skin ulcers, or from sputum may provide evidence of extraintestinal amebiasis. (Cultures of *E. histolytica* are feasible in commercially available media but cannot supplant meticulous microscopic examination.) Duodenal fluid (obtained easily by string capsules) may sometimes contain motile trophozoites of *Giardia lamblia* of rhabditiform larvae of *Strongyloides stercoralis* when examination of the feces has failed to reveal the infection.

IMMUNOLOGIC TESTS

Serology may provide the only diagnostic evidence of infection due to viruses and rickettsiae. In most bacterial and parasitic diseases, identification of the organisms rather than serology will be of most importance. Through the development of highly specific, refined antigens and reliably sensitive techniques (especially fluorescent-antibody staining, gel-diffusion methods and ELISA techniques, serodiagnosis has become useful and practical in the recognition of several important parasitic infections. Although of greater value in surveys of disease prevalence than in individual case diagnosis, immunologic tests are currently available for diagnosis of malaria, amebiasis, American trypanosomiasis (Chagas disease), trichinosis, cysticercosis, and echinococcosis. The results of all serologic tests should be interpreted critically and used with discrimination in the individual patient whose "positive" test may reflect prior exposure rather than active disease. Titers of acute and convalescent sera must always be determined to identify recent exposure to the etiologic agent.

BIOHAZARDS

Attending physicians, nurses, and laboratory personnel may be at considerable risk in handling fresh specimens and living cultures taken from patients with undiagnosed disease contracted in other parts of the world. The well-documented experiences with smallpox and with the virus of Lassa fever and other related arenaviruses afforded telling examples of the hazard even to highly trained persons. Hepatitis, rabies, most arboviral and rickettsial diseases, psittacosis, anthrax, coccidioidomycosis (infectious arthrospores), plague, and tularemia may be dangerous to the unwary. Attempts

to isolate the causative organism should be made only by experienced workers with special high-containment laboratory facilities.

TREATMENT OF GEOGRAPHIC ILLNESSES

The treatment of bacterial, mycobacterial, fungal, and viral illnesses has been discussed elsewhere in the text. Treatment of common parasitic infections, for example pinworm and ascarid infections in children, may be relatively safe and straightforward. Therapy of the less familiar parasitic diseases, however, may require medications that are seldom used and may be toxic. The initial decision of whether to treat or not must be weighed carefully. Attention must be given to age, body size, nutritional status, and intercurrent disease when deciding the therapeutic regimen. Consultation should be sought if experience is lacking.[1,4,7]

Current therapeutic recommendations for the most important protozoal and helminthic infections are given in Table 9.16–1 with dosages appropriate for adults in otherwise good health. Dosages for children and debilitated adults should be determined with due care. Some immunobiologic and chemotherapeutic agents are currently available only through the Centers for Disease Control, and this agency should be consulted regarding the use of these drugs.

PREVENTION OF GEOGRAPHIC ILLNESSES

In addition to being able to recognize disease in persons traveling from areas where these diseases may be acquired, physicians should also be able to give advice about prevention of some of these illnesses to persons traveling abroad, particularly to developing countries.[2,7] Advice to travelers for prophylaxis should include the following:

1. *Avoidance of fresh fruits and vegetables (unless peeled) in all areas where sanitation is in question.*
2. *Care in drinking only water that can be ascertained as being potable.*
3. *Immunizations appropriate to the geographic areas.* The major required immunization for travel now is yellow fever. A few countries still require cholera vaccination, although there is no rational basis for doing so. Effective vaccines are available against diphtheria, tetanus, poliomyelitis, and typhoid and should be given as necessary (either as primary or booster immunizations) to travelers to the developing world. Additional immunizations (rabies, hepatitis B, meningococcus, Japanese encephalitis) should be considered for travelers who may experience special risks.
4. *Passive protection against hepatitis A,* which can be given with globulin injections immediately prior to travel. This should be considered for all travelers to the developing world. The suggested dose for adults is 2 ml intramuscularly for a visit less than 3 months and 5 ml for a longer stay.
5. *Malaria prophylaxis for persons traveling to areas known to have malaria.* Chloroquine is the drug to be used in all malarious areas. The standard chloroquine regimen is 500 mg (300 mg base) once weekly beginning 1 week before arrival until 6 weeks after leaving the endemic area. Short-term travelers

to areas with chloroquine-resistant *Plasmodium falciparum* (these are continually expanding) should also take with them an emergency treatment dose of Fansidar (3 tablets) to use if symptoms of malaria develop while taking chloroquine. Long-term visitors to these areas also may take Fansidar (1 tablet, which contains 25 mg pyrimethamine and 500 mg sulfadoxine) on a regular weekly basis along with chloroquine. Severe adverse reactions have been noted with Fansidar, and its use is not recommended routinely. Primaquine (15 mg base) given daily for 14 days during the last 2 weeks of chloroquine prophylaxis is only recommended for long-term visitors leaving areas endemic with *P. vivax* and *P. ovale,* to prevent relapses.

6. *Diarrhea prophylaxis for short-term travelers.* Because of the known adverse effects of the drugs, routine prophylaxis is not indicated. In specific instances, however, for short term travel of less than 3 weeks, in which the travelers are willing to accept these risks, doxycycline (100 mg daily with food) or trimethoprim-sulfamethoxazole (1 double strength tablet daily) can be used, which will prevent most (70 to 80 percent) cases of travelers' diarrhea.

   For most travelers, early treatment of travelers' diarrhea is the preferred method; travelers must carry the medication with them and be instructed in how and when to use it. This consists of (1) replacement of fluids lost in the stool by glucose-electrolyte packets, which are commercially available, (2) the use of antimotility agents or bismuth-subsalicylate for mild symptomatic treatment if desired, and (3) the use of antimicrobials for specific therapy of moderate to severe diarrhea. The latter (trimethoprim-sulfamethoxazole, 1 double-strength tablet bid, or doxycycline, 100 mg bid) given for 3 days will shorten the illness to one of only 24 to 36 hours duration, rather than 3 to 4 days if not treated.

7. *General instructions about avoiding known hazards, such as swimming in fresh water in areas endemic for schistosomiasis.*

REFERENCES

1. Drugs for parasitic infections. Med Lett Drugs Ther 28:9, 1986
2. DuPont HL, Reves RR, et al: Treatment of travelers' diarrhea with trimethoprim/sulfamethoxazole and with trimethoprim alone. N Engl J Med 307:841, 1982
3. Health Information for International Travel 1985: U.S. Department of Health and Human Services Publication No. (CDC) 85-8280. Atlanta, Georgia, Centers for Disease Control
4. Immunizations and Chemoprophylaxis for travelers. Med Lett Drugs Ther 27:33, 1985
5. Sack RB: Treatment and prevention of travelers' diarrhea. In Holmgren J, Lindberg A, Mollby R (eds): Development of Vaccines Against Diarrhea, 11th Nobel Conf., Stockholm, 1985, p 289, Studenlitteratur, Lund, Sweden, 1986 (A comprehensive review of all controlled studies of prophylaxis and treatment.)
6. Vaccination Certificate Requirements and Health Advice for International Travel: Situation as on 1 January 1986. Geneva, Switzerland, World Health Organization
7. Warren KS, Mahmoud AAF: Tropical and Geographical Medicine. New York, McGraw-Hill, 1984

Disturbances in water and electrolyte metabolism are produced by a variety of factors, some intrinsic and some extrinsic, which affect the intake, output, or distribution of water and electrolytes. They may be the primary cause of illness, but more commonly they occur as by-products of some other disorder. Their recognition in some cases depends upon the detection of such obvious manifestations as edema or dehydration, but in other cases they are brought to light only by physical or chemical measurements. Alertness to the possible presence of these disorders in particular clinical settings facilitates early correct diagnosis. These settings are those in which either (1) the normal regulating mechanisms are upset by disease or (2) the fluid losses or excesses are so great that even normal regulating mechanisms cannot cope with them. Successful management depends upon (1) a correct diagnosis, (2) accurate quantitative information concerning the magnitude of the deficit or surplus to be corrected, and (3) a working knowledge of the principles underlying the regulation of water and electrolytes.

Appropriate identification and management of these problems require that the physician recognize that they are not unique diseases but rather occur as manifestations of a great many diseases or disorders and that their rate of development and severity are often determined by the disease setting in which they occur. The diagnosis and treatment of the underlying disease is, as always, dependent upon a careful evaluation of the history, physical examination, and laboratory data.

A semiquantitative estimate of the state of over- or underhydration can usually be made from careful analysis of information obtained from the history when adequate historical data are available. This estimate can be supplemented by the physical signs of abnormal hydration. Intelligent recruitment of information from blood and urine examinations should permit more accurate recognition and quantification of water or salt disturbances.

The physician then pays attention to correction of the specific disturbances of water and electrolyte balance. General principles in the management of water and electrolyte disturbances will be emphasized in this section, with presentation of specific illustrative cases in Chapter 10.4 accompanied by a discussion of therapeutic management.

The physician should determine to what degree the patient's regulating mechanisms can be relied upon for assistance in correcting the disturbance. In particular, the physician should assess the functional capacity of the cardiovascular system, especially to gauge how safely and at what rate water and salt can be administered without provoking congestive heart failure. This estimation of function can be very simple; adequate evaluation is accomplished by a careful history and physical examination that includes assessment of venous pressure. This appraisal is repeated as often as necessary during the course of fluid therapy, that is, the patient is examined several times a day for signs of early failure. The presence of pulmonary rales is an important sign, since increased venous pressure, hepatomegaly, and edema may not appear until later.

The physician should also assess *renal function*. The first step is to be sure that the patient can eliminate urine. If there is no spontaneous urination, the bladder is percussed, and if it is enlarged, urine should be obtained by catheterization for the determination of specific gravity and examination of the urinary sediment.

In the following chapters disturbances of water, sodium, potassium, and pH will be considered. Although each of these is first considered separately as though each were an isolated abnormality with all other constituents normal, they are in fact so interrelated that isolated disturbances occur rarely. It is important therefore to reconstruct the events that beset the patient and to disentangle from them the basic defect that set the disturbance in motion so that one can see clearly what alteration needs most urgent correction. It is the aim of this section to guide the physician to that goal.

REFERENCES

1. Brenner BM, Rector FC Jr (eds): The Kidney, 3d ed. Philadelphia, WB Saunders, 1986
2. Kurtzman NA, Martinez-Maldonado M (eds): Pathophysiology of the Kidney. Springfield, Ill, Charles C Thomas, 1977
3. Moore FD, Oleson KH, et al: The Body Cell Mass and Its Supporting Environment. Philadelphia, WB Saunders, 1963 (A compilation of data on variations in fluid and electrolyte content of the body in health and disease.)
4. Schrier RW (ed): Renal and Electrolyte Disorders, 3d ed. Boston, Little, Brown, 1986
5. Valtin H: Renal Dysfunction: Mechanisms Involved in Fluid and Solute Balance. Boston, Little, Brown, 1979
6. Wesson LG: Physiology of the Human Kidney. New York, Grune & Stratton, 1969 (A valuable source text for studies in man.)

CHAPTER 10.1
Disturbances of Water and Sodium Metabolism

W. Gordon Walker and William E. Mitch

Water is the chief constituent of the body, representing about 60 percent of body weight. Disturbances in the amount and distribution of body water are both serious and common. Frequently, however, these are unrecognized, often to the detriment of the patient. Three aspects contribute to the failure of early recognition. First, these disturbances are encountered much more frequently as a complication of some underlying disease than as isolated deficits in otherwise healthy individuals. Second, reliable physical signs develop relatively late in water balance disturbances; thus major emphasis must be placed upon careful historical evaluation of the patient's status, and many patients who are at high risk for the development of water disturbances may be unable to give a reliable history. Third, the regulation of body water content is very closely linked physiologically to the regulation of body sodium content, and separate identification and quantitation of changes in these two major constituents of the body is often difficult, requiring skillful interpretation of historical information, physical findings, and laboratory data.

In this chapter the physiology of water regulation is considered together with isolated disturbances in water balance, and this is followed by consideration of the physiology of sodium regulation and disturbances in sodium balance. Finally, the interaction between these two is considered, and the clinical and laboratory findings which are of value in diagnosis and management are reviewed.

PHYSIOLOGIC ASPECTS OF WATER METABOLISM IN MAN

DISTRIBUTION OF BODY WATER[2,10,17,21]

Approximately two thirds of the water is located within the cells, and the remaining one third is extracellular (Fig. 10.1–1). Water moves freely back and forth across virtually all cellular membranes and across the capillaries that separate the intravascular water from that of the interstitial fluid. This unrestricted movement of water allows for rapid establishment and maintenance of osmotic equilibrium between the interstitial compartment of body water and that fraction of the body water within cells in response to gain or loss of either water or solutes. This freedom of movement of water is not shared by the major solutes of the body. Sodium and its anions occupy a position that is almost exclusively extracellular, while potassium and its attendant anions are largely confined to the intracellular compartment. As a consequence, the distribution of water reflects the distribution of solute within and outside the cells, and it is the quantity of solute within and outside the cells that governs the volume of cellular and extracellular water. There are approximately 4000 mOsm (mainly sodium chloride and sodium bicarbonate) occupying the extracellular space and approximately 8000 mOsm (largely potassium and anions) in the intracellular space.

Because of the marked disparity between the permeance exhibited by water and that by the major solutes of body fluid, osmotic equilibrium is achieved by water shifts between the extracellular and intracellular compartments. Thus, loss of water, as for example during prolonged sweating, represents water lost initially from the plasma and extracellular fluid. This water loss within the extracellular compartment, however, results in a corresponding increase in solute concentration in this compartment. The water within the cell then exists at a higher concentration than in the extracellular fluid, and consequently a water shift from within the cell to the extracellular fluid occurs until osmotic equilibrium is reestablished and the total solute concentration (osmolality) is identical inside and outside the cell (Fig. 10.1–2). Similarly, if sodium is lost in excess of water from the extracellular compartment, the solute concentration falls in this compartment, resulting in a shift of water into the cells to reestablish osmotic equilibrium; excess intracellular potassium loss results in a corresponding shift in the opposite direction. Such fluid shifts operate to maintain osmotic equilibrium across the cellular membrane in the normal state as well as in a wide variety of abnormal conditions.

The rate at which osmotic equilibrium is reestablished between plasma and interstitial fluid is much more rapid than that between cellular water and interstitial fluid. A new steady state between plasma and interstitial fluid is usually achieved within one-half hour after disruption of osmotic equilibrium, but reestablishment of osmotic equilibrium between cellular and interstitial fluid may require more than 3 to 4 hours.

REGULATION OF BODY WATER[1,4,10,18,19,23]

The two effector mechanisms responsible for regulation of the volume of body water are thirst, which regulates water intake, and the level of circulating antidiuretic hormone (ADH), which controls the volume of urine output. Both effects are modulated by a chain of events arising from alterations in plasma osmolality or plasma volume or from changes in osmolality and volume in some compartment of body fluid that is directly and closely related to plasma volume and osmolality. As illustrated in Figure 10.1–3, both thirst and ADH release are altered by changes in either osmolality or volume. Under ordinary physiologic conditions, plasma osmolality is the variable most closely regulated; changes of less than 2 percent are capable of altering plasma ADH levels from minimal to maximal values. The body water of a healthy individual continually oscillates between a narrow range of slight excess and slight deficit as a result of the operation of these control mechanisms (Table 10.1–1, Fig. 10.1–4). This physiologic regulation is achieved primarily through osmoreceptor-mediated ADH control and associated thirst regulation in normal subjects, with volume regulation making only a minor contribution.

The effectiveness of the kidney in conserving water results from its capacity to produce a urine that is hypertonic to plasma in response to ADH.[23] The mechanism by which the urine is concentrated in response to the stimulus of ADH is presented in detail in Chapter 11.1. Since this mechanism is activated by ADH released after only a modest water deficit has occurred, it serves to retard the rate of further water loss. Concomitant stimulation of the thirst mechanism leads to increased water intake, which repairs the deficit.

The individual can tolerate disturbances in ADH release much better than disturbances in the thirst mechanism. In the absence of ADH the kidney excretes large volumes of dilute urine, with daily output often exceeding 6 to 8 L. The resultant persistent thirst easily increases intake to equal this loss. In the absence of a normally functioning thirst mechanism, such a rate of loss can lead to development of a severe water deficit in only a few hours. Any disorder that interferes with intake, such as disturbance of consciousness, disorientation in the elderly, etc., effectively disrupts the thirst mechanism and removes the most important defense against development of water deficit. Disturbances of either mechanism, however, can lead to serious and at times life-threatening abnormalities in water balance.

Volume-mediated stimuli that produce ADH release and sustain thirst may play a prominent and at times dominant role in some of the disturbances encountered in the regulation of body water. The volume-sensitive regulatory mechanism (Fig. 10.1–3)

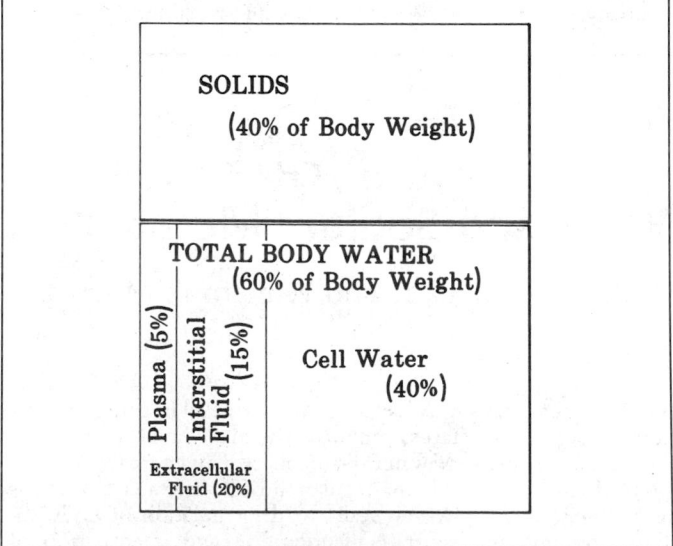

Figure 10.1–1. Distribution of body water.

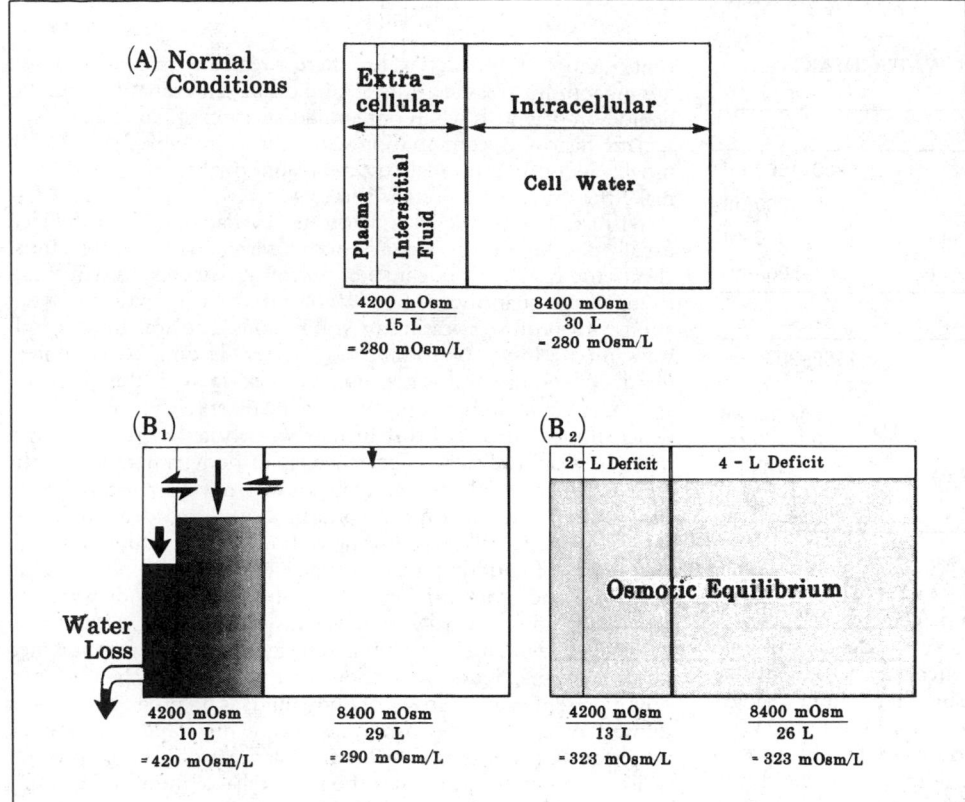

Figure 10.1–2. A. Compartments of body water under normal conditions are shown. Extracellular fluid compartment is composed of interstitial water plus plasma water. Relative size of intracellular and extracellular compartments is determined by total solute content of each compartment. **B_1, B_2.** Sequence of changes that result from water loss (6 L) from body compartments without accompanying solute loss (as, for example, in diabetes insipidus) is illustrated. Initial loss in urine represents loss of fluid delivered to kidney by blood. This loss is rapidly shared by interstitial fluid, resulting in rapid drop in total extracellular fluid volume and corresponding increase in solute concentration in ECF. Marked difference between intracellular and extracellular solute concentration resulting from this ECF water loss results in slower shift of water from intracellular to extracellular compartment **(B_1)**. This shift continues until solute concentrations are again equal. At this point loss is shared by both ECF and ICF **(B_2)**. Distribution of deficit is determined by proportion of solute inside and outside cell; 4-L deficit is intracellular and 2-L deficit extracellular.

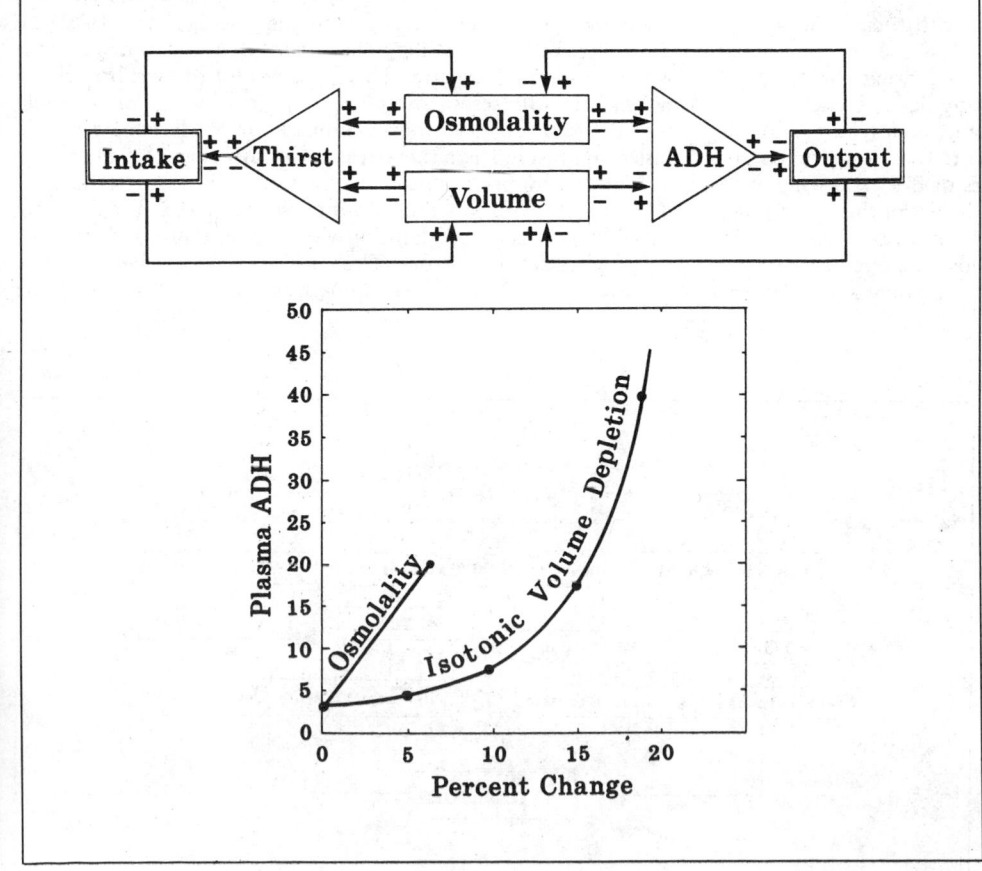

Figure 10.1–3. Regulatory mechanisms controlling body water. Two variables sensed to provide feedback signal are osmolality and volume of body fluids. Graph below summarizes experimental data indicating linear increase in ADH in plasma with small increases in plasma osmolality.[19] In the human this type of change results in maximal urinary concentration when plasma osmolality increases about 1 percent. When volume changes occur in absence of changes in osmolality, stimulus for ADH release is negligible with small changes but becomes much more marked with larger changes in volume and may in fact serve to override stimulus which results from osmolality changes when the two operate in opposing directions. This persistent stimulus to ADH release, which results from presence of persistent volume deficit, can lead to hypoosmolality and hyponatremia as result of persistent volume deficit.

TABLE 10.1–1. USUAL DAILY SOURCES OF WATER INTAKE AND LOSS FOR THE AVERAGE ADULT

Intake	
Fluid intake	1200–1800 ml
Water content of ingested food	700–1000 ml
Water of oxidation	250–300 ml
Total	2000–3000 ml
Output	
Urine	1500–2000 ml
Insensible loss	
Skin	300–600 ml
Lungs	200–400 ml
Gastrointestinal loss (water content of feces)	100 ml
Total	2000–3000 ml

does not play a significant role until volume changes (deficits) approach or exceed 5 percent. Since this is a greater change in volume of body compartments than is ordinarily encountered under usual physiologic circumstances, it is not surprising that volume changes influence day-to-day fluctuations in water balance very little. With changes much in excess of 5 percent, however, the influence of the volume-mediated stimulus assumes a dominant role and may completely override osmoreceptor-mediated stimuli.[7,18]

RECOGNITION OF WATER DEFICITS AND EXCESSES[1,2,5,10,18]

CLINICAL FEATURES OF WATER DEFICITS

The clinical features of water deficit vary with the severity of the deficit. In the conscious and alert patient, loss of 1 to 2 percent of the body water produces severe and unrelenting thirst. Quite often, however, in the disorders where water deficit is encountered clinically, the patient is disoriented for some other reason, and this important symptom may not be apparent. It is common to encounter patients who have water deficits of 5 to 7 percent who exhibit no identifiable physical signs of a deficit of this magnitude. This is particularly true in the elderly, in whom the inelastic skin and the changes of aging make recognition of altered skin turgor difficult. With a greater degree of water loss, approaching 10 per-

cent or more of the body water, there is regularly poor skin turgor, dry mucous membranes, stupor, and ultimately coma. Despite difficulties in diagnosis when only mild deficits exist, careful and systematic history documentation, as outlined in Table 10.1–2, will usually identify abnormal losses or abnormalities in intake that make the existence of a deficit likely.

Isolated water deficits, without associated sodium deficits, usually develop slowly over a period of several days and are almost always the result of poor intake, except in diabetes insipidus. Although large quantities of body water may be lost rapidly in association with profuse sweating or voluminous diarrhea, these are always mixed losses of sodium and water, leading to combined deficits of sodium and water discussed elsewhere in this chapter.

Changes in body weight provide the most reliable physical evidence in support of a disturbance in water balance. Acute changes in body weight always reflect changes in body water. When the patient's usual weight is accurately known, a weight at the time of the physical examination can confirm a suspected deficit of body water. Similarly, daily monitoring of body weight is the most reliable means of confirming the accuracy of intake and output measurements and of identifying significant changes in body water. In the healthy adult the daily basal weight (early morning weight after voiding and defecation and before eating or drinking) is maintained nearly constant. Sudden deviations that exceed more than ±1 percent represent gains or losses of body fluid, as do progressive trends upward or downward with time. Daily measurement of body weight in all patients in whom fluid balance problems are present, or likely to develop, provides the most reliable means of assessing day-to-day changes.

LABORATORY FEATURES

The most reliable laboratory evidence of a water deficit may be obtained by direct measurement of the serum osmolality, or measurement of the serum sodium concentration (Table 10.1–3). In the absence of renal disease these two tests provide equivalent information. In the presence of azotemia, measurement of serum osmolality can be misleading unless "corrected" by subtracting the osmolar equivalent of urea. This is accomplished by subtracting 1 mOsm from the serum osmolality for each increment of 3 mg/dl in the serum urea nitrogen. Similarly, hyperglycemia can yield misleading results. For these reasons measurement of the serum sodium concentration is probably the most reliable single indicator of the presence of a water deficit. It must be stressed that the serum osmolality and serum sodium provide only a relative indication of an excess or deficit of water. Thus it is possible to have a lowered serum sodium concentration, indicating a relative excess of water

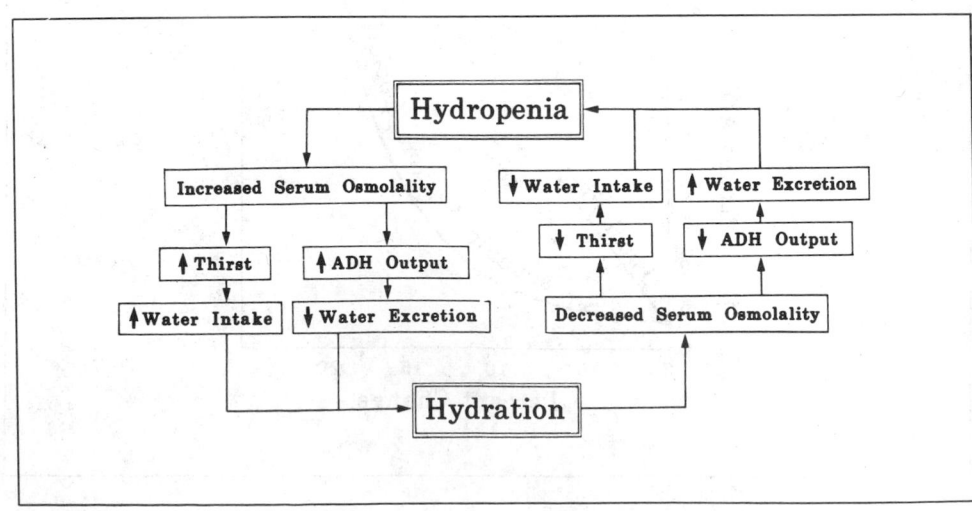

Figure 10.1–4. Regulation of water balance in normal man. This regulatory mechanism is dependent upon continuous sensing of plasma osmolality. In normal individual it regulates body water within such narrow limits that osmolality varies only 1 percent between hydropenia and hydration. Though volume change also leads to changes in ADH and in thirst, this mechanism is slow and insensitive and plays very little part in day-to-day regulation of water balance.

TABLE 10.1–2. HISTORICAL INFORMATION SOUGHT IN ASSESSING WATER BALANCE

Intake	Output
Average daily intake of water and other fluids	**Skin losses**
	Sweating[a] (duration and severity)
Recent alterations in intake pattern and cause (nausea or vomiting, inability to swallow, etc.)	Abnormalities of environment leading to excessive losses
	Lungs
Recent weight changes (acute changes in weight over period of several days are always caused by changes in body water)	Abnormal rate of breathing
	Excessively dry ambient air
	Gastrointestinal
	Diarrhea or vomiting[a] (estimate frequency and amount)
	Fistulas, enteric or biliary[a] (attempt quantitative estimate)
	Gastrointestinal intubation[a] (quantify drainage)
	Renal
	Frequency and volume of urination
	History of renal disease (including conditions impairing concentrating ability)

[a]Represent sources of loss of both water and electrolytes.

in the presence of a deficit in total body water (hypotonic contraction).

The hematocrit does not provide any measure of water deficit. It shows relatively little change during the development of a pure water deficit even when the deficit is large enough to be life-threatening (Table 10.1–3). For example, loss of 20 percent of the body water would result in elevation of the hematocrit from 42 to 43 percent, a change of no diagnostic value. *The presence of a significant elevation of the hematocrit in association with other data such as hypernatremia or hyperosmolality is strong evidence for the coexistence of a sodium deficit.*

Table 10.1–3 presents data on plasma osmolality and corresponding findings in water deficits of increasing severity. Water losses that exceed 10 percent of the total body water are usually associated with a progressive disturbance in central nervous system (CNS) function, and, unless the deficit is corrected, disorientation, stupor, and coma ensue. Water losses that exceed 20 percent of body weight are associated with an imminent demise.

CAUSES[10]

Reduced Water Intake[25]

Water deficits caused by decreased or absent water intake are ordinarily seen only in the very young, the very old, and those who are too enfeebled to satisfy their own water needs. The unique features of fluid and electrolyte disorders in infancy have not been considered in this section. Most commonly, pure water deficits are encountered in the elderly, particularly during hot weather. When the major source of water loss is perspiration, significant quantities of sodium may also be lost; a symptomatic sodium deficit that is masked by the hypernatremia resulting from water loss should always be considered in this circumstance. The demonstration of a significant rise in the hematocrit is most helpful in recognizing a coexisting sodium deficit.

Defective Thirst[1]

Gross disturbances in the thirst mechanism are quite rare but may be seen following head injuries or some neurosurgical procedures. In such patients progressive hypernatremia may develop despite an ability to concentrate the urine adequately. Such individuals, who may otherwise appear able to function reasonably well, are totally unable to respond to a water deficit because they have no sensation of thirst. They must be placed on a regular schedule of water administration. Such a defect may persist for several years.

Excess Solute

A common disturbance of intake encountered in elderly individuals relates to excess solute intake rather than reduced water intake. The elderly victim of a cerebral vascular accident who is being fed by nasogastric tube may be given a formula whose solute load requires a greatly increased water intake. For instance, tube feeding containing 120 g protein and 10 g salt will result in the excretion of more than 1000 mOsm of solute. This requires the obligatory excretion of a volume of urine between 1200 and 1500 ml when the kidney is capable of concentrating normally. Since elderly individuals often have significant impairments in renal concentrating ability, water loss as urine may exceed 2000 to 2500 ml per day. Such an individual would require 3 to 4 L of water per day simply to meet the increased demand created by this high solute intake. Failure to provide such patients with the increased water intake needed will result in a progressive water deficit that may rapidly become critical. *It is imperative that the physician know the complete composition of the tube feeding formulas used in incapacitated patients and gauge water intake accordingly.*

Water deficits may develop in other clinical situations, such as

TABLE 10.1–3. CLINICAL AND LABORATORY FEATURES OF WATER DEFICIT[10,21,22]

Clinical Severity	Symptoms	Signs	Serum Na (mEq/L)	Serum Osmolality (mOsm/kg)	Hct[a]	Magnitude of Deficit (L)	% Body Water Lost
Normal	—	—	144	285	42	—	—
Mild	Thirst[b]	None	149–151	294–298	42	1.5–2	3–4.5
Moderate	Thirst[b]	Dry mucous membranes	152–158	299–313	42.2	2–4	4.5–10
Severe	Thirst[b] Weakness	Above plus doughy skin	159–166	314–329	42.5	4–6	10–15
Very severe	Disorientation Severe weakness Fainting	Postural hypotension CNS changes Stupor Coma	>166	>330	43–44	>6	>15

[a]Note that these calculated changes are not clinically detectable.
[b]Requires that patient be alert and communicative.

severe myasthenia gravis, where the patient is simply too weak to maintain an adequate water intake; extensive oral herpes, where the painful condition of the mucous membranes precludes adequate fluid intake; and other disturbances leading to mechanical or neuromuscular difficulties that interfere with drinking. The physician should be alert to the possibility of inadequate water intake in any seriously ill patient who is too weak to drink.

Sweating
Among the possible sources of body water loss, severe and prolonged sweating probably represents the greatest threat to maintenance of the normal body water in the healthy individual. Because sweating varies from nil to quantities in excess of 8 L per day depending upon the environment, water loss from this source can on occasion lead to the rapid development of severe water deficits. Working in an extremely hot environment, vigorous body contact sports such as football in hot weather, and prolonged exposure to direct sunlight may all produce sweating at near maximal rates and may lead rapidly to the development of water deficits in the absence of adequate intake (Table 10.1–4).

Renal Loss[10]
Renal water losses contribute only minimally to the development of a water deficit in the absence of impairment of renal concentrating function. The normal kidney under the influence of antidiuretic hormone acts promptly to retard the rate of development of water deficit when any significant loss elevates plasma osmolality.

In the absence of the antidiuretic hormone, diabetes insipidus appears and may lead to extraordinarily large water losses from the kidneys (see Chapter 11.1).

Patients with impaired renal concentrating mechanisms are more likely to develop water deficits than are normal individuals. Indeed, seemingly minor reductions in water intake or increases in water loss may precipitate serious deficits. Among the disorders that impair the renal concentrating ability are the nephropathy associated with sickle cell anemia, hypercalcemia, hypokalemia, and nephrogenic diabetes insipidus (see Chapter 11.1). All but nephrogenic diabetes insipidus result in only moderate increase in the daily urine volume, since the kidney is usually able to excrete urine that is at least isotonic to plasma in these disorders. The minimum urinary volume in these patients is determined primarily by the solute output per day, a solute load of 600 mOsm requiring approximately 2 L for its excretion. This increased obligatory water loss renders the kidney relatively ineffective at conserving water if a deficit in body water develops.

Patients who have end-stage renal disease with glomerular filtration rates below 6 to 8 ml/min are particularly susceptible to development of water deficits. They often have an added obligatory water loss that results from their inability to produce hypertonic urine even when maximally stimulated with ADH. Some of these individuals excrete persistently hypotonic urine, and thus

their water deficit may be aggravated by large solute loads that lead to substantial increases in urine flow.

This discussion has dealt with the mechanisms of development of an isolated water deficiency and its recognition (Table 10.1–5). Mixed disturbances are considered below and in Chapter 10.4.

CLINICAL FEATURES OF WATER EXCESS

Diagnostic recognition of water excess requires a careful history to identify sources and amounts of water intake and an accurate appraisal of water output. Headache, blurred vision, muscle cramps, and twitches are seen in moderate water intoxication. Water excess does not occur under normal physiologic conditions, requiring for its production either persistent or inappropriate levels of circulating ADH or reduced water excretion. Although the patient who is otherwise awake and alert may experience headache and some gastrointestinal disturbance with as little as 5 to 7 percent excess body water, significant CNS symptoms are unusual until much more marked degrees of the disturbance are encountered.

Physical examination is rarely helpful. Pitting edema is virtually never seen in the presence of pure water excess. There may on occasion be some scleral edema. Increased body weight provides confirmation of the suspected water excess only in profound water intoxication (increase in body water by 15 to 20 percent or more), and disorientation, stupor, and convulsions are commonly seen. Table 10.1–6 lists the prominent clinical findings and expected laboratory data associated with water intoxication of increasing severity. The hematocrit changes represent calculated values and are included to emphasize that the hematocrit does not change significantly even in profound water intoxication when unassociated with other electrolyte disturbances.

LABORATORY FEATURES

The most important single laboratory observation is measurement of the serum sodium concentration supplemented by information

---

TABLE 10.1–4. POSSIBLE ABNORMAL DAILY LOSSES OF WATER[a]

Sweat[b]	6000–8000 ml
Upper gastrointestinal losses (vomiting or intubation)	2500–5000 ml
Diarrhea	500–10,000+ ml
Bile	500 ml
Urine	
Excluding diabetes insipidus[b]	4000–5000 ml
Diabetes insipidus[b]	5000–10,000+ ml

[a]Note that all these sources of loss represent combined losses of water simultaneously with variable quantities of sodium and potassium. Only diarrheal fluid losses approximate isotonic losses, while diabetes insipidus is associated only with water loss.
[b]Hypotonic losses, leading to hyperosmolality of body fluid.

TABLE 10.1–5. CLINICAL CONDITIONS LEADING TO AN ISOLATED WATER DEFICIT

Type of Disturbance	Clinical Setting
Disordered Intake	
Water deprivation	Elderly feeble patients Central nervous system disorders Unavailability of water Mechanical difficulties interfering with swallowing mechanism
Absence of thirst	CNS disorders
Increased solute intake	Nasogastric tube feeding containing high protein and NaCl content
Increased Losses	
Diabetes insipidus	Pituitary or hypothalamic disorder
Nephrogenic diabetes insipidus	Hereditary renal disorder associated with marked water loss via the kidney; unresponsive to ADH
Osmotic diuresis	Diabetes mellitus Hypertonic tube feedings
Sweating	Prolonged exposure to heat—usually associated with moderate sodium deficit
Renal disease (acquired nephrogenic diabetes insipidus)	Nephropathy of hypokalemia and hypercalcemia Nephropathy of sickle cell anemia Rarely pyelonephritis and other diffuse renal diseases after advanced renal failure supervenes

TABLE 10.1–6. CLINICAL AND LABORATORY FEATURES OF WATER EXCESS

Clinical Severity	Symptoms	Signs	Serum Na (mEq/L)	Serum Osmolality (mOsm/kg)	Hct[a]	Magnitude of Excess (L)	% Body Water Excess
Normal	—	—	144	285	42	—	—
Mild	Headache	—	139–132	275–261	41.8	1.5–4	3–8
Moderate	Headache Drowsiness Weakness	—	131–127	262–251	41.8	4–6	8–13
Severe	Above plus disorientation	Cramps Rarely seizures	126–118	250–233	41.6	6–10	13–22
Very severe	Stupor Coma, convulsions	Seizures	<118	<233	41.6–41.5	>10	>22

[a]Change not clinically detectable.

about change in body weight. Hematocrit is usually unchanged, but a low serum sodium concentration is a prerequisite to making the diagnosis of water excess. It is very rare to encounter significant symptoms until the serum sodium concentration drops below 125 mEq/L. For this reason the group of disorders associated with water excess are sometimes called "asymptomatic hyponatremia."

CAUSES

Water intoxication requires a persistent excess of intake over output for a sustained period. The scheme depicted in Figures 10.1–3 and 10.1–4 is so sensitive to changes in plasma osmolality and the kidney is capable of excreting excess water at such rapid rates that water excess is never encountered as a result of increased intake unless there is some associated disturbance in regulation of water balance. Thus, the individual who is a compulsive water drinker, the classic example of excess water intake, almost never develops water intoxication unless there is some intercurrent event that leads to increased ADH output that persists for several hours.

Nonphysiologic or inappropriate secretion of ADH may be seen in patients receiving opiate drugs for analgesic purposes in the presence of persistent severe pain and in several pulmonary and CNS disorders with resultant water intoxication of varying degrees of severity. Tumors producing polypeptide substances resembling ADH may also lead to inappropriate water retention. These abnormalities of ADH secretion are commonly encountered and are referred to collectively as the "syndrome of inappropriate secretion of ADH (SIADH)."

In summary, most cases of water excess represent (1) increased intake in circumstances associated with continued ADH output or (2) primary renal disturbances that interfere with renal water excretion. It is rare that this latter circumstance leads to pure water excess.

Table 10.1–7 lists some of the conditions that may be associated with water excess, in some of which the primary disorder is associated with increased intake and in others with decreased output. Not all are instances of isolated water excess, however. In some of these, such as congestive heart failure and cirrhosis, the primary disturbance is in sodium regulation. Hence, a clear understanding of the physiology of sodium regulation is also essential for appropriate diagnosis and management.

DISTURBANCES OF SODIUM METABOLISM

REGULATION OF BODY SODIUM CONTENT[6,10,12,20]

Sodium is the principal cation of the extracellular fluid of the body. Figure 10.1–5 indicates the predominant extracellular location of this important fraction of the body sodium. The difference be-

tween exchangeable and nonexchangeable sodium is that the majority of sodium present in bone and cartilage is deep in the matrix of these tissues and is not readily available for equilibration with the remainder of the body sodium. Therefore, in clinical situations, alteration in body sodium is synonymous with alteration in exchangeable sodium. The mean value for adult males is 41 mEq of exchangeable sodium per kilogram of body weight; for females, 40.

Significant symptoms are produced by either excesses or deficits in the sodium content of the body; too much sodium may lead to circulatory congestion and ultimately to pulmonary edema, while too little sodium leads to progressive circulatory collapse and shock. Either disturbance may terminate fatally if not appropriately recognized and treated.

The normal subject can vary sodium intake from less than 5 mEq per day to quantities in excess of 350 mEq per day, but the total body sodium content varies by no more than 150 mEq, or about 2 mEq/kg body weight over this intake range. The average intake during health usually ranges between 150 and 200 mEq per day, depending upon the individual's taste and dietary habits. As little as 5 mEq per day are adequate to sustain maximal growth during childhood; hence the average sodium consumption is far in excess of minimal daily requirements. The adult can survive without difficulty on less than 1 mEq per day for long periods in the absence of abnormal losses.

TABLE 10.1–7. CONDITIONS LEADING TO WATER INTOXICATION

Conditions	
Disturbances of Intake	*Clinical Setting*
Compulsive water drinking	Hyponatremia likely only with associated illness, e.g., pneumonia
Iatrogenic water administration	Excess fluid administration following major surgery
Disturbances of Output	*Clinical Setting*
Syndrome of inappropriate ADH secretion	Seen in carcinoma of the lung, CNS disorders, pulmonary tuberculosis, sarcoidosis
Renal impairment	Acute renal failure with oliguria Chronic renal failure
Congestive heart failure[a]	Seen in severe congestive failure when underperfused kidney cannot excrete water load
Cirrhosis of liver[a]	Occurs in presence of severe ascites

[a]Condition here included is dilutional hyponatremia resulting from retention of water in excess of NaCl. See Chapters 10.4, 11.1, and 11.2.

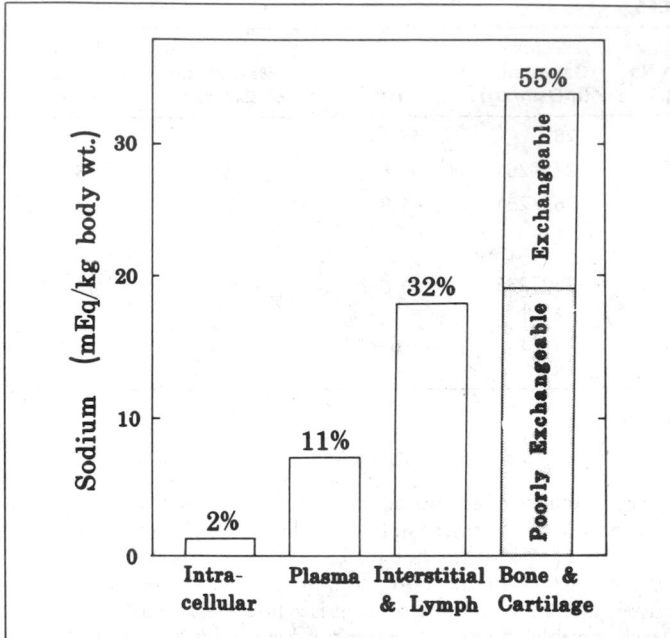

Figure 10.1–5. Distribution of exchangeable sodium within various spaces and tissues of body.

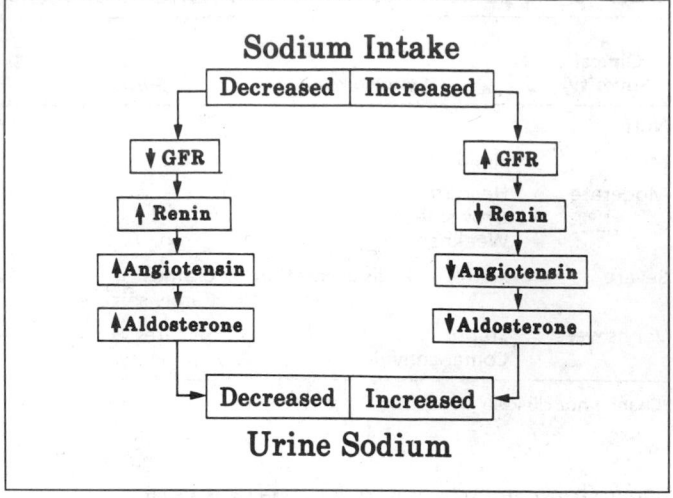

Figure 10.1–6. Role of renin-angiotensin-aldosterone system in regulation of sodium balance. Expansion of extracellular fluid and blood volume that results from increased intake of sodium increases glomerular filtration and reduces renin output with reduction in angiotensin production and aldosterone secretion. This reduces renal tubular reabsorption of sodium and increases urinary sodium. Reduction of salt intake reverses this sequence of events, leading to reduction in urine sodium.

Sodium loss occurs in the urine, sweat, and feces (Table 10.1–8). In the normal individual, regulatory mechanisms operate to reduce these losses to very low levels when the intake is reduced for any reason. Urine [Na] may decrease to less than 1 mEq/L of urine in the absence of sodium intake or in the presence of significant sodium deficits caused by losses from extrarenal sources. Sodium conservation in sweat is less efficient, but in the individual acclimated to heat, the sodium concentration in sweat is usually less than 15 mEq/L. Normally, these adjustments of sodium concentration require 2 to 4 days following change in the sodium intake, and it is during this short interval that the modest changes in the sodium content of the body occur in normal individuals when sodium intake is changed.

The renal mechanisms for regulation of sodium excretion include (1) hemodynamic alterations in response to variations in sodium intake, (2) the humorally mediated renin-angiotensin-aldosterone mechanism, and (3) atrial natriuretic factor.[6,12,20,24]

Increased sodium intake results in transient expansion of the plasma volume and interstitial fluid volume and an associated increase in glomerular filtration that increases the quantity of sodium filtered. These events lead to suppression of renin release and reduction in the rate of aldosterone secretion (Fig. 10.1–6) and release of atrial natriuretic factor, which results in decreased tubular reabsorption of sodium. Conversely, when sodium intake is reduced or stopped altogether, the sodium excretion that continues for a short period results in a decrease of extravascular volume as well as plasma volume, a reduction in the glomerular filtration rate and renal blood flow with resultant decrease in the quantity of sodium filtered at the glomerulus. This is associated with an in-

crease in renin release and increased sodium reabsorption. When sodium intake ceases, these mechanisms are so efficient that the kidney produces urine virtually free of sodium.

The colon, like the nephron, is capable of transporting sodium against a large gradient, thereby reducing sodium in the fecal contents to low levels. This transport mechanism has a relatively limited capacity, however. In the presence of diarrhea, the sodium concentration in the fecal fluid rises sharply and in extreme cases approaches the concentration in plasma. Hence, sodium loss in the feces is directly related to the total quantity or volume expelled by this route. In formed stool it rarely exceeds 10 mEq per day. In contrast, voluminous watery diarrhea may lead to losses that exceed 250 mEq per day when fecal volume exceeds 2.5 to 3 L per day.

In the normal individual, sweat represents the greatest potential source of sodium loss in the face of continued sodium restriction. Although the sodium concentration in sweat varies with variation in sodium intake, the normal subject cannot elaborate sweat with a sodium concentration of less than 15 mEq/L. This small concentration may produce continuing sodium loss and large deficits even in the normal individual when sweating continues at a significant rate and intake is inadequate.

SODIUM DEPLETION[8,13–15,22]

ROLE OF SODIUM LOSS

Severe sodium depletion occurs only as the result of excessive loss, not of reduced sodium intake. Rational management of sodium depletion, therefore, requires evaluation of the nature and time course of the sodium loss and an understanding of the compensatory responses to abnormal losses of sodium from the body.

EXPERIMENTAL SODIUM DEPLETION[13–15]

McCance's classic studies in man demonstrated two distinct phases of sodium depletion. In these experiments normal individuals were

TABLE 10.1–8. ROUTES OF NORMAL SODIUM LOSS FROM THE BODY

	Range of Loss in 24 Hours
Kidney	<1 to 150+ mEq
GI tract	<1 to 10+ mEq
Skin (sweat)	<15 to 70 mEq/L of fluid lost

subjected to persistent sweating and sodium restriction but not water privation. Sweating produced a greater loss of water than sodium, since it contains less sodium than does extracellular fluid (Fig. 10.1–7). The thirst mechanism, however, maintained the osmolality (and sodium concentration) constant as previously described. Thus, during the first phase there were equivalent net losses of sodium and water, producing isotonic contraction of the extracellular fluid volume.

Only when the losses exceeded 400 mEq of sodium did the situation change. In the second phase further sodium loss evoked attempts to maintain volume by water retention. Only in this phase of hypotonic contraction did the serum concentration fall.

CLINICAL PHASES OF SODIUM DEPLETION[13]

When one considers the possible sources of body sodium loss (Table 10.1–9, Fig. 10.1–7), that is, the various sodium-containing fluids that can be lost from the body, one recognizes that all such fluids have sodium concentrations that are either less than or equal to plasma sodium concentration. The most common events that lead to sodium loss from extrarenal routes (vomiting, diarrhea, and sweating) all represent fluid loss in which the sodium concentration is much less than that in plasma. Under extreme conditions, the sodium concentration in some excreted fluids may approach that in the plasma. Such an occurrence is limited almost exclusively to small bowel fistulas, ileostomies, or fulminant diarrhea as in cholera. Here, in the most severe cases, the sodium concentration of the fecal fluid may be virtually identical with that seen in plasma. The sequence encountered clinically in sodium depletion is in most instances similar to the experimental findings of McCance described above. Because of this it is useful to consider these two sequential phases of isotonic and hypotonic contraction in response to sodium loss as acute and chronic stages of sodium depletion and to review the clinical findings during each phase of the disorder.

TABLE 10.1–9. ROUTES OF ABNORMAL SODIUM LOSS FROM THE BODY

Source of Na Loss	Etiology	"Effective" Osmolality of Lost Fluid
Kidney	Diuretics	Hypotonic
	Osmotic diuretics	Hypotonic
	Acidosis	Hypotonic
	Salt wasting nephritis	Hypotonic
	Renal tubular acidosis	Hypotonic
	Adrenal insufficiency	Hypotonic
GI tract	Diarrhea	Hypotonic
	Ileostomy	Isotonic
	Small bowel fistula	Isotonic
	Chronic laxative ingestion	Hypotonic
	Vomiting	Hypotonic
	Nasogastric suction	Hypotonic
	Villous adenoma	Hypotonic
Skin	Sweating (excessive)	Hypotonic

ACUTE SODIUM DEPLETION (SODIUM DEPLETION WITHOUT HYPONATREMIA)[13,22]

Regardless of the route and rate of sodium loss, the body responds initially to restore solute concentration to normal. When intake of both salt and water are adequate, that is, of course, accomplished by retaining the quantity of salt that was lost and the corresponding amount of water. In the absence of sodium intake, however, the body adjusts the quantity of body water in a manner that returns the sodium concentration to normal. This leads to a net isotonic loss of extracellular fluid despite the fact that the initial sodium loss may have been as part of a hypotonic solution. As in the experimental example, the patient who loses a large quantity of sodium by sweating will lose much more water than sodium, and the fluid loss will be hypotonic. With adequate fluid intake, however, water is retained until the sodium concentration is returned to its original normal level. Serial measurement of the body weight during an event of this sort reveals that the net result is significant loss of body weight with the loss representing the loss of sodium and water in isotonic proportions. At this point the serum sodium concentration is normal. Thus *isotonic contraction* is the result of acute sodium depletion. This is so regardless of whether the sodium loss occurs through the kidneys, the gastrointestinal tract, or the skin.

The symptoms, physical findings, and laboratory data under these conditions all reflect a reduction in the extracellular fluid volume. With increasing losses, progressive weakness and lassitude are followed by postural hypotension and, on occasion, syncope. Examination reveals a low blood pressure with a striking postural hypotension. Poor skin turgor and, less often, decreased intraocular tension, relatively dry mucous membranes, and muscular cramps are present. On occasion, particularly when the sodium loss is quite rapid, this picture may progress to that of frank shock.

An additional feature of sodium depletion well supported by experimental studies is a disproportionately large decrease in plasma volume. This feature is most easily explained by the decrease in the circulating mass of plasma proteins which, in turn, probably represents some sequestration of protein in the interstitial space as a result of the decreased lymph flow that accompanies sodium depletion. This excessive reduction in plasma volume results in hemodynamic consequences and an increase in hematocrit beyond that to be expected from a simple isotonic contraction of the extracellular fluid volume.

The laboratory data are those to be expected whenever isotonic contraction of the extracellular fluid volume occurs. There is an elevation of the hematocrit and an increase in the serum urea

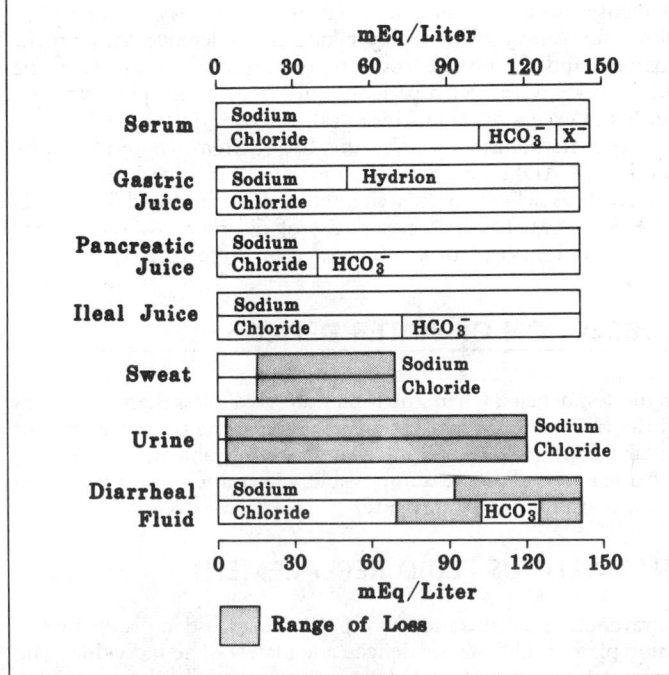

Figure 10.1–7. Sodium concentration in various body fluids and excreted fluids. Shaded areas identify variations that may be encountered in some of these fluids.

nitrogen and in serum creatinine concentrations. The serum sodium concentration is normal, however, in this circumstance.

Occasionally, quantities of sodium greatly in excess of 400 mEq may be lost, with persistence of the picture of isotonic contraction. This situation is particularly likely to occur in fulminant diarrhea, where several liters of fluid may be rapidly lost via the lower digestive tract during a very short period and unassociated with any water intake. Under such circumstances, the loss may exceed 5 L of isotonic fluid (more than 700 mEq of sodium). In the untreated patient this leads rapidly to profound shock, which occasionally terminates fatally. This sequence is quite common in those areas of the world where cholera is endemic. Table 10.1–10 gives a partial list of the clinical disorders that may be associated with acute sodium depletion. They may also produce chronic sodium depletion as outlined below.

CHRONIC SODIUM DEPLETION (SODIUM DEPLETION WITH HYPONATREMIA)[3,8,13]

In the presence of continuing net sodium loss, the homeostatic mechanisms of the body attempt to maintain the extracellular fluid volume by water retention. Figure 10.1–8 illustrates this phenomenon in a patient who was treated too vigorously with diuretics. He exhibits the sequence described in the preceding section; his losses were isotonic initially, resulting in no change in the serum sodium concentration. When the diuretic was stopped and rigid sodium restriction was maintained, however, he proceeded to dilute the body fluid compartments by water retention leading to hyponatremia.

For comparison, data from McCance's original sodium depletion studies, in which sodium depletion was produced by sustained sweating, are presented in similar format in Figure 10.1–9. The similarities are readily apparent.

Weakness, loss of appetite, giddiness, syncopal attacks, and muscle cramps are common and persistent. If the hyponatremia becomes sufficiently severe, disorientation may develop, followed by lethargy and, on occasion, convulsions. Physical findings include hypotension exaggerated by posture change. The skin turgor is poor. There may be a decrease in intraocular pressure and dry mucous membranes, but it is rare that the subjective complaint of thirst can be elicited.

The laboratory data are similar to those described above with more acute sodium loss with the exception that the serum sodium concentration is always depressed in the patient with chronic sodium depletion. On occasion it may be below 120 mEq/L. Loss of extracellular sodium results in movement of fluid into the intra-

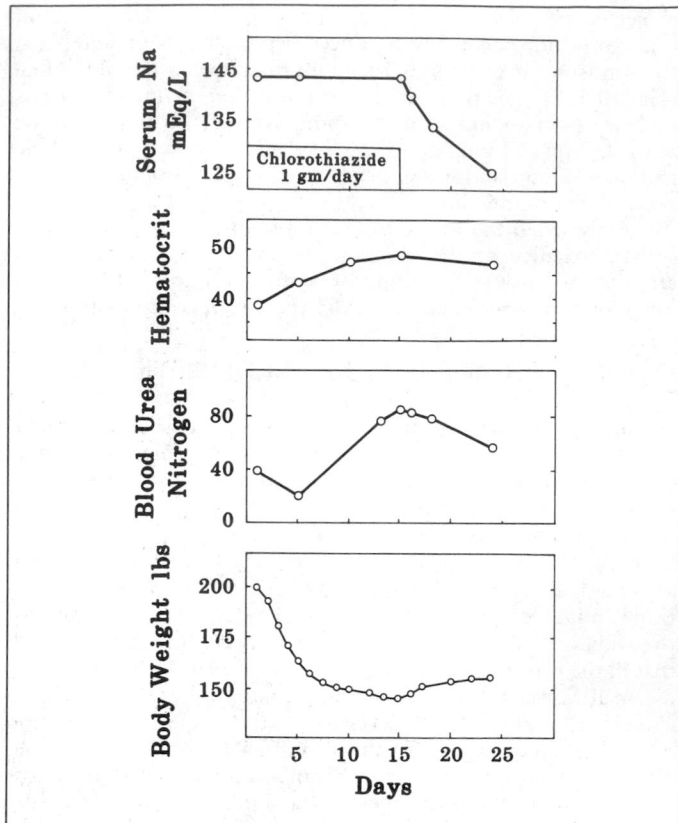

Figure 10.1–8. Sodium depletion produced by excessive diuretic therapy. Initial decline in weight was unassociated with changes in serum sodium concentration, but both hematocrit and blood urea nitrogen rose. Subsequently water retention and increase in weight were associated with a decrease in serum sodium concentration.

cellular space to readjust solute concentrations so that no osmotic gradient exists across the cell. An estimate of the *concentration deficit* of sodium can be obtained by taking the difference between the observed and the normal sodium concentration and multiplying this by body water. Such patients will, on occasion, prove to have deficits in excess of 700 or more mEq of sodium.

The mechanism whereby this hyponatremia is produced by continuing ADH output in response to the volume deficit was discussed elsewhere in this chapter and is illustrated in Figures 10.1–3 and 10.1–10. A partial list of disorders associated with chronic sodium depletion is presented in Table 10.1–10.

CORRECTION OF WATER DEFICITS

In modest deficits, where the total water loss is less than 10 percent of the body water, replacement is simple if the patient is capable of taking fluids orally. Should nausea be a problem, or if for any other reason oral intake is impossible, replacement must be undertaken by the intravenous route.

INTRAVENOUS FLUID REPLACEMENT

Intravenous administration of 5 percent dextrose in distilled water will replace modest water deficits adequately. The individual who can metabolize carbohydrate normally converts the dextrose in the fluids to glycogen, making solute-free water available for correcting the water deficit. Diabetic patients or patients with hyperosmolarity (see Chapter 14.7) can be more effectively treated by giving 2.5

TABLE 10.1–10. DISORDERS ASSOCIATED WITH CHRONIC SODIUM DEPLETION

Renal	Chronic diuretic use associated with decreased sodium intake
	Salt-losing nephritis
	Medullary cystic disease
	Renal tubular acidosis
Endocrine	Hypopituitarism
	Hypoadrenalism
	Inappropriate secretion of antidiuretic hormone
GI tract	Chronic nasogastric suction or vomiting
	Ileostomy or small bowel fistulae with decreased sodium intake
	Biliary fistulae
	Chronic diarrhea
	Villous adenoma
Skin	Chronic heat exposure and sweating with decreased sodium intake
	Burns with slow healing

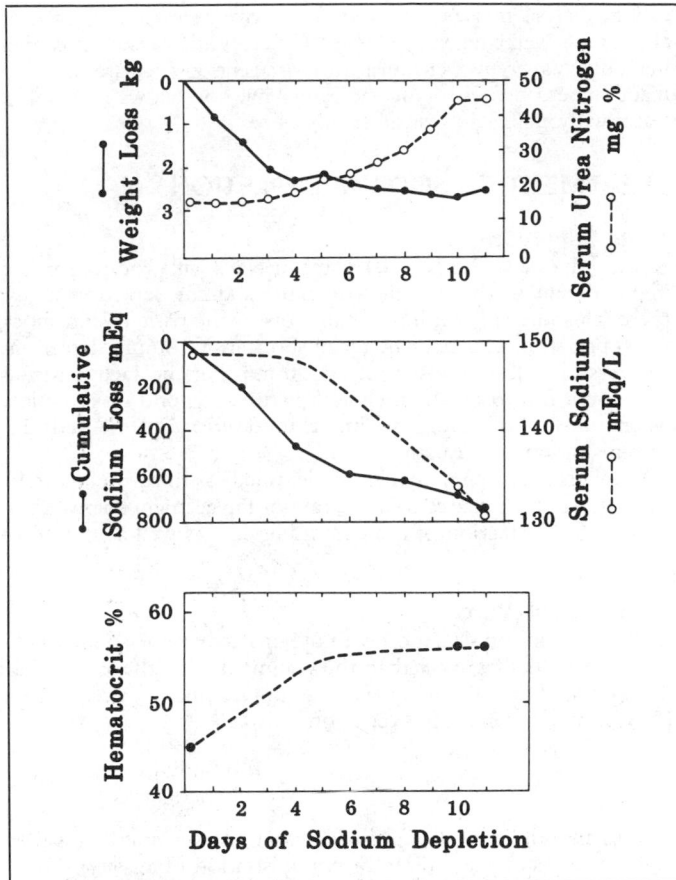

Figure 10.1–9. Experimental sodium depletion. Changes depicted in body weight, urea nitrogen, serum sodium, hematocrit, and cumulative sodium loss are drawn from data of McCance.[13] During first 3 days losses were isotonic with a 2-kg decrease in weight being associated with loss of about 300 mEq of sodium.

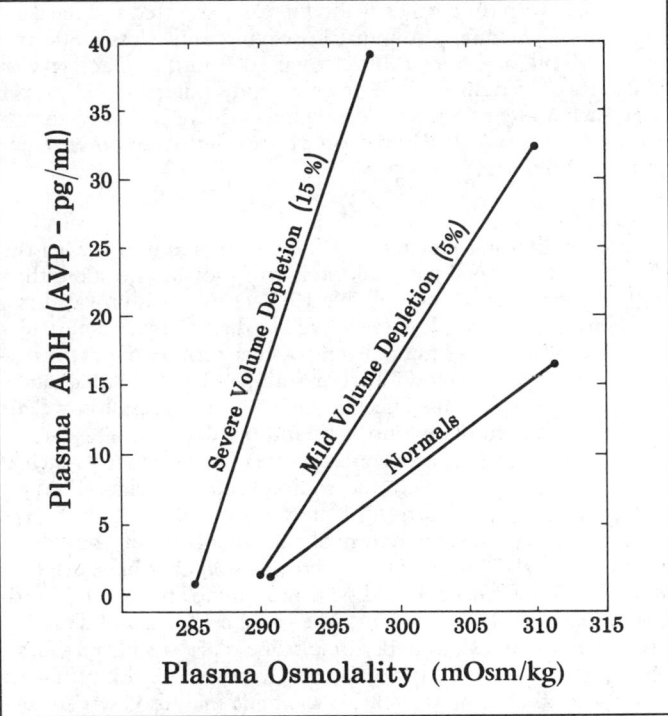

Figure 10.1–10. Influence of volume depletion on acute response of plasma ADH to osmotic stimulation. Effect of progressive volume depletion is much more rapid rise in circulating ADH for a given increment in osmolality. Slope relating rise in ADH to increase in osmolality increases threefold following large volume depletion. Thus combination of osmotic increment and volume deficit produce much more vigorous ADH response.

percent dextrose in distilled water. The use of 2.5 percent dextrose in distilled water or 2.5 percent dextrose in a solution containing 35 mEq of sodium and chloride per liter will provide adequate water replacement while avoiding the hemolysis that may result from the rapid administration of a more dilute solution.

When specific choice of fluid may depend very much on the individual case, as a guiding principle of therapy in the treatment of hyperosmolarity, no fluid should be administered that exceeds the osmolality of normal plasma. Osmolalities of some commonly used solutions of parenteral fluid are shown in Table 10.1–11.

Rate of Replacement

Patients with severe water deficits appear to respond more satisfactorily when the therapy is planned to restore body water to normal over a period of 24 to 36 hours. For this reason, when the estimated deficit exceeds 6 to 7 L, therapy should be planned to restore about half the total deficit in the first 24-hour period.

Estimation of Deficit

In a pure water deficit the solute content of the body fluid compartments does not change; the change in concentration of the solute (or serum sodium concentration) can be used to estimate the deficit quantitatively:

$$\frac{\Delta \text{ Body } H_2O}{\text{in liters}} = 0.6 \times \frac{\text{Body weight}}{\text{in kilograms}} (1 - 144/[Na_{obs}])$$

where $[Na_{obs}]$ is the abnormal serum sodium concentration observed in the patient to be treated. This calculation provides only an approximation; disturbances of consciousness or lack of knowledge by the patient concerning his usual weight introduces some uncertainty, as does the use of 0.6 as the fractional representation of body water. It does, however, provide an adequate estimate of the deficit that permits rational planning of therapy. For treatment of water excess in instances of "pure" water excess, the same equation is useful in estimating the size of the water excess. It must again be stressed that this equation assumes a pure water disturbance (deficit). It provides misleading information if a deficit or excess of sodium also exists.

CORRECTION OF WATER EXCESS

Fluid Restriction

Effective therapy requires appropriate reduction in fluid intake. The rate at which this decreases body water depends upon the dif-

TABLE 10.1–11. OSMOLALITY OF COMMONLY EMPLOYED PARENTERAL FLUIDS

Fluid	Osmolality (mOsm/kg H_2O)
2.5% Dextrose	139
2.5% Dextrose in 0.034 molar (0.2%) NaCl	207
5% Dextrose in distilled H_2O	280
5% Dextrose in 0.155 molar (0.9%) NaCl	560
Normal plasma	280
Plasma with 20% water deficit	350

ference between the total daily fluid intake permitted and the daily fluid losses. Assuming minimal losses (insensible losses 500 ml, urine 400 ml, and feces 100 ml; total 1000 ml), a total intake of 500 ml would result in a decrease in body water by 500 ml per day. Such a rate of loss would require a 12-day period to correct a water excess of 6 L. Correction of water intoxication by water restriction alone is a slow process.

Diet

Restriction of water intake to 500 ml per day requires altering the diet so that the total daily caloric intake provides no more than 200 ml of preformed water (Table 10.1–1). If this is provided as a high-protein, low-fat, low-carbohydrate diet, the water of oxidation is kept at a minimum. Even so, this permits the patient to drink only about 150 to 200 ml of fluid per day if the total intake is to be kept at 500 ml. Effective therapy should result in weight loss of one-half to three-fourths pound per day.

Water loss can be accelerated by use of osmotic agents such as urea, mannitol, or hypertonic sodium chloride, since all these agents will lead to excretion of more water than sodium by the kidney with consequent return of the osmolality of body fluids toward normal. The hazards of overexpansion or volume overload during such treatment should be kept in mind, particularly in patients with cardiac impairment. The concomitant use of diuretics, such as furosemide and hypertonic saline replacement, provides a therapeutic approach that reduces or removes the risk of further overexpansion during therapy. Furosemide may also exert antagonistic activity to ADH and, thus, further enhance its usefulness in treating water intoxication. Both lithium and demeclocycline, which antagonize the peripheral action of ADH, are potentially useful in treatment of inappropriate ADH excess. The hazard of toxicity with long-term use of lithium limits its potential usefulness, but demeclocycline appears promising.

Hypertonic Fluids

Water intoxication with severe CNS symptoms such as stupor, coma, or convulsions requires more rapid correction of the water excess than can be achieved by fluid restriction alone. Hypertonic saline with an additional osmotic agent such as urea or mannitol, plus a diuretic such as furosemide, is indicated under these circumstances.

Three percent sodium chloride solution (510 mEq/L, or about 1020 mOsm/L) will directly elevate the osmolality of body fluids and raise the serum sodium concentration even in the absence of any excretion of the excess water. Thus, it is the treatment to be considered first in severe water intoxication but only after careful evaluation of the cardiac status of the patient. Since administration of such hypertonic solutions rapidly expands ECF, it can rapidly overload the cardiovascular system. Because of this risk furosemide or some other potent loop diuretic should always be used as part of any treatment regimen that includes osmotic diuresis. The administration of 5 to 10 ml of 3 percent NaCl solution per kilogram body weight (2.5 to 5 mEq/kg body weight) will raise the osmolality of the body fluids about 7 to 14 mOsm/L when given slowly over a period of 2 to 4 hours and usually leads to significant improvement of the CNS disturbance. Greater quantities should be employed with great caution and only in patients with adequate renal function and a normal cardiovascular system.

The use of mannitol carries the same risks of cardiovascular overload as does hypertonic sodium chloride when given intravenously and in addition leads to further decrease in the electrolyte concentrations in the extracellular fluid as a result of fluid shifts. When given on a daily basis to patients with the syndrome of inappropriate antidiuretic hormone secretion, it is useful in increasing renal excretion of excess water. Administration of about 0.75 g/kg body weight as a 20 percent solution intravenously, given over a 6- to 8-hour period, should increase the daily urine volume by about 1 L per day in the average size adult.

In those individuals with seriously compromised cardiovascular function who exhibit severe CNS symptoms from water intoxi-

cation, dialysis may be necessary to remove excess water. In general, excess water may be removed either by ultrafiltration during hemodialysis or by peritoneal dialysis using a dialysate solution made hypertonic with glucose. Either method allows removal of water without ECF expansion.

TREATMENT OF SODIUM DEPLETION

Acute Depletion

A solution of 2 to 2.5 L of 0.155 molar NaCl will produce marked improvement in the patient with acute sodium depletion unless there is a source of continuing fluid loss or the patient is in shock when first seen. Patients who are in shock from sodium depletion, with systolic blood pressure below 90 mm Hg and tachycardia as prominent features of their clinical picture, respond more rapidly when infusions of isotonic sodium chloride are supplemented with administration of plasma.

Where continuing losses are identified, as in severe diarrhea, these must be measured and the rate of replacement increased to provide for correction of the continuing loss as well as the initial deficit.

Chronic Depletion

In chronic sodium depletion with hyponatremia, the sodium deficit is substantially greater than the volume deficit; this excess may be estimated from the observed serum sodium concentration, $[Na]_{obs}$, by the following expression:

$$Na\ deficit = (144 - [Na]_{obs}) \times \frac{0.6\ Body\ weight}{in\ kilograms}$$

In an individual with normally functioning kidneys, it is preferable to replace the sodium by administration of an *isotonic* solution of sodium chloride. When the hyponatremia is so severe that abnormalities of CNS function are present, initial therapy is more effective in correcting these abnormalities if a *hypertonic* solution such as 0.510 molar (3 percent) sodium chloride is given. Replacement of one third to one half the deficit within a 12-hour period will usually reverse the neurologic manifestations.[3]

When the patient is sufficiently alert and able to take medication by mouth, the oral route usually suffices to achieve restoration of sodium balance, provided renal function is normal. This must be done slowly because of the marked gastric irritation produced by taking more than 1 to 1.5 g of salt orally in one dose. In general, if the deficit has developed over a protracted period and is not associated with mental aberrations, it is sufficient to plan replacement gradually over a period of several days, and the oral administration of sodium chloride usually suffices.

Asymptomatic Hyponatremia

Hyponatremia unassociated with sodium deficit and caused by a primary disturbance in water metabolism have been discussed. The following additional specific situations merit comment.

Hyperlipidemia produces hyponatremia caused by a decrease in the aqueous phase of the plasma. Because of the high lipid content of the plasma, the water content is reciprocally reduced. If the correction is made for this reduction in plasma water, sodium concentration in the serum water is normal.

Hyperproteinemia rarely is associated with hyponatremia. This may be seen in multiple myeloma but only when the total protein concentration exceeds 11 or 12 g/dl. The mechanism here is similar to that outlined above in hyperlipidemia. This change as well as that in hyperlipidemia is not associated with symptoms, and no attempt should be made to correct the hyponatremia.

Hyperglycemia, when extreme, reduces plasma sodium concentration as a result of ECF expansion associated with intracellular dehydration. In diabetes, where glucose fails to enter the cells, osmotic equilibration results in a proportional lowering of the sodium concentration in the extracellular fluid. Thus, an increase in the serum glucose by 180 mg/dl will result in reduction in the

serum sodium by approximately 5 mEq/L. Extreme degrees of hyperglycemia may be accompanied by severe water deficit secondary to the associated osmotic diuresis, and under these circumstances the serum sodium concentration is unpredictable. In addition, such patients may have also developed a significant sodium deficit caused by the sustained osmotic diuresis engendered by the severe hyperglycemia.

Administration of osmotic agents such as *mannitol* may result in lowering of the plasma sodium concentration. The mechanism is similar to that with hyperglycemia. It may be encountered when one attempts to correct the oliguria of impending acute renal failure by mannitol administration or when mannitol is used to sustain an osmotic diuresis during the treatment of certain instances of drug overdosage.

The most important distinction to be made, from the standpoint of appropriate treatment, is between the dilutional hyponatremia of congestive heart failure and chronic sodium depletion. The differentiation is readily made on the basis of the presence or absence of dependent edema. Although either condition may be encountered in congestive heart failure, chronic sodium depletion resulting from too vigorous use of diuretics is less common than is the hyponatremia of congestive heart failure that appears when the heart failure is so severe that the patient is unable to excrete a dilute urine in response to water ingestion. *The presence of demonstrable pitting edema excludes the diagnosis of chronic sodium depletion.*

SODIUM EXCESS

The retention of abnormal quantities of sodium occurs most commonly in renal disease, cardiovascular disturbances leading to congestive heart failure, and cirrhosis of the liver. This is discussed elsewhere in this book in the context of the specific diseases in which it is encountered.

REFERENCES

1. Anderson R: Regulation of water intake. Physiol Rev 58:582, 1978
2. Austin MG, Berry JW: Observations on 100 cases of heat stroke. JAMA 161:1525, 1956
3. Ayus JC, Olivero JJ, Frommer JP: Rapid correction of severe hyponatremia with intravenous hypertonic saline solution. Am J Med 72:43, 1982
4. Brenner BM, Rector FC Jr (eds): The Kidney, 3d ed. Philadelphia, WB Saunders, 1986
5. Cooke CR, Turin M, Walker WG: The syndrome of inappropriate antidiuretic hormone secretion (SIADH): Pathophysiologic mechanisms in solute and volume regulation. Medicine 58:240, 1979
6. deBold AJ: Atrial natriuretic factor: A hormone produced by the heart. Science 230:767, 1985
7. Dunn FL, Brennan TJ, et al: The role of blood osmolality and volume in regulating vasopressin secretion in the rat. J Clin Invest 52:3212, 1973
8. Edelman IS, Liebman J, et al: Interrelations between serum sodium concentration, serum osmolality and total exchangeable potassium and total body water. J Clin Invest 37:1236, 1958
9. Haber E: Renin inhibitors (editorial). Hypertension 8:1093, 1986
10. Kokko J, Tannen RL (eds): Fluid and Electrolyte. Philadelphia, WB Saunders, 1986
11. Kurtzman NA, Martinez-Maldonado M (eds): Pathophysiology of the Kidney. Springfield, Ill, Charles C Thomas, 1977
12. Lang RE, Tholken H, et al: Atrial natriuretic factor: A circulating hormone stimulated by volume loading. Nature 314:264, 1985
13. McCance RA: Experimental sodium chloride deficiency in man. Proc R Soc, Series B 119:245, 1936
14. McCance RA: Medical problems in mineral metabolism. II. Experimental human salt deficiency. Lancet 1:823, 1936
15. McCance RA: Medical problems in mineral metabolism. II. Sodium deficiencies in clinical medicine. Lancet 1:704, 1936
16. Miller M, Moses AM: Drug induced states of impaired water excretion. Kidney Int 10:96, 1976
17. Moore FD, Oleson KH, McMurrey JD, et al: The Body Cell Mass and Its Supporting Environment. Philadelphia, WB Saunders, 1963
18. Robertson GL: Thirst and vasopressin function in normal and disordered states of water balance. J Lab Clin Med 101:351, 1983
19. Robertson GL, Athar S: The interaction of blood osmolality and blood volume in regulating plasma vasopressin in man. J Clin Endocrinol Metab 42:613, 1976
20. Sancho JR, Burton J, et al: The role of the renin-angiotensin-aldosterone system in cardiovascular homeostasis in normal human subjects. Circulation 53:400, 1976
21. Schrier RW (ed): Renal and Electrolyte Disorders, 3d ed. Boston, Little, Brown, 1986
22. Valtin H: Renal Dysfunction: Mechanisms Involved in Fluid and Solute Balance. Boston, Little, Brown, 1979
23. Verney EB: Gustonian Lectures on polyuria. Lancet 2:16, 539, 645, 751, 1929
24. Wright FS: Intrarenal regulation of glomerular filtration rate. N Engl J Med 291:135, 1974
25. Zierler KL: Hyperosmolality in adults: A critical review. J Chronic Dis 7:1, 1958

CHAPTER 10.2
Disorders of Potassium Metabolism

W. Gordon Walker and Daniel G. Sapir

Disorders of potassium metabolism occur in a variety of clinical problems, for the mammalian organism is more vulnerable to either losses or gains in potassium (K^+) than to similar changes in sodium (Na^+). In the presence of stimuli to conserve both sodium and potassium, sodium is conserved more efficiently. In abnormal states associated with aldosterone excess, this sodium conservation may be achieved at the expense of a progressively increasing potassium deficit. The body is subject to marked disturbances in potassium metabolism not only in disease but also as a complication of some therapeutic regimens.

Severe disturbances in body content of potassium may lead to life-threatening alterations in the function of cardiac, skeletal, and smooth muscles, leading to arrhythmias, sudden paralysis, or severe ileus. Such disturbances may also produce disorders in cell function that include cessation of growth in the young and a sustained catabolic state with exaggerated nitrogen losses in the adult. Potassium disturbances often lead to changes in composition and pH of body fluids as well.

Many of the pathophysiologic effects of these disturbances in potassium content are caused by the unique distribution of potassium within the body. More than 97 percent of the total body content of potassium is located within the cells.

NORMAL DISTRIBUTION AND MOVEMENT OF POTASSIUM WITHIN THE BODY[2-4,9,27,29]

DISTRIBUTION[3,27]

Potassium is the major intracellular cation of the body (>150 mEq/L of cell water). The total exchangeable potassium, measured by isotope dilution, differs significantly between males and females, with an average value of 38 mEq/kg body weight in the female and 48 mEq/kg in the male. As shown in Figure 10.2–1, only about 2 percent is located in the extracellular fluid, the remainder being confined within cells. There is a significant quantity of potassium within the bone, but this is not readily exchangeable and is not reflected in the above estimates of total exchangeable potassium.

TRANSCELLULAR K+ MOVEMENT[3,7,9,24,25]

There is a slow efflux of potassium from the resting cell throughout the day. The net flux of potassium, however, demonstrates a substantial diurnal fluctuation. Net flux during the day is outward, but this is reversed at night with net entry into cells. At its peak the resting potassium efflux adds as much as 15 mEq/hr (0.5 percent of intracellular potassium per hour) to the extracellular fluid (ECF). Since this rate of accumulation in the extracellular fluid could lead to an intolerable doubling of the extracellular potassium concentration in only 3 to 4 hours (Fig. 10.2–1), the importance of a renal mechanism for preventing this net rise in plasma extracellular potassium concentration is evident.

The resting K^+ efflux is greatly accentuated by glycogen breakdown, both metabolic and respiratory acidosis, and other metabolic activities that produce excess organic anions within the cell. Conversely, such metabolic activities as glycogen production, glucose uptake under the influence of insulin, and alkalosis produce a net influx of K^+ and an increase in intracellular K^+ concentration.

In addition to the resting flux and the flux influenced by metabolic activity, in muscle a rapid superimposed and transient potassium efflux associated with the electrical depolarization is responsible for muscle contraction. This is followed by equally rapid influx during repolarization.

More than one transport process is involved in transmembrane K^+ movement. Selective disturbances in some of these processes may be associated with specific disease states. There is evidence that one moiety of potassium transport is influenced by ouabain, and that this transport process may behave in an abnormal fashion in patients with essential hypertension. In fact, recent studies have been interpreted to provide support for the proposal that the primary defect, or at least one of the primary defects, in essential hypertension may be an abnormality in this transport process, leading to a progressive depletion of intracellular potassium and an increase in systemic vascular resistance as a result of the accompanying increase in smooth muscle tone.[21,30,31]

METABOLIC FUNCTIONS OF K+[13,14,24,25,31]

Potassium, as the major intracellular solute, determines the osmotic equilibrium across the cell surface and thus determines the volume of intracellular fluid. Potassium within the cell is usually in a constant ratio to cellular protein; the body contains 2.7 mEq of potassium for each gram of nitrogen or each 6.25 g of protein. Increase in the body store of protein (positive nitrogen balance) leads to potassium retention within the body, and conversely catabolic states (negative nitrogen balance) result in potassium loss. An adequate source of potassium is necessary for tissue growth, so potassium deficiency in the young leads to growth failure. A number of the enzymatic processes within the cell are critically dependent upon $[K^+]$, and this may be the mechanism responsible for failure of anabolic processes in potassium-deficient states. In addition, the electrical activity of cells is critically dependent upon the intracellular/extracellular concentration ratio, $[K_i^+]/[K_o^+]$, of potassium across cell membranes. An increase in this ratio leads to an increase in the potential difference or hyperpolarization of the cell and a decreased concentration leads to hypopolarization. Both of these abnormal states result in disturbances of the electrical activity exhibited by excitable cells and are primarily responsible for the adverse effects seen in cardiac and skeletal muscle function in potassium disturbances.

Disturbances in potassium content of the body may thus be responsible for clinical manifestations that range from diminished tendon reflexes to muscular paralysis, pH disturbances of the body fluids, and, in most extreme cases, cardiac arrhythmias and cardiac standstill.

REGULATION OF BODY POTASSIUM CONTENT[3,9]

Changes in the body potassium content result from a disparity between potassium intake and potassium excretion. In the normally growing child, the intake always slightly exceeds the output because of the need for progressive accumulation of potassium and protein to support growth. In adults both the concentration and amount of potassium in the body are closely regulated. Thus, intake and output are closely balanced.

INTAKE

Potassium is present in all natural foods, and its abundance precludes the development of potassium deficiency as long as food intake is adequate. Only when intake is sharply curtailed for long periods, as in anorexia nervosa, starvation, or chronic alcoholism, can a deficient intake lead to serious potassium deficiency. The

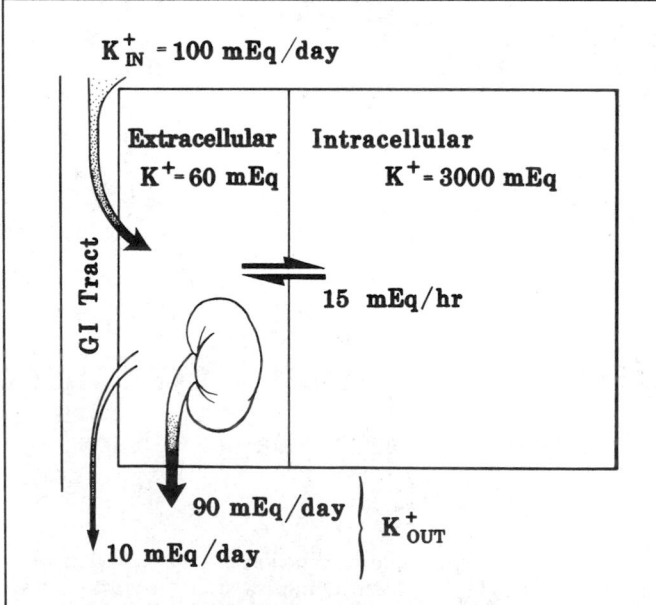

Figure 10.2–1. K+ distribution and exchange in average adult human. Total K+ in extracellular space is only about 60 mEq or approximately 2 percent of intracellular K+. Exchange between cells and ECF is approximately 15 mEq/hr under basal conditions and can increase markedly in response to exercise, anoxia, acidosis, and other stimuli. Thus, the body is extremely susceptible to hyperkalemia when kidneys do not function adequately, since they are responsible for excretion of about 90 percent of the ingested potassium.

practice of clay eating, or geophagia, can result in increased binding within the gastrointestinal (GI) tract and lead to K^+ deficits as a result of defective absorption. This is more frequent in the South, where geophagia is common in some locales. Since the body conserves potassium with much less efficiency than it retains sodium, modest reductions in dietary potassium intake, if sustained over long periods, may contribute substantially to the development of a potassium deficit. This should be kept in mind when searching for an explanation for obscure causes of hypokalemia.

The average dietary intake of potassium in the United States ranges between 50 and 90 mEq per day for an adult. There are marked regional differences, however, and daily intakes as low as 25 to 30 mEq have been documented for some subgroups in certain regions of the country.[10,28] In addition, some racial differences have been identified in the relation between sodium and potassium balance at extremes of intake. Blacks who take in very large quantities of sodium tend to lose more potassium in the urine than do whites.[30,32]

EXCRETION

Potassium excretion occurs by three routes: the skin, the GI tract, and the kidneys (Table 10.2–1). Skin losses are trivial. The concentration of potassium in sweat rarely exceeds 15 or 20 mEq/L, so that large volumes of sweat lead to only modest potassium losses by this route.

Gastrointestinal Excretion

The GI tract is not a significant source of potassium excretion in the normal individual. Although the potassium concentration in fecal water may significantly exceed the plasma potassium concentration, the small quantity of water in feces under normal circumstances (<250 ml per day) limits this source of potassium excretion to a few milliequivalents per day.

Diarrhea can lead to significant potassium losses from the GI tract. The concentration of potassium in diarrheal fluid may rise to 20 to 25 mEq/L. When the volume of diarrheal fluid exceeds 3 to 4 L per day, the total daily loss may be 100 mEq, a tenfold increase.

In advanced renal failure the GI tract may function as a major route of potassium excretion, with more than 60 to 80 percent of ingested potassium being excreted in the feces. Patients in this condition are particularly susceptible to potassium depletion when diarrhea occurs.

Renal Excretion[2,3,8–10]

The mechanisms involved in the renal transport of potassium include filtration, reabsorption, and secretion in exchange for Na^+. Potassium is freely filtered at the glomerulus and is probably reabsorbed passively, although active transport may also be involved to a minor degree. Most, if not all, of the potassium that is excreted reaches the urine by a secretory process located in the distal tubule. Maintenance of electroneutrality within the urine requires that this potassium secretion be balanced by net movement of cation in the opposite direction. Hence, the result of this secretory process is an exchange of K^+ for an equivalent amount of Na^+.

TABLE 10.2–1. NORMAL ROUTES OF POTASSIUM LOSS FROM BODY

Site	Average Rate of Loss (mEq/day)
Skin	<5
Gastrointestinal tract	5–10
Kidneys	80–100
Total	86–110

TABLE 10.2–2. INFLUENCES ON RENAL TRANSPORT AND EXCRETION OF POTASSIUM

Physiologic Stimuli Influencing Renal Potassium Transport
- K^+ intake
- Aldosterone
- Rate of Na^+ excretion
- H^+ excretion

Factors That Lead to Increase in Renal Potassium Excretion
- Increased K^+ intake
- Increased serum $[K^+]$
- Increased Na^+ excretion
- Increased anion excretion
- Decreased H^+ excretion
- Decreased NH_4^+ excretion
- Increased plasma cortisol level
- Increased plasma aldosterone level

REGULATORY MECHANISMS

In the normal subject there is no mechanism for modulating potassium balance that operates to reduce intake or to alter GI absorption. Even though the organism responds to alteration in the intake of potassium, the kidney is the effector organ in regulating potassium balance. Table 10.2–2 shows the factors that modify the rate of potassium output within the distal tubules.

Generally, the potassium excretion is increased whenever the quantity of *sodium* presented to the distal tubule is increased. Conversely, potassium excretion is restricted by a reduction in the quantity of sodium presented to the distal tubule. Since sodium delivery to the distal exchange site is thought to be adequate for the potassium excretion even when the rate of urinary sodium loss is low, the variation in potassium excretion with distal tubular sodium load has been ascribed to the effects of urinary flow rate in this region.

Potassium excretion is also increased by an increased distal tubular load of poorly reabsorbed *anions*. The ketoacids excreted in increased quantities in diabetic acidosis thus lead to increased potassium excretion. Intake of anions, such as sulfates, which are poorly reabsorbed by the kidney, may also lead to increased potassium loss.

Distal tubular *hydrogen ion secretion* has also been shown to change the rate of potassium output. In most instances there is a reciprocal relationship in the excretion of these two ions, so that an increased output of one will lower the excretion of the other. This reciprocal effect is thought to be responsible for the acceleration of potassium secretion observed in metabolic alkalosis.

An additional important element of control of potassium/hydrogen output is the direct effect of potassium on *renal ammonium ion production*. Production of ammonia, the major urinary buffer, is decreased by potassium loading, and it is increased by potassium depletion. An increase in renal ammonia genesis will generally lead to a higher hydrogen ion output and reduced potassium excretion.

Rate of potassium output is also subject to *diurnal variation* and influenced by potassium intake and the secretory rates of the mineralocorticoid hormones (Fig. 10.2–2). The pattern of diurnal variation in potassium excretion coincides with the pattern of diurnal flux across cell membranes described above.[4,5,8,9]

POTASSIUM DEFICITS AND HYPOKALEMIA[3,13–17,29]

CAUSES

Table 10.2–3 lists the causes of potassium deficiency, or hypokalemia. Potassium losses originate from within the GI tract or the kidneys. Many of the conditions leading to increased renal loss are primarily metabolic disorders and have been listed separately.

Figure 10.2–2. Influence of Na$^+$ and K$^+$ intake on aldosterone secretion. Two feedback mechanisms exist that, although independent, are capable of interaction. Plasma K$^+$ influences aldosterone directly without necessity for intact renin-angiotensin system.[4,5] Elevated plasma K$^+$ is also capable of suppressing renin output by kidney directly. Thus, this system monitors and regulates both sodium and potassium content of the body, but sodium is much more efficiently regulated than potassium. This coordinated regulatory system leads to prompt (usually within 72 hours) elaboration of urine that is virtually sodium free when Na$^+$ intake ceases abruptly. Body K$^+$ stores are not so effectively guarded. Despite cessation of potassium intake, urinary K$^+$ does not fall below plasma K$^+$ until large deficits in body potassium have accrued.

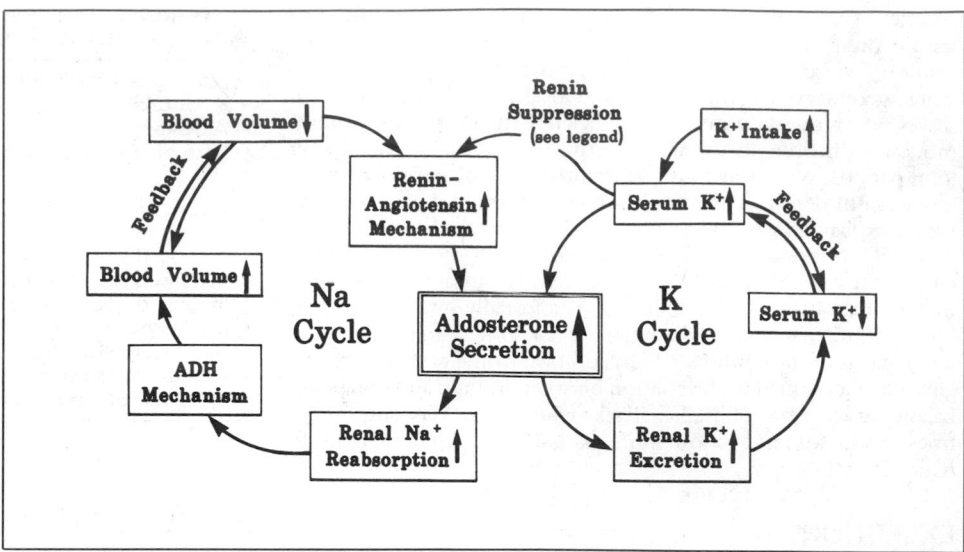

Deficient Intake

Clinically recognizable potassium deficiency caused exclusively by reduced intake rarely occurs except when potassium intake is severely restricted for prolonged periods. Since renal conservation of potassium lowers output below 10 mEq per day only with great difficulty, a chronic deficit regularly occurs when intake is persistently nil. Alcoholism may present with this form of potassium deficiency and is probably the most common cause for large K$^+$ deficits caused by deficient intake. Alcoholism is thus capable of producing clinically significant potassium deficits of sufficient severity to produce many of the clinical manifestations listed in Table 10.2–4.

Recent surveys in large numbers of people indicate that many individuals may have persistently low and probably inadequate potassium intake. Some individuals regularly take in less than 25 mEq/24 hr in contrast to the usual adult intake in this country of about 85 mEq/24 hr. Although no acute symptoms have been identified in association with such low intakes, the groups of individuals who have been documented to have such persistently low potassium intakes exhibit an unusually high prevalence of elevated blood pressure.[10,15,29,30,32,33] The role of this decreased potassium intake in the pathogenesis of hypertension remains to be determined, but most reported studies have demonstrated that the administration of potassium to hypertensive individuals is associated with a significant reduction in blood pressure.[12,16,20] None of these hypertensive patients exhibit any of the clinical manifestations of hypokalemia listed in Table 10.2–4, but whether such low intakes have significant long-term effects on the status of the individual's health constitutes an important but still unresolved question. The current information is sufficiently consistent to warrant recommendation of a low-sodium diet that includes an abundance of foods high in potassium.[33]

Gastrointestinal Loss

Gastrointestinal losses associated with vomiting, diarrhea, or fistulae usually lead to slow development of hypokalemia. The process

---

TABLE 10.2–3. CAUSES OF HYPOKALEMIA

Gastrointestinal
- Vomiting
- Diarrhea
- Gastrointestinal fistulae
- Villous adenoma
- Ureterosigmoidostomy
- Ileostomy
- Chronic laxative ingestion
- Prolonged absence of K$^+$ intake (alcoholism, geophagia, anorexia nervosa, dietary fads)

Metabolic
- Diabetic acidosis
- Respiratory alkalosis
- Adrenocortical excess
  ACTH-producing tumors
  Cushing syndrome
  Primary aldosteronism
    Adrenal adenomas
    Adrenal hyperplasia
  Steroid administration
  Thyrotoxicosis
  Familial periodic paralysis

Renal
- Renal tubular acidosis
- Diuretic therapy
- Potassium-losing nephropathy (Bartter syndrome, Fanconi syndrome)
- Acidosis
- Alkalosis
- Secondary aldosteronism
  Cirrhosis
  Nephrosis
  Bartter syndrome

TABLE 10.2–4. CLINICAL MANIFESTATIONS OF HYPOKALEMIA

Acute	Chronic
Weakness	Weakness
Hyporeflexia	Weight loss
Ileus	Polyuria
Flaccid paralysis	Growth retardation
Postural hypotension	Hyporeflexia
ECG abnormalities	Episodic paralysis
Respiratory distress	Postural hypotension
	ECG abnormalities
	Azotemia

may be hastened by the presence of conditions leading to associated increased renal losses, such as aldosterone excess stimulated by an associated sodium deficiency. Two conditions producing hypokalemia that are often not promptly recognized are chronic laxative abuse and villous adenoma of the colon. Patients abusing the use of laxatives are often unreliable historians, denying laxative use or liquid bowel movements. The presence of severe hypokalemia and very low concentrations of potassium in the urine should always raise suspicion of laxative abuse. Patients with villous adenoma typically give a history of frequent passage of mucoid secretions per rectum with intermittent liquid diarrhea. Since most gastrointestinal conditions leading to hypokalemia are associated with losses of rather large volumes of fluid by this route, associated sodium deficits are commonly seen.

Metabolic Disorders[7,14,24,31]

Metabolic disturbances producing increased urinary potassium losses usually result from mineralocorticoid excess or increased renal excretion of organic acids. The hypokalemia or mineralocorticoid excess may first be recognized as a result of what appears to be an inappropriate response to diuretics, with severe manifestations of hypokalemia occurring after only one or two doses of a diuretic that increases potassium excretion. This is a particularly valuable diagnostic feature in situations where overt stigmata of Cushing syndrome are not obvious on physical examination.

Diabetic acidosis with progressively increasing rate of ketoacid excretion may also lead to severe and rapidly developing potassium deficits that can exceed 500 mEq after only 3 or 4 days of acidosis.

The causative factors in the loss of potassium during diabetic acidosis are similar to those producing potassium loss in other forms of acidosis. Increased excretion of acetoacetate and β-OH butyrate is not equaled by the rise in the generation and excretion of ammonium, a process that requires several days to reach maximal efficiency. The result is that potassium and sodium are excreted in excess to maintain urinary electroneutrality. Contraction of the extracellular volume incident to continued losses of sodium leads to excess mineralocorticoid hormone release and increased potassium wastage. Two of these factors, lag in ammonium production and aldosterone excess stimulated by volume deficit, are factors responsible for potassium losses in other forms of metabolic acidosis.

Renal Loss[2,8,9,31]

Renal loss of potassium in renal tubular acidosis is seen in both distal (type I) and proximal (type II) forms of disease. It results from a failure of the hydrogen-secreting mechanism in both types of disease and may be quite severe. As with diabetic acidosis, the rate of potassium loss is accentuated by excess aldosterone but promptly diminishes when the acidosis is corrected.

Diuretic agents may also produce potassium losses. Two mechanisms are involved. First, potassium losses increase as the rate of urinary sodium excretion increases, a reflection of increased exchange of potassium for luminal sodium as increasing quantities of sodium reach the distal segments of the nephrons. This is accentuated by aldosterone excess. Second, since many diuretics produce a chloride deficiency and hypochloremic alkalosis, this increases potassium loss further. Renal potassium wastage is increased when metabolic alkalosis occurs.

Internal Shifts

The disorders covered in the preceding paragraphs are all associated with hypokalemia attributable to increased potassium losses from either the kidneys or the GI tract. There are disorders, however, in which hypokalemia occurs without either increased potassium loss or decreased intake. Familial periodic paralysis is the classic example of this type of acute hypokalemia.[24] It is associated with acute and profound decreases in plasma [K$^+$] and accompanying paralysis. The episodes of hypokalemic paralysis are precipitated either by excessive exercise or ingestion of a high-carbohydrate meal. In this condition the low serum potassium is a result of in-creased movement of this ion into the intracellular compartment and not of external losses. Similar episodes may also occur during the course of hyperthyroidism.

RELATION BETWEEN MAGNESIUM DEFICITS AND K$^+$ DEFICIENCY

Since Cotlove's[6] initial report that skeletal potassium loss occurs in magnesium depletion was confirmed by Whang and Welt,[34] a large body of experimental and clinical evidence has documented a significant role for magnesium depletion in the development and manifestations of some cases of hypokalemia. Magnesium deficiency is regularly associated with a decrease in intracellular potassium of a magnitude that may exceed 20 percent under experimental circumstances.[22,23,34] Moreover, repair of such coexisting potassium deficits is extremely difficult unless the magnesium deficit is corrected concomitantly. This is of importance clinically in the malabsorption syndrome, which is often associated with chronic magnesium depletion in addition to potassium depletion, and in severe alcoholics who have been demonstrated to have remarkable degrees of magnesium depletion at times associated with refractory hypokalemia. Perhaps the most important circumstance clinically is the magnesium depletion produced by long-term usage of furosemide and bumetamide, two potent diuretics that have been demonstrated to increase urinary magnesium losses and lead to profound magnesium depletion with chronic or persistent usage in congestive heart failure. Aldosterone produces a combined magnesium and potassium deficit, and perhaps the hyperaldosteronism seen in congestive heart failure also contributes to the development of hypomagnesemia in these heart failure patients. Various surveys upon hospitalized patients have reported an incidence of hypomagnesemia that varies between 7 and 30 percent depending upon the characteristics of the patients included in the survey.[22] Thus hypomagnesemia is evidently a common clinical problem and one that should always be kept in mind during the diagnostic investigation of hypokalemia. When both are identified, treatment of the two deficits should proceed concurrently.

CLINICAL MANIFESTATIONS OF HYPOKALEMIA

The diagnosis of potassium deficiency and hypokalemia must depend primarily upon a high index of suspicion. The disorders or conditions listed in Table 10.2–3 should always alert the physician to this possibility, and appropriate tests should be undertaken to diagnose or exclude potassium disturbance. Table 10.2–4 shows the signs and symptoms commonly associated with potassium deficits. The relation of these findings to the severity of the hypokalemia may be quite variable. Acute lowering of plasma [K$^+$] may produce profound disturbances at levels that, in chronic situations, may be associated only with weakness. Clinical manifestations are most likely to be hyperacute and catastrophic in situations where the plasma [K$^+$] is falling rapidly, as in diabetic acidosis during the early stages of treatment or in familial periodic paralysis.

Confirmation of the presence of a potassium deficit rests primarily on the measurement of the serum potassium. This generally falls with loss of potassium and is progressively depressed with larger degrees of negative potassium balance. Unfortunately, the correlation between potassium loss and depression of the serum potassium concentration is poor, so that the magnitude of deficiency cannot be accurately assessed from plasma [K$^+$]. Plasma K$^+$ does decrease with increasing K$^+$ deficits, however. A rough guide is that a decrease of 1 mEq in plasma K$^+$ reflects a total body K$^+$ deficit between 200 and 300 mEq. This does not hold absolutely; the distribution of potassium between extracellular and intracellular compartments is also governed by such factors as extracellular pH and renal function. Thus elevations of the serum potassium may occur in the presence of total body potassium depletion when acidosis is present. Alkalosis, in contrast to acidosis, can produce a depression of the serum potassium by causing increased move-

ment of extracellular potassium into intracellular fluid. These factors affecting the serum potassium make ancillary laboratory testing and clinical judgments important in the decision concerning the presence and magnitude of potassium deficiency. The presence of symptoms of potassium deficiency, associated with evidence of metabolic, endocrine, renal, or gastrointestinal lesions that cause potassium loss, constitutes important historical data in assessing the state of potassium stores.

The ECG changes of potassium deficiency, lowered T waves, and prolongation of the QT interval (these may ultimately lead to cardiac arrest) are also helpful signs in the diagnosis of potassium deficiency (Fig. 10.2–3). There is low correlation between ECG changes and the magnitude of potassium depletion.

Regardless of how hypokalemia is first recognized, one must assume that it is a manifestation of underlying disease. Judicious interpretation of the history, physical findings, and laboratory information is necessary to arrive at a final diagnosis. The association of hypokalemia and a history of vomiting suggests a GI disorder as the underlying cause. Hyperchloremia and decreased plasma [K+] suggest renal tubular acidosis or complication of acetazolamide therapy. Metabolic alkalosis with hypokalemia in the absence of GI signs or symptoms suggests either mineralocorticoid excess or diuretic-induced (chlorothiazide, furosemide, or ethacrynic acid) potassium depletion, or Bartter syndrome.

Alkalosis is seen in conjunction with hypokalemia when the underlying cause is persistent vomiting caused by upper GI obstruction; chronic laxative abuse; primary, secondary, or iatrogenic mineralocorticoid excess; or the administration of saliuretic diuretic agents such as chlorothiazide or furosemide.

Acidosis associated with hypokalemia is seen in the presence of severe diarrhea of relatively short duration, diabetic acidosis, renal tubular acidosis, chronic acetazolamide administration, ureterosigmoidostomy, and occasionally with diversion of the urinary stream into an ileal loop.

PATHOLOGIC CHANGES ASSOCIATED WITH POTASSIUM DEPLETION

In the presence of long-standing potassium depletion, structural changes occur in the kidney and in skeletal and cardiac muscles. Vacuolization within the renal tubular cells and peritubular scarring in the region of the distal tubules and collecting ducts represent the characteristic lesion of hypokalemic nephropathy. The scarring probably accounts for the loss of the renal-concentrating function that is seen regularly in potassium deficits of several weeks' duration. Vacuolization and fragmentation of fibers may be seen in both skeletal and cardiac muscle with long-standing potassium depletion.

TREATMENT

No reliable guides are present for estimating the magnitude of the potassium deficit in a given situation. Plasma [K+] below 2.5 mEq/L may be associated with deficits ranging from 400 mEq to more than 1000 mEq. The usual approach is to continue potassium administration until the plasma [K+] has returned to the normal range and until an adequate oral intake of food gives additional assurance that normal potassium balance will be maintained. The oral route of potassium repletion is preferable if the GI tract is functioning adequately. Administration of potassium by mouth has the advantage of being safer and requiring less monitoring than intravenous administration. (Initially 120 mEq may be given orally as a 10 percent solution of potassium chloride, preferably in orange or tomato juice.) When the potassium is less than 2.5 mEq/L, this dose can be safely repeated within 4 hours. Once the serum potassium rises, the rate of administration can be slowed and supplements of 80 to 120 mEq per day can be given in addition to potassium present in the diet (note that this applies only to patients with *normal renal function*).

In patients with advanced renal impairment and hypokalemia a much more cautious approach is mandatory. No more than 80 mEq should be given on the first day of therapy, and thereafter supplemental oral K+ should not exceed 30 to 40 mEq/24 hr. Even so, careful monitoring of the serum K+ is essential under these circumstances (Table 10.2–5).

If a malfunctioning GI tract precludes oral therapy, or if the severity of the hypokalemia makes intravenous replacement desirable, no more than 30 mEq of potassium chloride should be administered hourly, and this rate should not be achieved except in acute situations such as may be encountered in diabetic acidosis.

Under all other circumstances it is probably safer to keep the rate of administration at or below 10 to 15 mEq/hr. As repletion continues and gastrointestinal motility improves, oral therapy can replace the intravenous route. Extensive drug surveillance studies in several hospitals have all shown that hyperkalemia complicating potassium administration is one of the most common and dangerous complications of hospital drug usage.[18,19] It is particularly likely to occur when both oral and intravenous route of administration are used in the same patient. *Careful monitoring of all patients receiving potassium is mandatory.*

The ECG is useful in monitoring the results of parenteral potassium administration. It should always be used to monitor the earlier therapy of severe diabetic acidosis, since plasma [K+] may change so rapidly that it is not practical to rely upon serum [K+]

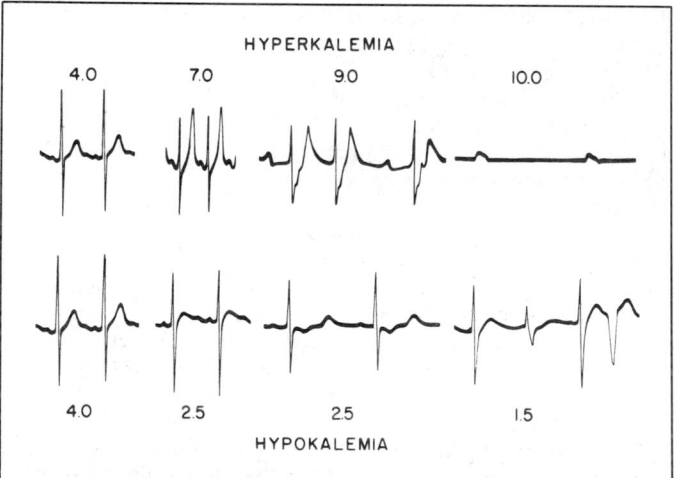

Figure 10.2–3. *Hyperkalemia:* ECG lead V₄ illustrating abnormalities encountered with progressive elevation of serum potassium. One of earliest changes is tall, peaked, and symmetrical T waves. As serum potassium rises further (to 9 mEq/L) P-R interval and QRS duration are prolonged. Both atrial and ventricular ectopic beats may occur. At levels of serum potassium near 10 mEq/L, P waves disappear and slow heart rate with wide QRS complexes is noted. This is followed by development of total asystole. *Hypokalemia:* ECG lead V₄ illustrating changes which may result as serum potassium is progressively lowered. At levels below 3 mEq/L, T-wave amplitude decreases and U wave appears or increases in magnitude. U wave may become very prominent and ST segment sagged or frankly depressed. Further lowering of serum potassium may result in ectopic activity in atria and ventricles, especially if patient has received digitalis. Ventricular fibrillation may develop.

TABLE 10.2–5. SOME PRINCIPLES OF POTASSIUM REPLACEMENT

- Use oral route whenever possible
- Give parenterally at less than 10 mEq/hr except in extreme emergency
- Never exceed 30 mEq/hr intravenously
- When parenteral K+ replacement exceeds 10 mEq/hr, ECG monitoring is necessary
- Never give K+ parenterally to patients with renal failure (GFR <10 ml/min)

measurements. As potassium balance improves, U waves disappear, T-wave amplitude increases, and the QT interval shortens. When acidosis is present together with hypokalemia, potassium can be given with bicarbonate to correct both the acidosis and potassium depletion. It must be reemphasized that a severe acidosis may mask significant potassium deficits if the plasma [K$^+$] is relied upon to exclude potassium deficiency. Great caution should be exercised in the treatment of severe acidosis by bicarbonate administration even in the presence of an initially normal plasma [K$^+$]. Sudden correction of the acidosis may acutely lower plasma [K$^+$] to life-threatening levels as improvement in the acidosis results in marked shifts of potassium into the cells. When alkalosis and hypokalemia are present, there usually is an associated chloride deficit, and both potassium and chloride are necessary to completely correct the alkalosis.[13]

Adequate work-up of the patient with potassium deficiency includes the identification or exclusion of sources of continuing potassium loss. In situations where potassium loss continues, as in steroid therapy, Cushing syndrome, or other disturbances associated with continuing renal or GI loss of potassium, supplemental therapy must be continued if recurrence of the hypokalemia is to be prevented.

HYPERKALEMIA[1,25]

Since the total quantity of potassium present in the extracellular fluid in a 70-kg man is 80 to 90 mEq, very small increases in the extracellular fluid potassium may result in large elevations of serum potassium. Hyperkalemia may thus occur swiftly.[1]

CLINICAL MANIFESTATIONS

With increases in extracellular fluid potassium the resting potential of cells is lowered and results in neuromuscular irritability. Irritability of muscle may progress to a state of depolarization block resulting in paralysis if the potassium continues to rise in ECF. This occurs in both cardiac and skeletal muscle. Figure 10.2–3 shows sequential ECG changes that occur with increases in serum potassium. Peaking of the T waves is the most reliable measure of hyperkalemic effects upon the heart. Although it may be first seen at different [K$^+$] in different patients and in different clinical situations, it is nonetheless the earliest and most reliable indicator of cardiotoxicity caused by hyperkalemia.

CAUSES

The most common clinical settings in which hyperkalemia occurs are renal failure and acidosis (Table 10.2–6). Acidosis may cause hyperkalemia when renal function is entirely normal. Hyperkalemia may be observed both early and late in the oliguric phase of acute renal failure.[25] It usually occurs late during the course of chronic renal failure when the glomerular filtration rate has fallen below 5 ml/min. This level of renal function is usually adequate to achieve excretion of the usual daily load of ingested potassium. The imposition of an additional load, either exogenously from increased intake or endogenously from increased catabolism caused by infection, hemorrhage, tissue necrosis, or acidosis, may exceed the capacity of the severely diseased kidney to excrete potassium, thereby leading to acute hyperkalemia.

Elevation of the serum potassium may also occur with mineralocorticoid deficiency, as is seen in Addison disease or isolated deficiency of aldosterone. This results primarily from failure of renal secretion of potassium in the absence of aldosterone.

Drug-related Hyperkalemia

Increasing numbers of drugs currently in wide use that alter potassium metabolism either directly or secondarily make this an increasingly important cause of hyperkalemia in hospitalized patients.[18,19,26] Since the introduction of spironolactone as an

TABLE 10.2–6. CAUSES OF HYPERKALEMIA

Disease Related
- Renal failure
  Acute
  Chronic
- Severe acidosis
- Addison disease
- Hereditary episodic adynamia[7]
- Iatrogenic
  K-retaining diuretics
  Inappropriate K administration

Spurious
- Hemolyzed blood sample
- Thrombocytosis
- Time lapse between drawing blood and separating cells
- Leukocytic distintegration in leukemia

aldosterone antagonist that suppresses renal K$^+$ secretion, two other widely used diuretic agents are well recognized to produce a major reduction in the rate of renal potassium secretion. These two agents, triamterene and amiloride, are both capable of producing hyperkalemia in normal individuals and have been documented to produce life-threatening hyperkalemia in individuals with preexisting renal impairment. While most such cases in the literature represent individuals who were inadvertently receiving supplemental potassium plus a potassium-sparing diuretic, the potential danger of these drugs is such that they should not be used in individuals with significant impairment of renal function (glomerular filtration rate <40 ml/min).[18]

Pharmacologic blockade of the beta-adrenergic receptors is now well recognized as an intervention that inhibits cellular uptake of potassium and thereby can produce acute hyperkalemia. Since it appears that this effect is a manifestation of blockade of the beta$_2$-adrenergic receptor system, such drugs should be avoided in conditions where the risk of hyperkalemia is significant, as in impaired renal function.

Of the other agents known to elevate the plasma potassium, cyclosporins, heparin, and angiotensin-converting enzyme inhibitors are probably not associated with risks as great as that which may be encountered with the use of succinylcholine. Since this muscle relaxant is used in anesthesia, it should be avoided in all patients undergoing anesthesia who have impaired kidney function and who may thus be acutely susceptible to acute and large elevations of potassium in the plasma.

TREATMENT

Since serious and potentially fatal elevations of the serum potassium result from small additions of this cation to the extracellular fluid in the absence of adequate renal function, successful therapy may be predicated on the removal of small amounts of potassium from this body fluid compartment (Table 10.2–7). A decrease in the serum potassium may be accomplished by the transfer of this cation from the extra- to the intracellular fluids, the removal of potassium from the body, or administration of an agent that has an antagonistic effect to the action of potassium on cell membranes. In clinical situations where the serum potassium is found or suspected to be significantly increased, an ECG should be obtained immediately and treatment started promptly upon recognition of increasing amplitude of the T wave. Frequent ECG monitoring during therapy is essential. Demonstration of widening of the QRS complex is particularly ominous and requires vigorous therapy if the patient's life is to be saved.

Calcium administration in the form of the chloride or gluconate salt is the most successful means of acutely counteracting the cardiac effects of hyperkalemia. This agent antagonizes the effects of potassium on all membranes. Administration of 1 to 2 g of calcium gluconate intravenously over 3 to 5 minutes partially reverses the characteristic ECG changes of hyperkalemia within minutes. Continuous calcium infusion at a rate of 1 g/hr may be used to

TABLE 10.2–7. TREATMENT OF HYPERKALEMIA

Temporary Measures
- Ca gluconate or CaCl$_2$ intravenously 1 g given over 10–15 min period
- Correction of acidosis (if present) with NaHCO$_3$
- 2.5% ($\approx$1000 mOsm/L) NaCl intravenously as slow infusion at 0.2–0.5 ml/min
- Glucose and insulin intravenously 3–4 g glucose with each unit of insulin

Permanent (Corrective) Measures
- Administration of Na polystyrene sulfonate resin, 25–75 g/day in 15–25% sorbitol orally or as retention enema (*Note:* This removes K$^+$ and replaces an equivalent amount of Na$^+$)
- Peritoneal dialysis (do not add K$^+$ to first 6–8 exchanges, then use dialysate containing 1 mEq K/L)
- Hemodialysis (use dialysate containing 2 mEq K/L)

control further cardiovascular toxicity of hyperkalemia. In the presence of acidosis, sodium bicarbonate can be given intravenously to increase the serum pH and transfer potassium into cells in exchange for hydrogen (see Chapter 10.3). Insulin and glucose are also effective in transferring potassium into the cells. Generally 1 U of regular insulin is given together with 3 to 4 g of glucose, the latter administered intravenously as a 10 percent glucose solution. At least 50 to 100 g of glucose may be given in this situation. All of these forms of therapy may be given concurrently to patients with marked elevation of the serum potassium. All these measures are effective when first used. Their effectiveness rapidly diminishes, however, in the presence of recurring hyperkalemia.

If hyperkalemia is refractory to the foregoing therapy, or if it occurs in the presence of poor renal function where potassium elevation may recur, dialysis is necessary. Initially peritoneal dialysis without addition of potassium to the first six to eight exchanges effectively reduces plasma [K$^+$]. The other measures described previously should also be continued until the serum potassium is normal. Peritoneal dialysis is relatively inefficient, however, at removing potassium (no more than 4 to 6 mEq/hr even when the entering dialysate contains no potassium). Hemodialysis is capable of removing K$^+$ at more than twice this rate under optimal conditions.

Administration of Kayexelate, a polystyrene sulfonate resin that removes potassium from the body through exchange for sodium across the lumen of the small and large bowel, can be used to control elevations of the serum potassium. It may be given by mouth together with sorbitol (to prevent fecal impaction) or as an enema. It has a maximum binding capacity of 4 mEq K$^+$/g of resin, but more than 50 percent binding is rarely achieved in practice. Although it may be used effectively for short periods, it suffers the disadvantage of replacing the potassium with equal quantities of sodium. Thus, in the patient with virtually absent renal function, sodium overload may become a serious problem if this form of therapy is continued for long periods.

REFERENCES

1. Bedford PD: Acute potassium intoxication. Lancet 2:268, 1954
2. Berliner RW: Renal mechanisms for potassium excretion. Harvey Lect 55:141, 1961
3. Cheng JT, Sapir DG, et al: A comparison of potassium bicarbonate and potassium chloride in the repair of potassium deficiency. Johns Hopkins Med J 133:299, 1973
4. Cooke CR, Horvath JS, et al: Modulation of plasma aldosterone concentration by plasma potassium in anephric man in the absence of a change in potassium balance. J Clin Invest 52:3028, 1973
5. Cooke CR, Ruiz-Maza F, et al: Regulation of plasma aldosterone concentration in anephric man and renal transplant recipients. Kidney Int 3:160, 1973
6. Cotlove E, Holliday MA, et al: Effects of electrolyte depletion and acid base disturbance on muscle cations. Am J Physiol 167:665, 1951
7. Gamstorp I: Adynamia episodica hereditaria. Acta Paediatr Scand (Suppl) 45:108, 1956
8. Giebisch GH: Renal potassium excretion. In Rouillen C, Muller AF (eds): The Kidney. New York, Academic Press, 1971, vol 3, p 329
9. Giebisch G, Malnic G, Berliner RW: Renal transport and control of potassium excretion. In Brenner BM, Rector FC Jr (eds): The Kidney, 2d ed. Philadelphia, WB Saunders, 1981
10. Grimm CE, Luft FC, et al: Racial differences in blood pressure in Evans County, Georgia: Relation to sodium and potassium intake and plasma renin activity. J Chron Dis 33:87, 1980
11. Hollifield J: Potassium and magnesium abnormalities: Diuretics and arrhythmias in hypertension. In Whelton P, Whelton A, Walker WG (eds): Potassium in Cardiovascular and Renal Medicine. New York, Marcel Dekker, 1986, p 261
12. Holly JMP, Goodwin FJ, et al: Reanalysis of data in two Lancet papers on the effect of dietary sodium and potassium on blood pressure. Lancet 2:1384, 1981
13. Kassirer JP, Berkman PM, et al: The critical role of chloride in the correction of hypokalemic alkalosis in man. Am J Med 38:172, 1965
14. Kassirer JP, Harrington JT: Diuretics and potassium metabolism: A reassessment of the need, effectiveness and safety of potassium therapy. Kidney Int 11:505, 1977
15. Khaw KT, Barrett-Connor E: Dietary potassium and stroke-associated mortality: A 12-year prospective population study. N Engl J Med 316:235, 1987
16. Khaw KT, Thorn S: Randomized double-blind crossover trial of potassium on blood pressure in normal subjects. Lancet 2:1127, 1982
17. Kurtzman NA, Martinez-Maldonado M (eds): Pathophysiology of the Kidney. Springfield, Ill, Charles C Thomas, 1977
18. Lawson DH: Adverse reactions to potassium chloride. Q J Med 43:433, 1974
19. Lawson DH, Henry DA, et al: Severe hypokalemia in hospitalized patients. Arch Intern Med 139:978, 1979
20. MacGregor GA, Smith SJ, et al: Moderate potassium supplementation. Lancet 2:567, 1982
21. Meyer P, Garay RP, Nazaret C, et al: Inheritance of abnormal erythrocyte cation transport in essential hypertension. Br Med J 282:1114, 1981
22. Ryan MP: The role of magnesium in K deficiency. In Whelton P, Whelton A, Walker WG (eds): Potassium in cardiovascular and renal medicine. New York, Marcel Dekker, 1986, p 23
23. Sheehan J, White A: Diuretic associated hypomagnesemia. Br Med J 285:1157, 1982
24. Shy GM, Wanko T, et al: Studies in familial periodic paralysis. Exp Neurol 3:53, 1961
25. Steinmetz PR, Kiley JE: Hyperkalemia in renal failure. JAMA 175:689, 1961
26. Tannen RL: Drug interactions causing hyperkalemia. In Whelton P, Whelton A, Walker WG (eds): Potassium in Cardiovascular and Renal Medicine. New York, Marcel Dekker, 1986, p 467
27. Valtin H: Renal Dysfunction: Mechanisms Involved in Fluid and Electrolyte Balance. Boston, Little, Brown, 1979
28. Voors AW, Berenson GS, et al: Racial differences in blood pressure control. Science 204:1091, 1979
29. Walker WG: Relationship between potassium and blood pressure in normotensive and untreated hypertensive subjects. In Whelton P, Whelton A, Walker WG (eds): Potassium in Cardiovascular and Renal Medicine. New York, Marcel Dekker, 1986, p 345
30. Walker WG: Relationships between sodium and potassium intake and blood pressure. In Joosens JV, Kesteloot H (eds): Epidemiology of Arterial Blood Pressure. Boston, Martinus Nijhoff, 1980, p 297
31. Walker WG, Sapir DG, et al: Potassium homeostasis and diuretic therapy. In DeWardener H (ed): Modern Diuretic Therapy in the Treatment of Cardiovascular and Renal Disease. International Congress Series #268. Amsterdam, Excerpta Medica, 1973, p 331
32. Walker WG, Whelton PK, et al: Relation between blood pressure and renin, renin substrate, angiotensin II, aldosterone and urinary sodium and potassium in 574 ambulatory subjects. Hypertension 1:287, 1979
33. Walker WG, Whelton PK, Whelton A: Perspectives on some important public health issues related to potassium balance. In Whelton P, Whelton A, Walker WG (eds): Potassium in Cardiovascular and Renal Medicine. New York, Marcel Dekker, 1986, p 537
34. Whang R, Welt L: Observations in experimental magnesium depletion. J Clin Invest 42:305, 1963

Acid–Base Disturbances

Daniel G. Sapir and W. Gordon Walker

In the normal individual, the daily production of hydrogen ion exceeds 12,000 mEq. Despite this large production the hydrogen ion concentration is maintained between 3.5×10^{-8} and 4.5×10^{-8} moles per liter in the plasma and interstitial fluid. The *buffers* in blood, interstitial and intracellular fluid, and the excretory functions of the *lungs* and *kidneys* are responsible for maintenance of the hydrogen ion concentration within these limits. Their actions, in concert, permit production and elimination of these large quantities of hydrogen ion with only very small changes in hydrogen ion concentration in body fluids. The lungs serve as a principal route of elimination of hydrogen ion when H_2CO_3 is converted to the CO_2 excreted in expired air. The kidneys provide a second route for hydrogen ion excretion that is quantitatively much smaller but is of prime importance in restoring the buffer capacity of the body fluids (Fig. 10.3–1). Without the great excretory capacity of the lungs and kidneys, the buffers would be quite inadequate to regulate hydrogen ion concentration and fatal acidosis would develop in a very short time. For convenience, pH is used to represent hydrogen ion concentration and is defined as:

$$pH = -\log [H^+] \qquad (1)$$

PHYSIOLOGY OF pH REGULATION[8,11,14,15]

SOURCES OF HYDROGEN ION PRODUCTION

The sources of hydrogen ion are shown in Figure 10.3–2. The major source is the production of CO_2 from metabolic processes (about 12,000 mEq per day). Metabolism of phospholipids, as well as of proteins that contain phosphate and sulfate, yields phosphoric and sulfuric acids. These latter substances account for no more than 80 to 100 mEq of hydrogen ion per day in normal individuals. Although quantitatively these sources yield only a very small fraction of the daily production, they are of special significance because the hydrogen ion thus formed is associated with nonvolatile anions, phosphate and sulfate, and must be eliminated via the kidney.

ROLE OF BUFFERS[2,11,13,14]

The buffers of the body fluids transport the hydrogen ion formed by all these processes from the production sources in the tissues to the lungs and kidneys for excretion.

The chemical buffering action that occurs within the body fluids is provided by mixtures of poorly dissociated weak acids and their highly ionized salts. Such buffer pairs minimize pH change by converting a strong, highly dissociated acid to a weak, poorly dissociated one, thereby reducing the concentration of hydrogen ion.

In the presence of a solution containing a buffer pair, such as carbonic acid–sodium bicarbonate, the hydrogen ion concentration of the solution is given by the relation:

$$[H^+] = K \frac{[H_2CO_3]}{[HCO_3^-]} \qquad (2)$$

This can also be expressed in its logarithmic form, the Henderson–Hasselbalch equation:

$$pH = pK + \log \frac{[HCO_3^-]}{[H_2CO_3]} \qquad (3)$$

The constant, pK, is related to the dissociation constant of the weak acid (K, in Eq. 2) and identifies the pH at which buffering is most effective (where pH change is smallest when a given quantity of hydrogen ion is added). It is also evident from Equation 3 that it is the pH at which the concentration of the acid and its salt are equal ($\log_{10} 1 = 0$).

The concentration of CO_2 in solution is related to $[H_2CO_3]$ by the following reaction:

$$H_2CO_3 \leftrightharpoons CO_3 + H_2O$$

The concentration of CO_2 is approximately 700 times greater than the carbonic acid concentration at equilibrium. Therefore, dissolved CO_2 represents virtually all the H_2CO_3 available, and the concentration of dissolved CO_2 can be taken as a measure of the $[H_2CO_3]$. The concentration of CO_2 is determined by its partial pressure, P_{CO_2}, and its solubility coefficient for plasma, α. Thus Equation 3 can be written in a more clinically useful form:

$$pH = pK' + \log \frac{[HCO_3^-]}{\alpha P_{CO_2}} \qquad (4)$$

The apparent pK' is 6.1. Since the pH of extracellular fluid is 7.4, the ratio of carbonic acid to bicarbonate can be calculated from the equation to be 1:20, a ratio quite unfavorable for optimum buffering action. The utility as an effective buffer depends, however, upon the speed and facility with which the lungs and kidneys act to restore this ratio when it has been altered by addition or removal of hydrogen ion.

The four principal buffer systems of the extracellular fluid and blood expressed in terms of Equation 2 are

$$\frac{[H_2CO_3]}{[HCO_3^-]} \qquad \frac{[H_2PO_4^-]}{[HPO_4^-]}$$

$$\frac{[H^+\ Protein^-]}{[Protein^-]} \qquad \frac{[H^+\ Hemoglobin^-]}{[Hemoglobin^-]}$$

Of these the carbonic acid–bicarbonate buffer system is most important because it is present in the greatest concentration, and both respiratory and renal action operate to maintain the ratio of the buffer pair constant.

ROLE OF LUNGS

The lungs perform two functions in regard to acid–base regulation. First, the lungs are the *excretory route* for the major acid-producing substance, carbon dioxide. Second, they serve an important pH *regulatory function* through their control of P_{CO_2}.

Carbon dioxide is generated by the body at the rate of 10 mEq/min and is excreted by the lungs at the same rate. The effect of CO_2 on $[H^+]$ is readily seen from the following reactions:

$$CO_2 + H_2O \leftrightharpoons H_2CO_3 \leftrightharpoons HCO_3^- + H^+$$

Routes of H⁺ Excretion:

| | LUNGS | KIDNEYS | |
	as CO₂	as Titratable Acid	as NH₄⁺
Basal Rate mEq/Day	12,000	30	60
Maximal Rate mEq/Day	30,000	150	700

Figure 10.3–1. Basal and maximal rates of hydrogen excretion by kidneys and lungs.

If CO_2 is permitted to accumulate, the $[H^+]$ will rise and pH will fall.

At pH 7.4 the $[H_2CO_3]$ is 1.3 mEq/L throughout the body fluids, *representing less than 0.01 percent of the daily CO_2 production, or the amount produced in about 5 seconds.* Thus, a large quantity of CO_2 is produced and fed into this small pool and equally rapidly removed by the respiratory system. The concentration of CO_2 (or carbonic acid) in the body fluids is determined by the balance between production of CO_2 by the tissues and excretion by the lungs. In contrast to other solutes (such as sodium, chloride, and bicarbonate ions), it is insensitive to changes in volume of body fluids and responds only to changes in respiratory rate or CO_2 production rate or to both.

The responsiveness of the carbonic acid concentration to changes in ventilatory rate provides the respiratory system with effective control over the regulation of pH of the body fluids. For example, a drop in pH (acidosis) stimulates an increase in alveolar ventilation, which increases the excretion rate of CO_2. This decrease in PCO_2, or $[H_2CO_3]$, restores the carbonic acid–bicarbonate ratio toward normal and returns pH toward normal [see Eq. 4 and Fig. 10.3–3]. It is this rapid response (half-time less than 15 minutes) of $[H_2CO_3]$ to changes in respiratory rate that makes the carbonic acid–bicarbonate system an effective buffer at pH 7.4 despite the fact that this is far above this system's most effective buffering range. This increased ventilation with lowering of PCO_2 and increase in pH is the initial response to acidosis resulting from increased hydrogen ion production. Partial compensation is thereby achieved with return of pH toward normal but with reduced values for the concentration of both H_2CO_3 and HCO_3^-. Restoration of these values to their normal physiologic ranges is ultimately dependent upon the renal responses to acidosis.

RENAL REGULATION OF pH[11,14,16]

The kidney restores the pH of the blood and body fluids to normal by secreting H^+ into the urine. By this process the filtered HCO_3^- is first reabsorbed within the proximal tubule. As H^+ secretion continues, the net content of H^+ in the urine increases (titratable acid and NH_4^+), with resulting generation and reabsorption of an equimolar quantity of bicarbonate as sodium bicarbonate. The reabsorption of filtered bicarbonate maintains the existing $[HCO_3^-]$ in extracellular fluid, and the net urinary excretion of H^+ restores bicarbonate to normal levels (see Fig. 10.3–3). These processes are discussed in more detail in Chapter 11.1. The net result of this exchange is an increase in bicarbonate concentration within the body fluids and a return of the $[H_2CO_3]/[HCO_3^-]$ to normal (Fig. 10.3–3).

ACID–BASE DISORDERS: CLINICAL AND LABORATORY CLASSIFICATION[1,4,6,8,9]

All the buffer systems in the body equilibrate rapidly. The gain or loss of hydrogen ion alters not only the $[H_2CO_3]/[HCO_3^-]$, but the pH change associated with this gain or loss determines the state of all the other buffer systems within the body. Because the gain or loss of either hydrogen or hydroxyl ion is quickly reflected in corresponding changes in the CO_2/HCO_3^- system, it is most convenient to characterize acid-base disturbances as gains or losses of CO_2 (carbonic acid), or bicarbonate. For clinical purposes, all primary or simple changes in hydrogen ion concentration within the body fluids may be placed in either one or the other (or both) of two categories: *respiratory* and *metabolic*. The primary clinical and chemical changes associated with each of these fundamental disorders is shown in Table 10.3–1. Also shown is a brief listing of the clinical features of acidosis and alkalosis in both categories. A more detailed study of the clinical aspects is given in chapters that consider the specific disease process responsible for the disturbance. For the present we are concerned with distinguishing between the two primary categories of pH disturbance—*respiratory* versus *metabolic*—and the recognition of simple or pure instances of a disturbance. We must distinguish pure respiratory acidosis produced by CO_2 retention from mixed disturbances that may occur in an individual with an underlying primary respiratory acidosis caused by chronic obstructive lung disease as well as a metabolic acidosis or alkalosis from another cause.

The Henderson–Hasselbalch equation (Eq. 4) identifies the variables that can be measured and used to diagnose the acid–base disturbance present. The variables routinely used in conjunction with clinical data to characterize the given pH disturbance are (1) direct pH measurement, (2) measurement of bicarbonate ion concentrations, (3) measurement of carbonic acid concentration, (4)

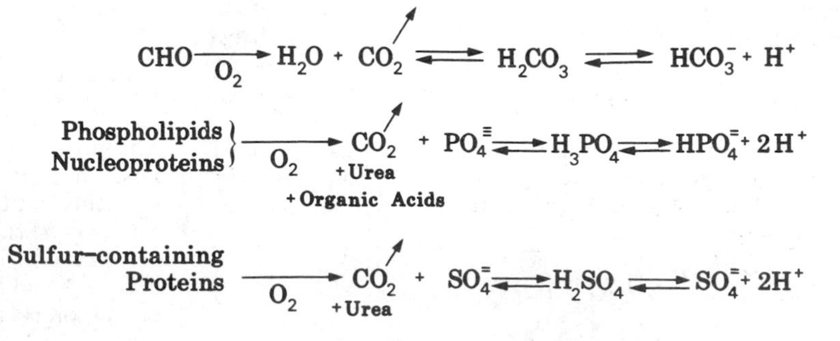

Figure 10.3–2. Dietary and metabolic sources of hydrogen ion production.

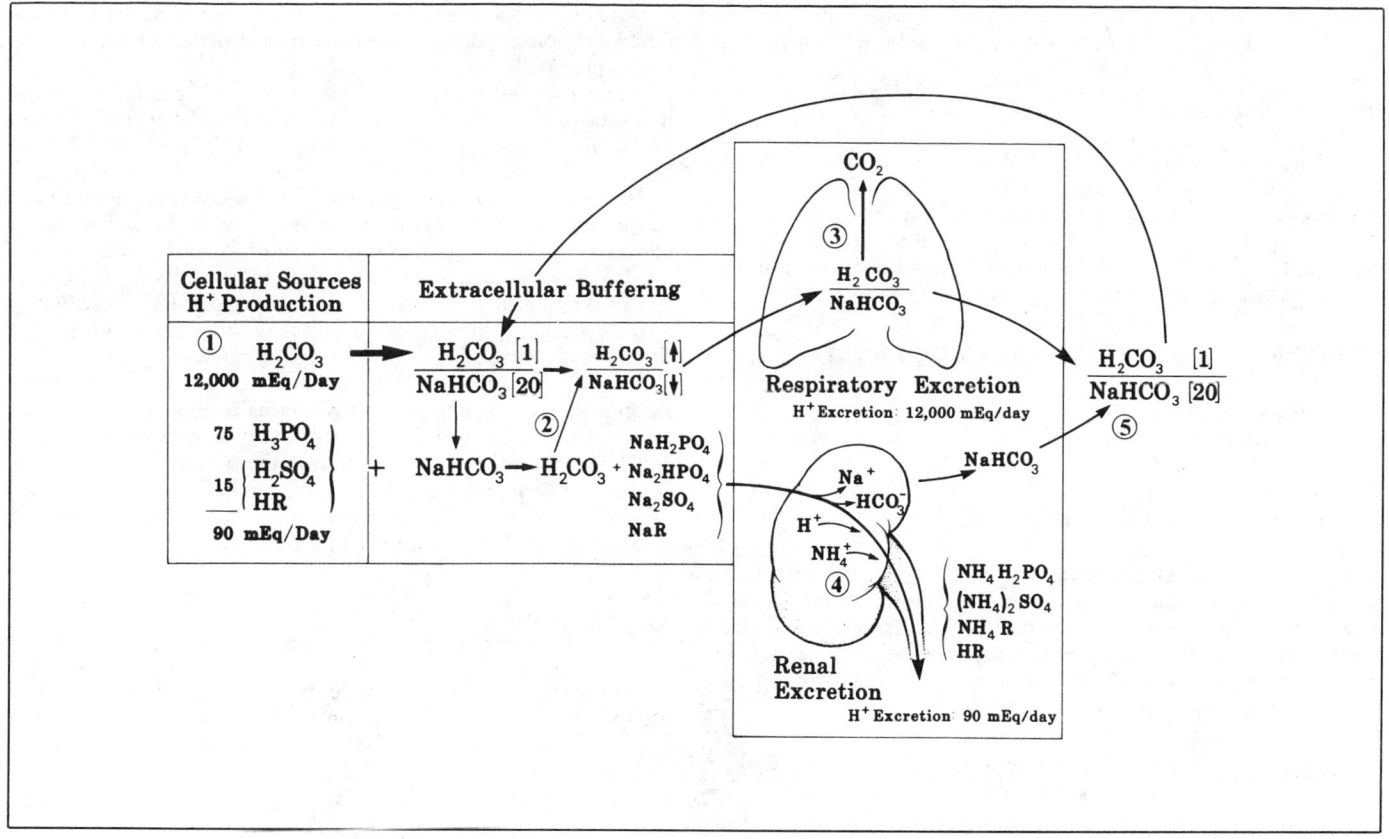

Figure 10.3–3. Buffering and excretion of daily acid production by the body. ① Acid is produced within the cell, almost all as carbonic acid. Only about 90 mEq per day are generated as a result of production of nonvolatile acids. These strong acids cannot exist as acids at physiolgic pH, hence they require immediate buffering. ② When they enter the extracellular fluid they immediately displace or lower bicarbonate concentration with production of H_2CO_3 and sodium salts of acids. ③ The H_2CO_3 is excreted quantitatively by the lung as CO_2 with resulting lowering of carbonic acid concentration (Pco_2). ④ Nonvolatile anions are excreted by the kidney in association with hydrogen ion or NH_4 or both. Secretion of hydrogen ion is associated with reabsorption of an equimolar quantity of $NaHCO_3$. ⑤ This $NaHCO_3$ is returned to the blood and restores carbonic acid–bicarbonate ratio to normal, thereby restoring buffering capacity of body fluids.

TABLE 10.3–1. PRIMARY OR SINGLE DISTURBANCES OF ACID–BASE BALANCE: CLINICAL AND LABORATORY CHARACTERISTICS

Primary Disturbance	Acute Primary Change	Bicarbonate Ratio Changes	Arterial pH	Serum K^+	Unmeasured Anions (AG)	Clinical Features
Respiratory						
Acidosis	CO_2 retention	$\uparrow Pco_2/\uparrow HCO_3^-$	$\downarrow$	$\uparrow$	N	Dyspnea, polypnea, respiratory outflow, obstruction, $\uparrow$ A-P diameter, chest, musical rales, wheezes—in severe cases, stupor, disorientation, coma
Alkalosis	CO_2 depletion	$\downarrow Pco_2/\downarrow HCO_3^-$	$\uparrow$	$\downarrow$	N or $\downarrow$	Anxiety, occasional complaint of breathlessness, frequent sighing, lungs usually clear to exam, positive Chvostek and Trousseau signs
Metabolic						
Acidosis	HCO_3^- depletion	$\downarrow Pco_2/\downarrow HCO_3^-$	$\downarrow$	$\uparrow$ or $\downarrow$	N or $\uparrow\uparrow$	Weakness, air hunger, Kussmaul respiration, dry skin and mucous membranes, poor skin turgor in severe cases, coma, hypotension, death
Alkalosis	HCO_3^- retention	$\uparrow Pco_2/\uparrow HCO_3^-$	$\uparrow$	$\downarrow$	N	Weakness, positive Chvostek and Trousseau signs, hyporeflexia

measurement of sodium, chloride, and potassium concentrations, and (5) calculation of the unmeasured anions, or anion gap.

pH MEASUREMENT[1,3,6,11]

Direct measurement of the pH of arterial blood drawn anaerobically and measured immediately will identify the presence of acidosis or alkalosis but does not provide information about the cause of the disturbance. To distinguish between metabolic and respiratory causes of the disturbance, measurement of bicarbonate or carbonic acid concentrations or both are necessary.

CARBONIC ACID CONCENTRATION (P_{CO_2})[11]

As mentioned in the discussion of Equation 4, the $[H_2CO_3]$ is determined by the partial pressure of carbon dioxide (P_{CO_2}) in the body fluids, as defined by the reaction:

$$CO_2 + H_2O \leftrightarrows H_2CO_3$$

At equilibrium, $[CO_2]$ greatly exceeds $[H_2CO_3]$ and is readily measurable. Hence, in practice the carbonic acid concentration is measured directly in arterial blood by means of specially adapted electrodes and is expressed as partial pressure of CO_2 (P_{CO_2}) in millimeters of mercury. The normal range of P_{CO_2} for arterial blood is 36 to 44 mm Hg.

BICARBONATE CONCENTRATION

The normal range for $[HCO_3^-]$ in arterial blood is 24 to 26 mEq/L. In practice, venous blood is usually used and is about 1.5 mEq higher (26.5 to 28.5 mEq/L) because of addition of carbon dioxide to the blood in transit through the tissues and the attendant increase in $[HCO_3^-]$ that results from the buffering action of the blood. The "standard bicarbonate," a commonly used value derived from measurement of pH of arterial blood after equilibration with two or more different CO_2 tensions, has no inherent advantage over the use of arterial bicarbonate in the assessment of clinical problems.

SERUM ELECTROLYTES AND THE ANION GAP[4,8-10,12]

Correct diagnosis of acid-base disturbance is facilitated by simultaneous measurement of sodium, potassium, chloride, and calculation of the unmeasured anions. These data, interpreted in conjunction with the arterial pH and P_{CO_2} measurements and bicarbonate concentration, are useful in corroborating the presence of respiratory or metabolic disturbances. In addition, they are essential for the correct diagnosis of mixed disorders (see page 708). In both circumstances the variables of primary interest are the *serum potassium* and the unmeasured anion estimate, or *anion gap*.

Potassium, as the major intracellular cation, plays an important role in maintaining electroneutrality across the transcellular membrane. Movement of H^+ ions into the cell (or excess production of H^+ within the cell) requires movement of K^+ out of the cells to maintain electroneutrality. Conversely, when H^+ moves out of the cell as a result of extracellular alkalosis, there is a comparable net shift of K^+ into the cells. Hence, alkalosis should always be associated with an abnormally low serum potassium, regardless of whether the primary cause is respiratory or metabolic. In acidosis with the associated outflux of K^+ from the cells as H^+ enters, the situation may be more complex, and serum $[K^+]$ may be either increased or decreased, depending upon the rate at which the kidney is excreting the K^+ that is being added to the extracellular fluid by this outflux. Thus, in renal tubular acidosis, the $[K^+]$ is usually decreased in plasma because of the increased urinary losses, whereas

in acute diabetic acidosis, the efflux of K^+ is much greater and renal function is often compromised, so that hyperkalemia is virtually always present.

The *anion gap*, or unmeasured anion in the plasma, is a useful indicator of the presence or absence of metabolic acidosis. It may be calculated either as $[Na] - ([Cl] + [HCO_3])$ or as $([Na] + [K^+]) - ([Cl] + [HCO_3])$. Both values serve the same purpose and are useful guides to the presence of an increase in some anionic constituent of the plasma other than Cl^- or HCO_3^-. It must be remembered, however, that the range of normal is different depending on the expression used. For the first $[Na] - ([Cl] + [HCO_3])$ the average difference is approximately 12 mEq/L (range 8 to 16 mEq/L); these values are all increased about 4.5 mEq/L if the expression includes K^+ as one of the cations.

The most commonly observed aberration is an increase in the anion gap. Possible anionic contributions to this increase include lactate, acetoacetic and β-OH butyric acids, phosphate, sulfate, and hyperalbuminemia. In addition, the anion gap may be increased by exogenous anions including salicylates, formate, carbenicillin, and other exogenous organic acids that may be ingested accidentally, as drugs, or in suicide attempts.

ACIDOSIS[4,6,8]

Alterations leading to an increase in hydrogen ion concentration may be identified from inspection of the equilibrium reaction for carbonic acid, the major buffer system in the extracellular fluid, where:

$$[H^+] = K \frac{[H_2CO_3]}{[HCO_3^-]}$$

Either (1) addition of H_2CO_3 (elevation of P_{CO_2}) as a result of alveolar hypoventilation, (2) the addition of hydrogen ion, or (3) the removal of HCO_3^- from body fluids could increase hydrogen ion concentration. All three situations are encountered clinically (Table 10.3–2). The acidosis associated with a primary rise in the carbonic acid is referred to as "respiratory acidosis" and the last two events are the basic causes of a "metabolic acidosis." These three mechanisms leading to the production of acidosis provide a convenient basis for classifying the types of acidosis encountered clinically, since they bear directly on the management of acidosis.

METABOLIC ACIDOSIS[1-6]

Causes

Increased hydrogen ion production shifts the equilibrium reaction toward H_2CO_3 with resulting drop in $[HCO_3^-]$. The accompany-

TABLE 10.3–2. CAUSES OF METABOLIC ACIDOSIS

Exogenous	Endogenous
Gain of Hydrogen Ion	
Aspirin	Renal failure
Methanol	Renal tubular acidosis[a]
Ethylene glycol	Diabetes
Ammonium chloride[a]	Lactic acidosis
Paraldehyde	
Loss of HCO_3^-	
Carbonic anhydrase–inhibiting diuretics[a]	Diarrhea[a]
	Biliary or pancreatic fistulae[a]
	Ureterosigmoidostomy[a]
	Ureteroileostomy

[a]Characterized by a normal anion gap.

ing decrease in pH stimulates ventilation and results in a drop in the [H₂CO₃] or (PCO₂). These changes lead to the characteristic findings in metabolic acidosis: decrease in pH, decrease in [H₂CO₃] (measured as decreased arterial PCO₂), and decreased [HCO₃⁻]. Respiratory compensation, the increased ventilatory response that lowers the PCO₂, moderates the decrease in pH and may, in the presence of only mild acidosis, succeed in restoring the pH to normal. In this circumstance, only a lowered [HCO₃⁻] and lowered PCO₂ will be observed. As the acidosis increases in severity, complete compensation cannot be achieved, and the pH then falls progressively as the severity of the acidosis increases. The renal response, operating much more slowly than the ventilatory response, again tends to retard the decrease in pH by addition of HCO₃⁻ to the body fluids.

Metabolic acidosis may result from endogenous or exogenous sources of hydrogen ion (Table 10.3–2). Such metabolic derangements as overproduction of ketoacids in diabetes mellitus, excess production of lactic acid in the presence of sustained anoxia of the peripheral tissues, and excess lactic acid production by exogenous agents (methanol and ethylene glycol) all result in addition of excess quantities of hydrogen ion to body fluids.

These acids (β-hydroxybutyric acid, acetoacetic acid, lactic acid) react with $NaHCO_3$ to form H_2CO_3 and the sodium salt of the added organic acid. The added anion is not measured in routine clinical chemical procedures, so that the anion gap, defined as the sum of measured cations minus the sum of measured anions, $([Na^+] + [K^+]) - ([Cl^-] + [HCO_3^-])$, is widened. This increased difference between the sums of anions and cations is a useful point in corroboration of a suspected metabolic acidosis (Fig. 10.3–4).

Decreased hydrogen ion excretion leads to the other major type of endogenous metabolic acidosis. It results from a failure of acid excretion by the kidneys. Ingestion of protein in the diet and its metabolic dissimilation and subsequent degradation as a source of energy yields urea plus phosphate and sulfate as metabolic end products (Fig. 10.3–2). The latter substances react with the buffer systems of the body to form H_2CO_3 and to decrease [HCO₃⁻] (see Fig. 10.3–3). These nonvolatile anions, existing as neutral salts of strong mineral acid at physiologic pH, must be excreted by the kidney and a comparable quantity of $NaHCO_3$ regenerated and returned to the blood to restore the normal pH of the body fluids. Since hydrogen ion is exchanged for sodium ion either directly (as titratable acid) or as NH_4^+, this reaction requires an intact tubular mechanism for the secretion of hydrogen ion. The rate of production of hydrogen ion from ingested foodstuffs never exceeds the capacity of the normal kidney to secrete hydrogen ion. In chronic or acute renal failure, however, hydrogen ion secretion is limited, and a fraction of these strong mineral acids is retained instead of excreted as net acid. This daily retention produces an acidosis that is also associated with widening of the anion gap by the retained sodium sulfate and phosphate salts of the inorganic acids (Fig. 10.3–4).

Bicarbonate loss via the urine or other body fluids will also produce acidosis. Normally, the kidney reabsorbs all the filtered HCO₃⁻ plus an additional amount equal to the amount of titratable acid plus the NH_4^+ produced. This process, accomplished through hydrogen ion secretion, is deficient in some patients with renal failure, so that relatively large amounts of bicarbonate will be excreted in the urine despite systemic acidosis. When the bicarbonate wasting is accomplished by retention of chloride (through reabsorption with sodium), the increased anion gap characteristic of patients who have renal failure and low glomerular filtration rates may be absent. This type of disturbance is referred to as hyperchloremic acidosis. Hyperchloremic acidosis may be encountered in advanced renal failure but is also seen in a primary form of renal disease known as "renal tubular acidosis."

"Renal tubular acidosis" is the term applied to the group of disorders that result from defective hydrogen ion transport in one or more segments of the tubule. Two basic defects are currently recognized; one involves the distal segment and the other the proximal segment. The *classic* or *distal* (type I) *renal tubular acidosis* is characterized by an abnormally elevated urine pH, hyperchloremia with resultant decrease in the anion gap, and usually mild systemic acidosis in the presence of a normal or only moderately reduced glomerular filtration rate. Restoration of plasma bicarbonate to normal is usually associated with only mild increase in urinary bicarbonate (rate of loss rarely exceeds 2 percent of glomerular filtration rate). *Proximal* (type II) *renal tubular acidosis* is characterized by more severe systemic acidosis (plasma HCO₃⁻ usually less than

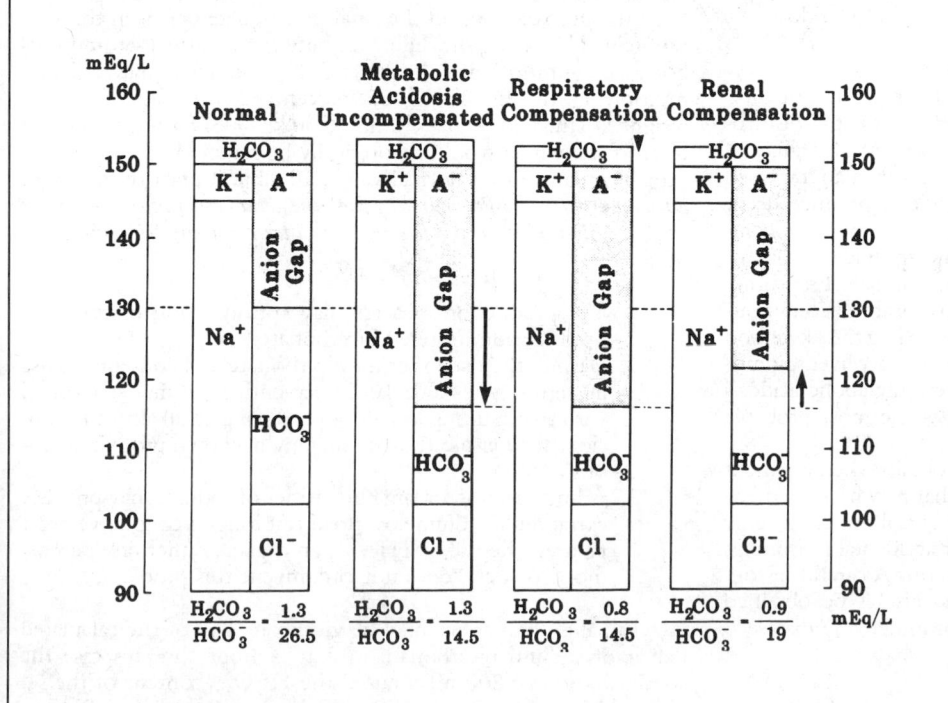

Figure 10.3–4. Recognition of unmeasured anions in metabolic acidosis. Since determination of organic anions in the blood is not a routinely available clinical procedure, the most helpful laboratory information is the difference between sum of cations and sum of anions. Shown here is normal value for anion gap, which is difference between ([Na] + [K]) − ([Cl] + [HCO₃]). Values in excess of 20 are associated with some increase in nonvolatile anion such as lactate or ketoacids. Also shown is response to production of this unidentified anion. Initially this accumulation displaces bicarbonate, and resultant decrease in pH stimulates respiration. Resulting drop in PCO₂ restores pH partially to normal, although concentration of nonvolatile anions in plasma remains unchanged. Renal compensation restores bicarbonate toward normal as the nonvolatile anion is excreted.

15 mEq/L in untreated patients), hyperchloremia, and a urine pH usually within the normal range (<5.0) in untreated patients. Return of plasma HCO_3^- toward normal by HCO_3^- administration results in markedly alkaline urine long before systemic pH is returned to normal. Return of plasma HCO_3^- to normal by infusion of sodium bicarbonate results in profound rate of loss of urinary bicarbonate with rate of HCO_3^- excretion often exceeding 20 percent of the filtered load of bicarbonate. Incomplete or mild defects are recognized in both types and mixtures of the two defects have also been described. These disorders are considered more fully in Chapter 11.6.

Gastrointestinal loss of bicarbonate leading to metabolic acidosis is present in pathologic conditions involving the small and large bowel. An excellent example is the severe bicarbonate-wasting diarrhea commonly affecting children, with a less frequent incidence in adults. Other conditions of the intestine leading to bicarbonate wastage include biliary and pancreatic fistulas, ureterosigmoidostomies, and poorly functioning ileal loops used as bladder replacements. In the latter instance, bicarbonate loss results from urinary chloride exchange for bicarbonate across the ileal loop membrane. Regardless of source of bicarbonate loss, the changes in composition of body fluid are similar, and hyperchloremia is usually a prominent feature of the acidosis resulting from gastrointestinal disturbances.

Increased intake of hydrogen ion from exogenous sources may also produce metabolic acidosis. Ammonium chloride, salicylates, methanol, and lysine hydrochloride are among the more common substances that may produce metabolic acidosis when ingested in large quantities. The acidosis that results from ammonium chloride, for example, results from the metabolic events that follow absorption; the ingested NH_4^+ is converted into urea by the liver, leaving an equivalent amount of HCl in the body fluids. This is immediately buffered with production of NaCl and with corresponding reduction in $[HCO_3^-]$. In general, clinical difficulties are encountered with ammonium chloride therapy only in patients with underlying hepatic or renal insufficiency. Other toxic agents that produce an organic acidosis of a poorly defined nature are included in Table 10.3–2.

Some drugs produce acidosis as a result of their pharmacologic action. The most widely used agent of this type is acetazolamide (Diamox), largely because of its utility in treating glaucoma. This drug produces metabolic acidosis by inhibiting bicarbonate reabsorption within the kidney. As a result of the urinary HCO_3^- loss, it produces a clinical picture resembling renal tubular acidosis.

Clinical Recognition of Metabolic Acidosis

Clinical features of metabolic acidosis are similar regardless of etiology. Signs and symptoms are related to severity of the pH disturbance rather than to specific cause of the acidosis. Mild degrees of acidosis may be associated with no changes other than an increased ventilatory rate. More severe degrees of acidosis produce deep, rapid respirations (Kussmaul breathing), dryness of mucous membranes, somnolence, stupor, and coma. The specific etiology of the acidosis can only be suspected from historical data. Preexisting diabetes, renal disease, and recurrent renal stones are all conditions that should increase the index of suspicion regarding the likelihood of acidosis. In a clinical setting where there is primary liver, pulmonary, neoplastic, or cardiac disease and where metabolic acidosis exists, lactic acidosis should be considered as the most probable underlying pathophysiologic event.

A clear-cut history is often difficult to obtain when a patient presents with acidosis of an unknown type that may have followed a toxic ingestion. Methanol and ethylene glycol are mistakenly taken by alcoholics, and suicide attempts or accidental poisonings in the younger age-groups often involve aspirin. A careful history of possible drug or toxin ingestions should always be obtained when acidosis is diagnosed in the absence of underlying disease.

Management of Metabolic Acidosis

In every case of acid–base disturbance, the physician's attention should be directed to the specific etiology as well as to the precise characterization of the accompanying metabolic alterations. Although the principles of therapy for the generalized electrolyte alterations occurring during metabolic acidosis are applicable in every case, knowledge of the etiology may enable the clinician to institute more effective means of treatment. The use of insulin in diabetic acidosis is an obvious example of this principle. The therapy of a case of metabolic acidosis may be illustrated by the following case presentation.

Case Presentation of Metabolic Acidosis

An 18-year-old male with severe uremia was admitted for chronic dialysis and transplantation. After several hemodialyses, a pericardial friction rub was heard, and within 24 hours he developed signs of pericardial tamponade. On examination his pulse rate was 120/per min, blood pressure was 80/50 mm Hg with marked pulsus paradoxus, respirations were 20/min and Kussmaul in character. Central and peripheral cyanosis was present and the extremities were cool. The jugular venous pressure was elevated (32 cm H_2O).

The clinical impression of an acute pericardial effusion resulting in tamponade was confirmed, and 400 ml of bloody fluid was removed by pericardiocentesis. His condition improved promptly and venous pressure fell to 22 cm. The systemic blood pressure rose to 110/70 mm Hg. Within a short time after the procedure the patient became semiconscious and respirations again were deep and rapid. Blood chemistries included a total CO_2 of 6 mEq/L, sodium 140 mEq/L, chloride 105 mEq/L, and potassium 6.6 mEq/L. The blood pH was 7.2, Pco_2 18 mm Hg, and the lactate level was 10 mmol/L. A blood glucose determination was 140 mg/dl, and there was no detectable ketonemia.

Discussion of Management

The appearance of a sudden metabolic acidosis characterized by a widened anion gap (140 − [105 + 6] = 29 mEq/L), in a patient who exhibited signs of circulatory insufficiency strongly pointed to the diagnosis of lactic acidosis (Fig. 10.3–4). Confirmation was obtained by the identification of the added anion as lactate. This chemical determination is not routinely done on a clinical service, so that diagnosis depends on the recognition of the clinical setting and the finding of a widened anion gap. Lactic acidosis is found in patients with circulatory insufficiency and hypoxia or in those with serious renal, hepatic, or pulmonary disease. It has also been reported in diabetic patients maintained on oral hypoglycemic agents.

An approximation of the total bicarbonate deficit in this case is obtained by taking the difference between a normal serum bicarbonate of 24 mEq/L and the patient's bicarbonate of 6 mEq/L and multiplying this figure by 35 percent of the patient's body weight.[13] Thus (24 − 6) × 0.35 × 60 kg = 378 mEq of sodium bicarbonate which would theoretically be required to raise the serum bicarbonate to a normal value. In clinical practice *this calculated quantity may differ markedly from the actual amount of bicarbonate needed or that which can safely be administered* for the following reasons:

1. The production of acids may continue and increase the need for administered bicarbonate.
2. Despite the rise in serum bicarbonate and consequent rise in serum pH, alveolar hyperventilation may continue, with the resulting low Pco_2 producing an alkalosis. Injudicious further bicarbonate therapy may then produce a serious alkalosis.
3. Administration of large quantities of sodium may produce extracellular volume overload resulting in congestive heart failure. The use of THAM, an organic buffer, itself an osmotic particle, does not circumvent this problem.

Initially, the patient may be given one half of the calculated deficit of sodium bicarbonate in 3 to 4 hours (in this case the administration of 200 mEq raised the HCO_3^- content of the serum to 17 mEq/L and the pH to 7.28), and a repeat assessment may then be made of the acid–base status. Coincident with the

amelioration of the systemic acidosis the patient became fully conscious. In view of the patient's clinical improvement and the continued absence of the initial cause of the acidosis (tamponade leading to shock), no further bicarbonate was given. Within 6 hours the oxidation of the circulating lactate had increased the total serum CO_2 to 23 mEq/L.

If the initial intravenous bicarbonate administered had not resulted in a rise in the blood pH and an improvement in the patient's condition, more vigorous therapy would have been required. Bicarbonate administration could be increased by (1) speeding the infusion rate, (2) instituting peritoneal dialysis, using a solution containing acetate which on oxidation yields an equimolar quantity of bicarbonate, and (3) employing hemodialysis with acetate or solutions containing HCO_3^-. More vigorous treatment of the acidosis by peritoneal dialysis can be effected by use of a solution made by mixing appropriate intravenous fluids containing 2 L of water, 77 mEq/L of sodium chloride, and 66 mEq/L of sodium bicarbonate, and 25 g glucose as the dialyzing fluid. Careful attention must then be directed to the maintenance of normal serum calcium, magnesium, and blood sugar concentrations. The use of some form of dialysis in the primary treatment of metabolic acidosis is indicated in patients who cannot receive added sodium.

A stable state of chronic metabolic acidosis often accompanies chronic renal failure or is seen in cases of renal tubular acidosis. This is caused either by daily retention of small quantities of hydrogen ion or bicarbonate-wasting, or both. In order to compensate for this progressive acid load, body buffers (mainly from bone in the form of CO_3^{2-}) are called upon to maintain acid–base balance. This cumulative demand upon bone buffers plays a major role in the production of renal osteodystrophy and constitutes the major reason for therapeutic intervention, as the decline in pH is often not severe enough to produce clinical symptoms.

The oral administration of citrate, lactate, or CO_3^{2-} as sodium or calcium salts may produce the desired rise of plasma $[HCO_3^-]$. Major problems with this form of therapy include (1) gastric intolerance to these agents and (2) inherent difficulties with the cation of the administered salt, which include volume expansion with sodium or the production of hypercalcemia when calcium is given.

In the treatment of this type of acidosis, the aim of therapy should be the gradual return to normal pH over a period of several days. Acute administration of large quantities of bicarbonate often results in the creation of a metabolic alkalosis with *tetany* and, on occasion, *seizures*. Acute hypokalemia may also be precipitated in this circumstance, since many of these patients, particularly those with renal tubular acidosis, have a latent or overt potassium deficiency.

RESPIRATORY ACIDOSIS

Cause

Respiratory acidosis is always caused by *impaired alveolar ventilation*. Failure of pulmonary ventilation results in CO_2 retention and elevation of H_2CO_3 concentration (increased arterial P_{CO_2}). From inspection of the H_2CO_3 equilibrium reaction it is clear that CO_2 retention will produce an increased hydrogen ion and HCO_3^- concentration but that the rise in $[HCO_3^-]$ will be quite small. The rise in hydrogen ion concentration produces a significant fall in pH.

Any pathologic condition involving the lung, tracheobronchial tree, chest wall, or central nervous control of respiration can result in respiratory acidosis. The rise in H_2CO_3 will produce a small but definite rise in plasma bicarbonate from the action of body buffers:

$$CO_2 + H_2O \leftrightharpoons H_2CO_3 \leftrightharpoons HCO_3^- + H^+$$
$$+$$
$$Buffer^-$$
$$\downarrow\uparrow$$
$$H\ Buffer$$

As more of the hydrogen ion is buffered by extra- and intracellular substances that bind hydrogen more tightly than H_2CO_3, the equilibrium is shifted to the right, with resulting HCO_3^- generation. Figure 10.3–5 demonstrates the rise in plasma bicarbonate that occurs with acute increases in P_{CO_2} in the normal individual. The extra- and intracellular buffers involved in this reaction include hemoglobin and other proteins.

Manifestations of Acute Respiratory Acidosis

The clinical circumstances in which uncomplicated acute respiratory acidosis occurs are often dramatic. The presence of severe respiratory outflow obstruction should always arouse suspicion of the existence of respiratory acidosis. Only measurement of the pH and P_{CO_2} will adequately define the magnitude of the acid–base changes.

In general, the patient will appear acutely ill, complaining of dyspnea and making a greater respiratory effort to increase alveolar ventilation. Hypoxemia manifested as cyanosis is a common accompanying sign of respiratory acidosis. Disorientation, stupor, and finally coma occur when the P_{CO_2} is markedly elevated.

Management of Acute Respiratory Acidosis

Therapy in uncomplicated acute respiratory acidosis is directed toward treatment of the underlying cause, for example, airway obstruction, chest wall trauma, or cardiorespiratory arrest. Mechanically assisted ventilation is the treatment of choice when the initial measures do not suffice to correct the CO_2 retention. Often the severity of the patient's distress in respiratory acidosis requires treatment before the quantitative alterations in the blood pH and P_{CO_2} are known. These measurements may usually be obtained at a later time as a check on the adequacy of therapy.

Manifestations of Chronic Respiratory Acidosis

Long-standing obstructive pulmonary disease results in acid–base changes that differ from those seen with acute CO_2 retention. Within several days after the elevation of P_{CO_2}, the kidneys begin to excrete increasing amounts of net acid and to reabsorb correspondingly increased amounts of bicarbonate. Figure 10.3–5 shows the portion of the elevated plasma bicarbonate that is attributable to augmented renal absorption. As can be seen by analysis

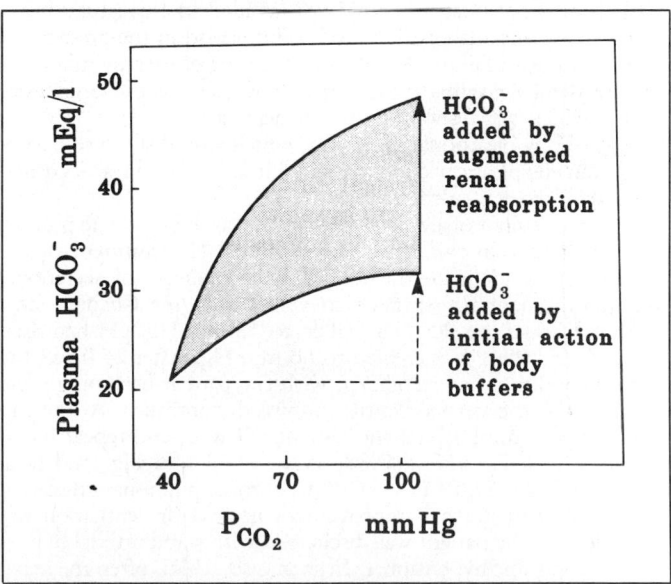

Figure 10.3–5. Relative roles of body buffers and renal response in adjusting to respiratory acidosis. Lower curve identifies bicarbonate generated by buffer systems in response to elevated P_{CO_2}, and upper curve identifies steady-state bicarbonate concentration after renal compensation. (*Redrawn from Schwartz et al.* [12])

of the equilibrium or Henderson–Hasselbalch equations, the increased $[HCO_3^-]$ reduces hydrogen ion concentration and increases the pH.

Management of Chronic Respiratory Acidosis

The goal of therapy, namely, the relief of CO_2 retention by improvement of ventilation, is the same in chronic as in acute respiratory acidosis. In uncomplicated acute respiratory acidosis, however, removal of the underlying cause will permit the P_{CO_2} to return to normal, whereas in the patient with chronic lung disease, therapeutic efforts may not overcome the underlying structural damage, so that a return to a chronic stable state of respiratory acidosis will be the therapeutic endpoint. Indeed, in many cases, the patient seen with pulmonary disease has developed a superimposed acute impairment of ventilation resulting in a combined acute and chronic respiratory acidosis. In this instance, therapy is dictated as much by the clinical state of the patient as by the blood gas abnormalities.

Case Presentation of Chronic Respiratory Acidosis

A 57-year-old male was admitted in a confused and somnolent state. He had smoked heavily for many years and had a chronic productive cough. For the past 2 to 3 years he had noted increasing exertional dyspnea and slight ankle edema.

On examination, his pulse was 132/min and regular, temperature 101F, blood pressure was 105/70 mm Hg, and respiratory rate was 26/min. There was central and peripheral cyanosis and an emphysematous configuration to the chest; the respirations were labored, with expiratory wheezing audible over the entire chest. Harsh respiratory rales and dullness to percussion were present over the whole of the left lower lobe. A forceful right ventricular impulse was present over the precordium, and there was cervical venous distension.

The hematocrit was 52 percent, and the white blood cell count 18,000/mm³. Electrolytes included a serum sodium of 134 mEq/L, potassium 5.7 mEq/L, HCO_3^- 39 mEq/L, and chloride 89 mEq/L. Measured blood gases included a P_{O_2} of 47 mm Hg, P_{CO_2} 78 mm Hg, and pH 7.29. The chest film showed a left lower lobe infiltrate.

Discussion of Management

The history and physical findings were compatible with bronchitis and emphysema. A recent period of further decompensation is suggested by the patient's stupor presumably caused by a left lower lobe pneumonia. The blood gas measurements indicated the presence of hypoxemia coupled with a respiratory acidosis. Increased renal bicarbonate reabsorption accounted for the elevated $[HCO_3^-]$. Bicarbonate therapy was avoided in this situation. It would represent a large additional sodium load in the presence of right-sided heart failure. Moreover, this type of therapy might aggravate the hypoxemia by (1) further depressing the respiratory center, which was responding to the acidosis, and (2) rapidly correcting pH by bicarbonate infusion, which would shift the oxyhemoglobin dissociation curve to the left, resulting in a decreased delivery of oxygen to the tissues.

Improvement of alveolar ventilation was therefore the primary goal of therapy in this case. This included (1) treatment of the infection, (2) adequate tracheobronchial drainage of secretions, and (3) mechanical assistance to ventilation (see Chapter 3.6). Within 4 hours the P_{CO_2} had fallen to 65 mm Hg, pH had risen to 7.34, and the P_{O_2} increased to 60 mm Hg. After 24 hours the clinical condition had stabilized, with the patient becoming more alert, so that the assisted ventilation was discontinued. At the end of 10 days in the hospital the patient felt well, and repeat blood studies revealed a pH of 7.38, P_{CO_2} of 55 mm Hg, and total HCO_3^- of 32 mEq/L. In view of his chronic pulmonary disease it was felt that no further improvement in alveolar ventilation was possible, and the patient was discharged with stable arterial hypoxemia and chronic hypercapnia. In such cases, this is often the maximum benefit that can be achieved.

In respiratory acidosis the compensation produced by bicarbonate retention will never be sufficient to return the serum pH to completely normal levels. An apparent state of total compensa-

tion with arterial pH above 7.44 is *always* the result of a mixed pH disturbance, with the secondary alteration being a metabolic alkalosis. This may be encountered, for instance, when diuretic therapy has led to superimposition of hypokalemic, hypochloremic metabolic alkalosis.

ALKALOSIS[12,13,16]

TYPES AND CAUSES

Alkalosis results from a decrease in the hydrogen ion concentration of the extracellular fluid. The carbonic acid equilibrium reaction identifies the mechanism for production of alkalosis (see Eq. 2). A decrease in the P_{CO_2} secondary to increased alveolar ventilation decreases $[H_2CO_3]$. This in turn gives rise to a decrease in hydrogen ion concentration and $[HCO_3^-]$ and is known as "respiratory alkalosis." *Metabolic alkalosis* results from either loss of hydrogen or a gain of bicarbonate, or both. A brief outline of the more common causes of alkalosis is shown in Tables 10.3–3 and 10.3–4. The two most common causes of metabolic alkalosis are vomiting with loss of hydrochloric acid and diuretic therapy that produces excessive chloride and potassium loss.

RESPIRATORY RESPONSE

Respiratory compensation for metabolic alkalosis produces an elevation in P_{CO_2} that virtually never exceeds 55 mm Hg, and it is not unusual to find a normal or only slightly elevated P_{CO_2} in these patients. When a steady state has been achieved, metabolic alkalosis is characterized by a decrease in the hydrogen ion concentration (increased pH), an increase in the bicarbonate concentration, and a normal or slightly elevated H_2CO_3 concentration.

BUFFER RESPONSE

The immediate buffering response that acts to minimize the pH change in alkalosis is achieved by the release of hydrogen ion from intracellular and extracellular buffers. This outward shift of hydrogen from intracellular stores is accompanied by an inward movement of sodium and potassium. Although quantitatively small, this sudden shift in potassium may lead to acute lowering of plasma potassium concentration, with the resulting cardiovascular effects of hypokalemia (see Chapter 10.2). This shift is particularly hazardous in patients with a preexisting potassium deficit from some other cause.

RENAL RESPONSE

The response of the kidneys to alkalosis does not represent simply a bicarbonate loss with concomitant retention of hydrogen. Alkalosis is usually associated with a decrease in sodium stores as, for example, in diuretic-induced alkalosis. In this situation chloride and sodium are lost from the extracellular fluid without any bicarbonate loss. There occurs a contraction of the extracellular fluid

---

TABLE 10.3–3. CAUSES OF METABOLIC ALKALOSIS

- Vomiting of gastric contents
- Administration of diuretics which cause virtually equal losses of Na and Cl (thiazides, mercurials, ethacrynic acid, furosemide)
- Hyperaldosteronism
- Hyperadrenocorticism
- Administration of alkali such as antacids
- Posthypercapneic alkalosis

TABLE 10.3–4. CAUSES OF RESPIRATORY ALKALOSIS

- Vigorous respirator therapy
- Acute hyperventilation syndrome
- Diffuse liver disease
- Diffuse CNS disease
- Drug induced (salicylates)

volume around the unchanged bicarbonate stores. This results in an increased bicarbonate concentration and frank alkalosis. Renal compensation with loss of bicarbonate through the urine can occur only with a significant loss of sodium. The stimulus to retain sodium in this situation is, however, maximal so that virtually all filtered sodium will be reabsorbed. Since the available chloride in the glomerular filtrate is limited (decreased extracellular fluid [Cl^-]), an increased fraction of the sodium must be reabsorbed through tubular exchange mechanisms. Sodium is exchanged for hydrogen, with resulting tubular reabsorption of $NaHCO_3$ and maintenance of [HCO_3^-] at an elevated level. The alkalosis is thereby maintained. Because of the increased exchange of hydrogen ion for sodium in these circumstances, a "paradoxically" acid urine is often observed in the presence of a systemic metabolic alkalosis. The hypokalemia commonly seen in alkalosis is caused by increased urinary potassium losses, which result from tubular exchange of potassium for sodium, and frequently by extrarenal losses, as in persistent vomiting.

CLINICAL FEATURES OF METABOLIC ALKALOSIS

The symptoms and signs of alkalosis are relatively few, and the clinical setting in which alkalosis occurs is often one in which symptoms of other electrolyte disorders predominate. Latent or overt tetany may be produced by an acute increase in the pH of the blood, but few other symptoms or signs can be attributed to the alkalosis per se. Metabolic alkalosis almost always occurs in association with varying degrees of sodium and potassium depletion, and often these disturbances dominate the clinical picture (see Chapters 10.1 and 10.2).

Case Presentation of Metabolic Alkalosis

A 53-year-old man was admitted to the hospital complaining of pernicious vomiting of 2 weeks' duration, weakness, and shortness of breath. He had undergone treatment for a stomach ulcer 8 years previously but developed recurrent abdominal pain 6 months before admission. Vomiting began 3 months later, and for the past 2 weeks he had had continued emesis with very poor food intake.

On examination the blood pressure was 80/40 mm Hg, pulse was 140/min and thready, respirations were 30/min, and body weight was 132 pounds (59.9 kg). The patient was cachectic, with poor skin turgor. The upper abdomen was distended, and a succussion splash could be elicited. Latent tetany in the form of positive Trousseau and Chvostek signs were present. The reflexes were hypoactive.

Laboratory data: hematocrit, 55 percent; white blood cell count, 7500/mm³; urinalysis, 1+ protein; specific gravity, 1.028; and pH, 5.5. Serum sodium was 132 mEq/L; potassium, 1.9 mEq/L; HCO_3^-, 48 mEq/L; and chloride, 75 mEq/L. Calcium was 7.8 mg/dl; SUN, 40 mg/dl. Arterial blood studies revealed a pH of 7.62; PCO_2, 48 mm Hg; and standard bicarbonate of 43 mEq/L; 24-hour urine chloride concentration was 33 mEq/L.

The history and physical findings together with the hypochloremic, hypokalemic alkalosis, and sodium depletion (indicated by the elevated hematocrit) were all consistent with pyloric obstruction, and appropriate x-rays revealed apparently complete obstruction at the pylorus with marked gastric dilation.

Discussion of Management

Gastric intubation with suction drainage was instituted to decompress the stomach and permit more accurate recording of intake and output. The hypotension, tachycardia, poor skin turgor, and high hematocrit represented evidence of decreased extracellular

fluid volume caused by sodium depletion. The hypoactive reflexes, generalized muscle weakness, and marked hypokalemia indicated the presence of a severe potassium deficit. The latent tetany was attributed to the alkalosis. Thus the disturbances requiring correction were sodium depletion, potassium depletion, and hypochloremic alkalosis.

As an approximation for planning therapy the magnitude of the chloride deficit can be equated with the estimated bicarbonate excess, that is, the quantity of chloride that was lost and replaced with bicarbonate. The chloride loss estimated in this fashion [(48 mEq/L − 25 mEq/L) × 0.35 × 60 kg] was 483 mEq. In the presence of adequate renal function, administration of chloride ion in combination with either sodium or potassium will lessen the alkalosis by the two following mechanisms: (1) Increase in serum chloride concentration increases chloride in the glomerular filtrate and permits increased renal tubular sodium chloride reabsorption. This reduces the exchange of hydrogen for sodium (which supported the increased sodium bicarbonate reabsorption and maintained the alkalotic state). As sodium retention restores a normal extracellular volume, a portion of the sodium becomes available for the urinary excretion of the excess bicarbonate. (2) Reexpansion of the extracellular volume with 0.155 molar chloride reduces the serum bicarbonate by dilution.

In this patient, 300 mEq of sodium chloride in combination with 60 mEq KCl were given intravenously during the first day of therapy. Oral replacement was impossible because of Levin tube drainage. The next morning the patient's serum bicarbonate was 44 mEq/L, potassium 2.2 mEq/L, and chloride 78 mEq/L. Latent tetany was still present. A urine chloride concentration of 89 mEq/L was recorded at this time.

When chloride loss is the primary event in alkalosis, chloride repletion alone without repair of potassium deficiency will correct the alkalosis. The values at the end of the first day's therapy indicate that a very small and clinically insignificant correction occurred despite administration of 360 mEq of chloride. Alkalosis in combination with significant chloruresis suggested that severe potassium depletion with intracellular acidosis was sustaining $NaHCO_3$ reabsorption despite adequate chloride intake. On the second hospital day 150 mEq of sodium chloride were given together with 150 mEq of potassium chloride, and the resulting serum electrolytes included a bicarbonate of 36 mEq/L, potassium 2.6 mEq/L, chloride 83 mEq/L, and sodium 140 mEq/L. It was now apparent that a severe degree of potassium depletion led to the initial resistance of the alkalosis to repair with sodium chloride. Over the next several days continued potassium chloride supplementation led to full correction of the alkalosis and potassium depletion. The precise role of potassium depletion in maintenance of metabolic alkalosis remains unclear. Hypokalemia is almost always present to some degree in metabolic alkalosis. For the clinical well-being of the patient, repair of potassium deficiency should routinely be undertaken as part of the treatment for metabolic alkalosis.

One additional feature merits comment. As in this case, metabolic alkalosis usually develops over a period of several days or weeks and is relatively well tolerated by the patient. Because of this, it is satisfactory and desirable to plan repletion over a period of several days, thereby avoiding rapid administration of large quantities of sodium and potassium. In fact, the oral route for potassium repletion is preferred when this is feasible.

CLINICAL FEATURES AND MANAGEMENT OF RESPIRATORY ALKALOSIS

Respiratory alkalosis occurs as a result of alveolar hyperventilation, which reduces the H_2CO_3 concentration (PCO_2) in the blood. Initial compensatory mechanisms include the reduction of extracellular bicarbonate by its combination with hydrogen released from extracellular and intracellular buffers. A diuresis of sodium bicarbonate also serves to moderate the increase in pH but may not be

seen when a strong stimulus to conserve sodium exists. The major clinical conditions associated with respiratory alkalosis are seen in Table 10.3–4.

Usually only the pH disturbance occurring with artificial mechanically assisted ventilation is severe, and it requires immediate control by the reduction of the minute volume of the respirator or increase in the dead space of the mechanical device if it is necessary to sustain the high rate to provide adequate oxygenation. The other clinical circumstance requiring treatment is encountered in the patient with an anxiety attack who hyperventilates and develops tetany as a consequence of the raised blood pH. Rebreathing into a paper bag or breath holding will usually suffice to increase the P_{CO_2} to a value sufficient to correct the disturbance. Milder forms of respiratory alkalosis are seen in hepatic and central nervous system disease and usually do not require therapeutic intervention.

The compensatory decrease of the serum bicarbonate may be misinterpreted as representing a mild metabolic acidosis in such patients if concurrent measurements of arterial pH and P_{CO_2} are not obtained.

MIXED ACID–BASE DISORDERS[3,5,8–10]

Frequently a patient will exhibit more than one acid–base disorder. Thus, an individual with chronic obstructive airway disease may develop both an acute respiratory acidosis and a superimposed metabolic acidosis or alkalosis. Conversely, an individual who has developed a metabolic acidosis from salicylate ingestion may develop a superimposed alkalosis because of CNS-induced hyperventilation. Recent studies defining the expected levels of compensation (first by body buffering and then by renal bicarbonate transport) in each of the primary acid–base disturbances (see Fig. 10.3–5) permit one to suspect the existence of mixed acid–base disturbances from a study of the relationship between the measured values for P_{CO_2}, arterial pH, and bicarbonate concentration. In the sections to follow, several relationships are presented that will serve as useful guides in clinical recognition of mixed acid–base disorders. For a more detailed development of these relationships, consult the review by Narins and Emmett.[8]

In metabolic acidosis, for example, there is a linear relationship between the decrease in bicarbonate concentration and the reduction in P_{CO_2}, until a minimal value of 8 mm Hg is reached. This relationship can be expressed by the following equation:

$$\text{Expected } P_{CO_2} = 1.5 \times (\text{measured } HCO_3^-) + 8 \pm 2 \quad \text{(a)}$$

If the directly measured P_{CO_2} is higher than this calculated value of P_{CO_2} based upon the bicarbonate concentration, then a coincident respiratory acidosis is present. If the measured P_{CO_2} is less than the expected value, a coincident respiratory alkalosis is present.

In metabolic alkalosis the degree of compensation caused by a rise in the P_{CO_2} is less predictable than the relationship described above for changes in P_{CO_2} observed in metabolic acidosis. Nonetheless, careful scrutiny of the measured P_{CO_2} value can provide some information about whether more than one simple disturbance is likely to be present. A P_{CO_2} value less than 37 mm Hg should lead to the suspicion of a coexisting respiratory alkalosis. Conversely, a value greater than 55 mm Hg should lead one to suspect a superimposed respiratory acidosis.

The contributions of buffering by the body fluids have been separated from those of renal buffering for both respiratory acidosis and respiratory alkalosis. Predictably the increase in hydrogen ion concentration (ΔH^+) that occurs following an acute rise in P_{CO_2} when only body fluid buffering has had an opportunity to modulate this is substantially greater than the increase seen after the kidneys have had an opportunity to increase bicarbonate reabsorption, thereby decreasing the elevation in hydrogen ion concentration. In *acute* respiratory acidosis and alkalosis the relationship between change in hydrogen ion concentration and change in P_{CO_2} is given by the following equation:

$$\Delta H^+ \text{ (nEq/L)} = 0.8 \, (\Delta P_{CO_2}) \quad \text{(b)}$$

For example, when a patient exhibits a P_{CO_2} of 70 mm Hg and this reflects the development of acute respiratory acidosis before any significant renal buffering has occurred, the pH should be 7.20, assuming a normal value for P_{CO_2} of 40 mm Hg ($\Delta P_{CO_2} = 70 - 40$), and a normal hydrogen ion concentration equal to 40 nEq/L:

$$\Delta H^+ = 0.8(30)$$
$$\Delta H^+ = 24$$
$$H^+ = 40 + 24 = 64 \text{ nEq/L}$$
$$pH = 7.20$$

Thus, in a patient with acute respiratory acidosis whose blood gas analyses yielded a P_{CO_2} of 70 mm Hg, if the simultaneously *measured* pH is less than 7.2, the diagnosis of a mixed disturbance that includes metabolic acidosis should be entertained. A pH value higher than the calculated value (greater than 7.2) would most probably represent partial compensation as a result of increased bicarbonate reabsorption by the kidney.

In the case of a patient with acute respiratory alkalosis where the P_{CO_2} is 20 mm Hg, the pH will be 7.61, as illustrated by the following calculations:

$$\Delta H^+ = 0.8(20)$$
$$\Delta H^+ = 16$$
$$H^+ = 40 - 16 = 24 \text{ nEq/L}$$
$$pH = 7.61$$

In similar fashion a measured pH that is less than 7.61 would signify a coexisting metabolic acidosis, whereas a higher value would identify a coexisting metabolic alkalosis. These calculations are quite helpful in dealing with both acute respiratory acidosis and alkalosis insofar as the recognition of coexisting metabolic acidosis is concerned. There is greater uncertainty, however, if the comparison between the calculated and measured pH values point toward a metabolic alkalosis; this could simply reflect partial renal compensation.

Once renal compensation has been achieved through bicarbonate reabsorption, the increased plasma concentration produces a new relationship between hydrogen ion and P_{CO_2}, but this new relationship is also linear. It is described by the following equation:

$$\Delta H^+ = 0.3 \, (\Delta P_{CO_2}) \quad \text{(c)}$$

Thus, if the clinical data indicate a *chronic* respiratory acidosis, a series of calculations undertaken for a P_{CO_2} of 70 mm Hg would reveal that the expected pH should be 7.31. A measured pH higher than this would provide strong support for the presence of a coexisting metabolic alkalosis; a lower pH would signify coexisting metabolic acidosis.

In *chronic* respiratory alkalosis, the diminution of renal hydrogen ion output reduces plasma bicarbonate concentration. In this instance also, the relationship between H^+ and P_{CO_2} is linear. Thus

$$\Delta H^+ = 0.17 \, (\Delta P_{CO_2}) \quad \text{(d)}$$

For example, a patient with a P_{CO_2} of 20 should have a pH of 7.43. A value below this would indicate coexisting metabolic acidosis. A higher value would signify metabolic alkalosis.

Early recognition and correct diagnosis of mixed acid–base disturbances require being alert to the clinical circumstances in which these are likely to occur. Table 10.3–5 lists some of the more common clinical settings that predispose to such mixed disorders. In arriving at a correct diagnosis and in determining which disturbance is primary and which secondary, the arterial pH is most useful

TABLE 10.3–5. CLINICAL SITUATIONS IN WHICH MIXED ACID–BASE DISTURBANCES MAY OCCUR

Respiratory Acidosis plus Metabolic Acidosis
Obstructive pulmonary disease with:
- Diabetic ketoacidosis
- Lactacidemia
- Exogenous toxic substances (ethylene glycol, paraldehyde, methanol salicyclate and other substances metabolized to nonvolatile organic anions)
  Respirator-controlled ventilation (Critical Care Units) associated with above complicating illness or sepsis, acute renal failure, hypotension with hypoxia.

Metabolic Acidosis with Superimposed Respiratory Alkalosis
Usually transient and occurs with:
- Rapid and excessive treatment of metabolic acidosis
- Acute severe salicylate intoxication
- Inappropriate use of mechanical ventilation in metabolic acidosis

Metabolic Alkalosis plus Respiratory Acidosis
Obstructive pulmonary disease complicated by:
- Persistent vomiting
- Nasogastric suction
- Laxative abuse
- Chronic diarrhea
- Vigorous diuretic usage
- Chronic alkali ingestion
- Mineralocorticoid excess, either endogenous or iatrogenic

in deciding whether the primary disturbance is an alkalosis or acidosis. Equations a to d on page 708 may then be used with the measured P_{CO_2} and HCO_3^- to identify a complicating secondary disturbance and to gauge its severity.

These simple relationships offer two useful results. The first is validation of the determination by establishing that all the measured values are consistent with a simple acid–base disorder. Second, when the calculation fails to confirm this, the possibility of a mixed acid–base disturbance must be considered. The first step to be taken when these laboratory values suggest a mixed disturbance must be to confirm the correctness of the laboratory data. *No ther-*

apy of acid–base disturbance should be undertaken until the physician is certain of the reliability of the observations on which he is basing therapy.

REFERENCES

1. Albert MD, Dell RB, Winters RW: Quantitative displacement of acid–base equilibrium in metabolic acidosis. Ann Intern Med 66:312, 1967
2. Bishop RL, Weisfeldt ML: Sodium bicarbonate administration during cardiac arrest: Effect on arterial pH, pCO$_2$ and osmolality. JAMA 235:506, 1976
3. Fagan TJ: Estimation of hydrogen ion concentration (letter). N Engl J Med 288:915, 1973
4. Gabow PA, Kaehny WD, et al: Diagnostic importance of an increased serum anion gap. N Engl J Med 303:854, 1980
5. Hamm L, Jacobson HR: Mixed acid–base disturbances. In Kokko JP, Tannen RL (eds): Fluids and Electrolytes. Philadelphia, WB Saunders, 1986
6. Kassirer JP: Serious acid–base disorders. N Engl J Med 291:733, 1974
7. Kassirer JB, Bleich HL: Rapid estimation of plasma carbon dioxide tension from pH and total carbon dioxide content. N Engl J Med 272:1067, 1965
8. Narins RG, Emmett M: Simple and mixed acid–base disorders: A practical approach. Medicine (Baltimore) 59:161, 1980
9. Oh MS, Carroll HJ: The anion gap. N Engl J Med 297:814, 1977
10. Orringer CE, Eustace JC, et al: Natural history of lactic acidosis after grand-mal seizures. A model for the study of an anion-gap acidosis not associated with hyperkalemia. N Engl J Med 297:796, 1977
11. Schwartz WB, Brachett WC, Cohen JJ: The response to graded degrees of chronic hypercapnia: The physiologic limits of the defense of pH. J Clin Invest 44:291, 1965
12. Schwartz WB, Van Ypersele de Strihou C, Kassirer JP: Medical progress. Role of anions in metabolic alkalosis and potassium deficiency. N Engl J Med 279:630, 1968
13. Singer RB, Clark JK, et al: The acute effects in man of rapid intravenous infusion of hypertonic sodium bicarbonate solution. Medicine (Baltimore) 34:51, 1955
14. Valtin H: Renal Function: Mechanisms Preserving Fluid and Solute Balance in Health, 2d ed. Boston, Little, Brown, 1983
15. Valtin H: Renal Dysfunction: Mechanisms Involved in Fluid and Solute Imbalance. Boston, Little, Brown, 1979
16. Winters RW, Dell RB: Acid–Base Physiology in Medicine, 3d ed. Boston, Little, Brown, 1982

CHAPTER 10.4
Water and Electrolyte Derangements in Practice

W. Gordon Walker

Previous chapters have dealt almost exclusively with the clinical characteristics of isolated deficits, representing solitary discrete disturbances in body water or in the exchangeable sodium or potassium in the body. Isolated deficits are not commonly encountered in clinical practice. More often the physician is faced with a complex situation involving derangements in both body water and several of the major inorganic solutes. Because of the complexity of these disturbances, it is desirable to use an explicit diagnostic terminology that avoids such terms as "dehydration" and instead characterizes the abnormality in terms that describe the alterations in volume and composition of body fluids. Volume changes may be identified as representing *expansion* or *contraction* and compositional changes can be described as producing *hypotonicity, hypertonicity*, or, when only volume changes, *isotonicity*. This permits definition of six categories of disturbance in volume and composition of body fluids. Table 10.4–1 shows the expected clinical and laboratory findings and lists major examples in each category. These categories, *isotonic expansion or contraction, hypotonic expansion or contraction*, and *hypertonic expansion or contraction*, cover the pri-

mary disturbances encountered in derangements of the body fluids.

Isotonic contraction primarily represents acute sodium and water loss in isotonic proportions. Sodium concentration and serum osmolality are normal, but the hematocrit is elevated, reflecting isotonic loss from the extracellular fluid space. If the condition persists for several days, serum urea nitrogen (SUN) and creatinine are also elevated. Probably the most common cause is diarrhea that continues for a period of 1 or 2 days or more and is associated with inadequate intake. In certain situations, as in acute severe diarrhea, acidosis may also be present because of excessive loss of bicarbonate in the fecal fluid. Other examples include moderate sodium loss from any source, but usually from the gastrointestinal tract or skin (sweating). Losses from the extracellular fluid compartment may occur without being identifiable as external losses. In severe ileus, for example, several liters of fluid may be pooled in the dilated gastrointestinal tract. A progressive increase in hematocrit may be one of the earliest signs of such fluid sequestration.

Isotonic expansion is caused by retention of sodium and water

TABLE 10.4–1. CLASSIFICATION OF CLINICAL WATER AND ELECTROLYTE DISTURBANCES

Type of Derangement	Body Weight	Hematocrit	Serum Sodium	Serum Osmolality	Serum[a] Urea Nitrogen	Urine[b] Sodium	Urine Osmolality	Common Clinical Examples
Isotonic contraction	↓	↑	N	N	N or ↑	± or ↓	↑	Fluid loss from diarrhea, overtreatment with diuretics, other conditions associated with acute sodium loss
Isotonic expansion	↑	N or ↓	N	N	N or ↓	±	±	Congestive heart failure, cirrhosis, nephrosis, acute glomerulonephritis, preeclampsia, iatrogenic
Hypotonic contraction	↓	↑	↓	↓	↑	↓	↑	Addison disease, severe sodium depletion of relatively long-standing from variety of causes
Hypotonic expansion	↑	N or ↓	↓	↓	N or ↓	±	↑	Acute water intoxication, syndrome of inappropriate ADH secretion, congestive heart failure, cirrhosis
Hypertonic contraction	↓	N or ↑	↑	↑	↑	± or ↓	↑	Severe sweating, inadequate fluid intake, diabetes mellitus
Hypertonic expansion	usually ↑	↓	↑ or ↓[c]	↑	± of no diagnostic value	±	±	Mannitol administration, ingestion of large quantities of NaCl

[a]All these disturbances may be superimposed upon renal disease.
[b]Urinary sodium determination is the least helpful laboratory test for diagnostic confirmation of these disorders.
[c]Depending upon whether solute responsible for expansion is NaCl or some nonelectrolyte solute.
N = normal, ↑ = increase; ↓ = decrease; ± = variable.

in isotonic proportions (1 L of water retained for each 145 mEq of sodium retained). It is most commonly seen in heart failure, cirrhosis, and nephrosis but also occurs in many other situations, including acute glomerular nephritis, as well as toxemia of pregnancy and preeclampsia. It may also be produced iatrogenically. Characteristically, the plasma sodium concentration and osmolality are normal. Body weight is increased and the hematocrit may be decreased, depending upon the circumstances. Persistent isotonic expansion such as that encountered in heart failure and cirrhosis is usually associated with a normal hematocrit. When the isotonic expansion develops more acutely, the hematocrit is reduced in proportion to the severity of the expansion.

Hypotonic contraction is usually initiated by a sodium loss that exceeds 5 mEq/kg body weight or exceeds 400 mEq in the average 70-kg adult. It is characterized by a decrease in skin turgor, serum sodium concentration, and serum osmolality. There is a variable increase in the serum urea nitrogen and hematocrit; the magnitude of change in these laboratory data is proportional to the severity of the deficits. Because of the circumstances under which such a derangement is likely to occur, potassium depletion is commonly seen, and alkalosis may be encountered. Clinical examples include chronic diarrhea, chronic adrenal insufficiency, sodium depletion resulting from sweating with inadequate salt intake, and excessive treatment with diuretics.

Hypotonic expansion is primarily the result of retention of excess water caused either by persistent antidiuretic hormone excess or some other cause of impaired water excretion as in severe congestive heart failure. In certain circumstances, such as the syndrome of inappropriate ADH secretion, the resultant expansion may increase sodium excretion and lead to development of a moderate sodium deficit. In other situations, such as congestive heart failure and cirrhosis, excessive sodium is retained, but the water excess exceeds sodium excess and hypo-osmolality results. The characteristic laboratory findings include lowered serum sodium concentration and lowered plasma osmolality. The clinical manifestations depend upon the severity of the hypotonicity. In edematous states such as heart failure and cirrhosis, the hypotonic expansion may be associated with other electrolyte disturbances resulting from vigorous diuretic usage. In the syndrome of inappropriate ADH secretion, serum urea nitrogen is often low, frequently below 7 or 8 mg/dl.

Hypertonic contraction is produced by loss of water in excess of solute. Typically it is seen in severe and acute sweating with inadequate intake of both water and salt. It may also follow prolonged periods of inadequate fluid intake where sodium loss has also occurred, as for example diarrhea with poor water intake. Laboratory findings include, most characteristically, an elevated serum sodium and serum osmolality. Where significant sodium loss is associated with the hypertonic contraction, the hematocrit will also be elevated. Since this disorder is commonly encountered in elderly indi-

viduals, the hematocrit at the time the patient is initially seen may be misleading if a preexisting anemia was present.

Finally, *hypertonic expansion* is virtually always iatrogenic. The two most common circumstances leading to its development include administration of 5 percent dextrose in 0.155 molar (0.9 percent) sodium chloride in diabetics who are unable to metabolize the sugar adequately and mannitol administration. The increasingly frequent administration of a hypertonic solution of mannitol as, for example, in an attempt to force diuresis when impending acute renal failure is suspected may lead to severe hypertonic expansion. The laboratory data that support this diagnosis depend upon the circumstances surrounding the production of the hypertonic expansion. Thus in the former case when sodium chloride and 5 percent dextrose are given in excess, there may be only a slight reduction in the plasma sodium concentration, but the osmolality of the plasma will be increased. Production of hypertonic expansion with mannitol will usually result in a much more dramatic decrease in the sodium concentration, largely because of the tendency to use solutions of mannitol that are quite hypertonic (15 to 20 percent solutions). The hematocrit is always markedly reduced. A third condition that may lead to hypertonic expansion is ingestion of large quantities of sodium chloride or intravenous administration of a hypertonic solution of sodium chloride.

ILLUSTRATIVE CASES

The following cases illustrate the clinical manifestations of these disorders and the approach to diagnosis and therapy. All of these cases summarize cases actually encountered on a large inpatient medical service. They are arranged so that the reader may attempt to arrive at his own diagnosis and treatment plan. The actual treatment employed with results and pertinent comments are included in the section following the case presentations. As an exercise, the reader should first attempt to arrive at the correct diagnosis of the fluid and electrolyte disorder and, when relevant, the type of pH disturbance present and the pathophysiologic events responsible for the abnormalities. As a final part of the exercise, the reader should develop a quantitative formulation of the appropriate treatment when indicated.

Case 1

A 29-year-old male was admitted to the hospital after a severe gastroenteritis of 36 hours' duration. Food and fluid intake had been poor because of persistent nausea and occasional vomiting, but his primary complaint was severe abdominal cramping and diarrhea with recurrent watery bowel movements. Physical examination revealed a blood pressure of 110/70 mm Hg, pulse of 98/min, and respiration of 26/min. The urine was unremarkable except for a specific gravity of 1.029; the hematocrit was 51 percent; and serum electrolytes revealed a sodium concentration of 142 mEq/L, chloride 104 mEq/L, HCO_3^- 22.5 mEq/L and a SUN of 31 mg/dl.

Case 2

A 52-year-old male with known hypertension and a history of a myocardial infarction 3 years previously was seen in the outpatient department complaining of breathlessness of sudden onset that awakened him at night and swelling of the legs of 3 weeks' duration. Physical examination revealed a blood pressure of 160/100 mm Hg, a pulse rate of 94/min, respiration of 22/min, weight 204 pounds (92.5 kg). The patient exhibited mild respiratory distress after walking only 20 to 30 paces. The neck veins were distended; auscultation revealed bilateral rales in lung bases, the heart was large with a gallop rhythm, the liver was felt 3 fingerbreadths below the costal margin, and there was 3+ pitting edema extending up to the knees. Diagnosis of congestive heart failure was made, and it was elected to treat the patient as an outpatient. He was given digitalis and furosemide 40 mg twice daily. He returned after 5 days complaining of weakness and giddiness on standing. He had

experienced two episodes of syncope. Supine blood pressure was 105/85 mm Hg and on standing dropped to 95/80. His weight was 168 pounds (76.22 kg). There was now no evidence of venous hypertension. The lungs were clear to auscultation and percussion. The gallop rhythm was no longer heard. The liver was not palpated, and there was no edema. Laboratory data revealed hematocrit 59 percent, SUN 50 mg/dl, sodium 145 mEq/L, chloride 95 mEq/L, bicarbonate 29 mEq/L, and potassium 5.1 mEq/L.

Case 3

A 37-year-old white male with known diabetes of 22 years' duration and with a history of repeated episodes of poor control and acidosis presented at the emergency room breathing rapidly and complaining of weakness. There was a strong odor of acetone on the breath. The blood pressure was 130/70 mm Hg, the pulse was 112/min, the skin was warm and dry, and the face was flushed. The patient was breathing rapidly with increased depth of respirations and complaining of thirst. Urinalysis revealed 4+ sugar and 3+ acetone, and the hematocrit was 48 percent. Blood chemical examinations revealed a glucose of 480 mg/dl, a serum sodium of 146 mEq/L, chloride 102 mEq/L, bicarbonate 15 mEq/L, and SUN 35 mg/dl. Because the patient was alert and in no acute distress, except for the increased respiratory rate, it was elected to treat him in the emergency room with intravenous fluids. An infusion of saline was begun, and he was given 10 U of crystalline zinc insulin. During the next 12 hours he received 6 L of 0.155 molar sodium chloride solution and a total of only 40 U of crystalline zinc insulin. At the end of this time the urine sugar remained 4+ and the acetone was persistently positive. Because of the persistent findings, he was admitted to the ward, where physical examination at that time revealed some neck vein distension to the angles of the mandible with the patient sitting. There were a few moist rales in both lung bases and prominent presacral pitting edema. The hematocrit at this time was 33 percent, and blood determinations revealed a glucose of 380 mg/dl, sodium of 143 mEq/L, chloride of 110 mEq/L, and bicarbonate of 17 mEq/L.

Case 4

A 33-year-old truck driver with known rheumatic heart disease, aortic insufficiency, and mitral insufficiency was admitted in heart failure with marked cardiomegaly, rales at both lung bases, hepatomegaly with the liver felt four fingerbreadths below the costal margin, and 3+ pitting edema. He was maintained on digitalis, placed on a diet containing 2 g of salt, and given 250 mg of chlorothiazide four times daily. On this regimen he lost 14 pounds (6.4 kg) while in the hospital, his symptoms of heart failure disappeared, and he felt well. He was given instructions for maintaining a 2 g salt diet and was discharged on a regimen of 250 mg of chlorothiazide four times daily and 50 mg of spironolactone twice daily. His weight at discharge was 125 pounds (56.7 kg). His serum sodium was 143 mEq/L, and his serum potassium was 4.6 mEq/L. He returned in one month complaining of marked weakness. Members of his family had noted some confusion and disorientation at times. His weight was 107 pounds (48.5 kg). There was questionable decrease in skin turgor. The lungs were clear on auscultation and percussion. The heart had decreased markedly in size, but the murmurs persisted. The liver was not felt, and there was no pitting edema. Serum electrolytes revealed a sodium concentration of 111 mEq/L and potassium of 5.6 mEq/L. The marked decrease in cardiac size was confirmed by chest x-ray.

Case 5

A 48-year-old male with remote history of three hospital admissions for tuberculosis was admitted complaining of severe back pain, occasional night sweats, and a 25-pound weight loss. Thoracic spine x-rays revealed a Pott abscess in the region of T-10, and a surgical drainage procedure was scheduled. When induction of anesthesia was begun, he became hypotensive and the procedure was terminated. Medical consultation was obtained at that time, and evaluation revealed blood pressure of 90/60 mm Hg, a pulse

of 120/min, a temperature of 99F, and respirations of 22/min and shallow. Buccal pigmentation was present, and there was impressive pigmentation in both the axilla and inguinal skin folds. There was moderate evidence of muscle wasting. Laboratory data revealed a hematocrit of 38 percent, a serum sodium concentration of 122 mEq/L, chlorides of 88 mEq/L, bicarbonate 26 mEq/L, and a potassium of 5.3 mEq/L. Review of abdominal x-rays previously obtained revealed flecks of calcium situated just above the upper poles of both kidneys.

Case 6

A 19-year-old male with a 2-year history of breathlessness on exertion and occasional hemoptysis was admitted with a diagnosis of mitral stenosis. Weight on admission was 132 pounds (59.9 kg), and he exhibited the classic physical findings of mitral stenosis. He underwent mitral commissurotomy, and postoperatively he received 2500 ml of fluid per day given intravenously as 5 percent dextrose in distilled water. On the third day following surgery, he appeared somewhat somnolent, and serum electrolytes revealed sodium concentration of 130 mEq/L and potassium 4.8 mEq/L. His urine output during this period had never exceeded 400 ml per day.

Case 7

A 49-year-old male was admitted because of disorientation and some inappropriate behavior. He had been in an automobile accident 3 years previously and received a severe blow on the head, resulting in loss of consciousness. A basilar skull fracture was diagnosed at that time, but he recovered apparently without incident. Following recovery, he was in reasonable health until the present illness. His confusion had been first noted 3 days prior to admission. On admission, his physical examination revealed a blood pressure of 125/70 mm Hg, pulse of 94/min, weight 158 pounds (71.7 kg); temperature and respirations were normal, and the general physical examination revealed little except poor mental function. No localizing neurologic signs were identified. Laboratory data revealed urine specific gravity of 1.022 and hematocrit of 43 percent. Serum electrolytes revealed sodium concentration of 112 mEq/L, chlorides of 79 mEq/L, bicarbonate of 29 mEq/L, and potassium concentration of 4.1 mEq/L. Measurement of urinary electrolytes revealed a sodium concentration of 60 mEq/L and a total 24-hour urine volume of 550 ml. The urine osmolality was 725 mOsmol/kg H_2O. The patient was given 1500 ml of 0.155 molar sodium chloride and responded with a prompt increase in urine volume. The following day the serum electrolytes were essentially unchanged, with a sodium concentration 114 mEq/L. Urinary electrolytes had increased markedly, however, and on the day of the second infusion the urinary sodium concentration was 110 mEq/L with a total urinary volume of 1600 ml for that day. Osmolality of this urine was 530 mOsmol/kg H_2O.

Case 8

An elderly man was brought to the emergency room in semicoma. No further history was available. On physical examination he responded to pain but was unable to speak. The blood pressure was 120/80 mm Hg; the pulse was 104/min. Respirations were 16/min, and he weighed 136 pounds (61.7 kg). The skin turgor appeared poor, but this was difficult to judge because of his loose, inelastic skin. Pertinent physical findings were limited to left-sided hyperreflexia, moderate in degree. Urine specific gravity was 1.017, and the blood studies revealed a hematocrit of 55 percent, serum sodium concentration of 163 mEq/L, chloride concentration of 121, and bicarbonate concentration of 24 mEq/L, SUN 48 mg/dl, and serum osmolality of 339 mOsmol/kg H_2O.

Case 9

A 37-year-old male with a long-standing history of heavy alcohol ingestion was admitted because of a severe, poorly localized pain in the upper abdomen that radiated through to the back. He had vomited once 8 hours previously at the onset of the pain without subsequent recurrence of vomiting or diarrhea. The pain had steadily increased in severity, and at the time of admission he was in acute distress. His blood pressure was 110/70 mm Hg, pulse 115/min, and temperature 101F. The skin was moist from perspiration. Remainder of the pertinent physical signs were confined to the abdomen. There was generalized abdominal tenderness with rebound tenderness present. Only an occasional bowel sound was heard. The remainder of the physical examination contributed little. Laboratory data revealed a marked leukocytosis, hematocrit of 48 percent, serum sodium concentration of 145 mEq/L, potassium 3.9 mEq/L, and bicarbonate of 22 mEq/L. Urinalysis revealed a specific gravity of 1.024 and a trace of protein. His condition deteriorated over the next 8 hours with increasing tachycardia and hypotension and persistence of the severe abdominal pain. The abdomen became silent. Repeat laboratory studies showed a hematocrit of 64 percent, but the serum electrolytes remained unchanged. An amylase drawn at this time was 425 units. An upright x-ray of the abdomen showed several air-fluid levels, all thought to be within the lumen of the gut.

Case 10

This patient, who had a long history of cigarette smoking, was admitted with increasing cough, dyspnea, and peripheral edema. A diagnosis of chronic obstructive lung disease had been established 7 years previously. Admission arterial blood gas values included a PO_2 of 42 mm Hg, PCO_2 of 62 mm Hg, pH 7.38, and $[HCO_3^-]$ of 35 mEq/L. Therapy was begun using nasal oxygen, bronchodilators, and diuretics. Twelve hours after admission he became increasingly combative, cyanotic, and clammy and was found to have a blood pressure of 90/50 mm Hg as compared to an admission value of 160/70 mm Hg. At this time his arterial blood gas values were PO_2 22 mm Hg, PCO_2 73 mm Hg, pH 7.21, and $[HCO_3^-]$ 29 mEq/L.

Case 11

This patient was admitted with an acute asthmatic episode. On examination a pulsus paradoxus of 30 mm Hg was noted, as well as accessory muscle use and marked pulmonary wheezes. Admission blood gases were PO_2 45 mm Hg, PCO_2 40 mm Hg, pH 7.40, and $[HCO_3^-]$ 24 mEq/L. After 12 hours of vigorous bronchodilator and oxygen therapy, the patient appeared tired and somewhat somnolent. At this point, the arterial blood gases were PO_2 35 mm Hg, PCO_2 56 mm Hg, pH 7.28, and $[HCO_3^-]$ 26 mEq/L.

COMMENTS ON DIAGNOSIS AND TREATMENT OF CASES

Case 1

The normal serum sodium concentration and elevated hematocrit in an individual with a history of severe diarrhea of 36 hours duration identifies the fluid disturbance as *isotonic contraction* with probable mild metabolic acidosis (HCO_3^- 22.5 mEq/L). Because of the story of continued fluid loss 2 days prior to admission, he was given 4000 ml of fluid the first day, 2000 ml of which were given as 0.155 molar (0.9 percent) sodium chloride. On the second day he received 3500 ml of fluid, 1500 ml of which were given as 0.155 molar sodium chloride. By the third day he was able to tolerate food and fluids without difficulty. At this point, his weight had increased 2 kg over admission, his hematocrit had dropped to 41 percent, and the serum sodium concentration was 146 mEq/L. The SUN was 19 mg/dl.

Comment. At presentation the patient was thought to have both a sodium and water deficit, largely because of persistent diarrhea in the face of inadequate intake. The elevated hematocrit and urea nitrogen tended to support the diagnosis, and the presence of a normal serum sodium concentration identified this as an instance of *isotonic contraction*. During the first 2 days the patient was given

moderate excesses of both sodium and water. This represents quite acceptable therapy when renal function is adequate, since the kidneys excrete any excess sodium or water administered. His weight gain during this 2-day period, associated with the drop in hematocrit to 41 percent, indicates that he retained approximately 2 L of isotonic fluid.

Case 2

This patient developed an elevated hematocrit and serum urea nitrogen associated with a marked reduction in weight resulting from diuretic therapy. As in Case 1, the serum sodium concentration was normal, indicating *isotonic contraction*. The diagnosis of diuretic-induced sodium depletion was made. Because of the patient's cardiovascular disease, treatment consisted of increasing his oral intake of salt. He was placed at bed rest and given a diet allowing an ad lib. salt intake. On this regimen he gained 6 pounds (2.7 kg) in 4 days, and his symptoms disappeared. Laboratory data obtained on the fifth day revealed a hematocrit of 47 percent, SUN of 30 mg/dl, serum sodium of 144 mEq/L, chloride of 101 mEq/L, and bicarbonate of 25 mEq/L. Following this improvement, sodium intake was again reduced and his diuretic dosage schedule reduced.

Comment. The deficit in this case was a result of vigorous diuretic therapy. The mild elevation of bicarbonate probably represented an alkalosis that resulted from disproportionate loss of sodium and chloride. Although the deficit here was as great as that in the previous case, parenteral therapy was avoided because of the hazard of overexpansion attendant upon intravenous sodium chloride administration. On oral intake he retained sodium and water progressively and corrected the deficit. It should be emphasized that oral therapy is a perfectly appropriate, safe, and convenient means of treating sodium depletion. It should be regarded as the route of choice in all patients with cardiovascular disease unless there is some contraindication to oral administration, or unless severe signs of sodium deficit are present.

Case 3

As a result of inappropriate therapy, this patient accumulated a large excess of fluid administered as an isotonic solution of sodium chloride *(isotonic expansion)*. Despite this, his diabetic acidosis remained uncontrolled. Following his admission, insulin dosage was increased on a sliding scale so that he received up to 45 U/hr depending upon the urinary glucose and the ketone concentration (see Chapter 14.7). On this regimen his glucosuria and ketonuria cleared during the third hour following admission to the ward. He subsequently diuresed so that his weight dropped by 4.9 kg. His hematocrit returned to normal, and he felt well.

Comment. This case illustrates the hazards of attempting to treat diabetic acidosis when the patient cannot be carefully watched. The hazard of overexpansion by excess sodium chloride administration is ever present in the management of diabetic acidosis, particularly when the insulin dosage is inadequate and the patient is not carefully monitored. The laboratory data are all consistent with overexpansion, including the considerable drop in the hematocrit and the moderate hyperchloremia that developed. Appropriate treatment at this point depends mainly upon the condition of the patient. If he is sufficiently stable to permit such therapy, control of the acidosis and ketosis with insulin without additional fluid administration is preferable. If the patient has reasonably normal renal function, he will usually be able to excrete the excess sodium in a short period.

Case 4

Striking improvement in this patient's cardiovascular status with disappearance of all manifestations of heart failure associated with the marked decrease in weight suggested a diagnosis of hyponatremia caused by chronic sodium depletion *(hypotonic contraction)*. Oral repletion was attempted, and he was given 205 mEq of sodium orally on each of 2 successive days. Thereafter he was maintained on a 25 mEq sodium diet. Throughout this period the urinary sodium did not exceed 6 mEq per day. During the 2 days of supplemental administration of sodium, his weight did not increase; in fact he lost 1 pound. His serum sodium concentration, however, over this 2-day period, rose from 111 to 127 mEq/L, representing an estimated increase in the sodium content of the extracellular fluid of 480 mEq. His diet plus supplemental intake during that period was estimated to be 470 mEq. Thus he appeared to retain all the administered sodium, a fact corroborated by measurement of urinary sodium, which totaled 12 mEq over these 2 days. His mental confusion disappeared, and he exhibited marked improvement over the next 7 days on increased dietary sodium alone. His sodium concentration rose further to 139 mEq/L. Throughout this period his weight changed very little, increasing only 3 pounds to 110 pounds (49.9 kg) at the end of the 10-day hospitalization.

Comment. Careful questioning of this patient revealed that he had been extremely careful about his dietary intake and had probably maintained himself on as little as 2 or 3 g of salt in the diet per day. On such limited salt intake the diuretic regimen proved to be too vigorous, and he developed a severe sodium deficit. Estimation of the deficit at the time of admission (based on the initial serum sodium concentration) revealed that he had lost more than 900 mEq of sodium after discharge. Replacement of about half of this deficit, however, resulted in complete clearance of the mental symptoms and marked improvement in his general well-being. This case illustrates the hazard of producing severe sodium depletion when a patient who has also been subjected to careful sodium restriction is given vigorous diuretic therapy with one of the strong nonmercurial oral agents. The necessity of observing such patients closely is well illustrated. Again, as in Case 2, it is perfectly clear that oral therapy is both safe and satisfactory in treating such patients.

Case 5

A diagnosis of Addison disease was made with associated *hypotonic contraction*, and the patient was given 100 mg of cortisol intravenously immediately followed by 2000 ml of isotonic sodium chloride over the next 2 hours. Continuous intravenous cortisol therapy was maintained at the rate of 100 mg every 8 hours given in 1000 ml of isotonic sodium chloride. By the following day, the patient's blood pressure had risen to 130/85 mm Hg, his pulse was 100/min, and his temperature was 98F. He appeared comfortable and was able to take food and fluid orally. His hematocrit measured at this time was 28 percent and persisted in this range for the next several days.

Comment. The Addisonian pigmentation was unrecognized at the time of initial physical examination, and it was only after the hypotensive episode at the time of surgery that the diagnosis became clear. Laboratory data are consistent with *hypotonic contraction;* however, his hematocrit was maintained at a level of 38 percent, indicating that his underlying anemia had masked a significant rise in the hematocrit. This illustrates one of the difficulties associated with use of the hematocrit as a guide for sodium depletion in patients who are anemic. This patient exhibited only modest hyperkalemia, not severe enough to warrant treatment beyond adequate hormonal replacement therapy and provision of an adequate salt intake.

Case 6

Water intoxication resulting in *hypotonic expansion* was diagnosed, and on the basis of the lowered serum sodium concentration, it was estimated that he had accumulated an excess of 3.6 L of water. His total fluid intake was limited to 400 ml per day. On this regimen he lost approximately 2 pounds of weight (0.9 kg) per day, and over the ensuing 4 days his serum sodium concentration returned to normal.

Comment. This case illustrates the hazard of continued excessive intake of water in individuals who have had extensive surgical procedures. On occasion the antidiuretic state may persist for 2 or 3 days, particularly when the patient is experiencing a great deal of pain. More appropriate therapy should have been based on monitoring the patient's output and daily weight, providing him with fluid adequate to cover urinary losses plus insensible losses, and keeping his weight nearly stable. In such a situation it is desirable to avoid weight gains of more than 1 kg unless there is a specific indication for more vigorous fluid therapy, as, for instance, hypotension, evidence of continued bleeding, or accumulation of fluid in the chest. In the present case, recognition of the water intoxication when the serum sodium had fallen to only 130 mEq/L warranted no more vigorous therapy than careful fluid restriction. When this condition occurs immediately following surgery, it is often caused by sustained release of ADH that persists for only a relatively short period and is followed by a water diuresis that hastens recovery from water intoxication.

Case 7

On the basis of the hyponatremia, hypo-osmolality, and hypertonicity of the urine with increased urinary sodium loss, the diagnosis of inappropriate antidiuretic hormone secretion leading to *hypotonic expansion* was made. The patient was placed on a regimen of rigid fluid restriction, total intake being kept below 600 ml per day. On this regimen he lost approximately 1.5 pounds per day (0.7 kg) for the next 5 days. His confusion cleared, and he felt well. His serum sodium concentration at this time was 125 mEq/L. Because of this improvement, his fluid intake was increased to a total of 1000 ml per day. As a result his rate of weight loss decreased to approximately 0.5 pound (0.2 kg) per day, but the plasma sodium continued to rise slowly and had returned to within normal range on the 14th hospital day. Further neurologic study revealed no space-occupying lesion of the central nervous system, so he was discharged on fluid restriction to total 2000 ml per day. He was advised to maintain a daily record of his weight and to be observed regularly by a physician.

Comment. This patient had developed *hypotonic expansion* as a result of progressive water retention produced by the persistent elaboration of ADH. The criteria for making this diagnosis include demonstration of hypotonicity or hypo-osmolality of the plasma (as compared to normal values) and hypertonic urine. He illustrates the efficacy of fluid restriction in such patients. On occasion, such patients will excrete sufficient quantities of sodium in the urine following their hypotonic expansion to develop a serious sodium deficit. This may subsequently become symptomatic and require therapy. In the present patient, if such a deficit existed, it was sufficiently mild that it was corrected by dietary sodium intake. The failure of the hematocrit to reflect changes in body water is well illustrated in this patient. The case also illustrates the prime importance of carefully determined daily weights in monitoring therapy.

Case 8

The diagnosis of water deficit with resulting *hypertonic contraction* was made. On the basis of serum sodium concentration of 163 mEq/L, this deficit was estimated at 5 L. The patient received half of this total replacement during the first 4 hours. Because of the presumption that the elevated hematocrit reflected a significant sodium deficit, the first 4 L of fluid were given as 2.5 percent dextrose in 0.034 molar (0.20 percent) sodium chloride, thus providing him with 120 mEq of sodium during the first 6 hours. Over the next 3 days he received 3000 ml of dextrose 5 percent in water and 1000 ml of 0.155 molar sodium chloride per day. He responded slowly, and at the end of the third day, when he had received a total quantity of water that exceeded his deficit plus estimated continued losses, he was still somnolent. Although he could be aroused, he could not speak. He showed slow improvement during the next 5 or 6 days and became oriented and able to com-

municate verbally. His serum sodium concentration decreased to 145 mEq/L, and his hematocrit fell to 41 percent. His weight increased to 154 pounds (69.8 kg).

Comment. This is a typical setting for the occurrence of *hypertonic contraction*. This elderly individual who lived alone probably had a mild cerebral vascular accident and became unable to maintain his fluid intake. Because of the hot environment, the most likely cause of the associated sodium depletion was persistent perspiration. Fluids chosen for replacement therapy were dictated by the need to keep the osmolality of the solution being infused well below that of his plasma osmolality. The fact that he had a significant sodium deficit is reflected in the marked decrease in his hematocrit as therapy progressed. Final hematocrit and the body weight indicate that he retained approximately 450 mEq of sodium and 8 L of water. The difference between the estimate of the water deficit made on the basis of the elevated serum sodium concentration and the total quantity of water retained represented the water that was retained with sodium as an isotonic solution.

Case 9

The single laboratory finding in this case of pancreatitis that pointed to progressive *isotonic contraction* was the *progressive rise in the hematocrit*. The value of following the hematocrit closely in situations where "hidden" fluid losses develop cannot be overemphasized. The abdominal film confirmed the diagnosis of paralytic ileus with pooling of fluid in the gut. Intravenous replacement therapy was begun promptly upon recognition of the contracted state. He received 3000 ml of 0.155 molar saline and 500 ml of plasma over a period of 3 hours. His blood pressure rose to 135/75 mm Hg, and his pulse dropped to 100/min. Peroral intubation of the duodenum with a Cantor tube with gentle suction yielded 2500 to 3000 ml per day for the succeeding 3 days. Replacement therapy consisted of giving a quantity of 0.155 molar sodium chloride solution equal to the duodenal drainage each day plus 2000 ml of 5 percent dextrose in 0.034 molar (0.20 percent) sodium chloride solution. Signs and symptoms of pancreatitis abated slowly, and his hematocrit, which had returned to normal the first day, remained in the normal range.

Comment. This case illustrates two points. Hidden fluid losses, such as accumulation of fluid in the gastrointestinal tract, rapid development of ascites, acute swelling of an extremity as is sometimes seen with an ischemic crush injury, all can lead to severe depletion of the functional extracellular fluid volume. They are extremely difficult to recognize, and the physician must be alert to the situations where such losses are likely to occur. The hematocrit is the only useful laboratory test for confirmation of the development of isotonic contraction under these circumstances. Second, maintenance therapy is as important as initial replacement therapy. In the present case, continued loss of fluid via the gastrointestinal tract would have rapidly led to a return of contraction of the extracellular fluid space with hypovolemia had not the losses been quantified by measuring and replacing the Cantor tube drainage.

Case 10

The elevated admission P_{CO_2} indicated the presence of respiratory acidosis. The increase in P_{CO_2} from a normal value of 40 was 22 mm Hg. Had the respiratory acidosis been chronic, then multiplying the change in P_{CO_2} by 0.3 would have yielded a figure of 6.6 nEq/L for the change in hydrogen ion concentration in a patient with chronic respiratory failure. Adding this number to the normal hydrogen ion of 40 nEq/L yields a hydrogen ion concentration of 47, or a pH of 7.33. Thus in chronic respiratory acidosis a steady state of P_{CO_2} of 62 mm Hg would be expected to produce a pH of 7.33. The initial value of 7.38 in this patient is slightly high and may indicate a mild degree of metabolic alkalosis induced by diuretic therapy.

The next blood gas, obtained following the appearance of signs of acute circulatory insufficiency, documented a significant

increase in the P_{CO_2} and a fall in the $[HCO_3^-]$. The increase in P_{CO_2} reflected the presence of a complicating acute respiratory acidosis. The fall in $[HCO_3^-]$, a directional change *opposite* to one expected after acute or chronic CO_2 retention, indicated the presence of an acute metabolic acidosis. The hypoxemia and signs of circulatory collapse pointed to the presence of lactic acidosis, suggested also by the finding of a widened anion gap. The clinical event probably responsible for these acute changes was an acute pulmonary embolus.

Comment. This case illustrates two important points in the diagnosis and management of acid–base disturbances. First, it is essential that the laboratory observations be validated. When the $[H^+]$ is estimated from the equation relating $[H^+]$ to P_{CO_2} in chronic respiratory acidosis, as outlined on page 708, it is evident that this is more than just chronic respiratory acidosis. The unexpectedly high arterial pH identifies the coexistence of metabolic alkalosis. This combination of respiratory acidosis and metabolic alkalosis could make interpretation of plasma potassium measurements difficult and could well serve to mask development of significant potassium deficits if diuretic usage is continued.

The second lesson taught by the events in this case is the importance of reevaluating the acid–base status when the clinical course differs from expectations. The paradoxical decrease in $[HCO_3^-]$ immediately heralds the appearance of a new complicating disturbance. The correct diagnoses could not have been made in this case without critical interpretation of accurate sequential analyses of arterial blood for pH, P_{CO_2}, $[HCO_3^-]$, and P_{O_2}.

Case 11

The presence of a normal P_{CO_2} on admission in an asthmatic patient should alert the physician to a very serious clinical condition inasmuch as most asthmatic patients exhibit alveolar hyperventilation and a low P_{CO_2}. The seriousness of the problem was confirmed by the patient's subsequent clinical deterioration and elevation of the P_{CO_2}. Had the respiratory acidosis been acute, then the change in P_{CO_2} of 16 ($56 - 40$ multiplied by 0.8) should have yielded a $\Delta [H^+]$ of 12. The new H^+ concentration would thus have been $40 + 12$, or 52 nEq/L, yielding a pH of 7.28, exactly the value found by measurement. Inasmuch as the patient's clinical condition was worsening rapidly, artificial ventilation would be the treatment of choice.

Comment. In this instance the blood gas analysis provided the necessary evidence that the only acid–base disturbance in this case was related to the acute asthmatic attack. This directs therapy toward more vigorous ventilatory support to relieve the asthmatic attack and offers reassurance that no complicating event or illness has resulted in a mixed acid–base disturbance.

CHAPTER 11.1
Pathophysiology of Uremia and Clinical Evaluation of Renal Function

W. Gordon Walker and William E. Mitch

Urine is formed by the nephron, a structure composed at its proximal end of a capillary tuft closely covered by epithelium that is continuous with the tubule of epithelial cells leading to the collecting system. This constitutes the primary functional unit of the kidney, and in healthy individuals each kidney contains approximately 1 million such nephrons. Each nephron has its own blood supply, and so long as this blood supply and the structure of the nephron are intact, the nephron functions independently as a single unit. Approximately 90 μl of plasma ultrafiltrate is made daily to elaborate a volume of urine that averages between 0.2 and 0.8 μl under normal conditions. Virtually all forms of diffuse renal disease result in progressive loss of these nephrons, whereas undamaged nephrons function normally or supranormally to regulate body fluids and maintain a balance between intake and output of various dietary constituents. Thus the impairment of renal function accompanying damage to the kidney associated with diffuse renal diseases is a result of progressive loss of nephrons. Accurate documentation of the rate of destruction necessitates a quantitative measure of the number of residual functioning nephrons. Clinical tests designed to assess the residual quantity of functioning renal tissue (functioning nephrons) provide the primary data that allow the clinician to estimate the severity of the disease and the rate of destruction of renal function. In particular, renal function can be most conveniently monitored by quantifying the renal clearance of creatinine. For this reason, the relationship between the serum creatinine, renal creatinine clearance, and the glomerular filtration rate is reviewed in detail. Once a precise understanding of these aspects of renal physiology is achieved, the clinical evaluation of renal function can proceed from a solid foundation.

QUANTITATIVE MEASUREMENTS OF RENAL FUNCTION

RENAL CLEARANCE

The principal means of studying renal function quantitatively in humans is to measure the excretion rates of substances appearing in the urine and then to relate these rates to plasma concentrations of the substances measured. This technique, termed "clearance" by Addis, provides a valuable means for relating renal function to plasma composition; it can be used to assess the kidney's capacity to maintain the constancy of the fluid environment of the cells and tissues.[7,25] For ease of understanding it is convenient to consider calculation of clearance as a special instance of the Fick principle (Fig. 11.1–1). For a substance that only traverses the kidney but is not synthesized, metabolized, or excreted, renal arterial input equals renal venous output. When a portion of the substance is excreted in the urine, arterial input equals renal venous output plus urine output. Stated symbolically:

$$A_S \times RPF = V_S \times RPF + U_S V \qquad (1)$$

where A_S denotes arterial concentration of substance s, V_S represents renal venous concentration of substance s, RPF is renal plasma flow, U_S denotes urinary concentration of s, and V equals urine flow. This restatement of the principle of conservation of mass allows partitioning of the arterial input of substance s into the portion leaving by way of the urine and that leaving by the renal vein. As illustrated in Figure 11.1–1, it can be restated to express the urinary excretion rate as the volume of plasma cleared of substance s in unit time, and the expression $U_S V/A_S$ is the expression for clearance. Because the concentration in renal arterial plasma (A_S) does not, in most instances, differ greatly from that in peripheral venous plasma (P_S), the latter is used and the equation

$$\text{Clearance} = U_S V/P_S \text{ or } UV/P \qquad (2)$$

is the usual means of defining clearance.

The chief virtue of this concept is the ease with which it makes possible the quantitative description of renal function in the intact human. In general, it is convenient to think of renal clearances of various endogenous and exogenous substances as falling into two categories. "Fixed" clearances, such as those of inulin, urea, mannitol, creatinine, or p-aminohippurate (PAH) remain relatively constant from day to day and provide an overall measure of the functional capacity of the kidney. "Variable" clearances of such substances as sodium, potassium, water, phosphate, calcium, and others reflect the regulatory activity of the kidneys and may change rapidly over a short period of time as a result of change in the individual's environment, or intake.

GLOMERULAR FILTRATION RATE (GFR)

Because urine formation begins with an ultrafiltrate of plasma formed in the glomerulus, it follows that the clearance technique can be used to measure the rate of glomerular filtration. This is contingent on the availability of a substance that is freely filtered at the glomerulus and is neither secreted nor reabsorbed in transit through the tubule. Inulin is such a substance and the quantity filtered at the glomeruli is identical to the quantity appearing in the urine. This may be expressed quantitatively as

$$GFR \times P_{INULIN} = U_{INULIN} V$$

and hence

$$GFR = U_{INULIN} V/P$$

The clearance of inulin is thus an accurate measure of the glomerular filtration rate and can be used to assess residual renal function; quantitatively it is related directly to the total number of functioning nephrons. Inulin clearance provides an accurate measure of glomerular filtration rate but is time consuming and costly and thus unsuited for routine clinical use. The most widely used clearance

For substance s confined to plasma during renal transit, i.e., neither metabolized, stored, nor excreted by kidney, input = output;

$$[A_s] \cdot RPF = [V_s] \cdot RPF$$

for substance excreted by the kidney

$$A_s \cdot RPF = [V_s RPF] + [U_s \cdot Urine\ Flow]$$

$$\underset{mg/min}{Arterial\ Input} = \underset{mg/min}{Venous\ Output} + \underset{mg/min}{Urinary\ Excretion}$$

or

$$[A_s - V_s] \cdot RPF = U_s V\ (Fick\ Equation)$$

If substance completely excreted by the kidney $V_s = 0$ and,

$$A_s \cdot RPF = U_s V$$

If substance partially excreted by the kidney

$$A_s \cdot E \cdot RPF = U_s V$$

where

$$E = \frac{A_s - V_s}{A_s} = Extraction\ Efficiency$$

thus,

$$RPF\ (ml/min) = \frac{U_s V\ (mg/min)}{A_s\ (mg/ml) \cdot E} \quad (if\ V_s = 0,\ E = 1.0)$$

Figure 11.1–1. Illustration of clearance as an application of Fick principle. $[A_s]$ = arterial concentration of substances; $[V_s]$ = renal venous concentration; $[U_s]$ = urinary concentration; RPF = renal plasma flow; and V = urine flow in milliliters per minute. For many substances (inulin, urea, creatinine) arterial and peripheral venous concentrations do not differ greatly, and hence peripheral venous concentrations $[P_s]$ may be used as an approximation of $[A_s]$.

substance is creatinine; the measure of glomerular filtration rate that it provides is quite adequate for clinical use.

RENAL PLASMA FLOW (RPF)

If simultaneous measurements of arterial and renal venous blood indicate that all of a substance (such as PAH) reaching the kidney is removed from the plasma and appears in the urine without significant storage or metabolism in the kidney, then V_S in Equation 1 becomes zero and the equation simplifies to:

$$A_S \times RPF = U_S V \tag{3}$$

yielding a means of measuring renal plasma flow: thus

$$RPF = U_S V / P_S \tag{4}$$

PAH clearance can be used in this manner to measure renal plasma flow (Table 11.1–1).

The renal blood flow (RBF) can be estimated if the hematocrit is known:

$$RBF = RPF/(1 - Hct) \tag{5}$$

where Hct is the hematocrit expressed as a fraction.

Not only does application of the clearance technique provide a means of measurement of glomerular filtration rate, renal plasma flow, and renal blood flow, it can also be used to characterize the regulatory functions of the kidneys. Table 11.1–1 contains normal values for renal hemodynamic data, plus a listing of the common urinary constituents and their mean clearance values; where appropriate, standard deviations are given to provide a measure of the range encountered in normal subjects. Data are also included on the fractional excretion rate of these substances. For the major electrolytes found in body fluids, the wide range of clearance reflects the kidneys' regulatory capacity or ability to vary secretion widely in order to maintain the body content within narrow limits. Table 11.1–2 contrasts some of these ranges seen in healthy subjects with those encountered in the presence of advanced renal failure.

There is an inverse relationship between clearance and plasma concentration (Eq. 2). For substances that are also handled by tubular transport, this relationship can be modified and, indeed, may be difficult to demonstrate until renal function has been extensively compromised. For substances handled largely or exclusively by glomerular filtration, the relationship is readily demonstrated over the entire range of clearance values. It is this relationship between plasma concentration of the substance and its clearance that is of primary clinical importance. This importance is most clearly illustrated by urea or creatinine, two substances whose plasma concentrations are used nearly exclusively to provide clinical informa-

TABLE 11.1–1. RANGE OF CLEARANCE VALUES AND SOME FRACTIONAL EXCRETION RATES IN ADULTS[6,7,18,26]

		Mean Value ±1 SD (ml/min)	Mean Value 1.73 m² BSA (ml/min)	Fractional Excretion Rates (Cx/GFR)
Effective renal plasma flow	Males		655±96	
	Females		600±90	
Renal blood flow (ERPF/(1 − Hct))	Males		1300	
	Females		1100	
Glomerular filtration rate	Males		130±23	
	Females		120±17	
Creatinine clearance	Males	110±20		
	Females	92±13		
Urea clearance[a]	Males	40−83		
	Females	35−60		
Sodium[a]				<0.001−0.02
Potassium[a]				0.006−0.09
Calcium[a]				<0.002−0.015
Phosphate[a]				0.05−0.20
Uric acid[a]				0.10−0.20

[a]Ranges only given for these variables.

tion regarding overall renal function. Urea is of particular value because its plasma concentration reflects both protein intake and renal function; creatinine provides the most accurate information about renal function.

Urea, like inulin, is freely filtered at the glomerulus, but urea diffuses back across the tubular cells from the tubular fluid, with the result that only about 50 to 60 percent of the urea that is filtered is ultimately excreted in the urine. Hence the urea clearance is only about 50 percent of the simultaneously measured inulin clearance. Nevertheless the plasma urea exhibits an inverse relationship that is readily demonstrable over the entire range of glomerular filtration so long as protein intake remains constant. Figures 11.1–2 and 11.1–3 illustrate this inverse relationship and the manner in which alterations in dietary protein intake influence the plasma urea concentration at any given rate of glomerular filtration. It is evident that fluctuations in protein intake can produce very wide fluctuations in plasma urea without any change in the glomerular filtration rate. For this reason, monitoring of the blood urea nitrogen does not produce useful and reliable information regarding constancy of renal function; it is better used for monitoring protein intake.

Because protein is 16 percent nitrogen, a normal subject eating 100 g of protein daily will have almost 14 g of urea nitrogen to excrete per day; the remaining 2 g of nitrogen will be excreted as nonurea nitrogen.[8] If he is in nitrogen balance, his renal excretory rate ($U_{UREA}V$) will be 10 mg/min. From this, one can predict his plasma urea level, assuming a urea clearance of about 60 percent of GFR, or 70 ml/min:

$$C_{UREA} = \frac{U_{UREA} \cdot V}{P_{UREA}}$$

$$P_{UREA} = \frac{U_{UREA} \cdot V}{C_{UREA}} = \frac{10 \text{ mg/min}}{70 \text{ ml/min}}$$

$$P_{UREA} = 0.14 \text{ mg/ml} = 14 \text{ mg/dl}$$

It is evident from this calculation that doubling the protein intake in this circumstance would result in doubling the concentration of urea in the plasma.

If renal disease destroys half of the nephrons, urea clearance

TABLE 11.1–2. CONTRASTING FUNCTION OF THE NORMAL AND SEVERELY IMPAIRED KIDNEY[7,18,23]

Parameter of Renal Function	Normal	Severely Impaired GFR <5% of Normal
Glomerular filtration rate (L/day)	180	7
Maximum urinary volume (L/day)	25	2
Minimum urinary volume (L/day)	0.50	1.4
Maximum solute concentration (mOsmol/kg H₂O)	1200	375
Maximum free water clearance (L/day)	24	1
Maximum free water reabsorption (L/day)	8	0.4
Maximum total hydrogen ion secretion (mEq/day) (HCO₃ reabsorption + titratable acidity + ammonia)	5000	150
Titratable acidity (mEq/day)[a]	150	15
Ammonia production (mEq/day)[a]	350	40
Average solute excretion per day (μOsm/min)[b]	600	400
Average solute excretion per deciliter GFR (μOsm/dl GFR)	342	6000

[a]Maximum values developed in the presence of persistent systemic acidosis.
[b]This is determined primarily by solute intake.

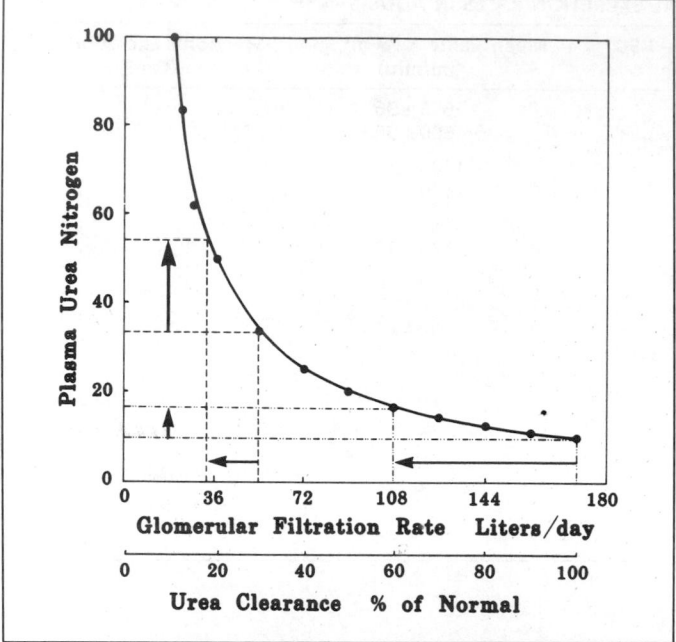

Figure 11.1–2. Relation of plasma concentration of urea to changes in glomerular filtration rate (GFR) or urea clearance. In normal subjects a 40 percent decrease in GFR from 180 to 108 L per day elevates the plasma or blood urea nitrogen only about 5 mg/dl. In advanced renal impairment, however, when GFR is only about 25 percent of normal, the same percentage decrease raises the plasma concentration of urea nitrogen 20 mg/dl. Thus large changes in GFR in the presence of previously normal renal function may not raise plasma levels beyond those usually considered normal. For this reason, blood urea nitrogen measurement is of limited value in monitoring changes in renal function.

will be halved. Under these circumstances, plasma urea concentration will be doubled even though protein intake is unchanged:

$$P_{UREA} = \frac{U_{UREA} \cdot V}{C_{UREA}} = \frac{10 \text{ mg/min}}{35 \text{ ml/min}}$$

$$P_{UREA} = 0.28 \text{ mg/ml} = 28 \text{ mg/dl}$$

It is apparent that if protein intake is reduced from 88 to 44 g per day, the urea excretory rate will be reduced from 10 to 5 mg/min, and plasma concentration can return to 14 ml/dl.

These important relationships between clearance, plasma concentration, and dietary protein are illustrated in Figures 11.1–2, 11.1–3, and 11.1–4.

Serum creatinine concentration provides a better assessment of the constancy of renal function because it is influenced much less by dietary fluctuations, since nearly all the creatinine that appears in the urine is produced at an essentially constant rate from creatinine and creatinine phosphate in muscle.[15] Because of this, serum creatinine permits detection of changes in normal renal function as small as 15 to 20 percent if measured with adequate precision in the clinical chemistry laboratory. In the presence of advanced renal disease, it can identify changes in renal function as small as 5 to 10 percent. The usefulness and limitations of the plasma concentration in creatinine and creatinine clearance as clinical indicators of renal function are considered later in this chapter.

REGULATION OF WATER EXCRETION AND OSMOLALITY OF BODY FLUID

Isotonic glomerular filtrate is formed at a rate of about 125 ml/min, or 180 L per day, in the average healthy adult. In contrast, urine output ranges usually between 500 ml and 1 L per day. The kidneys must thus reabsorb very large quantities of water and solute. The fraction of 180 L per day of filtered water and solute that finally appears as urine is determined by water and solute in-

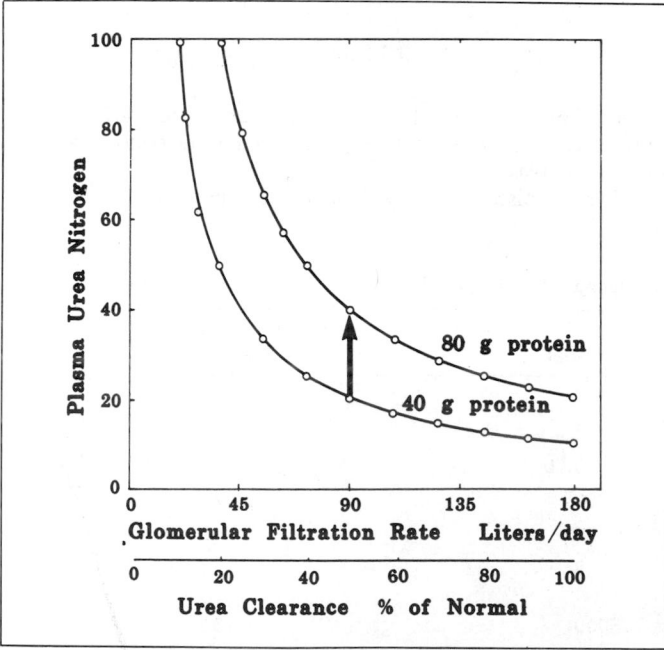

Figure 11.1–3. Variations in protein intake may produce significant changes in plasma concentration of urea in the absence of change in glomerular filtration rate. In general, when clearance is constant, the plasma or blood urea nitrogen is directly related to protein intake so that a doubling of protein intake doubles the plasma urea concentration. Conversely, halving protein intake reduces the plasma urea by half.

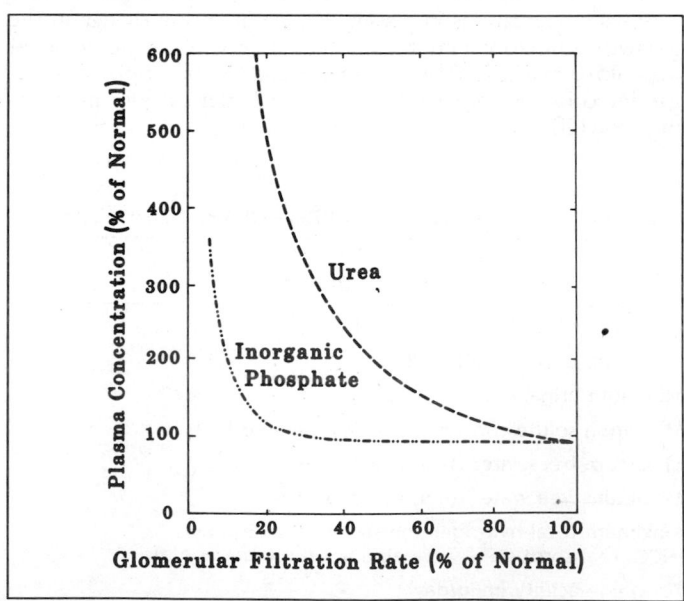

Figure 11.1–4. Schematic representation of relation between decrease in glomerular filtration rate and plasma concentration of substances handled by filtration (urea) and by filtration plus active reabsorption (inorganic phosphate). The ability of the kidney to alter the rate of phosphate reabsorption maintains phosphate near normal plasma levels despite extensive loss of renal function.

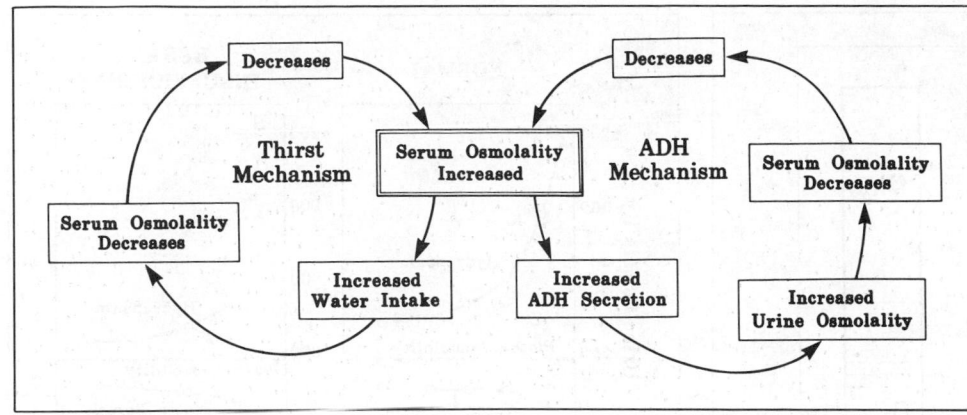

Figure 11.1–5. Sequence by which thirst mechanism and antidiuretic hormone output regulate serum osmolality. There is evidence that the thirst mechanism is mediated by a renin-angiotensin system, perhaps self-contained within the central nervous system.

take or, more precisely, the total quantity of water and solute requiring excretion. Regulation of absorption is so precise that the volume and solute concentrations of the body fluids remain constant. This is achieved in such elegant fashion that the solue concentration (osmolality) of body fluids varies little more than ±0.5 percent. To achieve this regulation, the kidney has the capacity to vary the rate of output of water and solute independently. Given an excess of body water, the kidney produces a urine that contains a much lower solute concentration than that in body fluids. Because urine formation begins as isotonic fluid, the kidney reabsorbs a hypertonic fluid in this situation. The result of this dual activity of excreting more water than solute and reabsorbing a hypertonic fluid rapidly corrects the hypotonicity (water excess) of the body fluids. Conversely, when a deficit of water is present in body fluids, the kidney produces a markedly hypertonic urine and reabsorbs a fluid that is hypotonic to body fluids, thus serving to correct or repair the water deficit. The mechanisms whereby the kidney achieves this remarkable regulation depend on integrated behavior of the intrarenal concentrating mechanism, the modulating influence of the antidiuretic hormone, and water intake. These interrelationships are examined below.

CONTROL OF OSMOLALITY

The osmolality of the plasma is controlled by two mechanisms: thirst, which leads to increased water intake, and antidiuretic hormone (ADH or vasopressin), which stimulates solute free water reabsorption.[2] Both mechanisms respond to changes in osmolality (Fig. 11.1–5; see also Chapter 10.1) as a primary stimulus and to changes in volume of body fluids as a secondary stimulus.[10,23] Conversely, increased water intake reduces plasma osmolality, thereby abolishing thirst and inhibiting ADH release. Inhibition of ADH leads to a prompt production of hypotonic urine, providing a mechanism for excreting the excess water that is ingested.[12,19] This regulatory mechanism is so sensitive that it responds to changes in plasma osmolality that are as small as 0.5 percent or less.

The kidneys are the effectors in this control system. Under ADH stimulus, they are capable of producing a urine with solute concentration up to four times as great as that found in plasma. This permits the kidney to excrete the necessary solutes resulting from daily intake plus metabolic activity with minimal loss of water. Under maximal stimulation by ADH the normal kidney can usually excrete an average daily solute load in a volume of less than 500 ml. The remarkable efficiency of this water-conserving process is achieved by the countercurrent multiplier and exchanger system in the renal medulla and has been the subject of several excellent reviews.[5,11] That renal disease can seriously impair the patient's ability to defend against physiologic changes in water, and solute is thus a logical corollary.

QUANTITATIVE ASPECTS OF WATER AND SOLUTE EXCRETION

The quantitative description of water conservation and excretion by the kidney is somewhat obscured by the terminology presently accepted as standard (Fig. 11.1–6). The concepts are simple, however, and derive from the clearance concepts discussed earlier.

Osmolal Clearance (C_{osm})

The kidneys under normal circumstances must excrete about 600 mosm per day. Solute excretion rate can be expressed in terms of milliosmoles per minute and may be calculated from the total solute concentration in the urine (U_{osm}) and the rate of urine excretion (V):

$$\text{Total Solute Excretion Rate} = U_{osm} \cdot V$$

For a given daily solute load the urine flow required to excrete solute at a constant rate will depend, of course, on the solute concentration. With high urinary solute concentrations (hypertonicity), small flows will be adequate, whereas at low concentrations high flows will be required. In dealing with this problem it is useful to determine the urine flow required to excrete this amount of solute if the urine were isotonic to plasma. This is $(U_{osm} \cdot V)/P_{osm}$, where the P_{osm} is the concentration of solute in plasma. This expression is also the definition of clearance:

$$\text{Osmolal Clearance} = C_{osm} = U_{osm} \cdot V/P_{osm}$$

When it is necessary to conserve water by excreting hypertonic urine, the observed urine flow rate (V) will be less than if isotonic urine were excreted (C_{osm}). Conversely, when it is necessary to lose water by excreting a hypotonic urine the observed flow (V) will exceed C_{osm} (Fig. 11.1–6). These differences between observed flows and the flows calculated for the formation of isotonic urine serve as important measures of the kidneys' ability to concentrate and dilute solute and provide a convenient means for quantitative definition of the rate at which the kidney is conserving or excreting solute free water.

Free Water Clearance (C_{H_2O})

Free water clearance is defined as the rate at which water is excreted without solute during the production of hypotonic urine (Fig. 11.1–6):

$$C_{H_2O} = V - C_{osm}$$

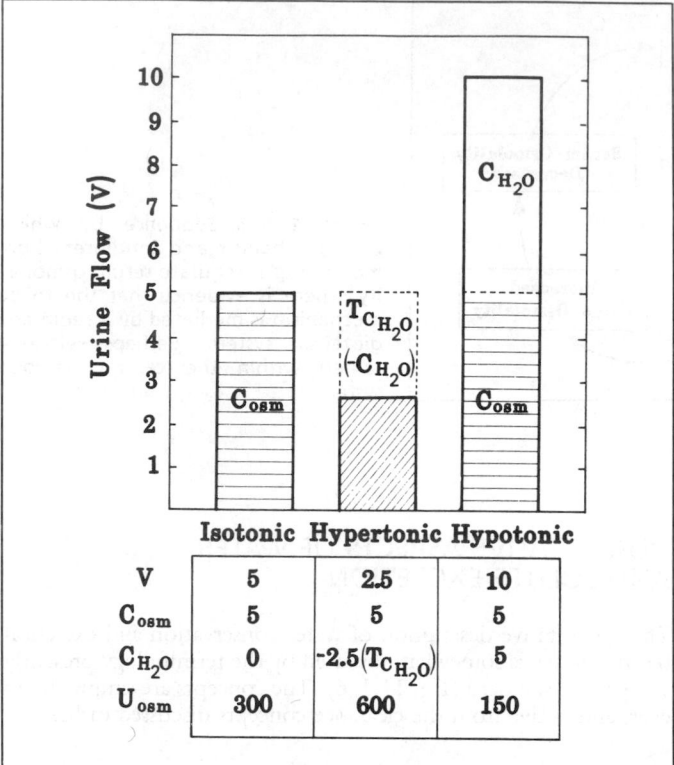

Figure 11.1–6. Renal conservation and excretion of water during formation of hypertonic and hypotonic urine. The relationships between urine osmolality, urine flow, osmolar clearance, and free water clearance are represented schematically. Note that when urine is hypertonic, free water clearance is negative and often designated TC_{H_2O}.

Negative Free Water Clearance (TC_{H_2O})

Negative free water clearance is the rate at which water is reabsorbed from tubular fluid during the production of hypertonic urine (Fig. 11.1–6):

$$TC_{H_2O} = C_{osm} - V$$

LIMITS OF WATER CONSERVATION AND EXCRETION IN NORMAL SUBJECTS AND IN SUBJECTS WITH SEVERE RENAL IMPAIRMENT

The rate at which solute-free water can be excreted (C_{H_2O}) may under certain circumstances reach 25 ml/min or more. The rate of reabsorption of solute-free water reaches its maximum rate at a much lower value, approximately 6 ml/min. These maximal rates are determined by two factors: (1) at lower rates of solute excretion the limits of water reabsorption and excretion are set by the maximal or minimal osmolar concentration that the kidney can develop, and (2) at higher rates of osmolal clearance (osmotic diuresis) they are set by the maximal rate at which water can move across the tubular membranes. These relationships are illustrated in Figure 11.1–7.

In chronic renal failure the concentrating function of the kidney fails steadily, with the urine tending toward the osmolality of plasma in much the same way as it does in the normal state under a progressively increasing osmotic diuresis. Most patients with advanced chronic renal failure produce a urine that is at or only slightly above isotonicity, even when sustained hydropenia results in maximal production of ADH. The impaired concentrating ability is probably a result of the virtual destruction of the countercurrent system, with obliteration of medullary hypertonicity

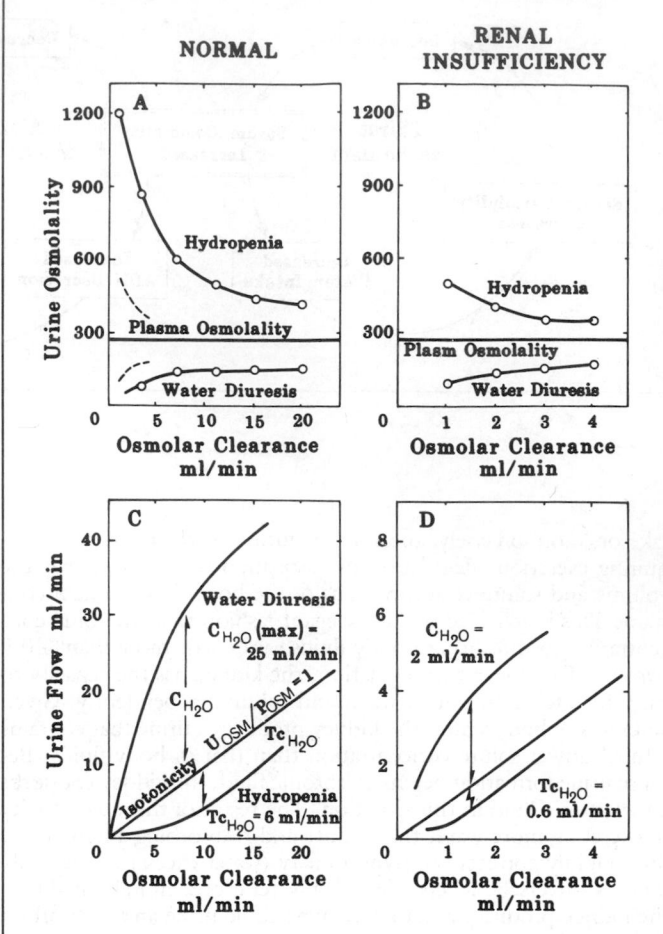

Figure 11.1–7. Relation between maximum range of renal concentrating and diluting function and urinary solute load in health and disease. The figures compare urine osmolality and solute-free water handling in the normal kidney and in the kidney in which renal function has been reduced to 10 percent of normal. **A.** Relation between urine osmolality and osmolar clearance in normal kidney during hydropenia and water diuresis. As solute clearance increases, urine osmolality approaches plasma osmolality in both cases. **C.** Rate at which solute-free water is excreted (C_{H_2O}) or reabsorbed (TC_{H_2O}) with increasing solute clearance during water diuresis and hydropenia. Water excretion and conservation are greatest at high solute loads despite the fact that the urine osmolality is less different from plasma than with low rates of osmolar clearance. **B, D.** Similar relationships in the presence of severe renal impairment (GFR 10 percent of normal), assuming that concentrating function of remaining nephrons is unimpaired. Note the different scale for osmolar clearance due to renal insufficiency. The marked restriction of maximum values for osmolality and solute-free water transfer set narrow limits on the diseased kidney with respect to conserving or excreting solute free water. The range of urinary osmolality in the presence of severe renal disease, as shown on the expanded scale in **B,** is also drawn in on **A** as the interrupted line.

plus mild impairment in sodium transport in the distal nephron. The severity of this concentrating impairment is closely related to the severity of the renal impairment, and in advanced uremia (GFR < 10 ml/min) the urine is frequently persistently hypotonic, despite maximal levels of circulating antidiuretic hormone.[23]

This impairment makes the patient with end-stage renal disease likely to develop serious water deficits and water intoxication. Because severe reduction in GFR in advanced failure limits the daily maximal water excretion (C_{H_2O}) to the range of 2 to 2.5 L and because the severe osmotic diuresis imposed by the increased urea

load per nephron requiring excretion by a reduced number of nephrons sets the minimal urinary volume at about 2 L per day, the patient must regulate fluid intake within a relatively narrow margin to avoid serious water deficit on the one hand and dilutional hyponatremia on the other.

SPECIFIC DISORDERS ASSOCIATED WITH IMPAIRED CONCENTRATING MECHANISM

In addition to the severe disruption of the concentrating process in advanced renal failure, there are several conditions that cause specific disturbances in the concentrating mechanism and are likely to result in excessive water loss at a relatively early stage in the loss of renal function. These conditions, including hypokalemia, hypercalcemia, sickle cell disease, and, in rare instances, pyelonephritis, result in production of a markedly hypotonic urine and profound polyuria.

Normally much more water is reabsorbed in concentrating distal tubular fluid to isotonicity than is conserved during concentration of isotonic distal fluid by the collecting duct. For example, a solute output of 600 mOsm per day would require only 2 L of urine if excreted as an isotonic solution, but a fixed solute concentration of 50 mOsm/L would require an output of 12 L per day. By first reducing this fluid to isotonicity, 10 L of water are conserved. Further concentration of distal tubule fluid to a value twice the solute concentration of plasma would save only an additional liter of water. Hence the diseased kidney that can only produce a markedly hypotonic urine may have an obligatory solute-free water loss of several liters per day. This condition is usually termed nephrogenic diabetes insipidus, regardless of the underlying renal disease responsible for disruption of the concentrating mechanism. These conditions are uncommon but occur rarely in hypercalcemia and potassium depletion as well as amyloidosis, Sjögren syndrome, lithium intoxication, and with the use of demeclocycline, amphotericin, and some other drugs.[19,23] As with other causes of diabetes insipidus, the total quantity of daily water loss varies with solute intake (Fig. 11.1–7C and D) so that diets with a high solute load aggravate this defect, whereas low-solute diets diminish it.

REGULATION OF ELECTROLYTE EXCRETION AND HYDROGEN ION BALANCE

Each day the normal kidneys filter approximately 25,000 mEq of sodium, 18,000 mEq of chloride, and 4500 mEq of bicarbonate in a volume of roughly 180 L. About 1 percent of the water and less than 1 percent of the electrolytes filtered are excreted, the remainder being absorbed by the renal tubules. The daily volume of glomerular filtrate is about 12 times as large as the extracellular fluid volume. Thus, the kidney filters and reabsorbs a volume of fluid equal to the extracellular fluid volume every 2 hours. By varying the composition of the reabsorbed fluids, the kidney effectively and rapidly regulates the electrolyte composition of the interstitial fluid. This control is impaired in severe renal disease. For instance, a kidney retaining only 10 percent of normal functional capacity would filter only 18 L per day and reabsorb no more than 16. Thus, nearly 24 hours would be required for one cycling of the interstitial fluid and perhaps as long as 2 or 3 days before a new steady state could be established. The principal mechanisms for the renal regulation of the composition of the extracellular fluid are the reabsorption of sodium, chloride, and bicarbonate in varying proportions and, in addition, the secretion of hydrogen ion and potassium.[4,17] These mechanisms are schematically presented in Figure 11.1–8.

SODIUM AND CHLORIDE

The principal urinary solutes are sodium, chloride, and urea. The daily output of sodium chloride varies normally over a wide range depending on intake but is usually about 140 mEq (8 g). Balance studies indicate that the normal kidney responds to variation in sodium intake ranging from less than 1 to more than 20 g in a manner that permits the total exchangeable sodium within the body to vary no more than 150 to 175 mEq despite these wide fluctuations in intake.[17] The normal adult kidney is capable of producing a sodium-free (<1 mEq/L) urine over periods of months without any deleterious effects on the individual so long as no ex-

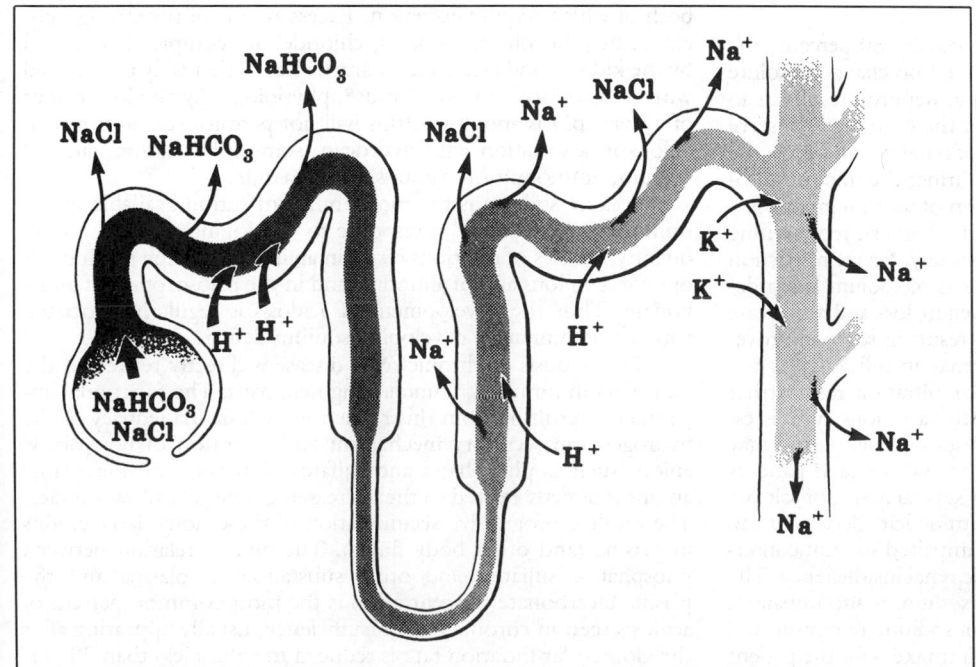

Figure 11.1–8. Mechanisms of renal sodium reabsorption. Sodium is reabsorbed in proximal segment of nephron as sodium chloride and as sodium bicarbonate in exchange for hydrogen ion. In the more distal segments of the nephron, both potassium and hydrogen ions are secreted into the urine as counter ions to maintain electroneutrality as sodium is reabsorbed. These transport processes together permit the normal kidney to excrete urine that may be virtually sodium free in response to a sustained stimulus to conserve sodium.

trarenal sodium losses occur. The mechanisms whereby the kidney achieves this regulation include (1) variation of filtered Na load by changes in GFR, (2) variation in renal transport of sodium by alterations in the renin-aldosterone system and (3) alterations in atrial natriuretic hormone.[2,8,18,29,32]

Atrial natriuretic factor is the most recent natriuretic hormone candidate. It is a small peptide isolated from atrial granulocytes and detected in the blood of humans and experimental animals with different conditions associated with volume expansion.[2] In experimental animals, it produces a fourfold to fivefold increase in sodium excretion and a prompt and sustained increase in glomerular filtration without an increase in renal blood flow. The natriuresis, however, cannot be attributed entirely to changes in glomerular filtration, and certain experiments suggest a direct effect on sodium reabsorption by distal nephron segments. Besides changing renal function, the factor has a vasorelaxant effect on preconstricted vessels in nonrenal vascular beds and on nonvascular smooth muscle.[2] The aorta, renal artery, and certain veins seem more sensitive to this vasodilatory effect than coronary or hindlimb vessels. Although these properties suggest that atrial natriuretic factor may exert an important regulatory influence on the control of body fluid volumes and blood pressure, its physiologic importance in normal humans and in patients with different diseases has not been established.

Aldosterone increases the renal reabsorption of sodium and chloride, with consequent expansion of the extracellular fluid volume; conversely, in the absence of aldosterone, extracellular fluid volume decreases as a result of renal loss of sodium and chloride. Aldosterone also increases reabsorption of sodium chloride and potassium secretion into distal tubular fluid.

The solute diuresis produced by poorly reabsorbed substances, such as mannitol and a number of anions, or by an excess of glucose in untreated diabetes mellitus results in increased excretion of sodium chloride because of reduction in proximal tubular sodium reabsorption and a resulting increase in distal delivery. This natriuresis of an osmotic diuresis persists even after the combination of increased sodium excretion and administration of large quantities of fluid has depressed the serum sodium concentration below the normal range. Under conditions of extreme osmotic diuresis, 10 to 15 percent of the filtered load of sodium and chloride may appear in the urine.

SODIUM AND CHLORIDE EXCRETION IN CHRONIC RENAL DISEASE[8,17]

When the functioning nephrons are reduced by 50 percent, the solute load per nephron is doubled (assuming no change in solute intake). This increase in solute excretion per nephron results in an osmotic diuresis that impairs the ability of the kidney to conserve sodium adequately. In advanced degrees of renal insufficiency, the kidney can no longer excrete sodium-free urine; the minimum sodium concentration in urine after restriction of sodium intake may be no lower than 10 mEq/L (and frequently higher), representing an obligatory loss of more than 25 mEq per day. Severe restriction of dietary salt will result in a progressive loss of sodium and a decrease in extracellular fluid. This causes weight loss and a decrease in the glomerular filtration rate that may result in some improvement of sodium conservation. When renal insufficiency is advanced, however, this drop in glomerular filtration rate further aggravates uremic symptoms. Consequently, a vicious cycle is established that can produce a pronounced sodium deficit and may be life-threatening.[17] In general, the dietary salt of such patients should not be restricted, and an intake of several grams of salt per day is prescribed to avoid creating a sodium deficit. Because it can lead to further deterioration of function, impaired sodium conservation is a very important aspect of chronic renal insufficiency. The diseased kidney's ability to excrete excess sodium is also impaired, and administration of salt may result in sodium retention and edema. The simplest means of assessing salt intake is for the patient to keep a daily weight record because acute changes in weight reflect changes in retention of salt and water. If serum bicarbonate is normal (see p. 725), salt intake should be regulated to maintain body weight with none or only a trace of edema.[17]

Renal sodium-wasting may be further intensified by failure of the mechanism responsible for exchanging hydrogen for sodium within the tubular lumen. This is more prominent in renal diseases characterized by disproportionate tubular damage and is manifested clinically as a hyperchloremic acidosis. The tubular impairment may produce cases of renal insufficiency that are dominated by salt-wasting. The clinical characteristics are extreme sensitivity to dietary salt deprivation, leading rapidly to weakness, hypotension, and clinical shock, with marked deterioration of renal function that may terminate in death. In such cases, the kidney may be unable to reduce the urinary sodium concentration below 40 or 50 mEq/L. Salt-wasting of this degree is unusual and is seen most often in pyelonephritis, medullary cystic disease, and other types of cystic renal diseases. Relatively large quantities of sodium chloride are required to restore the sodium deficit and maintain sodium balance.

Patients with these disorders have been shown to have persistently elevated secretion rates of aldosterone while on high salt intake. This failure of adequate tubular reabsorption of sodium in spite of excess aldosterone points to a predominantly tubular lesion. Although the difficulty may be aggravated by the osmotic diuresis of renal insufficiency or an increased rate of glomerular filtration per nephron, a specific tubular impairment (e.g., tubular atrophy) must also be present because the defect cannot be produced by solute-loading patients with a comparable degree of renal insufficiency but without such marked salt-wasting tendencies.

HYDROGEN ION REGULATION[1]

The net quantity of hydrogen ions excreted by the kidney (150 to 300 mEq per day) is very small compared to that excreted by the lungs as CO_2 (15,000 mEq per day). Hence, disturbances in pulmonary function may result in acidosis within minutes, whereas several days of complete anuria are required for acidosis to develop. The principal renal mechanism for maintaining body pH is the regulation of bicarbonate reabsorption and, hence, control of the ratio of carbonic acid to bicarbonate (see Chapter 10.3).[1,25,26] A second renal mechanism for regulating body pH is excretion of nonvolatile anions. The addition of an acid to the extracellular fluid provides excesses of hydrogen ion and its associated anion, both of which require excretion. Excess anions of the strong mineral acids (phosphates, sulfates, chloride) are completely excreted by the kidney, and electroneutrality demands that they be excreted with an associated cation. Because, physiologically the lower limit of urinary pH is about 4.5, this will not permit excretion of such anions in association with hydrogen; some other cation, such as sodium, ammonium, or potassium, is required.

Because sodium is the most abundant cation available in the urine, it is the first lost in response to developing acidosis. Subsequently, a series of reactions result in an increase in the production of hydrogen ions and of ammonia and in the reabsorption of bicarbonate. Thus the development of acidosis is regularly associated with a concomitantly developing sodium deficit.

The acidosis of chronic renal disease is directly related to the reduction in number of functioning nephrons. The functional impairments resulting from this reduction include inadequacy of the hydrogen ion secretory mechanism and retention of nonvolatile anions such as phosphates and sulfates. Retention of nonvolatile anions is directly related to the decreased glomerular filtration rate. The result is progressive accumulation of these nonvolatile anions in plasma (and other body fluids). The inverse relation between phosphates, sulfates, and other substances in plasma and the plasma bicarbonate concentration is the most common pattern of acidosis seen in chronic renal insufficiency, usually appearing after the glomerular filtration rate is reduced to values less than 20 per-

cent of normal. Because high-protein foods contain phospholipids, phosphoproteins, and sulfur-containing amino acids, the metabolic acidosis is aggravated by increased protein intake. Reduction in protein intake and substitution of carbohydrate as a food source improves this type of acidosis.

Acidosis due to defective hydrogen ion excretion, recognized clinically as hyperchloremic acidosis, is seen less commonly as a pure form of acidosis in chronic renal disease. The prime example is renal tubular acidosis (Chapter 11.6), which may be seen in a variety of renal disorders associated with renal insufficiency. Clinically, acidosis is usually compensated but may be symptomatic, with plasma chloride concentration exceeding 120 to 125 mEq/L. Plasma bicarbonate concentration is correspondingly low and plasma phosphate is usually normal. Ammonium production and titratable acidity are reduced.

FACTORS REGULATING BICARBONATE REABSORPTION

When presented with comparable loads of excess nonvolatile anions or acid loads, the major difference between the response of the normal kidney and the severely impaired kidney is in the rate at which these substances are excreted and the pH disturbance is repaired. The initial systemic effect is the same in both situations; an appropriate shift in the state of the buffer pairs minimizes the change in pH. One important result is the lowering of plasma bicarbonate. Of the three renal transport processes operating to maintain the concentration of bicarbonate of body fluids within normal limits or to return it to normal levels following an acid load, renal reabsorption of filtered bicarbonate is quantitatively much more important than urinary excretion of titratable acid or ammonia production. The rate at which plasma bicarbonate returns to normal is determined by the rate at which the kidney reabsorbs a tubular fluid with higher bicarbonate concentration than plasma. This is possible because total bicarbonate reabsorption equals hydrogen ion secretion. Thus bicarbonate concentration can be raised because it equals bicarbonate reabsorption plus titratable acid plus ammonia production divided by volume of fluid reabsorbed per unit time. This may be expressed quantitatively:

$$[HCO_3]T.R. = \frac{(HCO_3 \text{ filtered} - HCO_3 \text{ excreted} + \text{titr. acid} + NH_4) \text{ mEq/min}}{\text{Volume of tubular fluid reabsorbed (L/min)}}$$

This gives the bicarbonate concentration in milliequivalents per liter that would be found in extracellular fluid when the kidney has completely recycled the extracellular fluid. The normal kidney is capable of filtering and reabsorbing a volume of fluid equal to extracellular fluid volume in approximately 2 hours. As the glomerular filtration rate falls, however, the time required for completion of this operation varies in a reciprocal manner. Thus, the kidney with a glomerular filtration rate less than 10 percent of normal would require 20 hours. The increased time required for repair of a deficit in plasma bicarbonate concentration by the severely impaired kidney tends to make the effect of ingestion of dietary nonvolatile anions cumulative, producing progressive acidosis and other manifestations of the uremic syndrome. The secondary decrease in plasma bicarbonate concentration results in a corresponding decrease in the amount of filtered bicarbonate that is available for reabsorption. Although the formation of titratable acid and the production of ammonia are stimulated, they do not offset the net effect of the diminution in the filtered load of bicarbonate. As shown in Table 11.1–2, these quantities represent only 37 percent of maximum hydrogen ion secretion (total bicarbonate reabsorption) in chronic renal failure. Administration of bicarbonate is useful in combating progressive acidosis in patients with normal kidney function, because once the kidney is presented with a normal

bicarbonate concentration in the glomerular filtrate it has little difficulty in maintaining it at this level. For patients with chronic renal failure, sodium bicarbonate administration should be coupled with dietary protein restriction to reduce the intake of nonvolatile anions.

This bicarbonate deficit seen in the acidosis of chronic renal disease may be manifested as hyperchloremic acidosis even after excess loads of nonvolatile anions such as sulfate and phosphate have been excreted.[12] The reduced filtered load of bicarbonate results in a proportionately greater concentration of chloride than bicarbonate in the proximal tubular fluid than that which exists normally. The two forces that operate to maintain electroneutrality in response to active sodium reabsorption in the proximal convoluted tubule are chloride reabsorption and hydrogen ion secretion (exchange of $H+$ for $Na+$). The principal proton acceptor within the tubular lumen is bicarbonate, and its lowered concentration in acidosis restricts the quantity of hydrogen ion added to tubular fluid. As a result, a greater quantity of chloride accompanies the reabsorbed sodium. The net effect of this disparity is an increased concentration of chloride in the fluid reabsorbed by the proximal nephron. It is likely that the increased sodium loss—a regular feature of the acidosis of chronic renal disease—stimulates aldosterone secretion, resulting in increased sodium chloride reabsorption and further accentuation of the hyperchloremia. The administration of bicarbonate elevates plasma bicarbonate concentration and corrects the acidosis. Once this is accomplished, dietary restriction of protein may prevent recurrence of metabolic acidosis in chronic renal disease. In specific disorders of hydrogen ion transport such as renal tubular acidosis, maintenance therapy with some form of alkalinization therapy is necessary to prevent recurrence of acidosis (Chapter 11.6).

POTASSIUM

In the healthy individual, the average daily urinary excretion of potassium varies between 50 and 100 mEq/day, depending on dietary intake. Potassium excretion depends almost entirely on secretion by distal tubular cells and under appropriate circumstances may be twice the rate at which potassium is filtered at the glomerulus.[4]

The severely impaired kidney usually has more difficulty with potassium excretion than with sodium conservation. The potassium concentration in the urine becomes nearly fixed because of the limitations imposed by the tubular damage. Thus, potassium secretion must continue at a nearly maximal rate in order to excrete the daily intake of potassium. Because of the limited capacity of the diseased kidney, patients with severe chronic renal insufficiency are prone to the development of hyperkalemia or hypokalemia. An excess of dietary potassium or the Type IV renal tubular acidosis often associated with moderate chronic renal failure and caused by decreased renal renin production and associated hypoaldosteronism (Chapter 11.6) lead to hyperkalemia. On the other hand, chronic dietary potassium restriction coupled with continued renal potassium losses can lead to significant potassium deficits.[17] In this latter case, the stimulus for distal nephron sodium retention caused by metabolic acidosis-induced sodium losses (plus dietary salt restriction) causes persistent potassium secretion and hence excess potassium excretion. The potassium stores of chronic renal failure patients, therefore, are much more dependent on dietary potassium compared to normal subjects.

CLINICAL EVALUATION OF RENAL FUNCTION

Many diseases of the kidney are completely asymptomatic until advanced renal damage occurs; they may be detected in their early phases only by an adequate examination of the urine. A complete urinalysis on a freshly voided urine that demonstrates no abnor-

malities and a serum creatinine that is in the normal range represent the minimal requisite data to establish normal renal function. If one or the other is abnormal, it is necessary to establish a specific diagnosis of the renal disease present and to obtain a quantitative assessment of renal function. Only after a specific diagnosis is established can effective management be planned and a reasonably accurate prognosis offered. Although some diffuse diseases of the kidney are characterized by exacerbations and remissions without much loss of renal function, the majority of diffuse diseases of the kidney that present in the adult are associated with progressive loss of renal function. The rate of loss varies greatly for different diseases of the kidney, and the same disease may exhibit wide variations in rate of progression in different individuals. In a given individual, the rate of loss of renal function is usually constant or nearly so.[15,16] When this rate is established for a given individual, it is possible to predict with reasonable certainty when renal function will reach the point when support by dialysis, transplantation, or both become essential. Characterization of the rate of loss of renal function also permits anticipation of the appearance of clinical manifestations of uremia. In Table 11.1–2, the functions of the normal kidney and the severely diseased kidney are contrasted. These represent extremes, but it is feasible to assess intermediate levels of impairment and functional loss by appropriate clinical testing. The remainder of this chapter deals with those tests that are essential for adequate clinical evaluation of renal function.

EXAMINATION OF URINE

Examination of the urine provides the data of most value in establishing the presence or absence of renal disease. It should include measurement of specific gravity and pH, testing for the presence of protein, and careful examination of the urine sediment.[2,14] Examination of freshly voided, concentrated urine provides more useful information than does study of a dilute specimen. Formed elements, particularly red blood cells and casts, lyse quickly in dilute urine; proteinuria may escape detection, and no information is provided about the concentrating ability of the kidney. It is most desirable to obtain the first specimen voided in the morning, which should be examined promptly. No reliance should be placed on microscopic study of the urine sediment when more than 2 hours have elapsed between collection and examination. If the specific gravity of the urine is below 1.010, microscopic examination should be conducted immediately following collection.

SPECIFIC GRAVITY

Specific gravity in excess of 1.025 in otherwise normal urine usually signifies normal or adequate renal function. Specific gravity of urine is linearly related to its osmolality, but because it measures urine directly relative to the density of water, it may exhibit wide fluctuations at any given urine osmolality depending on the nature of the major solutes in the urine. For example, glucose in the urine produces a much higher specific gravity than an equiosmolar quantity of urea. Accurate assessment of renal concentrating ability can only be provided by direct measurement of urine osmolality. The range of maximal solute concentration that the normal human kidney can achieve varies between 750 and about 1100 mOsm/kg H_2O, depending on dietary intake of solutes and water and ADH status. The urinary specific gravity provides a clinically useful estimate of this function when the urine does not contain abnormal quantities of such high-density substances as glucose, phosphates, or radiocontrast dyes.

Casual measurement of the specific gravity in a randomly voided urine is of little value unless the fluid intake has been controlled. Overnight fluid restriction results in urinary solute concentration that is about three quarters of the maximum concentration achieved following 24 hours of fluid deprivation. Overnight water deprivation that results in the production of urine that is persistently hypotonic (less than a specific gravity of 1.010) provides

strong evidence for an impairment of the concentrating mechanism, as is seen with diabetes insipidus, sickle cell anemia, nephrogenic diabetes insipidus, and other rare disorders such as renal amyloidosis, lithium intoxication, and related disturbances.

URINARY pH

Measurement of pH on random urine samples is of little clinical importance because pH varies with time of day and with dietary intake. It may, however, yield valuable information in specific circumstances (as for example, renal tubular acidosis), because in the presence of systemic acidosis, a urine pH above 6.0 in the absence of urinary tract infection signifies impairment of the renal acidification mechanism. Urine infected with organisms capable of splitting urea to ammonium may give false high pH values, because the pH of ammonium is 9.2.

URINARY PROTEIN

The quantity of protein in normal urine is usually less than 50 mg per 24-hour period, representing an average concentration of less than 5 mg/dl. This concentration is too low to be detected by the usual clinical laboratory methods. The heat and acetic method, as well as the sulfosalicylic method, however, will regularly detect concentrations above 5 to 10 mg/dl. Although mild degrees of proteinuria may on occasion be observed in the absence of renal disease, its detection by these methods should always be taken as presumptive evidence of renal disease.[2] The urine used in testing must have a specific gravity greater than 1.010 or cases of mild proteinuria will be overlooked. It is important to test for Bence Jones proteinuria in all urine that yields a positive screening test for protein.[13]

Qualitative precipitation reactions (heat and acetic acid, and sulfosalicylic acid methods) are useful for screening purposes. They are not satisfactory as a means of following cases of proven renal disease, however, because the total quantity of protein excreted per 24 hours is a product of protein concentration in the urine and urine volume. Hence, wide variations in volume may produce remarkable changes in protein concentration in the presence of a constant daily protein excretion.

MICROSCOPIC EXAMINATION OF URINARY SEDIMENT

The importance of obtaining fresh urine for appropriate examination of the urinary sediment has already been stressed. The significant abnormal components of urine sediment are red cells, leukocytes, epithelial cells, and casts.[19]

Red blood cells may be seen in extremely small numbers in normal urine, particularly following strenuous exercise. Centrifuged urine from healthy persons rarely shows more than two or three erythrocytes on the usual microscopic slide preparation. Erythrocytes are present in considerable numbers, however, in almost all types of diffuse renal disease. A characteristic appearance of those associated with glomerular disease is their relatively small size and greater refractility when compared to red cells shed from the lower urinary tract. Although it may be possible to suspect the presence of renal disease from the appearance of the red cells alone, red cell casts are a specific index of the presence of glomerular disease. When glomerular disease is suspected as the cause of hematuria, repeated examination of early-morning, concentrated urine specimens may be necessary to confirm the diagnosis by demonstrating red cell casts.

There are several types of casts found regularly in renal diseases. With proper identification casts are of considerable diagnostic aid (Table 11.1–3).

TABLE 11.1–3. FORMED ELEMENTS FOUND IN URINE IN VARIOUS RENAL DISEASES

	Normal	Glomerulo-nephritides	Pyelonephritis	Amyloid	Arteriolo-sclerosis	K-W
Formed elements						
RBC	Rare	+	+	±	+	±
WBC	Rare	+	+	±	+	±
Epith. cells	Rare	+	+	±	+	+
Casts						
Hyaline	Rare	+	+	+	+	+
Granular	0	+	+	+	+	+
Cellular	0	+	+	0	0	Rare
WBC	0	+	+	0	0	0
Epith. cells	0	+	Rare	0	0	+
RBC	0	+	0	0	0	0
Waxy	0	+	Rare	0	0	+
Fatty	0	+	0	0	0	+

+ = present; 0 = absent; K-W = Kimmelstiel-Wilson syndrome.

QUANTITATIVE ASSESSMENT OF RENAL INSUFFICIENCY

Two questions can be asked when quantifying the degree of renal insufficiency. First, what is the value of the glomerular filtration rate as an index of the remaining number of nephrons? A precise answer to this question using standard tests is difficult to obtain. The second question, how rapidly is renal insufficiency progressing, is answerable using standard laboratory tests.[15]

The most commonly used quantitative measures of renal function are the determinations of plasma constituents that reflect changes in clearances or direct measurement of the endogenous creatinine clearance. The most extensively used plasma constituent measurements are the blood urea nitrogen (BUN) and serum creatinine concentrations. These provide screening measures to detect grossly impaired renal function, that is, a decrease in the glomerular filtration rate. The serum creatinine concentration provides a more precise measure of the level of glomerular function than the BUN. The reasons for the uncertainty associated with interpreting the BUN have been reviewed (Fig. 11.1–3). There are also inherent difficulties in interpreting the significance of small changes in serum creatinine values. Figure 11.1–9 indicates that in the average clinical chemistry laboratory, the 95 percent confidence limits for replicate measurement of creatinine values in the normal range are greater than ± 0.35 ml/dl, thus spanning a range of 0.7 mg/dl. As is evident from Figure 11.1–9, it is difficult to be certain that a change of less than 0.4 mg/dl is significant. Because this represents a 40 percent change in GFR at a normal creatinine value of 1.0 mg/dl, this is not a sensitive means of detecting small changes in renal function and is a poor estimate of the glomerular filtration rate. Though considerably greater sensitivity and precision are obtainable with currently available analytic procedures for creatinine, the ranges quoted here reflect the usual performances in clinical chemistry laboratories.

An equally important variable that must be considered in interpreting serum creatinine values is the marked variation that occurs with age (Table 11.1–4). Creatinine production, and hence plasma creatinine values, increase during the first two decades of life.[22] During and after the fifth decade, creatinine production declines as muscle mass decreases, but there is a concomitant decline in glomerular filtration rate that offsets this effect, and the serum creatinine value changes little in healthy elderly adults.

Fortunately, there is a more reliable means of identifying trends in directional changes in renal function in the individual patient with progressive renal insufficiency.[15,16] A plot of the reciprocal of the serum creatinine versus time (Fig. 11.1–10) identifies the direction of change in renal function and allows reasonable projection of the future appearance of renal failure. When all available serum creatinine values are used to construct this plot, the precision and utility of serum creatinine improve greatly.

This relationship means that renal function is being lost at a constant rate, and that creatinine clearance and the glomerular

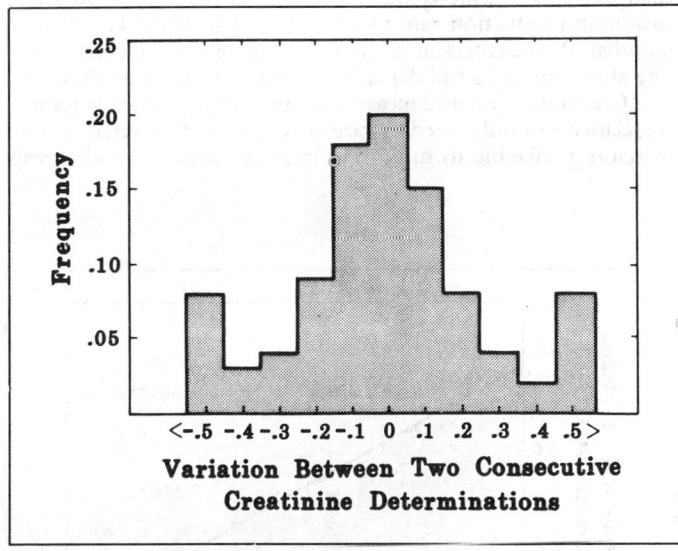

Figure 11.1–9. Distribution frequency of the difference between consecutive measurements of creatinine in 115 patients following renal transplantation (data represent 2500 creatinine measurements). The values included in the small peaks at the extremes are clearly significant differences and, thus, identify real changes in renal function. The larger proportion of differences appear to be normally distributed about a difference of zero with a standard deviation of 0.15 mg/dl. Considering two standard deviations (the 95 percent confidence limits), these data indicate that it is difficult to attach significance to changes in serum creatinine as great as ±0.3 mg/dl. At the normal creatinine value in the plasma of 1 mg/dl, this means that a ±30 percent change in renal function cannot be detected reliably. A single value of serum creatinine is therefore not a particularly sensitive means of detecting small changes in renal function.

TABLE 11.1–4. VARIATIONS AND RANGES IN PLASMA CREATININE AS FUNCTION OF AGE[22]

Age	Height (cm)	True Plasma Creatinine			
		Mean (mg/dl)	Range ± 2 SD (mg/dl)	Mean (μmol/L)	Range ± 2 SD (μmol/L)
Cord blood		0.75	0.51–0.99	66.3	45.1–87.5
0–2 wk	50	0.50	0.34–0.66	44.2	30.0–58.3
26 wk–1 yr	70	0.32	0.18–0.46	28.3	15.9–40.7
4 yr	101	0.37	0.25–0.49	32.7	22.1–43.3
8 yr	126	0.48	0.31–0.65	42.4	27.4–57.4
12 yr	147	0.59	0.41–0.78	52.2	36.2–69.0
Adult male	174	0.97	0.72–1.22	85.7	63.6–107.9
Adult female	163	0.77	0.53–1.01	68.1	46.8–89.3

filtration rate are decreasing linearly.[15,16] There are two potential difficulties in using this approach: In advanced renal insufficiency, renal creatinine secretion might be affected independently of changes in glomerular function. Secondly, a decrease in dietary meat can reduce creatinine production, which can decrease serum creatinine, even though creatinine clearance is unchanged. Fortunately, these do not create serious problems if steady-state considerations are always used when interpreting changes in the reciprocal serum creatinine relationship. In the steady state, creatinine secretion and production are constant, so changes in serum creatinine (or its reciprocal) reflect changes in renal function. The half-time to achieve a new steady state of creatinine excretion following a change in the amount of dietary meat is 41 days.[15] This is the result of the fact that a constant, 1.7 percent of the total creatinine pool is converted to creatinine each day. Thus, if dietary protein changes markedly, more than 90 percent of the new, steady-state creatinine production rate will be reached in three half-lives (4 months). Any changes in serum creatinine or its reciprocal occurring after 4 months will depend on changes in renal function.

Creatinine clearance measurements yield reproducible results, are relatively uninfluenced by variations in urine flow rates, and are therefore preferable to measuring inulin clearance. Simultaneous measurements of inulin and endogenous creatinine clearances yield values that agree reasonably well and, for an individual subject, replicate measurements show remarkable constancy. Consecutive measurements of the 24-hour creatinine clearance show a coefficient of variation of about 7 percent. In advanced renal impairment, as the plasma creatinine concentration rises, the fraction secreted by the tubules increases so that creatinine clearance exceeds the glomerular filtration rate. Consequently, creatinine clearance is an inaccurate estimate of the glomerular filtration rate.[15] In spite of this fact, it remains a useful technique for following renal function quantitatively if urine collections are accurately timed and complete.

A reasonably accurate measure of the glomerular filtration rate is essential for adjustment of dosage of potentially toxic drugs that are excreted by the kidney. Because such measurements are time consuming, creatinine clearance can be estimated from serum creatinine using a nomogram such as that developed by Siersbaek–Nielsen and others[6,9,24] or standardized formulas based on the age, weight, and sex of the patient. These methods have limitations, and whenever possible, serum or plasma concentrations of the drugs should be followed to avoid toxicity. The basis for estimating the creatinine clearance in this fashion and the potential errors associated with such estimates are illustrated in Fig. 11.1–11. The uncertainty is so great when the creatinine is nearly normal that use of a creatinine clearance estimated by this method is of little value in adjusting drug dosage and should be avoided. Conversely, when serum creatinine value exceeds 8 to 10 mg/dl, small changes in creatinine clearance may be associated with large changes in plasma concentrations of substances excreted largely by glomerular filtration; hence, estimated creatinine clearance should not be used as the final determinant of drug dosage adjustment in renal failure. In such circumstances, direct monitoring of plasma drug concentrations is to be preferred. If this is not possible, careful measurement of creatinine clearance is essential.

OTHER USEFUL DIAGNOSTIC TESTS

The tests described in the preceding section are designed to provide quantitative or semiquantitative data on adequacy of renal function. There also are diagnostic tests designed to establish the normality of genitourinary system structure. These include sonography and a number of radiographic procedures, both with and without the use of radiocontrast media.

Sonography uses ultrasound to identify interfaces or abrupt structural changes within the body, thereby defining or delineating the structures in a given two-dimensional cross-sectional plane of the body. It is of value in defining kidney size and identifying deformities such as cysts or masses. It is very helpful in guiding procedures such as cyst aspirations or renal biopsies. Its chief virtue is that it is noninvasive and without risk. Interpretation of patterns

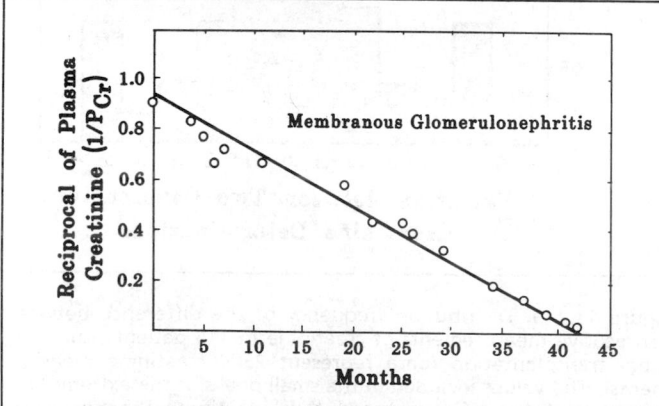

Figure 11.1–10. Monitoring change in renal function with reciprocal of serum creatinine. The graph of reciprocal of creatinine concentration (1/Cr) versus time in an individual with glomerulonephritis and vasculitis depicts a linear decrease with time. The slope is directly proportional to the rate of progression of disease (or rate of loss of renal function). This graphic representation of serial creatinine data permits more accurate assessment of the change in renal function than does measurement of a single value for creatinine of a small number of such measurements.[15,16]

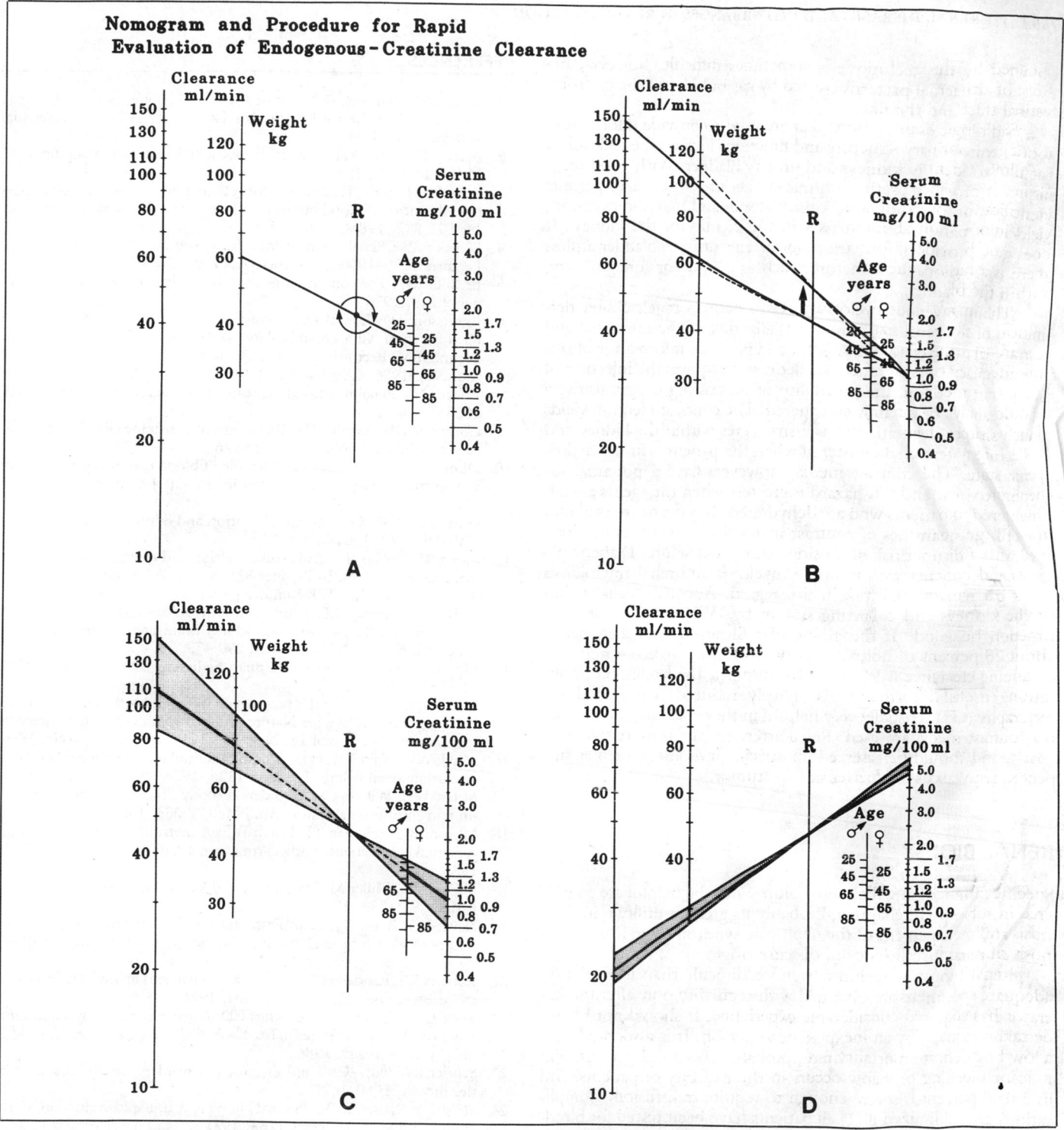

Figure 11.1–11. Utility and limitations of Siersbaek–Nielsen nomogram for estimation of creatinine clearance from serum creatinine. **A.** First, identify the axis along the reference line (R) around which the relation between serum creatinine and creatinine clearance rotates; this is a function of the age and weight of the patient. This nomogram is based on the assumption that an increase in weight represents mainly an increase in lean body mass. **B.** This illustrates the substantial error introduced into the estimate when a weight increase reflects obesity rather than increased lean body mass. A 45-year-old, 60-kg male has an estimated creatinine clearance of approximately 82 ml/min if serum creatinine is 1 mg/dl, but an increase in obesity to 120 kg would yield a creatinine clearance of 160 ml/min with the same plasma creatinine value, according to this nomogram. Thus obesity can introduce an error of nearly 100 percent in this estimate of the creatinine clearance. Even without this uncertainty the confidence limits for the estimate of creatinine clearance from the normal creatinine value spans a range nearly as large. **C.** The 95 percent confidence interval for the estimate of creatinine clearance (8 to 155 ml/min) is shown for an adult with normal renal function. The mean and standard deviation for plasma creatinine are taken from Table 11.1–4. In normals, estimation of creatinine clearance on this basis from the measured value for plasma creatinine has such a large uncertainty that it is virtually valueless for any type of quantitative work such as dosage estimation for drugs excreted primarily by glomerular filtration. Fortunately this is not true in the presence of advanced renal impairment, as shown in **D.** Creatinine clearance of such patients estimated from the nomogram yield values that differ little from the standard deviation for the normal range of serum creatinine. As illustrated, a serum creatinine of 5 mg/dl has a 95 percent confidence interval that extends from 19 to 21 ml/min (neglecting uncertainty due to obesity). Thus the nomogram yields a much more accurate estimate in the presence of moderate to moderately severe impairment. It probably should not be relied upon when the creatinine clearance falls below 15 ml/min (or when the serum creatinine exceeds 5 mg/dl).

obtained by this technique is sometimes difficult, however, because of artifactual patterns created by gas bubbles in the gastrointestinal tract and the like.

Radiologic examinations that are used to provide information about genitourinary structure and functions include the abdominal flat film to identify kidneys and urinary bladder. With good technique, it provides useful information about kidney size, permits identification of radiopaque kidney stones and may, on occasion, yield information about masses in the vicinity of the kidney. It does not provide information about the urinary bladder unless there is a radiopaque structure, such as a stone or foreign body, within the bladder.

The intravenous pyelogram (IVP) permits much clearer definition of the renal size, allows visualization of the intrarenal and extrarenal urine collecting system, and provides information about the adequacy of renal function. Because it requires the injection of a contrast medium, the possibility of preexisting drug sensitivity should always be carefully considered. The contrast medium yields much sharper delineation of the structures within the kidney and collecting system if administered when the patient is in the hydropenic state. The contrast media, however, have a potential for nephrotoxicity, and this hazard is greatest when the agents are administered to patients who are dehydrated. It must be stressed that use of large quantities of contrast material in ill patients is associated with a distinct risk of causing acute renal failure. Diabetic patients and patients with multiple myeloma and renal amyloidosis are at particularly high risk in this regard. Adequate visualization of the kidneys and collecting system by IVP requires that renal function be good. If the glomerular filtration has fallen below about 25 percent of normal (serum creatinine exceeds 4 mg/dl or creatinine clearance is less than 25 ml/min), the likelihood of obtaining useful information is sharply reduced. Computed tomography (CT) is usually very helpful in these patients, even when no contrast media are used. Renal arteriography is more risky and costly, and should be reserved for specific indications such as suspected renovascular hypertension or tumor.

RENAL BIOPSY

Specific instances in which renal biopsy may be helpful are considered in subsequent chapters. Probably its greatest utility is in diagnosis and management of the nephrotic syndrome and in the diagnosis of renal insufficiency of obscure origin.

Renal biopsy is technically more difficult than liver biopsy; adequate specimens are obtained with regularity only after the operator has acquired considerable experience. It should not be undertaken casually by an inexperienced person. It is associated with a low but definite mortality rate, probably about 0.2 percent. Significant bleeding probably occurs in the majority of patients, and in 2 to 3 percent is severe enough to require transfusion. Complications are minimized if (1) all patients have been tested for bleeding, clotting, and prothrombin times before biopsy (abnormalities of any of these should preclude biopsy); (2) biopsies are not performed on patients with a hemorrhagic diathesis, even if the previously mentioned tests are normal; and (3) following biopsy, the patient is kept in bed and watched carefully for 24 hours and kept on limited activity for 2 weeks.

REFERENCES

1. Alpern RJ, Warnock DG, Rector FC: Renal acidification mechanisms. In Brenner RM, Rector FC Jr (eds): The Kidney, 3d ed. Philadelphia, WB Saunders, 1986
2. Alyea EP, Parrish AH Jr: Renal response to exercise. Urinary findings. JAMA 167:807, 1958
3. Atlas SA, Laragh JH: Atrial natriuretic peptide: A new factor in hormonal control of blood pressure and electrolyte homeostasis. Ann Rev Med 27:397, 1986
4. Berliner RW: Renal mechanisms for potassium excretion. The Harvey Lectures 1959–1960. New York, Academic Press, 1961
5. Berliner RW: The concentrating mechanism in the renal medulla. Kidney 9:214, 1976
6. Bjornsson TD: Use of serum creatinine concentrations to determine renal function. Clin Pharmacokinet 4:200–222, 1979
7. Brenner BM, Rector FC Jr (eds): The Kidney, 3d ed. Philadelphia, WB Saunders, 1986, Chapters 3 and 4
8. Bricker NS: Renal function in chronic renal disease. Medicine 44:263, 1965
9. Cockcroft DW, Gault MH: Prediction of creatinine clearance from serum creatinine. Nephron 16:31, 1976
10. Dunn FL, Brennan TJ, et al: The role of blood osmolality and volume in regulating vasopressin secretion in the rat. J Clin Invest 52:3212, 1973
11. Gottschalk CW: Osmotic concentration and dilution of the urine. Am J Med 36:670, 1964
12. Hogg RJ, Kokko JP: Urine concentrating and diluting mechanisms in mammalian kidneys. In Brenner BM, Rector FC Jr (eds): The Kidney, 3d ed. Philadelphia, WB Saunders, 1986
13. Isobe T, Osserman EF: Patterns of amyloidosis and their association with plasma cell dyscrasia, monoclonal immunoglobulins and Bence Jones proteinuria. N Engl J Med 290:473, 1974
14. Lippman RW: Urine and the Urinary Sediment, 2d ed. Springfield, Ill, Charles C Thomas, 1957
15. Mitch WE: Measuring the progression of renal insufficiency. In Mitch WE (ed): The Progressive Nature of Renal Disease, Contemporary Issues in Nephrology, vol 14. New York, Churchill Livingstone, 1986
16. Mitch WE, Walser M, et al: A simple method of estimating progression of chronic renal failure. Lancet 2:1326, 1976
17. Mitch WE, Wilcox CS: Disorders of body fluids, sodium and potassium in chronic renal failure. Am J Med 72:536, 1982
18. Moroni BJ, Steinman TI, Mitch WE: A method for estimating nitrogen intake of patients with chronic renal failure. Kidney Int 27:58, 1985
19. Moses AM, Miller M: Drug induced dilutional hyponatremia. N Engl J Med 291:1234, 1974
20. Navar LG, Burke TJ, et al: Distal tubular feedback in the autoregulation of single nephron glomerular filtration rate. J Clin Invest 53:516, 1974
21. Roberts KE, Randall HT, et al: Renal mechanisms involved in bicarbonate reabsorption. Metabolism 5:404, 1956
22. Rock RC, Walker WG, Jennings CD: Nitrogen metabolites and renal function. In Tietz NW (ed): Textbook of Clinical Chemistry. Philadelphia, WB Saunders, 1986
23. Schrier RW (ed): Renal and Electrolyte Disorders, 2d ed. Boston, Little, Brown, 1980, p 27
24. Siersbaek-Nielsen K, Molholm-Hansen J, et al: Rapid evaluation of creatinine clearance. Lancet 1:1133, 1971
25. Valtin H: Renal Function: Mechanisms Preserving Fluid and Solute Balance in Health. Boston, Little, Brown, 1973
26. Wesson LG Jr: Physiology of the Human Kidney. New York, Grune and Stratton, 1969
27. Wright FS: Intrarenal regulation of glomerular filtration rate. N Engl J Med 291:135, 1974

The Proteinurias and Hematurias

W. Gordon Walker and Kim Solez

Diffuse renal disease is most often discovered as a result of routine examination of the urine. Because it is routine practice to accept a normal urine as excluding significant diffuse renal disease, an adequate specimen must be examined (Table 11.2–1), and the examination must include a careful microscopic examination of the urine. The abnormality signifying the existence of diffuse renal disease may be proteinuria, hematuria, or combinations of the two. Usually one of these two manifestations predominates and is responsible for focusing the physician's attention on the kidney as the source of disease.

The World Health Organization Committee on Renal Disease has proposed a detailed classification of glomerular disease that depends on whether the disease is limited to the kidney (primary) or is associated with primary vascular disease, metabolic disorders, or other systemic diseases.[14] The classification is based primarily on the histologic findings, including electron microscopy and immunofluorescence, and thus is of limited value to the clinician who is presented initially with an undiagnosed type of renal disease with no histologic information for guidance to the correct diagnosis. It is most helpful to take the two major modes of presentation, proteinuria and hematuria, and develop a systematic approach to the evaluation of these two findings. A careful examination of the urine is the most important prerequisite to the development of a diagnostic approach that is cost-effective and devoid of unnecessary and superfluous laboratory examinations.

When proteinuria exceeds 3 to 4 g per day, it produces a characteristic constellation of clinical findings irrespective of the nature of the underlying renal disease. For this reason the presentation to follow considers (1) the clinical features of the protein-losing kidney, (2) the specific diseases of the kidney that can give rise to this lesion, and (3) their management. This is followed by a similar examination of the renal disorders that may present with hematuria as the predominant urinary abnormality. Although significant overlap occurs and it is rare to see hematuria as a manifestation of diffuse renal disease without some accompanying proteinuria, the division is nevertheless a useful one insofar as it facilitates the differential diagnostic process.

Currently the differential diagnosis of many diffuse renal diseases is complicated by the lack of a single clinical entity corresponding to a unique morphologic picture and vice versa. There are many well-defined histopathologic entities that do not have a unique presentation but may be encountered in a variety of clinical situations.[14] These histopathologic findings are usually based on light microscopic, immunofluorescent, and ultrastructural changes that together present a distinctive and easily recognizable picture, but often there is no unique set of clinical findings that can be reproducibly associated with such findings. Crescentic glomerulonephritis, for example, may be seen in systemic lupus erythematosus, Schönlein-Henoch purpura, Wegener granulomatosis, polyarteritis, and in primary renal disease as Berger disease without involvement of other organ systems.[25,29,33] Identical immunofluorescent staining of glomeruli may be seen in membranous glomerulonephritis with nephrotic syndrome, systemic lupus erythematosus, and renal lesions associated with such different conditions as hepatitis and neoplasms. Conversely, cases of the nephrotic syndrome with identical clinical and urinary findings may show a wide range of histopathologic findings. This overlap makes establishment of diagnosis on a purely histologic or morphologic basis difficult indeed unless clinical information is available. Because clinical data must be so heavily relied on in reaching a diagnosis, we have divided the diffuse renal diseases into those in which

proteinuria predominates and those exhibiting hematuria as the principal abnormality.

THE PROTEINURIAS

Minor degrees of proteinuria are readily overlooked in a very dilute specimen; a specimen is suitable for excluding proteinuria only when the specific gravity exceeds 1.010, conditions usually met by examination of the first voided morning specimen. Under these conditions, proteinuria is probably the most sensitive indicator of diffuse renal disease.

The list of conditions that may cause proteinuria is extensive, and benign causes should be excluded before concluding that serious renal disease is present (Table 11.2–2).

A routine check for *postural proteinuria* should be made in all patients who have proteinuria without significant changes in the urinary sediment. This is done by having the patient empty his bladder immediately before retiring and then collecting the first specimen voided immediately upon arising in the morning. This must be compared with a specimen collected later in the day, after the patient has been up and about for several hours. When protein appears intermittently, even while the patient is upright, a possible relation to vigorous exercise should be sought.[3] Febrile proteinuria and mucus contamination from the genital tract should always be excluded as possible causes of minor degrees of proteinuria.

The practice of grading proteinuria as trace, 1+, 2+, and so on is inadequate. Quantitative measurement of urine protein excretion is essential for adequate diagnosis and management. It should be obtained on a 24-hour urine collection. When benign causes are excluded, persistent proteinuria in excess of 0.5 g per day is unequivocal evidence of renal disease, and diagnostic renal biopsy should be considered at this point.

CAUSES OF RENAL PROTEIN LOSS

The list of diseases presented in Table 11.2–2 emphasizes the almost universal occurrence of proteinuria as a manifestation of diffuse renal disease. In many of these entities the amount of protein lost may vary from a few hundred milligrams to over 20 g daily. Other clinical features may indicate the specific diagnosis, but the proteinuria may result in the same physiologic disturbances regardless of the underlying disease. The severity of clinical manifestations secondary to proteinuria can almost always be correlated well with the severity of the protein loss. Secondary manifestations usually do not appear unless the loss exceeds 2 to 3 g daily.[29]

Proteinuria is nearly always caused by a disturbance in the permeability of the glomerular basement membrane. An exception is the Bence Jones proteinuria of multiple myeloma, an instance of filtration of large quantities of a protein of low molecular weight. In general, the clearance of various species of plasma proteins is inversely related to their molecular weight or molecular size, a relation that holds over a wide range of rates of protein loss. More recently the studies of Brenner and others have shown that the glomerular basement membrane is polyanionic and that it is this relatively dense concentration of negative charges that tends to repel the plasma protein.[10] Glomerular injury is associated with a reduction in the net negative charge on the membrane, and as a consequence the permeability of the membrane is altered, permitting larger molecular sizes to pass. By measuring the clearance of

TABLE 11.2–1. STEPS TO BE OBSERVED IN CHECKING FOR PROTEINURIA

1. Examine first specimen voided in AM if possible
2. Examination should always include microscopic examination on *fresh* urine
3. Urine should have sp gr of 1.010 or greater
4. In females, urine should be obtained as clean catch specimen
5. Testing for protein should include either heat and acetic, or sulfosalicylic acid methods
6. Patients exhibiting proteinuria should be routinely checked for postural or orthostatic proteinuria
7. *Do not rely on dye-impregnated paper strips as an adequate screening procedure unless positives are confirmed by procedures under No. 5.*

proteins of progressively higher molecular weight, an index of glomerular permeability to protein can be obtained. In this fashion it is possible to characterize the permeability of the normal glomerular membrane and to show that disease processes that lead to increasing proteinuria also produce progressive deterioration in the permeability of the basement membrane. As this permeability increases, it can permit the urinary loss of extraordinarily large quantities of protein.[13]

The continuing drain on the protein stores of the body initiates a series of changes that result in the appearance of the *nephrotic syndrome*. This may occur in any patient if the rate of protein loss is sufficiently great. Hence, the nephrotic syndrome may be a feature of a number of renal diseases of different etiology. Urinary loss in excess of 3 g per day is evidence of severe glomerular disease, and recognition of its existence should not await the appearance of all clinical features of nephrotic syndrome. Early diagnosis is facilitated by the daily quantitative determination of urinary protein excretion. Patients with unexplained proteinuria that exceeds 0.5 g per day should be subjected to renal biopsy.

NEPHROTIC SYNDROME

The nephrotic syndrome is characterized clinically by edema of variable degree, heavy proteinuria, hypoalbuminemia, hypercholesterolemia, and hyperlipemia. The edema, even when severe, is associated with few or no complaints other than easy fatigability and local discomfort caused by the edema, unless there are large pleural effusions embarrassing respiration. The nephrotic syndrome may be diagnosed in the absence of one or more of these findings, and it is currently accepted that when proteinuria exceeds 3 g daily, the nephrotic syndrome will become clinically manifest at some time. The mechanism by which proteinuria progresses to the nephrotic syndrome is shown schematically in Fig. 11.2–1. If the proteinuria continues, it will eventually deplete body nitrogen and decrease albumin production by the liver, which will cause the plasma albumin concentration to fall. This decreases plasma oncotic pressure and allows transudation of fluid into the interstitial spaces. The decrease in circulating plasma volume and increase in aldosterone production promotes increased reabsorption of sodium and water and leads to progressive edema. The mechanism

TABLE 11.2–2. PROTEIN EXCRETION RATES OF VARIOUS RENAL DISORDERS[a]

	Protein Excretion Rate (mg/day)			
	50–100	150–1000	1000–3000	> 3000
Benign Proteinuria				
• Exercise proteinuria	+			
• Febrile proteinuria	+			
• Postural proteinuria	+	+		
Primary Glomerular Diseases				
• Lipoid nephrosis		+	+	+
• Focal glomerular sclerosis		+	+	+
• Membranous glomerulonephritis		+	+	+
• Membranoproliferative glomerulonephritis		+	+	+
• Acute glomerulonephritis	+	+	+	+
• Rapidly progressive glomerulonephritis		+	+	+
Glomerular Disease Associated with Systemic Illness				
• Systemic lupus erythematosus	+	+	+	+
• Anaphylactoid purpura	+	+	+	+
• IgA nephropathy	+	+	+	Rare
• Sickle cell disease	+	+	+	+
• Goodpasture syndrome	+	+	+	Rare
• Glomerulonephritis	+	+	+	
• Shunt nephritis	+	+	+	
• Malarial nephropathy		+	+	+
• Multiple myeloma[b]		+	+	+
• Diabetic glomerulosclerosis		+	+	+
• Polyarteritis nodosa	+	+	+ (Rare)	
• Nephrosclerosis				
Benign	+	+ (Rare)		
Malignant	+	+	+ (Rare)	
• Systemic sclerosis	+	+	+ (Rare)	
• Amyloidosis		+	+	+
Toxic Nephropathies				
• Acute	+	+		
• Chronic (heavy metals)	+	+	+	+

[a]Approximate ranges of daily protein excretion in some common disease of the kidney. Divisions should be taken as a guide, rather than absolute range of excretion in these diseases.
[b]Does not refer to Bence Jones proteinuria but to more general proteinuria frequently seen in multiple myeloma. On occasion, excretion of Bence Jones protein may exceed 8 to 10 g daily.

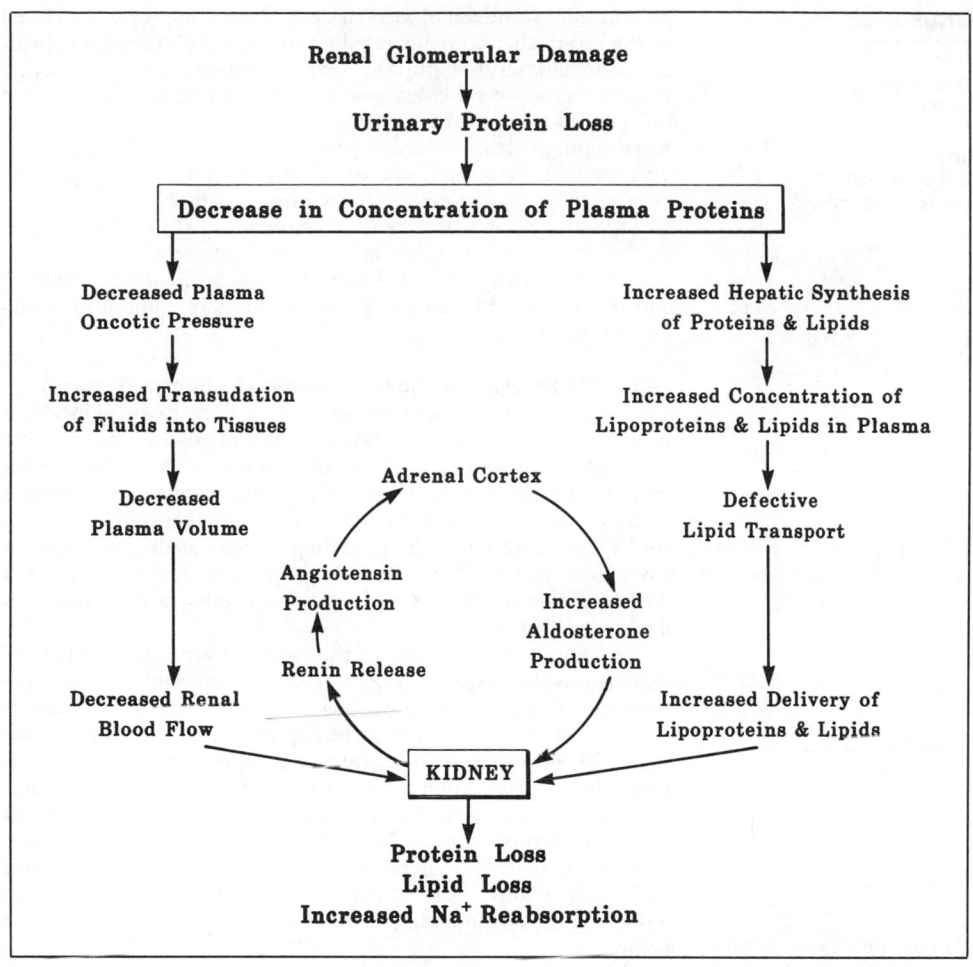

Figure 11.2–1. Sequence of events leading to the nephrotic syndrome.

for this increased aldosterone production is not completely settled, but it is likely that the primary stimulus is related to a drop in renal blood flow, consequent on the fall in plasma volume. The kidney in turn increases renin production, which stimulates liberation of angiotensin; the latter exerts a direct stimulatory effect on the zona glomerulosa of the adrenal cortex, resulting in increased production of aldosterone. This chain of events continues until (1) a new steady state is reached with respect to the distribution of intravascular and extravascular fluid, permitting the patient to maintain a normal plasma volume, or (2) fluid accumulation reaches disabling proportions. Lymphatic flow is increased and, in patients with marked fluid retention, dilated lymphatics can be identified over the lateral region of the buttocks and flank.

The principal protein found in the urine of nephrotic patients is albumin, despite the fact that its concentration may be greatly reduced in the plasma. Even though the renal clearance of albumin is much greater than that of the other larger plasma proteins, the increased glomerular permeability allows significant loss of gamma globulin, often leading to hypogammaglobulinemia. The differential permeability of the glomerular membrane results in proportionately greater losses of the plasma proteins of smaller molecular weight.[13,23] The net effect is a selective concentration of plasma proteins of larger molecular weight, such as the lipoproteins, which contribute to the lipidemia characteristic of nephrosis. Because these lipoproteins are intimately concerned with cholesterol transport, the plasma cholesterol content rises. There is also increased cholesterol synthesis by the liver. Thus, the hyperlipidemia and hypercholesterolemia result from a combination of differential retention of these substances at the glomerulus and their increased production by the liver.

Lipiduria is recognized by the presence of fatty casts in great numbers, as well as by cells that appear to be shed by the kidney. Occasionally, lipid is seen as free droplets or as small particles in the urine. Fat- or lipid-containing droplets can be readily identified by microscopic examination of urine under polarized light, which renders them doubly refractive. They probably arise as a result of increased filtration of some of the smaller lipoprotein molecules and cholesterol esters.

Although the total number of diseases that may occasionally be responsible for the protein-losing lesion associated with the nephrotic syndrome is large, over two thirds represent primary renal diseases (Table 11.2–2). Differentiation between them may be impossible on clinical grounds and often can only be made histologically. This is particularly true in those individuals discovered during a routine examination to have proteinuria. The primary renal diseases that exhibit significant protein-losing lesions at some time during their course are lipoid nephrosis or nil disease, membranous glomerulonephritis, mesangioproliferative glomerulonephritis, acute glomerulonephritis, and membranoproliferative glomerulonephritis. Less commonly, the nephrotic syndrome may be seen in systemic lupus erythematosus, amyloidosis, multiple myeloma, renal vein thrombosis, and diabetic glomerulosclerosis, as well as in those conditions caused by an impressive list of nephrotoxins, allergenic agents, and drugs (Table 11.2–3).

Percutaneous renal biopsy is of great value in establishing a diagnosis. Amyloidosis, for example, is readily recognized by this means, as is diabetic glomerulosclerosis. In addition, renal biopsy permits distinction between membranous glomerulonephritis, chronic proliferative glomerulonephritis, and the other diffuse glomerulonephritides.

TABLE 11.2–3. CAUSES OF NEPHROTIC SYNDROME[1,4,7,17,27,29]

Primary Renal Diseases
- Lipoid nephrosis (minimal change or nil disease)
- With glomerular mesangial hypercellularity
- Membranous glomerulonephritis
- Membranoproliferative glomerulonephritis
- Focal sclerosing glomerulonephritis (focal sclerosis)
- Acute glomerulonephritis (less than 10 percent of cases)
- Renal vein thrombosis

Nephrotoxins and Allergens
- Inorganic mercury and mercury compounds
- Bismuth
- Gold
- Insect stings
- Poison ivy
- Tridione
- Paradione
- Captopril
- Snakebites

Systemic Illness
- Diabetes with diabetic glomerulosclerosis
- Systemic lupus erythematosus
- Amyloidosis
- Multiple myelosis
- Syphilis
- Malaria
- Sickle cell anemia
- Schönlein-Henoch purpura
- Goodpasture syndrome

PRIMARY RENAL DISORDERS AND NEPHROTIC SYNDROME

The primary renal diseases that may present as the nephrotic syndrome can be divided into two groups on the basis of the findings obtained from the initial history and physical examination and urinalysis. The importance of careful microscopic examination of the urine must be stressed.

The largest group consists of those patients who present with the nephrotic syndrome and massive proteinuria but with relatively unimpressive urinary sediment. Fatty casts and granular casts are almost always present but usually not in great numbers. Red cell casts are not seen, and few or no erythrocytes are present. In the majority of cases, the onset of the disease is preceded by a mild upper respiratory illness, but no evidence can be obtained for beta-hemolytic streptococcal infection. Renal biopsies from these patients may exhibit one of three types of changes. Lipoid nephrosis (nil disease) is characterized by essentially normal histologic findings on routine examination by light microscopy. Membranous glomerulonephritis shows marked thickening of the glomerular basement membrane, including virtually all the glomeruli; there is little or no associated hypercellularity. Focal sclerosing glomerulonephritis is characterized by patchy involvement and does not affect all glomeruli (Fig. 11.2–2). Early in the course of the disease it may show abnormalities in only a very few tufts in a larger number of glomeruli. It is thus on initial biopsy frequently confused with lipoid nephrosis. It differs in response to therapy and, more importantly, in its clinical course. The prognosis with this disorder is generally poor; young people particularly often progress from a state of normal renal function to end-stage renal disease in a period of less than 1 or 2 years. The pathologic changes include focal segmental sclerosis and the presence of pink-staining hyaline exudative lesions. These changes are not specific; similar lesions may be seen in diabetes, arteriosclerosis, and in the sclerosing phase of the glomerulonephritis associated with Schönlein-Henoch purpura, polyarteritis, subacute infective endocarditis, and other systemic diseases exhibiting renal involvement.

The nephrotic patient with prominent hematuria and many granular and some red blood cell casts in the urine is readily placed in the group that contains rapidly progressing glomerulonephritis and acute glomerulonephritis. Further justification for considering these as a group is provided by the histologic findings encountered on renal biopsy. All these patients show a picture that varies in severity but is characterized as primarily proliferative. These disorders are considered in more detail in the section on hematurias because they usually present in circumstances in which other clinical features predominate; more often than not, the typical features of the nephrotic syndrome are absent. Hypertension of variable severity, frequently associated with evidence of circulatory overload and progressive renal failure, is a more common clinical presentation in this group.

Lipoid Nephrosis (Nil Disease, Minimal Change Disease)

Lipoid nephrosis, thought initially to be a disease of childhood, is now recognized to occur in both adults and children but is more common in the latter. Recent studies indicate that it accounts for more than three fourths of cases of nephrotic syndrome in patients under 6 years of age and perhaps 15 to 30 percent of cases seen in adults. As indicated in the preceding section, it does not exhibit any unique features that permit its recognition and separation as a distinct entity at the time of initial onset unless a renal biopsy is performed (Fig. 11.2–2).

A characteristic feature of the natural history of this type of nephrosis is the frequency of exacerbations and remissions and the relatively favorable long-term prognosis. There may be as many as ten or more typical episodes of the nephrotic syndrome distributed over a 15- or 20-year period. Despite this protracted course punctuated by clinical evidence of recurrent activity, renal function may remain essentially normal. The distinguishing feature of this disorder is the completeness of the remission. Protein usually diminishes to less than 100 mg per day and often becomes undetectable during remissions. Adrenal corticosteroids are clearly of value in inducing and maintaining remissions in lipoid nephrosis (see below).

Only a small percentage of patients with lipoid nephrosis shows evidence of progression to chronic renal insufficiency. Hypertension is rarely a significant problem. Azotemia of moderate degree may be seen in association with exacerbations but appears to be due largely to the hypovolemia that accompanies the marked reduction in plasma albumin. It disappears concomitantly with reduction in proteinuria and edema.

Nephrotic Syndrome and Glomerular Mesangial Hypercellularity

In about one fifth of adult patients with primary renal disease presenting as the nephrotic syndrome, a distinctive histologic lesion is present, characterized by hypercellularity confined exclusively to the mesangial cells. Whether this change identifies a single etiologic entity is doubtful, but the patients with this lesion do exhibit a consistent clinical pattern. They present with heavy proteinuria, normal renal function, and no blood pressure elevation. Microscopic hematuria is present in less than one third of cases, but casts are rare and there is no evidence of prior streptococcal infection. Except for the proteinuria, renal functional impairment is rare.

This disorder, like lipoid nephrosis, tends to relapse. It may exhibit spontaneous remissions, and in the majority of cases favorable response is obtained with steroid therapy. Sustained remissions occur in more than three fourths of these patients. Further study and long follow-up will be necessary to determine whether this is a separate and completely different entity from lipoid nephrosis. At present no distinction can be made in management or prognosis based on the finding of mesangial hypercellularity.

Focal Sclerosing Glomerulonephritis[1,4,14]

Focal sclerosing glomerulonephritis is a particularly ominous pathologic category, even though its initial clinical presentation is indistinguishable from nil disease or lipoid nephrosis. The disease is characterized histologically by focal lesions within the glomerulus

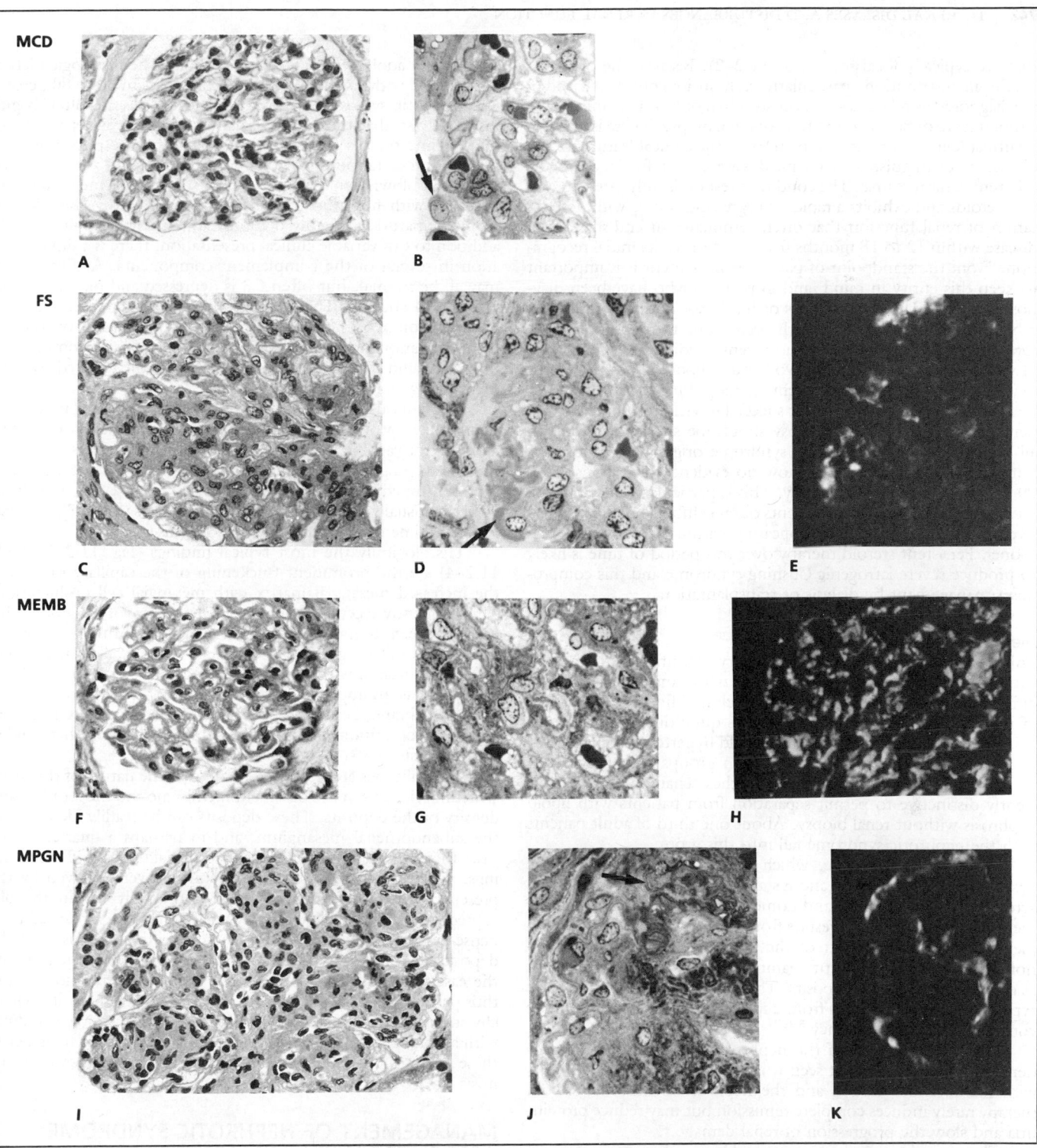

Figure 11.2–2. Characteristic glomerular changes seen in paraffin sections stained with hematoxylin and eosin (×330, left panels), plastic sections stained with toluidine blue (×750, middle panels), and frozen sections stained with fluorescein-tagged antisera (×410, right panels). In minimal change disease (MCD) glomeruli are essentially normal (**A**). High-power examination shows slight enlargement of epithelial cells (arrow in **B**). Immunofluorescence studies are negative. In focal sclerosing glomerulonephritis (FS) portions of glomeruli are solidified (bottom of **C**) with the remainder being normal. Hyaline exudative lesions may be seen in scarred regions (arrow in **D**) and these stain with IgM (**E**). In membranous glomerulonephritis (MEMB), capillary loops are diffusely thickened (**F**); punctate deposits are seen on the outside of capillary loop basement membranes (arrow in **G**); and these stain with IgG (**H**). In membranoproliferative glomerulonephritis (MPGN) there is increased lobulation of the glomeruli with mesangial hypercellularity and a patchy thickening of capillary loops (**I**). "Double contours" with bandlike subendothelial deposits are seen in the peripheral capillary loops (arrows in **J**); these peripheral capillaries stain with C3 (**K**). (The differences in size of the glomeruli in the left-hand panels are due in part to variation in how near the center of the glomerulus the section was taken and in part to glomerular enlargement in MPGN.)

that are typically focal scars (Fig. 11.2–2). Because the disease is patchy in distribution, particularly early in its course, it is often misdiagnosed as nil disease, especially when only a small number of glomeruli are obtained at the time of renal biopsy. There is nothing identifiable in the urinary sediment or in the clinical features of the disease to distinguish it from nil disease except for its markedly different clinical course. The condition responds only rarely to corticosteroids and exhibits a rapidly progressing course with deterioration of renal function that often terminates in end-stage renal disease within 12 to 18 months from the time of its initial recognition. From the standpoint of patient management it is important to keep this entity in mind, and in patients who have been diagnosed as having lipoid nephrosis or nil disease and who fail to exhibit the expected response with prednisone therapy, a *repeat biopsy should be done.* Immunofluorescent studies are occasionally of value in distinguishing the two because lipoid nephrosis almost never exhibits immunofluorescent staining, but this also may not be helpful if the biopsy does not succeed in yielding glomeruli that demonstrate the lesion. Rebiopsy should be standard practice in all patients with the nephrotic syndrome originally diagnosed as minimal change disease who show no evidence of response after 90 days of corticosteroid therapy. This is particularly important in focal sclerosis because these patients often exhibit a rapidly progressive course with renal failure appearing within 1 to 2 years, often sooner. Persistent steroid therapy over this period of time is likely to produce severe iatrogenic Cushing syndrome and this compromises management by dialysis or transplantation.

Membranous Glomerulonephritis[1,25,33]

This descriptive histopathologic category identifies a subgroup of patients with the nephrotic syndrome who cannot otherwise be differentiated from lipoid nephrosis on clinical findings at the time of initial presentation. The prognosis is quite different, however, as is the response to steroid therapy. Mild hypertension and microscopic hematuria are more common in groups of patients with membranous glomerulonephritis, but these changes are not sufficiently distinctive to permit separation from patients with lipoid nephrosis without renal biopsy. About one third of adult patients with the nephrotic syndrome fall into this group.

The histologic change, which appears as thickening of the basement membrane on H and E staining (Fig. 11.2–2) and a characteristic argentaffin spike and dome pattern within the basement membrane by silver stain, results from deposition of immune complexes on the outer aspect of the basement membrane. Immunofluorescent studies identify gamma globulins and complement as constituents of these deposits. This is cited as evidence that this type of renal disease results from deposition of circulating immune complexes within the kidney.[5,21,24,26,30,32,33]

The clinical course of the nephrotic syndrome in these patients is different from that seen with lipoid nephrosis. In patients with membranous lesions and the nephrotic syndrome, steroid therapy rarely induces complete remission but may reduce proteinuria and slow the progression of renal damage.[15]

The natural history is characterized by slowly progressive renal impairment with the nephrotic syndrome persisting for many years. Survival for periods in excess of 10 years is not uncommon, and occasionally, spontaneous complete remission occurs. The majority, however, progress slowly to terminal or end-stage renal disease with the clinical course characterized by the nephrotic syndrome that fluctuates in severity. Hypertension appears relatively early in the course of the disease and may be quite severe. Early and effective treatment of this manifestation of the disease is important.

Membranoproliferative Glomerulonephritis[14]

This subset of the nephrotic syndrome, so named because of the histologic findings of both basement membrane thickening and mesangial cell proliferation, is generally associated with a poor prognosis. It may be seen in any age group but is probably most common in adolescence and young adults. The histologic picture is associated with a variable clinical expression. In 60 to 80 percent the nephrotic syndrome is present, and the disease often begins insidiously so that there may actually be substantial renal damage by the time the disease is first recognized by the physician. The mode of presentation is variable, however, and may vary from that of the full-blown nephrotic syndrome to typical acute glomerulonephritis with hematuria that is at times grossly visible. Microscopic hematuria is readily demonstrable in virtually all cases. In addition to this variable clinical presentation, there is a similar variation in several of the complement components. At times these may all be normal, but often C3 is depressed and on occasion so is C1q, C4 and C2. These changes are often associated with the identification of C3 nephritic factor, a globulin capable of complement activation. It may be responsible for excessive complement utilization and thus indirectly responsible for the lowered complement values that occur at times.

The clinical course varies in its rate of progression; on occasion significant improvement in all manifestations of the disease occurs and lasts for variable lengths of time. Nearly all patients, however, ultimately progress to terminal renal failure, with the period of time consumed by this progression varying from several months to 10 years. Usually, however, renal failure appears within 3 to 5 years from the time of first recognition of the disease.

Histologically the most typical findings (Fig. 11.2–2; Table 11.2–4) are the prominent thickening of the capillary loops and the increased mesangial matrix with mesangial cell proliferation. This frequently accentuates the lobular structure of the glomerulus and has been termed "lobular glomerulonephritis" as well as "mesangiocapillary glomerulonephritis." The capillary wall thickening is associated with deposits and mesangial interposition, and often there is the appearance of duplication or splitting of the basement membrane, best demonstrated with silver stains. On the basis of histologic findings this clinical subset has been further divided into three subtypes.

The subtypes are defined according to the nature of the ultrastructural changes in the basement membrane and the location and density of the deposits. These deposits can be readily identified in the subendothelial mesangium, and in perhaps a quarter of the cases they may also be found as subepithelial deposits. These findings, which define type I, are occasionally overshadowed by the presence of extensive deposits located primarily within the disrupted lamina densa (type III). Type II has also been referred to as dense-deposit disease because of the extraordinary density of the deposits that are identifiable in the basement membrane. Despite the ease with which these histologic features are recognized and thus permit ready classification into the three categories, it is virtually impossible to associate a particular set of histologic findings with a unique clinical course. Thus, until it is possible to associate these findings with differences in therapeutic response or prognosis, their value to the clinician is limited.

MANAGEMENT OF NEPHROTIC SYNDROME ASSOCIATED WITH PRIMARY RENAL DISEASES[1,9,11,15,23,38]

General measures are directed toward treatment of the hypoproteinemia and the attendant edema. The persistent proteinuria characteristic of the disorder results in a marked nitrogen deficit that reduces the capacity of the liver to replace the plasma proteins lost in the urine.[9] Positive nitrogen balance can be maintained for prolonged periods of time when protein intake is increased (Fig. 11.2–3). Patients can usually tolerate up to 2 or 2.5 g of protein per kilogram body weight per day for long periods, and the clinical features of the nephrotic syndrome can occasionally be reserved by this therapy despite continued heavy proteinuria. It is occasionally difficult to get the patient to maintain this high protein intake if sodium is rigidly restricted. When unpalatability appears to reduce protein intake, it is preferable to liberalize sodium

TABLE 11.2–4. IMMUNOFLUORESCENCE IN GLOMERULONEPHRITIS[6,25,30,32,33,35]

Disease	IgG	IgA	IgM	C_3	C_4	C_{1q}	Fibrinogen
Acute glomerulonephritis	++	−	−	+	−	−	−
Glomerulonephritis associated with infection	++	−	+	++	+	++	−
Membranoproliferative glomerulonephritis							
Type 1	+	−	+	+++	+	++	−
Type 2 (dense deposit disease)	−	−	−	+++	−	−	−
Mixed cryoglobulinemia with nephritis	+++	−	+++	++	+	++	−
SLE with nephritis	+++	+	+	+	++	+++	−
Schölein-Henoch[a]	+	+++	−	+	−	−	+++
Berger disease[a]	+	+++	−	+	−	−	−
Malaria nephropathy	++	+	+				
Focal sclerosing glomerulonephritis	−	−	+ Focal	+ Focal	−	−	−
Goodpasture syndrome	+++ Linear	−	−	+	−	−	+
Polyarteritis nodosa	+	−	−	−	−	−	++

[a]Immunofluorescence found in mesangium.

intake to counter this. Under these circumstances diuretics may be relied upon to control edema.

On occasion, nephrotic "crises" characterized by anorexia, nausea, vomiting, and abdominal pain occur in association with profound anasarca and severe hypoalbuminemia. The cause of this clinical picture is not clear, but symptomatic improvement can on occasion be achieved by administration of intravenous albumin and the concomitant administration of diuretics. Relief often appears to be proportional to the quantity of fluid lost in response to this therapy. Its effect is transient because the administered protein is rapidly excreted in the urine. It may succeed in providing patient comfort, however, because transient diuresis almost always occurs, particularly if the albumin is given in conjunction with a diuretic such as furosemide.

Both adults and children with lipoid nephrosis (nil disease) will respond to corticosteroid therapy in approximately 80 to 90 percent of cases. Complete remissions occur in two thirds. The data from the International Study of Kidney Disease in Children reveal that 85 percent of patients treated with prednisone responded within 6 weeks, and of these over three quarters had had a remission within 3 weeks of beginning therapy. Of those responding, approximately one quarter have frequent relapses. *There is no good evidence from controlled trials to indicate that the use of maintenance corticosteroid therapy for long periods of time has any particular advantage over intermittent treatment when relapse appears.* Controlled trials have demonstrated that these results are not improved when azathioprine is added to the prednisone therapy. The use of cyclophosphamide, however, may add some advantage. This drug appears to diminish the number of patients who exhibit early relapses and, within the group of patients relapsing after cyclophosphamide therapy, the frequency of relapses is reduced. These results were achieved with cyclophosphamide therapy that lasted for 2 to 3 months. Similar results, albeit with smaller numbers of subjects, have been obtained in controlled trials of these therapeutic regimens in adults. The incidence of remissions with nil disease or lipoid nephrosis is approximately the same for adults and children. In both adults and children, the use of cyclophosphamide as adjunctive therapy in those patients with lipoid nephrosis who failed to respond to prednisone alone does not increase the number of "late" responders, that is, those respond-

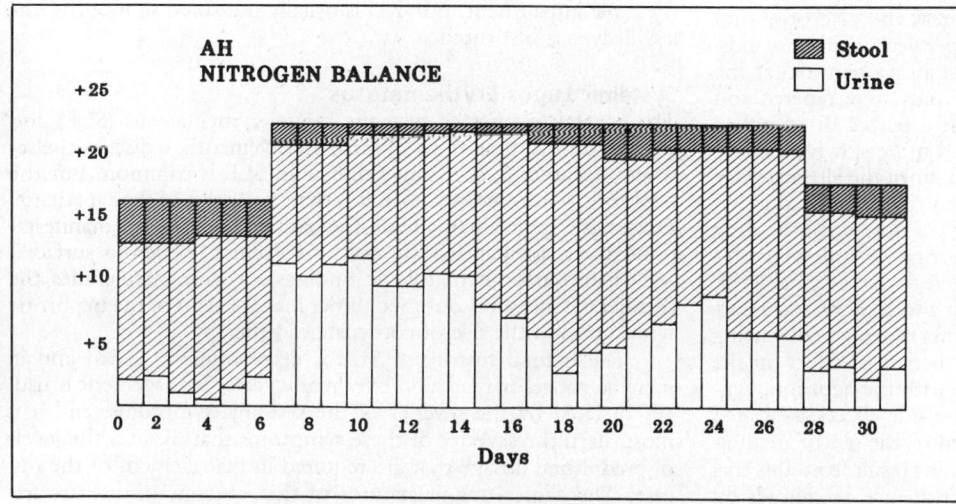

Figure 11.2–3. Nitrogen balance data on patient with lipoid nephrosis and severe proteinuria. Ordinate values are grams of nitrogen per day. Intake is plotted upward from zero and total shaded portion of each bar represents total nitrogen output for that day. Patient was studied during nitrogen intakes of 16, 23, and 18 g per day corresponding to daily protein intakes of 100, 143, and 112 g per day, respectively. White portion of each bar represents positive nitrogen balance achieved on that day. As protein intake increased, quantity of nitrogen retained each day increased. Protein loss in urine varied between 16 and 25 g per day throughout the period of study.

ing after 2 months. It does appear, however, that late responses are hastened somewhat when cyclophosphamide therapy is used.

The most appropriate treatment regimen for lipoid nephrosis should include a high-protein (2 g/kg body weight per day), low-salt (20 to 30 mEq Na per day) diet and initial treatment with prednisone (0.75 to 1 mg/ kg per day) for 6 weeks. If a satisfactory response is obtained (expected in approximately 85 percent), the prednisone should be tapered and stopped. The course should be repeated if relapse occurs. For those who fail to respond a longer course of prednisone therapy should be given and a full dosage schedule maintained for at least 3 months. If no remission is achieved with this regimen, the added risk of more prolonged therapy with this corticosteroid dosage outweighs the small likelihood of any significant benefit occurring from further prolongation of steroid therapy. Because the risk of death is relatively small in patients with lipoid nephrosis, the use of cyclophosphamide should be restricted, because the drug is not without serious side effects. In particular, gonadal atrophy poses a real threat that offsets the other benefits likely to be gained by the use of this drug. The relatively frequent occurrence of chemical cystitis associated with cyclophosphamide administration and undefined risk of neoplasms represent additional sources of concern.

For those patients showing no evidence of remission, the wisest course of management is to taper and then withdraw steroids while maintaining judicious supportive management, which includes a high-protein intake, selective use of diuretics, and early treatment of even minor infections. Because no data exist documenting that steroids, with or without such agents as cyclophosphamide, prolong survival in lipoid nephrosis, it is unwise to expose these patients to the increased risks associated with prolonged iatrogenic Cushing syndrome.

Membranous nephritis has a less favorable outcome regardless of the type of treatment used. Earlier clinical trials reported modest benefits characterized typically by some reduction in proteinuria in perhaps one fourth to one third of steroid-treated patients, but this appeared to be offset by a slightly higher mortality rate in the steroid-treated group.[8,11,12] The most instructive information regarding treatment in membranous glomerulonephritis comes from a controlled 5-year trial that compared prednisone treatment (125 mg on alternate days) with a placebo in a randomized, double-blind fashion.[15] The individuals were given prednisone or placebo on an alternate-day regimen for 8 weeks. Steroid dosage was 125 mg every other day for individuals whose weight was between 45 and 80 kg; below this range individuals received 100 mg of prednisone on alternate days and those with higher weights received 150 mg on alternate days. Only six of the prednisone-treated group had any significant period when their urine was free of protein, and in only two instances did this period of complete remission exceed 1 year. The most remarkable evidence for a beneficial effect of treatment, however, was the slowing of the rate of decline in renal function. In individuals receiving steroid therapy, the GFR declined at a median rate of 2 percent per year, whereas the placebo group exhibited a median decline of 10 percent per year. For those individuals exhibiting no response (no decrease in proteinuria) at the end of the initial 8 weeks of therapy, steroids were tapered and withdrawn over the following 4 weeks. If a partial or complete remission was achieved, tapering proceeded more slowly; the rate of reduction was 25 mg per dose each week until the alternate-day dose had diminished to 25 mg. Beyond this the rate of reduction was slowed to weekly decrements of 5 mg per dose until the drug was withdrawn. If there was a relapse during or following this withdrawal, the steroid dosage was returned to the original level, with the treatment continued for 1 month and then retapered according to the same schedule. This represents the most convincing evidence that prednisone has a significant beneficial effect on the course of membranous glomerulonephritis with the nephrotic syndrome. It is likely that the reduction in the side effects associated with steroid therapy in this trial was related to the use of an alternate-day dosage regimen. The most significant result from this trial was the documentation of the retarding influence of steroids on

the rate of loss of renal function. It may be inferred from this that steroids, used in this fashion, significantly prolong the period of adequate renal function in patients afflicted with this disorder, thereby delaying the point at which maintenance dialysis becomes essential.

There is considerable anecdotal information suggesting that immunosuppressive agents such as azathioprine and cyclophosphamide offer some additional benefit when combined with prednisone therapy in the treatment of the nephrotic syndrome caused by lipoid nephrosis, membranous glomerulonephritis, membranoproliferative glomerulonephritis, and diffuse proliferative glomerulonephritis. The numbers of cases on which these reports have been based are too small to permit clear evaluation of their utility.[1,11,27,38] Cyclophosphamide given at a dosage level of 5 mg/kg per day is commonly associated with leukopenia and thus represents a significant hazard to the patient. The usually recommended dosage is 2.5 mg/kg per day for a period of 6 weeks. Severe cases of hemorrhagic and cicatricial cystitis have been reported with the use of this drug. Because of these adverse effects and because the combination of cyclophosphamide and prednisone clearly increases risk of infection and compromises the patient's ability to deal with infection, great care should be exercised in the use of this combination.

NEPHROTIC SYNDROME ASSOCIATED WITH SYSTEMIC DISEASE[14,17]

Diabetic Glomerulosclerosis (Chapter 14.7)

The nephrotic syndrome occurs in association with insulin-dependent diabetes mellitus in 10 to 20 percent of reported cases. Clinically, this group can readily be distinguished from patients with membranous glomerulonephritis. In addition to evidence of preexisting diabetes that may have been present from 1 to 20 years, retinal microaneurysms are regularly found, diastolic hypertension is almost always present, and superimposed congestive heart failure is frequently noted. Renal function is reduced, with moderate to marked azotemia. Renal biopsy reveals diffuse intercapillary glomerulosclerosis, and concentric hyaline masses are frequently seen to distend capillary loops (Kimmelstiel-Wilson lesion). The diffuse intercapillary glomerulosclerosis appears to be the significant pathologic lesion because not all patients exhibit the nodular hyaline masses, and conversely, hyaline nodules may be seen in the glomeruli of diabetics without any evidence of the nephrotic syndrome.

Treatment is disappointing. Corticosteroid therapy is contraindicated. The severity of the renal insufficiency may be such that even modest increases in protein intake produce or aggravate preexisting acidosis. Salt restriction and cautious use of diuretics may be the only therapeutic measures that can be safely used. Treatment of hypertension is essential, but any sudden lowering of blood pressure must be avoided because it frequently worsens the renal impairment. Survival is usually measured in months unless dialysis is instituted.

Systemic Lupus Erythematosus

The general features of systemic lupus erythematosus (SLE) and the clinical manifestations of renal involvement are discussed elsewhere (Chapter 8.2). Kidney disease in SLE is common, but the nephrotic syndrome occurs in less than 5 percent of these patients. Diagnosis is generally made on the basis of the systemic manifestations (fever, arthralgias, skin rash, involvement of serous surfaces, and characteristic hematologic findings). Treatment includes the therapeutic measures outlined under management of the nephrotic syndrome and the use of corticosteroid therapy.

The natural history of SLE is extraordinarily varied and in many instances may extend over many years. Management is usually dictated by the severity of the systemic symptoms, and it is most often the severity of these symptoms that dictates the levels of prednisone dosage that are required in management of the disease. The clinical manifestations of this systemic disease are fre-

quently confined to the kidney. In such patients the use of long-term high-dose steroids should not be condoned. Maintaining the cushingoid state in such patients for periods of years produces numerous problems that accentuate the risk of both dialysis and transplantation. For this reason, when lupus nephritis is not associated with other significant systemic symptoms, it is far wiser to follow the steroid regimen proposed previously for the nephrotic syndrome caused by membranous nephritis and to continue tapering the steroids so long as the systemic symptoms of the disease do not appear to be exacerbated.

Amyloidosis

Amyloidosis is a disorder characterized by widespread deposition or accumulation of an extracellular eosinophilic proteinaceous material in the tissues or organs of the body (Chapter 6.20). The symptomatology is determined by the organs predominantly involved. Renal amyloidosis may be asymptomatic throughout the course of the disease, the only manifestation being proteinuria of modest degree. On occasion, extensive accumulation of amyloid material in the kidney results in renal insufficiency leading to death in uremia. This is particularly true in the form of the disease seen in association with chronic suppuration (secondary amyloidosis). The disease presents less often as the nephrotic syndrome. The incidence in reported series varies between 5 percent and more than 40 percent of those cases of amyloidosis showing renal involvement.[40]

In addition, renal amyloidosis with clinical features of the nephrotic syndrome may occur in association with renal vein thrombosis. This suggests that amyloid involvement of the kidney may predispose to renal vein thrombosis. Amyloidosis of the kidney is also seen in multiple myeloma presenting as the nephrotic syndrome. The diagnosis of renal amyloidosis is established by renal biopsy, this procedure appearing to be relatively safe in these cases.

Treatment should be confined to the general measures outlined for treatment of the nephrotic syndrome. Corticosteroids appear to be ineffective.

THE HEMATURIAS[2,17,20,21]

Hematuria is a manifestation of many local diseases of the kidney and lower urinary tract, as well as a constant finding in a number of diffuse renal processes. The distinction between local hematuria and hematuria due to diffuse renal disease is of practical importance, and certain clinical and microscopic features serve to distinguish between the two (Table 11.2–5). Local hematuria is virtually always sufficiently profuse to produce visible discoloration of the urine, and microscopic examination reveals erythrocytes with little or no evidence of distortion. Blood added at the glomerulus is almost always accompanied by red cell casts, and the erythrocytes exhibit marked distortion with crenated red cells and small, highly refractile microcytes. Proteinuria may accompany the local forms of hematuria if these are severe, but it is virtually always associated with hematuria of diffuse renal disease. The excretion of protein rarely exceeds a few hundred milligrams per day when associated with local disorders of the genitourinary tract. In diffuse renal disease it varies from a few hundred milligrams to more than 10 g per day, the latter value being associated with the nephrotic syndrome.

DIAGNOSTIC EVALUATION OF HEMATURIA

When hematuria is associated with pain and burning on micturition or suprapubic discomfort with frequency and urgency on urination, the lower urinary tract is the probable source. When the hematuria is noted only at the beginning or end of micturition, the urethra or bladder is usually the source. Hematuria associated with acute renal colic is most likely to be produced by nephrolithiasis, although clots themselves can produce renal colic on occasion when the clots form in the pelvis and are passed down the ureter.

In contrast, the hematuria of diffuse kidney disease is usually painless, is usually identifiable only by microscopic examination, and the blood is always uniformly distributed in the urine. Red blood cells that appear large and of normal morphology except for slight to moderate crenation are almost always associated with local disease somewhere in the urinary tract. When the source of the hematuria is the glomerulus or some site in the tubules, the red cells undergo considerable distortion (probably because of exposure to marked osmotic gradients during transit through the tubule). One characteristic form seen in hematuria of glomerular origin is the small, round microcyte that is one-half the size of a normal erythrocyte and exhibits increased refractility. Red cell casts, a characteristic feature of the hematuria of diffuse renal disease, unmistakably identify the nephron as the source of bleeding.

In most disorders, the severity of the hematuria varies greatly. Careful microscopic examination of freshly voided urine is necessary to establish the presence of hematuria in both local and diffuse disease and is a useful guide to further diagnostic studies. When red blood cell casts indicate that the hematuria results from diffuse parenchymal disease, renal biopsy is the procedure most likely to establish the diagnosis. Gross hematuria without casts or significant proteinuria indicates a localized disease of the collecting system or a bleeding disturbance. Exclusion of the former requires the use of all available diagnostic aids, including a flat radiograph of the abdomen, which may visualize radiopaque calculi, intravenous pyelography, renal arteriography, and cystoscopy with retrograde pyelography. The evaluation of hemorrhagic disorders is discussed elsewhere (Chapters 6.8 and 6.9), but it is worth noting here that several of the abnormal hemoglobins are associated with recurrent hematuria and should be excluded when painless hematuria unassociated with proteinuria or casts is encountered.

Careful studies should be made to exclude such correctable lesions as nephrolithiasis, tumors, and other surgically treatable disorders. Hematuria is frequently the last finding to disappear during the convalescent phase of acute glomerulonephritis. Patients seen initially during this stage of their illness may have little to point to a recent attack of acute glomerulonephritis. Even when the diagnosis is suspected, if no red cell casts are identified and the hematuria does not subside promptly, diagnostic evaluation as outlined previously should be undertaken. After all studies are exhausted, a few instances of hematuria will remain undiagnosed, and for these the only course is continued observation.

IMMUNOLOGIC INJURY AND DIFFUSE RENAL DISEASE

In many diffuse renal diseases immunologic injury as the basis for renal damage is suggested by certain features of the clinical course of the illness plus demonstration of deposits within the kidney that contain constituents of an antigen-antibody reaction. The nature of the events directly responsible for renal injury remain unknown, but animal studies have defined two models of immunologic injury to the kidney that require complement fixation as the cytotoxic event. Both models, one involving production of antibodies to glomerular basement membrane and the other associated with circulating immune complexes, lead to deposition of immune globulins and complement in the kidney and result in progressive renal damage. Based on experience with immunofluorescent histopathology in these animals, the demonstration of gamma globulin plus one or more components of complement in any of the human glomerulonephritides have been viewed as acceptable evidence for an immunologic mechanism underlying the renal injury in these disorders. In practice, interpretation of the results of immunofluorescent studies on renal biopsies is more difficult (Table 11.2–4).

Identification of antigen plus antibody and complement fixation by immunofluorescent identification of the constituents of this reaction is complicated by the fact that there are two pathways for activating complement by immune reactions, and reported studies have not always been complete.[24,26,30,33,39,41] Nevertheless,

TABLE 11.2–5. CLASSIFICATION OF HEMATURIA

Disorder	Urinary Findings	Clinical Features
I. Local Disorders of Kidney and Genitourinary Tract		
Exercise	Microscopic hematuria	History of vigorous exercise immediately preceding the examination
Trauma	Hematuria varying from microscopic to gross	History of trauma to region of kidney
Cystitis	WBC and clumps Proteinuria (mild) Bacteriuria No casts	Urgency, frequency, dysuria
Renal, calculi	No casts or protein unless pyelonephritis present	Flank pain varying from dull ache to severe renal colic; occasionally gross hematuria
Genitourinary tumors	Hematuria of variable severity	Local symptoms depending on tumor location
Heritable disorders Hemoglobinopathies Osler–Weber–Rendu disease Polycystic disease	Hematuria usually grossly visible No casts	Usually no symptoms Occasionally mild flank pain Rarely, severe flank pain
Thrombocytopenic purpura	Only RBC in urine, no casts	No symptoms
II. Diffuse Renal Lesions[2,5,14,17,21,24]		
Glomerulonephritis, acute Rapidly progressing glomerulonephritis MP glomerulonephritis	RBC casts, WBC, proteinuria, granular casts	Smoky urine Occasionally clinical features of uremia only or heart failure or hypertension
Glomerulonephritis, chronic	RBC casts, WBC, proteinuria, granular casts and cellular casts	Few symptoms until malignant hypertension or uremia supervene
Systemic lupus erythematosus	May resemble those in acute glomerulonephritis	Fever and joint pain are most prominent features but many systems may be involved
Polyarteritis	Telescoped urine sediment with all types of casts plus RBC and WBC	May present as acute glomerulonephritis with uremia but no hypertension; fever, anemia and CNS involvement common
Goodpasture syndrome	RBC casts, gran. casts, proteinuria	Severe recurrent hemoptyses precede onset of symptoms of uremia
Allergic nephropathies Schönlein-Henoch purpura	Uringary findings of acute glomerulonephritis with gross hematuria	Gastrointestinal and joint manifestations of this type of purpura
Thrombotic thrombocytopenic purpura	Proteinuria and RBC casts	Fever Neurologic manifestations Hemolytic anemia, jaundice
Focal embolic glomerulitis	RBC casts Mild proteinuria	Subacute bacterial endocarditis usually present; mild renal insufficiency
Malignant hypertension	Rarely gross hematuria	Headache, decreasing vision and other manifestations of severe hypertension
Chemical or drug-induced Carbon tetrachloride	RBC casts, protein	Progressive uremia, jaundice, hepatomegaly
Sulfonamides	Crystals in urine	Occasionally progressive renal insufficiency
Anticoagulants	Hematuria	Other manifestations of bleeding diathesis
Benign essential hematuria	Hematuria, often gross, RBC casts, proteinuria <1 g/day	Hematuria, few or no symptoms, benign course (see text)

such reports provide presumptive evidence for an immunologic basis for the renal diseases listed in Table 11.2–4.

Despite much effort to associate specific patterns of immunoglobulin deposition within the glomerulus with specific disease categories, no unique associations have been observed to date (Table 11.2–4). Although it has been well documented that one or the other mode of complement activation may be seen most often in a particular type of renal disease, no unique clinical features or specific prognostic associations have emerged as characteristic features of a particular immunofluorescent pattern.

Acute Glomerulonephritis[2,5]

Clinical Features. The clinical features of severe acute glomerulonephritis are so striking that the disease may be recognized even before the urine is examined. The sequence of events characteristically begins with a sore throat associated with fever. This subsides in 4 to 8 days, to be followed in 2 to 3 weeks by the appearance of smoky urine, usually with reduction in urinary volume and swelling of face and ankles. The swelling is most marked in the morning and subsides during the day, only to be replaced by swelling of the ankles as evening approaches. These abnormalities are followed by progressive shortness of breath, weakness, lassitude, and anorexia. Breathlessness may be followed by acute pulmonary edema or other manifestations of circulatory congestion, particularly in older people. All the signs of uremia may soon appear and may lead to coma and convulsions. On physical examination, the facial edema is most readily apparent in the periorbital region. The dependent edema in other areas is associated with tight rubbery

consistency of the overlying skin, characteristic of rapid development of edema beneath skin of normal turgor and elasticity. There is usually evidence of hyperactive circulation with full bounding pulses and variable hypertension, the diastolic blood pressure occasionally exceeding 115 to 120 mm Hg. Generalized venous hypertension may be readily apparent clinically and can be confirmed by measurement of the venous pressure. Moist rales are found in the lungs, and pleural effusions may be noted; cardiomegaly and hepatomegaly may be present. Costovertebral angle tenderness is frequently noted and, on occasion, pain in this area may be of such severity as to suggest acute renal colic.

The urine is usually turbid and has a characteristic brown or smoky color; it is rarely grossly bloody. The amount of protein in the urine usually exceeds 100 mg/dl, and microscopic examination reveals numerous red blood cells and variable numbers of casts, including red blood cell casts. Anemia is usually present, its severity varying directly with the severity of the azotemia. The blood urea nitrogen and serum creatinine are elevated and, occasionally, plasma protein concentrations are lowered, with reversal of the A/G ratio. Antistreptolysin O (ASO) titer usually exhibits a rise some time during the course of the disease and may be the only evidence of antecedent beta-hemolytic streptococcal infection.

Course. The subsequent course is variable, but it is usually relatively short, with complete recovery in several weeks to 2 or 3 months. With appropriate treatment the symptoms of congestion subside and the fluid retention disappears after the first few days. Proteinuria may persist for several weeks and microscopic hematuria for several months, even in those patients who recover completely. In a small number of cases, the urinary findings show no tendency to clear. Fluid retention of variable severity persists, and the subsequent course is one of gradual deterioration—the development of progressive renal insufficiency leading to death in uremia within a few months. More often, when the urinary abnormalities fail to disappear, the acute illness is followed by a latent period of several years during which the only identifiable abnormalities are proteinuria and hematuria. This may be followed within from 1 to more than 20 years by the appearance of the nephrotic syndrome, usually refractory to therapy, which progresses slowly to uremia and death. Alternatively, the latent period may terminate in chronic renal insufficiency and uremia without appearance of the nephrotic stage. About 5 percent of patients die during the fulminant acute phase as a result of such conditions as acute pulmonary edema, acute encephalopathy, or uremia. Recovery rates are approximately the same for adults and children.

Not infrequently, the initial episode is so mild as to go unrecognized unless the patient happens to be under medical care for his initial pharyngitis. The only manifestations may be microscopic hematuria and red cell casts in the urine. The disease may be discovered fortuitously as a result of urinalysis done as part of a routine examination. Questioning may reveal a recent history of upper respiratory infection; however, efforts to uncover a history of an antecedent upper respiratory infection are frequently unsuccessful, and the diagnosis cannot be excluded on the basis of the absence of such a finding.

Etiology. There is no satisfactory etiologic classification of the sporadic cases of acute glomerulonephritis. The majority of cases arise as late sequelae of infections due to nephritogenic strains of beta-hemolytic streptococci. Although these infections usually involve the upper respiratory tract, they may also involve the skin or other tissues. Glomerulonephritis proven by biopsy has also been associated with pneumococcal infections and subacute infective endocarditis, usually due to the staphylococcus and sometimes viral infections.

The frequency of acute glomerulonephritis following streptococcal epidemics is related to specific types of the Group A beta-hemolytic streptococci. Types 12, 4, 1, and Red Lake have been identified as nephritogenic strains. Epidemics due to these types are associated with a relatively high incidence of acute glomerulo-

nephritis. Those patients who exhibit hematuria during the acute phase of the streptococcal infection appear to be more likely to develop acute glomerulonephritis subsequently than are those who do not. The importance of routine urine examination in patients with suspected streptococcal infection and the implications with respect to convalescent follow-up are self-evident.

Incidence. Acute glomerulonephritis may occur at any age but is rare under the age of 2. It is more common in children but is being recognized with increasing frequency in adults. The diagnosis is probably missed more often in adults because of the greater likelihood of attributing the accompanying renal insufficiency to other diseases, such as hypertensive vascular disease with nephrosclerosis. Its occurrence in *all* age groups cannot be overemphasized, and acute glomerulonephritis should be considered as a possible cause in *any* case of undiagnosed uremia of short duration. Its higher incidence in men than in women remains unexplained.

Pathology. The commonest lesion is proliferation of cells indigenous to the glomerular tuft. The earliest change is a proliferation of the endothelial cells. When severe, it may lead to complete occlusion of the majority of the capillary lumina. A characteristic feature of the poststreptococcal variety is the involvement of almost every glomerulus. Exudation of polymorphonuclear leukocytes is frequently seen. An interstitial reaction occasionally predominates. Later, as the reaction begins to subside, the pattern of hypercellularity exhibits a focal distribution, being found mainly in the axial regions of the glomerulus. The cells involved appear to be the mesangial cells. Proliferation of epithelial cells is also noted later in the disease but may be present within 3 weeks of onset. These latter changes are seen in patients who recover completely and are not necessarily associated with a bad prognosis.

Immunofluorescent staining of the renal biopsy material obtained from patients with poststreptococcal glomerulonephritis demonstrates the presence of IgG and complement (C3) as interrupted deposits on the epithelial side of the glomerular basement membrane (GBM). Occasionally, only complement can be demonstrated. Electron microscopy of the GBM also confirms the presence of large subepithelial deposits ("humps"). In studies where these accumulations in the GBM have been eluted from human renal tissue, it has been possible to demonstrate the presence of antistreptococcal antibody as part of the immune complex material removed from the GBM.

In the chronic stage of the disease, glomerular destruction and fibrosis develop with varying degrees of interstitial inflammation and scarring. As progressive destruction of renal tissue occurs, the remaining tubules become dilated and hypertrophied.

Treatment. Because of the relation between specific types of streptococci and nephritis, it is wise to treat all cases of acute glomerulonephritis with penicillin (600,000 units per day for 8 days). Exposed members of the family should receive prophylactic penicillin therapy for a similar period.

All patients should be kept in bed during the acute phase and at rest until the urine clears. This usually requires 3 to 4 weeks. Minimal proteinuria and hematuria are not contraindications to ambulation, but should the urinary abnormalities show a persistent increase with activity, the period of bed rest must be extended. Patients with persistent heavy proteinuria and hematuria but otherwise stable urinary function should be kept at rest for 6 weeks to 2 months before ambulation is undertaken. Subsequent physical activity should be restricted as long as the urinary abnormalities persist. This advice is based on the clear relationship that appears to exist between increasing activity and increasing urinary abnormalities.

Edema and hypertension call for rigid salt restriction. When this regimen is instituted promptly, acute hypertensive encephalopathy with convulsions can usually be avoided so that emergency measures to lower blood pressure will not be required. It is doubtful that digitalization is effective in combatting the circulatory con-

gestion of acute nephritis. If pulmonary edema develops, some form of dialysis must be considered.

There is no need to restrict protein intake unless there is severe oliguria, azotemia, and acidosis. The management of acute uremia in these patients does not differ from that of other forms of acute renal failure.

Rapidly Progressive Glomerulonephritis[14]

In a small percentage of patients with acute glomerulonephritis, there is no demonstrable tendency toward improvement, but instead there is a relatively rapid deterioration with end-stage renal failure occurring within 6 to 12 months of the initial onset of the disease. This course of glomerulonephritis, also termed "subacute" or "crescentic" glomerulonephritis, does not appear to have a unique etiology; some of the cases have been clearly identified as poststreptococcal, whereas others have been failed to yield any evidence for antecedent streptococcal infection. The renal biopsy is particularly helpful in identifying this group of patients. The presence, on biopsy specimens, of extensive crescent formation involving more than 50 percent of the glomeruli identifies this group and heralds a guarded prognosis. These patients do not respond to steroid or immunosuppressive therapy and require chronic dialysis or renal transplantation during the first year of illness.

GLOMERULONEPHRITIS ASSOCIATED WITH INFECTION

Several types of infection have an increased incidence of associated glomerulonephritis. The disturbance is seen particularly with staphylococcal sepsis of various sorts but most commonly as a complication of staphylococcal subacute infective endocarditis. This type of glomerulonephritis is frequently characterized by rapidly progressive renal insufficiency with all of the attendant manifestations described under acute glomerulonephritis except that hypertension is less striking. The microscopic examination of the urine shows the typical urinary sediment of acute glomerulonephritis with much hematuria, red cell casts, and numerous granular casts. This is an immune complex type glomerulonephritis, and it tends to improve, usually reversing completely when the infection is eradicated.[14,21,25] This entity is distinct from the focal embolic glomerulitis or glomerulonephritis that is a common accompaniment of subacute infective endocarditis regardless of the type of organism involved. The latter entity rarely is associated with any substantial degree of renal impairment and usually is characterized by the finding of microscopic hematuria and, rarely, red cell casts but little in the way of clinical manifestations. This type of glomerulonephritis has also been seen with staphylococcal endarteritis and other types of chronic staphylococcal sepsis.

Membranoproliferative (Hypocomplementemic) Glomerulonephritis

Membranoproliferative glomerulonephritis presents much more commonly as the nephrotic syndrome (Table 11.2–3). In approximately one third of cases, however, it is characterized by hematuria, azotemia, and some proteinuria without clinical manifestations of the nephrotic syndrome. It must therefore be kept in mind when considering the patients who present with hematuria and no stigmata of the nephrotic syndrome. It occurs in both children and adults and pursues a course that is usually relentlessly progressive and terminates in renal failure within 3 to 6 years. The disease is associated with characteristic histopathologic lesions in the glomerulus, and the patients also have persistently low levels of complement. The prognosis is guarded and the course is variable, often following an accelerated pattern. Treatment with prednisone, immunosuppressive agents, and anticoagulants has been unimpressive.

In addition to the three types of membranoproliferative glomerulonephritis considered previously, there is a fourth type that should perhaps be included here. The *mixed cryoglobulinemia* as-

sociated with renal disease exhibits a pathologic picture of membranoproliferative glomerulonephritis that is indistinguishable from those mentioned previously, and the course and prognosis are similar.[42] Treatment, including prednisone, anticoagulation, and immunosuppressive agents, has been disappointing.[42]

Systemic Lupus Erythematosus

Systemic lupus erythematosus is a disease of varied clinical manifestations that may involve—simultaneously or at different times—the skin, joints, pleura, pericardium, spleen and lymphatic system, and kidneys (Chapter 8.2). Renal involvement is probably the leading cause of death, but SLE rarely presents with renal disease alone. The diagnosis is usually clinically evident before kidney involvement is identified, though renal disease may dominate the clinical picture and on occasion the majority of the clinical course of the illness is manifested by renal involvement and minor joint abnormalities.

Renal disease usually occurs early in this disorder and manifests itself in proteinuria and microscopic hematuria. The urinary sediment may be indistinguishable from that of acute glomerulonephritis. The disease may present as the nephrotic syndrome, with heavy proteinuria in addition to hematuria and red cell casts. The picture of acute severe glomerulonephritis with oliguria, azotemia, acidosis, and clinical manifestations of uremia may be the predominant manifestation. Although such cases are rare, early recognition is imperative because treatment of SLE differs from that of acute hemorrhagic glomerulonephritis.

Pathology. There are four histologic categories of renal involvement in systemic lupus: (1) minimal glomerular involvement with mild mesangial proliferation; (2) focal glomerulonephritis (lupus glomerulitis); (3) an extramembranous ("membranous") form of lupus nephritis with subepithelial deposits; and (4) "diffuse proliferative" lupus nephritis with subendothelial deposits. In the proliferative form, hypercellularity is seen in one or more regions of a glomerulus, with hyaline thrombi and necrosis of portions of glomerular tufts. Very thick capillary loops ("wire loops") are seen in regions of the glomerulus that show less proliferation. The hematoxylin bodies that are generally considered to be pathognomonic of the nephritis of SLE can be demonstrated in only a small proportion of biopsies. The presence of antigen-antibody complexes in these membranous lesions has been clearly established, and such complexes have been eluted and identified as anti-DNA-DNA complexes. It appears likely that deposition of these complexes within the kidney represents one of the early initiating events in the production of lupus nephritis.[30] Electron micrographs have been reported to show an extraordinarily high incidence of viruslike particles in the glomeruli of patients with SLE as well as characteristic fingerprintlike whorling patterns within some of the deposits.[22,40] The etiologic significance and therapeutic implications of this finding remain to be evaluated.

Treatment. The general measures outlined in the section on treatment of acute glomerulonephritis also apply here. In addition, the use of corticosteroids has been shown to have a beneficial effect, although they are rarely successful in producing a remission of renal involvement except in early focal glomerular involvement.

The combination of azotemia and nephrotic syndrome heralds a poor prognosis. Focal glomerular lesions without such severe clinical manifestations, however, carry a more favorable prognosis. It also appears that long-term maintenance on high steroid dosage is not necessary to sustain a remission after the activity of the disease process has been arrested. The addition of azathioprine to the therapeutic regimen for lupus nephritis appears to offer some additional advantage.

Polyarteritis

Polyarteritis is a multiple system disorder exhibiting a variety of clinical manifestations that depend on the location of the vascular lesions (Chapter 8.3). The symptoms and signs may be related to

the joints, the gastrointestinal tract, the kidneys, and the peripheral and central nervous systems, among others. This involvement of many organ systems is usually the clinical feature arousing suspicion of the disease. On occasion, however, the predominant manifestations may indicate disease of a single system.

The kidneys are involved to a variable extent in the majority of cases. The renal lesions are of two types: (1) arteritic lesions of the medium-sized renal arterioles similar to those seen elsewhere in the vascular tree and (2) a diffuse type of glomerulonephritis. The first type may produce only microscopic hematuria without clinical evidence of renal insufficiency. In the usual case, other symptoms overshadow renal involvement, or at least are of sufficient magnitude to suggest the correct diagnosis. Less often, it presents as a primary renal disease, and differentiation from acute glomerulonephritis may be difficult.[16,40] Fluid retention and signs of circulatory congestion associated with clinical manifestations of uremia of variable severity are seen, and the disease may pursue a fulminant course leading to uremia and death. Absence of hypertension in the early acute phase of polyarteritis is the most helpful characteristic distinguishing this illness from acute glomerulonephritis. As the disease progresses, hypertension appears and may be severe. Patients presenting with milder forms of the disease may enter a chronic phase with progressive hypertension that may ultimately become malignant and result in death.

Urinary Sediment. The urinary findings are similar to those in acute glomerulonephritis. Proteinuria is variable but usually exceeds 100 mg/dl. Hematuria is almost always present, and numerous red blood cell casts and cellular casts are seen. The urinary sediment has been said to represent a "telescoped" picture of all the formed elements seen in the various stages of ordinary glomerulonephritis. When the renal involvement is confined to the larger vessels in the kidney, there may be only a trace of protein and a few red cells in the urine, the latter being present only intermittently.

Pathology. The majority of the polyarteritic lesions occur in the arcuate vessels. The histologic features of the nephritis include proliferative and destructive glomerular involvement. In the early stages, microthrombi are frequently seen, involving one or two capillary loops of the glomerulus. There may also be fibrinoid changes involving all or part of the tuft. Adhesions to Bowman's capsule are common and may be associated with epithelial proliferation and crescent formation. Hemorrhage may occasionally be seen in the capsular spaces or in the tufts, but the glomerular capillaries usually are bloodless and exhibit variable degrees of polymorphonuclear infiltration. In older lesions, complete hyalinization of glomeruli is common, and it is usual to find lesions showing virtually all stages of glomerular damage and destruction within the kidney, some glomeruli being completely spared. Immunofluorescent staining of the glomeruli and electron microscopy of the GBM indicate that the glomerular damage noted in polyarteritis is in large part caused by immune complex deposits in the GBM. In about one third of the cases so examined, hepatitis B antigen appears to be the antigenic component in the immune complex.

Treatment. The administration of adrenal steroids results in suppression of the acute inflammatory and necrotic arteriolar lesions. In some patients, the evidences of renal involvement may greatly improve or disappear altogether. The prognosis appears to be determined by the extent and stage of the renal lesions before treatment is initiated (Chapter 8.3). Even if no new lesions develop after steroids are given, the existing renal damage may be so severe that hypertension has already appeared. Hypotensive agents may be indicated in this case. Prompt institution of steroid therapy and maintenance of full suppression as long as evidence of active arteritis exists is necessary for optimal results.

Thrombotic Thrombocytopenic Purpura
Thrombotic thrombocytopenic purpura is characterized by a decrease in the number of circulating platelets associated with purpura, hemolytic anemia, signs of central nervous system involvement, and renal disease (Chapter 6.9). The onset is usually acute, with malaise, headache, fatigue, and myalgia occurring frequently. Fever, nausea, vomiting, and abdominal pain are common. Mild jaundice is often seen, and hepatosplenomegaly with generalized lymph node enlargement has been observed. There may be signs of congestive heart failure. Central nervous system manifestations include confusion, delirium, psychotic behavior, and stupor, along with focal neurologic signs. The anemia is hemolytic, and the abnormally shaped red blood cells are called "helmet cells" or "schizocytes"; leukocytosis is common, and a leukemoid reaction may be seen.

The kidneys are frequently involved, and signs of renal disease occasionally dominate the clinical picture. Examination of the urine reveals proteinuria, gross or microscopic hematuria, and frequently red blood cell, as well as granular, casts. Renal insufficiency and moderate azotemia are common, and severe uremia may develop. Histologic examination reveals eosinophilic thrombi in the arterioles of the kidney and locally within segments of the glomerular capillaries. Dramatic remissions have been induced by large doses of adrenocortical steroids, but in general the prognosis has been poor. The question of the efficacy of plasmapheresis remains unsettled. Anecdotal evidence suggests that this procedure has therapeutic value and should be considered in all cases exhibiting evidence of progressive deterioration of renal function.

Hemolytic-Uremic Syndrome
Hemolytic-uremic syndrome characteristically appears in previously healthy infants and young children. The clinical features are sudden onset of severe hemolytic anemia, renal failure associated with thrombocytopenia, and an associated characteristic appearance of the blood smear with helmet cells and schizocytes, burr cells, microspherocytes, moderate leukocytosis, and nucleated red cells. This constellation of findings on the blood smear, termed "microangiopathic change," has been reported also in persons with cardiac valvular prostheses and occasionally in disseminated carcinomatosis.

Azotemia appears early, and severe symptomatic uremia usually appears in the most severe cases within 3 to 5 days. Typically the urine contains moderate to large quantities of protein, red blood cells and red blood cell casts, and varying degrees of oliguria with a substantial portion of patients exhibiting complete anuria. The disease is endemic in the western United States and several other areas of the world, but epidemics have also been described, some in the wake of viral and bacterial infections.

Unless dialysis is instituted early, the mortality rate among the anuric patients may approach 50 to 75 percent. Uremia is the usual cause of death, and prompt institution of dialysis is effective in decreasing the mortality rate. Although substantial improvement in renal function occurs in most patients who are managed by early and adequate dialysis, long-term follow-up indicates that the majority have some persistent renal impairment and associated hypertension. In rare instances neurologic deficits may persist.

Histologically the changes occurring within the kidney closely resemble the ones described in thrombotic thrombocytopenic purpura, including thickened glomerular capillary walls, obstruction of variable numbers of afferent and efferent arterioles by homogeneous eosinophilic hyaline thrombi containing large quantities of fibrin. This patchy vascular occlusion leads to infarction of complete glomeruli, and in some instances infarctions of larger areas of the kidneys are seen. The primary pathogenesis appears to be related to intravascular coagulation, but the repeated documentation of association with viral epidemics and with sporadic cases of viral infection raises the question of an underlying infectious cause. At present, management is confined to treatment of the uremia and early institution of dialysis. Because of the extensive intravascular coagulation numerous reports of the beneficial effects of systemic heparin have appeared, but these are difficult to evaluate because a substantial portion of the patients recover with improvement in renal function without any treatment other than dialysis.

Goodpasture Syndrome

The essential features of Goodpasture syndrome are profuse and persistent hemoptysis, followed by the development of rapidly progressive renal insufficiency, often leading to death within a few months. Hemoptysis may be the only initial manifestation, antedating all clinical evidence of renal disease by several weeks or more. Urine examination at this time usually shows albuminuria, hematuria, and red blood cell casts.

The glomerular lesion varies in severity, depending on the stage of the patient's clinical illness. These early lesions are of a focal nature that then become more extensive with crescent formation in the glomeruli, localized foci of necrosis in the capillary loops, and deposition of fibrin in Bowman's space. Immunofluorescent studies demonstrate the homogenous linear deposition of IgG along the basement membrane of the glomerular capillary loops.

This is the classic example of glomerular disease induced by the presence of antiglomerular basement membrane antibody. Common antigenic properties of the basement membrane of the lung and glomeruli have been identified and probably are responsible for the pulmonary involvement in the condition.[17]

Clinically, the disease usually progresses rapidly to end-stage renal disease, but high doses of corticosteroids may slow or arrest the progression of the disease in a few instances. Chronic dialysis and subsequent renal transplantation are of value. In some instances, bilateral nephrectomy after beginning dialysis has been associated with prompt cessation of hemoptysis. Recently, plasmapheresis combined with vigorous immunosuppression has been shown to be of some benefit in arresting the progress of the renal damage, with some reports emphasizing dramatic cessation of pulmonary hemorrhage following such treatment.

Nephritis Associated with Schönlein-Henoch Purpura[14,35]

Progressive renal disease may be associated with recurrent allergic purpura, evidenced by the early appearance and persistence of microscopic hematuria. In perhaps 25 percent of the cases the hematuria persists even after the acute skin changes have cleared. There is usually an exacerbation of the urinary findings associated with recurrence of the dermal lesions. The renal disease is slowly progressive, and the associated clinical manifestations are similar to those seen in chronic glomerulonephritis. Proteinuria accompanies the hematuria, and occasionally the nephrotic syndrome develops. Patients exhibiting persistent proteinuria, and hematuria when dermal manifestations are quiescent, usually develop hypertension and uremia eventually.

Histologic examination of the kidney usually demonstrates a focal lesion in the glomerulus and a characteristic increase in the mesangial matrix. The focal cellularity tends to increase as the disease increases. Immunofluorescence studies reveal fairly heavy depositions of IgA confined largely to the mesangial area. Smaller quantities of IgG are demonstrable, and complement deposition can usually be demonstrated.

The dermatologic manifestations of the disease usually respond promptly to treatment with corticosteroids. Such treatment also suppresses acute activity in the kidney, but it is doubtful whether the ultimate outcome of the renal disease is influenced. In many respects, the renal involvement in this disorder is similar to that seen in IgA nephropathy (Berger disease), although it is distinguished by appearance at an earlier age and more rapid progression.

IgA Nephropathy (Berger Disease)

This disease typically presents in adolescence and early adulthood and is almost always characterized initially by gross hematuria associated with proteinuria that is usually mild but may at times be quite heavy. Characteristically the attacks of gross hematuria are episodic and usually widely separated in time, but it is almost always possible to identify persistent microscopic hematuria during the intervals between attacks. It afflicts men more commonly than women and is usually associated with slowly progressing renal impairment. The circulating levels of immunoglobulin IgA are elevated, and it has been possible to demonstrate increased quantities of aggregated IgA or large-molecular-weight complexes containing IgA.[31]

Renal biopsy early in the disease reveals focal nephritis with some glomeruli showing localized areas of hypercellularity—presumably due to proliferation of endothelial and mesangial cells. Adhesions and crescents are frequent. In other instances, an entire glomerulus may show these changes of hypercellularity while adjacent glomeruli appear normal. These acute lesions are replaced by generalized or focal glomerular scars, and later in the disease nearly all glomeruli are affected, with changes resembling severe diffuse glomerulonephritis. Immunologic staining and electron microscopic evaluation of the glomeruli demonstrate, in particular, the presence of changes in the mesangial or stalk portions of the glomerular tuft. IgG, IgA, C3, and fibrinogen are frequently noted in the electron-dense deposits in the mesangium and contiguous segments of the peripheral capillary loops.[34]

No treatment capable of arresting the progression of the disease has been demonstrated, though phenytoin has been demonstrated to reduce the IgA aggregation in the plasma.[31] Whether this exerts any influence on the progressive renal impairment remains to be demonstrated. There are several very interesting parallels between this renal disease and that encountered in Schönlein-Henoch purpura.[19,35,36] The prevalence varies between countries, with France and Japan exhibiting remarkably high instances of IgA nephropathy and Schönlein-Henoch purpura. The prevalence ranges from 25 to 40 percent in these countries to a low of 3 percent in the United States for IgA nephropathy. In France, where the most detailed prevalence data are available, the incidence of IgA nephropathy is approximately twice that of Schönlein-Henoch nephropathy.[6,19] Histologically the appearance of the kidney is similar, with virtually identical immunofluorescence findings. In all cases, however, the IgA deposition is more intense in Schönlein-Henoch purpura than in IgA and is not confined to the mesangium in the former but very often can also be seen densely deposited along the capillary loops. One may speculate that these two apparently different disorders are both related to immune complex disturbances involving IgA as the primary immunoglobulin in the circulating complexes and that the difference merely relates to the severity of the disease.[19,35] Until the antigens responsible for these circulating complexes can be identified and measured this is only speculation.

CONTRIBUTION OF GLOMERULONEPHRITIS TO EPIDEMIOLOGIC CHARACTERISTICS OF END-STAGE RENAL DISEASE IN THE U.S.

Most of the diseases discussed in this chapter ultimately terminate in end-stage renal disease and require maintenance dialysis. It was long thought that these diseases, together with other entities such as polycystic renal disease, interstitial renal disease, and chronic pyelonephritis, contributed the major portion of patients to dialysis programs in this country and elsewhere. The Health Care Financing Administration has maintained statistics on the rate of entry and growth of the dialysis population in the United States since the national program of financing for dialysis began. This includes classification of end-stage renal disease according to diagnosis. Total end-stage renal disease enrollment in dialysis programs quadrupled nationwide between the years 1974 and 1981[18]; it is now documented that the United States has one of the highest incidence rates of end-stage renal disease in the world.

Table 11.2–6 presents the data on end-stage renal disease incidence nationally for the years 1978 through 1980. Incidence rate is expressed as new cases per year per one million population. Virtually all the diagnostic entities considered in this chapter are included in the diagnostic category glomerulonephritis in Table 11.2–6. It is apparent that glomerulonephritis accounts for only

TABLE 11.2–6. INCIDENCE RATES BY DIAGNOSTIC CATEGORY FOR END-STAGE RENAL DISEASE PATIENTS ENTERING DIALYSIS IN THE U.S. BETWEEN 1978 AND 1980

Diagnosis	No. per Million Population		
	1978	*1979*	*1980*
Glomerulonephritis	15	16	16
Hypertensive nephropathy	16	17	19
Diabetic nephropathy	13	15	18
Interstitial nephritis	6	6	6
Polycystic kidney disease	5	5	5
Collagen vascular disease	1	1	1
All cases	71	78	82

Modified from Eggers PW, Connerton R, McMullan M: Health Care Financing Rev 5:69, 1984.[18]

about 20 percent of the total number of cases. Interestingly, this has remained virtually unchanged during the 3 years examined here. In contrast, both hypertensive nephropathy and diabetic nephropathy are increasing at rates that range from 5 to 10 percent per year. Diabetic nephropathy in particular appears to be increasing in incidence at a rate that is approximately 20 percent per year. Thus hypertension and diabetes are accounting for an increasingly large proportion (nearly half) of the total number of patients who present each year with newly recognized terminal renal failure. In contrast polycystic kidney disease has remained unchanged at five cases per million population per year, as would be expected if ascertainment is virtually complete for each year.

Of additional interest is the remarkable difference in racial incidence that emerged from these national data. For most diagnostic categories the incidence in males was nearly 40 percent higher than in females. Of greatest significance, however, was the finding that the overall incidence rate for blacks was 2.8 times that seen among white people. The greatest difference was seen in hypertensive nephropathy; black entrants exhibited an incidence rate more than six times as great as that of whites. These findings emphasize that the glomerulonephritides considered as a group account for only a minority of the total cases of end-stage renal disease and that the contributions made by hypertension and diabetes mellitus need much more careful attention if appropriate preventive measures are to be identified. General confirmation of these findings has appeared in the Canadian Renal Failure Registry where, for the year 1985, glomerulonephritis of all types accounted for only 22 percent of the newly diagnosed patients with end-stage renal failure, and diabetic nephropathy accounted for 20 percent.[37]

REFERENCES

1. Abramowicz M, Barnett HL, et al: Controlled trial of azathioprine in children with nephrotic syndrome. Lancet 1:959, 1970
2. Addis T: Haemorrhagic Bright's disease: Natural history. Johns Hopkins Med J 49:203, 1931
3. Alyea EP, Parrish AH Jr: Renal response to exercise. Urinary findings. JAMA 167:807, 1958
4. Barnett HL: The natural and treatment history of glomerular diseases in children. In Giovannetti S, Bonomini V, D'Amico G (eds): Proceedings of the Sixth International Congress of Nephrology. Basel, Karger, 1975, p 470
5. Bates RC, Jennings RB, Earle DP: Acute nephritis unrelated to group A hemolytic streptococcus infection. Am J Med 23:510, 1957
6. Berger J, Noel L–H, Yanerva H: Complement deposition in the kidney. In Hamburger J, Crosner J, Maxwell M (eds): Advances in Nephrology, vol 4. Chicago, Year Book Medical Publishers, 1974
7. Berman LB, Schreiner GE: Clinical and histologic spectrum of the nephrotic syndrome. Am J Med 24:249, 1958
8. Black DAK, Rose G, Brewer DB: Controlled trial of prednisone in adult patients with the nephrotic syndrome. Br Med J 3:421, 1970
9. Blainey JD: High protein diets in the treatment of the nephrotic syndrome. Clin Sci 13:567, 1954
10. Brenner BM, Rector FC Jr (eds): The Kidney, 2d ed. Philadelphia, WB Saunders, 1981, vols 1 and 2
11. Cameron JS, Chantler C, et al: Long-term stability of remission in nephrotic syndrome after treatment with cyclophosphamide. Br Med J 4:7, 1974
12. Cameron JS, Turner DR, et al: The nephrotic syndrome in adults with minimal change lesions. Q J Med 43:461, 1974
13. Chinard FP, Lawson HE, et al: A study of the mechanism of proteinuria in patients with the nephrotic syndrome. J Clin Invest 33:621, 1954
14. Churg J, Sobin LH: Renal Disease. Classification and Atlas of Glomerular Diseases. New York, Igaku-Shoin, 1982
15. Coggins CH, Pinn V, et al: A controlled study of short-term prednisone treatment in adults with membranous nephropathy. N Engl J Med 301:1301, 1979
16. Davson J, Ball J, Platt R: Kidney in periarteritis nodosa. Q J Med 17:175, 1948
17. Earley L, Gottschalk C (eds): Strauss and Welt's Diseases of the Kidney, 3d ed. Boston, Little, Brown, 1979
18. Eggers PW, Connerton R, McMullan M: The medicare experience with end-stage renal disease: Trends in incidence, prevalence, and survival. Health Care Financing Rev 5:69, 1984
19. Egido J, Sancho J, et al: Immunopathogenetic aspects of IgA nephropathy. Adv Nephrol 12:103, 1983
20. Ellis A: Natural history of Bright's disease: Clinical, histological and experimental observations. Croonian Lectures. Lancet 1:1, 1942
21. Germuth FD Jr, Rodriguez E: Immunopathology of the Renal Glomerulus. Immunocomplex Deposit and Antibasement Membrane Disease. Boston, Little, Brown, 1973
22. Grausz H, Earley LE, et al: Virus-like particles in glomerular endothelium of patients with SLE. N Engl J Med 283:506, 1970
23. Gregoire F, Malmendier C, Lambert PP: The mechanism of proteinuria, and a study of the effects of hormonal therapy in the nephrotic syndrome. Am J Med 25:516, 1948
24. Habib R, Loirat C, et al: Morphology and serum complement levels in membranoproliferative glomerulonephritis. In Hamburger J, Crosner J, Maxwell M (eds): Advances in Nephrology, vol 4. Chicago, Year Book Medical Publishers, 1974
25. Heptinstall RH: Pathology of the Kidney, 2d ed. Boston, Little, Brown, 1974, vol 1, p 273
26. Herdman RC, Pickering RJ, et al: Chronic glomerulonephritis associated with low serum complement activity (chronic hypocomplementemic glomerulonephritis). N Engl J Med 283:506, 1970
27. Hopper J, Ryan P, et al: Lipoid nephrosis in 31 adult patients: Renal biopsy study by light, electron and fluorescence microscopy with experience in treatment. Medicine 49:321, 1970
28. Hunsiker LG, Ruddy S, et al: Metabolism of third complement component (C3) in nephritis. Involvement of the classical and alternate (properdin) pathways for complement activation. N Engl J Med 287:835, 1972
29. Kark RM, Pirani CL, et al: The nephrotic syndrome in adults: A common disorder with many causes. Ann Intern Med 49:751, 1958
30. Koffler D, Kunkel HG: Mechanisms of renal injury in systemic lupus erythematosus. Am J Med 45:165, 1968
31. Lopes-Trascasa M, Egido J, Sancho J: Evidence of high polymeric IgA in serum of patients with Berger's disease and its modification with phenytoin treatment. Proc Eur Dial Transplant Assoc 16:513, 1979
32. Michael AF, McLean RH: Evidence for activation of the alternate pathway in glomerulonephritis. In Hamburger J, Crosner J, Maxwell M (eds): Advances in Nephrology, vol 4. Chicago, Year Book Medical Publishers, 1974
33. Morel-Maroger L, Leathem A, Richet G: Glomerular abnormalities in non-systemic disease. Am J Med 53:170, 1972
34. Muller-Eberhard HJ: The complement system and nephritis. In Hamburger J, Crosner J, Maxwell M (eds): Advances in Nephrology, vol. 4. Chicago, Year Book Medical Publishers, 1974
35. Nakamoto Y, Asano Y, et al: Primary IgA glomerulonephritis and Schönlein-Henoch purpura nephritis. Clinicopathological and immunohistological characteristics. Q J Med 47:495, 1978
36. Nomoto Y, Sakai H, et al: Immunopathologic and histologic studies on benign recurrent hematuria. Clinicopathologic similarities with IgA nephropathy. Am J Pathol 94:51, 1979
37. Posen GA: Canadian Renal Failure Register: 1985 Report. Toronto, The Kidney Foundation of Canada, 1986, p 73
38. Report of Medical Research Council Working Party. Controlled trial of azathioprine and prednisone in chronic renal disease. Br Med J 2:239, 1971

39. Ruley EJ, Forrestal J, et al: Hypocomplementemia of membranoprolif-erative nephritis. Dependence of nephrotic factor reaction on proper-din factor. Br J Clin Invest 52:896, 1973
40. Walker WG, Solez K: Renal involvement in disorders of connective tissue. In Earley LE, Gottschalk GW (eds): Strauss and Welt's Diseases of the Kidney. Boston, Little, Brown, 1979
41. Westberg NG, Naff GB, et al: Glomerular deposition of properdin in acute and chronic glomerulonephritis with hypocomplementemia. J Clin Invest 50:642, 1971
42. World Health Organization Scientific Group. The role of immune complexes in disease. Geneva, World Health Organization Technical Report Series H606, 1977

CHAPTER 11.3

Chronic Pyelonephritis and Other Tubulointerstitial Nephropathies

W. Gordon Walker

The original reports of Weiss and Parker[34] and Raaschou[28] proposed that more than half of the deaths due to uremia during the preantibiotic era could be attributed to chronic pyelonephritis. Their diagnoses were based primarily on histopathologic findings. Subsequent studies indicate that the histopathologic entity that they designated "chronic pyelonephritis" is in fact a group of diseases exhibiting more or less interstitial inflammation with edema and variable tubular damage as the primary tissue abnormality. Extensive clinical, bacteriologic, histologic, and epidemiologic data have established that only a small number of these cases can be attributed to chronic bacterial infection. The characteristic histologic picture exhibited by this group of disorders may be reproduced by drug reactions, heavy metal poisonings, allergic phenomena, metabolic disturbances, and some hereditary disorders. The more general term "tubulointerstitial nephropathy" has been used to designate this histopathologic entity. Accurate diagnosis and treatment requires a knowledge of the various agents that can produce this picture as well as a clear understanding of the difference between urinary tract infection, chronic pyelonephritis, and the noninfectious causes of interstitial inflammatory disease of the kidney. Table 11.3–1 contains a list of the more common causes of tubulointerstitial nephritis. The major groups are discussed below.

CHRONIC PYELONEPHRITIS[3,28,34]

The typical clinical presentation of acute pyelonephritis constitutes fever, often exceeding 38C; chills; flank pain; dysuria; and marked pyuria, including numerous clumps of white blood cells as well as white blood cell casts in the urine. This disorder is seen most commonly in women during the child-bearing years and is often first noted during pregnancy. Azotemia rarely develops in association with acute uncomplicated pyelonephritis. When the disease complicates diabetes, however, the risk of renal papillary necrosis is significant, and progressive deterioration of renal function may ensue.

This process or disease was long considered to represent a complication of lower urinary tract infection that ascended from the bladder through the ureters to the kidneys. The corollary, that recurrent urinary tract infections were associated with a high risk of pyelonephritis leading to progressive renal damage, was also generally accepted. Although this may indeed be the route of spread that results in the development of acute pyelonephritis, recent evidence indicates that it is rare that this leads to a chronic infection that progresses to renal failure with uremia. Several long-term follow-up studies of persistent or recurrent bacteriuria have failed to identify such a connection. Freedman[11,12] found no evidence for progressive renal failure or hypertension during a 12-year follow-up of 250 women with urinary tract infection. Similar results were reported by Asscher.[2] Freeman[13] conducted a similar study in 249

men and was only able to identify progressive loss of renal function in patients who had severe underlying urologic disease. Even those patients who had abnormal pyelograms did not provide any evidence for progressive loss of renal function unless the course was complicated by hypertension, diabetes mellitus, or analgesic abuse.

More recent pathologic studies[11,17,27] have questioned whether most of the cases exhibiting signs of tubulointerstitial nephropathy at postmortem examination were in fact attributable to infection. In the study of Murray and Goldberg,[27] none of their 100 cases of chronic interstitial nephritis could be attributed to infections as the primary cause of the renal damage. Abnormalities of the urinary tract, analgesic abuse, and obstruction were the primary disturbance in more than half the cases. In perhaps a third of these, infection was reported as an important secondary factor. Thus in adults there is little evidence that recurrent urinary tract infection leads to pyelonephritis that becomes a chronic and progressive disease terminating in uremia, unless there is some underlying abnormality of the genitourinary system or serious systemic illness.

The situation is somewhat different in childhood. Early difficulty with urinary tract infection (before the age of 4 or 5 years) is frequently associated with vesicoureteral reflux. This condition predisposes to retrograde infection of the kidneys and the development of progressive renal scarring, atrophy, and loss of function. In fact, many of these individuals display evidence of scarring of the kidneys before age 5 and in the extreme case also show evidence of the characteristic deformity of the Ast-Upmark kidneys.[19] During subsequent follow-up these patients usually exhibit evidence of progressive loss of renal function. A more detailed treatment of this problem can be found in the pediatric literature. It should be emphasized that this difference in the course of urinary tract infections in children requires a different therapeutic approach[7,24,29] with earlier and more vigorous attempts to identify or exclude underlying reflux or other abnormalities.

Bacteriuria during pregnancy deserves special attention because these women are at high risk for the development of complications, including acute pyelonephritis, which require hospitalization and vigorous treatment.[3,22,25] There is some question whether the risk of maternal toxemia and neonatal prematurity may be increased under these circumstances. The increase in fetal wastage, the greater frequency of low-birth-weight infants, and the possible increased risk of maternal toxicity underscore the importance of regular checkups that include urine cultures and prompt treatment of bacteriuria in pregnant women.

TREATMENT

Patients with overt clinical pyelonephritis should be hospitalized for parenteral antibiotic therapy, and because nearly one fifth of such cases exhibit resistance to penicillin derivatives, initial therapy

TABLE 11.3–1. CLASSIFICATION OF TUBULOINTERSTITIAL NEPHROPATHY

Acute
- Bacterial
- Viral
- Drug-induced

Chronic
Chronic Bacterial Pyelonephritis
- Vesicoureteral reflux
    With infection
    Without infection
- Tuberculous pyelonephritis

Drug-induced Chronic Tubulointerstitial Nephropathy
- Analgesic nephropathy
- Penicillins
- Nonsteroidal anti-inflammatory agents

Metabolic Disorders
- Hypercalcemia
- Hyperoxaluria
- Hyperuricemia
- Cystinosis

Heavy Metals
- Lead
- Cadmium
- Mercury
- Gold

Hereditary Disorders (Chapter 11.6)
- Medullary cystic disease
- Familial interstitial nephritis

Miscellaneous
- Balkan nephropathy
- Sarcoidosis

should include an aminoglycoside. Such parenteral therapy should be continued for 4 to 7 days, or longer if the patient does not recover promptly during this period. Antibiotic treatment should be continued orally for 4 to 6 weeks. If an aminoglycoside is used, however, blood levels should be monitored at regular intervals to avoid toxicity. This drug should be discontinued and some oral agent to which the organism is sensitive substituted as soon as the acute manifestations are under control.

When the infection is complicated by the presence of renal stone or obstruction, these problems should be dealt with as soon as the acute infection is under control. It is extremely unlikely that the infection can be cured without relief of obstruction or removal of the stone, because it has been demonstrated that the organisms actually reside within stones. In this event even substantial blood levels of bactericidal drugs are unsuccessful in completely eliminating the infection.[31] The new technique of *lithotripsy* as a means of achieving dissolution and passage of these infected stones may greatly facilitate management in these difficult cases.

Radiologic and detailed urologic evaluation of these patients with recurrent urinary tract infections remains controversial. Recent studies,[8,9,10] including a total of nearly 500 women with recurrent urinary tract infections, revealed an incidence of abnormality that ranged from 3 to 5 percent, but these findings did not influence clinical management. Nevertheless, since as noted previously the risk of infection is much greater in those patients with stone and obstruction, it is essential to search for these factors, particularly in individuals who develop acute pyelonephritis as a complication of the urinary tract infection. A high index of suspicion for either of these conditions is essential so that proper measures to detect them can be instituted.

Men have relatively little difficulty with urinary tract infection until they pass age 50, when prostatic disease increases bacteriuria. It should also be stressed that men who have symptomatic urinary tract infections almost always have some predisposing anatomic abnormality of the genitourinary tract, the most common being bladder neck obstruction associated with prostatic enlargement. Distinguishing between prostatic infection and bladder infection in men is best done with the three-glass test.[26] The first voided portion (glass 1) reflects the bacterial flora of the urethra; the midstream, or glass 2, identifies material from the bladder; and glass 3, obtained by voiding immediately after prostatic massage, reflects the bacterial flora of the prostate. A sufficiently large volume of urine should be cultured to detect low concentrations of bacteria.

The treatment of uncomplicated lower urinary tract infection has been developed in a way that provides further useful diagnostic information.[20] Ingelfinger et al demonstrated that the simple, uncomplicated lower urinary tract infection could be treated successfully with a single dose of agents such as ampicillin or trimethoprim-sulfamethoxazole.[20] If, however, cure was not achieved by a single dose, there was a high incidence (80 percent) of radiologic abnormality on subsequent investigation. In contrast, conventional therapy given three times daily for periods of 10 days failed to discriminate between individuals with and without radiologic abnormalities. These authors proposed that for the simple and uncomplicated lower urinary tract infection, single-dose therapy should be tried first. Moreover in follow-up they found it important to characterize the organisms as completely as possible so the physician could establish whether reappearance of infection was simply a recrudescence of the preexisting infection or a new infection caused by a different organism. The former circumstance makes it much more likely that obstruction, stone, or some other complicating abnormality is present, indicating the necessity for further investigation.

RENAL TUBERCULOSIS

The natural history of renal tuberculosis is so distinct that it is unlikely to be confused with other forms of chronic bacterial pyelonephritis. It is such a significant and severe form of bacterial infection of the kidney, however, that it should always be entertained as a diagnostic possibility in patients presenting with hematuria and "sterile" pyuria.

Spread of renal tuberculosis occurs virtually always from a primary pulmonary focus. Early studies revealed the presence of miliary tubercles in the kidney of one fourth of patients dying of the disease. Approximately one fifth of these patients had already developed cavitary and fibrotic-renal tuberculosis. The currently accepted pathogenesis characterizes renal tuberculosis as resulting from blood-borne bacilli arising from the pulmonary lesion. These tend to lodge primarily in the glomeruli, resulting in miliary foci of tuberculosis, but some rupture into tubules, thereby producing both bacilluria and hematuria. The subsequent course is one of relentless and fairly rapidly progressive destruction of renal tissue with spread to the ureter and bladder and, in men, the epididymal structures as well.

The patient presents most often with asymptomatic microhematuria or sterile pyuria. On occasion the course at this early stage of the disease may be punctuated by intermittent gross hematuria. As the lesion extends and the bladder becomes involved, cystitis with urgency, frequency, and strangury may dominate the clinical picture. This is particularly true in women. Because hematuria and sterile pyuria often precede any identifiable abnormality of the collecting system or deformity of the renal shadow in excretory urograms, it is essential to culture the urine of all patients with microscopic hematuria for *Mycobacterium tuberculosis* if a definitive diagnosis has not been established by other means.

The incidence of renal tuberculosis has decreased, but the disease is not a rarity. Careful studies in the United Kingdom and in the United States show that the incidence of renal tuberculosis is about 10 percent of the incidence of pulmonary tuberculosis. It is still decreasing at a rate of about 10 percent per year, but it remains sufficiently common that the diagnosis should be entertained in all patients presenting with unexplained hematuria or pyuria. Successful treatment is more difficult than in pulmonary tuberculosis, and

antibiotics should be continued for longer periods. Isoniazid produces bactericidal concentrations in the urine, as do rifampin and pyrazinamide. The current recommendation is to use at least three drugs capable of achieving concentration levels that are bactericidal against *M. tuberculosis* in the urine. The combination of isoniazide, rifampin, and either ethambutol or pyrazinamide is recommended. The prevailing evidence indicates that a minimum of 2 years of continuous therapy with at least two drugs is essential to minimize recurrence. Although more recent reports suggest that the use of three drugs for shorter periods may be curative, these data are based on studies of patients with pulmonary tuberculosis, and no long-term follow-up of renal tuberculosis after as little as 6 months of therapy with three drugs is yet available. Until such time as persuasive information on this point is available, prudence dictates the longer course of treatment.

Patients with renal tuberculosis are highly infectious; 25 percent of children living with parents with genitourinary tuberculosis develop positive tuberculin reactions, even in families whose only source of bacterial exposure is the urine. Appropriate precautions therefore should include isolation of the bed clothes.

Long-term follow-up is an important part of management. After therapy ends, all patients should have careful microscopic examinations of the urine every 2 months with culture. At semiannual intervals they should have cystoscopy for the first 5 years and then yearly for another 10. Even when the disease is detected and treated early, a very careful watch for development of strictures over this extended period is essential. Eight to ten percent of patients develop ureteral stricture, and perhaps as many as a third of these progress to complete ureteric occlusion.

OTHER TYPES OF INTERSTITIAL NEPHROPATHY

DRUG-INDUCED ACUTE TUBULOINTERSTITIAL NEPHRITIS

The syndrome of rapidly progressing renal failure associated with hematuria, pyuria, mild proteinuria, and often eosinophiluria associated with the clinical picture of fever, rash, and eosinophilia called attention to the type of renal impairment that was thought at first to be specifically related to methicillin. It is now clear that this was the first of a large number of such reactions associated with other penicillin derivatives as well as a variety of other drugs (Table 11.3–2). Biopsy reveals infiltration of the renal parenchyma by inflammatory cells with accompanying interstitial edema and patchy tubular degeneration. This type of drug reaction occurs three times more often in men. The basis for this male preponderance remains unclear.

Most patients with drug-related, acute tubulointerstitial nephropathy develop some degree of renal failure. It may be nonoliguric or oliguric. The majority of cases do not show any significant diminution in urine volume. The only distinctive feature on examination of the urine is eosinophiluria.[14] In careful examination of the urine sediment of 52 patients with acute renal failure, however, only nine patients with penicillin-related interstitial nephropathy exhibited this finding. It should also be noted here that the urinary sodium:creatinine ratio in acute interstitial nephritis resembles that seen in acute renal failure of other causes. Gallium scanning of the kidney has revealed intense uptake in some instances, but this may also occur in many other renal disorders. Its diagnostic value is thus of limited usefulness.

Disturbances of renal tubular function may be seen, including abnormal urinary acidification with a picture resembling that of distal renal tubular acidosis, abnormalities of potassium excretion, and disorders of the concentrating mechanism. These are not striking clinical features of drug-induced acute tubulointerstitial nephritis, however, and the most common presentation is that of rapidly progressing renal failure.

The histopathology is characterized by an irregular but usually

TABLE 11.3–2. DRUG-INDUCED ACUTE INTERSTITIAL NEPHROPATHY

Antibiotics
- Penicillins
- Cephalothins
- Vancomycin
- Rifampin
- Ethambutol

Diuretics
- Thiazides
- Furosemide
- Chlorthalidone

Miscellaneous
- Sulfonamides
- Phenindione
- Phenytoin
- Cimetidine
- Allopurinol
- Sulfinpyrazone

Nonsteroidal Antiinflammatory Drugs
- Indomethacin
- Phenylbutazone
- Fenoprofen
- Naproxen
- Ibuprofen

extensive infiltration of the renal interstitium by an inflammatory exudate and associated edema. The kidneys do not usually exhibit the fibrosis seen with long-standing or chronic interstitial nephritis. The cellular types include lymphocytes and eosinophilia, though the presence of eosinophilia is not necessary for the diagnosis.[14,18] Although the pathologic findings are usually attributed to an allergic or hypersensitivity reaction and often are associated with systemic manifestations of allergy including rash and fever, this is not uniformly the case. Some, but not all, cases have demonstrable antibodies that react with tubular basement membranes. Immune complexes have been demonstrated in tubular basement membrane deposits that contain IgG and complement.[4] The current view, however, is that the disturbances depend primarily on a cell-mediated mechanism and that antibody formation and reaction are secondary phenomena.[1]

Treatment includes immediate withdrawal of the offending agent and treatment of uremia, including early dialysis when necessary. If continued antibiotic treatment is essential, it is important to avoid drugs that may exhibit cross-reactivity. Benefits associated with the use of corticosteroids have been reported, but this issue has not been subjected to prospective randomized clinical trial. Galpin et al[14] reported the most dramatic shortening of duration of penicillin-induced renal failure in rsponse to corticosteroid administration.

Numerous other drugs have been reported to produce acute interstitial nephritis (Table 11.3–2). Reports of this syndrome due to trimethoprim-sulfamethoxazole, rifampin, and the majority of available nonsteroidal anti-inflammatory agents represent the most frequent and convincing documentation that numerous drugs are capable of producing acute and usually reversible episodes of renal failure associated with interstitial nephropathy. As with penicillin, clinical evidence of systemic allergic reactions to the offending agent may not be present, and a high index of suspicion is necessary if early diagnosis is to be made. Early drug withdrawal appears to improve the likelihood of reversal of the renal damage. The principles of management of all these other drug-induced interstitial nephropathies are similar to the approach outlined in the penicillin-induced disease and consist of withdrawal of the drug and conservative management of renal failure (Chapter 11.5), supplemented with hemodialysis as necessary.

INTERSTITIAL NEPHROPATHY INDUCED BY HEAVY METALS

Acute renal failure as one of the major clinical manifestations of heavy metal poisoning is widely recognized, and mercury was once the most commonly encountered cause. There is, however, equally impressive evidence for interstitial nephritis as a complication, as chronic heavy metal exposure dates back to the last century.[33] Progressive renal failure associated with interstitial nephritis is a consequence of long-standing lead exposure. Patients at risk for the development of this progressive chronic renal disorder include children who are exposed to lead poisoning from eating paint (pica), as well as numerous workers who are exposed to lead fumes or other lead exposure. Though the entity has been publicized because of association of lead toxicity with consumption of illicitly distilled "moonshine" whiskey, recognition of lead toxicity in the workplace is in fact quite difficult in the absence of exposure to sufficiently high concentrations to produce acute lead toxicity. The use of the lead mobilization test (the administration of calcium disodium ethylenediamine tetra-acetic acid [EDTA], which mobilizes lead that has been deposited in bone and increases urinary lead excretion) is an effective means of identifying increased lead stores within the body.[33] When such tests are used on individuals who have some occupational exposure to lead, over 80 percent exhibit the response of increased lead excretion. Most of these individuals also demonstrate varying degrees of reduced renal function. In a few patients, renal biopsies have revealed typical focal interstitial nephritis.

The only keys to accurate diagnosis are a careful history of possible occupational exposure and the use of the EDTA lead mobilization test to document increased lead stores. In early renal involvement, urinalysis provides little helpful information. Proteinuria, even minimal proteinuria, is a very late manifestation of many cases of lead nephropathy, and the diagnosis must rest on a strong index of suspicion coupled with the mobilization test. Measurement of plasma lead does not provide a sensitive indication of increased body stores. The diagnosis early in the course of lead nephropathy is important; Wedeen and his colleagues have shown that treatment with EDTA (1 g intramuscularly three times weekly) actually produced a progressive increase in glomerular filtration rate in four of eight individuals who were documented to have chronic interstitial nephritis associated with increased lead stores.[33]

Other heavy metals have not been as well studied as lead, but cadmium, gold, and platinum have all been reported to produce chronic progressive renal failure.

ANALGESIC NEPHROPATHY

Spuhler and Zollinger[30] called attention initially to a marked increase in prevalence of chronic renal disease in individuals with a history of long-term use of analgesics, noting that many individuals with chronic progressive tubulointerstitial disease had such a history. These findings were confirmed by other workers.[16,21,23,27] The disease is more common in women and is associated with impaired renal function and abnormalities in intravenous pyelogram that include papillary necrosis in over half the cases. Hypertension is common, as is pyuria, but heavy proteinuria is rare. The disease tends to be progressive and ultimately terminates in end-stage renal disease and uremia requiring maintenance dialysis. Histologically the tubulointerstitial lesions are most concentrated in the medullary region, and papillary necrosis is a very prominent feature; it often leads to sloughing of the papillary tip, which may on occasion produce complete ureteral obstruction. Despite extensive documentation in the literature, the responsible agent has not yet been identified, although early studies focused attention on phenacetin as the common component of all of the analgesic preparations incriminated. It has been demonstrated that acetaminophen, the principal metabolite of phenacetin, is concentrated in the renal papilla and medulla, as is aspirin,[5,15] but the specific contribution of these agents to the pathogenesis of the clinical entity termed "analgesic nephropathy" remains unclear. The association between ingestion of large quantities of combination analgesics and the prevalence and progression of chronic interstitial nephritis is sufficiently strong, however, to warn against the use of analgesics in more than minimal doses in patients with any type of renal impairment. Patients who have renal impairment and who take in significant quantities of analgesics or nonsteroidal anti-inflammatory drugs should have their renal function monitored carefully.

INTERSTITIAL NEPHROPATHY DUE TO METABOLIC DISTURBANCES

Interstitial inflammatory reaction has been described repeatedly in association with hypercalciuria, hyperoxaluria, and hyperuricemia.

Persistent hypercalcemia is well recognized as a cause of progressive renal impairment. The functional effects of excess hypercalcemia on the kidney include progressive reduction in glomerular filtration rate and renal blood flow, impairment of concentrating ability, and calcium deposition within the kidney. In more advanced stages of nephrocalcinosis, disruption of tubular cells and severe tubulointerstitial nephritis may be seen. Experimental data indicate that this process is aggravated by increased phosphorus intake and slowed markedly by vigorous phosphate restriction. Walser, Mitch, and Collier[32] have demonstrated that dietary restriction of phosphorus slows the rate of loss of renal function in human renal disease. Because virtually all the changes in renal function associated with hypercalcemia are reversible if recognized early, careful evaluation of renal function should always be undertaken when hypercalcemia is recognized so that the hypercalcemia can be controlled before extensive renal destruction occurs.

The occurrence of interstitial nephropathy in association with gout and with increased oxalate excretion has been well documented, although the precise mechanism remains unclear. It has been suggested that, at least in the case of gouty nephropathy, the interstitial nephropathy is a manifestation of associated lead toxicity.[33]

REFERENCES

1. Appel GB, Kunis CL: Acute tubulo-interstitial nephritis. In Cotran RS, Brenner BM, Stein H (eds): Tubulo-Interstitial Nephropathies. New York, Churchill Livingstone, 1983
2. Asscher AW, Chick S, et al: Natural history of asymptomatic bacteriuria in non-pregnant women. In Brumfitt W, Asscher AW (eds): Urinary Tract Infection. London, Oxford University Press, 1973
3. Brumfitt W, Asscher AW: Urinary Tract Infection. London, Oxford University Press, 1973
4. Cogan MC, Arieff AI: Sodium wasting, acidosis and hyperkalemia induced by methicillin interstitial nephritis. Am J Med 64:500, 1978
5. Duggin GC, Mudge GM: Analgesic nephropathy: Renal distribution of acetaminophen and its conjugates. J Pharmacol Exp Ther 199:1, 1976
6. Edwards B, White RHR, et al: Screening methods for covert bacteriuria in school girls. Br Med J 1:463, 1975
7. Edwards D, Norman ICS, et al: Disappearance of reflux during long-term prophylaxis of urinary tract infection in children. Br Med J 2:285, 1977
8. Engel G, Schaeffer AI, et al: The role of excretory urography and cystoscopy in the evaluation and management of women with recurrent urinary tract infection. J Urol 123:190, 1980
9. Fair WR, McClennan BL, Jost RG: Are excretory urograms necessary in evaluating women with urinary tract infection? J Urol 121:313, 1979
10. Fowler JE Jr, Pulaski ET: Excretory urography, cystography, and cystoscopy in the evaluation of women with urinary tract infection. A prospective study. N Engl J Med 304:462, 1981
11. Freedman LR: Chronic pyelonephritis at autopsy. Ann Intern Med 66:697, 1967
12. Freedman LR, Andriole V: The long-term follow-up of women with

urinary tract infections. In Villarrela H (ed): Proceedings of the Fifth International Congress of Nephrology. Basel, S. Karger, 1972

13. Freeman RB, Smith WM, et al: Long-term therapy of chronic bacteriuria in men. US Public Health Service Cooperative Study. Ann Intern Med 83:133, 1975
14. Galpin JE, Schinaberger JH, et al: Acute interstitial nephritis due to methicillin. Am J Med 65:756, 1978
15. Gault MH, Blennerhassett J, Muerhcke R: Analgesic nephropathy—A clinico-pathologic study using electron microscopy. Am J Med 51:740, 1971
16. Grimlund K: Phenacetin and renal damage at a Swedish factory. Acta Med Scand 174(suppl 405):1, 1963
17. Heptinstall RH: Pathology of the Kidney, 2d ed. Boston, Little, Brown, 1974, p 837
18. Heptinstall RH: Interstitial nephritis. A brief review. Am J Pathol 83:214, 1976
19. Hodson CJ, Cotran RS: Vesicoureteral reflux, reflux nephropathy and chronic pyelonephritis. In Cotran RS, Brenner, BM, Stein JH (eds): Contemporary Issues in Nephrology: Tubulo-Interstitial Nephropathies. New York, Churchill Livingstone, 1983
20. Ingelfinger JR, Avner ED, et al: Single-dose amoxicillin treatment of uncomplicated urinary tract infections. As effective as conventional therapy. Pediatr Res 15:694, 1981
21. Kincaid-Smith P: Analgesic nephropathy in Australia. Contrib Nephrol 16:57, 1979
22. Kunin CM: Detection, Prevention, and Management of Urinary Tract Infections. Philadelphia, Lea and Febiger, 1979

23. Larsen K, Moller CE: A renal lesion caused by abuse of phenacetin. Acta Med Scand 164:53, 1959
24. Lenaghan D, Whitaker JG, et al: The natural history of reflux and long-term effects of reflux on the kidney. J Urol 115:728, 1976
25. McFadyen IR: Pregnancy bacteriuria and E. coli. J Soc Med 73:227, 1980
26. Meares EM, Stamey TA: Bacteriologic localization patterns in bacterial prostatitis and urethritis. Invest Urol 5:402, 1968
27. Murray T, Goldberg J: Chronic interstitial nephritis: Etiologic factors. Ann Intern Med 82:453, 1975
28. Raaschou F: Studies of Chronic Pyelonephritis with Special Reference to the Kidney Function. Copenhagen, Ejnar Munksgaard, 1948, p 260
29. Savage DCL, Howie G, et al: Controlled trial of therapy in overt bacteriuria in childhood. Lancet 1:358, 1975
30. Spuhler O, Zollinger HV: Die chronische interstitielle Nephritis. Z Klin Med 151:1, 1953
31. Stamey TA: Urinary tract infections in the female: A perspective. In Remmington JS, Swartz MN (eds): Current Clinical Topics in Infectious Diseases. New York, McGraw-Hill, 1980
32. Walser M, Mitch WE, Collier VU: The effect of nutritional therapy on the course of chronic renal failure. Clin Nephrol 11:66, 1979
33. Wedeen RP, Mallik DK, Batuman V: Detection and treatment of occupational lead nephropathy. Arch Intern Med 139:53, 1979
34. Weiss S, Parker FJ: Pyelonephritis: Its reaction to vascular lesions and to arterial hypertension. Medicine 18:221, 1939

CHAPTER 11.4
Oliguria and Acute Renal Failure

W. Gordon Walker
and Andrew Whelton

Acute renal insufficiency associated with suppression or cessation of urine formation constitutes a most important segment of renal disease. Because the lesions responsible are usually reversible, prompt recognition and appropriate management are vital.

The minimum volume of urine necessary for adequate solute excretion on a normal intake is approximately 450 ml/day, provided renal function is normal. This value varies moderately in healthy individuals, depending on the type and quantity of solute. A sustained urinary output of less than 15 ml per hour in an adequately hydrated adult with previously normal renal function is evidence of significant oliguria. Although this figure is arbitrary, it provides a basis for diagnosis at an early stage. A variety of abnormalities may result in the development of oliguria or anuria (Table 11.4–1). An orderly approach to appropriate management is facilitated by dividing these into three groups: (1) *prerenal* azotemia denotes suppression of urine formation due to inadequate perfusion of an anatomically and physiologically normal kidney and collecting system; (2) *postrenal* oliguria results from obstructive lesions of the collecting system at some point below the calyceal system; and (3) *renal* disturbances are the most common causes of oliguria, because many disorders of the kidneys are associated with failure of urine formation.

PRERENAL AZOTEMIA

Prerenal azotemia may result from any of several disturbances that lead to temporary reduction or cessation of urine formation persisting long enough to permit azotemia to develop. The most common causes are prolonged dehydration and sodium depletion. A typical example of such rapidly reversible azotemia may be seen in diabetic acidosis that has persisted for several days and resulted in severe dehydration. The fluid and sodium losses produce a depletion of extracellular fluid volume and decreased renal perfusion. This, coupled with the catabolic response to the uncontrolled diabetes, leads to rapid development of azotemia. Similar changes occur with severe diarrhea or recurrent vomiting. With adequate fluid and salt replacement, the azotemia promptly disappears, and no stigmata of acute renal failure develop.

The distinctive difference between the prerenal oligurias and those associated with structural change in the kidney (acute renal failure) lies in the rapidity with which the abnormalities are reversed with appropriate therapy in prerenal azotemia. In addition to electrolyte disturbances, persistent hypotension, severe congestive heart failure, rapidly developing ascites, and other conditions that tend to deplete plasma or extravascular fluid volume or both may result in prerenal azotemia. It is possible that the sequence of events may also be triggered by some reflex action. Anuria or marked oliguria may persist for relatively long periods following major surgical procedures; in some instances this occurs despite maintenance of adequate hydration at all times.

When the disturbance resulting in prerenal azotemia is correctly diagnosed and effectively treated, renal function is promptly restored to normal. Unless prompt therapy is instituted, however, protracted renal ischemia may result in renal failure. For this reason, prerenal causes should be sought in all cases that present initially with oliguria or anuria. As a rough diagnostic guide, oliguria associated with a urinary sodium concentration of less than 10 mEq/L or urinary osmolality of greater than 500 mOsm/kg H_2O is more likely to represent prerenal azotemia. This approach to differentiation between prerenal azotemia and acute renal failure has been extended to the definition of a "renal failure index" as the

TABLE 11.4–1. CAUSES OF ACUTE OLIGURIA OR ANURIA

Prerenal Azotemia
- Shock
- Acute hypovolemia
- Gastrointestinal fluid loss
- Severe dehydration
- Addisonian crisis
- ?Reflex anuria
- Postoperative antidiuresis
- Segregated fluid accumulations

Acute Renal Failure
Nephrotoxic Agents
- Aminoglycosides
- Radiographic contrast media
- Heavy metals (Hg, As, Ur, Au)
- Ethylene glycol
- Carbon tetrachloride
- Sulfonamides
- Kanamycin, neomycin

Circulatory Insufficiency
- Vascular insufficiency
- Blood loss and shock
- Acute sodium depletion
  Diarrhea and vomiting
  Heat stroke
  Diabetes mellitus
- Trauma and crush injury
- Transfusion reactions
- Burns

Other Disorders
- Acute glomerulonephritis
- Malignant hypertension
- Polyarteritis
- Wegener granulomatosis
- Eclampsia
- Bilateral renal cortical necrosis
- Infections
- Acute interstitial nephritis

Postrenal Obstruction
- Renal calculi
- Acute pyelonephritis
- Cancer of pelvic organs
- Irradiation, edema, and fibrosis
- Prostatic obstruction
- Surgical accidents

ratio of urinary sodium to plasma sodium concentration divided by the corresponding urine-to-plasma ratio for creatinine:

$$(U/P)Na/(U/P)Cr \times 100$$

In prerenal azotemia this ratio is less than 1 but usually exceeds a value of 2 in acute renal failure.[8] This diagnostic index is of considerable value in acute situations in which renal function was normal before the onset of acute oliguria. It is unreliable in patients who had substantial chronic impairment of renal function before the acute injury or insult and in patients who have recently been given diuretics. Examination of the urinary sediment may contribute further diagnostic information because an active sediment with renal tubular epithelial cells, tubular cellular casts, and granular casts occurs in acute renal failure but is unusual in prerenal azotemia. None of the renal function tests in use for distinguishing between prerenal and renal failure is entirely satisfactory, and the final decision must be based on clinical judgment and evaluation of the patient's response to therapy designed to overcome the prerenal abnormality. The treatment of hypovolemia, sodium depletion, and other conditions leading to lowered urine output have been covered in the section on fluid and electrolyte metabolism (see Section 10).

The infusion of 40 to 50 g of mannitol as a hypertonic solution or the use of a strong diuretic such as furosemide on suspicion of acute renal failure has gained wide acceptance as the early treatment of choice for oliguric patients. The general utility of this approach is considered in more detail in the section on management of acute renal failure. Although the approach is of considerable utility in differentiating prerenal azotemia from acute renal failure, *it must not be considered as a diagnostic or therapeutic intervention until the patient has received adequate fluids* (0.155M physiologic saline or Ringer lactate) to correct any documented or presumed fluid deficit that may be contributing to volume depletion and prerenal oliguria. *Use of mannitol or a potent diuretic before adequate volume replacement is achieved is dangerous and risks converting acute prerenal azotemia with oliguria to acute renal failure by aggravating volume deficits that are already serious enough to produce oliguria.*

POSTRENAL OBSTRUCTION

There are relatively few conditions that lead to complete cessation of urine formation as a result of urinary tract obstruction. If only one kidney or its ureter is obstructed, the remaining normal kidney is capable of adequately performing the necessary excretory function. There is no appreciable drop in urine output, and the associated symptoms are not those of renal failure but of local obstruction. Obstruction of the lower urinary tract leading to anuria is most frequently caused by prostatic enlargement, and the discomfort resulting from overdistension of the bladder usually calls attention to this cause. Bilateral ureteral obstruction is rare and may be associated with carcinoma of the bladder, prostate, colon, or cervix. Such obstruction may result from direct invasion by the tumor, from inflammation induced by local irradiation, or from dense periureteritic fibrosis, as is often seen with carcinoma of the prostate. Pain is variable with this type of obstruction and may even be absent. Inadvertent ureteral ligation should always be considered when postoperative anuria complicates gynecologic surgery or other pelvic surgery.

Complete absence of urine formation is rare in cases of renal failure due to intrinsic renal disease, so that distinguishing between acute renal failure and postrenal obstruction is seldom difficult. Obstruction should be suspected in all patients with *complete anuria*. Occasionally, obstruction of the ureters by uric acid crystals is encountered, particularly with the marked uricosuria that follows treatment of the lymphomas with one of the cytolytic antitumor agents.

Diagnosis of these conditions can only be established unequivocally by ureteral catheterization. This procedure is not without risk; infection is likely to be introduced and may be particularly difficult to manage if the cause of oliguria is not obstruction. Sonography is a highly reliable and noninvasive procedure that can identify even modest degrees of caliectasis. It is doubtful that catheterization is ever indicated to exclude obstruction if sonography fails to identify dilation of the upper collecting system. Sonography is also of great value in guiding percutaneous antegrade catheterization of the upper collecting system when retrograde catheterization of the ureter is unsuccessful.

In obstruction of relatively long standing, relief may be followed by profuse diuresis; urine flow rates may approach 50 percent of the glomerular filtration rate.[3] Presumably this is attributable to tubular atrophy resulting from back pressure caused by the obstruction, and the attendant solute load (principally urea), which acts as a solute diuretic. This diuresis may lead to such profound water and sodium losses that shock supervenes quickly. Appropriate fluid and sodium replacement alleviates these symptoms, and the condition is usually reversible, although weeks may be required before function restoration is complete. The management of this problem is outlined in Table 11.4–2.

TABLE 11.4–2. MANAGEMENT OF POSTOBSTRUCTIVE DIURESIS

1. If urine flow <50 ml/30 min (after hydronephrotic rush slows) manage conservatively.
   a. Oral fluids and added salts.
   b. Monitor blood pressure and 24-hr urine output.
2. If urine flow 50–100 ml/30 min, measure urine Na and K.
   a. Replace urine losses with 0.075 M NaCl in 50% dextrose at rate equal to urine flow for first 24 hr.
   b. If weight stable on second day, reduce infusion rate by 50%; if weight remains stable, switch to oral fluids on day 3.
   c. If weight loss ≥1 kg, continue (a) for second 24 hr and try (b) on day 3.
3. If urine flow >100 ml/30 min, start 0.075 M NaCl in 5% dextrose immediately at rate equal to urine flow (if urinary [Na] exceeds 75 mEq/L, increase [Na] in infusate accordingly).
   a. Continue this rate for at least 48 hr.
   b. Proceed as under 2(c). Watch BP and body weight carefully.
   c. If BP stable and weight stable, proceed with further reduction of IV fluids.
4. If initially measured urine flow rate >150 ml/30 min, wait at least 96 hr before proceeding as under 3(b), but infusion rate should only be reduced by 25%.

ACUTE RENAL FAILURE

The causes of acute renal failure are numerous (Table 11.4–1), but in most general hospitals, nephrotoxicity attributable to aminoglycoside toxicity or toxicity of nonsteroidal anti-inflammatory agents or of intravenous x-ray contrast media accounts for more than three quarters of cases seen on the medical and surgical services. Regardless of the condition causing the acute renal failure, only two mechanisms appear responsible for the structural changes in the kidney. Each mechanism has been demonstrated experimentally, and the histologic changes have been classified as *nephrotoxic* or *ischemic*. Although for many years it has been stated that the predominant lesion in both is necrosis of the tubular epithelium, there is usually a striking disparity between the minimal evidence of necrosis that can be demonstrated histologically and the gross derangement of renal function that often results in almost complete anuria.[11]

The nephrotoxic changes produced by specific toxic agents or chemicals (Table 11.4–1) include necrosis of the epithelium lining the tubules, with relatively complete preservation of the basement membrane. The glomeruli appear to be uninvolved. Regeneration of the epithelial cells can be demonstrated after about 2 weeks. When the tubular basement membrane is not damaged by the nephrotoxin, the epithelium grows to cover it completely, thereby reestablishing continuity of the tubule. When the basement membrane is disrupted by the necrotic process, continuity is not reestablished during regeneration and the tubule does not regain its function. In experimental studies, the length of time required for regeneration, as well as its adequacy, are directly related to the dosage of nephrotoxic substance. In general, regeneration is nearly complete by the 21st through the 25th day after the initial insult. In clinical situations, regeneration may take longer, and slowly increasing renal function may be demonstrated over a longer period.

In the *ischemic* form of acute renal failure, the histologic findings have for many years been described as those of acute tubular necrosis. In fact, the typical change is conversion of the tubular cells to low cuboidal epithelium, with only minimal evidence of scattered foci of mild necrosis. It is doubtful that these sporadic changes are responsible for the associated gross aberration of renal function. Development of techniques that allow identification of changes in total renal and intrarenal blood flow patterns have considerably increased our understanding of the sequence of events that culminates in ischemic acute renal failure.[6]

Studies in humans with acute oliguric renal failure from various causes reveal that total renal blood flow is decreased, usually one-half to one-third the normal flow rates. Changes in intrarenal blood flow occur with marked reduction in cortical flow and increase in the inner cortical or juxtamedullary flow. Afferent arteriole vasoconstriction develops, and net filtration pressures fall to levels commensurate with production of only minimal amounts of filtrate and clinical evidence of oliguria or anuria. Residual renal blood flow is adequate to prevent cellular necrosis.

If the initial cause of hypotension and renal ischemia is not corrected within approximately 2 to 12 hours, protracted oliguria sometimes lasting for weeks may result from the ischemia. This oliguria is associated with persistence of the pattern of decreased intrarenal blood flow over the next several days or 2 to 4 weeks, despite restoration of adequate circulating volume and return of systemic blood pressure to normal levels. The humoral and local factors responsible for this persistent reduction in renal blood flow remain to be clearly identified. The renin-angiotensin system and catecholamines have been implicated in some experimental situations, but their role in human disease remains to be defined.[9]

CLINICAL FEATURES

The clinical course of acute renal failure is characterized by three more or less distinct phases: the oligemic, the oliguric or anuric, and the diuretic.[2]

The *oligemic* phase is variable, and in a substantial number of cases is not recognizable. Clinically, this stage is characterized by hypotension and the signs of shock associated with reduction or complete cessation of urine formation. Prompt recognition and treatment at this time may prevent the development of the full course of acute tubular necrosis.

The oligemic phase is followed by the *oliguric* phase after a variable period of time. Urine flow may increase briefly (for 12 to 20 hours) following correction of the hypovolemia and then begins to decrease. The persistence of urine flow of less than 20 ml per hour in the face of adequate hydration is strong presumptive evidence of acute renal failure. The duration of this phase is variable and depends on the severity of kidney damage. It may last from 2 or 3 days to more than 4 weeks in patients who ultimately recover completely. If oliguria persists for 6 to 8 days or more, signs of uremia become increasingly severe. As uremia progresses and the patient becomes obtunded, gastrointestinal disturbances including nausea and vomiting appear, and there is increasing difficulty in handling respiratory secretions. The hazard of infection increases and is a more common cause of death at this stage than the uremia itself. The principal life-threatening consequences of the uremia are hyperkalemia, acidosis, and overhydration.

The *diuretic* phase may begin from 5 to 30 days after onset but is usually seen after 10 days to 2 weeks. In general, it is characterized by a urine output that at first increases slowly for 3 to 4 days and that may then suddenly increase to 6 to 8 L or more per day. During the first 3 to 4 days of this period, the signs, symptoms, and laboratory evidence of uremia may continue because the increasing urine flow indicates the function of only a small number of nephrons.

As recovery continues, more and more nephrons become active, with a correspondingly greater increase in urine output. This urine at first has a composition that reflects the limited ability of the tubules to function. It is characterized principally by a high sodium and chloride content, the concentration of sodium frequently being greater than 50 percent of that in the plasma. There is a correspondingly low concentration of urea. This state of affairs usually persists for a week to 10 days, gradually subsiding as tubular function improves. The clinical disorders that develop at the peak of the diuretic phase are related to obligatory losses of water and solutes in the urine. Thus, severe deficits of sodium, potassium, or water may be encountered.

MANAGEMENT

The prognosis of acute renal failure depends almost entirely on adequate management. Meticulous attention to the details of day-to-day care of the patient is essential.

If the patient is first seen at the very onset of the oliguria, attention should be directed toward the state of hydration. Because ischemic renal failure is usually due to reduction in blood and extracellular fluid volume, any deficit in either should be promptly replaced. Sources of blood loss should be identified quickly. Initially, it may be difficult to assess the state of hydration and sodium balance. If the available evidence fails to provide the needed information about fluid loss, a therapeutic trial of fluid administration may be necessary. It is most important that such treatment not be overdone. The rapid loss of more than 2 L of extracellular fluid usually produces severe hypotension; therefore, in the absence of continuing loss, it is unwise to give more than 1500 ml of isotonic saline intravenously. Isotonic losses (decrease in extracellular fluid volume) are most likely to lead to oliguria. Water loss alone or hypertonic dehydration, unless profound, does not produce oliguria, and under these circumstances severe hypernatremia is usually present. In managing oliguria, fluids should not be administered rapidly unless the patient is in shock. Slow administration lessens the likelihood of acute circulatory overload in the event that an error has been made in clinical evaluation of the state of hydration. If 1500 ml of fluid produces no significant change in the urinary output, one should adopt the plan of management outlined below.

The role of mannitol in the earliest phases of acute renal failure has not received an adequate clinical trial. There is, however, substantial experimental evidence that it can reduce, and may at times interrupt, the vicious cycle of anoxia, cell swelling, and increased local vascular resistance, leading to more anoxia, further cell swelling, and ultimately cell death. Mannitol or furosemide, given very early in the course of acute renal failure, may initiate an osmotic diuresis and convert oliguric to nonoliguric renal failure. Because the prognosis of nonoliguric renal failure is more favorable than that of oliguric renal failure, this is a desirable change. Intravenously administered mannitol given rapidly is not without danger, particularly in elderly individuals; it is probably safer and wiser to attempt this conversion with furosemide rather than mannitol.[4,5,13,14]

Successful management of the oliguric phase requires careful monitoring of the intake of calories, water, and salt and expert nursing care (Table 11.4–3). Fluid (water) requirements may vary,

TABLE 11.4–3. MANAGEMENT OF OLIGURIC ACUTE RENAL FAILURE

Fluid Management
- Record total intake and output of fluid.
- Keep fluid intake at 400 ml/day plus measured losses.
- Weigh daily; patient should lose 0.1 to 0.2 kg daily.

Diet
- Protein intake less than 0.4 g/kg body weight.
- Sodium intake ≤15 mEq/day.
- Potassium intake ≤15 mEq/day.
- Total caloric intake 1200–1500/day.

Management of Acidosis
- Maintain protein and phosphate intake at low levels.
- Replace any sodium losses as Ringer lactate or bicarbonate.

Dialysis
- Begin promptly for hyperkalemia, weight gain, acidosis, blood urea nitrogen >100 mg/dl (50–60 mg/dl if patient is catabolic).
- If complicating illness prevents adequate restriction of fluid intake, dialysis should be started early in course of oliguria.

depending on the presence or absence of sweating, the ambient air temperature, fever, or other factors that may increase insensible water loss. *A daily record should be kept of the patient's weight.* Because the catabolic response results in progressive loss of body tissue, under the regimen described above, a weight loss of approximately 0.2 to 0.3 kg per day is to be expected if proper fluid balance is being maintained. If this occurs, there should be no difficulty with circulatory overload or water intoxication. If unforeseen circumstances result in overhydration, the intake figures should be reduced to increase the rate of weight loss. It must be stressed that the patients' chances for recovery are optimum when all clinical manifestations of uremia are prevented. Because in many situations, particularly in traumatic and surgical cases, other aspects of patients' illness may require acute measures that prevent the parsimonious approach to fluid therapy previously outlined, *early and frequent dialysis is the hallmark of a good therapeutic regimen for acute renal failure.*

Hyperkalemia is a common problem. The rapidity with which it appears is variable and is related to the rate of catabolism. It is a special hazard in acute renal failure following hemorrhage, an enhanced catabolic response associated with extensive surgical procedures, extensive traumatic or crushing injuries, and myoglobinuria associated with oliguria. In these situations, frequent extracellular fluid (ECF) monitoring for progressive T-wave elevation is desirable. The appearance of peaking of the T waves is sufficient evidence of hypokalemia to warrant immediate therapy (Chapter 10.2). Both hyperkalemia and acidosis are absolute indications for dialysis. In the presence of severe and rapidly developing hyperkalemia, it may be essential to use glucose and insulin and other measures to combat the elevated potassium while preparing the patient for dialysis.

The administration of carbohydrate reduces protein catabolism; if oral intake is not possible, carbohydrate should be given intravenously. In healthy individuals a maximum protein-sparing effect is probably achieved with only 100 g per day. In patients with acute renal failure, however, larger amounts are probably necessary to bring about a maximal reduction in the rate of protein breakdown. The protein-sparing effect can be enhanced by administration of anabolic steroids (testosterone and its congeners).

The use of parenteral amino acid mixtures has been proposed as a means of minimizing catabolism and retarding the rate of development of uremia; hypertonic glucose plus essential amino acids was reported to lessen the degree of renal failure.[1] Hyperalimentation has also been said to have a beneficial effect on morbidity and mortality of acute renal failure when glucose and amino acids are used as a caloric source.[10] Recent experimental evidence reveals that this approach has an adverse effect on survival in animals, with acute renal failure produced by nephrotoxic substances.[12] Such regimens should thus be used with caution and only in patients who are optimally dialyzed.

The two most common causes of death during oliguria are infection and gastrointestinal hemorrhage. Prophylactic antibiotic treatment is of questionable value and probably should not be used. If obvious systemic infection has developed, appropriate antibiotic therapy, based on sensitivity testing, should be instituted. Because of the impaired excretory function of the kidney, careful attention to alterations in antibiotic dosage schedules is mandatory.[15,16] Early treatment of uremia reduces the likelihood of infection and decreases the morbidity and mortality associated with the syndrome. The decision to institute dialysis therapy should not be based solely on the blood chemistry findings but should be made in conjunction with the patient's clinical signs and symptomatology. Acceptable guidelines for the initiation of dialysis therapy are a serum urea nitrogen of 100 to 120 mg/dl and a serum creatinine value greater than 8 to 10 mg/dl. The aim of dialysis and the conservative techniques of patient management is to maintain the patient's health in the best state possible. Hemodialysis every 48 to 72 hours is usually effective in maintaining a patient with acute renal failure in a sufficiently stable function. The

TABLE 11.4–4. PROGNOSIS IN ACUTE RENAL FAILURE[2,6,7]

Etiology	Total Cases	No. Surviving	%
Traumatic (surgical)	2510	1051	42
Nephrotoxic (medical)	452	292	65

techniques of the various modalities of dialysis are described in Chapter 11.5.

The *diuretic* phase appears after a variable period of time, and the urinary output begins to increase slowly. Large quantities of sodium and potassium may be lost in the urine due to inadequate tubular activity during the first several days of this diuretic phase. The sodium concentration is rarely below 60 to 70 mEq/L and, because urine output usually exceeds 2 L, the patient may lose 120 to 140 mEq of sodium per day. Inadequate sodium replacement may lead to shock, further damage to the kidneys, and interruption of a beginning diuresis. The development of hypokalemia is less frequent. The diuretic phase, during which the kidney is unable to regulate the composition of the urine adequately, may persist for several days to 2 weeks or longer. In severe cases, renal function does not always return completely to normal, but virtually always reaches a level that permits the kidney to regulate the volume and composition of body fluids adequately.

The prognosis in acute renal failure is influenced by the underlying cause of the renal failure. In general, those cases associated with trauma do poorly, the mortality rate in some series exceeding 60 percent. Nontraumatic cases usually exhibit a survival rate that exceeds 75 percent.[6] The prognosis appears best in obstetric cases,[7] and cases arising in surgical or traumatic settings exhibit the poorest prognosis (Table 11.4–4).

REFERENCES

1. Abel RM, Beck CH Jr, et al: Improved survival from acute renal failure after treatment with intravenous essential 1-amino acids and glucose. N Engl J Med 288:695, 1973
2. Bleumle LW, Webster GC Jr, Elkinton JR: Acute tubular necrosis: Analysis of 100 cases with respect to mortality, complications and treatment with and without dialysis. Arch Intern Med 194:180, 1959
3. Bricker NS, Shwayri ER, et al: Abnormality in renal function resulting from urinary tract obstruction. Am J Med 23:554, 1957
4. Flores J, DiBona DR, et al: The role of cell swelling in ischemic renal damage and the protective effect of hypertonic solute. J Clin Invest 51:118, 1972
5. Frega N, DiBona DR, Leaf A: Ischemic renal injury. Kidney Int 10:517, 1976
6. Friedman EA, Eliahou HE (eds): Proceedings: Conference on Acute Renal Failure. D.H.E.W. Publication No. (NIH) 74-608, Washington, DC, U.S. Government Printing Office, 1973
7. Kleinknect D, Jungers P, et al: Factors influencing immediate prognosis in acute renal failure with special reference to prophylactic hemodialysis. In Hamburger J, Crosnier J, Maxwell MH (eds): Advances in Nephrology, vol 1. Chicago, Year Book Medical Publishers, 1971
8. Miller TR, Anderson RJ, et al: Urinary diagnostic indices in acute renal failure: A prospective study. Ann Intern Med 89:47, 1978
9. Mitch WE, Walker WG: Plasma renin and angiotensin II in acute renal failure. Lancet 2:328, 1977
10. Schrier RW, Conger JD: Acute renal failure: Pathogenesis, diagnosis and management. In Schrier RW (ed): Renal and Electrolyte Disorders, 3d ed. Boston, Little, Brown, 1986, p 423
11. Solez K, Morel-Maroger L, Sraer JD: Morphology of "acute tubular necrosis" in man: Analysis of 57 renal biopsies and comparison with the glycerol model. Medicine 58:362, 1979
12. Solez K, Stout R, et al: Adverse effect of amino acid solutions in aminoglycoside-induced acute renal failure in rabbits and rats. In Eliahou H (ed): Acute Renal Failure. London, John Libbey and Son, 1982
13. Stern JR, Eggleston LV, Hems R, Krebs HA: Accumulation of glutamic acid in isolated brain tissue. Biochem J 44:410, 1949
14. Vertel RM, Knochel JP: Non-oliguric acute renal failure. JAMA 200:598, 1967
15. Whelton A: Antibacterial chemotherapy in renal insufficiency: A review. Antibiot Chemotherap 18:1, 1974
16. Whelton A, Solez K: Aminoglycoside nephrotoxicity (editorial). J Lab Clin Med 99:148, 1982

CHAPTER 11.5
Management of Progressive and End-Stage Renal Disease

William E. Mitch, Walter L. Bender, Jr.
and W. Gordon Walker

It is misleading to speak of the management of progressive renal disease as a single therapeutic endeavor because that implies all renal diseases should be managed in a similar fashion. Although this is very nearly true after the decision is made to begin maintenance dialysis, the conservative management of the patient during the interim between the onset of renal failure and the point at which dialysis becomes necessary requires a multidisciplinary approach. This approach may vary considerably, depending on the nature of the disease responsible for progressive renal destruction. There are, however, certain principles of management that apply to nearly all forms of progressive renal disease. These management strategies are considered in this chapter.

DEFINITION OF END STAGE

Three objectives should be completed before planning the treatment of a patient with chronic renal failure. The first is to establish a specific diagnosis. If the clinical manifestations are made inadequate to support a unique diagnosis, a renal biopsy should be performed to confirm the diagnosis; a renal biopsy is not advised in patients with advanced renal insufficiency and small, scarred kidneys. In such patients, the risk outweighs the potential benefit of establishing a histologic diagnosis. The second objective is to determine the magnitude of renal insufficiency. As discussed in Chapter 11.1, it is difficult to measure the glomerular filtration rate (GFR) precisely using standard laboratory tests, although a reasonable estimate can be obtained from the 24-hour creatinine clearance. The third objective is to determine how rapidly renal function is being lost. If prior values of serum creatinine are available, this objective can be accomplished by plotting serial values of the reciprocal of serum creatinine with time. The slope of the relationship can be used to predict the future course of renal insufficiency. Even with such data, it is difficult to determine when derangements in homeostasis will initiate the development of uremic symptoms and signal the need for initiating dialysis or transplantation.

Detailed studies that have examined the clinical course of patients with different types of renal diseases once the plasma creatinine has reached 5 or 10 mg/dl, respectively, are particularly instructive. The various types of glomerulonephritis comprised the largest segment in both studies, but patients with polycystic renal disease, obstructive nephropathy, diabetic glomerulopathy, and other disorders were also represented. A creatinine of 5.0 mg/dl indicated that, on average, terminal uremia would be present in 10 to 11 months.[2] The median time before dialysis was necessary for 76 patients who had a serum creatinine concentration of 10 mg/dl was about 2 months in one study, whereas in another study of 132 patients, the median time varied between 2 and 8 months.[15,17] Rapidly progressive glomerulonephritis sometimes runs its course in weeks, whereas polycystic kidney disease may be associated with a slow rate of progression, indicating that specific diseases do influence prognosis. These average figures serve as useful guides and illustrate the enormous variability in rates of progression among various causes.[21] Such data also emphasize the importance of determining the rate of progression for each patient.

MANAGEMENT OF MANIFESTATIONS

A creatinine concentration of 5 mg/dl corresponds to a GFR of approximately 15 to 20 ml/min per 1.73 m² of body surface area. At this level of impairment, the kidney is incapable of excreting the daily ingested loads of a number of substances, and the concentration of these substances becomes elevated in the plasma and other body fluids. At this point, careful and effective conservative management is essential if the dialysis-free interval is to be extended. Reduction in protein intake is the most important step; regulation of fluid, sodium, potassium, and phosphate intake also is essential. Each of these is considered in more detail below, as are other important general approaches to the management of the patient.

AZOTEMIA

Evaluation of the blood urea nitrogen and creatinine are usually detected first in progressive renal failure. Despite the fact that many of the clinical manifestations of uremia occur regularly and predictably at specific levels of azotemia, there is considerable uncertainty about the degree to which urea contributes to the toxic manifestations of uremia.[5,14,16] Urea production, however, is directly related to protein intake, and dietary protein restriction alleviates uremic symptoms, so a rise in the blood urea level will reflect the buildup of all putative uremic toxins in body fluids.[16] These products include cyanate, a degradation product of urea, and various guanidinium compounds, including guanidinosuccinic acid, guanidinopropionic acid, methylguanidine, and creatinine. Some of these compounds have been demonstrated to be toxic in the experimental animal at levels ordinarily encountered in uremia and may contribute to the clinical manifestations of uremia, but there is no direct and unambiguous evidence establishing these compounds as major uremic toxins in humans.[16]

Restricting protein intake not only decreases the rate of urea formation and the production and circulating levels of guanidinium compounds, it also decreases phosphate intake and reduces endogenous acid production. This results in lessening or amelioration of uremic symptoms and retards and perhaps prevents the development of secondary hyperparathyroidism and the associated bone disease that is seen in uremia.[5,14] The amelioration of the manifestations of uremia is accelerated by reducing protein intake further, but this requires a supplement of essential amino acids or the ketoacid analogs of these amino acids to ensure neutral nitrogen balance and prevent protein malnutrition.[22]

At what stage of renal failure dietary protein restriction should be implemented is unknown. At creatinine levels exceeding 3 mg/dl, impaired or reduced renal hydrogen ion transport capacity has been well documented. There also is impaired regulation of calcium and phosphorous metabolism and in some instances impairment in the sodium transport. All these are associated with increased accumulation of urea and byproducts of protein metabolism that are found at much lower levels in subjects with normal kidneys. Reducing daily protein intake 0.6 g/kg body weight with dietary protein of high biologic value will largely reverse the abnormalities resulting from renal impairment of this magnitude (creatinine approximately 5 mg/dl).

A diet containing 0.6 g of protein per kilogram of body weight per day will provide the minimum daily protein requirement for healthy adults and will be sufficient to maintain neutral nitrogen balance and prevent protein wasting for patients with renal failure. It should be emphasized that at this level of dietary protein, foods containing a high proportion of essential amino acids (high-quality protein) should make up the bulk of dietary protein in order to meet essential amino acid requirements.[22] If the diet contains less protein, negative nitrogen balance will occur unless a supplement of essential amino acids or their alpha-ketoanalogs (ketoacids) is provided.[22] With supplemented regimens, protein intake can be reduced safely to approximately 0.3 g of protein per kilogram per day, a level that will be associated with a greater reduction in the accumulation of urea and other protein-derived waste products. Moreover, foods rich in protein are almost always rich in phosphorus, so protein-restricted diets also are useful for preventing the increase in serum phosphorus with the accompanying tendency to develop secondary hyperparathyroidism and the disabling bone disease renal osteodystrophy.[5,14,28] In fact, renal osteodystrophy can be so disabling that it is wise to withdraw milk and milk products from the diet of patients with progressive renal disease once the serum creatinine has exceeded 2.5 mg/dl. If hyperphosphatemia cannot be controlled by reducing dietary phosphates, then phosphate binders such as aluminum hydroxide or calcium carbonate should be used.

Whenever protein-restricted diets are prescribed, a supplement of calcium carbonate should be given to provide a total calcium intake of 1.5 g per day.[14] This level of calcium will be sufficient to promote neutral calcium balance and therefore blunt the tendency to develop renal osteodystrophy. Patients treated with low-protein diets also should receive a daily vitamin supplement containing vitamins B and C and folic acid. Supplemental vitamin A is not necessary because plasma vitamin A levels are high in patients with chronic renal failure.[22] At present, the indications for vitamin D include persistent hypocalcemia and advanced renal osteodystrophy, but it should not be prescribed until the serum phosphorus level is normal. This is necessary because vitamin D will increase intestinal absorption of calcium and phosphorus, causing a rise in their plasma levels and a tendency for soft-tissue calcification. In fact, when the product of the concentrations of plasma calcium and plasma phosphorus exceeds 60, there is a substantial risk for calcification of the kidney, heart, blood vessels, and other organs.[22] This is another reason for ensuring that the serum phosphorus of patients with renal insufficiency is kept within the normal range.

PROGRESSION OF CHRONIC RENAL INSUFFICIENCY

Besides reducing the accumulation of urea and other waste products, a low-protein diet may provide another benefit, delaying the progression of chronic renal failure. Results from Europe and the United States have provided evidence that a diet containing the minimum daily protein requirement (0.6 g protein per kilogram per day) can slow the deterioration of renal function in many patients who begin the diet at serum creatinine values below 5 mg/dl.[20,22] Similar beneficial results have been reported when patients with more advanced renal insufficiency are treated with diets containing less protein but supplemented with a mixture of essential amino acids or ketoacids. Several points should be emphasized. First, before beginning treatment with low-protein diets, it is wise

to establish that a patient is losing renal function, that is, has a progressive rise in serum creatinine, a progressive fall in the reciprocal of serum creatinine (see Chapter 11.1), or a progressive fall in creatinine clearance.[21] Second, it is preferable to establish the rate of loss of residual renal function in an individual patient before therapy so that the results after beginning therapy can be compared to judge the effectiveness of treatment.[20,22] A third important task is to assess compliance with the low-protein diet and prevent the development of protein malnutrition. This requires a simple and reliable method for estimating protein intake. Fortunately the rate of urea production is closely related to the amount of protein eaten. In the steady state, the daily rate of urea nitrogen production equals the daily rate of urea nitrogen excretion.[22] The other components of nitrogen excretion, fecal nitrogen, and nitrogen in urinary creatinine, uric acid, and unmeasured nitrogen vary minimally with protein intake; an average value for the total nonurea nitrogen excretion is 0.031 g N/kg body weight.[18] Consequently, the total nitrogen excretion can be estimated from the 24-hour urinary urea nitrogen excretion plus 0.031 g N/kg/day and compared to the prescribed nitrogen intake, calculated as 16 percent of protein intake (Table 11.5–1). For assessment of dietary compliance a patient is asked to collect urine for 24 hours; the urea nitrogen content, body weight, and BUN are then measured. If these values are stable, the estimated nitrogen excretion is compared with the prescribed value (Table 11.5–2). When the two values differ, the patient should undergo additional dietary counseling or investigation for causes of increased nitrogen losses, that is, the presence of catabolic illness.

The presence of more than 5 g of protein per day in the urine makes it more difficult to prescribe the amount of dietary protein that will prevent negative nitrogen balance and protein-wasting. Unfortunately, the amount of extra dietary protein needed to maintain nitrogen balance is not known, but it is reasonable to add 1 g of dietary protein for each gram of proteinuria. Patients with heavy proteinuria must be observed frequently to detect early signs of protein malnutrition, including a progressive fall in body weight, serum albumin, or transferrin concentrations and a loss of muscle mass as estimated from anthropometric measurements.[22] If any of these occur, dietary protein should be raised by at least 0.1 g of protein per kilogram per day.

Three hypotheses have been proposed to explain the beneficial effect of dietary protein restriction on progressive renal insufficiency. The mechanism that has the most secure experimental basis is that the adaptation to chronic renal failure includes an increase in blood pressure and flow in glomerular capillaries that raises glomerular filtration and minimizes the accumulation of waste products. This "hyperfiltration" response ultimately leads to glomerular sclerosis and progressive renal insufficiency.[10] Reducing dietary protein lowers the intraglomerular capillary pressure and protects the kidneys of rats from developing progressive sclerosis. The second proposed mechanism is linked to the abnormalities in calcium and phosphorus metabolism characteristic of chronic renal failure.[5,20] Because calcium phosphate deposition in the kidney, which is regularly associated with hyperparathyroidism, can excite an inflammatory response, it could lead to interstitial nephritis and progressive renal failure. Certain experimental studies in rats have suggested that the lower phosphorus intake associated with dietary protein restriction blunts the development of hyperparathyroidism and decreases the concentration product of plasma calcium and phosphorus, thereby contributing to the beneficial effects of these diets on progressive renal insufficiency.[20] Finally, it is possible that low-protein diets decrease the accumulation of a nephrotoxic substance that is derived from dietary protein. To date, a specific toxin has not been identified. It is not known whether any of these mechanisms apply to the beneficial effects of low-protein diets on progressive renal failure in humans.

PHOSPHATE INTAKE

In patients with chronic renal failure, serum inorganic phosphorus levels rise because of the inability of the damaged kidney to excrete dietary phosphates without a concomitant elevation of the plasma level. This appears to be a major factor responsible for the development of progressive hyperparathyroidism, but there also is a defect in the production of the most active vitamin D metabolite, 1,25-dihydroxy vitamin D_3.[5,14,28] This is due not only to the loss of functioning renal tissue but also to the high plasma phosphate causing inhibition of the renal enzyme that converts the moderately active 25-hydroxy vitamin D_3 to the most potent 1,25-dihydroxy molecule. The combination of these abnormalities leads to profound and, at times, disabling renal osteodystrophy.

Effective therapy consists of limiting protein and hence phosphorus intake. If this is not feasible because of heavy proteinuria, then it is important to use proteins that reduce phosphate intake to as low a level as possible (milk and milk products must be avoided under all circumstances), and it may be necessary to use phosphate binders to promote fecal excretion of phosphate. It should be reemphasized that limiting dietary phosphate must be the major goal; administration of phosphate binders alone will not be sufficient and may be hazardous. The most widely used phosphate binder, aluminum hydroxide, is associated with gradual accumulation of aluminum because chronic renal failure patients excrete aluminum poorly.[24] With progressive aluminum accumulation, there is deposition in bone, which can lead to defective calcification and a type of vitamin D–resistant osteomalacia. The prevalence of this type of bone disease is unknown. It has been observed mainly in dialysis patients and is very difficult to treat, requiring intravenous therapy with desferrioxamine to chelate aluminum.[24] To avoid these problems, serum phosphorus must be kept in the normal range using the least amount of aluminum-based phosphate binders possible. An alternative phosphate binder is calcium carbonate. Calcium carbonate therapy can also be beneficial because it increases calcium intake. Unfortunately, doses as large as 10 g per day are necessary to produce a clinically significant decrease in serum phosphorus. Most patients find it difficult to take this many tablets, and such high doses increase the risk of hypercalcemia. When this quantity of calcium carbonate is administered in the presence of hyperphosphatemia, the risk of soft tissue calcification is increased significantly.

HYDROGEN ION

The progressive reduction in the capacity of the kidney to secrete hydrogen ion results in accumulation of excess hydrogen ion in the body. Bone is primarily responsible for buffering this excess hydrogen ion, resulting in demineralization of bone. Because the requirements of the kidney for protein secretion are determined largely by the phosphate and sulfate content of the diet, the most

TABLE 11.5–1. DIETARY PROTEIN REQUIREMENTS FOR NORMAL SUBJECTS AND PATIENTS WITH RENAL FAILURE[7,9,21,37]

Patients	Minimum Requirements	Safe Level[a]
	(g/kg/day)	
Normal infants (3 mo–3 yr)		1.9–1.2
Normal children (3–12 yr)		1.0
Normal young adults		1.0
Adults		
Normal	0.6	0.8–1.5
Predialysis	0.6	0.8
Hemodialysis	1.0	1.0
Peritoneal dialysis	1.0	1.4

[a]Safe level is the amount that will meet the requirement of 97.5% of patients.

TABLE 11.5–2. ESTIMATION OF PROTEIN INTAKE OF PREDIALYSIS PATIENTS[18] [a]

Example 1: A 70-kg patient with stable weight and BUN excretes 6 g urea nitrogen per day.

$$B_N = I_N - U - NUN = 0$$
$$I_N = U + NUN$$
$$I_N = 6 \text{ g N/day} + (70 \text{ kg} \times 0.031 \text{ g N/kg/day})$$
$$I_N = 6 + 2.17 = 8.17 \text{ g N/day}$$

Protein intake: 8.17 ÷ 0.16 = 51 g protein/day.
Comment: Because BUN and weight are stable, there is no change in the urea nitrogen pool, and the urea appearance rate equals the daily urinary urea nitrogen excretion.

Example 2: A 70-kg patient with a BUN of 80 mg/dl excretes 7 g urea nitrogen per day, but is edematous and is treated with a diuretic. Seven days later, he has no edema, and his weight is 68 kg; his BUN is 70 mg/dl and 24-hour urine urea nitrogen is 6.5 g nitrogen per day.

$$B_N = I_N - U - NUN = 0$$
$$I_N = U + NUN = U_{UN}V + \Delta + NUN$$
$$I_N = (7.0 + 6.5) \div 2 + ([68 \text{ kg} \times 0.6 \times 0.7 \text{ gN/L}] - [68 \times 0.6 + 2L] \times 0.8) + 7 + 68 \times 0.031$$
$$I_N = 6.75 + (28.6 - 34.2) + 7 + 2.11$$
$$I_N = 6.75 - 0.81 + 2.11 = 8.05 \text{ gN/d}$$

Protein intake: 8.05 nitrogen per day ÷ 0.16 = 50.3 g protein per day.
Comment: To calculate the urea nitrogen appearance rate, the average urea nitrogen excretion rate is added to the change in the urea nitrogen pool or is calculated as the final pool size (60% of nonedematous weight × BUN in grams per liter) minus the initial pool size (60% of nonedematous weight plus edema weight × BUN in grams per liter) divided by the number of days between the observations. The calculated value of U plus that for NUN equals total nitrogen excretion that can be converted to protein.

Assumptions are that patients are in nitrogen balance, that 60% of body weight is the volume of distribution of urea,[23] that the nonurea nitrogen excretion (e.g., the nitrogen in feces, urine creatinine, uric acid) averages 0.031 g N/kg/d[18] and that protein is 16% nitrogen.

[a] Abbreviations: B_N, nitrogen balance; I_N, nitrogen intake; U, urea nitrogen appearance rate (the sum of urea nitrogen [$U_{UN}V$]) and the change in the urea nitrogen pool (Δ); NUN, nonurea nitrogen excretion. All values are in grams of nitrogen per day.

important initial measure in controlling acidosis is to reduce protein intake. When systemic acidosis develops, administration of sodium bicarbonate or some substance that is converted quantitatively to sodium bicarbonate (e.g., sodium citrate, sodium lactate) is essential. Alkali therapy should not be substituted for dietary protein restriction because patients who present with a plasma bicarbonate level of 15 mEq/L or below may exhibit a dramatic response to reduction of protein intake to a low level of 0.6 g/kg body weight, making supplementary alkalinization unnecessary. Although most patients who require supplement will respond to 15 to 30 mEq of sodium bicarbonate daily, some forms of renal tubular acidosis may require larger amounts (see Chapter 11.6). For some patients, dietary salt may need to be adjusted downward if the extra sodium aggravates edema or hypertension.

SODIUM INTAKE

A healthy subject can excrete sodium-free urine or 300 to 400 mEq sodium daily for protracted periods, according to the diet. As renal failure progresses, however, the kidney becomes unable to reabsorb the filtered sodium because of the osmotic diuresis accompanying the excretion of urea and other byproducts of metabolism. The distal tubular hydrogen ion excretory mechanism may also be impaired and cause further sodium losses. Consequently, it is incorrect to assume that patients with renal failure must follow a sodium-restricted diet.[23] Most patients with GFRs below 10 ml/min have sodium concentrations in the urine ranging from 10 to 25 mEq/L even when placed on sodium-free intakes. Because this will cause salt depletion and further compromise renal function, sodium intake should be repeatedly monitored in patients with end-stage renal disease. A serial record of body weight and a dietary history is usually sufficient to avoid salt depletion. Should the patient exhibit accumulation of edema, sodium intake should be reduced. In general, for most commercial foods, the sodium added in processing makes it difficult to reduce dietary sodium below 60 to 80 mEq per day. Fortunately, this is usually adequate to prevent sodium depletion in renal failure.

Two categories of renal disease require special attention. The group exhibiting edema and severe hypoalbuminemia as a part of the nephrotic syndrome have great difficulty excreting sodium chloride until the terminal stages of renal failure appear. Because rigid sodium restriction (< 10 mEq per day) is difficult to achieve, it is more effective to use an appropriate diuretic. For individuals who have glomerular filtration rates below 25 ml/min (serum creatinine greater than 5 mg/dl), furosemide, bumetanide, or ethacrynic acid are the only diuretics that will work dependably; the first two are the most effective and least toxic.[23] Potassium-sparing diuretics should not be given because they may produce life-threatening hyperkalemia when given to patients with impaired renal function.[32] The second category of renal disease requiring special attention to sodium intake, a salt-wasting renal disease, usually presents with insidious onset of uremia and no history of the nephrotic syndrome.[33] These patients may have marked pigmentation of the skin and usually have evidence of substantial volume depletion, including postural hypotension and poor skin turgor. The pertinent laboratory data are hyponatremia and urine [Na] in excess of 40 to 45 mEq/L. Daily intake of 250 mEq of sodium or more is often necessary to achieve sodium balance. This is a rare condition, but a high sodium intake produces such remarkable clinical improvement that the disturbance should always be considered for patients presenting with severe uremia and no history of acute renal disease.

POTASSIUM

The capacity of the normal kidney to secrete potassium exceeds the daily potassium intake by a substantial margin. Because of this, difficulty is not often encountered until the GFR declines to 1 to 2 percent of normal. Thus, dietary potassium restriction is usually not necessary until the patient nears the stage requiring dialysis in the immediate future or urine volume decreases sharply. Although potassium excretion may decline as acidosis progresses, this is usually corrected by correction of acidosis. Persistent elevation of potassium in the patient who has already reduced dietary protein and potassium is an indication for initiating maintenance dialysis. Hyporeninemic hypoaldosteronism of type IV renal tubular acidosis

is an exception. This disturbance, seen most commonly in diabetics with progressive diabetic nephropathy, is characterized by a persistently high serum potassium that is not responsive to the usual measures. When the diagnosis is confirmed by finding of low values for these hormones, treatment with 9-α-fluorohydrocortisone in addition to potassium restriction can correct serum potassium.[35]

WATER

The sustained osmotic diuresis of chronic renal failure impairs the concentrating process of the kidney. Solutes excreted by the kidney are at or near an isotonic concentration and, consequently, the average urinary volume ranges between 1600 and 2000 ml per day. When fluid intake is curtailed, output cannot fall until dehydration has resulted in a further reduction in GFR.[23] Because the loss of renal function is often only partially reversible, patients with renal failure should avoid significant dehydration. Should any intercurrent event or illness such as gastroenteritis supervene, prompt parenteral fluid therapy is essential if poor fluid intake or weight loss occurs.

Risk of dehydration and further renal impairment is particularly great in some diseases because of selective damage to the concentrating mechanism. These include the renal insufficiency of hypercalcemia, multiple myeloma, sickle cell disease, amyloidosis, and rarely some instances of advanced chronic pyelonephritis.

Restriction of water intake is almost never necessary in renal disease; indeed, hyponatremia is the only indication for restricting water intake. The patient should be told of the risks of dehydration and should be cautioned to seek medical advice promptly whenever diarrhea, nausea, and vomiting occur, even if they are mild.

HYPERTENSION

Hypertension is common and frequently hazardous in advanced renal failure. Severely hypertensive patients are at increased risk for all of the complications of high blood pressure and usually exhibit accelerated deterioration of renal function. Patients with end-stage renal disease who are about to begin hemodialysis often have an expanded extracellular fluid volume and inappropriately high levels of plasma renin activity. At different levels of salt intake, plasma renin activity is nearly always substantially higher in patients with end-stage renal disease compared to people with normal kidney function.[34] This suggests that the renin-angiotensin system is an important factor in the hypertension of end-stage renal disease. In the rare patient with end-stage renal disease in whom all forms of conservative management fail, bilateral nephrectomy should be considered as appropriate therapy.[34]

Because most hypertension in end-stage renal disease is associated with hyperreninemia, treatment should be directed at reducing renin levels. Beta-adrenergic blockade with propranolol, atenolol, or other agents is probably the safest initial step because renin release by the kidney is inhibited in addition to other, hypotensive, actions. Angiotensin-converting-enzyme (ACE) inhibitors should be used with great caution and begun at reduced dosage. A rapid fall in blood pressure resulting from overdosage with antihypertensive medications can precipitate prompt and on occasion irreversible anuria. Prudence dictates that the patient with a diastolic pressure above 115 mm Hg should be hospitalized.

If there is reason to suspect substantial renovascular disease associated with hypertension in renal insufficiency, ACE inhibitors are contraindicated if the serum creatinine is at or above 4 to 5 mg/dl. Deterioration of renal function may result from even modest doses of angiotensin-converting-enzyme inhibition under these circumstances.[12] The combination of ACE inhibition plus diuretic usage represents a particularly hazardous therapeutic regimen in the presence of impaired renal function.

ANEMIA

Anemia is a regular feature of advanced renal insufficiency, and the fall in hematocrit roughly parallels the diminution in renal function. The kidney produces a hormone, erythropoietin, that stimulates red cell production, and this hormone is decreased or absent in chronic renal disease. In addition, red cell survival time is shortened. These two factors may reduce the hematocrit to values less than 20 percent in severe uremia and cause prominent symptoms. Chief among these is weakness and easy fatigability, but the high cardiac output produced by anemia may lead to cardiac decompensation and coronary insufficiency. Patients being treated with low-protein diets or by dialysis should receive 1 mg folic acid daily and periodic measurement of serum ferritin concentration to detect evidence of iron depletion.[19] Although ferritin can be influenced by an acute illness and by protein malnutrition, a progressive decline in the serum level is consistent with iron deficiency. Although synthetic androgenic steroids have been shown to increase erythropoiesis and produce modest increases in the hematocrit in some uremic patients, their continued use is associated with signs of masculinization and a significant risk of hepatic toxicity. In addition to the usual hazards of blood transfusion, red cell destruction can result in hyperkalemia due to the increased plasma potassium present in stored blood. An even more common problem is acute circulatory overload, especially in patients who have a tendency to develop salt retention and congestive heart failure. If the symptoms of anemia require a transfusion, packed cells should be infused until the hematocrit is above 30 percent. Transfusion may improve fatigue and cardiac symptoms and may produce natriuresis. When transfusions become necessary, repeated investigation for evidence of gastrointestinal bleeding is mandatory because advanced uremia can impair clotting.[11]

USE OF DRUGS IN RENAL FAILURE

Many drugs in the original, metabolized, or conjugated form are excreted by the kidney. For this reason, recommended dosage ranges of many drugs may not be appropriate for this group of patients. In considering this problem, drugs can be divided into three groups: (1) Those that are metabolized in some extrarenal site or sites and excreted by the liver can be used in their usual dosages. (2) Those that are cleared so rapidly by the kidney that difficulty is encountered only when renal failure is far advanced. For example, ampicillin, carbenicillin, cephalosporins, para-aminosalicylic acid, and other organic acids have such high clearance values that their dosage need not be changed until creatinine clearance or GFR is reduced to less than 10 percent of normal.[3] Those excreted mainly by the kidney reach toxic levels when renal function has been only moderately impaired. This group includes the aminoglycosides, vancomycin, and colistimethate. For the latter two groups, therapy can be adjusted by reducing the dosage without changing the dosage interval or by extending the time interval between doses. The new dosage interval may be calculated from the ratio of the patient's creatinine clearance to the normal value for creatinine clearance.[3,31]

$$\text{Required dose interval} = \text{Normal dose interval} \times \frac{1}{f(K_f - 1) - 1}$$

where f is fraction of drug excreted by the normal kidney and K_f is the ratio of patient's creatinine clearance to normal creatinine clearance. Alternately, the dosage can be calculated:

$$\text{Required dose} = \text{Normal dose} \times \frac{f(K_f - 1) + 1}{1}$$

These calculations require measured or estimated values for the creatinine clearance. *For potentially toxic drugs with a low therapeutic index, the estimated creatinine clearance is never sufficiently accurate to permit safe dosage correction* (see Fig. 11.1–11); careful measurement of creatinine clearance is essential but still may be misleading because of fluctuations in GFR in seriously ill patients. If at all possible, drug dosage should be guided by repeated determination of plasma drug concentration, particularly when using toxic drugs such as the aminoglycosides. Table 11.5–3 lists some of the drugs exhibiting altered excretion in renal failure and the level of renal impairment at which dosage adjustment becomes necessary.

THERAPY OF END-STAGE RENAL FAILURE

Many patients (particularly those who are quite elderly) may not benefit materially from dialysis or transplantation. The patient with diabetes mellitus and extensive complications of peripheral vascular disease, cardiac disease, cerebral atherosclerosis, and loss of mental function or the patient with severe cerebral vascular disease and poor mental function probably will not benefit from chronic dialysis if their major symptoms are not related to uremia. The decision to forgo dialysis should be reached only after extensive discussion with the family and consultation with other physicians and the patient if he is capable of mental function. Perhaps the most useful criterion is the answer to the question: Is there a reasonable expectation that the quality of the patient's existence will be improved if dialysis is used to control uremia?

TREATMENT OF CHRONIC UREMIA BY DIALYSIS

Dialysis treatment has completely altered the prognosis for most forms of end-stage renal disease. Survival of patients has been extended from a period of months (see Fig. 11.5–2) to more than a decade. The dialysis procedure depends on the manipulation of osmotic and hydrostatic forces operating across a semipermeable membrane to remove waste substances, end products of metabolism, excesses of electrolytes and minerals, and water. Both peritoneal dialysis and hemodialysis are effective, and each has certain advantages and disadvantages.

TABLE 11.5–3. COMMONLY USED DRUGS AND REQUIREMENTS FOR DRUG MODIFICATION IN RENAL FAILURE

Drugs Requiring No Modification
- Clindamycin
- Erythromycin
- Isoxazolyl penicillins (Oxacillin, Nafcillin, Cloxacillin, Dicloxacillin)

Drug Dosage Modified When GFT < 50% of Normal
- Aminoglycosides (Amikacin, Gentamicin, Kanamycin, Tobramycin, Neomycin, Streptomycin)
- 5-Fluorocytosine
- Colistimethate
- Vancomycin

Drug Dosage Modified When GFT 10–20 ml/min
- Penicillins (Amoxicillin, Ampicillin, Methicillin, Carbenicillin, Ticarcillin, Penicillin G)
- Cephalosporins (Cephalothin, Cephamandol, Moxalactam, Cefotaxime)
- Lincomycin
- Sulfisoxazole
- Sulfamethoxazole-trimethoprim
- Isoniazid
- Ethambutol
- Metronidazole

PERITONEAL DIALYSIS

Peritoneal dialysis uses the peritoneal surface as a dialyzing membrane to exchange between the interstitial fluid and dialysis fluid infused into the peritoneal space.[8,25] The kinetics of this exchange are illustrated in Figure 11.5–1.

The optimum rate of peritoneal clearance obtained under ideal conditions is about 35 ml/min and is adequate to correct virtually all the symptoms of uremia within 24 hours.

Net fluid removal from the interstitial space and plasma will continue as long as the osmolar concentration of fluid infused in the peritoneal cavity exceeds that of plasma. Complete osmotic equilibrium between peritoneal fluid and interstitial fluid occurs in 2 to 4 hours. Until the two fluids become isosmolar, there is a continuing net shift of fluid from interstitium to peritoneal cavity. Even after isosmotic equivalence is achieved, complete equilibrium of the dialysate and interstitial fluids is not achieved. Glucose will be more concentrated and the concentrations of small solutes (e.g., urea, electrolytes) will be below plasma or interstitial concentrations. Thus, when dialysate is exchanged during the first 2 to 3 hours after installation, the net result is removal of water at a rate dependent on the concentration of glucose in the initial dialysate fluid. Except for this elevated glucose, the composition of dialysis fluid should be close to an ideal interstitial fluid except for the lack of potassium, urea, phosphate, and other substances to be removed. A solution containing 1.5 percent dextrose (373 mOsm/

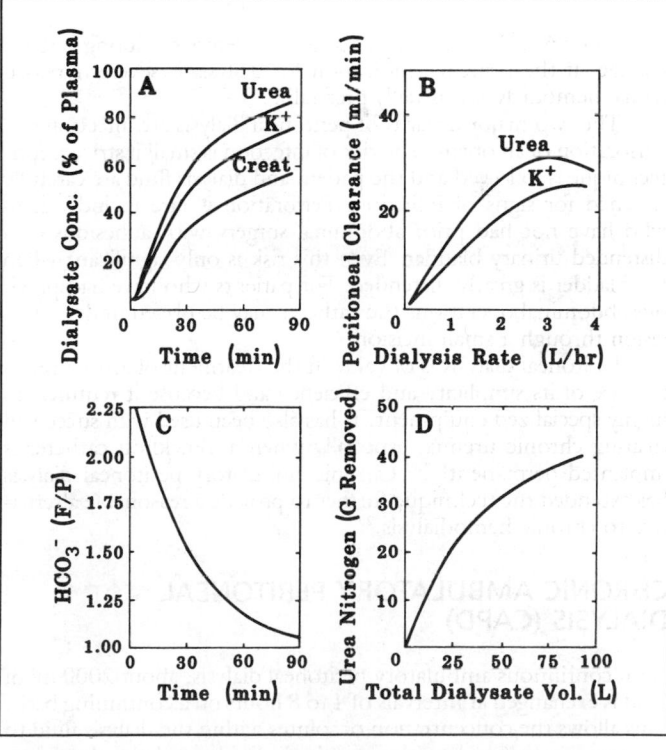

Figure 11.5–1. Kinetics of peritoneal dialysis. **A.** Rate at which plasma urea, potassium, and creatinine equilibrate with dialyzing fluid as a function of time remaining in abdomen. Quantitatively, the greatest net movement occurs in first 30 minutes. **B.** Peritoneal clearance as function of rate of dialysis. The drop at rates for dialysis in excess of 3 L per hour represents inadequate time for mixing and equilibration. **C.** Relatively rapid movement of bicarbonate from peritoneal cavity into body fluids. F/P refers to ratio of [HCO₃] in dialysate to that in plasma. **D.** An approximation of quantity of urea removed as function of total volume of dialyzing fluid. This varies with the initial level of urea. (*After Boen.*[8])

kg water) is adequate to achieve effective dialysis unless rapid fluid removal is the mean objective. In this case, 4 percent dextrose is more effective because it has an osmolality slightly in excess of 500 mOsm/kg of water.

The technique for performing peritoneal dialysis is to insert a polyvinyl catheter with multiple perforations into the right or left lower peritoneal cavity. Positioning is facilitated if insertion of the catheter is preceded by infusing a liter of fluid in the peritoneum through a small polyethylene catheter inserted through an 18-gauge needle. After the catheter is positioned, a normal-sized adult can usually tolerate 2 L of the fluid in the peritoneal cavity even when infused rapidly. In some patients with severe impairment of pulmonary function, only 1 L should be infused to avoid respiratory compromise. The fluid should be warmed to body temperature before infusion and should be left in the abdomen for 1 hour. Twenty minutes are usually required to withdraw fluid equal to that introduced, and 10 minutes is necessary to reintroduce new fluid. An exchange of 60 L over 40 hours is usually adequate.

Several points require emphasis:

1. *Acidosis:* the rate of bicarbonate movement across the peritoneum is sufficient to correct acidosis more promptly than with hemodialysis.
2. *Extracellular fluid overexpansion:* continuous and accurate recording of net fluid removal and changes in weight are necessary to avoid large excesses or deficits in body fluids.
3. *Hyperkalemia:* with potassium-free dialysis fluid, the potassium concentration will reach approximately 50 to 60 percent of the plasma concentration and may attain values as high as 3 to 4 mEq/L but is usually below this.[26]

Thus only 6 to 10 mEq of potassium are removed during one exchange: if the principal indication for dialysis is severe hyperkalemia, hemodialysis is usually preferable.

The two major hazards of peritoneal dialysis are infection and perforation of an organ. The risk of infection is small if strict aseptic technique is followed and the patient and dialysis fluid are carefully watched for signs of infection. Perforation is rare in individuals who have not had prior abdominal surgery with adhesions or a distended urinary bladder. Even this risk is only significant when the bladder is greatly distended. For patients who have had previous abdominal operations the catheter may be placed under direct vision through a small incision.

Peritoneal dialysis is of value in the treatment of acute uremia because of its simplicity and efficiency and because it requires no highly specialized equipment. It has also been used with success in treating chronic uremia, especially when a Tenckhoff catheter is implanted permanently.[30] Chronic ambulatory peritoneal dialysis has extended the technique further to provide a reasonable alternative to chronic hemodialysis.[25]

CHRONIC AMBULATORY PERITONEAL DIALYSIS (CAPD)

With continuous ambulatory peritoneal dialysis, about 2000 ml of fluid is exchanged at intervals of 4 to 8 hours on a continuing basis. This allows the concentration of solutes within the dialysis fluid to become nearly equal to those in body fluids, and the slower removal of fluid and solutes tends to minimize fluid shifts while chronically removing waste products.[26]

The fact that the peritoneal membrane has a different permeability than artificial membranes allows some large molecules, including the potentially toxic "middle molecules," to be removed at a significantly greater rate than in hemodialyzers. The increased "porosity" of the peritoneal membrane is further reflected in the substantial quantities of albumin found in the peritoneal dialysate. This may result in loss of more than 3 to 6 g of albumin per day. The loss of protein and amino acids during CAPD raises the dietary protein requirement to 1 to 1.4 g/kg per day.[7]

CAPD represents an important therapeutic option for managing end-stage renal disease and has proven particularly beneficial for children. It also is useful for diabetics who often do poorly with hemodialysis. The major limitation is the development of peritonitis.

CHRONIC HEMODIALYSIS

The continuing success of chronic dialysis depends on an adequate arteriovenous (A-V) communication in the form of an internal shunt or an internal fistula. Either form allows repeated access to blood flowing at a sufficiently high rate to achieve an adequate removal of waste products. An A-V fistula is usually preferable in younger individuals with good arterial vessels that are relatively free of atheromatous change. In the elderly, clotting of the fistula occurs much more readily, and better results are usually achieved with an internal synthetic (Goretex) communication between the artery and vein. To allow sufficient time for healing, it is desirable to create an A-V fistula (or insert a synthetic shunt) 2 to 3 months before dialysis is to start.

Maintenance Regimen

The dialysis patient may have no significant excretion of water and solutes except that provided by intermittent dialyses. For this reason, careful regulation of fluid and food intake is of primary importance. In general it is desirable to remove approximately 1.5 to 2 kg from the patient as fluid during the course of a single dialysis to allow the patient sufficient fluid intake. Removal of larger quantities usually produces hypotension, cramps, nausea, vomiting, and severe malaise. If the patient gains more than 1.5 kg between dialyses or has already accumulated excess fluid, more rigid restriction of fluid intake will be necessary in addition to dialysis.

The diet should be planned to provide a protein intake of 1 g/kg of body weight daily (Table 11.5–1). The additional protein is required because the stress of dialysis and loss of amino acids by the nonselective dialytic process raises protein requirements.[9] A lower protein intake requires less frequent dialysis.[21] The sodium intake should be between 1 and 2 g a day, and the potassium intake should be kept as low as possible according to palatability of the diet.

Knowledge of the metabolism and half-lives of drugs is necessary for safe and efficient therapy of these patients.[3,31] Drugs and drug metabolites excreted by the kidney exhibit variable dialysance depending on protein binding, type, and duration of dialysis and whether drug metabolism changes significantly in uremia.[3] Dialyzability of maintenance drugs is always an important issue in patients on maintenance dialysis because it influences both dosage and time and frequency of drug administration in relation to dialysis. Table 11.5–4 indicates the dialyzability of some of the more commonly used drugs in patients with end-stage renal disease. Where plasma levels are critical, as in maintenance of bactericidal levels of antibiotics, this information should be supplemented with frequent determination of plasma levels of drug whenever possible.

Complications of Long-Term Dialysis

Anemia is one of the most prevalent and characteristic features of hemodialysis patients. The primary cause appears to be reduced or absent erythropoietic activity, but folate or iron deficiency and blood loss may aggravate the anemia. Folic acid and other water-soluble vitamins should be given because hemodialysis removes water-soluble vitamins. Blood for laboratory determinations and blood remaining in the dialyser make it necessary to monitor iron stores periodically; if low values are found, iron therapy must be instituted. It is essential to check stool guaiac frequently in such instances to exclude blood loss as a factor.

Frequent blood transfusions increase the risk of hepatitis and the antibody response to foreign HLA antigens. This can reduce the likelihood of successful tissue matching, but there is evidence that patients who have many transfusions and then are successfully

TABLE 11.5–4. DIALYZABILITY OF DRUGS COMMONLY USED IN PATIENTS WITH RENAL FAILURE

Dialyzable	Nondialyzable
Amoxicillin	Cloxacillin
Ampicillin	Nafcillin
Penicillin G	Vancomycin
Ticarcillin	Clindamycin
Gentamicin	Erythromycin
Amikacin	Doxycycline
Tobramycin	Clonidine
Cephalosporins	Hydralazine
Sulfonamides	Propranolol
Methyldopa	Amphotericin
Minoxidil	Ketoconazole
Captopril	Miconazole
Enalaprilat	

tissue matched are more likely to have a successful transplantation with a cadaver kidney.[27]

Recently the gene for human erythropoietin has been molecularly cloned, and through recombinant DNA technology, biologically active erythropoietin can now be produced in adequate quantities. Preliminary clinical trials indicate that recombinant human erythropoietin can correct the anemia associated with end-stage renal disease, and in the future erythropoietin therapy should abolish the need for red cell transfusions in this situation.

Hyperkalemia represents the most serious threat to chronic dialysis patients. This is such a problem that patients with regular predialysis values in excess of 5 mEq/L should be treated with dietary potassium restriction and, if this is inadequate, with potassium exchange resins (Kayexalate). If hyperkalemia cannot be controlled effectively by these measures, then more frequent dialysis or more efficient dialysis is necessary.

Fluid overload and hypertension are other difficult problems. Because it is difficult to remove more than about 1.5 kg of fluid during dialysis, fluid intake should be limited to 400 ml per day or less to prevent fluid overload.

Hypertension is closely related to fluid overload and is aggravated markedly by excess salt and water intake. Although hypertension may be controlled by removing fluid in some instances, severe hypertension persists despite removal of 8 or 10 kg of fluid. In individuals who do not respond to salt and water removal and aggressive drug therapy, bilateral nephrectomy may be necessary.

Renal osteodystrophy[5,13,24,28], which is characterized as a combination of osteomalacia and osteitis fibrosa, has been attributed to vitamin D deficiency and secondary hyperparathyroidism. Symptomatic osteodystrophy with bone pain, gross evidence of bone resorption, and pathologic fractures requires therapy with 1,25-dihydroxy vitamin D_3 and, if this is unsuccessful, parathyroidectomy. Although a recent report[29] suggests that intravenous 1,25-dihydroxy vitamin D_3 may be especially effective treatment for hemodialysis patients, control of hyperphosphatemia is essential. Therapy should include a low-phosphate diet, phosphate binders such as aluminum hydroxide gels and calcium carbonate, and adequate dialysis.

RENAL TRANSPLANTATION

Successful renal transplantation represents the most effective means of correcting uremia. It is now clear that transplantation between members of the same family produces superior results, but cadaver kidneys also produce acceptable results.

Tissue typing based on identification of human leukocyte antigens permits selection of siblings with apparent identity of histocompatibility antigens. A renal transplant between these individuals has a 5-year survival rate exceeding 90 percent, substantially better than results of transplantation between siblings who share only two of the four HLA antigens or transplants of cadaver kidneys.[1]

Continuous immunosuppression is necessary to maintain stable renal function in transplant patients. A combination of prednisone and azathioprine is effective but adds risk of infection, aseptic necrosis of joints (particularly the hips and knees), cataracts, and an increased incidence of malignant neoplasms. The new drug, cyclosporine, is neither cytotoxic nor myelosuppressive but acts by blocking production of, and responsiveness to, the T-lymphocyte lymphokine, interleukin-2. By suppressing T-lymphocyte activation it has provided more effective immunosuppression and improved the survival rate of transplanted cadaver kidneys.[6] Unfortunately, cyclosporine is nephrotoxic, and determining whether a posttransplant decline in renal function is due to rejection or cyclosporine-induced renal damage is occasionally quite difficult. Its nephrotoxicity also limits long-term use.

Despite these problems, results with dialysis and transplantation are sufficiently good to permit considerable optimism regarding the treatment of chronic uremia. Results with both therapies continue to improve.

PROGNOSIS[36]

It has been estimated that the death rate among patients with chronic uremia who are maintained on chronic dialysis is approximately 10 percent per year. Of those who are adequately treated by dialysis, somewhere between one half and two thirds are able to return to work and may be regarded as rehabilitated. Figure 11.5–2 shows survival data for a large regional program and illustrates the improvement in survival offered by the combined approach of dialysis and transplantation. Individuals who receive a renal transplant that functions normally with modest dosages of immunosuppressive drugs are capable of leading normal lives. Pa-

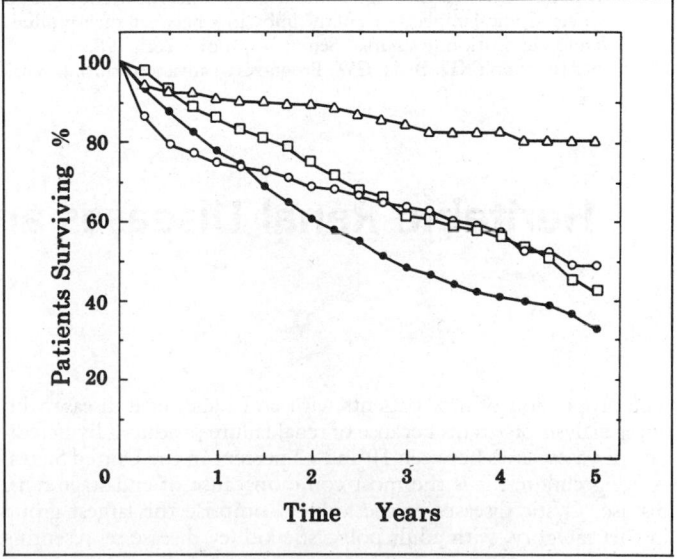

Figure 11.5–2. Survival percentage derived by the standard life-table method plotted against time for related transplant patients (△; N = 173), cadaver transplant patients (○; N = 402), home dialysis patients (□; N = 261), and all center dialysis patients (●; N = 2,396). (*Reprinted with permission, Kidney Int 21:78 1982.*)

tients who elect to dialyze themselves at home at night or in the evening may return to full-time employment with relatively little interference caused by their renal failure.

REFERENCES

1. Advisory Committee to the Renal Transplant Registry: The thirteenth report of the Human Renal Transplant Registry. Transplant Proc 9:9, 1977
2. Ahlmen J: Incidence of chronic renal insufficiency. A study of the incidence and pattern of renal insufficiency in adults during 1966–1971 in Gothenberg. Acta Med Scand entire Suppl 582, 1975
3. Anderson RJ, Bennett WM, et al: Fate of drugs in renal failure. In Brenner BM, Rector FC Jr (eds): The Kidney, 2d ed. Philadelphia, WB Saunders, 1981, vol 2, p 2659
4. Arieff AI, Guisado R, et al: Central nervous system pH in uremia and the effects of hemodialysis. J Clin Invest 58:306, 1976
5. Arnaud CD: Hyperparathyroidism and renal failure. Kidney Int 4:89, 1973
6. Bennett WM, Norman DJ: Action and toxicity of cyclosporin. Ann Rev Med 37:215, 1986
7. Blumenkrantz MJ, Kopple JD, et al: Metabolic balance studies and dietary protein requirements in patients undergoing continuous ambulatory peritoneal dialyses. Kidney Int 21:849, 1982
8. Boen ST: Kinetics of peritoneal dialysis, a comparison with the artificial kidney. Medicine 40:243, 1961
9. Borah MF, Schoenfeld PY, et al: Nitrogen balance during intermittent dialysis therapy of uremia. Kidney Int 14:491, 1978
10. Brenner BM, Meyer TW, Hostetter TH: Dietary protein intake and the progressive nature of kidney disease. N Engl J Med 307:652, 1982
11. Deykin D: Uremic bleeding. Kidney Int 24:698, 1983
12. Hricik DE, Browning PJ, Kopelman R, et al: Captopril-induced functional renal insufficiency in patients with bilateral renal artery stenosis or renal artery stenosis in a solitary kidney. N Engl J Med 308:373, 1983
13. Johnson WJ, Goldsmith RS, et al: The influence of maintaining normal serum phosphate and calcium in renal osteodystrophy. In Norman AW, Shaefer K, et al (eds): Vitamin D and Problems Related to Uremic Bone Disease. New York, Walter de Gruyter, 1975
14. Johnson WJ, Hagge WH, et al: Effects of urea loading in patients with far-advanced renal failure. Mayo Clin Proc 47:21, 1972
15. Johnson WJ, O'Kane HO, et al: Survival of patients with end-stage renal disease. Mayo Clin Proc 48:18, 1973
16. Kelly RA, Mitch WE: Creatinine, uric acid and other nitrogenous waste products: Clinical implications of the imbalance between their production and elimination in uremia. Semin Nephrol 3:286, 1983
17. Maher JF, Nolph KD, Bryan CW: Prognosis of advanced chronic renal failure. Unpredictability of survival and reversibility. Ann Intern Med 81:43, 1974
18. Maroni BJ, Steinman TI, Mitch WE: A method for measuring nitrogen intake of patients with chronic renal failure. Kidney Int 27:58, 1985
19. Mirahmadi KS, Paul WL, et al: Serum ferritin level: Determinant of iron requirement in hemodialysis patients. JAMA 238:601, 1977
20. Mitch WE: Nutritional therapy and the progression of chronic renal insufficiency. Ann Rev Med 35:249, 1984
21. Mitch WE: Measuring the progression of renal insufficiency. In Mitch WE (ed): The Progressive Nature of Renal Diseases. Contemporary Issues in Nephrology, vol 14. New York, Churchill Livingstone, 1986
22. Mitch WE, Walser M: Nutritional management of the uremic patient. In Brenner BM, Rector FC Jr (eds): The Kidney, 3d ed. Philadelphia, WB Saunders, 1986
23. Mitch WE, Wilcox CS: Disorders of body fluids, sodium and potassium in chronic renal failure. Am J Med 72:536, 1982
24. Nebeker HG, Coburn JW: Aluminum and renal osteodystrophy. Ann Rev Med 37:79, 1986
25. Nolph KD, Miller F, Rubin J: New directions in peritoneal dialysis concepts and applications. Kidney Int 18(suppl 10):5111, 1980
26. Nolph KD, Twardowski ZJ, Popovich M: Equilibration of peritoneal dialysis solutions during long dwell exchanges. J Lab Clin Med 93:246, 1979
27. Opelz G, Terasaki PI: Enhancement of kidney graft survival by blood transfusions. Transplant Proc 9:121, 1977
28. Slatopolsky E, Bricker NS: The role of phosphorus restriction in the prevention of hyperparathyroidism in chronic renal disease. Kidney Int 4:141, 1973
29. Slatopolsky E, Weerts C, et al: Marked suppression of secondary hyperparathyroidism by intravenous administration of 1,25 dihydroxycholecalciferol in uremic patients. J Clin Invest 74:2136, 1984
30. Striber GE, Tenckhoff HA: A transcutaneous prosthesis for prolonged access to the peritoneal cavity. Surgery 69:70, 1971
31. Tozer TN: Nomogram for modification of dosage regimen in patients with chronic renal function impairment. J Pharmacokinetic Biopharm 2:13, 1974
32. Walker BR, Capuzzi DM, Alexander F: Hyperkalemia after triamterene in diabetic patients. Clin Pharmacol Ther 13:642, 1972
33. Walker WG, Jost LJ, et al: Metabolic observations on salt wasting in renal disease. Am J Med 39:505, 1965
34. Weidmann P, Beretta-Picoli C, et al: Hypertension in terminal renal failure. Kidney Int 9:294, 1976
35. Weidmann P, Reinhart R, Maxwell WH: Syndrome of hyporeninemic hypoaldosteronism and hyperkalemia in renal disease. J Clin Endocrinol Metab 36:965, 1973
36. Weller JM, Port FK, et al: Analysis of survival of end-stage renal disease patients. Kidney Int 21:78, 1982
37. Young VR: Some metabolic and nutritional considerations of dietary protein restriction. In Mitch WE (ed): The Progressive Nature of Renal Diseases, Contemporary Issues in Nephrology, vol 14. New York, Churchill Livingstone, 1986

CHAPTER 11.6

Heritable Renal Diseases and Disorders of Tubular Function

W. Gordon Walker

The proportion of new patients with end-stage renal disease who enter dialysis programs because of renal failure produced by hereditary diseases varies between 10 and 12 percent in the United States. Among children it is the most common cause of end-stage renal disease. Cystic diseases of the kidney comprise the largest group in this category, with adult polycystic kidney disease representing approximately 10 percent of patients entering dialysis. The various categories of medullary cystic disease or nephronophthisis are responsible for the majority of end-stage renal disease in childhood and adolescence.

In this chapter are considered those heritable diseases and disturbances of renal function that are most likely to be encountered in adults and older adolescents. No attempt has been made to provide a comprehensive presentation of all hereditary renal disorders. Instead the presentation focuses on those heritable renal disorders that are more commonly encountered plus those in which correct diagnosis is essential for appropriate and specific therapy.

POLYCYSTIC KIDNEY DISEASE[6,12,19]

Polycystic kidney disease is by far the most prevalent hereditary disease of the kidneys and accounts for about one tenth of all pa-

tients requiring maintenance hemodialysis for end-stage renal disease. There are in fact two distinct polycystic kidney diseases with different patterns of inheritance: The more common or adult form of polycystic disease, which exhibits an autosomal dominant pattern of inheritance, and the much less common childhood polycystic kidney disease, which is inherited as an autosomal recessive trait.

ADULT POLYCYSTIC DISEASE

Adult polycystic disease presents most commonly with abdominal pain, usually in the third or fourth decade of life, although it is not uncommon to have males present in the late teenage years with severe flank pain and hematuria as a result of modest trauma. Additional patterns of clinical presentation include gross hematuria, bilateral flank masses, hypertension, and rare instances of salt-wasting or of intracranial hemorrhage. Occasionally azotemia with advanced renal failure is the presenting picture with no significant clinical manifestations before the renal failure. Most commonly, symptomatic renal failure appears in the fifth or sixth decade but in some instances may present later.

There is little that can be done to prevent the appearance and progressive enlargement of the cysts, and this progressive enlargement is responsible for the inexorable development of renal failure. The process is hastened by recurrent urinary tract infections and by inadequately treated hypertension. Consequently, all patients with polycystic kidneys should be watched carefully for signs of recurrent infection or hypertension. In addition to accelerating the kidney disease, the hypertension increases the risk of intracranial hemorrhage because of the strong association between polycystic kidney disease and berry aneurysms of the cerebral circulation. Postmortem studies have demonstrated berry aneurysms in as many as 10 percent of the patients dying from polycystic kidneys.

CHILDHOOD POLYCYSTIC DISEASE

Childhood polycystic disease is a separate hereditary disturbance that has a frequency of about 1 in 10,000 births. In the majority of instances bilateral flank masses are evident at birth and are associated with a protuberant abdomen. Hepatomegaly is readily demonstrated at birth because of cystic involvement of the liver associated with substantial renal failure at the time of delivery. Death occurs within the first year of life. The disorder is mentioned here because occasionally some patients survive into adolescence. The disease has been divided into four subcategories.

The *perinatal form* of childhood polycystic kidney disease presents with severe renal impairment at birth and death occurs within 6 to 8 weeks after delivery. The *neonatal form* of the disease has slightly less intense renal impairment from the cystic kidneys, but death from renal failure occurs virtually always within the first year of life if no attempt is made to support renal function by dialysis. The *infantile subcategory* of the disease has more striking hepatomegaly at birth, but kidney function is sufficient to support growth for a number of years. Occasionally individuals survive into adolescence and present with uremia at this time. The diagnosis is readily made by physical examination because of the large liver, usually with identifiable chemical evidence of hepatic dysfunction as well as progressive uremia. Finally, the *juvenile polycystic* form has liver involvement as the predominant disturbance, and death is often related to the liver involvement.

MEDULLARY CYSTIC DISEASE[12]

Medullary cystic disease is probably the most common cause of end-stage renal disease among children. The clinical presentation is characterized by polyuria and polydipsia at an early age followed by growth retardation, weakness, pallor, azotemia, and early death, usually in the second decade of life unless dialysis is used to maintain life.

Gardner[12] has called attention to the fact that there are four closely related types of medullary disease and has proposed the term "nephronophthisis-cystic renal medullary complex" to encompass them.

Juvenile nephronophthisis presents earliest and accounts for roughly half of all juvenile and adolescent cases of end-stage renal disease. The clinical presentation is as noted previously. The kidneys are characteristically quite small on sonography, and it is only on microscopic examination that cysts may be demonstrated in the medullary and corticomedullary junction. On occasion no cysts are demonstrated.

Renal-retinal dysplasia exhibits a similar clinical pattern but is associated with some form of retinitis, usually retinitis pigmentosa, with progressive loss of vision being associated with the renal manifestations of the disease. Renal-retinal dysplasia represents 15 percent of all the cases included in the nephronophthisis-renal medullary complex entity. *Adult-onset medullary cystic disease* accounts for about 20 percent of all cases and is usually recognized in the late years of the second decade or the early part of the third decade. In addition, perhaps 15 to 20 percent of cases have been termed sporadic because no family history can be obtained, and examination of the other family members fails to identify any evidence of similar renal disease.

Renal salt wasting is a prominent feature of this category of heritable disease. It has been found in over two thirds of those individuals who have been adequately studied for salt wasting. This is a matter of substantial therapeutic significance because the volume depletion further aggravates the renal failure. Many of the patients require sodium intakes in excess of 350 to 400 mEq per day to prevent acute decline in renal function.

Maintenance hemodialysis and renal transplantation have markedly altered the prognosis in this once uniformly fatal group of diseases. It is important to stress that these individuals are at particularly high risk for the development of renal osteodystrophy shortly after beginning dialysis, because they often have had very long-standing hyperphosphatemia and elevated levels of parathyroid hormone. They thus have had a much longer time to develop diffuse osseous changes, and in fact often show some stigmata of renal osteodystrophy before beginning dialysis. In general, however, effective control of phosphate intake with maintenance of serum phosphate within a normal range will reverse any bone damage that may have already occurred and allow progressive healing of the osteodystrophy if a normal phosphorus is maintained in the presence of an adequate calcium intake.

HEREDITARY NEPHRITIS (ALPORT SYNDROME)[3,23]

This heritable form of glomerulonephritis is associated with progressive renal damage and terminates in renal failure that requires maintenance dialysis or transplantation for survival. Clinical presentation is similar to other forms of nephritis, with all patients exhibiting microscopic hematuria and about 15 percent or more having episodes of gross hematuria. Red cell casts are demonstrable in 30 to 40 percent of patients. Proteinuria is always present and reaches nephrotic ranges in about 10 percent of patients with this disease.

Most reports containing information on more than one generation have proposed that the trait is an autosomal dominant trait and male-to-male transmission to offspring has been documented. There are some reports suggesting that the disease occasionally exhibits sex-linked dominant inheritance. It tends to be milder in females in some kindreds. Renal failure usually begins in childhood in affected males but often at a significantly later period in time in affected females. Progressive deafness is a commonly associated but not universally present disturbance.

No effective treatment is available for slowing or arresting the

disease, but maintenance dialysis and transplantation have been quite effective in prolonging life.

FABRY DISEASE[8]

Fabry disease is characterized by unique skin lesions; it was originally described under the title "angiokeratoma corporis diffusum." It presents usually in early childhood in males with severe pains in the extremities, often erroneously diagnosed as arthritis; frequent episodes of fever (which may alternately lead to the diagnosis of rheumatic fever); and hypohidrosis and evidence of progressive dysfunction of both sympathetic and parasympathetic neural systems.

The disease is inherited as an X-linked dominant disorder, so that all sons of male hemizygotes are free of the disease and all daughters are obligate carriers. Half of the male offspring of female carriers will be expected to have the disease, and half are free of the defective allele.

The metabolic defect is a deficiency of a lysosomal hydrolase, α-galactosidase A. The result is the accumulation of the lipid substrate of this enzyme, a ceramide trihexoside. This accumulates in cells within the kidney, producing the characteristic fat-laden cells, which distort the glomeruli and blood vessels. Comparable changes can also be found throughout the vascular bed and in the skin lesions, the peripheral nerves, and the central nervous system. The disease is progressive, and renal failure in males usually appears in the third decade of life. The disease is much less severe among females because their heterozygosity is associated with reduced rather than absent levels of α-galactosidase A.

Treatment of the hemizygote males has been disappointing. The hope that renal transplantation would provide them with an adequate source of enzyme has in general been clinically disappointing, although some transient decreases in the circulating levels of the ceramide trihexoside have been reported. Enzyme replacement by intravenous administration of purified enzyme has produced transient lowering of the circulating substrate. Perhaps the most encouraging aspect of this therapeutic approach is the failure to develop an immune response to the purified enzyme; thus long-term treatment with the enzyme appears to be at least a theoretical possibility. Plasmapheresis has been associated with removal of only modest quantities of the substrate. Although dialysis and transplantation have altered the outlook somewhat after renal failure occurs, the systemic manifestations of the disease are progressive, and the patients usually become progressively more incapacitated from other manifestations of the disease. Hence some form of enzyme replacement appears to be the only real hope for effective therapy at present.

HEREDITARY AMYLOIDOSIS[14,36]

Several forms of amyloidosis have been described that are associated with amyloid infiltration of the kidney and may produce nephrotic syndrome, progressive renal damage, and chronic renal failure. *Muckle Wells syndrome* is associated with severe, recurrent urticaria, which is usually associated with fever and limb pains. Renal involvement is manifested by increasing proteinuria, nephrotic syndrome, and ultimately renal failure. *Ostertag amyloid nephropathy* exhibits prominent hematuria in association with the proteinuria. Hepatosplenomegaly is usually present, and the course is slowly progressive, with uremia appearing in the fourth decade of life or later. In addition, *familial Mediterranean fever* is probably the most common manifestation of hereditary amyloidosis. In contrast to other forms of hereditary amyloid disease that exhibit autosomal dominant patterns of inheritance, familial Mediterranean fever is an autosomal recessive disorder that progresses to renal failure relatively early.

Other kindreds with hereditary amyloidosis have been re-

ported, not all of whom had renal involvement as a prominent feature of the disease. Once renal amyloid appears, however, it progresses inexorably to end-stage renal disease.

Until relatively recently only dialysis and transplantation could be offered as treatment for the uremia of amyloidosis; more recently, however, it appears that colchicine is of value in preventing progression of the renal failure, at least in those patients who have familial Mediterranean fever.[36]

RENAL TUBULAR ACIDOSIS

Renal tubular acidosis (RTA) is a syndome characterized by systemic hyperchloremic metabolic acidosis of variable severity that results from impaired urinary acidification. Two distinct genetic or familial types are recognized. Type I (classic) RTA is an autosomal dominant heritable disorder caused by a defect in distal tubular hydrogen ion secretion that decreases ammonium ion and titratable acid in the urine.[24] Type II (proximal) RTA is associated with defective proximal reabsorption of filtered bicarbonate.[1] Both types result in systemic hyperchloremic acidosis, but other clinical manifestations differ. The typical clinical syndromes as originally described are both examples of inherited disorders of tubular transport. More recently it has become evident that many disorders can interfere with hydrogen ion secretion in either the distal or proximal region of the nephron and produce a hyperchloremic acidosis typical of distal (type I) or proximal (type II) renal tubular acidosis. Because treatment of the two types is different, correct diagnosis is of practical importance.

A third type of defective acidification is encountered in diffuse renal disease when the functioning tubular mass is reduced to a level that interferes with hydrogen transport and leads to defective proximal bicarbonate reabsorption and total hydrogen ion secretion.[26] This is usually transient and occurs in the setting of advanced diffuse renal disease; the hyperchloremia is present only for a short period. It is superseded by an increase in nonvolatile anions (increased anion gap) as renal failure worsens.

A fourth type (type IV RTA) is of greater clinical significance, persists for longer periods of time, exhibits unique features, and is probably the most common encountered form of renal tubular acidosis. Type IV RTA is associated with impaired renal tubular function and characterized by hyperchloremic acidosis and hyperkalemia. It usually occurs in a setting of impaired renal function but has been recognized in subjects who have a normal glomerular filtration rate.[29] It occurs as one of the clinical features of several complex heritable disorders and in several acquired diseases associated with impaired renin secretion or defective aldosterone production or responsiveness. Because renal potassium transport is quite different in this group of disorders from that seen in type I or type II RTA, early recognition is essential if appropriate treatment is to be started and the risk of worsening hyperkalemia by inappropriate therapy avoided.

TYPE I DISTAL RENAL TUBULAR ACIDOSIS

This disease is most commonly recognized clinically in the second and third decades of life but may be diagnosed in virtually any age group.[10,31] Presenting symptoms may include renal stone, hematuria, periodic paralysis, or skeletal abnormalities. Presently, with the widespread use of screening laboratory determinations, the disorder is most often recognized by detection of unsuspected hyperchloremic acidosis.

The specific defect is an inability to transport hydrogen ions against a gradient comparable to that developed by the normal kidney in the presence of systemic acidosis (Table 11.6–1). This inability to lower the pH of the urine reduces both titratable acid and ammonia excretion. As a result, the kidney is forced to excrete abnormally large quantities of potassium, calcium, and sodium to maintain electroneutrality. This continuing drain of cations, par-

TABLE 11.6–1. DIAGNOSIS OF RENAL TUBULAR ACIDOSIS[1,2,4,10,18,21,22,24,26,35]

	Plasma HCO$_3$ (mEq/L)	Urinary pH	Titratable Acidity[a] (μEq/min)	NH$_4$ Production[a] (μEq/min)	Total H^{+}[a] Production
Normal subjects	23–25	4.8–5.2	30–40	50–60	80–100
Type I RTA (distal)	20–23	6.7–6.9	12–18	15–30	30–50
Type II RTA (proximal)	15–18	4.8–5.5	30–40	40–60	80–100

[a] Values represent responses to ammonium chloride loading (0.1/kg) as described by Wrong and Davies,[35] or values obtained during untreated systemic acidosis.

ticularly potassium and calcium, can lead to profound skeletal abnormalities and in some instances hypokalemia of such severity as to produce episodic paralysis. This failure of ammonia excretion and of titratable acid leads to a corresponding reduction in bicarbonate reabsorption that produces a decrease in serum bicarbonate, systemic acidosis, and hyperchloremia. The associated cation losses are responsible for the development of rickets or osteomalacia and may in some instances produce hypokalemic paralysis. Thus, hyperchloremic acidosis, hypokalemia, rickets or osteomalacia, and nephrocalcinosis, usually with recurrent renal stones, represent the hallmarks of untreated distal or type I renal tubular acidosis. When the disease presents clinically during childhood, these findings are also associated with a marked reduction in the rate of growth.

It has been demonstrated in one well-studied kindred that there was a much greater frequency of hypercalciuria than of a demonstrable acidification defect. In at least one instance a progression from hypercalciuria to nephrocalcinosis and final renal tubular acidosis was observed in a member of the kindred who exhibited only hypercalciuria when first seen during childhood.[2] It may be that some of the clinically recognized cases of distal tubular damage and resultant renal tubular acidosis represent changes secondary to long-standing hypercalciuria and associated nephrocalcinosis. The persistent hypercalciuria and progressive nephrocalcinosis seen in hyperparathyroidism can lead to an acidification defect and hyperchloremic acidosis.[2,29,31] Because of the different presentations and varied clinical courses exhibited by different kindreds reported to date, it has been suggested that there are several heritable disorders that present as distal or type I RTA.[21]

In addition to the genetic form of the disease that may be inherited without any other associated abnormalities, there are a number of disorders, some inherited, some acquired, that exhibit defective distal acidification. As with classic type I (distal) RTA, the characteristic feature is an inability to lower urinary pH. Ammonium ion production is adequate or normal for the level of urinary pH achieved. Among the genetic disorders exhibiting this type of acidification defect are patients with Ehlers-Danlos syndrome, hereditary elliptocytosis, and sickle cell anemia, as well as some cases of medullary cystic disease.[4,31] Hyperchloremic acidosis with inappropriately high urinary pH has also been described in association with hypergammaglobulinemia, Sjögren syndrome, chronic active hepatitis, systemic lupus erythematosus, and chronic biliary cirrhosis. Nephrocalcinosis, including primary hyperparathyroidism and vitamin D intoxication, is also associated with distal RTA.[31]

TYPE II PROXIMAL TUBULAR ACIDOSIS

In Type II proximal tubular acidosis the primary problem is failure of proximal reabsorption of filtered bicarbonate. As a consequence, the fluid reabsorbed by the kidney has a lower concentration of bicarbonate, and a systemic acidosis results. Once a steady state is reached at a lower bicarbonate level, however, the distal renal tubular mechanisms operate adequately. In this circumstance, the individual has a systemic metabolic acidosis characterized by a marked hyperchloremia, but with a normal urine pH. Thus, at this reduced level of bicarbonate concentration within the

body fluids, the acidification mechanism within the kidney works satisfactorily, yielding normal values for titratable acid and ammonia excretion. As a result, these patients do not have a continuous drain on the cation stores of the bone, and skeletal abnormalities are not usually seen.

When treatment of type II RTA is undertaken, two characteristic features are observed. First, large quantities of bicarbonate (up to 10 mEq/kg body weight per day) are required to return the plasma bicarbonate to normal levels and to maintain the concentration within this range. Urine pH becomes very alkaline long before the plasma bicarbonate returns to normal levels. Second, as bicarbonate administration is begun, there is a marked increase in potassium loss. Frequently, quite large quantities of supplemental potassium are required to maintain potassium balance and prevent severe hypokalemia.

Etiologically spontaneously occurring and hereditary forms of proximal (type II) renal tubular acidosis have been recognized. Much more commonly, the defect is associated with Fanconi syndrome or with evidence of tubular damage secondary to various toxic agents such as heavy metals, amphotericins, and other organic compounds.[29,31] It has also been reported as a feature of Lowe syndrome, and hereditary fructose intolerance. Patients with multiple myeloma and monoclonal gammopathy exhibit classic type II proximal renal tubular acidosis on occasion. In addition, a number of drugs have been recognized as producing this disturbance, including outdated tetracycline, sulfonamides, and streptozotocin.[31]

Differential Diagnosis—Type I and Type II

The features of all forms of renal tubular acidosis that call attention to the problem are hyperchloremia and acidosis with a normal anion gap. The principal diagnostic features that distinguish type I and type II renal tubular acidosis are (1) the urinary pH during systemic acidosis, (2) the severity of potassium wasting, and (3) the pattern of renal bicarbonate loss as plasma bicarbonate is progressively increased. As noted in Table 11.6–1, the patient with classic type I (distal) RTA has an abnormally elevated urine pH even when systemic acidosis is present. Thus a urine pH of greater than 6.5 in the presence of systemic hyperchloremic acidosis is diagnostic of type I RTA. Some patients labeled as having incomplete RTA do not present with hyperchloremia or have only borderline hyperchloremia and acidosis. Such patients may require a challenge with an acidifying agent such as ammonium chloride to see whether their urinary pH can be successfully lowered below 6.5.[35] The urine in patients with type II (proximal) RTA is capable of maximal acidification; when they present with hyperchloremic acidosis, the urine pH exhibits the normally low pH expected with acidosis (usually 5 or less). This acidification occurs only after the inadequately compensated systemic acidosis has developed, and the plasma bicarbonate has decreased substantially (Table 11.6–1). Administration of bicarbonate to such patients results in a prompt alkalinization of the urine, with loss of large quantities of bicarbonate in the urine long before the systemic acidosis has been corrected (in contrast to acidotic individuals with normal renal function). Thus patients with type II RTA become "renal bicarbonate-losers" before their systemic acidosis is corrected. Moreover the bicarbon-

ate administration identifies another distinctive difference between type I and type II RTA. Bicarbonate administration in type I RTA produces a decrease in potassium excretion; the kaliuresis in type II RTA is greatly exaggerated by bicarbonate administration, and indeed this often produces severe problems with hypokalemia before the acidosis is controlled. If this latter type of the disease is suspected, it is important to begin potassium replacement before attempting to return the plasma bicarbonate toward normal levels.

TREATMENT—TYPE I AND TYPE II

In general, type I RTA is much more easily treated than type II. In type I, administration of as little as 0.5 to 1.0 mEq of sodium bicarbonate per kilogram of body weight per day is adequate to maintain normal arterial pH and to stop the renal losses of cations such as calcium and potassium.

Successful correction of the acidosis of type II RTA often requires large amounts of alkali. In an individual with high bicarbonate levels in the proximal tubule and nearly normal glomerular filtration rate, more than 10 mEq/kg body weight per day may be required. Even then such vigorous treatment is only partially successful in correcting the acidosis. Smaller quantities may be effective in the presence of advanced renal failure when there is marked reduction in glomerular filtration rate. In both circumstances, however, the maximal stimulus to distal cationic exchange mechanisms (a constant feature of type II RTA) results in marked accentuation of urinary potassium loss as the bicarbonate loss increases. It is often necessary to supplement the potassium intake in these patients with large quantities of potassium, at times exceeding 75 to 100 mEq of potassium per day. The use of diuretics such as hydrochlorothiazide or furosemide can enhance the proximal reabsorption of bicarbonate, but this invariably accentuates further the potassium loss and it is doubtful whether diuretic administration is justified because of the risk of profound hypokalemia.

TYPE IV RENAL TUBULAR ACIDOSIS

A form of hyperchloremic acidosis with persistent hyperkalemia has been reported with increasing frequency. The feature that usually calls attention to the disturbance is hyperchloremia. As with other forms of RTA, but in sharp contrast to the electrolyte disturbances in type I and type II RTA, *hyperkalemia* is a persistent feature of the electrolyte abnormalities encountered in these patients. Perhaps the most important subgroup in this category contains diabetic patients who develop persistent hyperchloremia and hyperkalemia as diabetic renal disease progresses. Such patients exhibit hyporeninemic hypoaldosteronism, and they appear to have some problem with the production or secretion of renin; the major fraction of their circulating renin is inactive.[7] The consequent reduction in aldosterone production leads to impaired renal secretion of potassium.

The disorder is not confined to patients with diabetic nephropathy, because hyperkalemic hyperchloremic acidosis has also been reported in patients with interstitial nephropathy, congenital enzymatic defects leading to mineralocorticoid deficiency, other instances of mineralocorticoid deficiencies such as Addison disease, isolated hypoaldosteronism, or a failure of the kidney to respond adequately to mineralocorticoid excess.

These patients are difficult to treat. In addition to requiring some form of alkali therapy to correct the hyperchloremic acidosis, treatment of the hyperkalemia may be quite difficult. In patients such as the diabetic patients with hyporeninemic hypoaldosteronism, administration of 9-α-fludrocortisone may both improve acid secretion and facilitate potassium excretion, but accompanying sodium retention may seriously compromise management of hypertension in many of these patients. If the combination of treatment with mineralocorticoid and a potent diuretic such as furosemide is unsuccessful in controlling the hyperkalemia, dietary potassium reduction and the use of cation exchange resins such as Kayexalate

become necessary, and the patient must be monitored closely to assure compliance.

PHOSPHATE-LOSING NEPHROPATHY AND HERITABLE DISORDERS OF VITAMIN D METABOLISM[25]

Because dietary (vitamin D deficit) rickets is now a rare disease in the United States, hereditary phosphate-losing nephropathy and heritable disorders of vitamin D metabolism represent the leading causes of rickets in the United States. The disorder in all these genetic disturbances presents during early childhood, usually when weight-bearing first begins. Unless the disease is recognized and treated promptly, marked rachitic deformities of the skeleton occur.

Phosphate-losing nephropathy, or *familial hypophosphatemic rickets,* is characterized by a remarkably high urinary clearance of inorganic phosphate and associated hypophosphatemia. Characteristics are slow growth and marked deformity of the lower extremities, frequently anterior bowing of the tibias, and marked varus or valgus changes in the knees. Measurements of 1,25-dihydroxycholecalciferol have yielded values that are low-normal or moderately low; however, treatment with this vitamin is without benefit unless large quantities of phosphate are administered simultaneously. Effective therapy is usually achieved by the use of 1 to 2 g of neutral oral phosphate daily with 1 to 3 μg per day of 1,25-$(OH)_2D_3$. The phosphate should be given in four to six divided doses to prevent the occurrence of diarrhea from the osmotic effect of the phosphate load. Such optimal combined therapy will lead to normal growth rates and prevent further progression of skeletal deformity. Concomitantly, healing of the rickets and osteomalacia can be demonstrated radiographically.

The disease is inherited as an X-linked dominant trait. A rare form of the disease is also recognized, which presents in late childhood or in adult life. The clinical picture is that of osteomalacia without any evidence of rachitic deformity. This form of the disease is also characterized by hypophosphatemia and increased renal phosphate loss but is inherited as an autosomal recessive trait. Treatment of this form of the disease is identical with that of the juvenile form of the disease.

In addition there are two other hereditary forms of rickets that appear to be associated with a disturbance in the metabolism of vitamin D. One type (type I) vitamin D–dependent rickets, presents early in life with the skeletal manifestations previously described, but in addition, hypotonia, tetany, and convulsions are virtually always present. Plasma levels of 25-hydroxycholecalciferol concentrations are normal but 1,25-$(OH)_2D_3$ is low. It is thought to be related to a deficiency of renal 1-α-hydroxylase, which is responsible for synthesis of 1,25-$(OH)_2D_3$ from 25-hydroxycholecalciferol. The disease is corrected by small doses of 1,25-$(OH)_2D_3$ (1 to 3 μg/day): Tetany is promptly reversed and growth and skeletal development return to normal.

There is also a disorder indistinguishable clinically from the type I variety of vitamin D–dependent rickets but frequently associated with alopecia totalis and a failure to respond to administration of 1,25-$(OH)_2D_3$. In fact, circulating levels of this compound are usually elevated in type II vitamin D–dependent rickets. Although further studies are essential to clarify the specific defect in this last category of vitamin D–dependent rickets, the fact that appropriate therapeutic responses have occasionally been observed with pharmacologic doses of vitamin D (on occasion as high as 1.5 million units of ergocalciferol given intramuscularly at weekly intervals) raises the possibility that this is some form of abnormality in vitamin D metabolism that has not yet been adequately defined. Whether type II represents a single disturbance or may indeed represent several disorders, including perhaps defective receptor mechanisms, remains to be determined.

NEPHROGENIC DIABETES INSIPIDUS[5,20]

The primary lesion of nephrogenic diabetes insipidus resides in the kidney.[20] The clinical features of the disease are similar to those of diabetes insipidus associated with deficiency of the antidiuretic hormone, but the kidney fails to respond to exogenously administered vasopressin. The disease presents in infancy with signs of severe dehydration, fever, and plasma hyperosmolality, sometimes accompanied by convulsions; the dehydration may be so severe that polyuria is not recognized, although the urine is hypotonic to plasma. The diagnosis is established by the failure of administered vasopressin to induce a reduction in urine flow after adequate hydration. The disease is inherited, with the greatest frequency in males of affected kindreds.

Therapy consists principally of supportive care. Solute intake should be kept low in order to reduce obligatory water loss. Restriction of protein intake in children is limited by nutritional requirements, but strict reduction in salt ingestion also lowers solute intake effectively. Chlorothiazide and other diuretics will reduce urine flow by producing sodium depletion and diminishing glomerular filtration rate. This increases the proportion of filtered fluid reabsorbed in the proximal tubule, thereby reducing the rate of delivery of tubular fluid to the distal diluting segment, with a fall in total urine volume. This therapy may be hazardous because it leads to moderate sodium depletion that may be acutely aggravated by vomiting or diarrhea from any cause. Chlorothiazide induces potassium loss in the urine so that hypokalemia may develop. As these patients become older, management is less difficult because they can attend to their own water requirements.

AMINO-ACIDURIAS AND RELATED METABOLIC DISTURBANCES INVOLVING THE KIDNEY[11,13,14,16,17,21,22,30,32,33,37]

The free amino acids found in the plasma appear in the glomerular ultrafiltrate and are, for the most part, nearly completely reabsorbed by the tubules. The only amino acids that appear in the urine of healthy individuals in significant quantities are alanine, glycine, serine, histidine, and taurine. Excretory rates for all of these exceed 60 mg per day in the average adult. Of the other amino acids, only a few milligrams are excreted in 24 hours, despite the fact that between 1 and 5 g per day of each are filtered.

The term "amino-aciduria," as used clinically, may denote either the appearance of an abnormal quantity of a normal constituent amino acid or the appearance of an abnormal amino acid in the urine. Because renal transport involves filtration and reabsorption, amino-aciduria could be expected to result from filtration of increased quantities of normal or abnormal amino acids or from impairment of the tubular reabsorptive mechanisms for the normal amino acid constituents of glomerular filtrate. In fact, examples representing each of these possibilities have been recognized. Those resulting from an increase in quantity filtered are termed "overflow amino-aciduria," and are usually, but not always, associated with elevated plasma levels of amino acids. Occasionally, the compound may have no tubular reabsorptive mechanisms and, hence, filtration and excretion occur at such a rapid rate that plasma levels remain undetectable, as for instance β-amino-isobutyric aciduria.

Many of the amino-acidurias represent heritable disturbances in metabolism that result in overproduction of one or more such agents. Although these appear in the urine, they are unassociated with any definable defect in renal function. In contrast, there are instances in which defective renal transport exists as in cystinuria or the metabolic disturbance leads to defect in renal function. Table 11.6–2 presents some of the more important disturbances that lead to some derangement in renal function.

PRIMARY HYPEROXALURIA[33]

Primary hyperoxaluria is a relatively rare heritable metabolic disorder. Type I leads to the overproduction and excretion of oxalic acid and increased quantities of glyoxylic and glycolic acids in the urine. In type II oxalate plus large amounts of L-glyceric acid are found in the urine. The inheritance of both types appears to be autosomal recessive.[33]

Clinical presentation of the disease usually occurs early in childhood, most often before the age of 5 and occasionally during the first year of life. One of the earliest manifestations is recurrent calcium oxalate nephrolithiasis with typical renal colic, often associated with gross hematuria. Some of the patients have had acidosis early during the course of the disease as well as features consistent with secondary renal tubular acidosis. Over 80 percent of the patients die of renal failure before reaching the age of 20, and clinical manifestations have usually been present for 10 years or less at the time of end-stage renal disease.

The disease is associated with widespread deposition of calcium oxalate throughout the tissues of the body. A heavy concentration is found in the kidneys and is associated with progressive renal damage. This renal damage leads inexorably to uremia and requires maintenance dialysis. Although the initial response is encouraging, progressive accumulation of oxalate continues in other tissues of the body and the patients fare poorly. Attempts to reduce the availability of the major precursor of oxalate—glycine—by means of protein restriction has not been particularly successful. Similarly, attempts to provide partial enzyme replacement by renal transplantation have met with only transient benefit because of the rapid deposition of oxalate within the tissues of the transplanted kidney.

OTHER HERITABLE FAMILIAL DISEASES[14,15,27]

Although there are numerous other hereditary diseases that have been reported to manifest some degree of renal involvement that may at times terminate in renal failure, the more common ones have already been covered in this chapter. Perhaps it is wise to point out that there may be another aspect of genetics of great importance to renal disease. Glassock[14] calls attention to the third report of the HLA and Disease Registry, which identifies a marked increase in susceptibility to certain diseases associated with particular patterns of human leukocyte antigens. For example, patients with the HLA antigen DRw2 are 13 times as likely to develop Goodpasture syndrome as individuals who do not have this antigen. Similarly, individuals who possess antigen DRw3 are 12 times more likely to develop membranous glomerulonephritis than are comparable individuals who do not possess this antigen. Even more impressive is the fact that individuals possessing this antigen (DRw3) exhibit a relative risk for the development of penicillimine- or gold-induced nephropathy that is more than 30 times greater than individuals without this antigen. Lipoid nephrosis is encountered more than 25 times as frequently in individuals with HLA-B12.

Although the mechanism responsible for these remarkable associations remains to be clarified, their existence extends the concept of genetically determined diseases into the domain of heritable susceptibility to particular diseases. It is quite probable that continued pursuit of such associations and critical examination of the molecular characteristics of the antigens may provide further important insights into the role of these genetic factors in the pathogenesis of some of the most important and common renal diseases. It is of particular interest that virtually all of the diseases of the kidney that exhibit very marked increases in risk associated with a particular HLA antigen or antigens have an underlying immunologic mechanism as the primary pathogenetic event leading to the progressive destruction of renal tissue. The foregoing is only a partial list of the renal diseases associated with particular HLA anti-

TABLE 11.6–2. RENAL DISORDERS ASSOCIATED WITH AMINOACIDURIAS AND RELATED HERITABLE METABOLIC DEFECTS

Syndrome	Urinary Metabolite(s)	Clinical Features	Associated Disturbances of Renal Function
Specific Renal Tubular Transport Defects[9,16,32,37]			
Cystinuria	Cystine Lysine Ornithine Arginine	Recurrent stone formation	Occasionally infection and chronic pyelonephritis
Xanthinuria	Xanthine Hypoxanthine	Renal stone formation	
Glycinuria	Glycine	Recurrent renal stones	
Amino-Aciduria Associated with Generalized Tubular Dysfunction[11,13,17,21,22,30,31]			
Lignac-Fanconi syndrome	Generalized aminoaciduria with normal plasma amino acid levels	Vomiting, poor intake Polyuria Rickets Malnutrition Hepatosplenomegaly Cystine deposits in tissue	Glycosuria Impairment in acidification Increased uric acid and phosphate clearance
Adult Fanconi	Generalized aminoaciduria	Osteomalacia most striking feature No cystine deposits in tissues	Glycosuria Increased uric acid and phosphate clearance Frequently defective acidification
Lowe syndrome	Generalized aminoaciduria Increased phosphate clearance	Mental retardation Congenital glaucoma Nystagmus, photophobia Hypotonia	Concentrating defect Impairment in acidification Glycosuria Keto-acids in urine
Heavy metal damage Lead Uranium Cadmium	Reversible aminoaciduria	Variable	Variable
Hereditary fructose intolerance	Generalized aminoaciduria Fructosuria	Hypophosphatemia Hypokalemia Acidosis	RTA type II

gens. Increased risk of developing systemic lupus erythematosus, diabetes mellitus, and a number of other diseases have also been associated with specific HLA antigens.

REFERENCES

1. Brenes LG, Brenes JN, Hernandez MM: Familial proximal renal tubular acidosis. Am J Med 62:244, 1977
2. Buckalew VM Jr, Purvis ML, et al: Hereditary renal tubular acidosis. Medicine 53:229, 1974
3. Chazan JA, Zacks J, et al: Hereditary nephritis, clinical spectrum and mode of inheritance in five new kindreds. Am J Med 50:764, 1971
4. Cogan MG, Rector FC Jr, Seldin DW: Acid-base disorders. In Brenner BM, Rector FC Jr (eds): The Kidney, 2d ed. Philadelphia, WB Saunders, 1981
5. Culpepper RN, Hebert SC, Andreoli TE: Nephrogenic diabetes insipidus. In Stanbury JB, Wyngaarden JB, Fredrickson DS, et al (eds): The Metabolic Basis of Inherited Disease, 5th ed. New York, McGraw-Hill, 1983
6. Dalgaard OZ: Bilateral polycystic disease of the kidneys. A follow-up of 284 patients and their families. Acta Med Scand 158(suppl 328), 1957
7. DeLeiva A, Christlieb AR, Melby JC, et al: Big renin and biosynthetic defect in aldosterone in diabetes mellitus. N Engl J Med 295:639, 1976
8. Desnick RJ, Sweeley CC: Fabry's disease: Alpha-galactosidase A deficiency. In Stanbury JB, Wyngaarden JB, et al (eds): The Metabolic Basis of Inherited Disease, 5th ed. New York, McGraw-Hill, 1983
9. DeVries A, Kochwa S, et al: Glycinuria, a hereditary disorder associated with nephrolithiasis. Am J Med 23:408, 1957
10. Elkinton JR, Huth EJ, et al: The renal excretion of hydrogen ion in renal tubular acidosis. Am J Med 29:554, 1969
11. Fanconi G: Tubular insufficiency and renal dwarfism. Arch Dis Child 29:1, 1954
12. Gardner KD: Cystic diseases of the kidney. In Massry SG, Glassock RJ (eds): Textbook of Nephrology. Baltimore, Williams & Wilkins, 1983
13. Gitzelman R, Steinmann B, Vanden Berghe G: Essential fructosuria, hereditary fructose intolerance and fructose-1-6-diphosphatase deficiency. In Stanbury JB, Wyngaarden JB, et al (eds): Metabolic Basis of Inherited Disease, 5th ed. New York, McGraw-Hill, 1983
14. Glassock RJ: Other heredo familial diseases. In Massrey SG, Glassock RJ (eds): Textbook of Nephrology. Baltimore, Williams & Wilkins, 1983
15. Gubler MC, Lenoir G, et al: Early renal changes in hemizygous and heterozygous patients with Fabry's disease. Kidney Intern 13:223, 1978
16. Holmes EW, Wyngaarden JB: Hereditary xanthinuria. In Stanbury JB, Wyngaarden JB, Fredrickson DS (eds): Metabolic Basis of Inherited Disease, 5th ed. New York, McGraw-Hill, 1983
17. Hover JR, Michael AF, et al: Renal disease in nail-patella syndrome: Clinical and morphological studies. Kidney Intern 2:231, 1972
18. Hulter HN, Ilnicki LP, et al: Impaired renal H+ secretion and NH3 production in mineralocorticoid-deficient glucocorticoid replete dogs. Am J Physiol 232:F136, 1977
19. Lieberman E, Salinas-Madrigal L, Gwinn JL: Infantile polycystic disease of the kidneys and liver. Medicine 50:277, 1971
20. Macdonald WG: Congenital pitressin resistant diabetes of renal origin. Pediatrics 15:298, 1955
21. Morris RC Jr, Sebastian AA: Renal tubular acidosis and Fanconi syndrome. In Stanbury JB, Wyngaarden JB, Fredrickson DS, et al (eds): Metabolic Basis of Inherited Disease, 5th ed. New York, McGraw-Hill, 1983
22. Mudge GH: Clinical patterns of tubular dysfunction. Am J Med 24:785, 1958
23. O'Neill WM, Atkin CL, Bloomer HA: Hereditary nephritis: A reexamination of its clinical and genetic features. Ann Intern Med 88:176, 1978
24. Randall RE Jr: Familial renal tubular acidosis revisited. Ann Intern Med 66:1024, 1967

25. Rasmussen H, Anast C: Familial hypophosphatemic (vitamin D resistant) rickets and vitamin D dependent rickets. In Stanbury JB, Wyngaarden JB, Fredrickson DS, et al (eds): The Metabolic Basis of Inherited Disease, 5th ed. New York, McGraw-Hill, 1983

26. Relman AS: Renal acidosis and renal excretion of acid in health and disease. Adv Intern Med 12:295, 1964

27. Ryder LP, Anderson E, Svejgarrd A (eds): HLA and Disease Registry: Third Report. Copenhagen, Munksgaard, 1979, p 1

28. Rodriguez-Soriano R, Biochis H, et al: Proximal renal tubular acidosis. A defect in bicarbonate reabsorption with normal urinary acidification. Pediatr Res 1:81, 1967

29. Schambelan M, Sebastian A, Hulter HN: Mineralocorticoid excess and deficiency syndromes. In Brenner BM, Stein JH (eds): Acid-Base and K-Homeostasis, Contemporary Issues in Nephrology, vol 2. New York, Churchill-Livingstone, 1978, p 232

30. Schneider JA, Schulman JD: Cystinosis. In Stanbury JB, Wyngaarden JB, et al (eds): Metabolic Basis of Inherited Disease, 5th ed. New York, McGraw-Hill, 1983

31. Sebastian A, McSherry E, Morris RC Jr: Metabolic acidosis with special reference to the renal acidoses. In Brenner BM, Rector FC Jr (eds): The Kidney. Philadelphia, WB Saunders, 1976

32. Segal S, Thier SO: Cystinuria. In Stanbury JB, Wyngaarden JB, et al (eds): Metabolic Basis of Inherited Disease, 5th ed. New York, McGraw-Hill, 1983

33. Williams HE, Smith LH: Primary hyperoxaluria. In Stanbury JB, Wyngaarden JB, et al (eds): Metabolic Basis of Inherited Disease, 5th ed. New York, McGraw-Hill, 1983

34. Winters RW, Graham JB, et al: A genetic study of familial hypophosphatemia with vitamin D resistant rickets with a review of the literature. Medicine 37:97, 1958

35. Wrong O, Davies HEF: The excretion of acid in renal disease. Q J Med 28:259, 1959

36. Zemer D, Pras M, et al: Colchicine in the prevention of the amyloidosis of familial Mediterranean fever. N Engl J Med 314:1001, 1986

37. Zinneman HH, Jones JE: Dietary methionine and its influence on cystine excretion in cystinuric patients. Metabolism 15:915, 1966

CHAPTER 11.7
Renal Calculi

W. Gordon Walker

Renal colic and hematuria are cardinal manifestations of nephrolithiasis. The hematuria is usually microscopic, but on occasion grossly bloody urine may be produced. The pain associated with renal stones is a characteristically agonizing flank pain that waxes and wanes in intensity. It may radiate along the course of the ureter to the groin and, occasionally, into the suprapubic area and urethra. Nephrolithiasis may, however, persist for years without any associated pain, and radiopaque kidney stones may be discovered incidentally as a result of abdominal x-rays made for some other purpose. Regardless of the manner in which attention is first called to the existence of renal calculi, good medical management requires that both the cause of the stone formation and the composition of the stone be identified.

COMPOSITION OF KIDNEY STONES

Well over 95 percent of renal calculi are composed of one or more of the following substances: calcium, phosphate, oxalate, uric acid, cystine, magnesium, and ammonium.[3,6,12,15,18] The majority of these substances are found normally in the urine in concentrations that quite often exceed their solubility in water. Under certain circumstances the urine is supersaturated with respect to one or more of these constituents and is thus in a highly metastable state, that is, it will sustain rapid growth of crystals or stones already present, or when provided with a nidus or nucleation point, it will form new crystals. Indeed, calcium oxalate, calcium phosphate, uric acid, and (under certain circumstances) cystine crystals may precipitate out of the urine on standing. It is this metastable state of supersaturation that predisposes to renal stone formation.

In the absence of coexisting infection, renal stones usually tend to consist exclusively or predominantly of a single compound. Table 11.7–1 shows the more common crystalline substances that are found as major or exclusive components of renal stones and presents average figures for their incidence. Virtually all these substances are so insoluble in water that it is difficult to understand why stones are not a constant threat to all. Available evidence indicates that there are substances present in the urine that inhibit this tendency to precipitation and crystal formation. The tendency toward stone formation in some individuals probably reflects a deficit or absence of these inhibitory substances. Low-molecular-weight substances that have been demonstrated to possess potent inhibitory action in preventing aggregation and crystal formation include pyrophosphate, citrate, magnesium, and phosphocitrate, as well as other cations and anions.[2,5,14,19] In addition, mucopolysaccharide and other macromolecules have been demonstrated to possess inhibitory activity. The relative physiologic importance of all of these substances remains to be clarified, and the role of deficiency of one or more in predisposing to recurrent stone formation is unclear.[2,7,9,10,13,14,19]

Complete decalcification of stones leaves a residue of organic material that is highly structured and exhibits uniform staining properties and a regular architecture. Whether this material is important in the formation of a nidus or nucleus for beginning crystal precipitation and subsequent stone growth remains a matter of some speculation. Consideration of the usual concentration, physicochemical properties, and rate of excretion of the substances representing the principal constituent of stones makes it evident that even modest increases in the concentration or excretion rate increases the risk of crystal formation and subsequent stone growth. The substances listed in the preceding paragraph are all usually present in concentrations approaching supersaturation; hence it is not surprising that stones are rarely pure crystalline deposits of a single compound but are more often composed predominantly of one substance, with small quantities or traces of a number of other poorly soluble substances. The most common combination stone encountered in uninfected urine is a mixture of calcium oxalate and calcium phosphate. More than a third of the stones encountered in the United States are of this mixed type.[4,6,15,18] Therapy is designed to lower the concentration of these substances, with particular attention directed toward the substance believed to play the primary role. Table 11.7–1 also contains a partial list of the causes of the common types of stones as well as the urinary pH usually associated with formation of each of these stones.

CALCIUM STONES

Excluding stones that occur in infected urine and are mixtures of salts of calcium, magnesium, and ammonium (struvite stones), calcium stones of one type or another constitute about 90 percent of all the remaining stones. The most common variety is a mixture of

TABLE 11.7–1. COMPOSITION AND PREVALENCE OF COMMON VARIETIES OF RENAL STONES[3,5,12,15,18]

Type of Stone	Predisposing Urine pH	Causes	Prevalence (%)

Mixed calcium oxalate and calcium phosphate	Variable	Concentrated urine
		Secondary hypercalciuria
		  Vitamin D excess
		  Hyperparathyroidism
		  Sarcoidosis
		  Bony metastases
		  Primary bone tumors
		  Osteoporosis
		Idiopathic hypercalciuria
		Renal tubular acidosis
		Mild-alkali syndrome
			35

Calcium oxalate	Variable	As above	25
Calcium phosphate	Variable	Renal tubular acidosis Alkali ingestion	<10
Magnesium, ammonium, calcium phosphate (struvite)	Alkaline	Infection	20
Uric acid	Acid	Hyperuricaciduria Gout Hyperuricemia High purine diet Urinary hyperacidity Cancer chemotherapy	5
Cystine	Acid	Cystinuria	2

calcium oxalate and calcium phosphate, but pure stones of calcium oxalate are also common. Stones containing only calcium phosphate are much less common, representing less than 10 percent of all calcium-containing stones. Conditions that predispose to the formation of calcium stones include hypercalciuria, hyperuricosuria, hyperoxaluria, persistently alkaline urine, and low urine volumes. When all the foregoing predisposing factors are excluded, however, a significant incidence of calcium stone remains. Possible additional predisposing events could include elevated ionized calcium, abnormally high calcium concentrations at some point along the source of the nephron, reduction in naturally occurring urinary inhibitors or excessive supersaturation of one or more of the poorly soluble urinary constituents. It may well be that all of these are a consequence of persistently low urinary volume and its attendant effects of such supersaturation.

Modest increases in oxalate excretion have been documented in patients who form calcium stones and, in some, hyperexcretion of uric acid has been associated with recurrent formation of calcium stones. It has been postulated that the presence of uric acid crystals may serve as a nidus for the growth of calcium stones.[5]

Oversaturation, whatever the cause, creates favorable circumstances for precipitating calcium from the urine. Though spontaneous precipitation is relatively rare in the absence of some nidus or focus around which crystallization can occur, in the presence of such a focus, oversaturation is the driving force for stone growth. This is true whether the oversaturation results simply from a relative deficit of the aqueous phase (poor fluid intake) or increased urinary excretion of one or more of the constituents of calcium-forming stones. Nearly half of individuals who recurrently form calcium stones exhibit persistent hypercalciuria. The cause of this increased urinary calcium excretion is variable. After conditions known to produce hypercalciuria are excluded (sarcoidosis, renal tubular acidosis, hyperthyroidism, malignant tumors, rapidly progressive bone disease, bed rest, Paget disease, Cushing syndrome, medullary sponge kidneys, and administration of certain diuretics), there exists a substantial number of individuals with normal plasma calcium values who exhibit increased calcium excretion. These examples are labeled idiopathic hypercalciuria.[17]

Hypercalciuria is frequently associated with formation of calcium stones. In the absence of ingestion of foods rich in calcium, urinary calcium should not exceed 200 mg per day. Hypercalciuria

regularly accompanies hyperparathyroidism, vitamin D excess or intoxication, renal tubular acidosis, the bone resorption that follows osseous metastases of neoplasia, and very high calcium intake, such as ingestion of large quantities of milk. Most commonly, however, hypercalciuria is encountered unassociated with any of these specific disturbances and has been termed *idiopathic hypercalciuria*. It is usually encountered in healthy young men who give a history of recurrent calcium stones. In these individuals the serum calcium concentration is normal, and serum phosphate concentration is normal despite the persistent hypercalciuria. Hypercalciuria is frequently associated with formation of calcium stones. Definition has varied, but the ranges that are generally accepted in healthy individuals eating normal diets are values of 250 mg per day for women and 300 mg per day for men. Values exceeding these limits are generally accepted as diagnostic of hypercalciuria. The excretion rate has also been defined in terms of body weight as a normal range that is less than 4 mg of urinary calcium per kilogram of body weight per day. An alternate approach has been measurement of urinary calcium while on some limitation in calcium intake. It has been proposed that urinary calcium that exceeds 200 mg per day while an individual is on a known diet of 400 mg of calcium per day establishes the diagnosis of hypercalciuria. Urinary calcium excretion varies with dietary calcium intake in healthy subjects, with the urinary calcium increasing by about 6 percent of the corresponding increase in dietary intake. Thus for all of the proposed values cited here, the diagnosis of hypercalciuria should not be made before careful dietary review of the stone-forming patient is undertaken. The relation between calcium intake and the range of urinary calcium excretion in healthy subjects and in idiopathic hypercalciuria is shown in Figure 11.7–1. When the diagnosis of hypercalciuria is made, further study allows separating these into three categories: absorptive, reabsorptive, and renal hypercalciuria.[11,17]

Absorptive hypercalciuria, as implied by the name, results from increased gastrointestinal absorption of calcium. It is diagnosed by demonstrating that oral administration of calcium results in an increase in urinary excretion.[3] Serum calcium and phosphorus are normal. Calcium balance studies, if done, are virtually always positive, and dietary reduction of calcium reduces the rate of urinary calcium excretion.

Resorptive hypercalciuria represents excretion of calcium that has

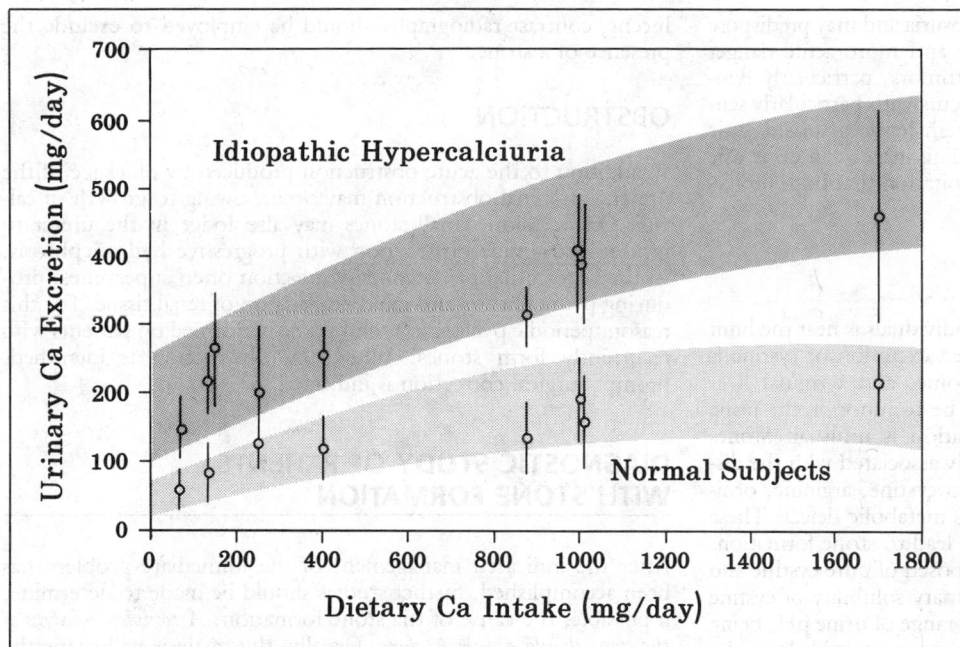

Figure 11.7–1. Relation between calcium intake and urinary calcium excretion in healthy subjects and in idiopathic hypercalciuria. (*Drawn from composite data from published studies compiled by Lemann.*[11])

been resorbed from bone. Most commonly, this is caused by hyperparathyroidism, particularly when overt cases of neoplastic bony metastases are excluded. Most such patients (>75 percent) have elevated serum calcium concentrations and are thus easily distinguished from patients with other forms of hypercalciuria. From the standpoint of accurate differential diagnosis, recognition of those cases of hyperparathyroidism with *normal* serum calcium values is a greater challenge. These patients exhibit elevated levels of urinary cyclic AMP and elevations in circulating levels of parathormone. They also exhibit a persistently negative calcium balance and decreasing bone density with time, in contrast to patients with absorptive hypercalciuria who show no changes in bone density, normal or low values for parathyroid hormone, and no evidence of persistently negative calcium balance.

Surgical treatment is indicated in those cases of resorptive hypercalciuria that are due to parathyroid adenoma. In patients exhibiting hypercalcemia as well as hypercalciuria, elevated urinary cyclic AMP, and renal lithiasis, diagnosis presents little difficulty and surgery is curative. In those cases with recurrent stones, elevation of urinary calcium, cyclic AMP, and elevated parathormone levels in the plasma but normal calcium values, surgical exploration is probably also the preferable therapeutic approach. It is wise, however, to see whether the elevated parathormone levels can be suppressed by calcium administration before recommending surgery.

Renal hypercalciuria represents persistent loss of calcium via the urine as a result of a renal "leak." The classic example is renal tubular acidosis. In at least one kindred with renal tubular acidosis, an increased incidence of hypercalciuria with renal stones was reported in other members of the kindred.[4] In two patients with renal hypercalciuria studied in detail, normal serum calcium, elevated parathormone levels, negative calcium balance, elevated cyclic AMP, and reduced bone density were demonstrated. The elevated parathormone levels in this condition have been suppressed by calcium administration and by thiazide administration.

Because the therapeutic regimen selected depends on the distinction between these types of hypercalciuria, patients presenting with calcium stones and hypercalciuria should be studied in sufficient detail to permit categorization of the urinary calcium loss. Table 11.7–2 summarizes the distinguishing features of each of these types of hypercalciuria.

URIC ACID STONES

Uric acid stones develop in association with excessive excretion of uric acid or with normal excretion when the urine has a persistently acid pH (below 6.0). The principal reason for increased uric acid excretion is hyperuricemia from a variety of causes. Less than 20 percent of uric acid stones is associated with gout. Increased intake of purines may lead to increased excretion of uric acid and predisposes to stone formation. A list of the disorders associated with formation of uric acid stones is given in Table 11.7–1.

Urate stones may be found without hyperuricemia or hyperuricaciduria. This may occur as an heritable disorder with autosomal dominant inheritance, or sporadic cases may be encountered in which no familial aggregation can be demonstrated. Because the disease is associated with abnormally low renal NH_3 production by the kidney and an excessively low or acid urine pH, it is easily treated by alkalinizing the urine and being certain that it is kept in the alkaline state.

Chronic myelogenous leukemia and myeloproliferative disor-

TABLE 11.7–2. DIFFERENTIATION OF TYPES OF HYPERCALCIURIA

Type	Serum Ca	Serum P	Ca Balance	Bone Density	Serum PTH	Urinary cAMP
Absorptive	NORM	NORM	POS or 0	NORM	↓	↓
Resorptive	↑ or NORM	NORM or ↓	NEG	↓	↑	↑
Renal	NORM	NORM	NEG	↓	↑	↑

ders are usually associated with hyperuricosuria and may predispose to uric acid stone formation. A greater and more acute danger arises following chemotherapy of large tumors, particularly lymphomas. The massive cell necrosis that occurs with particularly sensitive tumors results in extraordinarily high levels of plasma uric acid and corresponding hyperuricosuria. This increase in urine uric acid may lead to such marked urate precipitation that both ureters can become completely occluded.

CYSTINE STONES

The cystine content of urine in healthy individuals is near the limit of solubility of this amino acid. Increased excretion of cystine is seen in Wilson disease, Fanconi syndrome, and terminal liver failure. Although crystals of cystine may be common in the urine under these circumstances, stone formation is unusual. Stones composed of cystine are almost exclusively associated with the disorder in cystine transport. In addition to cystine, arginine, ornithine, and lysine are also excreted in this metabolic defect. These substances are so soluble that they never lead to stone formation. Hence, stones are practically always composed of pure cystine and exhibit a bright golden-yellow color. Urinary solubility of cystine varies nearly fivefold over the physiologic range of urine pH, being most insoluble in acid urine. Thus, stones are more likely to develop when the urine is persistently acid.

CLINICAL FEATURES OF NEPHROLITHIASIS

Renal colic and hematuria are the cardinal manifestations of nephrolithiasis, but the clinical spectrum may vary from an asymptomatic opaque stone discovered incidentally on radiographic examination to a fulminant pyelonephritis. The physician's responsibility includes care of the acute attack, definition of the underlying condition leading to stone formation, and the taking of preventive measures designed to reduce the likelihood of subsequent stone formation.

RENAL COLIC

Typical renal colic is an excruciating, lancinating pain that begins in the flank—posteriorly or laterally—and radiates downward along the course of the ureter and, at times, into the testis or urethra. It is one of the more severe, frightening pains encountered in medical practice. Renal colic compares with the pain of dissecting aneurysm or angina pectoris in severity. The pain may remain unrelieved even by as much as 16 mg of morphine, so that analgesic overdosage may result if vigorous therapy with opiates is used. The spectrum of pain associated with the passage of renal calculi is great. Patients with extensive nephrocalcinosis who frequently pass renal stones may have only slight to moderate discomfort for a short period.

Once the stone has entered the ureter, it must either be extruded by the peristaltic action of the ureter or extracted surgically because, if left in place, the resulting obstruction and stasis will rapidly lead to progressive loss of renal function. No invariable rules can be established for the timing of surgical intervention, but appropriate diagnostic procedures should determine promptly whether there is significant obstruction. If such obstruction is found, early surgical intervention is necessary. *It is doubtful that a kidney can regain significant function if the ureter has been completely obstructed for 2 weeks or more.*

HEMATURIA

The presence of red blood cells in the urine, in the absence of other formed elements, should always raise suspicion of renal lithiasis and should be investigated thoroughly. Because some stones are radiolucent, contrast radiography should be employed to exclude the presence of a stone.

OBSTRUCTION

In addition to the acute obstruction produced by blockage of the ureter, intrarenal obstruction may occur, owing to growth of calculi. On occasion, small stones may also lodge in the ureter to produce low-grade obstruction with progressive hydronephrosis. In the latter situation, secondary infection often supervenes, producing pyonephrosis and rapid destruction of renal tissue. For this reason, periodic pyelography should be performed on patients who recurrently form stones. When the obstruction is identified, prompt surgical correction is indicated.

DIAGNOSTIC STUDY OF PATIENTS WITH STONE FORMATION

After the indicated management of the immediate problem has been accomplished, further studies should be made to determine, if possible, the cause of the stone formation. *A complete analysis of the stone should always be done.* Usually, this analysis will shape the course of the subsequent diagnostic workup. If the stone is of calcium origin, 24-hour urinary calcium excretions followed by the studies outlined in Table 11.7–2 permit categorization of the type of hypercalciuria. Appropriate management depends on the results of these studies. In similar fashion, if stone analysis results in identification of uric acid or cystine stones, subsequent efforts should be directed toward defining the conditions necessary to maintain the urine at a sufficiently high pH to prevent crystallization and stone formation by these substances. Mixed stones (containing Ca^{2+}, Mg^{2+}, NH^+, PO^{3-}, oxalate) virtually always signify infection. Subsequent efforts should be directed toward being certain that all remaining stones are removed, if possible, and that the infection is controlled.

TREATMENT OF NEPHROLITHIASIS

Treatment of an acute attack of renal colic depends on the particular circumstances surrounding the attack. The first objective in evaluating the patient with renal colic is to decide whether the stone is obstructing the ureter. If no obstruction exists, expectant treatment with analgesia and hydration will usually result in passage of the stone. *Complete obstruction of the ureter is an indication for early surgery if the stone cannot be mobilized by retrograde or antegrade catheterization.* In addition, acute infection associated with a stone in the ureter is an indication for surgery. Chills and fever are ominous signs and usually herald generalized sepsis unless the obstruction is relieved and the stone removed promptly. Once infection complicates nephrolithiasis, it is virtually impossible to eradicate unless the stone is removed.

Surgical treatment is the treatment of choice for large stones in the upper collecting system, even when they are asymptomatic, if their location permits removal without extensive damage to the kidney. The long-term outlook for the patient is much better if this is done before management is complicated by a superimposed infection. Infection leads inevitably, and often rapidly, to the development of a staghorn calculus, and the results of treatment for this type of infected stone are poor regardless of whether a surgical or medical approach is chosen. Recurrence of infection and stone, progressive loss of renal function, and ultimately loss of the kidney occurs in nearly half of such cases.[20,21,22] Surgical intervention before infection supervenes is much to be preferred. The small stone situated in a minor calyx is difficult to approach surgically and is often small enough that it can be passed through the ureter. In

such instances careful observation, with other measures designed to retard stone growth and facilitate passage, is the preferable means of management.

Adequate conservative management includes maintaining a high urine output, which minimizes the concentration of the substances responsible for stone growth. The specific corrective measures listed in Table 11.7–3 should also be instituted if the composition of the stone has been established with enough certainty to permit rational selection. In general, all of these therapies are designed to reduce the concentration of the offending substance in the urine or to maintain the pH of the urine at or near the range where solubility of the components of the stone is greatest. Once infection has become established and urinary pH has become constantly alkaline as a result of the infection, stones of any basic composition tend to grow rapidly by the accretion of calcium and magnesium ammonium phosphate in alkaline solution. For this reason, eradication of the infection is imperative whenever possible. If not, every attempt to suppress the infection and acidify the urine should be made. In all patients with recurrent stone formation, regular supervision and periodic urine checks are vital. The physician must be certain that the prescribed regimen is followed.

The diagnosis of hypercalciuria during the workup for calcium stone merits special attention. Absorptive hypercalciuria is most appropriately managed by reducing calcium intake (exclusion of milk and milk products) and the use of cellulose phosphate as a calcium binding agent to further reduce calcium absorption.

A diagnosis of resorptive hypercalciuria implies excess parathormone from a parathyroid adenoma when occult neoplasm has been excluded. Ordinarily, surgery is indicated, but in those few cases with normal serum calcium values and little evidence of adverse effect, if the initial decision is to observe rather than carry out neck exploration, patients should probably not be given orthophosphates but watched carefully. A propensity toward recurrent stone formation should force reconsideration of surgical exploration.

Renal hypercalciuria is best managed with thiazides, high fluid intake, and moderate reduction in dietary calcium after parathyroid adenoma is excluded.

Occasionally, dissolution of stones already formed may occur under appropriate therapy. When urinary pH is carefully maintained above 7.0, both uric acid and cystine stones may dissolve. In attempting to achieve this persistent alkalinization, patients' personal habits become important. The physically active individual who engages in vigorous sports such as tennis, basketball, or jogging virtually always excretes a urine of pH 5 or less following such exercise. If this is to be avoided, it is imperative that the individual take a large quantity of alkali (3 to 4 g of $NaHCO_3$ or 20 to 30 ml Shohl solution) just before exercising. Allopurinol may further facilitate dissolution of uric acid stones by reducing the quantity of uric acid in the urine bathing the stone and thereby maintaining a gradient more favorable to solution of the stone. Excretion of a dilute urine is of added benefit under these circumstances.

REFERENCES

1. Albright F, Reifenstein EC: Parathyroid Glands and Metabolic Bone Disease. Baltimore, Williams & Wilkins, 1948
2. Bisaz S, Felix R, et al: Quantitative determination of inhibitors of calcium phosphate precipitation in whole urine. Mineral Electro Metab 1:74, 1978
3. Boyce WH, Garvey FK: Incidence of urinary calculi among patients in general hospitals, 1948 to 1952. JAMA 161:1437, 1956
4. Buckalew VM, Purvis ML, et al: Hereditary renal tubular acidosis. Medicine 53:229, 1974
5. Coe FL: Clinical stone disease. In Coe FL, Brenner BM, Stein JH (eds): Contemporary Issues in Nephrology: Nephrolithiasis. New York, Churchill Livingstone, 1980
6. Coe FL: Nephrolithiasis: Pathogenesis and Treatment. Chicago, Year Book Medical Publishers, 1978
7. Fleisch H: Inhibitors and promoters of stone formation. Kidney Intern 13:361, 1978
8. Griffith DP, Gibson JR, et al: Acetohydroxamic acid: Clinical studies of a urease inhibitor in patients with staghorn renal calculi. J Urol 119:9, 1978
9. Howard JE: Studies on urinary stone formation: A saga of clinical investigation. Johns Hopkins Med J 139:239, 1976
10. Howard JE: Urinary stone. Can Med Assoc J 86:1001, 1962
11. Lemann J Jr: Idiopathic hypercalciuria. In Coe FL, Brenner BM, Stein JH (eds): Contemporary Issues in Nephrology: Nephrolithiasis. New York, Churchill Livingstone, 1980, p 88
12. Melick RA, Henneman PH: Clinical and laboratory studies of 207 consecutive patients in a kidney stone clinic. N Engl J Med 259:307, 1958
13. Myer JL, Smith LH: Growth of calcium oxalate crystals. I. A model for urinary stone growth. Invest Urol. 13:31, 1975
14. Myer JL, Smith LH: Growth of calcium oxalate crystals. II. Inhibition of natural urinary crystal growth inhibitors. Invest Urol. 13:36, 1975
15. Nordin BEC, Hodgkinson A: Urolithiasis. In Dock W, Snapper I (eds): Advances in Internal Medicine. Chicago, Year Book Medical Publishers, 1967, p 1
16. Pak CYC, Hayashi Y, et al: Estimation of the state of saturation of brushite and calcium oxalate in urine: A comparison of three methods. J Lab Clin Med 89:891, 1977
17. Pak CYC, Ohata M, et al: The hypercalciurias, causes, parathyroid functions and diagnostic criteria. J Clin Invest 54:387, 1974
18. Prien EL: Studies in urolithiasis. J Urol 61:821, 1949
19. Robertson WG, Knowles F, Peacock M: Urinary acid mucopolysaccharide inhibitors of calcium oxalate crystallization. In Fleisch H, Robertson WG, Smith LH, Vahlensieck W, (eds): Urolithiasis Research. New York, Plenum Press, 1976
20. Singh M, Chapman R, et al: The fate of unoperated staghorn calculi. Br J Urol 45:581, 1973
21. Stamey TA: Urinary Infections. Baltimore, Williams & Wilkins, 1972
22. Wojewski A, Zajaczkowski J: The treatment of bilateral staghorn calculi of the kidneys. Int Urol Nephrol 5:249, 1974

TABLE 11.7–3. THERAPY FOR NEPHROLITHIASIS

Type of Stone	Treatment
Uric acid	Low purine diet High urine volume (>3000 ml/day) Urinary alkalinization (pH >7.4) Allopurinol
Cystine	Alkalinization (pH >7.4) High urine volume (>3000 ml/day)
Mixed stone	Most important to eradicate infection. Continuous suppression necessary if this is not achieved. Surgical therapy usually required.
Calcium stone	
Absorptive hypercalciuria	Low calcium diet Cellulose phosphate
Resorptive hypercalciuria	Parathyroid surgery High urine volume (>3000 ml/day)
Renal hypercalciuria	Chlorothiazide 500 mg bid High urine volume (>3000 ml/day)

DISEASES OF THE GASTROINTESTINAL TRACT

Section Editor: Thomas R. Hendrix

The major symptoms of alimentary tract disease are dysphagia, heartburn, abdominal pain, bleeding, nausea and vomiting, diarrhea, and constipation. All these symptoms arise from disordered function, but their description in physiologic terms is limited because our knowledge of normal alimentary tract function is so incomplete.

The alimentary tract has many functions, but its raison d'être is absorption. It is not, however, the disorders of absorption and secretion that give rise to most alimentary tract symptoms but, rather, disorders of motor function. With increased understanding of gastrointestinal function, and particularly of motor activity, it will be possible to describe gastrointestinal symptoms in more physiologic terms. Empiric therapy may be expected to give way to treatment directed at the correction of the primary disorder.

The diagnosis of, and therapeutic approach to, gastrointestinal disorders will be discussed under the following topics: (1) dysphagia and heartburn; (2) abdominal pain; (3) peptic ulcer and dyspepsia (4) gastrointestinal bleeding; (5) diarrhea and constipation; and (6) malabsorption. Important clinical examples will be given in each category. Although nausea and vomiting are very common symptoms, in reaching a diagnosis it is not particularly helpful to consider them alone.

REFERENCES

1. Granger DN, Barrowman JA, Kvietys PR: Clinical Gastrointestinal Physiology. Philadelphia, WB Saunders, 1985
2. Greenberger NJ: Gastrointestinal Disorders: A Pathophysiological Approach, 3d ed. Chicago, Year Book Medical Publishers, 1986
3. Hendrix TR: The absorptive function of the alimentary canal; The secretory function of the alimentary canal; The motility of the alimentary canal. In Mountcastle VB (ed): Medical Physiology, 14th ed. St. Louis, CV Mosby, 1980, vol 2
4. Sleisenger MD, Fordtran JS: Gastrointestinal Disease, 3d ed. Philadelphia, WB Saunders, 1983
5. Sircus W, Smith AN: Scientific Foundations of Gastroenterology. Philadelphia, WB Saunders, 1980
6. Spiro HM: Gastroenterology, 3d ed. New York, Macmillan, 1983
7. Yardley JH, Morson BC, Abell MR: The Gastrointestinal Tract. Baltimore, Williams & Wilkins, 1977

CHAPTER 12.1
Dysphagia and Heartburn

William J. Ravich and Thomas R. Hendrix

Dysphagia, difficulty in swallowing, is one of the most reliable of alimentary tract symptoms. It indicates an abnormality of the swallowing mechanism and hence requires careful evaluation. Although dysphagia is often associated with anxiety, anxiety is usually the consequence, rather than the cause, of dysphagia. Psychogenic dysphagia, if it ever occurs, is a rare disorder.

The patient with dysphagia initially becomes aware of swallowing and later notes interference or discomfort during passage of the bolus. This latter sensation may be localized anywhere from the oropharynx to the epigastrium.

It is useful to classify dysphagia as oropharyngeal or esophageal in origin because the symptoms and the diagnostic and therapeutic approaches are different. Oropharyngeal dysphagia is most frequently due to neurologic or neuromuscular diseases affecting function of striated muscle (Table 12.1-1). Esophageal dysphagia may be due to neuromuscular disorders affecting smooth muscle, but structural lesions obstructing the lumen are more frequently responsible (Table 12.1-2).

PHYSIOLOGY OF NORMAL SWALLOWING

Swallowing consists of elaborately coordinated contractions of the striated muscles of the mouth, pharynx, and upper esophagus and of the smooth muscles of the middle and lower esophagus.

Coordination is provided by the "swallowing center," a collection of neurons associated with the nucleus tractus solitarius and the nucleus ambiguus in the brain stem. Afferent impulses are supplied to it from the oropharynx by cranial nerves V, IX, and X, as well as from cortical centers involved in the voluntary aspects of mastication and deglutition. Efferent signals are transmitted via cranial nerves V, VII, IX, X, and XII. Damage to any component of this transmission and integration system can result in swallowing difficulties.[8]

Between swallows the nasopharynx and larynx are in open communication with the oropharynx, while the esophageal lumen is separated from the pharynx by a tonically contracted muscle, the upper esophageal sphincter (UES). This permits breathing to occur while limiting the volume of the respiratory dead space. At the lower end of the esophagus, another tonically contracted muscle, the lower esophageal sphincter (LES), prevents reflux of potentially irritating gastric contents into the esophagus (Fig. 12.1-1). Tonic contraction of both the UES and the LES is produced by continuous neural stimulation.

The first phase of swallowing—the propulsion of the bolus from the mouth into the pharynx—is voluntary, whereas subsequent events are involuntary. As the tongue forces the bolus into the pharynx, the nasopharynx is closed by elevation of the soft palate and contraction of the superior pharyngeal constrictor muscles. Airway penetration is prevented by inhibition of respiration, elevation of the larynx, approximation of the vocal cords (glottal closure), and deflection of the bolus by the epiglottis. The presence of multiple mechanisms for airway protection emphasizes the importance of prevention of pulmonary soilage. Failure of any one mechanism alone, as occurs, for example, after epiglottectomy for cancer, usually does not result in penetration of the swallowed bolus.

At the time of closure of the nasopharynx and larynx, inhibition of neural stimulation to the UES results in its relaxation, permitting a broad moving ring of contraction (pharyngeal peristalsis) to push the swallowed bolus into the esophagus unimpeded. The peristaltic wave continues down the length of the esophagus (esophageal peristalsis). Before arrival of the bolus in the distal

TABLE 12.1–1. CLASSIFICATION OF OROPHARYNGEAL DYSPHAGIA NEUROLOGIC AND NEUROMUSCULAR DISEASE

Site of Abnormality	Example
Sensory	Any oropharyngeal lesion affecting sensory receptors (e.g., glossitis, pharyngitis, retropharyngeal abscess, Vincent angina, thrush, Plummer-Vinson syndrome) Disorders of cranial nerves V, IX, X
Central control	Pseudobulbar palsy (e.g., multiple infarcts, multiple sclerosis, amyotrophic lateral sclerosis) Extrapyramidal disease (e.g., Parkinson disease, Huntington disease) Brain-stem lesions (e.g., infarct, trauma, neoplasm, multiple sclerosis)
Motor	Lower motor neuron disease (e.g., amyotrophic lateral sclerosis, bulbar poliomyelitis) Disorders of cranial nerves VII, IX, X, XIII; disorders of neuromuscular transmission (e.g., myasthenia gravis, botulism) Myopathy (e.g., polymyositis, hyperthyroidism, hypothyroidism, myotonic dystrophy, oculopharyngeal muscular dystrophy)
Isolated UES dysfunction	Incoordination of UES relaxation Incomplete UES relaxation

Anatomic Abnormalities	Example
Pharyngeal diverticula	Lateral pharyngeal pouches, Zenker diverticulum
Intrinsic lesions	Pharyngeal webs (e.g., Plummer-Vinson syndrome), cancer of the oral cavity or hypopharynx, surgical resection
Extrinsic impression	Thyromegaly, cervical osteophytes, soft tissue tumor

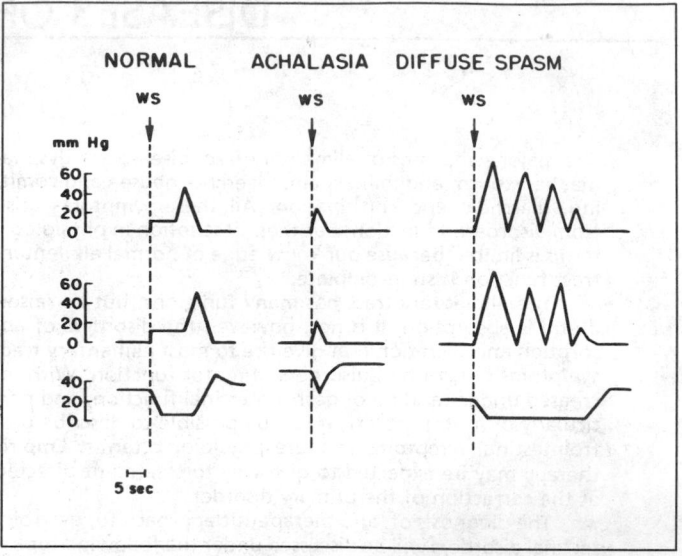

Figure 12.1–1. Esophageal manometric records from patients with normal esophageal function, achalasia, and diffuse esophageal spasm. Intraluminal pressure recordings from the LES (bottom tracings) and 5 cm (middle) and 10 cm (upper tracings) above the LES are shown. In *normal function* a swallow of water (WS) is followed by relaxation of the LES, and then the esophagus is swept clear by the peristaltic wave that is followed by contraction of the sphincter. In *achalasia,* the resting pressure in the LES is elevated and does not relax completely in response to a swallow. The simultaneous elevation of pressure at both esophageal recording sites is caused by the pharynx propelling the bolus of water into a *closed esophagus.* In *diffuse spasm,* a swallow initiates a series of high-amplitude, repetitive esophageal contractions. In this record, LES relaxation is normal but prolonged because of continuation of motor activity in the body of the esophagus. Some patients with diffuse spasm have intermittent sphincter dysfunction similar to that seen in achalasia.

esophagus, cessation of firing of vagal excitatory nerves and activation of vagal inhibitory nerves to the LES relax the sphincter, permitting easy passage of the bolus into the stomach.

DIAGNOSIS OF DYSPHAGIA

CLINICAL EVALUATION

The clinical history holds a key place in the assessment of dysphagia. Often the history accurately identifies the level of dysfunction and suggests the type of evaluation that will most likely lead to the correct diagnosis. In addition, minor abnormalities of motor function of the pharynx and esophagus are relatively common, and correlation with the patient's symptoms is necessary to ensure that such abnormalities are pertinent to the patient's complaints.

Disorders of the swallowing mechanism may cause a variety of symptoms. By careful analysis of the patient's history, the clinician can reach an accurate diagnosis in a large percentage of cases. The following symptoms require special consideration: dysphagia, choking or coughing, odynophagia, heartburn, chest pain, regurgitation, and the globus sensation.

Dysphagia
Dysphagia, the symptom of delayed transit of a swallow, is usually described by the patient as food "sticking," "holding up," or "going down slowly." Symptoms of dysphagia are often referred proximal to the site of the lesion. For example, in about one third of patients with a distal esophageal obstructive lesion, symptoms

are localized to the level of the substernal notch or above. On the other hand, localization of symptoms distal to the lesion is rare.

Dysphagia for solids only suggests structural abnormality narrowing the pharynx or esophagus, such as mucosal web, benign stricture, or neoplasm. Symptoms may initially be intermittent and involve foods that are difficult to chew. As the luminal diameter diminishes, symptoms become more frequent, and eventually dysphagia also occurs with liquids.

Dysphagia associated with motility disorders (abnormalities of muscle contraction) usually involve both liquids and solids and rarely involve solids alone. In esophageal spasm, symptoms tend to be intermittent and are frequently associated with chest pain.

TABLE 12.1–2. CLASSIFICATIONS OF ESOPHAGEAL DYSPHAGIA

	Examples
Esophageal dysmotility	Achalasia Aperistalsis (e.g., scleroderma, Raynaud phenomenon) Diffuse esophageal spasm
Narrowing of lumen	Inflammatory disease (e.g., reflux, candidiasis, herpes) Extrinsic compression (aberrant artery, mediastinal mass, enlarged heart) Malignancy (e.g., squamous carcinoma or adenocarcinoma) Inflammatory stricture (e.g., reflux, lye ingestion) Benign tumor (e.g., leiomyoma) Esophageal web (e.g., Schatzki ring)

In disorders of pharyngeal motility, which are usually the result of neurologic or myogenic disease, symptoms are more persistent and are often associated with symptoms of coughing or choking, resulting from entrance of a portion of the swallowed bolus into the larynx.

Choking or Coughing

Choking or coughing while eating usually indicates a disorder affecting the oral or pharyngeal phase of swallowing, although at times esophageal spasm or a high obstructing lesion of the esophagus can produce this symptom. Occasionally pulmonary symptoms can be the presenting complaint, and the patient is unaware of any difficulty in swallowing. Recognition that aspiration is the underlying cause of chronic or recurrent pulmonary symptoms requires a high index of suspicion.

Choking or coughing after meals may be due to either oropharyngeal or esophageal disorders. When these symptoms occur during sleep, the cause may be gastroesophageal reflux or prolonged retention of food in a Zenker diverticulum or in an obstructed esophagus (e.g., achalasia).

Odynophagia

"Odynophagia" refers to pain that specifically occurs during the act of swallowing and that may be localized to either the throat or chest. Although odynophagia may result from a motility disturbance, it is usually associated with mucosal inflammation.

Heartburn

Heartburn is the typical symptom of gastroesophageal reflux. It is usually described as a burning sensation located behind the sternum and is often felt to radiate toward the neck. It is a very common symptom and does not always imply significant disease.

Chest Pain[1]

Chest pain is a common symptom that may be associated with disorders in a variety of organs, including the heart, chest wall, gallbladder, and peripheral nervous system, as well as in the esophagus. Chest pain in patients with dysphagia strongly suggests an esophageal cause—most often esophageal spasm. Esophageal pain is not necessarily limited, however, to the time of swallowing. In many patients with spasm the chest pain is not related temporally to swallowing and hence is not associated with dysphagia.

Chest pain resulting from esophageal disease may be sharp or squeezing in character. It is located retrosternally and often radiates into the back. However, radiation into the neck and left arm can occur. The pain can, therefore, mimic that of myocardial ischemia and may respond to sublingual nitroglycerin, further confusing the clinical picture. All too often an esophageal cause of chest pain is considered only after coronary angiography shows no abnormality.

Regurgitation

The return of previously swallowed food or liquid, or of gastric contents, to the pharynx or mouth is referred to as regurgitation.

Regurgitation of undigested food during a meal may result from dysphagia of any cause. Late regurgitation of undigested material (i.e., regurgitation more than a few minutes after the meal is concluded) strongly suggests either a diverticulum, most commonly located in the hypopharynx (i.e., Zenker diverticulum), a tight obstructing lesion of the distal esophagus (e.g., an esophageal stricture or achalasia), or rumination (the effortless return of food to the mouth, with subsequent rechewing and reswallowing).

Regurgitation of sour or bitter-tasting food or liquid has different implications. It indicates that regurgitation is occurring from the stomach, rather than the esophagus (i.e., gastroesophageal reflux). The combination of heartburn with the regurgitation of sour or bitter material into the mouth is pathognomonic for gastroesophageal reflux. It is important, however, to distinguish between reflux and vomiting. Regurgitation is not associated with the abdominal muscle contractions that occur with vomiting.

The Globus Sensation

The globus sensation refers to a sensation of a lump or fullness in the throat. This symptom tends to be chronic. It is not usually associated with dysphagia; indeed the patient often indicates that the sensation is momentarily improved by swallowing.

Although this symptom is commonly assumed to be hysterical in origin ("globus hystericus"), studies have failed to demonstrate neurotic tendencies in most of these patients. The symptom has been attributed to a variety of causes, including sinus conditions, UES dysfunction, and gastroesophageal reflux. Obviously in patients with associated dysphagia, evaluation should proceed as indicated for the latter symptom. Although the diagnostic yield with this approach is probably substantially less than in patients with the globus sensation without dysphagia (true "globus"), evaluation along the same lines is advisable to rule out a serious lesion such as a neoplasm.

The physical examination of the oropharynx is often given too little attention in the evaluation of oropharyngeal dysphagia. The oral cavity should be carefully examined for evidence of cancer or inflammatory disease. Because chewing is vital for proper preparation of food, dental hygiene and denture fit should be assessed. Evaluation of muscle strength and tone and of oral sensation is important. Loss of tongue mass, asymmetry of the oropharynx, or fasciculations of the tongue are clues to a neurologic cause. Voice quality should be assessed. A wet or bubbly voice suggests laryngeal soiling, whereas a hoarse or weak voice indicates vocal cord dysfunction and should be evaluated by laryngoscopy by an experienced examiner. The neurologic examination may indicate the presence of specific neurologic disease associated with oropharyngeal dysfunction.

The physical examination is less helpful in esophageal dysphagia. Exceptions include the uncommon and late appearance of left supraclavicular lymphadenopathy (Virchow node), which is associated with esophageal or gastric cancer and the skin changes indicating Raynaud phenomenon or scleroderma.

RADIOLOGIC ASSESSMENT

Although a routine chest radiograph is essential for the assessment of pulmonary disease that might be caused by aspiration, it also occasionally reveals a dilated esophagus behind the heart shadow, thus providing a clue to the presence of achalasia.

Barium studies are central in the evaluation of dysphagia. Routine barium swallows are the first diagnostic procedure to employ in the evaluation of esophageal dysphagia. A good-quality study will reveal most structural lesions sufficient to cause obstruction to the flow of food or liquids. Occasionally the use of a barium-impregnated marshmallow will result in detection of an obstruction missed with liquid barium. In addition, the radiologist may be able to observe esophageal dysmotility. Unfortunately, the intermittency of esophageal spasm does not permit the fluoroscopist to rule out spasm if dysmotility is not noted.

Free reflux of barium witnessed on fluoroscopic examination is convincing evidence that the patient has significant gastroesophageal reflux disease. However, reflux can be documented by fluoroscopy in only about 40 percent of patients demonstrated to have clinically significant reflux by other diagnostic tests. The presence of a small sliding hiatal hernia—formerly thought to support the diagnosis of gastroesophageal reflux—is by itself of little or no clinical significance. Many patients with reflux do not have a hiatal hernia, whereas others with hiatal hernias have no evidence of reflux at all.

Although routine barium swallow studies are usually adequate for the evaluation of the esophagus, the rapidity of events in the oropharynx during swallowing makes cineradiographic evaluation mandatory in patients with oropharyngeal dysphagia. Significant constricting lesions of the pharynx and upper esophagus may be missed by fluoroscopy and can be identified only by review of the cinefilms of swallows. In addition, the frequency with which mus-

cular dysfunction produces oropharyngeal dysphagia makes a dynamic cineradiographic study of the oropharyngeal phase of swallowing essential. These films should be assessed for tongue motion, evidence of penetration of barium into the nasopharynx or larynx, asymmetry of the pharynx, the presence of lateral or posterior pharyngeal pouches, the presence of the pharyngeal peristaltic wave, and the completeness of opening of the pharyngoesophageal segment (the UES), as well as for structural lesions.

ESOPHAGEAL MOTILITY

Manometric studies are often helpful in patients with symptoms of dysphagia in whom no abnormality is noted on contrast radiography. In this situation the motility study offers a second chance to look for dysmotility without additional radiation. In addition, certain types of esophageal dysmotility are associated with contractions of very high amplitude but with normal progression of the peristaltic waves. These can be detected only by manometric evaluation.

ENDOSCOPY

Endoscopy with biopsy provides the most effective means of establishing the nature of anatomic abnormalities observed on barium studies. In addition, endoscopy is essential in any patient with dysphagia in whom no explanation is found by barium study. The presence of esophageal spasm may prevent full distension of the esophagus, thereby masking the presence of a significant structural lesion. Since obstruction is an important cause of spasm, the demonstration of esophageal spasm on radiography may require endoscopic evaluation to rule out an additional abnormality. In patients with heartburn, endoscopy with biopsy provides the only means to assess esophageal mucosal damage; however, actual inflammation of the esophagus occurs in only a minority of patients with gastroesophageal reflux. Reflux symptoms are so common that endoscopy of all patients with heartburn is unnecessary and impractical.

CLINICAL EXAMPLES OF DYSPHAGIA

OROPHARYNGEAL DYSPHAGIA[8,11]

Cerebrovascular Accidents

Brain-stem strokes can produce a variable pattern of swallowing dysfunction depending on the extent of damage to the swallowing center, and to the associated cranial nerve nuclei, or to both (see Chapters 15.6 and 15.13).

Although a careful assessment of oropharyngeal sensation and of oral muscle strength and function, as well as a general neurologic examination, is important, a detailed cineradiographic evaluation of swallowing is necessary if the specific pattern of dysfunction is to be determined. Studies should be initiated with care until the severity of airway penetration is appreciated. The absence of paroxysms of coughing during swallowing does not necessarily rule out significant airway penetration, because the cough reflex also may be impaired as a result of the stroke.

Therapy for dysphagia due to a stroke should be expectant initially. Gradual improvement can occur, although many months may pass before return to an acceptable diet can be achieved. In the meantime, measures should be instituted to ensure adequate hydration and nutrition. If the patient is unable to take adequate food and water by mouth, alternate means of hydration and nutrition must be used. The long-term choices include nasogastric intubation or an endoscopically placed feeding gastrostomy.

Rehabilitation therapists experienced in swallowing disorders can occasionally help patients sufficiently to avoid gastrostomy. Alterations in the consistency and volume of food ingested, and con-

scious adjustments in the pattern of swallowing, may produce sufficient improvement in swallowing to permit adequate intake without jeopardizing the airway. Often patients are unable to swallow liquids and yet are able to handle semisolids such as gelatin or pudding without aspiration. If necessary, complete nutrition and hydration can be maintained with gelatinized liquid nutrition. Depending on the specific pattern of dysfunction, alterations in head position or breathing pattern in relation to swallowing can be helpful.

Myasthenia Gravis

Myasthenia gravis is a neuromuscular disorder of striated muscle in which muscle weakness and easy fatigability result from a decreased number of functioning acetylcholine receptors on the motor endplate (see Chapter 15.15).

Of all neuromuscular causes of oropharyngeal dysphagia, myasthenia gravis is the most responsive to therapy. Characteristically, these patients find chewing and swallowing more difficult as the meal progresses. They tend also to have more difficulty during the evening meal than breakfast. Nasal regurgitation and coughing during eating are common.

Cineradiography demonstrates weakness of the tongue in pushing food into the pharynx, along with weakness of soft-palate elevation, laryngeal elevation, and pharyngeal peristalsis.

If the most prominent symptom is dysphagia, confirmation of the diagnosis can be obtained by cineradiography before and after the edrophonium (Tensilon) test.

Dysphagia associated with polymyositis, hyperthyroidism, or hypothyroidism is also responsive to drug therapy.

Idiopathic UES Dysfunction and Zenker Diverticulum

Isolated abnormalities of UES function are often implicated as the cause of oropharyngeal dysphagia. Radiographically, UES dysfunction is suggested by the incomplete opening of the pharyngoesophageal segment or by premature closure of this segment, resulting in division of the barium column during transit. Although manometric study may confirm failure of relaxation or incoordination of the pharynx and UES, pharyngeal weakness may be the primary cause of dysphagia in these patients. If the abnormality is truly restricted to the UES, cricopharyngeal myotomy may be beneficial.

Zenker diverticulum is an outpouching of the posterior wall of the hypopharynx through an area just above the UES in which the muscle layer is sparse. Although it is commonly held that UES dysfunction results in increased pharyngeal pressure, which in turn is responsible for the development of the diverticulum, several manometric studies have failed to provide support for this view.

Patients with Zenker diverticulum are typically elderly and have dysphagia for liquids and solids. Regurgitation of undigested food and liquid into the pharynx can occur many hours after eating and often produces paroxysms of coughing. Aspiration may be particularly severe at night.

Cineradiography reveals a barium-filled outpouching just above the pharyngoesophageal junction that remains filled after the remainder of the barium has passed into the esophagus.

Therapy involves surgical removal of the diverticulum or suspension of the apex of the diverticulum in conjunction with a cricopharyngeal myotomy. However, myotomy is contraindicated in the presence of severe gastroesophageal reflux disease.

ESOPHAGEAL DYSPHAGIA

Esophageal Stricture

Esophageal strictures may be malignant or benign. A benign stricture is most commonly a consequence of severe esophageal reflux disease or of a suicidal or accidental ingestion of a caustic material such as lye. Occasionally a drug in tablet form (e.g., quinidine, potassium, tetracycline, iron, or anti-inflammatory drugs) is not swept out of the esophagus by peristalsis and an ulcer with subsequent stricture may develop at the site.[7] Malignant strictures are

usually squamous cell carcinomas, but adenocarcinomas arising in the cardia or in the distal esophagus lined with columnar epithelium (Barrett esophagus) also produce obstruction of the esophagus. Peptic strictures in the squamous epithelium are usually found in the distal esophagus. Peptic strictures associated with Barrett esophagus occur at the squamocolumnar junction, which may be at any site in the distal two thirds of the esophagus. Pill-induced strictures are usually at the level of the aortic arch or in the distal esophagus.

Strictures cause symptoms by narrowing the esophageal lumen. Severity of symptoms will vary with diet and the care with which the patient chews his food. Often patients are surprisingly asymptomatic as a result of subconscious avoidance of tough and fibrous solids and careful oral preparation of food.

Barium swallow reveals a narrowed, noncompliant esophageal segment. If the lumen is severely compromised, an air-fluid level may be noted when the patient is in the upright position as a result of food retention above the stricture. A barium-impregnated marshmallow may demonstrate a site of obstruction not demonstrated by the liquid barium swallow. Malignant strictures characteristically are irregular in contour, whereas benign peptic strictures are smooth, symmetric, and have a tapering proximal margin. Pill-induced strictures occasionally mimic malignant strictures. Endoscopy with biopsies and brushing for cytologic study is necessary, however, to confirm the radiologic diagnosis.

Benign strictures can be managed by dilation.[9] Symptoms will recur, however, if the underlying cause is not removed and the ulcerated area does not reepithelialize. Patients with gastroesophageal reflux disease should be treated vigorously to prevent ongoing esophageal damage. Dilation provides effective palliation for malignant strictures, although the risk of perforation is substantial. Because the chance of cure in esophageal cancer by any therapy is remote, dilation with or without placement of a Silastic tube to maintain lumen patency is frequently the appropriate treatment choice in patients with advanced disease. Recently, laser therapy has been successfully used to provide a functional lumen through obstructing tumors.

Cancer restricted to the distal esophagus is usually treated by resection if the tumor appears to be localized. Irradiation may provide useful palliative therapy for middle- and upper-third lesions. Computed tomographic scanning is an aid in determining whether a malignancy is resectable. Five-year survival rates for patients with esophageal cancer in reported series vary from 0 to 10 percent.[6]

Achalasia

Achalasia is a disorder of esophageal motor function in which the LES fails to relax adequately and peristalsis is lost in the smooth-muscle portion of the esophagus. In addition, the average resting pressure in the LES is greater than in normal persons. The result is a functional obstruction at the level of the esophagogastric junction. Patients may have slowly progressive dysphagia, episodes of regurgitation, chest pain during eating, or unexplained pneumonia. Weight loss may occur, especially as the disease progresses. Untreated, the obstruction causes retention of food and liquid in the esophagus, which becomes massively dilated (the "sigmoid esophagus") late in the disease. Regurgitation into the mouth of previously consumed food often occurs hours after ingestion. If regurgitation occurs at night, the patient may awaken from sleep with paroxysms of coughing due to aspiration.

Although a dilated, fluid-filled esophagus with an air-fluid level seen on a chest radiograph occasionally provides the first clue to the diagnosis of achalasia, it is the barium swallow that demonstrates the diagnostic features: (1) a dilated esophagus with an air-fluid level that fails to empty; (2) absence of peristalsis (in some patients forceful, segmental contractions are seen—"vigorous achalasia"); and (3) a smoothly tapering obstruction of the distal esophagus—a "bird beak" appearance. The diagnosis is confirmed by fiberoptic endoscopy when it is found that the endoscope can be passed into the stomach easily, thus establishing that the obstruction at the cardia is functional and not anatomic.

Achalasia is caused by the idiopathic degeneration of ganglion cells in the myenteric plexus of the esophagus. Rarely, carcinoma of the cardia produces secondary achalasia by tumor invasion of the enteric nerve plexuses of the esophagus. In parts of South and Central America, Chagas disease, a chronic infection with *Trypanosoma cruzi*, leads to widespread ganglion cell degeneration with the development of achalasia usually in association with other abnormalities (e.g., megacolon, megaureter).

Esophageal manometric findings in achalasia are characteristic but are not necessary for the diagnosis. The pressure in the LES is usually, but not invariably, elevated. With swallowing, LES relaxation is incomplete and peristalsis is absent. These abnormalities are the consequence of degeneration of myenteric ganglion cells in the esophagus and neurons of the dorsal nucleus of the vagus.

In the absence of any method for reestablishing normal LES relaxation, therapy aims at weakening the LES to decrease the barrier to flow from the esophagus to the stomach.[13] Reduced sphincter tone is achieved by forceful dilation of the LES with a pneumostatic balloon dilator or by surgical myotomy in which the muscles in the area of the esophagogastric junction are severed down to the mucosa. Pneumostatic dilation is preferred, because (1) morbidity is less, (2) hospitalization is shorter, and (3) gastroesophageal reflux with esophagitis, which may occur after surgical myotomy, does not occur after dilation.

Although success has been reported with pharmacologic therapy (e.g., long-acting nitrites or calcium-channel blockers, such as with nifedipine), these agents are useful as adjunctive rather than primary therapy. If symptoms recur after an initial good response, the most probable explanations are (1) recurrence of achalasia, (2) carcinoma, which has been reported in some series to occur with increased frequency in achalasia, and (3) peptic stricture. Peptic stricture is seen almost exclusively after surgical treatment. Patients with achalasia can keep the esophagus free of retained food by drinking a carbonated beverage after each meal and at bedtime, thus avoiding aspiration during sleep.

Symptomatic Diffuse Esophageal Spasm and Related Disorders

Symptomatic diffuse esophageal spasm (SDES) is an esophageal motility disorder that is characterized by intermittent chest pain or dysphagia, or both, and that is associated with abnormal nonperistaltic esophageal contractions in the absence of any other disorder, such as gastroesophageal reflux. In about half the instances, pain appears while eating. A diagnosis of angina pectoris is often made in patients when pain appears independently of meals. The frequent response of this chest pain of esophageal origin to nitroglycerin is often perceived as confirmation that the chest pain is due to myocardial ischemia. One third of SDES patients have LES dysfunction consisting of high resting pressure and incomplete relaxation. An occasional patient with SDES evolves over a period of years into typical achalasia. For clinical purposes the feature distinguishing these two disorders is whether the esophagus empties while the patient is in the upright position.

The diagnosis of SDES is made from the characteristic history, absence of gastroesophageal reflux or of an anatomic cause for chest pain such as coronary artery disease and demonstration of abnormal esophageal motility by barium swallow or manometric study. The manometric tracings characteristically demonstrate high-amplitude, long-duration, repetitive, and nonperistaltic contractions. Normal peristalsis is often interspersed with these abnormal responses.

The treatment is reassurance and instructions to eat in a deliberate manner. If symptoms are not controlled, agents that relax smooth muscle, such as nitrites or calcium-channel blockers, may be useful.[13]

Many asymptomatic individuals are found to have esophageal motor abnormalities ranging from simultaneous contractions, low-amplitude contractions, or aperistalsis to those seen in SDES. Finally, in some patients, chest pain is found in association with high

amplitude peristaltic waves (as high as 400 mm Hg), the so-called nutcracker esophagus.

Systemic Sclerosis

In systemic sclerosis (SS) the esophagus is involved in 85 percent or more of patients.[3] The typical motility findings of low (or absent) LES pressure and aperistalsis predispose affected individuals to severe reflux and its complications such as esophagitis and stricture. Although these motor abnormalities are characteristic of SS, they are encountered in other collagen vascular diseases associated with Raynaud phenomenon (see Chapter 8.5). Reflux symptoms do not correlate well with the reflux severity. Indeed, dysphagia due to a peptic stricture is often the first indication that the patient has reflux disease. All patients with SS should be considered at risk for reflux and its complications. Therefore routine screening of asymptomatic patients with SS for objective evidence of esophageal involvement (by barium studies) or of reflux (by pH probe studies) should be done. Prophylactic reflux therapy should be instituted in those with documented esophageal reflux in an effort to limit esophageal mucosal damage.

Gastroesophageal Reflux Disease[2]

Heartburn is the most common sympton of gastroesophageal reflux. Typically, heartburn is described as a burning sensation that radiates upward retrosternally toward the neck. It is often associated with the oral regurgitation of a sour or bitter liquid. Heartburn associated with regurgitation is virtually pathognomonic of gastroesophageal reflux. Symptoms are exacerbated by eating, especially overindulgence. It is also made worse by lying down, bending over, or lifting heavy objects. Relief is often obtained by standing up and drinking liquids, especially antacids. When symptoms are not typical, differentiation from idiopathic esophageal spasm, angina pectoris, cholelithiasis, or peptic ulcer disease may be difficult. Rarely, patients have pulmonary symptoms resulting from aspiration without the typical symptoms of reflux.

The esophageal epithelium is protected from damage due to reflux of gastric contents by three mechanisms: (1) an antireflux barrier attributed primarily to the strength and responsiveness of the lower esophageal sphincter, (2) secondary peristalsis that sweeps reflux material back into the stomach, and (3) the acid-neutralizing effect of swallowed saliva. The major abnormality in patients with reflux is a weak, unresponsive lower esophageal sphincter.[5] However, abnormalities of esophageal clearance and of gastric emptying often contribute to esophageal reflux. Patients with scleroderma are at particularly high risk of developing esophageal damage (esophagitis and stricture) because all of these protective mechanisms are lost in the course of the disease.

Acid alone, or in combination with pepsin, which is activated at a pH less than 4, is generally assumed to be the main damaging agent in reflux disease. However, bile acids and pancreatic enzymes regurgitated into the stomach from the duodenum are equally capable of producing damage to the esophageal mucosa. There is evidence that reflux may produce a vicious cycle in which refluxed gastric contents impair esophageal clearing and LES tone, thereby facilitating further reflux. Reflux leads to an increased rate of loss of esophageal epithelial cells. When cell loss exceeds the ability of the germinal layer to provide replacements, erosions and ulcerations will develop. If healing is not prompt, a peptic stricture may form or the destroyed squamous epithelium may be replaced by a more acid-resistant columnar epithelium growing up from the stomach, leading to the development of the Barrett esophagus.[10]

Diagnosis. In the face of typical symptoms of heartburn associated with oral regurgitation of a sour- or bitter-tasting liquid, no laboratory studies are necessary. However, patients with atypical symptoms or those with symptoms that do not respond promptly to therapeutic intervention will require documentation that gastroesophageal reflux is in fact responsible for symptoms. There are three clinically important questions to be answered: (1) Is the esophagus the origin of the pain? (2) Is reflux actually occurring?

(3) Has reflux been severe enough to lead to esophagitis (which is the precursor of the serious complications of reflux, i.e., stricture formation and ulceration)? Unfortunately, no readily available laboratory test is capable of answering all of these questions. A combination of tests is therefore often used in assessment for reflux and its consequences.

The standard test of acid sensitivity is the acid perfusion test (Bernstein test), in which the blinded symptomatic responses to perfusion of the esophagus with 0.1N hydrochloric acid and with saline solution are compared. The test result is positive if the infusion of hydrochloric acid reproduces the patient's symptoms and the infusion of saline solution does not. Pain unlike that for which the patient is being evaluated indicates acid sensitivity but does not prove that acid reflux is the cause of the patient's symptoms. The test demonstrates acid sensitivity in about 15 percent of apparently normal individuals and in about 35 percent of patients with peptic disorders other than reflux disease. For this reason, although the acid perfusion is a useful screening test for patients with chest pain, it is necessary to confirm that reflux is occurring before it can be assumed that symptoms are reflux induced.

The most readily available test to evaluate reflux is the barium swallow. Unfortunately it documents only about 40 percent of clinically significant cases of reflux. The standard acid reflux test using an intraesophageal pH probe (Tuttle test) confirms reflux in about 90 percent of the patients with typical symptoms, and false-positive results are unusual. Intraesophageal pH is measured after intragastric infusion of 300 ml of dilute hydrochloric acid. After a period of basal recordings with the patient supine, the patient is put through a series of maneuvers designed to stress the antireflux barrier. Although this test measures reflux, it is performed under nonphysiologic conditions and does not demonstrate that the patient's symptoms are the result of reflux. A radionuclide scintiscan technique has been advocated as an alternative means of confirming the presence of reflux. This test appears to be less sensitive than the pH probe test but does not require intubation.

Continuous intraesophageal pH monitoring has provided important insights into the pathogenesis of reflux disease.[4] This test permits evaluation of reflux as it occurs under near-physiologic conditions. Correlation of symptoms with reflux episodes allows conclusions about the origin of these symptoms. In this sense, continuous pH monitoring is both a test confirming the presence of reflux and a means of evaluating the relationship of reflux to symptoms. In addition, it is the first test that permits objective assessment of the effect of therapy on the control of severity reflux.

Endoscopy with biopsy is the test to evaluate reflux-induced mucosal damage. The histologic findings in biopsy specimens of the esophageal mucosa in patients with reflux symptoms range from evidence of increased rate of turnover of the squamous epithelium without any inflammatory infiltrate, to leukocytic infiltration, and finally to frank ulceration. Esophagitis properly encompasses the latter two categories, although the term is frequently used inappropriately to designate reflux symptoms.

An additional endoscopic finding of importance is the presence of a columnar-lined mucosa in the esophagus itself (Barrett esophagus). This abnormality is recognized as a visible displacement of the esophagogastric junction into the tubular esophagus. In biopsy specimens the mucosa is composed of columnar epithelium similar to that found in the stomach, and this mucosa frequently undergoes intestinal metaplasia. It is now appreciated that Barrett esophagus is the result of chronic reflux damage that causes loss of squamous epithelium with subsequent replacement by columnar epithelium. Barrett esophagus, which has dysplastic changes, carries a significant risk of malignant transformation. Although the average reported prevalence of adenocarcinoma in Barrett esophagus is 10 percent,[10] in patients with Barrett esophagus but no associated carcinoma when diagnosed, the incidence of adenocarcinoma in subsequent study was approximately six cases per 1000 patient-years of follow-up.[12] In this series, fewer deaths resulted from Barrett associated cancer than from complications of esophageal surgery, carcinoma of the lung, and liver disease. If the

patient has Barrett esophagus without dysphagia, adequate follow-up consists of esophagoscopy with biopsy and cytologic study every 3 to 5 years. If low-grade dysphagia is found, yearly endoscopy is recommended; high-grade dysphagia warrants surgical resection.

Treatment of Reflux. The aim of therapy is to relieve symptoms and heal esophagitis if present. Therapy is directed at increasing LES competence, increasing esophageal clearing, and improving gastric emptying, as well as diminishing the irritant quality of refluxed gastric contents. The initial therapy should be intensive in order to interrupt the vicious cycle initiated by reflux and to establish whether or not symptoms are responsive to therapy. Failure of symptoms to respond should lead to a reconsideration of the diagnosis, and laboratory evaluation should be done if reflux has not previously been confirmed.

No special diet is indicated, but because the success of therapy is judged by relief of symptoms, the patient should avoid foods and beverages associated with dyspepsia. Large meals should be avoided. Coffee intake is usually limited, and the intake of foods that are known to diminish LES pressure, such as chocolate and fatty foods, should be decreased or eliminated. Obesity increases symptoms of reflux, and patients often report a correlation with the appearance of symptoms and weight gain. Weight reduction should, therefore, be encouraged in symptomatic, overweight patients.

Because reflux is often most severe in the supine position, patients should avoid lying down within 2 hours of eating. In addition, they should elevate the head of the their bed on 6-inch blocks to diminish the amount of reflux as well as to hasten esophageal clearing during sleep.

Initial treatment should consist of the use of H_2 receptor antagonists (cimetidine, 300 mg four times daily, or ranitidine, 150 mg twice daily) to decrease gastric acid secretion and antacids after meals and at bedtime. If after 2 weeks the symptoms have been controlled, treatment should be simplified by first decreasing the H_2 antagonists to a single bedtime dose. If symptoms remain uncontrolled, drugs to increase esophageal clearing, elevate LES pressure, and accelerate gastric emptying may bring symptoms under control. Bethanechol, 25 mg, or metoclopramide, 10 mg, before meals and at bedtime are the most frequently used agents.

If medical therapy is unsuccessful, antireflux surgery may be considered. The most effective procedure is fundoplication, in which the fundus of the stomach is wrapped around the distal esophagus. In general, surgery should be restricted to patients with evidence of reflux-induced esophageal damage that has failed to heal or that returns when medical therapy is decreased or stopped. Debilitating symptoms that fail to respond to intensive medical therapy without evidence of esophageal damage should raise the question of the accuracy of the diagnosis. A continuous pH study should be obtained before sending such a patient to surgery. Fewer than 5 percent of patients with significant reflux symptoms should require surgical intervention.

REFERENCES

1. Brand DL, Ilves R, Pope CE II: Evaluation of esophageal function in patients with central chest pain. Acta Med Scand (Suppl) 64:53, 1981
2. Castell DO, Wu WC, Ott DJ: Gastroesophageal Reflux Disease: Pathogenesis, Diagnosis, and Therapy. Mount Kisco, NY, Futura, 1985
3. Clements PJ, Kadell B, et al: Esophageal motility in progressive systemic sclerosis (PSS). Dig Dis Sci 24:369, 1979
4. Demeester TR, Johnson LF, et al: Patterns of gastroesophageal reflux in health and disease. Ann Surg 184:459, 1976
5. Dodds WJ, Dent J, et al: Mechanisms of gastrocsophageal reflux in patients with reflux esophagitis. N Engl J Med 307:1547, 1982
6. Earlam R, Cunha-Melo JR: Oesophageal squamous cell carcinoma. I. A critical review of surgery. Br J Surg 67.31, 1980
7. Kikendall JW, Friedman AC, et al: Pill-induced esophageal injury: Case reports and review of the medical literature. Dig Dis Sci 28:174, 1983
8. Kilman WJ, Goyal RL: Disorders of pharyngeal and upper esophageal sphincter motor function. Arch Intern Med 136:592, 1976
9. Lanza FL, Graham DY: Bougienage is effective therapy for most benign esophageal strictures. JAMA 240:844, 1978
10. Sarr MG, Hamilton SR, et al: Barrett esophagus: Its prevalence and association with adenocarcinoma in patients with symptoms of gastroesophageal reflux. Am J Surg 149:187, 1985
11. Seaman WB: Pharyngeal and upper esophageal dysphagia. JAMA 235:2643, 1976
12. Speckler SJ, Robbins AH, et al: Adenocarcinoma and Barrett esophagus an overrated risk? Gastroenterology 87:927, 1984
13. Vantrappen G, Hellemans J: Treatment of achalasia and related motor disorders. Gastroenterology 79:144, 1980

CHAPTER 12.2
Abdominal Pain

Thomas R. Hendrix, Gregory B. Bulkley, and Marvin M. Schuster

Abdominal pain is a frequent and often baffling symptom. Many of the diseases with abdominal pain as a symptom require prompt surgery; accurate differentiation is therefore important.

ORIGIN OF ABDOMINAL PAIN

A review of the origins of abdominal pain is a useful introduction to its differential diagnosis.[3] Although 80 to 90 percent of the nerve fibers in the vagus nerves are afferent, all visceral pain stimuli reach the central nervous system via the splanchnic nerves.

The alimentary tract from the esophagus to the anal canal is insensitive to many stimuli that produce pain in somatic structures. Mucosal biopsies produce acute ulcers but never produce pain at the time of biopsy or during the healing phase, whereas similar lesions in the buccal mucosa are very painful. The intestine can be cut, crushed or burned without pain. In contrast, if the intestine is distended or if its muscle coat contracts with spasm, pain is felt. As a general rule, only three phenomena are capable of producing pain in the alimentary tract: tension in the wall, ischemia, and inflammation of the serosa (peritoneum).

PAIN DUE TO TENSION

Colic, the wavelike pain associated with forceful peristaltic contractions, is the most characteristic type of pain arising from the viscera. Powerful peristalsis may be initiated by an irritant substance, such as the oxalic acid from green apples, or by an attempt to force the luminal contents through an obstruction. Other disorders,

such as ulcers or ischemia, produce painful spasm that is steady and continuous.

Tension on the mesentery and acute stretching of the capsule of a solid organ such as the liver, spleen, or kidney, also produce pain. Stretch receptors similar to those in muscle presumably are the source of these impulses interpreted as pain.

PAIN DUE TO ISCHEMIA

Ischemia of somatic, cardiac, or visceral muscle produces pain. The most common cause of intestinal ischemia is strangulation of the bowel due to an adhesion, hernia, or volvulus. Less frequently, ischemic pain is caused by mesenteric vascular occlusion.

PAIN DUE TO PERITONEAL IRRITATION

Inflammation of the peritoneum is the third major source of abdominal pain. Initially, the inflammation is usually limited to the serosa covering the inflamed organ (e.g., appendix or gallbladder), a visceral peritonitis. As the inflammatory process extends to the adjacent parietal peritoneum, localized peritonitis is produced and the pain becomes more severe and is referred to the corresponding area on the abdominal wall. Parietal peritonitis causes reflex spasm of the overlying muscles, resulting in rigidity and pain or tenderness of the abdominal wall. Generalized peritonitis may be sterile when gastric juice, pancreatic juice, or bile leaks into the peritoneal cavity, or it may be septic when the cavity becomes contaminated with contents of the colon or an abscess.

LOCATION OF ABDOMINAL PAIN

Pain arising from parietal structures is usually well localized. For example, pain associated with appendicitis becomes localized in the right lower quadrant of the abdomen only when the inflammation involves the contiguous parietal peritoneum. If the involved organ has migrated from its original embryonic position, the location of the pain may not correspond to the location of the organ. For example, diaphragmatic irritation leads to shoulder pain, and the discomfort caused by the involvement of gut alone is usually felt anteriorly in the midline.

The study of visceral pain responses in human subjects has provided useful information about localization:

1. Distension of the stomach or duodenum usually produces pain between the xiphoid and umbilicus in the midline or slightly to the right. The nearer the stimulus is to the third portion of the duodenum, the nearer the pain is to the umbilicus.
2. Stimulation of the small intestine typically results in periumbilical pain, but ileal pain may also be referred to the right lower quadrant.
3. Pain originating from the colon is usually referred to the midline between the umbilicus and the pubic symphysis; pain from the ascending or descending colon or from the hepatic and splenic flexures may also be localized to the side involved, presumably because of pressure on adjacent structures.
4. Rectosigmoid distension characteristically produces suprapubic pain, and distension of the rectum usually leads to pain in the area of the sacrum and perineum. Bladder distension also produces suprapubic pain.
5. Gallbladder distension or inflammation produces midepigastric pain radiating to the right upper quadrant or to the right scapular area as the distension increases. With common bile duct distension, pain often is felt in the midepigastrium and sometimes radiates to the shoulders.
6. Pancreatic pain is typically midepigastric. The pain radiates

laterally and to the back, when the posterior parietes become involved.

ACUTE ABDOMINAL PAIN

There are few situations in clinical medicine that demand decisive action as frequently as acute abdominal pain.[3] "Acute surgical abdomen" is medical jargon used to indicate the constellation of history and physical findings usually associated with those diseases requiring prompt surgical treatment. The failure to immediately recognize an "acute surgical abdomen" may result in a critical delay in initiating definitive treatment. For example, the results of prompt surgery for acute appendicitis are almost uniformly excellent, with minimal morbidity and almost no mortality. In contrast, if recognition is delayed until a perforation has occurred, postoperative morbidity is frequent and the chance of death is greatly increased. Although the physician should always attempt to make a specific diagnosis at the time of initial evaluation, the primary goal in the evaluation of patients with acute abdominal pain is to determine whether or not a "surgical abdomen" exists. A more specific diagnosis can be made promptly at the time of laparotomy and the definitive surgical treatment determined at that time. The operative procedure should not be delayed to determine more accurately the cause of the "surgical abdomen."

HISTORY

Careful documentation of the onset, location, nature, and subsequent course is an important aid in determining the cause of acute abdominal pain.

Onset of Pain
Sudden onset is most frequently caused by the perforation of a viscus, such as the perforation of a peptic ulcer. Acute intestinal ischemia, such as that caused by a superior mesenteric artery embolus, can also result in sudden pain. In conditions causing the obstruction of a hollow viscus or an inflammation of its walls, such as bowel obstruction, appendicitis, cholecystitis, and diverticulitis, the onset of pain is more gradual, taking several hours to reach its peak.

Character of Pain
Colic is the most characteristic type of abdominal pain and is often a manifestation of increased peristalsis proximal to an obstruction of a hollow viscus. Colic, an intermittent "wavelike" pain, should be distinguished from the continuous, steady pain produced by peritoneal irritation. This distinction is often critical; hence the patient should be specifically queried as to the presence or absence of a colicky component of the pain. Pleuritic pain is present when the inflammatory process involves the diaphragm or when the movement of the diaphragm brings the inflamed organ against the peritoneum. Patients may also describe their abdominal pain as sharp, dull, burning, tearing, or aching, but unfortunately these terms give little insight into the nature of the underlying disorder.

Location and Radiation of Pain
Severe abdominal pain that rapidly becomes generalized is often caused by the leakage of an irritating fluid into the peritoneal cavity. The irritating material may be gastric juice, bile, blood, or pus. Pain that is more localized may give help in indicating what organ is involved in the disease process. For example, midepigastric pain is associated with structures innervated by thoracic spinal nerves T6 to T8, namely, the stomach, duodenum, pancreas, liver, and biliary tree. Periumbilical pain is related to innervation from T9 to T10, including such structures as the small intestine, appendix, upper ureters, testes, and ovaries. Lower abdominal pain has its origin in structures innervated by T11 and T12, such as the colon, bladder, lower ureters, and uterus. Localization of pain to a point

on the abdominal wall may represent irritation of the underlying parietal peritoneum. Although this localization may provide an important clue as to the diagnosis (e.g., the localization of pain in the right lower quadrant suggesting appendicitis), it is well to remember that any other inflamed intra-abdominal organ in contact with that area of abdominal wall may be the cause of the pain. Thus an inflamed diverticulum in the redundant sigmoid colon that has flopped over into the right side of the pelvis may produce right lower quandrant pain, rather than pain localized in the left lower quandrant, the more characteristic location.

Associated Vomiting

Vomiting is a common accompaniment of abdominal pain. It may be a manifestation of intestinal obstruction or a visceral reflex caused by abdominal pain. In patients with intestinal obstruction, it may occur early if the obstruction is high but late or not at all if the obstruction is low. Although vomiting usually is not a symptom that helps define the specific cause of the abdominal pain, its presence is a good but not infallible indicator that the pain is of visceral rather than somatic origin.

PHYSICAL EXAMINATION

Observation of the Patient

In the performance of a physical examination on an acutely ill patient, there is often a tendency to cut corners and to center attention on the obvious. It is important, however, first to observe the patient carefully to evaluate the gravity of his illness. Is there evidence to suggest impending shock or vascular collapse? Is the patient restless, as is commonly seen with colic, or does he lie immobile in bed, as is commonly seen with peritonitis or advanced ischemia of the bowel? The initial examination of the patient often fails to establish the diagnosis of a "surgical abdomen" with sufficient certainty to proceed with laparotomy. The answer is provided by repeating the examination and assessment at regular intervals because the changing pattern may be as important as the signs themselves.

Signs of Impending Vascular Collapse

In many disorders associated with acute abdominal pain, such as peritonitis, acute pancreatitis, and intestinal obstruction, there is striking hypovolemia caused by a large and rapid translocation of fluid from the vascular space to the peritoneal cavity or the intestinal lumen. The signs of shock are rapid, weak pulse; hypotension; cold, moist skin; and restlessness. A clue to incipient vascular collapse that has been masked by compensatory homeostatic mechanisms is provided by a drop in blood pressure and a rise in pulse rate when the patient assumes the sitting position. Early recognition of these signs and vigorous replacement of fluid will improve the prognosis, regardless of the nature of the underlying disorder.

Examination of the Abdomen

The abdominal examination should provide answers to specific questions:

1. Are there signs of peritonitis? The single most reliable indicator of parietal peritonitis is the presence of involuntary guarding, that is, the presence of involuntary spasm of the abdominal wall musculature in the area in question. This must be carefully distinguished from voluntary guarding, due to the patient's pain or, more often, to the patient's fear that the examiner will worsen the pain by a too-vigorous palpation. It is therefore of critical importance that the palpation of the abdomen be slow and extremely gentle. The presence of guarding is determined by gentle palpation of the abdominal wall, not by deep palpation of the underlying organs. Next, if peritonitis is present, is it localized or diffuse?

2. What is the character of the bowel sounds? Are they hyperactive and do they come in rushes, as is typical of intestinal obstruction, or are they absent, as is characteristically seen with peritonitis, advanced ischemia, or strangulation of the bowel? It is important to allow time to elapse for the character of the bowel sounds to be determined. The bowel sounds may be present early in the course of ischemia and strangulation but may disappear as the process evolves.

3. Are there any masses to be seen or felt? Occasionally a dilated loop of bowel or a distended gallbladder is more clearly seen than felt. Care should be taken to exclude inguinal and femoral hernias.

4. Is there evidence of free fluid in the abdomen? For example, the presence of fat droplets or a high amylase content in the aspirate usually is indicative of pancreatitis but also may accompany a perforation of a duodenal ulcer. Gross blood suggests a ruptured aneurysm or spleen or an ectopic pregnancy; cloudy, dirty fluid is present after perforation of the bowel.

Pelvic and Rectal Examinations

The pelvic and rectal examinations help to differentiate disorders of the female reproductive tract from inflammatory diseases of the bowel. Occasionally, the abdominal examination reveals no abnormality in cases of appendicitis or diverticulitis even though the rectal examination demonstrates a tender localized mass. In addition, a bimanual pelvic and rectal examination allows for the direct palpation of the uterus and adjacent peritoneum.

Other Important Observations

The presence of fever makes the diagnosis of an acute inflammatory condition more likely. On the other hand, a rectal temperature above 102F is less frequently found in association with abdominal than with acute pulmonary and renal infections. If fever of this magnitude is associated with abdominal pain, consideration should be given to the possibility that the pain is being referred from an extra-abdominal site. Pulses should be evaluated in all four extremities to avoid overlooking a dissecting aneurysm.

LABORATORY AIDS

Hematologic Determinations

The hematocrit provides important information in patients with acute abdominal pain. When elevated, it suggests hemoconcentration and hypovolemia, and when it is low, intra-abdominal hemorrhage should be considered. However, a normal hematocrit does not exclude an acute massive hemorrhage for which the body has not yet compensated. Leukocytosis is indicative of inflammation and often accompanies disorders that require surgery.

Urine Examination

In addition to providing evidence of urinary-tract infections, calculi, or acute glomerulonephritis, urinalysis may provide the first indication of diabetes mellitus, which can occur in acute abdominal pain. Bilirubinuria may provide the first clue to the presence of hepatobiliary disease. Finally, examination of the urine for porphobilinogen is the simplest way to establish the diagnosis of porphyria.

Stool Examination

Blood in the stool suggests that the abdominal pain originates in the gut. It is usually seen with intussusception, mesenteric vascular occlusion, and obstructing neoplastic or inflammatory lesions.

Serum Chemical Determinations

Serum determinations of amylase and bilirubin should be obtained if involvement of the pancreas or biliary tract seems possible. For the interpretation of the laboratory results, it is important to know when in the course of the illness the blood sample was examined.

For example, the serum bilirubin and alkaline phosphatase levels may be normal early in the course of acute biliary tract obstruction. In addition, the serum amylase level frequently returns to normal 48 hours after the onset of pain in patients with pancreatitis, even though they are still symptomatic.

Lactescent or hyperlipemic serum may be found in as many as 20 percent of patients with acute pancreatitis. Hyperlipemia may obscure the diagnosis because the serum amylase level is often normal in its presence. Serum electrolytes and urea nitrogen should also be determined so that imbalances can be corrected, particularly if surgery is anticipated.

Radiographic Examination

A flat and an upright radiograph of the abdomen and a chest radiograph should always be obtained when one is evaluating a patient with an acute abdomen. Findings that may provide an explanation of the patient's abdominal pain include lower lobe pneumonia, free air under the diaphragm indicating a perforated viscus, absent psoas shadows suggesting retroperitoneal bleeding, abscess, displaced stomach or bowel gas shadows, small-bowel air fluid levels suggesting a paralytic or mechanical ileus, large-bowel gas or air fluid levels suggesting an ileus, volvulus, or obstruction, and pancreatic, biliary, or urinary calcifications.

If an emergency barium enema is performed to define the site and nature of a colonic obstruction, the full amount of barium is not necessary because the location of the obstructing lesion, rather than a detailed study of the mucosa, is the desired result. A water-soluble contrast medium should be used if a perforation of the colon is considered to be a possibility. Barium should not be given by mouth if an obstruction of the colon is suspected, but its use to confirm the presence of a small-bowel obstruction is perfectly safe and preferable to water-soluble contrast media.

CLINICAL EXAMPLES

Appendicitis[5,8,10]

Acute appendicitis is a condition wherein the importance of early and accurate diagnosis is paramount, for the consequences of delay are a substantial increase in the chance of complications or death.

A consideration of the clinical course of appendicitis illustrates the importance of serial observation of the patient. The first symptom of acute appendicitis frequently is epigastric discomfort attributed to indigestion. When epigastric symptoms predominate, there may be no tenderness in the right lower quadrant. In other patients the first symptom will be a colicky periumbilical pain; if the pain is associated with diarrhea, the patient will conclude, and the physician will most likely agree, that gastroenteritis is the cause of the symptoms. Anorexia, nausea, and vomiting are common at this stage. In a matter of hours, however, the pain shifts to the right lower quadrant. Frequently, but by no means invariably, tenderness on deep palpation is elicited at McBurney point. A fever of a degree or two appears, together with leukocytosis. If the patient remains untreated, a perforation will occur, followed by generalized peritonitis or periappendiceal abscess. The accurate diagnosis of appendicitis would not be so difficult if it regularly followed this pattern, but probably no more than one fifth of the patients with the disease manifest this characteristic course. The variable clinicial picture seen in patients with acute appendicitis is caused in part by the mobility of the cecum and appendix and by the consequent absence of contact between the inflamed appendix and the parietal peritoneum in the right lower quadrant. In large series of cases of acute appendicitis the most common sign was localized abdominal tenderness, which unfortunately is not sufficiently specific. The physical signs of appendicitis evolve slowly and are frequently atypical, thus making early diagnosis difficult. When the cecum resides high in the midabdomen, appendicitis may simulate cholecystitis or pyelonephritis. When the appendix lies deep in the right lower quadrant, appendicitis may mimic Crohn disease, psoas abscess, ureteral calculus, or even hip disease. In the pelvis, an inflamed appendix may produce bladder symptoms or, in women, symptoms suggesting disease of the right tube or ovary. A particularly difficult distinction is that which must be made between the pelvic peritonitis of pelvic inflammatory disease and acute appendicitis. Most of this confusion can be resolved by careful serial examinations of the patient, including rectal, pelvic, and urinary examinations.

Acute Diverticulitis[7]

The spectrum of diverticular disease of the colon extends from multiple asymptomatic diverticula involving the entire colon to a few diverticula in the sigmoid colon, associated radiographic evidence of spasm and irritability, and symptoms of irritable bowel syndrome. Diverticula associated with chronic or recurring symptoms can be shown to be associated with increased motor activity and striking elevation of intraluminal pressure. Acute diverticulitis most frequently involves the sigmoid colon and may appear with no premonitory symptoms, or it may be superimposed on longstanding symptoms of constipation and left lower quadrant pain. The pathologic process is a microperforation of the mucosa of a single diverticulum leading to peridiverticulitis, rather than diffuse inflammation of the wall of the diverticulum. The symptoms are pain in the left lower quadrant with severe constipation, nausea, and, uncommonly, vomiting. The patient becomes febrile and has leukocytosis. It is not surprising that this has been called "left-sided appendicitis." Frequently, the stool sample obtained by rectal examination will be positive for occult blood, but gross bleeding is not associated with diverticulitis. Usually the attack subsides in a few days and, unlike appendicitis, usually does not proceed to free perforation or pericolic abscess.

The diagnosis should be suspected with the clinical findings of left lower quadrant pain, fever, and leukocytosis in an elderly patient. If peritoneal signs suggest a perforation or an abscess, an abdominal computed tomographic (CT) scan should be obtained to determine the extent and nature of the pericolic inflammation, or a limited radiographic study with water-soluble contrast media to detect its presence outside the lumen, indicating bowel perforation. Care must be taken to avoid attributing narrowing of the lumen, mucosal irregularity, and blood in the stool to diverticulitis, when in fact carcinoma of the colon is present. After the acute attack subsides, this difficult differentiation is made most directly by fiberoptic sigmoidoscopy, which permits direct inspection of the lesion and mucosal biopsy.

Therapy for acute attack is the administration of broad-spectrum antibiotics and intravenous fluids. In most cases, oral intake should be withheld, and often nasogastric aspiration is useful for several days. After the attack subsides, the bulk in the diet should be increased by supplements of bran or a bulk laxative so that the stools are soft and constipation is avoided. If attacks with fever and leukocytosis are recurrent, or if pericolic abscess complicates the picture, resection is indicated.

Acute Cholecystitis[4,17]

In acute cholecystitis, pain occurs in the epigastrium and the right upper quadrant of the abdomen. Initially, the pain may be colicky; it then becomes steady and increases in intensity for several hours. Obstruction of the cystic duct by a stone initiates the attack. As the stone attempts to pass the cystic duct, pain is also felt at the inferior angle of the right scapula. If the attack is severe, nausea, vomiting, and a low-grade fever appear. Later, signs of irritation of the parietal peritoneum develop in the right upper quadrant. Leukocytosis is usual, and mild bilirubinemia and bilirubinuria are occasionally found after 24 hours. Constipation and mild paralytic ileus with an air-filled jejunal loop (sentinel loop) seen on an abdominal radiograph often accompany attacks of cholecystitis.

Gallstones are found in 85 to 95 percent of patients with cholecystitis, but unfortunately for diagnostic purposes, less than one fifth are radiopaque. Cholecystitis was formerly thought to be caused by an infection of the gallbladder, but present evidence indicates that cystic duct obstruction, usually by a gallstone, is the

most frequent precipitating factor, and then, if interference of gall-bladder emptying occurs, acute cholecystitis develops as the consequence of distension and chemical irritation. Bacterial infection is therefore a secondary phenomenon, rarely appearing in less than 48 hours.

The diagnosis of acute cholecystitis is supported by the presence of gallstones and a dilated gallbladder detected by ultrasonography. Cholecystitis is almost certain when the technetium-99m-labeled HIDA scan of the hepatobiliary tract fails to demonstrate the gallbladder. After intravenous injection, this labeled aminoacetic acid derivative normally is rapidly taken up by the liver and excreted into the biliary tract, thus visualizing the gallbladder. Acute cholecystitis should be distinguished, if possible, from acute cholangitis, with which it may be associated. Patients with cholangitis are at extreme risk from gram-negative sepsis and associated cardiovascular collapse. The treatment is intravenous broad-spectrum antibiotics and early decompression of the biliary tree, usually by percutaneous drainage or by surgery.

Immediate surgery is the treatment of choice for acute cholecystitis unless there are other medical problems that greatly increase the operative risks. It avoids the small risk of perforation and makes a second hospitalization for elective cholecystectomy unnecessary. If perforation does occur, usually it is contained in a well-localized abscess, but occasionally it leads to bile peritonitis or to one of the rare complications, such as the passage of a large stone into the intestine, with a subsequent obstruction at the ileocecal valve (gallstone ileus), or a permanent fistula (cholecyst-duodenal or cholecyst-colonic) with a chronic retograde infection of the biliary tract.

Acute Pancreatitis[1,9,11]

The clinical presentation of pancreatitis is as variable as the setting in which it occurs, ranging from a sudden acute abdominal catastrophe with shock and cyanosis to mild episodes of deep epigastric pain and vomiting. It is common in the latter situation, since it occurs too frequently in alcoholics, to attribute the episodes to "alcoholic gastritis." A patient may be carried on the emergency room records as having "gastritis" for several attacks until an elevated serum amylase level is found during an acute attack.

There is no specific clinical feature that allows the clinician to make the diagnosis of pancreatitis. The measurement of amylase is the most specific aid to the diagnosis, but often it is only transiently elevated and may return to normal in 48 to 72 hours even in the presence of continuing clinical activity. In addition, as many as 20 percent of the patients with acute pancreatitis have either normal or only borderline elevation of the serum amylase level. Striking elevations are almost always caused by pancreatitis if mumps can be excluded. Mild to moderate elevations are seen in a variety of situations, such as with a perforated viscus, strangulated bowel, mesenteric thrombosis, and renal insufficiency. Differentiation from pancreatitis will be difficult in 5 percent of cases. The administration of morphine can also produce mild elevations of the serum amylase level.

Enlargement of the pancreas detected by ultrasonography or CT scan increases the likelihood that pancreatitis is the cause of an attack of acute abdominal pain. Unfortunately, early in an attack, when help is most needed, changes in the pancreas are infrequently great enough to be diagnostic. These diagnostic procedures, however, are extremely accurate in the diagnosis of late complications such as pseudocysts and abscesses.

Other manifestations of pancreatitis include bilirubinemia and bilirubinuria (see in about one fifth of patients), hyperglycemia (seen in about one fourth of patients), and hypocalcemia. In severe cases the serum calcium level falls between the third and tenth days, occasionally low enough to cause tetany.

Acute pancreatitis simulates the complete clinical picture of an "acute surgical abdomen," including fever, leukocytosis, severe pain, sterile peritonitis, and frequently cardiovascular collapse. Indeed, it is the only condition with this clinical presentation that does not require immediate surgery. The recognition of pancreatitis is, therefore, critical to management. In cases where the diagnosis is unclear, it has been shown to be safer to surgically examine the patient to exclude other causes of an acute abdomen. If pancreatitis is encountered, the abdomen may be closed and the patient treated appropriately.

The pathogenesis of pancreatitis in man is not known, and it seems unlikely that there is a single pathogenic mechanism. Pancreatitis, like pneumonia, is a clinicopathologic syndrome that may be seen in association with a variety of conditions. The most common association by far is alcohol abuse, followed by cholelithiasis, hyperlipidemia, trauma, drugs, and hypercalcemia.

Regardless of antecedent factors, the final common pathway in the pathogenesis of pancreatitis is the liberation of activated pancreatic juice into the tissues of the pancreas. In the mildest form of pancreatitis, only edema develops, but it clears without residual changes in the structure or function of the pancreas. In the most severe form, tissue destruction extends to the blood vessels, leading to hemorrhagic pancreatitis, a disease with a fatality rate of 50 to 85 percent. In more severe cases, and especially with repeated attacks, there is a loss of acinar tissue and islets of Langerhans, with the development of pancreatic insufficiency with steatorrhea or diabetes or both.

The treatment of acute pancreatitis is supportive. Since hypovolemia may be severe, the restoration of the blood volume is imperative. Elderly patients and patients with signs indicating a serious or grave prognosis (e.g., leukocyte count $>16,000/mm^3$, blood glucose level >200 mg/dl, tachycardia >130 beats/min, adult respiratory distress syndrome, low urine output, falling hematocrit value, or falling serum calcium level) should be admitted to the intensive care unit for central venous pressure monitoring, aggressive fluid replacement, administration of oxygen, and liberal analgesia. The continued secretion of pancreatic juice into the substance of the pancreas increases tissue damage; therefore an effort to suppress pancreatic secretion should be made by withholding oral intake. A host of treatments (e.g., the use of glucagon, antitrypsins, anticholinergic agents, nasogastric suction, somatostatin, steroids, antibiotics, peritoneal dialysis), have been used to improve chances of survival, but in controlled trials these treatments have failed to show clear benefit. Because severe pancreatitis precludes oral caloric intake, many patients have nutritional deficiencies, and they have striking protein loss and catabolism; parenteral hyperalimentation should, therefore, be started early. The patient is followed closely to identify other possible causes of the acute condition of the abdomen and to detect complications of pancreatitis.

The complications of acute pancreatitis are numerous and include pseudocyst formation, renal failure, massive pleural effusion, hypocalcemia, pancreatic abscess, and pancreatic ascites.

Perforation of Peptic Ulcer[13]

In approximately 5 to 10 percent of patients with duodenal ulcer, perforation occurs. Perforation of a gastric ulcer is much less common. Most patients give a history of periodic dyspepsia compatible with the diagnosis of a peptic ulcer antedating the perforation. In a few patients, however, the sudden, severe, prostrating pain of perforation is the first indication of peptic ulcer disease.

With the escape of gastric contents into the peritoneal cavity, there is an immediate chemical peritonitis, which causes severe pain that appears first in the epigastrium and then rapidly spreads over the entire abdomen. The patient appears critically ill, with shallow thoracic respirations; he has a rigid, boardlike abdomen and is reluctant to move. As fluid pours out from the peritoneal surface, the pain may lessen, but this should not be misinterpreted as a sign of recovery. Fluid becomes detectable in the flanks, and liver dullness may be lost if a large amount of air escapes into the peritoneal cavity (more likely with the perforation of a gastric than of a duodenal ulcer).

About 80 percent of the patients with perforations can be shown by radiography to have free air in the peritoneal cavity. An upright chest radiograph is most likely to demonstrate free air un-

der the diaphragm. If the patient cannot stand, a left lateral decubitus film of the abdomen will usually demonstrate free air. Free air in the abdomen may come from other causes, such as perforation of the bowel, either spontaneous or traumatic. It is regularly found for several days after laparotomy. Finally, pneumatosis cystoides intestinalis may cause a benign asymptomatic pneumoperitoneum. The diagnosis may be suspected by a finding of localized collections of air along segments of the bowel wall.

As soon as a perforated peptic ulcer is suspected, the patient should be readied for laparotomy. This entails aggressive replacement of fluid lost from the intravascular space into the peritoneal cavity. Recurrence rates as high as 60 to 70 percent after simple ulcer closure have been reported, even in the absence of a history suggesting chronic ulcer disease. Unless the perforation has been present for an excessive period (greater than 12 hours) or the patient is elderly or extremely ill, definitive surgical therapy for peptic ulcer, rather than simple closure, should be carried out.

Intestinal Obstruction[12]

The hallmarks of intestinal obstruction are abdominal pain, distension, vomiting, and obstipation. All four symptoms are not always present in every case, and the severity of each of these clinical manifestations varies with the level and type of obstruction. When an obstruction is high in the small intestine, vomiting characteristically appears early and may be copious; distension may be minimal. In a colonic obstruction, distension may be marked and vomiting may not occur at all. Obstipation may be overlooked because the patient has two or three bowel movements early in the course of intestinal obstruction until the bowel distal to the point of obstruction is evacuated. On physical examination the abdomen is usually distended and bowel sounds typically are high pitched and occur in rushes.

Intestinal obstruction is most usefully classified into small- and large-bowel obstruction. Within each of these two categories the obstruction may be (1) simple obstruction, in which the lumen of the bowel is obstructed but with the blood supply intact, (2) strangulation obstruction, in which there is compromise of the blood supply to the intestine, as well as blockage of the lumen, and (3) closed-loop obstruction, in which the blood supply may or may not be interfered with but the egress of the intestinal contents is blocked both proximally and distally, causing rapid distension of the loop with the risk of both strangulation and perforation.

There are many causes of intestinal obstruction. These include extrinsic lesions, such as adhesions or an intra-abdominal abscess; intrinsic lesions, such as neoplasms of the bowel wall; and intraluminal masses, such as a bezoar, gallstone, or fecal impaction. In years past, incarcerated inguinal hernias were the most common cause of small-bowel obstruction. In recent years, however, with the ready access of hernia repair and with the increasing amount of abdominal and pelvic surgery being done, postoperative adhesions have become the most frequent cause of small-bowel obstruction. Incarcerated hernias probably remain the second most common cause, with other disorders such as Crohn disease, intussusception, volvulus, internal hernias, and small bowel neoplasms, following thereafter. The predominant cause of large-bowel obstruction is carcinoma, with diverticulitis second and volvulus (cecal or sigmoid) third.

Large-bowel obstruction should always be treated as an urgent situation because of the danger of cecal distension and consequent perforation. This is particularly true when there is a competent ileocecal valve, producing a closed-loop obstruction. Early surgical decompression with a colostomy is the indicated procedure. Small bowel obstruction is a less urgent situation, and more time can be taken to prepare the patient for surgery with the passage of a long intestinal tube and administration of intravenous fluids. However, unless there are extenuating clinical circumstances, surgery should not be delayed beyond 12 to 24 hours. This is because of the substantial risk (about 30 percent) of strangulation. Studies have shown that even the experienced clinician is unable to differentiate strangulation from simple obstruction on the basis of symptoms, physical signs, and laboratory studies. A decision to manage a patient with small-bowel obstruction nonoperatively, therefore, cannot be based reliably on the clinical impression that strangulation is not present. Such an impression has been shown to be wrong about one third of the time.

Differentiation of Mechanical Obstruction from Paralytic Ileus[3]

The differentiation of a mechanical obstruction of the bowel from paralytic ileus (failure of propulsive motor activity) requires careful serial observations. Typically in paralytic ileus there are no bowel sounds, but feeble sounds may be heard early in the course of the episode. The early stage of a mechanical obstruction is associated with strong, high-pitched, active bowel sounds. Later, bowel sounds may decrease or disappear as dilation of the bowel, strangulation, or peritonitis develops. Paralytic ileus can be found in association with any severe disease and is regularly present temporarily after anesthesia and abdominal surgery. It is frequently caused by peritonitis or by severe electrolyte disturbance, especially potassium deficiency, and may follow the use of anticholinergic and ganglion-blocking drugs. The treatment of paralytic ileus is supportive (intestinal decompression and restoration of fluid and electrolyte balance). If the primary disorder is correctable, the ileus is self-limiting.

Acute Mesenteric Ischemia[2]

Occlusion of the mesenteric blood supply leads to infarction of the intestine. If necrosis of the intestine is to be avoided and the life of the patient saved, early diagnosis and surgical correction are vital. Miraculous recoveries are possible, and patients who lose a large percentage of the small intestine may do surprisingly well.

Infarction of the bowel may be caused by either arterial or venous occlusion. With the former, the symptoms are usually acute in onset. Pain is characteristically colicky at first, rapidly progressing to a steady, severe ache as tissue damage appears. On physical examination, bowel sounds are initially hyperactive but rapidly become greatly diminished or absent. There may be only mild or even no tenderness. Characteristically, the severity of pain is disproportionate to the physical finding of abdominal tenderness. Hemoconcentration and a striking leukocytosis are usually found. With supportive care the patient's condition may appear stable for 2 to 4 days until necrosis, perforation, and peritonitis occur. If the patient is to survive, the diagnosis must be confirmed early by superior mesenteric arteriography and surgery performed within hours of the occlusion. Most superior mesenteric artery occlusions are caused by emboli in patients with atrial fibrillation or a recent myocardial infarction. If surgery is performed early, embolectomy or revascularization may be possible; otherwise massive bowel resection is necessary.

The symptoms associated with mesenteric venous occlusion are usually subtler and slower to evolve, symptoms often being present for days or even weeks. Because the clinical picture is less dramatic, diagnosis may be more difficult. The cause of venous occlusion is not usually determined. Often the patients have polycythemia. The extent of bowel involvement may be more limited than with arterial occlusion, but postoperative extension is frequent and anastomic disruption common.

Intestinal infarction can also be caused, in the absence of major vascular occlusion, by reflex vasospasm of the mesenteric resistance vessels, as a response to severe physiologic stress and administration of splanchnic vasoconstrictive agents, including sympathomimetics and the digitalis glycosides. This condition, termed nonocclusive mesenteric ischemia, is usually seen in severely ill patients after a hypotensive episode associated with sepsis, myocardial infarction, major surgery, respiratory insufficiency, or hypovolemic shock. Unlike occlusive mesenteric ischemia, its symptoms and initial clinical presentation are often mild and ob-

scured by obtundation. At an early stage of the disease, when the ischemic damage to the intestine is still reversible, specific physical signs and alteration in laboratory test results are not present. The diagnosis can be made only by angiography, obtained at this stage on the basis of a high index of suspicion in the vulnerable patient population. Treatment consists of pharmacologic reversal of the vasospasm with intra-arterial administration of vasodilators. Surgery is reserved for the later resection of infarcted bowel and should not be undertaken as the initial therapeutic step without prior angiography and vasodilator therapy. (See the discussion of ischemic colitis in Chapter 12.5.)

SURGERY IN ACUTE ABDOMINAL DISEASE

In some diseases in which acute abdominal pain is the presenting symptom, the prognosis worsens if operative intervention is delayed. A perforated viscus (duodenal ulcer), a bowel with compromised blood supply (strangulation obstruction), and inflammatory disease that is apt to lead to necrosis and perforation (appendicitis) are common examples. With the exception of a perforated peptic ulcer, the history is usually not of great value in making the decision that immediate surgery is necessary. The anteroposterior chest radiograph or upright abdominal radiograph can predict the urgency if free air is seen. Laboratory data can be confirmatory, but rarely does the decision to operate rest on a laboratory value. The decision in most instances rests on the findings obtained by physical examination. The diagnosis of an "acute surgical abdomen" depends on the presence of "peritoneal signs," that is, signs of parietal peritoneal irritation. These include rebound tenderness—pain elicited by sudden release of *gentle* pressure over an area of the abdomen remote from the area of pain. To the experienced clinician, the most reliable indication of underlying peritonitis is the presence of involuntary guarding: reflex spasm of the abdominal wall musculature on gentle, superficial palpation that does not abate when the patient relaxes his abdominal wall. Markedly decreased or absent bowel sounds generally accompany peritoneal signs in a "surgical abdomen." Making a precise diagnosis is secondary to the determination of whether an "acute surgical abdomen" is present. The single most valuable diagnostic test for the evaluation of a possible "acute surgical abdomen" is repeated physical examination by the same physician over an extended period.

DISEASES WHICH MIMIC THE ACUTE SURGICAL ABDOMEN

There are a variety of diseases that can mimic an "acute surgical abdomen."[16] Unnecessary surgical intervention can be avoided only if they are considered in the differential diagnosis. These conditions are as diverse as acute pyelitis, hepatitis, acute hepatic congestion caused by congestive heart failure, abdominal crisis associated with sickle cell anemia, and tabes dorsalis, diabetic ketosis, lactic acidosis, and acute porphyria. Although acute pancreatitis often produces frank signs of peritonitis, little can be accomplished by laparotomy.

CHRONIC ABDOMINAL PAIN

Many patients with chronic abdominal pain are not found to have any significant organic disease; hence they are said to have "functional" or "psychophysiologic" disorders. On the other hand, many patients with serious organic diseases, when first seen, have symptoms that are equally nonspecific. If such diseases are to be diagnosed correctly and promptly, each patient must be carefully evaluated and the diagnosis of functional disorder used only as a diagnosis of exclusion.

HISTORY

A careful history gives direction to the diagnostic workup. As new diagnostic possibilities arise, the patient should be questioned further, since decisive topics are unlikely to be pursued with sufficient tenacity if a specific diagnosis is not suspected.

Onset
Pain whose onset can be accurately dated is significant. The explanation may be organic, as in the case of pain caused by an intermittent intestinal obstruction or by porphyria, or the pain may have its origin in emotional problems precipitated by a stressful event. On the other hand, pain that has been present for years, or pain that the patient cannot remember ever being free of, is unlikely to be caused by a specific organic or psychologic factor.

Location of Symptoms
Radiation or spread of the pain may give diagnostic clues. For example, if the distress radiates up into the retrosternal region, it may well be that the reflux of gastric contents into the esophagus is responsible. If the pain radiates through to the back, the posterior penetration of an ulcer or a pancreatic lesion is suggested. Radiation to the right upper quadrant or through to the tip of the right scapula suggests the involvement of the gallbladder or the bile ducts.

The location of the symptoms is not an infallible guide to the location of the involved organ. For example, the initial symptoms of a carcinoma of the body and tail of the pancreas are usually indistinguishable from those of irritable bowel syndrome.

Type of Pain
It is important to distinguish colic from other forms of pain. Beyond this, the characterization of abdominal pain is so subjective and hence variable from patient to patient that it is of little help in diagnosis.

Timing of Symptoms
Several points are sufficiently helpful in differential diagnosis for their presence or absence to be specifically determined:

1. Pain that awakens a patient an hour or two after he goes to sleep is indicative of organic disease, usually a duodenal ulcer or gastroesophageal reflux, and should never be labeled "functional."
2. Pain relieved by eating is highly suggestive of the presence of a peptic ulcer (see Chapter 12.3). However, if eating initiates distress, then biliary tract disease, pancreatitis, carcinoma of the stomach, or esophageal reflux should be suspected. In addition, some patients with peptic ulcers, especially gastric ulcers and ulcers causing pyloric obstruction, have pain initiated or exaggerated by eating.
3. Pain before breakfast is infrequent with a peptic ulcer and is more likely to be a manifestation of the functional gastrointestinal disorder. It is not safe, however, to ignore this symptom, because it may be a presenting symptom of carcinoma of the stomach.
4. An inquiry into what type of food causes pain is rarely illuminating. Certainly the presence of indigestion after eating fatty foods or cabbage is not specific for gallbladder dysfunction. True epigastric colic, however, appearing within a half hour after a meal, especially if the meal contained fatty foods, strongly suggests biliary-tract dysfunction.
5. Periumbilical colic appearing after meals is a characteristic sign of an obstructing lesion of the small bowel or, rarely, intestinal angina. The typical history of intestinal angina is that the patient has no abdominal pain if he fasts or eats sparingly. With larger meals, colicky pain appears within a half hour of eating and lasts 1 to 2 hours. This sequence

leads to diminished intake and weight loss; hence a diagnosis of chronic intestinal angina is not tenable in the absence of weight loss.

6. If abdominal distress or colic is relieved by defecation, the responsible lesion is likely to be in the colon or distal ileum.

ASSOCIATED FINDINGS

Heartburn indicates the reflux of gastric juice into the esophagus, and it may accompany an exacerbation of a variety of gastrointestinal disorders (see Chapter 12.1)

Aerophagia with eructation is regularly increased by indigestion from any cause; hence it is no more characteristic of cholecystitis, for example, than of functional disorders.

Anorexia and Weight Loss
Anorexia and weight loss are indicative of serious underlying disease until proved otherwise. The underlying disease need not be neoplastic, however, because many patients with benign gastric ulcers have greater weight loss than patients with carcinoma of the stomach.

Constipation and Obstipation
A change in bowel function should receive careful attention. It may be constipation in a patient who paid no attention to bowel function in the past. It may be alternating diarrhea and constipation; or it may be such severe obstipation that the patient resorts to enemas. It is generally recognized that these symptoms suggest an obstructing lesion in the bowel, especially in the colon. It is not, however, well recognized that severe obstipation is often the initial symptom of such extracolonic disorders as carcinomas of the stomach, gallbladder, and pancreas.

PHYSICAL EXAMINATION

Physical findings, such as jaundice, a palpable gallbladder, and hepatomegaly, direct attention to the liver, bile ducts, and pancreas as possible sources of the pain. A succussion splash indicates gastric retention. An epigastric mass or a left upper quadrant mass suggests a tumor of the stomach or pancreas. Although the finding of an abdominal mass always brings to mind neoplastic disease, one should always rule out inflammatory diseases, which have a better prognosis and may be responsive to specific therapy.

Visible peristalsis, hyperactive bowel sounds, and visible or palpable distended loops of the bowel point to an obstructing lesion of the intestine.

Signs of ascites should be carefully sought; if they are present, an examination of the fluid may indicate the diagnosis and eliminate the necessity for expensive diagnostic procedures.

If fever is present, it must be explained. Even though abdominal pain is the presenting symptom, if it is associated with fever, the cause may be a systemic disease.

LABORATORY AIDS

The initial choice of laboratory studies will be determined by the diagnostic impression gained from the history and physical examination. Differential diagnosis based on clinical information has not been adequately analyzed if a barium enema, gastrointestinal tract radiographic series, abdominal sonogram, and CT scan are all requested as part of the initial diagnostic study.

In addition to the routine examination of blood and urine, evidence for partial obstruction of the biliary tract should be sought by testing the urine for bilirubin and by determining the bilirubin and alkaline phosphatase levels in the serum. If the problem is one of recurrent abdominal pain, then serum amylase and urine porphobilinogen determinations, sickle-cell preparation, and

serologic tests for syphilis are important aids in the differential diagnosis. Blood in the stool indicates a mucosal lesion and should be investigated by endoscopic or radiographic studies or both.

Radiographic Examination
A plain film of the abdomen, with both upright and supine views, is the first roentgenographic examination. The films should be reviewed for any evidence of renal, pancreatic, or biliary calculi. Dilated loops of bowel or abnormal gas shadows may indicate the site and nature of intrinsic bowel disease. Displaced gastric or colonic gas pattern may be produced by a mass. An air-fluid level or lucency in the mediastinum may be an indication of a large hiatal hernia. Only after the abdominal films have been carefully studied should more elaborate radiographic examinations be undertaken.

Ultrasonography
Ultrasonography, a technique that involves no x-ray exposure or side effects, is the best method for screening for cholelithiasis. In addition, it is ideally suited for identification of cystic lesions throughout the abdomen and for evaluation of the intrahepatic and extrahepatic biliary tract, as well as the urinary tract. It is particularly useful in the pelvis, an area less well visualized by conventional radiography. Finally, guided-needle aspiration or biopsy, under sonographic control, often provides the means to make a definitive diagnosis of mass lesions in the liver, pancreas, kidney, and retroperitoneum.

Computed Tomography
CT scanning provides the best imaging of soft tissue structures throughout the abdominal cavity. In the retroperitoneum it is particularly useful to delineate the pancreas. With and without the use of contrast material, it provides an enormous increase in diagnostic capability. It is best employed to confirm a diagnosis that has been suggested by other evidence.

Proctoscopy
Lower-abdominal symptoms should be investigated by proctoscopy and fiberoptic sigmoidoscopy before barium enema. Endoscopic examination should be completed first because (1) it is simpler to perform and more easily tolerated, (2) endoscopy examines the rectum more adequately than a barium enema, and (3) if a lesion is found by proctoscopy, biopsy can be performed and a tissue diagnosis obtained.

PATIENTS WITH NORMAL STUDY RESULTS

If results of all studies are either normal or inconclusive in a patient with recurrent abdominal pain, an arrangement should be made for reexamination *at the time of the next attack*. This will allow the physician to determine whether the pain is associated with any diagnostic clues; it will also permit the physician to get a clear idea of the onset and pattern of the pain while these features are fresh in the patient's mind; and finally it will provide an opportunity to obtain laboratory and radiographic studies at a time when they are most likely to show an abnormality.

CLINICAL EXAMPLES OF CHRONIC AND RECURRENT ABDOMINAL PAIN

The most important causes of chronic and recurrent abdominal pain, excluding peptic ulcer (see Chapter 12.3), are discussed here.

CHRONIC CHOLECYSTITIS AND CHOLELITHIASIS[4,17]

Gallstones are formed from precipitated pigment (bilirubin) or cholesterol. Pigment stones occur in patients with increased biliru-

bin excretion (as in hemolytic disorders such as sickle-cell disease). Cholesterol gallstones form from "lithogenic bile." In lithogenic bile, the concentrations of bile acids and lecithin are not sufficient to maintain the cholesterol in solution, especially when the bile is concentrated in the gallbladder. Stasis and changes in the gallbladder epithelium also appear to play a role. Gallstones may intermittently obstruct the cystic duct and thus produce cholecystitis or recurrent biliary colic.

The symptoms attributed to chronic cholecystitis and gallstones range from recurrent attacks of biliary colic, fever, and jaundice to nonspecific symptoms that are indistinguishable from functional dyspepsia.

Typical biliary colic appears in the epigastrium, with radiation to the right upper quadrant and subscapular regions. In about one fourth of the cases the pain also radiates to the left upper quadrant or left subscapular area, and occasionally, left-sided discomfort may be the most prominent feature. The pain builds up to a peak intensity in 15 to 45 minutes and subsides over several hours, but the patient may be aware of residual soreness for a day or two. Not all clinically significant gallbladder disease is associated with biliary colic, however. Because the gallbladder is stimulated to contract by humoral (cholecystokinin) and neural (vagus) stimuli released by eating, biliary colic typically appears 1 to 3 hours after a meal.

Frequently, the diagnosis of chronic cholecystitis rests on a history of pain after fatty food is eaten and on the absence of abnormalities in the gastrointestinal tract radiographic series. The impression is strengthened if the gallbladder fails to be visualized on a cholecystogram or if gallstones are found. There are, however, several flaws in this formulation.

1. Because gallstones and inflammation of the wall of the gallbladder are increasingly common with advancing age, postmortem examination reveals gallbladder disease in as many as 50 percent of persons who were in the seventh decade of life. These pathologic changes cannot be equated with a clinical syndrome with any regularity.

2. The dyspepsia and eructation associated with the eating of fatty food, cabbage, and so on have traditionally been considered characteristic of chronic cholecystitis. A number of investigations have shown that these symptoms are not specific. Indeed, if a history of intolerance of fatty food is elicited, the patient is more likely to have a functional gastrointestinal disease than gallbladder disease.

3. A distressing number of patients who have had cholecystectomies for chronic cholecystitis return with symptoms similar to their preoperative symptoms. Although often labeled "postcholecystectomy syndrome," these patients' symptoms are usually caused by one of the following conditions: (a) an unrecognized peptic or functional gastrointestinal disease, with symptoms erroneously attributed to gallbladder disease, (b) retained stones remaining in the common duct or cystic duct, (c) a partial obstruction of the common duct, or (d) associated pancreatitis. Before advising surgery for chronic cholecystitis, one should give serious consideration to the possibility that the patient's symptoms might be the result of one of these other conditions.

Since practically all clinically significant cases of chronic cholecystitis are associated with gallstones, the presence of gallstones should be demonstrated before this diagnosis receives serious consideration. Approximately 15 to 20 percent of all gallstones can be seen on a plain radiograph of the abdomen. Ultrasonography provides the most accurate means for the detection of gallstones.

Confidence that gallbladder disease is the cause of the patient's symptoms is increased if there is a history of biliary colic, fever, jaundice, or an elevated alkaline phosphatase level. The latter two symptoms are caused by transient obstruction of the common bile duct by stones being passed out of the gallbladder. If the patient has symptoms leading to the suspicion of gallbladder disease,

if other diseases that may mimic gallbladder disease have been excluded, if evidence of gallstones is found, and if the patient does not have some underlying illness that increases the hazard of a cholecystectomy, the treatment of calculous gallbladder disease is surgical excision. However, the case for cholecystectomy in the treatment of asymptomatic gallstones remains controversial. Although the risks of an elective cholecystectomy are small and the likelihood of the patient's developing symptomatic gallbladder disease is said to be 20 percent, the risk to life from elective surgery occurs on the day the surgery is performed, whereas the "silent" stone may not become symptomatic for another 5 to 20 years. If, however, surgery is delayed until the patient develops a complication such as common duct stones with jaundice, surgery will carry a several times greater risk than if it had been performed electively.

Much interest has been generated in gallstone dissolution therapy. It has been shown that feeding one (chenodeoxycholic acid), but not the other (cholic acid), primary bile acid leads to the dissolution of cholesterol gallstones. Initial enthusiasm for this treatment has decreased because (1) the overall dissolution rate after 2 years of treatment is 25 percent, (2) in only 20 to 30 percent of patients found to have gallstones are their stones likely to respond to dissolution, and (3) half the patients in whom stones dissolved will have recurrent stones in 5 years. Other therapies, such as direct percutaneous injection of solvents into the gallbladder and fragmentation of stones by shock waves (lithotripsy), are in the experimental stage.

CHRONIC RELAPSING PANCREATITIS[11]

The most common form of recurrent pancreatitis appears as episodes of acute pancreatitis associated with bouts of alcoholism. An elevated serum amylase concentration may be found, especially if the blood sample is drawn early in the attack. With each succeeding episode, however, pancreatic exocrine function decreases and the likelihood of finding an elevated amylase level diminishes. In patients without diagnostic pancreatic calcifications seen on an abdominal radiograph, several recently introduced procedures may be useful in establishing the presence of chronic pancreatic disease. Ultrasonography is a useful screening procedure for demonstrating enlargement of the pancreas, dilated ducts, pseudocysts, and small calcifications. Endoscopic pancreatography enables visualization of the characteristic abnormalities of pancreatic ducts. Finally, CT scanning gives the most detailed views of the pancreas. Although chronic pancreatitis is characterized by a triad consisting of pancreatic calcification, diabetes mellitus, and steatorrhea, the complete syndrome is present in no more than one third of the cases. Pancreatic exocrine insufficiency is discussed in Chapter 12.6.

There is no specific medical treatment for chronic pancreatitis, but patients are told to abstain from the use of alcohol and are usually placed on a regimen of antacids or H_2 receptor antagonists, with the aim of decreasing acid stimulation of pancreatic secretion. Recently it has been shown that pancreatic extract therapy provides relief of pain independent of any effect on malabsorption.[15] Many surgical procedures have been advocated (e.g., sphincteroplasty, caudal and longitudinal pancreaticojejunostomy, and 95 percent pancreatectomy), primarily for control of pain, but most have been given inconstant results. The major reason for failure is that most cases of recurrent pancreatitis are associated with alcoholism, and no operation has been devised that will permit these patients to drink with impunity. Ninety-five percent pancreatectomy, with a rim of pancreas left in the duodenal C-loop, has the greatest success rate, with 85 percent good results. This operation requires no anastomosis between ducts and intestine and hence has a low operative mortality rate. Roughly half of the patients not diabetic before surgery, however, require insulin thereafter. In some patients, pancreatitis is associated with cholelithiasis, peptic ulcer, hyperparathyroidism, or hyperlipidemia. The correction of these conditions is associated with an amelioration or cessation of the attacks of pancreatitis.

INTERMITTENT OR CHRONIC INTESTINAL OBSTRUCTION

Postoperative adhesions are frequently blamed for chronic or recurrent abdominal pain. Adhesions cause pain by producing partial or complete intestinal obstruction. Before an operation is undertaken to "lyse the adhesions," therefore, objective evidence of partial intestinal obstruction should be demonstrated. An intermittent incomplete volvulus is occasionally the cause of recurrent abdominal pain but can be diagnosed only if abdominal radiographs are taken during an attack. The most common inflammatory lesion of the bowel that produces partial intestinal obstruction and chronic abdominal pain is Crohn disease (see Chapter 12.5).

Neoplastic lesions are a frequent cause of chronic obstructive symptoms. The most common is carcinoma of the colon, especially on the left side. Lymphoma of the small bowel also produces symptoms of progressive obstruction. Intestinal polyps, such as those found with the Peutz-Jeghers syndrome, and carcinoid of the small intestine give rise to intermittent obstructive symptoms, usually by causing intussusception.

Intestinal ischemia, in addition to producing acute abdominal pain when there is an acute mesenteric vascular occlusion, may also produce symptoms of intestinal obstruction. A short ischemic segment produces partial obstruction as, in the process of healing, it becomes narrowed and fibrotic.

Intestinal pseudo-obstruction[14] is a rare intestinal motor abnormality with episodic abdominal distension and vomiting. Abdominal radiographs show dilated intestinal loops with air-fluid levels that may be interpreted as indicating the presence of a mechanical obstruction, but at laparotomy no obstructing lesion is found. To avoid unnecessary operation, careful small-bowel contrast studies should be done if a site of obstruction is not clear.

CHRONIC PERITONITIS

Chronic peritonitis caused by a tuberculous infection causes chronic diffuse abdominal pain, minimal tenderness, and low-grade fever. It may occur with or without ascites. When associated with cirrhosis and ascites, the diagnosis of tuberculous peritonitis is difficult to establish and is frequently overlooked or made unexpectedly at laparotomy.

SYSTEMIC DISEASES AND INTOXICATIONS WITH RECURRENT ABDOMINAL PAIN

Systemic diseases and intoxications in which chronic or recurrent abdominal pain is a presenting symptom are too numerous to discuss in this section. Included in this group are diseases as dissimilar as polyarteritis nodosa, systemic lupus erythematosus, lead poisoning, hypercalcemia, diabetic acidosis, ketoacidosis, porphyria, hyperlipemia, and tabes dorsalis.

CARCINOMA OF THE STOMACH

Although steadily decreasing in incidence in Western cultures over the past several decades, gastric carcinoma is still the seventh leading cause of cancer deaths in the United States and remains an important cause of abdominal pain. Intestinal metaplasia is associated with hypochlorhydria, achlorhydria, and gastric ulcer; hence it is not surprising they all are found in association with gastric cancer. Unfortunately, the clinical manifestations of gastric carcinoma can be so vague that a tumor may develop and become inoperable despite the fact that a patient is being followed up closely by a physician. Weight loss, anorexia, vomiting, and pain are the most common but unfortunately not early, symptoms. Weakness and dizziness resulting from chronic blood-loss anemia also may be the initial symptoms. A palpable mass is present in only one third of the patients and usually is a sign of incurability. Fiberoptic

gastroscopy, with endoscopic biopsies and cytologic brushings, is the first diagnostic test to be ordered in patients with suspected gastric malignancy. Surgery is the therapy for gastric carcinoma, but the 5-year survival rate is only 25 percent if "curative" surgery can be performed and only 10 percent for all patients. The disease-free environment appears to be prolonged somewhat by multiple chemotherapy combinations.

CARCINOMA OF THE PANCREAS[6]

Whereas gastric cancer is decreasing, cancer of the pancreas is increasing to the point that it is now the fifth most common cause of cancer death. To make matters worse, early diagnosis usually is made only by accident and as a result the 5-year survival rate is no more than 1 percent. Even when the tumor is in the head of the pancreas and jaundice is an early symptom, the survival rate is less than 10 percent. Pain is the most common presenting symptom, being noted by three fourths of the patients with carcinoma of the head of the pancreas and by practically all patients with involvement of the body and tail of the pancreas. Usually the pain is a dull ache in the epigastrium that may radiate to the right upper quadrant of the abdomen if the tumor is in the head and to the left if it is in the body and tail. In addition, patients frequently note sharp, intermittent epigastric pain. Many have crampy lower abdominal pain, and since over three fourths of the patients with carcinoma of the body or tail also have severe constipation, many are initially thought to have the irritable-bowel syndrome. A steady pain in the back or in the lower lumbar region is found in one fifth of the patients as the presenting complaint or as a second pain separate from the epigastric distress.

Seventy percent of patients with carcinoma of the head of the pancreas have jaundice, whereas fewer than 15 percent of the patients with involvement of the body of the pancreas are jaundiced. Not more than 50 percent of the patients show any displacement of the gastrointestinal tract by radiography. The only two diagnostic procedures that have any promise of leading to earlier diagnosis and, as a consequence, an increased chance of survival are CT scanning and endoscopic cannulation of the pancreatic duct, or endoscopic retrograde cholangiopancreatography (ERCP). Isolated examples of early diagnosis have been reported, but to date there is no evidence of improvement in the overall grim picture presented by pancreatic cancer. By the time the mass has grown large enough to show characteristic compression of the duodenum on barium studies or changes in pancreatic vessels on angiography, the chance for long-term survival is past. In most cases, surgery provides palliation with bypass of the gastric outlet and the biliary tract obstruction. Radiation treatment and alcohol injection of the celiac ganglia provide pain control in some patients. The tumor is not responsive to chemotherapy or radiation therapy.

IRRITABLE BOWEL SYNDROME[18]

"Irritable bowel syndrome," "functional bowel disorder," and "spastic colon" are all terms used to designate the most common cause of chronic or recurrent abdominal pain, as well as the most common gastrointestinal disorders. The pain is most frequently localized to the left lower quadrant of the abdomen or to the hypogastrium. When located in the left upper quadrant, it is often referred to as "splenic flexure syndrome" and when in the right upper quadrant as "hepatic flexure syndrome." It is thought that distention and spasm result from gas collecting in these two areas. Splenic flexure symptoms are sometimes confused with the pain of coronary artery disease, but they are relieved by the passing of flatus. Hepatic flexure symptoms may mimic symptoms of gallbladder dysfunction, and pain in the left lower quadrant may be attributed to diverticulitis. The diagnosis of irritable bowel syndrome is based on the presence of abdominal pain with altered bowel habits and the absence of detectable structural changes. The altered bowel

habit may consist of constipation or diarrhea, but more often there is alternating constipation and diarrhea with one of the two predominating. Abdominal bloating and distention are a frequent complaint, and hyperresonance to percussion is a frequent finding. Eating often aggravates the pain, and defecation may provide some relief, but defecation is frequently felt to be incomplete. Upper gastrointestinal tract symptoms of dyspepsia, bloating, belching, aerophagia, and anorexia may be part of the clinical picture, but vomiting is rare. Significant weight loss is unusual and cannot be attributed to this functional disorder unless accompanied by severe depression. Nocturnal awakening by the symptoms rarely occurs. The patient generally appears healthy, and the findings of physical examination are normal except for a tender, cordlike sigmoid colon and hyperresonance over other areas of the abdomen. A palpable sigmoid colon itself is not significant, because stool within the colon often is palpable, but significant tenderness is meaningful. Proctoscopy may reveal spasm and sometimes mucus on the mucosa, but there is never bleeding and mucosal biopsy specimens are always normal. Routine diagnostic studies, including complete blood cell count, determination of erythrocyte sedimentation rate, stool examinations for white blood cells, ova, and parasites; and blood chemistry studies, show normal results, as do colonoscopy and barium enema radiography.

Irritable bowel syndrome usually begins in early adulthood and rarely appears as a new entity after the age of 55 years. The condition is more common in women. Symptoms are often precipitated by meals or by stress, and they are attributed to spastic and incoordinated muscle contractions of the colon.

An acute attack of diarrhea due to a bacterial or viral infection, parasitic infestation, or antibiotic use may initiate symptoms of irritable bowel syndrome. In these instances it is thought that these factors trigger irritable bowel syndrome in patients who have a predisposition to the disorder but are barely compensated when these precipitating factors supervene.

Management includes reassurance, which is partially provided by the detailed interview under relaxed circumstances and by the diagnostic procedures. The syndrome should be described to the patient as a specific entity, with emphasis on the fact that it is a real disorder of motility, usually involving the colon and the more proximal gastrointestinal tract, that results from intestinal spasm triggered by a number of stimuli, most often stress, fatigue, or meals. Therapy includes the use of a high-fiber diet or bulk agents, such as psyllium hydrophilic mucilloid, to interrupt the constipation diarrhea cycle and to reestablish regular bowel habits. Anticholinergic agents are sometimes helpful in relieving painful spasm. Antidiarrheal agents, such as loperamide or diphenoxylate HCl, may be used to control diarrhea. Antidiarrheal agents are used only for severe diarrhea and must be prescribed with caution to avoid inducing constipation in patients who have a tendency to develop alternating diarrhea and constipation. Dietary restriction and manipulation have been grossly overemphasized in the management of this syndrome. Lactose and milk intolerance, however, should be ruled out as a contributing factor whenever the diagnosis is suspected, since lactose intolerance can mimic completely or aggravate the symptoms of irritable bowel syndrome.

REFERENCES

1. Bank S, Wise L, Geisten M: Risk factors in acute pancreatitis. Am J Gastroenterol 78:637, 1983
2. Clark RA, Gallant TE: Acute mesenteric ischemia: Angiographic spectrum. Am J Roentgenol 142:555, 1984
3. Cope Z: The Early Diagnosis of the Acute Abdomen, 15th ed. New York, Oxford University Press, 1979
4. Dowling RH: Cholelithiasis: Medical treatment. Clin Gastroenterol 12:125, 1983
5. Gilmore OJA, Brodribb AJM, et al: Appendicitis and mimicking conditions: A prospective study. Lancet 2:421, 1975
6. Hermann RE, Cooperman AM: Current concepts in cancer: Cancer of the pancreas. N Engl J Med 301:482, 1979
7. Hulnick DH, Megilow AJ, et al: Computed tomography in the evaluation of diverticulitis. Radiology 152:491, 1984
8. Lewis FE, Holcroft JW, et al: Appendicitis: A critical review of diagnosis and treatment in 1000 cases. Arch Surg 110:677, 1975
9. Mallory A, Kern F Jr: Drug-induced pancreatitis: A critical review. Gastroenterology 78:813, 1980
10. Owens BJ, Hamit HF: Appendicitis in the elderly. Ann Surg 187:392, 1978
11. Sarles H, Sarles JC, et al: Observations on 205 cases of acute pancreatitis, recurring pancreatitis and chronic pancreatitis. Gut 6:545, 1965
12. Sarr MG, Bulkley GB, Zuidema GD: Preoperative recognition of intestinal strangulation obstruction: A prospective evaluation of diagnostic capability. Am J Surg 145:176, 1983
13. Sawyers JL, Herrington JL Jr, et al: Acute perforated duodenal ulcer. Arch Surg 110:527, 1975
14. Schuffler D, Lowe MC, Bill AH: Studies of idiopathic intestinal pseudo-obstruction. 1. Hereditary visceral myopathy: Clinical and pathological studies. Gastroenterology 73:327, 1977
15. Slaff J, Jacobson D, et al: Protease-specific suppression of pancreatic exocrine secretion. Gastroenterology 87:44, 1984
16. Steinheber FU: Medical conditions mimicking the acute surgical abdomen. Med Clin North Am 57:1559, 1973
17. Stubbs RS, McLoy RF, Blumgart LH: Cholelithiasis and cholecystitis: Surgical treatment. Clin Gastroenterol 12:179, 1983
18. Whitehead WE, Engel BT, Schuster MM: Irritable bowel syndrome: Physiological and psychological differences between diarrhea-predominant and constipation-predominant patients. Dig Dis Sci 25:404, 1980

CHAPTER 12.3
Peptic Ulcer and Dyspepsia

Richard S. Johannes
and Thomas R. Hendrix

"Dyspepsia," originally meaning difficulty in digestion, now refers to a variety of symptoms associated with the ingestion of food. Such symptoms range from postprandial bloating, distension, and eructation to gnawing or burning epigastric pain. Most patients find accurate description of these symptoms difficult, and they often come to use terms learned while being questioned by physicians.

Peptic ulcer is the most common organic cause of dyspepsia.

The generic term "peptic ulcer" is applied to ulcers caused directly or indirectly by active gastric juice, that is, containing acid and pepsin. These ulcers may be found in the esophagus, stomach, and duodenum; at the site of a gastroenterostomy (marginal ulcer); in the jejunum at multiple levels (as seen at times in the Zollinger-Ellison syndrome); and in ectopic gastric mucosa in a Meckel diverticulum. Of these locations, the duodenum and stomach are the most common.

EPIDEMIOLOGY[11,14,23]

There is presently great interest in the changing epidemiologic features of peptic ulcer disease. This illness has shown a steady fall as a cause of death since the early 1960s. Annual hospital admission rates have decreased approximately 17 percent and 36 percent for duodenal ulcer and gastric ulcer, respectively, from 1958 to 1972. The enhanced interest in peptic ulcer disease epidemiology has helped to clarify some of the potential risk factors for peptic ulcer. The genetic influence has been recognized since the demonstration of an increased risk associated with group O blood type and the failure to secrete ABO blood substances in saliva. Less well known is the threefold increased incidence in first-order relatives and the 50 percent concordance rate among identical twins. There are documented differences in prevalence both within nations and across international borders. The data collected in the United States, United Kingdom, Nigeria, India, and Australia reveal notable regional differences, but to date no holistic way of interpreting these data is known. Other medical conditions that predispose to peptic ulcer include cirrhosis, renal failure, and chronic bronchitis. Smoking and alcohol are often cited, but data incriminating alcohol as a risk factor are weak. Smoking does seem to adversely affect the rate of ulcer healing. In fact, one estimate has suggested that as much as 50 percent of the attributable risk of death in ulcer disease is due to smoking. Smoking does not appear to be a major risk factor for ulcer development, however.

With regard to foods, there has been a steady movement away from a belief that spiced foods are gastric irritants. Evidently what is hot to the palate and what is hot to the gastric mucosa are different. Drugs, too, on closer analysis may be a lesser risk factor than was once believed. Even aspirin, which unquestionably leads to increased measurable fecal hemoglobin levels, may have a lesser clinical consequence than was once thought. In the Boston Collaborative Drug Study, only 10 hospitalizations could be traced to aspirin in a population of 100,000 long-term heavy aspirin users. Last, the data from both the United States and England now suggest that peptic ulcer is more common in lower than in higher socioeconomic groups, forcing reevaluation of the model of the highly stressed executive as the prototypic ulcer patient. A recent and still somewhat controversial finding in ulcer epidemiology is the finding of a cohort effect in both duodenal and gastric ulcer disease. The generation born from 1870 to 1900 showed the highest risk. The risk for duodenal ulcer lagged behind the risk for gastric ulcer by 10 to 30 years. It appears that this effect begins at a surprisingly young age, less than 5 years.

CLINICAL PRESENTATION

The onset of dyspeptic symptoms in relation to food intake and their duration, relief by antacids, nature, location, and radiation are helpful in determining the cause of the dyspepsia. None of these symptoms is specific, however, and they must be regarded only as clues to the diagnosis, which must be established by more definitive means. In addition to peptic disease, dyspepsia may be the presenting symptom of a variety of disorders, including gastric and pancreatic carcinoma, cholelithiasis, pancreatitis, abdominal angina, intestinal obstruction, functional disorders, and depression.

NATURE OF THE PAIN

Location of Pain
The pain of a peptic ulcer is referred to the epigastrium. If it is associated with a component radiating through to the back, a posterior perforation or at least inflammation extending posteriorly is strongly suggested.

Type of Pain
In its mildest form, ulcer pain is best described as hunger pain. It slowly builds up, is steady for $\frac{1}{2}$ to 2 hours, and then gradually subsides. As the pain becomes more severe, such adjectives as "gnawing" and "burning" are used to describe it, but the pattern of onset and disappearance remains the same.

Time of Pain
At first the ulcer patient may note hunger distress only before the evening meal, but as symptoms progress in intensity, he becomes aware of pain from 30 minutes to 4 hours after other meals determined in part by the size and content of the meal. Pain that awakens the patient from sleep 1 to 2 hours after he retires is so characteristic of a peptic ulcer, and especially of a duodenal ulcer, that this must be considered to be the diagnosis until convincing evidence to the contrary is presented. Conversely, pain before breakfast is so infrequent that this symptom strongly suggests that the patient's dyspepsia is not caused by a peptic ulcer.

Relief of Pain
The pain of a peptic ulcer is promptly relieved by the taking of food or antacids. Traditionally, milk is thought to be most effective, but almost any food gives temporary relief. Vomiting or the removal of the gastric contents by aspiration also is followed by subsidence of the pain. Patients with gastric ulcers may not give such clear stories of prompt improvement with the taking of food or antacids; in gastric ulcer the relief is usually less and pain is sometimes actually worsened by eating. As a result, anorexia and weight loss with dyspepsia favors a diagnosis of gastric ulcer, whereas increased food and milk product intake, sometimes with weight gain, favors that of duodenal ulcer. If a history is obtained of a typical food–pain relief pattern that changes so that eating can no longer be depended on to help, and may even exaggerate the pain, partial pyloric obstruction or deep penetration of the ulcer should be suspected.

LESS COMMON SYMPTOMS OF DUODENAL ULCER ACTIVITY

Constipation is a symptom commonly associated with ulcer activity, and a small percentage (about 5 percent) of the patients with chronic duodenal ulcers have predominantly colonic symptoms. Heartburn and eructation are also commonly associated with ulcer activity. Occasionally, heartburn is so prominent that the primary disease is thought to be esophageal.

LABORATORY EVALUATION

Routine Laboratory Evaluation
A measure of hematologic status (e.g., a hemoglobin determination or a hematocrit) and a measure of evidence for gastrointestinal blood loss (e.g., hemoccult slides) should be considered routine. The selection of further routine laboratory study will depend on the particular indications. For example, in recurrent peptic ulcer, measurement of serum gastrin levels or basal acid secretion might be warranted.

Radiographic Studies[15]
Upper gastrointestinal tract barium radiography remains the most readily available and least expensive method of diagnosing peptic ulcer. Best estimates suggest that upper gastrointestinal tract series have a 10 to 30 percent false-negative rate and a 5 to 10 percent false-positive rate. Thus radiographic examination does have limitations:

1. It is unable to define mucosal disease (e.g., gastritis).
2. It is not definitive in differentiating benign from malignant gastric ulcer.

3. It cannot delineate superficial, subacute gastric or duodenal erosions that have not yet developed well-defined craters.
4. It is unable to define complete healing of an ulcer.

Furthermore, as an ulcer heals, the surrounding tissue, especially in the duodenum, becomes scarred and deformed, and radiologic assessment of activity of the ulcer becomes more difficult.

Endoscopic Studies

For the reasons listed above and because it can provide visual, cytologic, and histologic information, endoscopy is playing the dominant role in the differential diagnosis of patients with dyspepsia. In addition, endoscopy provides accurate assessment of the healing of gastric and duodenal ulcers. Endoscopy should be employed to establish benignity of any gastric ulcer and is the only method of establishing healing of a duodenal ulcer.

PATHOGENESIS

There are many reasons for considering a duodenal ulcer and simple gastric ulcer as different diseases. They have a different sex distribution; different genetic distributions, as indicated by blood types; different age and socioeconomic distributions; different gastric secretory responses; and differences in their responses to medical and surgical treatment. Duodenal ulcer characteristically is associated with a high rate of gastric secretion, not only after a meal, but in the fasting state as well.

If gastric hypersecretion alone were the whole explanation for peptic ulcer disease, diffuse rather than localized ulceration would be expected. Additional factors are operative. One such factor is the striking tendency for peptic ulcers to occur at mucosal junctions, for example, at the esophagogastric, fundopyloric, and pyloroduodenal junctions. Another weakness in the concept that "acid hypersecretion equals ulcer" is that, although duodenal ulcer patients as a group secrete twice as much acid as do normal individuals, there is a striking overlap in the amounts of acid output of the two groups. In addition, patients with gastric ulcers tend to secrete less acid than do normal individuals. For these reasons, the measurement of gastric secretion has no value in the differential diagnosis of dyspepsia. Alterations in the microvasculature of the organ provide mechanisms that can operate independently of gastric acid secretion to increase the risk of peptic ulcer. The observed pattern of occurrence of ulcers in the upper gastrointestinal tract correlates well with breaks in the submucous vascular plexus. The knowledge that these are sites of potential ischemia because they seem vulnerable to vasomotor, endocrine, and mechanical insult is revitalizing interest in the role of the microvasculature in ulcer pathogenesis.[21]

The striking frequency of the association between duodenal ulcer and *Campylobacter* gastritis (75 to 100 percent in reported series) has added a new factor to be explained in pathogenesis of peptic ulcer disease (see Gastritis, p. 798).[2] It is known that patchy gastric metaplasia of the duodenal mucosa is practically universal in duodenal ulcer disease. This may be viewed as a protective adaptation to the increased acid production characteristic of patients with duodenal ulcer. When *Campylobacter pylori* infects the gastric mucosa, it colonizes the patches of gastric metaplasia in the duodenal bulb. As a consequence, the protection afforded by gastric metaplasia is lost, thus setting the stage for the development of a duodenal ulcer.

Not only is the pathogenesis of peptic ulceration unresolved, but the simpler question of how peptic ulcer pain is produced is also unanswered. From direct observation studies, it is known that neither mechanical pinching nor acid bathing is associated with pain in the normal stomach. If, however, the mucosa is inflamed, then either acid, alkali, or alcohol evoked the pain. The two major views are as follows:

1. Pain is produced directly when acid irritates exposed nerve endings in the ulcer.
2. Pain is produced indirectly by an increase in the tone of the wall of the duodenum and gastric antrum. The second view has more appeal, but it has not been proved. In addition, patients with and without demonstrable ulcers may have identical symptoms—hence the suggestion that the symptoms are not dependent on the presence of an ulcer. It may be that a combination of both views, with factor 2 leading to a change in the threshold for potentially painful stimuli, may be the most accurate.

CONTROL OF GASTRIC SECRETION[1,3,7]

An understanding of the physiology of gastric secretion is valuable even though the measurement of gastric secretion provides few data of diagnostic or prognostic value in peptic disease. Since therapy for peptic ulcer is aimed, in the main, at limiting gastric acidity, understanding of the normal control of gastric secretion is useful in the design of medical and surgical therapy.

Normal Secretion

Hydrochloric acid is secreted by the parietal cells of the proximal four fifths of the stomach by a mechanism involving H^+/K^+ ATPase and a cotransporter for K^+ Cl^- at the apical surface of stimulated parietal cells. The epithelium of the stomach stringently limits the diffusion of ions and is capable of maintaining a concentration gradient of 1 to 1 million for H^+ between plasma and gastric juice. Parietal cells secrete acid in response to three interacting endogenous stimuli: (1) acetylcholine from cholinergic neurons, (2) gastrin, the peptide hormone of the gastric antrum, and (3) histamine.

In man, the fasting acid secretory rate is about 15 percent of the maximal rate and shows diurnal variation, with a peak in the evening (10 PM) and low point in the morning (8 AM). Physiologic control of gastric secretion is divided into three interrelated phases. First is the cephalic phase, in which vagal efferent pathways, activated by the anticipation, smell, and taste of food, stimulate the parietal cells directly through the release of acetylcholine and indirectly by stimulating the G (gastrin-containing) cells of the antrum to release gastrin. Second is the gastric phase, in which distension of the stomach leads to direct (neural) and indirect (hormonal) stimulation of acid secretion through vagovagal and intramural reflexes. In addition, contact of the epithelium with the products of protein digestion also leads to direct and indirect stimulation of the parietal cells. Calcium increases the responsiveness of both the parietal cells and the G cells. The responsiveness of the G cells is decreased as the pH in the antrum falls, thus providing a negative feedback control for gastric secretion. Third is the intestinal phase, in which the release of duodenal gastrin and other intestinal hormones stimulate gastric secretion. The intestine also exercises a negative feedback control over gastric secretion. A number of duodenal and intestinal hormones released in response to acid, hyperosmolar fluid, and products of digestion inhibit gastric secretion and emptying. The list includes secretin, cholecystokinin, enteroglucagon, gastric inhibitory peptide (GIP), and vasoactive intestinal peptide (VIP). The relative importance of these hormones in normal control of gastrointestinal tract function remains to be determined.

The concentration of acid in the stomach is determined by three factors:

1. The rate of gastric secretion
2. The buffering capacity of gastric contents
3. The rate of gastric emptying

Although the rate of gastric secretion is the greatest in the first hour after a meal, the concentration of H^+ falls because of the

buffering capacity of the food. During the second and third hour after a meal, the H^+ concentration rises in spite of decreasing acid secretion, because the buffering capacity of the gastric contents decreases owing to saturation of proton acceptors of the food and loss of buffer from the stomach by gastric emptying. As a consequence, the highest rate of delivery of acid into the duodenum occurs in the second hour after eating. The pH of the duodenal contents is raised as a result of neutralization of acid by bicarbonate secreted by the pancreas, liver, and duodenum in response to secretin, which also limits gastric secretion and emptying. Hence the control of gastric and duodenal pH, as well as of gastric emptying, is the result of a complex series of interacting "feedback" mechanisms.

Hypersecretion

Average normal basal (fasting acid) output is 2 mEq/hr, with an upper range of normal about 5 mEq/hr, but basal secretion as high as 10 mEq/hr is occasionally found in patients without symptoms or obvious disease. Average normal maximal acid output is 20 mEq/hr, with an upper limit of 40 mEq/hr. Hypersecretion, or secretion above these "normal" levels, is found in the following:

1. Five percent of asymptomatic individuals
2. Twenty-five percent of patients with duodenal ulcer
3. Patients with hypergastrinemia due to the following:
   a. Gastrinoma of the pancreas (Zollinger–Ellison syndrome), duodenum, or antrum
   b. Hyperplasia of G cells of antrum or pancreas
   c. Retained antrum in which a portion of the antrum is left with the duodenal stump at the time of surgery (partial gastrectomy with gastrojejunostomy) (The retained antral G cells no longer bathed with gastric acid are removed from normal inhibition and release large amounts of gastrin.)
4. Portacaval shunts presumably due to failure of hepatic inactivation of histamine and other gastric secretagogues from the intestine
5. Small-bowel resection possibly due to removal of gastric inhibitory factors of intestinal origin
6. Pyloric obstruction possibly stimulating acid secretion through stimuli evoked by antral distension
7. Hypercalcemia of any origin
8. Malignant carcinoid, systemic mastocytosis, and basophilic leukemia due to hyperhistaminemia
9. Severe brain damage leading to increased vagal discharge
10. Pancreatitis or pancreatic duct obstruction

Hyposecretion[8,11]

Hyposecretion of gastric acid is the result of (1) decreased parietal cell secretion, (2) back-diffusion of secreted acid through an abnormal mucosa, or (3) a combination of these two factors. The gastric atrophy of pernicious anemia involves the acid-producing mucosa but spares the antrum. Not only is the secretion of intrinsic factor necessary for vitamin B_{12} absorption lost, but also the ability to secrete acid and pepsin. The more common form of gastritis involves the antrum and, to a lesser degree, the fundus. Although there is decreased secretion of acid with antral gastritis, probably of more importance is the damage to the mucosa that allows back-diffusion of acid, in turn leading to more mucosal damage. The damaged mucosa may be replaced with intestinal metaplasia, a very permeable epithelium that is unable to maintain a normal hydrogen gradient. A variety of agents lead to disruption of the gastric mucosal barrier: bile acids and lysolecithin refluxed from the duodenum, and drugs such as aspirin and alcohol and infection of the mucosa with *Campylobacter pylori*. Their role in the pathogenesis of antral gastritis is unknown. Finally, benign gastric ulcer and gastric carcinoma are usually associated with antral gastritis and gastric hyposecretion.

MUCOSA PROTECTION[5]

Gastric Mucus

Gastric mucus has been suggested as playing a role in protecting the stomach epithelium. Although gastric bicarbonate production is only 5 to 10 percent of the stomach's hydrogen ion production, the increased local concentration of bicarbonate in the mucus layer is believed to play an important role in protection of the mucosa. Of note, alcohol and aspirin, which are damaging to the gastric mucosa, result in reduced mucus thickness. On the other hand, prostaglandins, which appear cytoprotective, increase the production of gastric mucus.

Gastric Epithelial Repair

The gastric epithelium is very active. Only bone marrow produces cells more rapidly than the gastrointestinal tract epithelium. The epithelium appears to respond to a number of trophic influences, including gastrin and epithelial growth factor. Epithelial restitution is rapid after injury. It begins within 5 minutes and can resurface large areas in 30 to 60 minutes. The role of impairment of the restitution process in the pathogenesis of ulcer disease has not been defined.

Prostaglandins

The initial speculation about the role of prostaglandins in gastric mucosal protection was due in part to the observation that aspirin and nonsteroidal anti-inflammatory agents, both of which are associated with gastric ulceration, are known inhibitors of prostaglandin synthesis. Prostaglandins of the E series have been shown to be effective in lower animals in preventing ulcers as a result of administration of such agents as aspirin or indomethacin. Several prostaglandin E analogs have been developed and are being tested for medical therapy.

THERAPY FOR PEPTIC ULCER

MEDICAL THERAPY FOR PEPTIC ULCER

The treatment of peptic ulcer is still empiric and is based on the assumption that the mechanism of symptom relief and ulcer healing is through the neutralization of acid gastric juice.

Diet

The patient with a peptic ulcer should eat a normal diet with three meals a day and should avoid only those foods that he has found to cause dyspepsia. None of the so-called ulcer diets has been shown to hasten relief of symptoms or rate of healing. All meals stimulate gastric secretion by distention of the stomach and their protein content. Although protein stimulates acid secretion, it also buffers the pH of gastric contents.

After the symptoms have come under control, the use of coffee or alcohol with meals is not contraindicated unless it results in a recurrence of symptoms.

When the patient has severe, constant pain or vomiting, therapy should be initiated in the hospital by a period of 24 to 48 hours of continuous gastric suction. Then the patient may be placed on a regimen consisting of liquid or soft feedings. This regimen needs to be maintained only for a day or so if the patient has an appetite for a regular diet.

H_2-Receptor Antagonists[18]

H_2-receptor antagonists—cimetidine, ranitidine, and famotidine—are potent inhibitors of gastric acid secretion because they block histamine stimulation of the parietal cell. Histamine's action is mediated through two types of receptors: H_1 receptors, which are blocked by traditional antihistamine drugs, and H_2 receptors,

which are unaffected by antihistamines but are responsible for histamine-mediated stimulation of gastric secretion. Blocking the H_2 receptor on the parietal cell also blunts its response to the other physiologic stimuli (e.g., acetylcholine and gastrin). The basal and nocturnal acid secretion is reduced by 90 to 95 percent with clinically used doses, and food-stimulated acid secretion is reduced by 70 percent. Anticholinergic drugs, which were employed extensively in the past in the treatment of peptic ulcer disease, reduce food-stimulated acid secretion by only 25 to 30 percent. In a series of randomized trials, healing as determined by endoscopy was complete in 4 weeks in 75 percent of patients with duodenal ulcer treated with H_2-receptor antagonists, in comparison with 40 percent of placebo-treated patients. Ninety-five percent of H_2-antagonist–treated patients heal in 8 weeks. Studies indicate that suppression of nocturnal acid secretion is of prime importance in duodenal ulcer healing. As a consequence, a single evening dose (800 mg cimetidine, 300 mg ranitidine, or 40 g famotidine) is sufficient to achieve healing and to enlist maximal patient compliance. During the year after healing and cessation of the antagonist therapy, 60 to 80 percent of duodenal ulcers will recur, compared with only 10 percent in patients maintained on a single nighttime dose (half that used to produce healing) of an H_2-receptor antagonist. Since these drugs are rapidly excreted by the kidneys, dosage must be decreased if a patient has renal insufficiency.

The use of cimetidine has been associated with infrequent and reversible side effects, including gynecomastia and mild elevations of serum creatinine and aminotransferases. In elderly persons, especially those with renal insufficiency, reversible confusion and coma have been reported when the dose has not been scaled down. The second-generation H_2 antagonists, ranitidine and famotidine, seem to be free of the antiandrogen properties occasionally seen with cimetidine use. They do, however, slow metabolic clearance of a number of other drugs. This property should be considered when a patient is also using warfarin-related anticoagulants, phenytoin, propranolol, and theophylline.

Antacids[3,6,10]

Nonabsorbable antacids have been the cornerstone of medical therapy for the past 25 years. Their effectiveness is determined by the rate of gastric emptying and by their capacity to buffer gastric acid. Recent studies have shown that an intensive antacid regimen of 210 ml per day (30 ml of antacid [aluminum-magnesium hydroxide] with an in vitro buffering capacity of 123 mEq HCl per dose, 1 and 3 hours after meals and at bedtime) was as effective as cimetidine in healing duodenal ulcers. After 4 weeks of treatment, 64 percent of ulcers treated with cimetidine were healed as demonstrated by duodenoscopy, in comparison with 52 percent of those treated with the intensive antacid regimen.[11] Although antacid therapy is as effective as cimetidine, in practice fewer patients complete the full course. Thus fewer have their ulcers healed, in part because of the inconvenience of taking medicine seven times a day after symptoms have disappeared. It is noteworthy that if taken in full doses, the cost of antacids is more than that of H_2-receptor antagonists. Soluble antacids, such as sodium bicarbonate and calcium carbonate, are the most effective. However, in large doses they produce alkalosis, and with prolonged use in some individuals they lead to the milk alkali syndrome (hypercalcemia, renal insufficiency, and alkalosis). In addition, calcium-containing antacids produce acid rebound to a secretory rate twice that of basal acid secretion. For this reason, nonabsorbable antacids, such as aluminum hydroxide gel and magnesium trisilicate gel, are usually employed.

Since aluminum hydroxide is extremely constipating, most antacids containing this substance also contain varying amounts of magnesium oxide (milk of magnesia). Intensive antacid regimens based on magnesium oxide–containing preparations cause diarrhea in 25 percent of patients. This is corrected by a change to an antacid containing less laxative.

Sucralfate[20]

Sucralfate, a basic aluminum salt of a sulfated disaccharide, is a recent addition to the antiulcer armamentarium. It has been shown to be more effective than placebo or low-dose antacids and is as effective as the H_2-receptor antagonist cimetidine. The drug appears to work locally at sites of inflamed mucosa. There are two possible mechanisms for its action. First, by forming a barrier to further acid-pepsin attack, it produces a more benign microenvironment that fosters healing. Second, by directly inhibiting the action of pepsin, healing is enhanced. The impact of this second mechanism is speculative and the efficacy of the *barrier* mechanism is the prevalent belief. Controlled clinical trials suggest that 4 g daily of sucralfate is as effective as cimetidine in the treatment of acute duodenal ulcer. In addition, continued treatment with 1.25 g daily is effective in preventing recurrence of duodenal ulcer. Efficacy of maintenance therapy is in the same range as that of cimetidine maintenance but requires four daily doses, rather than one.

Anticholinergic Drugs[4]

Anticholinergic drugs decrease gastric acid secretion, but the dosages required produce other undesirable effects, such as dry mouth, blurred vision, and urinary retention. At present the uses of anticholinergics in the treatment of peptic ulcer disease are to augment the antisecretory effect of H_2 antagonists in the medical treatment of Zollinger-Ellison syndrome and other peptic ulcers not responding to conventional treatment.

Sedation

Sedatives should be given only on specific indication, rather than as a routine part of the ulcer regimen. The tricyclic antidepressant doxepin is a weak inhibitor of acid secretion and has been shown in an open clinical trial to have efficacy in the healing of duodenal ulcers. Pirenzepine is structurally related to the tricyclic agents. It has unique antimuscarinic binding properties and has been found in some trials to have an efficacy comparable to that of cimetidine. Experience is limited with this agent, but it may have a place when used in conjunction with H_2-receptor antagonists.

Long-Term Management[9]

The advent of H_2 antagonists has simplified medical therapy for peptic ulcer. On the basis of current experience, patients with uncomplicated duodenal ulcer should be treated for 6 to 8 weeks with an evening dose of an H_2 antagonist. Because of its convenience, more patients continue therapy to healing with H_2 antagonists than continue with other therapies. As a consequence, the frequency of the complications of ulcer has decreased. If the patient has a recurrence within 6 months, a second 8-week course of a H_2 antagonist should be instituted and serum gastrin measured to exclude hypergastrinemia as the cause of the ulcer disease. Because delayed healing and early recurrence are associated with smoking and *Campylobacter pylori*–associated gastritis, cessation of smoking should be strongly urged; the *C. pylori* gastritis should be treated with bismuth subsalicylate (Pepto Bismol, see Gastritis, p. 798). With recurrence of this type, healing should be documented by duodenoscopy. If the ulcer has healed, maintenance therapy will decrease the chance of recurrence. If, on the other hand, the ulcer has not healed, H_2-receptor antagonist therapy should be supplemented with an antacid, an anticholinergic agent, or both. If the patient is thought to be at high risk for recurrence of ulcer activity, maintenance therapy can be begun immediately after the first 8-week course. No clear guidelines currently exist regarding the length of maintenance therapy.

There is less agreement concerning the role of H_2 antagonists in the treatment of gastric ulcer. Although treatment with these drugs has not been shown to be more effective than intensive antacid therapy, patients are able to comply fully with the H_2-antagonist regimen; hence more have healing of their ulcers with H_2 antagonists than with traditional antacid therapy. H_2 antagonists

should be given on a twice-daily schedule when gastric ulcers are treated. Healing of gastric ulcers should be documented by endoscopy before therapy is discontinued. The concern for complete healing of a gastric ulcer is prompted by the high rate of recurrence; by the risk of complications of a chronic, incompletely healed gastric ulcer; and by the risk of undetected carcinoma in a partially healed gastric ulcer.

New Agents

Prostaglandins. As noted earlier, prostaglandins of the E class have a variety of effects on the gastric mucosa. They reduce gastric secretion by inhibiting the histamine-stimulated conversion of adenosine triphosphate (ATP) to cyclic adenosine monophosphate (cyclic AMP). Besides the antisecretory effects, these agents may exert a cytoprotective effect through the following:

1. Stimulation of mucus and bicarbonate
2. Maintenance of mucosal blood flow
3. Strengthening of the cell membrane
4. Provision of a surface-active, or surfactant, effect

Two synthetic prostaglandin E analogs, enprostil and misoprostol, are being tested in clinical trials for both duodenal and gastric ulcer. Both show improved response over placebo. When compared directly with cimetidine, they show slightly lower response rates, but these differences were not significant.

Substituted Benzimidazoles (Omeprazole). The final common pathway of gastric acid secretion is the H^+/K^+ ATPase proton pump. A substituted benzimidazole, omeprazole, is currently the only agent available that works at this site. Although H_2-receptor antagonists are potent inhibitors of acid secretion, omeprazole renders patients virtually achlorhydric. The healing rate with this agent is in the 80 to 90 percent range when used for 4 weeks at doses of 20 to 60 mg daily. This rate currently appears to be higher than that for cimetidine and suggests that omeprazole may now be the most efficacious drug for ulcer therapy. An investigational drug in the United states, it has had few reported side effects. Because omeprazole produces achlorhydria, in interrupts negative feedback inhibition of gastrin release. As a consequence, hyperplasia of the enterochromaffin-like (ECL) (histamine-producing) cells occurs with long-term treatment in animals and may progress to carcinoid tumors. A similar sequence occurs in pernicious anemia.

SURGICAL THERAPY FOR PEPTIC ULCER

The aim of the surgical treatment of peptic ulcer is to decrease gastric secretion to a level at which healing will occur and recurrences will be eliminated, while interfering as little as possible with alimentary tract function. Four types of operation have been employed:

1. Subtotal gastrectomy, in which the antrum and a substantial part of the body of the stomach (the acid-producing mucosa) are resected
2. Vagotomy and antrectomy, designed to remove both the neural and humoral stimuli of gastric secretion
3. Vagotomy and pyloroplasty, in which the neural stimuli are interrupted and the resulting gastric retention is minimized by pyloroplasty
4. Parietal cell or highly selective vagotomy, which denervates the acid-secreting portion of the stomach, and leaves the innervation and motor function of the antrum intact. (This operation has the lowest frequency of long-term side effects. In experienced hands a 5-year cure rate of 80 to 90 percent is reported.)

In the first two procedures, gastrointestinal tract continuity is reestablished by either gastroduodenostomy (Billroth I) or gastroenterostomy (Billroth II).

In general, the greater the gastric resection, the greater are the frequency and severity of postgastrectomy dumping symptoms. Postgastrectomy malabsorption tends to be more severe after gastroenterostomy than after gastroduodenostomy. The incidence of recurrent ulcer is greater in patients treated with vagotomy and pyloroplasty than in those treated with vagotomy and antrectomy. Vagotomy with antrectomy has the lowest recurrence rate of disease.

COMPLICATIONS OF THERAPY

Medical Therapy

The four main complications of medical therapy—diarrhea, delayed gastric emptying, hypophosphatemia, and the milk–alkali syndrome—are disappearing as H_2-receptor antagonists become the preferred treatment for peptic ulcer disease.

Surgical Therapy

Surgery provides completely satisfactory relief of ulcer symptoms in 80 percent of patients. In 10 to 20 percent of patients so treated, the results are unsatisfactory, and in a few the complications may be more severe than the original ulcer symptoms.

Dumping Syndrome.[16] The dumping syndrome is experienced in mild form by many patients after a partial gastrectomy. In most, symptoms disappear within a month, but in a few patients these symptoms continue to be prominent and on rare occasions disabling. Within 15 minutes of eating the patient becomes aware of an epigastric fullness, at times associated with nausea. If the attack is severe, tachycardia, sweating, and weakness appear. These symptoms may be followed by abdominal cramping and a loose stool or two. The attack is aggravated by walking about and relieved by lying down.

When the stomach and duodenum are anatomically and functionally intact, gastric emptying is controlled so that the intestinal contents never become hypertonic. In the postgastrectomy dumping syndrome, this control is lost. The appearance of hypertonic fluid in the intestine calls forth a rapid secretion of fluid into the jejunum. The resulting distension of the intestine causes a sensation of epigastric fullness and stimulates intestinal motility and diarrhea. The abrupt shift of water from the blood to the intestinal lumen gives rise to symptoms of hypovolemia—that is, tachycardia, sweating, and syncope.

The dumping syndrome can be minimized by small, frequent feedings that are low in carbohydrates and by separating the solid and liquid portions of the meal by 1 hour. Initially it may be necessary to lie down for 30 minutes after meals.

Postprandial Hypoglycemia Syndrome. The symptoms of the postprandial hypoglycemia syndrome are sweating, palpitations, and at times syncope 2 to 3 hours after meals. When the stomach empties rapidly, glucose is absorbed quickly and the blood sugar reaches hyperglycemic levels. The result is a compensatory release of insulin that overshoots, resulting in hypoglycemia.

Afferent Loop Syndrome.[19] The afferent loop syndrome is caused by a partial obstruction of the afferent loop of the gastroenterostomy. As a result, bile and pancreatic juice accumulate. When the loop empties, usually after the meal has passed into the efferent loop, the stomach is flooded with the retained duodenal fluid, and bilious vomiting occurs. *It is worth noting that the above-mentioned three postoperative complaints are essentially obviated by highly selective vagotomy.*

Postgastrectomy Anemia. A variety of factors contribute to postgastrectomy anemias, among them the following:

1. Bleeding from the stomach or jejunum
2. Decreased absorption of iron

3. Least commonly, decreased absorption of vitamin B_{12}, caused by the failure of the stomach to produce intrinsic factor (Patients who have had total gastrectomy regularly develop a vitamin B_{12} deficiency.)

Marginal Ulcer. Peptic ulcers may form in the jejunum adjacent to a gastroenterostomy. They rarely occur when the surgery is performed for a gastric ulcer, but depending on the procedure employed, they appear in about 1 to 10 percent of the patients with duodenal ulcers treated surgically. The first concern in the patient with a marginal ulcer is the adequacy of the surgical procedure. On occasion the vagotomy is incomplete or antral tissue is left in with the duodenal stump. In these patients, as well as in others in whom ulcer disease is poorly controlled by routine treatment, unusual forms of peptic ulcer disease, such as Zollinger-Ellison syndrome, should be looked for.

Postgastrectomy Malabsorption. See Chapter 12.6 for a discussion of postgastrectomy malabsorption.

COMPLICATIONS OF PEPTIC ULCER

In 20 percent of patients with chronic peptic ulcer, there is progression of the disease or the development of complications because of failure of medical therapy or failure of compliance with recommended treatment.

HEMORRHAGE

Hemorrhage complicates the disease course in 16 percent of patients with duodenal ulcers and in 12 percent of those with gastric ulcers (see Chapter 12.4). If hemorrhage is massive and is not brought under control in 12 to 24 hours, of if rebleeding occurs, surgical therapy should be considered.

PERFORATION[24]

Perforation occurs in 6 to 10 percent of peptic ulcers (see Chapter 12.2). All such patients require surgery.

OBSTRUCTION[13]

Obstruction complicates the disease course in 7 percent of patients with duodenal ulcers and in less than 0.5 percent of those with gastric ulcers.

Minor degrees of pyloric obstruction are common in patients with duodenal ulcers; indeed, much of the intractability seen in chronic disease has been attributed to partial pyloric obstruction. In fully developed pyloric obstruction, vomiting is the most characteristic symptom. Before this stage, the patient notes that meals aggravate his distress rather than relieve it.

In ulcer patients with these symptoms, a succussion splash, or clapotage, may be elicited, confirming the suspicion of gastric retention. Clapotage is a splashing sound heard in the epigastrium when the abdomen is gently rocked to and fro. This sign should not be elicitable from a normal stomach more than 1 hour after a glass of water has been drunk or 3 hours after a meal.

The differentiation between benign and malignant obstruction can best be established by endoscopy with cytologic study and biopsy. Adult pyloric hypertrophy is a rare cause of pyloric obstruction.

Endoscopy to establish the cause of gastric retention should not be performed until the patient has been on a regimen of gastric aspiration for 24 hours. If the obstruction is benign, the patient should be started on a regimen of small feedings daily (soft diet) and an H_2-receptor antagonist.

After 3 days the adequacy of gastric emptying can be assessed by aspirating and measuring the gastric contents 4 hours after the evening meal. If gastric emptying has returned to normal, less than 200 to 300 ml of gastric juice should be recoverable. Another simple test is performed by instilling 750 ml saline solution into the stomach and withdrawing the residue after 30 minutes. Ninety percent of normal individuals have less than 200 ml remaining, whereas patients with gastric retention have more than 400 ml. The initial episodes of pyloric obstruction are due to edema and spasm caused by ulcer activity. They can be treated satisfactorily with an ulcer treatment regimen. Recurrent episodes indicate that the ulcer is resistant to medical therapy or that scarring has led to irreversible narrowing. In either case the treatment is surgical.

INTRACTABLE OR RECURRENT PEPTIC ULCER

The words "intractable" and "recurrent" have come to have more specific meaning as a result of the experience of giving treatment with H_2-receptor antagonists. "Intractable" describes the ulcers of those patients who do not respond to primary therapy. Currently, this would mean approximately 20 percent of patients treated with 1 g of cimetidine for 4 weeks. "Recurrent" describes the ulcers of those patients who have a relapse after successful primary therapy. For patients who are not maintained on H_2-receptor antagonists, the relapse rate is about 8.5 percent per month. For those who receive maintenance therapy the relapse rate will be lower, about 2.5 percent. There are a number of factors that contribute to poor healing, including the following:

- Male sex
- Smoking
- Older age
- Ulcer size
- Maximum stimulated acid secretory rate
- *Campylobacter pylori*–associated gastritis

Most intractable or recurrent ulcers are a manifestation of the severity of the ulcer diathesis or the inability of the patient to follow an effective regimen, or of both. Before this formulation is accepted, however, several questions should be considered:

- Have other causes of dyspepsia been excluded?
- Is the patient receiving optimal ulcer therapy?
- Are the patient's symptoms truly due to the ulcer or to an associated unresolved emotional problem?
- Are complications related to the ulcer, such as obstruction or penetration through the wall, causing symptoms?
- Have all specific causes of gastric hypersecretion been ruled out?

The approach to such patients has not been studied in a controlled manner. Nonetheless, the clinical approach is simply to make a change in the manner of treatment. Because a variety of agents with different mechanisms but comparable efficacy are now available, making such a change is relatively easy to accomplish. Regimen changes can include combinations of the following:

1. Increase the dose of the original H_2-receptor antagonist.
2. Change to a different H_2-receptor antagonist.
3. Change to, or add, something completely different.
   a. Antacids
   b. Bismuth salts
   c. Sucralfate
   d. Anticholinergic agents
   e. Synthetic prostaglandins
   f. Omeprazole
   g. Surgery

ZOLLINGER-ELLISON SYNDROME AND RELATED DISORDERS[12,17,22]

Originally Zollinger and Ellison called attention to a group of patients with jejunal ulcers and gastric hypersection associated with non-beta-cell islet tumors of the pancreas. These tumors are composed of G cells and secrete large amounts of gastrin, which causes gastric hypersecretion and peptic ulcers. As experience has accumulated, it has been recognized that 75 percent of ulcers caused by gastrinomas are in locations expected in uncomplicated peptic ulcer disease. Zollinger-Ellison (Z-E) syndrome should be suspected in patients with intractable ulcer disease, giant or multiple ulcers, or rapid recurrence after surgery. In addition, the following findings should lead to a consideration of Z-E in the differential diagnosis:

- Gastric hypersecretion (More than two thirds of patients with Z-E syndrome have basal secretory rates over 10 mEq/hr, and half are greater than 15 mEq/hr.)
- Diarrhea or even steatorrhea (In more than one third of patients, diarrhea is a prominent symptom.)
- Hypertrophy of gastric rugae, seen with endoscopy or radiographic studies

The diagnosis is confirmed, however, by finding an elevated serum gastrin level (>500 pg/ml). In patients with Z-E syndrome with intermediate elevation (200 to 500 pg/ml), secretin infusions lead to striking elevations of serum gastrin. Ultimate proof of the diagnosis is demonstration of a non-beta-cell tumor in the pancreas at the time of surgery. These tumors are frequently multiple, and over half are malignant. Hence resection provides cures in only 10 to 15 percent. Total gastrectomy to remove the end-organ had been the treatment of choice. Now both medical therapy with H_2-receptor antagonists and primary tumor resection, which has had a resurgence of interest, appear to be viable. Medical therapy has been shown to be so effective in removing the threat to life from intractable ulcer disease that the major threat is now delayed malignant invasion from the tumor. Z-E syndrome has been shown to respond to cimetidine. Two thirds of the patients have their disease controlled by the usual dose of 1200 mg per day, but 85 to 90 percent will respond to cimetidine at doses of 2.5 to 5.0 g per day, or to the addition of an anticholinergic agent. In Z-E syndrome, cimetidine must be given continuously to keep the ulcer disease under control. The newer and more potent H_2-receptor antagonists (ranitidine and famotidine) have been shown to be effective and to have fewer side effects. Finally, omeprazole appears to be more effective than H_2-receptor antagonists. Since there are now better methods of localizing tumors, and since tumors are being found earlier, consideration of primary resection is being readdressed in selected patients.

A Z-E-like syndrome has been seen with gastrinomas of the antrum and duodenum and with G cell hyperplasia of the antrum and pancreas. In addition, gastrinomas may be one of the abnormalities encountered in familial multiple endocrine adenomas, or Wermer syndrome. Since as many as 20 percent of patients with Z-E syndrome have other endocrine adenomas, it has been suggested that Z-E syndrome is really only one manifestation of the so-called Wermer syndrome.

OTHER CAUSES OF DYSPEPSIA

NONULCER DYSPEPSIA

Patients with dyspepsia for which no organic cause is demonstrated are arbitrarily put into one of two groups. The first consists of patients whose symptoms simulate those associated with organic disease of the upper gastrointestinal tract, such as peptic ulcer, cholecystitis, and peptic esophagitis. In this group the symptoms probably result from a motor disturbance of the gastroduodenal segment, alterations in gastric secretion, emotional overlay or other poorly understood factors, rather than from anatomic abnormalities. At present, the techniques for studying gastroduodenal motility are not refined to the point that this hypothesis has been tested.

In patients with dyspepsia who have negative findings on an upper gastrointestinal tract radiography study and no other apparent cause for their symptoms, the use of fiberoptic endoscopy has provided new insight. In these patients, gross endoscopic or histologic abnormalities are found in approximately 75 percent. The more common findings include unsuspected gastric or duodenal ulcers, atrophic gastritis, antral gastritis, and duodenitis. It is not clear how these mucosal abnormalities are related to or cause dyspepsia. This clinical state is sometimes referred to as Moynihan disease. The symptoms in these patients usually respond to the same therapy given to ulcer patients.

Patients in the second group have symptoms that are bizarre compared with those of patients with known organic disease. It is thought that these patients are describing their emotional disturbances in somatic terms. The following is a list of markers believed to be of value in the diagnosis of nonorganic dyspepsia:

- Symptoms are out of proportion to clinical well-being.
- Symptom descriptions are not convincing and are inconsistent.
- Symptoms do not conform to recognized pathophysiologic or disease states.
- Abdominal pains are poorly localized or occur at several sites.
- Pain is continuous and often described as occurring daily without remission.
- Pain occurs on waking (distinct from peptic ulcer) and rarely interferes with sleep.
- When vomiting occurs, patients report being unable to eat for several hours thereafter.
- Anorexia without weight loss may occur.
- The patient may have had previous psychiatric contact.
- Abdominal pain may have been present in childhood.

This group of patients generally obtain less relief from symptomatic therapy and usually need formal psychotherapy.

GASTRITIS

Gastritis, or inflammation of the stomach, is a very common finding in mucosal biopsy specimens. It has been tempting to equate the pathologic change with the common symptoms of dyspepsia and flatulence, but unfortunately no simple relationship has been defined. There are several distinctive pathologic patterns of gastritis and multiple etiologic factors:

1. Nonspecific gastritis is typically most severe in the antrum. It was attributed in the past on the basis of frequent association to a variety of factors, e.g., hyperchlorhydria, bile reflux, drugs, especially nonsteroidal anti-inflammatory agents, alcohol, etc. The recent discovery that nonspecific gastritis is frequently (62 to 95 percent in reported series) accompanied by an infectious organism,[2] *Campylobacter pylori*. This organism attaches only to gastric epithelium and in its presence polymorphonuclear leukocytes are found in the inflammatory exudate, hence the frequently used term chronic active gastritis. The cause and effect relation is strengthened by the observation that the acute inflammatory cells disappear from the gastric mucosa when the *C. pylori* infection is eradicated. These observations require that the primary role of other factors in the pathogenesis of gastritis be re-examined. Bile reflux produces a characteristic form of "nonspecific" gastritis. Un-

like *C. pylori*-associated gastritis, it is inactive; that is, inflammation is minimal, but there is fibrosis, vascular congestion and proliferation of smooth muscle cells and surface mucin cells are present in the mucosa.

2. Atrophic gastritis is characterized by inflammation and loss of glands. It has been subdivided into two types on the basis of epidemiologic, clinical and pathogenic mechanisms. The first, autoimmune or type A, involves the body and fundus of the stomach, the parietal cell region. As a consequence of the loss of gastric glands with their parietal cells, secretion of acid and intrinsic factor disappears, leading to pernicious anemia. The second subtype (type B) involves the antrum primarily and has been called environmental because it has a variable geographic distribution and increases in frequency with age. Environmental atrophic gastritis has a high correlation with gastric ulcer and adenocarcinoma of the stomach. Both types of atrophic gastritis are associated with intestinal metaplasia of the gastric mucosa. There are a variety of less frequent forms of gastritis such as eosinophilic gastritis, Crohn disease associated gastritis, and syphilitic gastritis to mention only a few.

CHRONIC CHOLECYSTITIS

See Chapter 12.2 for a discussion of chronic cholecystitis.

REFERENCES

1. Black T, Hole D, Rhodes J: Bile damage to gastric mucosal barrier: The influence of pH and bile concentration. Gastroenterology 61:178, 1971
2. Blaser MJ: Gastric *Campylobacter*-like organisms, gastritis, and peptic ulcer disease. Gastroenterology 93:371, 1987
3. Deering TB, Malagelada JR: Comparison of an H_2 receptor antagonist and a neutralizing antacid on postprandial acid delivery onto the duodenum in patients with duodenal ulcer. Gastroenterology 73:11, 1977
4. Feldman M, Richardson CT, Peterson WL: Effect of low-dose propantheline on food-stimulated gastric acid secretion: Comparison with an "optimal effective dose" and interaction with cimetidine. N Engl J Med 297:1427, 1977
5. Flenstom G, Turnberg LA: Gastroduodenal defense mechanisms. Clin Gastroenterol 13:327, 1984
6. Fordtran JS, Collyns JA: Antacid pharmacology in duodenal ulcer. Effects of antacid on postcibal gastric acidity and peptic activity. N Engl J Med 274:921, 1966
7. Forte JG, Forte TM, et al: Correlation of parietal cell structure and function. J Clin Gastroenterol 5(Suppl 1):17, 1983
8. Geall MG, Phllips SF, Summerskill WHJ: Profile of gastric potential differences in man: Effects of aspirin, alcohol, bile, and endogenous acid. Gastroenterology 58:437, 1970
9. Gunmand-Hoyer E, Jensen KB, et al: Prophylactic effect of cimetidine in duodenal ulcer disease. Br Med J 1:1095, 1978
10. Ippoliti AF, Sturdevant RAL, et al: Cimetidine versus intensive antacid therapy for duodenal ulcer: A multicenter trial. Gastroenterology 74:393, 1978
11. Isenberg JI: Peptic ulcer. Disease-a-Month 27:7, 1981
12. Jensen RT, Gardner JD, et al: Zollinger–Ellison syndrome: Current concepts and management. Ann Intern Med 98:59, 1983
13. Kreel L, Ellis H: Pyloric stenosis in adults: A clinical and radiological study of 100 consecutive patients. Gut 6:253, 1965
14. Kurata JH: Epidemiology of peptic ulcer disease. Clin Gastroenterol 13:289, 1984
15. Laufer I: Assessment of the accuracy of double contrast gastroduodenal radiology. Gastroenterology 71:844, 1976
16. LeQuesne LP, Hobsley M, Hand BH: The dumping syndrome. I. Factors responsible for symptoms. Br Med J 1:141, 1960
17. McGuigan JE, Wolfe MM: Secretin injection test in the diagnosis of gastrinoma. Gastroenterology 79:1324, 1980
18. Misiewicz JJ: Clinical pharmacology and therapeutic potential of H_2-receptor antagonists. In Truelove SC, Ritchie JA (eds): Topics in Gastroenterology. Oxford, Blackwell, 1976
19. Mitty WF Jr, Grossi G, Mealon TF Jr: Chronic afferent loop syndrome. Ann Surg 172:996, 1970
20. Nakazawa S, Renpei N, Samloff M: Selective binding of sucralfate to gastric ulcer in man. Dig Dis Sci 26:297, 1981
21. Piasecki C: The microcirculation of the stomach and duodenum. In Truelove SC, Willoughby CP (eds): Topics in Gastroenterology. Oxford, Blackwell, 1979
22. Richardson CT, Peters MN, et al: Treatment of Zollinger–Ellison syndrome with exploratory laparotomy, proximal gastric vagotomy and H_2-receptor antagonists: A prospective study. Gastroenterology 89:357, 1985
23. Sonnenberg A: Geographic and temporal variations in the occurrence of peptic ulcer disease. Scand J Gastroenterol (Suppl) 110:11, 1985
24. Walker C: Complications of peptic ulcer disease and indications for surgery. In Sleisenger MH, Fordtran JS (eds): Gastrointestinal Disease. Philadelphia, WB Saunders, 1983

CHAPTER 12.4
Gastrointestinal Bleeding

David R. Kafonek, H. Franklin Herlong,
Francis M. Giardiello,
and Thomas R. Hendrix

Gastrointestinal bleeding may occur as a life-threatening emergency, with hematemesis, hematochezia, or melena, or, at the other extreme, it may be occult and chronic and discovered only in a search for the cause of anemia.[17] The mortality rate from acute gastrointestinal bleeding has not decreased from the range of 10 percent in recent decades, despite more accurate diagnosis and new therapeutic measures.[1] The failure of more accurate diagnosis and better supportive measures to improve the mortality rate is generally attributed to the higher average age of our population and, as a consequence, the increase in the number of patients with associated disease. Perhaps of more importance has been the failure to develop more accurate measures of blood loss and adequacy of volume replacement. The successful management of a gastrointestinal hemorrhage requires the close cooperation of the physician, radiologist, and surgeon.

ACUTE GASTROINTESTINAL BLEEDING

Acute gastrointestinal bleeding appears unexpectedly, and its source is usually uncertain. The volume of blood lost and the rate of continued bleeding are difficult to determine. The evaluation and management of acute gastrointestinal bleeding can be divided into three overlapping phases: (1) supportive: estimate blood loss and provide adequate volume replacement, (2) diagnostic: estab-

lish the source of the bleeding, and (3) therapeutic: institute specific and nonspecific treatment of bleeding lesion.

SUPPORTIVE MANAGEMENT

Estimate of Blood Volume Deficit
The lack of a simple reliable test to provide serial measurements of functional blood volume makes it necessary for the clinician to employ a series of indirect observations to provide an estimate of blood volume deficit. From this estimate the rate, volume, and type of initial fluid replacement are determined.

Hematemesis, Melena, and Hematochezia. The greater the rate of bleeding and the higher the lesion in the gastrointestinal tract, the more likely it is that the patient will vomit blood. The patient who has had a massive hematemesis should be considered to have lost one third to one half his blood volume. If blood replacement is based on this assumption, the chances of underestimating the blood loss and of suddenly finding it necessary to combat severe vascular collapse will be minimized.

As little as 50 to 80 ml of blood introduced into the upper gastrointestinal tract will turn the stools black. Thus, in evaluating a patient with melena, the physician must use other signs to estimate the volume of blood lost. Hematochezia, the passage of blood from the rectum, also does not provide a useful estimate of the volume of blood lost.

Blood Pressure and Pulse. Features of shock (hypotension, tachycardia, and cold, clammy skin), if present when the patient is recumbent, are indicative of at least a 50 percent loss of the blood volume. If signs of shock are present only when the patient assumes an upright position, a loss of at least 20 percent of the blood volume should be assumed.

The blood pressure is not a reliable indicator of the extent or rate of bleeding because it may be maintained at near-normal values until vasoconstrictor capacity is exceeded; further blood loss then leads to sudden and severe vascular collapse. On the other hand, a recumbent systolic blood pressure below 100 mm Hg or a pulse above 110 beats per minute usually indicates that more than 40 percent of the normal blood volume has been lost. Half the patients with systolic blood pressure below 100 mm Hg on admission have had a massive hemorrhage requiring more than 2.5 L blood replacement, whereas only 13 percent of patients requiring less than 2.5 L have an admission blood pressure below 100 mm Hg. A rising pulse rate also is an ominous sign. A steady pulse rate, however, is not a reliable indication that the blood volume is being maintained in a safe range. Measurement of blood pressure and pulse in both the recumbent and the erect positions gives valuable indications of the volume of blood loss. A fall in systolic blood pressure of greater than 15 mm Hg, coupled with a rise in pulse rate of greater than 20 beats per minute, is a reliable indicator of blood loss in excess of 20 percent of normal blood volume.

Most gastrointestinal hemorrhages, especially those of arterial or variceal origin, occur in episodes lasting about 30 minutes. After each bleeding episode the patient's blood pressure and pulse stabilize, and the physician may be lulled into a false sense of security. Each recurrent episode of bleeding, however, depletes the patient's vascular reserve, and if blood replacement is inadequate, further bleeding leads to vascular collapse.

Urine Output. One of the early indications of a decrease in blood volume is a fall in urine output, a decrease in urine sodium concentration, and a rise in urine specific gravity. With a 20 percent decrease in functional blood volume, urine output falls from the normal level of 50 ml/hr to 20 to 30 ml/hr. With greater deficits, there is a further fall in urine output (e.g., urine output of 5 to 15 ml/hr is associated with a 30 percent deficit [1500 ml] and little or no urinary output with a 40 to 50 percent deficit [2000 to 2500 ml]).

When volume replacement is adequate, output rises to 50 ml/hr and specific gravity returns to the range of 1.010.

Central Venous Pressure.[2,14] Central venous pressure (CVP) is determined by the balance between the volume of blood returning to the right atrium and the capacity of the right ventricle to pump the blood into the pulmonary circulation. A low CVP (<5 cm H_2O) is associated with hypovolemia, and a high CVP (>12 cm H_2O) indicates overtransfusion or right ventricular failure.

CVP is the most accurate indicator of functional blood volume but requires the insertion of a catheter into the superior vena cava. Because the largest fraction of the blood volume is in the venous compartment, one of the first indications of decompensation is a falling CVP. In a study of gastroduodenal hemorrhage a rapidly falling CVP (2 mm H_2O per minute with an overall fall of 5 cm H_2O) was always found to be associated with arterial bleeding. This event should alert the clinician to the likelihood that emergency surgery will be required.[2] Since the range of normal CVP is wide, 5 to 12 cm, the direction and rate of change are of more significance than is the initial pressure. Monitoring CVP also helps guard against overtransfusion, because the CVP rises before pulmonary congestion and edema occur. Overtransfusion, especially in patients with portal hypertension, leads to further increase in portal pressure and may induce rebleeding from esophageal varices. Blood volume is usually replaced to bring the CVP to 6 to 10 cm H_2O. In general, CVP is used to monitor blood volume in high-risk patients and those with orthostatic changes in blood pressure and pulse (i.e., patients estimated to have a loss of blood greater than 20 percent of blood volume).

Hematocrit.[18] The hematocrit is not a useful index of the extent of gastrointestinal bleeding. It tells only what percentage of the blood volume is composed of red cells and provides no accurate measure of blood volume in the bleeding patient. The hematocrit determined soon after the initial hemorrhage will be near normal. A period of 24 to 72 hours or more is required after a hemorrhage for hemodilution to be complete; therefore the hematocrit provides no guide to volume replacement.

Volume Replacement
The first priority in the management of gastrointestinal hemorrhage is the rapid restoration of the blood volume to a level that will preclude shock if an additional bleeding episode occurs. A large-caliber (14- to 16-gauge) intravenous line should be placed immediately and a rapid infusion (500 to 1000 ml in 30 minutes) of Ringer lactate or saline solution started. If the patient is in shock, two lines should be inserted. Since crystalloid-containing fluids rapidly equilibrate with the extravascular spaces, the volume infused needs to exceed the estimated deficit twofold to threefold. To avoid fluid overload, the physician should change the infusion fluid to a colloid (Plasmanate or albumin), which retains fluid in the vascular compartment. If the hematocrit value is below 30 percent, packed red blood cells should be added. It is not necessary to raise the hematocrit above 30 percent because tissue hypoxia in hemorrhage is due to decreased perfusion (hypovolemia) and not to insufficient oxygen-carrying capacity of the blood. Blood should be given if the blood loss is greater than 25 percent of the normal blood volume. Patients in shock should receive oxygen by nasal catheter at a flow rate of 4 to 6 liters per minute to improve oxygenation until volume replacement produces adequate tissue perfusion.

Flowchart
All clinical data should be recorded on a flowchart at the patient's bedside. Included should be pulse, blood pressure, urine output, CVP if a catheter is in place, volume and type of fluid infused, and loss of blood as manifested by hematemesis or the passage of blood-containing stool through the rectum. The frequency of recording should be every 15 minutes in the unstable patient and

may be extended to hourly when the patient is stable and shows no evidence of active bleeding. Each set of observations should lead to an estimate of volume deficit.

DIAGNOSIS

The aim of diagnostic procedures in the bleeding patient is to ascertain three factors: (1) site of bleeding (upper or lower gastrointestinal tract), (2) type of bleeding vessel (arterial, venocapillary, or variceal), and (3) nature of the bleeding lesion (e.g., ulcer, vascular anomaly, or neoplasm).

Site of Bleeding
As soon as measures have been instituted to correct hypovolemia, clues suggesting the location of the lesion should be sought by history and physical examination. The first step is to determine whether the bleeding originates in the upper or lower gastrointestinal tract so that appropriate diagnostic and therapeutic procedures can be employed. If the patient vomits blood, the bleeding lesion is almost always proximal to the ligament of Treitz.

Gastric Intubation.[12] If the patient has not vomited blood, a tube should be passed into the stomach. If the gastric aspirate contains blood, then the bleeding site is above the ligament of Treitz. If the stomach is free of blood, there are three possibilities: (1) the site of bleeding is below the ligament of Treitz; (2) bleeding has stopped and all the blood has passed into the intestine; or (3) rarely, the site of bleeding is distal to the pylorus and proximal to the ligament of Treitz (e.g., duodenal ulcer), but at the time of intubation the bleeding was not brisk enough to cause reflux of blood into the stomach.

Rectal examination should be done in all patients with gastrointestinal bleeding to assess the stool color and document the presence of blood. If a tarry stool is passed, the lesion is rarely lower than the ileocecal sphincter. Passage of red blood by rectum usually indicates a bleeding site within the colon. However, with massive hemorrhage and rapid intestinal transit, red blood passed through the rectum can emanate from a bleeding lesion as high as the esophagus. Thus the color of the blood passed is as much a function of the rate of bleeding and passage through the gastrointestinal tract as it is an indication of the site of bleeding. In general, the larger the hemorrhage, the more rapid is the passage through the gut.

History. The history should answer several questions. First, are there recent or remote symptoms of peptic ulcer disease? Peptic ulcer is the most common cause of massive upper gastrointestinal tract hemorrhage (Table 12.4–1). Statistical data, however, cannot be relied on to provide the correct diagnosis in the individual patient.

Next, is there a history of recent heavy alcohol intake or of drug ingestion, especially of aspirin, corticosteroids, phenylbutazone, or anticoagulants? The recent ingestion of any of these substances suggests the possibility of diffuse gastric erosions, an acute peptic ulcer, or an iatrogenic bleeding disorder. A history of blood appearing only after vomiting, especially after an alcoholic binge, should lead to a consideration of the Mallory-Weiss syndrome, in which retching leads to a longitudinal mucosal tear at the gastroesophageal junction.

Historical evidence of liver disease should be sought. Of course, not every alcoholic patient has cirrhosis, not everyone with cirrhosis has varices, and, certainly, not every cirrhotic patient with varices bleeds from this site. Indeed, in patients with demonstrated varices and upper gastrointestinal tract bleeding, up to 50 percent are found to be bleeding from other lesions.

Physical Examination. Signs of chronic liver disease (e.g., spider angioma, palmar erythema, splenomegaly, jaundice, and ascites)

TABLE 12.4–1. CAUSE OF BLEEDING IN 2225 PATIENTS FROM NATIONAL ASGE SURVEY ON UPPER GASTROINTESTINAL BLEEDING[15]

Duodenal ulcer	24.3%
Gastritis	23.4%
Gastric ulcer	21.3%
Varices	10.3%
Mallory-Weiss tear	7.2%
Esophagitis	6.3%
Erosive duodenitis	5.8%
Neoplasm	2.9%
Stomal ulcer	1.8%
Esophageal ulcer	1.7%
Arteriovenous malformation	0.5%
Other	6.3%

should be sought. Many of the rare causes of gastrointestinal hemorrhage are associated with characteristic physical findings that may be missed unless they are specifically looked for (see Chapter 17.7). These findings include the following: (1) Melanin spots on the lips and buccal mucosa, found in the Peutz-Jeghers syndrome, may be associated with bleeding from intestinal polyps. (2) Telangiectatic lesions of Osler-Weber-Rendu disease (hereditary hemorrhagic telangiectasia), seen on fingers, face, lips, and mucous membranes, may be associated with bleeding from similar vascular lesions in the gastrointestinal tract. (3) Characteristic "plucked chicken" skin changes of pseudoxanthoma elasticum are associated with vascular lesions, especially in the stomach, which may bleed. (4) Less commonly, café au lait spots may be associated with bleeding neurofibromas of the intestinal tract. Cutaneous "caviar" vascular lesions, "pinch" purpura with amyloidosis, and hyperextension of joints with Ehlers-Danlos syndrome may all be associated with bleeding gastrointestinal vascular anomalies. Finding manifestations of these rare diseases, however, cannot be taken as proof that they are the cause of gastrointestinal hemorrhage. (5) Purpura, ecchymoses, or bleeding gums, which can be overlooked easily if not specifically sought, are evidence of a bleeding diathesis.

Acute Upper Gastrointestinal Tract Hemorrhage
Peptic ulcer, erosive gastritis, and esophageal varices are the most common causes of upper gastrointestinal tract hemorrhage. Because the therapies for these disorders may differ radically, it is important to make a specific diagnosis (e.g., persistent arterial bleeding from a gastric or duodenal ulcer can be treated promptly and effectively by surgery, whereas surgery has little to offer in the care of gastric erosions, and although variceal bleeding may be controlled by surgical portasystemic shunting, the combined stress of hemorrhage and surgery is often more than the diseased liver can tolerate.

Endoscopy.[15] If the clinical evidence favors an upper gastrointestinal source of the bleeding, endoscopy should be performed after hypovolemia has been corrected. Fiberoptic endoscopes make it possible to examine the esophagus, stomach, and first part of the duodenum with ease and safety. To ensure that the lesion is visualized, blood is removed by gastric lavage through a large-bore gastric tube (36 French). Endoscopy will provide an accurate determination of the bleeding site in over 90 percent of patients with upper gastrointestinal tract bleeding. Even if a clear diagnosis cannot be made at endoscopy, certain diagnoses should be excluded if possible, particularly bleeding from esophageal varices, diffuse erosive gastritis, and peptic ulcer.

Angiography.[3] If endoscopy has failed to identify the source of bleeding, or if bleeding is so rapid that the stomach cannot be cleared of blood sufficiently for endoscopy and brisk bleeding continues, angiography should be considered. Selective visceral arteriography not only localizes the site of bleeding but may be employed to control hemorrhage by the infusion of vasoconstricting drugs or embolic occlusion of the bleeding vessel. A catheter is introduced percutaneously into the femoral artery and guided by fluoroscopy into the celiac, superior mesenteric, and/or inferior mesenteric arteries. Active bleeding is indicated by the extravasation of contrast material into the bowel lumen. The rate of bleeding must be greaer than 0.5 ml/min for consistent identification of the source. Arterial bleeding is episodic, and it slows or stops as hypovolemia occurs. If the likelihood of identifying the source of bleeding by angiography is to be increased, it is important to do the study when the blood volume deficit has been restored. Despite such measures, angiography often fails to identify the site of major hemorrhage. Occasionally a patient with recurrent gastrointestinal hemorrhage that has eluded diagnosis is shown by angiography to have vascular tumor or malformation of the intestine, or bleeding from a Meckel diverticulum that can be resected.

Barium Studies. Barium studies have no role in the evaluation of massive gastrointestinal hemorrhage because they rarely provide a definitive diagnosis and preclude the more accurate techniques of endoscopy and angiography until the barium is cleared from the gastrointestinal tract.

Lower Intestinal Tract Hemorrhage
Proctosigmoidoscopy. If the clinical findings suggest that the lower bowel is the source of bleeding, proctosigmoidoscopy with a rigid sigmoidoscope should be the first diagnostic procedure. This procedure is performed with the patient in the head-down position and permits better visualization of the mucosa of the rectum than does fiberoptic endoscopy, because blood can be cleared from the rectum more effectively. It can thus be determined whether the bleeding is from the rectum or anal canal or from the more proximal bowel. Bleeding lesions commonly identified include diffuse mucosal lesions, such as ulcerative and ischemic colitis; local vascular lesions, such as hemorrhoids; and tumors, such as polyps or cancer.

Angiography. If proctosigmoidoscopy fails to identify the source of bleeding and bleeding continues at a rapid rate, angiography of the superior and inferior mesenteric arteries is the most effective method of localizing the source of the bleeding. With more frequent use of angiography in patients with colonic hemorrhage, the necessity for emergency surgery has diminished, because local infusion of vasoconstrictor agents through the angiographic catheter controls the bleeding in most patients. Angiography has shown vascular ectasia or angiodysplasia of the colon to be commonly associated with massive as well as chronic colonic bleeding.[4] For the site of bleeding to be identified, the patient must be actively bleeding at the time the angiographic contrast material is injected.

Fiberoptic Endoscopy. If the bleeding has stopped or is not rapid and the patient is stable, flexible fiberoptic sigmoidoscopy or colonoscopy can be performed after the bowel has been prepared with whole gut lavage (Golytely, a sodium sulfate–polyethylene glycol solution, is used). Fiberoptic endoscopy makes it possible to visualize vascular ectasias, diverticula, and neoplastic and inflammatory lesions of the colon. Colonoscopy should not be attempted if fulminant colitis or colonic perforation is suspected. If ischemic bowel disease is the most likely diagnosis, endoscopy should be carried out with caution because distending the bowel with air may add to the vascular compromise.

Radionuclide Scintigraphy. For a solution to the problem of identifying the location of acute intermittently bleeding lesions, radionuclide scintigraphy has been advocated. The patient's red blood cells are labeled in vivo and returned by intravenous infusion. Abdominal scintiscans then are obtained at regular intervals during the following 24 hours. When investigation of a previous bleeding episode was unproductive, starting with a radionuclide study when the patient is admitted with a subsequent hemorrhage may localize the bleeding site.

If the patient is young, under the age of 30 years, the possibility of bleeding ectopic gastric mucosa in a Meckel diverticulum should be tested by scintigraphy after injection of ^{99m}Tc-labeled pertechnetate. This is the most common cause of massive lower intestinal tract hemorrhage in younger persons.

Barium Studies. Barium studies are not performed in the acute phase of lower intestinal tract bleeding because they are not capable of demonstrating the most common cause (i.e., vascular ectasias), and they make it impossible to perform more definitive studies, such as angiography or endoscopy. However, barium enema often is the simplest way to identify ischemic colitis with bleeding.

THERAPY

Upper Gastrointestinal Tract Bleeding
The vigorous approach to the identification of the source of gastrointestinal hemorrhage is advocated so that if bleeding continues or recurs, definitive therapy can be promptly instituted. In addition, the definitive therapy for an arterial bleeding lesion (e.g., duodenal or gastric ulcer) is different from that for bleeding from esophageal varices or gastric erosions. Patients at high risk for a poor outcome should be identified to ensure optimal supportive care and timely institution of definitive therapy[4] (Table 12.4–2).

Arterial Bleeding. Arterial lesions bleed rapidly for 15 to 30 minutes; then, as the blood volume is depleted, intense vasoconstriction of the splanchnic vessels allows a clot to form. Over the next 1 to 4 hours the blood volume is replenished by fluid absorbed from the intestine and drawn from the extravascular spaces. As splanchnic blood flow and pressure rise with increasing blood volume, another episode of arterial bleeding will occur if the clot in the artery does not hold. Rarely, even with an aortoduodenal fistula, does exsanguination occur with the first episode of arterial bleeding. Usually two or more bleeding episodes occur before signs of shock appear.

Peptic (gastric and duodenal) ulcer is the most common cause of severe upper gastrointestinal tract bleeding. Nevertheless, 60 to 70 percent of bleeding peptic ulcers do not bleed again once the patient has been admitted to the hospital. Such patients require no treatment other than that designed to heal the ulcer[19] (see Chapter 12.3). Two endoscopic findings are predictive of recurrent bleeding in peptic ulcer disease: (1) a spurting arterial lesion and (2) a visible vessel.[13] Treating these lesions with endoscopic hemostasis (laser, electrocautery, or thermal probe) has been shown to decrease the frequency of recurrent bleeding, the need for emergency surgery, and incidence of death.[9,16] Recurrent bleeding of a peptic ulcer after attempted endoscopic hemostasis is an indication for surgical treat-

---

TABLE 12.4–2. PREDICTORS OF POOR OUTCOME IN ACUTE UPPER GASTROINTESTINAL TRACT HEMORRHAGE

- Elderly: >75 years of age
- Concurrent disease, especially liver, heart, lung, and kidney diseases
- Blood pressure ≤100 mm Hg during first hour in hospital
- Fresh blood in gastric aspirate during first hour in hospital
- Ascites
- Abnormal prothrombin time
- ''Visible vessel'' (actually, a clot protruding from the bleeding vessel) seen during endoscopy
- Arterial bleeding seen during endoscopy

ment. In poor-risk patients, angiographically directed embolization of the bleeding vessel may be tried before one resorts to surgery.

Bleeding from Mallory-Weiss tears may be arterial but usually stops spontaneously. If bleeding continues, several techniques have been used to stop hemorrhage, including endoscopic electrocautery or laser coagulation, angiographic infusion of vasopressin or embolization, and surgery.

Variceal Bleeding. Esophagogastric varices are the second most common source of massive upper gastrointestinal tract hemorrhage but have the greatest mortality rate. One fourth of patients with cirrhosis who bleed from varices do not leave the hospital alive, and only 40 percent survive 1 year. This high mortality rate is most often due to the inability of the cirrhotic liver to stand the stress of hemorrhage, rather than exsanguination per se. In a comparison of survival rates of patients bleeding from varices caused by cirrhosis and by portal vein thrombosis without cirrhosis, none of the patients with cirrhosis survived 5 years after the initial hemorrhage, whereas 90 percent of those with variceal hemorrhage and portal vein thrombosis were still alive. A major factor in the increased sensitivity of the cirrhotic liver to hemorrhage is the altered blood supply to the regenerating nodules that make up the bulk of the functioning hepatic parenchyma. The blood supply to regenerating nodules is arterial, rather than the normal contribution of 75 percent from portal blood and 25 percent from arterial blood to the total hepatic blood flow. Thus the parenchyma of the cirrhotic liver is susceptible to ischemic necrosis when hemorrhage leads to hypovolemia with resultant arterial hypotension. Secondary effects of variceal hemorrhage include (1) ascites due to loss of albumin and impaired hepatic synthesis (ascites may contribute to portal hypertension, thus increasing the risk of hemorrhage); (2) impaired coagulation due to inability of the liver to replace lost clotting factors; (3) hepatic encephalopathy due to increased absorption of nitrogenous products from the large protein (blood) load in the gut and decreased removal caused by portasystemic shunting and decreased hepatic and renal perfusion; and (4) renal failure due to the hepatorenal syndrome or acute tubular necrosis (see Chapter 13.3).

The tendency to bleed from esophageal varices correlates poorly with portal pressure, although bleeding from varices is uncommon when the portal pressure is less than 12 mm Hg (measured by wedged hepatic vein technique). Which varices bleed, however, correlates better with their diameter, as determined by endoscopy, than with the level of portal pressure, because variceal wall tension is a major determinant of hemorrhage.[10]

Emergency Treatment for Variceal Bleeding. In the patient with suspected bleeding from varices, blood volume must be restored promptly to minimize ischemic hepatic injury. It is preferable to restore the circulating blood volume with packed red blood cells and fresh frozen plasma, because this combination provides not only increased oxygen-delivering capacity but also coagulation factors that are usually deficient.

Although bleeding stops spontaneously in some patients with bleeding varices, over 50 percent continue to bleed or rebleed after admission to the hospital. In such patients, the initial treatment is intravenous vasopressin, which decreases portal pressure and flow by constricting splanchnic arteries, thus decreasing the volume entering the portal system. Vasopressin is infused into a large peripheral vein at the rate of 0.4 units per minute. After bleeding is controlled, the rate of vasopressin infusion is decreased by 0.1 unit per minute every 12 hours. Vasopressin constricts other arteries as well and may lead to ischemia, especially if the blood volume has not been restored. Myocardial ischemia is the most important side effect, but intestinal cramps and hyponatremia that is caused by reduced renal free water clearance may complicate vasopressin therapy.

If vasopressin fails to control hemorrhage, or if hemorrhage recurs while vasopressin is being infused, direct tamponade with the Sengstaken-Blakemore tube should be employed to control the bleeding varices. The Sengstaken-Blakemore tube contains gastric and esophageal balloons and a distal aspiration port. It is inserted through the nose and passed into the stomach. The gastric balloon is inflated with air and pulled snugly against the gastroesophageal junction, with the tube held in place by traction. Correct positioning of the gastric balloon should be confirmed radiographically. The inflated gastric balloon controls hemorrhage by compressing the coronary and short gastric veins against the diaphragm and reducing blood flow into the esophageal varices. Successful control of hemorrhage will lead to disappearance of fresh blood from the gastric aspirate. If the patient continues to bleed after the gastric balloon has been successfully inflated and accurately positioned, the esophageal balloon is inflated for further compression. After 24 hours of tamponade, both the esophageal and gastric balloons are deflated and the tube is left in place for an additional 24 hours before removal.

Complications of use of the Sengstaken-Blakemore tube are (1) gastric and esophageal erosions that increase in frequency with an increase in the length of time the balloons remain inflated; (2) esophageal rupture due to improper placement and inflation of the gastric balloon; and (3) aspiration of blood accumulating proximal to the esophageal balloon, due to failure to control esophageal bleeding. Once hemorrhage from esophagogastric varices has been controlled, it is important not to overtransfuse the patient, because unnecessary expansion of the intravascular volume will lead to an increase in portal blood flow, causing renewed bleeding from the varices. Maintaining the CVP at between 5 and 8 cm of water produces adequate filling pressure of the right heart without an excessive increase in portal pressure.

Acute esophagogastric or duodenal erosions may coexist with varices and are the most common source of bleeding in patients with portal hypertension. If erosions are present, antacids and H_2-receptor antagonists should be added. Patients with tense ascites should have a therapeutic paracentesis to reduce portal pressure, respiratory compromise, and the risk of aspiration. Diuretic therapy for ascites may be dangerous in the setting of an acute hemorrhage and should be withheld until the patient has been stabilized. Prophylactic measures to prevent the development of hepatic encephalopathy (e.g., emptying of the gut of blood with a cathartic agent or enemas and the administration of lactulose) should be instituted (see Chapter 13.3).

Treatment After Variceal Bleeding Has Stopped. The most widely employed technique for preventing recurrent bleeding from esophageal varices is endoscopic sclerotherapy.[6,7] Although the results of some studies have suggested that sclerotherapy be used to stop hemorrhage in patients who are actively bleeding from varices, most reports have advocated its use in preventing recurrent hemorrhage in patients whose initial bleeding stopped with less invasive measures. Repeated sclerotherapy sessions are required to inject all the varices. Patients are susceptible to recurrent bleeding until the varices are completely obliterated. Complications of sclerotherapy include esophageal strictures, leading to dysphagia, and necrosis and perforation of the esophageal wall, leading to mediastinitis.

Propranolol, a general beta-adrenergic blocker, reduces portal pressure when administered to patients with cirrhosis. In some patients, long-term administration of propranolol at a dose that reduces heart rate by 25 percent prevents recurrent bleeding from gastroesophageal varices.[11]

Surgical Management of Portal Hypertension. There are two surgical approaches to the management of portal hypertension complicated by bleeding esophagogastric varices: (1) direct transabdominal ligation of the varices, which temporarily controls bleeding but usually requires more definitive surgery later, and (2) creation of an anatomic shunt between the hypertensive portal system and the low-pressure systemic venous system to lower the portal pressure. Esophagogastric varices disappear, and other complications of portal hypertension, including hypersplenism, may

improve after portasystemic shunting. Portal blood flow to the liver, however, falls after portacaval shunt, leaving the liver even more dependent on its arterial blood supply. A variety of anastomoses have been advocated: (1) The end-to-side portacaval shunt, in which the distal portal vein is anastomosed to the side of the inferior vena cava, can be used. This totally diverts blood from the portal vein to the systemic circulation. Although it does prevent recurrent variceal hemorrhage, it also severely depresses liver function and produces a high incidence of hepatic encephalopathy. (2) The mesocaval shunt, which involves placement of a graft between the superior mesenteric vein and the vena cava, is the most widely used shunt. Its relative simplicity makes it applicable to both emergent and elective situations. (3) The distal splenorenal shunt is the most complicated operation. The coronary vein through which blood flows from the portal vein to the gastroesophageal varices is ligated. Blood then flows from the varices via the short gastric veins to the spleen and via the splenic vein to the renal vein through a surgically created anastomosis and ultimately into the vena cava. This procedure not only decompresses varices but also preserves portal blood flow to the liver. In several clinical trials, this procedure has been associated with a lower incidence of hepatic encephalopathy than other shunt operations.[8]

The role of portasystemic shunts remains controversial despite extensive experience. Technically satisfactory shunts decrease portal pressure and prevent recurrent bleeding from varices. Hence these operations find their greatest application in patients with severe or repeated variceal hemorrhage. Shunt surgery does not, however, prolong survival. The decreased mortality rate among patients who have undergone variceal hemorrhage shunt surgery is offset by an increase in deaths from hepatocellular failure.

Patient selection and prediction of outcome of any shunt operation are related to the patient's liver function and general physical condition. Ideally, patients should have compensated liver disease, with serum bilirubin only slightly elevated, if at all, a normal serum albumin level, and an absence of ascites or hepatic encephalopathy. Age greater than 50 years at the time of surgery or necrosis and inflammation on liver biopsy indicate a poor prognosis. When therapeutic shunts have been compared with endoscopic sclerotherapy to control bleeding, prevention of bleeding and survival rates are approximately equal. In most centers, elective shunts are only performed in patients who have not benefited from endoscopic sclerotherapy.

Emergency portasystemic shunts are sometimes used when variceal hemorrhage has not been controlled by any other form of medical therapy. The operative mortality rate is often greater than 50 percent.

Arteriolar-Capillary Bleeding. Erosions of the gastroduodenal mucosa, by definition, do not penetrate below the lamina muscularis mucosae. The most clearly recognized clinical associations are with (1) drug and alcohol ingestion, (2) extensive burns (Curling ulcer), (3) intracranial operations or trauma (Cushing ulcer), and (4) sepsis, trauma, postoperative complications, and myocardial infarction. Erosions with the latter three associations are often referred to as "stress ulcers" and may at times lead to a true ulcer when necrosis extends through the muscularis mucosae and into the submucosa or deeper. Erosions of all types are the result of a failure of mucosal protection and of epithelial cell renewal. The common etiologic factor in the latter three categories is hypoperfusion of the mucosa. Drugs, such as aspirin, nonsteroidal anti-inflammatory agents, and alcohol, damage the mucosa by decreasing the production of bicarbonate and mucus by the epithelial cells, by increasing mucosal permeability, or both.

Bleeding from erosions associated with drugs or alcohol is usually self-limiting if the offending agent is discontinued. Maintaining gastric pH above 4.0 with the frequent use of antacids or of antacids in combination with H_2-receptor antagonists decreases the frequency of stress ulcer. If bleeding does not stop with hourly administration of antacids, selective infusion of vasopressin into the left gastric artery is associated with cessation of bleeding in over 75 percent of patients. Endoscopic cauterization of erosions is usually impractical because they are so numerous, but if the bleeding seems to be primarily from one or several erosions, cautery should be tried. Surgery should be avoided because the mortality rate is as high as 40 percent. The majority of these deaths are attributable, however, to the underlying disorders that set the stage for "stress ulcers."

Lower Intestinal Tract Bleeding

Most lower intestinal tract hemorrhages cease spontaneously. If not, angiography of the superior and inferior mesenteric arteries not only may identify the source of bleeding but also may provide an opportunity to control the bleeding by infusion of vasoconstrictors such as vasopressin. When active bleeding slows or stops, colonoscopy should be performed in an attempt to locate the site of bleeding. It also provides a means of treating localized lesions such as angiodysplasia, which are usually found in the right colon, with electrocautery or laser.[5] Bleeding associated with diverticula is arterial. If bleeding cannot be controlled by infusion of vasoconstrictors into the mesenteric artery, resection of the segment containing the bleeding diverticulum may be necessary. Unfortunately, in patients with massive lower bowel bleeding requiring surgery, the site of bleeding usually is not established despite the use of all diagnostic procedures. As a consequence, major bowel resection may have to be performed in an attempt to ensure that the bleeding site has been removed.

CHRONIC GASTROINTESTINAL BLEEDING

Chronic gastrointestinal bleeding may be intermittent or continuous. The rate of bleeding may be so slow that there is no visible change in the stools and yet exceed the capacity of iron absorption to maintain body stores. The resultant anemia provides the first indication of gastrointestinal bleeding. The lesions responsible range from the simple, such as hemorrhoids or anal fissures, to the ominous such as carcinoma of the colon.

SITE OF BLEEDING

If the first evidence of chronic gastrointestinal bleeding is blood on the stool, in the toilet bowl, or on the toilet paper, early examination of the patient gives the greatest chance of identifying the source. The first examination should be a rectal examination, followed by standard proctoscopy without preparatory enemas or cathartics. If no mucosal lesion such as colitis is seen, if the patient has seen blood with the passage of a stool, and if stool sampled from the upper part of the rectum or the sigmoid colon is negative for occult blood, the source of bleeding is almost certainly in the anal canal. In these circumstances, bleeding may be demonstrated by leaving a cotton swab in the rectum as the proctoscope is removed and then withdrawing the swab to simulate the passage of a stool. A telltale streak of blood will often appear on the swab. With this information it is easy to locate the source of bleeding by anoscopy. On the other hand, if stool from the rectosigmoid region is positive for blood, the diagnostic approach used for the detection of occult bleeding should be followed.

Because the majority of lesions that cause chronic occult gastrointestinal bleeding are in the colon, either air-contrast barium enema radiography or colonoscopy should be performed if proctoscopy fails to demonstrate an anorectal source of bleeding. Colonoscopy is preferred because it enables the examiner to visualize vascular lesions such as angiodysplasia and, if indicated, to perform endoscopic cautery.

If colonoscopy fails to reveal a source of bleeding, examination of the upper gastrointestinal tract is negative, and the patient continues to have occult blood in the stools, a "bleeder tube" (a mercury-weighted small-caliber tube that is allowed to pass to the cecum) should be used to identify the site of bleeding. The fluid

that has collected in the tube is aspirated every 4 hours and tested for the presence of blood. When the level of bleeding has been identified, contrast material may be injected through the tube to determine whether a gross lesion is present.

Finally, the upper gastrointestinal tract may be the source of chronic bleeding. The common lesions are esophagitis, drug-induced gastritis, and carcinoma of the stomach.

THERAPY

The treatment of chronic gastrointestinal bleeding is the treatment of the primary lesion if one is found. In all patients, particularly elderly ones, in whom no lesion is found, oral iron replacement should be instituted and supplemented by parenteral iron if necessary. In patients with striking anemia and limited cardiovascular reserve, it may be necessary to give transfusions with packed red blood cells.

CARCINOMA OF THE COLON AND RECTUM

Colorectal cancer is the major serious cause of occult blood in the stool (see Chapter 6.23). This malignancy deserves special comment because of (1) its frequency (second only to skin cancer, and second to lung cancer as a cause of death), (2) its potential for cure (although the 5-year survival rate is only 50 to 60 percent, it approaches 90 percent in patients with early tumors confined to the bowel wall), and (3) its precursor, the colonic adenomatous polyp, which antedates the appearance of malignancy by 5 to 15 years. Unlike many other precursor lesions, these polyps are easy to identify and simple to remove in toto. Only half of patients with colorectal cancer reach definitive surgical therapy before the tumor has extended through the bowel wall or metastasized to regional lymph nodes. Moreover, prognosis is dependent on the depth of wall invasion and the presence or absence of lymph node and hepatic metastases The five-year survival rate in those with spread beyond the bowel wall is only 14 percent. To improve these results, more effective screening for colorectal cancer is needed. Seventy-five percent of colorectal cancer occurs in patients over 55 years of age, and 95 percent after age 40 years. In addition, other high-risk groups need to be brought under close surveillance (e.g., patients with ulcerative colitis, familial polyposis, Gardner syndrome, previous polyps or colorectal cancer, a family history of colorectal cancer, or a member of a family with the familial cancer syndrome).[20]

It was hoped that, when first described, carcinoembryonic antigen (CEA), would provide a serologic screening test for colorectal cancer. Although test results are positive in 90 percent of patients with metastatic colorectal cancer, the test is not specific for colonic or malignant disease; on a more practical note, however, results are rarely positive in early disease. The major use of CEA is to follow postsurgical patients for evidence of recurrent tumor.

All patients over the age of 40 years should have a series of three stool specimens examined for occult blood annually. These examinations have been greatly facilitated by the development of Hemoccult slides, on which the specimens can be collected at home and mailed to the physician.

The Hemoccult test relies on the peroxidase activity of hemoglobin to cause a change in the reagent. Many foods (e.g., red meats and such vegetables as radishes, horseradish, cantaloupe, and cauliflower) have peroxidase activity. It is usually recommended that these foods be eliminated from the diet for 3 days before and during stool testing, to avoid false-positive results. When patients with positive Hemoccult test results are examined, 50 percent are found to have neoplastic lesions (12 percent carcinomas, 38 percent adenomatous polyps), if anal causes of bleeding such as hemorrhoids and fissures are excluded.

Patients with positive Hemoccult test results without documented anal bleeding should be evaluated with colonoscopy (colonoscopy is more sensitive than barium enema radiography in detecting colonic neoplasms). In the past, sigmoidoscopy and barium enema radiography usually preceded colonoscopy in the workup of patients with positive Hemoccult test results. Because both the finding of a lesion on sigmoidoscopy or barium enema and the absence of findings on these studies have led to colonoscopy, the workup can be abbreviated by moving directly to colonoscopy.

All patients over the age of 40 years should also be screened yearly with a series of three stool samples for the detection of occult blood and with a digital rectal examination. Further, flexible sigmoidoscopy should be performed every 3 to 5 years. Any polyps encountered should be removed, because most cancers evolve from previously benign adenomatous polyps.

Symptoms suggesting colorectal cancer (e.g., a recent change in bowel habits involving either constipation or diarrhea; a sense of incomplete evacuation; crampy abdominal pain; or anal pain or mass) should also be evaluated for colorectal cancer. First, these patients should undergo sigmoidoscopy, preferably with a flexible sigmoidoscope, which in most cases allows visualization of the rectum, sigmoid, and descending colon, where up to 70 percent of colon cancers are encountered. If polyps are seen, on sigmoidoscopy or barium enema radiography, colonoscopy should be performed to remove the polyps and to look for small cancers or other polyps. If a carcinoma is found, the primary treatment is surgical resection.

The best available evidence indicates that colorectal cancer does not arise de novo but, rather, passes through a stage of adenomatous growth, then epithelial atypia, and finally invasive carcinoma. It has been estimated that of 1000 colonic polyps, only 100 are neoplastic; of these, 10 will be large adenomatous polyps and 2 to 3 will be an invasive carcinoma. Thus it can be seen that there should be ample opportunity to make an early diagnosis of carcinoma if the tools available are used regularly.

REFERENCES

1. Allan R, Dykes P: A study of factors influencing mortality rates from gastrointestinal haemorrhage. Q J Med 45:533, 1976
2. Anderson D: The use of measurement of central venous pressure in the selection of patients with massive gastroduodenal haemorrhage for emergency operation. Scand J Gastroenterol 5:25, 1970
3. Athanasoulis CA, Waltman AC, et al: Angiography: Its contribution to the emergency management of gastrointestinal hemorrhage. Radiol Clin North Am 14:265, 1976
4. Bordley DR, Mushlin AI, et al: Early clinical signs identify low risk patients with acute upper gastrointestinal hemorrhage. JAMA 253:3282, 1985
5. Bosley SJ, Brandt LJ: Vascular ectasia of the colon—1986. Dig Dis Sci 31:265, 1986
6. Cello JP, Gendell JH, et al: Endoscopic sclerotherapy versus portacaval shunt in patients with severe cirrhosis and variceal hemorrhage. N Engl J Med 311:1589, 1984
7. Conn HO: Endoscopic sclerotherapy: An analysis of variants. Hepatology 3:769, 1983
8. Conn HO, Resnick RH, et al: Distal splenorenal shunt vs portal systemic shunt: Current status of a controlled trial. Hepatology 1:151, 1981
9. Fleischer D: Endoscopic therapy of upper gastrointestinal bleeding in humans. Gastroenterology 90:217, 1986
10. Lebrec D, Defleury P, et al: Portal hypertension, size of esophageal varices and risk of gastrointestinal bleeding in alcoholic cirrhosis. Gastroenterology 79:1139, 1980
11. Lebrec D, Poynard T, et al: A randomized controlled study of propranolol for prevention of recurrent gastrointestinal bleeding in patients with cirrhosis: A final report. Hepatology 4:355, 1984
12. Luk GD, Bynum TE, Hendrix TR: Gastric aspiration in localization of gastrointestinal hemorrhage. JAMA 241:576, 1979
13. McLeod IA, Mills PR: Factors identifying probability of further haemorrhage after acute upper gastrointestinal haemorrhage. Br J Surg 69:256, 1982
14. Northfield TC, Smith T: Central venous pressure in clinical management of acute gastrointestinal bleeding. Lancet 2:584, 1970
15. Persing J: Symposium, The National ASGE Survey on Upper Gastroin-

testinal Bleeding. I. Study design and baseline data. II. Clinical prognostic factors. Gastrointestinal Endosc 27:73, 1981

16. Silverstein FE, Feld AD, Gilbert DA: Upper gastrointestinal tract bleeding. Arch Intern Med 141:322, 1981

17. Spechler SJ, Schimmel EM: Gastrointestinal bleeding of unknown origin. Arch Intern Med 142:236, 1982

18. Tudhope GR: The loss and replacement of red cells in patients with acute gastrointestinal hemorrhage. Q J Med 27:543, 1958

19. Welch R, Douglas A, et al: Effect of cimetidine on upper gastrointestinal hemorrhage. Gastroenterology 80:1313, 1981

20. Winawer SJ, Schottenfeld O, Sherlock P: Screening for colorectal cancer: The issues. Gastroenterology 88:841, 1985

CHAPTER 12.5
Diarrhea and Constipation

Theodore M. Bayless, Marvin M. Schuster, and Thomas R. Hendrix

Diarrhea is caused by increased water in the stools. Normally 100 to 150 ml of water is lost in the stools daily, but when the volume of water increases, the stools lose their form and diarrhea results. Increased fluid in the stools can be caused by impaired absorption, increased secretion, or a combination of these factors. In addition, the disorder may involve the small intestine or colon singly or in combination.

PHYSIOLOGY OF INTESTINAL FLUID AND ELECTROLYTE MOVEMENT

The alimentary tract normally is presented with a fluid load of over 10 L per day derived from exogenous sources (dietary) and endogenous sources (salivary, gastric, biliary, pancreatic, and intestinal secretion). In healthy individuals all but 1500 to 2000 ml is absorbed by the time the cecum is reached, and the colon then absorbs all but 100 to 150 ml of the remaining fluid. Since the colon has a limited absorptive capacity, about 2.5 to 4.0 L per day, diarrhea appears if a larger volume is presented to the colon by the small intestine.[8]

The volume of fluid presented to the colon by the small intestine is increased (1) if there is a failure of intestinal absorption, for example, diffuse mucosal disease such as celiac disease, deficiency of a digestive enzyme such as lactase, or ingestion of a nonabsorbable solute such as magnesium sulfate (Epsom salt) or (2) if there is increased fluid secretion (e.g., toxin induced, such as toxigenic *Escherichia coli* or *Vibrio cholerae* infections, or hormone induced, such as vasoactive intestinal peptide [VIP] in pancreatic cholera or prostaglandin in medullary carcinoma of the thyroid). Similarly, the cause of diarrhea may be disordered colonic function such as (1) decreased colonic absorption due to diffuse mucosal disease (e.g., ulcerative colitis, collagenous colitis, or shigellosis) or (2) increased colonic secretion induced either by the entry of unabsorbed bile salts or fatty acids into the colon or caused by a fluid-secreting tumor, such as a villous adenoma.

The content of the intestine at each level has a characteristic composition: jejunum—Na^+ 148, K^+ 5.6, Cl^- 138, HCO_3^- 15 mEq/L; ileum—Na^+ 146, K^+ 5.7, Cl^- 121, HCO_3^- 42 mEq/L; and stool—Na^+ 55, K^+ 90, Cl^- 20, HCO_3^- 7.0 mEq/L. The greatest change in ionic composition occurs during passage through the colon. Since the colon's absorptive capacity is limited, stool electrolyte composition approaches ileal composition as the volume of diarrhea increases.

To design definitive therapy for diarrhea, the physician must determine the site and nature of the intestinal abnormality, as well as the volume and composition of the fluid lost.[2] It is convenient to categorize diarrhea on the basis of the onset and duration of the illness: (1) acute diarrhea with sudden onset and short duration and (2) chronic diarrhea, often with an insidious onset and a long duration.

ACUTE DIARRHEA

Infectious agents (viral, bacterial, or parasitic), toxins, poisons, and drugs are the major causes of acute diarrhea (Table 12.5–1). Enteric infections are discussed in Chapters 9.8, 9.12, and 9.13. Enterotoxins produced by noninvasive bacteria, most often toxigenic *E. coli* (in this country) and viral enteritis, are the most common causes of acute diarrhea. Since simple, specific diagnostic tests for these infections are not generally available, their diagnosis in clinical practice is by exclusion. Acute diarrhea due to infectious proctitis, colitis, or enteritis, encountered in male homosexuals as a sexually transmitted disease, is caused by a variety of organisms, including *Campylobacter* organisms, shigellae, chlamydiae, gonococci, herpes viruses, amebae, and *Giardia* organisms. Opportunistic agents, such as cytomegalovirus (CMV) and *Cryptosporidium*, frequently cause diarrhea in patients with a depressed immune system (e.g., graft-versus-host disease and acquired immunodeficiency syndrome [AIDS]). At times, ulcerative colitis occurs as an acute, fulminant illness. If unnecessary colectomies are to be avoided, it is important to stress that specific, curable infections (e.g., shigellosis, amebiasis, and antibiotic-associated pseudomembranous colitis) can mimic fulminant ulcerative colitis. Other inflammatory causes of acute diarrhea include appendicitis and diverticulitis. Causes of drug- and diet-related diarrhea are listed in Table 12.5–1. Ischemic colitis and partial intestinal obstruction also may result in diarrhea. Psychogenic stress is another important cause of acute diarrhea.

Evaluation
A schema for the evaluation and management of acute diarrhea is outlined in Figure 12.5–1.

Stool Examination. The initial diagnostic procedure should be a Wright stain or methylene blue stain of a fecal smear to determine whether fecal leukocytes are present.[18] In enteric inflammatory disorders, both those caused by specific invasive organisms and idiopathic inflammatory bowel disease, the fecal leukocytes are predominantly polymorphonuclear. In typhoid fever, mononuclear cells predominate. If few leukocytes are seen, the diarrhea is most likely viral or toxigenic. In addition, the stools should be examined for amebae and blood.

Proctoscopy. Proctoscopy should be performed, especially if there is blood in the stool. Direct smear of mucus obtained will reveal the presence of amebae, and biopsy of the mucosa will help to

TABLE 12.5–1. DRUG- AND DIET-RELATED DIARRHEA

Drug
Osmotic overload
- Magnesium-containing antacids
- Lactulose (in treatment of hepatic coma)
- Cathartics

Mucosal injury
- Cancer chemotherapy
- Antibiotic-associated colitis (pseudomembranous colitis—clindamycin, lincomycin, and cephalin most common)
- Colchicine
- Neomycin (causes steatorrhea)

Alteration of motility
- Parasympathomimetic agents
- Thyroid hormone
- Cardiovascular drugs (digitalis, quinidine, ganglionic-blocking drugs)

Diet
Osmotic overload
- Lactose-containing food (in lactase-deficient patients)
- Dumping syndrome
- Elemental diets

Increased secretion or mucosal injury, or both
- Caffeine (secretion)
- Food poisoning
  Bacterial (staphylococci, clostridia, salmonellae, shigellae, *Vibrio parahaemolyticus*)
  Toxin (mushroom, staphylococcus enterotoxin, botulism)
- Fat in patients with steatorrhea
- Heavy metals (mercury, arsenic, cadmium, lead)

determine the nature of the inflammatory process. This examination should be done without enema preparation, because an enema may make it difficult to identify amebae or to culture the causative pathogen and may obscure subtle histologic findings. Gonococci are sometimes found to be the cause of a heavy purulent exudate.

Special Diagnosis. If the history suggests that contaminated food might be the source of the infection, food samples should also be cultured. Enzyme-linked immunosorbent assay (ELISA) and other special techniques for detection of viruses, as well as enterotoxins including *Clostridium difficile* toxin, are discussed in Chapter 9.8.

Therapy
Most acute diarrheal episodes are self-limiting and do not require specific therapy. If, on the other hand, the patient is dehydrated, and especially if vomiting occurs, parenteral fluid replacement with Ringer lactate solution, supplemented with potassium to a total concentration of 15 mEq/L, should be instituted[4] (see Chapter 9.8). Agents that both decrease intestinal peristalsis and to a lesser degree enhance fluid and electrolyte absorption, such as deodorized tincture of opium (DTO), 5 drops after each movement (not more than five doses per day), paregoric, 5 ml after each movement (up to five doses per day), diphenoxylate hydrochloride with atropine sulfate (Lomotil), 2.5 to 5 mg, or loperamide, 2 mg four or five times per day, may be given provided that the diarrhea is not bloody, the patient has no fever, and there is no increase in leukocytes in the stool. Because diarrhea is a defense mechanism to wash away offending organisms, antidiarrheal agents should not be given early in the course of acute infectious diarrhea caused by an invasive organism.

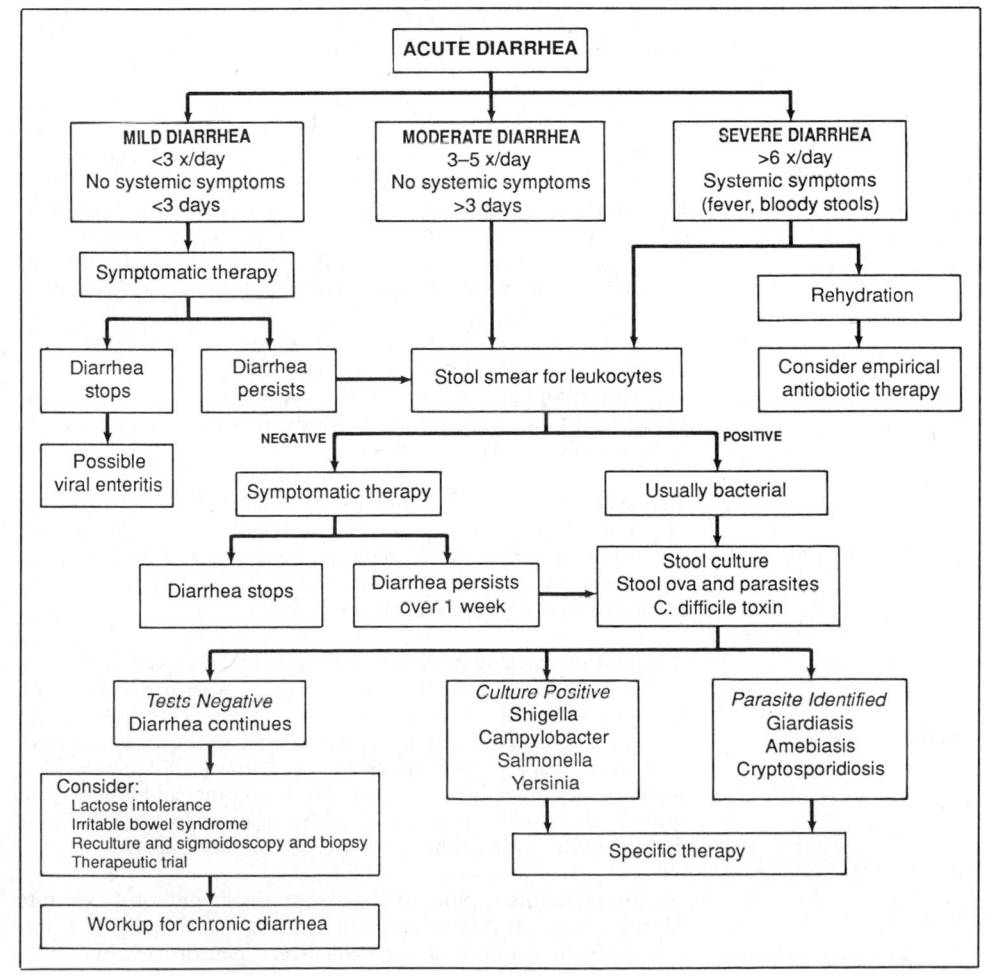

Figure 12.5–1. Evaluation and management of acute diarrhea.

CHRONIC DIARRHEA

Diarrhea that has persisted for several weeks usually requires a detailed diagnostic investigation. A classification of chronic diarrhea based on the predominant pathophysiologic mechanism is presented in Table 12.5–2. In some disorders, such as Crohn disease (regional enteritis), there are a number of physiologic derangements occurring at the same time—for example, increased exudation of fluid and protein as a result of inflammation, decreased absorption, and increased secretion and motility. In others, for example, giardiasis and ''food allergy,'' no satisfactory hypotheses are available. Indications of whether the lesion causing diarrhea is in the small or the large bowel are to be found in the patient's history. Crohn disease of the small bowel and celiac disease are examples of chronic diarrhea originating in the small intestine. Although the material entering the right colon is more voluminous than normal because of impaired small-intestine absorption, the reservoir and absorptive capacity of the colon are still intact and the patient may therefore have only one or two large bowel movements a day. If abdominal discomfort occurs, it is usually worse after meals or just before bowel movement. A barium enema with ileal reflux, a small-bowel series, and screening tests for malabsorption should confirm the clinical suspicion of small-bowel disease. In contrast, ulcerative colitis involving the descending colon and rectum illustrates the clinical findings of large-bowel diarrhea. Inflammation of the rectum lowers the threshold for stimulation by bowel contents, and small amounts of stool produce the urge to defecate. This symptom complex of frequent small stools, urgency, and blood and mucus in the stools points toward large-bowel diarrhea.

Evaluation

The findings from the history and physical examination should provide the basis for planning the search for the cause of chronic diarrhea. There are clinical features that aid in the differential diagnosis of diarrhea. At times, these signs and symptoms may be the presenting problem, and diarrhea may not be a major complaint.

Weight Loss. Weight loss is an important symptom, indicating a serious underlying disease until proved otherwise. Diarrhea and marked weight loss may be caused by the following conditions: (1) those that cause anorexia, (2) those that result in partial intestinal obstruction, with postprandial pain and a resultant decrease in food intake, as in ileal Crohn disease, (3) malabsorption syndromes, and (4) generalized diseases that affect the intestinal tract, such as hyperthyroidsm, Addison disease, diabetes with autonomic neuropathy, lymphoma, leukemia, polyarteritis, systemic lupus erythematosus (SLE), scleroderma, carcinoid syndrome, AIDS, and tuberculosis. Weight loss is not part of irritable bowel syndrome (functional bowel disease).

Malabsorption. The typical patient with intestinal malabsorption has weight loss and bulky, light-colored, greasy, foul-smelling stools. Secondary deficiencies due to the malabsorption of specific substances—such as calcium; iron; vitamins B, D, and K; folic acid; and proteins—and not diarrhea may dominate the clinical picture. Malabsorption should be considered in the differential diagnosis of unexplained weight loss, anemia, or edema even when diarrhea is not a prominent symptom (see Chapter 12.6).

Arthritis. Arthritis may occur in patients with chronic diarrhea but particularly in those with Crohn disease, ulcerative colitis, polyarteritis, SLE, and Whipple disease.

Skin Manifestations. Skin manifestations of diagnostic significance associated with diarrheal diseases include (1) flushing, in the carcinoid syndrome and VIP secreting tumors, (2) hyperpigmentation that spares the mucous membranes, in Whipple disease, (3) generalized pigmentation, in Addison disease, (4) dermatitis, in pellagra, (5) urticaria pigmentosa, with mast-cell tumors, (6) dermatitis herpetiformis, coexisting with celiac disease, (7) erythema nodosum, with Crohn disease or ulcerative colitis, (8) pyoderma gangrenosum, with ulcerative colitis, and (9) dermatomyositis. Glossitis and cheilosis occur most commonly with vitamin deficiencies and malabsorptive states. Clubbing occurs with Crohn disease and cirrhosis. Thrombophlebitis migrans may occur with intra-abdominal malignancies, including carcinoma of the pancreas. Kaposi sarcoma is commonly associated with AIDS.

Fistula or Sinus Tract. A fistula or sinus tract in the lower abdomen or perianal region is a common presentation of Crohn disease, but it may also be seen with tuberculosis and actinomycosis. Peri-intestinal abscesses caused by perforations due to foreign bodies or diverticulitis also produce fistulas on occasion.

Severe Abdominal Pain. Severe abdominal pain preceding the onset of diarrhea occurs with ischemic colitis, with perforation of a gallstone into the intestine, or with a marginal or gastric ulcer forming a gastrocolic fistula. Patients with severe ulcer diathesis associated with the Z–E syndrome (gastrinoma) frequently have diarrhea and may have steatorrhea. Cramping abdominal pain often is the initial symptom of Crohn disease. In fact, only one fifth of adults with Crohn disease have diarrhea initially.

Nocturnal Diarrhea. Nocturnal diarrhea usually indicates a definite organic disease. It may be associated with any severe disorder, but it is especially common in diabetic visceral neuropathy, hyperthy-

TABLE 12.5–2. PATHOPHYSIOLOGIC CLASSIFICATION OF CHRONIC DIARRHEA

Decreased Absorption (see Chapter 12.6)
Small intestine
- Generalized malabsorption
  Mucosal damage (celiac disease, graft-versus-host disease)
  Impaired intraluminal digestion (pancreatic insufficiency)
  Bacterial overgrowth (bile salt deconjugation and mucosal injury–scleroderma)
- Specific malabsorption
  Enzyme deficiency (disaccharidases)
  Transport defect (chloridorrhea, glucose-galactose malabsorption)
  Nonabsorbable solute (magnesium, lactulose)

Colon
- Idiopathic inflammatory bowel disease
  Ulcerative colitis
  Crohn disease
- Specific inflammatory bowel disease
  Amebiasis
  Ischemic colitis
  Radiation colitis

Increased Secretion
Small intestine
- Dumping syndrome
- Gastric hypersecretion (Z-E syndrome)
- Endogenous secretagogues (vasoactive intestinal peptide, prostaglandins, serotonin, etc.)

Colon
- Unabsorbed fatty acids
- Bile acids (failure of ileal reabsorption)
- Unabsorbed carbohydrates (lactase deficiency)
- Fluid secreting tumor (large villous adenoma)

Motor Disturbances (Decreased Mixing Activity)
Small intestine and colon
- Carcinoid syndrome
- Postvagotomy diarrhea
- Hyperthyroidism
- Diabetic visceral neuropathy
- Scleroderma

Colon
- Irritable bowel syndrome

roidism, and ulcerative colitis. It is unusual for the patient with functional diarrhea to be awakened at night by the urge to defecate.

Incontinence. Fecal incontinence can be devastating to a patient's self-esteem and disrupting to social life, so much so that patients often do not bring up the issue unless directly questioned. Incontinence is the result of one or several of the following: (1) loss of anorectal sensation, a factor in diabetic visceral neuropathy, (2) loss of anal sphincter strength, seen as a complication of anal surgery and neuromuscular diseases, and (3) loss of the reservoir capacity of the rectum, as seen in inflammatory disease of the rectum and lesions of the sacral cord or pelvic nerves. Obviously, the presence of diarrhea magnifies the problems of incontinence.

Immune Deficiency Disorders. Diarrhea is a common symptom in patients with hypogammaglobulinemia, graft-versus-host disease, and AIDS. Specific infectious agents are often the cause, and some, but not all, can be treated effectively.

Diagnostic Procedures

Stool Examination. The first step in determining the cause of diarrhea is examination of the stool. Blood, gross or occult, indicates ulceration of the mucosa or a neoplasm. An increase in fecal leukocytes (visualized by Wright or methylene blue stain) also indicates an inflammatory lesion in the colon. Examination for ova and parasites should be performed. Giardiasis has been the most common parasitic cause of diarrhea in this country, but cryptosporidiosis is being found with increasing frequency, especially in the immunocompromised host. If the stools contain fat as indicated by a positive test for split fats (Sudan III stain), malabsorption is the likely cause of the diarrhea[10] (see Chapter 12.6). Finally, if a fecal smear turns red on alkalinization, the patient has been taking phenolphthalein laxatives and the diarrhea may be factitious.

Proctosigmoidoscopy. A proctosigmoidoscopic examination should be performed on every patient with chronic diarrhea before radiographic studies are done. The examination is carried out without an enema preparation because hypertonic cleansing solutions produce edema, hyperemia, and an excessive secretion of mucus that may be mistaken for early ulcerative colitis. Enemas may also wash away the mucus containing amebic trophozoites and decrease the likelihood of seeing these organisms in a smear of rectal mucus or in a rectal biopsy. The use of fiberoptic flexible sigmoidoscopy, although requiring more skill to perform, makes it possible to examine the entire sigmoid colon and usually the descending colon. This extended view is particularly useful in establishing the diagnosis of Crohn disease and evaluating the source of blood in the stool.

The normal rectal mucosa is smooth, translucent, and covered with a thin, shiny layer of mucus, so that the submucosal vessels are clearly visible. Abnormalities range in severity from hyperemia and edema, which obscure the mucosal vascular pattern, to friability (small bleeding points in response to minor trauma such as rubbing with a cotton swab), to frank ulceration. Punched-out ulcers in an inflamed mucosa are more common in Crohn disease than in ulcerative colitis. In ulcerative colitis the ulcers are usually small, superficial, and stellate. Isolated ulcers are also seen in amebiasis and in the solitary rectal ulcer syndrome. Normal rectal mucosa sparing with colitis in the sigmoid colon and above is suggestive of Crohn disease. Finally, irregular ulcers of ischemic colitis sometimes extend down into the rectum. In addition, polyps may be seen that may be adenomas (true neoplasia) or "pseudopolyps." The latter are heaped-up masses of hyperplastic disordered epithelium and inflamed granulation tissue that represent an unsuccessful attempt to repair severe mucosal damage. Pseudomembranes of antibiotic-associated diarrhea appear as characteristic yellow plaques.

Rectal Biopsy. Rectal biopsy is useful (1) as a diagnostic tool in the evaluation of diarrheal diseases, (2) to provide follow-up informa-

tion concerning the activity of inflammatory bowel disease and response to therapy, and (3) to detect dysplasia (a marker of increased risk of colon cancer) in patients with ulcerative colitis.

Rectal biopsy specimens should be taken from any abnormal mucosa and even from normal mucosa in those patients in whom the diagnosis is in doubt, because the findings may give clues to the presence of disease such as Crohn disease, Whipple disease, amyloidosis, schistosomiasis, cystic fibrosis, collagenous colitis, and microscopic colitis.

Tests of Malabsorption. See Chapter 12.6 for a discussion of tests of malabsorption.

Roentgenologic Examination. Roentgenologic examination of the gastrointestinal tract is often helpful in unraveling the puzzle of chronic diarrhea. First, a plain film of the abdomen, without contrast medium, may reveal evidence of large- or small-bowel obstruction, pancreatic calcification, calcified tuberculous lymph nodes, "thumbprint" shadows that indent the air-filled bowel of ischemic bowel disease, or the colonic dilation of fulminant ulcerative colitis.

In most situations it is best to order a barium enema before proceeding with studies of the upper gastrointestinal tract and small bowel. Severe ulcerative colitis and Crohn colitis are exceptions; a barium enema should not be performed until the patient improves, lest toxic megacolon be induced. The barium enema, in addition to filling the entire colon, provides good visualization of the terminal ileum and of gastrocolic fistula. Double-contrast barium enema provides the best radiographic method for demonstrating early epithelial ulceration in inflammatory bowel disease. At times, the postevacuation films from a single contrast study will provide clues to the presence of mucosal disease not suspected on the basis of films of the barium-filled bowel.

An upper gastrointestinal tract series will show those forms of peptic ulcer disease commonly associated with diarrhea, such as the Z-E syndrome and pyloric stenosis. Gastrocolic fistulas or inadvertently created gastroileal fistulas after partial gastrectomy may also be demonstrated. Nodularity of the mucosa of the duodenal bulb may provide a clue to the presence of celiac disease. Gastroduodenal inflammatory changes of Crohn disease although often difficult to distinguish from peptic disease may be associated with nausea, vomiting, early satiety, and weight loss.

A small-bowel study normally reveals delicate intestinal folds, with continuity of the barium column and with no dilated segments. The small-bowel pattern is abnormal in over 90 percent of all patients with intestinal malabsorption due to mucosal involvement, as in celiac disease or tropical sprue (Chapter 12.6). Coarsening of the mucosal pattern is associated with mucosal infiltration (e.g., Crohn disease, Whipple disease, *Myobacterium avian-intercellulare* infection, intestinal lymphangiectasia, amyloidosis, lymphoma) and with villus hypertrophy caused by increased trophic hormones such as those produced by a glucagonoma. Dilution of barium in the small bowel by excessive intestinal secretion is often an important clue to the presence of chronic secretory diarrhea, such as in the pancreatic cholera syndrome.

In Crohn disease, the small-bowel changes may be localized to the terminal ileum, with narrowing of the lumen ("string" sign); affect separate segments, including the jejunum, duodenum, and colon, with narrowing and proximal dilation ("skip" areas); or involve the entire small bowel (ileojejunitis). At times only a small-bowel clysis (introducing the contrast material directly into the duodenum by tube) will give satisfactory delineation of multiple areas of inflammation.

Colonoscopy. Fiberoptic instruments have made it possible to examine visually the entire colonic mucosa and to determine by biopsy the histologic nature of any abnormalities seen. Colonoscopy is particularly helpful in differentiating inflammatory from neoplastic masses. Less frequently, it is used to obtain histologic evidence to support the diagnosis of Crohn disease, when rectal biopsy spec-

imens are normal and barium enema yields inconclusive evidence of abnormality, and to determine the extent of involvement in ulcerative colitis. The usefulness of the information obtained by colonoscopy should be weighed against the small but possible risk of perforation in acute inflammatory bowel disease. Collagenous colitis and microscopic colitis may be unexpected findings in colonic biopsy specimens taken from a normal-appearing colon or areas of mild inflammation in patients with unexplained watery diarrhea.

Stool Volume. Measurement of daily stool volume while the patient is on a regular diet and during a 48-hour fast (fluid intake maintained by intravenous infusion) is helpful in distinguishing endogenous from exogenous secretory stimuli. For example, if diarrhea is caused by an endocrine-secreting tumor, such as a VIP-secreting pancreatic adenoma, fecal volume will not fall significantly when the patient fasts. On the other hand, if diarrhea is caused by some dietary component that is not absorbed, such as lactose or fat, or by a dietary secretagogue such as caffeine, fecal volume will decrease strikingly during the fast.

Unexplained Diarrhea
It would be misleading to suggest that the employment of the diagnostic tests discussed above always leads to a diagnosis. An explanation can be found in only half of the patients referred to a medical center with no detectable cause of diarrhea. The most common examples in this group are microscopic colitis–collagenous colitis, surreptitious laxative use, Crohn disease, giardiasis, cryptosporidiosis, and anal sphincter dysfunction with incontinence.[14]

DIARRHEAL DISEASES

The examples of diarrheal diseases selected for presentation include idiopathic inflammatory bowel diseases, amebiasis, humorally mediated diarrheal syndromes, osmotic gradient–induced diarrhea, and functional diarrhea (Table 12.5–3).

INFLAMMATORY BOWEL DISEASES

Ulcerative Colitis
Ulcerative colitis[6,7] is a chronic inflammatory disease of unknown cause involving the mucosa of the colon.

Although genetic factors may play a role, the cause of the epithelial destruction and mucosal inflammation is unknown. It is unclear whether the damage is in response to some unique agent or material from the lumen of the colon or whether the damage is the consequence of some exaggerated immunologic response of the host to a common stimulus.

Clinical Manifestations. Ulcerative colitis occurs in persons of all ages, including infancy and old age, but the majority of those affected are young adults at the time of onset.

The incidence in family members of patients with ulcerative colitis and in the Jewish population is greater than in the general population, whereas black persons are less frequently affected. In the mildest form, called ulcerative proctitis, only the rectal mucosa is involved. Often the only symptom is blood in the stool that initially is erroneously attributed to hemorrhoids. In this limited form of the disease, inflammation almost never extends to the proximal portion of the colon. At the other extreme, the entire colon has already been irreparably damaged when the patient is first seen, and the damage may progress to life-threatening toxic megacolon with perforation.

The onset of ulcerative colitis may be insidious, with vague abdominal discomfort, anorexia, lassitude, and a gradual change in bowel habits. Rectal bleeding, with or without diarrhea, frequently is the first symptom that brings the patient to the doctor. The majority of patients with ulcerative colitis have frequent small bowel movements containing pus, blood, and mucus mixed with small amounts of fecal material. As rectal involvement progresses, the threshold for stimulation by fecal contents is lowered and the patient experiences urgency and tenesmus. Cramping lower abdominal pain relieved by defecation is a common complaint. One third of the patients have an abrupt onset, with bloody diarrhea, fever, anorexia, and weakness.

In two thirds of the patients, ulcerative colitis is intermittently symptomatic, but in the others the disease is continuously active. In about 5 percent the disease has an extremely rapid and progressive (fulminant) course. Acute fulminant manifestations may develop initially or appear in the course of established disease. Rectal discharge is almost constant, and bleeding may be massive. Fever, hypovolemia, tachycardia, and hypoproteinemia are important findings. Toxic megacolon and colonic perforation are highly lethal complications.

Diagnosis. Ulcerative colitis is a diagnosis of exclusion. When the onset is acute, it is essential to exclude infective colitis caused by shigellae, *Campylobacter* organisms, invasive *E. coli*, *Yersinia* organisms, salmonellae, gonococci, and amebae, as well as antibiotic-associated colitis and ischemic colitis. In the setting of possible

TABLE 12.5–3. DIFFERENTIAL DIAGNOSIS OF COLITIS

	Ulcerative Colitis	Crohn Disease	Amebic Colitis	Ischemic Colitis
Onset	Gradual or abrupt	Gradual	Abrupt or gradual	Abrupt
Symptoms	Rectal bleeding and diarrhea	Diarrhea with little or no bleeding	Diarrhea Streaks of blood	Sudden pain Rectal bleeding
Perianal inflammation	Occasionally	Common; at times presenting symptom	None	None
Proctoscopy	Diffuse with friability	Normal, or focal, discrete ulcers, or diffuse	Diffuse or isolated ulcers	Usually normal
X-ray distribution	Distal, continuous segmental	Right side most frequent, often discontinuous and asymmetric	Sigmoid or cecum	Segmental, splenic flexure often
Ileal involvement	Normal or dilated	Sometimes normal, often narrowed	Normal	Occasionally involved
Pathologic findings	Diffuse involvement of mucosa	Involvement of mucosa, muscularis and serosa with deep fissures	Mucosa and submucosal	Mucosa or transmural
Fistula	None	Common	None	None

sexually transmitted disease, as with homosexual men, syphilis, gonorrhea, *Chlamydia* infection, and herpes are other causes of proctitis that should be considered. Although no single finding is pathognomonic of idiopathic ulcerative colitis, the prime diagnostic procedure is sigmoidoscopy with mucosal biopsy. In mild active ulcerative colitis, the rectal mucosa is hyperemic, edematous, granular, and, characteristically, friable. Small mucosal bleeding points appear when the mucosa is rubbed with a cotton swab. In more severe disease, purulent exudate, spontaneous bleeding, and small superficial ulcerations are seen. Microscopic examination of the exudate for leukocytes, bacteria, and amebae, and culture of the exudate and stools, are essential because the endoscopic findings are nonspecific. An essentially normal mucosa at the time of proctoscopic examination in the presence of severe chronic diarrhea should lead to consideration of Crohn disease or collagenous colitis. The latter disease is especially common in women over age 50.

Rectal biopsy is a useful confirmatory measure.[21] The inflammation and crypt abscesses are characteristic but not specific for ulcerative colitis. The crypt abscess begins with infiltration of the crypt epithelium with neutrophils that spill into the crypt as the epithelium is destroyed. The lamina propria is densely infiltrated with acute and chronic inflammatory cells. As the crypts are destroyed, normal mucosal architecture is lost. Scarring leads to shortening and narrowing of the colon. Histologic features suggestive of Crohn disease (focal inflammation, the presence of granulomas, or both), ischemic colitis, antibiotic-induced pseudomembranous colitis, amebiasis, schistosomiasis, tuberculosis, and lymphogranuloma venereum should be looked for, because these diseases may sometimes have the same clinical picture as ulcerative colitis.

A barium enema is not required to make the diagnosis of ulcerative colitis and should not be done in acutely ill patients, lest toxic megacolon be induced. It does, however, indicate the extent of the disease and is useful in determining the prognosis. Careful review of an abdominal film occasionally provides an indication as to the extent of the colitis.

The air-contrast barium enema will result in abnormal findings in almost all patients with ulcerative colitis except those with ulcerative proctitis or disease limited to the rectosigmoid colon. Early changes include granularity and blurring of the bowel margins in the distal portion of the colon and obliteration of haustral folds. As the disease progresses, ulcerations appear and are seen on double-contrast barium enema radiographs as fine serrations and irregularities along the colon wall. If destruction of the mucosa is severe, the islands of remaining mucosa appear as pseudopolyps. With scarring there is a shortening and narrowing of the bowel, with the further loss of haustra. The involvement of the colon in ulcerative colitis is continuous from the rectum proximally, whereas in Crohn disease it may be segmental. The smooth colon without haustral folds, characteristic of chronic ulcerative colitis, may be simulated by the changes produced by chronic purgation with laxatives.

Treatment. Medical therapy is usually effective in suppressing disease activity in ulcerative colitis, but less than 5 percent of patients are "cured," or have no recurrences. Colectomy with an ileostomy, a continent ileostomy (a Koch pouch), or an ileal pouch with anal anastomosis is eventually required in about 20 percent of these patients. Adrenal corticosteroids and sulfasalazine (Azulfidine) are the mainstays of medical treatment. The aim of therapy is to produce and maintain a symptomatic remission. This is best accomplished by starting the patient on a regimen of full doses of steroids (60 mg prednisone per day) and tapering to a maintenance dose (15 to 30 mg on alternate days) when the desired clinical response is achieved. Sulfasalazine, a combination of sulfapyridine and salicylic acid (3 g per day orally), is used as an adjunct in the treatment of active disease and for maintaining a remission. If the patient is allergic to the sulfapyridine portion of the sulfasalazine, desensitization or use of oral 5-aminosalicylic acid will be helpful.

In ulcerative proctitis and mild disease localized to the rectum

and sigmoid colon, local administration of hydrocortisone, 100 mg, in the form of small retention enemas at night is often effective. A new rapidly metabolized steroid, tixocortal pivalate, administered as an enema produces equal local anti-inflammatory action without systemic steroid effects. Sulfasalazine may be given as an enema in the treatment of ulcerative proctitis. Its effect is believed to be due to the release by bacterial action of 5-aminosalicylate, which decreases the local release of prostaglandins and leukotrienes. Early experience with 5-aminosalicylate enemas indicates their usefulness in the treatment of proctitis that is resistant to other forms of treatment as well as in untreated proctitis.

The establishment of a strong patient-physician relationship is an important part of the long-term treatment of ulcerative colitis. The National Foundation for Ileitis and Colitis provides helpful patient-education materials through its national office, as well as hospital visitors and patient-support programs through its local chapters.

Fulminant ulcerative colitis requires intensive care in the hospital. The initial therapy is directed at correcting the large fluid and electrolyte losses that result from severe diarrhea. Parenterally administered hydrocortisone, 300 mg/day, or adrenocorticotropic hormone (ACTH) is usually effective. If toxic dilation of the colon appears, these same measures are used, plus parenteral feedings, intestinal aspiration by tube, use of antibiotics, avoidance of narcotics, and careful observation for signs of impending perforation. If the patient with severe fulminant colitis has not improved within 48 hours, total colectomy with ileostomy should be performed. The surgical mortality rate with an urgent operation is about 7 percent, whereas it is over 20 percent if a perforation occurs.

Surgery cures ulcerative colitis. In all but exceptional cases, the procedure should be either total colectomy with ileostomy or one of the recently developed ileostomy alternatives, the continent ileostomy (Koch pouch) or the rectal mucosal stripping with ileal pull-through and ileoanal anastomosis. When colectomy is done as an elective procedure, the mortality rate is about 1 percent. The indications for this procedure include (1) failure to respond to medical therapy, (2) life-threatening complications, such as toxic megacolon, impending perforation, bleeding, chronic malnutrition, and, in children, growth failure, (3) severe extracolonic complications, persistent and incapacitating arthritis, progressive ocular disease, progressive hepatobiliary dysfunction, or unresponsive pyoderma gangrenosum (the effect on skin and hepatobiliary complications are unpredictable), (4) strictures of the colon or extensive perirectal complications, and (5) high-grade dysplasia, widespread dysplasia, or dysplasia overlying a mass or stricture and carcinoma itself. The aim of therapy is to have the patient live a full and active life. If this cannot be accomplished by medical measures, then surgery should be employed. The use of well-fitted appliances and disposable bags has lessened the burden of self-care of an ileostomy. Many patients have found ostomy societies helpful in their adjustment to the inconvenience and psychologic problems associated with an ileostomy. "Continent ileostomies," which free the patient of the necessity of wearing an ileostomy appliance, provide an alternative to help some patients accept an indicated colectomy. The bowel is evacuated by inserting a catheter into the stoma periodically. With an ileoanal anastomosis, the patient must retrain his bowel to develop continence and an acceptable frequency of bowel movements.

Complications. The incidence of carcinoma of the colon not only is increased in ulcerative colitis but also occurs at a younger age (average, 40 years) than in the general population (average, 60 years). Factors associated with a high incidence of carcinoma of the colon are (1) involvement of the entire colon, (2) long duration, even if inactive, and (3) dysplasia in colonic biopsies. The risk of developing a carcinoma is not significantly greater than in age-matched control subjects in the first 5 years of the disease, but by the time the patient with pancolitis has had the disease for 15 years, the incidence may be as high as 1 in 25. Only 3 to 5 percent of all patients with ulcerative colitis including ulcerative proctitis

will develop colon cancer as a consequence of their colitis. This risk is more than 10 times that of the general population. Regular follow-up rectal and colonscopic biopsies with particular attention to dysplastic changes are useful in identifying those patients destined to develop carcinoma of the colon. Patients with dyplasia are advised to have a colectomy.[21]

The *extracolonic complications* of ulcerative colitis are varied and may be severe. In general, they occur when the colitis is active. *Skin lesions* are occasionally seen, including pustules, erythema multiforme, erythema nodosum, and pyoderma gangrenosum. *Arthritis* may affect either large or small joints, but it is especially likely to involve the knees and ankles. There is also an increased incidence of rheumatoid spondylitis in patients with ulcerative colitis, and spine changes may precede the recognized onset of colonic disease. *Ocular complications,* such as iritis, conjunctivitis, and uveitis, infrequently appear and usually coincide with colonic, skin, or joint disease activity.

Liver involvement in ulcerative colitis may take several forms. Mild diffuse fatty change is frequent but usually without clinical effect. Hepatitis, chronic active hepatitis, postnecrotic cirrhosis, biliary cirrhosis, sclerosing cholangitis, and bile duct cancer have been described in association with ulcerative colitis. The latter two complications have occurred even after the diseased colon has been removed by colectomy. Intermittent fever, liver tenderness, and elevation of the serum alkaline phosphatase concentration have been attributed to pericholangitis, possibly resulting from bacterial drainage from the colon. This hepatic disease may be related to sclerosing cholangitis. The effect of colectomy on the course of sclerosing cholangitis is unpredictable but not often helpful (see Chapter 13.2). Liver transplantation has been successful in a number of patients with sclerosing cholangitis and inflammatory bowel disease.

Prognosis. Eighty-eight percent of the patients with ulcerative colitis have at least one subsequent attack during the 5 years after the initial episode. The severity of the first attack and the extent of involvement influence both the short-term and the long-term prognosis. Eighty percent of patients with ulcerative proctitis can expect a benign recurrent course, usually responsive to local medication and without increased risk of colon cancer. Ten percent are unresponsive to topical corticosteroids and sulfasalazine therapy but respond to topical 5-aminosalicylate. Long-term treatment is required however. Another 10 percent develop more extensive ulcerative colitis, usually within the first or second year of illness. Among patients with left-sided or pancolitis, 70 percent run an acute intermittent course that often can be kept in remission with a long-term regimen of sulfasalazine, low-dose, alternate-day corticosteroids, or both. About 20 percent of patients with extensive ulcerative colitis have chronic unremitting disease activity that eventually requires colectomy. The mortality rate has continued to decrease with the use of steroid therapy, earlier surgery for severe and fulminant disease, and, more recently, surveillance for dysplasia to decrease the deaths from cancer of the colon.

Crohn Disease[7]

Crohn disease (also called regional enteritis, regional ileitis, or granulomatous colitis) is an inflammatory disease of unknown cause most commonly affecting the terminal ileum or colon, but it can involve any part of the gastrointestinal tract, from the mouth to the rectum. It is a chronic, recurrent illness affecting adolescents and young adults, with abdominal cramps, diarrhea, loss of weight, fever, anemia, right lower quadrant abdominal mass, and perianal fistulas as the most common symptoms. As with ulcerative colitis, there appears to be a high familial incidence of Crohn disease, and its occurrence in the Jewish population is greater than expected by chance.

Pathology. The gross pathologic changes are limited to the terminal portion of the ileum in one third of the patients. Several sharply demarcated "skip" areas separated by normal bowel occur in the others. Involvement of the proximal part of the colon and the terminal part of the ileum occurs in about 40 percent of the patients. Isolated lesions of the duodenum or stomach are much less common. In addition, Crohn disease may involve only the colon in 15 percent of cases. The colonic lesions are often segmental and sometimes spare the rectum. The differential diagnostic features of Crohn disease and ulcerative colitis are listed in Table 12.5–3. About 10 percent of chronic inflammatory bowel disease restricted to the colon cannot be clearly classified as either ulcerative colitis or Crohn disease and hence is called "indeterminate."

On gross examination, the involved intestine is thickened in Crohn disease. The mesentery contains numerous hyperplastic lymph nodes and is also thickened, with mesenteric fat extending up over the bowel. The lumen is narrowed and the mucosa is ulcerated with intervening edematous areas, causing a cobblestone appearance. The microscopic pathologic changes include focal mucosal inflammation and ulceration, with chronic inflammation extending through all layers of the bowel. Noncaseating granulomas (hard tubercles) can be found in 30 to 50 percent of the resected specimens. Deep fissures extend into the areas of inflammation and can lead to fistulas. Histologic alterations including focal inflammatory reactions are commonly found in areas of the bowel that appear normal on gross examination. This widespread involvement with microscopic disease may account, in part, for the high rate of recurrence in Crohn disease after surgical resection of all grossly apparent disease. In later stages, scarring leads to strictures, especially in the small intestine. It takes about 8 to 10 years of disease activity in the small bowel to produce a fixed, scarred obstruction requiring surgery.

Fistulas develop through fissures in the thickened bowel and often originate in the proximal portion of a stenotic area, thus decompressing the obstructed bowel.

No unified hypothesis is available to explain the pathogenesis of Crohn disease and its characteristic inflammatory pattern. It has been suggested that an infectious agent from the lumen initiates the disease in individuals with an unusual inflammatory response. Unexplained, however, are the segmental distribution of the inflammatory process, its predilection for the terminal part of the ileum and right colon, and the frequency of perianal disease.

Clinical Manifestations. The disease usually begins in the teens and twenties, with over 10 percent appearing before age 15 years, 50 percent beginning in the third decade, and over 90 percent before age 40 years. An insidious onset and a long course before a specific diagnosis is made are characteristic, the average duration of symptoms before diagnosis being 2½ years.

Another feature of the disease is the variation in the clinical picture. In the early phase, patients with ileal involvement may notice a gradual decrease in their sense of well-being and a vague, cramping abdominal pain. The discomfort, which is caused by partial obstruction of the small bowel, may be localized to the periumbilical area or to the right lower quadrant of the abdomen. It often occurs 1 or 2 hours after meals, may be preceded by audible bowel sounds, and may be relieved by defecation or vomiting. Because of anorexia, nausea, or the fear of abdominal cramps, food intake is decreased, and weight loss almost invariably results. In prepubescent adolescents a decrease in growth rate occurs in over three fourths of patients and may precede the appearance of intestinal symptoms by 1 to 2 years. In small-bowel Crohn disease, there is usually some moderate increase in the number of bowel movements, rarely over five per day, and stools become soft and unformed. As many as one fifth of the patients with ileal disease deny having diarrhea, and thus the intestinal origin of the disease remains obscure until other manifestations appear. An unexplained low-grade fever may be the only objective evidence of disease for many months. Some patients have iron deficiency anemia and occult blood in the stool. In a 20-year follow-up study of patients originally evaluated because of fever of undetermined origin, Crohn disease was the second most common final diagnosis. In children, since fever and arthralgia are often the presenting symp-

toms, many are initially thought to have rheumatic fever or juvenile rheumatoid arthritis.

Rectal bleeding and diarrhea are symptoms of Crohn colitis. Gross hemorrhage is rare, however. The colonic involvement may be segmental or diffuse and in the latter may be difficult to distinguish from ulcerative colitis.

Complications of Crohn Disease. The complications of Crohn disease often bring the patient to medical attention. At least half the patients form fistulas—internal, perianal, vaginal, vesical, or cutaneous through an appendectomy or laparotomy scar. On the other hand, free perforation is rare. These fistulas may make their appearance as abscesses or tender masses. Toxic megacolon may complicate the course of Crohn disease involving the colon, especially in adolescents.

Extensive ileal involvement or lengthy resections will produce impaired ileal absorption of bile salts and depletion of the bile salt pool with resultant steatorrhea. Malabsorption may also be produced by bacterial overgrowth in patients with Crohn disease. The frequency of oxalate renal calculi due to hyperoxaluria, gallstones, and vitamin B_{12} deficiency has been found to be increased. Arthritis and ankylosing spondylitis occasionally occur. Eye manifestations include iritis and episcleritis. Erythema nodosum is not uncommon with colonic involvement. Patients with perianal abscesses or fistulas should always be examined for the possibility of Crohn disease.[5]

Diagnosis. The diagnosis of Crohn disease is made on the basis of the combination of clinical, radiologic, and pathologic findings, and confidence in the diagnosis is strengthened as the patient's course is followed. In any patient with suspected Crohn disease, flexible sigmoidoscopy and colorectal biopsies should be performed. Often on histologic examination, suggestive abnormalities consisting of focal inflammation or even granulomas will be found even though no gross findings were encountered. A barium enema radiograph can demonstrate the right colon and the terminal part of the ileum, the areas most frequently involved in Crohn disease. The loss of mucosal detail and cobblestone filling defects and aphthous ulcers may be seen. The ileal lumen may be narrowed by spasm or scarring, producing the classic "string" sign. In acutely ill patients or in those with a suspected abscess in whom preparation for barium enema radiography may seem unwise, a small-bowel series with colon follow-through will usually provide adequate information for making diagnostic and therapeutic decisions. Small-bowel radiography demonstrates the proximal extent of disease, "skip" areas, and stenosis and dilation indicating a partial obstruction. The abdominal CT scan is an excellent way to look for intra-abdominal abscesses and fistulas.

Other diseases having the distribution of Crohn disease include ileal or ileocecal tuberculosis, yersinosis, lymphoma, carcinoid tumors, actinomycosis, carcinomas of the cecum, and amebic involvement of the cecum. In tuberculosis the cecum is usually fibrotic and narrowed. In about half of the patients, there is evidence of pulmonary tuberculosis. Typical calcified abdominal nodes are seen in a small percentage of cases with intestinal tuberculosis. Culture and histologic studies should be performed on colonoscopic biopsy specimens and on material from fistulae, if present, to rule out tuberculosis and actinomycosis. When a positive tuberculin skin test and other clinical features make tuberculosis a possibility, treatment with antituberculosis drugs may be desirable. At times, a laparotomy is necessary to establish a diagnosis before therapy is undertaken.

Treatment.[9,20] The aims of therapy should be to suppress active inflammatory disease with medical treatment and to try to conserve the small bowel by reserving surgery for the complications of fistulas and abscesses and for a "fresh start" in patients with obstruction.

Adrenocortical steroids (prednisone, 40 to 60 mg per day) in combination with sulfasalazine, 3 g/day, or antibiotics produce symptomatic improvement in the majority of patients treated during the first few years of their disease. Patients with predominantly ileal involvement are the most responsive. If there are deep fissures in the involved bowel, an antibiotic such as metronidazole or tetracycline is added. Symptoms such as fever, anorexia, crampy pain, and abdominal tenderness should abate. As soon as clinical improvement is apparent, the steroids are tapered over a 2- to 3-month period to a maintenance dose of 20 to 30 mg every other day. If symptoms do not respond promptly, the presence of an obstruction or abscess or an error in diagnosis must be carefully considered. Patients who require anti-inflammatory therapy, but who cannot tolerate steroids because of side effects or have failed to respond, sometimes respond to azathioprine or 6-mercaptopurine, 1 to 1.5 mg/kg per day) or metronidazole, 250 mg four times a day. Extensive colonic disease is less predictable and may be less responsive to steroid therapy. Metroidazole and azathioprine or 6-mercaptopurine have been useful in colonic Crohn disease and poorly responsive small-bowel disease. "Bowel rest" with total parenteral nutrition may help obtain a remission in Crohn colitis, in the 6 to 8 weeks that may be required for an immunosuppressive agent to have an effect. With small bowel Crohn disease, elemental diets have been useful by providing temporary relief while medical therapy is being instituted.

If there is obstruction caused by a fibrotic, stenotic segment, little relief can be expected from steroids. Forty to sixty percent of patients with ileal Crohn disease will require surgery during the first 10 years after the onset of symptoms, most frequently between 6 and 8 years. Surgery is employed for the complications of Crohn disease in the fibrotic stage: obstruction, abscess, and fistula. Crohn disease tends to recur after surgery—at a rate of 50 to 80 percent in some series with ileal disease—and over a 10-year period 40 to 50 percent of the patients will require a second operation. Abscesses require drainage, but it is wise to delay the definitive resection of the involved bowel or of fistulous tracts until the inflammatory reaction is controlled.

Intravenous hyperalimentation or enteral feedings with elemental diets have been useful in preparing seriously ill patients for surgery by improving nutrition and by putting the bowel at "rest" so that the inflammatory process may subside. In some patients, fistulas have closed, particularly if the bowel was not deformed by fibrosis; in some with colonic disease or uncomplicated obstruction, improvement was so striking that surgery has been postponed indefinitely. If a surgical resection is performed while the disease is clinically active, the early recurrence rate approaches 50 percent.

AMEBIASIS

Infestation with *Entamoeba histolytica* may cause an asymptomatic carrier state, chronic mild diarrhea, or acute diarrhea if the infestation is heavy or if the patient is malnourished and debilitated. Amebiasis has become an important sexually transmitted disease in homosexual men.

The typical proctoscopic findings in amebic colitis are irregular, punched-out ulcers with relatively normal mucosa between the ulcerations. Rectal involvement may not be distinguishable from ulcerative colitis, Crohn disease, shigellosis, or *Campylobacter* infections, but the uncertainty should be resolved by rectal biopsy.

Results of serologic tests (hemagglutination) are usually positive in the presence of tissue invasion and approach 100 percent with extracolonic disease such as liver abscess (see Chapters 9.8 and 9.13).

HUMORALLY MEDIATED SECRETORY DIARRHEAL SYNDROMES

An uncommon but important cause of chronic secretory diarrhea is hormone-producing tumors. The release of these secretagogues is not under normal physiologic control and hence is uninfluenced

by meals or fasting. In these disorders, diarrhea, usually over 1 L per day, continues unabated when oral intake is eliminated and fluid intake is provided via the intravenous route. The stool osmolality is approximately equal to that of plasma and is accounted for by the normal ionic constituents. In secretory diarrhea the sum of the concentration of sodium and potassium in the stool multiplied by 2 approximates the osmolality of the stool.[8] Except for Z-E syndrome (which is characterized by peptic ulcer), there is no histologic alteration in the gastrointestinal mucosa and hence no blood, leukocytes, or fat in the stool.

Non-Gastrin-Secreting Adenomas of Pancreas

These tumors have been associated with massive watery diarrhea and hypokalemia. The terms "pancreatic cholera," "watery diarrhea syndrome," "WDHA syndrome" (watery diarrhea, hypokalemia, achlorhydria), "Verner-Morrison syndrome," and "VIP oma" have been applied to this disorder. Decreased gastric acid secretion, flushing, hypercalcemia, and hyperglycemia are encountered in some patients. Vasoactive intestinal peptide (VIP) has been isolated from some of these tumors and is believed to account for the diarrhea by activation of intestinal adenylate cyclase. In others, prostaglandins seem to be the secretory agents. These tumors usually originate in the pancreas but also are found in the duodenum or stomach. Ganglioneuromas, ganglioneuroblastomas, and bronchogenic carcinoma also can secrete VIP and other intestinal secretagogues, and produce this syndrome. If the tumor can be completely resected, diarrhea disappears. Unfortunately, complete resection often is not possible, in which case antitumor chemotherapy with agents such as streptozocin may provide temporary control. Medical therapy is also directed at lessening fluid secretion. A variety of agents, for example, clonidine, adrenocorticosteroids, nicotinic acid, indomethacin, somatostatin analog, and lithium carbonate, have been helpful in some patients.

Medullary Carcinoma of Thyroid

Medullary carcinoma of the thyroid with metastasis is commonly associated with watery diarrhea. The diarrhea decreases with resection of large amounts of tumor tissue, suggesting the presence of a humoral agent. These tumors are sometimes associated with an overproduction of prostaglandins, whereas others have high calcitonin or VIP content.[12] If resection fails to control the diarrhea, the treatment listed earlier for pancreatic cholera should be tried.

Malignant Carcinoid Syndrome

Malignant carcinoid syndrome is frequently associated with diarrhea. These patients have increased blood levels of both serotonin and bradykinin. Serotonin increases smooth muscle contractions and intestinal motility and stimulates intestinal secretion. The diarrhea can usually be controlled by serotonin antagonists such as methysergide, cyproheptadine, or ketanserine, a selective 5-HT antagonist. Recently the inhibitory neural peptide somatostatin has been reported to be effective in patients with carcinoid and watery diarrhea.

Gastrin-Secreting Adenomas of Pancreas

Diarrhea or steatorrhea occurs in one third of patients with the Z-E syndrome. The mechanisms for diarrhea include the cathartic effects of excessive gastric secretion, acid inactivation of pancreatic enzymes, acid-induced mucosal damage, and increased fluid and electrolyte secretion by the pancreas and small bowel. Patients or family members may have other endocrine adenomas. Histamine-2-receptor antagonists such as cimetidine or ranitidine, total gastrectomy, or removal of the tumor, if solitary, will control the diarrhea. The most effective control, however, is achieved by an investigational drug, omeprazole, which blocks H^+/K^+ ATPase, the element responsible for the final step in acid secretion by the stomach. A highly selective vagotomy (parietal cell vagotomy) performed at the time of laparotomy seeking a solitary gastronoma has helped lessen the need for high dose antisecretory agents.

OSMOTIC GRADIENT–INDUCED DIARRHEA

Osmotic gradient–induced diarrhea is caused by the ingestion of a poorly absorbed solute. Impaired absorption of the solute may be due to (1) a deficiency of a digestive enzyme (e.g., lactase deficiency), (2) absence of a transport protein (e.g., glucose-galactose malabsorption), (3) generalized malabsorption with impaired absorption of all solutes (e.g., celiac disease), or (4) divalent ions (e.g., the saline cathartic $MgSO_4$). Because the bowel contents are iso-osmotic to plasma, and because water moves only in response to solute movement, water will be retained in the intestinal lumen whenever a nonabsorbable solute is present.

Lactase Deficiency and Milk Intolerance

Some otherwise healthy people experience gastrointestinal symptoms after drinking milk despite the fact that they drank milk without difficulty as children. One to four hours after consuming one or two glassfuls, they have abdominal bloating, cramps, and even diarrhea, although they can tolerate small amounts of milk as used in cooking or with cereal or coffee. This milk intolerance is caused by low levels of lactase, the brush-border enzyme that hydrolyzes lactose into its absorbable subunits, glucose and galactose. As a consequence, the unabsorbed lactose holds fluid in the small intestine. When this sugar reaches the colon, it is rapidly metabolized to lactic acid and other short-chain volatile acids with the release of carbon dioxide and hydrogen, which can be detected as a rise in breath hydrogen.[17]

Intestinal lactase falls to low levels in all mammalian species after weaning. This also occurs in most ethnic groups of man. Lactose intolerance is found in 2 to 8 percent of adults of Scandinavian or Western European extraction, whereas the prevalence is 70 to 100 percent in adult American Indians, African Bantus, Japanese, Thais, Filipinos, American black persons, Greek Cypriots, Arabs, and Ashkenazi Jews. Most of these lactose-intolerant people drink little or no milk, although they can use milk in a fermented form, such as cheeses and yogurt, without symptoms. In these foods the bulk of the lactose has been converted to lactic acid in preparation, or, in the case of yogurt, bacterial lactases pass through the stomach without losing activity and complete lactose hydrolysis in the small intestine. In addition to this genetically determined, acquired lactase deficiency, any patient with a disease that produces diffuse mucosal damage, for example, celiac disease or tropical sprue, may acquire clinically significant lactase deficiency that is reversible if the mucosal lesion heals. Finally, congenital lactase deficiency is encountered rarely in infancy.

Milk intolerance should be suspected if symptoms appear when milk intake is increased and in patients with unexplained abdominal distension, cramps, or diarrhea. It can be a contributing factor to the symptoms of patients with inflammatory bowel disease, malabsorption syndromes, postgastrectomy dumping syndrome, and the irritable bowel syndrome. Milk intolerance is assumed to be due to lactose intolerance if the patient develops symptoms after receiving 50 g of lactose in a tolerance test and improves on a low lactose diet. Inadequate hydrolysis of lactose can be documented (1) by a failure of the blood glucose level to rise during the tolerance test, (2) by a rise in breath hydrogen concentration after lactose ingestion, which is produced when the anaerobic bacterial flora of the colon metabolizes the unabsorbed lactose delivered from the small intestine, or (3) by demonstrating low levels of lactase in intestinal mucosa biopsy specimens. A patient administered tolerance test with two glasses of skim milk is sufficient to determine whether lactose-containing foods can be blamed for some of the patient's symptoms.

Treatment consists of decreasing the intake of milk and ice cream to amounts that can be tolerated without symptoms, using fermented dairy products, or adding a source of lactase to hydrolyze the lactose in milk before it is drunk. Yogurt and lactose-hydrolyzed milk are available commercially.

Other Carbohydrate Intolerances

Sucrose intolerance due to sucrase deficiency is a rarely encountered disorder with symptoms similar to those of lactose intolerance.

Fructose, now the major sweetener in soft drinks, is not well absorbed in man when used in large amounts. Excess fructose ingestion should be considered in patients with diarrhea, bloating, and flatulence who are ingesting apple juice, grapes, honey, or "soft drinks." Similarly, *sorbital,* the poorly absorbed carbohydrate used in dietetic gum and mints, may cause bloating or a laxative effect. Wheat starch is hydrolyzed less well than rice starch. Ingestion of large amounts of wheat products produces increased flatulence in many individuals. Finally, there is some evidence that older individuals have a decreased capacity to hydrolyze and absorb carbohydrates.[13]

FUNCTIONAL DIARRHEA

Functional diarrhea, unlike irritable bowel syndrome, is painless and can be looked on as an accentuation and a prolongation of the normal responses of the colon to stimuli such as emotional stress and meals. Unlike the diarrhea of irritable bowel syndrome, which occurs in association with long periods of life stress, functional diarrhea is more intimately associated with a stressful episode, such as a final examination, a court trial, or an oral presentation. In patients who are chronically anxious or in circumstances that are chronically stressful, diarrhea may occur daily.

Typically this type of diarrhea is manifested by the urgent passage of soft, watery stools, usually after meals or during periods of stress. The frequency of bowel movements may vary from three or fewer stools per day (which falls within the normal limits for the general population) to six or more per day. The total daily fecal output, however, does not exceed the normal limits of 200 g/day. Rapid transit through the small intestine and the inability of the colon to accommodate and absorb volumes that normal colons can handle are believed to be important factors in the pathogenesis of this disorder.[1]

Some patients benefit from hydrophylic colloids, which bind water and solidify stools, whereas others are helped by anticholinergic drugs, such as dicyclomine hydrochloride (Bentyl) or, in resistant cases, antidiarrheal agents such as diphenoxylate or loperamide. Anticholinergic or antidiarrheal drugs should be taken orally 30 minutes to 1 hour before anticipated diarrhea to allow the drug time to achieve effective blood levels.

CONSTIPATION

It is clinically useful to divide patients with constipation into the following types: (1) those with imaginary constipation, (2) those with spastic constipation, (3) those with hypotonic constipation or colonic inertia, and (4) those with dyschezia. In the first category are those patients whose stools appear normal by ordinary standards and yet who are concerned because their bowel movements do not measure up to their expectations.

The second category is composed predominantly of patients with irritable bowel syndrome (see Chapter 12.2) who have abdominal pain in addition to constipation, but it also includes a small number of people with painless constipation. These patients pass small, hard stools with effort and experience a sense of incomplete evacuation. It is thought that sigmoid spasm delays the passage of fecal material from the colon to the rectum for evacuation.

The third category consists of patients with a motility disturbance that results in stasis of stool throughout most or all of the colon. Plain films of the abdomen show stool filling the colon. The stool in the rectum is usually soft. This type of constipation can be documented by demonstrating the delayed passage through the colon of small radiopaque pellets swallowed by the patient and followed through the colon with serial plain radiographs of the abdomen.[19]

Treatment of this type of constipation is difficult. Because stools are already large and soft, bulk agents are rarely helpful. Treatment relies, instead, predominantly on colonic stimulation with agents such as senna capsules and bisacodyl in association with exercise (particularly the toning up of the extra-abdominal musculature), adequate fluid intake, and bowel training. Training consists of reinforcing a gastrocolic response by asking the patient to attempt to have a movement after either breakfast or supper, depending on his or her previous bowel habits. The patient is asked to attempt evacuation within 10 minutes of that meal and to try for 10 minutes to evacuate the bowel. If unsuccessful in 1 or 2 days, patients may initially need an assist with a suppository (glycerin preferably or bisacodyl) or an enema to initiate the movement. The goal is to condition the colon to empty itself in response to a particular meal each day. The success of this program correlates more with the age of the patient than with the duration of constipation. Young people who have been constipated for many years generally have better success than do elderly persons who have been constipated for shorter periods. Attempts should be made to wean the patients gradually from reliance on laxatives, suppositories, or enemas, but sometimes this may not be possible.

"Dyschezia," the term used to describe the fourth category of constipation, refers to difficulty in evacuation of stool from the rectum.[11] In dyschezia the radiopaque markers discussed above aggregate in the rectal area. In these patients, rectal evacuation is prevented by paradoxical contractions of the external sphincter during attempts to evacuate. Normally, the external sphincter relaxes during voluntary defecation. Biofeedback training directed at teaching patients to relax the sphincter during these efforts is often successful in managing this type of constipation.[15]

It is not known how this paradoxical response originates, although in some instances it appears to be related to a previous history of painful anal conditions such as fissures or hemorrhoids. In other instances, dyschezia is associated with anatomic abnormalities such as rectocele, rectal prolapse, or an accentuation of puborectalis contraction. A rectocele (herniation of the rectal wall anteriorly) is more likely to occur in women than in men. It can be demonstrated by defecatory proctogram, in which about 150 ml of barium is used to outline the rectum while the patient is performing defecatory maneuvers. After instillation of the barium, the patient attempts to evacuate in a sitting position during fluoroscopy so that the rectal defect can be seen to protrude into the vagina.

Defecatory proctography can also demonstrate an accentuation of the puborectalis muscle protruding into the anterior part of the rectum and the failure of this muscle to relax during defecation, thus preventing the straightening of the rectum that occurs during normal defecation.

Internal intussusception of rectal mucosa, which is the earliest stage of rectal prolapse, or prolapse itself can also impede evacuation of stool by acting as a mechanical barrier filling the rectal lumen.

Surgical correction of these mechanical factors may be required to improve bowel function.

Although chronic constipation is a common complaint and patients receive relief from its correction, with the exception of patients with hypothyroidism or one of the various forms of dyschezia, it is rarely a productive clue to important organic disease. A change in bowel habits, however, frequently is. For example, in carcinoma of the pancreas, carcinoma of the colon, lead poisoning, and porphyria, a change in bowel pattern is often the presenting symptom. Every patient who complains of the appearance of constipation or constipation alternating with diarrhea must be evaluated by a stool examination and proctosigmoidoscopy.

REFERENCES

1. Cann PA, Read NW, et al: Irritable bowel syndrome: Relationship of disorders in the transit of a single solid meal to symptom patterns. Gut 24:405, 1983

2. Fordtran JS, Santa Ana CA, et al: Pathophysiology of chronic diarrhea: Insights derived from intestinal perfusion studies in 31 patients. Clin Gastroenterol 15:477, 1986

3. Giardiello FM, Bayless TM, et al: Collagenous colitis: Physiologic and histopathic studies in 7 patients. Ann Intern Med 106:46, 1987

4. Gertler S, Pressman J, et al: Management of acute diarrhea. J Clin Gastroenterol 5:523, 1983

5. Greenstein AJ, Janowitz HD, Sachar DB: The extraintestinal complications of Crohn's disease and ulcerative colitis: A study of 100 patients. Medicine (Baltimore) 55:401, 1976

6. Janowitz HD, Sachar DB: Inflammatory bowel disease. Adv Intern Med 27:205, 1982

7. Kirsner JB, Shorter RC: Recent developments in "nonspecific" inflammatory bowel disease. N Engl J Med 306:775, 837, 1982

8. Krejs GJ, Fordtran JS: Diarrhea. In Sleisenger MH, Fordtran JS (eds): Gastrointestinal Disease: Pathophysiology, Diagnosis, Management. Philadelphia, WB Saunders, 1983, p 257

9. Lennard-Jones JA, Powell-Tuck J: Treatment of inflammatory bowel disease. Clin Gastroenterol 8:187, 1979

10. Luk GD, Hendrix TR: Microscopic examination of stool as a screening test for steatorrhea. Gastroenterology 74:1134, 1978

11. Martelli H, Devroede G, et al: Mechanisms of idiopathic constipation: Outlet obstruction. Gastroenterology 75:623, 1978

12. Ramband J-C, Hantefeuille M, et al: Diarrhoea due to circulating agents. Clin Gastroenterol 15:603, 1986

13. Ravich WJ, Bayless TM: Carbohydrate malabsorption. Clin Castroenterol 12:335, 1983

14. Read NW, Krejs GJ, et al: Chronic diarrhea of unknown origin. Gastroenterology 78:264, 1980

15. Read NW, Timms JM, et al: Impairment of defecation in young women with severe constipation. Gastroenterology 90:53, 1986

16. Riddell RH, Goldman H, et al: Dysplasia in inflammatory bowel disease: Standardized classification with provisional clinical applications. Hum Pathol 14:931, 1983

17. Solomons NW, Garcia-Ibanex R, Viteri FE: Hydrogen breath test of lactose absorption in adults: The application of physiological doses and whole cow's milk sources. Am J Clin Nutr 33:545, 1980

18. Stoll BJ, Glass RI, et al: Value of stool examination in patients with diarrhea. Br Med J 286:2037, 1983

19. Watier A, Devroede G, et al: Mechanisms of idiopathic constipation: Colonic inertia. Gastroenterology 76:1267, 1979

20. Whittington PF, Barnes HV, Bayless TM: Medical management of Crohn's disease in adolescence. Gastroenterology 72:1338, 1977

21. Yardley JH, Donowitz M: Colo-rectal biopsy in inflammatory bowel disease. In Yardley JH, Morson BC (eds): The Gastrointestinal Tract. Baltimore, Williams & Wilkins, 1977

CHAPTER 12.6
Malabsorption

Gordon D. Luk and Thomas R. Hendrix

Steatorrhea, increased fat in the stool, is the characteristic symptom of malabsorption. It is important to emphasize, however, that the majority of patients with malabsorption have a variety of symptoms, many the consequence of deficiencies of essential nutrients, and only a minority have obvious steatorrhea.

Impaired absorption (i.e., malabsorption) may involve the absorption of a single compound such as lactose in lactase deficiency or vitamin B_{12} in pernicious anemia, or it may involve all elements of the diet, as encountered in a diffuse mucosal abnormality such as celiac disease. Presenting symptoms of malabsorption may be voluminous, malodorous stools and weight loss, in which case there is no diagnostic uncertainty. At the other extreme, the presentation may be subtle and associated with no diarrhea and only nonspecific complaints of weakness, fatigue, and abdominal bloating, and it may be erroneously attributed to psychosomatic causes.

The clinical manifestations of intestinal malabsorption include (1) caloric deficiency resulting in weight loss, (2) specific deficiencies causing anemia, tetany, glossitis, or bleeding, and (3) intestinal dysfunction, leading to diarrhea or steatorrhea, or both.

For effective treatment of malabsorption, the deranged step or steps in the digestive-absorptive process must first be identified. The digestive-absorptive process involves three phases: (1) an intraluminal phase, during which the chemical and physical states of the nutrients are altered in preparation for absorption, (2) an epithelial phase, concerned with surface hydrolysis at the brush border, uptake, and preparation for extrusion into the lamina propria, and (3) a transit phase, during which absorbed material is removed from the lamina propria by lymph and blood flow.

PHYSIOLOGY OF DIGESTION AND ABSORPTION

An understanding of the normal physiology of digestion and absorption[3,4] is necessary to classify the cause of malabsorption and plan rational therapy.

The preparation of food for absorption begins in the mouth with the partial conversion of starch to dextrins and maltose by salivary amylase. In the stomach, food is homogenized and emulsified, and pepsin exerts its proteolytic action by cleaving proteins to peptides.

In the duodenum, the arrival of acidified chyme from the stomach causes the release of the hormones cholecystokinin (CCK) and secretin, which, in turn, stimulate the gallbladder to contract and empty bile into the duodenum and stimulate the release of digestive enzymes and bicarbonate by the pancreas. Conjugated bile salts form micelles, which carry the products of lipolysis, cholesterol, and lipid-soluble vitamins in micellar solution to the absorbing surface of the intestine. The lipids pass into the epithelial cells while the bile salts remain in the lumen to continue to transport lipids. Finally, the bile salts are absorbed by the ileum and carried in the portal blood to the liver to be excreted again into the bile. This enterohepatic circulation of bile salts is 95 percent efficient, so each day the liver has only to synthesize enough bile acid to replace the small amount lost into the colon. In the process of absorbing a meal, the bile-salt pool completes two or more enterohepatic cycles.

Pancreatic amylase continues the hydrolysis of polysaccharides to disaccharides. The hydrolysis of disaccharides to monosaccharides is accomplished by enzymes (disaccharidases) on the brush border of the small-intestinal epithelium. Glucose absorption releases gastric inhibitory peptide (GIP) from the intestinal mucosa, which in turn stimulates insulin release and inhibits gastric secretion. The pancreatic proteolytic enzymes are secreted in an inactive form. An intestinal enzyme, enterokinase, converts trypsinogen into active trypsin, which in turn converts the other proteolytic proenzymes into their active forms—chymotrypsin, elastase, carboxypeptidases, and so on. The major products of intraluminal protein digestion are small polypeptides and amino acids. Brush border peptidases hydrolyze large peptides to dipeptides and tripeptides, which are actively absorbed by a peptide transport carrier. In addition, there are amino acid transport carriers.

The motor activity of the small intestine mixes and churns the chyme and the digestive enzymes and brings the products of

digestion in contact with the absorbing surfaces of the intestine. The normal propulsive activity prevents stasis of the intestinal contents and consequent multiplication of bacteria that interfere with absorption, in part by deconjugating bile salts. Overgrowth of bacteria also interferes with the absorption of vitamin B_{12} because the bacteria use the vitamin before it reaches its site of absorption in the ileum.

The second phase of the absorptive process is the actual transfer of the products of digestion from the intestinal lumen to the blood and lymph. The absorption of nutrients occurs chiefly in the duodenum and jejunum, whereas bile salts and vitamin B_{12} are absorbed in the ileum.

The epithelial cells of the villi are the functional units in intestinal absorption, with those at the tips playing the major role. Some materials, such as some water-soluble vitamins, nucleic acid derivatives, and urea, pass through the intestinal cells by simple diffusion. Lipids enter the cells by nonionic diffusion. The majority of foodstuffs, however, are absorbed by more efficient and often highly specialized active transport processes. For example, glucose and galactose share the same sodium-coupled active transport mechanism, whereas fructose enters through another pathway by carrier-facilitated diffusion. Although there are at least four specific

amino acid transport mechanisms, amino acids are also absorbed as peptides, with hydrolysis to amino acids being completed within the absorbing cell. The intestinal absorption of some materials, such as iron, copper, calcium, and magnesium, involves specific and complex regulatory systems.

The portal blood is the primary route for all absorbed materials except lipids. The absorbed fatty acids and monoglycerides are reesterified within the absorbing cells. These triglycerides, along with other absorbed lipids, are packaged with a protein coat and extruded from the cell as chylomicrons, which are carried from the intestine by the lymphatic vessels.

CLASSIFICATION OF MALABSORPTION

Diseases of malabsorption are grouped according to the alterations in the normal digestive and absorptive physiology that cause malabsorption (Table 12.6–1).

CLINICAL MANIFESTATIONS OF MALABSORPTION

The clinical manifestations of malabsorption result from the following: (1) unabsorbed food substances affecting other intestinal functions, such as fat and fatty acids producing foul, bulky diarrhea; (2) secondary deficiencies of specific nutrients that, although eaten, are not absorbed, as exemplified by tetany secondary to calcium and vitamin D malabsorption; and (3) systemic symptoms, including anorexia and weight loss.

DIARRHEA

Diarrhea is usually a major complaint of patients with malabsorption, but those with mild steatorrhea may sometimes notice no change in their stools. Since the reservoir capacity of the colon is intact and there is no rectal disease to cause urgency or tenesmus, the patient with celiac disease or pancreatic insufficiency may have only a few bowel movements per day. However, there may be exacerbations of diarrhea, with 6 to 12 movements per day, especially when there are intercurrent respiratory or intestinal infections. Patients with gastrocolic or gastroileal fistulas may have frequent diarrhea and the passage of undigested food in the stool several minutes to several hours after eating. Because bloating (caused by unabsorbed gas and liquid) and diarrhea may be accentuated by eating, some patients voluntarily decrease their food intake to avoid discomfort.

Unabsorbed fats and fatty acids cause the stools to be bulky and voluminous. In addition, fatty acids, particularly after bacterial hydroxylation, stimulate colonic fluid secretion, thus increasing the water content of the stools and producing diarrhea. If increased amounts of bile salts enter the colon because of ileal dysfunction or resection, fecal water is increased because bile salts also stimulate colonic fluid secretion.[5] Rancid fats impart a particularly offensive odor to flatus and feces. In patients with disaccharidase deficiencies, unabsorbed carbohydrates act as an osmotic load that interferes with fluid reabsorption in the ileum and colon (see Chapter 12.5). It is important to inspect the stool personally, since the patient's description is rarely adequate. If there ever was a situation in which one look is worth a thousand words, it is in the evaluation of abnormal stools.

WEIGHT LOSS

Weight loss and weakness are often the patient's chief complaints and occur in part because calories are lost, especially in the form of fats, but also because anorexia is an accompaniment of malabsorption. Prolonged and severe malabsorption states, such as Whipple disease, intestinal fistulas, and celiac disease, may manifest

---

TABLE 12.6–1. PATHOPHYSIOLOGIC CLASSIFICATION OF MALABSORPTION

Failure of Digestion (Intraluminal Phase)
Decreased pancreatic enzymes
- Pancreatic insufficiency (pancreatitis, cystic fibrosis, protein deficiency, and pancreatic cancer)
- Inactivation of pancreatic enzymes by gastric hypersecretion (Z-E syndrome and ileal resection)
- Failure to convert proenzyme to active form (enterokinase and trypsinogen deficiencies)

Impaired bile-acid micelle formation
- Impaired bile-acid synthesis (severe hepatocellular disease)
- Interrupted enterohepatic circulation (ileal resection, bile duct obstruction, or biliary cirrhosis)
- Bile acid deconjugation (bacterial overgrowth)
  Stasis due to motor abnormality (scleroderma, intestinal pseudo-obstruction, diabetic visceral neuropathy)
  Stasis due to anatomic abnormalities (multiple diverticula, strictures, and blind loops, including long afferent loop of a gastrojejunostomy)
  Small-bowel contamination (gastrocolic and jejunocolic fistula)
- Inadequate mixing of food, bile, and pancreatic enzymes (gastrojejunostomy)

Failure of Absorption (Mucosal Phase)
- Inadequate absorptive surface (intestinal resection, intestinal bypass for obesity, inadvertent gastroileostomy)
- Damaged absorbing surface (cancer chemotherapy and radiation therapy, celiac disease, tropical sprue, hypogammaglobulinemia, giardiasis)
- Biochemical defect without anatomic alteration
  Disaccharide deficiency (lactase and sucrase deficiency)
  Transport deficiency
    Carbohydrate (glucose-galactose malabsorption)
    Lipid (a-β-lipoproteinemia)
    Amino acids (cystinuria, Hartnup disease, methionine malabsorption)
    Vitamin B_{12} malabsorption
- Infiltration of intestinal wall (Whipple disease, lymphoma, amyloid, Crohn disease)

Impaired Lymph and Blood Flow (Transit Phase)
- Developmental abnormality (intestinal lymphangiectasia, Milroy disease)
- Lymphatic obstruction (lymphoma, Whipple disease, tuberculosis)
- Mesenteric vascular insufficiency (rare if ever)

themselves as advanced malnutrition, often with secondary hypo-pituitarism and amenorrhea. These cachectic patients have been mistakenly considered to have a neoplasm.

EDEMA

Hypoalbuminemia and peripheral edema result from the prolonged malabsorption of protein and from the increased loss of serum proteins into the lumen of the intestine. This latter form of protein loss accompanies intestinal lymphangiectasia, constrictive pericarditis, portal hypertension, and a variety of diseases involving the mucosa, such as Menetrier disease, Crohn disease, Whipple disease,[2] and tropical sprue.[1] Gastric neoplasms may also cause excess protein loss and edema.

TETANY AND BONE DEMINERALIZATION

Tetany from the prolonged malabsorption of vitamin D, calcium, and magnesium may occur but is uncommon. Trousseau and Chvostek signs are seen more often. In patients with extensive ileal resections, magnesium depletion appears to be the major factor in the production of tetany. The serum phosphorus value is low in primary malabsorptive disorders, in contrast to elevated values in hypoparathyroidism. Osteoporosis and osteomalacia with bone pain and pathologic fractures may be the presenting features of celiac disease, postgastrectomy steatorrhea, or chronic obstructive jaundice. Secondary hyperparathyroidism may complicate chronic hypocalcemia, with a resultant osteitis fibrosa cystica.

BLEEDING

Patients with steatorrhea may have a bleeding diathesis, usually manifested by ecchymoses but occasionally by melena or hematuria. This is caused by malabsorption of fat-soluble vitamin K and the resultant hypoprothrombinemia. In megaloblastic anemia, as seen in tropical sprue, thrombocytopenia does occur but is rarely a cause of bleeding. Retinal hemorrhages can occur with any severe anemia. The parenteral administration of vitamin K corrects a prothrombin deficiency caused by malabsorption.

ANEMIA

In the malabsorption syndrome, anemia may be caused by the impaired absorption of iron, folic acid, or vitamin B_{12}, singly or in combination.

RENAL CALCULI

Patients with malabsorption and diarrhea frequently have concentrated urine. In addition, they tend to have hyperoxaluria because they absorb a larger proportion of dietary oxalate than normal. These two findings explain the greater-than-expected incidence of renal calculi in patients with steatorrhea. Normally, much of the dietary oxalate is precipitated in the lumen as calcium oxalate. In the presence of steatorrhea, calcium soaps are formed, leaving oxalate in solution to be absorbed.

OTHER MANIFESTATIONS

Other clinical manifestations include peripheral neuropathy, presumably a result of vitamin deficiency; night blindness caused by a lack of vitamin A; and nocturia caused by the delayed absorption of water. Skin pigmentation and chronic arthritis are common in Whipple disease.

Milk (lactose) intolerance, characterized by bloating, cramps, and watery, frothy diarrhea, may result from a genetically determined lactase deficiency or from deficiency resulting from mucosal damage, as in celiac disease and tropical sprue.

Other items in a patient's history that should alert the physician to the possibility of malabsorption include chronic cholestatic liver disease; chronic alcoholism; recurrent upper or midabdominal pain; diabetes with or without peripheral neuropathy; previous surgery, especially gastrectomy, gastroenterostomy, vagotomy, or intestinal resection; severe peptic ulcer diathesis with watery diarrhea; sudden onset of diarrhea and weight loss after prolonged peptic ulcer activity; childhood history of diarrhea, anemia, potbelly, or failure to thrive; previous residence or travel in a tropical area where sprue or giardiasis is endemic; and previous antibiotic therapy, especially with broad-spectrum antibiotics.

DIAGNOSTIC PROCEDURES IN SUSPECTED MALABSORPTION[13]

The symptoms, appearance of the stool, evidence of secondary deficiencies, or an abnormal small-bowel radiograph should lead to the suspicion that malabsorption is present, but confirmation of the diagnosis requires diagnostic tests. The investigative steps used are outlined in Figure 12.6–1.

PROVING THE PRESENCE OF STEATORRHEA

The microscopic examination for stool fat is an easy, convenient, rapid in-office screening examination that can demonstrate the presence of symptomatic steatorrhea. In many instances, it can also separate pancreatic insufficiency from other causes of steatorrhea. The presence of neutral fats indicative of pancreatic steatorrhea is detected by Sudan III–stained fat globules with warming of a stool sample on a microscope slide; the detection of split fats, indicative of nonpancreatic steatorrhea, requires first acidifying the stool sample with acetic acid. Measurements of radioactive label in the breath, serum, or stool after C-14 fat ingestion have also been suggested as potentially useful screening tests for steatorrhea.[8,14]

The determination of the blood level of fat-soluble materials, such as carotene, is also a useful screening test. Ninety percent of the patients with steatorrhea have subnormal levels. A low serum carotene level does not prove malabsorption is present, because it is also found when the intake of carotene-containing foods (vegetables) is decreased. Subnormal blood levels of other materials, such as vitamin A, cholesterol, prothrombin, calcium, phosphorus, albumin, iron, folic acid, and vitamin B_{12}, may be clues to the presence of malabsorption.

For an accurate assessment of fat absorption or the success of a therapeutic trial, all stools are collected for 3 days, and an average daily value of fecal fat excretion is determined. In addition, the patient should be ingesting a normal amount of fat (70 to 120 g per day) before and during the collection period. Normal fecal fat with this intake is less than 6 g per day.

RADIOGRAPHIC EXAMINATION OF THE SMALL BOWEL[15]

An abnormal small-bowel pattern discovered during radiographic examination of the upper gastrointestinal tract may provide the first clue that malabsorption is the basis for the patient's symptoms. The radiographic malabsorption pattern is, however, a nonspecific finding, and 50 percent of patients with a malabsorption pattern do not have malabsorption on subsequent testing. In addition, a small-bowel radiographic series may be useful in suggesting which category of disorders is the most likely cause of the intestinal malabsorption. Dilated small-bowel loops are common in celiac disease and scleroderma. Nodular thickened folds are common in Whipple disease, intestinal lymphoma, amyloidosis, and granu-

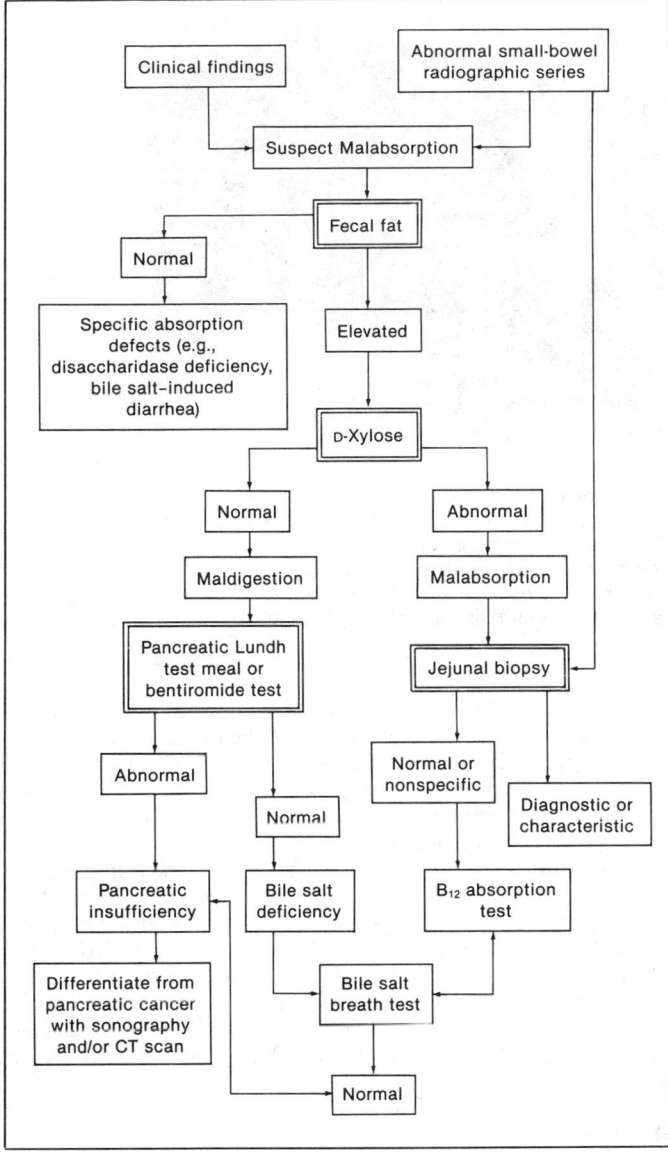

Figure 12.6–1. Evaluation of malabsorption.

measure of the absorbing capacity of the upper part of the small intestine. The normal 5-hour urinary excretion after the ingestion of 25 g of D-xylose orally is greater than 4.5 g. Serum D-xylose measurement may be used if complete urine collections are difficult to obtain. The test result is clearly abnormal in over 90 percent of patients with malabsorption caused by diffuse mucosal disease of the duodenum and jejunum, such as in celiac disease or tropical sprue. In contrast, normal results are obtained in 95 percent if the defect is in intraluminal digestion, as in chronic pancreatitis with pancreatic insufficiency or bile acid deficiency. Urinary excretion may be decreased in patients with bacterial overgrowth syndrome, because intraluminal bacteria metabolize the xylose before it can be absorbed.

Bentiromide Test[10]
Bentiromide (NBT-PABA; N-benzoyl-L-tyrosyl-p-aminobenzoic acid), a synthetic tripeptide when taken orally, is specifically cleaved by the pancreatic enzyme chymotrypsin. The released p-aminobenzoic acid (PABA) is rapidly absorbed from the small intestine, conjugated by the liver, and excreted in the urine. The amount of PABA recovered in the urine reflects the amount and activity of pancreatic chymotrypsin in the intestinal lumen and hence provides a measure of pancreatic exocrine function. An oral dose of 500 mg and a 6-hour urine collection have been shown to provide optimal sensitivity. As in the urinary D-xylose excretion test, a higher water intake to promote diuresis is important. The sensitivity is in the range of 60 to 90 percent, and the specificity is up to 60 percent; both are improved in patients with severe pancreatic insufficiency. The test is simple, noninvasive, inexpensive, and widely available. Results compare favorably with other tests of pancreatic exocrine function (e.g., Lundh test meal and secretin stimulation test).

Pancreatic (Lundh) Test Meal[10]
The Lundh test meal is the most physiologic test of pancreatic insufficiency. After intubation of the jejunum the patient drinks a 300-ml test meal containing protein, carbohydrate, and fat. The jejunal contents are aspirated in four half-hour samples and concentration of one of the pancreatic enzymes is measured. Failure of pancreatic enzyme levels to rise in response to a meal may be due to (1) inadequate release of hormonal stimulants (secretin and CCK), most frequently encountered in patients with a gastrojejunostomy because the meal does not come in contact with the duodenum and upper jejunum, which contain the highest concentration of cells that release these hormones; (2) obstruction of the pancreatic duct by a tumor or stone; (3) pancreatic exocrine insufficiency due to pancreatitis, cystic fibrosis, or pancreatic atrophy; or (4) inactivation of pancreatic enzymes by low duodenal pH, most commonly encountered in the Z-E syndrome but occasionally found in patients with gastric hypersecretion after ileal resection. Pancreatic secretory function can also be measured by the secretin test, in which the volume and bicarbonate content of duodenal aspirate is measured after parenteral administration of secretin.

Bile-Salt Breath Test[8]
The second intraluminal step in lipid assimilation is micellar solubilization. If the intestinal concentration of conjugated bile salts is below the critical micellar concentration (2 to 3 mmol/L), lipids are not solubilized and as a consequence diffusion to the absorbing surface is severely limited. Bile salt deficiency may be caused by (1) impaired hepatic synthesis and secretion of bile salts in severe chronic liver disease or (2) interruption of the enterohepatic circulation of bile salts by (a) obstruction of the common bile duct, (b) ileal disease, most often Crohn disease or resection, or (c) intraluminal precipitation of bile salts. The latter is caused by (1) deconjugation and hydroxylation of bile salts by an overgrowth of bacteria in the small intestine, (2) low intestinal pH due to extreme gastric hypersection, or (3) binding to drugs such as neomycin and

lomatous diseases. In most instances the small-bowel barium study only indicates the likelihood of a diagnosis but does not establish or exclude it. For example, the small-bowel series is usually normal in patients with pancreatic insufficiency, but an occasional patient with pancreatic insufficiency has clearly abnormal radiographs.

DISTINGUISHING MALDIGESTION FROM MALABSORPTION

D-Xylose Test
The ability of the intestine to absorb specific substances can be evaluated by measuring the appearance of an orally administered test substance in the blood or in the urine. The pentose, D-xylose, is used most commonly to distinguish maldigestion from malabsorption because it does not require digestion before absorption and because a large portion of the absorbed sugar is excreted unmetabolized in the urine. If the liver and renal functions are normal and there is no delay in gastric emptying, the determination of the urinary excretion after ingestion of D-xylose is an adequate clinical

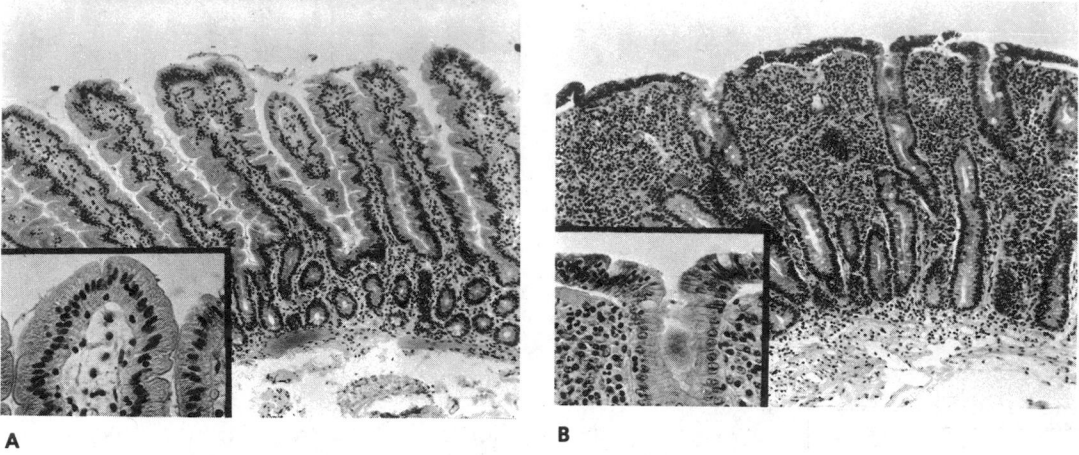

Figure 12.6–2. Jejunal biopsy specimen. **A.** Photomicrograph of a normal jejunal biopsy specimen. Villi are long and slender, covered by tall columnar epithelium (shown in detail in the inset). **B.** Photomicrograph of a typical biopsy specimen from a patient with a celiac disease is shown below. There are no recognizable villi, and there is apparent lengthening of the crypts of Lieberkühn. The lamina propria is infiltrated with plasma cells and lymphocytes. The surface epithelium is flattened and infiltrated with lymphocytes, whereas the crypt epithelium is normal (shown in inset).

cholestyramine. The role of interruption of the enterohepatic circulation of bile salts in the pathogenesis of steatorrhea can be assessed clinically by the bile-salt breath test. The test is performed by measuring $^{14}CO_2$ in the expired air after the oral administration of glycocholate with the glycine moiety labeled with ^{14}C. If the enterohepatic circulation is intact, less than 5 percent of the bile salt escapes reabsorption and enters the colon, where bacteria remove the glycine and convert it to the carbon dioxide that is absorbed and excreted in the breath. If there is ileal dysfunction or overgrowth of bacteria in the small intestine, the increased deconjugation of glycocholate will be manifested by increased appearance of $^{14}CO_2$ in the breath. Recent studies show that the ^{14}C-xylose breath test may be more sensitive and specific for the detection of bacterial overgrowth than the bile-salt breath test.[8]

Peroral Small-Bowel Biopsy[11]

The development of techniques for obtaining biopsy of the small-intestinal mucosa by the oral route was a major advance in the diagnostic approach to malabsorption. The procedures are safe and well tolerated.

The jejunal biopsy specimen has diagnostic features in a group of disorders, most of which are rare (Table 12.6–2). The characteristic abnormality may be missed in some of these disorders, such as intestinal lymphoma and amyloidosis, because the lesion does not involve the intestine uniformly. Whipple disease and giardiasis,

the two diseases on the list for which there is the most successful therapy, can always be identified by jejunal biopsy.

The jejunal biopsy result associated with celiac disease is not diagnostic, but in temperate regions the vast majority of patients with the characteristic biopsy specimen shown in Figure 12.6–2 will respond to a gluten-free diet.

The finding of a normal jejunal biopsy specimen in a patient with steatorrhea indicates that one of the intraluminal steps is at fault. Most commonly it is ileal dysfunction or bacterial overgrowth that has been misinterpreted as mucosal disease. To resolve this question, the bile-salt breath test should be done and vitamin B_{12} absorption measured. Normal jejunal biopsy specimens are obtained also in pancreatic insufficiency, postgastrectomy states, jejunal diverticulosis, pernicious anemia, diabetic visceral neuropathy, and scleroderma.

Therapeutic Trial

The development of specific therapies for many of the diseases causing malabsorption has increased the importance of making a definitive diagnosis in these patients. The therapeutic trial, such as a gluten-free diet in celiac disease, pancreatic enzyme replacement in pancreatic insufficiency, and tetracycline use in bacterial overgrowth, is used to confirm the specific cause of malabsorption but is not a substitute for a logical, step-by-step diagnostic process as outlined above.

TABLE 12.6–2. INTERPRETATION OF JEJUNAL BIOPSY SPECIMENS

Diagnostic	Characteristic	Nonspecific Abnormalities	Normal
Whipple disease	Celiac disease	Crohn disease	Pancreatic insufficiency
Giardiasis	Tropical sprue	Bacterial overgrowth	Bacterial overgrowth
Amyloidosis	Eosinophilic gastroenteritis		Bile salt deficiency
α-β-Lipoproteinemia	Dermatitis herpetiformis		
Lymphoma	Dysglobulinemia		
Coccidiosis			
Mast cell disease			
Lymphangiectasia			
Macroglobulinemia			

CLINICAL EXAMPLES

MALDIGESTION (INTRALUMINAL DEFECTS)

Pancreatic Insufficiency

Chronic relapsing pancreatitis is the commonest cause of pancreatic insufficiency. In other patients, pancreatic insufficiency appears insidiously in the absence of clinically recognizable pancreatitis; for this reason, it has been called "silent pancreatitis" or "idiopathic pancreatic atrophy." In still others, it is one of the presenting manifestations of carcinoma of the pancreas. In children and young adults, cystic fibrosis is the most frequent cause of pancreatic insufficiency. In children and young adults with pancreatic insufficiency, a sweat test should be performed to determine whether cystic fibrosis is the underlying cause.

Clinical Manifestions. The main clinical manifestations of exocrine pancreatic insufficiency are steatorrhea, abdominal bloating, and weight loss. Steatorrhea may be massive. Some patients excrete over 80 g of fat per day (normal less than 6 g). A helpful distinguishing feature from other malabsorptive disorders, such as celiac disease and Whipple disease, is the excellent appetite and lack of cachexia that might otherwise be expected with this degree of steatorrhea.

Diagnosis.[10] The methods of differentiating maldigestion and malabsorption are outlined in Figure 12.6–1. In addition, a plain film of the abdomen will show pancreatic calcifications in 40 to 50 percent of the patients with severe pancreatic steatorrhea; 25 percent will be diabetic, and in addition, in 60 percent a glucose tolerance test will indicate diabetes. On radiographs of the upper gastrointestinal tract, a distortion of the pattern of the second and third portions of the duodenum may be seen with chronic pancreatitis or with a carcinoma of the head of the pancreas. Neoplasms or pseudocysts are best demonstrated by sonography or CT scan. A therapeutic trial with pancreatic enzyme replacement is also a useful diagnostic procedure but does not establish the cause of the pancreatic insufficiency. With adequate replacement, steatorrhea will decrease but rarely disappears.

Treatment.[12] The management of pancreatic exocrine insufficiency involves the adequate replacement of the deficient digestive enzymes. There are several potent pancreatic enzyme preparations available. They are best given at least three to six times a day and have their optimal effect if given just before meals. For maximal effect, it is suggested that up to 12 g per day be given. The administration of antacids or cimetidine just before the pancreatic enzyme preparation may lessen the destruction of the enzymes during their passage through the acid environment of the stomach. As steatorrhea decreases and nutrition improves, pancreatic function often improves and the need for pancreatic enzyme replacement may diminish.

Bile-Salt Deficiency

Ileal Insufficiency.[5] Extensive ileal inflammation (particularly Crohn disease), surgical resection, or bypass of the ileum interrupts the enterohepatic circulation of bile salts and interferes with vitamin B_{12} absorption. With small resections, less than 100 cm, the liver is able to replace most of the bile acids lost, steatorrhea is mild (less than 10 g per day), and the diarrhea is primarily due to bile salts stimulating fluid secretion by the colon. Diarrhea in this circumstance can be controlled by the use of cholestyramine, a resin that binds bile salts. With larger resections, the liver is unable to synthesize sufficient bile salts to compensate for those lost into the colon. In these patients with a diminished bile-salt pool, the bile-salt concentration in the upper part of the intestine exceeds the critical micellar concentration only at breakfast. Fat absorption after the other meals is greatly impaired. Increased fatty acids pass-

ing into the colon also stimulate colonic fluid secretion. Limitation of fat intake will control diarrhea but may lead to caloric deficiency and weight loss. Supplementation of the diet with medium-chain triglycerides (fatty acid chain length C8–C10) may help. These fats are water soluble and hence do not require bile salts for the solubilization necessary for absorption of long-chain fatty acids.

Massive resection of the small bowel, usually necessitated by infarction, presents a major therapeutic challenge. Patients have survived with as little as 6 to 18 inches of jejunum beyond the ligament of Treitz, especially if the ileocecal sphincter and right colon can be preserved. In some patients in whom oral alimentation does not meet the caloric needs, long-term parenteral and enteral hyperalimentation have been successful.[6]

Bacterial Overgrowth Syndromes.[9] Bacterial deconjugation of bile salts in the small bowel is the second major cause of bile-salt deficiency. The normal small intestine is sparsely populated with bacteria, in part because the acid environment of the stomach is lethal to many bacteria but more importantly because the motility of the fasting intestine keeps it swept clean. Abnormalities of the intestine conducive to stasis of small-bowel contents favor the massive proliferation of bacteria to levels in excess of 10^6 organisms per milliliter of intestinal contents. The bacterial population is a colonic flora, including obligate anaerobes in large numbers and facultative anaerobes such as *E. coli* and *Streptococcus faecalis*. Situations that cause stasis include blind loops; a single large diverticulum or multiple small intestinal diverticula; strictures; afferent loop obstruction after a gastrojejunostomy; enteroenteric anastomosis or fistula; gastrocolic fistula; radiation enteritis; and generalized atony of the upper part of the small bowel, as in scleroderma or diabetic visceral neuropathy. In addition to steatorrhea from bile-salt deficiency, the bacterial overgrowth syndromes are characterized by vitamin B_{12} malabsorption that is not corrected by the addition of intrinsic factor. Vitamin B_{12} is used by the bacteria before it reaches the absorptive site in the ileum.

The results of xylose and bile-salt breath tests are positive in these patients. The low D-xylose excretion, which is the consequence of two factors (metabolism of D-xylose by the abnormal intestinal flora and spotty nonspecific epithelial damage, found in the bacterial overgrowth syndrome), may interfere with absorption.

Therapy for bacterial overgrowth includes eliminating the cause of stasis, if this is readily correctable, or, if not, antibiotic administration to decrease or change the bacterial flora. The responses to treatment are variable and depend on the extent, location, and severity of the abnormality; the types of bacteria present; their sensitivity to antibiotics; and the extent of the bile-salt deconjugation. Antibiotics that have been most useful are tetracycline and ampicillin. Neomycin should not be used because it precipitates bile salts.

The malabsorption that follows subtotal gastric resection and gastroenterostomy has multiple origins. First, food emptied directly into the jejunum is unlikely to be mixed adequately with pancreatic enzymes and bile. Second, release of bile salt and pancreatic enzymes may be suboptimal because the duodenum and upper jejunum, which contain the greatest concentration of secretin and CCK-secretory cells, are bypassed. Finally, bile salts may be precipitated and pancreatic enzymes may be inactivated by low pH because the rate of gastric emptying may exceed the rate of bicarbonate production by the pancreas.

MALABSORPTION (MUCOSAL DEFECTS)

Celiac Disease[16]

Celiac disease (gluten-induced enteropathy) is a chronic, probably hereditary, illness of unknown cause occurring in both children and adults and manifested by steatorrhea and deficiencies produced by intestinal malabsorption. The disordered absorption results

from damage to the proximal small-intestinal mucosa by the digestion products of gluten, a protein contained in grains, especially wheat, but not corn or rice. When food derived from these grains is avoided (gluten-free diet), a complete remission with improvement in the jejunal lesion occurs. Reintroduction of gluten causes a relapse and a worsening of the jejunal mucosa. The characteristic mucosal lesion of celiac disease (Fig. 12.6–2) is caused by intraepithelial T-lymphocyte-mediated damage to the epithelial cells absorbing gluten peptides. The accelerated loss of cells from the villus crests leads to compensatory crypt hyperplasia.[17] The mechanism of the gluten-induced damage is unknown. No specific defect in gluten hydrolysis has been identified. It has been suggested that some interaction between the absorbing epithelial cells and gluten peptides renders the cells subject to immune system attack.

Celiac disease has been recognized chiefly in temperate climates. The highest prevalence of the disease is in Ireland, where the rate has been projected to be 1 in 300 live births. Female patients outnumber male patients in most reports. Almost all patients are white, but occasionally black patients may have the disease. There is a 10 percent incidence of celiac disease in the siblings and relatives of celiac patients, and a dominant inheritance with incomplete penetration has been suggested. A striking relation between celiac disease and certain HLA haplotypes (B8, DR3, DR7, and DC3) has been found.

Diabetes mellitus or a history of diabetes in a close relative is common in celiac disease. Patients with dermatitis herpetiformis have been found to have a high incidence of a celiac-like lesion on intestinal biopsy that heals when gluten is removed from the diet. On the other hand, these patients do not have clinical malabsorption. Since patients with typical celiac disease do not have an increased incidence of dermatitis herpetiformis, it is possible that the gluten-induced lesion in dermatitis herpetiformis is caused by a defect at a different step in gluten handling than is the celiac lesion.

Clinical Manifestations. The symptoms and signs of celiac disease may first appear in childhood, as early as 8 to 12 months of age.

Diarrhea, weight loss, failure to thrive, wasting of the musculature, potbelly, and anemia are the main clinical features. The disease may remit spontaneously in the middle of the first decade. Careful study shows that these children may have occasional diarrhea, an abnormal jejunal mucosa, malabsorption, and some delay in growth and body development. Most patients with celiac disease are asymptomatic in the late teens and early twenties. Some remain in apparent remission, but others have a return of symptoms in their late twenties and thirties. Other patients first develop the clinical manifestations of malabsorption between the third and sixth decades without a childhood history of celiac disease. In some adults the disease first becomes clinically apparent after gastric surgery. All these patients have the same jejunal biopsy lesion and a similar excellent response to a gluten-free diet. The main symptoms in adults include bulky, light-colored stools, abdominal bloating, weight loss, weakness, and easy fatigability. Before specific deficiencies appear, these patients are frequently considered to have a functional bowel disease. As the effects of malabsorption become more pronounced, iron deficiency or megaloblastic anemia, bleeding tendencies, peripheral edema, or tetany may occur. Milk intolerance has also been noted in some patients because lactase levels are decreased in the damaged epithelium of the jejunum. An increased incidence of adenocarcinomas and lymphomas of the small intestine has been reported in patients with celiac disease. Intestinal ulceration and perforation have also been seen as fatal complications of celiac disease.

Diagnosis. At the time of the initial diagnosis, most patients have steatorrhea, low serum carotene levels, abnormal D-xylose absorption, and an abnormal small-bowel radiograph. The diagnosis is verified by the finding of a flattened mucosa on jejunal biopsy and by the subsequent clinical and histologic improvement with a gluten-free diet.

Treatment. Adults and children with celiac disease improve rapidly on a diet free of wheat, rye, oats, and barley gluten. The improvement is clinical, biochemical, and histologic. Symptoms usually decrease in the first week, and most patients are in remission within 2 months. Weight gain is rapid, averaging over 20 pounds in the first 2 months. The absorption of fat and D-xylose returns to normal. The absorption of all food substances improves rapidly, and secondary deficiencies are eventually corrected without specific replacement. If needed, calcium, potassium, vitamin K, iron, folic acid, or vitamin B_{12} can be given as emergency supportive therapy. The surface epithelium of the jejunum improves very rapidly, reaching the normal height in 7 to 10 days. Later, the villus pattern improves, and after a year or more the mucosa approaches a normal appearance if the patient continues to follow his diet. Minor dietary indiscretions may be tolerated without producing symptoms, but if they continue, mucosal damage and malabsorption will reappear. Adrenal corticosteroids produce improvement of the surface epithelium despite continued gluten ingestion, but the remission obtained is usually incomplete.

Tropical Sprue[16]

Tropical sprue is an endemic disease of unknown cause that occurs in certain tropical areas of the world (West Indies, India, and Southeast Asia). Patients with tropical sprue have also been recognized in temperate areas, such as New York, Boston, and London. These patients were either natives or former residents of endemic tropical areas, but their illness did not appear until several months or years after they left the tropics. The signs and symptoms are the result of malabsorption caused by a lesion of the small-intestinal mucosa. Unlike celiac disease, in which the greatest damage to the mucosa is in the jejunum, both the jejunum and ileum are equally involved in tropical sprue. In addition, the epithelial injury is less striking than in celiac disease, and truly "flat biopsy specimens" are not seen. Although many of the clinical manifestations of tropical sprue resemble those of celiac disease, they are two distinct diseases. The differentiation is based on the history (i.e., exposure to a tropical endemic region, a characteristic biopsy specimen, and the characteristic response to therapy, with tropical sprue responding to tetracycline). Although folate and vitamin B_{12} deficiencies, which are characteristic of tropical sprue, are eventually corrected with tetracycline treatment, patients become asymptomatic more rapidly if these vitamins are added to the regimen.

LYMPHATIC OBSTRUCTION

Whipple Disease[2]

Whipple disease has been converted from a progressive, fatal disease of unknown cause to one that is known to be caused by a bacterium, can be readily diagnosed by jejunal biopsy, and can be successfully treated with antibiotics.

Clinical Manifestations. Whipple disease occurs predominantly in white men whose average age at the time of diagnosis is 43 years. Migratory arthritis or arthralgia, affecting large joints and usually without deformity, occurs in 60 percent of the patients. The arthritis may be part of a generalized polyserositis and precedes the onset of diarrhea and steatorrhea. Other manifestations in the prodromal stage may include pleuritis, low-grade fever, abdominal swelling, uveitis, ascites, and central nervous system disorders.

The effects of malabsorption often dominate the picture when the disease enters a progressive phase. Weight loss, emaciation, and asthenia may be severe. Skin pigmentation, usually sparing the buccal membranes, occurs in two thirds of these patients. This combination of chronic ill health, weakness, hypotension, diarrhea, and skin pigmentation may result in an erroneous diagnosis of Addison disease. Other findings include a chronic cough (30 percent) and fever (25 percent). Lymphadenopathy, either generalized or localized, is noted in 50 percent of the patients. Enlarged

mesenteric and retroperitoneal nodes cause palpable abdominal masses in some patients. Uveitis, ocular palsies, dementia, and other central nervous system manifestations occasionally are the presenting symptoms or may be the major symptoms of relapse after antibiotic therapy.

Laboratory tests in the period of clinical activity may show leukocytosis, normocytic or hypochromic anemia, increased erythrocyte sedimentation rate, occult blood in the stools (30 percent), steatorrhea, low serum carotene and cholesterol levels, hypoalbuminemia, prolonged prothrombin time, and decreased D-xylose absorption. Small-bowel radiographs often show marked coarsening of the mucosal folds, especially in the jejunum, as well as the alterations associated with malabsorption (e.g., flocculation, segmentation of the barium column, and dilation of the lumen).

Diagnosis. Although the characteristic PAS-positive macrophages are found in many tissues, including the lymph nodes and rectal mucosa, Whipple disease is most readily and conclusively diagnosed by intestinal biopsy. The characteristics of the intestinal biopsy are as follows: (1) infiltration of the lamina propria with the foamy PAS-positive macrophages, with the infiltrate sometimes so dense that the villi are distorted; (2) lymphatics in the villi often grossly dilated with fat; and (3) a normal intestinal epithelium. Malabsorption results, in part, from the blockage of the lamina propria and the lymphatic channels by the granule-laden macrophages.

Electron microscopic studies have demonstrated bacteria in the intestinal mucosa and have shown that the PAS-positive granules are derived from ingested "bacillary bodies." The bacteria and the PAS-positive granules gradually disappear after successful antibiotic treatment. Immunofluorescence studies show that the bacteria in intestinal biopsy specimens from different patients are antigenically as well as morphologically similar, so that one as-yet-unidentified organism seems to be responsible for this unusual infection.

Treatment.[7] Because central nervous system relapse is resistant to antibiotic therapy, optimal treatment should consist of 2 weeks of penicillin, 1.2 million units, and streptomycin, 1 g administered intramuscularly, followed by maintenance therapy with a broad-spectrum antibiotic that crosses the blood-brain barrier, such as trimethoprim-sulfamethoxazole. The adequacy of the therapy is best gauged by follow-up intestinal biopsies showing continued absence of bacteria and decreasing numbers of the PAS-positive macrophages from the lamina propria of the intestine.

Protein-Losing Gastroenteropathy[3]

The term "protein-losing gastroenteropathy" is used for disorders in which there is an excessive loss of serum protein, into either the stomach or intestinal tract. The albumin loss can be documented by the intravenous administration of isotopic chromium-labeled albumins, followed by the measurement of the amount of radioactivity appearing in the stool. If the albumin loss exceeds the rate of synthesis by the liver, hypoalbuminemia and edema result. This "weeping" of protein occurs with (1) localized inflammation, as with Menetrier disease or gastric carcinoma; (2) diffuse inflammatory conditions of the bowel, including Crohn disease, ulcerative colitis, celiac disease, and tropical sprue; and (3) increased pressure in the lymphatics draining the bowel, including Whipple disease, intestinal lymphangiectasia, Milroy disease, congestive heart failure, constrictive pericarditis, and cirrhosis with portal hypertension.

Intestinal lymphagiectasia, a developmental abnormality of the intestinal lymphatic channels, is seen in adults and young children and may occur with peripheral edema that is sometimes asymmetric; serous and chylous effusions; hypoalbuminemia; or diarrhea. Some of the patients also have mild steatorrhea. There may be a family history of Milroy disease. On small-bowel radiographs one can see a coarsening of the folds of the jejunal mucosa and hypersecretion of fluid. Jejunal biopsies characteristically reveal dilated lymphatic channels in the mucosa with distortion of the villi. Lymphangiograms may reveal a generalized extraintestinal lymphatic involvement, and abnormalities of the lymphatic channels are seen at laparotomy.

The use of a low-fat diet or a medium-chain triglyceride as the fat source has been shown to be an effective method of decreasing protein loss by decreasing intestinal lymph flow in the inadequate and abnormal lymphatic channels.

REFERENCES

1. Bayless TM, Wheby MS, Swanson VL: Tropical sprue in Puerto Rico. Am J Clin Nutr 21:1030, 1968
2. Feldman M: Whipple's disease. Am J Med Sci 291:56, 1986
3. Freeman HJ, Sleisenger MH, Kim YS: Human protein digestion and absorption: Normal mechanisms and protein-energy malnutrition. Clin Gastroenterol 12:357, 1983
4. Glickman RM: Fat absorption and malabsorption. Clin Gastroenterol 12:323, 1983
5. Hofmann AF: Role of bile acid malabsorption in pathogenesis of diarrhea and steatorrhea in patients with ileal resection. I. Response to cholestyramine or replacement of dietary long-chain triglyceride by medium-chain triglyceride. Gastroenterology 62:918, 1972
6. Jeejeebhoy KN: Therapy of the short gut syndrome. Lancet 1:1427, 1983
7. Keinath RD, Merrell DE, et al: Antibiotic treatment and relapse in Whipple's disease: Long-term follow-up of 88 patients. Gastroenterology 88:1867, 1985
8. King CE, Toskes PP: The use of breath tests in the study of malabsorption. Clin Gastroenterol 12:591, 1983
9. Mathias JR, Clench MH: Review: Pathophysiology of diarrhea caused by bacterial overgrowth of the small intestine. Am J Med Sci 289:243, 1985
10. Niederau C, Grendell JH: Diagnosis of chronic pancreatitis. Gastroenterology 88:1973, 1985
11. Owen RL, Brandborg LL: Mucosal histopathology of malabsorption. Clin Gastroenterol 12:575, 1983
12. Perry RS, Gallagher J: Management of maldigestion associated with pancreatic insufficiency. Clin Pharmacol 4:161, 1985
13. Ryan ME, Olsen WA: A diagnostic approach to malabsorption syndromes: A pathophysiologic approach. Clin Gastroenterol 12:533, 1983
14. Thorsgaard-Pedersen N, Halgreen H: Simultaneous assessment of fat maldigestion and fat malabsorption by a double-isotope method using fecal radioactivity. Gastroenterology 88:47, 1985
15. Weigman Z, Stringer DA, Durie PR: Radiologic manifestations of malabsorption: A nonspecific finding. Pediatrics 74:530, 1984
16. Westergaard H: The sprue syndromes. Am J Med Sci 290:249, 1985
17. Yardley JH, Bayless TM, et al: Celiac disease: A study of the jejunal epithelium before and after a gluten-free diet. N Engl J Med 267:1173, 1962

The liver is the largest organ in the body. Its weight of 1500 g accounts for approximately 2 percent of the normal adult body weight. Situated in the right upper quadrant of the abdomen and bordered by the diaphragm, abdominal wall, and other abdominal organs, the liver is inaccessible to palpation except over its lower anterior surface. The many metabolic functions of the liver are facilitated by its rich blood supply, its extensive reserve capacity, its regenerative ability, and its position between the absorptive surface of the intestinal tract and the systemic circulation.

The broad range of normal and abnormal hepatic function and the methods of study of liver disease will be considered in Chapter 13.1. The principal manifestations of liver disease—jaundice, portal hypertension with ascites, and hepatic encephalopathy—are discussed in Chapters 13.2 and 13.4. Additionally, the major categories of hepatic disease are presented: acute hepatocellular disease including viral hepatitis and drug-induced liver disease (Chapter 13.3), circulatory and focal liver disease (Chapter 13.5), and chronic liver disease (Chapter 13.6).

REFERENCES

1. Popper H, Schaffner F: Progress in Liver Diseases. New York, Grune & Stratton, 1962, 1965, 1970, 1972, 1976, 1979, 1982, Vols 1–7
2. Schiff L, Schiff ER: Disease of the Liver, 6th ed. Philadelphia, Lippincott, 1987
3. Sherlock S: Diseases of the Liver, 7th ed. Philadelphia, FA Davis, 1985
4. Wright R, Alberti KGMM, et al: Liver and Biliary Disease. London, WB Saunders, 1979
5. Zakim D, Boyer TD: Hepatology: A Textbook of Liver Disease. Philadelphia, WB Saunders, 1982

CHAPTER 13.1
Normal and Abnormal Hepatic Physiology; Biochemical and Radiologic Assessment of the Liver; and Classification of Diseases of the Liver

H. Franklin Herlong

NORMAL HEPATIC PHYSIOLOGY AND ITS INVESTIGATION

In normal man, the liver receives approximately 1500 ml blood per minute. This rich blood supply is consistent with the central role of the organ in metabolism. Two thirds of the blood flow to the liver is via the portal vein and the remainder by way of the hepatic artery. The portal vein is a unique conduit linking the capillary bed of the splanchnic system to that of the hepatic sinusoids. Venous blood from the splanchnic system transports the products of absorption from the gut to the liver by the portal vein. Blood in the portal vein normally has a slightly higher pressure and increased oxygen content than that found in systemic veins. Once in the hepatic sinusoids, the portal blood is mixed with hepatic arterial blood and exposed to the extensive highly permeable sinusoidal surfaces of the hepatic cells. After traversing the sinusoids, blood leaves the liver by the hepatic veins.

In addition to an abundant blood supply, each liver cell has access to an excretory system through small bile canaliculi. Bile, which is the principal hepatic secretory product, is produced at a rate of 1000 to 1500 ml/day.

Table 13.1–1 enumerates several of the functions of the normal liver and their derangements in disease. Carbohydrate metabolism, protein metabolism, and lipid metabolism are all intimately dependent on proper hepatic function. The maintenance of serum glucose concentration, either from breakdown of glycogen stores or from gluconeogenesis, is a vital hepatic anabolic function. The normal liver contains 5 to 7 percent glycogen by weight. This stored glycogen is sufficient to maintain normal blood glucose concentrations for approximately 24 hours in the absence of exogenous carbohydrate. Hypoglycemia may be seen in severe acute liver damage when glycogen reserves are depleted and gluconeogenesis is impaired.

Both body growth and regulation of intravascular volume are dependent on hepatic synthesis of proteins. Certain proteins that participate in the coagulation process are manufactured by the liver, and reduced synthesis is indicated by prolongation of the prothrombin time and a bleeding tendency.[8] Amino acid metabolism by the liver is important in protein synthesis and in the conversion of amino acids to carbohydrates and lipids. The conversion of ammonia to urea occurs in the liver (Krebs-Henseleit cycle). Excess ammonia and other nitrogenous products in the blood may be associated with the development of hepatic encephalopathy. Abnormal serum concentrations of many amino acids are found in a variety of liver diseases. In chronic liver disease, plasma concentrations of aromatic amino acids (tyrosine, phenylalanine, tryptophan) are increased while branched-chain amino acids (leucine, isoleucine, valine) are decreased. In severe acute liver disease, all plasma amino acids are increased except the branched-chain amino acids, which are normal.

The liver contains lipids in many forms, including cholesterol, free fatty acids, triglycerides, and phospholipids. It participates broadly in lipid metabolism by converting free fatty acids to triglycerides, manufacturing cholesterol and the enzyme LCAT (lecithin cholesterol acyl transferase), which esterifies cholesterol in the bloodstream, producing bile salts and synthesizing lipoproteins. Abnormalities at any of these steps may lead to the accumulation of fat in the liver. Abnormal lipid metabolism as evidenced by fatty liver is an important manifestation of liver disease produced by ethanol and other toxic agents.

The catabolic functions of the liver are also important in hepatic metabolism. The liver is a major site for metabolism and biotransformation of drugs and hormones. The role of the liver in the

TABLE 13.1–1. SELECTED NORMAL FUNCTIONS OF THE LIVER AND CLINCIAL MANIFESTATIONS IN DISEASE

Function	Clinical Manifestations in Liver Disease
Metabolic	
Anabolic	
1. Maintenance of serum glucose	Hypoglycemia
a. Glycogenolysis	
b. Gluconeogenesis	
2. Synthesis of proteins	
a. Albumin synthesis	Hypoalbuminemia ($\downarrow$ oncotic pressure)
	Edema, ascites
b. Synthesis of coagulation proteins (factors II, V, VII, IX, and X)	Bleeding diathesis
c. Manufacture of haptoglobin, fibrinogen, ceruloplasmin, etc.	
3. Lipid metabolism	
a. Uptake of plasma free fatty acids and conversion to triglycerides	Fatty liver (multifactorial)
b. Lipoprotein synthesis and release	Hypercholesterolemia in obstructive jaundice
c. Cholesterol synthesis and production of lecithin cholesterol acyl transferase (LCAT)	$\downarrow$ Cholesterol esters in hepatocellular disease
d. Synthesis (LCAT) and excretion of bile salts	Steatorrhea—malabsorption syndrome ($\downarrow$ bile salts in gut)
	Pruritus ($\uparrow$ bile salts in serum)
Catabolic	
1. Conjugation, solubilization, glucuronidation, and deamination of drugs	Acute liver injury—generally prolonged duration of drug action
	Chronic administration of certain drugs (e.g., phenobarbital) leads to induction of drug metabolizing enzymes and $\uparrow$ clearance
2. Conjugation and excretion of bilirubin	Jaundice
3. Conversion of ammonia to urea	$\uparrow$ Blood ammonia; $\downarrow$ Urea
4. Steroid metabolism; decreased degradation of aldosterone	Hyperaldosteronism
5. Processing of antigens (bacterial, dietary) absorbed from the gut	Hyperglobulinemia
Storage Activities	
1. Fat-soluble vitamins (A, D, E, and K)	D deficit—osteomalacia
	A deficit—night blindness
	K deficit—coagulation defect
2. Vitamin B$_{12}$	Decreased B$_{12}$ reserve
3. Metals	
a. Iron	Increased storage in hemochromatosis and hemosiderosis
b. Copper	Increased hepatic copper—Wilson disease; primary biliary cirrhosis
Reticuloendothelial Function	
1. Phagocytosis	Abnormal hepatic scan ^{99m}Tc
Maintenance of Plasma Volume and Electrolyte Concentrations	
1. Water homeostasis	Decreased renal free water clearance
2. Sodium excretion	Increased sodium reabsorption
3. Plasma volume	Increase in chronic liver disease with portal hypertension

metabolism of drugs is complex and variable. The liver conjugates many water-insoluble drugs to water-soluble compounds that can then be excreted into bile or urine. Other metabolic steps include drug inactivation by oxidation, reduction, hydroxylation, and glucuronidation. Prolongation of the effects of a drug may occur in patients with acute liver-cell injury (e.g., viral hepatitis). Many drugs (e.g., phenobarbital, alcohol) however, induce a proliferation of the smooth endoplasmic reticulum and its drug-metabolizing enzymes (especially the cytochrome P-450 microsomal mixed-function oxidase system) and thereby increase their own rate of metabolism as well as that of other drugs.

The liver serves as a storage depot for the fat-soluble vitamins A, D, E, and K, and in chronic liver diseases, especially those associated with cholestasis, deficiency syndromes of these vitamins may develop. In addition, the intestinal absorption of fat-soluble vitamins is dependent on bile salts. A decrease in vitamin K absorption, with its concomitant bleeding tendency, is the most frequent and clinically important vitamin deficiency encountered.

The reticuloendothelial cells (Kupffer cells) lining the hepatic sinusoids have an important phagocytic role.

HEPATIC REGENERATION

Among the most important characteristics of liver tissue is its ability to regenerate.[4] When liver cells are damaged by toxins, by interference with blood supply, or by obstruction to biliary flow, the remaining cells rapidly regenerate. The exact stimulus to regeneration is unknown, but several studies suggest that humoral agents are responsible. Insulin, glucagon, and epidermal growth factor are trophic substances for liver regeneration.[4] In the rat, surgical removal of two thirds of the functioning liver is followed by nearly complete restoration in a matter of days. Similar regeneration occurs in humans subjected to partial hepatectomy after trauma or in an attempt to resect tumor. Older animals and presumably man have reduced capacity for liver regeneration. Restoration of normal architecture can be obtained even with severe liver injury such as occurs with fulminant hepatitis. Complete restoration is not possible, however, when the major blood vessels and bile duct scaffold of the liver are damaged. In this circumstance the reticulin fibers coalesce, active fibrogenesis is promoted, and scar tissue is formed. Hypertrophy of remaining cells occurs in nonuniform fashion, causing the formation of nodules of regenerating liver. The regenerative nodule obtains its blood supply from vessels that encircle its periphery much like fingers around a ball. As the nodule enlarges, pressure constriction of the blood supply may develop that can limit the extent of regeneration and also result in the development of portal hypertension (see Chapter 13.4).

The blood flow to areas of regenerating nodules is predominantly arterial, and therefore the regenerating nodule is more vulnerable to fluctuations in arterial pressure than is normal liver tissue and is more likely to be damaged in situations associated with

a decrease in the arterial blood pressure (e.g., gastrointestinal hemorrhage).

LABORATORY ASSESSMENT OF LIVER DISEASE
(Table 13.1–2)

Numerous biochemical and radiologic tests are available to study hepatic function. These tests, properly employed, are of value in detecting hepatic disease, in evaluating the nature and extent of dysfunction, in following the progression of disease, and in assessing the effects of therapy. The spectrum of functions performed by the liver is so broad that no one test is sufficient. The proper use of the biochemical tests of liver function requires a knowledge of the specificity and sensitivity of tests designed to evaluate several functions. Of particular importance is the recognition that impairment of function in hepatic disease may be highly selective. For example, a reduced ability to synthesize urea is a manifestation of late and very severe dysfunction, whereas clearance of bile salts may be abnormal with minimal injury to the liver. Repeated observations over a period of time and a critical interpretation of results for technical error are important. Clinical decisions should not rest on one unconfirmed study. In this section, selected individual tests are described. Determination of serum bilirubin concentration and its interpretation are discussed in Chapter 13.2.

Safety of Tests
Discussion of tests of the liver must begin with a comment concerning safety to the patient. The examination of blood, stool, and

TABLE 13.1–2. APPROPRIATE TESTS FOR THE STUDY OF THE HEPATIC CIRCULATION, BILIARY TRACT, AND PARENCHYMAL DISEASE OF THE LIVER

Hepatic Circulation	
Portal circulation	
Anatomic evidence of portal vein patency	Venous phase of superior mesenteric arteriography
Evidence of portal to systemic collateral vessels	Barium esophagogram Esophagoscopy
Pressure measurements	Wedged hepatic venous pressure (WHVP) (indirect)
Hepatic venous circulation	
Anatomic evidence of patency and determination of pressure	Hepatic venous catheterization with measurement of WHVP
Hepatic artery	
Anatomic evidence of patency and distribution	Celiac arteriography
Biliary Tract	
Gallbladder function	
Anatomic evidence	Oral cholecystography
Common bile duct patency	
Anatomic evidence	Ultrasonography Endoscopic retrograde cholangiography Transhepatic cholangiography ^{99m}Tc HIDA scan
Functional evidence	SAP and 5′-nucleotidase measurement
Parenchymal Disease	
Acute liver cell disease	
Anatomic evidence	Liver biopsy
Functional evidence	
Synthetic ability	Serum albumin and prothrombin
Ability to conjugate and excrete	Bilirubin
Evidence of inflammation	
Functional	Aminotransferases

urine is of no risk to the patient. The use of cholangiographic dye has been associated rarely with severe reactions, including anaphylaxis and death. Liver biopsy and percutaneous transhepatic cholangiography are occasionally complicated by intraperitoneal hemorrhage, bile peritonitis, or sepsis. There is a risk of septicemia or pancreatitis associated with retrograde endoscopic cannulation of the bile ducts.

Determination of Aminotransferase Levels
The aminotransferases are a group of intracellular enzymes that are present in large quantities in the liver and are released into the blood after cell injury. The two principal aminotransferases are aspartate aminotransferase (AST) and alanine aminotransferase (ALT), which were formerly designated serum glutamic oxaloacetic transaminase (SGOT) and serum glutamic pyruvic transaminase (SGPT), respectively. Cell death is not required for enzyme release, and elevated levels may result from altered cell permeability. Serum aminotransferase determinations are most helpful in diagnosing early or nonicteric hepatitis and in serially following the course of acute liver injury. Very high serum concentrations of AST and ALT are characteristic of ischemic liver disease, viral hepatitis, and toxic hepatitis (from acetaminophen overdose). A prolonged elevation of the aminotransferases for greater than six months suggests chronic hepatitis. A precipitous drop in the level of aminotransferase enzymes in a patient who is clinically deteriorating may be indicative of such severe necrosis of liver cells that no more enzymes are available to be released. In patients with obstructive jaundice, the aminotransferase levels are rarely greater than ten times normal. The pattern of aminotransferase elevation may help determine the cause of liver disease. Patients with alcoholic hepatitis have a ratio of AST to ALT greater than 2:1. In addition, the AST is modestly elevated and the ALT is frequently normal. AST is also present in high concentration in heart and skeletal muscle. ALT is more specific for the liver. Marked elevation of only the AST suggests rhabdomyolysis or acute myocardial infarction. Other enzymes such as lactate dehydrogenase (LDH) and xanthine oxidase offer no advantage over the aminotransferases in diagnosis.

Determination of Serum Protein Levels
The liver produces the majority of serum proteins, including albumin, fibrinogen, certain coagulation factors (II, V, VII, IX, and X), and the α- and β-globulins. γ-globulins are produced by the cells of the reticuloendothelial system.

Albumin is quantitatively the most important protein produced by the liver. The serum albumin concentration is an important regulator of intravascular volume. The normal albumin level of 3.5 to 5.0 g/dl is maintained by hepatic synthesis in the endoplasmic reticulum of approximately 120 to 200 mg/kg/day.[9] The half-life of serum albumin is 14 to 20 days. The serum albumin is usually decreased in patients with chronic liver disease. In patients with cirrhosis and portal hypertension, at least part of the decreased serum level is explained by an expansion of the plasma volume.

The serum globulins are produced in the reticuloendothelial system and are elevated in many liver diseases associated with continuing cell necrosis. In diffuse hepatocellular diseases such as cirrhosis or chronic active hepatitis, the serum albumin level is depressed and the globulin fraction elevated. Occasionally in chronic active hepatitis, levels of serum globulin over 5 g/dl, such as are encountered in sarcoidosis and myeloma, are found. The absolute levels of albumin and globulin are of importance in following the course of hepatic diseases. The albumin/globulin ratio is of no value. Serum protein electrophoresis in patients with chronic liver disease may demonstrate a polyclonal gammopathy. A diminution of the α₁-globulin fraction is characteristic of α₁-antitrypsin deficiency, which may be associated with chronic liver disease.

Many chronic liver disorders have associated abnormalities in serum immunoglobulins. Although not often of specific use in differential diagnosis, an elevation in IgG is characteristic of idiopathic chronic active hepatitis, elevated IgA of alcoholic liver disease, and elevated IgM of primary biliary cirrhosis.

Determination of Serum Prothrombin Time

The one-stage prothrombin time determination is a measure of multiple clotting factors, of which factors II, V, VII, IX, and X are proteins manufactured by the liver.[8] A persistently long prothrombin time after the parenteral administration of vitamin K is usually indicative of liver-cell disease. Prolongation of the prothrombin time to more than twice normal is an ominous prognostic sign in severe hepatic necrosis because death may ensue.

Determination of Serum Alkaline Phosphatase Levels

The serum alkaline phosphatases (SAP) are a group of isoenzymes manufactured by bone, liver, intestine, and placenta. The normal range for SAP varies with age and sex. Normally SAP is derived in almost equal proportions from bone and liver. Although isoenzyme analysis is available, it is not routinely employed in clinical practice. The SAP level is most frequently elevated in diseases associated with obstruction of the bile ducts or bone destruction and remodeling. Obstruction of bile flow causes an increased synthesis of alkaline phosphatase within the liver, with subsequent regurgitation of the newly formed enzyme into the serum.[2] Because normal SAP activity is unusual in obstructive biliary disease, determination of the SAP level is a useful test when bile duct obstruction is suspected. Elevation of the SAP level, with a normal or nearly normal serum bilirubin level is characteristic of granulomatous diseases of the liver, such as sarcoidosis or tuberculosis, and is often present in metastatic tumors and amyloidosis. The half-life of SAP is approximately 7 days. Levels may therefore remain elevated for several days after an obstruction has been relieved.

Determination of Serum 5′-Nucleotidase and γ-Glutamyl Transpeptidase Levels

5′-Nucleotidase is an enzyme that catalyzes the hydrolysis of nucleotides and is found predominantly in the bile canaliculi and sinusoidal membranes of the liver. The enzyme is also present in the placenta but not in bone. In liver diseases, 5′-nucleotidase has a spectrum similar to that of serum alkaline phosphatase. The test is most useful in determining whether an elevated SAP level is of bone or liver origin.

γ-Glutamyl transpeptidase (GGTP) is an enzyme that catalyzes transfer of the γ-glutamyl group of peptides and L-amino acids. The activity of the enzyme is high in kidney, liver, and pancreas. Elevation of GGTP is a sensitive indicator of hepatobiliary disease, with a spectrum similar to that of SAP and 5′-nucleotidase. GGTP may be used instead of the 5′-nucleotidase to determine whether an elevated SAP level is of hepatic origin.

A lack of specificity limits the usefulness of the GGTP value. Agents that induce microsomal enzymes can elevate the GGTP level in the absence of liver disease. Moderate consumption of alcohol leads to an increase in GGTP when all other tests of liver function are normal. Medications such as phenytoin and phenobarbital are associated with an elevated GGTP level.[1]

Bile Acid Tests

Bile acids are synthesized by the liver, secreted into bile, and subsequently reabsorbed from the ileum in an efficient enterohepatic circulation. Serum bile acid concentrations are determined by radioimmunoassay or chromatographic methods. In liver diseases, there may be decreased removal of bile acids from portal blood because of cell injury or hepatic bypass resulting from the development of portal hypertension and collateral vessels. Elevations of serum bile acids is a sensitive indicator of liver damage. Determination of the 2-hour postprandial bile acid level has been suggested to be the most sensitive test available to detect liver damage.[3]

Radiologic, Endoscopic, and Laparoscopic Procedures

Esophagogastric endoscopy in patients with liver disease often provides the earliest evidence of the presence and extent of varices in the lower esophagus and the stomach. Endoscopic procedures also allow assessment of other gastrointestinal lesions that are found with increased frequency in patients with liver disease—peptic ulcer, gastritis, and Mallory-Weiss lesions.

The development of the technique for endoscopic retrograde cannulation of the ampulla of Vater is useful in evaluation of the common bile duct.

Percutaneous transhepatic cholangiography is a worthwhile adjunct in the differential diagnosis of extrahepatic versus intrahepatic obstructive jaundice.[7] A long, thin needle is inserted into the liver and slowly withdrawn until bile is aspirated. Cholangiographic dye is then injected to outline the biliary system. Bile ducts that have become dilated as a consequence of obstruction are easily punctured. In the presence of intrahepatic obstruction, the bile ducts are small and less easily entered. Direct visualization of the surface of the liver and guided biopsy of focal lesions are available with laparoscopy. This technique allows the additional opportunity to examine the peritoneal surface for tumor implants or tuberculosis and to assess the other intraabdominal organs (e.g., gallbladder).

Determination of wedged hepatic venous pressure may be of considerable importance in the evaluation of portal hypertension, and the technique and interpretation are described in Chapter 13.4.

Ultrasonography

Ultrasonographic evaluation of the bile ducts and liver is an important noninvasive test. Ultrasonography is useful in detecting dilation of the bile duct and focal lesions in the liver. In addition, ultrasonographic guidance facilitates drainage of hepatic abscesses or cysts and is useful in directing liver biopsy and determining the presence of ascitic fluid. Ultrasonography is also useful in the detection of gallstones.

Computed Tomography (CT)

CT of the liver is useful in diagnosing focal masses in the liver and in the differential diagnosis of abdominal masses. Magnetic resonance imaging (MRI) of the liver is helpful not only for identifying focal lesions but for evaluating the hepatic vasculature.

Angiography

Selective angiography of the hepatic artery is useful in evaluating mass lesions within the liver and in defining vascular lesions such as hemangiomas. The venous phase of superior mesenteric arteriography allows determination of the patency of the portal vein.

Radioisotope Liver Scans

Technetium-99 is a gamma-emitting radioisotope selectively taken up by the reticuloendothelial cells and is useful in determining hepatic size, configuration, and the presence of filling defects. Hepatic scans are not accurate in determining nodules of less than 3 cm, and false-positive scans for filling defects are frequently found in the presence of alcoholic liver disease and cirrhosis. Technetium-

TABLE 13.1–3. CLINICAL USEFULNESS OF LIVER BIOPSY

Differential Diagnosis
- Hepatomegaly
- Jaundice
- Abnormal liver function test results

Detection of Intrahepatic Neoplasm

Recognition of Systemic Inflammatory or Granulomatous Disorders
- Tuberculosis
- Sarcoidosis
- Brucellosis
- Evaluation of prolonged fever of unknown origin

Evaluation of Effectiveness of Therapy
- Removal of copper (Wilson disease) or iron (hemochromatosis)
- Effect of corticosteroid or immunosuppressive therapy in management of liver disease

TABLE 13.1–4. LIVER BIOPSY

Contraindications
Absolute
- Uncooperative patient
- Bleeding tendency
   Prothrombin time <50%
   Bleeding time prolonged
- Infection in right pleural space
- Serious consideration of echinococcal disease
- Presumed hemangioma

Relative
- Obstruction to the extrahepatic biliary system
- Ascites

Complications
Minor
- Pain at site of biopsy needle entry
- Epigastric discomfort
- Vasovagal reaction

Serious
- Intraperitoneal hemorrhage—usually within 24 hours—rare
- Bile peritonitis—rare

99m iminodiacetic acid (HIDA) and related compounds are isotopes taken up by liver cells and subsequently excreted in the bile. Their major use is in determining patency of the cystic duct and common bile duct. Gallium-67 is a radionuclide that is concentrated in liver abscesses and hepatocellular carcinomas.

Needle Biopsy of the Liver

Needle biopsy of the liver is a safe, simple procedure of considerable importance in the diagnosis of liver disease. In addition to providing material for light microscopy, this procedure supplies specimens for electron microscopy, tissue culture, and heavy-metal analysis. The liver biopsy is particularly useful in the differential diagnosis of hepatomegaly and jaundice, in the search for hepatic neoplasms, in the evaluation of prolonged fevers, and in the evaluation of the course of liver disease and the effect of therapy (Table 13.1–3). The procedure is contraindicated in an uncooperative or stuporous patient, in the presence of a bleeding tendency, or when there is infected fluid in the right pleural space (Table 13.1–4). When these procedures are performed by experienced physicians, less than one biopsy in 1000 should be associated with a serious complication.

USE OF LIVER FUNCTION TESTS

In all patients with definite or suspected liver abnormalities, the following determinations should be made:

1. Serum bilirubin levels—total and direct-reacting fractions
2. Serum aminotransferase levels—AST and ALT
3. Serum alkaline phosphatase level
4. Total serum protein with determination of albumin and globulin levels
5. Prothrombin time
6. Urine bilirubin levels

In patients with an isolated elevation of alkaline phosphatase, a 5'-nucleotidase or GGTP value may provide added evidence that the rise is associated with hepatobiliary disease. After the initial clinical and laboratory assessment, liver biopsy is often the single most useful test. Percutaneous transhepatic cholangiography, endoscopic retrograde cholangiography, laparoscopy, and laparotomy are reserved for special instances in which the differential diagnosis of extrahepatic versus intrahepatic biliary tract obstruction is not possible by the use of simpler and more conventional means.

TABLE 13.1–5. CLASSIFICATION OF LIVER DISEASES

Disorders of Circulation
- Passive congestion from heart failure and cardiac cirrhosis
- Hepatic vein thrombosis (Budd-Chiari syndrome)
- Veno-occlusive disease
- Portal vein thrombosis
- Disorders of the hepatic artery (e.g., polyarteritis nodosa, hepatic artery aneurysms)

Disorders Due to Biliary Obstruction
Extrahepatic biliary obstruction
- Tumors of the bile duct, gallbladder, pancreas, ampulla of Vater, duodenum
- Choledocholithiasis
- Bile duct strictures, diverticula, etc.
- Sclerosing cholangitis

Intrahepatic biliary obstruction
- Intrahepatic bile duct stone or tumor
- Cholangitis
- Intrahepatic cholestasis (e.g., drugs)
- Primary biliary cirrhosis

Parenchymal Disorders
Focal liver disease
- Abscess (pyogenic, amebic); other suppurative processes (e.g., actinomycosis)
- Neoplasms (primary and secondary)
- Cysts (e.g., echinococcal, congenital), gummas
- Granulomas (sarcoidosis, tuberculosis, berylliosis, histoplasmosis, etc.)

Diffuse liver disorders
- Inborn errors of bilirubin metabolism
   Gilbert syndrome
   Dubin-Johnson and Rotor syndromes
- Hepatitis
   Viral hepatitis (A; B; non-A, non-B)
   Leptospirosis
   Drug-induced hepatitis
   Chronic active hepatitis
- Cirrhosis
   Portal (Laennec)
   Postnecrotic
   Hemochromatosis
   Wilson disease
   Primary biliary cirrhosis
   α_1-Antitrypsin deficiency
- Infiltrative diseases
   Fatty liver
   Amyloidosis, Gaucher disease, Neimann-Pick disease
   Leukemia, lymphoma

CLASSIFICATION OF LIVER DISEASES
(Table 13.1–5)

Diseases of the liver are classified most satisfactorily on the basis of cause (often presumed) or, lacking a specific etiologic agent, on the basis of morphologic changes. Three major categories of liver disease will be considered: disorders due to circulatory abnormalities, disorders due to biliary obstruction, and disorders due to parenchymal liver disease.

REFERENCES

1. Goldberg DM, Martin JV: Role of gamma-glutamyl transpeptidase activity in the diagnosis of hepatobiliary disease. Digestion 12:232, 1975
2. Kaplan MM: Alkaline phosphatase. N Engl J Med 286:200, 1972
3. Korman MG, Hofmann AF, Summerskill WHJ: Assessment of activity in chronic active hepatitis: Serum bile acids compared with conventional tests and histology. N Engl J Med 290:1399, 1974

4. Leffert HL, Koch KS, et al: Hormonal control of rat liver regeneration. Gastroenterology 76:1470, 1979
5. Matloff DS, Selinger MJ, Kaplan MM: Hepatic transaminase activity in alcoholic liver disease. Gastroenterology 78:1389, 1980
6. Menghini G: One-second biopsy of the liver—problems of its clinical application. N Engl J Med 283:582, 1970
7. Okuda K: Endoscopic/cholangiographic imaging and treatment. Semin Liver Dis 2:1–86, 1982
8. Roberts HR, Cederbaum AI: The liver and blood coagulation: Physiology and pathology. Gastroenterology 63:297, 1972
9. Rothschild MA, Oratz M, Schreiber SS: Albumin metabolism. Gastroenterology 64:324, 1973

CHAPTER 13.2
Jaundice

H. Franklin Herlong

Manifestations of liver disease include jaundice, ascites, esophageal variceal hemorrhage, and the mental status changes of hepatic encephalopathy. Significant liver disease may, however, be present with only nonspecific constitutional symptoms such as anorexia, fatigue, weight loss, nausea, or fever. The general deterioration of health so often encountered in liver disease frequently cannot be explained by the failure of any single hepatic function. Associated disease such as carcinoma or nutritional deficits, as seen in chronic alcoholism, may be more important than the liver disease itself in the production of the patient's symptoms.

Jaundice is the most common specific symptom of liver disease and results from accumulation of bilirubin in tissues. When the serum bilirubin level exceeds 2 to 4 mg/dl, visible staining of tissues, especially skin, mucous membranes, and sclerae, becomes detectable. A lesser elevation of serum bilirubin is detected only by biochemical means and is designated "subclinical jaundice." Bilirubin may be present in plasma and tissues in both unconjugated and conjugated forms. Conjugated bilirubin preferentially stains tissues with high elastin content, such as the sclerae or mucous membranes. Jaundice is more apparent in sunlight than in artificial light and is less apparent in edematous areas because of the low protein content of edema fluid. It is important to distinguish the yellow coloration of jaundice from the similar colors of several other substances. Neither carotene nor quinacrine causes scleral discoloration. Occasionally, with prolonged jaundice, particularly of the conjugated type, the patient has a greenish color, reflecting the oxidation of tissue bilirubin stores to biliverdin. Jaundice is not a sensitive sign of liver disease. Many patients with cirrhosis, hepatitis, or tumor have a normal bilirubin level because of the reserve capacity of the liver to excrete bilirubin.

METABOLISM OF BILIRUBIN[9] (Fig. 13.2–1)

Seventy to eighty percent of serum bilirubin is derived from the breakdown of senescent red blood cells in the reticuloendothelial system. The remaining 20 to 30 percent is derived from catabolism of other heme compounds such as cytochrome enzymes, catalases, peroxidases, or abortive preerythrocytic precursors in the bone marrow. In normal man, approximately 6.25 g of hemoglobin is released from aged red blood cells each day, with the formation of 250 to 350 mg of bilirubin. An additional 10 to 30 mg of bilirubin comes from nonerythropoietic sources.

In the phagocytic cells of the reticuloendothelial system of the spleen, bone marrow, and liver, bilirubin is produced from the breakdown of hemoglobin. The enzyme heme oxygenase cleaves the porphyrin ring of heme to yield IX-α biliverdin. This reaction requires molecular oxygen and releases carbon monoxide. Biliverdin reductase converts biliverdin to bilirubin, a water-insoluble, unconjugated compound that is rapidly and tightly bound to serum albumin. The unconjugated bilirubin-albumin complex is not filtered by the glomerulus. Several compounds, including sulfona-mides and ampicillin, can displace bilirubin from albumin. At the liver cell membrane, bilirubin is separated from its albumin carrier and is taken up by the liver cell (Figure 13.2–2). Once inside the cell, transfer of bilirubin from the plasma membrane to the endoplasmic reticulum is facilitated by Y protein (ligandin) and Z protein (fatty acid–binding protein). At the endoplasmic reticulum, bilirubin is conjugated with UDP-glucuronic acid to form a nontoxic water-soluble compound. This reaction involves the enzyme bilirubin UDP-glucuronyl transferase and is inducible with phenobarbital. Some studies suggest that bilirubin monoglucuronide is produced in the smooth endoplasmic reticulum and is subsequently converted to bilirubin diglucuronide in a subcellular fraction rich in plasma membranes. Conjugated bilirubin is then actively secreted across the canalicular membrane of the hepatocyte into the bile. This active transport of conjugated bilirubin is the rate-limiting step in the excretory pathway of bilirubin. With injury to the hepatocyte or obstruction to bile flow at the level of the canaliculus or beyond, conjugated bilirubin is regurgitated into the plasma. Regurgitated conjugated bilirubin is bound to albumin—but much less tightly than unconjugated bilirubin. Approximately 1 percent of the bilirubin-glucuronyl-albumin complex is excreted by glomerular filtration. With very high plasma levels of conjugated bilirubin, renal excretion becomes a major pathway for bilirubin elimination. When, therefore, impaired renal function is superimposed on jaundice, bilirubin levels may rise. After secretion into the biliary tree, conjugated bilirubin traverses the intestinal tract to the distal portion of the small intestine and colon, where conjugated bilirubin is catabolized by bacteria to colorless urobilinogens that are subsequently oxidized to colored urobilins. These urobilins give stool its characteristic brown coloration. Urobilinogen is efficiently reabsorbed by an enterohepatic circulation, with the majority reexcreted into the bile. Normally, approximately 1 percent of uribilinogen escapes reuptake by the liver and is detectable in the urine. An increased urine urobilinogen level is found in patients with an increased pigment load from hemolysis.

Urine urobilinogen is also elevated in hepatocellular disease, presumably because its normal removal from the blood by hepatic cells is impaired. An absence of urobilinogen in the urine suggests interruption of the intrahepatic circulation of bile pigments and is found in common bile duct obstruction. The urine urobilinogen level may be decreased when antibiotic therapy suppresses gut flora.

The van den Bergh reaction is the most frequently used test for serum bilirubin. Carotene, picrates, and quinacrine do not affect this reaction. In the van den Bergh reaction, bilirubin combines with diazotized sulfanilic acid to form chromogenic dipyrroles. The total serum bilirubin level is determined by eliciting the diazo reaction in the presence of alcohol, with both conjugated and unconjugated bilirubin. When the diazo reaction occurs in an aqueous medium, it measures only the water-soluble (conjugated) bilirubin, which is designated the direct-reacting fraction. The indirect-reacting (unconjugated) fraction of bilirubin is determined

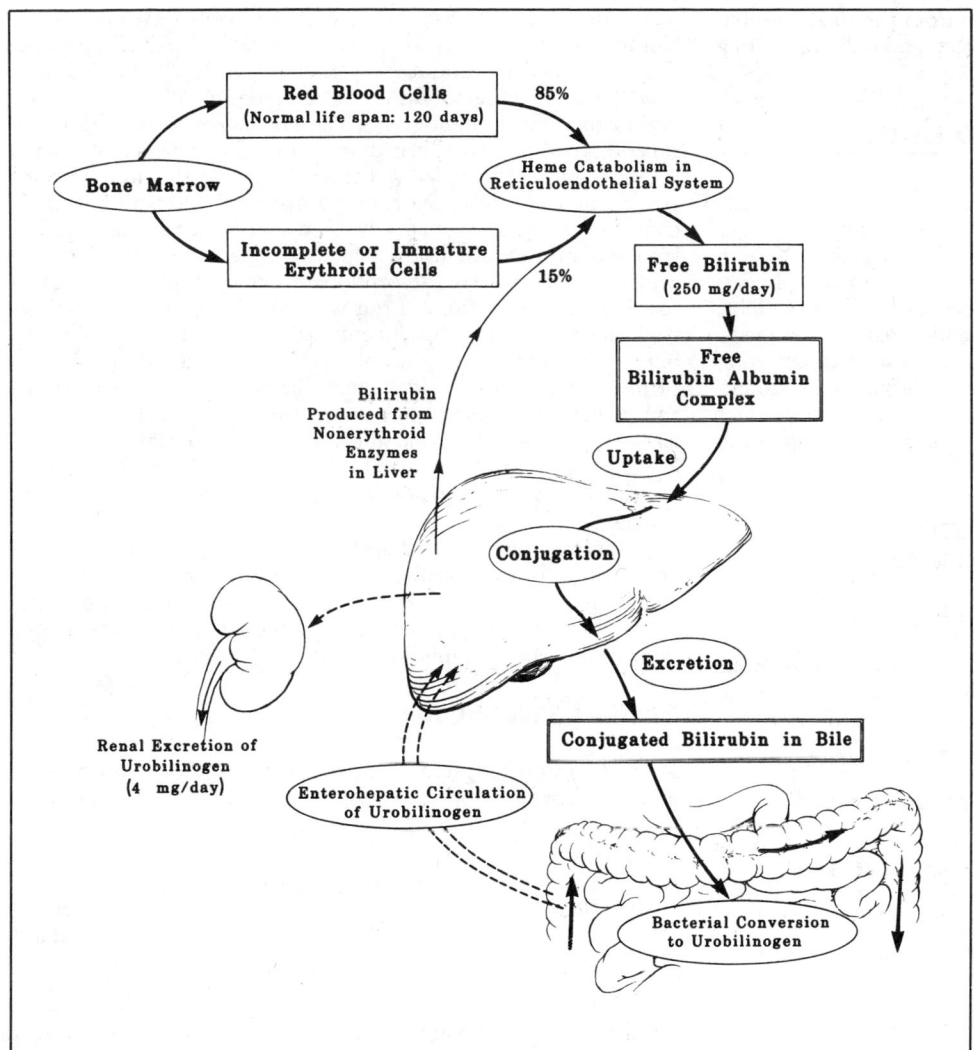

Figure 13.2–1. Metabolism of bilirubin. Breakdown of aged or injured red blood cells in reticuloendothelial system accounts for 70 to 80 percent of bilirubin production. A small percentage of bilirubin (20 to 30 percent) is derived from immature erythroid cells in bone marrow or from nonerythroid enzymes in the liver. Bilirubin released from hemoglobin is water insoluble (free or unconjugated bilirubin) and is transported in serum as bilirubin-albumin complex that is not filtered at the renal glomerular membrane. At the hepatic cell membrane, bilirubin-albumin complex is dissociated with selective uptake of bilirubin, conjugation in smooth endoplasmic reticulum and plasma membranes (see text) to diglucuronide, and active secretion into bile. Once in the intestine, conjugated bilirubin is catabolized by bacteria to urobilinogens that are reabsorbed into enterohepatic circulation, with majority excreted by liver into bile. Small amount (about 4 mg per day) of urobilinogen is filtered at glomerular membrane and excreted into urine.

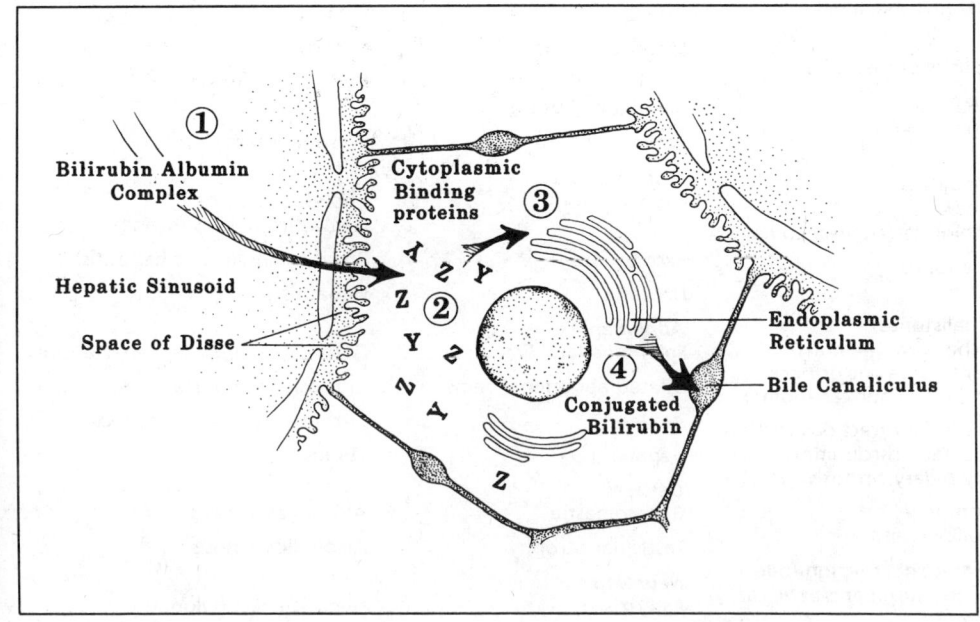

Figure 13.2–2. Pathway for movement of bilirubin through liver cell. ① Unconjugated bilirubin tightly bound to albumin is delivered to hepatic sinusoidal membrane, where unconjugated bilirubin is separated from albumin and selectively taken up into cytoplasm of hepatic cell. ② Once in cell, free bilirubin is bound to cytoplasmic acceptor proteins (Y and Z). ③ Subsequently, bilirubin is conjugated to a diglucuronide in smooth endoplasmic reticulum (see text). ④ Conjugated bilirubin is then secreted by active process into bile canaliculus. Jaundice may occur from (1) overproduction of free bilirubin, (2) defective uptake and cell storage, (3) defective conjugation, (4) defective excretion of conjugated bilirubin.

by subtracting the direct-reacting fraction from the total bilirubin value. The separation of bilirubin into direct- and indirect-reacting fractions is often clinically useful.

APPROACH TO THE JAUNDICED PATIENT[4,7]

The initial approach to the jaundiced patient requires attention to specific aspects of the history. Table 13.2–1 summarizes important historical features that are useful in establishing the cause of an elevated bilirubin. Detecting certain signs from the physical examination helps to characterize the liver disease further (Table 13.2–2). Finally, laboratory tests provide additional information to aid in differential diagnosis (Table 13.2–3). A useful classification system for jaundice is based on whether conjugated or unconjugated bilirubin accumulates in the blood. Quantitating the amount of the two bilirubin fractions is the first step in an orderly approach to the differential diagnosis of jaundice.

JAUNDICE WITH PREDOMINANTLY UNCONJUGATED HYPERBILIRUBINEMIA (Table 13.2–4)

Unconjugated hyperbilirubinemia suggests either an increase in the pigment load presented to the liver or a defect in the uptake or conjugation of bilirubin. Patients with this disorder do not have bilirubinuria. The reserve capacity of the normal liver to excrete bilirubin is considerable, and a marked increase in pigment production is required to produce hyperbilirubinemia. Plasma bilirubin concentrations in hemolysis do not exceed 4 mg/dl, provided that hepatic bilirubin clearance is normal. Higher concentrations imply superimposed hepatocellular dysfunction. Some degree of anemia is usually present with severe hemolysis, but an elevated reticulocyte count in the absence of anemia may be found with low grade compensated hemolytic anemia. A decreased serum haptoglobin level and an increased urine hemosiderin level provide additional evidence of hemolysis. Resorption of hemoglobin from areas of tissue trauma, infarction, or burns may lead to an elevation of unconjugated bilirubin. Defective uptake and conjugation of bilirubin may be hereditary or acquired. Certain medications, such as rifampin, can interfere with uptake and conjugation. In newborn and premature infants, immaturity of both the glucuronyl transferase system and the cytoplasmic protein receptors leads to unconjugated hyperbilirubinemia. This "physiologic" jaundice reaches its peak within 2 to 5 days of delivery and usually disappears within 2 weeks.

Impaired delivery of bilirubin to the liver from congestive heart failure is a common cause of unconjugated hyperbilirubinemia. In patients with surgical or endogenous portasystemic shunts, bilirubin can pass directly from the spleen into the systemic circulation, causing a mild unconjugated jaundice.

GILBERT SYNDROME[3,6]

Idiopathic unconjugated hyperbilirubinemia, or Gilbert syndrome, is a benign disorder transmitted as an autosomal dominant

TABLE 13.2–1. HISTORY IN THE JAUNDICED PATIENT

Family history	Wilson disease
	α_1-Antitrypsin deficiency
	Hemochromatosis
	Familial cholestasis
Current medications	Drug-induced cholestasis (chlorpromazine)
	Hepatitis (isoniazid)
	Budd-Chiari syndrome (estrogens)
	Gallstones (estrogens)
Travel history	Viral hepatitis
	Amebic liver abscess
	Echinococcal disease
Sexual contacts	Viral hepatitis
	Syphilitic hepatitis
	Atypical mycobacterial infection
Alcohol abuse	Alcoholic liver disease
Intravenous drug abuse	Viral hepatitis
	Pyogenic abscess
Employment history	
Health care worker	Viral hepatitis
Environmental toxins	Berylliosis
	Vinyl chloride (angiosarcoma)
Exposure to blood or blood products	Viral hepatitis
Pain	Colic (gallstones)
	Dull ache (viral hepatitis)
	Constant epigastric or back pain (pancreatic carcinoma)
Pruritus	Chronic biliary tract obstruction (pancreatic carcinoma)
	Primary biliary cirrhosis
Fever	Cholangitis
	Alcoholic hepatitis
"Acholic" stools	Biliary tract obstruction (bile duct stricture pancreatic carcinoma)
	Drug-induced cholestasis

TABLE 13.2–2. PHYSICAL EXAMINATION OF THE PATIENT WITH JAUNDICE

Head	
Kayser-Fleischer ring	Wilson disease
	Primary biliary cirrhosis
Lacrimegaly; parotid gland enlargement	Alcoholic cirrhosis
Xanthelasma	Primary biliary cirrhosis
	Bile duct stricture
Hands	
Clubbing	Cirrhosis (cholestatic)
Dupuytren contracture	Cirrhosis
Palmar erthema	Cirrhosis
Spider angiomata	Cirrhosis
Muehrcke lines (white-banded nail beds)	Hypoalbuminemia
Azure nail beds	Wilson disease
Extremities	
Pigmentation	Cholestasis (chronic)
	Hemochromatosis (bronze)
Excoriations	Pruritus (cholestatic hepatitis)
Urticaria	Hepatitis B
Abdomen	
Splenomegaly	Cirrhosis with portal hypertension
Dilated abdominal veins	Cirrhosis with portal hypertension
Ascites	Cirrhosis with portal hypertension
Hepatic rub	Tumor
General	
Gynecomastia	Alcoholic cirrhosis
Testicular atrophy	Alcoholic cirrhosis
Neurologic	
Asterixis	Hepatic encephalopathy
Hyperreflexia	Hepatic encephalopathy

TABLE 13.2–3. LABORATORY STUDIES IN PATIENTS WITH JAUNDICE

| Disorder Causing Jaundice | Liver Function Studies | | | | | | | Urine Bilirubin |
| | Bilirubin | | | | | Heme | | |
	Indirect	Direct	Alk. Phos.	AST	ALT	WBC	Hct	
Hemolytic anemia	↑	N	N	N	N	N	↓	0
Gilbert syndrome	↑	N	N	N	N	N	N	0
Viral hepatitis	↑	↑↑	N–↑	↑↑	↑↑	N–↓	N	+
Alcoholic hepatitis	↑	↑↑	N–↑	↑ (2:1)	N–↑	↑	N–↓	+
Drug-induced cholestasis	↑	↑↑	↑↑	↑–N	N–↑	N	N	+
Common bile duct obstruction	↑	↑↑	↑	N–↑	N–↑	↑	N	+
Primary biliary cirrhosis	↑	↑↑	↑↑	↑	↑	N	N	+

Alk. Phos. = Alkaline phosphatase; AST = aspartate aminotransferase; ALT = alanine-amino transferase; WBC = white blood cell count; Hct = hematocrit.

trait. It is found in 3 to 7 percent of the adult population, with a higher expression in men than women. An elevation of unconjugated bilirubin is found in 16 percent of the parents, and in 27 percent of the siblings, of patients with this disorder. The serum bilirubin level is usually less than 6 mg/dl and is often first noted on routine physical examination or blood screening. Jaundice is intermittent and more pronounced during the second and third decades. The bilirubin level fluctuates and may be increased by fasting, intercurrent infection, and strenuous exercise.

The liver is histologically normal, as are other biochemical test results of liver function. The hyperbilirubinemia in Gilbert syndrome is multifactorial. Hepatic glucuronyl transferase activity is reduced, and alterations in membrane fluidity impair the uptake of bilirubin by the liver cell. Some patients have a mild compensated hemolysis. This condition is benign, and the physician should reassure the patient that serious liver disease is not present. Patients with Gilbert syndrome have a normal life expectancy and require no specific treatment.

CRIGLER–NAJJAR SYNDROME[6]

The Crigler–Najjar syndrome is a rare form of severe unconjugated hyperbilirubinemia due to an absence of glucuronyl transferase. The prototype, type I, has an autosomal recessive pattern of inheritance and is associated with severe hyperbilirubinemia (20 to 31 mg/dl), kernicterus, and colorless bile. These patients have no response to phenobarbital therapy. Severe jaundice usually begins 3 to 4 days after birth, with bilirubin encephalopathy usually developing within 18 months. Patients with the type II form of the syndrome have a lower serum bilirubin level (9 to 17 mg/dl), do not acquire kernicterus, and have some bile color. The inheritance pattern suggests an autosomal dominant trait. The serum bilirubin in these patients responds to administration of phenobarbital, suggesting some glucuronyl transferase is inducible.

TABLE 13.2–4. EVALUATION OF PATIENT WITH UNCONJUGATED (INDIRECT) HYPERBILIRUBINEMIA, AN ELEVATED SERUM INDIRECT BILIRUBIN LEVEL, AND *NO* BILIRUBINURIA

Disorders and Causes of Increased Bilirubin	Pertinent Observations
Evidence of hemolysis? Overproduction	Increased reticulocyte count, anemia, positive Coombs test result, decreased haptoglobin, increased urine hemosiderin level
Extravasation of blood? Overproduction	Evidence of trauma, postoperative state
Abnormal erythropoiesis? Overproduction	Abnormal Schilling test result (pernicious anemia)
Gilbert syndrome? Decreased uptake with conjugation	Increased bilirubin with fasting, positive family history
Crigler-Najjar syndrome Type I? Absent glucuronyl transferase	Kernicterus, early death
Type II? Absent glucuronyl transferase	Decreased bilirubin with phenobarbital
Congestive heart failure? Decreased delivery	
Portacaval shunt? Escape through collateral vessels	
Cirrhosis? Escape through collateral vessels Increased production	Hypersplenism, portal hypertension

JAUNDICE ASSOCIATED WITH PREDOMINANTLY CONJUGATED HYPERBILIRUBINEMIA (Table 13.2–5)

Elevation in the conjugated bilirubin level is evidence of a defect in the excretory pathway of bilirubin. The defect may be due to primary dysfunction of the liver cell (hepatocellular jaundice) or obstruction to bile flow from the level of the canaliculus down to the common bile duct (cholestatic jaundice). There are two important clinical questions to ask in evaluating a patient with conjugated hyperbilirubinemia. First, does the patient have hepatocellular or cholestatic jaundice? Second, once it has been decided that the jaundice is due to biliary tract dysfunction, is the problem due to mechanical obstruction of the large bile ducts or to intrahepatic cholestasis? Liver function tests other than the bilirubin determination are useful in the differential diagnosis of patients with conjugated jaundice (Table 13.2–3). Elevated aminotransferase levels suggest hepatocellular disease, whereas predominant elevation in the alkaline phosphatase level suggests biliary tract injury. It is important to point out that individual laboratory tests alone are not sufficient to allow an accurate diagnosis in most patients. Instead, a clinical impression should be derived from information obtained from the history, physical examination, and screening laboratory data.

TABLE 13.2–5. EVALUATION OF PATIENT WITH CONJUGATED HYPERBILIRUBINEMIA

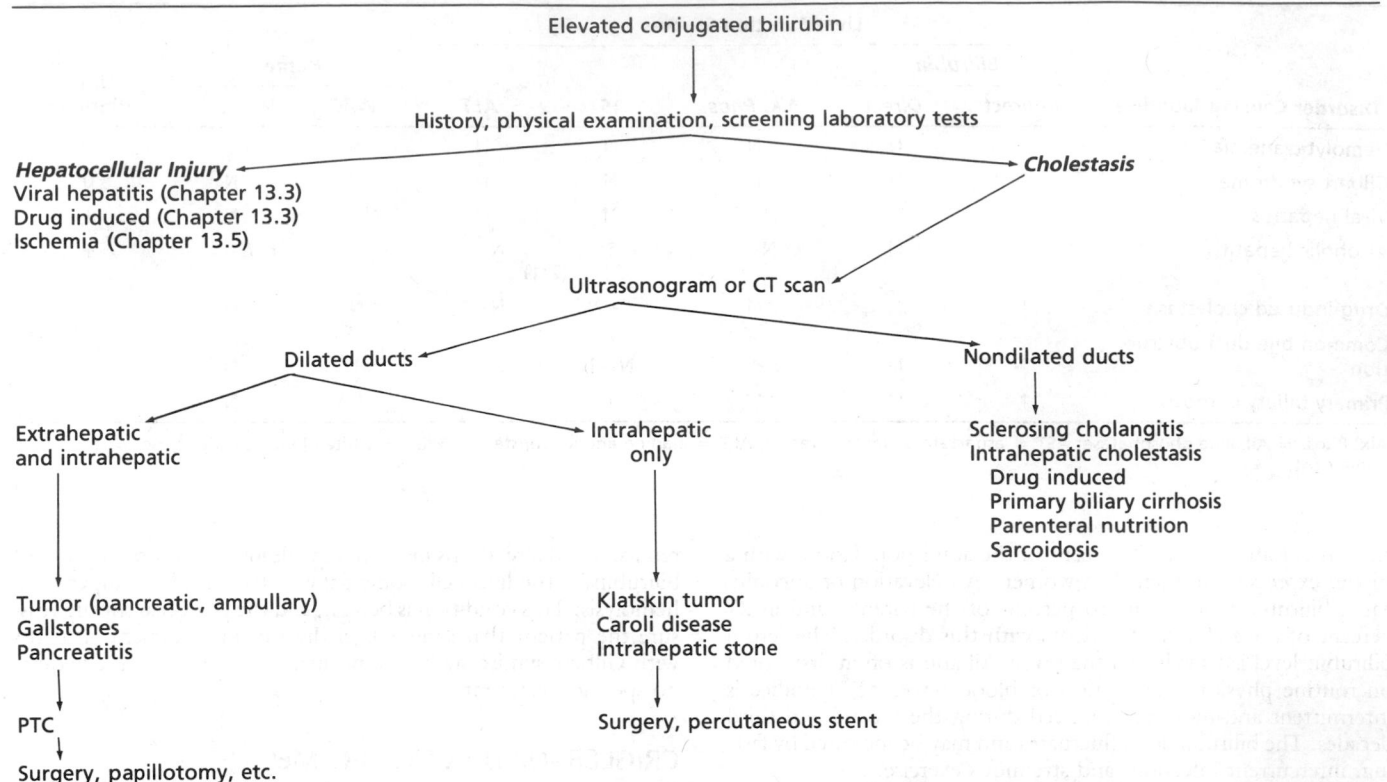

If extrahepatic biliary tract obstruction appears likely, then visualization of the bile ducts is necessary. Ultrasonography and CT scanning provide simple, noninvasive techniques for the detection of dilated biliary radicles. Dilated intrahepatic and extrahepatic ducts suggest obstruction of the distal common bile duct because of tumor (ampullary carcinoma, pancreatic carcinoma), pancreatic disease, gallstones, or a distal duct stricture. If the common bile duct is normal but the intrahepatic ducts are dilated, the cause may be cholangiocarcinoma at the duct bifurcation (Klatskin tumor), an intrahepatic gallstone, or Caroli disease, which causes cystic dilation of the intrahepatic bile ducts. Extrahepatic biliary obstruction without ductular dilation is characteristic of sclerosing cholangitis.

Direct visualization of the biliary tree is frequently necessary to establish a specific site of obstruction. Percutaneous transhepatic cholangiography (PTC) is most useful when intrahepatic ducts are dilated. At the time of PTC, silastic stents can be placed to drain the obstructed bile ducts. Endoscopic retrograde cholangiopancreatography (ERCP) is most useful when extrahepatic obstruction is suspected, but no ductal dilation is seen on an ultrasonogram or a CT scan. Sphincterotomy, with retrieval of common duct stones or dilation of distal duct strictures, can be performed at the time of ERCP. Definitive therapy for many patients with extrahepatic biliary tract obstruction requires surgical intervention.

INTRAHEPATIC CHOLESTASIS

Once radiographic visualization of the extrahepatic biliary tree has excluded mechanical obstruction, then the clinician must determine whether jaundice is related to hepatocellular disease or disorders of the intrahepatic bile ducts. Viral hepatitis and toxic liver injury result in impaired excretion of conjugated bilirubin into the canalicular bile. Metabolic disturbances such as ischemia or sepsis commonly impair liver cell excretory functions. Cholestasis may develop from septal or interlobular bile duct injury in primary biliary cirrhosis or compression from granulomatous hepatitis or tumor. Intrahepatic cholestasis occasionally occurs during pregnancy,

especially during the third trimester, and results from increased sensitivity to estrogenic compounds. The cholestatic jaundice of pregnancy is often reproduced by the administration of birth control pills. A careful history of complications of pregnancy should be taken in any woman in whom jaundice begins to develop while she is using an oral contraceptive.

Rare intrahepatic causes of defective excretion of conjugated bilirubin include the Dubin-Johnson syndrome, Rotor syndrome, and benign recurrent cholestasis. Inherited as an autosomal recessive trait, Dubin-Johnson syndrome is associated with a normal uptake and conjugation of bilirubin but an impaired secretion of conjugated bilirubin into the bile. Conjugated bilirubin regurgitates into the plasma and can be detected in the urine. Biliary excretion of other organic anions, such as indocyanine green, is also impaired. In the Dubin-Johnson syndrome the liver appears black because of melanin pigment, which accumulates as a result of the conversion of retained metanephrine glucuronide. There is a diagnostically significant abnormality in urinary coproporphyrin excretion in the Dubin-Johnson syndrome, with affected patients excreting 90 percent of their urinary coproporphyrins as coproporphyrin isomer I, whereas in normal persons, at least 70 percent of urinary coproporphyrin is in the isomer III form. This disorder, like Gilbert syndrome, is benign and requires no specific treatment. Rotor syndrome is similar to Dubin-Johnson syndrome, but hepatic pigmentation is lacking and coproporphyrin I excretion is normal. Benign recurrent cholestasis is characterized by recurrent bouts of intrahepatic cholestasis. During attacks, the patient may itch but have no other evidence of hepatic dysfunction. Between attacks, the liver is functionally and morphologically normal.

COMPLICATIONS OF CHOLESTASIS[1]

Clinical symptoms from impaired excretion of bile may develop regardless of the site of obstruction. They tend to be more severe with prolonged cholestasis. Impaired secretion of bile salts leads to inadequate micelle formation, causing fat malabsorption with

secondary fat-soluble vitamin deficiency states, including night blindness (vitamin A), osteomalacia (vitamin D), and coagulopathy (vitamin K). Prompt correction of the prothrombin time after parenteral vitamin K administration implies cholestasis rather than hepatocellular synthetic dysfunction. With chronic cholestasis, cholesterol levels are increased because of augmented hepatic cholesterol synthesis. When cholesterol levels exceed 1000 mg/dl, xanthomas and xanthelasma develop. Pruritus is the most common symptom of chronic cholestasis and results from retention of bile salts and other pruritogens normally excreted in the bile.

Anatomic changes in the hepatic cells in cholestasis are related to the duration of obstruction to bile flow. The earliest changes are degeneration of cells adjacent to the terminal hepatic venule with bile plugging. Electron microscopic studies reveal vacuolization of the Golgi apparatus, flattening and disappearance of biliary epithelial microvilli, and an increase in lysosomes and pericanalicular vesicles. If obstruction goes on for several weeks, necrotic cells in the periportal region are replaced by fibrous bands that may slowly progress to first a biliary and later a macronodular cirrhosis.

Complete obstruction to bile flow leads to a gradual accumulation of bilirubin in the serum for a period of 2 to 3 weeks. The bilirubin level usually does not exceed 30 mg/dl from obstruction alone. At this level, alternate pathways of bilirubin excretion provide for maintenance of a constant level. Relief of the obstruction within 1 month or 6 weeks is usually associated with a gradual and often complete resolution of biochemical as well as histologic abnormalities.[2]

REFERENCES

1. Badley BWD, Murphy GM, et al: Diminished micellar phase lipid in patients with chronic liver disease and steatorrhea. Gastroenterology 58:781, 1970
2. Dixon JM, Armstrong CP, et al: Factors affecting morbidity and mortality after surgery for obstructive jaundice: A review of 373 patients. Gut 24:845, 1983
3. Foulk WT, Butt HK, et al: Constitutional hepatic dysfunction (Gilbert's disease): Its natural history and related syndromes. Medicine (Baltimore) 38:25, 1959
4. O'Connor KW, Snodgrass PJ, et al: A blinded prospective study comparing four current noninvasive approaches in the differential diagnosis of medical versus surgical jaundice. Gastroenterology 84:1498, 1983
5. Okuda K: Endoscopic/cholangiographic imaging and treatment. Semin Liver Dis 2:1, 1982
6. Reichen J: Familial unconjugated hyperbilirubinemia syndromes. Semin Liver Dis 3:24, 1983
7. Scharschmidt BF, Goldberg HI, Schmid R: Current concepts in diagnosis: Approach to the patient with cholestatic jaundice. N Engl J Med 30:1515, 1983
8. Wolkoff AW, Chowdhury JR, Arias CM: Hereditary jaundice and disorders of bilirubin metabolism. In Stanbury JB, Wyngaarden JB, Fredrickson DS, et al (eds): The Metabolic Basis of Inherited Disease. New York, McGraw-Hill, 1982, p 1385
9. Wolkoff AW (ed): Bilirubin metabolism and hyperbilirubinemia. Semin Liver Dis 3:1, 1983

Acute Diffuse Hepatocellular Disease: Viral Hepatitis and Drug-Induced Liver Disease

H. Franklin Herlong
and Mack C. Mitchell

Viral hepatitis, caused by one of several viruses, is the most common cause of acute hepatocellular injury. Less frequent but of considerable importance is the acute hepatitis resulting from therapeutic drugs and environmental toxins. The mode of onset of disease, clinical course, physical manifestations, and biochemical findings are often similar in acute hepatocellular diseases of diverse causes. Malaise, anorexia, and weakness are frequent early symptoms of little differential diagnostic value. Evaluation of acute hepatocellular disease should include a meticulous history of possible contact with jaundiced persons, evidence of use of illicit or therapeutic drugs, contact with known drug abusers, use of alcohol, place of work, recent hospitalization or dental procedures, and travel experience.

VIRAL HEPATITIS

Viral hepatitis is an acute systemic disease caused by one of several viruses, with predominant clinical and pathologic manifestations related to hepatocellular necrosis. Studies of transmission of viral hepatitis have demonstrated at least three clinically similar but epidemiologically distinct types, hepatitis A, hepatitis B, and non-A, non-B hepatitis. Hepatitis A was formerly known as "infectious hepatitis" or "short-incubation hepatitis," and hepatitis B was known as "serum hepatitis" or "long-incubation hepatitis." Major advances in virology have identified and characterized the viruses that cause types A and B. The agent or agents that cause non-A, non-B hepatitis have not yet been identified. Other viral agents that cause acute hepatitis and should be considered in the differential diagnosis of acute hepatitis, especially in immunocompromised hosts, include Epstein-Barr virus, cytomegalovirus, and herpesvirus.

HEPATITIS A[8]

Hepatitis A, formally known as infectious hepatitis, accounts for about 20 percent of clinical hepatitis in this country, but the number of cases is decreasing. The hepatitis A virus (HAV) is a 27 nm spherical ribonucleic acid (RNA) enterovirus. It is the first hepatitis virus to be successfully grown in tissue culture. Hepatitis A is transmitted predominantly by fecal-oral routes. It occurs sporadically or in epidemics where inadequate sewage disposal and decreased attention to personal hygiene allow fecal contamination of water supplies. Outbreaks occur most commonly in day care centers for children, mental institutions, and military installations. There is an increased frequency of hepatitis A in homosexuals. Transmission of HAV by blood transfusion or other parenteral means is extremely rare. HAV may be transmitted by raw or partially cooked shellfish harvested from sewage-contaminated waters.

The usual incubation period for hepatitis A is 15 to 40 days. HAV is detected in the feces late in the incubation period and early during the acute disease. HAV appears transiently in the blood during the late incubation period. Antibody to HAV (anti-HAV) develops near the time of onset of the acute illness, and its ap-

pearance is associated with a decline in fecal shedding of HAV (Figure 13.3–1). The initial anti-HAV is an IgM antibody that disappears after several months. An IgG anti-HAV appears later and persists. The presence of IgM anti-HAV indicates acute or very recent infection and is diagnostic of acute hepatitis A, whereas IgG anti-HAV signifies previous infection and immunity to reinfection.

Hepatitis A is usually an acute, self-limited mild illness. Nonspecific "flu-like" symptoms of malaise, fatigue, and anorexia are usual. However, the majority of patients with HAV infection are asymptomatic without jaundice. The mortality rate from hepatitis A is very low, although fulminant hepatitis has been reported. There is no chronic carrier state for hepatitis A and no evidence that it causes chronic active hepatitis or cirrhosis.

HEPATITIS B[4]

Hepatitis B accounts for the majority of cases of viral hepatitis in American adults. The hepatitis B virus (HBV), formerly termed the Dane particle, is a 42 nm spherical DNA virus belonging to a new class of animal viruses called hepadna viruses. It has a 7-nm-thick lipoprotein outer envelope that expresses the hepatitis B surface antigen (HBsAg, Australia antigen) and a 27-nm-electron-dense inner core that contains the hepatitis B core antigen (HBcAg). This inner core contains a single molecule of circularized double-stranded DNA with a single-stranded region. Most other human viruses are entirely single or double stranded. Also unlike many other human viruses, HBV has an endogenous DNA polymerase. Viral subtypes of HBV (d, y, w, r) have been identified. No differences in virulence or tendency toward chronic infection have been associated with the various subtypes of the virus. Viruses similar to HBV have been found to cause liver disease in woodchucks, ground squirrels, and Peking ducks.

Hepatitis B Surface Antigen (HBsAg)
Three circulating particles are known to express HBsAg: the intact 42 nm virus particle, a small, spherical 20 to 22 nm particle, and a tubular particle of variable length. The smaller spherical and tubular forms represent excess viral coat and are immunogenic but not infectious. In the blood they may outnumber intact virus by a ratio of 10 million to one. HBsAg exists in glycosylated and non-glycosylated forms and has been found in blood, saliva, semen, urine, feces, and bile. Anti-HBs, a marker of previous infection, indicates recovery from infection and immunity to reinfection.

Hepatitis B Core Antigen (HBcAg) and DNA Polymerase
HBcAg is a component of the inner core of HBV and is found in the nuclei of hepatocytes infected with HBV. HBcAg is found only in the liver and cannot be detected in the blood, because it is always immunologically sequestered within a shell of HBsAg. Anti-HBc can be detected by radioimmunoassay in the blood shortly after HBsAg appears. The initial response is made up primarily of IgM anti-HBc. During convalescence, IgM anti-HBc titers decline and IgG anti-HBc titers rise. Eventually the IgM component disappears. IgG anti-HBc usually persists for life. Persistence of IgM anti-HBc implies ongoing hepatitis B infection. During the early recovery period of acute hepatitis B, IgM anti-HBc may be the only marker of hepatitis B infection.

During the early phase of active viral replication, DNA polymerase is detected in the blood. This enzyme is responsible for adding nucleotides to the single-stranded portion of the viral DNA to close its gap, making the virus completely double stranded and capable of replication. Detecting DNA polymerase in the blood implies active viral replication.

Hepatitis B e Antigen (HBeAg)
HBeAg is a soluble, electrophoretically heterogeneous antigenic material. It is immunologically distinct from HBcAg, HBsAg, and DNA polymerase. It is found only in HBsAg-positive serum. HBeAg appears transiently in the serum early in the course of hepatitis B, and its presence is correlated with circulating intact virus and increased infectivity. The persistence of HBeAg is more common in patients who become chronic HBsAg carriers. The presence of anti-HBe suggests lower infectivity and less frequent development of HBsAg carrier state or chronic hepatitis.

Transmission
Although HBV is clearly transmitted by parenteral routes (blood transfusions, contaminated needle), many patients with hepatitis B have no history of any apparent parenteral exposure. Nonparenteral or inapparently parenteral transmission is frequent and accounts for the majority of the acute hepatitis B cases seen in adults. Transmission of HBV by personal contact such as sexual intercourse is the major route of transmission for most sporadic cases. This route of transmission is generally associated with a longer incubation period than when HBV infection is acquired from parenteral inoculation.

There is a risk of intrafamilial spread of HBV during acute hepatitis. Spouses have a 20 to 25 percent risk of developing hepatitis B infection. Many of these patients have asymptomatic seroconversion. Children and other household contacts are at considerably less risk. The potential for transmission of HBV from an infected mother (especially an HBeAG-positive mother) to her baby is a serious problem. Because the incubation period for neonatal hepatitis B infection is about 2 months after birth, it appears that transmission does not represent transplacental infection but, rather, results from exposure of the baby to maternal blood during birth or close postnatal contact. This mode of transmission accounts for the high carrier rate in many developing countries. Although the incidence of hepatitis B antigen–positive persons is extremely low in a normal North American population (0.1 percent), population studies in tropical countries and Southeast Asia have demonstrated HBsAg in a significant number (4 to 20 percent) of persons, many of whom have no signs of liver disease.

Clinical Course of Acute Hepatitis B[11]
The usual clinical course and interpretation of various patterns of hepatitis B markers are outlined in Figure 13.3–2. The incubation

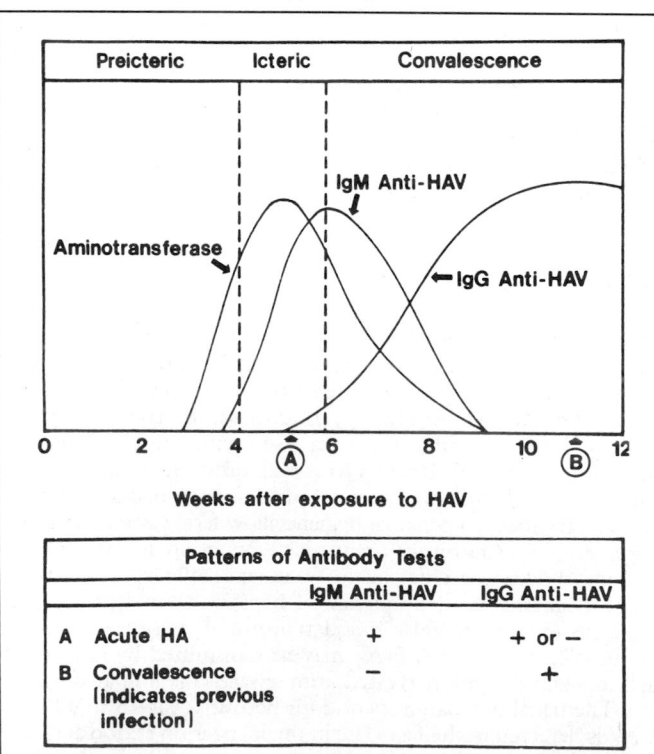

Figure 13.3–1. Usual pattern of serologic changes in hepatitis A (HA).

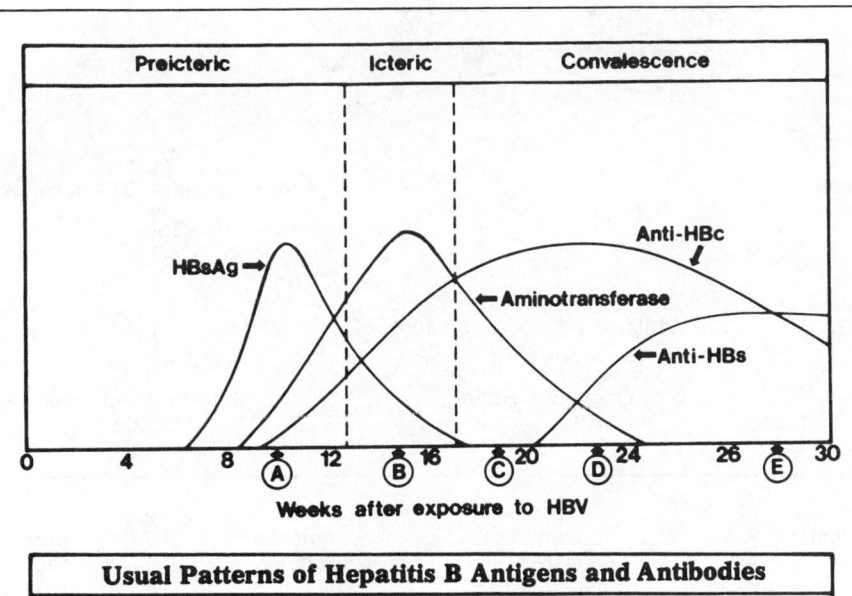

Usual Patterns of Hepatitis B Antigens and Antibodies			
	HBsAg	**Anti-HBc**	**Anti-HBs**
(A) Very Early	+	+ or − (IgM)	−
(B) Acute	+	+ (IgM)	−
(C) Active HB with high titer Anti-HBc ("window")	−	+ (IgM)	−
(D) Convalescence	+	+ or − (IgM)	+
(E) Recovery	−	+ or − (IgG)	+

Figure 13.3–2. Usual pattern of serologic changes in hepatitis B.

period for hepatitis B varies from 30 to 180 days. There is an inverse correlation between the dose of the inoculum and the incubation period. Early in the course there is active viral replication, and DNA polymerase accompanies HBsAg in the serum. Deposition of immune complexes and complement accounts for prodromal symptoms such as arthritis, urticaria, and angioneurotic edema. A few patients develop glomerulonephritis related to immune complex deposition. The typical symptomatic period after the prodromal phase is characterized by malaise, fatigue, myalgias, headache, and nausea. Anorexia, right upper quadrant abdominal pain, and dysgeusia may also be prominent features. Low-grade fever is often present. Physical examination reveals mild, tender hepatomegaly in addition to jaundice. Transient enlargement of the spleen is found in 10 to 20 percent of patients, and posterior cervical lymphadenopathy may also be present. Occasionally spider angiomas appear transiently during acute hepatitis. Laboratory findings in viral hepatitis include hyperbilirubinemia with bilirubinuria, marked aminotransferase elevations (>300 IU/L), and a mild rise in the alkaline phosphatase level. The leukocyte count is usually normal, with a relative lymphocytosis. Prolongation of the prothrombin time (>5 seconds beyond control values) suggests severe hepatitis that may become fulminant.

Outcome of Hepatitis B[16]

Figure 13.3–3 summarizes potential outcomes of hepatitis B infection. Because the hepatitis B virus is not directly cytopathic, the outcome of infection with this virus depends largely on the host's immunologic response to its presence. Fortunately, the prognosis is excellent in acute symptomatic hepatitis B occurring in young, previously healthy persons. Fulminant hepatitis is the rarest of all outcomes and is characterized by encephalopathy appearing within a few days to 4 weeks after the onset of hepatitis. The liver may rapidly decrease in size, an event associated with prolongation of the prothrombin time and worsening jaundice. Hypoglycemia, se-

vere generalized bleeding, cerebral edema, superimposed bacterial infections, and renal failure contribute to an overall mortality rate of greater than 75 percent in fulminant hepatitis B. Survival from fulminant hepatitis is age dependent, with the highest survival rate in patients less than 20 years old.

Chronic HBV infection, defined as the persistence of HBsAg for greater than 6 months, develops in about 10 percent of individuals after acute hepatitis B. Predisposing factors for a chronic carrier state include (1) the clinical expression of the acute disease (anicteric hepatitis is more likely to become chronic), (2) the age when infection occurs (90 percent of infected neonates become carriers) (3) gender (the male/female ratio is 5:1), and (4) immune status (immunocompromised hosts are more likely to become carriers). Disappearance of HBsAg in chronic carriers is unusual, occurring at a rate of about 1 percent per year. Patients who are chronically HBsAg-positive and have normal aminotransferase values are designated "asymptomatic chronic carriers." If there is no change in their immune status or coinfection with other viruses (e.g., delta agent), then these patients do not develop significant hepatitis. No therapy is indicated, but they should be advised to take precautions to reduce the risk of infecting others with HBV. Patients who remain HBsAg-positive for longer than 6 months and have elevated aminotransferase levels have some form of chronic hepatitis. In most of these patients a liver biopsy is necessary to determine the severity of the hepatitis. On the basis of the histologic appearance, chronic viral hepatitis is classified as chronic persistent hepatitis, chronic lobular hepatitis, or chronic active hepatitis. The liver biopsy in chronic persistent hepatitis shows a mild periportal infiltrate of mononuclear cells. The architecture of the liver is preserved and there is no fibrosis. Laboratory tests reflect mild hepatocellular injury. The prognosis for patients with chronic persistent hepatitis is good.

Some patients with chronic hepatitis B have a mild illness characterized by recurrent symptoms of acute hepatitis associated

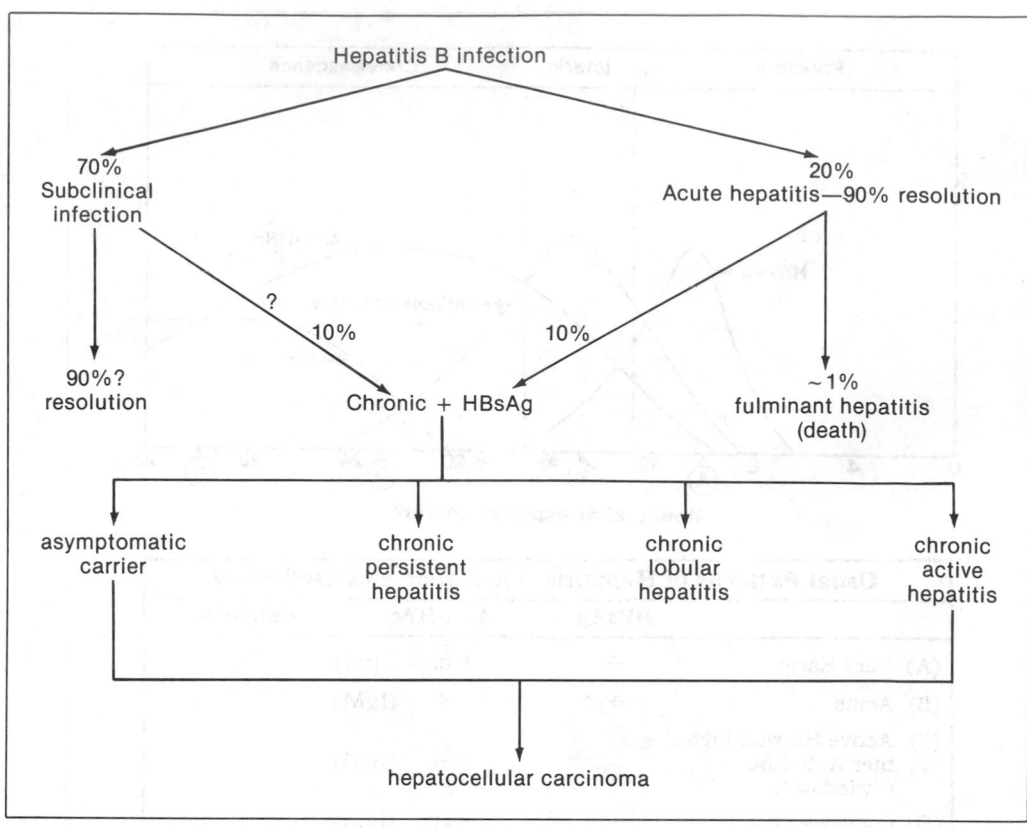

Figure 13.3–3. Outcomes of hepatitis B infection.

with fluctuating aminotransferase elevations. The liver biopsy specimens in these patients show portal inflammation with focal necrosis and mononuclear infiltration throughout the lobule. These patients have chronic lobular hepatitis. Like chronic persistent hepatitis, this illness carries a favorable prognosis and needs no specific therapy.

Chronic active hepatitis develops in about 3 percent of individuals infected with the HBV. This serious liver disease progresses in many cases to cirrhosis, portal hypertension, and death. Chronic active hepatitis can follow an acute symptomatic illness or be discovered incidentally when abnormal liver enzyme values are found. The liver biopsy specimens show marked infiltration of portal areas with mononuclear cells frequently associated with fibroinflammatory bridging. Fibrous septa isolate groups of liver cells, and there is erosion of the limiting plate. These patients are frequently symptomatic, with anorexia, malaise, and fatigue. Some may already have cirrhosis, with signs of portal hypertension at initial presentation. An important consequence of persistent hepatitis B infection is the development of primary hepatocellular carcinoma. In the world, hepatocellular carcinoma is the most prevalent nondermatologic carcinoma in humans. Although cirrhosis is commonly present in patients with persistent hepatitis B and primary hepatocellular carcinoma, this tumor can develop in patients without cirrhosis. The key steps in the progression from persistent HBV infection to hepatocellular carcinoma involve the integration of hepatitis B DNA into the genome of the host's live cell. This integration leads to alteration in cellular gene expression, with transformation into clones of cells that become autonomous and ultimately neoplastic.

NON-A, NON-B HEPATITIS[3]

The term "non-A, non-B viral hepatitis" refers to the liver disease caused by hepatotropic viruses other than HAV, HBV, and other specific viruses, including the delta agent, cytomegalovirus,

Epstein-Barr virus, and a variety of unusual agents, including the Marburg virus and the yellow fever virus. Non-A, non-B hepatitis accounts for over 90 percent of the cases of posttransfusion hepatitis. Posttransfusion non-A, non-B hepatitis develops in about 10 percent of multitransfused patients, with a frequency of about 5 cases per 1000 units transfused. The agent that causes non-A, non-B hepatitis has not yet been identified, and the diagnosis depends on the exclusion of both nonviral causes of hepatitis and the other known hepatitis viruses. Non-A, non-B hepatitis accounts for 20 to 40 percent of cases of sporadic hepatitis. Many of these cases are thought to be acquired through sexual contact. Several waterborne epidemics of non-A, non-B hepatitis have been reported. These epidemics have had a high attack rate for adults and unusually high mortality rates (a case fatality rate of 10 percent) in pregnant women. Clinical features of non-A, non-B hepatitis are similar to other types of viral hepatitis, with some minor exceptions. As a rule, acute non-A, non-B hepatitis tends to be less severe than hepatitis B. The peak levels of serum aminotransferases and bilirubin are lower, and the percentage of asymptomatic cases is higher. Extrahepatic manifestations of hepatitis B, such as arthritis and skin rash, are less common with non-A, non-B hepatitis. A characteristic feature of non-A, non-B hepatitis is episodically fluctuating aminotransferase elevations. At times the AST and ALT levels may even fall to normal, only to rise again within days. This biochemical pattern makes it difficult to assess convalescence in patients with non-A, non-B hepatitis. Most of the cases of hepatitis-associated aplastic anemia have occurred after non-A, non-B hepatitis. Perhaps the most disturbing feature of non-A, non-B hepatitis is its tendency to cause chronic liver disease. Combining all reported series, persistent aminotransferase elevations for longer than 6 months were detected in approximately 40 percent of cases. Although many of these patients have chronic persistent hepatitis, a significant number have chronic active hepatitis, cirrhosis, or both. At present, no reliable tests are available to detect non-A, non-B viruses or their antigens. Preliminary reports of interferon therapy for chronic non-A, non-B hepatitis are promising.

DELTA HEPATITIS (TYPE D)[12]

The delta agent is a defective hepatotropic RNA virus. It is pathogenic only in the presence of the HBV, which provides it with envelope protein and allows it to replicate. Since the delta agent is inextricably linked to its helper virus, its mode of transmission is similar to that of HBV. The outcome of delta infection depends on whether the host is infected simultaneously with the delta agent and the HBV (coinfection) or the delta agent superinfects a chronic hepatitis B carrier. Coinfection by the delta agent and hepatitis B produces a biphasic acute hepatitis that is often very severe. Approximately 30 percent of cases of fulminant hepatitis B represent coinfection with the delta agent. Because the delta agent cannot outlive the hepatitis B virus, delta infection always terminates with the clearance of hepatitis B infection.

When a chronic carrier becomes superinfected with the delta agent, there usually is a relapse of symptoms of hepatitis, which are often severe. Asymptomatic carriers may then develop a serious case of hepatitis that can be fatal.

MANAGEMENT OF VIRAL HEPATITIS

No specific therapy is available for acute viral hepatitis. The patients tend to get well, given time, rest, and adequate diet. Indications for hospitalization of a patient with acute viral hepatitis include (1) evidence of significantly impaired coagulation function (prothrombin time >16 seconds), (2) encephalopathy, (3) ascites, or (4) dehydration resulting from nausea and vomiting. Hepatitis in patients without these criteria can be managed on an outpatient basis.

Bed rest is a time-honored therapy in viral hepatitis. Patients with hepatitis are often weak, and bed rest seems a logical recommendation. Studies in previously healthy military personnel, however, demonstrated no deleterious effects of moderate or even forced exercise in the ultimate recovery of patients with hepatitis. On the other hand, the outcome observed in previously healthy young patients may not apply to an older and more heterogeneous civilian population. A reasonable approach is to encourage rest during active phases of hepatitis with gradual ambulation as the symptoms subside. An adequate supply of calories and protein is important in the management of acute hepatitis. A high-calorie, high-protein diet (1 g/kg body weight of protein) appears to reduce the duration of illness in patients with viral hepatitis. Adjustment of calorie intake to provide much of the diet in the morning, when nausea is often less severe, may be useful. A mild antiemetic such as diphenhydramine (Benadryl) may be helpful in controlling nausea. Should signs of encephalopathy develop, dietary protein should be restricted. Specific vitamin deficiencies must be corrected, but there is no need for routine vitamin supplementation in acute hepatitis. In patients with severe cholestasis, parenteral vitamin K is indicated.

Specific Therapy
At present there is no specific therapy of proved efficacy in the treatment of acute or chronic viral hepatitis. Corticosteroid therapy is not indicated in acute viral hepatitis regardless of cause or severity. In controlled trials of the treatment of patients with chronic viral hepatitis, long-term steroid therapy has not shown benefit compared with placebo. Antiviral agents alone have also not proved clinically efficacious in the treatment of acute or chronic viral hepatitis. The use of immunosuppressive agents in combination with antiviral agents is currently being tested. Successful liver transplantation has been performed in patients with fulminant viral hepatitis and in patients with chronic active viral hepatitis, but this form of therapy is currently not routinely available.

Prevention and Prophylaxis of Viral Hepatitis[2]
Prevention of hepatitis A is best accomplished by general hygienic measures that prevent contact with fecally contaminated water or foods. The shedding of virus during the prodromal period and the frequency of anicteric cases make prevention of spread difficult. Immune serum globulin (ISG) given to the contacts of patients with hepatitis A does provide protection against development of overt hepatitis but not against subclinical infection. ISG should be given to close personal contacts of patients with hepatitis A and to travelers in countries where hepatitis A is endemic.

Passive immunization against hepatitis B is possible through the use of hyperimmune serum globulin (H-BIG Hepatitis B Immune globulin [Human]). This preparation should be given as soon as possible after exposure to individuals with HBsAg-positive blood. It is also indicated for babies born to HBsAg-positive mothers. Prophylaxis for sexual contacts with HBV remains an area of controversy. Protection against HBV infection is possible through the use of hepatitis B vaccines such as Heptavax B, which is prepared from the blood of hepatitis B carriers. The plasma is treated with a number of steps that inactivate all infectious agents. Hepatitis B vaccine administered intramuscularly induces an antibody response in about 95 percent of healthy people who complete the immunization schedule. These individuals are protected against acute hepatitis B, subclinical hepatitis B, and asymptomatic seroconversion. Groups recommended to receive hepatitis B vaccine in this country include health care workers exposed to blood or other body fluids, hemodialysis patients, parenteral drug abusers, heterosexual contacts of HBsAg carriers, homosexually active men, and infants born to HBsAg-positive mothers. Recombinant DNA technology has been used to produce a hepatitis B vaccine. A yeast-derived recombinant vaccine has an efficacy similar to that of plasma-derived vaccines.

HEPATIC INJURY INDUCED BY DRUGS AND OTHER CHEMICALS

Liver damage from drugs and chemical exposure is becoming an increasingly common cause of both acute and chronic liver diseases. Adverse drug reactions involving the liver produce a wide variety of manifestations ranging from asymptomatic elevation of aminotransferase levels to clinically apparent diseases such as acute hepatitis, chronic hepatitis, granulomatous hepatitis, cirrhosis, hepatic tumors, and fulminant hepatic necrosis. Hepatic drug reactions can be classified according to the histologic features of liver injury (Table 13.3–1) or to the mechanism of injury (Table 13.3–2).

CLASSIFICATION BY HISTOLOGIC TYPE OF INJURY

Acute hepatocellular injury due to drugs is usually indistinguishable from acute viral hepatitis on the basis of clinical, laboratory, and histologic findings. Occasionally the finding of zonal, particularly centrilobular necrosis in the absence of inflammation on liver biopsy suggests a drug-induced cause. Most often acute hepatitis due to therapeutic agents resembles acute viral hepatitis but may be patchy rather than diffuse. Since there are no direct tests to confirm the diagnosis of drug-induced hepatocellular injury, known causes such as hepatitis A (IgM anti-HAV) and hepatitis B (HBsAg), as well as non-A, non-B viruses such as cytomegalovirus, should be excluded.

Drug-induced liver damage may also mimic biliary obstruction. For example, chlorpromazine may result in painless jaundice associated with pruritus, light stools, absent or low urine urobilinogen level, and increased serum alkaline phosphatase level. The absence of dilated intrahepatic or extrahepatic bile ducts helps distinguish this cause of cholestasis from that produced by a tumor obstructing the common bile duct.

Numerous drugs, including phenylbutazone, quinidine, allopurinol, hydralazine, and phenytoin, have been reported to cause hepatic granulomas.[10,17] Steatosis and steatohepatitis occur as a

TABLE 13.3–1. CLASSIFICATION OF DRUG-INDUCED LIVER DISEASE BY HISTOPATHOLOGIC FINDINGS

Type of Injury	Biochemical Abnormalities ($\times$ normal)		Examples
	Aminotransferase	*Alkaline Phosphatase*	
Hepatocellular			
Acute necrosis	10–500$\times$	1–2$\times$	Acetaminophen, carbon tetrachloride
Acute hepatitis	10–200$\times$	1–2$\times$	Isoniazid, α-methyldopa, aspirin, phenytoin
Chronic hepatitis	5–50$\times$	1–2$\times$	Isoniazid
Steatosis	5–10$\times$	1–3$\times$	Tetracycline, valproate, corticosteroids
Cholestasis	5–10$\times$	1–3$\times$	Ethanol, amiodarone, perhexiline maleate
Inflammatory	1–10$\times$	3–10$\times$	Chlorpromazine, erythromycin
Noninflammatory	1–5$\times$	1–5$\times$	Oral contraceptives, rifampin
Granulomatous inflammation	5–25$\times$	2–10$\times$	Numerous
Vascular			
Peliosis hepatitis	1–2$\times$	1–2$\times$	Anabolic steroids, oral contraceptives
Hepatic vein thrombosis	2–5$\times$	1–2$\times$	Oral contraceptives
Veno-occlusive disease	2–5$\times$	2–5$\times$	Several antineoplastic agents
Tumors			
Hepatic adenomas	Variable	1–3$\times$	Oral contraceptives
Hepatocellular carcinoma	Variable	1–3$\times$	Anabolic steroids, oral contraceptives
Angiosarcoma	Variable	1–3$\times$	Vinyl chloride

consequence of heavy ethanol ingestion but have also been reported in patients taking amiodarone, perhexiline maleate, valproic acid, and corticosteriods. Rarely, hepatic vascular injury occurs as a consequence of drug toxicity. Veno-occlusive disease of the liver and the Budd-Chiari syndrome may result in rapid development of portal hypertension with hepatomegaly and ascites, as discussed in Chapter 13.4.

Tumors due to drug and chemical exposure have become a growing cause for concern since the recognition of the association of exposure to the vinyl chloride monomer and the development of angiosarcoma in chemical workers.[1]

CLASSIFICATION BY MECHANISM OF INJURY

Classification of drug-induced liver damage based on the mechanism of injury may be helpful not only in understanding the pathogenesis but also in establishing a rational basis for therapy. Injury can be divided into two broad categories: direct and idiosyncratic hepatotoxicity. Direct hepatotoxins characteristically cause reactions that are reproducible, are dose dependent, occur in the majority of exposed individuals, and are usually manifested within

TABLE 13.3–2. CLASSIFICATION OF DRUG-INDUCED LIVER DAMAGE BY MECHANISM OF INJURY

Mechanism	Example
Intrinsic Toxins	
Direct	Carbon tetrachloride, arsenic
Metabolism-mediated	Acetaminophen, carbon tetrachloride, chlorpromazine
Idiosyncratic Toxins	
Hypersensitivity	Phenytoin, sulfonamides, para-aminosalicyclic acid, halothane
Host idiosyncrasy metabolic	Phenytoin(?), valproate, isoniazid(?), halothane(?)

several days of exposure. By contrast, idiosyncratic hepatotoxins, which are unpredictable and poorly reproducible, affect only a minority of exposed individuals, may or may not be dose dependent, and usually require several weeks of exposure before initial manifestations arise. In addition, true hypersensitivity, or allergic features, including fever, lymphadenopathy, arthralgias-arthritis, rashes, and eosinophilia, may accompany some idiosyncratic reactions. However, these features are not requirements for establishing the diagnosis of idiosyncratic hepatotoxicity.

With both direct and idiosyncratic hepatotoxins, either the parent drug itself or one of its metabolites may be responsible for initiating damage. Although the liver carries out a large number of biotransformation reactions, oxidation is the one pathway most often responsible for producing hepatotoxic metabolites. Oxidation can produce chemically reactive electrophilic metabolites or radical species of drugs that produce either alkylation or peroxidation of vital macromolecules. Important cellular defense mechanisms against this potential damage include, for example, glutathione-S-transferases, peroxidase, epoxide hydrolase, and glucuronyl transferase. It should be immediately apparent how genetic defects in any of these detoxification or activation pathways might render an individual uniquely susceptible to drug-induced injury.

APPROACH TO DIAGNOSIS AND MANAGEMENT OF DRUG-INDUCED LIVER DAMAGE

Since most adverse drug reactions are idiosyncratic, it is often difficult to recognize drug-induced damage with certainty. Thus a high index of suspicion is important, particularly in patients with a history of previous drug reactions and in patients receiving a medication for the first time.

Most often the physician is confronted with hepatic biochemical abnormalities in a patient who is asymptomatic. In this setting one should exclude other possible causes of the abnormalities, such as viral hepatitis, hemochromatosis, or α_1-antitrypsin deficiency. Once these other disorders have been excluded, the physician must decide whether the drug is being used to treat a potentially life-threatening illness, such as arrhythmias, or whether the

drug can be safely discontinued for a short time. The majority of patients with drug-induced liver damage show distinct improvement within 2 to 3 weeks after discontinuation of the offending agent. Rechallenge does not invariably produce a recurrence of abnormalities within a short time, because some drug hepatotoxicity is related to metabolites that require time to accumulate. Furthermore, rechallenge may be hazardous, producing an exaggerated, even fatal outcome in patients with drug hypersensitivity.

Therapy for most adverse hepatic drug reactions is limited to discontinuation of the agent. In a few instances specific therapy, as discussed below, is available. In general, corticosteroids are not useful in the treatment of drug-induced liver damage.

Acetaminophen-Induced Hepatic Necrosis. Ingestion of excessive doses (>10 g) of acetaminophen causes dose-related hepatic necrosis. The therapeutic index is usually high, with toxic effects occurring only at doses more than 10 times the usual therapeutic dose of 1 g. Acetaminophen is metabolized by several pathways in the liver. Approximately 90 percent is converted to nontoxic glucuronides and sulfates, whereas the remaining 10 percent is oxidized by cytochrome P-450 to a potentially toxic intermediate. At low doses this intermediate is detoxified uneventfully by further conjugation with glutathione. After large doses, however, hepatic glutathione stores are rapidly depleted and the toxic intermediates formed subsequently bind covalently to cellular macromolecules, leading to cell injury and death. Once this critical threshold has been exceeded, dose-related hepatic necrosis occurs and in some cases may be fatal. Suicide attempts and accidental ingestion of large doses by children account for most cases of acetaminophen hepatotoxic effects. Alcoholics and patients receiving anticonvulsants such as phenobarbital, which enhance cytochrome P-450 activity, may be at risk with lower doses.[13] Prompt recognition and treatment of patients with *N*-acetylcysteine, a precursor for the formation of glutathione, can prevent hepatic necrosis. For maximal effectiveness, treatment must be instituted within 12 hours of ingestion and is ineffective more than 24 hours after overdose.

Isoniazid-Induced Hepatic Necrosis. Isoniazid (INH) has been extensively administered in both the treatment and chemoprophylaxis of tuberculosis. Approximately 10 percent of patients receiving isoniazid alone in chemophylactic programs develop moderate increases in serum aminotransferase levels and have minimal nonspecific inflammation on liver biopsy. A few patients (approximately 1 percent) develop clinically apparent hepatitis from isoniazid.[7,9] The duration of therapy before the onset of symptoms may be several weeks to 6 months. Prodromal symptoms of hepatitis, such as malaise, fatigue, nausea, and vomiting, are usual, and continuation of the drug after appearance of these symptoms may worsen the hepatitis. As in other instances of drug-induced hepatitis, there is often a discrepancy between a relatively well appearing patient and liver biopsy changes of bridging and multilobular necrosis. The pathogenesis of isoniazid-induced hepatitis most likely involves the production of toxic intermediates of isoniazid, but components of individual susceptibility or sensitization reactions cannot be excluded. Management of isoniazid-induced hepatitis consists of drug withdrawal and supportive care. Corticosteroids are not of proved benefit.

There appears to be an increased frequency of adverse reactions in patients receiving isoniazid and rifampin (rifampicin). In this situation it is thought that rifampin induces the drug-metabolizing enzyme system and thereby promotes an increased production of isoniazid toxic intermediates. Rifampin alone has been a very rare cause of hepatic injury.

Halothane-Induced Hepatic Necrosis. Adverse hepatic reactions ranging from mild subclinical derangement of liver function on biochemical tests to fulminant hepatic failure have been associated with the administration of the fluorinated hydrocarbon anesthetic agent halothane.[15] There is a large body of evidence to implicate this agent in hepatic necrosis. The frequency of the reaction is low.

The mechanism of halothane-induced injury is apparently by an idiosyncratic reaction, although evidence of direct toxicity in a metabolite has been reported. Although 25 percent of cases occur after the first exposure to the agent, the importance of multiple administration of halothane in the development of liver injury has been established. Approximately three fourths of patients who have developed fulminant hepatic failure after halothane anesthesia give a history of postoperative fever, often occurring 1 to 2 weeks after an earlier exposure to the agent. The adverse reactions to halothane do not appear to be related to the type of surgery. There is no greater incidence after operations on the liver or biliary tract. Obese women appear to be more susceptible. The clinical course is similar to that found in severe viral hepatitis. Liver biopsy is of particular value in separating these patients from those with postoperative jaundice caused by shock or sepsis. Therapy is mainly supportive. Cirrhosis may occur from repeated bouts of halothane-induced hepatitis. There is no evidence that halothane causes chronic active hepatitis. The nature of the reaction with fever and eosinophilia suggests that corticosteroids should be useful, but the effectiveness of this therapy has not been established.

Phenytoin-Induced Hepatic Necrosis. Phenytoin may induce a severe and even fatal hepatic necrosis. Affected patients often have fever, exfoliative dermatitis, lymphadenopathy, eosinophilia, and leukocytosis. The interval between introduction of therapy and appearance of injury is from 1 to 8 weeks. Although many features of phenytoin-induced injury suggest an idiosyncratic sensitization reaction, some evidence suggests a role for toxic intermediates in pathogenesis.[14] The prognosis for patients with the full syndrome is poor.

Drug-Induced Chronic Hepatitis. Chronic active hepatitis has been produced by reactions to several drugs, including methyldopa, dantrolene, and nitrofurantoin. The clinical illness, biochemical findings, and liver histologic findings in these patients may closely resemble chronic active hepatitis from other causes. In patients with nitrofurantoin-induced injury, as in patients with idiopathic chronic active hepatitis, hyperglobulinemia, antinuclear antibodies, and female predominance are common findings. There is no evidence that corticosteroids are useful in drug-induced chronic hepatitis.

Chlorpromazine Jaundice. Clinically apparent cholestatic hepatitis occurs in 1 to 2 percent of patients taking the phenothiazine tranquilizer chlorpromazine. Serial biopsy and biochemical studies have revealed minor hepatic morphologic and functional changes in many patients receiving this agent. The mechanism of injury is thought to be toxic damage to the bile secretory mechanism by chlorpromazine metabolites. The syndrome of overt hepatitis characteristically appears in the second to fourth week after institution of the drug and has a prodromal phase of fever, chills, malaise, and anorexia similar to that found in viral hepatitis.[5] Pruritus, arthralgias, and lymphadenopathy may dominate the clinical picture. Several days after the onset of constitutional symptoms, jaundice appears. It is unusual for liver damage to be manifested during the first week of drug administration or to appear after the patient has taken the agent for more than 5 weeks. Both liver function tests and liver biopsy reveal cholestatic hepatitis. The course of the disorder is one of gradual resolution of liver function abnormalities over a 2- to 8-week period after withdrawal of the drug, but progression of the cholestatic reaction, even to frank biliary cirrhosis, has been reported. Resolution of the hepatitis while the patient continues to take the drug suggests occasional spontaneous desensitization. Instances of cross-reactions to other phenothiazine derivatives have been observed.

Hepatic Effects of Oral Contraceptives. Several of the important side effects of contraceptive use involve the liver.[17] Minor abnormalities in liver function are found in many women receiving these agents. A syndrome of contraceptive steroid jaundice and choles-

tasis usually has its onset in susceptible women within the first six cycles of therapy and may appear in the first month. Pruritus usually precedes jaundice. The serum bilirubin level rarely exceeds 10 mg/dl. The serum alkaline phosphatase and aminotransferase levels are often slightly elevated. Typical liver biopsy findings are those of minimal cholestasis without inflammation. The jaundice usually subsides within 1 month of drug withdrawal. Susceptible women are also likely to develop a similar syndrome during pregnancy.

Liver cell adenoma is a benign tumor found almost exclusively in women receiving oral contraceptives, and the association is firmly established.[6,17] The adenoma may be found as an asymptomatic mass discovered on routine examination (50 percent) or as a tender right upper quadrant abdominal mass (30 to 35 percent). There may be few if any biochemical abnormalities. Occasionally, the adenoma ruptures and causes an intra-abdominal hemorrhage. Some liver cell adenomas regress when the contraceptives are discontinued. Other important considerations in the differential diagnosis of intrahepatic masses are hepatocellular carcinomas, which may be associated with contraceptive usage, and focal nodular hyperplasia, which although found predominantly in women is not clearly associated with contraceptive usage.

Hepatic vein thrombosis (Budd-Chiari syndrome) has been associated with contraceptive use and is described in Chapter 13.5.

REFERENCES

1. Berk PD, Martin JF, et al: Vinyl-chloride associated liver disease. Ann Intern Med 84:717, 1976

2. Centers for Disease Control: Recommendations for protection against viral hepatitis. MMWR 34:313, 1985
3. Dienstag JL: Non-A, non-B hepatitis: Recognition, epidemiology and clinical features. Gastroenterology 85:437, 1983
4. Hoofnagle JH, Shafer DF: Serologic markers of hepatitis B infection. Semin Liver Dis 6:1, 1986
5. Ishak KG, Irey NS: Hepatic injury associated with phenothiazines: Clinicopathologic and follow-up study of 36 patients. Arch Pathol Lab Med 93:283, 1972
6. Klatskin G: Hepatic tumors: Possible relationship to use of oral contraceptives. Gastroenterology 73:386, 1977
7. Maddrey WC, Boitnott JK: Isoniazid hepatitis. Ann Intern Med 79:1, 1973
8. Mijch AM, Gust ID: Clinical serologic and epidemiologic aspects of hepatitis A infection. Semin Liver Dis 6:42, 1986
9. Mitchell JR, Zimmerman HJ, et al: Isoniazid liver injury: Clinical spectrum, pathology and probable pathogenesis. Ann Intern Med 84:181, 1976
10. Ochner RK: Drug-induced liver disease. In Zakim D, Boyer TD (eds): Hepatology, 1st ed. Philadelphia, WB Saunders, 1982, p 691
11. Redeker AG: Viral hepatitis: Clinical aspects. Am J Med Sci 270:9, 1975
12. Rizetto M: The delta agent. Hepatology 3:724, 1983
13. Seeff LB, Cuccherini BA, et al: Acetaminophen hepatotoxicity in alcoholics: A therapeutic misadventure. Ann Intern Med 104:399, 1986
14. Spielberg SP, Gordon GB, et al: Predisposition to phenytoin hepatotoxicity assessed in vitro. N Engl J Med 305:722, 1981
15. Touloukian J, Kaplowitz N: Halothane-induced hepatic disease. Semin Liver Dis 1:134, 1981
16. Weissberg JI, Andres LL, et al: Survival in chronic hepatitis B. Ann Intern Med 101:613, 1984
17. Zimmerman HJ, Maddrey WC: Toxic and drug-induced hepatitis. In Schiff L, Schiff ER (eds): Diseases of the Liver, 5th ed. Philadelphia, Lippincott, 1982, p 621

CHAPTER 13.4

Portal Hypertension: Ascites, Spontaneous Bacterial Peritonitis, Hepatorenal Syndrome, and Hepatic Encephalopathy

H. Franklin Herlong

PORTAL HYPERTENSION

The portal vein is formed by the superior mesenteric vein, which drains the intestinal capillaries, and the splenic vein. Blood in the portal vein normally has a slightly higher pressure (5 to 10 mm Hg) and a higher oxygen content than that in the systemic veins. Because there are no valves in the portal vein, the pressure in the portal system is normally dependent on resistance to blood flow through the liver. When the portal vein reaches the liver, it divides into many small branches that deliver the blood to the extensive sinusoidal system. The hepatic artery usually arises from the celiac axis and enters the liver adjacent to the portal vein. The arterial blood supply also perfuses the hepatic sinusoids. After percolating through the sinusoids, the blood is re-collected and discharged into the inferior vena cava via the hepatic veins. Portal hypertension is present when the portal pressure exceeds the inferior vena caval pressure by 5 mm Hg. It results from anatomic or functional obstruction to blood flow in the portal venous system at any point from its origin in the splanchnic bed to its exit into the systemic circulation via the inferior vena cava. Obstruction to blood flow may result from compression or thrombosis of the extrahepatic portal vein, inflammatory obliteration of intrahepatic portal and hepatic vein radicles, or distortion of intrahepatic architecture by

collapse, infiltrations, and regenerating nodules. Rarely, the major hepatic veins are blocked (Budd-Chiari syndrome), often in conjunction with obstruction in the inferior vena cava. Increased blood flow in the portal venous system may cause portal hypertension in patients with massive splenomegaly or arteriovenous fistulas or may contribute to portal hypertension in patients with other chronic liver diseases such as cirrhosis.

Portal hypertension is conveniently divided into two major categories on the basis of whether the obstruction to flow occurs before (presinusoidal), or in and beyond (sinusoidal and postsinusoidal), the hepatic sinusoid. Measuring the wedged hepatic venous pressure (WHVP) gives an estimate of the portal venous pressure and helps to determine the type of portal hypertension in an individual patient. The WHVP is measured by wedging an end-hole catheter, usually introduced percutaneously via a femoral vein, into a peripheral hepatic venule. The catheter in the wedged position creates stasis in the hepatic vasculature that extends to the point of anastomotic collateral runoff into the hepatic sinusoids. An elevation in WHVP suggests increased resistance to collateral flow in the sinusoidal bed.

Presinusoidal portal hypertension is characterized by an elevated portal venous pressure and a normal WHVP, since the sinusoidal pressure is not elevated. Portal vein thrombosis, schistosomiasis, and arteriovenous fistulas in the splanchnic bed are

examples of causes of presinusoidal portal hypertension. Increased blood flow in the portal venous system in patients with massive splenomegaly contributes to presinusoidal hypertension. An elevated portal pressure and elevated WHVP are characteristic of sinusoidal or postsinusoidal obstruction to portal flow and are most commonly encountered in patients with cirrhosis. There is a close correlation between the WHVP and the portal pressure measured directly in patients with both alcoholic liver disease and postnecrotic cirrhosis. A classification of the causes of portal hypertension based on the site of obstruction to blood flow is presented in Table 13.4–1. Occasionally a complex situation may exist, such as portal vein thrombosis complicating hepatic cirrhosis.

The physiologic consequences of portal hypertension are related both to a decrease in the blood supply to the liver via the portal vein and to the shunting of products of intestinal origin around the liver into the systemic circulation. The decrease in the portal component of the hepatic blood flow is associated with a compensatory increase in the hepatic arterial component in an attempt to maintain total liver blood flow at or near normal. The liver thereby becomes more dependent on arterial blood. The most important consequences of portal hypertension are (1) the development of a collateral circulation that bypasses the liver and links the portal and systemic venous systems, (2) the shunting of products of intestinal origin around the liver, (3) the development of splenomegaly, and (4) the formation of ascites. Collateral blood vessels linking the portal and systemic veins commonly develop between the coronary vein of the portal system and the azygos veins of the caval system in the submucosa of the lower esophagus and upper part of the stomach. These thin-walled vessels (esophagogastric varices) are poorly supported by the underlying connective tissue and are a frequent site of major hemorrhage in patients with portal hypertension.[7] One third of patients with cirrhosis die because of variceal hemorrhage (see Chapter 12.4). Although gastroesophageal varices most often result from an elevation in the portal pressure, an occasional patient may have varices from superior vena cava or azygos vein obstruction.

Abdominal collateral vessels are prominent in some patients with portal hypertension and are arranged radially from the umbilicus like the spokes of a wheel (caput medusae). Occasionally these collateral vessels are large and associated with a vascular bruit (Cruveilhier-Baumgarter syndrome). Dilated abdominal vessels may also appear because of obstruction of either the superior or inferior vena cava. Observation of the direction of blood flow in the collateral vessels is important for diagnosis. In superior vena cava obstruction, the flow in the collateral vessels is downward from the chest toward the lower half of the body, with the converse true for inferior vena cava obstruction. In abdominal collateral vessels associated with portal hypertension, the blood flow is away from the umbilicus.

Splenomegaly is common in patients with an elevated portal venous pressure, but the size of the spleen often does not correlate with the degree of the portal hypertension. Thrombocytopenia, leukopenia, and anemia may complicate splenomegaly, but the severity of pancytopenia does not correlate well with the size of the spleen.

ASCITES

Ascites, fluid in the peritoneal cavity, may be seen as an isolated clinical finding or in a setting of generalized fluid retention with edema. The most common disorders associated with ascites are cirrhosis, tumors, and congestive heart failure. Tuberculous peritonitis, the nephrotic syndrome, and pancreatitis are less frequent causes. Small amounts of ascitic fluid (< 1000 ml) may be difficult to detect, especially in obese patients. Both a high index of suspicion and careful physical examination are necessary for diagnosis. Bulging of the flanks and shifting percussion dullness of the abdomen when the patient turns to one side are important physical signs that suggest ascites but may not be present until a considerable amount of fluid has accumulated. The accuracy of the physical examination in detecting ascites is only about 50 percent, related to a low specificity. Ultrasonography of the abdomen is therefore helpful in detecting small amounts of ascites and determining the best site for paracentesis.

Examination of the ascitic fluid by a diagnostic paracentesis should be performed when ascites is initially detected or in patients with known ascites in whom there has been a marked increase in fluid or development of fever. Complete fluid analysis includes determination of the protein and glucose content, LDH and amylase levels, blood cell counts and differential count, bacterial culture, fungal and acid-fast bacillus (AFB) cultures, and cytologic examination. On the basis of the protein concentration, ascitic fluid may be separated into two broad categories: transudate, in which the protein content is less than 3 g/dl, and exudate, in which the protein concentration is greater than 3 g/dl. Disorders associated with inflammatory reactions, such as tuberculosis, tumors, and peritonitis, are most frequently exudative in nature. Ascitic fluid with a high protein content may occur in patients with myxedema. Chronic liver disease, congestive heart failure with constrictive pericarditis, and the nephrotic syndrome are common causes of transudates. Rarely, transudative ascites complicates ovarian disease (Meigs syndrome). There is considerable overlap in the classification of ascites based on protein content, and in general the total protein content has poor discriminating value in the differential diagnosis of ascites (Table 13.4–2).

Bloody ascitic fluid, containing more than 50,000 red blood cells/mm³, suggests neoplasm or pancreatic ascites.[5] Chylous ascites refers to the presence of milky fluid containing chylomicrons and may result from lymphatic obstruction most commonly due to trauma to the thoracic duct, tuberculosis, or to a mediastinal tumor. An acidic fluid with pH less than 7.35 suggests tumor or

---

TABLE 13.4–1. CLASSIFICATION OF PORTAL HYPERTENSION

Portal Hypertension Due to Increased Resistance to Blood Flow
Prehepatic (presinusoidal)
  Portal venous thrombosis
  • Idiopathic
  • Neonatal sepsis
  • Tumor compression
  • Blood dyscrasias (e.g., polycythemia vera)

Hepatic
  Presinusoidal
  • Congenital hepatic fibrosis
  • Schistosomiasis
  • Sarcoidosis (rare)
  • Myeloproliferative disorders (rare)

  Sinusoidal and postsinusoidal[a]
  • Cirrhosis
    Alcoholic
    Posthepatitis
    Hemochromatosis
    Biliary
    Hepatolenticular degeneration (Wilson disease)
    α_1-Antitrypsin deficiency
  • Veno-occlusive disease

Posthepatic (postsinusoidal)
  • Hepatic venous obstruction (Budd-Chiari syndrome)
  • Constrictive pericarditis
  • Congestive heart failure

Portal Hypertension Due to Increased Flow in the Portal Vein
  • Arteriovenous anastomoses
  • Increased flow from massive splenomegaly

---

[a] In patients with acute and chronic liver cell disease such as hepatitis or cirrhosis, elements of both presinusoidal and postsinusoidal portal hypertension may be present. Occasionally, patients with cirrhosis develop portal vein thrombosis.

TABLE 13.4–2. CAUSES OF ASCITES

Exudative Ascites
1. Inflammatory diseases of peritoneum—peritonitis
   a. Ruptured viscus with or without intra-abdominal abscess: peptic ulcer, diverticulitis, appendicitis, cholecystitis, intestinal infarction, etc.
   b. Tuberculous peritonitis
   c. "Spontaneous" bacterial peritonitis
   d. Pancreatitis
   e. Bile peritonitis due to ruptured gallbladder, needle penetration of dilated bile duct, etc.)
2. Tumors
   a. Metastatic to liver, peritoneal lining, or both
   b. Leukemia, lymphoma, myeloid metaplasia
   c. Primary hepatocellular carcinoma and cholangiocarcinoma
3. Hypothyroidism

Lymphatic Obstruction with Chylous Ascites
1. Trauma to thoracic duct in chest
2. Mediastinal tumors
3. Filariasis
4. Tuberculosis (occasionally)
5. Cirrhosis (occasionally)

Transudative Ascites
1. As part of generalized fluid retention with hypoalbuminemia
   a. Nephrotic syndrome
   b. Protein-losing gastroenteropathy
2. Failure of return of blood to right side of heart
   a. Congestive heart failure
   b. Tricuspid insufficiency
   c. Constrictive pericarditis
3. Blockage of hepatic veins, vena cava, or both
   a. Budd-Chiari syndrome, tumor, webs, etc.[a]
   b. Veno-occlusive disease
4. Diffuse hepatic disease with portal hypertension
   a. Cirrhosis—all forms (Table 13.6–1)
5. Infiltrative processes of liver
   a. Tumors, lymphomas, myeloid metaplasia, etc.[a]
   b. Granulomatous disease (occasionally sarcoidosis, schistosomiasis)
6. Portal vein obstruction (rare)

Conditions that May Mimic Ascites
1. Pregnancy
2. Ovarian cyst
3. Pancreatic cyst
4. Mesenteric cyst

[a]Ascites may have characteristics of an exudate.

infection. The ascitic fluid LDH concentration helps differentiate ascites caused by uncomplicated cirrhosis and nonhepatic disorders. A fluid LDH value less than 400 IU and an ascitic fluid serum LDH ratio less than 0.6 implies uncomplicated cirrhosis. Characteristics of ascitic fluid analysis and the major causes of ascites are outlined in Table 13.4–3.

In patients with chronic liver disease and cirrhosis, ascites represents an intraperitoneal expansion of the extracellular fluid compartment. Important factors in the pathogenesis of the ascites in a patient with cirrhosis include elevation of the portal venous pressure, decrease of the serum colloid osmotic pressure as evidenced by a decreased serum albumin level, and retention by the kidney of both salt and water. The low serum albumin level reflects both impaired protein synthesis by the liver and the dilutional effect of a marked expansion of plasma volume in a patient with portal hypertension. The combination of obstruction to blood flow through the liver and low serum albumin level drives fluid out of the intrahepatic sinusoids and splanchnic bed into the peritoneal cavity (Starling hypothesis). The increase in intrahepatic sinusoidal pressure resulting from cell loss, fibrosis, and regenerative nodules leads to an increased movement of fluid into hepatic lymphatic vessels. Some of the excessive fluid escapes from the hepatic lymphatic vessels into the intraperitoneal space. When the rate of fluid production exceeds the capacity of the visceral peritoneal lymphatic vessels to reabsorb the fluid, ascites develops.

Rarely is elevation of portal pressure alone sufficient to cause ascites. In extrahepatic obstruction of the portal vein, a disorder characterized by portal hypertension and normal liver functions, ascites is unusual.

Characteristic abnormalities of salt and water metabolism contributing to ascites in chronic liver disease include increased sodium reabsorption in the proximal renal tubule, decreased free water clearance, and hyperaldosteronism.[1] Patients with liver disease and ascites usually have increased reabsorption of sodium in the proximal renal tubules. The factor or factors responsible for enhanced proximal sodium reabsorption have not been identified, but a humoral agent is suspected. Free water clearance is markedly reduced because of inappropriate release and decreased degradation of antidiuretic hormone. Hyperaldosteronism with increased distal reabsorption of sodium is a nearly constant factor in patients with chronic liver disease and ascites. Impaired metabolism of aldosterone, with decreased rate of aldosterone degradation, is present. As a result of these complex derangements in portal pressure, in plasma colloid osmotic pressure, in hepatic lymph production, and

TABLE 13.4–3. LABORATORY ANALYSIS OF ASCITIC FLUID

Diagnosis	Fluid Analysis			Other Laboratory Features
	WBC (mm³)	RBC	Protein (g/dl)	
Cirrhosis	<250 (mono)	Few	<3.0	LDH (fluid:serum) <0.6 fluid LDH <400 IU (pH >7.4)
Congestive heart failure	Few	Few	<2.5	
Nephrotic syndrome	Few	Few	<2.5	
Infection				
Bacterial	>500 (poly)	Few	>3.0	pH <7.35
Tuberculous	>500 (mono)	Few[a]	>3.0	pH <7.35
Tumor	Few	Many	>3.0	pH <7.35 (tumor cells present)
Pancreatitis	>500 (poly)	Many	>2.5	Fluid amylase >1000 IU/L
Pseudomyxoma peritonei	Few	Few	<2.5	Gelatinous fluid, occasionally with tumor cells
Chylous ascites	Few	Few	Variable	Fluid triglycerides elevated >400 mg/dl

[a]Occasionally many.

in abnormalities in salt and water balance, the total extracellular volume expands and ascites develops.

Edema commonly accompanies ascites in patients with liver disease, particularly in the presence of severe hypoalbuminemia. A pleural effusion occurs in approximately 5 percent of patients with ascites. The pleural effusion is usually in the right thorax and occurs in part from the direct escape of ascites from the peritoneal cavity into the chest via anatomic defects in the diaphragm. These pleural effusions occasionally develop in the absence of clinically detectable ascites.

The appearance or worsening of ascites in a patient with known cirrhosis may signify a deterioration in the status of the underlying liver disease. Other complications of cirrhosis that may cause ascites include (1) hepatocellular carcinoma, (2) tuberculous peritonitis, and (3) spontaneous bacterial peritonitis. Ascites with or without abdominal pain may be the initial presentation of any of these conditions. Fever with ascites may result from the underlying liver disease but should alert the clinician to the possibility of tuberculous or bacterial peritonitis. Pancreatic ascites with direct leakage of pancreatic fluid from a disruption of the pancreatic duct may cause ascites in a patient with chronic alcoholism and is suggested by the finding of an elevated amylase level in the abdominal fluid.

SPONTANEOUS BACTERIAL PERITONITIS

Spontaneous bacterial peritonitis (SBP) occurs in approximately 5 percent of patients with chronic liver disease, particularly alcoholic cirrhosis. Although bacterial infection of ascites may occur from many causes, including empyema of the gallbladder, rupture of a colonic diverticulum, or perforation of a peptic ulcer, the entity most often encountered is designated as "spontaneous" in that no entry site from the gut to the peritoneal cavity is found. In most instances a single organism, usually an aerobic gram-negative bacillus, causes SBP; anaerobic organisms are rarely a cause. SBP may result from septicemia, with gut bacteria entering the portal vein, bypassing the liver, and disseminating via the systemic circulation, or from direct movement of gut bacteria across the edematous gut wall into the ascites. Occasionally a nonenteric bacterial organism is found, and in this situation the ascites most likely became infected from septicemia. If fluid cultures grow multiple organisms, especially anaerobes, direct seeding from a large-bowel source (e.g., diverticulitis) should be suspected. Although SBP is characterized by rapidly accumulating ascites, fever, and abdominal pain, it is important to recognize that the disorder may appear with little or no fever and none of the usual signs of peritoneal inflammation.

The ascitic fluid in SBP is characteristically cloudy because of an increased leukocyte count (>300 cells/mm^3), with predominantly polymorphonuclear cells. The pH is less than 7.35. Organisms are seen on Gram stain in about one fourth of patients. Therapy for presumptive bacterial peritonitis should not await fluid culture results. Empiric antibiotic coverage directed toward gram-positive organisms, streptococci and staphylococci, and gram-negative bacilli should be instituted immediately. If an aminoglycoside is used, careful monitoring for aminoglycoside nephrotoxicity is necessary because patients with cirrhosis are predisposed to this complication.

MANAGEMENT OF ASCITES IN PATIENTS WITH UNDERLYING LIVER DISEASE

The recognition that ascites is a result of liver disease and portal hypertension, and not a disease entity itself, is a prerequisite to effective management. There is little but trouble to be gained if an effort is made to clear the ascites at a time when there has been no abatement of the underlying liver disease. Hospitalization is recommended for beginning therapy in most patients. A careful search is made for precipitating causes of the ascites, with particular reference to occult gastrointestinal hemorrhage, increased dietary sodium intake, and medications that increase renal sodium retention. Once complicating extrahepatic conditions have been excluded or treated, therapy may be directed specifically toward mobilization of ascites. The initial steps in the management of these patients are careful assessment of the status of the liver, bed rest, and restriction of dietary sodium. The maximum amount of ascites that can be mobilized in 24 hours is 700 to 900 ml.[12] If diuretic-induced fluid losses exceed this amount, the extra fluid is removed at the expense of the intravascular space, and hypoperfusion may ensue. The goal in treating ascites is to use the simplest regimen that will induce a diuresis of about 900 ml (1 to 1½ pounds per day). Patients who have peripheral edema in addition to ascites can tolerate greater fluid losses. One of the most important factors in the development of ascites is renal retention of sodium. Quantitation of renal sodium excretion is therefore valuable in planning a specific therapeutic regimen. Table 13.4–4 includes dietary sodium and diuretic recommendations based on renal excretion of sodium. In general, fluid restriction is not necessary unless the patient develops hyponatremia.

In most patients, ascites can be successfully treated with a combination of salt restriction and diuretics. Refractory ascites is defined as an inability to induce diuresis (less than 10 mEq of sodium in 24 hours) despite maximum diuretic doses and salt restriction. In these patients the tendency to form ascites is so severe that diuretic therapy sufficient to mobilize the ascites leads to volume depletion and prerenal azotemia. Alternative therapies in these patients include therapeutic paracenteses and peritoneovenous shunts.

TABLE 13.4–4. MANAGEMENT OF ASCITES IN PATIENTS WITH LIVER DISEASE

Determination of Cause of Ascites
1. Diagnosis of liver disease established
2. Tuberculosis, bacterial peritonitis, neoplasm, etc., ruled out

Direct Management: Therapy for Underlying Liver Disease

General Management
1. Bed rest
2. Measurement of urinary sodium excretion

Therapy
1. If 24-hr urine sodium value exceeds 50 mEq/24 hr, restrict dietary sodium to 2.0 g/day.
2. If 24-hr urinary sodium value equals 25–50 mEq/24 hr, add spironolactone (100–350 mg/day).
3. If 24-hr urine sodium value equals 10–25 mg/24 hr, restrict dietary sodium to 1 g/day and add furosemide (40–160 mg/day) or bumetanide (2–8 mg/day).
4. If 24-hr urine sodium value is less than 10 mEq/day use maximal diuretic dose. Consider therapeutic paracenteses or LeVeen shunt.

Assessment of Improvement by Daily Weight
1. Loss of ½–1½ lb/day satisfactory

Complications of Diuretic Therapy
1. Hyponatremia: nearly always from overretention of water (total body sodium normal or increased)
   a. Record of intake-output and avoidance of overhydration intravenously or orally
   b. Restriction of fluids to 500 ml/day or less
2. Hypokalemia—total body K+ usually decreased in liver disease
   a. Spironolactone to minimize losses
   b. Supplementation of 60–150 mEq/day K+ often required
3. Hypochloremic alkalosis
   Replace with chloride in form of KCl
4. Progressive rise of and oliguria ("hepatorenal syndrome")
   a. Stop all diuretics.
   b. Use intravenous albumin to replete intravascular volume.
   c. Monitor venous pressure; avoid overexpansion of intravascular space.

Repeated therapeutic paracenteses have been used in patients with severe ascites and markedly impaired urinary sodium excretion. Paracenteses of up to 4 L in 24 hours were not associated with more complications than were potent diuretic regimens.[11] The peritoneojugular, or LeVeen, shunt is a surgical approach to the management of resistant ascites. In this procedure, ascites is siphoned from the peritoneal cavity through a long Silastic subcutaneous tube to the jugular vein or right atrium. The device is equipped with a one-way pressure-operated valve so that when the intra-abdominal pressure from the ascites is greater than 3 cm over the venous pressure, the valve opens and ascitic fluid flows from the peritoneal cavity into the systemic circulation. The peritoneal jugular shunt may be dramatically effective in reducing ascites. Complications of the procedure may, however, be severe and life threatening. They include clotting of the Silastic tube with blood or debris, infection, and disseminated intravascular coagulopathy. If the reinfusion of ascites exceeds the ability of the kidney to excrete the fluid, hypervolemia may result, leading to congestive heart failure or bleeding from esophageal varices.[6]

PROGRESSIVE RENAL FAILURE IN LIVER DISEASE (HEPATORENAL SYNDROME)[10]

Transient renal insufficiency may develop in patients with liver disease after a gastrointestinal hemorrhage, overvigorous diuresis, or intercurrent infection. In some patients with severe liver disease, however, progressive renal failure develops and no specific cause is found. This form of renal failure is called the hepatorenal syndrome and is associated with azotemia, oliguria, and hyponatremia. It is a frequent terminal event in patients with decompensated hepatic disease. The pathogenesis of the hepatorenal syndrome is unknown. The kidneys are histologically normal and have been used successfully as donor organs in human renal transplantation.

Abnormalities in the volume and distribution of renal blood flow have been demonstrated, with a marked decrease in renal cortical perfusion, suggesting active intrarenal vasoconstriction. Secondary reduction in glomerular filtration leads to marked sodium retention, oliguria, and azotemia. Urinary and plasma electrolyte measurements can help differentiate the hepatorenal syndrome from acute tubular necrosis. The urine osmolarity in the hepatorenal syndrome is normal, but the urine contains very little sodium (<5 mEq/24 hr). The urinary/plasma creatinine ratio is greater than 30. In contrast, with acute tubular necrosis, the urinary/plasma creatinine ratio is approximately 1, and significant urinary sodium excretion is found (>30 mEq/L). Treatment of the hepatorenal syndrome is unsatisfactory, and few patients survive. In some patients, renal function improves if the liver disease abates. Plasma expansion with albumin or blood is indicated if the central venous pressure is less than 6 cm H_2O. Vasoactive drugs have all generally failed to reverse this disorder. Treatment must be directed toward the correction of underlying precipitating factors and the maintenance of salt and water balance. Care must be taken to avoid the use of prostaglandin synthetase inhibitors such as nonsteroidal anti-inflammatory agents. Impaired synthesis of renal vasodilators by these agents may precipitate or accentuate renal failure in patients with cirrhosis. A few patients have apparently recovered from the hepatorenal syndrome after construction of a portal-systemic shunt or insertion of the peritoneojugular shunt, but these therapies must be considered unproved.

HEPATIC ENCEPHALOPATHY[3,4]

Hepatic encephalopathy is a complex neuropsychiatric disorder occurring in patients with acute and chronic liver disease. It is characterized by disturbances in consciousness, personality, behavior, and neuromuscular function. The individual components of the syndrome are nonspecific. Early manifestations include reversal of sleep patterns, hypersomnia, irritability, neglect of personal appearance, and forgetfulness. In later stages, delirium and deep coma may occur. Neurologic signs include hyperreflexia, generalized rigidity, and myoclonus. Asterixis, a nonrhythmic flapping tremor of the wrist and metacarpophalangeal joints, best demonstrated with the arms outstretched and the hands dorsiflexed, is commonly seen but is not specific for hepatic encephalopathy. It may be found in uremia, chronic congestive heart failure, and chronic lung disease. Seizures are uncommon in hepatic encephalopathy. Biochemical abnormalities in hepatic encephalopathy include hyperammonemia and an increase in cerebrospinal fluid glutamine concentration. The cerebrospinal fluid is otherwise normal. Hepatic encephalopathy is associated with abnormalities in plasma amino acid concentrations, including elevated levels of methionine, phenylalanine, and tyrosine, and decreased concentrations of the branched-chain amino acids valine, leucine, and isoleucine. Pathologic changes in the brain are nonspecific, with only a generalized increase in protoplasmic astrocytes. The electroencephalogram shows nonspecific slow-wave activity (delta waves less than 4 Hz) found predominantly over the frontal regions. Triphasic waves are seen in many patients but are not pathognomonic for hepatic encephalopathy.

Factors important in the pathogenesis of hepatic encephalopathy include the shunting of blood around the liver cells into the systemic circulation and the presence of hepatocellular dysfunction. In most patients, both factors are present. The shunting of portal blood around the liver cells may be through extrahepatic or intrahepatic shunts. It is assumed that the neurologic syndrome is produced by presentation to the systemic circulation of one or more toxic products of intestinal origin normally metabolized by the liver.[13]

Abnormalities of ammonia metabolism are most frequently incriminated in the pathogenesis of hepatic encephalopathy. Ammonia is normally produced in the gut by bacterial ureolysis and is transported via the portal vein to the liver, where it is converted to urea. Evidence in favor of ammonia as a principal toxin in hepatic encephalopathy includes (1) an elevated arterial or cerebrospinal fluid ammonia level in most patients with this disorder, (2) induction of hepatic encephalopathy in susceptible patients by administration of ammonium salts, (3) relief of the syndrome after therapy directed toward reduction of the blood ammonia level, and (4) presence of hepatic encephalopathy in children with genetically determined deficiencies of the enzymes of the Krebs-Henseleit cycle, leading to hyperammonemia.

Evidence against ammonia as the only toxin includes (1) the absence of a close correlation between blood ammonia levels and the clinical degree of encephalopathy and (2) the occurrence of the disorder in some patients in whom the blood ammonia level is not elevated. Other compounds implicated as possible toxins in producing hepatic encephalopathy include endogenous benzodiazepine-like substances, mercaptans derived from the metabolism of methionine, and biogenic amines (e.g., γ-aminobutyric acid) that affect neurochemical transmission in the brain. Most likely, several toxins act in combination to cause hepatic encephalopathy.

Hepatic encephalopathy may arise without an apparent precipitating cause in the course of acute or chronic hepatic disease or may have a clearly identifiable precipitating factor. Exogenous factors of importance include increased dietary protein, the administration of certain drugs (sedatives and analgesics in particular), overzealous use of diuretics leading to hypovolemia and hypokalemia, azotemia, infection, and gastrointestinal hemorrhage. Gastrointestinal hemorrhage may precipitate hepatic encephalopathy not only because of decreased liver perfusion due to hypovolemia but because blood in the gut is a rich source of ammonia. One hundred milliliters of blood contains about 20 g of protein. The particular susceptibility of patients with hypokalemia and alkalosis to hepatic encephalopathy results from two factors. Ammonia moves across membranes in its nonionic form, NH_3. With its pK at 9.1, only a small percentage of ammonia in the blood is in the nonionic form.

When the patient becomes alkalotic, more ammonia is present in the NH_3 form and is therefore available for translocation into cells. In addition, hypokalemia significantly reduces renal excretion of ammonia. Hypoxia and intercurrent infections have been implicated in coma. The increased response of the brain to drugs may be demonstrated by giving susceptible patients a small dose of parenteral morphine. A rapid and marked disorganization of the electroencephalogram occurs, with slow-wave activity over the frontal areas.

MANAGEMENT OF HEPATIC ENCEPHALOPATHY

The objective of management of heptic encephalopathy consists of (1) lowering the levels of ammonia and other toxic substances by reducing protein or excluding it from the diet and (2) cleansing nitrogenous materials from the gut. An additional benefit may be obtained by reducing colonic bacteria with nonabsorbable antibiotics. General support of the confused or comatose patient, combined with aggressive efforts to detect factors such as gastrointestinal hemorrhage, dietary indiscretion, and drugs that may have precipitated or worsened the syndrome, is required. Alternative

TABLE 13.4–5. MANAGEMENT OF HEPATIC ENCEPHALOPATHY

Careful Search for Precipitating Factors
A. Excess nitrogen load
   1. Gastrointestinal hemorrhage
   2. Excess protein in diet
   3. Increased enterohepatic circulation of urea in azotemia
B. Electrolyte abnormalities
   1. Hypokalemia (especially hypokalemic alkalosis induced by diuretics)
   2. Hypovolemia (gastrointestinal hemorrhage, paracentesis, diuresis)
C. Drugs
   1. Narcotics, tranquilizers, and sedatives (particularly dangerous)
   2. Diuretics
      a. Via hypovolemia and hypokalemia
      b. Increased renal production of ammonia
D. Infection
E. Surgical procedures

Management
A. For minimal encephalopathy
   1. Reduction of dietary protein to 20–40 g/day
   2. Lactulose, 30 ml every 4–6 hr (to promote two soft bowel movements per day) or neomycin, 1 g orally bid or qid
   3. Follow patient with:
      a. Handwriting chart
      b. Mental status examination
      c. Repeated search for precipitating factors in item I, above
B. For moderate to marked encephalopathy
   1. Removal of all protein from diet
   2. Vigorous catharsis—enemas and oral magnesium citrate
   3. Calories—1000–1500/day—provided as carbohydrate (orally or intravenously)
   4. Lactulose or neomycin as in item II-A-2, above
   5. Follow-up of patient as in item II-A-3, above
C. Once improvement occurs
   1. Reinstitution of dietary protein in 10 g increments every 3–5 days
   2. Continuation of lactulose as tolerated or neomycin until patient can tolerate a 50 g protein diet; then withdrawal of lactulose or neomycin considered

explanations for coma and depressed mentation in patients with liver disease must not be overlooked. Subdural hematoma, hypoglycemia, meningitis, and sedative overdose should be excluded before specific therapy for hepatic encephalopathy is instituted. A plan for the management of hepatic encephalopathy is outlined in Table 13.4–5.

Cleansing of the gut with enemas may dramatically improve the mental status. Protein should be excluded from the diet until control of the encephalopathy has been obtained. Protein is gradually reinstituted in daily 10 g increments. The potential hazard in using any drug in a patient with liver disease must be recognized. Analgesics and sedatives are especially dangerous. Volume depletion and electrolyte disturbances should be corrected.

Lactulose is the most important drug in the management of hepatic encephalopathy. It is a synthetic disaccharide that is degraded by intestinal bacteria, acidifying the contents of the lower gut. It also produces an osmotic, fermentative diarrhea. Lactulose can be administered orally or by retention enema. Lactulose regularly reduces blood ammonia levels and is associated with a reduction in the frequency of episodes of encephalopathy in patients with chronic disease. Alternatively, the nonabsorbable antibiotic neomycin may be used. Neomycin leads to bacteriostasis with inhibition of urea-splitting and deaminating bacteria. The dangers of long-term administration of neomycin are well documented and include ototoxic effects, production of malabsorption, and renal tubular toxic effects. In some patients the combination of lactulose and neomycin is more effective than either used alone.

Other experimental therapeutic approaches to the management of chronic hepatic encephalopathy include the use of L-dopa or bromocriptine and attempts to increase the low levels of branched-chain amino acids by administration of these compounds either as the amino acids themselves or as their ketoanalogs.

In patients with encephalopathy that develops as part of fulminant hepatic failure, the approach outlined in Table 13.4–5 is generally employed but with less success. Other manifestations of fulminant hepatic failure (hypoglycemia, cerebral edema, and secondary infection) may contribute to coma and must be addressed.

REFERENCES

1. Arroyo V, Bosch J, et al: Plasma resin activity and urinary sodium excretion as prognostic indices in nonazotemic cirrhosis with ascites. Ann Intern Med 94:198, 1981
2. Cattau EL, Benjamin SB, et al: The accuracy of the physical examination in the diagnosis of suspected ascites. JAMA 247:1164, 1982
3. Conn HO, Lieberthal MM: The Hepatic Coma Syndromes and Lactulose. Baltimore, Williams & Wilkins, 1979, p 1
4. Crossley IK, Wardle EN, William R: Biochemical mechanisms of hepatic encephalopathy. Clin Sci 64:247, 1983
5. DiSitter C, Rector WG: The significance of bloody ascites in patients with cirrhosis. Am J Gastroenterol 79:136, 1984
6. Epstein M: The LeVeen shunt for ascites and hepatorenal syndrome. N Engl J Med 302:628, 1980
7. Galambos JT: Esophageal variceal hemorrhage: Diagnosis and an overview of treatment. Semin Liver Dis 2:711, 1982
8. Hoefs JC, Canawati HN, et al: Spontaneous bacterial peritonitis. Hepatology 2:399, 1982
9. Pappas SC, Jones EA: Methods for assessing hepatic encephalopathy. Semin Liver Dis 3:298, 1982
10. Papper S: Hepatorenal syndrome. In Epstein M (ed): The Kidney in Liver Disease. New York, Elsevier, 1983, p 87
11. Quintero E, Arroyo V, et al: Paracentesis versus diuretics in the treatment of cirrhotics with tense ascites. Lancet 1:611, 1985
12. Shear L, Ching S, et al: Compartmentalization of ascites and edema in patients with hepatic cirrhosis. N Engl J Med 282:1391, 1970
13. Zieve L: The mechanism of hepatic coma. Hepatology 1:360, 1981

Hepatomegaly: Focal and Circulatory Disorders

Mack C. Mitchell

HEPATOMEGALY

The span of the normal liver averages 8 to 10 cm in adults and can usually be palpated at the right costal margin. The upper edge of hepatic dullness determined by percussion is at the fifth to sixth intercostal space. Extension of the normal-sized liver below the costal margin may occur in thin persons during deep inspiration or in patients with pulmonary hyperinflation. In obese patients and patients with ascites, ultrasonography and CT scanning may be helpful in determining hepatic size.

Complete evaluation of the liver on physical examination includes determination not only of hepatic size but also of the texture and contour of the liver surface and border. Gross nodularity suggests either tumor or cirrhosis, whereas soft, tender hepatomegaly suggests congestion or steatosis. Tenderness may also be present in patients with viral or alcoholic hepatitis, hepatic abscess, biliary obstruction, or tumor.

Enlargement of the liver occurs not only in patients with hepatocellular diseases but also in patients with focal and circulatory disorders. The causes of hepatomegaly are outlined in Table 13.5–1. A systematic approach is required to determine the underlying cause of hepatomegaly. Massive (>10 cm below the right costal margin) hepatomegaly usually occurs as a consequence of tumor infiltration, fatty infiltration, congestion, or amyloidosis. Radiographic visualization of the liver by ultrasonography, CT scanning, or MRI is useful in distinguishing focal disease from diffuse hepatocellular disease. Liver biopsy is often indicated to confirm the diagnosis of malignancy or to distinguish between causes of diffuse enlargement.

FOCAL LIVER DISORDERS

The finding of a liver mass in a patient with or without hepatomegaly requires further evaluation to determine the nature of the mass. Ultrasonograms and CT scans can distinguish cystic masses from solid ones and reliably differentiate hepatic abscesses from other cystic lesions.

HEPATIC CYSTS

Nonparasitic hepatic cysts may be solitary or multiple and may also be associated with cysts in other organs.[15] The majority of hepatic cysts, particularly solitary cysts, are asymptomatic and are found during ultrasonography or CT scanning for other abdominal complaints. In some patients, cysts may become symptomatic during a period of enlargement or after hemorrhage into the cyst. Pain in the right upper quadrant of the abdomen and hepatomegaly are the most common findings. Multiple cysts may be found in the liver as a manifestation of adult polycystic disease, in which renal cysts are commonly found. The cysts originate in the bile duct but usually do not communicate with extrahepatic bile ducts. In most patients these cysts remain asymptomatic and do not require treatment. Occasionally, large cysts may be aspirated under ultrasonography guidance to relieve pain.

Caroli disease is a disorder characterized by multiple choledochal cysts that communicate with extrahepatic bile ducts. Often there is an increase in portal fibrous tissue. The combination of fibrosis with or without choledochal cysts or bile-duct hamartomas is referred to as congenital hepatic fibrosis.[15] These patients may have portal hypertension and develop biliary cirrhosis and hepatic failure resulting from obstruction due to choledochal cysts. Jaundice and recurrent episodes of ascending cholangitis occur in patients with Caroli disease and congenital hepatic fibrosis. Long-term antibiotic suppression is indicated in those patients with documented recurrent cholangitis.

PYOGENIC LIVER ABSCESS

The majority of liver abscesses occur as a complication of biliary tract obstruction and ascending cholangitis. Biliary obstruction may be due to gallstones, tumor, ductal stricture, or choledochal cysts. Trauma, both blunt and penetrating, may result in hepatic abscess. Occasionally, portal septicemia may be the source of infection, usually as a complication of other intra-abdominal abscesses. Certain organisms such as *Actinomyces* have a predilection for hepatic abscess formation. Rarely abscesses result from dissemination of bacterial endocarditis or other arterial sites of infection.

Liver abscesses often contain a mixed flora, predominantly aerobic gram-negative rods and anaerobic organisms. *Staphylococcus aureus* occasionally is found, but most often after surgical exploration of the abdomen or biliary tract. Interference with blood supply, impaired biliary drainage, and decreased host resistance to infection are important risk factors in the pathogenesis of liver abscesses.

The clinical manifestations of hepatic abscess include fever, either low grade or spiking with chills; vague discomfort in the entire abdomen or in the right upper quadrant; anorexia; inanition; and weight loss. The liver is enlarged and tender, and occasionally a friction rub may be heard over the lower ribs. Jaundice is usually absent or slight unless there is high-grade biliary obstruction, and ascites is rare. Leukocytosis, anemia, and elevation of the serum alkaline phosphatase level are common.

Management of liver abscess requires recognition and treatment of underlying conditions such as biliary tract disease, endocarditis, or extrahepatic intra-abdominal infection. Broad antibiotic coverage, often for a prolonged time, is required but may be ineffective without proper surgical drainage. The mortality rate from multiple abscesses remains high because of the difficulty in achieving adequate drainage.

AMEBIC ABSCESS

Entamoeba histolytica is an important worldwide cause of both dysentery and liver abscess. After invasion of amebae through the colon, the organisms are transported to the small portal radicles in the liver. Proteolytic enzymes secreted by the amebae cause local tissue destruction and abscess formation.

Amebic liver abscesses usually cause insidious symptoms such as vague pain in the right upper quadrant of the abdomen, malaise, fever, and night sweats. A history of dysentery or active colitis is found in approximately 20 percent of patients. Mild to moderate leukocytosis and anemia are common, whereas jaundice is rare. Results of biochemical tests of liver function, including determination of the serum alkaline phosphatase level, are often normal. Ultrasonography, technetium liver scans, and CT scans are useful to identify the presence of an abscess. Indirect hemagglutination tests are the most reliable method for establishing the diagnosis.[11] Amebic

TABLE 13.5–1. CAUSES OF HEPATOMEGALY

Venous Congestion of Liver
- Congestive heart failure
- Constructive pericarditis
- Tricuspid insufficiency
- Obstruction of hepatic veins (Budd-Chiari syndrome) with or without obstruction of the inferior vena cava

Diffuse Hepatomegaly Without Infection
- Cirrhosis
- Hepatitis due to drugs or toxins
- Infiltrative processes
   - Fatty liver
   - Amyloidosis
   - Hemochromatosis
   - Sarcoidosis (occasionally)
   - Metabolic defects (glycogen storage diseases)
- Primary biliary cirrhosis

Hepatomegaly Associated with Infection
- Abscess (may be localized enlargement)
   - Amebic
   - Pyogenic
- Viral hepatitis (A; B; non-A, non-B)
- Leptospirosis
- Other infections (syphilis, tuberculosis, brucellosis, actinomycosis, echinococcosis, schistosomiasis

Obstruction to Bile Ducts
- Gallstones
- Common bile duct stricture
- Tumors (pancreas, ampulla of Vater, bile ducts)
- External pressure (enlarged lymph nodes, pancreatitis)
- Sclerosing cholangitis

Neoplasms
- Lymphomas and leukemia
- Metastatic tumors
- Primary tumors (hepatocellular carcinoma, cholangiocarcinoma)

liver abscess may rupture into the chest, pericardium, or peritoneum. These complications, although uncommon, may cause serious illness and even death.

Management of amebic abscess is usually medical. Metronidazole is the drug of choice and is given in high doses (750 mg three times daily for 7 to 10 days). Intestinal amebicides such as iodoquinol or chloroquine are also recommended. Aspiration is usually unnecessary, except in left lobe involvement, in which the risk of rupture into the pericardium is higher. Amebic pus is almost always sterile and has a thick consistency and a color that resembles anchovy paste.

PRIMARY LIVER TUMORS

Hepatocellular Carcinoma

Hepatocellular carcinoma (HCC) is one of the most common tumors worldwide. It is most frequently found in sub-Saharan Africa, Southeast Asia, Japan, China, and the South Pacific islands. In North America, it is still a rare tumor, although the frequency may be increasing. Chronic hepatitis B virus infection is the single most important risk factor in the development of HCC. The worldwide occurrence of hepatitis B and that of HCC overlap almost identically. Furthermore, the hepatitis B virus genome has been found to be incorporated into the host genome in human HCCs.[12] Integration of viral DNA into the hepatocyte DNA is thought to be an important step in malignant transformation. Other secondary factors, such as host immune response, exposure to cocarcinogens such as aflatoxins and hepatotoxic chemicals, and exposure to tumor promoters, possibly alcohol, may play a role in the ultimate development of HCC.

Cirrhosis due to α_1-antitrypsin deficiency and chronic active hepatitis also increases the risk of HCC. In these patients the process of chronic injury and regeneration may be important in pathogenesis. Whether oral contraceptives or androgenic steroids increase the risk for developing HCC is controversial.[9] α-Fetoprotein is elevated in approximately 75 percent of patients with HCC, regardless of the causative agent. Because there are few false-positive results, an elevated α-fetoprotein level (>500 mg/ml) is highly suggestive of HCC in a high-risk patient.

HCC should be considered in any patient with cirrhosis who develops weight loss, a rapidly enlarging liver, unexplained deterioration in liver function, or ascites, particularly if blood tinged. Both hepatic friction rubs and bruits may be heard over the liver. Paraneoplastic syndromes, including erythrocytosis, porphyria cutanea tarda, dysfibrinogenemia, and hypercalcemia, may be present in patients at the time of diagnosis.[8] Hypoglycemia is a common preterminal manifestation that is probably related to large metabolic requirements of the tumor.

BENIGN TUMORS OF THE LIVER

Cavernous hemangiomas of the liver are often found at autopsy examination of the liver but are rarely symptomatic. Occasionally hepatic hemangiomas are found as a cold spot on a liver scan or as a calcified mass in the liver on a radiograph. Hemangiomas rarely result in infarction or rupture but may require resection.

Focal nodular hyperplasia (FNH) is a benign tumor often found in women. It generally occurs as an asymptomatic intrahepatic mass that is discovered accidentally. There is no definite association of FNH and the use of oral contraceptives. The lesion has a characteristic central scar, contains Kupffer cells, concentrates technetium-99m (^{99m}Tc) and rarely ruptures. Hepatic resection may be required for patients with right upper quadrant abdominal pain or for the rare patient with hemorrhage.

Liver cell adenomas are hepatic tumors that are definitely associated with oral contraceptive use.[9] The lesion may occur as an asymptomatic intrahepatic mass, as a painful mass in the right upper quadrant of the abdomen due to hemorrhage in or around the lesion, or as intra-abdominal hemorrhage. The liver cell adenoma characteristically has no portal tracts and no Kupffer cells and therefore does not take up ^{99m}Tc. Hepatic resection is required for adenomas that bleed. Asymptomatic adenomas become smaller or disappear if oral contraceptives are discontinued, and the size of the lesion is followed by imaging techniques.

Secondary Tumors of the Liver

Metastatic tumors in the liver are common. Dissemination of the tumor to the liver is most often by the bloodstream, with contiguous or lymphatic spread occurring less frequently. When the liver is involved with metastatic tumor, multiple lesions are the rule. The liver that harbors metastatic tumor may attain gigantic size.

Clinical features of secondary tumors in the liver may be overshadowed by symptoms of the primary tumor, but hepatomegaly, abdominal pain, or an abnormal biochemical test result may be the first indication of the presence of tumor. Systemic symptoms of lassitude, weight loss, and anorexia are frequent. Discomfort of the abdomen in the right upper quadrant is common, and pain in the region of the liver also occurs, particularly if metastases involve the capsule of the liver. Portal hypertension manifested by splenomegaly, abdominal collateral vessels, and esophagogastric varices may develop but is usually of no clinical importance. Bile duct obstruction or portal venous thrombosis caused by the tumor may occur. Surprisingly few biochemical test abnormalities are encountered in even large livers extensively replaced by tumor. The most constant changes are elevation of the serum alkaline phosphatase level and moderate increases in serum aminotransferase levels. Jaundice, when present, is usually mild. The diagnosis is often apparent when an enlarged, nodular liver occurs in a setting of a known tumor, but massive hepatic replacement may foreshadow evidence of primary tumor (e.g., malignant melanoma). Hepatic scintiscanning, CT scanning, and ultrasonography are useful in the

evaluation of the presence and extent of metastatic tumor. Liver biopsy is indicated to confirm the diagnosis. Even in patients with no signs or symptoms that suggest hepatic involvement, liver biopsy uncovers approximately 20 percent of metastases. A liver biopsy directed by ultrasonography or CT scan may improve the diagnostic yield.

Management of these patients is largely supportive. An occasional solitary metastasis has been successfully removed by hepatic lobectomy. Results with arterial infusion of chemotherapeutic agents are generally unsatisfactory.

GRANULOMAS OF THE LIVER

Granulomas have been reported in from 3 to 10 percent of large series of liver biopsies. The differential diagnosis of these granulomas may require extensive investigation, encompassing bacterial, viral, fungal, allergic, physical, and neoplastic causes.[4,13] An exact cause for many hepatic granulomas is never found. The histologic pattern of an individual granuloma is usually of little diagnostic value, although special stains and culture of liver biopsy material for acid-fast and fungal organisms may assist in making an exact diagnosis. Table 13.5–2 presents several of the common disorders associated with granulomas, with an outline of principal associated features and diagnostic methods. An elevated serum alkaline phosphatase level is frequent in granulomatous liver disease, but other biochemical tests of the liver are often normal. The discovery of granulomas in liver biopsy material may be a focal point of significant value in directing the investigation of patients with unexplained fever, hepatomegaly, lymphadenopathy, pulmonary infiltrates, or weight loss. Hepatic granulomas are frequently found in patients with primary biliary cirrhosis and may also be the first clue to the diagnosis of Hodgkin disease.

Liver biopsy is of considerable value in the diagnosis of sarcoidosis, with granulomas found in almost all patients with the disease. The granulomatous liver disease in sarcoidosis has on occasion been associated with severe hepatocellular involvement, portal hypertension, and bleeding esophageal varices.[7] The usefulness of liver biopsy in investigating miliary tuberculosis is likewise established, with virtually all these patients having granulomas on biopsy. Granulomas of the liver are common in patients with both histoplasmosis and brucellosis. A disorder characterized by hepatosplenomegaly and hepatic granulomas is found in workers exposed to beryllium compounds in aircraft manufacturing and metallurgy industries and is confirmed by determination of urinary beryllium.

CIRCULATORY DISORDERS

Elevation of right atrial pressure increases hepatic venous pressure because the major hepatic veins enter the inferior vena cava just below the diaphragm. Both acute and chronic forms of congestive heart failure commonly cause obstruction to hepatic venous outflow. Constrictive pericarditis is a rare but treatable cause of hepatic venous obstruction. Decreased venous outflow, in turn, produces sinusoidal dilation and congestion within the liver lobule, particularly in the region surrounding the terminal hepatic venules. Hepatocyte dysfunction and even frank necrosis may result from impaired circulation.[4] Long-standing elevation of right atrial pressure can lead to hepatic necrosis and eventually to cirrhosis with portal hypertension. Whether the injury is a consequence of arterial hypoxemia, decreased arterial flow leading to ischemia, increased venous pressure, or a combination of these factors is unclear.

Hepatomegaly, which is often accompanied by tenderness of the liver, and right upper quadrant abdominal pain are the most frequent clinical manifestations of congestive liver disease. Ascites and splenomegaly are infrequently seen but, if present, suggest portal hypertension. Characteristically the protein content of ascitic fluid is high (>2.5 g/dl) despite the absence of inflammation. This high protein content may reflect the more distal obstruction to portal flow in these patients (postsinusoidal) in comparison with portal hypertension complicating cirrhosis (sinusoidal). The usually normal serum albumin level is another factor that may explain the higher protein content of ascitic fluid. Although aminotransferase levels (ALT and AST) are often moderately elevated (100 to 300 IU), the alkaline phosphatase concentration remains normal in the majority of patients. Mild hyperbilirubinemia, both conjugated and unconjugated, occurs in one third of patients and may be due to either decreased delivery of bilirubin to the liver cells or to hepatocyte dysfunction as a consequence of elevated right atrial pressure and ischemia.

Acute hepatic arterial ischemia causes a prompt rise in serum aminotransferase level that may reach values as high as 10,000 to 20,000 within 24 hours.[3] The levels fall rapidly because the injury does not continue in most cases. Although the AST level is initially higher than the ALT level, the shorter serum half-life of AST results in values reaching normal more rapidly than for ALT. This pattern may be diagnostically useful if serial values are monitored. Histologic examination demonstrates bland centrilobular necrosis without inflammation. This lesion resembles that seen in toxic injury to the liver from acetaminophen. Hypoprothrombinemia may

TABLE 13.5–2. GRANULOMATOUS LIVER DISEASE

Etiology[a]	Associated Features	Diagnostic Procedures
Tuberculosis	Chest infiltrates; hemoptysis, pericarditis; meningitis; etc.	Tuberculin skin tests, sputum and biopsy examinations, and culture for acid-fast bacilli
Sarcoidosis	Bilateral hilar adenopathy; chest infiltrates; lymphadenopathy, uveitis	Diagnosis of exclusion Kveim test positive in 80% Demonstration of noncaseating granulomas in two organs in patient with compatible history
Histoplasmosis	Residence in endemic area Chest infiltrates	Histoplasmin complement fixation test Fungal stains and culture of sputum, liver, and bone marrow
Brucellosis	Occupational exposure (farmer, packing-house worker, veterinarian) Acute or chronic febrile illness, often with hepatosplenomegaly	Brucella skin test Complement fixation test Culture of blood, liver, and bone marrow
Berylliosis	Occupational exposure	Skin patch test Urinary beryllium test

[a]All these disorders have a similar presenting clinical picture of wasting, malaise, and fever. Pulmonary involvement is frequent and often is the major manifestation of disease.

occur early in the course but usually improves within several days, whereas conjugated hyperbilirubinemia may develop as other parameters are improving. The diagnosis of ischemic hepatitis is established from the characteristic clinical and laboratory findings. Liver biopsy is seldom necessary and treatment is supportive. Ischemic hepatitis may be a devastating, potentially fatal occurrence, particularly in patients with underlying chronic liver disease.

HEPATIC VEIN THROMBOSIS (BUDD-CHIARI SYNDROME)

Thrombosis of the major hepatic veins, thereby blocking outflow of blood from the liver (Budd-Chiari syndrome), is a rare disorder that may occur alone or in association with inferior vena cava thrombosis. In many patients no cause of the thrombosis is found, but associations with polycythemia vera, paroxysmal nocturnal hemoglubinuria, use of oral contraceptives, renal cell carcinoma, and hepatocellular carcinoma are all established.[10] Membranous webs in the inferior vena cava obstructing the ostia to the hepatic veins that may be surgically removed have been a reported cause of hepatic vein obstruction.

Hepatic venous thrombosis may occur suddenly with a rapidly enlarging liver, ascites, abdominal pain, and often watery diarrhea, rapidly followed by hepatocellular failure and coma. The chronic form usually occurs with progressive ascites. There is a wide range of reported ascitic fluid protein concentrations. In most patients there is only a slight increase in aminotransferase levels. Portal hypertension with hematemesis from bleeding esophageal varices may occur. Liver biopsy characteristically reveals intense congestion with necrosis and atrophy of hepatocytes around the terminal hepatic venule, often in association with large hemorrhagic areas. There is scant inflammatory reaction. ^{99m}Tc liver scans may reveal no uptake in those areas behind the blocked veins. Inferior vena caval and hepatic venography establishes the diagnosis.

Anticoagulants and streptokinase have been employed in acutely developing cases but with little success. Most patients die with hepatocellular failure and hepatic coma. Side-to-side portacaval shunt operations or grafts from the superior mesenteric vein to the inferior vena cava (mesocaval shunt) may be helpful in allowing the portal vein to become an outflow vessel, relieving part of the intrahepatic congestion. In patients with hepatic vein thrombosis and inferior vena cava thrombosis, a mesoatrial shunt may be required.[10] The peritoneojugular shunt may relieve the ascites but does not correct the underlying problem.

VENO-OCCLUSIVE DISEASE

The clinical manifestations of acute or subacute obstruction of the small interhepatic veins and venules resembles Budd-Chiari syndrome. The disorder was first observed in children in the West Indies who had consumed herbal teas brewed from plants containing pyrrolidine alkaloids.[2] In some patients the disease is rapidly fatal, whereas in others the course is chronic, eventually leading to nonportal cirrhosis with portal hypertension. Although the condition is rarely seen in otherwise healthy patients, it is a recognized complication of bone marrow transplantation.[6] Veno-occlusive disease usually occurs within the first 2 to 3 weeks after marrow transplantation. It appears to be a separate entity from graft-versus-host disease and may be related to irradiation or chemotherapy given before marrow transplantation. It has also been reported in some patients with leukemia treated with chemotherapy. In most of these patients the course is relentlessly progressive. The majority of patients die as a result of hepatic failure or complications related to accompanying portal hypertension.

PORTAL VEIN THROMBOSIS

Extrahepatic obstruction of the portal venous system may result from neonatal umbilical sepsis, pylephlebitis, abdominal trauma, pancreatitis, or HCC, or it may be a complication of cirrhosis.[14] The usual presentation for such patients is with sudden, unheralded massive hematemesis. Recurrent episodes of bleeding are typical. Splenomegaly is a constant feature. Results of biochemical tests of the liver are usually normal. In general, these patients do not develop significant ascites or hepatic encephalopathy after a hemorrhage. When portal vein thrombosis occurs as a complication of cirrhosis, however, ascites may occur. The end-to-side portacaval shunt procedure is precluded by the obstructed portal vein, and alternative operations, including mesocaval shunts or devascularization procedures, are employed.

OTHER CIRCULATORY DISORDERS

Sinusoidal packing with abnormal red blood cells leads to focal intrahepatic thromboses in patients with sickle-cell anemia. Occasionally this disorder may result in fulminant hepatic failure or lead to serious chronic liver disease with fibrosis, cirrhosis or both.[1] Diseases of the hepatic arteries are rare and include occasional instances of polyarteritis nodosa, aneurysms of the hepatic artery, embolism from subacute infective endocarditis, or inadvertent ligation of the hepatic artery at surgery.

REFERENCES

1. Bauer TW, Moore GW, Hutchins GM: The liver in sickle cell disease. A clinicopathologic study of 70 patients. Am J Med 69:833, 1980
2. Bras G, Hill KR: Veno-occlusive disease of the liver: Essential pathology. Lancet 2:161, 1956
3. Bynum TE, Boitnott JK, Maddrey WC: Ischemic hepatitis. Dig Dis Sci 24:129, 1979
4. Dunn GD, Hayes P, et al: The liver in congestive heart failure: A review. Am J Med Sci 265:174, 1973
5. Klatskin G: Hepatic granulomata: Problems in interpretation. Ann NY Acad Sci 278:427, 1976
6. MacDonald GB, Sharma P, et al: Veno-occlusive disease of the liver after bone marrow transplantation: Diagnosis, incidence and predisposing factors. Hepatology 4:116, 1984
7. Maddrey WC, Johns CJ, et al: Sarcoidosis and chronic hepatic disease: A clinical and pathologic study of twenty patients. Medicine (Baltimore) 49:375, 1970
8. Margolis S, Homcy C: Systemic manifestations of hepatoma. Medicine (Baltimore) 5:381, 1972
9. Mays ET, Christopherson W: Hepatic tumors induced by sex steroids. Semin Liver Dis 4:147, 1984
10. Mitchell MC, Boitnott JK, et al: Budd-Chiari syndrome: Etiology, diagnosis and management. Medicine (Baltimore) 61:199, 1982
11. Patterson M, Healy GR, Shabot JM: Serologic testing for amoebiasis. Gastroenterology 78:136, 1980
12. Shafritz DA, Shouval D, et al: Integration of hepatitis B virus DNA into the genome of liver cells in chronic liver disease and hepatocellular carcinoma. N Engl J Med 305:1067, 1981
13. Simon HB, Wolff SM: Granulomatous hepatitis and prolonged fever of unknown origin: A study of 13 patients. Medicine (Baltimore) 52:1, 1973
14. Webb LJ, Sherlock S: The aetiology, presentation and natural history of extrahepatic portal venous obstruction. Q J Med 48:627, 1979
15. Witzlebin CL: Cystic diseases of the liver. In Zakim D, Boyer TD (eds): Hepatology, 1st ed. Philadelphia, WB Saunders, 1982, p 1193

Chronic Liver Disease: Alcoholic Liver Disease, Chronic Hepatitis, and Cirrhosis

Esteban Mezey

Diffuse hepatic diseases characterized by (1) evidence of present or past hepatic cell necrosis, (2) fibrosis involving all parts of the liver, and (3) the presence of regenerating nodules are grouped under the term "cirrhosis." By definition, nonuniform liver diseases such as hepatic abscesses are excluded.

Leading known causes of cirrhosis include alcohol, viral hepatitis (B and non-A, non-B), toxic or idiosyncratic drug-induced injury, biliary obstruction, long-term hepatic congestion, schistosomiasis, hemochromatosis, porphyria cutanea tarda, hepatolenticular degeneration (Wilson disease), and α_1-antitrypsin deficiency (Table 13.6–1). It is notable that hepatitis A does not cause chronic active hepatitis or cirrhosis. In many patients with cirrhosis there is no clearly demonstrable cause of their disease. The morphologic classification of cirrhosis into small nodular (micronodular, portal) or large nodular (macronodular, postnecrotic) varieties is of limited usefulness.

The clinical manifestations of cirrhosis are variable and may reflect the loss of hepatic cells with jaundice, wasting, hypoalbuminemia, and a bleeding tendency, or they may be due to scarring and architectural distortion of the liver, resulting in portal hypertension, often with ascites and hepatic encephalopathy. Occasionally cirrhosis is completely asymptomatic and discovered only at autopsy.

The major problems facing the clinician in the management of a patient with cirrhosis are to (1) establish an exact etiologic diagnosis and remove, insofar as possible, the inciting agent, (2) assess the nature and extent of complications, and (3) estimate prognosis. The most common causes of cirrhosis and the methods used to establish the etiology are listed in Table 13.6–2. In this chapter the major types of cirrhoses (alcoholic, postnecrotic, biliary, cardiac, schistosomiasis, hemochromatosis, porphyria cutanea tarda, hepatolenticular degeneration [Wilson disease] and α_1-anti-

trypsin deficiency) are presented, along with a discussion of chronic hepatitis and hepatocellular carcinoma.

ALCOHOLIC LIVER DISEASE

Excessive alcohol ingestion in man is related to the development of (1) fatty liver, (2) alcoholic hepatitis, and (3) alcoholic (Laennec) cirrhosis.[13] Cirrhosis related to alcoholism is the most common form of chronic liver disease found in the United States, and its incidence has roughly paralleled the per capita consumption of alcohol.[12] During the Prohibition era, deaths from cirrhosis decreased and after the repeal of the law began to rise again. The majority (80 to 90 percent) of patients with alcoholic cirrhosis give a history of years of heavy alcohol use.

Although the amount of alcohol ingested is established as the most important factor in the development of alcoholic cirrhosis, several observations suggest that undefined constitutional or genetic factors are also of importance. Individual susceptibility to the development of cirrhosis shows considerable variability. In epidemiologic studies, only a small percentage (approximately 8 percent) of chronic alcoholics develop cirrhosis.

MECHANISM OF ALCOHOL-INDUCED LIVER DISEASES

The relative contributions of alcohol as a hepatotoxin and the protein-vitamin–deficient diet so characteristic of the chronic alcoholic to the development of cirrhosis are areas of continuing study. Malnutrition of proteins or vitamins alone often results in fatty liver but has not been demonstrated to lead to cirrhosis in man.[13] Cirrhosis does not develop in the most severe form of protein malnutrition, kwashiorkor. Alcohol has direct hepatotoxicity apart from any dietary deficiencies. Short-term administration of alcohol to volunteers induced both fatty changes and ultrastructural abnormalities such as distorted mitochondria and vesiculated rough endoplasmic reticulum.[20] Direct toxic effects of alcohol on liver cells are the most likely mechanisms of injury, but associated malnutrition may contribute to the liver damage. The presence of protein-calorie malnutrition correlates with the severity of the alcoholic liver disease.[15] The inflammatory lesion of alcoholic hepatitis is apparently the most important precursor of alcoholic cirrhosis.

CLINICAL FEATURES

Fatty liver is the most frequent hepatic abnormality noted in alcoholics.[11] A combination of increased influx of fatty acids from adipose stores, enhanced hepatic synthesis of triglycerides from fatty acids derived from the diet, and decreased fatty acid oxidation are all of apparent importance in pathogenesis.

Fatty liver in the patient with alcoholism may be clinically silent or may mimic more severe hepatic disease. Hepatomegaly, often associated with hepatic tenderness, is frequent. Jaundice is unusual, but an occasional patient may have cholestatic jaundice and hepatic tenderness that closely resembles extrahepatic biliary obstruction. Liver biopsy is required to make the diagnosis of fatty liver. Fatty liver without concomitant alcoholic hepatitis has an

---

TABLE 13.6–1. CAUSES OF CIRRHOSIS

Acquired
- Alcohol
- Hepatitis viruses (B and non-A, non-B)
- Hepatotoxins (e.g., vinyl chloride)
- Drug reactions (e.g., methyldopa; nitrofurantoin)
- Biliary cirrhosis
  Primary biliary cirrhosis
  Secondary biliary cirrhosis
    Sclerosing cholangitis
    Bile duct stricture
    Bile duct tumors
- Cardiac cirrhosis
- Infiltrative diseases (sarcoidosis—rare)
- Infectious diseases
    (?) Schistosomiasis
    Brucellosis—rare

Genetically Determined
- Hepatolenticular degeneration (Wilson disease)
- Hemochromatosis
- Porphyria cutanea tarda
- α_1-Antitrypsin deficiency
- Galactosemia
- Cystic fibrosis

TABLE 13.6–2. AN APPROACH TO ESTABLISH THE CAUSE OF CIRRHOSIS

Presumed Cause	History	Histology	Additional Diagnostic Tests
Alcohol	Long-term (years) heavy ingestion	Fatty infiltration; Mallory bodies; portal (usual) or postnecrotic pattern	None
Hepatitis B and non-A, non-B	Exposure to jaundiced persons or drug addicts; history of blood transfusion; intravenous drug abuse	Postnecrotic pattern with areas of collapse; often active hepatocellular necrosis	Presence of HBsAg
Hepatotoxic or drug idiosyncratic reactions	Exposure	Postnecrotic cirrhosis; biliary cirrhosis	None
Cardiac congestion	Recurrent congestive failure; tricuspid and mitral valve disease	Congestion and fibrosis, predominately around the terminal hepatic venule	Demonstration of elevated venous pressure
Biliary obstruction			
Primary biliary cirrhosis	Middle-aged women; pruritus	Chronic nonsuppurative destructive cholangitis; granulomas (40%)	Presence of antimitochondrial antibodies (>85%); increased serum IgM
Secondary	History of biliary tract surgery	Biliary cirrhosis	Visualization of extrahepatic duct system by endoscopic retrograde bile duct cannulation or transhepatic cholangiography
Metabolic disorders			
Hepatolenticular degeneration	Positive family history; neurologic abnormalities	Postnecrotic cirrhosis; increased hepatic copper	Serum ceruloplasmin; hepatic copper
Hemochromatosis	Positive family history; diabetes; hyperpigmentation	Portal (usual) or postnecrotic cirrhosis; increased hepatic iron	Serum iron and iron-binding capacity; serum ferritin
Porphyria cutanea tarda	Cutaneous hypersensitivity to light, blisters, hyperpigmentation, scarring	Fibrosis Cirrhosis	Elevated urinary uroporphyrins and coproporphyrins
Granulomatous disorders (rare causes of cirrhosis)			
Schistosomiasis	Endemic areas	Pipestem fibrosis; granulomas	Demonstration of ova in liver or rectal biopsy
Sarcoidosis	Pulmonary disease; skin rash; lymphadenopathy	Diffuse granulomas and inflammation	Kveim test of occasional use

excellent prognosis, with the fat usually diminishing over a 4- to 6-week period of adequate diet and abstinence from alcohol.[11] Although fatty liver is often found in the patients with alcohol-induced cirrhosis, progression of the fatty lesion alone to cirrhosis has not been demonstrated.

Alcoholic liver disease with cell necrosis (alcoholic hepatitis) may occur as an acute illness during a prolonged bout of heavy alcohol intake or may be discovered when a liver biopsy is performed in an otherwise asymptomatic alcoholic patient with biochemical test abnormalities. Abdominal pain, an enlarged tender liver, nausea, vomiting, and jaundice are common presentations of alcoholic hepatitis. Fever is present with active hepatic necrosis in the absence of infection. Other manifestations of alcoholism, such as pancreatitis, gastritis, peripheral neuritis, Wernicke encephalopathy, malnutrition, or intercurrent infection, often first lead the patient to seek medical attention.

Laboratory abnormalities may include hyperbilirubinemia, elevated serum AST (100 to 300 mIU), and a decrease in serum albumin. The degree of aminotransferase elevation does not reflect the extent of hepatocellular injury. The ALT level is usually much lower than the AST level in patients with alcoholic hepatitis. Leukocytosis may be pronounced. Hypokalemia is frequent in these patients and may represent gastrointestinal losses, decreased oral intake, or increased urinary excretion. The serum IgA level is often elevated. Liver biopsy reveals fatty infiltration and cell necrosis. Perinuclear eosinophilic inclusions designated alcoholic hyaline or Mallory bodies are typical. Occasionally, patients with acute alcoholic disease have fever, pruritus, and a predominant elevation in the serum conjugated bilirubin level, suggesting extrahepatic obstruction of the biliary system. Bouts of alcoholic hepatitis in patients with established cirrhosis are designated florid cirrhosis or active Laennec cirrhosis.

Alcoholic cirrhosis is most often a disease of middle-aged persons with a history of alcohol use for 5 to 15 years. Although malnutrition and a past history of pancreatitis, gastritis, gross neglect, and previous bouts of acute alcoholic hepatitis are common, advanced alcoholic cirrhosis may develop in asymptomatic, well-nourished patients. In many patients, cirrhosis has an insidious onset and is recognized only after the development of weight loss, ascites, confusion, or the occurrence of an upper gastrointestinal tract hemorrhage.

Physical examination reveals the signs of chronic hepatocellular failure, such as palmar erythema, spider angiomas, jaundice, Dupuytren contractures, peripheral neuritis, and enlargement of the parotid and lacrimal glands. Clinical evidence of hypogonadism and overt feminization, with gynecomastia and development of a female escutcheon and body habitus, is frequently found in men with cirrhosis. The pathogenesis of the changes is complex.[29] Male cirrhotics have a decreased production of testosterone and a slight increase in circulating estrogen levels, but these changes do not correlate well with the clinical manifestations. There is evidence to suggest a hypothalamic defect, with abnormal hypothalamic-pituitary secretion of gonadotropins.

The liver is generally enlarged and firm early in the course of

alcohol-induced cirrhosis but later may be of normal size or even small. Nodularity of the liver edge or surface may be detected on palpation. Abnormalities in biochemical test results are variable and depend on the activity of the disease. Anemia, leukopenia, and thrombocytopenia are often present. Liver biopsy is important in establishing the diagnosis and in staging the disease. The histologic pattern may be that of fatty infiltration, present or past cell necrosis, diffuse fine scarring linking portal triads and central veins, inflammatory infiltrates, or any combination of these. Occasionally the liver in patients with long-standing alcoholic cirrhosis has a macronodular pattern with large, irregular nodules. Histologically significant cirrhosis may be discovered only incidentally ("compensated cirrhosis") when abnormal liver test results are observed and liver biopsy is performed in the course of evaluating other complaints. A number of instances of alcoholic cirrhosis are discovered for the first time at autopsy. Sometimes a patient with apparent alcohol-induced liver disease has hepatic histopathologic features compatible with chronic active hepatitis. Whether the two disorders coexist or whether alcohol can induce chronic active hepatitis, which persists after the removal of alcohol, has not been established.

PROGNOSIS AND SURVIVAL IN ALCOHOLIC CIRRHOSIS

The course and prognosis in alcholic and other forms of cirrhosis are dependent on the ability of the liver to heal and regenerate. The most important determinant of healing and survival in patients with Laennec cirrhosis is abstinence from alcohol. In a study of 278 patients with biopsy-proved Laennec cirrhosis, Powell and Klatskin[17] observed a 63 percent overall 5-year survival rate in the 93 patients who stopped drinking, as opposed to a 40.5 percent 5-year survival rate in the 185 patients who continued to drink.

An apparent overall improved survival rate among patients with cirrhosis in the past 30 years may relate to emphasis on abstinence from alcohol, nutritious diet, improved understanding of the management of fluid and electrolyte disturbances, antibiotics for control of intercurrent infections, and more successful treatment of ascites and hepatic encephalopathy. Associated vitamin deficiencies are more common in these patients. Liver biopsy often reveals evidence of coexisting acute and chronic disease. Patients with jaundice and liver abnormalities in a setting of acute alcoholism often benefit from evaluation in the hospital. Other complications of alcoholism, such as decreased resistance to infection, electrolyte abnormalities, gastritis, and delirium tremens, further complicate management. Corticosteroid therapy for patients with alcoholic hepatitis has shown varying degrees of success. Therapy aimed at improving nutrition such as the parenteral administration of amino acids may improve the chance of survival in severely ill patients.

POSTNECROTIC CIRRHOSIS AND CHRONIC AUTOIMMUNE HEPATITIS

POSTNECROTIC CIRRHOSIS

Grouped under the heading of postnecrotic cirrhosis are a number of liver diseases of both known and unknown cause that are characterized pathologically by large areas of collapse, suggesting previous significant but nonuniform liver cell damage, broad scars, and regenerating nodules of up to several centimeters in diameter. Injury to the liver by such diverse processes as hepatitis viruses, as in chronic active hepatitis, hepatotoxins (e.g., methyldopa and nitrofurantoin), and hepatolenticular degeneration is implicated in the etiology of postnecrotic cirrhosis. In many patients, no cause can be established. The pathologic pattern of postnecrotic cirrhosis may be predominant in many patients with long-standing alcoholic liver disease.

Postnecrotic cirrhosis may be a clinically silent disorder or may be manifested by hepatocellular insufficiency and the complications of portal hypertension. Patients with active cellular disease are indistinguishable from those with the later stages of chronic active hepatitis, with predominant manifestations of jaundice, ascites, and hepatic encephalopathy. In a patient with a small, shrunken liver and no history or physical evidence of hepatocellular disease, the cirrhosis may first be diagnosed after an episode of hemorrhage from esophagogastric varices. These patients may also have unexplained bouts of abdominal pain or ascites. Hepatocellular carcinoma develops in 15 to 20 percent of patients with postnecrotic cirrhosis and should be considered whenever there is clinical deterioration in a previously stable patient.

The onset is usually insidious, with the appearance of jaundice and fatigue as major symptoms. In other cases, the onset can be acute, resembling acute viral hepatitis; however, the patient never recovers and remains jaundiced and symptomatic.[24] Amenorrhea is a common feature.

CHRONIC AUTOIMMUNE HEPATITIS

One type of chronic active hepatitis has no established cause and encompasses all cases not associated with viral infection, drug-induced liver injury, or metabolic or inherited disorders.

Several clinical and laboratory features suggest that many of these idiopathic cases are the result of altered immune reactivity. No viral agent has been identified, and the HBsAg is uniformly absent. The majority of this group (75 percent) are women, with many having the onset of disease during adolescence. Hyperglobulinemia is usually found, the lupus erythematosus (LE) cell preparation is occasionally positive (15 percent), and smooth muscle and antinuclear antibodies are frequent. Antimitochondrial antibodies occur in some of these patients (5 to 10 percent). Extrahepatic manifestations of disease, including amenorrhea, Hashimoto thyroiditis, pleurisy, pulmonary hypertension, polyarthritis, Coombs-positive hemolytic anemia, Sjögren syndrome, chronic diarrhea, or ulcerative colitis, may also be present and further suggest a role for altered immunity. There is an apparent increased incidence of idiopathic chronic active hepatitis in patients with histocompatibility antigens HLA-A1 or HLA-B8. On physical examination these patients usually have hepatomegaly; they often have splenomegaly and ascites. Jaundice, acne, diffuse rashes, and a bleeding tendency with purpura may be apparent.

The pathologic features of chronic autoimmune hepatitis are variable. All patients show evidence of ongoing cell necrosis; portal and periportal inflammation with mononuclear and plasma cells; diffuse fibrosis; and often widespread focal hepatitis. In many patients, bridging areas of necrosis connecting portal and central areas of the lobule are the dominant features. Whole lobules may be collapsed (multilobular necrosis). Postnecrotic cirrhosis may be present at the time of diagnosis in many patients and develops subsequently in the majority.

The course is variable and in untreated patients may be one of continuous deterioration with early death or intermittent bouts of acute hepatitis interspersed with temporary apparent remissions. Treatment with corticosteroids has been clearly established as effective therapy only in patients with autoimmune idiopathic chronic active hepatitis. In these patients, treatment with corticosteroids should be promptly instituted once the diagnosis has been established. Prednisone or prednisolone, 40 to 60 mg, is given initially to suppress the activity of the disease and then tapered slowly, usually over a period of 1 to 3 months to a maintenance dose of 15 to 20 mg.[26] Symptomatic improvement followed by a fall in serum aminotransferase levels and a rise in the serum albumin level occurs in the first 4 weeks. Histologic transformation to a lesion of persistent hepatitis will occur in some patients within a 2-year period. Repeated liver biopsies are helpful in determining the effectiveness of therapy. Immunosuppressant drugs (e.g., azathioprine) have not been demonstrated to be effective in therapy alone, as are corticosteroids, but may be useful adjunctive agents, particularly in

patients who develop severe side effects from corticosteroids. Treatment with corticosteroids is discontinued in patients who attain remission. Approximately 50 percent of the patients who enter remission have a relapse within 6 months of cessation of therapy, which requires restarting corticosteroid therapy. Continuous treatment beyond 4 years is not recommended because the prospect of remission diminishes while the risk of side effects increases.[5]

Patients with postnecrotic cirrhosis and no evidence of ongoing necrosis may have bleeding from esophagogastric varices. In these patients the prognosis is dependent on the success in managing hematemesis and its sequelae. These patients often are suitable candidates for a portal systemic shunt operation.

BILIARY CIRRHOSIS

Prolonged stasis of bile is often associated with portal and periportal inflammation, which, over a period of months to years, leads to fibrosis. Biliary cirrhosis results from linkage of periportal areas of fibrosis. The site of biliary obstruction may lie in the major extrahepatic ducts (secondary biliary cirrhosis) or in the small intrahepatic biliary radicles, as in primary biliary cirrhosis. The characteristic clinical features of biliary cirrhosis develop slowly and are direct consequences of the interruption of bile flow.

PRIMARY BILIARY CIRRHOSIS

Primary biliary cirrhosis (PBC) is a disease predominantly of women (90%), often in the age range of 30 to 55 years, who have pruritus, dark urine, and hepatomegaly.[9,21] Occasionally more than one member of a family is affected. Pruritus may precede other symptoms by many months and occasionally years. Most patients feel well during the early years of the disorder, complaining only of pruritus. The disorder occasionally has its onset during pregnancy. From its insidious beginnings, the disease slowly progresses to a characteristic picture of xanthomas, bone pain, hyperpigmentation, and cirrhosis. Most patients die within 5 to 10 years from the onset of jaundice. Signs of hepatocellular insufficiency such as spider angiomas, palmar erythema, ascites, and bleeding from esophagogastric varices are late occurrences. Many asymptomatic middle-aged women with only an elevated alkaline phosphatase level are initially found to have a positive antimitochondrial antibody and histologic findings comparable with those of PBC. Many of these patients have an asymptomatic illness that does not progress even when followed up for many years. When the serum bilirubin level begins to rise and exceeds 2 mg/dl, the disease is entering a progressive phase, and when the serum bilirubin level exceeds 10 mg/dl, the prognosis is very unfavorable.[9]

The cause of primary biliary cirrhosis is not known. No virus has been isolated, and an increased incidence of hepatitis B antigen has not been found. Occasionally patients have had the onset of clinically typical primary biliary cirrhosis while taking phenothiazines, with continuing activity of the liver disease after the drugs are stopped. An association with the CRST syndrome (calcinosis, Raynaud phenomenon, sclerodactyly, and telangiectasia) and with Sjögren syndrome and renal tubular acidosis suggests links with other disorders of presumed disturbed immunity.[19] Certain laboratory findings strongly suggest altered immune responses in primary biliary cirrhosis.[28] The serum immunoglobulin M (IgM) level is elevated in 80 to 90 percent of patients, and plasma cells in the portal and periportal region have been demonstrated to contain IgM. Immunofluorescence studies have demonstrated a circulating antibody directed against mitochondria (antimitochondrial antibody) in more than 85 percent of patients with primary biliary cirrhosis.[10] These antibodies are rarely positive in patients with extrahepatic bile duct obstruction but are found in 10 to 15 percent of patients with chronic active hepatitis and postnecrotic cirrhosis. The interrelationship of these disorders remains unclear.

Laboratory features of symptomatic primary biliary cirrhosis include hyperbilirubinemia, with the serum bilirubin level usually from 4 to 10 mg/dl. The alkaline phosphatase level is markedly elevated, and hypercholesterolemia of an extreme degree (greater than 2000 mg/dl) may be present. The serum aminotransferase enzyme levels are usually only slightly (100 to 200 mIU) increased. Liver biopsy in primary biliary cirrhosis characteristically shows portal inflammation and nonsuppurative destruction of bile ducts in the portal triads. The plasma cells in the portal areas are predominantly producing IgM. Ductular proliferation may be a dominant feature, and granulomas are often found in and around the damaged ducts. Patients with granulomas in the liver biopsy apparently have a better prognosis than those without this finding. Bile stasis and periportal fibrosis may be prominent. Actual cirrhosis is a late finding.

The major complications of primary biliary cirrhosis are bone pain, fractures due to vitamin D deficiency and osteoporosis, and occasionally bleeding disorders associated with decreased absorption of vitamin K. Xanthomatous involvement of peripheral nerves may cause neuritis. The management of the disorder is supportive. Cholestyramine may be useful in controlling pruritus. Vitamin A deficiency is frequent in PBC, and abnormalities in dark adaptation common. Vitamin D or its derivative 25-hydroxycholecalciferol may be helpful in the management of bone pain. Corticosteroid therapy is not useful in primary biliary cirrhosis and may accelerate the bone disease. Treatment with D-penicillamine, azathioprine, and cyclosporine has also been found to be ineffective. Trials with colchicine have shown no effect on liver histologic features but variable results in regard to survival. Further studies and better therapeutic agents are needed. Patients with marked worsening of their hepatic function (rising bilirubin: >10 mg/dl in the absence of complicating hemolysis) should be considered for hepatic transplantation.[2]

SECONDARY BILIARY CIRRHOSIS

Secondary biliary cirrhosis may result from choledocholithiasis, bile duct strictures developing after biliary tract surgery, or slow-growing carcinoma of the bile ducts. It is important to rule out a secondary, possibly correctable, cause of bile duct obstruction in any patient with biliary cirrhosis. In most instances, endoscopic retrograde cholangiography or percutaneous transhepatic cholangiography is required for diagnosis. In secondary biliary cirrhosis, the antimitochondrial antibody test is negative.

SCLEROSING CHOLANGITIS

Sclerosing cholangitis is a rare cause of chronic obstructive jaundice characterized pathologically by diffuse thickening and obliteration of the major bile ducts. Sclerosing cholangitis may result from recurrent cholangitis associated with recurrent choledocholithiasis or may follow bile duct injury during surgery. Sclerosing cholangitis with no previous history of choledocholithiasis or surgery (primary sclerosing cholangitis) is a disorder of unknown cause; it may be associated with ulcerative colitis, Crohn disease, or retroperitoneal fibrosis. The diagnosis of sclerosing cholangitis is established by demonstration of irregular, diffusely narrowed bile ducts by endoscopic retrograde cholangiography or transhepatic cholangiography. It is generally difficult, or impossible, to distinguish sclerosing cholangitis from slow-growing carcinomas of the bile ducts. There is no satisfactory medical therapy for sclerosing cholangitis.

Vitamins D, A, and K and cholestyramine may be useful in managing complications. Corticosteroid therapy and long-term antibiotics are of doubtful value. In some patients the placement of stents in the damaged bile ducts is an effective means of reinstituting bile flow.

CARDIAC CIRRHOSIS

Congestive heart failure is frequently associated with liver dysfunction but rarely causes cirrhosis.[6] The pathogenesis of the liver dysfunction involves both decreased perfusion due to forward failure and increased pressure on the outflow of blood from the liver in cases of right-sided heart failure. The liver is enlarged and tender, pressure over the liver distends the veins in the neck (hepatojugular reflux), and ascites may be present. Jaundice is rare, but a rise in the serum bilirubin level is common. Other laboratory abnormalities are a mild rise in serum aminotransferase levels and occasionally the alkaline phosphatase level. Serum albumin is usually reduced. Liver biopsy reveals dilation of the central veins, and of the sinusoids draining into them, and degenerative changes, sometimes with frank necrosis of the hepatocytes in the central areas. Cardiac cirrhosis develops only after prolonged and severe cardiac failure, usually due to valvular disease, particularly tricuspid incompetence, or in patients with constrictive pericarditis. Jaundice, hepatomegaly, and ascites are prominent features, but the diagnosis can be established with certainty only by liver biopsy. The therapy is directed toward the management of heart failure.

HEPATIC SCHISTOSOMIASIS

Hepatic schistosomiasis may occur in persons from tropical areas who have been infected by schistosome cercariae while swimming or walking in infested waters. The liver disease is due to the deposition of ova of *Schistosoma mansoni* in the portal areas with the development of an inflammatory reaction, often with granuloma formation, and periportal fibrosis.[18] The parenchymal cells outside the immediate portal area remain normal, and there are no regenerating nodules. The principal manifestation of hepatic schistosomiasis is portal hypertension complicated by bleeding esophageal varices. The most common laboratory abnormality is an increase in the serum alkaline phosphatase level. There may be mild elevations of the serum bilirubin and aminotransferases, but jaundice is uncommon. The diagnosis of active infection is made by demonstrating mobile schistosome ova on fresh examination of a rectal biopsy, and the diagnosis of liver involvement is made by showing the presence of oval capsules on liver biopsy. The present drug therapy of choice is with praziquantel if the infection is still active. This drug, which is given in three doses 1 week apart, has mild gastrointestinal side effects but no serious toxicity. The course of therapy can be repeated after 2 to 3 months, if necessary.

HEMOCHROMATOSIS

Hemochromatosis is a rare disorder of iron metabolism characterized by the gradual accumulation of excessive tissue iron stores associated with parenchymal damage and fibrosis. The principal organs involved are the liver, pancreas, heart, and gonads. Total body iron stores are increased from the normal 4 g to as much as 60 g. The pathogenesis of hemochromatosis is apparently an increase in iron absorption from the gut, with both genetic and environmental factors of importance. Hereditary hemochromatosis is inherited as an autosomal recessive trait, with partial biochemical expression in heterozygotes. It is often associated with HLA types A_3 and B14.[25] Environmental factors associated with an increased iron uptake include ingestion of alcoholic beverages (especially wine), cooking in iron pots, and long-term administration of medicinal iron in refractory anemias.[14]

The majority of patients with hemochromatosis are male (80 percent), and in most the disease becomes manifest between the ages of 40 and 60 years. The disease develops earlier in men, probably because of menstrual loss of iron in women. The disorder is rare under the age of 20 years. Constitutional symptoms of lassitude and weakness are frequent. The major involved organ is the liver, which usually is large, firm, and frequently tender. Cirrhosis is usually present when the diagnosis is first established in a family. The spleen is usually enlarged. Esophagogastric varices and other signs of portal hypertension are less common than in alcoholic or postnecrotic cirrhosis. Ascites and hepatocellular failure are late manifestations. Diabetes mellitus occurs in the majority of patients, and insulin therapy is required. Abnormalities in carbohydrate metabolism occur in 80 percent of patients. The major diabetic complications of retinopathy, nephropathy, and neuropathy may occur. The diabetes results from the deposition of iron in the pancreatic islet cells. The carbohydrate abnormalities associated with the development of cirrhosis and portal hypertension may also be contributing factors. Cardiac involvement may be manifested by congestive heart failure or by arrhythmias from involvement of both the myocardium and the cardiac conduction system (particularly the atrioventricular node). Heart block may occur. The congestive failure in hemochromatosis may be relatively resistant to digitalis therapy. Increased skin pigmentation with a slate-gray color is the result of melanin deposition in the basal layers of the thinned epidermis and is best seen over exposed areas, in the axillae and groin, and in scars. In some patients, iron deposited in the corium adds to the pigmentation. Impotence is frequent and associated with testicular atrophy and fibrosis. Less common manifestations include arthritis from synovial deposition of iron and evidence of anterior pituitary insufficiency, which may also contribute to the impotence. Chondrocalcinosis (pseudogout) is found in 25 to 50 percent of patients and may be manifested as an acute arthritis in weight-bearing joints or in the wrist or metacarpophalangeal joints. Hepatocellular carcinoma develops in 25 to 40 percent of patients with hemochromatosis.

The diagnosis of hemochromatosis is established by finding an elevation of the serum iron level (greater than 220 μg/dl), saturation of the serum transferrin (greater than 75 percent), an elevated serum ferritin level, and demonstration of increased tissue iron stores on liver biopsy.[16] The combination of high transferrin saturation and an elevated serum ferritin level is 94 percent sensitive and 86 percent specific in the diagnosis of hemochromatosis.[1] In most patients there is a good correlation between the extent of iron stores and the serum ferritin level, although there have been reports of a few patients with hemochromatosis and normal serum ferritin levels. Biochemical tests of the liver often show nearly normal results even when considerable tissue damage is present. Diagnostic tests with iron chelating agents such as desferrioxamine are useful in demonstrating increased body stores of iron but are seldom required for diagnosis.

The goal of therapy in hemochromatosis, removal of the excess tissue iron, is accomplished by repeated phlebotomy. Removal of 500 ml of blood rids the body of approximately 250 mg of iron and mobilizes iron from the tissue stores. Because the amount of iron stored in tissue may be 20 to 60 g, phlebotomy of 500 ml per week may be required for up to 2 years. The effectiveness of the therapy is ascertained by determining the serum iron transferrin saturation, and serum ferritin levels, and by results of follow-up liver biopsy. Decrease in iron stores during therapy can be monitored by CT scans or nuclear magnetic resonance. Therapy, when effective, will decrease hepatomegaly and hyperpigmentation and at least stabilize the diabetes and cardiac involvement.[3] There will be little improvement of testicular function, portal hypertension, arthropathy, or the tendency to develop hepatocellular carcinoma. Rarely will the liver damage diminish.

For patients with hemochromatosis due to chronic refractory anemic states, phlebotomy is not possible, and therapy with chelating agents (deferoxamine) is instituted. Up to 200 mg of iron can be mobilized per day in patients receiving subcutaneous deferoxamine infusions over 8- to 12-hour periods.[8] Relatives of patients with hemochromatosis should be evaluated regularly with determination of serum iron levels, transferrin saturation, and serum ferritin levels. Therapy to remove iron should be instituted in asymptomatic relatives of patients with hemochromatosis when an

elevation in iron stores is found. Identification of homozygotes at risk requires HLA typing of the family members once the haplotype of the proband has been determined.[25] This determination is done when the diagnosis is in doubt or to identify young individuals before the development of heavy iron overload.

Difficulty may arise in differentiating hemochromatosis from alcoholic cirrhosis, because iron deposition is common in this disease and patients with hemochromatosis often give a history of heavy alcohol intake. The difference may be apparent in liver biopsy: in hemochromatosis, iron deposition precedes fibrosis and is often excessive in the presence of a low degree of fibrosis, and the iron is found mainly in the hepatocytes. In the alcoholic patient, marked iron deposition is seen only in advanced cirrhosis and, when present, is found chiefly in the Kupffer cells. Determination of liver iron concentration clearly separates alcoholic cirrhosis from cirrhosis due to hemochromatosis. In a recent study, all patients with hemochromatosis, but none of the alcoholic patients, had liver iron concentrations greater than 1000 μg/100 mg.[4] There is evidence that chronic use of alcoholic beverages increases iron absorption. Emphasis on the abstinence from alcohol is important in treatment. After abstinence is followed, and if the patient is not anemic, phlebotomy therapy may be required.

PORPHYRIA CUTANEA TARDA

Porphyria cutanea tarda is probably the most common form of porphyria. It is characterized by cutaneous hypersensitivity to light, resulting in the formation of blisters, hyperpigmentation, scarring, and sclerodermoid changes in association with chronic liver disease.[7] The disease is often manifested after chronic alcohol consumption or after the intake of estrogen in women. Common laboratory abnormalities are mild elevation of the serum aminotransferase levels and an elevated serum iron. Liver biopsy reveals portal inflammation with fibrosis or cirrhosis. Stainable iron is increased, and a red fluorescence can be detected under ultraviolet light because of the high hepatic content of uroporphyrin. The disease is inherited as an autosomal dominant trait, and the metabolic abnormality is a deficiency of uroporphyrinogen decarboxylase, which converts uroporphyrinogen to coproporphyrinogen. The diagnosis is made by demonstrating increased urinary excretion of uroporphyrin and coproporphyrin, but normal urinary excretion of δ-aminolevulinic acid and porphobilinogen. Treatment with weekly phlebotomy is usually effective in producing clinical and biochemical remission of the disease in 6 to 12 months. Cloroquine, which causes hepatic depletion of hepatic uroporphyrins, should be reserved for patients with severe illness because of its potential serious hepatotoxic effects.

HEPATOLENTICULAR DEGENERATION (WILSON DISEASE)

Hepatolenticular degeneration (Wilson disease) is a rare inherited disorder of metabolism characterized by accumulation of copper in the liver, central nervous system, cornea, kidneys, and other tissues.[30] The disorder is inherited as an autosomal recessive trait and becomes apparent most frequently during adolescence. Liver and neurologic disease, separately or in combination, are usually present. Wilson disease may be manifested by slight biochemical abnormalities or by a chronic active hepatitis in an adolescent or young adult with no evidence of neurologic disease.[22] Some patients have fulminant hepatic failure when first seen. The most frequent neurologic symptoms are those resulting from basal ganglia damage, with rigidity, choreoathetoid movements, and ataxia. Less common presentations include hemolytic anemia or renal disease with aminoaciduria, uricosuria, and phosphaturia (acquired Fanconi syndrome). The persistent phosphaturia may cause osteomalacia. Of particular diagnostic importance is the presence of Kayser-Fleischer rings, which are brownish rings of pigment at the periphery of the cornea due to copper deposition in Descemet membrane.

The pathogenesis of Wilson disease is most likely an inability to excrete copper into the bile, possibly through abnormalities in hepatic lysosome function. The major biochemical manifestations of Wilson disease are a deficiency in ceruloplasmin (the plasma copper-binding protein), an increase in hepatic copper, and an increase in urinary copper excretion. The total serum copper level is generally reduced, but the free (unbound) copper level is markedly increased.

The diagnosis of Wilson disease is established by the demonstration of a reduction in plasma ceruloplasmin, an increase in urinary copper, and an increase in hepatic copper (greater than 250 μg/g dry weight). Lifetime therapy with D-penicillamine to chelate the excess copper may be required in patients with Wilson disease and in presymptomatic relatives with evidence of excessive copper stores. There is no indication for corticosteroid therapy in Wilson disease. Patients with fulminant hepatitis or those with decompensated cirrhosis, who are not responding to therapy, should be considered for liver transplantation.[27]

α_1-ANTITRYPSIN DEFICIENCY

α_1-Antitrypsin (AAT) is a glycoprotein that is synthesized by the liver and accounts for the majority of serum α_1-globulin. Inherited deficiencies of serum AAT lead to pulmonary emphysema and to a variety of liver disorders, including neonatal hepatitis, chronic active hepatitis, cryptogenic cirrhosis, and hepatocellular carcinoma.[23] AAT serves as a protease inhibitor (Pi), and there are multiple alleles in the Pi system controlling AAT production. The most frequent (normal) allele is designated M, and normal individuals have Pi MM. The inheritance is as an autosomal codominant trait. Most patients with liver disease have Pi ZZ, with only 15 to 20 percent of normal serum AAT. There are molecular abnormalities in the AAT produced by the variant alleles. The diagnosis of AAT deficiency is suggested by the absence of the serum α_1-globulin peak and is confirmed by demonstrating a low value of AAT in the serum and by Pi typing. Characteristic changes on liver biopsy are the presence of multiple round acidophilic PAS-positive, diastase-resistant bodies in the cytoplasm of hepatocytes. The bodies are accumulations of AAT within the rough endoplasmic reticulum. Presumably the inability to transfer the abnormal AAT from its site of synthesis in the liver to the serum is important in pathogenesis.

Cirrhosis develops in 10 to 15 percent of adults with Pi ZZ. The liver disease may be present as a cholestatic illness. Whether heterozygotes for Pi Z (e.g., Pi MZ) are at increased risk of developing chronic autoimmune hepatitis and cirrhosis is uncertain. Hepatocellular carcinomas have been reported in patients with Pi ZZ and cirrhosis. There is no accepted therapy for ATT-related liver diseases. Corticosteroid therapy is not indicated. Patients with advanced liver disease from AAT deficiency may be candidates for liver transplantation.

REFERENCES

1. Bassett ML, Halliday JW, et al: Diagnosis of hemochromatosis in young subjects: Predictive accuracy of biochemical screening tests. Gastroenterology 87:628, 1984
2. Beswick DR, Boyer JL: Primary biliary cirrhosis. Hepatology 4:295, 1984
3. Bomford A, Williams R: Long-term results of venesection therapy in idiopathic haemochromatosis. Q J Med 45:611, 1976
4. Chapman RW, Morgan MY, et al: Hepatic iron stores and markers of iron overload in alcoholics and patients with idiopathic hemochromatosis. Dig Dis Sci 27:909, 1982
5. Czaja AJ, Ludwig J, et al: Corticosteroid treated chronic active hepatitis

in remission: Uncertain prognosis of chronic active hepatitis. N Engl J Med 304:5, 1981

6. Dunn GD, Hayes P, Breen KS: The liver in congestive heart failure: A review. Am J Med Sci 265:174, 1973

7. Grossman ME, Bickers DR, et al: Porphyria cutanea tarda: Clinical and laboratory findings in 40 patients. Am J Med 67:277, 1979

8. Hoffbrand AV, Gorman A, et al: Improvement in iron studies and liver function in patients with transfusional iron overload with long-term subcutaneous desferrioxamine. Lancet 1:947, 1979

9. Kapelman B, Schaffner F: The natural history of primary biliary cirrhosis. Semin Liver Dis 1:273, 1981

10. Klatskin G, Kantor FS: Mitochondrial antibody in primary biliary cirrhosis and other diseases. Ann Intern Med 77:533, 1972

11. Leevy CM: Fatty liver: A study of 270 patients with biopsy proven fatty liver and a review of the literature. Medicine (Baltimore) 41:249, 1962

12. Lelbach W: Cirrhosis in the alcoholic and its relation to volume of alcohol abuse. Ann NY Acad Sci 252:85, 1975

13. Lieber CS: Metabolism and metabolic effects of ethanol. Semin Liver Dis 1:203, 1981

14. MacDonald RA: Primary hemochromatosis: Inherited or acquired? In Brown EB, Moore CV (eds): Progress in Hematology. New York, Grune & Stratton, 1966, vol 5, p 324

15. Mendenhall CL, Anderson S, et al: Protein-calorie malnutrition associated with alcoholic hepatitis: Veterans Administration Cooperative Study Group on alcoholic hepatitis. Am J Med 76:211, 1984

16. Powell LW, Halliday JW, Cowlishaw JL: Relationship between serum ferritin and total body iron stores in idiopathic haemochromatosis. Gut 19:538, 1978

17. Powell WJ Jr, Klatskin G: Duration of survival in patients with Laennec's cirrhosis. Am J Med 44:406, 1968

18. Prata A: Schistosomiasis mansoni. Clin Gastroenterol 7:49, 1978

19. Reynolds TB, Denison EK, et al: Primary biliary cirrhosis with scleroderma, Raynaud's phenomenon and telangiectasia. Am J Med 50:302, 1971

20. Rubin E, Lieber CS: Alcohol-induced hepatic injury in nonalcoholic volunteers. N Engl J Med 278:869, 1968

21. Schaffner F, Popper H: Clinical-pathologic relations in primary biliary cirrhosis. In Popper H, Schaffner F (eds): Progress in Liver Diseases. New York, Grune & Stratton, 1982, vol 7, p 529

22. Scott J, Gollan JL, et al: Wilson's disease, presenting as chronic active hepatitis. Gastroenterology 74:645, 1978

23. Sharp HL: Alpha-one-antitrypsin, an ignored protein in understanding liver disease. Semin Liver Dis 2:314, 1982

24. Sherlock S: Chronic hepatitis. Gut 15:581, 1974

25. Simon M, Bourel M, et al: Idiopathic hemochromatosis: Demonstration of recessive transmission and early detection by family HLA typing. N Engl J Med 297:1017, 1977

26. Soloway RD, Summerskill WHJ, et al: Clinical, biochemical, and histological remission of severe chronic active liver disease: A controlled study of treatments and early prognosis. Gastroenterology 63:820, 1972

27. Sternlieb I: Wilson's disease: Indications for liver transplants. Hepatology 4:155, 1984

28. Thomas HC: Potential pathogenic mechanisms in primary biliary cirrhosis. Semin Liver Dis 1:338, 1981

29. Van Thiel DH, Gavaler JS, et al: Is feminization in alcoholic men due in part to portal hypertension: A rat model. Gastroenterology 78:81, 1980

30. Williams DM, Lee GR: Hepatolenticular degeneration (Wilson's disease). In Powell LW (ed): Metals and the Liver. New York, Marcel Dekker, 1978, p 241

Principles of Clinical Endocrinology and Metabolism

Paul W. Ladenson and Simeon Margolis

Clinical endocrinology[3,8] is the subspecialty of internal medicine concerned with understanding, diagnosing, and treating disorders of the endocrine glands. Endocrinology also encompasses the study and treatment of disorders involving other organs that secrete hormones affecting distant tissues: the neuroendocrine systems of the hypothalamus (secreting vasopressin, oxytocin, pituitary hormone-releasing and inhibitory factors, and endogenous opioids); gastrointestinal peptides (e.g., gastrin, vasoactive intestinal peptide); renin and erythropoietin from the kidney; growth factors (e.g., somatomedins produced by the liver); and atriopeptins from the heart. In addition, endocrinologists are concerned with paracrine and autocrine interactions, which involve the production of factors affecting, respectively, adjacent cells (e.g., somatostatin effects on insulin-producing beta cells within pancreatic islets) or the elaborating cell type itself (e.g., lymphokines from T lymphocytes).

Metabolism[3,7] is a closely related discipline principally concerned with the investigation and clinical management of disorders relating to intermediary metabolism of carbohydrates (e.g., diabetes mellitus, hypoglycemia) and lipids (hyperlipidemias). Metabolism also deals with nutritional problems encountered in clinical practice (e.g., obesity, malnutrition). The disorders arising from abnormal metabolism of amino acids, uric acid, and nucleic acids are discussed in Chapters 5.3, 8.10, and 5.3, respectively.

MECHANISMS OF ENDOCRINE PATHOPHYSIOLOGY

Three basic pathophysiologic mechanisms lead to virtually all clinical disease states involving endocrine glands: (1) deficiency of hormone action on target tissues, (2) excessive hormone production and action, and (3) neoplasia. These underlying processes may be seen in combination, for example, functioning endocrine tumors that secrete excessive hormone (Table 14.1–1).

DEFICIENT HORMONE ACTION

Deficiency of hormone action is most commonly caused by an abnormally low level of biologically active hormone reaching target tissues. Inadequate hormone production may occur as a result of primary gland failure. Endocrine gland hypofunction may be congenital, caused by complete failure of gland development (e.g., hypoparathyroidism in the DiGeorge syndrome), a mutant gene encoding the structure of a hormone (e.g., diabetes mellitus resulting from genetic insulin variants), or an enzyme responsible for hormone biosynthesis (e.g., adrenal insufficiency arising from complete 21-hydroxylase deficiency).

Endocrine gland failure may also be acquired as a consequence of physiologic atrophy (e.g., menopausal ovarian failure), replacement by tumor, surgical extirpation, effects of pharmacologic or environmental agents, or inflammation (e.g., chronic lymphocytic thyroiditis). Infection (e.g., adrenal tuberculosis) and autoimmune disorders (e.g., idiopathic adrenal failure) are the most common inciting factors for inflammation. Inflammatory disorders of the thyroid gland may also present with local and constitutional symptoms such as neck pain, fever, and malaise. Some types of glandular injury may transiently increase hormone release (e.g., lymphocytic thyroiditis) before development of glandular hypofunction.

Primary failure may involve more than one endocrine gland (Table 14.1–2). Polyendocrine deficiency syndrome type I usually begins in childhood and is characterized by hypoparathyroidism, adrenal insufficiency, and mucocutaneous candidiasis. Less frequently, primary gonadal failure, autoimmune thyroid disorders (autoimmune thyroiditis or Graves disease), and insulin-dependent diabetes mellitus may also occur in these individuals. Polyendocrine deficiency syndrome type II typically presents in the third or fourth decades of life with adrenal insufficiency and autoimmune thyroid disease (Schmidt syndrome). These individuals may also have insulin-dependent diabetes mellitus, and primary or secondary gonadal failure. An autoimmune basis for these syndromes is strongly suggested by the presence of circulating antibodies against involved glands, abnormalities in suppressor T cell function, and linkage with certain histocompatibility alleles (e.g., HLA-B8) in these patients and their relatives.[2]

Other causes of decreased hormone action in target tissues are encountered less frequently. Deranged physiologic control of pituitary gland function causes secondary glandular failure, which can be either congenital (e.g., idiopathic hypogonadotropic hypogonadism) or acquired (e.g., adrenal insufficiency secondary to pituitary ablation). Impairment of hormone release may result in glandular hypofunction (e.g., hypoparathyroidism caused by hypomagnesemia). Defective postsecretory hormone activation (e.g., vitamin D-resistant rickets with decreased renal 1-hydroxylation of 25-hydroxyvitamin D) or accelerated hormone metabolism (e.g., osteomalacia induced by diphenylhydantoin) may result in abnormally low hormone activity.

Hormonal deficiency states, despite normal or even elevated concentrations of biologically active hormone in the circulation, may be due to target-tissue resistance. Resistance can be congenital (e.g., familial thyroid hormone resistance) or acquired (e.g., non-insulin-dependent diabetes mellitus). This failure of target tissue responsiveness may be due to an abnormality of hormone receptors[1] or in postbinding signaling of the hormone-receptor interaction (e.g., absence of the guanine nucleotide stimulatory subunit in pseudohypoparathyroidism). Receptor abnormalities may be attributed to a quantitative deficiency in the number of receptors (e.g., obese type II diabetics) or a qualitative defect in receptor function (e.g., some androgen resistance states).

EXCESSIVE HORMONE ACTION

Excessive hormone action in peripheral tissues can be caused by several pathophysiologic processes. Autonomous hyperfunction due

TABLE 14.1–1. MECHANISMS OF ENDOCRINE PATHOPHYSIOLOGY

Deficient hormone action
- Primary glandular failure
    Congenital: aplastic and biosynthetic defect
    Acquired: physiologic atrophy, tumor, surgery, drug-induced, inflammation (infectious, autoimmune)
- Secondary gland failure
- Disordered hormone release or activation
- Accelerated hormone metabolism
- Target-tissue resistance to hormone action

Excess hormone production and action
- Gland autonomy: neoplasia or hyperplasia
- Abnormal stimulation of gland function
- Ectopic hormone production
- Altered hormone metabolism
- Target-tissue hypersensitivity to hormone action

Neoplasia
- Benign and malignant
- Functional and nonfunctional
- Ectopic hormone production by tumors
- Sporadic and familial, including the multiple endocrine neoplasia syndromes

to neoplasia arising within the endocrine gland is a common etiology of glandular hyperfunction (e.g., acromegaly due to a growth hormone-secreting pituitary adenoma). Hormonal hypersecretion may also result from hyperplasia of secretory cells without a true neoplasm (e.g., hyperparathyroidism due to parathyroid hyperplasia). In some conditions, an abnormal stimulator of glandular function causes hyperplasia and overproduction of hormone (e.g., thyroid-stimulating immunoglobulins in Graves disease). Ectopic hormone production by tumors may also cause hormonal excess.[4,6] In some cases, the tumor is believed to express the physiologic hormone itself (e.g., lung carcinoma secreting adrenal corticotropic hormone). In other syndromes, such as hypercalcemia of malignancy, the tumor product shares certain biologic properties with parathyroid hormone. Altered hormone metabolism in non-

TABLE 14.1–2. DISORDERS INVOLVING MULTIPLE ENDOCRINE GLANDS

Multiple endocrine neoplasia (MEN) syndromes
MEN I (Wermer syndrome)
- Hyperparathyroidism
- Pituitary adenoma
- Pancreatic adenoma or carcinoma

MEN II (MEN IIa, Sipple syndrome)
- Hyperparathyroidism
- Medullary carcinoma of thyroid
- Pheochromocytoma

MEN III (MEN IIb)
- Medullary carcinoma of thyroid
- Pheochromocytoma
- Mucosal neuromas
- Marfanoid habitus

Polyendocrine failure syndromes
Type I
- Hypoparathyroidism
- Adrenal insufficiency
- Mucocutaneous candidiasis
- Other associated conditions: hypogonadism, autoimmune thyroid diseases, type I diabetes mellitus

Type II
- Adrenal insufficiency
- Autoimmune thyroid disease
- Other associated conditions: type I diabetes mellitus, primary or secondary gonadal failure

glandular tissues may produce excessive hormone levels either by increasing hormone activation (e.g., activation of vitamin D in sarcoidosis) or reducing hormone degradation (e.g., gynecomastia in cirrhosis due to decreased estrogen metabolism). A few syndromes of true tissue hypersensitivity to physiologic circulating hormone concentrations have been recognized (e.g., normoprolactinemic galactorrhea).

NEOPLASIA OF ENDOCRINE GLANDS

Endocrine gland tumors are more commonly benign than malignant. For example, most palpable thyroid nodules and radiologically detected adrenal and pituitary tumors are benign. The broad spectrum of clinical behavior among endocrine malignancies is exemplified when the indolent growth and frequent cure of well-differentiated thyroid carcinoma is contrasted with the rapid progression and almost invariably fatal outcome in anaplastic thyroid cancer.

Functional endocrine tumors secrete a hormonal product. Nonfunctional tumors cause disease by compromising normal glandular function (e.g., hypopituitarism due to pituitary macroadenoma), local extension (e.g., visual field loss with suprasellar extension), or distant spread. Because functional tumors typically lack physiologic regulatory mechanisms, autonomous hormone production causes clinical syndromes of hormonal excess (e.g., virilization due to adrenal carcinoma). Neoplasms of both endocrine and nonendocrine origin can secrete biologically active hormones. The resulting syndromes of ectopic hormone excess must be distinguished from primary endocrine disorders (e.g., Cushing syndrome) and may be among the most distressing manifestations of the primary tumor (e.g., hypercalcemia of malignancy).

Neoplasia of the endocrine glands may be sporadic or may occur with a familial predisposition (e.g., medullary carcinoma of the thyroid). Familial endocrine tumors may involve a single gland or present as part of a syndrome of tumors involving multiple endocrine glands (Table 14.1–2). Three specific syndromes transmitted by autosomal dominant inheritance have been recognized. Multiple endocrine neoplasia I (MEN I, Wermer syndrome) includes parathyroid hyperplasia and hyperparathyroidism, pancreatic islet cell tumors (secreting gastrin, insulin, glucagon, or vasoactive intestinal peptide), and pituitary adenomas, which may or may not be secretory. Multiple endocrine neoplasia II (MEN II or IIa, Sipple syndrome) is characterized by hyperparathyroidism, medullary carcinoma of the thyroid, and pheochromocytoma. Individuals with the closely related MEN III (or IIb) have medullary thyroid cancer and pheochromocytoma in association with mucosal neuromas and Marfanoid habitus. Patients with crossover syndromes have been described rarely.

PATHOPHYSIOLOGIC MECHANISMS IN METABOLIC DISEASES

Disordered carbohydrate and lipid metabolism may have a single definable underlying cause or a complex, multifactorial pathophysiologic basis. Primary endocrine diseases may cause secondary metabolic disturbances. Hyperglycemia, for example, may be the result of Cushing syndrome or acromegaly. Similarly, hyperlipidemia may be secondary to hypothyroidism.

Inherited traits play a central role in the development of many metabolic disorders. Familial hypercholesterolemia, for example, is a consequence of a dominantly transmitted defect in the membrane receptor for low-density lipoproteins. The pattern of inheritance for other metabolic disorders such as diabetes mellitus is less well understood. Evidence suggests an interaction between genetic and environmental factors, for example, obesity and viral infection, in the development of diabetes. Nutrition and body weight are

important environmental factors leading to expression of these and other metabolic disorders. Dietary intake of total calories and saturated fats can be pivotal determinants of the disorder's expression and severity. Neuropsychiatric factors appear to play a central pathogenetic role in the development of the metabolic disorders of obesity and anorexia nervosa. Behavioral factors also contribute significantly to the expression and management of metabolic diseases.

CLINICAL APPROACH TO ENDOCRINE AND METABOLIC DISEASES

CLINICAL ASSESSMENT

The spectrum of biochemical and clinical severity of endocrine and metabolic diseases typically ranges from total absence of clinical manifestations to pathognomonic symptoms and signs. Moreover, the clinical manifestations of endocrine disorders are often quite nonspecific and may be encountered more commonly in nonendocrine illness. For these reasons, a high index of suspicion for endocrine and metabolic disorders is warranted. The physician should remain especially alert to laboratory clues suggesting these disorders (e.g., eosinophilia in adrenal insufficiency, hyperphosphatemia in acromegaly) when interpreting conventional diagnostic tests requested in the assessment of nonspecific complaints. The possibility of endocrine disease should be entertained much more frequently than it is ultimately established as the diagnosis.

Once an endocrine or metabolic disorder is suspected, this diagnostic hypothesis must be tested by additional clinical and laboratory observations. Other than the chief complaint, does the patient have symptoms or signs consistent with the suspected disorder? For example, does the anxious patient also have weight loss despite good appetite, heat intolerance, tremor, and palpitations—findings that might indicate hyperthyroidism? If not, is the limited symptomatology still consistent with some portion of the known clinical spectrum for the disease?

LABORATORY AND RADIOLOGIC ASSESSMENT[5]

Laboratory investigations of endocrine and metabolic disorders can be categorized as (1) screening tests that reliably exclude the suspected disorders, (2) diagnostic tests that definitively establish the presence of disease, and (3) localizing tests that characterize the specific etiology and site of the responsible disorder.

Direct measurement of circulating hormone concentrations is vital for the accurate diagnosis of most endocrine diseases. Fortunately, highly sensitive and specific tests permit precise quantitation of most hormones in blood despite their low concentrations (10^{-9} to 10^{-12} mol/L). Foremost among these techniques is the competitive protein-binding assay. Radioimmunoassay (RIA), the most widely employed form of this procedure,[9] utilizes a radioactive hormone (tracer) to compete with known concentrations of hormone (standards) or test samples for the high-affinity binding sites of specific heterologous immunoglobulins, for example, rabbit antisera to human prolactin. It is important to remember that an RIA actually measures immunoreactivity (the ability of a hormone to be recognized by a specific immunoglobulin), not true biological activity (the competence of hormone to bind to target-tissue receptors and initiate hormone actions). Although unusual, dissociation between the immunologic and biologic activities of a hormone represents a possible source of confusion in the clinical interpretation of RIA results. Another potentially confounding issue arises because many circulating hormones are partially bound to protein with only a fraction of their total blood concentration available to interact with target tissues. The total hormone concentration measured by RIA may be particularly misleading if the con-

centration of binding protein changes under physiologic, pathophysiologic, or pharmacologic influences (e.g., thyroxine-binding globulin increase due to estrogen). As a consequence, a variety of methods have been devised to determine the concentrations of unbound or free hormones in blood.

Because endocrine and metabolic parameters are by their very nature dynamically responsive to both internally generated rhythms and external stimuli, circulating levels of hormones and metabolic substrates often fluctuate considerably in the absence of disease. Appropriate timing of laboratory tests is therefore important, particularly with regard to factors such as preceding meals (e.g., serum glucose and insulin), time of day (e.g., serum cortisol), and the menstrual cycle (e.g., serum estradiol).

In subtle endocrine and metabolic disturbances, it is not unusual for measurement of hormonal and metabolic parameters to yield equivocal results in the basal state. This is particularly true of endocrine systems with physiologic fluctuations in circulating hormone concentrations, such as diurnally cycling adrenal-glucocorticoid secretion. Provocative endocrine test procedures are designed to accentuate differences between normal and pathophysiologic states by manipulating physiologic regulatory mechanisms, such as the negative feedback system which characterizes the hypothalamic-pituitary-adrenal axis (Fig. 14.1–1A). As a general rule, if a deficiency of hormone production is suspected, a stimulation test is instructive, whereas excessive or autonomous hormone secretion is revealed by suppression testing. An example of a stimulation test is the evaluation of possible primary adrenal insufficiency by administration of ACTH with serial blood sampling for measurement of the anticipated serum cortisol response (Fig. 14.1–1B). A suppression test is exemplified by the use of dexamethasone, a potent synthetic glucocorticoid, to evaluate negative feedback on the hypothalamus and pituitary (Fig. 14–1C). Dexamethasone would normally suppress corticotroph function and reduce ACTH release; but suppression does not occur, for example, in the presence of an autonomously functioning adrenal adenoma.

Localization of the primary abnormality responsible for an endocrine or metabolic disorder is accomplished by several approaches. Different etiologies may have characteristic "fingerprints" with provocative endocrine test procedures (e.g., differentiation of central versus nephrogenic diabetes insipidus, or pituitary versus adrenal Cushing syndrome). Regional blood sampling for determination of local hormone concentrations may lead to a specific pathogenetic diagnosis as well as the site of involvement (e.g., selective venous sampling in the differentiation of parathyroid hyperplasia from adenoma). Finally, both noninvasive and invasive radiologic studies are an important aid in the identification of the pathogenesis and location of disease. Radionuclide scanning, in particular, provides valuable functional and morphologic information (e.g., iodine-123 thyroid scan, iodo-131 cholesterol scan of the adrenal cortex). Computed tomography (CT) and magnetic resonance imaging (MRI) have revolutionized the approach to localization of pituitary and adrenal disorders. Because benign nonfunctioning neoplasms of the endocrine glands are relatively common, radiologic findings must be interpreted with great caution in patients with possible or even proven endocrine disease. It is preferable, in general, to establish a diagnosis based on hormonal laboratory data before requesting any localizing radiologic studies.

Pathologic studies play a role, of course, in establishing the specific diagnosis in patients with endocrine disease. Routine histopathology distinguishes benign from malignant neoplasms in most cases, especially when there is clear invasion of the gland capsule, blood vessels, or adjacent structures. Endocrine tissues, however, may exhibit considerable overlap between the pathologic features of normal tissue, hyperplasia, benign neoplasia, and malignancy. These distinctions may ultimately be based more on hormonal secretory patterns, gross surgical findings, response to therapy, and long-term behavior of the endocrine condition than on histologic appearance. Cytologic diagnosis of material obtained by biopsy has nonetheless proven valuable in the evauation, for example, of thy-

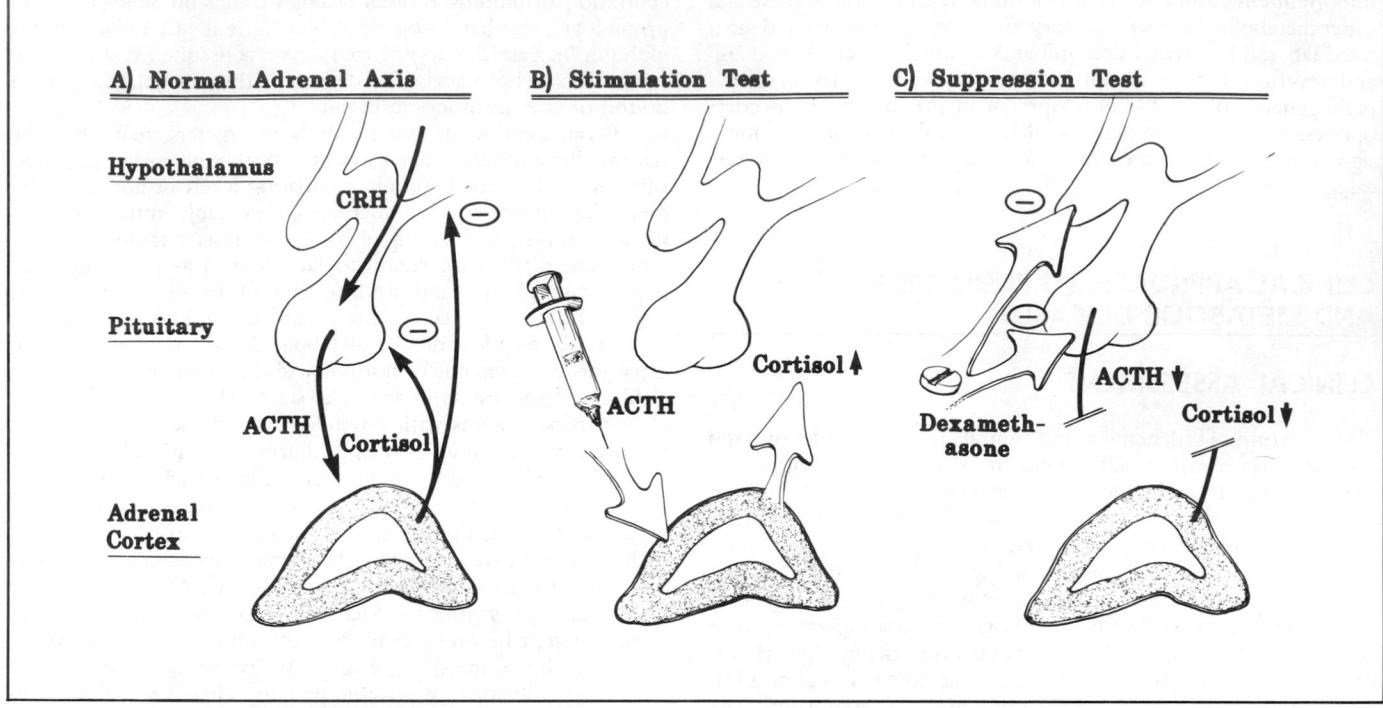

Figure 14.1–1. A. Hypothalamic-pituitary-adrenal axis. **B.** ACTH stimulation test for adrenal insufficiency. The serum cortisol concentration is measured before and 30 minutes after adrenal cortical stimulation by exogenous administration of synthetic ACTH. **C.** Dexamethasone suppression test. Oral administration of this potent synthetic glucocorticoid assesses the integrity of glucocorticoid inhibitory feedback on the hypothalamus and pituitary.

roid nodules. Immunochemical techniques, using antisera against hormonal antigens, permit the identification of specific hormonal products in specimens of endocrine tissue. This information may be extremely valuable in establishing a precise diagnosis or in designing a therapeutic strategy (e.g., thyroglobulin staining of pulmonary metastasis from an unknown primary site).

THERAPEUTIC PRINCIPLES IN ENDOCRINOLOGY AND METABOLIC DISORDERS

The paramount goal of treating endocrine and metabolic disorders is the restoration of a normal hormonal and metabolic substrate milieu in the tissues. This includes establishing normal concentrations of these substances in the blood and tissues and simulating their physiologic excursions with meals, stress, and other life events. For example, insulin treatment must be coordinated with the patient's patterns of caloric intake and physical exercise. Glucocorticoid replacement must be adjusted to mimic the physiologic increase in adrenal glucocorticoid secretion that would normally accompany the response to illness. Particularly in metabolic disorders, appropriate modifications in diet, physical activity, and body weight are often the first line of treatment. This approach is often the only intervention required in the management of type II diabetes mellitus or certain hyperlipidemias, for example. Because endocrine therapy almost invariably alters the laboratory parameters needed to establish the diagnosis, it is vital to obtain adequate samples for testing before the initiation of treatment.

REFERENCES

1. Clayton RN (ed): Receptors in health and disease. Clin Endocrinol Metab 12(1), 1983
2. Eisenbarth GS, Wilson PW, et al: The polyglandular failure syndrome: disease inheritance, HLA type, and immune function: Studies in patients and families. Ann Intern Med 91:528, 1979
3. Felig P, Baxter JD, et al (eds): Endocrinology and Metabolism, 2d ed. New York, McGraw-Hill, 1987
4. Mendelsohn G, Baylin SB: Ectopic (inappropriate) hormone production by tumors: Mechanisms involved and the biological and clinical implications. Endocrinol Rev 1:45, 1980
5. Ney RL (ed): Investigations of endocrine disorders. Clin Endocrinol Metab 14(1), 1985
6. Odell WD: Humoral manifestation of cancer. In Wilson JD, Foster DW (eds): Williams Textbook of Endocrinology, 7th ed. Philadelphia, WB Saunders, 1985
7. Stanbury JB, Wyngaarden JB, et al (eds): The Metabolic Basis of Inherited Disease, 5th ed. New York, McGraw-Hill, 1983
8. Wilson JD, Foster DW (eds): Williams Textbook of Endocrinology, 7th ed. Philadelphia, WB Saunders, 1985
9. Yalow RS: Radioimmunoassay: A probe for the fine structure of biologic systems. Med Phys 5:247, 1978

Disorders of Hypothalamus and Pituitary Gland

Gary S. Wand and David S. Cooper

The hypothalamus and pituitary form a physiologic unit that regulates the functions of the thyroid, adrenal cortex, and gonads, as well as somatic growth, lactation, and renal water excretion. Through an intricate feedback system, peripheral hormones can in turn influence hypothalamic-pituitary secretion (Fig. 14.2–1).

HYPOTHALAMIC NEUROSECRETORY UNIT

The hypothalamus is located at the base of the brain (Fig. 14.2–2) superior and posterior to the optic chiasm and superior to the pituitary gland. The inferior portion of the hypothalamus contains the *median eminence,* which forms the floor of the third ventricle. The pituitary stalk, or *infundibulum,* is a direct extension from this region. The hypothalamus is composed of specialized neurons, neurosecretory cells, which in addition to having the functional and structural properties typifying all neurons, synthesize and secrete the hormones that regulate anterior pituitary function. The hypothalamus has been called a "neuroendocrine transducer" because it translates neural activity into hormonal output. These hypothalamic neurosecretory cells are in turn regulated by numerous converging inputs from higher brain centers. The median eminence thus is the switching center, where nerve endings from higher centers terminate, and in response hypothalamic factors are delivered into the portal veins of the pituitary stalk to modulate the function of pituitary cells.

Five hypothalamic peptides are known to stimulate or inhibit the release of anterior pituitary hormones[2] (Table 14.2–1). Some of these peptides also are found in other regions of the CNS and in the gastrointestinal tract. Thyrotropin-releasing hormone (TRH) stimulates production of both thyroid-stimulating hormone (TSH) and prolactin (although endogenous TRH probably does not play a major role in the regulation of prolactin secretion). Growth hormone–releasing hormone (GRH) promotes growth hormone release. Gonadotropin-releasing hormone (GnRH) stimulates both luteinizing hormone (LH) and follicle-stimulating hormone (FSH) secretion. Corticotropin-releasing hormone (CRH) stimulates release of ACTH, β-endorphin, and related peptides of pro-ACTH/endorphin. Somatostatin is a potent inhibitor of growth hormone and TSH release. It is also found in the pancreatic islets and may modulate insulin and glucagon secretion. Dopamine, the one nonpeptide hypothalamic hormone, is the most im-

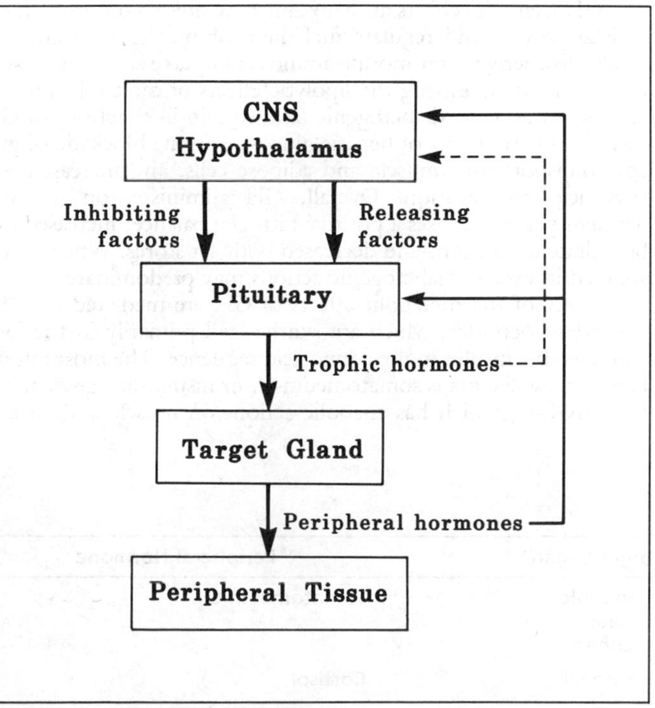

Figure 14.2–1. Specific nuclei within hypothalamus synthesize and secrete hormones that regulate anterior pituitary hormone secretion. In turn, trophic hormones released by pituitary affect peripheral target glands. Through a system of feedback loops, peripheral hormones such as cortisol, L-thyroxine, and gonadal steroids can modulate hypothalamic and pituitary function.

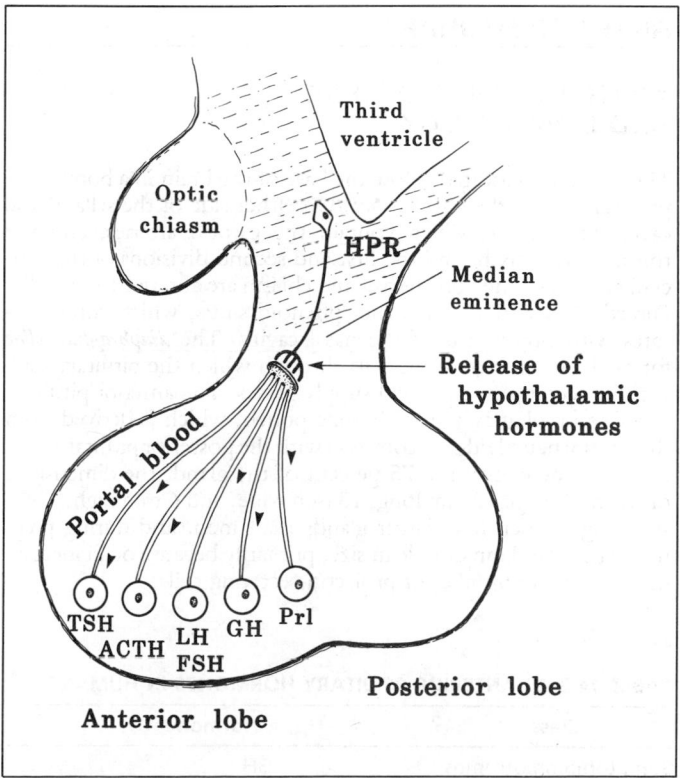

Figure 14.2–2. Hypothalamic neuroendocrine cells are diffusely distributed throughout mediobasal hypothalamus in region known as hypophysiotropic region (HPR). These secretory cells terminate on fenestrated capillary endothelium of medium eminence. It is here that hypothalamic hormones are released into pituitary portal vasculature, which serves as a conduit for hormone passage to specific pituitary cell membrane receptors. TSH = thyroid-stimulating hormone; ACTH = adrenocorticotropic hormone; LH = luteinizing hormone; FSH = follicle-stimulating hormone; GH = growth hormone; Prl = prolactin.

TABLE 14.2–1. HYPOTHALAMIC HORMONES THAT REGULATE ANTERIOR PITUITARY FUNCTION

Hypothalamic Hormone	Anterior Pituitary Hormone
Thyrotropin-releasing hormone	Stimulates TSH and prolactin
Growth hormone–releasing hormone	Stimulates GH
Gonadotropin-releasing hormone	Stimulates LH and FSH
Corticotropin-releasing hormone	Stimulates ACTH and other peptides of the pro-ACTH/endorphin family
Somatostatin	Inhibits GH (TSH and others)
Dopamine	Inhibits prolactin (and TSH)
Prolactin-releasing factor[a]	Stimulates prolactin

[a]Vasoactive intestinal peptide is a likely candidate for a prolactin-releasing factor; other physiologic factors are yet to be determined.

portant physiologic inhibitor of prolactin in addition to its role as a neurotransmitter. Thus, the hypothalamic hormones are stimulatory to the pituitary, except for dopaminergic inhibition of prolactin secretion. Pituitary stalk interruption, therefore, causes decreased secretion of all pituitary hormones except prolactin, the secretion of which actually increases. All of these hypothalamic hormones (TRH, GnRH, CRH, and GRH) can be employed clinically to assess the qualitative and quantitative responses of the anterior pituitary.

ANTERIOR PITUITARY

ANATOMIC RELATIONSHIPS AND EMBRYOLOGY

The pituitary is located below the base of the brain in a bony compartment called the sella turcica. On either side of the sella lie the cavernous sinuses, which contain the carotid arteries, and the third, fourth, sixth, and the first and second divisions of the fifth cranial nerves. The optic nerves and chiasm are anterior to the sella. Directly below the sella is the sphenoid sinus, which communicates with other parts of the nasal cavity. The *diaphragma sellae* forms the dural roof of the sella through which the pituitary stalk with its accompanying blood supply passes. The anterior pituitary arises embryologically from Rathke pouch, which is derived from the ventral neural ridge in common with the posterior pituitary. The anterior lobe constitutes 75 percent of the gland, the dimensions of which average 10 mm long, 13 mm wide, and 6 mm high. Menstruating women have larger glands than men, and during pregnancy the gland can double in size, primarily because of an increase in the size and number of prolactin-secreting cells.

ANTERIOR PITUITARY CELLS AND THEIR HORMONES

Five distinct cell types in the anterior pituitary secrete six physiologically important hormones (Table 14.2–2), which can be classified by their chemical structure: (1) somatomammotropin hormones: growth hormone (GH) and prolactin, (2) pro-ACTH/endorphin derived hormones: ACTH and related peptides, and (3) glycoprotein hormones: LH, FSH, and TSH. Specific radioimmunoassays are available to measure plasma concentrations of all these pituitary hormones.

Somatomammotropin Hormones

Somatotrophs and Growth Hormone. The growth hormone secreting cells, which compromise 50 percent of anterior pituitary cells, are located predominantly in the lateral portions of the lobe. GH is a single-chain polypeptide of 191 amino acids; it shares common amino acid sequences with prolactin and human placental lactogen. Approximately 90 percent of pituitary and circulating GH has a molecular mass of 22,000 daltons. A 20,000-dalton GH variant, with a 15-amino-acid deletion, is of clinical interest because it lacks the hyperglycemic and diabetogenic activity of the 22,000-dalton GH but possesses the same growth-promoting activities.

The hypothalamic neurons regulate GH production by secreting GRH and somatostatin which stimulate and inhibit GH secretion, respectively. Plasma levels of GH vary widely, with bursts of secretion occurring principally during the first few hours of sleep. Basal levels are higher and these flucuations are more pronounced in children and menstruating women. GH secretion is affected by nutrients, exercise, and physical and emotional stress (Table 14.2–3). Estrogens increase GH responsiveness to various provocative agents, whereas glucocorticoids decrease somatotroph responsiveness. Basal plasma GH levels are usually less than 5 ng/ml in adults. Spontaneous secretory pulses of GH as high as 30 to 50 ng/ml can be seen in young adults.

GH exerts its effects at many different sites to promote linear skeletal growth and regulate fuel metabolism. Acutely, GH has insulin-like activity, promoting amino acid uptake and protein synthesis, and antagonizing the lipolytic effects of catecholamines in adipose tissue. The diabetogenic (anti-insulin-like) actions of GH include enhancement of hepatic glucose output, blockade of glucose transport into muscle and adipose cells, and increased free fatty acid mobilization. Overall, GH administration to GH-deficient patients causes a positive nitrogen balance, increased carbohydrate utilization, and decreased body fat stores. When GH is secreted in excess, diabetogenic actions may predominate.

Many of the metabolic affects of GH are mediated by GH-dependent peptides, which are synthesized primarily in the liver and resemble insulin in the amino acid sequence. The most important of these factors is somatomedin-C, or insulin-like growth factor I (IGF-I), which has anabolic actions on muscle and fat and

TABLE 14.2–2. ANTERIOR PITUITARY HORMONES IN HUMANS

Class	Hormone	Target Organ	Peripheral Hormone
Somatomammotropins	GH Prolactin	Multiple Breast (Others?)	Somatomedin-C
Pro-ACTH/endorphins	ACTH β-Endorphin β-LPH γ_3-MSH	Adrenal ? ? ?	Cortisol
Glycoproteins	LH	Gonad	Testosterone or estradiol
	FSH	Gonad	Spermatogenesis or ovum maturation
	TSH	Thyroid	L-T_4, L-T_3

TABLE 14.2–3. REGULATORS OF GROWTH HORMONE RELEASE

Stimulants	Inhibitors
Physiologic	• Somatostatin
• Sleep	• Glucocorticoids
• Newborn period	• Fatty acids
• Stress	• Hyperglycemia
• Exercise	• Alpha blockers
• Amino acids	
• Decrease in fatty acids	
• Hypoglycemia	
Pharmocologic	
• GRH	
• Dopamine agonists	
• Alpha agonists	

promotes growth by stimulating proliferation of chondrocytes and the synthesis of cartilage matrix.

Lactotrophs and Prolactin. The lactotrophs and somatotrophs are probably derived from a common stem cell; the lactotrophs are also located predominantly in the lateral portions of the pituitary gland. Prolactin is a single-chain polypeptide containing 198 amino acids; it circulates in three major forms (molecular weights 170,000, 48,000, and 22,500) with the low-molecular-weight form prolactin accounting for more than 80 percent of the total.

Because prolactin is under tonic inhibitory control, lesions of the hypothalamus, median eminence, or pituitary stalk can cause an increase in prolactin secretion. Dopamine is believed to be the physiologic prolactin-inhibiting factor. A portion of the GnRH precursor molecule may be an even more potent inhibitor of prolactin secretion; however, its physiologic role is yet to be defined. TRH and vasoactive intestinal peptide (VIP) are two hypothalamic peptides that cause prolactin release, but it is doubtful that they are the only physiologic mediators of prolactin secretion.

Prolactin levels fluctuate with four to nine pulses per day, especially during sleep, after meals, and in times of stress. The only established role for prolactin in humans is the initiation and maintenance of lactation, although prolactin receptors are present in the kidney, liver, adrenal glands, heart, and gonads. Prolactin levels, stimulated by placental estrogens, rise progressively during pregnancy, and, along with placental lactogen, estrogen, and progesterone, mediate breast growth and milk production. Prolactin specifically stimulates the biosynthesis of certain milk proteins, as well as the enzyme catalyzing the production of lactose from glucose and galactose. Lactation occurs when estradiol levels fall at the time of parturition. Prolactin levels rise sharply with each suckling episode, but gradually become blunted over the ensuing months if nursing continues. The pathway regulating this rise in prolactin includes afferent fibers from the nipple, thoracic nerves to the spinal column, and less well characterized pathways in the hypothalamus. Some nonparous women may lactate after prolonged nipple

stimulation or with chest wall trauma or inflammation (e.g., herpes zoster) because of activation of this neural pathway (Table 14.2–4).

Basal plasma prolactin levels are less than 25 ng/ml in women and 20 ng/ml in men. During the third trimester of pregnancy, prolactin levels normally rise to 150 to 300 ng/ml.

Corticotrophs and Pro-ACTH/Endorphin-Derived Peptides

The corticotrophs comprise about 15 to 20 percent of the anterior pituitary cells and lie in the anteromedial and posterolateral regions of the gland. They produce ACTH, a 39-amino-acid peptide that is synthesized as part of a larger precursor molecule, pro-ACTH/endorphin (also called pro-opiomelanocortin, POMC). This prohormone is also the precursor for other neuropeptides—endorphins, lipotropin, and melanotropins—which are the result of posttranslational cleavage of the prohormone (Fig. 14.2–3). β-Lipotropin and β-endorphin are secreted in an equimolar ratio to ACTH.

The circadian rhythm of pulsatile ACTH release is predominantly under hypothalamic CRH regulation. Plasma ACTH levels (10 to 80 pg/ml) are lowest in the evening and highest in the early morning at about the time of awakening. Physical and psychic stress cause increased ACTH secretion, a process mediated by CRH and other hypothalamic and peripheral hormones. ACTH stimulates adrenal cortical hormone synthesis and secretion; after a short lag period, plasma cortisol values follow the ACTH rhythm closely. Cortisol in turn inhibits hypothalamic CRH and pituitary ACTH synthesis and secretion. While ACTH is the predominant regulator of adrenal glucocorticoid and androgen biosynthesis and secretion, it plays only a minor role in mineralocorticoid secretion. An amino-terminal fragment of the prohormone γ_3-MSH may be important in the regulation of mineralocorticoids.

Glycoprotein Hormones

Thyrotrophs and TSH. The thyrotrophs that secrete TSH are located in the anteromedial region of the pituitary and comprise only 5 percent of anterior pituitary cells. TSH is a protein with a molecular weight of approximately 26,000, which, like LH and FSH, is composed of a peptide core containing noncovalently linked alpha and beta subunits to which are attached carbohydrate side chains. These carbohydrate moieties probably influence the bioactivity and stability of the peptide in plasma. The protein cores of TSH, LH, FSH, and the placental hormone human chorionic gonadotropin (hCG) have identical alpha subunits. The specific biologic action of each hormone is conferred by the uniqueness of its beta subunit.

TSH controls thyroid hormone biosynthesis and secretion by the thyroid gland. TSH secretion is stimulated by hypothalamic TRH and is inhibited by thyroid hormone in a typical negative-feedback loop. The pituitary thyrotroph is exquisitely sensitive to plasma thyroid hormone levels, and minute increases or decreases in thyroid hormone concentrations can suppress or stimulate TSH secretion, respectively. In primary hypothyroidism, the thyrotrophs may undergo marked hypertrophy, hyperplasia, and histologic changes indicative of increased secretory activity. Whether

TABLE 14.2–4. CAUSES OF HYPERPROLACTENEMIA

Physiologic	Pharmacologic	Pathologic
• Pregnancy	• TRH	• Prolactin-secreting tumors
• Suckling	• Vasoactive intestinal peptide	Macroadenoma
• Newborn	• Psychotropic drugs, metoclopramide	Microadenoma
• Estrogens	(dopamine-blocking agents)	• Acromegaly (25–30%)
• Stress	• Catecholamine-depleting drugs	• Hypothalamic disease (e.g., sarcoidosis)
• Exercise	(e.g., reserpine)	• Hypothyroidism
• Sleep	• Serotonin	• Renal failure
• Postprandial	• Cimetidine (intravenous)	• Chest wall trauma
• Hypoglycemia	• Verapamil (intravenous)	• Idiopathic hyperprolactinemia
		• Polycystic ovary disease (15–30%)

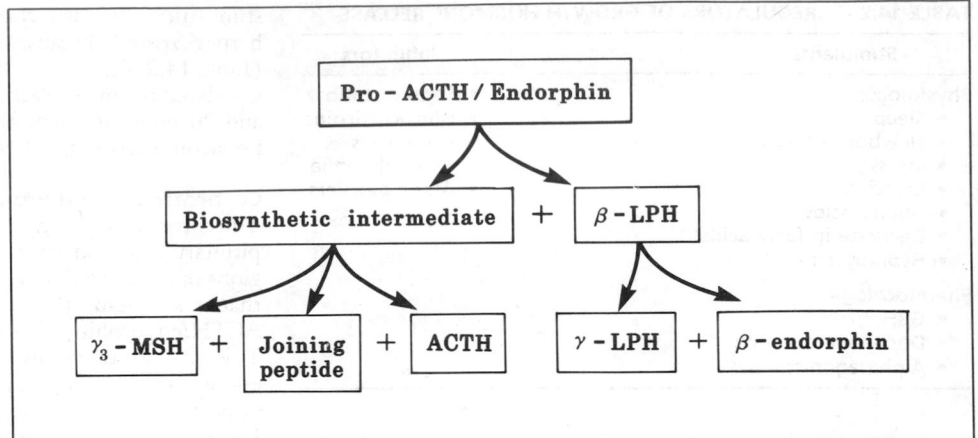

Figure 14.2–3. Peptides derived from the prohormone pro-ACTH/endorphin in the anterior pituitary. The mature peptides are secreted into plasma in a coordinated, equimolar fashion.

thyroid hormones also act on the hypothalamus directly to modulate TRH secretion.

Gonadotrophs and LH and FSH. Gonadotrophs secrete both LH and FSH and constitute only 3 to 5 percent of anterior pituitary cells. Their numbers increase appropriately following castration or primary gonadal failure, and decrease during pregnancy secondary to the production of hCG, which stimulates estrogen secretion by the placenta. LH and FSH are composed of a common alpha subunit and a hormone-specific beta subunit. Pulsatile hypothalamic GnRH release stimulates the episodic release of both pituitary gonadotropins. The stimulatory effect of GnRH is modified by plasma levels of estrogen, progesterone, and testosterone. In women, estrogen can have either a positive or negative-feedback effect on gonadotropin release. The midcycle surge in gonadotropins is thought to reflect either increased sensitivity of the gonadotrophs to GnRH or a stimulatory effect of estrogen on hypothalamic GnRH secretion. On the other hand, chronic estrogen administration (e.g., oral contraceptives) decreases gonadotroph sensitivity to GnRH and may also depress hypothalamic GnRH secretion directly. Similar negative-feedback effects are seen in men after estrogen or testosterone administration.

HYPOPITUITARISM

Pituitary Failure Due to Hypothalamic Dysfunction
In the early part of this century, clinicians recognized that pituitary dysfunction could occur when the hypothalamus was affected by certain disease processes. In addition to organic lesions that destroy the hypothalamic neurosecretory cells, functional or psychic disturbances can cause abnormal pituitary function. A striking example of the latter is "psychogenic" or hypothalamic amenorrhea, a reversible form of amenorrhea that affects certain women during times of stress.

Because hypothalamic projections are generally not lateralized, unilateral damage to the hypothalamus seldom results in significant hypopituitarism. Hypopituitarism due to hypothalamic disease is most commonly seen, therefore, with diseases that diffusely infiltrate the hypothalamus or masses that extend across the midline (Table 14.2–5).

The clinical approach to the work-up of hypopituitarism and clues for distinguishing hypothalamic disease from hypopituitarism will be discussed in this section.

Hypopituitarism Due to Pituitary Disorders
Hypopituitarism[1] may be caused by a number of disease processes (Table 14.2–6). Primary pituitary tumors in adults and craniopharyngiomas in children are the most common causes of hypopituitarism, which can be partial or complete. The clinical presentation varies with the extent of pituitary damage, the specific etiology of the disorder, the age of onset, and how rapidly the process evolves. The abrupt onset of hypopituitarism usually signifies extensive hormonal loss, including the corticotrophs and thyrotrophs. In patients with more insidious presentations, there may be sequential loss of anterior pituitary hormones, with LH, GH and prolactin deficiency preceding the onset of ACTH and TSH deficiency. General clinical features of chronic hypopituitarism include pale, finely wrinkled skin with decreased turgor, particularly in the periorbital region. Men may have an adolescent hairline. As a consequence patients appear paradoxically both youthful and prematurely aged. Patients may have psychiatric manifestations, including impaired mentation, apathy, and occasionally psychosis.

Specific Hormone Deficiencies
Growth Hormone Deficiency. In the adult, GH deficiency is not associated with any clinical manifestations. Inadequate GH in the child is characterized by short stature (height generally being less than the third percentile), abnormal growth velocity (less than 4 cm/yr), delayed bone age, and in the infant, a tendency to fasting hypoglycemia (Table 14.2–7). A number of conditions cause GH deficiency, idiopathic growth hormone deficiency (IGHD) being the most common. IGHD is really a heterogeneous group of disorders that can be classified on a metabolic, hormonal, or hereditary basis. The majority of patients with IGHD have a GH response to (GRH), implying that deficiency of hypothalamic GRH is the primary cause of the problem.

TABLE 14.2–5. HYPOTHALAMIC DISEASES THAT AFFECT PITUITARY FUNCTION

Hypothalamic disease associated with hypopituitarism
- Tumor/mass (e.g., craniopharyngioma)
- Infiltrative disorders (e.g., sarcoidosis)
- Genetic disorders (e.g., Prader-Willi syndrome)
- Midline defects (e.g., Kallmann syndrome)
- Radiation
- Trauma
- Meningitis-encephalitis

Hypothalamic disease associated with hyperpituitarism
- Hamartoma (e.g., precocious puberty)
- Pineal tumor (e.g., precocious puberty)
- Gangliocytoma (e.g., acromegaly)

Functional hypothalamic or CNS disease
- Anorexia nervosa
- Depression
- Psychosocial dwarfism
- Hypothalamic amenorrhea

TABLE 14.2–6. MAJOR CAUSES OF HYPOPITUITARISM

- Pituitary tumors
  Intrasellar (e.g., secretory or nonsecretory adenoma or craniopharyngioma)
  Parasellar (e.g., meningioma)
- Pituitary apoplexy (e.g., hemorrhagic infarction of a pituitary tumor)
- Ischemic necrosis (e.g., Sheehan syndrome)
- Aneurysm
- Cavernous-sinus thrombosis
- Infiltrative disease (e.g., sarcoidosis)
- Irradiation to sella
- Surgical damage
- Infectious disease (e.g., fungal)
- Idiopathic (e.g., monohormonal deficiency)

Prolactin Deficiency. Failure of postpartum lactation is the only known consequence of a prolactin-deficient state. Classically, this clinical syndrome has suggested postpartum pituitary necrosis (Sheehan syndrome), caused by extensive hemorrhage and shock during labor. Sheehan syndrome may also be accompanied by partial or complete loss of other pituitary hormones. Fortunately, this syndrome is now rarely seen, because of advances in obstetrical care.

ACTH Deficiency. ACTH deficiency and consequent adrenal glucocorticoid lack is accompanied by nonspecific symptoms such as fatigue, weakness, anorexia, and vomiting. Volume depletion and hyperkalemia seen in Addison disease (primary adrenal insufficiency) rarely occur, since aldosterone secretion is maintained via the renin-angiotensin pathway independent of ACTH. Orthostatic hypotension is common, however, as glucocorticoids are important for the maintainance of vascular tone. Hyponatremia is seen in both primary and secondary adrenal insufficiency caused by the effects of glucocorticoid deficiency on renal free-water clearance. Lack of the pigmenting properties of ACTH and related peptides leads patients with secondary adrenal insufficiency to appear pale and to tan poorly.

TSH Deficiency. Manifestations of hypothyroidism resulting from damage to the pituitary or hypothalamus are similar to the classic features of primary hypothyroidism, although they are usually less severe. Patients complain of fatigue, weight gain, cold intolerance, constipation, and dry skin but rarely become frankly myxedematous. Isolated TSH deficiency is rare, and hypogonadism or secondary adrenal insufficiency are often present. When the latter occurs, the patient can become profoundly ill if treated with thyroid hormone without concomitant replacement with glucocorticoids (see below).

Gonadotropin Deficiency. Hypogonadotropic hypogonadism before puberty prevents the development of secondary sexual charac-

teristics and is accompanied by infertility and a eunuchoidal appearance. In adult men, the absence of testosterone causes loss of libido and potency, a decrease in testicular volume, slowed growth of androgen-dependent hair (beard, pubic, and axillary hair), and loss of muscle mass. Adult women with decreased estrogen levels have amenorrhea, often with decreased vaginal secretions, dyspareunia, hot flushes, decreased libido, and breast atrophy. Osteoporosis is another consequence of chronically low estrogen levels. Hypogonadotropic hypogonadism is often the first sign of an expanding pituitary mass, and in that context, is often associated with other trophic hormone deficiencies. The most common form of isolated hypogonadotropic hypogonadism is Kallmann syndrome, a familial condition characterized by primary GnRH deficiency and a variety of midline defects including anosmia and cleft palate.

Evaluation of Hypopituitarism

The history and physical examination are often helpful in establishing the etiology of hypopituitarism. For example, a history of headaches and a bitemporal visual field deficit suggest the presence of a sellar mass lesion. Anosmia suggests the diagnosis of Kallmann syndrome or an olfactory groove meningioma. High-resolution CT and MRI are the best tools to determine the specific etiology of hypopituitarism.

Clinical observations must be confirmed by radioimmunoassay determinations of circulating hormone concentrations. This information is useful to: (1) distinguish primary endocrine end-organ failure from hypothalamic-pituitary disease and (2) to establish a patient's need for various hormonal replacement therapies. The initial endocrine assessment should test for hyposecretion of each anterior pituitary hormone. In addition to basal hormone concentration, provocative testing of pituitary hormone reserve should be performed in many instances (Table 14.2–8).

Assessment of GH Deficiency. Multiple tests can evaluate potential growth hormone deficiency (Table 14.2–9). In adults, GH reserve can be effectively assessed during insulin-induced hypoglycemia (see section on ACTH deficiency). In a short child, the diagnosis of GH deficiency is made when GH fails to exceed 7 ng/ml in response to at least two stimuli for GH release.

Assessment of Prolactin Excess and Deficiency. A modestly elevated basal prolactin level (25 to 150 ng/ml), particularly in the presence of other features of hypopituitarism, may indicate a hypothalamic lesion causing anterior pituitary failure, or pituitary stalk compression from a nonsecretory sellar tumor or parasellar mass. Compression of lactotrophs by an intrinsic sellar lesion causes hypoprolactinemia and a blunted or flat prolactin response to TRH stimulation; normal subjects will demonstrate at least a doubling in prolactin after TRH.

Assessment of ACTH Deficiency. Tests of ACTH reserve can identify patients with defects in ACTH secretion that may not be apparent during basal hormone evaluation. These tests depend on

TABLE 14.2–7. CLASSIFICATION OF DWARFISM RESULTING FROM ABNORMALITIES IN THE HYPOTHALAMIC-PITUITARY-SOMATOTROPH AXIS

Type of Dwarfism	Serum GH RIA	Somatomedin RIA	Pathophysiology	Response to	
				GH	GRH
Hypothalamic	Low	Low	Defect in hypothalamic GRH synthesis or secretion	+	+
Pituitary	Low	Low	Defect in pituitary GH synthesis or secretion	+	–
Laron	High	Low	Failure of GH to generate somatomedin-C (GH resistance)	–	–
Abnormal GH	High	Low	Biologically inactive GH	+	–
Somatomedin resistance	Normal	High	Failure of somatomedin to produce growth-promoting activity	–	–

TABLE 14.2–8. PROVOCATIVE TESTS TO EVALUATE ANTERIOR PITUITARY HORMONE RESERVE

Test	Dose	Hormone Sampled	Sampling Intervals	Normal Response
TRH	200 μg IV	TSH Prolactin	0, 30, 60 min 0, 30, 60 min	6 μU/ml or twice basal value (should be standardized by individual laboratory)
GnRH	100 μg IV	LH and FSH	0, 30, 60 min	Twice basal value (should be standardized by individual laboratory)
Insulin	0.1–0.15 U/kg IV (regular insulin)	Cortisol	0, 30, 60, 90 min	Stimulated value greater than 18 μg/dl
Metyrapone	a) 750 mg PO q4h for 6 doses	Urinary 17-hydroxy-cortico-steroids	24-hr urine day before, day of, and day after metyrapone	Twice basal value
	b) 30 mg/kg at midnight	Cortisol 11-deoxycortisol	8:00 AM next day 0, 30, 60, 90 min	Cortisol: <5 μg/dl 11-deoxycortisol: >10 μg/dl
CRH	100 μg IV	ACTH Cortisol	0, 30, 60, 90 min	No established criteria

prior documentation of adequate adrenal responsiveness to ACTH, that is, exclusion of primary adrenal insufficiency. The evaluation of adrenal insufficiency and methods for distinguishing primary from secondary disease are discussed in Chapter 14.3.

The most definitive test for evaluating corticotroph function is insulin-induced hypoglycemia, a potent stimulus of hypothalamic CRH and, in turn, ACTH secretion. The test is performed after an overnight fast with measurements of cortisol values before and then 30, 45, 60 and 90 minutes after insulin (0.1 to 0.15 U/kg) has been administered intravenously. A fall in blood glucose to 40 mg/dl or less, accompanied by adrenergic symptoms, indicates an adequate response. During the procedure a physician should be in attendance and equipped to administer intravenous glucose if the patient develops severe neuroglycopenic symptoms. The test generally should not be performed in patients over 65 years of age or in patients with cerebrovascular disease, seizure disorder, or cardiovascular disease. It is also contraindicated in ill patients strongly suspected of having adrenal insufficiency because they can be exquisitely sensitive to insulin. A suboptimal response (Table 14.2–8) indicates secondary adrenal insufficiency.

ACTH reserve can also be evaluated by the metyrapone test. This competitive inhibitor of the adrenal enzyme 11-β-hydroxylase blocks conversion of 11-deoxycortisol to cortisol. The subsequent decrease in negative cortisol feedback is a potent stimulus to pituitary ACTH secretion, which stimulates adrenocortical steroidogenesis proximal to the site of enzyme inhibition. A normal pituitary response to metyrapone, therefore, causes a rise in serum 11-deoxycortisol or in urinary 17-OHCS, reflecting increased excretion of 11-deoxycortisol metabolites.

Corticotropin-releasing hormone (CRH) has more recently been used as a provocative agent for assessment of ACTH secretion. A normal response to CRH and an inadequate response to insulin hypoglycemia indicate hypothalamic rather than pituitary disease.

Assessment of TSH Deficiency. Hypothalamic or pituitary hypothyroidism should be suspected in any patient with symptoms of hypothyroidism, low serum total and free thyroxine concentration, and a TSH value that is not appropriately elevated. The TRH stimulation test assesses pituitary TSH reserve and, in some cases, may distinguish pituitary from hypothalamic hypothyroidism. In normal subjects, TSH increases at least 6 μU/ml, 20 to 30 minutes after the administration of TRH. In hypothalamic disease, the peak value may not occur until approximately 60 minutes after injection, and the 90-minute TSH value will be greater than the 30-minute value. Patients with intrinsic pituitary disease may display a normal, blunted, or flat response to TRH stimulation, or they may have a delayed response, similar to patients with hypothalamic disease. TRH may cause a mild metallic taste and a transient urge to urinate several minutes after injection. Rarely, hypotension or hypertension may occur, so that patients should be supine during testing.

Assessment of LH and FSH Deficiency. Where there is clinical hypogonadism and serum estrogen or testosterone values are low, basal serum LH and FSH determinations will distinguish primary from secondary hypogonadism. Low or low normal gonadotropin values indicate hypothalamic or pituitary dysfunction, whereas ele-

TABLE 14.2–9. PROVOCATIVE TESTS USED IN ASSESSMENT OF HYPOTHALAMIC-PITUITARY-SOMATOTROPH AXIS

Provocative Tests	Dose	Sampling Interval (min)	Normal Response
Physiologic Sleep		60, 90 (after clinically evident deep sleep)	GH >7 ng/ml
Exercise		0, 20, 40, 60 after 20 min strenuous exercise	GH >7 ng/ml
Pharmocologic Arginine	30 g of 10% solution of L-arginine monochloride infused over 30 min	0, 30, 60, 90	GH >7 ng/ml
Insulin	0.1–0.15 μ/kg IV (regular insulin)	0, 30, 45, 60, 90	GH >10 ng/ml
L-Dopa	500 mg PO	0, 30, 60, 90	GH >10 ng/ml
GRH	100 μg IV	0, 15, 30, 60	GH >7 ng/ml

vated gonadotropins are consistent with primary gonadal failure. Gonadotropin responses to gonadotropin-releasing hormone (GnRH) can also be determined. In normal subjects, GnRH will stimulate a three- to fivefold rise in serum LH concentrations in approximately 30 minutes. Patients with hypothalamic disease may initially have a blunted response to GnRH that improves after several days of repeated stimulation, whereas patients with pituitary disease usually have a blunted response after extensive GnRH priming.

Summary

Pituitary hormone reserve should be tested when there is clinical evidence of hypopituitarism, and after pituitary or hypothalamic surgery or irradiation. It is possible to assess simultaneously the reserve capacity of all six hormones by performing a combined insulin-tolerance TRH-GnRH stimulation test.[4] Insulin, TRH, and GnRH can be administered in bolus form: hypoglycemia will stimulate ACTH and GH, TRH will stimulate TSH and prolactin, and GnRH will stimulate LH and FSH.

Treatment

Because hypopituitarism often persists after the underlying cause has been corrected (e.g., surgical removal of a pituitary tumor), patients usually need lifelong hormonal replacement.

Treatment of GH deficiency in adults is never indicated. GH from human cadaver pituitaries has been the primary agent for treatment of short stature resulting from GH deficiency, but because of evidence of "slow virus" contamination (Creutzfeldt-Jakob disease) in earlier GH preparations, this form of GH is no longer available. Fortunately, recombinant human GH is now available and is now the treatment of choice for children with GH deficiency. Synthetic GRH, administered by subcutaneous infusion pump or intranasally, may supplant GH treatment for children with defects of hypothalamic GRH secretion.

ACTH deficiency is treated with hydrocortisone 20 mg each morning and 10 mg in the late afternoon (or an equivalent dose of another glucocorticoid), which mimics the normal diurnal variation of cortisol secretion. Mineralocorticoid replacement is not necessary because normal adrenal aldosterone secretion will be maintained by the renin-angiotensin system. The glucocorticoid dose must be increased two- or threefold during stress, such as a febrile illness. In the presence of nausea and vomiting, parenteral glucocorticoids should be given. For more severe stress (surgery or trauma) the patient will require 200 to 300 mg of hydrocortisone per day or its equivalent. All patients on steroids need to be educated about the nature of their replacement therapy and should wear medical identification indicating their condition.

TSH deficiency is treated with L-thyroxine (1.6 μg/kg). In older individuals or patients with cardiovascular disease, a small dose of L-thyroxine (0.025 mg/day) should be used initially and gradually increased. It is important to diagnose and correct any accompanying adrenal insufficiency before beginning thyroid replacement. Failure to do so may provoke adrenal insufficiency because thyroid hormone increases cortisol metabolism, leading to lower circulating cortisol levels.

Treatment of secondary hypogonadism may entail both hormonal replacement and possible treatment of infertility (see Chapter 14.5). Treatment of symptomatic hormonal deficiency is a much simpler task than restoring fertility. For men, testosterone replacement is achieved by intramuscular injections of a long-acting testosterone preparation (e.g., testosterone enanthate 200 mg every 3 to 4 weeks). Men with pituitary disease may have their infertility treated with FSH and human chorionic gonadotropin (hCG) therapy. If hypothalamic dysfunction is present, pulsatile GnRH therapy has been useful in achieving fertility.

For women, estrogen can be given in the form of ethinyl estradiol 5 to 20 μg/day or as Premarin (conjugated estrogens) 0.625 to 1.25 mg/day. In order to create cyclic bleeding, the estrogen compound is given for 25 days accompanied by a progestational agent for the last 10 to 13 days. Both hormones are then withdrawn

for 5 days to induce endometrial shedding. Women with pituitary disease may have fertility restored with combined gonadotropin preparations. If hypothalamic damage is present, clomiphene or chronic pulsatile GnRH therapy may induce ovulation.

PITUITARY TUMORS AND OTHER CAUSES OF ENLARGED SELLA TURCICA

The pituitary gland may be affected by the growth of an intrinsic pituitary mass (pituitary tumor or craniopharyngioma) or as a result of parasellar masses or tumors. Pituitary lesions (Table 14.2–10) can cause varying degrees of hypopituitarism, local neurologic abnormalities, and pituitary hormone hypersecretion.

Evaluation

Evaluation of pituitary mass lesions is necessary to (1) differentiate a pituitary tumor from parasellar disease, (2) assess tumor size and extent of local invasion, and (3) characterize possible associated hormonal abnormalities. Pituitary function testing is essential in the initial evaluation of a sellar lesion and is of particular importance after surgery or radiotherapy in documenting the necessity for hormonal replacement therapy. Computed tomographic technology with high-resolution imaging permits assessment of suprasellar extension of tumors, identification of microadenomas (tumors < 10 mm), and differentiation of an empty sella from a sellar mass. When an aneurysm is considered in the differential diagnosis, digital subtraction angiography or carotid angiography may be required. Magnetic resonance imaging may play an increasing role in sellar imaging. Finally, patients with a pituitary tumor should have formal visual field evaluation by Goldmann perimetry, which can be used serially to document responses to therapeutic intervention.

Craniopharyngioma

Craniopharyngiomas are squamous cell tumors thought to be derived from remnants of Rathke pouch. These tumors usually originate in the upper portion of the pituitary stalk and can extend down into the sella and upward toward the hypothalamus. Although the peak incidence of the disorder is the second decade of life, craniopharyngiomas are commonly recognized during adulthood. These tumors tend to be cystic, and in approximately two thirds of children and one third of adults are visible on routine radiographs of the skull because of calcifications within the mass.

Empty Sella Syndrome

The empty sella syndrome is a nontumorous enlargement of the sella that must be differentiated from a pituitary mass. The syndrome is thought to be initiated by a small arachnoid diverticulum that passes through the diaphragma sellae together with the pituitary stalk and allows CSF to enter the sella. The chronic pressure expands the sella and compresses the pituitary against the posterior sellar wall. Ninety percent of patients with empty sella syndrome

---

TABLE 14.2–10. CAUSES OF AN ENLARGED SELLA TURCICA

- Pituitary tumors
   Secretory
   Nonsecretory
- Craniopharyngioma
- Empty sella syndrome
- Aneurysm
- CNS tumors (e.g., meningioma)
- Metastatic tumors (e.g., breast cancer)
- Hypothalamic hamartoma
- Pituitary abscess
- Granulomatous disease (e.g., sarcoidosis)
- Primary hypothyroidism
- Primary gonadal failure

are women. Most patients are asymptomatic, although headaches may be present. The syndrome is most commonly seen in obese women and can be associated with pseudotumor cerebri and CSF rhinorrhea. On routine radiographs the sella is symmetrically enlarged, and focal erosions are generally not present. Endocrine abnormalities are rare despite pituitary compression. The diagnosis can usually be established by pituitary CT scanning. On occasion, metrizamide cisternography must be performed for definitive diagnosis. No treatment is necessary unless CSF rhinorrhea or pseudotumor cerebri is present. A partially empty sella is occasionally seen in association with past or present evidence of a pituitary tumor (e.g., acromegaly), presumably representing previous asymptomatic infarction of the tumor.

Nonsecretory Pituitary Adenomas

Pituitary tumors arise from the anterior lobe and account for 10 percent of all intracranial tumors. Nonsecretory tumors, that is, tumors without immunohistochemical staining for any of the six anterior pituitary hormones, comprise 20 percent of all pituitary adenomas. The incidence of nonsecretory pituitary tumors peaks in the fourth and fifth decades with males and females equally affected. Tumors may be large enough to cause compressive symtoms (e.g., visual field abnormalities) but usually are small and clinically silent. In 25 to 30 percent of people without known pituitary disease, a small adenoma is discovered at autopsy. Rarely, patients have pituitary adenomas associated with the multiple endocrine neoplasia syndrome, type I (MEN I), an autosomal dominant disorder including adenomas of the pituitary, parathyroids, and pancreas (see Chapter 14.1). MEN I patients can also develop secretory pituitary tumors.

Signs and Symptoms. The clinical features of nonsecretory pituitary adenomas are solely due to tumor expansion producing local neurologic damage and hypopituitarism. The signs and symptoms produced by the expanding tumor are related to the anatomical relationship of the sella turcica to nearby structures. Pituitary tumor growth generally takes the path of least resistance: the tumor extends superiorly with pressure on the diaphragma sellae and traction on nearby blood vessels, causing headache. The headache is usually dull with no characteristic distribution, is not associated with nausea or visual aura, and can usually be relieved by analgesics. Continued expansion of the tumor superiorly can compress the optic chiasm. Initially this may produce a unilateral or bilateral superior temporal field-cut with progression to bitemporal hemianopsia, amblyopia, optic atrophy, and permanent blindness. Further tumor growth rarely leads to hypothalamic damage and possible irregularities in thermal regulation, eating and sleeping patterns, and emotional behavior. If the third ventricle is compressed, hydrocephalus can develop. If the tumor expands inferiorly, it will erode through the sellar floor and enter the sphenoid sinus; an apparent "sinus" headache and CSF rhinorrhea may develop. Lateral extension of the tumor may damage structures contained within the cavernous sinus. Ophthalmoplegia and diplopia can develop if the third, fourth, or sixth cranial nerves are injured. The expanding adenoma can also seriously damage the normal pituitary gland, and varying degrees of hypopituitarism will ensue.

When the tumor expands rapidly, pituitary hemorrhage occurs. Known as *pituitary apoplexy,* this syndrome is heralded by sudden onset of severe headache, often associated with visual field defects or blindness, ophthalmoplegia, and signs of subarachnoid irritation. The CSF may be bloody, and a large suprasellar mass is seen on CT scan. Significant hypopituitarism can develop. If ACTH and TSH deficiencies go unrecognized, stupor, hypotension, and hypothermia can appear within days or weeks. In most patients, surgical evacuation of the sellar contents is essential for decompression of the mass and restoration of visual function. Glucocorticoid coverage is mandatory in such patients until secondary adrenal insufficiency has been ruled out.

Treatment. Treatment of pituitary tumors is indicated to limit or prevent extrasellar expansion and hypopituitarism. Pituitary surgery through the nasal cavity and sphenoid sinus (transsphenoidal route) is the current approach. Only rarely, when significant suprasellar extension is present, is a transfrontal approach required. Adrenal insufficiency and hypothyroidism, if present, should be corrected before surgery. The operative mortality is less than 1 percent; major complications are rare but include diabetes insipidus, CSF rhinorrhea, and wound infection.

Adjunctive radiation therapy is generally employed because total tumor removal is usually not possible. Radiation therapy can also be used as the primary therapy in patients at high operative risk. Because of delayed treatment effects, radiation is a less attractive initial form of therapy. It is also not the initial mode of therapy when visual field defects are present because postirradiation edema can worsen vision. There are two forms of radiation therapy, conventional high-energy (supravoltage) or heavy particle (proton beam). Supravoltage therapy is widely available. During this treatment, 4500 to 5000 rad are delivered to the pituitary over a 5-week period. Varying degrees of hypopituitarism may occur 6 months to 10 years after therapy in 20 to 50 percent of patients. Currently, there is no effective pharmacologic treatment for nonsecretory pituitary tumors.

HORMONE-SECRETING PITUITARY TUMORS

In addition to causing neurologic defects and hypopituitarism, 80 percent of pituitary tumors secrete an excess of one or more of the anterior pituitary hormones.

Prolactin-secreting Pituitary Tumors

Prolactinomas are the most frequently occurring secretory pituitary tumors (60 to 70 percent). Hyperprolactinemia and its clinical consequences may be seen in a number of disorders (Table 14.2–4) but is most often due to a pituitary tumor. Pituitary tumors arbitrarily are referred to as macroadenomas if by CT scan their size is greater than 10 mm, and microadenomas if less than 10 mm. The vast majority of prolactin-secreting tumors are microadenomas. Hyperprolactinemia without radiologic evidence for tumor and no other identifiable cause for excess prolactin secretion is common and is referred to as "idiopathic hyperprolactinemia." Microadenomas and idiopathic hyperprolactinemia may represent different stages of the same disease. These tumors are most frequently recognized in women between 20 and 35 years of age.

Signs and Symptoms. In women, hyperprolactinemia may cause galactorrhea, amenorrhea, oligomenorrhea or other menstrual disturbances, and infertility. Secondary amenorrhea is most often the presenting complaint, and 15 to 20 percent of all patients with this problem will be found to have hyperprolactinemia. Menstrual irregularities are thought to result from increased hypothalamic dopaminergic tone that interferes with normal pulsatile GnRH secretion. Consequent hypoestrogenemia may cause diminished libido, hot flushes, decreased vaginal secretions, and dyspareunia. Mild hirsutism in association with increased adrenal androgen production has been observed as well. Galactorrhea is present in 50 to 80 percent of hyperprolactinemic patients; it is defined as milk secretion occurring at a time other than the postpartum period. Its absence does not exclude hyperprolactinemia, and the severity of galactorrhea does not correlate with serum prolactin levels. Furthermore, many women with galactorrhea in the absence of amenorrhea do not have hyperprolactinemia: such normoprolactinemic galactorrhea is common in parous women and is not indicative of an endocrine disorder. The physical examination in hyperprolactinemic women is characterized by galactorrhea, demonstrated by massaging the outer areolar region centrally toward the nipple. True galactorrheal discharge is lactescent or opalescent; in doubtful cases the fluid should be Sudan-stained for fat droplets.

Prolactinomas in men appear most often in the fifth to sixth decade and are usually macroadenomas associated with headaches and visual field defects. As in women, a defect in GnRH secretion causes chemical and clinical hypogonadism. Because men often

have large tumors, actual destruction of gonadotrophs can also be the cause of hypogonadism. Men with hyperprolactinemia will usually complain of loss of libido, impotence, and infertility. Galactorrhea is rare in men, even in those who have very high serum prolactin levels. Gynecomastia may be present and is indicative of a hypogonadal state.

Approach to Diagnosis. Determination of the serum prolactin concentration is central to the differential diagnosis in patients with menstrual disorders, galactorrhea, infertility, or hypogonadal symptoms (decreased libido, impotence). Hyperprolactinemia is not necessarily indicative of a prolactin-secreting pituitary tumor. Pregnancy, hypothyroidism, drug-induced hyperprolactinemia, and other causes of hyperprolactinemia (Table 14.2–4) must also be considered. The basal prolactin level may be helpful in the differential diagnosis; mild hyperprolactinemia is often seen in patients with large nonsecretory pituitary tumors secondary to stalk compression. Prolactin levels less than 150 ng/ml are of little use in distinguishing among the various causes of hyperprolactinemia, whereas levels greater than 150 ng/ml are almost always indicative of a prolactin-secreting pituitary tumor. Indeed, the prolactin level correlates well with tumor size. In general, patients with prolactin tumors will have a blunted serum prolactin response to TRH, while patients with nontumorous hyperprolactinemia will usually demonstrate greater than a twofold increase. This distinction is not uniformly reliable and the test is seldom employed in the differential diagnosis of hyperprolactinemia.

If the prolactin level is elevated in the absence of any identifiable nonpituitary cause for hyperprolactinemia, a high-resolution CT scan should be obtained. This will often reveal a pituitary tumor and determine its size. Unless the tumor is a macroadenoma, detailed testing for hypopituitarism is not necessary; patients with microadenomas almost always have normal pituitary function.

Treatment of Prolactin-secreting Microadenomas. The dopamine agonist bromocriptine is used in the treatment of hyperprolactinemic disorders.[10] It rapidly lowers the serum prolactin level, restores reproductive function, reverses galactorrhea, and shrinks the majority of prolactin-secreting tumors. For the patient with idiopathic hyperprolactinemia or a microadenoma, bromocriptine is usually all that is required. Better therapeutic results (normalization of prolactin levels and reversal of symptoms) will not be obtained by surgical intervention or radiation therapy. Most patients require small doses (2.5 to 7.5 mg/day). Therapy should begin with 1.25 mg at bedtime to minimize side effects, which include nausea, dizziness from postural hypotension, headache, and nasal congestion. Hyperprolactinemia and tumor regrowth usually follow discontinuation of bromocriptine, and long-term therapy may be required. Spontaneous remission occurs in 10 percent of patients with hyperprolactinemic microadenoma. Thus, the dose should be tapered periodically in order to identify such patients.

Treatment for Macroadenomas. In more than two thirds of patients with prolactin-secreting macroadenomas, bromocriptine will reduce tumor size by 50 to 75 percent within 6 months of therapy. It is, therefore, reasonable to initiate pharmacologic therapy in patients with macroadenomas, even when visual field defects are present. If significant tumor shrinkage occurs and neurologic deficits are corrected, bromocriptine treatment can be continued indefinitely. The patient must be followed for evidence of tumor regrowth. Tumor enlargement can occur with therapy despite decreasing serum prolactin levels. Careful monitoring with CT scans and visual field assessments, therefore, is essential.

For the macroadenoma unresponsive to bromocriptine, transsphenoidal surgery can reduce tumor mass and correct visual field abnormalities. Because surgery is not usually followed by permanent normalization of prolactin levels, bromocriptine may need to be continued postoperatively. Radiation therapy is relatively ineffective and slow in normalizing prolactin levels.

Prolactin Tumors and Pregnancy. Bromocriptine alone usually restores fertility in women with prolactinomas, regardless of size. Prolactin-secreting tumors may enlarge, however, during a subsequent pregnancy, under the influence of placental estrogens. Consequently, visual field deficits, headache, and diabetes insipidus occur in 15 to 20 percent of pregnant women with macroadenomas and in <5 percent of women with microadenomas. These complications are rapidly reversible with reinstitution of bromocriptine, which is then continued through term. There is no current evidence that bromocriptine is teratogenic. Prophylactic radiation therapy or surgery before induction of pregnancy has been advocated to avoid complications in macroadenoma patients. Women with microadenomas who become pregnant rarely develop problems and require no special prophylactic therapy. All women with prolactinomas should be followed closely throughout pregnancy and monitored expectantly for symptoms and signs of tumor expansion.

Growth Hormone-secreting Tumors: Acromegaly

The most common cause of acromegaly is a growth hormone-secreting pituitary tumor. A subset of these tumors may be due to hypothalamic dysfunction (ectopic GRH secretion) rather than an intrinsic pituitary abnormality. Rarely, this syndrome may be caused by carcinoid tumors, which ectopically produce GRH, leading to pituitary somatotroph hyperplasia.[9] If GH excess occurs before the completion of puberty, gigantism develops. After epiphyseal closure, excess GH increases only periosteal bone growth. In the adult, it is the resulting enlargement of bones and soft tissue—especially facial features, hands, and feet—that characterizes acromegaly.

Signs and Symptoms. The onset of signs and symptoms of GH hypersecretion are insidious and may be present for 1 to 2 decades before recognition. The patient and close associates may not be aware of the slow emergence of acral enlargement. The presenting symptoms are most often related to (1) physical changes—skeletal, soft tissue, visceral, or skin—produced by GH excess, (2) metabolic abnormalities resulting from GH excess, and (3) neurologic defects caused by an expanding sellar mass, especially visual field defects.

Symptoms of acromegaly include fatigue, excessive sweating, and weakness. Soft-tissue swelling leads to the characteristic changes in facial features (nose, ear lobes, lips, tongue) and fleshy, spade-like enlargement of hands and feet. The patient may complain of increasing shoe, glove, hat, and ring size. The skin becomes thickened and coarse with sebaceous cyst formation and papillomas (skin tags). Mandibular growth results in prognathism and overbite, and maxillary growth produces a widened jaw and separation of the teeth. As a consequence, patients may develop increasing dental caries and temporomandibular joint dysfunction. Hypertrophy of the frontal sinuses leads to frontal bossing. Laryngeal cartilage growth and a thickened tongue can cause sleep apnea and make tracheal intubation difficult. Vocal cord and sinus hypertrophy deepen the voice. Connective tissue growth may lead to nerve entrapments, especially carpal tunnel syndrome. Thickening of synovial membranes and articular cartilage may cause arthralgias and degenerative arthritis.

Excess GH causes enlargement of many visceral organs, including the thyroid, heart, kidneys, lungs, colon, liver, spleen, and gonads. Although the incidence of cardiomegaly, hypertension, and heart failure is increased in acromegaly, the existence of a specific acromegalic cardiomyopathy is controversial. Electrocardiographic abnormalities may include left ventricular hypertrophy, conduction defects, and ectopic ventricular beats. Thyroid enlargement with nodule formation is common, but thyroid function is usually normal. Colonic polyps and carcinomas are more common in acromegalic patients.

Metabolic Abnormalities. Chemical glucose intolerance is seen in 50 percent of acromegalics, and frank diabetes mellitus occurs in 20 to 30 percent of patients. Diabetic microangiopathy is uncommon, however, even in longstanding acromegaly. Excess GH increases

renal tubular phosphate absorption resulting in hyperphosphatemia, and an increase in intestinal calcium absorption leads to hypercalciuria. Hypercalcemia should suggest the possibility of MEN-I. Hyperprolactinemia, caused by mixed prolactin-GH secreting tumors, is seen in 20 to 30 percent of acromegalics and can cause galactorrhea and menstrual disturbances in women and loss of libido and impotence in men.

Diagnosis. Once acromegaly is suspected on clinical grounds, serial review of old photographs may reveal the slow emergence of acromegalic features. A markedly elevated basal serum GH concentration is seen in many acromegalic adults, but because GH is episodically secreted in both normal subjects and acromegalics, a single basal GH sample is often nonspecific, particularly in children and young adults. The oral glucose suppression test is the simplest and most reliable provocative test. A serum GH concentration greater than 5 ng/ml 1 hour after the administration of 75 g of oral glucose confirms the presence of autonomous GH secretion, whereas normal subjects will suppress serum GH below this level (Table 14.2–11).

The TRH test can also be useful, because 70 to 80 percent of acromegalics display a paradoxical elevation in serum GH following TRH, whereas normal subjects do not respond. The TRH test is useful if glucose administration gives ambiguous results or when assessing potential cure following surgery or radiotherapy. Plasma somatomedin-C levels are generally elevated in acromegalics, even when basal GH values are at the upper limit of the normal range, and may correlate better with disease activity than basal GH measurements. Somatomedin-C may also prove to be a reliable screening test for the diagnosis of acromegaly.

Cranial CT scanning demonstrates a pituitary tumor in most acromegalics. In one half of patients the tumor is confined to the sella, while one third will present with evidence of suprasellar extension.

Therapy. Surgery, radiotherapy, and pharmacologic treatment all have a role in therapy for the acromegalic patient and are often employed in combination. Assessment and management of hypopituitarism and neurologic deficits are similar to those described for nonsecretory pituitary tumors. Cure of acromegaly is defined by (1) cessation of progressive clinical features, (2) normalization of basal GH and somatomedin-C levels, (3) suppression of GH by glucose, and (4) disappearance of a paradoxical GH response to TRH.

The results of transsphenoidal surgery depend on tumor size and GH levels. GH levels may return to normal in 70 to 90 percent of patients with small tumors, but surgical cure is seldom achieved if the tumor is greater than 2 cm in diameter or the GH level is greater than 100 ng/ml. Radiotherapy gradually reduces GH levels to normal over 1 to 10 years. Radiotherapy is indicated after surgery or when surgery is contraindicated.

Bromocriptine reduces GH levels in up to 70 percent of acromegalics but will normalize GH levels in only 15 to 20 percent. Only a small percentage (10 to 20 percent) of acromegalic patients will have tumor shrinkage with bromocriptine. To achieve these results, doses up to 60 mg per day may be required, and side effects

are frequent. Bromocriptine plays only an adjunctive role, therefore, and is most useful when given temporarily after operative or primary radiation therapy. The promising role of somatostatin analogues for controlling GH secretion and tumor size is under investigation.[5] In any patient with acromegaly, consideration should be given to the rare situation in which the disease is caused by ectopic GRH secretion, usually by a carcinoid tumor. Plasma GRH levels are elevated in this situation, and therapy should be directed toward the primary tumor rather than the pituitary gland.

ACTH-secreting Tumors: Cushing Disease

Cushing disease is hypercortisolism caused by semiautonomous ACTH secretion by a pituitary tumor, in most cases a microadenoma.[7] Cushing disease accounts for 80 percent of endogenous cases of hypercortisolism, is more common in females, and usually affects individuals 20 to 40 years of age. Rarely, hypothalamic CRH hypersecretion and tumors secreting CRH ectopically may induce corticotroph hyperplasia and Cushing disease.

Signs and Symptoms. Details of the clinical presentation are discussed in Chapter 14.3. Like all patients with hypercortisolism, patients with Cushing disease may develop truncal obesity; moon facies with plethora; pigmented striae; hirsutism; acne; menstrual irregularities; a dorsal fat pad; and thin, easily bruised skin. Mental status changes are frequent, including depression and psychotic symptoms. Prolonged hypercortisolism can cause proximal muscle wasting, diabetes mellitus, hypertension, and osteoporosis.

Diagnosis. The diagnostic assessment of Cushing disease is discussed in Chapter 14.3. The presence of hypercortisolism must first be established and then pituitary-dependent hypercortisolism distinguished from other diseases that result in excess cortisol secretion. Measurement of 24-hour urinary free cortisol (UFC) is the most reliable screening test for patients suspected of having hypercortisolism. If the 24-hour UFC is elevated ($>125 \mu g/24$ hour), dexamethasone suppression testing is performed. Normal subjects receiving low-dose dexamethasone (2 mg/day for 2 days) will suppress serum cortisol below 5 $\mu g/dl$, urine 17-hydroxycorticosteroids below 3 mg/24 hour (or UFC $<20 \mu g/24$ hour), whereas patients with hypercortisolism will not. Patients with pituitary-dependent hypercortisolism will suppress urinary 17-hydroxycorticosteroids or plasma cortisol by at least 50 percent with high-dose dexamethasone (8 mg/day for 2 days). In contrast, even high-dose dexamethasone will not suppress cortisol secretion if it is the result of an adrenal tumor secreting excess cortisol, or more commonly, a tumor secreting ACTH ectopically. On occasion, further studies are needed to distinguish pituitary-dependent Cushing disease from nonpituitary hypercortisolism. Patients with pituitary-dependent hypercortisolism usually demonstrate an exaggerated ACTH response to exogenous CRH administration, whereas adrenal or ectopic Cushing patients display no ACTH response after receiving CRH. In difficult cases, selective venous sampling of both inferior petrosal sinuses can demonstrate a central ACTH gradient in patients with an ACTH-secreting pituitary adenoma and thus secure the diagnosis. Such sampling can also assist in localizing the tumor within the pituitary gland. Unfortunately, even high-resolution cranial CT scanning will not reveal 60 to 70 percent of ACTH-secreting microadenomas.

Therapy. Transsphenoidal surgery is the most effective treatment for Cushing disease, with high cure rates (85 to 95 percent) in expert hands. Although bilateral adrenalectomy is virtually always curative, it is associated with higher morbidity and the potential for inducing Nelson syndrome. The normalization of serum cortisol levels by bilateral adrenalectomy apparently unleashes the growth potential of the ACTH-secreting tumor in about 10 percent of cases. The resulting Nelson syndrome is characterized by rapid expansion of the pituitary tumor, high plasma ACTH levels (often greater than 1000 pg/ml), and progressive hyperpigmentation. These tumors are aggressive and often difficult to treat.[6]

TABLE 14.2–11. GROWTH HORMONE RESPONSES IN ACROMEGALY AND NORMALS

Test	Acromegaly	Normal
Glucose (75 g PO)	Moderate decrease (>5 ng/ml) Unchanged Paradoxical rise	GH <5 ng/ml
TRH	Increase in GH (70–80%)	No response
Dopamine agonists	Decrease in GH (60–70%)	Increase in GH

Radiotherapy is a valuable treatment for Cushing disease in children, with cure in 80 percent. In adults, a lower cure rate of 20 to 60 percent and a slow response make radiotherapy a less acceptable primary therapy.

Pharmacologic managment of Cushing disease can block adrenal steroidogenesis or inhibit ACTH secretion. Metyrapone, aminoglutethamide, trilostane, and ketoconazole all decrease cortisol secretion by blocking cortisol biosynthesis. Although these drugs are not routinely used for primary treatment of Cushing disease, they can be administered to patients who are not able to tolerate immediate surgical therapy, or they can be coupled with radiotherapy. The serotonin antagonist cyproheptadine, the dopamine agonist bromocriptine, and the γ-aminobutyric acid (GABA) agonist valproate sodium have all ameliorated the clinical and chemical manifestations of Cushing disease in some patients, presumably by inhibiting ACTH secretion directly or by affecting hypothalamic neurotransmitter function. Response rates are low, 5 to 10 percent, and remissions are rarely sustained.

Glycoprotein Hormone-secreting Pituitary Tumors

Pituitary tumors uncommonly produce the glycoprotein hormones (TSH, LH, FSH, or alpha subunit).[8] The exact prevalence is unknown, but pituitary adenomas previously thought to be nonsecreting may have, in fact, produced gonadotropins or the alpha subunit. The frequent absence of specific associated clinical manifestations probably accounts for underestimation of the true frequency of this type of pituitary tumor. Patients with pituitary tumors that secrete TSH have clinical hyperthyroidism, with elevated total and free thyroid hormone levels that are associated with an inappropriately detectable TSH level. These patients may be mistakenly treated for Graves disease. At the time of presentation, these tumors are usually large and have produced visual field abnormalities. Half of TSH-secreting pituitary tumors have also been associated with acromegaly or hyperprolactinemia. These tumors require surgical intervention and often adjunctive radiation therapy. The manifestations of hyperthyroidism must be controlled pharmacologically before surgery.

Gonadotropin-secreting tumors occur mostly in older men, some of whom may have elevated serum testosterone levels, whereas hypogonadism may be present in other cases. In postmenopausal women, the diagnosis is difficult to establish because elevated serum gonadotropin concentrations are expected. Common presenting complaints are headache and visual field defects. These tumors are usually large, with significant suprasellar extension. Surgery followed by adjunctive radiotherapy is usually required.

POSTERIOR PITUITARY

The posterior lobe of the pituitary, or neurohypophysis, secretes the peptide hormones vasopressin (VP) and oxytocin. Unlike anterior pituitary hormones, VP and oxytocin are synthesized in two discrete hypothalamic regions, the supraoptic and paraventricular nuclei. The two hormones are packaged into neurosecretory granules and transported from their hypothalamic sites of synthesis along axons that terminate in the posterior lobe, where they are stored awaiting appropriate signals for secretion into blood. Vasopressin has both antidiuretic and vasopressor activity. In the nipple, oxytocin stimulates periductal smooth muscle contraction, is required for ''milk-let-down,'' and is involved in parturition by stimulating uterine muscle contraction.

Vasopressin regulates renal water excretion by binding to specific receptors on distal renal tubule cells and stimulating cAMP production. This second messenger alters the plasma membrane to increase permeability of the renal tubular cell to water, with consequent concentration of tubular fluid along the renal medullary gradient. Vasopressin secretion is controlled by three principal factors: plasma osmolality, blood volume, and blood pressure. Plasma osmolality is normally confined to a narrow range (285 to 290 mOsm/kg H_2O). Anterior hypothalamic osmoreceptors are exquisitely sensitive to alterations in plasma osmolality. When plasma osmolality rises above 290 mOsm/kg H_2O, the osmoreceptors normally trigger VP secretion. A thirst center located in the anterior hypothalamus assists in control of plasma osmolality. Thirst is stimulated when plasma osmolality exceeds 294 mOsm/kg H_2O. Baroreceptors that sense changes in blood volume and blood pressure by alterations in wall tension in the left atrium and aorta also regulate VP secretion. These receptors are connected to neural pathways that terminate in the hypothalamus. Hypovolemia and hypotension can stimulate VP release, resulting in the production of a concentrated urine and a decrease in the free H_2O clearance, as well as vasoconstriction. A number of other factors regulate VP secretion, including stress, pain, emotional stimuli, and certain drugs (Table 14.2–12). Atrial natriuretic factor, which is produced in the brain as well as the atria, also inhibits VP release.

CENTRAL DIABETES INSIPIDUS

Diabetes insipidus is a polyuric syndrome characterized by the excessive excretion of a dilute urine followed by secondary polydipsia. It can result from either hypothalamic-pituitary or renal pathology. Central diabetes insipidus occurs when the pituitary fails to secrete adequate amounts of VP, which may be the result of a number of disorders (Table 14.2–13). Most cases of central diabetes insipidus are idiopathic, and present with the sudden onset of polyuria and polydipsia. Head trauma, CNS infection, and CNS inflammatory disorders (e.g., sarcoidosis) are less common causes. Primary pituitary disease is rarely the cause of central diabetes insipidus, because the neurohypophysis is merely a VP storage site, whereas VP synthesis occurs in the hypothalamus. The presence of diabetes insipidus accompanying anterior pituitary hormone failure

TABLE 14.2–12. DRUGS AND OTHER FACTORS AFFECTING VASOPRESSIN RELEASE

Stimulation	Inhibition
• Chlorpropamide	• Phenytoin
• Nicotine	• Alcohol
• Clofibrate	• Narcotic antagonists
• Vincristine	• Alpha agonists
• Cyclophosphamide	• Atrial natriuretic factor
• Carbamazepine	
• Barbiturates	
• Opiates	
• Stress	
• Pain	

TABLE 14.2–13. CAUSES OF DIABETES INSIPIDUS

Central	Nephrogenic
• Idiopathic	• Familial
• Postneurosurgical	• Acquired
• Infiltrative disorder (e.g., sarcoidosis)	Sickle cell anemia
	Potassium deficiency
• CNS tumor (e.g., craniopharyngioma)	Hypercalcemia
	Amyloidosis
• Head trauma	Sjögren syndrome
• Familial	Multiple myeloma
• Vascular	• Drugs
• Infectious	Demeclocycline
	Lithium carbonate

suggests that hypothalamic disease may be present. When central diabetes insipidus occurs following transsphenoidal surgery, there is classically a triphasic VP response. Immediately following injury, the neurohypophyseal tract may transiently stop secreting VP for hours or 1 to 3 days with consequent polyuria. The second phase occurs when injured axon terminals degenerate and release VP with resulting oliguria and possible hyponatremia. With death of these neurons, permanent diabetes insipidus may then return in a complete or partial form. In the postoperative setting, polyuria or oliguria secondary to abnormal fluid balance or anesthesia can be difficult to differentiate from abnormalities in hypothalamic VP release.

Differential Diagnosis

Polyuria is not unique to central diabetes insipidus, and other conditions must be considered when a patient presents with complaints of excessive urination and thirst (Table 14.2–14). Nephrogenic diabetes insipidus refers to a group of disorders characterized by renal tubular unresponsiveness to appropriate levels of plasma VP. The condition can be familial or acquired as a result of electrolyte abnormalities (hypokalemia and hypercalcemia), diseases of the renal interstitium that disrupt medullary concentrating mechanisms, or drugs that affect renal tubular function.

Compulsive water drinking (psychogenic polydipsia) is a condition that produces primary polydipsia and secondary polyuria. Chronic ingestion of excess water results in the loss of normal renal medullary hypertonicity, which then impairs urine concentration despite appropriate plasma VP levels. Primary polydipsia is usually diagnosed in young women with known psychiatric disease. Rarely, a neurologic lesion in the hypothalamus will precede this behavior. Polyuria also occurs, of course, in disorders that promote an osmotic diuresis; common causes include hyperglycemia (diabetes mellitus) and diuretic therapy.

Diagnosis

In approaching the patient with polyuria, causes of osmotic diuresis should first be excluded. Then central and nephrogenic diabetes insipidus and primary polydipsia must be differentiated. Pertinent historical and laboratory information can exclude diabetes mellitus, primary renal abnormalities, drugs, electrolyte disturbances, and systemic diseases affecting renal interstitial function (e.g., sickle cell anemia, amyloidosis, multiple myeloma, Sjögren syndrome). In general, patients with true diabetes insipidus (central or nephrogenic) will have elevated fasting overnight plasma osmolality and inappropriately low urine osmolality, while compulsive water drinkers will have a low plasma osmolality.

A water-deprivation test generally is necessary to diagnose diabetes insipidus and distinguish central diabetes insipidus from nephrogenic diabetes insipidus. In the hospital, it is probably safest to do the test during the daytime. Body weight and urine osmolality are measured before and hourly after all liquids are withheld. When urine osmolality plateaus and varies less than 30 mOsm/kg H_2O per hour or when 3 percent or more of body weight is lost, 5 units of aqueous VP are given subcutaneously. Urine osmolality is then determined after 30, 60, and 120 minutes. In response to water deprivation, normal subjects will have a rise in urine osmolality exceeding plasma osmolality by two- to fourfold. Their endogenous VP is maximally stimulated, and no further concentration of urine is seen after exogenous VP is administered. Patients with complete central diabetes insipidus will not have concentrated

urine despite a rise in plasma osmolality to 298 to 320 mOsm/kg H_2O, and their urine osmolality will remain below plasma osmolality. In response to exogenous VP, the urine of patients with complete central diabetes insipidus will increase in osmolality by at least 50 percent. Even in partial central diabetes insipidus, urine osmolality will increase more than 9 percent. Patients with nephrogenic diabetes insipidus will also maintain a dilute urine despite dehydration, but their urine osmolality will not rise above plasma osmolality even when exogenous vasopressin is administered.

Although the water-deprivation test is usually definitive, distinguishing patients with partial diabetes insipidus from those with primary polydipsia may occasionally be difficult. Patients with primary polydipsia often have a diluted renal medullary gradient and their urine does not concentrate in response to dehydration despite maximally stimulated VP secretion. Exogenous VP administration usually results in less than a 5 percent rise in urine osmolality. When uncertainty remains, other features may clarify the diagnosis: (1) Polyuria in primary polydipsia is usually of gradual onset whereas in patients with diabetes insipidus it is sudden. (2) Patients with primary polydipsia usually have a random plasma osmolality below 285 mOsm/kg or dilutional hyponatremia. Patients with diabetes insipidus replace their water losses but usually do not overcompensate. (3) Patients with primary polydipsia may have less significant nocturia whereas patients with diabetes insipidus usually have a constant urine output. Vasopressin radioimmunoassay determination can often resolve the differential diagnosis. Plasma VP levels are normal relative to plasma osmolality in patients with primary polydipsia but are low in patients with central diabetes insipidus.

When central diabetes insipidus is diagnosed, a cranial CT scan should be obtained to examine the hypothalamic and pituitary regions for evidence of a tumor or infiltrative disease of the hypothalamus.

Therapy

In cases of mild diabetes insipidus, treatment may not be necessary as long as patients have an intact thirst mechanism and access to water. If diabetes insipidus is severe and the patient is temporarily deprived of access to water, circulatory collapse and/or hypertonic encephalopathy may rapidly develop. Treatment is usually indicated when urine volumes are greater than 5 L per day.[3]

Vasopressin is the treatment of choice for central diabetes insipidus; several preparations are available (Table 14.2–15). DDAVP (1-desamino-8-D arginine VP) is a long-acting synthetic analogue of VP; its antidiuretic properties are enhanced, and vasopressor activity has been eliminated. The drug is administered by nasal insufflation starting with 5 to 10 μg taken at bedtime. An additional afternoon dose may be required. This compound is also available for subcutaneous administration for use in acute settings, such as after transsphenoidal pituitary surgery. Aqueous VP is a short-acting preparation, which can be administered subcutaneously. It is ideal in the immediate postoperative period for neurosurgically induced diabetes insipidus, but its short half-life limits its usefulness in chronic treatment. Pitressin tannate in oil is a long-acting preparation, which has been largely replaced by DDAVP for three reasons: (1) Careful warming and mixing of the ampule is required to adequately suspend the hormone in oil. (2) Because of variable absorption, timing of administration is more variable; patients can easily be overtreated with this preparation, resulting in dilutional hyponatremia and possible seizures. (3) Sterile abscesses may form at the injection site. Pitressin in oil should not be used in the immediate postoperative period when central diabetes insipidus may be transient.

If patients with partial central diabetes insipidus require treatment, they can often be successfully managed with chlorpropamide, which augments VP release and potentiates its action on the renal tubule. Patients with normal glucose tolerance can usually tolerate the drug in doses up to 250 mg per day without developing symptomatic hypoglycemia. Clofibrate and carbamazepine can also augment VP release but are less often used.

TABLE 14.2–14. COMMON CAUSES OF POLYURIA

- Central diabetes insipidus (see Table 14.2–13)
- Nephrogenic diabetes insipidus
- Primary polydipsia (compulsive water-drinking)
- Osmotic diuresis (diabetes mellitus)

TABLE 14.2–15. POTENCY OF HORMONE PREPARATIONS FOR THE TREATMENT OF DIABETES INSIPIDUS[a]

Drug	Antidiuretic	Pressor	Duration of Action (hr)	Route
Aqueous VP	100	100	2–6	IV or subcutaneous
Lysine-VP	60	70	2–6	Nasal
Pitressin in oil	100	100	24–48	IM
DDAVP	290	0.14	6–20	Nasal or subcutaneous

[a]Relative to aqueous VP equivalent of 100.

SYNDROME OF INAPPROPRIATE VASOPRESSIN SECRETION

Excessive secretion of VP, with the development of hyponatremia and hypo-osmolality, is usually referred to as the syndrome of inappropriate secretion of antidiuretic hormone (SIADH) (Table 14.2–16).[2] In small cell carcinoma of the lung and several other malignancies, ectopic secretion of VP may occur. SIADH also occurs with a wide variety of neurological disorders, pulmonary diseases, and after treatment with a number of drugs. Cardinal features of the syndrome are hyponatremia with serum hypo-osmolality and inappropriately high urine osmolality in the absence of volume depletion, edema, intrinsic renal, adrenal, or thyroid dysfunction. Patients with SIADH usually retain 2 to 5 L of excess water. Few clinical signs may be present if the SIADH is mild. With serum sodium below 130 mEq/L, patients may become anorexic and confused, and experience nausea and muscle cramping. When the serum sodium falls below 115 mEq/L, obtundation, muscle-twitching, seizures, and death may ensue. The severity of symptoms depends on the degree of hypo-osmolality and the rate at which overhydration occurs.

To establish the diagnosis of SIADH, other causes of hyponatremia must be excluded (Table 14.2–17). Pseudohyponatremia may be secondary to hyperlipidemia, or hyperproteinemia. A clinical evaluation should exclude cirrhosis, congestive heart failure, dehydration, drug ingestion, neoplasia, and endocrine, pulmonary, and neurological disorders. On physical examination, patients with SIADH appear euvolemic. If edema is present, congestive heart failure, cirrhosis, or nephrotic syndrome should be considered. Poor skin turgor and postural hypotension suggest volume contraction, which may be due to diuretics, laxatives, vomiting, or adrenal disease. Although it is still uncertain whether hypersecretion of VP is always responsible, patients with glucocorticoid or mineralocorticoid deficiency or hypothyroidism often develop hyponatremia in association with impaired water excretion. Patients with hyponatremia secondary to hypothyroidism are usually severely myxedematous.

In SIADH, urine sodium is generally greater than 20 mEq/L, whereas in states of intravascular volume contraction or decreased effective plasma volume (e.g., congestive heart failure, cirrhosis, nephrotic syndrome) the urine sodium is usually less than 20 mEq/L. The BUN and uric acid are low in SIADH, whereas they are elevated in volume-contracted states. Lastly, in SIADH, the urine osmolality will be less than maximally dilute (50 to 100 mOsm/kg) despite plasma hypo-osmolality, but need not be actually greater than the plasma osmolality.

The aims of therapy for SIADH are to correct the underlying disorder and the hyponatremia. For mild to moderate cases in which the patient is relatively asymptomatic and serum sodium is greater than 115 mEq/L, water restriction to 500 to 1000 ml per day will correct hyponatremia at a rate of approximately 5 mEq/L per day. Dietary sodium chloride (3–5 g per day) will correct the total body sodium deficit, while insensible losses will reduce excess body water. Attempts to correct the hyponatremia with normal saline infusions are ineffective because sodium will promptly be excreted in the urine. For chronic SIADH, demeclocycline 600 to 1200 mg per day will often normalize the serum sodium concentration. Like lithium, demeclocycline inhibits the renal action of VP and produces partial nephrogenic diabetes insipidus. Lithium is rarely used because it is associated with greater toxicity.

TABLE 14.2–16. COMMON CAUSES OF SIADH

CNS disease
- Meningitis-encephalitis
- Head injury
- Brain abscess
- Subarachoid hemorrhage
- Psychosis
- Hydrocephalus

Pulmonary disease
- Abscess
- Pneumonia
- Cavitation
- Tuberculosis
- Positive-pressure breathing

Tumors
- Carcinoma of the bronchus, duodenum, pancreas, prostate
- Thymoma
- Lymphoma

Drugs
- Vincristine
- Chlorpropamide
- Clofibrate
- Carbamazepine
- Nicotine
- Phenothiazine
- Cyclophosphamide

TABLE 14.2–17. MAJOR CAUSES OF HYPONATREMIA

Pseudohyponatremia
- Hyperlipidemia
- Hyperproteinemia

Deficiency of total body sodium
- Addison disease
- Salt-losing nephropathy
- Gastrointestinal loss
- Diuretics

Excessive body water
- SIADH
- Primary polydipsia
- Hypothyroidism

Hyponatremia associated with increased total body sodium
- Congestive heart failure
- Cirrhosis
- Nephrotic syndrome

If the serum sodium falls below 110 mEq/L, or if significant neurologic symptoms are present, more rapid correction of the hyponatremia is indicated. This can be accomplished by administering hypertonic saline (3 to 5 percent). When given as 5 percent saline at the rate of 3 ml/kg per hour, plasma sodium will increase at a rate of 2 percent per hour. If hypertonic saline is used, assiduous attention to the patient's volume status is required to prevent volume overload. The combination of hypertonic saline plus furosemide (40 mg intravenously) may be useful in patients with marginal cardiac reserve and will also correct hyponatremia more rapidly than hypertonic saline alone. Rapid correction to levels greater than 135 mg/L should be avoided, however, because it may be associated with irreversible brain damage (central pontine myelinolysis).

REFERENCES

1. Abbond C: Laboratory diagnosis of hypopituitarism. Mayo Clin Proc 61:35, 1986
2. Bartter F, Schwartz W: The syndrome of inappropriate secretion of antidiuretic hormone. Am J Med 42:790, 1967
3. Cobb W: Management of neurogenic diabetes insipidus with dDAVP and other agents. In Reichlin S (ed): The Neurohypophysis. New York, Plenum, 1984, p 115
4. Cohn R, Bonquier S, et al: Pituitary stimulation by combined administration of four hypothalamic releasing hormones in normal men and patients. J Clin Endocrinol Metab 62:892, 1986
5. Ikuyama S, Nawata H, et al: Plasma growth hormone responses to somatostatin in pituitary adenomas in acromegalic patients. J Clin Endocrinol Metab 62:729, 1986
6. Kasperlik-Zaluska A, Nielubowicz J, et al: Nelson's syndrome: Incidence and prognosis. Clin Endocrinol 19:693, 1983
7. Krieger D: Physiopathology of Cushing's disease. Endocr Rev 4:22, 1983
8. Ridgway EC: Glycoprotein hormone production by pituitary tumors. In Black P, Zervas B, Ridgway EC, Martin J (eds): Secretory Tumors of the Pituitary Gland. New York, Raven Press, 1984, p 343
9. Thorner M, Perryman R, et al: Somatotroph hyperplasia: Successful treatment of acromegaly by removal of a pancreatic islet tumor secreting growth hormone releasing factor. J Clin Invest 70:965, 1982
10. Vance M, Evans W, Thorner M: Bromocriptine. Ann Intern Med 100:78, 1984

CHAPTER 14.3
Disorders of Adrenal Gland

Gary S. Wand and Bruce P. Hamilton

The adrenal glands are paired structures located superomedially to the kidneys. Each gland is composed of a cortex and medulla which are embryologically and functionally distinct. The cortex contains three histological zones. The outermost portion, the zona glomerulosa, secretes aldosterone, the principal mineralocorticoid. Internal to the zona glomerulosa is the zona fasciculata, which produces the glucocorticoid cortisol. Adrenal androgens are synthesized in the innermost layer of the cortex, the zona reticularis (Fig. 14.3–1). The medulla is derived from neural crest cells, which differentiate into chromaffin tissue. These cells are the principal site for epinephrine production.

Clinical adrenal disorders are the result of excess or insufficient hormone production as well as specific enzyme deficiencies leading to aberrant patterns of steroid synthesis. Accurate clinical and laboratory diagnosis is essential to distinguish these relatively unusual disorders from more common conditions with which they may be confused.

DYNAMICS OF HYPOTHALAMIC-PITUITARY-ADRENAL AXIS

Adrenal cortisol secretion is stimulated by pituitary ACTH which is in turn under the control of hypothalamic corticotropin-releasing hormone (CRH). Cortisol feeds back on the pituitary and hypothalamus to inhibit secretion of ACTH and CRH.

CRH, a 41-amino-acid peptide, is a potent stimulator of ACTH secretion.[1] Although CRH is found throughout the central nervous system (CNS), only the CRH synthesized in the paraventricular nucleus of the hypothalamus is involved in ACTH regulation. After neural stimulation, CRH is secreted into the pituitary portal circulation and transported to specific receptors on the corticotroph (ACTH-secreting cell) membrane. Acting through the second messenger, cyclic AMP, CRH stimulates both the synthesis and secretion of pituitary ACTH.

ACTH is a 39-amino-acid, single-chain peptide synthesized as part of a larger precursor molecule referred to as pro-ACTH/ endorphin or pro-opiomelanocortin (POMC) see Chapter 14.2. In healthy individuals, plasma levels of ACTH range from less than 10 pg/ml to approximately 80 pg/ml. ACTH secretion displays a distinct diurnal pattern; lowest levels occur around midnight while peak values occur early in the morning (5 to 8 AM) about the time of awakening. After a short lag period, plasma cortisol follows the ACTH rhythm closely.

In addition to the normal diurnal fluctuation in ACTH and cortisol secretion, the hypothalamic-pituitary-adrenocortical (HPA) axis is activated by stress, for example, hypotension, acute infection, surgical or accidental trauma, and psychic stress. During such stress, plasma ACTH values can increase tenfold and override negative feedback by cortisol. CRH, in combination with vasopressin, catecholamines and other secretogogues, may have a synergistic role in the stress-mediated release of ACTH.

SYNTHESIS, AND ACTION OF ADRENAL STEROIDS

The pathway for the synthesis of adrenal steroids begins with cholesterol. A series of enzymatic steps converts cholesterol into steroids with glucocorticoid, mineralocorticoid, or androgen activity (Fig. 14.3–1). Specific inherited enzyme deficiencies result in the aberrant synthesis of cortisol, aldosterone, and adrenal androgens.

Cortisol (hydrocortisone), the major glucocorticoid in humans, has important metabolic effects on most body tissue. Cortisol has potent gluconeogenic action and is an important regulator of intermediary fuel metabolism. In addition, cortisol has effects on calcium metabolism, renal water excretion, CNS function, inflammatory processes, and immune responses.

The normal cortisol production rate ranges from 10 to 25 mg per day and is related to body mass; obese subjects have elevated rates of cortisol production and degradation but normal plasma cortisol values. Approximately 90 percent of secreted cortisol is bound by plasma proteins, principally corticosteroid-binding glob-

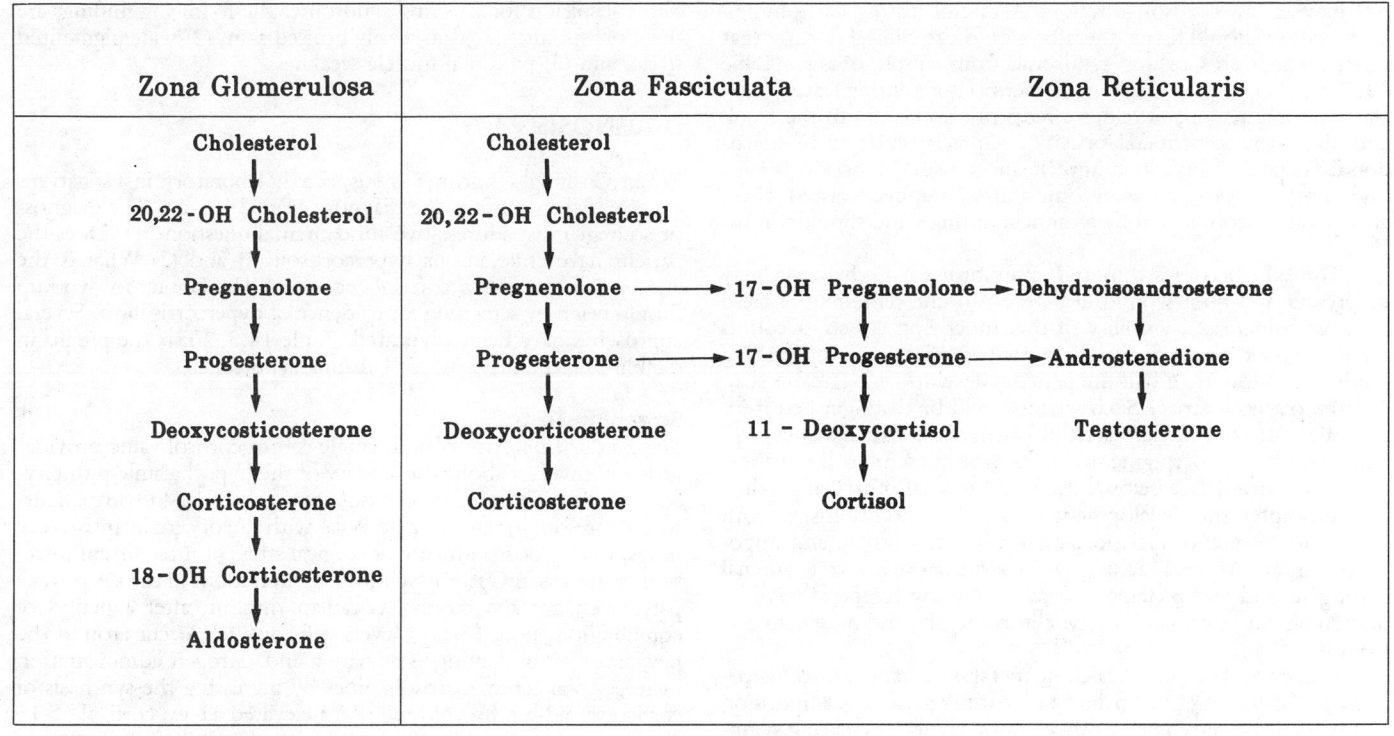

Figure 14.3–1. Outline of synthetic pathways for glucocorticoids, mineralocorticoids, and adrenal androgens. Because pregnenolone is a common precursor for all three classes, relative or absolute blockade of one pathway results in overflow synthesis of the other adrenal steroids.

ulin. Only the free or unbound fraction of plasma cortisol is physiologically active.

The adrenal cortex also synthesizes androgenic steroids, dehydroepiandrosterone sulfate (DHEA-S) and androstenedione. Although DHEA-S and androstenedione have low intrinsic androgen activity, they are converted to testosterone or estradiol in the periphery. Thus, these adrenocortical precursors are the major sources for the minor sex steroids in both sexes, testosterone in women and estradiol in men. In women, conversion of androstenedione to testosterone accounts for 60 percent of total testosterone production, whereas in men, only 5 percent of testosterone is from extratesticular sources. Adipose tissue and muscle aromatize this androstenedione to estradiol. This is the principal route of estrogen production in postmenopausal women and in men. Although ACTH can stimulate adrenal androgen production, the exact mechanism underlying physiologic control of adrenal androgen secretion has not been established.

Aldosterone, the principal mineralocorticoid, plays an important role in sodium and potassium homeostasis. Deoxycorticosterone is a weaker mineralocorticoid that can have physiologic significance when secreted in excessive amounts. The renin-angiotensin system is the major regulator of aldosterone secretion. In addition, ACTH, hyperkalemia, and hyponatremia can also stimulate the glomerulosa cell to produce aldosterone. The major effects of aldosterone are on the distal tubule of the nephron, where it promotes sodium reabsorption and potassium excretion.

CUSHING SYNDROME: HYPERCORTISOLISM

The clinical manifestations of chronic cortisol excess are referred to as Cushing syndrome. Administration of exogenous glucocorticoids to treat nonendocrine disease is now the most frequent cause (iatrogenic Cushing syndrome). Spontaneous Cushing syndrome, from the overproduction of endogenous cortisol, occurs in three distinct pathogenetic states: excessive pituitary ACTH secretion (Cushing disease), autonomous cortisol production by benign or malignant adrenal tumors, and ectopic production of ACTH by a variety of extrahypophyseal neoplasms.

Pituitary Cushing disease accounts for about two thirds of all cases of endogenous hypercortisolism. The vast majority (90 percent) of patients are premenopausal women. Cushing disease is usually caused by an ACTH-secreting pituitary adenoma, which is less responsive than the normal pituitary to negative feedback by cortisol. Most of these tumors are small (several millimeters in diameter), and approximately 70 percent cannot be identified even by cranial computerized tomography (CT). A small percentage of patients with Cushing disease secrete excessive amounts of hypothalamic or ectopic CRH; the resulting chronic stimulation of corticotrophs may lead to the secondary development of a microadenoma.

Adrenal tumors account for 25 percent of the cases of Cushing syndrome. The tumor may be an adenoma and is usually single and surrounded by a narrow rim of atrophic cortical tissue; the contralateral gland is atrophic. Malignant tumors are less frequent. Adrenal carcinomas are aggressive with a tendency to invade the adrenal vasculature and metastasize to the liver and lung. Adrenal cancer is often associated with excessive secretion of both cortisol and adrenal androgens.

In 15 percent of cases, Cushing syndrome is due to ectopic production of ACTH by neoplasms arising in organs other than the pituitary gland. Tumors commonly associated with this syndrome are small cell carcinoma of the lung, islet cell tumors of the pancreas, medullary carcinoma of the thyroid, pheochromocytoma, and thymic carcinoma; less commonly the syndrome has been associated with a wide variety of other tumor types.

CLINICAL FEATURES

The presentation of a patient with hypertension, obesity, and diabetes mellitus should raise suspicion of Cushing syndrome. This triad, however, appears more frequently in obese patients who do

not have excess cortisol secretion. A careful history and physical examination should focus, therefore, on those clinical features that often distinguish Cushing syndrome from simple obesity (Table 14.3–1). Weight gain is the most common presenting feature, and classically the patient develops a redistribution of fat to the trunk and abdomen (centripetal obesity), supraclavicular and cervicodorsal fat pads ("buffalo hump"), and a round ("moon") face. Over time the extremities become thin and appear wasted; these changes are accompanied by weakness of thigh and shoulder muscles.

The skin becomes thin and easily bruised. Ecchymoses may be present and poor wound healing can occur. Thinning of facial skin, with increased visibility of the underlying vessels, accounts for the red or plethoric facial appearance often seen in Cushing syndrome. More than half the patients develop wide (greater than 1 cm) violaceous striae. Such striae should be distinguished from the paler "stretch marks" seen in other obese patients and pregnant women. Hyperpigmentation can be present in the ectopic ACTH syndrome (see below). Increased adrenal androgen production promotes the development of acne and folliculitis in both sexes, hirsutism and oligo- or amenorrhea in women, and impotency in men. Adrenal carcinomas in particular may secrete adrenal androgens and virilize female patients, causing temporal balding, deepening voice, breast atrophy, clitoromegaly, and muscle hypertrophy.

Excess cortisol alters calcium metabolism and causes osteoporosis. Bone and back pain from pathological or compression fractures of the vertebrae or other bones may be presenting symptoms. Enhanced calcium mobilization from bone causes hypercalciuria and an increased incidence of renal calculi. Children with Cushing syndrome exhibit early closure of epiphyseal plates and a marked diminution in linear growth. Enhanced gluconeogenesis from hypercortisolism may cause diabetes mellitus or worsen preexisting disease. Accompanying hypersecretion of mineralocorticoids can produce hypertension, peripheral edema, and hypokalemia. Potassium-wasting is particularly common in the ectopic ACTH syndrome (see below).

Approximately two thirds of patients with Cushing syndrome have reversible psychiatric manifestations ranging from emotional lability to frank psychoses. An agitated depression is most common.

Although many signs and symptoms should arouse the clini-

cian's suspicion for Cushing syndrome, the following findings are the most specific: (1) thin, easily bruised skin, (2) wide pigmented striae, and (3) proximal muscle weakness.

DIAGNOSIS

When Cushing syndrome is suspected, laboratory investigations are essential to confirm the diagnosis (Fig. 14.3–2).[5] The diagnostic strategy must address two fundamental questions: (1) Does the patient have endogenous hypercortisolism? and (2) What is the etiology of the excess cortisol secretion? The laboratory workup should begin by screening for evidence of hypercortisolism. Several approaches have been advocated. Table 14.3–2 lists the pitfalls in establishing the diagnosis of Cushing syndrome.

Screening Tests

Plasma Cortisol. An isolated, single serum cortisol value provides little information about the activity of the hypothalamic-pituitary-adrenal axis. The diurnal cortisol rhythm can be lost in patients with depression or anorexia nervosa, with use of certain antiseizure drugs, during posttraumatic or surgical stress or intercurrent infection, as well as in Cushing syndrome. Alterations in the sleep-wake pattern change the cortisol circadian rhythm; after a period of equilibration, peak cortisol levels will routinely occur around the new hour of awakening. Pregnancy and estrogen administration increase total serum cortisol values by increasing the synthesis of corticosteroid-binding globulin. An elevated 11 PM cortisol (>15 μg/dl) does suggest Cushing syndrome, but other confirmatory screening tests must be obtained before pursuing an etiologic diagnosis.

Overnight Dexamethasone Suppression Test. Dexamethasone is a synthetic glucocorticoid that is 30 times more potent than cortisol. When given in small amounts, it does not interfere with measure-

---

TABLE 14.3–1. CLINICAL-METABOLIC CORRELATES IN CUSHING SYNDROME

Metabolic effects
A. Fat metabolism
  • Truncal obesity, widening of mediastinum
  • Hypercholesterolemia, accelerated atherosclerosis
B. Protein metabolism
  • Muscle-wasting with proximal myopathy
  • Fragility of skin—ecchymoses, striae
  • Growth hormone unresponsiveness
C. Carbohydrate metabolism
  • Latent or overt diabetes mellitus
D. Electrolyte balance
  • Aldosterone or DOC excess with hypertension
  • Hypokalemic alkalosis

Endocrine effects
A. 1,25 Dihydroxycholecalciferol antagonism—secondary PTH excess and osteopenia
B. Growth hormone suppression—growth failure
C. MSH excess—hyperpigmentation
D. Androgen excess—hirsutism, amenorrhea, and infertility

Neurologic effects
A. Psychosis or emotional lability

DOC = deoxycorticosterone; MSH = melanocyte-stimulating hormone; PTH = parathyroid hormone.

TABLE 14.3–2. POTENTIAL ERRORS IN LABORATORY DIAGNOSIS OF CUSHING SYNDROME

Urinary free cortisol, overnight and low-dose dexamethasone suppression test
False positives
• Alcohol-induced pseudo-Cushing syndrome
• Depression-induced pseudo-Cushing syndrome
• Enhanced metabolism of dexamethasone (e.g., Dilantin)
• Stress (e.g., hospitalization; overnight dexamethasone only)
• Increased CBG (e.g., estrogen administration; overnight dexamethasone only)

False negatives
• Periodic hormonogenesis:[a] Quiescent phase
• Creatinine clearance, 10 ml/min (UFC only)
• Technical error (incomplete urine collection, failure to take dexamethasone, taking dexamethasone at the wrong time)
• Increased pituitary sensitivity to dexamethasone compared to the "typical" case of Cushing disease (overnight and low-dose dexamethasone)

High-dose dexamethasone suppression test
Cushing disease without suppression during high-dose dexamethasone
• Periodic hormonogenesis[a]: Active phase
• Enhanced metabolism of dexamethasone (e.g., phenytoin [Dilantin])
• Decreased pituitary sensitivity to dexamethasone compared to "typical" case of Cushing disease (usually larger tumors)

Suppression during high-dose dexamethasone other than in Cushing disease
• Dexamethasone-suppressible ectopic ACTH syndrome (e.g., pulmonary carcinoids)

---

[a]A subset of patients with Cushing syndrome episodically secrete cortisol. Laboratory results are difficult to interpret if testing coincides with an active or quiescent phase of cortisol secretion.

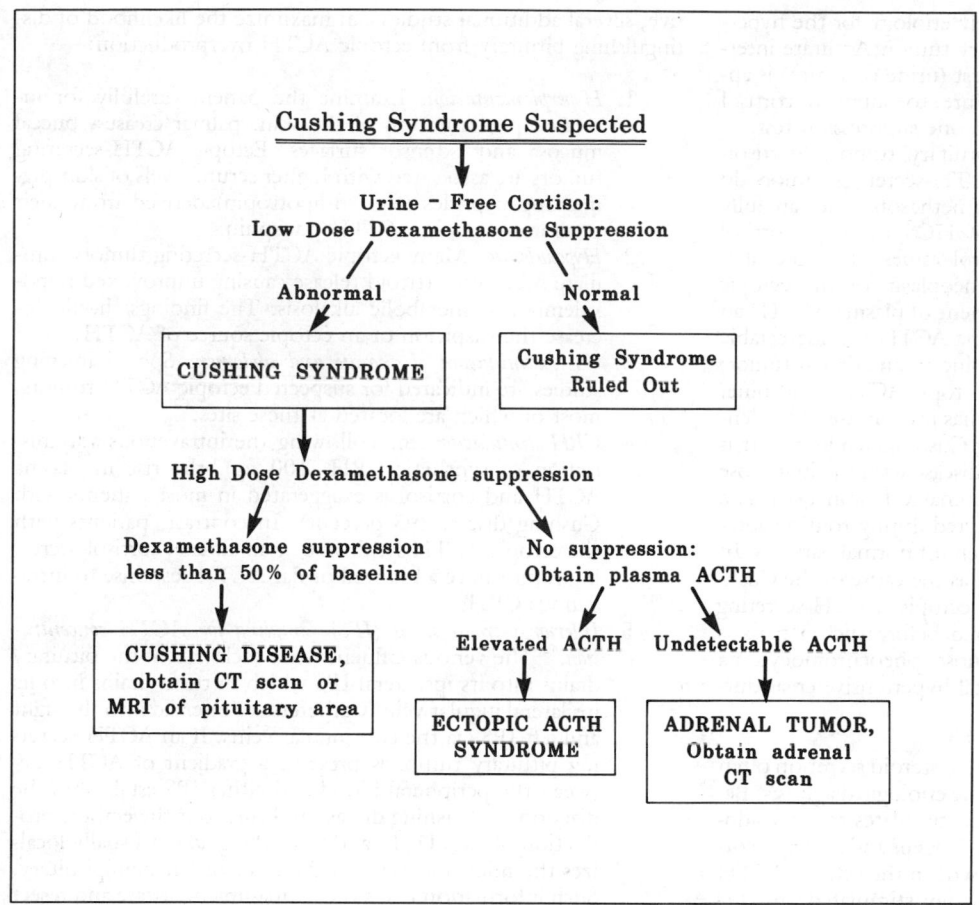

Cushing Syndrome Suspected

Urine - Free Cortisol:
Low Dose Dexamethasone Suppression

Abnormal → **CUSHING SYNDROME**

Normal → Cushing Syndrome Ruled Out

High Dose Dexamethasone suppression

Dexamethasone suppression less than 50% of baseline → **CUSHING DISEASE, obtain CT scan or MRI of pituitary area**

No suppression: Obtain plasma ACTH

Elevated ACTH → **ECTOPIC ACTH SYNDROME**

Undetectable ACTH → **ADRENAL TUMOR, Obtain adrenal CT scan**

Figure 14.3–2. Laboratory evaluation of Cushing syndrome. See text for potential diagnostic pitfalls.

ments of cortisol or its metabolites in plasma or urine. Administration of 1 mg of dexamethasone at bedtime to a normal individual should suppress ACTH secretion so that the plasma cortisol level is less than 5 μg/dl at 8 to 9 AM the following morning. If Cushing syndrome is present, plasma cortisol values are usually not suppressed to less than 10 μg/dl. False positives are seen during stress, depression, alcoholism, and when dexamethasone is rapidly metabolized (e.g., with dilantin therapy; Table 14.3–2).

Urinary Free Cortisol. Only a fraction of plasma cortisol is excreted in the urine as unmetabolized free cortisol; less than 125 μg/24 hr in normal adults. Urinary free cortisol (UFC) levels are nearly always elevated in patients with Cushing syndrome. In contrast to urinary 17-hydroxycorticosteroids (17-OHCS), the UFC is not elevated in obesity. Measurement of UFC is the most sensitive and specific screening test for Cushing syndrome.

Low-dose Dexamethasone Suppression Test. When UFC levels are elevated or the overnight dexamethasone suppression test is abnormal, a low-dose dexamethasone suppression test should be done to confirm or refute the diagnosis of Cushing syndrome. The test is performed as follows. A basal 24-hour urine is collected and assayed for UFC or 17-OHCS. Then two additional 24-hour urines are obtained while the patient receives 0.5 mg of dexamethasone every 6 hours for 2 days. If adrenal function is normal, the UFC will fall below 25 μg/24 hr by the second day of dexamethasone administration. UFC will remain above this level whenever spontaneous Cushing syndrome of any etiology (pituitary, adrenal, or ectopic) is present. If urinary 17-OHCS is measured instead of UFC, adequate suppression is indicated only when 17-OHCS falls below 1 mg/g creatinine. (Expressing 17-OHCS levels per gram of creatinine corrects for the elevations in 17-OHCS seen in simple obesity.)

Etiologic Diagnosis

Once the diagnosis of Cushing syndrome has been confirmed, its etiology must be established.

If steroid or ACTH administration can be excluded by history, the goal is to differentiate among three different forms of spontaneous Cushing syndrome: an ACTH-secreting pituitary tumor, an adrenocortical adenoma or carcinoma, or the ectopic ACTH syndrome.

Patients with pituitary ACTH-secreting tumors are responsive to glucocorticoid suppression, but they have an altered set-point for cortisol feedback. The negative feedback system of the tumor is deranged and will respond only to higher circulating levels of cortisol. In this form of Cushing syndrome, therefore, cortisol secretion is not adequately suppressed by the administration of 2 mg of dexamethasone per day, but suppression can be demonstrated with higher doses. The standard procedure for identifying this situation, the high-dose dexamethasone suppression test, is the cornerstone for distinguishing pituitary Cushing disease from other forms of Cushing syndrome.

High-dose Dexamethasone Suppression Test. This test differs from the low-dose suppression test only by the administration of 2 mg of dexamethasone, instead of 0.5 mg, every 6 hours for 2 days. If the UFC or 17-OHCS measurements fall to 50 percent of control values, the most likely etiology for the hypercortisolism is an ACTH-secreting pituitary tumor. The high-dose suppression test can also be performed by monitoring plasma cortisol values. This approach is less costly and avoids hospitalization but requires a cooperative, reliable patient. An 8 AM blood sample is obtained for serum cortisol measurement. That evening the patient receives 8 mg of dexamethasone between 11 PM and midnight, and a second blood sample is obtained the next day at 8 AM for plasma cortisol measurement. If the cortisol level falls to 50 percent of the control

(predexamethasone) value, the most likely etiology for the hypercortisolism is an ACTH-secreting pituitary tumor. Accurate interpretation of the high-dose suppression test (urine or serum) is appropriate only after demonstrating failure to suppress cortisol adequately during a low-dose dexamethasone suppression test.

In contrast to ACTH-secreting pituitary tumors, cortisol-secreting adrenal tumors and ectopic ACTH-secreting tumors do not generally respond to any dose of dexamethasone; they are fully autonomous. If urinary free cortisol, 17-OHCS, or serum cortisol levels do not fall to 50 percent of control values, therefore, it is likely that the patient has an adrenal neoplasm or the ectopic ACTH syndrome. Subsequent measurement of plasma ACTH can help distinguish these two entities. Plasma ACTH is undetectable in patients whose Cushing syndrome is due to an adrenal tumor; ACTH levels are clearly elevated in the ectopic ACTH syndrome. In addition, CT scanning of the adrenals has proven useful in identifying adrenocortical neoplasms causing Cushing syndrome. It is important to rule out pituitary Cushing disease with the high-dose suppression test before obtaining an adrenal CT scan because a nonfunctional adrenal mass may be detected during routine adrenal CT scanning in approximately 1 percent of normal patients. In addition, if an adrenal mass is discovered as the cause of the Cushing syndrome, the possibility of an ectopic ACTH-secreting pheochromocytoma should be considered before such a mass is approached surgically. Failure to diagnose pheochromocytoma preoperatively can lead to potentially fatal hypertensive crisis during adrenalectomy.

Pattern of Steroid Secretion.   The pattern of steroid secretion often provides useful information concerning the etiologic diagnosis. Because ACTH excess (pituitary or ectopic) stimulates the steroidogenic pathway at an early step, cortisol, androgens and mineralocorticoid metabolites are significantly increased. In the ectopic ACTH syndrome, the adrenals are often maximally stimulated and 17-OHCS excretion may be more than fourfold above normal. 17-Ketosteroid excretion is also high, but the increase is less dramatic. In pituitary Cushing disease both 17-OH and 17-ketosteroid excretion are modestly elevated. When Cushing syndrome is caused by a benign adrenal adenoma, the androgen pathway is not stimulated because ACTH is low and 17-ketosteroid excretion may be normal. The biosynthetic sequence is generally more deranged in adrenal carcinoma than in adenoma; exaggerated secretion of adrenal androgens is common and urinary 17-ketosteroids are typically increased more than the 17-OHC steroids.

Challenges in Diagnosis of Cushing Syndrome

Proper use of the endocrine laboratory and adrenal CT scanning makes it relatively easy to distinguish between adrenal and pituitary tumors. It is occasionally difficult, however, to determine whether pituitary or ectopic ACTH production is the cause of Cushing syndrome.

Small cell carcinoma of the lung accounts for more than half of all cases of ectopic ACTH production. Almost invariably, the diagnosis of cancer predates the clinical manifestations of Cushing syndrome. In fact, these patients often do not develop the full-blown features of Cushing syndrome. Instead, they primarily demonstrate marked metabolic consequences of their hypercortisolism and hyperaldosteronism (potassium-wasting, metabolic alkalosis, and polyuria). Performance of the low- and high-dose dexamethasone suppression tests will usually confirm the diagnosis.

In contrast, when ectopic ACTH secretion arises from an occult tumor, for example, bronchial carcinoid or other tumors of foregut origin, the clinical and biochemical features of Cushing syndrome may be noted long before the neoplasm is detected. Furthermore, many of these tumors mimic the laboratory findings in pituitary Cushing disease, (e.g., cortisol suppression with high-dose dexamethasone). Unfortunately, a cranial CT or MRI scan is usually not helpful because most ACTH-secreting pituitary microadenomas are too small (only 2 or 3 mm in diameter) to be detected by such scans. Although no single test is completely effective, several additional studies can maximize the likelihood of distinguishing pituitary from ectopic ACTH overproduction:

1. ***Hyperpigmentation.*** Examine the patient carefully for increased pigmentation of the skin, palmar creases, buccal mucosa and extensor surfaces. Ectopic ACTH-secreting tumors are associated with higher serum levels of skin-pigmenting peptides (e.g., β-lipotropin) derived from their prohormone, pro-ACTH/endorphin.

2. ***Hypokalemia.*** Many ectopic ACTH-secreting tumors stimulate mineralocorticoid release causing unprovoked hypokalemia and metabolic alkalosis. The findings should increase the suspicion of an ectopic source of ACTH.

3. ***CT examination of thorax and abdomen.*** Special imaging studies are indicated for suspected ectopic ACTH tumors, most of which are located at these sites.

4. ***CRH stimulation test.*** Following the intravenous administration of synthetic CRH (100 μg), the rise in plasma ACTH and cortisol is exaggerated in most patients with Cushing disease (95 percent). In contrast, patients with the ectopic ACTH syndrome or an adrenal cortisol-secreting tumor have a blunted or flat ACTH response to intravenous CRH.

5. ***Inferior petrosal sinus (IPS) sampling for ACTH concentration.***[14] The venous effluent from each half of the pituitary drains into its ipsilateral IPS which in turn, drains into its ipsilateral jugular vein. Catheters are inserted into the right and left IPS via the two jugular veins. If an ACTH-secreting pituitary tumor is present, a gradient of ACTH between the peripheral blood and either IPS establishes the diagnosis of Cushing disease and rules out the ectopic production of ACTH. In addition, the gradient usually localizes the microadenoma to the right or left hemipituitary. Such information helps the neurosurgeon locate and resect these small tumors, which are often difficult to find. This procedure requires an experienced angiographer.

Alcoholic Pseudo-Cushing Syndrome and Depression

Patients with alcoholism or depression may manifest certain clinical and laboratory features of Cushing syndrome, including a Cushingoid appearance in the alcoholic patient.[13] Frequently these patients have elevated cortisol levels in plasma and urine. The plasma cortisol circadian rhythm may be absent, and often cortisol fails to suppress adequately with low-dose dexamethasone. The mechanism of this form of hypercortisolism may be hypersecretion of hypothalamic CRH. These patients must be distinguished from patients with Cushing syndrome.

Several laboratory responses help to distinguish Cushing syndrome from depression or alcoholic pseudo-Cushing syndrome. Although UFC levels may be elevated in depression or alcoholism, they rarely exceed 300 μg/24 hour whereas higher values strongly suggest true Cushing syndrome. When the UFC values are between 150 and 300 μg/24 hour, an insulin tolerance test may be helpful (see Chapter 14.2). In general, patients with Cushing syndrome have a blunted cortisol response to insulin-induced hypoglycemia; the cortisol response is usually normal in depressed or alcoholic patients. When the correct diagnosis remains elusive, observation over time is warranted. Cushing syndrome is a progressive disease; in alcoholics and depressed patients the hypercortisolism waxes and wanes and may resolve with time. The hypercortisolism seen in depression may improve after antidepressant drug treatment or psychotherapy; clinical and biochemical features of alcoholic pseudo-Cushing syndrome resolve when the patient abstains from alcohol.

TREATMENT

Cushing syndrome is a serious disorder. Its morbidity and mortality are determined by the severity of steroid excess as well as host

factors, such as the presence of other illness. The approach to therapy depends on the underlying pathology.

Therapy of Cushing Disease

Selective transsphenoidal microadenomectomy is a major advance in the treatment of Cushing disease.[9] When employed by an experienced neurosurgeon, this procedure has a primary cure rate of approximately 90 percent and is now the first choice for treatment of Cushing disease. Potential complications include varying degrees of hypopituitarism, diabetes insipidus, rhinorrhea, and infection. Provocative tests are usually employed (see Chapter 14.2) postoperatively to assess anterior pituitary function. Preoperative hypercortisolism invariably suppresses the nontumorous pituitary corticotrophs. Successful surgery, therefore, causes transient ACTH deficiency, which requires glucocorticoid replacement for 1 to several months. Periodically, attempts are made to taper glucocorticoid therapy, and patients are assessed for the normal recovery of their pituitary-adrenal axis.

Pituitary irradiation has been employed to treat Cushing disease. With supervoltage techniques that deliver 4000 to 5000 rad to the pituitary, approximately 40 to 50 percent of patients are cured. The results of irradiation have been more favorable in children and adolescents, and in many centers this is the preferred treatment in these age groups. When pituitary irradiation is successful, the benefits are much slower in onset than with transsphenoidal surgery. Significant side effects are uncommon, although varying degrees of hypopituitarism may develop even many years after the initial therapy. Radiotherapy should be used if surgery has failed or if the patient is not a surgical candidate.

Bilateral adrenalectomy was previously the first-line treatment for Cushing disease, and cure rates approached 100 percent. Transsphenoidal surgery is now preferred, however, for several reasons. It is associated with less morbidity and mortality, and bilateral adrenalectomy requires lifelong replacement therapy. Bilateral adrenalectomy predisposes the patient to the development of aggressive pituitary tumors (Nelson syndrome; see Chapter 14.2). It is currently difficult to justify bilateral adrenalectomy as the first treatment for Cushing disease when a complete cure is possible by other techniques.

Pharmacologic therapy for Cushing disease can be directed at the adrenals or the pituitary. Several drugs can induce a "medical adrenalectomy." Metyrapone inhibits cortisol biosynthesis (11-hydroxylase step) and can lower plasma cortisol values. It is generally well tolerated if taken with food. The daily dose ranges from 750 to 4000 mg per day and must be individually adjusted. The drug is less effective in Cushing disease because of escape from the 11-hydroxylase blockade. The adrenolytic drug o,p'-DDD (mitotane) is cytotoxic to the cells of the adrenal zona fasciculata and zona reticularis. The dose ranges from 2 to 6 g per day. This drug was initially used to treat adrenal carcinoma but can be effective in Cushing disease. It takes longer to achieve normal cortisol levels with mitotane than metyrapone. A number of side effects of mitotane (CNS and intestinal) can limit its usefulness. Other adrenal blocking drugs include aminoglutethimide, trilostane, and ketoconazole. Although effective, aminoglutethimide commonly is associated with a skin rash.

The adrenal blocking drugs are not used as primary therapy. These drugs may be used to reduce hypercortisolism before surgical intervention, to improve wound healing—minimizing risk of infection—or to reverse psychiatric symptoms. They can also be used in combination with pituitary irradiation to lower cortisol levels more rapidly. Periodically, the drug should be tapered to determine if radiotherapy has induced a permanent cure.

Two drugs, cyproheptadine (serotonin antagonist) and bromocriptine (dopamine agonist) directly affect pituitary ACTH secretion. Cyproheptadine (14 mg/day) may induce clinical remission in a subset of patients. Weight gain and increased appetite are common side effects. Bromocriptine has not proven effective for most patients with Cushing disease.

Therapy of Cushing Syndrome Due to Adrenal Neoplasm

Cushing syndrome caused by adrenocortical adenomas can usually be treated successfully by unilateral adrenalectomy. On occasion, bilateral adenomas make it necessary to remove both glands. Inhibitors of adrenal steroid biosynthesis, such as metyrapone, can successfully ameliorate Cushing syndrome due to an adenoma, either in preparing a patient for surgery or when surgery is contraindicated. Unlike the situation in Cushing disease, ACTH secretion is suppressed in most patients with adenomas. Hence, reflex mechanisms that tend to push ACTH to high levels in response to adrenal inhibitors, and thus overcome the blockade, are not operative in the case of adrenal neoplasms.

The therapy of adrenocortical carcinomas includes surgical removal of tumors when possible and the use of adrenal inhibitors to ameliorate Cushing syndrome when the tumor is unresectable. Because mitotane is cytotoxic, there has been particular interest in its use for the chemotherapy of adrenocortical carcinoma. In some patients, large doses of the drug have reduced tumor mass. Its use has been limited, however, by its toxicity, unpredictable responsiveness, and lack of evidence that the drug prolongs life.

Therapy of Cushing Syndrome Due to Ectopic Production of ACTH

Initial treatment is aimed at localization and, if possible, surgical removal of the tumor producing ectopic ACTH. Radiotherapy and chemotherapy are directed at inoperable tumors according to the usual protocols employed for the given tumor. Many neoplasms associated with ectopic ACTH production cannot be cured by any available treatment, and excessive ACTH production and the metabolic consequences of Cushing syndrome represent serious clinical problems. These patients can be treated with adrenal inhibitors such as metyrapone or mitotane.

ADRENAL INSUFFICIENCY (ADDISON DISEASE)

Adrenal insufficiency is a rare disorder that frequently must be considered in the differential diagnosis of more commonly encountered disorders (Table 14.3–3). Fever, hypotension, nausea, vomiting, and abdominal pain must all raise suspicion of adrenal insufficiency because adrenal crisis demands prompt recognition and treatment for the patient's survival. In less seriously ill patients, insidious development of adrenal insufficiency should be considered as the possible cause for asthenia, anorexia, and weight loss.

TABLE 14.3–3. CLINICAL FEATURES IN ADDISON DISEASE

Grouped Category	Possible Presenting Signs or Symptoms
I. Asthenia	Decrease in strength and work capacity Irritability, drowsiness, and restlessness Paralysis (hyperkalemic)
II. Cardiovascular	Hypotension, small heart
III. Gastrointestinal disorder	Weight loss Food idiosyncrasy, poor appetite Anorexia, nausea, vomiting, diarrhea, abdominal pain
IV. Salt wastage	Salt-craving Muscle cramps Dizziness and syncope (hypotension)
V. Hypoglycemia	Coma
VI. Pigmentation	Recent scars, buccal mucosa, knuckles, elbows, palmar creases
VII. Miscellaneous	Loss of sex characteristics in female

ETIOLOGY

When first described, Addison disease was most frequently attributable to infection of the adrenals by tuberculosis. Autoimmune destruction and adrenal hemorrhage are now the most common causes of primary adrenal insufficiency in this country. Eighty to 90 percent of adrenocortical tissue must be destroyed before adrenal reserve is so impaired that adrenal insufficiency occurs.

Idiopathic adrenal atrophy is now attributed to autoimmune adrenal inflammation.[12] Circulating antiadrenal antibodies can be detected in many individuals with this condition during the course of the disease. Histology of the adrenals shows mononuclear cell infiltration that progresses to atrophy involving all three zones of the cortex, although the medulla remains intact. Occasionally, such patients have a family history of adrenal insufficiency. These patients and their families may also develop autoimmune failure of the thyroid and gonads. Diabetes mellitus and hypoparathyroidism associated with cutaneous candidiasis may also occur (see Chapter 14.1). Vitiligo is seen more frequently in Addison disease than in other autoimmune endocrinopathies. The risk of Addison disease is ten times greater in people with HLA-Dw3 and nearly four times greater in those with HLA-B8 histocompatibility haplotypes.

Hemorrhagic destruction of the adrenal may arise iatrogenically, as a complication of anticoagulant therapy or as a consequence of fulminant infections, for example, meningococcal or staphylococcal septicemia. Hemorrhagic destruction of the adrenal may appear suddenly during anticoagulation therapy in myocardial infarction. The acute onset of hypotension, nausea, and vomiting can be mistaken for an extension of the infarction. Granulomatous, neoplastic, or other infiltrative disorders may also lead to adrenal insufficiency. In addition to tuberculosis, fungal infections, such as histoplasmosis and blastomycosis can also produce adrenal failure. Metastatic tumors, for example, from the breast or lung, can infiltrate both adrenals as can amyloidosis.

Adrenal glucocorticoid deficiency may be secondary to diseases that alter the function of the hypothalamus or pituitary and thus reduce ACTH production. Although the adrenal gland is not directly affected by the primary disease process, lack of trophic stimulation by ACTH leads to glucocorticoid deficiency (see Chapter 14.2).

CLINICAL FEATURES

Chronic Adrenal Insufficiency

History. The manifestations of slowly emerging adrenal insufficiency are nonspecific. The most common complaints are anorexia, weight loss, fatigability, and lightheadedness. Most patients also experience myalgias, arthralgias, and muscle weakness. Many patients develop hypersensitivity of taste, smell, and hearing. There is often a history of salt-craving. Acute prostration, hypotension, fever, and hypoglycemia may be precipitated by a relatively minor intercurrent infection or stress.

Physical Findings. Hypotension, particularly in the upright posture, is typically present. Orthostatic hypotension is due to sodium loss and volume depletion as well as a mineralocorticoid deficit. Hyperpigmentation of the skin, a frequent occurrence in primary adrenal insufficiency, is caused by increased production of peptides derived from the ACTH precursors, pro-ACTH-endorphin, which have melanocyte-stimulating activity. Characteristically, they produce diffuse tanning of both unexposed and exposed parts of the body. The skin appears dirty, particularly over the knees, elbows, and other pressure points. Other common sites of increased pigmentation are the anogenital region, areolae, and recent scars. Small black freckles appear, especially over the forehead, face, and neck. Patients with autoimmune adrenal insufficiency may have islands of vitiligo in the areas of greatest pigmentation. Hyperpigmentation may also involve the mucous membranes with dark pigmented areas on the lips, gums, buccal, rectal, and vaginal surfaces. It is important to recognize that although such hyperpigmentation warrants attention in whites, it is often normally found in blacks and American Indians.

Muscle weakness, delayed deep-tendon reflexes, and myasthenia-like fatigability can often be demonstrated. Hyperkalemia and cortisol deficiency may in part be responsible for these manifestations.

Laboratory Abnormalities. The laboratory findings reflect glucocorticoid and mineralocorticoid deficiency. Hypoglycemia may be present, and failure to recognize it will increase morbidity and mortality. As a consequence of the mineralocorticoid deficit, patients may exhibit hyponatremia, hyperkalemia, and metabolic acidosis. Salt loss and volume depletion lead to a fall in glomerular filtration rate and a rise in serum urea nitrogen and creatinine. Changes in the formed elements of the blood include eosinophilia and anemia (which may become more readily apparent after the patient is rehydrated). A small heart is often noted on chest radiograph.

Several features distinguish Addison disease from secondary adrenal insufficiency, for example, decreased or absent ACTH (see Chapter 14.2). The hyperpigmentation characteristic of Addison disease is absent in secondary adrenal insufficiency because of the low levels of circulating ACTH in the latter condition. Patients with absent or low levels of ACTH are usually not dehydrated and lack signs of volume depletion. Aldosterone secretion is reasonably well-preserved in these patients because aldosterone is primarily regulated by the renin-angiotensin system. Despite intact aldosterone secretion, patients with secondary adrenal insufficiency may exhibit postural hypotension and hyponatremia as a reflection of the requirement for cortisol to preserve vascular tone and to maintain excretion of a free water load by the renal tubules, respectively. Finally, patients with secondary adrenal insufficiency as a result of hypopituitarism usually have deficiencies of other pituitary hormones, such as TSH, LH, or FSH. Clinical evidence for concurrent hypothryoidism and hypogonadism should be sought.

Laboratory Diagnosis. An ACTH stimulation test should be performed in suspected cases of adrenal insufficiency (Fig. 14.3–3). The best initial screen is the rapid ACTH stimulation test in which cortisol is measured before and 1 hour after an intravenous dose of 250 μg of a synthetic ACTH that contains the first 24 amino-terminal amino acids of ACTH. Primary adrenal insufficiency is excluded if the rise in plasma cortisol exceeds 7 μg/dl and the final value is greater than 18 μg/dl. (If secondary adrenal insufficiency is suspected, insulin-induced hypoglycemia or a metyrapone test is performed; see Chapter 14.2.) If the adrenal is unresponsive to acute administration of ACTH, a 3-day ACTH stimulation test is done to confirm the results of the rapid screening test and to distinguish Addison disease from secondary adrenal insufficiency. In this procedure a basal 24-hour urine collection is followed by 24-hour urine collections for 3 additional days, whereas synthetic ACTH (500 μg) is administered daily over an 8-hour infusion period. Healthy individuals have a two- to fourfold increase in urinary 17-OHCS or free cortisol during the first day of ACTH stimulation. Patients with primary adrenal insufficiency demonstrate little or no rise in urinary 17-OHCS throughout the 3 days. In patients with secondary adrenal insufficiency, the urinary 17-OHCS response is deficient on day 1 but increases two- or threefold above control values by the 3rd day of ACTH infusion. Alternatively, measurement of plasma ACTH may be employed to distinguish Addison disease from secondary adrenal insufficiency. In Addison disease, ACTH values are elevated (>100 pg/ml), reflecting loss of cortisol feedback on ACTH secretion. In contrast, low or normal ACTH values are seen in secondary adrenal insufficiency.

Therapy. Patients with primary adrenal insufficiency can be satisfactorily treated by the oral administration of cortisone acetate, 25

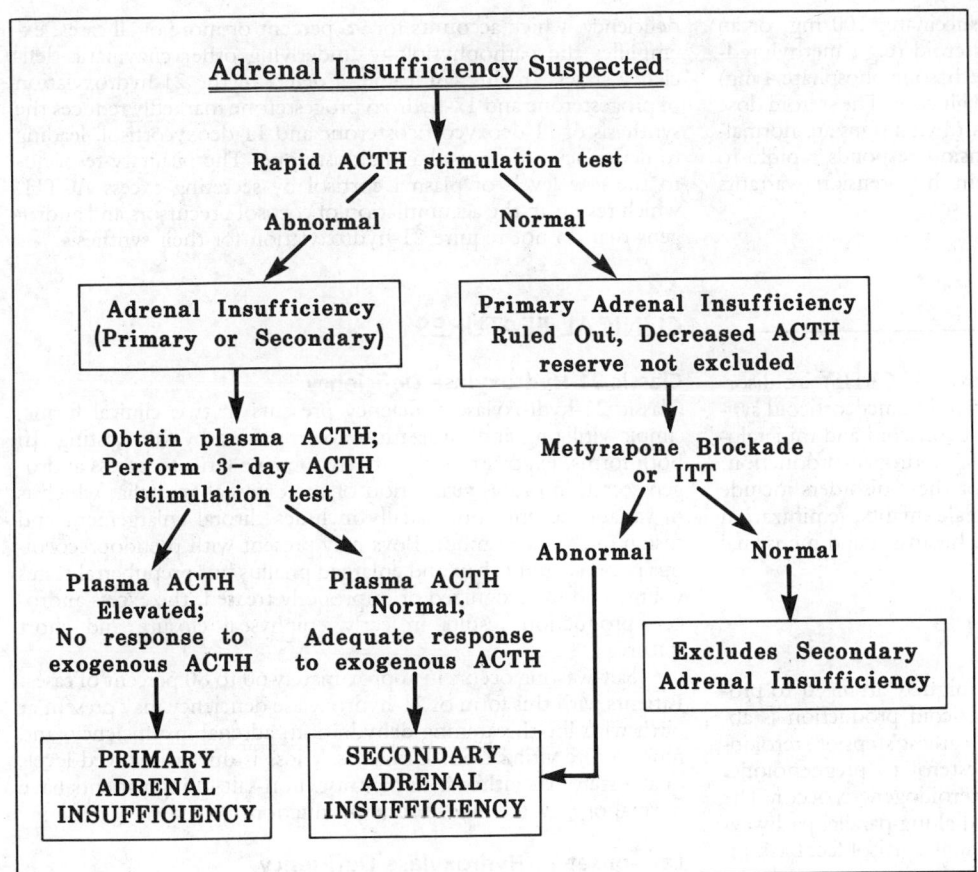

Figure 14.3-3. Laboratory evaluation of suspected adrenal insufficiency. ITT = insulin-tolerance test.

to 37.5 mg daily. Hydrocortisone or synthetic glucocorticoids can be used equally well if appropriate adjustments in the quantities administered are based on their relative potencies. A salt-retaining steroid, for example, 9α-fluorocortisol (0.05 to 0.1 mg daily), is usually added for mineralocorticoid effects. Patients rapidly attain a sense of well-being after therapy is begun. Some patients with preexisting renal disease or hypertension may not require mineralocorticoid replacement if cortisone is used but may require mineralocorticoid if a synthetic glucocorticoid with little salt-retaining activity is employed.

Addisonian patients should wear an identifying bracelet and be instructed to increase their glucocorticoid replacement twofold to threefold during any serious stress such as infections, or trauma. At home, patients should keep injectable steroid available in the event that intercurrent illness associated with vomiting prevents taking an oral steroid supplement. When such patients require surgery, it is necessary to administer supraphysiologic amounts of glucocorticoid by a parenteral route. For example, the patient can be given hydrocortisone hemisuccinate, 100 mg intramuscularly, 1 hour before major surgery; another 100 mg intravenously during surgery; and an additional 100 mg every 8 hours postoperatively. These doses can be progressively tapered on each postoperative day. Usually patients also require 1 L of normal saline intravenously daily until they can take oral fluids. The dosage of other steroid preparations (e.g., methylprednisolone phosphate) available for parenteral use must be adjusted according to their potency (Table 14.3–4).

Acute Adrenal Insufficiency (Addisonian Crisis)
Minor infections or surgical procedures may provoke crisis in patients with untreated or inadequately treated adrenal insufficiency. Addisonian crisis is a medical emergency. The patient should be

TABLE 14.3–4. PREPARATIONS OF ADRENOCORTICAL STEROIDS

Preparation (mg)	Route	Biological Half-Life (hr)	Relative Antiinflammatory Potency	Relative Mineralocorticoid Potency	Approximate Equivalent Dose
Cortisol	O/I/T	8–12	1.0	1.0	20
Cortisone	O/I	8–12	0.8	0.8	25
Prednisone	O	12–36	4.0	0.8	5
Methylprednisolone	I	12–36	5.0	0.5	4
Dexamethasone	O/T	36–72	25	0	0.75
Dexamethasone sodium succinate	I/T	36–72	25	0	0.75

O = oral; I = injectable; T = topical.
(From Gilman AG, et al (eds): Goodman and Gilman's The Pharmacological Basis of Therapeutics, 7th ed. New York, MacMillan, 1985, with permission.)

given intravenous hydrocortisone hemisuccinate, 100 mg, or an equivalent amount of another soluble steroid (e.g., methylprednisolone hemisuccinate 20 mg or dexamethasone phosphate 4 mg) along with intravenous normal saline and glucose. The steroid dose should be repeated every 6 to 8 hours until vital signs are normalized and the patient is stable. Hypotension responds rapidly to fluid and steroid replacement. Persistent hypotension warrants search for another underlying etiology.

CONGENITAL ADRENAL HYPERPLASIA SYNDROMES

The congenital adrenal hyperplasia syndromes (CAHS) are disorders of specific enzymatically catalyzed steps in glucocorticoid synthesis resulting in varying degrees of glucocorticoid and mineralocorticoid deficiency and increased adrenal androgen production. The spectrum of clinical presentations for these disorders include neonatal adrenal crisis, virilization of female infants, feminization of male infants, precocious puberty, and hirsutism and menstrual disorders in postmenarche women.

PATHOPHYSIOLOGY

Steroidogenesis in the adrenal cortex is uniquely arranged to promote androgen secretion when glucocorticoid production is abnormal (Fig. 14.3–1). ACTH acts at the earliest steps of steroidogenesis, stimulating conversion of cholesterol to pregnenolone. Beyond this step the major branches of steroidogenesis occur. The earliest steroid precursors may be shunted along parallel pathways leading to androgen synthesis when deficient cortisol feedback increases ACTH levels. Both pregnenolone and progesterone are good substrates for the 17-hydroxylase enzyme. In turn, both of the 17-hydroxyl derivatives of these steroids are good substrates for the desmolase enzymes that cleave the carbon 20,21 side chain to produce dehydroandrosterone and androstenedione, respectively. Although these two steroids are only weak androgens, they are readily converted by liver and other tissues into testosterone, dihydrotestosterone, and the biologically active androstenediols. Thus, any distal defects in steroidogenesis that cause a rise in ACTH are likely to exaggerate androgen production by the adrenal. A number of specific inborn errors of steroid synthesis have been identified. Each presents with unique abnormalities depending upon the site of the lesion (Table 14.3–5). The 21-hydroxylase

deficiency, which accounts for 95 percent or more of all cases, exemplifies the pathophysiology underlying other enzymatic deficiency states. In this syndrome, a defect in the 21-hydroxylation of progesterone and 17-hydroxyprogesterone markedly reduces the synthesis of 11-deoxycorticosterone and 11-deoxycortisol, leading to deficiencies in cortisol and aldosterone. The pituitary responds to the low levels of plasma cortisol by secreting excess ACTH, which results in the accumulation of cortisol precursors and androgens that do not require 21-hydroxylation for their synthesis.

CLINICAL FEATURES

Classic 21-Hydroxylase Deficiency
Classic 21-hydroxylase deficiency presents in two clinical forms, simple virilizing and virilization accompanied by salt-wasting. In both forms, exposure of the affected female fetus to excess androgen secretion causes virilization of the external genitalia, which is of variable severity but usually includes clitoral enlargement and fusion of the labia minor. Boys may present with pseudoprecocoious puberty (pubic hair and enlarged phallus but prepubertal testes volume). If unrecognized or improperly treated, the excess androgen production results in early epiphyseal closure and short stature.

Salt-wasting occurs in approximately 60 to 80 percent of cases. Patients with this form of 21-hydroxylase deficiency may present at birth with life-threatening dehydration, adrenal insufficiency, and more severe virilization. Urinary salt loss is due to reduced levels of aldosterone synthesis. In contrast, non-salt-losing patients have normal or elevated aldosterone production.

Late-onset 21-Hydroxylase Deficiency
A delayed or attenuated form of 21-hydroxylase deficiency is characterized by virilization or hirsutism, menstrual irregularities (oligo- or amenorrhea) and biochemical features of a 21-hydroxylase block. Unlike classical congenital adrenal hyperplasia, clinical abnormalities in the late-onset form are frequently not observed until after menarche.

DIAGNOSIS

Diagnosis of congenital adrenal hyperplasia involves answering the two critical questions: (1) Is there clinical evidence of a specific enzyme defect (ambiguous external genitalia, hypertension, salt-

TABLE 14.3–5. ENZYME DEFECTS IN ADRENOGENITAL SYNDROME

Defect	Clinical Features	Steroid Patterns
21-Hydroxylase	Mild, simple virilism Severe virilism and salt-wasting	*Urine:* elevated 17-ketosteroids and pregnanetriol *Plasma:* elevated 17-OH progesterone, progesterone, and testosterone
11-Hydroxylase	Virilism and hypotension	*Urine:* elevated 17-hydroxysteroids (tetrahydros) *Plasma:* elevated 11-deoxycortisol, deoxycorticosterone, and testosterone
3-β Dehydrogenase	1° adrenal insuffiency Ambiguous genitalia in both sexes	*Urine:* elevated 17-ketosteroids and pregnenetriol *Plasma:* elevated pregnenolone, 17-OH pregnenolene, and DHA
17-Hydroxylase	Hypertension Delayed puberty in females Ambiguous genitalia in males	*Urine:* decreased 17-OH and 17-ketosteroids *Plasma:* elevated progesterone, deoxycorticosterone and corticosterone
20,22-Hydroxylase	Female phenotype regardless of genotype Massively enlarged adrenals High mortality	?
18-Oxidase	Salt-wasting	*Urine:* normal 17-OH and 17 ketosteroids *Plasma:* elevated 18-OH corticosterone and corticosterone; low aldosterone

wasting, hyperpigmentation, hirsutism, adrenal insufficiency)? (2) Is there biochemical evidence for the accumulation of adrenal steroid precursors and products as a result of ACTH stimulation? The laboratory findings in classical 21-OH deficiency include elevated levels of 17-hydroxyprogesterone, progesterone, and ACTH in the plasma. Elevated ketosteroids and pregnanetriol, a metabolite of 17-OH progesterone, are found in the urine. Plasma cortisol is normal or decreased. Patients with the delayed-onset type of 21-OH deficiency may have normal or only modestly elevated levels of 17-hydroxyprogesterone. In such cases, the diagnosis is confirmed by performing a rapid ACTH stimulation test.[7] Synthetic ACTH analog administration to these patients causes an exaggerated rise in 17-hydroxyprogesterone. In all cases, final proof for the syndrome requires suppression of elevated steroid values by dexamethasone administration. Prenatal diagnosis of the classical syndrome has been reported using measurements of amniotic fluid 17-OH progesterone values.

TREATMENT

When an enzyme defect leads to inefficient cortisol synthesis, the androgen excess is corrected by suppression of the pituitary-adrenal axis with physiologic doses of glucocorticoid. Excessive doses of glucocorticoid must be avoided in the growing child to prevent early epiphyseal closure and ensure growth to normal stature. The preferred treatment for growing children is hydrocortisone (10 to 20 mg/m²/day) in divided doses, which takes advantage of the increased suppressibility of pituitary ACTH later in the day. During episodes of intercurrent illness, trauma, or surgery, a glucocorticoid supplement is needed as for patients with adrenal insufficiency. Equally important in the classical forms of 21-OH deficiency is careful assessment of the mineralocorticoid requirement. Even when they are not overt salt-losers, most patients have elevated plasma renin activity as an indication of increased total urinary sodium loss. The accompanying hypovolemia stimulates ACTH secretion, and the increased production of adrenal androgens may be misinterpreted as a need for more glucocorticoids. Additional glucocorticoid treatment in this setting could slow linear growth or possibly cause iatrogenic Cushing syndrome. Instead, appropriate treatment is mineralocorticoid replacement (9α-fluorocortisol), which will normalize plasma renin activity, correct hypovolemia, and lower ACTH values.

PHARMACOLOGIC ROLE OF GLUCOCORTICOIDS

Physiologic concentrations of glucocorticoids are often used to treat patients with primary or secondary adrenal insufficiency. Glucocorticoids are also administered in pharmacologic doses to control a variety of diseases such as asthma, inflammatory bowel disease, collagen-vascular disorders, sarcoidosis, nephrotic syndrome, and hypersensitivity reactions. Although such therapy can be beneficial, potential ill-effects of long-term use of glucocorticoids must be weighed against this benefit. Clinicians must be familiar with the variety of glucocorticoid preparations available and their potencies, duration of action, and special applicability in particular clinical situations. The clinician must also understand the potential complications of steroid therapy, be aware of ways to minimize the total dosage without compromising the therapeutic benefit, and most important, exercise judgment in the decision to initiate such therapy. Finally, the clinician must know the physiology of the HPA axis in order to understand the time course of its suppression and recovery.

CHOICE OF PREPARATIONS

Glucocorticoid preparations vary in their relative glucocorticoid and mineralocorticoid potency and their durations of biological activity (Table 14.2–4). Both aspects have important therapeutic implications. For example, a glucocorticoid with low mineralocorticoid activity (e.g., dexamethasone) is preferable when pharmacologic doses are used to treat nonendocrine disease. Such a choice will minimize sodium retention, edema, hypokalemia, and hypertension. On the other hand, hydrocortisone administration is more appropriate than dexamethasone during the acute treatment of adrenal insufficiency; the mineralocorticoid activity of hydrocortisone is beneficial in this setting. For poorly compliant patients, a preparation that has a long duration of action and can be taken once daily (e.g., prednisone or dexamethasone) may be preferable to a shorter-acting steroid (hydrocortisone or cortisone acetate) that requires a twice daily or three times daily schedule. The chemical structure of the glucocorticoid may also influence the choice of preparations. For example, cortisone and prednisone are 11-ketosteroids that lack glucocorticoid activity before their conversion by the liver into biologically-active 11-hydroxyl steroids. This chemical conversion may not occur in patients with significant liver disease. The clinician should also know which preparations can be administered parenterally when oral treatment is impossible.

COMPLICATIONS OF THERAPY

The chronic administration of supraphysiologic doses of glucocorticoids can be hazardous. Clinical features of Cushing syndrome may emerge during sustained treatment. Because the complications of glucocorticoid therapy are time- and dose-dependent, the smallest possible dose should be employed for the shortest period of time. Many of the clinical features of iatrogenic and endogenous Cushing syndrome are similar. These include truncal obesity, psychiatric symptoms, easy bruising, poor wound healing, hypertension, diabetes mellitus, proximal muscle weakness and osteoporosis. Patients may require insulin and antihypertensive therapy as well as calcium and vitamin D supplements. Signs and symptoms that are unique to iatrogenic Cushing syndrome include posterior subcapsular cataracts, pancreatitis, aseptic necrosis of bone, and benign intracranial hypertension. In contrast, the adrenal androgen-related complications of hirsutism, virilization, and menstrual disturbances are features of endogenous but not iatrogenic Cushing syndrome.

Alternate-day therapy may minimize the side effects of exogenous glucocorticoids, thus reducing steroid-induced complications and suppression of the HPA axis. Unfortunately, some diseases (e.g., giant cell arteritis) cannot be treated effectively by this mode of therapy. If patients cannot tolerate alternate-day therapy, glucocorticoids should be administered each morning as a single dose whenever possible. This schedule mimics the diurnal rhythm of the normal HPA axis and produces less suppression than a divided dosage schedule.

SUPPRESSION AND RECOVERY OF HYPOTHALAMIC-PITUITARY-ADRENAL AXIS

In addition to producing the clinical features of Cushing syndrome, exogenous glucocorticoids can suppress the HPA axis. When steroids are stopped abruptly or an intercurrent illness occurs, the suppressed HPA axis cannot meet the increased glucocorticoid requirements. As a result the patient may quickly develop symptoms of secondary adrenal insufficiency (fatigue, weakness, arthralgias, anorexia, nausea, hypotension, and hypoglycemia). The degree of HPA-axis suppression is related to both the dose and duration of glucocorticoid therapy. Although there is variability among individuals, it is prudent to assume HPA-axis suppression in any patient who has received 20 to 30 mg per day of prednisone (or its equivalent) for more than a week.

All patients maintained on glucocorticoids should wear a medical alert tag indicating that they are steroid-dependent. The patient must understand the importance of compliance with the medical regimen and appreciate the need for increased glucocorti-

coid dose during times of stress. The patient should receive an additional 100 mg of hydrocortisone per day during febrile illnesses and before dental work, outpatient surgical procedures, or endoscopy. The patient must receive 100 mg of hydrocortisone intravenously every 6 to 8 hours during periods of major stress (surgery or trauma). The dosage is gradually tapered back to a maintenance level when the patient stabilizes.

When it is time to stop glucocorticoid therapy, the physician must follow a course of cautious drug withdrawal. As the dose is gradually reduced, the patient is carefully monitored both for activity of the underlying disease and for signs and symptoms of adrenal insufficiency. Pharmacologic doses of glucocorticoids are first tapered to physiologic levels, a maintenance dosage. The patient is then switched to a glucocorticoid preparation with a short half-life, such as hydrocortisone (20 mg each morning). After several weeks at this dose, an 8 AM plasma cortisol value is obtained. A plasma cortisol value greater than 10 µg/dl generally indicates that the patient is secreting enough cortisol for basal (nonstressed) function; the hydrocortisone dose can then be quickly tapered and stopped. If the plasma cortisol is less than 10 µg/dl, maintenance hydrocortisone is continued until the morning plasma cortisol exceeds 10 µg/dl. Until an appropriate dynamic pituitary test confirms that the HPA axis can respond appropriately to stressful stimuli (see below), the patient must still be treated with additional steroids at times of increased stress.

The time required for full recovery of the HPA axis ranges from weeks to months. Tests of basal adrenal function are often misleading; a normal morning plasma cortisol, 24-hour urinary free cortisol or urinary 17-OHCS value does not guarantee that the HPA axis is capable of responding to stressful stimuli. A dynamic test is necessary to demonstrate full recovery. The patient should be challenged with one of the following: insulin-induced hypoglycemia, metyrapone blockade, or a rapid ACTH stimulation test (see Chapter 14.2). The rapid ACTH test is more convenient but is associated with more false-positive and false-negative test results.

Occasionally as steroids are tapered patients may complain of symptoms that are similar to those of adrenal insufficiency. If the tapering process is too rapid the symptoms may reflect inadequate levels of glucocorticoids. Some patients experience such symptoms without biochemical evidence of deficient adrenal secretion, however. This steroid-withdrawal syndrome[16] occurs in patients who are receiving physiologic doses of steroids or whose HPA axis has fully recovered. The most prominent features are anorexia, lethargy, malaise, myalgias, weight loss, headache, and fever. If severe symptoms persist for more than a few days, the steroid dose should be increased to its former level. After symptoms have resolved, the dose can be tapered again using smaller decrements and over a longer period of time.

Currently there is no proven means of hastening the recovery of the suppressed HPA axis. ACTH therapy is not helpful. The potential role of CRH in assessing or enhancing the recovery of the HPA axis remains to be defined.

MINERALOCORTICOID DISORDERS

Aldosterone is the adrenal steroid that regulates sodium and potassium balance. It is also a part of a vital system controlling blood pressure and extracellular fluid volume—the renin-angiotensin-aldosterone (RAA) system (see Chapter 2.10).

Renin is a proteolytic enzyme released from juxtaglomerular cells lying along the afferent arteriole of the renal glomerulus in response to upright posture, decreases in renal perfusion pressure, or extracellular fluid volume.

Renin in the circulation generates the production of angiotensin II, a potent systemic and renal vasoconstrictor that also stimulates the zona glomerulosa of the adrenal to synthesize aldosterone. Aldosterone, in turn, stimulates renal sodium reabsorption and thus expansion of extracellular fluid volume. As a result, renin

secretion is suppressed. The RAA system, therefore, provides a defense against a fall in blood pressure or blood volume by angiotensin II-mediated vasoconstriction and aldosterone-mediated volume expansion. Aldosterone-mediated increases in distal renal tubule reabsorption of sodium favors the movement of hydrogen and potassium into the tubular lumen and subsequent excretion.

In aldosterone deficiency states such as Addison disease and the syndrome of hyporeninemic hypoaldosteronism (see below), hyperkalemia and metabolic acidosis are typical and volume depletion with postural hypotension may occur. With aldosterone excess, potassium depletion and alkalosis develop with increased production of ammonia. Potassium depletion produces muscle weakness, decreased carbohydrate intolerance, resistance to the urine-concentrating effects of vasopressin, and blunting of circulatory reflexes (postural hypotension) (see Table 14.3–6).

In addition to angiotensin II, other stimuli important in aldosterone secretion are ACTH, potassium excess, and sodium depletion. There is also evidence of a role for certain derivatives of the pituitary hormone precursor POMC (pro-ACTH/endorphin) and other unidentified factors including a glycoprotein from the anterior pituitary termed ''aldosterone-stimulating factor'' (ASF). Dopamine may modulate aldosterone secretion, and it inhibits the angiotensin II-mediated stimulation of aldosterone during sodium depletion. This may work through inhibition of ASF.

HYPORENINEMIC HYPOALDOSTERONISM

The syndrome of hyporeninemic hypoaldosteronism (SHH)[15] is the commonest cause of mineralocorticoid deficiency in adults. The hypoaldosteronism appears to be secondary to insufficient stimulation of the adrenal gland by the renin-angiotensin system. Plasma renin activity (PRA) is low or borderline in the basal state and shows subnormal stimulation with upright posture or volume depletion. Plasma aldosterone is also usually low and is poorly stimulated by ACTH and angiotensin II infusion. Glucocorticoids, however, respond normally to ACTH stimulation. The pathogenesis has not been clarified, but the low and unresponsive aldosterone plasma levels are mainly the consequence of prolonged hyporeninemia. Explanations for low PRA include damage to the juxtaglomerular apparatus, impaired conversion of renin precursors to active hormone, insufficient sympathetic stimulation of renin-producing cells, inhibition of renin release by hyperkalemia or volume expansion, and altered synthesis of renal prostaglandins.

Most patients with SHH are over 50 years of age and suffer from mild renal insufficiency (serum creatinine 2 to 4 mg/dl). This is most frequently due to diabetes mellitus but may be caused by other tubulointerstitial renal diseases such as chronic pyelonephritis, nephrolithiasis, analgesic abuse, and hypertensive nephrosclerosis. Despite mineralocorticoid deficiency, hypertension is frequently present. The diagnostic clue to SHH is hyperkalemia (5.6 to 6.5 mEq/L) in disproportion to the mild degree of renal failure. The hyperkalemia is usually chronic and asymptomatic but may be provoked by hyperglycemia in diabetics, reduced sodium intake,

TABLE 14.3–6. CLINICAL FEATURES OF PRIMARY ALDOSTERONISM

Due to hypertension
- Asymptomatic
- Ischemic heart disease, congestive heart failure
- Stroke

Due to hypokalemia
- Muscle: weakness, paralysis
- Autonomic reflexes: orthostasis
- Renal: nephrogenic diabetes insipidus-polyuria, hypernatremia; metabolic alkalosis, paresthesias
- Insulin secretion: carbohydrate intolerance

and drugs such as spironolactone and nonsteroidal anti-inflammatory agents. Hyponatremia and hyperchloremic acidosis are present in about 60 percent of cases. The anion gap is normal in this form of acidosis; the urine pH is between 5 and 6 and responds normally to acidification.

The major cause of the metabolic acidosis is defective renal ammonia production (renal tubular acidosis [RTA], type IV) due to hyperkalemia. Defective sodium ion–hydrogen ion exchange in the renal tubule because of aldosterone deficiency also contributes.

Administration of a mineralocorticoid such as 9α-fluorohydrocortisone in high doses (0.1 to 0.2 mg/day) is effective in correcting the hyperkalemia and metabolic acidosis. This agent can be used effectively in combination with the loop diuretic furosemide, which also promotes increased potassium and net acid excretion. In patients with hypertension or volume expansion, mineralocorticoids are contraindicated, but furosemide can be used alone.

SECONDARY HYPERALDOSTERONISM

Hyperaldosteronism is commonly encountered in clinical medicine through stimulation of the renin-angiotensin axis. The common stimulus is a low effective intravascular volume or renal perfusion pressure. This may occur with chronic liver disease, cardiac failure, or volume depletion due to diuretic therapy. In the condition of renal artery stenosis, renin secretion is also stimulated because of the lowered renal perfusion pressure. Because renin is stimulated primarily and aldosterone secondarily, these conditions are categorized as secondary hyperaldosteronism, and both PRA and aldosterone are elevated. The hyperaldosteronism produces potassium depletion and hypokalemia. Because the serum sodium correlates inversely with PRA, hyponatremia is often also present and is a useful clue to the secondary nature of the hyperaldosteronism.

PRIMARY ALDOSTERONISM (CONN SYNDROME)

Primary aldosteronism[8,17] is a hypertension syndrome produced from the autonomous excessive secretion of aldosterone by the adrenal cortex. It is an uncommon condition found in 1 to 2 percent of the general hypertensive population.[2] A unilateral, benign adrenocortical adenoma is found in about 60 percent of cases and bilateral adrenocortical hyperplasia in the remainder. Rare causes are adrenal carcinoma and a form of bilateral hyperplasia in which the abnormalities can be corrected with glucocorticoids.

Patients with primary aldosteronism present with hypertension and hypokalemia. This disorder has a peak incidence in the third and fourth decades but may develop at any age. Adenomas are more frequent in women, whereas bilateral hyperplasia is equally divided between the sexes. Frequently there are no clinical features that distinguish this syndrome from other forms of hypertension. Most symptoms are related to the degree of potassium depletion and may be induced or aggravated by diuretics. Headache, nocturia, weakness, and fatigue are common nonspecific complaints. Occasionally thirst, polyuria, intermittent paresthesias, and cardiac arrhythmias are reported. With severe potassium depletion, flaccid paralysis has occurred.

The degree of hypertension can vary from mild to severe, and there may be vascular complications such as myocardial infarction and cerebrovascular accident. Retinopathy, however, is mild and fundal hemorrhages are rare. A postural fall in blood pressure without a concomitant rise in pulse rate may be a diagnostic clue, but this occurs only when severe potassium depletion interferes with adrenergic reflexes. As primary hyperaldosteronism develops, the hypertension is initially associated with normal peripheral vascular resistance and increased intravascular volume. Subsequently, volume status gradually returns to normal and peripheral vascular resistance rises. Edema is virtually never seen. Because of hypokalemia, deep-tendon reflexes may be absent. Metabolic alkalosis may produce positive Trousseau and Chvostek signs, and brief

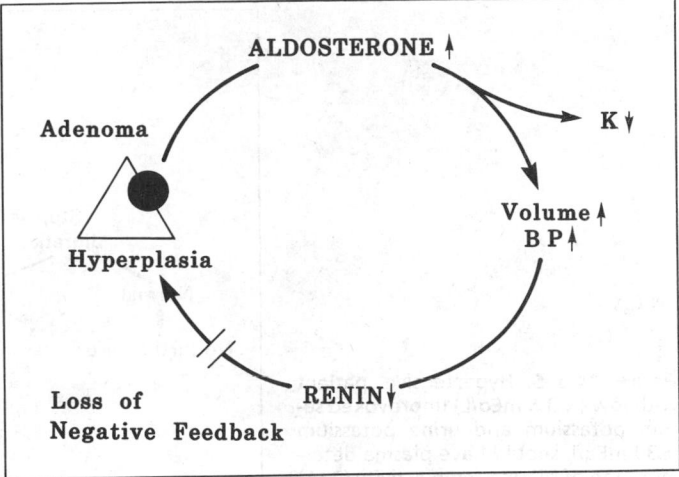

Figure 14.3–4. Aldosterone secreted autonomously from aldosterone-producing adenoma (APA) or from idiopathic hyperaldosteronism (IHA) is unresponsive to negative feedback of renin-angiotensin axis suppressed by aldosterone-mediated extracellular fluid volume expansion. *(From Biglieri EG: Cardiovasc Rev Rep. 3:734, 1982.)*

hyperventilation and excitement can lead to frank tetany (see Table 14.3–6).

Screening Laboratory Studies

The hallmarks of primary aldosteronism are hypertension, hypokalemia, increased aldosterone production, and suppression of the renin-angiotensin system (Fig. 14.3–4). Adrenal glucocorticoid production is normal. All hypertensives should be screened for hypokalemia before treatment (Fig. 14.3–5). If hypokalemia is absent, no further evaluation for hyperaldosteronism is indicated. With this approach, only occasional patients with bilateral adrenal hyperplasia are missed initially, and these can be subsequently detected when they develop spontaneous or diuretic-induced hypokalemia. The vast majority of patients with essential hypertension are thus spared the considerable expense and discomfort of a needless hyperaldosteronism work-up.

Hypokalemia due to excessive urinary potassium loss, the characteristic feature of primary hyperaldosteronism, may be masked by a low sodium intake. When there is less sodium available for reabsorption in the kidney, coupled potassium secretion is reduced and potassium losses are minimized. A practical approach in excluding a falsely normal serum potassium is to place the patient on an unrestricted salt diet plus a supplement of 1 g of sodium chloride with each meal for 4 days. If the fasting serum potassium is normal on the fifth morning in a specimen without hemolysis or difficulty with the venipuncture, hyperaldosteronism is excluded.

Previous diuretic therapy complicates the interpretation of a low serum potassium level. Although this is seldom due to primary aldosteronism, in some cases hypokalemia develops only in this way. If diuretics are the sole cause, when they are discontinued normal dietary potassium intake should restore the serum potassium to normal in 3 weeks.

Hypokalemia in a hypertensive patient should be interpreted in conjunction with a 24-hour urinary potassium determination. If the urinary potassium is above 30 mEq/24 hour in the presence of hypokalemia, then the presence of a renal potassium-losing state is established. In addition to primary aldosteronism, the causes of renal potassium wastage that must be considered are: (1) primary renal diseases with tubular dysfunction, (2) other conditions with increased mineralocorticoid activity—secondary hyperaldosteronism (see above), Cushing syndrome, secretory adrenal tumors, excessive ingestion of licorice (which contains glycyrrhizinic acid),

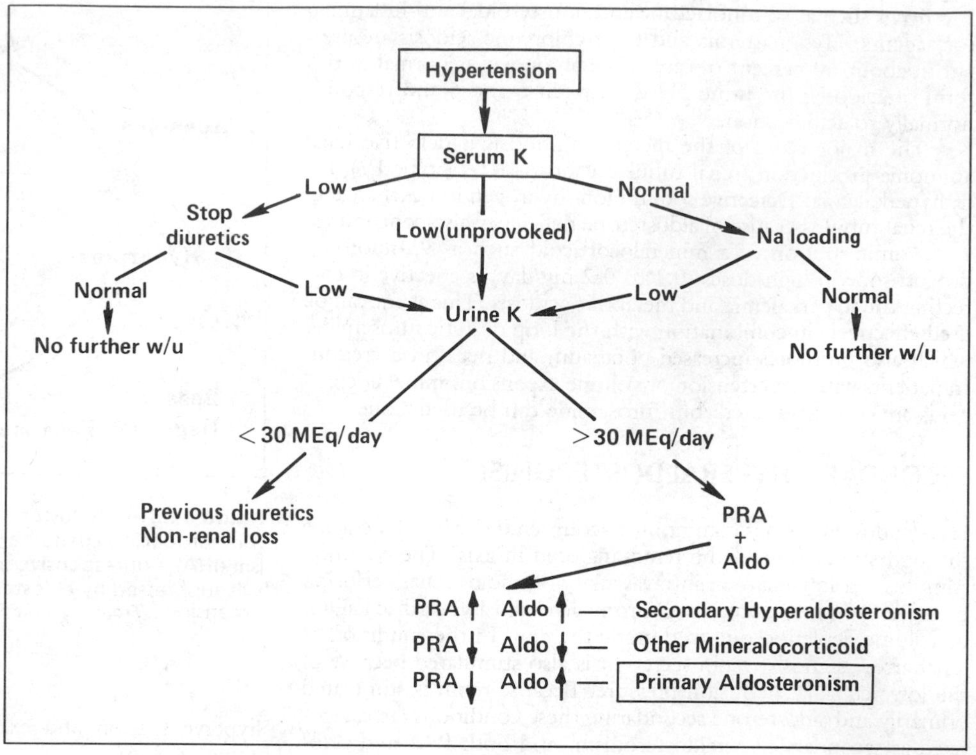

Figure 14.3–5. Hypertensive patient with low (<3.5 mEq/L) unprovoked serum potassium and urine potassium >30 mEq/L should have plasma determination of plasma renin activity (PRA) and aldosterone. If both are elevated, secondary hyperaldosteronism is likely; if both are suppressed, another unmeasured substance with mineralocorticoid activity may be responsible. If PRA is suppressed and aldosterone is elevated, primary aldosteronism should be further investigated as described in the text. (*From Kaplan NM: Clinical Hypertension, 4th ed. Williams & Wilkins, 1986.*)

and rarely other adrenal mineralocorticoid excess states. These disorders are differentiated from primary aldosteronism by measurement of PRA, cortisol, and aldosterone (see below). Before embarking on these studies, it is important to correct potassium depletion with potassium supplements because hypokalemia lowers aldosterone and raises plasma renin activity levels and thus may obscure the diagnosis.

Potassium deficiency accounts for other abnormalities in the initial laboratory evaluation. Metabolic alkalosis is attributable to urinary hydrogen ion loss. Carbohydrate intolerance, due to impaired insulin release, is present in about half of the cases. A defect in urinary concentration unresponsive to vasopressin (nephrogenic diabetes insipidus) accounts for the thirst and polyuria. Excessive renal water loss explains the high serum sodium (139 to 152 mEq/L), which is a useful distinguishing feature from secondary hyperaldosteronism, in which the serum sodium is frequently less than 139 mEq/L. Potassium depletion also produces morphological changes in the kidney with vacuolar degeneration of the proximal tubules and susceptibility to pyelonephritis. Electrocardiographic changes including signs of mild left ventricular hypertrophy and potassium depletion may be clues to the diagnosis.

Definitive Diagnosis

The definitive diagnosis of primary aldosteronism depends on the demonstration of high nonsuppressible aldosterone production and suppressed PRA that cannot be stimulated (Fig. 14.3–6).

Many procedures have been designed to test the appropriateness of aldosterone and plasma renin activity responses to extracellular fluid volume contraction and expansion. A relatively simple test is measurement of the PRA and aldosterone, with the patient standing, 4 hours after 80 mg of oral furosemide (Lasix) is given at 8 AM. A baseline PRA that is suppressed (below 1 ng/ml/hour) and is not stimulated by this volume-depleting maneuver is characteristic of primary aldosteronism. This pattern also occurs in low-renin essential hypertension (25 percent of all hypertensives), and some patients with primary aldosteronism, especially those with bilateral adrenal hyperplasia, may show minimal PRA stimulation. This test

is particularly valuable, however, in excluding secondary hyperaldosteronism in which PRA is high (Fig. 14.3–6).

It also is essential to demonstrate high autonomous aldosterone production in the face of extracellular fluid volume expansion. To do this, plasma aldosterone is measured before and after 2 L of saline infused over 4 hours. In primary aldosteronism the plasma aldosterone level remains above 10 ng/dl (Fig. 14.3–6). In low-renin essential hypertension the aldosterone is suppressible. Elevated aldosterone levels related to physiologic stimulation through the renin-angiotensin axis will also suppress with this rapid volume expansion.

Differentiation of Adrenal Adenoma from Bilateral Hyperplasia

Once the diagnosis of primary aldosteronism is established, patients with bilateral adrenal hyperplasia, also known as idiopathic hyperaldosteronism (IHA), must be distinguished from those with aldosterone-producing adenomas (APA). This differentiation is important and has major therapeutic implications. Surgery is usually indicated for APA but is contraindicated in IHA.

APA is associated generally with a greater metabolic disturbance, a higher mean plasma aldosterone and bicarbonate, and lower serum potassium and PRA. There are also differences between these disorders in hormonal diurnal variation and changes with posture. As already described, primary aldosteronism is largely unresponsive to manipulations of sodium balance. Yet it is very sensitive to ACTH, and patients with APA often show a diurnal variation in aldosterone that parallels cortisol. Patients with IHA may show the same diurnal changes when supine, but in contrast to APA patients, also show an increased sensitivity to angiotensin-II stimulation, reflected in a rise in plasma aldosterone with upright posture. In practice, after overnight recumbency, a blood sample is drawn at 8 AM with the patient supine and again at noon in the upright position. In patients with APA, the plasma aldosterone at 8 AM is above 20 ng/ml and falls at noon, reflecting diurnal variation in ACTH secretion. In those with IHA, the 8 AM plasma aldosterone is less than 20 ng/ml but rises sharply in the noon sample, because of the effect of posture. This test is not foolproof,

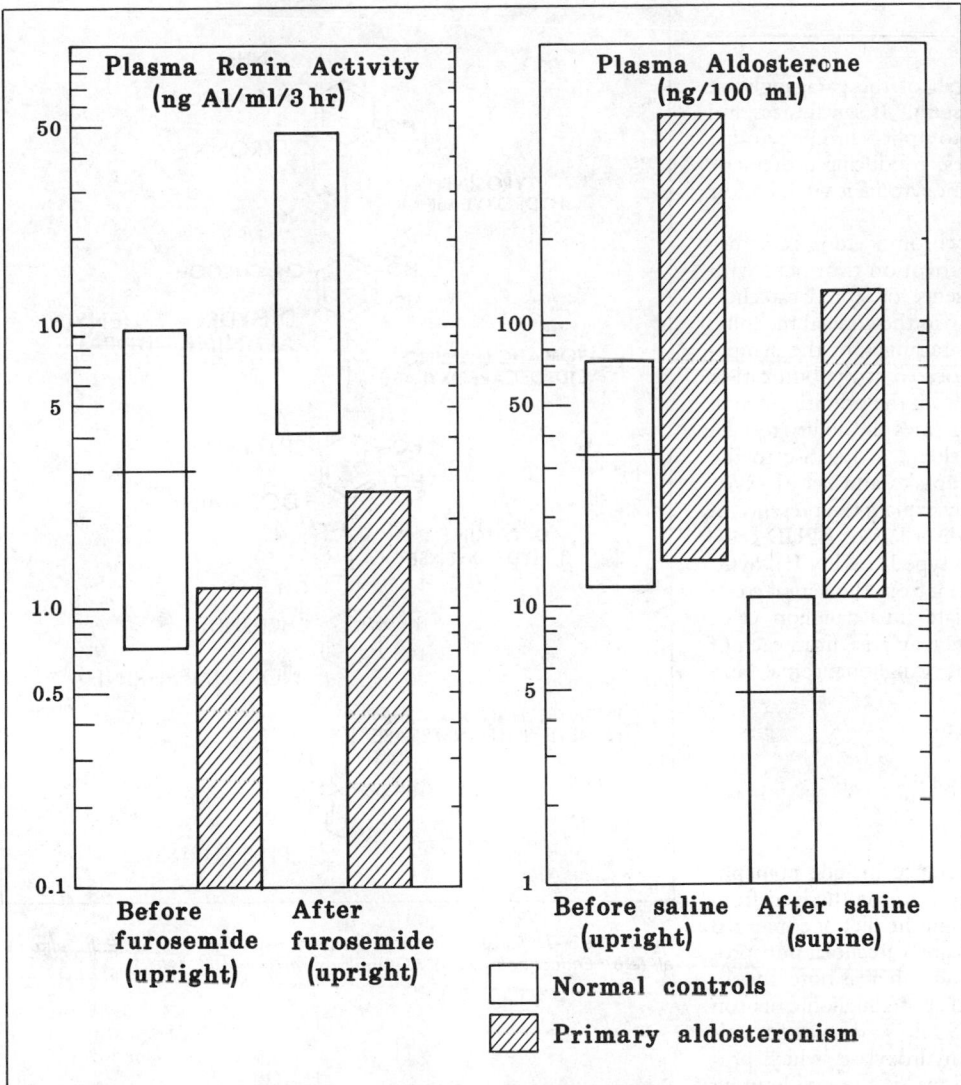

Figure 14.3–6. PRA response to furosemide and posture stimulation (*left panel*) and plasma aldosterone response to saline infusion (*right panel*) in primary aldosteronism and normal controls. Note overlap of baseline measurements but differentiation with stimulation and suppression tests (see text). (*From Weinberger MH, et al: Ann Intern Med 90:386, 1979.*)

and the aldosterone in some APA patients may rise with posture, but a decrease in aldosterone at noon is very suggestive of APA. Measurement of serum 18-hydroxycorticosterone, a precursor of aldosterone, is also useful. This is significantly higher in APA than IHA, and shows a postural rise paralleling aldosterone in IHA.

The most conclusive test used in differentiating an adrenal adenoma from hyperplasia is bilateral adrenal venous catheterization. This procedure should be performed by a radiologist highly skilled in invasive techniques. Samples from the venous effluent of both adrenal glands and from the inferior vena cava are collected and assayed for aldosterone to determine if overproduction is unilateral (adenoma) or bilateral (hyperplasia). If the sampling catheter has been correctly placed in the adrenal veins, cortisol and epinephrine levels will also be high, ensuring the validity of the sampled aldosterone levels. Adrenal venous catheterization is the most accurate test available and the only means of localizing small adenomas. The initial localizing procedure of choice, however, is CT scanning, which has a 90 percent accuracy rate and can detect adrenal adenomas 1 cm in diameter. If IHA is present, both adrenals may appear enlarged or normal in size. CT scanning is generally replacing iodocholesterol radioisotope scintigraphy because it is faster, more accurate, less expensive, and involves lower radiation dosage. As it becomes more widely available MRI will also be extremely useful in adrenal adenoma localization.

Treatment

The treatment of APA is surgical excision of the adenoma whenever possible. More than 50 percent of patients are cured, and in an additional 25 percent there is improvement in the hypertension. Preoperatively, patients are prepared with spironolactone (200 to 400 mg per day) for 1 to 3 months. By its unique action at the level of the mineralocorticoid receptor, spironolactone (1) restores the blood pressure to normal (and therefore gives an indication of the probable response to surgery), (2) corrects the volume expansion and potassium deficits, and (3) reactivates the chronically suppressed renin-angiotensin axis so that postoperative hypoaldosteronism and resultant hyperkalemia are rare.

If surgery cannot be performed, patients can be managed medically with spironolactone. Initially a dose of 400 mg per day may be necessary; spironolactone is associated with impotence, gynecomastia, and menstrual dysfunction. After 6 to 12 weeks, however, when the blood pressure and serum potassium have been controlled, the dose can often be gradually reduced to 100 to 150 mg per day.

Unfortunately, the results of treating IHA are not as rewarding (and therefore there is less emphasis on identifying this disorder). Surgery is of little or no benefit, and although spironolactone in large doses corrects the hypokalemia, treatment of the hypertension often requires additional medication.

THE ADRENAL MEDULLA

The adrenal medulla is a specialized organ of the paraganglionic extension of the sympathetic nervous system.[6] It synthesizes and secretes catecholamines and may give rise to a pheochromocytoma, a tumor that also secretes catecholamines, producing a dramatic clinical picture. Detection of a pheochromocytoma is vital, and its treatment is often a medical emergency.

The chromaffin cell from which pheochromocytomas arise derives its name from the ability to stain brown on treatment with chromium salts. This is due to the presence of stored catecholamines. Chromaffin cells are found mainly in the adrenal medulla, but also appear along the ganglia and paraganglia of the sympathetic chain and organs of Zuckerkandl located at the bifurcation of the aorta. Chromaffin cells are derived from the primitive neural crest and share with other neural crest cell lines the ability to take up amine precursors and decarboxylate them, giving rise to the acronym APUD cells (*a*mine *p*recursor *u*ptake and *d*ecarboxylation). This relationship of APUD cells may explain the presence of pheochromocytoma as a part of familial disorders of APUD cells, for example, multiple endocrine neoplasia type II (MEN II). Sympathogonia, the primordial stem cells arising from the neural crest, migrate out of the CNS and differentiate into ganglion cells, neuroblasts, and chromaffin cells. Tumors may arise from each of these cell lines, namely neuroblastoma, ganglioneuroma, and pheochromocytoma.

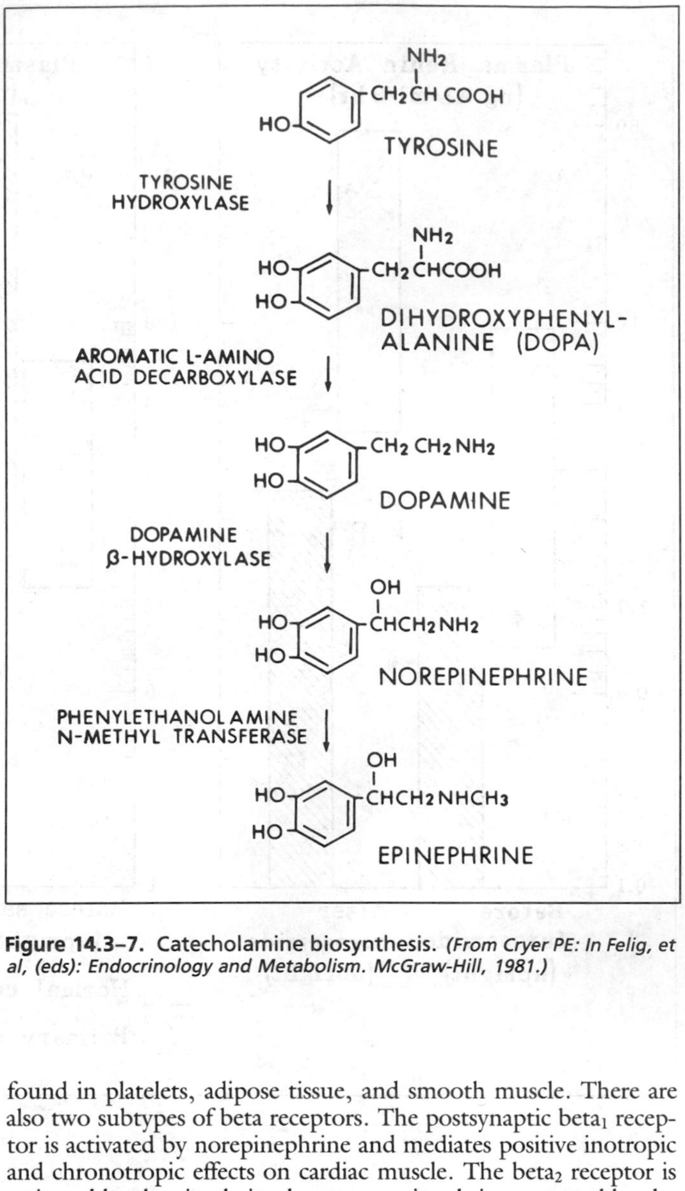

PHYSIOLOGY AND METABOLISM OF CATECHOLAMINES

The catecholamines of physiologic importance include epinephrine, norepinephrine, and dopamine. These are synthesized from tyrosine (Fig. 14.3–7), which is consumed in the diet or converted from phenylalanine in the liver. The major catecholamine produced in the adrenal medulla is epinephrine, whereas norepinephrine is released principally from sympathetic postganglionic neuron axon terminals. The neurons of the CNS release dopamine, epinephrine, and norepinephrine. Tyrosine hydroxylase, which promotes the hydroxylation of tyrosine to dopa, is the rate-limiting enzyme in catecholamine biosynthesis. The adrenal medulla also contains the enzyme phenylethanolamine *N*-methyl transferase (PNMT), which catalyzes the *N*-methylation of norepinephrine to epinephrine. PNMT is induced by glucocorticoids, which are present in high concentration in the adrenal medulla because of a portal venous blood supply from the adrenal cortex. This requirement for glucocorticoids in the synthesis of epinephrine probably explains why norepinephrine is the dominant catecholamine synthesized by extraadrenal pheochromocytomas.

Experimentally, a hemodynamic response to epinephrine is obtained at plasma concentrations of 50 to 100 pg/ml, and these levels occur frequently under stressful situations. In contrast, a plasma level of norepinephrine of 1500 to 2000 pg/ml is required to produce a response, and only rarely are these levels reached under physiologic conditions. It seems, therefore, that norepinephrine functions primarily as a local synaptic neurotransmitter and epinephrine is the mediator of the stress reaction or "fight and flight."

Adrenergic Receptors

Both epinephrine and norepinephrine exert their effects through alpha- and beta-adrenergic receptors on the surface of their target cells. Two subtypes of alpha-adrenergic receptors have been identified. Postsynaptic alpha$_1$ receptors mediate vasoconstriction in vascular smooth muscle. Presynaptic alpha$_2$ receptors are found on nerve endings where they facilitate reuptake of norepinephrine released into the synaptic cleft. By this mechanism further norepinephrine release is inhibited. Alpha$_2$ receptors have also been

Figure 14.3–7. Catecholamine biosynthesis. *(From Cryer PE: In Felig, et al, (eds): Endocrinology and Metabolism. McGraw-Hill, 1981.)*

found in platelets, adipose tissue, and smooth muscle. There are also two subtypes of beta receptors. The postsynaptic beta$_1$ receptor is activated by norepinephrine and mediates positive inotropic and chronotropic effects on cardiac muscle. The beta$_2$ receptor is activated by the circulating hormone epinephrine, secreted by the adrenal medulla. It mediates smooth-muscle relaxation in the bronchi, blood vessels, and uterus. Receptors constitute an important site of regulation of adrenergic activity, and the number of target tissue receptors can be reduced by the binding of an agonist, a phenomenon referred to as "down-regulation." This reduces the sensitivity of an effector cell to high levels of circulating agonist. The reverse occurs with a low level of agonist, in which "up-regulation" of receptors occurs, increasing the sensitivity of the target cell. Hormones other than those binding to the receptor can also alter the interaction between catecholamine agonist and adrenergic receptor. Thyroid hormones increase the number of myocardial beta receptors.

Cardiovascular Effects

Important changes in cardiovascular function are mediated through adrenergic reflexes and triggered via baroreceptors in the heart and great vessels. When blood pressure falls, peripheral anteriolar vasoconstriction (alpha$_1$ receptors) and increase in cardiac output and heart rate (beta$_1$ receptors) are reflexly stimulated. When blood pressure rises, heart rate and cardiac output are reflexly lowered (alpha$_1$) and peripheral vasodilatation may occur (beta$_2$). With sustained peripheral vasoconstriction there is a rapid reduction in intravascular volume because of reduced capacity of the constricted arterial and venous beds.

Extravascular Smooth Muscle Effects

In addition to cardiovascular effects, catecholamines produce relaxation (beta$_2$) and contraction (alpha$_1$) of the uterus and the smooth muscle of the trachea and sphincters of the intestine and bladder.

Metabolic Effects

In humans metabolic effects appear to be mediated through the beta$_2$-adrenergic receptor. Catecholamines increase oxygen consumption and heat production. They also regulate glucose production from storage sites in heart, skeletal muscle and liver, and stimulate lipolysis.

Catecholamines in Regulation of Other Hormonal Systems

Catecholamines are involved in the regulation of the hormonal system both centrally and peripherally. Centrally, they act as neurotransmitters in the control of peptidergic-releasing factors. Dopamine is the prolactin inhibitory factor, and other anterior pituitary hormones are under similar adrenergic influences. Peripherally, norepinephrine stimulates renin production from the juxtaglomerular apparatus of the kidney (beta$_1$). Epinephrine stimulates insulin production from pancreatic islets (beta$_2$), and stimulation of alpha receptors at this site inhibits insulin production. Similar effects have been noted on glucagon secretion from pancreatic A cells. Catecholamines are associated with the increased release of thyroxine, calcitonin, parathyroid hormone, and gastrin—all by a beta$_2$-receptor mechanism.

DEGRADATION OF CATECHOLAMINES

Catecholamines are degraded by two principal enzyme systems (Fig. 14.3–8). Catechol-o-methyl transferase (COMT) and monoamineoxidase (MAO). In the presence of COMT and the methyl donor S-adenosyl methionine, norepinephrine and epinephrine are converted to normetanephrine and metanephrine, which in turn, are converted in the presence of MAO to 3-methoxy-4-hydroxy mandelic acid. This is the major end product of norepinephrine and epinephrine degradation and is usually known as vanillylmandelic acid (VMA). An alternative degradation pathway may also occur where norepinephrine and epinephrine are converted initially in the presence of MAO to 3-,4-dihydroxymandelaldehyde. Dopamine undergoes a similar degradation pathway, except that the metabolites of dopamine lack the hydroxyl group that is present on the beta-carbon of norepinephrine and epinephrine. The end product of this degradation is homovanillic acid. The measurement of the metabolites, VMA, and metanephrines in the urine is a very useful index of catecholamine secretion.

PHEOCHROMOCYTOMA[3,10,11]

Eighty to 90 percent of pheochromocytomas arise from the adrenal glands, but they may be located anywhere along the sympathetic chain and rarely in aberrant sites. Extraadrenal pheochromocytomas are sometimes called paragangliomas, and those arising from specialized chemoreceptor tissue in the carotid body, glomus jugulare, and aortic body have been separately classified as chemodectomas. About 10 percent of pheochromocytomas are malignant with distant metastases, which most commonly involve paraaortic lymph nodes and less frequently liver, lungs, and bone. Malignancy cannot be determined by histology alone, and benign tumors may invade the pheochromocytoma capsule. Ten percent of adrenal pheochromocytomas are bilateral. In the case of familial pheochromocytoma, however, pheochromocytomas commonly occur bilaterally even though one side may present years before the other (Table 14.3–7). In the familial pheochromocytoma that is part of MEN-II there is a precursor stage of adrenal medullary hyperplasia that is also associated with catecholamine overproduction.

Pheochromocytomas are rare; they have been detected in all

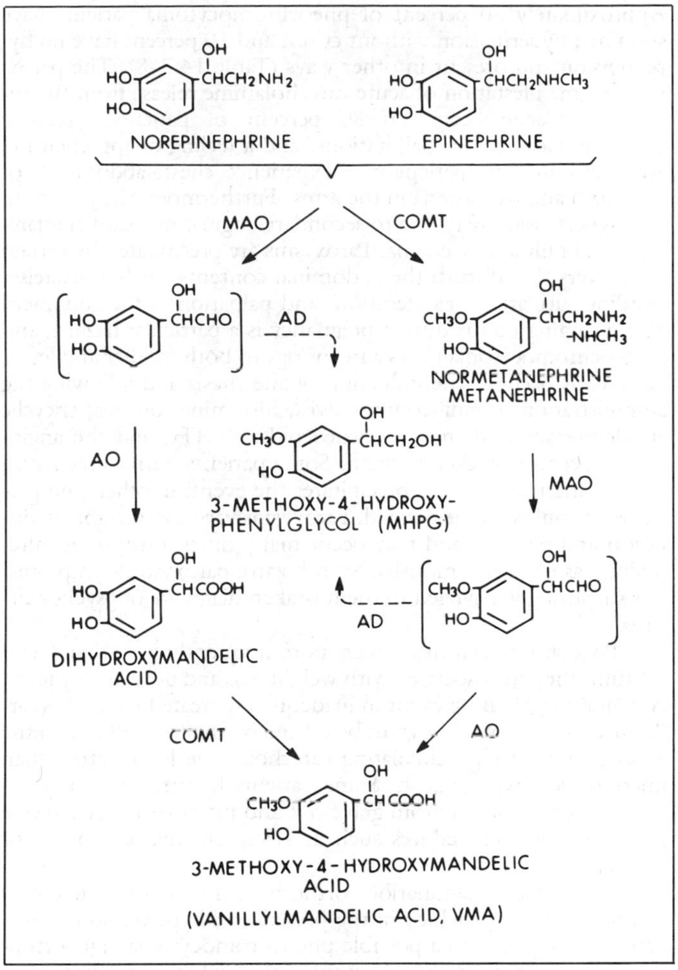

Figure 14.3–8. Catecholamine degradation. COMT = Catechol-*O*-methyl transferase; MAO = monoamine oxidase; AO = aldehyde oxidase; AD = alcohol dehydrogenase. *(From Cryer PE: In Felig, et al, (eds): Endocrinology and Metabolism. McGraw-Hill, 1981.)*

age groups, but occur in only 1 of every 500 hypertensive patients. Screening of every hypertensive would not be cost-effective, therefore, and other clinical clues must be taken into account.

The classic clinical feature of a pheochromocytoma is the paroxysmal hypertensive crisis, which occurs in 60 percent of cases.

TABLE 14.3–7. FAMILIAL PHEOCHROMOCYTOMA SYNDROMES (AUTOSOMAL DOMINANT)

Multiple endocrine neoplasia (MEN) (pheochromocytoma in 75% or more)

MEN-II (Sipple syndrome)
• Pheochromocytoma
• Medullary carcinoma of the thyroid
• Hyperparathyroidism

MEN-III (mucosal neuroma syndrome)
• Pheochromocytoma
• Medullary carcinoma of the thyroid
• Mucosal neuromas
• Ganglioneuromatosis of gut

Phakomatoses
• Von Recklinghausen neurofibromatosis (pheochromocytoma in about 1%)
• von Hippel-Lindau disease (pheochromocytoma in 5–10%)

Approximately 30 percent of pheochromocytoma patients have sustained hypertension without crises, and 10 percent have no hypertension and present in other ways (Table 14.3–8). The paroxysm is a manifestation of acute catecholamine release from the tumor. Headache occurs in 80 percent of patients; excessive sweating, facial pallor, palpitations, and a feeling of apprehension are common. The patient may experience chest, abdominal, or back pain and paresthesia in the arms. Furthermore, the paroxysm and hypertension may lead to secondary angina, myocardial infarction, and pulmonary edema. Paroxysms are precipitated by certain maneuvers that disturb the abdominal contents, such as exercise, bending, urination or defecation, and palpation of the abdomen. The enlarging uterus during pregnancy is a particular hazard, and a pheochromocytoma poses a major risk to both mother and fetus. Paroxysms occur at the induction of anesthesia and following the administration of radiocontrast dyes, histamine, opiates, tricyclic antidepressants, adrenal glucocorticoids, ACTH, and the angiotensin receptor blocker saralasin. Some patients learn to recognize that a particular stimulus precipitates the event; in others, no particular stimulus can be defined. Paroxysms vary considerably in duration and severity, and may occur many times a day or as infrequently as every few months. Such bizarre paroxysmal symptoms, not surprisingly, have led to the mistaken diagnosis of psychoneurosis.

Pheochromocytomas occur more frequently in patients who are thin; they are associated with weight loss and occasionally fever. A major complicating event in inadequately treated patients is cardiomyopathy. This appears to be caused by the toxic effects on the myocardium of high circulating catecholamine levels rather than uncontrolled hypertension. Some patients have few or no symptoms, but are not free from grave risk and may experience a severe paroxysm with procedures such as arteriography, anesthesia, or surgery.

On physical examination, orthostatic hypotension may be a prominent finding, which in the presence of hypertension constitutes a strong clue to a possible pheochromocytoma. The orthostasis is caused by reduced intravascular volume resulting from chronic vasoconstriction and reduced sensitivity of baroreceptors and adrenergic reflexes caused by down-regulation of adrenergic receptors secondary to high circulating catecholamine levels. Severe hypertensive retinopathy is frequently detected and is observed more frequently than in essential hypertension. Surprisingly, renal damage does not parallel the retinopathic changes and tends to be minimal. The features of familial syndromes that are associated with pheochromocytoma may be present (Table 14.3–7).

Routine laboratory tests may show nonspecific abnormalities. A high hematocrit is attributable to reduced intravascular volume and, in some cases, to ectopic production of erythropoietin and a true increase in red cell mass. An elevated leukocyte count without a left shift is consistent with demargination of white cells secondary to generalized vasoconstriction. The plasma glucose may also be elevated, reflecting suppression of insulin secretion and stimulation of liver glycogenolysis by catecholamines.

Electrocardiographic changes have been reported and if transient during a paroxysm are particularly suggestive of a pheochromocytoma.

Sudden death in patients with pheochromocytoma may be due to cardiac arrhythmia. Myocardial infarction, acute pulmonary edema, and thrombotic or hemorrhagic stroke are all frequent complications of a paroxysm. Pheochromocytoma is also associated with cholelithiasis, ectopic ACTH syndrome, and secondary hyperaldosteronism from compression of a renal artery. Hemorrhagic necrosis of a pheochromocytoma may be a disastrous event. This can mimic an acute abdomen or cardiovascular catastrophe and necessitates prompt removal of the tumor.

In contrast to the intermittent nature of clinical symptoms, most pheochromocytomas secrete catecholamines continuously. Paroxysms are presumably due to a sudden, acute surge in this catecholamine secretion. Clinically detected small tumors tend to secrete intact epinephrine and norepinephrine that produce symptoms, whereas larger tumors tend to release biologically inactive catecholamine metabolites with less symptomatic effects. Most pheochromocytomas produce both norepinephrine and epinephrine. Epinephrine production points to a location in the adrenal medulla but has been associated with extraadrenal pheochromocytoma on occasions. Predominant or isolated epinephrine secretion is rare and may produce a distinctive clinical picture with symptoms and signs of a metabolic nature such as weight loss and hyperglycemia and less impressive hypertension.

Diagnosis

The diagnosis of a pheochromocytoma is made by demonstrating elevated levels of catecholamines or their metabolites in the blood and urine (see normal values, p. 1222). Localization procedures and exploratory surgery should be undertaken only after such biochemical confirmation of the diagnosis, not because of clinical suspicion alone. One carefully collected, acid-preserved 24-hour urine specimen assayed for VMA, total metanephrines, or total free catecholamines constitutes an excellent screening test with a reliability of 95 percent, if drug interference is excluded. Metanephrines are more consistently elevated than VMA in pheochromocytoma, and there are less interfering factors with the assay. Urinary free catecholamines are less reliable, but can be fractionated into epinephrine and norepinephrine moieties. A high epinephrine level suggests that the pheochromocytoma is located in the adrenal medulla and is a sensitive screening procedure for the familial pheochromocytoma which is part of MEN-II. Basal plasma catecholamines have comparable diagnostic accuracy to 24-hour urinary catecholamines and metabolites but are generally reserved for the validation of urinary tests or to catch a burst of catecholamine secretion during an intermittent paroxysm. Considerable care must be practiced in obtaining the blood sample. The patient should lie quietly and the needle inserted with a heparin lock 30 minutes before the sample is obtained. Plasma levels are also used in provocative testing and in selective venous catheterization for localization of a pheochromocytoma (see below).

A number of pharmacologic tests for the diagnosis of pheochromocytoma have been reported, both stimulatory (inducing a hypertensive response) and suppressive (inducing a fall in blood pressure). Histamine, tyramine, and phentolamine tests have become obsolete because of the danger and the high incidence of both false-negative and false-positive results. Two tests that are safe and more reliable measure both the blood pressure response and

TABLE 14.3–8. COMMON SYMPTOMS AND SIGNS OF PHEOCHROMOCYTOMA

	(% of Cases)
Hypertension	>90
Sustained	(30)
Sustained with crises	(30)
Paroxysmal	(30)
Headache	80
Sweating	70
Palpitations	65
Pallor	45
Nausea with or without vomiting	40
Nervousness	35
Funduscopic changes	30
Weight loss	25
Epigastric or chest pain	20

Data derived from Hermann H, Mornex R: Human Tumors Secreting Catecholamines. New York, Macmillan, 1964[10] and based on 507 cases.

the change in plasma catecholamines. In patients with a pheochromocytoma, glucagon 0.5 to 1.0 mg intravenously induces a blood pressure rise of at least 20/15 mm Hg in excess of that seen with a cold pressor test, and at the blood pressure peak plasma catecholamines are increased threefold above baseline or to over 2000 pg/ml. The alpha₂-adrenergic agonist *clonidine* inhibits the release of catecholamines from nerve terminals and thus the elevated levels associated with sympathetic nervous system activity but has no effect on the autonomous catecholamine production from pheochromocytomas. Plasma catecholamines are measured basally and 3 hours after clonidine 0.3 mg orally. In a positive clonidine test plasma levels fail to suppress significantly or to fall below 500 pg/ml. Pentolinium, a preganglionic blocking agent, has been used in a similar fashion. Clonidine is the safest pharmacological test when the patient is hypertensive, and glucagon may be used as a substitute if the patient is normotensive at the time of testing.

Localization

Once the presence of a pheochromocytoma has been confirmed by biochemical testing, it is necessary to localize the tumor or tumors. No localizing procedure should be performed until a biochemical diagnosis has been made. The best test available is the abdominal CT scan, which is capable of detecting tumors 1 cm in diameter or greater and has an overall accuracy of more than 90 percent in the diagnosis of pheochromocytoma. Ultrasonography is less accurate, and intravenous pyelogram (IVP) with or without tomograms of the suprarenal areas is outmoded except where other modern procedures are unavailable. CT scanning is not as reliable in the detection of tumors outside the renal-adrenal area, and it may be necessary to sample venous blood in the great veins at many sites from the neck to the pelvis. A step-up in plasma catecholamine concentration would then identify a site that can be further studied by arteriography or CT scanning. Arteriography is infrequently required but may provide additional information about blood supply to the tumor, especially when it is at the hilum of the kidney close to the great vessels. Arteriography, of course, is an invasive procedure that may precipitate a hypertensive crisis, and patients must be prepared with alpha-adrenergic blocking agents beforehand.

Radionuclide iodine-131 scanning with metaiodobenzylguanidine, an analog of norepinephrine that is specifically concentrated in adrenergic vesicles, is also employed. The normal adrenal medulla is not visible, but most tumors of all sizes, in the adrenals and elsewhere, both benign and malignant, are located easily. Tumors too small to be seen by CT scan and even adrenal medullary hyperplasia have been visualized. The use of diagnostic and localization techniques is summarized in Figure 14.3–9.

Treatment

Surgical excision remains the only satisfactory method of treating pheochromocytomas. The preoperative and intraoperative period, however, can be associated with large swings in blood pressure and life-threatening arrhythmias. Postoperatively profound hypotension may occur. Considerable skill and experience is mandatory in the coordinated medical, anesthesia, and surgical care of these cases.

Once the diagnosis is made, treatment is begun with alpha-adrenergic blockade (Table 14.3–9). Phenoxybenzamine, 10 mg orally, is given twice daily and the dose increased slowly up to a maximum of 20 mg four times a day to attain blood pressure control. Alpha blockade provides relatively stable blood pressure through further evaluation procedures such as arteriography, induction of anesthesia, and surgery. By reversing peripheral vasoconstriction, it also allows blood volume to be restored preoperatively, and catastrophic postoperative hypotension is thus avoided. To facilitate blood volume expansion, intravenous fluids are given over the preoperative period, and in some centers, two to three units of whole blood are added 12 to 18 hours before the operation. Beta blockade may also be used if tachycardia or a cardiac arrhythmia is present. It should never be started until full alpha blockade has been achieved because a paradoxical pressor response

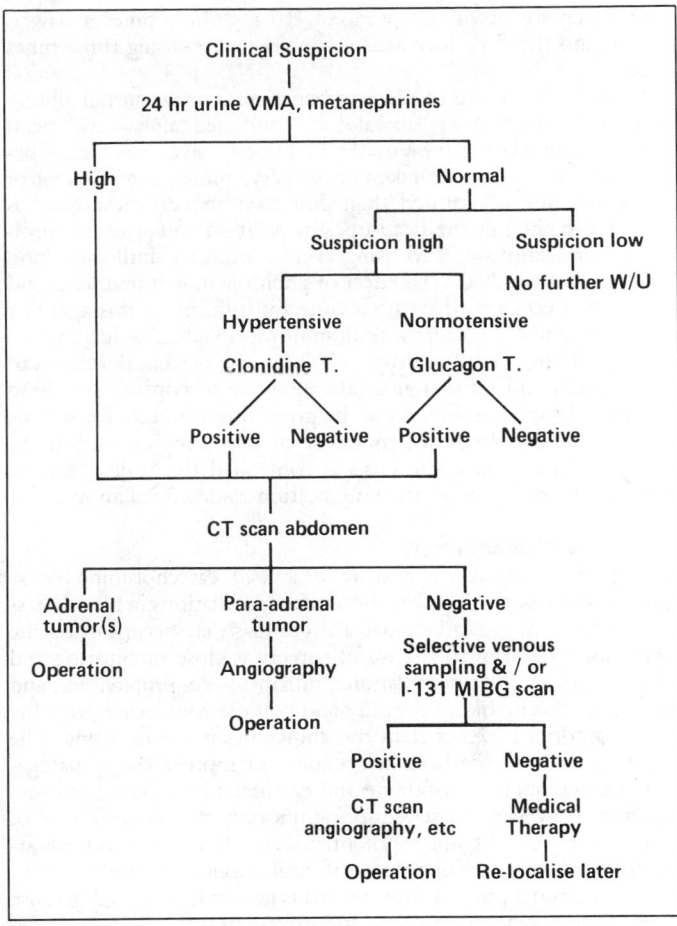

Figure 14.3–9. Flow chart for investigation and localization of a possible pheochromocytoma. (*From Welbourn RM, et al: Tumors of the Neuroendocrine System. Current Problems in Surgery, August 1984, Year Book.*)

TABLE 14.3–9. DRUGS IN MEDICAL MANAGEMENT OF PHEOCHROMOCYTOMA

Alpha-adrenergic blockers
Acute
• Phentolamine, 2–5 mg IV
Chronic
• Phenoxybenzamine, 10–20 mg tid to qid
• Prazosin, 1–5 mg bid

Beta-adrenergic blockers (after alpha blockade)
Acute
• Propranolol, 1–2 mg IV
• Labetalol (alpha + beta), 20–40 mg IV
Chronic
• Propranolol, 10–40 mg qid or other β blocker
• Labetalol, 200–600 mg bid

Catecholamine-synthesis inhibitors
• Alpha-methyl p-tyrosine (metyrosine), 250 mg to 1 g bid

For hypertensive crisis
• Phentolamine, IV 2–5 mg (bolus) *or* 100 mg in 500 ml 5% dextrose (infusion)
• Nitroprusside, 100 mg in 500 ml 5% dextrose (infusion)

For hypotension
• Norepinephrine infusion

For arrhythmias
• Lidocaine, 50–100 mg IV (20–50 mg/min)
• Propranolol, 0.5–2 mg IV

may otherwise occur. Propranolol, 10 mg three times a day, is started and the dose increased gradually up to 40 mg three times a day.

As an alternative to phenoxybenzamine, prazosin (an alpha$_1$-adrenergic blocker) or labetalol (a combined alpha- and beta-adrenergic blocker) can be used. If a hypertensive crisis occurs before the patient can be taken to surgery, more acute control of blood pressure is required than described above. The patient is then maintained in the head-upright position and given phentolamine intravenously, 2 to 5 mg every 5 minutes until the blood pressure is controlled. The effect of phentolamine is transient, and it may be necessary to set up a constant infusion of this agent or of the peripheral vasodilator sodium nitroprusside. A solution containing 100 mg of either drug in 500 ml of 5 percent dextrose can be prepared and infused at a rate adequate to control the blood pressure. Propranolol may also be given intravenously for serious tachycardia or arrhythmias in a dose of 1 to 2 mg over a 5 to 10 minute period. Once the crisis is controlled the patient can be switched to oral preoperative medication as described above.

Operative Management

Despite the preoperative measures described, catecholamine blockade is usually not complete, and marked oscillations in blood pressure, hypotension, and cardiac arrhythmias may occur during the operation. The key to successful surgery is close monitoring and ready availability of phentolamine, nitroprusside, propranolol, and lidocaine. Precise blood pressure and volume control are probably more important factors than the choice of anesthetic agent. The halogenated hydrocarbon halothane and more recently halogenated ethers such as isoflurane and enflurane have been used successfully, however. These reduce significantly the pressor action of catecholamines but may potentiate catecholamine-induced arrhythmias. An anterior transperitoneal surgical approach for an intra-abdominal pheochromocytoma is generally preferred because these tumors may be multiple and extra-adrenal.

Postoperatively, hypotension may be a serious problem. The factors possibly involved include continued blood loss with inadequate replacement, down-regulation of adrenergic receptors with insensitivity of adrenergic reflexes, and persisting effects of preoperative alpha- and beta-adrenergic blockade (e.g., with phenoxybenzamine and propranolol). Rigorous monitoring should be continued in the postoperative period with continued attention to blood-volume replacement. Hypertension may also occur, as a result of fluid overload, residual pheochromocytoma tissue, or inadvertent ligation of a renal artery. Severe hypoglycemia has been reported, presumably because of the sudden reduction in catecholamine levels and the associated inhibition of glycogenolysis.

Prognosis

The 5-year survival rate after successful resection of benign pheochromocytomas is 96 percent; 75 percent of patients are rendered normotensive. Some patients remain hypertensive without evidence of residual tumor. Patients with sporadic tumors should be followed for at least 2 years, and should have urine collections at least once a year to rule out late recurrence. In familial cases, yearly follow-up should be continued indefinitely because of the possibility of a second pheochromocytoma on the contralateral side.

The treatment of malignant pheochromocytomas also involves surgery with radical removal of the primary lesion and involved lymph nodes and further excision of recurrent tumor when detected at follow-up. Chemotherapy has generally been disappointing, but a combination of cyclophosphamide, vincristine, and dacarbazine may be the best current combination available. Radiation therapy is also ineffective. Although it may not be possible to eradicate these tumors totally, it is still appropriate to treat patients medically and control symptoms related to catecholamine secretion. As with benign pheochromocytomas, alpha and, in some cases, beta blockade is used as well as the agent metyrosine, which blocks tyrosine hydroxylase and thus norepinephrine synthesis. Metyrosine, 250 mg twice a day, is gradually increased by 250 to 500 mg per day up to a total dose of 3 g per day. This provides satisfactory blood pressure control and reduction in blood catecholamine levels.

REFERENCES

1. Antoni F: Hypothalamic control of ACTH secretion: Advances since the discovery of 41-residue corticotropin-releasing factor. Endocr Rev 7:351, 1986
2. Biglieri EG: Adrenocortical components in hypertension. Cardiovasc Rev Rep 3:734, 1982
3. Bravo EL, Gifford RW Jr: Pheochromocytoma: Diagnosis, localization and management. N Engl J Med 311:1298, 1984
4. Bravo EL, Tarazi RC, et al: The changing clinical spectrum of primary aldosteronism. Am J Med 74:641, 1983
5. Carpenter P: Cushing's syndrome: Update of diagnosis and management. Mayo Clin Proc 61:49, 1986
6. Cryer PE: Physiology and pathophysiology of the human sympathoadrenal neuroendocrine system. N Engl J Med 303:436, 1980
7. Dewailly D, Vantyghem-Haudiquet M, Sainsard C: Clinical and biological phenotypes in late-onset 21-hydroxylase deficiency. J Clin Endocrinol Metab 63:418, 1986
8. Ferris JB, Beevers DJ, et al: Low-renin (''primary'') hyperaldosteronism. Am Heart J 95:375, 641, 1978; 96:97, 1978
9. Hardy J: Cushing's disease—50 years later. Can J Neurol Sci 9:375, 1982
10. Hermann H, Mornex R: Human Tumors Secreting Catecholamines. New York, Macmillan, 1964
11. Manger WM, Gifford RW Jr: Pheochromocytoma. New York, Springer-Verlag, 1977
12. Neufeld M, Maclaren N, Blizzard R: Two types of autoimmune Addison's disease associated with different polyglandular autoimmune syndrome. Medicine 60:355, 1981
13. North R, Walter R: The effects of alcohol on the endocrine system. Med Clin North Am 68:133, 1984
14. Oldfield E, Chrousos G, et al: Preoperative lateralization of ACTH-secreting pituitary microadenomas by bilateral and simultaneous inferior petrosal venous sinus sampling. N Engl J Med 312:100, 1985
15. Phelps KR, Lieberman RL, et al: Pathophysiology of the syndrome of hyporeninemic hypoaldosteronism. Metabolism 29:186, 1980
16. Sullivan J: Steroid withdrawal syndromes. South Med J 75:726, 1982
17. Weinberger MH, Grim CE, et al: Primary aldosteronism. Ann Int Med 90:386, 1979

Disorders of Thyroid Gland

Paul W. Ladenson

Diseases of the thyroid gland are commonly encountered, challenging to diagnose, and satisfying to treat because of usual good results. Some disorders cause excessive production of thyroid hormones (hyperthyroidism); others cause insufficient production (hypothyroidism). Thyroid gland enlargement may be generalized (goiter) or focal (nodule) and may be caused by functional impairment, inflammation (thyroiditis), or neoplasia.

Several comprehensive texts provide detailed discussions of all aspects of thyroid physiology and pathophysiology.[3,6]

CLINICAL ANATOMY

Thyroid tissue differentiates at the base of the tongue and migrates caudally to its midline position anterior to the trachea at the level of the sternal notch. Ectopic thyroid tissue may be found either above or below the gland's normal position, as a lingual thyroid, in the superior mediastinum, or anywhere in between. Thyroglossal duct cysts may develop later in life along the course of the gland's embryologic migration and may be complicated by infection or malignancy.

The normal thyroid has two lobes, which are draped over the lateral aspects of the trachea and connected by a slender isthmus. A pyramidal lobe projects superiorly in 10 percent of normal individuals and is often palpable in enlarged glands. Congenital absence of one thyroid lobe (hemiagenesis) occurs rarely but does not cause hypothyroidism because the remaining lobe develops compensatory hypertrophy. Complete or partial thyroid agenesis occurs in 1 per 4000 births and causes fetal and neonatal hypothyroidism which, if untreated, leads to cretinism.

The gross anatomic relationships of the thyroid gland are clinically important. Thyroid enlargement (goiter) may compress the trachea or esophagus producing local symptoms of dyspnea, cough, or dysphagia. The recurrent laryngeal nerves, which pass beneath the thyroid, may be compressed or invaded by thyroid disease or may be injured during thyroid surgery. Resulting vocal cord paralysis causes hoarseness or aspiration if unilateral, and dyspnea, stridor, or respiratory insufficiency if bilateral. The parathyroid glands lie deep to the thyroid and may be inadvertently removed or devascularized during thyroid surgery.

Thyroid epithelial cells are oriented around a follicular lumen containing colloid composed of the thyroid hormone precursor thyroglobulin. The thyroid also contains parafollicular cells (C cells), which produce calcitonin and give rise to medullary carcinoma of the thyroid. The gland is surrounded by a fibrous capsule endowed with afferent sensory fibers. Stretching, inflammation, or invasion of the capsule may cause pain in the anterior neck or referred pain in the mandible, ears, or throat. The thyroid gland is highly vascular, and increased blood flow in some forms of hyperthyroidism may cause a bruit or thrill over the gland.

CLINICAL PHYSIOLOGY

CONTROL OF THYROID GLAND FUNCTION

Thyrotropes in the anterior pituitary gland secrete thyrotropin (thyroid-stimulating hormone, TSH), the principal stimulus to thyroid hormone biosynthesis and secretion. TSH is a glycoprotein comprising an alpha subunit, which is virtually identical to that in the gonadotropins, and a unique beta subunit, which confers biologic specificity. TSH acts on follicular epithelial cells by binding to cell membrane receptors, which are coupled to adenylate cyclase. TSH is essential for normal thyroid function, and TSH deficiency predictably results in secondary (thyroprivic) hypothyroidism.

Pituitary TSH production is chiefly controlled by two factors, stimulation by hypothalamic thyrotropin-releasing hormone (TRH) and inhibition by thyroid hormones (Fig. 14.4–1). TRH is a tripeptide synthesized in the medial basal hypothalamus, released into the hypothalamic-hypophyseal portal venous system, and bound to membrane receptors on thyrotropes where it promotes TSH synthesis and release by modulating intracellular calcium fluxes. TRH deficiency due to hypothalamic disease or pituitary stalk interruption causes tertiary hypothyroidism.

Negative feedback on the pituitary by thyroid hormone decreases TSH production. Even modest thyroid gland hyperfunction suppresses pituitary TSH release, and conversely a small decrement in circulating thyroid hormone causes higher circulating TSH levels. This exquisite thyrotrope sensitivity renders the serum TSH concentration an extremely valuable measure of thyroid function.

THYROID HORMONE BIOSYNTHESIS

Thyroid follicular epithelial cells synthesize the two biologically active thyroid hormones, thyroxine (T_4; 3,3′,5,5′-L-tetraiodothyronine) and triiodothyronine (T_3; 3,3′,5-L-triiodothyronine) (Fig. 14.4–2). The normal North American diet contains 300 to 1000 μg of iodine per day of which approximately 10 to 30 percent is trapped by a transport system in thyroid cell membranes. Thyroid cells also synthesize thyroglobulin, a unique protein (molecular mass, 660,000 daltons) not produced by other tissues. Thyroglobulin is normally sequestered within the thyroid follicles so that its release into the circulation is a useful marker of thyroid disease. An enzyme present in the apical membrane, thyroid peroxidase, catalyzes oxidation of iodine and its covalent linkage to tyrosines in thyroglobulin, a process called *organification,* to produce monoiodotyrosine and diiodotyrosine. Thyroid peroxidase also promotes the *coupling* of certain iodinated tyrosines brought into close apposition by the tertiary structure of thyroglobulin to form the iodothyronines, T_4 and T_3. These thyroid hormone precursors are secreted into the follicular lumen bound to thyroglobulin. When stimulated, follicular epithelial cells reabsorb colloidal thyroglobulin by pinocytosis. Iodothyronines are hydrolyzed off, and T_4 and T_3 are released into the circulation. The normal human thyroid gland synthesizes ten times as much T_4 as T_3 and secretes them at the same relative rates: T_4 80 to 90 μg per day and T_3 8 μg per day. Iodine is salvaged within the thyroid and recycled for organification by *deiodination* of iodotyrosines and other iodothyronines, which are not normally detected in plasma. Thyroid hormone production is regulated by TSH and by iodine itself. TSH stimulates all steps in thyroid hormone synthesis and release. Iodine exerts several distinct effects on thyroid gland function. Moderate dietary iodine deficiency (<100 μg per day) causes TSH-dependent compensatory thyroid enlargement, whereas severe sustained iodine deficiency (<20 μg per day) alone can lead to hypothyroidism, particularly in the fetus and neonate. In contrast, a pharmacologic iodine load (>30 mg per day) actually interferes with the trapping and organification of iodine and with the release of stored thyroid hormones. Iodine-induced inhibition of organification, called the

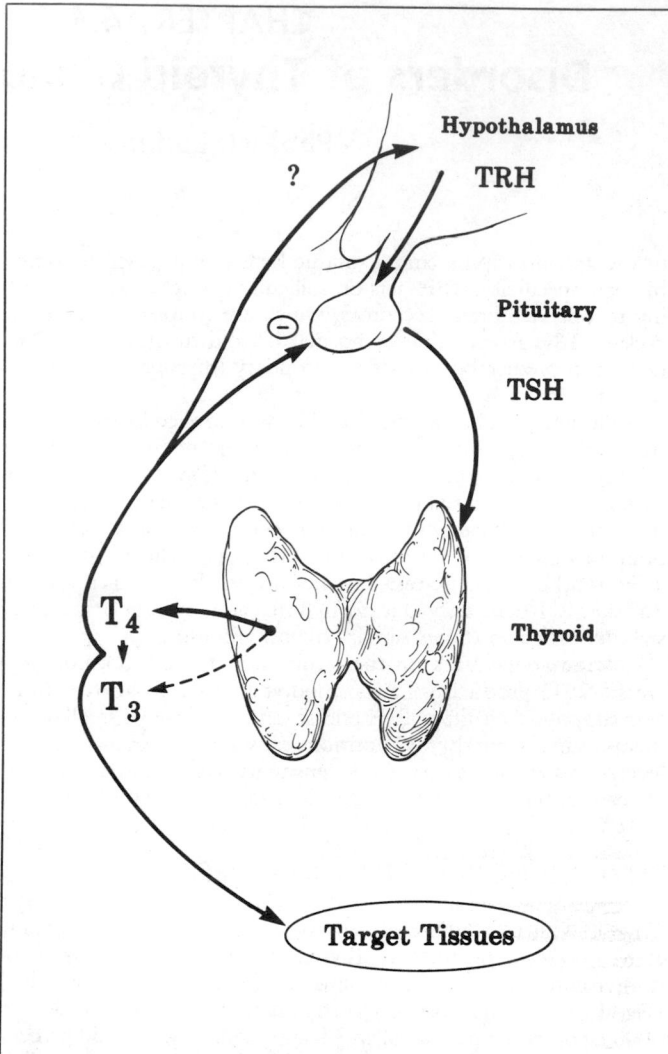

Figure 14.4–1. Hypothalamic-pituitary-thyroid axis. Hypothalamic thyrotropin-releasing hormone (TRH) stimulates pituitary thyrotropin production. TSH regulates thyroid gland growth and the biosynthesis and release of thyroid hormones (thyroxine [T_4] and triiodothyronine [T_3]), which act on target tissues, including the pituitary where negative feedback inhibits TSH production.

Wolff-Chaikoff effect, is a transient phenomenon in normally functioning thyroid glands, lasting 2 to 3 weeks followed by escape and resumption of iodine organification. These effects of iodine on thyroid hormone biosynthesis have been termed "autoregulation" because they uncouple dietary iodine intake from thyroid hormone production. In certain thyroid diseases, iodine and other cations (e.g., lithium and perchlorate) may cause sustained thyroid dysfunction—hypothyroidism in autoimmune thyroiditis and hyperthyroidism[4] in nodular goiter (see below).

THYROID HORMONE TRANSPORT AND METABOLISM[9]

Thyroxine (T_4) is 99.97 percent bound to three classes of plasma proteins: thyroxine-binding globulin (TBG, 75 percent), thyroxine-binding prealbumin (TBPA, 15 percent), and albumin (10 percent). Triiodothyronine (T_3) is bound to a lesser extent (99.7 percent) and almost exclusively to TBG. The small free fractions of circulating T_4 (0.03 percent) and T_3 (0.3 percent) readily enter cells. In certain tissues, some bound thyroid hormone may also be available for intracellular exchange.

The presence of these plasma thyroid hormone-binding proteins has several clinically important consequences. Quantitative and qualitative abnormalities in the binding proteins alter the serum total T_4 and total T_3 concentrations but do not affect the biologically active, free thyroid hormone fraction, which is principally responsible for expression of thyroid hormone action. States of altered thyroid hormone-binding proteins may, however, be confused with true thyroid dysfunction if only total serum thyroid hormone concentrations are considered. Because T_4 is relatively more protein-bound, it is normally present in an approximately 50-fold higher plasma concentration, has a longer serum half-life (7 days) than T_3 (1 day), and is more extracellular in its distribution.

Thyroid hormones are metabolized by deiodination and deacetylation in target tissues, and conjugated metabolites are secreted in bile. Metabolic clearance of thyroid hormone may be altered by physiologic, pathophysiologic, and pharmacologic factors. Thyroxine metabolism is reduced by 50 percent in the elderly. Many nonthyroidal systemic illnesses and some drugs cause dissociation of thyroid hormones from binding proteins and increase their clearances. Some pharmacologic agents, for example, phenytoin, directly enhance hepatic metabolism of thyroid hormones.

Outer ring monodeiodination of T_4 in extrathyroidal tissues accounts for 80 percent of daily T_3 production in humans (Fig. 14.4–3). The conversion of T_4 to more biologically active T_3 contributes significantly to the intranuclear T_3 available for interaction with thyroid hormone receptors, particularly in the anterior pituitary and central nervous system (CNS). Several circumstances reduce T_4-to-T_3 conversion, including systemic illness, fasting, and some pharmacologic agents (Table 14.4–1). In all of these states, reduced tissue-T_3 concentration may cause a compensatory decrease in rates of protein catabolism and tissue oxygen consumption. The inner ring monodeiodination of T_4 yields reverse T_3 (3,3′,5′-triiodothyronine, rT_3), a biologically inactive compound. Because rT_3 monodeiodination to diiodothyronine is catalyzed by the same enzyme facilitating T_4-to-T_3 conversion, factors causing low serum T_3 typically produce a reciprocal increase in rT_3.

THYROID HORMONE ACTIONS IN TARGET TISSUES[8]

Thyroid hormone crosses cellular and nuclear membranes of target cells by simple diffusion or facilitated transport. Within the nucleus, T_3 is bound with high affinity by specific receptors. T_4 is also bound with lower affinity. Nuclear thyroid hormone receptors are composed of a nonhistone chromatin protein that is intimately associated with DNA. In some kindreds with resistance to thyroid hormone action, there is abnormally decreased receptor number or affinity for thyroid hormone. Thyroid hormone binding to its receptor promotes expression of specific messenger RNA (mRNA) molecules that define the translation of specific proteins (Fig. 14.4–4). In experimental systems several proteins have been identified that exemplify this mode of thyroid hormone action. In myocardium, for example, thyroid hormone increases beta-adrenergic receptor number and promotes production of the myosin isoenzyme species that more rapidly hydrolyze ATP and cross-link with actin filaments.

It has long been appreciated that thyroid hormone increases the rates of many cellular metabolic processes. Whether these ac-

TABLE 14.4–1. CIRCUMSTANCES THAT DECREASE T_4-TO-T_3 CONVERSION

- Fetus and neonate
- Systemic (nonthyroidal) illness (e.g., surgery, sepsis, myocardial infarction, renal or hepatic failure)
- Poor caloric intake
- Drugs: propylthiouracil, glucocorticoids, beta-adrenergic blockers, amiodarone, radiocontrast dyes

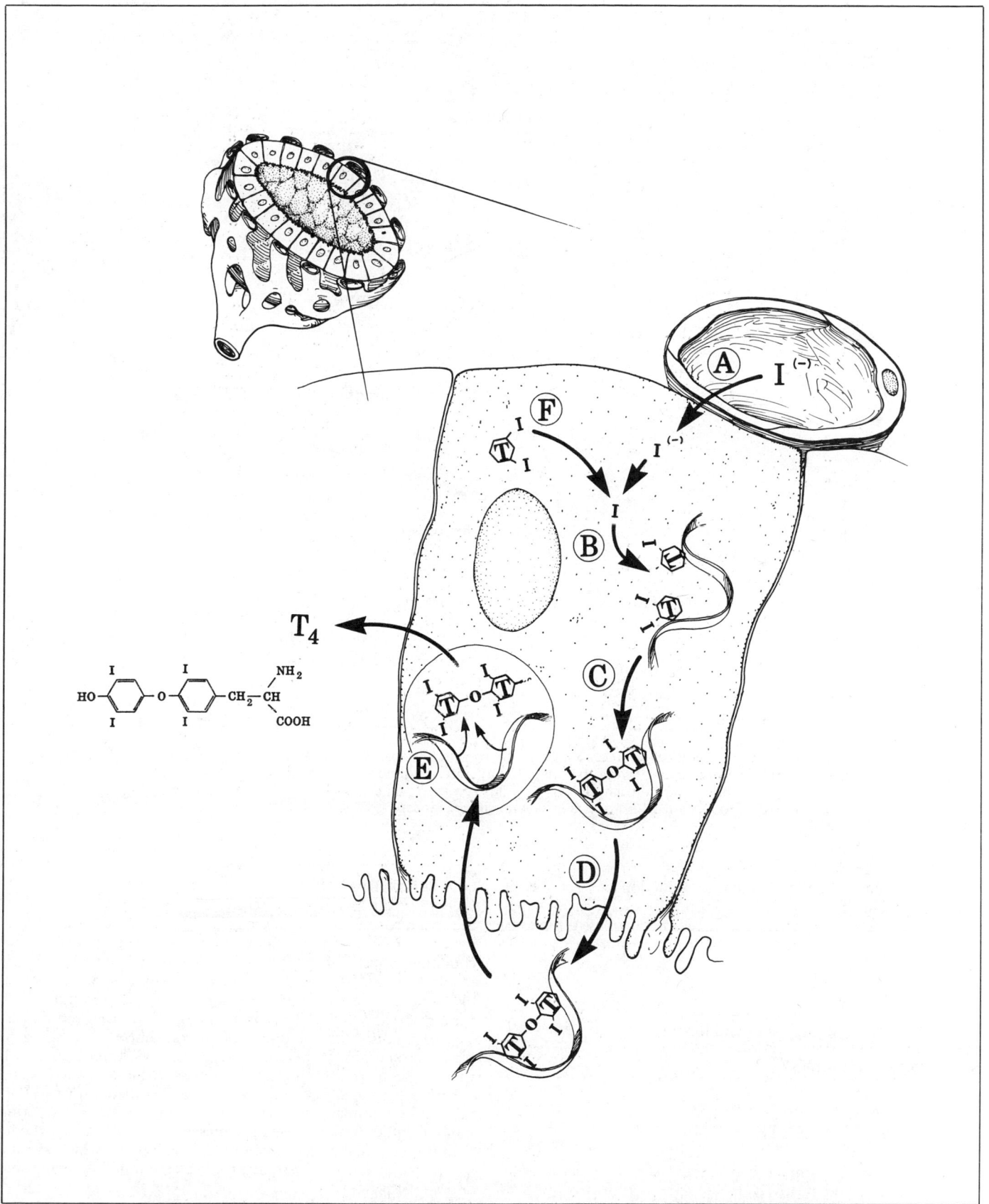

Figure 14.4–2. Biosynthesis of thyroid hormones. Iodine is trapped by follicular cells *(A)* and organified, i.e., linked to tyrosines on thyroglobulin *(B)*, two of which are coupled *(C)* to form iodothyronines. Iodinated thyroglobulin is stored *(D)* as colloid in the follicular lumen before pinocytosis, hydrolysis, and release *(E)* of thyroid hormones into blood. Intrathyroidal deiodination *(F)* scavenges iodine from inactive iodinated compounds. All steps are stimulated by thyrotropin (TSH).

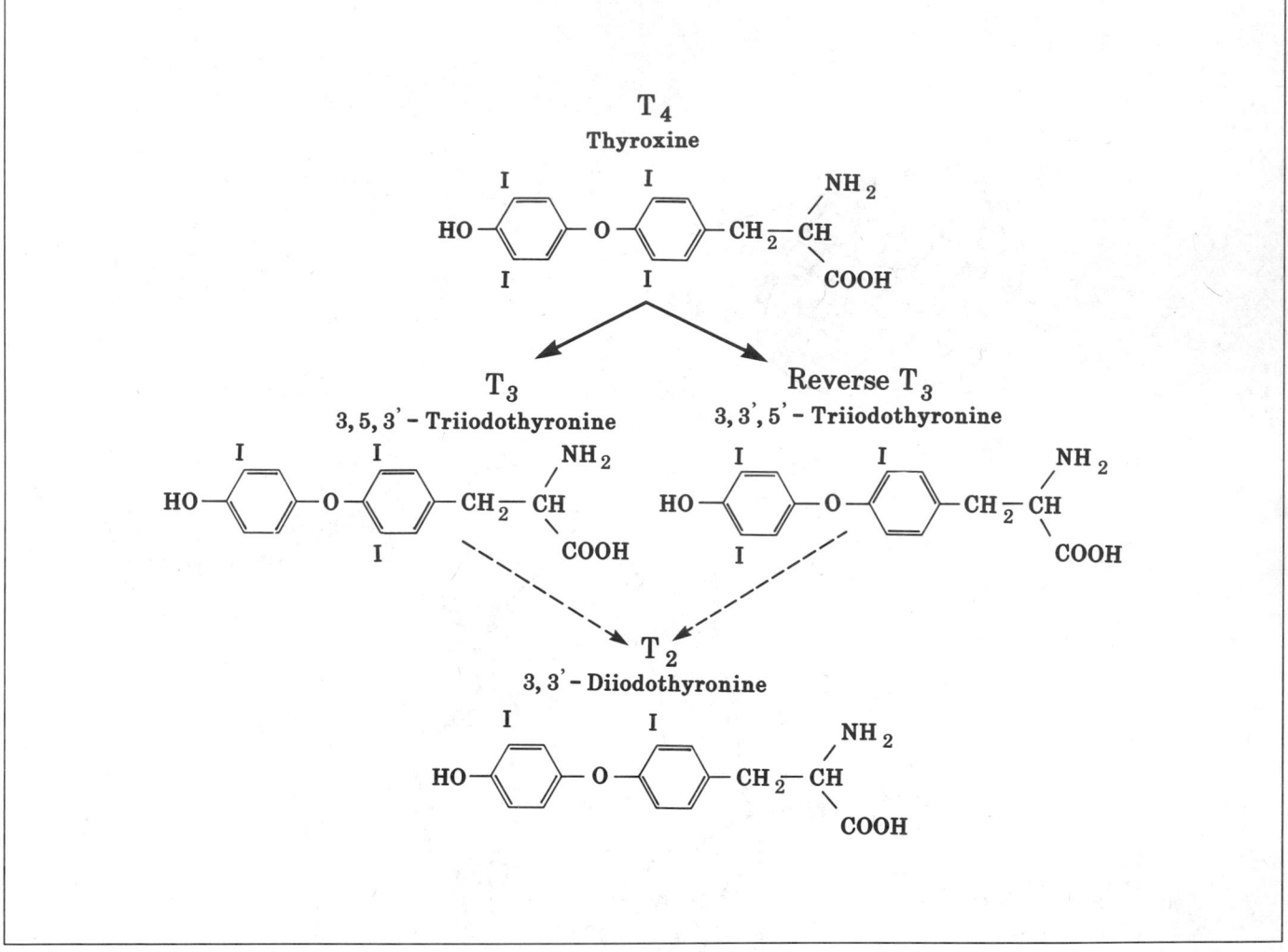

Figure 14.4–3. Deiodinative metabolism of thyroid hormones. Thyroxine (T₄) is enzymatically converted to more potent triiodothyronine (T₃) by outer-ring monodeiodination in target tissues and thyroid. Inner-ring deiodination of T₄ yields reverse T₃ (rT₃), which is biologically inactive. Decreased T₄ to T₃ conversion occurs in several circumstances (see Table 14.4–1).

tions will ultimately be attributable to induction of a few specific proteins remains uncertain. Furthermore, thyroid hormone-binding sites have also been identified in cell membranes, cytoplasm, and mitochondria, although their biologic relevance remains less clear.

TESTS OF THYROID FUNCTION AND MORPHOLOGY[7]

MEASUREMENT OF THYROID HORMONE CONCENTRATIONS

Circulating thyroid hormone concentrations can be measured by accurate, rapid, and relatively inexpensive competitive protein-binding assays, which are sufficiently sensitive to diagnose or exclude hyperthyroidism or hypothyroidism under most clinical circumstances. Because serum T₄ and T₃ levels may also be altered by a variety of nonthyroidal diseases and drugs, abnormally elevated or decreased thyroid hormone concentrations are not, however, always specific for thyroid gland dysfunction.

Low Serum Total Thyroxine Concentration

Hypothyroxinemia is characteristic of hypothyroidism, whereas the serum total T₃ level often remains normal in mild to moderate hypothyroidism. In the patient with a low serum total T₄, other conditions must also be considered in the differential diagnosis (Table 14.4–2). Decreased circulating TBG may be due to several diseases and drugs. In all of these conditions, TBG-bound T₄ and the measured serum total T₄ concentration is low. Low serum total T₄ also results from inhibition of thyroid hormone binding to plasma proteins by drugs or endogenous factors. Interference with the T₄-TBG interaction minimally increases the free T₄ fraction and enhances both feedback inhibition of TSH-mediated thyroid hormone production and the metabolic clearance of T₄. A circulating inhibitor of T₄-protein binding is present in sera of some patients with nonthyroidal systemic illness[9] This substance, which may be a free fatty acid, causes a striking fall in the serum T₄ level in some critically ill patients.

High Serum Total Thyroxine Concentration

The serum total T₄ concentration is increased in most cases of hyperthyroidism—the remaining patients having T₃ toxicosis, that is, an isolated increase in the serum T₃ level. There are numerous other conditions, however, that are associated with a high serum

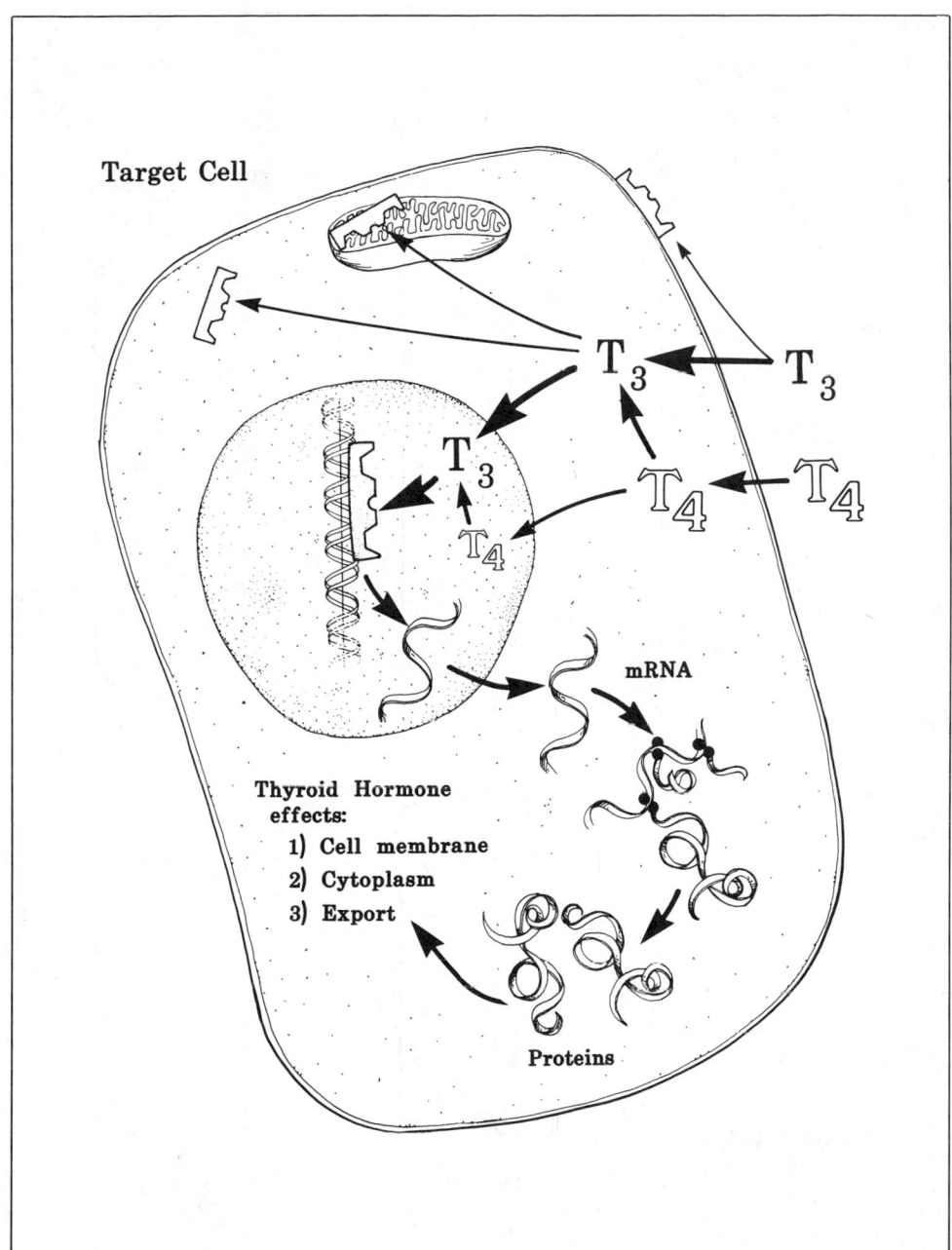

Figure 14.4–4. Thyroid hormone receptors and modes of action. Thyroid hormones enter the cell and nucleus, where more T_4 is converted to T_3. T_3 binds to its DNA-associated receptor and induces transcription of specific mRNAs, which direct translation of proteins effecting thyroid hormone actions. Other thyroid hormone receptors in the cell membrane, mitochondria, and cytoplasm have also been described.

T_4 concentration in the absence of hyperthyroidism, that is, euthyroid hyperthyroxinemia[1] (Table 14.4–2). Increased T_4 binding by all three classes of the plasma thyroxine binding proteins has been described. TBG excess is most commonly due to an estrogen-induced decrease in TBG degradation, as in pregnancy or with exogenous estrogens. In these conditions the serum total T_4 concentration and, to a lesser extent, the total T_3 level are increased, but the free T_4 and T_3 values are generally normal. Direct serum TBG measurement confirms this diagnosis. Less commonly, congenital abnormalities of TBPA and albumin binding can cause hyperthyroxinemia. Illnesses and drugs impairing T_4 degradation may produce modest hyperthyroxinemia.

Peripheral tissue resistance to thyroid hormone is a familial disorder characterized by elevated serum thyroid hormone concentrations, goiter, and clinical euthryoidism or hypothyroidism. Typically the concentrations of both total and free T_4 and T_3 are elevated. This rare condition should be suspected in hyperthyrox-

inemic patients who are not clinically hyperthyroid or who are hyperthyroxinemic with an inappropriately elevated or normal serum TSH concentration. Isolated pituitary resistance to thyroid hormone is an even rarer disorder in which there is only impaired thyroid hormone feedback on the pituitary, resulting in both clinical and chemical hyperthyroidism but an inappropriately increased circulating TSH level. In some families with thyroid hormone resistance, but not in others, abnormal T_3 binding to tissue receptors has been demonstrated.

Measurement of Serum Free T_4 and T_3 Concentrations

Because the free thyroid hormone fractions reflect their biological activity and total thyroid hormone concentrations may be altered by nonthyroidal factors, techniques for free T_4 and T_3 measurement have been developed. Equilibrium dialysis measures the partition of labeled thyroid hormone across a membrane with pores small enough to permit free, but not protein-bound, hormone to

TABLE 14.4–2. CAUSES OF ABNORMAL SERUM TOTAL THYROXINE CONCENTRATION

Low serum total thyroxine
Hypothyroidism

Decreased serum-protein binding
- Decreased TBG production
    Inherited TBG deficiency
    Chronic liver disease
    Excessive TBG loss
    Nephrosis and renal dialysis
    Protein-losing gastroenteropathy
- Systemic illness
- Drugs: androgens, L-asparaginase, glucocorticoids

Inhibition of T_4-protein binding
- Systemic illness
- Drugs: salicylates, phenytoin

T_3 *(Cytomel)*

High serum total thyroxine
Hyperthyroidism

Increased serum-protein binding
- Increased TBG concentration
    Inherited
    Endogenous estrogen (pregnancy, neonate, estrogen-
      secreting tumors)
    Liver disease
    Acute intermittent porphyria
    Hydatidiform mole
    Drugs: estrogens, 5-fluorouracil, clofibrate, methadone,
      heroin
- Increased albumin and TBPA binding
    Familial dysalbuminemic hyperthyroxinemia
    TBPA excess (inherited, ectopic neoplastic)
- Anti-T_4 immunoglobulins (artifactual increase)

Transient hyperthyroxinemic states
- Acute systemic illness
- Acute psychiatric illness
- Hyperemesis gravidarum
- High altitude exposure
- Drugs: amphetamines, amiodarone, beta-adrenergic blockers,
  iodinated radiocontrast dyes

Peripheral tissue resistance to thyroid hormones

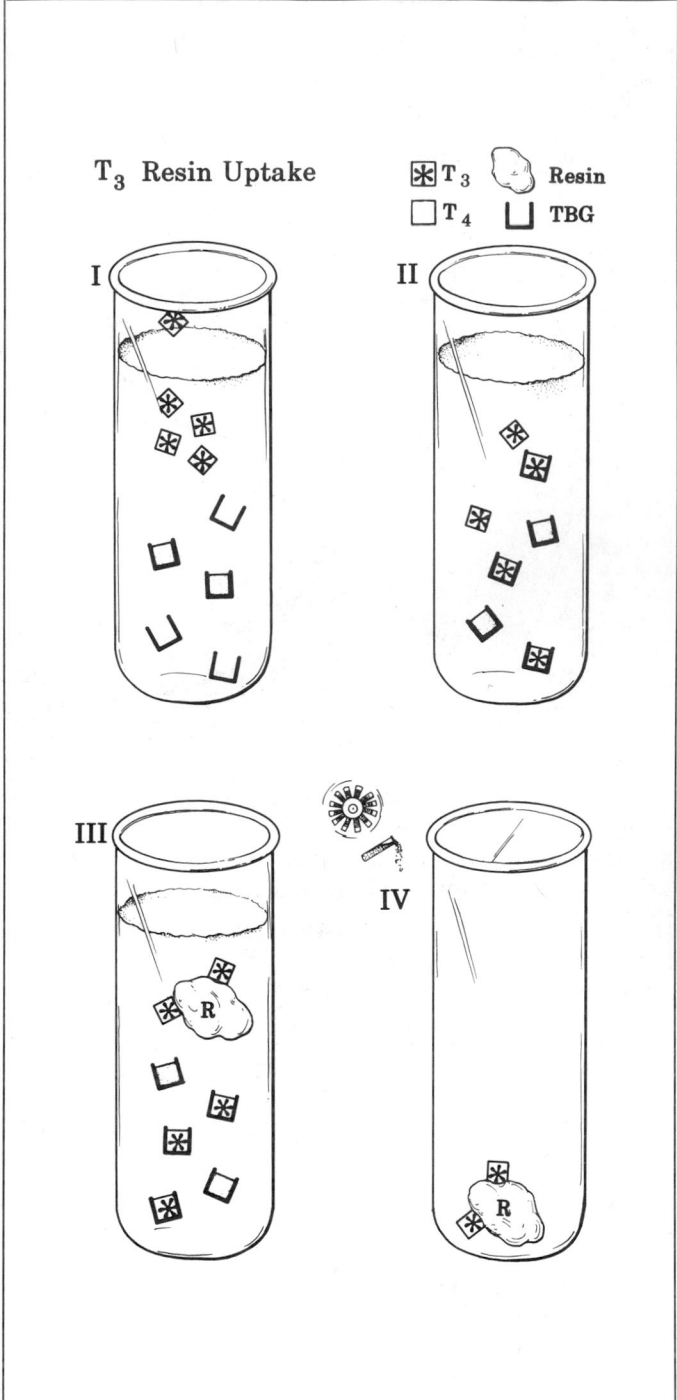

Figure 14.4–5. T_3 resin uptake. T_3 resin uptake is determined by incubating test serum with a tracer quantity of radiolabeled T_3 (*T_3), which interacts with available binding sites on TBG. At equilibrium between bound and free *T_3, an insoluble resin is added and free *T_3 is adsorbed. Resin is separated from serum by centrifugation, and the resin-associated *T_3 activity is quantified.

diffuse across. Although it remains the theoretical gold standard for free hormone measurement, the technique is unnecessarily complex for clinical use.

The T_3 resin uptake is a simple, rapid, and inexpensive test that indirectly estimates the free T_4 concentration (Fig. 14.4–5). Resin-absorbed T_3 tracer activity is inversely proportionate to the number of unoccupied binding sites on serum proteins. The free T_4 index (FT$_4$I) is then calculated by multiplying the total T_4 concentration by the T_3 resin uptake. In doing so, abnormal binding protein concentrations are corrected for, whereas true thyroid function abnormalities are accentuated. The FT$_4$I is less accurate, however, in accounting for the presence of circulating inhibitors of protein binding. The T_3 resin uptake should not be confused with the direct RIA measurement of T_3 in serum.

Newer RIA techniques permit direct measurement of free T_4 and free T_3 concentrations. Values provided by these assays generally distinguish between true thyroid dysfunction and TBG abnormalities but can be misleadingly low in euthyroid patients with systemic illness.

Reverse T_3 and Other Iodothyronines and Iodotyrosines

Serum rT_3 RIA has been proposed as an approach to distinguish hypothyroid patients from those with nonthyroidal illness. Specific RIA for other iodinated thyronine and tyrosine compounds are available but are used only rarely to investigate patients with defective thyroid hormone biosynthesis.

MEASUREMENT OF SERUM THYROTROPIN CONCENTRATION

Negative feedback of the thyroid hormones on the hypothalamic-pituitary axis makes serum TSH measurement valuable in recognizing centrally mediated forms of thyroid dysfunction, diagnosing

subtle forms of hyperthyroidism and hypothyroidism, and monitoring treatment of thyroid disorders.

Serum TSH in Hypothyroidism

An elevated serum TSH concentration accompanies primary hypothyroidism due to increased pituitary TSH production. In very mild thyroid gland failure, the serum TSH rises even while serum T_4 and T_3 levels remain within the normal range, a condition known as subclinical hypothyroidism. Pituitary (secondary) or hypothalamic (tertiary) hypothyroidism are usually associated with low-normal or undetectable serum TSH levels. Differentiating primary from central (thyrotropoprivic) hypothyroidism is essential because patients with the latter may have other elements of hypopituitarism, such as adrenal insufficiency, requiring treatment.

Syndromes of Inappropriate TSH[11]

When the serum TSH level is inappropriately elevated in the face of normal or increased serum total and free thyroid hormone concentrations, several unusual disorders should be considered (Table 14.4–3). Rarely, a TSH-secreting pituitary adenoma may cause hyperthyroidism. Generalized target-tissue thyroid hormone resistance and isolated pituitary resistance to thyroid hormone, an even rarer syndrome, also cause inappropriately increased serum TSH concentrations (see section on high serum total thyroxine above). An additional, less exotic cause of inappropriate serum TSH elevation is partial or intermittent compliance with thyroid hormone treatment for hypothyroidism. Reinstitution of L-thyroxine medication just before a medical appointment may acutely restore the serum T_4 concentration to normal but not promptly suppress serum TSH.

TRH-stimulation Testing

In normal individuals, synthetic TRH (100 to 500 μg IV) stimulates pituitary TSH release with the peak serum TSH concentration occurring after 20 to 30 minutes. This test is primarily used to rule out hyperthyroidism in patients with equivocal clinical and basal laboratory findings. Excess thyroid hormone feedback on the pituitary thyrotrope inhibits basal and TRH-stimulated TSH release, yielding a "flat" response with no rise in serum TSH concentration. A normal TSH response to TRH excludes all common forms of hyperthyroidism. A number of other endocrine and nonendocrine conditions and several drugs may also cause abnormal TSH responsiveness to TRH (Table 14.4–4).

RADIONUCLIDE EVALUATION OF THYROID STRUCTURE AND FUNCTION

Because the thyroid concentrates iodide and some other anions (e.g., pertechnetate and perchlorate), glandular function and morphology can be assessed directly by radioisotopic scintigraphy, employing radioactive isotopes of iodine (I-123 or I-131) or technetium pertechnetate ($^{99m}TcO_4$) (Table 14.4–5).

TABLE 14.4–3. CAUSES OF INCREASED SERUM THYROTROPIN CONCENTRATION

Appropriately increased TSH
- Primarily hypothyroidism
- Subclinical hypothyroidism

Inappropriately increased TSH
- TSH-secreting pituitary adenoma
    TSH secretion alone
    Associated growth hormone or prolactin secretion
- Generalized target-tissue resistance to thyroid hormone
- Isolated pituitary resistance to thyroid hormone

TABLE 14.4–4. CAUSES OF ABNORMAL TSH RESPONSE TO TRH

Increased thyroid hormone feedback
- Hyperthyroidism
- Autonomously functioning thyroid tissue without overt hyperthyroidism

Pituitary or hypothalamic dysfunction
- Thyrotropoprivic (control) hypothyroidism

Other disorders
- Endocrine disorders
    Cushing syndrome
    Acromegaly
- Nonendocrine diseases
    Depression
    Systemic illness

Drugs
- Glucocorticoids
- Dopamine
- Beta-adrenergic blocking agents

Technical problems
- Failed administration of TRH
- Insensitive TSH assay

Thyroidal Radioisotopic Uptake

The fractional radioactive iodine uptake (RAIU) 24 hours after an oral dose reflects principally iodide trapping and organification. Release of iodothyronines normally contributes significantly to uptake only after 24 hours but does so earlier in hyperfunctioning glands. Since pertechnetate is not organified, the technetium uptake is lower and is usually determined 20 minutes after intravenous administration of the tracer.

Radioisotopic uptake determinations are sometimes useful in differentiating among the causes of hyperthyroidism or hypothyroidism, but the radionuclide uptake cannot be equated with the patient's clinical status or circulating thyroid hormone levels. For example, hyperthyroidism may occur with a high radioisotopic uptake (as in Graves disease) or a low value (as in lymphocytic thyroiditis), and hypothyroidism may be accompanied by a low (as in postablative hypothyroidism) or an elevated uptake (as in severe dietary iodine deficiency).

A number of compounds interfere with concentration of radioisotopes by the thyroid. Stable iodine blocks the subsequent thyroidal uptake of radioactive tracers. Following radiologic studies with iodinated contrast dyes (e.g., intravenous pyelography), the RAIU may be decreased for several weeks.

Thyroid Scintiscan

The thyroid gland can also be imaged by scintigraphy. Radionuclide thyroid scans provide valuable information about the size

TABLE 14.4–5. RADIOISOTOPES FOR THYROID SCINTIGRAPHY

Agent	Normal Uptake (%)	Advantages	Disadvantages
Tc-99m	0.4–1.0 (20 min)	Inexpensive 1-day procedure Lowest thyroid dose	Tests only trapping Higher background
I-123	10–30 (24 hr)	Tests trapping and organification Low thyroid dose	2-day procedure Expensive
I-131	10–30	Same as I-123	Higher thyroid dose

and location of thyroid tissue and the character of thyroid nodules. Thyroid scanning is also useful in localizing metastases from well-differentiated thyroid carcinoma. Thyroid scintiscan and radioisotopic uptake tests can be combined with classic endocrine suppressive and stimulatory maneuvers. T_3 or T_4 suppression tests, in which thyroid hormone administration is followed by assessment of radioisotope uptake, identify autonomously functioning thyroid tissue.

QUANTIFICATION OF PERIPHERAL TISSUE THYROID HORMONE EFFECTS

The most useful thyroid function tests are theoretically those measuring effects of thyroid hormones in peripheral tissues. Available techniques (e.g., basal metabolic rate and pulse-wave arrival time), however, lack sufficient specificity and sensitivity for routine diagnostic use. These tests remain valuable in assessing unusual thyroid disorders such as thyroid hormone resistance, in which there is discordance between the patient's clinical status and circulating thyroid hormone concentrations. Thyroid hormones affect concentrations of a number of routinely measured substances in blood (Table 14.4–6), which may occasionally be the first clue suggesting thyroid dysfunction.

TESTS FOR SPECIFIC THYROID DISORDERS

Detection of immunoglobulins against thyroid cell antigens is often important in diagnosing or assessing the activity of autoimmune thyroid disorders. Thyroglobulin is released from the gland in a number of inflammatory and neoplastic thyroid conditions and is measurable by RIA. Thyroid biopsy is central to the definitive, conservative assessment of nodular thyroid disease. Other imaging techniques [sonography, computed tomography (CT), and magnetic resonance (MRI)], are occasionally useful in evaluation of certain thyroid conditions. (For discussion, see specific disorders to which tests apply.)

SYNDROMES OF ABNORMAL THYROID HORMONE PRODUCTION

A number of diseases cause the thyroid gland to produce an excess or deficiency of thyroid hormones. Both hyperthyroidism and hypothyroidism have a broad spectrum of clinical severity, ranging from subtle or absent clinical findings with mild chemical abnormalities to characteristic and potentially life-threatening clinical syndromes. Because many symptoms and signs of thyroid dysfunction are nonspecific, it is essential that appropriate diagnostic tests be used to distinguish true thyroid function abnormalities from deranged laboratory values that may accompany nonthyroidal illnesses. Finally, it is essential to differentiate among the specific causes of thyroid dysfunction to plan effective treatment.

HYPERTHYROIDISM (THYROTOXICOSIS)

Clinical Manifestations

Many clinical features of hyperthyroidism can be characterized as sympathomimetic or hypermetabolic. Some thyrotoxic symptoms mimic increased catecholamine activity, for example, palpitations, tremulousness, diaphoresis, and anxiety. Related physical signs include tachycardia, systolic hypertension, prominent cardiac apical impulse, staring gaze, and lid lag (a delay in closure of the upper eyelid with downward gaze). The exact pathogenesis of these symptoms is incompletely understood. Circulating catecholamine concentrations are decreased in hyperthyroidism, but increased beta-adrenergic receptor number has been observed in some tissues and may account for the enhanced catecholamine responsiveness observed by some investigators.

The calorigenic actions of thyroid hormones cause hyperthyroid patients to experience heat intolerance, a sensation of inordinate warmth, and preference for cool environments. Hypermetabolism classically produces weight loss despite a hearty appetite. Weight gain due to hyperphagia is relatively common, however, particularly in younger patients, and anorexia may be present in the elderly. Fatigue, increased sweating, and dyspnea are additional findings attributable to hypermetabolism.

Other clinical features of hyperthyroidism reflect excessive thyroid hormone action in specific organ systems (Table 14.4–7). Several forms of myopathy are associated with hyperthyroidism: (1) a limb girdle myopathy, (2) thyrotoxic periodic paralysis (occurring particularly in oriental males), (3) a rare bulbar myopathy, and (4) extraocular myopathy in patients with Graves disease. Pruritus, urticaria, hyperpigmentation, hair loss, and onycholysis (separation of the fingernail from its bed) are dermatologic features. Hyperthyroidism causes increased bone turnover, which results in osteoporosis, hypercalcemia, hypercalciuria, and rarely nephrolithiasis.

Symptoms and signs of hyperthyroidism may be masked or atypical in some patients, particularly the elderly. In individuals with so-called apathetic thyrotoxicosis, sympathomimetic symptoms are absent and clinical features may be limited to a single organ system. For example, patients may have only atrial fibrillation and heart failure, or manifest a cachectic syndrome of weight

TABLE 14.4–6. ALTERED SERUM CONSTITUENTS WITH THYROID DYSFUNCTION

Hyperthyroidism	Hypothyroidism
Increased	
Calcium	Cholesterol (LDL, VLDL)
Sex hormone-binding globulin	Triglycerides
Angiotensin-converting enzyme	Creatine phosphokinase[a]
Alkaline phosphatase	Lactic dehydrogenase
Ferritin	Carcinoembryonic antigen
Factor VIII	
Decreased	
Cholesterol	Hemoglobin
	Sodium
	Osmolarity

[a]Predominantly skeletal muscle (MM) isoenzyme form.
LDL = Low density lipoprotein; VLDL = very low density lipoprotein.

TABLE 14.4–7. CLINICAL MANIFESTATIONS OF HYPERTHYROIDISM

Organ System	Symptoms	Signs
Metabolic	Hyperphagia	Weight loss (or gain)
	Heat intolerance	Warm, moist skin
	Diaphoresis	
Cardiopulmonary	Palpitations	Tachyarrhythmias
	Chest pain	Systolic hypertension
	Dyspnea on exertion	Systolic murmur
Gastrointestinal	Hyperdefecation	
	Nausea, vomiting	
Genitourinary	Polyuria, nocturia	
	Decreased libido	
	Men—impotence	Gynecomastia
	Women—oligo-menorrhea	
Musculoskeletal	Weakness	Proximal myopathy
		Osteoporosis
Neuropsychiatric	Fatigue	Distal tremor
	Nervousness	Staring gaze and lid lag
	Insomnia	
	Depression	

loss, weakness, gastrointestinal complaints, and depression suggesting malignancy. The absence of goiter in 40 percent of elderly thyrotoxic patients makes diagnosis an even greater challenge.

Causes (Fig. 14.4–6)

The most common forms of hyperthyroidism are due to overproduction of thyroid hormones by a thyroid gland functioning autonomously. This may be caused by immunologically mediated thyroid stimulation, that is, Graves disease, or by intrinsic glandular autonomy, that is, toxic nodular goiter. Certain forms of thyroiditis produce hyperthyroidism by causing transient, excessive release of thyroid hormones from an inflamed gland. There are numerous other, rarer causes of hyperthyroidism (Table 14.4–8).

Graves Disease (Diffuse Toxic Goiter). This most common cause of hyperthyroidism occurs more frequently in women than in men (10:1). The disorder may develop at any age but does so most often between 20 and 40 years of age. Patients usually present with obvious clinical manifestations of hyperthyroidism, although thyrotoxicosis may be masked, particularly in the elderly. Typically the thyroid gland is diffusely enlarged with a smooth or lobular contour; a pyramidal lobe is frequently palpable. In severely thyrotoxic

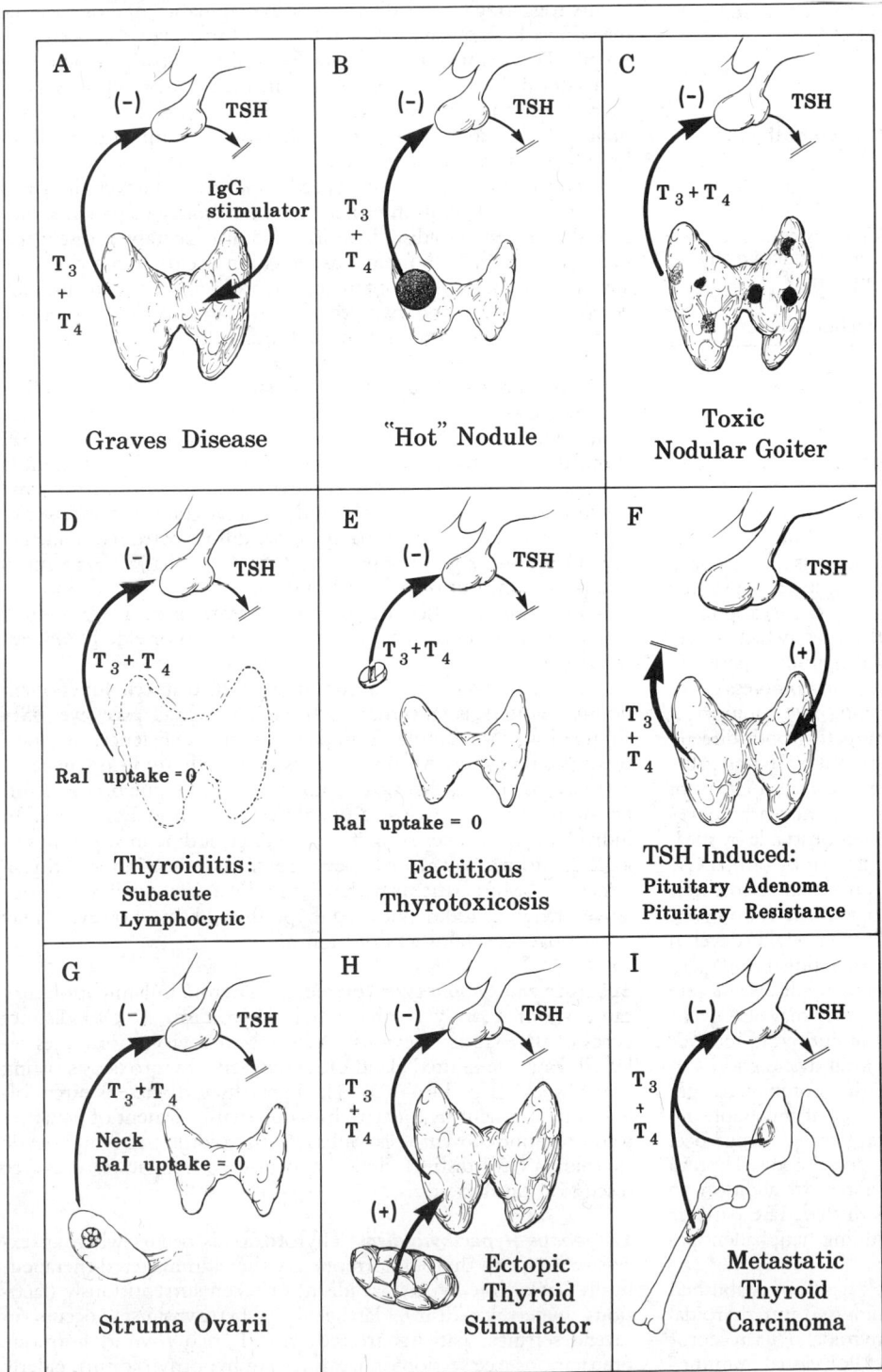

Figure 14.4–6. Pathogenesis of various forms of hyperthyroidism. **A.** Graves disease (diffuse toxic goiter). **B.** Toxic adenoma. **C.** Toxic multinodular goiter. **D.** Thyroiditis, subacute or lymphocytic (postpartum). **E.** Exogenous hyperthyroidism (iatrogenic and factitious). **F.** TSH-secreting pituitary adenoma. **G.** Struma ovarii. **H.** Choriocarcinoma, molar pregnancy, embryonal carcinoma. **I.** Metastatic follicular carcinoma of the thyroid. (*From Daniels GH, Maloof F: In Frohlich ED (ed): Pathophysiology. Philadelphia, JB Lippincott, 1976.*)

TABLE 14.4–8. DISEASES CAUSING HYPERTHYROIDISM

Disorder	Pathogenesis
Graves disease	Thyroid-stimulating immuno-globulins and T lymphocytes
Toxic nodular goiter • Solitary toxic adenoma • Toxic multinodular goiter	Autonomously functioning follicular cells
Thyroiditis • Subacute (de Quervain) • Lymphocytic (postpartum)	Hormone discharge from inflamed gland Viral Unknown
Drug-induced • Thyroid hormone prepara-tions • Iodine (iodides, amiodarone, iodinated contrast dyes)	Iatrogenic, factitious usually in nodular goiter[4]
TSH-mediated • TSH-secreting pituitary tumor • Isolated pituitary resistance to thyroid hormone	TSH stimulation of thyroid function
Other rare forms • Struma ovarii • Choriocarcinoma, molar pregnancy, embryonal carci-noma • Metastatic follicular cancer	Ectopic follicular epithelium Gonadotropin-mediated thy-roid stimulation Ectopic functioning metastases

patients, a bruit is often audible over the lateral lobes because of increased blood flow.

In addition to thyroid dysfunction, Graves disease has unique ophthalmologic and dermatologic aspects not found in other forms of hyperthyroidism. Graves ophthalmopathy is characterized by inflammatory swelling of extraocular muscles, increased orbital fat, and increased retroocular pressure. This may cause exophthalmos (proptosis), a forward protrusion of the eyes, which is frequently asymmetric. Orbital congestion may also produce periorbital edema, limitation of extraocular motility, and compression of the optic nerve with potential threat to vision. The conjunctiva and cornea are inflamed in Graves ophthalmopathy, both directly and as a consequence of increased exposure caused by staring gaze, proptosis, and loss of Bell phenomenon (the upward rotation of the eyes accompanying eyelid closure). Most patients with Graves disease have some degree of opthalmopathy demonstrable by measurement of intraocular pressure on upward gaze or by orbital CT. Only a minority (10 percent) suffer severe functional or cosmetic complications requiring specific ophthalmologic therapy, however. Graves ophthalmopathy and hyperthyroidism generally develop within a few months of one another but may then pursue independent courses with persistence or exacerbation of eye disease despite control of thyrotoxicosis. Graves ophthalmopathy may also occur in patients with autoimmune thyroiditis or in euthyroid individuals who often prove to have subclinical thyroid dysfunction.

Pretibial myxedema, an unusual but pathognomonic feature of Graves disease, is a subcutaneous infiltration of mucopolysaccharide that produces a painless, sharply circumscribed orange-peel induration over the anterior lower leg or dorsal foot. Thyroid acropachy—distal finger clubbing—is even rarer. In addition to these classical eye and skin signs of Graves disease, rare patients may have other atypical presentations, including lymphadenopathy, splenomegaly, and urticaria.

An autoimmune basis for Graves disease[10] has been established by recognition of circulating immunoglobulins and intrathyroidal T lymphocytes capable of binding to the thyroidal TSH receptor and mimicking TSH action (Fig. 14.4–6A). Polyclonal immunoglobulins in the sera of patients with Graves disease have been shown to induce physiologic follicular cell responses, including promotion of thyroid cell growth, stimulation of iodine uptake, induction of thyroid hormone synthesis and release, and competitive inhibition of TSH membrane binding. The thyroid-stimulating immunoglobulin (TSI) assay, which measures the cyclic adenosine monophosphate response of thyroid tissue to test sera, is the most sensitive and specific assay. TSI is detectable in 90 percent of Graves patients, and TSI titer correlates relatively well with disease activity. There is a clear familial predisposition for autoimmune thyroid diseases, and individuals with certain histocompatibility antigen haplotypes, for example, B8 and Dr3, are more susceptible. Other autoimmune disorders, such as type I diabetes mellitus, vitiligo, and pernicious anemia, are also known to occur more frequently in patients with Graves disease. Although the precise events triggering Graves disease remain enigmatic, viral or bacterial infections, high dietary iodine intake, and stress have all been proposed. The pathogenesis of Graves ophthalmopathy is less well understood. Postulated mechanisms include cross-reaction of antithyroid antibodies with extraocular muscle antigens or lymphatic drainage of thyroid antigen-immunoglobulin complexes to the orbit where inflammation ensues.

The natural history of hyperthyroidism in Graves disease is quite variable. The disorder persists in a majority of patients with relapsing hyperthyroidism if antithyroid drug therapy is discontinued. In a minority, spontaneous remission occurs after a period of antithyroid therapy. Spontaneous hypothyroidism can also develop after treatment of hyperthyroidism, particularly with ablative therapies but even after antithyroid drugs alone.

Toxic Adenoma and Toxic Multinodular Goiter. Hyperthyroidism may be caused by benign neoplasia of thyroid follicular epithelium, which functions autonomously, that is, independently of TSH stimulation. In toxic adenoma, hyperfunctioning tissue is limited to a single benign tumor with suppression of extranodular thyroid function (Fig. 14.4–6B). Toxic multinodular goiter is composed of more than one toxic adenoma or a more diffuse pattern of follicular cell autonomy (Fig. 14.4–6C). Nodular goiter has a clear familial predisposition, but only a small fraction (≤ 1 percent) of individuals with this condition develop hyperthyroidism. Toxic nodular goiter develops most frequently in middle-aged or elderly individuals.

The pathogenesis of autonomous follicular cell function in nodular goiters is uncertain, although previous excessive TSH stimulation, for example, from dietary iodine deficiency, may be a predisposing factor. Autonomy causes hyperthyroidism whenever the mass of independently functioning thyroid tissue becomes sufficient to produce excessive quantities of thyroid hormones. In individuals with preexisting nodular goiter, iodine in supraphysiologic quantities may incite hyperthyroidism (iodine-induced thyrotoxicosis).[4] Most patients with toxic nodular goiter will require ablative therapy. Iodine-induced hyperthyroidism, however, may resolve over several weeks or months.

Subacute and Lymphocytic Thyroiditis. Thyroid inflammation may cause spontaneously resolving hyperthyroidism in two distinct types of thyroiditis. Previously synthesized thyroid hormones released from the injured gland cause transient thyrotoxicosis lasting 2 to 8 weeks (Fig. 14.4–6D). The hyperthyroid phase is often followed by transient hypothyroidism due to impairment of new thyroid hormone biosynthesis. Subacute thyroiditis and lymphocytic thyroiditis have distinct clinical and histopathologic features (see discussion on thyroiditis).

Exogenous Hyperthyroidism. Thyrotoxicosis occurs when an excessive dose of a thyroid hormone is either administered therapeutically (iatrogenic hyperthyroidism) or taken surreptitiously (factitious hyperthyroidism). Iatrogenic hyperthyroidism occurs in several settings: patients treated with T_3-rich thyroid hormone preparations (see section on treatment of hypothyroidism), elderly individuals whose metabolism of thyroid hormones is reduced,

and patients requiring TSH suppression in the treatment of thyroid neoplasms. Factitious hyperthyroidism is encountered predominantly in women who mistakenly believe thyroid hormone to be effective for weight reduction. Rare epidemics of exogenous hyperthyroidism have followed contamination of meat with thyroid tissue. In exogenous hyperthyroidism, both the thyroid radionuclide uptake (Fig. 14.4–6E) and serum thyroglobulin are suppressed—features which differentiate these disorders from common types of thyrotoxicosis.

Rare Causes of Hyperthyroidism. Autonomous pituitary TSH production is responsible for two rare forms of hyperthyroidism: TSH-secreting pituitary adenoma (Fig. 14.4–6F) and isolated pituitary resistance to thyroid hormone (see discussion of syndromes of inappropriate TSH above). In these patients, the serum TSH level is not suppressed, as would be expected in common types of hyperthyroidism. Placental and testicular neoplasms producing large amounts of hCG, which mimics TSH action, may cause hyperthyroidism (Fig. 14.4–6G). Struma ovarii, an ovarian teratoma containing thyroid tissue, may rarely produce enough thyroid hormone to cause hyperthyroidism (Fig. 14.4–6H). In women with this condition, thyrotoxicosis is accompanied by absent thyroidal radioisotopic uptake with tracer localization in the pelvis. In rare cases, extensive functioning metastases from follicular thyroid carcinoma produce hyperthyroidism (Fig. 14.4–6I).

Laboratory Diagnosis and Differential Diagnosis
Hyperthyroidism is usually accompanied by elevated circulating total and free concentrations of both T_4 and T_3. The relative degrees of T_4 and T_3 elevation vary in different forms of thyrotoxicosis. In Graves disease and toxic nodular goiter, serum T_3 is typically more elevated than serum T_4. A minority (5 percent) of these patients have isolated T_3 toxicosis. In contrast, thyroiditis and iodine-induced hyperthyroidism may cause a predominant T_4 elevation. Isolated T_4 toxicosis may occur in these patients or in any thyrotoxic patient with coexisting systemic illness that impairs extrathyroidal T_4-to-T_3 conversion. Mild hyperthyroidism may be present with serum thyroid hormone concentrations in the upper portion of the laboratory normal range. In such cases, basal and TRH-stimulated TSH concentrations may be required to establish or exclude hyperthyroidism (see discussion on TRH-stimulation testing above).

When the etiology of hyperthyroidism is not obvious on clinical grounds, the thyroidal radioactive iodine uptake and radionuclide scan are highly useful in differentiating, for example, between Graves disease and lymphocytic thyroiditis. These tests must not be used, however, to establish the general diagnosis of hyperthyroidism. Detection of Graves immunoglobulins may occasionally be helpful in differential diagnosis. The erythrocyte sedimentation rate is typically increased during the initial phase of subacute thyroiditis. Serum thyroglobulin RIA assists in identifying patients with factitious hyperthyroidism because elevated thyroglobulin levels occur only in endogenous forms of thyrotoxicosis.

Treatment
Hyperthyroidism can be effectively treated even though the underlying cause of thyroid dysfunction is often not directly corrected. Tissue effects of excess thyroid hormones can be blocked, thyroid hormone production can be inhibited, and abnormally stimulated or autonomous thyroid tissue can be ablated. For a particular type of hyperthyroidism, some approaches may be well-suited and others entirely inappropriate. The choice of treatment modalities can often be tailored to accommodate the patient's associated medical problems and personal preferences.

Beta-adrenergic Blocking Agents. Beta blockers promptly relieve many clinical manifestations of hyperthyroidism. Tremor, palpitations, diaphoresis, and anxiety are decreased within hours. Some other less frequent clinical features of hyperthyroidism such as hypercalcemia, periodic paralysis, and bulbar myopathy also may be improved by beta blockade. The metabolic consequences of thyrotoxicosis, for example, weight loss, heat intolerance, and proximal myopathy, are not well controlled by beta blockers alone, however. In addition to their sympatholytic activity, some beta blockers, propranolol, for example, partially inhibit conversion of T_4 to T_3. For common forms of sustained hyperthyroidism, beta blockers represent useful adjuncts to definitive therapy. For the spontaneously resolving types of hyperthyroidism, a beta blocker alone is the preferred treatment. Propranolol, 10 to 80 mg every 6 to 8 hours, is used for relief of symptoms or control of tachycardia ($<$100 beats per minute). Longer-acting beta blockers (e.g., nadolol 40 to 80 mg, metoprolol 50 mg, or long-acting propranolol 80 to 320 mg per day) are also effective and may ensure greater compliance. Beta-adrenergic blockade can be tapered as soon as underlying hyperthyroidism is controlled. Patients may play an active role in determining their requirement for beta blockade but should not discontinue their drug abruptly because rebound symptoms may mimic recrudescent hyperthyroidism. Beta-adrenergic blocking agents should be avoided or used with caution in thyrotoxic patients with coexisting bronchospasm, bradycardic conducting-system disorders, or heart failure. In thyrotoxic patients with high-output heart failure, beta blocker use should be limited to control of hemodynamically deleterious tachyarrhythmias. No attempt should be made to normalize heart rate completely because drug toxicity may be encountered first.

Thionamide Antithyroid Drugs. The two thionamide antithyroid drugs available in the United States, methimazole (Tapazole) and propylthiouracil (PTU), are well absorbed after oral administration and are actively concentrated in the thyroid gland. Both agents block thyroid hormone biosynthesis-inhibiting thyroglobulin iodination and iodotyrosine coupling. PTU, but not methimazole, also reduces extrathyroidal T_4-to-T_3 conversion. It has recently been shown that thionamides may also have immunosuppressive properties in patients with Graves disease.

Antithyroid drugs ameliorate forms of hyperthyroidism in which there is overproduction of thyroid hormones by the gland. Two to six weeks of therapy are required to control hyperthyroid Graves disease or toxic nodular goiter because the agents do not interfere with release of previously synthesized thyroid hormones or their target-tissue actions. Thionamides are obviously inappropriate for management of hyperthyroidism caused by the self-limited release of thyroid hormones from an inflamed gland. For patients with mild to moderate hyperthyroidism, methimazole is the drug of choice because its longer duration of action permits less frequent dosing and greater compliance. Low-dose ($\leq$30 mg per day) methimazole may also have a lower incidence of severe side effects. Methimazole 10 to 30 mg may be prescribed as a single daily dose; for more severe thyrotoxicosis, 20 mg two or three times daily may be required. To be effective, antithyroid drugs must be taken faithfully, and treatment failure is almost invariably due to noncompliance. For patients with very severe thyrotoxicosis, PTU 100 to 200 mg every 6 hours may be preferable because this drug blocks T_4-to-T_3 conversion. In critically ill patients, thionamides can be administered by nasogastric tube, and methimazole can be given rectally or intravenously. The duration of antithyroid drug therapy depends on the clinical setting. The majority of patients with Graves disease and virtually all with toxic nodular goiter will relapse when the drugs are discontinued.

Thionamide therapy is occasionally complicated by rash and fever (5 percent). Mild skin eruptions and pruritus may subside despite continued drug administration and can be controlled with diphenhydramine 25 to 50 mg every 4 to 6 hours. In general, however, it is best to switch to the other thionamide or another treatment modality. Mild dose-related neutropenia is common and does not necessitate stopping the drug. Rarely, antithyroid drugs may cause life-threatening agranulocytosis (0.3 percent), hepatitis, or vasculitis. These side effects are more common with higher medication doses, in the elderly, and within the first 3 months of therapy. The onset of agranulocytosis is precipitous, and routine moni-

toring of the leukocyte count is not useful. All thionamide-treated patients should be cautioned that high fever, pharyngitis or other signs of infection, and jaundice or other symptoms of hepatitis require immediate discontinuation of the drug and prompt consultation with their physician.

Iodides and Other Agents. Iodide (>15 to 30 mg per day) promptly blocks thyroid hormone release from the gland and interferes with hormone synthesis by inhibiting iodine uptake and organification by the follicular cell. Ordinarily, the inhibitory effects of iodides are short-lived, and escape occurs in 10 to 20 days, making them primarily useful as adjuncts in the early management of severe hyperthyroidism. Previous iodine-131 therapy prolongs these actions of stable iodide therapy so that its sustained use is reasonable after radioactive iodine treatment of Graves disease. In hyperthyroidism caused by thyroiditis, iodides are not helpful, and in toxic nodular goiter, their use may actually exacerbate thyrotoxicosis. Iodide (50 to 500 mg/day) is administered orally as a saturated solution of potassium iodide (SSKI), 40 mg per drop, or Lugol's solution, 8 mg/drop. Sodium iodide (1 to 2 g/day) may be administered intravenously when needed for severely thyrotoxic patients. Hypersensitivity reactions to iodides include fever, rash, and rarely vasculitis.

Several other drugs inhibiting thyroid hormone release or metabolism have been used to treat hyperthyroidism under special circumstances. Glucocorticoids partially inhibit T_4-to-T_3 conversion and may ameliorate the immunologic processes responsible for thyroiditis and Graves disease. Dexamethasone (8 mg/day) has been shown to lower the serum T_3 concentrations in these disorders, and full stress-dose glucocorticoids (300 mg hydrocortisone or its equivalent) have often been advocated as part of the management of thyroid "storm." Lithium carbonate (300 to 600 mg/day) blocks release of preformed thyroid hormones from the gland but is used only when there are contraindications to iodide.

Ablative Therapies: Iodine-131 and Thyroidectomy. In toxic nodular goiter, patients typically experience recurrent hyperthyroidism on discontinuation of drug therapy. Permanent control of Graves disease requires its spontaneous resolution (which occurs in less than 30 percent of cases after 1 year of antithyroid drug therapy), continued antithyroid drug therapy, or ablation of thyroid tissue. Sodium iodine-131 is administered orally on an outpatient basis. It is concentrated almost exclusively in thyroid cells and, therefore, delivers tissue-specific radiation therapy. Treatment is rarely complicated by mild transient thyroiditis or exacerbation of thyrotoxicosis. Hyperthyroidism is permanently cured in 70 percent of patients with a single dose, and repeated therapy at 4- to 6-month intervals is invariably effective. Actual control of thyrotoxicosis requires 4 to 12 weeks, during which adjunctive therapy must be continued. Hypothyroidism is a common consequence of radioactive iodine treatment for Graves disease (50 to 70 percent), but occurs less often (25 percent) in toxic nodular goiter. Long-term follow-up studies have shown that radioactive iodine treatment is not associated with thyroid or extrathyroidal malignancies.[5] In women of child-bearing age there is no evidence that the low level of ovarian radiation received, which is comparable to many diagnostic radiologic studies, for example, barium enema with fluoroscopy, is associated with teratogenesis or infertility. Concurrent pregnancy or nursing are the only absolute contraindications to radioactive iodine therapy.

Surgical thyroidectomy effectively controls hyperthyroidism in 95 percent of patients with Graves disease and virtually all patients with toxic adenomas. Hyperthyroidism must be controlled preoperatively. Surgery entails hospitalization, anesthetic risk, modest discomfort, and a surgical scar for all treated patients. Hypothyroidism occurs in 50 percent of operated Graves' patients. Unusual severe complications of thyroid surgery include hypoparathyroidism and recurrent laryngeal nerve injury, which, if unilateral, causes hoarseness and, if bilateral, causes laryngeal obstruction. Surgery is an appropriate option for patients with toxic adenomas and large, locally obstructive toxic multinodular goiters. The role of surgical thyroidectomy in management of Graves disease, particularly in adults, has diminished. It is vital that thyroidectomy be performed only by surgeons experienced in the procedure because complication rates are clearly higher in less skilled and practiced hands.

Treatment of Hyperthyroidism in Pregnancy. PTU is the drug of choice for Graves disease or toxic nodular goiter in pregnancy. Although PTU crosses the placenta, maternal hyperthyroidism can be controlled without fetal hypothyroidism or goiter if the smallest dose required to maintain a high-normal or minimally elevated serum free T_4 level is employed. Methimazole therapy has rarely been associated with congenital scalp defects but can be employed in patients with previous PTU reactions. Combined thionamide and L-thyroxine treatment is inadvisable because T_4 crosses the placenta poorly. Patients should be monitored clinically and chemically every 4 to 8 weeks. Beta-adrenergic blocking agents are an effective temporary adjunct for symptom control and are essential if severe thyrotoxicosis is present at the time of delivery. Surgical thyroidectomy during the second trimester may be the only alternative for patients with severe thionamide hypersensitivity reactions or grossly negligent compliance with medication. Stable iodide causes fetal goiter and compressive complications and is contraindicated in pregnant patients. Radioactive iodine administered after 10 weeks of gestation may cause fetal hypothyroidism and earlier in pregnancy has potential teratogenic effects. Neonatal Graves disease is transient hyperthyroidism, which occurs in approximately 10 percent of children born to mothers with active Graves disease, and can occur even in a euthyroid mother previously treated with ablative therapy.

Hyperthyroidism in Systemically Ill and Elderly Patients. Because thyrotoxicosis can exacerbate cardiopulmonary disease and because Graves disease and toxic nodular goiter are the causes of hyperthyroidism most commonly encountered in these patients, definitive radioactive iodine treatment is ultimately desirable in virtually all cases. Before iodine-131, however, a 2- to 4-week course of antithyroid drug therapy is important to control thyrotoxicosis promptly and to avoid the potential of transiently worsened hyperthyroidism after radioactive iodine.

Preparation of Hyperthyroid Patients for Surgery. To decrease risk of perioperative complications, at least 2 weeks of antithyroid drug treatment is advisable before surgery with the addition of iodides (SSKI 6 to 12 drops twice daily) 10 to 14 days before surgery. Residual sympathomimetic manifestations of hyperthyroidism can be ameliorated with beta blockers.

HYPOTHYROIDISM

Clinical Manifestations (Table 14.4–9)

The features of severe thyroid hormone deficiency (myxedema) are often obvious, but clinical manifestations of mild to moderate hypothyroidism can be quite subtle, insidious in onset, and nonspecific. Decreased calorigenesis accounts for the classical complaints of cold intolerance and weight gain despite poor appetite. In elderly patients, however, weight loss may occur. Tissue mucopolysaccharide accumulation and impaired lymphatic clearance of interstitial proteins cause other common complaints: hoarseness, headache, periorbital swelling, and paresthesias attributable to the carpal tunnel syndrome. Serous effusions may involve the pericardial, pleural, joint, and peritoneal spaces.

All major organ systems are affected by thyroid hormone deficiency (Table 14.4–9). The cardiovascular manifestations of thyroid hormone deficiency are due to both decreased tissue metabolic demands and direct effects of thyroid hormone deficiency to slow sinus node depolarization, diminish myocardial contractility, and increase peripheral vascular resistance. Although heart failure

TABLE 14.4–9. CLINICAL MANIFESTATIONS OF HYPOTHYROIDISM

Organ System	Symptoms	Signs
Metabolic	Cold intolerance	Weight gain (or loss)
Cardiopulmonary	Dyspnea	Bradycardia Diastolic hypertension Cardiac rub or soft heart tones caused by pericardial effusion
Gastrointestinal	Anorexia Hypogeusia, dysgeusia Constipation	Ileus
Genitourinary	Decreased libido Menorrhagia, amenorrhea Oliguria	Galactorrhea Urinary retention
Musculoskeletal	Arthralgias Myalgias, muscle stiffness and cramps	
Dermatologic	Dryness	Loss of brow and scalp hair Yellow (carotinemic) skin
Neuropsychiatric	Fatique Depression Irritability Impaired concentration and memory Paresthesia	Psychosis Coma Carpal tunnel syndrome
Hematologic	Pallor	Anemia

is rarely the result of hypothyroidism alone, thyroid hormone deficiency often exacerbates intrinsic cardiac disease. Dyspnea is common, ventilatory responsiveness to hypercapnia and hypoxia may be blunted, and sleep-apnea syndrome can occur. Impaired gastrointestinal motility causes constipation frequently and ileus rarely. Gastric achlorhydria and pernicious anemia are both associated with autoimmune thyroid failure. Impaired renal excretion of free water can cause hyponatremia and hypo-osmolarity. Anemia is relatively common and may also be due to marrow hypoplasia or iron deficiency.

Secondary metabolic and endocrine abnormalities may complicate hypothyroidism. Hypercholesterolemia is due to decreased low-density and very low-density lipoprotein clearance. Hyperprolactinemia and consequent galactorrhea may occur. Women often experience menstrual dysfunction, most commonly menorrhagia but also amenorrhea. Growth failure and precocious or delayed puberty can occur in hypothyroid children. Profound hypothyroidism causes a reversible blunting of the hypothalamic-pituitary-adrenal (HPA) axis response to stress. Adrenal insufficiency can, of course, also accompany hypothyroidism in Schmidt syndrome of polyendocrine failure and in hypopituitarism.

Myxedema coma is a life-threatening syndrome characterized by profound, usually longstanding thyroid hormone deficiency and consequent multiple organ system failure. Its clinical features may include obtundation, hypothermia, heart failure, hypotension, ventilatory failure, ileus, hypo-osmolarity, coagulopathy, and a propensity to develop occult infection and drug toxicity.

Causes (Table 14.4–10)

Thyroid gland failure is usually caused by autoimmune thyroiditis[10] or thyroid ablation. Autoimmune thyroiditis (chronic lymphocytic thyroiditis, Hashimoto thyroiditis) is distinctly more common in women and typically has its onset during the second to fifth decades of life. Evidence supporting an autoimmune pathogenesis for the disorder includes the presence of circulating antithyroid antibodies in most patients, lymphocytic infiltration of the gland, and associations with other autoimmune endocrine and nonendocrine disorders. Postablative hypothyroidism may be the consequence of previous surgical thyroidectomy or radioactive iodine therapy for hyperthyroidism or may be a complication of neck surgery and radiotherapy for neoplastic disease.

Several less common causes of hypothyroidism occur in adults.

Subacute and lymphocytic thyroiditis produce transient hypothyroidism (see discussion on thyroiditis). Pharmacologic agents such as iodine, lithium, and aminoglutethimide may cause reversible thyroid dysfunction, particularly in individuals with underlying autoimmune thyroiditis. Thyrotropoprivic hypothyroidism is due to interruption of the normal hypothalamic-pituitary control of thyroid function and is usually attributable to primary or metastatic tumors involving the pituitary or CNS (see Chapter 14.2).

Laboratory Diagnosis and Differential Diagnosis

Suspected hypothyroidism must always be confirmed in the laboratory. Primary (thyroidal) hypothyroidism is typically associated with low serum total and free thyroxine (T$_4$) concentrations and an elevated serum TSH. Hypothyroxinemia is not, of course, pathognomonic of hypothyroidism (Table 14.4–2). In hypothyroidism the T$_3$ resin uptake is typically decreased but may be elevated or normal if TBG is deficient or a circulating inhibitor of thyroid hormone binding is present. Serum TSH determination is mandatory in every patient with hypothyroidism. The serum TSH value

TABLE 14.4–10. DISEASES CAUSING HYPOTHYROIDISM IN ADULTS

Disorder	Pathogenesis
Autoimmune thyroiditis (chronic lymphocytic thyroiditis, Hashimoto disease)	Antithyroid antibodies and T lymphocytes
Postablative	Destruction of thyroid tissue by previous surgery or radiation
Thyroiditis Subacute (de Quervain) Lymphocytic (postpartum)	Transient inflammatory disruption of hormone synthesis ? Autoimmune
Drug-induced: iodine, lithium, aminoglutethimide, polybrominated biphenyls	Persistent blockade of organification and hormone release in glands with autoimmune thyroiditis
Secondary (central; thyrotropoprivic)	Lack of TSH stimulation of thyroid function

confirms the significance of hypothyroxinemia and differentiates between primary thyroid disease and thyrotropoprivic (central) hypothyroidism due to pituitary (secondary) or hypothalamic (tertiary) disorders. It is important that patients with central hypothyroidism be identified so that their underlying disease can be defined and other aspects of hypopituitarism can be recognized and treated.

Hypothyroxinemic patients with systemic illness pose the greatest challenge in diagnosing hypothyroidism. Many nonthyroidal conditions, for example sepsis, myocardial infarction, hepatic and renal dysfunction, as well as surgery and simple starvation, have been associated with low serum thyroid hormone concentrations. Measurement of serum TSH is the single most useful laboratory test for differentiating primary hypothyroidism from systemic illness in a euthyroid patient. Although TSH secretion can be modestly increased or decreased by systemic illness, these alterations are rarely sufficient to obscure the diagnosis of primary hypothyroidism. Two settings in which TSH determination may not be definitive are (1) patients receiving intravenous dopamine, which inhibits pituitary TSH secretion, and (2) patients with potential pituitary or hypothalamic hypothyroidism in which an elevated TSH is not expected.

Some patients with very mild thyroid gland dysfunction may have an elevated serum TSH concentration in association with serum thyroid hormone levels within the normal range. This syndrome, termed subclinical hypothyroidism, is commonly encountered in individuals with autoimmune thyroiditis or previous thyroid ablative therapy. Subtle thyroid dysfunction in these patients will only be recognized if TSH is measured.

Although the etiology of hypothyroidism is generally obvious clinically, other studies are occasionally helpful in differential diagnosis. Antimicrosomal and antithyroglobulin antibodies are detected in serum of most patients (95 percent) with autoimmune thyroiditis but may also be present in Graves disease and transiently positive in subacute or lymphocytic thyroiditis.

Treatment
Sodium L-thyroxine (levothyroxine) is the treatment of choice for hypothyroidism. L-thyroxine is reliably absorbed and has a 7-day half-life, providing a stable circulating level with a single daily dose. T_4 can provide completely physiologic thyroid hormone replacement by virtue of conversion to T_3. Biologic thyroid hormone formulations (USP desiccated thyroid and thyroglobulin [Proloid]) may have variable potency. Furthermore, both biologic preparations and synthetic T_4 plus T_3 combinations (liotrix, [Thyrolar] and [Euthroid]) contain T_3 and often cause T_3 toxicosis. Pure T_3 (liothyronine [Cytomel]) has limited usefulness when its shorter 1-day half-life is desirable, for example, in discontinuation of suppression therapy for scanning or iodine-131 treatment.

Patient weight is the most important factor in estimating the appropriate L-thyroxine dosage (~ 1.8 μg/kg per day). A lower initial dosage should be employed in the elderly, who metabolize thyroid hormone less rapidly. Thyroid hormone therapy in hypothyroid patients with ischemic heart disease has the potential of increasing myocardial oxygen consumption. In both cardiac patients and the elderly, it is prudent to initiate treatment with a low T_4 dose (25 to 50 μg/day), which can be increased in 12.5 to 25 μg increments at 4- to 6-week intervals until clinical euthyroidism is restored.

The best thyroid hormone therapy for critically ill myxedematous patients with cardiopulmonary or neurologic complications is controversial. The most widely advocated regimen is intravenous L-thyroxine, 100 to 200 μg per day, which some would precede with a 500-μg loading dose. The alternative is T_3 therapy, 50 to 100 μg per day, which has a more rapid onset of action and circumvents the uncertainties of impaired T_4-to-T_3 conversion, but may be more likely to induce myocardial ischemia or arrhythmias. Prevention and management of the multisystem complications that accompany severe hypothyroidism are probably more important determinants of outcome than the particular thyroid hormone treatment regimen selected.

A common therapeutic conundrum is posed by the critically ill patient with possible clinical evidence of hypothyroidism and hypothyroxinemia. While awaiting definitive diagnosis based on the serum TSH, medical management should be adapted to deal with the special concerns in myxedema. Whether thyroid hormone should be started depends on the strength of the clinical evidence for myxedema, the severity of the systemic pathophysiology attributable to hypothyroidism, and the probability of coexisting ischemic heart disease. There is currently no convincing evidence that thyroid hormone therapy is indicated for patients with nonthyroidal systemic illness, even if profound hypothyroxinemia is present.

THYROIDITIS

Thyroid inflammation may cause local neck symptoms, constitutional complaints, and abnormalities of thyroid hormone production. The pathologic, clinical, and laboratory features of the various forms of thyroiditis are well described (Table 14.4–11), although their pathogeneses are only partially understood.

Subacute (de Quervain) Thyroiditis
Subacute thyroiditis is believed to be caused by viral infection of the thyroid gland and is often preceded by a prodromal upper respiratory syndrome. The cardinal symptom of subacute thyroiditis is thyroid pain, which may be referred to the throat, ear, or lateral neck (Table 14.4–12). Constitutional symptoms including fever, sweats, fatigue, and malaise are often present. The thyroid gland is typically exquisitely tender, firm, and moderately enlarged. Hyperthyroidism occurs during the initial phase of the illness (2 to 8

TABLE 14.4–11. FORMS OF THYROIDITIS

Disorder	Pathogenesis	Clinical Features	Laboratory Data
Subacute (de Quervain)	Viral	Painful goiter; fever, constitutional symptoms; hyperthyroidism followed by hypothyroidism	Elevated ESR; increased, then decreased T_4; low RAI uptake
Lymphocytic (postpartum, painless, silent)	?Autoimmune	Hyperthyroidism often followed by hypothyroidism in postpartum women; small painless goiter	Increased then decreased T_4; low RAI uptake; normal ESR
Autoimmune (Hashimoto)	Autoimmune	Hypothyroidism; goiter; associated autoimmune disorders	Elevated TSH ± low T_4; antithyroid antibodies
Riedel (chronic sclerosing)	Unknown	Large, hard, locally compressive goiter; ± hypothyroidism	
Acute (suppurative, infectious)	Bacterial	Fever; painful thyroid swelling	Leukocytosis; focally decreased thyroidal radionuclide uptake

TABLE 14.4–12. CAUSES OF PAINFUL THYROID

Commonly cause pain
- Subacute thyroiditis
- Hemorrhage within thyroid nodule
- Thyroid malignancy
- Suppurative thyroiditis

Uncommonly cause pain
- Autoimmune thyroiditis
- Graves disease

weeks) as the result of hormone release, predominantly T_4, from the gland (Fig. 14.4–6D). Defective thyroid hormone synthesis then often induces transient hypothyroidism. Thyroid function usually returns to normal, although permanent hypothyroidism rarely occurs. Recurrent episodes occur in a small minority of patients.

The diagnosis of subacute thyroiditis is confirmed by detection of abnormal thyroid hormone concentrations, an elevated ESR, and a markedly decreased thyroidal radioactive uptake. Antithyroid antibodies are often transiently present in low titer, and serum thyroglobulin is typically detectable. Thyroid biopsy, which is seldom required for diagnosis, reveals an inflammatory infiltrate comprised of polymorphonuclear leukocytes, lymphocytes, and macrophages with granuloma formation.

Inflammatory and constitutional symptoms are best treated with aspirin 600 mg every 4 to 8 hours. If this regimen and other nonsteroidal anti-inflammatory agents (e.g., indomethacin 50 mg three times daily) fail, glucocorticoid therapy (e.g., prednisone 20 mg twice daily) is invariably effective but must generally be tapered slowly over 3 to 4 weeks to avoid provoking a flare-up of the disorder. No treatment may be required for thyroid dysfunction, but transient hyperthyroidism can be managed with beta-adrenergic blocking agents and hypothyroidism reversed by temporary L-thyroxine therapy.

Lymphocytic (Postpartum, Silent, Painless) Thyroiditis

Lymphocytic thyroiditis occurs predominantly in young women, particularly 4 to 24 weeks after delivery when it may be confused with postpartum depression or somatization. The illness is initially typified by clinical manifestations of hyperthyroidism without features of local thyroid inflammation. Hyperthyroidism resolves spontaneously over several weeks and, in half the cases, is followed by a period of transient hypothyroidism. Although the etiology of lymphocytic thyroiditis is unknown, the disorder may be a form of autoimmune thyroid inflammation because it occurs in women with previous Graves disease and may evolve into typical autoimmune thyroiditis and permanent hypothyroidism. Treatment is limited to managing symptoms associated with transient thyroid function abnormalities. Recurrent episodes should be anticipated following subsequent pregnancies.

Rare Forms of Thyroiditis

Suppurative thyroiditis is caused by the spread of bacterial infection from contiguous structures. This rare disorder is characterized

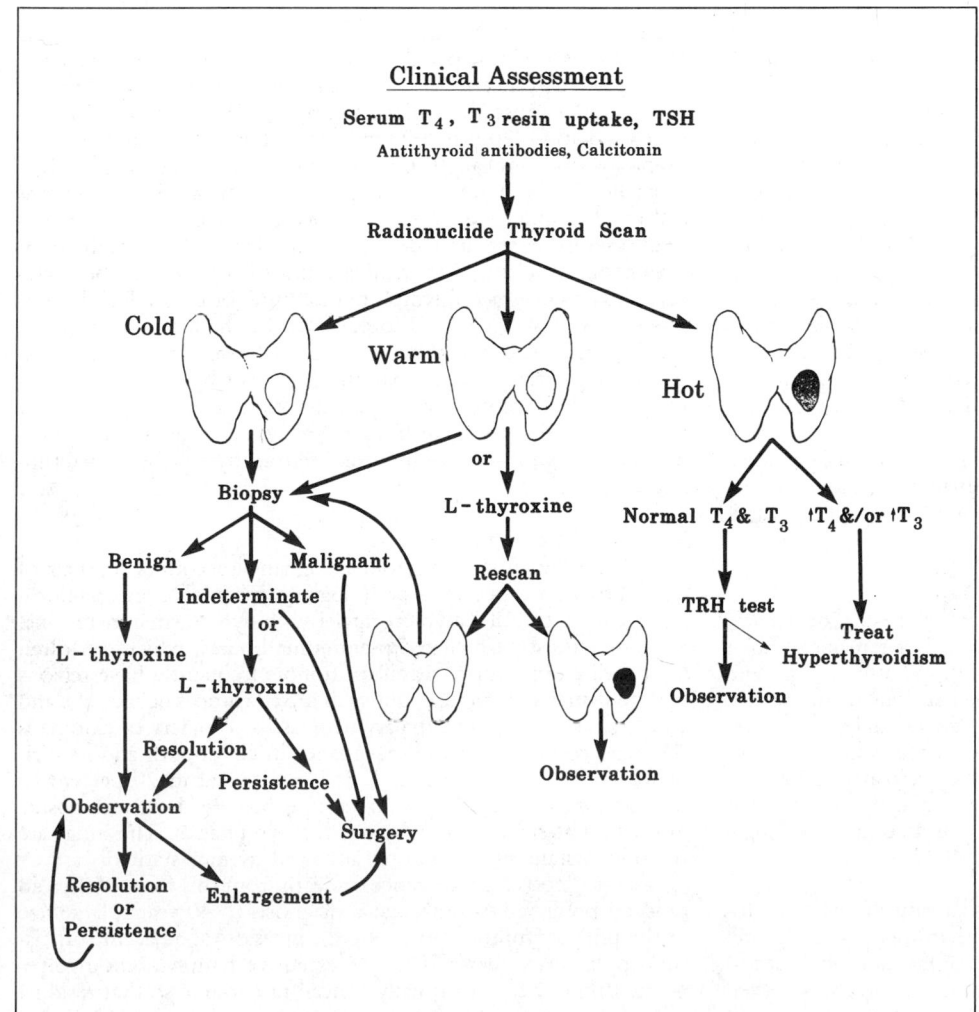

Figure 14.4–7. Diagnostic evaluation of patient with thyroid nodule. After clinical evaluation and serum thyroid function tests a radionuclide thyroid scan is performed. Nonfunctioning (cold) and possibly functioning (warm) nodules are biopsied. Cytologically malignant nodules are excised, and a trial of L-thyroxine is begun for cytologically benign nodules. Indeterminate nodules are either excised or subjected to a 3- to 6-month trial of thyroid hormone suppression with surgery if the nodule does not regress completely.

by high fever, systemic manifestations of sepsis, and intense thyroid pain and inflammatory signs. The diagnosis is generally established on clinical grounds. Thyroid scintigraphy may demonstrate a focal hypofunctioning region, and needle biopsy can yield purulent material that can be Gram stained and cultured.

Riedel thyroiditis (chronic sclerosing thyroiditis) is a rare form of thyroiditis most often affecting middle-aged men. The gland is progressively replaced by fibrous tissue that is densely adherent to adjacent structures. Clinical manifestations are related to compression of adjacent structures and occasionally hypothyroidism. Open biopsy is generally required for diagnosis and differentiation from thyroid malignancy. Treatment is the surgical relief of compressive complications and L-thyroxine therapy for hypothyroidism.

Other rare forms of thyroiditis may be caused by external or iodine-131 radiation therapy, direct trauma, sarcoidosis, tuberculosis, or fungal infections.

GOITER AND THYROID NEOPLASIA

GOITER

Thyroid enlargement, or goiter, can be classified by its incidence, physical characteristics, functional status, or etiology. When goiter affects 10 percent or more of a population, it is endemic, whereas a lower incidence is termed sporadic. Goiters are categorized as multinodular or diffuse (simple) based on physical examination or radiologic findings. Although certain diseases typically cause nodularity while others produce diffuse enlargement, there is considerable variability in expression of disorders causing thyromegaly, most of which can progress from diffuse to multinodular enlargement. Goiter may be associated with hyperthyroidism (e.g., toxic nodular goiter and Graves disease), euthyroidism (e.g., nontoxic nodular goiter), or hypothyroidism (e.g., autoimmune thyroiditis). The diagnosis and management of thyroid function disorders have been discussed previously. Other clinical problems encountered in patients with goiter are local compressive phenomena and thyroid malignancy. Regardless of the underlying etiology, goiter may cause dysphagia, dyspnea, and cosmetic dissatisfaction. Pain and hoarseness may be encountered with benign disease, but these complaints should raise suspicion of malignancy. Severe compressive phenomena, such as tracheal narrowing and venous obstruction, are actually encountered most often with benign multinodular goiters, which extend substernally into the superior mediastinum, where they must be differentiated by thyroid scan from lymphoma, teratoma, and thymoma. Most thyroid neoplasms present as focal thyroid enlargement, or nodules, the management of which will be discussed. Some thyroid malignancies, however, do cause generalized glandular enlargement, for example, lymphoma, anaplastic carcinoma, and multifocal papillary carcinoma.

Endemic Goiter
Endemic goiter is usually caused by dietary iodine deficiency, which no longer occurs in North America, but remains a major international health problem causing goiter, hypothyroidism, and cretinism in mountainous underdeveloped regions of the world. Exposure to goitrogens in water supplies, for example, resorcinol, may also be responsible for endemic goiter. Treatment of endemic goiter, that is, provision of dietary iodine or avoidance of environmental goitrogens, is usually straightforward medically but has often proved to be an enormous economic and political challenge.

Sporadic Goiter
Sporadic or benign multinodular goiter is a relatively common disorder affecting women more frequently than men, typically presenting in the third through fifth decades of life, and often occurring in families. Although the condition can be caused by inherited defects in thyroid hormone synthesis and by childhood neck irradi-

ation, in the vast majority of cases the cause is unknown. In these thyroid glands, follicular epithelial cells grow and, in some cases, produce thyroid hormone autonomously, that is, without regard for TSH regulation. The pathogenesis of this phenomenon remains unclear, although it has been suggested that in some patients a thyroid growth-stimulating immunoglobulin may be responsible. Pathologically, the gland typically contains multiple nodules, which are cellular or colloid-laden adenomas or hemorrhagic cysts with fibrotic or calcified walls, or both.

Treatment. Thyroid hormone suppression therapy is the preferred initial approach for relief and prevention of the local compressive or cosmetic complications associated with goiter. In otherwise healthy individuals, L-thyroxine can be started in a dose expected to suppress TSH secretion completely, approximately 1.8 $\mu g/kg$ per day. A lower dosage should be employed in the elderly, in patients with cardiopulmonary disease, and in persons who may have autonomously functioning thyroid tissue within their glands. Six to 12 months may be required to appreciate any treatment response. For patients with further goiter progression or persistent symptoms, partial thyroidectomy may be required, particularly for goiters with significant substernal extension. Patients with nontoxic nodular goiter should avoid pharmacologic iodine doses, which may incite hyperthyroidism (iodine-induced thyrotoxicosis).[4] (The treatment of toxic nodular goiter has been described in the discussion on hyperthyroidism.) Although radioactive iodine is useful in treating hyperthyroidism, it has no established role in management of locally compressive nontoxic goiter.

THYROID CARCINOMA

Thyroid malignancies have a broad spectrum of behavior, from clinically insignificant papillary carcinomas to relentlessly progressive anaplastic cancers, which are almost invariably fatal. Thyroid cancer can be caused by radiation of the gland, particularly by low-dose irradiation (200 to 2000 rads) in childhood. Medullary carcinoma may be familial. In most cases of thyroid carcinoma, however, the cause is unknown. Thyroid cancer most often presents as a thyroid nodule, which may produce local symptoms or be entirely asymptomatic and detected only at routine examination. Less commonly, the first manifestation of disease may be metastatic lesions in regional lymph nodes, lung, or bone. The diagnosis of thyroid malignancy is complicated by the fact that there is a much higher incidence of benign than malignant thyroid nodules. Although treatment of thyroid cancer is beset by a number of unresolved controversies, most patients have a good or excellent prognosis, and sensitive techniques are available for tumor follow-up, that is, iodine-131 scanning and serum thyroglobulin determination.

Papillary Carcinoma
This well-differentiated thyroid malignancy accounts for half of clinical thyroid cancers. Its pathologic features include papilliform arrangement of cells, atypical nuclei with cytoplasmic inclusions, and characteristic lamellated psammoma bodies, which can often be identified on biopsy. Papillary tumors frequently have regions with follicular architecture, but such mixed tumors behave like and are classified with pure papillary neoplasms. Papillary carcinoma is the most common thyroid malignancy in childhood, and its incidence increases in older adults. It is multifocal in 20 percent of cases and typically spreads by extension through the gland capsule into adjacent structures or by regional lymphatics. The lungs are the only distant site commonly involved by metastatic disease. A poorer prognosis for recurrence or death from this form of thyroid cancer is predicted by older age at diagnosis (>40 years), large size of the primary tumor (>3 to 4 cm), invasion of adjacent soft tissues, pulmonary metastases, and extensive lymph node involvement. Papillary tumors usually concentrate iodine so that residual tumor after surgery can often be treated with iodine-131.

Follicular Carcinoma

One fourth of thyroid cancers have a follicular appearance that is differentiated from benign thyroid neoplasms primarily by invasion of the capsule and blood vessels, features that are often inapparent in biopsy specimens. Follicular carcinoma occurs most commonly in the middle-aged and elderly. In addition to local invasion and regional lymphatic spread, these malignancies metastasize hematogenously, particularly to lung and bone. Distant metastases may retain the ability to concentrate iodine, rendering them amenable to radioactive iodine therapy. Poor prognostic factors include extensively invasive tumor, distant metastases, and absence of radioactive iodine uptake in metastatic lesions.

Medullary Carcinoma

Tumors arising from parafollicular C cells are most often sporadic but may be familial as part of the MEN II or III syndromes (Chapters 14.1 and 14.6). Production of calcitonin by these tumors permits their immunohistochemical diagnosis and their follow-up with serum calcitonin measurements.

Anaplastic Carcinoma

This poorly differentiated thyroid malignancy is almost exclusively a disease of the elderly. The tumor invariably pursues a rapidly progressive course with local invasion by tumor and blood-borne distant metastases. Except for occasional reports of success with regimens of combined radiation and chemotherapy, there is no effective treatment.

Lymphoma and Other Malignancies

Lymphoma may involve the thyroid gland primarily or as part of systemic disease. Thyroidal lymphoma is more frequently encountered in patients with preexisting autoimmune thyroiditis. Squamous cell carcinoma may arise from or secondarily involve the thyroid. Extrathyroidal malignancies, particularly renal cell carcinoma, may metastasize to the thyroid. Such metastatic lesions are usually suspected on a clinical basis, and their presence may be confirmed by needle biopsy.

Treatment

Well-differentiated thyroid carcinomas should be generously excised. Although the performance of partial versus total thyroidectomy remains controversial, near total thyroidectomy is preferred for invasive follicular carcinoma to facilitate subsequent radioactive iodine scanning and therapy, and for medullary carcinoma, which is often bilateral. Radical neck dissection does not improve the prognosis of patients with well-differentiated thyroid cancer. Surgery has only a palliative role in anaplastic carcinoma and a diagnostic role in lymphoma.

Postoperative thyroid hormone therapy prevents hypothyroidism and suppresses TSH, decreasing the likelihood of tumor recurrence. The ideal L-thyroxine dose completely inhibits TSH secretion, including the TSH response to exogenous TRH, while avoiding iatrogenic hyperthyroidism. Routine postoperative radioactive iodine ablation of thyroid remnants is debatable. For patients with a high risk of recurrent papillary carcinoma or possible metastatic follicular cancer, iodine-131 ablation is generally believed valuable but must be administered after temporary withdrawal of thyroid hormone suppression. Radioactive iodine is agreed to be the treatment of choice for iodine-concentrating metastases from well-differentiated thyroid cancers, but has no proven benefit in management of medullary or anaplastic carcinomas. Conventional radiation therapy and chemotherapy have limited usefulness in treatment of thyroid malignancies with the exception of lymphoma, for which these modalities are often curative.

EVALUATION OF THYROID NODULE PATIENT

Thyroid nodules are present in more than 6 percent of women and almost 2 percent of men in the United States. The vast majority of these patients are euthyroid and have benign nodules which will not produce significant compressive problems. The challenge for the physician is to recognize the minority of patients with thyroid dysfunction or cancer, with minimal risk and expense. Clinical evaluation can identify patients at higher risk of thyroid malignancy. Nodules developing over weeks or months are more likely to reflect the typical growth pattern of malignant neoplasms than those emerging over days or years. Nodules producing local symptoms, particularly pain, hoarseness, or hemoptysis, warrant greater concern. A history of childhood neck irradiation for thymic enlargement, tonsillitis, or other indications, increases risk of thyroid cancer, whereas a family history of benign thyroid nodules is relatively reassuring. On physical examination, hard fixed nodules associated with regional lymphadenopathy are clearly alarming, but even soft mobile nodules may prove malignant. Solitary thyroid nodules should be approached with greater suspicion than multinodular glands, which are more often benign. A dominant nodule, that is, one enlarging more rapidly or creating more local symptoms in a multinodular gland, deserves the same attention as a solitary nodule, however. Clinical or laboratory evidence of hyperthyroidism or hypothyroidism is relatively reassuring and suggests the presence of benign toxic adenoma or autoimmune thyroiditis, respectively.

Radionuclide thyroid scanning is useful to categorize thyroid nodules as nonfunctioning (cold), autonomously functioning (hot), or possibly functioning (warm) (Fig. 14.4–7). Cold and warm nodules require additional investigation. Thyroid biopsy plays a central role in the contemporary evaluation of these thyroid nodules. Indeed, thyroid biopsy may be employed as the initial diagnostic procedure. Fine-needle (20 to 25 gauge) aspiration biopsy is easily performed and complication-free but provides cytologic specimens that require special expertise for proper interpretation. Cutting-needle (12- to 16-gauge) biopsy is technically more demanding and associated with greater risk of injury to adjacent structures but yields a better specimen for histopathologic study. Benign lesions, for example, colloid adenoma, autoimmune thyroiditis, and cysts, can usually be diagnosed with both techniques, thereby avoiding surgery. The sensitivity of needle biopsy for thyroid malignancy is 95 percent, but categorization of follicular neoplasms in particular is problematic. For patients with benign nodules on biopsy, a subsequent trial of thyroid hormone suppression therapy is usually prudent. Shrinkage of the nodule after administration of L-thyroxine further supports pursuit of a conservative nonsurgical approach. On the other hand, nodule enlargement despite medical therapy warrants consideration of definitive surgical excision or at least repeat biopsy of the nodule.

Ultrasonography has limited applications in the investigation of thyroid nodules. Solid nodules can be distinguished from pure or complex cysts, and, in a gland with a solitary palpable nodule, ultrasonography frequently demonstrates the presence of other nodules escaping clinical detection. The technique cannot, however, exclude malignancy in most patients because only small, simple cysts (< 4 cm) can be assumed benign. Ultrasonography is most useful for monitoring the change in thyroid nodule size with thyroid hormone suppression therapy or simple observation. CT is helpful in defining the extent of thyroid malignancies and large nodular goiters, particularly when they extend substernally, but CT has no other special value in the work-up of patients with a thyroid nodule.

REFERENCES

1. Borst GC, Eil C, Burman KD: Euthyroid hyperthyroxinemia. Ann Intern Med 98:366, 1983
2. Chopra IJ (moderator), Hershman JM, et al: Thyroid function in nonthyroidal illnesses. Ann Intern Med 98:946, 1983
3. DeGroot LJ, Larsen PR, et al (eds): The Thyroid and Its Diseases, 5th ed. New York, John Wiley and Sons, 1984
4. Fradkin JE, Woolf J: Iodide-induced thyrotoxicosis. Medicine 62:1, 1983

5. Graham GD, Burman KD: Radioiodine treatment of Graves' disease: An assessment of its potential risks. Ann Intern Med 105:900, 1986
6. Ingbar SH, Braverman LE (eds): The Thyroid: A Fundamental and Clinical Text, 5th ed. Philadelphia, Lippincott, 1986
7. Ladenson PW: Diseases of the thyroid gland. In Ney RL (ed): Investigations of Endocrine Disorders. Clin Endocrinol Metab 14:145, 1985
8. Oppenheimer JH: Thyroid hormone action at the nuclear level. Ann Intern Med 102:374, 1985
9. Schimmel M, Utiger RD: Thyroid and peripheral production of thyroid hormones: Review of recent findings and their clinical implications. Ann Intern Med 87:760, 1977
10. Volpe R: Autoimmunity in thyroid disease. In Volpe R (ed): Autoimmunity in Endocrine Diseases. New York, Marcel Dekker, 1985
11. Weintraub BD (moderator): Inappropriate secretion of thyroid stimulating hormone. Ann Intern Med 95:339, 1981

CHAPTER 14.5
Gonadal Disorders

Patrick C. Walsh and Howard A. Zacur

The entire spectrum of reproductive system disorders can be attributed to abnormalities occurring at one of the milestones in sexual maturation. Abnormalities in utero present with abnormal sexual differentiation. Abnormalities occurring between infancy and puberty may present as precocious maturation with appropriate or inappropriate secondary sexual characteristics. At the time of puberty, the commonest problems are delay of puberty or abnormalities in the maturation process (gynecomastia in men, asymmetry of breast development or virilization in women). Postpubertal gonadal disorders include menstrual abnormalities, infertility, inappropriate virilization or feminization, and premature gonadal failure.

The great variety and complexity of gonadal disorders stem from the fact that the male and female reproductive organs develop from the same fetal anlage, respond to the same pituitary tropic hormones, and synthesize steroidal hormones in similar fashion. These disorders are best understood if each is approached with knowledge of the effects of the sex hormones, the complex reciprocal pituitary-gonadal relationships, and the normal sequence of reproductive development.

SEXUAL DIFFERENTIATION

The undifferentiated fetal gonad, which is formed between 3 and 5 weeks of gestation, is bipotential in sexual differentiation. Early in gestation, both wolffian and müllerian ducts are present in both sexes. Male sexual development requires the presence of testes, whereas female sexual development occurs in their absence.

MALE SEXUAL DIFFERENTIATION

Chromosomal determinants direct differentiation of the indifferent gonad into either a testis or an ovary. A gene on the short arm of the Y chromosome, testis-determining factor, plays the major role in the differentiation of the gonadal anlage into a testis. Müllerian-inhibiting substance (MIS), produced by fetal Sertoli cells, causes ipsilateral regression of the müllerian ducts. Testosterone secretion promotes differentiation of the wolffian structures into the epididymis, vas deferens, and seminal vesicle.

The fetal external genitalia are also sexually bipotential. In the male, androgens promote differentiation of the urogenital sinus into the prostate and the genital tubercle into the glans penis. The genital swellings merge and migrate inferiorly to form the scrotum. Testosterone exerts these effects only after local conversion by the enzyme 5-α-reductase to dihydrotestosterone, which binds to a specific cytoplasmic protein receptor. This receptor binds to an acceptor on nuclear chromatin to induce transcription of specific gene products.

FEMALE SEXUAL DIFFERENTIATION

The genes that determine ovarian formation have not been identified. In the normal female, testosterone is not secreted and the wolffian ducts regress. In the absence of MIS, the müllerian ducts differentiate into the fallopian tubes, uterus, and upper vagina. The lack of androgen secretion by the fetal ovary maintains the appropriate female external genitalia.

ABNORMAL SEXUAL DIFFERENTIATION

Disordered sexual differentiation is most commonly due to (1) sex chromosomal abnormalities; (2) defective androgen production or action in the male, producing feminization of the genitalia (male pseudohermaphroditism); or (3) excessive androgen production in the female, causing virilization of the external genitalia (female pseudohermaphroditism) (Table 14.5–1).

DISORDERS OF MALE SEXUAL DIFFERENTIATION

Chromosomal Abnormalities
Klinefelter syndrome (46,XXY), the most common disorder of gonadal differentiation in men, affects 1 out of 500 newborn males. In its classic form men present with gynecomastia, small firm testes, azoospermia, decreased facial hair, and increased mean body height with eunuchoid proportions. Plasma luteinizing hormone (LH) and follicle-stimulating hormone (FSH) levels are high, and plasma testosterone levels are only 50 percent of normal. About 30 other karyotypic varieties have been described including XXYY, XXXY, XXXXY, and a variety of mosaics such as XY/XXY. Diagnosis of the classic form can be made from the buccal smear, which shows a nuclear chromatin clump (Barr body) inappropriate for the male cell. The mosaic forms require chromosomal analysis to confirm the diagnosis.

True hermaphrodites have both ovarian and testicular tissue. Differentiation of the external genitalia is variable, and 75 percent of patients have been reared as males because of the phallic size. About two thirds of these individuals have a 46,XX karyotype. Patients with *mixed gonadal dysgenesis* have a unilateral streak gonad, a testis on the other side, a uterus, at least one fallopian tube, and widely variable appearance of the external genitalia. Because most of these patients are poorly virilized, more than half have been reared as females. The most common karyotype is 46X/46,XY. Adult infertility is due to a lack of germinal elements in seminiferous tubules, and more than 25 percent of the patients develop testicular tumors, typically gonadoblastomas.

TABLE 14.5–1. CLASSIFICATION OF INTERSEXUALITY

Disorder	Gonads	Internal Ducts	External Genitalia	Sex Chromatin	Karyotype
Disorders of gonadal differentiation					
Klinefelter syndrome	Bilateral testes	Wolffian	Male	Positive	47,XXY
Turner syndrome	Bilateral streaks	Müllerian	Female	50% negative	45,XO
True hermaphroditism	Testes + ovary	Mixed	Variable	80% positive	46,XX;46,XY; mosaics
Mixed gonadal dysgenesis	Testis + streak	Mixed	Variable	Negative	45,XO/ 46,XY;46XY; other mosaics
Female pseudohermaphroditism					
Congenital adrenal hyperplasia Prenatal virilization from drugs Virilizing disorder of mother Idiopathic	Bilateral ovaries	Müllerian	Variable virilization	Positive	46,XX
Male pseudohermaphroditism					
Defective androgen production 3-β-hydroxysteroid dehydrogenase deficiency 17-hydroxylase deficiency 17-ketosteroid reductase deficiency 20,21-desmolase deficiency 17,20-desmolase deficiency	Bilateral testes	Wolffian	Variable virilization	Negative	46,XY
Defective androgen action Testicular feminization	Bilateral testes	Absent	Female	Negative	46,XY
Incomplete androgen insensitivity	Bilateral testes	Variable Wolffian differentiation	Variable	Negative	46,XY
5-α-reductase deficiency	Bilateral testes	Wolffian	Variable virilization	Negative	46,XY
Defective Müllerian regression (persistent Müllerian duct syndrome)	Bilateral testes	Müllerian and Wolffian	Male	Negative	46,XY

Male Pseudohermaphroditism

In these disorders, genetic males (46,XY) with bilateral testes differentiate partially or completely as phenotypic females. This disorder can result from defects in androgen synthesis, androgen action, or müllerian regression. A defect in any of the five enzymatic steps in the conversion of cholesterol to testosterone, giving rise to inadequate testosterone synthesis in utero, may result in incomplete virilization and ambiguous genitalia in male infants. The diagnosis is based on the demonstration of inadequate testosterone synthesis, elevated gonadotropin levels after puberty, and the accumulation of elevated steroids proximal to the particular metabolic block.

Three distinct familial forms of defective androgen action can be identified (Table 14.5–1).

Patients with *testicular feminization syndrome* (androgen insensitivity) are phenotypic females with absent pubic and axillary hair but normally developed breasts and a shallow blind-ending vagina. The disorder, which may present as primary amenorrhea in an apparently normal female, is inherited as an X-linked recessive trait and is the most complete form of androgen resistance. Testosterone synthesis is normal and the primary defect is an abnormal amount or function of the androgen receptor.

Reifenstein syndrome (incomplete androgen insensitivity) refers to a group of patients presenting as males with hypospadias, azoospermia, incomplete virilization at the time of puberty, gynecomastia, and a family history of similar traits transmitted in a pattern consistent with X-linked inheritance. Subjects have either a decreased number of normal androgen receptors or qualitatively abnormal receptors.

In the rare condition *5-α-reductase deficiency*, phenotypic females have normal wolffian duct structures, severe perineal hypo-

spadias, variable masculinization at puberty, and a family history consistent with autosomal recessive inheritance. A defect in dihydrotestosterone formation is the fundamental defect.

In *persistent müllerian duct syndrome* (hernia uteri inguinale), phenotypic males with cryptorchidism have a rudimentary uterus, bilateral fallopian tubes, and a variable development of the vasa deferentia. Failure of MIS production or action is suspected as the cause.

DISORDERS OF FEMALE SEXUAL DIFFERENTIATION

Chromosomal Abnormalities

The most common disorder of gonadal differentiation in females is *Turner syndrome* (gonadal dysgenesis), which most commonly is associated with the 45,X karyotype and occurs in 1 of 2700 newborn females. Classically, these patients have nonfunctional streak gonads and associated somatic abnormalities such as short stature, wide (shield) chest, brachydactyly, cubitus valgus, web neck, low hairline, lymphedema, coarctation of the aorta, and intestinal telangiectasia. Other X chromosome abnormalities are also associated with gonadal dysgenesis. About 40 percent are mosaics; XX/XO is the most common.

Turner syndrome must be distinguished from *46,XX pure gonadal dysgenesis* and from *Noonan syndrome* (pseudo-Turner syndrome), both of which have a normal 46,XX karyotype. The former are entirely normal females except for bilateral streak gonads. Most stigmata of Turner syndrome, including short stature, can be present in Noonan syndrome. The associated cardiovascular abnor-

mality is usually pulmonic stenosis, however, and the hypogonadism is partial.

Treatment of patients with Turner syndrome can include anabolic steroids (oxandrolone) between 11 and 13 years of age to avoid short stature; estrogen replacement is then indicated to promote female secondary sexual characteristics and prevent premature osteoporosis.

Female Pseudohermaphroditism

These patients are genetic females (46,XX) with bilateral ovaries. Their external genitalia are virilized by intrauterine exposure to excessive androgen. Because they have normally developed ovaries and müllerian derivatives, they are all potentially fertile. Depending on the time of exposure to androgen, the degree of masculinization varies from clitoral hypertrophy to true phallic-urethral formation with labioscrotal fusion. The most common cause is congenital adrenal hyperplasia (see Chapter 14.3). Other causes of female pseudohermaphroditism include prenatal virilization from drugs, maternal virilizing, and an idiopathic form.

TESTICULAR ANATOMY AND PHYSIOLOGY

The normal adult testis measures 4.6 cm in length (range, 3.6 to 5.5 cm) and 2.6 cm in width (range, 2.1 to 3.2 cm) and weighs about 21 g. Beneath the white outer capsule of the testis, lobules separated by fibrous septa contain the coiled, U-shaped seminiferous tubules, which have a central lumen, a stratified epithelium composed of Sertoli and spermatogenic cells, and a thin outer basement membrane. Because over 75 percent of the total testicular mass consists of seminiferous tubules, isolated tubular damage causes the testes to become small and soft. Leydig cells, found in the loose connective tissue stroma between the tubules, constitute only 12 percent of the testicular volume. Leydig cells, the principal source of testosterone, secrete about 7 mg per day, which is transported bound to albumin and testosterone-estradiol-binding globulin (TEBG). Only unbound testosterone, less than 5 percent of the total, is available to the androgen target cells.

The testes are regulated by the gonadotropins LH and FSH, which are synthesized and stored in the anterior pituitary. Their release is regulated by the hypothalamic decapeptide, gonadotropin-releasing hormone (GnRH), which itself is controlled by neurotransmitters in the CNS. GnRH is secreted at 60- to 100-minute intervals, and this pulsatile release is necessary for normal episodic secretion of LH and FSH. LH stimulates Leydig cells to secrete testosterone. FSH binds to the Sertoli cells and facilitates the maturation of spermatids to mature spermatozoa.

The hypothalamic-pituitary-testicular axis is a closed-loop, negative-feedback system in which testicular hormones inhibit the secretion of LH and FSH. Testosterone is the primary regulator of gonadotropin secretion. Castration results in an elevation of both LH and FSH, whereas selective germ cell damage produces an elevation of serum FSH alone. The testes also produce inhibin, a polypeptide that inhibits FSH release.

OVARIAN ANATOMY AND PHYSIOLOGY

The ovaries are the paired female gonadal glands, measuring approximately 3 by 2 by 1.5 cm. Beneath their surface covering of coelomic mesothelium (also known as germinal epithelium) is a layer of connective tissue, the tunica albuginea. Blood is supplied by the ovarian artery (by the abdominal aorta) and branches of the ascending uterine artery. Venous blood drains directly into the inferior vena cava from the right ovary and into the left renal vein from the left ovary.

The ovary itself consists of a thick outer cortex surrounding an inner medulla. Follicles in different stages of development and

corpora lutea are present in the cortex. Connective tissue and large blood vessels are located in the medulla.

EARLY MATURATION OF THE FOLLICLE

The human ovary develops between weeks 5 and 10 of fetal life when germ cells migrate from the yolk sac to the gonadal ridges. Recognizable ovarian development is evident by 16 weeks when the germ cells, or oogonia, intermingle with ovarian cortical cells. Oogonia undergo mitosis until 6 to 7 million are present at 20 weeks. Oogonia then enter prophase of the first meiotic division to become oocytes but do not complete the first stage of meiosis until ovulation. No further mitosis of oogonia occurs postnatally, and the prenatal onset of oocyte atresia leaves only 1 to 2 million oocytes at birth.

Follicle development accompanies growth and differentiation of the oocyte (Fig. 14.5–1). A newly formed oocyte is surrounded by flattened ovarian cortical cells (granulosa cells) resting on a basement membrane, creating a structure known as the primordial follicle located in the ovarian cortex beneath the tunica albuginea. Only a few primordial follicles are recruited during each menstrual cycle to become primary follicles. In this process, the oocyte enlarges and acquires a covering membrane called the zona pellucida. The surrounding granulosa cells become cuboidal and increase in number. Primary follicles are formed when the developing primordial follicles migrate toward the ovarian medulla and become covered by ovarian thecal cells arranged in inner (theca interna) and outer (theca externa) layers.

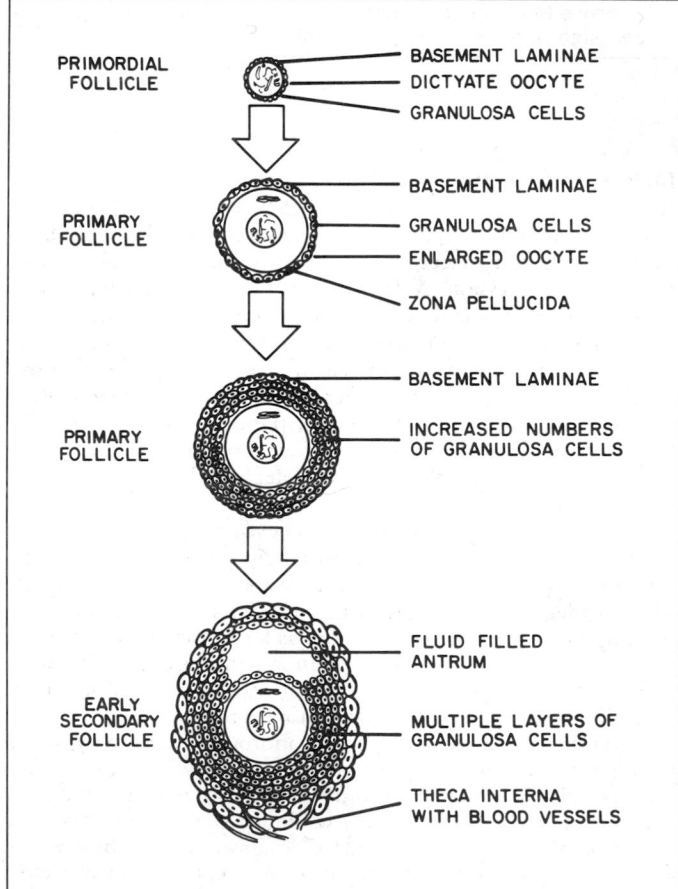

Figure 14.5–1. Stages in follicular development. (*Modified from Erickson GF: Clin Obstet Gynecol 21:31, 1978.*)

THE MENSTRUAL CYCLE

The human menstrual cycle[11] involves a repetitive sequence of hormonal changes that result in episodic uterine bleeding. *Menarche* is the initial menstrual cycle in reproductive life. *Menopause* is the termination of cyclic menses.

Normally, each menstrual cycle has a mean interval of 21 to 35 days, conventionally beginning with the first day of menstrual flow and ending on the day before the next onset of bleeding. Variation in the menstrual cycle interval is greatest during the first 7 years after menarche and during the last 7 years before menopause. Duration of the menstrual flow is usually 2 to 6 days with loss of 20 to 60 ml of blood. Menstrual blood loss exceeding 80 ml is called *menorrhagia*.

The menstrual cycle is divided into follicular and luteal phases, each corresponding to changes occurring in the ovary. These phases may also be described as proliferative or secretory, corresponding to changes observed in the uterine endometrium. Variations in the length of the cycle are usually due to alterations in the follicular phase, because the luteal phase length remains relatively constant at 12 to 16 days.

Ovarian and Hormonal Changes
During the Menstrual Cycle

A characteristic sequence of hormonal changes, reflecting specific events within the ovary, recur during each menstrual cycle (Fig. 14.5–2).

During the follicular phase several primary follicles are recruited for further growth and development. Granulosa cells in primary follicles possess FSH and estradiol receptors. Upon FSH stimulation, granulosa cells produce aromatase. This enzyme converts the androgens androstenedione and testosterone, made in response to LH by thecal cells, to estrone and estradiol, respectively. Granulosa cells respond to estradiol by undergoing mitosis to increase the number of granulosa cells and estradiol production. By day 7 of the cycle, one enlarging primary follicle is selected by unknown processes to be the follicle that will release the oocyte at ovulation. This follicle is called the dominant follicle and produces the additional estradiol found during the late follicular phase of the cycle.

As the number of granulosa cells increases, fluid accumulation forms a cavity or antrum within the dominant follicle[4] and creates a secondary follicle, which grows primarily because of increasing fluid accumulation. Before ovulation, the large secondary or preovulatory follicle reaches a diameter of 20 mm.

The midcycle rise in plasma estradiol stimulates the large midcycle LH surge. Late in the development of the secondary follicle, LH receptors appear on the surface of its granulosa cells.

The midcycle LH surge triggers resumption of meiosis within the oocyte and luteinization of the granulosa cells within the preovulatory follicle. Immediately before ovulation, the outer follicular wall begins to dissolve and an oocyte is released approximately 24 to 36 hours from the onset of the LH surge.

After ovulation, granulosa cells and the surrounding theca cells enlarge, accumulate lipid, and become transformed into lutein cells. These cells form a new vascularized structure called the corpus luteum, which secretes estradiol and progesterone. LH maintains the corpus luteum during the luteal phase and, acting via the adenyl cyclase system, stimulates progesterone production. If the oocyte is fertilized, the corpus luteum continues to be hormonally active but requires pituitary LH for its maintenance during the first 6 weeks of pregnancy. After that time placental secretion of hCG maintains corpus luteum progesterone secretion. If pregnancy does not occur, lutein cells degenerate, and diminished hormone secretion precedes menstruation.

Menstruation is immediately followed by the onset of another menstrual cycle. From the fixed complement of oocytes present at birth, it has been estimated that only 400 oocytes are released throughout reproductive life. The remainder undergo the unex-

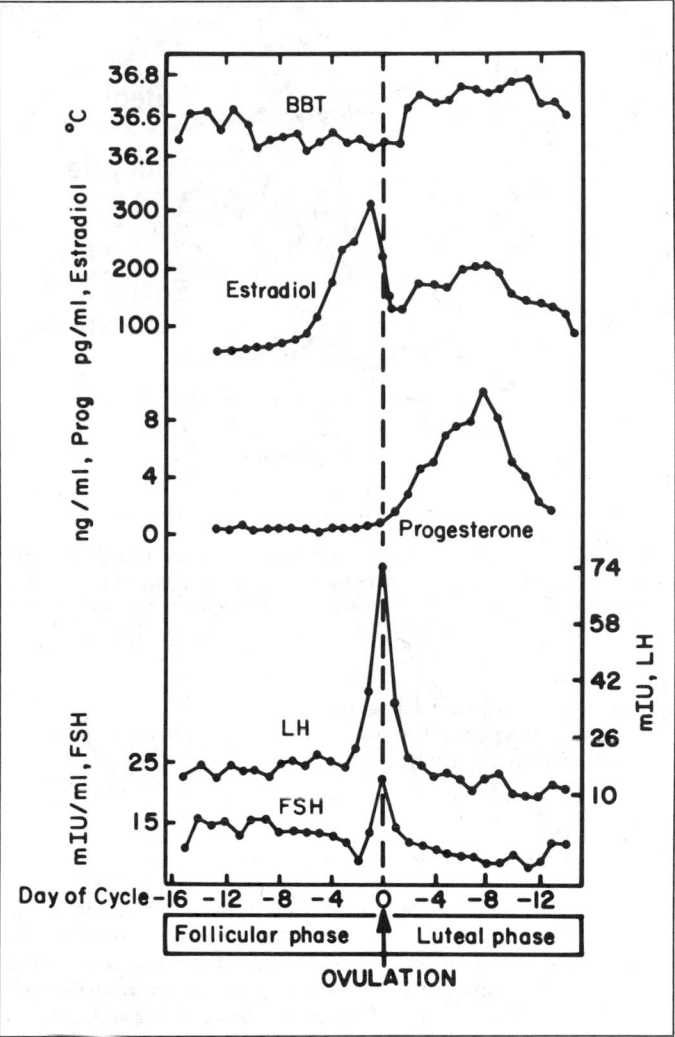

Figure 14.5–2. Changes in basal body temperature (BBT), estradiol, progesterone, LH, and FSH occurring during the normal human menstrual cycle.

plained process of atresia. Loss of all ovarian oocytes results in menopause.

Gonadotropin-releasing Hormone and the Menstrual Cycle

Pituitary-ovarian communication depends upon pituitary LH and FSH and ovarian estradiol and progesterone. Throughout the menstrual cycle LH and FSH levels exhibit an oscillating pattern that is most pronounced for LH. This pattern is called a circhoral rhythm since the peaks or valleys of LH concentration occur at approximately hourly intervals. During the follicular phase, LH peaks exhibit a periodicity of 60 to 90 minutes (Fig. 14.5–3). As ovulation approaches at midcycle, the interval between the LH peaks shortens and their amplitude increases. During the luteal phase LH peaks decrease in frequency but increase in amplitude. Progesterone appears to be responsible for this effect.

Experiments in subhuman primates suggest the existence of a fixed pulse generator for GnRH secretion within the hypothalamus. Whether ovarian sex steroids or other substances modulate the pulse generator for GnRH remains controversial. Other factors may also change peripheral LH concentrations. For example, shifts in pituitary portal blood flow or changes in pituitary cell binding or responsiveness to GnRH could be responsible.

An understanding of the effects of pulsatile GnRH release on

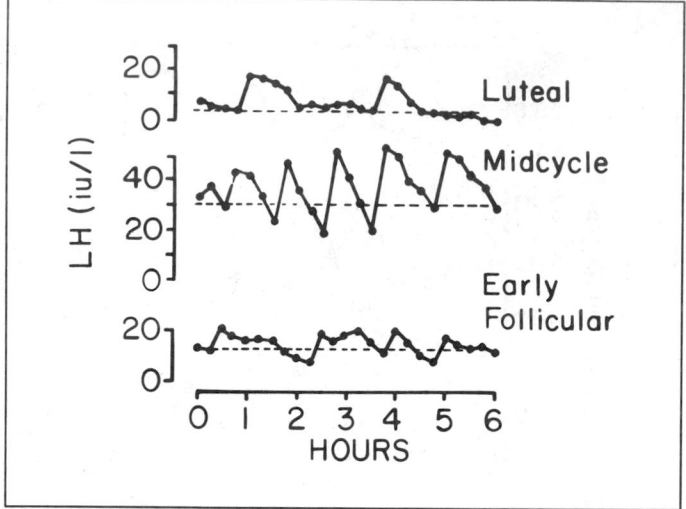

Figure 14.5–3. Changes in LH concentrations observed during different phases of the human menstrual cycle. (*Modified from Yen SSC, Vandenberg G, et al: In Ferin M, et al (ed): Biorhythms and Human Reproduction. New York, John Wiley, 1974.*)

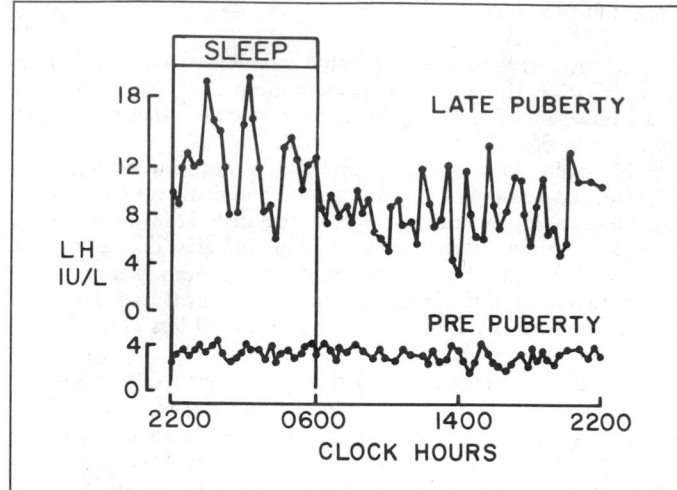

Figure 14.5–4. Observed changes in LH concentrations during puberty in the human female. (*Modified from Katz JL, Boyar RM, et al: In Sachar EJ (ed): Hormone Behavior and Psychopathology. New York, Raven Press, 1976.*)

pituitary LH secretion has allowed the use of GnRH to induce ovulation and to stimulate and complete the development of secondary sex characteristics.

PUBERTY

Puberty represents the complex transition from sexual immaturity to maturity. Attainment of reproductive capacity is accompanied by development of secondary sexual characteristics, acceleration of somatic growth, and psychological changes. Factors controlling the initiation of puberty remain uncertain, but genetic and environmental influences are involved. In prepubertal children levels of gonadotropins and sex hormones are low, and administration of exogenous GnRH evokes the release of subnormal amounts of gonadotropins. As the hypothalamic-pituitary-gonadal axis is reset toward the beginning of puberty, increased secretion of LH and FSH, initially during sleep and later in a sustained fashion, augments the secretion of testosterone in boys and estradiol in girls (Fig. 14.5–4). The enhanced release of pituitary gonadotropin is believed to result from either increased release of GnRH or increased pituitary sensitivity to GnRH.

GROWTH SPURT AND SECONDARY SEXUAL DEVELOPMENT

Maturation of the hypothalamic-pituitary axis is accompanied by a growth spurt and development of secondary sexual characteristics. In girls this is manifested by enlargement of the breasts (*thelarche*), growth of pubic and axillary hair, and enlargement of the labia majora and minora. Boys undergo testicular enlargement, growth of pubic and axillary hair, and enlargement of the penis. The age of onset of these changes and their progression varies widely (Table 14.5–2). States of development of breasts, female pubic hair, and male genital and pubic hair have been described (see Chapter 17.4).

PRECOCIOUS PUBERTY

Onset of puberty earlier than two standard deviations from the mean ages depicted in Table 14.5–2 is considered precocious. This may be incomplete when only one pubertal event occurs, for ex-

ample, breast development, or complete if all secondary sexual characteristics develop prematurely. Isosexual precocious puberty denotes precocious development consistent with genetic sex; heterosexual precocious puberty refers to pubertal changes characteristic of the opposite sex.

Heterosexual precocious puberty in girls can be caused by congenital adrenal hyperplasia, androgen-secreting tumors of the adrenal or ovary, or on rare occasions exposure to exogenous androgen. Feminizing adrenal tumors and estrogen ingestion are the main causes of heterosexual precocity in boys. In these patients, it is necessary to differentiate their feminizing signs from the "physiologic" gynecomastia of isosexual precocious puberty.

Complete isosexual precocious puberty[8] may be divided into true and pseudo forms. In both types serum sex hormone levels (estradiol or testosterone) are elevated, but only the true form has adult levels of gonadotropins and the capacity for reproduction.

Table 14.5–3 shows the features of the most common types of true isosexual precocious puberty, constitutional or idiopathic, and those resulting from CNS disorders. Identification of CNS disorders has been aided by the use of CT and MRI scans. Sexual precocity can also occur in hypothyroidism in which the bone age is markedly retarded, and sexual development usually regresses following thyroid replacement. *McCune-Albright syndrome,* characterized by precocious puberty, café-au-lait pigmentation of the skin, and polyostotic fibrous dysplasia, occurs predominantly in females. Only 10 percent of patients with complete precocious puberty have pseudoisosexual precocious puberty (Table 14.5–3).

TABLE 14.5–2. AGE AT ONSET OF PUBERTAL STAGE

	Mean (yr)	SD
Girls		
Breast budding	11.2	1.1
Pubarche	11.7	1.2
Menarche	13.5	1.0
Boys		
Testicular growth	11.6	1.1
Penile growth	12.8	1.0
Pubarche	13.4	1.1

From Marshall WA, Tanner JM: Arch Dis Child 44:291, 1969 and 45:13, 1970.

TABLE 14.5–3. COMPLETE ISOSEXUAL PRECOCIOUS PUBERTY

True isosexual precocious puberty
Constitutional or idiopathic
- 80% of girls and 50% of boys with true precocious puberty
- Frequent abnormal EEG patterns

CNS disorders
- Neoplasms (astrocytoma, neurofibroma, hamartoma, histiocytosis X)
- Infections (meningitis, encephalitis)
- Phakomatoses (tuberous sclerosis, neurofibromatosis, Sturge–Weber syndrome)
- Developmental defects (aqueduct stenosis, craniostenosis)
- Trauma

Hypothyroidism

McCune–Albright syndrome

Pseudoisosexual precocious puberty
Ovarian
- Estrogen-secreting tumors (e.g., granulosa-thecal cell)
- Teratomas (secrete hCG, which stimulates ovarian estrogen production)

Testicular
- Leydig cell tumors
- Teratomas (hCG secreting)

Adrenal
- Androgen-secreting tumors
- Estrogen-secreting tumors

Diagnosis of the type of precocious puberty is facilitated by a careful history to exclude drug ingestion or head trauma; examination for ovarian or testicular masses; measurements of serum gonadotropins, plasma estrogen, testosterone, and TSH; and a CT or MRI scan to exclude intracranial lesions. Occasionally hCG levels help to exclude embryonic tumors, and elevated levels of dehydroepiandrosterone sulfate (DHEA-S) may identify patients with adrenal tumors.

Administration of GnRH (GnRH test) may distinguish between the two forms of precocious puberty. A pubertal pattern of LH and FSH release is seen in children with true precocious puberty; those with the pseudo form demonstrate a prepubertal response.

Surgery should be considered in cases of hCG-producing tumors (hepatoblastoma, chorionepithelioma, teratoma). Surgery, radiation, and chemotherapy must be considered when intracranial tumors produce signs of compression. Periodic observation may suffice if the intracranial lesion is self-limited, nonprogressive, and asymptomatic.

In cases of idiopathic isosexual precocious puberty, medical therapy might be indicated, particularly if the child is quite young, to avoid short stature as an adult. Recently an investigational long-acting GnRH analogue has successfully suppressed gonadotropins and reduced sex hormone secretion in these patients.

Incomplete precocious puberty is defined by the occurrence of isolated premature pubertal events. Premature adrenarche and pubarche refer to the appearance of axillary or pubic hair, respectively, before age 8 in females and 10 in males. They are usually associated with an increased secretion of adrenal androgens, such as androstenedione and dehydroepiandrosterone (and its sulfate). Peripheral conversion of androstenedione to testosterone may also elevate levels of this hormone. Slightly advanced bone age and increases in urinary 17-ketosteroid secretion may occur. Premature adrenarche is a benign condition requiring no specific treatment. Premature thelarche refers to the isolated premature development of breast tissue, which is usually bilateral but can be unilateral. Bone age may be slightly advanced, and the vaginal smear shows no significant estrogen effect. Plasma estrogen levels are generally in the normal prepubertal range but may be mildly elevated. This condition

is also benign and requires no treatment. A presumptive diagnosis of incomplete precocious puberty requires close follow-up to determine that the premature pubertal event is isolated.

DELAYED PUBERTY

Delayed onset of puberty may be assumed if testicular enlargement has not occurred by age 14 in boys and menarche has not occurred by age $16\frac{1}{2}$ years in girls. Delayed puberty may result from a failure in the production of gonadotropins (hypogonadotropic hypogonadism) or sex steroids (hypergonadotropic hypogonadism) or may be a temporary condition (constitutional delay). Adolescents with constitutional delay, a diagnosis made by exclusion, have prepubertal levels of gonadotropins, low sex steroid hormone levels, and a bone age compatible with chronologic age. The causes of delayed puberty in boys and girls are discussed below under the headings Hypogonadism and Amenorrhea, respectively.

GONADAL DISORDERS IN MEN

Men with gonadal dysfunction may present with signs of hypogonadism (e.g., lack of beard), infertility, impotence, gynecomastia, undescended testes, hypospadias, or scrotal masses. The history should seek information about congenital anomalies (hypospadias, undescended testes), age at onset of puberty, adequacy of the four elements of male sexual function (libido, erection, emission of fluid, orgasm), exposure to physical agents that may alter testicular function (radiation, chemotherapeutic agents, high temperature), ingestion of drugs (alcohol, estrogen, spironolactone, antihypertensives) and infertility. Inquiry should also address symptoms of other endocrine diseases, such as hypothyroidism or hypopituitarism, and other organic derangements such as uremia and significant psychic disturbances.

The examination must evaluate the extent of virilism; the presence or absence of subclinical gynecomastia; and the size, consistency, and structure of the phallus, testes, and prostate. The sense of smell should be tested because Kallmann syndrome is associated with anosmia. A careful ophthalmologic examination should exclude findings associated with sellar mass lesions.

If hypogonadism is suspected, measurement of serum testosterone, LH, FSH, and prolactin are essential (Table 14.5–4). Because episodic fluctuations of serum LH and testosterone levels broaden the range of normal values, borderline values should be repeated.

HYPOGONADISM

Hypogonadism in men may present as delayed puberty, incomplete virilization at puberty, postpubertal gonadal failure, or infertility. Because androgens have a major influence on sexual desire in men, the presenting complaint may be loss of libido. The cause of androgen deficiency, either hypogonadotropism or faulty testosterone secretion by the testes, can be distinguished easily by plasma

TABLE 14.5–4. SERUM GONADOTROPIN AND TESTOSTERONE LEVELS IN MALE HYPOGONADISM

	LH	FSH	Testosterone
Primary testicular failure	High	High	Normal or low
Gonadotropin deficiency	Normal or low	Normal or low	Low
Isolated seminiferous tubular failure	Normal	High	Normal

testosterone and gonadotropin measurements. Because the testosterone required to maintain libido is often less than the amount necessary for full stimulation of the prostate and seminal vesicles, loss of libido because of endocrine factors is generally accompanied by decreased semen volume. A normal libido and semen volume, therefore, make endocrine factors an unlikely cause for the sexual dysfunction. On examination, hypogonadism is suggested by female habitus (narrow shoulders, wide hips, fat chest), absence of beard and poor secondary sex hair growth, arm span greatly exceeding height, small phallus, atropic testes (less than 4 cm), small prostate, and gynecomastia.

Laboratory evaluation of these patients generally includes measurement of serum gonadotropins, testosterone, and prolactin; a chromosomal analysis; and a sperm count. The broadest classification of hypogonadism is based on the level of pituitary gonadotropins. In patients with clinical hypogonadism and low plasma testosterone levels, elevated LH and FSH values indicate primary testicular disease, whereas low gonadotropin levels (hypogonadotropic hypogonadism) suggest pituitary or hypothalamic disease. Occasionally, the clomiphene stimulation test may be useful when the results are equivocal. Clomiphene, a nonsteroidal compound with antiestrogenic activity, interferes with the negative feedback of testicular steroids on the pituitary and hypothalamus. In normal patients 50 mg clomiphene twice a day for 7 days increases the serum LH and FSH over control levels by 30 and 22 percent, respectively. To distinguish between defects in the hypothalamus and pituitary, treatment with GnRH (100 μg IV) has been advised. Unfortunately, this test is unreliable because the pituitary must be exposed to GnRH for prolonged periods to achieve a normal adult response in patients with hypothalamic deficiency.

Hypogonadotropic Hypogonadism

The history will help diagnose chronic systemic disorders such as pituitary or CNS trauma, tumor, or inflammatory processes in these patients (Table 14.5–5). They require a full evaluation of pituitary structure and function, including at least CT or MRI scanning of the sellar region, and laboratory assessments of the serum prolactin, cortisol, TSH, and thyroxine. Hyperprolactinemia due to a secretory pituitary tumor, pituitary stalk interruption, or drugs (e.g., phenothiazines, reserpine) interferes with hypothalamic GnRH release and secondarily causes hypogonadotropic hypogonadism as well as occasional galactorrhea and gynecomastia. Congenital syndromes with various midline CNS abnormalities can cause hypogonadotropic hypogonadism. In Kallmann syndrome atrophy of the olfactory tracts results in anosmia or hyposmia. The "fertile eunuch syndrome" is an incomplete variant of Kallmann syndrome. The Bardet-Biedl syndrome is characterized by retinitis pigmentosa, obesity, mental deficiency, and polydactyly. Perinatal muscular hypotonia is characteristic of Prader-Willi syndrome, which also includes obesity, disproportionately small hands and feet, and mental deficiency. In septo-optic dysplasia, hypoplastic optic discs and absent septum pellucidum accompany the hypopituitarism.

Hypergonadotropic Hypogonadism

This form of hypogonadism may be caused by an abnormal karyotype, developmental anomalies, or acquired testicular defects (Table 14.5–6).

Treatment of Male Hypogonadism

In testicular failure, exogenous testosterone must be provided to achieve masculinization in adolescence or to maintain it in adults. Oral testosterone is rapidly catabolized in the gastrointestinal tract and has a short half life when absorbed. To reduce the metabolic clearance, steroids substituted in the 17 position are used. Methyltestosterone can be given sublingually (5 mg three times daily) or orally (10 mg three times daily). Fluoxymesterone (Halotestin) is also given orally (2 mg three times daily). Unfortunately, these agents have limited potency, and large amounts can alter liver function and cause cholestatic jaundice or rarely hepatic tumors. For these reasons, intramuscular preparations such as testosterone cypionate and enanthate are preferred. These long-acting preparations are given at doses of 100 to 200 mg at 1- to 3-week intervals. Patients usually learn how to titrate their required dosage, based on their degree of libido and other subjective feelings, and to inject themselves, attaining more independence practically and psychologically.

Patients with hypogonadotropic hypogonadism may be treated with exogenous androgens to induce or maintain masculinization but need LH and FSH treatment to induce spermatogenesis. Two gonadotropin preparations are available: human menopausal gonadotropins (HMG) and hCG. Both hCG and HMG are necessary to induce spermatogenesis. Once spermatogenesis has been initiated, however, it can usually be maintained by hCG alone. In patients with GnRH deficiency, synthetic GnRH can be administered chronically by a pump that provides subcutaneous doses every 60 to 90 minutes.

TABLE 14.5–5. HYPOGONADOTROPIC HYPOGONADISM IN MALES

Chronic systemic disorders
- Malnutrition
- Respiratory and cardiovascular problems
- Renal tubular acidosis
- Crohn disease

Inflammatory processes
- Encephalitis
- Granulomas (lupus, sarcoidosis, histiocytosis)

Neoplasia
- Craniopharyngioma
- Hypothalamic tumors

Head trauma
- Fracture
- Hemorrhage

Congenital anomalies
- Panhypopituitarism
- Isolated LH/FSH deficiency
- "Fertile eunuch" (isolated LH deficiency)
- Pituitary aplasia or hypoplasia
- Kallmann syndrome
- Bardet–Biedl syndrome
- Prader–Willi syndrome
- Septo-optic dysplasia

Suppression of gonadotropin secretion by
- Exogenous steroid hormones
- Pituitary tumor producing prolactin

TABLE 14.5–6. HYPERGONADOTROPIC HYPOGONADISM IN MEN

Abnormal karyotype
- Klinefelter syndrome (XXY and variants)
- XO/XY mosaic with male genitalia

Congenital anomalies
- Del Castillo syndrome (Sertoli cells only)
- Vanishing testes syndrome (congenital anorchia)
- Male Turner syndrome (Noonan syndrome)
- Myotonic dystrophy
- Cystic fibrosis

Testicular failure due to
- Bilateral orchitis (mumps, gonorrhea)
- Trauma, torsion, irradiation
- Drugs (cyclophosphamide, spironolactone, narcotics, alcohol)
- Systemic diseases (liver disease, renal failure)

HYPOSPADIAS AND CRYPTORCHIDISM

Hypospadias, which occurs in 0.2 percent of newborn males, is classified according to the location of the urethral meatus as coronal, penile, penoscrotal, or perineal. Most cases are not associated with endocrine abnormalities; however, 25 to 50 percent of patients with either hypospadias or cryptorchidism have a disorder of sexual differentiation (see section on abnormalities of male sexual differentiation). Cryptorchidism, defined as nonpalpable testes, is unilateral in 80 percent of cases. It is the most common disorder of male sexual differentiation, occurring in 0.8 percent of men. A careful examination is necessary to differentiate true cryptorchidism from the more common and benign condition of retractile testes. Because patients with cryptorchidism have an increased incidence of infertility and malignant testicular tumors, placement of the testes into the scrotum is desirable before 2 to 4 years of age.

MALE INFERTILITY

Approximately 10 percent of marriages in the United States are barren and another 10 percent result in fewer children than desired. The husband is the cause of infertility in about a third of those marriages. Infertility can be due to disorders of the hypothalamic-pituitary system, the testes, or the ejaculatory system. The physician should collect information about the duration of infertility, fertility in prior marriages of both partners, the presence of acquired or congenital disease that may lead to infertility, technique and frequency of intercourse, and family history of infertility. The examination should evaluate distribution of body hair, presence of gynecomastia, development of the scrotum and penis, location of the urethral meatus, presence of normal vasa deferentia and epididymides, and size of the testes. A reduction in testicular size (less than 4 cm in length) indicates a severe deficiency in spermatogenic function. Finally, with the patient standing, the Valsalva maneuver is used to test for a varicocele.

Semen analysis is next undertaken to obtain a semiquantitative estimate of the severity of the dysfunction. The findings are usually considered normal if the semen coagulates and then liquefies, volume is 2 to 5 ml, count exceeds 20 million per milliliter, and more than 60 percent of the sperm are actively motile and have normal morphology. If no sperm are present, the term *azoospermia* is used; if the sperm count is less than 20 million per milliliter, the patient is considered to have oligospermia. In azoospermic males, the differential diagnosis includes hyalinization of the seminiferous tubules, the "Sertoli cell only syndrome," gonadotropin deficiency, ductal obstruction, or maturation arrest. In patients with hyalinization of the seminiferous tubules, LH and FSH are elevated and plasma testosterone is low or borderline. Patients with Sertoli cell only syndrome usually have normal LH and testosterone levels, but characteristically FSH levels are elevated. In gonadotropin deficiency, LH, FSH, and testosterone are low. All studies are normal in ductal obstruction or maturation arrest, and a testicular biopsy is necessary to distinguish between them. In oligospermic patients, laboratory tests are unlikely to define the etiology if the history and physical examination are normal. These patients are usually classified in the large group termed "idiopathic oligospermia."

GYNECOMASTIA

Gynecomastia, or enlargement of the male breasts, may be unilateral (more frequently on the left) or bilateral; gynecomastia is always mediated by estrogens and results from a disturbance of the normal ratio of active androgen to estrogen in plasma or within the breast itself. Gynecomastia occurs when androgen production is decreased or estrogen formation is increased.

Physiologic gynecomastia occurs in the newborn secondary to maternal or placental estrogens, at adolescence, and with aging.

TABLE 14.5–7. CAUSES OF PATHOLOGIC GYNECOMASTIA

Deficient production or action of testosterone
- Chromosomal abnormalities with decreased testosterone secretion, Klinefelter syndrome
- Male pseudohermaphroditism, e.g., partial gonadal dysgenesis, partial defects in testosterone biosynthesis, androgen-insensitivity syndrome
- Secondary testicular failure (orchitis)

Increased estrogen production
- Elevated production: True hermaphroditism, testicular tumors, carcinoma of lung and choriocarcinoma (hCG), feminizing adrenal tumors
- Increased substrate for peripheral aromatase: Adrenal disease, liver disorder, starvation, thyrotoxicosis
- Increased peripheral aromatase

Drugs
- Hormones: Estrogens, hCG
- Antiandrogens: Cimetidine, spironolactone, flutamide, digitalis, marijuana, heroin
- Tricyclic antidepressants

Forty percent or more of aged men have gynecomastia. The causes of pathologic gynecomastia are shown in Table 14.4–7.

SCROTAL MASSES

Careful physical examination allows classification of a scrotal mass into one of four categories: (1) mass in the spermatic cord, (2) fluid within the tunica vaginalis (hydrocele), (3) epididymal mass, or (4) testicular mass.

The most common abnormality in the spermatic cord is a varicocele. Retrograde filling of the internal spermatic vein and pampiniform plexus produces a "wormlike" mass in the scrotum that is palpable in the upright position. Ninety percent are on the left side. They can cause infertility. The sudden development of a varicocele in an adult should suggest inferior vena cava obstruction, such as that due to invasion of the renal vein by renal cell carcinoma.

Hydroceles, the most common cause of scrotal swelling, usually obscure all normal anatomical landmarks within the scrotum. Transillumination is usually necessary to confirm the diagnosis.

An epididymal mass is usually benign; a mass in the testis is malignant until proven otherwise. The most common epididymal abnormalities are cysts, spermatocele, epididymitis (tuberculous or other bacterial causes), and rare benign tumors.

Testicular tumors can arise from the germ cells, the specialized gonadal stroma, or both. The malignant germ cell tumors of the testis in order of decreasing prognosis are seminoma, teratocarcinoma, embryonal carcinoma, and choriocarcinoma. Although sonography may provide some help in evaluating testicular masses, most patients require surgical exploration. The prognosis of testicular tumors has improved with the development of new diagnostic and therapeutic techniques: tumor markers (beta-chain hCG and α-fetoprotein), accurate staging techniques (chest tomography, lymphangiography, CT scanning), improved surgical procedures for lymphadenectomy, and new chemotherapeutic agents (e.g., cis-platin).

PROSTATIC DISEASES

The adult prostate weighs approximately 20 g and is situated at the base of the bladder surrounding the proximal urethra. Although it provides approximately 20 percent of ejaculate volume, the physiologic function of prostatic secretion is not clear; it appears to play no essential role in male fertility. Most men become aware

of the existence of the prostate only if they develop inflammatory or neoplastic disturbances that most often give rise to difficulties with urination. Between puberty and age 50, prostatitis is the most common prostatic disorder. Beyond the fifth decade benign prostatic hyperplasia and prostatic carcinoma predominate.

Prostatitis

Prostatitis[6] refers to any condition associated with prostatic inflammation. The disease can be acute or chronic and can have bacterial or nonbacterial causes. Clinically, it can be divided into three discrete disorders. *Acute bacterial prostatitis* is a fulminating bacterial infection characterized by fever, chills, and perineal pain with intense irritative voiding symptoms. On rectal examination the prostate is usually tender, swollen, and firm. Prostatic discomfort and the risk of bacteremia make prostatic massage unwise in the acute phase. Because bacterial cystitis usually accompanies the disease, the pathogen can be identified by culture of a voided urine specimen. The response to antibacterial agents is often dramatic. Chronic *bacterial prostatitis* is one of the most common causes of relapsing urinary tract infection in men. Most patients complain of irritative urinary symptoms and perineal discomfort; by the time symptoms appear, usually significant bacteriuria has developed. The diagnosis is based upon quantitative bacterial localization studies confirming the prostate as the source for the infection. Although antimicrobial agents may sterilize the urine and cause symptoms to disappear, the organism often persists in prostatic fluid. When therapy is discontinued, reinfection of the urine and reappearance of symptoms may occur. *Nonbacterial prostatitis* is now the most common type of prostatitis. The symptoms are similar to those of chronic bacterial prostatitis, and the expressed prostatic secretion frequently exhibits pyuria. Patients with nonbacterial prostatitis have no history of urinary tract infections, however, and cultures fail to confirm an infectious etiology. The cause of this disorder and its treatment are unknown. Finally, patients with *prostatodynia* have symptoms that mimic prostatitis, but characteristically no white blood cells are present in the expressed prostatic secretion and urine cultures are negative.

Benign Prostatic Hyperplasia[10]

Benign prostatic hyperplasia (BPH) is probably the most common neoplastic growth in men. The disease characteristically occurs in men older than age 40; in those older than 50 years the frequency of symptomatic BPH varies from 50 to 75 percent. A 40-year-old man has about a 20 to 25 percent probability of requiring an operation for BPH if he lives to age 80. The etiology of the disorder is unknown.

As the prostate enlarges, patients develop a symptom-complex called "prostatism": diminution in the caliber and force of the urinary stream, hesitancy in initiating voiding, inability to terminate micturition abruptly causing postvoid dribbling, a sense of incomplete emptying of the bladder, and occasional urinary retention. As the amount of residual urine increases, the patient may note nocturia, diurnal urinary frequency, a mass in the lower abdomen, and outflow urinary incontinence. Patients with slowly progressive obstruction may gradually adjust to the symptoms that develop with "silent prostatism." These patients may present with a lower abdominal midline mass, representing a distended bladder and renal insufficiency.

Usually there is no difficulty in establishing the diagnosis of BPH. Before examination the physician should observe the patient voiding to completion to document the decrease in the size and force of the urinary stream. The prostate is palpated with attention to size, consistency, and shape. Hyperplasia usually produces a smooth, firm, and elastic enlargement of the prostate. The size of the prostate on rectal examination may not correlate with the degree of bladder neck obstruction, however. Patients with marked prostatic enlargement may have no urinary obstruction while those with a large intravesical median lobe may have marked outflow obstruction without palpable enlargement of the gland.

Laboratory tests include urinalysis and urine culture to detect infection, serum creatinine to evaluate renal function, and serum acid phosphatase (preferably drawn before prostatic examination). When the disease is in an early stage and symptoms are mild, no further studies are necessary. In men with marked outlet symptoms, however, several other conditions should be considered: carcinoma of the prostate, bladder neck contracture, urethral stricture, bladder calculus, and neurogenic bladder.

Surgery is presently the only effective treatment for BPH. The general indications for surgical relief of prostatic obstruction are acute urinary retention, hydronephrosis, recurrent urinary tract infection aggravated by residual urine, severe hematuria, and obstructive symptoms of sufficient concern to the patient. Simple prostatectomy can be performed in a variety of ways; transurethral resection has the least morbidity.

Carcinoma of the Prostate

Prostatic carcinoma[3] is one of the two most common cancers in men, occurring in approximately 9 percent. Although eunuchs do not develop prostatic carcinoma, no other evidence suggests a direct relationship between it and hormone levels. Similarly, there is no relationship between prostatic cancer and the development of BPH, exposure to carcinogens, cigarette smoking, alcohol use, circumcision, weight loss, height, blood group, hair distribution, or sexual activity. More than 95 percent of all prostatic carcinomas are adenocarcinomas which can spread by lymphatic or hematogenous dissemination or by local extension to the urethra, bladder neck, seminal vesicles, and the trigone. The most common sites of lymph node metastases are to the pelvic lymph nodes and periaortic lymph nodes. Osseous metastases constitute the most common form of hematogenous spread. Visceral metastases, mostly to the lung and liver, are rare. Pulmonary metastases are detected in less than 6 percent of patients.

A careful rectal examination is the only means of detecting prostatic cancer at an early stage before the development of urinary outflow obstruction or bone pain. Carcinoma of the prostate characteristically is felt as a region of dense induration with a hard consistency within the substance of the prostate. When the tumor penetrates the capsule, the margins of the prostate may become obscured and tumor may be palpated extending to the seminal vesicles and region of the bladder neck. Other causes of prostatic induration include focal regions of BPH, prostatic calculi, granulomatous prostatitis, and postoperative changes. A needle biopsy should be performed if a prostatic nodule is palpated because about half of them are malignant. A positive biopsy dictates further studies—serum acid phosphatase, intravenous pyelogram, bone scan, and chest radiograph.

The prognosis of patients with prostatic cancer correlates well with the stage of the tumor (Table 14.5–8). Stage A disease is detectable only by pathologic examination following prostatectomy. Stage B tumors are limited to the prostate. Stage C tumors extend beyond the prostatic capsule but have not metastasized. Stage D represents metastatic carcinoma of the prostate and includes any patient with an elevated serum acid phosphatase level.

There is considerable debate concerning the best mode of therapy for each stage of prostatic carcinoma. The threat of the tumor to the quality of life and the likely duration of survival must be considered in each patient as the physician selects a form of treatment that provides the proper balance between efficacy and morbidity. Although several types of treatment are relatively effective, accurate information on their relative efficacy is limited and all are associated with undesirable side effects. Recommended treatment for each stage of prostatic cancer is indicated in Table 14.5–8. Hormonal therapy (bilateral orchiectomy or treatment with a GnRH analogue or estrogen) is the preferred initial treatment for stage D disease. Reactivation of symptoms following an initial response to hormonal therapy usually indicates that the tumor is no longer under hormonal control. Attempts at further endocrine therapy (adrenalectomy, hypophysectomy, or antiandrogen therapy) are usually disappointing. At present, chemotherapy is the only hope for treatment of such patients.

TABLE 14.5–8. PROSTATIC CANCER STAGING AND TREATMENT

Stage	Definition	Treatment
A	No induration; found by histopathology	
A_1	<5% cancer, well-differentiated	Observation, except for young patients
A^2	>5% cancer, moderate, poor differentiation	Radical prostatectomy
B	Palpable induration limited to prostate	
B_1	Induration <1 lobe prostate	Radical prostatectomy
B^2	Induration ≥1 lobe prostate	Radical prostatectomy *or* radiation therapy
C	Extension beyond prostate	Radiation therapy
D	Metastatic disease	
D_1	Pelvic lymph nodes only	
D^2	Bony metastases	Hormonal therapy

SEXUAL DYSFUNCTION IN MEN[5]

Male sexual dysfunction (Table 14.5–9), often termed "impotence," can be manifested by a disorder in one or more of the four normal sexual functions in men: libido, erection, ejaculation, and orgasm.

Loss of Libido

Because androgens have a major influence on sexual desire in men, decreased libido may indicate androgen deficiency arising from either pituitary or testicular disease. Stress or depression can also cause a loss of libido.

TABLE 14.5–9. DISORDERS OF SEXUAL FUNCTION

Loss of libido
- Hypogonadism
- Depression/stress

Loss of erection
Neurogenic
- Diabetic neuropathy
- Spinal cord injury or tumor
- Injury to parasympathetic nerves, e.g., radical prostatectomy
- Polyneuropathy

Vascular
- Leriche syndrome
- Previous priapism
- Peyronie disease

Drugs
- Anthihistamines
- Antihypertensives
- Anticholinergics
- Psychogenic agents
- Narcotics/alcohol

Loss of emission
- Retrograde ejaculation, e.g., bladder neck surgery or autonomic dysfunction
- Sympathetic denervation, e.g., retroperitoneal lymphadenectomy
- Androgen deficiency
- Alpha-adrenergic blocking agents

Loss of orgasm
- Psychiatric disorder

Loss of Erection

Erection is a primary neurologic event that results in increased blood flow to the penis, causing engorgement. The common organic causes for loss of erection are neurologic, vascular, and drug related (Table 14.5–9). Sensory fibers to the penis arise from the pudendal nerve; autonomic fibers from the pelvic plexus provide both parasympathetic and sympathetic innervation. Because the bladder receives similar innervation, when neurologic disorders produce impotence patients commonly have bladder dysfunction as well. The internal pudendal artery, a terminal branch of the hypogastric artery, provides the major blood supply to the penis. Obstruction of the distal aorta at the bifurcation of the common iliac causes buttock claudication and impotence (Leriche syndrome). Drugs can also produce a loss of erection (Table 14.5–9).

Loss of Emission

Ejaculation is controlled by the sympathetic nervous system, which regulates contraction of the smooth muscle in the vas deferens, prostate, seminal vesicles, and the bladder neck. Causes for the absence of emission are listed in Table 14.5–9.

Absence of Orgasm

Orgasm is a cortical sensory phenomenon and is purely psychic. Orgasm can occur without either an erection or emission of fluid. If libido and erectile function are normal, the absence of orgasm is almost always due to a psychogenic disorder.

Evaluation of Impotence

A careful history should include pubertal development, the age at onset of erections and nocturnal emissions, the specific nature of the disorder (loss of libido, erection, etc.), the emotional stability of the patient and presence of stress, the relationship with a sexual partner, drug use and alcohol consumption, and the timing of the onset of sexual dysfunction. An abrupt onset of impotence suggests a psychogenic disorder, whereas gradual loss over many months is more suggestive of organic dysfunction. Because nocturnal erections occur normally during rapid-eye-motion sleep from the time of childhood, a history of turgid erections under any circumstances (often when awakening in the morning) suggests that the dysfunction is due to a psychogenic disorder. The presence of nocturnal penile tumescence can be confirmed by recordings with a strain gauge. The examination should include steps to detect hypogonadism, palpation of peripheral pulses, and a careful neurologic evaluation. If a neurologic disorder is suspected, a cystometrogram should be performed, because most patients with a neurologic etiology for impotence have an abnormal cystometrogram. Vascular abnormalities can be detected by using a Doppler technique to measure simultaneously the penile and brachial artery blood pressures. The penile-brachial index is determined by dividing the penile by the brachial blood pressure. An index over 0.75 is normal; one less than 0.6 suggests impotence due to vascular disease. Alternately, a combination of papaverine and phentolamine can be injected directly into the corpora cavernosa. Failure of an erection to develop confirms the diagnosis of vasculogenic impotence. If an erection occurs but disappears rapidly, venous insufficiency is suspected as a cause for impotence. The evaluation for endocrine dysfunction has been described previously.

GONADAL DISORDERS IN WOMEN

Gonadal disorders in postpubertal women usually cause menstrual abnormalities. Either menses do not begin (primary amenorrhea) or they stop prematurely (secondary amenorrhea). Primary amenorrhea is defined as the failure to initiate menses by $16\frac{1}{2}$ years of age; secondary amenorrhea is defined as the absence of menses for 6 months or longer after menarche has occurred. The evaluation is similar for patients with either primary or secondary amenorrhea.

PRIMARY AMENORRHEA

Primary amenorrhea may result from the lack of sex hormone stimulation of the uterine endometrium, absence of the uterus, or obstruction of the uterovaginal outflow tract. The complete absence of sex hormone exposure is associated with the failure to develop secondary sexual characteristics. Transient exposure to small amounts of sex steroids may result in patients with primary amenorrhea having incomplete secondary sexual characteristic development. The other causes of primary amenorrhea are accompanied by completely normal secondary sexual development. Thus the presence or absence of secondary sexual characteristics and the presence of a uterine cervix are important considerations in the evaluation of primary amenorrhea (Table 14.5–10). All patients with primary amenorrhea should have karyotypic analysis to exclude certain genetic causes of amenorrhea.

Primary Amenorrhea Without Secondary Sexual Characteristics

This form of primary amenorrhea with the cervix present can arise from CNS abnormalities that cause hypothalamic or pituitary failure (hypogonadotropic hypogonadism) or from genetic or ovarian abnormalities causing gonadal failure (hypergonadotropic hypogonadism). Hypogonadotropic hypogonadism is characterized by low levels of LH, FSH, and estradiol; in hypergonadotropic hypogonadism, LH and FSH are elevated and estradiol levels are low. Estrogen deficiency in both conditions accounts for the absence of secondary sexual characteristics.

Hypogonadotropic hypogonadism may result from failure of either hypothalamic release of GnRH or pituitary secretion of LH and FSH. In Kallmann syndrome, the most common example of the former condition, patients exhibit anosmia due to olfactory bulb agenesis. It is a genetic disorder more frequent in men than in women. GnRH deficiency may also result from other genetic causes or may be acquired as a result of histiocytosis, inflammatory disorders, vascular lesions, or irradiation of the hypothalamus. Chronic systemic illness, such as malnutrition, renal, cardiovascular, or hepatic diseases, may also reduce GnRH release. Excessive levels of prolactin may prevent pulsatile gonadotropin release.

Destructive lesions of the pituitary, such as craniopharyngioma, germinoma, or pituitary adenoma, diminish the secretion of gonadotropins along with other pituitary hormones so that isolated gonadotropin deficiency is rarely encountered. The condition responsible for hypogonadotropic hypogonadism may be identified by a thorough history and physical examination, CT or MRI scans, and GnRH stimulation tests.

Treatment with exogenous sex steroids will produce maturation of secondary sexual characteristics. Oral conjugated estrogens, 1.25 mg daily from days 1 to 25 each month, and medroxyprogesterone acetate 10 mg daily from days 13 to 25 each month, are usually sufficient.

When fertility is desired, exogenous hormone replacement is stopped and menotropins (LH and FSH obtained from the urine of menopausal women) are administered to induce ovulation. Alternatively, ovulation may be induced with continuous administration of pulsatile GnRH when pituitary gonadotropin stores are adequate and the patient is willing to utilize an intravenous or subcutaneous infusion line connected to a small infusion pump.

The absence of gonadal function during puberty results in primary amenorrhea without secondary sexual characteristics. Such gonadal failure results either from the lack of normal ovarian development (gonadal dysgenesis) or from postnatal damage to the ovary. Turner syndrome, a common cause of gonadal dysgenesis, is easily recognized clinically (short stature, webbed neck, shield chest, cubitus valgus) and by karyotypic analysis. Certain XY individuals who lack stigmata of Turner syndrome can develop streak gonads and female genitalia rather than male internal and external reproductive tract structures. This condition, termed "Swyer syndrome," may result from failure of the undifferentiated gonad to produce a testes-inducing agent. Multiple genetic aberrations involving sex chromosomes (XX/X mosaicism, XXX, deletions of the long or short arms of the X chromosome) may also cause primary amenorrhea. The term "pure gonadal dysgenesis" is applied to those rare individuals who are sexually infantile, lack stigmata of Turner syndrome, and possess streak gonads with an XX karyotype.

Prepubertal gonadal injury may result from infection, surgery, irradiation, or exposure to chemotherapeutic drugs for childhood neoplasia. Occasionally autoimmune oophoritis, occurring alone or in association with other autoimmune disorders, sufficiently damages the gonad to produce primary amenorrhea. Galactosemia may cause primary amenorrhea as a result of a direct toxic effect of galactose or its metabolites on the ovary.

The treatment of primary amenorrhea due to gonadal failure is identical to that described for hypogonadotropic hypogonadism except that pregnancy is not possible. In patients with gonadal dysgenesis who possess a Y chromosome, surgical removal of both gonads is indicated because of the high risk of gonadal tumors (gonadoblastoma, germinoma). Hormonal replacement therapy is instituted following surgery.

Primary Amenorrhea with Normal Secondary Sexual Characteristics

Cervix Absent. These patients all require a complete evaluation, including a pelvic examination. Abnormalities of the reproductive outflow tract, such as a transverse vaginal septum or imperforate hymen, must be considered. Patients with an absent uterus on gynecologic examination may have a form of müllerian agenesis (Rokitansky-Küster-Hauser syndrome) or androgen insensitivity. Androgen insensitivity ("testicular feminization") results from abnormal target tissue responsiveness to androgens. This diagnosis must be considered in a phenotypic female with normal secondary

---

TABLE 14.5–10. EVALUATION OF PRIMARY AMENORRHEA

Lack of secondary sexual characteristic development (cervix present)

CNS abnormalities
- Kallmann syndrome (anosmia with absence of GnRH)
- Neoplasms (craniopharyngioma, hamartoma, etc)
- Hypothalamic amenorrhea (exercise, weight loss, systemic illness)
- Hyperprolactinemia
- Hypopituitarism

Genetic causes of gonadal dysgenesis
- Turner syndrome (45,X)
- Swyer syndrome (46,XY)
- X chromosome abnormalities (isochromosome, ring chromosome, deletions)
- Pure gonadal dysgenesis (46,XX)

Ovarian abnormalities (excluding gonadal dysgenesis)
- Infection, irradiation, and chemotherapy

Presence of secondary sexual characteristic development (cervix absent)

Genital tract abnormalities
- Vaginal septal defects and imperforate hymen
- Rokitansky-Kuster-Hauser syndrome

Genetic causes
- Testicular feminization
- Enzyme defects in steroidogenesis (17-α-hydroxylase deficiency, 17-β-hydroxysteroid oxidoreductase deficiency, 5-α-reductase deficiency)

Presence of secondary sexual characteristic development (cervix present)
- CNS abnormalities (as indicated above)
- Ovarian resistance to gonadotropin stimulation
- Congenital adrenogenital syndrome
- Chronic anovulation

sexual characteristics but with absent or scanty pubic and axillary hair and a shallow, blind-ending vagina. Inguinal masses, the testes, may be palpated in some. Enzyme defects within the testes, resulting in deficient testosterone secretion at critical times of sexual differentiation, may allow the development of female external genitalia, despite the presence of male internal reproductive structures.

Cervix Present. Some patients with primary amenorrhea have normal secondary sexual characteristics and a palpable uterus. They may have similar CNS causes for primary amenorrhea as do patients without secondary sexual characteristics. Different degrees of secondary sexual development may reflect the time of onset of the CNS disturbance. For example, early onset would prevent any stimulation of the hypothalamic-pituitary-ovarian axis. Onset of the CNS disorder following activation of the hypothalamic-pituitary-axis but before menarche would result in secondary sexual characteristics.

Ovarian resistance to gonadotropins occurs in a few individuals. These patients have primary amenorrhea, normal secondary sexual characteristics, normal-appearing ovaries on laparoscopic examination, and elevated levels of plasma gonadotropins. A defect in ovarian receptors to gonadotropins or antibodies to these receptors may be responsible.

Untreated congenital adrenogenital syndrome may result in primary amenorrhea. Adrenogenital syndrome may present as ambiguous genitalia in infants and in early childhood. Mild forms are often not detected until puberty. These patients are usually short in stature because excessive androgen production causes premature closure of the epiphyses. Chronic suppression by increased androgen production results in an immature hypothalamic-pituitary-ovarian axis.

Individuals with chronic ovulation or polycystic ovarian syndrome may present with primary amenorrhea. Secondary sexual characteristic development is normal. Diagnosis and therapy of chronic ovulation is discussed under Secondary Amenorrhea below.

Treatment of this type of primary amenorrhea depends on its etiology. Abnormalities of the outflow tract or forms of müllerian agenesis are treated surgically to prevent cryptomenorrhea and to allow intercourse. Therapy for androgen insensitivity and congenital adrenal hyperplasia has been discussed previously.

SECONDARY AMENORRHEA

Secondary amenorrhea may result from disorders of the hypothalamus, pituitary, ovary, or uterus, or from chronic disease (Table 14.5–11). The most common cause of secondary amenorrhea is pregnancy. As a rule, a patient with secondary amenorrhea should be considered pregnant until proven otherwise by a sensitive pregnancy test.

Once pregnancy has been excluded, evaluation should include a thorough history, with particular emphasis on the endocrine system, and a complete physical examination, including the pelvic examination. Especially important in the history are the setting of the amenorrhea, emotional stress, gain or loss of weight, acute and chronic illness, accidents or injuries, relationship to pregnancy, temperature intolerance, changes in bowel habits and energy, hirsutism, family history of menstrual disturbances, infertility, autoimmune endocrine disease, and tuberculosis.

Secondary amenorrhea may result from abnormalities of the hypothalamic-pituitary axis, ovaries, or uterovaginal outlet. It is useful to focus on the specific causes of amenorrhea occurring at each organ level.

Central Nervous System Dysfunction
Hypothalamic tumors or destructive lesions must be considered. Hypothalamic dysfunction may be the basis for amenorrhea in polycystic ovarian disease or hyperprolactinemia. Severe stress is often associated with functional hypothalamic amenorrhea, a diag-

TABLE 14.5–11. CAUSES OF SECONDARY AMENORRHEA

Genetic
- Abnormalities in the X chromosome

CNS
- Tumors of brain or pituitary
- Trauma
- Metabolic disease
- Hyperprolactinemic disorders
- Weight loss or gain
- Exercise-induced

Ovarian
- Infection, irradiation, chemotherapy
- Autoimmune
- Tumors
- Insensitive ovary

Uterine
- Infection
- Uterine synechiae (Asherman syndrome)

Unclassified
- Polycystic ovarian disease

nosis of exclusion. Typical stresses include marital disturbances, leaving home to attend school, and unresolved conflicts with family or friends. Several explanations have been suggested for the exercise-associated amenorrhea observed in ballerinas and distance runners. These include decreased body fat stores, resulting in decreased extraovarian estrogen production, and an effect of elevated endorphin levels on hypothalamic-pituitary function.

The secondary amenorrhea due to weight loss exceeding 20 percent of ideal body weight, such as in anorexia nervosa (see Chapter 16.8), may be due to the same factors contributing to exercise amenorrhea. Patients with exercise-induced amenorrhea or anorexia nervosa have reduced estrogen levels. Because persistent amenorrhea correlates with decreased bone density, estrogen replacement therapy has been advocated to reduce further bone loss in these individuals.

Secondary amenorrhea may result from pituitary infarction following postpartum hemorrhage (Sheehan syndrome), or pituitary or suprasellar tumors.

Gonadal Disorders
Ovarian disorders causing secondary amenorrhea include ovarian failure, ovarian tumors, and ovarian resistance. Ovarian failure, the most common disorder, is due to the loss of all ovarian follicles from genetic, toxic, autoimmune, or idiopathic causes. Ovarian failure may also result from chemotherapy, irradiation, infection, or autoimmune processes that reduce the number of ovarian follicles. A tentative diagnosis is made by documenting a persistent elevation in serum gonadotropins. Conclusive evidence requires an ovarian biopsy to demonstrate afollicular ovaries. Karyotypic analysis is recommended in all women suspected of having ovarian failure under age 35. Identification of an abnormal karyotype (e.g., XX/XO mosaicism) will explain the elevated gonadotropins and obviate the need for an ovarian biopsy.

Functioning ovarian tumors may produce excessive amounts of sex steroids, which suppress gonadotropin secretion and cause secondary amenorrhea. Most functional tumors produce either androgens or estrogens; as a general rule, however, granulosa and theca cell tumors produce estrogen, whereas arrhenoblastomas, hilar cell and adrenal rest tumors cause virilization by producing excess amounts of androgen. Ovarian tumors are treated surgically.

Finally, the insensitive ovary syndrome may be associated with either primary or secondary amenorrhea. This syndrome may be due to blocking antibodies to ovarian gonadotropin receptors. Gonadotropin levels are also elevated in this disorder; therefore, differentiation of this condition from premature ovarian failure may require an ovarian biopsy. Individuals with insensitive or resistant

ovaries may be given exogenous menotropins or temporary estrogen suppressive therapy in an attempt to induce ovulation if fertility is desired.

Uterine Disorders

Damage to the uterine endometrium may prevent a response to cyclical hormonal changes and cause amenorrhea. Tubercular infection or trauma are the most common types of uterine injury that cause amenorrhea. Endometrial scarring and adhesions (Asherman syndrome) may follow aggressive curettage of the uterine cavity. Tubercular infection frequently requires hysterectomy and intensive antibiotic therapy. Asherman syndrome is best treated by hysteroscopic lysis of uterine adhesions and oral estrogen therapy.

Unclassified Disorders

Polycystic ovary syndrome (PCO) is a major cause of secondary amenorrhea. PCO is a more general term, replacing Stein-Leventhal syndrome, which described patients with bilateral polycystic ovaries, hirsutism, amenorrhea, and unexplained abdominal pain. PCO presents after menarche and persists throughout reproductive life. Patients with PCO classically have normal FSH levels but chronically elevated concentrations of LH, testosterone, and androstenedione, presumably resulting from LH stimulation of ovarian theca cells. Also observed is heightened LH responsiveness to GnRH. The cause of PCO remains obscure; ovarian, adrenal, and hypothalamic-pituitary causes have been suggested.

The term "PCO" is confusing since it implies ovarian pathology. The cystic ovaries result, however, from an inability of preovulatory follicles to complete their maturation because of elevated androgen levels. Multiple ovarian cysts and thickening of the ovarian capsule or tunica albuginea also occur in normal women given high doses of androgens. Biopsies of normal and PCO ovaries have shown no enzyme defects in steroidogenic pathways. Because these findings make an ovarian etiology for PCO unlikely, use of the term "chronic anovulation" has been encouraged in lieu of PCO. Other endocrine disorders that elevate androgen levels may mimic this condition. These include Cushing syndrome, congenital adrenal hyperplasia, hyperprolactinemia, and androgen-producing tumors of the ovary or adrenal. Interestingly, rapid weight gain, the "stress-obesity syndrome," may produce a clinical picture identical to that of PCO. Weight loss restores cyclic menstruation in these patients.

A hypothalamic cause for PCO currently seems most likely because before menarche young women who later develop PCO exhibit elevated LH levels during the day rather than at night.

Treatment depends upon the type of amenorrhea and additional concerns of the patient, that is, menopausal symptoms or fertility. Menopausal symptoms (hot flashes, mood swings, vaginal dryness) are frequent in patients with premature ovarian failure who are also at risk for accelerated bone loss. Replacement therapy with conjugated estrogens and progestins is recommended.

Selection of therapy for patients with PCO depends on whether fertility, resumption of regular withdrawal bleeding, or hirsutism is of utmost concern. If infertility is the major complaint, induction of ovulation with oral clomiphene citrate may be tried initially with 50 mg per day for 5 days. Clomiphene-induced ovulation generally occurs 5 to 10 days after the last tablet is taken. If this regimen fails to produce ovulation, the dosage is increased by 50 mg up to 250 mg per day in subsequent cycles. Failure to respond to clomiphene citrate may necessitate menotropin or GnRH therapy. Menstrual regulation may be desired or even required in those patients with PCO who do not desire fertility. Estrogen concentrations (principally estrone) are elevated in 90 percent of PCO patients and may result in endometrial hyperplasia. To reduce the risk for endometrial neoplasia caused by prolonged unopposed estrogen stimulation, cyclic therapy is prescribed with oral medroxyprogesterone acetate, 10 mg for 10 to 13 days each month. An endometrial biopsy should be taken before instituting therapy to evaluate pretreatment histology. While on cyclic progestin therapy patients are advised that they may ovulate at unexpected intervals

and that progestin therapy is contraindicated during pregnancy. Barrier contraception is recommended in sexually active individuals. Alternatively, oral contraceptive therapy is highly effective in regulating menses and treating hirsutism in PCO patients.

DYSFUNCTIONAL UTERINE BLEEDING

Dysfunctional uterine bleeding[1] differs from normal bleeding in frequency, duration, or amount without an apparent organic cause. A careful history permits categorization of abnormal uterine bleeding (Table 14.5–12). Age of the patient and ovulatory status are important criteria for diagnostic and therapeutic purposes. Whether the patient's dysfunctional uterine bleeding occurs during ovulatory or anovulatory cycles is determined by using a menstrual calendar and a chart of daily basal body temperature. Oral temperature upon awakening follows a biphasic pattern due to the thermogenic effects of progesterone during the luteal phase of the menstrual cycle in ovulatory individuals (Fig. 14.5–2).

Common organic causes for abnormal bleeding include complications of pregnancy, malignancy, cervical or vaginal trauma, presence of a foreign body, and obvious cervical-vaginal pathology, for example, infection or polyps. These conditions all should be excluded. A pregnancy test and a careful pelvic examination, including pap smear and cervical cultures for gonorrhea and chlamydia, are performed initially. Administration of progesterone to determine whether withdrawal bleeding occurs has been advocated by some but is not usually required. Premature use of a progestin challenge may actually delay diagnosis by altering gonadotropin levels and the uterine endometrium.

Anovulation is quite common during the first 7 years following menarche. Occasional missed menses are followed either by spotting before the onset of the next menses or excessive bleeding during the subsequent menses. Diagnosis of this disorder may be made with menstrual calendar and temperature chart. Reassuring the patient is usually all that is required.

PCO should be suspected when young women complain of persistent irregular menses associated with heavy vaginal bleeding. A chart of basal body temperatures coupled with measurement of serum gonadotropins and testosterone usually suffice to make this diagnosis. Treatment consists of hormonal regulation of the menses both for the patient's comfort and to protect her from an increased risk of uterine malignancy resulting from chronic unopposed estrogen exposure. Cyclical therapy with 10 mg of oral medroxyprogesterone acetate for 10 to 13 days each month is usually effective. Alternatively, therapy with a low estrogen oral contraceptive may be prescribed.

TABLE 14.5–12. DISORDERS OF MENSTRUAL CYCLE

Term	Definition
Oligomenorrhea	Infrequent and irregular bleeding occurring at intervals greater than 35 days
Polymenorrhea	Frequent and regular bleeding occurring at intervals of 21 days or less
Menorrhagia	Profuse bleeding occurring at regular intervals
Menometrorrhagia	Excessive bleeding occurring at frequent and irregular intervals
Hypomenorrhea	Diminished bleeding occurring at regular intervals
Intermenstrual (pseudopolymenorrhea)	Light bleeding occurring regularly at midcycle
Premenstrual staining or spotting	Light uterine bleeding immediately preceding onset of usual menstrual flow

When excessive vaginal bleeding occurs in young women who ovulate regularly, presence of coagulation defects should be investigated by measuring the platelet count and clotting times.

From age 20 to 35 years, the menstrual interval is regular in most women, and benign organic conditions are usually responsible for any menstrual disturbances. Complications of pregnancy, such as ectopic pregnancy and threatened or incomplete abortion, should be suspected if the pregnancy test is positive.

Leiomyomata or benign smooth-muscle tumors of the uterus, which are frequently responsible for dysfunctional uterine bleeding in ovulatory women, may be detected by a careful bimanual examination of the uterus. Polyps or leiomyomata within the uterine cavity can cause midcycle spotting or bleeding in ovulatory women. Hysterosalpingography or hysteroscopy may be required for diagnosis. Treatment consists of polyp removal by dilation and curettage or operative removal of the myomas. In certain cases hysterectomy may be necessary. Medical therapy of leiomyomata with either progestins or an analogue of GnRH has been described.

After age 35 concern increases about uterine malignancy in patients with dysfunctional uterine bleeding. Sampling of the uterine endometrium is recommended in addition to the pregnancy test, pelvic examination, and pap smear. Anovulation is the most common cause of dysfunctional uterine bleeding during the last 7 years before menopause. These patients can be reassured only after a formal work-up that includes endometrial sampling. Follow-up may require periodic endometrial biopsies.

Rare patients with dysfunctional uterine bleeding may present with acute and extremely heavy vaginal bleeding. Therapy should be supportive as these episodes are usually self-limited. If intervention is required, a dilation and curettage almost always proves effective.

Gynecologic consultation is frequently requested to help manage bleeding in patients with low platelet counts due to chemotherapy. Continuous high-dose progestin therapy is usually effective. Ablation of the uterine endometrium with laser applied through the hysteroscope or ovarian destruction by irradiation are rarely required. In younger individuals without other contraindications, therapy with a low-dose oral contraceptive may occasionally prove useful.

HIRSUTISM[7]

The number of hair follicles in human skin is fixed at birth and differs between ethnic groups but remains the same between sexes within the same race. Hair grown from follicles in the adult can be vellus (thin, soft, lightly pigmented) or terminal (thick, coarse, darkly pigmented). Terminal hair growth is androgen-dependent and found on the face (beard area), back, chest, lower abdomen, and upper arms and legs. Terminal hair growth present in women outside of the axillary and pubic regions is called hirsutism. Interestingly, elevated plasma androgen levels cause both hirsutism, by stimulating terminal follicles throughout the body surface, and loss of hair from terminal follicles in the scalp. The reason for this effect on scalp hair remains unknown.

Increased hair growth from follicles throughout the body with minimal coarsening of the hair shaft is termed "hypertrichosis." Phenytoin, diazoxide, streptomycin, or minoxidil frequently cause hypertrichosis by an unknown process.

Terminal hair growth from androgen-sensitive follicles is dependent upon dihydrotestosterone formation from testosterone within the hair follicle. In women, testosterone is secreted by the ovaries and adrenal glands but is also synthesized peripherally from androstenedione. Circulating testosterone is 95 to 99 percent bound to testosterone-binding globulin, which is synthesized by the liver. Ovarian and adrenal contributions to circulating androgen concentrations are listed in Table 14.5–13.

Once hirsutism is diagnosed, an attempt is made to identify the elevated androgen and locate its source. Possible causes of hirsutism are listed in Table 14.5–14. Idiopathic hirsutism, a term

TABLE 14.5–13. OVARIAN AND ADRENAL CONTRIBUTIONS TO CIRCULATING ANDROGEN LEVELS

	Percent (Approximate)
Ovary contribution	
Androstenedione	50
Testosterone	5–20
DHEA	20
DHEA-S	10
Adrenal contribution	
Androstenedione	50
Testosterone	0–30
DHEA	80
DHEA-S	90

used when hirsutism is associated with normal androgen levels, may result from either increased sensitivity to androgens by the hair follicles or alterations in androgen metabolism that cannot currently be detected.

Virilism must be distinguished from excessive terminal hair growth. Decreased breast size, lowering of the voice, increased muscularity, and clitoral enlargement are seen in the virilized patient. Most commonly, ovarian or adrenal tumors are responsible when virilism accompanies hirsutism.

Rate of progression of the hirsutism may aid in differentiating a benign process from a neoplastic one. Gradual worsening of hirsutism over many years suggests a functional disorder whereas rapid appearance of symptoms suggests an underlying ovarian or adrenal neoplasm.

Evaluation of Hirsutism

A detailed medical history and thorough physical and pelvic examination are the important initial steps. Age at onset, progression of the hirsutism, and use of medications are important features of the history. Extent of the hirsutism, presence or absence of virilization, and the existence of adnexal masses should be determined by examination.

TABLE 14.5–14. CAUSES OF HIRSUTISM AND SIMPLIFIED LIST OF DIAGNOSTIC AIDS

Polycystic ovarian syndrome	Elevated serum LH; normal serum FSH; elevated testosterone and androstenedione
Hyperthecosis	Hormonal pattern identical to that of the PCO patient
Partial adrenal enzyme deficiencies (21-hydroxylase, 3-β-hydroxysteroid dehydrogenase and 11-β-hydroxylase)	ACTH stimulation testing
Cushing syndrome	Dexamethasone-suppression test
Adrenal tumors	Extremely elevated DHEA-S concentration; abnormal adrenal CT scan
Ovarian tumors (arrhenoblastoma, lipoid cell, hilar cell, pseudomucinous cystadenoma or cystadenocarcinoma, and in pregnancy luteoma)	Extremely elevated testosterone concentration; abnormal pelvic exam or pelvic sonogram

Hormonal Evaluation[9]

Gonadotropins and Prolactin. Laboratory studies may be limited or extensive depending upon the individual patient. The ratio of LH/FSH is usually 1.0 in ovulatory patients, but usually exceeds 2.0 in chronically anovulatory patients. To avoid erroneous results due to the circhoral pattern of gonadotropin release, an average concentration is determined from three blood samples taken at 20-minute intervals. Measurement of the plasma prolactin concentration is also advised because 10 to 20 percent of patients with chronic anovulation have hyperprolactinemia, which alone can be associated with an elevation in the adrenal androgen dihydroepiandosterone sulfate (DHEA-S).

Steroid Hormone Determinations. Measurement of testosterone, 3-α-androstanediol, androstenedione, and DHEA-S may be performed to identify the androgen responsible for hirsutism. Plasma assays for testosterone usually measure both bound and free hormone. Measurement of the free testosterone fraction may be needed when the total testosterone and other plasma androgen concentrations are normal in the hirsute patient.

In patients with normal androgen levels, hirsutism may be caused by increased conversion of testosterone to dihydrotestosterone within the hair follicle. These patients may be identified by measuring plasma 3-α-androstanediol, a metabolite of dihydrotestosterone.

Measurement of androstenedione is recommended because this hormone and testosterone are usually elevated in patients with PCO.

DHEA-S is secreted almost exclusively by the adrenal gland. Although not greatly affected by diurnal variation, DHEA-S levels increase at puberty and decline after menopause. Because of its reliability, measurement of DHEA-S may be substituted for urinary 17-ketosteroid determination as a marker of adrenal androgen production.

Adrenal Stimulation and Suppression Tests. An overnight dexamethasone-suppression test can exclude Cushing syndrome as a cause of hirsutism. ACTH stimulation testing has been advocated to identify adult patients with congenital virilizing adrenal hyperplasia. These patients present with a clinical picture indistinguishable from that of PCO. A defect in 21-hydroxylase, or much less commonly 3-β-hydroxysteroid dehydrogenase, or 11-β-hydroxylase may cause excessive adrenal androgen production, hirsutism, and cystic ovarian enlargement. Baseline levels of precursor steroids for the defective enzyme are frequently normal in patients with partial adrenal enzyme dysfunction and, therefore, are of limited use in screening. There is no widespread agreement concerning the best ACTH stimulation test to identify the adrenal enzyme defects. A simple ACTH stimulation test has been described, however, to detect individuals with partial 21-hydroxylase dysfunction, the most common enzymatic defect. This test is described in Table 14.5–15.

Radiologic Studies

Ultrasonography. Pelvic ultrasonography may be particularly helpful to identify ovarian enlargement in obese hirsute patients. In patients of normal weight, a well-performed pelvic examination usually can exclude the presence of adnexal enlargement.

Computed Tomography. CT scan of the adrenals to identify tumors and adenomas has replaced many of the hormonal tests previously utilized as diagnostic aids. This technique is quite sensitive but need not be routinely employed when evaluating patients whose only problem is hirsutism. In contrast, CT scans of the adrenals should be requested to evaluate virilized hirsute patients.

Therapy

PCO accounts for 70 to 80 percent of cases of hirsutism. If there are no contraindications, oral contraceptive therapy with any low-dose, combination birth control pill is very effective. Therapy low-

TABLE 14.5–15. ACTH STIMULATION TESTING

Procedure:
Administer 1 mg ACTH IV in the fasting state during the follicular phase of the cycle if the patient is ovulating.

Measurements:
Measure plasma progesterone and 17-OH progesterone before ACTH administration and at 30 min after ACTH administration.

Calculation:
1. Subtract the basal value of plasma progesterone in nanograms per deciliter from the value obtained 30 min after ACTH injection to obtain Δ progesterone, i.e., Time 30 progesterone − Time 0 progesterone = Δ progesterone. Perform the same calculation for 17-OH progesterone to obtain Δ 17-OH progesterone, i.e., Time 30 17-OH progesterone − Time 0 17-OH progesterone = Δ 17-OH progesterone.
2. Calculate the sum of Δ progesterone + Δ 17-OH progesterone and divide by 30 min (ignore units). If the value is 6.5 or less, the test is normal.

Adapted from Gutai JP, Kowarski AA, Migeon CJ: The detection of the heterozygous carrier for congenital virilizing adrenal hyperplasia. Pediatrics 90:924, 1977.

ers gonadotropin levels and decreases ovarian androgen production. The estrogen component of the pill also increases levels of testosterone-binding globulin and thereby diminishes the availability of free androgen to the hair follicle. The progestin allows regular withdrawal bleeding and diminishes the risk of endometrial cancer.

Recent studies have shown that spironolactone reduces the plasma androgen concentration and decreases terminal hair shaft diameter after 3 to 6 months of therapy. Although not currently approved for the treatment of hirsutism, oral administration of 100 to 200 mg of spironolactone in divided doses for 6 to 12 months has proven effective. Spironolactone apparently acts both by blocking androgen receptors and decreasing androgen production. Patients should avoid pregnancy since transplacental passage of spironolactone could feminize a male fetus.

Partial adrenal enzyme deficiencies may be treated with glucocorticoids. Oral prednisone 5 mg or dexamethasone 0.5 to 0.7 mg given nightly are particularly effective. Fasting plasma cortisol levels are monitored at periodic intervals to identify pituitary-adrenal insufficiency. The 8 AM cortisol level should be kept above 2 μg/dl.

Combination oral contraceptives, prednisone, and spironolactone are equally effective in the treatment of hirsutism caused by PCO, partial adrenal enzyme defects, or idiopathic factors. Approximately 70 to 75 percent of hirsute patients respond to treatment with any one of these agents. When patients fail to respond to a single agent, combinations of oral contraceptives or dexamethasone with spironolactone have been effective. The combination of oral contraceptives with glucocorticoids is not recommended because contraceptive pills decrease the clearance of total and unbound cortisol.

Other medications used to treat hirsutism include cimetidine and cyproterone acetate, which presumably act by blocking androgen receptor sites. Cimetidine has been given in large doses (300 mg five times per day). Cyproterone acetate is not available for clinical use in the United States. Both drugs may prevent masculinization of male fetuses when given during pregnancy.

Response to therapy for hirsutism should be evident after 3 to 6 months of treatment. Response is assessed primarily by the cessation of new growth of terminal hair follicles. Follicles present before the onset of therapy may decrease in hair-shaft diameter but will not disappear. Electrolysis is required to destroy the terminal hair follicle.

In patients who are unable to take medications or have minimal hair growth, shaving, bleaching, or use of depilatory creams may be adequate therapy.

Plasma testosterone levels exceeding 200 ng/dl, despite a nor-

mal pelvic examination, prompt concern for a small androgen-producing ovarian tumor. Diagnosis may be possible only through surgical exploration. Surgery should not, however, be undertaken unless an adrenal source has been excluded. Alternatively, pelvic exploration should always be given strong consideration in hirsute patients with unilateral adnexal enlargement even if the testosterone level is only mildly elevated.

MENOPAUSE

Menopause[2] is defined as the last menstrual period; the climacteric refers to associated perimenopausal changes which include vasomotor symptoms, urogenital atrophy, and diminished bone density. The age at menopause appears not to depend upon the age at menarche, socioeconomic status, race, weight, or height. On average, it occurs between 49 and 51 years of age. During the 7 years before menopause mildly elevated levels of FSH may cause more rapid follicular growth and development and thus shorten the follicular phase. Later in the perimenopausal period the luteal phase interval also shortens. Skipped or irregular menses account for increased variability in the menstrual cycle length before menopause. With the onset of menopause, serum levels of FSH and LH increase 20fold and three- to fivefold, respectively. These elevations result primarily from a marked decline in estradiol levels from 120 ng/L premenopausally to 18 ng/L after menopause. The loss of ovarian follicles at menopause is responsible for this decline. The greater elevation in FSH results from its decreased metabolic clearance and relatively increased pituitary secretion. Loss of inhibin from ovarian follicles may contribute to increased FSH secretion.

Menopausal symptoms are strongly associated with the decline in circulating estradiol. Hot flushes are a particularly troublesome vasomotor symptom characterized by increased skin temperature, peripheral vasodilation, a transient increase in heart rate, and sweating. The onset of the hot flush is heralded by facial redness, which spreads to the anterior chest wall. Approximately 85 percent of perimenopausal women experience hot flushes, and 80 percent of them have symptoms for 1 year after menopause. Less than 25 percent of menopausal women have vasomotor symptoms for more then 5 years after the menopause. A surge in plasma LH concentrations may reflect a hypothalamic cause for the vasomotor symptoms. LH itself is not responsible because hot flushes occur in hypophysectomized women.

Estrogen loss causes epithelial thinning and foreshortening of the vagina and the urethra during menopause. Vaginitis from these atrophic changes is common and may on occasion produce a blood-tinged vaginal discharge. Dysuria, frequency, and urgency are typical complaints resulting from epithelial changes in the urethra.

Bone density decreases in both men and women after age 40, but the rate of decline is greater in women than men. White women of slight build who smoke and are sedentary are at increased risk for osteoporosis. Bone loss accelerates after ovarectomy or as a consequence of menopause.

Estrogen administration is the usual treatment for menopausal symptoms. Conjugated estrogens are most commonly used. They are derived from pregnant mares' urine and predominantly consist of estrone sulfate and the horse estrogens equilin sulfate and 17-α-dihydroequilin. Conjugated estrogens provide relief from hot flushes, restore epithelium of the urogenital tract, and retard further loss in bone density. A dosage of 0.3 mg given daily for 24 days each month usually provides relief from hot flushes and restores urogenital epithelium; however, at least 0.625 mg given daily for 25 days each month is required to prevent bone loss.

Continuous administration of unopposed estrogen during the menopause is a risk factor for the development of adenocarcinoma of the endometrium. For this reason concomitant progestin therapy is recommended when estrogens are administered to menopausal women who have not had a hysterectomy. Medroxyprogesterone acetate (10 mg) given simultaneously with estrogen for the last 13 days of the 25-day course of estrogen therapy is advised.

REFERENCES

1. Aksel S (guest ed), Speroff L (ed): Dysfunctional Uterine Bleeding. Semin Reprod Endocrinol 2:307, 1984
2. Buchsbaum HJ (ed): The Menopause. New York, Springer-Verlag, 1983
3. Catalona WJ, Scott WW: Carcinoma of the prostate. In Walsh PC, Gittes RF, et al (eds): Campbell's Urology, 5th ed. Philadelphia, WB Saunders, 1986
4. Hodgen GD: The dominant ovarian follicle. Fertil Steril 38:281, 1982
5. Krane RJ: Sexual function and dysfunction. In Walsh PC, Gittes RF, et al (eds): Campbell's Urology, 5th ed. Philadelphia, WB Saunders, 1986
6. Meares EM Jr: Prostatitis and related disorders. In Walsh PC, Gittes RF, et al (eds): Campbell's Urology, 5th ed. Philadelphia, WB Saunders, 1986
7. Rittmaster RS, Loriaux DL: Hirsutism. Ann Intern Med 106:95, 1987
8. Root AW, Shulman DI: Isosexual precocity: Current concepts and recent advances. Fertil Steril 45:749, 766, 1986
9. Speroff L, Glass RH, Kase NG: Clinical Gynecologic Endocrinology and Infertility, 3d ed. Baltimore, Williams & Wilkins, 1983
10. Walsh PC: Benign prostatic hyperplasia. In Walsh PC, Gittes RF, et al (eds): Campbell's Urology, 5th ed. Philadelphia, WB Saunders, 1986
11. Yen SSC, Jaffe RB (eds): Reproductive endocrinology, 2d ed. Philadelphia, WB Saunders, 1986

CHAPTER 14.6
Disorders of Bone and Mineral Metabolism

Michael A. Levine

Bone is tissue composed of actively metabolizing cells whose principal role is the continuous remodeling of the skeleton to permit growth and repair. Throughout the latter process, interchange of the principal ions, calcium and phosphorus, takes place between bone and extracellular fluid under the control of parathyroid hormone, vitamin D, and calcitonin. Because the secretory rates of these hormones are regulated by the ambient concentration of plasma calcium, an intimate relationship exists between these ions, hormones, and the skeleton, such that derangements of one may induce abnormalities in another.

CALCIUM HOMEOSTASIS[23]

There is 1 to 2 kg of calcium in the average adult body, of which 99 percent is present in the skeleton. Calcium at the bone surface is in dynamic equilibrium with the remaining 1 percent in soft tissue and blood. Blood levels are normally regulated within a range of 9 to 10.5 mg/dl despite wide variations in dietary intake, the demands of the skeleton during growth, and losses during pregnancy and lactation. The calcium in the plasma is in three

forms: ionic calcium (45 percent); diffusible calcium complexed principally with citrate, carbonate, and phosphate (10 percent); and protein-bound calcium (γ-globulin [5 percent] and albumin [40 percent]). Calcium binding to albumin is pH-dependent. Alkalosis increases binding and decreases ionized calcium. Aberrations in serum proteins, especially albumin, readily cause changes in the total plasma calcium, while not affecting the concentration of ionic calcium.

The exchangeable calcium in bone and the calcium in the extracellular fluid are in continuous interchange. The kinetics of this flux are mediated by three calcium-regulating hormones: PTH, calcitonin, and vitamin D. Ionic calcium, in turn, regulates their rates of production.

Finally, changes in concentrations of the three common calcium-complexing ions (phosphate, citrate, and carbonate) can affect calcium flux. Factors that affect calcium movement in bone produce similar changes in these ions as well.

ABSORPTION AND EXCRETION OF CALCIUM

Calcium is absorbed by the small bowel by both passive diffusion and active transport (Fig. 14.6–1). The average daily intake is between 600 and 1200 mg but this may vary between far greater extremes. To prevent wide oscillations in plasma calcium, a greater proportion of calcium is absorbed when the diet is deficient and a lesser proportion when intake is high. This control is largely mediated by a specific intestinal calcium-binding protein which is regulated by 1,25-dihydroxycholecalciferol (1,25(OH)$_2$D$_3$). Net absorption of the dietary calcium consumed is approximately 100 to 200 mg per day.

In the presence of normal vitamin D metabolism, calcium absorption increases during periods of rapid skeletal growth (e.g., childhood and adolescence) and during periods of increased calcium demand (e.g., pregnancy and lactation). Conversely, the decrease in calcium absorption that accompanies advancing age may be related to defective production of 1,25(OH)$_2$D$_3$.

Factors other than vitamin D also affect calcium absorption. Absorption is enhanced by acid conditions, which permit greater solubility of calcium salts; excessive lactose, which forms soluble complexes with calcium; and high-protein diet. Conversely, absorption is impaired by a high intake of fats, oxalates, and alkali, all of which promote the formation of insoluble compounds. In addition, strontium, magnesium, and phosphorus, which inhibit vitamin D metabolism, may likely reduce absorption.

Severe dietary deficiency or malabsorption of calcium can result in a negative calcium balance despite maximal renal calcium conservation. In this setting, maintenance of normal extracellular fluid calcium concentrations will be achieved by accelerated mobilization of calcium from bone in response to increased secretion of PTH. This is one consequence of calcium malabsorption in progressive skeletal demineralization.

Calcium is lost from the body primarily in the feces as a result of both nonabsorption and active secretion. This loss constitutes approximately 80 to 90 percent of the dietary intake when the body is in normal calcium balance. The remaining 10 to 20 percent is excreted in the urine but is under exacting control. Of the approximately 10 g of calcium handled by the renal tubules a day, 97 to 99 percent is reabsorbed. When plasma calcium values fall below 8 mg/dl, little is excreted, and when plasma levels are excessive, losses may be high. These changes are largely mediated by PTH. Urinary excretion of calcium is also increased by high-salt or high-protein diets and by chronic acidosis.

BONE PHYSIOLOGY[3]

The skeleton is a vital organ composed of cells, minerals, and organic matrix. Bone is constantly undergoing a process of "remodeling," wherein previously calcified areas are absorbed and replaced by new bone deposition. Chemically, bone consists of approximately 65 to 70 percent crystalline hydroxyapatite. The remaining 30 to 35 percent is organic matrix composed of collagen (95 percent) and other proteins, carbohydrates, and polymers of these hexosamines and glucuronic acid. The major noncollagen proteins include a glutamic acid (GLA)-containing protein, osteocalcin, and a glycoprotein called "osteonectin." Bone collagen is capable of initiating nucleation of crystals of hydroxyapatite. These crystals are small hexagonal rods, distributed over the collagen surface, which in humans has been estimated to be 100 acres. All this surface, however, is not in equilibrium with the surrounding fluid. As crystals of hydroxyapatite form on collagen, they displace the water molecules that make up the sphere of hydration surrounding individual collagen fibrils. As the crystal population increases and the sphere of hydration decreases, the facility with which ions can

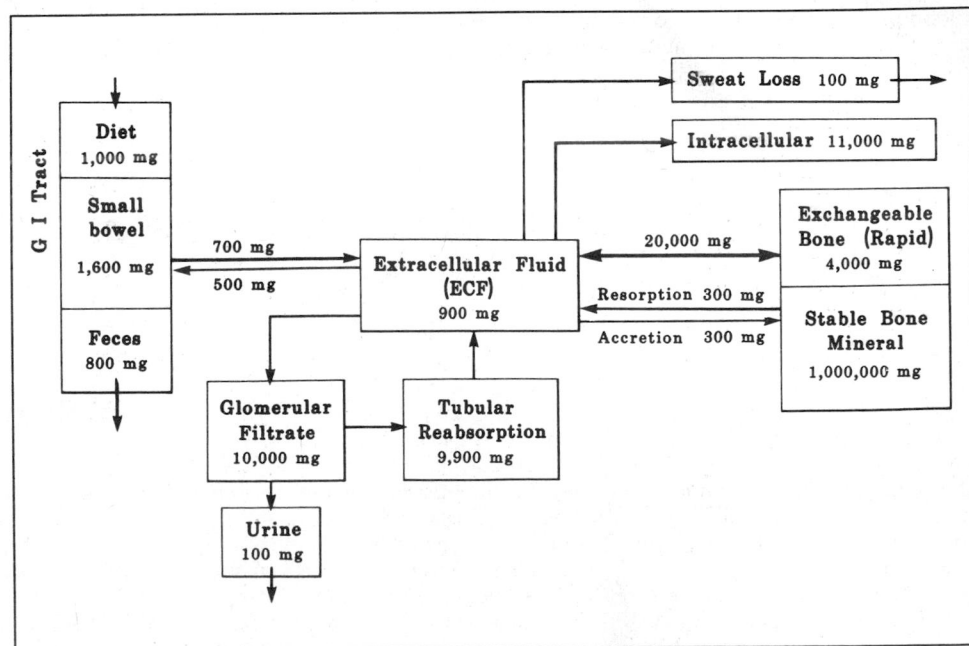

Figure 14.6–1. Functional pools of calcium distribution, showing size and magnitude of flux between them.

enter is impaired and crystal formation stops. The structural characteristics of the relationship of hydroxyapatite crystals to collagen explain why less than 1 percent of bone mineral is freely exchangeable. Presumably only those collagen fibrils that do not have their full complement of crystals are capable of presenting surfaces upon which exchange can readily take place. Conditions that interfere with either collagen synthesis, the calcium-phosphate solubility coefficient, or mucopolysaccharide formation will likewise affect hydroxyapatite deposition and the ability of mineral ions to participate in exchange reactions.

The collagen molecules are longitudinally oriented within the basic microscopic unit of bone, the osteon, or Haversian system. The osteon is an irregular cylindrical structure about 150 μm in external diameter. Within its center is a narrow lumen, the Haversian canal, which has its own nutrient artery. Branching from the Haversian canal are multiple interconnecting canalicules. These serve as conduits for the microcirculatory system connecting the central Haversian canal with lacunae, or concentrically located housing units for the bone cells.

There are three types of bone cells: osteoblasts, osteocytes, and osteoclasts. The osteoblasts arise from mesenchymal precursor cells during early development of the skeleton. They synthesize the collagen and glycoproteins of bone matrix, contain bone alkaline phosphatase, and secrete bone GLA protein, which may initiate mineralization of the uncalcified matrix osteoid. With growth, the osteoblasts become surrounded by osteoid and develop into osteocytes. The osteocytes continue to lay down matrix, which eventually becomes mineralized. The osteocytes remain connected with the osteoblasts covering the external surface of bone by cytoplasmic processes that extend radially from each cell in the canalicules. The osteocytes are arranged concentrically within the Haversian systems and maintain already formed bone by local resorption, accretion, and transport of nutrients and waste products. Additional bone resorption is carried out by multinucleated osteoclasts, which arise from a primitive hematopoietic stem cell related to the mononuclear phagocyte series. Osteoclasts promote local bone dissolution by the elaboration of lytic enzymes and organic acids. These cells line the surface of the marrow cavity. Stimulation of osteoclasts is followed by formation of a ruffled border membrane and production of an acid environment in the adjacent extracellular space, which helps to solubilize the mineralized bone undergoing resorption. The activity and possibly the differentiation of all three types of bone cells—osteoblasts, osteocytes, and osteoclasts—are, at least in part, hormone-dependent.

Physiologic factors that alter bone resorption and accretion rates include the following:

1. *Hormones and growth factors.* Bone activity is also influenced by hormones with specific effects on mineral metabolism (e.g., PTH, calcitonin, $1,25(OH)_2D_3$), as well as those with generalized anabolic or catabolic activity. Osteoblasts may be stimulated to produce matrix by several bone-derived growth factors, somatomedins, beta-transforming growth factor, and a poorly characterized glycoprotein termed "bone morphogenetic protein."
2. *Changes in blood vessels.* Alterations in blood supply, produced by anatomic, nervous, or biochemical processes, will alter the nutrition of the osteons.
3. *Nutrients in the blood.* Because bone matrix is composed of collagen and mucopolysaccharides, protein deficiencies may have adverse effects on bone formation.
4. *Ions.* Increases in plasma phosphate promote deposition of calcium in bone and inhibit bone resorption. As a consequence, plasma calcium and phosphate are inversely related. Other ions may affect crystallization of hydroxyapatite. Of particular note is fluoride, which may affect both crystal size and solubility.
5. *Pyrophosphate.* Naturally occurring pyrophosphate plays a role as an inhibitor of both bone accretion and resorption. It acts by replacing phosphate in the crystal surface,

thereby altering exchange properties. Its physiologic importance is poorly understood because of its rapid intracellular degradation.
6. *Mechanical stress.* Weight-bearing and the functional activity of muscles as they relate to the forces they exert on bone at their insertions generate local differences in piezoelectric fields in bone. These may play a role in the distribution of osteoclasts and osteoblasts in bone, thereby altering the effects of hormones on bone determining morphology and the rate of bone remodeling.

In general, bone is of two types: cortical or compact bone, which is highly calcified but relatively inactive metabolically, and spongiosa, which is more metabolically active and composed of trabeculae. Both are surrounded by an endosteal membrane consisting of osteoblasts and their precursors, which act as calcium pumps in controlling the local concentration of calcium in the fluid surrounding bone.

In growing children, bone may develop either by replacement of previously calcified cartilage (endochondral bone formation) or by de novo formation (intramembranous bone formation). In adult bone, epiphyses have closed, and growth in length ceases. Remodeling of bone continues through life, however, and is accomplished by formation of bone at periosteal surfaces and by resorption at endosteal surfaces. Osteoblasts cover actively forming bone surfaces and secrete osteoid. An osteoid "seam," or layer of uncalcified bone, results from the physiologic delay in mineralization of the newly formed organic matrix. In general, resorption precedes formation and is more intense, but it does not persist as long as formation. During normal remodeling of mature bone the rate of formation exceeds or equals that of resorption. An index of the rate of osteoid formation and mineralization can be determined by analysis of a nondemineralized specimen of bone obtained by biopsy from an individual who has received two courses of tetracycline separated by a drug-free interval. The distance between the two fluorescent bands (normally less than 12 μm) reflects the new bone formed during the period between administration of the two tetracycline "labels."

CALCIUM-REGULATING HORMONES

Of the three principal hormones that affect calcium metabolism, the earliest to evolve were calcitonin and vitamin D. Their initial function may have been to conserve phosphate. With the development of terrestrial forms of life, they were probably adapted to regulate calcium homeostasis. To facilitate more efficient remodeling of the skeleton, PTH evolved later as an adjunctive control.

PARATHYROID HORMONE (PTH)[7]

The gene for preproPTH has a remarkable degree of interspecies conservation for both protein structure and gene organization. PTH is synthesized in the parathyroid glands as a preprohormone (115 amino acids), converted to a prohormone (90 amino acids) by intracellular enzymes, and stored and released principally as a single-chain, 84-amino-acid peptide. Biologic activity requires the continuous amino acid sequence extending from residue 2 to residue 6 in the amino terminus of the polypeptide. PTH is produced at a rate inversely proportional to the ambient serum ionic calcium concentration. Changes in calcium of as little as 1 percent acutely affect secretion of newly synthesized as well as preformed pools of PTH. The precise mechanism by which calcium controls secretion of PTH is unknown. High concentrations of calcium may decrease PTH synthesis by reducing transcriptional activity of the PTH gene. There is no evidence that calcium influences translational events or conversion of proPTH to PTH, although it does increase the rate of intracellular degradation of the mature hormone.

Glucocorticoids, vitamin D metabolites, magnesium, and

other ions also modulate elaboration of PTH. Glucocorticoids transiently augment PTH secretion, indirectly by lowering plasma calcium as a consequence of inhibiting bone resorption and decreasing calcium absorption from the gut, and by directly stimulating the parathyroid glands. Vitamin D metabolites also may have both direct and indirect effects. By inducing hypercalcemia consequent to increasing bone resorption and calcium absorption, they indirectly inhibit PTH secretion. Elevated levels of $1,25(OH)_2D$ also directly decrease PTH gene transcription. Although less effective than calcium, magnesium in high concentrations inhibits secretion. In severe magnesium deficiency, however, hypocalcemia parodoxically develops due to impaired secretion and possibly altered end-organ response. Lithium increases secretion and decreases the sensitivity of the parathyroid cell to inhibition by calcium.

In addition to the major form of biologically active PTH secreted from the parathyroid gland (1–84), carboxy-terminal (and possibly amino-terminal) fragments are also released. The proportion of C-terminal fragments released is increased in hyperparathyroidism. Circulating, PTH is rapidly degraded by the liver and kidney. As a consequence of both secretion and degradation, marked heterogeneity of PTH is present in blood. Because clearance of the intact hormone from blood is more rapid than that of carboxy-terminal fragments, the principal circulating form of PTH immunoreactivity is the biologically inert carboxy-terminal peptide against which most antisera used in currently available RIAs are directed. As a consequence, such assays in fact measure predominantly biologically inactive fragments in blood. Hence, changes in PTH immunoreactivity may result from either an altered rate of hormone secretion or a change in the generation or clearance of carboxy-terminal fragments. For example, in renal insufficiency clearance of biologically inert PTH fragments is decreased, and plasma PTH immunoreactivity may far exceed concentrations of the biologically active peptide.

PTH acts directly on bone and kidney and indirectly, through $1,25(OH)_2D$, on the gut, to raise serum calcium levels.

PTH regulates both mineral homeostasis and bone remodeling. Acute changes in plasma calcium are counteracted by the effects of PTH on calcium release from bone. On the other hand, chronic maintenance of normal plasma calcium reflects the PTH effects on $1,25(OH)_2D$ levels and on gastrointestinal calcium absorption. PTH directly affects the activity of osteoclasts, increasing their ruffled borders and their citric acid and lytic enzymes, both of which promote bone resorption. Chronically PTH regulates the size and number of osteoclasts, which remodel bone. In hyperparathyroidism, the rate of bone accretion is usually less than that of resorption, causing net bone loss. The increase in both functions leads to an increased bone turnover rate, and therefore increases urinary hydroxyproline excretion and plasma alkaline phosphatase activity.

PTH has three effects on the kidney: (1) it enhances renal tubular reabsorption of calcium; (2) it increases urinary excretion of phosphate, bicarbonate, potassium, sodium, and amino acids; and (3) it enhances conversion of $25(OH)D$ to the more active $1,25(OH)_2D$. The hormone appears to have different actions in different parts of the renal tubule: the predominant effect on phosphate is mediated by changes in the proximal tubule, whereas the main effects on calcium are mediated through changes in the distal tubule.

Parathyroid hormone exerts its effects on its target organs, bone, and kidney, by binding to specific membrane receptors, thereby stimulating adenylate cyclase and increasing tissue concentrations of cAMP. Cyclic AMP activates cytosolic protein kinases causing specific enzymatic reactions that produce the physiologic effect of PTH.

Vitamin D[21]

This sterol increases bone resorption and absorption of both calcium and phosphate from the intestine. These actions are me-

diated by its polar metabolite, 1,25-dihydroxycholecalciferol $(1,25(OH)_2D_3)$, the production of which is exquisitely controlled in order to effect regulation of serum calcium, facilitate growth, and maintain the normal skeleton. The production of $1,25(OH)_2D_3$ is dependent upon the availability of precursors and the subsequent hydroxylation of these, first in the liver and then in the kidney.

The daily requirement for calciferol is about 100 IU. To prevent vitamin D deficiency the National Research Council of the United States has recommended an intake of 400 IU per day. In the United States, however, endogenous synthesis of cholecalciferol (vitamin D_3), promoted by sunlight, generally provides more calciferol than does dietary intake of ergocalciferol (vitamin D_2) or cholecalciferol from fortified milk, breads, and cereals. Absorption of calciferol from the intestinal lumen requires bile-mediated micelle information. If bile production is impaired, vitamin D deficiency may result. Once internalized, vitamin D is incorporated into chylomicra and transported via the lymphatics to the liver. Transportation of the lipophilic sterol is facilitated in the circulation by vitamin D-binding protein (transcalciferol). Although cholecalciferol is present in animal products, notably butter, eggs, and fish oils, precursor requirements are met primarily by conversion of 7-dehydrocholesterol (provitamin D_3) in the skin under the influence of ultraviolet light, the amount of sunlight being a critical determinant of the rate of cholecalciferol production.

In humans, vitamin D_2 and vitamin D_3 are similarly metabolized. In the liver, vitamin D is hydroxylated to 25-hydroxycholecalciferol $(25(OH)D)$ by a microsomal enzyme. This conversion is only loosely regulated by a product feedback inhibition, and is unaffected by serum calcium, phosphorus, or PTH. The major circulating metabolite of vitamin D, $25(OH)D$, generally reflects dietary intake or endogenous production of vitamin D. Some $25(OH)D$ is conjugated in the liver, excreted in bile, and reabsorbed from the gut. Large amounts can be lost in malabsorption states. The only role of $25(OH)D$ is as a substrate for conversion to $1,25(OH)_2D$. Because only a small fraction of $25(OH)D$ is converted to $1,25(OH)_2D$, extensive liver damage must be present before impaired production becomes apparent.

In the renal cortex, $25(OH)D$ is further modified by one of two mitochondrial enzymes, $25(OH)D$-1-hydroxylase and $25(OH)D$-24-hydroxylase. Although $25(OH)D$-1-hydroxylase activity has been localized principally to the proximal renal tubule, similar enzyme activity has been identified in bone cells, placenta, and sarcoid granulomas.[4,13] The reaction mediated by renal $25(OH)D$-1-hydroxylase is stringently regulated. Its activity is enhanced by (1) hypophosphatemia directly, and (2) hypocalcemia indirectly as mediated by PTH; its activity is inhibited by hyperphosphatemia and $1,25(OH)_2D$. Each of these initiates appropriate correction of plasma calcium, phosphate, and $1,25(OH)_2D$ levels toward normal. $1,25(OH)_2D$ is far more active than either vitamin D itself or $25(OH)D$ in stimulating intestinal calcium absorption.

A second renal cortical enzyme, $25(OH)D$-24-hydroxylase, is also present in skin fibroblasts, intestinal cells, and pituitary cells. Activity of this enzyme is increased by $1,25(OH)_2D$. The production of $1,25(OH)_2D$ and $24,25(OH)_2D$ is conjointly regulated by the ambient calcium and phosphate levels such that when either is low, $1,25(OH)_2D$ is elaborated and, conversely, when either is high, $24,25(OH)_2D$ is produced. In this way, the appropriate product is secreted to maintain normal serum calcium and phosphate levels. Under normal conditions, approximately 100 times more $24,25(OH)_2D$ than $1,25(OH)_2D$ is present in the circulation. The biologic role of $24,25(OH)_2D$ in humans is not determined, but it may be involved in bone metabolism.

Vitamin D and its biologically active metabolites, $25(OH)D$ and $1,25(OH)_2D$, act on intestine and bone. Calcium is absorbed by the gut primarily in the distal portion of the small bowel by passive diffusion. A significant amount can be actively absorbed in the duodenum, however, when calcium deprivation elevates levels of $1,25(OH)_2D$, which stimulates the synthesis of a calcium-binding protein in duodenal cells. The active metabolites of vitamin D

directly increase the rate of bone resorption. This effect is enhanced by PTH. Whether vitamin D alters renal tubular transport of calcium or phosphate is not known.

CALCITONIN

Calcitonin is secreted in humans by the parafollicular or "C-" cells of the thyroid. In lower species, similar cells are found in the ultimobranchial bodies. Secreting cells originate from the neural crest and migrate during early development to the last pharyngeal pouch, which subsequently participates in the formation of the thyroid gland. The hormone is a 32-amino-acid, single-chain polypeptide. The calcitonin gene is located on chromosome 11 in the general region of the PTH and insulin genes, and generates distinct mRNAs encoding both calcitonin and a novel neuropeptide referred to as calcitonin gene-related peptide (CGRP). Contrary to PTH, calcitonin is secreted in response to elevations in plasma calcium, its rate of secretion being directly proportional to the concentration of this cation. It acts to inhibit bone resorption and prevents egress of calcium from bone while allowing calcium from blood to enter bone. Secretion of calcitonin may, in part, be mediated by gastrin under physiologic conditions. In experimental animals, gastrin is secreted in response to a calcium meal, prompting secretion of calcitonin before calcium is absorbed, thereby protecting against postprandial hypercalcemia. The physiologic significance of other secretagogues for calcitonin, including secretin, glucagon, strontium, and magnesium, remains in doubt.

In bone, calcitonin has a direct and immediate effect on osteoclasts. Within minutes after its administration, the ruffled border of these cells retracts from the surface of adjacent bone undergoing resorption. Subsequent effects include a reduction in the rate of osteoclast production. For this reason, calcitonin is a useful therapeutic agent in reducing exaggerated osteolysis in such conditions as Paget disease of bone.

Calcitonin in pharmacologic doses promotes the renal excretion of phosphate, sodium, and potassium. The mechanism of action of calcitonin remains unknown but appears to involve activation of adenylate cyclase in renal tubular cells and osteoclasts.

In animals, calcitonin subserves three functions: (1) protection against postprandial hypercalcemia, (2) prevention of excessive skeletal demineralization during times of extreme demand for calcium, such as pregnancy and lactation, and (3) modulation of plasma calcium homeostasis and bone remodeling. This activity may be particularly important during growth by permitting the calcium-conserving activity of vitamin D and PTH on gut and kidney, respectively, while preventing excessive bone resorption.

A physiologic role of calcitonin in humans remains to be demonstrated. Two observations suggest that the hormone is not important in calcium homeostasis: (1) In patients with medullary carcinoma of the thyroid in whom high concentrations of plasma calcitonin are present, little or no aberration in plasma calcium levels is seen. (2) After thyroidectomy without obvious impairment of PTH secretion, deficiency of calcitonin does not overtly impair handling of calcium loads. These findings, however, do not constitute definitive proof that calcitonin is inactive in humans. It can be argued that in medullary carcinoma the effects of excessive amounts of the hormone are prevented by concomitant increases in PTH secretion. In patients who lack a thyroid gland, the fall in plasma calcium following a calcium infusion may be delayed, and this delay may result in excessive renal loss of the ion, leading ultimately to a deficiency of calcium. The present view is that if calcitonin is physiologically active in calcium regulation in humans, it plays a lesser role than either PTH or vitamin D.

OTHER FACTORS THAT MAY AFFECT MINERAL METABOLISM

Other hormones and metabolically active substances influence calcium and phosphate metabolism. These include somatomedins, glucocorticoids, insulin, estrogens, androgens, thyroid hormone, osteoclast-activating factor, and prostaglandins.

The growth-promoting effects of growth hormone on the skeleton are indirectly mediated through the production of somatomedins (see Chapter 14.2). These substances, produced primarily in the liver, are peptides that stimulate DNA and RNA synthesis in osteoblasts and promote the uptake of amino acids required by these cells for the production of collagen. When in excess they may induce gigantism or acromegaly; conversely, deficiencies of these substances or end-organ failure in children may result in short stature.

Glucocorticoids are essential for normal skeletal growth. In high concentration, however, they promote loss of bone mass. States of glucocorticoid excess are associated with decreased bone formation and increased bone resorption. Multiple factors may be involved, including inhibition of osteoblast function, impaired synthesis of collagen, interference with vitamin D metabolism, and inhibition of intestinal calcium transport independent of vitamin D.

Insulin likewise is required for normal development of the skeleton. It promotes the rate of collagen synthesis. The osteoporosis in patients with diabetes mellitus has been attributed, in part, to insulin deficiency.

Estrogens and androgens hasten epiphyseal closure at puberty and inhibit bone resorption. High plasma levels before puberty prevent attainment of full growth potential and low levels in postmenopausal women may contribute to the development of osteoporosis by leaving the effects of PTH on the skeleton unopposed.

Thyroid hormones increase the rate of both bone accretion and bone resorption, thereby augmenting bone turnover. Deficiencies in these hormones in early childhood may result in dwarfism.

Prostaglandins, principally PGE_2, stimulate bone resorption. They may play a significant role in the genesis of hypercalcemia associated with some malignant tumors.

Osteoclast-activating factor (OAF) likewise is a potent stimulator of bone resorption. It is present in leukocytes and may induce hypercalcemia in lymphoproliferative disorders, especially multiple myeloma.

PHOSPHATE HOMEOSTASIS

Eighty-five percent of the phosphate in the body is in bone. The remainder is widely distributed in soft tissues, where it is found principally as a component of nucleic acids, enzymes, and high-energy intermediates of carbohydrate metabolism. In the blood phosphorus is present as inorganic orthophosphate. Unlike calcium, it exists mostly as the free ion (88 percent). Its concentration varies markedly during the course of the day, with oscillations as wide as 50 percent from baseline. Most of these changes are induced by dietary carbohydrate, which provokes falls in blood phosphorus levels. Superimposed on these changes is a natural diurnal rhythm that parallels the rate of ACTH secretion and is brought about by rises in renal threshold consequent to variations in cortisol secretion.

ABSORPTION AND EXCRETION OF PHOSPHATE

Approximately 1 g of phosphate is ingested in the normal daily diet. This is more than twice that required by the body. Phosphorus absorption is relatively efficient. About 70 percent of intestinal phosphorus is absorbed under normal conditions and up to 90 percent if dietary phosphorus is restricted.

Because most foods are rich in phosphate, deficiency is rarely secondary to inadequate intake. Low levels of phosphate are not even provoked by prolonged fasting because phosphate is released by catabolized tissues.

Transport across the gut takes place principally by active trans-

port. This system is energy dependent, concentrative, carrier mediated, and stimulated by $1,25(OH)_2D$. The phosphate diffusional system is of minor quantitative importance. Phosphate absorption is increased under mildly alkaline conditions in the gastrointestinal tract, whereas above pH 8.0, absorption is partially prevented by the formulation of insoluble salts.

Phosphate reabsorption by the proximal tubule of the kidney is a high-affinity system operating near saturation. This sodium-dependent process is inhibited by PTH. When filtered phosphate rises above a threshold concentration, the overflow is virtually completely excreted into urine. PTH decreases the renal threshold, an action mediated by activation of adenylate cyclase in proximal tubule cells. Increased intracellular concentrations of cAMP lead to inhibition of phosphate reabsorption in the proximal tubule, inducing phosphaturia. Tubular reabsorption of phosphate is increased by vitamin D and its metabolites. Whether or not this is a direct effect remains uncertain. A number of other factors promote phosphaturia. These include estrogen, thyroid hormone, cortisol, insulin, diets high in phosphate, potassium, magnesium, expansion of the extracellular fluid volume, metabolic acidosis, and most diuretics.

CONSEQUENCES OF HYPERPHOSPHATEMIA AND HYPOPHOSPHATEMIA

Chronic hyperphosphatemia occurs with hypoparathyroidism, hyperthyroidism, and chronic renal failure. When serum phosphate levels are high, ionic calcium levels in the blood are low, thereby stimulating secretion of PTH.

Hypophosphatemia is rarely caused by inadequate phosphate intake but can occasionally result from decreased intestinal absorption due to excessive ingestion of aluminum hydroxide antacids. Hypophosphatemia occurs usually as a result of a reduction in renal tubular reabsorption of phosphate. This can be caused by respiratory alkalosis, large carbohydrate loads, cirrhosis, magnesium deficiency, diabetic ketoacidosis, and hyperalimentation. At levels below 2.0 mg/dl, hypophosphatemia may provoke bone pain secondary to osteomalacia, hypercalciuria as a consequence of hypercalcemia, impaired cardiac contractility, skeletal muscle weakness, rhabdomyolysis, and abnormalities in blood cell function due to deficiencies in ATP and 2,3-DPG.

DISORDERED CALCIUM HOMEOSTASIS

HYPERCALCEMIA

Hypercalcemia may result from many pathologic states as well as from inappropriate blood sampling and laboratory errors. Such errors may be avoided by the use of cork stoppers and by using either acid-washed or calcium-free disposable blood collection materials. The total serum calcium is also directly influenced by the level of binding proteins, primarily albumin and globulin. Certain hyperproteinemic states may result in modest elevations of total serum calcium, with no increase in ionized calcium. Hemoconcentration secondary to prolonged application of the venipuncture tourniquet, profound dehydration, and prolonged fasting can also result in elevations of total serum calcium. Adjusted approximation can be made because an elevation of the albumin of 1 g/dl will increase total serum calcium by 0.8 mg/dl. Direct measurement of ionized calcium is preferred, however, when serum protein abnormalities are present. When the serum calcium is only marginally elevated multiple samples should be obtained. Once true hypercalcemia is established, its cause (Table 14.6–1) should be determined.

The signs and symptoms of hypercalcemia are nonspecific, protean, and often severe. Furthermore, clinical manifestations may derive from the hypercalcemia alone or may represent other features of the underlying primary disorder. Physical examination is rarely helpful in recognizing hypercalcemia except when areas of

TABLE 14.6–1. CAUSES OF HYPERCALCEMIA

Hyperparathyroidism
- Primary hyperparathyroidism
- Hyperparathyroidism of renal failure
- Familial hypocalciuric hypercalcemia
- Parathyroid carcinoma

Neoplasia
- Humoral hypercalcemia of malignancy
- Tumor osteolysis

Medications
- Vitamins A and D
- Thiazide
- Lithium

Endocrinopathies
- Hyperthyroidism
- Adrenal insufficiency
- Pheochromocytoma

Granulomatous diseases

Miscellaneous causes
- Immobilization
- Milk-alkali syndrome
- Recovery phase of acute renal failure
- Idiopathic hypercalcemia of infancy

calcification within the corneal limbus of the eye (band keratopathy) are observed.

Contractility of skeletal, smooth, and cardiac muscle, excitability of nervous tissue, and cerebral function are all depressed by elevations in extracellular calcium ion concentration. Lassitude or fatigue are early signs of altered cerebration and may presage lethargy or somnolence. Generalized rather than localized neurologic signs are typical and may be accompanied by an electroencephalographic pattern characterized by a diffusely slow pattern consistent with a metabolic disturbance.

Mental and behavioral disturbances can be attributed to hypercalcemia, ranging from confusion and depression to mania and psychosis. In many cases there is a positive correlation between the degree of mental dysfunction and serum calcium.

Hypercalcemia may also be associated with neuromuscular abnormalities. Generalized muscle weakness and depressed deep tendon reflexes are not uncommon. In addition, hypercalcemia can cause a nonspecific proximal myopathy that correlates poorly with other symptoms.

The effects of hypercalcemia upon cardiovascular function include hypertension and alterations in cardiac excitability and contractility. Severe hypercalcemia (serum levels greater than 13 mg/dl) is accompanied by decreased conduction velocity and shortened refractory period and produces electrophysiologic effects that are similar to and synergistic with the inotropic and toxic manifestations of digitalis. Electrocardiographic findings include slight P-R interval and QRS complex prolongation and S-T segment shortening, which produces a short Q-T interval. The decreased conduction velocity, decreased automaticity, and shorter refractory period of hypercalcemia predispose to cardiac arrhythmias.

Hypercalcemia impairs renal sodium transport and water conservation, and may result in a clinical picture of polyuria, polydipsia, and nocturia, which resembles nephrogenic (vasopressin-resistant) diabetes insipidus. In addition, hypercalciuria may be accompanied by either nephrolithiasis or nephrocalcinosis. The latter, due to deposition of calcium in the renal parenchyma, may result in potassium-wasting and hypokalemia, albuminuria, hyposthenuria, and eventually, azotemia.

The gastrointestinal effects of hypercalcemia include constipation, dyspepsia, anorexia, nausea, and vomiting. Abdominal pain is a common presenting symptom and may be nonspecific or indicative of pancreatitis or peptic ulcer disease.

TABLE 14.6–2. BIOCHEMICAL AND RADIOLOGIC FINDINGS IN HYPERCALCEMIA

Diagnosis	sCa	sPO₄	uCa	25(OH)D	1,25 (OH)₂D	Alkaline Phosphatase	Urinary Cyclic AMP	iPTH	Bone Survey
Primary hyperparathyroidism	↑	↓	n/↑	n	↑	↑	↑↑	↑↑	Osteitis fibrosa cystica
Osteolytic malignancy	↑	↑	↑↑	n	↓	↑↑	↓	↓	Lytic lesions
Humoral hypercalcemia of malignancy	↑	↓	↑↑	n	↓	n	↑↑	↓	n
Sarcoidosis	↑	↑	↑↑	n	↑↑	↑	↓	↓	Punched-out lesions or cortical thinning
Vitamin D intoxication	↑	↑	↑↑	↑↑	n	n	↓	↓	n
Familial hypocalciuric hypercalcemia	↑	↓	↓	n	n	n	↑	↑	n

Differential Diagnosis (Table 14.6–2)

The diagnostic approach to the patient with hypercalcemia (Fig. 14.6–2) begins with a complete history and physical examination and proceeds to a thorough laboratory evaluation (Table 14.6–3). Primary hyperparathyroidism and malignancy are the two most common conditions that cause hypercalcemia (Table 14.6–1) and can often be distinguished from one another on a historical basis; a long, relatively benign clinical history and the laboratory finding of associated hypophosphatemia are characteristic of primary hyperparathyroidism.

Primary Hyperparathyroidism

Primary hyperparathyroidism is characterized by hypersecretion of parathyroid hormone. It is a common disorder, occurring with an estimated incidence of 25/100,000 of the general population, with more than 50,000 new cases each year in the United States. The disease most commonly occurs in adults, with a peak incidence in the sixth decade of life. Women are affected more frequently than men (3:2). Among women over 65, the annual incidence is estimated at 10 times the overall figure, or 250/100,000. The biochemical etiology is unknown, but the disorder can be produced by a single adenoma, chief cell hyperplasia of all parathyroid glands, or carcinoma.

A solitary adenoma of one of the parathyroid glands is most

TABLE 14.6–3. DIAGNOSTIC SCREENING TESTS OF HYPERCALCEMIA

Serum tests
- Fasting calcium and phosphate
- Serum urea nitrogen and creatinine
- Electrolytes
- Serum protein electrophoresis
- Alkaline phosphatase
- Magnesium
- PTH, T₄, T₃

Urine tests
- 24-hour urinary calcium excretion
- Urinary cAMP
- Tubular reabsorption of phosphate

Radiographic evaluations
- Chest radiograph
- Intravenous pyelogram
- Bone scan
- Bone radiograph

commonly (80 to 90 percent) the cause of primary hyperparathyroidism. So-called double or multiple adenomas probably represent asymmetric chief-cell hyperplasia because removal of "double adenomas" is often followed by recurrence of hyperparathyroidism. Chief cell hyperplasia is a disorder of all the parathyroid glands and constitutes about 15 percent of cases. It may occur sporadically or as a familial disorder. It is often difficult to differentiate adenoma and chief-cell hyperplasia histologically, and thus it is often necessary to rely upon the gross pathology of the glands observed at surgery. Hyperparathyroidism in families or in the multiple endocrine neoplasia (MEN) syndromes is almost invariably due to involvement of all of the parathyroid glands (see discussion of hypercalcemia in families).

Carcinoma of the parathyroid glands is rare, and less than 1 to 2 percent of hyperfunctioning glands are carcinomatous as judged by histology, gross appearance, or biologic behavior.

The clinical presentation of primary hyperparathyroidism tends to segregate into three overlapping syndromes: (1) Fifty percent or more of patients are asymptomatic and diagnosed serendipitously by a routine determination of serum calcium. (2) In 10 percent, nephrolithiasis is the clinical presentation of primary hyperparathyroidism. Although primary hyperparathyroidism is present in less than 5 percent of all patients who have nephrolithiasis, it is still advisable to consider the diagnosis. Interestingly, nephrolithiasis and nephrocalcinosis rarely are present in the same patient. (3) A third syndrome of primary hyperparathyroidism is characterized by marked hypercalcemia, weight loss, debility, and bone pain, sometimes accompanied by pathologic fracture. In this form of the disease, hyperparathyroidism may be so aggressive as to suggest a malignancy. The symptoms and signs of primary hyperparathyroidism have been said to constitute a syndrome of "stones, bones, abdominal groans, and psychic overtones." When symptoms do occur in patients with primary hyperparathyroidism, they can be generally attributed to hypercalcemia with associated hypercalciuria or osteitis fibrosa cystica. As previously mentioned, hypercalcemia may cause neurologic, muscular, gastrointestinal tract, and genitourinary tract complaints. Bone disease in hyperparathyroidism can be demonstrated by radiologic examination or by special histologic techniques in bone biopsy specimens in most patients. Symptomatic bone disease is now uncommon, possibly due to earlier discovery and treatment of hyperparathyroidism. Osteitis fibrosa cystica, the unique bone lesion in hyperparathyroidism, may cause diffuse bone pain or pathologic fracture through an area of a bone cyst. Radiologic manifestations range from generalized osteopenia to localized bone cysts, "brown tumors," epulis of the jaw, loss of the lamina dura about the teeth, and erosion of

Critical Questions:
1. Is drug or diet involved?
2. Is there a family history of hypercalcemia or endocrinopathy?

Recommendations:
1. History and physical exam
2. Screening tests (Table 14.6-3)

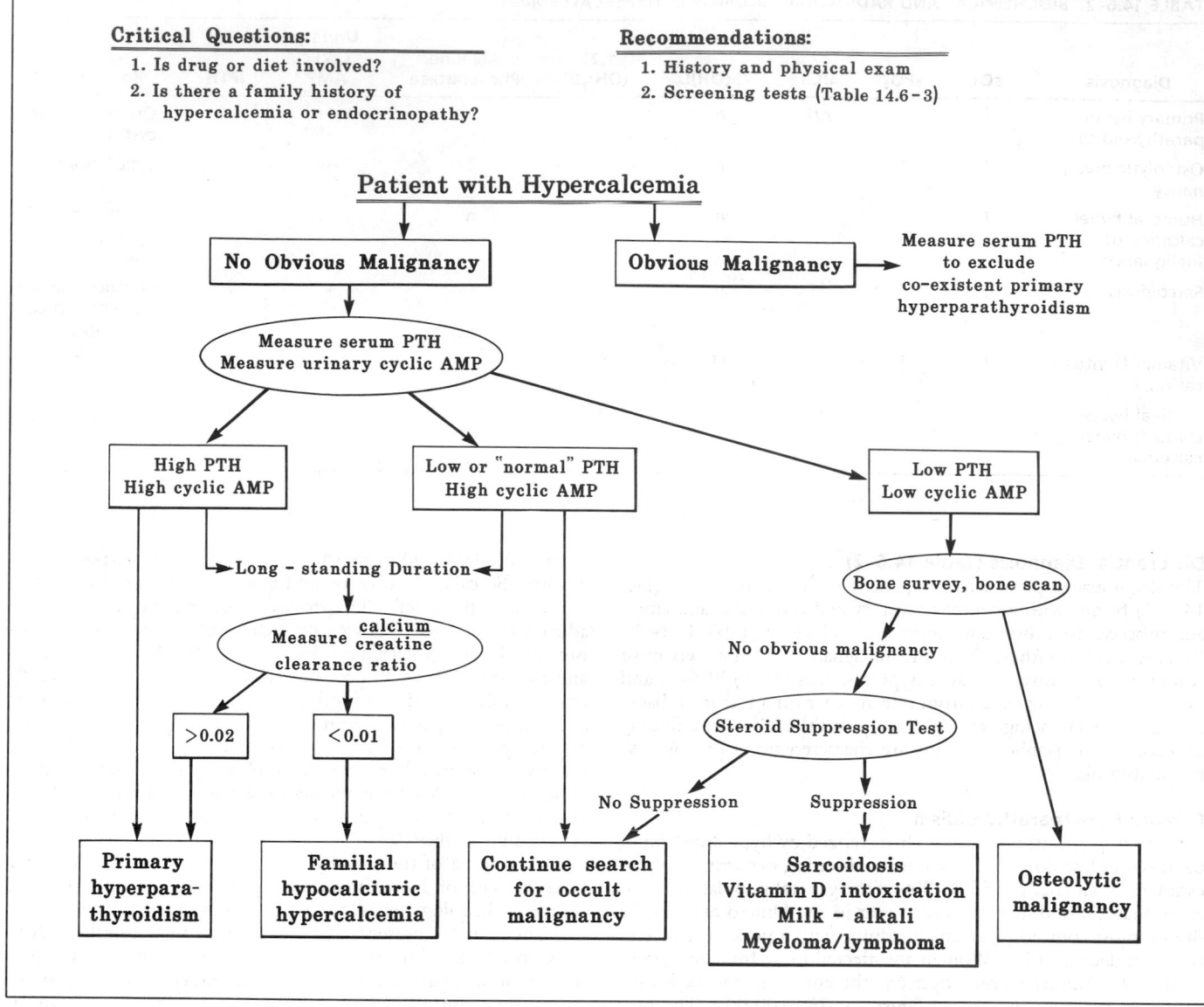

Figure 14.6–2. An approach to differential diagnosis of hypercalcemia.

distal phalangeal tufts, cortical margin of the digits in the hand, or the lateral ends of the clavicles (subperiosteal resorption).

Progressive loss of bone and osteopenia are often documented using improved techniques for measuring bone mineral density (e.g., computed tomography [CT] or dual photon absorptimetry of the spine).

Other symptoms may be more vague and include headache, pruritus, pseudogout (chrondrocalcinosis), gout, dry skin, and malaise.

Physical findings are few and nonspecific. Hypertension is common and frequently is unimproved by correction of hyperparathyroidism. Neuromuscular findings may include, in order of frequency, proximal muscle weakness, cranial nerve abnormalities (especially fasciculations of the tongue), and sensory loss for pain and vibration. Progressive kyphoscoliosis and epulis of the jaw are unusual and seen only in far advanced disease.

Radiologic findings may include ectopic calcification in the skin, eye (band keratopathy), lungs, arteries, and kidneys with long-standing hypercalcemia, especially if renal function is impaired and serum phosphate levels are elevated. Radiologic evaluation of the skeletal system is occasionally useful, particularly when

serum alkaline phosphatase levels for osteitis fibrosa cystica are elevated.

In uncomplicated primary hyperparathyroidism biochemical abnormalities may include:

1. Hypercalcemia (constant or intermittent)
2. Hypophosphatemia
3. Serum bicarbonate less than 24 mEq/L
4. Serum chloride greater than 107 mEq/L
5. Hypercalciuria
6. Serum uric acid greater than 6.8 mg/dl

These laboratory abnormalities are consequences of the hypersecretion of PTH and can be attributed to an acceleration of the normal physiologic actions of PTH on bone and kidney. Elevated levels of alkaline phosphatase activity in plasma and of hydroxyproline excretion in urine are common in patients with significant bone disease and represent increased rates of bone formation and resorption, respectively. In the kidney, PTH enhances the urinary excretion of phosphate and bicarbonate. In the absence of renal failure, urinary calcium excretion is increased in approximately 25

percent of patients. Because PTH enhances calcium reabsorption by the renal distal tubules, however, urinary excretion of calcium is less in hyperparathyroidism than in hypercalcemia resulting from other causes.

The diagnosis of hyperparathyroidism is best supported by serum PTH values that are elevated relative to the concentration of ionized calcium. Hypercalcemia is almost always present in primary hyperparathyroidism but may be documented only intermittently in some patients with early or mild disease. Highly sensitive and specific radioimmunoassays of PTH in serum have been developed in several laboratories and are commercially available.

Unfortunately, measurement of serum immunoreactive PTH in the evaluation of hypercalcemia is not a uniformly reliable diagnostic index for primary hyperparathyroidism. The fact that PTH exists in heterogeneous forms in the peripheral circulation introduces uncertainties in the interpretation of any particular radioimmunoassay.

Following secretion from the gland, intact PTH undergoes rapid degradation to fragments in the periphery. The biologically active "amino-terminal" fragment of the hormone has a short half-life ($t_{1/2} < 5$ minutes) and is rapidly cleared from blood. The principal fragment(s) present in the peripheral circulation, therefore, is derived from the carboxyl terminus of the molecule. These fragments have a long survival time ($t_{1/2} \approx 60$ minutes) and thus are present in greater quantity than either intact or amino-terminal fragments. Although carboxyl-terminal fragments are biologically inert, serum levels of these fragments generally reflect the rate of PTH secretion. Thus, assays that are specific for carboxyl-region fragments generally give much higher values and provide greater diagnostic discrimination between normal and excessive secretion of PTH than amino-region assays. A notable exception occurs in chronic renal disease, when the clearance of carboxyl-terminal fragments from the blood is impaired and immunoreactive fragments accumulate out of proportion to hormone secretion.

Accurate determination of biologically active PTH in the serum by radioimmunoassay requires the use of an antiserum that is both amino-terminal-region specific and highly sensitive. Such radioimmunoassays are becoming commercially available.

Several other tests are helpful adjuncts in the diagnosis of hyperparathyroidism and are based on the known physiologic action of PTH on the kidney. In part, PTH exerts its effects on its target organs by activating adenylate cyclase and causing thereby an increase in tissue concentration of cyclic AMP. Approximately 50 percent of the cyclic AMP excreted in the urine is derived from the renal tubular cell and is almost entirely under the control of PTH. This component of urinary cyclic AMP, termed nephrogenous cAMP, is elevated in approximately 80 percent of patients with primary hyperparathyroidism. Because the total amount of urinary cyclic AMP represents cyclic AMP cleared from the circulation plus that derived from the kidney, determination of nephrogenous cyclic AMP requires simultaneous measurement of plasma and urinary cyclic AMP and creatinine. In practice, however, measurement of total urinary cyclic AMP excretion has been found to be nearly as accurate. The urinary cyclic AMP index can be applied to random urine samples, enabling clinicians to quantitate in vivo PTH effect.

PTH decreases the tubular resorption of phosphate (TRP) and promotes the urinary excretion of phosphate. In patients with hyperparathyroidism, phosphate clearance may be increased and TRP may be as low as 50 to 60 percent (normal greater than 85 percent). Determination of the TRP in a patient with suspected hyperparathyroidism is infrequently performed now, having largely been supplanted by direct measurement of urinary cyclic AMP excretion. Recently, however, the reliability of elevated levels of urinary cyclic AMP as a specific indicator of primary hyperparathyroidism has been challenged by the recognition that certain nonparathyroid malignancies producing hypercalcemia are associated with high rates of nephrogenous cAMP excretion. Thus the failure of this index to discriminate between primary hyperparathyroidism and nonparathyroid malignancy greatly limits its usefulness as a diagnostic adjunct.[32]

The corticosteroid suppression test may be useful in distinguishing patients with vitamin D intoxication, milk-alkali syndrome, sarcoid or other granulomatous diseases, and certain lymphoproliferative diseases. In many of these disorders hypercalcemia is in part secondary to increased absorption of calcium from the gastrointestinal tract. The levels of serum calcium in these patients may decrease substantially in 7 to 10 days with daily administration of 100 to 120 mg of cortisone acetate or its equivalent. The hypercalcemia of primary hyperparathyroidism and many malignancies is generally resistant to the effects of this treatment.

Despite the usefulness of the foregoing tests (Fig. 14.6–2), the diagnosis of primary hyperparathyroidism is often made on the basis of a history of long standing hypercalcemia, nephrolithiasis, or bone lesions, or by exclusion of other causes of hypercalcemia.

Management. Surgical excision of the hyperfunctioning parathyroid gland or glands is the definitive treatment. Surgery may not be of significant or equal benefit to all patients with primary hyperparathyroidism, however. Although large-scale randomized prospective clinical trials have not been undertaken, the natural history of the disease has been studied in several centers to establish rational guidelines for recommending surgery. Based on these studies, it is generally accepted that surgical treatment should be undertaken in the following patients: (1) those with a plasma calcium level greater than 1 mg/dl above the upper limit of normal; (2) those with symptoms secondary to hyperparathyroidism or hypercalcemia; (3) those who have evidence of substantial or progressive bone loss (or osteitis fibrosa cystica); (4) those who have nephrocalcinosis, nephrolithiasis, progressive loss of renal function, or significant hypercalciuria. In addition, surgery is often considered appropriate for patients with mild disease who are relatively young and who would otherwise face lifelong exposure to the risks of hyperparathyroidism as well as the expense of monitoring. Finally, no decision regarding surgery can be made without considering social, general health, and psychological factors. Patients who may have difficulty with long-term longitudinal follow-up or who would be unable to deal emotionally with the diagnosis should also be considered surgical candidates.

Surgical exploration should be performed only by an experienced operator. Localization and removal of abnormal parathyroid tissue is successful in greater than 90 percent of cases when performed by an experienced surgeon. Preoperative localization techniques should be reserved for patients who require a second parathyroid exploration or who have had prior unrelated neck surgery (e.g., thyroid surgery). Noninvasive techniques, such as ultrasonography, differential radionuclide scanning after thallium and technetium administration, and computed tomography of the neck and mediastinum, are available in most hospitals and detect abnormal parathyroid tissue in 50 to 70 percent of cases. Greater success is possible with invasive techniques, particularly selective intra-arterial angiography and selective venous catheterization of the veins that drain the thyroid plexus, mediastinum, and adjacent areas, coupled with radioimmunoassay for PTH; these procedures are available, however, in only a few highly specialized centers.

Many surgeons perform a bilateral neck exploration and attempt to visualize all four glands, with identity confirmed by examination of frozen sections of tissue. This strategy advocates the resection of a single enlarged parathyroid gland in the case of adenoma, or removal of all parathyroid tissue except approximately 50 mg of the most normal-appearing gland in multiple gland hyperplasia. Alternatively, some surgeons will not explore both sides of the neck if an adenoma and a normal gland are found on the same side.

Nonsurgical treatment of primary hyperparathyroidism is reserved for patients who are unwilling to undergo surgery or are suboptimal surgical candidates or for asymptomatic patients who fail to meet any of the surgical guidelines presented above. There is currently no way to predict in which asymptomatic patients renal or skeletal deterioration will occur.

Several generalized recommendations can be made regarding the medical management of hyperparathyroidism. Patients should

be monitored at 6- to 12-month intervals for evidence of biochemical progression, renal function deterioration, or skeletal demineralization. Patients should be instructed to maintain adequate hydration and encouraged to remain active. Diuretics should be avoided, and thiazide-type diuretcs should not be used at all. Calcium gluttony should be discouraged, but calcium restriction will be of little benefit except to those patients with hypercalciuria or recurrent nephrolithiasis.

Specific recommendations for medical treatment of hyperparathyroidism are controversial. Oral neutral phosphate (1 to 1.5 g elemental phosphorus per day) will usually lower serum calcium and reduce urinary calcium excretion and should reduce the incidence of renal stone complications.[5] Careful follow-up of renal function is essential, as progressive renal failure is the principal complication of this therapy. In postmenopausal females estrogen replacement (0.625 to 2.5 mg/day of conjugated estrogens or 30 μg/day of ethinyl estradiol) may lower serum calcium levels and reduce urinary calcium excretion. Interestingly, serum levels of PTH remain stable while urinary hydroxyproline and serum alkaline phosphatase levels improve. Although bone turnover decreases, the histologic abnormalities of bone do not improve.[28] Several newer-generation bisphosphonates reduce serum calcium concentrations when administered orally and when available may become a practical alternative in patients who must be treated medically.[29]

Special Problems Associated with Management of Primary Hyperparathyroidism

Hypercalcemic Crisis. Occasionally patients with hyperparathyroidism may present with progressive and severe hypercalcemia (in excess of 15 mg/dl) accompanied by dehydration, mental deterioration, and marked weakness. Hypercalcemic crisis leads to uremia and coma within a short period, and it should be treated vigorously medically to reduce the serum calcium before surgery.

Thiazide-associated Hypercalcemia. Transient hypercalcemia may be secondary to decreased extracellular fluid volume following diuresis. Sustained and significant hypercalcemia is unusual. Persistent hypercalcemia while a patient is taking a thiazide diuretic suggests an underlying disorder of mineral metabolism, most frequently primary hyperparathyroidism. The drug should be discontinued and appropriate evaluation begun.

Normocalcemic Hyperparathyrodism. This variant of primary hyperparathyroidism is generally suspected in patients with renal stones or osteoporosis. In general, mild hypercalcemia alternates with normocalcemia, and serum levels of PTH are elevated. Hyperparathyroidism in these patients is either mild or complicated by vitamin D deficiency. Although surgery may benefit those with active stone disease not controlled by medical therapy, it is currently unknown if parathyroidectomy in patients with involutional osteoporosis complicated by hyperparathyroidism results in improvement of the osteopenia.

Persistent or Recurrent Hyperparathyroidism. Persistent or recurrent hyperparathyroidism following an initial surgical approach may be secondary to inadequate surgical technique, failure to recognize multiglandular hyperplasia, or incorrect preoperative diagnosis. It is best not to proceed with mediastinal exploration at the time of initial neck surgery, because although mediastinal tumors account for approximately 20 percent of parathyroid adenomas, 95 percent of them are readily removable through the routine neck exploration. Before proceeding with a second operative procedure, one should attempt to localize the abnormal parathyroid gland(s). Ultrasonography, CT of the neck and mediastinum, selective arteriography of the inferior and superior thyroid arteries, and selective venous catheterization and parathyroid hormone radioimmunoassay on samples collected therefrom should be performed before undertaking further parathyroid surgery.[17]

Postoperative Complications of Parathyroidectomy. Recurrent laryngeal nerve palsy is a rare complication of parathyroid surgery. A decline in blood calcium levels generally occurs within 12 to 24 hours after successful surgery. Hypocalcemia is usually mild and transient, with a return to normal calcium values as the remaining normal parathyroid tissue resumes hormone secretion, usually after 3 to 6 days.

When hyperparathyroidism is complicated by osteitis fibrosa generalisata, removal of the adenoma will usually result in profound hypocalcemia. Presumably calcium and phosphorus available in the serum are taken up into the "hungry bones" for bone formation.

Transient mild hypocalcemia is common, is usually well tolerated, and seldom requires treatment. Symptomatic hypocalcemia and tetany may be treated acutely with oral calcium supplementation and rapid-acting vitamin D metabolites (e.g., $1,25(OH)_2D_3$). Rarely is tetany severe, and intravenous infusion of calcium is required.

Hyperphosphatemia and profound hypophosphaturia are excellent indices of successful surgery. A rapid fall in urinary cyclic AMP can serve as an intraoperative index of successful parathyroidectomy. Determination of urinary cyclic AMP in the postoperative period allows differentiation of hypocalcemia secondary to hypoparathyroidism from that secondary to hungry bones. Permanent hypoparathyroidism occurs in less than 2 percent of cases. Its management is outlined in the section on hypoparathyroidism. Other postoperative complications may include hypomagnesemia and attendant hypoparathyroidism, pancreatitis, gout or pseudogout, and worsening of metabolic acidosis.

Secondary Hyperparathyroidism

The pathogenesis of secondary hyperparathyroidism is low serum ionized calcium in individuals who initially had normally functioning parathyroid glands. Precipitating conditions include insufficient vitamin D intake or production, calcium malabsorption, $1,25(OH)_2D$-deficiency secondary to renal disease, vitamin D malabsorption from the gut, and inborn errors of vitamin D metabolism. Prolonged stimulation of the parathyroids by persistent hypocalcemia may result in hypertrophy of all the glands.

The pathogenesis of hyperparathyroidism secondary to renal failure is complex. With progressive loss of nephrons, there is retention of phosphate. Hyperphosphatemia causes hypocalcemia both by reciprocal reduction in serum calcium by physicochemical mechanisms and by inhibition of the synthesis of $1,25(OH)_2D$, which is already decreased because of loss of functioning renal tissue. Prolonged hypocalcemia leads to hypersecretion of PTH and hypertrophy of the glands. Treatment consists of oral aluminum hydroxide or aluminum carbonate gels to bind phosphate in the gut and hence lower serum phosphate, restriction of dietary phosphate intake, administration of $1,25(OH)_2D_3$, dialysis if necessary, and management of the underlying renal disease. In a few patients, sustained hypercalcemia develops after the renal failure is corrected, especially following renal transplantation. In these instances, involution of the secondary hyperparathyroidism may be incomplete (tertiary hyperparathyroidism). Parathyroidectomy may be necessary in fewer than 10 percent of patients.

Hypercalcemia Associated with Malignant Disease[19]

Hypercalcemia is a common complication of malignant disease. In a survey of 439 patients admitted for radiotherapy of cancer, 9.1 percent had hypercalcemia. The estimated incidence of hypercalcemia associated with malignancy is 150 new cases per million persons per year, and compares with an annual incidence of primary hyperparathyroidism of approximately 250 new cases per million persons.[19] In most instances, the hypercalcemia appears abruptly and late in the course of the disease when the diagnosis is already obvious. In some patients, however, tumor may be occult, and a careful search for the neoplasm is necessary.

Hypercalcemia is not associated with all types of neoplasms. Certain malignancies rarely cause hypercalcemia (e.g., carcinoma of

the female genital tract or carcinomas of the gastrointestinal tract), whereas other malignant tumors are commonly associated with hypercalcemia (e.g., epidermoid cell carcinomas of the head, neck, and lung, and breast carcinoma).

Malignant tumors can produce hypercalcemia by several mechanisms, but in most cases accelerated net bone resorption is believed to be the source of the hypercalcemia. For convenience, malignancy associated hypercalcemia has been classified into three clinical categories on the basis of different underlying pathogenetic mechanisms.

Solid Tumors: Direct Osteolysis by Tumor Cells Metastatic to Bone.
In approximately 40 percent of patients with the hypercalcemia of cancer the mechanism of hypercalcemia is presumably related to the excessive osteolytic destruction that accompanies direct invasion of the bone endosteal surface by metastatic tumor. Although there is evidence that in some cases tumor cells may directly phagocytose bone (e.g., some breast carcinomas), in most instances it is assumed that the tumor cells secrete locally-acting bone-resorbing or osteoclast-activating factors. Several implicated substances, which all stimulate osteoclastic bone resorption, include tumor necrosis factor alpha, lymphotoxin, interleukin-1, and prostaglandin E2.

The most common tumor in this group is breast carcinoma, which accounts for about 50 percent of all patients with hypercalcemia of malignancy. Although most patients display widespread skeletal involvement as evidenced by radiographs or radionuclide bone scans, in some individuals diagnosis may require direct histologic examination of bone or bone marrow. In rare cases tumor cell invasion of bone may be recognized only at postmortem examination.

Solid Tumors: Humoral Hypercalcemia of Malignancy.
The second major group of patients with malignancy associated hypercalcemia are patients with solid tumors without bone metastases. This syndrome, termed the "humoral hypercalcemia of malignancy" (HHM), is responsible for hypercalcemia in about 30 to 40 percent of patients with cancer. It occurs most commonly in patients with squamous cell carcinomas of the head, neck, esophagus, and lung; carcinoma of the pancreas; carcinoma of the ovary; and carcinoma of the kidney or bladder.[32] The cumulative evidence indicates that hypercalcemia is due to production by the malignant cells of humoral factor(s) that increase distant bone resorption.

Because hypercalcemia associated with these tumors is often accompanied by hypophosphatemia and increased excretion of nephrogenous cAMP, which are features of excessive parathyroid hormone, the condition has been called "ectopic hyperparathyroidism." The suggestion that ectopic secretion of parathyroid hormone is responsible for tumor-associated hypercalcemia arose from the early observations that patients with malignant disease and hypercalcemia have increased immunoreactive PTH in the circulation or in tumor extracts. More recent studies have failed to confirm these findings, however, and have documented low or normal serum levels of immunoreactive PTH in several series of hypercalcemic patients. Further evidence against the role of PTH as a mediator of the HHM syndrome is the failure to detect PTH mRNA in tumors from five hypercalcemia patients.[30]

The factor or factors responsible for HHM are currently unknown. Prostaglandins probably do not play a major role. Some patients with HHM show increased excretion of urinary cAMP (consistent with increased PTH-like activity) but are relatively hypercalciuric and have low serum levels of $1,25(OH)_2D$ (both in contrast to the expected PTH-like effects). PTH-like adenylate cyclase–stimulating proteins have been identified by several groups in tumors derived from patients with HHM. These proteins can activate adenylate cyclase in renal and skeletal tissues through interaction with the PTH receptor. One recently characterized 141 amino acid protein has considerable homology to human PTH.

A second class of bone-resorbing factors that have been impli-cated as possible mediators of HHM are the transforming growth factors of the alpha and beta classes.[19] These peptides share some of the mitogenic and osteoclastic properties of epidermal growth factors and platelet-derived growth factors.

Hematologic Malignancies.
Hematologic malignancies are a heterogeneous group of malignancies, in which hypercalcemia may have several causes. Most common is myeloma: hypercalcemia develops in about 30 percent of patients with myeloma, particularly those who have extensive bone destruction. Bone involvement may take the form of osteolytic lesions or diffuse osteopenia. Myeloma cells present in the bone marrow secrete an osteoclast-activating factor that stimulates osteoclasts to resorb bone. This factor (or factors) is a locally-acting lymphokine that is similar to (or identical with) osteoclast-activating factor produced by normal activated lymphocytes. Other hematologic malignancies associated with hypercalcemia and release of an osteoclast-activating factor include Burkitt lymphoma, lymphosarcoma, and adult T cell lymphoma (HTLV I retrovirus).

Patients with lymphoma, primarily of the histiocytic type, may develop hypercalcemia as a result of elevated plasma concentrations of $1,25(OH)_2D_3$.[26] In these cases it is suspected that activated lymphocytes in the lymphoma tissue can, as in sarcoidosis, convert $25(OH)D$ to $1,25(OH)_2D_3$ in an excessive and unregulated manner, causing endogenous vitamin D intoxication.

Finally, coexisting primary hyperparathyroidism may be responsible for hypercalcemia in a patient with a malignancy, and this treatable disorder should not be overlooked.

Vitamin D Intoxication
Vitamin D intoxication is a rare disorder that occurs if doses of vitamin D in excess of 50,000 IU per day are given to normal individuals. The sequence of events may be as follows: (1) increased gastrointestinal absorption of calcium and increased bone resorption, (2) increased serum calcium, (3) suppression of PTH, (4) decreased urinary phosphorus excretion, and, when renal function deteriorates, (5) hyperphosphatemia, and (6) ectopic calcification in soft tissue and viscera. The clinical picture is usually one typical of hypercalcemia. Nausea, vomiting, and dehydration may be prominent, and pruritus is common. The combination of hypercalcemia, hyperphosphatemia, azotemia, and mild alkalosis may be a valuable clue to the diagnosis. The serum levels of $25(OH)D$ are on average five to ten times above normal. Interestingly, serum levels of the active metabolite, $1,25(OH)_2D_3$, are only modestly elevated. Hypercalcemia is attributable to the high levels of $25(OH)D$ and the supranormal levels of $1,25(OH)_2D$. Rarely, hypercalcemia persists as long as 1 year after vitamin D has been stopped. Response to glucocorticoids is usually prompt.

Milk-alkali Syndrome
An unusual complication of peptic ulcer therapy is hypercalcemia consequent to excessive intake of milk (1.5 quarts or greater a day) and absorbable alkali, usually as calcium carbonate. The amount of calcium and alkali reported to produce the syndrome is poorly defined, ranging from 4 to 60 g of calcium carbonate per day. In advanced cases, significant renal failure, phosphate retention, band keratopathy, and ectopic calcification may be present. Renal damage is usually reversible following exclusion of milk and alkali. When hypercalcemia is severe enough to cause alteration of consciousness, glucocorticoids may be required in addition to hydration.

Both the milk-alkali syndrome and vitamin D intoxication are diagnosed by taking a careful history of dietary habits and medications. Medicines obtainable without prescriptions, such as Tums, and vitamin preparations are often not regarded as "medicine" by patients. When possible, family members should be questioned because hypercalcemia can affect the patient's memory.

Sarcoidosis
Hypercalcemia (15 percent) and hypercalciuria (30 percent) are frequently associated with sarcoidosis (see Chapter 3.5). Hyper-

calcemia may also infrequently occur in association with many granulomatous diseases, including tuberculosis, histoplasmosis, cytomegalovirus infection, and the granulomatous reaction to silicone implants. In sarcoidosis the mechanism appears to be excessive, systemic production of $1,25(OH)_2D_3$. The finding of elevated levels of $1,25(OH)_2D$ in an anephric patient with sarcoidosis suggests that 25-hydroxy-1-α hydroxylase activity may be present in sarcoid granulomas.[4] Subsequent studies have demonstrated conversion of $25(OH)D$ to $1,25(OH)_2D_3$ by sarcoid-derived pulmonary alveolar macrophages and lymph node homogenates. In contrast to the tightly regulated activity of the renal 25-hydroxy-1-α hydroxylase, conversion of $25(OH)D$ to $1,25(OH)_2D_3$ in granulomatous tissue appears exclusively substrate-dependent. Thus exposure to small amounts of dietary vitamin D or to solar irradiation, which leads to a physiologic increase in circulating levels of $25(OH)D$, can precipitate hypercalcemia due to excessive production of $1,25(OH)_2D_3$. Patients appear to have hypervitaminosis D: calcium absorption from the gut is enhanced and urinary calcium excretion exaggerated. It is unusual to find sarcoidosis in the process of evaluating a patient with cryptic hypercalcemia. More often, the patient has typical lesions of the skin and lungs, mediastinal adenopathy, or cystic changes in bones, characteristically in the hands. Suspicion of the disorder is raised by finding hyperglobulinemia, hypercalciuria, on an elevated serum angiotensin-converting enzyme level. The diagnosis is confirmed with a Kveim test and biopsy of the involved organ. Glucocorticoid therapy is effective.

Hyperthyroidism

Mild hypercalcemia is associated with hyperthyroidism in 5 to 20 percent of patients as a result of accelerated turnover of bone. When present it is often accompanied by hypercalciuria, phosphaturia, elevation of serum alkaline phosphatase and suppressed levels of serum PTH. Calcium homeostasis is restored when thyrotoxicosis is controlled, and coexistent hyperparathyroidism needs to be considered only if hypercalcemia persists after a euthyroid state is achieved.

Acute Adrenal Insufficiency

Acute adrenal insufficiency may be accompanied by hypercalcemia and hypophosphatemia. The clinical picture is dominated by the features of adrenal steroid deficiency. Hypercalcemia may also appear with acute withdrawal of exogenous corticoids. The cause of the hypercalcemia is not known, but profound dehydration is one of the contributing factors. It resolves with steroid treatment.

Hypercalcemia of Immobilization and Osteoporosis

Hypercalcemia, hypercalciuria, and osteoporosis may occur when patients with active turnover of bone are immobilized. This can be observed in young people and in patients with thyrotoxicosis, Paget disease, or hyperparathyroidism, with immobilization occasionally unmasking previously unsuspected disease. Enhanced bone resorption is responsible for hypercalcemia and hypercalciuria in immoblized patients. Consonant with this mechanism are the findings of elevated calcium excretion, increased fractional renal phosphorus threshold, and suppression of the parathyroid–$1,25(OH)_2D$ axis. If bed confinement is unavoidable, hydration should be maintained, but dietary calcium restriction is without obvious benefit.[31]

Hypercalcemia in Families

Hypercalcemia occurs in several distinct genetic disorders: multiple endocrine neoplasia (MEN) type I, MEN type IIA, and familial hypocalciuric hypercalcemia (FHH) (see Chapter 14.1). Hyperparathyroidism in these autosomal dominant disorders is virtually always attributed to hyperplasia of the parathyroid glands. Distinction among these categories may be made on the basis of information shown in Table 14.6–4. Familial parathyroid hyperplasia without additional endocrine involvement may occur as a distinct genetic entity, but it is likely that variable penetrance and inade-

TABLE 14.6–4. HYPERCALCEMIA IN FAMILIES

	MEN I	MEN IIA	MEN IIB	FHH
Parathyroid hyperplasia	90%	90%	—	>90%
Pancreatic tumor	5%			
Pituitary tumor	65%			
Carcinoid	<5%			
Lipoma	5%			
Adrenal cortical adenoma	5%			
Medullary thyroid carcinoma		90%	90%	
Pheochromocytoma		20%	50%	
Multiple mucosal neuroma			90%	
Marfanoid habitus			90%	

quate evaluation of the patient (and kindred) may explain the absence of other components of the MEN I syndrome. MEN I (Wermer syndrome) is associated with hyperplasia of neuroendocrine cells located principally in the pituitary, pancreas, and parathyroids. Pancreatic tumors in MEN I are frequently multiple and most commonly secrete gastrin, producing the Zollinger-Ellison syndrome (see Chapter 12.3) or insulin, producing profound hypoglycemia (see Chapter 14.8). The pancreatic tumors differ markedly from the other elements of the MEN I syndrome, as gastrinomas and insulinomas may take a malignant course. Pituitary tumors in female patients with MEN I most frequently secrete prolactin. Other pituitary tumors may be nonfunctioning, or, rarely, may secrete ACTH or growth hormone.

A second genetic polyendocrine syndrome associated with parathyroid hyperplasia is Sipple syndrome (MEN IIA). Although parathyroid disease occurs in Sipple syndrome, medullary carcinoma of the thyroid and pheochromocytoma are clinically more worrisome. Whereas parathyroid hyperplasia is a common histologic finding in MEN IIA, hypercalcemia may be present in only 40 percent of patients. Hyperparathyroidism is uncommon in MEN IIB, a similar but genetically distinct syndrome. Pheochromocytomas occurring in association with MEN II may not become obvious until many years after the diagnosis of medullary thyroid carcinoma. Adrenal medullary hyperplasia is a frequent predecessor of the pheochromocytomas seen in MEN II, and is probably responsible for the high (>70 percent) incidence of bilateral and multicentric tumors, in contrast to the solitary adrenal lesion that occurs in sporadic pheochromocytoma.[8]

Another genetic syndrome associated with hypercalcemia is FHH. It is most important to recognize FHH because of its generally benign prognosis and refractoriness to surgical intervention. It is characterized by the following features: (1) autosomal dominant inheritance, with nearly complete penetrance for hypercalcemia before age 10 years, (2) mildly hyperplastic parathyroid glands and generally normal or only mildly elevated serum levels of PTH (lower than in typical primary hyperparathyroidism), and (3) low renal clearance of filtered calcium and magnesium and relative hypocalciuria as a constant finding. The most useful index for diagnosis of FHH is the ratio of the renal clearance of calcium to the renal clearance of creatinine (Ca_{cl}/Cr_{cl}). Patients with FHH typically have Ca_{cl}/Cr_{cl} values that are less than 0.01.[18]

Other Conditions Associated with Hypercalcemia

Hypercalcemia may occur following lithium administration, secondary to vitamin A intoxication, or during the course of acute renal failure secondary to rhabdomyolysis.

Treatment[20]

The decision to treat chronic hypercalcemia should be based on symptoms rather than degree of hypercalcemia, as patients vary considerably in ability to tolerate a given elevation of serum calcium. Acute hypercalcemia and rapidly progressive hypercalcemia (hypercalcemic crisis) can be life threatening, and management constitutes a medical emergency. The most important therapeutic measure, irrespective of the cause, is hydration. Rapid rehydration with normal saline (usual recommendation, 3 L over 9 hours) is important. Sodium enhances calciuria by competitively inhibiting tubular reabsorption of calcium. Calcium excretion can be further enhanced by use of a loop diuretic (e.g., intravenous furosemide, 20 to 80 mg every 2 to 4 hr), after loading with 1 to 2 L of saline and with continued fluid and electrolyte replacement. Because potent loop diuretics can, in poorly hydrated individuals, decrease glomerular filtration rate and actually worsen hypercalcemia, these agents should be used only in patients with an expanded intravascular volume. They are most useful in patients whose cardiovascular tolerance to saline is limited. Thiazide diuretics should never be used because they decrease renal excretion of calcium.

If cardiac or renal function is poor, hydration alone is ineffective and may be hazardous. Plicamycin (mithramycin) is useful in the management of patients with severe hypercalcemia and in those who require urgent therapy. The usual dose is 15 to 25 μg/kg body weight given intravenously as a single bolus injection. It strikingly inhibits bone resorption, producing within 48 hours its hypocalcemic effect, which may persist for several days. If necessary, repeated doses can be given, but toxic effects on bone marrow, liver, and kidney are more likely to develop.

High doses of glucocorticoids (200 mg cortisone or greater per day) are most effective in treating the hypercalcemia of vitamin D intoxication, sarcoidosis, milk-alkali syndrome, lymphoma, breast cancer, multiple myeloma, and, of course, adrenal insufficiency. Generally the onset of action of the steroid is slow. Glucocorticoids increase urinary calcium excretion and decrease intestinal calcium absorption. In addition, glucocorticoids may be effective as antitumor agents. Calcitonin is another hypocalcemic agent that has some use in the management of hypercalcemia. Calcitonin, like plicamycin, inhibits osteoclastic bone resorption; it also increases urinary excretion of calcium. Theoretically it should be an ideal agent; however, when used by itself, it is rarely effective. The concomitant administration of glucocorticoids may prevent "escape" from calcitonin action. The usual dose is 50 to 100 units given subcutaneously at intervals of 6 to 12 hours. Its effect is short-lived and often not marked unless the rate of bone turnover is unusually high. When hypercalcemia is associated with hyperphosphatemia, however, it may be the agent of choice because it also promotes urinary phosphate excretion.

Intravenous infusion of phosphate (1500 mg phosphorus given over 6 to 8 hours) can effectively and reliably reduce serum calcium, primarily by precipitating calcium into bone and soft tissue. Because widespread metastatic calcification, fatal arrhythmias, and irreversible renal damage have been reported as complications of this treatment, it should be used only as a last resort. Oral phosphate therapy has no important role in the acute management of hypercalcemia. Oral administration of phosphate is attended by less acute elevations of serum phosphate and can be used chronically with less danger of soft-tissue calcification.

EDTA administered intravenously effectively lowers ionized calcium by chelation. It too may cause severe renal toxicity. Because therapeutic alternatives are available, its use is no longer warranted. Indomethacin and salicylates in usual therapeutic doses may occasionally be effective in controlling hypercalcemia.

Newer bisphosphonates (e.g., dichloromethylene bisphosphonate) as well as the currently available ethane-1-hydroxy-1, 1-bisphosphonate (EHDP, Didronel) may be useful in treating hypercalcemia secondary to increased bone resorption, that is, hyperparathyroidism or malignancy. The bisphosphonates are analogues of pyrophosphate and thus have a high affinity for bone, particularly in areas of high turnover. Once concentrated in an area of intense metabolic activity, the bisphosphonates are taken up by osteoclasts and inhibit the action of these cells by an unknown mechanism. EHDP is effective in reducing serum calcium levels to the normal range in 75 percent of patients when administered intravenously (7.5 mg/kg) with 3 L of saline as daily infusions for 3 days. Although oral EHDP alone is rarely effective in the treatment of hypercalcemia, when administered orally (5 mg/kg per day) after intravenous EHDP, it can be beneficial in maintaining normocalcemia.[6]

The major agents that lower plasma calcium are listed in Table 14.6–5. In general, a combination of hydration with one of these agents is recommended to manage hypercalcemic crisis.

Patients with far-advanced, well-documented, incurable neoplasms may present with life-threatening hypercalcemia. In such patients, the somnolence induced by hypercalcemia may be a welcome development. The decision to treat, therefore, should depend upon the relative advantages and disadvantages of alternative palliatives and the patient's prognosis. Mild hypercalcemia of malignancy may be left untreated because it may serve as a marker to assess the effects of chemotherapy.

HYPOCALCEMIA

Hypocalcemia develops when either PTH or vitamin D is deficient or defective or when their target tissues fail to respond. Proof of sustained hypocalcemia requires multiple serum calcium determi-

TABLE 14.6–5. COMMONLY USED AGENTS FOR THE MANAGEMENT OF HYPERCALCEMIA

	Onset of Action	Dosage	Comments
Saline hydration and furosemide	Rapid	3 L/9 hr 20 to 80 mg/hr	Reduce serum calcium 2–3 mg/dl but rarely normalize serum calcium, may precipitate congestive heart failure
Mithramycin	Rapid	25 μg/kg body weight, IV push	Effective in all types of hypercalcemia associated with increased bone resorption; toxic to bone, liver, and kidney
Calcitonin	Rapid but not sustained	50–100 MRC U, subcutaneously; aqueous form can be given IV	Ideal for hypercalcemia associated with hyperphosphatemia
Phosphate	Rapid	1500 mg phosphorus given IV 6–8 hr (In-Phos or Hyper-Phos-K)	Effective but may cause soft-tissue calcification
Glucocorticoid	Slow	200–300 mg cortisone acetate	Most useful for vitamin D intoxication, milk-alkali syndrome, myeloma, lymphoma, breast cancer, leukemia
Indomethacin	Slow	100–150 mg/ day	Effective for prostaglandin-associated hypercalcemia

nations. Because serum albumin levels and serum pH can influence the values of serum calcium they should be measured concomitantly for meaningful interpretations. If serum albumin is normal, symptoms of hypocalcemia may not be apparent until serum calcium falls below 7.5 mg/dl. The cardinal clinical manifestation is tetany. Characteristically an attack of tetany is heralded by perioral or acral paresthesias. This may be followed by a feeling of stiffness in the limbs. Muscle cramps and carpopedal spasm next develop. The hands assume a characteristic posture, with the thumbs forced into adduction while the fingers are firmly pressed together with the metacarpophalangeal joints flexed ("obstetrician's hand"). Rarely, laryngeal stridor and seizures may occur. Psychoneurotic manifestations associated with hypocalcemia include emotional lability, anxiety, delirium, and frank psychosis. Symptoms of extrapyramidal or cerebellar lesions, that is, tremor, athetosis, and ataxia, have have reported. Papilledema with or without increased CSF pressure may occur. Long-term complications of untreated hypocalcemia include dry or coarse skin, brittle nails, and growth and mental retardation. Dental and enamel hypoplasia and absence of adult teeth, indicate that hypocalcemia has been present since childhood. Calcification of the basal ganglia and cataracts are noted with hypocalcemia associated with elevated serum levels of phosphate, as occurs in individuals with untreated hypoparathyroidism.

With mild hypocalcemia, spontaneous tetany is usually absent; however, carpopedal spasm may be elicited by compression of nerves in the arm with a sphygmomanometer inflated above the systolic pressure for at least 3 minutes (Trousseau sign). Increased neuromuscular irritability can also be demonstrated by eliciting twitching of facial muscles by tapping the facial nerve (Chvostek sign). Latent tetany may also be precipitated by menstruation, pregnancy, lactation, and exercise. Chvostek sign is present in 10 to 30 percent of normal persons. Serial examinations, therefore, including preoperative evaluation of patients undergoing neck surgery, are often helpful.

Symptoms of overt or latent tetany are dependent on altered muscle membrane stability, which may be mimicked by systemic alkalosis. Accordingly, tetany may also occur with hyperventilation syndrome, alkali ingestion, hypokalemia, and magnesium deficiency. Serum electrolytes and a careful history usually suffice to differentiate the causes (Fig. 14.6–3).

Causes

Hypocalcemia usually reflects deficient PTH secretion, deficient generation of active vitamin D metabolites, or both. Less commonly, hypocalcemia may be a manifestation of reduced target-organ sensitivity to these hormones or the result of secretion of ineffective PTH. Hypocalcemia of diverse and uncertain etiology may also accompany acute medical events such as pancreatitis, fat embolism, rhabdomyolysis, sepsis, or hepatic failure. Hypermagnesemia may cause hypocalcemia because this divalent cation inhibits PTH secretion. Paradoxically, hypomagnesemia of any cause may also be associated with hypocalcemia, because of reversible interference with either parathyroid gland secretion or target-tissue responsiveness to PTH.[2] The clinical and biochemical features of hypocalcemia depend on the nature of the underlying abnormality, but the disorder can usually be assigned to one of six general classifications (Table 14.6–6). Hypocalcemia secondary to low serum albumin does not present a clinical problem because ionized calcium levels are usually normal. Simultaneous measurement of serum proteins should always be obtained to exclude such pseudohypocalcemia. A normal ionized serum calcium level excludes true hypocalcemia. Hypocalcemic agents, such as mithramycin, calcitonin, phosphate, and EDTA, can cause hypocalcemia when used inappropriately.

Hypoparathyroidism.[22] Primary hypoparathyroidism occurs most commonly following parathyroid, thyroid, or neck cancer surgery and in patients who develop idiopathic disease. Transient hypoparathyroidism and hypocalcemia are frequent after parathyroidectomy, especially in patients with markedly hyperfunctioning parathyroid glands (see section on postoperative complications of parathyroidectomy). In addition, thyroid surgery for cancer or

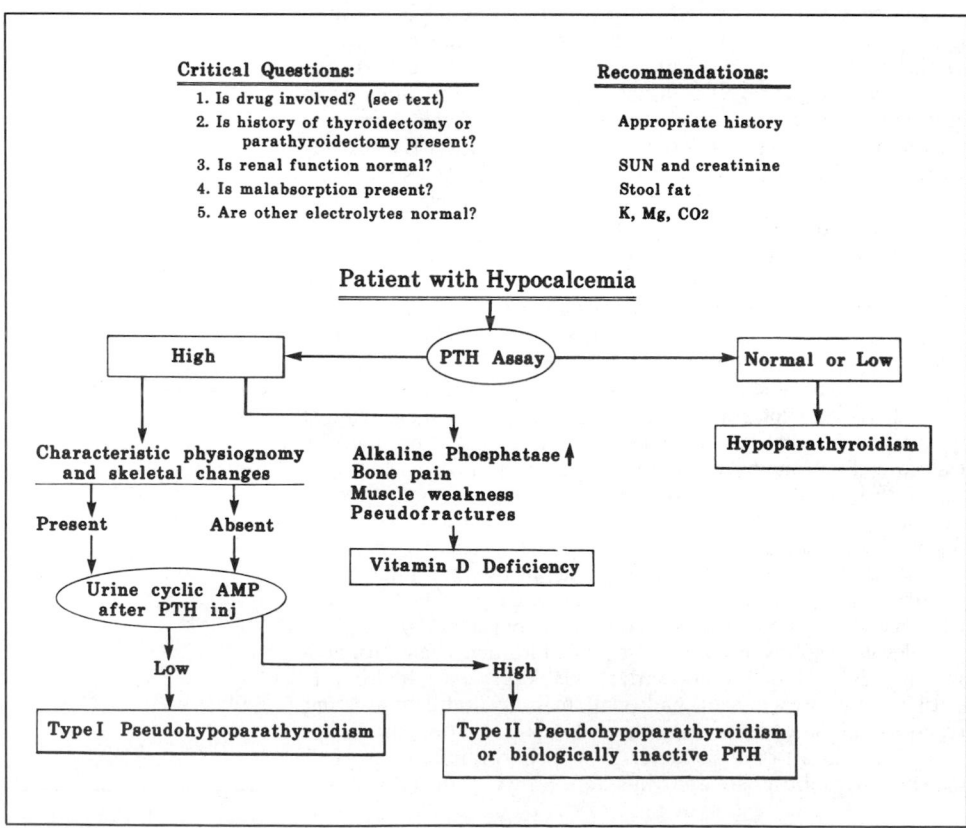

Figure 14.6–3. Differential diagnosis of hypocalcemia. Extensive study is usually not necessary in patient with surgical hypoparathyroidism.

TABLE 14.6–6. BIOCHEMICAL CHARACTERISTICS IN CATEGORIES OF HYPOCALCEMIA

Diagnosis	Serum PTH	Serum Phosphate	Urinary cAMP	Serum 25(OH)D	Serum 1,25(OH)$_2$D
PTH deficiency	Low[a]	High	Low	Normal	Low
PTH resistance (PHP type I)	High[a]	High	Low[a]	Normal	Low
cAMP resistance (PHP type II)	High[a]	Normal to high	High[a]	Normal	Low
25(OH)D deficiency	High	Low	High	Low[a]	Low to normal
1,25(OH)$_2$D deficiency	High	Low	High	Normal	Low[a]
1,25(OH)$_2$D resistance	High	Low	High	Normal	High[a]

[a]Critical index for diagnosis

Graves disease is frequently accompanied by mild hypocalcemia. Spontaneous recovery is the rule, but hypocalcemia may recur and become permanent many months or years later. The incidence of surgical hypoparathyroidism is decreasing and in experienced hands is probably less than 2 percent. Idiopathic hypoparathyroidism may be an autoimmune phenomenon analogous to autoimmune thyroiditis and adrenal failure, because antibodies to parathyroid tissue have been demonstrated. This entity is usually detected in childhood. It has been reported in sibs and may occur as a component of type I polyglandular autoimmune syndrome, in which it may be associated with primary adrenal insufficiency, moniliasis, diabetes mellitus, hypothyroidism, pernicious anemia, chronic hepatitis, malabsorption, and hypogonadism. In some patients the onset of idiopathic hypoparathyroidism may occur in adult life. Recent evidence suggests that some patients possess antibodies that inhibit the secretion of PTH rather than cause parathyroid gland destruction. Congenital absence of the parathyroids and thymus, resulting from maldevelopment of the third and fourth branchial pouches, occurs in DiGeorge syndrome. Rarely the parathyroid glands are affected by infiltrative processes, for example, metastatic disease and hemochromatosis.

In the absence of PTH, serum phosphorus rises and both factors contribute to impaired 1-α-hydroxylation of 25(OH)D. In these circumstances, calcium absorption from the gut is low, the rate of bone resorption is decreased, and calcium fails to be normally resorbed by the renal tubules. As a consequence, hypocalcemia results.

Hypoparathyroidism Due to Defective PTH. This disorder apparently results from production of an immunogically active but biologically inactive form of PTH. Clinically, it is indistinguishable from hypoparathyroidism except that PTH is detected by radioimmunoassay. This condition is not associated with autoimmune endocrinopathies.[1]

Familial Hypoparathyroidism. Hypoparathyroidism caused by deficient secretion of PTH occurs rarely as a distinct genetic syndrome. Patients do not have evidence of an autoimmune disorder, associated endocrinopathies, or a secondary destructive process of the parathyroid glands. The onset of hyperphosphatemia and hypocalcemia is usually within the first decade of life, but clinical recognition may be delayed until later. The cause of hypoparathyroidism is at present unknown but may involve heterogeneous defects in synthesis, production, or secretion of PTH. The pattern of inheritance may be X-linked, autosomal recessive, or autosomal dominant. In some individuals hypoparathyroidism may be caused by an alteration in or near the structural gene for PTH.[1]

Secondary Hypoparathyroidism. Hypomagnesemia reversibly inhibits PTH secretion. When profound, it produces typical hypocalcemia and hyperphosphatemia, and tetany may result. An element of peripheral resistance to PTH and vitamin D may also be present in some patients. Measurement of serum magnesium is, therefore, essential in the evaluation of all hypocalcemic patients.[2]

Pseudohypoparathyroidism. The term "pseudohypoparathyroidism" (PHP) is used for a group of diverse endocrine syndromes that share the feature of resistance of the target organs, bone and kidney, to the biologic actions of PTH. Patients with PHP display the biochemical features of hypoparathyroidism, hypocalcemia, and hyperphosphatemia, despite circulating levels of PTH, which are generally high. In addition, patients do not respond to exogenous parathyroid hormone with hypercalcemia or phosphaturia. The biologic action of PTH is mediated by cyclic AMP, and patients with PHP type I exhibit a markedly blunted nephrogenous cyclic AMP response to intravenous infusion of PTH in comparison with normal individuals and patients with other forms of hypoparathyroidism. This observation suggests that PHP type I is caused by a biochemical defect proximal to cyclic AMP generation, that is, in the plasma-membrane-bound hormone receptor-adenylate cyclase complex. Integral components of the adenylate cyclase complex are the guanine nucleotide-binding regulatory (G or N) proteins that couple hormone receptors to the catalytic unit of the enzyme. At least two G proteins are associated with adenylate cyclase, one of which (Gs) mediates stimulation of enzyme activity, while the other (Gi) is responsible for inhibition. Although hormone receptors are target-cell-specific, the G proteins appear to be common to the adenylate-cyclase complex of most tissues. Patients with PHP type Ia have reduced Gs in membranes prepared from many tissues.[8,14] Deficient membrane Gs activity is associated with decreased responsiveness of diverse tissues (e.g., kidney, thyroid, gonad, and liver) to tropic hormones (e.g., PTH, TSH, gonadotropin, and glucagon) that act via activation of adenylate cyclase and lead to reduced accumulation of intracellular cyclic AMP in response to hormonal stimulation. Patients with PHP type Ia manifest a syndrome of hormone resistance generalized to multiple tissues, presumably on the basis of a genetic deficiency of Gs. Patients with normal Gs activity (PHP type Ib) generally manifest hormone resistance limited to PTH target tissues. The defect in PHP type Ib may reside in the PTH receptor.[15]

Another variant of PHP is one in which patients respond to PTH with a brisk increase in nephrogenous cyclic AMP excretion but fail to increase their excretion of phosphate. These patients are probably resistant to cAMP. This disorder is called type II pseudohypoparathyroidism, and hormone resistance appears to be limited to PTH.

In addition to the biochemical abnormalities, many patients with PHP exhibit a unique somatic appearance, referred to as Albright hereditary osteodystrophy (AHO), which encompasses multiple developmental defects: (1) round face, short neck, and stocky build; (2) one or more short metacarpals or metatarsals; and (3) foci of subcutaneous ossification. Patients who show the features of AHO but who lack any evidence of hormone resistance are considered to have pseudo-pseudohypoparathyroidism (PPHP). Patients with PPHP who are members of a PHP Ia kindred also have reduced Gs levels, thus suggesting that a single gene may be responsible for both disorders.[20]

There is failure of 1-hydroxylation of 25(OH)D in PHP. As a result, absorption of calcium is decreased and osteomalacia may

develop. The impaired formation of $1,25(OH)_2D$ from $25(OH)D$ suggests that the suppressive effects of hyperphosphatemia can override the stimulatory effects of PTH on the 1-hydroxylation or that tissue resistance to PTH includes a refractoriness of renal $25(OH)D-1$-hydroxylase activity. The fact that osteomalacia, osteitis fibrosa, or subperiosteal resorption may develop in a small number of patients indicates that bone cells are not always totally refractory to PTH. This conclusion is supported by the observation that administration of $1,25(OH)_2D_3$ to patients with PHP restores the normal skeletal response to PTH.

Variable expressivity and inadequate family studies have complicated analysis of the genetics of PHP. Examples of both X-linked and autosomal patterns of inheritance have been reported and probably reflect the genetic heterogeneity of this group of disorders.

Vitamin D and Hypocalcemia. Vitamin D deficiency, due to diet or impaired conversion of vitamin D to $1,25(OH)_2D$, can result in failure of bone to mineralize normally. Profound hypocalcemia is unusual in vitamin D-deficient disorders because compensatory hyperparathyroidism occurs. Severe forms may present with diffuse bone pain and muscle weakness. Suggestive laboratory findings include hypophosphatemia, hyperphosphatasia, and low to low-normal serum and urinary calcium. Radiologically, osteopenia or biconcave-shaped vertebrae may be evident, but the most characteristic finding is the presence of Looser zones, also known as pseudofractures or Milkman lines. The major conditions related to vitamin D deficiency are listed in Table 14.6–7. In the United States, dietary vitamin D deficiency is not a major cause of osteomalacia. It is a well-recognized complication, however, of intestinal malabsorption, gastric surgery, chronic laxative abuse, hepatic disease, renal failure, and long-term treatment with either phenytoin or barbiturates.

Treatment

Acute severe hypocalcemia associated with tetany or seizures requires intravenous administration of calcium. In the adult, symptoms are usually relieved by a single bolus of 10 to 20 ml of 10 percent calcium gluconate injected slowly intravenously. There-after 0.5 to 2.0 mg calcium/kg body weight may be infused per hour with serum calcium levels closely monitored.

Chronic hypoparathyroidism is treated with a combination of oral calcium and vitamin D. Elemental calcium, 1.5 to 2.0 g per day, is given as lactate, gluconate, or carbonate salts. To provide 1 g of elemental calcium, 8 g of calcium lactate, 11 g of calcium gluconate, or 2.6 g of calcium carbonate must be administered. In the absence of PTH and in the presence of hyperphosphatemia, pharmacologic doses of vitamin D of the order of 50,000 IU (1.25 mg) per day (but this may vary from 25,000 to 200,000 IU per day) are required to control hypocalcemia. The daily therapeutic dosage of $1,25(OH)_2D_3$ is much lower: 0.5 to 1 μg. The dose of vitamin D may have to be reduced if the patient is concomitantly receiving thiazide diuretics or if hyperthyroidism or adrenal insufficiency is present. Higher doses may be necessary when the patient is on a diet rich in phosphate or is taking tranquilizers or estrogen preparations.

The therapeutic goal is to relieve symptoms of hypocalcemia (tetany) and maintain serum calcium in low to normal range (8.5 to 9.5 mg/dl). In the absence of PTH, tubular reabsorption of calcium is diminished and nephrocalcinosis and deterioration of renal function subsequent to massive hypercalciuria may occur if the treatment is too vigorous. To maintain eucalcemia without inducing hypercalciuria, 50 mg per day of chlorthalidone orally plus a low-salt diet (50 mEq/day) appears to be an effective alternative or adjunct to vitamin D in some patients with hypoparathyroidism.

Osteomalacia or hypocalcemia in epileptics taking anticonvulsants may be initially managed with 50,000 to 75,000 units of vitamin D per week in divided doses plus supplemental calcium. After normalization of biochemical and skeletal abnormalities, patients can be maintained on 5000 to 10,000 units of vitamin D per week. Acute hypomagnesemia can be managed by the intravenous administration of 1 to 2 g of magnesium (usually in the form of magnesium sulfate) as a 10 percent solution. Oral magnesium is best given in the form of magnesium oxide, 35 to 70 mEq per day. Dietary vitamin D deficiency can be treated with as little as 100 IU of vitamin D per day.

TABLE 14.6–7. CAUSES OF OSTEOMALACIA SYNDROMES

Disorders of vitamin D

Inadequate vitamin D supply
- Dietary deficiency
- Malabsorption syndrome (gastric surgery, laxative abuse, pancreatic insufficency, cholestyramine)

Impaired metabolism of vitamin D
- 25-Hydroxylation defect
  Phenytoin, barbiturate administration
  Cholestatic liver disease
- 1-Hydroxylation defect
  Hypoparathyroidism and pseudohypoparathyroidism
  Renal failure
  Hereditary vitamin D–dependent rickets
  Oncogenous osteomalacic syndrome

Target-organ resistance to $1,25(OH)_2D$
- Uremia
- Phenytoin and barbiturate administration
- Primary resistance to $1,25(OH)_2D$

Phosphate deficiency
- Familial hypophosphatemic rickets
- Acquired hypophosphatemic rickets

Hypophosphatasia

Defects in formation of bone matrix

Drug-induced
- Fluorides
- Diphosphonate

METABOLIC BONE DISEASE

Disorders that alter the bone remodeling process lead to abnormal bone structure. Metabolic bone disease, therefore, can be produced by abnormalities of any of the following: (1) $1,25(OH)_2D$; (2) PTH; (3) phosphorus metabolism; (4) calcium metabolism; (5) collagen synthesis; (6) osteoprogenitor cell activity; (7) osteocyte activity; and, probably, (8) calcitonin.

In most instances there is a single principal cause of a metabolic disorder. The interrelationships between factors controlling bone and mineral metabolism, however, may obscure this cause when homeostatic mechanisms come into play that produce their own biochemical abnormalities.

CLASSIFICATION

Metabolic bone disease includes any disorder in which the process of bone remodeling is altered to the extent that abnormal bone structure results. Radiographically it may present as porous or dense bone. The most common osteopenic conditions are osteoporosis (loss of bone mass), osteomalacia (failure of calcification of osteoid), and osteitis fibrosa cystica (see section on hyperparathyroidism). Radiographically dense bone is observed in osteopetrosis, osteosclerosis, and Paget's disease. Polyostotic fibrous dysplasia is another disease of unknown etiology. Radiologic examination of bone characteristically shows patchy, cystlike lesions in the cortex or ground-glass appearance in the expanded cortex.

LABORATORY EVALUATION[3]

Metabolic bone disease can be evaluated:

1. radiographically to demonstrate gross alterations in bone
2. histologically by examining nondecalcified sections of bone that have been "labeled" at mineralization zones with tetracycline
3. biochemically by measuring serum and urine calcium, phosphorus, and magnesium
4. by measuring serum levels of osseous alkaline phosphatase (index of the pyrophosphatase activity of the osteoblast) to assess bone formation, and urinary hydroxyproline excretion rate to evaluate bone resorption
5. by measuring humoral factors that regulate bone remodeling, such as vitamin D and its metabolites, PTH, calcitonin, and prostaglandins

The serum alkaline phosphatases are enzymes that originate in bone, liver, kidney, gut, and placenta. Elevated serum alkaline phosphatase activity is found in normal growing children and in pregnancy, but when due to disease it is most commonly from bone or liver. Although enzyme thermostability can be used to distinguish bone- (heat-labile) and liver- (heat-stable) derived isoenzymes of alkaline phosphatase, the most practical method of discrimination is to measure serum 5′ nucleotidase activity. Hepatobiliary disorders that elevate hepatic alkaline phosphatase are also associated with increased serum 5′ nucleotidase activity. Accordingly, an increased serum alkaline phosphatase and a normal 5′ nucleotidase indicate that the alkaline phosphatase activity originates from bone. Hydroxyproline-containing peptides are released and excreted in the urine as a consequence of collagen breakdown. As the skeleton contains 55 to 60 percent of total body collagen, increased bone resorption is invariably associated with an increase in the rate of urinary hydroxyproline excretion. Care in the interpretation of values is essential. Excretion normally varies with age, being greatest in the first year and at puberty and lowest in adulthood (15 to 50 mg/24 hr). It may be raised when dietary intake of gelatin or collagen is high or with increased extraskeletal collagen turnover secondary to burns, Cushing syndrome, or psoriasis.

OSTEOMALACIA AND RICKETS[10]

In the adult, failure to mineralize bone osteoid results in soft and pliable bones. These abnormally calcified bones are termed "osteomalacic." Rickets refers to a similar condition in children in which mineralization is defective in both bone and cartilage. Because endochondrial skeletal growth is incomplete in growing children, rickets frequently results in clinically recognizable bone deformities. Parietal flattening and frontal bossing of the skull and softening of the calvaria (craniotabes) may be present. Prominence of the costochondral junctions ("rachitic rosary") and indentations of the lower ribs (Harrison grooves) may impair respiration. Because linear bone growth has ceased in the adult, gross skeletal abnormalities are rare in osteomalacia. The clinical manifestations of osteomalacia are subtle and often difficult to recognize. Moderate to severe forms may present with diffuse muscle weakness and bone pain. In extreme instances of vitamin D deficiency, hypocalcemia may produce tetany. In the elderly, osteomalacia may occur with senile osteoporosis. Because uncomplicated osteoporosis is usually painless, the presence of pain in a patient with radiographic evidence of osteopenia suggests that osteomalacia may also be present. Radiographically, generalized porosity of bone and biconcave-shaped vertebral bodies may be present, because of associated osteoporosis.

Looser zones are infrequently seen but are almost pathognomonic of osteomalacia. Looser zones represent areas of linear decalcification along the course of large blood vessels and are frequently found symmetrically distributed in the scapulae, pelvis, and proximal long bones. When secondary hyperparathyroidism persists, bone changes such as subperiosteal erosions, cysts, and osteitis fibrosa cystica may occur. In children, there is a widening and irregularity of the epiphysis. Cupping of the metaphysis, fractures, and bowing of bones may develop. Definitive diagnosis of osteomalacia or rickets is made by examination of nondecalcified sections of bone. To determine the rate and extent of calcification of bone matrix, tetracyline is administered to the patient in two pulses prior to bone biopsy in order to "label" the areas of active osteoid mineralization. Characteristic findings include (1) widened osteoid seams, (2) decreased rate of osteoid mineralization, and (3) a low appositional rate.

The defect in mineralization that occurs in osteomalacia may arise from lack of $1,25(OH)_2D$ or its effects, deficiency of calcium or phosphate, or a defect in production of alkaline phosphatase and bone matrix (Table 14.6–7). The laboratory findings in rickets and osteomalacia vary with the different underlying disorders. The serum calcium may be normal or low, serum phosphorus may be normal or low depending upon the absence or presence of secondary hyperparathyroidism, and serum alkaline phosphatase activity is generally elevated. Secondary hyperparathyroidism develops in vitamin D deficiency or resistance, and serum levels of immunoreactive PTH will be increased. Serum levels of $25(OH)D$ and $1,25(OH)_2D_3$ may be normal, elevated, or reduced depending upon the underlying pathophysiology.

Nutritional Osteomalacia

The daily requirement of dietary vitamin D is approximately 100 IU. In the United States and many other industrialized nations dairy products are fortified with vitamin D, and nutritional deprivation of this vitamin has not been regarded as an important cause of osteomalacia. In the absence of an exogenous supply, vitamin D must be formed endogenously through UV irradiation of the precursor 7-dehydrocholesterol in the skin. In elderly persons who have eaten sparingly and have little or no exposure to sunlight, osteomalacia may be more common than generally appreciated. Clearly, vitamin D deficiency occurs in patients with intestinal malabsorption, gastrectomy, pancreatic insufficiency, chronic obstructive jaundice, laxative abuse, and long-term administration of cholestyramine. Interruption of enterohepatic circulation of $25(OH)D$ may be an important mechanism of vitamin D deficiency associated with gastrointestinal and hepatobiliary disease. Serum levels of $25(OH)D$ are generally reduced. Circulating levels of $1,25(OH)_2D_3$ are generally reduced, but may be normal (because of secondary hyperparathyroidism and increased activity of renal $25(OH)$-1-α-hydroxylase) in some patients with intestinal malabsorption. In these patients hypocalcemia may also occur as a result of inadequate intestinal absorbing surface.

Disorders of Vitamin D Metabolism

Abnormal availability or effectiveness of $1,25(OH)_2D$, the active metabolite of vitamin D, can arise as the result of disease in three organs:

1. The liver, where 25-hydroxylation of cholecalciferol occurs
2. The kidney, where 1-hydroxylation of $25(OH)D$ takes place
3. The intestine, where $1,25(OH)_2D$ stimulates calcium absorption

Defects of 25-Hydroxylation of Vitamin D. The serum concentration of $25(OH)D$ is dependent primarily on diet and exposure to sunlight. Severe hepatic disease can diminish the production of $25(OH)D$ in one of two ways: by disrupting its enterohepatic circulation or by destruction of tissue that normally produces 25-hydroxylase. Osteomalacia is an infrequent complication of liver disease, but serum $25(OH)D$ concentrations are low in some patients with parenchymal and cholestatic disease. Although the dis-

eased liver is usually able to convert some administered vitamin D to its 25-hydroxylated metabolite, complete healing of undermineralized osteoid may require oral administration of 25(OH)D.

Patients on long-term anticonvulsant treatment with phenytoin and phenobarbital may develop osteomalacia. In many, circulating levels of serum 25(OH)D are decreased, presumably because of accelerated metabolic destruction of both cholecalciferol and 25(OH)D. Serum levels of 1,25(OH)$_2$D are usually normal, however. Therefore, osteomalacia is most likely secondary to either a direct suppressive effect of anticonvulsants on the action of 1,25(OH)$_2$D on gut absorption of calcium or a deficiency of 25(OH)D, which may also be required to promote normal mineralization of bone.

Defects of 1-Hydroxylation of 25(OH)D

Renal Osteodystrophy. Metabolic bone disease is inevitable in patients with chronic renal failure. In approximately 50 to 80 percent of patients, the bones show pathologic changes that are a complex mixture of varying degrees of osteomalacia, osteitis fibrosa generalisata, and osteosclerosis. The pathogenesis of renal osteodystrophy remains unclear, but it is certain that impaired metabolism of vitamin D and secondary hyperparathyroidism play a role.

Plasma levels of 25(OH)D are normal in most patients with renal failure but the concentrations of 1,25(OH)$_2$D are usually low. The severely damaged kidney is incapable of synthesizing adequate amounts of 1,25(OH)$_2$D, despite elevated levels of serum PTH. Renal 25(OH)D-1-hydroxylase activity is reduced by the inhibitory effect of chronic hyperphosphatemia and by a deficiency of enzyme secondary to loss of renal parenchyma. As a result, intestinal calcium absorption is decreased, hypocalcemia develops, and PTH secretion is stimulated. Although this cascade of events accounts for the presence of osteomalacia and osteitis fibrosa in renal osteodystrophy, it does not explain why osteomalacia is inconsistently observed. That a defect in 1-hydroxylation of 25(OH)D exists is consistent with the dramatic improvement in uremic patients after administration of 1,25(OH)$_2$D$_3$. Nearly physiologic doses of 1,25(OH)$_2$D$_3$ (about 1 µg/day) will correct calcium malabsorption and return serum calcium and PTH to normal. However, frequently the improvement in osteomalacia is only partial. In some patients with sufficient functioning renal tissue, vigorous control of hyperphosphatemia alone may result in return of 1,25(OH)$_2$D levels to normal.

Patients with renal osteodystrophy can have predominately hyperparathyroid bone disease, low-turnover osteomalacia, or mixed uremic osteodystrophy. Even though these groups do not represent fully separate entities, it is worthwhile to distinguish the dominant bone lesion so that therapy can be prescribed according to the underlying pathophysiology. In many patients with renal osteodystrophy, stainable aluminum may be found at the bone mineralization front. Aluminum may accumulate in other tissues as well, including the parathyroid glands, where it can result in decreased PTH secretion and suppression of bone turnover. Possible sources of aluminum include drinking water or water used for dialysis, prescription of aluminum hydroxide gels as phosphate binders, and other foods.

Optimally treatment of renal osteodystrophy should begin before the patient develops severe bone disease. Secondary hyperparathyroidism can be prevented by careful maintenance of normal serum levels of calcium and phosphate. Hyperphosphatemia may be controlled by reducing dietary phosphate intake and decreasing intestinal absorption of phosphate. Calcium carbonate may be as effective as aluminum hydroxide in decreasing phosphate absorption and has the benefit of avoiding aluminum toxicity. Oral administration of 1,25(OH)$_2$D$_3$ or dihydrotachysterol, vitamin D compounds that do not require renal metabolism for bioactivity, should be used with calcium supplements to maintain normal serum calcium levels and to prevent or reverse secondary hyperparathyroidism. Surgical reduction of parathyroid mass may be necessary in debilitating predominant hyperparathyroid bone disease, particularly if accompanied by spontaneous hypercalcemia, hyper-

phosphatemia, or progressive extraosseous calcifications. Low-turnover osteomalacia may develop after total parathyroidectomy or subtotal parathyroidectomy in patients with excessive bone aluminum. Because low-turnover osteomalacia is associated with severe aluminum accumulation in bone, intravenous therapy with deferoxamine should be beneficial for these patients.

As uremia progresses, muscle weakness, bone pain, and arthralgias may become prominent; parathyroid gland hyperplasia develops; and serum phosphate may become inappropriately elevated relative to calcium levels. As a consequence, there is a predisposition for metastatic calcification to occur in subcutaneous tissues and conjunctivae. Calcium phosphate crystals in the conjunctivae are responsible for the "red eyes" observed in patients with far-advanced uremia. Successful renal transplantation results in a return of 1,25(OH)$_2$D levels to normal, but parathyroid hyperplasia may persist and cause posttransplantation hypercalcemia. Whether pretreatment with 1,25(OH)$_2$D$_3$ to restore calcium homeostasis to normal can prevent the occurrence of hypercalcemia after transplantation remains to be seen.

Hypoparathyroidism and Pseudohypoparathyroidism. Deficiency of, or resistance to, PTH is attended by reduced concentrations of 1,25(OH)$_2$D.

Two mechanisms are responsible for the lower capacity of the renal 25(OH)D-1-hydroxylase system in patients with functional hypoparathyroidism: (1) loss of the stimulatory effect of PTH and (2) direct inhibition of enzyme activity by elevated levels of phosphate. Aberrant vitamin D metabolism probably accounts for the fact that patients with these conditions are relatively resistant to vitamin D. Whereas correction of hypocalcemia requires pharmacologic doses of ergocalciferol, physiologic amounts of 1,25(OH)$_2$D$_3$ are effective. Despite low blood levels of 1,25(OH)$_2$D in hypoparathyroidism, osteomalacia is rare. Conceivably, elevated serum levels of phosphate may prevent osteomalacia. Alternatively, full expression of the bone lesion may require PTH.

Hereditary Disorders of Vitamin D Metabolism. Vitamin D dependency (pseudo–vitamin D deficiency) is an uncommon autosomal recessive disorder. Affected individuals clinically manifest the typical abnormalities of early-onset nutritional rickets, with hypocalcemia, secondary hyperparathyroidism, and hypophosphatemia. Patients with vitamin D dependency are unresponsive, however, to amounts of exogenous vitamin D or 25(OH)D that are effective in nutritional vitamin D deficiency. In the type I disorder, physiologic amounts of 1,25(OH)$_2$D$_3$ (1 µg) are sufficient to correct the metabolic abnormalities. These findings, together with the observation that blood levels of 1,25(OH)$_2$D are low in these patients, suggest that the basic defect in this disorder is the failure of 1-hydroxylation of 25(OH)D. In type II vitamin D-dependent rickets circulating levels of 1,25(OH)$_2$D are elevated. This represents a decrease or absence of target sensitivity to 1,25(OH)$_2$D. Most cases exhibit total alopecia and autosomal recessive transmission.

Target-tissue Resistance to 1,25(OH)$_2$D. Osteomalacia may result from target-tissue (intestine, bone, and kidney) unresponsiveness to 1,25(OH)$_2$D. In uremic patients, in addition to deficient production of 1,25(OH)$_2$D, intestinal response to 1,25(OH)$_2$D is diminished. Similarly, elevated levels of glucocorticoids can lead to intestinal resistance to 1,25(OH)$_2$D. Another example of end-organ unresponsiveness to vitamin D is in patients treated with anticonvulsants, particularly phenobarbital and phenytoin. Both drugs, in addition to altering the metabolism of vitamin D, inhibit bone resorption that is normally stimulated by PTH and 1,25(OH)$_2$D. As noted above, type II vitamin D-dependent rickets may result from resistance to 1,25-(OH)$_2$D$_3$.[16]

Therapeutic Implications of Metabolic Disorders of Vitamin D Metabolism

1,25(OH)$_2$D$_3$ is clinically effective in most vitamin D-resistant conditions. This compound has the following advantages:

1. Its onset of action is rapid (normocalcemia may be restored in 3 to 7 days in contrast to 4 to 8 weeks for ergocalciferol).
2. Its toxic effects subside more quickly than other vitamin D preparations (3 to 5 days in contrast to 6 to 18 weeks for ergocalciferol and 4 to 12 weeks for 25(OH)D).
3. It bypasses vitamin D hydroxylation abnormalities that may exist in the liver or kidney.

Only in patients with end-organ resistance and in some patients with renal osteodystrophy are suboptimal responses observed.

The recommended daily dose of $1,25(OH)_2D_3$ is 0.25 to 0.50 μg. This, however, may be increased to 1 to 2 μg per day, depending on the clinical indications.

Another useful agent is dihydrotachysterol (DHT). This synthetic substance is a sterol that has a 3-hydroxyl group sterically positioned in such a way that it mimics the position of the 1-hydroxyl of $1(OH)D$ and $1,25(OH)_2D$. DHT requires 25 hydroxylation in the liver but is fully active in the absence of functioning kidneys. It has proved to be a useful substitute for the active derivatives of cholecalciferol. A daily dose of 1 mg of DHT is usually sufficient.

Osteomalacia of Phosphate Deficiency

Chronic hypophosphatemia may lead to florid rickets or osteomalacia. Hypophosphatemia often accompanies Fanconi syndrome or other defects in proximal tubular function. Most commonly, however, chronic fasting hypophosphatemia is secondary to the disorder X-linked hereditary hypophosphatemia (XLH; also termed "vitamin D-resistant rickets" or "phosphate diabetes"). In XLH serum levels of PTH as well as serum concentration of both 25(OH)D and $1,25(OH)_2D$ are normal. Because the level of $1,25(OH)_2D$ might be expected to be elevated in the presence of hypophosphatemia, however, a defect in regulation of renal 25(OH)-1-hydroxylase has been suggested to be an additional component of this syndrome. XLH usually presents in childhood with growth failure and rickets.

Patients with XLH rarely manifest muscular weakness, and in some patients spontaneous clinical (but not histological) remission may occur in adulthood. Aggressive therapy with inorganic phosphorous and high doses of $1,25(OH)_2D_3$ (2-4 μg/day) will often reverse osteomalacia. Despite administration of $1,25(OH)_2D_3$, in some patients secondary (or primary) hyperparathyroidism develops in response to phosphate.

Nonfamilial adulthood hypophosphatemic osteomalacia is rare. In contrast to XLH, myopathy is often present. Presenting symptoms include muscle weakness, bone pain, and frequent fractures of long bones. Because slow-growing tumors such as angiomas, sarcomas, and hemangiomas can produce a similar condition, even when small, a search should be carried out to exclude them. The treatment is inorganic phosphate salts at doses equivalent to 1 to 4 g of elemental phosphorous per day at 4-hour intervals. The concomitant administration of physiologic doses of $1,25(OH)_2D_3$ improves bone mineralization and enables the use of lower amounts of phosphate.

Tumor Osteomalacia

A number of neoplasms, including giant cell, mesenchymal, angiomatous, and sarcomatous tumors, produce hypophosphatemic rickets and osteomalacia clinically indistinguishable from hereditary hypophosphatemic rickets. Usually the tumors are benign. Analogous disturbances have also occurred in patients with fibrous dysplasia of bone, neurofibromatosis, and metastatic carcinoma of the breast or prostate. The metabolic bone lesions heal upon removal of the tumor but also regress with administration of high doses of $1,25(OH)_2D_3$. Characteristically, blood levels of 25(OH)D are normal but $1,25(OH)_2D$ values are low. These tumors of connective-tissue origin may produce a substance that inhibits 1-hydroxylation of 25(OH)D.

Familial Hypophosphatasia

Hypophosphatasia is a rare metabolic bone disease of variable severity. Its most severe form, infantile hypophosphatasia, is an autosomal recessive trait, which is frequently fatal by age 1 to 2 years. Childhood hypophosphatasia, a less severe form of the disorder, presents after 6 months of age and causes retarded growth, premature loss of deciduous teeth, pseudofractures, and rickets with a highly variable course. An autosomal dominant adult type of hypophosphatasia is the least severe form of the disorder and is characterized by loss of deciduous teeth in childhood and early loss or extraction of adult teeth and osteomalacia. Skeletal disease may not be clinically apparent in some patients.

A low serum concentration of alkaline phosphatase is characteristic of all forms of hypophosphatasia and is secondary to reduced activity of the bone isoenzyme. Total serum alkaline phosphatase activity may be intermittently normal in some affected individuals. Biochemical features include a marked increase in serum and urinary phosphorylethanolamine and lesser increases in pyrophosphate. Urinary hydroxyproline excretion rate is abnormally low.

No satisfactory treatment for hypophosphatasia is available.

Calcium-wasting Osteomalacia

Intestinal malabsorptive states commonly are complicated by insufficient absorption of both calcium and vitamin D. Occasionally hypomagnesemia is also present, and magnesium replacement may be required to facilitate restitution of calcium homeostasis.

The pathogenesis of so-called idiopathic hypercalciuria has been partially resolved.[11] It is now thought that excessive excretion of calcium can have two causes. In one form, the primary defect is inability of the kidney to conserve calcium. With loss of calcium, secondary hyperparathyroidism develops. Excess PTH, in turn, promotes phosphaturia and enhances 1-hydroxylation of 25(OH)D and hence intestinal calcium absorption. The cause of calcium-wasting by the kidney is unknown. Patients with this disorder usually present with renal stones and are found to have normal serum calcium, low phosphorus, increased serum levels of PTH and $1,25(OH)_2D$, increased urinary cyclic AMP, and reduced tubular reabsorption of phosphorus. Radiologic evidence of osteopenia is rare. Their stone-forming tendency can be managed with chlorothiazide and neutral phosphate.

The second cause of idiopathic hypercalciuria is increased intestinal absorption of calcium that is unrelated to secondary hyperparathyroidism. Two subpopulations of patients have been identified: (1) those with normal levels of $1,25(OH)_2D$, whose hyperabsorption of calcium is probably caused by a primary intestinal defect, and (2) those with high levels of $1,25(OH)_2D$, who invariably have hypophosphatemia secondary to unexplained renal phosphate-wasting. The hypophosphatemia stimulates formation of $1,25(OH)_2D$, which enhances the intestinal absorption of calcium. Low serum PTH concentration reduces tubular reabsorption of calcium, thereby further promoting hypercalciuria and renal stone formation. In those patients with hypophosphatemia, oral phosphate is effective therapy because it reduces circulating $1,25(OH)_2D$ and therefore urinary calcium excretion. Osteomalacia is not a feature of this disorder, because presumably osteoid is mineralized in the presence of excess $1,25(OH)_2D$.

Renal Tubular Dysfunction and Osteomalacia

Osteomalacia or rickets may occur in patients with renal tubular dysfunction. Bone disease in these patients is disproportionate to the degree of renal failure. Various inborn or acquired disorders of the proximal tubule produce a characteristic pattern of renal wastage of phosphate, glucose, bicarbonate, and amino acids (Fanconi syndrome). In addition to phosphate depletion, deficient production of $1,25(OH)_2D$ has been implicated as a cause of osteomalacia in these syndromes. Distal tubular dysfunction produces a gradient renal tubular acidosis in association with hypercalciuria and nephrocalcinosis. Metabolic acidosis that occurs in these disorders as well as following ureterosigmoidostomy may contribute to

the production of a rachitic state. Skeletal manifestations can be corrected or prevented by treatment with sufficient bicarbonate to normalize the serum pH. Adequate treatment of bone disease in Fanconi syndrome requires the administration of $1,25(OH)_2D_3$ as well as bicarbonate.

OSTEOPOROSIS

Osteoporosis, the most common metabolic bone disease, is defined as an absolute decrease of bone mass and is associated with an increased frequency of certain types of fractures. Osteoporotic bone shows a significant decrease in cortical thickness and in the number and size of the trabeculae. There is no known abnormality in the structure of the organic matrix (osteoid), nor is there any defect in mineralization. Thus, osteoporosis can be readily distinguished histologically from osteomalacia, in which mineralization of osteoid is impaired and the ratio of organic matrix to mineral is increased. The term "osteopenia" is frequently used to describe the condition of individuals who have osteoporosis without fractures. To minimize confusion it is preferable to use the term "asymptomatic osteoporosis" when referring to this condition, and to reserve the term osteopenia for the nonspecific description of any state of decreased bone mass, without regard to its histological diagnosis or pathophysiological basis.

A decrease in bone mass is a natural consequence of aging. Skeletal growth is nearly complete by the end of adolescence, but even after closure of the endochondral growth plate, bone mass increases by radial growth until peak bone mass is achieved at about age 35. After a short interval of balanced bone metabolism, bone resorption begins to exceed bone formation and skeletal mass decreases. The rate of bone loss differs for different areas of the skeleton. Thus, after age 35 individuals of both sexes begin to lose bone mass from cortical bone at a rate of about 0.5 percent per year and, because of its higher metabolic activity, from trabecular bone at a rate of about 1.5 percent per year. In postmenopausal women, the loss of estrogen is accompanied by a transient phase of accelerated bone loss. This accelerated rate subsides over time, so that after 8 to 10 years the rate of bone loss is similar to the premenopausal rate. Thus, compared with her maximal bone mass, the average woman will lose about 50 percent of trabecular and 35 percent of cortical bone mass. Men lose only about two thirds of these amounts. The mechanism responsible for the accelerated rate of bone loss that accompanies estrogen withdrawal is unknown. Estrogen appears to inhibit bone resorption in general and to decrease PTH-directed bone resorption in particular. Alternatively, the effects of estrogen on bone may be indirect and mediated by other hormones.

In addition to the loss of bone that accompanies aging and menopause, other factors that may be related to the pathogenesis of osteoporosis have been recognized. Genetic and constitutional considerations are important determinants of peak bone mass and may influence the rate of bone loss. In general, white and Asian women have a greater risk of osteoporosis than black women, and white men have a greater risk than black men. One explanation may be that blacks have a greater bone mass at skeletal maturity than whites and may lose bone mass at a slower rate. Patients with osteoporosis are frequently less muscular, have lower average body weight, and have a lighter frame with thinner bones than individuals without osteoporosis. Among whites and Asians, lactase deficiency occurs more frequently in individuals with osteoporosis than in control subjects. Other risk factors for osteoporosis are modifiable and reflect the influence of life-style. Thus, cigarette smoking, which is associated with reduced circulating levels of estrogen and an earlier menopause, is a significant risk factor. A high alcohol and possibly caffeine intake may also contribute to excess bone loss. A sedentary life-style is also a risk factor for osteoporosis. Immobilization in bed and weightlessness during space flight are associated with increased bone turnover and resorption. In bed-rested subjects, the process of bone loss appears to be self-limiting,

and restoration of bone mass follows renewed ambulation. Whether this is true in space flight has not been determined. Conversely, weight-bearing exercise and physical activity are associated with increased bone formation and can reverse bone loss in some patients with osteoporosis.

The role of the calciotropic hormones that influence bone formation or resorption has yet to be defined. Most studies have not shown an alteration in serum calcitonin levels in patients with osteoporosis. Several studies indicate that patients with osteoporosis have lower (albeit normal) serum $1,25(OH)_2D_3$ levels. PTH may be decreased or increased.

Nutrition has been implicated in the pathogenesis of osteoporosis. Experiments with laboratory animals have established that calcium deficiency can cause osteoporosis by decreasing peak bone mass. Comparable studies in patients are incomplete or conflicting, and a consensus regarding the role of calcium in the pathogenesis of osteoporosis, or its usefulness in preventing bone loss or fracture, is lacking. It does appear, however, that for some ethnic groups an increased calcium intake during skeletal growth and development is associated with an increased peak bone mass at skeletal maturity, and if a high calcium intake is maintained, a decreased incidence of hip (but not wrist) fractures. Calcium supplementation may decrease the rate of bone loss from some sites, particularly those that consist primarily of cortical bone.

Involutional osteoporosis has been divided into two distinct syndromes on the basis of clinical and hormonal features and the pattern of bones affected.[24] Type I osteoporosis, also termed "postmenopausal" osteoporosis, may affect 25 percent of white women. This disorder characteristically occurs 10 to 15 years after menopause in women who are 51 to 65 years of age. Hypogonadal men may develop an equivalent disorder. There is an accelerated and disproportionate loss of trabecular bone as compared to cortical bone. The most common clinical manifestations are vertebral crush fractures, distal wrist (Colles) fractures, and mandibular resorption with increased tooth loss. It has been proposed that accelerated bone resorption and mobilization of skeletal calcium leads to decreased secretion of PTH, which causes decreased conversion of $25(OH)D$ to $1,25(OH)_2D_3$. Reduced serum levels of $1,25(OH)_2D_3$ are thought to be responsible for decreased intestinal absorption of calcium, which may further aggravate bone loss. Patients usually present with back pain that is caused by a vertebral compression fracture. The most frequently affected vertebrae are those from T6 to L3, and complete compression is more characteristic than anterior wedging. Fractures typically occur with minimal or no trauma. Some patients may develop chronic back pain and height loss after collapse of several or more vertebrae. Occasional patients may experience progressive height loss and deformity without pain. There is a marked female predominance (6:1) in type I osteoporosis.

Type II osteoporosis is termed "senile" osteoporosis. Patients with type II osteoporosis show a proportionate loss of trabecular and cortical bone, and bone-density values are usually in the lower part of the normal range. This disorder generally occurs in both women and men (2:1) who are 70 years of age or older and is primarily manifested by hip, pelvic, and vertebral fractures. Vertebral fractures are characteristically of the wedge type and lead to progressive dorsal kyphosis ("dowager's hump"). The pathogenesis of this disorder may be related to decreased osteoblast function and impaired production of $1,25(OH)_2D_3$. Decreased circulating levels of $1,25(OH)_2D_3$ lead to reduced intestinal absorption of calcium and mild secondary hyperparathyroidism.

Osteoporosis becomes clinically significant when bone mass is reduced to the extent that the skeleton is insufficient to perform its normal function. Generalized skeletal pain is uncommon, and between fractures most patients are free of symptoms. Although the disorder is generally progressive, after one or two fractures a patient may not experience further bone problems for many years. Because extreme variability appears to be characteristic of osteoporosis, it is often difficult to predict the course of the disorder or assess the effects of treatment in any one individual.

In the absence of a typical fracture, the diagnosis of osteoporosis can be established by demonstration of decreased bone mass. Because standard radiographs may fail to disclose less than a 30 percent decrease in bone density, this technique provides an insensitive indicator of bone loss. Several features of the osteoporotic vertebral body may be appreciated by radiographic examination, however, including an increased prominence of vertical striations and end plates and the development of "codfish" vertebrae resulting from the expansion of the intervertebral disks into the weakened subchondral plates. Schmorl nodes, which arise from the protrusion of the nucleus pulposa of the disc into the vertebral body, are pathognomonic. Looser zones are absent unless there is coexisting osteomalacia.

Newer procedures are available to establish whether an individual has lost sufficient bone mass to be at risk of fracture. These include quantitative single- and dual-energy CT, single- and dual-photon absorptiometry, and neutron activation analysis of total-body calcium. It is important to note that measurement of bone density at one site generally cannot be used to predict the bone density at a different site. Only CT and dual-photon absorptiometry techniques can measure bone density of the hip and spine. Dual-photon absorptiometry has the advantage of a significantly lower radiation exposure to the patient. Routine bone density screening of asymptomatic patients by any of these techniques is to be discouraged, because of their limited sensitivity and specificity in detection of osteoporosis.

Decreased bone mass may be secondary to a number of systemic diseases (Table 14.6–8) and these conditions must be excluded before the diagnosis of type I or type II primary osteoporosis can be established. Malignancies of various types, particularly multiple myeloma, can masquerade as osteoporosis. Similarly, radiologic evidence of osteoporosis is not uncommon in patients who have primary hyperparathyroidism, iatrogenic or endogenous hyperthyroidism, or glucocorticoid excess. Other metabolic bone diseases, such as Paget disease or osteomalacia, may coexist with or mimic osteoporosis, and bone biopsy may be required to establish the correct diagnosis.

Laboratory studies in primary osteoporosis, including serum calcium, phosphorus, alkaline phosphatase, PTH, and vitamin D metabolites, are nearly always normal. Mild hypercalciuria may be found in some patients, but usually the excretion rates of calcium, phosphorus, and hydroxyproline are normal.

TABLE 14.6–8. CONDITIONS ASSOCIATED WITH OSTEOPOROSIS

Primary
- Involutional
- Osteoporosis of juveniles

Secondary
- Cushing syndrome
- Hyperthyroidism
- Hypogonadism
- Diabetes mellitus
- Hyperparathyroidism
- Malnutrition
- Chronic liver disease
- Immobilization
- Heparin therapy
- Alcoholism
- Myeloma, lymphoma
- Calcium deficiency
- Scurvy
- Chronic obstructive pulmonary disease
- Mastocytosis

Heritable disorders
- Homocystinuria
- Osteogenesis imperfecta
- Menkes syndrome

Management

Successful measures to prevent or to treat osteoporosis remain elusive. Patients who suffer from fractures and are in acute pain will frequently require hospitalization. Collaboration between internist, orthopedist, and physical therapist is essential. Local heat and analgesias are helpful, and as soon as pain permits the patient should be encouraged to get out of bed. Programmed exercise and physical activity to increase muscle tone and bulk are useful, but frequent rest periods must be observed. Proprietary or custom-made braces or corsets can be used to provide support, relieve discomfort, and improve posture. It must be kept in mind that not every pain in the area where osteoporosis is present necessarily arises from the condition.

Calcium supplements, vitamin D and vitamin D metabolites, estrogen, calcitonin, and sodium fluoride have been used to treat osteoporosis with variable results. The most effective agent in the treatment of type I osteoporosis is estrogen replacement. Estrogens decrease the rate of bone resorption; in some studies the combination of estrogen and a progestin has resulted in modest increases in bone mass. Although the major role of estrogen is in preventing osteoporosis in menopausal women, estrogen replacement can be effective in retarding further bone loss and decreasing new fractures even when administered 10 to 15 years after the menopause. The use of unopposed estrogens is associated with a significantly increased risk of endometrial carcinoma. Estrogen should be combined, therefore, with a progestin when prescribed to a woman who has an intact uterus. Various cyclic and noncyclic protocols have been proposed; one frequently used regimen consists of conjugated estrogens, 0.625 mg per day for the first 25 days of each month, with the addition of medroxyprogesterone, 5 to 10 mg per day from days 13 to 25 of the month. Endometrial biopsy is recommended before beginning estrogen replacement and should be performed after any episode of unexplained bleeding.

All patients with types I and II osteoporosis should maintain a calcium intake of 1000 mg per day (1500 mg/day if postmenopausal and not receiving estrogen replacement). This can be provided from dietary sources, but in patients who are unable to meet this goal calcium supplements can be used. A daily calcium intake in excess of these recommendations has not been shown to be of greater benefit or efficacy and may result in hypercalciuria or hypercalcemia. Therapy with vitamin D or any of its more active metabolites may accelerate bone destruction and should be reserved for patients with specific disorders of vitamin D metabolism.

Sodium fluoride is currently not approved for the treatment of osteoporosis. Experimental treatment with sodium fluoride has demonstrated stimulation of new bone formation. Although this bone is poorly mineralized and histologically abnormal, it is associated with a decreased incidence of fractures.[25] Sodium fluoride in doses between 40 to 80 mg per day is an effective regimen when combined with a calcium intake of 1500 mg per day plus vitamin D, 50,000 IU weekly. Patients may note improved well-being in 9 to 12 weeks, although the vertebral fracture rate does not generally decrease within the first year of treatment. Only about 75 percent of patients will respond to sodium fluoride. In addition, nearly one third of patients may develop gastric irritation or an acute lower extremity pain syndrome. The absorption of sodium fluoride is decreased by simultaneous ingestion of calcium.

Calcitonin therapy is an expensive alternative when estrogen therapy is contraindicated or not tolerated. In appropriate subjects, particularly young men or women who have high bone turnover or idiopathic osteoporosis, calcitonin 100 MRC units every other day subcutaneously can be highly effective.

Patients with type II osteoporosis may have already lost all the bone mass they will ever lose. In addition, their bone density does not differ significantly from peers who have not sustained fractures. There is no evidence that estrogen or calcitonin therapy is effective in these patients, and sodium fluoride will not prevent hip fractures. Treatment should be directed towards elimination of unnecessary or excessive medications that increase bone loss or tendency

to fall and correction of any underlying coexisting medical conditions. Calcium supplementation and institution of measures that decrease the risk of falls are recommended.

Glucocorticoid-associated Osteoporosis

Glucocorticoid therapy and adrenal hypercorticism commonly produce osteoporosis and hypercalciuria. Radiographic evidence of skeletal loss is found in about 50 percent of patients with obvious Cushing syndrome. Postmenopausal women, immobilized subjects, adolescents, and patients with emphysema appear more susceptible to the adverse skeletal effects of glucocorticoids. Glucocorticoid excess accelerates catabolism of $1,25(OH)_2D$, decreases calcium absorption from gut, and prolongs the time necessary for completion of each bone modeling unit. Glucocorticoids alone depress collagen synthesis and decrease rates of both bone formation and bone resorption. The development of mild secondary hyperparathyroidism accelerates bone resorption, however, and a net loss of bone mass results. Catabolic effects of glucocorticoids lead to inadequate formation of bone matrix and delay in healing of bone fractures. Alternate-day administration of glucocorticoids is not associated with a reduced risk of developing significant bone disease.

Management of glucocorticoid-associated osteoporosis should be directed at correction of the endogenous cause or reduction of the dose of steroid. Because it is not always possible to reduce the dose of glucocorticoid because of the underlying illness, 50,000 IU of vitamin D twice weekly plus supplemental calcium should be given to those patients requiring long-term treatment. Alternatively, $25(OH)D$ in doses of 20 to 40 μg per day may be used. It is important to measure serum and urinary calcium before initiating therapy and to prescribe a thiazide-type diuretic if hypercalciuria is present. Thereafter, serum and urinary calcium should be monitored at intervals of 2 to 4 months.

Other Hormone-related Causes of Osteoporosis

The rate of bone turnover is increased in thyrotoxic patients. Serum alkaline phosphatase and urinary hydroxyproline excretion are increased, and serum PTH may be decreased. Marked bone resorption can occur in some patients, producing mild hypercalcemia, and hypercalciuria is common. Clinically significant bone loss may occur in patients with long-standing unrecognized hyperthyroidism.

Osteoporosis is associated with Klinefelter, Kallman, and Turner syndromes. Sex steroid replacement may be effective in decreasing the rates of bone loss in patients with these conditions. The incidence of osteoporosis is also increased in patients with diabetes mellitus, acromegaly, and primary hyperparathyroidism.

Disuse Osteoporosis

Mechanical stress plays an important role in the maintenance of normal bone mass. Immobilization leads to rapid mobilization of bone mineral, produces hypercalciuria, an increase in urinary excretion of hydroxyproline, and occasionally hypercalcemia. Loss of skeletal mass results from a decrease in osteoblastic bone formation and an increase in osteoclastic resorption. Secretion of PTH is generally suppressed, and serum levels of PTH and $1,25(OH)_2D$ may be reduced. When a limb is immobilized by a cast, local osteoporosis may develop.

Patients must be mobilized as soon as conditions permit. Hydration is essential because hypercalciuria is common.

Osteoporosis of Deficient Collagen Synthesis

In severe malnutrition, scurvy, and chronic illnesses complicated by protein-wasting, osteoporosis may develop. In these conditions newly formed bone may be defective.

Certain heritable disorders of connective tissue may be associated with osteoporosis. In osteogenesis imperfecta deficient bone mass may be severe. In this disorder, of which several forms are recognized, the synthesis and organization of collagen in bone and skin are abnormal. The bones may be severely deformed and frag-

ile. The numbers of osteoblasts and osteoclasts are normal, but turnover of bone is high, with the balance favoring resorption.

Osteoporosis is also a common finding in patients with homocystinuria. The diagnosis is established by determining homocystine in urine. Homocystine or its metabolites interfere with the formation of the intermolecular cross-links that are necessary to stabilize collagen.

Idiopathic Osteoporosis

This disorder is seen primarily in males under 40 years of age or in premenopausal women in whom no other etiologic factor is detected. It differs from primary osteoporosis in several respects: hypercalciuria is common, urinary hydroxyproline may be elevated, and histologically there appears to be increased activity of bone cells. The etiology of this disorder is unknown. Some patients may have mild osteogenesis imperfecta or adult-onset hypophosphatasia.

INCREASED DENSITY OF BONE

Osteopetrosis

Increased density of bone is observed in only a few diseases. The term "osteopetrosis" is usually reserved for Albers–Schönberg disease (marble bone disease), an inherited disorder characterized by generalized and marked increase in bone density. Patients with the autosomal recessive form of the disease are most severely affected. There may be obliteration of the bone marrow cavity, severe deformities of the skull, and compression of the cranial nerves. Death occurs in childhood from severe anemia, bleeding disorders, extramedullary hematopoiesis, and increased intracranial pressure.

In patients who have mild cases and who survive, there is short stature, a propensity to develop fractures, and increased density of bone radiographically. Patients are prone to develop osteomyelitis, particularly in the mandible. In nearly 50 percent of patients with the autosomal dominant form, the disorder may be clinically asymptomatic. Histologically, there is evidence of reduced bone resorption and osteoclasts are absent. Serum calcium, phosphate, and alkaline phosphatase are normal but acid phosphatase activity is often elevated. The basic defect is unknown. In mice with a disorder apparently homologous to the severe autosomal recessive form of osteopetrosis, there is evidence that a stem cell defect results in deficiency of osteoclasts. In several cases of this "malignant" form of osteopetrosis, bone marrow transplantation has been performed to restore osteoclasts. The differential diagnosis of osteopetrosis includes vitamin A intoxication, fluorosis, and myelosclerosis.

Osteosclerosis is occasionally observed in patients with renal osteodystrophy. This condition is characterized by increased bone density, which is particularly prominent in the metaphyseal regions of the vertebrae. Skeletal radiographs show sclerotic foci within bones ("endobones") and sclerotic vertebral end-plates ("rugger-jersey spine"). Its etiology remains unknown, although some evidence suggests that PTH or elevated serum phosphate may be causative factors. More commonly, aberrations in phosphate, PTH, and vitamin D lead to the development of osteomalacia and osteitis fibrosa cystica, which may be present concomitantly with osteosclerosis.

Paget Disease of Bone (Osteitis Deformans)

Paget disease is a disorder of locally increased bone remodeling. The clinical manifestations depend upon the extent and location of the lesions as well as the presence of associated complications. Many patients are asymptomatic, and their lesions are usually detected during radiographic evaluation of unrelated illness. Local pain and joint stiffness, often described as rheumatic, gouty, or neuralgic, are common complaints. Because the spine, pelvis, skull, and femur are the usual sites of involvement, hip pain, lower back pain, headaches, and tinnitus are frequent symptoms. Pathologic fractures may be the initial presentation. Basilar skull invag-

ination in advanced cases may lead to progressive ataxia and tetraplegia, as a result of compression of the cerebellar tonsils. Paraplegia is probably caused by concentric narrowing of the spinal canal or shunting of blood away from the spinal cord through hypervascular skin and bone. The most common neurologic complication is hearing loss of combined conductive and sensorineural type. A marked increase in bone blood flow is well recognized. Cardiac output may be markedly increased when involvement of the skeleton is extensive. Hyperkinetic circulation may aggravate preexisting cardiac dysfunction and hasten the development of congestive heart failure in the elderly.

Physical findings, when present, include an enlarged skull with prominent superficial veins, hearing impairment, progressive kyphosis with shortening of stature, and deformity of long bones. The skin temperature overlying a lesion may be elevated, and flow murmurs are sometimes audible. Angioid streaks of the retina have been observed in some patients.

Paget disease is more common in the elderly than generally appreciated. European autopsy and radiographic studies suggest that about 3 percent of the adult population is affected. By the ninth decade, the incidence may be as high as 5 to 11 percent. The basic pathologic process is an accelerated resorption of bone caused by excessive osteoclastic activity, followed by osteoblastic regeneration and formation of new bone. The newly formed bone under these circumstances is defective, however, and often deformed. Sarcomatous degeneration of the bone lesions occurs but fortunately affects no more than 1 percent of Paget patients. The etiology of this disorder remains obscure. Attention has been drawn to the familial occurrence of the disease.

Serum calcium and phosphorus are normal but hypercalciuria is common. During immobilization for severe pain or fractures, excessive bone resorption continues whereas the rate of new bone formation is diminished. Such a distortion of the balance between bone resorption and formation occasionally leads to hypercalcemia.

The laboratory approach to the diagnosis of Paget disease can be divided into two major categories: (1) anatomic delineation of the lesion and (2) assessment of the activity of the disease. In the absence of bone histology, the anatomic evaluation can be made by conventional radiography and radioisotopic scanning. The bone changes noted on radiographs need not reflect active disease. About 85 percent of bone lesions are detectable by both radiography and scan, 10 percent are visualized by radiograph alone, and the remaining by the scan alone. The lesions detected by bone scan are usually symptomatic.

Measurements of serum alkaline phosphatase activity and total urinary hydroxyproline are both sensitive indices of the activity of Paget disease of bone. They are also useful "markers" to assess treatment. Elevation of serum acid phosphatase activity also occurs in severe Paget disease.

Paget disease is usually amenable to treatment with pharmacologic doses (50 to 100 MRC units per day) of calcitonin given subcutaneously. Salmon calcitonin, by virtue of its long half-life in humans, has proved to be more potent than the porcine or human hormone. In some instances in which remission has not been sustained, development of neutralizing antibodies to calcitonin or an escape of the bone cells from the effects of the hormone have been incriminated. Human calcitonin can be used in these patients with restoration of responsiveness. Calcitonin restores normal bone remodeling, is safe for long-term use, and has only trivial side effects. Its principal disadvantages are its cost and that it can be given only by injection.

Sodium etidronate is also available for the management of this disease. This compound binds strongly to crystals of hydroxyapatite to slow bone-turnover rate. The usual dose is 5 mg/kg per day given orally. The effectiveness of this agent is similar to that obtained by calcitonin injection. The duration of treatment generally should not exceed 6 months because significant impairment of mineralization of both normal and diseased bone occurs thereafter. Patients with lytic bone lesions should not receive sodium etidro-

nate because it may precipitate fracture through the area of weakened bone.[12] Other agents that have been used include mithramycin, actinomycin D, and glucagon.

Mild Paget disease may be managed with salicylate or indomethacin. The indications for more specific treatment include significant bone pain, prevention of further deformity, neurologic compromise, operative preparation for joint replacement, hearing loss, and high-output congestive heart failure.

POLYOSTOTIC FIBROUS DYSPLASIA (ALBRIGHT SYNDROME)[33]

This is a disease of unknown etiology. The classic triad of this syndrome consists of skin pigmentation, bone lesions, and precocious sexual development. The brownish skin pigmentation tends to be unilateral, flat, and multiple, with irregularly indented margins. The bone lesions are results of fibrous dysplasia.

Radiologically, the bone lesions appear as cystic lesions in the cortex or ground-glass change in expanded cortex. As with the skin lesions, the bone involvement is usually unilateral, often on the same side as the skin pigmentation. Precocious puberty is the best-known endocrine disorder associated with this syndrome, but other reported conditions include goiter, hyperthyroidism, acromegaly, Cushing syndrome, gynecomastia, and parathyroid enlargement. It has been postulated that a congenital abnormality of the hypothalamus causes excessive production of hypothalamic-releasing hormones in this syndrome.

REFERENCES

1. Ahn TG, Antonarakis SE, et al: Familial isolated hypoparathyroidism: A molecular genetic analysis of 8 families with 23 affected persons. Medicine 65:73, 1986
2. Anast CS, Winnacker JL, et al: Impaired release of parathyroid hormone in magnesium deficiency. J Clin Endocrinol Metab 42:707, 1976
3. Avioli LV, Krane SM (eds): Metabolic Bone Disease, vol 1. New York, Academic Press, 1977
4. Barbour GL, Coburn JW, et al: Hypercalcemia in an anephric patient with sarcoidosis: Evidence for extrarenal generation of 1,25-dihydroxy-vitamin D in man. J Clin Invest 69:722, 1982
5. Broadus AE, Magee JS, et al: A detailed evaluation of oral phosphate therapy in selected patients with primary hyperparathyroidism. J Clin Endocrinol Metab 56:953, 1983
6. Canfield RE (ed): Etidronate disodium: A new therapy for hypercalcemia of malignancy. Am J Med 82(2A):1, 1987
7. Cohn DV, MacGregor RR: The biosynthesis, intracellular processing, and secretion of parathormone. Endocrinol Rev 2:1, 1981
8. Deftos LJ, Catherwood BD, Bone HG III: Multiple endocrine disorders. In Felig P, Baxter JD, et al (eds): Endocrinology and Metabolism. New York, McGraw-Hill, 1981
9. Farfel Z, Brickman AS, et al: Deficiency of receptor-cyclase couple protein in pseudohypoparathyroidism. N Engl J Med 303:237, 1980
10. Habener JF, Mahaffey JE: Osteomalacia and disorders of vitamin D metabolism. Annu Rev Med 29:327, 1978
11. Haussler MR, McCain TA: Basic and clinical concepts related to vitamin D metabolism and action. N Engl J Med 297:974, 1977
12. Krane SM: Etidronate disodium in the treatment of Paget's disease of bone. Ann Intern Med 96:619, 1982
13. Lambert PW, Stern PH, et al: Evidence for extrarenal production of 1,25-dihydroxyvitamin D in man. J Clin Invest 69:722, 1982
14. Levine MA, Downs RW Jr, et al: Deficient activity of guanine nucleotide regulatory protein in erythrocytes from patients with pseudohypoparathyroidism. Biochem Biophys Res Commun 94:1319, 1980
15. Levine MA, Jap T-S, et al: Activity of the stimulatory guanine nucleotide-binding protein is reduced in erythrocytes from patients with pseudohypoparathyroidism and pseudopseudohypoparathyroidism: Biochemical, endocrine, and genetic analysis of Albright's hereditary osteodystrophy in 6 kindreds. J Clin Endocrinol Metab 62:497, 1986
16. Liberman UA, Eil C, Marx SJ: Resistance to 1,25-dihydroxyvitamin D. Association with heterogeneous defects in cultured skin fibroblasts. J Clin Invest 71:192, 1983

17. Mallette LE, Gomez L, Fisher RG: Parathyroid angiography: A review of current knowledge and guidelines for clinical application. Endocrinol Rev 1:124, 1981
18. Marx SJ, Attie MF, et al: The hypocalciuric or benign variant of familial hypercalcemia: Clinical and biochemical features in fifteen kindreds. Medicine 60:397, 1981
19. Mundy GR, Ibbotson KJ, et al: The hypercalcemia of cancer: Clinical implications and pathogenic mechanism. N Engl J Med 310:1718, 1984
20. Mundy GR, Wilkinson R, Heath DA: Comparative study of available medical therapy for hypercalcemia of malignancy. Am J Med 74:421, 1983
21. Norman AW, Roth J, Orci L: The vitamin D endocrine system: Steroid metabolism, hormone receptors, and biologic response (calcium binding proteins). Endocrinol Rev 3:331, 1982
22. Nusynowitz ML, Frame B, Kolb FH: The spectrum of the hypoparathyroid states: A classification based on physiologic principles. Medicine 55:105, 1976
23. Raisz LG, Mundy GR, et al: Hormone regulation of mineral metabolism. In McCann SM (ed): International Review of Physiology, Endocrine Physiology II, vol. 16. Baltimore, University Park Press, 1977
24. Riggs BL, Melton LJ III: Involutional osteoporosis. N Engl J Med 314:1679, 1986
25. Riggs BL, Seeman E, et al: Effect of the fluoride-calcium regimen on vertebral fracture occurrence in post-menopausal osteoporosis. Comparison with conventional therapy. N Engl J Med 306:446, 1982
26. Rosenthal N, Fusogna KL, et al: Elevations in circulating 1,25-dihydroxyvitamin D in three patients with lymphoma-associated hypercalcemia. J Clin Endocrinol Metab 60:29, 1985
27. Scholz DA, Purnell DC: Asymptomatic primary hyperparathyroidism: 10-year prospective study. Mayo Clin Proc 56:473, 1981
28. Selby PL, Peacock M: Ethinyl estradiol and norethindrone in the treatment of primary hyperparathyroidism in post-menopausal women. N Engl J Med 314:1481, 1986
29. Shane E, Baquiran DC, Bilezikian JP: Effects of dichloromethylene diphosphonate on serum and urinary calcium in primary hyperparathyroidism. Ann Intern Med 95:23, 1981
30. Simpson EL, Mundy GR, et al: Absence of parathyroid hormone messenger RNA in nonparathyroid tumors associated with hypercalcemia. N Engl J Med 309:325, 1983
31. Stewart AF, Adler M, et al: Calcium homeostasis in immobilization: An example of resorptive hypercalciuria. N Engl J Med 306:1136, 1983
32. Stewart AF, Horst R, et al: Biochemical evaluation of patients with malignancy-associated hypercalcemia; evidence for humoral and non-humoral groups. N Engl J Med 303:1377, 1980
33. Warrick CK: Some aspects of polyostotic fibrous dysplasia: Possible hypothesis to account for associated endocrinologic changes. Clin Radiol 24:125, 1973

CHAPTER 14.7
Diabetes Mellitus

Christopher D. Saudek

Diabetes mellitus is defined by inappropriate hyperglycemia, although it is a disease with multiple causes, manifestations, and complications. In all cases, insulin secretion is inadequate to normalize glucose metabolism either because of peripheral tissue resistance to insulin action, reduced insulin secretion, or both. A series of metabolic abnormalities result from insulin insufficiency, and these cause complications that remain a major cause of morbidity and mortality.

About 11 million Americans have diabetes, almost half of them undiagnosed.[17] In the United States, the chronic complications of diabetes cause 40 to 50 percent of all nontraumatic amputations, 30 percent of all end-stage renal failure, and almost 6,000 new cases of blindness each year. Diabetic patients account for 10 percent of all acute-care hospital days, and the economic impact of diabetes is estimated to be $14 billion annually. The incidence of diabetes is increasing; about 500,000 new cases are diagnosed per year.

Primary, or idiopathic, diabetes is divided into two major categories: insulin-dependent diabetes mellitus (IDDM, type I diabetes), and noninsulin-dependent diabetes mellitus (NIDDM, type II diabetes). These types are defined on the basis of the patient's tendency to develop ketoacidosis, but the two diseases differ fundamentally in their etiology and pathogenesis as well as their susceptibility to ketoacidosis. Other types of diabetes are due to specifically identified causes of pancreatic beta-cell deficiency or peripheral insulin resistance.

The underlying abnormality in all diabetes is insufficient insulin, although there may also be excess production of counterinsulin hormones such as glucagon, cortisol, or growth hormone. Insulin insufficiency causes a clinical state that is largely independent of the etiology or type of diabetes. In many respects, a common therapeutic approach is appropriate for all types of diabetes.

The first treatment objective is to keep the patient free from acute symptoms and acute complications of hyperglycemia. Beyond this minimum goal, good management can avoid or treat many of diabetes' chronic complications. But in approaching these therapeutic goals, the side effects of therapy, particularly incapacitating hypoglycemic reactions or intolerable life-style restrictions, must be avoided.

PATHOPHYSIOLOGY

Insulin is the hormone of carbohydrate availability, directing the utilization of circulating glucose as metabolic fuel while storing lipid and glycogen. There are many insulin secretagogues (including amino acids, glucagon, and beta-adrenergic stimulation), but hyperglycemia is the primary signal for insulin secretion. Insulin binds to specific cell membrane receptors and, by a complex sequence of intracellular events, promotes glucose entry into the cell. Simultaneously, insulin protects and repletes endogenous stores of both glycogen and adipose tissue triglyceride. Glycogenesis is promoted, while glycogenolysis and gluconeogenesis are inhibited by insulin. Insulin stimulates the synthesis of adipose tissue triglyceride from circulating fatty acids and inhibits lipolysis of adipose tissue triglyceride.

In the postabsorptive state (6 to 24 hours of fasting), low insulin and high glucagon concentrations change the pattern of fuel production and utilization. Glucose is provided by glycogenolysis and gluconeogenesis; free fatty acids are released from adipose tissue and become a major source of metabolic fuel. If fasting continues beyond 24 hours, limited sources of glucose (primarily muscle amino acids) are further protected by reducing glucose utilization to a minimum. Free fatty acids become the predominant energy substrate.

Reduced insulin effect makes uncontrolled diabetes metabolically similar in some respects to fasting. Cellular glucose metabolism is diminished; gluconeogenesis, glycogenolysis, and lipolysis are activated. The normal homeostasis of fasting, however, runs amok because of inadequately metabolized dietary glucose, the failure to diminish gluconeogenesis, ketogenesis which may exceed ketone-body utilization, and dehydration from osmotic diuresis. The result is hyperglycemia, inefficient utilization of calories, dehydration, and, with complete insulin lack, ketoacidosis.

Counterregulatory hormones, such as glucagon, growth hormone, and cortisol, which oppose insulin's action, may be elevated in some forms of diabetes. The importance of increased, or nonsuppressed, glucagon has been widely debated. It probably plays a role in ketogenesis, but insulin insufficiency is the primary defect in diabetes.

DIAGNOSIS AND CLASSIFICATION

CRITERIA

The diagnosis of diabetes requires documentation of hyperglycemia meeting any of three criteria[16] (Table 14.7–1). Random hyperglycemia ≥ 200 mg/dl plasma glucose along with symptoms attributable to hyperglycemia establishes the diagnosis without further work-up. Likewise, fasting hyperglycemia ≥ 140 mg/dl makes the diagnosis. If neither of the above criteria is met, an oral glucose tolerance test (OGTT) may be useful.

ORAL GLUCOSE TOLERANCE TEST

A 2-hour OGTT is indicated if the index of suspicion is high, but diabetes is not diagnosed by random or fasting hyperglycemia (Table 14.7–2). Patients with strongly predisposing factors, such as obesity, syndromes associated with diabetes, or complications that appear typical of diabetes may require glucose tolerance testing. OGTT is unnecessary if the diagnosis is already established. OGTT is not used to follow treatment.

Results of the OGTT that do not meet the criteria for diagnosing diabetes may be normal, equivocal, or indicate impaired glucose tolerance.

CLASSIFICATION

Once diabetes is diagnosed, the patient should be classified in order to guide therapy and to ensure that a correctable cause of diabetes is not ignored.

The accepted classification of diabetes[16] distinguishes IDDM, NIDDM, "other types," and gestational diabetes (Table 14.7–3).

TABLE 14.7–1. THE ORAL GLUCOSE TOLERANCE TEST (OGTT): Diagnostic Criteria for Normal, Impaired Glucose Tolerance (IGT), Diabetes Mellitus, and Gestational Diabetes Mellitus (GDM)

	Plasma Glucose (mg/dl)				
		After 75 g Oral Glucose[a]			
	Fasting		$\frac{1}{2}$, 1, or $1\frac{1}{2}$ hr		2 hr
Normal[b]	<115	and	<200	and	<140
IGT[c]	<140	and	≥200	and	140–200
Diabetes mellitus[d]	≥140	or	≥200	and	≥200
	After 100 g Oral Glucose				
	Fasting	1 hr	2 hr	3 hr	
GMD[e]	>150	>190	>165	>145	

[a]Subjects should have at least 150 g carbohydrate intake per day for 3 days and be ambulatory before test.
[b]Values between normal and IGT are considered borderline and nondiagnostic.
[c]IGT and diabetic responses to OGTT should be demonstrated on more than one occasion to be considered diagnostic.
[d]Diabetes mellitus is diagnosed without OGTT if the patient has classic symptoms and random plasma glucose ≥200 or fasting plasma glucose ≥140 mg/dl.
[e]GDM is diagnosed if two or more of these values are exceeded.

TABLE 14.7–2. CLINICAL USE OF ORAL GLUCOSE TOLERANCE TEST[a]

- Testing suspected diabetes with fasting plasma glucose (PG) <140 mg/dl
- Screening pregnant women at weeks 24–28 of gestation[b]
- Documenting reactive hypoglycemia (see Chapter 14.8)[c]

[a]75 g oral glucose, with PG at 0, 30, 60, 90, 120 min.
[b]50 g oral glucose: if 1 hr postglucose PG ≥ 150 mg/dl, proceed with 100 g OGTT (Table 14.7–1).
[c]5-hr test.

IDDM, type I, was formerly called "juvenile-onset diabetes." NIDDM, type II, was referred to as "maturity-onset diabetes." Other types of diabetes were called secondary, that is, those forms with a relatively well-defined cause. Gestational diabetes is defined by the first diagnosis during pregnancy. The categories of glucose intolerance, equivocal OGTT, previous history of diabetes, and statistical risk classes[16] should not be designated diabetes, although they do confer an increased risk of developing diabetes.

CLINICAL TYPES OF DIABETES

INSULIN-DEPENDENT DIABETES MELLITUS

Insulin-dependent diabetes mellitus (Table 14.7–4) is a disease of insulin deficiency, defined as that form of diabetes that requires exogenous insulin to avoid ketoacidosis in the basal state.[16] Many people with IDDM, however, pass through a "honeymoon period" lasting up to a year after the initial diagnosis during which they may not be prone to ketoacidosis or even need insulin. Peripheral insulin resistance may also be present in IDDM. The clinical onset is usually abrupt, but subtle evidence of impending diabetes may be present for years before the clinical presentation. New cases of IDDM are more common in winter months. Patients are usually normal weight or underweight, and the family history is often negative for diabetes. Ketoacidosis, the hallmark of IDDM, may be avoided by early diagnosis and appropriate therapy; when ketoacidosis is not documented, IDDM is diagnosed on the basis of other characteristics of the disease (Table 14.7–4).

IDDM was called "juvenile-onset diabetes" because the peak incidence occurs in early adolescence, although the disease may occur at any age. The capacity for endogenous insulin secretion, as indicated by C-peptide measurements, is diminished or entirely absent. The etiology of this beta-cell failure is unknown, but it is clear that IDDM is an autoimmune endocrinopathy with some

TABLE 14.7–3. CLASSIFICATION OF DIABETES AND OTHER CATEGORIES OF GLUCOSE INTOLERANCE

Diabetes mellitus
- Type I: insulin-dependent
- Type II: noninsulin-dependent
- Other types:
  Pancreatic disease
  Hormonal
  Drug or chemically induced
  Insulin receptor abnormalities
  Certain genetic syndromes
  Other types

Impaired glucose tolerance (IGT)

Gestational diabetes (GDM)

Statistical risk classes
- Previous abnormality of glucose tolerance
- Potential abnormality of glucose tolerance

TABLE 14.7–4. CLINICAL COMPARISON OF IDDM (TYPE I) AND NIDDM (TYPE II)

	IDDM (Type I)	NIDDM (Type II)
Former name	Juvenile-onset diabetes	Maturity-onset diabetes
Without exogenous insulin	Ketosis	No ketosis
Age of onset	Usually <40, may be at any age	Usually >40, may be younger
Endogenous insulin secretion	Reduced or absent	Normal or increased
Peripheral insulin resistance	Yes or no	Yes
Obesity	Rare	Common
HLA association	Yes	No
Requires insulin to avoid hyperglycemia	Yes	Yes or no

genetic predisposition.[7] Autoimmunity is indicated by the association of IDDM with other autoimmune endocrinopathies (especially Hashimoto thyroiditis and Addison disease) and by the demonstration of anti–islet cell antibodies in up to 85 percent of patients with IDDM, often antedating the onset of diabetes. More than 90 percent of IDDM patients in the United States have HLA-DR3 and/or -DR4, indicating a probable relationship to genetically-mediated immune mechanisms. Monozygotic twin studies show about 50 percent concordance for diabetes, but sibs of children with IDDM have only about a 2 percent chance of developing IDDM (although the chance is increased markedly if the sib shares the high-risk HLA haplotype). The precise interplay between genetic predisposition, environmental factors (such as viruses), and autoimmunity remains to be defined.

NONINSULIN-DEPENDENT DIABETES MELLITUS

NIDDM (Table 14.7–4) is a disease of insulin resistance and abnormal beta-cell responsiveness. While exogenous insulin may be required to avoid hyperglycemia, patients with NIDDM do not, by definition, develop ketoacidosis in the basal, unstressed state. The diagnosis of NIDDM does *not* depend on whether the patient takes insulin to treat hyperglycemia; about 25 percent of people with NIDDM require insulin therapy to control hyperglycemia. The diagnosis of NIDDM may be made on the basis of typical clinical features, including older age of onset (usually >40 years old), obesity (in over 80 percent of cases), and blood glucose levels that are less labile than in IDDM. There is usually a strong family history of diabetes and over 90 percent concordance rate for NIDDM among monozygotic twins. The end-stage acute complication of NIDDM is hyperosmolar nonketotic coma rather than ketoacidosis.

Endogenous insulin secretion in NIDDM prevents patients from becoming ketotic and is responsible for their relatively stable course. Plasma insulin concentration may even be higher than normal because of peripheral insulin resistance. If the cause of insulin resistance can be eliminated, for example by achieving normal body weight, endogenous insulin secretion may be adequate to maintain normal glucose tolerance. Because insulin secretory capacity usually decreases with age, NIDDM may gradually worsen, often causing "secondary failure" to oral hypoglycemic agents and the requirement for exogenous insulin replacement. If beta-cell function ultimately fails entirely, patients become ketosis-prone and thereby have IDDM by definition. This common sequence is a weakness of the current system of classification, because most of these older patients with progressive loss of beta-cell capacity probably do not

have the same autoimmune disease as typical young IDDM patients.

The etiology of insulin resistance in NIDDM is a subject of intensive research.[3] Abnormal pancreatic insulin responsivity to glucose may also be the initial event that causes hyperinsulinemia and peripheral insulin resistance. Insulin secretion, as well as peripheral response to insulin, are clearly improved by establishing normal blood glucose. Cell surface insulin receptors are usually diminished in number in NIDDM, but intracellular postreceptor events that mediate insulin action may be more important in conferring cellular resistance.

OTHER TYPES OF DIABETES

A long list of syndromes and medications are known to be diabetogenic (Table 14.7–5). Relatively common causes include treatment with drugs that inhibit insulin secretion (such as thiazide duiretics or alpha-adrenergic agonists), excess counterregulatory hormones (from endogenous or exogenous hypercortisolism, acromegaly, and glucagon-secreting tumors of the pancreas), or direct pancreatic insufficiency (e.g., after pancreatectomy or with infiltrative diseases of the pancreas such as hemochromatosis, amyloidosis, or chronic relapsing pancreatitis). An unusual but fascinating series of patients have severe insulin resistance associated with acanthosis nigricans and virilization due to one of several peripheral cell defects. One such syndrome includes reduced insulin receptors while another has circulating antibody against the insulin receptor.

TABLE 14.7–5. OTHER TYPES OF DIABETES[a]

Pancreatic disease
- Neonatal, congenital
- Neonatal, transient
- Acquired
    Traumatic, neoplastic, infectious, pancreatitis
- Inherited
    Cystic fibrosis, hemochromatosis

Hormonal
- Hypoinsulinemic
    Pheochromocytoma, somatostatinoma, aldosteronoma, glucagonoma, hypoparathyroidism, type I isolated growth hormone deficiency, Laron dwarfism, hypothalmic lesions
- Hyperinsulinemic (insulin resistance)
    Excessive secretion of glucocorticoids, progestins, estrogens, growth hormone, acromegaly; type II isolated growth hormone deficiency
    Associated endocrine and autoimmune disorders
        Thyrotoxicosis, Hashimoto disease, primary hypothyroidism, hypoparathyroidism, Addison disease, Schmidt syndrome, myasthenia gravis, pernicious anemia, polyendocrine disorders

Drugs and chemicals
- Diuretics (thiazides, furosemide), antihypertensives (clonidine), psychoactive drugs (tricyclics, phenothiazines), beta blockers (propranolol), miscellaneous (phenytoin, L-dopa, morphine, marijuana)

Insulin receptor abnormalities
- Receptor defect
    Congenital lipodystrophy, virilization, acanthosis nigricans
- Antibody to insulin receptor

Genetic syndromes
- Hemochromatosis, Turner syndrome, Werner syndrome, Klinefelter syndrome, optic atrophy-diabetes mellitus-diabetes insipidus syndrome, Laurence-Moon-Biedl syndrome, Friedreich ataxia, ataxia-telangiectasia, Refsum syndrome, glycogen storage I, myotonic dystrophy, Down syndrome

Other types
- Malnourished populations

[a] A complete list is found in Ref. 16.

DIABETES IN PREGNANCY

Gestational diabetes mellitus is defined by first diagnosis during pregnancy. Pregestational diabetes refers to preexisting diabetes in a pregnant woman. It is important to make the diagnosis of diabetes in pregnancy because of its adverse effects on fetal development.[10] High-risk women include those with a history of prior miscarriage, a previous baby with >10 lb birth weight, obesity, or a strong family history of diabetes. But all pregnant women should be screened during the 24th to 28th weeks of pregnancy. A plasma glucose ≥140 mg/dl 1 hour after 50 g oral glucose should be followed by a 100-g OGTT (Table 14.7–1). The modified plasma glucose criteria take into account the normal changes in glucose tolerance during pregnancy.

Diabetes during pregnancy causes significant and avoidable fetal morbidity. Poor diabetic control in the first trimester is associated with an increased incidence of congenital malformations. Later in pregnancy, maternal blood glucose crosses the placenta while maternal insulin does not, causing the fetal pancreas, continuously exposed to hyperglycemia, to become hyperplastic. Fetal hyperinsulinism results in excessive adiposity (macrosomia), neonatal hypoglycemia, and a variety of other perinatal complications.

Seventy-five percent of women with gestational diabetes mellitus regain normal glucose tolerance postpartum, but about 30 to 40 percent of them will again become diabetic within 10 years. Weight control is a particularly important preventive measure in these women.

IMPAIRED GLUCOSE TOLERANCE (IGT)

This mild abnormality in glucose tolerance, not meeting the criteria for diabetes mellitus,[16] progresses to diabetes in only about 25 percent of cases. Patients with IGT, however, are at greater than normal risk for atherosclerosis.

STATISTICAL RISK CATEGORIES

A variety of conditions is associated with an increased risk of developing diabetes.[16] Among these is a previous history of abnormal glucose tolerance, having a monozygotic twin with diabetes or the same HLA phenotype as a sibling with diabetes, or belonging to a high-risk group such as the Pima Indians. Despite the increased risk, however, there is no justification for calling such persons "prediabetic" or "latent diabetic."

CLINICAL MANIFESTATIONS

ACUTE SIGNS AND SYMPTOMS

The acute complications of diabetes (Table 14.7–6) are directly and immediately due to hyperglycemia or other metabolic sequelae of insulin insufficiency such as ketosis.

Glycosuria ensues as the renal threshold for glucose is exceeded, at about 180 mg/dl plasma glucose. The associated osmotic diuresis causes loss of free water and dehydration. Hyperglycemia itself adds 5.5 mOsm/L to serum osmolarity for every 100 mg/dl plasma glucose. The glucosuria and osmotic diuresis cause polyuria (increased volume of urine), while the hyperglycemia and dehydration cause thirst and polydipsia (increased fluid intake).

Weight loss is the result of inefficient utilization of ingested calories with urinary loss of glucose. Patients with poorly controlled diabetes also report fatigue, poor wound-healing, and, occasionally, increased caloric intake (hyperphagia) without weight gain.

Vaginitis, usually monilial, is common in uncontrolled diabetes and is often unresponsive to therapy until the hyperglycemia is improved. Periodontal disease may be severe. Visual blurring results from osmotic changes in the optic lens when blood glucose is fluctuating rapidly. Because diabetics in unstable control have transient changes in lens refraction, glasses should not be prescribed until their diabetes is stable.

The signs and symptoms of uncontrolled diabetes occur only with severely elevated plasma glucose, usually above 300 mg/dl. There is a considerable range of hyperglycemia, therefore, which is abnormal although asymptomatic. The clinician should be aware that lack of symptoms does not indicate good control of diabetes.

LONG-TERM COMPLICATIONS

Long-term complications cause most of the morbidity and mortality associated with diabetes. Although they are well-classified (Table 14.7–7) and well-described pathologically, their causes and clinical variability remain a mystery. Usually long-term complications are not found until after at least 5 years of diabetes, but occasionally they are seen upon initial presentation. Any complication can develop in any form of diabetes, regardless of etiology. This suggests that the hyperglycemia or other metabolic abnormalities of diabetes—rather than some feature of the disease independent of the metabolic state—is responsible.

Although the duration and severity of hyperglycemia are strongly correlated with chronic complications, there is great var-

TABLE 14.7–6. ACUTE SIGNS AND SYMPTOMS OF DIABETES

Hyperosmolarity	Polyuria
	Polydipsia
	Blurred vision
Infections	Vaginitis
	Periodontitis
	Urinary tract infections
Constitutional	Fatigue
	Weight Loss
	Polyphagia
	Hyperphagia
	Slow healing
	Dehydration
Clinical emergencies	Ketoacidosis
	Hyperosmolar nonketotic coma

TABLE 14.7–7. LONG-TERM COMPLICATIONS OF DIABETES

Macrovascular
- Peripheral vascular disease
- Coronary artery disease
- Cerebrovascular disease

Dermopathies
- Necrobiosis diabeticorum
- Shin spots

Musculoskeletal
- Tendon contractures
- Bursitis
- Charcot joints
- Osteomyelitis

Microvascular
- Retinopathy (see Table 14.7–8)
- Nephropathy

Cataracts

Neuropathies (see Table 14.7–9)

Cardiomyopathy

iability in their onset and severity, often not entirely explained by diabetic control.

A number of possible mechanisms have been proposed. Non-enzymatic glycosylation of tissue proteins, resulting in chronic hyperglycemia, has been implicated as a cause of microvascular and macrovascular complications. The polyalcohol myo-inositol is reduced in tissues of diabetic animals and humans. Sorbitol accumulation, the result of noninsulin-dependent aldose reductase activity, damages, at least, the optic lens and peripheral nerve tissue. These findings have prompted clinical interest in aldose reductase inhibitors that block sorbitol synthesis. Documented abnormalities in multiple aspects of lipid metabolism may promote accelerated large vessel atherosclerosis. None of the above theories, however, has been conclusively proven to explain the long-term complications of diabetes.

Diabetic Microangiopathy

Microangiopathy is manifested clinically by ophthalmopathy and nephropathy, although neither eye nor kidney disease is due solely to microangiopathy. It is debatable whether the small vessel disease of diabetes also contributes to ischemic complications of the lower limbs and heart. The pathophysiology of microangiopathy is uncertain. Hemodynamic changes are receiving increasing attention as factors in the pathogenesis of both retinal and glomerular lesions.[20] Thickened capillary basement membranes are early hallmarks of microangiopathy.

Diabetic Nephropathy. Kidney disease in diabetes may affect all levels of the urinary tract. Kimmelstiel-Wilson syndrome, or intercapillary glomerulosclerosis, is virtually pathognomonic for diabetes but is by no means the only diabetic glomerular lesion. Diffuse glomerulosclerosis is a common cause of nephropathy, and both exudative and hyalinizing glomerular lesions are described. Capillary occlusion and arteriolar hyaline sclerosis may affect blood flow to the glomerulus. Tubular lesions are usually secondary to either glomerular pathology or pyelonephritis; the latter is a major consideration in diabetic renal failure. Renal papillary necrosis is more common in diabetics than in nondiabetics but is nevertheless rare. Neurogenic bladder with reflux hydronephrosis is an important cause of renal insufficiency, particularly when associated with chronic urinary tract infections.

Creatinine clearance is often elevated in poorly controlled diabetes, returning to normal either with improved control or developing nephropathy. Even with normal creatinine clearance, persistent proteinuria (>500 mg protein or about 25 mg albumin per 24 hours) is usually the first sign of nephropathy; occasionally nephropathy presents as nephrotic syndrome. About a third of diabetics have persistent proteinuria 15 years after the onset of diabetes; those who develop IDDM after puberty are at risk after a shorter course of diabetes. Azotemia develops an average of 3 to 5 years after proteinuria, and 6 to 10 years later most diabetics will have progressed to end-stage renal disease. Many diabetics, however, never develop proteinuria or detectable nephropathy. Hypertension is intimately related to nephropathy, as a cause, an effect, or both.

Diabetic Ophthalmopathy. The other major microangiopathy, diabetic retinopathy, is the most common form of diabetic eye disease but not the only form. Posterior lenticular cataracts develop in poorly controlled diabetics, and the incidence of both senile cataracts and glaucoma is increased. Ocular nerve palsies may occur.

Diabetic retinopathy is the leading cause of new blindness in people under 65 years of age in the United States.[17] It is clinically evident much earlier in the course of diabetes than is nephropathy. With careful observation and fundus photography, the first lesions of diabetic retinopathy (usually microaneurysms or intraretinal hemorrhages) are seen in half of patients with IDDM after 5 to 8 years. The initial event(s) may involve areas of focal deoxygenation because of abnormal erythrocyte aggregation, microthrombi, or primary capillary wall (mural cell) abnormalities.[18] Early lesions

usually do not threaten useful vision, however, and some patients never progress beyond simple background retinopathy. The major threat to vision occurs with capillary leakage, ischemic areas, and, ultimately, gross vitreous hemorrhage interfering with central macular function. A guide to the classification and treatment modalities is presented in Table 14.7–8.

Diabetic Macrovascular Disease

Diabetes accelerates large vessel atherosclerosis, causing an increased incidence of peripheral vascular, coronary artery, and cerebrovascular disease.[5] About 60 percent of people with NIDDM die of atherosclerotic cardiovascular disease; about 25 percent die of stroke.[17] The increased incidence of atherosclerosis in NIDDM over IDDM probably reflects the more advanced age of NIDDM patients. Coexisting risk factors for atherosclerosis—especially smoking, hypertension, and increased low-density lipoprotein (LDL) cholesterol or decreased high-density lipoprotein (HDL) cholesterol—add greatly to the risk of atherosclerosis in diabetes.

Stroke is about twice as common in diabetics as in nondiabetics, the small arteries being often more affected in diabetes, although major cerebral vessels are also involved. Lacunar strokes are common. Thrombotic strokes, however, are to be distinguished from cranial or peripheral mononeuropathies.

Peripheral vascular disease is usually more diffuse and more severe in diabetics than in nondiabetics, making reconstructive vascular surgery and interventional radiologic procedures more difficult. Symptoms of intermittent claudication should be carefully distinguished from neuropathic pain. The most reliable indications of poor distal circulation are absent dorsalis pedis and posterior tibial pulses, especially when such pulses were present on previous examination. Cool feet, distal hair loss, thin skin, dependent edema, and pallor on elevation are less reliable signs of peripheral vascular disease.

Sensory neuropathy often causes blisters or foot trauma to go unnoticed, and neuropathy also inhibits the normal local vasodilatory response to early infection. Thus, peripheral vascular disease and neuropathy act in concert to increase the incidence of serious foot infections and amputation.

Cardiac neuropathy may cause myocardial infarctions to be painless. Diabetic cardiomyopathy may decrease cardiac output or cause frank congestive heart failure even in the absence of coronary artery disease.

Diabetic Neuropathies

Diabetes affects the peripheral nervous system in a variety of ways (Table 14.7–9). An acute drop in nerve conduction velocity occurs with hyperglycemia and is correctable by controlling the blood glucose, but this acute metabolic change in nerve function probably

TABLE 14.7–8. CLASSIFICATION AND TREATMENT OF DIABETIC RETINOPATHY

Classification	Signs	Treatment
Background	Microaneurysms	Observation
	Intraretinal hemorrhages	Observation
	Hard exudates	Observation
	Macular edema[a]	Photocoagulation
Preproliferative	Venous beading	Photocoagulation
	Soft exudates	Photocoagulation
	Intraretinal microvascular abnormalities (IRMA)	Photocoagulation
	Extensive intraretinal hemorrhages	Photocoagulation
Proliferative	Neovascularization on disk or elsewhere	Photocoagulation
	Vitreous hemorrhages	± Vitrectomy
	Scarring, retina detached	± Vitrectomy

[a]Macular edema is sometimes classified as a more advanced stage of retinopathy.

TABLE 14.7–9. CLASSIFICATION OF DIABETIC NEUROPATHY

Neuropathy	Manifestations
Peripheral symmetrical polyneuropathy	Gradual onset, paresthesias, hyperesthesia, numbness, decreased vibratory and pin sensation, interosseal wasting, neuropathic ulcer, absent ankle and knee jerks
Mononeuropathies	
Peripheral	Acute onset involving single nerve; intense pain in lower or upper extremity, abdomen, or back; occasional motor involvement; resolves in several months
Cranial	CN III (with pupillary sparing), IV, VI, and occasionally VII; motor involvement; resolves gradually
Mononeuropathy multiplex	Several nerve trunks involved asymmetrically, rapid onset, sometimes painful
Autonomic neuropathies	
Impotence	Gradual onset, waxes and wanes, retrograde ejaculation
Neurogenic bladder	Residual postvoid urine, chronic infection, hydronephrosis, abnormal cystometrics
Orthostatic hypotension	Symptomatic on arising, syncope
Gastroparesis	Bloating, nausea, early satiety, vomiting, slow food absorption
Enteropathy	Intermittent diarrhea, especially postprandial and nocturnal; incontinence; intermittent constipation
Esophageal	Dysphagia
Abnormal sweating	Hemianhydrosis (usually lower body with upper body hyperhydrosis)
Cardiac neuropathy	Decreased R-R interval variation, "silent" myocardial infarction
Diabetic amyotrophy	Gradual onset; asymetric proximal muscle-wasting and pain, usually pelvic girdle and thigh; increased CSF protein and ESR; usually resolves in 3 to 6 months

does not reflect the nerve damage of long-term diabetes. Rather, the pathologic changes seen as a long-term diabetic complication include segmental demyelination of the peripheral sensory, motor, and autonomic nerves. It is unclear whether this is a primary Schwann cell lesion or is secondary to axonal degeneration. Spinal roots may be involved, and there is a propensity for involvement of small sensory nerve fibers.

Clinically, the diabetic neuropathies may be classified as peripheral symmetric polyneuropathy, mononeuropathy, autonomic neuropathy, or the amyotrophy syndrome (Table 14.7–9). Peripheral symmetric polyneuropathy is the most common. Absent deep tendon reflexes in the ankle and loss of proprioception are usually the first clinical signs. The neuropathy is predominantly sensory. Symptoms are extremely variable, from mild paresthesias or numbness to burning or lancinating pain. Pain usually resolves as the feet become progressively numb.

The mononeuropathies are single or multiple (mononeuropathy multiplex) and cranial or peripheral. Evidence is strong that the mononeuropathies result from a local vascular insufficiency. They occur suddenly, consistent with an acute vascular insult, and usually resolve in 1 to 6 months. Cranial neuropathies most often affect nerves III, IV, or VI. The third nerve palsy characteristically lacks papillary involvement. Cranial mononeuropathies involve only motor deficits. In contrast, peripheral mononeuropathies are generally painful and occur in the distribution of a large nerve bundle. The syndrome of diabetic amyotrophy is rare but presents a striking picture of asymmetric proximal muscle weakness, pain, and cachexia. It is considered to result from multiple mononeuropathies of the sacral plexus and, as with other mononeuropathies, usually resolves in about 6 months.

Autonomic neuropathy has a wide variety of manifestations but is usually not seen in the absence of significant peripheral symmetrical polyneuropathy. Sexual impotence and changes in bowel motility are the most common forms of autonomic neuropathy. Gastroparesis, atonic bladder, postural hypotension, cardiac denervation, and abnormal sweat patterns are also common manifestations.

TREATMENT

GENERAL PRINCIPLES

The first goal of diabetic therapy is to keep the metabolic state as close to normal as possible, consistent with an acceptable life-style and an acceptable incidence of treatment side effects such as hypoglycemia. Normalization of the metabolic status will eliminate acute complications and is likely to minimize or avoid the long-term complications. If such complications do occur, however, the goal of treatment is to prevent their progression.

While there is considerable circumstantial evidence that improved glycemic control will reduce the occurrence of long-term diabetic complications, rigorous proof is lacking. It is unclear exactly what level of glycemic control is necessary, that is, whether there is a continuous direct correlation between control and complications or whether there is a plateau above which complications occur. At present, clinicians should act on the evidence that good control does have a positive effect in avoiding complications.

Because diabetes is in most cases a lifelong illness, with fluctuations of metabolic status on an hour-to-hour basis, adequate therapy requires cooperation between the patient and the treating professional. Thorough education of the patient as to principles and specifics of self-care is integral to treatment. Full, open communication, positive attitudes, and support systems are essential.

The initial evaluation should include a careful history, eliciting information that will confirm the diagnosis of diabetes and classify the diabetic as IDDM, NIDDM, other, or gestational. History and physical examination document the status of risk factors (especially hypertension) and of diabetic complications. Laboratory evaluation should evaluate diabetic control with glycosylated hemoglobin (see below). This assay (or hemoglobin A_1c) is used both to assess diabetic control initially and to follow control longitudinally. Laboratory evaluation should also assess plasma lipid abnormalities and complications such as proteinuria.

All diabetic therapy begins with diet. Pharmacologic agents

may be added, but not to replace sound dietary management. If IDDM is diagnosed, insulin is started immediately. In NIDDM, there is usually time to try diet alone, progressing to oral hypoglycemic agents and, if necessary, to insulin. Most NIDDMs with fasting plasma glucose >250 mg/dl will require oral agents or insulin. Gestational diabetes requires stringent control promptly, either with diet alone or with insulin.

MONITORING DIABETIC CONTROL

Throughout the lifetime of a diabetic, regular monitoring of glycemic control should be used to adjust therapy. Occasional assays of fasting blood or urine glucose are of virtually no value, because glycemia changes markedly from hour to hour. Approaches to monitoring—self-monitoring of blood glucose and glycosylated hemoglobin assay—have progressed dramatically in recent years.

Urine glucose testing, still used by many diabetics, is distinctly inferior to self-monitoring of blood glucose, but it may be the only acceptable approach for some patients. The technique has many limitations: (1) Glucosuria occurs only when the blood glucose exceeds the renal threshold for glucose (normally 180 mg/dl, but extremely variable). A negative urine glucose does not indicate normoglycemia, but only the absence of severe hyperglycemia. (2) Urine testing provides no information about frank or borderline hypoglycemia. (3) Urine glucose reflects preexisting rather than a current plasma glucose. (4) The technique measures urinary glucose concentration, not the absolute amount. Recent water intake reduces urinary glucose concentration markedly while affecting blood glucose very little. A 24-hour collection of urine may provide an indication of poor diabetic control but still remains subject to all variables mentioned above except the last. Urine glucose is therefore not the recommended approach to monitoring.

About one quarter of all diabetics now perform self-monitoring of blood glucose. A spring-loaded lancet is used to prick the side of the distal phalanx of the finger. A drop of blood is applied to a reagent stick impregnated with glucose oxidase, and a color change may be read either visually or, preferably, with a reflectance meter. The technique is accurate if performed with careful attention to timing. It is relatively simple, well-accepted by most patients, and has revolutionized diabetic self-care.

It is important for patients to keep accurate records of all monitoring to allow appropriate modifications in the treatment regimen. Record-keeping is now facilitated by automatic memory devices in some reflectance meters. These devices also provide the physician with various statistical representations of the monitored data.

Another advance in glycemic monitoring is the use of glycosylated hemoglobin or hemoglobin A_{1c} assays.[2] As hemoglobin circulates in the erythrocyte, some is nonenzymatically and permanently glycosylated. If the plasma glucose is chronically elevated, more hemoglobin is glycosylated. Improvement in glycemic control is reflected by decreased glycosylated hemoglobin only as old erythrocytes are replaced with new cells containing less glycosylated hemoglobin. This slow responsiveness is the clinical strength of the test, because glycosylated hemoglobin thereby reflects the average glycemia over the previous 6 to 10 weeks. The test is used as a rough indication of control and as a tool for longitudinal follow-up.

The adequacy of blood glucose control is a matter of judgment. Guidelines presented in Table 14.7–10 are offered with the understanding that some "brittle" patients will never achieve consistently excellent or even good control, and that social instability or difficulty adhering to a regimen make even "fair" control too risky a goal in some patients. In the reliable and motivated patient, however, excellent control may be a reasonable target. It should always be the goal in pregnancy.

THE DIABETIC DIET

The diabetic diet includes adequate caloric intake to establish or maintain normal body weight, avoidance of concentrated sucrose,

TABLE 14.7–10. CRITERIA FOR ADEQUACY OF DIABETIC CONTROL

Control	Plasma Glucose (mg/dl)		
	Fasting and Preprandial	**1 hr Postprandial**	**Glycosylated Hemoglobin (%)[a]**
Excellent	70–120	100–140	<7.5
Good	121–140	141–160	7.6–9
Fair	141–160	161–200	9.1–11
Poor	>160	>200	>11

[a]Normal values for glycosylated hemoglobin vary markedly according to method used and laboratory standards.

distribution of calories in a reasonable pattern, increased fiber, and regularity of food intake.[8] The diet can be very palatable and nutritious and is best planned with the help of a trained nutritionist. Simply giving the patient printed instructions is inadequate.

Weight reduction is the most important goal for the obese diabetic. For children and pregnant women, caloric intake should be adequate to establish normal growth. The calories necessary to maintain body weight in the normal adult may be roughly estimated by multiplying the ideal body weight in pounds by 10 to approximate basal caloric expenditures and then adding either 33 percent for light activity, 50 percent for moderate activity, or 75 percent for heavy activity. Caloric requirement decreases with age, and obese individuals usually have lower energy requirements per unit body weight. There are about 3,500 calories in 1 pound of adipose tissue. A diet that is 500 calories per day less than that needed for weight maintenance therefore will result in loss of about 1 pound of adipose tissue per week.

Complex carbohydrates (potato, bread, rice, etc) require enzymatic cleavage in the gut to monosaccharides and disaccharides for absorption and enter the circulation more slowly than simple sugars. Different complex carbohydrates produce slightly differing degrees of glycemia. The "glycemic index" reflects these differences. It quantitates the glycemic response to fixed portions of various carbohydrates compared to that of white bread. In practice, however, glycemic excursions depend on many variables, such as the mix of fat and carbohydrate in a meal and gastric motility. The glycemic index is of little practical value, therefore, and self-monitoring of blood glucose should be used to determine the effects of diet.

Concentrated sources of sucrose (candy, cake, and nondiet soft drinks, etc) are avoided in the diabetic diet because they cause an abrupt and unpredictable rise in blood glucose. Carefully limited amounts of simple sugar may be included in the diabetic diet if treatment regimen is adjusted (e.g., by increasing short-acting insulin) to avoid unacceptable hyperglycemia. Noncaloric sweeteners and diet beverages are acceptable. Caloric sweeteners such as fructose, xylose, and sorbitol should be counted as caloric intake, although they raise plasma glucose more slowly than does sucrose. Alcohol in strict moderation may be included in the diabetic diet, counted as fat calories. Alcohol, however, may cause hypoglycemia in insulin-treated diabetics.

For patients treated with intermediate or long-acting insulins, the timing of meals must be regular to avoid hypoglycemia before a delayed meal or hyperglycemia from an early meal. The regularity of food portions is most important in insulin-treated patients and is easily accomplished using exchange lists. This ingenious system allows considerable dietary variety while maintaining approximately equal amounts of carbohydrate, fat, and protein.

The diabetic diet should not restrict complex carbohydrate. Indeed, 50 to 60 percent of total calories should be in the form of complex carbohydrates. Diets high in complex carbohydrates may improve insulin sensitivity in NIDDM patients and may smooth out blood glucose excursions in IDDM, allowing safe and accurate insulin dosage. A reduction of total fat to about 30 percent of calories, and of protein to 10 to 20 percent of calories, together

with a polyunsaturated to saturated fat ratio of 1:1 and a cholesterol intake of < 300 mg per day, are prudent goals for the diabetic to help control plasma cholesterol.

Finally, evidence has accumulated that a high intake of dietary fiber, especially bran and guar gums, may improve diabetic control, probably by delaying carbohydrate absorption. When diabetics are acutely catabolic or have serious metabolic complications, multivitamin supplementation may be indicated; the stable diabetic diet, however, should not require added vitamins.

EXERCISE

Exercise enhances insulin action and thus is potentially of specific benefit in controlling blood glucose as well as reducing cardiovascular risk factors and body weight.[6] Regular exercise is to be strongly recommended for the healthy diabetic but must be undertaken with certain precautions: (1) The hypoglycemic effect of exercise sometimes lasts as long as 8 to 12 hours. Exercise should be covered with extra dietary carbohydrate if blood glucose is near normal. (2) Particularly in the diabetic over 35 years of age, thorough evaluation of cardiac status should precede initiating of any exercise regimen. (3) Special precautions should be taken to avoid blisters and other foot problems, especially if peripheral neuropathy is present. (4) Excess strain or jarring is sometimes contraindicated for people with diabetic retinopathy.

With these precautions, a gradually progressive, carefully supervised exercise regimen is recommended.

ORAL HYPOGLYCEMIC AGENTS

Oral hypoglycemic agents may be useful in the treatment of NIDDM and some other types of diabetes. All currently available oral hypoglycemic agents are sulfonylureas; they all stimulate endogenous insulin secretion and potentiate peripheral insulin action.[12] Sulfonylureas are never a substitute for good dietary management. A high proportion of patients progress from oral hypoglycemic agents to insulin ("secondary failures") over 5 to 10 years.

Specific types of oral hypoglycemic agents, dosage, and routes of metabolism and clearance are summarized in Table 14.7–11. In addition to the rare allergic reaction and occasional (1 to 3 percent) gastrointestinal (GI) intolerance seen with all sulfonylureas, chlorpropamide has two specific side effects. First is the potentiation of antidiuretic hormone action, occasionally causing the syndrome of inappropriate ADH secretion. Second, 15 to 30 percent of patients taking chlorpropamide note a marked facial flush when they ingest alcohol—the "chlorpropamide-alcohol flush." Third, any sulfonylurea may induce hypoglycemia; but chlorpropamide, because it is renally excreted as active drug, is the longest acting sulfonylurea and may cause prolonged or recurrent clinical hypoglycemia.

A "second generation" of sulfonylureas was introduced in the United States in 1984. These agents, glyburide and glipizide, are more potent than the earlier sulfonylureas on a milligram for milligram basis (Table 14.7–11). Dosage range is thus 2.5 to 40 mg daily for the new agents, as compared to 250 mg to 1.5 g for the "first-generation" agents.

It is not yet clear whether the new sulfonylureas offer specific advantages over the older agents. The dosage range is somewhat wider, and there may be a reduced incidence of drug-drug interactions, such as the potentiation of coumadin anticoagulants. There is little evidence that the second-generation agents will be effective in patients who are unresponsive to first-generation agents. The cost of the new agents is generally competitive with that of the older drugs.

A long-term prospective trial conducted in the 1960s, the University Group Diabetes Program (UGDP), clouded the issue of sulfonylurea therapy. An increased cardiovascular mortality rate was found in mild NIDDM patients taking tolbutamide when compared with placebo or insulin therapy. A prolonged and exhaustive debate ensued, without resolution. Clinicians may evaluate the study for themselves, but reasonable conclusions would be that (1) oral hypoglycemic agents should not be used when control can be achieved with diet alone or given to pregnant women and (2) patients should be informed of the results of the UGDP. It is mentioned as a warning in the patient package insert.

Because sulfonylureas have a peripheral effect on insulin sensitivity, they might be considered beneficial in conjunction with exogenous insulin. There is no conclusive evidence, though, that combining insulin therapy with oral hypoglycemic agents is of clinical benefit.

INSULIN

By definition all IDDM patients require exogenous insulin. Many NIDDM patients also need insulin for glycemic control. In normal or underweight patients with NIDDM, the decision to start insulin therapy is relatively easy. Insulin is indicated when inadequate control is achieved with diet and exercise or when maximum doses of oral hypoglycemic agents have failed. The decision to start insulin is more difficult in the obese patient, because large doses are usually required (often >100 U/day), and appetite is stimulated by insulin therapy. The underlying problem in obesity-related NIDDM is clearly insulin resistance caused by obesity, not lack of endogenous insulin. Weight reduction, not insulin, is, therefore, the treatment of choice.

Commercial insulin preparations vary in species of origin, purity, concentration, and duration of action.[11]

Species of Origin
Standard commercial insulin preparations in the United States are prepared from mixed beef and pork pancreases (beef/pork insulin) (Table 14.7–12). Purified pork, purified beef, and human insulin are now also available. People treated with nonhuman insulin (i.e., beef/pork, beef, or pork) regularly develop antibodies to these insulins, which differ in structure from human insulin. The antibodies are clinically significant, however, only when they cause insulin allergy or marked insulin resistance. Pork insulin is less antigenic

TABLE 14.7–11. ORAL HYPOGLYCEMIC AGENTS

Drug	Daily Dosage	Route of Metabolism	Duration of Action (hr)	Comments
Tolbutamide	1.5 g	Inactivated in liver	6–8	Short-acting, tid dosage
Chlorpropamide	0.1–0.5 g	Excreted by kidney	36	Longest-acting, qd
Acetohexamide	0.25–1.5 g	Liver and kidney	12–18	Single or divided dose
Tolazamide	0.25–1.5 g	Liver and kidney	12–14	Single or divided dose
Glyburide	1.25–20 mg	Liver and kidney	24	Single or divided dose
Glipizide	5–40 mg	Liver and kidney	12–24	Single or divided dose

TABLE 14.7–12. VARIATIONS IN INSULIN PREPARATIONS

Species of origin	Beef/pork
	Pork
	Beef
	Human[a]
Purity	Standard (<25 ppm contaminants)
	Purified (<10 ppm contaminants)
Concentration	100 U/ml (U-100)
	500 U/ml (U-500)
	80 U/ml (U-80)
	40 U/ml (U-40)
Duration of action (see Table 14.7–14)	

[a]"Human" insulin is synthesized either by chemical modification of pork insulin or by recombinant DNA technology.

in humans than beef insulin because its amino acid structure is closer to that of human insulin. Although less antigenic than either beef or pork insulin, human insulin does elicit detectable antibody response in some patients. Because variable levels of anti-insulin antibody interfere with the radioimmunoassay of insulin, it is usually pointless to measure plasma insulin levels in patients who have been taking insulin.

Standard beef/pork insulin may be continued in patients already treated with these preparations in the absence of marked resistance (>200 units per day) or insulin allergy. Human insulin is preferable in certain circumstances (Table 14.7–13). Its cost is about 30 percent higher than beef/pork and about the same as purified pork insulin.

Purity

Standard beef/pork insulin is less pure (<25 ppm contaminants) than purified beef or pork insulins (<10 ppm contaminants) (Table 14.7–12), although all insulin preparations are purer than they were some years ago. Degree of purity is clinically significant only in the setting of insulin allergy or resistance.

Concentration

Insulin should be used routinely in the concentration of 100 U per ml (U-100). Still available U-40 and U-80 preparations are confusing and unnecessary. U-500 preparations are available for extreme insulin resistance. Insulin syringes must match the insulin concentration. "Low dose" U-100 insulin syringes contain only $\frac{1}{2}$ cc (50 units) when full, allowing more legible numbers and more accuracy if patients take less than 50 units per injection.

Duration of Action

The duration of action of insulin preparations varies according to the rate of absorption from subcutaneous tissues (Table 14.7–14). Modifications are accomplished either by changing crystal size (in the case of lente insulins) or by adding protamine (in the case of NPH or protamine zinc insulins). In practice, however, the duration of insulin action is affected in unpredictable ways by local factors at the site of injection (heat, vascularity, depth of injection) and systemic factors such as insulin antibody titer, nephropathy, and stress. The classic times of action presented in Table 14.7–14, therefore, are only rough approximations. Each patient's regimen must be individually tailored.

TABLE 14.7–13. INDICATIONS FOR USE OF HUMAN INSULIN

- Diabetics newly treated with insulin
- Marked insulin resistance (>200 U/day)
- Systemic insulin allergy (may require desensitization)
- Anticipated intermittent insulin therapy (e.g., surgery or pregnancy)

TABLE 14.7–14. DURATION OF ACTION OF INSULIN PREPARATIONS

Type of Action	Protein Additive	Buffer	Peak Action (hr)	Duration of Action (hr)
Rapid-acting				
• Crystalline zinc (regular)	None	None	2	5–7
• SemiLente	None	Acetate	2	8–16
Intermediate-acting				
• NPH	Protamine	Prosphate	6–12	18–24
• Lente	None	Acetate	6–12	18–24
Long-acting				
• Protamine zinc	Protamine	Phosphate	8–14	24–36
• UltraLente	None	Acetate	12–16	24–36

Initiation and Adjustment of Insulin Therapy

Table 14.7–15 provides an algorithm for initiating insulin therapy. In most insulin-requiring patients, it is advisable to mix a short-acting insulin preparation in the same syringe with an intermediate-acting preparation for morning administration; otherwise, there is unlikely to be sufficient coverage of breakfast. The morning dose of mixed insulins is increased until consistent hyperglycemia is broken. Insulin dosage should be increased in increments of 2 to 4 units ordinarily, or about 10 percent of the total dose, whichever is greater. The dosage should not be raised more frequently than every 2 to 4 days because the full effect of the new dose may not be seen in less time.

Once the patient no longer has continuous hyperglycemia or glucosuria, additional insulin injections may be added to establish

TABLE 14.7–15. GUIDELINES FOR INITIATION OF INSULIN THERAPY

One daily dose
Initial dose: 0.2–0.3 U/kg body weight before breakfast
- Preferably as mixed insulins[a]
- Increase total dose until persistent hyperglycemia is overcome
- Increase Regular insulin to treat prelunch hyperglycemia
- Increase NPH or Lente insulin to treat presupper hyperglycemia
- Add second daily dose to treat persistent fasting or bedtime hyperglycemia

Two daily doses
To treat fasting hyperglycemia:
- Switch about $\frac{1}{3}$ total daily dose to NPH or Lente given at bedtime
- Continue about $\frac{2}{3}$ total daily dose as mixed insulin before breakfast

To treat bedtime hyperglycemia:
- Switch about $\frac{1}{3}$ total daily dose to Regular before supper
- Continue about $\frac{2}{3}$ total daily dose as mixed insulin before breakfast

To treat persistent bedtime or fasting hyperglycemia despite the second daily dose, add a third daily dose

Three daily doses
- Treat fasting hyperglycemia with NPH or Lente insulin at bedtime
- Treat bedtime hyperglycemia with presupper Regular insulin

More intensive regimens
For more intensive insulin regimens, progress to external insulin pump or four times daily insulin, using about $\frac{1}{3}$ daily dose as UltraLente, $\frac{2}{3}$ daily dose divided into premeal injections of Regular insulin.

[a]Mixed insulin combines, in one syringe, NPH or Lente insulin (about $\frac{2}{3}$ of total dose) with Regular insulin (about $\frac{1}{3}$ of total dose).

adequate glycemic control throughout the day and night. The second daily dose may consist of Regular insulin with a small amount of NPH (ratio about 2:1 Regular to NPH) used before supper to control bedtime hyperglycemia; or NPH alone may be given at bedtime to control fasting hyperglycemia. An alternative intensive regimen combines one daily dose of long-acting insulin (protamine zinc or UltraLente) with short-acting (regular of semiLente) before each meal.

"Sliding scale" Regular insulin dosage is customarily used in acutely unstable, hospitalized patients, although it is preferable to add NPH as soon as the patient stabilizes. For the knowledgeable diabetic, sliding scales may be written for outpatient management. Ordinarily, the amount of Regular insulin is adjusted by 2 to 6 units according to blood glucose before a meal. For example, a patient taking 15 units NPH with 5 units Regular each morning may be instructed to increase the Regular to 7 units if blood glucose is >150 mg/dl and to 10 units for blood glucose >250 mg/dl.

Insulin Infusion Devices

A variety of external insulin pumps are available. All are open loop, i.e., without the ability to sense blood glucose, and all are worn on a belt with insulin delivery via a catheter to a needle placed subcutaneously in the abdomen and changed every 2 to 3 days. Basal infusion rates are established for overnight and between meals; bolus additions are triggered by the patient at each mealtime according to the current blood glucose and the meal about to be ingested.

Reasonable prerequisites for consideration of insulin pump therapy are established (Table 14.7–16). It is clear that insulin pumps are not useful and may be dangerous in patients with suboptimal motivation. Knowledge of diabetes and ability to adjust insulin dosage according to frequent self-monitoring of blood glucose are essential.

Implantable open-loop pumps are in an experimental stage, and glucose sensors await future development.

Complications of Insulin Therapy (Table 14.7–17)

Hypoglycemia is by far the most common complication of insulin therapy. Insulin reactions cause a range of symptoms from vague, mild auras to coma or death. All insulin-treated diabetics should know the symptoms of hypoglycemia, wear a Medic Alert tag, and carry a source of glucose for self-treatment. Mild, occasional insulin reactions are not necessarily harmful, but patients who experience severe reactions, impairing mentation, should have insulin doses adjusted downward. Because of the normal endogenous counter-regulatory response to hypoglycemia, unnecessary hyperglycemia may result if the patient overtreats (e.g., with large amounts of sugar added to orange juice). The patient and the family should learn to treat an insulin reaction without overcorrection, usually with 8 oz orange juice, milk, or hard candy.

Failure of counterregulatory response occurs, especially when autonomic neuropathy is present. This may predispose patients to more severe hypoglycemia while blunting the adrenergic symptoms. If patients are unable to detect hypoglycemia in time to self-treat, that is, if confusion is the first sign of insulin reactions, then goals for blood glucose control may have to be relaxed.

Somogyi effect consists of hypoglycemia, usually nocturnal,

TABLE 14.7–16. PREREQUISITES AND INDICATIONS FOR INSULIN PUMP TREATMENT

- Inadequate diabetic control on conventional therapy
- Demonstrated ability to perform glucose self-monitoring
- Reliability in dietary compliance
- Close contact with treating professionals
- Motivation and realistic expectations
- Careful in-hospital initiation

TABLE 14.7–17. COMPLICATIONS OF INSULIN THERAPY

- Hypoglycemia
- Dermatologic
  Lipoatrophy
  Lipid hypertrophy
  Local allergy
- Systemic allergy
- Insulin resistance
- Sodium retention

followed by significant hyperglycemia caused by counterregulation. It should be suspected when (1) wide swings of glycosuria are noted, (2) nocturnal sweating is followed by morning ketonuria, or (3) increasing doses of insulin appear to worsen rather than improve diabetic control.

Several local dermatologic complications of insulin are common. Loss of subcutaneous adipose tissue (lipoatrophy) causes large (5- to 10-cm) areas of depression. Conversely, lipid hypertrophy results in rounded elevations of subcutaneous tissue. These complications are minimized by rotation of injection sites and the use of purified or human insulins.

Erythema and itching at the site of insulin injection are common in newly treated diabetics. This local allergy usually resolves in several weeks and is not an indication to switch insulins, desensitize, or discontinue therapy. Local allergy must be carefully distinguished from systemic insulin allergy, however.

Urticaria remote from the site of insulin injection, generalized pruritus, periorbital edema, or bronchospasm may indicate systemic insulin allergy, potentially a medical emergency. Insulin should be changed to a human preparation, and symptomatic therapy with antihistamines should be initiated. If symptoms persist, patients should be hospitalized and desensitized with progressive doses of purified insulin, obtainable as a kit from Eli Lilly Co in Indianapolis. Anaphylactic shock is rare in this IgE-mediated allergy, but intravenous insulin should be strictly avoided.

Insulin resistance is defined as a basal daily requirement of >200 units or >3 units/kg. Such high insulin requirements are usually secondary to elevated titers of IgG antiinsulin antibody or excessive counterregulatory hormones, as seen in Cushing syndrome or acromegaly. Unusual causes of insulin resistance include decrease in the number of insulin receptors or defective intracellular translation of the insulin message in patients with acanthosis nigricans, lipotrophic diabetes, and other syndromes.

Patients treated for acute ketoacidosis with large amounts of saline often develop transient edema (called "insulin edema"), not clinically significant unless the sodium retention precipitates cardiovascular decompensation. This is the result of the antinatriuretic effect of insulin combined with the saline delivered therapeutically.

TREATMENT OF SPECIFIC DIABETIC COMPLICATIONS

Diabetic Ketoacidosis

In diabetic ketoacidosis (DKA), circulating insulin concentrations are inadequate to inhibit the release of free fatty acids from adipose tissue. Hepatic reesterification of these long-chain fatty acids is suppressed, and ketogenesis is promoted by an elevated glucagon/insulin ratio.[9] Ketone-body synthesis exceeds peripheral utilization, and poor renal perfusion reduces excretion of organic acids. The acidosis causes hyperventilation (Kussmaul respiration) as a compensatory mechanism. Nausea, vomiting, and circulatory collapse may follow. True coma from DKA is uncommon, however, and should suggest other causes such as hypoglycemia or stroke. Extreme glucosuria and osmotic diuresis can cause serious dehydration with extracellular fluid deficits, which average 6 liters. Potassium is shifted extracellularly by the acidosis, so that total body

potassium deficit from kaliuresis is masked by normal to elevated serum potassium. Serum potassium falls predictably with correction of acidosis and the shift of potassium back into the cells. Serum phosphate is similarly elevated by acidosis, and also falls with normalization of acid-base status. Other abnormal laboratory values seen in DKA include elevated amylase, serum transaminases, and increased hematocrit and SUN from dehydration.

A definite etiology cannot be identified in most cases of DKA. Infections of all sorts may be present without fever and are further obscured by the leukocytosis (even >20,000 WBC/mm³), which may accompany DKA even in the absence of infection. Decompensated diabetes can lead to signs of peritoneal inflammation, which along with leukocytosis can mimic appendicitis or acute biliary tract disease. In the presence of significant hyperglycemia or acidosis, therefore, every effort should be made to correct the metabolic status prior to surgery.

Because the underlying cause of DKA is insulin lack, insulin replacement is the basis of therapy (Table 14.7–18). Associated volume and electrolyte depletion, and precipitating or coexisting diagnoses, also guide appropriate treatment. The intensity of therapy is determined by the degree of hyperglycemia, dehydration, acidosis, and coexisting conditions such as myocardial infarction or sepsis. Insulin delivery is most conveniently and effectively accomplished by primed continuous intravenous infusion. While some insulin adheres to glass and plastic surfaces of the infusion apparatus, the infusion rate is adjusted according to clinical response, so loss of bound insulin may be ignored. A priming bolus of insulin followed by continuous intravenous infusion (Table 14.7–18) establishes a steady hyperinsulinemia, which ideally will lower plasma glucose to 200 to 250 mg/dl within 8 to 12 hours. If plasma glucose has not declined after 2 hours, the rate of infusion is increased 50 percent and further in stepwise fashion every hour until plasma glucose falls. Very high rates of insulin infusion (e.g., 0.3 U/kg) may be required initially. With severe hyperglycemia, hydration is as important as insulin in correcting plasma glucose.

Fluid deficits should be replaced over about 12 to 24 hours. Whether to use isotonic (0.9 percent) or hypotonic ("half normal," 0.45 percent) saline is controversial. Isotonic saline is preferable, however, in the setting of intravascular hypovolemia with shock, in order to expand the intravascular volume more rapidly. On the other hand, the possibility of cardiovascular decompensation from too vigorous fluid replacement must be considered, and a central venous pressure line should be placed when cardiovascular compromise is suspected. If serum potassium is normal or low on admission, potassium phosphate or chloride (20 mEq/L) should be infused. If serum potassium is high initially, potassium replacement therapy should begin when it has fallen into the normal range, anticipating the above-mentioned reduction of serum potassium as acidosis is corrected. The use of intravenous sodium bicarbonate is restricted to those cases in which acidosis itself threatens cardiovascular status. For example, severe acidosis with pH <7.10 may be an indication for bicarbonate therapy. Even with a higher pH, if respiratory compensation is extreme (e.g., P_{CO_2} <18 mm Hg), correction of the acidosis with bicarbonate is indicated because minor degrees of respiratory decompensation could quickly lower pH to dangerous levels.

The treatment of DKA should be gradual. Attempts to normalize plasma glucose and acidosis within a few hours invite both overcorrection (hypoglycemia and/or metabolic alkalosis) and the possibility of cerebral edema or paradoxical worsening of cerebrospinal fluid (CSF) acidosis. When plasma glucose falls to <250 mg/dl, insulin administration should be slowed to maintain glucose at about that level. Nitroprusside, used in bedside measurement of urine or blood acetone, reacts only to acetoacetate, although the predominant ketone body in DKA is beta-hydroxybutyrate. As acidosis is corrected, β-hydroxybutyrate is converted to acetoacetate. The nitroprusside reaction will remain positive, therefore, even as total ketone-body concentration and acidosis improve. Arterial pH and venous bicarbonate concentrations, as well as the patient's clinical state, are the best parameters to follow.

DKA is still a common cause of hospitalization in IDDM, costing $120 million in direct care per year and accounting for 9 to 10 percent of deaths among people with IDDM.[17] Complicating myocardial infarction or infections are the most common causes of death in DKA.

Hyperosmolar Nonketotic Coma

Hyperosmolar nonketotic coma results from severe, uncontrolled hyperglycemia. Ketosis is not seen because lipolysis is suppressed by low but present circulating insulin.

In hyperosmolar nonketotic coma, plasma glucose is always over 1000 mg/dl, and serum osmolarity exceeds 360 mOsm/L. Massive osmotic diuresis depletes total body water, often producing hypernatremia despite total body sodium depletion. Profound urinary potassium loss occurs. With hypovolemia, and often underlying renal disease, glomerular filtration rate falls and failure of the "escape valve" function of glucosuria further exacerbates hyperglycemia. The end result is uncontrolled elevation of blood glucose with dehydration, more from lack of water than insulin. Changes in mental status are well correlated with serum osmolarity, which may be estimated using the following formula:

$$\text{Osmolarity (mOsm/L)} = 2\,[\text{Na}^+ + \text{K}^+ \text{ mEq/L}] + \frac{\text{PG}}{18}\,\text{mg/dl} + \frac{\text{SUN}}{2.8}\,\text{mg/dl}$$

where PG = plasma glucose.

Stupor and coma occur only when serum osmolarity is >350 to 400 mOsm/L. Treatment is accomplished with rapid (1 L/hr) infusion of 0.9 percent saline for the first 2L, followed by 0.45 percent saline. The infusion rate may be halved after the first 2 liters. As with DKA, the central venous pressure should be monitored if there is a question of cardiac decompensation. Insulin administration is usually indicated, but low doses may be adequate (3 U/hr by intravenous infusion). The plasma glucose will fall more in

TABLE 14.7–18. TREATMENT OF DIABETIC KETOACIDOSIS

- Establish venous access with 20-gauge needle
- Draw venous blood for glucose, urea nitrogen, electrolytes; bedside test for glucose and acetoacetate; arterial blood gases; ECG
- Insulin: 10–20 U regular insulin by bolus intravenously, then 5–10 U/hr diluted in IV fluids; increase by 50% every 2 hr until plasma glucose begins to fall
- Fluids: 0.9% saline solution at 1 L/hr for 2 hr, then 500 ml/hr until hydration is established
- Nasogastric tube placement if patient is comatose; central venous pressure line if cardiovascular status is questionable
- Keep flow sheet of mental status, insulin, fluids, urine output, laboratory results
- Monitor mental status, cardiovascular, renal and blood chemistry status at least every 2 hr; may use T-waves on ECG to monitor serum potassium
- Bicarbonate: Add 45 mEq (1 ampule)/L fluid if arterial pH <7.10; give 1–2 amps bolus IV if pH <7.00, or cardiorespiratory arrest
- Potassium phosphate or chloride: Add to IV fluids if serum potassium is normal or low
- Check urine output; catheterize bladder only if patient unable to void; discontinue catheter within 24 hr if possible
- Add 5 or 10% dextrose by IV infusion when blood glucose is <200 mg/dl
- Discontinue IV insulin when chemistries have been normal for 6 hr
- Begin intermediate-acting insulin usually within 24 to 48 hr of admission; do not maintain regular insulin alone when patient is stable

response to hydration than to insulin. Potassium replacement is usually necessary. Restoration of normal plasma glucose should be gradual, over 12 to 24 hours.

Diabetic Pregnancy

Whether diabetes is newly diagnosed in pregnancy (gestational diabetes) or antedates pregnancy, tight plasma glucose control is indicated for the well-being of the fetus (see above).[10] Early in pregnancy, insulin requirements may decrease, probably on the basis of diminished food intake. After midpregnancy, however, the insulin requirement rises progressively, often to twice the prepregnancy dose. It is important during this phase to increase insulin replacement because diabetic ketoacidosis in pregnancy is associated with severe fetal wastage. Furthermore, normal maternal nutrition and weight gain require adequate insulinization. Immediately postpartum, patients usually return to their prepregnancy insulin requirement.

The timing of delivery is controversial, but current management principles would allow an uncomplicated diabetic pregnancy to progress to at least 37 weeks; delivery should be based on tests of fetal maturity. With evident complications of pregnancy, delivery may be earlier, again depending on evidence of fetal maturity.

In women with IDDM, pregnancy may exacerbate diabetic retinopathy, and any preexisting nephropathy may cause toxemia. Borderline cardiac status may be decompensated by pregnancy. Patients may be advised against pregnancy, therefore, if late-stage complications of diabetes are present. The well-controlled diabetic with mild preexisting complications, however, has a good chance for a normal pregnancy without harm to mother or fetus. The risk of diabetes in the offspring of a diabetic mother is no greater than if the father is diabetic (i.e., about 1 to 5 percent).

Surgery in the Diabetic

For elective major surgery in the diabetic, the objective is to avoid extremes of either hyperglycemia and acidosis or hypoglycemia. Usually, 33 to 50 percent of the daily insulin dose is given as an intermediate-acting preparation on the morning of surgery. Blood glucose is checked every 2 to 4 hours during and for 24 hours after surgery. Five percent dextrose (about 200 cc/hr) is infused intravenously. Regular insulin should be given postoperatively to maintain plasma glucose usually between 100 and 200 mg/dl.

In NIDDM, insulin should not be started just for surgery unless ketoacidosis develops. With dietary management and oral hypoglycemic agents, most non-insulin-treated patients will withstand surgery adequately. There is an elevated incidence of later insulin allergy following intermittent insulin treatment.

Large-vessel Atherosclerosis

Coronary artery and cerebrovascular disease in diabetics generally require the same treatment approaches used in nondiabetics. Risk factors such as smoking, hypertension, and elevated serum lipids must be treated vigorously. Beta-adrenergic blocking agents should be used with caution because they may blunt counterregulatory responses and predispose to insulin reactions.

With peripheral vascular disease in the lower extremities, the diffuse and severe nature of the atherosclerotic process requires education of the patient in preventive approaches to avoid amputation. Diabetics should be taught to avoid foot trauma at all costs, by breaking in new shoes slowly, never going barefoot, avoiding extremes of heat, and inspecting their feet daily. When foot deformities exist, specially designed therapeutic shoes may reduce the chance of pressure ulcers.

Open foot lesions must be treated vigorously, often with hospitalization, bed rest, and intravenous antibiotics.[14] Angiograms are helpful in deciding when to attempt interventional radiological procedures and reconstructive vascular approaches. Toe or trans-metatarsal amputations are sometimes effective in treating isolated areas of gangrene, but healing is slow and more proximal amputations often become necessary, especially if pockets of infection exist.

Retinopathy

Laser photocoagulation treatment is available for diabetic retinopathy[15] (Table 14.7–8). Randomized, prospective trials have shown conclusively that photocoagulation reduces the incidence of visual impairment when used to treat proliferative retinopathy or clinically significant macular edema. Consequently, every diabetic should have a thorough examination of the fundus at least yearly by an ophthalmologist. Vitrectomy—the surgical removal of vitreous—may be possible for diabetics with visual loss from the vitreous hemorrhage and its complications. This technique is by no means always successful and is usually indicated only as a last resort. Hypophysectomy is no longer used to treat retinopathy. A variety of support services may enhance the quality of life of the blind or severely visually impaired diabetic.

Hypertension in the Diabetic

Hypertension and diabetes pose a particularly dangerous combination of cardiovascular risk factors.[4] Hypertension may result from diabetic nephropathy but may also accelerate the progress of renal disease in a vicious cycle that can adversely affect retinopathy and large vessel disease as well. Hypertension associated with nephropathy is often of the volume-expanded, low-renin type. This suggests that diuretic therapy is indicated as the first line of treatment. The hyperglycemic effect of thiazide diuretics appears to be secondary to urinary potassium-wasting and the suppression of endogenous insulin secretion by hypokalemia. If blood pressure does not respond to diuretic therapy, second- and third-line antihypertensives should be added, including angiotensin-converting-enzyme inhibitors. Special considerations in the diabetic include (1) the effect of hypokalemia on endogenous insulin secretion and (2) the ability of beta-adrenergic blocking agents such as propranolol to suppress hypoglycemic symptoms and physiologic counter-regulation of blood glucose. Insulin-treated diabetics are more susceptible to unrecognized insulin-induced hypoglycemia when treated with beta-adrenergic blocking agents.

Nephropathy

Diabetic nephropathy occurs at a relatively predictable rate in some but not all diabetics.[13] Control of hypertension is the only treatment known to be effective in early stages of nephropathy. Some studies with animals suggest that control of plasma glucose may also slow or even reverse the early glomerular lesions of diabetic nephropathy. Controversy exists as to whether diminished dietary protein is indicated early in nephropathy, but increased dietary protein (over 100 g/day) is necessary in the setting of nephrotic syndrome, with excessive urinary protein losses and hypoalbuminemia. Conversely, as uremia progresses, a reduced dietary protein load (less than 40 g/day) and treatment with phosphate binders will probably delay the development of end-stage renal disease.

Renal dialysis is now more successful in diabetics than in previous years, with chronic ambulatory peritoneal dialysis often the treatment of choice. Nevertheless, there is a significantly increased incidence of complications when diabetics are dialyzed, and kidney transplantation is a preferred approach.

Diabetic Neuropathy

The management of peripheral symmetric polyneuropathy is a therapeutic dilemma.[20] Pain may be reduced by avoiding strenuous activity but is often worse at night. Phenytoin is of no value, whereas carbamazepine (200 mg two to four times daily) and other analgesics are sometimes effective. Phenothiazines, particularly when an element of depression is present, are advocated. Patients should be reassured that pain usually eases, albeit as neuropathy worsens and numbness supervenes.

Autonomic neuropathy is also treated symptomatically depending on its manifestations. Penile implants of various types are available if impotence is a major problem; androgen therapy is useless. In diabetic enteropathy with diarrhea, a 2-week course of tetracycline may help if bacterial overgrowth is a factor. Otherwise, diphenoxylate (Lomotil) or opiates are used, recognizing that diabetic diarrhea characteristically remits within weeks to months.

Gastroparesis may respond to metoclopramide (10 to 15 mg four times daily).

REFERENCES

1. Bliss M: The Discovery of Insulin. Toronto, McClelland and Steward, 1982
2. Bunn HF: Evaluation of glycosylated hemoglobin in diabetes patients. Diabetes 30:613, 1981
3. Caro JF, Ittoop O, et al: Studies on the mechanism of insulin resistance in the liver from humans with noninsulin-dependent diabetes. J Clin Invest 78:249, 1986
4. Christlieb RA: Hypertension in the diabetic patient. In Marble A, Krall L, et al (eds): Joslin's Diabetes Mellitus, 12th ed. Philadelphia, Lea & Febiger, 1985
5. Collwell JA (ed): Workshop on insulin and atherogenesis. Metabolism 34(suppl 1), 1985
6. DeFronzo RA (ed): Exercise and diabetes. Diabetes/Metab Rev 1:317, 2:1, 1986
7. Eisenbarth GS: Type I diabetes mellitus: A chronic autoimmune disease. N Engl J Med 314:1360, 1986
8. Flood TM, Halford BN, et al: Dietary management of diabetes. In Marble A, Krall L, et al (eds): Joslin's Diabetes Mellitus, 12th ed. Philadelphia, Lea & Febiger, 1985
9. Foster DW, McGarry JD: The metabolic derangements and treatment of diabetic ketoacidosis. N Engl J Med 309:159, 1983
10. Freinkel N, Dooley SL, Metzger BE: Care of the pregnant woman with insulin-dependent diabetes mellitus. N Engl J Med 313:96, 1985
11. Galloway JA, DeShazo RD: The clinical use of insulin and the complications of insulin therapy. In Ellenberg M, Rifkin H (eds): Diabetes Mellitus: Theory and Practice, 3d ed. New Hyde Park, NY, Exerpta Medica Co, 1983
12. Gerich JE: Sulfonylureas in the treatment of diabetes mellitus—1985. Mayo Clin Proc 60:439, 1985
13. Krolewski AJ, Warram JH, et al: The changing natural history of nephropathy in type I diabetes. Am J Med 78:443, 1986
14. LoGerfo FW, Coffman JD: Vascular and microvascular disease of the foot in diabetes. Implications for foot care. N Engl J Med 311:1615, 1984
15. Murphy RP: Current status of treatment of nonproliferative and proliferative diabetic retinopathy. In Friedman EA, L'Esperance FA (eds): Diabetic Renal-Retinal Syndrome, vol 2. New York, Grune & Stratton, 1982
16. National Diabetes Data Group: Classification and diagnosis of diabetes mellitus and other categories of glucose intolerance. Diabetes 28:1039, 1979
17. National long-range plan to combat diabetes. NIH Publication No. 87-1587 by National Diabetes Advisory Board. September, 1987, p ix
18. Patz A: Studies on retinal neovascularization. Invest Ophthalmol Vis Sci 19:1128, 1980
19. Pfeifer MA, Greene DA: Diabetic neuropathy. Current Concepts. Kalamazoo, Michigan, Upjohn Co., 1985
20. Zatz R, Brenner BM: Pathogenesis of diabetic microangiopathy. The hemodynamic view. Am J Med 80:443, 1986

CHAPTER 14.8
Hypoglycemia

Angeliki Georgopoulos and Simeon Margolis

Chemical hypoglycemia, often defined arbitrarily as a plasma glucose level less than 50 mg/dl, is not uncommon, particularly in women. Less frequently, low plasma glucose triggers symptomatic hypoglycemia. Evaluation of a patient for possible hypoglycemia poses two diagnostic problems: demonstration that hypoglycemia produces the patient's symptoms and identification of the underlying cause for the abnormally low plasma glucose.

The degree of hypoglycemia required to produce symptoms varies widely, as do the clinical manifestations reported by different patients. A similar pattern of symptoms generally recurs, however, in any one individual. The hypoglycemic symptoms result from sympathetic (adrenergic) activation and impaired central nervous system (CNS) function (neuroglucopenia). Symptoms consequent to sympathetic activation usually occur when plasma glucose falls rapidly. They include sweating, palpitations, tremor, nervousness, hunger, acral and perioral numbness, faintness, and weakness. These important clues to the presence of hypoglycemia may be blunted or absent in patients treated with beta-adrenergic blocking agents and in some patients with long-standing diabetes. Hypoglycemia also impairs the CNS, which requires an adequate supply of glucose for normal function. Central nervous system symptoms, which can mimic a wide variety of neurologic and psychiatric abnormalities, usually predominate when plasma glucose levels decline slowly and reach lower levels (40 mg/dl or below). Common symptoms include headache, diplopia, confusion, inappropriate affect, motor incoordination, and with extreme hypoglycemia, seizures, coma, and ultimately death. Convulsions are particularly common in children. Signs of severe hypoglycemia include hypothermia, conjugate deviation of the eyes, extensor rigidity of the limbs, trismus, and Babinski sign. In patients with cerebral vascular disease, symptoms may occur at higher plasma glucose levels, and localized neurologic findings may correlate with underperfused regions of the brain. The symptoms and signs of hypoglycemia are generally reversible, but permanent brain damage can result from prolonged, severe hypoglycemia.

Glucose values vary with the method of measurement. Although many reports are based on values obtained from whole blood, most laboratories now employ automated methods to measure *plasma glucose,* values of which are 10 to 15 percent higher than blood glucose values. Thus, a blood glucose of 50 mg/dl corresponds to a plasma glucose of about 57 mg/dl, and such differences are significant in the definition of chemical hypoglycemia.

MAINTENANCE OF GLUCOSE HOMEOSTASIS

Hypoglycemia results when the removal of glucose from the bloodstream by peripheral tissues exceeds glucose delivery from the diet or the liver. In the normal state, a number of hormones, through their actions on both the exit and entry of glucose, maintain the level of plasma glucose within fairly constant and narrowly defined limits.

Immediately after food intake, absorbed glucose and amino acids, together with hormones released from the intestinal mucosa, promote insulin secretion by pancreatic beta cells. Insulin stimulates glucose translocation into muscle and adipose tissue cells where glucose is utilized for energy or stored after conversion to glycogen or triglycerides. As much as 25 percent of ingested glucose is retained by the liver, where insulin promotes glycogen storage and inhibits the synthesis of glucose (gluconeogenesis) from amino acids, lactate, and glycerol. As blood glucose falls, prompt

cessation of insulin secretion, along with increased release of glucagon and epinephrine, normally prevents a fall in plasma glucose to hypoglycemic levels. If hypoglycemia occurs despite these hormonal changes, cortisol and growth hormone secretion is triggered. Epinephrine release is responsible for most symptoms of postprandial hypoglycemia; it also acts rapidly to stimulate glycogen breakdown and fatty acid mobilization and to inhibit insulin secretion and glucose uptake in peripheral tissues.

Early in fasting, plasma glucose levels are maintained through increased glucose release from the liver. Glycogen breakdown predominates in the first 24 hours of fasting. During a more prolonged fast, peripheral glucose utilization is decreased, and hepatic gluconeogenesis becomes the sole source of plasma glucose. Gluconeogenesis is regulated by hormonal control of the activity of hepatic enzymes as well as the release of substrates from muscle (amino acids) and adipose tissue (glycerol). The most significant hormonal alteration is a marked reduction in levels of circulating insulin. Insulinopenia decreases peripheral glucose utilization; allows mobilization of glycerol, fatty acids (the major energy source during fasting), and amino acids; diminishes hepatic glycogen synthesis; and permits glycogenolysis and gluconeogenesis in the liver. The secretion of counterregulatory hormones also helps to maintain plasma glucose levels. Thus, glucagon promotes glycogen breakdown in the liver; glucagon and cortisol stimulate hepatic gluconeogenesis; growth hormone and cortisol impede glucose entry into muscle. Glucocorticoids also increase the availability of amino acids for gluconeogenesis, and, along with growth hormone, stimulate triglyceride breakdown in adipose tissue.

Based on their relation to food intake, two major patterns of hypoglycemia can be defined: (1) postprandial hypoglycemia and (2) fasting hypoglycemia. Postprandial hypoglycemia is provoked by food ingestion and does not occur in the fasting state. Fasting hypoglycemia can be due to endogenous causes or can be induced by drugs or poisons (exogenous hypoglycemia). Although they usually follow a period of fasting, some forms of fasting hypoglycemia, especially those due to exogenous causes, can occur in the postprandial period. Classifications of postprandial and fasting hypoglycemia are presented in Tables 14.8–1 and 14.8–2.

SYMPTOMATIC HYPOGLYCEMIA OCCURRING ONLY IN THE POSTPRANDIAL STATE[2,8,9,11]

Lay publications have popularized the notion that hypoglycemia is a common disorder that produces a wide variety of often vague complaints. In contrast, some experts have questioned whether hypoglycemia in the postprandial state exists at all. The truth lies somewhere between. Although symptomatic postprandial hypoglycemia is uncommon, food ingestion does induce hypoglycemic symptoms during the subsequent 1 to 6 hours in some individuals. In rare hereditary abnormalities seen in children, hypoglycemia may follow the ingestion of fructose, galactose, or leucine; in adults, hypoglycemia is usually related to glucose intake. Symptoms of postprandial hypoglycemia are caused by sympathetic activation and catecholamine release. Significant CNS symptoms are uncommon in the adult; seizures and coma are rare. The symptoms usually subside within 30 minutes even if no therapy is un

TABLE 14.8–1. CLASSIFICATION OF POSTPRANDIAL HYPOGLYCEMIAS

- Induced by glucose
  - Reactive
  - "Diabetic"
  - Alimentary
  - Hormonal
- Induced by fructose, galactose, or leucine (pediatric)

TABLE 14.8–2. CLASSIFICATION OF FASTING HYPOGLYCEMIAS

Endogenous (spontaneous)
- Hepatic
  - Extensive liver disease
  - Enzyme defects (pediatric)
- Hormonal
  - Insulin excess
    - Insulinoma, other islet cell tumors
    - Autoimmune hypoglycemia
  - Growth hormone deficiency
  - Glucocorticoid deficiency
- Hypoglycemia associated with serious medical illness
  - Renal disease
  - Malnutrition
  - Sepsis
  - Congestive heart failure
- Extrapancreatic tumors

Exogenous (drug-induced)
- Insulin
- Sulfonylureas
- Alcohol
- Salicylates
- Propranolol
- Poisons (plants, hepatotoxic substances)

dertaken because catecholamine release raises the plasma glucose levels. Because adrenergic symptoms are not specific and can be encountered in situations other than hypoglycemia, it is important for the diagnosis of postprandial hypoglycemia to show that the symptoms are associated with low blood glucose levels (Fig. 14.8–1). The repetition of a particular constellation of symptoms, which have a fairly constant relationship to food intake and occur commonly late in the morning or afternoon, is suggestive of postprandial hypoglycemia. Minimal food intake, such as sugar-containing fruit juices or sodas, can trigger hypoglycemic symptoms, especially if the person is on a low-carbohydrate diet. Thus, it is important to obtain a careful dietary history and to assess the carbohydrate content of the diet. In addition the patient is instructed in the use of a glucose oxidase strip reagent (Chemstrips bG) to measure the blood glucose at the time of the symptoms. The strips are brought to the office within a week to have the reading verified by the physician or another health professional. No further work-up is necessary if these glucose levels are greater than 80 mg/dl. If the glucose level is below 80 mg/dl, the diet is modified to contain at least 50 percent of calories as carbohydrates, and simple sugars are severely restricted. If symptoms persist and are accompanied by Chemstrip glucose values less than 80 mg/dl, a 6-hour glucose tolerance test is performed.

To avoid false-positive and false-negative results, the test must be done after a standard protocol. The patient should avoid drugs known to affect glucose tolerance and ingest at least 250 g of carbohydrates for 3 days before the test. The standard dose of glucose (1.75 g/kg ideal body weight, but not to exceed 100 g total) is given as a 50 percent solution. Because the plasma glucose nadir is often transient, blood samples are obtained at 30-minute intervals throughout the test. In addition, the patient is instructed to record the time and nature of any symptoms and to notify the technician so that an immediate blood sample can be obtained. Moreover, the technician can be trained to recognize and record signs of hypoglycemia (tremor, pallor, perspiration, tachycardia, bounding pulse). Although no single value is uniformly accepted as evidence of chemical hypoglycemia, a plasma glucose greater than 60 mg/dl rules out the diagnosis and a level less than 50 mg/dl, in association with appropriate symptoms, confirms the diagnosis of symptomatic hypoglycemia. Normal individuals occasionally exhibit values below 50 mg/dl without symptoms. Because the rapidity of blood glucose fall also contributes to the development of adrenergic symptoms, the hypoglycemic index,[5] which takes into account

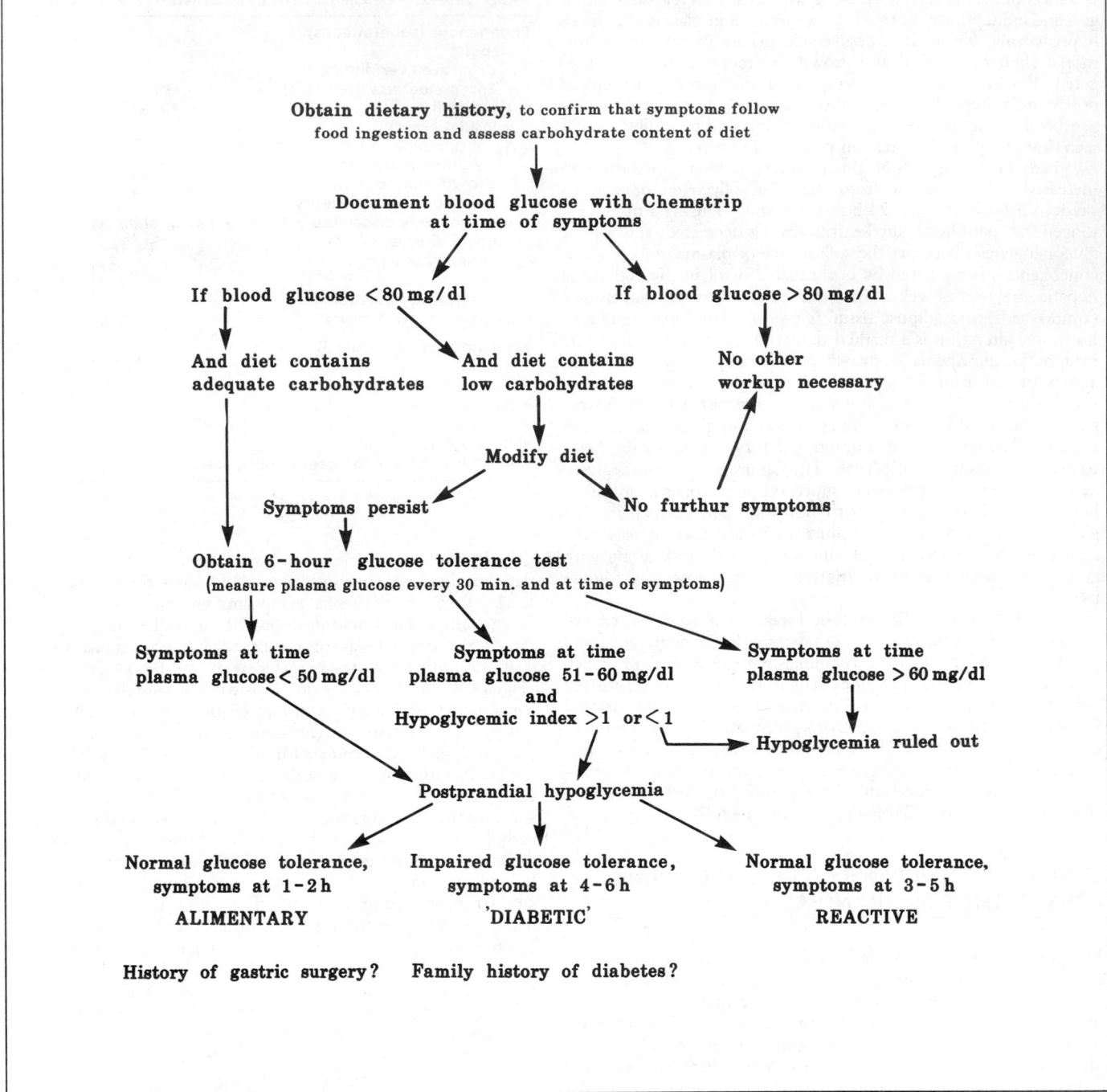

Figure 14.8–1. Flow chart for diagnosing postprandial hypoglycemia.

both the rate of decline and the nadir of plasma glucose, can be used as an additional diagnostic criterion in patients who are symptomatic during the test and have a measured plasma glucose between 50 and 60 mg/dl. The hypoglycemic index = $(P_{GN-90}-P_{GN})/P_{GN}$, where P_{GN} is the plasma glucose nadir and P_{GN-90} is the plasma glucose 90 minutes before P_{GN}. A value greater than 1 strongly supports the diagnosis; a value below 1 rules out the diagnosis.

Historical information and the glucose tolerance test also help to distinguish among the types of postprandial hypoglycemia. Based on the timing of symptoms and the profiles of plasma glucose and insulin, four types of glucose-induced postprandial hypoglycemia can be identified (Table 14.8–1). The three most common forms are reactive, diabetic, and alimentary. In addition,

deficiencies of growth hormone, cortisol, or thyroxine may cause postprandial symptoms in rare patients. In such cases hypoglycemia is just one of the symptoms associated with abnormal levels of these hormones. In some patients the pattern may change over the years from reactive hypoglycemia to the "diabetic" form.

REACTIVE, FUNCTIONAL, OR IDIOPATHIC HYPOGLYCEMIA

This syndrome is the most common of the postprandial hypoglycemias. Although abnormal secretion of a number of hormones, including gastrointestinal hormones, has been suggested by various

investigators, the pathogenesis is still unclear. It is noteworthy that intravenous glucose does not produce symptoms in these patients. Glucose tolerance is not impaired and serum insulin responses are heterogeneous. In some patients, serum insulin levels are appropriate for the plasma glucose (Fig. 14.8–2), but occasionally serum insulin concentrations are excessively high. Most often the insulin response is delayed in onset but normal in magnitude. Symptoms, which usually appear 3 to 5 hours after a meal, may be limited to mild anxiety and restlessness, but some patients describe more severe complaints associated with blatant sympathetic activation. Because a faulty diet, high in simple sugars and low in complex carbohydrates, can also promote the development of hypoglycemic symptoms in even normal subjects, a careful dietary history is an important part of the work-up for reactive hypoglycemia.

"DIABETIC" HYPOGLYCEMIA

The term "diabetic" hypoglycemia is a misnomer. Some patients with normal fasting plasma glucose but impaired glucose tolerance (at least one plasma glucose level exceeding 200 mg/dl during the first 2 hours of the glucose tolerance test and a 2-hour value between 140 and 200 mg/dl) develop hypoglycemia 4 to 6 hours following glucose ingestion (Fig. 14.8–2). Only a small fraction of these patients later become diabetic, and postprandial hypoglycemia does not occur in patients with overt diabetes. The hypoglycemia is attributed to excessive and delayed insulin response to the glucose load; as a result insulin levels are elevated at a time when plasma glucose is falling.

ALIMENTARY HYPOGLYCEMIA

Alimentary hypoglycemia, which usually presents with the most characteristic clinical picture and test results, may occur in patients with thyrotoxicosis or rapid gastric emptying of unknown cause. Most often, however, the syndrome follows gastrectomy, gastrojejunostomy, or vagotomy and pyloroplasty. As illustrated in Figure 14.8–2, a precipitous rise in plasma glucose levels, resulting from the rapid entry of large amounts of glucose into the small intestine, provokes dramatic secretion of insulin and subsequent hypoglycemia, which occurs earlier (1 to 2 hours after glucose ingestion) than in other forms of postprandial hypoglycemia. The dumping syndrome (see Chapter 12.3), rather than hypoglycemia, may cause symptoms in many individuals following gastrointestinal surgery.

THE "NONHYPOGLYCEMIA" SYMPTOMS[3,10]

In cases of severe adrenergic symptoms not associated with low blood sugars, the differential diagnosis should include thyrotoxicosis, pheochromocytoma, and anxiety attacks. It has long been stressed that individuals with reactive hypoglycemia tend to be asthenic, hyperkinetic, obsessive-compulsive persons who are tense and often emotionally labile. Psychologic tests have shown similar personality profiles, however, in patients with all types of symptomatic postprandial hypoglycemia.[4] It should also be made clear that lack of energy, chronic anxiety, lethargy, mental dullness, and similar complaints rarely result from hypoglycemia. Yet a large number of patients persistently blame hypoglycemia for such symptoms, which they attempt to control by a variety of dietary measures. The physician performs a valuable service by demonstrating that symptoms have been incorrectly attributed to hypoglycemia. Because plasma glucose may fall below 50 mg/dl in normal individuals during a glucose tolerance test, a diagnosis of symptomatic hypoglycemia can be made only if chemical hypoglycemia and characteristic symptoms coincide.

TREATMENT OF POSTPRANDIAL HYPOGLYCEMIA[2,11]

The management of patients with postprandial hypoglycemia is hampered by a lack of controlled clinical trials and objective measures to quantify therapeutic effectiveness. A number of unproven modes of treatment have been employed. Rational therapy, which includes both dietary modification and drugs, is directed toward timing of meals, proper selection of foods, and attempts to delay glucose absorption. High-protein, carbohydrate-restricted diets were stressed in the past, but studies suggest little benefit, and possibly increased symptoms, from a low carbohydrate intake. Instead, emphasis should be placed on the ingestion of complex carbohydrates (such as starches) and elimination of simple sugars and fruit drinks. It is important to recognize, however, that different starch-containing foods evoke variable responses in plasma glucose and insulin levels. The inclusion of fiber and some fat in every meal will delay gastric emptying and lessen postprandial hypoglycemia. Fructose can be used as a sweetening agent since it produces a smaller response in blood levels of glucose and insulin than does glucose or sugar. The dietary measures described above, as well as a pattern of multiple small feedings, may be helpful in any type of postprandial hypoglycemia. In patients with diabetic hypoglycemia reduction to ideal body weight is an important goal.

If dietary treatment is not totally satisfactory, symptoms may be controlled by anticholinergic drugs that slow gastric emptying and intestinal motility and inhibit vagal stimulation of insulin re-

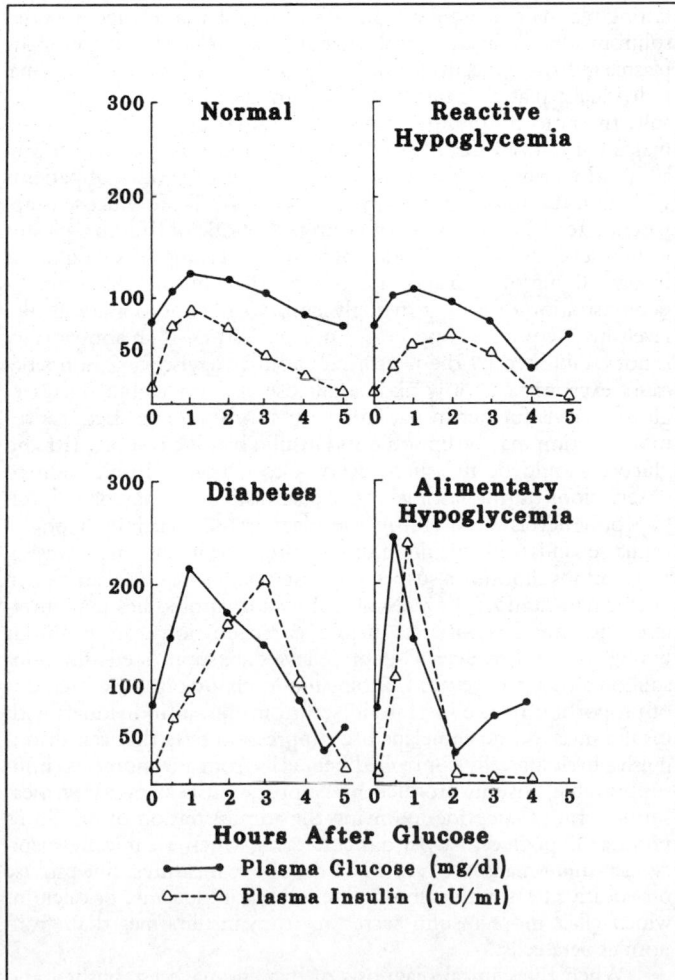

Figure 14.8–2. Comparison of glucose and insulin levels in normal subjects and individuals with various types of postprandial hypoglycemia during a 5-hour glucose tolerance test.

lease. Tincture of belladonna (10 to 15 drops), atropine sulfate (0.5 to 1 mg), or probantheline bromide (Pro-Banthine, 7.5 mg) 30 minutes before each meal have all proven effective in some patients. Most success has been achieved in reactive hypoglycemia, but symptoms may also respond in alimentary hypoglycemia. If symptoms persisted in the latter group, improvement was observed in some patients following reversal of the jejunal segment of the bowel. The sulfonylurea hypoglycemic agents may ameliorate hypoglycemic symptoms in patients with diabetic hypoglycemia by stimulating the early secretion of insulin. If symptoms do not improve despite dietary compliance and the use of drugs, treatment for coexisting anxiety attacks should be considered. Because there is evidence for abnormal personality profiles in patients with all types of postprandial hypoglycemia, psychotherapy may help by addressing their psychiatric problems, including symptoms generated by anxiety attacks.

SYMPTOMATIC HYPOGLYCEMIA IN THE FASTING STATE[2,8,11]

The overnight fasting glucose level, rather than a glucose tolerance test, is the most useful screening test for fasting hypoglycemia. Fasting plasma glucose values must be interpreted carefully, especially in women, because prolonged fasting causes a much greater fall in plasma glucose in healthy young women than in men.[9] Thus, a fasting plasma glucose level below 50 mg/dl in a man should raise strong suspicion of significant hypoglycemia. In women the lower limit of plasma glucose is not defined with certainty; however, a level below 40 mg/dl is highly suspicious. Plasma glucose levels after a prolonged fast are lower in women 16 to 22 weeks pregnant than in nonpregnant women. In all individuals, concomitant symptoms are just as important for the diagnosis of symptomatic hypoglycemia as the absolute level of plasma glucose.

Because the underlying disorder is more serious in the fasting than in the postprandial hypoglycemias, it is imperative to identify the abnormality. Fasting hypoglycemia is generally caused by reduced glucose release by the liver. Sometimes peripheral glucose utilization is also increased. The major causes of fasting hypoglycemia are listed in Table 14.8–2.

ENDOGENOUS HYPOGLYCEMIA

Hepatic Causes

Primary Liver Disorders. Despite the central role of hepatic gluconeogenesis in maintaining normal fasting levels of plasma glucose, liver disease is an infrequent cause of symptomatic hypoglycemia. Severe hypoglycemia usually does occur immediately after extensive surgical resection of the liver unless preventive measures are taken. Hypoglycemia can also follow acute, fulminant hepatic necrosis of viral or toxic origin.

Symptomatic hypoglycemia may occur in some severe cirrhotics. If the hypoglycemia is not due to ethanol intake, the physician should be especially alert to the presence of a hepatoma when repeated hypoglycemia is noted in the course of cirrhosis. Most commonly a poorly differentiated hepatoma is associated with severe anorexia, marked weight loss, and hypoglycemia as a late complication. In a few patients with well-differentiated hepatomas, hypoglycemia begins many months before their death, whereas loss of appetite and weight develop late in their illness. The cause of hypoglycemia in these patients is not clear, but the hypoglycemia can occur without massive replacement of normal liver.[7] Rarely, hypoglycemia is associated with biliary tract disease.[8]

Inborn Hepatic Enzyme Defects. Hypoglycemia also occurs in several rare disorders, each resulting from the deficiency of a specific hepatic enzyme required for normal carbohydrate metabolism. In these diseases, which include glycogen storage diseases, galacto-

semia, and hereditary fructose intolerance, symptoms of hypoglycemia usually begin in infancy and are less prominent in affected adults.[2]

Hormonal Causes
Insulin Excess

Insulinomas. Insulinomas[6] are rare tumors that occur at all ages and with equal frequency in men and women. They are diagnosed most commonly in individuals in the fourth through seventh decades. Multiple insulinomas are present in approximately 10 percent of the cases and a similar number are malignant.

Because nonspecific complaints, such as malaise, profound fatigue, confusion, or headaches upon arising, often predominate in early stages of the disorder, symptoms have generally been present for a long time before a correct diagnosis is made. Amnesia and impaired judgment may make it difficult to obtain a reliable history from the patient. With increasing size of the tumor, symptoms of acute hypoglycemia become more prominent. Hunger and compulsive eating occasionally lead to weight gain. In addition to symptoms of sympathetic activation, the patient may develop reversible paralysis or a seizure disorder. Because the clinical picture can mimic a wide variety of neuropsychiatric disorders, patients are often admitted to neurologic or psychiatric wards. In one series, 40 percent of patients with insulinomas had neuropsychiatric symptoms. After successful removal of the tumor, half of the patients had persistent, irreversible neuropsychiatric complaints that were attributed to the duration of symptoms before appropriate therapy.

The diagnosis of an insulinoma requires the demonstration of fasting plasma glucose levels below 50 mg/dl and relative hyperinsulinism, that is, insulin levels that are inappropriately high for the plasma glucose concentration. During continued fasting by normal individuals, plasma glucose and insulin decline together. As a result, the ratio of immunoreactive insulin (IRI) to glucose (G) remains constant. In one study, fasting IRI/G was less than 0.3 in all healthy nonobese men tested. In the great majority of patients with an insulinoma, an abnormal ratio of insulin to glucose is apparent after 12 to 14 hours of fasting. As a rule of thumb a plasma insulin level >20 μU/ml associated with a fasting plasma glucose below 50 mg/dl is diagnostic of hyperinsulinism. Occasionally, demonstration of fasting hypoglycemia with inappropriate insulin levels may require as long as 72 hours of fasting. If an abnormality is not established by then, subjects should exercise for 2 hours because exercise raises low plasma glucose in normals but decreases glucose levels further in patients with an insulinoma. Because tumor secretion may be episodic and insulin half-life is short, IRI and glucose should be measured every 4 to 6 hours. In addition to observations during fasting, other diagnostic tests may be helpful. C-peptide levels are useful in the diagnosis of factitious hypoglycemia secondary to insulin administration or in the rare occasion when an insulinoma is suspected in an insulin-treated diabetic. In both circumstances the presence of insulin antibiodies may interfere with accurate plasma insulin determinations. In factitious hypoglycemia, however, C-peptide levels are suppressed and in insulinoma they are elevated. Proinsulin levels are often elevated out of proportion to the increase in serum insulin in individuals with insulinomas. Some clinicians use suppression tests that can distinguish physiologically controlled beta cells from autonomous (nonsuppressible) insulin production. Suppression is assessed by measuring serum C-peptide following the administration of insulin to produce hypoglycemia. In difficult cases, when a clinically suspicious insulinoma is not verified by the above measures, one can use provocative tests with tolbutamide, glucagon, leucine, or calcium, which elicit more insulin secretion from insulinomas than from normal beta cells.[8]

When the clinical diagnosis of insulinoma is established and surgery is anticipated, efforts are made to determine whether the tumor is malignant and to localize it. Serum levels of chorionic gonadotropin, or its alpha or beta subunits, are elevated in about two thirds of patients with functioning malignant insulinomas but

not in those with benign or inactive tumors. A liver scan may detect metastases and thus avoid unnecessary surgery. Tumors larger than 2 to 3 cm can be detected by ultrasonography or computed tomography, but angiography is more sensitive for small tumors. About half of the tumors can be identified before surgery by celiac and superior mesenteric arteriography. If the tumor is not located by radiography or direct palpation at surgery, surgeons at some centers perform progressive pancreatic resection, beginning at the tail and proceeding toward the body, with frequent monitoring of blood glucose levels and the pathologic specimens. A very successful but quite specialized procedure used at some centers is percutaneous transhepatic portal venography with selective blood sampling for insulin measurements from the portal and pancreatic veins.

If surgery fails to restore normoglycemia or a malignant tumor has spread, attempts are made to control hypoglycemic episodes with medical therapy. Frequent high-carbohydrate feedings may be sufficient. In cases of more profound hypoglycemia, pharmacologic agents have been used with variable success. Diazoxide, 200 mg daily in two equal doses, together with thiazides may help to control intractable hypoglycemia in some patients with insulinoma. The hyperglycemic effect of diazoxide is believed to result from inhibition of insulin release and enhanced secretion of catecholamines. Diazoxide may also increase hepatic glycogenolysis through direct effects on the liver. Thiazides are administered to counteract the side effect of sodium and fluid retention, which may precipitate congestive heart failure. Additional side effects of diazoxide include diabetic ketoacidosis, hyperosmolar nonketotic coma, nausea, vomiting, and hirsutism. The antibiotic streptozotocin destroys beta cells of the pancreas. In one study, intravenous administration of streptozotocin, 1 g/m² body surface area per week for 4 weeks, improved hypoglycemic symptoms and survival in about half of those treated. Almost all patients had significant side effects of therapy, the most serious being irreversible renal failure. Administration of zinc glucagon or glucocorticoids reduces hypoglycemic manifestations, but their action is short-lived and glucocorticoid treatment is accompanied by undesirable side effects.

Other Islet Cell Tumors. As shown in Table 14.8–3, a variety of clinical syndromes result from functioning islet cell tumors. Most commonly, the tumors secrete insulin, with resultant hypoglycemia, or gastrin, which causes the Zollinger-Ellison syndrome (Chapter 12.3). Diarrheal syndromes (Chapter 12.5) may result from tumor production of vasactive intestinal peptide (VIP), gastrin, secretin, or prostaglandin E. ACTH secretion by islet cell tumors may cause Cushing syndrome. Some pancreatic tumors produce serotonin and consequently the carcinoid syndrome.

Several types of islet cell tumors are associated with hyperglycemia. Glucagon-secreting tumors have been documented in numerous instances. The most common clinical manifestations of glucagonoma include glucose intolerance, dermatitis, and weight loss without accompanying anorexia. Glossitis or stomatitis occurs in about one third of the patients, and a few have diarrhea. The tumor is more common in women and is malignant in about 80 percent of reported cases. When suspected on clinical grounds, the diagnosis is made by demonstrating high levels of circulating glucagon; the tumor may be localized by angiography. In a few cases hyperglycemia has resulted from somatostatin secretion by D-cell tumors of the pancreas. VIP-producing tumors, in addition to causing watery diarrhea, may cause hyperglycemia and hypercalcemia.

Symptoms caused by the simultaneous production of other hormones by islet cell tumors may complicate the recognition of insulinoma-induced hypoglycemia. Moreover, insulinomas may coexist with other nonpancreatic tumors as part of the syndrome of multiple endocrine adenomatosis (type I MEA).

Autoimmune Hypoglycemia (Table 14.8–2). On rare occasions severe hypoglycemia occurs in patients who have antibodies to insulin without any previous administration of exogenous insulin. Even rarer patients with autoantibodies to insulin receptors can develop overwhelming, refractory hypoglycemia.[8]

Pituitary Disorders. Growth hormone and ACTH both play important roles in the regulation of glucose metabolism. Growth hormone acts on both the liver and peripheral tissues, whereas ACTH deficiency produces hypoglycemia through the resultant secondary adrenal insufficiency. Because evidence indicates that the peripheral actions of insulin are antagonized by growth hormone, deficiency of this hormone probably produces hypoglycemia because of peripheral glucose overutilization when insulin effects are unopposed by growth hormone. Absence of both growth hormone and ACTH can lead to hypoglycemia in patients with all types of acquired pituitary insufficiency. With glucocorticoid replacement, episodes of symptomatic hypoglycemia are uncommon in adults but occur in about 10 percent of patients with panhypopituitarism that begins in childhood. Hypoglycemia can also occur in patients with pituitary dwarfism caused by a gentic defect in the secretion or structure of growth hormone. Many such patients, however, have a compensatory insulinopenia, and hypoglycemia is clinically important only in young children.

Glucocorticoid Deficiency. Symptomatic hypoglycemia commonly follows a period of fasting in patients with diminished glucocorticoid secretion (Addison disease). The low plasma glucose probably results from diminished glucose output during fasting because cortisol is required for optimal hepatic gluconeogenesis. Occasionally, patients with glucocorticoid deficiency exhibit hypoglycemic symptoms late in the postprandial period. Adequate steroid replacement, including increased doses with stress and pregnancy, completely prevents attacks of hypoglycemia.

Hypoglycemia Associated with Serious Medical Illness (Table 14.8–2)[8]

Some patients with chronic renal failure develop hypoglycemia. The hypoglycemia has been variously attributed to decreased gluconeogenesis in liver and kidney, reduced availability of amino acid precursors of glucose, congestive heart failure, and rarely hyperinsulinism. Hypoglycemia can also occur following hemodialysis.

Severely malnourished children and adults can present with significant hypoglycemia. The prognosis is particularly poor if edema is also present. Severe hypoglycemia can also occur with infection and sepsis. Direct effects of endotoxin on the liver, decreased liver perfusion and hyperinsulinism have been postulated as the cause.

TABLE 14.8–3. FUNCTIONING ISLET CELL TUMORS

Product	Clinical Manifestations
Glucagon	Hyperglycemia, skin lesions, weight loss
Insulin	Fasting hypoglycemia
Somatostatin	Hyperglycemia
ACTH	Cushing syndrome
Gastrin	Gastric hypersection, peptic ulcer, diarrhea
Vasoactive intestinal peptide (VIP)	Watery diarrhea, hypokalemia, hyperglycemia
Secretin	Pancreatic hypersecretion, diarrhea
Serotonin	Carcinoid syndrome
Prostaglandin E	Diarrhea

Transient hypoglycemia occasionally complicates congestive heart failure or pericardial disease, presumably because poor perfusion of the liver limits the supply of amino acids needed for gluconeogenesis. Recognition of hypoglycemia can be difficult in this situation where symptoms may be misinterpreted as evidence of cerebral anoxia.

Extrapancreatic Tumors[6,8]

Hypoglycemia can occur in patients with tumors of virtually any histopathologic type. Most frequently described are mesenchymal tumors, massive fibromas, or sarcomas located (in decreasing order of frequency) in the retroperitoneal, intrathoracic, and intraabdominal spaces. Hypoglycemia may also complicate the course of other nonislet cell tumors, including hepatoma, adrenocortical tumors, and gastrointestinal, bronchial, and exocrine pancreatic carcinomas. The causes of tumor-related hypoglycemia are not known, and they probably vary from case to case. Clearly, these tumors do not synthesize or store insulin, and circulating insulin levels are low during hypoglycemic episodes. Some attribute hypoglycemia to elevated levels of nonsuppressible insulinlike activity (NSILA), measured by radioimmunoassay; yet NSILA levels are normal in a sizable fraction of these hypoglycemic patients, whereas some cancer patients have elevated NSILA levels without hypoglycemia. Some tumors are thought to lower plasma glucose by converting large amounts of glucose to lactate; other investigators have suggested that these tumors secrete a substance that inhibits hepatic gluconeogenesis and enhances glycolysis. A report of intractable hypoglycemia in a patient with a somatostatinoma suggests that the failure of counterregulatory hormone response could contribute to hypoglycemia in patients with tumors.

Extrapancreatic tumors are usually distinguished from an insulinoma by elevated plasma insulin levels in the latter. In some cases, however, the clinical picture in patients with extrapancreatic tumors may closely resemble the hypoglycemia of islet cell tumors.

Because of their large size, extrapancreatic tumors associated with hypoglycemia are generally not resectable, and management has been directed toward raising blood glucose levels through frequent feedings, glucose infusions, and treatment with pharmacologic agents like diazoxide and prednisone.

EXOGENOUS (DRUG-INDUCED) HYPOGLYCEMIA[8] (Table 14.8–2)

Insulin Administration

Insulin overdosage in diabetics is the most common cause of hypoglycemia. Most diabetics learn to recognize their own particular symptoms and to abort attacks by carbohydrate ingestion. Defective secretion of glucagon and epinephrine can occur, however, in patients with long-standing insulin-requiring diabetes mellitus who have severe autonomic neuropathy, especially when they are treated with beta-adrenergic blockers. The combined lack of these two hormones, coupled with continuous insulin absorption from subcutaneous depots, can result in the development of dangerous hypoglycemia (plasma glucose < 35 mg/dl).[1] For that reason, intensive insulin therapy is contraindicated in such patients. Occasionally a nondiabetic may self-administer insulin and produce symptoms of recurrent hypoglycemia. Such is most commonly observed either in family members of insulin-dependent diabetics or in hospital personnel, who have ready access to insulin and syringes. An individual suspected of this type of malingering must be examined carefully for injection marks, and his or her hospital room should be searched for hidden insulin and syringes. The detection of insulin antibodies in a nondiabetic supports the suspicion of self-administration of insulin, but insulin autoantibodies occur in some individuals who have not received exogenous insulin. As mentioned earlier, measurement of serum or urinary levels of C-peptide, which will be low relative to serum insulin in patients with factitious insulin injection, is helpful in making this diagnosis.

Oral Hypoglycemic Agents

All of the sulfonylureas have produced hypoglycemia, but the longer-acting drugs, such as chlorpropamide, are more commonly the causative agents. Nondiabetics may use oral hypoglycemic agents to induce hypoglycemia. Clinical settings that favor the development of drug-induced hypoglycemia include decreased food intake or malnutrition, impaired liver or renal function that prolongs the action of sulfonylureas, decreased adrenocortical activity, and extremes of age. Concomitant use of ethanol or other drugs, especially salicylates, also augments the hypoglycemic effect of the sulfonylureas. Sulfonylurea ingestion can cause protracted and severe hypoglycemia. After an initial injection of 50 percent glucose, the patient should be hospitalized and plasma glucose levels maintained over 100 mg/dl with continuous intravenous glucose. Glucose infusions are cautiously slowed and finally discontinued when the patient's plasma glucose level is stable on an oral intake of at least 300 g of carbohydrate daily.

Alcohol Ingestion[10]

Most commonly, ethanol causes hypoglycemia in chronically malnourished alcoholics who stop their intake of food and alcohol 10 to 20 hours earlier. Neither liver disease nor hepatic glycogen depletion is necessary, however, because hypoglycemia can follow a short drinking spree in healthy adults or children. Alcohol usually produces fasting hypoglycemia, but some individuals may develop hypoglycemic symptoms in the postprandial period when significant amounts of alcohol are consumed with a meal, especially one containing simple sugars. Normal amounts of liver glycogen provide some protection against alcoholic hypoglycemia, which results mainly from blockage of hepatic gluconeogenesis by products of ethanol metabolism. Reduced nicotinamide adenine dinucleotide (NADH) accumulates in the liver during ethanol oxidation. The consequent increase in the ratio of NADH to NAD prevents the entry of substrates, such as alanine, lactate, and glycerol, into the gluconeogenic pathway. Patients with reactive postprandial hypoglycemia and diabetics using insulin or sulfonylureas are especially susceptible to ethanol-induced hypoglycemia. In contrast, obese subjects are less sensitive to the hypoglycemic effects of ethanol.

Ethanol ingestion is probably the most frequent cause of fasting hypoglycemia, especially in urban centers, but its manifestations are often mistakenly attributed to drunkenness. To improve the recognition of alcoholic hypoglycemia, plasma glucose should be determined in all symptomatic patients with a history of significant alcohol intake. Although hypoglycemic symptoms usually respond promptly to intravenous glucose infusions, glucose administration must be continued for a number of hours to prevent recurrence of hypoglycemia. The tendency for ethanol to produce hypoglycemia is diminished if nutrients containing fiber, fat, or protein are ingested together with the ethanol.

Other Drugs and Poisons

Hypoglycemia can be induced by beta blockers, salicylates, and other drugs that interfere with glucose metabolism in the liver. In most cases the exact mechanism is unclear. Drug-induced hypoglycemia is most common in children, diabetics treated with insulin or sulfonylureas, and patients with compromised renal function. Ingestion of certain poisonous plants, such as mushrooms and Ackee fruit, as well as hepatotoxins, can cause fatal hypoglycemia in humans.

DIAGNOSTIC APPROACH TO SYMPTOMATIC FASTING HYPOGLYCEMIA

The most important step in the diagnosis of symptomatic fasting hypoglycemia (Table 14.8–4) is to document that chemical hypoglycemia and typical symptoms occur at the same time during a spontaneous attack or a provocative test. Moreover, prompt relief of symptoms by ingestion or infusion of glucose may provide a valuable clue.

TABLE 14.8–4. DIAGNOSTIC APPROACH TO FASTING HYPOGLYCEMIA

A. Prove that hypoglycemia is responsible for symptoms during spontaneous or provoked attack by showing:
   1. Typical symptoms
   2. Plasma glucose <50 mg/dl
   3. Prompt relief of symptoms by glucose ingestion or infusion
B. Measure plasma glucose and insulin levels after an overnight fast
C. If glucose <50 mg/dl and
   1. Insulin <20 μU/ml:
      Differentiate between causes other than hyperinsulinism by:
      a. History and physical examination
      b. Liver function tests
      c. Urinary or plasma cortisol levels
      d. Growth hormone levels
      e. Work-up for extrapancreatic tumors
   2. Insulin >20 μU/ml:
      Hyperinsulinism is present; insulinoma is the most likely cause. Measure insulin antibodies, sulfonylurea levels, C-peptide, and proinsulin in selected patients
D. If glucose >50 mg/dl but hypoglycemia is strongly suspected:
   1. Begin 72-hour fast with repeated determinations of plasma glucose and insulin. Exercise patient at end of the fast if hypoglycemia is not documented
   2. In difficult cases:
      a. Suppression test: administer commercial insulin and measure C-peptide response
      b. Provocative tests: measure glucose and insulin reponse to tolbutamide, calcium, leucine, or glucagon
E. Once chemical tests establish the diagnosis of insulinoma, localize tumor by selective celiac angiography or transhepatic venography

When suggestive symptoms occur, efforts should be made to document hypoglycemia by measuring plasma glucose levels after an overnight fast. Once symptomatic fasting hypoglycemia is demonstrated, the physician must measure plasma insulin levels (C-peptide determinations are substituted in diabetics with insulin antibodies) to distinguish between hyperinsulinism and other causes of hypoglycemia. Hyperinsulinism is identified by plasma insulin >20 μU/ml in association with a plasma glucose <50 mg/dl following an overnight fast. If hyperinsulinism is absent in a patient with documented fasting hypoglycemia who is not seriously ill, the differential diagnosis should include hormonal factors, liver disease, drug-induced hypoglycemia, and extrapancreatic tumors (Table 14.8–2). When clinical evidence suggests hypoadrenalism or hypopituitarism, growth hormone and cortisol levels are measured (Table 14.8–4). Ingestion of alcohol, drugs, or toxins and severe liver disease can generally be distinguished by history, physical examination, and liver function tests. Blood levels of drug can be measured when sulfonylurea ingestion is suspected. If the clinical findings and specific laboratory tests do not support one of the above conditions, the patient should be worked up for extra-

pancreatic tumor. Severe wasting or an abdominal mass favors the diagnosis of extrapancreatic tumor. If hyperinsulinism is present and self-administration of insulin is suspected, insulin antibodies and C-peptide levels are measured.

When glucose and insulin levels fail to establish a diagnosis after a 12-hour fast but insulinoma is still strongly suspected (Table 14.8–4), these measurements can be continued during a prolonged period of starvation (48 to 72 hours), terminated with an exercise period. This approach will establish the diagnosis in most patients. During such periods of fasting, the physician must monitor the patient closely and intervene promptly if symptomatic hypoglycemia occurs.

On occasion, recognition of an insulinoma may require measurement of proinsulin and C-peptide levels following insulin injection to show the failure of beta cells to suppress. Rarely, provocative agents may be used to stimulate insulin secretion (Table 14.8–4). After chemical tests have established the diagnosis, insulinomas can often be localized by the appearance of an abnormal collection of vessels or a tumor blush during selective angiography or transhepatic venography. In summary, the preoperative diagnosis of insulinoma proceeds in four steps: (1) documentating symptomatic fasting hypoglycemia, (2) demonstrating spontaneous hyperinsulinism, (3) localizing the tumor, and (4) attempting to determine whether it is benign or malignant.

Despite all diagnostic efforts, laboratory tests may yield equivocal results in some patients. Under these circumstances, the physician has the option of continued observation and retesting the patient after an interval or proceeding immediately to exploratory laparotomy. This decision must be based in part upon the intensity of the patient's symptoms.

REFERENCES

1. Cryer PE, Gerich JE: Glucose counterregulation, hypoglycemia and intensive insulin therapy in diabetes mellitus. N Engl J Med 313:232, 1985
2. Ensinck JW, Williams RH: Disorders causing hypoglycemia. In Williams R (ed): Textbook of Endocrinology, 6th ed. Philadelphia, WB Saunders, 1981, p 856
3. Fajans SS, Floyd JC Jr: Fasting hypoglycemia in adults. N Engl J Med 294:766, 1976
4. Ford CV, Bray GA, Swerdloff RS: Psychiatric study of patients referred with a diagnosis of hypoglycemia. Am J Psychol 133:290, 1976
5. Hadji-Georgopoulos A, Schmidt MI, et al: Elevated hypoglycemic index and late hyperinsulinism in symptomatic postprandial hypoglycemia. J Clin Endocrinol Metab 50:371, 1980
6. Laurent J, Derby G, Floquet J: Hypoglycemic tumors. Amsterdam, Exerpta Medica, 1971
7. Margolis S, Homcy C: Systemic manifestations of hepatoma. Medicine 51:381, 1972
8. Marks V, Rose F: Hypoglycemia. St Louis, Blackwell Scientific, 1981
9. Permutt MA: Postprandial hypoglycemia. Diabetes 25:719, 1976
10. Service JF (ed): Hypoglycemic disorders: Pathogenesis, diagnosis and treatment. Boston, Mass, Hall Medical Publishers, 1983
11. Sherwin RS, Felig P: Hypoglycemia. In Felig P, Baxter JD, et al (eds): Endocrinology and Metabolism. New York, McGraw-Hill, 1981

Disorders of Plasma Lipids and Lipoproteins

Simeon Margolis

The major plasma lipids are transported in combination with proteins to form the plasma lipoproteins. Hyperlipidemia, defined as an elevation of plasma cholesterol or triglycerides, is always associated with an increased concentration of one or more of the plasma lipoproteins. The type of hyperlipidemia is determined by the type of lipoprotein present in excess. The primary clinical manifestation of hyperlipidemia is premature atherosclerotic disease. In addition, severe hypertriglyceridemia may cause recurrent attacks of acute pancreatitis. Xanthelasmas and xanthomas, the nonlaboratory clues to the presence of hyperlipidemia, may pose cosmetic problems.

Some uncommon types of hyperlipidemia result from deficiencies in enzymes that metabolize the lipid components of lipoproteins, from defects in their proteins, or from defective receptors for lipoprotein uptake by cells. Such protein abnormalities also cause several rare types of hypolipidemia.

LIPOPROTEIN STRUCTURE, NONMENCLATURE, AND COMPOSITION (Table 14.9–1)[8]

The plasma lipoproteins are composed of a central core of apolar lipids, triglycerides, and cholesterol esters, surrounded by a surface coat of proteins and more hydrophilic lipids, cholesterol and phospholipids (mainly lecithin). The size and density of each lipoprotein are both determined by the amount of lipid in its central core. Lipoproteins with the most core lipids are largest in size and lowest in density; as the percentage of core lipid decreases, the lipoprotein density and the proportion of surface protein increase. These density differences are used to separate four distinct classes of lipoproteins by centrifugation (Table 14.9–1). Largest and least dense are the chylomicrons; progressively smaller in size and greater in density are very low (VLDL), low (LDL), and high (HDL) density lipoproteins. A second nomenclature for the lipoproteins is based on their electrophoretic mobility. VLDL is identical with pre-β, LDL with β, and HDL with α lipoproteins. In normal individuals chylomicrons are never found in overnight fasting plasma. Intermediate products of chylomicron and VLDL metabolism (remnant particles or β-VLDL) are present only transiently and in small concentrations.

Each lipoprotein has a characteristic composition (Table 14.9–1). Triglycerides are the major component of chylomicrons (85 to 90 percent) and VLDL (55 to 65 percent). Cholesterol, about two thirds as esters, comprises about half of LDL. The protein content increases from about 2 percent in chylomicrons to 50 percent in HDL. These protein components, called apoproteins, impart water solubility to the core lipids, mediate lipoprotein uptake by binding to cellular receptors, and activate enzymes that metabolize the lipid moieties of the lipoproteins. The apoproteins differ in each lipoprotein class (Table 14.9–1). HDL contains the two apo A proteins, A-I and A-II. The sole protein of LDL is apo B_{100}. VLDL has the most complex composition. The small apo C proteins comprise about half its protein mass; apoproteins B_{100} and E account for about 35 and 10 percent of VLDL protein, respectively. Apo B_{48} and apo C are the major proteins of chylomicrons. Because apoproteins A, C, and E exchange readily between lipoproteins other than LDL, VLDL and chylomicrons carry small amounts of apo A; and HDL contains apo C and E, as well as the quantitatively minor, but functionally important apoprotein D.

PHYSIOLOGY OF LIPID TRANSPORT (Figs. 14.9–1 and 14.9–2)[4]

Triglyceride transport is one of the major functions of the plasma lipoproteins; chylomicrons and VLDL carry triglycerides from the intestine and the liver, respectively. The major digestion products of dietary triglycerides, fatty acids and monoglycerides, are resynthesized to triglycerides within mucosal cells of the small intestine. These triglycerides are combined with small amounts of other lipids and proteins to form chylomicrons, which are synthesized exclusively in the intestine after fat-containing meals. The intestine also produces small amounts of VLDL, but this lipoprotein is synthesized mainly in the liver. Apo B_{48} and B_{100} are needed to trans-

TABLE 14.9–1. PLASMA LIPOPROTEIN CLASSES

Lipoprotein	Electrophoretic Migration	Major Components	Apoprotein[a]	Important Features
Chylomicron	Origin	Triglycerides (85–90%) derived from dietary fat	B_{48}, C (A)	Float during overnight refrigeration of plasma Synthesized in intestinal mucosal cells Not present after overnight fast in normal individuals
Chylomicron and VLDL remnants (β-VLDL)	Beta	Triglycerides (35%) Cholesterol esters (35%)	B_{48}, B_{100}, E	Rapidly cleared after binding to apo E receptors in the liver
Very low density (VLDL)	Prebeta	Triglycerides (55–65%) derived from endogenous synthesis	B_{100}, C, E (A)	Synthesized mainly in the liver, but also in the intestine Apo C-II activates lipoprotein lipase
Low density (LDL)	Beta	Cholesterol (50%)	B_{100}	Mainly formed during metabolism of VLDL
High density (HDL)	Alpha	Protein (50%)	A (C, D, E)	May transport cholesterol from peripheral tissues to the liver Apo A-I activates LCAT

[a]Minor apoproteins are shown in parentheses.

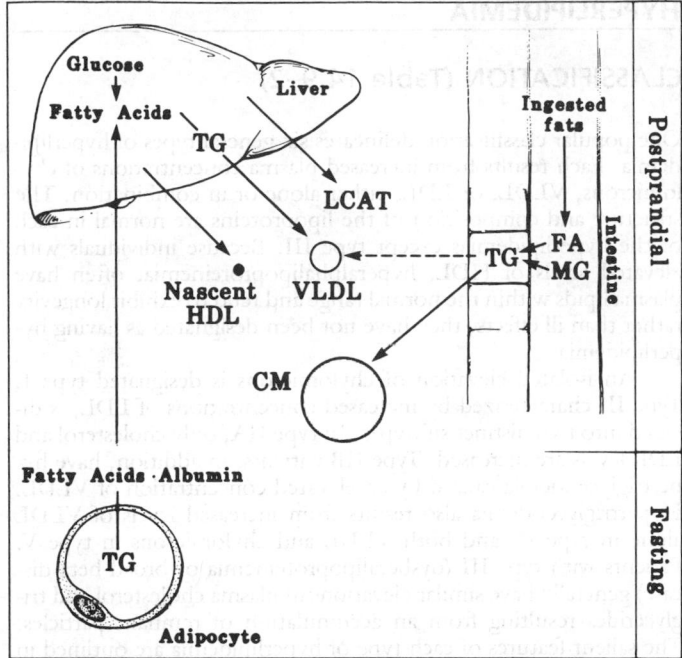

Figure 14.9–1. Overall scheme for lipoprotein formation: Ingested fats are broken down in the intestinal lumen to form fatty acids (FA) and monoglycerides (MG), which are absorbed into the mucosal cell. Triglycerides (TG) are resynthesized and released into the lymphatics on chylomicrons (CM), which enter the general circulation. Following a meal, hepatic FA synthesized from glucose are used to form TG. During fasting periods, FA released from adipose tissue are the source of hepatic TG. TG are released from the liver on VLDL. The intestine also synthesizes VLDL. Nascent HDL and LCAT are secreted by the liver. Nascent HDL is converted to HDL₃ by the accretion of cholesterol from peripheral tissues.

port triglycerides out of cells of the intestinal mucosa and the liver, respectively. VLDL carries endogenous triglycerides formed in the liver from fatty acids derived mainly from de novo hepatic synthesis, from carbohydrates postprandially, and from unesterified fatty acids released from the adipose stores during fasting.

The enzyme lipoprotein lipase, located in the capillary endothelium of adipose tissue and muscle, removes triglycerides from chylomicrons and VLDL by splitting them into their constituent fatty acids. These fatty acids may be stored as triglycerides in adipose tissue or utilized directly as an energy source by peripheral tissues, such as muscle. Lipoprotein lipase requires apo C-II for activation. After triglyceride removal, VLDL and chylomicrons contain redundant cholesterol, phospholipids, and apoproteins on their surface. These excess surface components are transferred to HDL, where the enzyme lecithin:cholesterol acyltransferase (LCAT), released into the blood from the liver, forms cholesterol esters and lysolecithin from cholesterol and lecithin. Apo A-I and a cholesterol ester transport protein (probably apo D) participate in LCAT action. The apo A-I on HDL activates LCAT, and apo D transfers the product cholesterol esters to VLDL and LDL. The other product, lysolecithin, is removed by albumin. The action of lipoprotein lipase produces chylomicron remnants that are rapidly removed from the circulation after binding to apo E receptors in the liver. These enzymatic reactions, accompanied by the action of a hepatic triglyceride lipase and the loss of apo A and apo C peptides, also convert VLDL to LDL (Fig. 14.9–2). Thus, LDL arises predominantly as a product of VLDL catabolism. Some LDL is also synthesized directly in the liver.

A second major function of the plasma lipoproteins is the transport of cholesterol, an essential component of cell membranes and the precursor of steroid hormones. Tissue cholesterol arises from dietary sources and endogenous synthesis, primarily in the liver and intestinal mucosa. VLDL secretion from these sites, its conversion to LDL, and the subsequent cellular uptake of LDL serve to supply cholesterol to tissues such as the adrenal gland for use in steroid hormone formation or lymphocytes where the

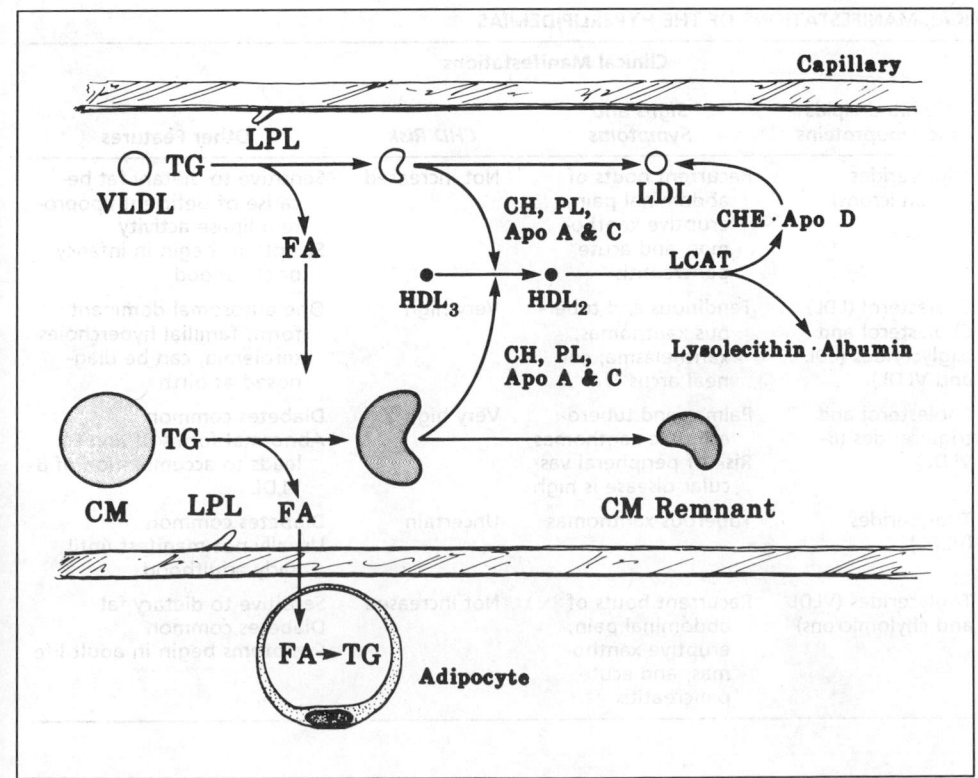

Figure 14.9–2. Chylomicron (CM) and VLDL metabolism in peripheral tissues: As CM and VLDL traverse adipose tissue (or muscle), lipoprotein lipase (LPL) bound to the capillaries splits their triglycerides (TG) to form glycerol and fatty acids (FA). FA enter the adipocyte, where TG are resynthesized. Excess surface cholesterol (CH), phospholipids (PL), and apoproteins are transferred from CM and VLDL to HDL₃ to form HDL₂. LCAT converts CH and PL to cholesterol esters (CHE) and lysolecithin. The former are transferred to VLDL and LDL by apo D; the latter are picked up by albumin. In concert, LPL and LCAT convert CM to CM remnants and VLDL to LDL. CM remnants are removed after binding to apo E receptors in the liver. LDL is cleared by LDL receptors in liver and peripheral tissues.

cholesterol is incorporated into cell membranes. LDL is removed from the circulation after binding to LDL receptors (apo B-E receptors) in peripheral tissues and liver.[2] Bound LDL is internalized into lysosomes where the apo B and cholesterol esters are hydrolyzed. The rise in intracellular free cholesterol stimulates cholesterol esterification, slows the formation of apo B receptors, and reduces cholesterol synthesis by inhibiting β-hydroxy-β-methylglutaryl coenzyme A (HMG CoA) reductase, the rate-limiting enzyme in cholesterol formation. In this manner, the free cholesterol content of the liver cell controls its cholesterol synthesis and esterification and LDL uptake.

On the usual American diet, between 200 and 350 mg of cholesterol per day are carried from the intestine on chylomicrons. Cholesterol ester-rich remnants formed during the catabolism of chylomicrons are taken up by the liver. Lipoproteins also transport cholesterol from peripheral tissues to the liver, the only organ that can eliminate cholesterol from the body by direct secretion into the bile or by conversion of cholesterol to bile acids. Interruption of the enterohepatic recirculation of bile acids, such as by T-tube drainage of bile or by cholestyramine treatment, stimulates cholesterol synthesis and LDL uptake in the liver. HDL is secreted from both liver and intestine as a disc-shaped, *nascent* lipoprotein composed primarily of apo A-I and phospholipids. Nascent HDL removes cholesterol from peripheral tissues; the accumulation of cholesterol and its esterification by LCAT converts nascent HDL to a spherical particle called HDL_3. The cholesterol esters of HDL are transferred to VLDL and LDL for return to the liver. During the metabolism of chylomicrons and VLDL by lipoprotein lipase, the transfer of lipids and apoproteins to HDL_3 converts it to a larger, less dense form of HDL, HDL_2.

When lipoproteins are present in high concentrations or are abnormal in structure, they are taken up by scavenger cells in the arterial wall and in other tissues where they can produce xanthomas, lymphadenopathy, or hepatosplenomegaly.

HYPERLIPIDEMIA

CLASSIFICATION (Table 14.9–2)

One popular classification delineates six general types of hyperlipidemia. Each results from increased plasma concentrations of chylomicrons, VLDL, or LDL, either alone or in combination. The structure and composition of the lipoproteins are normal in each of the hyperlipidemias except type III. Because individuals with elevated levels of HDL, hyperalphalipoproteinemia, often have plasma lipids within the normal range and tend to exhibit longevity rather than ill effects, they have not been designated as having hyperlipidemia.

An isolated elevation of chylomicrons is designated type I. Type II, characterized by increased concentrations of LDL, is divided into two distinct subtypes. In type IIA, only cholesterol and LDL levels are increased. Type IIB patients, in addition, have hypertriglyceridemia caused by an elevated concentration of VLDL. Hypertriglyceridemia also results from increased levels of VLDL alone in type IV and both VLDL and chylomicrons in type V. Patients with type III (dysbetalipoproteinemia or broad beta disease) generally have similar elevations in plasma cholesterol and triglycerides resulting from an accumulation of remnant particles. The salient features of each type of hyperlipidemia are outlined in Table 14.9–2.

Assignment of a specific type to each hyperlipidemic patient may aid in prognosis and management, but the typing scheme has serious deficiencies. Endocrine abnormalities or treatment with diet or drugs may alter the lipoprotein pattern. Because distinctions are based entirely on phenotypic manifestations, the same type of hyperlipidemia may result from different underlying primary disease, environmental factors, or genetic defects. Three common forms of hyperlipidemia can be inherited as autosomal

TABLE 14.9–2. CLASSIFICATION AND CLINICAL MANIFESTATIONS OF THE HYPERLIPIDEMIAS

Type	Prevalence	Appearance of Plasma on Overnight Refrigeration	Elevated Lipids and Lipoproteins	Clinical Manifestations		Other Features
				Signs and Symptoms	CHD Risk	
I	Rare	Creamy layer over clear infranatant	Triglycerides (chylomicrons)	Recurrent bouts of abdominal pain, eruptive xanthomas, and acute pancreatitis	Not increased	Sensitive to dietary fat because of deficient lipoprotein lipase activity; Symptoms begin in infancy or childhood
IIA IIB	Common Common	Clear; Clear or cloudy	Cholesterol (LDL); Cholesterol and triglycerides (LDL and VLDL)	Tendinous and tuberous xanthomas; xanthelasma; corneal arcus	Very high	One autosomal dominant form, familial hypercholesterolemia, can be diagnosed at birth
III	Uncommon	Clear or cloudy	Cholesterol and triglycerides (β-VLDL)	Palmar and tubero-eruptive xanthomas; Risk of peripheral vascular disease is high	Very high	Diabetes common; Abnormal forms of apo E leads to accumulation of β-VLDL
IV	Common	Clear or cloudy	Triglycerides (VLDL)	Tuberous xanthomas	Uncertain	Diabetes common; Usually not manifest until early adulthood
V	Uncommon	Creamy layer over cloudy infranatant	Triglycerides (VLDL and chylomicrons)	Recurrent bouts of abdominal pain, eruptive xanthomas, and acute pancreatitis	Not increased	Sensitive to dietary fat; Diabetes common; Symptoms begin in adult life

CHD = coronary heart disease.

dominant traits. Patients with familial hypercholesterolemia and familial hypertriglyceridemia have types II and IV, respectively. In most patients with type II or IV hyperlipidemia, however, the underlying cause is polygenic or environmental. In the United States the estimated incidence of both familial hypercholesterolemia and hypertriglyceridemia is between 0.1 and 0.2 percent. The most common monogenic form of hyperlipidemia is familial combined hyperlipidemia. Affected family members have type IIA, IIB, or IV patterns with about equal frequency.

PATHOPHYSIOLOGY

Hyperlipidemia results from either increased synthesis or diminished removal of plasma lipoproteins and their constituent lipids. Increased availability or production of lipids or excessive formation of apoproteins may enhance lipoprotein synthesis. Abnormalities in the enzymatic metabolism of the lipids or the interactions of apoproteins with specific tissue receptors retard the removal of lipoproteins. The complex nature of lipoprotein metabolism and the hormonal regulation exerted at several steps may account for the frequency of secondary hyperlipidemia as a complication of other diseases. In diabetes, for example, overproduction of VLDL has been implicated as the major cause of elevated triglyceride levels; but marked insulin depletion can reduce the synthesis of lipoprotein lipase so that delayed triglyceride cleavage produces severe hypertriglyceridemia.

Primary Hyperlipidemia

Although the precise pathogenesis is unknown for most hyperlipidemias, considerable progress has been made in the basic understanding of several genetic forms of hyperlipidemia where lipid or lipoprotein removal rates are reduced. Severe hypertriglyceridemia with chylomicronemia occurs in individuals with defective formation of lipoprotein lipase (type I hyperlipidemia) or an inability to synthesize its activator, apo C-II; the latter are a small subset of all patients with type V hyperlipidemia. Patients with type III (dysbetalipoproteinemia) have a variety of abnormal forms of apo E that bind poorly to apo E liver receptors and impede the clearance of remnant particles, leading to their accumulation in the plasma. Some other factor must be present for the expression of type III because 1 percent of the population has abnormal forms of apo E while the incidence of type III is far lower.

Familial hypercholesterolemia is due to abnormal cellular uptake of LDL. Homozygotes with familial hypercholesterolemia have absent or defective cell membrane receptors for LDL or an internalization abnormality. Resultant failure of specific LDL binding or internalization interferes with LDL degradation and also results in overproduction of cholesterol in the liver.

Although the abnormality is not clearly defined, familial hypertriglyceridemia results from both increased synthesis and reduced catabolism of VLDL. Familial combined hyperlipidemia is due to overproduction of VLDL and apoprotein B, with a resultant elevation in plasma levels of LDL apo B, which may account for the increased risk of premature coronary artery disease in these patients.

Secondary Hyperlipidemia

In addition to its occurrence as a primary inherited disorder, secondary hyperlipidemia is a common finding (Table 14.9-3). Secondary hyperlipidemia may present as any of the types, but type IV is most common. An abnormal, cholesterol-rich lipoprotein (lipoprotein X) is found in patients with hypercholesterolemia resulting from obstructive liver disease. Chylomicron levels may be increased because of a deficiency in the activity of tissue lipoprotein lipase in hypothyroidism, severe insulin deficiency, or chronic glucocorticoid administraton. Estrogen treatment can cause severe hypertriglyceridemia when given to patients with modest triglycer-

TABLE 14.9–3. MAJOR CAUSES OF SECONDARY HYPERLIPIDEMIA

- Obesity
- Diabetes mellitus
- Hypothyroidism
- Renal disease
    Chronic renal failure
    Nephrotic syndrome
    Maintenance dialysis
- Glycogen storage disease
- Dysgammaglobulinemias (multiple myeloma, macroglobulinemia, systemic lupus erythematosus)
- Acute intermittent porphyria
- Obstructive liver disease
- Acute stress states (trauma, burns, sepsis, myocardial infarction)
- Drugs
    Thiazide diuretics
    Beta-blocking agents
    Estrogens
    Corticosteroids
    Retinoids

ide elevations. Several drugs commonly used in the management of patients with heart disease (thiazide diuretics and beta blockers) may also raise triglyceride levels.

Although severe degrees of hyperlipidemia are invariably the result of a metabolic abnormality or are secondary to some demonstrable disease, modest elevations of plasma lipids may occur in subjects who are overweight or ingest large amounts of animal fat. Such diet-induced hyperlipidemia is more frequent in countries with a high standard of living. In general, the hyperlipidemia in such subjects responds well to dietary measures.

CLINICAL MANIFESTATIONS (Table 14.9–2)

Xanthomas (see Chapter 17.7) are the only overt manifestation of hyperlipidemia. Xanthelasmas are common in type II, but about 60 percent of patients with xanthelasmas have normal serum lipids. Patients with type II may also have premature arcus senilis and tendon xanthomas. Tendon xanthomas are almost always diagnostic of familial hypercholesterolemia and the accumulation of cholesterol esters. Tendon xanthomas also occur, however, in two other rare hereditary conditions: plant sterols are stored in sitosterolemia and patients with cerebrotendinous xanthomatosis have a block in bile acid synthesis that leads to accumulation of cholestanol. Treatment with ion-exchange resins may prevent the premature coronary heart disease found in patients with sitosterolemia. Chenodeoxycholic acid (250 mg twice daily) may retard progression of neurologic disease in cerebrotendinous xanthomatosis. Type III is characterized by planar xanthomas in the palmar creases and tuberoeruptive xanthomas. Tuberous xanthomas can occur in types II, III, and IV. When plasma triglycerides reach especially high levels and chylomicronemia is present, patients may develop eruptive xanthomas and lipemia retinalis.

Heterozygotes for familial hypercholesterolemia exhibit plasma cholesterol values between 300 and 500 mg/dl (usually type IIA but occasionally type IIB), tendinous xanthomas, and symptomatic coronary artery disease 10 to 15 years earlier than normolipidemic peers of the same sex. The disorder is much more severe in homozygotes; plasma cholesterol often exceeds 800 mg/dl, tendon and planar xanthomas are evident in the first decade, severe coronary atherosclerosis is invariably present, aortic stenosis is common, and death usually results before age 20.

Dysbetalipoproteinemia is associated with both premature coronary and peripheral vascular disease. The risk of coronary heart disease is high in patients with familial combined hyperlipidemia but not in familial hypertriglyceridemia. Severe hypertriglyceride-

mia (>1000 mg/dl) may produce eruptive xanthomas, hepatosplenomegaly, and severe abdominal pain caused by acute pancreatitis. Chylomicronemia can also cause arthritic symptoms, dryness of eyes and mouth, emotional lability, and tingling in the extremities. Type I and apo C-II deficiency (manifest as type V) can be identified in childhood. Most often, type V is first manifested in adult years and is frequently associated with diabetes. Hyperuricemia occurs in more than half the patients with hypertriglyceridemia.

RATIONALE FOR TREATMENT

The major goal in the treatment of hyperlipidemia is the prevention of premature vascular disease. Epidemiologic studies have shown that hypercholesterolemia is a major risk factor for coronary heart disease caused by the atherogenic potency of LDL, the major carrier of plasma cholesterol. Recent studies have clearly demonstrated that a reduction in plasma cholesterol and LDL levels is associated with decreased manifestations of coronary heart disease (a 2 percent decrease in manifestations for every 1 percent reduction in plasma cholesterol)[7] and a slowed progression of angiographic lesions in the coronary arteries.

Elevated concentrations of LDL apo B, even in the absence of increased LDL cholesterol, are strongly associated with coronary heart disease. β-VLDL is also highly atherogenic. In contrast, HDL, particularly HDL_2, is a protective lipoprotein. HDL may exert its protective effects against atherosclerosis through its role in transporting cholesterol from the arterial wall to the liver or by partially blocking the uptake of LDL cholesterol by endothelial or smooth muscle cells of large arteries. In general, plasma triglyceride elevations are not an independent risk for premature coronary artery disease. Hypertriglyceridemia is usually associated with reduced levels of HDL, however, which may predispose to coronary heart disease. Moreover, hypertriglyceridemic patients with the genetic pattern of familial combined hyperlipidemia are at increased risk. Thus, strong evidence supports the value of improving the plasma lipid and lipoprotein profile. The goals are to reduce plasma LDL, β-VLDL, and possibly VLDL while raising levels of HDL.

A second reason for treating hyperlipidemia is to prevent attacks of acute pancreatitis provoked by severe hypertriglyceridemia, usually associated with the chylomicronemia of type I or V. Reduction of fasting plasma triglycerides to less than 500 mg/dl may completely prevent further attacks in these patients.

APPROACH TO DIAGNOSIS (Table 14.9–4)[9,10]

Because of the serious consequences of coronary heart disease and the availability of effective therapy for most hyperlipidemic patients, plasma lipids should be screened at an early age in all individuals. Screening is particularly important in those individuals with other major risk factors for coronary heart disease (cigarette smoking, hypertension, diabetes).

The initial screening tests, which do not require a fasting sample, are a plasma cholesterol and examination of plasma after overnight refrigeration. Expanded testing is undertaken in those individuals indicated in Table 14.9–4. These expanded tests require a 12-hour fast and include plasma cholesterol, triglycerides, HDL

TABLE 14.9–4. APPROACH TO THE DIAGNOSIS OF HYPERLIPIDEMIA

Question	Comments

I. Is hyperlipidemia present?	• The only overt manifestation is the presence of xanthomas:
	  Tendon: familial hypercholesterolemia (FH)
	  Palmar: type III
	  Tuberous: FH or hypertriglyceridemia
	  Tuberoeruptive: type III
	  Eruptive: severe hypertriglyceridemia with chylomicronemia
	 • Turbid fasting plasma is diagnostic of hypertriglyceridemia

A. Who should be tested?	• *Routine screen:* all young adults • *Expanded screen:* Individuals at increased risk from routine screening[10]

Age (yr)	Cholesterol Value (mg/dl)
20–29	>200
30–39	>220
40+	>240

	• Turbid plasma in refrigerated specimen. • Premature atherosclerotic disease (before the age of 50 in men or 60 in women) in the individual or a first-degree relative • Unexplained pancreatitis • Presence of xanthomas or lipemia retinalis • Settings associated with secondary hyperlipidemia • If tests are normal, repeat every 5 years
B. What tests should be done?	• *Routine screen:* Cholesterol and refrigerated plasma. Patient need not be fasting • *Expanded screen:* 12-hour fasting serum for cholesterol, triglycerides, HDL_{ch}, and refrigerated plasma
C. When are tests abnormal?	• LDL_{ch}: see Table 14.9–5 • HDL_{ch}: less than 30 mg/dl in men or 40 mg/dl in women • LDL_{ch}/HDL_{ch}: >4.0 • *Triglycerides:* >250 mg/dl
II. What is the type of hyperlipidemia?	• Delineate the lipoprotein present in excessive concentration (Table 14.9–2).
III. Is hyperlipidemia primary or secondary?	• Carry out diagnostic tests for the causes of secondary hyperlipidemia (Table 14.9–3).
IV. Are other family members affected?	• Because hyperlipidemia is often inherited, screen other family members • Familial hypercholesterolemia can usually be detected at birth or shortly thereafter • Hypertriglyceridemia is often not manifest until late teens or early twenties.

cholesterol (HDL$_{ch}$), and examination of refrigerated plasma. If the results of the initial or expanded screening tests are normal, they should be repeated at 5-year intervals.

It is critical to consider the method used in the laboratory when interpreting the results of cholesterol determinations. The values given in Tables 14.9–4 and 14.9–5 are based on those obtained using the methods of the Lipid Research Clinics (LRC). The methods used in most clinical laboratories yield cholesterol values 6 to 8 percent higher than those determined in the LRC. Using the results obtained in most laboratories, therefore, could mistakenly identify many individuals as being at moderate or high risk.

Physicians may also be misled by relying solely on plasma total cholesterol levels. Some patients may have elevated LDL or depressed HDL levels despite normal values for total cholesterol. Conversely, a high total cholesterol may be due to increased HDL concentration. LDL cholesterol (LDL$_{ch}$) can be measured directly in special laboratories or estimated as follows:

$$LDL_{ch} = \frac{Total\ plasma}{cholesterol} - HDL_{ch} - \frac{Plasma\ triglycerides}{5}$$

This formula is applicable whenever the plasma triglycerides are less than 600 mg/dl and the patient does not have type III.

Individuals are considered at moderate or high risk when their LDL$_{ch}$ exceeds the 75th or 90th percentiles, respectively (Table 14.9–5). Moderate risk dictates dietary management; drug treatment may be needed as well in those at high risk.

Mean HDL$_{ch}$ levels below the 10th percentile (30 mg/dl in men and 40 mg/dl in women) also indicate high risk. The ratio of LDL$_{ch}$ to HDL$_{ch}$ can also be used to evaluate risk. Because few measures are available to raise HDL$_{ch}$ appreciably, an LDH$_{ch}$/HDL$_{ch}$ ratio greater than 4.0 is another useful criterion for the initiation of efforts to lower LDL$_{ch}$.

When normal triglycerides are associated with high LDL$_{ch}$ levels, type IIA can be distinguished without further tests. Fibroblast studies in specialized laboratories can confirm the diagnosis of familial hypercholesterolemia. The presence of hypertriglyceridemia dictates further studies. Examination of overnight refrigerated plasma will often delineate the type of hyperlipidemia. Thus, a floating creamy layer demonstrates the presence of chylomicrons, which indicate either that the patient was not fasting or has type I or V hyperlipidemia. Chylomicrons float on top of otherwise

clear plasma in type I and above a turbid infranatant in type V and in some patients with type III. When patients with types IIB, III, or IV have significant hypertriglyceridemia, the plasma generally shows diffuse turbidity without a chylomicron layer. Lipoprotein electrophoresis is rarely helpful in distinguishing between the types of hypertriglyceridemia. Additional tests are required to make a diagnosis of type III, which is suspected whenever the plasma cholesterol and triglycerides are elevated to about the same degree. The diagnosis requires the use of a specialized laboratory to demonstrate the presence of β-VLDL (beta-electrophoretic mobility of VLDL isolated by ultracentrifugation) and a ratio of VLDL cholesterol to total plasma triglycerides that exceeds 0.3.

Apoprotein concentrations can now be obtained from a number of laboratories. In the near future such determinations will undoubtedly be used more widely because apo A-I levels apparently predict the risk of coronary heart disease better than HDL$_{ch}$, and elevated apo B is a risk factor even in the setting of normal LDL$_{ch}$.

Because treatment of the underlying disorder in patients with secondary hyperlipidemia (Table 14.9–3) may return plasma lipid values to normal, appropriate studies should be carried out to eliminate these conditions as a cause of the hyperlipidemia. To avoid misinterpretaton caused by the secondary effects of acute illnesses, such as myocardial infarction, lipid tests should be deferred or repeated after 6 weeks.

Ideally, at least three lipid profiles, obtained at weekly intervals during a period of stable weight, are needed to confirm the diagnosis of hyperlipidemia and to establish a pretreatment baseline.

Finally, all types of hyperlipidemia may be genetically determined; therefore, first-degree relatives should be screened for abnormal plasma lipids to identify the genetic disorder and to initiate treatment before irreversible vascular changes occur. Familial hypercholesterolemia can be detected in affected children at the time of birth. In contrast, hypertriglyceridemia is often not manifest until the late teens or early twenties.

MANAGEMENT

General Principles

As detailed earlier, the need for treatment to lower LDL$_{ch}$ is based on the presence of elevated levels of LDL$_{ch}$ or the LDL$_{ch}$:HDL$_{ch}$ ratio. Special efforts should be made to reduce LDL$_{ch}$ in young individuals and in those positive for other major risk factors, such as hypertension, cigarette smoking, or diabetes mellitus. Dietary management, the initial treatment for all hyperlipidemic patients, is generally the only measure employed in patients at moderate risk. In high-risk patients drugs are added when the diet is ineffective or cannot be followed by the patient.

Because a 3-month period is generally sufficient to determine the effectiveness of a dietary regimen, a medication may be started if dietary measures fail over such a time period. If serum lipids do not fall adequately after 2 months of treatment with maximal doses of the drug, the initial drug is discontinued and another is tried in a similar manner. A combination of lipid-lowering agents may be required in some hyperlipidemic patients. Because patients should not be maintained for long periods on an ineffective drug or combination of drugs, lipid and lipoprotein values must frequently be compared with baseline levels during the period of treatment. Follow-up values will also determine when a beneficial effect on the atherogenic lipoproteins is accompanied by an undesirable fall in HDL$_{ch}$.

Dietary Therapy (Table 14.9–6)[5]

The main dietary measures for the treatment of hyperlipidemia are reduced intake of saturated fats, decreased dietary cholesterol, and weight loss. The first two measures decrease cholesterol levels; weight control is the most effective way to lower triglycerides. An increase in the intake of soluble dietary fibers, namely those found in vegetables, fruits, legumes, and oats, can also improve lipid lev-

TABLE 14.9–5. LDL CHOLESTEROL LEVELS FOR 75TH AND 90TH PERCENTILES IN WHITE MEN AND WOMEN

Age (yr)	Men (Percentile)		Women (Percentile)	
	75 (mg/dl)	90 (mg/dl)	75 (mg/dl)	90 (mg/dl)
10–20	110	125	110	130
20–24	120	140	120	140
25–29	140	160	125	150
30–34	145	165	130	150
35–39	155	175	140	160
40–44	160	175	145	165
45–49	165	185	150	175
50–54	165	185	160	185
55–59	170	190	170	200
60–64	165	190	170	190
65–69	170	200	185	205
≥70	165	180	170	190

TABLE 14.9–6. MANAGEMENT OF HYPERLIPIDEMIA

| Type | Dietary[a] | Drug | |
		1st Choice	2nd Choice
I	Limit fat intake to 25–30 g/day	None	

IIA and IIB	Total fat intake <30% of calories
	P/S = 1
	Cholesterol <300 mg/day
	Weight reduction
	Increase fiber intake
		Anion-exchange resins (cholestyramine 12 g bid, colestipol 10 g bid)
		Nicotinic acid
		    Initial dose: 100 mg tid
		    Maintenance: 1–2 g tid
		Anion-exchange resin + nicotinic acid
			Probucol 500 mg bid
			Lovastatin 40 mg bid

III and IV	Weight reduction Total fat intake <30% of calories P/S = 1 Cholesterol <300 mg Replace simple sugars with complex carbohydrates Limit alcohol	Clofibrate 1 g bid Gemfibrozil 600 mg bid Nicotinic acid	
V	Weight reduction Total fat intake <25% of calories Replace simple sugars with complex carbohydrates Limit alcohol	Clofibrate Nicotinic acid Gemfibrozil	Medroxyprogesterone acetate (women) 5 to 10 mg/day Oxandrolone (men) 2.5 mg tid

[a]Dietary measures are listed in order of efficacy.

els. Exercise is also recommended to control weight, raise HDL levels, and lower triglycerides.

The current North American diet contains about 40 percent of calories as fat, with 15 percent of total calories coming from saturated fat. Cholesterol intake averages about 500 mg/day. The prime dietary measure in hypercholesterolemic patients is to reduce saturated fat intake to 10 percent of calories or less. This aim can be accomplished by lowering total fat intake to 30 percent of calories, by replacing fat calories with carbohydrates, and by partially substituting mono- or polyunsaturated fats for saturated ones. Although there is debate about the special value of polyunsaturated fats, the common recommendation is to achieve a ratio of polyunsaturated (P) to saturated (S) fats (P:S ratio) of 1.0. Most polyunsaturated fats in the American diet are derived from vegetable oils that contain omega-6 polyunsaturates. The omega-3 polyunsaturated fats, found almost exclusively in seafood, lower LDL equally well and may exert other beneficial effects on atherosclerosis by reducing platelet aggregation. Dietary cholesterol intake should be reduced to less than 300 mg/day.

The major features of a cholesterol-lowering diet are a reduced intake of animal meats, dairy products, egg yolks, and commercially baked products along with the greater use of fish, poultry, and low-fat dairy products. Also recommended is a concurrent increase in the intake of low-fat, high-fiber foods such as vegetables, grains, and fruit. Several studies showing an association between large intakes of coffee and elevated cholesterol levels await confirmation.

These recommended dietary changes lower total and LDL cholesterol by 5 to 20 percent, depending on the patient's previous diet. In highly motivated patients, plasma cholesterol can be reduced even more by greater restrictions of saturated fat and a decrease in dietary cholesterol to 100 mg/day (phase III of the American Heart Association diet). This stringent diet requires significant discipline but is worthy of consideration before introducing drugs.

Triglyceride levels may be reduced dramatically by dietary modifications, which generally lower triglyceride-rich lipoproteins (chylomicrons, VLDL, and β-VLDL) more than plasma cholesterol and LDL. Weight loss is particularly effective in lowering triglycerides; weight goals are defined by weight gained since reaching full maturity. Alcohol is also restricted in diets aimed at reducing triglycerides. The intake of simple sugars is limited, but complex carbohydrates are not restricted. Fasting chylomicronemia (types I and V) requires more severe restriction of dietary fat. Triglyceride levels in these patients may respond to the use of omega-3 polyunsaturated fats. Supplementation with 30 to 40 g of medium chain triglycerides, which are broken down and transported in the portal blood rather than as chylomicron triglycerides, can make these fat-restricted diets more palatable.

Patient understanding of and compliance with diets can be improved by referral to a trained dietician. The dietician will translate seemingly complex dietary recommendations into practical advice and adjust the dietary plan to the patient's life-style, while considering other dietary requirements imposed by concurrent medical conditions. The cost of dietary consultation is far less than that of drugs. The patient's spouse should be included in dietary counseling whenever possible, and the physician must reinforce dietary changes.

Nondietary Reduction of Plasma Cholesterol and LDL Levels (Table 14.9–5)[9,11]

When plasma cholesterol and LDL remain elevated despite the dietary measures outlined above, drugs should be added to the regimen of high-risk patients. The initial drugs of choice are nicotinic acid and the anion-exchange resins, cholestyramine and colestipol. Nicotinic acid lowers plasma cholesterol and LDL by 15 to 25 percent, lowers triglycerides, and raises HDL significantly. This efficacy is counterbalanced by a high frequency of troublesome side effects. The resins reduce cholesterol and LDL levels by 20 to 30 percent. Although these agents are inconvenient to take and often produce gastrointestinal side effects, major adverse reactions are rare. The combination of anion-exchange resins with nicotinic acid has proven highly effective in controlling LDL and raising HDL levels in heterozygotes with familial hypercholesterolemia. Probucol is usually well tolerated but decreases plasma cholesterol by only 10 to 15 percent and lowers HDL significantly. Although the fibrozils (clofibrate and gemfibrozil) lower plasma cholesterol by 5 to 10 percent in type IIA, they are not recommended for use in these patients.

Neomycin, 1 g twice daily, is effective in lowering LDL_{ch} by 20 to 30 percent but is not yet approved for this use. A number of clinical trials are now in progress to evaluate several promising

drugs that block cholesterol synthesis by inhibiting the activity of HMG CoA reductase. Lipid-lowering drugs are discussed in more detail later.

Partial ileal bypass should be considered in severely hypercholesterolemic patients who do not respond to the measures outlined above. By interfering with the reabsorption of bile acids, ileal exclusion lowers plasma cholesterol and LDL by an average of 40 percent. Because the bypassed segment is considerably shorter than in the jejunoileal procedure used for the treatment of massive obesity, most of the complications of the latter procedure have not occurred in patients bypassed for hypercholesterolemia. The major side effect is an increase in stool frequency in the majority of patients. Partial ileal bypass is ineffective in patients with homozygous familial hypercholesterolemia. Frequent plasmapheresis or portacaval shunt is currently the treatment of choice for lowering plasma cholesterol in such patients.

Treatment of Hypertriglyceridemia (Table 14.9–6)[6,9,11]

The goal in the treatment of types IIB, III, and IV is the prevention of premature vascular disease. In types I and V efforts are made to reduce serum triglycerides sufficiently to prevent episodes of acute pancreatitis. An NIH Consensus Conference[9] recommended that no treatment is necessary when triglyceride levels in adults are less than 250 mg/dl. When triglycerides exceed 500 mg/dl, treatment with diet, and drugs if necessary, is required to prevent attacks of acute pancreatitis. Management of patients with triglycerides between 250 and 500 mg/dl is determined by individual circumstances. All are candidates for dietary measures. Drugs should be added if dietary management fails in those with a personal or family history of premature coronary heart disease, other major risk factors (hypertension, cigarette smoking, diabetes), dysbetalipoproteinemia, or familial combined hyperlipidemia.

Weight reduction and maintenance of ideal body weight are the most important measures for the treatment of all forms of hypertriglyceridemia except type I. Drugs should be started only after maximal efforts to control triglyceride levels by dietary measures. Nicotinic acid and the fibrozils are effective in lowering triglyceride levels in all forms of hypertriglyceridemia except type I. The fall in triglycerides produced by clofibrate or gemfibrozil is often accompanied by a rise in LDL levels. When type V patients do not respond adequately to diet or other drugs, progestational agents or anabolic steroids may be used in women or men, respectively.

Diabetes is often associated with types III, IV, and V, and good control may lower triglyceride levels. When insulin deficiency is profound, some diabetics may accumulate excessive chylomicrons. Insulin treatment will rapidly clear the chylomicronemia in such patients. Many diabetics also have inherited a predisposition to primary hypertriglyceridemia that requires additional specific therapy. Because of their high risk for coronary and peripheral vascular disease, a cholesterol-lowering diet is recommended for all diabetics.

Oral contraceptives and postmenopausal estrogens should not be prescribed for women with types IV or V. Estrogen causes chylomicronemia and the appearance of a type V pattern in patients with type IV and accentuates the hypertriglyceridemia in those with type V. The mechanism of this estrogen effect is uncertain, but the hormone depresses hepatic triglyceride lipase activity. Attacks of acute pancreatitis may complicate the severe hypertriglyceridemia resulting from oral contraceptive use or poorly controlled diabetes.

Type I disorder is treated by restricting fat intake to about 30 g daily. Drugs are not helpful.

Measures to Raise HDL Levels

Weight loss, cessation of cigarette smoking, increased physical activity, and moderate alcohol intake increase HDL levels. It is also important to monitor the effects of dietary and drug treatment of hyperlipidemia on HDL levels. Diets rich in carbohydrates (low-fat diets), excessively high in polyunsaturated fats, or low in choles-

terol content tend to lower plasma HDL at the same time that they decrease LDL levels. Nicotinic acid, clofibrate, and gemfibrozil raise plasma HDL, but it is reduced by probucol or oxandrolone treatment. Present evidence indicates that all of the factors mentioned, with the possible exception of alcohol, affect plasma HDL2, the HDL component linked with protection against coronary heart disease. No drug can be recommended for use solely to raise HDL. Estrogen administration raises HDL levels and is probably responsible for the higher plasma HDL in women compared with men. Estrogen use in men has been associated with increased manifestations of coronary heart disease, however, perhaps related to the adverse effects of estrogen on clotting factors.

Plasma HDL and triglyceride levels are inversely related, and hypertriglyceridemic patients usually exhibit depressed HDL levels. Although control of plasma triglycerides in type V patients generally raises their plasma HDL, measures that lower plasma triglycerides in type IV are often not accompanied by a rise in HDL levels.

Lipid-lowering Drugs (Table 14.9–6)

Cholestyramine and *colestipol* are anion-exchange resins that bind bile acids and remove them in the stools. The fecal loss of bile acids lowers the cholesterol content of liver cells and thus stimulates the hepatic uptake of LDL cholesterol and its conversion to bile acids. Although cholesterol synthesis is also enhanced, the net effect is a reduction in plasma cholesterol and LDL levels. The resins may raise plasma triglycerides, especially in patients with type IIB. Side effects are minimized by slowly increasing drug intake to the usual dose of 12 g twice daily for cholestyramine and 10 g twice daily for colestipol. Because these agents are not absorbed, systemic manifestations rarely occur; gastrointestinal effects are common, however. Constipation, the most frequent and troublesome side effect, is often ameliorated by a stool softener. Epigastric discomfort and bloating usually disappear after a short period of treatment with the drug. Resins may impair the absorption of many drugs, such as salicylates, cardiac glycosides, warfarin derivatives, thiazides, and thyroxine; therefore, other drugs should be taken at least 1 hour before the resins. Resin use may also interfere with the absorption of folate and iron. Malabsorption of fat and fat-soluble vitamins occurs only at daily doses greater than 28 g. Poor compliance and expense are the major limitations of these agents. A positive attitude by the physician is critical for good compliance.

Nicotinic acid is effective in the treatment of patients with elevated cholesterol or triglycerides. The primary action of nicotinic acid is to reduce fatty-acid release from adipose tissue. The decreased availability of fatty acids to the liver diminishes VLDL synthesis. Consequently, nicotinic acid lowers both plasma LDL and triglycerides (VLDL); the drug also raises HDL levels. Upon first taking this drug, patients may experience flushing, pruritus, and gastric distress within 30 to 60 minutes after each dose. These adverse effects can be minimized by introducing the medication slowly and with meals. An initial dose of 100 mg three times a day is increased weekly by 300 mg/day to a full therapeutic dose of 1 to 2 g three times a day. Administration of 300 mg of aspirin 60 minutes before the nicotinic acid may ameliorate persistent flushing episodes, which appear to be mediated by prostaglandins. Nicotinic acid may activate peptic ulcer disease and augment the hypotensive effects of ganglionic blocking agents. Nicotinic acid may also impair glucose tolerance and should not be used in insulin-dependent diabetics. Other side effects of nicotinic acid include reversible elevations of serum transaminase levels and uric acid.

Probucol, in its usual dose of 500 mg twice daily, lowers plasma cholesterol by 10 to 15 percent with little change in triglycerides. The drug is incorporated into the lipid portion of LDL and speeds its removal from the circulation. Because probucol is concentrated in adipose tissue, its peak action is reached after 3 to 7 weeks of treatment and effects continue for several weeks after the drug is stopped. The fall in plasma cholesterol results from a nearly equivalent percentage reduction in LDL and HDL. None-

theless, studies on the regression of atherosclerosis in monkeys and xanthomas in patients, as well as on the incidence of myocardial infarction, suggest that probucol may decrease tissue concentrations of cholesterol. The drug is well tolerated. Diarrhea, the most common side effect, occurs in about 10 percent of patients. Although arrhythmias have not been reported during probucol treatment in humans, the drug sensitizes the dog myocardium to epinephrine-induced ventricular fibrillation. Accordingly, probucol should be used with caution in patients with arrhythmias.

Clofibrate, 1 g twice daily, is effective in most patients with hypertriglyceridemia, particularly in those with type III, where even smaller doses may normalize cholesterol and triglyceride levels. Clofibrate also may reduce triglycerides by 15 to 50 percent in patients with type IV and by as much as 60 percent in those with type V. During clofibrate treatment of hypertriglyceridemic patients, both HDL and LDL concentrations tend to rise. Although clofibrate lowers LDL by 5 to 10 percent in some patients with type II, it is not recommended for such individuals because of concerns regarding its long-term side effects. Clofibrate has multiple effects, but its major action is to increase VLDL clearance. Enhanced cholesterol excretion in the bile leads to a doubling of the incidence of gallstones with clofibrate treatment. A multicenter trial showed that the drug reduced the incidence of nonfatal myocardial infarction, but there was a significant increase in overall mortality in the clofibrate-treated group, mainly from gallstones and gastrointestinal cancer. Short-term tolerance of clofibrate is good. Weight gain, mild nausea, decreased libido, or skin rash may occur in a few patients. Rarely, a reversible myositis, accompanied by high levels of serum creatinine kinase, may require discontinuation of the drug. This problem is especially common in patients with the nephrotic syndrome or chronic renal failure. Because clofibrate potentiates warfarin anticoagulants, the dosage of these drugs should be halved when clofibrate is started, and prothrombin time and clotting parameters must initially be monitored closely. Because of its long-term complications, clofibrate should be used to treat hypertriglyceridemia only when significantly elevated triglyceride concentrations persist despite maximal efforts at dietary management and when the patient is at high risk for pancreatitis or atherosclerosis.

Gemfibrozil, which is structurally similar to clofibrate, is used at a dose of 600 mg twice daily. The major mechanism for the lipid-lowering effect of gemfibrozil is enhanced clearance of VLDL. The drug is at least as effective as clofibrate in lowering triglyceride levels, has a greater positive effect on HDL, and appears less likely to cause gallstones. Like clofibrate, gemfibrozil lowers LDL levels by about 5 to 10 percent in hypercholesterolemic subjects and may raise LDL in those with type IV. Gemfibrozil is generally well-tolerated. Gastrointestinal symptoms are the most common adverse effect. Other rare side effects include skin rash, anemia, leukopenia, myositis, and blurred vision. Gemfibrozil also potentiates the action of warfarin anticoagulants. Because gemfibrozil resembles clofibrate chemically, it is possible that the two drugs will demonstrate similar long-term adverse effects.

Progestational agents, such as norethindrone acetate or medroxyprogesterone acetate, are used to lower plasma triglycerides only when other measures fail in adult women with type V. These agents probably work by increasing lipoprotein lipase activity. The usual dose is 5 to 10 mg daily. Progestational agents may lower plasma triglyceride levels by 50 percent or more. Because they may cause congenital anomalies in the fetus, progestational agents should not be used in the first 4 months of pregnancy. The drug is also contraindicated in women with a history of thrombophlebitis, thromboembolic disorders, and known or suspected malignancy of the breasts or uterus. Abnormal uterine bleeding and fluid retention are common. Occasional patients exhibit cholestatic jaundice, nausea, mental depression, or tenderness and enlargement of the breasts.

Oxandrolone is an anabolic steroid that increases the activity of hepatic triglyceride lipase. Use of the drug is limited to adult men with type V because it may cause virilization in women. At a dose of 2.5 mg three times daily, the drug may lower plasma triglycerides by as much as 50 percent in responsive patients and has produced normal triglyceride levels in some. Although this agent is usually well tolerated, occasional side effects include sodium retention, edema, leukopenia, and abnormal liver function tests. Oxandrolone should be used with caution in men with cardiac, renal, or hepatic disease and should not be used concomitantly with adrenal corticosteroids or ACTH. Caution is warranted in the long-term use of oxandrolone because it causes profound reduction in HDL levels.

Lovastatin blocks cholesterol synthesis by inhibiting the enzyme HMGCoA reductase. Although quite effective in lowering plasma cholesterol with few short-term side effects, the drug is presently considered a second line agent because it has been used in relatively few subjects. The full dose is 40 mg twice daily.

OTHER FORMS OF DYSLIPOPROTEINEMIA[3,11]

Earlier sections have described dyslipoproteinemias resulting from defects or absence of apo C-11 (type V hyperlipidemia), apo E (type III), and the enzyme lipoprotein lipase (type I). Other disorders, mostly rare, are caused by abnormalities of apo A-I or apo B (abetalipoproteinemia) and by deficiency of LCAT.

HDL DEFICIENCY

The most common deficiency of HDL is familial hypoalphalipoproteinemia, which is inherited as an autosomal dominant trait. Levels of HDL_{ch} below the 10th percentile are associated with premature coronary heart disease. The underlying defect is not known.

Tangier disease results from the failure to convert secreted proapoprotein A-I (apo A-I Tangier) into the mature form of apo A-I. Apo A-I Tangier does not associate normally with lipoproteins. Consequently, apo A-I and HDL constituents are catabolized at an excessive rate, and their plasma levels fall to about 1 percent of normal. The ratio of apo A-I to apo A-II in HDL is normally about 3:1; in Tangier disease the ratio is 1:12. Transmitted as an autosomal recessive trait, the disease is recognized by very low levels of HDL, decreased LDL, and slightly increased VLDL.

Deposition of cholesterol esters in reticuloendothelial cells of homozygotes may produce hepatosplenomegaly and lymphadenopathy; the most dramatic clinical finding is grossly enlarged, orange-colored tonsils. Lipid deposits also cause mild corneal opacification. Systemic manifestations are generally minor although premature coronary heart disease and mild transient peripheral neuropathy may develop.

To date, seven variants of apo A-I have been recognized with a single amino acid substitution. Heterozygotes for these mutant forms of apo A-I occur in approximately 0.2 percent of the population. Several of these mutants have associated reductions in HDL and elevated triglycerides. Absence of apo A-I and C-III, marked HDL deficiency, xanthomas, premature coronary heart disease, and mild corneal opacification are found in homozygotes with DNA rearrangements in the adjacent apo A-I and apo C-III gene loci. Striking corneal opacification and low HDL levels occur in fish-eye disease. The defect has not been identified.

APO B DEFICIENCY

Apo B deficiency occurs in at least three different forms: abetalipoproteinemia (autosomal recessive), familial hypobetalipoproteinemia (autosomal codominant), and normotriglyceridemic abetalipoproteinemia. Homozygotes for the first two disorders have similar laboratory and clinical features. Inability to synthesize apo B leads to plasma cholesterol and triglyceride levels below 50 mg/dl and

virtual absence of chylomicrons, LDL, and VLDL. The clinical manifestations include fat malabsorption with steatorrhea and triglyceride deposition in cells of the intestinal mucosa, fatty liver, growth retardation, ataxic neuropathy, acanthocytosis, and atypical retinitis pigmentosa. High doses of vitamin E can prevent further neurologic and retinal damage. Supplementary vitamin A and K may also be useful. Fat restriction may reduce diarrhea, especially in children. Heterozygotes have normal lipoprotein levels in abetalipoproteinemia and about half normal levels of VLDL and LDL in hypobetalipoproteinemia.

Patients with normotriglyceridemic abetalipoproteinemia can synthesize apo B_{48} in the intestine but not apo B_{100} in the liver. They manifest plasma lipoprotein levels similar to those of abetalipoproteinemia in the fasting state, but chylomicrons are produced after a fat-rich meal. These patients have mental retardation and vitamin E deficiency.

LECITHIN:CHOLESTEROL ACYLTRANSFERASE DEFICIENCY

In patients with a deficiency of the enzyme lecithin:cholesterol acyltransferase (LCAT), all plasma lipoproteins exhibit structural or compositional abnormalities caused by an increased content of cholesterol and phospholipids along with decreased cholesterol esters. Hemolytic anemia is associated with an increased cholesterol content of red blood cells. Lipid deposition in the cornea and glomeruli cause marked corneal opacification and proteinuria progressing to renal failure, respectively. These patients may benefit from a low-fat diet.

REFERENCES

1. Blank DW, Hoeg JM, et al: The method of determination must be considered in interpreting blood cholesterol levels. JAMA 256:2867, 1986
2. Brown MS, Goldstein JL: A receptor-mediated pathway for cholesterol homeostasis. Science 232:34, 1986
3. Dargel R: Classification of primary dyslipoproteinemias. Exp Pathol 27:67, 1985
4. Eisenberg S: Plasma lipoprotein conversions: The origin of low density and high density lipoproteins. Ann NY Acad Sci 348:30, 1980
5. Grundy SM: AHA special report: Recommendations for the treatment of hyperlipidemia in adults: A joint statement of the Nutrition Committee and Council on Arteriosclerosis of the American Heart Association. Arteriosclerosis 4:445A, 1984
6. Hoeg JM, Gregg RE, Brewer HB Jr: An approach to the management of hyperlipoproteinemia. JAMA 255:512, 1986
7. Lipid Research Clinics Coronary Primary Prevention Trial Results. I. Reduction in incidence of coronary heart disease. JAMA 51:351, 1984
8. Mahley RW, Innerarity TL, et al: Plasma lipoproteins: apolipoprotein structure and function. J Lipid Res 25:1277, 1984
9. National Institutes of Health Consensus Conference on the Treatment of Hypertriglyceridemia. JAMA 251:1196, 1984
10. National Institutes of Health Consensus Conference Statement: Lowering blood cholesterol to prevent heart disease. JAMA 253:2080, 1985
11. Schaefer EJ, Levy RI: Pathogenesis and management of lipoprotein disorders. N Engl J Med 312:1300, 1985

CHAPTER 14.10
Nutritional Disorders

Simeon Margolis and James V. Sitzmann

Adequate nutritional intake is necessary not only to maintain good health but also to compensate for the additional requirements imposed by pregnancy, lactation, disease, and growth in children. Despite their decreased incidence in this country, primary disorders of malnutrition are still prominent in poor, elderly, and alcoholic persons, and there is greater recognition of the importance of nutritional problems in both acutely and chronically ill patients. Many studies show that malnutrition is common among hospitalized patients and that nutritional status often declines during the hospital stay.

The physician must understand the nutritional requirements of healthy individuals and the effects of disease states on these requirements. He or she should be able to identify deficiencies through an assessment of nutritional status and to initiate measures to restore nutritional balance. The latter requires the ability to calculate the needs for repletion and maintenance, as well as a knowledge of alternative approaches to delivery of nutritional requirements. The physician must also recognize the need for special diets in the management of some diseases in which malnutrition is not the primary problem.

NUTRIENT REQUIREMENTS

Maintenance of normal body mass, composition, physiologic function, and growth in children requires the intake of adequate amounts of energy (calories), protein to supply the eight essential amino acids, a polyunsaturated fatty acid, 11 vitamins, at least 14 inorganic elements, and water. The vitamins and inorganic ions, except for the bulk minerals sodium, potassium, calcium, magnesium, phosphorus, and chloride, are all micronutrients, that is, their requirement is less than 100 mg daily. The needs for these nutrients are often expressed as the recommended daily allowances (RDAs), defined as the mean requirement, plus two standard deviations, for healthy adults.[8] Because the RDAs are estimated with a large margin of safety, individuals are not necessarily malnourished when they ingest less than the RDA. Conversely, the RDAs may be inadequate during illness because of the additional nutritional requirements imposed by disease.

ENERGY

Caloric intake must be sufficient to meet energy needs. Carbohydrates and protein (4 kcal/g), alcohol (7 kcal/g), and fat (9 kcal/g) provide energy for basal metabolic requirements as well as for physical activity. Basal energy needs vary with body size, sex, age, and environmental temperature. Energy required for the assimilation of protein, the "specific dynamic action," increases the metabolic rate after each meal. Basal metabolic needs are about 22 kcal/kg of ideal body weight (see Table 14.11–3). Caloric demands are raised by about 30, 50, and more than 100 percent by mild, moderate, and strenuous activity, respectively. Caloric expenditure is also increased by fever, trauma (especially burns), infections, organ failure, and hyperthyroidism. Inadequate dietary calories, caused by poor intake or malabsorption, lead to weight loss (cachexia) in

adults and weight loss accompanied by failure of growth in children.

Most energy requirements are met by carbohydrate and fat; each supplies about 40 to 50 percent of the calories in the usual North American diet. Most nutritionists now recommend a more prudent diet containing no more than 30 percent of calories from fat and about 55 percent of calories from carbohydrates, especially complex carbohydrates. Foods containing complex carbohydrates provide vitamins, iron, and fiber, whereas simple sugars serve only as an energy source. The minimal requirement for fat is about 3 g per day of a polyunsaturated fatty acid, mostly ingested as linoleic acid, to avoid essential fatty acid deficiency.

PROTEIN

In addition to their use as an energy source, proteins provide the amino acids and nitrogen necessary for protein synthesis. Dietary protein must supply the eight essential amino acids (isoleucine, leucine, lysine, methionine, phenylalanine, threonine, tryptophan, and valine) because their carbon backbones cannot be synthesized by humans. Arginine and histidine are also considered essential amino acids in children and may be limiting in some disease states. Dietary protein requirements vary with the quality or biologic value of the proteins and with caloric intake.

The biologic value of a protein depends on its digestability, absorption, and content of essential amino acids. In general, animal products (particularly milk and eggs) have proteins with the highest biologic value; vegetable proteins are poorer in quality because they are deficient in one or more of the essential amino acids. This poor quality can be overcome by the ingestion at the same meal of two "complementary" proteins, each deficient in different essential amino acids. For example, methionine is limited in soy beans, and lysine, threonine, and tryptophan are deficient in corn. Meals containing the complementary foods, soy beans and corn, will provide protein of adequate biologic value.

The RDA for protein, 50 g per day in adults, assumes the intake of protein of high biologic value. The daily protein requirement is higher when vegetables are the major protein source. Protein requirements are increased in growing children and during pregnancy and lactation, as well as by disease states, such as fever, trauma, infection, or malabsorption. Protein requirements are further increased when caloric intake is inadequate because amino acids are then used as a source of energy by serving as precursors of glucose. Kwashiorkor develops when protein intake is severely deficient relative to calories.

EFFECTS OF DISEASE ON NUTRIENT REQUIREMENTS

As shown in Table 14.10–1, energy and protein needs are significantly raised by malabsorption or the increased utilization of nutrients caused by fever, trauma, infection, or hyperthyroidism. Additional intake of fat-soluble vitamins, calcium, magnesium, iron, and phosphorus may be needed in patients with malabsorption. Efforts to replenish tissue losses in cachectic patients require greater than normal intake of vitamins and minerals as well as attention to energy and protein needs. Physicians should also be aware of the need for increased intake of specific nutrients in certain disease states, for example, folic acid in hemolytic anemias, vitamin D in renal disease, B vitamins in liver disease, and protein in severe nephrosis. A variety of drugs may cause depletion of nutrients by altering their metabolism or absorption. Thus, anticonvulsants may deplete vitamin D and folate stores by altering their metabolism while cholestyramine and antacids may cause malabsorption of fat-soluble vitamins and phosphorus, respectively.

Restricted intake of specific amino acids is necessary in certain inborn errors, such as in phenylketonuria and maple syrup urine disease. Protein-restricted diets in patients with chronic renal failure and chronic liver disease are discussed in Chapters 11.5 and

TABLE 14.10–1. EFFECTS OF DISEASE STATES ON NUTRITIONAL REQUIREMENTS

Mechanism	Disease States	Increased Requirements For
Increased nutrient utilization	Fever, trauma, infection, hyperthyroidism	Calories, protein
	Hemolytic anemia, cancer	Folic acid
	Repletion of cachexia	Calories, proteins, vitamins
Malabsorption	Multiple	Calories, protein, linoleic acid, fat-soluble vitamins, calcium, magnesium, phosphorus, iron
Inability to convert nutrient to active form	Renal disease	Vitamin D
	Liver disease	Folate, thiamine, pyridoxine
Nutrient losses	Renal disease Diarrhea Nasogastric suction Dialysis Burns Blood loss	Sodium, potassium, energy, proteins, phosphorus
Drug treatment	Methotrexate	Folate
	Cholestyramine	Folate, vitamin D

Mechanism	Disease States	Reduced Tolerance To
Impaired catabolism or excretion	Renal failure	Protein
	Liver failure	Protein
	Inborn errors, e.g., phenylketonuria	Phenylalanine
Excessive absorption	Wilson disease	Copper
	Hemochromatosis	Iron
	Hypercalciuria	Calcium

13.6, respectively. There are growing efforts to use selected essential amino or keto acids in the treatment of these two disorders as well as in the rare hyperammonemias of infants.

THE NORMAL DIET

Many different dietary styles and food choices can supply adequate amounts of all required nutrients if the diet is balanced and contains enough calories. A balanced diet involves selections from each of the four major food groups: (1) milk and milk products; (2) fruits and vegetables; (3) bread and cereals; and (4) meat, fish, eggs, and legumes. Although a balanced diet assures nutritional adequacy, normal nutritional status can be maintained despite the intake of an unbalanced diet. Only the bread and cereal group and dark green vegetables are indispensable. Thus, proper selection of foods will prevent nutritional deficiencies even in those vegetarians who eat only foods from these two groups.

There is a widespread belief that the usual North American diet fails to promote good health. For example, some feel that the use of additives and refined foods is dangerous. In fact, most food additives are essential to prevent spoilage of food and have been carefully checked for safety. "Natural" foods have no demonstrated advantages. Others hold the view that the usual diet contains inadequate nutrients, especially vitamins and minerals. Dietary deficiencies do occur in this country, but most often they result from socioeconomic problems that lead to an inadequate intake of energy. Strict vegetarianism can also produce protein deficiency unless care is taken to use complementary foods appropriately. If healthy individuals ingest an adequate amount of calories,

however, they have to persevere with an extremely unusual diet to become deficient in any nutrients other than iron and calcium. Nonetheless, vitamin and mineral supplements are widely used by North Americans, who have apparently succumbed to the advertising of the health food industry, in an effort to "improve their health," "reduce fatigue," or "increase their resistance to disease."[10] Such supplements do not benefit healthy adults unless they have made a deliberate effort to avoid whole classes of foods.

The diets of many menstruating women are deficient in iron, and the inadequte calcium intake in this country may be an important factor in the high frequency of osteoporosis, especially in older women. Clearly, dietary supplementation is also required during pregnancy, lactation, and in many disease states. There is also growing evidence for the benefits of including more fiber in the diet.

More important than dietary deficiencies as a health problem in the United States is the excessive intake of total calories (Chapter 14.11), cholesterol and saturated fat (Chapter 14.9), salt (Chapter 2.10), and sugar. A major risk of refined sugar, in addition to its high caloric content, is dental caries.

PROTEIN-ENERGY MALNUTRITION

Protein-energy malnutrition can be primary, arising solely from a poor diet, or result predominantly as a secondary consequence of other illnesses. As many as one quarter of Africans and Asians suffer from protein-energy malnutrition because they lack ample supplies of high-quality food. In the United States, poverty, alcoholism, and vegetarianism are the major causes of primary protein-energy malnutrition, often of mild degree. More severe malnutrition can develop rapidly in chronically ill patients, especially in those with a prior borderline nutritional status, and is often overlooked in the hospital setting. Table 14.10–2 delineates the patient characteristics suggesting protein-energy malnutrition and indicates the disease states and therapeutic situations contributing to this problem.

Two distinct syndromes of protein-energy malnutrition can be identified, but mixed forms are common. Marasmus is due mainly to caloric deficiency and is characterized by diminished growth rate in children, a striking decrease of both fat and lean body mass, and the absence of edema. In kwashiorkor the diet is adequate in calories, but deficient in protein. Children fail to grow normally, but weight is maintained by preservation of adipose tissue and the accumulation of edema. In mixed forms of protein-energy malnutrition, the balance between the features of marasmus and kwashiorkor is determined by the relative degree of caloric and protein deficiency. Protein-energy malnutrition is often accompanied by vitamin and mineral deficiencies and complicated by infections.

When protein deficiency predominates, patients exhibit peripheral edema; ascites; hepatomegaly; temporal wasting; skin lesions that resemble those of pellagra; hair that is brittle, dry, straight, poorly pigmented, and falls out easily; cold extremities; and hypothermia. They are apathetic, fatigue easily, and have a poor appetite. In contrast, marasmic individuals tend to be alert and hungry.

Hematocrit, albumin, and transferrin levels are usually reduced in patients with kwashiorkor but remain relatively normal in those with pure marasmus. Serum amino acid concentrations are decreased in patients with kwashiorkor, as are urinary levels of urea and creatinine. Serum lipids are low, and blood glucose levels may occasionally fall into the hypoglycemic range. Impaired cellular immunity, reflected in decreased lymphocyte counts and cutaneous anergy, along with diminished numbers and bactericidal function of polymorphonuclear cells, leads to higher susceptibility to infections with common and opportunistic organisms. Delayed wound healing complicates surgery.

Hepatomegaly is due to massive fat accumulation in kwashiorkor. The gastrointestinal mucosa atrophies, and the content of mucosal enzymes and production of pancreatic enzymes decline. Heart size and cardiac output are reduced in proportion to the smaller lean body mass, but the heart may be unable to respond adequately when infections or other acute stresses impose a demand for increased output.

Women may manifest amenorrhea and infertility. Pregnant women are at particular risk for protein-energy malnutrition. Infants born to mothers who are protein-energy deficient have lower birth weights, and their nutrition is further impaired by poor maternal lactation.

Prevention is the obvious approach to protein-energy malnutrition. Physicians must be able to recognize both subclinical and overt protein-energy malnutrition. Vigorous nutritional support, using enteral or parenteral nutrition when necessary, should be initiated in the early stages of malnutrition especially when anticipated stresses of surgery or chronic illness are likely to further impair nutritional status. In addition to the provision of ample protein, the management of kwashiorkor demands careful attention to hydration, electrolyte status, intercurrent infections, and repletion of needed vitamins and minerals.

VITAMINS

With the exception of ascorbic acid, all of the water-soluble vitamins are chemically modified in the body to serve as cofactors in various enzymatic reactions. Three fat-soluble vitamins (A, D, and K) also require chemical modification in vivo before they are active, but only vitamin K acts as an enzyme cofactor. Deficiency of fat-soluble vitamins often accompanies fat malabsorption because bile salts and micelle formation are essential for the absorption of these vitamins. Table 14.10–3 details the requirements, sources, and physiologic and biochemical functions of the vitamins associated with deficiency states in humans (Table 14.10–4). In the developed countries, vitamin deficiencies are rarely caused by a poor diet alone; rather they are complications of alcoholism or other disorders or occur during periods of unusual dietary need, such as pregnancy and lactation, when the requirements for most vitamins are increased. Pantothenic acid and biotin are not included because deficiency syndromes have not been identified in humans. These two vitamins are recommended, however, for patients on total parenteral nutrition. The rapidity of development

TABLE 14.10–2. PROTEIN-ENERGY MALNUTRITION

Patient characteristics suggesting protein-energy malnutrition
- Alcoholism, poverty, chronic disease, drug dependency, inadequate dentition, social isolation, food faddism
- Body weight <85% ideal weight
- Recent loss of >10% of usual weight
- Midarm muscle or fat area <15th percentile
- Lymphopenia (<1200/μl), cutaneous anergy
- Serum albumin <3.2 mg/dl, serum transferrin <150 mg/dl

Disease states contributing to protein-energy malnutrition
- Acute febrile illness
- Infection
- Organ failure
- Major trauma
- Burns
- Gastrointestinal disorders
- Neoplasia
- Central nervous system disease
- Coma

Therapeutic situations contributing to protein-energy malnutrition
- Gastrointestinal surgery
- Bowel rest
- Corticosteroids
- Cancer radiation or chemotherapy
- Prolonged 5% dextrose infusions

TABLE 14.10–3. VITAMIN REQUIREMENTS, SOURCES, PHYSIOLOGIC, AND BIOCHEMICAL FUNCTIONS[7,8]

Vitamin	RDA (Adults)		Sources	Physiologic Functions	Biochemical Mechanisms	Comments
Thiamin (B₁)	*Men:*	1.4 mg	Widely distributed in foods, but rapidly destroyed during cooking	Energy metabolism	Thiamin pyrophosphate is a coenzyme for (1) oxidative decarboxylation reactions involving pyruvate, ketoglutarate, and branched-chain ketoacids and (2) utilization of pentoses in the hexose monophosphate shunt	
	Women:	1.1 mg (P&L: 1.5 mg) Requirement increases with caloric intake				
Riboflavin (B₂)	*Men:*	1.4–1.7 mg	Leafy vegetables, milk, meat, and fish Destroyed by cooking	Energy metabolism	Cofactor or prosthetic group (FMN, FAD) of flavoproteins involved in oxidative metabolism	
	Women:	1.2 mg (P&L: 1.6– 1.8 mg)				
Niacin, (nicotinic acid, nicotinamide)	*Men:*	16–19 mg	Whole grain cereals, nuts, meats and fish are rich sources of niacin Tryptophan is converted to niacin—60 mg of tryptophan is equivalent to 1 mg of niacin	Energy metabolism	Nicotinamide is a component of two coenzymes (NAD and NADH) that play essential roles in oxidation-reduction reactions	
	Women:	13–15 mg (P&L: 15– 20 mg)				
Pyridoxine, pyridoxal, pyridoxamine (B₆)	*Men:*	2.2 mg	Meats, vegetables, whole grain cereals	Amino acid metabolism Hemoglobin synthesis	Pyrodoxal phosphate is cofactor for a number of enzymes of amino acid metabolism	
	Women:	2.0 mg (P&L: 2.6 mg)				
B₁₂		——————————————— See Chapter 6.4 ———————————————				
Ascorbic acid (C)			Citrus fruits, fresh vegetables	Collagen synthesis	Biochemical role is linked to the capacity of ascorbate to undergo reversible oxidation and reduction. Exact function of the vitamin is unclear, but it is required for hydroxylation of proline in collagen	
Folic acid		——————————————— See Chapter 6.4 ———————————————				
A (Retinol)		(As retinol)	Preformed vitamin A is present in animal foods β-carotene of plants is abundant precursor	Essential for growth, reproduction and maintenance of normal epithelium Required for night vision	Unknown Vitamin A aldehyde (retinal) is structural component of the visual pigment rhodopsin	β-carotene is converted to retinol in the intestine Retinol is transported in the plasma on retinol-binding protein Vitamin A is stored in the liver as retinyl esters
	Men:	1 mg				
	Women:	0.8 mg (P&L: 1–1.2 mg)				
D		200–400 IU	D₂ (ergocalciferol) is used to fortify milk and other foods D₃ (cholecalciferol) present in fish, egg yolk, butter Ultraviolet light converts 7-dehydrocholesterol of skin to vitamin D	Maintains plasma Ca and PO₄ levels, thus supporting bone mineralization	*Intestine:* stimulates active transport of Ca and PO₄ probably by enhancing synthesis of mucosal calcium-transport protein *Bones:* mobilizes bone Ca and PO₄ (parathyroid hormone required) *Kidney:* increases Ca reabsorption in distal tubule	Vitamin D itself is inert The active form of vitamin D, 1,25-dihydroxyvitamin D, is synthesized by sequential hydroxylations at the 25 position in the liver and the 1 position in the kidney
E		(As α-tocopherol)	Oils, margarines, fruits, vegetables, whole-grain products are rich sources of α-tocopherol	Required for normal function of central nervous system, red cells, muscle and vascular tissue	Serves as an antioxidant to protect tissue polyunsaturated fatty acids from peroxidation by free radicals	
	Men:	10 mg				
	Women:	8 mg (P&L: 10 mg)				
K		—	Vegetables are abundant food source Synthesis by intestinal bacteria is another major source	Required for normal blood clotting	Vitamin K is cofactor for a liver carboxylase that activates factors II (prothrombin), VII, IX, and X by the conversion of specific glutamate residues to γ-carboxyglutamate	Warfarin anticoagulants act by blocking vitamin K modifications needed to activate clotting factors

P&L = Pregnancy and lactation.

TABLE 14.10–4. VITAMIN DEFICIENCY STATES

Vitamin	Major Causes of Deficiency	Manifestations of Deficiency	Comments

Thiamin	*Inadequate diet:*
	• Alcoholism—poor diet is coupled with impaired thiamin absorption
	• Diets with refined grain as major caloric source (thiamin is especially rich in outer layers of grains)
		Beriberi
		  Paresthesias, diminished reflexes, muscle fatigue and cramps, foot and wrist drop
		  Peripheral vasodilatation produces state of high cardiac output and tachycardia; myocardial failure; sodium and water retention with edema
		Wernicke-Korsakoff syndrome—see Chapter 17.5
			Blood pyruvate and lactate levels rise with deficiency
			Raw seafood contains thiaminase, which destroys thiamin

Riboflavin	*Inadequate diet for 3 to 8 mo:* • Alcoholism, malignancies	Soreness and burning of mouth and tongue, cheilosis (fissures at the angles of the mouth), seborrheic dermatitis, glossitis, photophobia, conjunctivitis, sore throat, anemia	Commonly associated with protein-calorie malnutrition and other B vitamin deficiencies
Niacin	*Inadequate diet:* • Alcoholism • Reduced dietary niacin coupled with an imbalanced intake of amino acids	Pellagra: dermatitis, dementia, diarrhea 1. Symmetrical bilateral dermatitis due to photosensitivity 2. Fatigue, apathy, disorientation, memory loss, organic psychosis 3. Diarrhea	Corn is low in niacin and tryptophan content; a portion of the niacin is protein bound, making it unavailable for absorption
Pyridoxine	• Alcoholism: ethanol interferes with the metabolism of pyridoxal phosphate • Pregnancy • Drugs: isoniazid, dopamine, penicillamine, estrogens	Nausea, vomiting, dizziness, cheilosis, glossitis, convulsions	Pyridoxine deficiency in the United States is most commonly due to the use of drugs which act as pyridoxine antagonists
B_{12}	See Chapter 6.4		
Ascorbic acid	*Inadequate diet*	Scurvy Perifollicular hemorrhages, purpura, bleeding in muscles and joints, poor wound-healing, gum disease with swelling, bleeding and loosening of teeth	
Folic acid	See Chapter 6.4		
A	*Developed countries:* • Malabsorption • Parenteral nutrition *Underdeveloped countries:* • Dietary deficiencies of vitamin A, β-cartotene, or proteins and calories	Loss of night vision Xerophthalmia—dryness of the conjunctiva and cornea Bitot spots—small plaques begin on the exposed conjunctiva, then enlarge and spread to the cornea Keratomalacia—ulceration of the cornea leading to perforation, prolapse of the iris, and panophthalmitis Dryness of the skin and hyperkeratinization	Protein-calorie malnutrition leads to vitamin A deficiency due to inadequate synthesis of retinol-binding protein Vitamin A deficiency is a major cause of blindness in underdeveloped countries Except for keratomalacia, all manifestations of vitamin A toxicity are readily reversible with adequate replacement
D	• Inadequate exposure to sunlight • Failure to ingest vitamin D–supplemented foods • Malabsorption • Parenteral nutrition	Osteomalacia due to failure of bone mineralization Symptoms of hypocalcemia: muscle cramps, decreased muscle tone and strength, seizures	Although patients with liver or renal disease may require 25-hydroxy- or 1,25-dihydroxyvitamin D, individuals with simple deficiency should be treated with vitamin D itself
E	• Premature infants whose formulas contain large amounts of polyunsaturated fats and iron • Chronic biliary obstruction, cystic fibrosis, abetalipoproteinemia	1. Edema, anemia 2. Areflexia, reduced proprioception and vibratory sense, gait disturbance, and ophthalmoplegia	There is no evidence that increased vitamin E intake improves sexual function or prevents premature coronary artery disease
K	• Excessive amounts of warfarin anticoagulants • Malabsorption • Parenteral nutrition	Bleeding disorders	Synthetic, water-soluble forms of vitamin K, such as menadione, require modification in the liver before thay are active; therefore, always use natural vitamin K to treat bleeding due to an overdose of warfarin anticoagulants

of deficiency states varies from vitamin to vitamin. Although an inadequate diet can provoke symptoms of folate deficiency after a few months, the large body stores of vitamins A, D, and B_{12} may delay clinical symptoms for more than 2 years.

Intake of pyridoxine or vitamin D that far exceeds their RDAs is necessary in a number of inherited disorders of pyridoxine metabolism or for conditions characterized by vitamin D resistance. Otherwise there is no benefit from the ingestion of large amounts of any vitamin. For example, controlled trials have not demonstrated that large doses of vitamin C are useful in preventing or ameliorating the common cold. Megavitamin intake is generally safe, albeit expensive, but excessive use of vitamins A or D or pyridoxine can cause distinct toxic manifestations.

Chronic vitamin A toxicity is characterized by dryness of the skin, itching, desquamation, hair loss, weakness, fatigue, loss of appetite, headaches, and blurred vision. Symptoms of hypervitaminosis A occur most often in individuals taking more than 20,000 IU of vitamin A daily but can also complicate the use of new pharmacologic derivatives of vitamin A to treat patients with severe acne or ichthyosis. Acute vitamin A intoxication, manifested by nausea and vomiting, violent headaches, dizziness, extreme lethargy, and desquamation, has resulted when explorers have ingested polar bear liver. Massive intake of foods rich in β-carotene can produce hypercarotenemia, with a yellowish appearance of the skin over the palms and soles, but not hypervitaminosis A. Reversible neurologic complications, manifested by progressive sensory ataxia with impaired position and vibratory sensation, have occurred in individuals taking pyridoxine in amounts exceeding 500 mg per day. The metabolism of ascorbic acid to oxalate may contribute to the formation of calcium oxalate stones in association with large excesses of vitamin C. The findings in vitamin D toxicity are described in Chapter 14.6.

INORGANIC ELEMENTS[6,8]

Almost all physiologic and biochemical processes require inorganic ions. With the exception of magnesium, the need for the bulk minerals is discussed elsewhere in this book. Trace elements are present in only minute concentration, micrograms to picograms per gram of tissue. The essential nature of some trace elements for humans is evident either because they are constituents of body proteins or because clinical manifestations result from deficiencies. Deprivation of other trace elements produces specific deficiency states in experimental animals, but their requirement for humans has not yet been determined. RDAs have been established for only a few inorganic elements. These RDAs for adults are as follows: calcium and phosphorus, 800 mg; magnesium, 350 mg in men and 300 mg in women; iron, 10 mg in men and postmenopausal women and 18 mg in menstruating women; zinc, 15 mg; and iodine, 150 μg.

Manifestations of deficiencies of trace elements, other than iron or iodine (described in Chapter 6.3 and 14.4, respectively), are rare in humans except in patients on parenteral nutrition. An increased intake of one mineral may alter the needs for another. For example, an elevated intake of copper raises the requirement for zinc because both metals compete for sites on the same binding proteins. Finally, excessive intake of most inorganic ions can produce toxic side effects. Thus, nausea, vomiting and diarrhea are manifestations of zinc toxicity, while nausea, vomiting, gastrointestinal bleeding, and liver necrosis can occur with acute copper poisoning.

Table 14.10–5 lists the functions and major causes and manifestations of deficiency of magnesium and eight trace elements that play a role in human nutrition.

NUTRITIONAL THERAPY

Successful management of many acute and chronic diseases often requires nutritional modification. Some diseases, such as the vitamin deficiency syndromes or obesity, result directly from deficits or excesses of nutrients. Other disorders, such as malabsorption, increase certain nutrient requirements. In other instances, a normal diet produces disease manifestations because of nutrient intolerance (e.g., celiac disease), and dietary restrictions are necessary (Table 14.10–1). Finally, protein-energy malnutrition may complicate many clinical situations, either as a primary predisposing condition or as a secondary consequence of various diseases and their therapy. Newer nutritional support techniques can prevent or reverse protein-energy malnutrition in most cases, thereby promoting faster recovery and minimizing nutrition-related complications.

NUTRITIONAL ASSESSMENT

The goals of nutritional assessment are to identify candidates for nutritional support and to monitor nutritional therapy. The initial step involves establishing the diagnosis of malnutrition or the risk of malnutrition in a given patient. As with any disease state, the diagnosis is established by history, physical examination, and laboratory tests. Patients with advanced malnutrition are easy to recognize by loose, ill-fitting clothing; muscle-wasting; thin, brittle hair; dermatologic changes; and characteristic physical and mental lethargy. By contrast, patients with borderline nutritional status can escape the detection of even the careful physician, especially on initial examination. Yet such patients are vulnerable to the nutritional complications of serious illness and hospitalization.

Nutritional assessment should be incorporated into the initial evaluation of most hospitalized patients[4] (Table 14.10–6). Poverty, alcoholism, drug abuse, or previous serious illness and its therapy should prompt especially close scrutiny. Reported weight changes are important clues, but a history of stable body weight does not ensure good nutritional status because marked alterations in body composition may occur without net change in weight. For example, in patients on a regimen of corticosteroids, depletion of lean body mass is masked by accumulation of fat and extracellular fluid. A diet history by a trained nutritionist is of great value; the physician should at least obtain the information outlined in Table 14.10–6. A review of the systems involved in food ingestion helps to identify patients who may have chronic undernutrition because of poor intake.

Every hospitalized patient must have height and weight measured (rather than reported by the patient) on admission. Frame size is determined by measuring wrist circumference and referring to published tables[3]; ideal body weight for sex, height, and frame size is estimated from the Metropolitan Life tables (see Table 14.11–1). Many dietitians are trained in anthropometry: measurement of midarm circumference and triceps skin fold thickness allows calculation of midarm muscle and fat areas by standard formulas. These values can be compared to published tables[2] giving percentile values[5] for the US population. These measurements, although imprecise, are helpful baselines for future reassessment. The careful clinician will be alert to physical signs of protein-energy malnutrition or specific vitamin deficiencies, especially in the skin, hair, eyes, mouth, limbs, and neuromuscular system.

Laboratory screening need not be extensive (Table 14.10–6), and abnormal values must be interpreted in light of possible nonnutritional causes. Creatinine excretion is related to muscle mass in patients with normal renal function, and available tables give standards for healthy individuals of various heights (creatinine/height ratio).[3] Expensive tests of serum vitamin levels are not useful because they frequently do not reflect tissue stores. Delayed hypersensitivity, assessed by skin testing with recall antigens, is frequently impaired in protein-energy malnutrition but may also be affected by the underlying disease, independent of nutritional status. A simpler method of assessing immune competence is the total lymphocyte count. A count below 1500 is a strong indication of malnutrition in the absence of a nonnutritional disease state affecting immune competence.

Current methods of nutritional assessment do not produce a

TABLE 14.10–5. FUNCTIONS AND DEFICIENCY STATES FOR INORGANIC ELEMENTS

Inorganic Element	Function	Major Causes of Deficiency	Manifestations of Deficiency
Magnesium[a]	Major constituent of bone Required for neuromuscular contraction, protein synthesis, and reactions involving ATP	Alcoholism, diuretic use, kwashiorkor, malabsorption, diabetic ketoacidosis, parenteral nutrition	Muscle irritability and tetany, weakness, confusion, coma, tremor, seizures, arrhythmias (plasma Mg may be normal though tissue levels are low)
Copper[a]	Essential for connective tissue metabolism, heme synthesis, and nerve function. Bound to ceruloplasmin and metallothionein. A component of several oxidative enzymes	Nephrotic syndrome, malabsorption, kwashiorkor, parenteral nutrition High-fiber diets decrease copper absorption	Pancytopenia. Bone marrow shows increased megaloblasts and sideroblasts with maturation arrest
Zinc[a]	Required for normal growth and development. Essential component of a number of enzymes and the salivary protein gustin	Diets limited largely to whole wheat bread and beans (dietary phytate binds zinc and decreases its absorption) Acrodermatitis enteropathica, an autosomal recessive disorder	Dwarfed males with hypogonadism, anemia, lethargy, hepatosplenomegaly, geophagia Severe chronic diarrhea; thickened, ulcerated skin on limbs and around mouth and anus Loss of normal taste sensation
Chromium[a]	Glucose tolerance factor, a low-molecular-weight organic complex, is needed in some animal species for normal glucose metabolism. Low chromium levels have been reported in some diabetics, but the role of chromium in human diabetes is unclear.		
Cobalt	Cobalt is a component of vitamin B_{12}. Cobalt deficiency has not been reported in humans. Cardiomyopathy has resulted from the addition of cobalt to beer. Other toxic manifestations of cobalt include nausea, vomiting, diarrhea, tinnitus, and hearing loss.		
Fluoride	Fluoride is incorporated into bone and teeth. Addition of fluoride to water supplies low in this element reduces the incidence of dental caries. Excessive fluoride causes mottling of dental enamel, gastrointestinal symptoms, tetany, and cardiovascular collapse.		
Manganese[a]	Manganese is a cofactor for several enzymes and a component of bone and several metalloenzymes. Manganese deficiency has not yet been described in humans.		
Molybdenum	Molybdenum is a constituent of some oxidases. No deficiency state is known in humans.		
Selenium	Selenium is a component of glutathione peroxidase and may function, like vitamin E, to protect against intracellular peroxides. A fatal cadiomyopathy in Chinese children has been attributed to selenium deficiency.		

[a]Inorganic elements commonly included in parenteral nutrition solutions.

single score of nutritional well-being and mainly serve to guide the clinician in the judicious use of nutritional support. A widely used guideline for establishing a diagnosis of malnutrition in hospitalized patients includes a weight loss of 10 percent or greater, a serum albumin of less than 3.5 mg/dl, or a total lymphocyte count less than 1500. The diagnosis is further supported by findings of depressed serum transferrin or creatinine:height index, or an abnormal anthropometric examination. The most helpful measurements to monitor nutritional therapy are weight, intake and output measurements (see below), hydration status, and reexamination of abnormal laboratory tests noted in the baseline assessment.

Nitrogen Balance

Because protein-energy malnutrition is the most prevalent nutritional problem in US hospital patients, nitrogen balance studies are useful to follow their progress. Nitrogen balance is the net difference between total nitrogen intake and excretion: in catabolic states, nitrogen excretion exceeds intake and the nitrogen balance is negative; in growing children and patients recovering from depletion, intake exceeds excretion and the nitrogen balance is positive. Because urinary urea is the major route of excretion for amino nitrogen, nitrogen balance can be estimated from accurate measurements of protein intake and of urea nitrogen and protein in 24-hour urine collections (Fig. 14.10–1).

Nitrogen balance depends upon an adequate supply of both protein and energy. A diet inadequate in protein causes muscle catabolism which releases essential amino acids to provide substrates for synthesis of key enzymes and circulating proteins. By contrast the released nonessential amino acids are not efficiently reutilized for protein synthesis. In addition, when energy requirements are not satisfied, amino acids become gluconeogenic precursors. Utilization of the carbon skeleton of amino acids for glucose synthesis results in the excretion of their nitrogen, mainly as urea. Thus, inadequate intake of protein and energy is signaled by negative nitrogen balance. The goal of nutritional repletion is a positive nitrogen balance of at least 2 to 5 g per day. Positive nitrogen balance is a more specific indicator of effective nutritional therapy than an increase in body weight, which is markedly influenced by hydration status.

SELECTION OF PATIENTS FOR NUTRITIONAL SUPPORT

Treatment of specific nutrient deficiencies or dietary modification for nutrient intolerance depends on recognition of the deficiency or underlying disease process. For example, dietary management of celiac disease is straightforward once the diagnosis is established (see Chapter 12.6). Malnourished patients often manifest multiple vitamin deficiency syndromes simultaneously, and complete vitamin supplementation is appropriate in such patients. Deciding when to begin nutritional support for protein-energy malnutrition is often more difficult.

Evaluation of patients for nutritional support must include consideration of their preexisting nutritional status, the impact of the present illness on nutritional status and nutrient intake, and the nutritional side effects of planned medical or surgical therapy

TABLE 14.10–6. DATA BASE FOR NUTRITIONAL ASSESSMENT OF HOSPITALIZED PATIENTS

History

General	Age, life-style, socioeconomic status, alcoholism, drug dependency, recent illness or surgery, pregnancy, lactation, chronic disease, medications
Weight	Usual weight, weight changes, fit of clothing
Diet	Usual diet, last 24 hours diet, food preferences and aversions, dietary fads or myths, supplements Previous therapeutic diet
Food ingestion	General—appetite, nausea, chronic pain Oral cavity—taste, teeth, mucous membranes, chewing, swallowing Esophagus—dysphagia, painful swallowing Stomach—early satiety, pain, vomiting, postprandial symptoms Intestines—diarrhea, malabsorption, cramping, surgery

Examination

Habitus	Height, weight, percent ideal weight
Anthropometry	Wrist circumference (frame size), midarm muscle area, midarm fat area
Hydration	Skin turgor, edema
Skin	Pallor, pellagrous or flaky paint dermatosis, xerosis, follicular hyperkeratosis or hemorrhage, ecchymoses, hair (pigment, pluckability)
Eyes	Xerosis, keratomalacia, corneal vascularity, Bitot spots
Oral cavity	Dentition, mucous membranes, tongue color and texture, gums, cheilosis, angular stomatitis
Cardiovascular	Cardiomegaly, heart failure
Abdomen	Hepatomegaly, ascites
Neuromuscular	Alertness, orientation, memory, strength, spontaneous activity, reflexes, muscle wasting

Laboratory

Blood	Hemoglobin, hematocrit, red cell indices, lymphocyte count
Serum	Albumin, transferrin, prealbumin
Plasma	Prothrombin time
Other	Delayed hypersensitivity, 24-hr urinary creatinine excretion, creatinine/height ratio

(Table 14.10–2). It is better to identify patients at risk for developing hospital malnutrition and prevent its occurrence than to wait until advanced protein-energy malnutrition has developed. For example, in patients with extensive burns, nutritional support is usually begun promptly even in patients with good premorbid nutritional status.

Even mild intercurrent illness may necessitate nutritional support in malnourished patients to prevent nutritional decline and secondary complications. Well-nourished patients may tolerate a brief serious illness without nutritional support. If response to therapy and restoration of normal feeding are not prompt, however, well-nourished patients will also benefit from nutritional support. In general, hospitalized patients become malnourished because effective nutritional support modalities are not utilized.

When patients are unable to ingest a diet that satisfies nutrient requirements, nutrient intake must be augmented. Initial efforts may be directed towards increasing voluntary food intake. Patients with simple anorexia may benefit from counseling or frequent small feedings of high nutrient density. Previous food restrictions, such as salt or cholesterol, should be relaxed when possible. Chronic pain and depression suppress appetite and should be aggressively treated. No drugs are universally effective in stimulating appetite, although alcohol with meals is sometimes useful. Anabolic steroids are of no value if nutrient intake is inadequate.

Home-cooked meals can be enriched in nutrients by adding eggs or powdered milk, and most experienced dietitians can provide recipes to help outpatients with feeding problems. Many commercially available liquid meal replacements, flavored for oral feeding (Table 14.10–7), can occasionally improve a marginal diet into one that satisfies requirements. When attempts to augment voluntary intake fail, enteral (tube) feeding techniques or parenteral nutrition should be utilized. The choice between the two depends on the functional state of the gastrointestinal tract. The first principle of nutritional support is "if the gut works, use it." Parenteral nutrition is used only when nutritional requirements cannot be satisfied by enteral feeding.

ENTERAL NUTRITION

Anorexia or other causes of poor intake are major components in the development of protein-energy malnutrition in the setting of acute or chronic disease. Enteral nutrition can satisfy nutritional requirements in patients with sufficient intestinal function and has many advantages over the parenteral route.[1] Hormonal responses (insulin, intestinal hormones) to feeding are preserved; metabolic processes in the intestinal mucosa, such as transamination, are not bypassed; total costs are much lower; nutrient requirements are more firmly established; enteral formulas are generally more nutritionally complete (containing essential fatty acids and iron, for example); and enteral feeding is generally safe and better maintains the structure and function of the gut mucosa.

Appropriate patients for enteral nutritional support include many with burns, trauma, organ failure, CNS disorders, cancer, intestinal fistulas, or primary malnutrition. Contraindications include intractable vomiting, ileus, intestinal obstructions that cannot be bypassed, and proximal intestinal fistulas. Malabsorption and inflammatory bowel disease are not necessarily contraindications.

Recent improvements in nasoenteral tubes and formulas and the introduction of feeding pumps have greatly improved the acceptance and effectiveness of tube feeding.

FEEDING TUBES

Most patients require the placement of some type of tube. Nasal or oral enteric tubes can be inserted in a straightforward bedside procedure. There are few indications for oral-gastric tubes, which are uncomfortable and cause frequent gagging and poor oral hygiene. In addition, the tube can be chewed by a confused or disoriented patient. Small-bore tubes with weighted tips, passed transnasally using a removable stilet, are well tolerated for prolonged periods, even months. Some patients learn to pass the tubes themselves for nightly feeding at home. Tubes placed in the stomach allow the use of high-osmolality solutions and bolus feedings. Such placement is safe in alert patients with a good gag reflex. The drawbacks of a nasogastric tube are the risks of aspiration and tube dislodgement. Current technology now allows very flexible Silastic or polyethylene mercury-weighted tubes to be passed into a postpyloric position. This placement bypasses proximal obstructions or fistulas and reduces the risks of tube displacement and aspiration. Feeding formulas requiring little or no digestion are then used (see below). Because such formulas tend to be hyperosmolar, bolus feedings provoke cramping and osmotic diarrhea. Regulation of

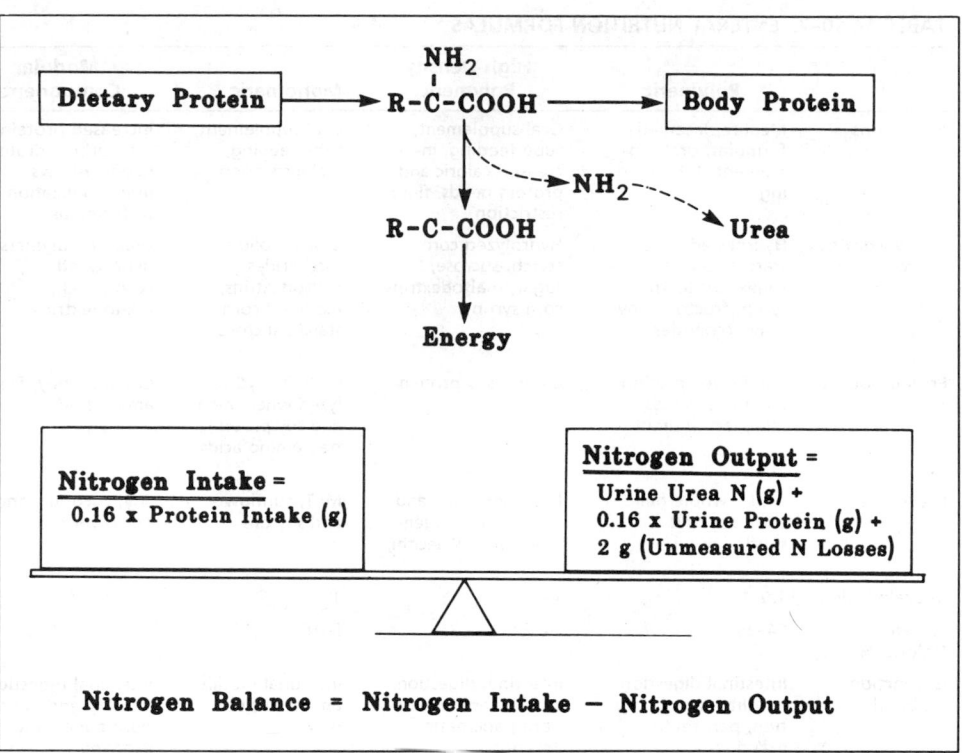

Figure 14.10–1. Nitrogen balance. When energy needs are unmet, amino acids (from dietary or body protein) are deaminated and the carbon skeleton used for energy production. When protein needs are unmet, body protein is catabolized to supply essential amino acids; nonessential amino acids are deaminated. Unutilized amino nitrogen is excreted largely as urea. Nitrogen intake can be calculated with good accuracy from measurements of the volume and composition of the administered solution [total daily nitrogen (g) = total daily amino acids (g) × 0.16]. Urea nitrogen and protein measurements in an accurate 24-hour urine collection provide a good estimate of urinary nitrogen excretion; a factor of 2 g per day is used to estimate nonurinary nitrogen losses in the usual TPN patients with normal or reduced stool volume and no other major protein losses.

the infusion rate with a simple pump and the use of longer infusion times produce the most satisfactory results.

Patients who need prolonged tube feeding should have an operative procedure to place a gastrostomy or jejunostomy tube. Usually these are large-bore tubes that allow the use of inexpensive blenderized foods administered by continuous pump. Occasionally, a needle-catheter jejunostomy is placed; because of its small caliber, only an elemental diet can be administered.

ENTERAL NUTRITION FORMULAS
(Table 14.10–7)

A bewildering array of formulas is available for oral and tube feedings; however, they can be divided conveniently into six groups, and most physicians will employ only products from the first three groups in Table 14.10–7, that is, polymeric, high-density polymeric, or monomeric formulas.

Polymeric diets are whole-protein, meal-replacement formulations. Their advantages, compared with amino acid or peptide (monomeric) formulas, are lower cost, reduced osmolarity, and increased palatability. These products can be given through small-bore feeding tubes but not through jejunostomy catheters. They can be used as an oral supplement. Obviously, an intact functioning gut is required for digestion and absorption.

High-density polymeric diets are identical with polymeric diets except that fat is used as a major energy source to increase caloric density to 1.2 to 2.0 kcal/ml. These formulas require essentially normal gut function and are indicated in patients with increased energy requirements or reduced fluid tolerance.

Monomeric (elemental) diets are popular but have limited indications. The protein source is amino acids or partially hydrolyzed peptides. Carbohydrate is supplied as partially hydrolyzed corn starch, maltose, sucrose, or glucose. Fat is given as medium-chain triglycerides (MCT) or, in some cases, as soy, safflower, or corn oil. The purpose of such formulations is to provide a nutritionally complete diet that requires little or no digestive function of the gut and is very low in residue. In theory, feeding an elemental formula would result in complete absorption by mid- to distal jejunum and require little intestinal function other than absorption. In addition, because of their low viscosity, they are the only formulas that can reasonably be administered through needle-catheter jejunostomies. Their use as oral supplements is limited by high cost, low fat content, and unpalatable taste. Their major indications are in patients with inflammatory bowel disease or distal bowel fistulae, where low-residue diets are of theoretic advantage. They are also used in patients whose digestive function is impaired by the short-gut syndrome or pancreatic exocrine insufficiency.

Modular component diets are combinations of the individual nutrient components of either monomeric or polymeric diets. Thus, the protein component is either hydrolyzed proteins or amino acids. Carbohydrate modules are either multidextrin, corn starch, or hydrolyzed corn starch (monomeric). Fat modules are either safflower oil or MCT. In theory, these components can be mixed to form a nutritionally complete diet with a ratio of protein to calories selected by the physician; however, the cost of doing so is prohibitive. Instead, a modular component is more often added to an already composed polymeric diet to alter its protein to calorie ratio. For example, a carbohydrate module is added to lower the protein to calorie ratio in patients with renal failure, or a protein module is added to increase the protein to calorie ratio in trauma patients.

Blenderized diets are the least expensive and simplest of all enteral feeding. They can be purchased or prepared at home. Their major drawbacks are the need for normal gastrointestinal function and a large-bore feeding tube (22 French or greater) to prevent clogging.

Special formulations are monomeric (elemental) formulations with altered amino acid composition. They have an increased content of either branched chain (valine, leucine, isoleucine) or essential amino acids. In theory, they reproduce special parenteral solutions (hepatamine, nephramine), and the only argument for their use is the somewhat controversial evidence supporting their parenteral cousins. There is no good evidence that they are superior to modular-supplemented diets, and their cost is the highest of all the enteral formulations.

TABLE 14.10–7. ENTERAL NUTRITION FORMULAS

	Polymeric	High-Density Polymeric	Monomeric	Modular Components	Blenderized Feedings	Disease-Specific Products
Indications	Meal replacement formulas, oral supplement, tube feeding	Oral supplement, tube feeding, increased caloric and/or protein needs, fluid restriction	Oral supplement, tube feeding, malabsorption	Increased protein, fat, carbohydrate needs. Allows individualization of formulas	Tube feeding May use table food[b]	Hepatic failure Renal failure Trauma
Carbohydrate source	Hydrolyzed corn starch, sucrose, maltodextrins, corn syrup, fructose, soy polysaccharides	Hydrolyzed corn starch, sucrose, sugar, maltodextrins, corn syrup	Glucose oligosaccharides, maltodextrins, modified corn starch, sucrose	Glucose polymers, hydrolyzed corn starch, maltodextrins	Hydrolyzed cereal solids, vegetable purees, nonfat milk, maltodextrins, fruit puree, juices	Maltodextrins, sucrose
Protein source	Casein, soy protein, egg white solids; milk; lactalbumin	Casein, soy protein	Partially hydrolyzed whey, meat and soy protein; free amino acids	Casein, whey, free amino acids	Beef puree, milk, casein	Free amino acids with increased branched chain, or essential amino acids
Fat source	MCT[a]; whole milk; corn, soy and sunflower oils	MCT; corn, soy and partially hydrogenated soy oils; lecithin	MCT, sunflower and soy oils	Soy, coconut, and safflower oils	Beef puree, corn oil, partially hydrogenated soy oil	Soy bean oil, lecithin, mono and diglycerides, sunflower oil
Kilocalories/ml	1.0–1.1	1–2	1		1[c]	1–2
Protein (calorie %)	14–26	14–22	8–18		14–16	4–11
GI function required	Intestinal digestion, motility and absorption; pancreatic exocrine	Intestinal digestion, motility and absorption; pancreatic exocrine	Intestinal motility and absorption only	Intestinal digestion, motility and absorption; pancreatic exocrine	Intestinal digestion and absorption; pancreatic exocrine; gastric mixing	Intestinal absorption and motility
Formulas available	Ensure, Enrich, Osmolite, Isocal, Meritene, Precision Isotonic, Sustacal, Travasorb, Travasorb MCT, Precision LR, Citrotein, Ross SLD, Fortison, Portagen	Ensure Plus, Ensure HN, Ensure Plus HN, Osmolite HN, Isocal HCN, Magnacal, Precision High Nitrogen, Sustacal HC, Isotein HN, Traumacal, Pulmocare, TwoCal HN, Travasorb HN, Fortical	Vital HN, Criticare HN, Vivonex, Vivonex TEN, Stresstein, Pepti-2000	*Carbohydrate:* Polycose, Moducal, Sumacal, Nutrisource Carbohydrate *Protein:* Propac, Promix, Casec, ProMod, Nutrisource Amino Acids, Nutrisource HBC amino acids, Nutrisource Protein *Fat:* MCT, Microlipid, Nutrisource Lipid; Long-chain triglycerides	Compleat,[d] Compleat Modified Formula, Vitaneed	Hepatic-Aid, Amin-Aid, Travasorb Renal, Travasorb Hepatic, Travin-aid HBC

[a]MCT = medium-chain triglycerides.
[b]Information provided is for commercially available formulas only; home preparation will vary.
[c]May be further concentrated. Available in powder form.
[d]Contains lactose.

ADMINISTRATION

After proper tip placement has been confirmed radiographically, tube feedings are administered either as intermittent bolus feedings or as a constant infusion. Patients with nasogastric or gastrostomy tubes generally tolerate bolus feedings (60 to 100 ml every 4 to 6 hours) unless their gastric outlet function is impaired. The volume is increased as tolerated until the intake satisfies nutrient requirements. If small volumes of hypertonic formulas produce symptoms, the formula may be diluted to isotonicity.

Most patients tolerate duodenal or jejunal infusions if isotonic formulas are initially administered slowly (30 to 50 ml per hour). Around-the-clock, continuous infusion, regulated if necessary by an enteral feeding pump, usually prevents the diarrhea, bloating, and cramping associated with large bolus feedings. As patient tolerance is demonstrated, the infusion rate is increased in increments of 20 to 50 ml per hour every 6 to 12 hours until the total intake is adequate. Many patients require additional fluid (25 to 50 percent of the daily volume of tube feeding).

As voluntary oral intake improves, tube feedings can be tapered by extending the interval between bolus feedings or eliminating the daytime infusion. In this way, the patient's appetite is stimulated and he or she is free to eat more normally. The nighttime infusion is continued until oral intake is adequate.

MONITORING

Patients should be closely monitored for signs of intolerance to enteral feeding and for their response to nutritional therapy, particularly in the early stages of the program. Gastric residuals are checked before each bolus feeding and after every 6 to 8 hours of continuous infusion. Complaints of cramping, distension, or pain should be evaluated. Diarrhea is not a normal or acceptable consequence of tube feeding. Rather, the cause should be identified and corrected. Persistent diarrhea should be treated pharmacologically, if necessary. Hydration status is especially vulnerable in patients with large fluid losses and those who cannot express thirst. Serum electrolytes and proteins are measured weekly in stable patients and more frequently in those who are acutely ill.

Effectiveness of nutritional support is evaluated by daily measures of weight and intake and output, and by periodic reassessment of anthropometric measurements and nitrogen balance.

COMPLICATIONS

Mechanical, metabolic, and psychologic problems can complicate tube feeding. The most frequent mechanical difficulty, tube clogging, can be avoided by routinely flushing the tube (especially be-

tween bolus feedings or after an interruption of the infusion). Soft, Silastic tubes help to prevent mucosal irritation while weighted tips reduce the risk of tube displacement when the patient coughs or sneezes. Polyurethane tubes afford more protection from tube dislodgement and are usually well-tolerated. The risk of aspiration is reduced by keeping the head of the bed elevated and by ensuring that the tube is placed correctly in the stomach or beyond the pylorus before instituting tube feeding.

The most common metabolic problem, diarrhea, is often preventable by slowing the feeding rate. Diarrhea may also result from intolerance to some component in the formula (e.g., lactose or long-chain fats). A change in the formula is usually effective treatment. Because bacterial contamination of the formula can also cause diarrhea, the formula should be refrigerated between bolus feedings, and only a volume sufficient for an infusion of 6 to 8 hours should be placed in the input container at any one time.

Some patients develop constipation from prolonged inactivity, the chronic use of minimal-residue formulas, or narcotics. Distension, nausea, and vomiting are uncommon unless the feeding administration rate is too rapid or the formula is excessively hypertonic. Fluid imbalances and electrolyte abnormalities must be detected and treated promptly.

Patients' initial lack of enthusiasm for tube feedings can usually be overcome when time is taken to relieve anxieties and answer questions. Proper care and hygiene of the nasal and oral cavities make the patient more comfortable. Finally, because a visible feeding tube can be embarrassing, gastrostomies or feeding enterostomies should be considered in patients requiring tube feedings for a prolonged period.

PARENTERAL NUTRITION

Total parenteral nutrition (TPN) provides total nutrition requirements by a nongastrointestinal route.[3] Intravenous feeding bypasses gastrointestinal digestive and absorptive functions by supplying all nutrients in a directly utilizable form (amino acids, monosaccharides, fat emulsions, and the like). TPN is not only able to supplement patients whose nutrient requirements exceed the functional capacity of their gastrointestinal tract, but also to sustain indefinitely patients with total gastrointestinal failure.

The risks of TPN are minimized by careful attention to patient-management protocols, and a favorable risk-benefit ratio can be achieved by appropriate selection of patients. Like other specialized support services, TPN produces its best results when physicians, nutritionists, pharmacists, and nurses collaborate closely as a team.

INDICATIONS

TPN is considered whenever gastrointestinal feeding cannot maintain an adequate nutritional status. The approach to the individual patient must involve a careful estimation of four interrelated issues: patient nutritional status, nutrient requirements, gastrointestinal function, and the duration of any abnormal states. Initially well-nourished patients will tolerate moderate periods of undernutrition, but TPN should be considered when interruption of enteral feeding is expected to exceed 10 days and nutritional requirements are increased by illness. In nutritionally depleted patients, a shorter interval of interrupted enteral feeding should prompt consideration of TPN.

PARENTERAL NUTRITION SOLUTIONS

Amino Acids
Commercially available amino acid solutions are formulated from synthetic L-amino acids in various concentrations to provide a mixture of essential and nonessential amino acids.[3] Among the commercial mixed amino acid solutions, the small differences in content of essential (39 to 53 percent of total amino acids), nonessential, and branched-chain (16 to 25 percent of total) amino acids probably have little clinical significance.

In acute renal failure, TPN utilizing restricted protein intake and high calorie-to-nitrogen ratios (750:1) improves nutritional status and lowers serum urea nitrogen by decreasing the catabolism of endogenous protein.[3] Despite theoretic advantages, there are limited indications for use of costly solutions of essential amino acids in patients with renal failure. Also rarely needed are the solutions with reduced aromatic amino acids and increased branched-chain amino acids marketed for patients requiring protein restriction for hepatic failure. Both solutions should be employed only in patients who cannot tolerate balanced amino acid solutions in suitably reduced amounts.

The use of nitrogen-free, alpha-keto analogues of essential amino acids in patients requiring nitrogen restriction because of renal or hepatic failure is discussed in Chapters 11.1 and 13.6. Such solutions are investigational and not available commercially.

Most TPN patients achieve satisfactory nitrogen balance on 0.75 to 1.5 g/kg per day (120 to 240 mg/kg/day as nitrogen) of mixed amino acids if also given 120 to 200 nonprotein calories per gram nitrogen. Amino acid requirements may exceed 2.5 g/kg per day, however, in severely stressed patients with protein losses or metabolic derangements interfering with normal protein economy.[3] To verify satisfactory nitrogen retention, a series of simple nitrogen balance studies should be performed on TPN patients (Fig. 14.10–1) once predicted requirements are reached. The amount (or occasionally the composition) of the TPN solution is adjusted until a positive nitrogen balance of 2 to 5 g per day is reached.

Energy
In the United States, commercial energy sources for TPN are limited to glucose (dextrose), xylitol, and fat emulsions. Xylitol, evaluated extensively in Europe, offers no convincing advantage over glucose.[7]

Nondiabetic adults can metabolize intravenous glucose at a rate of 0.3 to 0.5 g/kg per hour or higher. Provision of energy solely as glucose requires infusions that are extremely high in either volume or osmolarity. For example, more than 15 L of 5 percent dextrose would be needed to provide 3000 kcal per day; a 25 percent dextrose solution delivers 3000 kcal in about 3.5 L but has an osmolarity of 1400 mosm/L. In practice, when glucose is used as the nonprotein energy source in TPN, hypertonic solutions are infused through an indwelling catheter into a central vein with high blood flow.

Fat emulsions, on the other hand, are isotonic and can be safely administered by peripheral vein.[7] Commercial lipid solutions are triglyceride emulsions stabilized with egg phospholipids and made isotonic with glycerin. Fatty-acid source and composition differ somewhat, but the available products appear clinically equivalent. Fat emulsions prevent essential fatty acid deficiency and are an attractive energy source because of their high caloric density (1.1 to 2.0 kcal/ml).

Because nitrogen balance depends on an adequate supply of nonprotein calories, the nitrogen balance technique can be used to verify satisfactory energy intake once nitrogen requirements are satisfied. Because protein and energy requirements are so interrelated, it is common clinical practice to provide solutions of mixed amino acids and nonprotein energy (glucose with or without fat) in a calorie-to-nitrogen ratio of 120 to 200 kcal/g and adjust the daily volume of feeding until positive nitrogen balance is attained.

Electrolytes
Electrolyte requirements depend on such factors as nutritional status, protein-energy intake, renal and nonrenal losses, and preexisting deficiencies or excesses (Table 14.10–8).

During periods of undernutrition the release of intracellular ions (potassium, magnesium, phosphate) by catabolism of lean

TABLE 14.10–8. DAILY ELECTROLYTE REQUIREMENTS DURING TPN IN ADULTS

Electrolyte	Daily Requirement (Range)[a]	Provided as
Sodium	60–120 mEq	Sodium chloride or acetate
Chloride	60–120 mEq	Sodium or potassium chloride
Potassium	75–150 mEq	Potassium chloride, acetate, or phosphate
Magnesium	15–30 mEq	Magnesium sulfate
Phosphate	10–40 mmole	Potassium phosphate, sodium hypophosphate
Calcium	8–24 mEq	Calcium gluconate
Acetate	0–60 mEq	Sodium or potassium acetate

[a]Electrolyte losses in intestinal fluids, chest tube drainage, etc., must be replaced; electrolyte requirements can vary markedly in patients with renal, hepatic, or cardiac disease.

TABLE 14.10–9. RECOMMENDED DAILY INTRAVENOUS ADMINISTRATION OF VITAMINS AND TRACE MINERALS IN ADULTS[a]

Vitamins[b]	Recommended
A	3300 IU
D	200 IU
E	10 IU
Ascorbic acid	100 mg
Folacin	400 μg
Niacin	40 mg
Riboflavin	3.6 mg
Thiamin	3.0 mg
B_6 (pyridoxine)	4.0 mg
B_{12} (cyanocobalamin)	5.0 μg
Pantothenic acid	15 mg
Biotin	60 μg

Trace Minerals[b]	Recommended
Zinc	2.5–4.0 mg[c]
Copper	0.5–1.5 mg
Chromium	10.0–15.0 mg
Manganese	0.15–0.8 mg
Selenium	20–40 μg

[a]Nutrition Advisory Group, American Medical Association.
[b]Iron and vitamin K are given by intramuscular injection.
[c]Additional zinc should be given to patients with either acute catabolic illnesses or excessive intestinal losses.

body mass supplies a large part of the daily requirements for these electrolytes, and their serum concentrations remain relatively normal. In contrast, by inhibiting catabolism and promoting anabolism, TPN markedly increases the requirements for exogenous potassium, magnesium, and phosphate. Deficiencies of intracellular ions are dangerous in themselves and also may limit nitrogen retention even when protein and energy needs are met.

The major extracellular ions (sodium, chloride, bicarbonate, and calcium) are less affected by nutritional status than by renal function and regulatory hormones (cortisol, renin, and so on). Serum measurements are more useful to monitor requirements for bicarbonate and calcium than for sodium and chloride. Sodium and chloride excesses are much more common than deficiencies, while the opposite is true for bicarbonate. The serum calcium level is influenced by serum albumin and phosphate concentrations and by vitamin D administration; intravenous requirements for calcium are not well established. In some cases, electrolyte balance studies can establish requirements more accurately. The 24-hour urinary excretion of the important electrolytes, quantitated in the same urine collected for nitrogen measurements, is compared to the 24-hour intravenous intake. Positive nitrogen balance is always accompanied by positive balance of the major intracellular ions. Zero balance of the major extracellular ions argues against unsatisfied needs. Poor renal conservation of potassium and magnesium sometimes explains apparently excessive requirements to maintain normal serum concentrations.

Vitamins and Trace Minerals

Vitamin requirements by the intravenous route, especially in disease states in which TPN is used, are not well established. Published RDAs for vitamins pertain specifically to oral intake and take into account such factors as intestinal absorption and metabolism. Moreover, serum or urinary measurements are poor guides to body vitamin stores and thus of little therapeutic help. Finally, deficiencies, especially of water-soluble vitamins, can develop rapidly during the repletion phase of TPN and may be difficult to detect in already seriously ill patients.

Supplemental zinc, copper, chromium, and manganese are recommended during TPN.[7] The trace element selenium is probably necessary for health, and minimal requirements have recently been established. It is unnecessary to replace selenium, however, unless patients are receiving long-term TPN. Patients able to take any food by mouth or receiving periodic transfusions of blood products rarely develop clinical signs of deficiency of trace elements other than zinc. Current guidelines to vitamin and trace mineral requirements during TPN are shown in Table 14.10–9.

SOLUTION ADMINISTRATION

The proper route for administration of a TPN solution depends largely on its final osmolarity. Prolonged infusion of hyperosmolar solutions (>650 mOsm/L in adults) by peripheral veins produces chemical thrombophlebitis. In contrast, administration into a central vein allows chronic infusion of even very hyperosmolar solutions.

Because of its potential dangers, central venous catheterization should only be performed by skilled and experienced personnel using strict aseptic technique after appropriate patient education and correction of intravascular volume deficits and hemostatic defects. Correct catheter tip placement must be verified radiographically, and the TPN catheter should never be used for any purpose other than TPN.

Peripheral veins can be used for TPN if the osmolarity of the solution is not excessive. Thus, fat emulsions are usually a major calorie source in peripheral vein solutions in order to minimize daily fluid volume.

Patient Monitoring

Routine physical measurements and laboratory studies in the uncomplicated patient on TPN are outlined in Table 14.10–10. In patients with severe acute illness, renal failure, or hepatic or cardiac disease, such measurements are repeated more often. In general, TPN solutions should not be ordered more than 24 hours in advance in such patients because frequent adjustments in electrolyte composition may be necessary.

Complications

Mechanical injuries associated with central venous catheters are minimized when catheter placement is performed only as an elective procedure by experienced personnel. The most common technical complications are pneumothorax, hemothorax, subclavian ar-

TABLE 14.10–10. GUIDELINES FOR MONITORING TPN PATIENTS

Procedure or Test	Frequency	
	Initial	After Stabilization
Body weight	Daily	Daily
Intake and output	Daily	Daily
Serum:		
• Electrolytes (Na, K, Cl, HCO₃)	Daily	1–3 times weekly
• Albumin, total protein, transferrin	Weekly	Weekly
• Glucose, creatinine, SUN	Daily	1–3 times weekly
• Ca, PO₄, Mg	3 times weekly	Weekly
• Hepatic enzymes, bilirubin	Weekly	Weekly
• CBC, prothrombin time	Weekly	Weekly
• Cholesterol, triglycerides	Weekly	Weekly[a]
Urine:		
• Sugar and acetone	Each void	Daily
• 24-hr collection for urea N, protein	Daily	Weekly
• Na, K, Cl, Mg, PO₄	[b]	[b]

[a]Patients receiving fat emulsions.
[b]When needed to determine requirements.

TABLE 14.10–11. REPRESENTATIVE TPN SOLUTIONS FOR CENTRAL VEIN AND PERIPHERAL VEIN ADMINISTRATION

TPN Solution	Central Vein	Peripheral Vein
Composition		
• Carbohydrate:		
50% dextrose	500 ml	—
10% dextrose	—	500 ml
• Lipid:		
20% fat emulsion	—	500 ml
• Amino acids:		
8.5% amino acid	500 ml	500 ml
• Electrolytes (mEq/L):		
Na^+	20	20
K^+	80	40
Cl^-	30	26
Mg^{++}	16	8
Ca^{++}	14	10
HPO_4^-	20	10
Acetate	110	77
• Vitamins, trace minerals: See Table 14.10–9		
Nutrient analysis		
• Carbohydrate	250 g (850 kcal)	79 g[a] (269 kcal)
• Lipid	—	100 g (900 kcal)
• Amino acids	42.5 g	42.5 g
• Total nonprotein energy	850 kcal	1169 kcal
• Nonprotein calorie-to-nitrogen ratio (kcal/g)	130:1	178:1
Final osmolarity	1893 mosm/L	637 mosm/L
Total volume[b]	1000 ml	1500 ml

[a]Includes 29 g glycerin from fat emulsion.
[b]Excluding 50–100 ml additional volume for addition of electrolytes, vitamins, and trace minerals.

tery puncture, great-vein thrombosis (often due to incorrect position of the catheter tip), brachial plexus injury, and air embolism.[9] Complications of long-term venous catheterization are sepsis and vessel thrombosis. Sepsis, which occurs in 5 to 10 percent of these patients, requires removal of the catheter and appropriate antibiotic treatment. To reduce the risk of catheter-related sepsis, scrupulous sterile technique should be used while changing solutions, and the catheter site should be cleaned on a daily basis by experienced nurses. To prevent contamination of the line, the catheter should not be used to draw blood or to administer other fluids or blood products. Solution contamination can be entirely eliminated by preparing TPN solutions only in the pharmacy and by prohibiting any subsequent additions to the container.

Metabolic complications of TPN, although more common in patients with metabolic derangements, are usually iatrogenic. They can be minimized by careful baseline assessment and conscientious monitoring. The most common deficiencies are potassium, magnesium, phosphate, bicarbonate, and essential fatty acids. Declining serum concentrations of these electrolytes signal deficiencies before clinical signs and symptoms develop; electrolyte concentrations in the TPN solution should be increased until serum concentrations are normal. Because of solubility problems, bicarbonate is given as its precursor, acetate. Essential fatty acid deficiency usually occurs only when patients receive fat-free solutions exclusively for weeks or months. Because glucose infusions stimulate insulin secretion and thus prevent mobilization of body fat (which contains 12 percent linoleic acid), deficiency can develop despite abundant adipose tissue.

The most common excesses are fluid, sodium, chloride, and glucose. Hyponatremia is almost never symptomatic and invariably results from water excess rather than sodium deficiency. Glucose intolerance is common in stressed patients, but its sudden appearance in a febrile TPN patient suggests sepsis. Diabetics can be managed on TPN by substituting a fat emulsion for some of the glucose or by adding exogenous insulin to the TPN solution so that any interruption will halt the glucose and insulin infusions simultaneously. In nondiabetic patients interruption of the TPN solution can occasionally cause hypoglycemia; thus whenever a TPN infusion is interrupted, a 10 percent dextrose infusion is given until TPN is resumed. Other metabolic complications include acid-base disturbances and deficiencies or excesses of vitamins and trace elements.

Hepatic function abnormalities can vary from transient increases in liver enzymes to severe fatty infiltration of the liver with marked elevations of alkaline phosphatase and bilirubin levels. Fatty liver can be caused by essential fatty acid deficiency or excessive administration of fat (typically heralded by hypertriglyceridemia) or glucose (>7mg/kg/min). Patients who receive TPN for 6 weeks or more may develop TPN-induced gallstones.

Representative TPN Solutions

Table 14.10–11 shows some representative TPN solutions for central and peripheral vein infusion. Appropriate modifications of the electrolyte and protein content are made for patients with renal, cardiac, or hepatic disease.

REFERENCES

1. Freeman JB, Fairfull-Smith RJ: Current concepts of enteral feeding. Adv Surg 16:75, 1983
2. Frisancho AR: New norms of upper limb fat and muscle areas for assessment of nutritional status. Am J Clin Nutr 34:2540, 1981
3. Grant JP: Handbook of total parenteral nutrition. Philadelphia, WB Saunders, 1980
4. Grant JP, Custer RR, Thurlow J: Current technique of nutritional assessment. Surg Clin North Am 61(3):437, 1981
5. Gray GE, Gray LK: Anthropometric measurements and their interpretation: Principles, practices and problems. J Am Dietet Assoc 77:534, 1980
6. Mertz W: The essential trace elements. Science 213:1332, 1981
7. Phillips GD, Odgers CL: Parenteral nutrition: Current status and concepts. Drugs 23:276, 1982
8. Recommended Dietary Allowances, National Research Council. Washington, DC, National Academy of Sciences, 1980
9. Sitzmann JV, Townsend TR, et al: Septic and technical complications of central venous catheterization. Ann Surg 202:766, 1985
10. Yetiv JR: Popular Nutritional Practices: A Scientific Appraisal. Toledo, Ohio, Popular Medicine Press, 1986

Obesity is a common medical and public health problem in the United States, health implications of which surpass undernutrition in importance. A recent national survey showed the presence of obesity sufficient to increase mortality risk in more than 34 million Americans.[1] Morbidity, both physical and emotional, impairs performance in countless others. Although clearly defined metabolic abnormalities play an etiologic role in some patients, little progress has been made in detecting metabolic aberrations that cause obesity in the great majority. In many, psychologic factors appear to be paramount; for them overeating may represent a form of substance abuse. Effective therapy must combine metabolic, nutritional, psychologic, and sometimes surgical approaches. Few individual physicians are adequately trained in all of these disciplines. This accounts in part for the poor results of treatment in the usual office setting.

ASSESSMENT OF EXTENT OF OBESITY

Obesity is defined simply as an excess of body fat, but the actual quantification of adipose tissue mass is difficult. In the research laboratory adipose tissue mass is estimated from body density measurements or by isotope dilution techniques. These methods are cumbersome, and consequently height-weight tables are most commonly used clinically to quantify obesity (Table 14.11–1). The degree of obesity is frequently expressed as *relative weight,* the percentage of actual to ideal weight. In fact, this index does not reflect obesity specifically, but rather *overweight,* which can result from an excessive mass of muscle, bone, fluid, or fat. Various ratios of weight to height are also employed to quantify obesity. Best correlated with the actual amount of body fat is the body mass index, where

$$\text{Body mass index} = \frac{\text{Weight (kg)}}{\text{Height}^2 \ (\text{m}^2)}$$

A man of ideal body weight (Table 14.11–1) will have a body mass index of approximately 22.9, a woman 22.6. The body mass index can be used to calculate a patient's relative weight; for men

$$\text{Relative weight} = \frac{\text{Body mass index} \times 100}{22.9}$$

Ideal body weight can also be calculated:

$$\text{Ideal body weight} = \text{Height}^2 \times 22.9$$

(For women the constant 22.6 is substituted for 22.9 in calculating relative and ideal body weights.) These equations conveniently eliminate the need for a height-weight table. Individuals are considered obese when relative weight is more than 120 percent of ideal, corresponding to a body mass index of 27.5 for men and 27.1 for women. Weights above this benchmark are associated with increased mortality.[10] Another practical method for estimating body fat is skin-fold thickness, particularly in the subscapular and triceps areas. Obesity is present when the sum of subscapular and triceps skin-fold thicknesses exceeds 38 mm in men and 52 mm in women. This corresponds to the upper 15 percent of values in the general population aged 20 to 29 years.

CLASSIFICATION

There is no uniform method for classifying obesity, but several categorical distinctions may be useful in predicting both the results of therapy and the presence of increased mortality risk. In this context obesity can be *hypertrophic* or *hyperplastic* depending on whether fat cells are increased in size or number. Adult-onset obesity tends to be hypertrophic, central in distribution, and more easily controlled than hyperplastic obesity but is frequently associated with factors that increase cardiovascular risk. Hyperplastic obesity is characteristically early in onset and both central and peripheral in distribution. It is associated with a poor prognosis for long-term control, but cardiovascular risk factors are less frequently present. When weight gain in adult years is massive, some degree of fat-cell hyperplasia accompanies hypertrophy. Individuals may also be classified by the severity of their weight problem, that is, as having mild-moderate, severe, or morbid obesity when body weight exceeds ideal by 20 to 40, 40 to 100, or more than 100 percent, respectively. For therapeutic purposes it is convenient to divide obesity into primary (idiopathic) and secondary obesity resulting from a known medical disorder. In the latter instance treatment must obviously be directed toward the underlying disorder.

TABLE 14.11–1. IDEAL BODY WEIGHT ACCORDING TO SEX AND HEIGHT[a]

Height (inches)	Men		Women	
	Ideal Weight (lb)	Acceptable Range	Ideal Weight (lb)	Acceptable Range
57			112	99–128
58			114	100–131
59			117	101–134
60			119	103–137
61	131	123–145	122	105–140
62	133	125–148	125	108–143
63	135	127–151	128	111–148
64	137	129–155	131	114–152
65	140	131–159	134	117–156
66	143	133–163	137	120–160
67	146	135–167	140	123–164
68	149	137–171	143	126–167
69	152	139–175	146	129–170
70	155	141–179	149	132–173
71	159	144–183	152	135–176
72	162	147–187		
73	166	150–192		
74	169	153–197		
75	174	157–202		

[a]Weights at ages 25–59 based on lowest mortality. Weights are without clothes, and heights are without shoes.
Adapted from Metropolitan Life Insurance Company, 1983. (Source of basic data 1979 Build Study of Actuaries and Association of Life Insurance Medical Directors of America, 1980.)

Rare patients have lipodystrophy with very unusual patterns of fat distribution.

EPIDEMIOLOGY

Obesity correlates importantly with such epidemiologic variables as age, sex, race, and economic status.[10] Among whites, the percentage of men with obesity increases with age to a peak of 30 percent at about 50 years, then declines. Obesity in women continues to increase through age 70 years to a peak of 36 percent. Consequently, obesity is more common in men before age 45 and in women after age 55. The same relationships between age, sex, and obesity apply for blacks; however, black women of all ages are more often overweight than are black men or white women of comparable age. Affluence also affects weight, but principally among women. Those living above the poverty line are substantially thinner than those below. For men the reverse is true, although weight differences between affluent and poor men are small. Race and affluence affect weight independently. National origin affects weight. Americans of Eastern European descent are heavier than those of Western European origin. Nine percent of American women of British descent are obese compared to 27 percent of Italian origin. Obesity declines with increasing number of generations a family has lived in the United States. While genetic factors undoubtedly exert a powerful influence on weight (see below), these epidemiologic correlations confirm an important role for environmental factors as well. Morbid obesity may be a separate category that does not correlate with these epidemiologic variables.

ADIPOSE TISSUE IN OBESITY

Among young adults of average weight who do not participate regularly in vigorous physical activity, adipose tissue constitutes approximately 15 percent of total body weight in males and 25 percent in females. More than 90 percent of body energy is stored in 10 to 20 kg of adipose tissue triglycerides. Most adults gradually gain weight because of an increase in adipose tissue. Moreover, because lean body mass decreases with age, there is a concomitant increase in body fat even in those adults who are weight-stable.

Two factors finally determining adipose tissue mass are the number and size of fat cells. Early in life adipose tissue grows by an increase in both the size and number of adipocytes. Obesity developing during this time is associated with an increased number (hyperplasia) of fat cells. After adolescence, accretion of fat cell mass initially is due to an increase in size (hypertrophy) of existing fat cells. When the upper limit of fat-cell size is reached, adipocyte proliferation is triggered. In adults, therefore, obesity may be almost exclusively hypertrophic when mild and both hypertrophic and hyperplastic when severe. Because fat cells have a long lifespan, adipose tissue hyperplasia persists indefinitely and weight loss occurs only from a reduction in fat-cell size. This type of obesity is relatively more refractory to dietary control. In hypertrophic obesity, alterations in the metabolism of adipocytes seem to correlate with their size and the associated relationships of membrane surface-to-cell volume. Abdominal fat cells readily become hypertrophic; thus, such metabolic abnormalities as glucose intolerance and hypertriglyceridemia tend to be associated with hypertrophic, centrally distributed obesity. Hypertension is also associated with this type of obesity.[1] Hence, mortality risk is increased in such patients.

REGULATION OF ENERGY BALANCE

Most normal adults maintain a relatively constant weight because caloric intake closely approximates energy requirements. When caloric ingestion exceeds expenditure, energy is stored as triglycerides in adipose tissue. In both animals and nonobese adult men, weight changes during experimental forced feeding or starvation are rapidly reversed when access to food is normalized. These observations imply a capacity to regulate caloric intake, energy expenditure, or both to maintain relative constancy of adipose tissue mass. An elevated "set-point" for adipose tissue mass in obese patients has been postulated but not established and is in fact inconsistent with the wide fluctuations in body weight characterizing the obese.

CALORIC INTAKE

Food intake is influenced by internal or physiologic mechanisms and by learned or cognitive responses to external environmental stimuli. Physiologic mechanisms, although poorly understood, are both central and peripheral. One important component of central regulation resides in the hypothalamus. The ventromedial hypothalamus is often referred to as the "satiety center" because its destruction produces hyperphagia and obesity in experimental animals. The hyperphagia may result from increased secretion of insulin, mediated by signals from the vagus and sympathetic nerves, because destruction of the ventromedial hypothalamus is rapidly followed by enlargement of the islets of Langerhans and hyperinsulinemia. Application of alpha-adrenergic agents to the ventromedial hypothalamus also stimulates food intake. In contrast, lesions of, or injection of beta-adrenergic drugs into, the lateral hypothalamus ("feeding center") cause decreased food intake, and electrical stimulation of this area increases food intake. While these hypothalamic nuclei are important in the neural control of appetite and weight, they are actually part of a much more extensive system involving the limbic system and cortex. It is, therefore, an unwarranted oversimplification to attribute the central regulation of feeding and satiety to the hypothalamus alone.

Peripheral factors also regulate food intake. Gastric distention may delay the initiation or terminate the intake of food. Opposite effects are observed when the stomach is empty. Various nutrients are delivered from the stomach into the duodenum at the rate of 1.2 kcal per minute until the concentration of nutrients becomes very dense, at which point the control of caloric release breaks down and excess calories leave the stomach. Plasma concentrations of glucose or amino acids may be stimuli for the cessation of food intake while circulating levels of fatty acids, glycerol, or ketone bodies may affect appetite by serving as signals for the amount of calories stored in adipose tissue. Appetite suppression by high plasma concentrations of ketone bodies in some patients is particularly noteworthy. Insulin tends to increase appetite; glucagon and cholecystokinin appear to suppress food intake.

Cognitive factors affecting eating include the taste, odor, and appearance of specific foods, perceptions of their nutritive and caloric content, time of day, and feeling states surrounding the eating process. These influences may override internal physiologic drives of hunger and satiety. The principal consequence of overeating, the development of obesity, also modifies eating behavior in a fashion specific for humans because of the associated social and health implications. Many of the cognitive factors that influence food intake and hence weight are uniquely human. Thus, the extrapolation to humans of data from studies of eating behavior and weight patterns in animals, and in particular animal models of obesity, is hazardous.

ENERGY EXPENDITURE

Energy is used for basal metabolism, nutrient digestion and absorption, physical activity, and heat production. Energy used under basal conditions fuels such processes as membrane transport, protein synthesis, and cardiac and respiratory muscle contraction. Basal metabolism, measured under carefully controlled conditions of rest and environmental temperature, is dependent on size (surface area), age, and gender. Basal metabolic rate decreases with age and is lower in women than men. This is explained largely by dif-

ferences in body composition, because muscle is metabolically more active than adipose tissue. Relative to fat, muscle mass is greater in men and diminishes with age. Thyroid hormone also accelerates basal metabolic rate. Basal metabolism decreases with caloric restriction to an extent greater than can be accounted for by the loss of tissue mass, contributing to the slowing of weight loss in patients on a hypocaloric diet. Nutrient digestion and absorption is associated with an increase in heat production (and caloric utilization) of about 10 percent of ingested calories for a meal of mixed nutrient composition. Sixty to 75 percent of calories utilized daily cover basal needs, 10 percent the thermic effect of food, and virtually all of the rest are used for physical activity in the average person. This latter component is the only one potentially under conscious control. Obese individuals require more energy in performing a given task than do lean subjects because of their increased weight. In certain small mammals heat produced by mitochondria-rich brown adipose tissue is important in maintaining body temperature in a cold environment and in mediating the increase in thermogenesis associated with overfeeding ("adaptive thermogenesis"). The role of "adaptive thermogenesis" in energy balance in humans is debated.

ETIOLOGY AND PATHOPHYSIOLOGY

Genetic and psychosocial factors, along with increasing age, appear to be most important in producing obesity. As with many other disorders, the greatest effect occurs when environmental factors are added to a physiologic predisposition. Further, the relative contribution of these etiologic factors may vary significantly with the type of obesity. Although rigorous evidence is lacking, age and psychosocial factors probably play the greatest role in mild to moderate obesity, whereas inheritance probably makes the greater contribution in severe and morbid obesity.

Both animal and human studies have demonstrated genetic contributions to obesity. Genetic factors are of prime importance in a few rare disorders. In the Bardet-Biedl syndrome obesity accompanies mental retardation, retinitis pigmentosa, and polydactyly. Patients with the Prader-Willi syndrome, who often possess an abnormality of chromosome 15, exhibit mental retardation, short stature, hypotonia, and hypogonadism as well as lifelong hyperphagia and obesity. Studies of twins and adopted children[9] document the primacy of inheritance in more common forms of obesity. In addition to inheritance, such epidemiologic observations as the influence of socioeconomic class on weight confirm an important role for environmental influences. In this context animal studies show that obesity can be induced simply by enhancing the palatability of the diet.

The etiology of primary obesity remains obscure. Excessive caloric intake is certainly a major factor in most patients. Unsuccessful attempts have been made to identify abnormalities in the set-points for an appetite-controlling chemical, a physical sensor for glucose or other circulating metabolites, heat production, or mass of adipose tissue. Increasing attention has been directed to the possibility that obese individuals gain weight because they are more efficient in their use of ingested calories.[7] Animal experiments raise the as yet unproved possibility that obesity may result from decreased heat production by brown fat or through reduced activity of futile enzyme cycles that waste energy as heat. A decrease in physical activity has been demonstrated in obese adults.

Physicians occasionally play a role in producing obesity through the type of diet, activity, or medication they prescribe. The smallest contribution to obesity is probably from underlying medical diseases (see below), but it is important to recognize and treat secondary obesity with appropriate specific measures.

Although the possible etiologic role of hormonal or metabolic abnormalities remains unclear, obesity regularly provokes several hormonal and metabolic alterations that are generally reversible with return to normal weight.[8] These include increased glucocorticoid production, hyperinsulinism, and diminished release of growth hormone in response to stimuli. Glucagon levels are unaffected. In obesity, basal insulin levels and the insulin response to glucose or amino acid loads are markedly increased. The presence of normal glucose tolerance despite elevated insulin levels, as well as other more direct evidence, indicate that liver, muscle, and adipose tissue are at least partially resistant to the actions of insulin in obese patients. The reduced number of insulin receptors on the surface of large fat cells in obesity accounts in part for insulin resistance.[6] In addition, the relative proportions of dietary fat and carbohydrate can alter insulin sensitivity. Consequently, diabetes may develop in obese patients who are genetically predisposed. Normalization of adipocyte size and insulin receptor number results in improved glucose tolerance when obese diabetics lose weight.

PSYCHOLOGY AND BEHAVIOR OF OBESE INDIVIDUALS

No simple psychologic explanations for obesity have proved valid. Numerous studies of large general populations have failed to reveal consistent differences between obese and nonobese individuals in the presence of significant psychiatric disturbances.[11] On the Minnesota Multiphasic Personality Inventory obese individuals show minor elevations in the depression scale but are not different from control patients presenting to a large general medical clinic for treatment of a broad range of other medical and surgical conditions. Disparagement of body image is, however, a characteristic of the obese, particularly in juvenile-onset obesity. While significant psychopathology, as measured by currently used objective tests and interview techniques, is not present in obese individuals as a group, many suffer from severe anxiety and depression.

There is some evidence that obese people are hyperresponsive to external cues and relatively unresponsive to internal physiologic signals (hunger and satiety). Although this hypothesis has been challenged in recent years, the sight of extremely tempting foods is clearly the most powerful external stimulus for eating, and once eating is "turned on," the obese patient does not simply eat, but overeats. Dysphorias (anxiety and depression) are potent eating stimuli for the obese, particularly after periods of dieting. Dieting itself often induces anxiety or depression in obese individuals. A vicious cycle can result; dietary deprivation produces anxiety or depression and leads the patient to overeat for relief. The resultant weight gain then evokes additional emotional distress and more overeating.

Several specific eating syndromes have been described in the obese. In the "night-eating syndrome," evening hyperphagia and nocturnal insomnia are followed by morning anorexia. This occurs in about 10 percent of obese patients, especially women, when experiencing continuing stress. The "binge-eating syndrome" is characterized by a subjective sense of compulsion to eat large amounts of food, usually in the setting of an identified stressful precipitant. In one study of patients more than 30 percent above ideal weight, 22 percent reported binging at least once a week. The similarities between this pattern of eating and the abuse of other addictants (e.g., alcohol) are compelling: emotion-initiated ingestion followed by loss of control, physically destructive binging, and ultimately extreme remorse and self-hatred. Frustratingly, the sequence may be initiated by attempts to treat the addiction.

Weight loss after ileal bypass surgery or gastroplasty is usually accompanied by an improved psychologic state, including improved mood, increased self-esteem, and decreased food intake. Thus, the dysphorias that often accompany dieting relate more to the sense of deprivation than to weight loss itself.

OBESITY SECONDARY TO MEDICAL ILLNESS

Central Nervous System Disease
Obesity associated with central nervous system disease is generally due to destructive lesions in the ventromedial nucleus of the hypothalamus. Both hyperphagia and reduced activity may play a role in hypothalamic obesity. Solid tumors, particularly craniopharyn-

giomas, are the most common lesion. Inflammatory diseases or trauma may also produce hypothalamic obesity. Obesity may occasionally result from increased intraventricular pressure.

Endocrine Disorders

Although many patients ask physicians whether their obesity is due to an endocrine problem, relatively few people develop obesity on this basis. In hypothyroidism, added adipose tissue and myxedema fluid may contribute to weight gain, but few hypothyroid patients are truly obese. Obesity occurs commonly in Cushing syndrome; central distribution of fat in these patients is typical. Significant obesity results only occasionally from the hyperphagia caused by high insulin levels in patients with an insulinoma. Women with the polycystic ovary syndrome and eunuchoid males tend to be obese.

IATROGENIC OBESITY

Obesity may result from prescribed medical treatments. Neuroleptic agents, such as phenothiazines and butyrophenones (haloperidol) used to treat schizophrenia and other disorders, are often associated with weight gain. Tricyclic antidepressants not only improve the anorexia accompanying depression but may in addition promote excessive weight gain. Corticosteroids in high doses may produce Cushing syndrome with severe obesity. Women using birth control pills may gain weight for a variety of reasons, including increased appetite and fluid retention. Cyproheptadine, a serotonin and histamine antagonist, promotes weight gain but to a lesser degree than the corticosteroids or neuroleptics.

Prescribed diets may lead to obesity when the total calories exceed the patient's nutritional requirements. Some physicians still prescribe frequent small feedings of bland foods, especially dairy products, for peptic ulcer disease, and obesity may result. Frequent small meals are often recommended for gastroesophageal reflux, especially for hiatal hernia, and also for reactive hypoglycemia, not infrequently diagnosed to explain nonspecific symptoms in young women without adequate documentation by glucose tolerance testing.

OTHER MEDICAL DISORDERS ASSOCIATED WITH OBESITY

Adiposis dolorosa (Dercum disease) is a disorder of painful irregular masses of subcutaneous fat, peripheral neuropathy, endocrine adenomas, and sometimes generalized obesity. In addition, several lipodystrophies are characterized by abnormal regional lipid deposits, for example in the legs, with deficiency of fat of the trunk, arms, and face.

CONSEQUENCES

Although serious limitations are recognized in the retrospective and unrepresentative nature of the data, life insurance statistics show an association between obesity and early mortality. Increased mortality is evident in subjects 20 percent or more above ideal body weight (Table 14.11–1), or when body mass index exceeds 27.1 and 27.5 in women and men, respectively. Coronary and cerebrovascular disease are responsible for most of the excess mortality. The increase in vascular disease can be attributed in large measure to the adverse effects of obesity on blood pressure, blood glucose, and serum lipids (increased total cholesterol, decreased HDL cholesterol, and increased triglycerides). Weight reduction can improve these risk factors. Obesity also exerts an adverse effect on overall cardiovascular mortality independent of these risk factors.[4] Mortality rates for diabetes, cholecystitis, and some forms of cancer (uterus, ovary, gallbladder, and breast in women, and colon and prostate in men) are increased in obese individuals. As indicated in Table 14.11–2, a number of other diseases occur with

increased frequency in obese patients. Moreover, obesity complicates the management of and diminishes the likelihood of recovery from many illnesses. In general, mortality rates, as well as the frequency and severity of medical complications, are proportional to the degree of obesity.

Extreme adiposity in the thoracic and abdominal regions can impair the mechanics of ventilation enough to cause cardiorespiratory failure. This *Pickwickian syndrome* is characterized by alveolar hypoventilation. Clinical features include hypoxia, hypercarbia, somnolence, periodic breathing, cyanosis, secondary polycythemia, right ventricular hypertrophy, and cor pulmonale. Prompt recognition of this syndrome is imperative because sudden respiratory arrest can occur in the presence of an apparently stable clinical condition. *Sleep-apnea syndrome* is also associated with obesity. Periods of apnea during sleep are associated with hypoxia and potentially fatal cardiac arrhythmias. Daytime hypoxia and hypersomnolence also occur. This syndrome is most often due to airway obstruction in the region of the hypopharynx (obstructive sleep apnea), though hyporesponsiveness of the medullary respiratory center is the cause in some (central sleep apnea). Weight reduction is effective for both the Pickwickian and sleep-apnea syndromes. Oxygen and respiratory stimulants, such as progestational agents,

TABLE 14.11–2. INITIAL EVALUATION OF THE OBESE PATIENT

Onset and Progression	Etiology	Complications
History		
Age of onset	Symptoms of	Symptoms of
Weight at milestones	• Hypothyroidism	• Diabetes
• High school graduation	• Hypogonadism	• Hypertension
• College graduation	• Polycystic ovary	• Congestive heart failure
• Marriage	• Hypoglycemia	• Pickwickian syndrome
• Discharge from service	• Intracranial mass	• Sleep apnea
• Pregnancy	Psychiatric problems	• Degenerative joint disease
• Menopause	• Depression	• Gout
Weight-reduction efforts	• Anxiety	• Gallstones
	Drug use	• Esophageal reflux
	• Tricyclics	• Menstrual irregularity
	• Phenothiazines	• Depression
	Exercise level	
	Obesity in family	
Physical examination		
Height	Slow reflexes, goiter	Hypertension
Weight	Striae, buffalo hump, central fat distribution	Right upper quadrant tenderness
Skin-fold thickness (subscapular, triceps)	Hirsutism	Varicose veins, phlebitis
	Small testes	Asterixis, facial rubor, somnolence
	Papilledema	Intertrigo
	Retinitis pigmentosa, polydactyly (Bardet-Biedl syndrome)	Joint tenderness or deformity
	Hypotonia, mental retardation (Prader-Willi syndrome)	
Laboratory[a]	24-hr-urine free cortisol	GTT
	Testosterone	Blood gases
	FSH, LH	Radiographs of back, knees, hips
	Androstenedione	Gallbladder sonogram
	CT scan of head	

[a]A minimum laboratory evaluation includes a CBC, urinalysis, spirogram, ECG, chest radiograph, serum thyroxine, TSH, multichannel blood analysis (glucose, creatinine, electrolytes, uric acid, liver function studies), triglycerides, and HDL and LDL cholesterol. Additional studies listed are performed when specifically indicated.

may also be used. Tracheostomy may be required in obstructive sleep apnea (see Chapter 3.7).

In addition to its direct effects on physical health, obesity causes social problems. Obese individuals are often subject to social ridicule, may be discriminated against in the job market, and have difficulty getting into college. Obese patients are frequently dealt with in an unsympathetic manner by physicians who are frustrated both by the patients' self-destructive behavior and their refractoriness to treatment.

MANAGEMENT

EVALUATION

The physician's major concern is the patient with obesity sufficient to constitute a significant physical or emotional health hazard. Many patients seek medical guidance for weight control when adiposity is minor and only a cosmetic concern. A comprehensive history, physical examination, and laboratory evaluation must precede the initiation of treatment (Table 14.11–2). In a small number of patients an underlying disease can be identified as the cause of obesity, and obviously specific therapy is directed toward the primary condition. Weight-related risk factors (hypertension, diabetes, lipid abnormalities) or symptoms (e.g., shortness of breath, dependent edema, somnolence) are identified. It is important to emphasize their reversibility to the patient, because this will buttress the patient's motivation to follow a weight-reduction program. The weight history focuses on the age at onset of the obesity, periods of rapid weight gain and their association with major life stresses, and the results of previous efforts at weight reduction. During the physical examination, the degree of obesity is assessed from weight and height measurements. Evidence for complications of obesity is sought primarily in the cardiovascular, pulmonary, and musculoskeletal systems. Laboratory determinations include plasma glucose, LDL and HDL cholesterol, triglyceride, thyroid hormone, and TSH levels. Some patients may require a 24-hour urinary free cortisol determination or an overnight dexamethasone-suppression test. Other tests of hypothalamic, pituitary, or gonadal function are performed when specifically indicated. When obesity is substantial, arterial blood gases should be measured. Overweight patients often believe that a metabolic defect is responsible for their obesity and are convinced that their caloric intake is not excessive. Thus, shortcuts in their medical evaluation can jeopardize the physician's credibility when dieting rather than hormonal therapy is recommended as the basic therapeutic approach.

TREATMENT

An approximate weight goal is established before the onset of treatment. All patients should be encouraged to achieve a weight within 20 percent of ideal to normalize mortality risk. If this goal is reached, the medical need for further weight reduction is determined by reassessing risk factors and weight-related symptoms. Even in the absence of a clear-cut medical indication, patients may desire more weight loss for cosmetic reasons. The physician should discourage target weights that are inappropriately low because failure and frustration may trigger overeating. Overconcern about weight can lead to excessive dieting and the syndrome of anorexia nervosa, particularly in young women.

Weight loss requires a reduction in caloric intake to a level below caloric utilization. When caloric utilization exceeds intake, the breakdown of adipose tissue triglycerides provides most of the energy deficit and results in the loss of fat tissue. The initial period of weight loss must ultimately give way to a prolonged period of caloric balance, where intake and output are equal, in order to maintain a stable and lower weight. Ideally, the latter period is lifelong. Caloric utilization at a reduced weight is less than at the pretreatment weight. This decline in caloric requirement follows from the loss of metabolizing tissue (mainly adipose tissue), the

reduced work load, and a fall in basal metabolic rate beyond that accountable for by the loss of metabolizing tissue. Because the patient presenting for weight reduction has already demonstrated an appetite for calories in excess of metabolic need, it is evident that maintenance of a lower weight will require continuous effort, a point that should be made clear at the outset. A short period of dieting, followed by a return to previous eating habits, will inevitably and inexorably lead to weight gain. Patients should be followed at weekly or biweekly intervals throughout the period of weight loss and well into weight maintenance to monitor progress, make dietary adjustments, and provide encouragement. Thereafter, continued though less frequent follow-up is desirable. Treatment is best accomplished by a team comprising a physician, nutritionist, and behavioral psychologist. Needless to say, fundamental changes in eating behavior can seldom be accomplished merely by giving the patient general advice to ingest a certain number of calories or by providing printed diet instructions.

Diet

Dieting is the mainstay of weight reduction because exercise alone rarely produces a negative caloric balance large enough to cause significant weight loss. The patient's daily caloric requirement is first estimated; this varies with age, sex, surface area (height and weight), and physical activity, as shown in Tables 14.11–3 and 14.11–4. The caloric content of a diet aimed at achieving the desired rate of weight loss can then be calculated on the assumption that a deficit of 3500 kcal is necessary to lose one pound of fat. A

TABLE 14.11–3. BASAL ENERGY NEEDS FOR MEN AND WOMEN

Height (inches)	Weight (lb)	Kilocalories/day by Age Group		
		20–35	36–50	51–65
Men				
60–63	160[a]	1690	1560	1490
	186	1800	1670	1590
	213	1900	1760	1690
64–67	172	1820	1680	1610
	200	1940	1790	1720
	229	2055	1910	1830
68–71	186	1970	1820	1750
	217	2100	1950	1870
	248	2230	2050	1970
72–75	204	2130	1970	1890
	238	2280	2100	2010
	272	2410	2230	2140
Women				
58–60	139	1370	1340	1280
	162	1460	1420	1370
	186	1550	1510	1450
61–63	150	1470	1430	1370
	175	1570	1530	1460
	200	1650	1610	1550
64–66	161	1570	1530	1460
	188	1670	1620	1560
	214	1760	1710	1650
67–69	172	1660	1620	1550
	200	1780	1730	1660
	229	1880	1830	1750
70–72	182	1730	1690	1620
	213	1880	1830	1750
	243	1990	1940	1860

[a]The three weights given for each height range represent values approximately 20, 40, and 60 percent above ideal (Table 14.11–1). Weight undressed and height without shoes should be used.
Adapted from Rynearson EH, Gastineau CP: Obesity. Springfield, Ill, Charles C Thomas, 1949.

TABLE 14.11–4. FRACTIONAL INCREASE OVER BASAL ENERGY NEEDS FOR ACTIVITY[a]

Activity	Kilocalories/day	
	Men	*Women*
Light (office worker, most professionals)	0.59	0.36
Light to moderate (industrial worker, student, custodial worker)	0.76	0.49
Moderate to heavy (farmer, dancer, unskilled laborer)	1.06	0.76
Heavy (blacksmith, lumberjack, construction worker)	1.35	1.03

[a]To calculate total daily caloric requirement estimate the basal requirement (Table 14.11–3) and multiply by 1 plus the appropriate fractional increase over basal for activity.
Adapted from Jequier E, Schutz Y: In Cioffi LA, James WPT, Van Itallie TB (eds): The Body Weight Regulatory System: Normal and Disturbed Mechanisms. New York, Raven Press, 1980, pp. 89–96.

45-year-old man, 71 inches tall, who weighs 220 lb and engages in light activity would require about 3430 kcal per day to maintain weight. Thus, a reduction of intake to 2400 kcal per day should result in the loss of about 2 pounds of fat weekly. (Weight loss is actually slightly slower because of the decrease in basal metabolic rate associated with dieting and weight loss.)

The standard low-calorie diet most commonly prescribed is well balanced with respect to carbohydrate, protein, and fat content. A wide variety of foods is offered by grouping those of comparable nutritional composition in seven exchange lists. The patient is then given a fixed number of selections daily from each exchange list. The transition from weight reduction to weight maintenance is made simply by expanding the number of exchange list selections to the isocaloric point. Lay organizations such as Weight Watchers and TOPS (Take Off Pounds Sensibly), which combine this diet with regular follow-up, are probably at least as effective as physicians. Although a standard low-calorie diet is eminently logical and often effective with mild degrees of obesity, fewer than 30 percent of patients following such a regimen lose over 20 pounds. Because variety is preserved, this diet permits obese patients to consume small amounts of certain foods that they may find highly palatable. Unfortunately, binges may ensue because an inability to control quantity, especially when confronted with these attractive foods, is precisely the problem for moderately to severely obese patients.

Alternative dietary approaches tend to limit variety and are often called "fad" diets. When patients are refractory to management by the standard low-calorie diet, variety-restricted diets should be considered. They can be effective for moderately to severely obese patients because common binge stimulators (sweet foods in particular) are usually eliminated. Boredom with the permitted foods may lead the dieter to consume less than the allowed ration. Weight loss is generally rapid, reinforcing the dieting effort. Books addressed to the lay public have popularized a number of fad diets whose safety and efficacy have not been subjected to rigorous scientific scrutiny.

One of the best studied and most widely used of the variety-restricted diets is the protein-sparing modified fast. This diet seeks to circumvent the negative nitrogen balance and loss of muscle mass that accompany total starvation. A daily intake of 50 to 75 g of hydrolyzed protein provides amino acids as the only caloric source (200 to 300 kcal per day). Vitamins, minerals, and noncaloric fluids are also given. This diet produces dramatic weight loss in the majority of moderately to severely obese patients. Appetite is suppressed in many by the ketosis resulting from the absence of dietary carbohydrate. Vigorous salt and water diuresis may lead to symptomatic postural hypotension, but this can be corrected by salt supplementation. Hyperuricemia can provoke attacks of gout, which can be controlled with colchicine. Deaths caused by myocardial degeneration and refractory arrhythmias have been reported in patients undergoing the protein-supplemented modified fast for more than 2 months. These deaths were generally associated with the use of protein hydrolyzates of poor nutritional quality. Because nitrogen balance remains negative in many patients, this diet has been supplemented with carbohydrate (up to 50 g/day) for its protein-sparing effect. Deaths have been reported, however, even with the use of diets containing high-quality protein and enriched with carbohydrate. The protein-sparing modified fast should be undertaken, therefore, only under close supervision and for periods not exceeding 2 months.

An alternative type of variety-restricted diet limits dietary carbohydrate to less than 50 g per day by utilizing foods rich in protein, such as poultry, fish, cheese, and eggs, along with leafy vegetables as bulk. Vitamin and mineral supplementation are also needed. Compliance is improved both by the appetite-suppressing effect of the accompanying ketosis and the absence of foods that commonly stimulate binges. The content of saturated fats and cholesterol is potentially high and may raise serum levels of LDL cholesterol, but the diet is rarely followed long enough for this to be of concern. Weight loss itself tends to compensate by lowering LDL and raising HDL cholesterol. The brisk diuresis caused by ketogenic diets results in large initial weight losses; patients may become discouraged when weight reduction slows after the first week or even plateaus with subsequent periods of fluid retention. Because chest, waist, hip, thigh, and biceps circumferences are unaffected by fluid changes, weekly measurements of these body dimensions can provide psychologic support by demonstrating continued fat loss despite a plateau in weight. The management of patients on a variety-restricted diet mandates familiarity with specific side effects, the potential for nutritional deficiencies, and the psychologic impact of substantial weight loss. The physician must assess the risk-benefit ratio for each patient.

Ultimately, the variety-restricted diet must be liberalized for nutritional reasons. A suitable time for this transition is when the objective of treatment changes from weight reduction to weight maintenance. This transition period is difficult because the expansion of food choices introduces appetizing foods that may stimulate binging. It is particularly hazardous for patients whose intake has been limited exclusively to synthetic supplements because this type of diet does not facilitate identification or correction of the dieter's poor eating habits. Such patients are particularly likely to regain lost weight. Adjunctive supports are discussed below.

All dieters should be encouraged to keep a record of foods consumed and their caloric content. This familiarizes the patient with the basic nutritional information necessary to make food choices. Such self-scrutiny also helps to restrain eating.

Drugs

Drugs to promote weight loss fall into two categories: those that may enhance caloric utilization, such as thyroid hormone and human chorionic gonadotropin (hCG), and appetite suppressants. Pharmacologic doses of thyroid hormone should not be used because they cause loss of muscle, and human chorionic gonadotropin has not been effective in controlled studies. The appetite suppressants, which are all chemically related to the catecholamines, reduce appetite and stimulate the central nervous system in animals and humans. The many agents in common use appear to be equally potent in facilitating weight loss for periods up to 6 months. Effectiveness for more than 6 months has not been established. Stimulation of the central nervous system can lead to abuse of these drugs, especially amphetamines, which therefore should not be used. Side effects include insomnia, palpitations, hallucinations, and blood pressure elevation; depression may follow abrupt withdrawal. The use of appetite suppressants should be temporary, limited to the faltering dieter, and comprise only one component of a more comprehensive weight control program.

Alteration of Eating Behavior

Overweight patients frequently eat to relieve emotional distress, such as anxiety, depression, or boredom, and lose control over food intake once eating has begun. In addition, dieting itself can induce depression, frustration, impatience, self-pity, and the additional distress of adjusting to a new and lower weight. (Many of these features characterize other forms of substance abuse, e.g., alcohol.) It is essential, therefore, to include a psychological component in the treatment of obesity. The technique of behavioral modification has been extensively employed for this purpose in recent years. The diet diary is a central feature; data include the time and place of eating, the foods consumed, triggering stimuli, and emotional states associated with eating. An attempt is then made to deal more directly with dysphoric states or to redirect the patient's response from eating toward less destructive behavior, such as exercise or ventilating emotions with a friend or therapist. External cues—for example, foods that stimulate binges—are identified and eliminated. It is customary to limit the permissible times and locations of eating. A system of rewards may be developed to recognize the attainment of specific eating-related goals. Typically, a group format is used; regular group meetings offer the patient an opportunity to explore eating behavior in a sympathetic and supportive setting. Although behavioral modification has improved short- and intermediate-term results, recidivism rates continue to be high over the long term. Other forms of psychologic therapy include self-help groups and couples training.

Exercise

Exercise must be encouraged in all patients, particularly for weight maintenance, to compensate for the decline in caloric utilization that accompanies weight loss. Strenuous exercise, like jogging, increases caloric utilization by 10 to 15 kcal per min (Table 14.11–5). Most patients, however, will not exercise enough to accelerate weight loss significantly. On the other hand, 20 minutes of vigorous exercise three times a week for a year, or alternatively, a 1-mile walk daily, can burn the equivalent of 10 to 15 pounds of fat yearly and thereby make an important contribution to long-term success. Sustained low-intensity exercise is as effective at increasing caloric output as short periods of high intensity exercise. The former is recommended because of less risk and discomfort. In the sedentary patient a regular exercise program should be started at an early stage of dieting when motivation and enthusiasm are greatest. Increased exercise is a consistent characteristic of patients who have been successful at maintaining substantial weight loss. In humans, no consistent effect of exercise on appetite has been demonstrated.

Some young women may develop amenorrhea as a result of strenuous exercise that decreases their percentage of body fat significantly even without a change in body weight. Body weight in general, and percentage of adipose tissue in particular, must exceed specific limits for menses to occur.

Surgery

Two types of surgical procedures, intestinal bypass and gastric restriction, have been used for the treatment of obesity. Surgical management is limited to grossly obese patients, usually less than 50 years of age, who are twice ideal weight or at least 100 lb above ideal weight and have been unsuccessful at dieting. Other indications include significant medical or psychosocial problems that will not improve without major weight loss. Patients must understand the hazards of the procedure.

Following jejunoileal bypass, most patients achieve a large and permanent weight loss because of decreased food intake and malabsorption. Benefits include better social and psychologic adjustment, decreased blood pressure, reduced total cholesterol and triglycerides, and improved glucose tolerance. Although operative mortality and immediate postoperative morbidity are low, some long-term complication of bypass occurs in almost every patient.[3] The more common complications are electrolyte disturbances (hypokalemia, hypocalcemia), calcium oxalate kidney stones, migratory polyarthralgias, intractable diarrhea, and two gastrointestinal syndromes due to bacterial overgrowth. Pseudo-obstructive megacolon causes intermittent symptoms of colonic obstruction and abdominal distention. Less common is bypass enteritis, characterized by fever, abdominal pain, and distention. Oral antibiotics may provide temporary improvement in both syndromes. Liver disease, which may progress to cirrhosis and fatal liver failure in a small number of patients, is the most serious complication of bypass surgery. Because of the frequency and severity of long-term complications, bypass surgery is done rarely now.

The various gastric restriction procedures are all based upon the formation of a small gastric pouch with a restricted outlet.[2] As a result, patients may experience abdominal pain or vomit after ingesting a large meal. The original technique involved gastric transection with a gastrojejunostomy. Procedures that create a small reservoir by stapling across the stomach have recently become more popular. Operative mortality is low, but immediate postoperative sequelae are common because of technical difficulties. When successful, the magnitude of weight loss with these techniques approaches that of bypass surgery. Severe, persistent vomiting may be an ongoing problem, but the frequency and seriousness of late complications are much less than for bypass surgery. Unfortunately, the failure rate, defined by insufficient weight loss or inadequate maintenance of weight loss, may exceed 30 percent. Success requires a significant modification of eating habits. The repeated ingestion of large amounts of food at a single meal leads to frequent vomiting and dilatation of the gastric pouch and stoma. Alternatively, patients may defeat the purpose of the procedure by constant nibbling or eating many small meals.

An innovative new technique to discourage overeating involves the endoscopic introduction of a balloon into the stomach. The balloon is then inflated and left in the stomach for up to 4 months. Preliminary results show appetite suppression and significant weight reduction. Gradual balloon deflation and possible gastric irritation and ulcer formation mandate endoscopic reassessment after 4 months. Reballooning is then possible, but as yet this technique has not been employed for over 8 months.

TABLE 14.11–5. CALORIES USED FOR EACH MINUTE (IN KCAL/MIN) OF CONTINUOUS EXERCISE

Activity	Weight (lb)					
	120	150	170	200	220	250
Walking, 3 mph	3.2	4.0	4.6	5.4	5.9	6.8
Bicycling, 5.5 mph	3.8	4.7	5.3	6.3	6.9	7.9
Calisthenics	3.9	4.9	5.6	6.6	7.2	8.2
Walking, 4 mph	4.6	5.8	6.6	7.8	8.5	9.7
Aerobics	4.6	5.8	6.6	7.8	8.5	9.7
Tennis, singles	6.0	7.5	8.5	10.0	10.9	12.5
Bicycling, 10 mph	6.5	8.1	9.2	10.8	11.9	13.6
Swimming, crawl	6.9	8.7	9.8	11.6	12.7	14.5
Jogging, 11-min mile	7.3	9.1	10.4	12.2	13.4	15.3
Racquetball	7.6	9.5	10.7	12.7	13.9	15.8
Running, 8-min mile	11.3	14.1	16.0	18.8	20.7	23.5

Figures developed under standardized conditions at the Human Performance Research Center at Brigham Young University, Provo, Utah. Factors such as ambient temperature and clothing can affect values.

PREVENTION

Whenever possible good medical practice stresses prevention rather than treatment. The nutrition of infants is a balance between avoidance of adipocyte hyperplasia and the dangers of overly restrictive diets. Thirty-six percent of infants in the 90th percentile or greater for weight become overweight adults. In contrast, only 14 percent of infants who are average or below average in weight become obese adults.[5]

In most cases, treatment of overweight infants is best postponed until after 1 year of age. Although the use of skim milk appears to be a healthy dietary habit, it should be avoided too early in life because of its low fat content, unphysiologically high concentration of protein, and excessive solute load. Beginning at about 1 year of age, however, a gradual transition may be started to dairy products with reduced fat content. Especially to be encouraged are the use of social praise for good nutritional habits, the avoidance of concentrated sweets and fats, and the use of food for nutritional purposes only rather than as a reward for good conduct or a substitute for affection.

The fact that 80 percent of obese adolescents become obese adults emphasizes the need for attention to weight problems in adolescence. Adolescents have special needs because of the social pressures to conform to idiosyncratic patterns of eating. Formal nutritional education should begin in school at this age. Realistic teaching of ''survival skills'' in fast-food chains is helpful. School physical education programs would do well to promote physical fitness through aerobic exercises that are enjoyable and not excessively demanding. The traditional preoccupation with competitive athletics and team sports often alienates overweight adolescents who then believe themselves to be incapable of meaningful exercise. While increasing intensity of exercise is necessary for physical conditioning, this is not the case for calorie utilization.

REFERENCES

1. Bjorntorp P: Regional patterns of fat distribution. Ann Intern Med 103:994, 1985
2. Dickerman RM: Gastric exclusion surgery in the management of morbid obesity. Ann Rev. Med 33:263, 1982
3. Hocking MP, Duerson RN, et al: Jejunoileal bypass for morbid obesity. Late follow-up in 100 cases. N Engl J Med 308:995, 1983
4. Hubert HA, Feinleib M, et al: Obesity as an independent risk factor for cardiovascular disease: A 26 year follow-up of participants in the Framingham Heart Study. Circulation 67:968, 1983
5. Johnston FE: Health implications of childhood obesity. Ann Intern Med 103:1068, 1985
6. Kolterman OG, Insel J, et al: Mechanisms of insulin resistance in human obesity: Evidence for receptor and postreceptor defects. J Clin Invest 65:1272, 1980
7. Leibel RL, Hirsch J: Diminished energy requirements in reduced-obese patients. Metabolism 33:164, 1984
8. Sims EAH, Danforth E Jr, et al: Endocrine and metabolic effects of experimental obesity in man. Recent Prog Horm Res 29:457, 1973
9. Stunkard AJ, Sorenson TIA, et al: An adoption study of human obesity. N Engl J Med 314:193, 1986
10. Van Italle TB: Health implications of overweight and obesity in the United States. Ann Intern Med 103:983, 1985
11. Wadden TA, Stunkard AJ: Social and psychological consequences of obesity. Ann Intern Med 103:1062, 1985

CHAPTER 15.1
Introduction to Disorders of the Nervous System

Hamilton Moses III

Neurologic complaints are ubiquitous. Symptoms referable to the nervous system account for about 10 percent of outpatient visits to a physician. Neurologic disease is present in about 15 percent of patients hospitalized on a general medical service and in 12 percent of patients seen in a busy city hospital's emergency room.[3] Furthermore, neurologic diseases, especially stroke, Parkinson disease, epilepsy, multiple sclerosis, and chronic pain, account for more long-term disability than all other conditions combined. Every physician will have a large number of patients with headache, dizziness, back or neck pain, and weakness or insomnia, which represent a group of symptoms that may or may not be associated with significant underlying abnormalities of the nervous system. Thus, it is essential that all physicians have an organized approach for evaluation of neurological abnormalities.

The epidemiology of neurologic disease is not immutable, and several recent changes are noteworthy (Table 15.1-1). The incidence of stroke, particularly hypertensive hemorrhage, has shown dramatic and sustained decline over the past decade, most probably caused by changes in the American diet and vigorous control of hypertension. Conversely, apparently new diseases have emerged, for example, the variegated neurologic manifestations of acquired immunodeficiency syndrome (AIDS), which can mimic many other conditions. The most important changes have occurred—and will continue to occur—in those conditions directly related to age, such as dementia, Parkinson disease, and motor neuron disease. As the population ages, the physician will encounter these conditions more frequently.

Therapeutic options have likewise expanded, and many once untreatable conditions are now amenable to effective therapy. Since the previous edition of this book, new neurologic therapies include acyclovir for herpes simplex encephalitis, calcium channel antagonists for migraine, plasmapheresis for the Guillain-Barré syndrome, and a proven role of immunosuppression for certain forms of multiple sclerosis. Conversely, controlled trials have cast doubt on the utility of some modalities that were formerly standard therapies, such as external carotid–internal carotid bypass surgery for ischemic stroke, and there is increasing skepticism about carotid endarterectomy in patients who are asymptomatic or who have only minor carotid stenosis. Although neurology has been considered by many a field with only limited therapeutic options, one need only view the dramatic and demonstrable success of therapy in epilepsy, Parkinson disease, migraine, subarachnoid hemorrhage, myasthenia gravis, and certain peripheral neuropathies to conclude that neurology compares most favorably with other medical disciplines.

NEUROLOGICAL HISTORY AND EXAMINATION

General aspects of obtaining clinical information have been discussed in Section 1. Several principles are especially impor for patients who have neurologic symptoms.

Assessment of a patient with any disease begins at the moment of first meeting the physician. The patient may betray an aphasia or dysarthria when first saying "hello." One may suspect an ocular motor paresis by the tilt of the head or see facial weakness with the first smile. The patient may not try to smile and have difficulty arising from the chair to enter the examining room, displaying two of the cardinal elements of parkinsonism. There may be a limp, showing weakness or pain in the leg, or one may hear the double foot slap that occurs with distal weakness from polyneuropathy.

The ability to make clinical observations and assemble them so that an understandable pattern is formed requires conscious effort, a knowledge of the disease process, and proficiency in examination. While this is true for all medical disciplines, it is especially true in neurologic diagnosis. Although neurology is complex and requires knowledge about neuroanatomy and neurophysiology, the student should not be daunted by arcane terminology, historical eponyms, or overly complex explanations. Fortunately, the principles of neurologic diagnosis can be simplified so that the patterns of disease can be more easily recognized. The goals of neurologic evaluation are three: (1) define the *anatomy* of the lesion, (2) discern in what way normal *physiology* is altered, (3) judge what the *etiology* is likely to be. Only after information about those three areas has been obtained by history-taking and neurologic examination can proper additional diagnostic studies be undertaken and therapy prescribed. In reaching a tentative diagnosis, the history is of prime importance, the examination second, and ancillary studies clearly third. Experienced neurologists estimate that about two thirds of all diagnoses can be reached by information supplied in the history primarily, that the examination adds about one fourth, and that all ancillary studies add only a small increment to defining a neurological problem.

NEUROLOGICAL HISTORY

The aim of the history is to document the abnormalities noticed by the patient (or other observers) together with the circumstances under which they developed. This relies on the skills outlined in Section 1, but there are certain other aspects to be emphasized in neurology.

1. What is the *pattern of disease?* Many disease processes result in similar neurologic manifestations and disabilities, in part because dysfunction of a particular region of the nervous system will lead to predictable symptoms. The timing, rate, and pattern of progression are usually very distinctive, however. Several examples of the patterns of disease are given in Figure 15.5–1.

2. Can we *bracket the lesion?* By that we mean, "What is the highest and what is the lowest point in the nervous system that can account for the dysfunction?" Do the symptoms suggest a single lesion or multiple lesions?

3. Where should we *concentrate our efforts?* A detailed examination of all possible neurologic functions is lengthy, dull, and unrewarding. Proper interpretation of the history should steer the physician to the parts of the neurologic examination that require greater attention. For instance, symptoms of memory loss or hallu-

TABLE 15.1–1. CURRENT NEUROLOGIC BURDEN OF ILLNESS AND INJURY IN THE UNITED STATES

| Disorder | Approximate Rates per 100,000 Population | | Approximate Years Duration[a] |
	Annual Incidence	Prevalence	
Migraine and other severe headache	450	3500	40
Spinal osteoarthritis	335	910	3
Severe head or brain injury	350	830	4
Epilepsy	50	650	13
Acute cerebrovascular disease	150	600	4
Ménière disease	50	300	6
Dementias	50	250	5
Parkinsonism	20	200	10
Transient ischemic attacks	30	150	5
Multiple sclerosis	3	60	35
Congenital malformations CNS	7	70	10
Mental retardation	12	60	NA
Subarachnoid hemorrhage	15	50	3
Meningitis-encephalitis	30	25	1
Polyneuropathy	40	20	0.5
Malignant primary or metastatic brain tumor	20	20	1
Motor neuron disease	2	6	3
Bell palsy	25	5	0.2
Myasthenia gravis	0.4	4	10

NA = Not applicable.
[a]Approximate time of onset to time of maximal functional recovery or death.
Adapted from Kurtzke JF: Neurol 32:1207, 1982.[6]

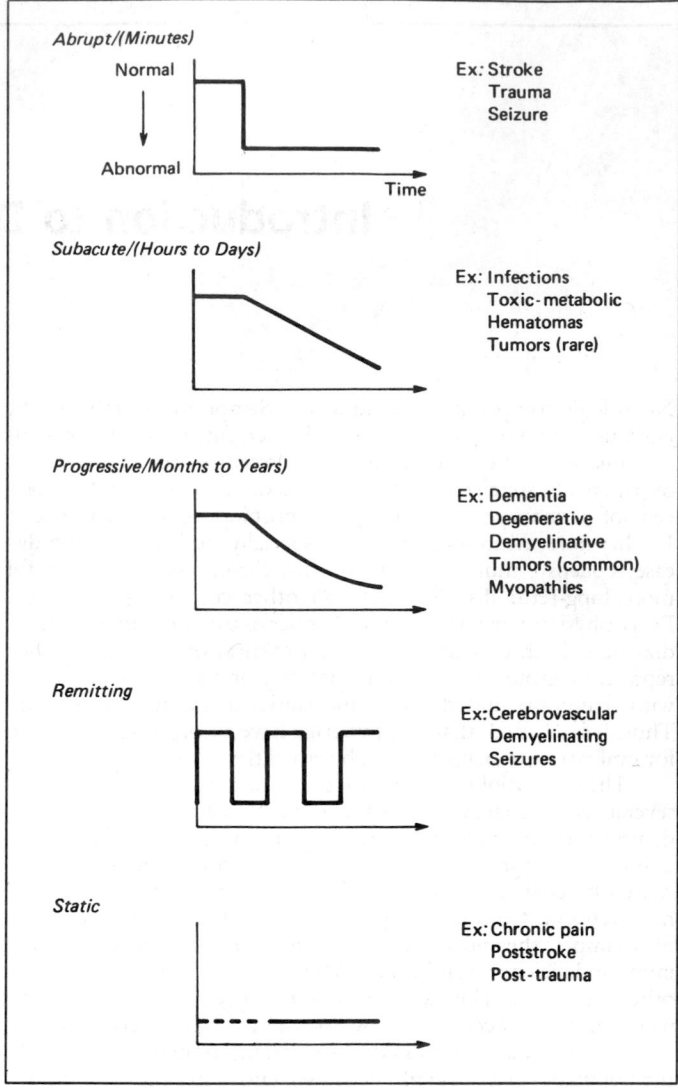

Figure 15.1–1. Patterns of progression of neurologic illness.

cinations would indicate more detailed examination of the mental state, while paresthesias or numbness would suggest that sensory examination should be emphasized.

4. Is the *patient aware* of the dysfunction? In many instances of acute disease such as strokes or seizures, the patient is totally unable to report what has happened. In these circumstances, important observations about the onset and pattern require the report of another person. In eliciting this outside information, one should be aware that sudden disruption of neurologic function can be an extremely frightening event for witnesses. Thus, comments on subjects such as the duration or degree of unresponsiveness should be interpreted cautiously.

5. Is there an *underlying disease?* Many treatable conditions affecting the nervous system are manifestations of systemic illnesses. Thinking of the nervous system in isolation from the rest of the body can lead to serious errors in diagnosis and management. For instance, overlooking a subtle nodule in the breast when an intracranial mass is obvious will cause one to miss the diagnosis of metastatic breast cancer. This principle applies to all underlying diseases, but patients with neoplastic, metabolic, toxic, connective tissue, and cardiac diseases are particularly likely to present initially with neurologic manifestations.

Information about occupation and hobbies is very important in patients with neurologic disease, as both toxic exposures and trauma may predispose to certain illness (for instance, seizures or polyneuropathy) and because neurologic dysfunction may jeopardize the patient's safety at work or at home.

The family history is also of particular importance, for many inherited conditions that have neurologic implications are easily overlooked. This is especially true for abnormalities that begin in adolescence or early adulthood, but it is also so in mid- or late life. For example, proper diagnosis of Huntington disease, which usually begins in mid-life, largely depends upon the discovery of other family members with characteristic psychiatric or neurologic abnormalities. Also, once a neurologic diagnosis has been established, the implications for the family should likewise be considered, both when the condition is familial and when it is not. Many families will fear, for instance, that they or subsequent generations will be at risk for epilepsy, Parkinson disease, or stroke, even when inherited factors and risks are few.

NEUROLOGIC EXAMINATION

Examination of the nervous system begins at the moment the patient is first seen. It is most logically performed methodically while the general physical examination is being performed. Special areas

of emphasis—for instance, the mental state, sensory, or visual examination—can later be added, either during the same session or after an interval. An interval for rest is particularly important when either the patient or examiner is fatigued. Used in this regional manner, neurologic testing becomes concrete, automatic, and no longer artificial.

Many guides to specific aspects of neurologic examination are available. Those of Denny-Brown,[4] Haymaker,[5] The Medical Research Council,[8] and Strub[12] are particularly recommended.

REFERENCES

1. Adams RD, Victor M: Principles of Neurology, 3d ed. New York, McGraw-Hill, 1986
2. Baker AB, Baker LH: Clinical Neurology, vols 1–4. Hagerstown, Md, Harper & Row, 1986
3. Brust JCM: Neurology in a municipal teaching hospital. Semin Neurol 5:32, 1985
4. Denny-Brown D: Handbook of Neurological Examination and Case Recording. Cambridge, England, Cambridge University Press, 1957
5. Haymaker W: Bing's Local Diagnosis in Neurological Disease. St. Louis, CV Mosby, 1969
6. Kurtzke JF: The current neurological burden of illness and injury in the United States. Neurol 32:1207, 1982
7. Mancall EL: Alper's and Mancall's Essentials of the Neurologic Examination, 2d ed. Philadelphia, FA Davis, 1981
8. Medical Research Council: War Memorandum No 7: Aids to the Investigation of Peripheral Nerve Injuries. London, Her Majesty's Stationery Office, 1978
9. Montgomery ED, Wall M, Henderson V: Principles of Neurologic Diagnosis. Boston, Little, Brown, 1986
10. Rowland LP: Merritt's Textbook of Neurology, 7th ed. Philadelphia, Lea & Febiger, 1986
11. Samuels MA (ed): Manual of Neurologic Therapeutics. Boston, Little, Brown, 1986
12. Strub R, Black FW: The Mental Status Examination in Neurology. Philadelphia, FA Davis, 1977
13. Vinken PJ, Bruyn GW: Handbook of Clinical Neurology, vols 1–35. Amsterdam, North-Holland, 1969–1979
14. Youmans SR: Neurological Surgery, vols 1–5. Philadelphia, WB Saunders, 1982

CHAPTER 15.2

Use of Ancillary Neurologic Tests

Hamilton Moses III

Anatomic, biochemical, and physiologic derangements of the nervous system can be demonstrated by a number of different diagnostic procedures. The physician should know what each procedure can and cannot do, the relative risks of each procedure, and the most effective and efficient sequence of tests for a particular clinical problem. In addition, the physician should be clear about what question needs to be elucidated, for the technique of the procedure often needs to be varied depending upon the type of information sought.

When possible, the most specific test for a clinical problem should be chosen and performed first, avoiding less specific tests. In general, one proceeds from the simpler examinations, which have little risk or discomfort, to more complex tests, which often have greater risk. The sequence of tests is often very important, for certain procedures make the performance or interpretation of subsequent procedures more difficult. For instance, a lumbar puncture should be deferred in a patient considered for myelography, for the tear in the arachnoidal membrane may allow myelographic contrast to escape from the subarachnoid to the subdural space.

NEURORADIOLOGY[5]

Indications for various neuroradiologic procedures are given in Table 15.2–1.

SKULL FILMS

Skull films may indicate disruption or distortion of the bony structures of the skull, the location of normally calcified structures such as the pineal and choroid plexus, or the presence of abnormal calcifications. Although skull films continue to be indicated in cases of direct trauma to the skull, they have been largely replaced by computed tomography (CT) and magnetic resonance imaging (MRI) for most other neurologic conditions.

COMPUTED TOMOGRAPHY (CT SCANNING)

Rapid and safe images of the skull, cerebrospinal fluid, and the different densities of white and gray matter in the brain parenchyma are easily obtained via this technique. Herniations, ventricular size, and the nature of other intracranial structures can be seen at once, with the etiology—whether infarct, hemorrhage, edema, abscess, or tumor—usually easily determined. The integrity and distribution of the vasculature can be demonstrated by "enhancement," which is obtained by performing a CT scan after intravenous injection of an iodinated dye.

Areas of Usefulness
The CT scans largely replace pneumoencephalography, arteriography, and isotopic brain scanning as the primary diagnostic procedure for investigation of patients with acute or chronic intracranial processes. It plays a particular role in neurologic trauma, dementia, developmental defects, stroke, and the diagnosis of intracranial neoplasms.

Risks[4]
The patient is exposed to dosage of irradiation approximately equivalent to that of a skull series. Anaphylaxis after intravenous iodinated dye is the major concern. With the nearly universal availability of CT scanning, overinterpretation of CT scans has become a problem. Physicians should be cautious of reported abnormalities that do not correspond to the patient's neurologic signs and symptoms. Artifacts do occur on CT scans and can best be checked by repeating the procedure. False-negative CT scans occur with small lesions near the base of the skull; in the orbits, the parasellar region, and the posterior fossa; and at the craniocervical junction. Consultation with the radiologist before the study can guard against these false-negative results. Special views are often necessary when conditions in those locations are suspected.

TABLE 15.2–1. VALUE OF NEURORADIOGRAPHIC PROCEDURES

	Skull Radio-graph	CT Scan	MRI Scan	Angio-gram	Isotopic Scan
Skull					
Fracture	+				
Bone density	+	+	±		
Bone erosion	+	±	±		
Intracranial calci-fication	+	+			
Ventricular system					
Size		+	+	±	
Displacement		+	+	±	
CSF dynamics					+
Brain substance					
Atrophy		+	+	±	
Masses		+	+	±	+
Infarction		+	+		
Hematoma		+	+	±	±
Vascular pattern					
Patency		±	+	+	
Displacement				+	
Malformation		±	+	+	±
Aneurysm				+	

MAGNETIC RESONANCE IMAGING (MRI SCANNING)

Clinically useful images of extraordinarily high quality can be obtained by the emerging technology of magnetic imaging. In these devices, the patient is surrounded by a high-strength magnetic field through which pulses of radio frequency (RF) irradiation are projected, thereby exciting the nuclei of hydrogen, phosphorus, oxygen, or other elements. Coils within the scanner are placed quite close to or on the patient's body and serve as antennae for the altered RF signal that is produced as the nuclei relax after stimulation. Computer manipulation of the data thus acquired using imaging algorithms produces a clinically useful image. By varying the strength of the magnetic field, the frequency and energy of the radio frequency stimulation, and the timing of the stimulation pulses, selected images of many biologic materials can be discerned in the living patient. In particular, differences between white and gray matter, lesions within white matter, structures of the brain that are in close proximity to bone (such as the skull base and within the spine), and the distinction among cerebral infarction, edema, and neoplasm are all aided by MRI.

Risks[4]

The patient receives no ionizing radiation, and there is no evidence of biologic effects of the magnetic or radio frequency fields as they are used. MRI is therefore recommended when repeated examinations in a single patient are required, and for use in pregnancy. Metallic intracranial clips (because of the fear of displacement) and the presence of a cardiac pacemaker are the only absolute contraindications to MRI, although magnetic materials in other parts of the body, for instance, certain prosthetic cardiac valves or orthopedic prostheses, may represent risk because of heating. These relative risks are currently being investigated.

Areas of Usefulness

MRI is expected to replace CT scanning for the diagnosis of multiple sclerosis, for the early detection of cerebral infarction, and for the early diagnosis of intracranial neoplasms. It is eventually likely to replace CT for the diagnosis of many intracranial conditions, although CT will continue to be important for staging many diseases.

NUCLIDE BRAIN SCANNING

CT and MRI have largely replaced scintillation scanning of the head in nearly all conditions including early cerebritis, early herpes simplex encephalitis, and major abnormalities in cerebral blood flow to the hemispheres.

Cisternal scans are used to demonstrate the patency of pathways of cerebrospinal fluid (CSF) flow and CFS reabsorption. Radioactive material is injected in the lumbar subarachnoid space, and serial scans of the head are performed at periodic intervals for up to 72 hours. Normally, little isotope enters the ventricles, the majority going over the convexities of the cortical surface as CSF is reabsorbed. In communicating hydrocephalus secondary to block in reabsorption of CSF, the isotope enters the ventricular system to an abnormal degree and may persist for 24 to 72 hours (ventricular stasis). Cisternography is also useful for detecting the site of a CSF leak in patients with recurrent meningitis or after head injury.

ANGIOGRAPHY

Cranial angiography is usually performed via retrograde insertion of a femoral or brachial catheter through which injections into the carotid arteries, either vertebral artery, or the aortic arch may be directed. Radiographic images are sequentially obtained. Digital imaging is increasingly replacing conventional film screen techniques, allowing reduction in the amount of injected dye, a particular attraction in patients who require multiple injections or who have significant cardiovascular or renal disease. Transvenous digital subtraction angiography (with injection of a large volume of iodinated contrast material) is useful for imaging the great vessels and major intracerebral branches, although it provides considerably less detail (and possibly no less risk) than intra-arterial injections. Progress is rapidly being made in digital technology, which has made angiography a considerably faster, safer, and more pleasant procedure than in past years.

Areas of Usefulness

Angiography demonstrates processes that obstruct, disrupt, or displace the normal vascular patterns. Thus, local obstruction secondary to atherosclerotic disease can be demonstrated. Selected catheterization may be required to demonstrate the origin of major vessels from the aortic arch and the carotid bifurcations (see Chapter 15.13).

In subarachnoid hemorrhage, careful angiography is essential for demonstrating the site of bleeding, whether from aneurysm or arteriovenous malformation. It is extremely important that careful coordination among neurologic, neurosurgical, and neuroradiologic personnel be achieved so that the correct assessment of surgical feasibility is reached. Special views are often required to demonstrate the exact shape and position of an aneurysm. *Balloon occlusion and embolization* via catheter play an increasing role in the definitive treatment of arteriovenous malformations, large congenital vascular anomalies of the skull and brain, and acquired carotid-cavernous fistula.

CT and MRI have replaced angiography for the delineation of intracranial masses and other cerebral lesions.

Risks[4]

Angiography via retrograde catheter injection has decreased the rate of complications. In most large series, a 0.5 percent risk of serious neurologic complications and a 5 to 7 percent risk of transient reversible neurologic signs or symptoms is cited. In patients with cerebrovascular disease, however, the risk may be higher by a factor of two to three times those rates, while the risk may be

decidedly lower in the young. Meticulous technique, coordination between the primary physician and the neuroradiologist, and clear indications for performing the study are required before angiography is undertaken. Hematoma or vascular spasm at the site of injection are usually self-limited complications. The most serious problems are emboli, either from the end of the catheter or dislodged from the vessel wall, dissection of an artery, and hypersensitivity reactions to the dye. In elderly patients with known arteriosclerotic vascular disease, the increased risk of angiography should be weighed against the feasibility and efficacy of possible subsequent therapeutic steps, e.g., carotid endarterectomy.

MYELOGRAPHY AND IMAGING OF THE SPINE

The bony spinal column lies in close relation to important neurologic structures that include the spinal cord, spinal roots, and blood vessels, as well as the subdural and epidural spaces, epidural fat, and intervertebral ligaments and discs. Imaging of these structures has undergone major improvement in recent years. CT scanning supplements myelography with water-soluble radiopaque material, while MRI often obviates the need for invasive studies. Conventional oil-based radiopaque dye (pantopaque) has been largely replaced by water-soluble radiographic dye (metrizamide, iopamidol). An injection of dye is made either into the lumbar or cisternal space after which conventional x-ray films are taken of suspected regions. After several hours have elapsed to allow complete mixing of contrast, CT images of particular areas are obtained. Improvement in myelographic technique, especially the use of small amounts of contrast, has allowed most lumbar and some cervical myelography to become standard outpatient procedures.

Areas of Usefulness
Myelography is used for demonstrating external compression of the spinal cord and roots by masses such as protruding intervertebral discs, osteoarthritic bone, tumors, or abscesses. In addition, the size of the spinal cord can be easily determined to allow differentiation of intramedullary processes, such as syringomyelia or neoplasms, from other causes of myelopathy. Myelography can also demonstrate large vascular malformations of the spinal cord, although spinal angiography via intercostal arteries is usually required to identify the blood supply of spinal malformations. Magnetic resonance imaging will probably replace conventional myelography and spinal CT scanning in these conditions, however. At present, myelography with CT scanning is superior for demonstrating details of nerve roots and their relation to the neural foramen and overgrown bone, which are of special importance in osteoarthritis of both the cervical and lumbar regions.

Risks[4]
Myelography is a safe procedure. Occasionally patients with a mass impinging on the spinal cord will develop further compression following myelography. A neurosurgeon should therefore, be consulted before myelography when a large mass is suspected. Spinal headache follows myelography in about one fifth of patients, but it can usually be prevented by the precautions described below. Metrizamide myelography causes nausea and vomiting in about one quarter of patients; while severe, these side effects routinely resolve within 24 hours of the procedure. Seizures after myelography with metrizamide occur in about 1 percent of patients, particularly those with preexisting epilepsy, intracranial masses, or inflammation of the CSF; they may be prevented by premedication with diazepam. With metrizamide, phenothiazines (promethazine) should be avoided because they lower the seizure threshold, although other antiemetics can be used (trimethobenzamide). The use of small spinal needles and low concentrations of contrast material reduces the risk of these complications.

POSITRON EMISSION TOMOGRAPHY (PET)

Positron emission tomography is an investigational tool that has not yet become routinely available clinically. Along with electroencephalography, PET scanning is one of the few modalities that indicate the physiologic function of the brain. Radioactive energy substrates, such as glucose or oxygen, or ligands of neurotransmitters are injected into an awake patient. Images are obtained from positrons that are emitted from brain as radioactive material binds or is consumed within the parenchyma. Both the rate of consumption (or binding) and location can thereby be deduced. Selection of appropriate substrates or ligands allows imaging of highly specific physiologic systems, such as dopaminergic neurons, or those that use abnormally high amounts of energy, such as epileptogenic regions. Although PET is currently largely an investigational tool, it plays an important role in the delineation of seizure foci, the distinction of normal brain from neoplastic tissue, and the elucidation of the border zone of ischemia that surrounds areas of cerebral infarction. It is likely that knowledge gained from PET will allow improved interpretation of information obtained from MRI in the future.

ELECTROENCEPHALOGRAPHY[3]

The electroencephalogram (EEG) records electrical activity generated near the surface of the cerebral cortex. Newer techniques, including EEG telemetry, prolonged ambulatory EEG monitoring, and combined video-EEG monitoring, are important in the evaluation of syncope and seizures (see Chapter 15.5).

AREAS OF USEFULNESS

The EEG is the only widely available technique for determining the physiological activity of the brain. Focal or generalized disruption of the normal rhythms of the awake and sleeping brain occurs as a result of most of the alterations to which the cerebral cortex is predisposed. For instance, general metabolic derangements that result in delirium, stupor, or coma reliably produce generalized slowing of the EEG record, while withdrawal from depressant drugs commonly activates the record. The EEG is especially useful for the characterization of epileptic disorders. Discrete sharp waves and spikes are seen with focal seizure discharges; three per second spike and wave abnormalities suggest subcortical discharges, as does bilateral symmetrical frontal activity. It is possible, however, for seizure activity, particularly coming from the temporal lobes, not to be reflected as an abnormality in scalp recordings. Sleep deprivation, hyperventilation, photic stimulation, and certain special electrodes (nasopharyngeal) may make certain seizure discharges more evident.

While the EEG may be helpful in detecting intracranial masses (owing to the appearance of slow delta waves) or subdural hematoma (locally decreased amplitude), CT and MRI are far superior. A normal EEG by no means excludes an intracranial mass lesion.

The EEG is commonly used for ongoing physiologic monitoring of the state of the brain during anesthesia, in cardiac and intracranial surgery, for ongoing assessment of the state of drug intoxication, metabolic encephalopathies, diffuse infections, and in severe trauma. An electrically silent or flat EEG has become an almost universal prerequisite for the diagnosis of brain death (see Chapter 15.3).

TECHNIQUE

The electroencephalographer must know which medications the patient is taking and the nature of the diagnostic problem because these influence the techniques that will be employed and the interpretation of the result. For example, if temporal lobe seizures are

suspected, recordings during sleep or specially placed electrodes may be required.

There are no significant risks to electroencephalography, although the patient who receives sedation for the recording should not drive for several hours thereafter.[4]

CORTICAL EVOKED POTENTIALS[1]

Stimulation of the visual, auditory, or somatosensory pathways produces transient potentials that can be recorded by electrodes along the sensory pathways, especially electrodes applied to the scalp. These potentials that are time-locked to the stimulus may be recorded by an electroencephalograph and averaged by computer. The evoked potentials thereby derived have a highly reproducible amplitude, latency, and waveform. Each peak or wave corresponds to a particular sensory relay, and alterations of the timing or amplitude of the wave reflect an abnormality at a certain anatomic site.

Visual evoked potentials were discovered first and are the most easily recorded. A flashing light or alternating light and dark pattern is displayed to the patient who fixates on the object with one eye alternately covered. The evoked potentials are recorded over the occiput. Visual evoked potentials give information about the eye, optic nerve, lateral geniculate, and occipital cortex but are most useful for abnormalities of the optic nerve itself. The detection of asymptomatic lesions in multiple sclerosis, evaluation of visual acuity in the very young or the retarded, and the distinction of blindness from malingering are particular indications.

Brain stem auditory evoked potentials (BSAER) are recorded over the scalp after a tone or click is introduced unilaterally into an earphone. The pathways measured include the auditory nerve itself, cochlear nucleus, olivary lateral lemniscus, inferior colliculus, thalamus, and auditory radiations of the temporal lobe. In practice, information about the peripheral auditory apparatus and brain stem may be derived from analysis of the potentials. BSAERs are particularly useful in the assessment of eighth nerve tumors, further characterization of audiometric abnormalities, the assessment of lesions that are placed ventrally in the pons and medulla (which include brain stem tumors), plaques in multiple sclerosis, and trauma to the brain stem.

Somatosensory evoked potentials are produced by stimulation of a peripheral nerve and recorded over the neck and scalp. Relays include the spinal cord, thalamus, and somatosensory cortex; the technique is most useful for disorders of the spinal cord and brain stem. Intraoperative recording of somatosensory potentials now routinely occurs during orthopedic and neurosurgical procedures to ensure integrity of the spinal cord or brain stem while they are manipulated. Maintenance of evoked potentials may be of prognostic value in cases of spinal trauma (see Chapter 15.19). They are also useful in following progress of patients with a variety of intraspinal abnormalities, particularly syringomyelia, intramedullary tumors, and spinal vascular malformations.

EXAMINATION OF THE CEREBROSPINAL FLUID[2]

Cerebrospinal fluid (CSF) is formed within the ventricular system by secretion from the choroid plexus and transudation of cerebral interstitial fluid. This fluid circulates through the ventricular foramina, down over the surface of the spinal cord and roots, and up through the basal cisterns to the sites of reabsorption over the surface of the brain. One ordinarily samples the spinal subarachnoid fluid via lumbar puncture to obtain information about intracranial pressure, composition of the CSF, and evidence of infection, infiltration, or cellular reaction from meningeal irritation.

AREAS OF USEFULNESS

Changes in the CSF may be diagnostic of intracranial infections or subarachnoid hemorrhages. Unless there is clear contraindication (coagulopathy or evidence of increased intracranial pressure), the CSF should be examined in anyone suspected of having meningitis, patients with a positive serologic test for syphilis, or those suspected of having neurosyphilis. Examination of the CSF is also important in many patients who have leukemia or lymphomas, certain solid tumors, or systemic vasculitis and in those who are immunocompromised, to ascertain involvement of the nervous system. Changes in the CSF are also important for diagnosing many primary diseases of the nervous system including multiple sclerosis, inflammatory neuropathies, and many inherited and degenerative neurological diseases. Often, a normal spinal fluid is an important pertinent negative finding, such as in the diagnosis of Alzheimer disease, metabolic encephalopathy, and idiopathic epilepsy. Stroke may cause red cells or xanthochromia, which indicates past intracranial bleeding, but it must be remembered that normal CSF findings do not exclude thrombosis, embolism, parenchymal intracranial hemorrhage, or epidural and subdural hematoma. The diagnosis of intracranial masses can be aided by finding either elevated protein or increased pressure, although primary diagnosis is more directly and safely accomplished by CT or MRI scans.

TECHNIQUE

Cerebrospinal fluid is usually sampled from the lumbar subarachnoid space, and proper positioning of the patient is essential for easy entry. The patient should lie on the side with the neck flexed and head supported by a pillow. The thighs should be flexed on the abdomen with the plane of the back perpendicular to the bed. The L4-L5 interspace may be identified by an imaginary line connecting the iliac crests. After the skin is cleaned with iodine and after the antiseptic has been removed with alcohol, the skin and intraspinous ligament are infiltrated with a local anesthetic and the lumbar puncture needle advanced. It should be kept parallel to the bed with the bevel turned upward to pass through the longitudinally running fibers of the dura. There is usually a distinct "pop" as the dura is penetrated. The stylet should be withdrawn periodically as the needle is advanced to determine if CSF is flowing. A stylet in the needle should always be used to avoid introduction of cutaneous tissue that can produce an intraspinal epidermoid inclusion cyst many years later.

After the needle has entered the subarachnoid space, particularly with an anxious or uncooperative patient, it is wise to remove a few drops of fluid for cell count before moving the patient. The patient is then allowed to extend the neck and thighs slowly to avoid spurious increase in the pressure measurement. The manometer is attached and the initial pressure measured. After removal of appropriate fluid for studies, a final pressure is determined and the needle withdrawn.

If the pressure is unexpectedly high, there will be enough fluid within the manometer for cell count, culture, and chemistries. It is important in this situation that no excess fluid be removed. Jugular compression (manometrics) may be useful to demonstrate spinal subarachnoid block but has receded from use as imaging techniques have improved.

The patient should be instructed to lie prone for 3 hours following lumbar puncture to allow the dural rent to close. Consuming fluids liberally may aid rapid replacement of CSF that has been removed.

RISKS[4]

Headache

The incidence of headache approached 25 percent in older series, but newer techniques (especially the use of 22- or 25-gauge small

spinal needles) has lowered the rate to about 10 percent. The size of the dural rent best predicts loss of CSF and subsequent headache. The headache is usually generalized, usually bifrontal and temporal, occasionally strictly occipital, and rarely unilateral. Nausea is occasional and vomiting very rare. Usually all symptoms disappear in a few hours following lumbar puncture, but they may persist for several days. Persistence for longer than a week suggests continuing CSF leak and requires further investigation. Pathophysiology of headache is presumed to be irritation of the basal meninges and blood vessels caused by "sagging" of the brain following removal of CSF.

Pain and Paresthesias

Radicular pain and paresthesias occur at the time of lumbar puncture in 10 to 15 percent of individuals but persist in about 0.1 percent, usually resolving within 1 year. Cranial nerve palsies, especially of the abducens, may immediately follow lumbar puncture or may appear after several weeks; they are thought to be caused by stretching of the long intracranial sixth nerve. Arachnoiditis occurs very rarely unless foreign materials (iodine, anesthetic agents, or adulterants) have been inadvertently introduced into the spinal subarachnoid space.

Cerebral Herniation

This is the most dreaded complication of lumbar punctures. Similarly, compression of the spinal cord can be precipitated by removing CSF below a block. Both complications can be prevented by performing CT or MRI scanning before the procedure. Clinical deterioration is a threat both when a mass is known to exist or when one can be expected to evolve rapidly, for instance in the stage of cerebritis before brain abscess. The risk is currently judged to be between about 10 and 20 percent when a mass is known to exist. Rapidly evolving lesions (brain abscess, parenchymal hemorrhage, and malignant tumors with extensive edema) and those in the posterior fossa are most likely to deteriorate, while slowly progressive lesions (small benign tumors, chronic subdural hematomas) are less likely to deteriorate (see Chapter 15.10). Occasionally, when meningitis is thought to coexist with a mass, lumbar puncture may be unavoidable. Alternatively, empiric treatment with antibiotics may be justified when a mass is large. Lumbar puncture with a known mass requires expert judgment, and consultation with the neurologist or neurosurgeon is mandatory.

EXAMINATIONS

Normally, the fluid is crystal clear, contains fewer than five mononuclear cells, and has a protein content of 45 mg/dl or less, of which 14 percent or less is gamma globulin; its glucose concentration is greater than half of the blood glucose, and it is under less than 180 mm of H_2O pressure.

Certain examinations should always be performed on the CSF, including description of its appearance, cell count and protein determination. Bacterial culture and glucose determinations are indicated when a white cell pleocytosis is found or infection otherwise suspected. Simultaneous blood sugar should also be obtained for comparison with CSF glucose. When infection, CSF inflammation, or subarachnoid hemorrhage is suspected, cell count should be performed immediately (in less than 15 to 30 minutes), as cells may rapidly lyse, causing ambiguities in interpretation.

Special studies of the CSF are indicated in certain circumstances: cytologic examination in a patient with cancer or certain fungal infections; myelin basic protein assay in multiple sclerosis and degenerative diseases of white matter; oligoclonal banding of IgG in multiple sclerosis, vasculitis, and infections; syphilis serology when serum serology is positive or when suspicion is high.

Specific patterns of cerebrospinal fluid abnormalities are discussed in appropriate chapters, including infections (Chapter 9.11), tumor (Chapter 15.10), cerebrovascular disease (Chapter 15.13), peripheral neuropathy (Chapter 15.16), and multiple sclerosis (Chapter 15.18).

NEUROPSYCHOLOGIC ASSESSMENT

Techniques derived from cognitive and sensory psychology may be applied to patients with neurologic disease. Patients who complain of failing memory, intellectual deterioration, spatial disorientation, a variety of sensory alterations, aphasia, agnosia, and apraxia may have their abnormalities characterized by careful neuropsychological study (see Chapter 15.4). The examinations themselves are complex and must be administered by a psychologist, neurologist, or psychiatrist who is experienced and has intimate knowledge of the patterns of neurologic disease. Unless the examination is tailored to the precise question being considered, misleading findings usually result. These findings are, however, frequently helpful in determining unsuspected cognitive abnormalities and may also provide reassurance for the patient or physician who fears an abnormality in the cognitive sphere when none actually exists.

Projective and nonprojective personality tests are helpful in the evaluation of patients who have neurologic symptoms that do not have a clear origin. In hysteria, somatization disorders (hypochondriasis), with the "worried well," and in conditions causing chronic pain, personality testing may indicate the roots of the problem and provide a fruitful rationale for therapy (see Chapter 16.4).

BIOPSY

Brain biopsy is used for the definitive diagnosis of brain tumor and for certain types of inflammatory, degenerative, or infectious diseases. Peripheral nerve biopsy, usually of the sural (a purely sensory) nerve, is valuable in specific diagnosis of familial, inflammatory, and certain metabolic defects of nerve, for example, metachromatic leukodystrophy and amyloidosis (see Chapter 15.16). Muscle biopsy is a routine, simple, and often essential part of the evaluation of patients with weakness (see Chapter 15.14). Fibroblasts derived from the conjunctiva or skin may be used to assay for specific enzymes and are used for the diagnosis of a variety of metabolic diseases in children and adults (see Section Five).

REFERENCES

1. Chiappa KH: Evoked Potentials in Clinical Neurology. New York, Raven Press, 1983
2. Fishman RA: Cerebrospinal Fluid and Diseases of the Nervous System. Philadelphia, WB Saunders, 1980
3. Kiloh LG, McComas AJ, et al: Clinical Electroencephalography, 4th ed. London, Butterworth, 1981
4. Moses H: Neurological complications of diagnostic and therapeutic procedures. In Asbury AK, McKhann GM, McDonald WI (eds): Diseases of the Nervous System. Philadelphia, WB Saunders, 1986
5. Newton TH, Potts DG (eds): Modern Neuroradiology, vols 1 and 2. San Anselmo, Calif, Clavadel Press, 1983

The Management of the Unconscious Patient

Hamilton Moses III

Stupor and coma are common medical conditions. Surgical anesthesia produces a controlled and readily reversible state of unconsciousness, whereas many general systemic derangements and diverse primary neurologic abnormalities produce coma, which may or may not be reversible. Nearly 5 percent of admissions to a busy hospital's emergency room are for stupor or coma, most commonly from drug intoxication and closed-head injuries. Of these, about three fifths are ultimately proved to have metabolic encephalopathy, one fifth supratentorial mass lesions, with the remaining fifth having subtentorial lesions or hysteria.[5]

The patient who presents in coma has a medical emergency. Chance of recovery often depends on the speed that specific therapy is begun; time must not be wasted. All physicians should have an organized approach to the unconscious patient that will ensure that: (1) Life-threatening metabolic derangements are treated, including hypotension, inadequate ventilation, and hypoglycemia. (2) The etiology of coma is determined by a brief but focused general examination of the body and assessment of neurologic integrity, with particular attention to functioning of the brain stem, and simultaneous additional history. (3) Steps are taken to avoid aspiration, sepsis, pulmonary embolism, and other risks to which patients in coma are predisposed.

DEFINITIONS

Consciousness may be defined as awareness of oneself and one's environment. Coma is a state in which the patient lies with the eyes closed and shows no psychologically understandable response to external stimuli or internal need. Between coma and full wakefulness lies a range of altered consciousness, including obtundation and stupor. These have in common an alteration in the *arousal* of consciousness that should be distinguished from delirium, dementia, and psychosis, in which the *content* of consciousness is disturbed.

Patients in *stupor* are initially unresponsive but can be aroused sufficiently to verbalize and demonstrate purposeful motor activity. *Coma* is a state of sleeplike unarousable unconsciousness without verbalization or purposeful motor response. The distinction of deep stupor from light coma is arbitrary, but these definitions provide workable nomenclature for use at the bedside.

PHYSIOLOGY OF CONSCIOUSNESS

Normal wakefulness requires the proper functioning of vital structures in the brain stem and one cerebral hemisphere. The critical brain stem structures for consciousness in man lie in the paramedian tegmental zone, which is ventral to the ventricular system, extending from the posterior hypothalamus to the midbrain-pontine junction. This area of the brain stem contains the ascending reticular formation, which projects to most areas of the cerebral cortex. Quite close to these brain stem structures lie nuclei and pathways important for certain brain stem reflexes, particularly those controlling oculomotor function, the pupils, facial movement, and skeletal muscle tone. Reflexes served by the lower brain stem (caudad to the midpons), particularly respiration, may be impaired in deep coma.

One, but not both, of the cerebral hemispheres is required for preservation of consciousness. Rarely, a large dominant hemispheral lesion may produce brief unconsciousness; generally, however, coma caused by cerebral cortical abnormalities implies a bilateral and diffuse (usually metabolic) depression of the hemispheres. Commonly, an expanding lesion of one cerebral hemisphere may impair the function of the opposite cerebral hemisphere or of the brain stem by a shift of intracranial structures. These cerebral *herniations* are fully discussed in Chapter 15.10.

MECHANISMS

Metabolic coma is produced by a variety of general systemic conditions and many intoxications (Table 15.3–1). In only a few instances is the precise pathophysiologic cause understood. For most metabolic processes it remains unresolved whether a generalized defect occurs simultaneously throughout many areas of the brain or whether a more selective abnormality of a specific neuronal system (such as the reticular activating system or basal forebrain) is responsible. Generalized impairment of energy metabolism is important in hypoxia and hypoglycemia, which lead to immediate neurologic deficit from lack of energy substrate. Deficiency of vitamin cofactors (particularly thiamine), hypothyroidism, and carbon monoxide poisoning also interfere with energy metabolism. Acidosis, alkalosis, hypokalemia, and the hypo- and hyperosmolar states produce enzymatic and membrane abnormalities that interfere with both normal metabolism and neurotransmission. In most of the common causes of coma, such as diabetic ketoacidosis, uremia, hepatic coma, and the coma that occurs with sepsis, however, the pathophysiologic mechanism is unclear. In these conditions, neuronal membrane abnormalities, interference with synaptic transmission, and certain vascular alterations have all been indicted. Many "depressant" drugs such as alcohol, barbiturates, benzodiazepines, and anticonvulsants exert their primary effect via inhibition of neuronal firing by depressing membrane excitability. Selective blockade of neurotransmitters without general metabolic or membrane effect can be implicated with anticholinergic (central muscarinic antagonist, atropine-like drugs).

Transitory mechanical disruption in neural pathways, particularly those in the brain stem, produces coma, as with the concussion of closed head injury (see Chapter 15.9). Axonal processes are particularly vulnerable to shearing forces. Mass lesions produce direct pressure on critical brain stem structures through herniations. They also exert a variety of secondary metabolic defects at some distance from the primary mass. Local ionic alterations and ischemia produced by abnormalities in cerebral blood flow are particularly important examples. Although the mechanisms that produce coma are diverse, clinical signs occur in highly predictable patterns, and a proper diagnosis can usually be derived from just a few quickly obtainable bedside observations.

CLINICAL EXAMINATION[2]

The vital signs should be quickly measured and appropriate steps for resuscitation immediately begun if any are impaired. The physician should particularly guard against hypoxia, hypercarbia, and

TABLE 15.3–1. CLINICAL FEATURES OF DISORDERS THAT COMMONLY CAUSE COMA

Disease Process	Common Clinical Features
Focal Structural Lesions	
Supratentorial	Commonly characterized by the syndrome of uncal herniation: dilated pupil proceeding to full third nerve palsy; ipsilateral or contralateral hemiparesis; finally, brain stem signs appear
Intrahemispheric hemorrhage	Apoplectic onset of hemiplegia, aphasia, or hemianopia followed by coma
Subdural hematoma	Hemianopia uncommon; trauma, anticoagulants, coagulopathy all predispose
Infarction	Lateralizing neurologic signs are followed by coma if cerebral edema causes shift of intracranial contents or if metabolic derangement occurs
Tumor (primary or metastatic)	Syndrome of uncal herniation is common; sudden deterioration may occur with hemorrhage into tumor
Abscess	Headache and fever may precede obtundation; cyanotic congenital heart disease, alcoholism, pneumonia, sepsis, sinus infections or direct trauma predispose; lumbar puncture is especially hazardous
Trauma	Coma may be due to concussion, subdural hematoma, epidural hematoma, cerebral laceration, brain stem injury
Infratentorial	
Compressive lesions (cerebellar hemorrhage, infarction, tumor)	Occipital headache, vertigo and vomiting leading to coma with gaze palsy, facial palsy, and irregular respiration; surgical treatment may be life saving
Intrinsic lesions (pontine hemorrhage or infarction)	Apoplectic onset, pinpoint pupils, ocular bobbing; quadriplegia, bifacial weakness, early respiratory failure; distinguish from locked-in syndrome
Diffuse Brain Disease	
Drug intoxications	Pupillary light responses preserved except for glutethimide, atropine and massive barbiturates; small reactive pupils characteristic of narcotic overdose; vestibulo-ocular reflex often abnormal; respiration often depressed except for hyperventilation in salicylism
Metabolic disturbances	Tremor, asterixis, multifocal myoclonus, abnormal respiratory patterns are common findings; pupillary and vestibulo-ocular reflexes usually preserved
Hypoglycemia	Coma may be preceded by bizarre behavior, restlessness, anxiety and sweating; hypothermia is common; tachycardia may be absent
Uncontrolled diabetes mellitus	Usually caused by hyperosmolality or sometimes lactic acidosis, when patient is usually in shock
Hypernatremia	Often iatrogenic (e.g., tube feeding and failure to hydrate adequately); requires slow correction to avoid cerebral edema
Hyponatremia	Often iatrogenic (from diuretics or volume overload) or as part of the syndrome of inappropriate ADH secretion; seizures are commonly an early feature
Renal failure	Coma may be from uremia or dialysis dysequilibrium syndrome
Hypercalcemia	Common in patients with cancer; coma preceded by mental changes
Hypocalcemia	Convulsions and tetany are features
Myxedema	Hypothemia and pseudomyotonic stretch reflexes are characteristic
Pulmonary insufficiency	Asterixis and multifocal myoclonus are common; papilledema may occur
Nutritional deficiency	Thiamine deficiency (Wernicke encephalopathy) characterized by abnormal eye movements, memory loss, and delirium progressing to coma
Disturbance of body temperature	
Hyperthermia	Heat stroke characterized by sudden disturbance of consciousness and convulsions
Hypothermia	Pale skin, shallow respiration; no shivering occurs if body temperature falls below about 30C
Global hypoxia or ischemia	
Cardiopulmonary arrest, pulmonary embolism	Sudden onset; convulsions and extensor posturing are common; may be precipitated by sedative drugs
Strangulation or drowning	
Widespread emboli (e.g., fat emboli)	(Follows fractures of long bones; petechiae frequently present over chest)
Widespread thrombosis (e.g., thrombotic thrombocytopenic purpura)	
Encephalitis and meningitis	Fever; stiff neck; coexistent site of infection
Subarachnoid hemorrhage	Stiff neck (note: though neck stiffness may be prominent in an awake or stuporous patient, in coma it may disappear)
Seizures and the postictal state	Motor convulsions may be slight or absent
Psychogenic Unresponsiveness	Blepharospasm; nystagmus response to minimal caloric stimulation of vestibuloocular reflex; variable signs over short periods of observation

hypotension as the damaged brain is unduly sensitive to even minor alterations (see Chapter 4.9). An odor about the patient may suggest diabetic ketoacidosis, fetor hepaticus, or the smell of alcohol. The skull and body should be searched for signs of obvious external trauma. Examination of the chest may reveal signs of pneumonia (indicating aspiration or a cause of primary sepsis); cardiac examination may reveal signs of pulmonary edema (often coexisting with acutely increased intracranial pressure), valvular heart disease, or endocarditis. Hepatic enlargement, abdominal masses, or signs of abdominal catastrophe may all point to a systemic cause of coma.

Three sets of neurologic observations are especially important in the examination of the unconscious patient: the level of responsiveness, the brain stem reflexes, and vegetative functions (see Table 15.3–2). These observations may be carried out within just a few minutes at the bedside and when properly interpreted may enable the distinction of supratentorial lesions, infratentorial lesions, or metabolic encephalopathy.

LEVEL OF CONSCIOUSNESS

The patient should be briefly observed from a distance, with spontaneous eye opening, motor responses, and verbalization noted. If there is no spontaneous movement he or she should be repeatedly called, touched, or vigorously shaken, or firm pressure applied to the supraorbital ridge or nail bed. Excessively noxious stimuli should be avoided, as they rarely provide additional information. The examiner should carefully note the verbal, motor, or autonomic response to each of these maneuvers. The patient may make a purposeful action (open the eyes, look to the examiner, and remove the stimulated limb) or may be capable of only stereotyped reflex movements, such as posturing accompanied by autonomic arousal.

Motor responses to stimuli should be carefully evaluated with particular attention to response of the upper limbs. Extension of the neck, extension of the arms at the elbows, accompanied by extension of the leg, is often called "decerebrate" posturing but probably localizes only to the low brain stem. Extension of the

TABLE 15.3–2. SYSTEM FOR EXAMINATION OF UNCONSCIOUS PATIENT

Level of consciousness
- Eye opening
- Motor response
- Verbal response

Brain stem reflexes
- Pupillary light reflex
- Corneal reflex
- Vestibulo-ocular reflex

Vegetative functions
- Respiration
- Blood pressure
- Pulse
- Temperature

Motor examination
- Muscle tone
- Deep tendon reflexes
- Plantar responses

General examination
- Ocular fundus
- Skull
- Ears (gross and otoscopic)
- Spine
- Chest
- Heart
- Skin

neck, flexion of the arms at the elbows, with extension of the legs has been called "decorticate" posturing and usually implies diencephalic or bilateral hemispheral abnormalities. Extension of the upper limbs accompanied by flexion at the hips and knees suggests a structural lesion of the pons. The terms "decerebrate" and "decorticate" are inaccurate; it is best to describe the specific motor reactions.

The verbal response of the patient to noxious stimuli should be graded as being absent, incomprehensible (verbalization with no recognizable words), inappropriate, or normal.

BRAIN STEM REFLEXES

Although asymmetry of the stretch reflexes may be of lateralizing value, the brain stem reflexes are usually more important in the diagnosis of coma. The neural circuits responsible for the pupillary light reflex, corneal reflex, and vestibulo-ocular reflex lie close to those tegmental structures responsible for consciousness. Loss of any of these reflexes may enable the clinician to identify the level of the brain stem at which disease is present.

The size and shape of the pupils should be noted with their response to bright light. Pinpoint pupils strongly suggest a pontine lesion. A unilaterally fixed pupil suggests *uncal* herniation and compression of the peripheral third nerve. This sign may precede disturbance of consciousness or any motor deficit (see Chapter 15.10). Bilaterally dilated, fixed pupils suggest a tectal lesion. Pupillary responses are important in differentiating structural from metabolic or toxic diseases. With the exception of glutethimide and massive poisoning with central nervous system (CNS) depressants, the pupils usually remain reactive to light in metabolic or toxic encephalopathy.

The *corneal reflex* tests the V, VII, and III cranial nerves. Bell phenomenon—upward deviation of the globes with eye closure—implies intact connections from the trigeminal to the oculomotor nucleus and intact lid closure implies integrity of the connections between the trigeminal and facial nuclei. In most unconsciousness patients, the eyelids are tonically closed, and if they are opened by the examiner, they slowly close again. Sudden closing or blepharospasm suggests either psychogenic unresponsiveness or mild metabolic encephalopathy.

Eye movements are most important in evaluation of coma. In light coma, spontaneous, slow, usually horizontal movements occur; these are called *roving eye movements*. Sustained lateral conjugate deviation of the eyes suggests disease of the ipsilateral cerebral hemisphere or contralateral pons. Downward deviation of the eyes with convergence is seen with thalamic lesions. Ocular bobbing (rapid downward movement followed by slow return to primary position) classically occurs with pontine lesions. After noting spontaneous movements, the eyes should be induced to move by stimulating the *vestibulo-ocular reflex*. This can be done in two ways. The first consists of rotating the head from side to side, the so-called doll's eyes maneuver. *This should not be performed if there is a suspicion of trauma to the neck or spine until a fracture has been excluded.* In light coma, the eyes make a full horizontal conjugate excursion, but if the level of consciousness deteriorates, these movements may become less, and eventually the eyes are fixed to midposition. Internuclear ophthalmoplegia (Chapter 15.6) is evident by slow or restricted movements of the adducting eye compared with the abducting eye. A second method of stimulating the vestibulo-ocular reflex consists of irrigating the external auditory meati of the ears with cold water. The tympanic membrane should first be checked and then initially 10 ml of ice water should be introduced slowly. In mild impairment of consciousness or psychogenic unresponsiveness, nystagmus may be present with the rapid phase away from the side of caloric stimulation. In coma, caloric stimulation may produce a tonic deviation of the eyes toward the side of the stimulated labyrinth. Sometimes this tonic response is disconju-

gate, owing to internuclear ophthalmoplegia. Up to 100 ml of iced water should be infused before the caloric response can be pronounced as absent. If the vestibulo-ocular reflex is abnormal, but other brain stem or motor responses are preserved, disease of the pons or medulla should be considered. Isolated disturbance of the vertical doll's eye maneuver implies disease of the midbrain. In contrast to the pupillary light response, the vestibulo-ocular reflex is readily depressed by sedative and tranquilizing drugs.

VEGETATIVE FUNCTIONS

Disturbance of respiration is very common in unconscious patients. Metabolic encephalopathy is often distinguished by abnormal respiratory pattern such as Kussmaul breathing from diabetic ketoacidosis; hyperventilation is also seen with other causes of metabolic acidosis, such as salicylate intoxication and sepsis. Structural lesions in the nervous system also cause abnormal respiration. Bilateral cortical dysfunction, as with hypotension, sedative drug intoxication, and direct vascular lesions, produces periodic (Cheyne-Stokes) respiration. Midbrain damage is associated with rapid regular respiration (central neurogenic hyperventilation). Lesions of the pontine-medullary junction may cause irregular or ataxic breathing. Medullary lesions produce hypoventilation or apnea, which is very commonly associated with secondary systemic hypotension or cardiac arrhythmias.

Hypotension may be encountered in severe sedative drug intoxications, usually when coma is deep and after respiratory depression has occurred. *Hypertension* may reflect the disease process responsible for the coma or concomitant hypoxia, or it may be the result of brain stem dysfunction itself (see Chapter 15.6). The Cushing response, which consists of an increase in systemic blood pressure accompanied by bradycardia secondary to a rise in intracranial pressure, is more common with compressive lesions in the posterior fossa and acute increases in intracranial pressure; it is most frequently encountered in children.

Fever may reflect disease processes causing coma, such as meningitis or anticholinergic overdose, or it may reflect an abnormality of hypothalamic or brain stem function, particularly following severe head injury and subarachnoid hemorrhage.

TABLE 15.3–3. IMMEDIATE MANAGEMENT OF COMA[a]

First aid
- Assure airway and respiration: Observe for stridor, cyanosis, intercostal retraction; intubate trachea when in doubt; place in lateral decubitus position; clear mouth of foreign material; suction or place nasogastric tube with caution; intubate trachea first
- Assure circulation: Mean pressure of 80–90 mm Hg is sufficient in nearly all adults; elevate feet, expand volume, use pressors to reach this range; correct cardiac dysrhythmias
- Correct hypoglycemia: Give 50 ml of 50 percent glucose in water intravenously *after first drawing blood* for laboratory evaluation; do not wait for blood measurements; do not rely on bedside strip estimates. Extra glucose will do no harm. (Glucose should be avoided in ischemic infarction)
- Lower elevated intracranial pressure (Chapter 4.9)
- Control seizures (Chapter 4.8)
- Treat infection (Chapter 9.11)
- Restore normal body temperature (Chapter 4.11)
- Correct electrolytes and acid–base disturbance (Chapter 10.4)
- Administer thiamine (Chapter 17.5)
- Consider specific antidotes, especially naloxone if opiate poisoning is suspected (Chapter 4.10)

Obtain a history
- Talk to family, witnesses, ambulance crew

Rapid examination: See Table 15.3–2

Adapted from Plum F, Posner J: The Diagnosis of Stupor in Coma. Philadelphia, FA Davis, 1980.[5]

IMMEDIATE MANAGEMENT

Most unconscious patients require immediate measures to protect the airway and maintain oxygenation and adequate circulation (Table 15.3–3). Endotracheal intubation should be performed if there is any doubt about the patient's ventilatory ability, or if the patient is at risk of aspiration, such as when vomiting. Suctioning or an attempt at passing an intragastric tube can precipitate vomiting. Endotracheal intubation should be done first; it is easier and safer when done electively, more hazardous when done as an emergency.

Hypotension may produce coma by bilateral cerebral ischemia. This may occur when the systolic blood pressure falls below 60 mm Hg in the young adult or 80 or about 90 mm Hg in an older individual. Hypotension should be treated by elevation of the legs, volume expansion, use of pressor agents, and treatment of the cause of systemic hypotension (see Chapter 4.3).

Hypoglycemia is another acute threat that should be treated by intravenous administration of 50 ml of 50 percent glucose in water. As an intravenous line is being established, blood should first be drawn and sent for glucose and other estimations (Table 15.3–4). Glucose should be given, however, without waiting for the results of laboratory tests, unless a vascular lesion or mass is strongly suspected from the history.

Other emergency measures include treatment of seizures, restoration of normal body temperatures, reduction of elevated intracranial pressure, correction of electrolyte and acid–base disturbance, and consideration of specific treatments: thiamine for Wernicke encephalopathy and naloxone for opiate poisoning.

If trauma is known or suspected, all manipulations of the patient should be done with caution, particularly avoiding movement of the head and neck to avoid further spinal injury.

TABLE 15.3–4. LABORATORY TESTS FOR THE EVALUATION OF COMA

Venous blood tests
- Glucose[a]
- Electrolytes[a]
- Urea[a] and creatinine[a]
- Osmolality[a]
- Ammonia
- Liver enzymes
- Hematocrit[a]
- White blood count with differential platelet estimate[a]
- Toxicology screen (also urine toxicology screen)
- Arterial blood gases[a]
- Electrocardiogram[a]

CT scan
Particularly valuable in unexplained coma, where neurological signs are present to suggest a structural cause

Lumbar puncture
Safe when focal neurological signs are absent and the fundi are normal; must be performed *without delay* when a meningeal infection is suspected; if a CT scan is immediately available, do it first, but do not delay lumbar puncture if meningitis is strongly suspected
- CSF examination[a]
- Glucose, protein
- Cell counts
- Gram stain

Electroencephalogram
Usually not helpful immediately; may help distinguish metabolic from structural causes; limited prognostic value

Evoked potentials
Unproven value; adds little to bedside examination, but may have some prognostic value in prolonged coma

[a]Tests to be considered first.

As all of these emergency measures are being carried out, a history should be obtained from the patient's family and friends. Such information is vital, and if it cannot be obtained from witnesses, then sometimes telephone calls to the patient's family or physician will provide important data. The patient's belongings should be carefully searched for medications and other clues. Ideally, an unconscious patient should receive emergency therapy from one physician, an initial examination from another, while a third person is obtaining history from other parties.

Once emergency measures have been performed and vital signs are stable, a more detailed examination of the patient, further blood studies, and appropriate radiographic examinations may be performed.

A CT scan plays an important role in the definitive diagnosis of the cause of coma and should be performed promptly unless a toxic or metabolic cause is evident from the history and the initial examination. If focal abnormalities are present, if a reliable history is unavailable, or if clinical information seems conflicting a CT scan should be performed. A CT scan is mandatory for a patient in coma who has had obvious head trauma; it should also be performed in the patient who is at risk of having previously had unapparent trauma, such as the alcoholic and those patients who are old, demented, or have systemic abnormalities that would predispose to secondary intracranial abnormalities (endocarditis, coagulopathy, cancer).

Early in the evaluation of the unconscious patient, a decision must be made whether to perform a lumbar puncture. The most pressing indication for lumbar puncture in coma is the suspicion of central nervous system infection. The latter may be suggested by fever or neck stiffness, although signs of meningeal irritation are usually absent in very young or very old patients as well as in those in deep coma. If meningitis is strongly suspected on the basis of history (as discussed in Chapter 9.11), lumbar puncture should be performed without delay. If the history is ambiguous or if focal neurological abnormalities are evident on examination, lumbar puncture should be postponed until after the CT scan. If CT scanning is not immediately available, empirical therapy should be begun immediately with the choice of antibiotics made on the basis of the most likely causative organism (see Table 9.11–3).

DETERMINING THE PROGNOSIS IN THE UNCONSCIOUS PATIENT[1,3,4]

Whether a patient will fully or partially recover from a disease that causes coma depends on how quickly resuscitative measures are begun as well as the nature and severity of the underlying process. For instance, a patient with ischemic encephalopathy from hypotension caused by hypovolemia may fully recover if treated promptly and the coma is short. Likewise, a patient with bacterial meningitis may fully recover if the diagnosis is immediately recognized and appropriate antibiotics are begun. In contrast, the patient with pontine infarction, severe and prolonged hypoxia, or head injury may have prolonged coma and never fully recover.

Because of the variability of recovery from coma, several prospective studies have been undertaken to determine the prognosis of coma secondary to neurologic disease and head trauma. Several clinical signs may be used early in coma to indicate the likely outcome. Thus patients who, 24 hours after entering in coma, still lack corneal, pupillary, and vestibulo-ocular reflexes, are most unlikely to regain independent function. Conversely, patients who within 24 hours have intact brain stem reflexes, open their eyes, and make purposeful motor reactions have a favorable prognosis for recovery of intellectual function and independent existence. Exceptions to these prognostic indicators do occur, particularly when patients are young and have suffered head trauma. Particular care should be taken to exclude the effects of drugs, hypothermia, and secondary systemic illnesses (such as sepsis, fluid or electrolyte

abnormalities, or hypothermia) that depress brain stem reflexes and may therefore make the neurologic injury seem more severe. When such secondary processes are corrected, the prognosis may be excellent. Current neurologic methods allow prediction of the outcome of coma with a certainty of between 5 and 10 percent, although new observations and continuing study of these patients may improve certainty. Because of this level of uncertainty, however, dogmatic predictions about individual patients are not warranted and have limited clinical utility.

The electroencephalogram is of limited prognostic value. Auditory evoked potentials do provide confirmation of brain stem integrity, but they are not superior to bedside clinical examination.

A small number of comatose patients (usually after ischemic lesions or trauma) recover consciousness but remain in a *vegetative state*. These patients have spontaneous eye opening and maintain sleep-wake cycles. They show certain spontaneous motor activity, such as saccadic eye movements and chewing movement; nevertheless, they behaviorally show no psychologically understandable response. Bilateral frontal lesions or lesions of the rostral midbrain commonly produce the vegetative state. These patients may slowly improve over some months, but they rarely achieve functional recovery, proper use of language, or movements other than the most primitive.

THE LOCKED-IN SYNDROME

Some patients with pontine lesions appear to be in coma but are actually awake and alert, suffering from paralysis of eye movements and quadriplegia. Lesions of the pontine base that spare the tegmentum interrupt decending motor fibers and the centers of horizontal eye movement, while allowing vertical eye movements, producing a patient who is fully awake but who is "locked in" his own body. Vascular occlusions, brain stem encephalitis, vasculitis, and rarely trauma may lead to this syndrome. It should not be overlooked and may be suspected when motion of the eyelids and vertical eye movements persist. Respiratory function is variably affected, but locked-in patients are nearly always mute; some have established effective communication by indicating Morse code with their eyes.

BRAIN DEATH

Over the last three decades great advances in resuscitation, life support, and the use of antibiotics have allowed the heart, lungs, kidneys, and other parenchymal organs to work well while the brain has become irreversibly and totally damaged. Patients who have suffered cardiac arrest, severe hypotension, anesthetic or surgical misfortunes, as well as trauma and major strokes commonly suffer irreversible brain damage, resulting in cessation of all cerebral hemisphere and brain stem activity. These patients can be maintained on respiratory and vascular support for days, weeks, or months after their injury. After a variable interval, however, failure of the systemic organs inexorably follows, although the time may be prolonged and the anguish great. As failure of systemic organs is reliably predicted by irreversible total brain failure, most physicians, legal authorities, religious groups, and philosophic scholars have agreed that total and irreversible failure of the brain is sufficient to diagnose death. Many states have enacted statutes recognizing the certainty of this prediction.

Brain death can be diagnosed if certain criteria are met: the cause, nature, and duration of coma must be specifically known (Table 15.3–5). Metabolic derangements, drug intoxications, and hypothermia must be excluded. The patient must be observed by a responsible physician, usually a neurologist or neurosurgeon, over a period of time (usually 6 to 24 hours). Examination must show no motor responses to noxious stimuli, and brain stem re-

TABLE 15.3–5. CRITERIA FOR BRAIN DEATH

Prerequisites
1. Known and untreatable structural damage to the brain.
   Note: Excludes patients who are dead on arrival or who suffer out of hospital cardiac arrest.
      or
2. Irreversible systemic metabolic derangement.
   Note: Some authors hesitate to diagnose brain death that arises from metabolic causes as these sometimes prove capriciously reversible, particularly when present for only a short time.
3. Absence of hypothermia.
4. Absence of cardiovascular shock.
5. Observation and repeat examination after 6 hours.
   Note: The duration of observation has been gradually shortened. Six hours is the current standard, though 12 to 24 hours is required in some centers.

Clinical criteria
1. Absent brain stem function.
   a. Fixed and dilated pupils.
      Note: Requiring dilated pupils is an added safety to exclude inadvertent drug intoxication.
   b. No oculovestibular response to 100 ml of instilled ice water (ice water calorics).
   c. Absent corneal and pharyngeal reflexes.
   d. Apnea (with hypercarbic stimulation).
2. Absent cerebral function.
   a. No behavioral or reflex response to noxious stimuli that imply function above the level of the foramen magnum. (Note: Spinal reflexes may be preserved and their presence does not preclude diagnosis of brain death.)
      Note: Areflexia is common after severe brain injury. However, as the duration of absent cerebral function lengthens, it becomes more likely for spinal reflexes to reappear.
   b. Electroencephalogram isoelectric for 30 minutes at high sensitivities. (Performed by a qualified electroencephalographer, under the direction of the director of electroencephalography laboratory, using the accepted World Health Organization technique.)

Special cases:
1. Brain death in children is controversial. Many authors have recommended that conventional criteria for death be used in children since no criteria for brain death have been validated in them.
2. When the patient is a potential donor of organs for transplantation, the patient's primary physician should solicit consultation with a neurologist or neurosurgeon, who should examine the patient, coordinate the ancillary investigations, and document them in the chart. The primary physician has first and final responsibility for all aspects of care and for pronouncing death.
   Note: It is imperative for the primary physician to remain in charge. No primary physician should abrogate his position concerning management, the time of death, or prospective transplantation.
3. Therapeutic drug-induced coma. Absent cerebral blood flow as measured by bilateral carotid and arch angiography precludes functioning of the brain and will be required.

flexes must be absent (this is a point of minor controversy, as some centers allow spinal reflexes to be preserved). Patients must have apnea in the presence of elevated carbon dioxide tension, thus assuring adequate respiratory drive. Ancillary neurologic tests are of confirmatory value. Particularly, the electroencephalogram should be isoelectric for 30 minutes with recordings obtained by a qualified electroencephalographer at high sensitivities. Absent brainstem-evoked potentials and absent cerebral blood flow, as determined by bilateral carotid angiography, CT, or radionucleid methods, are currently under investigation. They may also prove to be of confirmatory value.

If these criteria are met, the physician may diagnose brain death even if the systemic circulation is maintained or spinal reflexes persist. The physician primarily responsible for the patient has an obligation to the patient and the patient's family to apply these criteria properly in a timely manner and with attention to the details of the bedside clinical examination and the performance of ancillary investigations. In practice, most centers require consultation of the neurologist and neurosurgeon, particularly when organ transplantation or medical-legal issues coexist.

REFERENCES

1. Caronna JM, Levy DE: Neurological manifestations of cardiac disease. In Asbury AK, McKhann GM, McDonald WI (eds): Diseases of the Nervous System. Philadelphia, WB Saunders, 1986, p 1449
2. Fisher CM: The neurological examination of the comatose patient. ACTA Neurol Scand 36(Suppl):1, 1966
3. Jennett E, Teasdale G, et al: Prognosis of patients with severe head injury. Neurosurg 4:283, 1979
4. Levy DB, Caronna JM, et al: Prognosis in non-traumatic coma. Ann Intern Med 94:293, 1981
5. Plum F, Posner J: The Diagnosis of Stupor in Coma. Philadelphia, FA Davis, 1980

Aphasia and Disorders of Cognitive Function

Barry Gordon and Hamilton Moses III

NORMAL LANGUAGE PROCESSING

To understand what happens in disease, it is important to understand how the brain normally processes language.

Speech and language depend upon the left cerebral hemisphere in almost all right-handed and most left-handed people (Fig. 15.4–1). Specific areas of the cortex have more or less specific functions. The primary auditory cortex (on the dorsal aspect of the temporal lobe, Fig. 15.4–1) receives the acoustic input and passes it on to Wernicke area and adjacent cortical areas (the supramarginal and angular gyri). There, the sound waves are transformed as meaningful speech sounds (phonemes) and then into their actual meanings. The angular gyrus is probably also where visual symbols (written words) are translated into their meanings. It is not understood where our own inner speech originates, but it is probably also channeled through these centers. To speak, language information is transmitted by the arcuate fasciculus (and probably other paths) to Broca area in the inferior frontal lobe, where it is converted into motor commands. The commands are sent from Broca area to nearby areas in the motor strip, which are the cortical areas for control of the speech musculature. These areas in turn control the brain stem nuclei of the cranial nerves and the centers of respiration to orchestrate the speech act. Overall, we can think of these processes as the input (receptive), central, and output (expressive) functions necessary for normal speech.

Damage or interference with the function of these brain regions will disrupt speech. This disruption can have a number of possible etiologies: ischemia, hemorrhage, tumor, or even seizure or migraine-associated vasospasm, to give some examples. As with any neurologic disorder, proper diagnosis depends upon accurate recognition of the patient's symptoms, knowledge of their time course, and the approximate anatomic assignment that this outline can give.

EXAMINATION AND DIAGNOSTIC SYNDROMES[2,4]

The most important first steps of the examination are to obtain the history of what happened, either from the patient or other observers, and the background information about the patient: handedness, education, ability to read and write. Knowing the temporal evolution of the problem will help define its etiology; knowing the patient's background will help determine which aspects of speech predate the immediate problem (for example, stuttering or inability to read and write), and which represent new problems.

The next vital step (which can often be done while getting the history) is to *listen* to the patient's speech (see Table 15.4–1).

How the patient's speech is produced is important information. Note whether the individual speech sounds are distorted or slurred (dysarthria) or whether they are being produced correctly despite other speech problems. At this point, it is important to distinguish between *dysarthria* and *aphasia*.

Dysarthria is difficulty with articulation caused by impaired motor control of the tongue, lips, palate, pharynx, larynx, and respiratory muscles. Dysarthria can therefore be caused by a wide variety of lesions of either or both cerebral hemispheres, the basal ganglia, the brain stem, cerebellum, or the muscles themselves. Some features of dysarthric speech that can be appreciated clinically often permit a broad functional grouping that narrows the etiologic possibilities (Table 15.4–2).

Aphasia (dysphasia) is a true disturbance of language and therefore implies a cerebral lesion, usually on the left, and usually cortical. Aphasia implies a deficit in more than one modality. There are three common patterns of aphasic disorder, which correspond to the distinction between receptive and expressive speech processes: Broca aphasia (expressive aphasia), Wernicke aphasia (receptive aphasia), and mixed aphasia (features of both other types) (see Table 15.4–3).

To help gauge the *expressive* component of the patient's speech, continue listening to the speech output. Note the degree of effort the patient uses to speak, the rate of speech, and its rhythm. In *Broca (expressive) aphasia*, there is relatively little speech produced, and the remaining speech is produced with great effort, slowly and haltingly, without the normal rhythms and flow of speech (nonfluent aphasia). Speech is often dysarthric as well. Although relatively few words can be spoken, the ones produced are usually nouns or verbs so that the patient's intended meaning can often be understood ("telegraphic speech"). In *Wernicke (receptive)*

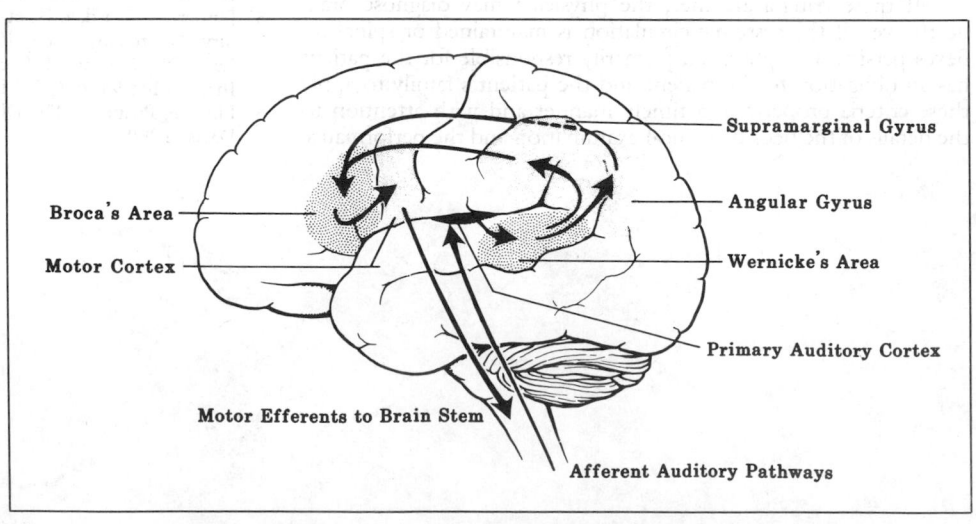

Figure 15.4–1. Speech and speech-related areas of left hemisphere.

TABLE 15.4–1. CLINICAL EXAMINATION OF APHASIA

Clinical Task	Observation

Spontaneous speech	Pronunciation/dysarthria
	Rate (fast, slow, or normal)
	Effort
	Rhythm (prosody)
	Content:
	  Phonemic (literal) paraphasias:
	    sound substitutions
	  Semantic (verbal) paraphasias:
	    word substitutions
	  Neologisms
	  Types of words preserved/
	    omitted

Comprehension of spoken language: Yes-no questions, simple commands, pointing to objects	Kinds of difficulty and types of errors (controlling for expressive difficulties)
Repetition: Digits, words, sentences	Abilities/inabilities and types of errors
Naming objects, body parts	Abilities/inabilities and types of errors
Reading aloud Comprehension: Written commands, questions, etc.	Reading aloud may be impaired by both receptive and expressive problems Reading comprehension requires only receptive abilities
Writing	Difficulty with letter production Difficulty spelling Neologisms Omission of words Disorganization of words

aphasia, by contrast, speech is usually of normal speed and rhythm (fluent), and there is usually no expressive motor deficit. (Sometimes, a patient will have a great deal of difficulty finding the words to say—*anomia*.) This is common, for example, in fatigue, and more pronounced in metabolic encephalopathies (see Chapter 16.7). Speech in anomia is often slow and halting, too.

What the patient is able to say is also important. Does the patient get the meaning across with the few words he is able to say (telegraphic speech, characteristic of an expressive or Broca aphasia), or are there a number of apparently mispronounced, mischosen, or completely unintelligible words that generally make it difficult, if not impossible, to understand the patient? These distortions are termed paraphasias (when the sounds or the words are mischosen) and neologisms (when the sound is not a real word at all). Paraphasias and neologisms can be normal when they are occasional or rare errors; they occur in a wide variety of aphasias, but are particularly characteristic of Wernicke aphasia. At times, the Wernicke speech is so distorted that it sounds like a foreign language (jargon aphasia).

The next part of the examination is to test *receptive* speech functions by checking how well the patient obeys spoken commands, answers yes-no questions, or understands questions, for example, "Can cows fly?" or "Is there ice in Antarctica?" Be careful not to give the patient hints as to the intended response by gesturing or giving the words special emphasis, as is often natural. In Broca aphasia, comprehension of spoken and written speech is fairly good clinically. By contrast, in Wernicke aphasia, comprehension of speech is typically very poor.

Repetition tests how well speech input and output work without asking for comprehension. It is tested by asking the patient to repeat digits, words, and sentences. In Broca aphasia, repetition will be fairly accurate, but slow, halting, and probably dysarthric. In Wernicke aphasia, the patient will probably not be able to repeat or will give a fluent but hopelessly garbled rendition of what was asked.

Finally, reading, writing, and object naming can be checked to determine the status of other input and output routes from the cerebral language areas. Have the patient read a paragraph from a newspaper and report on its meaning; have him write a brief description of the room; show him common items and parts of common items (a watch, the watchband) and ask for their names. In Broca aphasia, naming is often slow but fairly accurate (although corrupted by dysarthria); reading is slow, but comprehension is good; writing is slow, laborious, and poorly done when it can be done at all (with the left hand). In Wernicke aphasia, naming is often rapid but inaccurate (paraphasic or neologistic); reading is very poor or impossible; writing is fluent, but the words or letter combinations make no sense.

TABLE 15.4–2. DYSARTHRIA: DISORDERED ARTICULATION

Type	Site/Nature of Lesion	Associated Features	Common Causes
Inarticulate/slurred	Paralysis or incoordination of tongue, pharynx		Brain stem or hemispheral lesion (either side); local lesions of tongue, mouth; intoxication by drug, alcohol
Nasal	Soft palate; IX or X cranial N. or nuclei	Nasal regurgitation; dysphagia	Local myopathy; myasthenia gravis; polyneuritis; motor neuron disease; brain stem lesions
Hoarse	Larynx; unilateral X or recurrent laryngeal N. damage	Dysphagia and discomfort only with local lesions; otherwise none	Laryngitis and regional tumor; surgical trauma; mitral stenosis; aortic aneurysm; mediastinal lesions
Weak	Larynx; bilateral X or recurrent laryngeal N. damage; intercostal, diaphragmatic weakness	Dysphagia; pharyngeal regurgitation; dyspnea; weak cough; stridor; may extend to aphonia	Surgical trauma; polyneuritis, motor neuron disease; local laryngeal disease, e.g., cancer of esophagus, larynx; mediastinal, cervical adenopathy
Hesitant	Bilateral pyramidal tract damage above midpons; pseudobulbar palsy	Indistinct: aphonic if severe; dysphagia; emotional lability; faulty tongue movement; brisk jaw jerk	Motor neuron disease; vascular lesions; tumor; encephalitis
Slow, weak	Corpus striatum; substantia nigra	Monotonous; weak; slurred; other features of parkinsonism	Parkinson disease; Wilson disease; rigid Huntington chorea
Ataxic	Cerebellum and brain stem connections; other basal ganglia	Explosive; scanning; other signs of cerebellar damage, chorea, athetosis	Heredofamilial cerebellar disorders; demyelinating disease; brain stem or cerebellar vascular disease; chorea; athetosis

TABLE 15.4–3. APHASIA: DISTURBANCE OF LANGUAGE

	Expressive Aphasia	Receptive Aphasia	Conduction Aphasia
Name(s)	Broca aphasia Anterior aphasia Motor aphasia Nonfluent aphasia	Wernicke aphasia Posterior aphasia Sensory aphasia Fluent aphasia Jargon aphasia (when severe)	Auditory-verbal, short-term memory disorder
Characteristics			
Spontaneous speech	Nonfluent, effortful, dropping of small, grammatical words, retaining meaningful words, may be poor pronunciation, dysarthria	Fluent, little effort, high output of words, often poor in meaningful words with many circumlocutions, often paraphasias (substitutions of different sounds or words) or neologisms (completely uninterpretable sounds), pronunciation normal, no dysarthria	Spontaneous speech, fluent, often with paraphasic errors
Comprehension	Usually fairly good, or normal	Poor	Usually good, or normal
Repetition	Poor (consistent with spontaneous speech)	Poor	Very poor
Naming	Better than spontaneous speech	Poor, often paraphasic	Often paraphasic
Reading	Poor reading aloud, often good reading comprehension	Poor reading aloud, little or no comprehension	Poor reading aloud, good reading comprehension
Writing	When possible, often poorly formed letters and words	Letters well-formed, but poorly combined into words, words often jumbled	Spelling errors
Localization	Anterior: inferior frontal lobe (often extensive and more posterior as well)	Posterior, superior temporal gyrus (Wernicke area) and inferior parietal lobe	Posterior temporal and/or inferior parietal regions (arcuate fasciculus)
Associated Signs	Right hemiplegia and facial weakness	Often no other signs May have right-sided sensory deficit, constructional apraxia, hemiparesis	Variable, as with receptive aphasia

LOCALIZATION

Broca aphasia is associated with anterior lesions damaging to Broca area and the nearby expressive motor areas. Often the lesion is quite extensive; lesions restricted to Broca area typically produce only a transitory expressive aphasia. The most common cause is infarction in the territory supplied by the upper main division of the middle cerebral artery, which is often the result of embolism from more proximal vessels. Because of this, these patients almost always have right-sided facial weakness and a hemiparesis, or hemiplegia, and even a hemisensory deficit.

In *Wernicke aphasia*, the lesion is posterior, damaging the primary auditory areas, Wernicke area, and the other surrounding speech reception areas. The etiology is frequently infarction in the territory supplied by the inferior division of the middle cerebral artery. Thus, Wernicke aphasia may be accompanied by other signs of damage in this region: parietal-type sensory deficits, difficulty with drawings (contructional apraxia), or hemiparesis. However, there are often no appreciable accompanying deficits.

MIXED APHASIAS AND VARIABILITY

The categories of expressive (Broca) and receptive (Wernicke) aphasia are prototypes; most aphasias cannot be classified so neatly, especially when they are acute. In the fairly typical case of infarction in the territory of the left middle cerebral artery, many patients will have (acutely) a *mixed* expressive and receptive aphasia. Usually, the expressive component tends to dominate the clinical picture because it is so obvious and because the patient often circumvents comprehension problems by attending to nonspeech aspects of the conversational situation, e.g., the general context and gestures. When severe, the picture of markedly impaired expression together with disrupted comprehension is called *global* aphasia. Fortunately, most patients are not so severely impaired.

The physician should recognize how difficult it may be to classify a particular patient and that aphasic symptomatology varies both in *type* (the mixture of disorders) and in *degree* (how severe the disorders are). Some patients will have only mild expressive aphasias; some will find it almost impossible to utter a sound. One reason for this variability of expression is differences in both the size and location of the lesions (see below). Another reason for the diversity is that the lesion—whether infarction, tumor, trauma, or other cause—frequently involves several functional areas. Yet another reason is that people probably differ somewhat in how language is represented in their brain. All these reasons indicate that one patient's aphasia can be mild and transient (for example, after embolism into a branch of the middle cerebral artery), while another's can be severe (for example, after a massive hemorrhage destroying almost all the speech areas). Furthermore, expect to see different patterns of aphasia at different times in the same patient as the original problem resolves, and his brain adjusts. Typically, the *mixed* aphasias become more exclusively *expressive*, and the expressive and *receptive* aphasias tend to become less pervasive and milder. Ultimately, the aphasia may resolve to a state of slight word-finding difficulty or disappear entirely. Also, expect to see variability caused by stress (both mental and physical, such as fever) as well as on a day-to-day basis without known cause. (The physician should also be alert to the possibility that the underlying lesion itself is worsening.)

OTHER DISORDERS

There are many other types of language disruption, such as conduction aphasia and the disconnection syndromes. In *conduction aphasia,* spontaneous speech and comprehension are relatively well preserved, but the patient is strikingly unable to repeat items such as digits or sentences. The classic explanation is a disconnection between the receptive and expressive centers (a lesion of the arcuate fasciculus), but some cases seem to be caused by an impaired memory for the material. In the *disconnection syndromes,* major functional areas are cut off from each other. For example, both the visual and language centers may be intact, but visual information can be prevented from getting to the language areas. Although such a patient is able to speak and write normally, he is completely unable to read, even his own writing (alexia without agraphia). The many different varieties of aphasia are discussed more completely in the references.[1-3]

DIAGNOSTIC AND THERAPEUTIC MANAGEMENT

ETIOLOGIC DIAGNOSIS

The clinical examination will help define how language is being disrupted and to some extent determine the location of the disturbance. Other features of the history and examination will help define the etiology. Aphasia of sudden onset is usually vascular, that is, infarction. Slowly progressive deficits may be vascular (hours to days), caused by mass lesions (days to weeks or longer), or even caused by focal degenerative conditions. The nature of the disturbance may be suggested by associated signs or symptoms. A hemianopsia helps to support the diagnosis of a localized cerebral lesion. Conversely, speech impairment as part of a global confusional state of dementia does not necessarily represent a focal lesion. Typically, in metabolic encephalopathies causing delirium, word finding is impaired (anomia), and the patient may produce phonemic and semantic paraphasias. The major focal syndrome to be excluded in such cases is usually Wernicke aphasia. Fortunately, the marked variability (with good peak performance) and absence of a firm pattern of deficits usually helps rule out a focal lesion in such cases.

Brain scanning, CT scanning, and other tests should be used where appropriate to further define the location and nature of the lesion(s) (Table 15.4–4).

TREATMENT AND PROGNOSIS

Whenever possible, the best form of treatment for aphasia is one that specifically addresses its underlying cause, such as anticoagulation or vascular surgery for certain types of stroke (see Chapter 15.13).

TABLE 15.4–4. LABORATORY EVALUATION OF APHASIA

Laboratory Test	Findings/Usefulness
EEG	Focal slowing will help confirm localization
Brain scan	
Flow study	Suggest carotid disease
Static scan	Localize lesion (not usually positive until 7–10 days after ischemic infarct; may not show hemorrhage or small lesion)
CT scan, MRI scan	Localize lesion and suggest nature of lesion, particularly good for hemorrhage; may not show early or very small infarctions
Arteriography	Directly visualize arterial disease; help determine whether lesion is operable

Speech Therapy

There is definite evidence that speech therapy can help many patients improve faster; it is not known if their ultimate performance is improved. Speech therapy is also beneficial to many patients because of the social contact and understanding that the speech therapist provides.

Prognosis depends upon the patient's age (the younger the patient, the better; children often recover full function even after severe aphasia), the location of the lesion (anterior lesions may be less disabling and more likely to recover), the size of the lesion (based on other neurologic signs or the brain or CT scan), and the patient's handedness and sex (left-handed persons and women have a somewhat better prognosis). However, prediction on an individual basis is hazardous. Much of the potential improvement occurs in the first 6 to 8 weeks, but the maximum possible recovery may not occur for 12 to 18 months or even for many years; thus, the physician should be wary of giving a bleak prognosis early in the patient's course.

APRAXIAS, AGNOSIAS, AND NEGLECT

The terms *apraxia* and *agnosia* encompass a variety of clinical abnormalities that may be seen with either focal or diffuse cerebral dysfunction. *Apraxia* is most commonly defined as a disorder of learned, skilled movements *not* caused by any simple sensory or motor problem or by failure of comprehension of the task. *Agnosia* refers to a difficulty with recognition that similarly *cannot* be attributed to a simple sensory or language deficit. Both terms are commonly abused in clinical practice. For example, when confronted with a patient who is unable to draw, the examiner fails to rule out the basic sensory or motor deficits or other explanations that could account for the problem, and labels it a "constructional apraxia" instead. However, other explanations are often more common, e.g., never having learned to draw, or are more localizing, for example, a dense visual field defect or impaired fine finger movements. Several disorders are either fairly common or very distinctive. Others may require a specialist to identify. Emphasis here is on the former.

HEMISPATIAL NEGLECT

The full-blown picture of a hemi-inattention deficit is striking. It is typically associated with a right (nondominant) parietal lobe lesion, usually an infarction. Associated focal signs (hemianopsia, hemiparesis, hemisensory deficit) may or may not be present. The inattention deficit proper is a failure to appreciate anything occurring on that side of space. The patient ignores anything on the left—the examiner, his family, his own limbs, his clothes, his food—or mislocalizes it to somewhere on the right. An examiner speaking from that side of the bed may be ignored or vainly searched for on the right. Even direct visual, auditory, or tactile stimulation on the left may not be appreciated or may only be perceived as long as there are no competing stimuli on the right; e.g., double simultaneous stimulation leads to extinction on the left. Even when shown their own arm, they may insist it does not belong to them. Their left side may therefore appear to be more paretic than it actually is. Maximum motor ability on the left might be elicited only when the right side is restrained, with painful stimuli to the left, or both. With dense inattention, patients can be completely unaware of any problems at all with their left side (anosognosia, or agnosia for their own agnosia). It may be impossible to convince them that anything is wrong. Such patients often insist on leaving the hospital and wonder why they cannot move when they try, or they may come to an intellectual appreciation of their stroke but still not emotionally appreciate their problem.

Dense inattention deficits are usually seen only after acute right (nondominant) parietal or thalamic lesions. Less dense and

less pervasive inattention syndromes affecting the contralateral side can occur with right frontal lesions, or with left-sided lesions, particularly parietal lesions. Typically, inattention is a relatively transient problem that greatly diminishes or disappears after just a few weeks.

CONSTRUCTIONAL APRAXIA

Constructional apraxia refers to any difficulty with drawing or with constructing, for example, with blocks, that *cannot* be attributed to a more elementary perceptual problem (such as a visual field loss or cortical blindness), to a more elementary motor problem (hemiparesis or clumsiness), or to lack of intrinsic ability. Typical tests are drawing a clock or a house from an example supplied by the examiner or drawing these from memory. Drawing from memory is a more difficult task that can bring out more subtle deficits. Two typical patterns of poor performance are *neglect* of one side

(usually the left) (see Fig. 15.4–2), and *visuospatial disorganization,* or jumbling up of the elements (see Fig. 15.4–2). The neglect is usually seen with right (nondominant) parietal lesions. Visuospatial disorganization can be seen after lesions of either inferior parietal lobe but is most often associated with lesions in the right, nondominant side or with bilateral lesions. This disorganization may also be part of more diffuse lobe disease, such as Alzheimer or delirium.

In *ideomotor apraxia,* a task cannot be performed on comand or in "make believe," but can be performed automatically or if a real object is present. One example is not being able to purse the lips voluntarily but being able to whistle or blow out a match. This particular example is commonly seen as part of expressive aphasia. The references give other examples.

Ideational apraxia implies an inability to carry out a multistep command, even though each step can be performed normally by itself. The *three-step command* is a common clinical test for this. For

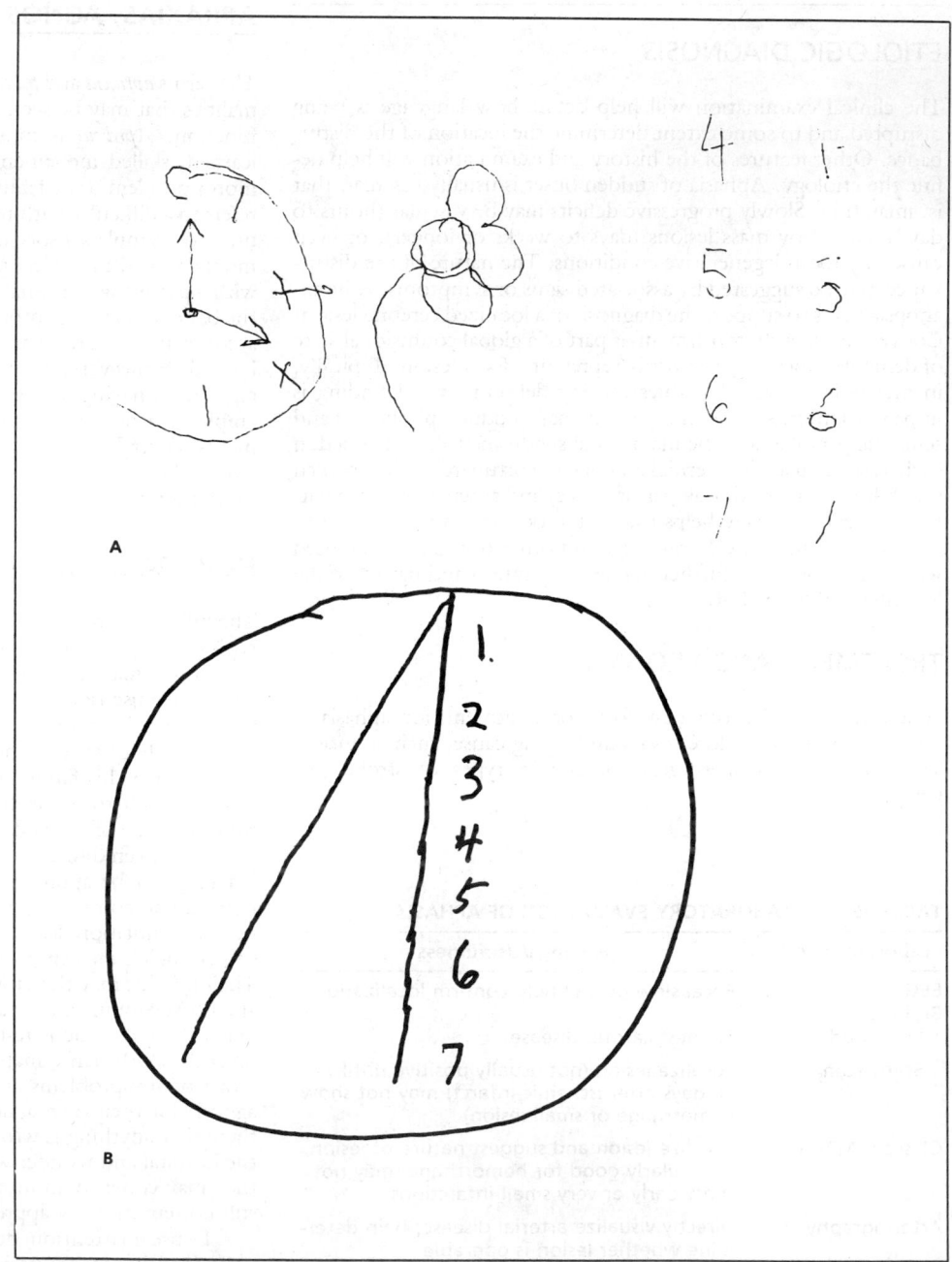

Figure 15.4–2. A. Left-sided neglect in patient with right parietal infarct. **B.** Example of marked visuospatial disorganization in spontaneous clock drawing in patient with Alzheimer disease.

example, ask the patient to close his eyes, raise his left hand, then open his mouth. If the patient can truly carry out each individual step without difficulty (which is often not the case) but cannot really do all three together, then the usual explanation is poor attention or poor memory. These are themselves nonspecific problems, but delirium or dementia are typical causes.

VISUAL AGNOSIA

Visual agnosia, failure to recognize objects properly, despite normal visual perceptual ability, is quite rare in its pure form. Incomplete cortical blindness is a common cause.

REFERENCES

1. Benson D, Geschwind N: The aphasias and related disturbances. In Baker AB, Joynt RT (eds): Clinical Neurology. Philadelphia, Harper & Row, 1985
2. Heilman KM, Valenstein E (eds): Clinical Neuropsychology, 2d ed. New York, Oxford University Press, 1985
3. Mesukam M (ed): Principles of Behavioral Neurology. Philadelphia, FA Davis, 1985
4. Poeck K: The clinical examination for motor apraxia. Neuropsychologia 24:129, 1986
5. Wertz RT, Weiss DG, et al: Comparison of clinic, home, and deferred language treatment for aphasia. Arch Neurol (Minn). 43:653, 1986

CHAPTER 15.5
Syncope, Seizures, and Other Episodic Disorders

Hamilton Moses III and Robert S. Fisher

Many patients experience peculiar and transient symptoms of brief duration. They may use words such as dizzy, unsteady, nearly fainting, lightheaded, blurred vision, feeling drunk, fuzzy headed, or almost blacking out to describe them. Some may feel as if they are about to lose consciousness but do not do so; others actually do lose consciousness. Some may have an aura or warning before loss of consciousness occurs; others have the experience begin abruptly with no warning. This chapter discusses those patients who have an acute but transient disturbance of consciousness. Chapter 15.7 contains an approach to patients who have dizziness *without* alteration in consciousness.

These transient symptoms may be quite difficult for the physician to evaluate properly. Careful attention to the details of the history, often checked with a reliable witness, noting the chronology of symptoms, and a thorough general and neurologic examination with the proper use of ancillary diagnostic studies will usually lead to proper diagnosis.

Some causes (see Table 15.5–1) of episodic symptoms are trivial, although disabling, for instance, a patient with mild orthostatic hypotension after bedrest. Others, such as pulmonary embolism, hypoglycemia, or cardiac arrhythmias, may produce only mild symptoms and yet have a clear and immediate threat to life. Every clinician must therefore have an organized approach to this common clinical problem.

APPROACH TO THE PATIENT

The physician should ask the patient (and any witnesses) about three phases of the symptoms: what happened before the attack, during the attack, and what was the manner of recovery afterward. Table 15.5–1 enumerates the significance of several observations. Three patterns are particularly common.

ABRUPT ONSET AND ABRUPT RECOVERY

Patients with arrhythmias (Stokes-Adams attacks), orthostatic hypotension, and hysteria often report that they lose consciousness "as if the lights went out," thereupon to abruptly awaken, usually immediately becoming fully alert.

ABRUPT ONSET AND PROLONGED RECOVERY

Subarachnoid hemorrhage, other intracranial hemorrhages, cerebral infarction, complex partial and primary generalized convulsions, and severe orthostatic hypotension all may cause immediate loss of consciousness (in seconds), with a delayed recovery (over minutes to hours), because of significantly altered cerebral metabolism.

GRADUAL LOSS OF CONSCIOUSNESS WITH GRADUAL RECOVERY

This is the most common pattern. Mild or progressive hypotension (blood loss), hypoglycemia, hypoxia, hypercapnea, serious electrolyte disturbance (especially when multiple), hysteria, drug intoxication, increased intracranial pressure, and nervous system infections all cause this pattern. When unconsciousness is prolonged (the patient is in coma) the evaluation and management should proceed as outlined in Chapter 15.3.

Observations before and during the ictus are helpful, although not infallible. For instance, palpitations suggest arrhythmia; purposeful movements, hysteria; stereotyped movements, complex partial seizures; tonic movements or focal weakness, transient ischemic attacks. Sleeplike unconsciousness is of no diagnostic value, however.

SYNCOPE[2,6,14]

Syncope is a loss of consciousness that begins abruptly and lasts for a finite length of time (usually less than a few minutes). A warning or aura may not be present and, if recalled, is usually quite short. Full recovery, although often abrupt, may be prolonged in certain circumstances. Syncope must be distinguished from delirium, where the content of consciousness is altered, but the person is awake; from stupor, where the person appears asleep but can be aroused; and from coma, where the person appears asleep and cannot be aroused. *Near syncope,* or impending syncope, is a state of transient dizziness caused by any of the conditions that can cause frank syncope. Near syncope is far more common than true syncope; most persons (for example, those with transient postural lightheadedness) probably do not report the problem to their phy-

sicians. The physiologic changes leading to the two problems are identical; they are simply shorter in duration or less severe, and the person soon becomes dizzy without actually losing consciousness.

TABLE 15.5–1. CAUSES OF EPISODIC DISORDERS

1. **Circulatory**
   A. Vasovagal syncope
   B. Hypotension
      • Hypovolemia
      • Medication induced
      • Post bedrest
      • Autonomic insufficiency
      • Peripheral vasodilation
         Neurogenic
         Anaphylactic
         Septic
   C. Decreased cardiac output
      Valsalva
         Micturition
         Defecation
         Tussive
      • Myocardial infarction
      • Pulmonary embolus
      • Arrythmia
         Sinus bradycardia (including carotid sinus)
         Tachyarrhythmias
         Heart block (Adams-Stokes)
         Frequent ectopic beats
      • Valvular heart disease
         Mitral valve prolapse
         Aortic stenosis
      • Tension pneumothorax
      • Pericardial tamponade
      • Fluctuating congestive failure
   D. Cerebrovascular
      • Vertebrobasilar ischemia
      • Hemorrhage
         Subarachnoid
         Intraparenchymal
         Subdural or epidural
      • Migraine with "vasospasm"
      • Transient global amnesia
      • Drop attacks
2. **Respiratory**
   A. Hypoxic
   B. Hyperventilation
3. **Endocrinologic**
   A. Hypoglycemia
   B. Hyperthyroid
   C. Pheochromocytoma
   D. Carcinoid
4. **Vestibular**
   A. Benign positional vertigo
   B. Vestibular neuronitis
   C. Meniere disease
   D. Acoustic neuroma
   E. Brain stem lesion
5. **Sleep disorder**
   A. Narcolepsy
   B. Cataplexy
6. **Epileptic**
   A. Partial complex seizures
   B. Generalized tonic-clonic seizures
   C. Generalized absence seizures
7. **Increased intracranial pressure**
   A. Brain stem compression
   B. Acute ventricular obstruction
8. **Psychiatric**
   A. Conversion
   B. Panic attacks
   C. Malingering
9. **Miscellaneous neurologic**
   A. Demyelination
   B. Episodic movement disorder

Normal wakefulness requires the proper functioning of one, but not necessarily both, cerebral hemispheres and of the ascending reticular formation of the brain stem (see Chapter 15.3). Unconsciousness therefore implies that either both cerebral hemispheres are impaired or that critical structures in the brain stem have failed. Syncope occurs when there is temporary impairment of the reticular formation or of both cerebral hemispheres.

Most syncopal patients have failure of systemic circulation as the cause. This accounts for about 70 percent of syncope. Heart disease and intracranial disease account each for 10 percent, while metabolic disorders and a miscellany of other causes account for about 5 percent each (see Table 15.5–2).

CIRCULATORY FAILURE

Autoregulation of cerebral blood flow protects normal functioning of the brain over a wide range of blood pressures. In normal persons, critical decreases in central nervous system (CNS) blood flow do not occur until the mean blood pressure falls below 50 to 60 mm Hg. In elderly people, those who receive vasodilating drugs, and those who have been hypertensive, the critical mean pressure may be much higher, thereby allowing syncope to occur with only a moderate fall in systemic blood pressure, making these individuals more sensitive.

SIMPLE FAINT (VASOVAGAL SYNCOPE)

The simple faint often affects young people and is apt to occur in a setting of anxiety, tension, fatigue, or during venipuncture or other painful procedures. An early theory suggested that bradycardia caused by vagal overactivity was the initial event. It is now believed that venous pooling caused by peripheral arterial constriction with concomitant venous dilatation first occurs, with bradycardia occurring only after the faint itself. Vasovagal attacks nearly always occur while the patient is upright but may occur when seated, rarely when recumbent; consciousness is nearly always regained promptly when the patient becomes recumbent. There is often a prodrome lasting a minute or two, during which the patient feels dizzy, lightheaded, often hot or flushed, and has palpitations, tinnitus, dimming of vision, often with a tightness in the throat or mild nausea. A patient who becomes recumbent during this stage may not lose consciousness. An observer will note cold hands, pale skin, and tachycardia before the patient loses consciousness. An occasional death has occurred if the patient cannot become recumbent, as for instance in a telephone booth, or if he is held upright during the spell. Bradycardia may persist for several minutes after the faint. Aside from bradycardia and pallor, the examination is normal unless there has been secondary trauma or aspiration.

Autonomic Impairment

Autonomic impairment causes syncope by producing orthostatic hypotension. This is easily confirmed by measuring the blood pressure while supine, sitting, and upright. Blood pressure should also be measured after exercise in patients with venous insufficiency or who have any antihypertensive medications prescribed.

Autonomic neuropathy should be suspected in patients who have diabetes, amyloidosis, parkinsonism, other peripheral neuropathies, or tabes; it also occurs in an idiopathic form rarely. In addition to syncope, the patient often will have noted constipation, diarrhea, or impotence. Physical examination will reveal abnormal pupils, alteration in sweating, and abnormal Valsalva response, as well as orthostatic hypotension. Sympathetic failure can be successfully treated by cautioning the patient to stand slowly after sitting for some minutes beside the bed or chair, volume expansion with salt, the use of mineralocorticoids (9α-fluorohydrocortisone), and the use of supportive hose.

Decreased intravascular volume may be caused by hemorrhage,

TABLE 15.5–2. CLINICAL ATTRIBUTES OF EPISODIC DISORDERS

Timing	Observation	Significance	Comment
Before ictus	Abrupt onset (no warning)	Generalized seizures	See text
		Cardiac arrhythmia	Chapter 2.9
		Severe orthostatic hypotension	
		Valsalva	See text
		Pulmonary embolism	Chapter 3.8
		Subarachnoid hemorrhage	Chapter 15.13
		Hysteria	Chapter 16.4
	Gradual onset (with aura)	Focal seizure (motor, sensory, psychomotor)	See text
		Orthostatic hypotension	See text
		Hemorrhage	Chapter 4.3
		Hypoglycemia	Chapter 14.8
		Hypoxia-hypercapnia	Chapter 4.7
		Vertebrobasilar ischemia	Chapter 15.13
		Cardiac disease (esp. valvular, obstructive)	Chapter 2.3
During ictus	Onset with change in position	Orthostatic hypotension	See text
		Ventricular obstruction	Chapter 15.10
	Sleeplike unconsciousness	No diagnostic value	
	Tonic or tonic-clonic movements	Generalized convulsions	Convulsions may occur with any cause of unconsciousness (see text)
		Hypoglycemia	
		Hypotension	
		Cardiac arrhythmia	
		Transient ischemic attack	
		Severe hypoxia	
	Purposeful movements	Hysteria	Chapter 16.4
	Stereotyped movements	Complex partial seizure	See text
	Skeletal weakness without impairment of consciousness	Periodic paralysis	
		Atlantoaxial dislocation	Chapter 15.13
		Vertebrobasilar ischemia	Chapter 15.17
		Hysteria	
After ictus	Abrupt recovery	Cardiac obstruction, arrhythmia	
		Hysteria	
		Orthostatic hypotension	
		Ventricular obstruction	
	Prolonged recovery	Drug intoxication	Recovery may be delayed for hours or days after the abnormality is corrected (see text)
		Severe hypotension	
		Hypoglycemia	
		Severe hypercapnia, hypoxia	
		Electrolyte derangement	
		Subarachnoid hemorrhage	
		Increased intracranial pressure	
	Headache	Intracranial hemorrhage	
		Generalized or complex partial seizure	
		Hypercapnia	
		Hypoglycemia	
	Focal weakness or other focal neurological signs	Cerebral infarct	
		Focal or generalized seizure	
		Trauma	Chapter 15.19
		Severe metabolic derangement	

salt or water loss, for example, from gastroenteritis, heat exposure, diuretics, etc., and is recognized by the combination of orthostatic hypotension with tachycardia and an associated reason for the volume deficit. Hot weather and exercise, prolonged fasting (as in anorexia nervosa or fad diets), adrenal insufficiency, hypoalbuminemia, or chronic disease may coexist. Treatment is effected by immediate volume expansion with salt and water (carefully observing for congestive heart failure) plus definitive treatment of the underlying condition.

Venous pooling prevents return of blood to the heart, lowering cardiac output and thereby systemic blood pressure. Syncope may occur after exercise or prolonged standing, as in recruits standing at attention. Severe dependent varicose veins or the compression of pelvic veins by a fetus or large tumor may predispose. Supportive elastic stockings and slow ambulation may be of aid.

Orthostasis of the aging is quite common, with a 30 mm Hg fall in systolic pressure found in approximately 10 percent of healthy older persons. The pathophysiology of this is not understood but probably represents a combination of autonomic insufficiency plus patulous peripheral veins. It is ameliorated by following the steps recommended for patients convalescing from bed rest.

Syncope after bed rest is caused by venous pooling, relative hypovolemia, and probably some lowered sensitivity of the baroreceptor reflex. It occurs very commonly in people who have been at bed rest for more than a few days. It may persist for 1 to 2 weeks after ambulation. Orthostatic symptoms may be minimized by having the patient gradually stand only after several minutes of sitting on the bed with the legs dependent.

Tussive syncope may follow a prolonged or severe bout of coughing in otherwise normal individuals. It more often occurs in per-

sons with obstructive airways disease. Abnormalities of the pulmonary and pleural vagal receptors in those individuals produce bradycardia and hypotension with coughing; decreased venous return from increased pleural pressure is another mechanism.

Micturition syncope often occurs in older men with large bladders and some prostatic obstruction as well as in younger men who waken with a very full bladder in the middle of the night.

Hypersensitivity of the carotid sinus occurs in older patients with long-standing and severe hypertension or with coronary or carotid atherosclerosis. Older men who wear tight collars, women with cumbersome necklaces, or patients having large masses in the neck are predisposed. Although some authorities recommend provoking syncope by unilateral or bilateral carotid massage, this may be a dangerous maneuver and should be performed only when material for resuscitation is immediately available; it should be avoided in patients with carotid stenosis.

Pulmonary embolism leads to syncope in about 15 percent of the cases. Prolonged unconsciousness may occur, and seizures are quite common, even when paradoxical embolization has not occurred.

Severe pain arising from any site, but particularly the viscera, may be followed by a faint through the vasovagal mechanism.

Cardiac Abnormalities

Rhythm disturbances (Stokes-Adams attacks) particularly heart block may reflect ischemic, infiltrative, or neoplastic lesions of the heart. Similarly, brady- or tachyarrhythmias without block may lead to cerebral symptoms or syncope. Cardiac arrhythmia should be strongly considered in older patients or when unconsciousness occurs nocturnally or while seated or recumbent. Drugs may also predispose (especially quinidine, digitalis, tricyclic antidepressants, or neuroleptics). Cardiac syncope may occur without warning, although an aura (grayout) is common; palpitations are notoriously unreliable. The resting ECG may be normal or, at most, with minor PR or QT prolongations present. Therefore, 24-hour cardiac monitoring is essential to confirm this diagnosis (see Chapter 2.9).

Aortic stenosis, whether calcific or rheumatic, may lead to syncope in older individuals, almost always following exertion and usually associated with chest pain or arrhythmia. *Hypertrophic cardiomyopathy* may lead to syncope in patients of any age. Very rarely *left atrial myxoma* may lead to syncope or peripheral embolization. *Cyanotic congenital heart disease* produces syncope after exercise or during hypoxia, as during an airplane flight. *Myocardial infarction* causes syncope at its onset because of hypotension or arrhythmia. Embolization from mural thrombus should be considered when syncope occurs during recovery from myocardial infarction and in those with cardiomyopathy.

Metabolic Abnormalities

Hypoglycemia can produce unconsciousness when the blood glucose falls below 40 mg/dl. Hunger, palpitations, sweating, and anxiety nearly always occur just before the patient loses consciousness, unless beta-blockers have been prescribed. Episodes of confusion, bizarre behavior, or irritability may be the only manifestations of mild attacks. Permanent damage occurs when blood glucose below 20 mg/dl persists for more than just a few minutes. Administration of glucose is warranted therefore in anyone who remains unconscious long enough for the physician to prepare the solution of 50 percent dextrose and water. Convulsions and incontinence commonly accompany hypoglycemic coma, and neurological abnormalities may persist after recovery (see Chapter 14.8).

Hypocapnia from hyperventilation may lead to syncope caused by the secondary decrease in cerebral blood flow (see Chapter 4.7). Athletes preparing to race, musicians playing wind instruments, or anyone who is fearful or anxious may develop syncope in this way. Tetany or carpopedal symptoms may precede cerebral symptoms. Recovery is prompt when ventilation is slowed after consciousness is lost. *Hypoxemia* may occur because of obstruction of the upper airway, severe anemia, poisoning with carbon monoxide, or in patients with lung disease. Seizures are very common in patients with acute hypoxemia, and neurologic sequelae are the rule after unconsciousness lasting more than 1 or 2 minutes. Management depends entirely on a prompt and accurate diagnosis of the disorder causing the hypoxemia.

Intracranial Abnormalities

Cerebral embolism or thrombosis may cause a brief or prolonged unconsciousness if the basilar artery is affected. Rarely a carotid occlusion may cause unconsciousness initially, even if the remaining vessels are patent. Premonitory neurologic signs (basilar: hemianopia, diplopia, dysarthria, vertigo; carotid: aphasia, hemiplegia, hemisensory abnormalities) are the rule and may persist after recovery of consciousness (see Chapter 15.13).

Subarachnoid hemorrhage may begin with a brief period of unconsciousness. The constellation of headache, confusion, and neck stiffness follows shortly after the syncopal episode. Any patient who is confused and who develops headache during the initial evaluation should have subarachnoid hemorrhage excluded, even if meningismus has not yet developed.

Increased intracranial pressure, whether caused by tumor, trauma, or ventricular obstruction, may lead to syncope when a Valsalva maneuver is performed, such as during straining at stool or bending over. Preexisting symptoms, papilledema, or neurologic signs usually coexist (see Chapter 15.10).

Brain stem compression may lead to unconsciousness caused by a displaced fracture of C_1 or of the odontoid process or from tumors or cystic abnormalities of the posterior fossa. Unconsciousness often occurs with movement of the neck. Associated neurologic signs are the rule (see Chapter 15.6).

SEIZURES[3,4,11]

A seizure is an episodic event of variable duration, consisting of abnormal movements, sensation, or consciousness caused by abnormal electrical discharges in the brain. The term "epilepsy" refers to a condition characterized by recurrent spontaneous seizures. Seizures occur in about 5 percent of the American population, whereas 0.5 to 1 percent will have epilepsy. Thus, the prevalence of epilepsy is second only to that of stroke among the serious neurologic diseases.

The underlying pathophysiologic mechanism of epilepsy is only partially understood. Evidence from various animal models and simple cellular systems suggests that seizures result from a relative excess of excitatory processes versus inhibitory processes. In some models, a decrease of cellular synaptic inhibitory potentials is most evident. In other models, large paroxysmal depolarizing shifts are recorded within neurons, probably reflecting excessive excitatory communication among neural networks. Rapidly firing "pacemaker" neurons may play some role in epileptogenesis, as may changes in the brain ionic microenvironment. Experimental models have not yet led to an understanding of how seizures start, why they take the pattern of spread that they do, why they stop, and why they recur with seemingly random incidence over time. Thus, therapy for epilepsy is predominantly empirical.

CLASSIFICATION OF SEIZURES[4,15]

A standardized classification for seizures, referred to as the "International Classification," is based primarily upon the appearance of a seizure to a hypothetical qualified observer (Table 15.5-3). Seizures are categorized by their character at onset as partial (focal) or generalized. Partial seizures are further subdivided into partial simple, without loss of consciousness, and partial complex, with loss or blunting of consciousness.

TABLE 15.5–3. CLASSIFICATION OF SEIZURES

Partial (focal)
- Simple
  - Motor
  - Sensory
  - Psychic
  - Autonomic
  - Mixed
- Complex

Generalized
- Absence, typical
- Absence, atypical
- Tonic-clonic
- Tonic
- Clonic
- Atonic
- Myoclonic

Secondary generalized

Unclassified

Partial Seizures

Manifestations of *partial simple seizures* depend upon their site of brain origin. The most common type has an origin in motor cortex, resulting in focal jerking of the face or limb. In some instances the electrical discharge may spread to contiguous regions of the motor homunculus, resulting in a "Jacksonian march," named after John Hughlings Jackson, who first described this phenomenon. Partial simple seizures in the somatosensory area may present with abnormal tingling sensations that are difficult to distinguish from transient ischemic episodes. Partial simple seizures in the occipital or parietal regions may give rise to visual manifestations similar to those seen as prodromes of migraine headaches. Partial simple seizures with visceral, autonomic, or cognitive features may occur with origin in the temporal or frontal lobes and most often present as auras for partial complex seizures.

Partial complex epilepsy was previously referred to as "temporal lobe epilepsy," "psychomotor epilepsy," or "limbic epilepsy." This is the most common form of epilepsy seen in the majority of adult seizure clinics. As with all seizures, partial complex seizures are relatively stereotyped and clearly demarcated in time. In addition, these seizures contain the following elements: aura (in approximately 50 percent), blunting or loss of consciousness (by definition in all), and automatism (in the majority). The term "aura" refers to the partial simple aspect of this seizure before blunting of consciousness. Most commonly, this takes the form of a general discomfort in the abdomen or chest, tingling or flushing sensations, cognitive abnormalities such as a sense of déjà vu or emotional intrusive experiences, or distorted perceptions including abnormal smells, visions, sounds, or vestibular sensations. The blunting of consciousness frequently takes the form of a fugue or dreamlike state, with partial preservation of ability to function. Incomplete recall of the event after it is over is not inconsistent with this seizure type, but amnesia is usually present. Automatisms are robot-like, semiautomatic fragments of behavior, such as lip-smacking, repetitive mouthing of words, walking in circles, raising and lowering an arm, or buttoning and unbuttoning clothing. Automatisms vary a great deal from person to person, but within a given person they tend to be fairly replicable. Autonomic features of partial complex seizures are often prominent, with pupillary dilation, flushing, sweating, and tachycardias. The typical partial complex seizure lasts 15 to 120 seconds and is followed by recovery over many minutes.

Any partial seizure may secondarily generalize to a full tonic-clonic convulsion involving four limbs. These are also known as "major motor" convulsions. Tonic-clonic seizures are discussed below.

Generalized Seizures

The second large category in the International Classification is generalized seizures. The traditional grand mal and petit mal seizures have been renamed tonic-clonic and absence.

Tonic-clonic generalized seizures appear to begin from all sites in the cortex simultaneously. No specific aura is recalled by the patient afterwards, and the episode is generally a complete blank in memory. Observers report a sudden cessation of activity, eyes rolling up or to the side, expiration of air, sometimes with an associated involuntary cry. This is then followed by four-limb stiffening, known as the tonic phase, and extension alternating with flexion synchronously in the four limbs, known as the clonic phase. The entire tonic-clonic sequence lasts about 1 minute, leading to a period of flaccid unresponsiveness called the "postictal state." Tongue-biting and incontinence are frequent in this seizure type. The patient almost invariably falls, sometimes with secondary injuries. Clear-cut origin of abnormal movements on one side of the body and face or, alternatively, residual paralysis postictally on one side (Todd paralysis) indicates a partial onset of the seizure with secondary generalization. Postictal sleepiness and confusion usually last several minutes to several hours after a tonic-clonic seizure. When Todd paralysis is severe, it may be difficult to distinguish from a minor stroke or transient ischemic attack (see Chapter 15.13).

Absence seizures are generalized seizures presenting as brief staring spells. These seizures typically last only a few seconds and are accompanied by very few motor or behavioral abnormalities. The event is not recalled by the patient, and observers generally have an impression of frequent inattentiveness or daydreaming. When absence seizures are prolonged beyond 10 to 15 seconds, automatisms such as eyelid fluttering or mouth movements become increasingly a part of the seizure, and distinction from partial complex seizures may be difficult on behavioral grounds alone. In general, recovery from typical or atypical absence seizures is fairly quick and automatisms relatively minor in comparison with loss of awareness.

Other generalized seizures include *myoclonic seizures* with sharp nonrhythmical jerking of the limbs or head and atonic seizures where tone is suddenly lost, resulting in a fall to the ground.

Unclassified Seizures

Because seizures are classified largely on the basis of their onset, a seizure must remain unclassified if it is impossible to determine whether it began focally or nonfocally.

Etiology

Proper classification of seizures permits establishing the etiology, which is generally idiopathic or metabolic for the primary generalized epilepsies and structural for the partial epilepsies. In addition, seizure classification gives clues to prognosis and to the most likely effective therapeutic agents.

The common etiologies of seizures are listed in Table 15.5–4. Each seizure type and etiology is age dependent (see Table 15.5–5). Seizures in infants are usually secondary to hypoxia, birth trauma, intraparenchymal or intraventricular hemorrhage, hypoglycemia, hypocalcemia, or infection. For children in the age range 1 to 12 years, seizures are most often caused by high fevers, genetic epilepsy, infections, metabolic causes such as hypoglycemia, hyponatremia, hypocalcemia, aminoaciduria, tumor, or developmental-degenerative diseases. In adolescents and young adults, seizures are most often genetic or idiopathic. Scarring of the temporal lobe—known as "mesial temporal sclerosis"—is presumed to be the etiology for the partial complex seizures originating at this age. Infections, toxins or drugs, drug or alcohol withdrawal, metabolic abnormalities, trauma, tumor, intracranial hemorrhage, eclampsia, organ system failure, vasculitis, and multiple sclerosis all play roles in this age group. Young and middle-aged adults who newly develop partial seizures are at high risk for an underlying tumor or posttraumatic scar. In the elderly, cerebrovascular disease becomes the most important etiology for seizures, but all those listed above

TABLE 15.5–4. COMMON CAUSES OF SEIZURES

Infants	*Children*
• Hypoxia	• Febrile
• Birth trauma	• Idiopathic
• Hemorrhage	• Psychogenic
• Hypoglycemia	• Infection
• Hypocalcemia	• Hypoglycemia
• Infection	• Hyponatremia
	• Hypocalcemia
	• Aminoaciduria
Young Adults	• Tumor
• Idiopathic	• Developmental
• Mesial temporal sclerosis	• Degenerative
• Psychogenic	
• Infection	
• Toxins—drugs	*Elderly*
• Hypoglycemia	• Cerebrovascular
• Hypocalcemia	• Tumor
• Hyponatremia	• Trauma
• Trauma	• Hemorrhage
• Tumor	• Toxins—drugs
• Hemorrhage	• Renal failure
• Eclampsia	• Hypocalcemia
• Renal failure	• Hyponatremia
• Vasculitis	• Hypoglycemia
• Multiple sclerosis	• Psychogenic
	• Idiopathic

may play a role. At any age, excepting that of the infant, idiopathic epilepsy and psychogenic seizures stand prominently on the list of etiologies.

DIAGNOSIS OF EPILEPSY

Clinical Approach
The key to diagnosing epilepsy is elicitation of a careful description of the attack by the patient and observers. The episodes should have the characteristics of seizure defined above and should be distinguishable from several common imitators of the epilepsies, listed in Table 15.5–5. In practice, the most difficult differential diagnosis is usually partial complex seizures or generalized tonic-clonic versus psychogenic seizures. This distinction may require direct observation in a hospitalized setting, often with medicines withdrawn and with specialized concurrent electrical studies.

Diagnostic Tests[4,12]
Laboratory studies in epilepsy are directed primarily to ascertaining the site of origin of seizure discharges in the brain and to specifying an etiology. Blood tests such as white blood count, differential, serum glucose, sodium, calcium and magnesium, urinalysis, and serum urea nitrogen may point to infectious, circulatory, toxic, or metabolic causes for the seizures.

The *electroencephalogram (EEG)* is the most important single test in the evaluation of patients with epilepsy, but it is frequently misused and misinterpreted. Each seizure type has a relatively characteristic pattern of EEG electrical discharges. Partial seizures show

TABLE 15.5–5. IMITATORS OF EPILEPSY

• Syncope	• Migraine
• Presyncope	• Vertigo
• Transient ischemic attack	• Tremor or tick
• Transient global amnesia	• Breath-holding spells
• Cardiac arrythmia	• Narcolepsy-cataplexy
• Hypoglycemia	• Functional

large paroxysmal "spikes" or "sharp waves" lasting up to 70 milliseconds and with amplitude usually well above the background. In partial complex seizures these spikes or sharp waves are usually found over the temporal or inferior frontal lobes. Generalized tonic-clonic (grand mal) seizures show spikes diffusely, usually with frontocentral maximum. Typical absence (petit mal) is almost always associated with three to four per second spike-wave discharges diffusely. The EEG may therefore help in making a diagnosis of epilepsy, in classifying the seizure type, and in helping to localize the seizure focus.

Unfortunately, interictal records, that is, those taken in the interval between clinically observable seizures, may fail to show any abnormality in as many as one of three cases. With a good clinical history for a seizure, negative EEG findings should not negate the impression of underlying epilepsy. If the EEG is recorded during a clinical seizure, abnormal seizure discharges should almost always be visible (very focal seizures are an exception), and their lack should be grounds for considering a nonepileptic cause. Conversely, EEG patterns resembling spikes, sharp waves, and spike-wave complexes should never be grounds for treatment in the absence of a clinical history for epilepsy, since they may be seen in 1 to 5 percent of the normal population.

Activating procedures for the EEG include hyperventilation, photic stimulation, and sleep. Each of these may bring out abnormalities not evident in the unstimulated waking state. Diagnostic problems may require prolonged ambulatory EEG monitoring or concurrent EEG monitoring with video observation.

Usually CT scans of the brain are performed in all patients with focal epilepsies and are found to be abnormal in about one of three for partial complex seizures and two of three for focal motor seizures. The rate of CT scan abnormality falls to 5 to 10 percent in patients with primary generalized epilepsies, usually consisting only of nonspecific atrophy. Rarely, silent structural lesions giving rise to apparently nonfocal epilepsies are discovered. This yield is vanishingly small for children with typical tonic-clonic and absence seizures. Magnetic resonance imaging may show greater sensitivity in identification of structural lesions giving rise to seizures. Its role remains to be determined. Positron emission tomographic scanning is able to delineate metabolic activity of the brain associated with seizures or the interictal state; it is still primarily a research tool. Arteriography is done in special cases in which seizures are suspected to be secondary to vascular problems or highly vascularized tumors. If meningitis is suspected, a lumbar puncture is mandatory. Usually CT scanning is performed first to demonstrate lack of increased intracranial pressure, which would contraindicate a lumbar puncture.

Pseudoseizures (Hysterical, Factitious, Hystero-Epilepsy)
Many patients, particularly older children, adolescents, and young adults, have ictal events that resemble seizures. The behavior most often takes the form of apparent major motor or grand mal convulsions or absence spells. While pseudoseizures may be a conscious mimicking of a seizure (a form of malingering), more often the patient displays the behavior without conscious effort (hysteria). Moreover, many patients often have an active epileptic disorder or have had seizures in the past, thus often making correct diagnosis very difficult. Frequently, patients with pseudoseizures have significant emotional or social difficulties that are provoked by their underlying disorder. Others use pseudoseizures as an attention-getting device. Toxic levels of anticonvulsants may predispose to pseudoseizures.

Diagnosis depends upon careful observation of the ictal event and watching for voluntary activity during the episode. This is not infallible, however. For this reason, EEG telemetry, long-term mobile EEG recordings, or simultaneous video and EEG recordings are required. Occasionally, suggestion or coaxing may produce pseudoseizures while a routine EEG is being obtained, during which the tracing is normal.

THERAPEUTIC MANAGEMENT[1,5,7,9,10]

Medical Therapy[7,8,13]

The vast majority of patients with epilepsy are manageable by medications. Approximately two out of three patients will have a satisfactory degree of seizure control with minimal toxicity, provided several basic principles are followed. These are listed in Table 15.5–6. The first principle is to decide when to treat. Single unprovoked seizures are nonrecurrent in two out of three patients followed for at least 3 years. Unless there is strong desire for treatment on the part of patient and family, most experts advise withholding treatment until after the second seizure, which generally predicts further recurrences.

The second principle is to choose the best drug for the particular seizure type. Table 15.5–7 summarizes the major anticonvulsant drugs, doses, desired serum levels, and side effects. Controlled comparative studies are few, so choice of anticonvulsants often depends upon physician familiarity, drug costs and side effects, and ease of administration. For partial seizures, including partial complex, most experts now recommend carbamazepine or phenytoin. These two agents are also effective for primary generalized tonic-clonic seizures. Valproic acid is particularly effective for absence seizures, primary generalized tonic-clonic seizures, and myoclonic seizures. Barbiturates, such as phenobarbital, and primidone exhibit a broad spectrum of anticonvulsant coverage but are probably not as effective as the newer drugs listed above.

The next principle is to start drugs slowly and build up to a therapeutic level. Toxicity of anticonvulsants may be overwhelming when the drug is started full dose. A common cause of treatment failure is poor compliance. The regimen should be as simple as possible: phenobarbital, phenytoin, and ethosuximide may usually be given once per day, preferably upon retiring; other anticonvulsants, two or three times per day, unless seizures or side effects require more frequent dosing. Serum levels may be checked for documentation of compliance, adequate total dose, and analysis of possible toxicity. Serum levels need not be obtained upon every visit once control has been effected.

Therapy with a single drug is preferable to polypharmacy because of the likelihood of multiple drug interactions and unnecessary toxicity when more than one agent is used. Despite this goal, some patients cannot be controlled by a single anticonvulsant and require two or three anticonvulsants.[13]

The last principle is to decide how long to treat. Children with primary generalized epilepsy and no underlying structural lesion often "outgrow" their seizures during their adulthood. A person who has been seizure free for 2 to 4 years, is generally well and without continuing cause for seizures, and has a normal EEG may be a candidate for tapering off of medications. Approximately one out of two will fail such a medication taper, despite all positive indices. Patients should understand and be willing to accept this risk. Medicines should be tapered one at a time and slowly, for example, over 1 to 2 months for each anticonvulsant.

The goal of medical therapy for epilepsy is no seizures and no medication toxicity. For at least two out of three patients this goal should be obtainable. Some of the individuals whose seizures are not controllable with medications will be candidates for surgical ablation of their seizure focus.

TABLE 15.5–6. PRINCIPLES FOR ANTICONVULSANT THERAPY

- Decide when to treat
- Choose the best single drug
- Start drugs slowly
- Use simple regimens
- Monitor compliance
- Use serum levels selectively
- Add other drugs when necessary
- Decide how long to treat

Indications for Reevaluation

Several warning signs indicate the need for reevaluating a diagnosis of idiopathic epilepsy. These most often apply for patients with focal seizures and include (1) a failure to respond to medication or a recurrence of previously controlled seizures, (2) a change in clinical pattern of seizures, (3) the appearance of previously absent neurologic symptoms or signs, including behavior changes, and (4) changing laboratory data, such as a more focal electroencephalographic abnormality or a lesion appearing on CT or MRI scans.

Surgery for Epilepsy

Surgery for epilepsy is considered in patients who are not adequately controlled by good regimens of medicine, administered in accordance with the principles listed above. In addition, the seizure focus must be well localized and surgically accessible. In most cases, candidates are individuals with intractable partial complex seizures and a seizure focus in the anterior temporal lobe. The focus should be unilateral, since bilateral anterior temporal lobectomy produces severe memory registration difficulties. Unilaterality of the focus is verified by repeated surface EEGs, prolonged intensive monitoring in specialized units, new studies, such as PET scanning, and in some instances recordings made with wires implanted into the depth of the brain. Ablation of the anterior 4 to 5 cm of temporal lobe on the speech-dominant side or up to 7 cm on the nondominant side generally leaves no major neuropsychological deficit in this group of patients. With proper selection, cure of partial complex epilepsy may be expected in 50 percent and a substantial benefit in another 25 percent. Morbidity and mortality is less than 5 percent in experienced centers. Newer methods of seizure localization and surgical technique may improve these standard figures.

Other operations for epilepsy include local cortical resection of seizure foci, partial hemispherectomy in children with widespread epileptogenic brain injuries, and resection of the corpus callosum to interrupt bilateral synchrony associated with atonic seizures. Indications for seizure operations, other than anterior temporal lobectomy, are not well established. Patients should be informed that all seizure surgery is elective, unless there is a progressive underlying lesion.

Social Issues

Epilepsy is a disease with an unfortunate social stigma. Patients and family should be informed that epilepsy will not lead to a shortened life span, mental retardation, or insanity. Family and friends should be instructed how to behave during a seizure. No folk therapy can shorten the duration of a seizure. Observers should remain calm, loosen the patient's clothing, move him or her away from sharp corners and precipitous drops, and turn the head to the side to avoid aspiration. Attempts should not be made to force the mouth open, since such maneuvers usually result in broken teeth and bite injuries. It is impossible to swallow the tongue. Suffocation or death during a seizure is exceedingly rare. During partial complex seizures patients may wander and be confused and irritable, but they do not exhibit directed violence. They should simply be kept from harm's way, without active physical restraint. In most cases, a physician should be contacted after a seizure, unless its benign nature has previously been well established.

People with epilepsy should be encouraged to go to school and to work and to raise families. Certain common sense restrictions may be required, but these are usually fairly minimal. People with frequent seizures should not work on dangerous heights or around machinery that would injure them should there be a lapse of attention. They may swim with company or supervision sufficient to keep their head above water during a seizure. Contact sports and vigorous exercise are generally allowed and encouraged; several great athletes have had epilepsy.

Each state has its own set of driving regulations pertaining to epilepsy. Some states require physician reporting of seizures to motor vehicle administrations; others do not. Physicians should in all

TABLE 15.5–7. ANTICONVULSANT DRUG DOSES

Agent	Indication	Typical Daily Dose	Serum Level (μg/ml)	Common Side Effects
Phenytoin	Partial Tonic-clonic	200–500 mg qd	10–20	Cosmetic Ataxia Rash Sedation
Phenobarbital	Partial Tonic-clonic	60–180 mg qd	15–35	Sedation Hyperactivity Mood change
Carbamazepine	Partial Tonic-clonic	200–400 mg bid–qid	6–12	Diplopia GI upset Ataxia Blood changes
Valproic acid	Absence Tonic-clonic Myoclonic Mixed	250–750 mg bid–qid	50–100	GI upset Sedation Ataxia Alopecia Weight gain
Primidone	Tonic-clonic Partial	250 mg bid–qid	6–12	Sedation Hyperactivity Mood change
Ethosuximide	Absence	500–1500 mg qd	50–100	GI upset Sedation Headache Dizziness
Clonazepam	Myoclonic Mixed	0.5–3 mg tid	0.05–0.7	Sedation Ataxia Dizziness Mood change

cases give patients their best medical opinion about the safety of driving and inform them of the local state regulations.

Counseling

A seizure is a frightening experience for the patient, family, and colleagues. There are still many misconceptions and superstitions regarding seizures. It is important to explore together the patient's ideas and concerns about seizures and the need for continuing medications. Patients will have many questions regarding restrictions of their pattern of living, such as driving, riding a bicycle, working conditions, swimming, pregnancy, or long-term effects of medications. It is difficult to generalize because seizures are a symptom rather than a specific disease. Guidelines can be offered, however.

Common questions include:

1. Are seizures hereditary? Except for certain well-characterized conditions, such as tuberous sclerosis or disorders of amino acid, carbohydrate, or lipid metabolism, seizures are not genetically determined. Although certain families seem to have a genetic predisposition to seizures, expression is variable from generation to generation, making genetic counseling difficult.

2. Is pregnancy a special risk? Generalized tonic-clonic convulsions present a clear risk to the unborn child, causing mechanical (pressure) forces on the abdomen and fetus, hypoxia, and acidosis, which are all factors leading to increased fetal loss and possibly congenital anomalies. Anticonvulsants also introduce the risk of teratogenic effects, especially in early pregnancy. While it is known that certain anticonvulsants have relatively specific effects (phenytoin and phenobarbital with orofacial, digital, and cardiac anomalies; valproic acid with neural tube defects), the safety of most anticonvulsants in pregnancy has not been adequately determined.

It is generally accepted that the risk to both mother and child of frequent generalized motor convulsions during pregnancy substantially exceeds the risk posed to the fetus by anticonvulsants. Before pregnancy is contemplated, mothers who take anticonvulsants should be reevaluated using the principles described above to determine if anticonvulsants can probably safely be discontinued. Mothers who remain on anticonvulsants should be specifically counseled about the effects. Antenatal testing (α-feto-protein) is important for mothers on valproic acid. Both counseling and antenatal testing can best be performed by an experienced obstetrical or pediatric group.

3. Will anticonvulsants interfere with my intellect? All anticonvulsant medications have the potential for decreasing cognitive function in a dose-dependent, reversible fashion. The barbiturates are most troublesome in this regard, followed by benzodiazepines, valproic acid, phenytoin, and carbamazepine. The clinical effect on intellect, memory, and cognitive functioning is usually not severe with drug levels in the therapeutic range. If impairment is severe, blood levels should be monitored.

4. Can I take other drugs? Anticonvulsants potentiate the effects of alcohol and most other sedative drugs. Other drugs can alter the metabolism of anticonvulsants, often in unpredictable ways. Patients should be cautioned about the use of alcohol, but most patients may drink in moderation. If new drugs are introduced, repeat determination of anticonvulsant drug levels should be performed.

OTHER EPISODIC DISORDERS

HYSTERICAL FAINT

Fainting was common during the Victorian era. Today it occurs less commonly but is often more complex. Dramatic fainting usually happens in a manner that avoids injuries; the patient crumples to the ground, often on a carpet or in soft surroundings. The body becomes limp and respirations are shallow. A period of unconsciousness is usually brief and recovery is quite abrupt, with full consciousness occurring immediately as the eyes open. The hysterical faint may be embellished with movements resembling seizures,

incontinence, tongue biting, a prolonged "twilight state," or paralysis, all of which may be diagnostically vexing. Often these patients will betray their state by having complete or partial memory of the spell, by showing purposeful movements during the episode, or by reproducing the spell when coaxed or when asked to hyperventilate (see Chapter 16.4 for guides to management).

DROP ATTACK

Drop attacks occur because of an abrupt loss of tone in the extensor muscles of the legs and trunk. This loss of tone is produced by ischemia to the central midbrain or pons, causing an abrupt and transitory ischemia of the descending vestibulospinal and pyramidal motor tracts. The precise pathophysiology of the spells is unclear. Drop attacks are frequently stereotyped and very brief. The patient is usually older, at risk for arteriosclerotic disease, and is often hypertensive. He describes a sudden loss of muscle power so that he crumples to the ground but recovers immediately. Incontinence is rare. These attacks are distinguished from syncope because loss of consciousness does not occur. The patient can, in fact, give a vivid account of the details of each spell. Such patients should be managed identically to those with transient ischemic attacks occurring in the posterior circulation (see Chapter 15.13).

NARCOLEPSY AND CATAPLEXY

Narcolepsy (see Chapter 15.8) causes sleep at unpredictable times during the day. An incomplete form of narcolepsy may exist in which a person feels irresistibly sleepy without actually falling asleep. Attacks of *cataplexy* (spells similar to drop attacks, causing the patient to fall to the ground with a loss of muscle tone but without loss of consciousness) are often associated with narcolepsy. They are often triggered by laughing, sneezing, or a sudden startle. Sleep paralysis (paralysis of the limbs for a moment or two upon awakening) and a peculiar visual hallucination on awakening or before falling asleep may also accompany narcolepsy and cataplexy.

TRANSIENT GLOBAL AMNESIA

This peculiar disorder has been only recently recognized. Transient global amnesia describes an episode lasting several hours (or rarely half a day) when the patient becomes confused, bewildered, and disoriented because of a defect in memory. The patient is fully awake and alert but cannot recall events even immediately before the attack and has a defect of ongoing memory coding during the episode. During the attack routine motor skills are maintained, as

mowing the lawn, driving an automobile, or walking about may continue. The episode terminates abruptly, and afterward the patient can recall nothing of what transpired during the spell.

The pathophysiologic basis for transient global amnesia is not understood. It has a predilection for middle-aged and elderly individuals, particularly men. An epileptic disturbance was at first thought to be responsible, but more recent studies suggest a vascular basis. Similar episodic amnesia occurs in epilepsy (complex partial seizures), transient ischemic attacks affecting small branches of the posterior cerebral arteries, in migraine and intermittent hydrocephalus. These disorders may be suspected when other symptoms occur suggesting them, but a pure episodic amnesia in an older individual points to this disorder.

REFERENCES

1. Annegers JF, Hauser WA, Elveback LR: Remission of seizures and relapse in patients with epilepsy. Epilepsia 20:729, 1979
2. Bannister R (ed): Autonomic Failure: A Textbook of Clinical Disorders of the Autonomic Nervous System. Oxford, Oxford University Press, 1983
3. Delgado-Escueta AV: Epileptogenic paroxysms: Modern approaches and clinical correlations. Neurology 29:1014, 1979
4. Dreifuss FE: Proposal for revised clinical and electroencephalographic classification of epileptic seizures. Epilepsia 22:489, 1981
5. Elwes RDC, Johnson AL, et al: The prognosis for seizure control in newly diagnosed epilepsy. N Engl J Med 311:944, 1984
6. Gilliatt RW, Roberts C: Syncope. In Asbury AK, McKhann GM, McDonald WI (eds): Principles of Neurology, Philadelphia, WB Saunders, 1987
7. Gram L, Bentsen KD, et al: Controlled trials in epilepsy: A review. Epilepsia 23:491, 1982
8. Hart RG, Easton JD: Carbamazepine and hematological monitoring. Ann Neurol 11:309, 1982
9. Hauser WA, Anderson VE, et al: Seizure recurrence after a first unprovoked seizure. N Engl J Med 307:522, 1982
10. Juul-Jensen P: Frequency of recurrence after discontinuance of anticonvulsant therapy in patients with epileptic seizures: A new follow-up study after 5 years. Epilepsia 9:11, 1968
11. Masland RL: Commission for the control of epilepsy. Neurology 28:861, 1978
12. Ramirez-Lassepas M, Cipolle RJ, et al: Value of computed tomographic scan in the evaluation of adult patients after their first seizure. Ann Neurol 15:536, 1984
13. Shorvon SD, Chadwick D, et al: One drug for epilepsy. Br Med J 1:474, 1978
14. Wayne HH: Syncope: Physiologic considerations and an analysis of the clinical characteristics in 510 patients. Am J Med 30:418, 1961
15. Zielinsky JJ: Epidemiology. In Laidlaw J, Richens A (eds): A Textbook of Epilepsy. New York, Churchill Livingstone, 1982, p 16

CHAPTER 15.6
Brain Stem Dysfunction

David S. Zee

The brain stem of an adult is in essence a cylinder 2 to 4 cm in diameter and 8 cm long (Fig. 15.6–1). Ascending and descending sensory and motor fiber tracts course through it longitudinally, and cranial nerve nuclei and reticular formation (tegmental) nuclei are arranged within it. Lesions can be precisely localized, since the combined manifestations of nuclear involvement and tract involvement give information about the axial and lateral location of the lesion, respectively. Furthermore, some kind of lesions, for example, occlusion of the vertebral artery with infarction of the lateral medulla (Table 15.6–1), produce highly characteristic clinical patterns.

CRANIAL NERVE SIGNS[3]

Although cranial nerve dysfunction per se does not localize lesions to the brain stem, certain patterns of involvement suggest intrinsic involvement of either the cranial nerve nuclei or their intramedullary nerve fibers. In general, either multiple or bilateral cranial nerve involvement points to a proximal and often intrinsic lesion. This is especially true if the affected cranial nerves exit the skull through different bony foramina. For example, isolated involvement of cranial nerves IX, X, and XI usually reflects a lesion at the

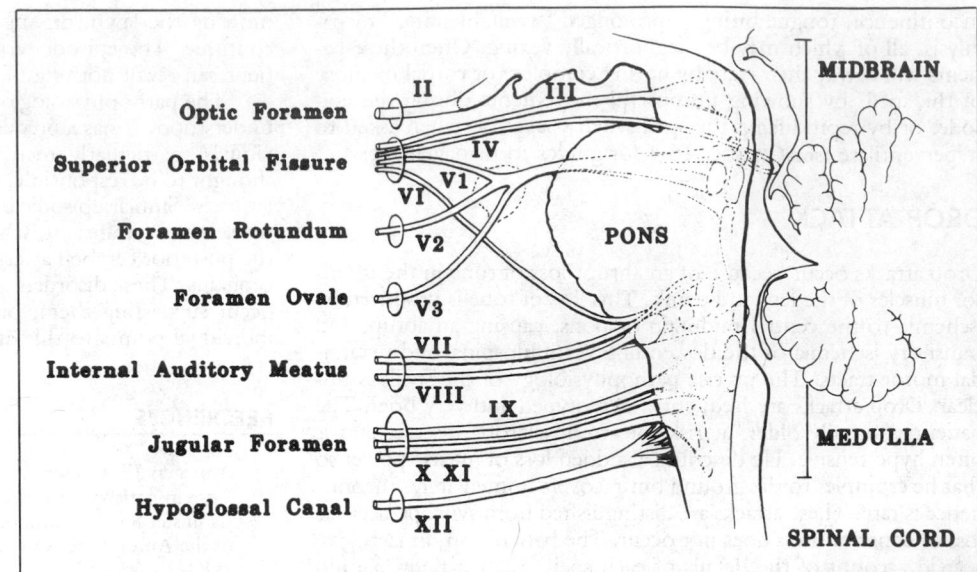

Figure 15.6–1. Diagram showing different adjacencies of cranial nerves in brain stem and as they exit skull. This provides useful information about site of lesions. See text.

level of the jugular foramen, while a combined VI and VII nerve paresis usually indicates a lesion within the pons (Fig. 15.6–1).

A partial loss of cranial nerve function may be of even more localizing value. Dissociated sensory loss (loss of response to pain and temperature, preservation of touch) on the face suggests a lesion of the descending tract and nucleus of the trigeminal nerve within the pons or medulla, for these structures subserve only pain and temperature modalities (see Table 15.6–1B). Similarly, an onion-skin pattern of sensory loss (loss of sensation around the nose and mouth with preservation of sensation more peripherally on the face) points to a brain stem lesion (often a syringobulbia). Loss of taste over both anterior and posterior portions of one side of the tongue (the anterior two thirds is usually innervated by VII and the posterior one third by IX) with preservation of the function of other structures innervated by the facial and glossopharyngeal nerves indicates an intrinsic lesion involving the tractus solitarius in the upper medulla (See Table 15.6–1C).

The combination of signs of cranial nerve involvement with signs of a motor or sensory deficit in the trunk or limbs suggests that the lesion is in the brain stem, involving both the cranial nerve nucleus and the long ascending or descending fiber tracts. For example, a single lesion in the midbrain can involve the intramedullary portion of the III nerve and the cerebral peduncle on the same side, causing an ipsilateral III nerve paresis and contralateral hemiparesis (Weber syndrome) (see Table 15.6–1A). This pattern of crossed hemiplegia can occur with any of the cranial nerves.

Hemisensory loss (either complete or dissociated) with cranial nerve signs has the same localizing significance as crossed hemiplegia. Since the intramedullary portions of the motor cranial nerves do not course as close to the ascending sensory fiber tracts as they do to the pyramidal tracts, however, an isolated cranial nerve motor loss with a contralateral hemisensory loss occurs infrequently. In contrast, a single lesion interrupting the descending tract of the trigeminal nerve and the ascending spinothalamic tract on the same side does occur frequently (see Table 15.6–1B). It causes loss of pain and temperature sensation on the ipsilateral face and contralateral trunk and extremities.

Descending sympathetic fibers also course through the brain stem, and ipsilateral Horner syndrome (ptosis, miosis, enophthalmos, with hypohydrosis) often occurs with brain stem lesions.

EYE SIGNS[1,2,3]

Disorders of ocular motility frequently provide the best clues to precise brain stem localization. The first step in diagnosis is to lo-

calize the lesion either to the peripheral ocular motor apparatus (motor neurons, nerve, or muscle) or to the intramedullary structures mediating supranuclear eye movement control. Peripheral involvement can usually be recognized by the pattern of extraocular muscle involvement. For example, a III nerve paralysis causes paresis of adduction and elevation of the globe, often with associated ptosis and pupillary mydriasis. Depression (IV cranial nerve) and abduction (VI cranial nerve) of the globe are spared. Special causes of peripheral ocular motor palsies are considered in Chapter 17.6. On the other hand, if the pattern of involvement does not conform to a peripheral ocular motor paralysis, and especially if the peripheral apparatus can be shown to be intact for some but not other types of eye movements, a supranuclear disorder is suggested.

There are four major types of eye movements: saccadic, smooth pursuit, vestibular, and vergence. *Saccades* are rapid refix eye movements that bring the images of objects seen in the periphery onto the fovea. They may be reflex (quick phases of nystagmus) or under voluntary control (saccades). *Smooth pursuit* movements are lower-velocity, smooth, following eye movements that enable one to track moving targets. *Vestibular* movements function to stabilize images upon the retina during head movements. The *vestibulo-ocular reflex* moves the eye in the orbit (slow phase of vestibular nystagmus) an amount exactly equal and opposite to a head movement to maintain clear vision. Quick phases of *vestibular nystagmus* are rapid resetting movements that keep the eye from reaching extreme degrees of deviation in the orbit. *Vergence* movements are slow disjunctive movements that keep images of the target on the fovea of each eye as the object approaches or recedes from the face.

DISORDERS OF EYE MOVEMENTS

NYSTAGMUS

Nystagmus is an involuntary rhythmic movement of the eyes. It may consist of a slow drift in one direction (slow phase) followed by a rapid corrective move in the other (quick phase), in which case it is called "jerk nystagmus." If oscillations are smooth and sinusoidal, it is designated "pendular nystagmus." Jerk nystagmus can be induced in normal individuals by rotating them in a chair for 30 to 60 seconds and then suddenly stopping the chair (postrotatory vestibular nystagmus) or by passing a band of stripes across the patient's visual field (optokinetic nystagmus). The latter consists of a smooth following eye movement (slow phase) in the di-

TABLE 15.6–1. BRAIN STEM LESIONS

A. Midbrain Lesions

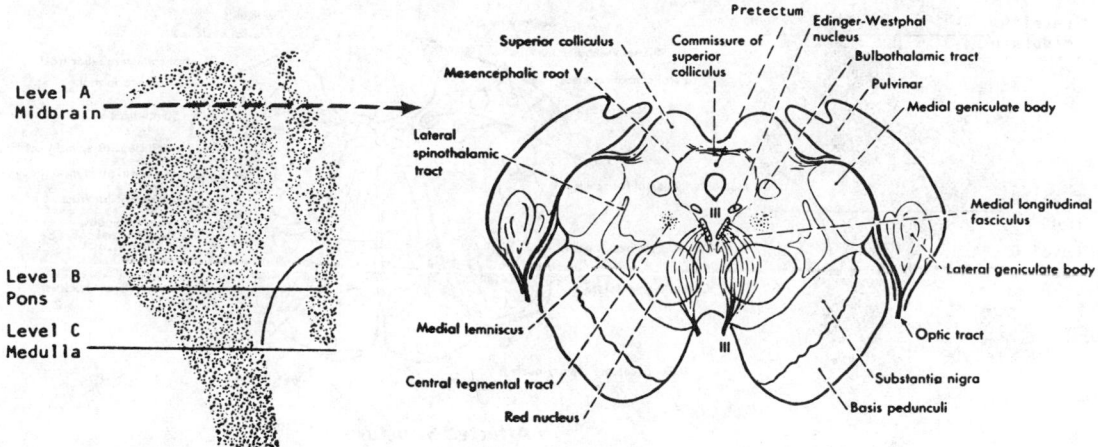

Neurologic Sign	Affected Structure
Ipsilateral	
Paresis eye adduction, elevation	C.N. III
Paresis depression	C.N. IV
Paresis upward gaze	Pretectum
Paresis downward gaze	Ventral-mesencephalic-diencephalic junction
Horner syndrome	Descending sympathetic
Ataxia and tremor	Superior cerebellar peduncle
Contralateral	
Ataxia and tremor	Red nucleus
Hemiparesis	Corticobulbar and spinal tracts
Hemihypesthesia	Medial lemniscus, spinothalamic, and quintothalamic tracts

B. Pontine Lesions

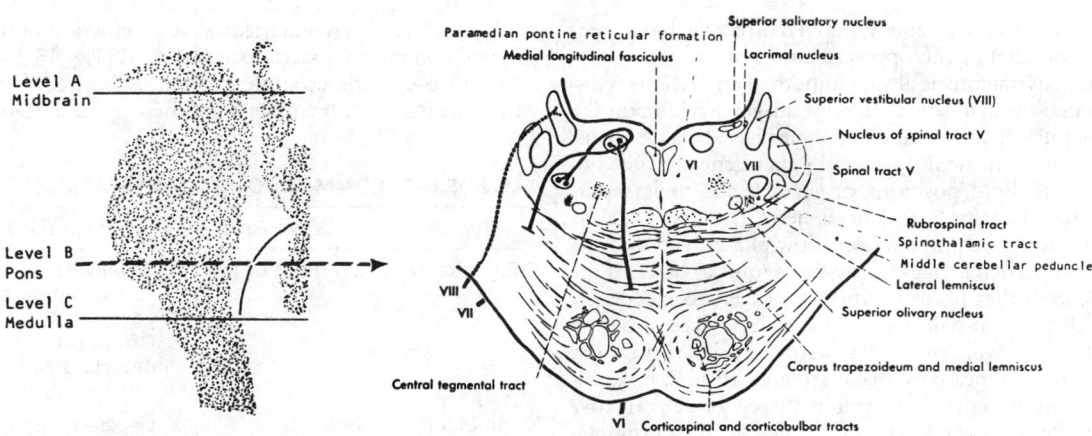

Neurologic Sign	Affected Structure
Ipsilateral	
Paresis eye abduction	C.N. VI
Paresis conjugate gaze	Paramedian pontine reticular formation (PPRF)
Internuclear ophthalmoplegia	Medial longitudinal fasciculus
Nystagmus	Vestibular nuclei, PPRF
Facial paresis	C.N. VII
Deafness	C.N. VIII
Ataxia	Middle cerebellar peduncle
Facial hypesthesia	C.N. V
Paresis chewing	C.N. V
Horner syndrome	Descending sympathetic
Contralateral	
Hemiparesis	Corticobulbar and spinal tract
Hemihypesthesia	Medial lemniscus, spinothalamic tract

(continued)

TABLE 15.6–1. BRAIN STEM LESIONS (Continued)

C. Medullary Lesions

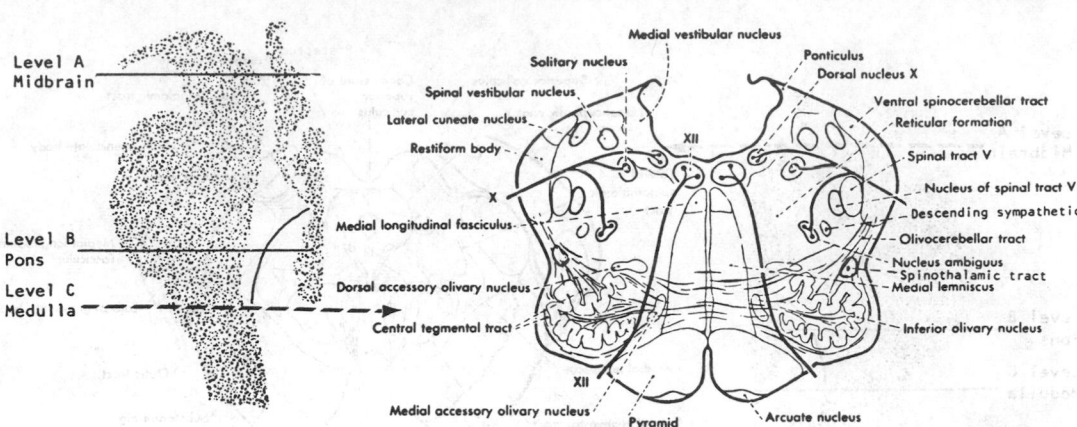

Neurologic Sign	Affected Structure
Ipsilateral	
Paresis of tongue	C.N. XII
Facial hypalgesia	Spinal tract C.N. V
Ataxia	Inferior cerebellular peduncle
Nystagmus	Vestibular nuclei
Horner syndrome	Descending sympathetic
Loss of taste	Tractus solitarius
Dysphagia, dysarthria	Nucleus ambiguus, C.N. IX and X
Contralateral	
Hemiparesis, arm, leg	Corticospinal tract
Hemihypesthesia, arm, leg	Medial lemniscus, spinothalamic tract
Crossed monoplegia	
Paresis of one upper extremity and opposite lower extremity	Decussation of pyramids

From Haymaker W: Bing's Local Diagnosis in Neurological Diseases, 15th ed. St Louis, CV Mosby, 1969.

rection of stripe movement and a rapid corrective movement (quick phase or saccade) in the opposite direction.

Spontaneous nystagmus is always abnormal and reflects a disorder of the neural mechanisms that keep images stable upon the retina. Both the pursuit and vestibular systems have balanced tonic inputs to the brain stem neural networks that generate the constant innervation to hold positions of gaze. If the tonic inputs from either system become unbalanced, jerk nystagmus results. The eyes continuously drift off fixation (slow phase), and saccades are required to bring back images to the fovea (quick phase). If the neural network itself that holds positions of gaze becomes defective, however, the patient will not be able to hold eccentric positions of gaze. The eyes will drift back toward the primary position, and the patient must repeatedly make saccades to look eccentrically. The continuous centripetal drift with repetitive corrective saccades is called "gaze-evoked nystagmus." Table 15.6–2 summarizes some distinguishing features of different types of nystagmus.

PARESIS OF HORIZONTAL GAZE

The portion of the reticular formation lying just ventral to the medial longitudinal fasciculus between the IV and VI cranial nerve nuclei (paramedian pontine reticular formation, or PPRF) and the abducens nucleus region itself are important for production of ipsilateral horizontal conjugate eye movements (Fig. 15.6–2). Patients with a unilateral lesion in the PPRF near the abducens nucleus or in the abducens nucleus itself (Fig. 15.6–2, Lesion 2) are unable to make any type of conjugate eye movement (saccade, quick phase, pursuit, or vestibular) into the ipsilateral hemifield. With more rostral PPRF lesions, vestibular movements may be spared. Cerebral hemispheral lesions may also cause abnormalities in conjugate horizontal eye movements, but the pattern of involvement is different.

With a unilateral cerebral lesion, the production of ipsilateral pursuit and contralateral saccades is impaired (Fig. 15.6–2, Lesion 1). Table 15.6–3 outlines some differences between conjugate gaze palsies arising from brain stem and hemispheral lesions.

TABLE 15.6–2. COMMON FORMS OF NYSTAGMUS

Type	Wave Form	Special Features
Congenital	Pendular or jerk	Usually horizontal Persists on up and down gaze Often associated with visual defects, strabismus or head turn
Vestibular	Jerk	Decreased by fixation If purely vertical or purely torsional, it indicates central vestibular involvement
Acquired	Pendular	Associated with a lesion in dentatorubro-olivo pathway and with palatalmyoclonus, also seen with multiple sclerosis
Gaze-evoked (inability to hold eccentric gaze)	Jerk	Small amount may be observed in normal subjects on lateral gaze May occur with lesions in lower brain stem or cerebellum Most common cause is drug side effects (sedatives, anticonvulsants)

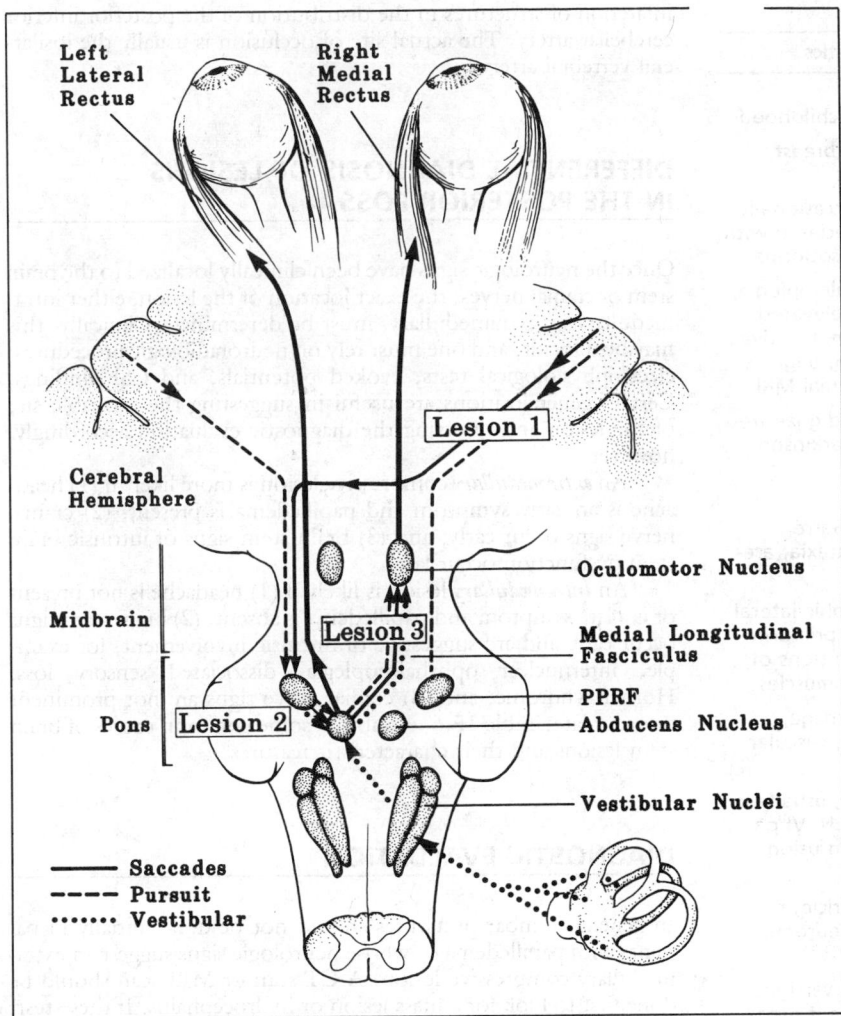

Figure 15.6–2. Control of horizontal conjugate eye movements. This explains manifestations of hemispheral lesions (Lesion 1), pontine lesions involving paramedian pontine reticular formation, paramedial pontine reticular formation (PPRF) or abducens nucleus (Lesion 2), and lesions involving medial longitudinal fasciculus (Lesion 3). See text for full description.

INTERNUCLEAR OPHTHALMOPLEGIA

The medial longitudinal fasciculus (MLF) carries fibers that mediate impulses from the abducens nucleus region to the contralateral oculomotor nucleus for adduction of the eye during conjugate horizontal gaze.

A lesion interrupting the MLF (Fig. 15.6–2, Lesion 3) causes (1) paresis of adduction of the eye ipsilateral to the side of the lesion during all types of conjugate movements, (2) sparing of adduction during convergence, and (3) jerk nystagmus in the abducting eye. This syndrome is called "internuclear ophthalmoplegia"

and is pathognomonic for a lesion of the MLF in the caudal midbrain or pons. When bilateral, it is often associated with multiple sclerosis; if unilateral, with vascular disease.

PARESIS OF VERTICAL GAZE

Vertical eye movements depend upon midbrain structures. Lesions in the region of the posterior commissure cause a paralysis of upward gaze (Parinaud syndrome). Associated signs in Parinaud syndrome are retractory and convergence nystagmus, lid retraction, and loss of pupillary reactions to a light but not to a near stimulus. Downward eye movements are more diffusely represented in the midbrain, and bilateral lesions at the ventral midbrain-thalamic junction (in the so-called rostral interstitial nucleus of the MLF) cause paresis of downward gaze. Vertical gaze disorders frequently are the earliest signs of compressive lesions arising in the region of the pineal gland (pinealoma, teratoma). Hemispheral lesions rarely cause defects in vertical gaze except as a secondary phenomenon due to, for example, transtentorial herniation from a mass lesion.

SPECIFIC BRAIN STEM SYNDROMES[1,3]

Table 15.6–1 outlines the common neurologic signs and symptoms of lesions at different levels of the brain stem. A number of eponyms have been attached to various combinations of signs and symptoms, but they serve no useful purpose in diagnosis. Only

TABLE 15.6–3. HORIZONTAL CONJUGATE GAZE PALSIES

| | Location of Lesion | |
	Brain Stem	Cerebral Hemisphere
Motor signs	Eyes deviate toward side of hemiparesis	Eyes deviate away from side of hemiparesis
Defect	All ipsilateral conjugate movements (vestibular, saccades, and pursuit) Lesion 2, Fig. 15.6–2	Contralateral saccades, Ipsilateral pursuit Vestibular spared Lesion 1, Fig. 15.6–2
Duration	Permanent	Transient

TABLE 15.6–4. COMMON BRAIN STEM LESIONS

Lesion	Characteristics
I. Intrinsic Disorders	
Primary tumors	Glioma common in childhood
Metastatic tumors	Carcinoma of lung, breast, melanoma frequent
Brain stem encephalitis	Etiology obscure, occasionally paraneoplastic, associated with myocolonus and opsoclonus
Multiple sclerosis (Chapter 15.18)	Internuclear ophthalmoplegia, nystagmus, ataxia, elevated CSF gamma globulin, positive myelin basic protein, oligoclonal bands, abnormal MRI
Progressive supranuclear palsy (Steele-Richardson-Olszewski syndrome) (Chapter 15.12)	Paresis of downward gaze frequently first sign, Parkinson syndrome
Fisher syndrome (Chapter 15.16)	Variant of Guillain-Barré Ophthalmoplegia, ataxia, areflexia
Progressive bulbar palsy (Chapter 15.16)	Variant of amyotrophic lateral sclerosis C.N. VII-XII primarily involved, often with signs of denervation in limb muscles
Cerebrovascular disease (Chapter 15.13)	Thrombosis, hemorrhage, aneurysm, vasculitis, vascular malformation
Wernicke syndrome (Chapter 17.5)	Thiamine deficiency, usually in alcoholics, ataxia, C.N. VI paresis, nystagmus, confusion
II. Extrinsic Disorders	
Tumors (Chapter 15.10)	Cerebellum, IV ventricle, pinealoma, acoustic neuroma, chordoma, metastatic
Cerebellar hemorrhage, abscess (Chapter 15.10)	Often presents with vertigo, surgically remediable if diagnosed early
Congenital abnormalities	Basilar invagination, Arnold-Chiari malformation
Vascular anomalies (Chapter 15.13)	Especially basilar aneurysm or tortuous, dilated basilar artery
Basilar meningitis (Chapter 9.11)	Especially *Listeria*, tuberculosis, fungus, syphilis, sarcoidosis, meningeal carcinomatosis

one, Wallenberg syndrome (lateral medullary infarction), occurs with any frequency or consistency. Patients develop acute symptoms of involvement of the lateral medulla (ipsilateral loss of facial sensation, ataxia, nystagmus, vertigo, vomiting, hiccough, dysphagia, dysarthria, and contralateral hemisensory loss) secondary to infarction of structures in the distribution of the posterior inferior cerebellar artery. The actual site of occlusion is usually the ipsilateral vertebral artery.

DIFFERENTIAL DIAGNOSIS OF LESIONS IN THE POSTERIOR FOSSA

Once the neurologic signs have been clinically localized to the brain stem or cranial nerves, the exact location of the lesion, either intramedullary or extramedullary, must be determined. Clinically, this may be difficult, and one must rely on neuroradiologic procedures, electrophysiological tests, evoked potentials, and CSF findings. Certain generalizations are useful in suggesting the probable site of the lesion and directing the diagnostic evaluation accordingly, however.

An *extramedullary* compressive lesion is more likely if (1) headache is an early symptom and papilledema is present, (2) cranial nerve signs occur early, and (3) brain stem signs of intrinsic brain stem dysfunction occur late.

An *intramedullary* lesion is likely if (1) headache is not present or is a late symptom and papilledema is absent; (2) brain stem signs occur early and are suggestive of intrinsic involvement, for example, internuclear ophthalmoplegia, dissociated sensory loss, Horner syndrome; and (3) cranial nerve signs are not prominent or occur late. Table 15.6–4 outlines some common causes of brain stem lesions and their characteristic features.

DIAGNOSTIC EVALUATION

In general, lumbar punctures should not be done initially in patients with papilledema or whose neurologic signs suggest an extramedullary compressive lesion. A CT scan or MRI scan should be done first to look for a mass lesion or hydrocephalus. If these tests are negative, a lumbar puncture can be safely performed. Brain stem auditory evoked potentials may also help localize the site of pathology. In patients in whom the site of the lesion is unclear, arteriography should be performed.

REFERENCES

1. Haymaker W, Kuhlenbeck H: Disorders of the brainstem and its cranial nerves. In Baker AB, Baker LN (eds): Clinical Neurology, vol 3. Hagerstown, Md, Harper & Row, 1974
2. Leigh RJ, Zee DS: The Neurology of Eye Movements. Philadelphia, FA Davis, 1983
3. Vinken PJ, Bruyn GW: Localization in clinical neurology. In Vinken PJ, Bruyn GW (eds): Handbook of Clinical Neurology, vol 2. Amsterdam, Elsevier-North-Holland, 1969

Dizziness, Vertigo, and Hearing Loss

David S. Zee and Leonard R. Proctor

Patients may use a variety of words, such as dizziness, giddiness, lightheadedness, swaying, or vertigo, to describe a sensation of imbalance or disequilibrium. Many of these patients do not have a primary disorder of vestibular function but have their symptoms secondary to any of a number of nonneurological, nonotological diseases (Table 15.7–1). Dizziness and vertigo, however, may indicate the presence of a condition specifically affecting the inner ear or the more central neurologic components of the vestibular system. Three sensations—vertigo, oscillopsia, and impulsion—should be explicitly defined and distinguished from vague giddiness, since the presence of any of these is suggestive of a primary disorder of the vestibular system, either peripherally or centrally. *Vertigo* is the illusion that either the patient or the environment is rotating or moving. *Oscillopsia* is the visual illusion that the environment is moving back and forth or up and down. *Impulsion* is the sensation that one is being forcibly propelled or pulled within the environment. Precipitation or exacerbation of these sensations by head movements is further evidence of vestibular system involvement.

PATHOPHYSIOLOGY OF VESTIBULAR DISORDERS

The vestibular system functions through two phylogenetically old responses, the vestibulospinal and vestibulo-ocular reflexes. The vestibulospinal reflex uses information from both the semicircular canals and the otolith organs (utricle and saccule) to determine the orientation of the head with respect to the ground and to promote appropriate postural adjustments to keep the body upright. The vestibulo-ocular reflex uses information from the semicircular canals to detect rotational movements of the head and to generate appropriate compensatory eye movements that are exactly equal and opposite to head movements. This reflex permits one to maintain ocular fixation during head movements.

For both systems there is a tonic discharge from each vestibular end organ that is perfectly balanced in the central nervous system (CNS). When the head is tilted or rotated in one direction, the labyrinthine output from one side increases while the other decreases, and it is this temporary imbalance of sensory input that elicits the compensatory motor commands for vestibulospinal and vestibulo-ocular reflexes. If, for some reason, the tonic inputs from the peripheral labyrinths becomes imbalanced or the central processing of labyrinthine inputs becomes disordered, inappropriate motor responses are elicited.

Vestibulospinal dysfunction is manifested by a tendency to fall or by the sensation of impulsion. With acute unilateral loss of labyrinthine function the patient will fall or feel propelled toward the side of the lesion. In the vestibulo-ocular system inappropriate oc-

ulomotor responses are manifested as oscillopsia during head movements, vertigo, and spontaneous nystagmus. Since the tonic input from each labyrinth tends to drive the eyes in the opposite direction, removal of one labyrinth causes jerk nystagmus with a slow drift (slow phase) toward the affected ear and a rapid corrective movement (quick phase) toward the intact ear. Nystagmus arising from the peripheral vestibular apparatus must be distinguished both from nystagmus of central vestibular origin (Table 15.7–2) and from nystagmus caused by other CNS lesions (Chapter 15.6).

APPROACH TO THE PATIENT WITH VERTIGO[1,2]

On the basis of the history and physical examination, it is necessary to establish whether the patient's symptoms are caused by direct involvement of the vestibular system (inner ear, vestibular nerve, or more central portions in the brain stem, cerebellum, or cerebral cortex). In a patient whose history reveals vague giddiness or dizziness without vertigo, oscillopsia, or impulsion and whose neurologic and auditory review of systems and examination are completely normal, further neurologic or otologic work-up is not initially indicated. Instead, a careful search for nonneurologic causes of dizziness (Table 15.7–1) should be made. If either the history or examination suggest auditory, vestibular, or neurologic involvement, however, special tests of vestibular and auditory function should be performed to localize the site of origin of the patient's symptoms to the labyrinth, VIII cranial nerve, or CNS (Table 15.7–2).

ANCILLARY DIAGNOSTIC TESTS[1]

CALORIC TEST (Table 15.7–3)

The most important test of peripheral vestibular function is the caloric examination. When an external auditory canal is irrigated with water above or below body temperature, convection currents induce displacement of the endolymph of the semicircular canals. The movement of the fluid mimics labyrinthine stimulation by head rotation, with the exception (and the advantage) that each labyrinth can be tested individually. If cold water is used and the head positioned such that the lateral canal is in the vertical plane (with the patient recumbent and the head elevated 30° above the horizontal), horizontal nystagmus is induced, with the slow phase directed toward the stimulated ear. Hot water induces nystagmus with the slow phase directed away from the stimulated ear. At the bedside, a small amount of ice water (0.1 to 0.3 ml) can be infused into the exterior auditory canal to elicit a vestibular response. Nystagmus can be best observed using Fresnel glasses (+ 20 diopter lenses). Since the patient's vision is blurred, he is less able to use fixation to suppress nystagmus. The caloric test can be standardized by carefully controlling water temperature, volume, and duration of irrigation. Responses can be quantified by measuring the frequency and duration of nystagmus under direct observation. For more precise measurements eye movements can be recorded with electronystagmography, and responses to both caloric and rotational stimuli can be quantified.

TABLE 15.7–1. COMMON NONNEUROLOGIC CAUSES OF DIZZINESS

- Hyperventilation, anxiety
- Syncope
- Anemia
- Postural hypotension
- Hypoglycemia
- Cardiac arrhythmia
- Hypothyroidism
- Drug side effects
- Hypertension

TABLE 15.7–2. APPROACH TO THE PATIENT WITH DIZZINESS AND VERTIGO

Variable	Observation
History	Establish presence or absence of vertigo, oscillopsia, impulsion, decreased hearing or tinnitus
Physical examination	
Vestibulospinal reflex (with eyes closed patient stands with feet together or tandem walks)	Falling or veering to one side Patient falls to side of acute peripheral lesion
Vestibulo-ocular reflex (head rotation)	Presence and characteristics of spontaneous nystagmus, positional nystagmus Patient will develop oscillopsia during head movement
Hearing	Weber, Rinne tests
Localization of the defect	
Labyrinth	Associated auditory dysfunction; no other neurological findings
VIII nerve	Auditory and vestibular dysfunction Brain stem or cerebellar compression with large masses
Brain stem	Auditory function normal, other neurological findings, pure vertical or torsional nystagmus indicates central lesion
Ancillary tests	
Caloric stimulation with recording of responses (electronystagmography)	See Table 15.7–3
Audiometry	See Table 15.7–4
Brain stem auditory evoked potential (BAER)	Good screening test for VIII nerve tumors
EEG	Vertigo secondary to seizures
Skull radiographs	
CT scan	Erosion of internal auditory meatus with acoustic neuroma, tumor in petrous bone
MRI scan	Delineation of VII and VIII cranial nerves as well as other intracranial structures
CT scan (with air or metrizamide)	Demonstration of mass in cerebellopontine angle or porous acousticus
Cerebral angiogram	Demonstration of vascular lesions
Lumbar puncture	Protein may be elevated with acoustic neuroma, inflammatory processes, chronic or neoplastic meningitis

HEARING TESTS

Assessment of hearing is essential in the evaluation of patients with vestibular dysfunction because any associated disturbances of hearing or the presence of tinnitus may be of key diagnostic importance in the evaluation of the dizzy patient.

Audiometric tests are used primarily to localize lesions peripheral to the brain stem. Sensorineural (cochlear or retrocochlear) deafness can easily be distinguished from conductive (middle ear) deafness by relative preservation of bone-conducted hearing in the latter. Clinically this is detected by the Rinne test, in which a vibrating tuning fork is held against the mastoid process until the sound fades, then is placed near the ear. Normal subjects hear the sound about twice as long by air as by bone. Conversely, patients with a conductive loss can hear the bone-conducted sound longer than the air-conducted sound. The Weber test compares bone-conducted hearing between the two ears. A vibrating tuning fork is placed at the center of the head. In conductive hearing losses the sound lateralizes to the abnormal ear; in sensorineural hearing losses, to the normal ear. Table 15.7–4 outlines common causes of disorders of hearing, and Table 15.7–5 outlines the basic patterns of hearing loss in cochlear and retrocochlear lesions.

TABLE 15.7–3. CALORIC TESTS

Lesion	Response
Peripheral	Decreased on side of lesion Fixation decreases induced nystagmus
Central	Relatively normal Fixation may not decrease induced nystagmus

AUDIOMETRY

The patient's threshold for detection of pure tones at various frequencies is the key test in audiometric evaluation. Tones are presented through earphones (air conduction) or by a vibrator applied to the mastoid process (bone conduction) in a soundproof room. The results are marked on a chart (audiogram) showing the loudness in decibels (db) required for detection of tones at 500, 1000, 2000, 4000, and 8000 hertz. Each ear is tested separately. Certain patterns on the audiogram may point to a specific diagnosis, such as a more pronounced loss at lower frequencies in Menière disease.

The speech discrimination test involves presentation of single words through the earphones and scoring the number of words correctly identified. "Recruitment" is an abnormal sensitivity to increments of loudness; this finding suggests a disorder of the cochlear hair cells. Recruitment can be demonstrated by the "Short Increment Sensitivity Index" (SISI) test or by the loudness balance test (wherein loudness of a pure tone in the affected ear is balanced by the patient to a specific loudness level in the good ear).

"Tone decay" is tested by maintaining a pure tone at a specific level until it seems to the patient that it has faded away. Patients with retrocochlear lesions often have an abnormally rapid tone decay.

The acoustical impedance of the middle ear can be measured through tiny probes inserted into the external ear canal. In this way, reflex contraction of the stapedius muscle to loud tones presented in the same or opposite ear can be detected. In some cases this provides helpful information about the stapedius reflex arc (auditory nerve, brain stem interneurons, facial nerve).

Auditory evoked responses to clicks can be detected by computerized signal averaging. The responses are a reflection of neural

TABLE 15.7–4. COMMON DISORDERS OF HEARING

Type	Examples	Distinguishing Characteristics
Conductive	Obstruction in external canal (cerumen) Damage to tympanic membrane Middle ear infection or fluid accumulation Otosclerosis	Hearing loss usually spares high frequencies Sounds are muffled with paracusis (hear better in noisy background) and a low-pitched, fluctuating tinnitus; with otosclerosis, tinnitus is usually whistling and constant
Sensorineural	Hereditary Congenital (rubella, erythroblastosis) Presbycusis Trauma (occupational, skull fractures)	
	Infections: postmeningitic (*H. influenzae*, meningococcal), viral (mumps, measles, herpes zoster); rickettsial (murine typhus) Drug toxicity (quinine, salicylate, dihydrostreptomycin, gentamycin, kanamycin, arsenic)	Hearing loss usually affects high frequencies; must differentiate retrocochlear from cochlear pattern (Table 15.7–5) Acoustic trauma usually gives a specific loss of hearing at 4000 Hz Facial palsy often occurs with herpes zoster
	Menière syndrome	Menière syndrome may be mimicked by hypothyroidism, neurosyphilis, perilymph fistula, and vasculitis
	Lesions of the VIII nerve	See Table 15.7–8

TABLE 15.7–5. EVALUATION OF HEARING LOSS

Cochlear	Retrocochlear
Pure tone loss proportional to speech discrimination loss	Pure tone loss much less than speech discrimination loss
Recruitment (sudden abnormal loudness growth as sound intensity is slowly increased)	No recruitment
High SISI (short increment sensitivity index, pathologic ability to detect slight increases in loudness)	Low SISI
Minimal tone decay	Pronounced tone decay

often associated with positional vertigo. It can be elicited by rapidly moving the patient from the sitting to the lying position with the head turned toward one side. Positional nystagmus can be caused by either peripheral or central lesions. If of peripheral origin, it usually occurs predominantly in only one head position and begins after a short delay (2 to 10 seconds) after assuming the recumbent position. Typically there is a crescendo of predominantly torsional nystagmus associated with vertigo. It dies out within a minute, and it becomes more difficult to elicit with repeated testing. In contrast, positional nystagmus of central origin usually occurs in more than one head position, begins with no delay, and does not fatigue upon repeated testing.

CENTRAL VESTIBULAR DISORDERS

Vertigo of central origin may arise from lesions anywhere in the vestibular nuclei or their cerebellar connections (Table 15.7–7). Hence, pontine, medullary, or cerebellar lesions all may cause vertigo, but patients usually have additional neurologic symptoms or signs pointing to the location of the lesions. Occasionally, vertigo is part of temporal lobe seizures or is associated with a migraine syndrome. Patients with recent onset of an extraocular muscle paresis may also complain of mild degrees of vertigo.

Acute, severe vertigo occurs with brain stem lesions such as multiple sclerosis or brain stem infarction. Positional vertigo and nystagmus are more characteristic of chronic processes such as posterior fossa neoplasms, spinocerebellar degenerations, or congenital malformations.

The distinction between acute attacks of vertigo and transient ischemic attacks of the brainstem may be difficult. Persistent vertigo, without other neurologic signs or symptoms, is seldom secondary to brainstem ischemia.

VIII NERVE TUMORS

Early diagnosis of acoustic nerve tumors has become increasingly important because of the comparatively low morbidity and mortality of surgical removal if the tumor is small. Every patient with unexplained unilateral hearing loss or vague dizziness and imbalance must be considered a tumor suspect and evaluated accordingly.

Although acoustic neuroma is the most common lesion of the VIII nerve, a number of other lesions may have a similar clinical presentation (Table 15.7–8). Patients usually complain first of insidious hearing loss or tinnitus and, if specifically asked, they may describe a vague feeling of unsteadiness. At this point, however, caloric testing and brain stem auditory evoked responses (Chapter 15.2) may be abnormal despite a paucity of symptoms. As the tumor enlarges, patients may have headache; retroaural discomfort; facial numbness, pain, or paresthesias; ataxia; loss of taste; dyspha-

activity within the auditory nerve and brain stem. This test is very sensitive and has been found useful in detecting the presence of acoustic neuromas or demyelinating disorders affecting brain stem auditory pathways.

PERIPHERAL VESTIBULAR DISORDERS

With the exception of acoustic neuromas, disorders of the peripheral vestibular system usually present acutely. The common causes are indicated in Table 15.7–6. Patients may be severely ill, with incapacitating vertigo, impulsion, nausea, vomiting, and prostration. Nystagmus is usually present at the onset of illness and is usually horizontal, but varying degrees of torsional or vertical components may be present. The direction of the horizontal component of nystagmus in peripheral disorders usually reflects the measure of a hypoactive labyrinth—consequently the slow phase is directed toward the affected ear, for example, acute vestibular neuritis. Occasionally, when there is some ongoing recovery of function, the slow phase may be directed away from the affected ear, for example, following an attack of Menière syndrome, or a lesion may be irritative, for example, purulent labyrinthitis. In peripheral disorders, auditory symptoms and signs may be present, but other evidence of neurologic involvement is absent. Caloric tests usually show decreased responses in the involved ear.

Positional nystagmus is a special form of vestibular nystagmus

TABLE 15.7–6. PERIPHERAL VESTIBULAR DISORDERS

Disorder	Characteristics	Auditory	Caloric	Nystagmus	Neurologic Symptoms and Signs
Menière syndrome	Paroxysmal vertigo, tinnitus, fluctuating but eventually progressive permanent hearing loss Recurrent attacks occasionally associated with hypothyroidism, otosclerosis, syphilis, collagen vascular disease	Cochlear pattern of hearing loss (occasionally bilateral), worse for low frequencies	Minimally abnormal	Only at peak of attack Usually horizontal	None
Benign paroxysmal positional vertigo	Only positional vertigo Severe, usually self-limited, often secondary to trauma	Normal	Usually normal	Positional nystagmus is of peripheral type Mixture of vertical and torsional Elicited with affected ear down	None
Vestibular neuritis and labyrinthitis	Acute onset, of vertigo, may also be exacerbated by positional changes, usually self-limited, etiology unknown	Usually normal	Marked hypoactivity	Horizontal-torsional Slow phase toward bad ear	None

Drug toxicity
  Tobramycin
  Streptomycin
  Kanamycin
  Gentamicin
  CIS platinum
	Insidious onset
	Often irreversible
	Bilateral
		Usually not affected	Decreased bilaterally	Usually absent	None

Blood dyscrasias (hemorrhage into labyrinth)	Acute	Normal	Absent on side of lesion	Horizontal torsional Slow phase toward bad ear	None
Acoustic neuroma	Insidious onset Vertigo unusual Commonly imbalance, vague dizziness with unilateral hearing loss or tinnitus	Retrocochlear pattern of hearing loss	Hypoactive responses	If present, usually horizontal with slow phase in either direction	Decreased corneal response Trigeminal sensory loss Gait ataxic Mild facial nerve involvement

TABLE 15.7–7. CNS DISORDERS IN WHICH VERTIGO MAY BE A PROMINENT FEATURE

Disease	Comment
Multiple sclerosis	Acute vertiginous episode may be first manifestation; oscillopsia frequent
Syringobulbia	Pure torsional nystagmus common
Lateral medullary infarction (Wallenberg syndrome)	Severe lateropulsion to side of lesion, nystagmus, and vertigo
Cerebellar hemorrhage	Severe nausea and vomiting, gait ataxia, surgically remediable
Transient ischemic attacks	Usually associated with brain stem symptoms and signs
Posterior fossa tumors	Positional nystagmus of central type, gaze-evoked nystagmus
Arnold-Chiari malformation	Vertical oscillopsia, downbeat nystagmus Positional nystagmus of central type
Basilar migraine	Other signs of brain stem involvement, headache
Temporal lobe epilepsy	Usually with loss of consciousness and other automatisms suggestive of a seizure

gia; or dysarthria. Early in the course of the condition, neurologic examination may be normal except for hearing loss, but eventually patients show signs of involvement of other cranial nerves, the cerebellum, and the brain stem. Papilledema and lower cranial nerve dysfunction are late signs and indicate a large tumor.

If the neurologic examination shows any abnormality, or caloric or audiometric tests reveal an abnormality suggestive of an VIII nerve tumor, the patient should have a CT scan with special attention to the internal auditory meatus or an MRI scan, which nicely delineates the VII and VIII cranial nerves as well as the other posterior fossa structures. If the routine CT scan or MRI is negative, a contrast (air or metrizamide) CT scan should be performed and, at the same time, the CSF protein level determined, since it may be elevated in acoustic tumors. If all tests are negative, careful follow-up examination is still indicated with audiograms, caloric tests, CT scans, and MRI scans as necessary.

Treatment is surgical. For small tumors, translabyrinthine removal is possible with minimal risk. For larger tumors, posterior fossa exploration is indicated, but with microsurgical techniques, the outlook is good.

TREATMENT[3]

While symptomatic treatment of vertigo is often helpful, therapy aimed at the underlying cause is most effective. Fortunately, most

TABLE 15.7–8. NERVE LESIONS

- Acoustic neuroma (if bilateral, von Recklinghausen disease)
- Cholesteatoma
- Meningioma
- Teratoma
- Metastatic carcinoma (especially lung and breast)
- Arachnoid cysts
- Vascular malformations and aneurysms
- Paget disease
- Glomus jugulare tumors
- Mononeuropathy (meningeal carcinomatosis, diabetes, vasculitis, herpes zoster, sarcoidosis)

TABLE 15.7–9. DRUGS USED IN THE TREATMENT OF VERTIGO

Sedatives	
Diazepam (Valium)	2–5 mg PO tid
Anticholinergics	
Atropine	0.4 mg sublingual prn
Scopalamine	0.1 mg PO, transdermal
Antiemetics	
Trimethobenzamide (Tigan)	200 mg PO or PR
Prochlorperazine (Compazine)	5–25 mg PO or PR
Antihistamines	
Dimenhydrinate (Dramamine)	50 mg PO tid
Meclizine (Bonine, Antivert)	25–50 mg PO tid

peripheral disorders are self-limited, and reassurance of the patient, along with judicious use of sedatives, antiemetics, and antivertiginous agents (Table 15.7–9), is indicated. These agents are more effective when used prophylactically between attacks than in an attempt to abort an attack already in progress. Benign paroxysmal positional vertigo can be effectively treated with vestibular exercises.[2]

Patients with intractable, incapacitating vertigo occasionally require destruction of either the labyrinth or portions of the vestibular nerve.

REFERENCES

1. Baloh RW, Honrubia U: Clinical Neurophysiology of the Vestibular System. Philadelphia, FA Davis, 1978
2. Brandt T, Daroff RB: Physical therapy for benign paroxysmal positional vertigo. Arch Otolaryngol 106:484, 1980
3. Zee D: Treatment of vertigo. In Johnson RJ (ed): Current Therapy in Neurologic Disease, 1985–86. Philadelphia, BC Decker, 1985

CHAPTER 15.8
Sleep Disorders

David Buchholz

NORMAL SLEEP[3]

There are three distinct states of human existence: wakefulness, rapid eye movement (REM) sleep, and non-REM sleep. Sleep is not a passive state, as both REM and non-REM sleep are actively generated by specific brain mechanisms.

Non-REM sleep is a quiet state that comprises 80 percent of sleep in the adult and is divided into four stages. Stage I is a transition between drowsiness and sleep; the electroencephalogram (EEG) slows, muscles relax, and slow rolling eye movements occur. Stage II has a distinctive EEG pattern, with sleep spindles and K-complexes. Stages III and IV (slow-wave sleep) are marked by profound EEG slowing.

In contrast, REM sleep resembles wakefulness in many ways. The EEG is fast, like an "alert" recording, and dreaming indicates active mental processes. Autonomic activity is high, with wide variations of heart rate, blood pressure, and respiration, and penile erections occur. Although limb muscles are generally paralyzed during REM sleep, intermittent limb twitches and rapid eye movements take place.

A typical adult's night of sleep lasts approximately 7 hours, with a normal range of 4 to 10 hours. Adequacy of sleep duration is determined by the extent of restoration of waketime alertness. Sleep latency (the time it takes to fall asleep) averages 5 to 30 minutes. During this time hypnic jerks (sudden limb movements) may startle a person, but such jerks are normal and should be distinguished from abnormal phenomena such as sleep-related myoclonus (see below) or seizures.

After sleep onset, stages I to IV of non-REM sleep take place successively. The first REM sleep period occurs approximately 90 minutes after sleep onset. Subsequent REM and non-REM sleep periods cycle throughout the night at 90-minute intervals, with REM sleep periods increasing in intensity and duration from 5 to 20 or more minutes. Thus, most slow-wave sleep occurs early, and most REM sleep occurs late in the course of a night's sleep.

Children have more slow-wave sleep and total sleep than adults. Further decreases in slow-wave sleep and total sleep in the elderly have been considered a continuation of this maturational trend, but these changes may represent increasing abnormality rather than normal physiology of sleep in the elderly.

The major sleep period is part of a daily sleep-wake schedule that is the dominant rhythm of the body. Most bodily functions, such as hormonal secretion and temperature homeostasis, have a cyclic pattern that is tightly synchronized with the sleep-wake schedule. Serious disruption of the sleep-wake schedule leads to disruption of subordinate bodily rhythms, and subsequent normalization of these rhythms may not occur for several weeks. Oddly, as demonstrated by experiments in which subjects live in environments without time cues, the endogenous sleep-wake cycle is about 25 hours long. This requires each of us to make a daily adjustment of our 25-hour internal clock to conform with the 24-hour solar day.

SLEEP DISORDERS[1,2,3]

Persistent sleep disorders affect 10 to 20 percent of the population and are life disrupting, sometimes life threatening, and largely unrecognized. Physicians must distinguish these serious problems from less important sleep disturbances such as transient insomnia caused by situational anxiety.

Four general categories of sleep disorders are recognized. These are *disorders of initiating and maintaining sleep* (insomnia), *disorders of excessive somnolence* (hypersomnia), *disorders of the sleep-wake schedule* (circadian rhythm disturbance), and *parasomnias* (miscellaneous abnormal behaviors in sleep). In evaluating a patient with

sleep complaints it is helpful to locate the primary complaint within this framework, although overlap is frequent. For example, patients with insomnia primarily report inadequate nocturnal sleep but may also note daytime fatigue. Patients with hypersomnia fall asleep at inappropriate times during the day, such as while conversing, working, or driving. Yet they may also complain of nocturnal awakenings caused by the underlying disorder that is fragmenting sleep and resulting in daytime sleepiness.

SLEEP APNEA[4]

The two basic types of sleep apnea (periodic cessation of respiration during sleep) are *central* sleep apnea (failure of respiratory effort during sleep) and *obstructive* sleep apnea (upper airway collapse in sleep). *Mixed* apnea is a central respiratory pause followed by upper airway obstruction. Normal subjects may have occasional brief apneas, especially in REM sleep, but by definition patients with sleep apnea have at least five episodes per hour of at least 10 seconds duration each. In fact, hundreds of episodes may occur per night, with individual episodes lasting as long as 1 or 2 minutes.

People of all ages may develop sleep apnea, and in infants it may be related to some cases of sudden infant death syndrome. Children are predisposed to obstructive sleep apnea by tonsillar hypertrophy or congenital deformities of the upper airway. The elderly have an increased incidence of sleep apnea caused by neurologic disease and normal age-related degeneration of central respiratory control.

The prototypical obstructive sleep apnea patient is a middle-aged male or postmenopausal female with normal breathing during wakefulness. The patient usually either complains of hypersomnia (irresistible sleepiness at work or while driving) or presents at the request of his bed-partner because of loud snoring, irregular breathing, and abnormal movements during sleep. The patient with obstructive sleep apnea is generally unaware of disturbed breathing or movements even though these events substantially disrupt nocturnal sleep and thereby cause daytime sleepiness. In contrast, the patient with central sleep apnea may awaken frequently with apneic episodes and complain of difficulty maintaining sleep. Long-term complications are largely related to severe episodic nocturnal hypoxemia and include systemic and pulmonary hypertension, cor pulmonale, cardiac arrhythmias, sudden nocturnal death, and motor vehicle accidents.

The etiology of sleep apnea in the typical middle-aged male patient is unknown, although various anatomic, neurologic, and hormonal factors have been implicated. Complete polysomnography (see below) is essential in determining diagnosis and appropriate therapy.

Initial treatment of sleep apnea includes weight loss (if appropriate), avoidance of CNS depressants, and caution about driving and operating machinery. Medication has a limited role in sleep apnea. Protriptyline 5 to 20 mg at bedtime suppresses REM sleep and may be useful when apneas occur mainly in REM sleep. Continuous positive airway pressure (CPAP), applied through a facial mask, acts as a "pneumatic splint" to maintain upper airway patency during sleep. Finally, severe sleep apnea may require surgical treatment with tracheostomy or uvulopalatopharyngoplasty (UPPP), a procedure in which excessive palatal and pharyngeal tissue is excised to create a more spacious oropharynx.

NARCOLEPSY[1,2]

Narcolepsy is partly genetically determined and presents in teenage or early adulthood. Classically it is defined by the tetrad of *sleep attacks, cataplexy, hypnogogic hallucinations,* and *sleep paralysis.* In reality, the full tetrad is rarely seen, and excessive sleepiness with or without cataplexy is the usual presentation. Sleep attacks are often irresistible, last up to 30 minutes, may be associated with dreaming, and typically leave the patient feeling refreshed. Cataplexy is transient muscle weakness without loss of consciousness, usually precipitated by an emotional outburst, such as laughter or anger.

Hypnogogic hallucinations are strange, vivid, dreamlike experiences occurring at sleep onset, and sleep paralysis is the transient inability to move while drifting off to sleep or upon awakening. Disturbed nocturnal sleep is common in narcolepsy, but it is an effect rather than a cause of the disorder.

Narcolepsy can be thought of as inappropriate intrusions of REM sleep phenomena into wakefulness. The sleep attacks are complete REM sleep episodes; cataplexy and sleep paralysis are REM-related muscle inhibition; the hallucinations are dreams in wakefulness. Multiple sleep latency testing (see below) reveals excessive sleepiness and premature onset of REM sleep during brief daytime naps. Treatment includes stimulants such as pemoline or methylphenidate for sleepiness and tricyclic antidepressants such as protriptyline or imipramine (which are REM sleep suppressants) for cataplexy. Patients with narcolepsy should take brief preventive naps during the day to reduce accumulation of sleepiness, and they should avoid CNS depressants.

SLEEP-RELATED MYOCLONUS[3]

Repetitive, sudden limb movements may occur in sleep either independently or in association with another sleep disorder such as sleep apnea. These movements should be distinguished from normal hypnic jerks that many individuals experience sporadically while falling asleep. The chief complaint may be either insomnia caused by awakenings from sleep or hypersomnia caused by partial arousals leading to fragmented, nonrestorative sleep. *Restless legs syndrome* and nocturnal leg cramps are often associated with sleep-related myoclonus. Some patients have an underlying condition such as uremia, folate or iron deficiency anemia, peripheral neuropathy, myelopathy, pregnancy, or caffeine abuse, but most cases are idiopathic. Treatment is directed at any identifiable cause and may also include medication if the movements are severely symptomatic. A benzodiazepine such as triazolam 0.125 to 0.5 mg or a narcotic such as codeine 30 to 60 mg or propoxyphene 65 mg at bedtime may suppress the limb jerks and/or the associated arousals.

DISORDERS OF THE SLEEP-WAKE SCHEDULE[4]

Disorders of the sleep-wake schedule represent asynchrony of the patient's circadian rhythm and the 24-hour clock on the wall. Transient disorders include *jet lag* and *rotating work shifts.* When traveling east to west, jet lag is readily managed by postponing sleep the appropriate number of hours. It is much easier to postpone sleep than to fall asleep prematurely, as is necessary with west-to-east travel, in which case a short-acting hypnotic medication such as triazolam 0.125 to 0.5 mg is useful.

Workers who regularly rotate shifts are prone to chronic insomnia *and* hypersomnia, especially if shift rotations are made too quickly to allow adjustment of the patient's sleep-wake schedule and other bodily rhythms. At least several weeks should pass between shift rotations, and rotations should always be made in a forward direction, for example, moving from a 7 AM to 3 PM shift to a 3 PM to 11 PM shift. Also, shift workers are well advised to avoid changing to their family's sleep-wake schedule on off-days, since this further disrupts the worker's own rhythms.

Persistent sleep-wake schedule disorders represent chronic failure to adjust the 25-hour endogenous sleep-wake rhythm to the 24-hour day. Some individuals seem unable to reset their internal clocks daily, and those individuals become asynchronous with the rest of society. Treatment is difficult and involves gradual synchronization of internal and external clocks followed by rigid adherence to the newly established sleep-wake schedule, a technique known as "chronotherapy."

PARASOMNIAS[3,4]

The parasomnias are a diverse group of abnormal behaviors in sleep too numerous to mention other than the three most common:

somnambulism (sleep walking), *night terrors,* and *enuresis.* These three disorders share certain features and are probably related. Onset is usually in early childhood, resolution generally occurs by adolescence, and other family members may be affected. Incomplete arousal from excessively deep slow-wave sleep seems to be a common factor among these disorders. Accordingly, they take place in the early hours of sleep, when most slow-wave sleep occurs. These conditions are considered benign in childhood, and recurrence in adulthood suggests an underlying psychiatric or neurologic condition. Treatment is usually conservative, such as protecting a sleepwalker from injury by gating stairs and locking windows, but benzodiazepines can be used to inhibit these parasomnias.

Night terrors are episodes of apparent awakening with inconsolable fright, screaming, and autonomic hyperactivity. Fortunately, the child has little or no memory of an episode after reawakening. Night terrors should be distinguished from nightmares, which are unpleasant dreams with vivid recall. Nightmares are related to REM sleep and therefore tend to occur in the late hours of sleep, unlike night terrors.

PSYCHOLOGIC AND PSYCHIATRIC PROBLEMS[2]

All individuals are susceptible to transient insomnia as a result of a temporarily stressful life situation. Persistent insomnia develops in some anxious individuals in whom repeatedly frustrated efforts to sleep cause ever greater concern about not sleeping. Chronic anticipation of poor sleep is a self-fulfilling prophecy known as "learned insomnia." This condition is treated with behavioral therapy, including *sleep hygiene* (Table 15.8–1) and psychotherapy. *Sleep restriction* is a behavioral approach to extinguishing the insomniac's preoccupation with inability to sleep. A patient who goes to bed at 11 PM but does not usually fall asleep until 2 AM is instructed to stay awake and out of bed until 2 AM. The patient's concern is thereby shifted from falling asleep to staying awake. The permitted bedtime is then very gradually reset from 2 AM to the desired hour of 11 PM.

Personality disorders, obsessions, compulsions, phobias, mania, and schizophrenia are often associated with insomnia. Alcohol and other abused substances may produce sleep and arousal disturbances associated with acute intoxication, chronic use, or withdrawal. *Depression* causes a variety of sleep disturbances, most characteristically early morning awakening. Patients with endogenous depression demonstrate reduced REM sleep latency during polysomnography, that is, the first REM sleep episode occurs within 30 rather than the usual 90 minutes. This finding is useful in evaluating depression as to both its type and its response to treatment, since conversion to normal REM sleep onset time occurs rapidly after effective antidepressant medication is begun and predicts eventual success of the medication in elevating mood.

TABLE 15.8–1. SLEEP HYGIENE

The following advice is of value for patients with insomnia, especially if behavioral factors are primary:
- Sleep in a comfortable place on a regular schedule. Get out of bed at the *same* time each morning, shortly after the final awakening.
- Large meals, heavy exercise, caffeine, and excessive alcohol should be avoided before sleep.
- If unable to sleep after 30 minutes in bed, get out of bed and engage in a restful activity or eat a light snack until sleepiness develops, then return to bed. Do *not* lie in bed and struggle to go to sleep.
- Avoid daytime naps if nocturnal sleep is a problem. Instead, substitute exercise.
- A bothersome mental concern can be "put to sleep" by writing it down and dealing with it in the morning.
- Use sedative and hypnotic medication sparingly, not regularly.
- Be assured that sleeplessness, distressing though it may be, will not cause permanent harm to body or mind.

SEDATIVE AND HYPNOTIC USE AND ABUSE[1]

Sedatives and hypnotics are often improperly prescribed for chronic insomnia. These medications are effective on a short-term basis in reducing sleep latency (time until sleep onset) and increasing total sleep time. Chronic use, however, results in drug accumulation, tolerance, and dependence. Rapid withdrawal from chronic hypnotic use produces temporary worsening of insomnia, thereby reinforcing the patient's and the physician's conviction that the medication is beneficial. In addition, chronic insomnia in some patients, especially the elderly, may be caused by important but unrecognized sleep disorders such as sleep apnea. These disorders may seriously worsen with hypnotic medication. Such medication should therefore, be restricted to short-term use in patients with transient insomnia.

Short-acting benzodiazepines such as triazolam 0.125 to 0.5 mg or temazepam 15 to 30 mg at bedtime are the safest and most effective prescription hypnotic medications. Sedating tricyclic antidepressants such as amitriptyline 25 to 100 mg at bedtime are often helpful, especially if depression is playing a role in insomnia. The over-the-counter hypnotics usually contain an antihistamine, and some patients with insomnia are helped by L-tryptophan 500 to 2000 mg at bedtime.

MEDICAL DISORDERS

Both insomnia and hypersomnia can result from a variety of medical disorders such as thyroid disease, hepatic and renal insufficiency, and cardiopulmonary dysfunction. Neurologic patients are at significant risk for sleep disorders related to CNS disease (affecting control of sleep and breathing) and neuromuscular disease (affecting pharyngeal and pulmonary muscle function). Insomnia can be caused by medications such as corticosteroids, theophylline, and beta-blockers, and hypersomnia can occur with the use of anxiolytics, antihistamines, and narcotics, among other drugs. The complete workup of a sleep disorders patient often includes medical, neurologic, and psychiatric history and examination, blood count, blood chemistries, thyroid function tests, ECG, and chest radiograph. Hypersomnia that remains unexplained after such a workup should be further evaluated by formal sleep studies (Tables 15.8–2 and 15.8–3).

SLEEP STUDIES[3]

Polysomnography, the simultaneous recording of multiple physiological functions in sleep, is the basic tool for clinical evaluation of sleep and its disorders. The patient sleeps in a private room for one or more nights with continuous monitoring. The monitoring devices include limited *EEG* (to determine sleep stages), *ECG* (to record arrhythmias associated with disorders such as sleep apnea), *chin electromyogram* (EMG; to record suppression of muscle tone in REM sleep), *leg EMG* (to record normal twitches of REM sleep as well as abnormal movements caused by seizure or sleep-related myoclonus), *nasal and oral thermistors* (to monitor air flow), *thoracic*

TABLE 15.8–2. APPROACH TO HYPERSOMNIA

- Determine that the complaint is true excessive sleepiness, not simply fatigue. Does the patient fall asleep during routine activities such as driving and working?
- Consider underlying medical conditions, medication effects, and substance abuse as causes of hypersomnia.
- Is nocturnal sleep too short? Try extending sleep by 1 to 2 hours each night for at least a few weeks.
- If hypersomnia persists, refer the patient to a sleep disorders center for polysomnographic evaluation of possible causes such as sleep apnea, narcolepsy, and sleep-related myoclonus.

TABLE 15.8–3. APPROACH TO INSOMNIA

- Consider underlying medical conditions, medication effects, and substance abuse as causes of insomnia.
- Give sleep hygiene advice (Table 15.8–1).
- Supervise a trial of sleep restriction (see text).
- Consider psychotherapy.
- Use hypnotic medication cautiously and briefly. Consider sedating antidepressant medication if depression is suspected.
- If insomnia is very difficult to manage, refer the patient to a sleep disorders center. Some patients with insomnia have an underlying sleep disorder such as sleep apnea or sleep-related myoclonus, and polysomnography is occasionally (but not often) indicated in the workup of insomnia.

and abdominal strain gauges or endoesophageal balloon (to monitor respiratory effort), and *ear oximeter* (to record capillary oxygen saturation). Minimal, if any, discomfort is involved, and the patient is easily disconnected and readily mobile.

The data obtained from polysomnography define the patient's night in bed including the timing of wakefulness and specific sleep stages as well as any attendant respiratory, cardiac, or neurologic pathology. Other measures can be studied during sleep, such as complete EEG in nocturnal seizure disorders or esophageal pH in gastroesophageal reflux. The recording of nocturnal penile tumescence has been very useful in the workup of persistent erectile impotence (see Chapter 16.10).

Another study performed in sleep disorders centers is multiple sleep latency testing (MSLT), which quantifies daytime sleepiness. The patient is instructed to lie down in a dark, quiet room during the day and try to sleep while being monitored to determine wakefulness or stage of sleep. Normal subjects require at least 10 to 15 minutes to fall asleep, but pathologically sleepy patients fall asleep within 5 minutes. Patients with narcolepsy characteristically enter REM sleep shortly after onset of a daytime nap. Using the MSLT, a complaint of excessive daytime sleepiness can be confirmed and quantified, and the effect of treatment upon a sleep disorder can be objectively evaluated.

Polysomnography and MSLT are essential studies in the proper evaluation of suspected sleep apnea, narcolepsy, and sleep-related myoclonus. There is no adequate alternative method of acquiring the data needed to effectively manage these problems. Any patient with excessive sleepiness unexplained by insufficient sleep duration, medication use, substance abuse, or medical illness should be considered for referral to a sleep disorders center for testing. On the other hand, sleep studies are not generally indicated for evaluation of insomnia unless there is specific evidence suggesting sleep apnea or sleep-related myoclonus as the cause.

REFERENCES

1. Buchholz D: Sleep disorders. In Bayless TM, Brain MC, Cherniack RM (eds): Current Therapy in Internal Medicine—2. Philadelphia, BC Decker, 1987
2. Hauri P: The Sleep Disorders. Kalamazoo, Mich, Upjohn, 1982
3. Parkes JD: Sleep and Its Disorders. London, WB Saunders, 1985
4. Riley TL (ed): Clinical Aspects of Sleep and Sleep Disturbance. Boston, Butterworth, 1985
5. Roffwarg HP: Diagnostic Classification of Sleep and Arousal Disorders. Sleep 2(1):1, 1979

CHAPTER 15.9
Headache

William G. Speed III and
Justin C. McArthur

Headache is ubiquitous. Nearly everyone occasionally experiences a "tension" or muscle contraction headache. Migraine occurs in 6 to 8 percent of the population, and headache is estimated to be chronic or recurrent in about 20 percent of the population.

The clinical implications of headache vary widely. It may herald a life-threatening disorder, for example, brain tumor, subarachnoid hemorrhage, or brain abscess, or it may simply be the result of a stressful day, for example, the headache associated with increased muscle tone. It may be so severe that total incapacitation occurs yet not be threatening to life (as exemplified by some cluster and migraine headaches). It may be so mild as to be only annoying and yet be a threat to life (such as the headache associated with some brain tumors.) Because headache is so common and because the implications vary from the relatively trivial to the catastrophic, each patient who has chronic or recurrent headache should have a carefully taken history, physical examination, and appropriately selected laboratory investigations.

Emotional factors are important. All patients with chronic or recurrent headaches have some disruption of their life, and in some there may be secondary emotional effects. The risk of dependence on or addiction to narcotic drugs is high in the patient with chronic head pain, and development of drug-seeking behavior, depression, and personality problems is common. Referral to a psychiatrist or other counselor may be appropriate when these problems are severe; nevertheless, referral cannot replace the receptive ear of a willing primary physician.

PATHOGENESIS OF HEAD PAIN[3,4,6] (Table 15.9–1)

EXTRACRANIAL CONDITIONS

Virtually all extracranial structures are sensitive to pain,[1] including the skin, subcutaneous tissues, muscles, arteries, fascia, and the periosteum of the skull. The eyes, ears, sinuses, and nasopharynx are all highly sensitive. The teeth are richly innervated by the lower two divisions of the trigeminal nerve. Head pain may result from dilatation or distension of extracranial blood vessels, from increased tone in the muscles attached to the skull, from localized inflammation, infection, or invasion by tumor.

INTRACRANIAL CAUSES

The nociceptive structures within the cranium include the main arterial structures, the venous sinuses, and their larger tributaries on the brain surface.[1] The dura lining the anterior, middle, and posterior cranial fossae are innervated by the trigeminal and glossopharyngeal nerves. These nerves, as well as the vagus and the upper cervical nerves, are also pain sensitive. The cranium, much of the pia-arachnoid, the dura, choroid plexus, ependyma, and the brain parenchyma are insensitive.

Most mechanisms of headache involve one or more of the

TABLE 15.9–1. CAUSES OF HEADACHE

Extracranial
- Muscle contraction
- Cervical arthritis
- Sinusitis
- Glaucoma
- Otitis media
- Dental abscess
- Nasopharyngeal carcinoma
- Cranial arteritis

Intracranial
Vascular
- Migraine
- Cluster
- Hypertension
- Subarachnoid hemorrhage

Infection
- Meningitis
- Encephalitis
- Brain abscess
- Systemic infection

Mass lesions
- Brain tumor
- Brain abscess

Trauma
- Subdural hematoma
- Posttraumatic syndrome

Other
- Pseudotumor cerebri
- Postspinal

Facial pain
- Trigeminal neuralgia
- Glossopharyngeal neuralgia
- Atypical facial pain

following: (1) distension, traction, or dilatation of vascular structures—this is the mechanism by which elevated intracranial pressure and mass lesions produce pain; (2) compression, distortion, or irritation of cranial or spinal nerves; (3) inflammation of the meninges; and (4) excessive contraction or spasm in the paraspinal or scalp musculature.

SPECIFIC TYPES OF HEADACHE (Table 15.9–2)

MUSCLE CONTRACTION

Muscle contraction headache (also called tension, psychogenic, or nervous headache) is usually described as a steady, nonpulsatile aching, tightness, pressure, or soreness. The pain is almost always bilateral and involves the frontotemporal vertex, or occipito-cervical regions, separately, in various combinations, or in toto. Sometimes there is the sensation of a bandlike constriction about the head. These pains may last a few hours, a few days, or much longer. Patients with this type of headache may describe constant headache for years. It is commonly associated with emotional stress and, in some patients, may represent a physiological response to anxiety, repressed hostility, or depression. In other patients, however, no psychological or emotional factors are identified.

The etiology of muscle contraction headache is unclear, especially since other types of headache may also be associated with excessive contraction in the muscles of the scalp. For example, sustained muscle contraction may also be a factor in the pain associated with vascular headache and with disease of the eye, ear, nose, paranasal sinuses, or cervical arthritis.

There are no characteristic physical findings, and diagnosis is based on the clinical description and exclusion of other etiological factors.

TABLE 15.9–2. COMMON FORMS OF HEADACHE

	Location	Duration	Onset	Associations
Muscle contraction	Temporal, frontal parietal, occipital posterior, cervical, or generalized	Hours to days (in the chronic form may be present for years)	Gradual	Emotional stress Unknown
Migraine	Any area May be unilateral and repetitive	Hours to days	Gradual or abrupt	Positive family history Aura secondary to vasoconstrictive events
Cluster	Temporal-ocular areas	Hours Groups of attacks 10–120 min (usually less than 60 min)	Abrupt	Ipsilateral nasal congestion and lacrimation; miosis; ptosis Often nocturnal
Postspinal	Occipital to frontal	Hours to days	Abrupt on standing	Relieved by lying down
Trigeminal neuralgia	One or more divisions of nerve V (unilateral)	Minutes	Abrupt	"Trigger" areas often present Occur in attacks
Subarachnoid hemorrhage	Postcervical Occipital Frontal	Hours to days	Abrupt	Very severe Nausea, vomiting, lethargy Localizing signs (partial III nerve paresis)
Meningitis and encephalitis	Postcervical Frontal	Days	Gradual	Fever, lethargy, seizures
Cranial arteritis	Temporal areas or generalized	Days, weeks, or months	Gradual—rarely abrupt	Painful vessels Systemic symptoms Increased erythrocyte sedimentation rate Ophthalmic arteritis
Hypertension	Occipital Frontal	Weeks	Gradual	Worse in morning

There are two varieties of muscle contraction headache. The *acute* type is relatively short in duration and is commonly precipitated by fatigue, emotional crisis, stressful workloads, driving under difficult conditions, or similar pressures. It invariably subsides with removal of the stress trigger. The *chronic* muscle contraction headache represents a very different entity. Such patients present with constant unremitting headaches that may be present for months, years, or decades. In addition to the characteristics of acute type muscle contraction headache, these patients may also describe scalp soreness, weightlike sensations and tight bands, a feeling of a tight skull cap, or even crawling sensations. Depression, personality problems, and excessive use of analgesics (which may lead to frank addiction) may contribute to the prolongation of the headache. Physical examination is usually unremarkable, and there is rarely an indication for laboratory studies. If, however, the pattern of headache is changed in a patient who had a stable pattern, if the neurologic examination is abnormal, or if the patient proves resistant to a management program, then a contrast computed tomographic (CT) scan is recommended.

Management

Acute muscle contraction headache usually subsides once the stress trigger is removed and, if not, is often relieved by simple analgesics.

The patient with *chronic* muscle contraction headaches, however, presents a difficult problem. Management of this variety depends on the source of the muscle contraction.[9] If it is secondary to ocular, nasal, paranasal, or temporomandibular joint disorders or to intracranial pathology, then specific treatment must be directed to these primary disorders. If there is underlying cervical arthritis, a nonsteroidal anti-inflammatory drug such as aspirin, indomethacin, or ibuprofen can be beneficial. Local heat, massage, and traction may be helpful. If paraspinal spasm is present, use of a muscle relaxant (cyclobenzaprine 10 mg tid) may be useful.

In the vast majority of individuals with chronic muscle contraction headache, however, a specific disorder will not be found. Many of these patients rely on frequent use of narcotic analgesics and become habituated to them even though they produce little or no benefit. Long-term use of nonnarcotic analgesics may lead to nephrotoxicity. Furthermore, the chronic use of analgesics may perpetuate these pains, and every effort should be made to have these patients discontinue their use. Tricyclic antidepressant compounds are the most useful of all agents for treating chronic muscle contraction headache. These compounds may be effective whether or not depression is overt. Side effects such as drowsiness, weight gain, or anticholinergic symptoms may preclude their use in some patients. Propranolol is sometimes beneficial, particularly when combined with tricyclic compounds. (For a discussion of side effects, see Migraine section.)

Muscle relaxants are usually less effective than their name might suggest.

Psychotherapy and regular counseling may be helpful in some patients. Because deep-seated emotional or psychological factors may be important in the development of chronic muscle contraction headaches, psychiatric referral may be necessary. Biofeedback is a useful therapeutic modality for the well-motivated individual with chronic muscle contraction headache. Two biofeedback-assisted methods have proved useful: thermodigital self-regulation and frontalis electromyographic self-regulation. Both techniques require repeated practice and may be time-consuming.

MIGRAINE[6,7,9]

Migraine is a neurovascular disorder characterized by recurrent episodic headache attacks, which are often unilateral and associated with nausea, vomiting, and neurological dysfunction. Fifty percent of all migraineurs will have their first attack before the age of 20; however, migraine can begin at any age. Women are affected somewhat more commonly than men, and a family history of migraine occurs in up to 70 percent. As with most types of headache, the diagnosis of migraine is dependent upon the characteristic manifestations and sequence of symptoms. Symptoms are not always typical, however, and may mimic other neurologic diseases including stroke. Close attention to historical detail and familiarity with the full spectrum of migraine is critical in avoiding misdiagnosis as well as unnecessary and potentially harmful investigations.

Pathophysiology

Although the precise etiology of migraine remains unknown, it is generally agreed that it is a vascular disturbance.[1,3] Whether the vascular changes are primary or secondary to neuronal influences has not yet been resolved. During a migraine attack, there is an initial phase of intracranial vasoconstriction followed by vasodilatation. The phase of vasoconstriction may precede vasodilatation, or they may occur simultaneously, affecting different areas of the cranial vasculature. The vasoconstriction may be entirely asymptomatic or may produce symptoms of cerebral ischemia. The pain of the migraine attack results from the dilatation plus sterile inflammation of the vessel wall. Cerebral blood flow studies have documented a spreading phase of vasoconstriction during the aura of a classic migraine attack.[7]

The role of vasoactive substances and neurotransmitters has been studied for decades. Despite numerous leads and observations, there is still no definite clue as to the primary biochemical or electrophysiological event that initiates a migraine attack. The available information relating to vasoactive substances in migraine suggests that:

1. Serotonin is released from platelets and taken up by vessels with subsequent fall in blood levels. It may act as a potent vasoconstrictor and heighten pain sensitivity.
2. The local release of neurotransmitters such as substance P from small nerve fibers linking the trigeminal ganglion with intracranial blood vessels may play an important mediating role in the pain of migraine. Other nociceptive agents, including serotonin, bradykinin, histamine, and prostaglandins, may be important in lowering pain thresholds locally.
3. Circulating substances such as norepinephrine, epinephrine, and acetylcholine may play a role in the pathogenesis of migraine, perhaps by their effects on vascular tone. Substances such as tyramine, prostaglandins, and histamine, if administered exogenously, may trigger migraine attacks in susceptible individuals.
4. There is evidence for platelet aggregation and a platelet release reaction in the cerebral circulation.

Manifestations

Migraine attacks occur in two phases: *Vasoconstriction* produces focal ischemia leading to transient neurologic deficits, including visual impairment, dysarthria, dysphasia, hemiparesis, hemianesthesia, transient global amnesia, vertigo, ataxia, impaired thought processes, or even disturbed consciousness. Visual phenomena are very common, including scotoma, scintillations, or zigzag lines. These visual phenomena may last from 5 to 20 minutes and typically precede the headache of the migraine attack.

Vasodilatation causes unilateral or bilateral pain in any area of the head, but particularly the frontotemporal area. It is frequently pounding and throbbing but may be dull, boring, or expanding. Sudden movements of the head, bending over, straining, and exposure to bright lights or loud noises may aggravate the pain. Anorexia, nausea, and vomiting are common accompanying symptoms. Patients may achieve some relief from direct pressure over the superficial temporal artery. The migraine attack may last from several hours to 2 or 3 days or, uncommonly, longer. In occasional individuals one migraine attack will lead immediately into another without any respite (status migrainosus).

Common migraine refers to a vascular headache that is unaccompanied by visual or neurologic symptoms. It is the most frequent type of migraine.

Classical migraine refers to a vascular headache preceded by painless sensory experiences, most often visual, including scotomata and field defects with scintillations or flashes of light.

Complicated migraine (hemiplegic, ophthalmoplegic, or basilar migraine) refers to a vascular headache that is accompanied by neurologic symptoms, often in a characteristic sequence. If neurologic symptoms occur alone without headache, the differential diagnosis may be broad. Such patients may indeed have migraine, but one must consider cerebral embolization, thrombosis, aneurysm, or seizures. The differential diagnosis of complicated migraine is often vexing, although ancillary investigations, particularly CT and angiography, are usually definitive. (See Chapters 15.2, 15.5, and 15.13.)

In some patients a severe migraine attack may be followed by permanent neurologic dysfunction, and there may be areas of cerebral infarction on CT.

Management (Table 15.9–3)

The treatment of migraine may be divided into two phases, management of the individual attack and prophylaxis.

Individual Attack. Vasoconstrictive agents have been used for decades to abort migraine attacks with the rationale that the pain is related to vasodilatation. Ergotamine tartrate is the treatment of choice. It has a direct vasoconstrictive effect on arterial smooth muscle. For best results ergotamine must be given immediately at the onset of headache. It may be given by mouth, by inhalation, rectally, or parenterally. The route of administration may depend on nausea, vomiting, severity of headache, and patient convenience. Vasovasora of the involved vessels also participate in the migraine syndrome, and dilatation of these vessels tends to produce edema of the wall of the vessel they are supplying. Ergotamine is less effective in constricting edematous vessels—hence the necessity that the patient take this medication at the first warning of headache. Although some patients may tolerate ergotamine on a daily basis for weeks, this is not recommended because of the risk for the development of ergot-dependent vessels, leading to chronic headache.

It is essential to discontinue ergot if there is aching of the extremities, intermittent claudication, decreased vascular pulsations, or hypertension. Ergot alkaloids are contraindicated in peripheral vascular disease, coronary artery disease, hypertension, impaired hepatic or renal function, hyperthyroidism, and pregnancy. They should probably be avoided in complicated migraine because of the potential for producing prolonged vasoconstriction and cerebral infarction.

Isometheptene mucate (Midrin), another vasoconstrictor, may be a useful alternative in patients intolerant of ergotamine.

A particularly severe migraine attack unresponsive to ergotamine may require the use of strong analgesics either given orally or parenterally, for example, meperidine 100 mg and promethazine 25 to 50 mg. Frequent use of such medications must be avoided because of the potential for narcotic addiction, as well as the potentiation of headache owing to chronic analgesic use.

Prophylactic Management. Selection of prophylactic therapy of migraine depends on the combination of frequency and duration of headache, as well as the severity of the attacks.[6]

Propranolol is a lipophilic beta-adrenergic blocker that is one of the most useful agents for migraine prophylaxis. Propranolol is currently the drug of choice for migraine prophylaxis but should be used cautiously or avoided in patients with asthma, chronic obstructive lung disease, congestive heart failure, marked bradycardia, peripheral vascular insufficiency, and Raynaud phenomena. The usual starting dose is 20 mg four times daily. An adequate trial, in terms of both duration and total daily dose, is important before discontinuing propranolol. The dosage may need to be advanced as high as 320 mg daily in some patients. A long-acting preparation of propranolol (Inderal LA) is now available and may be more con-

TABLE 15.9–3. MANAGEMENT OF MIGRAINE

Preparations	Indication and Use
Individual attacks	
Ergotamine tartrate (1 mg) and caffeine alkaloid (100 mg) (Cafergot)	Two tablets at onset of headache Two tablets every 30 min, to a maximum of 6 in 24 hr Maximum of 10 per week but under careful supervision may permit up to 18 in some weeks
Ergotamine tartrate (1 mg), caffeine (100 mg), belladonna (0.125 mg), and pentobarbital (30 mg) (Cafergot-PB)	Useful in patients with nausea
Suppositories	
Ergotamine tartrate (2 mg) and caffeine (100 mg) (Cafergot Rectal)	Useful in patients with nausea One immediately at onset of headache; repeat once in 1 hr, maximum of 2/day and 4/wk
Ergotamine tartrate (0.36 mg per compression) (Medihaler Ergotamine)	One inhalation at start of headache; repeat at 5-min intervals to maximum of 6/day and 15/wk
Dihydroergotamine mesylate (1 mg/ml) (DHE-45)	1 ml subcutaneously at onset of headache; may repeat once in 1 hr; maximum 2 ml/day or 4 ml/wk (usually)
Isometheptene mucate (65 mg), dichloralphenazone (100 mg), and acetaminophen (325 mg) (Midrin)	Two capsules at onset, one capsule every hour to maximum of 5 in 24 hours
Prophylaxis	
Propranolol (10, 20, 40, 60, 80, or 90 mg) (Inderal)	20 mg qid, maximum 320 mg/day
Amitriptyline (10, 25, 50, 75, 100, or 150 mg) (Elavil)	25–150 mg, average 75 mg/qhs
Verapamil (80, 120 mg) (Calan, Isoptin)	80–120 mg qid or tid
Methysergide (2 mg) (Sansert)	2 mg tid (see text for precautions)
Cyproheptadine (4 mg) (Periactin)	4 mg tid

venient for the patient. Other beta-blockers may be used for migraine prophylaxis.

Tricyclic compounds such as amitriptyline, doxepin, or imipramine are beneficial in some patients with migraine whether or not there is an associated depression. Tricyclic compounds inhibit the membrane pump mechanism responsible for norepinephrine and serotonin re-uptake into adrenergic neurons, thus potentiating their effects. The tricyclic compounds may be used as first-line prophylactic agents, particularly in an anxious or depressed individual. Tricyclic compounds and propranolol may be given together, and in some patients this combination may be more effective than either used alone. The side effects of the tricyclic compounds include weight gain, a "hangover" feeling, and anticholinergic effects such as dry mouth, urinary retention, and postural hypotension. Tricyclic compounds should be avoided in patients with a history of cardiac arrhythmias, ischemic heart disease, or glaucoma.

Calcium channel antagonists may provide effective prophylaxis in patients refractory to or intolerant of beta-blockers or tricyclic

compounds. The mode of action of calcium channel antagonists in migraine is unknown. Acting as relaxants of arterial wall smooth muscle, however, they may block the initial phase of vasoconstriction and, thus, may prevent a full-blown migraine from developing. Of the three currently available, verapamil (Calan or Isoptin) and diltiazem (Cardizem) appear better tolerated than nifedipine (Procardia) and may be more effective. Side effects are uncommon but include constipation and, rarely, rash. These compounds should be avoided in patients with heart block and hypotension. Because of the delay in action, an adequate trial should last at least 4 to 6 weeks.

Methysergide maleate is an antiserotonin compound and is rarely used as a first-line agent. It may, however, be beneficial in patients refractory to other prophylactic medications. Methysergide should be interrupted for 1 month out of every 4 to 6 months of therapy. Careful and repeated monitoring for development of bruits, cardiac murmurs, and signs of retroperitoneal fibrosis is essential for all patients taking methysergide.

Monoamine oxidase inhibitors may be effective in migraine prophylaxis by modifying serotonin levels. Their use should be restricted to patients who have failed adequate trials of the first-line drugs and should be prescribed only by experienced physicians (see Chapter 16.5).

Corticosteroid actions include stabilization of cell membranes and reduction in inflammation. The long-term use of prednisone for migraine prophylaxis is not indicated. A few patients who have severe migraine may respond to a short course of prednisone, however.

Other Therapy for Migraine. *Dietary restrictions* may be helpful. Certain vasoactive chemical substances found in food are capable of triggering migraine attacks in some individuals. These include phenylethylamine, tyramine, monosodium glutamate, and sodium nitrate and nitrite. The following foods should therefore be avoided: alcohol, chocolate, aged cheese, onions, citrus fruits, coffee, tea, chicken livers, fermented sausages, (salami, etc.), bananas, nuts, Chinese food, flavor enhancers, yogurt, canned figs, avocado, hot dogs, and processed meats. Dietary restriction needs to be continued for at least several weeks to determine its effectiveness.

Oral contraceptives and estrogens should be discontinued in the patient with migraine. These agents may precipitate migraine in a susceptible individual and may enhance the risk of permanent ischemic damage.

Biofeedback training is helpful in many patients with migraine, particularly if both electromyographic (EMG) and hand-warming techniques are used. It works best in younger people and in attentive, well-motivated individuals. About 50 to 60 percent of patients appropriately chosen may benefit.

Education and counseling play a very important role in the management of migraine (as in all chronic, recurrent headache). Patients should be reassured about the benign, although recurrent, course, and the rarity of serious underlying disease or neurologic occurrences. They should be warned that the goal of therapy should be to decrease the frequency of attacks and lessen their severity but that complete abolition of attacks of migraine will be unlikely, despite aggressive therapy. Psychotherapy may be useful for the (rare) patient with serious underlying emotional triggers.

CLUSTER HEADACHES[6,8,9]

Cluster headaches represent a distinct clinical syndrome that was first described in the early nineteenth century. They are described in the literature under various names such as sphenopalatine ganglion neuralgia, periodic migrainous neuralgia, histaminic cephalgia, migraine variant, and Horton syndrome.

Manifestations

Clusters occur frequently in spring or fall but are not limited to these times. They may vary in duration from weeks to months and occasionally may revert to a chronic or almost daily pattern.[8]

The individual attacks of pain are of short duration, lasting from 10 to 120 minutes, rarely longer. One to six attacks in 24 hours are common, and they often occur with clockwork-like predictability for an individual patient. Nocturnal onset is quite common, often awakening the patient in the early morning hours. The pain predominantly involves the temporal and ocular regions. It occasionally spreads to the face (including the teeth) and rarely the parietal, occipital or cervical regions. The pain is described as "excruciating" with a rapid peak developing within a few minutes of onset and with no aura. Ipsilateral nasal congestion, lacrimation, and conjunctival injection frequently accompany the pain. Nausea and vomiting are unusual. Neurological symptoms do not accompany cluster headaches. Ipsilateral oculosympathetic paralysis occurs occasionally and is usually transient.

Cluster headache can be distinguished from migraine on the basis of the historical description. Typically, cluster headaches affect middle-aged men, who are often heavy smokers; women are less commonly affected. The attacks are more frequent but shorter than those of migraine, and there may be a remission between clusters lasting for weeks, months, or years.

Cluster headache pain probably results from vasodilatation of branches of both the external and the internal carotid artery systems. The role of vasoactive amines in this disorder, if any, has not been established, although histamine blood levels appear to be elevated. There is no demonstrable fall of serotonin at the onset of an attack, as in migraine.

Management

A number of medications may be useful for aborting an individual attack or shortening a cluster. *Ergotamine tartrate* is often effective, particularly if the attacks occur at a predictable time. This makes it possible to give an appropriate dose of ergotamine shortly before the anticipated onset. For example, if most attacks are occurring 2 hours after going to sleep, ergotamine can be given at bedtime. With proper supervision, 4 to 6 mg can be used per 24 hours. In particularly severe clusters, self-administration of subcutaneous dehydroergotamine mesylate (DHE-45) can be taught. Appropriate amounts can be given once or twice a day within the limits previously described in the management of migraine (Table 15.9–3). Careful monitoring of the patient is essential if ergotamine is required over prolonged periods.

Oxygen inhalation (7 L/min for 15 min) starting immediately at the onset of a pain attack will occasionally abort it.

Adrenal corticosteroids may control some clusters, but if response does not occur within 2 or 3 days, the medication should be promptly discontinued. Prednisone may be given at an initial dose of 60 mg daily (sometimes 100 mg) with gradual appropriate reduction to a reasonable maintenance level. Fortunately, most patients with cluster headaches will have remissions in several weeks. For some patients, however, cluster headaches recur as the steroid dose is reduced. In these cases, the physician must give careful consideration to the potential side effects of continuing the corticosteroids.

Methysergide (Sansert) may be useful in the management of cluster in the same dose used for migraine; if effective, the response is likely to be apparent within 1 to 2 days.

Calcium channel antagonists have also been used; their effect in controlling cluster is delayed several weeks.

Antihistaminics are of little value.

Lithium carbonate, in doses of 300 mg three times daily, may benefit patients with refractory cluster. Lithium blood levels should be obtained and should not exceed 1 mEq/L (see Chapter 16.5).

The existence of a chronic variety of cluster headaches is now well recognized in patients with no significant remission for 6 to

12 months. A small percentage of these patients is extremely resistant to management. Forty percent of them will be controlled by lithium. Nonsteroidal anti-inflammatory drugs, for example, indomethacin (Indocin), are also sometimes beneficial. A variant of chronic cluster headache, chronic paroxysmal hemicrania, occurring predominantly in women and characterized by 16 to 18 attacks per day, is very responsive to indomethacin.

PSEUDOTUMOR CEREBRI[9]

Pseudotumor cerebri (idiopathic intracranial hypertension, benign intracranial hypertension) is an uncommon cause of headache characterized by the symptoms and signs of elevated intracranial pressure. Mass lesions and hydrocephalus are absent, and the cause may be related to an overproduction of CSF or inadequate absorption. Mental status is unaffected. Papilledema and occasionally a VI cranial nerve paresis may occur, however, decreased visual acuity is a late manifestation. A CT scan will show small ventricles, and lumbar puncture will be normal except for elevated opening pressure.

The headache is often improved after the initial diagnostic lumbar puncture, which may need to be repeated at intervals. Acetazolamide (Diamox), a potent carbonic-anhydrase inhibitor, will reduce production of CSF and decrease intracranial pressure in doses of 2 to 4 g daily. Obese patients should be given a weight-reduction diet. Rarely, lumbar thecoperitoneal shunts will be required in the patient refractory to Diamox.

FACIAL PAIN

TRIGEMINAL NEURALGIA[2]

Trigeminal neuralgia (tic douloureux) is a disabling cause of facial pain, more common in the elderly and in women. Pain occurs in brief lancinating jabs of great severity; the patient may wince—hence the name "tic." The pain is unilateral and localized to one or more divisions of the trigeminal nerve (usually maxillary or mandibular) and may spread to other divisions when severe. The pain may be precipitated by talking or chewing or touching a certain spot innervated by that division—a trigger area. The pain may recur in a series of jabs or episodes that can occur once or many times a day. Following a flurry of jabs, the patient may experience an afterburn or chronic ache. Exacerbations, during which pain recurs frequently, tend to last for weeks and may be separated by long periods free of pain.

The etiology of trigeminal neuralgia is unknown.[2] Cerebellopontine angle tumors can induce trigeminal distribution pain from local nerve irritation, but the pattern of pain rarely resembles that of a tic.

Diagnosis depends on the physician's recognition of these characteristics. On examination there are usually no abnormalities; rarely there is some tenderness of the skin, or hypesthesia.

Management
The initial management of tic is medical. Narcotic analgesics are not helpful, and their use should be avoided. Carbamazepine (Tegretol), 200 mg two to four times daily, may be effective. Blood counts and liver-function tests should be monitored at intervals. Phenytoin (Dilantin), 300 mg daily, appears to be helpful in some patients. Baclofen (Lioresal), 5 mg three times daily and increasing gradually to 60 mg daily in divided doses, may also be used either alone or in combination with these agents.

In the unresponsive patient, surgical therapy can be considered. The two principal procedures for tic are:

1. Gangliolysis, which can be performed either by percutaneous radiofrequency destruction or by glycerol injection.

2. Surgical decompression of the trigeminal nerve by suboccipital craniectomy, a major intracranial procedure. Many patients with tic will be found to have an artery compressing the trigeminal nerve that, if dissected free, will relieve the neuralgia.

GLOSSOPHARYNGEAL NEURALGIA

Although less common than trigeminal neuralgia, paroxysmal glossopharyngeal neuralgia is otherwise quite similar in its characteristics. The pain occurs in the pharynx or external auditory canal, and swallowing is usually the trigger. The same approach with medical management can be utilized, with surgical therapy reserved for the unresponsive patient.

ATYPICAL FACIAL PAIN

Atypical neuralgias involving the head and face may be seen in multiple sclerosis, angina pectoris, myocardial infarction, apical petrositis (Gradenigo syndrome), Raeder paratrigeminal neuralgia, intra- or extracervical spinal abnormalities (usually in the area of C1 to C3, but occasionally from lower spinal areas), postherpetic neuralgia, central pain from brain stem or thalamic area, temporomandibular joint dysfunction, lethal midline granuloma, intracranial aneurysm, inflammation of the teeth or gums, glaucoma, iritis, retrobulbar neuralgia, or cranial arteritis. Some are psychogenic and some are caused by migrainous or nonmigrainous vasodilatation. The diagnosis and treatment depend entirely on identifying the underlying source of pain by way of a detailed history, physical examination, and appropriate ancillary studies. Surgical intervention, as described for trigeminal neuralgia, is not helpful.

CRANIAL ARTERITIS[5]

Cranial arteritis is a disorder of old age; nearly all patients are over the age of 50, and most are over 60. When a headache begins for the first time in someone over the age of 50 or there is a change in a previous headache pattern, cranial arteritis should be considered. Women are affected somewhat more than men.[5]

Cranial arteritis is characterized by painful inflammation of the superficial temporal and other cranial arteries and is associated with generalized systemic signs and symptoms—malaise, weight loss, fever, sweating, and myalgias (see polymyalgia rheumatica, Chapter 8.3). Sometimes the symptoms are subtle, and a patient's complaints have been mistaken for depression or neurosis. The sedimentation rate is usually elevated, and there is frequently a mild to moderate elevation of the leukocyte count. The disorder may not be limited to the cranial arteries but may include the internal carotid artery, the aorta, innominate, subclavian, vertebral, pulmonary, and systemic arteries.

Although the etiology remains obscure, it may represent vasculitis associated with deposition of immune complexes in involved arteries.

Manifestations
The onset is often insidious, and the process may smolder for weeks or months before it is recognized. Occasionally, the onset is explosive. Headache is nonspecific, usually moderately severe, and involves the temporal area unilaterally or bilaterally. It may also be frontal, occipital, or generalized. It is often aching or throbbing. The intensity may vary, but its presence is likely to be persistent. Frequently, there is scalp tenderness along the course of the involved artery. The arterial wall may be palpably thickened or nodular and the pulsation decreased or absent. Jaw claudication, manifested by complaints of pain on chewing, may occur. Less commonly there will be mentation changes resulting from cerebral ischemia.

Blindness is the most dreaded complication of cranial arteritis; it occurs in about 50 percent of untreated cases, may involve one

or both eyes, and can be total and permanent. It is secondary to ophthalmic arteritis. Rarely, blindness may be the presenting complaint; hence, the diagnosis of cranial arteritis must be considered in the differential diagnosis of sudden onset of blindness in the elderly, with or without other related symptoms.

Management

In the patient presenting with suspicious symptoms, prednisone 60 mg daily should begin promptly. Diagnosis is confirmed by biopsy of the superficial temporal artery. Patients presenting with a characteristic clinical picture should be started on steroids without waiting for the biopsy. Normal sedimentation rate or a negative biopsy does not exclude the diagnosis. Response to steroids is usually dramatic, with disappearance of headache within 24 to 72 hours. If a response does not occur within 72 hours, then the diagnosis should be reassessed. Careful tapering of prednisone dosage, guided by relief of symptoms and normalization of the sedimentation rate, follows. The disease is self-limiting but may persist for months or years and may recur.

OTHER CAUSES OF HEAD PAIN

SINUSITIS

Sinus pain is usually dull and aching, occasionally throbbing. It is often described as a "painful fullness." When the maxillary antrum is involved, the discomfort appears over the antrum itself, the upper teeth, or the forehead. With ethmoiditis or sphenoid sinusitis, the pain is felt around the orbit or over the cranium. With frontal sinusitis the discomfort is localized to the supraorbital region and often associated with percussion tenderness. The pain is often worse when the patient awakens and improves with drainage during the day while in the erect posture. The pain is usually reduced by decongestants. Nasal congestion or discharge and local tenderness over the sinus are helpful clues to the diagnosis. Transillumination of the sinuses is a useful technique. Sinus radiographs, CT scan, and nasopharyngoscopy serve to establish the diagnosis.

If the headache persists after the involved sinuses drain, one should suspect osteomyelitis or parameningeal extension. Fever over 102F, delirium, or meningismus suggest a complicated sinusitis. Acute sinusitis can be responsible for headache, but it is uncommon for chronic recurrent headache to be related to sinusitis.

EYE DISEASE

Glaucoma, keratitis, or uveitis may cause headaches. Hyperopia, astigmatism, and muscle imbalance may occasionally do so as well. Pain of ocular disease may be dull without appreciable throbbing; it may be periorbital, retro-orbital, or referred to the forehead or temple. Chemosis, congestion, and periorbital inflammation should suggest cavernous sinus inflammation or infection.

EAR DISEASE

Head pains associated with inflammatory or infective conditions of the external auditory canal, middle ear, and mastoid air cells are usually localized but may be referred to the jaw or neck. There is often local tenderness and, in otitis, inflammation of the eardrum. Chronic infections can lead to osteomyelitis, cholesteatoma formation, subdural empyema, or venous thrombosis.

DENTAL DISEASE

Dental disease is not a common cause of chronic or recurrent head or facial pain. The pain may, however, be referred to the head or face because nerve fibers from the teeth are carried in the second and third divisions of the trigeminal nerve. Secondary muscle spasm may be a factor in headache associated with dental disease. There is always pain or discomfort in the tooth itself, however. Unless there is clearly a primary dental problem, headaches should never be attributed to dental disease.

The etiology of temporomandibular joint dysfunction is controversial, but the majority of patients have excessive muscle contraction. A small minority have malocclusion, for which expert dental intervention may be necessary.

REFERENCES

1. Dalessio DJ (ed): Wolf's Headache and Other Head Pain, 3d ed. New York, Oxford University Press, 1980
2. Framm GH, Terrence CF, Maroon JC: Trigeminal neuralgia, current concepts regarding etiology and pathogenesis. Arch Neurol 41:1204, 1984
3. Friedman AP: Research and Clinical Studies in Headache, vol 1. Baltimore, Williams & Wilkins, 1967
4. Friedman AP: Research and Clinical Studies in Headache, vol. 2. Baltimore, Williams & Wilkins, 1969
5. Huston KA, Hunder GG, et al: Temporal arteritis: A 25-year-epidemiologic, clinical, and pathologic study. Ann Intern Med 88:162, 1978
6. Lance JW: Mechanism and Management of Headache. London, Butterworth, 1973
7. Lauritzen M, Olesen TS, et al: Changes in regional cerebral blood flow during the course of classic migraine attacks. Ann Neurol 13:633, 1983
8. Mathew NT: Clinical subtypes of cluster headache and response to lithium therapy. Headache 19:26, 1978
9. Packard RC (ed): Neurologic Clinics: Headache, vol. 1. Philadelphia, WB Saunders, 1983, p 2

CHAPTER 15.10
Intracranial Masses

Henry Brem, Stuart A. Grossman, and Daniel F. Hanley

The term "intracranial mass lesion" is often used to refer only to primary and metastatic neoplasms of the central nervous system (CNS). It is of clinical importance, however, to include ischemic infarcts, intracranial hemorrhages, inflammatory disorders, aneurysms, and arteriovenous malformations (Table 15.10–5). These disorders may present in a manner similar to CNS neoplasms, are often amenable to curative therapy, and can progress rapidly if neglected.

SYMPTOMS FROM INTRACRANIAL MASS LESIONS

Intracranial mass lesions produce symptoms in three different ways (Table 15.10–1). *First,* the lesions may compress or destroy adjacent nervous system structures. The resulting neurologic symptoms depend upon the location of the lesion. Thus, craniopharyn-

TABLE 15.10–1. HOW CNS MASS LESIONS PRODUCE SYMPTOMS

- Compression or destruction of adjacent nervous structures
- Seizures
- Increased intracranial pressure
  - Mass lesion
  - Edema
  - Hydrocephalus

giomas produce visual disturbances; medulloblastomas result in cerebellar dysfunction; and malignant tumors of a dominant hemisphere cause Broca's aphasia. *Second,* the lesion can cause local irritation, which may result in either focal or generalized seizures. *Third,* CNS mass lesions often cause an increase in intracranial pressure, which may be a result of the expanding mass lesion, the accompanying edema, or obstruction of the normal flow of cerebrospinal fluid. The management of acutely increased intracranial pressure is discussed in Chapter 4.9. It is of utmost importance to recognize the signs that indicate increasing intracranial pressure and the herniation syndromes (Tables 15.10–2 and 15.10–3).

Herniation syndromes[8] can be grouped into two types: central herniation and temporal lobe (uncal) herniation. Both syndromes present initially as diminished levels of consciousness. Early clinical findings may include lethargy or the patient "just not being himself"; these may progress to obtundation and then coma. As intracranial masses enlarge, intracranial pressure becomes elevated. When the intracranial mass is near the midline in the supratentorial cerebral hemispheres, a central herniation syndrome occurs, in which obtundation is followed by bilateral pupillary dilatation and then signs of progressive thalamic, midbrain, and pontine dysfunction. This dysfunction is best characterized by serial evaluation of the behavioral response to pain. In the early stages of central herniation a painful stimulus to the limb often results in purposeful withdrawal. As the syndrome progresses, purposeful withdrawal is replaced by stereotyped flexor posture. When the lower midbrain and pons become involved, this response to pain becomes extensor posturing. Only at this time does localizing cranial nerve dysfunction uniformly appear. Irregular breathing patterns are also associated with these late stages. Central herniation syndromes occur over a period of minutes to hours with a relatively steady progression.

Temporal lobe herniations (uncal herniations) may occur when a mass lesion is in the lateral region of the cranial vault in or near the temporal lobe. The expanding mass exerts most of its force on the thalamus and midbrain. This results in obtundation or coma and rapid deterioration characterized by unilateral pupillary dilatation secondary to oculomotor nerve dysfunction and contralateral hemiparesis caused by compression of the corticospinal tract at the midbrain peduncle. If the herniation remains untreated, bilateral midbrain and pontine dysfunction usually occurs.

Both central and temporal lobe herniations are best treated by addressing the underlying cause and preventing progression. If a mass remains untreated and presents as a herniation syndrome, this represents an acute surgical and medical emergency that should be treated as described in Chapter 4.9.

EVALUATION OF INTRACRANIAL MASS LESIONS

The evaluation of a patient with a possible intracranial mass lesion begins with a detailed history and neurologic examination (Table 15.10–4). The new onset of seizures in an adult, the development of a focal neurologic deficit, or alterations in mental status should raise the possibility of a brain tumor and lead to further investigation.

A *computed tomography* (CT) scan of the brain is the most direct radiographic approach.[1,8] The noncontrast CT scan can identify the presence of hemorrhage, calcification, hydrocephalus, or a mass causing edema and shift. A contrast-enhanced CT scan can delineate brain tumors and abscesses and can be useful in identifying vascular lesions, such as aneurysms or arteriovenous malformations. *Magnetic resonance imaging* (MRI) may be used in conjunction with or instead of CT scanning. The MRI is especially useful in defining posterior fossa lesions, low-grade gliomas, and the extent of cerebral edema. In addition, MRI is useful in differentiating plaques of multiple sclerosis from brain tumors. Other diagnostic tests for mass lesions have been largely supplanted by CT and MRI.

Skull radiographs may demonstrate calcifications, erosion of normal bony structures, signs of increased intracranial pressure, or evidence of head trauma.

Angiography is used to distinguish a tumor from a vascular abnormality or to delineate the pathologic vascular anatomy before surgery. Technetium *brain scanning* has largely been replaced by CT and MRI. In some centers, *positron emission tomography* (PET)

TABLE 15.10–2. MANIFESTATIONS OF INCREASING INTRACRANIAL PRESSURE

	Early	Late	Severe
Symptoms			
Headache	Nocturnal or on awakening, worse with cough and head motion	Constant, dull	Constant, dull
Mental state	Lethargy Slowness of response	Stupor	Coma
Vomiting	May occur without nausea	Projectile	May be projectile
Signs			
Pupils	Unilateral irregularity or dilation	Unilateral dilation	Unilateral dilation
Fundi	Blurring of disc margins Loss of venous pulsations	Disc hyperemia Flame-shaped hemorrhages at disc margin	Disc margins obscured Hemorrhages in retina
Extraocular movements	Ptosis, unilateral	Unilateral III and VI nerves	Ophthalmoplegia Loss of vestibular-ocular reflexes
Motor	Normal	Hemiparesis (may be false localizing, see Table 15.10–3)	Bilateral hemiparesis
Arterial pressure	Normal	Normal	Elevated with widened pulse pressure
Pulse	Normal	Normal	Slow, irregular

TABLE 15.10–3. MANIFESTATIONS OF HERNIATION

Clinical Signs and Symptoms	Mechanism[a]
Right herniation	
Level of consciousness:	
Alert (early)	Cortical function normal
Stupor (rapidly progressing)	Decreased ascending reticular activating system (ARAs)
Unarousable (late)	Absent hemispheric or ARF activity; often associated with brain stem hemorrhages
Motor function:	
Withdrawal (early)	Cortical response normal
Unilateral decerebrate posture (late)	Removal of ipsilateral cerebral influence on posture
Flaccid (very late)	
Eyes:	
Unilateral dilatation, fixed (rt.)	Incomplete compression of oculomotor nerve
Ptosis (rt.)	
Ophthalmoplegia (rt.) (late)	Complete compression of oculomotor nerve
Vestibulo-ocular reflex normal	Absent cortical input
Absent vestibulo-ocular reflex (very late)	Brain stem dysfunction often associated with brain stem hemorrhages
Central herniation	
Level of consciousness:	
Stupor (early)	Bilateral hemisphere dysfunction
Unarousable (late)	ARF dysfunction
Motor function:	
Bilateral decorticate posture (early)	Bilateral hemispheric dysfunction
Bilateral decerebrate posture (late)	Removal of cerebral influence on posture
Flaccid (very late)	
Pupils:	
Bilateral miosis	Hypothalamic sympathetic disruption
Bilateral dilation, fixed	Compression of III nerve or brain stem damage
Oculomotor function:	
Voluntary movement normal (early)	Cortical response normal
Vestibulo-ocular reflex	Absent cortical input
Absent vestibulo-ocular reflex (very late)	Brain stem dysfunction often associated with brain stem hemorrhage

[a]See Chapter 15.3 for a detailed discussion.

scanning is used on an experimental basis to evaluate the metabolic activity of brain tumors. *Electroencephalography* (EEG) is instrumental in evaluating seizures that may accompany intracranial mass lesions.

Lumbar puncture should not be performed if the patient has papilledema in the presence of a mass or if there is a mass effect by CT scan or MRI. Spinal taps are generally reserved for patients with a history strongly suggestive of subarachnoid hemorrhage (sudden severe headache accompanied by a stiff neck) or of meningitis (stiff neck, fever, chills). The cerebrospinal fluid (CSF) of patients with pineal and posterior fossa tumors may contain markers helpful in diagnosis, for example, alpha-fetoprotein or human chorionic gonadotropin.

Evaluation of the patient with an intracranial mass lesion is usually not complete until tissue has been obtained for pathologic or bacteriologic examination (Table 15.10–5).[1] Three basic approaches are available for obtaining abnormal brain tissue. For patients with small tumors that are not causing mass effect and are located in critical regions, a CT stereotactic biopsy may be recommended. For larger lesions, an open biopsy, occasionally with the aid of ultrasonography or the operating microscope, is utilized to obtain tissue. Finally, tissue can be obtained at the time of tumor removal or decompression. In patients whose intracranial pressure is elevated because of obstructive hydrocephalus, ventricular decompression may be accomplished by means of a ventricular drain or a permanent shunt.

ETIOLOGY OF INTRACRANIAL MASS LESIONS (Table 15.10–5)

NEOPLASTIC LESIONS[7]

Metastatic Tumors

It has been estimated from autopsy studies that 18 percent of all patients with cancer develop intracranial metastases. About 67,000 patients annually in the United States present with brain metastases. Thus, metastatic lesions are far more common than primary brain tumors. Most metastases to the brain are from malignancies that originate in the lung, breast, kidney, and skin (malignant melanoma), but there are case reports of tumors from virtually every organ metastasizing to the brain. Most patients who present with brain metastases and an unknown primary tumor will eventually be found to have bronchogenic carcinoma. The most common route of spread of metastasis to the CNS is hematogenous. As a result, most patients have evidence of lung metastases on chest roentgenograms or computed tomographic studies at the time they present with brain metastases. Most cerebral metastases occur within 2 years of the primary tumor, but the interval may be much longer. Brain metastases are usually supratentorial and multiple. Computed tomographic scans with a double dose of intravenous contrast material or MRI may be required to demonstrate multiple lesions.

TABLE 15.10–4. EVALUATION OF POSSIBLE INTRACRANIAL MASSES

Procedure	Possible Findings
History	Change in mental status or neurological function
Neurologic examination	Evidence of localizing findings or increased intracranial pressure
CT scan	Mass lesion Ventricular size and position Cerebral edema or atrophy Contrast enhancement Evidence of herniation
MRI	May further delineate mass and surrounding edema
EEG	Focal slowing or seizure activity
Angiogram	Distortion of cerebral vessels Abnormal vessels
Lumbar puncture (only if CT scan shows no evidence of mass effect)	Increased pressure Elevated protein Evidence of infection, pleocytosis, low sugar, positive serological test for syphilis
Skull radiograph	Calcifications Evidence of new or old trauma Hyperostosis or erosions

TABLE 15.10–5. INTRACRANIAL MASS LESIONS

- Tumor
    Metastatic
    Primary
- Cerebrovascular disease
    Occlusive vascular disorders
    Hemorrhagic vascular disorders
    Arteriovenous malformations
    Aneurysms
- Abscess
- Focal encephalitis
    Herpes simplex, type II
    Toxoplasmosis

Primary Brain Tumors

The frequency distribution of the primary intracranial neoplasms in adults is presented in Table 15.10–6.

Astrocytomas. Low-grade astrocytomas (Grades I and II) have an unpredictable clinical course. Patients may present with long-standing seizures or, depending upon the location of the tumor, slowly progressive neurologic dysfunction. At the time of presentation 75 percent of patients complain of headaches, and one third have changes in mental status. These tumors usually occur in the cerebral hemispheres but can also occur in the cerebellum or spinal cord.

The two most important prognostic features are the histologic grade of the tumor and the age of the patient at the time of diagnosis. Histologically, distinctions between the grades of astrocytomas are not always clear. The problem is further compounded by sampling error. One portion of a biopsied tumor may show more or fewer malignant features than an adjacent portion that was evaluated histologically. The age of onset is an important prognostic

TABLE 15.10–6. FREQUENCY OF SOLITARY INTRACRANIAL MASS LESIONS IN SURGICAL SERIES

Supratentorial (75% in adults)
Glioma (40%)
- Glioblastoma
- Astrocytoma
- Oligodendroglioma

Meningioma (15%)
Metastatic carcinoma (20%)
- Lung
- Breast
- Melanoma
- Choriocarcinoma } Often present with hemorrhage
- Renal cell
- Thyroid
- Gastrointestinal

Infratentorial (15% in adults)
Metastatic carcinoma (5%)
Glioma (5%)
- Medulloblastoma
- Astrocytoma
- Ependymoma

Cranial nerve neuromas (5%)

Suprasellar (10% in adults)
Craniopharyngioma (3%)
Pituitary tumors (7%)
- Chromophobe adenoma
- Acidophilic adenoma
- Basophilic adenoma

factor. If the patient is under 30 years of age, the 5-year survival is 81 percent. By contrast, if the patient is older than 30 years, the 5-year survival is 15 percent.[10]

Grades III and IV astrocytomas (anaplastic gliomas and glioblastomas) are the most common primary intracranial neoplasms in adults and are much more aggressive than grades I and II.[1,7] Patients with these tumors also present with seizures, progressive neurologic dysfunction, changes in mentation, and increased intracranial pressure. The mass effect of the tumor is greatly augmented by surrounding edema, which may respond dramatically to corticosteroids.

Age is also an important prognostic factor, with patients over 45 having the poorest survival durations. The overall prognosis for patients with these tumors is poor, as the average survival in treated patients is only 9 to 12 months.

Meningioma.[9] Meningiomas, which constitute 15 percent of all intracranial tumors, are benign tumors derived from the meninges and have a characteristic dural attachment that is usually apparent on CT scan. They present predominantly (60 percent) in women, with a peak incidence at age 45. The most common locations of meningiomas are the parasagittal and falx regions (24 percent), convexity (18 percent), sphenoid ridge (10 percent), olfactory groove (10 percent), suprasellar (10 percent), posterior fossa (9 percent), and intraventricular regions (2 percent). Meningiomas usually compress rather than invade adjacent neural structures. Although meningiomas are often large and vascular, they can usually be removed with minimal morbidity. Prognosis for patients is related to the surgical accessibility of these tumors. Multiple meningiomas are found most frequently in association with von Recklinghausen neurofibromatosis.

Pituitary Tumors. Pituitary tumors present either by endocrine abnormality (hypersecretion or hypopituitary function) or by mass effect (such as optic nerve compression leading to visual field defects). The diagnosis and management of these tumors is discussed in Chapter 14.2. The most common of the pituitary tumors are the chromophobe and acidophilic adenomas.

Craniopharyngioma. Craniopharyngiomas are slow-growing suprasellar tumors that may be cystic and are potentially curable by surgical resection. Patients with these tumors usually present with visual or endocrine dysfunction because of the pressure on adjacent neural structures.

Cranial Nerve Sheath Tumors. The most common tumor of the sheaths of the cranial nerves is the acoustic neuroma. Patients with this tumor usually present with hearing loss, tinnitus, vertigo, facial weakness, and facial sensory loss (Chapter 15.7). These slow-growing tumors can compress CSF pathways and result in increased intracranial pressure. The treatment of choice is surgical resection.

Hemangioblastomas. Hemangioblastomas are benign, often cystic tumors that arise in the cerebellum and less frequently in the brain stem, spinal cord, and cerebral hemispheres. Multiple tumors may be associated with the hereditary syndrome of von Hippel–Lindau. Single lesions may be curable by surgery.

Medulloblastomas and Ependymomas. The medulloblastoma is an embryonal tumor originating from the external granular layer of the cerebellum. It is the most common brain tumor of children. Ependymomas, which are also primarily childhood tumors, are derived from the ependymal cells that line the cavities of the CNS and often involve the posterior fossa. Both medulloblastomas and ependymomas frequently metastasize by way of the CSF pathways and are usually treated with surgery and radiation therapy. The role of chemotherapy in these diseases appears to be expanding.

Oligodendrogliomas. Oligodendroglia are nonneuronal cells that are involved in the process of myelination. Tumors of these cells are usually slow growing, frequently are partially calcified, and often may have caused seizures for several years. Oligodendrogliomas may be pure or mixed with malignant astrocytes. The mixed tumors tend to have a poorer prognosis, although some pure oligodendrogliomas can also be extremely aggressive. Patients with oligodendrogliomas respond well to surgical decompression and may benefit from multiple resections over many years. Radiation therapy has also been successful in the palliation of symptoms in these patients.

Lymphoma. Diffuse histiocytic lymphoma of the CNS, previously referred to as microglial or reticulum cell sarcoma, is being diagnosed with increasing frequency. Patients who are severely immunosuppressed, such as patients with acquired immunodeficiency syndrome (AIDS) (Chapter 7.7) or organ transplant recipients, appear to be at particular risk. Surgery is required for a histologic diagnosis. These tumors usually respond to radiation therapy and steroids, but the long-term outlook remains poor.

NONNEOPLASTIC LESIONS

Cerebral Vascular Disease

Vascular disorders of the CNS are among the most frequently observed illnesses in hospitalized patients. These diseases are described in detail in Chapter 15.13. The diagnostic distinction between cerebral vascular events and neoplastic mass lesions is not always clear. The onset of neurologic symptoms in patients with brain tumors can be abrupt and similar to that of a stroke, if a cerebral vessel is occluded by the tumor or if there is hemorrhage into a tumor. Melanomas, renal cell carcinomas, and choriocarcinomas frequently present with intracranial bleeding, either within or around the tumor. CT scans of patients with recent cerebral vascular accidents complicated by mass effect and edema can be very difficult to differentiate from tumor. A repeat study 6 or more weeks after the neurologic event is sometimes required to distinguish the resolving changes of vascular disease from the persistent or progressive abnormalities of neoplastic disorders. MRI shows increasing promise in making the distinction as well. Aneurysms and arteriovenous malformations can present with seizures and neurologic dysfunction from mass effect. Hemorrhagic events in the CNS (intraparenchymal, subdural, epidural, and subarachnoid) can also cause increased intracranial pressure and produce focal neurologic symptoms from compression of normal structures.

Brain Abscesses[6]

Brain abscesses are most common in the first 5 decades of life. One third of these result from an adjacent focus of infection (such as dental, ear, or sinus), while the remainder are hematogenous in origin. Clinically, patients with brain abscesses usually present with headache, seizures, altered mentation, and focal neurologic findings. Since the course may be prolonged and fever may be absent in up to one half the cases, it may be difficult to distinguish a brain abscess from any other expanding mass lesion by clinical means. This is especially true for indolent organisms, such as fungal and parasitic infections. Surgery is required to confirm the presence of an abscess and to obtain an organism for culture. The abscess can be removed or merely drained and antibiotic therapy initiated. Computed tomography–directed stereotactic techniques now allow multiple aspirations to be performed without major complications. This technique can be particularly helpful when optimal antibiotic treatments do not provide resolution of the infection (see Chapter 9.11).

TREATMENT OF BRAIN TUMORS[4,11,12]

STABILIZATION

The first objective in the treatment of brain tumors is to stabilize the patient. Thus, seizures are treated with anticonvulsants (see Chapter 15.5). In addition, patients with supratentorial brain tumors in whom surgery is anticipated should be placed on a prophylactic regimen of anticonvulsants. Diphenylhydantoin (1 g as a loading dose given in divided doses, followed by 300 mg each day) is the most commonly prescribed anticonvulsant in this situation. Serum levels are then monitored. Glucocorticoids are prescribed for patients who have mass effect or peritumoral brain edema as evident on CT scan or MRI. The usual loading dose is 10 mg of dexamethasone followed by 4 mg every 6 hours, but higher doses may be necessary. Fluid restriction to 1800 ml/day may also help control cerebral edema. Renal function should be monitored concomitantly. Acetylsalicylic acid (aspirin) should be avoided, since it prolongs bleeding time; therefore, acetaminophen is usually given for pain. Narcotic analgesics should be avoided, since these agents may alter mental status, making the sequential evaluation of the patient difficult. In addition, they may depress respirations, thereby increasing PCO_2. An elevation of PCO_2 produces cerebral vasodilatation, which causes a further increase in intracranial pressure. Such an increase in intracranial pressure may initiate herniation in a tenuously stable patient (see Chapter 4.9).

EMERGENCY TREATMENT

Emergency treatment of increased intracranial pressure is indicated if the patient is deteriorating rapidly. These measures may include intubation with hyperventilation (to a PCO_2 of 25 mm Hg), dehydration with mannitol or furosemide, and ventricular drainage. These measures are temporary, however, and are generally followed by surgical decompression. The details of the emergency management of increased intracranial pressure are discussed in Chapter 4.9.

METASTATIC TUMORS[2,4]

Patients with metastatic brain tumors are initially treated with glucocorticoids. These agents frequently provide temporary alleviation of the patient's symptoms by reducing the edema surrounding most metastatic lesions. Radiation therapy generally palliates the CNS disease, and most patients eventually die of systemic (not CNS) progression.[2] Surgical therapy of metastatic CNS lesions is rarely indicated, except in the following circumstances:

1. There is no known primary tumor, and therefore a diagnosis is needed. The options include stereotactic biopsy or resection of the tumor.
2. There is a single CNS lesion in an accessible location, with a long time-interval from the identification of the initial tumor.
3. There are no other treatment options in a patient without progressive systemic disease who has a solitary accessible lesion causing CNS symptoms that continue to progress even after radiographic therapy.

Chemotherapeutic agents can cross the disrupted blood-brain barrier around brain tumors in a manner similar to the intravenous contrast material, and, in tumors sensitive to chemotherapy, responses to CNS metastasis have been reported.[4] Despite the ability to palliate neurologic disease, the overall prognosis of patients with brain metastases remains poor, primarily because of systemic disease progression.

PRIMARY BRAIN TUMORS

In patients with primary brain tumors, surgery establishes the diagnosis and may provide decompression. This appears to provide a longer symptom-free period and allows time for the initiation of radiation therapy or chemotherapy.[3] The use of high-dose glucocorticoids, CT stereotactic biopsies and aspirations, intraoperative ultrasonography, ultrasonic aspiration, and laser surgery has decreased morbidity and mortality associated with neurosurgical procedures in patients with brain tumors. Unfortunately, these new techniques have not significantly affected the duration of survival of these patients. Currently, patients with grade I and II astrocytomas treated with surgery and radiation therapy have an average survival of about 7 years.[7] The average survival of patients with grade III and IV astrocytomas treated similarly is about 40 weeks.[11,12] As a result, new therapeutic approaches to the management of patients with malignant astrocytomas, such as interstitial irradiation,[5] interstitial chemotherapy, and immunotherapy, are currently being explored.

REFERENCES

1. Burger PC: Pathologic anatomy in CT correlation in the glioblastoma multiforme. Appl Neurophys 46:180, 1983

2. Cairncross JD, Kim JH, Posner JB: Radiation therapy for brain metastases. Ann Neurol 7:529, 1980
3. Chang CH, Horton J, et al: Comparison of postoperative radiotherapy and chemotherapy in the multidisciplinary management of malignant gliomas. Cancer 52:997, 1983
4. Grieg NH: Chemotherapy of brain metastases: Current status. Cancer Treatment Rev 11:157, 1984
5. Gutin PH, Leibel SA, et al: Interstitial brachytherapy for recurrent malignant gliomas. J Neurosurg 67:864, 1987
6. Kaplan K: Brain abscess. Symposium of Infections of the Central Nervous System. Med Clin North Am 69:435, 1985
7. Kornblith PC, Walker MD, Cassady JR: Neoplasms of the central nervous system. In DeVita VT Jr, Hellman S, Rosenberg SA (eds): Cancer: Principles and Practice of Oncology, 2d ed. Philadelphia, JB Lippincott, 1985, p 1437
8. Plum F, Posner JB: The Diagnosis of Stupor and Coma, 3d ed. Philadelphia, FA Davis, 1982, p 337
9. Quest DO: Meningiomas: An update. Neurosurgery 3:219, 1978
10. Salcman M: Morbidity and mortality of brain tumors. Neurol Clin 2(3):229, 1985
11. Shapiro WR: Treatment of neuroectodermal brain tumors. Ann Neurol 12:231, 1982
12. Walker MD, Green SB, et al: Randomized comparisons of radiotherapy and nitrosources for the treatment of malignant glioma after surgery. N Engl J Med 303:1323, 1980

CHAPTER 15.11
Disorders of Movement

Mahlon R. DeLong and
Hamilton Moses III

Normal movement depends on the integrity of several areas of the brain. Together, the brain stem, basal ganglia, cerebellum, and motor and premotor cortex function to maintain posture and produce coordinated movements. When specific components of the motor system are damaged through disease or injury, characteristic abnormalities result. This chapter will provide an overview of these disturbances (Table 15.11–1).

ORGANIZATION OF THE MOTOR SYSTEM[1,2]

The major components of the motor system and their more prominent anatomic relationships are schematically shown in Figure 15.11–1. Certain simplifications and omissions have been made to emphasize the major features and the overall organization of the motor system.

All supraspinal motor systems ultimately exert influence upon a limited number of spinal circuits, which link each muscle with the spinal cord (segmental motor apparatus). Although these spinal circuits are capable of mediating simple reflexes, their activity is also controlled by descending motor pathways. One major pathway originates from the sensorimotor cortex and descends directly to spinal levels. This is the pyramidal or corticospinal tract. All other descending tracts originate in nuclei in the brain stem. The brain stem constitutes a major prespinal integrating center, regulated by higher centers including the cerebellum, basal ganglia, and the precentral motor fields.

As seen in Figure 15.11–1, both the cerebellum and the basal ganglia exert a direct influence on the brain stem, yet a major portion of the output from these two subcortical structures is directed to the precentral motor fields via the thalamus. The ascending

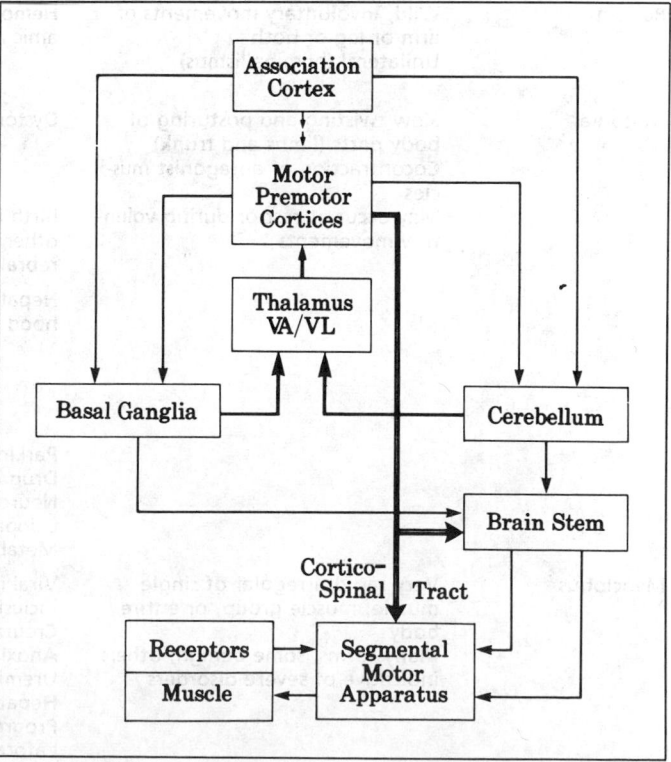

Figure 15.11–1. Schematic diagram of motor system showing current concepts of interactions between elements. See text for details.

TABLE 15.11–1. EXTRAPYRAMIDAL AND OTHER DISORDERS OF MOVEMENT

Disorder	Character	Cause	Distinguishing Features
Akinesia	Poverty and slowness of movement (bradykinesia) Maintenance of fixed postures Decreased associated movements	Parkinsonism (dopamine, deficiency in the striatum)	
Rigidity	Increased tone in all muscle groups throughout full range of passive movement ("leadpipe" or "plastic" quality)	Parkinsonism Huntington disease Neuroleptics Reserpine	
Chorea	Frequent, varied, irregular involuntary movements of the extremities, trunk, and face	Acute infections (Sydenham)	Often follows streptococcal infection Females:males (2:1) Onset insidious or acute Duration 4–6 wk Often associated with behavioral changes
		Gravidarum	Associated with pregnancy Often previous history of infectious chorea Reversible
		Vascular	Acute onset Usually unilateral May merge with ballistic movements Remission over several months May be manifestation of systemic vasculitis
		Huntington Hyperthyroidism Drugs (Levodopa, Phenytoin)	Organic mental change Psychiatric disturbance Dominant inheritance Males:females (1:1) Usually bilateral Associated with mental retardation and signs of cerebral displegia
Athetosis	Slow writhing movement of limbs, grimacing of the face	Perinatal insult (hypoxia) Posthemiplegia	
Ballism	Wild, involuntary movements of arm or leg or both Unilateral (hemiballismus)	Hemorrhage or softening in subthalamic nucleus	Sudden onset Usually subsides in a few weeks Rarely death may result from exhaustion
Dystonia	Slow twisting and posturing of body parts (limbs and trunk) Cocontraction of antagonist muscles May occur at rest or during voluntary movements	Dystonia musculorum deformans	Autosomal dominant and recessive forms Slowly progressive
		Birth injury, neonatal jaundice, or other condition causing nonfatal cerebral anoxia	
		Hepatolenticular degeneration (childhood variety of Wilson disease)	Insidious onset with gaping mouth, minor abnormal posturing Rapidly progressive course Progressive dementia Other features similar to adult variety
		Parkinson disease Drug induced Neuroleptics L-dopa Metabolic disorders	
Myoclonus	Very rapid, irregular of single muscle, muscle group, or entire body Many forms, some benign, others indicative of severe disorders	Viral infections acute and subacute inclusion body encephalitis Creutzfeldt-Jakob disease Anoxia Uremia Hepatic insufficiency Progressive myoclonic epilepsy Lafora body group System degenerations (Ramsey-Hunt) Benign essential myoclonus Nocturnal myoclonus	

(continued)

TABLE 15.11–1. EXTRAPYRAMIDAL AND OTHER DISORDERS OF MOVEMENT (Continued)

Disorder	Character	Cause	Distinguishing Features
Asterixis	Periodic, brisk, repetitive flapping of outstretched arms and hands due to sudden loss of muscle tone	Chronic cerebral hypoxia (in liver failure, chronic lung disease) Cerebral metabolic derangement (with liver or renal disease) Cerebral degenerations or diffuse infections	Sleep disturbance
Tics	Rapid, stereotyped movements	Unknown	Usually involves facial or neck musculature
	Simple or complex	Transient tic of childhood	Most common form lasts weeks to months
		Chronic tic	Constant frequency
		Tourette syndrome	Chronic multiple tic disorder Onset between 5 and 10 years, Males:females (4:1), family history often positive, vocal tics common Responds to Haloperidol or Clonodine
Tardive dyskinesia	Involuntary movements of lingual-facial-buccal muscles and sometimes limbs	Neuroleptics	Appears during therapy on withdrawal

pathways from the cerebellum and basal ganglia (via the thalamus) constitute the major inputs to the motor cortex and premotor areas from these subcortical structures. The motor cortex, instead of being at the highest level of the motor system (contrary to earlier notions), seems to occupy a position near the final output and is influenced by activity in other areas of cortex, cerebellum, and basal ganglia, rather than being the major controller itself.

CLINICAL MANIFESTATIONS

UPPER MOTOR NEURON LESIONS

Lesions of the motor cortex, subcortical white matter, internal capsule, brain stem, or spinal cord, regardless of cause, produce shock, paralysis, release phenomena, and reflex changes. These effects are caused in part by damage to other motor pathways. The term "upper motor neuron syndrome" is used to refer to the signs resulting from such combined damage.

SHOCK

With lesions of rapid onset, regardless of the level, some degree of spinal shock occurs. By shock is meant the widespread depression of neuronal activity, as evidenced by profound paralysis and decreased or absent muscle tone and tendon reflexes. Shock results largely from the removal of pyramidal tract influence, and it is generally commensurate with the severity and rate of onset of the noxious process. Shock is usually deep and long lasting with severe sudden physical trauma or a massive stroke, whereas it may be minimal or absent when the damage results from a slowly growing tumor or other mass lesion.

PARALYSIS

The paralysis or weakness that remains after recovery from an upper motor neuron lesion has certain characteristic features caused by interruption of the pyramidal tracts. The functional deficit is greatest in isolated, finely coordinated, delicate acts, particularly those involving the distal muscles of the hands and feet. Impairment of dexterity is disproportionate to the degree of weakness. Thus, individual movements of the fingers may be greatly impaired even though grasping movements are well preserved. Certain movements may be impaired on volition yet be present in reflex behaviors or in associated movements mediated by the spared subcortical motor mechanisms (such as the movement of a hemiparetic limb during yawning). Movements that are generally bilateral and symmetrical, involving the jaw, pharynx, larynx, thorax, and abdomen, are usually spared with unilateral upper motor neuron lesions. As one might expect, with unilateral lesions the contralateral hand musculature is most severely affected, the leg next, and, of the cranial musculature, only the lower face and to variable extent the tongue are involved. Finally, the weakness preferentially involves the extensors of the upper extremity and physiologic flexors of the lower extremity.

RELEASE PHENOMENA

Following upper motor neuron lesions *spasticity* gradually develops. Spasticity is characterized by increased tendon reflexes and resistance to passive muscle stretch in the antigravity muscles, that is, the flexors of the upper limbs and the physiologic extensors and adductors of the lower limbs. Characteristically, the arm is held in a posture of flexion and adduction and the leg in extension and adduction. The first sign of ensuing spasticity is generally the return and increase of the tendon jerks. A resistance to passive stretch then develops that at first is felt only with rapid stretching. Later the increased resistance is felt even with slow stretching, and near the end of the movement there is a sudden decrease in resistance (the clasp-knife reaction). Spasticity is often accompanied by *clonus,* which consists of rhythmic contractions in response to rapid application of a sustained stretch of the muscle.

CUTANEOUS REFLEXES

Abdominal and cremasteric reflexes are usually diminished or abolished following upper motor neuron damage. An extensor plantar response to stimulation of the lateral part of the sole of the foot (Babinski sign) is present immediately after injury. Babinski sign is

by far the most reliable indicator of upper motor neuron damage and may be present when other signs of upper motor neuron damage (increased tone, reflexes, and weakness) are minimal or lacking. The reflex is part of the generalized flexion response to noxious stimuli. When pronounced, it takes the form of a generalized flexion-withdrawal of the entire limb (the triple flexion response) and may be triggered by stimulation from a wide area of the foot.

MANAGEMENT OF A PATIENT WITH AN UPPER MOTOR LESION

ACUTE PHASE

In the acute phase, weakness and shock cannot be altered. Therapy is aimed at avoiding factors that will limit recovery. Contractures can be avoided by passive motion and the use of a footboard. There is no evidence, however, that any form of physical therapy actually speeds the recovery process.

RECOVERY PHASE

During recovery, the strength of proximal, large-bulk muscles returns first. Thus, standing and movements around the shoulder and around the hip can be encouraged. In most patients, spasticity is not a disabling symptom and may be of value in aiding standing. When spasticity is bilateral, however, it may disrupt locomotion and other movements. No drug specifically alters spasticity. Diazepam (Valium) 5 mg three times daily; dantrolene sodium (Dantrium), given in gradually increasing dosage to 100 mg four times

daily; or baclofen (Lioresal) given in increasing doses to 30 to 80 mg per day in divided doses may be of value in some patients. Physical therapy can be of benefit through gait training; in instructing patients in the use of slow, bulk movements to compensate for the loss of fine, distal movements; and in avoiding disuse of a limb and subsequent contractures.

TREMOR[4,6,8]

Tremor is a rhythmic oscillation of a body part resulting from alternating contractions of opposing muscle groups. It is convenient to classify tremors according to their relationship to movement and posture (Table 15.11–2). Thus, a tremor that is present when the limb is at complete rest is termed "static" or "resting tremor." Tremors present only during movement or during sustained maintenance of posture are referred to as "action tremors." Two types of action tremors are recognized: (1) postural tremor, which is present during sustained posture (such as holding the arms outstretched) and throughout the course of movement, and (2) intention tremor, which is absent during steady maintenance of posture but develops during movement of the limb, especially as the object is approached.

Physiologic Tremor

It should be recognized that in all normal individuals there is a physiologic action tremor (9 to 11/sec) present both during maintained posture and during movement. Although normally of low amplitude, it may be greatly heightened during states of anxiety, thyrotoxicosis, with fatigue, after injection of caffeine or other stimulants, during withdrawal from alcohol, and with certain drugs such as lithium or valproic acid. For individuals subject to

TABLE 15.11–2. TREMORS CLASSIFICATION

Type	Character	Cause	Age of Onset	Distinguishing Features
Static				
"Parkinsonian"	Present at rest 4–5/sec	Idiopathic parkinsonism Parkinson syndromes Reserpine CO or Mn poisoning	40+	Rigidity or akinesia usually present Responds to antiparkinson drugs, thalamotomy
"Rubral"	Present at rest but with action components 3–5/sec at rest	Damage to multiple pathways in the midbrain tegmentum including brachium conjunctivum	Any age	Tremor looks parkinsonian at rest but with intention component Absence of rigidity and akinesia
Postural				
Physiologic	Present normally Adults: 9–11/sec Children and aged: 6–8/sec		All ages	Increased with anxiety, effort, fatigue, thyrotoxicosis, caffeine, epinephrine, lithium, alcohol withdrawal, metabolic disturbance
Essential "familial"	5–9/sec	Unknown Often hereditary	Middle age or late life ("senile")	Bilateral, symmetric, best seen when hands are outstretched Not seen in legs Usually no intentional component Increased by stress Decreased by alcohol Responds to propranolol, Mysoline, or thalamotomy, if severe
Intention	Absent during maintained posture and first part of movement Worse with precise, goal-directed movements	Cerebellar damage: cortex or "outflow" (brachium conjunctivum) tumors, vascular disease, multiple sclerosis, Dilantin toxicity	Any age	When severe, the target may never be attained and has "wing-beating" character Proximal > distal

situational anxiety manifested as exaggerated physiological tremor, such as musicians before an audition, prophylactic treatment with propranalol (40 to 80 mg) 1 hour beforehand may be extremely beneficial.

Static Tremor

Static tremor (4 to 5 sec) is almost always caused by parkinsonism of one etiology or another. Parkinsonian tremor is most often confused with essential tremor (see below), which may in some cases be present at rest. The treatment of resting tremor is discussed in Chapter 15.12.

Action Tremors

Essential Tremor. Essential tremor often is an inherited disorder (autosomal dominant). It is therefore sometimes termed "familial tremor." A family history, however, is often lacking. Typically the tremor develops in middle age but may come on in childhood or in late life, when it is sometimes referred to as "senile tremor." The onset is gradual over many years. The anatomic and physiologic defect is unknown.

Essential tremor is a coarse tremor whose frequency (5 to 9/sec) is somewhat lower than that of physiologic tremor (9 to 11/sec). It is most noticeable in the distal upper extremities, usually sparing the lower extremities. While completely absent at rest, it is easily brought out by having the patient extend the arms. With movements of the arm the tremor may increase somewhat in amplitude, that is, there may be an intentional component. When severe, the tremor seriously interferes with writing, feeding, and fine movements. This form of tremor may also appear in the lips, tongue, face, and head and cause tremulous speech. Patients with essential tremor often find that the tremor is relieved by one or two drinks of alcohol. The tremor is exacerbated by emotional stress and often is a source of considerable embarrassment to patients. Patients are at increased risk of alcoholism because of alcohol's palliative effect.

The treatment of essential tremor has until recently been largely restricted to the beta-adrenergic antagonist propranalol; propranalol should be given in divided doses up to 300 mg per day. Recently the anticonvulsant Mysoline has been used successfully as well. The starting dose should be small (50 mg at bedtime) because some patients are extremely sensitive to the drug. Increases should be made gradually on a weekly basis up to 250 mg daily. In the most severe cases where medical management has failed, stereotactic thalamotomy can be performed with good results.

Intention Tremor. Intention tremor is distinguished from postural tremor in that the tremor does not appear unless the limb is used in goal-directed activity, such as reaching for an object or bringing an object to the mouth, as in eating and drinking. The tremor is absent at the onset of the movement but increases rapidly as the target is reached and greater precision is required. After reaching the target, the tremor abates. In the most severe instances, however, the target may never be attained. The tremor is frequently accompanied by ataxia and is sometimes referred to as "ataxic tremor." This type of tremor nearly always indicates disease of the cerebellum or its brain stem connections and is most often caused by lesions of cerebellar outflow, that is, the brachium conjunctivum or the lateral cerebellar hemisphere. It is seen most often in multiple sclerosis but may also be a manifestation of tumors and vascular and degenerative diseases of the cerebellum. Medical treatment is of little benefit. If the tremor is severe and incapacitating, thalamotomy may also be recommended to ameliorate it in the contralateral limbs.

Rubral Tremor. Although rubral tremor is often present at rest, it is greatly intensified with the maintenance of posture and movement. The resting component is usually of low frequency (3 to 5/sec), while the action component is of higher frequency. It is termed "rubral" tremor because of the presumed localization of the pathologic lesion in the red nucleus. It is now believed, however, that this tremor is caused by the interruption of several pathways in this region (including the brachium conjunctivum, which passes through the red nucleus) and other pathways crossing the midbrain tegmentum. The intention tremor appears to reflect involvement of the cerebellar outflow (brachium conjunctivum).

MYOCLONUS AND MYOCLONIC JERKS[4]

This movement disorder is characterized by rapid lightning-like muscle jerks, which are most often irregular and asynchronous. Myoclonus may be focal, generalized, or multifocal. It may occur spontaneously or be activated by voluntary movement (action myoclonus) or by sensory stimulation (reflex myoclonus). It is important to distinguish among (1) patients with a benign, nonprogressive myoclonus, (2) those with myoclonus secondary to an acute insult to the nervous sytem, such as anoxia, and (3) those in whom myoclonic jerks are an indication of a diffuse, progressive disease of the nervous system, such as subacute sclerosing panencephalitis or a lipidosis. After etiologic classification, consideration of symptomatic characterization is possible. Some success has been achieved in treating forms of epileptic myoclonus with anticonvulsants such as clonazepam and valproate (both of which appear to enhance GABAergic transmission). Also, serotonergic agents (such as 5-HTP) may be effective.

ATAXIA AND OTHER ABNORMALITIES OF CEREBELLAR FUNCTION

CLINICAL SYNDROMES[3]

Lesions of the cerebellum interfere with the programming of movements and important feedback mechanisms involved in motor control. They are marked in general by disorders of the rate, rhythm, force, and sequence of movements with little associated weakness. The clinical syndrome differs in relation to the temporal onset (acute vs. chronic) and the localization of the lesion (hemisphere, vermis, or flocculonodular lobe).

Hemisphere

Acute lesions of the cerebellar hemisphere cause disordered motor control of the ipsilateral extremities. This consists of a generalized decrease in muscle tone, dysmetria (inability to move to a given point precisely), intention tremor (tremor absent at rest that appears with movement), and dysdiadochokinesia (inability to make repetitive movements in a normal rhythmic fashion).

Vermis

Lesions of the cerebellar vermis result in truncal ataxia, with an unsteady, staggering, wide-based gait, difficulty sitting unsupported, and often dysarthric, "scanning" speech that has an explosive character resulting from an inability to coordinate the expulsion of air and movement of the larynx, palate, tongue, and lips.

DIAGNOSTIC EVALUATION

The evaluation of a patient with ataxia is indicated in Table 15.11–3. Unfortunately, we do not know enough about the neurophysiology and neurochemistry of ataxia to have a rational pharmacologic approach to its management. In severe cases, particularly where tremor is the disabling symptom, stereotactically placed lesions in the ventrolateral nucleus of the thalamus or dentate nucleus may be of help.

TABLE 15.11–3. EVALUATION OF ATAXIA

Procedure	Findings	Significance
History	Pattern of progression Drug usage Symptoms of systemic illness Other neurologic dysfunctions Family history	Acute vs. chronic (Tables 15.11–4 and 15.11–5) Toxic (Tables 15.11–4 and 15.11–5) Metabolic, malignancy, infection, toxic Multiple sclerosis, brain stem tumor Wilson disease, degenerative disease (Tables 15.11–5 and 15.11–6)
Physical examination	Truncal or limb involvement Symmetry, other neurologic signs Evidence of undelying systemic illness Papilledema	Hemisphere vs. vermis Diffuse or focal disease Metabolic, malignancy, infection, toxic Mass lesion (tumor, abscess, hemorrhage)
Cervical spine radiograph	Spondylosis, especially canal narrowing	Cord compression
CT or MRI scan	Ventricular size and position Abnormal cranial-cervical junction	Hydrocephalus Congenital malformations
Lumbar puncture (deferred if intracranial pressure is possibly elevated)	Elevated protein Elevated gamma globulin Increased CSF pressure Pleocytosis	Tumor Multiple sclerosis Stop, if elevated Evidence of infection
Metrizimide myelogram	Mass or atrophy	

TABLE 15.11–4. ATAXIAS OF ACUTE ONSET

Etiology	Characteristics	Therapy	Remarks
Toxic Ethanol[a] Anticonvulsants[a] (diphenylhydantoin) Sedatives (barbiturates)	Acute, truncal May have nystagmus Dose related, reversible	Withdrawal of toxin	Chronic toxicity may be irreversible Underlying lesion, such as Wernicke, may be missed
Organomercurials	Subacute, irreversible Associated with dementia	Withdrawal of mercurial	
Nutritional Wernicke encephalopathy[a]	Truncal ataxia Paresis of extraocular muscles Confusion Defects in recent memory Peripheral neuropathy	Thiamine, 100 mg	Underlying Korsakoff syndrome may be missed May not be reversible (Chapter 17.5)
Cerebrovascular Cerebellar hemorrhage[a]	Nausea and vomiting, headache Unsteadiness of gait, limb ataxia Long tract findings Nystagmus Gaze paresis Progressive obtundation	Surgical evacuation on emergency basis	History of hypertension or anticoagulation CT scan diagnostic Xanthochromic CSF (lumbar puncture contraindicated)
Vertebral-basilar artery ischemia[a]	Asymmetrical ataxia Associated brain stem signs (Chapter 15.6) Progressive deterioration in some patients (similar to hemorrhage)	Anticoagulation in some patients	Demonstrable by vertebral angiography
Parainfections Acute ataxia of childhood and young adults	Truncal and limb ataxia Nystagmus Lymphocytosis of CSF Self-limited	None	Associated with varicella, coxsackie, polio, and echo viruses
Landry-Guillain-Barré	Ascending motor weakness Areflexia Gait ataxia Decreasing respiratory function	Supportive (Chapter 15.16)	CSF protein elevated Often preceded by nonspecific respiratory infection
Demyelinating Multiple sclerosis	May be either part of first attack or of exacerbations CSF gamma globulin elevated in 70% of cases	ACTH or corticosteroids may shorten acute attacks (Chapter 15.18)	Neurologic lesions spread topographically and temporally

[a]Most common.

ACUTE CEREBELLAR ATAXIA

Causes of acute ataxia and their distinguishing features are indicated in Table 15.11–4. The involvement is usually diffuse, with the exception of cerebellar hemorrhage and multiple sclerosis, which are often asymmetrical in their involvement. Cerebellar hemorrhage is important to recognize because without the surgical evacuation that is made possible by prompt diagnosis, this condition may be fatal (see Chapter 15.13).

CHRONIC AND PROGRESSIVE ATAXIA

The causes and characteristics of chronic ataxia of cerebellar origin are indicated in Table 15.11–5. In the United States, the most

TABLE 15.11–5. CHRONIC AND PROGRESSIVE ATAXIA

Etiology	Characteristics	Therapy	Remarks
Toxic			
Alcohol[a]	Superior vermis involved Gait ataxia Slowly progressive	Abstinence	(See Chapter 17.5)
Phenytoin[a]	Gait ataxia Nystagmus	Decrease dosage	Associated with lethargy May be reversible
Organomercurials	Limb and gait ataxia Dementia Visual loss	Stop exposure	
Metabolic			
Wilson disease	Dyskinesia Choreoathetosis Kayser-Fleischer rings Elevated serum copper Decreased ceruloplasmin	Decrease copper (penicillamine)	Similar picture after portocaval shunt
Hypothyroidism	Ataxia Thickened, dry skin Cold intolerance Low T_4	Thyroid replacement	(See Chapter 13.6)
Metachromatic	Ataxia Dementia Dystonia Peripheral neuropathy Decreased arylsulfatase A	None	Occurs as a juvenile and adult form
Associated with Malignancy			
Metastasis[a]	Asymmetrical headache May be increased by intracranial pressure Abnormal brain scan or arteriogram	Surgery if single metastasis May be helped by steroids	Lung and breast common primaries
Cerebellar degeneration	Truncal ataxia (early) May be associated brain stem involvement	Removal of primary (especially lung, ovary, gastric)	May improve after removal of pituitary tumor

Primary tumor
  Astrocytoma
  Medulloblastoma
  Hemangioblastoma
  Ependymoma
	Usually asymmetrical
	Obstructive hydrocephalus
		Surgical removal radiation	More common in children (See Chapter 4.9)

Infection			
Abcess	Asymmetrical headache Increased intracranial pressure Abnormal brain scan or arteriogram	Surgical removal	Follows chronic otitis media, septicemia, subacute bacterial endocarditis or lung abscess
Spongiform encephalopathy	Ataxia Tremor Dementia Slowly progressive	None	Transmissable agent (See Chapter 16.7)
Demyelination			
Multiple sclerosis[a]	CSF gamma globulin elevated in 70%	Stereotactic surgery for tremor in some patients	(See Chapter 15.18)
Genetic	Other areas of nervous system are usually involved	Physical therapy, gait training	(See Table 15.11–6)
Idiopathic	Hemisphere usually	None	Probably a spectrum of disorders Diagnosis by exclusion

[a]Most common.

common causes in adults are alcoholism, cerebellar degeneration secondary to neoplasm, multiple sclerosis, and, for a large number of patients, no identifiable etiology.

CEREBELLAR AND SPINOCEREBELLAR DEGENERATIONS[5]

This group of processes is often called "system degenerations" because specific groups of neurons degenerate. The different entities are distinguished by age of onset, pattern of progression, and degree of involvement of the nervous system and other organs (Table 15.11–6) as well as their pattern of inheritance. Many of the conditions are genetically determined. Unfortunately, there is neither information about the basic mechanisms of these diseases nor effective therapy.

Friedreich ataxia is the best known and one of the more common of the spinocerebellar degenerations. The pattern of inheritance appears to be recessive. Partial or incomplete forms of the disease are common. Symptoms start in childhood, usually in the first decade of life. Patients commonly complain that they have never been able to run well or keep up in athletic activities. A progressive ataxia with muscle wasting and weakness and a profound loss of proprioception develops by the middle of the second decade. Pes cavus and kyphoscoliosis are usually present. The deep tendon reflexes are depressed or absent, but the plantars are extensor, indicating pyramidal tract involvement.

A cardiomyopathy is often present and may be evident on electrocardiogram well before clinical evidence of heart failure is noted. Most patients with Friedreich ataxia die from cardiac complications.

A number of cases clinically indistinguishable from the milder forms of Friedreich ataxia have been described in which there are decreased or absent beta-lipoproteins. Steatorrhea may be seen as an early manifestation, and in the recessively transmitted a-beta-lipoproteinemic cases acanthocytosis or erythrocytes and retinitis pigmentosa are usually present.

There is no effective treatment, and slow progression is usual.

Ataxia telangiectasia is a progressive degenerative disease of the cerebellum that is probably recessively transmitted. It begins in early childhood with ataxia and increased susceptibility to infections, followed by the appearance of conjunctival and cutaneous telangiectasia between 3 and 6 years of age. The serum gamma globulin may be decreased, perhaps accounting for the increased susceptibility to infection and the resulting decreased life span.

Olivopontocerebellar degeneration includes a number of closely related disorders that have in common degeneration of the inferior olivary nuclei, nuclei pontis, and cerebellum, with variable involvement of dorsal columns, spinocerebellar pathways, and other neuronal systems including the basal ganglia. Most of these appear to be transmitted as an autosomal dominant trait, but a few families display a recessive pattern, and sporadic cases are common. The age of onset ranges from infancy to advanced age; it may even vary widely within a given family.

The clinical characteristics are progressive ataxia, dysarthria, and clumsiness in the hands, with a variable degree of spasticity. In some families other neurologic signs, such as progressive visual loss, rigidity, or dementia are regular features of the condition. The

TABLE 15.11–6. CEREBELLAR AND SPINOCEREBELLAR DEGENERATIONS

Disease	Age of Onset	Progession	Life Expectancy	Neurologic Findings	Nonneurologic Findings	Inheritance	Eponym and Remarks
Ataxia telangiectasia	1–5 yr	Ataxia Mental retardation Pulmonary infections	25 years	Ataxia Choreoathetosis	Sinopulmonary infections Telangiectasia of sclera and skin Decreased IgG	Recessive	—
Friedreich ataxia	5–15 yr	Ataxia Scoliosis Cardiomyopathy	10–15 yr from onset	Ataxia Nystagmus Areflexia Extensor plantars	Scoliosis Cardiac failure Pes cavus	Recessive	Form fruste common
A-beta lipoproteinemia	Childhood to early adult	Ataxia Visual loss	May be normal	Ataxia Areflexia Extensor plantars Retinitis pigmentosa	Steatorrhea Acanthocytosis Absent beta lipoproteins	Recessive	Bassen-Kornzweig disease
Hypo-beta lipoproteinemia		Ataxia	May be normal	Ataxia Areflexia Extensor plantars	Decreased beta lipoproteins	Probably dominant with incomplete penetrance	—
Familial ataxia	Adult	Ataxia	May be normal	Ataxia	None	Mixed	Multiple forms
Olivoponto-cerebellar degenerations	Childhood and adult	Ataxia Visual loss Dementia	20+ yr from onset	Ataxia Bulbar dysfunction Posterior column dysfunction Parkinsonian features Retinitis pigmentosa Dementia		Mixed	Multiple forms

condition is slowly progressive, with many patients surviving 10 to 20 years.

Late cortical cerebellar atrophy is a heterogeneous group of degenerations of insidious onset, usually beginning in the fifties or sixties. It is occasionally familial and usually has a prolonged course. Patients have symptoms and signs of a progressive cerebellar hemisphere disorder. When the family history is negative, a careful search for an occult neoplasm (especially of lung or ovary), inapparent intoxication, past symptoms of multiple sclerosis, hypothyroidism, and malabsorption should be made.

SENSORY AND FRONTAL ATAXIA

Not all ataxia is caused by cerebellar dysfunction. Sensory ataxia occurs when there is insufficient sensory feedback about limb position and movement. The pathologic basis for sensory ataxia is lesions of posterior roots (tabes dorsalis or polyneuropathies) or of the posterior columns (pernicious anemia). In these patients the ataxia is much worse in the absence of visual cues (eyes closed), and the defect in position sense is clearly demonstrable (positive Romberg sign).

Frontal ataxia occurs with lesions of the frontal lobe such as tumors, occult hydrocephalus, multiple infarcts, or presenile dementia (Pick disease). Ataxia of frontal origin may be difficult to distinguish from ataxia of cerebellar origin. The presence of dysmetria and dysdiadochokinesia are indicative of cerebellar dysfunction.

PROBLEM OF GAIT DISTURBANCE IN THE ELDERLY

Older people generally have difficulty walking. Their gait becomes tentative and insecure, and their posture becomes progressively more flexed. Falls are common. Many conditions produce this caricature of old age. Most patients, however, do not have a specific abnormality but rather the combined effects of visual impairment (cataracts, macular degeneration), mild loss of proprioceptive sense in the legs, and impairment of vestibular reflexes. All these impairments are frequent and usual concomitants of aging, although specific lesions may underlie their occurrence. Regular exercise, proper nutrition, and a cane may help to ameliorate the gait disturbance.

Several specific diseases should be distinguished. Parkinsonism may cause disturbance of gait before other symptoms are evident (see Chapter 15.12). Falls are especially common. Cryptic frontal infarction leads to progressive gait ataxia, usually with mild pyramidal signs. Occult hydrocephalus (normal pressure hydrocephalus), while classically a triad of gait disturbance, dementia, and incontinence, may cause gait disturbance before other manifestations are evident. Slowly growing frontal or subfrontal neoplasms (especially meningiomas and astrocytomas) lead to apathy, dementia, and gait

disturbance in a varying order. Cervical spondylosis frequently produces a myelopathy, with spasticity and variable proprioceptive loss, often without significant pain. These conditions may be distinguished by careful neurologic examination and other simple ancillary techniques.

MANAGEMENT

Acute ataxia caused by toxins, Wernicke encephalopathy, neoplasms, and hemorrhage may be promptly and dramatically improved by appropriate therapy (see Table 15.12–4). Acute attacks of multiple sclerosis may similarly remit fully.

The chronic ataxias may in some instances be ameliorated by specific therapies. Fortunately, those caused by intoxication, occult neoplasms, and metabolic abnormalities may improve after removal of the toxin or specific therapy of the primary disorder. Experimental therapies for the inherited ataxias have been many, but none has clear benefit.

All patients with ataxia, however, may be aided by specific training of gait, physical therapy and occupational therapy designed for ataxia, and walking aids (cane, trailing cane, or walker) and by removal of other causes of impaired coordination. Special attention to visual impairment (refraction, removal of cataracts), proper lighting in bedroom and bathroom at night, and attention to loose carpets and stairs will make living easier and safer.

REFERENCES

1. Alexander GE, DeLong MR: Organization of supraspinal motor systems. In Asbury AK, McKhann GM, McDonald WI (eds): Diseases of the Nervous System. Philadelphia, Ardmore, 1986, p 352
2. DeLong MR, Alexander GE: Organization of the basal ganglia. In Asbury AK, McKhann GM, McDonald WI (eds): Diseases of the Nervous System. Philadelphia, Ardmore, 1986, p 379
3. Gilman S: Cerebellum and motor dysfunction. In Asbury AK, McKhann GM, McDonald WI (eds): Diseases of the Nervous System. Philadelphia, Ardmore, 1986, p 401
4. Hallet M, Ravits J: Involuntary movements. In Asbury AK, McKhann GM, McDonald WI (eds): Diseases of the Nervous System. Philadelphia, Ardmore, 1986, p 452
5. Harding AE: Hereditary ataxias and related disorders. In Asbury AK, McKhann GM, McDonald WI (eds): Diseases of the Nervous System. Philadelphia, Ardmore, 1986, p 1227
6. Marsden CD: Basal ganglia and motor dysfunction. In Asbury AK, McKhann GM, McDonald WI (eds): Diseases of the Nervous System. Philadelphia, Ardmore, 1986, p 394
7. Young AB, Penney JB Jr: Pharmacological aspects of motor dysfunction. In Asbury AK, McKhann GM, McDonald WI (eds): Diseases of the Nervous System. Philadelphia, Ardmore, 1986, p 423
8. Young RR: Tremor. In Asbury AK, McKhann GM, McDonald WI (eds): Diseases of the Nervous System. Philadelphia, Ardmore, 1986, p 435

CHAPTER 15.12

Parkinsonism and Other Disorders of Extrapyramidal Function

Hamilton Moses III

The most prominent manifestations of abnormalities in the basal ganglia (the extrapyramidal system) are *positive* symptoms, particularly involuntary movements such as chorea, athetosis, dystonia, hemiballismus, tremor, and rigidity. These adventitious movements characteristically disappear or markedly diminish during sleep and are made worse by emotional stress. The *negative* symptoms resulting from loss of neural function, however, are also seri-

ously disabling, as with the akinesia and bradykinesia of parkinsonism. Many disorders that affect the basal ganglia produce combinations of positive symptoms and negative symptoms as the disease progresses or is influenced by treatment. For instance, the rigid and akinetic parkinsonian may become choreatic after treatment with levodopa, and the choreatic patient with Huntington disease may become rigid and mute toward the end of the illness.

In contrast to upper motor neuron (pyramidal) lesions, weakness per se is not a prominent feature of the extrapyramidal disorders. Also, focal lesions such as neoplasms, stroke, and trauma very rarely give rise to extrapyramidal symptoms. Diseases that affect the basal ganglia are usually *system degenerations*[4] that slowly but relentlessly progress and often involve other neurologic systems, such as the autonomic nervous system, the cortex causing dementia, or the cerebellum.[5]

Information about the etiology, biochemical pathophysiology, and epidemiology of these disorders is increasing; but with almost no exception, definitive information is lacking. Palliative treatment is available for many of the disorders affecting the basal ganglia, yet specific therapies that alter progression of the diseases are not now known.

The characteristics of the disorders of the basal ganglia and their differential diagnosis are indicated in Table 15.11–1.

PARKINSONISM AND RELATED DISORDERS

PARKINSONISM

The terms "parkinsonism," "Parkinson disease," and "paralysis agitans" all refer to a neurologic disease characterized by akinesia, bradykinesia, rigidity, postural instability, and tremor. One manifestation, particularly tremor, may precede another by months or years. Early in the course, abnormalities are frequently asymmetrical and may be strictly unilateral or truncal. In addition, a minority of patients may have one or more of the characteristic manifestations of parkinsonism but have other neurologic abnormalities, distinctive functional lesions, and responses to drugs that are considered part of other system degenerations (see Table 15.12–1).

CLINICAL FEATURES

Idiopathic parkinsonism is a disease of the elderly, affecting about 1 percent of the population over the age of 60 and as many as 3 to 5 percent of the population older than 70 years. The disease occurs worldwide, slightly more frequently in men, less often among nonwhites, with peak onset in the late 50s and early 60s.

The *rigidity* of parkinsonism is the most common symptom, often presenting as a stiff gait with loss of the normal associated movements in the arms during walking. Rigidity usually involves the proximal arms and legs first, particularly the shoulders and neck, later spreading distally. The expressionless *masklike* facies, with infrequent blinking, is also called the "parkinsonian stare." Rigidity in the limbs is usually ratchet-like or "cogwheeling."

Akinesia refers to an inability to initiate and execute a movement. It is the most disabling manifestation of parkinsonism. Akinesia affects both fine motor movements, such as writing or buttoning one's clothes, and gross movements, such as walking, standing, and sitting. Not only are movements slow to begin, but they also are slow once started (*bradykinesia*).

TABLE 15.12–1. SYSTEM DEGENERATIONS ASSOCIATED WITH PARKINSON SYNDROME

- Shy-Drager syndrome (idiopathic postural hypotension)
- Progressive supranuclear palsy
- Striatonigral degeneration
- Olivopontocerebellar atrophy
- Creutzfeldt-Jakob disease
- Familial basal ganglia calcification
- Familial Parkinson disease
- Normal pressure hydrocephalus
- Huntington chorea
- Cerebral hemosiderosis
- Hallevorden-Spatz disease

Tremor is the initial manifestation of Parkinson disease in about 20 percent of individuals and occurs in over 90 percent by late stages. A patient with a parkinsonian syndrome but without tremor should be investigated for the presence of one of the other system degenerations. Parkinsonian tremor is generally of varying amplitude, present at rest, at a frequency of about 5 hertz, although more rapid fine postural and intention tremors occasionally also occur (see Chapter 15.11). Parkinsonian tremor is rarely seriously disabling but may be a great cosmetic nuisance and cause considerable embarrassment to the patient or family.

The *gait* is abnormal because of small, shuffling steps that gradually increase in speed, as if the patient is chasing the center of gravity (festinating gait), in addition to the paucity of associated movements. The patient becomes stooped, rigid, and progressively akinetic. Unpredictable falls occur because of loss of reflexes that are necessary to maintain a normally balanced upright posture. *Postural instability* may be an early symptom, often before akinesia, rigidity, or tremor are manifest; it is a common cause of broken bones in the elderly.

Early parkinsonism can easily be confused with spastic paraparesis caused by cervical spondylosis or occult hydrocephalus. The spastic patients usually have evidence of pyramidal involvement with hyperreflexia and extensor plantar responses. The truncal ataxia of cerebellar disease and sensory ataxia of neuropathy and spinal cord disease may also be confusing (see Chapter 15.11).

To the classical manifestations of parkinsonism should be added several recently recognized features.[6] *Dementia* affects 20 percent of the patients within the first 2 or 3 years of the disease and may appear before or coincidentally with the motor symptoms; 50 to 70 percent may be affected within 5 years of diagnosis. Impairment of memory, apraxia, and language disturbance are early manifestations. The clinical features are indistinguishable from senile dementia or Alzheimer disease (see Chapter 15.4). Pathologic findings are similar, including changes in the cerebral cortex and certain subcortical areas where cholinergic cortical projections originate. Dementia is now thought to be a manifestation of advanced parkinsonism per se and not the result of therapy with levodopa. Now that parkinsonian patients are able to live longer, dementia is a greater problem. *Depression* also occurs. Early, it is often overlooked, although the masked face may make it more obvious. Later, failure of treatment may accompany depression, but serious depression occurs at all stages of the disorder and may be treated simultaneously with standard therapy and levodopa. *Sleep* is disturbed in early and late parkinsonism; usually the patient falls asleep at his normal hour, only to awaken 2 or 3 hours into the night. Abnormalities in central serotonin pathways may underlie a sleep disturbance as well as depression and are currently under intense investigation.

ETIOLOGY

No clear etiology can be indicted for most cases of parkinsonism that begin late in life. The parkinsonian syndrome frequently arises from therapy with neuroleptics (major tranquilizers), which cause prominent akinesia and rigidity. Manganese poisoning, hypoxia, and carbon monoxide exposure all cause the syndrome, often after a delay of many years. Parkinsonism undeniably occurred after encephalitis lethargica during the 1915 to 1925 outbreak of that obscure illness. Most patients who now present with the disease, however, were not alive during that time. Conventional viruses, "slow viruses," and other unconventional agents have been investigated but have no proven relationship to idiopathic parkinsonism. Family influences are not a major factor, as less than 5 percent have a family history of the disease. Most cases of familial parkinsonism have an earlier age of onset (third to fifth decade), with associated cerebellar, pyramidal, brain stem, or other abnormal neurologic signs. No clear clusters have occurred in North America to suggest an infectious or toxic agent, although these are under scrutiny in certain Pacific islands (Table 15.12–2).

TABLE 15.12–2. CAUSES OF PARKINSON DISEASE

- Idiopathic
- Drug intoxication
  - Reserpine
  - Phenothiazines
  - UPTP
- Postencephalitic
- Manganese poisoning
- Hypoxia
- Carbon monoxide poisoning
- Iron intoxication
- Familial (rare)

TABLE 15.12–3. MEDICAL THERAPY OF PARKINSONISM

Drugs	Average Daily Dose
Primary	
Levodopa and carbidopa (Sinemet)	300–750 mg
Adjunctive (anticholinergics)	
Benztropine (Cogentin)	2–6 mg
Trihexyphenidyl HCl (Artane)	6–15 mg
Procyclidine HCl (Kemadrin)	15 mg
Biperiden (Akineton)	6 mg
Amantadine HCl (Symmetrel)	200 mg
Direct	
Bromocriptine (Parlodel)	5–15 mg

MANAGEMENT OF PARKINSONISM[2,7]

The symptoms of parkinsonism can be effectively ameliorated by specific therapy, forestalling for about a decade the complications of the illness that in earlier years led to premature death. Death rates were about three times greater at a given age (based on life-table analysis) before the use of levodopa in 1968, with the patient living on average about 5 years after diagnosis. Modern therapy, especially levodopa, has lowered death rates to about 1.3 times normal, with patients usually living 10 to 15 years after diagnosis. Most of the remaining excess mortality occurs in those patients who have significant dementia. Thus, the therapy of parkinsonism stands second only to the use of anticonvulsants for the epilepsies as testimony to the efficacy of new therapies in neurology.

Once the diagnosis is made, the patient should be counseled about the natural history of the disease, the generally favorable prognosis, and the effectiveness of available therapies. The goal of therapy should be to improve—but not completely abolish—symptoms. This is because all the currently available antiparkinsonian agents have adverse effects that limit therapy in late stages. There is growing suspicion that the duration of treatment and cumulative total dose of medications (especially of levodopa) best predict failure of medications in late stages of the illness (see below). Conservative treatment of parkinsonism therefore calls for using the fewest medications possible in the lowest effective doses for as long as possible.

Early parkinsonism usually responds to amantadine or anticholinergics, with the two often prescribed together as the disease advances. These drugs are generally effective for 6 months to 2 years, after which time the substitution of levodopa is generally necessary. The direct dopamine agonist, bromocriptine, is also effective in the early stages of the illness. Its early use to forestall late treatment failure is currently under investigation.

Late stages of parkinsonism are therapeutically challenging, usually requiring careful and frequent adjustment of the dose of levodopa, the addition of bromocriptine, and reintroduction of amantadine to minimize adverse effects and maximize efficacy. Unfortunately, a majority of patients with parkinsonism experience one or another adverse effect (especially delirium and dyskinesias) or periodic lack of efficacy (clinical fluctuation) within 5 years of the initiation of levodopa. In general, once the late stages of the illness have been reached, manipulation of the drug by an experienced neurologist is necessary.

The patient who shows little or no response to antiparkinsonian drugs when used in maximal doses should be strongly suspected of having another system degeneration rather than idiopathic parkinsonism, for example, progressive supranuclear palsy or a striatonigral degeneration.

Specific Drugs (Table 15.12–3)

Anticholinergics are particularly effective in ameliorating tremor and are less effective against akinesia, rigidity, and postural instability. Anticholinergics may be used alone when tremor is a cosmetic nuisance and may be added to levodopa if tremor is particularly promi-

nent. Diphenhydramine, trihexyphenidyl, benztropine, and others are equally effective (Table 15.12–3), although differences in absorption may make one more effective in an individual patient.

Amantadine has both central dopaminergic and anticholinergic properties and is useful as an adjunct to levodopa in patients with long-standing disease. It is also useful in early parkinsonism when used alone or in combination with an anticholinergic. The anticholinergics and amantadine share toxic effects, including delirium, confusion, nocturnal hallucinations, impairment of thermoregulation and sweating, paresis of accommodation, urinary retention, and edema (amantadine only). These are especially prominent with high doses, and an occasional patient will have them even at low dose.

Specific therapy with _levodopa_ soon followed the discovery of an abnormality in the dopamine-containing pathway originating in the substantia nigra, an area of the upper midbrain. Dopamine itself cannot cross the blood-brain barrier. Its precursor, levodopa (levo-dihydroxyphenylalanine), can cross the blood-brain barrier to replenish central dopaminergic stores. A decarboxylase in liver and brain metabolizes levodopa to dopamine, resulting in both central efficacy and peripheral side effects. Circulating dopamine causes anorexia, nausea, vomiting, and hypotension, thereby limiting the useful dose. Carbidopa (α-methyldopa-hydrazine) effectively blocks the liver (but not CNS) decarboxylase, decreasing peripheral side effects and increasing central levodopa concentration. Carbidopa, 75 to 125 mg daily, is maximally effective in most individuals and is administered with levodopa, 300 to 750 mg daily. It is formulated as a 1:4 or 1:10 ratio (Sinemet 25/100, 10/100, or 25/250). Treatment generally begins with three 25/100 tablets daily and may be slowly increased (over several months) up to total levodopa daily dose of 750 mg. Up to eight 25/250 tablets daily may be safely administered, although the strategy of limiting total lifetime exposure to the drug suggests that less than 750 mg daily be used if possible.

Not all symptoms are equally improved. Akinesia and bradykinesia respond promptly. Tremor responds as well, but rarely completely. Postural instability improves, especially when mild, but does not improve as much as akinesia or rigidity, often producing the paradox of a patient who is less rigid and more mobile and who is therefore predisposed to more unpredictable falls. Patients should be reminded to take extra care while walking because of this. A cane, two canes, or a platform cane with a regular cane may help.

Levodopa-carbidopa toxicities include anorexia, nausea and vomiting, hallucinations, delirium, and hypotention (see Table 15.12–4).

Bromocriptine is the only currently available direct-acting dopamine agonist. Unlike levodopa, bromocriptine does not rely on transformation by a presynaptic neuron but rather acts directly on the postsynaptic dopamine receptor. Bromocriptine may be effec-

TABLE 15.12–4. SYMPTOMS APPEARING IN PATIENTS TREATED WITH LEVODOPA

	Symptom	Remarks
Early	Dyskinesias	Usually dose related
	Anxiety	
	Hallucinations	
	Delusions	
Late	Dyskinesias	May be dose related
	Hallucinations	
	Somnolence	
	Akathisia	
	Abrupt changes in therapeutic benefit ("on-off" phenomenon)	Usually not dose related
		Probably related to progression of disease
	Postural dysequilibrium	
	Gait disturbances	Probably related to progression of disease
	Dementia	Alzheimer type

tive in early parkinsonism but plays an important role in the treatment of late stages and is now often prescribed in combination with levodopa to minimize the levodopa dose. The effective daily dose of bromocriptine varies over a wide range, 5 to 50 mg daily. Once a levodopa dose of 600 to 750 mg daily is reached, most neurologists advocate the addition of bromocriptine, 1.25 mg at bedtime (h.s.), thereafter slowly increasing the dose of bromocriptine at about 1-month intervals until improvement occurs (usually 5 to 15 mg daily). Bromocriptine shares all the adverse effects of levodopa; hypotension and delirium are especially likely to develop.

Limiting Effects

Prominent *motor fluctuations* (the "on-off effect") are puzzling and increasingly frequent. Such patients are mobile and fluid one moment, only to become rigid and akinetic the next. They may cycle rapidly between the extremes every few hours. Clinical fluctuations may occur soon after a dose or without relationship to the last dose of medication. *Dyskinesics* induced by levodopa or bromocriptine are choreoathetotic movements of the tongue, face, neck, hands, and legs, resembling those that occur with tardive dyskinesia. They usually occur soon after dose of levodopa and abate as the blood level falls. Lowering the dose of levodopa may ameliorate the dyskinesias, but they usually reappear eventually at the smaller dose. The mechanism of these paradoxical dyskinesias and the disabling clinical fluctuations are unclear, but they probably result from changes both in blood level and the sensitivity of central dopaminergic receptors. Lowering the dose of levodopa while raising that of bromocriptine, or adding amantadine, may provide relief in patients who have prominent clinical fluctuations.

A therapeutic drug holiday was frequently recommended for patients with clinical fluctuations or delirium. There is considerable doubt, however, about either its safety or utility for these indications, and it has now largely been abandoned. Omission of drugs is justified for the early patient when there is doubt about the diagnosis or if serious delirium with agitation occurs. Patients with advanced disease should be admitted to the hospital where all drugs may be stopped for 3 to 5 days and appropriate precautions observed for aspiration, dysphagia, severe akinesia, and rigidity that predictably will ensue.

Surgical procedures were once popular but have a limited role today. Tremor responds well to ventral lateral thalamotomy, but surgical lesions do not effectively alleviate akinesia, rigidity, or postural instability, which are the most disabling features of the disease. Highly selective thalamotomy is currently being performed at several surgical centers for patients who have unusually prominent tremor, especially for tremor that is present on intention. Stereotactic lesions are placed under control by MRI and CT, using physi-

ologic monitoring for additional localization. These techniques have improved safety so that the procedure is valuable in experienced hands.

PARKINSON-LIKE SYSTEM DEGENERATIONS[4]

A number of diseases have symptoms and signs of parkinsonism at some stage in their evolution. The most common degenerations are associated with autonomic disturbance, dementia, or ophthalmoplegia, and some are hereditary. The nosology of these disorders is complex and diagnosis often vexing, but proper diagnosis may be made by recognizing the pattern of the neurologic systems involved.

SHY-DRAGER SYNDROME[1]

Shy and Drager described intractable orthostatic hypotension combined with parkinsonian symptoms. Often other evidence of dysautonomia coexists, particularly segmental loss of sweating, Horner syndrome, fixed cardiac rate, reduced bowel motility, impotence, and bladder dysfunction. The parkinsonian symptoms (rigidity and bradykinesia) usually respond to levodopa. Postural hypotension does not and may require supplemental mineralocorticoids (9-α-fluorohydrocortisone, Florinef) and ephedrine. Tremor is an inconspicuous feature, but other features such as pseudobulbar palsy, and particularly emotional lability, are often prominent. Dysphagia and obstructive apnea are potential threats to life (see Chapter 15.8).

Pathologically, the abnormalities are a diffuse neuronal loss and gliosis involving the substantia nigra, striatum, cerebral cortex, and, most conspicuously, the intermediolateral column of the spinal cord.[1] Identical changes also occur in idiopathic parkinsonism, especially late in the disease, but are present unusually early in the patient with the Shy-Drager syndrome.

PROGRESSIVE SUPRANUCLEAR PALSY

This is a Parkinson-like disorder whose conspicuous feature is a progressive decrease in conjugate ocular movement, particularly vertical movement. Characteristically, downward conjugate movement of the eyes is affected first and remains the most severely impaired. Disturbance of upward movements then follows; finally lateral conjugate movements are restricted. The patient cannot voluntarily move the eyes, but the eyes move quickly when the head is turned (see Chapter 15.6).

Rigidity is very prominent in the muscles of the neck; rigidity and akinesia are prominent in the limbs, but tremor is rarely conspicuous. Dementia is the rule, and progressive bulbar palsy with disturbances of speech, swallowing, and palatal movement occur late. The disease occurs late in life and may be confused with idiopathic parkinsonism, especially early in its course.

None of the manifestations of progressive supranuclear palsy respond well to currently available therapy. Levodopa may work for a short time but rarely is of enduring value. Other medications are not useful.

HYPERKINESIAS

CHOREAS

Rheumatic Chorea (Sydenham Chorea)

This is an acute, usually benign disorder characterized by involuntary, rapid, nonrepetitive movements occurring focally or in a multifocal fashion, often associated with disturbance of behavior and mood. The movements may be strictly unilateral. The face, extremities, and trunk are variably involved. Other manifestations of

rheumatic fever may be evident, although chorea may first occur weeks or months after the rash and arthritis have resolved. Rheumatic chorea shares all the features of acute rheumatic fever, including peak age of onset between the ages of 5 and 20.

The disorder is usually benign and fully reversible over several weeks. Rarely it may persist for months. Behavioral manifestations, however, such as withdrawal, irritability, and emotional lability, often continue beyond the period of disordered movement. About one third of patients shows other evidence of rheumatic fever or rheumatic carditis.

The chorea can be modified in the acute phase by small doses of neuroleptics or phenobarbital, although medication is rarely required. Rheumatic chorea is an indication for long-term prophylaxis with penicillin.

Chorea may recur with subsequent streptococcal infections.

Chorea Gravidarum

Patients who have had rheumatic chorea may have return of the abnormal movements during pregnancy. Other women who have no history of rheumatic fever may develop chorea, especially early in pregnancy. The chorea remits immediately after delivery; medication should be avoided.

Symptomatic Choreas

Oral contraceptives induce chorea in a small number of women. Chorea occurs soon after they are first administered or if the dose of hormones is changed. It fully remits when medication is discontinued. As with chorea gravidarum, asymptomatic rheumatic fever may have occurred. *Hyperthyroidism* often produces chorea, particularly in older patients. Central hypersensitivity to dopamine appears to underlie this disorder. It fully remits when the hyperthyroidism resolves. *Systemic lupus erythematosus (SLE)* may have chorea as its initial manifestation, although transverse myelitis, dementia, or seizures are more common nervous system complications of SLE (see Chapter 8.2).

Huntington Chorea[8]

This familial disorder consists of chronic chorea plus prominent affective disturbance and dementia. It usually occurs in the latter half of life, usually the third to fifth decades. It is a hereditary disorder with a clear autosomal-dominant inheritance. The mutation rate is low and a family history is the rule, particularly if care is taken to inquire about family members who had depression, suicide, or other mental illness. As the onset is relatively late in life, after the childbearing years, the disease is perpetuated in unwary families. Unfortunately, presymptomatic detection is unreliable, and diagnosis must await recognition of the first manifestations of the disease. This dilemma is a source of much family and emotional stress.

The disorder is slowly progressive, appearing as either bizarre movements and postures or by symptoms of depression or dementia. Any of these expressions may predominate early in the course, but all usually occur before it ends. The disordered behavior presents the most serious problem in management and is usually the reason for custodial care. In each kindred, disease may be expressed to varying degrees, but members of the same family have about the same age of onset, pattern of symptoms, and rate of progression. A Parkinson-like rigidity and seizures are prominent in some families, particularly in members whose disease begins in childhood or adolescence.

Pathologic changes are generalized but invariably affect most conspicuously the caudate nucleus. Caudate atrophy is easily demonstrable by CT or MRI. Gliosis and neuronal loss also occur in the thalamus, cerebral cortex, and cerebellum, but the loss is milder. Other portions of the nervous system are spared.

No effective form of therapy exists. Prevention through genetic counseling is mandatory. Haloperidol, reserpine, and phenothiazines may reduce the severity of the movement disorder, but most patients find these medications undesirable because of rigidity and exacerbation of depression. Levodopa worsens the involuntary movements.

HEPATOLENTICULAR DEGENERATION (WILSON DISEASE)[3]

This process, caused by an abnormality in copper metabolism, has a characteristic triad of cirrhosis of the liver, signs of basal ganglia disease, and brownish green deposits of copper at the corneoscleral junctions of the eyes (Kayser–Fleischer rings).

The onset is usually during adolescence, but the process may begin before age 10 or after age 35 or 40. A few patients begin with symptoms of liver dysfunction, such as jaundice or ascites. The majority of patients, however, begin with abnormal movements, usually a coarse proximal tremor. Initially the tremor is brought out by movement or by attempts to maintain posture. Athetoid or dystonic contortions and myoclonic jerks may appear. As the disease progresses, transition from one pattern of involuntary movement to another may occur. In the late stages, generalized rigidity with contractures occurs. Speech becomes indistinct or even unintelligible. Dementia is a late manifestation, associated with emotional lability.

Evidence of liver damage, hepatomegaly, and aminoaciduria are variable. The Kayser-Fleischer ring is best demonstrated by tangential illumination of the cornea and most easily seen by slit-lamp examination.

The pathologic features are nodular cirrhosis of the liver and gliosis of the putamen and globus pallidus, often with cavitation. Nerve cell loss is widespread, including the basal ganglia, caudate nuclei, and cerebral cortex.

The disease is thought to be caused by an impaired ability to incorporate copper into a number of proteins, particularly ceruloplasmin, the protein to which copper is normally bound in serum. Unbound copper is subsequently deposited in tissues throughout the body.

With the full clinical picture, the diagnosis of hepatolenticular degeneration is generally easy. Variations, however, make it important to consider this entity whenever abnormal tone and postures or involuntary movements are encountered. Low serum ceruloplasmin levels and elevated serum copper, when present, are confirmatory. Copper deposits can be demonstrated in liver biopsy material. Untreated, the course is progressive.

The objectives of therapy are to diminish the absorption and to increase the excretion of copper. Absorption is decreased by avoiding foods rich in copper (such as liver) and by precipitating copper in the gastrointestinal tract with potassium sulfide in doses of 0.2 g, taken with each meal. Renal excretion is enhanced by chelating the copper with penicillamine, in a dose of 0.5 to 1.0 g taken three times daily. A gauge of the effectiveness of mobilization is the disappearance of the Kayser-Fleischer ring. Ideally, therapy should begin before there is much neural change—thus the importance of recognizing early cases. For some reason, treatment is less helpful in the juvenile variety, which progresses rapidly.

REFERENCES

1. Bannister R (ed): Autonomic Failure: A Textbook of Clinical Disorders of the Autonomic Nervous System. Oxford, Oxford University Press, 1983
2. Burton K, Calne DB: Pharmacology of Parkinson's disease. Neurolog Clin 2:461, 1984
3. Cartwright GE: Diagnosis of treatable Wilson's disease. N Engl J Med 298:1347, 1978
4. Fahn S: Parkinson's disease and other basal ganglion disorders. In Asbury AK, McKhann GM, and McDonald WI (eds): Diseases of the Nervous System. Philadelphia, WB Saunders, 1986
5. Forno LS: Pathology of Parkinson's disease. In Marsden CD, Fahn S (eds): Movement Disorders. London, Butterworth, 1982
6. Mayeux R: Depression and dementia in Parkinson's disease. In Marsden CD, Fahn S (eds): Movement Disorders. London, Butterworth, 1982
7. Moses H III: Parkinson's disease. In Johnson RT: Current Therapy in Neurologic Disease. Philadelphia, Decker, 1985
8. Shoulson I: Huntington's disease. In Asbury AK, McKhann GM, and McDonald WI (eds): Diseases of the Nervous System. Philadelphia, WB Saunders, 1986

Cerebrovascular Disorders

Thomas J. Preziosi and Barney J. Stern

Strokes are caused by abnormalities of the cerebral circulation and are usually characterized by a neurologic deficit of sudden onset. The impairment may be in motor, sensory, or mental function; the dysfunction may be major or minor, transient or permanent.

Other cerebrovascular disorders may present without neurologic deficits; a subarachnoid hemorrhage can cause headache and meningeal irritation, while internal carotid artery stenosis can cause a bruit in an otherwise asymptomatic individual.

It is important that all physicians be competent in the management of strokes for several reasons: (1) strokes are the most common serious disorder affecting the central nervous system (CNS), (2) other disorders may mimic strokes and vice versa, and (3) proper diagnostic and therapeutic management has a profound influence on the outcome.

Therapy obviously rests upon optimal diagnostic definition. Diagnosis, in turn, depends upon several factors:

1. Syndrome recognition: Various constellations of symptoms and signs are associated with different clinical entities.
2. Analysis of time course: Strokes of various etiologies often have distinctive temporal patterns.
3. Anatomic localization: The site of the lesion may provide information regarding the probable cause. Furthermore, a single lesion suggests different etiologies from those that cause multiple lesions.
4. Ancillary tests: The appropriate use of additional studies may reveal the diagnosis, while an unwise strategy can subject the patient to unnecessary risk and expense.

This chapter presents an approach to the management of the patient with cerebrovascular disease. Topics include (1) a description of the clinical entities that cause strokes, (2) a strategy for approaching the common modes of presentation, (3) comments on the situations that lead to incorrect management, and (4) the principles of therapeutic management.

STROKE SYNDROMES

Stroke syndromes may be broadly divided between predominantly ischemic or hemorrhagic processes. Although on pathologic examination there can be overlap between these categories, a distinction to guide further management can usually be made clinically. Furthermore, stroke syndromes are best regarded initially as clinical phenomena rather than as specific disease presentations; ultimately, thorough evaluation will usually permit a precise etiology to be established. For example, there is no essential difference between the clinical manifestations of a cerebral embolus caused by a ventricular mural thrombus following myocardial infarction or a left atrial thrombus associated with chronic atrial fibrillation. At other times, however, diligent investigation may fail to reveal the precise cause of the disorder.

ISCHEMIC PROCESSES

ARTERIAL OCCLUSION

Although ischemic stroke remains a common neurologic problem, the incidence has declined over the last few decades. This decrease is most probably a result of better therapy of hypertension. Improved management of the patient at risk for stroke may also contribute to the decreasing occurrence of stroke but not to the same degree attributable to control of hypertension.[26]

Occlusion of a vessel may produce effects that range from the disastrous to the undetectable (Table 15.13–1). The outcome depends upon the size and position in the vascular tree of the occluded vessel, the length of time over which the occlusion develops, the availability of collateral flow into the involved territory from neighboring vessels, the duration of the occlusion, and the nature of the occluding agent. Clinical effects reflect the locus and extent of the damaged tissue and not the exact vessels occluded or the etiology of the occlusions. Accordingly, not only are the major etiologic categories of embolus and thrombus frequently difficult to separate from one another, but it is also often difficult to infer the precise vascular territory involved in a particular patient. Detailed analysis of appropriate clinical features can, however, be helpful in defining the vessels affected as well as the varying etiologies of stroke (Table 15.13–2).

Carotid Territory Ischemia

The patient with carotid territory ischemia can manifest weakness, sensory loss, visual field deficits, aphasia, neglect syndromes, and visual loss. Of these phenomena, only aphasia and transient monocular blindness are pathognomonic for carotid territory ischemia; all the other findings can also occur with vertebrobasilar disease. Rarely are all these findings present in a single patient; however, the presence of weakness, sensory loss, and visual field defects affecting only one side of the body is highly suggestive of carotid territory disease.

Even after the patient is identified as having carotid territory disease, it can be difficult at the bedside to assign a more precise locus of involvement: the extracranial carotid artery bifurcation vs. the intracranial carotid artery (siphon) vs. the middle cerebral artery.[21] For instance, internal carotid artery disease can involve brain perfused by both the anterior and middle cerebral arteries and, therefore, affect strength and sensation throughout the contralateral side; often only the middle cerebral artery territory is involved, however, thereby causing principally contralateral face and hand dysfunction (see Fig. 15.13–1). Anterior cerebral artery lesions usually produce weakness in the contralateral lower extremity. Obstruction of the smaller, distal cortical branches of the middle cerebral artery lead to more isolated symptoms, especially involving speech or highly selective sensory or motor impairment. Disease involving the lenticulostriate arteries can result in other highly selective clinical findings such as pure motor or pure sensory loss contralateral to the infarction. Because of the close aggregation of white matter pathways in the internal capsule, lenticulostriate territory obstructions often cause disturbances involving the face, arm, and leg equally.

Vertebrobasilar Territory Ischemia

Vertebrobasilar territory ischemia can result from lesions at numerous sites: one or both vertebral arteries, the basilar artery, the large "named" branches of the vertebral and basilar arteries, and innumerable unnamed median and paramedian brain stem perforating vessels arising from the basilar artery, and the posterior cerebral arteries.[7] Clinical presentations are varied, and there is a relatively poor correlation between symptomatology and precise localization of vascular lesions. Several symptoms and signs do identify vertebrobasilar territory ischemia: bilateral, often asymmetric, weakness; ataxia; vertigo associated with other nonvestibular neurologic

TABLE 15.13–1. MAJOR SYMPTOMS AND SIGNS OF CEREBRAL ARTERIAL OCCLUSIONS

Artery	Motor and Sensory Signs	Cognitive Deficits

1. Middle cerebral	Contralateral hemiplegia
	Contralateral hemisensory loss
	Paresis of conjugate gaze to opposite side
	Contralateral homonymous hemianopia
		Dominant hemisphere
		  Aphasia
		  Dysgraphia
		  Dyslexia
		  Gerstmann syndrome
		Nondominant hemisphere
		  Neglect syndromes
		  Dyspraxias for constructions, dressing
		  Dysphasic syndromes

Lenticulostriates	Lacunes—contralateral "pure" motor hemiplegia, ataxic hemiparesis, etc.	Dementia with multiple lacunes
2. Posterior cerebral	Contralateral hemisensory loss, occasionally with "thalamic syndrome" of pain, dysesthesias Contralateral homonymous hemianopia, occasionally quadrantic defects	Occasional aphasias Memory loss Visual dysfunction Neglect syndromes
Thalamoperforators	Lacunes—"pure" sensory loss	Dementia with multiple lacunes
3. Anterior cerebral	Contralateral hemiplegia, leg predominating Grasp, suck reflexes; gegenhalten Urinary incontinence	Akinetic mutism Apraxia of limbs Apathy
4. Internal carotid	Any combination of the above Frequently disproportionate motor and sensory deficits referable to fingers, hand, arm	Any combination of the above
5. Vertebrobasilar	Cranial nerve deficits with contralateral (or bilateral) motor or sensory signs Cerebellar signs Visual disturbances	Dysarthria without aphasia Memory deficits Hallucinations Somnolence

signs; diplopia; bilateral visual disturbances; and "crossed syndromes" of ipsilateral facial numbness or weakness with contralateral numbness or weakness of the limbs (see Chapter 15.6). Phenomena associated with the "top of the basilar" syndrome such as somnolence, hallucinations, and memory loss suggest ischemia to the thalamus or ascending reticular activating system.[6]

Of the numerous historic eponymic syndromes of vertebrobasilar disease, Wallenberg (lateral medullary) syndrome is the most common. This is characterized by several cardinal features including vertigo, facial numbness with ipsilateral ataxia and Horner syndrome, and contralateral loss of pain and temperature sensation. Wallenberg syndrome is caused by occlusion of the ipsilateral vertebral or posterior inferior cerebellar artery. Typically the prognosis for recovery is good.

Basilar or bilateral intracranial vertebral artery stenosis or occlusion is associated with a poor prognosis. Although the neurologic symptoms associated with lesions in this vascular location vary, the worsening of neurologic function when the patient assumes an upright posture is highly suggestive of severe disease involving the basilar or vertebral arteries. Postural neurologic symptoms occurring without systemic hypotension imply intracranial hypoperfusion.

Small penetrating branch arterial occlusions in the posterior circulation cause highly selective neurologic deficits such as an internuclear ophthalmoplegia or oculomotor nerve palsy with contralateral hemiparesis (see Chapter 15.6). Hypertensive arteriolar deterioration causes a limited infarction, and only rarely does the patient develop more widespread ischemia from basilar artery disease.

EMBOLISM

Cerebral emboli may arise from cardiac mural thrombi associated with atrial fibrillation or myocardial infarction, valvular lesions complicating rheumatic heart disease, infective endocarditis, or mitral valve prolapse. Emboli are also associated with calcific plaques in the major extracranial arteries, thrombi from leg veins accessing the arterial circulation via a patent foramen ovale, left atrial myxoma, or entry of foreign bodies into the vascular system. No neurologic symptoms occur before the arrival of the embolus at the brain. Accordingly, embolic strokes typically appear suddenly. Emboli appear to be arrested at arterial bifurcations, after which they may fragment, passing into single or multiple vessels further along in the circulation. A major neurologic deficit may accompany blockage of a large artery but improve dramatically when the embolus breaks up and comes to rest in a small branch artery. Since individual cortical arteries may be the point of final embolic occlusion, isolated cortical deficits such as Broca or Wernicke aphasia (Chapter 15.4) are most easily attributable to emboli.

Fragmentation of emboli is also related to the propensity of emboli to cause a hemorrhagic infarction. Here a vascular territory, having become ischemic from an embolic occlusion, becomes hemorrhagic after the embolus disintegrates and the damaged region is exposed to greater blood perfusion.

Emboli are frequently difficult to find at autopsy. An arteriogram done immediately after an embolic episode may occasionally demonstrate an embolus no longer visible on a repeat arteriogram performed a day or more later. Emboli may occur sequentially, so

TABLE 15.13–2. VASCULAR TERRITORY SIGNS AND SYMPTOMS OF GOOD LOCALIZING VALUE

Carotid System	Vertebrobasilar System
Aphasia	Bilateral weakness
Transient monocular blindness	Ataxia
	Vertigo associated with other neurologic dysfunction
Face > arm > leg weakness and/or numbness	Diplopia
	Bilateral visual disturbances
	Facial weakness or numbness with contralateral weakness or numbness

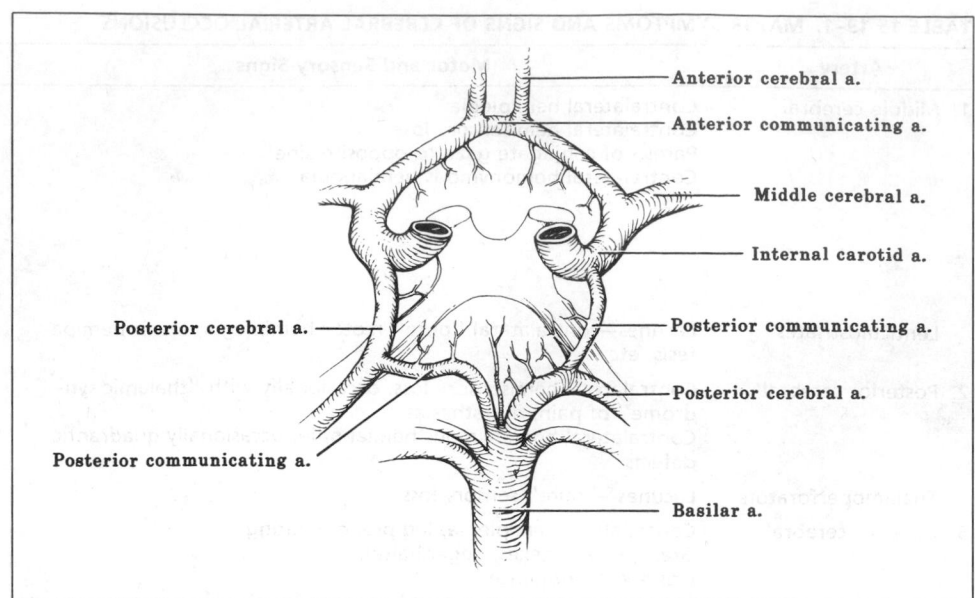

Figure 15.13–1. Circle of Willis. *(Modified from Peele: The Neuroanatomical Basis for Clinical Neurology. New York, McGraw-Hill.)*

that the clinical picture is that of multifocal neurologic deficits that vary in location with time. Other systemic embolic events can occasionally also be detected by examination for hematuria (renal embolus), occult blood in the stool (splanchnic embolus), newly absent peripheral pulses, and cutaneous petechiae; the patient may complain of abdominal or limb pain.

THROMBOSIS

Many conditions lead to thrombosis (Table 15.13–3). Although thrombosis, like embolism, may appear suddenly, thrombosis usually produces repeated progressive deficits in the same vascular territory over a period of hours or days.

Atheromatous Thrombosis
Atherothrombosis tends to involve the larger arteries, especially the extracranial carotid and vertebral arteries, and spare the individual cortical surface arteries. Neurologic symptoms can be caused by cerebral hypoperfusion distal to a hemodynamically significant arterial stenosis or occlusion and/or emboli originating from an atherosclerotic plaque or a thrombosis associated with an atherosclerotic lesion.

A cervical bruit in a middle-aged or elderly patient suggests turbulence caused by an atherosclerotic plaque near the carotid bifurcation. Finding a bruit in an ischemic stroke patient is therefore important. Because internal carotid artery stenosis typically develops slowly, collateral routes of flow can develop to maintain perfusion of the threatened hemisphere. Potential alternate pathways include the external carotid artery–ophthalmic artery–internal carotid artery circuit and increased flow through the posterior or anterior communicating arteries, via the basilar and anterior cerebral arteries around the circle of Willis. Increased flow in the external carotid artery is suggested by an exaggerated facial or temporal artery pulse demonstrable by palpation.

Atherosclerosis can involve only the intracranial arteries. Black and oriental patients are especially prone to intracranial atherosclerosis. The lack of evidence of extracranial occlusive disease, therefore, does not exclude the possibility of significant atherosclerotic disease in patients with cerebral infarction.

Thrombosis of Small Arteries
Occlusion of small penetrating arteries results from hypertension that produces lipohyalinosis.[18] These lesions commonly involve the vessels that penetrate the deep white matter of the frontal lobes, basal ganglia, internal capsule, thalamus, and pons. When the small arterioles are individually occluded, a small infarct, or lacune, results that can at times be detected by imaging studies. Specific clinical syndromes occur that are distinctive and only rarely observed with occlusion of large vessels. Lacunar syndromes include pure motor hemiplegia (paresis without sensory findings), pure hemisensory deficit, dysarthria with a clumsy hand, and hemiparesis with ipsilateral ataxia. Multiple infarcts may occur over months or years, producing a syndrome (the "lacunar state") of spastic gait, rigid limbs, emotional lability, and pseudobulbar palsy. Dementia, usually with subtle pyramidal signs, may occur when lacunes are particularly numerous. Atheromatous change is uncommon in such small vessels, although it may be present in larger, more proximal arteries. If a patient presents with a lacunar syndrome therefore, and no evidence of extracranial vascular disease is present, the patient may be spared arteriography. Treatment of hypertension is the mainstay of therapy; use of antiplatelet agents or anticoagulants is of no proven benefit.

WATERSHED INFARCTION

Systemic hypotension from any cause reduces cerebral arterial perfusion and produces its first effects in specific regions of the brain, the "watershed" regions.[24] These include the zones between the anterior and middle cerebral arteries and between the middle and posterior cerebral arteries. Watershed infarctions can also be caused by cerebral hypoperfusion secondary to severe internal carotid artery stenosis or occlusion. The leptomeningeal arteries overlying the watershed areas can be occluded with in situ thromboses or microemboli and thereby contribute to cerebral hypoperfusion.

Clinically, patients have difficulties with vision, cognition, and speech; weakness and fluctuating levels of consciousness can occur. If the patient recovers, a distinctive clinical state is found in which the patient behaves as if he were "a man in a barrel" with the arms paralyzed but the face and distal legs spared.

TRANSIENT ISCHEMIC EVENTS

Patients commonly present with transient cerebral ischemic events. These are often very brief, lasting seconds or minutes, may seem inconsequential, and yet are the first warning signs of impending stroke. Symptoms usually begin abruptly and last several minutes. By definition, total clinical resolution within 24 hours is needed

TABLE 15.13–3. CAUSES OF CEREBRAL ARTERIAL THROMBOSIS

Disease of the artery
- Atherosclerosis
- Lipohyalinosis
- Inflammation
  Infectious: Meningovascular syphilis, herpes zoster, septic embolism, arteritis secondary to pyogenic or granulomatous meningitis
  Noninfectious: Lupus erythematosus, rheumatoid arteritis, polyarteritis nodosa, granulomatous arteritis, giant-cell (temporal) arteritis, isolated cerebral angiitis
- Fibromuscular dysplasia
- Takayasu disease
- Moya moya disease

Mechanical processes affecting arteries
- Cervical spondylosis involving vertebral arteries
- Compression against bony prominences or dural folds caused by increased intracranial pressure, especially the posterior cerebral artery compressed against the tentorium
- Traumatic or spontaneous dissection

Prolonged vasoconstriction
- Subarachnoid hemorrhage
- Migraine
- Malignant hypertension

Inadequate cerebral perfusion
- Systemic hypotension from any cause

Hematologic disorders
- Sickle cell disease
- Polycythemia
- Dysproteinemias
- Coagulopathy—thrombotic, thrombocytopenic purpura, lupus anticoagulant, factor VIII excess
- Thrombocytosis

Miscellaneous
- Radiotherapy with radiation necrosis
- Drug abuse

Intracranial Venous and Sinus

Septic thrombosis
- Secondary to ear, mastoid, and paranasal sinus infections
- Secondary to pyogenic or inflammatory meningitis, brain abscess, or subdural empyema

Aseptic thrombosis
- Secondary to ear or mastoid infection
- Secondary to dehydration
- Hematologic disorders with hypercoagulability
  Sickle cell disease
  Polycythemia
- Postpartum and postoperative
- Oral contraceptives
- Carcinomatous meningitis
- Behçet disease

to classify an ischemic event as a transient ischemic attack (TIA). The natural history and clinical evaluation of cerebral ischemic events manifested for as long as several days, however, is identical to that of a TIA and, therefore, the 1-day limitation is arbitrary. The key point is that even the relatively prompt resolution of a clinical event implies that a more pronounced neurologic deficit may follow.[9]

The symptoms are often stereotyped. Transient monocular blindness (amaurosis fugax, Chapter 17.6), unilateral weakness or sensory changes, diplopia and dysarthria, or transient aphasia are particularly common presentations.

Transient ischemic events may be multiple; usually the history indicates transient ischemia in the territory of one or the other carotid artery or in the distribution of the basilar-vertebral system. It is important to identify the pathophysiologic cause underlying the transient ischemia, since management must be individualized for each patient. For example, when symptoms suggest ischemia in the carotid territory, many patients will have a surgically correctable extracranial lesion of the appropriate internal carotid artery. In contrast, patients with symptoms that suggest vertebrobasilar ischemia are much less likely to benefit from surgical intervention but do require medical management.

A single transient ischemic event may be caused by emboli originating from a cardiac or arterial site or be related to cerebral hypoperfusion caused by arterial stenosis or occlusion. When attacks are multiple and repetitive, the patient has a 30 percent probability of developing a major stroke within the next 4 to 5 years. It is therefore of extreme importance that the underlying cause be defined and managed before a stroke occurs. With multiple attacks, recurrence of the same symptoms often suggests an arterial origin, while the appearance of symptoms in different vascular territories implies recurrent cardiac emboli. Cardiac emboli, however, can cause multiple similar events. Rarely, an intracerebral neoplasm, subdural hematoma, or cerebral arteritis will produce transient neurologic deficits; these causes can be distinguished from thrombotic or embolic processes with computed tomography or angiography.

A variety of episodic deficits can be confused with transient ischemic events. Vasovagal syncope or Stokes-Adams attacks produce unconsciousness, a symptom rarely associated with transient focal cerebral ischemia. Isolated dizziness is often mistakenly associated with vertebrobasilar ischemia. Episodic behavioral abnormalities are seldom vascular in origin. Seizures may cause transient neurologic phenomena that need to be distinguished from vascular disease; however, on occasion, seizures may be the presenting feature of cerebrovascular disease, especially of emboli (Chapter 15.5).

VENOUS OCCLUSION

Thrombosis of the large cerebral veins is an uncommon but important cause of stroke (Table 15.13–3). The potential for collateral drainage is extremely good, so the resulting neurologic deficit is usually mild and frequently completely reversible. Occlusion of the deep venous system is, however, of grave consequence as few potential collaterals exist.

Cortical venous thrombosis, including superior sagittal sinus thrombosis, occurs in several settings. These include hypercoagulable states associated with the peripartum period, disseminated malignancy, systemic sepsis, severe dehydration, primary hematologic conditions, particularly Waldenström macroglobulinemia and polycythemia, Behçet disease, inflammation of the venous system, and mechanical obstruction of venous flow.[5] The process can simultaneously involve several scattered areas of cortex, and therefore the patient may display multifocal neurologic signs. Convulsions and headache occur as well as occasional papilledema, nuchal rigidity, and fever. The cerebrospinal fluid is usually blood tinged from hemorrhagic infarction, and the CSF pressure may be elevated. Neurologic abnormalities usually wax and wane over several days. Prompt treatment may ameliorate the course, but persistent seizures and variable neurologic sequelae commonly occur. Specific treatment of the primary systemic illness should be initiated as well as anticonvulsant therapy (Chapter 15.5) and treatment of raised intracranial pressure (Chapter 4.9). The role of anticoagulants is controversial, but they are occasionally effective in the deteriorating patient even in the presence of hemorrhagic infarction (see Chapter 6.24).

Pseudotumor cerebri (see Chapter 15.9) can arise from occlusion of the lateral sinus, occlusion of the internal jugular vein, or obstruction of the superior vena cava. Increased intracranial pressure will frequently resolve if an effective collateral drainage system develops. Lateral sinus thrombosis was a frequent accompaniment of purulent otitis media before antibiotic availability but is now uncommon.

SPINAL CORD STROKE

An ischemic insult to the spinal cord may follow systemic hypotension or occlusion of the small vessels supplying the cord.[22] Damage to the midthoracic region typically follows systemic hypotension and presents as a transverse myelopathy. Occlusion of arteries can be caused by atherosclerotic disease, aortic dissection, or any of the other causes of vessel occlusion. Typically, thrombosis of the artery of Adamkiewicz, which supplies the lumbar spinal cord, results in bilateral, flaccid leg weakness, bowel and bladder dysfunction, and pain and temperature loss with preservation of vibratory and position sense in the lower extremities (the syndrome of the anterior spinal artery).

SPECIAL PROBLEMS

Young Stroke Patients

Since atherosclerotic vascular disease is relatively less common, determining the etiology of an ischemic cerebral event in a young patient is often complex because of numerous diagnostic considerations.[13] Particular attention needs to be given to the possibility of migraine, rheumatic valvular disease, mitral valve prolapse, drug abuse, Takayasu disease, fibromuscular dysplasia, arterial dissection, vasculitides, sickle cell anemia, factor VIII elevation, and lupus anticoagulant.

Pregnant or Postpartum Patient

These patients are at relatively high risk for stroke or strokelike syndromes. Intracranial hemorrhage caused by aneurysm, arteriovenous malformation, or metastatic choriocarcinoma may occur. Cortical venous thromboses characteristically develop in the postpartum period as do "paradoxical" cerebral emboli caused by venous thrombosis in the legs or pelvis. Peripartum cardiomyopathy is a rare cause of cardiogenic cerebral embolus. Eclampsia also must always be considered as a cause of neurologic dysfunction.

Asymptomatic Patient

The patient may be asymptomatic but have abnormal vascular findings recognized by a physician. These physical signs include, most importantly, a bruit heard over the skull, orbit, or neck; a decreased carotid pulsation; or asymmetrical facial or superficial temporal pulses. Any of these signs may indicate a vascular abnormality.

Bruits are often multiple and are always a significant finding in adults, although they are commonly encountered in normal young children. A bruit must be distinguished from a cervical venous hum. The location, timing, and character of the sound should be noted so that subsequent examinations can be compared with the original observations.

An asymptomatic carotid bruit is a frequent clinical problem.[27] The patient should be questioned about symptoms of transient cerebral ischemia. The bruit should be considered a marker for generalized atherosclerosis so that pertinent risk factors may be managed appropriately. Patients with carotid bruits are at special risk for coronary artery disease. The risk of stroke in the territory of the diseased artery is low, and routine carotid endarterectomy is not justified. A subgroup of patients with hemodynamically significant stenosis may warrant prophylactic surgery, however, because of a higher stroke risk. The role of carotid surgery for the asymptomatic carotid bruit is, however, controversial.

An argument similar to the asymptomatic bruit protocol pertains to patients with incidentally discovered angiographic evidence of carotid disease or patients found to have a carotid bruit before cardiac or major vascular surgery. In the latter group, if carotid surgery is elected, it can be done after the patient has recovered from the primary operation.

Patients with asymptomatic carotid bruits or stenosis can develop transient cerebral ischemia over time; surgical intervention may then be warranted. Serial noninvasive vascular testing may

highlight the group of patients with progressive atherosclerosis who are at relatively high risk for ischemic stroke.

INVESTIGATION (Tables 15.13–4 and 15.13–5)

Asymptomatic Patient

The asymptomatic or intermittently symptomatic patient can be investigated electively. If transient neurologic deficits are frequent, severe, or of considerable duration, however, the investigation should be undertaken without delay. Investigation is aimed at a search for a treatable cause of the problem, such as a stenotic vessel, using bedside techniques as well as laboratory methods. The evaluation should consider systemic illnesses, hematologic and cardiac conditions, and vascular processes that cause stroke, contribute to the severity of the neurologic deficit, or predispose to future neurologic insults.[10]

A *CT scan* can identify a clinically silent ischemic stroke or discover a tumor or arteriovenous malformation (AVM) presenting with transient neurologic deficits. *Magnetic resonance imaging (MRI)* promises to be a more sensitive technique for detecting clinically silent lesions. An *electroencephalogram* (EEG) can highlight seizure discharges and raise the suspicion of seizure activity causing neurologic dysfunction. A noninvasive vascular examination is used to screen for atherosclerotic disease in the carotid artery system. "Direct" techniques assess the cervical carotid bifurcation employing *ultrasound imaging and Doppler flow analysis.* "Indirect" studies attempt to define the hemodynamic consequences of extracranial carotid disease by analysis, for instance, of the ophthalmic artery systolic blood pressure.

Arteriography is the definitive examination to define cerebral vascular anatomy (Fig. 15.13–2). Conventional arterial angiography is being replaced by intra-arterial digital subtraction angiography, which promises to be a safer technique because of the small amount of contrast agent and small catheter size required.

Occasionally a *CSF analysis* is helpful in searching for an inflammatory process or occult infection such as syphilis. Although a lumbar puncture is rarely indicated for elderly patients with a "typical" ischemic infarction, young stroke victims and patients with prominent headache or a systemic disease known to predispose to stroke warrant a CSF analysis.

Laboratory tests for syphilis, immunologic diseases, such as systemic lupus erythematosus, polycythemia, paraproteinemia, hyperlipidemia, and hypercoagulability can identify a systemic process predisposing to stroke. Ambulatory electrocardiography (Holter monitoring) can detect arrhythmias that predispose to cardiac emboli. Echocardiography, which characterizes valvular lesions, chamber function and size, and intracardiac masses, is best reserved for younger stroke patients, those with an abnormal cardiac examination by bedside observation, chest radiograph, or ECG, and those without an obvious atherosclerotic basis for their stroke.

Symptomatic Patient with Nonprogressing Deficit

The *symptomatic* patient with a *nonprogressing* neurologic deficit demands immediate attention. Diagnostic studies, as already described, need to be obtained; a CT scan is particularly important in distinguishing between ischemic and hemorrhagic processes. MRI can detect an ischemic infarction sooner than a CT scan but is not currently particularly effective, in contrast to CT, in separating a hematoma from an ischemic infarction early in the clinical course.

A complete data base is necessary to optimize patient management. Attention to factors thought to affect cerebral blood flow and neuronal integrity are particularly important for the acute management of the stroke patient.[20] These items include systemic blood pressure, blood glucose, hematocrit, and intracranial pressure.

TABLE 15.13–4. COMMON PRESENTATIONS OF STROKES

Condition When Seen	History	Likely Mechanism	Other Diagnosic Considerations
Intermittent symptoms	First episode of transient neurologic deficit (TIA)	Cardiogenic embolus Atherosclerosis/thromboembolism	Seizure Syncope Mass lesion Migraine Demyelinating disease Arteritis
	Repeated identical transient deficits (TIAs)	Atherosclerosis Emboli (rarely) Arteriovenous malformation	Seizures Migraine Tumor
	Repeated, different transient deficits (TIAs)	Emboli Atherosclerosis	Seizures Arteritis Demyelinating disease Meningeal inflammation
Symptomatic, not progressing	Sudden onset headache, no localizing findings	Subarachnoid hemorrhage	Meningitis
	Sudden onset, lateralizing	Embolus Thrombosis	Mass lesion, etc.—especially if headache
	Previous TIAs in same area	Thrombosis Arteriovenous malformation	Tumor with seizures
	Previous TIAs in different areas	Emboli	Arteritis Meningeal inflammation
Symptomatic, progressing	Headache, progression of signs	Parenchymal hemorrhage Arteriovenous malformation	Migraine Mass lesion Thrombosis
	Stepwise progression or signs from same area	Thrombosis	Migraine Seizures with postictal paralysis Tumor
	Progression, with different areas of involvement	Emboli	Multiple mass lesions
	Stepwise progression with headache and altered consciousness	Repeated subarachnoid bleeds and vasospasm Venous thromboses	Mass lesion Arteritis Meningitis

Patient with Progressive Deficit

The *symptomatic* patient with a *progressive* neurologic deficit requires emergency attention. Key to the recognition of this problem are serial neurologic examinations to document a fluctuating clinical course. Obtaining a CT scan is particularly important in searching for a possible hematoma or other mass lesion. Many patients with ischemic strokes have minor fluctuations in the neurologic deficit, especially over the first few days, that are usually attributed to brain edema and local variations in cerebral blood flow following loss of vascular autoregulation. Sudden stepwise worsening also occurs, however, because of further vascular occlusions caused by increased thrombus formation or new embolic events. Approximately 25 percent of patients with carotid territory thrombotic disease deteriorate within 48 hours of presentation, whereas 50 percent of patients with vertebrobasilar thrombosis fluctuate over 4 days. Close observation of the acute-stroke patient is therefore necessary to detect significant changes in the neurologic status.

GENERAL PRINCIPLES IN MANAGEMENT

The most serious error in diagnosis is to assume the patient has had a stroke, particularly one caused by atherosclerosis, when the underlying process is some other, potentially more treatable condition. In particular, the possibility of migraine, subdural hematoma, neoplasia, or seizure disorder should be considered. As discussed, the distinction between a primarily ischemic lesion and a hemorrhagic neurologic event needs to be made.

Patients with ischemic atherosclerotic cerebrovascular disease should be evaluated for appropriate risk factors: hypertension, hyperlipidemia, smoking, oral contraceptives, diabetes mellitus, etc. Furthermore, the patient with atherosclerotic cerebrovascular disease usually suffers from generalized atherosclerosis and is prone to coronary and peripheral vascular disease. In fact, the cause of death in most patients with atherosclerotic cerebrovascular disease is ischemic heart disease. The stroke patient's cardiac status should therefore be evaluated not only to assess a possible cardiac source for central nervous system ischemic events but also to detect clinically significant coronary artery disease amenable to life-prolonging interventions.[1]

Particular attention needs to be paid to the patient's blood pressure, serum glucose, and hematocrit, especially in symptomatic individuals. Extremes of blood pressure should be avoided. Excessively high blood pressure may exacerbate cerebral edema, whereas hypotension may worsen the neurologic deficit because of cerebral hypoperfusion. In general, careful downward titration of blood pressure should be achieved over days to weeks in severe hypertensives with careful monitoring of the neurologic status. Only in malignant hypertension should a rapid decrease in blood pressure be allowed and then only with careful monitoring of the neurologic examination. Hyperglycemia in the first few days after stroke has been associated with a poor outcome, possibly because of an associated high lactate concentration in ischemic tissue leading to cellular membrane destruction, and should be avoided. Last, a major determinant of blood viscosity, and hence cerebral perfusion, is the hematocrit.[23] Polycythemic patients should have

TABLE 15.13–5. DIAGNOSTIC EVALUATION OF STROKES

Procedure	Comment
History	Age Previous episodes Pattern of progression Associated symptoms Underlying disease
Examination	Vital signs Location of lesion Completeness of lesion Meningeal irritation Cardiac dysfunction Vascular status
Examination—repeat	Evidence of progression or regression
Hematology	Evidence of underlying systemic disease: glucose, sodium, hematocrit, platelets, sedimentation rate, serology, PO_2, clotting studies
Urinalysis	Hematuria or occult blood, signifying renal emboli or coagulopathy
CT or MRI	Evidence of hemorrhagic or ischemic lesion identifying and localizing the stroke Evidence of increased intracranial pressure Evidence of hydrocephalus Mass effect
Lumbar puncture	Evidence of intracranial bleed, increased pressure, infection, or inflammation
Noninvasive vascular studies	Anatomy of carotid bifurcation; hemodynamic effects of carotid disease
EEG	Regional cerebral dysfunction Seizure activity
Arteriography	Characterization of diseased vessel(s) Vasculitis, aneurysm, arteriovenous malformation
Cardiac monitoring	Abnormal recurrent arrhythmias with sudden interruption or decrease in cerebral blood flow or predisposition to emboli
Echocardiography	Abnormal left ventricular function, valvular disease, or mass indicative of source of cerebral emboli

isovolemic hemodilution to improve perfusion of ischemic brain. Recent data suggest that patients with hematocrits in the high-normal range may also benefit from isovolemic hemodilution; investigations are under way to further evaluate this procedure.[23]

SPECIFIC THERAPY

Antiplatelet Therapy

Inhibitors of platelet aggregation and adhesion have been shown to decrease the frequency of embolization from atheromatous plaques that lie within large arteries and to decrease the likelihood of in situ arterial thrombosis.[15] Since platelet aggregation is believed to be one of the most common pathogenic mechanisms for transient focal cerebral ischemia, treatment with antiplatelet agents has become an important addition to medical management. The most effective agent is acetylsalicylic acid (aspirin). Optimal dosage is not known, and advocates suggest doses from 1 mg/kg/day to 1300 mg/day. Aspirin is effective in decreasing the frequency of transient ischemic events and stroke, particularly in men. Aspirin also decreases the risk of reinfarction following an ischemic stroke. Patients with asymptomatic cerebrovascular disease are often treated with aspirin, as are patients following carotid endarterec-

tomy. Aspirin is also used to prevent recurrent cardiac emboli in patients with ischemic stroke associated with mitral valve prolapse.

Anticoagulation (See Chapter 6.24)

Anticoagulants are commonly used to treat symptomatic progressing ischemic infarction. The evidence that anticoagulation affects outcome in these patients is controversial. If anticoagulation is initiated with constant infusion of heparin, the issue then becomes the duration of therapy. Once the patient is neurologically stable for 5 to 7 days, and if the patient is not severely incapacitated, angiography should be obtained to define the vascular anatomy and guide further treatment. For instance, if severe extracranial stenotic disease is demonstrated, elective carotid endarterectomy may be indicated as definitive therapy; either aspirin or anticoagulants can be used before surgery. On the other hand, if severe basilar artery stenosis is present, long-term Coumadin therapy may be the best option. Last, and perhaps most important, if no significant vascular lesions are visualized and if there is no evidence of a cardiogenic embolus, aspirin therapy can be advised rather than more potentially dangerous long-term treatment with Coumadin.[17]

The risk of recurrent cardiogenic cerebral emboli can be decreased with anticoagulation. Embolic cerebral infarction, especially when large, however, can be hemorrhagic, and therefore care should be taken to minimize the risk of iatrogenic hemorrhage in these patients. A sensible protocol is to obtain a CT scan of a patient with a cardiogenic embolic stroke 24 hours after the ictus to attempt to visualize a hemorrhagic process. If no blood is seen, if there are no other contraindications to anticoagulation (such as severe hypertension), and if the patient does not have a large, potentially life-threatening neurologic deficit, anticoagulation can be initiated. If the patient is severely ill, therapy should be deferred 1 week and then begun only if there is no hemorrhagic lesion on another CT scan and if the patient does not have major morbidity from the stroke. If heparin is administered to a patient with a cardiogenic cerebral embolus, a loading bolus dose should be avoided; rather, a constant infusion of heparin is preferred.[11]

Arterial Surgery

Carotid endarterectomy is best performed if a significant atherosclerotic lesion near the carotid bifurcation has been identified and the patient's symptoms are appropriate to the diseased vessel. Transient ischemic events and stroke may be prevented by successful removal of an atherosclerotic lesion if emboli are originating from the diseased vessel or if there is a hemodynamically significant stenosis. Patients may also be selected for carotid surgery if there has been a functional recovery from an ischemic carotid territory stroke and arteriography demonstrates a localized cervical internal or common carotid artery stenosis. Endarterectomy is not successful when extensive intracranial atherosclerotic disease is present. Knowledge of the patient's general medical condition, particularly the health of the heart, is essential before recommending surgery. The combination of modern neurosurgical anesthesia and meticulous surgical technique does allow successful endarterectomy even in patients of advanced age and delicate health.[2]

The results of carotid endarterectomy must be compared with those obtained by antiplatelet agents and anticoagulation. This area is controversial. Surgical results compare admirably with medical therapy when the operating surgeon is experienced, pays close attention to technique, and is supported by proper anesthetic methods. Surgical results are not optimal, and often compare unfavorably to medical therapy, if expert patient care is not available.

Patients with severely stenotic carotid disease, with appropriate correlation to the neurologic signs or symptoms, are generally considered appropriate surgical candidates. Patients with less severe carotid stenosis are often first treated medically and subjected to surgery if symptoms continue. Noninvasive vascular evaluation may highlight those patients with severe, hemodynamically significant disease who may benefit most from surgery.

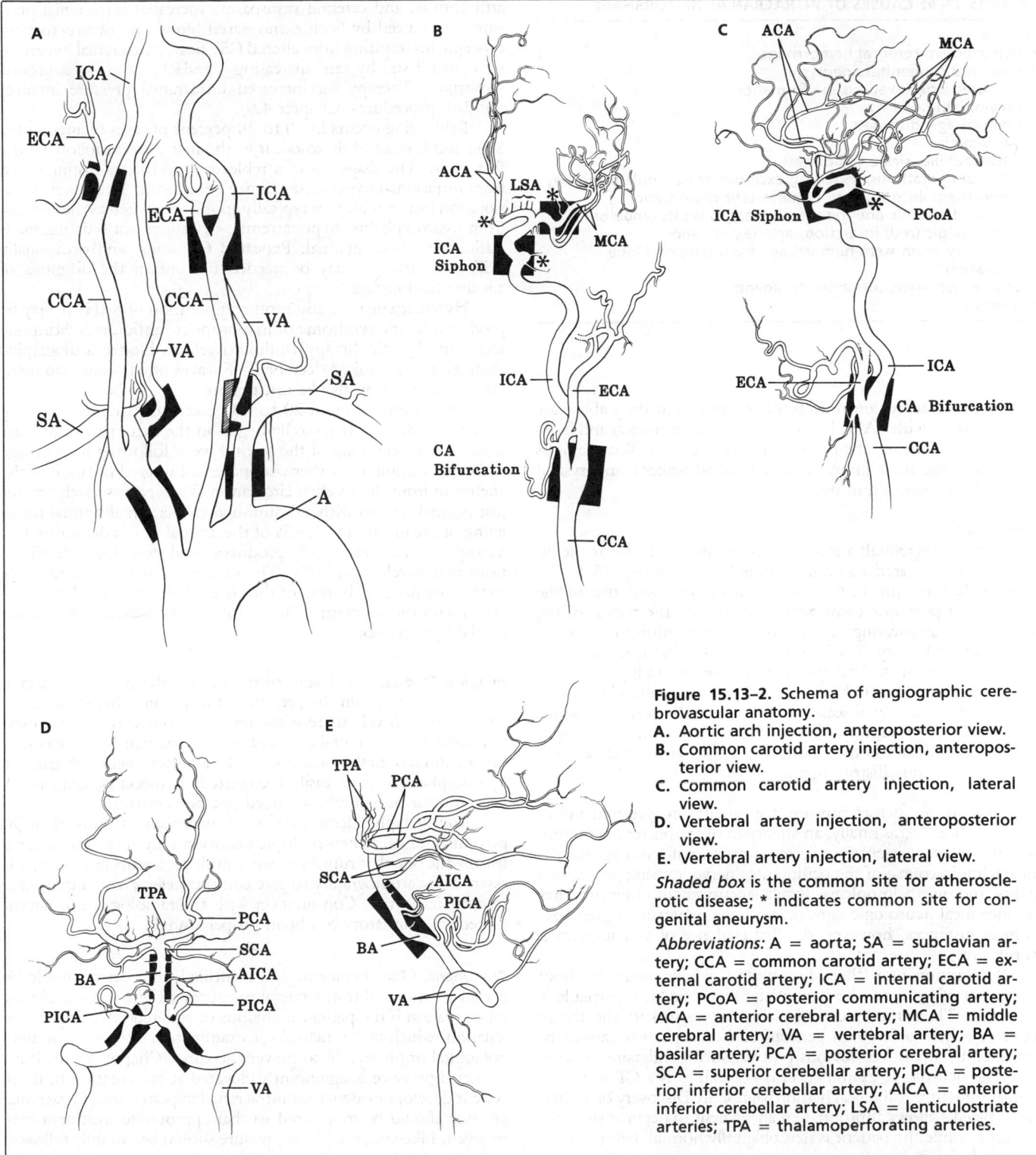

Figure 15.13–2. Schema of angiographic cerebrovascular anatomy.

A. Aortic arch injection, anteroposterior view.

B. Common carotid artery injection, anteroposterior view.

C. Common carotid artery injection, lateral view.

D. Vertebral artery injection, anteroposterior view.

E. Vertebral artery injection, lateral view.

Shaded box is the common site for atherosclerotic disease; * indicates common site for congenital aneurysm.

Abbreviations: A = aorta; SA = subclavian artery; CCA = common carotid artery; ECA = external carotid artery; ICA = internal carotid artery; PCoA = posterior communicating artery; ACA = anterior cerebral artery; MCA = middle cerebral artery; VA = vertebral artery; BA = basilar artery; PCA = posterior cerebral artery; SCA = superior cerebellar artery; PICA = posterior inferior cerebellar artery; AICA = anterior inferior cerebellar artery; LSA = lenticulostriate arteries; TPA = thalamoperforating arteries.

HEMORRHAGIC PROCESSES

Intracranial hemorrhage can involve bleeding into the subarachnoid space, brain parenchyma, or ventricular system. Any or all of these sites can be involved in a single patient, but typically one area is predominant by clinical or CT scan criteria. Overall, the most common cause of intracranial hemorrhage is severe head trauma (Chapter 15.19); this discussion will detail the various etiologies of spontaneous, nontraumatic hemorrhage (Table 15.13–6). The recognition and management of intracranial masses was discussed in Chapter 15.10.

SUBARACHNOID HEMORRHAGE

Subarachnoid hemorrhage (SAH) caused by leakage from a berry (congenital) aneurysm is a well-known cause of SAH, but hemato-

TABLE 15.13–6. CAUSES OF INTRACRANIAL HEMORRHAGE

Trauma
- Hypertensive cerebral hemorrhage
- Ruptured congenital aneurysm
- Ruptured arteriovenous malformation
- Amyloid angiopathy
- Hemorrhagic disorders
    Leukemia
    Hemophilia, sickle cell disease
    Bleeding diathesis, including excessive anticoagulant therapy
- Hemorrhage into primary or metastatic brain tumor
- Ruptured mycotic aneurysm secondary to septic embolism
- Hemorrhagic (red) infarction, arterial, or venous
- Secondary brain stem hemorrhage from temporal lobe herniation
- Drug abuse—sympathomimetic agents
- Arteritis

logic, inflammatory, and infectious processes and drug abuse are also associated with SAH. Usually appropriate historical and laboratory data will define the pathogenesis of the SAH. Because of its importance and the high mortality rate of 50 percent, aneurysmal SAH will be discussed in detail.

Aneurysm[14]

Most berry (congenital) aneurysms are saccular and arise at the bifurcations of the arteries forming the circle of Willis (Fig. 15.13–1). These include the junction of the internal carotid with the middle cerebral and posterior communicating arteries, the region of the anterior communicating artery, and the first bifurcation of the middle cerebral artery. The basilar artery and its branches occasionally show aneurysms. Aneurysms are frequently multiple.

Aneurysms occur in higher than expected numbers in patients with polycystic kidney disease, coarctation of the aorta, fibromuscular dysplasia, moya moya disease, Ehler-Danlos and Marfan syndromes, pseudoxanthoma elasticum, polyarteritis nodosa, and those with a family history of aneurysms.

Clinical Features. Before rupture, few aneurysms give evidence of their presence. Occasionally, an aneurysm of the posterior communicating artery, as it enlarges before rupture, will press against the subarachnoid course of the oculomotor nerve, causing ptosis, mydriasis, and ophthalmoplegia. Rarely, aneurysms at other sites may produce focal neurologic signs or headache by virtue of their size. In most instances, however, the first evidence of an aneurysm is its rupture.

Recognition of a "heralding bleed," which occurs in about 40 percent of patients who have a later severe SAH, is particularly important. The clinical picture is that of a patient with the abrupt onset of a new or atypical generalized headache that cannot be explained by any other obvious process, such as migraine or sinusitis. The neurologic examination is normal, as is a CT scan, but lumbar puncture will reveal hemorrhagic CSF. Discovery of a "heralding bleed" allows appropriate management to begin at the optimal time, while the patient is neurologically normal, before a catastrophic hemorrhage.

Rupture can occur during strenuous physical activity or at rest. Virtually every patient has an excruciating headache, "the worst headache of my life." On examination, meningismus is usually present and preretinal hemorrhages can occur. The clinical profile just described is virtually diagnostic of ruptured aneurysm. Since aneurysms rupture into the subarachnoid space directly and only infrequently directly into the brain substance, patients tend to show surprisingly few or no focal neurologic signs. Vomiting, restlessness, and drowsiness are common.

Complications of SAH include increased intracranial pressure, hydrocephalus, repeat SAH, hyponatremia, cardiac ischemia and

arrhythmias, and cerebral vasospasm. Increased intracranial pressure is produced by both extravasated blood and obstructive hydrocephalus resulting from altered CSF flow. Intracranial hypertension manifests by an increasing headache and a depressed sensorium. Therapy for increased intracranial pressure involves standard procedures (Chapter 4.9).

Rebleeding occurs in 10 to 20 percent of cases of aneurysmal SAH and is most likely to occur in the first 2 weeks following the first bleed. The diagnosis of a rebleed, especially as distinguished from intracranial hypertension, may be difficult. Neurologic deterioration from a rebleed is typically apoplectic, whereas the changes from hydrocephalus, hyponatremia, vasospasm, or sedating medications are more gradual. Repeated CT scans, and occasionally CSF examinations, may be needed to confirm the diagnosis of another hemorrhage.

Hyponatremia is a common complication of SAH. It may be produced by the syndrome of inappropriate antidiuretic hormone secretion, diuretic therapy, or fluid overload. Electrocardiographic changes such as peaked "cerebral" T-waves often occur, and myocardial damage may also be documented.

Vasospasm occurs in 20 to 30 percent of patients following aneurysmal SAH.[16] It typically begins in the latter part of the first week or the beginning of the second week following hemorrhage and often complicates otherwise successful surgical isolation of the aneurysm from the cerebral circulation. Vasospastic vessels are not just normal arteries with a diminished caliber; an abnormal thickening of the intima and media of the arterial wall is demonstrable. Vasospasm characteristically produces focal neurologic deteriorations that develop gradually. The neurologic deficits are referable to the vascular distribution of the affected artery. The edema associated with the resultant ischemic infarctions contributes to intracranial hypertension.

Imaging Studies. A CT scan of the head is the preferred imaging technique to ascertain the presence of intracranial hemorrhage. In most cases of SAH, there is subarachnoid blood in the basal cisterns or over the cerebral convexities. Less frequently, intraventricular or intracerebral blood is seen. In addition, acute obstructive hydrocephalus can be easily recognized. If blood is seen on CT scan, lumbar puncture often need not be performed.

Arteriography demonstrates an aneurysm in more than 90 percent of cases. When multiple aneurysms are seen, the larger is usually the one that ruptured. Since multiple aneurysms occur, it is essential for arteriography to give complete views of all intracranial vascular territories. Consultation with the radiologist and neurosurgeon is mandatory to obtain proper studies.

Treatment. Once hemorrhage is identified, the patient should be placed at strict bed rest. General measures include stool softeners, mild sedation if the patient is anxious or agitated (avoiding undue sedation, which makes neurologic examination difficult), and phenobarbital or phenytoin to prevent seizures (Chapter 15.5). If intracranial pressure is significantly elevated at presentation or if the patient develops evidence for intracranial hypertension, intracranial pressure should be monitored so that appropriate treatment may be given. Likewise, the blood pressure should be carefully followed and an acceptable range maintained; extremes of pressure are to be avoided. Serum sodium concentration should be determined and fluids administered appropriately.

Most cerebral aneurysms are surgically accessible. Since the natural history of aneurysmal subarachnoid hemorrhage is poor, neurosurgeons have had great enthusiasm for a number of procedures to isolate aneurysms from the circulation. Expert neurosurgical technique combined with proper facilities for preoperative evaluation and postoperative care, particularly neuroradiology and neurologic intensive care, all add to improved neurosurgical outcome. Currently, the most effective neurosurgical techniques involve clipping the neck of the aneurysm. The timing of surgery remains contro-

versial, although there is a trend to early surgical intervention if the patient is stable following SAH.

Medical management of subarachnoid hemorrhage with systemic hypotension is not preferred when surgical therapy is available and the patient can tolerate craniotomy. Increasingly, referral to specialized centers is becoming standard. Some investigators advocate treatment with ε-aminocaproic acid to decrease the likelihood of repeat hemorrhage, but this therapy may not alter the overall morbidity and mortality because of an associated increased risk of vasospasm.

Treatment of vasospasm is difficult. If possible, careful vascular volume expansion and moderate blood pressure elevation can be initiated, although this may well increase the risk of rebleeding if the aneurysm has not been surgically isolated from the circulation. Recent work with the calcium antagonist nimodepine suggests that it is effective in prophylaxis of vasospasm following subarachnoid hemorrhage.[3]

Asymptomatic Aneurysm. Occasionally an aneurysm is detected in an otherwise asymptomatic individual. Because of the risk of rupture, elective surgical therapy is advised in all but elderly patients if the aneurysm is greater than approximately 7 mm in its greatest dimension. The risk of rupture of asymptomatic aneurysms 7 mm or larger is 2 to 3 percent annually.

VASCULAR MALFORMATIONS

Vascular malformations include capillary telangiectasias, cavernous hemangiomas, venous angiomas, and arteriovenous malformations (AVM).[25] Although the first three types of malformations are usually clinically silent, an AVM can present with a seizure, hemorrhage, or fluctuating neurologic deficit. AVMs can leak, sometimes repeatedly, and should be suspected as the source of intracerebral bleeding in the younger, normotensive patient with SAH. Since malformations lie within the substance of the brain, there is frequently some form of focal neurologic deficit associated with their rupture. Fortunately the seepage of blood in an AVM is from a low pressure system, and therefore an explosive destruction of brain tissue does not occur. Many patients have repeated bleeds from an AVM with amazingly little neurologic residue. Giant malformations may involve the blood supply to the major portion of a cerebral hemisphere and produce a murmur that the patient can hear. Rupture of a giant AVM is often catastrophic and rarely amenable to therapy. Computed tomographic scan with contrast enhancement almost invariably identifies the existence of an AVM. Management involves anticonvulsant therapy for seizures and consideration of the various options to prevent bleeding. These include surgical resection, embolization, and radiotherapy. The long-term risk of bleeding from an AVM is 2 to 3 percent per year.

HYPERTENSIVE HEMORRHAGE[19]

Anatomy

In contrast to ruptured aneurysm, hypertensive hemorrhage arises from damaged small penetrating arteries deep in the brain substance. Two thirds occur in the putamen and thalamus; pontine, cerebellar, lobar, and caudate hemorrhage account for the remaining third. The artery involved can be thought of as "springing a leak," the resulting hemorrhage enlarging steadily over several minutes to a mass of varying size. Over the ensuing hours, secondary edema leads to progressive neurologic deterioration, increased intracranial pressure, and cerebral herniation (Chapter 15.10).

Clinical Features

Hypertensive hemorrhage usually occurs in older patients who have been moderately hypertensive or in young individuals who have accelerated hypertension. Onset is abrupt but not as explosive as in subarachnoid hemorrhage. The patient complains of head-

TABLE 15.13–7. CLASSICAL SYMPTOMS AND SIGNS OF HYPERTENSIVE HEMORRHAGE

Site	Ocular Signs	Other Signs
Putamen	Conjugate horizontal deviation of eyes toward side of lesion	Contralateral hemiplegia, hemisensory loss Aphasia in dominant hemisphere Neglect syndromes in nondominant hemisphere
Thalamus	Conjugate downward deviation of eyes	Contralateral hemisensory deficit, hemiplegia, hemianopsia Aphasia in dominant hemisphere
Pons	Impaired lateral ocular movement Pinpoint, reactive pupils	Abrupt onset Coma Bilateral motor, sensory signs
Cerebellum	Occasionally conjugate deviation of eyes away from side of lesion Small, reactive pupils	No motor or sensory deficit early Vomiting, ataxia, inability to stand and talk

ache and notes focal neurologic symptoms with signs evident on examination (Table 15.13–7) and may ultimately become lethargic and comatose, all with smooth progression over several hours.

Hemispheric hemorrhages produce hemiplegia, hemisensory loss, aphasia, visual field defects, neglect syndromes, and difficulties with ocular motility. *Brain stem hemorrhage* usually presents with early loss of consciousness, gaze palsy, facial palsy and quadriplegia. *Cerebellar hemorrhage* may be quite cryptic in its presentation but is especially important, as surgical intervention is often required. The neurologic findings may be very mild, with only ataxia of the trunk and an impairment of stance and gait as the earliest signs. Later, gait ataxia and dysmetria of the limbs appear. Compression of the brain stem can follow, causing paralysis of lateral gaze, bilateral facial palsies, and eventually quadriplegia and death. The signs of cerebellar hemorrhage may appear only over several hours, and the patient may not seem very ill initially, factors that commonly lead to errors in diagnosis.

Laboratory Findings

Intraparenchymal hemorrhage is easily diagnosed by CT scan. The hemorrhage appears as a high-density mass of varying size within the brain substance, sometimes with rupture into the ventricular system. The scan also identifies displacement and distortion of the ventricular system and edema. Lumbar puncture is rarely indicated in patients with an intraparenchymal hematoma and is contraindicated if a CT scan identifies a large intracerebral mass.

Computed tomographic examinations have indicated that intracerebral hemorrhages are not invariably catastrophic. They can be associated with deceptively mild neurologic signs and even present masquerading as a lacune with, for instance, ataxic hemiparesis.

Arteriography may also demonstrate a mass lesion but may be normal if the hemorrhage is small. Occasionally, the history, clinical signs, and CT scan may not distinguish between a hypertensive hemorrhage and a hemorrhage caused by an AVM or primary or metastatic malignant neoplasm; here, arteriography (showing abnormal blood vessels) may be definitive. Arteriography can also identify an arteritis as being the cause of a hemorrhage.

Prognosis

Patients with a massive intracerebral hemorrhage die as a direct result of the hemorrhage or from complicating medical conditions. In general, a patient who continues to deteriorate neurologically

after arrival at the hospital will most probably die unless some form of intervention is undertaken. Those who do survive a hypertensive hemorrhage usually never rebleed from the same site. This is quite different from subarachnoid hemorrhage, in which repeated hemorrhage from an aneurysm is common.

Treatment

Immediate management consists of general measures of medical support. Raised intracranial pressure should be identified, monitored, and treated (Chapter 4.9). Particular attention should be devoted to control of the blood pressure, as both extreme hypertension and relative hypotension should be avoided (Chapter 2.10). Although surgical treatment for cerebellar hemorrhage is often appropriate, the indications for surgery for hemorrhage at other sites remain controversial. A reasonable approach is to consider surgical evacuation of a putaminal or lobar hematoma, especially if it is in the nondominant hemisphere, the patient is worsening, and maximal attempts to control intracranial hypertension by medical means fail.

AMYLOID ANGIOPATHY

Elderly patients with intracerebral hemorrhages in sites atypical for hypertensive hemorrhage may have cerebral amyloid angiopathy as the cause of bleeding.[12] These patients typically are not hypertensive, or only mildly so, and can have repeated hemorrhages at varying hemispheric sites over time. Management considerations are similar to those outlined for hypertensive hemorrhage. The diagnosis can be confirmed premortem only by biopsy of the brain surrounding a hematoma and confirming the presence of congophilic material in the blood vessels. Since vessels containing amyloid are prone to rupture, however, surgical intervention is rarely pursued.

STROKE AND DRUG ABUSE

A variety of ischemic and hemorrhagic strokes are associated with drug usage.[8] Pathogenic mechanisms include foreign-body or air embolus, endocarditis-associated cardiogenic emboli, vasculitis, and the hemodynamic stress of hypertension. Prescription drugs such as Talwin and amphetamines, over-the-counter preparations such as sympathomimetic decongestants, and illicit agents such as heroin and cocaine are all implicated as causes of stroke. Intravenous injection of substances increases the likelihood of septic or foreign-body emboli. Sympathomimetics cause intraparenchymal hematomas that can be multiple, as well as vasculitis leading to ischemic infarction.

REHABILITATION

If a patient has a persistent neurologic deficit following stroke, rehabilitation becomes important. The immobile patient should be frequently turned and appropriate bedding supplied to prevent decubitus ulcers. Physical therapy should begin during the first days of paralysis to avoid contractures. The nursing staff and family should be involved in range-of-motion exercises. The patient should be positioned to avoid aspiration if there is bulbar dysfunction or depressed level of consciousness. Bladder hygiene is essential. Thrombophlebitis, a leading cause of death in neurologic patients who do not die of their primary neurologic disease, is a constant threat and should be guarded against, particularly during initiation of rehabilitation. When the patient is mobilized, orthostatic hypotension should be avoided. Rehabilitation options include intensive multidisciplinary inpatient services, outpatient facilities, and home programs. Emotional problems, especially depression, are common following stroke and, if left untreated, can hamper the rehabilitation process.[4]

REFERENCES

1. Adams HP Jr, Kassell NF, Mazuz H: The patient with transient ischemic attacks—Is this the time for a new therapeutic approach? Stroke 15(2):371, 1984
2. Allen GS, Preziosi TJ: Carotid endarterectomy: A prospective study of its efficacy and safety. Medicine 60(4):298, 1981
3. Allen GS, Ahn HS, et al: Cerebral arterial spasm—A controlled trial of nimodipine in patients with subarachnoid hemorrhage. N Engl J Med 308(11):619, 1983
4. Binder LM: Emotional problems after stroke. Stroke 15(1):174, 1984
5. Bousser MG, Chiras J, et al: Cerebral venous thrombosis—A review of 38 cases. Stroke 16(2):199, 1985
6. Caplan LR: Are terms such as completed stroke or RIND of continued usefulness? Stroke 14(3):431, 1983
7. Caplan LR: "Top of the basilar" syndrome. Neurology 30:72, 1980
8. Caplan LR: Treatment of cerebral ischemia—where are we headed? Stroke 15(3):571, 1984
9. Caplan LR: Vertebrobasilar disease. Time for a new strategy. Stroke 12(1):111, 1981
10. Caplan LR, Hier DB, Banks G: Current concepts of cerebrovascular disease—stroke: Stroke and drug abuse. Stroke 13(6):869, 1982
11. Cerebral Embolism Study Group: Immediate anticoagulation of embolic stroke: Brain hemorrhage and management options. Stroke 15(5):779, 1984
12. Cosgrove GR, Leblanc R, et al: Cerebral amyloid angiopathy. Neurology 35:625, 1985
13. Hart RG, Miller VT: Cerebral infarction in young adults: A practical approach. Stroke 14(1):110, 1983
14. Heros RC, Kistler JP: Intracranial arterial aneurysm—an update. Stroke 14(4):628, 1983
15. Hirsh J: Progress review: The relationship between dose of aspirin, side-effects and antithrombotic effectiveness. Stroke 16(1):1, 1985
16. Kassel NF, Sasaki T, et al: Cerebral vasospasm following aneurysmal subarachnoid hemorrhage. Stroke 16(4):562, 1985
17. Kassell NF: Size of intracranial aneurysms. Neurosurgery 12:291, 1983
18. Mohr JP: Lacunes. Stroke 13(1):3, 1982
19. Ojemann RG, Heros RC: Spontaneous brain hemorrhage. Stroke 14(4):468, 1983
20. Raichle ME: The pathophysiology of brain ischemia. Ann Neurol 13(1):2, 1983
21. Rodda RA: The arterial patterns associated with internal carotid disease and cerebral infarcts. Stroke 17(1):69, 1986
22. Silver JR, Buxton PH: Spinal stroke. Brain 97:539, 1974
23. Thomas DJ: Hemodilution in acute stroke. Stroke 16(5):763, 1985
24. Torvik A: The pathogenesis of watershed infarcts in the brain. Stroke 15(2):221, 1984
25. Wilkins RH: Natural history of intracranial vascular malformations: A review. Neurosurgery 16(3):421, 1985
26. Wolf PA: Risk factors for stroke. Stroke 16(3)359, 1985
27. Yatsu FM, Hart RG: Asymptomatic carotid bruit and stenosis: A reappraisal. Stroke 14(2):301, 1983

Weakness

Daniel B. Drachman

Any disturbance of the power to act may be reported by a patient as "weakness." However, motor impairment may represent the outward manifestation of a wide variety of disorders, only some of which involve the motor system. Underlying the patient's complaint of weakness may be (1) a disorder of the central nervous system (CNS), particularly the corticospinal pathways; (2) damage to the motor neurons in the spinal cord; (3) a disorder of the nerve roots or peripheral nerves; (4) a defect of neuromuscular transmission; (5) a disorder of muscles; (6) a painful affliction of the musculoskeletal system; (7) an unrelated systemic disease; or (8) a purely psychogenic cause.

The purpose of this section is to present an orderly approach to the problem of weakness, so that the physician can quickly sort out these possibilities.

From the standpoint of diagnosis, it is useful to distinguish three separate entities: *weakness, fatigue,* and *tiredness,* defined as follows:

Weakness is a reduction in the maximum force of muscle contraction. Clinical testing of muscles evaluates the maximum muscle force. True weakness always indicates an organic disorder.

Fatigue is a reduction in muscular force on repeated contraction. To some extent, muscle fatigue is a normal phenomenon. A normal person may fatigue after 15 or 20 push-ups and be unable to resume until he or she has rested the exercised muscles. In the presence of weakness, fatigue may occur more rapidly than normal. Muscular fatigue is especially prominent in myasthenia gravis.

Tiredness is a subjective sensation of listlessness and lethargy that follows muscular exertion. Like fatigue, it is experienced by normal individuals. As a presenting complaint, it is most often psychogenic, but it may accompany systemic disease.

APPROACH TO THE PATIENT

HISTORY

Weakness should be assessed against the background of the patient's usual activities. The interviewer should determine whether there has been a specific *change* in the patient's motor abilities. Often a direct question is useful, such as, "What can't you do now that you previously were able to do?" For a construction worker, the inability to lift a 200-pound sack of cement may represent a real change. Obviously, the same criterion could hardly apply to a high school girl. The *earliest manifestation* of weakness should be sought, since it may give an important clue to the true course of the disorder. A housewife may first have noticed difficulty in lifting the baby or in placing grocery packages on high shelves. A school boy may have had trouble in throwing a baseball or in carrying out exercises in gymnasium. If the patient has had no change in motor performance, has he or she merely noted a sensation of *tiredness,* or an unwillingness to undertake physical activity? If so, the problem is more likely not organic.

The *distribution* of weakness may often be ascertained from the history. The interviewer should determine which extremities are involved and whether the weakness is *symmetric* or *asymmetric.* Does it involve the *proximal* or the *distal* musculature? Proximal weakness of the lower limbs may first be noticed as difficulty in getting out of the bathtub or arising from a low chair. Proximal weakness of the upper limbs interferes with any heavy manual labor and may make shaving in men or brushing the hair in women

difficult. Distal weakness results in foot drop, or in "clumsiness" in the use of the hands.

If the "weakness" is universal and uniform, it is more likely to be psychogenic or systemic in cause rather than to be a disorder of the motor system. Proximal, symmetrical weakness suggests myopathy. A distal symmetrical distribution of weakness is often seen in neuropathic disorders.

Associated symptoms may provide important clues to the nature of the problem. If sensory loss or other neurologic symptoms are present, a disorder of the peripheral nervous system or CNS should be considered. Fever or weight loss would point to an underlying systemic disease. Local pain in the weak limb may be an important symptom. The patient's emotional status must be evaluated critically. Has depression or apathy preceded the onset of symptoms?

PHYSICAL EXAMINATION

Coordinated Actions

A great deal can be learned from observing the patient closely as he or she performs natural coordinated movements. For example, the patient's gait may be very revealing. A waddling gait, in which the pelvis tilts from side to side, suggests proximal muscle weakness. Weakness of the ankle extensors may be seen as a tendency to overlift the leg, so as to compensate for a slight degree of foot drop. In testing the proximal musculature, it is useful to watch the patient as he or she arises from a chair or from a seated position on the floor. Patients with proximal weakness may boost themselves by using the upper limbs for added support. In patients with minimal weakness, deep knee bends or push-ups may reveal a minor degree of impairment.

Formal Testing

When weakness is present, it should be evaluated as objectively as practicable by testing the function of individual muscles and rating the results according to a quantitative scale. This requires that the examiner know the action of each muscle tested. An illustrated manual on muscle testing published by the British Medical Research Council is available. Muscle strength is graded according to standardized criteria:

	Grade
No muscle contraction	0
Flicker of muscle contraction	1
Full range of motion, with gravity excluded	2
Full range of motion, against gravity only	3
Full range of motion, against gravity and some external resistance	4
Normal power	5

With this method of grading, many weak muscles will fall in the range of 4 to 5. Although this is not sensitive to detecting minor degrees of weakness, further refinements of grading are not reliable, since they depend too heavily on subjective impressions.

It must be emphasized that the purpose of individual muscle testing is to obtain an objective assessment of the degree and pattern of weakness. Beginners must be cautioned to avoid bogging down in the testing ritual; try to determine *patterns* of weakness if possible.

Hysteria and Malingering

When the examiner suspects that the patient may not be cooperating fully, he or she must try to distinguish between organic weakness and apparent weakness caused by hysteria or malingering. The following points are often helpful. (1) When the examiner overcomes the force of a genuinely weak muscle, he or she will notice that it yields smoothly to pressure. By contrast, the malingering or hysterical patient releases the muscle contraction in a stepwise or *jerky* manner. (2) When the muscle strength demonstrated in coordinated actions (especially when the patient is not aware that he or she is being observed) is greater than that found on formal muscle testing, the *disparity* may suggest that real weakness is not present. (3) The examiner may use *subterfuge* to elicit maximal effort from the patient. For example, some patients may pretend to be weak when moving the limb through a range of motion but will exert full power when directed to maintain a fixed posture.

Muscle Bulk

This may be evaluated by inspection or measurement of the muscles. In cachectic patients one must avoid confusing loss of subcutaneous fatty tissue with muscle atrophy. When measuring the circumference of a limb, it is necessary to specify the point at which the measurement is made. For example, the calf circumference may be measured at a level 8 to 12 cm below the tibial tubercle.

Muscle Fasciculations

These should be sought when denervation atrophy is suspected. The patient must be at complete rest and comfortably warm. Good lighting from the side, rather than overhead, is essential. Fasciculations are spontaneous twitching of *motor units* or parts of motor units. They are seen more commonly in disorders of the anterior horn cells or nerve roots than in the more distal peripheral neuropathies. It should be emphasized that fasciculations also occur occasionally in well over 90 percent of the normal population. They are particularly common in times of stress and fatigue and are aggravated by smoking and drinking coffee.

Fibrillations, or the spontaneous contraction of single muscle fibers, cannot be seen through the skin. They are visible only through the thin mucosa of the tongue and can best be seen with the tongue at rest within the mouth.

Reflexes

The deep tendon reflexes should be tested in all patients with weakness. Weakness associated with absent reflexes is usually suggestive of neuropathy rather than myopathy.

SPECIAL EXAMINATIONS

In most cases of neuromuscular disorders, muscle biopsy, electrodiagnostic testing (electromyography and nerve conductions), and determination of serum enzymes released from muscle are essential to establish a correct diagnosis.

Muscle Biopsy

This procedure discloses the histopathology of the affected muscle directly. Only one or at the most two muscles may be sampled in this way, however, and of necessity, only a small fragment of muscle is studied. It is important for the clinician to know what kind of information can be provided by proper interpretation of a muscle biopsy:

1. It can confirm the clinical diagnosis of myopathy. Often the biopsy findings do not permit any further statement about the specific kind of myopathy present. The severity and acuteness of the disease process in the muscle from which the specimen was taken can also be estimated.
2. It can occasionally provide a definitive diagnosis of a specific type of myopathy on the basis of pathognomonic histologic, histochemical, or electron microscopic findings.

Polyarteritis, sarcoidosis, and some of the "rare" myopathies may be identified by biopsy.

3. It can identify neurogenic atrophy caused by lesions of motor nerve cells or peripheral nerves and reliably distinguish it from myopathy.

A negative muscle biopsy is much less helpful. It may mean that (1) the clinical diagnosis of neuropathy or myopathy is incorrect; (2) the portion of muscle selected for the biopsy is not yet involved, although changes may be present elsewhere; or (3) the disorder is one that does not produce histologic lesions in muscles (metabolic myopathies, upper motor neuron lesions, psychogenic disorders, or systemic disease).

A detailed discussion of the histopathology of muscle is not possible here. The principles of diagnosis are very simple, however. In the *myopathies,* muscle fibers are attacked *at random* and show typical *destructive changes*. Thus, degenerative changes in muscle fibers scattered randomly throughout the biopsy specimen are typical of myopathy. Reactive changes, such as phagocytosis, fibrosis, and fatty infiltration, are also seen (Fig. 15.14–1).

By contrast, *denervation* produces a shrinkage of muscle fibers without destructive changes. Neighboring *groups* of muscle fibers formerly supplied by the damaged nerves (motor units) are affected (Fig. 15.14–2).

Electrophysiology

Electromyography (EMG) and nerve conduction studies provide information about the function, rather than the structure, of muscle and nerve.

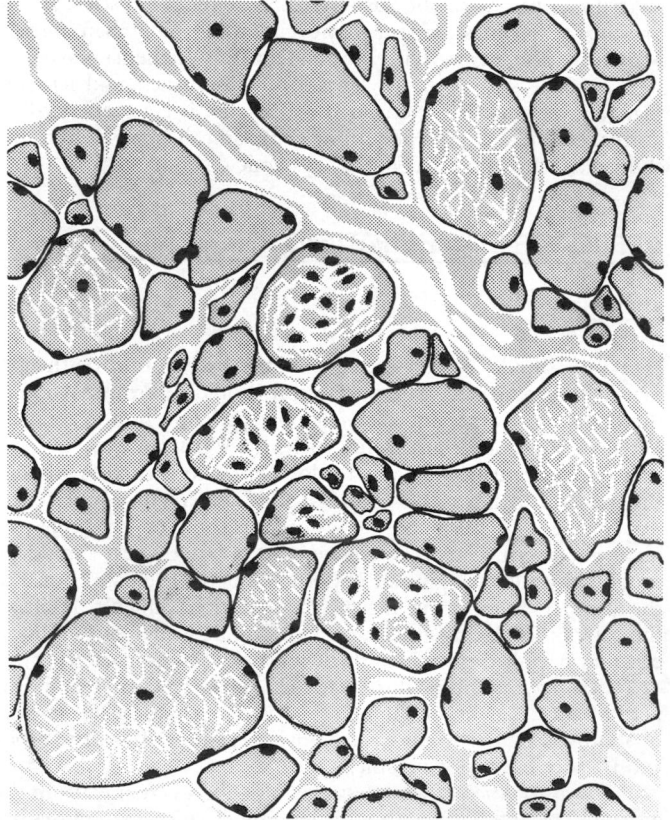

Figure 15.14–1. Drawing of myopathic changes in muscle biopsy (transverse section). There is random variation in muscle fiber size. Sarcolemmal nuclei are placed centrally rather than in their normal position immediately under sarcolemmal membrane. Several fibers are undergoing floccular degenerative changes. There is increase in endomysial connective tissue.

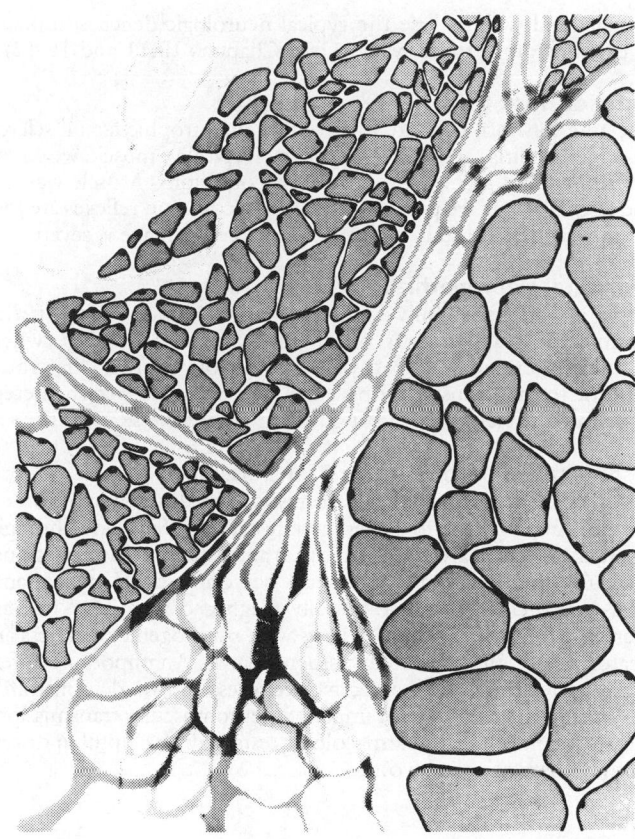

Figure 15.14–2. Neurogenic atrophy in muscle biopsy (transverse section). Groups of atrophic (small) muscle fibers are shown above to left. Group of muscle fibers to right is or normal size. Muscle nuclei remain peripheral in position. Degenerative changes are absent.

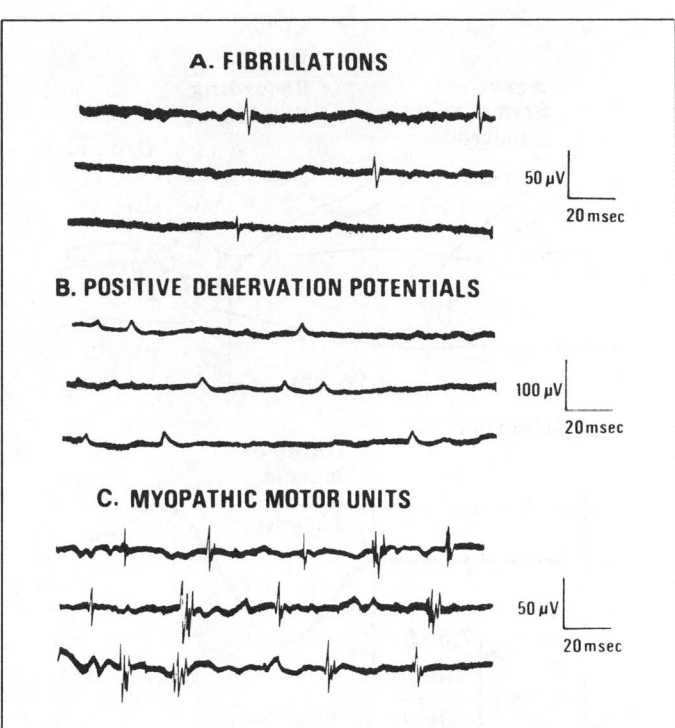

Figure 15.14–3. Electromyographic features. **A.** Fibrillations consist of spontaneous depolarization of single muscle fibers that have been denervated. They appear as short duration di- or triphasic potentials of low amplitude. **B.** Positive denervation potentials also occur spontaneously in denervated muscle fibers. They are larger in amplitude and longer in duration than fibrillations. There is initial rapid upward phase followed by slower return to baseline. **C.** Myopathic action potentials are low in amplitude and short in duration. They have characteristic ragged, polyphasic appearance.

By the use of needle electrodes, the electrical activity of muscle fibers is sampled and displayed on an oscilloscopic screen for viewing and photographic recording. Several different muscles can be tested at a single examination.

EMG patterns characteristic of myopathy, peripheral neuropathy, and anterior horn cell destruction can be identified. In the *neuropathies,* two defects are apparent: (1) Whole motor units are lost, and (2) denervated muscle fibers show spontaneous electrical discharges called fibrillations and positive denervation potentials (Fig. 15.14–3). In the *myopathies,* the total number of motor units available is not substantially decreased, but destruction of individual muscle fibers within the remaining motor units results in a diminution in the amplitude and duration of action potentials and a ragged (polyphasic) appearance to the potentials (Fig. 15.14–3).

In some peripheral neuropathies, damage to the myelin sheaths of nerve fibers results in *slowing* of their electrical conductivity. It is a simple matter to measure the speed of electrical conduction in certain superficial nerves, as outlined in Figure 15.14–4. In other neuropathies, loss of axons produces a reduction in the *amplitude* of the evoked muscle potential or nerve potential.

Serum Enzymes

The enzymes contained within the muscle fiber leak out when the muscle membrane is damaged and eventually reach the bloodstream. In the destructive myopathies the serum levels of certain enzymes may be elevated. These values are highest when the destructive process is most active. In contrast, disorders of the motor neurons or peripheral nerves seldom cause elevation of serum enzyme levels. The enzyme that it most useful in the diagnosis of muscle diseases is creatine kinase (CK). This enzyme is not present to any appreciable extent in liver or red blood cells, and its serum levels are unaffected by malignancy, hepatic disease, or in vitro hemolysis. Although the CK concentration may be raised in the acute stages of myocardial infarction, this rarely presents a problem in interpretation. When in doubt, the CK isoenzymes are determined: The MM isoenzyme is elevated in disorders of skeletal muscle, while the MB isoenzyme is raised in myocardial infarction. The chief value of serum enzyme determination is to confirm the diagnosis of myopathy. The serum CK levels should also be followed in assessing the efficacy of treatment (see Chapter 15.15).

CHARACTERISTICS OF WEAKNESS DUE TO VARIOUS CAUSES

Although a detailed description of the findings in each of the following conditions is beyond the scope of this section, the characteristics of the weakness and certain associated findings may be helpful.

Central Nervous System (CNS)

Lesions of the corticospinal (pyramidal) system usually produce spasticity, with hyperactive deep tendon reflexes and extensor plantar responses. The motor weakness may overshadow the other signs, however. The weakness is often most pronounced in the "physiologic flexor muscles," while there is relative sparing of the "antigravity" muscles. The physiologic flexors are those muscles which are flexed in withdrawing the foot from a noxious stimulus,

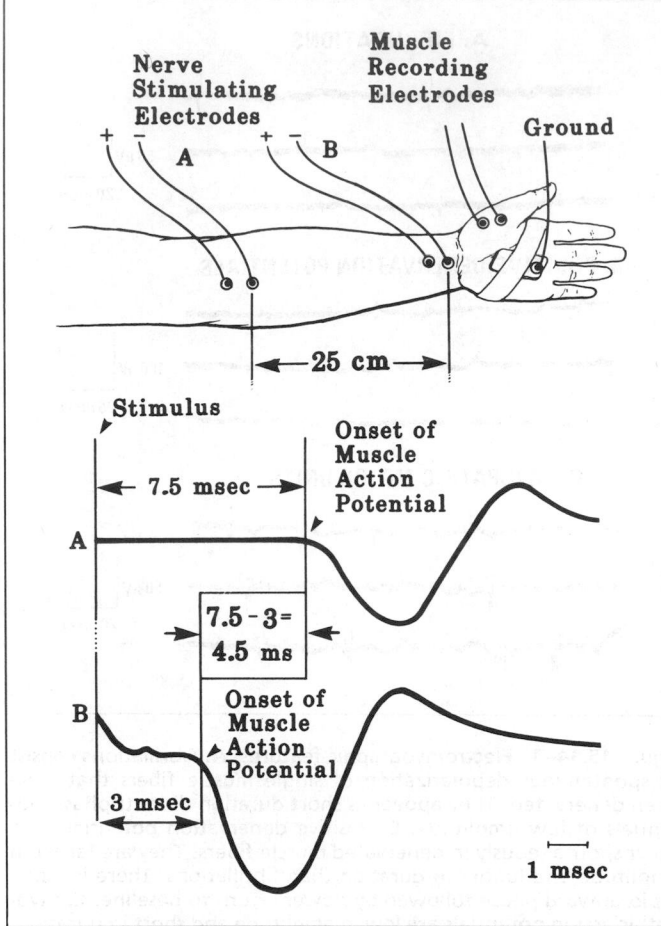

Nerve Stimulating Electrodes

Muscle Recording Electrodes

Ground

A

B

+ − + −

A B

← 25 cm →

Stimulus

Onset of Muscle Action Potential

← 7.5 msec →

A

7.5 − 3 = 4.5 ms

Onset of Muscle Action Potential

B

3 msec

1 msec

Figure 15.14–4. Median motor nerve conduction velocity. Recording electrodes are placed over thenar muscles. Two pairs of nerve stimulating electrodes are represented in A and B. In lower panel, tracing A represents muscle action potential evoked by nerve stimulation at elbow, while tracing B represents action potential evoked by stimulation of median nerve at wrist. Velocity of conduction in median nerve from point A to point B equals distance from A to B (25 cm or 0.25 m) divided by time it takes impulse to travel from A to B (7.5 msec − 3 msec = 4.5 msec). In this case velocity is normal, 55.6 m per second.

for example, when stepping on a tack, and include the iliopsoas, hamstrings, and tibialis anterior muscles. The antigravity muscles tend to support the lower limb, for example, when standing on tiptoes, and include the glutei, quadriceps, and gastrocnemius muscles.

The finding of weakness of the physiologic flexors often confirms the diagnosis. Corticospinal involvement may be unilateral or bilateral. It may affect only the lower extremities if the lesion is at the level of the spinal cord or may affect the upper extremities and face as well if the lesion is at a higher level.

Other disorders of the CNS involving the extrapyramidal system or cerebellum may be interpreted as "weakness" by the patient. Careful examination, however, will reveal that muscle power

is intact and will disclose the typical neurologic deficit secondary to dysfunction of these systems (see Chapters 15.11 and 15.12).

Anterior Horn Cells

The anterior horn cells are involved in amyotrophic lateral sclerosis, poliomyelitis, and other disorders. Typically, muscle weakness is scattered and asymmetrical in these conditions. Muscle wasting and fasciculations are prominent. The deep tendon reflexes are lost when weakness caused by anterior horn cell damage is severe.

Peripheral Neuropathies and Myopathies

These are discussed fully in Chapters 15.15 and 15.16. In the neuropathies, weakness is often distal. Sensory changes, when prominent, exclude myopathy as the cause of weakness. Electrodiagnostic testing, muscle biopsy, and serum muscle enzyme determinations are helpful in distinguishing among these conditions.

Disorders of Neuromuscular Transmission

A defect of neuromuscular transmission produces weakness and easy fatigability but no other manifestations. Since psychologic disorders are associated with tiredness and asthenic manifestations, these two groups of disorders may be confused. Many patients with myasthenia gravis are initially diagnosed as being "neurasthenic." Conversely, some patients with psychogenic weakness are treated as though they had myasthenia gravis. An important differentiating feature is that objective weakness can be demonstrated in virtually all patients with impaired neuromuscular transmission. Electrodiagnostic and pharmacologic tests may be helpful in distinguishing between the two.

Pain

Disorders that produce pain in the joints, bones, or muscles may limit the patient's ability to exert maximum muscle force. The apparent weakness may be beyond the patient's voluntary control. The finding of local tenderness in the affected part supports this diagnosis.

Systemic Disease

Any serious illness may cause weakness. The weakness is usually not localized but involves all muscle groups. There may be loss of muscle bulk as well as loss of subcutaneous fat. Those patients who present with weakness as the sole complaint pose difficult diagnostic problems. In most of these patients other manifestations of their disease can be found upon careful questioning or examination. In some, however, general weakness is the only evidence of disease on initial appraisal. This may be true in the weakness associated with endocrinopathies (hyperthyroidism, Addison disease, and hypopituitarism), in indolent infections (tuberculosis, subacute bacterial endocarditis), and in various neoplastic and metabolic diseases.

Psychologic Disorders

Psychologic problems are the predominant underlying disorders in any group of patients presenting with complaints of weakness and fatigue. As mentioned earlier, careful study will reveal that most of these patients are tired, not weak. This is particularly true of the patients who are depressed or psychoneurotic (neurasthenic). A psychogenic basis may be suspected when the weakness is inconstant or fits no physiologic pattern. Although it is not difficult to suspect or establish a diagnosis of emotional illness, it is difficult to be certain that the emotional illness is the *sole* cause of the weakness.

Diseases of Muscle

Daniel B. Drachman
and Hamilton Moses III

MYOPATHIES[16]

The term *myopathy* is used for those conditions that produce weakness by affecting muscle fibers without interfering with their nerve supply. By contrast, we speak of *neurogenic atrophy* or *neuropathy* when describing the changes in muscle that follow denervation, as for example, in poliomyelitis or peripheral neuropathy. The myopathies include conditions with or without known biochemical abnormalities and with or without any hereditary tendency.

It is useful to discuss this heterogeneous group of diseases together because of similarities in the clinical manifestations of weakness, the diagnostic methods used, and the management of patients.

CLINICAL RECOGNITION

The cardinal feature of myopathy is weakness. The weakness usually involves the proximal musculature in a symmetric pattern. Proximal weakness of the upper limbs may interfere with the patient's ability to maintain the arms abducted, as in shaving, brushing the hair, or placing objects on high shelves. Proximal weakness in the lower extremities may produce a waddling gait and results in difficulty climbing stairs and getting out of a bathtub or low chair. As a rule, pain and tenderness of the muscles are *not* presenting features, even in the inflammatory myopathies. If pain and tenderness are the only or the most prominent symptoms, one may suspect that myopathy is not the problem. Disorders such as polymyalgia rheumatica or polyarteritis more commonly produce severe pain.

On physical examination, the outstanding finding is weakness usually in the proximal muscles. If the patient is asked to arise from a seated position on the floor, he may "climb up himself" in a characteristic fashion (the Gower sign). The gait should be observed with the patient wearing only undergarments to determine whether the pelvis tilts from side to side. Individual muscle testing (as described in Chapter 15.14) is important in determining the distribution of weakness.

Apart from the muscle weakness, the remainder of the neuromuscular examination is normal. The tendon reflexes are usually obtainable until weakness is advanced (the Duchenne form of muscular dystrophy is an exception to this rule). Fasciculations are not present. The plantar responses are flexor. Sensation is normal. These negative findings are important in distinguishing myopathy from diseases of the central or peripheral nervous system.

Once it is recognized that a patient's weakness is probably myopathic in origin, attention turns to determining *which* myopathy afflicts the patient. As has been indicated, the similarity of the weakness seen in all these conditions renders weakness per se a poor feature for distinguishing one myopathy from another. Other clinical and laboratory features of the myopathies must be used. This evaluation should be done in an orderly and systematic fashion.

CLASSIFICATION

The myopathies have been classified in many different ways. From the clinical point of view, the separation into four groups—the muscular dystrophies, inflammatory myopathies, metabolic myopathies, and rare myopathies—has the virtue of combining simplicity with suggesting a rational approach to diagnosis (Table 15.15–1).

DIAGNOSTIC APPROACH

As indicated in Table 15.15–1, some myopathies have distinctive clinical characteristics that permit the knowledgeable physician to recognize the constellation of manifestations—syndrome recognition. Other disorders have nondescript manifestations but have distinctive histopathologic lesions. Still others, especially those associated with systemic diseases, have neither unique muscle manifestations nor unique lesions; these are diagnosed by demonstrating the underlying disease.

The remainder of the chapter is devoted to a description of the entities listed in Table 15.15–1 with emphasis on (1) those which are recognized by their clinical manifestations and (2) those which are amenable to therapy.

MUSCULAR DYSTROPHIES

The dystrophies are a group of myopathies classified together largely for historical reasons. In general, they are characterized by (1) a strong hereditary predisposition; (2) onset of weakness in the first to third decade, with varying rates of progression; and (3) fairly consistent clinical patterns.

There are exceptions to all these features, and cases without a clear family history and with uncommon patterns of muscular involvement may defy classification. There is a growing body of evidence to suggest that abnormalities of the cell membrane of muscle and other tissues may be present at least in some of the dystrophies.[10,14] At present there is no curative treatment for any of the dystrophies, and the efforts of the physician must be directed toward supportive measures. Nevertheless, it is of great importance to identify the dystrophy accurately so that the physician is able to give an accurate prognosis and undertake genetic counseling for the other members of the family. The forms of dystrophy are outlined in Table 15.15–2. Two forms, the pseudohypertrophic form and myotonic dystrophy, are discussed in greater detail.

Pseudohypertrophic (Duchenne) Form of Muscular Dystrophy

This is the most common and the most devastating form of muscular dystrophy. It is inherited as a sex-linked recessive trait and therefore affects only males, while being carried by females. The abnormal gene has been localized to the short arm of the X chromosome.[6,12] At present, there are many available cDNA probes; female carriers and affected fetuses can be identified with well over 90 percent accuracy in "informative" families (see Chapter 5.2).

This form of muscular dystrophy begins in childhood, often within the first few years of life. The earliest symptoms may be a tendency to walk on the toes, to be a slower runner than other boys of the same age, or to fall easily. The parents may first notice enlargement of the calves or of other muscles. Later, the child has difficulty in walking upstairs, develops lordosis, and has great difficulty in arising from a seated position on the floor. Eventually, the patient is reduced to a bed and wheelchair existence. Fortunately,

TABLE 15.15–1. CLASSIFICATION AND DIAGNOSTIC APPROACH TO THE MYOPATHIES

Classification and Examples	Approach to Diagnosis

I. Dystrophies
  1. Pseudohypertrophic (Duchenne)
  2. Facio-scapulo-humeral (Landouzy-Dejerine)
  3. Limb-girdle (Erb)
  4. Distal (Gower)
	• Syndrome recognition (see Table 15.15–2)
	• Genetic history
	• Biopsy and serum enzyme confirmation

5. Myotonic	Same plus demonstrable myotonia
6. Ocular myopathy	Syndrome recognition

II. Inflammatory (polymyositis, dermatomyositis)
  1. With malignancy
  2. With connective tissue disease (lupus, rheumatoid arthritis, systemic sclerosis, Sjögren syndrome)
	• Demonstrable confirmation on biopsy
	• Demonstration of underlying disease

3. With sarcoidosis	Diagnostic lesions in biopsy
4. Without associated disease	Diagnosis of exclusion in an inflammatory myopathy

III. Metabolic
  1. Adrenal steroid myopathy (iatrogenic and spontaneous)
  2. Dysthyroid myopathy
  3. Hyperparathyroid myopathy
  4. Hypoadrenal myopathy (Addison)
	Demonstration of the metabolic disorder

5. Periodic paralysis 6. Glycogen storage diseases (McArdle, Pompe, phosphofructokinase deficiency)	Syndrome recognition Demonstration of metabolic disorder

IV. Miscellaneous rarer causes
  1. Congenital myopathies (central core disease, rod or nemaline myopathy, mitochondrial and myotubular myopathies)
  2. Trichinosis
	Distinctive histopathology

3. Myositis ossificans	Same plus calcification on radiograph
4. Myotonia congenita (Thompsen)	• Syndrome recognition • Myotonia
5. Paroxysmal rhabdomyolysis (myoglobinuria)	• Syndrome recognition • Myoglobinuria
6. Drug-induced (chloroquine)	History

the distal musculature is relatively spared until late in the disease, and the patient is able to feed himself and perform other useful tasks with his hands. The cardiac musculature is affected in some patients, with the development of a wide variety of arrhythmias and electrocardiographic changes. Approximately 30 percent of patients with the Duchenne form of muscular dystrophy have associated mental retardation.

The *diagnosis* of the Duchenne form of muscular dystrophy is not difficult because of the remarkably consistent pattern of mus-

cular involvement, exclusive affection of males, and uniformly rapid progression of weakness. The serum CK levels are usually very high in this disorder. The muscle biopsy shows severe changes of myopathy.

Myotonic Dystrophy[16]
Myotonic dystrophy is characterized by difficulty in relaxing muscles after contraction and progressive weakness and wasting of muscles. The muscles of the face and jaw and the distal muscles of the

TABLE 15.15–2. CLINICAL FEATURES OF THE MUSCULAR DYSTROPHIES

Name	Distribution	Age of Onset	Progression	Inheritance	Remarks or Associated Conditions
Pseudohypertropic (Duchenne)	Generalized	Under age 8	Rapid	Sex-linked recessive	Pseudohypertrophy Cardiac involvement Mental retardation Death by adulthood
Benign pseudohypertrophic	Generalized	8–20 yr	Slow	Sex-linked recessive	Possible normal life expectancy
Facio-scapulo-humeral	Face, shoulders, legs	10–20 yr	Slow	Dominant or recessive (rare)	May "burn out" in adult life
Limb-girdle	Shoulder and pelvic musculature	10–30 yr	Slow (varies)	Varies	Heterogeneous group
Ocular myopathy	Eyelids and extra-ocular muscles	30+ yr	Slow	Varies	Retinal abnormalities Dysphagia
Distal dystrophy (Gowers)	Distal limb musculature	20+ yr	Slow	Dominant or sporadic	Heterogeneous group

limbs are affected first and involved most severely. Inheritance is as an autosomal dominant trait. The abnormal gene is located on chromosome 19, and cDNA probes have been prepared that are extremely close to, or directly at, the locus of the abnormal gene. The rate of progression varies, even among members of a given family. Some individuals may be able to live essentially normal lives, while others are severely disabled by the third or fourth decade. When the clinical manifestations of myotonic dystrophy are present at birth, a poor prognosis is the rule. In addition to the muscular defects, abnormalities of several other systems may be present. Cataracts, frontal baldness, testicular atrophy, and myocardial abnormalities are common. Some patients suffer from intellectual impairment that may progress and may constitute the major disability.

The diagnosis of myotonia may be made by percussion of the thenar eminence. Patients with myotonia show a delayed relaxation of the contraction. Myotonia may also prevent prompt relaxation of a firm hand grip. If troublesome, the myotonia may be treated with quinine, dilantin, or procainamide. When the distal weakness causes foot drop, braces are usually needed.

Treatment of the Dystrophies

At present there is no curative treatment for any of the forms of muscular dystrophy. For the most part, the treatment of these conditions must, therefore, be symptomatic. Treatment with adrenal corticosteroids, however, prolongs ambulation by an average of 2 years in Duchenne muscular dystrophy.

Patients with muscular dystrophy have a tendency to develop muscular contractures when immobilized for even short periods. It is therefore essential that they remain active as consistently as possible. Once put in a wheelchair, a child with muscular dystrophy may never get out. If confined to bed while recuperating from an orthopedic operation, the child may never resume his former level of activity. Physiotherapy, with passive and active stretching of muscles and tendons, is useful in preventing the development of contractures, but rigorous exercise is unnecessary. Bracing of limbs and various mechanical devices are often helpful in prolonging the patient's ability to ambulate or care for himself.

Genetic Counseling. One of the most important developments in the management of muscular dystrophy has been achieved through a greater understanding of the genetics of the dystrophies. With knowledge of the mode of inheritance and with the recent development of cDNA probes for some of the dystrophies, the physician can give the patient or his relatives an accurate prediction of the likelihood that future offspring will be affected by the disease (see Section Five).

METABOLIC MYOPATHIES[8]

Clinical Manifestations

Like the other myopathies, these disorders present with proximal weakness. The serum muscle enzymes and the muscle biopsy are, however, usually normal in these conditions. The electromyogram may be normal as well. The *absence* of confirmatory laboratory evidence in a patient with proximal weakness may first suggest a diagnosis of a metabolic myopathy.

Steroid Myopathy

Steroid myopathy is one of the most common endocrine-metabolic causes of muscle disease in the adult. The steroids may have been secreted by a hyperfunctioning adrenal cortex or more often prescribed by a physician for the treatment of some other condition. In either case, the patient develops proximal weakness closely resembling that found in the other myopathies. The halogenated steroids (triamcinolone and dexamethasone) are most likely to produce this syndrome. Differential diagnosis is especially difficult when a patient develops weakness in the course of a connective tissue disease for which he is receiving steroid therapy. It may be

necessary to discontinue the steroids temporarily or to switch from triamcinolone to dexamethasone or prednisone.

Thyrotoxic Myopathy

Chronic thyrotoxicosis is often accompanied by weakness of the proximal limb muscles. Although the manifestations of the hyperthyroid state are usually obvious by the time myopathy is manifest, they may be masked, especially in older patients. Tachycardia, fasciculations, and a fine tremor of the outstretched fingers may provide clues to the diagnosis. Biopsy and electromyography show relatively minor abnormalities. Serum thyroxin and radioactive iodine uptake tests establish the diagnosis.

Hyperparathyroidism

Hyperparathyroidism and hypophosphatemia are occasional causes of proximal muscle weakness in the adult. Although these conditions are uncommon, the symptoms they produce may be clinically indistinguishable from those of the inflammatory myopathies. The diagnosis is made on the basis of the characteristic abnormalities of calcium and phosphorus metabolism. Radiographic studies of the bones may be helpful.

Hypopituitarism

In Addison's disease muscular weakness is usually present but does not dominate the picture. The characteristic endocrine abnormalities readily identify this condition.

McArdle Disease[15]

This rare myopathy is so distinctive that its clinical recognition is simple once the physician considers the diagnosis. The underlying biochemical defect is a lack of the muscle enzyme phosphorylase. As a result, glycogen cannot be broken down, and the muscle is without a source of quick energy. Since the pathways of oxidative metabolism are intact, however, energy for muscle contraction can still be supplied at a slower rate.

In clinical terms, this metabolic defect results in the patient's inability to perform vigorous exercise for more than a brief period. Muscle strength may be normal or only slightly diminished, and the patient is able to carry out mild or moderate exercise normally. When he attempts to sustain a greater degree of muscular activity for a more prolonged period, however, he develops cramps and paralysis. If the cramps are particularly severe, there may be some muscle damage with myoglobinuria (dark urine).

Laboratory studies provide definitive confirmation of the diagnosis. Because of the lack of myophosphorylase, the patient with McArdle disease is unable to break glycogen down to lactate under anaerobic conditions. The ischemic exercise test is carried out by inflating a cuff around the patient's arm above systolic pressure and instructing him to clench his fist repeatedly for 40 seconds. The cuff is released, and blood samples are drawn at intervals after the exercise. Normal individuals show a marked rise in serum lactate concentration, while patients with McArdle disease show a flat curve. Other laboratory aids are now available, including histochemical and chemical measurements of the phosphorylase activity in muscle biopsy material.

The treatment of McArdle disease is the avoidance of excessive exercise.

Virtually identical clinical manifestations are seen in another metabolic disorder of muscle: phosphofructokinase (PFK) deficiency, or Tarui disease. In this condition the block in breakdown of glycogen occurs at a slightly later enzymatic step, but the clinical effects of limitation of exercise tolerance and cramps are the same.

Other Metabolic Disorders of Skeletal Muscles

During the past decade numerous disorders of carbohydrate, lipid, and energy metabolism of skeletal muscle have been reported, but detailed description of them is beyond the scope of this section. In general, they give rise to exercise intolerance, cramps, weakness, or myoglobinuria.

INFLAMMATORY MYOPATHIES[1,11]

This group of disorders includes dermatomyositis, polymyositis, and juvenile dermatomyositis. These conditions are thought by most authorities to differ with respect to their pathology, associated conditions, and prognosis, although their clinical manifestations are closely similar. The outstanding symptom of the inflammatory myopathies is weakness, which is usually symmetrical and proximal. For this reason they are often confused with the muscular dystrophies, especially those of late onset, and with metabolic myopathies. Proper diagnosis depends upon finding involvement of other organ systems, especially the skin, joints, or other connective tissue, as well as by characteristic serological abnormaliites. Electromyography reveals the findings characteristic of myopathy, to which may be added features of denervation, that is, fibrillations or positive denervation potentials. Muscle biopsy reveals "myopathic" changes (see Chapter 15.14). In some instances the appearance is indistinguishable from that of dystrophy; in others, destruction may be more severe and inflammatory changes more obvious.

The differential diagnosis and treatment of inflammatory myopathies was fully discussed in Chapter 8.4.

MYASTHENIA GRAVIS

Myasthenia gravis is a disorder of neuromuscular transmission characterized by weakness and fatigability of skeletal muscles. The basic defect is a reduction of available acetylcholine receptors (AChRs) at neuromuscular junctions produced by an autoimmune mechanism. Accurate diagnosis and effective therapy are now available for most patients with myasthenia gravis.

PATHOPHYSIOLOGY[3]

In normal individuals, each nerve impulse liberates acetylcholine (ACh) from the motor nerve terminal (Fig. 15.15–1). The ACh in turn combines with AChRs, resulting in depolarization of the endplate region of the muscle fiber. If the depolarization is sufficiently large, it triggers a muscle action potential and muscle contraction. The effect of ACh is quickly terminated by the hydrolyzing action of acetylcholinesterase (AChE) and by rapid diffusion of ACh away from the receptors.

In the myasthenic patient, this process fails at some neuromuscular junctions. ACh has too little depolarizing effect on the muscle endplate because there is a marked reduction of available AChRs.[4] This reduction of receptors accounts for the abnormalities in myasthenia, since experimental blockade of AChRs in animals has been shown to reproduce all the physiologic effects found in the disease.

There is extensive evidence that autoimmune mechanisms are involved in the pathogenesis of myasthenia gravis. Antibodies directed against AChRs are found in the serum of more than 80 percent of patients.[5,9] These antibodies have been shown to be pathogenic, since passive transfer of immunoglobulin G from myasthenic patients to mice reproduces the basic features of the disease in the recipient. The antibody molecules bind to AChRs at the neuromuscular junction and decrease the number of available AChRs by several different mechanisms: (1) AChRs with bound antibody are degraded at a more rapid rate than normal; (2) the active site of the AChR molecule, that is, the site that normally accepts ACh, may be blocked by the antibody; and (3) the postjunctional portion of the endplate may be damaged by the antibody, possibly by complement-mediated mechanisms.

CLINICAL FEATURES[13]

Myasthenia gravis may affect individuals in any age group, but there are peaks of incidence in young women in their 20s and 30s and in older males in their 50s and 60s. The cardinal features are weakness and fatigability of muscles. The weakness increases during repeated use of the muscle and may improve after rest. The course of myasthenia gravis is often variable. Exacerbations and remissions occur in some patients, but the remissions are rarely complete or permanent. Intercurrent infections or systemic disorders may aggravate the weakness.

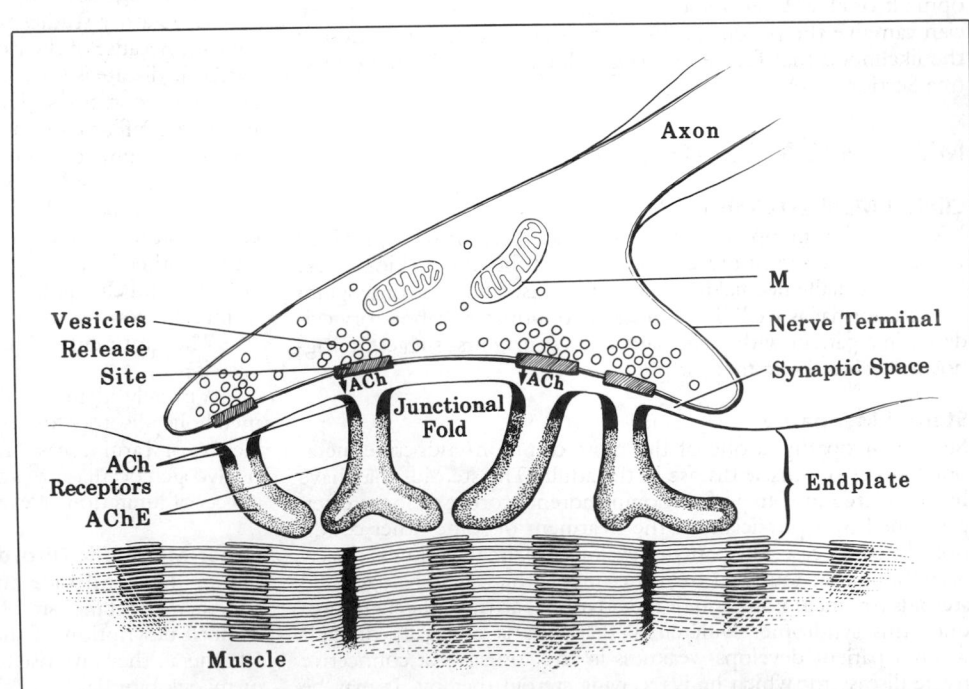

Figure 15.15–1. Diagram of neuromuscular junction. Vesicles release their acetylcholine (ACh) contents at specialized release sites. After crossing narrow synaptic space (path indicated by arrow), ACh reaches ACh receptors, which are most densely situated at peaks of junctional folds. Acetylcholinesterase (AChE) in clefts rapidly hydrolyzes ACh. M denotes mitochondia. *(Reprinted by permission of New England Journal of Medicine 298:136, 1978.)*

DISTRIBUTION OF MUSCLE WEAKNESS

Myasthenia gravis usually affects the cranial musculature early, while the limb muscles are often affected later, in more severe cases. Involvement of the ocular muscles, resulting in diplopia and ptosis, is a common initial complaint. Many patients may have symptoms restricted to ocular muscles during the early stages of their disease. Facial weakness leads to the "myasthenic snarl" upon attempting to smile. Weakness in chewing is most noticeable after prolonged effort, as in chewing meat. Difficulty in swallowing may be secondary to weakness of the palate, tongue, or pharynx. Speech may have a nasal quality caused by palatal weakness or a dysarthric quality resulting from tongue weakness. The limb weakness in myasthenia is often proximal and may be asymmetrical. The deep tendon reflexes are preserved.

DIAGNOSIS AND EVALUATION (Table 15.15–3)

The diagnosis is suspected on the basis of weakness and fatigability as described earlier. The suspected diagnosis should always be confirmed by one or more of the following diagnostic tests.

Trial of Anticholinesterase Drugs

The simplest and most frequently used method is the edrophonium (Tensilon) test. This test is based on the fact that Tensilon, an inhibitor of AChE, produces an improvement in the strength of myasthenic muscles. The beneficial effect begins within 30 seconds and is over in about 5 minutes. It is essential that an objective endpoint be used to evaluate the effect of edrophonium. The examiner should select an unequivocally weak muscle group and evaluate its strength in an objective manner. For example, it is often useful to determine how long the patient is able to maintain upward gaze before the lids become ptotic. Similarly, the time that the patient is able to maintain his or her arms in abduction is a useful measure. Weakness of extraocular muscles, impairment of speech, or other objective signs may also be followed. Two milligrams of edrophonium are administered intravenously. The patient is then asked to repeat the test maneuver. If objective improvements occur, the test is considered positive and is terminated. If there is no change, the patient is given an additional 4 to 8 mg intravenously. The dose is administered in two parts because some

TABLE 15.15–3. WORK-UP FOR MYASTHENIC PATIENTS

History
- Distribution of weakness
- Fluctuations with exercise and rest
- Respiratory or bulbar involvement
- Association with other autoimmune disorders: rheumatoid arthritis, systemic lupus erythematosus, thyroiditis, pemphigus
- Intercurrent medical problems: hyperthyroidism, infection, endocrine disturbance, etc.

Physical examination
- Distribution and degree of weakness:
    Arm abduction time
    Vital capacity
    Quantitative muscle testing

Diagnostic tests
- Tensilon test
- Repetitive nerve stimulation
- Anti-AChR antibody titer

Tests for associated conditions
- Thyroid function tests
- Rheumatoid factor, LE cell preparations, ANA
- Quantitative immunoglobulins
- Pulmonary function studies
- CT scan of anterior mediastinum (or radiographs of chest PA, lateral, obliques)

patients react to a small dose of edrophonium with unpleasant side effects such as nausea, diarrhea, excessive salivation, fasciculations, and, rarely, syncope. Atropine (0.6 mg) should be at hand for administration by vein, should these symptoms be troublesome.

False-positive tests occur in placebo-reactors and in rare patients with other neurologic disorders such as amyotrophic lateral sclerosis. False-negative or equivocal tests may also occur. In some cases, it is helpful to give a trial of a longer acting drug, such as pyridostigmine (Mestinon) or neostigmine (Prostigmin), orally. They permit more time for detailed strength evaluation.

Electrodiagnostic Tests

It is helpful to carry out electrodiagnostic tests, especially in doubtful cases. Electric shocks are delivered repetitively at rates of 3 to 5 per second to the ulnar, median, or axillary nerves, and action potentials are recorded from the appropriate muscles. In normal individuals the amplitude of the evoked muscle action potentials will not change at these rates of stimulation. In myasthenic patients, however, there is a rapid reduction in the amplitude of the evoked responses. A single dose of edrophonium prevents or diminishes this decremental reaction.

Antiacetylcholine Receptor Antibody

As noted earlier, anti-AChR antibody is detectable in more than 80 percent of myasthenic patients. The antibody titer corresponds only approximately to the patient's state, but the presence of anti-AChR antibodies is useful in the diagnosis. The test is a radioimmunoassay that is now widely available clinically. A negative test does not exclude the disease.

ASSOCIATED DISORDERS

Myasthenic patients have an increased incidence of several disorders. Thymic abnormalities are found in approximately 75 percent of patients. About 85 percent of the abnormal thymus glands are hyperplastic, while the other 15 percent are neoplastic (thymomas). Computed tomography of the anterior mediastinum is the best test for detecting thymomas. Hyperthyroidism may occur in 3 to 8 percent of patients and may aggravate the myasthenic weakness. Tests of thyroid function should be obtained. Blood tests for rheumatoid factor and antinuclear antibody and lupus erythematosus cell preparations should be carried out in all patients. Abnormalities of immunoglobulin levels should be determined by quantitative immunoglobulin measurements (not paper electrophoresis). Finally, measurements of ventilatory function are valuable because of the frequency and seriousness of respiratory impairment in myasthenic patients.

MEDICAL AND SURGICAL THERAPY[4]

The prognosis has improved markedly in the past few years as a result of improved therapy. Virtually all myasthenic patients can be returned to full productive lives with proper treatment (Table 15.15–4).

Anticholinesterase Medications

The most important medications used in the treatment of myasthenia gravis are the anticholinesterase (anti-ChE) agents, adrenal corticosteroids and other immunosuppressive agents (Table 15.15–5). Most myasthenics can be improved, but very few can be brought completely to normal by anti-ChE medication. In general, there is no difference in efficacy among the various anti-ChE drugs, but oral pyridostigmine bromide (Mestinon) seems to have the optimum duration of action for most circumstances. As a rule, the beneficial action of oral Mestinon begins within 15 to 30 minutes and lasts for 3 to 4 hours, but the individual patient's response may vary greatly from the average. Therapy is begun with a moderate dose, for example, 60 mg at 4-hour intervals, five times

TABLE 15.15–4. TREATMENT PLAN

I. Initial treatment
 A. Establish definite diagnosis
 B. Treat with anticholinesterase medication (pyridostigmine bromide), adjust dosage to obtain optimal effect
 C. If results are not satisfactory, consider thymectomy or corticosteroids

II. Thymectomy
 A. Indications
  1. Thymoma
  2. Generalized myasthenia gravis not satisfactorily controlled with anticholinesterase drugs
   a. Patients younger than 50 years
   b. Wait long enough to exclude early spontaneous remission (usually 6 months after onset of myasthenia)
 B. Preoperative preparation: If operation would pose risk because of patient's state of weakness, give course of plasmapheresis or corticosteroids until condition is satisfactory
 C. Surgical approach—median sternotomy, must be done in institution with facilities and experience for postoperative management of thymectomy patient

III. Corticosteroid therapy
 A. Indications
  1. After thymectomy for thymoma
  2. Any of the following in a patient not satisfactorily controlled by anticholinesterase drugs
   a. Older age group (older than 50 years of age)
   b. Declines to have thymectomy
   c. Status postthymectomy
   d. Purely ocular involvement when disability outweighs risks
 B. Method
  1. Optimal adjustment of anticholinesterase drugs
  2. Begin with daily administration of small dose (e.g., 12.5–20 mg of prednisone) and increase gradually to optimal response or as tolerated (maximum usually 50–60 mg of prednisone/day)
  3. Gradually switch to alternate-day schedule
  4. Maintain dose until improvement reaches plateau (usually 6–12 mo)
  5. Decrease very gradually: establish minimal maintenance dose
  6. Observe full precautions for side effects
  7. Anticholinesterase dosage may be cautiously decreased, as tolerated

daily. The dose is then increased until optimum strength is achieved. Adjustment of the dosage should be tailored to the patient's individual requirements throughout the day, based on carefully kept records of strength and motor abilities. For example, many patients are strongest in the morning and weakest in the late afternoon. They may therefore require a larger dose of Mestinon at 4 PM than at 8 AM. Patients with chewing and swallowing difficulties are often benefited by adjusting the time of medication to precede meals by 45 minutes so that optimal strength coincides with mealtime. Mestinon Timespan tablets, which have a prolonged effect, may be helpful at night but should not be used for daytime medication. The dose of these drugs should not be revised more frequently than every 2 days to permit the full effect of a given regimen to be seen. The maximum useful dose of Mestinon rarely exceeds 120 mg every 3 hours during waking hours. Overdosage with anti-ChE medication may cause weakness and other side effects.

Atropine

Atropine or atropine-like drugs are sometimes necessary to block the unpleasant "muscarinic" side effect produced by the anti-ChE medication (diarrhea, abdominal cramps, excessive salivation, nausea). Atropine blocks the autonomic effects without influencing the beneficial effects on skeletal muscle. It is, however, preferable to avoid masking these side effects, since they may provide important clues to anti-ChE overdosage. The use of atropine should therefore be limited to those patients who would otherwise be unable to tolerate the optimum dose of anti-ChE drugs.

Ephedrine

Ephedrine benefits some patients. The usual dose is 25 mg, three times daily. It occasionally causes excitement or nervousness, but insomnia can be avoided by giving the last dose before 6 PM.

Steroid Therapy

Adrenal corticosteroids in various dosage regimens have been used with beneficial effect in some patients with myasthenia gravis who do not respond fully to anticholinesterases. Early weakening seen with the abrupt onset of high-dose prednisone regimens can usually be avoided by beginning treatment with 25 mg per day and increasing the dose in steps (usually 2.5 mg at 3-day intervals), until there is marked clinical improvement or the dose of 50 mg is reached.[4] This dose is maintained for a month or more and then is gradually changed to an alternate-day regimen, over the course of several additional months, until the dosage of 100 mg on alternate days is reached. Some patients experience weakness on the "off day" and require 5 to 15 mg. The prednisone may eventually be reduced to levels of 30 to 60 mg every other day in most patients, but this usually takes many months or years to accomplish and must be monitored closely by both patient and physician. Few patients are able to do without prednisone entirely. Patients on long-term corticosteroid therapy must be carefully followed to avoid or treat adverse side effects.

Immunosuppressive Drugs

Immunosuppressive drugs such as azathioprine (Imuran) or occasionally cyclophosphamide (Cytoxan) have been found effective in myasthenic patients, including some who are refractory to other medical therapy or thymectomy. The full beneficial effect of these drugs may not be present for many months. Treatment with these immunosuppressive agents should be managed by physicians experienced in their use because of the possibility of adverse side effects, which include idiosyncratic allergic reactions and bone marrow depression.

TABLE 15.15–5. DRUGS USED IN MYASTHENIA GRAVIS

Drug	Preparation	Usual Dose	Comment
Pyridostigmine bromide (Mestinon)	60 mg tablet	60–120 mg/4 hr	Adjust dosage, as needed
Mestinon Timespan	180 mg tablet	180 mg	Only at night
Neostigmine bromide (Prostigmin)	15 mg tablet	15–30 mg/4 hr	Not in general use
Edrophonium hydrochloride (Tensilon)	10 mg/ml	0.2 ml + 0.8 ml	For diagnosis
Prednisone	5, 20, and 50 mg	up to 100 mg qid	Regimen in text
Azathioprine (Imuran)	50 mg	2–3 mg/kg	See cautions, in text

Thymectomy

Two separate problems should be distinguished: thymectomy as a treatment for myasthenia gravis and thymectomy for thymoma. Thymectomy has for many years been proposed as a therapeutic measure. The available evidence suggests that up to 85 percent of patients may benefit from thymectomy.[4] The improvement is, however, usually partial and may not occur for 1 to 10 years after surgery. The advantage of thymectomy is that it offers the possibility of long-term benefit, in some cases diminishing or eliminating the need for continuing medical treatment. We therefore recommend thymectomy in young adult patients with generalized disease of moderate to severe degree.

Thymectomy is the preferred method of treatment of thymoma because of the possibility of local tumor spread.

Plasmapheresis[2]

In view of the antibody-mediated pathogenesis of myasthenia gravis, plasma exchange, or plasmapheresis, has been used therapeutically. Modern plasmapheresis machines separate the plasma from blood cells. The plasma containing the pathogenic antibodies is removed, and the blood cells are returned to the patient in a suitable fluid medium. Plasmapheresis produces a short-term reduction in anti-AChR antibody levels followed by clinical improvement in many patients. Thus it is useful as a temporary expedient in seriously affected patients or to improve the patient's condition to withstand surgical thymectomy. The long-term treatment of myasthenic patients requires other methods of therapy outlined in this chapter.

Management of Myasthenic Crisis

Myasthenic crisis may be defined as an exacerbation of weakness of sufficient severity to endanger life. The common serious threats to life are respiratory failure caused by intercostal or diaphragmatic weakness and aspiration secondary to pharyngeal weakness. The possibility that the deterioration is the result of excessive administration of anticholinesterases ("cholinergic crisis") should be excluded. This is best accomplished by temporarily stopping treatment with anticholinesterase drugs. Treatment should be carried out in an intensive care unit staffed with physicians experienced in the management of myasthenia gravis, respiratory problems, infectious disease, and fluid management. Pulmonary infection occurs commonly and should be treated promptly because the mechanical and immunologic defenses of the patient may be impaired. Early and effective antibiotic therapy, respiratory assistance, and pulmonary physiotherapy are essentials of the treatment program and cannot be overemphasized.

OTHER DISORDERS OF THE NEUROMUSCULAR JUNCTION[13]

Eaton-Lambert Myasthenic Syndrome

Patients with Eaton-Lambert myasthenic syndrome have variable and fluctuating weakness, particularly of the arms and legs and often sparing the cranial musculature; prominent difficulty in walking; and often, autonomic abnormalities. This syndrome differs from myasthenia gravis in that in Eaton-Lambert syndrome, the cranial nerves are usually not or are only mildly affected; patients may have mild ptosis without ophthalmoplegia; and they may have mild bulbar weakness, although respiratory function is usually unimpaired. Diurnal variation is less common than in myasthenia gravis, although at times it may be prominent.

On examination, rapid fatigue on continuous muscle activity is not the rule, as compared with myasthenia gravis. Muscle strength is often improved during and after effort. Stretch reflexes, while usually present in myasthenia gravis, are usually absent in the Eaton-Lambert syndrome, although they may appear after exertion.

The clinical presentation often resembles that of a proximal myopathy, which is the major differential diagnostic issue, although the two can usually be distinguished both clinically and by neurophysiologic studies. In Eaton-Lambert syndrome, post-tetanic facilitation can be demonstrated after repetitive nerve stimulation at high rates; an *incremental* response occurs, unlike the decremental response seen in myasthenia gravis. Similarly, the electromyogram is usually normal, whereas in myopathy typical abnormalities are usually demonstrable.

The syndrome frequently occurs with an associated malignant neoplasm, especially small-cell (oat-cell) carcinoma of the lung. About 3 percent of patients with this tumor have myasthenic syndrome, and about two thirds of those with Eaton-Lambert syndrome will ultimately prove to have a tumor. Small-cell carcinoma has the most frequent association, but other tumors—including gastric, renal-cell, and thymic—have rarely been reported. The syndrome may precede identification of the tumor by as many as several years or may occur after a tumor is identified. All patients with this syndrome should have a careful search for a lung neoplasm with chest CT or MRI, which if negative should be repeated at regular intervals.

This myasthenic syndrome is thought to be produced by an IgG antibody that interferes with the release of acetylcholine at the neuromuscular junction. Unlike myasthenia gravis, in which the antibody is directed to the acetylcholine receptor, the antibody in myasthenic syndrome is directed at the mechanism releasing acetylcholine, probably through interference with calcium channels.

Therapy, which is usually only variably successful, includes treatment of the primary neoplasm if one is evident; 3,4-diaminopyridine (which enhances acetylcholine release); immunosuppression; and plasmapheresis.

Botulism

The very potent toxin of *Clostridium botulinum* causes a dramatic and striking weakness of both cranial nerves and skeletal muscles, usually with prominent gastrointestinal and autonomic abnormalities. Botulism usually follows ingestion of food that has been processed in a way allowing production of toxin by the organism. Poorly canned vegetables are usually implicated, but some outbreaks can be traced to meat or fish. After ingestion of toxin, symptoms occur between several hours and 2 or 3 days later. Because the toxin is irreversibly bound, weakness usually persists for many weeks. *Wound botulism* also occurs, producing a clinically similar illness several weeks after the organism infects a wound.

The patient usually presents with constipation, blurred vision or diplopia, ptosis, dysphagia with evidence of bulbar weakness, followed by progressive generalized skeletal weakness and respiratory embarrassment ensuing over a period of hours or days. Autonomic symptoms and signs are usually prominent with a dry mouth, urinary retention, abnormal response to Valsalva maneuver, and constipation. The diagnosis can usually be confirmed when distinctive neurophysiologic abnormalities are found. Identification of toxin in stool or from the wound is often successful.

Once the syndrome is recognized, trivalent antitoxin should be administered to prevent progression of the disease. Respiratory support in an intensive care unit with close monitoring of autonomic instability is mandatory in the early stages and until recovery ensues. Guanidine and 3,4-diaminopyridine may be of value; immunosuppression and plasmapheresis have no role. The prognosis for full recovery is excellent when the syndrome is promptly recognized and supportive measures are undertaken.

REFERENCES

1. Bohan A, Peter JB: Polymyositis and dermatomyositis. N Engl J Med 292:344, 1975
2. Dau PC (ed): Plasmapheresis and the Immunobiology of Myasthenia Gravis. Boston, Houghton Mifflin, 1979
3. Drachman DB: Biology of myasthenia gravis. Ann Rev Neurosci 4:195, 1981

4. Drachman DB: Myasthenia gravis. In Conn H (ed): Current Therapy. Philadelphia, WB Saunders, 1982, p 754

5. Drachman DB, Adams RN, et al: Functional activities of autoantibodies to anti-acetylcholine receptors and the clinical severity of myasthenia gravis. N Engl J Med 307:769, 1982

6. Epstein HF: Second MDA colloquim on mapping the X chromosome. Neurology 33:494, 1983

7. Hawley RJ, Cohen MH, et al: The carcinomatous neuromyopathy of oat-cell lung cancer. Ann Neurol 7:65, 1980

8. Kendall-Taylor, Turnbull: Endocrine myopathies. Br Med J 287:705, 1983

9. Lindstrom JM, Seybold ME, et al: Antibody to acetylcholine receptor in myasthenia gravis: Prevalence, clinical correlates, and diagnostic value. Neurology 26:1054, 1976

10. Lucy JA: Is there a membrane defect in muscle and other cells? Br Med Bull 36:187, 1980

11. Mastaglia FL, Ojeda VJ: Inflammatory myopathies: 1. Ann Neurol 17:215, 1985; 2. Ann Neurol 17:317, 1985

12. Monaco AP, Bertelson CJ, et al: Detections of deletions spanning the Duchenne muscular dystrophy locus using a tightly linked DNA segment. Nature 316:842, 1985

13. Newsom-Davis J: Diseases of the neuromuscular junction. In Asbury AK, McKhann GM, and McDonald WI (eds): Diseases of the Nervous System. Philadelphia, WB Saunders, 1986, p 269

14. Rowland LP: Biochemistry of muscle membranes in Duchenne muscular dystrophy. Muscle and Nerve 3:3, 1980

15. Trend P, Saint J, Wiles CM, et al: Acid maltase deficiency in adults. Brain 108:845, 1985

16. Walton JN, Gardner-Medwin D: Progressive muscular dystrophy and the myotonic disorders. In Walton JN (ed): Disorders of Voluntary Muscles. Edinburgh, Churchill Livingstone, 1981, p 481

CHAPTER 15.16
Peripheral Neuropathies

John W. Griffin and David R. Cornblath

The peripheral nerves provide the major interface between the central nervous system and the environment. In addition to somatic motor and sensory functions, the peripheral nervous system (PNS), through the autonomic nerves, is intimately involved in cardiovascular, thermoregulatory, and sexual function and in control of micturition and defecation. The peripheral nerves are susceptible to injury by a variety of known metabolic, toxic, inflammatory, vascular, physical, and infectious insults and are undoubtedly vulnerable to other agents yet to be identified.

The pathologic responses of the PNS in disease are limited, so specific etiologies usually do not produce distinctive pathologic changes. Normal function depends on the integrity of both the nerve fiber (axon) and its supporting elements, the Schwann cells with their myelin sheaths. Some processes selectively affect the Schwann cells or myelin, resulting in *demyelination;* examples are diphtheria and the Guillain-Barré syndrome. Other disorders primarily affect the nerve cell body or axon, resulting in *axonal degeneration,* as seen in the toxic neuropathies induced by vincristine or isoniazid, for example. Many of the most common metabolic and heritable neuropathies show evidence of both axonal degeneration and demyelination. This presumably reflects the mutual interdependence among cellular elements of the peripheral nervous system.[1,3]

CLASSIFICATION

A basic and clinically useful distinction is among mononeuropathies, multiple mononeuropathies, and polyneuropathies (Table 15.16–1).

SYMPTOMS AND SIGNS OF NEUROPATHIES[2,3,4,7]

ALTERATIONS IN SENSIBILITY

Patients with alterations in sensibility caused by peripheral nerve disease may use a remarkable variety of descriptions to communicate their subjective symptoms. It is helpful to encourage the patient to describe his symptoms in his own words: "numbness" may cover a host of meanings, but phrases such as "it feels as if I were walking on cotton wool" or "it's like walking on coals" cannot be misunderstood. Common types of complaints include: *paresthesias*—subjective tingling, "pins and needles"; *dysesthesias*—unpleasant perceptions of normally innocuous stimuli; and *hyperpathia*—a markedly painful experience of tactile or thermal stimuli. *Hypesthesia* describes an elevated threshold to perception of a stimulus; for example, a patient may appreciate the sharpness or painful quality of a pinprick only with considerable pressure. *Hyperesthesia* is a seemingly heightened sensibility, in that light stimuli will be experienced intensely. Careful testing will often reveal that the threshold stimulus is elevated above normal, but when the threshold is reached, an unusually intense perception is experienced. Finally, it should be added that occasional patients will show profound deficits in sensibility on examination with few subjective sensory symptoms and little functional deficit.

Many patients have loss of all sensory modalities—pain, temperature, light, touch, vibration, and joint movement (proprioception). It is helpful to look for selective loss, which often occurs in one or two patterns: selective loss of pain and temperature sensibility, or selective loss of joint position sense and vibratory sensibility. The significance of these selective functional deficits in differential diagnosis is discussed later.

MOTOR CHANGES

Flaccid weakness or paralysis of muscles results from involvement of motor fibers in the nerves. If motor fibers have been denervated for more than a few weeks, atrophy of the muscles will be apparent. The distribution of weakness is of major importance in accurate diagnosis, and often detailed individual muscle testing is required. In asymmetrical processes, particularly involving only one extremity, it is necessary to distinguish between lesions of a nerve root (radiculopathy), nerve plexus (brachial or lumbosacral), or nerve. For example, injury to the C5 root may produce marked weakness of the deltoid, supraspinatus, and infraspinatus and some weakness of the biceps. On the other hand, weakness of the opponens, short abductor, and short flexors of the thumb would suggest median nerve damage rather than a nerve root lesion. When weakness in such processes is mild, comparison of strength (and bulk) with the contralateral limb is helpful. A convenient guide to individual muscle testing and the innervation patterns of muscle is the "Aids to the Investigation of Peripheral Nerve Injuries."[5]

In polyneuropathies, weakness is usually greatest distally.

TABLE 15.16–1. CLASSIFICATION OF PERIPHERAL NEUROPATHIES

Form	Characteristics	Usual Mechanisms
Mononeuropathy	Involves a single nerve, e.g., ulnar, median, or peroneal	Trauma, pressure, compression, vascular
Multiple mononeuropathies	Involves two or more nerves, asymmetrical, stepwise progression	Involvement of small blood vessels (e.g., diabetes, vasculitis)
Polyneuropathy	Symmetrical, distal involvement, usually of feet and legs first	Multiple (see Table 15.16–3)

Early manifestations often include weakness of dorsiflexion of the toes and ankles. Atrophy may be seen in the short extensor of toes and in the anterior tibials. In the hands, the intrinsic muscles are often involved first; atrophy may be found in the thenar and hypothenar eminences and first dorsal interosseus muscles.

AUTONOMIC ABNORMALITIES

Autonomic dysfunction is frequently overlooked but is of considerable importance in differential diagnosis and management. Screening for autonomic involvement can quickly be accomplished at the bedside. *Cardiovascular* responses can be screened by testing for orthostatic hypotension and for slowing of pulse rate during the Valsalva maneuver. Abnormal patterns of *sweating* should be sought; often patients will have anhydrosis over large areas of the body. They may complain, however, of *excessive* sweating in those areas that are uninvolved. In a warm room, the pattern of sweating can be determined by passing the dorsum of the examiner's hand lightly over the skin, looking for the "drag" of moist skin. *Pupillary reactions* are easily examined; symptomatically, abnormalities may be associated with loss of accommodation or photophobia (caused by loss of the light reflex). *Gastrointestinal* symptoms may include constipation or diarrhea. *Bladder involvement* should be sought by specific questioning. Finally, it is essential to inquire for impotence in men; this is often an early manifestation of autonomic neuropathy and is rarely volunteered by the patient.

LABORATORY FINDINGS

Electrodiagnostic studies are useful in the evaluation of neuropathies. A variety of tests are available to evaluate the physiology of both nerve and muscle (see Chapter 15.14). Nerve conduction studies primarily test the state of the largest myelinated fibers. The major uses of these studies in evaluating polyneuropathies are to confirm the presence of nerve disease, to help differentiate multiple mononeuropathies from polyneuropathies, and to determine whether axonal degeneration of demyelination is the underlying basis of the disease. Axonal degeneration is characterized by preserved distal latencies, F-wave latencies, and conduction velocities but reduced evoked amplitudes. Conversely, studies indicative of demyelination have abnormal distal and F-wave latencies and conduction velocities with normal evoked amplitudes. Partly for this reason, there may be differences between the severity of the clinical disease and the degree of abnormality in the conduction velocities.

Electromyography can aid in confirming that weakness is caused by denervation and in demonstrating the distribution of involvement. Muscle biopsy can also confirm the presence of a denervation process and may be useful in evaluating for vasculitis.

In selected patients nerve biopsy can yield a specific diagnosis or allow determination of the type of lesion (acute demyelination, recurrent demyelination, axonal degeneration with large fiber or small fiber loss), thereby orienting further diagnostic evaluation. Its usefulness is limited by several factors. First, the tissue must be specially processed (plastic-embedded thin sections and electron microscopy) to provide maximum information. Second, only a sensory nerve (usually the sural) can be biopsied. Third, few neuropathies produce specific lesions; this lack of specificity reflects the limited pathologic responses mentioned previously. Specific diagnosis—including amyloidosis, sarcoidosis, vasculitis, leprosy, or some inherited metabolic disorders, such as metachromatic leukodystrophy—may be made by nerve biopsy, but often laboratory tests or biopsy of other tissues would more easily establish the diagnosis.

DIFFERENTIAL DIAGNOSIS OF POLYNEUROPATHIES

When faced with a peripheral neuropathy, especially one of the polyneuropathies, the physician may feel overwhelmed by the large number of possible underlying causes. It is useful to have a scheme for evaluation. Initially one should search the history for clues in diagnosis (Table 15.16–2). Next, one should use features of the neuropathy, such as distribution, time course, age at onset, selectivity of functional involvement, or electrodiagnostic data, to limit the differential diagnosis. Table 15.16–4 presents the differential diagnosis of polyneuropathies according to these schemes. The most common etiologies are given in italic type. Less common disorders are also listed for completeness; details of their clinical presentation may be found in neurology texts or specialized references.[2,3,7]

The approach to an individual patient with an undiagnosed polyneuropathy is often best begun by asking, "What is unusual or distinctive about this patient's neuropathy?" The unusual features may provide clues to orient further evaluation. In particular the age of onset, rate of progression, selectivity of functional involvement, distribution, and presence of associated neurologic disease should be sought.

The *rate of progression* may be difficult to ascertain in longstanding neuropathies, since neither the patient nor the family may have been aware of mild neuropathy in childhood. Often such patients will recall never having kept up with their peers in races and sports or always having been chosen last for teams. Often they have never engaged in sports of any sort for recreation. High-arched feet (pes cavus) with hammer-toe deformities are important indicators of childhood onset, since they are the consequence of long-standing muscle imbalances. Such patients usually have a form of heritable predominantly motor neuropathy (Charcot-Marie-Tooth).

Selective functional involvement is often particularly helpful. Some neuropathies are typically predominantly *motor* (see Table 15.16–4); of these, the inflammatory neuropathies (includ-

TABLE 15.16–2. EVALUATION OF NEUROPATHY FROM THE HISTORY

- Known medical illness: Diabetes, uremia, cancer
- Exposures: Lead, acrylamide, mercury, arsenic, thalium, solvents
- Residence abroad: Leprosy
- Medications: INH, vincristine, furantoins, disulfiram, dapsone, phenytoin, amiodarone
- Diet and nutritional state
- Alcohol use
- Smoking
- Family history

TABLE 15.16–3. MNEMONIC FOR PERIPHERAL POLYNEUROPATHIES: *DANG THERAPIST*

D	Diabetic	Polyneuropathy; sensorimotor in the setting of longstanding diabetes. May have "small fiber" pattern. Mononeuropathy: abrupt painful onset of III or VI nerve palsies, or subacute asymmetrical lumbosacral plexus dysfunction ("diabetic amyotrophy")
A	Alcoholic	Sensorimotor neuropathy with multiple nutritional deficiencies
N	Nutritional	Individual B-complex vitamins: thiamine, niacin, B_6, B_{12}
G	Guillain-Barré	The acute form of inflammatory neuropathy: immunologically mediated, chiefly motor, demyelinating. Respiratory, facial muscles may be involved. CSF protein often raised without pleocytosis.
T	Toxic	Drugs: furantoin; vincristine; cis-plantinum (sensory); isoniazid (B_6 antagonism); penicillamine; gold salts; vitamin B_6 (sensory neuropathy following massive doses); perhexilene Metals: lead (radial nerve palsies), arsenic; thallium (alopecia) Industrial and environmental agents acrylamide hexacarbon solvents (industry, glue sniffing); triorthocresyl phosphate
H	Hereditary	Charcot-Marie-Tooth disease (very slowly progressive, predominantly motor, with high arches, stork legs, often nerve enlargement, dominant inheritance) Dejerine-Sottas disease (childhood onset, severe hypertrophic neuropathy with high CSF protein, recessive inheritance) Refsum disease (ataxia, retinitis pigmentosa, hypertrophic neuropathy, deafness, elevated serum phytanic acid) Hereditary sensory neuropathy
R	Recurrent	Relapsing form of inflammatory neuropathy; often responds to steroids.
A	Amyloidosis	All forms include autonomic involvement. May result from circulating paraproteins (myeloma) Hereditary forms
P	Porphyric	Chiefly motor neuropathy, may progress rapidly: younger patients, with acute intermittent form of porphyria
I	Infections	Diphtheria, leprosy
S	Systemic	Associated with collagen diseases, uremia, sarcoidosis
T	Tumor	Carcinomatous neuropathies: pure sensory or sensorimotor neuropathy, may be combined with myopathy

ing Guillain-Barré syndrome), the heritable motor-sensory neuropathies (such as Charcot-Marie-Tooth disease), porphyric neuropathy, and those caused by some toxins, particularly lead, are the most frequent causes. Most neuropathies have both sensory and motor involvement, with sensation more severely affected than strength. Disorders with primarily sensory involvement and little motor involvement (Table 15.16–4, IIB) can be separated into those with loss of all modalities (global loss), dissociated loss of pain and temperature sensibility, and associated loss of proprioception and vibratory sensibility. The development of a rapidly evolving global, purely sensory neuropathy in an adult may be a remote manifestation of underlying malignancy. The responsible lesion is an inflammatory destruction of dorsal root ganglion cells (ganglioradiculitis). This syndrome is among the most distinctive of the malignancy-related neurologic syndromes; thorough search for tumor and long-term observation are indicated.

Neuropathies with prominent *autonomic* involvement may present with complaints of impotence, urinary hesitancy, constipation, or symptoms of orthostatic hypotension. Often autonomic neuropathies are associated with spontaneous pain and loss of pain and temperature sensibility. Strength, vibration, and proprioceptive sensibilities and tendon reflexes may be preserved. This picture represents a "small fiber" polyneuropathy and is seen as one of the manifold syndromes of diabetic neuropathy as well as in systemic amyloidosis and, occasionally, in association with paraproteinemia or cryoglobulinemia.

SPECIFIC NEUROPATHIES

Diabetic Neuropathy
The various manifestations of *diabetic neuropathies* cover in themselves nearly the full spectrum of peripheral nerve disease (Table 15.16–3).[3,6] Diabetic mononeuropathies and multiple mononeuropathies represent vascular insufficiency or infarction in nerve, presumably caused by small vessel disease. Their onset is typically abrupt and often painful. Cranial nerves III and VI, the femoral nerve, or other major nerves of the extremities may be involved. Occasionally, lumbosacral plexus involvement occurs, producing a picture often confused with intraspinal disease. There is often asymmetrical weakness of the hip girdles with little sensory loss. Although the initial manifestations may be incapacitating, the prognosis for eventual recovery in diabetic multiple mononeuropathies is usually good. Diabetic polyneuropathies include distal sensorimotor neuropathy and severe sensory neuropathy, which may be of the "large fiber" or "small fiber" types, the latter often associated with autonomic involvement. Diabetic polyneuropathies may be mild and asymptomatic; they are often progressive and are major causes of mobidity and disability in diabetes.

Inflammatory Demyelinating Neuropathies
The inflammatory neuropathies are a group of related disorders classified by time course into acute, chronic, and relapsing types. They are immunologically mediated and share the pathologic features of demyelination of spinal roots and peripheral nerves, with a variable degree of phagocyte-mediated myelin stripping and mononuclear cell infiltration within nerve. All produce predominantly motor involvement with reduced nerve conduction velocities and, in most patients, elevated spinal fluid protein without pleocytosis. In these aspects the disorders represent a clinical counterpart of experimental allergic neuritis, a disorder produced by immunization of susceptible animals against peripheral nerve myelin or its constituents. It is likely that these disorders represent a spectrum of a single process, but they are considered separately because of the differing approaches to treatment.

Acute Inflammatory Neuropathy (Guillain-Barré Syndrome). This disorder is the most common neuropathic cause of paralysis in the post–polio vaccine era. Sixty percent of cases follow some antecedent event such as viral infection, parturition, surgery, or neoplasm, particularly Hodgkin disease. Because of the alarming rapidity with

TABLE 15.16–4. DIFFERENTIAL DIAGNOSIS OF POLYNEUROPATHIES[a]

I. Course
- A. Acute (days)
  - *Guillain-Barré syndrome*
  - Porphyric neuropathy
  - Diphtheritic neuropathy
  - Some toxins (e.g., tri-orthocresyl phosphate)
- B. Subacute (weeks)
  - *Many toxins*
  - *Nutritional neuropathies*
  - Carcinomatous neuropathies
  - Uremic neuropathy
- C. Relapsing
  - Relapsing inflammatory neuropathy
  - Refsum disease
- D. Chronic (many months or years)
  - *Diabetic motor-sensory neuropathy*
  - Chronic inflammatory neuropathies
- E. Very chronic (childhood onset)
  - Heritable motor-sensory neuropathies (e.g., Charcot-Marie-Tooth disease)

II. Selective functional involvement[b]
- A. Predominantly motor
  - Guillain-Barré syndrome
  - Relapsing and chronic inflammatory neuropathy
  - Acute intermittent porphyria
  - Lead neuropathy
  - Heritable motor-sensory neuropathies (Charcot-Marie-Tooth)
- B. Predominantly sensory
  1. Global loss
     - *Diabetes*
     - *Carcinomatous sensory neuropathy (ganglioradiculitis)*
     - Paraproteinemic and cryoglobulinemic neuropathy
     - Tabes dorsalis
  2. Dissociated loss of pain and thermal sensibility
     - Diabetes (small fiber type)
     - Amyloidosis
     - Hereditary sensory neuropathies
     - Lepromatous leprosy
  3. Dissociated loss of joint position and vibration sensibility sensibility
     - Subacute combined degeneration
     - Friedreich ataxia
- C. Autonomic neuropathy
  - *Diabetes*
  - *Amyloid*
  - Acute, chronic, and relapsing pandysautonomia
  - Dysautonomia (Riley-Day)

III. Distribution[c]
- A. Proximal weakness
  - Guillain-Barré
  - Porphyria
  - Carcinomatous neuropathy with proximal weakness ("carcinomatous neuromyopathy")
  - Spinal muscular atrophies
- B. Proximal sensory loss
  - Porphyria
  - Tangier disease (analphalipoproteinemia)
- C. Temperature-related distribution
  - Lepromatous leprosy

IV. Age
- A. Childhood
  - *"Steroid-dependent" inflammatory neuropathies*
  - Giant axonal neuropathy
  - Krabbe disease
  - Metachromatic leukodystrophy
  - Neuroaxonal dystrophy
  - Heritable sensorimotor neuropathy (Dejerine-Sottas)

[a]The most common etiologies are set in italic.
[b]Most polyneuropathies produce sensory and motor disturbances.
[c]Most polyneuropathies produce distal involvement.

which weakness and respiratory insufficiency can develop, Guillain-Barré syndrome (GBS) should always be regarded as a potential medical emergency. The cornerstones of management are early diagnosis, careful observation, and supportive care. Back pain and leg pain with paresthesias are a common presenting manifestation, and at this stage trivial viral infections or functional complaints are often suspected. A clue to the gravity of the complaint is often the finding of depressed or absent reflexes. In most cases, weakness rapidly becomes the predominant problem. Weakness is generally symmetrical and may involve any distribution including cranial nerves; proximal as well as distal muscles are usually affected. The diagnosis is supported by demonstration of reduced conduction velocities, compatible with the demyelinating process, at some level of the peripheral nervous system. These changes may be present only in very distal nerve regions (measured as terminal latencies) or within spinal roots (measured as F-wave latency). An elevated spinal fluid protein is also supportive and may reach dramatic levels, but the rise of protein may follow onset of neuropathy by many days, so that a normal protein at the time of presentation is frequent. When patients present, one associated viral syndrome, infectious mononucleosis, can easily be sought. The remote possibility of acute intermittent porphyria should be excluded because of the implications for management.

All but the mildest cases should be hospitalized and the patient's respiratory status closely monitored. Autonomic involvement is a major contributing factor to death and complications and may be manifested by flushing, orthostatic hypotension, or cardiac rhythm changes.

Plasmapheresis has been shown in a prospectively controlled trial to be beneficial in the treatment of GBS. When performed on patients unable to walk unassisted and performed in the first 30 days of illness, plasmapheresis improves the degree of recovery at 1 month, shortens the time on a respirator, and shortens the time to independent walking. The potential complications from plasmapheresis are significant such that experience with both plasmapheresis and GBS is necessary.

This is not to de-emphasize the importance of supportive care, including good pulmonary toilet, prevention of thrombophlebitis, and prevention of corneal ulceration in patients with facial weakness. Although approximately 30 percent of patients require respirator assistance, the mortality with modern intensive care has been reduced to 2 to 5 percent. The nadir of the clinical course is usually reached within 2 to 4 weeks of onset, and improvement can be dramatic. In a severely affected patient, however, recovery may be very prolonged, and these 15 percent of patients have substantial residua.

Chronic and Relapsing Inflammatory Neuropathies. These disorders are among the most common previously undiagnosed neuropathies referred for intensive evaluation and represent a major indication for nerve biopsy in centers where appropriate handling is available. The suspicion is usually raised by the presence of a predominantly motor neuropathy with reduced conduction velocities and elevated spinal fluid protein. Because the onset and progression may be insidious, patients must be carefully distinguished from heritable motor-sensory neuropathies described below. The establishment of a diagnosis is important because these are among the most treatable peripheral nerve disorders. Initial therapy is with adrenal steroids. In patients with contraindications to steroids, plasmapheresis and immunosuppression appear to be of value. Patients with chronic inflammatory neuropathies who improve either spontaneously or in response to treatment are at risk for subsequent relapse. With this caution, the prognosis in steroid-responsive patients is good.

Hereditary Neuropathies. There are a large variety of inherited disorders of the peripheral nervous system; hereditary motor-sensory neuropathy (Charcot-Marie-Tooth disease) is the most common.

Because of the chronicity of the symptoms and the slow evolution, patients do not realize they have peripheral nerve disease until middle or old age. Weakness, particularly foot drop and hand weakness, is the most severe manifestation in most patients and may be associated with the foot deformities described previously, as well as marked thinness of the calf and anterior tibial muscles (stork legs). Most patients with Charcot-Marie-Tooth disease have a demyelinating neuropathy, with recurrent demyelination and remyelination, resulting in redundant Schwann cell processes. These so-called onion bulbs occupy space and contribute to a visible and palpable enlargement of nerves in many individuals (hypertrophic neuropathy). The diagnosis can usually be established by careful elicitation of a history of childhood onset and by examination of family members. Mildly affected individuals may have only foot deformities or slowed conduction velocities. Nerve biopsies showing marked onion bulb formation strongly suggest a heritable etiology. The disorder is dominantly inherited. The patients usually respond well to reassurance about the slow rate of progression and to appropriate physical therapy and rehabilitation measures, including ankle bracing.

Toxic Neuropathies. Finally, the *toxic neuropathies* require emphasis, both because of the increasing list of pharmaceutical, industrial, and environmental agents that can injure peripheral nerves and also because of the therapeutic importance of proper diagnosis. They may be subacute in evolution, as in vincristine or Furadantin neuropathy, or may be insidious and progressive as often seen in industrial exposure (for example, to solvents such as methy-*n*-butyl ketone). In the vast majority of toxic neuropathies, the lesion is degeneration of the distal regions of the longest or largest axons (dying back), so that early clinical involvement may involve blunting of sensation in the toes, loss of the Achilles tendon reflex, and weakness of the intrinsic muscles of the foot. Such a distal axonal degeneration may occur in the CNS as well and produce degeneration of the corticospinal tracts in the lumbosacral cord and of the gracile tract of the dorsal columns in the cervical cord. Such central involvement may be "masked" by the peripheral neuropathy when the patient is first seen and becomes apparent as a spastic paraparesis only when the neuropathy has recovered. Careful occupational and recreational history, and in some instances visits to home or place of work, may reveal the presence of toxic exposure.

TREATMENT

This section has emphasized diagnosis because the best treatment is directed toward the etiologic disorder. Unfortunately, of patients referred for evaluation of neuropathy, a substantial proportion remain without etiologic diagnosis after initial screening. Nonspecific therapeutic measures include maintenance of optimal nutritional status (with supplemental B vitamin preparations if the diet is suspect) and avoidance of potential neurotoxins, particularly alcohol, that might have a synergistic effect.

For neuropathic weakness, appropriate bracing is helpful. Daily activities such as eating, writing, or buttoning are often made easier by "built-up" (large) utensils.

The sensory deficits are often more bothersome. The small-fiber neuropathies are particularly difficult medical and psychologic problems. The diminished pain sensibility can lead to painless injuries (e.g., Charcot joints caused by traumatic arthropathy) and contribute to "trophic" ulcers, osteomyelitis, and ultimately spontaneous or surgical amputation. Prevention through education is paramount. Foot care, avoidance of trauma and pressure on anesthetic extremities, and prompt attention to early lesions are mandatory. The spontaneous pain that often accompanies the small-fiber neuropathies may respond to anticonvulsants such as phenytoin or carbamazepine; opiates are contraindicated because of the potential for addiction. Although neurogenic impotence cannot be satisfactorily corrected, understanding the neurologic cause of the impaired function may relieve considerable anxiety.

REFERENCES

1. Asbury A, Johnston P: Pathology of Peripheral Nerve. Philadelphia, WB Saunders, 1978
2. Dyck P, Thomas PK (eds): Peripheral Neuropathy. Philadelphia, WB Saunders, 1984
3. Griffin JW: Peripheral neuropathies. In Rosenberg R (ed): Clinical Neurosciences. New York, Churchill Livingstone, 1984
4. Haymaker W, Woodhall B: Peripheral Nerve Injuries: Principles of Diagnosis. Philadelphia, WB Saunders, 1953
5. Medical Research Council of Great Britain: Aids to the Investigation of Peripheral Nerve Injuries. London, 1984
6. Raff M, Asbury A: Ischemic mononeuropathy and mononeuropathy multiplex in diabetes mellitus. N Engl J Med 279:17, 1968
7. Schaumburg HH, Spencer PS, Thomas PK: Disorders of Peripheral Nerves. Philadelphia, FA Davis, 1983

CHAPTER 15.17
Diseases of the Spine and Spinal Cord

John Rybock and Hamilton Moses III

The majority of the disorders of the spine are the result of focal compression, displacement, or irritation of the spinal cord, spinal nerve roots, or spinal skeletal structures causing a varying combination of neurologic dysfunction and pain. Other causes of spinal cord and root dysfunction, such as inflammatory, infectious, and metabolic disorders, are considered in other chapters of this text.

Since the spinal cord is especially intolerant of compression or displacement and since reversibility of the resulting neurologic deficit is particularly dependent upon the duration of the pressure, a physician must be able to recognize cord lesions, identify the location and mechanism of the lesion, and institute prompt therapy. In addition, in view of the frequent occurrence of disability and suffering caused by lesions of spinal nerve roots and skeletal structures, the basic approach to such problems should be understood by all physicians.

MANIFESTATION OF SPINAL CORD LESIONS

ACUTE INJURY (Table 15.17–1)

The acuity of spinal cord damage will affect the clinical presentation. Sudden injury results in a period of spinal shock in which no spinal cord function is detectable caudal to the lesion. This usually follows fracture-dislocations of the spine or penetrating wounds

TABLE 15.17–1. ACUTE SPINAL CORD INJURIES AND DISEASES

Trauma
- Penetrating wounds
- Vertebral dislocations
- Herniation of intervertebral discs
- Whiplash injuries

Infection
- Epidural abscess
- Viral infection (poliomyelitis, coxsackie, herpes)
- Meningitis
    Bacterial

Vascular
- Occlusion of feeding arteries
    Anterior spinal artery occlusion
    Dissecting aortic aneurysm
- Arteriovenous malformation
- Hematomyelia

Demyelinative and inflammatory
- Transverse myelitis
- Multiple sclerosis
- Chemical meningitis

Neoplastic
- Metastatic
    Extradural
    Intradural

and often persists for 3 to 6 weeks, after which the chronic manifestations of spinal cord injury gradually occur. In more slowly developing lesions, there may be no detectable period of spinal shock (Table 15.17–2).

CHRONIC INJURY

The more common gradual compression or displacement of the spinal cord produces a variable mixture of motor and sensory dysfunction depending upon the level of involvement and the relative impairment of specific spinal tracts.

Motor dysfunction results from a combination of nerve roots and anterior horn cells (lower motor neurons) at the level of injury plus interference with tracts (upper motor neurons) subserving motor function caudal to the lesion. The upper motor neuron signs, including weakness without atrophy and hyperreflexia, are diagnostic of cord involvement, but the lower motor neuron signs, including weakness with atrophy and loss of reflexes, are often more useful in defining the exact level of involvement.

Sensory manifestations are produced at the level of the lesion by involvement of the posterior roots. The radicular symptoms correspond to one or more dermatomes and may include pain as well as cutaneous sensory loss. The pain is often aggravated by coughing, straining, and movement of the vertebral column.

Other sensory manifestations are produced below the lesion by interruption of the tracts serving the various sensory modalities. Of these modalities, pain is most reliably tested. Since fibers conveying pain ascend a short distance before crossing to the opposite side of the spinal cord, the observed level of response in partial injuries is often a few segments below the actual lesion. The transition between normal and impaired pinprick sensation is often abrupt, defining a sensory level. Touch and position sense, which ascend without crossing in the spinal cord, are less useful in providing localization of the level of injury.

Autonomic findings, such as decreased sweating, may be detected below the level of the lesion but seldom provide precise localizing information.

Incomplete lesions may present one of several patterns of neurologic deficit depending upon the source of the damage.

Small intrinsic lesions may predominantly destroy the crossing fibers of the spinothalamic tracts, producing a "dissociated" sensory loss, the isolated loss of pain and temperature sensation in the dermatomes related to the lesion. A larger central cord lesion will encroach upon the corticospinal tracts, producing greater motor loss in the arms (medial fibers) than the legs (lateral fibers). More extensive lesions may lead to almost complete loss of spinal cord function except for the most peripheral fibers, which subserve sacral sensation (sacral sparing).

Lesions involving only one side of the cord produce a Brown-Séquard syndrome. Upper motor neuron function is lost caudally on the side of the lesion, as is touch and proprioceptive sensation. Pain and temperature sensation, however, is lost from the opposite side of the body. Penetrating injuries, as well as compression from laterally placed tumors, often produce this syndrome.

Compression of the spinal cord anteriorly, as in a massive central disc herniation, produces a syndrome in which dorsal column function (touch and position sense) remains essentially intact with major loss of other motor and sensory functions.

TABLE 15.17–2. SUBACUTE SPINAL CORD DISEASES

Trauma or compression
- Cervical spondylosis
- Herniation of intervertebral discs
- Syringomyelia

Infections
- Chronic meningitis (syphilis, tuberculosis, or fungal)
- Epidural abscess (usually acute)

Inflammatory
- Arachnoiditis

Vascular
- Arteriovenous malformations
- Arteritis

Demyelination
- Multiple sclerosis

Neoplastic
- Meningioma
- Neurinoma
- Lymphoma or leukemia
- Metastatic
- Seeding from brain tumor

Metabolic
- Pernicious anemia

Degenerations
- Spinocerebellar
- Amyotrophic lateral sclerosis
- Peroneal muscular atrophy

MANIFESTATIONS OF SPINAL ROOT LESIONS

Each spinal nerve root provides the innervation for specific muscles or portions of muscles and carries sensation from a specific cutaneous band, its dermatome (see Figs. 15.17–1, 15.17–2 and Table 15.17–3). Additionally, efferent fibers of the sympathetic or parasympathetic system and sensation from proprioceptors and other deep receptors travel in the various nerve roots; these functions are seldom of diagnostic importance.

Milder lesions of nerve roots often cause only irritative symptoms, pain or paresthesias that are perceived in the corresponding dermatome. As the severity of the lesion increases, the irritative symptoms may persist, increase, or disappear.

More diagnostic of a spinal root lesion is a pattern of dermatomal sensory loss along with weakness in the muscle or muscles innervated by the same root. The weakness is of the lower motor neuron type with loss of tone, loss of reflexes, and atrophy. The

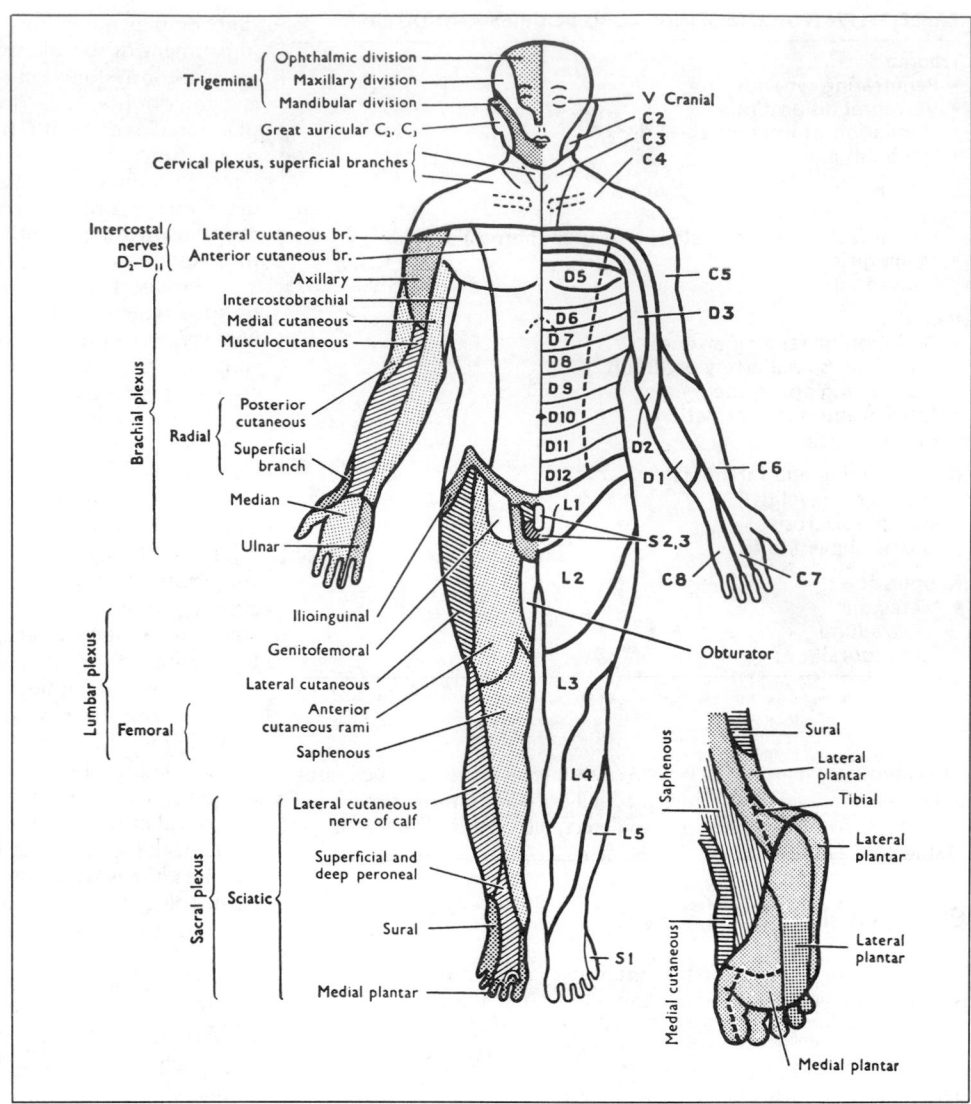

Figure 15.17–1. Anterior aspect. Cutaneous distribution of spinal segments (*right*) and peripheral nerves (*left*). (*From Brain: Clinical Neurology, 2d ed, Oxford University Press, 1964.*)

sensory loss affects all modalities, although this may be difficult to demonstrate fully because of dermatomal overlap and methodologic problems in testing. Pinprick testing is usually most helpful.

MANIFESTATIONS OF SKELETAL LESIONS

Lesions affecting the bony and ligamentous structures of the spine cause local pain and mechanical dysfunction. Local muscle spasm, tenderness to percussion, and limitation of motion are often present, and distant, or referred, pain may be noted. This pain, which may be perceived throughout the dermatomes in which the lesion is present, tends to be deep and aching in nature, less discrete than radicular pain, and, of course, has no associated neurologic deficit.

DIAGNOSIS OF NEUROLOGIC IMPAIRMENT OF SPINAL ORIGIN[4]

DIFFERENTIAL DIAGNOSIS

It is essential that spinal cord compression be differentiated from other lesions of the cord that cause paraplegia, namely, transverse myelitis, ischemic myelomalacia, syphilis, multiple sclerosis, subacute combined degeneration of the cord, and motor neuron disease. The extremities may also be involved in a hysterical paralysis, which may be accompanied by sensory loss but no involvement of bladder or bowel control and no alteration in the reflexes. Flaccid paraplegia occurs with lesions of anterior horn cells of the lumbosacral region, for example, poliomyelitis; with lesions of the cauda equina or the peripheral nerves, for example, polyneuritis; or as the result of primary muscle disease. Bilateral leg weakness may also result from a parasagittal intracranial meningioma as the pyramidal fibers from both leg areas of the motor cortex are involved. On occasion an early symptom of spinal compression is root pain, which may be confused with that caused by such visceral disorders as pleurisy, angina, cholecystitis, or peptic ulcer. Furthermore, these radicular pains may be mistaken for local joint disease.

Usually the distinction between a mass lesion and these other conditions can be made clinically. Whenever there is doubt, myelography with CT scanning or an MRI scan is carried out to exclude cord compression, especially in more treatable forms.

DIAGNOSTIC STUDIES

Roentgenograms of the spine may reveal loss of mobility, bony erosion, bony overgrowth, or narrowing of the intervertebral

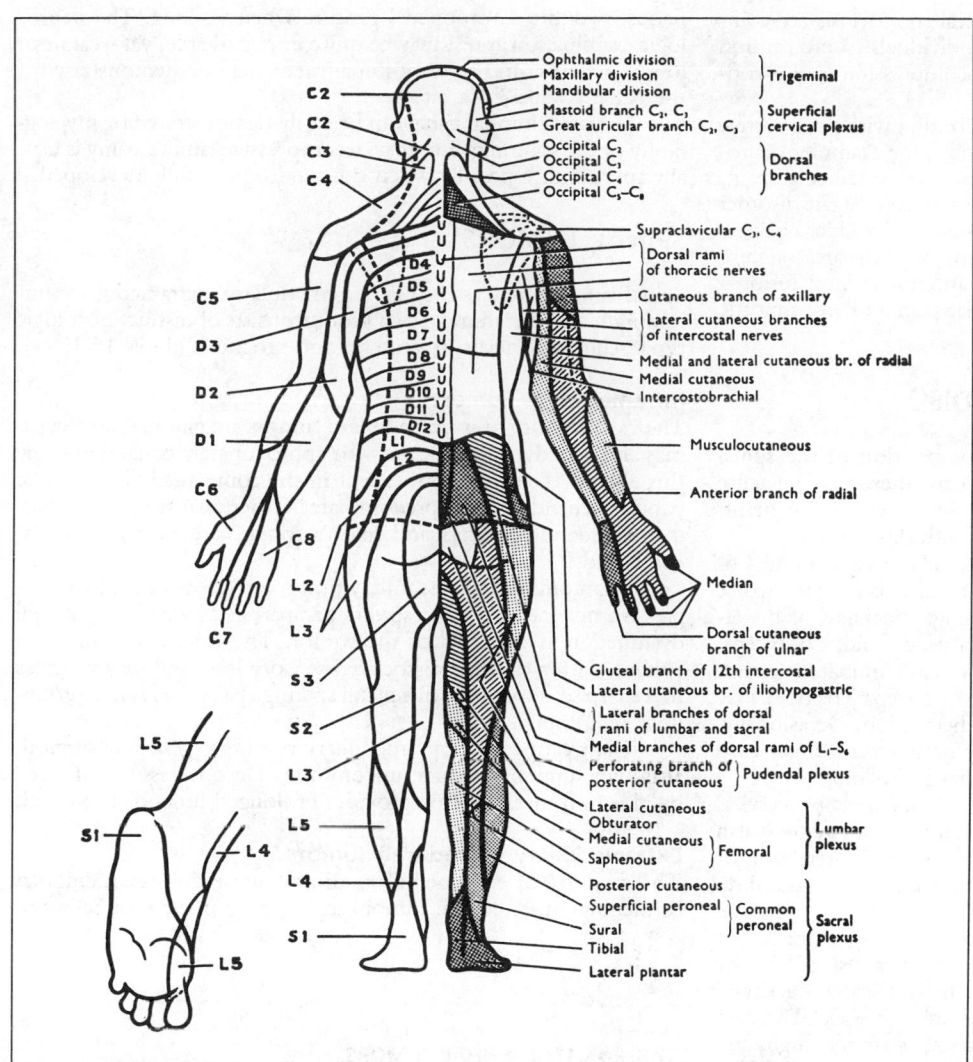

Figure 15.17–2. Posterior aspect. Cutaneous distribution of spinal segments (*left*) and peripheral nerves (*right*). (*From Brain: Clinical Neurology, 2d ed, Oxford University Press, 1964.*)

space. Lumbar puncture may reveal CSF abnormalities such as increased protein concentration and xanthochromia (Froin syndrome). All these studies should be performed for all patients seriously considered to have cord compression.

Myelography with CT scanning provides a definitive answer to the question of the presence or absence of a mass lesion and its location. These studies should be performed for all patients seriously considered to have cord compression. It appears that MRI may provide even better resolution of both intrinsic spinal cord lesions and some compressive lesions (see Chapter 15.2).

SPECIFIC DISEASE ENTITIES

CERVICAL SPONDYLOSIS[3]

Spondylosis in the cervical region is the most common cause of spinal cord compression occurring after middle life. The degeneration of one or more intervertebral discs, with the development of osteoarthritic changes, leads to compression not only of cord but also of spinal roots. The onset is usually insidious, but acute presentations do occur. There may be limitation of both active and passive movements of the head, and pain may radiate to the shoulders, upper extremities, and scapular region.

The clinical picture depends on the level or levels at which cord compression occurs and on the extent of the damage. There is often a mixture of symptoms, owing to upper and lower motor neuron involvement in the upper extremities and to upper motor neuron dysfunction in the lower limbs. No sensory loss may be apparent, but often there is diminished appreciation of light touch and of pinprick over the fingers and vibratory loss in the toes. The deep tendon reflexes may be diminished or increased in the arms and are usually increased in the legs with associated extensor plantar responses. Cerebrospinal fluid studies are usually normal.

TABLE 15.17–3. SPINAL ROOT LESIONS

Root	Pain/Sensory Loss	Weakness	Reflex Loss
C6	Digits 1 and 2, radial forearm	Biceps	Biceps
C7	Digits 2 and 3	Triceps	Triceps
C8	Digits 4 and 5, ulnar forearm	Wrist extensors, intrinsics of hand	None
L4	Anterior shin	Quadriceps	Knee jerk
L5	Lateral calf, medial foot	Toe extensors	None
S1	Posterior calf, lateral foot	Gastrocnemius	Ankle jerk

Since the radiologic features of cervical spondylosis are commonly detected in asymptomatic older individuals, some caution should be used in attributing spinal cord compression to this condition.

The first step in treatment is immobilization with a supportive collar. The indications for further evaluation, for example, neuroradiologic studies and surgery, are (1) intractable radicular pain, (2) progressive weakness and atrophy, (3) progressive gait disorder secondary to a spastic paraparesis, and (4) loss of bladder control. Surgery—either decompressive laminectomy or, if the area of compression is limited to one or two levels, anterior cervical fusion—is quite successful in relieving the radicular pain and arresting the progression of myelopathy.

HERNIATED INTERVERTEBRAL DISC

In contrast to the slowly progressing compression of the spinal cord or cervical roots in cervical spondylosis, there may be acute symptoms from herniated intervertebral discs. Thoracic disc herniations are rare and are usually associated with direct trauma.

Herniated cervical discs usually occur at the C5-C6 and C6-C7 levels. The first symptom is usually radicular pain, made worse by moving the neck, coughing, or straining. Weakness of the affected muscles (C5, rhomboid, supraspinatus, deltoid; C6, biceps, brachioradialis; C7, triceps; C8, intrinsic hand muscles) appears next. Depression of the biceps jerk (C6) or triceps jerk (C7) may often be useful in localizing the level of herniation. Occasionally, a midline protrusion of the cervical disc occurs with direct cord compression resulting in long-tract findings in isolation.

Treatment involves immobilization of the neck by cervical traction or a supportive collar and drug treatment of muscle spasm and pain. If the patient does not respond to cervical traction or develops signs of cord compression, myelography and surgical removal of the protruded disc material are indicated.

Herniated lumbar discs are often preceded by an injury or strain to the back accompanied by a feeling of a "snap" in the lower back. Nonlocalized pain appears in the lower back and makes it difficult for the patient to stand erect or walk. The pain then becomes more localized to the buttock, posterior thigh, and leg. Exacerbations of pain occur with bending, coughing, or lifting objects. Muscle weakness and absent knee jerk (L4-L5) or ankle jerk (L5-S1) may occur. Dermatomal sensory loss is present.

Treatment is bed rest and analgesics. Surgery may be required, but it is appropriate only after at least a 3-week trial of bed rest. Investigations including EMG, myelography, and CT scanning are indicated only in patients in whom the diagnosis is not certain or for whom surgery is intended.

LUMBAR STENOSIS

Many older patients complain of pain and weakness that begins after walking some distance or with standing for prolonged periods. Vascular claudication, caused by atherosclerosis of the large or small arteries of the leg, must be distinguished from neurogenic claudication, which arises because of spondylotic narrowing of the lumbar canal. In these patients, symptoms occur from compression of the cauda equina as a result of thickening of the ligaments, hypertrophy of the facet joints, and small disc protrusions superimposed on a shallow spinal canal.

These patients complain of pain in the back and legs after exertion or prolonged standing. The pain is usually bilateral but may be unilateral, and it is often anterior or deep in the thigh, unlike pain from vascular claudication, which is usually in the buttock or calf. If exercise continues, demonstrable weakness, falling, paresthesias, sensory loss, and urinary urgency or incontinence may occur. These symptoms are uncommon with vascular claudication. Both pain and the accompanying neurologic symptoms may be promptly relieved by flexing the spine, and many patients sponta-

neously assume a "stooped" posture when walking. The neurologic examination at rest may be quite unremarkable, yet weakness, loss of reflexes, and sensory impairment may be demonstrated if the patient walks for a bit.

The small lumbar canal can be easily demonstrated by myelography or CT scanning. Lumbar decompressive laminectomy is usually successful, especially when the syndrome is fully developed.

SPINAL TUMORS[4]

Spinal tumors are classified as intramedullary, extramedullary (intradural), and extradural. Each group consists of distinct histologic types, clinical patterns, treatment, and prognosis (Table 15.17–4).

Intramedullary Tumors
The vast majority of intramedullary tumors are gliomas; astrocytomas and ependymomas occur with approximately equal frequency throughout the spinal cord except in the conus medullaris, where papillary ependymomas predominate. Other glial tumors, including oligodendrogliomas and glioblastomas, are occasionally encountered.

Symptoms of intramedullary tumors are those of a slowly progressive myelopathy, with spastic paraparesis as well as segmental dysfunction at the level of the tumor. The tumor may mimic a sphinx, with a capelike dissociated sensory loss, and may progress to a sharp sensory level with sacral sparing. Pain is seldom a prominent symptom.

The treatment of intramedullary tumors is generally surgical, although surgical cures are uncommon. Decompression followed by radiation therapy often provides prolonged functional survival.

Extramedullary (Intradural) Tumors
The majority of extramedullary tumors are either neurilemomas or meningiomas, benign tumors arising from nerve root Schwann

TABLE 15.17–4. SPINAL TUMORS

	Intra-medullary	Extra-medullary (Intradural)	Extradural
Incidence	Least common	Less common	Most common
Types	Astrocytoma Ependymoma	Meningioma Neurillemoma	Metastatic carcinoma (breast, lung, prostate, kidney)
Symptoms	Slowly progressive painless myelopathy	Myelopathy with radicular pain	Local pain with rapidly progressing myelopathy
Radiographic findings	None	Enlarged intervertebral foramen	Bone destruction
Best test	MRI	CT or myelogram	CT or myelogram
Surgical treatment	Biopsy, rarely total excision	Total excision	Decompression or biopsy only
Adjuncts	Radiation	None needed	Radiation chemotherapy
Prognosis	Slow progression over years	Cure	Per primary disease

cells or arachnoid cells, respectively. Although the former is more likely to protrude through a neural foramen and form a "dumbbell" tumor and the latter is more common in females, preoperative distinction is often impossible. Lipomas, dermoids, and benign cysts occasionally occur in this location.

Extramedullary tumors often present with radicular pain caused by nerve root irritation. Progressive radicular deficit then occurs along with a progressive myelopathy. Since most tumors displace the cord laterally, a Brown-Séquard pattern is frequently present, although dorsally arising tumors may initially show selective loss of posterior column function.

Surgical therapy is usually curative. "Dumbbell" tumors may require a two-stage approach if a substantial portion projects into the chest or abdominal cavity.

Extradural Tumors

Most extradural tumors are metastases that have spread hematogenously into the epidural venous plexus or vertebral body. Lung, breast, prostate, and kidney are the most common locations of the primary tumor. Less commonly, primary bone tumors, myelomas, and lymphomas may invade the epidural space, causing cord compression.

Local pain is an almost invariable presenting symptom, generally deep and aching, as a result of skeletal and soft tissue involvement. Radicular pain, increased by coughing and straining, may be present. Symptoms of an evolving myelopathy then occur, with weakness and dorsal column sensory loss beginning in the legs and gradually ascending to involve the trunk and cervical segments. A sensory level may then appear. Bowel and bladder dysfunction soon follow. The evolution of the syndrome usually occurs over a number of weeks but may accelerate and evolve over just a few days.

Clinical suspicion may be substantiated by an elevated alkaline phosphatase, evidence of vertebral collapse, or blastic, destructive lesions on routine radiograph and a positive radionuclide bone scan. Spinal CT scans can clearly demonstrate destruction of bone and impingement of the epidural space. Myelography is usually required, however, to delineate fully the superior and inferior extent of the lesion. Magnetic resonance imaging is a promising alternative, but its role in epidural lesions is unclear at present.

Spinal epidural metastasis is an urgent condition that demands prompt treatment, as complete functional cord transection may occur quickly once myelopathy has begun. An acute abrupt deterioration often follows a long period of indolent, chronic progression. One must be very suspicious, therefore, when back or neck pain begins in a patient with known cancer.

Immediate treatment consists of corticosteroids. Radiotherapy should be immediately begun if the nature of the tumor is known and if it is radiosensitive. Decompressive laminectomy with biopsy of the mass should be performed if the diagnosis is in doubt or if the tumor is not radiosensitive.

SYRINGOMYELIA

In syringomyelia an elongated cavity lined with ependymal cells develops in close relationship to the central canal of the spinal cord, particularly in the cervicothoracic region, and on occasion in the medulla (syringobulbia). The cavitation destroys decussating pain and temperature fibers and compresses adjacent motor neurons as well as the long ascending and descending tracts. Although it is considered a congenital abnormality, clinical manifestations do not appear until early adult life.

The initial signs are usually confined to one hand and consist of wasting and weakness together with deficits of pain and temperature sensation. Scars resulting from painless burns or other traumas are frequently seen. Perception of light touch and position are usually spared; this dissociated sensory loss is characteristic. As the lesion progresses, the contralateral upper extremity becomes simi-

larly afflicted, and upper motor neuron signs and sensory disturbances appear in the lower limbs. Horner syndrome, dysarthria, dysphagia, and nystagmus may also occur. The course is slowly progressive, but spontaneous arrest may occur. Rarely, an acute exacerbation caused by a spontaneous or traumatic hemorrhage into the cavity occurs.

The diagnosis can be confirmed by either MRI or a myelogram followed by a delayed CT scan; the latter will usually demonstrate myelographic contrast within the syrinx cavity. Surgical insertion of a drainage tube into the cavity will usually arrest further progression.

BACKACHE[1]

Backache is one of the most common problems in general medicine. It is second only to upper respiratory infections as cause for days lost from work. Unlike the well-delineated entities involving the spine, spinal cord, and roots, where the pathophysiology is reasonably clear, backache often defies explanation.

ACUTE BACKACHE

Acute backache often begins after an injury or strain such as a fall, lifting a heavy object, or twisting suddenly. Many patients, however, "throw their backs out" without any apparent preceding events. Symptoms predominate in the lower back and consist of pain, paravertebral muscle spasm, and inability to bend. Coughing, straining, and bending make the symptoms worse. It is important to remember that most acute back episodes are caused by mechanical strain of the soft tissues of the back and not by disc herniation. In the latter case, sharp pain radiates down the leg into the calf, usually to the ankle. This "sciatica" appears within a few hours of onset of symptoms and usually overshadows the back pain; it is reproduced by straight-leg raising and is associated with radicular deficits.

Therapy for the patient with acute back pain, whether mechanical or disc related, is bed rest and analgesics. In many cases the pain begins to subside within a few days, and the patient may gradually increase activity. Unless demonstrating definite signs of a disc herniation, the patient should be encouraged to begin increasing activity after a few days even if some back discomfort persists, since prolonged disuse of the back muscles produces weakness that will delay full recovery. For the same reason, back braces are not recommended. Often weakness in the back muscles from underexercise is a contributory factor in the acute strain. Institution of an exercise program or referral to a physical therapist may be needed to complete the recovery.

If sciatica remains a prominent symptom, especially with neurologic deficit, bed rest should be continued for a longer period, at least 10 days. If progressive improvement is not seen, referral to a neurosurgeon is indicated.

CHRONIC BACKACHE[2]

Chronic backache usually arises from poor posture, sedentary lifestyles, and obesity, often in combination. Repeated minor trauma may play a role, as can prior back surgery. Backache may occur as a symptom of depression, and secondary gain in the form of industrial compensation or interpersonal benefits may cloud the diagnostic issues and make therapy more difficult.

The general and neurologic examinations are usually normal, aside from mild paravertebral muscle spasm and limitation of motion of the back. Varying degrees of spondylotic (degenerative) change may be seen on radiographs, but such changes are a normal part of the aging process and seldom cause significant back pain.

Therapy of these patients can be quite difficult. It must be

remembered that surgery is not indicated for chronic back pain without significant radicular pain or neurologic deficit, except in the presence of major structural abnormalities, such as subluxations. Even then, surgery should be approached with caution.

Empirically, the single most useful therapy for chronic back pain is a well-designed and monitored exercise program to stretch and strengthen the back muscles. Weight reduction is also important. Modifications in life-style to avoid activities that predictably aggravate the back, attention to good body mechanics, and a firm mattress can help. Muscle relaxants offer no benefit in chronic pain, and narcotic analgesics must be completely avoided. Many patients are done a disservice by physicians who feel it necessary to prescribe medications and provide repeated tests and active treatments rather than teach the patient to take responsibility for his own recovery, for example, by exercising and losing weight. The main accomplishment of most "back schools" and "pain clinics" is the teaching of this lesson.

REFERENCES

1. Finneson B: Low Back Pain, 2d ed. Philadelphia, JB Lippincott, 1980
2. Hendler NH, Long DM, Wise TN: Diagnosis and Treatment of Chronic Pain. Littleton, John Wright, 1982
3. Rothman R, Simeone F: The Spine, 2d ed. Philadelphia, WB Saunders, 1982
4. Youmans JR: Neurological Surgery, 2d ed. Philadelphia, WB Saunders, 1982

CHAPTER 15.18

Multiple Sclerosis and Other Demyelinating Diseases

Guy M. McKhann and
Justin C. McArthur

Demyelinating diseases of the nervous system include some of the most prevalent neurologic disorders occurring in childhood and young adult life. Multiple sclerosis (MS), for example, is the most common cause of disability among adults under the age of 40, after trauma and rheumatologic conditions. Demyelination can occur in the peripheral nervous system, producing inflammatory demyelinating neuropathies, such as the Guillain-Barré syndrome (see Chapter 15.16); however, discussion in this chapter is limited to demyelinating disorders of the CNS.

In the nervous system, myelin serves as a high-resistance insulator that increases conduction velocity along the axon of a neuron. Myelin sheaths are multilayered lamellae formed by apposition of the plasma membranes of processes of satellite cells that wind around axons. In the peripheral nervous system, the processes extend from Schwann cells; in the CNS, from oligodendrocytes.

Myelin can be damaged by a number of processes including ischemia, tumor, or infection; however, the term *demyelinating* disease is reserved for disorders in which myelin breakdown is the primary abnormality and neural elements, particularly axons, are relatively spared. Disorders with inherited defects in myelin metabolism involving either the synthesis or maintenance of myelin lipids or proteins are termed *leukodystrophies* (or dysmyelinating disorders). The leukodystrophies are more common in infancy and childhood and will not be discussed in detail in this chapter. A further classification of disorders of CNS myelin is presented in Table 15.18–1.

Demyelinating disorders of the CNS can be grouped into three etiologic categories: (1) immunopathogenic, (2) viral, and (3) secondary to systemic disease.

DEMYELINATING DISEASES— IMMUNOPATHOGENIC

MULTIPLE SCLEROSIS

Multiple sclerosis is a common neurologic disorder characterized by an immunologically mediated attack on myelin within the CNS. The disease is unpredictable, and multiple, discrete areas of the CNS may be involved episodically. In the United States 250,000 people have MS, with 8800 new cases diagnosed annually. Ninety percent of those affected are between the ages of 20 and 40. The case fatality rate is extremely low, and, on aggregate, there is little or no effect on expected life span. Prevalence in northern Europe and the northern United States is 30 to 80 per 100,000; in southern Europe and the southern United States, 6 to 14 per 100,000; and in the tropics, fewer than 1 in 100,000. Migrant studies have suggested that those who migrate after the age of 14 or 15 years carry with them the prevalence rate of their place of origin, whereas those migrating in early childhood assume the risk of their new home. There have also been clusters or "epidemics" of MS in localized areas, for example, the Faeroe Islands after British occupation in World War II, and most recently in Key West, Florida. These studies have strengthened the hypothesis that a viral infection, perhaps acquired in childhood and with a long latency period, is responsible for MS.

There are parallels between the CNS demyelination that occurs with MS and the inflammatory leukoencephalopathy that occurs in sheep infected by the lentivirus, visna. This virus can produce a slow infection with a relapsing course and areas of inflammation and demyelination in the CNS similar to those seen in MS. Another animal model for MS, experimental autoimmune encephalomyelitis (EAE), can be induced in a number of laboratory animals by immunization with myelin and shares pathologic features with MS. While both visna virus infection and EAE share many clinical and pathologic similarities with MS, the absence of an exact animal model has hindered advances in unraveling the pathogenetic secrets of MS.

Genetic factors are of importance, too; MS is 15 to 20 times more frequent in first-degree relatives of patients than in the general population. The concordance in identical (monozygotic) twins (28 percent) is higher than in fraternal (dizygotic) twins (2.5 percent), which approaches that in siblings (1.9 percent).[10] In MS patients with a European derivation, the frequency of the Class I histocompatibility antigens A3, B7, Dw2, and Dr2 is increased.

Currently, the most plausible explanation for the etiology of MS attempts to link much of the epidemiologic, genetic, and immunologic data. A genetically susceptible individual exposed during childhood to certain exogenous trigger factors, possibly viruses, may go on to develop MS after a latent period of 10 to 30 years.

Pathology

The characteristic pathology in MS is scattered plaques of demyelination of varying ages. Histologically, an acute plaque will show

TABLE 15.18–1. DISORDERS OF CENTRAL NERVOUS SYSTEM MYELIN

Demyelinating

Immunopathogenic
- Multiple sclerosis
- Neuromyelitis optica (Devic disease)
- Acute disseminated encephalomyelitis
- Transverse myelitis

Viral
- Progressive multifocal leukoencephalopathy
- Subacute sclerosing panencephalitis

Secondary to systemic processes
- Postanoxia
- Nutritional deprivation
- Hypothyroidism
- Chemo/radiotherapy

Leukodystrophy

Identified biochemical
- Metachromatic leukodystrophy (arylsulfatase A deficiency)
- Globoid cell leukodystrophy (β-galactosidase deficiency)
- Adrenoleukodystrophy (C24-C30 fatty acid excess)

Unidentified biochemical
- Alexander disease—fibrinoid leukodystrophy (autosomal recessive)
- Pelizaeus-Merzbacher disease (X-linked recessive)
- Canavan disease—spongy sclerosis (autosomal recessive)
- Neuroaxonal dystrophy (recessive, mainly females)

sparing of nerve cell bodies and axons, with perivascular cuffs of lymphocytes and areas of myelin dissolution in the presence of macrophages containing myelin debris. Both T4 (helper) and T8 (T suppressor-cytotoxic) cells are present. Intramyelinic edema may be present in acute plaques. In chronic plaques, there may be a loss of oligodendrocytes, particularly in the center, with a surrounding astrocytic response. There is accumulating evidence that remyelination can occur, although it appears to be delayed, incomplete, and limited to the periphery of lesions.[15] Electron microscopic studies have provided no convincing evidence of viral particles or inclusions.

Plaques can occur anywhere within the CNS, although the largest plaques are found within white matter, particularly the periventricular areas around the lateral ventricles, the optic nerves, brain stem, and spinal cord. The correlation between the distribution and number of plaques visualized at autopsy and clinical symptoms and signs is often quite poor. Magnetic resonance imaging (MRI) will often demonstrate large numbers of plaques that are "silent," or causing no symptoms.

Immunology

Increasing information points to an immune disturbance as the pathogenetic basis for MS. Evidence gathered over the past 10 years suggests that there is hyperactivity of the immune system, with a selective immunologic attack on CNS white matter.[21] There is no evidence that other organ systems are affected in MS. The major unanswered question is what specific trigger turns on this autoimmune process and what causes the disease to relapse and remit.

During acute attacks, some patients have been shown to have reduced numbers of circulating immunoregulatory T lymphocytes with a loss of T8 (suppressor) cells and preservation of T4 (helper) cells. These changes can precede clinical disease activity and are also present in about half the patients with chronic progressive disease. Similar changes may be present in the cerebrospinal fluid.[21] Such research tools, while potentially important in understanding the pathogenic mechanisms in MS, have no role in the day-to-day management of patients.

Clinical Features

Two characteristic features of MS are (1) an episodic course with exacerbations and remissions or a progressive course from onset and (2) the presence of multicentric involvement of the white matter of the CNS.

Relapsing/remitting MS, the most common form, is characterized by the acute onset of neurologic deficit over a period of a few hours or days, usually followed by a complete or nearly complete recovery over a period of weeks or months. This period of remission is followed, at unpredictable intervals, by other acute relapses. With each episode the neurologic residua may accumulate. From pathologic studies and from initial experience with MRI, it is clear that demyelination can continue without any clinical correlate. This increasingly recognized feature of MS, namely, the prevalence of subclinical disease, can lead to difficulties in interpreting the results of treatment trials, since almost all are based on the modification of clinical signs and symptoms. Future trials will have to take into account the newer imaging techniques, to link anatomic correlation with physical symptoms and signs. Patients with MS may develop transient symptoms or signs as a result of excessive fatigue or when overheated, for example, by an infection, or after strenuous exercise. These transitory symptoms do not represent a true exacerbation but are the result of conduction block developing in previously damaged myelin. There may be great difficulty in deciding whether an individual is having a definite exacerbation, and this has complicated the interpretation of many clinical trials, in that transient electrophysiologic changes may be misclassified as acute exacerbations. For definitional purposes, symptoms and signs must persist for longer than 48 hours to be classified as an exacerbation.

Clinical manifestations of MS vary widely from patient to patient.[16] With time, 25 to 40 percent will develop overt optic neuritis, with monocular blurring or blindness and often some pain on eye movement. Eventually 80 percent of patients will have signs and symptoms suggesting spinal cord involvement; in fact, the most common presentation in age groups over 40 is with a slowly progressive myelopathy.[13] The clinical features of cord involvement include bilateral leg weakness, which may be described by the patient as "stiffness" or "clumsiness." Numbness or loss of proprioception in the legs may add to gait difficulty. Bladder, bowel, and sexual dysfunction are frequent manifestations of spinal cord involvement.[19] At least 50 percent of patients will eventually demonstrate brain stem involvement with eye movement abnormalities such as internuclear ophthalmoplegia or VI cranial nerve paresis. Facial weakness, trigeminal neuralgia, dysarthria, and dysphagia are also symptoms reflecting bulbar disease. Cerebellar dysfunction, presenting as tremor, limb ataxia, or gait instability from truncal ataxia, can be particularly disabling. Painful sensory symptoms, which can be fleeting, migratory, or intermittent, may be the presenting complaint in 5 to 10 percent of patients with MS. Many of these individuals may have had these symptoms for years and may have been misdiagnosed as hysterics, depressives, or malingerers. A proportion of patients with MS will develop significant cognitive impairment, usually personality change or memory loss. Seizures occur only slightly more frequently than in the general population and are an uncommon feature.

Although MS is unpredictable and prognosis uncertain, several clinical points can be helpful:

1. The age of onset. As a general rule, persons between the ages of 20 and 35 have a better long-term outcome in terms of disability than those under the age of 20 or over 50.
2. Patients presenting predominantly with cerebellar, cognitive, or progressive motor symptoms fare worse than patients with visual or sensory complaints.
3. Patients who achieve complete remissions with resolution of neurologic symptoms and signs after each relapse have a better prognosis than patients with accumulating deficits after each relapse.

4. A steadily progressive course from onset implies little likelihood of remission and a high chance of subsequent disability.
5. The effect of pregnancy on the course of MS has been examined by several investigators. During the 9 months of pregnancy there is a reduced risk of relapse, probably because of the natural immunosuppression afforded by alpha-fetoprotein and the other natural hormones of pregnancy. During the 3 months of the puerperium, however, there may be an increased frequency of exacerbation. On aggregate, the effect of pregnancy on MS is minimal.
6. Multiple sclerosis has little effect on the course of pregnancy. Most women have normal pregnancies and are able to deliver vaginally. There is no increase in birth defects. The use of epidural anesthesia does not appear to provoke exacerbations of the disease.

The course of most patients can be categorized as either relapsing-remitting or chronic progressive. About 90 percent of patients will present initially with the relapsing-remitting form, but between 5 and 10 percent will annually convert to the progressive form. Table 15.18–2 gives some indication of the course of the disease for the two different categories.

Diagnosis

At present, the diagnosis of multiple sclerosis is primarily based on clinical criteria.[14] Laboratory and imaging studies can be corroborative and helpful in excluding other conditions, but they do not supplant detailed historical information and clinical examination. A definite diagnosis of MS requires a description of two or more episodes of neurologic symptoms affecting discrete areas of the CNS and evidence on examination of white-matter involvement in at least one area. Differentiation between MS and a functional disorder may be difficult in the early stages of the disease, particularly when sensory complaints predominate. If the patient's symptoms and signs suggest only a single lesion, ancillary studies may be helpful in disclosing subclinical disease in other CNS sites. Table 15.18–3 illustrates some of the conditions that may be misdiagnosed as MS.

Appropriate selection of ancillary studies is important to minimize the cost and morbidity of diagnostic evaluation. It is unnecessary, expensive, and potentially harmful to subject a patient to an unselected battery of tests. In general, only those tests that are required to corroborate the clinical diagnosis are indicated, and the use of serial studies is rarely justified. Neurodiagnostic studies may serve the following functions.

Evoked potential studies may demonstrate lesions that are not producing symptoms or signs (subclinical). Two are widely available—visual evoked potentials (VEP) and auditory evoked potentials (AEP). Somatosensory evoked potentials (SSEP) are technically more difficult, and their reliability and predictive value are uncertain. Visual evoked potentials are the most useful for the detection of subclinical lesions because of the frequency of involvement of the optic pathways and because the test is well standard-

ized. In patients with clinically definite MS, VEP will be abnormal in 70 percent.[5] There is little reason to perform VEPs in a patient presenting with unequivocal optic neuritis.

Imaging studies may demonstrate a multicentric process affecting predominantly white matter. MRI has now been proved a more sensitive technique for demonstrating demyelinating lesions within the brain and spinal cord and may render more invasive imaging techniques such as CT scan and myelography unnecessary.[20] MRI is, however, relatively nonspecific and may demonstrate focal white matter "lesions" even in the absence of clinical manifestations of MS. The significance of such findings has not yet been examined critically, and in the absence of clinical features suggesting MS, such "lesions" cannot alone point to a diagnosis of MS. In the elderly, periventricular white-matter abnormalities appear commonly. They most likely represent small areas of ischemia or infarction and should not be overinterpreted as representing MS unless there is a compatible clinical history. Where MRI is unavailable, a CT scan may detect demyelinating lesions within the brain, but the brain stem and spine are not well visualized. The use of double-dose contrast may increase the yield of visible

TABLE 15.18–3. DIFFERENTIAL DIAGNOSIS OF MULTIPLE SCLEROSIS: CONDITIONS THAT MAY MIMIC MS

Brain/brain stem
Cerebrovascular disease
- Multiple CVAs
- Vasculitis
- Arteriovenous malformation

Migraine

Tumor
- Multifocal primary
- Multiple metastases
- Lymphoma
- Paraneoplastic

Congenital/degenerative
- Olivopontocerebellar atrophy
- Arnold-Chiari malformation
- GM2 deficiency (hexosaminidase A or A and B deficiency)
- Wilson disease, adult form (pseudosclerosis)

Inflammatory/infective
- Acute disseminated encephalomyelitis
- Neurosarcoidosis
- Neurosyphilis
- Behçet
- Connective tissue disorders

Leukodystrophies
- Adrenoleukodystrophy
- Metachromatic leukodystrophy (adult type)

Somatiform disorders
- Somatization disorder (Briquet syndrome)
- Conversion disorder
- Hypochondriasis

Spinal cord
Extrinsic compression
- Spondylotic arthritis
- Herniated cervical/thoracic disc
- Spinal canal stenosis

Intrinsic cord lesions
- Syringomyelia
- Glioma, ependymoma
- Arteriovenous malformation

Inflammatory
- Transverse myelitis

Degenerative
- B$_{12}$ deficiency
- Hereditary spastic paraplegia

TABLE 15.18–2. COURSE OF MULTIPLE SCLEROSIS

	% of Patients	
	Relapsing-Remitting ⟶	Progressive
At diagnosis	90	10
At 10 years	50	50
Not disabled	80	40
Moderately disabled	20	30
Severely disabled/dead		30

plaques but may add to the risks of the procedure in terms of nephrotoxicity and dye reactions.

Studies may exclude other etiologies; for example, the demonstration of degenerative cervical disease and spinal canal stenosis might account for a myelopathy rather than MS. Magnetic resonance imagery is now the most sensitive technique to exclude syringomyelia.

Immunologic studies may demonstrate immunologic perturbations in the spinal fluid. Patients with MS may have nonspecific immunologic abnormalities within the CSF that can aid in diagnosis[8] (see Table 15.18–4). IgG is elevated in 70 percent of patients with clinically definite MS. The IgG index provides a measure of intrathecal synthesis of IgG. Subfractions of these immunoglobulins have indicated specific "oligoclonal bands" (OCB) that are present in 80 to 90 percent of patients with definite MS. Oligoclonal bands have been demonstrated in a number of other neurologic conditions, including Guillain-Barré syndrome, viral meningoencephalitis, tumors, and even stroke. Ebers estimates that 7.2 percent of these patients without MS have oligoclonal bands.[6] The bands persist between acute attacks and perhaps for life. The source of the IgG in the CSF is presumably plasma cells derived from B-cell clones within the brain. It is not known against which antigens these immunoglobulins are directed. Patients with MS may have elevated serum and CSF titers to a number of viruses, particularly measles, and the production of these antibodies may be a secondary phenomenon of the hyperactive immune system.

Myelin basic protein, a component of myelin, appears in the CSF during acute exacerbations and may be a useful, albeit nonspecific, indicator of disease activity. Myelin basic protein may be elevated in other disorders, including after head trauma, stroke, or with inflammatory conditions such as systemic lupus erythematosus.

The presence in the sera of patients with MS of circulating factors that could cause demyelination or block neuroelectric transmission has been demonstrated. At present such techniques are limited to research purposes and are not widely applied in the diagnosis or management of the MS patient.

Treatment

There is no proven cure for MS and as yet no proven therapy that will decrease the frequency or severity of relapses.[4] The comprehensive management of the patient with MS is best accomplished by an interdisciplinary approach among neurologist, rehabilitation specialist, urologist, and social worker. Education, counseling, empathy, and encouragement are critical elements in the overall approach to treatment. Certain issues arise frequently and are addressed in detail in several texts.[18]

Symptomatic treatment is important in maintaining and improving the quality of a patient's life. For example, suppression of cerebellar tremor with clonazepam (Klonopin) 0.5 to 1.0 mg three times daily can be helpful. Prompt treatment of bladder infections and the appropriate use of intermittent catheterization is important. Agents such as propantheline (Pro-Banthine) 15 to 30 mg four times daily or oxybutynin (Ditropan) 5 mg twice daily can reduce bladder urgency. A cystometrogram, or measurement of residua after voiding, may be useful in monitoring the management of bladder symptoms. In patients with marked limb spasticity or flexor spasms, baclofen (Lioresal) can be used in doses up to 80 mg daily. The drug is better tolerated if started at the dose of 5 mg three times daily and increments made only every few days.

Results of a collaborative study support the beneficial effect of ACTH in shortening the duration of acute relapses.[17] Although the role of corticosteroids has not been definitely proven, they are widely used for treatment of acute relapses. Synthetic glucorticoids—prednisone and methylprednisolone—avoid some of the mineralocorticoid effects of ACTH and are less expensive. Table 15.18–5 gives examples of regimens used in the treatment of acute relapses.[2] There is no indication for the long-term use of either ACTH or corticosteroids.

Currently a number of clinical trials are in progress to evaluate the efficacy of such agents as interferon, plasmapheresis, and a variety of immunosuppressive agents. Copolymer I is a synthetic peptide with some homology to myelin basic protein and, in preliminary trials has demonstrated a reduction in frequency and severity of acute relapses in relapsing-remitting disease.[3] In chronic progressive MS, the category with the worst long-term outlook, there have been promising results suggesting disease stabilization after courses of high-dose intravenous cyclophosphamide plus ACTH.[7]

All these proposed treatments have limitations from side effects, expense, or patient inconvenience.[4] The use of such treatments should be restricted to closely supervised research protocols until their benefit has been demonstrated and side effects defined. The efficacy of most experimental agents is based on clinical response, which may not reflect continuing subclinical disease.

ACUTE DISSEMINATED ENCEPHALOMYELITIS

Acute disseminated encephalomyelitis (ADE) is an acute, inflammatory, demyelinating disease affecting brain and spinal cord. It is usually associated with an antecedent infection (measles, mumps, chicken pox), vaccinations (smallpox and rabies), or antiserum administration (Table 15.18–6). Pathologically, there is edema, perivascular cellular infiltration, and patchy areas of perivascular demyelination. Evidence of viral replication within the CNS is absent. Because of the temporal relationship to antecedent infection or immunization and the pathologic similarities to the animal model, experimental allergic encephalomyelitis, an immunopathogenic mechanism is likely.[9]

Clinically, the picture is quite varied, ranging from a mild malaise and headache occurring 10 to 15 days after viral infection or

---

TABLE 15.18–4. DIAGNOSIS OF MULTIPLE SCLEROSIS

• History	Relapsing/remitting symptoms Progressive symptoms
• Examination	Multifocal involvement of CNS
• CT scan MRI	Multiple plaques—particularly periventricular
• Evoked potential studies	
Visual	Evidence of delayed central conduction
Brain stem Somatosensory	Useful for detecting subclinical lesions
• Cerebrospinal fluid	
Cells	Mononuclear pleocytosis 10–20/mm³
Protein	Slightly elevated, 40–60 mg/dl
Immunoglobulin G	Elevated in 70% of clinically definite MS
Oligoclonal bands	Present in 80–90% of clinically definite MS
Myelin basic protein	Elevated in acute attacks; a nonspecific indicator of disease activity

---

TABLE 15.18–5. TREATMENT OF ACUTE RELAPSES OF MULTIPLE SCLEROSIS

A. Ambulatory patient with mild/moderate symptoms:
Prednisone: 60 mg/daily × 5 days
           40 mg/daily × 5 days
           30 mg/daily × 4 days
           20 mg/daily × 3 days
           10 mg/daily × 3 days
           10 mg/every other day × 3 doses

B. Nonambulatory patient with severe symptoms:
Methylprednisolone (Solu-Medrol) 1 g IV daily for 3–7 days depending on clinical response. Follow by tapering course of prednisone as in A, above.

TABLE 15.8–6. ACUTE DISSEMINATED ENCEPHALOMYELITIS (ADE)

	Rate per 100,000	Case Fatality Rate (%)	Major Sequelae
Exanthemata			
Measles	100	20	Frequent
Varicella	10[a]	5	10%
Rubella	20[a]	20	Very rare
Nonexanthemata			
Mumps	Rare[a]	Rare	Rare
Epstein-Barr	Rare	Rare	Rare
Influenza	Rare	Rare	Rare
Vaccinations			
Vaccinia	0.5–1600[b]	25	Common
Rabies-Semple	100–333[c]	15	Common
Influenza	?[d]	Uncommon	Rare
Measles	4[d,e]	Rare	Rare
Rabies-DEV	?[d]	12	Common
Rabies-HDCV	None[f]	0	None

[a]The exact frequency of ADE is difficult to estimate because of the frequency of toxic encephalopathy or direct infection and the paucity of autopsy-proven cases.
[b]Vaccination no longer widely used. The wide variation in incidence is unexplained.
[c]Semple neural-tissue vaccine is still widely used outside the USA.
[d]The incidence of ADE is so low as to be indistinguishable from the background rate.
[e]Duck-embryo vaccine (DEV). No longer used in the USA.
[f]Human diploid cell vaccine (HDCV) has been used in the USA since 1980. Although two cases of neuroparalytic illness have been reported, there are no documented instances of ADE.
Modified from Johnson RT, Griffin DE, Gendelman HE: Semin Neurol 5:180, 1985.[9]

vaccination to a fulminant illness with severe headache, confusion, coma, fever, and vomiting. There is a period of relatively normal health between the viral infection or vaccination and the onset of neurologic symptoms. Meningismus, focal cerebral signs, and myoclonic jerks are common. Optic neuritis, brain stem signs, and myelitis may also be present. The CSF protein is elevated with increased gamma globulin and a mononuclear pleocytosis. Recovery over several weeks is usual, although there may be residual neurologic deficits including weakness, cognitive impairment, or subtle behavioral changes. Acute hemorrhagic leukoencephalitis is a severe and fulminant variant of ADE. Most patients die within 5 days of onset or are left with severe sequelae. The CSF is often hemorrhagic.

Despite the widespread use of corticosteroids, ACTH, and gamma globulin, there is no proven effective treatment. Aggressive supportive treatment is indicated, including antipyretics, maintenance of fluid balance without exacerbating cerebral edema, and ventilatory support.

DEMYELINATING DISEASES—SECONDARY TO SYSTEMIC DISEASES

POSTANOXIC ENCEPHALOPATHY

Seven to twenty-one days following any acute hypoxic episode, a small number of patients show signs and symptoms of a progressive encephalopathy. Pathologically, the brain shows diffuse, widespread demyelination in the hemispheres, with preservation of neurons. The basal ganglia are sometimes infarcted.

The clinical picture is that of a patient who is initially comatose after the hypoxic insult but usually awakens within 24 to 48 hours. Some patients with lesser degrees of hypoxia are initially only disoriented or dazed. The patient is next normal for 7 to 21

days but then develops irritability, confusion, diffuse spasticity, and rigidity. Some patients progress to coma or death, while others make a full recovery. The mechanism of demyelination is not known, but cerebral edema may play a role.

DEMYELINATION FOLLOWING CHEMOTHERAPY OR RADIOTHERAPY

A delayed complication of methotrexate therapy is leukoencephalopathy. It occurs more frequently in patients who also receive cranial irradiation and is manifested by a progressive encephalopathy months or years after treatment. It can result from both intrathecal and systemic use of high-dose methotrexate and is not reversible by leucovorin. Rarely, a subacute demyelinating illness will develop 2 to 3 months after radiation for head and neck tumors; the pathogenesis is unclear.

DEMYELINATING DISEASES—VIRAL INFECTIONS

There are two human demyelinating diseases in which viruses play a primary role. *Progressive multifocal leukoencephalopathy* (PML) occurs in patients with immunocompetence resulting from other diseases such as sarcoidosis, tuberculosis, and neoplasms, particularly lymphomas and leukemias. An increasingly common association is with acquired immunodeficiency syndrome (AIDS) (Chapter 9.15). Immunosuppressive drugs, either steroids or cancer chemotherapy, may also be linked with the development of PML. The etiologic agent is a papovavirus, JC virus (rarely SV-40). Patients develop progressive multifocal neurologic deficits including aphasia, hemiparesis, visual loss, or ataxia. Computerized tomographic scan or MRI may be helpful in diagnosis. A brain biopsy may be indicated when differentiation is difficult. No specific treatment is available, however, except reduction of doses of immunosuppressive drugs. Antiviral agents have not been beneficial.

Subacute sclerosing panencephalitis (SSPE) occurs primarily in children, particularly those who had measles when they were less than 3 years old, and is a persistent infection with the measles virus. The interval from acute measles to SSPE is usually 3 to 9 years. The risk of SSPE is far less following measles immunization than after natural measles infection. The symptoms of dementia, seizures, myoclonus, and ataxia progress to death over months. Electroencephalography may be useful in diagnosis, showing recurring bursts of spike and slow-wave complexes. There is no cure, although the antiviral agent amantadine (Symmetrel) may slow the deterioration.

LEUKODYSTROPHIES

These are listed in Table 15.18–1. Only one, adrenoleukodystrophy, will be discussed in detail.

ADRENOLEUKODYSTROPHY

Adrenoleukodystrophy (ALD) is classified with the dysmyelinating disorders and has demonstrable biochemical abnormalities. It is an X-linked recessive disorder characterized by CNS demyelination and adrenal insufficiency.[12] Studies of linkage analysis are close to identifying the exact position on the X chromosome of the defective gene.

Classical childhood adrenoleukodystrophy presents between 4 to 8 years of age with personality change, deterioration in school performance, skin pigmentation, cortical blindness, seizures, and bilateral hemiplegia. Relentless progression to death occurs over several months or years. Immunosuppressive therapy has been unsuccessfully tried, and dietary restriction is currently under study. Pathologically there is inflammation, extensive demyelination, and

gliosis in the white matter of the cerebral cortex. The cortex of the adrenal glands is atrophic. Excessive levels of long-chain fatty acids in serum are found and accumulation of unbranched saturated or monounsaturated C24-C30 fatty acids.

Uncommon variants of ALD have been noted, including a neonatal form and an adult type (adrenomyeloneuropathy) occurring in the third decade and manifest by spastic paraparesis and mild peripheral neuropathy.

REFERENCES

1. Allen JC: The effects of cancer therapy on the nervous system. J Pediatr 93:903, 1978
2. Barnes MP, Bateman DE, et al: Intravenous methylprednisone for multiple sclerosis in relapse. J Neurol Neurosurg Psych 48:157, 1985
3. Bornstein MB, Miller AI, et al: Clinical trials of copolymer I in multiple sclerosis. Ann NY Acad Sci 436:366, 1984
4. Brown JR: Therapeutic Claims in Multiple Sclerosis. New York: National Multiple Sclerosis Society (US), 1982
5. Chiappa KH, Ropper AH: Evoked potentials in clinical medicine. N Engl J Med 306:1140, 1205, 1982
6. Ebers GC: Oligoclonal banding in MS. Ann NY Acad Sci 436:206, 1984
7. Hauser SL, Dawson DM, et al: Intensive immunosuppression in progressive multiple sclerosis: A randomized three-arm study of high-dose intravenous cyclophosphamide, plasma exchange and ACTH. N Engl J Med 308:173, 1983
8. Johnson KP, Nelson BJ: Multiple sclerosis: Diagnostic usefulness of cerebrospinal fluid. Ann Neurol 2:425, 1977
9. Johnson RT, Griffin DE, Gendelman HE: Postinfectious encephalomyelitis. Semin Neurol 5:180, 1985
10. McFarland HF, Greenstein J, et al: Family and twin studies in multiple sclerosis. Ann NY Acad Sci 436:118, 1984
11. McFarlin DE, McFarland HF: Multiple sclerosis. N Engl J Med 307:1183, 1246, 1982
12. Moser HW, Moser AE, et al: Adrenoleukodystrophy: Survey of 303 cases: Biochemistry, diagnosis, and therapy. Ann Neurol 16:628, 1984
13. Noseworthy J, Paty D, et al: Multiple sclerosis after age 50. Neurology 33:1537, 1983
14. Poser CM, Paty DW, et al: New diagnostic criteria for multiple sclerosis: Guidelines for research protocols. Ann Neurol 13:227, 1983
15. Prineas JW, Kwon EE, et al: Continual breakdown and regeneration of myelin in progressive multiple sclerosis plaques. Ann NY Acad Sci 436:11, 1984
16. Reder AT, Antel JP: Clinical spectrum of multiple sclerosis. Neurol Clin 1:573, 1983
17. Rose AS, Kuzma JW, et al: Cooperative study in the evaluation of therapy in multiple sclerosis: ACTH vs. placebo—final report. Neurology (Minneap.) 20:1, 1970
18. Scheinberg LC: Multiple Sclerosis: A Guide for Patients and Their Families. New York, Raven Press, 1984
19. Schoenberg H: Bladder and sexual dysfunction in multiple sclerosis. Neurol Clin 1:601, 1983
20. Sheldon JJ, Siddhartan R, et al: MR imaging of multiple sclerosis: Comparison with chemical and CT examinations in 74 patients. ANJR 6:683, 1985
21. Weiner HL, Hauser SL: Neuroimmunology I: Immunoregulation in neurological disease. Ann Neurol 11:437, 1982

CHAPTER 15.19
Trauma to the Head and Neck

Hamilton Moses III

Each year in the United States, about 3,000,000 individuals have significant head trauma. For those with the most serious injuries, immediate mortality is about one third, while over half have serious persisting deficits. Serious injuries to the spine are far less common (about 3 per 100,000) but are usually more severe, often devastating, and usually produce persisting disability. As with many neurologic processes, the initial manifestations may seem trivial and may not even be remembered, yet be sufficient to give rise to serious neurologic sequelae.[4]

The initial management of patients who have had neurological trauma is usually within the province of the neurosurgeon, orthopedist, or general surgeon. However, the internist and general physician are often the first to evaluate the patient after minor head trauma, or may be called upon to evaluate the manifold late effects of serious head injury, especially of chronic subdural hematoma, post-traumatic headache, seizures, and dizziness. The general physician should be familiar enough with head and spine injury to be able to answer such questions as: When should the patient be hospitalized? What clues suggest a progressive disorder? What factors influence the prognosis? What symptoms that occur late after head injury can and cannot be related to the trauma?

HEAD INJURY (Table 15.19–1)

ACUTE EFFECTS

Trauma to the head takes three forms: *blunt trauma,* which occurs in falls or blows to the head; *penetrating head wounds,* as occur with bullets; and *indirect trauma,* as in blast injury or sudden flexion-extension movements of the neck (whiplash). In all instances, forces of deformation, acceleration, and deceleration are inflicted on a relatively movable brain that is limited by the fixed skull, dura, cranial nerves, blood vessels, and brain stem. In addition, with penetrating head wounds, the missile will impart a shock wave to the brain that will cause tearing of tissue some distance from the path of the object. A review of the possible underlying stresses associated with these forces has been provided by Walker.[5]

Skull Fracture

About 70 percent of skull fractures are *linear.* The location of brain injury may directly underlie the fracture, but more often the locus is distant (contra coup) or may be diffuse. A linear fracture that crosses the groove of the middle meningeal artery or one of the dural sinuses indicates high likelihood of subsequent epidural or subdural hematoma. Fractures of the cribriform plate or base of the skull may lead to cerebrospinal fluid (CSF) rhinorrhea or otorrhea and predispose to subsequent intracranial infection, particularly with pneumococcus (see Chapter 9.11).

Depressed skull fractures are nearly always associated with direct contusion and laceration of the underlying brain; they require immediate neurosurgical elevation.

Epidural Hematoma

This entity results from the rapid accumulation of blood between the skull and the dura, usually secondary to a linear skull fracture that tears the middle meningeal artery. The classic clinical presentation is a brief period of unconsciousness at the time of the injury, followed by an interval of lucidity that is then followed by progressive drowsiness, stupor, and eventually localizing neurologic signs

TABLE 15.19–1. SEQUELAE OF HEAD TRAUMA

Acute
- Skull fracture
- Epidural hematoma
- Subdural hematoma
- Concussion
- Contusion and laceration of brain
- Subarachnoid hemorrhage
- Headache

Subacute
- Amnesia and personality changes
- Cranial nerve dysfunction
- Focal neurologic deficit including aphasia
- Subdural hematoma
- Prolonged coma
- Seizures
- Headache

Chronic
- Seizures
- Focal neurologic deficits
- Defects in memory, judgment, and personality
- Psychoneurosis
- Headache

with evidence of herniation (see Chapter 15.10). Only about half of patients follow this classic course, however. Many have just progressive somnolence leading to eventual herniation.

The diagnosis should be strongly suspected in an individual with a linear fracture who has evidence of progressive neurologic abnormalities. CT scan usually provides confirmation of the diagnosis, although occasionally arteriography may be required when CT is ambiguous. Prompt surgical evacuation of the hematoma is mandatory. Because patients with epidural hemorrhages may decompensate very rapidly, medical means of lowering increased intracranial pressure are justified in the somnolent patient while surgery is being arranged (see Chapter 4.9).

Subdural Hematoma

Subdural hematomas can be either acute or chronic. The mode of presentation of the two types is quite different.

Acute subdural hematomas are caused by venous bleeding into the subdural space, usually from a torn dural sinus or bridging

meningeal vein. Clinical presentation is usually similar to an epidural hematoma but evolves over a longer period, usually several hours or a day or two.

Plain skull films may show a fracture, but a CT scan is usually definitive. Surgical evacuation, often on an emergency basis, is indicated.

Chronic subdural hematomas are frequently overlooked and should be suspected in any patient with a history of even minor or trivial head trauma. Some patients have a clear history of head trauma, unconsciousness, recovery, and the persistence of confusion, lethargy, and neurologic findings. Such a diagnosis is not difficult to make. More commonly, however, the patient or family considers the preceding trauma so minor that they do not recall or report it. Headache of recent onset, fluctuating confusion, apathy, and dementia (or worsening of pre-existing dementia) are typical clinical presentations. Localizing neurologic deficits, such as hemiparesis, aphasia, or hemianopia, are usually *absent,* even in the presence of other major neurologic dysfunction. Eventually, herniation with signs of brain stem compression will develop.

In certain groups of patients, such as the alcoholic, the elderly demented patient, or the patient receiving anticoagulant therapy, the presence of progressive general or localized neurologic signs and symptoms should be considered secondary to a subdural hematoma until proven otherwise.

The diagnosis depends primarily on a high index of suspicion. An approach to diagnostic management and sources of confusion are indicated in Table 15.19–2.

The therapy for most subdural hematomas is surgical evacuation. Occasionally, a small hematoma in a patient without neurologic abnormalities may be treated with corticosteroids, avoiding surgery. Such patients must be followed closely for signs of progression, however, with the active participation of a neurosurgeon.

Concussion and Contusion

The term *concussion* refers to the acute loss of neurologic function following head injury without demonstrable radiographic or pathologic abnormality. Some authors limit this term to patients who have had a loss of consciousness, no matter how brief, who then subsequently fully recover. Frequently, however, the patient will note symptoms of amnesia, both retrograde and anterograde, dizziness, diplopia, and headache, immediately following head trauma; these symptoms usually improve after several days or weeks. These symptoms have been called the *syndrome of posttraumatic nervous system instability* (see below).

TABLE 15.19–2. APPROACH TO THE PATIENT WITH SUSPECTED SUBDURAL HEMATOMA

Test	Findings	Pitfalls
History	Previous trauma Dementia	May be minimal or forgotten May be ascribed to other causes
Examination	Hemiparesis Aphasia Papilledema III-nerve paresis	May be ascribed to vascular disease May be missed Difficult to elicit in an uncooperative
Skull radiographs	Shift of pineal Previous fracture	Rarely abnormal
Lumbar puncture	Increased pressure Xanthochromia Increased protein	All of these may be absent
EEG	Decreased voltage and slowing on the side of the hematoma	Often, or nonspecifically, abnormal
CT	Abnormal absorbance, fracture	May be normal, especially 1–2 wk after trauma when other studies are ambiguous
MRI	Abnormal signal	Technically often difficult in an uncooperative patient; sensitivity unknown
Arteriography	Displacement of brain away from the inner table	Definitive test; should be done bilaterally

Contusion and laceration of brain nearly invariably lead to prolonged unconsciousness, slow recovery, persisting focal neurologic signs, and a high likelihood of immediate seizures.

The duration of unconsciousness and amnesia are the most salient indicators of the degree of brain injury. The prognosis is related both to the age of the patient (children recover generally to a much greater extent than adults) and the duration of coma and amnesia. Numerical description of traumatic coma has been standardized (the Coma Score), and prognosis can be quantified in statistical terms with a high degree of reliability.[2]

MANAGEMENT OF ACUTE HEAD INJURIES

The key to management is careful *observation*. Any patient with a period of unconsciousness must be watched closely for at least 12 hours for evidence of progressive deterioration. Any patient with neurologic findings or impairment of consciousness should undergo radiologic study. Important clinical variables are summarized in Table 15.19–3. Clinical findings should be recorded on a flow chart.

During the period of observation, sedatives, narcotics, or other drugs that may alter the level of consciousness should be generally avoided. One is ill-advised to use sedatives or mydriatics unless absolutely necessary. The patient should be kept quiet and given reassurance. The sleeping patient should be aroused at hourly intervals until it becomes clear that the patient's condition is stable or improving.

The severely injured patient, in a comatose or stuporous state, should also be carefully observed with particular attention to integrity of the brain stem so that the early manifestations of herniation will be recognized (see Table 15.19–3 and Chapter 15.3).

Seizures occur in approximately 10 percent of patients. Diazepam (Valium) or paraldehyde are less likely to depress respirations than high doses of barbiturates. Phenytoin is the drug of choice for maintenance.

TABLE 15.19–3. OBSERVATIONS TO MAKE IN A PATIENT WITH HEAD INJURY

Variable	Evidence of Deterioration
Mental state	
Arousal	Persistence of defect or inability to
Awareness	perform at previously tested level
Orientation	
Speech	
Comprehension	
Abstract thinking	
Pupillary responses	
Diameter at rest	Asymmetrical dilatation at rest or
Response to light	after exposure to light
Extraocular movements	
	Evidence of a N III or N VI paresis
Motor system	
Strength	Asymmetry of response
Tone	Increase in tone
Sensory system	
Pain	Asymmetry of response
Position	Presence of a sensory level
Reflexes	
Corneal	Asymmetry of response
Tendon jerks	Changing response
Babinski	Present
Vital signs	
Blood pressure	Changes indicate brain stem compression
Pulse	
Respiration	

Cerebral edema is usually generalized and may become the most life-threatening factor. Management has been outlined in Chapter 4.9. Therapeutic barbiturate-induced coma is of possible value for the control of severe generalized edema, although its efficacy has not been universally confirmed.

SUBACUTE AND CHRONIC EFFECTS

Seizures
Seizures after head trauma are related to both the severity and location of injury.[1] In patients with closed-head injuries without prolonged coma, the incidence is about 5 percent. Conversely, in patients with penetrating wounds, particularly those involving the precentral and postcentral gyri and temporal lobes, the incidence is about 50 percent. There may be an interval of months to years between the time of injury and subsequent appearance of seizures, although most occur between 6 months and 2 years after the trauma.

The chance of posttraumatic seizures may be minimized by avoiding anoxia, promptly treating cerebral edema, and aggressively treating repetitive seizures acutely at the time of injury. Potential epileptogenic cicatrixes may be prevented by decompression, debridement of grossly damaged brain tissue, and closure of dural lacerations. There is no convincing evidence that anticonvulsant drugs given prophylactically will prevent subsequent appearance of posttraumatic seizures. The management of posttraumatic seizures is similar to that of seizures from other causes (see Chapter 15.5). Patients with focal seizures from a discrete unilateral focus are candidates for the neurosurgical removal of the traumatic scar and should have aggressive neurologic evaluation.

Defects in Memory, Judgment, and Personality[3]
Patients who have had a significant head injury may take a very long time to recover. The ultimate prognosis is difficult to judge until at least 1 to 2 years after the injury, particularly in younger patients. The severity of the initial injury, presence of focal neurologic defects, for example, hemiparesis and aphasia, prolonged duration of coma, and severe agitation during the transition to alertness are all factors that have been associated with an increased incidence of residual behavioral abnormalities. Behavioral sequelae include conceptual disorganization, motor retardation, apathy, and emotional withdrawal. In addition, deficits in memory and cognition may be paramount, producing a dementia of varying degree. Formal psychometric testing often reveals that the deficits are multifocal in nature in a pattern that can usually be distinguished from dementia associated with Alzheimer disease (see Chapter 15.4).

In addition, a group of patients is often encountered who have very prominent neurologic symptoms, especially headache, dizziness, and irritability; who have neither major behavioral abnormalities nor an overt dementia; but who may be quite severely incapacitated. This symptom complex has been called the syndrome of *posttraumatic nervous system instability*, a somewhat cumbersome term for a syndrome that has been increasingly recognized as organic in origin. Such patients are irritable, have a short attention span, have lost confidence in their ability to perform, and may be emotionally quite labile. They often avoid stressful situations in which they cannot perform adequately and may be unable to return to work or other normal daily activities. The patients' recovery can be judged by their behavior in nonstressful situations and by serial psychologic testing. Unfortunately, issues of legal compensation often cloud both the patient's and physician's judgment about recovery and actual capacity, causing considerable ambiguity about the true prognosis. Prominent anxiety and both minor and major depressions are common in patients with these less severe posttraumatic syndromes and may require specific psychotherapy and pharmacologic management (see Chapter 16.5). Important aspects of treatment also include continuing reassurance, a struc-

tured daily routine, job retraining, and both occupational and physical therapy.

Posttraumatic Vertigo

Patients may develop true vertigo with prominent nausea and vomiting but without other brain stem or neurologic symptoms following minor head injury. Trauma is one cause of benign positional vertigo, discussed in Chapter 15.7. Although symptoms may be initially severe, their occurrence gradually becomes less frequent, although they may recur at irregular intervals for many years. Abnormalities of the otolith organs have been clearly implicated in this entity.

Posttraumatic Headache

Thirty to 50 percent of patients with head injury will develop chronic or recurrent posttraumatic headaches. There is no correlation between the severity of the headache and the severity of the initial head injury, as evidenced by the presence of coma (or its duration), the presence of amnesia, signs of focal brain injury, intracranial hemorrhage, cerebral edema, or electroencephalographic abnormalities. In fact, chronic headache may be less frequent after major cerebral injury than after a minor blow. Some of the most intractable cases of posttraumatic headache occur after only trivial injury.

Posttraumatic headache may mimic any type of chronic recurring headache. It may be constant or intermittent; may involve any area of the head, for example, frontal, temporal, vertex, or occipital, alone or in any combination; and may be unilateral, bilateral, or generalized. Patients may exhibit more than one type of headache. Some describe their headaches as a "band around the head" or as "an ache located deep inside the head." The pains are described variously as aching, pressing, squeezing, expanding, burning, stabbing, pounding, or throbbing.

A variety of mechanisms are responsible for posttraumatic headache. These may operate individually or in various combinations.

1. Muscle contraction: This is the most frequent cause of chronic posttraumatic headache. It is clinically indistinguishable from chronic muscle contraction headache unrelated to trauma.
2. Vasodilatation: These are pulsating, pounding headaches; some are nonmigrainous vascular headaches, but others clearly are those of migraine. Both classic migraine and common migraine have been precipitated by head injuries; presumably a blow to the head, even though trivial under some circumstances, is capable of activating this vascular abnormality. It is not clear, however, why the process continues to malfunction for a month or longer following head injury.
3. Scar formation: A focal scar may form in the soft tissues of the head as a result of localized injury. This mechanism is especially implicated in pain that recurs at the precise site of a blow or penetrating injury. Presumably, sensory nerve endings at the site of the injury are stimulated by the scar. Headache may be intermittent or continuous with exquisite tenderness to even light pressure.
4. Blood in the extradural, subdural, or subarachnoid space: This may play a role in the headache occurring in the first few days or weeks following injury but is not likely to be responsible for those headaches lasting for months or years.
5. Hydrocephalus: Increased intracranial pressure occurs both acutely, when the awake patient may complain of headache, and after months or years. Late hydrocephalus after head injury is especially common in patients who have had traumatic subarachnoid hemorrhage. Headache, dementia, gait disturbance, long tract signs, or incontinence occurring months or years after a serious head injury should trigger search for occult hydrocephalus (see Chapter 15.10).
6. Injuries to the neck: The popular term "whiplash injury" describes the sudden hyperextension of the neck followed by hyperflexion, usually as a result of a prominent acceleration, such as a rear-end automobile collision. The headache may be limited to the occipital area, or it may spread to involve the vertex and temporal, frontal, and even the thoracic and lumbar areas as well. It is usually a dull pressure or squeezing pain with throbbing components at times. Neck pain is considerably aggravated by head movement. Exacerbation of pre-existing osteoarthritis is often a factor. In some cases the occipital nerve–vascular bundle (made up of the occipital nerve, artery, and vein) may be directly traumatized at the time of injury or may be traumatized secondarily by prolonged muscle contraction or chronic vascular dilatation. The resultant headache from this condition is called "occipital neuralgia."
7. Psychological factors: Emotional factors must be considered in assessing the posttraumatic headaches. It is generally agreed that constitution, personality, pre-existing psychological abnormalities, and stressful life situations that existed at the time of injury strongly contribute to the occurrence of both posttraumatic headache and other chronic pain states, as well as to the syndrome of posttraumatic nervous system instability.

The management of posttraumatic headache depends on the underlying pathogenic mechanism (see Chapter 15.9 for details and drug management).

Posttraumatic Meningitis

Acute meningitis, cerebritis, and brain abscess are extremely common following penetrating head injury, when a variety of organisms may be implicated. The late occurrence of meningitis, weeks or months following injury, very strongly suggests the presence of a CSF leak caused by an unrecognized fracture of the skull base. Common sites include the cribriform plate (which may or may not produce CSF rhinorrhea); the temporal bone; and the sphenoid, ethmoid, and frontal sinuses. A single episode of pneumococcal meningitis soon after head injury, or recurrent meningitis with any organism, should trigger a diligent search for the location of CSF leak. Consultation with a neurosurgeon is mandatory, and meticulous examination by an otolaryngologist is required in addition to thin-section CT using bone windows. A variety of radioisotope studies may also be useful.

Pain States

Unfortunately, patients who have been injured have often seen a number of physicians in various medical specialties, especially neurosurgeons, orthopedists, physiatrists, pain specialists, and often a psychiatrist or psychologist, in addition to an internist or general physician. Many drugs and other treatments have often been prescribed, often in inadequate doses. Furthermore, minor tranquilizers, antidepressants, anticonvulsants, and many other drugs often exacerbate many of the abnormalities in balance, memory, and mentation that are frequently most disabling. Frequently, minor or major operations will have been recommended for the relief of pain, often without success. In general, therapeutic conservatism is warranted after head and other injuries with a minimum of medications prescribed in adequate doses for a long enough period to judge therapeutic response. Fortunately, especially after minor head trauma, most pain states and the many various minor neurologic symptoms usually gradually improve, although the time required may be quite lengthy. Unfortunately, medical-legal factors often complicate judging the degree of improvement and may actually inhibit prompt recovery from symptoms. For this reason, it is wise to recommend a prompt resolution of outstanding legal issues when symptoms are prolonged.

CERVICAL SPINE INJURY[6]

Injuries to the upper spine may be devastating and are easily overlooked. Any patient with head trauma should have a coexisting injury to the upper spine excluded. When there is any question of spine injury, the head and neck should be immobilized until proper radiographic studies can be obtained. Respiratory failure and hypotension caused by severe and immediate vasodilatation are common immediately following a serious spine injury, and diagnostic confusion can at times lead to an erroneous diagnosis of myocardial infarction, internal hemorrhage, or primary respiratory failure.

Both *direct penetrating trauma* and *indirect flexion-extension* injuries may lead to myelopathy. Penetrating injuries may coexist with vertebral fracture and dislocation. Careful radiographic study is mandatory, and operative reduction and fixation are usually required. Indirect injury through flexion-extension results in secondary vascular impairment (contusion). Older patients or those with degenerative spine diseases are predisposed to cervical injuries and may have severe myelopathy as a result of even relatively minor injury.

Despite the serious neurologic disabilities associated with spinal cord trauma, the large majority of patients survive. Spine injury centers and teams conversant with special problems of spinal injury have greatly improved the outcome. Of those with paraplegia who survive the first 3 months, nearly 90 percent are alive 10 years later; of those with quadriplegia, 80 percent are alive after 10 years.

Patients with chronic spine injuries are predisposed to a number of secondary medical complications, which include decubitus ulcers with secondary sepsis due to multiple drug-resistant organisms, urinary sepsis due to neurogenic bladder and hemodynamic instability with supine hypertension, and upright hypotension. The internist should beware of these frequent complications.

REFERENCES

1. Branch CL: Post-traumatic epilepsy. In Youmans JR (ed): Neurological Surgery, vol. 4. Philadelphia, WB Saunders, 1982
2. Jennette B, Teasdale G, et al: Prognosis of patients with severe head injury. Neurosurgery 4:283, 1979
3. Levin HS, Grossman RG: Behavioral sequelae of closed head injuries. Arch Neurol 35:72, 1978
4. Walker AE: Mechanisms of cerebral trauma and the impairment of consciousness. In Youmans JR (ed): Neurological Surgery, vol. 4. Philadelphia, WB Saunders, 1982
5. Walker AE, Caveness WF, Critchley M: The Late Effects of Head Injury. Springfield, Ill, Thomas, 1969
6. White RJ, Yashon D: General care of cervical spine injuries. In Youmans JR (ed): Neurological Surgery, vol. 4. Philadelphia, WB Saunders, 1982

CHAPTER 16.1
The Place of Psychiatry in Medicine
John B. Imboden and Joseph T. Coyle

The nature of medical practice is such that physicians are inescapably involved in the diagnostic assessment and management of patients who are suffering primarily from a psychiatric disorder or whose medical illness is significantly complicated by psychiatric features. The generalist or primary care physician is apt to see far more patients with primarily emotional disorders than any other specialist.

In recent years psychiatry has acquired even greater relevance to the general practice of medicine because of the advances in the management of patients with psychiatric disorders, notably, pharmacotherapy in the treatment of schizophrenic disorders, major depression, bipolar disorder, and the anxiety disorders.

The efficacy of pharmacotherapy, together with supportive psychotherapy in the treatment of depression, has made it feasible for the internist to manage some patients with this disorder in the office while referring other patients with a more severe or unresponsive form of the illness for specialized care. Furthermore, it is common for the psychiatrist to enlist the assistance of the internist in the medical evaluation of certain patients with major emotional disorders for whom the psychiatrist is considering pharmacologic management.

Over the last two decades a policy of deinstitutionalization of patients with serious, chronic forms of mental illness has been in effect throughout the United States. Consequently, the practitioner, whether in the office or in the emergency room of a general hospital, is increasingly likely to be consulted by patients with serious psychiatric illness who are experiencing an acute exacerbation, an incidental medical disorder, or, perhaps, side effects or complications of pharmacotherapy.

For these reasons, this section includes a succinct overview of the major psychiatric disorders. Accordingly, separate chapters are devoted to schizophrenia, affective disorders, anxiety disorders, and organic mental syndromes. In addition, the diagnosis and management of psychiatric problems commonly encountered in the office, on the hospital floor, and in the emergency room are emphasized.

CHAPTER 16.2
Psychological Reactions to Serious Physical Illness
Thomas N. Wise and John B. Imboden

Serious physical illness is a major stress for anyone. The success of the patient's strategies in coping with the complex situation that disease creates is measured by his ability to tolerate treatment and to achieve maximum recovery. Generally, the individual patient reacts to his illness as a unique subjective phenomenon that adversely affects his quality of life and promotes emotional distress.[19] Thus psychological issues are important elements in serious illness, and the physician must be concerned with them if he is to provide optimum patient care.

COPING WITH THE STRESSES OF SERIOUS PHYSICAL ILLNESS

The patient with a serious illness experiences a series of phases from symptom onset, diagnosis, and treatment to rehabilitation and recovery (Table 16.2–1). He or she must recognize the existence of a problem, take the necessary steps to obtain appropriate medical help, cooperate with necessary diagnostic investigations and treatment regimens, relinquish a customary social role if hospitalized, adapt to the complexities and uncertainties of life in a modern hospital, then relinquish the "sick role" during convalescence, and finally return to a preillness position in society to the extent that recovery allows. Psychological problems may arise at any of these stages to impede proper medical care and create personal distress for the patient.[10]

Usually this entire process goes smoothly, although apprehension and depression usually occur at one time or another in the course of illness. When painful emotional disturbances do occur, careful evaluation and psychiatric management are required.

THE ONSET OF ILLNESS

An individual with serious discomfort, functional impairment, or a perceptible change in his body will usually seek medical attention unless the initial awareness of becoming ill is accompanied by overwhelming fear or a sense of hopelessness. Such fear may promote denial of the physical illness itself, "doctor shopping," or noncompliance. The woman who finds a breast mass but does not seek help because she is overwhelmed by fear exemplifies an emotional reaction that delays proper medical attention. Such anxiety and behavioral paralysis are often fostered by misinformation or by experiences with friends or family who had similar symptoms. Knowledge of the patient's ideas, hopes, and fears about the symptoms are essential to understand fully the initial reaction.

An important factor that may be implicated in delayed recognition of an illness is *denial*. Denial is a dynamic process.[24,25] There

TABLE 16.2–1. STAGES IN THE COURSE OF AN ILLNESS

Stages	Impediments
1. Recognition of disease	Denial, lack of knowledge, impairment of cognitive or sensory function
2. Obtaining treatment	Fear, economic limitations, idiosyncratic meanings of illness
3. Hospitalization	Severe regression, significant anxiety, depression, noncompliance
4. Convalescence	Prolonged dependency, reluctance to relinquish sick role

must be knowledge of the illness for the "denier" to deny. Thus, the patient with essential hypertension cannot be said to deny the disorder until the condition is diagnosed and the patient is informed of it. Not all delay in seeking medical help is based on denial. The indigent, unemployed laborer with a chronic cough may not seek medical care because of the cost of outpatient evaluation. On the other hand, the physician who is a heavy smoker and begins coughing blood-tinged sputum but does not seek medical care is either denying the importance of the symptom or is acting out a self-destructive bent. Denial is a psychological "defense" that wards off anxiety. By elucidating the fears that foster denial, strategies may be developed to minimize denial if it conflicts with medical care. Sometimes, however, denial is adaptive and does not interfere with treatment. Indeed, the patient with inoperable carcinoma, undergoing palliative radiation, may adaptively use selective denial to prevent hopelessness and despair. Such a patient may focus on the positive effects of such treatment but may not be preoccupied with the reality that curative treatment is impossible.

Certain symptoms and signs, however, are frequently not observed by the patient even though they are readily apparent to relatives and close associates. This lack of awareness occurs particularly when a slowly progressive disease process destroys higher cerebral functions or organs of perception.[19] The patient with progressive deafness may be annoyed at others for mumbling while remaining unaware of his own difficulty in hearing. Bitemporal hemianopsia, unilateral blindness, blunting of affect, and gradual intellectual deterioration are among the disabilities that may either remain unnoticed or be denied by the patient although they are readily apparent to the physician on examination.

THE MEANINGS OF ILLNESS

If the patient has been able to observe initial signs of illness, his subsequent response is determined both by what these mean to him and by his habitual mode of responding to stress. Illness is almost always perceived as a threat, but in some circumstances it can also be seen as a promise.

ILLNESS AS A THREAT

The patient usually views serious physical illness as a potential loss. The most basic fear is loss of life, but the patient may also fear being left crippled, disfigured, or in some way less of a person and therefore less valued and loved. The primacy of the threat of loss helps to explain the depressive reactions frequently seen in the physically ill. If the illness or its treatment threatens to deprive the patient of a characteristic mode of behavior or life-style that has served important defensive purposes in the preservation of self-esteem, the patient may react with extreme anxiety, followed by depression. A person who is compelled to be very independent will react differently to the limitations imposed by a myocardial infarction than the person whose approach to life is not "driven" but

is flexibly related to the ever-changing demands of reality. The adolescent, with age-appropriate needs to defy authority and gain peer approval, may be more distressed at having diabetes, with its never-ending treatment regimen, than the mature adult, for whom independence and peer acceptance are no longer emotionally charged issues. In families with limited finances or inadequate health insurance, serious illness may present the threat of economic catastrophe. At times, a patient perceives his illness as something shameful. This attitude is reminiscent of the pariah status conferred by disease in ancient times when illness was regarded as a punishment.

ILLNESS AS A PROMISE

Illness may be welcomed by the individual for whom it provides an avenue of escape from a difficult situation. The prospect of being free of responsibilities and of being cared for may be viewed very positively by a person who has intense dependency needs.

The shades and nuances of the meaning of being seriously ill are by no means exhausted by this brief discussion. The sensitive physician will always want to ascertain the context in which the patient's illness developed and, through the establishment of rapport and trust, encourage the patient to communicate his feelings and expectations.

DIAGNOSIS AND TREATMENT

Once the patient seeks initial evaluation, there is usually a diagnostic period during which various examinations and tests are performed. The patient may be sent for consultation to specialists with whom he has no prior relationship. During this stage of unavoidable uncertainty some degree of anxiety and depression can develop with difficulty in concentration, irritability, and insomnia. The patient may wish to avoid tests such as computerized tomography or studies that are embarrassing, such as barium enemas, owing to fears of discomfort as well as anxiety about what the investigation will discover.

When a diagnosis has been made, the physician must discuss with the patient its meaning and implications for treatment and recovery. Patients often do not fully comprehend medical terminology, especially when anxious. Thus, explanations using simplified terms and diagrams can be most helpful. Allowing the patient time to ask questions is mandatory. When the diagnosis is grave, every patient must be given hope and assurance that he will receive adequate treatment to alleviate pain and suffering. If an illness is terminal, the physician must understand the patient's personality to inform him of the status of his condition. This does not mean deceiving the patient but rather giving him information in a manner that he can best manage both intellectually and emotionally.

HOSPITALIZATION

Many serious illnesses are evaluated and managed in a hospital setting, which has its own unique stresses. It is a rare person who does not experience some degree of both fear and depression upon entering the hospital.[23] The reasons for this are numerous:

Separation. Separation from family and friends promotes loneliness and fear. The hospitalized patient is deprived of his usual sources of satisfaction and familiar surroundings.

The Peculiarities of Hospital Life. The hospitalized patient is confronted with the prospect of placing himself almost totally in the care of people who, with the exception of his personal physician, are apt to be complete strangers. Further, he is subjected to a number of procedures that have a "leveling" effect: Certain personal belongings are removed for safekeeping; he is tagged with a wrist-

band and clothed in a short white gown more or less open in the back; he endures repeated history-taking and physical examination by house staff and students, has various body orifices inspected and probed, is carted around by wheelchair or stretcher for radiographs or tests, and, in general, is in a relatively passive position of having things done to him that he does not understand by people who are often in a hurry and who may seem to him to be concerned with patients who are more ill than he.

Uncertainty. There is always some degree of uncertainty in the patient's mind regarding the danger to life and limb, duration of hospital stay, likelihood of suffering, and ultimate outcome of his hospital experience.[18]

Regression. During the course of hospitalization, the seriously ill patient almost invariably undergoes some degree of regression. Regression is defined as return to earlier modes of behavior that are immature. Behavioral symptoms of regression are varied: irritability, inappropriate jocularity, withdrawal, extreme passivity, and demandingness. The actual dependency inherent in hospitalization combined with intense anxiety promotes regression, and some degree of it is both inevitable and temporarily helpful. Extreme regressive symptoms and behaviors, however, often herald the emergence of a psychiatric disorder that demands immediate treatment. Excessive regression is clearly demonstrated when a cooperative, sensible patient becomes excessively dependent and demanding, seems constantly to need someone to do something for him, and is unduly upset by minor provocations. The development of an organic brain syndrome is often accompanied by severe anxiety and regression, since the patient does not have his usual cognitive ability to cope with unfamiliar surroundings.

PSYCHOLOGICAL REACTIONS TO TREATMENT

In addition to the nuances of the actual hospital environment, diagnostic tests and treatments may stress the patient. Pain from venipuncture or fear of contagion may foster anxiety. Pain and nausea postoperatively enhance both anxiety and depression. The side effects of medications can cause a number of psychological symptoms. For example, some antihypertensive drugs may precipitate depression.[13] Corticosteroids may promote anxiety and insomnia.[15] Nausea from antineoplastic medications or pruritic rashes from allergic reactions can create dysphoric states. The cognitive impairment from a delirium secondary to medication may create misperceptions and anxiety in the patient who finds himself confused and disoriented.

SPECIAL SITUATIONS IN THE HOSPITAL

THE INTENSIVE CARE UNIT

Advances in medical technology have allowed the development of intensive care units, specifically equipped and staffed to provide lifesaving care for patients with acute myocardial infarction and other life-threatening conditions. As valuable as these units are, they may present significant psychological hazards to the patient. The patient is surrounded by complicated, sometimes frightening equipment; he may be immobilized, isolated from other people, and forced to endure long periods of sleep deprivation. He may hear other patients moaning or rambling incoherently, and he may observe or infer that a patient has died. It is relatively rare for patients in the intensive care unit to complain of anxiety or depression, but it is not rare for them to experience it.[6] Tremulousness, restlessness, palmar sweating, and talkativeness should alert the physician to the possibility of an anxiety reaction. Depression may be manifested by sad facies, disinterest, pessimism, slow speech,

and tearfulness. Delirium is demonstrated by fear, disorientation, incoherent speech, memory impairment, and sometimes visual hallucinations.

HEMODIALYSIS

The psychological stresses involved in chronic renal insufficiency requiring hemodialysis include (1) the individual's forced dependence upon the dialysis machine,[14] (2) the restrictive treatment schedule and strict dietary limitations, and (3) the experience of chronic fatigability or weakness. Feelings of depression, resentment, and intolerance of treatment may occur. As in other conditions, an individual's past history of coping will frequently indicate how well he will tolerate this difficult form of treatment. A sensible past dietary pattern, good work history, family support, and religious convictions all appear to be factors positively correlated with successful adaptation to the treatment regimen.[28]

SURGERY

Various surgical procedures can create psychological distress.[7,8] Cosmetic surgery such as rhinoplasty can result in difficult psychologic reactions if the individual's expectations are not met.[17] It is imperative, before deciding upon such surgery, to evaluate fully the patient's reasons for the procedure so that any unrealistic expectations may be discovered and corrected.

Other surgical procedures, particularly those involving sexual organs or disfigurement, can also create psychologic distress. Hysterectomies can precipitate depressive reactions in women who have precarious self-esteem.[20] Mastectomies also necessitate readjustment to an altered body image.[16] It has been noted that men frequently report sexual dysfunction following colostomy. Sexual dysfunction is usually organic after operations for carcinoma but may have a purely psychological basis in individuals with ulcerative colitis or regional ileitis, in which surgery does not interrupt nerve pathways to the genital system.[2]

CONVALESCENCE

During convalescence the patient is expected to relinquish the "sick role" and to return to normal duties and responsibilities.[10] This time is comparable to the transitional period of adolescence in that the patient is expected to remain cooperative with those taking care of him while at the same time becoming more independent of them. Among the factors influencing the convalescent process are the presence of "secondary gains," emotional illness, and the life situation to which the patient is returning.

"Secondary gain" refers to psychological or material gains associated with illness. In general, the longer the patient has been incapacitated, the more difficult it is to give up the gratification of regression and dependency. The "sick role" protects the person who feels inadequate from premorbid anxiety-provoking situations. More obvious gains associated with illness may result from financial compensation, pending litigation, and excessive attention from solicitous relatives.

Specific psychiatric syndromes may retard symptomatic recovery. Patients with conversion reactions unconsciously simulate physical illness; the depressed patient may complain of fatigue, weakness, and symptoms that may resemble those of the illness from which he is recovering.[11,29] The patient's attitudes toward recovery are also strongly influenced by his perception of the situations of his life to which he is returning. A stormy marital relationship, indebtedness, difficulties at work, and other troublesome situations may arouse considerable dread and anxiety in the convalescent patient.

EVALUATION AND MANAGEMENT

The foregoing discussion suggests that the variables helping to determine the patient's psychological reaction to serious illness fall into several categories: characteristics of the illness and its treatment, the life setting or psychosocial context in which the illness occurs, and the character of the patient. All these variables need to be taken into account when the physician assesses the patient's psychological reaction to illness and undertakes management of reactions that complicate the patient's illness.

An immediate tactical objective of management is to achieve a relationship in which the patient not only feels trust and confidence in the technical skill of the physician but also feels free to reveal feelings, fears, worries, and problems. An individual who is seriously ill, especially when hospitalized, finds himself unusually dependent upon others, particularly the physician. This dependence upon others for comfort and survival often evokes some measure of anxiety, more in some people than in others. This anxiety is partially allayed if the patient imputes to the physician the omniscient and omnipotent qualities reminiscent of those of his parents when he was dependent upon them as a small child. This displacement of feelings and attitudes from important childhood relationships to someone in the present such as the physician has been called "transference." It is not uncommon for a patient to be convinced that his physician is infallible, although he may in fact know very little about him. This type of transference, so commonly seen, is useful to the patient, and the physician does well simply to accept it.

There may, however, be transference reactions of a negative nature. Warning clues to this type of transference are obtained when the patient, in relating his history, is excessively critical of other physicians who have cared for him in the past. It may not be possible to prevent the development of negative transference, especially if the patient is excessively threatened by authority figures, even if they have the professional competence of a physician. Nevertheless, if the patient becomes resentful and critical, it is important to assess the possibly realistic justification for his feelings. If such an assessment leads to the conclusion that the patient's negative criticisms are overdone, it is likely that transference distortion is operative. Recognition of this fact helps the physician to be more tolerant of the patient's feelings and to engage him in discussion of them. As a rule, however, it is not helpful to attempt to interpret the origins of transference feelings to the patient.

When confronted with denial of illness or one of its features, the physician should proceed cautiously. If the denial is interfering with compliance to essential treatment, it may be necessary to point out tactfully aspects of the situation that are essential for the patient to understand. It may also be necessary to modify the treatment regimen to conform with the patient's ability to accept his situation. In an initial confrontation with adversity, some degree of denial may be useful, giving the time to muster resources and to prepare for what lies ahead.[9]

The observation of certain personality features in the patient gives the physician a basis for tailoring the approach to the patient's individual needs.[12] The controlled, intellectual, obsessive individual generally responds well to being given facts and explanations. Such a person should be allowed the opportunity to ask questions or to settle various possibilities and doubts that may have arisen. On the other hand, the excited, "hysterical" individual responds to an opportunity to ventilate feelings, yet needs supportive, matter-of-fact reassurance. He, too, needs to be informed, but at his own pace. In dealing with suspicious or paranoid persons, it is important to avoid incomplete or ambiguous messages; clear communication is essential. If one observes some overt evidence of distress, it may be necessary to engage the patient in open discussion of this matter. The schizoid individual is not particularly apt to pose a problem in management, but one should respect his need for privacy. The independent individual who is threatened by the prospect of immobilization and dependency may require

discussion of his conflict with the treatment regimen; it is often best to settle for a modified or compromise plan of treatment.

The individual who fulfills the criteria for a "borderline" personality disorder can create particular havoc on a medical or surgical unit.[4,5] These individuals may exhibit severe denial; intense feelings, especially of a hostile sort; and impulsive behavior. Under the stress of illness and hospitalization they may regress to transient psychotic episodes. These patients tend to react to staff members as though they were divided into "good" and "bad" groups and may stimulate disagreement among members of the treating team through manipulative behavior. Thus, open communication among the staff must be maintained so that the patient receives clear and unconflicting information. Firm, nonpunitive limits must also be set by the staff to control impulsive and hostile behavior. Making the patient aware that the staff acknowledges his distress because of his illness can help him to moderate his emotional reactions. The staff, however, should not attempt to gratify the patient's wish for dependency but should be aware that such an individual often feels entitled to special treatment, which may try the patience of the treating staff. Recognition of these dependent and manipulative behaviors and understanding the style of the borderline patient can help the physician to deal with these individuals early in treatment and to prevent complicated emotional difficulties.

In ambulatory settings, noncompliance is a major problem limiting effective care.[21] The various elements that contribute to noncompliance include an overly complex treatment plan, financial problems, lack of understanding, fear of side effects, and problems in the physician-patient relationship.[22] To enhance compliance systematically the physician should simplify drug regimens when possible and warn of possible side effects. The patient on a low-sodium diet may need instruction on alternative condiments to promote more pleasing taste. The construction worker whose low-back pain prevents work will need vocational retraining. If the patient's life situation is a complicating issue that is worrisome to the patient, it is often helpful not only to encourage the patient to discuss it but also to consult with members of the family who may be of help. The medical social worker is often of considerable assistance when the patient is apprehensive and feels helpless or guilty about family, financial, or occupational problems. Identification of psychiatric syndromes that impede compliance is important. The management of specific psychiatric syndromes is discussed in subsequent chapters.

REFERENCES

1. Balint M: The Doctor, His Patient and the Illness. New York, International Universities Press, 1972
2. Druss RG, O'Connor JF, et al: Psychological response to colectomy. Arch Gen Psychiatr 18:53, 1968
3. Engel GL: The clinical application of the biopsychosocial model. Am J Psychiat 137:535, 1980
4. Groves JE: Management of the borderline patient on a medical or surgical ward. Int J Psychiatr Med 6:337, 1975
5. Groves JE: Taking care of the hateful patient. N Engl J Med 298:883, 1978
6. Hackett TP, Cassem NH, Wishnie H: Detection and treatment of anxiety in the coronary care unit. Am Heart J 78:727, 1969
7. Hackett TP, Weisman AD: Psychiatric management of operative syndromes I. Psychosom Med 22:267, 1960
8. Hackett TP, Weisman AD: Psychiatric management of operative syndromes II. Psychosom Med 22:356, 1960
9. Hamburg DA, Adams JE: A perspective on coping behavior. Seeking and utilizing information in major transitions. Arch Gen Psychiatr 17:277, 1967
10. Imboden JB: Psychosocial determinants of recovery. Adv Psychosom Med 8:142, 1972
11. Imboden JB, Canter A, Cluff LE: Convalescence from influenza. Arch Intern Med 108:393, 1961
12. Kahana RJ, Bibring GL: Personality types in medical management. In

Zinberg NE (ed): Psychiatry and Medical Practice in the General Hospital. New York, International Universities Press, 1964, p 108

13. Klerman GL: Depression in the medically ill. Psychiatr Clin North Am 4:301, 1981
14. Levy NB: Psychological reactions to machine dependency. Hemodialysis. Psychiatr Clin North Am 4:351, 1981
15. Lewis DA, Smith RE: Steroid induced psychiatric syndromes. J Affect Dis 5:319, 1983
16. Lewis FM, Bloom JR: Psychosocial adjustment to breast cancer. Int J Psych Med 9:1, 1978–79
17. Meyer E, Jacobson WE, et al: Motivational patterns in patients seeking elective plastic surgery. Psychosom Med 22:193, 1960
18. Meyer E, Mendelson M: Psychiatric consultations with patients on medical and surgical wards: Patterns and processes. Psychiatry 24:197, 1961
19. Reading AJ: Illness and disease. Med Clin North Am 61:703, 1977
20. Roeske NCA: Quality of life and factors affecting the response to hysterectomy. J Fam Prac 7:483, 1978
21. Sackett DL, Haynes RB (eds): Compliance with Therapeutic Regimens. Baltimore, Johns Hopkins Press, 1976

22. Stoudemire A, Thompson TL: Medication noncompliance: Systematic approaches to evaluation and intervention. Gen Hosp Psychiatr 5:233, 1983
23. Strain JJ, Grossman S: Psychological Care of the Medically Ill: A Primer in Liaison Psychiatry. New York, Appleton-Century-Crofts, 1975, p 23
24. Weinstein EA, Kahn RL: Denial of Illness. Springfield, Ill, Charles C Thomas, 1955
25. Weisman AD, Hackett TP: Denial as a social act. In Levin S, Kahana SJ (eds): Psychodynamic Studies on Aging. New York, International Universities Press, 1967, p 79
26. Weisman AD: Coping behavior and suicide in cancer. In Cullen JW, Fox BH, Isom RN (eds): Cancer: The Behavioral Dimensions. New York, Raven, 1976, p 331
27. Wise TN: The emotional reactions of chronic illness. Prim Care 1:373, 1974
28. Wise TN: Pitfalls of diagnosing depression in chronic renal disease. Psychosomatics 15:83, 1974
29. Ziegler FJ, Imboden JB: Contemporary conversion reactions: II. A conceptual model. Arch Gen Psychiatr 6:279, 1962

CHAPTER 16.3
Psychiatric Emergencies

John B. Imboden
and John Chapman Urbaitis

Psychiatric emergency refers to any serious mental or emotional disorder that requires prompt intervention. A variety of conditions may arouse alarm in the patient himself as well as in others.[3,12] One of the most common emergencies is posed by the patient who has made a suicide attempt or who is judged to be in danger of doing so. Acute behavioral disturbances of an emergent nature include violent or assaultive behavior and sudden or recent changes in behavior associated with delirious or other psychotic states. Patients in a state of panic frequently have a fear of impending heart attack or death and seek the assistance of the emergency room physician.

THE SUICIDAL PATIENT

Few occurrences evoke a more intense welter of emotions in relatives and physicians than suicide. In fact, the physician, as a person dedicated to the alleviation of suffering and the preservation of life, often must come to grips with the intense ambivalence aroused in himself by a suicide attempt if he is to approach the patient with the same compassion and objectivity that he exercises in other medical emergencies.

In potential suicide and attempted suicide, the physician's difficult task is to determine the seriousness and immediacy of the current danger to the patient's life. Evaluation of suicidal risk and the associated psychiatric illness includes the assessment of a variety of personal, interpersonal, and circumstantial variables. This process usually necessitates interviews with relatives and friends as well as with the patient.

The assessment of suicidal risk can in certain instances be relatively easy; in others, it can be all but impossible. A number of statistical studies have revealed that certain variables are consistently correlated with the rate of completed suicides in the general population. Those variables which are positively correlated with suicide rate include being male, white, middle-aged or older, alcoholic, Protestant, single, and having a history of a previous suicide attempt and a history of suicide in the family. Knowledge of these variables is of limited use to the clinician who is dealing with an individual patient but may be of some value if used in conjunction with the total clinical picture.[1,2,13]

THE POTENTIAL SUICIDAL RISK

Among both completed and attempted suicides, the most commonly made diagnosis is depression.[4,7] It is therefore important to be alert to depressive illness in any patient and, if it is found, to assess the suicidal risk.[9] Affective disorders are discussed in Chapter 16.5. It is common for a depressed patient to focus primarily on physical symptoms and to rationalize his depressed mood as being secondary to them. In such cases the diagnosis may be easily missed.[5]

Once the diagnosis of depression is made, the assessment of suicidal danger is based upon the severity of the depression, the presence of hopelessness and guilt, prior history of suicide attempts, and present suicidal thoughts and intentions.

In the general adult population the incidence of relatively mild, transient periods of depressed mood is extremely high, perhaps universal. If, however, the degree of mood change is moderately severe and accompanied by other symptoms such as somatic complaints, insomnia, psychomotor retardation, anorexia, decrease in interest, and decreased ability to experience pleasure, the patient can be regarded as suffering from a depressive condition of significant severity.

In persons suffering from affective disorders, the lifetime risk of suicide has been estimated to be 15 percent. Although there are numerous exceptions, there is some correlation between severity of depression and suicidal risk. Paradoxically, however, apparent symptomatic improvement in the course of the illness does not necessarily mean that the risk of suicide has decreased. Some patients may seem to have improved because they have secretly made a decision to kill themselves, while others, who had been functionally incapacitated by severe depression, may become better able to carry out a suicide plan as their depression begins to lift.

The patient who feels that his future is bleak, his problems insoluble, his illness incurable, and that he is not worthy of relief

or of any other good fortune represents a greater suicidal risk than a person who, although depressed, has a hopeful outlook regarding his future. A hopeful, but nonetheless depressed, patient may make casual reference to future plans, thus implying that he intends to be around. A history of previous suicide attempts increases the probability that another attempt will be made.

A common error in dealing with a suspected suicidal patient is failure to ask him directly about his wishes and intentions regarding death and suicide. All depressed patients, at one time or another, probably feel a wish to die and have thoughts of suicide. It is important, however, to ask the patient directly if he has been preoccupied with death and suicidal thoughts, and if he has, whether he has actually intended to commit suicide. If the response to this inquiry is in the affirmative, the patient should also be asked to describe the method contemplated, whether he has procured the means to carry out the act, and other details.

The potentially suicidal patient may have an illness other than primary depression. In fact, any condition or situation that has resulted in a feeling of hopelessness may be associated with the danger of suicide. For example, persons confronted with public exposure of unethical behavior or evidence of incompetence or individuals with progressive, incurable disease may choose death in preference to a future that is perceived as laden with unbearable misery. The schizophrenic patient may attempt suicide in a moment of despair or in response to a hallucinated command. The delirious patient, while not necessarily intending suicide, may seriously or fatally injure himself in a variety of ways, such as leaving the room via a window. Alcoholism, especially if associated with depressive illness, increases the risk of suicide.

In the event that the physician has judged that the suicidal risk is grave, this should be discussed openly with the patient and his next of kin. Psychiatric consultation should be obtained without delay. There may be circumstances in which the physician decides upon immediate hospitalization and institution of suicidal observation while awaiting psychiatric consultation. In any event, precautions should be taken to prevent suicide until definitive therapy has taken effect. Management of associated illness, such as depression, schizophrenic illness, delirium, or alcoholism, should be initiated immediately.

THE SUICIDE ATTEMPT

In addition to the immediate medical or surgical management necessitated by the attempt itself, the physician must assess the seriousness of suicidal intent. To assist him in carrying out this assessment, it is advisable, for both clinical and legal reasons, to obtain the assistance of a psychiatric consultant.

Routine psychiatric hospitalization in every case of attempted suicide is impractical and probably unwise. The incidence of attempted suicides is conservatively estimated to be more than ten times that of completed suicides. The rate of attempted suicides (in contrast to completed suicides) is higher among women than men and reaches its peak in the third decade of life. These statistical differences, coupled with the fact that many persons who complete suicide have made previous attempts, suggest that although the attempted-suicide group is heterogeneous, it contains eventual members of the "completed" group; that is, as the members of the attempted-suicide group age, they contribute substantially to the completed-suicide group. The risk of suicide in the attempted-suicide group has been estimated at approximately 1 to 2 percent per year.[13]

In assessing the seriousness of intent, the principles regarding the depressed patient also apply to the suicidal one. In addition, it is helpful to take into account the lethality of the attempt, the circumstances surrounding it, precipitating factors, and consequences.

LETHALITY OF THE ATTEMPT

This refers to the danger to life posed by the act itself regardless of any mitigating circumstances. For example, the ingestion of a large number of barbiturate capsules and self-inflected gunshot wounds to the head or chest are highly lethal acts, whereas an overdose of chlordiazepoxide and superficial lacerations are not. If the attempt is judged to be highly lethal, that is, if death probably would have ensued in the absence of timely intervention, it is best to presume that the suicidal intent was extremely serious and remains so in the immediate postattempt period. This is a practical policy, even though it is recognized that an occasional patient may not be aware of the relative dangerousness of one type of attempt as opposed to another, for example, the lethality of barbiturate versus chlordiazepoxide overdosage. Obviously, the converse is not true: Low lethality does not necessarily point to low seriousness of intent.

SURROUNDING CIRCUMSTANCES

The following circumstances are positively correlated with seriousness of intent:

1. Being alone at time of attempt
2. Actively taking precautions against being discovered
3. Not anticipating rescue
4. Evidence of premeditation, such as a suicide note, recent increase in life insurance, recently written will, and acquisition of material or equipment specifically needed for the attempt

PRECIPITATING FACTORS

The attempt may have arisen out of hopelessness and guilt as part of a depressive illness or in association with some other illness or life situation. Not infrequently, however, the patient makes a suicide attempt, even a dangerous one, to bring about a change in his life. For example, the attempt may well be a "cry for help," an effort to arouse sympathetic concern by others or to change the direction in which an important relationship has been going. The attempt may be designed to punish someone, symbolically or actually, by evoking guilt. It may be an attempt to punish oneself.

It is therefore important to review with the patient what was going on in his life and in his mind at the time of the attempt. The patient should be asked if he had felt that the attempt would result in death. Had he thought that he might live, but that his life would be different? If so, how? Had he been angry and wanting to "get even" with someone? Had he felt guilty and that he deserved to be punished? Had he wanted to die?

CONSEQUENCES

A key question is, Does it appear that the suicide attempt will be followed by significant changes in the patient or in his circumstances? If the physician has been able to gauge the patient's original purposes, feelings, and expectations before the attempt, he may be able to ascertain its psychological and interpersonal results. For example, if one infers that the patient had sought to be less isolated, to be more accepted by family, to get help for his problems or his depression, does the attempt seem to achieve these goals? Does the patient seem unsurprised, perhaps even glad, that he is still alive? Does he seem to feel less guilty than before the attempt? Or did the suicide attempt achieve nothing as far as the patient is concerned? Does he now feel even less adequate and more isolated than before? Did he "wake up" to find a sullen, resentful spouse and an emergency room staff too harried with "real" emergencies to be very concerned with him?

All the above categories of factors have to be weighed in forming a decision as to the seriousness of intent and the continuing danger of suicide.

MANAGEMENT

It is wise to obtain psychiatric consultation for the patient who has made a suicide attempt or who is suspected of being at risk to harm

himself. If the patient is judged to be an imminent or serious suicide risk, psychiatric hospitalization is indicated with subsequent treatment of the depression or other associated psychiatric illness. In those instances where psychiatric hospitalization does not appear to be mandatory, outpatient psychiatric treatment should be recommended. Where feasible, it is helpful to include the patient's spouse or other close relatives in the planning of treatment so as to increase the likelihood of obtaining the patient's cooperation.

ACUTE BEHAVIORAL DISTURBANCES

More often than not, the patient who engages in aggressive, inappropriate, bizarre, or otherwise disturbing behavior does not seek medical attention on his own initiative because he is unaware of the abnormality of his behavior, unconcerned about it, or both. He may therefore be brought to the emergency room by a concerned relative or friend or by the police.

Acute behavioral disturbances may be characterized by one or more of the following:

1. Recent development of impulsive behavior or behavior that is "out of character" for the patient
2. Aggressive or violent behavior
3. Excessive activity, verbal or nonverbal
4. Inactivity, withdrawal
5. Bizarre, silly, or "crazy" behavior
6. Behavior characterized by evidence of confusion

THE VIOLENT PATIENT[6,11]

Although the diagnostic considerations that arise in the evaluation of violent behavior do not essentially differ from those of other kinds of disturbing behavior, the violent patient does require certain immediate steps. As with acute anxiety or panic, diagnosis and therapeutic management go hand in hand.

The excited, threatening, or combative patient instills fear in everyone in contact with him, including the physician. It is useful to assume that the patient himself is afraid of losing control of his own aggressive impulses. Thus, the physician attempts to establish verbal contact with the patient by assuring him that the physician and staff are there to help him. It may be useful to ask the patient what sorts of problems or fears concern him most. If the patient is too excited to be able to engage in conversation or if focusing on troubling problems seems to increase his emotional disturbance, it is wise not to press the issue. If the patient is actively excited or aggressive and does not respond to reassurance, it is important to have four or five male staff members present to place the patient in seclusion and, if necessary, in restraints under the supervision of the physician. The patient in locked seclusion or in restraints should be monitored regularly and frequently. As will be noted below, chemotherapy may be indicated to reduce excitement or aggressive behavior. In dealing with the actively or potentially assaultive patient it is important to ensure that neither the patient nor anyone in contact with the patient has any weapons on his person.

DIAGNOSTIC EVALUATION OF ACUTE BEHAVIORAL DISTURBANCE

A variety of behavior patterns may alarm the family and prompt them to seek immediate medical attention. A useful diagnostic approach is to determine if the acute behavioral disturbance is organic or functional, then to proceed toward a more specific diagnostic entity.

In general, acute disturbances of behavior in which organic factors play a major etiologic role, such as delirium or toxic psychosis, are associated with evidence of impaired intellectual functions: memory impairment, disorientation, rambling and incoherent speech, and difficulty in comprehension and abstract thinking.[10] In the hallucinating patient, a predominance of visual hallucinations favors an organic basis, although it may be a feature in early, acutely developing schizophrenic decompensation. A history of "spells" or repeated, discrete episodes of behavioral disturbance, with or without amnesia, may indicate a seizure disorder. The medical history should be carefully reviewed. Insulin-induced hypoglycemic reactions, for example, can be associated with confusional states and bizarre behavior. Careful review of the alcohol and drug history (including prescribed drugs, over-the-counter drugs, and illicit drugs) is important to determine the possibility of intoxication or withdrawal syndromes. The withdrawal syndrome associated with alcohol, benzodiazepines, or other central nervous system (CNS) depressants may be associated with marked confusion, hallucinations, excitement, and fear. Intoxication with drugs such as phencyclidine and amphetamines can produce psychotic states, excitement, and aggressive behavior.

Evidence in favor of an organic condition may indicate the need for prompt chemical determinations of blood and urine, skull radiograph, computed tomographic scan of head, electroencephalogram, repeated neurologic examination, and other diagnostic procedures.

The diagnostic characteristics of schizophrenic illness and manic states are discussed in Chapters 16.5 and 16.6. In general, these disorders are not associated with the type of intellectual impairment that produces defective recent memory and disorientation. Careful examination and judgment, however, may be required to determine that the patient has a clear sensorium. For example, the schizophrenic patient may give a bizarre response when asked to state where he is. Later in the interview he may indicate, in response to a more oblique inquiry, that he is clearly aware of his location. The severely depressed patient, or any patient who is self-absorbed and preoccupied, may appear to have a poor memory for recent events. For example, he may not recall what he had for breakfast because he was too preoccupied to have noticed.

MANAGEMENT

It is wise to obtain prompt psychiatric consultation in all cases of acute behavioral disturbance, including those in which an organic component is strongly suspected.

If the acute behavioral disturbance is based upon an organic condition, hospitalization is mandatory to manage the patient safely while the specific nature of the organic or toxic factors is being determined. Delirious patients must be carefully observed. Confusion and the likelihood of panic can be reduced, especially at night, by keeping the room well lighted; having a trained person in constant attendance; addressing the patient in clear, simple terms; and otherwise avoiding ambiguous environmental cues.

The patient's behavior may necessitate the temporary use of chemotherapeutic agents to allow further examination. If there is evidence of drug intoxication, it is desirable to choose an agent that will not adversely interact with the intoxicant, such as augmenting anticholinergic effects. Among the antipsychotic agents, haloperidol may be useful, as it has relatively little anticholinergic action compared with high-dose phenothiazines. Haloperidol may be administered in 5 mg doses intramuscularly, repeated in 1 or 2 hours for three or four doses, if necessary. Careful observation of the patient and monitoring of vital signs should be done when a relatively high dosage of antipsychotic medication is employed in these circumstances. The benzodiazepines, given orally or parenterally, may also be used in this circumstance, especially if the nature of the toxic drug is uncertain or if there is concern about drug interaction. The chemotherapeutic management of central nervous system–depressant withdrawal syndrome is discussed in Chapter 16.9.

Usually it is necessary to hospitalize the patient with acute functional psychosis who presents to the emergency room in a state of excitement or uncontrolled behavior. A patient who is not

suicidal or homicidal, responds well to the intramuscular administration of antipsychotic agents while under observation for several hours, and has one or more responsible relatives to care for him, may benefit from outpatient psychiatric treatment, initially on a daily basis.

SEVERE ANXIETY OR PANIC[8]

Regardless of the cause, all states of acute, severe anxiety are characterized by intense fear, restlessness, and various other symptoms and signs such as palpitations, a feeling of suffocating, blurring of vision, tachycardia, pallor, and sweating. The patient's fear commonly becomes localized or specific, for example, fear of death through suffocation or cardiac arrest, or of "going crazy." Sometimes the source of danger is projected onto the external world.

The most common conditions associated with severe acute anxiety or panic are anxiety disorder, a "bad trip" with a hallucinogenic agent, acute phase of a schizophrenic illness, amphetamine intoxication, and delirium.

Diagnosis and treatment of the acute attack must be managed in parallel. Having established the presence of acute anxiety, the physician should matter-of-factly discuss that finding with the patient. While acknowledging the patient's extreme discomfort, he should reassure him about specific fears, for example, that his condition will not cause his heart to stop. He should also reassure the patient that his fearfulness itself has momentarily affected his judgment. Usually, a patient with anxiety disorder will respond to sympathetic attention, reassurance, and an opportunity to discuss his feelings with the physician. The abatement of symptoms should provide evidence that the patient is not psychotic. In panic disorder, the patient may have a history of previous attacks.

If the panic state is part of a psychotic condition, the patient does not usually respond to psychological support as readily as the neurotic patient. As a general rule, acute schizophrenic illness and amphetamine intoxication are associated with a clear sensorium. The latter closely simulates paranoid schizophrenia and can be diagnosed definitively only by obtaining a history of excessive amphetamine ingestion. The "bad trip" resulting from ingestion of a hallucinogen may be associated with extreme anxiety. The patient will often reveal his drug history, particularly if the importance of doing so is explained to him. He may or may not be disoriented. Delirium from any cause may be associated with extreme fear. Chapter 16.5 presents further discussion of the differential diagnosis of anxiety disorders.

MANAGEMENT

Psychiatric consultation should be obtained. Chemotherapeutic intervention is often necessary in panic associated with psychosis, whether functional or toxic. The choice of drug is based upon the considerations mentioned in management of the violent patient and is discussed further in Chapter 16.6. Phenothiazines are usually not employed in treating intoxication with hallucinogenic substances. If the anxiety state is associated with an organic or toxic psychosis, hospitalization is indicated. In the event of functional psychosis, the decision to hospitalize is based upon the same factors discussed in the management of acute behavioral disturbances. For management of panic disorder, see Chapter 16.5.

REFERENCES

1. Beck AT, Resnik H, et al: The Prediction of Suicide. Bowie, Md, Charles Press Publishers, 1974
2. Dublin LI: Suicide. A Sociological and Statistical Study. New York, Ronald Press, 1963
3. Gerson S, Bassuk E: Psychiatric emergencies: An overview. Am J Psychiatr 137:1, 1975
4. Guze SB, Robins E: Suicide and primary affective disorders. Br J Psychiatr 117:437, 1970
5. Leeman CP: Diagnostic errors in emergency room medicine: Physical illness in patients labelled "psychiatric" and vice versa. Int J Psychiatr Med 6:553, 1975
6. Rada RT: The violent patient: Rapid assessment and management. Psychosomatics 22:101, 1981
7. Robins E, Gassner S, et al: The communication of suicidal intent: A study of 134 consecutive cases of successful (completed) suicide. Am J Psychiatr 115:724, 1959
8. Sheehan DV: Panic attacks and phobias. N Engl J Med 307:156, 1982
9. Sletten IW, Barton JL: Suicidal patients in the emergency room: A guide for evaluation and disposition. Hosp Commun Psychiatr 30:407, 1979
10. Strub RL: Acute confusional state. In Benson DF, Blumer D (eds): Psychiatric Aspects of Neurologic Disease, Vol. 2. New York, Grune & Stratton, 1982
11. Tupin J: The violent patient: A strategy for management and diagnosis. Hosp Commun Psychiatr 34:37, 1983
12. Urbaitis JC: Psychiatric Emergencies. Norwalk, Conn, Appleton-Century-Crofts, 1983
13. Weissman MM: The epidemiology of suicide attempts, 1960 to 1971. Arch Gen Psychiatr 30:737, 1974

CHAPTER 16.4

The Patient with Medically Unexplained Physical Complaints

Mark Teitelbaum

The management of patients with medically unexplained physical complaints is difficult for physicians and patients alike. The patient may be worried or fearful that he is physically ill despite adequate medical investigation and the reassurance by his physician to the contrary. This can lead to antagonism between patient and physician.

Other patients with medically unexplained physical complaints may seem curiously indifferent to their symptoms. The problem may be compounded by the fact that the patient has been told by previous physicians that he suffers from various physical conditions such as hypoglycemia, which cannot currently be substantiated. Additionally, the physician may have to cope with a patient who is pressuring him for an operation, is dependent upon narcotics, or is litigious. Terms such as "psychogenic," "functional," "psychosomatic," "hysterical," or "hypochondriacal" to describe the patient's illness or the person himself are sometimes used in a pejorative way. This is unfortunate, as these patients are genuinely suffering and in need of care.

EPIDEMIOLOGY

Unexplained somatic symptoms are extremely common: 60 to 80 percent of a normal population will experience one physical symp-

tom in a week, and from 20 to 80 percent of patients presenting to primary care physicians have unexplained physical symptoms.[5] Such patients account for about 20 percent of patients seen in psychiatric consultation at The Johns Hopkins Hospital. In a large survey of such patients seen consecutively in psychiatric consultation there, 77 percent were women and 87 percent were white. Their mean age was 41 years, and over one half had been referred from the medical service.[9]

CLINICAL FEATURES

At the initial visit, the physician might be confronted with someone who has become increasingly preoccupied with one or more of a variety of vague and ill-defined physical symptoms. Pain, fatigue, and weakness as well as vague neurologic symptoms and functional gastrointestinal symptoms are common complaints. In a survey of patients for medically unexplained bodily complaints, 51 percent involved unexplained pain; 23 percent, unexplained neurologic symptoms; and 5 percent, gastrointestinal symptoms.[9] Complaints referable to the head, abdomen, back, and chest accounted for 40 percent of cases. The patient may also describe growing difficulty in work, social functioning, and family relationships, all of which have deteriorated in proportion to a deepening assumption of the sick role. The patient may seem to be on a "medical pilgrimage," spending financial resources, time, and energy visiting a variety of physicians and hospitals in search of help, yet unwilling to be reassured. He may describe a growing sense of discouragement that the bodily source of his illness will be discovered.

DIFFERENTIAL DIAGNOSIS

UNRECOGNIZED PHYSICAL DISORDER

Physical disorders presenting with vague and ill-defined symptoms include multiple sclerosis, systemic lupus erythematosus (SLE), carcinoma of the pancreas, and myasthenia gravis. Long-term follow-up of patients with unexplained physical symptoms who were thought to be exhibiting hysterical behavior has shown that about one third were discovered subsequently to have a physical disorder, unrecognized at the time of initial presentation.

DEPRESSIVE DISORDER

Nearly a fifth of patients presenting with unexplained physical complaints are suffering from a depressive disorder.[4,10] Physical complaints are very common in depression. Lack of energy, fatigue, functional gastrointestinal symptoms, anorexia, weight loss, sexual dysfunction, vague pain complaints, or headache may be the patient's chief complaint. Typical findings of a low or dysphoric mood, poor self-attitude, feelings of hopelessness, and signs of slowed psychomotor activity support the diagnosis of depressive illness (see Chapter 16.5). The patient may report previous episodes of depression and a family history of depression. It is not fully understood why some patients with depressive illness present to physicians with primarily physical complaints while others do not. Such patients may be more neurotic, have different premorbid personalities, different early life experiences, or a different sociocultural background.

Case Example
A middle-aged business executive was admitted to the medical service because of fatigue and weakness of six months' duration. A thorough medical evaluation was unremarkable. Psychiatric consultation was requested because the patient's primary physician thought he might be depressed. The psychiatrist's interview revealed a normally ambitious, hard-driving, and energetic man who was quite successful in his work.

He described himself as "functioning ineffectively and thinking inefficiently" recently, yet he denied feeling sad. He stated he simply felt "disappointed" in himself and described a feeling of hopelessness about his chances of recovery despite the fact that no serious physical disorder had been diagnosed. Along with his lowered energy and vitality, he described significant changes in his appetite and sex drive. His overall enjoyment of life was diminished. Mental status examination revealed psychomotor retardation. Formal cognitive testing was entirely within normal limits. A diagnosis of major depressive disorder was made by the consultant and psychiatric treatment recommended.

ANXIETY DISORDER

Anxiety disorder accounts for nearly a tenth of patients with unexplained physical complaints.[2] Patients suffering from anxiety disorders who are seen in the general medical setting frequently present to the primary physician with somatic complaints. Chest pain, palpitations, dyspnea, weakness, light-headedness, dizziness, vertigo, tremor, diarrhea, or vomiting may be the patient's chief complaint. Typical findings of generalized tension, apprehension, fear or worry sometimes associated with difficulty in concentrating, insomnia, and fatigue, suggest a diagnosis of an anxiety disorder. Some patients may give a history of acute attacks of overwhelming panic with feelings of terror and fear of impending death accompanied by signs of sympathetic nervous system arousal. Some patients may report having developed secondary fears of being alone or leaving their homes and may have become essentially "housebound."

Case Example
A married woman in her 50s was hospitalized to evaluate lower extremity weakness and fear of walking for about 2 years. Her illness had begun acutely, within days after her mother's unexpected death. At that time, she had been alone in her house while her husband, an airline pilot, was away on an international flight. She was awakened suddenly from sleep with palpitations, dyspnea, light-headedness, weakness in her legs, and an overwhelming sense of terror and impending death. She called her family physician who came to her home, recognized her state of panic, and medicated her with an injection of barbiturate. He told her to "stay in bed until you feel better." She described falling asleep quickly. Upon waking the next day, she attempted to get out of bed but once again felt weak, light-headed, and fearful, and her legs collapsed under her. When her husband returned home the next day, he found her in bed, afraid to get up, fearful that she would "feel weak and fall." A series of hospitalizations with essentially negative evaluations occurred during the next 2 years. During this time, the patient spent most of her time in bed or in her swimming pool, reluctant to walk or go out of her house alone. Almost every attempt to do so precipitated a recurrence of symptoms identical to the original attack. Her illness required her husband's reassignment from flight duties to a desk job in his airline's local branch office so he could care for her. An extensive medical workup during the present admission was likewise unremarkable.

Psychiatric consultation was requested to investigate possible "psychogenic factors." After a series of interviews with the patient, the consulting psychiatrist came to the conclusion that the patient was suffering from an anxiety disorder with panic attacks. Her refusal to walk or go out alone was understood as related to her fears of having an attack with no one around to help.

SCHIZOPHRENIA

Undiagnosed schizophrenia is a rare cause of unexplained physical symptoms in hospitalized patients. In such cases, the patient's complaints center around a belief of ill health that is false, unshakeable, and idiosyncratic, i.e., delusional. He may believe that he is suffering from a bizarre or unusual infestation, poisoning, or metabolic derangement. The diagnosis of schizophrenia is supported by a history of previous episodes of hallucinations and delusions in clear consciousness as well as the presence of significant disturbances of expression of thought, emotion, and volition in a person who shows no evidence of coarse brain disease or depressive illness[7] (see Chapter 16.6).

Case Example

A middle-aged woman was admitted to the dermatology service with infected excoriations that covered a good deal of her skin. She admitted to almost continuous scratching. Because the patient "seemed strange" to her physician and because he thought she had no primary medical or dermatologic disorder to explain her itching, he requested psychiatric consultation. The psychiatrist found a disheveled and obese woman who admitted to several state hospital psychiatric admissions "because of voices" since her early 20s. Examination of her mental state revealed the delusional belief that her itching was caused by "small worms" that had infiltrated her skin. She scratched some skin debris from her arm and gave it to the psychiatrist, stating: "Send this stuff to the lab; you'll find them." Informing the patient that skin biopsy examinations had been negative was to no avail. The diagnosis of schizophrenia was established.

HYSTERIA

Over a third of patients presenting with unexplained physical complaints suffer from hysteria.[1,8] Hysteria involves the imitation of the behavior of a person suffering from a physical disorder. The behavior is undertaken to achieve a goal such as getting attention, love, compensation, relief of guilt or other unpleasant affect; to avoid responsibility; or to solve some life difficulty. The goal of the behavior is generally outside the patient's awareness, which distinguishes hysteria from factitious illness and malingering.

Hysterical behavior may begin abruptly in the setting of a stressful life situation and is termed "conversion disorder."[3] Marital difficulties, work-related stress, occupational or vehicular accidents, combat, separations, or bereavement may be involved. The particular choice of symptom may involve the unconscious copying of a symptom or sign demonstrated by a family member or other person known or seen by the patient when that other person was ill. The symptom or sign displayed may also convey something about the meaning of the person's distress, which is symbolically communicated through "body language." The diagnosis ultimately rests upon recognizing (1) a vulnerable personality, often with self-dramatizing, egocentric, emotionally labile, and immature features; (2) a situation understood as stressful and disruptive to the person involved; (3) symptoms or signs unexplained on the basis of physical disease that can be understood as symbolically meaningful communication; and (4) the purpose that the behavior serves in solving a life problem.

Case Example

An unmarried lawyer in his early 30s was admitted with a 1-month history of weakness of his legs and difficulty in walking. Neurologic evaluation was unremarkable, yet the patient persisted in a fearful worry that he had multiple sclerosis. Because his physician suspected that his complaints were "functional," psychiatric consultation was requested. His present illness had begun acutely, after he started a new job in a law firm where he felt fearful of a boss whom he perceived as critical and demanding. The "final straw" came after he had begun dating a woman from his office. Although he saw their relationship as casual and platonic, she had begun pressing him for more of a commitment. After a distressing discussion with her in a restaurant one night, he awoke the next morning feeling weak in his legs and unable to walk. By temperament he was a dramatic, perfectionist, and self-centered man who had been an excellent student and had graduated from law school at the top of his class. Examination of the patient's mental state did not reveal the phenomena of depressive illness, an anxiety disorder, or schizophrenia. His behavior was understood by the psychiatrist as motivated by fears of dealing with a difficult life situation that he wished to avoid and a desire to "save face" at the same time. His behavior appeared to serve the purpose of keeping him from having to "stand up" to his boss and "making the step" toward marriage without having to deal with either his boss or girlfriend directly. A diagnosis of conversion disorder was made.

SOMATIZATION DISORDER

Some patients with hysterical behavior have lifelong histories of multiple unexplained physical complaints involving multiple organ systems, usually starting in adolescence with exacerbations and re-

missions throughout life. These individuals suffer from somatization disorder.[5] They may be taking unneeded medications, be dependent upon narcotics, and have had multiple surgical procedures. Many have significant associated emotional disturbance and personality disorder with both histrionic and obsessional features. Long-term follow-up of such patients has shown that in 90 percent of cases, no new physical or psychiatric illness will appear within 6 to 8 years of diagnosis.

Case Example

A divorced woman in her 50s was admitted to the medical service with recurrent, vague abdominal pain. She had had poorly explained abdominal complaints since adolescence, having had her first surgery, an appendectomy, as a teenager. Over the years she had been operated upon many times for unexplained pain and more recently for intestinal obstruction caused by adhesions from previous surgeries. Her gall bladder as well as portions of her stomach and small and large bowel had been resected, all without documented evidence of physical disease. She was taking a variety of medications, including tranquilizers and narcotic analgesics. Psychiatric consultation was requested to evaluate a possible "psychogenic contribution" to the patient's pain.

The psychiatrist's interview revealed a woman who was carefully made up, seemed in no distress, and did not look at all sick. He learned that she had been ill "all her life." She had grown up in a home with marital discord, was married at a young age, and was currently divorced yet remained in an emotional battle with her ex-husband. Her mother had been "cold and distant," her father "loving." His death, approximately 10 years before, had occurred just before a marked increase in all her complaints, especially abdominal pain and a downhill course that involved multiple hospitalizations and surgery. Her preoccupation with symptoms and her emotional withdrawal from her family were major factors in the failure of her marriage and her alienation from her children, who refused to visit her in the hospital. She felt discouraged, lonely, and "hurt." Examination of her mental state did not reveal symptoms of depressive illness. It did illuminate, however, her anger at her husband and children for abandoning her as well as her rage at a number of previous physicians who "never really cared." Furthermore, multiple unexplained bodily complaints involving several organ systems were reported. The psychiatrist interpreted her behavior as being motivated by a desire for love, care, and attention from others that she could not ask for directly. A diagnosis of somatization disorder was made.

PSYCHIATRIC CONSULTATION

Psychiatric consultation is indicated for all patients with unexplained physical complaints to help in the diagnostic process and planning for management. Preparing patients for consultation is important but is often overlooked. The crucial elements in effective preparation of a patient for psychiatric consultation include a full and open discussion between the primary physician and the patient of the reasons for requesting consultation. The physician must provide enough time to listen for and deal with the patient's reactions. It is important for the primary physician to understand that psychiatric consultation can have a variety of meanings for a patient that may serve as obstacles to the patient's acceptance of the consultation. Although idiosyncratic issues, for example, a previous negative experience with a psychiatrist, occasionally are involved, certain common emotionally charged themes tend to recur.

The patient may interpret the recommendation for psychiatric consultation as an insult. Additionally, the patient may fear the physician's or some other significant person's disapproval should it be concluded that he is suffering from a psychiatric disorder. In some instances, the patient might be responding to a realistic perception of the physician's attitude toward psychiatric disorders and psychiatric patients. The physician can directly convey positive regard for the patient, thus supporting the patient's self-esteem. He can do this by openly sharing his empathic understanding of the patient's dilemma with him. For example, he might comment: "I know you feel hurt by my suggesting you might need psychiatric help. Because I'm concerned about you and want you to get the best care, I think it is important for you to go ahead and have

the consultation. Doing something that's difficult for you will only increase everyone's respect for you, not diminish it." The patient may be more likely to comply with the physician's recommendations if he feels that the physician likes and approves of him.

The patient may experience the recommendation for psychiatric consultation as a threatened abandonment. Some patients are extremely sensitive to rejection and will often resist psychiatric consultation because they feel that their relationship with their physician is being jeopardized. Occasionally, the patient might be responding to a realistic perception that the physician may be wanting to extricate himself from a relationship with a difficult patient. It is helpful for the physician to let the patient know directly that he will continue to follow the patient as his primary physician regardless of the recommendations that the psychiatrist may make as a result of the consultation. The physician could comment, for example: "You know, people who have psychiatric problems get physically ill sometimes and need a general physician they can count on to be there. You can count on me to be there as your primary doctor whether it turns out you need psychiatric help or not."

The patient may experience the recommendation for psychiatric consultation as being based on the physician's belief that the symptoms are "imaginary" or "all in his head," or that his suffering is not appreciated. He may feel betrayed and may suffer a loss of trust in his physician. The physician can convey his appreciation of the reality of the patient's suffering. He might say, for example: "I know that you are ill and are suffering greatly with your (pain, nausea, weakness, etc.) even though I have not found its cause. The purpose of psychiatric consultation is to explore all possible causes of your suffering, since emotional troubles and stress may cause symptoms such as yours and produce real suffering."

The patient may experience the recommendation for psychiatric consultation as a communication that his condition is hopeless, that nothing can be done, and that the referral to a psychiatrist is basically an "end-of-the-line" or "last-ditch attempt" to help. The inclusion of psychiatric consultation as an integral part of the evaluation process, right from the beginning of hospitalization or certainly as soon as the possibility of psychiatric disorder is suspected, may work to mitigate against this sense of hopelessness. The physician can share his realistic pessimism with the patient but should combat the unrealistic aspects of the patient's discouragement. For example, he might comment: "I share with you your pessimism about (discovering a bodily cause for your symptoms, curing your pain with more surgery, etc.). However, I do not share your hopelessness about getting well. It is very possible that psychiatric consultation may lead to a recommendation for treatment that could prove to be helpful."

The patient may experience the recommendation for psychiatric consultation as a disappointment in the physician and suffer the loss of him as an idealized figure. The patient may interpret the physician's asking for help as reflecting some inadequacy within the physician. Simply acknowledging his understanding of the patient's reaction can be supportive to the patient and rekindle the patient's faith in the physician, not as an all-knowing parent figure but perhaps as a more realistically perceived, competent, insightful, and caring professional. The physician might even comment that "everyone needs help sometimes, both doctors and patients alike!" Many patients are grateful to their physicians for requesting psychiatric consultation, and the primary physician-patient relationship is generally strengthened rather than undermined.

MANAGEMENT

If a specific psychiatric disorder is diagnosed after thorough workup of a patient with unexplained physical complaints, the first step is the presentation of the diagnosis to the patient and its implications for treatment. This is usually done by the primary physician, sometimes together with the consulting psychiatrist. To avoid any miscommunication, it is often of help to have appropri-

ate family members present when this "summing up" takes place. Clear and straightforward explanation that it is thought that the patient suffers from "emotional difficulties" or "stress" or "depression," or whatever is most accurate and acceptable to the patient, is warranted, plus the laying out of an appropriate treatment plan. Great care must be taken at this point by the physician to communicate his appreciation of the patient's suffering as real, despite the absence of a physical disorder to explain it. The psychiatrist might recommend treatment on an inpatient basis. This is often needed for a patient who is suffering from a serious depression with suicidal ideation, schizophrenia with marked delusional thinking, or hysteria where the symptom is incapacitating or is associated with drug dependence.

There should always be provisions made for ongoing general medical follow-up in addition to the recommended psychiatric treatment. The reasons for this are obvious. First, disrupting the primary physician-patient relationship in many instances will be a great loss to a patient who has counted on a particular physician over the years for his medical care. Second, patients diagnosed as hysterical when first seen may subsequently be discovered to be suffering from a physical disorder. Last, since psychiatric disorder and physical disorder seem to be associated at a frequency greater than chance, some patients with psychiatric disorder presenting with physical complaints are probably at greater risk than nonpsychiatrically ill patients for becoming physically ill in the future. For the collaboration to work, open lines of communication between psychiatrist and the primary physician should be maintained. The primary physician should be aware of the fact that during the course of psychiatric treatment, especially in its early stages, there are often crises in which the patient may wish to discontinue treatment and return to "doctor shopping." The primary physician can be of help during these periods in supporting the patient's continued efforts at psychiatric treatment and discouraging a renewed search for physical disease.

Limiting "doctor shopping" is an important goal of treatment for a patient with medically unexplained physical complaints. Both psychiatrist and primary physician should make every effort to persuade the patient to limit the number of physicians the patient sees. A good relationship between primary physician and patient, as well as between psychiatrist and patient, seems to reduce the risk of "doctor shopping."

Restricting unneeded diagnostic tests, procedures, and treatments is often an ongoing issue throughout treatment. Both psychiatrist and primary physician need to be actively involved in this endeavor. Additional investigative testing should be considered only with the appearance of new signs, and testing should be carefully limited. Potentially harmful treatments should also be strictly avoided. These patients are at risk for becoming iatrogenically addicted to narcotics, dependent upon psychotropic drugs, and subjected to unnecessary surgical procedures. Firm but kind limit-setting by the physician runs little risk of disrupting a good physician-patient relationship.

The treatment of depression and anxiety are discussed in Chapter 16.5, and of schizophrenia, in Chapter 16.6. The treatment of hysteria is essentially based upon persuasion through the medium of regularly scheduled interviews. Treatment on an "as-needed" basis tends to encourage an escalation of symptom complaints and should be avoided. The physician's aim is to encourage the patient gradually to talk about personal difficulties while gradually discouraging his focus on physical complaints. As a therapeutic alliance is forged and trust established, the task may become progressively easier, and opportunities may arise for both patient and physician to address the difficulties that are prompting the hysterical behavior in the first place and to search for more direct and satisfying solutions. Patients suffering from chronic hysteria are often resistant to such an undertaking. In such cases, a stable physician-patient relationship and the elimination of "doctor shopping," unneeded drugs, tests, and procedures may be more realistic goals. When a patient with medically unexplained physical complaints who has been diagnosed as suffering from a psychiatric disorder refuses referral for treatment by a psychiatrist, the pa-

tient's primary physician may elect to treat the patient himself with ongoing consultation from a psychiatrist.

PROGNOSIS

Prognosis depends upon the underlying condition discovered. With appropriate treatment, the outlook for recovery from an episode of depressive illness, an anxiety disorder, or conversion disorder is good. The prognosis for patients suffering from somatization disorder or schizophrenia is considerably more guarded.

REFERENCES

1. Kaminsky MJ, Slavney PR: Hysterical and obsessional features in patients with Briquet's syndrome (somatization disorder). Psychol Med 13:111, 1983
2. Katon W: Panic disorder and somatization, Am J Med 77:101, 1984
3. Lazare A: Conversion symptoms. N Engl J Med 305:745, 1981
4. Mathew RJ, Weinman ML, Mirabi M: Physical symptoms of depression. Br J Psychiatr 139:293, 1981
5. Monson RA, Smith GR: Somatization disorder in primary care. N Engl J Med 308:1464, 1983
6. Perley MJ, Guze SB: Hysteria—The stability and usefulness of clinical criteria: A quantitative study based on a follow-up period of six to eight years in 39 patients. N Engl J Med 266:421, 1962
7. Retterstol N: Paranoid psychoses with hypochondriac delusions as the main delusion. Acta Psychiat Scand 44:334, 1968
8. Slater ET, Glithero E: A follow-up of patients diagnosed as suffering from "hysteria." J Psychosom Res 9:9, 1965
9. Slavney PR, Teitelbaum ML: Patients with medically unexplained symptoms: DSM III diagnoses and demographic characteristics. Gen Hosp Psychiatr 7:21, 1985
10. Wilson DR, Widmer RB, et al: Somatic symptoms: A major feature of depression in family practice. J Affective Disord 5:199, 1983

CHAPTER 16.5
Affective Disorders and Anxiety Disorders

Joseph T. Coyle and John B. Imboden

Anxiety disorders and depression are the most common serious psychiatric disorders that the primary physician is apt to encounter. There is evidence that the affective and anxiety disorders may be more closely related than heretofore suspected. Genetic studies suggest the possibility of some degree of familial concurrence of panic disorder and major depression.[2,4,5,7,12] Many patients exhibit a mixture of depressive and anxiety symptoms. Finally, certain forms of anxiety disorder respond to antidepressant medication.

AFFECTIVE DISORDERS: CLASSIFICATION

Depression is a normal emotional response to adversity, particularly one that involves loss of some type, such as the death of a loved one, separation, divorce, or loss of job, money, physical health, or professional or social standing. A normal reaction to the vicissitudes of life must be distinguished from the sustained alterations of mood and self-attitude accompanied by other signs and symptoms that comprise the syndromes of depression. By convention, *major depressive disorder* refers to a syndrome in which depression is the prominent feature and in which there is no history of previous manic or hypomanic episodes. *Dysthymic disorder* describes a milder form of depression, which tends to be chronic, that is, lasting 2 years or more. The term *bipolar disorder* refers to a recurrent disorder in which the patient suffers from one or more episodes of mania as well as serious depression. *Cyclothymic disorder* describes a condition characterized by alterations in moods, but not of the severity to warrant diagnosis of major depressive disorder or of mania; it recurs over a period of at least 2 years.

MAJOR DEPRESSIVE DISORDER[1]

CLINICAL FEATURES

The clinical manifestations of major depressive disorder may be grouped as follows: (1) change in mood, (2) negative attitude toward self, (3) bleak outlook on the future, (4) psychomotor changes, and (5) physiologic symptoms and somatic complaints. Typically, the patient complains of feeling "sad," "down," "low," "blue," "despondent," or simply "depressed." This feel-

ing may exhibit diurnal variation, typically but not always being more severe in the morning. The patient may state that nothing interests him or gives him pleasure (anhedonia). Of particular importance diagnostically is the fact that these subjective symptoms of depression are sometimes minimized or denied by the patient, or they may be ascribed to some other cause, such as poorly defined physical symptoms.

To some degree, the depressed patient is inordinately self-deprecatory, indicating that he sees himself as inadequate or "bad." In severe depression, the debased self-concept may be stated explicitly, but sometimes it is expressed metaphorically in somatic delusions, such as a feeling of emitting noxious odors of "rotting." In addition, the patient may experience auditory hallucinations and paranoid delusions in which derision and accusations are directed at him by others. The patient may attempt to justify his feeling of inadequacy and guilt by ruminating about and inappropriately magnifying past failures and misdeeds.

Depending upon the severity of the depression, the patient feels mentally and physically sluggish and "slowed down." He finds it difficult to concentrate, and he lacks initiative and energy so that small tasks appear to require great effort. He typically withdraws from social and occupational activities. In severe cases, the patient may exhibit psychomotor retardation, tending to be silent, immobile, and seemingly unresponsive to his surroundings. In contrast, some patients suffer from agitation and marked restlessness punctuated by repeated pleadings for help. The patient's view of the future may vary from that of moderate pessimism to one of utter hopelessness. He may express the certainty that he will never feel well or happy again. Almost all seriously depressed patients have at least an occasional wish to die to be relieved of suffering. Some patients become actively suicidal, particularly if they believe their condition to be hopeless or if they feel unworthy of treatment.

Among the most common somatic complaints in depression are fatigue, an oppressive feeling over the chest, and nonspecific pains.[1] Several physiologic disturbances commonly occur in severe depression. Anorexia with substantial weight loss is common; however, occasionally a depressed patient eats excessively, especially at night. Insomnia is a frequent complaint, for which there is now evidence of disturbances on sleep electroencephalogram. While difficulties in getting to sleep and maintaining sleep occur, early morning awakening is typical for severe depression. A minor-

ity of patients suffer from hypersomnia. Decrease in sexual interest, impotence, and anorgasmia are common. Reduced gut motility with constipation also occurs.

DIAGNOSIS

When the above-mentioned constellation of symptoms is present, the diagnosis is usually apparent. Indeed, the patient may be well aware of the diagnosis, particularly if he has had prior episodes of depression. Sometimes, however, the patient is unaware of the altered mood state but focuses upon the somatic manifestations such as low energy, difficulty in sleeping, or persistent pain. In these instances the patient may have little insight and resist the diagnosis of a primary psychiatric disorder as the cause of his symptoms. The physician may easily be led to share this view.

Case Example
A 63-year-old engineer returned to the United States following a trip to North Africa. Upon his return, he began to experience general lassitude. Stool examination revealed a parasitic infestation, which was treated. In the ensuing months the patient gradually developed feelings of low energy, anhedonia, poor concentration, feeling of inadequacy, inappropriate guilt, insomnia, and anorexia. In spite of eradication of the parasites, all these symptoms continued to be ascribed to the earlier-diagnosed infection, and almost a year elapsed before the presence of depression was recognized. The patient was successfully treated with nortriptyline.

Unexplained vague aches and pains, anorexia, weight loss, insomnia, loss of libido, and fatigue should arouse suspicion of depression.[1] It is helpful to keep in mind that only rarely does a physical symptom or "depressive equivalent" completely replace or "contain" other features of depression. Careful assessment usually reveals the feelings of sadness, discouragement, subtle or indirect self-deprecation, and decline in interest and energy. A diagnosis of depression is further supported by a history of previous episodes in the patient. In light of the mounting evidence of genetic predisposition, a family history of episodic major mental disorder without deterioration also provides supportive evidence for the diagnosis.

In the elderly patient, depression may cause serious impairment of cognitive functions and memory, giving rise to the false impression of senile dementia. In these patients it is important to be alert to the symptomatic evidence of depression. Occasionally, it may not be possible to determine to what degree the impairment of cognition is based upon an organic dementia versus depression. In such cases it may be necessary to resort to a trial of pharmacologic treatment for depression to resolve the question.

It is important to keep in mind that depression can be precipitated by a variety of drugs or biologic factors associated with physical disorders and their treatment. Among the drugs that may be implicated in depression are methyldopa, guanethidine, propanolol, reserpine, levodopa, and cimetidine. A number of medical disorders, including hypothyroidism, pernicious anemia, carcinoma of the pancreas or colon, and parkinsonism, are sometimes associated with depression.[1]

ETIOLOGY

Genetic studies of families with probands suffering from major depression provide strong evidence for hereditary predisposition.[4,5,12] Thus, the incidence of affective disorders among parents and sibs of the proband is three to four times the prevalence rate in the general population; the concordance rate between fraternal twins is similar to that of sibs, whereas it exceeds 50 percent in identical twins. Recent studies using recombinant DNA methods have identified a polymorphism on chromosome 11, which is linked to a hereditary form of manic-depressive disorder.[7] Other studies have suggested possible biochemical abnormalities, perhaps involving a decrease in the functional activity of central aminergic systems, in-

cluding those which use serotonin and norepinephrine.[9,10] Abnormality of the pituitary-adrenal axis in about half of patients with major depressive disorder is suggested by failure in these patients of an oral dose of 1 mg of dexamethasone given at 11:00 PM to suppress plasma cortisol levels below 5 μg/dl at 4:00 PM the following day. As already noted, a number of antihypertensive drugs, which affect central catecholaminergic neurotransmission, can precipitate major depressions in susceptible individuals.

Psychological factors have been studied intensively. There is suggestive evidence that experience of traumatic loss early in life and the development of more than usual need for approval from others increases the likelihood of reacting to recurrent losses and disappointments with depression.[3,11] These developmental factors may play a greater role in the genesis of dysthymic disorder, which is more chronic, than in etiology of a major depressive disorder. Nevertheless, recent studies do point to the role of serious stress and recent losses in the recurrence of depression in patients suffering from major affective disorders.[13] Further, there is evidence that some patients with depression respond favorably to specific types of psychologic intervention, such as cognitive therapy.

MANAGEMENT

The primary physician must decide whether to treat the depressive patient himself, usually with a combination of supportive psychotherapy and pharmacotherapy, or refer the patient to a psychiatrist for management. The treating physician must also decide whether to initiate therapy on an inpatient or outpatient basis.

This decision must be based on the type and severity of the depression and the personal variables that may be relevant in contributing to the depression. It is also important to assess the degree to which the patient's current living situation will provide the support initially needed during the illness and following recovery. If the patient's depression is of mild to moderate degree, is of recent onset, and is not associated with serious suicidal risk, the primary physician may elect to manage the patient on an outpatient basis.

The assessment of suicidal risk requires explicit discussion with the patient about thoughts of death and suicide (see Chapter 16.3). The physician should not fear that this will precipitate suicidal thoughts; to the contrary, many patients are relieved to have the opportunity of discussing this often frightening preoccupation. Almost all depressed patients have experienced at least a passive wish to die to achieve relief from suffering. It is important, however, to ask the patient if he has been preoccupied with suicidal thoughts and if he has an intention or plans to end his life. The patient who feels that his condition is hopeless or believes that he is too evil to deserve treatment is particularly at risk for suicide. Other factors that predict increased risk for suicide include inability to articulate future plans, history of suicide in the family, alcohol or other substance abuse, previous suicide attempts, living alone, and lack of family or personal support.

Those patients who are suffering from a severe depression with or without psychotic symptoms, who have not responded to standard treatment, or who are deemed to be at risk for suicide should be referred to a psychiatrist. Psychiatric hospitalization is often indicated for the severely depressed patient, especially if the suicidal risk is deemed serious.

Antidepressants
There are currently no rigid criteria for determining which patients will respond optimally to treatment with antidepressant medications.[1] Most clinicians are inclined to offer a trial of supportive psychotherapy if the depression is mild and its onset is clearly related to an environmental stress or significant loss. There is growing evidence that many patients with dysthymic disorder or chronic depression may respond to treatment with antidepressants. Clearly, those patients with severe depression accompanied by suicidal preoccupation or physiologic symptoms such as diurnal variation in mood, anorexia, weight loss, loss of libido, constipa-

tion, psychomotor retardation or agitation, and anhedonia are candidates for somatic therapies. Evidence is now compelling that imminently life-threatening depression, particularly if the condition has not responded to other treatment, is most effectively treated by electroconvulsive therapy, which should be administered by an experienced psychiatrist in conjunction with an anesthesiologist.[6] A vast majority of depressed patients, however, are candidates for therapy with antidepressant drugs. For patients with severe depression who have a history of one or more manic episodes, the current depression may respond better to treatment with lithium. If an antidepressant is used to treat a patient with bipolar disorder, it may be advisable to administer lithium concomitantly as the antidepressant may precipitate a manic episode when given alone.

Two classes of antidepressants are available for treatment: monoamine oxidase inhibitors (MAOI) and non-MAOI antidepressants, of which the older tricyclic antidepressants (TCA) have been the mainstay of treatment over the last 30 years. The MAOI may be somewhat less effective than TCA in treating major depressive disorder. Treatment with MAOI renders the patient vulnerable to hypertensive crisis if he consumes foods containing substantial amounts of tyramine or phenethylamine, such as wines, aged meats, strong cheeses, and pickled herring. Nevertheless, MAOIs have proved effective in the treatment of many patients who do not respond to TCA and in certain atypical forms of depression in which chronic anxiety and phobic symptoms are prominent. Since the MAOIs are not recommended for use by the general physician, the present discussion will focus on the TCA.

Mechanism of Action. The mechanism of therapeutic action of TCA remains unclear. As a class, these drugs appear to enhance synaptic neurotransmission of the central serotonergic and noradrenergic neurons, primarily by inhibiting the high-affinity uptake process on their terminals that inactivates the released neurotransmitter. Some of the more recently developed, clinically effective antidepressants appear to exert their therapeutic effects by other mechanisms.

Use and Treatment. Although the usual daily dose for various TCAs has been established, this dose is at best an approximation. The therapeutic response may occur at doses well above or below the recommended dose because of considerable variation among individuals in the pharmacodynamic disposition of these drugs. Initially, low doses should be administered (one quarter of the recommended therapeutic dose), and the dose should be increased at quarterly increments every few days as tolerated (Table 16.5–1). Because of the long half-life of the drugs, administration of the total dose once per day will usually maintain adequate plasma levels throughout a 24-hour period, with the exception of trazodone. The drug is often taken at bedtime, which focuses the sedating side effects at an appropriate time and obviates the necessity of coprescription of sedatives.

The clinical response to antidepressant treatment is gradual, and the rate of improvement is inversely proportional to the severity of the depression. Whether the depression is mild or severe, one should not consider TCA treatment a failure until the patient has been on the recommended dose for about 3 or 4 weeks without significant improvement. The somatic symptoms of major depression generally respond more rapidly than the psychologic symptoms. The early effects on insomnia and anorexia may be used as predictors of positive clinical response. The delay in improvement of depressive mood, impaired interest, and pessimism may cause the patient to feel that he is not yet benefiting from the chemotherapy. Accordingly, it is useful to obtain corroborative information from family members or nursing staff on changes in activity, sleep pattern, and eating to document early signs of clinical response.

A number of studies have correlated clinical response with plasma levels of antidepressants. With regard to the tricyclic nortriptyline, the most extensively studied drug, plasma levels above 50 ng/ml and less than 200 ng/ml are associated with optimal improvement, whereas levels below or above, respectively, are associated with a lack of clinical response. Whether an upper limit of efficacy for other TCAs exists remains unclear; nevertheless, plasma levels in excess of 300 to 500 ng/ml are associated with an increased risk for toxic side effects. Although the average daily dose recommended in Table 16.5–1 should result in appropriate plasma levels in the majority of patients, the considerable variation among patients in their metabolism of TCA can result in plasma levels outside therapeutic range. For example, elderly patients tend to obtain higher steady-state plasma levels on a given dose than do younger patients. Accordingly, there is increasing emphasis on monitoring plasma levels of the antidepressant drugs in patients who exhibit poor response to treatment.

Side Effects. The atropine-like action of the TCA is primarily responsible for the peripheral and occasional central side effects accompanying their use. By blocking peripheral muscarinic cholinergic receptors, the drugs interfere with parasympathetic function, which results in decreased salivation, impaired visual accommodation, decreased gut motility, and difficulties in the initiation of micturition. For patients suffering from closed-angle glaucoma, TCA may dangerously elevate intraocular pressure. The vagolytic action of these drugs results in a consistent increase in heart rate. Because of their alpha-adrenergic blocking effects, the TCAs can also cause symptomatic orthostatic hypotension, a side effect to which the elderly are particularly vulnerable. Nevertheless, these drugs can interfere with the antihypertensive effects of drugs such as guanethidine and clonidine. With regard to central side effects, the anticholinergic properties of the TCA may produce delirious states, to which elderly patients are particularly susceptible. Behavioral deterioration and confusion herald this serious side effect; physostigmine, a central acetylcholinesterase inhibitor, can transiently reverse the confusional state, although this is not a recommended therapeutic strategy.

All the TCAs have quinidine-like effects and directly interfere with impulse conduction in the heart, which can result in prolongation of the QRS interval and produce ST- and T-wave abnormalities. Although such cardiac effects generally occur with plasma levels well above the therapeutic range, they have been observed in vulnerable patients at plasma levels within the therapeutic range. Thus, these drugs should be used cautiously in patients with preexisting cardiovascular disease. These effects on the heart are the primary cause of death in cases of overdose with TCA. The potential peripheral and central side effects of the TCAs indicate the serious toxic potential of these drugs. As little as a week's prescription of TCA, when ingested acutely, can prove fatal, rendering the TCA the most potentially lethal of the commonly used psychotropic

**TABLE 16.5–1. AVERAGE DOSE
OF NON-MAOI ANTIDEPRESSANTS**[a]

Generic Name	Proprietary Name(s)	Average Dose (mg/day)
Amitriptyline	Elavil	150
Nortriptyline	Pamelor	100
Imipramine	Tofranil	150
Desipramine	Norpramin, Pertofrane	125
Protriptyline	Vivactil	20
Doxepin	Sinequan, Adapin	150
Maprotiline	Ludiomil	150
Trazodone	Desyrel	200
Amoxapine	Asendin	200

[a]Studies of the relationship between plasma levels of parent drug and active metabolites and clinical response indicate that optimal dosage may vary by 50% or more from the recommended average dose.

TABLE 16.5–2. SIDE EFFECTS COMMONLY ENCOUNTERED WITH CYCLICAL ANTIDEPRESSANTS

Histamine (H1) blocking	Drowsiness
Anticholinergic action, peripheral	Impaired visual accommodation, increased intraocular pressure in patients with closed angle glaucoma, dry mouth, tachycardia, constipation, urinary retention
Anticholinergic action, central	Mental confusion or delirium
Alpha-adrenergic blocking	Orthostatic hypotension
Interference with impulse conduction in the heart	QRS prolongation, ST-T wave abnormalities
Drug interaction	Interference with antihypertensive effect of certain drugs such as guanethidine and clonidine; cyclical antidepressants should not be administered concomitantly with MAO inhibitors
Amoxapine has a degree of dopamine-blocking activity	Extrapyramidal symptoms; possibility of tardive dyskinesia

medications. Only limited amounts of these drugs should be prescribed at any one time for the suicide-prone patient, and appropriate care should be exercised to avoid accidental ingestion by children. The safety of antidepressant drugs in pregnancy and during lactation has not been established.

Recently, several structurally novel antidepressants have been introduced with the hope of reduced toxicity without the loss of efficacy. Trazodone, amoxapine, and maprotiline exhibit lower anticholinergic effects and are somewhat less cardiotoxic than are the other cyclical antidepressants. Nevertheless, each of these drugs has its own side effect profile and limitations. For example, maprotiline is associated with seizures, especially at higher doses; amoxapine has been reported to be associated with extrapyramidal side effects; and trazodone has been associated with the development of priapism. Table 16.5–2 summarizes many of the more common important side effects of the antidepressant drugs. No attempt has been made to review all the possible side effects or drug interactions.

MANIA

Bipolar affective illness is characterized by recurrent episodes of mania interspersed with episodes of depression. While the episodes of depression are virtually indistinguishable from those which occur in major depressive disorder, the history of elevated mood and its associated symptoms is critical in formulating the diagnosis of bipolar affective illness. The age of onset varies. The first episode often appears in the 20s, but symptoms may occur as early as preadolescence.

CLINICAL FEATURES

The patient suffering from bipolar affective illness often has a history of mood swings punctuated by periods of heightened activity, drive, and increased social interactions balanced by periods of withdrawal, depression, and inactivity. When a frank manic episode begins, the patient frequently has no insight into his condition. Several clinical features characterize the manic state. The patient experiences an alteration in mood; he may feel euphoric and exhilarated but also may become irritable and quite intolerant of reasonable constraints proposed by his family and colleagues. The patient typically exhibits excessive talkativeness, which is manifested by a

compulsion to converse with others. Speech may be incessant and rapid, and, in extreme cases, the patient may exhibit flight of ideas in which thoughts merge and are elliptical in presentation. This can be difficult to distinguish from the thought disorder of schizophrenia. The manic patient exhibits physiologic disturbances that are the converse of those seen in depression. He generally exhibits marked increase in activity, a lack of requirement for sleep, increased libido, and a reckless sense of optimism that can result in improvident behavior. In the extreme, the patient can suffer from delusions of grandeur and even experience hallucinations and paranoid delusions that are difficult to distinguish from those seen in schizophrenic psychoses.

DIFFERENTIAL DIAGNOSIS

The distinction of manic psychosis from schizophrenia is particularly important because of the differences in treatment and outcome. Usually this distinction is made on the basis of elevated mood or irritability, hyperactivity, and talkativeness, even in the presence of hallucinatory or delusional experiences that commonly occur in schizophrenia. Nevertheless, in some instances making this distinction may be difficult, and the history of recurrent episodes with periods of restoration to the premorbid state points to manic-depressive disorder. A careful history of drug usage is important in any patient who presents with a combination of euphoric and psychotic symptoms, since commonly abused drugs such as amphetamines, cocaine, and phencyclidine can produce a syndrome that mimics the manic psychosis.

MANAGEMENT

Generally, the manic patient should be referred to a psychiatrist for further evaluation and treatment. Hospitalization is often indicated until the patient's condition has been brought under control through treatment with psychotropic medications. Nevertheless, because of the increasing prevalence of the prophylactic use of lithium salts for preventing the recurrence of mood disturbances in manic-depressive illness, it is likely that the medical specialist will encounter patients receiving this drug who exhibit few if any psychiatric symptoms.

Lithium, an alkaline earth metal administered in the form of a salt, is the treatment of choice for manic-depressive illness. While lithium carbonate is effective in treating an acute manic episode, neuroleptics are often prescribed in the initial phases of treatment as their onset of therapeutic action is more rapid than that of lithium. More important, the maintenance of lithium significantly reduces the recurrence of mood disturbances in up to 80 percent of the patients. The mechanism of therapeutic action of lithium remains unknown. Basic studies indicate, however, that the ion selectively accumulates within the neurons, altering their electrophysiologic characteristics and their ability to release, inactivate, and respond to neurotransmitters. As an ion, lithium is not metabolized but is eliminated by excretion, primarily via the kidneys. Accordingly, the half-life of lithium is directly related to renal function. In addition, dietary sodium, diuretics, and nonsteroidal anti-inflammatory drugs can alter the rate of excretion of lithium.

Lithium is optimally effective in a rather narrow therapeutic range, between 0.6 and 1.5 mEq/L of plasma. In the initial phases of treatment patients may suffer from nausea and gastrointestinal distress that resolves as therapeutic levels are achieved. Within therapeutic levels many patients experience significant polyuria caused by a vasopressin-insensitive diabetes insipidus, a fine tremor, and occasionally a nontoxic goiter. Symptoms of toxicity generally appear at serum levels greater than 1.5 mEq/L, and potentially fatal toxicity occurs at three times this level (see Table 16.5–3). For the average adult with normal renal function, therapeutic levels can be achieved with a dose of lithium carbonate of approximately 300 to 600 mg administered three times per day. Because of the narrow range between therapeutic effects and toxicity, lithium carbonate

TABLE 16.5–3. SIDE EFFECTS OF LITHIUM[a]

Plasma Level	Symptoms
≤ 1.5 mEq/L (therapeutic)	Nausea (limited to initial period of treatment) Fine tremor Mild polyuria
>1.5<2.5 mEq/L	Vomiting and diarrhea Polyuria (concentration defect) Coarse tremor, ataxia Muscle weakness, fasciculations Sedation
>2.5 <4.0 mEq/L	Muscle hypertonia Choreiform movements Increased deep tendon reflexes Confusion and stupor Transient focal neurologic signs Seizures
>4.0 mEq/L	Coma Death

[a]The loss of sodium as a result of vomiting, diarrhea, polyuria, or the initiation of a sodium-restricted diet with diuretics reduces the clearance of lithium. Thus, under these conditions, much higher plasma levels of lithium will occur on a fixed dose of lithium carbonate.

is usually administered in three doses throughout the day to maintain plasma levels within the appropriate range. It is important that plasma levels of lithium be monitored at regular intervals and whenever a change in the patient's medical condition occurs that may affect renal function or electrolyte status. Recently, a slow-release form of lithium has been approved that reduces the necessity for frequent administration of the drug.

Lithium does have teratogenic effects and therefore should not be used during pregnancy, especially in the early months. Sexually active females in the childbearing period are advised not to become pregnant while taking lithium. Because of the risk of fetal distress, it should not be used near term. Since lithium is excreted in breast milk, it is advisable for the mother taking lithium not to breast-feed her infant.

ANXIETY DISORDERS

Included in this category are several conditions, all of which are characterized by various manifestations of anxiety as a major or central feature: panic and agoraphobic disorders, generalized anxiety disorder, obsessive-compulsive disorder, and posttraumatic stress disorder.[8] With the exception of the latter, these conditions usually first appear in young adulthood. They last for weeks to years and sometimes spontaneously remit.

Anxiety refers to a largely subjective state of discomfort that varies from relatively mild degrees of tenseness or apprehension to a state of panic or terror. As a subjective experience, it is indistinguishable from fear except that in anxiety states there is no actual external threat. A number of symptoms may occur with subjective apprehension, such as those associated with sympathetic discharge and muscle tension. These conditions in their severe form can result in much suffering and disability. Commonly, the patient may resort to alcohol or other substances to obtain relief and thereby develop a chemical dependency, which itself will require treatment. Many patients become discouraged or demoralized if the condition has persisted for a long period without adequate treatment. Anxiety disorder is commonly present in patients with depression.

PANIC AND AGORAPHOBIA[8]

The patient with panic disorder suffers from recurrent attacks of severe anxiety. In an acute attack the patient experiences a sudden onset of symptoms indistinguishable from intense fear or terror. There are signs and symptoms of peripheral sympathetic discharge, including tachycardia, palpitations, sweating, dry mouth, pupillary dilation, and blurring of vision. Transient discomfort over the precordium or in the upper left quadrant of the chest, not related to exertion, may also occur. The patient may show fine tremor of the hands and restlessness. He may complain of not being able to get a deep or satisfying breath or of having a suffocating feeling while objectively exhibiting tachypnea. Hyperventilation, in turn, may lead to respiratory alkalosis, resulting in paresthesias of the extremities and circumoral region, dizziness, or a feeling of weakness or faintness. Frank tetany with carpopedal spasm may occur rarely.

More often than not, the patient is not aware of any precipitating factor, but, once the attack has begun, he is apt to focus his apprehension upon something specific. This commonly takes the form of a fear that the perceived cardiac palpitation signals an impending heart attack and death. The patient may fear that he is "going crazy," that he will suffocate, or that something terrible that he cannot specify is about to happen to him. The attacks typically last a few minutes. The patient may have a single attack, an occasional attack, or a cluster of attacks over a period of several weeks.

Frequently, the patient suffering from panic attacks will develop fear of being in the setting in which the attacks initially occurred, such as at public meetings, in crowded shopping areas, or driving a car. The patient may begin to avoid these situations for fear of experiencing another attack. This anticipatory anxiety over the recurrence of attacks can lead to increasing avoidance behavior with resulting severe restriction of the patient's activities. The term "agoraphobia" applies to the condition in which anticipatory anxiety results in the patient's being more or less confined to home unless accompanied by a friend or member of the family. It is apparent from the foregoing description that there are varying degrees of phobic avoidance of everyday activities in patients with a history of panic attacks.

GENERALIZED ANXIETY DISORDER (CHRONIC ANXIETY STATE)

The patient suffering from chronic anxiety presents with a long history of being tense, worried, vaguely apprehensive, and sometimes irritable, "edgy," or impatient. The content of the patient's worry may involve a variety of issues such as personal health, family matters, or work. The patient usually reports a variety of somatic complaints, some of which appear to be secondary to musculoskeletal tension, such as bitemporal and occipital headaches, backache, or neckache. Increased sympathetic activity is suggested by moist palms, dry mouth, palpitations, fine tremor of the hands, and mild restlessness. He may complain of vague epigastric distress such as "butterflies in the stomach" and may experience episodes of diarrhea, frequent urination, lightheadedness, or hot or cold spells. Difficulty in getting to sleep is common, and the lack of restful sleep and a chronic sense of fatigue are often noted. These diffuse and poorly specified symptoms may wax and wane in severity, probably influenced by life events, and may be temporarily allayed when the patient becomes absorbed in some activity.

ETIOLOGY

The etiology of the anxiety disorders is not fully understood. There is evidence that strongly supports a genetic predisposition to generalized anxiety disorder and panic disorder.[5] Genetic studies also suggest a high incidence of generalized anxiety and panic disorder among depressed probands and an increased incidence of both anxiety and depression among the first-degree relatives of the depressed probands who have anxiety symptoms. Further, imipramine, widely used as an antidepressant, effectively blocks the occurrence of panic attacks. It has also been observed that sodium lactate infusion precipitates a panic attack in some patients with a history of panic disorder.[9] These and other observations, such as

the probable higher incidence of mitral valve prolapse in patients with panic disorder, point to as-yet-unknown physiologic and metabolic processes that may play an essential role in these disorders. Psychologic stress may well predispose to panic disorders. Clinical evidence points to the presence in many of these patients of relatively intense separation anxiety. In fact, many adult patients with panic disorder have a history of school phobia in childhood, that is, fear of separation from the mother.

DIAGNOSIS

In most instances the diagnosis of agoraphobia, panic attacks, and generalized anxiety is readily made on the basis of the characteristic features described above. Nevertheless, anxiety neurosis and acute panic attacks may be mimicked by a number of medical disorders. Indeed, the patient generally presents with the avowed fear that a serious medical condition is responsible for his symptoms.

Hyperthyroidism can produce a state of increased anxiety and irritability with subjective symptoms similar to those of anxiety disorder. The episodic tachycardia of anxiety disorder, however, generally reflects a sympathetic lability, whereas in hyperthyroidism the tachycardia tends to be more constant. Nevertheless, evaluation of thyroid status should be considered when signs and symptoms raise the possibility of hyperthyroidism.

Caffeinism, which is characterized by a fine tremor of the hands, irritability, tenseness, restlessness, and insomnia, is by no means rare. Notably, the vulnerability to caffeine appears to increase with age despite constant dietary habits. The diagnosis of caffeinism is supported by a history of drinking excessive amounts of coffee, tea, or caffeine-containing beverages and by the reduction of symptoms following abstinence or moderation in intake of these beverages. A similar picture may be seen with the use of indirectly acting sympathomimetics such as pseudoephedrine, dextroamphetamine, or methylphenidate.

Episodes of hypertension, tachycardia, and severe anxiety similar to panic attacks are associated with pheochromocytoma. As noted above, mitral valve prolapse can be associated with anxiety attacks. Acute hypoglycemic episodes, from whatever cause, may mimic anxiety attacks. Acute panic states can also be seen in association with the ingestion of hallucinogenic substances such as LSD or phencyclidine, intoxication with stimulants such as dextroamphetamine or cocaine, or as a symptom in other major psychiatric disorders such as schizophrenia.

Finally, the early stages of withdrawal from central nervous system–depressant drugs such as the barbiturates, benzodiazepines, and alcohol may produce symptoms virtually indistinguishable from those of the anxiety state. An accurate history of recent drug and alcohol use is therefore crucial in evaluating the symptoms, especially since many patients with anxiety disorders are prone to misuse alcohol and sedatives to control symptoms.

MANAGEMENT

The management of patients with anxiety disorders depends in part on the symptomatic manifestations at the time the patient is being seen by the physician. In the initial evaluation the physician must keep in mind that the patient probably fears that the symptoms result from a serious medical disorder. Accordingly, the physician should communicate a sense of reassurance by listening carefully to the patient's description of his experiences, obtaining a careful history, and performing the physical examination in a thorough but calm fashion. After medical causes for the symptoms have been ruled out, the patients should be reassured that their specific fears of physical illness are without foundation. The patient should be provided a simple and readily understandable explanation that some physical symptoms of anxiety reflect increased activity of the sympathetic nervous system.

The fundamental strategy for the management of anxiety disorders is to establish a relationship of confidence and trust with the patient. The patient should be encouraged to make observa-

tions about himself and his everyday experiences to see if he can detect some correlation between life events and the waxing and waning of symptoms. Such perceptions on the part of the patient not only afford him an increased opportunity to discuss anxiety-provoking experiences but also have the effect of making his anxiety symptoms seem less mysterious and foreign. Furthermore, such an approach will help the patient to accept referral to a psychiatrist when, in the physician's judgment, such a referral is indicated. The physician should consider referral for psychiatric treatment when the patient's symptoms remain unabated or persistently recur beyond a few weeks despite treatment.

A variety of psychotropic drugs have been recommended in the treatment of the chronic anxiety that waxes and wanes in association with stressful life events and in the anticipatory anxiety that may develop in the intervals between panic attacks. The benzodiazepines are clearly the drugs of choice. They are anxiolytic at doses that do not produce marked sedation. Although some patients do develop physical dependence to these agents after long-term, high-dose treatment, the risk of habituation and physical dependence is less than with the formerly used agents such as barbiturates. Significantly, fatal overdosage with benzodiazepines, when taken alone, is a rare occurrence.

Even with the benzodiazepines, some sedation accompanies the anxiolytic effects. Thus, patients should be cautioned against driving or performing hazardous tasks while taking these drugs. In addition, benzodiazepines potentiate the effects of sedatives or alcohol, which can result in fatal respiratory depression. Clinical evidence suggests that anxiolytic drugs may accentuate mood swings and may reduce impulse control. Discontinuation of the drug should be gradual, especially when high doses have been employed or treatment has continued for longer than a month. The range of daily dosages for commonly used benzodiazepines is shown in Table 16.5–4. Buspirone, a recently introduced anxiolytic, has a different mechanism of action and a more delayed onset of effects than the benzodiazepines.

The physician should carefully consider the context for prescribing benzodiazepines to a patient suffering from chronic anxiety or the symptoms of anxiety associated with the other neuroses. Benzodiazepine treatment should clearly be time limited, generally not exceeding 4 to 6 weeks. Persistent or escalating demands for anxiolytics should prompt the primary physician to refer the patient for psychiatric evaluation and treatment. It should be emphasized that anxiety is a common symptom in neurotic conditions that can serve as an impetus for exploring underlying conflicts and prompting positive changes in a patient's life; a too-ready reliance upon anxiolytics may subvert this motivation for change.

An effective strategy for the prevention of panic attacks is the administration of a TCA such as imipramine.[14] Antidepressant treatment generally results in the elimination of the panic attacks at doses approximately equivalent to those used in the treatment of major depressive disorder. Monamine oxidase inhibitors have also been found effective in eliminating panic attacks. Finally, the benzodiazepine alprazolam has been reported to be useful in the

TABLE 16.5–4. ANXIOLYTIC BENZODIAZEPINES

	Trade Name	Daily Dose (mg)	Half-Life[a] (hr)
Alprazolam	Xanax	0.5–4	12
Chlordiazepoxide	Librium	15–60	18
Clorazepate	Tranxene	30	100
Diazepam	Valium	4–40	60
Halazepam	Paxipam	60–160	50
Lorazepam	Ativan	2–6	15
Oxazepam	Serax	30–60	8
Prazepam	Centrax	20–40	100

[a]Half-life refers to parent compound and active metabolites; half-lives may vary considerably among individuals.

treatment of panic disorder, although most other benzodiazepines are not.

In the management of agoraphobia the elimination of panic attacks alone is usually not sufficient because it is necessary to assist the patient to overcome the anticipatory anxiety and the often-present situational anxiety that persists between panic attacks. Supportive psychotherapy, behavioral desensitization, and the administration of benzodiazepines are helpful in allaying the fear of leaving home and engaging in outside activities. It should be noted, however, that benzodiazepines alone, except for alprazolam, are not effective in preventing the panic attacks themselves. For a review of the dosage and side effects associated with TCA, the previous discussion of treatment of affective disorders should be consulted together with Tables 16.5–1 and 16.5–2.

POSTTRAUMATIC STRESS DISORDER

This disorder is apt to occur in individuals who have had a sudden, severely frightening or life-threatening experience such as combat, assault, rape, earthquakes, floods, and accidental injuries. Following the psychologically traumatic event, the patient may become somewhat emotionally withdrawn or "numb," tense, and easily startled and may tend to relive the experience in nightmares, memories of the event while awake, or both. Occasionally, the syndrome may be accompanied by symptoms of generalized anxiety and depression. This emotional state may last for weeks, months, or longer, but it tends slowly to attenuate with the passage of time. Psychologic support and reassurance are helpful. Antianxiety or antidepressant drugs may be indicated for symptoms of anxiety or depression.

OBSESSIVE-COMPULSIVE NEUROSIS

Obsessions are persistently recurrent, unwanted thoughts that are often described by the patient as being alien to his own values and sense of propriety. Disturbing obsessive thoughts may contain ideas of destruction, mutilation, death, or blasphemy, while others may seem superficially to be psychologically neutral, such as the recurrent title of a song. Compulsions refer to acts or rituals, such as counting, hand washing, or long prayers, that the patient must carry out to avoid anxiety. The anxiety in turn may be related to fear that an obsessive thought might, in some magical way, bring harm to someone.

In mild and transient form this neurosis is probably quite widespread. Indeed, it is likely that everyone is occasionally afflicted with a mild obsession, such as being haunted by doubts about whether one has turned off the stove even though one "almost" knows that he turned it off. In severe form obsessive-compulsive neurosis is relatively uncommon. When present in severe degree, the diagnosis is apparent from the patient's own description of his tormenting condition.

It is advisable to refer the patient with this disorder to a psychiatrist for further evaluation and treatment. In addition to psychotherapy, an antianxiety drug or an antidepressant may be indicated for symptoms of anxiety or depression in some cases.

REFERENCES

1. Baldessarini RJ: Biomedical Aspects of Depression and Its Treatment. American Psychiatric Press, 1983
2. Bertelson A, Harvald B, Hange M: A Danish twin study of manic-depressive disorders. Br J Psychiatr 130:330, 1977
3. Brown F: Depression and childhood bereavement. J Ment Sci 107:754, 1961
4. Cadoret RJ: Evidence for genetic inheritance of primary affective disorder in adoptees. Am J Psychiatr 135:463, 1978
5. Crow RR, Noyes R Jr, et al: A family study of panic disorder. Arch Gen Psychiatr 40:1065, 1983
6. Crowe RJ: Electroconvulsive therapy—A current perspective. N Engl J Med 311:163, 1984
7. Egeland JA, Gerhard DS, et al: Bipolar affective disorder linked to DNA marker on chromosome 11. Nature 235:783, 1987
8. Leckman JF, Weissman MM, et al: Panic disorder and major depression. Arch Gen Psychiatr 40:1055, 1983
9. Liebowitz MR, Fyer AJ, et al: Lactate provocation of panic attacks. I. Clinical and behavioral findings. Arch Gen Psychiatr 41:764, 1984
10. Maas J: Biogenic amines and depression. Arch Gen Psychiatr 32:1357, 1975
11. Paykel E, Myers J, et al: Life events and depression: A controlled study. Arch Gen Psychiatr 21:753, 1969
12. Schlesser MA, Altschuler KZ: The genetics of affective disorder: Data, theory, and clinical applications. Hosp Commun Psychiatr 34:415, 1983
13. Thompson KC, Hendrie H: Environmental stress in primary depressive illness. Arch Gen Psychiatr 26:130, 1972
14. Zitrin CM, Klein DF, et al: Treatment of phobias. I. Comparison of imipramine hydrochloride and placebo. Arch Gen Psychiatr 40:125, 1983

CHAPTER 16.6
Schizophrenia

Godfrey Pearlson and Joseph T. Coyle

Schizophrenia is a serious, chronic mental illness generally characterized by waxing and waning psychotic symptoms and a progressive deterioration in adaptive skills.[1] Because of the absence of pathognomonic physical or laboratory findings, schizophrenia is by necessity a diagnosis by exclusion based on clinical signs and symptoms. Nevertheless, the development of operational diagnostic criteria for the disorder has led to increased precision in diagnosis that has implications for management and outcome. Since the lifetime prevalence of schizophrenia in the general population is 1 percent and the number of patients chronically hospitalized in state facilities has decreased considerably, a growing number of patients suffering from schizophrenia will be seen by physicians in the community for the management of psychiatric and medical problems. The patient's status is likely to be complicated by the effects of neglect, poor personal hygiene, poor nutrition, and increased liability for abuse of drugs and alcohol. Thus, optimal treatment of these patients requires accurate diagnosis, effective management of their psychiatric symptoms, and attention to the medical complications of the disorder.[4]

CLINICAL FEATURES

Schizophrenia typically has its symptomatic onset in adolescence and early adulthood. Approximately half the patients have a premorbid history characterized by impairment in social and academic performance as well as personality traits of shyness, seclusiveness,

and a preoccupation with vague concepts. The onset of overt symptomatology is preceded by a prodromal phase involving weeks to months of gradual deterioration, typically characterized by social withdrawal and anxious bewilderment. Other symptoms at this stage can include self-neglect, loss of motivation, and a coarsening of personality with deterioration in social judgment and behavior. Since some of these behaviors can conceivably occur during normal adolescence, they may initially be misinterpreted in young patients. In this setting of anxiety and puzzlement, delusions often crystallize suddenly, appearing to provide the patient in a dramatic flash of insight with an explanation for his previous perplexing experiences. In a minority of patients florid delusions, hallucinations, and bizarre behavior emerge rapidly in full force in an individual with an unremarkable premorbid history. Such cases of acute onset are more likely to be associated with a favorable outcome and may represent a variant of affective disorder.

POSITIVE SYMPTOMS

During the acute, active phase of schizophrenia, "positive" symptoms are most prominent.[2] These include hallucinations, which are realistic perceptions in any sensory modality in the absence of external cause; delusions, which are fixed false beliefs idiosyncratic to the individual's culture that are not amenable to change by logical argument; and thought disorder, which involves abnormalities in the form of the patient's language and thinking. None of these symptoms is exclusive to schizophrenia and can occur in delirium, dementia, and affective disorders. Auditory hallucinations are the commonest type encountered in schizophrenia. Typically, they take the form of voices repeating the patient's thoughts out loud and commenting on the patient's behavior or two or more voices discussing the patient in the third person. The content of the hallucinations may be frightening or amusing and may prompt the patient to engage in bizarre and potentially dangerous behavior.

Delusions in schizophrenia are generally prominent and striking. They may be single and well encapsulated, such as the belief that one is infested with parasites, or multiple and occasionally organized into a complex hierarchy. While patients may occasionally discuss their delusional beliefs, they are generally secretive regarding them, especially those suffering from paranoid delusions. Certain types of delusions are commonly observed in schizophrenics. These concern the belief that the individual's mind or body is controlled by outside forces against his will, that thoughts are being inserted or removed from his mind, and that his thoughts are being broadcast to others at a distance. Such delusions, termed "passivity" experiences, may prompt the schizophrenic patient to present to the physician with odd physical complaints such as "a fungus is controlling my brain." It is therefore helpful on a routine basis to ask patients their interpretation of the cause of their medical symptoms.

Thought-disordered speech is characteristically vague with no logical thread connecting ideas. Words may be used idiosyncratically or are invented (neologisms). Typically, the replies to examiner's questions may be quite circumstantial and off the point. Motor abnormalities such as catatonia are occasionally seen as part of the disorder. It is important, however, to differentiate these from neuroleptic-induced extrapyramidal side effects, especially those such as rigidity or dystonic posturing (see below). Some patients will exhibit negativism (doing the opposite of what is asked), echolalia (repeating the examiner's words), echopraxia (repeating the examiner's actions), and perseveration.

Because the inner experiences of patients with schizophrenia can be bizarre, clinicians may tend to shy away from asking direct questions about the content of the hallucinations and delusions. One helpful approach to uncover these experiences is to begin by asking the patient about a neutral topic or acknowledged symptoms, then work toward the delusional and hallucinatory material, eventually asking directly about them in a factual and supportive manner.

NEGATIVE SYMPTOMS

"Negative" implies a loss or diminution of normal psychologic functions.[2] The balance between the predominance of positive and negative symptoms varies from one schizophrenic patient to another, but negative symptoms generally emerge and increase in severity in the course of recurrent, acute psychotic episodes. Although more subtle than positive symptoms, they can be quite disruptive to the patient's occupational and interpersonal functioning, leading to severe and chronic disability. Commonly encountered negative symptoms include blunting or impoverishment of the patient's emotions with a characteristic lack of spontaneity and warmth. There may be a reduction in the amount of speech, in the ideas conveyed in the patient's speech, and in the nonverbal gestures and emotional flavoring that normally accompany speech. Other negative symptoms include physical underactivity, lack of interest, and decreased energy. This loss of initiative and deteriorating interpersonal skills combines to make unemployment a significant problem and has led to the increasing representation of schizophrenics among "street people."

Neuropsychologic testing indicates that many schizophrenics have poorly sustained concentration and marked difficulty in switching cognitive "set" as manifested, for example, by the perseverance of elements of a preceding task into a current one. These constitute a mild but definite dementia syndrome. The negative symptoms and subtle dementia that accompany the schizophrenic syndrome may correlate with underlying structural abnormalities of the cerebral cortex and midbrain documented with computed tomography (CT) scans in up to half of all schizophrenics. Unlike positive symptoms, the negative symptoms respond poorly to neuroleptic treatment.

EPIDEMIOLOGY

Although the form of the symptoms—such as the characteristic hallucinations, delusions, and negative symptoms—appears constant across cultures, the content of these symptoms varies from culture to culture. The lifetime risk for schizophrenia is slightly in excess of 1 percent. The age-distributed risk of first hospitalization for schizophrenia is highest between 15 and 35 years of age. Onset occurs earlier in males, although women appear to "catch up" eventually.

Epidemiologic studies indicate that genetic factors are important in the expression of schizophrenia. Thus, a higher morbid risk exists for schizophrenia in close relatives of schizophrenics than in the general population. The closer the biologic relationship, the higher the risk. The lifetime risk for an individual with one schizophrenic parent is approximately 15 percent, which increases to 45 percent for one with two schizophrenic parents. The percentage risk for full siblings of schizophrenics is approximately 12 percent. Twin studies indicate that the proband concordance for dizygotic twins is 12 percent but for monozygotic twins approaches 65 percent. To separate genetic from environmental factors, studies of adoptees have been carried out. Offspring of a schizophrenic parent adopted into families without schizophrenia exhibit a considerably higher risk for developing schizophrenia than adoptees from nonschizophrenic biologic parents who are raised in a family in which one of the adoptive parents is schizophrenic. Nevertheless, these genetic studies indicate that schizophrenia does not fit any known classic Mendelian inheritance model, and the lack of complete concordance in identical twins suggests that environmental factors, such as perinatal insults, may contribute to the phenotypic expression of schizophrenia.

DIFFERENTIAL DIAGNOSIS

The diagnosis of schizophrenia is based upon operational inclusionary and exclusionary criteria that were established in the

**TABLE 16.6–1. DSM-III DIAGNOSTIC CRITERIA
FOR SCHIZOPHRENIA**

I. At least one of the following symptoms:
  A. Bizarre delusions of passivity or control
  B. Somatic, grandiose, or religious delusions
  C. Persecutory delusions
  D. Auditory hallucinations in the third person
  E. Auditory hallucinations incongruent with mood
  F. Disturbance in the logical sequence of thought associated
    with inappropriate affect; or delusion or hallucinations or
    grossly disorganized behavior
II. Deterioration from previous level of functioning
III. Duration of 6 months
IV. Not associated with an established affective disorder
V. Onset before age 45
VI. Absence of organic brain disorder or mental retardation

Diagnostic and Statistical Manual III (Table 16.6–1). These criteria result in a much more restricted use of this diagnosis than occurred in the past and have clearer implications with regard to treatment and outcome. Since there are no pathognomonic symptoms of schizophrenia, however, it is always necessary to exclude the presence of other conditions that can give rise to symptoms also seen in schizophrenia.[8] This leaves schizophrenia as a diagnosis of exclusion.

ORGANIC MENTAL DISORDERS

Patients with delirium, unlike schizophrenics, generally manifest reduced attention and concentration, fluctuating levels of consciousness, prominent disorientation, and an abnormal electroencephalogram (EEG). Patients with primary degenerative dementia generally demonstrate obvious global decline in cognitive function from a previously higher level, and evidence may be available for specific lesions within the brain.

AFFECTIVE DISORDERS

Clear alterations of mood in association with psychotic symptoms and a longitudinal course characterized by distinct episodes with return to normal between periods of illness helps differentiate the affective disorders from schizophrenia. Moreover, family history of affective disorder or suicide in first-degree relatives is strongly suggestive of an affective disorder and not of schizophrenia. Because affective disorder occurs in clear consciousness, it is probably the most difficult clinical entity to distinguish from schizophrenia. This difficulty is compounded by the fact that catatonic phenomena and florid hallucinations and delusions can also occur in affective disorder.[8] Nevertheless, the distinction is important because of the differences in pharmacologic management of schizophrenia as compared to affective disorder (see Chapter 16.5).

SYMPTOMATIC SCHIZOPHRENIAS

Several other clinical states can mimic acute schizophrenia, and a small number of patients can develop chronic schizophrenia-like illness. These "symptomatic schizophrenias" occur in association with several well-defined pathologic conditions and affect individuals with no familial or premorbid predisposition for schizophrenia. Neurologic disorders including sequelae of head injury, frontal brain tumors, encephalitis, or storage diseases such as metachromatic leukodystrophy can all on occasion give rise to hallucinations, delusions, and thought disorder in clear consciousness. Chronic use of amphetamines, cocaine, or phencyclidine (PCP) can also produce sympatomatic schizophrenia. It is therefore necessary to obtain a careful drug abuse history and to perform toxicologic screening when such abuse may be a contributory factor. Al-

coholic hallucinosis is a withdrawal state occurring after the cessation of heavy drinking and is characterized by auditory and/or visual hallucinations in clear consciousness. Finally, individuals with temporal lobe epilepsy, especially where the focus is in the dominant temporal-limbic area, can develop a chronic symptomatic schizophrenia that may appear more than a decade after the onset of seizures.

ETIOLOGY

The commonly accepted hypothesis for the cause of schizophrenia is the "stress-diathesis" model, according to which environmental stressors precipitate the disorder in the genetically predisposed individual. At present, neither the underlying causal disorder nor the mechanisms of clinical symptom production are clearly understood in schizophrenia. In vivo imaging with CT and postmortem neuropathologic studies indicate that nearly half of schizophrenics exhibit nonspecific cortical and subcortical atrophy as compared to age-matched controls. The cause of these changes remains obscure, but they appear to be present at the onset of the symptoms.

The most compelling hypothesis for the neurobiologic cause of positive symptoms of schizophrenia posits an excessive activity of limbic dopamine receptors.[6] This hypothesis is based upon several lines of evidence. Positive symptoms may be precipitated in normal individuals and exacerbated in schizophrenics by drugs such as cocaine and amphetamine that indirectly increase the stimulation of brain dopamine receptors. On the other hand, neuroleptic drugs, which reduce the positive symptoms of schizophrenia, act by means of blocking the dopamine D-2 receptor in the brain, and the clinical potency of these drugs correlates highly with their affinity for this receptor.[9] Recent studies have indicated an increased number of dopamine D-2 receptors in the caudate nucleus and the nucleus accumbens in brains of individuals who suffered from schizophrenia before death. Nevertheless, the confounding effects of chronic neuroleptic treatment have not been totally resolved with regard to these latter findings.

TREATMENT

It is advisable for the internist or family physician to refer the patient to the psychiatrist for treatment and management.

NEUROLEPTICS

The mainstay of treatment for schizophrenia is neuroleptic medications. Well-controlled studies have indicated that treatment with neuroleptics is more effective than any other form of therapy alone, including psychotherapy, milieu therapy, or electroconvulsive therapy. The neuroleptics are effective both in reducing the positive symptoms of an acute schizophrenic psychosis and, with chronic administration, in forestalling relapse. As a by-product of the efficacy of neuroleptics, the number of patients, primarily schizophrenic, who require long-term institutional care has been radically reduced.

Clinical and fundamental research over the last two decades has led to an understanding of the basic mechanism of action of neuroleptics. The neuroleptics are potent blockers of the brain receptors that mediate the effects of the neurotransmitter dopamine.[6,9] The clinical efficacy of the various neuroleptics, regardless of chemical structure, correlates with their affinity for the D-2 subtype of brain dopamine receptors. With regard to the therapeutic effects, the neuroleptics reduce and may even eliminate the positive symptoms of schizophrenia, including thought disorder, hallucinations, and delusions, but they have little impact on negative symptoms such as the amotivational state and affective blunting.

The fact that all available neuroleptics exert their antipsychotic effects by the same mechanism has important therapeutic implica-

tions. First, no neuroleptic is specifically effective in ameliorating any particular subset of psychotic symptoms such as thought disorder or paranoid thinking; all are equally effective. Second, there is little justification for using more than one type of neuroleptic to treat these psychotic symptoms. A single neuroleptic is as effective as a combination and may be associated with fewer side effects. There is, however, a considerable range of potency among the neuroleptics, varying over 100-fold (see Table 16.6–2). This variation of potency does not imply that one drug is superior to another but rather that the less potent medication must be used in higher doses to achieve equivalent clinical responses. The major differences among neuroleptics that dictate choice for treatment are the side effects associated with the various drugs. For example, the less potent thioridazine and chlorpromazine are rather sedating and can cause orthostatic hypotension because of their significant alpha-receptor-blocking activity, whereas the much more potent fluphenazine and haloperidol exhibit a greater propensity for causing acute neurologic side effects. Droperidol is a drug of high potency that has significant sedating action and thus has proved useful as an intramuscularly injected, rapidly acting, sedating neuroleptic for treating acutely agitated psychotic individuals.

The goal of neuroleptic therapy is to achieve remission of the positive symptoms of schizophrenia. The dosage requirements and the rate of remission vary among patients and are determined by titration of symptoms with drugs. Typically, therapy is initiated with a dose of neuroleptic equivalent to 50 to 100 mg of chlorpromazine administered orally four times a day (see Table 16.6–2 for dosage equivalents). The doses are increased progressively according to the response of the patient. Some patients may ultimately require the equivalent of 800 to 1600 mg of chlorpromazine per day before responding. In cases where behavior is extremely disruptive, more rapid control can be achieved by intramuscular injection of potent neuroleptics such as haloperidol or droperidol. Clinical reports indicate that administration of 5 mg of haloperidol intramuscularly every 1 to 2 hours will result in a marked reduction of psychotic behavior after two to four injections. This aggressive, high-dose therapy, however, must be accompanied by careful monitoring of the patient's vital signs and bears the risk of serious side effects. Behavioral improvement generally precedes the reduction in delusions and hallucinations. As the psychotic state begins to resolve, the sedating effects of neuroleptics may become much more prominent. At this point in treatment, the daily dosage of medication can be gradually and progressively reduced with careful monitoring of the patient for recurrence of symptoms.

In addition to their important role in reducing the positive symptoms of an acute psychotic episode of schizophrenia, neuroleptics have proven quite effective prophylactically to prevent relapse in chronic schizophrenics. In patients in whom the chronicity of the disorder has been established, discontinuation of neuroleptic treatment results in an exponential rate of relapse, with half the patients having relapsed by 6 months. For maintenance therapy, the lowest amount of neuroleptic that alleviates psychotic symptoms should be sought.[3] The average daily dose for maintenance therapy is usually equivalent to 100 to 300 mg of chlorpromazine. There is considerable variation among patients in terms of their drug requirements and even with a particular patient, depending upon life events.

Because of the prolonged half-life of neuroleptics, a single dose of medication is usually sufficient to maintain steady blood levels throughout a 24-hour period. A single daily dose reduces the expense of medication, simplifies the treatment schedule, and thus enhances compliance. When the neuroleptic is prescribed for evening administration, this strategy focuses the sedating effects at the appropriate time. For patients in whom compliance in taking medication is a serious problem, long-acting injectable forms of neuroleptic can be used. A single injection of approximately 25 mg of fluphenazine decanoate or 100 mg of haloperidol decanoate provides neuroleptic coverage for a period of 2 to 4 weeks without the requirement for oral medication.

Neurologic Side Effects (Table 16.6–3)

Neurologic symptoms resembling those seen in disorders of the extrapyramidal system are frequent side effects encountered with neuroleptic therapy. Parkinsonism, the most common of these side effects, is manifest by bradykinesia, rigidity, tremor, expressionless face, shuffling gait, and drooling. Dystonic reactions, which occur more frequently in younger patients, involve transient and recurrent contractions of axial and facial muscles. Typical dystonic symptoms include torticollis, oculogyric crisis (eyes fixed in an upward gaze), and opisthotonos. A diagnostically confusing side effect is akathisia, in which the patient experiences an inner tension and muscular discomfort that is relieved by movement. Thus, akathisia, depending upon its severity, can cause a range of symptoms from mild fidgeting to marked agitation with constant pacing. Akathisia should be distinguished from psychotic anxiety by the fact that the patient describes the discomfort as peripheral and because the symptom is exacerbated with increasing doses of neuroleptic.

TABLE 16.6–2. COMPARATIVE POTENCY OF NEUROLEPTICS

	Dose Equivalent (mg)
Phenothiazine	
• Chlorpromazine	100
• Thioridazine	100
• Perphenazine	10
• Trifluoperazine	5
• Fluphenazine	2
Thioxanthine	
• Chlorprothixene	100
• Thiothixene	3
Butyrophenone	
• Haloperidol	2
• Droperidol	1
Indolone	
• Molindone	10
Dibenzoxazepine	
• Loxapine	15

TABLE 16.6–3. SIDE EFFECTS OF NEUROLEPTICS

Neurologic

Acute
- Parkinsonism
- Dystonic reaction
- Akathisia
- Dyskinesia

Delayed
- Tardive dyskinesia
- Neuroleptic malignant syndrome

Endocrine
- Gynecomastia-galactorrhea
- Hyperprolactinemia
- Suppression of growth hormone secretion
- Obesity

Autonomic
- Orthostatic hypotension
- Dry mouth
- Blurred vision
- Impotence

Idiosyncratic
- Retinal degeneration (thioridazine)
- Photosensitivity
- Hepatitis and other allergic reactions

All three of these side effects are likely caused by neuroleptic blockade of dopamine receptors in the striatum. The neuroleptic-induced reduction in dopamine-receptor stimulation in the striatum results in part in the disinhibition of striatal cholinergic neurons (Figure 16.6–1). Accordingly, these side effects can be effectively reduced or eliminated by the administration of antiparkinsonian drugs that block central muscarinic acetylcholine receptors, including benzotropine, biperidin, and trihexiphenidyl. Since anticholinergic drugs cause their own spectrum of central and peripheral parasympathetic side effects, these drugs should not be administered unless the patient develops extrapyramidal symptoms or is at high risk for them. When treatment with anticholinergic drugs is indicated, the patient should be started on low, divided doses, which are progressively increased until the extrapyramidal symptoms are resolved or anticholinergic side effects become troublesome. These include dry mouth, visual blurring, constipation, and difficulty in urination. After a several-week course of treatment with anticholinergics, their dosage should be tapered to determine if continued use is required. In the case of acute dystonic reactions, which often require rapid intervention, intramuscular diphenhydramine (25 to 50 mg) or benzotropine (2 mg) generally results in the quick reversal of these painful and frightening symptoms.

A relatively irreversible neurologic side effect known as "tardive dyskinesia" can complicate long-term treatment with neuroleptics.[5] This side effect is characterized by oral and facial dyskinesias and writhing movements of the tongue. In severe cases choreoathetotic movements of the extremities and lordotic posture may occur. Prevalence studies suggest that approximately 10 percent of patients chronically treated with neuroleptics manifest symptoms of tardive dyskinesia. In aged, chronically institutionalized patients the prevalence may achieve 40 percent or more. The risk of tardive dyskinesia should therefore be carefully considered and discussed before engaging a patient in long-term neuroleptic treatment. Risk factors for tardive dyskinesia include exposure to high cumulative doses of neuroleptics; female gender; and pre-existing brain damage. The mechanism thought to be responsible for tardive dyskinesia appears to be an irreversible, neuroleptic-induced supersensitivity of striatal dopamine receptors. Accordingly, affected patients generally exhibit a transient improvement upon elevation of neuroleptic dosage and exacerbation on withdrawal of neuroleptics. Notably, neuroleptic treatment may obscure an underlying tardive dyskinesia syndrome. Finally, anticholinergic drugs generally exacerbate the symptoms of tardive dyskinesia in contrast to their ameliorating effects on acute extrapyramidal side effects.

An uncommon but potentially fatal neurologic side effect is the neuroleptic malignant syndrome.[7] Patients suffering from this disorder present with high fever, marked perspiration, striking rigidity, confusion, and rhabdomyolysis with elevated serum creatine kinase activity. The fever is associated with cardiovascular instability; the rhabdomyolysis, with acute renal failure; and the profound rigidity, with impairments in clearance of secretions and aspiration pneumonia. The disorder is associated with treatment with high-potency neuroleptics, but the symptoms can persist for a considerable period of time after neuroleptic discontinuation. Treatment with dantrolene rapidly reverses the rhabdomyolysis and fever; however, it is ineffective with regard to the rigidity. Accordingly, a direct dopamine agonist such as bromocryptine is also often administered to reverse the severe extrapyramidal symptoms. Since anticholinergics interfere with perspiration, these drugs are contraindicated because of their potential for exacerbating the fever.

Idiosyncratic Side Effects

By blocking dopamine receptors in the pituitary, neuroleptics cause an increased release of prolactin, which can result in galactorrhea in females. Interference with peripheral sympathetic function, seen especially with less potent neuroleptics, can cause orthostatic hypotension, blurred vision, and impotence. Thioridazine in doses in excess of 800 mg per day can cause retinal degeneration. Phenothiazine neuroleptics may cause photosensitivity dermatitis and pigmentation of the skin. Allergic reactions and cholestatic jaundice can occur rarely.

PSYCHOSOCIAL TREATMENT

Pharmacotherapy is one aspect of the overall management of patients with schizophrenia. Neuroleptics are of limited value in alle-

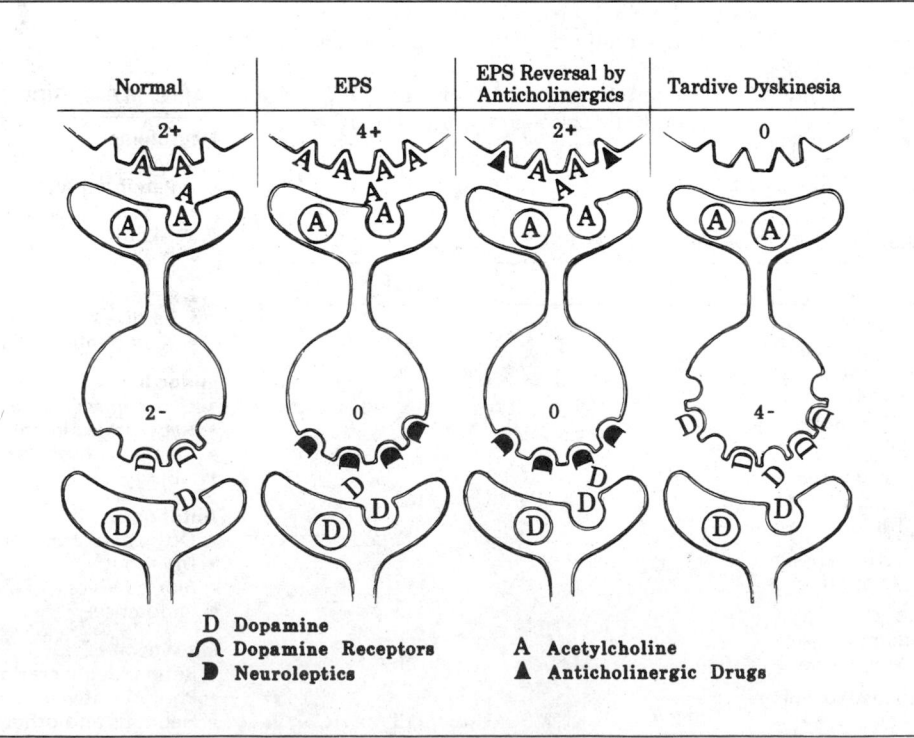

Figure 16.6–1. Drug interactions in the striatum in neuroleptic-induced extrapyramidal side effects. The synaptic relationship between the nigrostriatal dopaminergic terminals and the striatal cholinergic interneurons is presented. Dopamine inhibits the release of acetylcholine in the striatum by activating dopamine receptors. Neuroleptics block the dopamine receptors resulting in increased release of acetylcholine and emergence of acute extrapyramidal side effects. These neurologic symptoms can be counteracted by the anticholinergic drugs. In tardive dyskinesia, there is a pathologic increase in the density and sensivity of the dopamine receptors, resulting in the insufficient release of acetylcholine and emergence of dyskinetic symptoms.

viating the negative symptoms of the defect state. Like other chronically ill, impaired people, some schizophrenics are demoralized by repeated hospitalizations, lower standard of living, and stigmatization as "crazy, dangerous, and undesirable." Some patients retain insight into their loss of drive and motivation and are tormented by their inertia and social incompetence to the point of attempting suicide. Families are often confused by the dramatic change in their ill relative, may blame themselves for causing the disorder, or may respond to the symptoms with criticism, intrusiveness, and unrealistic demands. All these issues are to be addressed with an ongoing therapeutic relationship that focuses on current problems of daily living and supports the patient in his attempts at independent work and social interaction. Both the patient and family require education on the nature of the illness, the particular stressors that increase symptoms, early prodromal warning signs of exacerbations, the purpose of medication and possible side effects, and the need for a modest pace of clearly defined expectations that neither underestimates nor overwhelms the patient. There is now convincing evidence that therapeutic interventions that enhance communicational skills and reduce discord within the family can significantly decrease the rate of relapse in patients receiving optimal neuroleptic treatment.

Other adjunctive therapies can assist in reducing the disability suffered by the schizophrenic. Occupational therapy and day-hospital programs can provide structure and directed supervision that may partially overcome some of the emotional problems. Supervised living arrangements, halfway houses, and other group transi-

tional residences may combat the tendency toward reversal of sleep patterns and social isolation. Optimal care comes through a multimodal program coordinated by one person who can tailor the various elements to the individual needs of the patient.

REFERENCES

1. American Psychiatric Association: Diagnostic and Statistical Manual of Mental Disorders (DSM III-R). Washington, DC, APA Press, 1987
2. Crow TJ: Positive and negative symptoms and the role of dopamine. Br J Psychiatr 139:251, 1981
3. Davis J: Overview: Maintenance therapy in psychiatry: I. Schizophrenia. Am J Psychiatr 132:1237, 1975
4. Faloon IRH: Family Management of Schizophrenia. A Study of Clinical, Social, Family and Economic Benefits. Baltimore, Johns Hopkins University Press, 1985
5. Kane J, Smith J: Tardive dyskinesia. Prevalence and risk factors, 1959–1979. Arch Gen Psychiatr 39:473, 1982
6. Pearlson G, Coyle JT: The dopamine hypothesis and schizophrenia. In Coyle JT, Enna SJ (eds): Neuroleptics: Neurochemical, Behavioral, and Clinical Perspectives. New York, Raven Press, 1983, pp. 297–324
7. Pope HG, Keck PE, McElroy SL: Frequency and presentation of neuroleptic malignant syndrome in a large psychiatric hospital. Am J Psychiatr 143:1227, 1986
8. Pope HG, Lipinski J: Differential diagnosis of schizophrenia and manic depressive illness. Arch Gen Psychiatr 35:811, 1978
9. Snyder SH: Dopamine receptors, neuroleptics and schizophrenia. Am J Psychiatr 138:460, 1981

CHAPTER 16.7
The Cognitively Impaired Patient

Marshal Folstein, Barry Rovner,
Larry Tune, Andrew Warren,
and Jason Brandt

Cognitive impairment is frequently encountered by physicians because the prevalence is high: 5 percent in the general population, 20 percent among the elderly, and 25 percent of medical inpatients. The high prevalence among the elderly was once thought to represent a normal aspect of aging; however, it is now recognized that cognitive impairment in older patients often is caused by a number of different medical disorders, some of them reversible. Diagnosis and treatment of cognitive impairment depends on the same clinical method used in the rest of medicine. In other words, symptoms and signs elicited during a history-taking interview, a mental-state examination, and a physical examination are analyzed to formulate a diagnosis, a prognosis, and an appropriate treatment plan.

The term "cognitive impairment" indicates a diminished capacity to know and reason about the world. It can be viewed as a single dimension of impairment or as a mosaic of impairments of several discrete capacities. When viewed as a single dimension that can be quantified into various levels of impairment, it can be related to the general level of intelligence and described clinically as the capacity to think with accustomed speed and clarity and to grasp the essentials of a situation. The validity of the single-dimensional concept of cognition is confirmed by correlations between measures of cognitive impairment and standard measures of intelligence, and between these measures and the amount of pathologic damage—regardless of location—found in studies of diffuse brain diseases, stroke, and brain tumors.

When cognitive impairment is viewed as a mosaic of impairments, deficits in specific functions such as memory or language can be grouped into particular cognitive syndromes and related to

specific neural systems. This approach has some advantages in terms of both diagnosis and treatment. Although mental retardation is often defined by the single dimension of intelligence, it can also be assessed in terms of particular development or learning disabilities, such as dyslexia, and treatment can be more specifically tailored to the patient's needs.

Cognitive impairment has important consequences for the patient in school, at work, and in the courts, as well as at home. It also affects the patient's ability to follow medical directions in the treatment of other medical disorders that might require taking medications on schedule, adhering to special diets, and keeping outpatient appointments. These factors must all be taken into account by the treating physician. The physician must also comprehend and treat any associated abnormal moods, perceptions, ideas, and behaviors and understand the demoralization that can result from the limitations necessarily placed on the patient's life choices.

On the other hand, it is also important for the physician to appreciate the functions that are preserved in the patient that give meaning to the life of even the most severely impaired individual. Such functions include the capacity to love and to suffer. Too often the cognitively impaired individual is given low priority because it is assumed that human dignity depends only on intelligence.

RECOGNITION OF COGNITIVE IMPAIRMENT

The cognitively impaired patient does not always complain about his impairment. Sometimes family members notice the patient's

difficulties and bring him for evaluation; at other times the physician seeing the patient for other reasons must detect the problem. In these cases cognitive impairment can be measured quantitatively, and this should be done as a routine matter, just as checking blood pressure is a standard part of the physical examination. Only occasionally does the detection of impairment lead to the diagnosis of a reversible condition, but in all cases recognition of the patient's cognitive state will influence management.

Several quantitative screening batteries of brief psychologic tests are available to assess the cognitive state of the individual in the home or in the physician's office. With these tools physicians can detect cases of cognitive impairment in their patients who attend their clinics for other reasons. Like measurements of blood pressure or sedimentation rate, these cognitive measurements are not diagnostic but are useful indicators of the need for further evaluation or the need for special management. The Mini-Mental State Examination (MMSE) is one such quantiative method for grading the cognitive state of patients (Table 16.7–1). It is a brief battery of tests of different cognitive functions that can be grouped to define syndromes such as dementia or amnesia, or it can be scored as a single dimension of cognitive capacity. Thus, it can be used to analyze cognitive function as a single dimension of intelligence and also as a mosaic of functions.[1]

USE OF THE MINI-MENTAL EXAMINATION

Instructions

The test is introduced by asking the patient's permission to test his memory: "It is a routine part of the examination at this point to ask questions about memory. Is it all right if I test your memory?" The examiner tries to put the patient at ease and not correct errors, since this might lead to a catastrophic reaction or refusal to cooperate.

The subject is first asked to state the season, the date, the day of the week, the time, and the place.

Registration and recall are then tested by asking the patient to remember three objects (such as a pony, a quarter, an orange) presented at 3-second intervals and then asking him to repeat them. One point is given for each correct response. If all three objects are not repeated correctly, the patient is allowed to practice until he can remember them all and the number of trials can be recorded, but only the first trial is scored.

The patient is then asked to subtract 7 from 100 and then 7 from each subsequent remainder for five trials; the number of correct subtractions is scored one point for each. If the patient refuses this test, he can alternatively be asked to spell the word "world" backwards; however, this task is not given if the patient tries and fails the serial 7's task. At this time, the patient is asked if he can remember the three items he was previously asked to repeat, and each item recalled is scored one point.

The next section of the test samples the functions of naming, repetition, following a three-point command, reading a sentence, writing a sentence, and copying a design. This section differentiates the MMSE from most other screening tests because it samples aspects of aphasia and apraxia, abnormalities found in several syndromes that present significant management problems.

The number of correct responses is scored, with 30 points representing the perfect score. In addition, particular deficiencies and retained capacities are noted for purposes of diagnosis and management. For example, individuals who are unable to remember three objects after the serial 7's distraction but are able to perform calculations should be evaluated for the amnestic syndrome and the disorders that can cause it. Individuals who perform poorly on most tasks but are able to read can often understand written commands better than spoken commands.

The level of consciousness is not scored but is rated on an analogue scale labeled at one extreme as fully alert and at the other as comatose. This item serves to draw the examiner's attention to those cases where cognitive impairment associated with an altered state of consciousness would lead to the diagnosis of delirium.

The MMSE is recommended as a clinical tool because of its established reliability, validity, specificity, and sensitivity and because normative values by age, sex, and race for an urban community are known. Ninety-five percent of a representative sample of the population of Baltimore living at home scored higher than 23 on the test. Race and sex did not affect scores, but age and education did, with individuals who had less education and who were older scoring lower. Only 20 percent of an elderly population, who were mostly poorly educated, scored less than 23, however.

For clinical purposes, individuals scoring in the 0 to 23 range, or scoring 23 to 29 but showing signs of change in mental capacity, should be evaluated for cognitive dysfunction. Of these individuals, however, 33 percent will be found to have no currently diagnosable condition, while many individuals currently scoring in the normal range will eventually develop low scores as a result of progressive neurologic disease. Thus, as with any scored clinical test, diagnosis cannot be assumed from the score alone but must be deduced from the sum of the clinical evidence.

TABLE 16.7–1. MINI-MENTAL STATE EXAMINATION

Maximum Score	Score	
		Orientation:
5	( )	What is the (year) (season) (date) (day) (month)?
5	( )	Where are we: (state) (county) (town) (hospital) (floor)?
		Registration:
3	( )	Name 3 objects: 1 second to say each. Then ask the patient all 3 after you have said them. Give 1 point for each correct answer. Then repeat them until he learns all three. Count trials and record. (No. of Trials: _____)
		Attention and Calculation:
5	( )	Serial 7's. 1 point for each correct. Stop after 5 answers. Alternatively spell "world" backwards.
		Recall:
3	( )	Ask for 3 objects repeated above. Give 1 point for each correct.
		Language:
9	( )	Name a pencil, and watch (2 points).
		Repeat the following: "No ifs, ands, or buts." (1 point)
		Follow a 3-stage command: "Take a paper in your right hand, fold it in half, and put it on the floor." (3 points)
		Read and obey the following: "Close your eyes." (1 point)
		Write a sentence. (1 point)
		Copy this design. (1 point)

Total Score _____

Assess level of consciousness along a continuum.

Alert	Drowsy	Stupor	Coma

EXAMPLES FROM THE CLINIC

Alzheimer Disease

The MMSE becomes abnormal in most patients within the first year after definite complaints of memory impairment are noted. After 3 to 4 years of illness, scores of 14 to 15 are usual, although the course in individual patients can be variable. The orientation and memory items deteriorate first, and after 1 year of illness most patients will be unable to recall two of three items. Performance on the language items is better preserved until 3 to 4 years of illness, when aphasia and apraxia become prominent.

Delirium

Most patients meeting criteria for delirium will have MMSE scores in the abnormal range; however, 33 percent will score normally. The best method for the assessment of delirium is the analogue rating of level of consciousness found at the bottom of the MMSE form. This type of rating is a reliable and sensitive indicator of delirium.

Mental Retardation

The MMSE scores of mentally retarded individuals correlate with other measures of social function, such as the Adaptive Behavior Scale of the American Association of Mental Deficiency, and with intelligence scores. The sensitivity and specificity of the MMSE as a case-finding method for mental retardation has not been established. Abnormal scores, however, are usually found in those mentally retarded individuals who never were able to learn to read despite access to educational facilities.

NEUROPSYCHOLOGIC EXAMINATION[8]

Brief cognitive screening procedures such as the MMSE are useful for the identification and follow-up of individuals with moderate to severe cognitive impairments. Often, however, clinical care and patient management will necessitate more detailed neuropsychologic assessment. Such assessment can serve several purposes: (1) help to establish the existence of an abnormal mental state in mild cases or early in progressive illnesses, (2) assist in differential diagnosis, that is, help to identify the presence and localization of cerebral lesions, (3) be used to construct a profile of the patient's cognitive strengths and weaknesses to be used in directing treatment and rehabilitation and monitoring their effects, and (4) be used to predict the patient's adaptive functioning in his everyday environment. Patients suspected of having impaired cognition should be seen by the psychiatrist or neurologist for diagnostic assessment and possible referral to the clinical psychologist for neuropsychologic testing.

DELIRIUM: A DETERIORATION OF THE LEVEL OF CONSCIOUSNESS

Delirium is a syndrome characterized by cognitive impairment and an alteration of consciousness, but it is also associated with prominent noncognitive symptoms, such as depression, delusions, hallucinations, autonomic disturbances, and motor disturbances, which often are the presenting features. Delirium has two subtypes, which differ in their clinical presentation but often merge in particular clinical situations. The first type is characterized by a state of drowsiness and a diffusely slow electroencephalogram (EEG) and is exemplified by a variety of drug intoxications including alcohol and anticholinergic drugs. This type is sometimes called a "confusional state." The second is characterized by a vigilant state of altered consciousness and a normal or fast-frequency EEG and is exemplified by the delirium caused by alcohol withdrawal syndrome.

Delirium is common in medical inpatient wards, with a prevalence of approximately 10 percent, not including individuals recovering from anesthesia. The onset, course, and prognosis depend to a certain extent on the underlying disorder. The onset is acute or subacute, beginning over minutes to hours, although it often is not recognized until fully developed. The course is fluctuating from hour to hour and day to day. The prognosis is serious in that up to 25 percent of patients will not live through their hospital admission, but if the underlying disorder can be treated, the mental state returns to normal except for occasional residual symptoms, which will be discussed later.

DIAGNOSIS OF DELIRIUM

The diagnosis of delirium depends on the recognition of an altered state of consciousness in a patient with cognitive impairment. A disruption of the normal cycle of wakefulness and sleep is often present. The assessment of consciousness depends on a judgment of whether the patient is alert, aware, and normally responsive to ordinary conversation. The cognitive impairment of the delirious patient can be rated by the MMSE. A third of delirious subjects will score in the normal range, however, although repeated measures will often indicate an increase in score as the patient recovers. Special features of the cognitive impairment of delirium include slowness of visual perception time as well as disorientation, attentional deficits, a forgetting of the recent past, and a difficulty in learning new material. Delirious individuals are typically apraxic and occasionally aphasic. One simple useful measure of delirium is a daily handwriting chart in which the patient is asked to sign his name, write a sentence, or copy a design. The improvement in the delirium will be documented by the clarity of the written material.

Features

Anxiety, depression, delusions, and visual and auditory hallucinations are all prominently associated features of delirium. These symptoms appear in almost half of all cases. Suicidal behavior is occasionally seen. Delirium is regularly associated with tachycardia, but tachypnea, hypoventilation, and fever or hypothermia can also occur. The pupils may be fixed and dilated in anticholinergic delirium as well as in delirium associated with raised intracranial pressure. The skin can be hot and flushed or perspiring. The onset of tachycardia is often a useful clinical sign pointing to the onset of delirium. Connection of the onset of tachycardia with the clinical events of that period, including the prescription of new drugs, can suggest etiology.

Disturbances of the motor system are common and have important implications for diagnosis and management of the delirious patient. Delirious patients display regular rhythmic tremor and also an irregular asterixis or flapping tremor when they try to sustain a fixed posture. Widespread myoclonus also occurs. Nystagmus, dysarthria, ataxia, and a variety of other transient focal motor signs can be seen. The assessment of the patient's station and gait, with the examiner at his side to prevent falls, is a useful measure of the capacity of the delirious patient to be out of bed. The presence of these motor signs, particularly asterixis and myoclonus in a highly agitated patient, often provides a useful differential diagnostic clue in distinguishing delirium from mania and schizophrenia.

Differential Diagnosis

One of the most important clues in the differentiation of delirium from other psychiatric disorders is the frequency of the dominant rhythm of the EEG. In most cases of delirium the EEG is diffusely slower than the usual rate for that individual, and in most cases of other psychiatric disorders, the background activity of the EEG is not slow. Exceptions include those instances of drug-induced delirium and withdrawal where an excess of low-voltage, fast activity can predominate, although slow waves are usually present as well. Since in mild cases of delirium the state of consciousness can fluctuate, however, serial EEGs may be necessary.

COMMON CAUSES OF DELIRIUM

Because the epidemiology and cause of delirium are as yet unclear, the somatic disorders associated with delirium must be listed in a more or less unrelated series based in part on prevalence, such as cerebral injury, drugs, and seizures, and in part on those relatively rare events, such as hypoglycemia, which must be listed because of the treatment implications. In most cases of delirium, the etiology is likely to be mixed, since delirious patients often suffer from several chronic diseases that can affect the brain, and in addition, are taking multiple medications. One current hypothesis is that the final common pathway of many causes of delirium is the disruption in function of cholinergic neurons innervating the cerebral cortex.

Cerebral Injury

Patients suffering from structural central nervous system (CNS) damage are prone to delirium. This damage can be the result of stroke, Alzheimer disease, or head trauma. Often these same patients will suffer from seizures, which themselves can cause delirium after a single seizure or in the midst of a flurry of attacks. A special variant of delirium, termed a "twilight state," occurs after a series of temporal lobe seizures. This state is characterized by an altered, but not drowsy, state of consciousness with marked psychomotor retardation best demonstrated during the performance of a repetitive task such as the serial 7's task. These patients can also be unpredictably violent. Treatment consists of suppressing all seizure activity and protecting the patient and others around from his behavior during the period of days to weeks required for the state to subside. Because delirium can be caused by meningoencephalitis of viral, bacterial, or fungal origin, a lumbar puncture should be performed in the evaluation of the delirious patient.

Drug-Related Delirious States

Drugs can cause delirium when they are ingested or when they are withdrawn after chronic ingestion. The mechanism by which drugs produce delirium is not completely known, but recent evidence suggests that one mechanism is through their capacity to block brain cholinergic receptors. Many drugs have some anticholinergic properties (Table 16.7–2). While the dosage of one particular drug might not produce delirium, the combination of that drug with others having anticholinergic effects may symptomatically compromise brain cholinergic function. The evidence for this mechanism comes from the work of many investigators who have demonstrated that anticholinergic drugs such as scopolamine or atropine can affect memory and produce alterations of consciousness. The typical anticholinergic syndrome includes dry mouth, dilated pupils, tachycardia, flushed dry skin, disorientation, memory loss, and hallucinations. The treatment for drug-related (induced) delirium is reduction in the number and dosage of medications. In some cases physostigmine can be administered.

Abrupt discontinuation of alcohol, short-acting barbiturates, and benzodiazepines produces a characteristic withdrawal syndrome most commonly seen in the alcohol withdrawal syndrome, delirium tremens. Within hours after the last dose of drug patients become tremulous, and some develop seizures. In the first 2 days

after withdrawal, a hallucinatory state in clear consciousness sometimes develops, which occasionally becomes chronic and indistinguishable from schizophrenia. Two to three days after withdrawal, patients develop a hypervigilant state with disorientation, attentional deficits, memory loss, vivid hallucinations, delusions, marked anxiety, and depression. There is tachycardia, diaphoresis, fever, and sleeplessness. Although sedatives and beta-blockers can alter some of the symptoms, prevention is the best treatment. The syndrome can be prevented by the gradual withdrawal of the offending drug and the substitution of a benzodiazepine from which the patient is then withdrawn. Because of the patient's tolerance to drugs of this class, large doses are necessary. See Chapter 17.5 for details of management.

Management of the delirious patient begins with proper diagnosis. Since delirious patients can suffer from dramatic psychiatric symptoms, they are often misdiagnosed as schizophrenic or depressed. The disturbance in consciousness, cognitive deficit, and abnormal EEG are all useful in formulating the differential diagnosis. After the diagnosis is made and the underlying cause is treated or corrected, the patient may require days to weeks of psychiatric care during the period of rehabilitation. The provision of adequate nutrition, activity, and sleep patterns is useful. Reassurance that the condition is reversible is helpful for the patient and the family. Occasionally small doses of haloperidol (5 to 15 mg per day) for short periods are useful in treating agitation, delusions and hallucinations.

DEMENTIA

Dementia is a syndrome defined by a global deterioration of intellectual functioning in clear consciousness. This definition differentiates dementia from other syndromes that affect cognition. Since it is an acquired deterioration, it is differentiated from mental retardation—a lifelong impairment. Since it is global, it is differentiated from the amnestic syndrome, which is primarily a disorder of memory, and from aphasia, which is limited to the disorder of language. Since it occurs in clear consciousness, it is differentiated from delirium, which is a cognitive impairment with clouded consciousness. Dementia affects 5 to 10 percent of the general population over age 65 and 20 to 30 percent over age 85; it accounts for almost half the patients in nursing homes in the United States. As the population ages, dementia will become an increasingly serious public health problem.[3,7,11]

The many causes of dementia are listed in Table 16.7–3. In most cases there is no cure, but in some instances, notably depression, nutritional disorders, infectious diseases, and endocrinopathies, the condition may be reversible. Careful differential diagnosis is therefore crucial. It is helpful to distinguish the dementias in which aphasia ia a cardinal manifestation from those in which a lack of motivation is predominant.

TABLE 16.7–2. COMMONLY USED DRUGS WITH ANTICHOLINERGIC POTENTIAL

- Anesthetic agents (indirect)
- Analgesics
- Antidepressants
- Neuroleptics
- Antispasmodics
- Atropine and related drugs
- Barbiturates (indirect)
- Alcohol (indirect)
- Benzodiazepines (indirect)

TABLE 16.7–3. CAUSES OF DEMENTIA

Alzheimer disease	Depression
Multi-infarct disease	Hypothyroidism
Brain tumor	Hyperclasimia
Subdural hematoma	Deficiency of vitamin B$_{12}$, niacin, thiamine, folate
Dementia in alcoholics	Infection with fungus or *Treponema*
Occult hydrocephalus	Renal dialysis
Creutzfeldt-Jakob disease	Malabsorption
Huntington disease	Hepatic encephalopathy
Drug ingestion	

Diagnosis and management of dementia require a combined neurologic and psychiatric approach. Neurologic methods are necessary to determine the underlying cause of the disease, while psychiatric methods are most helpful in evaluating the presenting symptoms and directing patient care. Successful management of patients with dementias demands a commitment of the physician to continuity of the patients' care and support for the family throughout the long course of these diseases.

Because Alzheimer disease and multi-infarct dementia are the most common causes of dementia, they will be used to illustrate the diagnostic and therapeutic management. The same principles apply to the management of less common dementias whose distinguishing features are mentioned briefly.

ALZHEIMER DISEASE[2,5,9]

Alzheimer disease is the most common cause of dementia, accounting for about one half of all diagnosed cases. It is characterized by insidious onset and gradual, but relentless, worsening of cognitive defects over a period of years with the absence of motor paralysis or gait disorder until the later stages. The age of onset is from 25 to 90, but is usually between 70 and 80. The prevalence of this form of dementia is 2 percent of the population over the age of 65, rising with age to prevalence of 15 percent of the population over age 85. In most surveys there is a preponderance of females over males, but this observation is usually attributed to the greater rate of survival among females and the greater use of institutions by females.

Lesions and Etiology
The neuropathologic lesions consist of large numbers of neurofibrillary tangles in the frontal, temporal, and parietal lobes.[15] Senile plaques, which contain a unique protein known as "cerebrovascular amyloid," are numerous, and the brain is atrophic with a reduced weight.[6,15] Reduction in markers for cortical cholinergic, noradrenergic, and somatostatin-containing neurons has been well described.[11] The number of plaques and tangles and the severity of cholinergic neuronal loss are related to the severity of the dementia.

The etiology is unknown, but several theories are under investigation. A genetic basis is strongly suggested by evidence that many cases are familial and probably inherited. Studies of family pedigrees indicate that the disorder in many families is transmitted as an autosomal-dominant, age-dependent trait. In fact, a polymorphism on chromosome 21 has recently been shown to be linked to the gene responsible for a form of Alzheimer disease.[14] Notably, the gene that codes for cerebral vascular amyloid is also localized to chromosome 21. The suggestion of a viral origin is based on finding the lesions of Alzheimer disease in some family members of patients affected by Creutzfeldt-Jakob disease, which is an infectious disorder. Unlike Creutzfeldt-Jakob disease, however, Alzheimer disease has not been transmitted to animals.

Clinical Features
Alzheimer disease has a distinctive clinical course, and specific symptoms can be expected to appear at fairly predictable stages. Amnesia is usually one of the first symptoms to appear. In the early stages the patient often seems normal to the casual observer because of the patient's retained social facade. Only close family members, friends, or an employer may be aware of the first signs of forgetfulness. Soon, however, the patient's difficulty in remembering and learning becomes more obvious and incapacitating. Unlike the memory blurring that occurs in the benign forgetfulness of Kral, the memory deficit in Alzheimer disease is for major life events and results in serious behavior problems, such as forgetting the way home, losing money, and forgetting important events.

Difficulties in using language begin to occur 2 to 3 years after the onset of amnesia. At first, the family may notice only that the patient has difficulty entering the conversation at the dinner table. Thereafter, his capacity to understand and communicate deteriorates progressively and provides a benchmark in the progress of the disease. The ability to read and write is lost, and speech becomes anomic, empty, and aphasic and may include jargon. Apraxias appear 3 to 4 years after the onset of the disease. The patient loses the capacity to use common objects such as the telephone, the stove, and the checkbook and eventually becomes unable to dress, feed, or care for himself.

Agnosia is present about midway in the course of the disease. Although visual and auditory acuity remain relatively normal, the patient loses the ability to perceive the meaning of objects and can no longer recognize people around him. Gait disorder, incontinence, seizures, and myoclonus appear late in the course of the disease, and death occurs 8 to 10 years after onset.

Mood disturbances, especially depression and anxiety, occur in 20 percent of patients. As the disease progresses, the patient may become emotionally labile and develop a very low tolerance for demanding situations. Task failure or changes in the patient's environment can precipitate violent, emotional outbursts known as the "catastrophic reaction of Goldstein." Other psychiatric symptoms, such as delusions and hallucinations, occur in 30 percent of patients.

Differential Diagnosis
The distinction between dementia and delirium has been discussed. The next step is to determine the underlying pathologic condition associated with the dementia syndrome. In its early stages the diagnosis of Alzheimer disease can be difficult because gradually developing amnesia is characteristic of many dementing disorders, including benign ones such as Kral syndrome, and reversible ones, such as hypothyroidism, depression, hydrocephalus, brain tumors, and thiamine deficiency (see Table 16.7–3). As the disease progresses, however, its characteristic course makes it easier to diagnose with confidence.

Severe depression causing cognitive impairment can sometimes be difficult to distinguish from Alzheimer disease. The dementia of depression is characterized by an apathetic dementia of subacute onset of days to weeks. There may be a clear history of previous episodic depression, often a family history of depression, and aphasia is not present. The EEG is usually normal. When the distinction cannot be made with certainty, the patient should be given a therapeutic trial of antidepressants.

Alzheimer disease is differentiated from Pick disease, which is a lobar atrophy of the brain inherited as an autosomal-dominant disorder. In Pick disease the focal atrophy can be seen on the CT scan, and the EEG is often normal. Elderly patients can become progressively cognitively impaired from taking many drugs, including digitalis, antidepressants, and sedatives. To differentiate such conditions from Alzheimer disease often requires the discontinuation of suspect drugs. The most common problem of differential diagnosis is the distinction between Alzheimer disease and multi-infarct dementia. This distinction is complicated by the presence of both disorders in many patients.

Management
Currently, there is no cure for Alzheimer disease. Careful management can greatly diminish the suffering of both the patient and his family, however. The family of the patient with dementia needs special support if early institutionalization is to be avoided. This illness requires intensive, skilled care for 8 to 10 years and becomes a severe burden for families. In the early stages of the illness the family may need advice regarding the patient's legal status and his ability to drive a car or manage his finances. As the patient's faculties deteriorate, the family will need help managing his behavior. In the later stages advice in finding home help, day care, or a nursing home may be required. Behavior disturbances include awakening in the middle of the night, wandering out of the house, and searching through dresser drawers. The implementation of a schedule of daily events is often a great help in managing the patient's behavior. A regular routine can reduce anxiety in the patient

and will also be helpful to the family because it specifies the times that the patient will require supervision and enables the family to devise a series of regular activities to occupy the patient. A routine is also helpful in avoiding catastrophic reactions. The physician and family should recognize the patient's strengths and weaknesses so that situations that cause difficulty and frustration can be avoided. If irritability and emotional outbursts are a problem, a bedtime dose of 25 to 50 mg of thioridazine may be indicated. Mood disturbances can be treated with the appropriate medications, antidepressants for depression, and haloperidol 1 to 5 mg daily for elation.

Delusions and hallucinations are a significant problem for some patients with Alzheimer disease. Treatment with the ordinary neuroleptics such as haloperidol or fluphenazine must be approached cautiously because of the possibilities of undesirable sedation and extrapyramidal syndrome. Extrapyramidal side effects occur less frequently with thioridazine. The anticholinergic effects of these drugs can cause particular problems for the elderly, and a special inquiry must be made for the presence of glaucoma, prostate disease, and cardiac arrhythmia.

Sleep disturbance is a common problem, and sedatives such as chloral hydrate are helpful. In rare instances sedatives can produce excitement in the elderly. If the patient requires antidepressants or neuroleptics, however, these can be given at bedtime to avoid the use of a hypnotic. Associated medical problems must be carefully monitored and treated. Minor urinary tract infections or pulmonary infections can greatly worsen the mental state of patients with dementia, since these patients are particularly liable to develop delirium. Cardiovascular disorders must be treated with care because cardiotonic drugs and antihypertensives can contribute to the patient's confusional state.

MULTI-INFARCT DEMENTIA[4]

Multi-infarct dementia, the second most common cause of dementia, is a syndrome resulting from multiple cerebral infarctions and is characterized by sudden onset and a stepwise progression. It is seen in the context of cardiovascular disease and hypertension and may affect 2 percent of the population over 65. The presenting symptoms of multi-infarct dementia are often identical to those of Alzheimer disease and consist of a deterioration of intellectual function in clear consciousness. Unlike Alzheimer disease, however, multi-infarct disease has a sudden onset with periods of stabilization between attacks. Symptoms fluctuate from day to day and often are worse at night. The typical patient with multi-infarct dementia also complains of symptoms related to vascular disease, such as headache, dizzy spells, fatigue, and lethargy; he will often have symptoms and signs of focal cerebral infarctions, such as weakness and numbness of limbs.

Physical examination reveals signs of reflex asymmetry and the stigmata of vascular disease of the heart and peripheral blood vessels. Bruits may be heard in the neck, and arteriovenous nicking and hemorrhages are often seen in the retina (see Chapter 15.13). These signs have been formulated by several authors into a quantitative checklist known as the Hachinski Scale or the Modified Ischemia Scale. High scores in these rating scales are associated with the neuropathology of multiple cerebral infarctions.

In multi-infarct disease, efforts are made to avoid additional ischemic lesions (Chapter 15.13). In all other respects the management of the demented patient with multi-infarct disease is identical to that of the patient with Alzheimer disease.

AMNESIC SYNDROMES

DIAGNOSIS

The amnesic syndrome is characterized by a severe and incapacitating memory disorder in the face of relatively normal cognitive functioning in other domains. Thus, the patient with an amnesic syndrome is virtually unable to learn new information yet performs normally on tests of attention, perceptual processing, expressive and receptive language, and reasoning. Several diseases and disorders of the nervous system can produce a severe, isolated memory disorder (see Table 16.7–4). Common to the various causes of human amnesia is the site of neuropathology: In virtually every case of "pure" amnesia, lesions can be found in the hippocampal formation and/or amygdala or their projections to the diencephalon (mammillary bodies and thalamic nuclei).

KORSAKOFF SYNDROME

The prototype of the amnesic syndrome is alcoholic Korsakoff syndrome (see Chapter 17.5). This disorder is caused by very severe alcoholism coupled with vitamin deficiencies (especially lack of thiamine). It is characterized by a striking inability to establish new permanent memories (anterograde amnesia) with preservation of normal intelligence. Immediate memory capacity is normal, as measured, for example, by digit span or the ability to engage in conversation. The Korsakoff patient is also unable to remember events in his past (retrograde amnesia), although events of the remote past are remembered somewhat better than events of the recent past. Confabulation, a tendency to fill in memory gaps with fantastic stories, is often present early in the disease. Neuropathologically, the disease is characterized by hemorrhagic lesions of the dorsomedial thalamic nucleus and the mammilary bodies.

OTHER SYNDROMES

There is substantial heterogeneity in the psychologic characteristics of amnesic syndromes. For example, compared to patients with alcoholic Korsakoff syndrome, patients with bilateral temporal lobe lesions (involving the hippocampus and/or amygdala) usually have a much more rapid rate of forgetting and a much more limited retrograde amnesia. More circumscribed memory disorders can be seen in a variety of disorders. After unilateral temporal lobectomy, for example, mild material-specific memory disorders are often seen: verbal memory difficulties after dominant temporal lobe removal and spatial/configural memory difficulties after nondominant temporal lobe removal.

Amnesic syndromes may be temporary. Transient global amnesia refers to an acute episode of severe memory loss that lasts for a few minutes or hours and leaves no apparent residual deficits. These are typically thought to reflect vascular events, that is, transient ischemic attacks.

Occasionally, patients present with marked, although atypical, memory disorders for which a neurologic cause cannot be found. In these cases of "functional" or "psychogenic" amnesia, the retrograde memory loss is almost always more severe than the anterograde memory loss and may include loss of personal identity. Careful history-taking often reveals severe emotional trauma and/or a potential legal or financial motive. The possibility of malingering or factitious disorder should always be considered in these cases.

TABLE 16.7–4. COMMON CAUSES OF AMNESIC SYNDROMES

- Head trauma
- Chronic alcoholism
- Cerebral infarction
- Tumors
- Viral encephalitis (especially herpes simplex)
- Cerebral anoxia
- Surgical lesions
- Electroconvulsive therapy

MANAGEMENT

Clinical management of the amnesic syndromes involves, first, treatment of the underlying disorder, e.g., detoxification and vitamin supplements for the patient with Korsakoff syndrome, pharmacotherapy for the depressed patient. Compensation for the memory defect and reliance on intact cognitive skills is typically the major management strategy. For example, patients, their caretakers, and family members are encouraged to use memory aids, such as note pads and large, write-in calendars to remember day-to-day events. Cognitive retraining of memory skills appears to hold some promise for some types of patients, but there are still few well-controlled studies of this therapeutic modality. Research continues on the pharmacologic manipulation of memory, but there is not yet a clinically useful drug for the treatment of amnesic syndromes.

REFERENCES

1. Folstein MD, Folstein SE, McHugh PR: Mini-mental state: A practical method for grading the cognitive state of patients for the clinician. J Psychiatr Res 12:189, 1975
2. Folstein MF, McHugh PR: Dementia syndrome of depression. In Katzman R, Terry RD, Bick KL (eds): Alzheimer's Disease: Senile Dementia and Related Disorders. Aging, vol 7. New York, Raven Press, 1978
3. Gruenberg EM: Epidemiology of senile dementia. In Schoenberg BS (ed): *Advances in Neurology*. New York, Raven Press, 1978
4. Hachinski VC, Lassen NA, Marshall J: Multi-infarct dementia: A cause of mental deterioration in the elderly. Lancet 2:207, 1974
5. Heston LL, Mastri AR, et al: Dementia of the Alzheimer type. Clinical genetics, natural history and associated conditions. Arch Gen Psychiatr 38:1085, 1981
6. Kang J, Sermaire HG, et al: The precursor of Alzheimer's disease amyloid A4 protein resembles a cell surface receptor. Nature 235, 733, 1987
7. Kral VA: Senescent forgetfulness: Benign and malignant. Can Med J 86:257, 1962
8. Lezak MD: Neuropsychological Assessment, 2nd ed. New York, Oxford University Press, 1983
9. Mace NL, Rabins PV: The 36-Hour Day. Baltimore, Johns Hopkins University Press, 1982
10. McHugh PR, Folstein MR: Psychopathology of dementia: Implications for neuropathology. In Katzman R (ed): Congenital and Acquired Cognitive Disorders. New York, Raven Press, 1979
11. Perry EK, Tomlinson BE, et al: Correlation of cholinergic abnormalities with senile plaques and mental test scores in senile dementia. Br Med J 2:1457, 1978
12. Robinson RG, Szetela B: Mood change following left hemispheric brain injury. Ann Neurol 9:447, 1981
13. Squire LR, Butters N (eds): Neuropsychology of Memory. New York, Guilford Press, 1984
14. St. George-Hyslop PH, Tanyi RE, et al: The genetic defect causing familial Alzheimer's disease maps on chromosome 21. Science 235, 885, 1987
15. Tomlinson BE: Plaques, tangles and Alzheimer's disease. Psychol Med 12:479, 1982

CHAPTER 16.8

Anorexia Nervosa and Bulimia Nervosa

Arnold E. Andersen

Anorexia nervosa (self-induced starvation) and bulimia nervosa (overeating often followed by purging) are disorders of weight and eating that are primarily psychologic in origin but have profound physical consequences. Patients share the common features of a fear of fatness and a distortion of body image. Transitions between anorexia nervosa and bulimia are common, especially from the former to the latter.

ANOREXIA NERVOSA

Anorexia nervosa is a serious disorder. Some series in the past have reported mortality rates as high as 5 to 15 percent, although such figures overestimate the recent experience with current diagnostic and therapeutic approaches. Considerable morbidity results from both the emaciation and the abnormal behavior of these patients. The urgency of making a correct diagnosis is highlighted not only by the serious consequences of the disorder but also by its potentially treatable nature. The current sociocultural emphasis on slimness has greatly increased the incidence of anorexia nervosa (about 1 percent of college-bound teenage girls), although part of the increased incidence results from more accurate diagnosis.[1]

Patients with anorexia nervosa usually present first to internists and family physicians rather than to psychiatrists. The multiple guises of the disorder lead to referrals to various specialists. Gynecologists are often consulted for secondary amenorrhea. Physically active, thin, intense young women may present to endocrinologists with hyperthyroidism as a presumed explanation of their weight loss. Gastroenterologists consider malabsorption and often carry out a full radiologic evaluation of the gastrointestinal tract. Neurologists are consulted for symptoms that suggest a hypothalamic tumor.

DIAGNOSIS

The diagnosis of anorexia nervosa should be based on the clinical presentation and direct examination of the patient's mental state. Failure to recognize the characteristic features of anorexia nervosa often leads to unnecessary tests and considerable delay in diagnosis. Early diagnosis and treatment improve the outcome by decreasing the time during which symptoms become firmly and chronically fixed. Some medicolegal consequences may occur if accurate diagnosis is not made promptly. The three essential diagnostic criteria are (1) significant weight loss that is self-induced and unexplained by medical illness or other psychiatric disorders, usually in a woman 10 to 30 years of age, but occasionally in older individuals, and in males in about 10 percent of cases; (2) fear of fatness from the loss of control over eating; (3) amenorrhea in the female or loss of sexual interest in the male. The more specific diagnostic criteria of the American Psychiatric Association are presented in Table 16.8–1.

When the four criteria in Table 16.8–1 are met, it is rare to find a medical disorder to account for weight loss. Patients low in weight who binge and purge are classified as having anorexia nervosa with bulimic features. When they gain some weight but continue to binge and purge, the disorder is called bulimia nervosa[6] (Table 16.8–2). At times patients may conceal important aspects

TABLE 16.8–1. DIAGNOSTIC CRITERIA FOR ANOREXIA NERVOSA

A. Refusal to maintain body weight over a minimal normal weight for age and height, e.g., weight loss leading to maintenance of body weight 15% below that expected; or failure to make expected weight gain during period of growth, leading to body weight 15% below that expected

B. Intense fear of gaining weight or becoming fat, even though underweight

C. Disturbance in the way in which one's body weight, size, or shape is experienced, e.g., the person claims to "feel fat" even when emaciated, believes that one area of the body is "too fat" even when obviously underweight

D. In females, absence of at least three consecutive menstrual cycles when otherwise expected to occur (primary or secondary amenorrhea). (A woman is considered to have amenorrhea if her periods occur only following hormone, e.g., estrogen, administration)

Adapted from American Psychiatric Association: Diagnostic and Statistical Manual of Mental Disorders (DSM-IIIR), Washington, DC: American Psychiatric Association, 1987.[1]

of the full history for a variety of reasons, and this possibility should be sympathetically explored.

CLINICAL PRESENTATION

The typical adolescent patient with anorexia nervosa starts to diet when 5 to 10 pounds overweight. As the diet proceeds, the patient seeks an even lower weight but becomes increasingly fearful of losing control and becoming overweight. Many, but not all, patients have the perceptual distortion that they are fat even when emaciated. Weight loss is induced by a variety of techniques. More than half of patients simply decrease their caloric intake. They first eliminate foods with a high sugar or fat content, then decrease all foods, and finally reach weights as low as 25 kg. They often assist the weight loss by strenuous exercise; as a consequence, they appear more energetic than patients who attain low weights through medical illness. Diuretic or laxative abuse in some patients may produce severe hypokalemic alkalosis. Serum potassium levels below 2 mEq/L may occasionally lead to cardiac arrest. Some eat normal, or even greatly excessive, amounts of food but induce vomiting, which may add severe metabolic abnormalities to their weight loss. Anorexia-producing drugs are rarely employed.

The end results of starvation, binging, vomiting, exercising, and abuse of medications produce a variety of confusing manifestations: (1) The direct effects of starvation may produce hypotension, inanition, hypothermia, anemia, weakness, difficulty in intellectual concentration, and constipation. (2) The particular means of inducing weight loss confers other symptoms, for example, the hypokalemia of diuretic abuse or vomiting. (3) The reduced weight of patients with anorexia nervosa makes them more vulnerable to

TABLE 16.8–2. DIAGNOSTIC CRITERIA FOR BULIMIA NERVOSA

A. Recurrent episodes of binge eating (rapid consumption of a large amount of food in a discrete period of time)

B. A feeling of lack of control over eating behavior during the eating binges

C. The person regularly engages in either self-induced vomiting, use of laxatives or diuretics, strict dieting or fasting, or vigorous exercise in order to prevent weight gain

D. A minimum average of two binge eating episodes a week for at least three months

E. Persistent overconcern with body shape and weight

Adapted from American Psychiatric Association: Diagnostic and Statistical Manual of Mental Disorders (DSM-IIIR), Washington, DC: American Psychiatric Association, 1987.[1]

certain medical disorders. They often respond poorly to mycotic or bacterial infections but appear surprisingly resistant to viral infections. (4) Last, and speculatively, certain symptoms may be unique to anorexia nervosa. This possibility is suggested by the fact that about one third of women with anorexia nervosa lose their menses before their weight falls. Extensive endocrinologic investigations[7] suggest that dysfunction in temperature control and the partial diabetes insipidus of these patients may be unique. Bradycardia, found in many patients, appears to result from a combination of decreased activity of the sympathetic nervous system common in starvation and the effect of regular exercise. Other studies, however, conclude that all symptoms are caused by starvation. Elevated plasma cortisol levels are commonly found as a result of lowered weight and do not reflect primary endocrine disease. A positive dexamethasone suppression test will often be present, but without additional evidence it does not indicate the presence of major depressive illness. Starvation results in central hypogonadotrophic hypogonadism, subclinical T_3, increased reverse-T_3, and low-normal levels of T_4, all reversible with refeeding. Some probably reversible shrinkage of brain size occurs, and may contribute to the mental state.

ETIOLOGY

The cause of anorexia nervosa is unknown, but it is probably multifactorial in origin. Most patients have a perfectionistic and sensitive temperament before illness. They are often model students and children, as evidenced by high grades, obedience, and compliance toward parents. The highest incidence of anorexia nervosa occurs in families of upper-middle socioeconomic status. Only a few cases have been reported among nonwhites but these are increasing. Some experts believe that the family is the primary cause of anorexia nervosa, but this hypothesis has not been borne out empirically. The families are often stressed by internal or external conflicts, such as marital discord, lack of parenting skills, separation, or a change of location. In the absence of convincing etiologic data, it is presently best to view the disorder as occurring when weight loss from dieting (occasionally from a medical illness or romantic disappointment) occurs in a person with vulnerable temperament, stressed family, a genetic history of mood disorder, and perhaps preexisting dysfunction of biologic regulation. The increased incidence of depression in the families of these patients may also play a role, including the generation of obsessional personality characteristics and mood swings, which may be partially controlled by starvation or binges.

TREATMENT

All treatment programs seem to work better when patients are younger, less severely ill, acutely rather than chronically ill and motivated to improve, and have a relatively normal temperament and family structure before the onset of illness.[2] The prognosis is less favorable in those with atypical features, such as very young or old age of onset, and presence of more severe and enduring features of illness, especially eating binges and vomiting. In addition to weight gain, goals for treatment include achieving a relative absence of preoccupation with food and weight, normal menstrual function, return to school or work, and good working relationships with parents or other family members, normal mood, and age-appropriate activities.

A variety of treatment approaches have been tried, but none has been uniformly successful.[2] Strict psychoanalytic psychotherapy, independent of weight gain, has been classically used without demonstrable improvement in weight or psychologic function. Strict behavior modification, based on rewarding weight gain in a systematic way, produces short-term weight gain, but the long-term benefits are unknown. The phenothiazines, tricyclic antidepressants, and to some extent cyproheptadine encourage weight

gain; however, stimulation of appetite without alleviating the fear of fatness may produce only increased psychologic distress unless the morbid fear of fatness is decreased.

Individual psychotherapy or family therapy focused on relevant issues in the current life situations and behavioral patterns and attitudes can be conducted on an outpatient basis in relatively mild cases. Patients are usually referred for inpatient treatment when they meet any of the following criteria: (1) loss of 20 to 25 percent of body weight, (2) persistently low serum potassium levels, (3) threats or attempts at self-harm, and (4) lack of response to at least one-half year of well-designed outpatient treatment.

Perhaps the most effective inpatient management employs an empirical approach utilizing a team of psychiatrist or psychologist, nurse, and social worker.[5] Four stages are involved, beginning with nutritional rehabilitation that employs 24-hour nursing care but no nasogastric tubes or intravenous alimentation except on rare occasions when such treatment may be necessary in patients with life-threatening inanition. Dynamic psychotherapy techniques are not effective in the very starved person: Concentration is poor, and symptoms result from a mixture of starvation and pertinent psychologic issues. During this period, exercise is limited and the patient's nutritional needs are prescribed like medication. Fats and sugars are initially restricted and gradually introduced as gastrointestinal lipases and lactases regenerate. After nutritional status has improved, individualized psychotherapy is begun. The issues discussed in individual, group, and family therapy arise from the individual's personality, life situation, and experiences rather than from a theoretical construct. The next stage of therapy attempts to return the control of food, weight, and exercise to the patient's own choice. This period provides a chance for the patient to practice, under supervision and with encouragement, the information learned and explored in the second stage of treatment. Finally, the patient is followed in treatment after leaving the hospital. Reintroduction of the patient to the everyday environment results in predictable stresses and, occasionally, a return to the previous symptoms. Close follow-up and attention to structured programs of everyday activities and eating schedules increase the probability of maintained improvement. Symptoms of mood disorder may emerge on follow-up. Two to three years of outpatient treatment after hospitalization are generally recommended.

PROGNOSIS

Although mortality and morbidity are decreased when the disorder is recognized quickly and treated appropriately, few patients recover completely. Most are substantially improved by treatment but are left with some continuing preoccupation with food and weight, especially at times of stress. Menses may not return until the patient's weight exceeds by several kilograms her weight at the menarche; sometimes amenorrhea persists for months after the attainment of normal weight. Between 25 and 35 percent of patients remain chronically ill, with lowered weight and severe psychologic distress. In Theander's long-term follow-up, there was a death rate of 19 percent (half from starvation and half from suicide). Of the majority who survived, about 90 percent eventually improved.

BULIMIA NERVOSA

The widespread occurrence of binge eating followed by self-induced vomiting, compensatory fasting, purgation with laxatives, or salt and water loss with diuretics has only been recently recognized. Up to 15 percent of college students regularly use these methods for weight control.[4] Male gymnasts and wrestlers are especially vulnerable. Usually, weight is not lowered to the point where the patients meet diagnostic criteria for anorexia nervosa.

DIAGNOSIS

Diagnostic criteria are summarized in Table 16.8–2. The essential feature is the occurrence of episodes of rapid and compulsive consumption of large amounts of food. This behavior leads to guilt, physical discomfort or danger, increased fear of fatness, and methods to counteract the calories ingested, such as compensatory fasting or purging. The term "bulimia" is derived from the Greek words for "ox" and "hunger" (*bous* and *limos*) and refers to binge episodes. Vomiting or purging alone without binges is often incorrectly diagnosed as bulimic symptoms. Clinical indicators of possible undisclosed bulimia include (1) persistent hypokalemic alkalosis, (2) loss of dental enamel from tooth contact with gastric acid, (3) unexplained parotid gland enlargement, (4) scars on the knuckles where the teeth hit the hand when vomiting is induced, and (5) frequent unexplained fluctuations of more than 10 pounds in weight.

CLINICAL PRESENTATION

Since weight is often in the normal range, the diagnosis may not be apparent until the patient seeks help or the above-mentioned clinical signs are noticed. The individuals often live complicated, guilt-ridden lives, having to plan in advance how to dispose of food after social occasions. The most common triggers for the binge are hunger from attempted fasting or emotional distress of any kind, especially anxiety, depression, boredom, or anger. In contrast to anorectic patients, bulimic patients are usually more extroverted and more aware of their emotional distress and may be sexually experienced. Some are vulnerable to other impulse disorders, such as drug and alcohol abuse, shoplifting, or repeated attempts at self-harm. The binges, which begin as an unwanted response to hunger from food restriction, generalize to become an all-purpose mechanism to deal with distress of any kind, often causing an arrest in development of emotional maturity.

TREATMENT

Whenever possible, treatment should be in the outpatient setting. Some of the important phases of treatment include (1) decreasing the frequency and severity of binges by delay in responding to compulsive urges and alternative activities, (2) increasing weight to the normal range if it is lowered, and (3) helping patients to deal directly with their emotional distress and environmental stresses instead of indirectly with binges.[2] Antidepressants may be employed if patients meet criteria for depressive illness after the eating pattern and weight are returned to normal. There is no convincing evidence that antiseizure medications are of any help. Although some researchers have recommended tricyclic antidepressants as effective antibinge medications independent of antidepressant effect, there is no convincing evidence for this claim. Pharmacologic treatments of the eating disorders without associated psychotherapeutic and behavioral work are rarely effective.

PROGNOSIS

Because this disorder has only recently been defined and its natural history, especially for mild cases, remains unknown, the prognosis is not well known. Bulimic patients are at greater risk for suicide than anorectic patients, and they may die suddenly from hypokalemia-induced cardiac arrhythmias. The more severe the underlying personality disorder and the longer the illness has endured, the worse the prognosis. Many patients respond well to treatment, however, and are benefited by the recent improvement in treatment methods.

REFERENCES

1. American Psychiatric Association: Diagnostic and Statistical Manual of Mental Disorders (DSM-IIIR), 3d ed. Washington, DC, American Psychiatric Association, 1987
2. Andersen AE: Comprehensive Practical Treatment of Anorexia Nervosa and Bulimia. Baltimore, Johns Hopkins University Press, 1985
3. Fairburn C: A cognitive behavioral approach to the treatment of bulimia. Psych Med 11:707, 1981
4. Halmi KA, Falk JR, Schwartz E: Binge-eating and vomiting: A survey of a college population. Psych Med 11:698, 1981
5. Hedblom JE, Hubbard FA, Andersen AE: Anorexia nervosa: A multidisciplinary treatment program for patient and family. Social Work in Health Care 6:67, 1981
6. Russell G: Bulimia nervosa: An ominous variant of anorexia nervosa. Psych Med 9:429, 1979
7. Vigersky RA, Loriaux DL, et al: Anorexia nervosa: Behavioral and hypothalamic aspects. Clin Endocrin Metab 5:517, 1976

CHAPTER 16.9
Chemical Dependence

Donald Jasinski

Substance abuse accounts for a major portion of all illness in the United States. Some have estimated that 50 percent of hospital admissions are alcohol- or drug-related, many undiagnosed. In 1982, alcohol and drug addiction cost nearly $50 billion yearly in health-care costs, accidents, violence, and loss of productivity.[5] One partial consequence is increasing recognition and acceptance of the notion that the problems of substance abuse require medical rather than social or legal solutions.

Chemical dependence has been defined as a medical illness that includes both physical and psychic reliance on a chemical. Chemical dependence can develop to social drugs such as alcohol, tobacco, and coffee; licit prescription and over-the-counter drugs; and illicit drugs. The term "chemical dependence" encompasses alcoholism and drug addiction. In distinction, the term "problem use" is defined to include abuse, misuse, and overuse of chemicals short of dependence. Such problem use is also associated with significant morbidity and mortality.

Direct and indirect medical illnesses occur as a result of substance abuse. Direct illnesses result from transient or permanent alterations in brain and body functioning. Indirectly, trauma, infections, and malnutrition occur as a result of intoxication, inebriation, or self-injection. Of current concern is the finding that intravenous drug abusers are now the major vector for transmission of the acquired immunodeficiency syndrome (AIDS) virus.

The responsibility of the physician is the diagnosis, treatment, and prevention of chemical dependence. To make a diagnosis, the physician must recognize the behavioral and physical effects of various types of chemical dependence as well as the subtle and often presenting complaints of behavioral and social dysfunction. At a minimum, the physician must treat the alterations in brain and body function induced by drugs and then, most often, refer the patient for rehabilitation by other health-care professionals, including self-help groups. The best prevention is probably early diagnosis and intervention. As the prescriber of prescription drugs and advisor about over-the-counter drugs, the physician must recognize the abuse potential of drugs and prescribe and advise appropriately, especially to prevent iatrogenic dependence and diversion. Finally, the physician must educate and counsel patients about the appropriate use of all chemicals that may induce dependence.

PATHOPHYSIOLOGY OF DEPENDENCE

PHARMACOLOGIC MECHANISMS

Although chemicals that produce dependence may have differing pharmacologic modes of action, they share some common properties important in leading to abuse. The chemicals are psychoactive. All are euphoriants in that they produce feelings of well-being and elation. Dysphoric or undesirable effects usually accompany this euphoria. With repeated ingestion, tolerance and often physical dependence develop. The tolerant patient demonstrates persistent drug effects, some of which emerge and increase after repeated administration. Other effects diminish and cannot be recaptured by increasing the amount of drug taken. Physical dependence is manifested by the occurrence of a characteristic syndrome after termination of drug administration. This syndrome consists of changes in brain function reflected in dysphoric changes in mood, feelings, thinking, and perception; changes in autonomic function; and changes in behavior that include increased drug-seeking.

LEARNING MECHANISMS

Various types of learning are involved in the process of chemical dependence. First, these individuals often join subcultures and assume the behaviors and attitudes of the subculture. Operant psychologists have demonstrated that drugs which produce chemical dependence can act as reinforcers in operant paradigms. A reinforcer is an event that maintains, terminates, or postpones behavior. Such operant behavior can be scheduled, indicating that the amount of drug-acquisition behavior is independent of the strength of the drug reinforcer. At times, drug-acquisition behavior can be maintained by associated nondrug stimuli in the absence of the drug. Finally, it is recognized that the abstinence syndrome and drug-seeking can be conditioned. These conditioned responses to associated stimuli are important determinants in relapse, even in the absence of physical dependence.

PERSONALITY DISORDERS

Many workers have felt that the majority of patients who present with chemical dependence have an underlying disease that is responsible for drug-seeking and asocial behavior and that this underlying disease is reflected in a variety of personality disturbances. The predominant disorder, now termed "antisocial personality," has many dimensions, but most characteristic are egocentricity and narcissism, impulsiveness and inability to delay gratification, low mood and depressed feelings, and sociopathic behavior. Chronic drug administration may worsen the personality disturbance by disinhibition or improve the disturbance by suppressing unfulfilled needs and wants. Withdrawal may worsen the personality disorder, possibly by increasing needs and wants. A variety of other types of psychopathology is often encountered in chemically dependent patients.

SOCIOENVIRONMENTAL FACTORS

Availability of drugs, access to a subculture, cultural mores, and social attitudes are obvious contributors to the occurrence of chemical dependence. Low socioeconomic status, family and social instability, minority status, and other social problems are also factors, perhaps because they increase needs and wants.

CHEMICAL DEPENDENCE SYNDROMES

Specificity of chemical dependence syndromes results predominantly from the pharmacologic actions of the chemicals. Chemical dependence can be classified clinically. Alcohol dependence is a class of singular importance and is discussed separately (Chapter 17.5).

OPIOIDS

Fundamental knowledge of opioid dependence comes from studies of morphine, the prototype for other opioids.[6] In addition, the pathophysiologic model for morphine dependence is the standard to which all other forms of chemical dependence are compared and related. The major opioid of abuse, diacetylmorphine, or heroin, is rapidly metabolized to morphine with a resulting identical pharmacologic effect.

Clinical Manifestations
Initially, morphine administration produces euphoria. As tolerance develops, the feelings change to apathy and lethargy. Patients become tired, withdrawn, hypochondriacal, and resentful. Alteration in autonomic functions persists. Of these, miosis and constipation are clinically evident. Anemia, leukocytosis, and abnormal glucose tolerance occur.

Following abrupt withdrawal, the intensity of abstinence reaches a maximum within 2 days and then subsides. Although discomforting and dysphoric, this abstinence is not usually life threatening. This primary abstinence syndrome persists for approximately 5 weeks and is followed by the secondary or protracted abstinence syndrome, which persists for at least 6 months. A history of loss of energy, weakness, irritability, depressed feelings, and poor self-image may be obtained during secondary abstinence.

Relapse to opioid dependence is held to be related to the persisting psychopathology, the protracted abstinence, the conditioned abstinence and drug-seeking, and persistence of socioenvironmental factors.

Other opioids, such as methadone, propoxyphene, codeine, oxycodone, hydromorphine, and meperidine, produce similar dependence. Propoxyphene, meperidine, and methadone have additional toxic properties seen commonly with chronic administration. Propoxyphene is a convulsant, and seizures occur with the chronic administration of greater than therapeutic doses. Meperidine is strongly anticholinergic, and toxicity, including psychosis, occurs with repeated administration. Normeperidine, the major metabolite, has a longer half-life and is a convulsant; chronic meperidine administration is therefore characterized by preconvulsant and convulsant behavior. Methadone and morphine have similar analgesic and euphoric durations, yet the durations of the miotic, abstinence-suppressing, and respiratory-depressant actions, as well as the withdrawal syndrome of methadone, greatly exceed those of morphine.

Management
There are two fundamental and differing approaches to treatment of opioid dependence. The first is transfer of dependence to orally administered methadone (maintenance therapy) with attempts at rehabilitation. The other involves terminating drug administration (detoxification), followed by a program to prevent relapse, educate, and rehabilitate (abstinence counseling). The Federal Narcotic Addict Treatment Act proscribes the administration of opioids for maintenance or treatment, except for the use of methadone under special license. Detoxification can be accomplished by slow dose reduction. With illicit opiates, this is done by substituting methadone, usually in designated clinics. In the case of iatrogenic dependence in a patient with pain, dose reduction of the opioid is regarded as appropriate. In inpatient settings the opioid can be abruptly discontinued and the withdrawal treated with large doses of the alpha-adrenergic agonist clonidine, the only nonopioid shown to be effective. Side effects of orthostatic hypotension and sedation limit outpatient use of clonidine. Following detoxification, chronic administration of the competitive opioid antagonist naltrexone may be used to prevent relapse.

The mixed agonist/antagonist drugs are less toxic and have a lesser abuse potential than other opioids. One problem has been the abuse of mixtures of pentazocine and the antihistamine tripelenamine. In general, toxicity from acute or chronic administration is less with use of the agonist/antagonists than with other opioids, and the withdrawal syndrome is less active and shorter lived, usually 2 or 3 days. Treatment is directed toward abstinence.

BARBITURATE SEDATIVE HYPNOTICS

Chemical dependence that resembles alcohol dependence in many ways can develop to a diverse group of drugs used for sedation and antianxiety. The best-studied group are the barbiturates such as pentobarbital and secobarbital.

Clinical Manifestations
Chronic administration allays anxiety, sedates, and at times produces disinhibition. If doses are sufficient, ataxia, dysarthria, impairment of sensorium and judgment, and asynergy can develop. Respiratory, cardiovascular, and reflex depression may occur. Abrupt withdrawal is followed by disappearance of the signs of chronic intoxication and the occurrence of an abstinence syndrome that in intensity is roughly proportional to the dose administered. At the lower dose levels, autonomic hyperactivity, postural hypotension, loss of body weight, and tremulousness may be the only effects, subsiding within 2 to 5 days. More severe withdrawal consists of generalized grand mal seizures and/or psychoses resembling alcohol delirium tremens, effects that may persist for 2 weeks. Most severe is psychosis accompanied by hyperpyrexia, which can lead to death.

Nonbarbiturate sedatives and antianxiety agents such as glutethimide, ethinamate ethchlorvynol, methyprylon, meprobamate, and methaqualone produce dependence similar to the barbiturates; however, the effects of chronic intoxication on withdrawal have not been studied to the same degree as the barbiturates.

Management
Treatment is directed toward detoxification and rehabilitation. Maintenance therapy, per se, is not generally acceptable. The best-documented and useful procedure is the substitution of pentobarbital in doses of 100 or 200 mg orally or intramuscularly at frequent intervals to suppress all signs of abstinence, followed by slow dose reduction. Phenobarbital may also be used; however, because of the long half-life, steady states are not achieved until after 1 week. Consequently, loading doses of at least 300 to 500 mg of phenobarbital must be used in treating withdrawal.

NONBARBITURATE SEDATIVE HYPNOTICS

The prevalence of chemical dependence to barbiturates and nonbarbiturate sedative hypnotics has decreased as benzodiazepines have extensively replaced these drugs in therapeutics. Chemical de-

pendence to certain of the benzodiazepines is currently the most prevalent dependence among the abused sedative hypnotics.

Clinical Manifestations

Unlike barbiturates, chronic administration of the benzodiazepines does not generally produce ataxia or other psychomotor retardation or impairment. One effect of importance is disinhibition, which results in socially inappropriate behavior that is perceived as aggressiveness. The withdrawal syndromes, however, are generally similar to those of the barbiturates. The best studied are diazepam and chlordiazepoxide, two slowly eliminated benzodiazepines with biologically active metabolites. The onset of withdrawal consequently does not occur until the fifth or sixth day after drug termination and may last for at least 2 weeks or longer. Less studied are the rapidly eliminated benzodiazepines, which appear to have a time course similar to barbiturates such as pentobarbital. Benzodiazepines are not equivalent in their capacity to produce dependence or similar intensity of withdrawal. For example, experimental and epidemiologic evidence indicates that chlordiazepoxide and oxazepam have less abuse potential than diazepam.

Management

Treatment is usually detoxification and abstinence counseling. Rapidly eliminated benzodiazepines are best treated by dose reduction. Slowly eliminated benzodiazepines are treated with substitution and subsequent dose reduction of a rapidly eliminated benzodiazepine. Alternatively, phenobarbital may be given in loading doses before withdrawal and then discontinued after peak withdrawal. No consensus exists on maintenance therapy with benzodiazepines, since some workers advocate their use in certain patients, especially those with chronic anxiety.

COCAINE

Cocaine is ingested in various forms. The un-ionized base is extracted from coca leaf in alkaline solution usually described as cocaine paste. The ionized cocaine hydrochloride forms upon treatment with hydrochloric acid and can be crystallized from aqueous solution. Cocaine hydrochloride treated with alkali forms free base, which in solid form is referred to as "crack" or "rocks." Cocaine hydrochloride is snorted intranasally or injected intravenously. Vasoconstriction and surface area limit both the rate and the maximum amount of absorption of intranasal cocaine. Cocaine base vaporizes at relatively low temperatures, allowing the material to be smoked and absorbed rapidly through the lungs in relatively unlimited amounts.

Clinical Manifestations

Acute administration produces euphoria with signs of sympathomimetic activity followed by dysphoric effects. Repeated administration in sufficient dose produces dysphoric perceptual distortions, which in the extreme progress to visual, auditory, tactile, and olfactory hallucinations. Suspicious or paranoid ideation occurs, which in combination with hallucinations can actively lead to aggressive or violent behavior. Seizures and cardiac arrhythmias can occur. Anorexia and weight loss are prominent.

Upon abrupt withdrawal, these physiologic, behavioral, and perceptual changes subside spontaneously, usually after a few hours, and are followed by a withdrawal syndrome consisting of anxiety, depression, fatigue, hyperphagia, somnolence, and craving for cocaine. Within a few days, this withdrawal syndrome subsides except for the occasional craving for cocaine and depression.

Management

Treatment is directed toward abstinence, and patients are easily detoxified if placed in a cocaine-free situation. The reports of persistent craving and depression and a high relapse rate have led some workers to hypothesize that norepinephrine or dopamine deficiency is a cause of relapse. Amino acid precursors of catechol-amines, dopamine agonists, norepinephrine re-uptake blockers, and norepinephrine and dopamine releasers have consequently been advocated for treatment. To date, no controlled studies document the effectiveness of these treatments.

AMPHETAMINES

Amphetamines as well as methamphetamine, phenmetrazine, phentermine, methylphenidate, ephedrine, and other related centrally active sympathomimetic amines produce a type of chemical dependence resembling that of cocaine.

Clinical Manifestations

In general, these drugs are longer lasting than cocaine in all actions. On rare occasions, acute administration of a large dose of amphetamine produces a toxic psychosis with hallucinations. Chronic administration even of low doses may produce a paranoid psychosis with clear sensorium that is indistinguishable from paranoid schizophrenia. Abrupt withdrawal of these drugs is followed by diminution of the sympathomimetic effects and an abstinence syndrome characterized by somnolence with prolonged sleep, hyperphagia, and depression. The paranoid psychoses diminish slowly, lasting on occasion for 2 to 3 weeks. Phenothiazines suppress the paranoid psychosis.

Management

Treatment of chemical dependence to cocaine and amphetamine-like drugs for all practical purposes, consists of detoxification and abstinence counseling. Maintenance is not recommended, although there are reports of rare patients maintained on amphetamines. In this regard, chronic administration of methylphenidate is accepted as a treatment for hyperkinetic children.

PHENCYCLIDINE

Phencyclidine (PCP) is an analgesic and dissociative anesthetic that is a frequent cause of chemical dependence. The drug is taken orally, smoked, or injected.

Clinical Manifestations

Low doses are euphoric. With larger doses a varied profile of alterations in brain function occur. These include agitation, excitement, catatonic rigidity, nystagmus, hypertension, impairment of sensation and dissociation, diaphoresis, muscle twitching, seizures, and coma. Delirium or toxic psychosis is frequent. Patients become combative, have increased strength, and may experience increased symptoms in response to auditory, visual, or tactile stimuli. On occasion violent and bizarre behavior has been related to PCP intoxication. In contrast to other hallucinogens, the toxic psychosis may improve upon removal of environmental stimulation. Abrupt withdrawal is followed by slow diminution of effects over 24 to 48 hours. There are no clinically significant withdrawal symptoms. On occasion, a schizophreniform psychosis characterized by violent and aggressive behavior, paranoia, delusions, and hallucinations has been observed to persist for 2 to 4 weeks or longer.

Management

Because phencyclidine is almost completely ionized at pH 5.5, phencyclidine toxicity has been treated by acidification of the urine, forced diuresis, and continuous gastric suction. To suppress psychosis, haloperidol is recommended rather than phenothiazine neuroleptics. Treatment is directed toward detoxification and abstinence.

LSD-LIKE HALLUCINOGENS

LSD-25, mescaline, and psilocybin all produce a similar chemical dependence and have been the most thoroughly studied.

Clinical Manifestations

Euphoria, distortion of visual perception and body image, synesthesias, hallucinations, depersonalization, derealization, and paranoid delusions occur in a dose-related manner. Orientation and memory are intact, and the subjective changes can be minimized by engaging the patient in conversation or other activities. This is in contrast to PCP-induced psychosis. Physiologically, sympathomimetic effects are produced. Rapid and almost complete tolerance develops to the effects of LSD-like drugs. After drug termination, the toxic psychosis subsides within 8 to 10 hours, and no withdrawal phenomena of clinical significance are encountered. Other drugs such as N,N-dimethyltryptamine (DMT), 2,5-dimethoxy-4-methylamphetamine (DOM), 3,4-methylene-dioxyamphetamine (MDA), and 5-methoxy-3,4-methylenedioxyamphetamine (MMDA) produce a chemical dependence similar to that of LSD-25.

Management

Psychotic reactions respond to barbiturates, benzodiazepines, or phenothiazines. Treatment is directed toward abstinence.

ANTICHOLINERGIC AGENTS

Drugs with central anticholinergic action are occasionally abused. These include, among others, atropine, jimsonweed, and certain antihistamines.

Clinical Manifestations

These drugs produce a toxic delirium with memory impairment and peripheral inhibition of parasympathetic activity that can result in hyperpyrexia and death. No withdrawal syndrome of clinical significance is seen.

Management

Physostigmine given parenterally is a specific anticholinergic antagonist. Phenothiazine neuroleptics are not used because of additive anticholinergic effects. Treatment is directed toward abstinence.

CANNABIS

L-Δ^9-Tetrahydrocannabinol (THC) is the most active ingredient in various preparations of cannabis.

Clinical Manifestations

Experimental studies with THC indicate that low doses produce euphoria, immediate memory impairment, alteration in time sense, pointless laughter, and thinking disturbances accompanied by an appetite for sweets.

Larger doses can produce a toxic psychosis similar to that of LSD-25. Dose-related tachycardia, reddening of the eyes, diuresis, and mild orthostatic hypotension are the prominent physiologic changes. Experimental studies indicate that tolerance and physical dependence can develop to THC in large doses. The withdrawal syndrome as described is mild, lasting 72 hours. Chronic administration may be associated with apathetic sedation.

Management

Acute medical treatment for cannabis dependence is rarely required. Some workers ascribe this to consumption, in the United States primarily, of plant products with relatively low THC contents.

TOBACCO

Clinical Manifestations

Nicotine inhaled through smoking or taken intravenously is a euphoriant of 1 to 3 minutes' duration; intense learning thus occurs with multiple frequent ingestions. Rapid tolerance develops, but dysphoric effects may increase. Nausea, dizziness, cough, tachycardia, and increase in blood pressure are produced. Abrupt withdrawal is followed by an abstinence syndrome consisting of fatigue, feeling of loss or emptiness, nausea, headache, irritability, anxiety, and impairment of psychomotor performance persisting for 3 to 14 days or longer. Craving for tobacco and other symptoms persist for many months or years, suggesting the possibility of a protracted abstinence syndrome.

Management

The use of a nicotine-containing chewing gum (detoxification) in combination with education and counseling has been demonstrated effective in treating tobacco dependence in some smokers. Since the permanent cessation rate is less than 30 percent, smoking prevention deserves emphasis.

MIXED DEPENDENCIES

In the usual case, patients present with mixed dependencies that complicate the detoxification process.[1] The most frequent mixed dependency is alcohol in combination with other drugs. Each dependence must be assessed and treated individually. Alcohol and sedation hypnotic dependence, on the one hand, and opioid dependence, on the other, require different and distinct treatment for detoxification. Cocaine and cannabis usually do not need specific treatment if part of mixed dependence. Amphetamines and PCP usually require separate treatment if psychosis persists. Finally, the consumption of tobacco and caffeine often increases during detoxification from other dependence-producing chemicals. Withholding tobacco and caffeine can add to the withdrawal discomfort and inappropriate behavior.

XANTHINE-CONTAINING BEVERAGES

Coffee and other xanthine-containing beverages such as tea and cola produce elation, well-being, and elevated moods to which some tolerance occurs. Chronic administration may result in restlessness, anxiety, depression, disturbed sleep, myocardial stimulation, and gastrointestinal dysfunction. Abrupt withdrawal is often accompanied by a few days of headache and fatigue. Medical treatment is usually not necessary.

DIAGNOSIS AND MANAGEMENT

DIFFERENTIAL DIAGNOSIS

Chemical dependence or problem use of chemicals may present commonly as depression and social dysfunction. Alternately, substance abuse may be suspected when patients present with such illnesses as psychosis, trauma, violent behavior, hypertension, tachycardia, infections, gastrointestinal dysfunction, and a myriad of other illnesses and symptoms. Thus, substance abuse is the great mimic in medicine. The primary diagnostic measure is an appropriate history and physical examination by an astute examiner.

Recently, increased reliance has been placed on the detection of drugs or their metabolites in biologic fluids, especially urine. This has led to the use of mass urine screening to detect the presence of illicit drugs.[4] It is important to recognize that such tests are useful only if combined with a diagnostic examination. Drugs and their metabolites usually persist after the alterations in body and brain function. A positive test does not distinguish between use, problem use, and dependence. False negatives result from dilute urine, changes in pH, presence of interfering substances in urine, or substitution of urine. False positives occur because of operator error—especially in mass screening—and presence of other cross-reactive chemicals, especially those that are cross-reactive to antibodies used in immunoassay techniques. Codeine, for exam-

ple, binds to the morphine antibody so that legitimate use of codeine could be misconstrued as heroin dependence. Passive inhalation of marijuana smoke can result in a positive urine test for THC. If a positive urine test is critical in diagnosis, the test must be confirmed with more specific analyses and the patient interviewed.

THERAPEUTIC MANAGEMENT

Clinical management of patients with chemical dependence is frequently difficult and often trying for the physician. To plan treatment, the physician must distinguish among use, problem use, and chemical dependence. Failure to do so complicates management. Treatment involves acute management (detoxification and treatment of underlying illnesses) and chronic management (arranging for long-term rehabilitation needs). Drugs alter brain functioning and behavior so that the patient's true personality and level of psychosocial functioning can only be judged after complete detoxification. Failure to treat the patient objectively, empathetically, kindly, and nonjudgmentally exacerbates undesirable behavior, especially in those patients with personality disorders. Finally, the physician must be familiar with and able to call upon the health-care specialists treating chemical dependence and the various community resources, especially self-help groups.

Finally, chemical dependence is a chronic disease characterized by relapses and remissions. The goal of treatment often is to facilitate and prolong remission. Fortunately, when compared to most other chronic diseases, chemical dependence is highly treatable.

REFERENCES

1. Coleman JH, Tayen BJ, et al: Double diagnosis: Double dilemma, the polyaddictions: Alcoholism, substance abuse; smoking, gambling. Clin Psychiatr 45, Special Supplement Section, 1984, p 3
2. Jasinski DR, Henningfield JE, Johnson RE: Abuse liability assessment in human subjects. Trends Pharmacol Sci 5:196, 1984
3. Martin WR: Drug Addiction I & II. Berlin, Heidelberg, New York, Springer-Verlag, 1977
4. Morgan JP: Problems of mass urine screening for misused drugs. J Psychoactive Drugs 16:305, 1984
5. Stone S, et al: Health and Public Policy Committee American College of Physicians: Chemical dependence. Ann Int Med 102:405, 1985
6. Wikler A: Opioid Dependence. New York, Plenum Press, 1980

CHAPTER 16.10
Sexual Disorders
Chester W. Schmidt, Jr.

Although their exact incidence is not known, sexual disorders are common complaints. Several decades ago, the assumption was that 90 percent of such disorders were psychogenic, but currently it is thought that they are caused as often by organic as by psychologic processes. Often, both organic and psychologic factors interact to produce the disorder. Many sexual disorders can be readily evaluated and treated in a medical setting: those of mild to moderate severity, those of recent onset, and those which are secondary to physical illness, to side effects of medication, to the abuse of drugs or alcohol, and to psychologically caused dysfunction that is related to current life stresses.

Patients usually are willing to discuss their sexual problems. The physician must, however, indicate a willingness to listen to the complaint, to provide sufficient time for evaluation, and to create a climate of comfort for both the patient and himself. During the evaluation, it is helpful to obtain the patient's ideas about the cause of the problem and his expectations about the type of treatment required. Media attention to sexual disorders has contributed to public knowledge about sexual function, but it also has contributed to misunderstandings about rational treatment.

Sexual disorders can be divided into four groups: physical disorders, functional disorders, paraphilias, and gender-identity disorders. This chapter will focus primarily on physical disorders and functional disorders that can be treated in a medical setting. Because they are seen in practice less often, the paraphilias and gender-identity disorders will be discussed in less detail.

Two decades ago, most sexual disorders were lumped under the terms "impotence" (male) and "frigidity" (female). Because they are diagnostically imprecise and laden with negative connotations, these terms were an impediment to diagnosis and treatment. While "frigidity" has practically disappeared as a term in the scientific literature, "impotence" is still frequently used.

SEXUAL RESPONSE CYCLE

The studies of Masters and Johnson described four phases of a normal sexual-response cycle, creating a framework for more discrete evaluation and diagnosis of sexual dysfunction.[4] A description of those four phases follows.

DESIRE

The initial phase of the response cycle acknowledges *desire*, drive, or libidinal interest as a requisite for sexual activity. Sexual desire in men is influenced by circulating levels of testosterone. Hormonal control of drive in women has not been established. Cognition and fantasy also play an important role in stimulating and maintaining sexual desire in both sexes.

AROUSAL

The second component of the cycle, *arousal*, develops out of a series of physiologic and subjective responses to the pleasurable sensory stimuli (tactile, visual, auditory, olfactory) inherent in sexual experiences. Men and women identically experience increase in heart and breathing rate, the development of muscular tension throughout the body (most pronounced in the pelvic area and thighs), and vasocongestion in the pelvic and genital areas. These vascular changes are responsible for vaginal lubrication and for swelling of external genitalia in women and tumescence of the penis in men. Vasocongestion in both sexes is governed by two neurologic pathways: (1) a local reflex pathway initiated by tactile stimulation of the genitalia and mediated by sensory fibers entering

dorsal roots S-2 through S-4 and by parasympathetic fibers to the perivascular, prostatic (male), and cavernosus plexus (most ganglionic fibers from these plexuses go to the blood vessels of the corpora cavernosa and to the clitoral tissue)[3] and (2) a cortical pathway initiated by psychic stimuli and mediated by sympathetic fibers that originate at the thoracolumbar center (T-11 to T-12) of the spinal cord. At least one consequence of the action of these pathways is the promotion of the rapid inflow and retention of blood in the genitalia of both men and women.

ORGASM

The third phase of the cycle is *orgasm*. Arousal in both sexes increases in intensity, leveling off to a plateau subjectively experienced as a heightened state of pleasurable tension. The duration of time at plateau for men is usually brief and is followed rapidly by orgasm. Women appear to require longer periods of time at plateau before they are prepared for orgasm. The subjective experience of orgasm for both sexes is a sudden, intense, pleasurable release from a high level of tension. The physiologic manifestation of orgasm in men is ejaculation, a process mediated by the sympathetic nervous system and consisting of (1) emission resulting from contraction of the vas deferens, the prostate, and the seminal vesicles, and (2) ejaculation, resulting from rhythmic contraction from the muscles of the pelvic floor, closure of the internal sphincters of the bladder (thus preventing retrograde ejaculation), and propulsion of the semen through the external urethra. Physiologic response to orgasm in women is a rythmic contraction of the musculature of the outer third of the vagina, the perineal muscles, and the uterus.

RESOLUTION

During the last phase of the response cycle, *resolution,* there is a gradual return of heart rate, breathing rate, muscle tension, and vascular changes to baseline status. This phase of the cycle is accompanied by a sense of pleasure, well-being, and relaxation. Men are usually refractory to entering another cycle of sexual activity for varying periods of time (minutes in younger men and up to an hour or longer in older men). Women, however, can return to or maintain plateau levels of sexual excitement upon continued stimulation and experience multiple orgasms within a single cycle of activity.

SEXUAL DYSFUNCTION ASSOCIATED WITH ORGANIC DISORDERS

Because sexual behaviors involve the integrated function of several physiologic systems, many conditions (see Table 16.10–1), pathologic disorders, and medications may potentially interrupt normal sexual function (see Table 16.10–2). Diabetes mellitus is a frequent cause of sexual dysfunction. Approximately 25 to 40 percent of diabetic men report partial or total impairment of the ability to obtain or maintain an erection with sparing of capacity for ejaculation or at least emission. Female diabetics apparently may develop impairment of all phases of the sexual response cycle, although care must be taken to discern in them the psychosocial effects of chronic illness.[6] Hypertension with arterial narrowing may also cause sexual dysfunction but is more likely to affect men (erectile disorder) than women. Unfortunately, most classes of antihypertensive medications (excluding vasodilators and angiotensin-converting-enzyme inhibitors) are reported to affect sexual function adversely. Central acting sympatholytics (clonidine), alpha-blockers (prazosin), and peripheral sympatholytics (guanethidine) cause erectile disorders in men and inhibition of desire in both men and women. Occlusive vascular disease of large vessels (Leriche syndrome) is more likely to affect men (erectile disorder) than women.

Chronic debilitating illness and chronic pain syndromes inhibit desire and capacity for arousal in both men and women. Multiple sclerosis initially inhibits the arousal phase in men and the orgasmic phase in women and, with fatigue, commonly inhibits desire in both sexes. Painful intercourse (dysparunia) is often caused by infections of the prostate or urethra in men and infection of the vagina in women. Atrophic vaginitis secondary to estrogen deficiency may also cause painful intercourse in women. Peyronie disease, a fibrosis of the corpora cavernosa, often causes pain on tumescence secondary to mechanical torsion.

Medications can cause sexual dysfunction and can result in the patient's noncompliance with treatment. Sexual problems associated with the side effects of antihypertensive drugs have been discussed. Most psychoactive drugs have been reported to affect sexual function. Fortunately, the most adverse side effect, usually inhibition of desire in both men and women, occurs only with high doses. Mellaril (thioridizine) has been reported to cause retrograde ejaculation. Lithium carbonate may cause inhibition of desire and/or inhibited arousal in both men and women.

Alcohol, marijuana, narcotics, and cocaine have a variety of effects on sexual function. Small doses, which produce mild intoxication, may cause a disinhibition of sexual restraints and a loosening of social mores, thus giving rise to the claim of "aphrodisiac" properties. The belief that the substance predisposes one to acting sexually may "permit" an otherwise prohibited behavior. Even moderate intoxication, however, may lead to inhibited excitement and delayed or inhibited orgasm in both sexes.[7] Chronic abuse results in inhibition of all phases of the response cycle, secondary to both the pharmacologic action and the physical sequelae of chronic use, that is, debilitation, peripheral neuropathy, etc.

EVALUATION

The usual history of a sexual disorder associated with a physical condition is one of a persistent, progressive decline from a prior

TABLE 16.10–1. SOME ORGANIC FACTORS AFFECTING SEXUAL RESPONSE

Men	Women	Both
• Peyronie disease	• Atrophic vaginitis	• Chronic systemic disease
• Urethral infections	• Infections of the vagina	• Chronic pain
• Testicular disease	• Cystitis, urethritis	• Diabetes mellitus
• Hypogonadal androgen-deficient states	• Endometriosis	• Angina pectoris
• Hydrocele	• Episiotomy scars, tears	• Hypertension
• Lumbar sympathectomy	• Uterine prolapse	• Multiple sclerosis
• Radical perineal prostatectomy	• Infections of external genitalia	• Hyperprolactinemia
		• Spinal cord lesions
		• Alcoholism
		• Substance abuse

TABLE 16.10–2. DRUGS THAT MAY AFFECT SEXUAL RESPONSE

• Alcohol	• Digoxin
• Amphetamines	• L-Dopa
• Anxiolytics	• Lithium
• Antidepressants	• Marijuana
• Antihypertensives	• Narcotics
• Cimetidine	• Neuroleptics
• Cocaine	• Sedatives

level of trouble-free, satisfactory sexual function. The impairment is reported as pervasive, with function affected during all sexual experiences and with all stimuli. For example, the impairment is present with all sexual partners and with self-stimulation. Evaluation includes a medical history with a focus on the sexual complaint and an elaboration of the present illness, using the phases of the sexual response cycle as reference points for developing a differential diagnosis. In addition, a psychosocial history and mental-state examination should be obtained, with laboratory tests as indicated. In most cases, the relationship of the sexual dysfunction to the underlying organic disorder will be apparent as a result of the basic evaluation. Additional studies are required at times, including measuring prolactin levels of patients who complain of inhibited sexual desire (prolactin-secreting pituitary adenomas) and measuring morning testosterone levels of men who complain of inhibited sexual desire and/or erectile disorders (hypogonadism). Gynecologic and/or urologic consultations are often indicated, as are neurologic and occasionally vascular surgical consults. Nocturnal penile tumescence studies are helpful in differentiating organic dysfunction from psychologically based dysfunction in men with erectile disorders. Home monitoring devices are less expensive, but more unreliable than penile tumescence studies. Most recently, the injection of papaverine into the corpora cavernosa has been used diagnostically to establish the degree of penile vascular competency.

TREATMENT

Reversible Disorders

Desire, arousal, and orgasmic phase disorders secondary to the debilitation of chronic illness, to chronic pain, or to the side effects of medications are potentially reversible by a variety of medical interventions. Improvement of the patient's overall physical condition and relief of pain often restore sexual function. Drug holidays, change of medication, or discontinuance of medications may reverse dysfunction. Sexual disorders secondary to the acute effects of substance abuse usually remit once abuse is controlled. Abuse may, however, also mask the presence of primarily psychogenic sexual dysfunction. Prolactin-secreting microadenomas may be treated by resection or with bromocriptine. Men with hypogonadism who have inhibited desire and/or an erectile disorder usually return to normal function following the intramuscular administration of exogenous testosterone. Testosterone is not an effective treatment for inhibited desire or erectile dysfunction in men with normal testosterone levels. The efficacy of yohimbine in treating psychogenic erectile disorders in men has also not yet been established.

Irreversible Disorders

Even when sexual function is irreversibly impaired by disease processes, trauma, or the sequelae of surgery, patients can be helped to function sexually at levels that are psychologically, if not entirely physically, satisfying to themselves and their partners. Treatment, based on principles of rehabilitation medicine, consists of establishing realistic goals, assisting the patient to adapt to loss of function, and training the patient to maximize utilization of residual functional capacities. Patients can be taught sexual techniques that substitute for their lost function. The new technique must, however, be compatible with the patient's belief systems. Sexual techniques that are morally or experientially offensive will not be utilized by patients.

Even working within these restrictions, certain patients can experience rewarding physical and psychologic intimacy through kissing and caressing. When married, the impaired partner often derives enormous psychologic benefit from being able to share a sexual experience with the unimpaired partner. Many patient self-help associations have public forums and literature on sexual problems associated with specific conditions, for example, ostomies. Patients should be encouraged to avail themselves of these resources.

Erectile disorders are treatable surgically and nonsurgically. Two types of prostheses are available, paired silastic rods with malleable metal cores and inflatable devices, either of which is implanted in the corpora cavernosa of the penis. Medical treatments include the injection of vasodilating substances (papaverine) into the corpora cavernosa and suction devices that mechanically produce tumescence.[8] Papaverine injections have the obvious advantage of having a temporary result and do not cause permanent damage to the tissue structure of the penis. Patients can be taught with supervision to inject themselves painlessly with 28 gauge needles.

Currently, the only medical treatment available for women with organically caused arousal or orgasmic disorders is estrogen replacement for deficiency states.

PSYCHOSEXUAL DISORDERS

The sexual response cycle described by Masters and Johnson has become the conceptual basis for defining the common psychosexual disorders: sexual desire disorders, sexual arousal disorders, orgasm disorders, and sexual pain disorders.[1]

GENERAL CHARACTERISTICS

Estimates of lifetime incidence of the psychosexual disorders range from a high of 75 percent in marriages and other long-term relationships to a low of 25 percent. The exact incidence, however, is not known. Psychosexual dysfunctions may be experienced by heterosexual and homosexual individuals and couples. The onset may be any time during adult life. In some instances, psychologic and behavioral antecedents of these disorders can be identified in adolescent or childhood sexual behaviors and fantasies. Severe forms of these disorders appear to be associated with predisposing personality factors insofar as impairments in personality development contribute to the evolution of maladaptive sexual behaviors. In addition, religious beliefs, cultural values, and experience can generate negative attitudes about sexual function.

The course of these disorders is variable. Some patients experience dysfunction their entire adult lives, while others are episodically dysfunctional. Severity of symptomatology ranges from mild to severe. Good prognosis following treatment is associated with no past history of sexual dysfunction, recent onset of symptoms, mild to moderate severity, the presence of related situational stress factors, good psychologic health, past or current history of the ability to maintain long-term relationships, and a current relationship to which the partners are equally committed. Poor prognosis is associated with chronicity of symptoms, severe dysfunction, other psychopathology, and a history of unstable relationships.

The principal complications of these disorders are the inability to develop stable relationships, the disruption of existing relationships, and a reduction in the overall quality of one's life. Sexual dysfunction may give rise to symptoms of anxiety, depression, guilt, shame, or anger.

SEXUAL DESIRE DISORDERS

Diagnostic Criteria

Inhibition of sexual desire is diagnosed on the basis of a history of loss of sexual interest of sufficient degree to block repeatedly the patient's willingness to seek out and engage in sexual experience. Moderately severe forms of this dysfunction may be associated with the inhibition of sexual fantasies. The disorder may be situational: Loss of desire is experienced with one partner but not with another. Patients in heterosexual and homosexual relationships can suffer inhibition of desire as well as patients who engage solely in autoerotic sexual practices. Married bisexual patients may experience loss of desire for their spouse that may occasion a crisis in the marriage.

Evaluation

Assessment of the complaint of inhibited desire is documented by quantitating the decline in sexual drive. The current level of sexual activities should be compared with that at a point of time considered normal by the patient. Evaluation should include psychosexual and psychosocial histories and a mental-state examination. Since loss of sexual interest is a prominent symptom of depression, affective disorders should be ruled out as well as other psychiatric disorders less commonly associated with inhibited sexual desire. Loss of desire may be secondary to the anxiety and frustration of repeated sexual failure associated with other psychosexual disorders. The evaluation should also include the assessment of frequency of autoerotic experiences.

In practice, most patients presenting with this disorder are married, one or both partners reporting loss of sexual interest in the other. Evaluation requires an assessment not only of the chief complaint and present illness but also of the marital relationship. Substantial marital discord and anger will usually be revealed. Marital partners regularly fail to make a connection between their loss of sexual interest and their anger toward each other. Situational stress factors (loss of job, in-law problems, child-rearing practices, financial problems) generate tension and are common sources of discord.

The partners should be interviewed together and individually. Discrepancies in their descriptions of problems during the individual interviews may provide important clues to the origin of the marital strife. In all but the most complicated cases, the interview material will reveal precipitating stress factors and highlight the conflicts. Should extramarital relationships complicate the situation, they can be discussed openly if both partners are aware of the outside relationships. If an extramarital relationship is uncovered during individual interviews, however, the involved partner, not the physician, has the responsibility for deciding whether the extramarital relationship should be disclosed.

Treatment

Cases with a favorable prognostic profile can be managed in an office setting with brief counseling (see Table 16.10–3). Counseling should focus on lessening situational stress. For example, support and encouragement can be provided while a new job is being sought, or counseling can create a neutral environment in which a couple can explore their differences about child-rearing techniques. A series of two to five sessions of approximately 30 minutes is usually sufficient. Cases of inhibited sexual desire secondary to other psychiatric disorders or involving more complex marital dynamics most likely will require referral to an appropriate mental health professional.

TABLE 16.10–3. FAVORABLE PROGNOSTIC FACTORS FOR TREATING PSYCHOSEXUAL DISORDERS

- Recent onset of symptoms
- Mild to moderate severity
- No history of sexual dysfunction
- Related situational stress factors
- Absence of other psychopathology
- History of good long-term relationships
- Spouse or partner cooperative with evaluation

SEXUAL AROUSAL DISORDERS

Diagnostic Criteria

Arousal disorders are characterized by the inability to obtain and maintain a level of sexual excitement that permits a smooth and trouble-free progression from the beginning of a sexual experience to its completion. Specifically, this means in women the inability to obtain and maintain lubrication and the swelling response of the external genital; for men, the failure is the inability to obtain and maintain an erection. In both sexes this inability normally prevents the completion of the sexual act. In some cases women may accept penetration without sufficient lubrication, thereby experiencing discomfort or pain. Additionally, the clinician must be convinced that the patient complaining of this particular disorder experiences the problem during sexual activity that is adequate in focus, intensity, and duration and that the disorder is not secondary to a physical condition.

Evaluation

Evaluation of complaints of arousal disorders includes a history of the present illness, a psychosexual history, a psychosocial history, and a mental-state examination. The focus of the evaluation should be directed to identification of the patient's internal psychologic events and/or situational stress factors that are potential sources of psychologic interference of the normal progression of sexual arousal. A dramatic example of an external event that routinely causes a massive shift of attention away from sexual stimuli occurs with the ringing of a telephone next to the bed.

Persistent preoccupation about how well one is performing sexually is a common internal psychologic event. This experience is described as "performance anxiety" and "spectatoring." Although more subtle than the example of the ringing telephone, the effect on the natural progression of arousal is similar. These and similar events block one's ability to focus on the sexual stimuli that maintain arousal. When patients realize arousal is decreasing, they try to will arousal, psychologically shutting off their ability to respond to sexual stimuli.

The marital dynamics described in the section on sexual desire disorders associated with stressful life situations also contribute to the development of arousal disorders. Stress may cause frustration and anger, which eventually become an interference during lovemaking. In contrast to the history obtained from patients with organic impairment of the arousal phase or a gradual loss of ability, patients usually report a more rapid loss of their ability to be aroused. In addition, there is evidence of normal capacity for arousal with self-masturbation, fantasy, pornographic material, and sometimes with other partners. Men report nocturnal and early morning erections, and women may report arousal during sleep associated with sexual dreams.

Treatment

The selection of cases for treatment by the internist should be determined principally by matching the patient to a prognostic profile. The goal of counseling is to eliminate the negative effects of the identified interfering factors. Stressful life situations are managed by encouraging the patient to examine his or her situation and to create options and compromises that lead to a resolution of

the problem. Successful resolution usually results in the patient's return to baseline sexual function. Performance anxiety (an internal event) can be overcome by teaching the patient to relax and to focus on the enjoyment of the sexual stimuli that maintain arousal. Two to five sessions of approximately 30 minutes are usually sufficient to accomplish these treatment goals. Single patients or couples who do not meet the prognostic profile or do not respond to counseling should be considered for referral.

ORGASM DISORDERS

Diagnostic Criteria

Orgasm is considered inhibited if there is a history of recurrent and persistent inability to experience sexual release following a normal excitement phase that includes the achievement of plateau level of arousal. In women, orgasm is manifested by rhythmic contractions of the muscles of the outer third of the vagina, the perineal muscles, and the uterus. Orgasm in males is normally manifested by ejaculation.

Evaluation

The exact incidence of orgasm disorders in women is unknown, but studies estimate that 10 percent of the female population in the United States is anorgasmic to any sexual stimuli, and 30 to 50 percent of all married women are occasionally anorgasmic during intercourse. Psychogenic anorgasmia in men is a rare disorder. The evaluation of the disorder in both sexes includes an elaboration of the present illness, a psychosexual history, a psychosocial history, and a mental-state examination. The history should document that the patient has normal desire, routinely experiences arousal, and regularly reaches plateau (high) level of arousal before failing to experience orgasm. Since women generally require more time than men at plateau for preparation for orgasm, evaluation must document whether the routine sequence of coitus allows for that preparation. If the partner consistently reaches orgasm before the patient is ready for her release, the problem may be one of timing, or it is conceivable that the problem is the partner's rather than the patient's. It is also very important to document a history of orgasmic response with a partner and/or self-masturbation. Women who have been anorgasmic to all forms of sexual stimuli (primary anorgasmia) do less well with treatment than do women with a history of orgasmic response (secondary anorgasmia). Anorgasmia in men is associated with severe personality disturbances of two types: obsessive/compulsive character disorders and sadomasochistic character disorders. The evaluation should therefore focus on psychiatric aspects through history and mental state examination.

Treatment

Males with orgasm disorders should be referred, because they are difficult to manage. Women with secondary anorgasmia are candidates for brief counseling. The goals of counseling should be first to eliminate the impact of any stressful life situations as was discussed earlier and second to assist the patient to shift the focus of attention from concern about orgasm to enjoyment of the total sexual experience. The encouragement and support inherent in the counseling process will usually promote sufficient relaxation of concern to permit the patient to return to her baseline sexual function (which by history included orgasmic capacity). These goals are achievable in five 30-minute sessions.

PREMATURE EJACULATION

Diagnostic Criteria

There are many definitions of premature ejaculation, which include factors such as length of time of intercourse or number of thrusts, but a less potentially contentious definition is ejaculation that regularly occurs before the partner or the patient wishes. The clinician should take into account the duration of the excitement

phase, the novelty of the sexual partner, the state of the relationship, and the frequency of sexual experiences.

Evaluation

Premature ejaculation is a psychogenic disturbance with no confirmed physical causes. It is unusual for unmarried males to complain of this problem. In most instances, the patient is brought to evaluation by a frustrated, angry, complaining spouse. Invariably, the history of the present illness is that ejaculation occurs during or immediately after penetration. Patients with the most severe form of this disorder may ejaculate if their penis is touched by their partner, thus restricting foreplay as well as coital time. Most patients eventually reveal that they have experienced the dysfunction ever since they became sexually active. An occasional patient may report better control with one partner than with others. The female partner's description of the sexual encounters is essential because in many cases the patient is not aware of or does not believe that a sexual problem exists. Remarkably, couples will report they experienced trouble from the outset of their sexual relationships but either accepted the limitations or "worked around them."[5] Assessment of the general aspects of the marital relationship will reveal additional patient behavior and attitudes that irritate the spouse, of which the patient appears unaware. The general form of the patient's relationship with his spouse is passive-aggressive. Upon initial evaluation the spouse is usually considered free of any dysfunction. During therapy, however, at least 30 percent of the spouses will be found to have problems with sexual arousal and/or orgasm disorders. Occasionally, premature ejaculation may evolve into an erectile disorder.

Treatment

Behavioral methods of treatment that include the partner are usually successful in treating this disorder, especially when favorable prognostic features are present (Table 16.10–3). These methods are outside the scope of office practice and require specific expertise. In addition, the anger typically experienced by the woman and repressed by the patient usually complicates the marriage and necessitates marital therapy before sexually focused treatment.

FUNCTIONAL DYSPAREUNIA

Diagnostic Criteria

Functional or psychogenic dyspareunia is recurrent genital pain associated with intercourse, not caused by a physical condition, and not secondary to female arousal disorder.

Evaluation

The diagnosis of psychogenic dyspareunia should be made only after all physical causes have been excluded. Gynecologic and urologic examinations are essential, followed by psychosexual history, psychosocial history, and mental-state examination.

Treatment

Psychogenic dyspareunia is a rare disorder in both sexes. Patients who suffer dyspareunia often harbor significant psychopathology and require referral. An occasional patient with recent onset of dyspareunia who has other favorable prognostic features (Table 16.10–3) may be a candidate for brief counseling. Counseling should focus on the alleviation of anxiety, which is typically the cause of the symptom. The counseling techniques and strategies that bear on interpersonal dynamics already described are to be kept in mind.

FUNCTIONAL VAGINISMUS

Diagnostic Criteria

Vaginismus is a recurrent, involuntary spasm of the musculature of the outer third of the vagina not caused by a physical condition. Contraction of the musculature may be sufficiently severe to pre-

vent gynecologic examination with the smallest speculum. Spasm during attempts at coitus may prevent penile penetration.

Evaluation

The diagnosis of vaginismus is made frequently by gynecologists during routine pelvic examinations. Patients may complain of being unable to engage in intercourse because of difficulties with penetration. The clinician can differentiate the mechanical obstruction of vaginismus from the difficulty of penetrating secondary to lack of lubrication (female arousal disorder) by noting the patient's history with regard to gynecologic examinations and response to manual stimulation (by partner) of her vagina. Occasionally, this disorder may be uncovered as the cause of unconsummated marriages. Painful intercourse is occasionally the cause of the initial episode of vaginismus. A gynecological examination is therefore an important component of evaluation. Functional (psychogenic) vaginismus is rare and may be caused by anticipatory fears of being harmed through the act of penetration. It should be remembered that vaginismus is an involuntary reflex, much like that of an eye blink with an approaching object. Evaluation therefore should focus on the patient's psychosexual history with the identification of factors that historically contribute to the development of fear of penetration.

Treatment

Psychogenic vaginismus has been successfully treated using desensitization techniques that gradually allow the patient to accept penetration. In a prescribed series of exercises performed in privacy, the couples are instructed to engage in nonsexually demanding general body touching, excluding the genitals. The next session they repeat general touching but include genital touching. During following sessions they repeat the touching exercises but, in addition, pass graded-size dilators into the vagina until the dilator approximates the circumference of a penis. The penis can then be substituted for the dilator, permitting coitus. A similar technique can be offered to single patients who must pass the dilators themselves.

GENDER-IDENTITY DISORDERS

Diagnostic Criteria

Transsexualism is defined as a persistent sense of discomfort about one's anatomic sex accompanied by the determined wish to be rid of one's own genitals and to live as a member of the other sex. No physical or genetic condition should be present and, by definition, the condition is not associated with another mental disorder. Adult transsexualism is divided into asexual, heterosexual, and homosexual types. The definition of the gender-identity disorders of childhood similarly requires the persistent wish by a child to be of the opposite sex. Prepubertal children with this condition repudiate their genitals and insist they are going to grow up as a member of the opposite sex.

General Characteristics

Genetic or biochemical predisposing factors of these disorders have not been identified, although research continues on the effects of hormonal differentiation of the fetal brain and neonatal "critical periods" of development. Limited evidence suggests a relationship between confused sexual identity of parents and early childhood cross-dressing overtly or covertly condoned by parents or grandparents.[2] The disorder is rare; the male to female ratio is reported to be 2 to 1. Children have been reported to express cross-gender wishes at age 4 years. Onset of the adult form occurs in late adolescence or early adulthood, although in some cases (typically men) as late as age 40 or 50. The course of the disorder in children is as yet unknown, although an undetermined number of affected boys and girls may adopt a homosexual orientation during adolescence and as adults. The course in adults is variable; some patients consistently maintain their wish to live in the cross-gender role and eventually are surgically reassigned. Most patients follow an epi-

sodic course with the intensity of the desire and actual function (socially and vocationally) in the cross-gender role waxing and waning. Major complications associated with these disorders are the social and occupational problems associated with trying to function in the cross-gender role during the transitional phases of the course. In addition, there are difficulties developing and maintaining relationships. Failure to achieve the desired wish may lead to depressive episodes and suicide attempts. In rare instances, men who have not succeeded in being surgically reassigned have mutilated their own genitals.

Evaluation

Children are brought by their parents to evaluation, which necessitates combined child psychiatric and gender-disorder expertise. Adults enter the medical system at any point they believe they have the best chance of obtaining support for furthering their goals. A medical history and physical examination will typically reveal both males and females to be anatomically normal. An occasional patient may be found to be congenitally intersexed. Differential diagnosis should include schizophrenia (Chapter 16.6), transvestism and transvestism associated with major depressive disorder (see below).

Treatment

Children and adults with gender-identity disorders should be referred to mental health professionals.

Most university medical centers have specialized programs for the evaluation and treatment of transsexualism.

PARAPHILIAS

Diagnostic Criteria

The paraphilias are a group of disorders that have as their essential feature sexual interest toward objects other than human beings, toward sexual acts not usually associated with coitus, and toward coitus performed under bizarre conditions. Paraphilias are divided into the following forms: fetishism, transvestism, pedophilia, exhibitionism, voyeurism, sadism, and masochism.

Fetishism is the use of material objects as the preferred or exclusive means of achieving sexual excitement.

Transvestism is recurrent and persistent cross-dressing by heterosexual males or females who use the cross-dressing for the purpose of sexual excitement, at least when the cross-dressing first begins. This disorder should not be confused with transsexualism.

Pedophilia is the act or fantasy of engaging in sexual activity with prepubertal children as the preferred or exclusive method of achieving sexual excitement.

Exhibitionism is the repeated act of exposing one's genitals to an unsuspecting stranger for the purpose of achieving sexual excitement. There is no attempt at further sexual activity with the stranger.

Voyeurism is repeated episodes of observing unsuspecting people who are in the act of disrobing, who are naked, or who are engaging in sexual activity as a preferred or exclusive method of achieving sexual excitement.

Sadism and masochism is the act of inflicting pain or experiencing pain as a requisite for achieving sexual excitement. The spectrum of behavior included in this category is broad, ranging from humiliation and mental cruelty to extreme overt physical injury and, in some instances, murder.

General Characteristics

The etiology of these disorders is not known. A history of physical and/or sexual abuse during childhood appears in a number of cases. The prevalence of the disorder is unknown, and the sex ratio is predominantly male, with the exception of sexual sadism and masochism. The course is often lifelong, with peaks of activity occurring during periods of stress and accompanied by other psychiatric symptoms, most notably depression. The major complica-

tions of these disorders are the civilian and criminal consequences of forcing behavior on unconsenting partners or unwitting victims. In addition, patients with these disorders have significant difficulties in developing long-term, affectionate relationships.

Evaluation
A patient may reveal the practice of, or urge to experience, a paraphilia during a routine medical examination. Hypersexuality associated with paraphiliac behavior has been reported as associated with temporal lobe epilepsy. Abuse of alcohol or other substances may precipitate the manifestation of paraphilic behavior in patients who otherwise have control of paraphilic tendencies. Other psychiatric disturbances such as organic brain syndrome, mental retardation, and anxiety may be associated with episodes of paraphilic behavior, but these episodes should not be diagnosed as paraphilias.

Treatment
The treatment of paraphilias is difficult and should be carried out by psychiatrists with expertise in managing these disorders. Paraphilic behavior may expose patients to sexually transmitted diseases, a fact that should be taken into account during evaluation.

HOMOSEXUALITY

General Characteristics
Homosexuality itself is not classified as a mental disorder. Thirty years ago, Kinsey estimated that 10 percent of white American men and 5 percent of white American women were predominantly homosexual. Today, it is generally held that between 10 and 12 percent of the adult female population has had a homosexual experience. The principal feature of a homosexual orientation is the persistent requirement that sexual partners be of the same sex. Although there are many theories about the etiology of homosexuality, no studies have demonstrated genetic determinants, abnormal endocrine function, or confirmed psychosocial etiologies. Homosexuality is usually lifelong, with most individuals accepting a homosexual orientation during late adolescence or early adulthood. Despite the fact that complications associated with homosexual behavior have been significantly less in the past decades as the bias and stigma associated with homosexuality have lessened, many individuals and their families have significant adjustment problems in accepting a homosexual orientation.

Evaluation and Management
Patients who are concerned about homosexual fantasies or experiences should be given a chance to explore their feelings to determine the significance of their concerns. Heterosexual patients experience homosexual fantasies and may require reassurance about the normality of such thoughts. The patient who is exploring the acceptance of a homosexual orientation may need brief counseling to explore that option. The clinician can fill this therapeutic role or make a referral to a psychiatrist or mental health professional who is experienced in working with such patients. Most homosexuals prefer that their personal physician know of their homosexuality and indicate they are more satisfied with the care they obtain when their physician is aware. Homosexuals who have multiple partners may require special attention with regard to their routine medical care because of the problems associated with sexually transmitted diseases. The disorders that have been associated with promiscuity include acquired immunodeficiency syndrome (AIDS), Type B hepatitis, syphilis, gonorrhea, and giardiasis.

REFERENCES

1. American Psychiatric Association: Diagnostic and Statistical Manual of Mental Disorders-IIIR. Washington, DC: American Psychiatric Association, 1987
2. Halle E, Schmidt CW, Meyer JK: The role of grandmothers in transsexualism. Am J Psychiatr 137:497, 1980
3. Lepor H, Gregerman M, et al: Precise localization of the autonomic nerves from the pelvic plexus to the corpora cavernosa. A detailed anatomical study of the adult male pelvis. J Urol 133:207, 1985
4. Masters WH, Johnson VE: Human Sexual Response. Boston, Little, Brown, 1966
5. Schmidt CW: Sexual disorders in couples. In Meyer JK, Schmidt CW, Wise TN (eds): Clinical Management and Sexual Disorders, 2d ed. Baltimore, Williams and Wilkins, 1983, p 223
6. Schreiner EP, Schiavi RC, et al: Diabetes and female sexuality: A comparative study of women in relationships. J Sex Marital Therapy 11:165, 1985
7. Wilson GT: Alcohol, selective attention, and sexual arousal in men. J Studies Alcohol 46:107, 1985
8. Zorgniotti AW, LeFleur RS: Autoinjection of the corpus cavernosum with a vasoactive drug combination for vasculogenic impotence. J Urol 133:39, 1985

CHAPTER 17.1
Specific Complications of Medical Management

Craig R. Smith and Brent G. Petty

Diseases caused by diagnostic and therapeutic procedures are among the most disturbing consequences of medical practice. Since Hippocrates, who wrote "first do no harm" (*primum non nocere*), the importance of this problem has been repeatedly emphasized. Considerable effort is currently expended to develop safer methods of diagnosis and treatment as well as effective surveillance procedures to identify adverse reactions.[5]

The technologic advances of the past few decades have led to an expanding list of diseases associated with medical management. Development of iatrogenic diseases during hospitalization has been reported in as many as 36 percent of patients. For some patients, such as those in intensive care units or those undergoing cancer chemotherapy, the percentage may be higher. It has been estimated that 3 to 5 percent of all hospitalizations are caused by adverse drug reactions and that the fatality rate from these reactions may be as high as 0.1 percent. In the face of these problems physicians must maintain continued vigilance and must always weigh the potential risks of a procedure or medication againts its potential benefits.

ADVERSE EFFECTS OF DRUGS[5,8]

About 10 to 20 percent of hospitalized patients and 2 to 5 percent of outpatients develop adverse effects while taking medications. This frequency varies greatly, depending on the drug administered, the patient population treated, and the definitions of adverse effects.[4] Epidemiologic studies indicate that a small group of frequently used drugs accounts for the majority of adverse drug reactions. Since these drugs produce most of the problems, familiarity with their adverse effects is important (Table 17.1–1).

Adverse drug reactions may be classified into those caused by excessive intended pharmacologic effects and those caused by unintended actions. Adverse effects from excessive intended pharmacologic effects are all dose dependent. For example, hypoglycemia may be caused by excessive doses of insulin, hypotension by excessive doses of antihypertensives, and sodium and water depletion by excessive doses of diuretics. Altered drug pharmacokinetics are a frequent cause of dose-dependent adverse effects. For example, when the clearance of a drug is reduced, excessive drug concentrations may accumulate at the drug receptor and cause exaggerated pharmacologic effects.

Adverse effects caused by unintended actions of the drug may be categorized into those due to (1) the physical and chemical properties of the drug or its excipients, (2) the direct cytotoxic effects of the drug, (3) the induction of an abnormal immune response, and (4) heritable enzyme defects. The first category is usually caused by decomposition of the drug or effects of the excipients commonly used for stabilization or solubilization.

Probably the most common examples of unintended pharmacologic effects are those from the direct cytotoxic action of drugs. The production of reactive metabolites that covalently bind to tissue macromolecules is a frequent cause of cytotoxic effects. Hepati-

tis from isoniazid is an example, but many other "idiosyncratic" reactions may also have this mechanism.

Abnormal immune responses frequently cause adverse drug reactions. Although most drugs are poor antigens, virtually all drugs have been associated with allergic reactions. These reactions are usually caused by one of three mechanisms: (1) the drug binds to proteins or cells and directly induces an antibody response, (2) the drug alters tissue and induces an autoimmune response directed against the altered tissue, or (3) the drug induces the production of antibodies that are cross-reactive with other proteins or tissues.

Two patterns of immunologic responses may be induced by drugs: (1) immediate reactions mediated by IgE and characterized by urticaria, wheezing, rhinorrhea, skin rash, and, rarely, anaphylaxis, and (2) delayed reactions, or serum sickness, from IgG-mediated immune complex formation and characterized by arthralgias, lymphadenopathy, glomerulonephritis, arthritis, cerebritis, and vasculitis. Drugs may also suppress the immune system and lead to infectious complications that may be life threatening.

Adverse drug reactions resulting from heritable enzyme defects are fortunately unusual. Two examples are excessively prolonged neuromuscular blockade caused by succinylcholine in patients with pseudocholinesterase deficiency and hemolytic anemia induced by sulfonamides in patients with glucose-6-phosphate dehydrogenase deficiency (see Chapter 6.6).

Most adverse drug reactions occur soon after administration, although some, such as mutagenesis and teratogenesis, may not be manifest until months, years, or even generations after the drug is administered. Unfortunately, these latter effects are difficult to study. For the most part we must rely on in vitro studies of the effects of drugs on chromosomes and DNA, on the results of studies in experimental animals exposed to high drug concentrations, or on the results of epidemiologic studies. Because most drugs cross the placenta, fetal drug concentrations are directly related to maternal plasma levels. During the first trimester, when organogenesis is taking place, the risk of drug-induced defects is greatest but exposure anytime during pregnancy may delay or distort normal development. The evidence for teratogenesis is strong for antineoplastic agents, some hormones (corticosteroids, androgens), warfarin, phenytoin, inhaled anesthetics, tobacco, alcohol, phenothiazines, and tricyclic antidepressants. Despite being linked to teratogenic effects, all of these drugs have been given to pregnant women who have subsequently delivered normal children. Because the risks are inadequately defined for most drugs, establishing the risk-benefit ratio in pregnancy is difficult.

Carcinogenesis has been conclusively demonstrated for only a few drugs in clinical use despite extensive clinical investigation. An example of a carcinogenic effect is the development of vaginal carcinoma in the daughters of women given diethylstilbestrol during pregnancy. Antineoplastic agents such as cyclophosphamide have also been linked to the development of chromosomal damage and subsequent malignancy.

Certain patients may be at greater risk for developing adverse reactions to drugs. Common predisposing factors include advanced

TABLE 17.1–1. FREQUENT OR SERIOUS ADVERSE EFFECTS OF COMMONLY USED DRUGS

Drug	Adverse Effects
Penicillins and cephalosporins	Hypersensitivity reactions, injection site pain and inflammation, neutropenia, interstitial nephritis, pseudomembranous colitis, coagulation abnormalities
Aminoglycosides	Nephrotoxicity, ototoxicity, neuromuscular paralysis
Tetracyclines	Nausea, metallic taste, pseudomembranous colitis, photosensitivity, vertigo (doxycycline), *Candida* superinfections
Trimethoprim-sulfamethoxazole	Skin rash, nausea, diarrhea, neutropenia, thrombocytopenia
Aspirin	Nausea, epigastric discomfort, tinnitus, gastritis, prolonged bleeding time
Nonsteroidal anti-inflammatory agents	Nausea, epigastric discomfort, headache, gastritis, diarrhea, edema, interstitial nephritis, hepatitis, thrombocytopenia, neutropenia
Acetaminophen	Skin rash, leukopenia, hepatic necrosis, papillary necrosis
Digoxin	Anorexia, nausea, yellow-green vision, gynecomastia, cardiac arrhythmias, bradycardia
Warfarin	Anorexia, nausea, hematuria, hemorrhage, hemorrhagic necrosis of breast, skin, or toes
Furosemide	Hypovolemia, hypokalemia, hyponatremia, hyperuricemia, hyperglycemia, ototoxicity
Thiazides	Hypokalemia, hyperuricemia, hyperglycemia, hypercalcemia, thrombocytopenia, pancreatitis, pulmonary edema
Insulin	Hypoglycemia, allergic reactions, lipoatrophy
Prednisone	Osteoporosis, adrenal suppression, proximal muscle weakness, skin atrophy, vascular fragility, hyperglycemia, hyperlipidemia, centripetal obesity, edema, depressed cell-mediated immunity, pancreatitis, insomnia, psychosis, cataracts, glaucoma, hirsutism
Propranolol	Congestive heart failure, bronchospasm, bradycardia, fatigue, depression, impotence, vivid dreams
Oral contraceptives	Nausea, headache, breast tenderness, weight gain, thromboembolism, cholelithiasis, secondary amenorrhea
Tricyclic antidepressants	Somnolence, fatigue, orthostatic hypotension, headache, xerostomia, blurred vision, constipation, urinary retention, delayed ejaculation, glaucoma, seizures, parkinsonian-like syndrome, tardive dyskinesia, cardiac arrhythmias, congestive heart failure

age, female gender, severe underlying disease, previous drug allergy, hepatic dysfunction, renal failure, inherited enzyme deficiencies, and concomitant drug administration. Most of these factors result in increased risk because they alter drug pharmacokinetics. For example, compared to younger patients, aged patients have a lower glomerular filtration rate for the same concentration of serum creatinine; therefore, an older patient, given the same dose of a drug eliminated by the kidney as a younger person, may have reduced drug clearance and accumulate high plasma concentrations. These patient factors may be additive, making some individuals at particularly high risk for adverse effects. It is important to identify high-risk patients in order to most accurately estimate the risk-benefit ratio.

Another important cause for adverse drug reactions is drug-drug interaction.[9] Such interactions can be divided into those caused by the enhancement of the cytotoxic effects of one drug by another and those caused by alteration of the pharmacokinetics of one drug by another. Additive effects of two drugs on the same organ system may also be viewed as a drug interaction.

Medication errors may also cause adverse drug reactions. Errors may be made by many people, including the prescribing physician, nursing staff, pharmacists, and the patient. All of these individuals have a responsibility to take every possible precaution to prevent mistakes. The most serious error occurs when the wrong medicine is given. Physicians may erroneously prescribe the wrong medicine, but more often the wrong medicine is given because abbreviations or illegible handwriting is misinterpreted, because drugs have similar names, for example, acetohexamide and acetazolamide, or because drugs are packaged in similar containers. Even if the correct medication is dispensed, serious errors can still occur. Medications can be incorrectly formulated or given with incompatible drugs. Drugs may also be given by the wrong route, in the wrong dose, or in the wrong frequency. Two causes for a wrong dose are the improper placement of a decimal point and the use of incorrect units, for example, mg rather than mEq. An effective method for preventing errors due to overlooking a decimal point is to place a zero before the decimal, for example, 0.25 mg rather than .25 mg.

A broad spectrum of disease is produced by adverse drug reactions. The most common manifestations are skin rash, pruritus, fever, nausea, vomiting, dizziness, headache, and diarrhea. Other important and relatively frequent adverse effects include bone marrow suppression, hepatitis, nephrotoxicity, arrhythmias, and a variety of neuropsychiatric symptoms including hallucinations, somnolence, depression, and confusion. Since such a broad spectrum of diseases may be induced, adverse drug reactions should always be considered when investigating a patient's complaints.

Although establishing the diagnosis of an adverse drug reaction may be difficult, several criteria may be useful.[8] Perhaps the most important factor in identifying an adverse drug reaction is the temporal relationship between the reaction and drug administration. Careful attention should be given to establishing that the suspected drug was administered before the reaction under investigation began. If the reaction disappears when the drug is discontinued and reappears when the drug is readministered, an adverse drug reaction should be strongly suspected. Other features that may be helpful are reversal of the reaction by a specific drug antagonist, previous conclusive reports that the drug produces the suspected reaction, the detection of blood or tissue concentrations of the drug that are known to be toxic, an increase in the severity of the reaction when the drug dose is increased or a decrease in severity when the dose is decreased, and the previous occurrence of the same or similar reactions to the same or similar drugs.

Eliciting a drug history is an essential step in the diagnosis of adverse drug reactions. Patients should be questioned about all drugs they have recently taken or are currently taking as well as any

other drugs they have at home that they may have used. Attention should be directed to nonprescription as well as prescription drugs. Repeated questioning may be necessary since patients may not recall or may overlook a course of therapy they considered inconsequential.

The management of adverse drug reactions should be systematic and should be tailored to the severity of the reaction. When patients are taking multiple drugs and a severe reaction occurs, all drugs that are thought to be likely causes of the adverse effect should be stopped as well as all others that may be discontinued safely. The time course for the disappearance of the reaction is usually related to the clearance of the drug. Fortunately, most adverse effects disappear promptly when the offending drug is discontinued. If the reaction is severe and the drug has a prolonged duration of effect, measures to remove the drug from the body, such as dialysis or hemoperfusion, may be necessary.

After the adverse effect has disappeared, further drug therapy must be carefully considered. If no effective alternative is available for the treatment of a life-threatening disease, each essential drug that was discontinued should be readministered individually, in order of importance, while observing the patient carefully for recurrence of the reaction. If the reaction was allergic, readministration may be hazardous because anaphylaxis may develop. If therapy has to be continued after the development of an adverse effect, every effort should be made to treat or attenuate the reaction. Allergic reactions may often be lessened by antihistamines or corticosteroids, and dose-dependent adverse effects may be reduced by lowering the dose.

One of the most important aspects of managing adverse drug reactions is prevention. Because of the direct relationship between the frequency of adverse reactions and the number of medications administered, as few drugs as possible should be used. Physicians can play another role in preventing adverse drug reactions by reporting severe, unusual, or previously unrecognized reactions to the Food and Drug Administration. Although most adverse effects are recognized during the development of a new drug, postmarketing surveillance is needed to identify unusual reactions, drug interactions, and patient populations at increased risk.

ADVERSE EFFECTS OF BIOLOGIC PRODUCTS

The therapeutic use of biologic products has recently increased as the result of technologic advances in blood banking and cell separation, plasma fractionation, and vaccine production. The biologic products used most often are blood components (red cells, granulocytes, and platelets), plasma proteins (albumin, gamma globulin, and coagulation factor concentrates), and vaccines (Table 17.1–2).

The adverse effects of whole blood, packed red cell, and granulocyte transfusions are discussed in Chapter 6.24.

Plasma protein preparations used in clinical medicine include 5 percent plasma protein, albumin, gamma globulin, and coagulation factor concentrates. The most common reactions to these products are allergic and are usually manifest by flushing, urticaria, fever, rigors, and headache. Hypotension and pulmonary edema are unusual and anaphylaxis is rare. Plasma protein preparations contain Hageman factor fragments, which may cause release of kallikrein and bradykinin, which in turn may cause vasodilatation and hypotension. This mechanism may explain worsening hypotension in some patients being resuscitated with these materials. A variety of infections similar to those associated with blood transfusion, including acquired immunodeficiency syndrome (AIDS), may also be transmitted by protein preparations. Fortunately, the availability of screening tests for antibody to HIV has dramatically reduced this risk. Viral infections and AIDS are most likely to occur with coagulation factor concentrates, which are usually prepared by pooling donor plasma. Other complications of these preparations include thrombocytopenia, hemolysis, and thrombosis. Rarely, commercial factor VIII preparations may cause transient visual disturbances, presumably a result of microembolization of fibrin aggregates.

Many vaccines are now available for the prevention of serious diseases such as polio, smallpox, hepatitis B, measles, and rubella. Most of these vaccines are produced from live, attenuated organisms whereas pneumococcal vaccine is produced from purified capsular polysaccharides. Adverse reactions to these preparations are usually local, with pain, edema, urticaria, or pruritus at the injection site. Regional lymphadenopathy and systemic allergic reactions such as fever and skin rash may also occur, particularly in patients with egg hypersensitivity because most attentuated vaccines are produced in eggs. Because they are prepared from live, attenuated organisms, subclinical or mild cases of disease may be produced. In rare cases, meningoencephalitis associated with seizures and optic neuritis may develop. Transient suppression of cell-mediated immunity may also occur, as may a demyelinating peripheral neuropathy characteristic of Guillain-Barré syndrome. Patients with immune deficiency appear to be at greatest risk for adverse effects from vaccines.

Interferon preparations have been made available for intravenous use. Fever, pain on injection, and hypersensitivity reactions have been the most common adverse effects, but neutropenia, thrombocytopenia, elevation of hepatic enzymes, and hypotension have also occurred.

COMPLICATIONS OF DIAGNOSTIC PROCEDURES

The complications resulting from diagnostic procedures are diverse and include both local and systemic reactions. Specific local complications for each procedure are related to the site of the diagnostic study and the procedure used (Table 17.1–3). Systemic reactions to diagnostic procedures may also occur. For example, vasovagal reactions can accompany any procedure and are characterized by nausea, sweating, epigastric distress, hyperventilation, weakness, confusion, bradycardia, blurring of vision, and loss of consciousness.

Medications used to prepare patients for diagnostic studies, such as cathartics, analgesics, sedatives, and atropine, may cause adverse effects either from interaction with other drugs or excess pharmacologic effects. For example, patients are routinely not given anything by mouth for as long as 18 hours before some studies. In combination with the overzealous use of cathartics, patients may become dehydrated, and dehydrated patients are at increased risk for renal toxicity from parenteral iodinated contrast material. Thus, the routine preparatory measures used for some studies may

TABLE 17.1–2. ADVERSE EFFECTS OF BIOLOGIC PRODUCTS

Biologic Product	Adverse Effect
Blood transfusion	Hemolytic reaction, volume overload, infection, coagulation defect, electrolyte abnormality, hyperammonemia, hypothermia, reduced red cell 2,3-DPG, microemboli, hemosiderosis
Granulocyte transfusion	Fever, pulmonary insufficiency, viral infections, graft-versus-host disease
Plasma protein preparations	Allergic reactions, pulmonary edema, hypotension, infection, thrombocytopenia, hemolysis, thrombosis
Vaccines	Injection site reactions, regional lymphadenopathy, allergic reactions, meningoencephalitis, optic neuritis, Guillain-Barré syndrome, vasculitis, immunosuppression
Interferon	Fever, injection site reactions, allergic reactions, neutropenia, thrombocytopenia, elevated hepatic enzymes, hypotension

TABLE 17.1–3. COMPLICATIONS OF DIAGNOSTIC PROCEDURES

Procedure	Complications
Radiologic	
Upper gastrointestinal series	Barium impaction, hypovolemia
Barium enema	Perforation
Oral cholecystography	Nausea, vomiting, diarrhea, or headache in up to 50%
Bronchography	Bronchospasm
Iodinated contrast studies	Flushing, nausea, vomiting (20%), hypersensitivity reactions (5%), death (0.0013%), congestive heart failure, nephrotoxicity, seizures
Cardiac catheterization	Death (0.3%), infarction (0.3%), arrhythmia (1%)
Cerebral angiography	Transient (1%) or permanent (0–6%) neurologic deficits
Venography	Thrombophlebitis
Endoscopy	
Esophagogastroduodenoscopy	Aspiration, apnea, Mallory–Weiss laceration (0.1%), esophageal rupture (0.03%)
Endoscopic retrograde cholangiopancreatography	Pancreatitis, cholangitis, peritonitis
Sigmoidoscopy	Perforation (0.2%)
Colonoscopy	Perforation, excessive bleeding after polypectomy (1%)
Bronchoscopy	Hypoxemia, pneumothorax after biopsy (10%)
Laparoscopy	Cardiac arrest (0.1%), hypotension (0.15%), gas embolism (0.01%), significant bleeding (0.3%), bowel perforation (0.1%), uterine perforation (0.2%)
Cystoscopy	Infection, hemolysis with excessive water irrigation
Needle Aspiration	
Venipuncture	Local complications, vasovagal reactions
Arterial puncture	Pseudoaneurysm, median nerve compression
Lumbar puncture	Headache (30%), subdural hematoma with paraplegia (2%), severe back or radicular pain longer than 48 hours (2%), nerve root injury, uncal herniation
Thoracentesis	Pneumothorax, hemothorax, intercostal nerve injury, pulmonary edema, hypoxemia
Paracentesis	Intestinal perforation, hemoperitoneum, persistent ascitic fluid leak, hypotension
Arthrocentesis	Local complications
Pericardiocentesis	Laceration of coronary vessel or ventricle, infarction, tamponade
Transtracheal aspiration	Hemoptysis, vasovagal reaction, subcutaneous emphysema
Liver biopsy	Subcapsular hematoma, bile peritonitis
Renal biopsy	Hematuria (7%), retroperitoneal bleeding (2%), death (0.1%)
Thin-needle aspiration	Peritonitis, pancreatitis, malignant seeding of needle tract, pneumothorax

actually increase their morbidity. Reducing the risk of the "routine prep" involves individualizing the procedures employed before the diagnostic studies, providing intravenous fluids, if necessary, in order to reverse dehydration, and avoiding excessive doses of medications.

Bacteremia may occur with many diagnostic procedures but is most common when there is interruption of the normal mucosal barrier of a contaminated site. Efforts to sterilize the site, such as the use of alcohol on the skin before venipuncture or antiseptic enemas before transrectal prostatic biopsy, appear to reduce the incidence of bacteremia. Nevertheless, seeding of bacteria onto foreign bodies, for example, prosthetic heart valves, prosthetic joints, or arterial grafts, or onto damaged structures, for example, rheumatic valves or joints damaged by rheumatoid arthritis, remains a risk in spite of local antiseptic efforts. In certain situations, prophylactic antibiotics are recommended.

DIAGNOSTIC RADIOLOGY

Although radiation exposure may be teratogenic or mutagenic, most diagnostic radiologic procedures expose patients to negligible risk. For example, routine chest radiographs expose patients to about 5 millirads of radiation. This dose is approximately 5 percent of the average annual environmental radiation level to which we are all exposed and is probably inconsequential. In assessing risk from radiation it is generally assumed that carcinogenesis and mutagenesis occur as nonthreshold phenomena and that there is some probability of cancer induction at any dose, no matter how small. Compared to plain radiographs, barium and other contrast studies carry more risk since they expose patients to substantially greater amounts of radiation. Nevertheless, the radiation dose is still low, and unless such studies are performed repetitively over the course of years, they are not likely to pose a serious threat to the patient's health. Even though the overall risk of radiogenic injury from diagnostic radiographic procedures is 0.01 percent or less, one should not expose a patient to even this minute risk unless some benefit is likely to result.

An important concern regarding diagnostic radiation exposure is the potential teratogenicity or carcinogenicity for a fetus, especially early in pregnancy. The fetus is more sensitive to radiation than adults, and it appears that the risks from routine diagnostic procedures, while still low, are important. Retrospective studies indicate that the radiation from pelvimetry, abdominal radiographs, or placentograms may double the risk of leukemia during the first decade of the child's life. It has been recently estimated

that about 1000 millirads is required to double the risk of leukemia from in utero exposure. This is approximately the exposure from a single barium enema or ten abdominal radiographs. It seems clear that in pregnant patients one should be circumspect in the use of radiographic procedures, obtain them only when strongly indicated, provide as much lap shielding as the radiologic procedure will allow, and avoid studies associated with higher levels of exposure. In women with child-bearing potential abdominal radiation is safe during the 10 days following onset of menstruation but the precautions listed above should be observed thereafter unless effective contraception is being utilized.

Fertility is not affected by acute doses of radiation unless exposure exceeds 100 rads, a level not attained in diagnostic imaging. However, gametes may be damaged by as little as 1000 millirads, resulting in increased risk of genetic mutation. Men are at greater risk for this damage than women. As damaged gametes are eliminated over a period of months after exposure, the effect is reversible, but a period of several months should elapse between unprotected radiation exposure and conception. It is noteworthy that no detectable increase in genetic abnormalities has appeared among the children of Japanese who survived the two atomic bombings. Even though the risk of mutagenicity is low, it is appropriate to utilize radiation shields for procedures that expose the gonads of adults with child-bearing potential to radiation.

CONTRAST MATERIAL

Iodinated contrast material is now widely used in diagnostic radiology. It is generally safe and well tolerated, but generalized systemic reactions, seizures, cardiac toxicity, and renal toxicity may complicate its use. These adverse effects occur more frequently with intravenous than with intraarterial infusions. Iodinated contrast material predictably causes a flushing sensation when infused, and nausea and vomiting occur in up to 20 percent of patients. Hypersensitivity reactions, such as urticaria, bronchospasm, and pruritus, occurs in about 5 percent of patients. Cardiovascular collapse with hypotension and reflex tachycardia may also occur but is fortunately rare. Patients who have suffered a previous hypersensitivity reaction to iodinated contrast material may usually receive it again safely if pretreated with corticosteroids or antihistamines for 1 to 3 days before the study. The need for such pretreatment is disputed, but it seems prudent to utilize these medications as a precaution. Vasovagal reactions may be seen with iodinated contrast material and can be distinguished from hypersensitivity-induced hypotension because the latter is associated with tachycardia whereas the former causes bradycardia.

Because of the direct negative inotropic effect and high osmolality and sodium content of iodinated contrast material, congestive heart failure can be induced in patients with marginal cardiac function. Patients with normal cardiac function generally tolerate these effects without difficulty. Ventricular arrhythmias can occur but are usually seen only with coronary artery infusions.

The nephrotoxicity of iodinated contrast material is caused by a direct toxic effect on the tubules, leading to acute tubular necrosis. This is generally self-limited and resolves within 4 to 14 days. The most important risk factors for nephrotoxicity are dehydration, diabetes, proteinuria, and underlying organic renal disease. Careful attention to the hydration of the patient both before and after the study is the most important preventive measure.

ANGIOGRAPHY

Angiography has become an extremely useful radiographic tool. The risks of angiography are related to the contrast material and procedure used to introduce the catheter into the vessel. Venous studies are largely free of mechanical hazards, though thrombophlebitis can be induced. With arterial puncture the risk of hematoma is much greater and represents the most frequent local adverse effect. Current antiseptic practices make infections at the site

of vascular puncture uncommon. Vessel laceration and embolization of fibrin thrombi or atherosclerotic plaques are also infrequent. The overall death rate associated with thoracic, abdominal, and peripheral angiography is about 0.05 percent, and the overall complication rate for such studies is about 2 to 4 percent. The most common complications are vasovagal hypotension, arrhythmia, seizures, and stroke.

Recent studies are divergent in the assessment of the risk of cerebral angiography. One group found that 5 percent of their patients experienced a stroke after cerebral angiography; these were usually patients with previous ischemic episodes. The preponderance of data from several other groups indicates that the risk of stroke is only 0 to 2 percent, even in patients with critical stenosis of the carotid artery.

Cardiac catheterization with coronary angiography has become a routine procedure in most large institutions. Complications include arrhythmia, stroke, myocardial infarction, and death. The incidence of such complications, however, is remarkably low, despite use of the procedure in seriously ill patients. Patients at greater risk for complications are those with congestive heart failure, left main or severe coronary artery disease, hypertension, and unstable angina.

ENDOSCOPY

Esophagogastroduodenoscopy is usually safe and well tolerated. However, complications may be caused by the drugs used to produce sedation and analgesia during the procedure. Rarely apnea may occur when these drugs are infused rapidly or in excessive doses. Aspiration of secretions can occur during or after the procedure. Vasovagal responses with bradycardia and hypotension can also occur during the procedure, particularly in older individuals. Mallory-Weiss tears may complicate upper gastrointestinal endoscopy, especially in patients with hiatal hernias. These complications are, however, rare, and the procedure is performed safely in outpatients.

Sclerotherapy by means of endoscopy has become increasingly popular in recent years as an alternative to portosystemic shunting for the treatment of actively or recently bleeding esophageal varices. The most frequent complications of this procedure include chest pain, dysphagia, and bleeding. Sclerotherapy has become so safe in centers that do it often that many patients can receive initial and follow-up treatments as outpatients.[6]

Coagulation by endoscope has been used to treat safely vascular ectasias of the gastrointestinal tract. The use of laser photocoagulation for this procedure has recently been assessed.[1] About 11 percent of patients bleed with laser photocoagulation, but all of these hemorrhages stopped after continued photocoagulation at the same treatment session. Bowel perforation is infrequent, occurring in only about 2 percent of cases.

Bronchoscopy is associated with few adverse effects. Mild hypoxemia and vasovagal responses are the most frequent ones. When transbronchial biopsy is performed, pneumothorax occurs in less than 10 percent of cases. Hemoptysis following biopsy is usually mild and self-limited.

NEEDLE ASPIRATION

The most common needle aspiration is venipuncture, which is essentially risk free except for vasovagal reactions. When the state of the patient's peripheral veins requires femoral or brachial venipuncture, the adjacent artery may be punctured and lead to deep tissue bleeding. Even without arterial damage, aspiration of blood from these sites is associated with a risk of deep hematoma. Such hematomas can dissect proximally and involve the retroperitoneal space or axilla. These same problems can occur with arterial blood sampling if the femoral or brachial sites are used and inadequate compression is provided following the procedure. Arterial or venous puncture of these sites should be avoided in any patient with

an acquired or hereditary bleeding diathesis. In contrast, bleeding from arterial puncture of the radial artery is usually controlled easily. If substantial bleeding does occur it may cause compression of the median nerve in the carpal tunnel or compression of the artery itself with distal arterial insufficiency. Pseudoaneurysms are more likely to occur with repetitive punctures at the same site.

Complications after lumbar puncture are most likely if the patient has severe liver disease with defective coagulation, is therapeutically anticoagulated during or after the procedure, takes aspirin, or has a traumatic tap.

Percutaneous liver biopsy has become a routine procedure in the assessment of hepatomegaly, abnormal liver function tests, and some cases of jaundice. When the patient has a normal prothrombin time, partial thromboplastin time, platelet count, and bleeding time, the procedure is safe. The incidence of subcapsular hematoma, bile peritonitis, and other complications is low.

COMPLICATIONS OF MECHANICAL THERAPEUTIC PROCEDURES (Table 17.1–4)

Soft plastic catheters provide more secure intravenous access than can be obtained with metal needles. The major adverse effects associated with their use are phlebitis and infection. The incidence of these complications is proportional to the length of time the catheter is in place. Many hospitals have a policy routinely to remove intravenous catheters after 2 to 7 days and insert another at a differ-

ent site if intravenous access is still needed. Radial artery catheterization carries more risk in patients who are hypotensive, treated with vasoconstrictive medications, or have the catheter in place longer than 5 days.

Compared to peripheral venous catheters, central venous catheters carry more risk. Some published experience suggests that an internal jugular approach has fewer complications than a subclavian approach, whereas other results suggest no significant difference between the two routes. With more experience in performing the procedure, the incidence of complications falls.[10] Regardless of site of access, air embolism and vascular laceration are immediate risks whereas thrombosis of the superior vena cava is a later complication. Thrombosis is more frequent in patients with heart failure, particularly if the hemodynamic compromise continues for several days. The vascular complications may also be related to the composition of the catheter. Those composed of silicon, polyurethane, or Teflon are least likely to be associated with major thrombi. Erosion and perforation of the vessel may occur, especially when stiff catheters are left in place for prolonged periods, and can lead to hydromediastinum and hydrothorax. Air embolus during catheter placement is best prevented by placing patients supine with head down and legs elevated to keep venous pressure high in the vein being punctured. After the catheter is properly positioned, efforts to assure that the tubing remains connected are essential. Should the tubing become disconnected with the patient's trunk elevated, life-threatening air embolus can occur.

Indwelling bladder catheters are a portal of entry for bacteria into the urinary tract. Catheter-induced urinary tract infections are

TABLE 17.1–4. COMPLICATIONS OF MECHANICAL THERAPEUTIC PROCEDURES

Procedure	Complications
Catheters	
Peripheral venous catheters	Phlebitis, infection (2.5%), catheter fracture/embolism
Radial artery cannulation	Pseudoaneurysm, thrombosis, hematoma after removal (9%)
Central venous catheters	Pneumothorax (1–3%), hemothorax (1%), thrombosis (1–20%), air embolism (0.5%), vascular laceration, catheter fracture/embolism (0.2%)
Swan-Ganz catheters	Ventricular ectopy (15%), pulmonary artery rupture, pulmonary infarction, tricuspid damage, right bundle branch block, thrombosis
Temporary indwelling urethral catheters	Infection (16%), hematuria, bladder perforation
Chronic indwelling urethral catheters	Pyelonephritis, renal failure, bladder rupture, urethral stricture
Dialysis	
Hemodialysis	Hypotension, infection, aluminum intoxication, hepatitis B, depression, dysequilibrium syndrome, reduced HDL, hypertriglyceridemia
Peritoneal dialysis	Infection, aluminum intoxication dysequilibrium syndrome, fluid overload, atelectasis
Other Transvenous Procedures	
Hyperalimentation	Rebound hypoglycemia, hypophosphatemia, hypomagnesemia, vitamin deficiencies, sepsis
Temporary transvenous pacemakers	Ventricular ectopy (2%), right ventricular perforation (2%), percardial rub (5%), diaphragm stimulation (1%), phlebitis (0.6%)
Permanent transvenous pacemakers	Thrombosis—symptomatic (1%), asymptomatic (44%), perforation, ectopy, diaphragm stimulation
Pulmonary Procedures	
Artificial mechanical ventilation	Pneumothorax, infection, decreased cardiac output
Endotracheal intubation	Cuff necrosis, maxillary sinusitis (2%), oral or nasal trauma
Gastrointestinal Procedures	
Nasogastric intubation	Epistaxis, aspiration, pharyngeal or esophageal perforation, sinusitis, otitis media, laryngeal (arytenoid) edema (30%), vocal cord paralysis, intratracheal position
Intestinal (Cantor) tube	Obstruction, perforation, sinusitis, spillage of mercury
Esophageal variceal sclerotherapy	Bleeding (2–14%), chest pain (9–14%), dysphagia (2–6%), fever, esophageal perforation, mediastinitis, adult respiratory distress syndrome, stricture, bacteremia, death (0–7%)
Endoscopic laser photocoagulation	Bleeding (10%), perforation (2%)

the most common nosocomial infections. When these catheters are used for a short time in patients, they are safe, although about one fourth of patients develop bacteriuria. The risk of infection with these catheters is greatest in female, elderly, or critically ill patients who may develop a serious infection or bacteremia. The duration of cannulation, the type of catheter system, and the aseptic precautions employed all have a bearing on the development of a serious infection.

The condom catheter is sometimes used as an alternative to an indwelling catheter in men, but it is not without complications. Especially if it is secured too tightly it may cause penile necrosis, erosions, ulcerations, and urethrocutaneous fistula.

Transluminal balloon angioplasty has been developed as an alternative to surgery in patients with arterial stenosis. It has been utilized mainly in patients with coronary artery disease, but renal, subclavian, iliac, and other peripheral artery stenoses have been successfully treated with transluminal angioplasty. This procedure can be complicated by distal cholesterol embolization, vessel rupture, or severe intimal dissection with occlusion. In spite of these problems, transluminal angioplasty is an important nonsurgical alternative to the treatment of arterial stenosis.

Mechanical ventilation is sometimes associated with infection, pneumothorax, and complications from the endotracheal tube. The complications of intubation include cuff necrosis of the trachea and damage to the teeth, oral cavity, or nasal passage, depending on the route of insertion. Pneumothorax is more common when positive end-expiratory pressure (PEEP) is used. Although venous return may be reduced with PEEP, cardiac output is usually not reduced to a critical level unless the patient already has cardiac impairment.

Hemodialysis may be complicated by (1) hypotension; (2) infection; (3) aluminum intoxication, which may be related to the anemia, osteodystrophy, and encephalopathy of these patients; (4) hepatitis B infection; (5) increased risk of bleeding; (6) neutropenia; and (7) psychologic depression. Recent data suggest that intradialytic hypotension may be ameliorated by using dialysate with a relatively high calcium concentration (7.5 mg/dl). Hemodialysis may also be associated with hypertriglyceridemia and reduced serum levels of high-density lipoprotein. Aluminum intoxication may be more of a problem with peritoneal dialysis than with hemodialysis. The use of deionized dialysate reduces the incidence and severity of aluminum intoxication. The dysequilibrium syndrome may occur with hemodialysis or peritoneal dialysis and may be related to the development of edema of the basal ganglia, especially following rapid dialysis.[7]

COMPLICATIONS OF ANESTHESIA AND SURGERY

Despite remarkable advances in anesthesiology, complications may occur with the administration of any anesthetic. Even local anesthesia has some risk, including hypersensitivity reactions, dermatitis, convulsions, hypotension, or cardiac arrest. Convulsions and cardiovascular complications are usually caused by excessive doses, inadvertent intravenous injection, or altered drug pharmacokinetics. Spinal anesthesia frequently causes hypotension as a result of massive sympathetic blockade. Fluid and colloid loading or treatment with pressor agents may control this effect. Transient or permanent neurologic deficits may also occur following spinal anesthesia.

The risk of general anesthesia is not related simply to the potential toxic effects of the agents being used. Profound physiologic changes accompany general anesthesia and render the patient somewhat unstable, primarily as a result of effects on the autonomic nervous system. Issues related to the risks of general anesthesia and the identification and amelioration of risk factors are covered in Chapter 17.2.

COMPLICATIONS OF RADIATION THERAPY

Large doses of ionizing radiation are successfully employed in the treatment of many neoplastic disorders. Radiation therapy is associated with both acute and chronic adverse effects. All tissues exposed to the radiation beam are affected, although the degree of the effect on normal tissues may not be predictable.

Acute radiation reactions include generalized fatigue, anorexia, nausea, and vomiting. There may be local pain from radiation burns. If the mediastinum is in the radiation port, dysphagia is a common problem. These symptoms usually occur 1 to 2 weeks after the initiation of radiation therapy and are generally proportional to the dose of radiation and the rapidity with which the course is delivered. It may be several weeks or months after the radiation treatments are discontinued before these symptoms resolve.

Chronic radiation injuries are more serious, more likely to be permanent, and can be progressive. Radiation pneumonitis occurs in 5 to 20 percent of patients whose lungs are exposed to radiation therapy. The incidence of asymptomatic patients with only histologic changes may be greater than this. Although most patients who develop radiation pneumonitis recover from the dyspnea and nonproductive cough related to this entity, nearly all develop radiologic evidence of fibrosis. In a few patients, especially those with preexisting lung disease, this fibrosis will contribute to their pulmonary dysfunction and may cause chronic respiratory failure. The fibrosis may distort the architecture of the thorax, especially if the process is unilateral and retraction occurs. The loss of lung volume can induce a shift of the trachea or mediastinum and scoliosis may develop. Rarely, a small pleural effusion may appear and persist for years, but it usually disappears spontaneously.

The cardiac abnormalities resulting from radiation therapy include pericarditis with effusion (36 percent) and occasionally tamponade (5 percent), coronary artery fibrosis, constrictive pericarditis, and left ventricular dysfunction with restrictive cardiomyopathy (38 to 50 percent). Although some of these complications occur within 12 to 24 months after treatment, the development of pericardial effusion or left ventricular dysfunction may be delayed for years. Surgery may be required for relief of constriction. Adriamycin and radiation therapy appear to be synergistic in causing cardiotoxicity.

Radiation enteritis generally involves the small intestine and probably affects at least 1 to 10 percent of patients treated with radiation therapy for pelvic or abdominal carcinomas. The interval between radiation therapy and the diagnosis of radiation enteritis ranges from 3 months to as long as 20 years, and the incidence appears to be greater in patients with previous abdominal surgery. The symptoms may be minor and self-limited. In some patients the symptoms are more chronic and may improve with sulfasalazine and steroids. Some patients, however, develop intestinal obstruction or perforation requiring surgical therapy. Others have a syndrome that may include nausea, vomiting, diarrhea, malabsorption, weight loss, enteroenteric fistulae, or a combination of these. They may be refractory to medical or surgical therapy, and parenteral nutrition may be the only recourse.

Venoocclusive disease of the liver may follow radiation exposure and can resemble the Budd-Chiari syndrome, with rapid accumulation of ascites, hepatomegaly, and jaundice. It was reported in about 30 percent of patients given irradiation to the liver for metastatic disease, and about one fourth of these patients died of the radiation-induced liver disease.

Radiation therapy can also cause acute and chronic renal disease if the kidneys fall within the radiation port. Radiation cystitis occurs in 2 to 10 percent of patients receiving treatment for pelvic neoplasms, but in up to 80 percent of patients treated for bladder carcinoma.

In the past, radiation was used to treat hypertrophic tonsils and adenoids, pharyngitis, acne, and tinea capitis in children and young adults, and enlarged thymus glands in infants. These uses

of radiation have been associated with the development of benign and malignant neoplasms of the thyroid, parathyroid, and salivary glands, with latent periods between irradiation and diagnosis of about 30 years. Using radiation therapy as part of multimodality therapy for Hodgkin disease or other malignancies also seems to increase the risk of acute leukemia or second neoplasms in irradiated areas.

REFERENCES

1. Cello JP, Grendell JH: Endoscopic laser treatment for gastrointestinal vascular ectasias. Ann Intern Med 104:352, 1986
2. Dukes MNG: Meyler's Side Effects of Drugs: An Encyclopedia of Adverse Reactions and Interactions. 10th ed. Amsterdam, Excerpta Medica, 1984
3. Eknoyan G: Medical Procedures Manual. Chicago, Yearbook Medical Publishers, 1981
4. Jick H: Drugs—Remarkably nontoxic. N Engl J Med 291:824, 1974
5. Jick H: The discovery of drug-induced illness. N Engl J Med 296:481, 1977
6. Lewis M: Outpatient esophageal variceal sclerotherapy: Is it safe and cost-effective? Gastrointest Endosc 32:51, 1986
7. Maynard JC, Cruz C, et al: Blood pressure response to changes in serum ionized calcium during hemodialysis. Ann Intern Med 104:358, 1986
8. Naranjo CA, Busto U, et al: A method for estimating the probability of adverse drug reactions. Clin Pharmacol Ther 30:239, 1981
9. Shinn AF, Shewsbury RP: Evaluations of Drug Interactions, 3d ed. St. Louis, CV Mosby, 1985
10. Sznajder I, Zveibil FR, et al: Central vein catheterization: Failure and complication rates by three percutaneous approaches. Arch Intern Med 146:259, 1986

CHAPTER 17.2

Medical Assessment of the Preoperative Patient

Brent G. Petty

The management of patients with medical diseases during the perioperative period requires the coordinated efforts of the surgeon, the anesthesiologist, and the internist. The assessment of surgical benefit, operative risk, and intervention to reduce risk involves the combined perspectives of these physicians.

When a patient with a medical disease has a surgically treatable condition, the timing of the surgical procedure is a key question. In deciding whether to delay surgery the physician must weigh several opposing issues. For example, when the patient's medical condition is good and the potential benefits of surgery are great, surgery can proceed with confidence. When the patient's medical condition is poor and the benefits of surgery are minimal, surgery should not be performed. When the patient's medical condition is poor but the potential surgical benefits are great, surgery should be delayed if (1) it is possible to improve the patient's medical condition and thereby reduce risk and (2) the surgical condition will not substantially change during the postponement, which may be as short as a few days or as long as several months.

There are no absolute contraindications to surgery. Even the most serious underlying medical illness represents a relative contraindication if the patient's surgical condition is life threatening. On the other hand, when a decision to proceed with surgery is made, it should not be construed as a guarantee that no complications will occur. It means, rather, that the risks of surgery are understood, that the risks are minimized as much as possible within the time constraints imposed by the surgical condition, and that the potential benefits of surgery outweigh the risks.

The internist's usual role is (1) to assess surgical risk in light of the patient's medical disease(s), (2) to put these risks into perspective for the surgeon and anesthesiologist, (3) to take whatever measures will reduce the patient's surgical risk before the procedure, and (4) to assist in the postoperative care of the patient's known medical problems or new complications that may arise.

Patients undergoing anesthesia and surgical procedures of any sort have substantial associated physiologic stress. This stress particularly affects the cardiovascular and pulmonary systems. The evaluation of the patient who is to undergo surgery should be comprehensive, therefore, but with particular focus on these systems. The assessment follows the same general approach as any internal medicine evaluation. First, a careful history is performed, emphasizing cardiac and respiratory problems, significant past medical illnesses, and major recent changes in overall health. It is important to determine when the patient most recently underwent anesthesia and whether any problems were encountered at that time. Current medications must be reviewed, including self-administered medications such as aspirin, which can impair platelet function. If the patient is unlikely to resume oral consumption of food and medications soon after surgery, should each medication be eliminated during the perioperative period, or should it be administered by another route until oral intake resumes?

The history is followed by a thorough physical examination. Next, the physician should review both routine and special laboratory studies indicated by the nature of the patient's illnesses or intended surgery. Based on the data from these three sources—history, physical examination, and laboratory tests—the physician can make a final determination of the patient's medical condition, which can then be used to assess surgical risk.

CARDIOVASCULAR SYSTEM

Anesthesia has profound effects on the circulatory system. During intubation and the induction of anesthesia, there may be catecholamine release leading to arrhythmias and hypertension. General anesthetic agents, used during the remainder of an operation after induction, are negative inotropic agents and dilate the vascular bed. These effects lead to the hypotension that accompanies general anesthesia. Anesthetic agents are also arrhythmogenic themselves. Thus, the induction and then maintenance of general anesthesia have significant cardiovascular effects mediated in large measure by the sympathetic nervous system and always associated with the risk of arrhythmia. A large number of infarctions and arrhythmias occur up to several days after anesthesia, suggesting that autonomic instability may extend beyond the duration of the anesthetic effect of the agents used.

Spinal anesthesia is widely assumed to be safer than general anesthesia, but it may result in serious hypotension caused by sympathetic blockade. Overall, spinal anesthesia may present no less cardiovascular risk than general anesthesia.

The remainder of the chapter will be concerned with the problems that may be associated with general anesthesia.

Cardiovascular complications are the leading cause of perioperative mortality. In light of the physiologic effects mentioned earlier, it is not surprising that these complications take the form of ventricular arrhythmias, myocardial infarctions, and congestive

TABLE 17.2–1. RISK FACTORS FOR PERIOPERATIVE CARDIOVASCULAR COMPLICATIONS

Major	Moderate	Minimal or None
Myocardial infarction within 6 mo	Hypokalemia	Stable angina
Congestive heart failure	Hypoxemia	Diabetes
Age over 70 yr	Aortic stenosis	Mild or moderate hypertension
Rhythm other than sinus	Renal failure	Asymptomatic carotid bruits[a]
Reduced exercise capacity	Respiratory insufficiency	
	Elevated AST	
	Chronic liver disease	
	Bed-ridden patient	
	Emergency surgery	
	Thoracic or upper abdominal surgery	

[a]See Ref. 2.

heart failure, any of which may result in death. Studies comparing the preoperative medical conditions of patients undergoing surgery have identified several risk factors for the development of cardiovascular complications (Table 17.2–1).

The incidence of perioperative infarction in patients with a previous myocardial infarction appears to have decreased over the past 20 years. Whether this improvement in outcome is attributable to better case selection, better preparation, more extensive intraoperative monitoring, or improved postoperative care is hard to determine. Nevertheless, both the older and the more recent data reveal that if a patient has had an infarction, the risk of any surgery will be less if it is performed 6 months or more after the infarction.

The ability to do moderate exercise, long a clinical measure of surgical suitability, has recently been confirmed in a geriatric population to be an excellent identifier of patients with low cardiovascular risk.

Surgical risk can be reduced by eliminating or decreasing the severity of identified risk factors. Appropriate measures to reduce risk include the gradual correction of congestive heart failure and electrolyte abnormalities, the control of arrhythmias, and, if the surgical condition allows, delay of surgery pending recovery from myocardial infarction or acute renal failure. On the other hand, rapid reduction in blood pressure to the normal range in chronically hypertensive patients may make the patient's condition relatively unstable and increase the difficulty in managing reflex vasodilatation.

RESPIRATORY SYSTEM

Several factors related to surgery contribute to the development of pulmonary complications. General anesthesia of any sort decreases vital capacity. This effect is magnified in patients undergoing upper abdominal surgery as compared with patients having lower abdominal or extra-abdominal, nonthoracic surgery, because upper abdominal surgery induces diaphragmatic dysfunction, which leads to a restriction of lung expansion at the lung bases.

The use of postoperative analgesics and sedatives contributes to the hypoventilation caused by general anesthesia. Not only is there a reduction in the depth of breathing with general anesthesia, but also there is decreased clearing of secretions. Since smoking also reduces sputum clearing mechanisms, smokers are at substantially greater risk for pulmonary complications than nonsmokers. The combination of hypoventilation and reduced clearing of secretions can lead to atelectasis with ventilation-perfusion mismatches and consequent hypoxemia, respiratory failure, and pneumonia.

Various preoperative pulmonary function tests have been examined in an effort to determine which best predicts postoperative pulmonary complications.[4] It has been shown that patients with abnormal preoperative spirometry or arterial blood gas values who undergo upper abdominal surgery are at increased risk. Nevertheless, no studies have clearly delineated a minimum forced expiratory volume in 1 second (FEV_1) or forced vital capacity (FVC) below which the patient must not be subjected to surgery. Preoperative arterial blood gas studies may be beneficial, not only as a predictor of postoperative complications (Table 17.2–1), but also to establish a baseline for the patient.

Certain interventions will reduce perioperative pulmonary complications (Table 17.2–2). These interventions include treatment of acute exacerbations of bronchitis or other respiratory infections with antibiotics, incentive spirometry starting before surgery and continuing afterward, postoperative continuous positive airway pressure (CPAP) given at frequent intervals, psychologic preparation of the patient to anticipate the pain in the immediate postoperative period, elimination of smoking as long as 2 weeks before surgery, effective but not excessive narcotic analgesia to control pain, and early postoperative ambulation.

ENDOCRINE SYSTEM

There are several endocrine issues of importance for the surgical patient. The physiologic stresses involved with surgery lead to an increase in circulating cortisol, glucagon, growth hormone, and catecholamines. The increase in catecholamines puts increased work on the cardiovascular system, as mentioned earlier. Elevations of cortisol, glucagon, and growth hormone have a detrimental effect on glucose metabolism, leading to hyperglycemia, particularly in patients with diabetes.[7] In addition, the dose of oral hypoglycemic agents or insulin is routinely reduced immediately before surgery, so hyperglycemia in diabetics is further potentiated. Hyperglycemia may lead to several undesirable problems for the postoperative patient, such as dehydration, reduced wound healing rates, and reduced leukocyte function. While perioperative hypoglycemia should be scrupulously avoided, frequent blood

TABLE 17.2–2. EFFECTIVE INTERVENTIONS TO REDUCE PERIOPERATIVE PULMONARY COMPLICATIONS

- Early ambulation
- Smoking cessation 3–14 d before surgery
- Antibiotic treatment of acute bronchitis or pneumonia
- Incentive spirometry
- Intermittent administration of CPAP
- Effective but not excessive analgesia
- Psychologic preparation for postoperative pain

sugar determinations and appropriate supplemental short-acting insulin can be beneficial in bringing elevated blood sugar into control in the postoperative period, thereby reducing the risks incurred by hyperglycemia. Despite all of these potential problems, diabetes of itself, that is, not complicated by cardiac or renal disease, does not appear to substantially increase the morbidity or mortality of surgery with current management practices.

Hyperthyroidism represents a serious and well-recognized problem for surgery. It is in the setting of uncontrolled or undetected hyperthyroidism that general anesthesia can precipitate thyroid storm. If surgery cannot be delayed until the hyperthyroidism has been controlled with the usual medications, preoperative intravenous propranolol and iodides should be used to prevent thyroid storm. When surgery can be delayed, aggressive therapy will bring the overactive thyroid under control and then allow surgery to proceed without risk of thyroid storm.

Because of the importance of the thyroid gland in regulating metabolic activity, it seems reasonable to assume that hypothyroidism could cause serious problems in the perioperative period. Recent experience indicates that hypothyroidism does increase the incidence of intraoperative hypotension, perioperative heart failure, and postoperative ileus or constipation, but there was no increase in duration of hospitalization, arrhythmias, pulmonary complications, or mortality in hypothyroid patients compared to euthyroid patients.

A marked elevation in blood pressure at the induction of anesthesia can be a sign of pheochromocytoma, though the majority of patients in whom this blood pressure response occurs are not found to have pheochromocytoma. These blood pressure elevations probably relate to a sympathetic nervous system particularly sensitive to the normal perioperative increases in catecholamines or to an exuberant release of catecholamines by a normal adrenal medulla.

A common management problem is the patient receiving therapeutic doses of adrenocorticosteroids that suppress the pituitary-adrenal axis. This suppression prevents such patients from providing the usual glucocorticoid release in response to the stress of anesthesia, and without supplementation these patients can suffer acute adrenal insufficiency. It is important to give intravenous hydrocortisone to these patients, starting shortly before induction of anesthesia and continuing every 6 hours for 2 or 3 days and then returning to the usual steroid dose or providing the intravenous equivalent. The supplementation should be continued longer than 3 days only if postoperative complications arise, and it is not necessary to taper the dose back down to the preoperative dose.

THROMBOEMBOLISM

Thromboembolic disease can be a serious problem for patients during the postoperative period. The immobility associated with a recent surgical procedure makes this a potential complication for any patient, but some patients are at particular risk. Such patients include the obese; the elderly; those with malignancies; those who undergo prolonged surgical procedures; those likely to have prolonged postoperative immobility of the legs, for example, patients undergoing orthopedic surgery; and those with a previous history of thrombophlebitis.

Because of the frequency of thromboembolic disease in such patients, effective but also safe prophylactic measures are desirable. These measures include low-dose heparin therapy, platelet inhibitors, elastic stockings, and intermittent pneumatic leg compression systems[3] (see Chapter 6.25).

GASTROINTESTINAL SYSTEM AND NUTRITION

Gastrointestinal diseases in general do not constitute serious risks for surgery. Nevertheless, they become significant if they have resulted in malnutrition, anemia, or overall debility. For example, in patients who undergo elective surgery for Crohn disease, those with a serum albumin level below 3.1 g/dl have a higher incidence of complications. The incidence of surgical complications is also inversely correlated with serum total iron-binding capacity.[9] This relationship between serum albumin or total iron-binding capacity and the increased incidence of complications holds in other surgical populations as well.

In most cases when the surgery is elective, the reduced caloric intake during the perioperative period is of little consequence. In patients already suffering from poor nutrition, however, such as alcoholics or patients with cancer, further restriction of calories may aggravate their underlying condition. This may delay healing, impair host defense against infection, and prolong convalescence following surgery. Hyperalimentation may be advisable before and after surgery in some of these patients.

Liver disease, especially chronic liver disease, appears to be an important surgical risk factor. Both nutritional and hepatic status combine in Child's classification, which is a fairly reliable indicator of prognosis for patients who are to undergo portasystemic shunts. Patients with the combination of an albumin level less than 3 g/dl, serum bilirubin level over 3 mg/dl, severe ascites, encephalopathy, and generalized wasting have a 50 percent operative mortality for portasystemic shunts, whereas if none of these abnormalities is present the operative mortality is less than 1 percent. Chronic liver disease is also a risk factor for other surgical procedures. Acute viral hepatitis has been implicated as a serious perioperative risk factor, but the risk of general anesthesia in patients with alcoholic hepatitis is less clear.

Obesity increases perioperative morbidity in several ways. Obese patients are more prone to wound infections or dehiscence than nonobese patients. Obesity contributes to hypoventilation and consequent pulmonary complications in the postoperative period. Thrombophlebitis is more likely to occur in obese surgical patients. Severe obesity also presents mechanical problems for intubation and establishment of a patent airway.

HEMATOLOGIC SYSTEM

Because oxygen delivery to tissues depends in large part on the hemoglobin concentration in blood, anemia is undesirable in the surgical setting. Furthermore, if the patient's hematocrit is low before the operation, then there is less margin for safety with the blood loss that occurs as surgery proceeds. It is general practice to maintain or achieve a hematocrit of at least 30 percent before beginning surgery, except for minor surgical procedures or in patients who have chronic, compensated anemias and potential volume contraindications to preoperative transfusion, such as patients with chronic renal failure.

Severe thrombocytopenia may create problems with hemostasis. Platelet plug and clot formation are usually normal with platelet counts over $70,000/mm^3$, but at lower levels hemostasis becomes compromised, and at platelet counts of 20,000 or less there is the risk not only of increased bleeding at surgery but also of spontaneous bleeding unrelated to surgery. On the other hand, platelet function may be impaired despite a normal platelet count because of an underlying illness, for example, uremia, or exogenous factors, such as aspirin. Platelet function can be accurately assessed at the bedside by the bleeding time, but an abnormal bleeding time is not reliable in identifying patients who will develop excessive surgical blood loss.[1]

INFECTION

Postoperative infections are extremely common, and several factors contribute to their development. Normal skin integrity, an ex-

tremely important barrier to invasive pathogens, is lost at the site of surgical incision and this leads to a high incidence of perioperative wound infections. Invasive monitoring and support equipment also violate normal barriers to bacteria and act as portals of entry for infection. Anesthetic agents themselves have an adverse effect on neutrophils that makes them less active in killing bacterial invaders.[10] There is evidence that prolonged hyperglycemia in diabetics has similar and additional detrimental effects on the body's response to infection, and diabetics as a group are probably more likely than comparable nondiabetic patients to develop postoperative infections.

Antibiotic prophylaxis has been shown repeatedly to reduce the incidence of infections in elective abdominal, gynecologic, and other surgery. Antibiotics are especially effective in reducing wound infections and urinary tract infections. Surgical wound infections are more common after contaminated surgery, such as that for a ruptured abdominal viscus, than after noncontaminated procedures; in contaminated surgery, treatment with antibiotics should be started before surgery.

Antibiotic prophylaxis is also indicated in patients with valvular or congenital heart disease in whom the surgical procedure carries a likelihood of bacteremia. Transient bacteremia may be associated with such procedures as dental extraction, catheterization, and various types of endoscopy.

REFERENCES

1. Barber A, Green D, et al: The bleeding time as a preoperative screening test. Am J Med 78:761, 1985
2. Barnes RW, Nix ML, et al: Late outcome of untreated asymptomatic carotid disease following cardiovascular operations. J Vasc Surg 2:843, 1985
3. Fasting H, Andersen K, et al: Prevention of postoperative deep venous thrombosis: Low-dose heparin versus graded pressure stockings. Acta Chir Scand 151:245, 1985
4. Gass GD, Olsen GN: Preoperative pulmonary function testing to predict postoperative morbidity and mortality. Chest 89:127, 1986
5. Gerson MC, Hurst JM, et al: Cardiac prognosis in noncardiac geriatric surgery. Ann Intern Med 103:832, 1985
6. Goldman L: Cardiac risks and complications of noncardiac surgery. Ann Intern Med 98:504, 1983
7. Hjortrup A, Sorensen C, et al: Morbidity in diabetic and nondiabetic patients after abdominal surgery. Acta Chir Scand 151:445, 1985
8. Kammerer WS, Gross RJ (eds): Medical Consultation: Role of the Internist on Surgical, Obstetric, and Psychiatric Services. Baltimore, Williams & Wilkins, 1983
9. Lindor KD, Fleming CR, Ilstrup DM: Preoperative nutritional status and other factors that influence surgical outcome in patients with Crohn's disease. Mayo Clin Proc 60:393, 1985
10. Welch WD: Inhibition of neutrophil activity by volatile anesthetics. Anesthesiology 64:1, 1986

CHAPTER 17.3
Special Aspects of Care for the Aged

William R. Hazzard

Gerontology and geriatric medicine are related but distinguishable disciplines: gerontology is the study of the aging process, and geriatric medicine relates to the medical care of the aged. As such, geriatric medicine is a subdiscipline of geriatrics, which encompasses all of the relevant health sciences, such as the geriatric aspects of nursing, social work, nutrition, psychology, and dentistry, as well as still broader areas of law, the arts, economics, and political science as they apply to aging. Within geriatric medicine are relevant specialties, notably internal medicine, family medicine, psychiatry and behavioral science, physical medicine and rehabilitation, and the surgical subspecialties that are important in the care of the elderly, such as urology, ophthalmology, and orthopedics. Thus, geriatric medicine may seem nearly all-encompassing (excluding most obviously only obstetrics and pediatrics). Gerontology is still more comprehensive, as the study of aging is not confined to the elderly and, some would argue, is best studied in those who are not yet old so that the fundamental changes may be delineated before final common pathways of disease and death blur pathophysiologic mechanisms. Thus, ironically, much of the best gerontologic research has been performed by studying children suffering from disease processes, often monogenically determined, in which progression is accelerated, for example, coronary heart disease in children with homozygous familial hypercholesterolemia and various aspects of aging in those with progeria, a caricature of the aging process in multiple dimensions.

Understanding the aging process is an enormous challenge, as is caring for the needs of the elderly. Although such understanding would be enhanced ideally through the study of aging in the absence of disease (especially time-determined disease), it is becoming increasingly apparent that aging and physiologic dysfunction may be inseparable. Normal aging inevitably involves an increasing probability of dysfunction, to the point where the clinical threshold is passed and disease can be detected. Thus, the clinician will be left with the challenge of sorting out, in the individual patient, which aspects of the presentation are attributable to aging per se, to specific disease processes, or to the interaction between the two (Table 17.3–1).

THE DEMOGRAPHIC IMPERATIVE

When Osler wrote the first edition of this textbook, the distribution of the American population by age was triangular, that is, the largest proportion was in the youngest age group and the smallest proportion was in the oldest age group. This distribution is typical of developing nations even today, which are characterized by a high birth rate and a high infant mortality rate. However, as socioeconomic development has taken place—bringing improved nutrition, public and personal hygiene and sanitation, less crowded housing, and better education—a rectangularization of the population by age has occurred, a process that will be completed in the United States by about 2030, when the present bulge of young and middle-aged persons from the post–World War II baby boom has been fully assimilated. At that point the proportions under 20 and over 55 years of age will be equivalent, and the "dependency ratio" (those within in relation to those outside the work force) will be such that a substantial economic burden will rest on those who are employed to care for those at the ends of the age spectrum. The need for care will apply especially to those over 75 years (which one might arbitrarily, but conveniently, define as the lower age limit of geriatrics) and over 85 years, where the proportionate growth will be greatest.

The dimensions of this "demographic imperative" are yet greater than represented by the fourfold increase in the percentage over 65 years between 1900 and 2030. In absolute terms the el-

Organ System	Clinical Expression	Primary Age-related Change	Secondary Aging Factors (diseases and time-related, including iatrogenic, effects)
Skin	Wrinkling Purpura with minor trauma Susceptibility to pressure sores and slower healing Dry skin/pruritus Hair loss; hair graying	Atrophy (especially subcutaneous), decreased elasticity, increased vascular fragility/decreased extravascular tamponade; decreased sweating and sebaceous gland secretions; decreased hair and hair pigment	Sun exposure Chemical exposure Iatrogenic or self-induced changes in hair color or amount
Eyes	Presbyopia, decreased dark adaptation ?Cataract ?Glaucoma ?Macular degeneration	Altered lens elasticity Altered physiology of vitreous, retina	Diabetes ?Cataract ?Glaucoma ?Macular degeneration Drug effects (miosis)
Ears	Decreased hearing, especially high frequency Decreased sound discrimination Diminished position sense—"dizziness"	Diminished function of hair cells Diminished vestibular function	Traumatic hearing loss Ménière disease Drug toxicities "Benign positional vertigo"
Nose/mouth	Decreased taste and food enjoyment Dry mouth	Diminished olfaction Diminished number of taste buds and salivation	Zinc deficiency Periodontal disease Drug-induced dry mouth, salivation
Gastrointestinal tract	Dysphagia, gastric reflux Hypochlorhydria with bacterial overgrowth Constipation Retarded drug metabolism	Diminished esophageal motility and sphincter function Diminished acid, pepsin, trypsin Decreased intestinal motility Altered hepatic enzymes	Hiatus hernia Pernicious anemia Constipation secondary to low-residue diet Drug toxicities
Respiratory	Decreased vital capacity, FEV_1, maximum breathing capacity	Diminished lung elasticity Diminished respiratory musculature	Chronic obstructive pulmonary disease secondary to smoking, pollution
Cardiovascular	Diminished cardiac reserve (increased dependence on Frank-Starling mechanism), increased pulse pressure, increased vulnerability to hypotension and syncope Tissue ischemia	Diminished myocardial cell number, increased left ventricular and arterial resistance, diminished chronotropic response (especially maximum heart rate), diminished vascular baroreceptor (adrenergic) sensitivity ?Arteriosclerosis (without cholesterol accumulation)	Atherosclerosis-related ischemia, ventricular dysfunction, arrhythmias, CHF, hypertensive heart disease Atherosclerosis and related phenomena
Renal-urinary system	Decreased glomerular filtration rate, tubular reabsorption Obstructive uropathy Incontinence Vulnerability to urinary infection	Diminished number of nephrons; changes in basement membranes and tubular function Decreased bladder tone, decreased bladder capacity, diminished sphincter tone, prostatic hypertrophy (men), diminished pelvic muscular tone (women)	Drug-induced renal disease (aminoglycosides, nonsteroidal anti-inflammatory agents) Renal infections
Endocrine-metabolic system	Menopause (vasomotor symptoms, vaginal atrophy, osteoporosis in old age) Altered male libido, potency, sexual behavior Relative glucose intolerance Diminished thyroid reserve	Hypogonadism: Relatively abrupt (women) Relatively slow (men) Diminished insulin response to glucose load; decreased insulin sensitivity (increased adiposity) Diminished thyroid response	Accelerated osteoporosis with low calcium intake, smoking Increasing incidence of diabetes mellitus Autoimmune thyroiditis and hypothyroidism
Musculoskeletal	Decreased strength Increased vulnerability to fracture Joint stiffness and inflammation	Decreased muscle fiber and diameter Diminished bone mineral and osteoid Increased stiffness of tendons, connective tissue Diminished joint cartilage	Disuse atrophy (sedentary life-style) Diet, alcohol-, tobacco-, drug-related osteoporosis Drug-induced osteoarthritis (fluoride)
Neural regulation	Hypothermia Hyperthermia Dehydration	Diminished tolerance to temperature variation Diminished thirst and drinking	Hypothermia from hypothyroidism Hyperosmolar, nonketotic diabetes mellitus

(continued)

TABLE 17.3–1. PRIMARY VERSUS SECONDARY AGING: EXAMPLES OF AGE- AND TIME-RELATED DISEASE EFFECTS (Continued)

Organ System	Clinical Expression	Primary Age-related Change	Secondary Aging Factors (diseases and time-related, including iatrogenic, effects)
Neural regulation (Cont.)	Postural hypotension, "dizziness," syncope, falls	Diminished postural reflexes and autonomic regulation	Drug-induced dehydration; autonomic insensitivity
	Increased incidence of Alzheimer disease	Neuronal loss, nucleus basalis, decreased cholinergic neurotransmitters and choline acetyltransferase activity	Drug-induced cognitive dysfunction Delirium
	Slowness of movement	Diminished basal ganglia function	Drug-induced parkinsonism
	Parkinson disease	Diminished dorsal column function	Drug-induced ataxia
	Retarded positional correction, falls		Alcohol toxicity
	Altered sleep patterns		Alzheimer disease
			Parkinson disease
Immune system	Increased susceptibility to infections, malignancies	Diminished cellular immunity (decreased helper cells)	Nutritional deficiency, autoimmune diseases (thyroidosis), pernicious anemia
	Impaired response to immunization	Diminished primary antibody response	
	Increased autoantibodies	Increased abnormal immunoglobulin and autoimmunity	

From Burton JR, Hazzard WR: Geriatric medicine: Special considerations. In Barker LR, Burton JR, Zieve PD (eds): Principles of Ambulatory Medicine, 2d ed. Baltimore, Williams & Wilkins, 1986, p 80.

derly will have grown even more: 3 million Americans over 65 years in 1900 to 46 million in 2030. Furthermore, the progressive accumulation of "life's insults" parallels aging and, hence, increases the probability of disease and dysfunction. As a consequence, the elderly consume health-care resources at a rate far greater than their younger counterparts ($3593 per capita in 1983, nearly four times the figure for those under 65 years). By far the largest proportion of that support has been of governmental origin (notably Medicare for hospital and ambulatory care and Medicaid for long-term institutional care): the specter of an ever-increasing elderly population now threatens to bankrupt the Social Security system and is the subject of considerable anxiety within the health-care industry.

America has begun to recognize this imperative (long since addressed by societies more mature than ours, e.g., Sweden and the United Kingdom), and interest has grown rapidly in geriatrics, including geriatric medicine. An approach selected by other societies has been the definition of "geriatric medicine" as a distinct specialty, with separate facilities and separate academic departments. However, an alternative mode appropriate to the American health-care system may be the retention of geriatric medicine in the mainstream, eschewing perhaps the easier course of separation in favor of an integrated approach that capitalizes on the strengths of the system as it has evolved in the United States.

It seems appropriate to distribute gerontologic and geriatric content liberally throughout the undergraduate and postgraduate medical curriculum as well as throughout general medical textbooks, the approach chosen for this text. Hence this chapter will constitute but an overview of what might otherwise prove redundant and daunting. Here we shall confine the discussion to general principles in the care of elderly patients plus introductions to three areas of special concern in geriatric medicine not addressed in depth elsewhere in this text: urinary incontinence, nutritional disorders, and geriatric pharmacology.

CARDINAL FEATURES OF GERIATRIC MEDICAL PRACTICE

As the proportion of aged persons in the population increases, physicians must adapt their practice to the characteristics and needs of the elderly patient. This translates into certain behaviors and sensitivities:

1. The elderly patient is a survivor with proven resilience and resistance to the diseases that limit survival. For example,

the overweight elderly woman has proven her ability to live with her obesity (she may even have derived some benefit, as osteoporosis is uncommon among the obese). Prescription of a weight-losing diet is rarely indicated in the elderly (and weight loss is an ominous sign even among the obese). The elderly person not under a physician's care is likely to be the most fit; conversely, those who consult a physician, even if never having previously done so, are likely to be ill. In fact, elderly persons often put off seeing a physician until disease is far advanced, either because they have feared seeking help or have attributed dysfunction to "just being old," an unfortunate ageist attitude highly prevalent among today's elderly and often reinforced by insensitive physicians.

2. The elderly patient is highly vulnerable to collapse of homeostasis by virtue of multiple potential or real limitations; it is the multiplicity of such frailties and their synergism that account for the exponential rise in death rate with age, rather than any single physiologic parameter. The threats to this tenuous homeostasis include forces other than disease or age-related decrements: social disruption, death of a spouse, change of residence, economic deprivation, and nutritional deficiencies are just a few possible triggers for homeostatic collapse. Hospitalization per se is one such trigger and, hence, is not to be entered into lightly. The geriatrician seeks to prevent phenomena that may initiate a cascade of complications and death or decreased function. Preventive measures must have benefit in the near term, such as immunization against influenza or environmental alterations that may prevent a fall.

3. Given the time-limited definition of potential benefit and the increased probability of adverse reaction to any intervention, including diagnostic, therapeutic, and social, the therapeutic ratio narrows progressively with age, frequently dipping below unity. The rationale for "doing nothing," therefore, is often clear (the physician who so chooses is doing far from nothing but rather electing the wisest option from experience and judgment). In such circumstances (and even when the physician is actively intervening), attention is focused on patient comfort and "supporting the supporters," who must continue to help the patient to cope with pain, discomfort, and dysfunction. Although more time and personal involvement are involved in geriatric practice, these investments can yield great satisfaction in the gratitude of elderly patients and their families.

4. The geriatrician thinks multidimensionally, especially on the dimension of time in the diagnostic and therapeutic process. These dimensions include not only the traditional physical and psychologic but also and especially the social, all adding up to the central feature of geriatric evaluation: functional assessment.

The patient's ability to function is often more important than the specific disease or diseases present. The blind patient with diabetes may function perfectly well in the home until her husband, who has been drawing up the insulin in the syringe, dies and she is left alone. The man with Alzheimer disease may function adequately in his home until he develops incontinence or a deranged sleep pattern. The patient with advanced osteoarthritis may function well until developing renal failure from a nonsteroidal anti-inflammatory drug.

A number of assessment instruments have been developed to aid the physician or paraprofessional in functional assessment.[5,7] Although none is perfect, all help with diagnosis and management. One such instrument, emphasizing activities of daily living, is listed in Table 17.3–2.

5. The geriatrician assesses the disabilities peculiar to each elderly patient and adapts the management accordingly. This frequently requires changes in the interview and physical examination. The examining room light may be adjusted to shine brightly on the physician (not from behind or in the patient's eyes) to aid in visual communication. Speaking louder and especially more slowly and distinctly (and with amplification where appropriate) helps overcome deafness. The interview may have to proceed more slowly and possibly over multiple visits to adjust for the patient's limited endurance. The physical examination often takes longer and may similarly have to take place in parts at multiple visits. Information from other observers, especially family members and other care providers, is often critical (with appropriate adjustments for their biases). This requirement for outside information and verification has sometimes led the physician to short-circuit the patient, an unfortunate by-product of a hurried approach and the common lack of feedback from the patient. This must be consciously avoided; at the same time, since the caregivers themselves are frequently fatigued or frustrated, they too require support and patience, an effort that is amply rewarded by the maintenance of the patient in the home environment.

6. Given the multidimensional nature of geriatric dysfunction, therapy must be likewise multidimensional. This often translates into treatment variously involving nursing; social work; pharmacy; physical, occupational, and recreational therapy; nutrition; and a host of other disciplines (and the family or other supporters as well). The geriatrician, therefore, must be a skillful leader, formulating an appropriate diagnostic and therapeutic regimen (often with input from these disciplines) and supervising its implementation over time as required both legally and by the expectations of the patient and family. A critical attribute for success in this leadership is delegation to other members of the health-care team those functions appropriate to their disciplines and individual skills.

7. The effective geriatrician serves as an advocate for the elderly patient. This takes the form of a commitment over time to the patient's welfare. It may require bridging gaps in the continuity of care between levels, such as hospital, office, clinic, specialists' offices, home, and long-term care facility, gaps to which the elderly are especially vulnerable. It may mean imposing a judgment after consultation with specialists that "nothing further should be done" (after discussion with the patient and family). It may mean acceptance of the patient's death as preferable to prolonging the dying process by heroic interventions that may be inhumane; this requires acceptance of that death as something other than defeat; or it may mean indomitable efforts against the bureaucracy to see to the patient's needs for housing, health care, or economic assistance. All this must be delivered without an attitude of condescending paternalism or fatalism . . . a tall order for the physician involved.

It is apparent, then, that good geriatric medicine is good general medicine. An increment of about 10 percent in the knowledge and skills of the general internist may be required for the practice of geriatric medicine (and certain subspecialty skills relevant primarily to younger patients may be deducted). Redressing these deficiencies in knowledge and skills seems to be a relatively minor obstacle to facing the challenge posed by the "demographic imperative." Rather, the major impediment is likely to be resolving attitudinal problems. The requisite attitudes have been broadly described within this chapter, in the introductory chapters, and widely throughout this textbook. They are best summarized, however, in the words of Francis Peabody, "The secret of the care of the patient is in caring for the patient." Nowhere is this more applicable than in geriatric medicine.

NUTRITION AND NUTRITIONAL ASSESSMENT IN THE ELDERLY

Old age is characterized by the merging of physiologic and pathologic decline in certain final common pathways of disease and disability. Malnutrition is one such common pathway (depression is another).

Although much has been proclaimed regarding the prevalence, severity, and causes of malnutrition in old age, few careful studies have been reported. A fundamental cause of this uncertainty is the lack of firm information regarding nutritional requirements in the elderly; indeed, current recommended daily allow-

---

TABLE 17.3–2. AREAS AND LEVELS OF ASSESSMENT IN THE KATZ INDEX OF INDEPENDENCE IN ACTIVITIES OF DAILY LIVING

Bathing
- Receives no assistance
- Receives assistance in bathing only one part
- Receives assistance in bathing more than one part

Dressing
- Gets clothes and dresses without assistance
- Needs assistance in tying shoes only
- Needs assistance greater than above or stays undressed

Toileting
- Needs no assistance
- Needs assistance only in getting to toilet room or in cleaning self
- Does not go to toilet room

Transferring
- Needs no assistance from another person
- Needs assistance with transferring
- Does not get out of bed

Continence
- Continent
- Occasional accident
- Needs supervision, uses catheter, or is incontinent

Feeding
- Needs no assistance
- Needs assistance in cutting meat or buttering bread
- Needs more assistance or is tube or intravenously fed

From Burton JR, Hazzard WR: Geriatric medicine: Special considerations. In Barker LR, Burton JR, Zieve PD (eds): Principles of Ambulatory Medicine, 2d ed. Baltimore, Williams & Wilkins, 1986, p 83.

ances (RDAs) for macronutrients and micronutrients are constant for all adults above 50 years of age. Given the gradual decline in food intake with aging (attributable principally to decreased caloric expenditure and appropriate compensatory reduction in caloric intake), a progressive increase in the prevalence of inadequate intake of calories, vitamins, and minerals seems inevitable, but this is more apparent than real.

More threatening to homeostasis are the very real impediments to adequate nutrition that are prevalent in the elderly (see Table 17.3–1): diminished smell and taste, decreased salivation, poor dentition, difficulties with swallowing, impairment of esophageal sphincter function, decreased gastric secretion of acid and pepsin, diminished motility of small and large intestine, and, commonly, biliary tract dysfunction. Perhaps most threatening is the loss of social cues to consumption of an adequate diet: eating and living alone, the norm among widows, invites consumption of a lackluster, unbalanced diet. The prevalence of marginal nutrition, however defined, undoubtedly rises in old age, especially among the frail elderly and those living alone.

Of greater importance is the common superimposition of age-related diseases in the marginally nourished older patient. Anorexia (and weight loss) are cardinal manifestations of disease at any age; nowhere is this more evident than among the elderly. Curiously, the mechanism of this fundamental, common, ominous symptom is only beginning to be understood. Infection; malignancy (not just of the gastrointestinal tract); end-stage cardiac, pulmonary, and renal disease; and even psychiatric disease (especially depression) are all characterized by anorexia and weight loss. Further, such weight loss renders the patient more vulnerable to complications of infection (through immunocompromise) and delayed wound healing. Finally, iatrogenic anorexia is common: many drugs depress appetite (digitalis), others impair intake (antidepressants with anticholinergic side effects), and a therapeutic diet may invite malnutrition through tastelessness (salt restriction). Such malnutrition, commonly manifested by loss of both lean and adipose mass, has often already become far advanced by the time the patient seeks the advice of a physician. Weight loss greater than 10 percent is common and defines malnutrition. A decrease in subcutaneous skinfold thickness and arm circumference accompanies such losses. Review of dietary intake by a nutritionist will confirm the suspicion of malnutrition and may identify selective deficiencies in intake. Biochemical measures of malnutrition include decreased serum albumin, ferritin, and retinol-binding protein levels; a lymphocyte count less than 1500 is also suggestive. Low levels of folate and vitamin B_{12} are also common. However, these costly laboratory analyses add little to measurement of weight and, especially, documentation of weight loss in the diagnosis and management of malnutrition in elderly patients.

Nutritional therapy is commonly attempted in the elderly; often it is unsuccessful, and at times it prolongs the dying process in the terminally ill. Most frequently vitamin and mineral supplements are taken, usually without prescription. Most rational is the supplementation of the diet of women with calcium (currently recommended at 1500 mg/day), though maximum effectiveness would be achieved with the institution of this practice long before old age. The addition of liquid or semisolid, calorie-rich supplements may be helpful and at times clearly essential. This is most commonly employed in the patient requiring major surgery or chemotherapy, having an impediment to adequate intake, having lost muscle mass sufficient to impair mobilization, or with pressure sores. Many such liquid formulations are available; none is clearly superior to any other, providing that the intake of protein and calories is sufficient to permit reconstitution of lost tissue in addition to compensating for diminished intake secondary to the primary disease process.

The complications and cost of such artificial alimentation are substantial: long-term intravenous hyperalimentation is not appropriate for the elderly with devastating or progressive illness, and problems with venous access and infections commonly militate against such usage; enteral alimentation with nasogastric tubes invites aspiration and esophageal erosion. Early gastrostomy should, therefore, be considered among those with more than a short-term need for enteral alimentation.

PHARMACOLOGIC ISSUES IN THE ELDERLY

Iatrogenic illness is extraordinarily prevalent in the elderly, and pharmacologic misadventures contribute to this problem. Although aspects of aging physiology and anatomy per se contribute to the vulnerability of the aged to drug-induced illness (Table 17.3–3), noth-

TABLE 17.3–3. SUMMARY OF FACTORS AFFECTING DRUG DISPOSTION IN THE GERIATRIC PATIENT

Pharmacokinetic Parameter	Age-related Physiologic Changes	Pathologic Conditions
Absorption	Increased gastric pH Decreased absorptive surface Decreased splanchnic blood flow Decreased gastrointestinal motility	Achlorhydria Diarrhea Gastrectomy Malabsorption syndromes Pancreatitis
Distribution	Decreased cardiac output Decreased total body water Decreased lean body mass Decreased serum albumin Increased body fat	Congestive heart failure Dehydration Edema or ascites Hepatic failure Malnutrition Renal failure
Metabolism	Decreased hepatic mass Decreased enzyme activity Decreased hepatic blood flow	Congestive heart failure Fever Hepatic insufficiency Malignancy Malnutrition Thyroid disease Viral infection or immunization
Excretion	Decreased renal blood flow Decreased glomerular filtration rate Decreased tubular secretion	Hypovolemia Renal insufficiency

From Vestel RE: Clinical pharmacology. In Andres R, Bierman EL, Hazzard WR (eds): Principles of Geriatric Medicine. New York, McGraw-Hill, 1984, p 428.

TABLE 17.3–4. EXAMPLES OF DRUGS USUALLY GIVEN IN REDUCED DOSAGE IN THE ELDERLY[a]

Drug (or drug class)	Possible Consequences of Standard Dosage Regimen
Aminoglycosides	Ototoxicity and nephrotoxicity
Benzodiazepines	Unwanted CNS depression (more common with larger doses)
Carbamazepine	Drowsiness or ataxia possible
Chlormethiazole	Confusion possible with larger doses
Digoxin	Digitalis toxicity
Haloperidol	Extrapyramidal reactions
Levodopa	Hypotension common
Meperidine	Respiratory depression
Metoclopramide	Confusion common
Thioridazine	Confusion common
Thyroxine	Myocardial infarction
Vitamin D	Renal toxicity

[a]The drugs listed are examples only; this is not intended to be an exhaustive list.
From Vestel RE: Clinical pharmacology. In Andres R, Bierman EL, Hazzard WR (eds): Principles of Geriatric Medicine. New York, McGraw-Hill, 1984, p 439.

TABLE 17.3–5. PRINCIPLES OF GERIATRIC PRESCRIBING

1. *Evaluate the need for drug therapy.*
   a. Not all diseases afflicting the elderly require drug treatment.
   b. Avoid drugs if possible, but do not withhold because of age drugs that might enhance the quality of life.
   c. Strive for a diagnosis before treatment.
2. *Take a careful history of habits and drug use.*
   a. Patients often seek advice and receive prescriptions from several physicians.
   b. Knowledge of existing therapy, both prescribed and nonprescribed, helps one anticipate potential drug interactions.
   c. Smoking, alcohol, and caffeine may affect drug response.
3. *Know the pharmacology of drug prescribed.*
   a. Use a few drugs well, rather than many drugs poorly.
   b. Awareness of age-related alterations in drug disposition and drug response is helpful.
4. *In general, use smaller doses in the elderly.*
   a. Often the standard dose will be too large for the elderly patient.
   b. Although the effect of age on hepatic drug metabolism is less predictable, renal excretion of drugs and their active metabolites tends to decline.
   c. The elderly are particularly sensitive to drugs affecting central nervous system function.
5. *Titrate drug dosage with patient response.*
   a. Establish reasonable therapeutic end points.
   b. Adjust dosage until end points are reached or unwanted side effects prevent further increases.
   c. Use an adequate dose for the patient. This is particularly important in the treatment of pain associated with malignancy.
   d. Sometimes combination therapy is appropriate and effective.
6. *Simplify the therapeutic regimen and encourage compliance.*
   a. Try to avoid intermittent schedules. Once- or twice-daily dosage is preferred.
   b. Select a dosage form appropriate for the patient.
   c. Label drug containers clearly. When appropriate, specify standard containers.
   d. Give careful instructions to both patient and a relative or friend. Explain why the drug is being prescribed.
   e. Suggest the use of a medication calendar or diary.
   f. Encourage the return or destruction of old medications.

From Vestel RE: Clinical pharmacology. In Andres R, Bierman EL, Hazzard WR (eds): Principles of Geriatric Medicine. New York, McGraw-Hill, 1984, p 434.

ing is so important as the obvious: the elderly have multiple illnesses, begetting multiple drugs, begetting multiple (and commonly synergistic) adverse drug reactions.

Up to 90 percent of the ambulatory elderly take at least one medication, and the majority take two or more. Most commonly prescribed are cardiovascular drugs, antihypertensives, analgesics, anti-inflammatory agents, and psychotropic drugs. Over-the-counter drugs account for over 40 percent, a figure likely to rise as the list of prescription-free drugs increases, for example, nonsteroidal anti-inflammatory drugs. Those in long-term care facilities receive even more drugs, notably psychotropics (up to 25 percent) for the control of behavioral problems. Adverse drug reactions occur in 6 to 40 percent and are a leading cause of hospitalization. Risk factors to such reactions, in addition to advanced age and multiple drug regimens, are small body size, female sex, hepatic or renal insufficiency (reflecting problems in drug elimination), and previous drug reactions.

Problems in compliance with drug regimens (including overcompliance) also require consideration in the elderly: 25 to 50 percent fail to take their medications as prescribed, and multiple errors are common (especially among those at greatest risk, those above 75 years).

The clinician, thus, is commonly faced with a dilemma in treating the elderly patient: the therapeutic index for many drugs becomes increasingly small, yet the need for relief may be acute and unrelenting. Careful attention should be paid to drug choice and dosage (Table 17.3–4) and the principles of geriatric drug prescribing (Table 17.3–5). Most important, however, is the continual evaluation and reevaluation of the patient during treatment, the longitudinal application of geriatric assessment, a keystone of the art of geriatric medicine.

URINARY INCONTINENCE

Urinary incontinence is the repetitive involuntary (accidental) loss of urine from the bladder. It may be acute or chronic and may be mild or severe, ranging from one or two accidents to several hundred accidents per week. The volume of the urine may be small (dampness or spotting) or large (puddles or soaked clothing).

Urinary incontinence is a common problem of the elderly, affecting 10 to 15 percent of those living independently in the community. The prevalence in acute-care hospitals is nearly 20 percent in elderly patients. In nursing homes the prevalence of urinary incontinence is 50 percent, and frequently it is stated as one of the reasons precipitating admission. Strikingly, nearly 85 percent of patients with urinary incontinence have not been recognized as having this problem by their physicians. Urinary incontinence is accepted by many elderly as one of the "curses of aging," and they do not report it; however, physicians often do not inquire about this problem when taking a patient's history.

Urinary incontinence may lead to serious physical complications, such as skin maceration, urinary tract infections, or sepsis; just as important, however, are the profound psychologic and sociologic complications of social isolation and embarrassment.

PHYSIOLOGY OF MICTURITION

The urinary bladder is part of a spinal reflex arc connected to the spinal cord at the S2 to S4 level by efferent and afferent nerves. This reflex loop is modified by higher centers of the brain for augmentation or inhibition. An urge to void is normally sensed when

the bladder volume approaches 100 to 150 ml of urine. These higher centers permit the urge to void to be temporarily suppressed until a socially acceptable location to void can be located. In addition to these reflex loops, there are efferent and afferent connections to the tissues of the sphincters and perineal area that aid in the voiding process and in the inhibition and augmentation of micturition. Some of the neuroreceptors of these loops are adrenergic and others are cholinergic.

CLASSIFICATION OF URINARY INCONTINENCE

Urinary incontinence may be classified into two major groups: disorders of storage and disorders of emptying.

Disorders of Storage
Urge Incontinence. Urge incontinence is also called the uninhibited urinary bladder or detrusor hyperreflexia. In this condition the patient is unable to suppress the sensation of bladder fullness. When a certain urinary volume is achieved, therefore, voiding occurs often before the patient can get to a toilet. Urge incontinence is a dominant pattern in 50 to 60 percent of the elderly with urinary incontinence. It occurs because of diseases in the nervous system affecting cognitive function, in the brain stem, or in the spinal cord. Dementing illnesses or cerebrovascular events are two of the most common causes of this problem.

Reflex Incontinence. Reflex incontinence is caused by abnormal reflex activity in the spinal cord in the absence of sensation associated with the desire to void (urge). This problem develops because suprasacral spinal cord lesions have interrupted the spinal reflex center from high centers. Reflex incontinence is not common in the elderly; however, in patients with very severe cognitive impairment, urge incontinence may mimic reflex incontinence because the urge is not perceived.

Stress Incontinence. Stress incontinence is also called sphincter insufficiency. This problem occurs when there is inadequate sphincter resistance to an increase in abdominal muscular tone (stress), which is transmitted directly to the urinary bladder. This problem is very common in postpartum and postmenopausal women, but it also occurs in men who have had prostate surgery. Stress incontinence is the most common form of urinary incontinence in young women and occurs as the only incontinent pattern in 25 to 30 percent of elderly women. Often, it occurs in combination with urge incontinence in elderly women.

Disorders of Emptying
Overflow Incontinence. Overflow incontinence occurs when there is inadequate detrusor muscle function and/or inadequate sensory perception within the bladder wall or if there is a significant bladder outlet obstruction. The result is overdistension of the urinary bladder and eventually spontaneous detrusor contractions at a very high bladder volume. This disorder occurs commonly in men because of prostatic hypertrophy, but in both men and women overflow incontinence may also occur because of autonomic neuropathy, such as in diabetics.

Functional Incontinence. Functional incontinence occurs when continence is lost because of functional impairment such as decreased mobility or an increase in urinary volume from, for example, diuretics. An altered environment, such as with hospitalization, commonly precipitates this pattern of incontinence.

ACUTE CAUSES OF URINARY INCONTINENCE

When a patient has urinary incontinence, it is first important for the physician to perform an evaluation for acute or reversible causes. A useful mnemonic developed by Ouslander to help recall these causes is the word DRIP (Table 17.3–6).

TABLE 17.3–6. DRIP—MNEMONIC FOR ACUTE OR TRANSIENT CAUSES OF URINARY INCONTINENCE

D	Delirium
R	Restricted mobility; acute urinary retention
I	Infection of the urinary tract, vagina, or perineal area; impaction of feces
P	Pharmaceuticals; polyuria

Adapted from Kane RL, Ouslander JG, Abrass IB: Essentials of Clinical Geriatrics. New York, McGraw-Hill, 1984, p 116.

The most common reversible causes of urinary incontinence are changes in mental state for any reason, drug effects (especially diuretics, sedatives, neuroleptics, and anticholinergics), urinary tract infection, fecal impaction, and, in women, atrophic vaginitis. These problems should be considered routinely when initially evaluating a patient for urinary incontinence. In the instance of urinary tract infections, however, the treatment of the infection will eradicate the urinary incontinence in only an occasional patient, as in most instances the bacteriuria is an accompaniment of the incontinence rather than the cause of it.

EVALUATION OF PATIENTS WITH ESTABLISHED INCONTINENCE

History
Once reversible causes of urinary incontinence have been ruled out, it is important to establish the pattern of urinary incontinence by taking a careful history. Stress incontinence is characterized by episodes of small urine loss or of dribbling that occurs in association with increases in abdominal muscular tone (as with carrying groceries or coughing). Patients with urge incontinence have episodes of large volume losses occurring when the patient has an urge to void and is not able to reach a toilet in time. The physician should have a patient record his or her accidents. These records will serve not only as a guide to the diagnosis of the problem but also as a record of baseline function, thus helping the physician to judge the results of any therapeutic intervention. The physician may easily devise a daily record form and give a supply to the patient. Several examples the physician could use as a guideline for these records are available.[9]

In obtaining the history the physician should look for symptoms that suggest a cause of overflow incontinence (symptoms of prostatism or diabetes).

Physical Examination
The examination should include certain observations that will help in the classification of the incontinence. The lower abdomen should be carefully palpated for the presence of a distended urinary bladder. A palpable bladder strongly suggests overflow incontinence; the absence of a palpable bladder, however, does not rule out urinary obstruction. The anal sphincter tone and the sensation of the perineal area should be part of the neurologic examination in order to assess neurologic function associated with micturition. Also, in men, the bulbocavernosus reflex (contraction of the bulbus portion of the urethra caused by tapping the penis near the scrotum) should be tested.

A rectal examination is necessary to evaluate the possibility of fecal impaction and, in men, to assess the possibility of prostatic cancer, enlargement, or infection. In women a pelvic examination is necessary to evaluate for atrophic vaginitis, outlet relaxation, or related problems. During the pelvic examination a Bonney test may be performed: The patient while in the lithotomy position should cough with a full bladder. If stress incontinence is present, a small urine leak may result; if following the leak the incontinence can be prevented by lifting the urethra and the base of the bladder by two examining fingers, the diagnosis of stress incontinence is

established. Generally those patients who have a positive Bonney test corrected by the described maneuver have an excellent outcome after surgery if stress incontinence is the only mechanism involved.

Finally, a postvoid straight sterile catheterization of the urinary bladder should be accomplished. If the urinary volume is greater than 100 to 200 ml, overflow incontinence may be present. This is especially of concern when the residual volume is quite large (over 250 ml). It is important that this possiblity be diagnosed, because patients with overflow incontinence should be referred to a urologist for evaluation. Depending on the cause of the patient's condition, treatment may be surgical, by intermittent catheterization, or by drugs designed to increase detrusor activity (bethanechol).

The urine obtained from the straight catheterization should be analyzed to rule out infection or other abnormalities such as hematuria that might suggest another bladder problem, for example, a tumor.

Urodynamic Evaluation

Patients referred to a urologist, a continence clinic, or a geriatrician with a special interest in urinary incontinence may have urodynamic studies to classify more precisely the voiding disorder. Although this procedure is useful whenever there is a question of overflow incontinence and in research protocols, it is not yet of proven efficacy in all elderly patients with urinary incontinence. Further, not only are there insufficient resources to evaluate the many elderly patients with urinary incontinence in this manner, but also there are very many fragile elderly patients who are not candidates for any invasive evaluation. In most elderly patients, therefore, a careful history and physical examination are sufficient to establish a working diagnosis for urinary incontinence.

REFERRAL

In the frail elderly patient referral is often not possible because of the patient's condition or resistance to consultation; however, operations that are less stressful to the patient (e.g., endoscopic suspension of the bladder neck) are available. Further, 30 to 40 percent of elderly incontinent patients may have a mixed pattern (typically, in women, urge and stress), and correction of the stress component will not cure the problem.

TREATMENT

The physician must recognize that small therapeutic gains may be extremely important to the elderly patient and his family. Although cure is not usually accomplished, even a decrease in incontinent episodes is a welcome result that will improve the patient's sense of well-being and social confidence.

The physician should recognize that urinary incontinence in the elderly is usually a remediable condition, and perhaps as many as 60 to 70 percent of those with incontinence may be cured or significantly improved.

When filled in by the patient, the bladder record may provide an important clue to the treatment of the incontinence. The physician, on review of the record, might advise avoiding situations associated with accidents, such as carrying groceries without first emptying the bladder.

With patients who are felt to have stress incontinence, the physician can help greatly by explaining the mechanism of the incontinence to them. This will help the patients avoid increasing abdominal musculature tone without simultaneously contracting the external sphincters (see Kegel exercises, below).

If the incontinence is associated with polyuria, then fluid intake may be modified such that minimal fluids are taken 4 to 6 hours before the patient will be without easy access to a toilet.

The patient may be advised to begin a program in bladder retraining whereby he is asked to void at timed intervals, such as every 2 hours; as continence improves, these intervals can be slowly lengthened by an hour every 2 to 3 weeks until an acceptable voiding pattern occurs.

Kegel exercises to strengthen the external sphincter and perineal musculature may also be helpful in some women. When doing the pelvic examination, the physician places two fingers in the vagina and separates them as much as possible. The patient at that time is asked to squeeze her perineal muscles around the fingers. The physician will sense when the musculature has been properly contracted and should instruct the patient to practice repeatedly contracting the muscles in this group. Once the patient has learned how to contract this muscle group, she may practice many times a day, thereby strengthening the sphincter and perineal muscles.

Patients with mobility problems may have incontinence improved by moving the toilet, obtaining a lift chair, or acquiring a portable toilet. All these techniques increase accessibility to a toilet. Regardless of the mechanism of incontinence, sensitivity and concern by the physician to the enormity of the problem will create trust and understanding for which the patient and the family will be grateful. The problem then can be discussed, and frequently the physician will be able to make simple, commonsense suggestions. Currently, however, physicians often ignore the problem of urinary incontinence in the elderly, and this causes further discouragement and isolation for the patient.

Garments and external catheters have been improved dramatically in recent years and may be available to patients who do not respond to other forms of therapy.

Indwelling urinary catheters generally have no place in the treatment of urinary incontinence, except in instances where there is severe secondary skin maceration or a pressure sore has developed. In those instances the catheter should be used temporarily until those conditions have improved. Intermittent self-catheterization is a useful technique for a patient with an atonic bladder and overflow incontinence; however, the patient or caretaker must be able and willing to perform the procedure several times each day.

Preliminary results of biofeedback studies indicate considerable promise in treating incontinence in nondemented elderly patients, but referral centers for this treatment are not yet widely available.

Experimental surgical techniques creating artificial urinary sphincters and electric stimulators are under investigation, and as they improve, these may become available on a more widespread basis. Currently, however, they are considered investigational.

DRUG THERAPY

In the treatment of urinary incontinence only three drugs have been shown by controlled trials in the elderly to have significant efficacy: estrogen, imipramine, and oxybutynin.

Estrogen therapy for female patients with atrophic vaginitis has been beneficial in improving continence. At first it probably is simplest for the physician to prescribe topical estrogen cream, such as conjugated equine estrogen (Premarin) vaginal cream, or to administer oral Premarin, 0.625 mg each day. A 1-month trial should be adequate: If there is significant improvement, the physician should discuss with the patient the possibility of long-term estrogen therapy. It must be recognized that even topical estrogen therapy has a systemic effect, and the physician must be sensitive to the complication of uterine cancer from continuous progestin-unopposed estrogen therapy when given in relatively high doses for prolonged periods. In general, when the patient is to be treated with estrogen for a long time, it is best to prescribe the lowest dose possible, combining it with a progestin in the latter several days of a cycle. Such a regimen minimizes or eliminates the uterine cancer risk.

Imipramine (Tofranil), has been effective in some elderly patients with stress or urge incontinence. It is the only antidepressant carefully studied for this effect. The drug probably works by increasing bladder capacity and increasing sphincter tone. A dose of 25 mg orally is given every night, then increased every third night

to a maximum of 150 mg or until side effects occur. The most common side effects are postural hypotension, constipation, dizziness, and mucous membrane dryness. While the drug may be partially effective for 50 to 60 percent of patients, over half experience some side effects and approximately 20 percent will discontinue the medication because of intolerance.

Short-term studies have shown oxybutynin (Ditropan) to be effective when administered in patients with stress or urge incontinence. It probably works by increasing sphincter tone and increasing bladder capacity. Oxybutynin is administered orally in 5 mg tablets, three times daily. In the very frail only half of this dose should be used initially to minimize side effects. It is effective in approximately 50 percent of patients, but the side effects of dryness of the mouth, blurred vision, abdominal cramps, and constipation are encountered in nearly 50 percent. Twenty percent of patients using this drug discontinue it because of intolerance. A drug trial of 2 to 3 days at full or maximally tolerated dose may be considered in elderly individuals if imipramine fails. Long-term studies of this agent are not available.

REFERENCES

1. Andres R, Bierman EL, Hazzard WR (eds): Principles of Geriatric Medicine. New York, McGraw-Hill, 1985
2. Burgio KL, Whitehead WE, Engle BT: Urinary incontinence in the elderly. Ann Intern Med 103:507, 1985
3. Cape RDT, Coe RM, Rossman I (eds): Fundamentals of Geriatric Medicine. New York, Raven Press, 1983
4. Cassel CK, Walsh JR (eds): Geriatric Medicine. New York, Springer-Verlag, 1984
5. Kane RA, Kane RL: Assessing the Elderly: A Practical Guide to Measurement. Lexington, Mass, Lexington Books, DC Heath, 1981
6. Kane RL, Oslander JG, Abrass JB: Essentials of Clinical Geriatrics. New York, McGraw-Hill, 1984
7. Katz S, Ford AB, et al: Studies of illness in the aged: The index at ADL: Standardized measure of biological and psychosocial function. JAMA 184:94, 1986
8. Ouslander JG, Kane RL, Abrass IB: Urinary incontinence in elderly nursing home patients. JAMA 248:1194, 1982
9. Ouslander JG, Urman HN, Uman GC: Development and testing of an incontinence monitoring record. J Am Geriatr Soc 34:83, 1986
10. Resnick NM, Yalla SV: Management of urinary incontinence in the elderly. N Engl J Med 313:800, 1985
11. Sullivan DH, Lindsay RW: Urinary incontinence in the geriatric population of an acute care hospital. J Am Geriatr Soc 32:646, 1984
12. Vestel RE: Clinical pharmacology. In Andres R, Bierman EL, Hazzard WR (eds): Principles of Geriatric Medicine. New York, McGraw-Hill, 1984
13. Williams ME, Pannill FC: Urinary incontinence in the elderly. Ann Intern Med 97:895, 1982

CHAPTER 17.4
Special Aspects of Care for Adolescents

Catherine DeAngelis

This chapter, devoted to the care of adolescents, has been developed because of the increasing realization that their care often requires special expertise beyond that necessary for other age groups. The purpose is to discuss some of the characteristics and problems of the teen years in order to enable the physician and other health care providers to function more effectively with teenagers. This is especially important because adolescence is the time at which many lifelong health habits are established.

MANAGEMENT OF THE ADOLESCENT PATIENT

Adolescence is the time or process of maturation from childhood to adulthood. It includes the period of life between puberty and maturity, usually ages 12 through 19. In 1980, there were approximately 50 million adolescents in the United States, about 20 percent more than in 1970. Since that time there has been a gradual decrease. Differences in cultural, ethnic, geographic, and economic influences prevent teenagers from being a homogenous group. However, a number of characteristics common to all bind them together into a subculture with specific needs that require special understanding and management.

MORTALITY AND MORBIDITY

Injuries, homicides, and suicides are the three leading causes of death among adolescents. They account for about 70 percent of deaths in this age group. Individuals from 15 to 24 years of age are the only segment of the United States population for which an increase in mortality has been recorded within the last decade. Sadly, the vast majority of these deaths are preventable, and it is imperative for providers to consider these statistics when caring for adolescents.[1]

Almost 75 percent of teenage deaths result from injuries. Motor vehicle injuries are the number one cause of death. Concomitant use of alcohol is frequently associated with this mortality.

Teenagers should be urged to wear seat belts when driving a car, to wear helmets when riding on a motorcycle, and to refrain from alcohol use during either activity. Parents should be encouraged to wear seat belts, especially since use by adolescents appears to correlate with parental utilization. Since half of fatal automobile-induced injuries occur after 9 PM, discussions about when teenagers should drive are also appropriate.

Homicides are frequently a cause of death, especially among black males. In some populations, death rates from homicide exceed those from injuries. Guns and knives account for most of the homicides, with the pattern of offense generally involving a male victimized by another male acquaintance. Approximately one fourth of these deaths are also related to alcohol use.

Suicides also account for a large number of deaths, especially in white adolescent males. Many clinicians fear that asking a teenager about suicide may actually precipitate such an event; there are no data to support this. In fact, physicians must address the issue of teenager suicide if the suicide rate in this population, which has increased by 75 percent since 1968, is to be reduced. About one third of these suicides are related to drug or alcohol use.

It is estimated that for each successful suicidal death, there are one hundred attempts. Most individuals who commit suicide have previously communicated their intent to someone either through words or actions.

To the extent that a teenager expresses concrete ideas or plans about suicide, appropriate safeguards should be undertaken, ranging from psychiatric referral to immediate hospitalization. Suicide gestures, no matter how apparently innocuous, should be taken seriously. A full exploration of the factors leading up to the gesture should be made before discharging the patient. Hospitalization or alternative placement should be considered whenever the nature of the gesture appears related to factors still operative in the home

or when the parents or caretaker appear hostile or angry with the adolescent rather than supportive.

It is interesting to contrast the leading causes of adolescent mortality and morbidity as perceived by health professionals working in a medical setting with those problems as perceived by the teenagers themselves.

From a medical viewpoint, the problems most often identified with adolescence include scoliosis, slipped epiphysis, acne, sports injuries, infectious mononucleosis, body image problems, drug abuse, venereal disease, goiter, sexual dysfunction, delinquency, tumors, anorexia nervosa, hepatitis, primary amenorrhea, and learning problems in school. The problems intensified by adolescence are tuberculosis, automotive injuries, unwed pregnancy, attempted suicide, diabetes, inflammatory bowel disease, menstrual dysfunction, dental caries, abortion, gynecomastia, and mental retardation. The problems that often originate during adolescence are obesity, alcoholism, duodenal ulcer, hypercholesterolemia, labile hypertension, irritable colon syndrome, migraine headaches, and marital conflicts.[5]

This primarily disease-oriented list can be contrasted with those cited by teenagers. The problems and concerns ranked highest by adolescents were school, drugs, how far to go with sex, getting along with parents and other adults, birth control, venereal disease, pregnancy, menstrual periods, sadness and depression, acne, and weight problems.[24]

This disparity emphasizes the importance of identifying what the adolescent feels his problem is and what his concerns are.

ADOLESCENT GROWTH AND DEVELOPMENT

The development of an adolescent is a complex process that occurs within three overlapping spheres: biologic, sociocultural, and psychologic. Development in each area is influenced by, and in turn influences, development in the other two. Because of the variations within these spheres, considerable differences will occur among adolescents. Nevertheless, certain broad, general patterns do characterize the adolescent period.

PHYSICAL DEVELOPMENT

Adolescence is associated with the second accelerated growth in height and weight; the first occurs in the first 2 years of life. The adolescent growth spurt is accompanied by the appearance of sexual characteristics. Physically, adolescence is terminated by fusion of the epiphyses and metaphyses of bone and by the ability to reproduce, thereby completing the transition from childhood to adulthood.

Essentially, the sooner puberty occurs, the sooner will the rate of growth decline and finally stop.[32] The onset of puberty is better correlated with the mean height and weight than with chronologic age.[9] Growth may proceed an average of 3 inches, with a range of 1 to 7 inches, after the onset of menses. The comparable measure in boys is not known because a finite marker, like menses, does not exist in boys.

A normal growth spurt may begin as early as 9.5 years in girls and 10.5 in boys or as late as 14.5 years in girls and 16.0 years in boys.[33] For both sexes the acceleration, peak, deceleration, and fusion of bone usually span a period of approximately 2 years; the gain in height equals about 20 percent of adult height.

In general, adolescent weight changes parallel those in height but the incremental changes and variabilities are greater. The weight gain is usually steady throughout puberty in the nonobese adolescent, and the total weight gain during this period is approximately half that of the ideal adult body weight. Figures 17.4–1 and 17.4–2 show the height and weight growth curves for adolescent females and males. Change in the rate of growth from the begin-

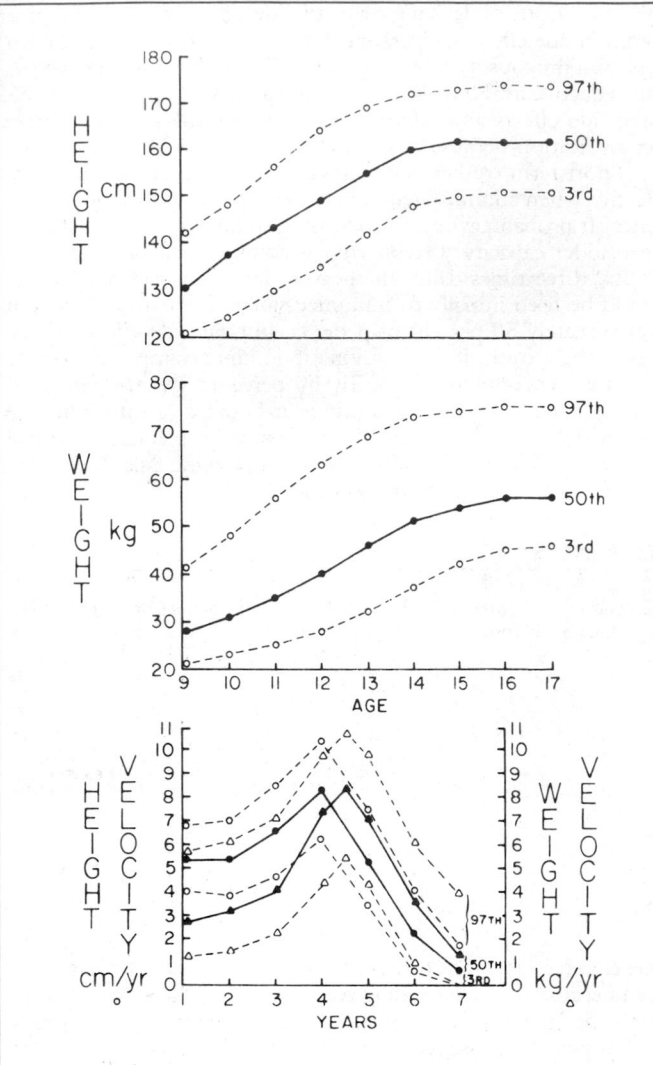

Figure 17.4–1. Cross-sectional female height and weight by chronologic age (3rd, 50th, 97th percentiles) and longitudinal values for height and weight during the year of peak height and weight velocity and the 3 years before and after peak height velocity and peak weight velocity (3d, 50th, 97th percentiles). (*Adapted from Tanner JM: Growth at Adolescence, 2d ed. Oxford, Blackwell, 1962.*)

ning to the end of the growth spurt is relatively abrupt for the individual teenager and covers a period of months, rather than years. Hence, the individual growth curve is not nearly as smooth as those depicted in the figures.

There is variation in the age at which the various sequences of puberty begin and considerable differences in the rapidity with which each individual progresses from one stage to the next. However, the sequences themselves are the same for all individuals. Tables 17.4–1 and 17.4–2 list the stages of sexual development for girls and boys.

The exact causes of the onset of puberty are not clearly known. However, various hormonal assays have correlated the relationship of increased levels of pituitary luteinizing hormone and follicle stimulating hormone with (1) the advancing stages of adolescent psychologic development, (2) gonadal growth and function, and (3) bony maturation.[4,28,30] Table 17.4–3 shows the hormones involved in puberty.

Over the past 140 years, menarche has occurred on the average of 3 months earlier each decade. Currently, menarche occurs at the average age of 13.5 years in the United States, with a range

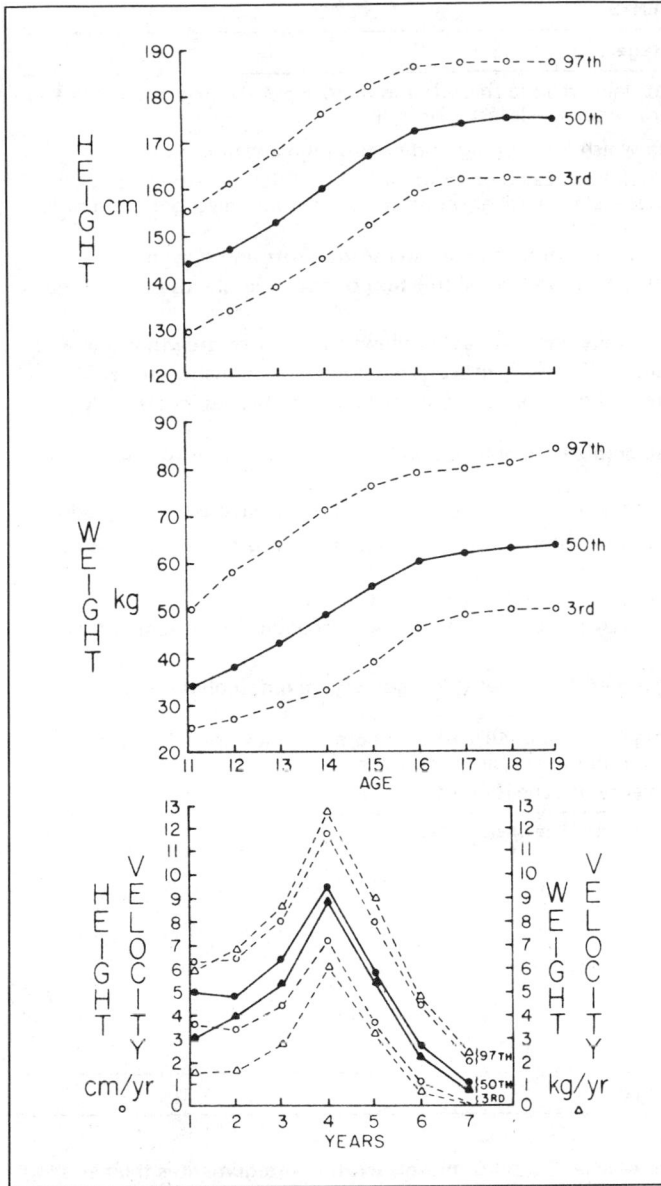

Figure 17.4–2. Cross-sectional male height and weight by chronologic age (3rd, 50th, 97th percentiles) and longitudinal values for height and weight during the year of peak height and weight velocity and the 3 years before and after peak height velocity and peak weight velocity (3d, 50th, 97th percentiles). (*Adapted from Tanner JM: Growth at Adolescence, 2d ed. Oxford, Blackwell, 1962.*)

of 6 to 17 years, with 95 percent of girls reaching menarche by 15.6 years.[26]

Socioeconomic factors play an important role in the age of onset of puberty. Generally, menses occurs earlier in young women from higher socioeconomic levels. Age of maternal menarche and race seem to have only minor influences. Factors, such as malnutrition, blindness, and chronic illness, tend to delay the onset of puberty in boys and girls.[34] Some other pathologic conditions associated with delayed or precocious sexual development are listed in Table 17.4–4.

EMOTIONAL DEVELOPMENT

Generally, three major developmental tasks must be accomplished by the adolescent before emotional adulthood can be achieved. The first is to become emancipated from parents and acquire skills

for future economic independence; the second is to learn to function in an adult, sexual role; and the third is to acquire a realistic, stable, and positive adult self-identity. Behavioral experimentation is the principal method used by adolescents to achieve these development tasks.

Early adolescence and mid-adolescence are times of strong peer group activities in what is commonly known as the adolescent subculture. During this phase, the adolescent has traded the safety of childhood identification with the parents for the safety of a peer group identity. The individual identity of the adult is a phenomenon of the future, but behavioral experimentation with adult-like roles, such as dating, part-time jobs, and acquiring special educational interests, is common. Developmental conflicts frequently occur because emotional ties with the peer group are often superficial and the teenager's individuality may be compromised. Risk-taking behavior, such as high-speed driving with an automobile or motorcycle and experimentation with sexual activity and drug usage, including alcohol and smoking, is common. For the most part, these are transient phases, but complications result when the adolescent has no friends, has poor peer-group ties, is multiply sexually active, or becomes involved in drug abuse, or when the initial experimentation with drugs ends in disaster.

The rebellion and withdrawal from adults, the heavy reliance on the group, and the constant, apparent changes in their value systems, which are reflections of their changing environment and behavioral experimentation, are often confounding to even the most patient parents. Helping teenagers and their parents work through these times can be a very rewarding experience for the health professional.

To function as a sexually mature adult, an adolescent must concurrently integrate personality with developing biologic and physiologic capabilities. Bryt describes four distinct factors that influence psychosexual growth during adolescence.[3] First in importance, and becoming increasingly significant from early adolescence onward, is the irresistible urge for active expression of sexual impulses. Before puberty only anger is nearly so compelling. The second factor is the effect of prevailing social mores. Adolescents' need to express themselves sexually may or may not be at odds with the community's current morality. The chances of a significant confrontation with social mores increases in the later teens. Third is the unconscious influence of family ethics that have been an environmental factor since childhood. The adolescent's actual, rather than apparent, personal value system is an integral part of how he or she will respond to the later experiences that are essential for psychosexual maturation. Fourth, the relationship between public and private morality may create and perpetuate internal conflicts and delay maturation in late adolescence. Gross discrepancies often exist between the two, and there is no readily available pattern after which the adolescent can model himself.

The availability of heterosexual peers is a necessary factor in the resolution of middle adolescent sexuality. Sociosexual experimentation such as dating, not sexual intercourse, is the vital ingredient. Currently, there seems to be inadequate limit-setting in this area for many teenagers, and pregnancy prevention has become a vital factor in allowing adolescents the time to work through the developmental tasks previously defined. Teenagers have had to develop new patterns to deal with the fact that sexual intercourse is an increasingly frequent part of mid-adolescence.

This developmental process takes time. Should it be abbreviated or interrupted by pregnancy or marriage, the result is often catastrophic.

GENERAL APPROACHES
TO THE TEENAGER

In addition to the concepts discussed in other sections of this textbook, certain key issues should be considered in the general approach to routine management of the adolescent patient.[27]

TABLE 17.4–1. STAGES OF SEXUAL DEVELOPMENT IN FEMALE ADOLESCENTS

Age (yr)	Stages
0–12	I. Preadolescent. Female pelvic contour evident; breasts flat; labia majora smooth and minora poorly developed; hymenal opening small or absent; mucous membranes dry and red; vaginal cells lack glycogen
8–13	II. **Breasts:** Elevation of nipple; small mound beneath areola which is enlarging and begins pigmentation
	Labia majora: become thickened, more prominent, and wrinkled. **Labia minora:** easily identified due to increased size along with clitoris; urethral opening more prominent, mucous membranes moist and pink; some glycogen present in vaginal cells
	Hair: First appears on mons and then on labia majora about time of menarche; still scanty, soft and straight
	Skin: Increased activity of sebaceous and merocrine sweat glands, and initial function of apocrine glands in axilla and vulva begin
9–14	III. Rapid growth peak is passed; menarche most often at this stage and invariably follows the peak of growth acceleration
	Breasts: Areola and nipple further enlarge and pigmentation more evident; continued increase in glandular size
	Labia minora: Well developed and vaginal cells have increased glycogen content; mucous membranes increasingly more pale
	Hair: In pubic region is thicker, coarser, often curly (considerable normal variation including a few girls with early Stage II at menarche)
	Skin: Further increased activity of sebaceous and sweat glands with beginning of *acne* in some girls; adult body odor
12–15	IV. **Breasts:** Projection of areola above breast plane and areolar (Montgomery) glands apparent (this development is absent in about 20% of normal girls); glands easily palpable
	Labia: Both majora and minora assume adult structure; glycogen content of vaginal cells begins cyclic characteristics
	Hair: In pubic area more abundant; axillary hair present (rarely present at Stage II, not uncommonly present at Stage III)
12–17	V. **Breasts:** Mature histologic morphology; nipple enlarged and erect; areolar (Montgomery) glands well developed; globular shape
	Hair: In pubic area more abundant and may spread to thighs (in about 10% of women it assumes "male" distribution with extension toward umbilicus); facial hair increased often in form of slight mustache
	Skin: Increased sebaceous gland activity and increased severity of *acne* if present before

From Lowrey GH: Growth and Development of Children, 7th ed. Chicago, Year Book Medical Publishers, 1978.

TABLE 17.4–2. STAGES OF SEXUAL DEVELOPMENT IN MALE ADOLESCENTS

Age (yr)	Stages
0–14	I. Preadolescent
10–14	II. **Testes and penis:** Increasing size is evident (testicle length reaches 2.0 cm or more); scrotum integument is thinner and assumes an increased pendulous appearance
	Hair: First appearance of pubic hair in area at base of penis
	Skin: Increased activity of sebaceous and apocrine sweat glands and initial function of apocrine glands of axilla and scrotal area begins
11–15	III. Rapid growth peak is passed; nocturnal emissions begin
	Testes and penis: Further increase in size and pigmentation apparent. Leydig cells (interstitial) first appear at Stage II; are now prominent in testes
	Hair: In pubic area more abundant and present on scrotum; still scanty and fine textured; axillary hair begins
	Breasts: Button-type hypertrophy in 70% of boys at Stages II and III
	Larynx: Changes in voice due to beginning of laryngeal growth
	Skin: Increasing activity of sebaceous and sweat glands with beginning of *acne;* adult body odor
12–16	IV. **Testes:** Further increase in size, length 4.0 cm or greater; increase in size of *penis* greatest at Stages III and IV
	Hair: Pubic hair thicker and coarser and in most ascends toward umbilicus in typical male pattern; axillary hair increases; facial hair increases over lip and upper cheeks
	Larynx: Voice deepens
	Skin: Increasing pigmentation of scrotum and penis; acne often more severe
	Breasts: Previous hypertrophy decreased or absent
13–17	V. **Testes:** Length greater than 4.5 cm
	Hair: Pubic hair thick, curly, heavily pigmented; extends to thighs and toward umbilicus; adult distribution and increase in body hair (chest, shoulders, thighs, etc.) continues for more than another 10 yr; baldness may begin
	Skin: Acne may persist and increase
	Larynx: Adult character of voice

From Lowrey GH: Growth and Development of Children, 7th ed. Chicago, Year Book Medical Publishers, 1978.

TABLE 17.4–3. HORMONES INVOLVED IN ADOLESCENT DEVELOPMENT

Luteinizing Hormone Release Factor

Activity	Stimulates pituitary to release gonadotropins (LH and FSH)
Source	Hypothalamus
Nature	Decapeptide

Luteinizing Hormone

Activity	Preparation and ripening of ovarian follicle, may stimulate release of progesterone, role not clear in prepubertal girl; in male stimulates interstitial (Leydig) cells of testes to secrete testosterone
Source	Pituitary
Name	LH, a glycoprotein

Follicle-Stimulating Hormone

Activity	In female, develops ovarian follicle to antrum stage, increases estrogen secretion from follicle; in male, matures sperm and may influence growth of seminiferous tubules
Source	Pituitary
Name	FSH, a glycoprotein

Estrogens

Activity	Feminizing; cause breast development, uterine growth, vaginal maturation, bone maturation; no effect on somatic growth
Source	Mainly ovarian but small and possibly significant amounts from adrenal cortex and testes
Names	Estrone, estradiol, estriol

Androgens

Activity	Virilizing; cause penile and prostatic development; promote hair growth of pubic, axillary, facial, and general body areas; bone maturation; laryngeal development; sebaceous and sweat gland development; stimulus to somatic growth
Source	Testicles, adrenal cortex, small amounts from ovary
Names	Dehydroepiandrosterone, testosterone, epitestosterone, androstenedione

Progesterones

Activity	Block estrogen effect on endometrium, stimulate endometrial gland secretion, stimulate lobule-alveolar breast formation and growth
Source	Mainly from ovarian corpus luteum, small amounts from testes and adrenal cortex (large amounts from placenta)
Names	Progesterone, pregnenolone

From Lowrey GH: Growth and Development of Children, 7th ed. Chicago, Year Book Medical Publishers, 1978.

HISTORY

A careful review of the *perinatal period* is essential. A teenage girl whose mother received diethylstibestrol during her pregnancy with the teenager should be examined and observed carefully to rule out vaginal adenocarcinoma.[14] Teenage boys with a similar history should be watched carefully for genitourinary anomalies.[13]

TABLE 17.4–4. PATHOLOGIC CONDITIONS ASSOCIATED WITH ABNORMALITIES OF SEXUAL DEVELOPMENT[a]

Conditions associated with *delayed onset* of puberty
- Pituitary dwarfism
- Hypothyroidism
- Hypogonadism (agenesis, atrophy, surgical or traumatic castration)
- Acromegaly (rare)
- Any severe chronic illness
- Hypothalamic lesions (Fröhlich syndrome)

Conditions associated with *precocious* sexual development
- Adrenal cortex tumors or hyperplasia
- Interstitial cell tumors of the testes
- Ovarian tumors (granulosa cell and thecoma)
- Pineal gland tumors (in males only)
- Third ventricle tumors of the brain
- Hydrocephalus (rare)
- Postencephalitis (rare)
- McCune-Albright syndrome (polyostotic fibrous dysplasia)

[a]Besides the endocrine glands, it will be noted that the central nervous system (hypothalamus) may also be involved.
From Lowrey GH: Growth and Development of Children, 7th ed. Chicago, Year Book Medical Publishers, 1978.

Immunization review is often neglected in teenagers. Consequently preventable, infectious diseases, such as rubeola, often occur in adolescents.

Nutritional history is important because of the increased energy and protein demands of rapid growth and development and accelerated physical activity. Generally, teenage girls require about 2400 calories per day and boys about 2900 calories per day.

Teenagers eat according to habits and attitudes learned early in life, and these are very difficult to alter. The motivation to eat well-balanced meals does not come naturally. Foods are chosen primarily because they are pleasing to the senses and are convenient to obtain. Consequently, many teenagers are junk food enthusiasts. Furthermore, the effects of good and bad nutrition are not easily demonstrated in the teen years, and the threat of illness from malnutrition seems so remote to an adolescent that the idea usually has little or no effect.[21]

The greatest demand for nutrients and energy occurs during the height of the adolescent growth spurt. Diet counseling should take into account the teenager's stage of growth, life-style, and schedule. For example, snacks and meals taken away from home might include juices, fruit, pizza, and cheeseburgers with lettuce and tomatoes rather than soda pop, pretzels, potato chips, and candy.

About 10 to 15 percent of American adolescents are obese. In addition to the possible subsequent cardiovascular problems in later life, many overweight adolescents are not well adjusted emotionally. Physical appearance is a very important teenage socializing factor. Obese adolescents tend to be depressed, to have poor body images, to have difficulty making friends, to be very dependent on family approval, and to have severe psychiatric disturbances requiring treatment. Obese applicants to college are less likely to be ac-

cepted than the nonobese, even though academic achievement, social class, and motivation are essentially equivalent.[6]

A complete *sexual history* should include degree of sexual activity, use of contraception, possibility of venereal disease, and, in girls, menarche and menses. Questions should be asked directly, specifically, and in a nonjudgmental manner.

Inquiries about the teenager's living and family situation; school history and performance; sleeping habits; hobbies and activities; social and peer relationships; and use of tobacco, alcohol, and drugs should be made. About 25 percent of all teenagers smoke, with 4 to 5 percent of them doing so on a regular basis.[1] Over the past few years the incidence has been decreasing somewhat. Teenagers who smoke can develop sputum production, cough, shortness of breath, and abnormally low expiratory flow rates that reflect small-airway obstruction.[29]

National surveys have shown that 70 percent of adolescents use alcohol monthly, and 28 percent do so on a weekly basis. Furthermore, national crime reports indicate that among 15- to 19-year-olds, the rate of drug abuse violations was 9.2 per 1000. Obviously, these problems exist among teenagers, and they can only be addressed if appropriate questions are part of the routine medical history.[15]

PHYSICAL EXAMINATION

Special attention should be given to the examination of *breasts* in both male and female adolescents. This is an excellent time to teach teenage girls how to examine their breasts for masses and to reassure boys with gynecomastia that it is a normal variant that will regress.[8,11]

Male teenagers should be taught self-examination of the *testes*. Most masses are benign varicoceles or hydroceles, but the incidence of malignant testicular tumors is highest during adolescence.[10]

Pelvic examinations should be performed on all sexually active women. Significant abnormalities such as specific infection, smears with atypical inflammatory cells, and dysplasia can occur.[7,22]

It is especially important to *examine the spine* of teenagers to rule out scoliosis and kyphosis. Kyphosis, or "round shoulders" is found in up to 8 percent of adolescents of both sexes, typically in the early teen and mid-teen years. Radiographs usually show an irregularity of the vertebral end-plates early. Later, the anterior surface of one or more vertebrae is narrowed by at least 5 degrees. Teenagers with this problem should be referred to an orthopedic surgeon for therapy.

Scoliosis, a lateral deviation or rotation of a series of vertebrae away from the normal spinal axis, is usually first observed as a lowering of one scapula when the teenager is standing up straight with both feet close together. When he bends over and allows his arms and hands to hang down loosely, one side of the back is elevated over the other. Diagnosis is confirmed by radiographs, and an orthopedist should be consulted.

It is essential to make the diagnosis in the early teen years, before or early in the onset of rapid growth. By menarche, all girls will have begun the decelerating phase of growth, and nonsurgical correction is impossible. On the other hand, if only a slight deviation is found after the onset of menses, referral is probably not warranted.

DIAGNOSTICS

Routine tests should include:

1. Hemograms in menstruating girls
2. Sickle cell screening in appropriate teenagers where genetic counseling is available
3. Tuberculin testing annually in tuberculin-negative teenagers who live in endemic areas or who have traveled in such areas, and every 3 years in others

4. Rubella titers in sexually active women who are not certain of their immune status for that disease

THERAPEUTICS

Diphtheria-tetanus vaccine (adult type) booster should be given every 10 years. Because most children receive their last childhood immunizations on entering school, teenagers usually require the vaccine.

Mumps vaccine should be given to any teenager who has no history of receiving the vaccine or of having had the disease. Fifteen percent of mumps occur after age 15 years, and 20 percent of these cases are associated with orchitis and a smaller percentage with salpingo-oophoritis.

Twenty-five percent of the cases of rubeola occur in teenagers. Anyone who has no history of having received the vaccine after 1 year of age or of having had the disease should receive *rubeola vaccine*. It should be noted however, that rubeola is often confused with other viral illnesses. Rubeola is associated with fever, conjunctivitis, cough, coryza, Koplik spots, and a generalized maculopapular rash that lasts 9 to 10 days.

Atypical measles occurs especially in those who have been immunized with killed measles vaccine, which was used in the United States from 1963 to 1967. When these individuals are later infected by the wild measles virus, a petechial, vesicular, or urticarial rash accompanied by peripheral edema and pneumonia with pleural effusions might result. A number of atypical measles epidemics have occurred on college campuses over the past few years.[23]

As much as 20 to 30 percent of rubella infections occur during adolescence. Sexually active teenage girls with no history of rubella infection or immunization and with a low rubella titer should receive the *rubella vaccine*. Pregnancy should be prevented for at least 2 months following the administration of the vaccine because of the risk of transmission of live virus to the fetus.

SPECIAL TYPES OF HEALTH FACILITIES AND PERSONNEL

Management of the types of problems associated with the adolescent years requires something other than the traditional, one-physician-to-one-patient relationship. The characteristics of a physician found to be most desirable by teenagers are a high degree of understanding, a good personality, and informality. Age, sex, and dress are of minor concern.[31]

Most teenagers consult a physician less than once a year, and these visits usually involve only a specific physical ailment. The vast majority of adolescents seek the help of other individuals such as nurses, teachers, school counselors, clergy members, social workers, community workers, and friends. In order to meet the health needs of teenagers better, care must be provided by the various types of health and other professionals and their assistants functioning as an integrated team. The team effort can help to alleviate gaps, prevent duplication, and decrease mixed and contradictory messages and advice.

The environment in which health care is provided should be designed especially for teenagers. The area does not require expensive decor, but the furniture, bulletin boards, magazines, and the like should be designed to appeal to teenagers. If at all possible, some clinic hours should be scheduled in the late afternoon or evening to prevent absence from school.

CONSENT AND CONFIDENTIALITY

Confidentiality is of utmost importance to ensure the trust of the adolescent, and his privacy and personal dignity must be preserved. It is therefore essential that guidelines be set and clearly explained regarding the involvement of parents and legal guardians in their care. Ideally, teenagers should be allowed to accept responsibility

for their own care if they choose to do so. However, they must not be forced into accepting this responsibility if they have not yet reached that stage of emancipation. In crisis situations, teenagers should be encouraged to involve their parents.

The degree to which adolescents can and should function independently of their parents raises profound legal and ethical issues for physicians and other health professionals. The legal system in the United States generally does not recognize an individual to be competent until his or her eighteenth birthday. However, since 1967, almost every state has enacted legislation allowing at least specific groups of teenagers to consent to their own care.[2,17] In 1973 the American Academy of Pediatrics' Committee on Youth published a model minor consent act.[12] The goals of the proposed act are to ensure quality health services of all minors by granting them self-consent in instances where they might not seek care if parental consent were required and to encourage health professionals to provide quality care without incurring legal liability.[16]

Failure to treat adolescents as adults might prevent them from seeking needed health care. Surveys in family-planning clinics have shown that many teenagers avoid medical facilities where confidentiality is not maintained. Many potential conflicts can be avoided if the physician meets with the parents during the first visit to discuss the rationale for according their teenager autonomy and confidentiality.

The financial aspect of providing care for adolescents bears some consideration. Currently, a number of federal programs provide funding for adolescent health services. However, most teenagers still must depend on their parents for support, and this makes it very difficult for them to receive care without their parents' permission or knowledge.

COMPLIANCE

One of the most exasperating areas of providing health care to teenagers involves poor compliance with suggested treatment and with follow-up appointments despite what appears to be elaborate individual and team counseling. The adolescent frequently misses appointments for no apparent reason and misuses or discontinues medications for what appear to be trivial reasons. For example, discontinuation of oral contraceptives may occur as a result of small, midcycle, vaginal spotting or because the teenager may suddenly decide it is not a ''natural process.''

When such situations occur frequently, there is a tendency for the health professional to retreat in despair and exasperation. However, it might be easier to maintain this important input if one considers two aspects of caring for adolescents. First, the teenager has the potential for over 50 more years of a healthy, happy life. Second, the behavior that often exasperates parents and health professionals is part of the normal developmental process toward adulthood and is self-limited.

Compliance is a complex phenomenon and is affected by characteristics of the provider and of the patient. Generally, the adolescent with poor self-esteem or with psychosocial problems is at increased risk for noncompliance. In contrast, behaviors consistent with autonomy, such as making his own appointments, correlate with compliance. Studies of provider-related characteristics show that teenagers do not comply with physicians who keep them waiting for long periods of time.

SPECIAL PROBLEMS OF ADOLESCENCE

The three major problem areas in adolescent medicine are (1) sexuality, (2) drug abuse, including alcohol and nicotine, and (3) trauma, including injuries, suicides, and homicides. The problems associated with drug abuse and trauma are discussed in Chapters 16.9 and 15.19, respectively.

Sexually transmitted infections (see Chapter 9.15), sexual problems in general (see Chapter 16.10), drug and alcohol dependence (see Chapters 16.9 and 17.5), adolescent suicide (Chapter 16.3), and similar behavior are also discussed elsewhere in this text. This discussion, therefore, will be limited to teenage pregnancy and contraception.

Providing family-planning and contraceptive advice and general, realistic, and pertinent sexual education is a major function of all health professionals who care for adolescents.

The pregnancy and birth rates for all ages have declined since 1966 except for the 15- to 19-year-old group, which has stabilized at an unacceptably high rate, and for the under-15-year-old group, which has continued to rise. Approximately 30,000 youngsters under 15 and over 1 million 15- to 19-year-olds become pregnant every year in the United States.

Over 60 percent of those teenagers who do not use contraceptives become pregnant annually compared to 30 percent of those who use them even inconsistently.

Generally, they become pregnant primarily because of ignorance regarding basic physiology and unexpected, unprotected intercourse. The desire for an infant is seldom the cause.[25,35]

PREGNANCY AND CONTRACEPTION

Teenage pregnancy is a serious problem. Maternal mortality is 13 percent higher for mothers from 15 to 19 and 60 percent higher for mothers under 15 than for mothers in their 20s. Infant mortality and low birth weight are twice as high for mothers under 15 years as for mothers in their 20s. Further, the surviving infants do not fare as well intellectually or physically, owing to prematurity and other factors.

The teenager mother is hampered in a number of respects. Physically, she is prone to iron deficiency anemia, cephalopelvic disproportion, and other problems of gestation and delivery. The teenager mother rarely has a chance to develop the normal independence that should be achieved during adolescence. She becomes emotionally and economically dependent. Her chance for social and economic advancement is hampered because her education is interrupted or ceases. In fact, pregnancy is the principal cause of school dropout for young women.

Very often, the father is also a teenager, and it is becoming more and more obvious that the emotional impact on the adolescent father is as serious as that on the mother. This is especially true as society moves away from placing the sole responsibility for contraception and unwanted pregnancy on women.

According to Lindemann,[19] the process whereby an adolescent moves from using no contraception to the consistent use of an effective contraceptive involves three stages: the natural, the peer, and the expert stages. During the *natural stage*, adolescents do nothing about contraception. Coitus is infrequent and unpredictable. There is a preference for the naturalness and spontaneity of sexual activity, and at this point, the adolescent is not willing to define herself as sexually active, capable of reproduction, or in need of contraception.

During the *peer stage*, adolescents acquire information from their peers and experiment with various methods of birth control. The longer a young woman remains in this stage, the more and various are the methods she uses. The variations in the use of contraception may increase the risk of pregnancy. Often pregnancy occurs as a result of a lack of skills and information, a change in the boy-girl relationship, or because the use of peer prescription methods interrupts the spontaneity of the natural stage and is deemed unacceptable. The frequency and predictability of sexual intercourse continue to condition birth control behavior, as does belief in the effectiveness of the methods being used and the lack of real commitment to nonmarital sexual intercourse.

A final and major step in the peer stage is the willingness of the adolescent to disclose his or her sexual activity if nothing more than by the need to purchase foam or condoms. This is often the psychosocial profile of the teenagers when they are identified as sexually active. During the peer prescription period, important

psychologic changes are occurring. The adolescent is moving from little to greater awareness, from noncommitment to commitment, from one self-concept to another, and from no birth control to planned birth control.

The *expert stage* involves the use of professionals for contraception advice. However, just because expert advice is sought, this does not imply that the teenager will comply with the advice.

Rapid psychologic and physiologic change is the hallmark of mid-adolescence. By definition, therefore, it is the norm rather than the exception to have wide fluctuations in effective birth control use. However, it is the responsibility of the health professionals who care for teenagers to provide them with information and means for contraception either directly or by referral. The type of birth control used should be individualized according to the stage of psychologic development and the environmental needs of the teenager. Adolescent misconceptions about birth control devices should be addressed. For example, adolescents should know that soda pop douches and using plastic wrap for condoms are not very effective and may be hazardous.

Spermatocides immobilize and kill sperm. In general, foams are more effective than creams, jellies, and suppositories, which do not disperse well. The spermatocide should be inserted into the vagina within 1 hour before each act of coitus.

Condoms generally are made of latex or the collagenous lining of sheep intestines and should always be used with a spermatocidal agent. They should not be stored for long periods of time, especially in warm, closed areas such as wallets and glove compartments. An added benefit of condom use is the barrier protection they provide against sexually transmitted diseases.

Diaphragms, which also should be used with spermatocidal agents, act as barriers to the cervical orifice and hold the spermatocide in place against the cervix. They are relatively easy to fit, and the clinician can learn the technique in a short period of time. The diaphragm may be inserted up to 2 hours before intercourse, and it should be left in for at least 6 hours after coitus. The diaphragm should be rechecked about 1 week after the initial fitting. It should then be rechecked annually to assure proper fitting, sooner if the woman has been pregnant, has had a pelvic operation, or has lost or gained a significant amount of weight.

Intrauterine devices (IUDs) are not one of the better types of birth control for adolescents, especially for those who have never been pregnant. Because of the prevalence of gonorrhea in teenagers, the IUD may place them at higher risk for pelvic inflammatory disease. The IUD may act as a foreign object and make treatment difficult. If an adolescent presents with pelvic inflammatory disease, the IUD should probably be removed and another type of contraceptive used, at least until the infection has cleared.

Oral contraceptive pills prevent ovulation by inhibiting release of the pituitary gonadotropins, follicle stimulating hormone, and luteinizing hormone. They also cause a decrease in secretion and an increase in viscosity of cervical mucus, thereby inhibiting sperm motility and penetration.

The combination oral contraceptives contain synthetic progestin and estrogen in each pill. In the 28-pill package, at least 7 pills are placebos. The first 14 pills contain estrogen only and the following 7 contain estrogen and progestin. In general, it is better to begin with low-estrogen-containing pills and increase the amount of estrogen as necessary.

Regardless of the contraceptive method used, constant reassurance and encouragement are necessary for the adolescent to remain motivated to continue use. It is not enough to write a prescription for pills or fit a diaphragm. The role of the clinician as confidante and motivator cannot be overemphasized. It is evident that premarital sexual activity is widespread among teenagers. It should be practiced in a manner that will not produce the added problems of pregnancy.

Sterilization has no place in contraception for adolescents. Their lives and ideas will probably change dramatically as they mature. They should not be burdened with a possible undesired infertility based on a decision made before full maturity has been reached.

Regardless of the amount of energy expended in the area of birth control for teenagers, pregnancies in this age group continue to occur.

When the pregnant teenager comes for care, it is essential to determine how far she has advanced into the pregnancy, how she and the father feel about it, and, if possible, why it occurred. An evaluation of the young woman's support system and current living situation is valuable in determining where she might receive assistance. If the father is known, he should be included in the decisions and counseling if at all feasible.

The teenage parents' physical and emotional welfares and their rights of privacy and confidentiality should be preserved. Their own parents should take an active part in the overall situation if at all possible. If the teenagers do not have a good relationship with their parents, they may be able to find support from other sources, such as their brothers, sisters, close friends, or members of the clergy. Ideally, the parents or others will be able to provide the reassurance and assistance necessary for the teenagers to go through the pregnancy. They might also be willing to help care for the infant or provide the necessary emotional and possible economic support.

In all cases, the adolescent parents should be encouraged to continue school and complete their educations as soon as feasible. The practitioner should advise the young parents about local agencies that may provide assistance and help to arrange for the initial contact with the proper agency if assistance is needed.

After an assessment of the resources available to the teenager, the alternatives should be discussed. Basically, there are three options: (1) the mother can keep the baby as a single parent or get married and keep the baby; (2) she can give the baby up for adoption; or (3) she can have an abortion.

If the teenagers feel that they want to keep the baby, it is important to discuss how a pregnancy will change or influence their lives and future goals. Many adolescents have unrealistic expectations and ideas about child rearing. Some young women feel that it is an act of emancipation to have a child, or perhaps they view the baby as someone who will love them unconditionally. It is often valuable to explore the adolescents' goals regarding child rearing and how they plan to meet them.

The options of adoption and abortion should also be discussed, and the feeling of the prospective grandparents about each alternative should be explored. If the teenagers know some individuals who have experienced adoption or abortion, they may wish to speak to them about the decision. The teenagers may have strong moral feelings about abortion or may be influenced by the values of friends and family.

Although some adolescents can intellectually understand the rationale for an abortion, they often have much difficulty with this concept emotionally. Besides the moral issues involved, other common concerns regarding abortion include the effect it will have on future children; the possibility of sterility, pain, and complications; and the financial cost. The abortion procedure and possible complications should be explained. If the primary clinician personally is unable to provide abortion advice because of religious or moral beliefs, the adolescent should be referred to someone who can provide the advice.

Unfortunately, abortion seems to be used by too many adolescents as the primary form of birth control. Currently 27 percent of adolescent pregnancies are aborted by induction; an additional 14 percent are spontaneously aborted. Stated another way, the abortion rate per 1000 live births is 1183 for 12- to 14-year-olds, 687 for 15- to 17-year-olds, and 602 for 18- and 19-year-olds.

Abortion should never be used to replace adequate preventive measures. Sex education and contraception should be provided to the potentially sexually active teenager long before abortion becomes an alternative.

The total care of the teenage parents and their child requires

all the resources of the health team, including obstetrician and local social service agencies. Even with this multidisciplinary approach, the long-range outlook for the teenage mother, father, and child is replete with possible physical and emotional problems. It is much better to have prevented the pregnancy.

CHRONIC DISEASE

The advent of modern therapy has made it possible for many children with illnesses such as cystic fibrosis to survive through adolescence. The problems of dealing with any chronic illness are compounded by the normal "developmental turmoil" of adolescence.

Diabetes mellitus can be used to illustrate this point. The adolescent characteristically has labile diabetes. Emotional stress may include temporary insulin insensitivity. Fluctuations in blood glucose levels may be caused by erratic eating habits, irregular hours, and bursts of physical activity.[18] Often, teenagers simply do not take their insulin as prescribed. Similar problems may be encountered with other chronic illnesses during adolescence.

It may be difficult or embarrassing for adolescents to take medication or to explain signs or symptoms of a chronic illness to their peers. Whenever possible, medical regimens should be sufficiently flexible to allow for normal socialization to occur. Finally, emotional support must be an integral component to any treatment of chronic illness in teenagers.

REFERENCES

1. Adolescent Behavior and Health. Washington, DC, Institute of Medicine, National Academy of Science, 1978
2. Brown RH: Consent. Pediatrics 57:414, 1976
3. Bryt A: Adolescent sex causes. Med Aspects Human Sexuality 20:8, Oct 1978
4. Burr IM, Sizon Enko PE, et al: Hormonal changes in puberty. I. Correlation of serum luteinizing hormone and follicle stimulating hormone with stages of puberty, testicular size and bone age in normal boys. Pediatr Res 4:25, 1970
5. Cohen MI, Litt IF: Health care for adolescents in a traditional medical setting. Youth Health and Social Systems Symposium, Washington, DC, April 1974
6. Cunning H, Mayer J: Obesity and its possible effects on college acceptance. N Engl J Med 275:1172, 1966
7. Delke I, Veridano N, et al: Abnormal cervical cytology in adolescents. J Pediatr 98:985, 1981
8. Foster S, Lang S, et al: Breast self-examination practices and breast cancer stage. N Engl J Med 299:265, 1978
9. Frisch RE: A method of prediction of age of menarche from height and weight at ages 9 through 13 years. Pediatrics 53:384, 1974
10. Goldenring J: Teaching testicular self-examination to young men. Contemp Pediatr 7:73, 1985
11. Greenwald P, Nasca P, et al: Estimated effect of breast self-examination and routine physical examinations on breast cancer mortality. N Engl J Med 299:271, 1978
12. Hazard SW, Allen RV, Eisner V: A model act providing for consent of minors for health services. Pediatrics 51:293, 1973
13. Henderson BE: Urogenital tract abnormalities in sons of women treated with diethyestilbesterol. Pediatrics 58:505, 1976
14. Herbst AL: Clear cell adenocarcinoma of the vagina and cervix in girls: Analysis of 170 registry cases. Am J Obstet Gynecol 119:713, 1974
15. Hoffman A: A Handbook on Drug and Alcohol Abuse. New York, Oxford University Press, 1975
16. Hoffman A: A rational policy toward consent and confidentiality in adolescent health care. J Adolesc Health Care 1:9, 1980
17. Hormann AD, Pilpel HF: The legal rights of minors. Pediatr Clin North Am 20:989, 1973
18. Laron Z: Treatment of diabetes in children: Revisited. Pediatr Ann 3:63, 1974
19. Lindemann C: Birth Control and Unmarried Women. New York, Springer, 1974
20. Lowrey GH: Growth and Development of Children, 7th ed. Chicago, Year Book Medical Publishers, 1978
21. Marino D, Kling J: Nutritional concerns during adolescence. Pediatr Clin North Am 27:125, 1980
22. Marks A, Cohen MI: Health screening and assessment of adolescents. Pediatr Ann 49:177, 1978
23. Martin D, Weiner L, et al: Atypical measles in adolescents and young adults. Ann Intern Med 90:877, 1979
24. Parcell GS, Nader PR, Meyer MD: Adolescent health concerns, problems, and patterns of utilization in a triethnic urban population. Pediatrics 60:157, 1977
25. Polit D, Kahn J: Early subsequent pregnancy among economically disadvantaged teenage mothers. Am J Pub Health 76:167, 1986
26. Prader A: Constitutional delay of growth and puberty. In Chiunello G, Laron Z (eds): Proceedings of the Scrono Symposia: Recent Progress in Pediatric Endocrinology. London, Academic Press, 1977
27. Rapp C: The adolescent patient. Ann Intern Med 99:52, 1983
28. Root AW: Endocrinology of puberty. J Pediatr 83:1, 1973
29. Seely J, Zuskin E, Bouhays A: Cigarette smoking: Objective evidence for lung damage in teenagers. Science 172:741, 1971
30. Sizon Enko PC, Burr IM, et al: Hormonal changes in puberty. II. Correlation of serum luteinizing hormone and follicle stimulating hormone with stages of puberty and bone age in normal girls. Pediatr Res 4:36, 1970
31. Sternlieb JJ, Munan L: A survey of health problems, practices, and needs of youth. Pediatrics 49:117, 1972
32. Stuart HC: Physical growth during adolescence. Am J Dis Child 74:495, 1947
33. Tanner JM: Growth at Adolescence, 2d ed. Oxford, Blackwell, 1962
34. Zacharias L, Wurtmann RJ: Age at menarche. N Engl J Med 280:868, 1969
35. Zuckerman B, Walker D, et al: Adolescent pregnancy: Biobehavioral determinants of outcome. J Pediatr 105:857, 1984

CHAPTER 17.5
Alcoholism and Associated Medical Problems

Mack C. Mitchell
and Esteban Mezey

The consumption of alcoholic beverages is widely accepted as a normal practice in almost all societies. Yet most individuals as well as societies recognize that the excessive consumption of alcoholic beverages is undesirable and potentially deleterious. This chapter explores briefly how one distinguishes between alcohol use, alcohol abuse, and alcoholism and discusses specific medical problems to which the abuse of alcohol may lead.

DEFINITION

Many definitions of alcohol abuse and alcoholism have been proposed. As is often the case with disorders for which there are multiple definitions, none is completely adequate. In some definitions, alcoholism is regarded as drinking patterns that deviate from an accepted norm, whereas others require demonstrable physiologic

addiction to alcohol. The World Health Organization has defined "alcohol-type drug dependence" as existing "when the consumption of alcohol exceeds the limits that are accepted by his culture; if an individual consumes alcohol at times that are deemed inappropriate within that outline, or intake of alcohol becomes so great as to injure his health or impair his social relationships."[7,18] Although this definition is one that might apply to many societies, it is too vague to be of value in the diagnosis or understanding of the problem.

By contrast, the American Psychiatric Association uses a more biologic definition and separately defines alcohol abuse and alcoholism. Alcohol abuse may be suspected when an individual shows evidence of psychologic dependence on alcohol or needs alcohol to continue daily functioning. Other pathologic patterns of use such as frequent episodes of intoxication, or continuous intoxication, or both may also be present. These events must persist for at least a month to avoid inclusion of transient problems that may occur in the life of any individual. Alcoholism is defined as alcohol abuse with evidence of physiologic addiction to alcohol.[1] This addiction is characterized by extreme degrees of tolerance and physical signs of withdrawal. Although tolerance develops over time in most drinkers, there may be some who exhibit an extreme degree of tolerance such that an individual appears sober with blood ethanol levels in excess of 200 mg/dl, twice the legal limits for driving a motor vehicle. Although objections may be raised about these definitions, their strengths lie in their emphasis on physiologic changes that occur in alcoholism.

Both definitions emphasize a pathologic response to alcohol consumption with subsequent loss of control over drinking and other behaviors. Importantly, no definition of alcoholism requires that medical complications of excessive alcohol use be present.

PHARMACOLOGY OF ETHANOL

Ethanol is a simple two-carbon alcohol that is rapidly and completely absorbed by the gastrointestinal tract in the fasting state. It is well recognized that ethanol absorption may, however, be slowed when ingested together with food, leading to lower than expected peak blood levels. After absorption, ethanol is oxidized to acetaldehyde and later to acetate primarily in the liver by the enzymes alcohol dehydrogenase (ADH) and aldehyde dehydrogenase (ALDH). During each metabolic step, the cofactor NAD^+ is converted to NADH stoichiometrically. This shift in the cellular redox status (increased NADH/NAD ratio) may result in important changes in metabolism and cellular function (Table 17.5–1).

Intoxication by ethanol has been known since Neolithic times, yet the mechanism by which intoxication occurs remains unsettled. Recent studies have suggested that ethanol may alter the fluidity of neural membranes in a manner similar to general anesthetics.[3] Effects of alcohol on membrane functions including altered ion transport and receptor function may be important in causing intoxication and other effects of alcohol.[17] In general, ethanol causes central nervous system depression. Extremely high blood concentrations of ethanol, usually in excess of 400 to 500 mg/dl, may even lead to respiratory depression and death, except in highly tolerant individuals. However, by depressing certain inhibitory pathways, the behavioral effects of ethanol may appear to be stimulatory or excitatory. With respect to understanding alcoholism, one of the most important pharmacologic actions of ethanol may be the development of tolerance and dependence. Long-term consumption of alcoholic beverages reduces the pharmacodynamic responses to ethanol when given acutely. This reduction in the magnitude of the effects of ethanol or an increase in the threshold for its effects such as intoxication is referred to as "tolerance." A detailed discussion of this concept has recently been published.[13] Although tolerance is believed to play some role in alcohol dependence, the nature of this relationship is uncertain.

TABLE 17.5–1. DISORDERS DUE TO ALCOHOL-INDUCED INCREASE IN NADH/NAD REDOX STATUS

Problem	Mechanism
Fasting hypoglycemia	Inhibition of gluconeogenesis Glycogen depletion
Alcoholic ketoacidosis	Decreased fatty acid oxidation with catabolism to acetic acid residues
Lactic acidosis	Reduction of pyruvate to lactate
Hyperuricemia	Decreased urinary excretion of uric acid as a result of lactate
Alcoholic fatty liver	Increased triglyceride synthesis Decreased fatty acid oxidation

ETIOLOGY OF ALCOHOLISM

The development of alcoholism in individuals who drink alcoholic beverages is an uncommon, although by no means rare, occurrence. The actual prevalence rate of alcoholism among all drinkers is thought to be between 5 and 10 percent. Alcoholism has been said to be a disorder in which a complex interaction exists between alcohol, the individual, and his environment.[11] Genetic factors are one important determinant of the risk for the development of alcoholism. For example, sons of alcoholics are at greater risk for the development of alcoholism, and the concordance rate for alcoholism is significantly higher in monozygotic than in dizygotic twins.[4] The roles of social factors and stress are less clear, but these may be important in certain individuals. These factors may favor continued drinking in alcoholics or promote an underlying predisposition to alcoholism, perhaps through development of pathologic patterns of alcohol use (abuse). The reason for the use of alcohol is another factor that may determine why loss of control of drinking and alcoholism develop in a given individual. Furthermore, reasons for an individual's drinking are not static but may change over time.

DIAGNOSIS AND MANAGEMENT OF ALCOHOL ABUSE AND ALCOHOLISM

DIAGNOSTIC MANAGEMENT

Diagnosis of alcohol abuse and alcoholism may be difficult, particularly at early stages of the problem. Alcoholism is a disorder with protean manifestations; therefore, the ways in which this disorder presents may be highly variable. Occasionally, the first recognition of a patient's alcoholism will be the result of hospitalization for an obviously alcohol-related disorder such as cirrhosis or withdrawal symptoms. Other patients or their families seek medical care or counseling for emotional or social problems resulting from drinking or compounded by this problem. More commonly, the problem is less obvious. Patients may appear healthy, neatly dressed, and coherent at routine examinations or for unrelated medical problems. Only after careful questioning and examination will the patient's problem with alcohol become known. At the initial interview, a careful medical and psychiatric history and physical examination should be performed. Particular attention should be given to eliciting the patterns of alcohol use and the quantity of alcohol consumed. Drinking patterns in the general population vary considerably, and it may be difficult to establish evidence of pathologic drinking patterns with certainty. In general, one *cannot* assume that there is no safe limit of intake of ethanol. In fact, evidence has accumulated in recent years to suggest that there may even be beneficial effects of moderate drinking. Data reviewed by Turner

et al. suggest that those individuals with problems related to alcohol consume more than 0.7 mg/kg of absolute ethanol daily (50 to 60 g for the average person, or 6.0 oz of 80 proof spirits).[18] When the patient is reluctant to discuss details of drinking or unable to remember facts clearly, family members may assist in providing information. It is important for the physician to be frank and nonjudgmental in approaching the patient in order to establish effective communication. Clues to pathologic drinking include frequent episodes of drinking to the point of intoxication, an inability of the individual to control his intake of alcohol, alcoholic "blackout" periods, and drinking despite strong social contraindications, such as job losses or marital discord resulting from drinking. Some of these clues are summarized in Table 17.5–2. A variety of screening questionnaires have been developed to assist in the diagnosis of alcoholism. Of these the Michigan Alcoholism Screening Test (MAST) is the best validated and most reliable. The questions of the MAST are shown in Table 17.5–3. The interpretation of the screening on this test is as follows: 10 or more: alcoholism; 5 to 9: 80 percent chance of alcoholism; 4: borderline; zero to 3: normal drinker. One important aspect of the approach to the patient is the exclusion of underlying intrinsic psychiatric disorders such as schizophrenia and manic-depressive illness (see Chapters 16.5 and 16.6).

LABORATORY STUDIES

Certain laboratory tests have recently been used as an aid to early detection of heavy alcohol intake. The serum gamma glutamyltransferase activity has been reported to be elevated frequently in alcoholics. However, this test is by no means specific for heavy alcohol consumption and may be abnormal in patients receiving anticonvulsants and in those with biliary tract disease. When elevated in the absence of other causes it may suggest heavy alcohol consumption. The red-cell mean corpuscular volume (MCV) is also increased in alcoholics and remains elevated even after correction of vitamin deficiencies.[24] Because of the wide range of disorders that elevate MCV, it is probably not of value as an isolated screening test. High-density lipoprotein (HDL) levels are elevated in moderate social drinkers as well. Parenthetically, this elevation in HDL may account for the reduction in incidence of coronary artery disease that has been observed in moderate drinkers.[6] Dependable biochemical or genetic markers for alcoholism are not yet available.

THERAPEUTIC MANAGEMENT

Despite present limitations, alcoholism can be diagnosed correctly by physicians using the aforementioned definitions and guidelines. A number of treatment options are available, but evaluation of their outcome is difficult because of an inherent bias in selection by both physician and patient. Continuation in any alcoholism program by the patient is usually considered to be a success. This implied need for continuation does suggest that in many individuals alcoholism is a chronic disorder characterized by periods of relapse and remission. Any physician treating alcoholics must recognize this fact and resist the natural tendency to become frustrated by relapses. The situation is analogous to management of any chronic medical problem such as diabetes, heart disease, or cancer. Involvement of a spouse or close family member with the treatment is essential. Long-term goals of treatment must be individualized to a degree. For the majority of alcoholics, abstinence is the goal of treatment. The rationale for this goal is that in those individuals who are physiologically dependent on alcohol, continued drinking at any level may lead to progression and recurrence of the illness. In some patients, modification of abnormal drinking patterns to moderate levels and responsible use of alcoholic beverages has been tried. Most of these efforts have been unsuccessful,

TABLE 17.5–2. DIAGNOSTIC CLUES FOR ALCOHOLISM

History
- Preoccupation with drinking
- Inability to "control" drinking
- Guilt about drinking or its consequences
- Drinking to alter emotions (e.g., reduce anxiety, boredom, etc.)
- Morning drinking (i.e., to avoid withdrawal)
- Social, occupational, or legal problems caused by drinking
- Drastic personality changes in response to drinking
- Memory loss for drinking episode (e.g., blackouts)
- Continued drinking despite serious physical disorders contraindicating use of alcohol (e.g., cirrhosis)

Laboratory
- Elevated blood alcohol concentration (>150 mg/dl) in an individual who appears sober
- Elevated gamma-glutamyltranspeptidase (GGT)
- Elevated red-cell mean corpuscular volume (MCV)
- Elevated uric acid
- Elevated aspartate aminotransferase (AST)
- Thrombocytopenia

and the validity of this approach has been questioned. At this time, it cannot be recommended.

Of the various treatment programs, Alcoholics Anonymous is perhaps the most widely recognized and claims the largest membership. In most of their "chapters" a group therapy approach is employed, with "reformed" alcoholics offering assistance to those who wish to cease drinking. Behavioral modification programs, both inpatient and outpatient, have been used with combinations of aversive and rewarding stimuli. In some individuals insight-oriented therapy has been used, but successes are perhaps the exception rather than the rule. A number of programs include use of disulfiram, a potent inhibitor of aldehyde dehydrogenase, as a primary or adjunctive therapy. This medication is given as a deterrent to further drinking because of the unpleasant effects of flushing, headache, sweating, palpitations, occasional chest pains, and vomiting that occur when alcohol is ingested while taking this medication. Unfortunately, its use is probably limited because more serious complications such as hypotension and coma may occur if heavy ethanol intake is continued. Patients should be fully informed of the potential adverse effects that occur from drinking while receiving disulfiram. The medication should not be given to patients with arteriosclerotic heart disease, serious liver disease, or known hypersensitivity. Further, because of a large number of potential drug-drug interactions, caution should be used in treating patients on other medications, particularly warfarin, tranquilizers, and anticonvulsants.

Often, short-term hospitalization is necessary in initial management of alcoholism because of the propensity for the development of alcohol withdrawal syndromes in patients with true physiologic addiction. Although some individuals may be withdrawn and still continue as outpatients, the majority require inpatient care either in an alcohol detoxification center or in a general hospital.

ALCOHOL WITHDRAWAL SYNDROMES

Occurrence of withdrawal symptoms after cessation of alcohol ingestion is firm evidence of physical dependency on alcohol. The majority of patients in whom alcohol withdrawal syndromes are observed have been drinking heavily (over 100 g ethanol per day) for at least 1 to 4 weeks before onset of withdrawal. Periodic or binge drinkers seem to be at greater risk for this complication, although chronic continuous abusers of alcohol are not immune to this problem. The manifestations and severity of the withdrawal syndromes vary considerably. Severity of withdrawal symptoms has

TABLE 17.5–3. MICHIGAN ALCOHOLISM SCREENING TEST

	Yes	No
0. Do you enjoy a drink now and then?	0	
1. Do you feel you are a normal drinker? (By normal we mean you drink less than or as much as most other people.)		2[a]
2. Have you ever awakened the morning after some drinking the night before and found that you could not remember a part of the evening?	2	
3. Does your wife, husband, a parent, or other near relative ever worry or complain about your drinking?	2	
4. Can you stop drinking without a struggle after one or two drinks?		2
5. Do you feel guilty about your drinking?	1	
6. Do friends or relatives think you are a normal drinker?		2
7. Are you able to stop drinking when you want to?		2
8. Have you ever attended a meeting of Alcoholics Anonymous (AA)?	5	
9. Have you gotten into physical fights when drinking?	1	
10. Has your drinking ever created problems between you and your wife, husband, parent, or other relative?	2	
11. Has your wife, husband (or other family member) ever gone to anyone for help about your drinking?	2	
12. Have you ever lost friends because of your drinking?	2	
13. Have you ever gotten into trouble at work or school because of drinking?	2	
14. Have you ever lost a job because of drinking?	2	
15. Have you ever neglected your obligations, your family, or your work for two or more days in a row because you were drinking?	2	
16. Do you drink before noon fairly often?	1	
17. Have you ever been told you have liver trouble? Cirrhosis?	2	
18. After heavy drinking have you ever had delirium tremens (DTs) or severe shaking or heard voices or seen things that really weren't there?	2[b]	
19. Have you ever gone to anyone for help about your drinking?	2	
20. Have you ever been in a hospital because of drinking?	5	
21. Have you ever been a patient in a psychiatric hospital or on a psychiatric ward of a general hospital where drinking was part of the problem that resulted in hospitalization?	5	
22. Have you ever been seen at a psychiatric or mental health clinic or gone to any doctor, social worker or clergyman for help with any emotional problem, where drinking was part of the problem?	2	
23. Have you ever been arrested for drunk driving, driving while intoxicated, or driving under the influence of alcoholic beverages? (If *yes*, how many times? _____)	2[c]	
24. Have you ever been arrested, or taken into custody, even for a few hours, because of other drunken behavior? (If *yes*, how many times? _____)	2[c]	

Scoring System: ≤4 Nonalcoholic
5–6 Suggestive of alcoholism
≥7 Definite for alcoholism

Programs using the above scoring system find it very sensitive at the 5-point level; it tends to find more people alcoholic than anticipated. However, it is a screening test and should be sensitive at its lower levels.

Most alcoholics score 10 points or more.

The MAST is reproduced for self-administered use with patients and clients.

[a] Indicates alcoholic response and points for scoring.
[b] 5 points for delirium tremens.
[c] 2 points for *each* arrest.

not been well studied in relationship to levels and duration of intake of alcohol.

EARLY WITHDRAWAL (TREMULOUSNESS)

In select individuals, a mild degree of tremulousness and nausea may occur within 6 to 8 hours of the last drink. This mild withdrawal state may even serve as a stimulus for continued drinking. Of note is the fact that such symptoms may develop before blood ethanol concentration has reached zero.[10,22] Intake of ethanol abolishes the withdrawal syndrome at this time, but if abstinence is maintained, symptoms usually progress. Tremor may be generalized and increase with activity, in some instances becoming severe enough to prevent the patient from standing. Accompanying symptoms include facial flushing, mild sweating, anorexia, nausea,

and mild tachycardia. Sleeping becomes difficult, and the patient appears to be hyperalert. Mild disorientation with respect to time is common, but overall awareness of the surroundings and situation remains intact. Although administration of alcohol reverses the syndrome, it is not usually a part of routine medical management.

HALLUCINOSIS

Hallucinations and illusions are present in approximately 25 percent of alcoholics suffering from the early withdrawal syndrome. These hallucinations occur despite the fact that the patient may otherwise be oriented and alert. Visual illusions are more frequent than auditory. For example, the patient may mistake an intravenous pole for a threatening person. In contrast to the schizophrenic, the alcoholic most often responds appropriately to these hallucinations by seeking to escape from or to protect self from threatening objects or noises. In this setting, it is imperative that the patient be prevented from harming self or others. Rarely the hallucinations may persist for prolonged periods (up to several weeks). Nightmares and milder hallucinations occurring at night may be related to disturbances in REM sleep.

In general, the early withdrawal syndrome characterized by tremulousness, with or without associated hallucinosis and other symptoms, usually resolves within 48 to 72 hours. In hospitalized patients, benzodiazepines such as chlordiazepoxide, diazepam, or oxazepam may be helpful in managing these symptoms (see Chapter 16.5). Careful attention should, of course, be given to the patient's overall metabolic state, including proper degree of hydration and replacement of vitamins and minerals, particularly potassium and magnesium.

ALCOHOL-RELATED SEIZURE DISORDERS

Grand mal seizures may occur within the first 12 to 48 hours following alcohol withdrawal. Characteristically, these seizures are generalized and are not preceded by an aura. Most patients have several brief bursts of seizure activity within a short time, rather than a single isolated seizure.[21] Focal seizures suggest a central nervous system (CNS) lesion and are not alcohol related. However, patients with idiopathic or posttraumatic epilepsy may have seizures during alcohol withdrawal even after short periods of drinking. The interval electroencephalogram (EEG) is normal in patients with alcohol-induced withdrawal seizures and can be helpful in distinguishing this group from those with idiopathic or posttraumatic epilepsy. Intravenous diazepam may be used to control seizure activity (see Chapter 4.8), and the incidence of seizures may be reduced by prophylactic treatment with chlordiazepoxide, 50 to 100 mg intramuscularly daily, during periods of alcohol detoxification.[15] Other benzodiazepines may also be effective, but their use is unproven. Prophylactic use of phenytoin, 300 mg orally daily, also decreases the incidence of alcohol-related seizures,[14] but its use is not widely accepted because these patients often stop taking their medication when they resume heavy drinking. Cessation of anticonvulsants may precipitate status epilepticus. In any event, long-term anticonvulsant treatment of alcohol-induced withdrawal seizures is unnecessary. Alcohol withdrawal seizures may herald the onset of delirium tremens in up to one third of patients.

LATE WITHDRAWAL (DELIRIUM TREMENS)

Delirium tremens is a serious, potentially lethal, syndrome that occurs in approximately 5 percent of all patients with alcohol withdrawal symptoms. Confusion, marked agitation, and disorientation are the hallmarks of this syndrome, but autonomic hyperactivity is frequently associated with it. Fever (up to 40C), marked tachycardia, diaphoresis, hypertension, mydriasis, and gross tremor are all common. Although the majority of patients show symptoms of early withdrawal, delirium tremens may begin abruptly between 2 and 5 days after alcohol withdrawal. The clinical course is variable and may continue for 1 to 6 days, averaging 3 days. Previous estimates of mortality were as high as 10 to 20 percent, although this figure has been reduced to approximately 1 percent in most hospitals as a result of improvements in management.

Sedation is required in all patients, and can usually be achieved by parenteral administration of diazepam (10 to 40 mg intravenously) or chlordiazepoxide (25 to 100 mg intravenously). These doses can be repeated at 15-minute intervals until adequate sedation is achieved. These drugs can then be given at 6- to 8-hour intervals. The dose given should be the lowest needed to provide adequate sedation, since accumulation of both the drug and its active metabolites occurs during repeated administration. Restraints may be required, but their use should be judicious. Patients must be monitored carefully to prevent aspiration or peripheral nerve injuries. Intravenous fluids are usually required with careful assessment of serum electrolytes and state of hydration. Thiamine and vitamin B complex are recommended as part of overall medical management. It is important to note that the prognosis of delirium tremens and the frequency of complications are most often related to other accompanying problems including serious trauma or medical illnesses. Judicious medical management is necessary in these seriously ill patients.

ALCOHOL-RELATED DISORDERS OF THE CENTRAL NERVOUS SYSTEM

One of the major organ systems commonly affected by chronic ingestion of alcohol is the CNS. Acutely, ethanol acts as a CNS depressant, producing intoxication that may progress to respiratory depression and even death, as mentioned earlier. Many of the disorders of the CNS commonly associated with alcohol consumption are caused by concomitant nutritional deficiencies and are discussed separately.

ALCOHOLIC CEREBELLAR DEGENERATION

Degeneration of the anterior, superior vermis of the cerebellum may develop in some alcoholics. Histologically, severe loss of Purkinje cells with narrowing of the granular and molecular layers is seen.[23] Clinically, ataxia affecting the lower extremities and gait is more commonly observed than upper limb or speech involvement or nystagmus. In mild cases, only abnormalities of tandem gait may be demonstrable. The pathogenesis of this syndrome is unclear and is either a direct result of alcohol or possibly related to thiamine deficiency.

ALCOHOLIC POLYNEUROPATHY

Loss of ankle jerks and a mild polysensory loss affecting the feet are seen in approximately 25 percent of hospitalized alcoholics. Occasionally, the sensory loss may be accompanied by severe dysesthesias and paresthesias. In the most severe cases, sensory loss in a stocking-glove distribution and even muscle weakness result. Pathologic changes of the myelinated nerve fibers show noninflammatory degeneration of large fibers with occasional segmental demyelination. Again, the pathogenesis is uncertain. Some patients improve with adequate nutrition, B vitamin supplementation, and abstinence. However, vitamin replacement alone does not correct the disorder in a substantial number of affected alcoholics.

ALCOHOLIC RHABDOMYOLYSIS

Rhabdomyolysis, characterized by increases in serum creatine kinase (CK) up to 50,000 IU and myoglobinuria are seen in some

alcoholics. Whether this disorder occurs more frequently is unknown, because it rarely causes alcoholics to seek medical attention. Often it is difficult to determine the role of seizures, cold exposure, and trauma in the development of this syndrome. Its direct relationship to alcohol or the possibility that it is a multifactorial problem is unclear, but prompt recognition is important because myoglobinuria may produce acute renal failure.

ALCOHOL-RELATED GASTROINTESTINAL AND HEPATIC DISORDERS

The liver is the major organ injured by excessive alcohol ingestion. Gastritis and pancreatitis also occur in alcoholics. (These disorders are discussed in detail in Chapters 12.4 and 13.6.) Although much research has been conducted on the metabolism of ethanol and its effects on the liver, the pathogenesis of alcoholic liver disease remains uncertain. Clearly the amount and duration of excessive alcohol ingestion are the most important factors that determine the risk of developing serious alcoholic liver damage. One study suggests, however, that significant alcoholic liver injury occurs more commonly in individuals who drink more than 160 g of absolute ethanol per day for approximately 7 to 10 years.[8] Another report indicates that there may be an increased risk of alcohol cirrhosis in individuals consuming greater than 40 g of ethanol per day,[12] although neither study presents conclusive data.

ALCOHOL-RELATED NUTRITIONAL DEFICIENCIES

Alcoholism is the most frequent cause of nutritional deficiencies in developed countries. The etiology of these deficiencies is multifactorial. Decreased nutrient intake occurs because of substitution of ethanol for other dietary caloric sources. Further, ethanol interferes with absorption, metabolism, and storage of vitamins and minerals, as well as increasing urinary losses of these nutrients. These effects may increase nutrient requirements in the alcoholic and compound problems of poor nutritional intake. Specific nutritional deficiency syndromes and corresponding treatment are discussed in Chapter 14.10. A few of the most frequently encountered deficiencies are discussed below in detail to illustrate specifically how alcoholism can lead to nutritional deficiencies.

THIAMINE DEFICIENCY SYNDROMES

Severe thiamine deficiencies occurring in alcoholics may produce a syndrome characterized by ophthalmoplegia, ataxia, and mental disturbances (Wernicke encephalopathy). Ocular signs in this syndrome are most frequently nystagmus (both horizontal and vertical) with or without associated sixth nerve palsies. With sixth nerve palsies there is a loss of abduction with impairment of lateral gaze bilaterally. Amnesia and confusion with confabulation are prominent features. Ataxia is similar to that described with alcoholic cerebellar degeneration. Administration of as little as 100 to 200 mg of thiamine intravenously results in dramatic reversal of the signs and symptoms of this disorder within hours. The pathogenesis of Wernicke encephalopathy is complex; however, some studies suggest that individuals with a hereditary deficiency of the enzyme transketolase are particularly susceptible to its development.[2] This enzyme requires thiamine pyrophosphate as a cofactor in catalyzing certain steps of the hexose monophosphate shunt. Thiamine should be given before any glucose-containing solutions are administered to the alcoholic because glucose may acutely deplete limited thiamine reserves and precipitate Wernicke encephalopathy.

Beriberi is another syndrome caused by thiamine deficiency and may occur in some alcoholics. Weakness, fatigue, myalgias, anorexia, and cardiac problems are the major clinical features. There may be high-output congestive heart failure with prominent tachycardia. Circulatory collapse and sudden death are potential complications that emphasize the importance of thiamine replacement therapy in the alcoholic.

FOLIC ACID

Alcoholics generally have a decreased intake of folate caused by poor nutrition. Alcohol also impairs folate absorption from the gut, and increases its hepatic storage in a polyglutamate form, and decreases its biliary excretion and enterohepatic circulation.[16] Folic acid deficiency is common in alcoholics and may lead to megaloblastic anemia in severe cases. However, alcohol also appears to increase the MCV independent of its effects on foliate metabolism. Suppression of all bone marrow elements may occur with large alcohol intake unrelated to folate deficiency. Replacement therapy in alcoholics should include 1.0 mg of folic acid daily given either orally or parenterally.

PYRIDOXINE (VITAMIN B₆)

Pyridoxine deficiency may also occur in alcoholics as a result of decreased nutritional intake. Further, acetaldehyde displaces the active circulating form, pyridoxal phosphate, from binding to albumin, causing its increased degradation by membrane-bound alkaline phosphatases.[9] Pyridoxine deficiency may lead to development of sideroblastic anemia and may also cause peripheral neuropathy. Its role in the alcoholic polyneuropathy described above is unclear. In patients with alcoholic liver disease, decreased hepatic content of pyridoxal phosphate may be responsible for the low serum alanine aminotransferase, compared to serum aspartate aminotransferase, which is characteristically observed in these patients.

OTHER ALCOHOL-RELATED DISORDERS

METABOLIC SYNDROMES (KETOACIDOSIS AND HYPOGLYCEMIA)

In some patients, nondiabetic ketoacidosis may occur with little or no blood glucose elevation. Some of these patients have "chemical diabetes" but most have no detectable glucose intolerance. The syndrome occurs in those patients who have had a recent period of prolonged, heavy ethanol ingestion followed by anorexia, hyperemesis, and starvation. Clinically these patients have metabolic acidosis with some respiratory compensation. Laboratory testing for ketonemia and ketonuria may underestimate the extent of ketosis since β-hydroxybutyrate levels are increased to a greater degree than acetoacetate, which is the primary ketone measured by the nitroprusside reaction (Ketostix, Acetest). Ketogenesis is the result of increased fatty acid synthesis accompanied by decreased fatty acid oxidation resulting in excess catabolism of fatty acids to acetic acid residues. Both of these metabolic derangements are favored by the intracellular redox shift caused by alcohol metabolism (Table 17.5–1).

Fasting alcoholic hypoglycemia develops in a small number of patients. Prolonged fasting or liver disease may result in decreased hepatic glycogen stores. As mentioned, large amounts of alcohol inhibit hepatic gluconeogenesis, which exacerbates the risk of hypoglycemia in fasting individuals. Although inhibition of gluconeogenesis is multifactorial, there is evidence that changes in the intracellular redox state may be important in pathogenesis. Under ordinary circumstances these factors are compensated by release of glucagon and glucocorticoids.[5] Adrenal insufficiency may also be a risk factor for development of this rare syndrome.

Awareness and prompt recognition of the possibility of hypoglycemia in obtunded alcoholics who otherwise seem intoxicated is vital. Patients should be given glucose, 50 g intravenously if blood Dextrostix testing is less than 50 mg/dl. If properly treated, most

patients recover promptly, but the syndrome may be fatal if unrecognized.

OTHER DISORDERS PRESUMED TO BE ALCOHOL RELATED

ALCOHOLIC CARDIOMYOPATHY

Low-output heart failure has been described in a small number of alcoholics. This syndrome, called alcoholic cardiomyopathy, is distinguished from beriberi, because it is unresponsive to thiamine and the cardiac output is reduced rather than increased. Pathologically, the heart becomes enlarged and dilated, but no specific changes allow definitive diagnosis. Most affected patients have come from lower socioeconomic groups with poor nutrition. Men appear to be more susceptible than women. Large amounts of alcohol depress myocardial contractility and may be arrhythmogenic. Thus, patients with underlying congestive heart failure should be advised to limit alcohol intake to small and moderate amounts, for example, two drinks (30 g) per day. The possibility of postviral cardiomyopathy has not been excluded.

HYPOGONADISM AND TESTICULAR FAILURE

Hypogonadism and gynecomastia have long been associated with cirrhosis. Recent studies suggest that this association is much more frequent in alcoholic cirrhotics than in those with postnecrotic cirrhosis. Further, there is a suggestion that reduction in serum testosterone levels and impotence may occur in alcoholics with or without significant liver disease. The basis for this observed reduction in testosterone and gonadal function is presently under investigation. Both Leydig cells and seminiferous tubules are abnormal in alcoholics. Current evidence suggests that there may be defects in both gonadal function and in the hypothalamic-pituitary axis as a result of excessive alcohol consumption.[19,20]

REFERENCES

1. American Psychiatric Association. Diagnostic and Statistical Manual of Mental Disorders, DSM-IIIR, 3d ed. Prepared by the Committee on Nomenclature and Statistics of the American Psychiatric Association, Washington, DC, 1987
2. Blass JP, Gibson GE: Abnormality of a thiamine-requiring enzyme in patients with Wernicke-Korsakoff syndrome. N Engl J Med 297:1367, 1977
3. Chin JH, Goldstein DB: Effects of low concentrations of ethanol on the fluidity of spin-labeled erythrocyte and brain membranes. Mol Pharmacol 13:435, 1977
4. Goodwin DW: Genetic determinants of alcoholism. In Mendelson JH, Mello NK (eds): The Diagnostic and Treatment of Alcoholism. New York, McGraw-Hill, 1979, p 59
5. Gordon GG, Southren AL, Lieber CS: The effects of alcohol and alcoholic liver disease on the endocrine system and intermediary metabolism. In Lieber CS (ed): Medical Disorders of Alcoholics. Philadelphia, WB Saunders, 1982, p 105
6. Klatsky AL, Friedman GD, Siegelaub AB: Alcohol consumption before myocardial infarction. Results from the Kaiser-Permanente Epidemiologic Study of Myocardial Infarction. Ann Intern Med 81:294, 1974
7. Kramer JF, Cameron DC (eds): A manual on drug dependence. Geneva, World Health Organization, 1975, p 107
8. Lelbach WK: Quantitative aspects of drinking in alcoholic liver cirrhosis. In Khanna JM, Isreal Y, Kalant H (eds): Alcoholic Liver Pathology. Ontario, Addiction Research Foundation of Ontario, 1975
9. Lumeng L, Li TK: Plasma B_6 metabolism in chronic alcohol abuse. Pyridoxal phosphate levels in plasma and the effects of acetaldehyde on pyridoxal phosphate synthesis and degradation in human erythrocytes. J Clin Invest 53:693, 1974
10. Mello NK, Mendelson JH: Experimentally induced intoxication in alcoholics: A comparison between programmed and spontaneous drinking. J Pharmacol Exp Ther 173:101, 1970
11. Mendelson JH, Mello NK: Diagnostic criteria for alcoholism and alcohol abuse. In Mendelson JH and Mello NK (eds): The Diagnosis and Treatment of Alcoholism. New York, McGraw-Hill, 1979, p 2
12. Pequignot G, Tuyns AJ, Buta JL: Acute cirrhosis in relation to alcohol consumption. Int J Epidemiol 7:113, 1978
13. Rigter H, Crabbe JC Jr (eds): Alcohol Tolerance and Dependence. Amsterdam, Elsevier/North-Holland, 1980
14. Sampliner R, Iber FL: Diphenylhydantoin control of alcohol withdrawal seizures: Results of a controlled study. JAMA 230:1430, 1974
15. Sellers EM, Kalant H: Alcohol intoxication and withdrawal. N Engl J Med 294:757, 1976
16. Steinberg SE, Campbell CL, Hillman RS: Effect of alcohol on hepatic secretion of methylfolate in bile. Biochem Pharmacol 30:96, 1981
17. Tabakoff B, Hoffman PL: Alcohol and neurotransmitters. In Rigter H, Crabbe JC Jr (eds): Alcohol Tolerance and Dependence. Amsterdam, Elsevier/North-Holland, 1980, p 201
18. Turner TB, Mezey E, Kimball AW: Measurement of alcohol-related effects in man: Chronic effects in relation to consumption. Johns Hopkins Med J 141:235, 1977
19. Van Thiel DH, Lester R, Sherins RJ: Hypogonadism in alcoholic liver disease: Evidence for a double defect. Gastroenterology 67:118, 1974
20. Van Thiel DH, Lester R, Vaitakaitis J: Evidence for a defect in pituitary secretion of luteinizing hormone in chronic alcoholic men. J Clin Endocrinol Metab 47:488, 1978
21. Victor M: The pathophysiology of alcoholic epilepsy. In The addictive states. Res Publ Assoc Res Nervous Mental Disease 46:431, 1968
22. Victor M, Adams RD: The effect of alcohol on the nervous system. In Metabolic and toxic disease of the nervous system. Res Publ Assoc Res Nervous Mental Disease 32:526, 1953
23. Victor M, Adams RD, Mancall EL: A restricted form of cerebellar degeneration occurring in alcoholic patients. Arch Neurol 1:577, 1959
24. Whitehead TP, Clarke CA, Whitfield AG: Biochemical and hematological markers of alcohol intake. Lancet 1:978, 1978

CHAPTER 17.6
Ophthalmology in Medicine

Robert P. Murphy, Neil R. Miller, and Douglas A. Jabs

Ocular disorders are important to the general physician in three ways:

1. Certain systemic diseases have important ocular manifestations, for example, the retinopathy associated with diabetes mellitus. In these disorders the physician needs to know how to detect the ocular involvement and to understand how these findings may alter the diagnostic or therapeutic management of the patient. He also needs to know whether the management requires early collaboration with an ophthalmologist.

2. Certain patients may present themselves to the physician with specific ocular symptoms, for example, pain or double vision. Here the physician needs to be able to assess

the clinical symptom correctly and develop a rational diagnostic plan. Here, too, he must determine whether management requires referral to an ophthalmologist.

3. Finally, there are clinical signs referable to the eye that may or may not be associated with ocular symptoms, such as pupillary abnormalities or retinal hemorrhages. In these situations the clinician needs an approach to the differential diagnosis. This requires an understanding of the diseases or conditions that may produce such findings. This chapter is organized to reflect these aspects of ocular disorders.

OCULAR MANIFESTATIONS OF SYSTEMIC DISEASES[1-7]

Many systemic diseases have ocular manifestations. Ocular motility may be disrupted by various systemic myopathies or neuropathies. In addition, the ocular fundus is the sole location in the body permitting observation of both arteries and veins. The retinal vessels may be affected by systemic diseases in the same way as the vasculature in other parts of the body.

DIABETES AND DIABETIC RETINOPATHY

Diabetic retinopathy is an important cause of blindness throughout the world, and it is the most frequent cause of blindness in patients under 60 years of age in the United States. The prevalence of diabetic retinopathy is directly correlated with the duration of the disease. After 6 years of diabetes, almost one fourth of patients have some degree of retinopathy, and after 25 years 95 percent have retinopathy. Retinopathy is frequently associated with generalized microangiopathy involving small vessels throughout the body. Most noteworthy are the vascular lesions of the renal glomeruli resulting in diffuse and nodular glomerulosclerosis.

Ophthalmoscopic Findings

Diabetic retinopathy is conveniently divided into a background stage, in which the vascular changes are contained within the retina, and a proliferative stage, in which new vessels proliferate through the inner surface of the retina (Table 17.6–1; Color Plate: Fig. 17.6–1A,B).* A more florid and advanced phase of *background* diabetic retinopathy is referred to as "preproliferative" retinopathy.[6]

Microaneurysms are the earliest signs of retinopathy. In *simple* background retinopathy, small microaneurysms along with dot-and-blot hemorrhages are usually scattered at random throughout the posterior retina. Hard exudates, small lipoprotein deposits, frequently take a ring or circinate pattern. Retinal edema is common in background retinopathy and can cause mild to moderate visual blurring (Color Plate: Fig. 17.6–1B).

In *preproliferative* background retinopathy, cotton-wool spots were previously thought to indicate an associated "hypertensive" component to the diabetic retinopathy. However, these areas (representing local retinal infarcts) occur commonly in normotensive diabetic patients with no history of hypertension. Venous beading consists of the irregular sausage-shaped changes in the appearance of the retinal veins. Intraretinal microvascular abnormalities—dilated capillary-shunt vessels in the retina—frequently develop around the focal areas of capillary nonperfusion. The triad of preproliferative retinopathy (cotton-wool spots, venous beading, and microvascular abnormalities) should alert the examiner to a more progressive and florid stage of retinopathy. Eyes with moderate or advanced preproliferative characteristics have a 50 percent chance of developing neovascularization within 1 year.

In proliferative retinopathy, the neovascularization can lead to visual loss by causing vitreous hemorrhage or the development of a fibrovascular scar. The latter (which is adherent to retina and

---

*Color Plate: Fig. 17.6–1A to L appears after page 1190.

TABLE 17.6–1. OPHTHALMOSCOPIC SIGNS OF DIABETIC RETINOPATHY

Background diabetic retinopathy
Simple
- Microaneurysms
- Dot-and-blot hemorrhages
- Hard exudates
- Macular edema

Preproliferative
- Soft exudates (cotton-wool spots)
- Beaded veins
- Intraretinal microvascular abnormalities
- Extensive intraretinal hemorrhages frequently present

Proliferative diabetic retinopathy
- Neovascularization emanating from disc area
- Neovascularization emanating from elsewhere in fundus
- Vitreous hemorrhage
- Traction retinal detachment

---

vitreous) can induce further hemorrhage or cause traction or tear-related (rhegmatogenous) retinal detachment, which can cause severe visual loss.

Therapy of Diabetic Retinopathy

Patients with background retinopathy do not generally require treatment unless significant macular edema is present. The therapeutic efficacy of photocoagulation and of aspirin in simple background retinopathy and in preproliferative retinopathy is under prospective study. Photocoagulation has been shown to reduce visual loss from macular edema and from high-risk proliferative diabetic retinopathy.

It is recommended that patients with any stage of diabetic retinopathy have routine ophthalmologic consultations. Patients with simple background retinopathy should have detailed eye examinations at least yearly. Patients with preproliferative changes should be promptly referred, and the ophthalmologist will usually observe these cases at approximately 3-month intervals. All patients demonstrating any form of proliferative retinopathy (neovascularization at the optic disc or elsewhere in the retina) should be promptly referred for consideration of photocoagulation therapy. Eyes with optic disc neovascularization or any neovascularization with vitreous hemorrhage are at high risk of developing severe visual loss. Prompt photocoagulation of these eyes can significantly reduce the risk of blindness.

Vitrectomy is often successful in selected cases of advanced proliferative diabetic retinopathy with dense vitreous hemorrhages or fibrous tissue causing traction detachment of the retina.

Control of Diabetes and Retinopathy

Although clinical reports of small populations of patients and animal studies suggest that multiple insulin injections with improved control of diabetes reduce the occurrence of diabetic retinopathy, neither the experimental nor the human studies can be considered conclusive. Nevertheless, there is sufficient evidence to recommend a strong effort to maintain good control of the diabetic patient.

Other Ocular Changes of Diabetes

Cataracts develop at an earlier age in diabetics than in the normal population. In children with very high blood sugars before the diabetes is regulated, a diffuse punctate opacification of the lens may occasionally occur, causing poor vision. *Neovascularization of the iris* (rubeosis iridis) is a serious complication of proliferative diabetic retinopathy and can cause a severe type of glaucoma.

HYPERTENSIVE AND ATHEROSCLEROTIC RETINOPATHY

Although mild retinal vascular abnormalities may occur in patients with atherosclerosis without associated systemic hypertension, the

TABLE 17.6–2. GRADING OF HYPERTENSIVE-ARTERIOSCLEROTIC RETINOPATHY

Grade I
- Slight generalized arteriolar narrowing
- Increased arteriolar light reflexes
- Mild arteriovenous (A-V) compression (nicking)

Grade II
- Copper wire arterioles
- Moderate A-V nicking
- A-V crossings at right angles

Grade III
- Silver-wire arterioles
- Flame hemorrhages
- Occasional soft exudates (retinal infarcts)
- Prominent A-V nicking

Grade IV
- Optic disc edema
- Silver-wire arterioles, perivascular sheathing
- Numerous soft exudates
- Flame hemorrhages, especially around the disc
- Marked A-V nicking
- Macular exudates—star pattern

most severe vascular changes are seen with systemic hypertension. It is convenient to provide a general grade to the fundus changes using the broader category of *hypertensive arteriosclerotic* retinopathy (Table 17.6–2).

Retinal examination is especially reliable in accelerated hypertension where cotton-wool spots and papilledema accurately reflect the hypertensive crisis. For lesser degrees of systemic atherosclerosis and arteriosclerosis, the retinal findings are a useful guide to the systemic vasculature but may not always reflect precisely the degree of generalized vascular disease.

Retinal changes associated with hypertension or atherosclerosis do not generally result in irreversible visual impairment; however, during hypertensive crises or as a result of atherosclerosis, the optic nerve may become ischemic, resulting in permanent visual loss. There is no specific treatment for hypertensive-atherosclerotic retinopathy, since it usually resolves once the underlying systemic disease is controlled.

In patients with either eclampsia or pheochromocytoma, fundus changes of severe hypertension may develop acutely. Generalized advanced arteriolar narrowing, cotton-wool spots, and diffuse retinal edema occur. In severe cases, bilateral retinal detachments result from fluid extravasation beneath the retina. Once the hypertension is controlled, the detachments subside, and the retinal vessels rapidly return to normal unless the hypertension has been long-standing. In the latter cases, arteriolar narrowing and arteriovenous compressions persist.

HEMATOLOGIC AND IMMUNOLOGIC DISORDERS

The eye may become involved in various hematologic disorders as well as in all of the blood dyscrasias (Table 17.6–3).

Patients who are immunodeficient or immunosuppressed are also prone to a variety of ocular infections. These include external infection of the eye with viruses, such as herpes zoster ophthalmicus, and infection of the retina (retinitis) or entire eye (endophthalmitis) with normally nonpathogenic organisms, including fungi such as *Candida* and viruses such as herpes simplex and cytomegalovirus. Any ocular infection that occurs in a debilitated or immunosuppressed patient should be managed by an ophthalmologist as soon as possible.

Graft-versus-Host Disease
After bone marrow transplantation (BMT), patients may develop either acute or chronic graft-versus-host disease (GVHD), which affects the skin, liver, and gastrointestinal tract. Patients with acute GVHD may develop a dry-eye syndrome caused by lacrimal gland involvement, or they may develop a pseudomembranous conjunctivitis associated with severe cutaneous GVHD. The majority of patients with chronic GVHD will develop a dry-eye syndrome that requires treatment with tear substitutes and bland ophthalmic ointments. While immunosuppressed, BMT patients may also develop ocular infections, particularly *Candida* retinitis.

TABLE 17.6–3. THE EYE IN HEMATOLOGIC DISORDERS

Disease	Cornea	Conjunctiva	Anterior Chamber	Vitreous	Retina	Orbit
Anemia (see Chapter 6.2)		Pallor			Hemorrhages	
Polycythemia (see Chapter 6.17)		Tortuous vessels			Hemorrhages Dilated veins	
Hemoglobinopathies (see Chapter 6.5) S-C and S-thal		Comma-shaped conjunctival vessel		Hemorrhages	Hemorrhages, scarring, neovascularization, detachment	
S-S and S-A					Hemorrhages	
Leukemias (see Chapters 6.15, 6.16) Lymphomas (see Chapter 6.18)	Peripheral infiltrates	Focal cellular accumulations	Uveitis Hemorrhages	Hemorrhages	Hemorrhages Roth spots	Chloroma
Lymphocytic					Infiltration[a]	
Histiocytic			Uveitis	Cellular accumulation	Infiltration[a] Hemorrhages	
Dysproteinemia (see Chapter 6.19)	Crystalline deposits	Focal cellular accumulations			Hemorrhages Dilated veins Macular edema	

[a]Usually in the form of specific masses, often involving the lacrimal gland.

Acquired Immunodeficiency Syndrome (AIDS)

A microangiopathy affecting the retinal blood vessels is seen in approximately 75 percent of AIDS patients and consists of cotton-wool spots with or without intraretinal hemorrhages. Although AIDS patients may develop any opportunistic infection of the eye, they are particularly prone to cytomegalovirus retinitis, which develops in approximately 25 percent of such patients.

RHEUMATOLOGIC DISORDERS

Joint Disease

Ocular involvement in rheumatologic disorders is common and often severe. Patients with adult rheumatoid arthritis (see Chapter 8.7) may develop either a dry-eye syndrome or scleritis. The Sjögren syndrome (see Chapter 8.6) is caused by inflammation of the lacrimal and salivary glands and produces a dry eye (keratoconjunctivitis sicca) in approximately 15 percent of patients with rheumatoid arthritis. Such patients often describe an irritated, sandy sensation in their eyes or complain that the eyes feel tired. The diagnosis of a dry eye is made by testing basal tear secretions and the integrity of the ocular surface. After a topical anesthetic has been placed in both eyes, Schirmer test strips are hooked over the lateral third of both lower lids. After 5 minutes the wetting of the strips is measured. Abnormal tear secretion with this test is less than 5 mm of wetting. The integrity of the ocular surface can be tested with rose bengal drops, which are placed on the eye and stain, in a punctate fashion, tissues damaged by drying. Such patients are best treated with artificial tear solutions and ointments used as often as needed to eliminate symptoms and preserve the integrity of the ocular surface. Drops may be required as frequently as every hour or more. If this treatment fails, soft contact lenses or occlusion of tear drainage pathways may be of benefit.

Scleritis is an inflammation of the white collagenous coat of the eye and may be a painful, erythematous, florid condition (anterior scleritis or posterior scleritis, which may decrease vision), or a quiet dissolution of the sclera with perforation (scleromalacia perforans). The cornea may also be involved peripherally as part of a sclerokeratitis. The treatment of scleritis involves the use of both topical corticosteroids and systemic anti-inflammatory agents such as indomethacin or corticosteroids.

Patients with juvenile rheumatoid arthritis (JRA) frequently develop uveitis. Older boys with oligoarticular JRA often have spondylitis, and these patients frequently develop an acute anterior uveitis. Young girls with an oligoarticular JRA, however, are subject to an insidious and often asymptomatic chronic anterior uveitis. These patients have a positive antinuclear antibody (ANA) test. For this reason, patients with JRA should be examined by an ophthalmologist at regular intervals.

The spondyloarthropathies are a group of related diseases, which include ankylosing spondylitis, the Reiter syndrome, and spondylitis in association with either inflammatory bowel disease or psoriasis (psoriatic spondylitis; see Chapter 8.9). Acute anterior uveitis occurs in approximately 25 percent of these patients and is generally manifested by a painful, photophobic red eye and blurred vision. When this occurs, the patient should be referred to an ophthalmologist for management. The treatment of uveitis involves depressing the inflammatory response with topical and, if necessary, systemic corticosteroids. Mydriatics are also used to relieve pain and prevent scarring, which may lead to secondary glaucoma. Patients with the Reiter syndrome may also develop a simple conjunctivitis.

Connective Tissue Disease

Involvement of the eye in connective tissue disease, such as systemic lupus erythematosus (SLE; see Chapter 8.2) and systemic sclerosis (see Chapter 8.5), is common. Ocular manifestations of SLE include involvement of the lids by cutaneous lupus, secondary Sjögren's syndrome with dry eye, retinal vascular disease, and neuroophthalmic lesions. The most common retinal vascular lesions are cotton-wool spots (Color Plate: Fig. 17.6–1C), which are microinfarcts of the nerve fiber layer of the retina that occur in 25 percent of hospitalized patients with SLE. Far less commonly, lupus patients may develop a retinal vasculitis, resulting in severe visual loss. Optic nerve involvement can occur in patients with lupus and may be seen either as an acute visual loss (optic neuritis, ischemic optic neuropathy) or as a slowly progressive visual loss. Ocular involvement in scleroderma includes sclerodermatous lid disease with corneal exposure, a dry-eye syndrome, and fine telangiectatic abnormalities of the conjunctival blood vessels. In the CREST syndrome (see Chapter 8.5; Calcinosis, Raynaud phenomenon, Esophageal dysmotility, Sclerodactyly, and Telangiectasis) the dry-eye syndrome appears to be secondary to lacrimal gland inflammation, whereas in progressive systemic sclerosis it may be caused by glandular fibrosis.

Systemic Vasculitis

Loss of vision in the patient with giant-cell (temporal) arteritis (see Chapter 8.3) is an ocular and medical emergency. Although systemic symptoms, such as fever, malaise, and polymyalgia rheumatica, frequently precede the ocular involvement, these symptoms may be ignored, and sudden loss of visual acuity in one or both eyes may be the presenting symptom. The suspicion of giant-cell arteritis by the internist demands immediate ocular assessment. Although high-dose systemic corticosteroid administration may abort visual loss in the second eye, recovery of vision in the involved eye is rare. Ocular involvement includes ischemic optic neuropathy, central retinal artery occlusion, and retinal ischemia.

Patients with polyarteritis nodosa (see Chapter 8.3) and Wegener granulomatosis may have ocular involvement with scleritis, sclerokeratitis, and corneal ulceration. Ocular involvement in Wegener granulomatosis is common and occurs in 50 to 60 percent of patients. Scleritis may be extremely severe (necrotizing scleritis), and corneal ulceration may lead to perforation. In addition, patients with vasculitis may develop involvement of the retinal vessels either with cotton-wool spots (Color Plate: Fig. 17.6–1C) or a more severe retinal vasculitis. Patients with Wegener granulomatosis may also have orbital involvement (orbital pseudotumor) as part of their granulomatous disease.

All patients with systemic vasculitis and ocular involvement should be observed closely by both the ophthalmologist and the internist. Treatment is usually a combination of topical and systemic corticosteroids, often with systemic immunosuppressive agents, and should be determined by the two physicians together.

SARCOIDOSIS

Ocular involvement by sarcoidosis is common and occurs in approximately 26 percent of these patients (see Chapter 3.5). The most common ocular finding is an anterior uveitis, which may be either acute or chronic. Patients with chronic sarcoid uveitis often have a "granulomatous" uveitis, characterized clinically by large collections of inflammatory cells on the corneal endothelium (keratic precipitates) seen on slit-lamp examination. Posterior uveitis with either involvement of the choroid by sarcoid granulomata or involvement of the retinal vessels (candle-wax dripping) may be seen. Although many patients with sarcoid uveitis can be treated with topical corticosteroids, those with chronic ocular inflammation or involvement of the posterior part of the eye may require treatment with systemic corticosteroids as well. Lacrimal gland involvement by sarcoidosis may result in either enlargement of the gland, simulating a tumor, or a dry-eye syndrome.

THYROID DISEASE

Patients with autoimmune thyroid diseases (Graves disease and chronic lymphocytic thyroiditis) may develop a characteristic set of ophthalmologic and orbital changes, which have been termed "dysthyroid" or "Graves ophthalmopathy" (see Chapter 14.4). These problems usually develop coincidentally with the thyroid disease, but they may occur before the onset of thyroid dysfunc-

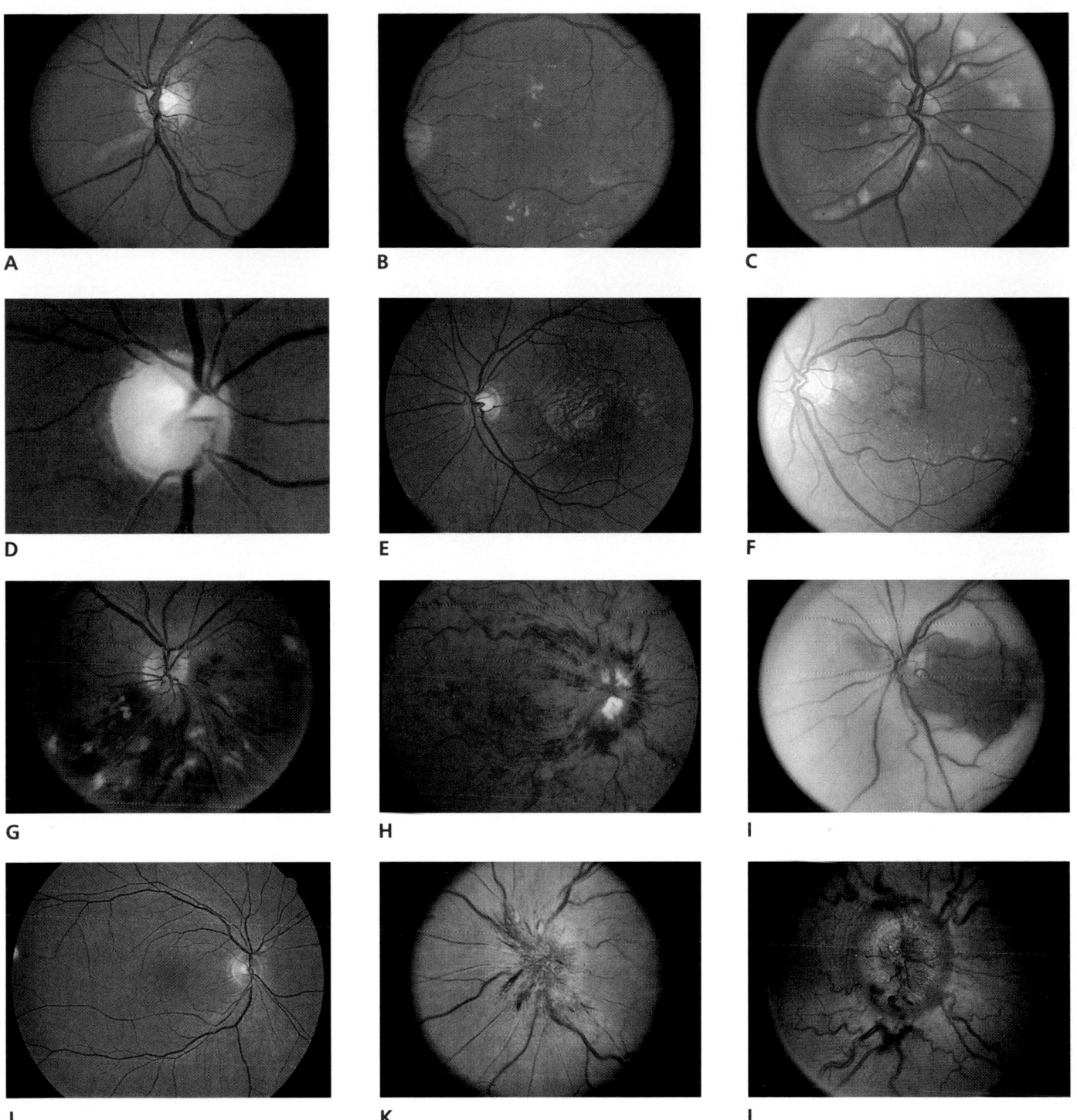

Figure 17.6–1. A. Proliferative diabetic retinopathy with extensive neovascularization of the optic nerve (NVD). **B.** Diabetic macular edema with hard exudates and thickening of the macula causing loss of transparency. **C.** Cotton-wool spots in patient with systemic lupus erythematosus. (Reproduced from Severe Retinal Vaso-Occlusive Disease in Systemic Lupus Erythematosus, *Archives of Ophthalmology,* 104:560, April 1986, Copyright 1986, American Medical Association) **D.** Chronic (open angle) glaucoma with extensive cupping of the optic disc. **E.** Atrophic macula in age-related macular degeneration. **F.** Choroidal neovascularization in age-related macular degeneration with subretinal fluid and hemorrhage coming from the abnormal choroidal vessels. **G.** Inferior branch retinal vein occlusion with segmental retinal hemorrhages and cotton-wool spots. **H.** Central retinal vein occlusion with extensive intraretinal hemorrhages. **I.** Central retinal artery occlusion with diffuse ischemic whitening of the retina, sparing the macula (which is supplied by a separate cilio-retinal artery). **J.** Multiple arteriolar emboli following coronary artery bypass surgery. **K.** Anterior ischemic optic neuropathy. Note the swelling of disc with dilated vessels and hemorrhages. **L.** Papilledema showing marked hyperemia and elevation of optic disc, blurring at the disc margin, and superficial peripapillary hemorrhages.

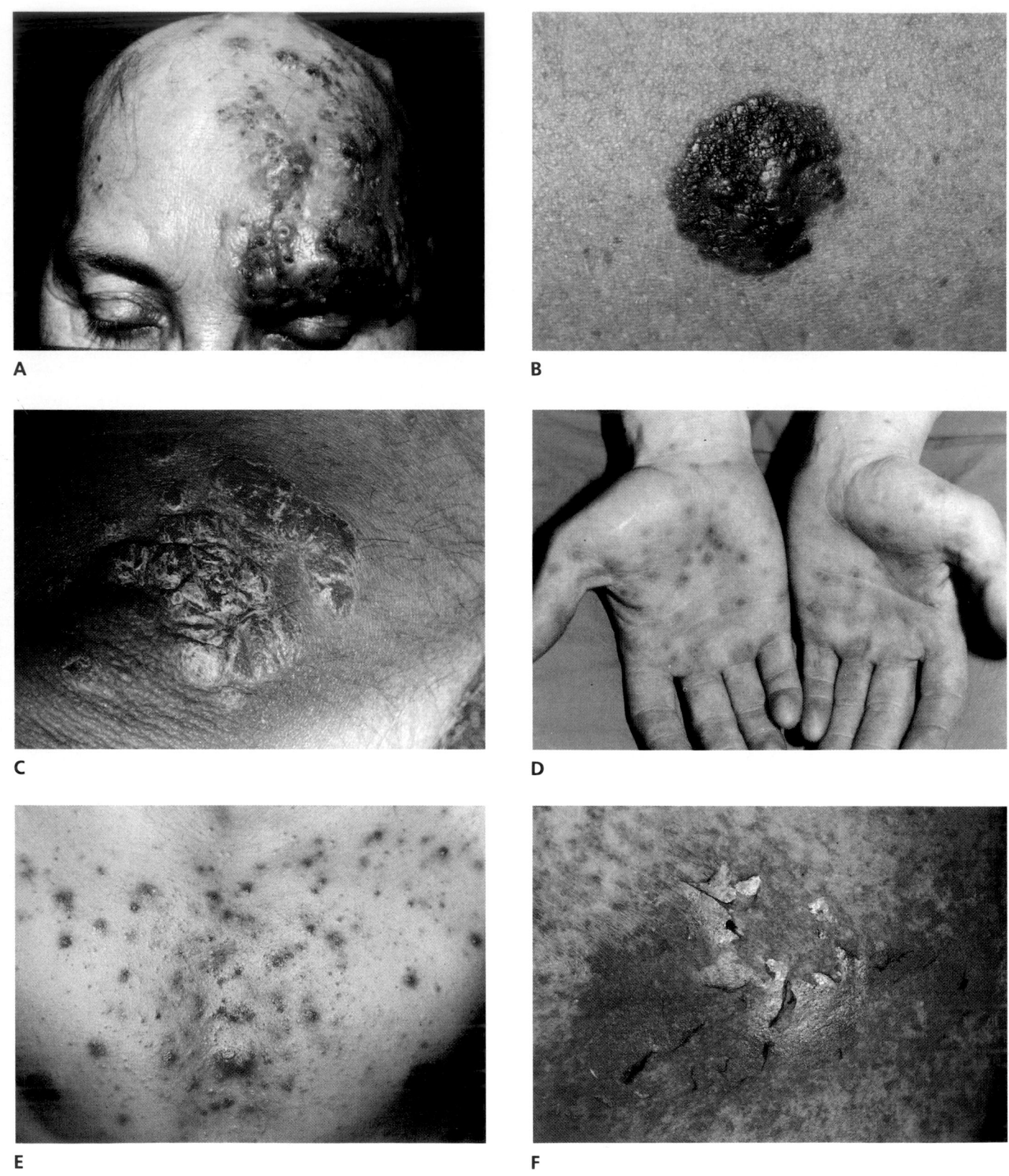

Figure 17.7–5. A. Severe herpes zoster involving the ophthalmic division of the trigeminal nerve. **B.** Variegated color in a cutaneous melanoma. **C.** Psoriatic plaque with classic silvery scale. **D.** Bull's eye lesions seen in erythema multiforme. **E.** Cysts, papulopustules, and comedones in a patient with moderately severe acne. **F.** Denuded skin in a patient with toxic epidermal necrolysis.

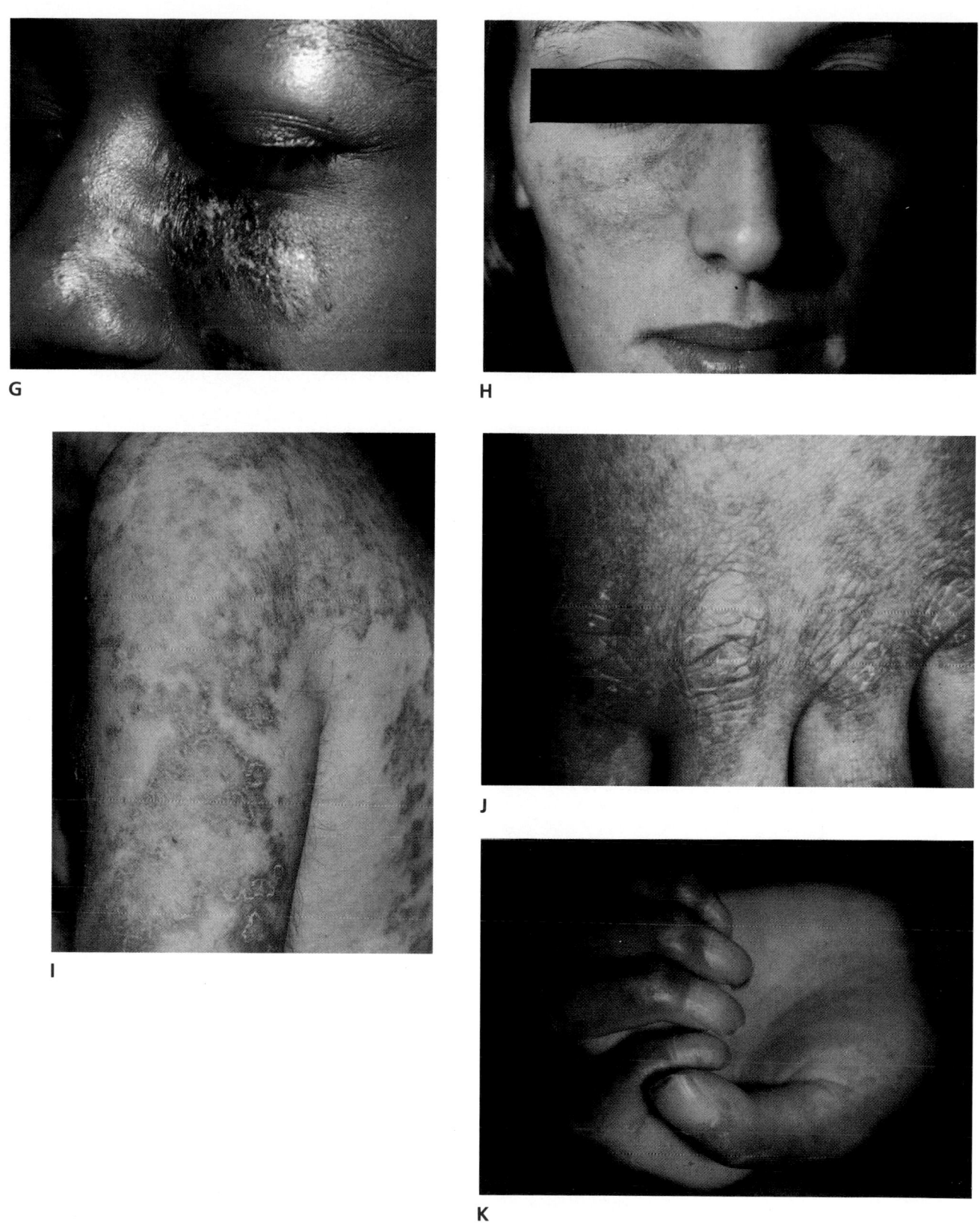

Figure 17.7–5. (Continued)
G. Scarring discoid lupus lesion. **H.** Classic malar distribution of butterfly rash in lupus. **I.** Polycyclic lesions in subacute cutaneous lupus erythematosus. **J.** Gottron papules in dermatomyositis. **K.** Marked flexion contracture and resorption of terminal phalanges in scleroderma.

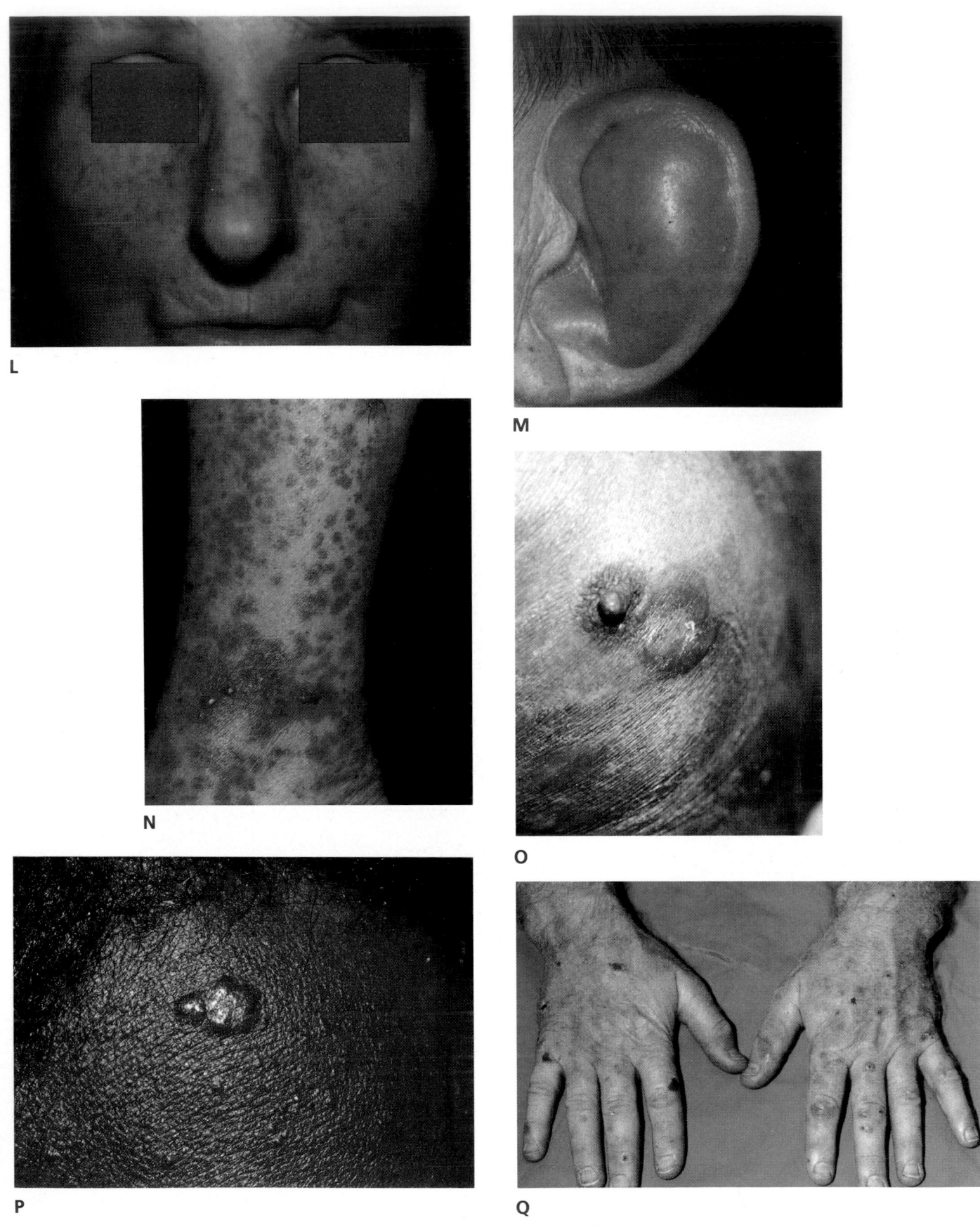

Figure 17.7–5. (Continued)
L. Characteristic telangiectatic mats in CRST syndrome. **M.** Marked ear involvement in relapsing polychondritis. **N.** Characteristic cutaneous features of vasculitis. **O.** Eroded plaques of mycosis fungoides. **P.** Skin colored nodule of sarcoidosis. **Q.** Characteristic hemorrhagic bullae on dorsa of hands in porphyria cutanea tarda.

tion or worsen when the thyroid disorder is under good control. Euthyroid Graves ophthalmopathy refers to the occurrence of this characteristic eye disease in the absence of any signs or symptoms of thyroid dysfunction. In many of these patients, however, a subtle abnormality of thyroid function may be revealed by TRH stimulation, T₃ suppression testing, or the detection of antithyroid antibodies.

The pathogenesis of dysthyroid ophthalmopathy is believed to be autoimmune. Both circulating antibodies and enhanced T cell reactivity specific to orbital antigens have been observed. Pathologically, there is infiltration of the orbital contents by mucopolysaccharide substances and chronic inflammatory cells, particularly lymphocytes. Swelling of the retroocular fat and extraocular muscles may result in protrusion of the eye (proptosis or exophthalmos), exposure keratitis, restricted ocular motility, and diplopia. In severe cases, infiltration of the extraocular muscles at their origin at the orbital apex causes compression of the optic nerve leading to progressive visual loss.

Treatment is directed at specific abnormalities as they arise (Table 17.6–4). Patients with significant dysthyroid ophthalmopathy should be observed by an ophthalmologist with regular measurements of visual acuity, intraocular pressure, and the degree of proptosis. Proptosis can be quantified with an exophthalmometer, a device that uses prisms to measure the distance from the lateral orbital rim to the corneal apex.

MYASTHENIA GRAVIS

Approximately 75 percent of patients with myasthenia gravis first complain of double vision (diplopia) or drooping of their eyelids (ptosis), and 90 percent of patients with the disease will eventually develop ocular signs and symptoms. Typically, the onset of either ptosis or diplopia is insidious, intermittent, and fatigue related. Ptosis is usually incomplete and asymmetric but may be bilateral and severe. Diplopia may be vertical, horizontal, or skewed. Differentiation from ocular motor nerve pareses is often extremely difficult unless other systemic signs and symptoms are present. As with other systemic manifestations of the disease, the diagnosis is based on a positive edrophonium (Tensilon) or neostigmine (Prostigmin) test (see Chapter 15.15).

The ocular signs of myasthenia gravis may be refractory to treatment with anticholinesterase agents, although they do tend to improve with systemic corticosteroid therapy. Devices to elevate the eyelids may be affixed to the patient's glasses in some cases to alleviate residual ptosis (ptosis crutches); however, some patients with severe, residual diplopia may need constant patching of one eye. Surgery of the ocular muscles is never indicated.

Approximately 10 percent of patients have a purely ocular form of myasthenia gravis. This diagnosis can only be made after the patient has been without systemic symptoms and signs for about 2 years. It is important to remember, however, that the vast majority of patients in whom myasthenia gravis presents with ocular symptoms and signs will develop systemic myasthenia within 18 months. For this reason, such patients should be closely observed not only by an ophthalmologist but also by an internist or a neurologist.

COMMONLY USED SYSTEMIC DRUGS AND THEIR OCULAR SIDE EFFECTS

Several commonly used systemic drugs have ocular side effects. In many cases, the effects are insignificant; however, in certain instances the ocular symptoms and signs are not only significant but also irreversible (Table 17.6–5).

COMMON OCULAR SYMPTOMS

Many patients with ocular disorders may first consult an internist with their symptoms. The physician should know which symptoms require immediate attention by an ophthalmologist and which symptoms are minor.

OCULAR PAIN

Most pain that occurs in or around the eyes is associated with ocular inflammation or irritation. The etiology is usually found within the eye or on its surface. On rare occasions, diseases that affect the trigeminal nerve, such as migraine or aneurysm, cause severe pain that is referred to the eye and orbit. Patients with severe ocular pain should first be examined carefully by an ophthalmologist. If no ocular abnormality is found, a neurologic evaluation should be undertaken.

DIPLOPIA

Although acquired diplopia may occur as a monocular phenomenon in rare patients with opacities of the ocular media and as a functional disorder, most patients with acquired diplopia have a misalignment of the eye caused by abnormalities in the ocular muscles or in their innervation. The diagnosis of binocular diplopia is made by covering either eye and noting disappearance of the double vision. Binocular diplopia may be myopathic or neuropathic in origin. It has already been mentioned that two systemic diseases that may produce diplopia are thyroid disease and myasthenia gravis. These entities should always be considered in a patient who develops double vision without other symptoms of neurologic disease. In addition to myopathic and neuromuscular disorders, diplopia is often caused by paralysis of one or more of the three ocular motor nerves (Table 17.6–6).

VISUAL LOSS

Loss of visual acuity is always a significant symptom and usually indicates major ocular disease. In assessing the patient with visual loss, the physician should pay careful attention to whether the visual loss has been intermittent or permanent, how long it has lasted, and whether there are any associated symptoms.

Although some of the disorders mentioned in Tables 17.6–7 to 17.6–10 are manifestations of systemic diseases, most of them are purely ocular disorders. As such, some of the more important ocular disorders require further comment.

TABLE 17.6–4. THYROID EYE DISEASE

Symptoms	Signs	Treatment
Tired, irritated eyes	Conjunctival redness	Tear substitutes
Lid swelling	Conjunctival and eyelid edema	Elevate head of bed at night
Prominent stare	Lid retraction and lag	Eyelid surgery
Prominent eyes	Proptosis	Depends on severity[a]
Double vision	Limitation of ocular motility	Prisms occasionally of benefit; surgical correction usually required
Pain and blurred vision	Corneal ulceration from chronic exposure	Tarsorrhaphy; tear substitutes; orbital decompression
Blurred vision	Optic nerve dysfunction (from orbital compression)	Systemic steroids; orbital decompression; radiation to posterior orbit

[a]There is no specific treatment for proptosis. Some physicians consider the cosmetic deformity alone an indication for orbital decompression. In most cases, treatment is directed toward the specific problems caused by the proptosis, for example, corneal exposure, diplopia, or compressive optic neuropathy.

TABLE 17.6–5. SYSTEMIC DRUGS AND THEIR OCULAR TOXICITY

Drug	Condition	Comments
Atropine	Blurred vision	Caused by paralysis of accommodation; systemic administration of atropine has *never* been shown to cause glaucoma[a]
Amiodarone	Corneal deposits	May cause occasional "halos" but usually not visually significant; reversible when drug discontinued
Chloramphenicol	Optic neuropathy	Rare; test visual acuity, color vision; usually reversible with withdrawal of drug
	Erythema multiforme bullosum (Stevens-Johnson syndrome)[b]	Variable scarring of conjunctiva causing dry eye syndrome. If mild, may respond to tear substitutes; however, if severe, irreversible blindness results
Chloroquine	Corneal deposits	Not clinically significant; disappear on withdrawal of drug
	Retinal degeneration	Visual function slowly lost; may be irreversible or progress after drug is withdrawn; regular testing of visual acuity, visual fields important
Corticosteroids	Cataracts	Related to length of use; irreversible; may progress despite steroid withdrawal; good prognosis with surgery
	Glaucoma	Dose and time-related; genetic predisposition; intraocular pressure returns to normal when drug is stopped. May require topical medication or surgery for control
Ethambutol	Optic neuropathy	Dose related; usually reversible if early withdrawal; not usually seen if dose kept at 15 mg/kg or less. Test visual acuity, color vision, and central visual field at 6-mo intervals
Oxygen	Retrolental fibroplasia	In premature infants; related to incomplete development of retinal vasculature; monitor arterial blood gases
Phenothiazines	Eyelid skin pigmentation Blurred vision	After long-term therapy; caused by either temporary accommodative paralysis or induction of myopia; transient and reversible
	Corneal deposits	Not significant; reversibility uncertain
	Lens opacities	Not significant
	Chorioretinopathy	Most significant side effect; almost exclusively with piperidines, such as Mellaril; dose and time related; usually partially reversible with low total doses; check visual acuity, visual fields, and electroretinogram (if indicated)
Tetracycline	Papilledema (pseudotumor cerebri)	Also seen with vitamin A intoxication and nalidixic acid; syndrome resolves once drug withdrawn; loss of visual acuity or field may result depending on duration and severity of papilledema

[a]Similarly, the belladonna alkaloids used for various gastrointestinal disorders do not cause or exacerbate glaucoma.
[b]May also be caused by sulfonamides and penicillin.

Glaucoma

Glaucoma is defined as an elevation of intraocular pressure that damages the optic nerve and may ultimately result in loss of peripheral visual field and central visual acuity. There are two principal types of glaucoma that are determined by the anatomic configuration of the anterior chamber and should be considered as completely separate entities.

TABLE 17.6–6. OCULAR MOTOR NERVE PALSIES[a]

Type	Signs	Probable Etiology
Third nerve palsy	Ptosis Limitation of elevation Limitation of depression Limitation of adduction May or may not have pupillary involvement	With pupillary involvement: aneurysm; tumor; trauma Without pupillary involvement: diabetes mellitus
Fourth nerve palsy	Hypertropia on side of palsy Often have head tilt to opposite side May notice torsional diplopia	Trauma; rarely diabetes mellitus or hypertension
Sixth nerve palsy	Limitation of abduction	Vascular; trauma; tumor, especially nasopharyngeal or metastatic carcinoma

[a]What appears to be a partial ocular motor nerve palsy may actually represent the effects of a systemic disorder, such as thyroid disease or myasthenia gravis.

Acute Narrow-angle Glaucoma. In patients with narrow angles, the access of the aqueous humor to the outflow channels of the eye is partially blocked by the iris root. When the pupil dilates, either in sustained darkness or in response to drugs, the angle becomes completely blocked, and intraocular pressure rises. The patient may initially note blurred vision and halos around lights as the pressure begins to rise. As the pressure continues to rise, the patient develops severe, deep ocular pain, often with nausea and vomiting. Vision becomes extremely blurred and may be completely lost. The eye itself becomes red with a hazy cornea and a nonreactive pupil (Table 17.6–11). During an acute attack of narrow-angle glaucoma, the intraocular pressure will range between 40 and 90 mm Hg compared to the normal range of 10 to 20 mm Hg. When the pressure is increased to these levels, digital palpation reveals a firm, hard globe compared to the other eye.

Prompt referral to an ophthalmologist for immediate therapy is essential. If an ophthalmologist is not readily available, the physician should institute treatment with pilocarpine drops every 10 minutes. In addition, either oral glycerin or intravenous mannitol should be used to lower the intraocular pressure. Definitive therapy consists of an iridectomy performed surgically or with a laser.

Chronic Open-angle Glaucoma. In open-angle glaucoma, the anterior chamber is of normal depth and the angle is open, allowing free access of aqueous humor to the drainage structures. A defect within the tissue of the drainage channels reduces the rate of drainage such that the intraocular pressure gradually rises to levels between 30 and 50 mm Hg. Unlike patients with acute narrow-angle glaucoma, patients with chronic open-angle glaucoma do not ex-

TABLE 17.6–7. ABRUPT (SECONDS–MINUTES) INTERMITTENT VISUAL LOSS

Cause	Clinical Findings	Management	Prognosis
Retinal emboli	Clear (platelets), white (calcific), or glistening yellow (cholesterol) Occlusive plug or plugs in retinal arterioles Segmental retinal pallor sometimes	Seek cardiac or vascular (esp. carotid) source of emboli If macula affected, treat as central retinal artery occlusion Possible surgical treatment of carotid disease	Good
Papilledema	Elevated optic discs Blurred peripapillary nerve fiber layer Splinter hemorrhages Exudate and other vascular changes Associated with raised intracranial pressure, pseudotumor cerebri, or hypertension	Diagnosis and treatment of underlying condition; see Table 17.6–12 and Chapter 15.10	Depends on etiology and duration
Migraine	Often precedes headache but can occur without headache Retinal arteries narrow often during attack	Treatment of migraine (see Chapter 15.9)	Good

TABLE 17.6–8. ABRUPT (SECONDS–MINUTES) PERMANENT VISUAL LOSS

Cause	Clinical Findings	Management	Prognosis
Central retinal vein occlusion	"Blood and thunder" retinal appearance Optic disc edema Venous vascular tortuosity and engorgement May be associated with hypertension, diabetes mellitus, or hyperviscosity states	Treatment underlying systemic disease Anticoagulation or photocoagulation may be of value in selected cases	Poor 25% develop secondary glaucoma
Pituitary apoplexy	Severe headache Progressive lethargy Ocular motor nerve palsies Occasional endocrine crisis	Immediate neurosurgical decompression	Dependent on duration of visual loss Usually good
Occipital lobe vascular accident	Homonymous hemianopia, unilateral or bilateral Associated posterior cerebral artery insufficiency signs Hypertension	See Chapter 15.13	Poor
Vitreous hemorrhage	Hazy vitreous; no view of retina Associated hypertension and diabetes mellitus Ocular trauma	Ultrasound to exclude other retinal disease Bed rest Vitrectomy in selected cases	Dependent on etiology
Central retinal artery occlusion	Retinal edema Macular cherry-red spot Attenuated arterioles, eventual optic atrophy May be associated with carotid artery occlusive disease, hypertension, or giant-cell arteritis	CO_2 inhalation Ocular massage Anterior chamber paracentesis Venous vascular tortuosity and engorgement	Poor

TABLE 17.6–9. PROGRESSIVE (HOURS–DAYS) VISUAL LOSS

Cause	Clinical Findings	Management	Prognosis
Acute keratoconus	Opaque central cornea Frequently conical cornea on other side	Observation	Good
Acute angle-closure glaucoma	Raised intraocular pressure Red eye Semidilated pupil with shallow anterior chamber Severe pain	Pilocarpine drops Diamox and oral or intravenous hyperosmotic agents Surgery	Dependent on duration of angle-closure glaucoma
Neovascularization in macular degeneration	Blood and lipid in macula Subretinal fluid	Laser treatment	Mixed; prognosis better with early detection and treatment; peripheral vision remains normal
Retinal detachment	Elevated retina Occasional vitreous hemorrhage	Surgical reattachment	Dependent on duration and location of detachment
Optic neuritis (including ischemic)	Pale, swollen, or normal disc Afferent pupil defect Decreased color vision May be associated with demyelinating disease or giant-cell arteritis	Use of systemic corticosteroids is controversial except in giant-cell arteritis	Dependent on etiology

TABLE 17.6–10. SLOWLY PROGRESSIVE (MONTHS–YEARS) VISUAL LOSS

Cause	Clinical Findings	Management	Prognosis
Corneal dystrophies	Corneal opacities bilaterally Frequent familial involvement	Corneal transplantation	Excellent
Chronic open-angle glaucoma	Quiet, nonpainful Characteristic visual field loss Raised intraocular pressure Optic nerve cupping	Parasympathomimetic or sympathetic blocking agents topically Diamox Ocular surgery	Dependent on duration of glaucoma
Cataracts	Lens opacities	Ocular surgery	Excellent
Atrophic macular degeneration	Circumscribed atrophy of maculae	No treatment	Poor for central vision but patients always maintain peripheral vision
Optic nerve compression	Optic atrophy Radiologic evidence of optic canal changes	Surgical exploration	Dependent on etiology and duration of compression

perience pain, discomfort, or acute visual loss. Rather, the sustained, moderately elevated intraocular pressure gradually results in loss of the peripheral visual field (Color Plate: Fig. 17.6–1D). The patient may, thus, be unaware of any visual difficulty until the disease is advanced. For this reason, early detection by routine measurement of intraocular pressure in all patients undergoing ophthalmologic examination is essential. Because open-angle glaucoma is most common in the age group from 40 to 70 years, all patients over age 40 should have their intraocular pressure measured yearly.

Open-angle glaucoma is generally treated medically with both topical and oral agents. When these are ineffective, surgery is required.

Age-related Macular Degeneration

Age-related macular degeneration is the commonest cause of legal blindness in patients over the age of 60 in the United States. It is most common in Caucasians and is uncommon in Blacks. These patients usually show scattered drusen (yellowish-white spots) in the posterior fundus before developing more advanced changes. The mild form with drusen is very common in patients over age 60 but is consistent with normal vision. In some patients with age-related macular degeneration, progressive atrophy of the outer layers of the retina and choriocapillaris leads to deterioration of central vision.

Only 10 percent of the patients who become legally blind (visual acuity 20/200 or worse) from macular degeneration do so because of these atrophic changes. Ninety percent of patients blinded by macular degeneration lose central vision because of a potentially treatable complication, the ingrowth of blood vessels and scar tissue in the macula (Color Plate: Fig. 17.6–1E,F). This complication begins with degeneration of Bruch membrane, the layer between the retinal pigment epithelium and choriocapillaris. Breaks in Bruch membrane allow ingrowth of choroidal vessels beneath the

TABLE 17.6–11. RED EYE: DIFFERENTIAL DIAGNOSIS

Sign	Conjunctivitis	Anterior Uveitis	Acute Glaucoma
Vision	Normal or intermittent blurring that clears with blinking	Slightly blurred	Marked blurring
Conjunctival injection	Diffuse	Circumcorneal (ciliary flush)	Diffuse and circumcorneal
Discharge	Significant, often with crusting of lashes	None	None
Pain	None or minimal	Moderately severe; stabbing or aching	Very severe; often nausea and vomiting
Pupil size	Normal	Normal or irregular	Mid-dilated and fixed
Pupillary response to light	Normal	Normal or irregular constriction	Minimal or no reaction
Intraocular pressure	Normal (sterilize tonometer after use)	Normal or slightly low	Elevated
Corneal appearance	Clear	Clear or slightly hazy	Steamy; opaque
Anterior chamber depth	Normal	Normal	Shallow
Comments[a]	If viral, spontaneous resolution; if bacterial, use topical bacteriocidal agent; if allergic or irritative, withdraw offending agent; all have good prognosis	Systemic workup indicated if recurrent; treat with topical steroids and cycloplegics	Immediate therapy with pilocarpine and osmotic agents; surgical or laser iridectomy is only definitive treatment; visual prognosis dependent on duration and severity of attack

[a]Topical steroid preparations should never be used to treat a red eye without a specific indication because they may cause the development of glaucoma, cataracts, or herpetic keratitis.

retina. Leakage of fluid and blood from these new vessels has a predilection for the macula, producing serious visual impairment. Organization of the hemorrhages results in fibrous scar tissue formation in the central macula with loss of central vision.

Laser treatment, when applied in the early stages of the neovascular form of macular degeneration, can significantly reduce the risk of visual loss by destroying the abnormal blood vessels. Treatment appears not to be effective once a central scar has formed. Because the new blood vessels can grow quickly and damage the center of the macula irreversibly, their appearance should be diagnosed and the patient referred to an ophthalmologist without delay. Early symptoms of this complication include blurriness or dimness of central vision in the affected eye. Straight lines appear curved or "wavy" because of the fluid in the macula. The presence of blood, lipid deposits, or fluid in the macula further support the diagnosis, which can be confirmed by fluorescein angiography of the fundus.

Retinal Vein Occlusion

Branch vein occlusion is the second most common cause, after diabetes, of retinal vascular disease observed in the United States. The obstruction occurs at an arteriovenous crossing where the artery and vein share a common adventitia. Distal to the obstruction, flame hemorrhages and retinal edema are common (Color Plate: Fig. 17.6–1G). In occasional cases, neovascularization develops several months after the occlusion. Anticoagulant therapy is of no value. Photocoagulation benefits patients with persistent macular edema. Photocoagulation is also effective for treating the secondary neovascularization.

Systemic hypertension is found in the majority of patients; however, a medical evaluation should also include a workup for diabetes.

Central vein occlusion produces the classic, vivid "blood-and-thunder" appearance to the entire posterior fundus (Color Plate: Fig. 17.6–1H). Extensive flame hemorrhages as well as dilation and tortuosity of all the branch retinal veins are present. Cotton-wool spots are frequently present and when extensive are a poor prognostic sign. In 1 to 3 months, approximately 50 percent of patients with cotton-wool spots and retinal ischemia will show iris neovascularization, which frequently leads to a severe form of glaucoma. This can often be prevented by laser treatment. All patients with central vein occlusion should have an immediate evaluation by an ophthalmologist.

Medical evaluation should rule out diabetes and systemic hypertension. It should also include hematologic evaluation, since the occlusion may be a manifestation of a variety of conditions such as polycythemia, macroglobulinemia, blood dyscrasia, or dysproteinemia. Chronic simple glaucoma is a contributing factor in a substantial number of these patients and should be ruled out by an ophthalmologist.

The role of anticoagulant therapy is highly controversial and adequate studies are lacking. The possible therapeutic role of fibrinolytic agents in early cases is under investigation.

A milder form of central retinal vein occlusion, occurring usually in younger patients without systemic or hematologic abnormalities, is termed "papillophlebitis" and has a favorable prognosis.

Retinal Arterial Occlusion

The obstruction may involve either the entire central retinal artery or one of its branches. The area of retinal occlusion takes on a pale, milky-white appearance. In central retinal artery occlusion the entire posterior retina is pale except for the center of the macula, which is not edematous and maintains its normal pinkish-red color, appearing as a cherry-red spot (Color Plate: Fig. 17.6–1I).

Causes of central or branch retinal artery occlusion include emboli from carotid artery disease or valvular heart disease and giant-cell arteritis (Color Plate: Fig. 17.6–1J). The condition also occurs in patients with hypertension.

Although some patients spontaneously improve, the majority do not. Treatment is usually unsatisfactory. Systemic vasodilator drugs generally have no effect on the retinal vessels and may in fact be deleterious by reducing ocular perfusion through a reduction of systemic blood pressure. Because CO_2 may dilate the retinal vessels, breathing into a bag or inhalation of a mixture of 95 percent O_2–5 percent CO_2 is advocated. Prompt referral to an ophthalmologist is advised for further management, which may include ocular massage or paracentesis of the globe.

Ocular Histoplasmosis (The Presumed Ocular Histoplasmosis Syndrome)

A significant part of the population throughout the Ohio River Valley (and to a lesser extent in the eastern and southern United States) has been exposed to *Histoplasma* infection. The exact pathogenesis of the ocular lesion remains unclear, but during the active systemic infection, which may be mild or unnoticed, focal ocular lesions may develop, leaving small atrophic spots in the fundus (histo-spots) or pigmented changes about the optic nerve. The histo-spots are of no visual significance per se except that years later choroidal neovascularization growing through a defect in Bruch membrane about the histo-spot may produce hemorrhage and scar tissue in the retina similar to that seen in senile macular degeneration. The triad of atrophic spots scattered about the fundus, pigmented scars about the disc, and hemorrhage near the macula constitutes the presumed ocular histoplasmosis syndrome. In the endemic areas the presumed *Histoplasma* syndrome with macular hemorrhage is a significant cause of visual impairment. A positive histoplasmin skin test further supports the diagnosis but is of little practical value in endemic areas, because the majority of the population are positive reactors.

No treatment is indicated for quiescent histo-spots. Corticosteroid therapy has been advocated for the active neovascularization by some investigators but has not been proven to be beneficial and is not recommended. Photocoagulation therapy for the neovascularization has been shown in a randomized clinical trial to reduce the risk of visual loss in selected patients.

COMMON OCULAR SIGNS

Certain ocular abnormalities that can be observed by the physician may or may not be associated with symptoms. The physician must, thus, be able to recognize the significance of these signs with respect to underlying ocular or systemic disease.

RED EYE

Disorders that irritate or inflame the eye result in redness of the conjunctiva (Table 17.6–11).

OPTIC DISC ABNORMALITIES

Optic Disc Swelling

Swelling of the optic disc may be produced by a wide variety of neurologic or systemic diseases (Table 17.6–12). Patients with optic disc swelling may present with acute visual loss, slowly progressive visual loss, or no visual complaints.

Regardless of the clinical presentation, however, ophthalmoscopic findings of optic disc swelling include hyperemia of the disc, blurred disc margins, blurring of the peripapillary retinal nerve fiber layer, and often small flame-shaped hemorrhages at the disc margin (Color Plate: Fig. 17.6–1K,L).

Patients with optic disc swelling should be referred immediately to an ophthalmologist for evaluation unless systemic signs and symptoms suggest increased intracranial pressure. In such cases, the patient should be immediately referred for neurologic evaluation (see Chapters 15.1 and 15.10).

TABLE 17.6–12. OPTIC DISC SWELLING

Type	Vision	Visual Field	Other Findings	Etiology
Papilledema	Normal	Full, enlarged blind spot	Headache, diplopia (sixth nerve palsy), nausea, vomiting	Intracranial mass, pseudotumor cerebri, hypertension
Anterior ischemic optic neuropathy	Usually acutely decreased	Altitudinal or arcuate defect	Sudden visual loss (hours), painless, most patients over age 55	Giant-cell arteritis, hypertension, diabetes mellitus, "idiopathic"
Anterior optic neuritis	Acutely decreased	Central scotoma	Sudden visual loss (hours to days), often with pain on ocular movement, most often in ages 15–45	"Idiopathic," multiple sclerosis
Compressive optic neuropathy	Slow, progressive decrease	Peripheral defect, rarely central scotoma	May have proptosis and/or limited eye movement	Orbital mass, such as meningioma or hemangioma
Toxic optic neuropathy	Slow, progressive decrease	Bilateral cecocentral scotomas	May have peripheral neuropathy or other evidence of toxicity	Nutritional, chloramphenicol, or ethambutol; lead
Hypotony	May be normal or decreased	Full	Low intraocular pressure	Intraocular surgery; trauma
Infiltrative optic neuropathy	May be normal or decreased	Variable	Other signs of inflammation or tumor, vitreous cells	Tumor, for example, lymphoma, leukemia; inflammation, for example, sarcoid, tuberculosis

Optic Atrophy

Optic atrophy results from damage to the fibers that comprise the optic nerve. The damage may occur to nerve fibers within the eye, as in central retinal artery occlusion and glaucoma, or to the fibers after they leave the eye, as in compression from intracranial and intraorbital masses. The atrophic disc may appear yellow or grey-white and devoid of visible capillaries; however, the appearance of the disc does not usually indicate the nature of the process that caused the atrophy. In dealing with a patient who has optic atrophy, the history of visual loss as well as any associated symptoms is of primary importance. In general, optic atrophy associated with a history of sudden visual loss suggests either an inflammatory or an ischemic process, whereas the same picture associated with slowly progressive visual loss suggests a compressive lesion.

In addition to a history of visual loss, characteristic defects in the visual field may suggest a specific etiology in patients with optic atrophy. Optic atrophy that occurs after an attack of optic neuritis generally is associated with a defect in the central visual field, the central scotoma, whereas optic atrophy from anterior ischemic optic neuropathy is usually associated with loss of the upper or lower portion of the visual field (an altitudinal visual field defect). Compression of the intracranial optic nerve may produce a variety of field defects; however, compression of the optic chiasm often produces a classic temporal defect in each eye with preservation of

visual acuity. A bitemporal hemianopia, associated with optic atrophy, indicates compression of the optic chiasm, most often from a pituitary adenoma, meningioma, aneurysm, or craniopharyngioma (Table 17.6–13).

Optic Disc Anomalies

Various congenital anomalies of optic nerve development may mimic acquired optic nerve defects or may be associated with various systemic abnormalities. Drusen of the optic disc, concretions of material that stain positively for calcium and mucopolysaccharide, may be visible on the optic disc surface as small, glistening, refractile globules; however, they may also develop beneath the surface of the disc, giving rise to a picture that is often confused with true optic disc swelling. The differentiation between true optic disc swelling and anomalous elevation of the optic disc may be extremely difficult and requires careful ophthalmoscopic examination. Other disc anomalies, such as optic disc tilting, dysplasia, and colobomas, may occur as isolated phenomena or may be associated with midline craniofacial abnormalities such as basal encephalocele. Optic nerve hypoplasia may occur as an isolated defect but is also found in children of diabetic mothers as well as in children whose mothers have taken various medications, such as quinine and antiepileptic drugs. The observation of an optic disc anomaly should

TABLE 17.6–13. OPTIC ATROPHY

History of Visual Loss	Visual Field Defect	Probable Etiology	Other Findings
Rapid (hours to days)	Central scotoma	Optic neuritis	Most common in ages 15–45 Often with pain on ocular movement
Rapid (hours to days)	Altitudinal or arcuate scotoma	Ischemic optic neuropathy	Usually over age 55
Progressive (weeks to months)	Bilateral cecocentral scotomas	Toxic	May have peripheral neuropathy
Progressive (months to years)	All types	Compression	Headache, anosmia
	Bitemporal hemianopia	Optic chiasmal compression	May have pituitary insufficiency, may have pituitary overactivity, e.g., acromegaly

alert the examiner to consider the possibility of other developmental abnormalities.

PUPILLARY ABNORMALITIES

Along with the appearance of the optic disc, pupillary abnormalities may be the only objective signs of neurologic dysfunction. For this reason, a knowledge of common pupillary abnormalities is essential. Iris movement is designed to control retinal illumination. Afferent impulses from the retina produce increased efferent impulses in the parasympathetic innervation of the iris and decreased activity in the sympathetic innervation. Both serve to constrict the pupil. A reduction in illumination reduces the afferent impulse, reduces parasympathetic activity, increases sympathetic activity, and causes dilation of the pupil. Figure 17.6–2 shows the pathways that mediate this reflex control and the effect of lesions at different sites. These findings are helpful in defining isolated pupillary abnormalities and in localizing the level of more general neurologic deficits.

The Afferent Pupillary Defect (Marcus Gunn Pupil)

Damage to the afferent arc of the parasympathetic system, such as in severe macular degeneration or optic neuritis, results in a characteristic pupillary abnormality commonly referred to as the Marcus Gunn pupil, or afferent pupillary defect. In such cases, shining a bright light in the normal eye produces a direct pupillary constric-

tion in that eye as well as a consensual response in the opposite eye; however, when the light is directed into the abnormal eye, the total amount of light entering the system is reduced, and both pupils redilate to a resting state determined by the amount of ambient light in the room. The observer, looking at the pupil of the abnormal eye, sees what appears to be a paradoxical dilation to light. Swinging the light back and forth between the two eyes results in the observation of pupillary constriction when the light is directed at the good eye and pupillary dilation when the light is directed at the bad eye.

Observation of an afferent pupillary defect is objective evidence of a significant lesion of the retina or optic nerve. It is never seen with cataract or corneal disease. If the retina appears normal in a patient with an afferent pupillary defect, an optic neuropathy is almost certainly present. Such patients should be referred to an ophthalmologist as soon as possible for evaluation and management.

The Fixed, Dilated Pupil

Interruption of the efferent arc of the parasympathetic pathway (the third nerve) results in a fixed, dilated pupil. When the third nerve is affected before the synapse of the pupillary fibers in the ciliary ganglion, other signs of third-nerve palsy are virtually always present (Table 17.6–6). In such cases, the pupil is generally mid-dilated. When a widely dilated, nonreactive pupil is the only ocular abnormality, either postganglionic parasympathetic fibers have been damaged or iris sphincter receptors paralyzed. The two most common causes for this ocular sign are damage to the ciliary ganglion (the tonic, or Adie, pupil) and a pharmacologically dilated pupil caused by the deliberate or inadvertent administration of a parasympatholytic agent, for example, atropine, to the eye (Table 17.6–14). The diagnosis can usually be established through the use of gradually increasing solutions of pilocarpine, because the tonic pupil is generally supersensitive to parasympathomimetic agents whereas the pharmacologically dilated pupil will not constrict to solutions that constrict the normal pupil.

The Argyll Robertson Pupil

Bilateral, small pupils that are irregular and are nonreactive to light but normally reactive to a near target almost always represent a manifestation of syphilis (Table 17.6–15).

Horner Syndrome

Damage to the sympathetic system produces a characteristic picture of ptosis and miosis known as Horner syndrome (Table 17.6–16). The diagnosis of Horner syndrome and subsequent lo-

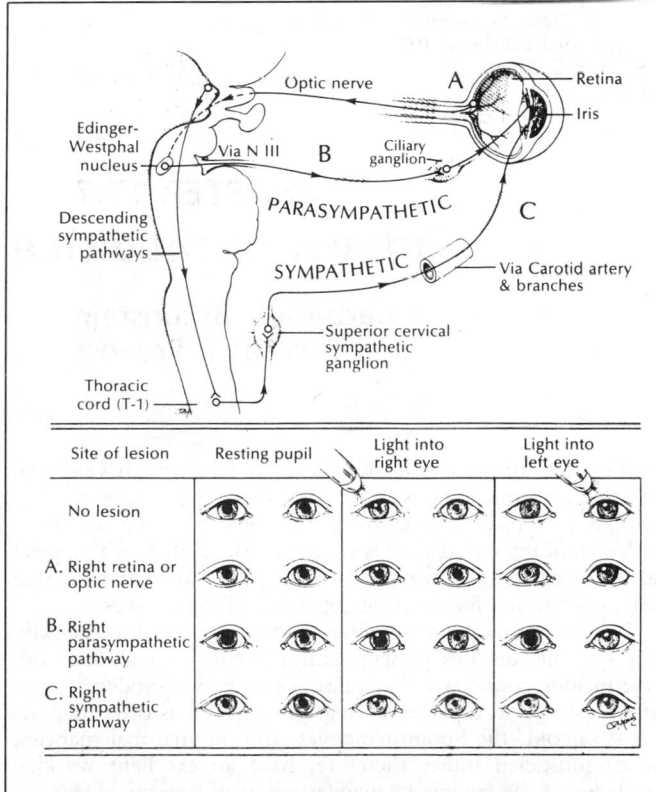

Figure 17.6–2. Pupillary reflex. The afferent pathway is from the retina via the optic nerve. The efferent parasympathetic pathway is from the Edinger-Westphal nucleus via the third nerve and the ciliary ganglion. The sympathetic efferent pathway is via the brainstem, thoracic cord, superior cervical ganglion and thence via the carotid and ophthalmic artery to the eye. The effect of a right-sided (A) lesion of retinal or optic nerve, (B) interruption of the parasympathetic pathway, and (C) interruption of the sympathetic pathway on the size of the resting pupil and the response to shining light into the right and left eyes are illustrated.

TABLE 17.6–14. THE FIXED, DILATED PUPIL

Characteristics	Tonic (Adie) Pupil	Drug Induced
Age	Usually in middle-aged adults	Usually teenagers or young adults
Sex	Females predominate	Usually females; often hospital personnel
Neurologic signs	Diminished deep tendon reflexes in about 75%	None
Diagnosis	Constricts with 0.125% pilocarpine	Will not constrict with pilocarpine solutions strong enough to constrict the normal pupil (1–4%)
Treatment	None; accommodation usually returns within months to years; reassurance	If inadvertent, reassurance; if deliberate, consider psychiatric referral

TABLE 17.6–15. ARGYLL ROBERTSON PUPIL

- Small irregular pupils
- Nonreactive to light
- React to near (accommodation) stimulus
- Generally bilateral
- Basic defect in dorsal midbrain
- Almost always associated with neurosyphilis

TABLE 17.6–16. HORNER SYNDROME

- Miotic pupil (more obvious in dim light)
- Reacts normally to light
- Variable ptosis
- Facial anhydrosis on same side (preganglionic only)
- Pupil fails to dilate with cocaine solution (4–10%)

calization of the lesion are extremely important, because lesions that affect the sympathetic fibers before their synapse at the superior cervical ganglion (preganglionic lesions) have a higher probability of being malignant than do lesions affecting the fibers after they synapse at the superior cervical ganglion (postganglionic lesions). The diagnosis of Horner syndrome and its location is based on two factors: (1) the clinical picture of unilateral mild, variable ptosis associated with an ipsilateral miotic but *normally reactive* pupil and (2) the inability of the Horner pupil to dilate on instillation of a 4 to 10 percent cocaine solution. Once the diagnosis of Horner syndrome has been established on clinical grounds, pharmacologic grounds, or both, a 1 percent hydroxyamphetamine solution (which releases norepinephrine from the postganglionic nerve ending) can be used to differentiate between preganglionic and postganglionic lesions.

Physiologic (Central) Anisocoria

In approximately 20 percent of the normal population, the size of the two pupils, which react normally to light and near stimuli, differs. This anisocoria is of no clinical significance. Physiologic anisocoria can be differentiated from Horner syndrome by the absence of other signs (ptosis, anhydrosis) and by the normal dilation of *both* pupils to cocaine solution.

RETINAL EXUDATES AND HEMORRHAGES

The appearance of retinal exudates or hemorrhages suggests an abnormality in the systemic vasculature. This may be a hematologic disorder (Table 17.6–3) or a systemic vascular disease such as hypertension or diabetes mellitus (Tables 17.6–1 and 17.6–2). Such patients should undergo a complete medical and hematologic evaluation.

REFERENCES

1. Burde RM, Savino PJ, Trobe JD: Clinical Decisions in Neuro-Ophthalmology. St. Louis, CV Mosby, 1985
2. Glaser JS: Neuro-Ophthalmology Symposium, vol 8. Miami, University of Miami and Bascom Palmer Eye Institute, 1977
3. Miller NR: Walsh and Hoyt's Clinical Neuro-Ophthalmology, vol 1, 4th ed. Baltimore, Williams & Wilkins, 1982
4. Miller NR: Walsh and Hoyt's Clinical Neuro-Ophthalmology, vol 2, 4th ed. Baltimore, Williams & Wilkins, 1985
5. Newell FW: Ophthalmology: Principles and Concepts. St. Louis, CV Mosby, 1982
6. Patz A: Current concepts in ophthalmology, retinal vascular disease. N Engl J Med 298:1451, 1978
7. Scheie HG, Albert DM: Textbook of Ophthalmology. Philadelphia, WB Saunders, 1977

CHAPTER 17.7
Cutaneous Medicine

Barbara L. Braunstein
and Thomas T. Provost

It has been estimated that approximately 15 to 20 percent of patients presenting themselves to a general practitioner do so for skin-related problems. It has also been estimated that approximately one third of the general population needs dermatologic care at least once during their lifetime. Two chronic skin diseases, atopic eczema and psoriasis, affect between 1 and 2 percent of the general population.

Since the advent of antibiotics and corticosteroids, great progress has been made in eliminating and controlling some of the more serious and at times lethal skin diseases, such as syphilis, tuberculosis, and pemphigus. However, when large areas of the skin are denuded, for example, in toxic epidermal necrolysis, third-degree burns, and pemphigus vulgaris, significant mortality does occur even today.

Although mortality from skin diseases is generally very low, skin diseases, especially those involving the hands and feet, create a great deal of morbidity; for example, the dentist who has developed allergic contact dermatitis on his hands from the acrylic monomers used in making dentures; the new mother with hand eczema; or the salesman with severe psoriasis of his scalp, face, and hands. These problems interfere with job performance, resulting in economic loss and interference with the quality of life. As a consequence, many dermatologic patients are emotionally upset, demonstrate a high degree of anxiety, or are depressed. Further,

advertisements promoting blemish-free skin raise patient's expectations, and communications that stress the potential dangers of excessive sun exposure create anxiety. We live in a vain society in which significant skin disease is viewed by the patient with a great deal of alarm and seriousness. To manage the patient with skin disease effectively, one must be cognizant of these issues.

In addition to the many diseases that are limited to the skin, many systemic diseases present with a cutaneous manifestation. These include connective tissue diseases such as scleroderma, dermatomyositis, and lupus erythematosus, as well as other diseases such as sarcoid, the lipoproteinemias, and internal malignancies. The diagnostician must, therefore, have an excellent working knowledge of the cutaneous manifestations of systemic diseases.

This chapter is designed to provide an overview of the structure and function of the skin; evaluation of dermatologic patients; the diagnosis and management of common dermatologic diseases; and the cutaneous manifestations of systemic diseases.

STRUCTURE OF THE SKIN

The skin is the largest organ in the body and is composed of three distinct layers. The deepest layer is the subcutaneous tissue, and

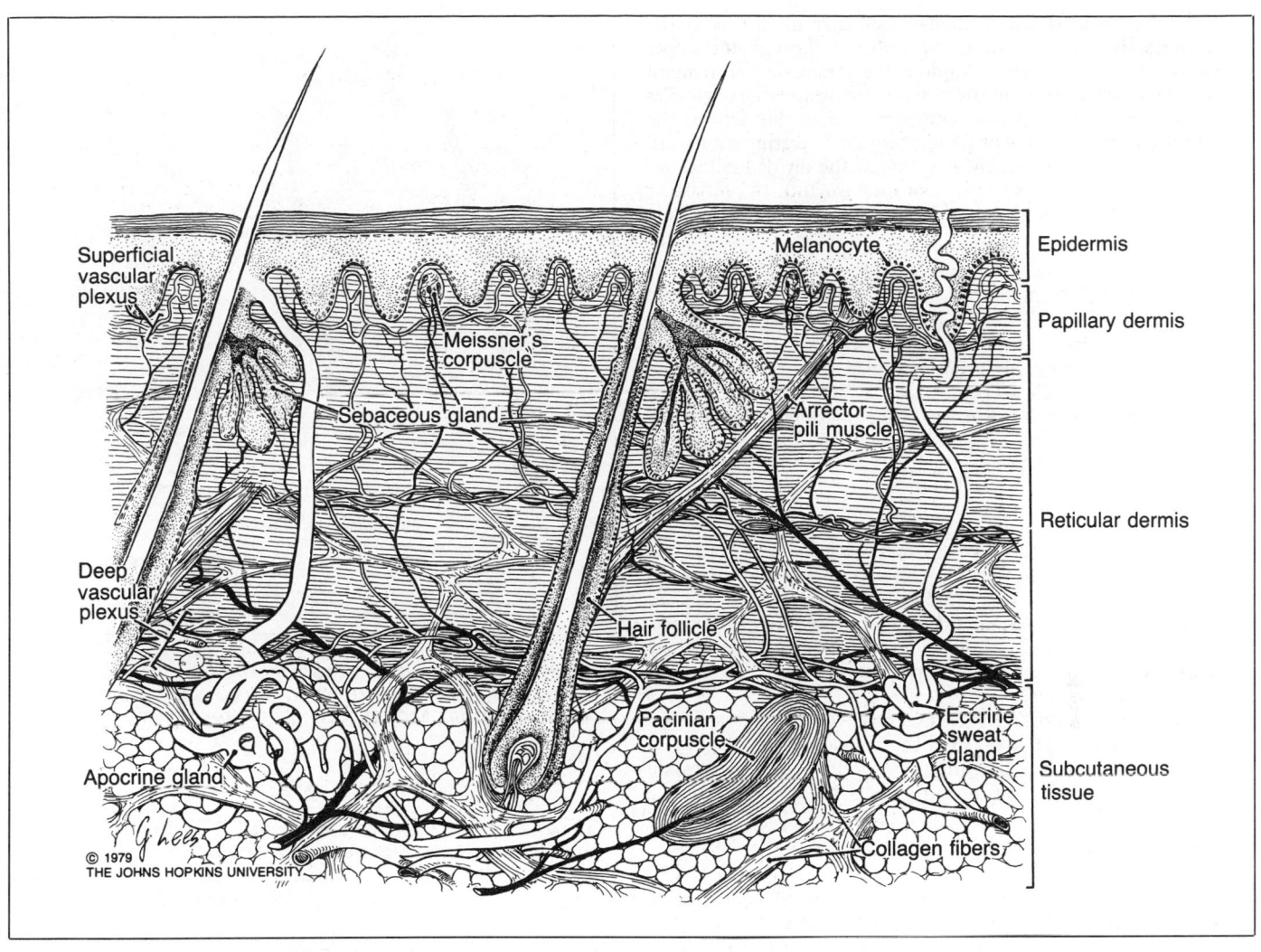

Figure 17.7–1. Cross section of the skin.

the outermost layer is the epidermis. Between the subcutaneous tissue and the epidermis is the dermis (Fig. 17.7–1).

SUBCUTANEOUS TISSUE

The subcutaneous tissue is composed of variable quantities of fat. The fat acts as a cushion, protecting internal organs, and also serves to insulate the body. This layer of skin contains blood vessels and nerves that pass through to the dermis. Sweat glands are found at the junction between the dermis and subcutaneous tissue, and deep hair follicles have their origin in the subcutaneous layer.

DERMIS

The dermis is composed of connective tissue and has a rich blood and nerve supply. The connective tissue is composed of elastic and reticular fibers and collagen strands. The collagen strands run through the dermis and subcutaneous tissue to fascial planes below. These fibers, especially the collagen fibers, provide the support and elasticity of the skin.

Within the dermis are a rich supply of cells including fibroblasts, histiocytes, mast cells, plasma cells, polymorphonuclear leukocytes, eosinophils, and lymphocytes.

The lower portion of the dermis is termed the "reticular portion"; the upper portion is designated "papillary." Between the papillary portion of the dermis and the epidermis is an undulating periodic acid–Schiff (PAS) positive basement membrance. In this complex PAS-positive basement membrane are many structures (recognized by electron microscopy), the function of which is to maintain the integrity of the epidermis with the dermis. Destruction of these structures by inflammatory processes, such as bullous pemphigoid or a genetic deficiency (epidermolysis bullosa), produces blister formation in which the epidermis separates from the dermis, resulting in widespread denuding of the skin.

EPIDERMIS

This is the outer layer of skin. The epidermis is composed of two distinct cell types, dendritic cells and keratinocytes.

The *dendritic cells* are of two types. Langerhans cells, which compose 3 to 5 percent of the epidermal cells, are bone marrow-derived macrophage cells capable of presenting antigens to lymphocytes. Melanocytes, cells derived from the neural crest, are capable of synthesizing and distributing melanin. The melanin is distributed to keratinocytes via dendritic processes.

The *keratinocytes* are biologically active cells derived from embryonic ectoderm. In addition to producing a fibrous protein, keratin, these cells have recently been shown to be capable of synthesizing other structural proteins, such as bullous pemphigoid antigen; hormones capable of activating lymphocytes (epidermal thymus activating factor [ETAF], interleukin I); as well as proteolytic enzymes.

The epidermis is very dynamic. Cell division occurs in the basal layers. Individual keratinocytes ascend through the upper portions of the epidermis, undergoing dramatic biochemical changes in which keratin fills the cells, replacing all other organelles and producing an amorphous, compact layer of skin termed the "stratum corneum." This process is termed "keratinization." In general, it takes approximately 4 weeks for the divided cell to migrate from the basal layer to the stratum corneum. In psoriasis, a disease of enhanced epidermal proliferation, this time lapse is only 4 days.

VASCULAR SUPPLY

An elaborate arterial and venous network perforates the subcutaneous and dermal tissues. This intense vascular network when dilated can shunt approximately 50 percent of the cardiac output into the skin, resulting in excessive heat loss and alterations in blood pressure.

NERVE SUPPLY

The nerve supply to the skin is very rich. Sensory nerves carry the sensations of touch, pain, itch, vibration, proprioception, and discriminative touch. The skin contains many specialized sensory end-organs (Merkel cells in the epidermis; Vater–Pacini and Wagner–Meissner tactile corpuscles in the dermis). The highest concentrations of these sensory nerve endings are in the hands, feet, and genital regions.

Sympathetic motor nerves innervate sweat and apocrine glands, arterioles, and skin smooth muscles. When the skin smooth muscles (erector pili muscles) contract, hair follicles are pulled into an upright position, producing "goose flesh."

APPENDAGES

Hair, a vestige of our primitive ancestors, covers the entire body with the exception of the palms, soles, dorsa of the terminal phalanges of the digits, glans penis, and the mucocutaneous junctions. Hair is different on different parts of the body. Hairs vary in structure, rate of growth, and response to various stimuli. For example, scalp hair, eyebrows, and eyelashes are not affected by sex hormones. On the other hand, facial, axillary, and pubic hair are.

There are two types of hair. The vellus hairs are fine, short, and colorless. This fine hair covers most of the body of youngsters and adults. By contrast, long, coarse, pigmented hairs (terminal hairs) develop most extensively on the scalp, eyebrows, extremities, axillae, pubes, and male beard.

Hair develops from hair follicles located most commonly in the dermis. The hair follicles arise from an invagination of the epidermis. Hair growth undergoes three distinct phases: anagen, catagen, and telogen (Fig. 17.7–2). The active growth phase of hair is termed "anagen" and is characterized by rapid mitotic activity in the hair bulb. During the anagen phase, the hair may grow by as much as 0.35 mm per day. The phase between active growth and the resting stage (telogen) is termed "catagen." The time period for transition from anagen to telogen is approximately 3 months. The most common type of transient hair loss is termed "telogen effluvium" and generally occurs approximately 3 months following a stressful situation, such as childbirth, severe illness (negative nitrogen balance), or stress. When the telogen hair is shed, an anagen hair takes its place.

NAILS

Nails are keratin structures and are also an evolutionary vestige, with little utility. Nails grow at approximately 0.1 mm per day. A fingernail is restored in approximately 3 months, whereas a toenail will take three times as long to regrow. The nail is produced by a

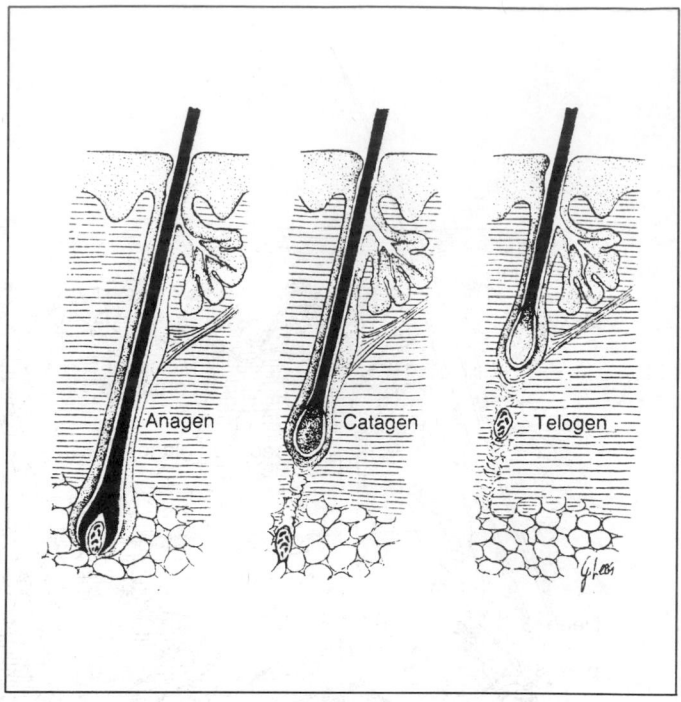

Figure 17.7–2. The hair cycle. The progressive changes from a growing hair (anagen) through catagen to the resting stage (telogen) affect the epithelial and connective tissue components.

nail matrix located at the base of the nail. Nail growth can be inhibited by illness and advancing age. Severe febrile illnesses may produce a partial or complete cessation in keratin synthesis, resulting in a characteristic transverse groove in the nail (Beau line).

GLANDULAR APPENDAGES

There are three glandular appendages in the skin. These are sebaceous glands, eccrine sweat glands, and apocrine sweat glands.

The sebaceous glands are branched glands whose secretory products are discharged through a sebaceous duct into a hair follicle. Sebaceous glands are found everywhere except the palms and soles. The scalp and face contain the most sebaceous glands. The sebaceous gland is composed of fully differentiated, anucleated sebaceous cells, and lipids. The lipid component is composed of free fatty acids, esterified fatty acids, waxes, sterol esters, and squalene. The sebum is mildly bacteriostatic and fungistatic and retards water evaporation. The sebaceous glands markedly increase in activity at puberty. The activity and size of the glands diminish with age.

Eccrine sweat glands are found all over the body and are most abundant on the palms and soles. These glands are of ectodermal origin and open directly onto the skin's surface. The eccrine sweat glands produce sweat in response to heat and emotional stress. A person exposed to high environmental temperatures may produce 2 to 3 L of sweat every hour. One liter of evaporated sweat removes approximately 585 kcal of heat from the body.

Apocrine sweat glands are of little biologic importance and are responsible for the production of body odor. These glands are responsive to emotional stresses and do not develop until the time of puberty. The apocrine sweat glands are found predominantly in the axillary and genital regions, but apocrine units are also found on breast areolae, the external ear canal (ceruminous glands), and eyelids (Moll glands). Apocrine secretion has no known function in humans. Bacteria present on skin surface act on apocrine secretions to produce ammonia, free fatty acids, and other odoriferous substances.

FUNCTIONS OF THE SKIN

The skin acts as a barrier separating the body from the external environment. This barrier function serves to protect the body from the penetration of foreign materials, for example, chemicals, bacteria, and ultraviolet irradiation, and to cushion the body from physical trauma. The skin also houses highly developed sensory neurons that provide the body with pain, temperature, light touch, and two-point discrimination. In addition to the barrier function, the skin plays a primary role in thermal regulation.

The barrier function of the skin resides in the epidermis, predominantly in the stratum corneum. The skin is relatively impermeable, although all molecules demonstrate some ability to pass through the skin. Following the successive removal of layers of the epidermis by adhesive tape, the permeability of the skin increases. With the complete removal of the epidermis, the skin loses its permeability barrier.

The skin displays remarkable ability to adjust to noxious external stimuli. For example, repeated mechanical trauma to the skin will result in epidermal proliferation with increase in the thickness of the stratum corneum (callus formation). Excessive ultraviolet light irradiation produces stimulation of the melanocytes, resulting in tanning, which protects the body from the effects of ultraviolet light.

The skin plays a dominant role in thermal regulation and responds to stimuli originating in the hypothalamus. With an increase in blood flow to the skin, heat is delivered to the skin surface and dissipates into the environment through convection and radiation. In addition, eccrine sweat glands deliver sweat to the surface, providing accelerated heat loss to the environment by evaporation. Excessive water loss from the skin can result in dehydration (heat prostration); eccrine sweat gland failure in the presence of excessive external heat can produce hyperthermia resulting in core body temperatures in excess of 41C. If the body is not immediately cooled, this hyperthermia can be lethal (see Chapter 4.11).

Heat is conserved by autonomic sympathetic nervous system stimulation, which causes vasoconstriction in the skin, reducing heat loss by conduction and radiation. This, coupled with the act of shivering, serves to increase the core body temperature.

Some diseases such as psoriasis, atopic eczema, and drug reactions may progress to erythroderma, in which there is marked vasodilation, resulting in a red, hot skin. Thermal regulation is lost, and the patients become poikilothermic (assume a body temperature of the environment). This can be associated with relatively wide fluctuations in core body temperature (e.g., 33C to 38C within an hour). The patients may alternately complain of being hot and cold and demonstrate shivering. Such a condition is associated with a decrease in peripheral blood vessel resistance, an increased pulse rate, a widening of the pulse pressure, an increase in cardiac output, and an increase in insensible water loss. Such a dramatic insult may result in high output cardiac failure, especially in the elderly patient.

APPROACH TO THE DERMATOLOGIC PATIENT

HISTORY

The history is an important part of the evaluation of a patient with a cutaneous disorder. The depth of the history taking will depend to an extent on the patient's primary complaint. Certain disorders such as warts do not require detailed histories. Other disorders such as heritable diseases or drug eruptions require detailed questioning. Date of onset, symptoms, previous therapy, history of exposure, family history, and medications are examples of some factors that may be important in a patient's history.

PHYSICAL EXAMINATION

In most instances, when a patient is being examined for the first time, it is recommended that the patient be completely undressed and covered with a loose-fitting gown or sheet. This allows the physician to examine the patient's entire skin surface, not only to search for clues that may aid in the diagnosis of the patient's primary complaint but also to discover any unrelated problems of which the patient may be unaware. This is especially important in the case of the life-threatening disease malignant melanoma.

Adequate lighting should be available when examining the skin. Natural window light gives the most accurate perception of color and is recommended whenever possible. Fluorescent lighting is the next best alternative. A gooseneck lamp is helpful for directed lighting. A penlight is recommended for side lighting of lesions with subtle elevation or depression, as well as for examination of the mouth.

The patient should be examined thoroughly and in an orderly fashion. The physician should palpate the skin to assess consistency or depth of a lesion.

DERMATOLOGIC TERMINOLOGY

Once the patient has been examined, it is important for the physician to be able to describe his findings using accurate morphologic terms. The description should include distribution, configuration, and morphology.

Distribution of an eruption may be generalized or localized, symmetric or asymmetric. The description of distribution should include precise terminology such as acral (distal extremities), truncal, perioral, periorbital, periungual, inguinal, facial, flexural, extensor surfaces, or periumbilical.

The configuration of lesions is the pattern in which they are arranged. Examples (Fig. 17.7–3) include:

1. Solitary: Only one lesion is present.
2. Linear: Lesions are arranged in a line.
3. Annular: Lesions form a circle.
4. Arcuate (arciform): Lesions form incomplete circles.
5. Polycyclic: Both annular and arcuate lesions are present.
6. Grouped: Lesions are arranged in a cluster.
7. Herpetiform: Grouped vesicles are present.
8. Zosteriform: Lesions follow a dermatome.
9. Serpiginous: Lesions form a serpentine pattern.
10. Target: Lesion forms a bull's-eye pattern.
11. Reticulated: Lesions form a netlike pattern.

The morphology is a description of an individual lesion and includes type of lesion, surface changes, color, shape, and consistency. Definitions and examples of morphologic terms used to describe types of lesions and surface changes (Fig. 17.7–4) are given in the following discussions.

Macule
A flat (nonpalpable), circumscribed area with altered coloration (If over 2 cm in diameter, the lesion is called a macular patch.); may be caused by melanin or vascular changes (vasodilation or extravasation of blood). *Examples:* Café au lait spot, freckles, vitiligo, petechiae, ecchymosis (purpura), erythema (e.g., sunburn).

Papule
A solid elevated lesion less than 1 cm in diameter; may be caused by epidermal, vascular, or melanocytic proliferation, dermal infiltration, or deposition of a solid substance. *Examples:* Nevus (mole), cherry angioma, molluscum contagiosum, sarcoid, eruptive xanthoma, vasculitis (palpable purpura).

Nodule
Similar to papule but larger both horizontally and vertically. (A tumor is similar to a papule or nodule but larger.) *Examples:* Gouty tophus, basal cell carcinoma, sarcoid.

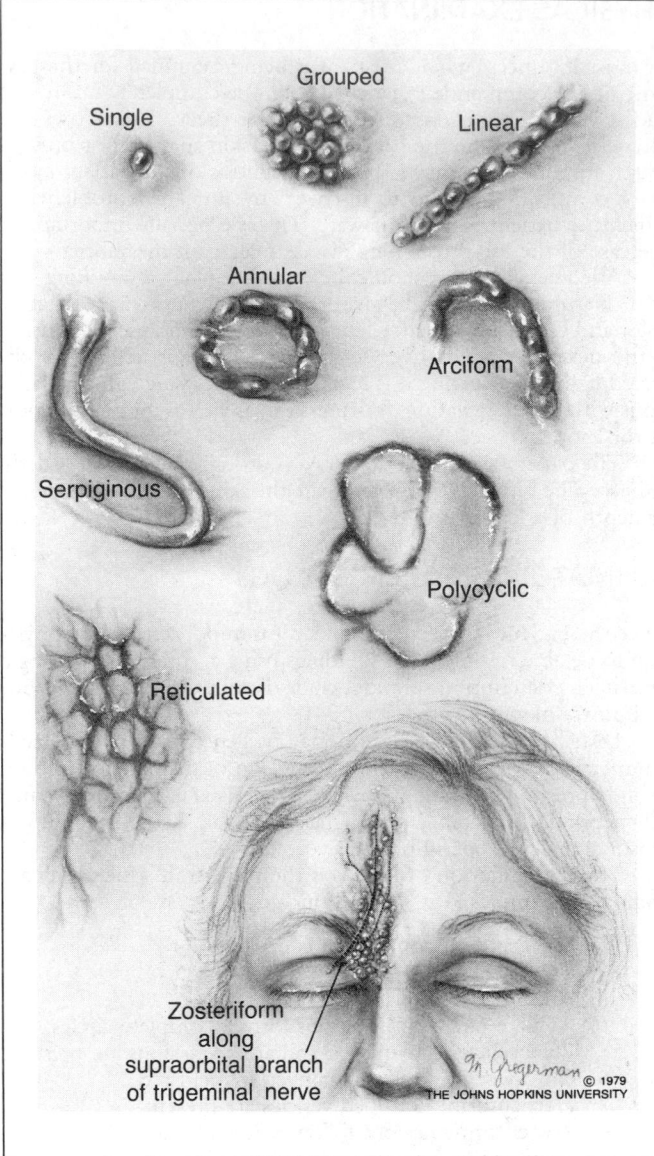

Figure 17.7-3. Configuration of skin lesions.

Morbilliform
Maculopapular; consisting of erythematous macules and papules (discrete and confluent). *Examples:* Drug rash, measles.

Plaque
A flat-topped, elevated (plateaulike) lesion that is over 1 cm (if less than 1 cm, a lesion is called a flat-topped papule); may be secondary to epidermal and/or dermal changes. *Examples:* Psoriasis, mycosis fungoides, lichen planus.

Wheal (Hives)
Erythematous, slightly raised lesion that results from vasodilation and edema. (Hives may present as papules, plaques, or arcuate or polycyclic lesions.) *Example:* Urticaria.

Vesicle
Fluid-filled lesion less than 0.5 cm in diameter; may be subcorneal (beneath the stratum corneum), intraepidermal, or subepidermal. *Examples:* Herpes zoster, herpes simplex, dyshidrotic eczema, dermatitis herpetiformis.

Bulla
Fluid-filled lesion greater than 0.5 cm in diameter (differs from vesicle only in size of lesion). *Examples:* Pemphigus vulgaris—intraepidermal blister, bullous pemphigoid—subepidermal blister.

Pustule
A papule containing a purulent exudate. *Examples:* Folliculitis (pustule is around a hair follicle), gonococcemia (purpuric pustule).

Cyst
An elevated dome-shaped lesion filled with semisolid or fluid material. *Example:* Epidermal inclusion cyst.

Atrophy
Depressed area produced by thinning of the epidermis, dermis, or panniculus (subcutaneous fat). *Examples:* Poststeroid injection atrophy, striae.

Erosion
Loss of superficial layers of skin (epidermis or mucous membrane). *Examples:* Infected eczema, stomatitis, excoriations.

Ulcer
Loss of deeper layers of skin (epidermis and dermis); ulcers heal with scarring. *Examples:* Pyoderma gangrenosum, statis ulcer.

Fissure
Linear ulcer. *Examples:* Perlèche, hand dermatitis (fissured).

Lichenification
Epidermal hypertrophy with thickening of skin and accentuated skin markings. *Example:* Lichen simplex chronicus.

Crusting
Results from dried fluid (serous or bloody exudate). *Example:* Impetigo.

Scaling
Dry white flakes of epidermis (stratum corneum). *Examples:* Ichthyosis, xerosis (dry skin), dandruff.

Verrcous
Marked hypertrophy of epidermis (especially stratum corneum). *Example:* Verruca vulgaris.

For examples of different colors, shapes, and consistency, see Tables 17.7-1 to 17.7-3.

DIAGNOSTIC PROCEDURES

POTASSIUM HYDROXIDE EXAMINATION

A potassium hydroxide (KOH) examination is performed to confirm or rule out the diagnosis of a fungal infection. Scale is scraped from the surface of an eruption, preferably from an active border, and is placed on a glass slide. When candidiasis is suspected, the contents of a pustule may be obtained. Ten to 20 percent KOH is added and a coverslip applied. The slide should be heated gently but not allowed to boil. The hyphae are sought first under low power and then confirmed at high power.

TABLE 17.7-1. EXAMPLES OF COLOR

• Red	• Tan	• Orange
• Pink	• Brown	• Salmon
• Erythematous	• Black	• White
• Yellow	• Blue	• Flesh colored
• Pearly	• Violaceous	• Slate gray
• Translucent	• Green	

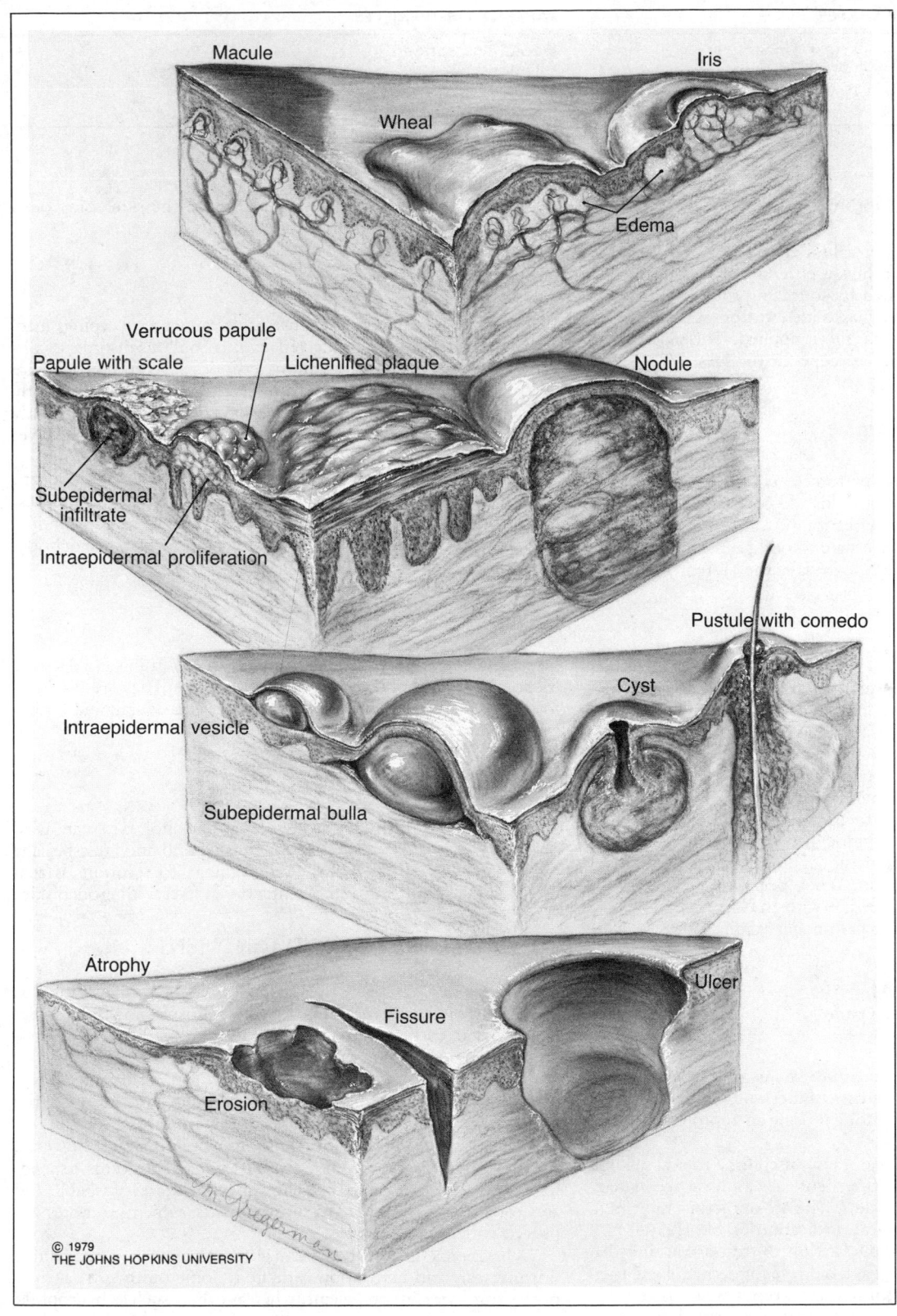

Macule

Iris

Wheal

Edema

Verrucous papule

Papule with scale

Lichenified plaque

Nodule

Subepidermal infiltrate

Intraepidermal proliferation

Pustule with comedo

Cyst

Intraepidermal vesicle

Subepidermal bulla

Atrophy

Ulcer

Fissure

Erosion

© 1979
THE JOHNS HOPKINS UNIVERSITY

Figure 17.7–4. Types of skin lesions.

TZANCK PREPARATION

A Tzanck preparation is performed to evaluate vesicular lesions that may represent a herpetic infection. The contents, base, and roof of a vesicle are scraped and applied to a glass slide. After fixing, the slide can be stained with various stains such as a Wright or Giemsa stain. If multinucleated giant cells are seen, the diagnosis of a herpetic infection is confirmed.

SCRAPING FOR MITES

A skin scraping for mites is performed to confirm a diagnosis of scabies. A burrow or nonexcoriated papule should be scraped vigorously using a no. 15 blade. A drop of oil can be added to the blade or skin to improve adherence of the scraping to the blade. The skin sample is then examined under the microscope for adult mites, eggs, or feces.

TABLE 17.7–2. EXAMPLES OF SHAPES

• Oval	• Linear
• Round	• Arcuate
• Annular	• Polygonal
• Dome shaped	

DARK-FIELD EXAMINATION

A dark-field examination is essential for the evaluation of an ulcer if the possibility of primary syphilis is entertained. Serous or serosanguineous exudate is obtained by squeezing the indurated base of the ulcer and is applied to a glass slide. A drop of nonbacteriostatic saline is added, and a coverslip is applied. The slide is then examined under a dark-field microscope for the presence of spirochetes.

IMMUNOFLUORESCENCE

Immunofluorescence testing is performed (1) on skin to examine for the deposition of immunoglobulin and complement at sites of lesions (direct immunofluorescence) or (2) on serum to examine for serum autoantibodies (indirect immunofluorescence) to aid in the diagnosis of certain disorders, especially the blistering disorders and connective tissue diseases.

SKIN BIOPSY

The skin biopsy is a simple procedure that is done when a diagnosis is unknown or needs to be confirmed. There are four different types of biopsy techniques: (1) shave biopsy, (2) punch biopsy, (3) incisional biopsy, and (4) excisional biopsy.

When the shave biopsy technique is used, only a superficial portion of a lesion is removed by shaving it off flush with the skin. When a punch biopsy is performed, a plug of skin 2 to 6 mm in diameter is removed using a cylindric instrument with a sharp cutting edge and a handle. For an incisional biopsy, a part of a lesion is removed with an elliptic excision. When performing an excisional biopsy, one removes the entire lesion with an elliptic excision. The specimen is then submitted for pathologic examination.

PRINCIPLES OF TOPICAL DERMATOLOGIC THERAPY[1]

Topical therapy plays a major role in the management of dermatologic patients. For this reason a basic understanding of the principles of topical therapy is critical for choosing an appropriate topical medication.

The vehicle (ointment, cream, etc.) used for a topical medication is frequently as important therapeutically as the active ingredient incorporated into that vehicle. There are numerous vehicles to consider when choosing a topical medication (Table 17.7–4).

When choosing a topical medication to treat a skin disorder, one should generally follow the age-old rule for dermatologic therapy, "If it's wet, keep it dry; if it's dry, keep it wet." If the skin disease is weeping, macerated, and exudative, one should treat with drying measures. If the skin is dry, scaly, lichenified, and hy-

TABLE 17.7–3. EXAMPLES OF CONSISTENCY

• Firm	• Cystic
• Soft	• Fluctuant
• Rock hard	• Rubbery
• Gelatinous	• Indurated

TABLE 17.7–4. VEHICLES

• Solutions, sprays	• Powders
• Lotions	• Pastes
• Creams	• Gels
• Ointments	

perkeratotic, the aim should be to lubricate the skin using ointments and emollient creams.

WET DRESSINGS

Wet dressings (compresses) are used to treat acute, weeping, macerated dermatoses such as infected eczema, bullous disorders, contact dermatitis, and intertriginous eruptions. Wet dressings are soothing, cooling, and drying; they serve to cleanse the skin gently and inhibit secondary bacterial infection. Examples of commonly used dressings include tap water, aluminum acetate, saline, silver nitrate, and acetic acid.

Patients are instructed to soak or compress the affected skin, using towels or gauze, several times daily for 20 to 30 minutes. Care should be taken to avoid excessive drying of the surrounding skin. Wet-to-dry dressings may be used if more aggressive debridement is desired.

POWDERS

Powders are drying, absorptive, cooling, and soothing and decrease friction between opposing surfaces of the skin. They are used primarily for macerated dermatoses on intertriginous skin and for hygienic purposes.

SOLUTIONS

Solutions are liquids that usually contain alcohol. They are used on "wet" dermatoses or when drying is desired and are especially useful for hair-bearing skin. A disadvantage to solutions is that they may cause stinging and burning on contact with eroded skin.

LOTIONS, CREAMS, AND OINTMENTS

Lotions are divided into either shake lotions or "milky" lotions. A shake lotion, such as calamine lotion, is a suspension of a powder in a liquid and serves to dry and cool the skin as the liquid evaporates and deposits the powder on the skin.

A milky lotion is an emulsion of oil droplets in water. Most over-the-counter moisturizers are milky lotions, but because of the high water content they are not very effective lubricants.

Creams, like lotions, are emulsions of oil in water; however, the oil content is higher. They are fair to good lubricants depending on the amount of oil present. They are water washable and are cosmetically acceptable to most patients, which promotes improved patient compliance.

Ointments are the best vehicle to choose when the skin is dry and scaly and lubrication is desired. Some ointments, such as petrolatum, are water repellent, whereas others such as hydrophilic petrolatum or Aquaphor, contain emulsifiers that enable them to take up water to form water-in-oil emulsions. Some ointments such as Eucerin "cream" are a mixture of water in oil plus emulsifiers.

Ointments are protective, soothing, and hydrating and are excellent vehicles for topical medications because they allow for maximum penetration of active ingredients through the skin. However, because they are messy and not water washable, they are less cosmetically acceptable to patients and therefore may lead to poorer patient compliance.

TABLE 17.7–5. SIDE EFFECTS OF TOPICAL CORTICOSTEROIDS

- Atrophy of the skin
- Telangiectasia
- Striae
- Easy bruising
- Rosacea
- Depression of the hypophyseal-pituitary-adrenal axis
- Hirsutism
- Glaucoma

TOPICAL CORTICOSTEROIDS

Topical corticosteroids are the most frequently prescribed topical medications for the treatment of skin disorders. They are used primarily for their antipruritic and anti-inflammatory effects. However, they are also helpful in the treatment of hyperplastic disorders such as psoriasis and infiltrative disorders such as sarcoid and granuloma annulare as well as for other unrelated diseases.

Unfortunately, there are many undesirable side effects related to topical steroid use. As the potency of the steroid is increased, the severity and likelihood of adverse side effects also increase (Table 17.7–5).

Depression of the hypothalamic-pituitary-adrenal (HPA) axis can occur if as little as 50 to 100 g/wk of a potent topical steroid is used for more than 2 weeks. This is a special concern in children.

There are seven classes of topical steroids based on their potency (Table 17.7–6). As a general rule, only the weaker steroids (1 percent hydrocortisone) should be used on the face and intertriginous skin, and in children, because of the potential for atrophy and telangiectasia.

In order to keep side effects to a minimum, patients should be instructed to apply only a thin layer of medication to the affected skin. When used on a long-term basis for chronic dermatoses, topical steroids are more effective if they are used intermittently.

COMMON CUTANEOUS DISORDERS[6]

COMMON INFECTIONS

Bacterial Infections

Most cutaneous bacterial infections are caused by group A β-hemolytic *Streptococcus* or *Staphylococcus aureus*. Of the cutaneous infections caused by these organisms, impetigo contagiosa is the most frequently encountered.

Impetigo is a superficial bacterial infection that may be caused by *Streptococcus* alone, by *S. aureus* alone, or by *Streptococcus* primarily with *S. aureus* present as a secondary invader. When *Streptococcus* is the causative agent, the lesions may be vesicular initially but rapidly become golden or yellow-crusted lesions. If the infection is caused by *S. aureus,* the initial vesicular lesion progresses rapidly to form a bullous lesion. On rupture of the bulla, a golden or brownish crust develops.

Impetigo is a highly contagious disorder that primarily affects children. Lesions frequently begin on the face and spread to other areas of the body by autoinoculation. The infection is superficial and does not cause scarring unless it has been allowed to progress to a deeper pyoderma. Rare complications include cellulitis or bacteremia. The most serious sequela of cutaneous group A *Streptococcus* infection is glomerulonephritis. The glomerulonephritis follows infection by nephritogenic strains of group A *Streptococcus* after a latent period of approximately 3 weeks.

Penicillin (1.0 g daily for 10 days) is the drug of choice in the treatment of impetigo caused by *Streptococcus*. If the patient is allergic to penicillin or if *S. aureus* is present in a cultured lesion, erythromycin (1.0 g daily for 10 days) will give adequate coverage for most staphylococcal as well as streptococcal infections.

Superficial Fungal Infections

Dermatophytosis. Dermatophytosis, also known as *tinea* or *ringworm*, is a superficial fungal infection that may affect the skin, hair, and nails. Dermatophyte infections are frequent in normal individuals, but the disease is usually more widespread, severe, and difficult to treat in patients who are debilitated, immunosuppressed, or atopic.

TABLE 17.7–6. TOPICAL STEROID CLASSIFICATION (SELECTED EXAMPLES)

Class	Generic Name	Brand Name	Potency
I	Hydrocortisone 1% Dexamethasone 0.05%	Synacort, Penecort, Nutraderm Decadron ophthalmic ointment	Low potency
II	Desonide 0.05% Locorten 0.03%	Tridesilon cream and ointment Flumethasone pivalate	Intermediate potency
III	Betamethasone valerate 0.1% Fluocinolone acetonide 0.025% Hydrocortisone valerate 0.2% Triamcinolone acetonide 0.025%	Valisone cream and lotion Synalar cream Westcort cream Aristocort cream	Moderately high potency (mid-potency)
IV	Fluocinolone acetonide 0.025% Hydrocortisone valerate 0.2% Triamcinolone acetonide 0.1%	Synalar ointment Westcort ointment Aristocort ointment	
V	Amcinonide 0.1% Betamethasone dipropionate 0.05% Betamethasone valerate 0.1% Triamcinolone acetonide 0.5%	Cyclocort cream Diprosone cream Valisone ointment Aristocort cream and ointment	
VI	Amcinonide 0.1% Betamethasone dipropionate 0.05% Desoximetasone 0.25% Fluocinonide 0.05% Halcinonide 0.1%	Cyclocort ointment Diprosone ointment Topicort ointment and cream Lidex cream and ointment Halog cream and ointment	High potency
VII	Betamethasone dipropionate 0.5% Clobetasol propionate 0.05%	Diprolene ointment Temovate cream and ointment	Very high potency

A lesion on the skin begins as a small scaly patch that gradually enlarges to form an annular lesion with erythematous, scaly borders and central clearing. Tinea pedis most often is seen as maceration and fissuring of the skin between the fourth and fifth toes. Tinea capitis is most commonly seen in children and presents as a localized or widespread scaling in the scalp. The hair becomes lusterless and fragile and may eventually be lost. The diagnosis is confirmed by the finding of fungal hyphae on a KOH preparation of scale from a lesion or an infected hair.

Mild infections of the skin usually respond to topical antifungal preparations alone. Tinea capitis, tinea unguium, and severe infections of the skin require systemic therapy. The initial drug of choice for systemic antifungal therapy is griseofulvin (250 to 500 mg twice daily until cure). For patients who are unresponsive to or unable to take griseofulvin, ketoconazole (200 to 400 mg daily until cure) is usually effective.

Candidiasis. Although *Candida albicans* is a normal inhabitant of the gastrointestinal tract, it may cause disease of the skin and mucous membranes, and under some circumstances systemic involvement may occur. Predisposing factors for candidiasis are pregnancy, oral contraceptives, diabetes mellitus, antibiotics, corticosteroids, debilitation, and immunosuppression.

Oral candidiasis, or thrush, presents as discrete, creamy white, friable patches on the mucous membranes. Cutaneous candidiasis involves primarily intertriginous areas and consists of marked erythema with papules and pustules that may form satellite lesions.

Chronic mucocutaneous candidiasis is a progressive candidal infection seen in individuals with an underlying T cell defect. Lesions are widespread and are generally resistant to therapy.

Systemic candidiasis is seen most frequently in hospitalized patients who are debilitated and immunosuppressed. The eruption consists of nonspecific erythematous macules, papules, and pustules that may become hemorrhagic. A skin biopsy of a lesion is needed to confirm the diagnosis of systemic candidiasis.

Most superficial candidal infections can be treated with topical antifungal preparations. Low-dose intravenous amphotericin B or oral ketoconazole is used to treat chronic mucocutaneous candidiasis; however, the disease invariably recurs when the medications are discontinued, and, therefore, maintenance therapy is required. Amphotericin B remains the drug of choice for systemic candidiasis. Ketoconazole and intravenous miconazole may also be effective.

Tinea Versicolor. Tinea versicolor is an extremely common superficial fungal infection caused by the organism *Pityrosporon orbiculare (Malassezia furfur)*. Some predisposing factors are warm climate, pregnancy, corticosteroids, and debilitation. Tinea versicolor is an asymptomatic or mildly pruritic eruption that involves primarily the neck, upper trunk, upper arms, and sometimes the groin. The lesions are scaly, hypopigmented or tan patches that coalesce as they enlarge. The diagnosis is confirmed by performing a KOH preparation on scale from a lesion. Characteristic hyphae and budding yeast are seen. Tinea versicolor can be treated with many different topical agents, including selenium sulfide lotion and antifungal creams. Maintenance therapy each month is usually needed to prevent recurrence. Widespread or resistant infections may be treated with a very short course of ketoconazole.

Viral Infections

Warts. Verruca vulgaris (warts) is an extremely common infection caused by the human papilloma virus. There are many different types of papilloma virus, some of which are known to be oncogenic. The immune responses leading to viral tumor regression are poorly understood but are believed to involve both a cell-mediated and a humoral immune response. Immunosuppressed patients are particularly susceptible to the development of widespread warts that are difficult to eradicate.

Numerous methods of treatment are available, including cryosurgery; electrocoagulation; and the topical application of cantharidin, trichloroacetic acid, and other acids. Severe, recalcitrant, and widespread warts may be treated with intralesional bleomycin or dinitrochlorobenzoic acid (DNCB). When DNCB is used, the patient is first sensitized to the DNCB, and then gradually increasing strengths of the DNCB are applied to the warts. This causes a localized severe allergic inflammatory reaction, which frequently leads to resolution of the warts. Genital warts (condyloma acuminatum) are usually treated with the application of 25 percent podophyllin with or without adjunctive cryosurgery.

Another type of wart, caused by a pox virus, is molluscum contagiosum. These are small, pearly, dome-shaped, or umbilicated papules that are seen most frequently on the face in children and in the genital area of adults. They can be treated quite simply with superficial curettage.

Widespread verruca vulgaris or molluscum contagiosum should alert the physician to the possibility of immunosuppressive diseases including the acquired immunodeficiency syndrome (AIDS).

Herpes Simplex. Herpes simplex is another viral disease of the skin characterized by the development of grouped vesicles on an erythematous base. The primary infection with herpes simplex usually occurs in childhood or adolescence. Infection of infants during the neonatal period is associated with dissemination and encephalitis resulting in severe morbidity and mortality. Infants do not acquire the ability to resist this DNA virus until they are several months old.

A primary infection usually involves the mouth, the lips, and the pharynx but can begin as a skin infection. Recurrent herpes simplex infections of the lips (cold sores) are a common condition. Recurrent herpes simplex infections in patients with atopic eczema may disseminate, causing eczema herpeticum, a widespread and sometimes life-threatening vesicular eruption. Recurrent herpes simplex infections of the genitalia can also be a very debilitating disease in normal individuals. Herpes simplex, like molluscum contagiosum and verruca vulgaris, can be sexually transmitted. Finally, it is important to note that indolent herpes simplex infections of the skin, especially of the genitalia and perianal region, are frequent cutaneous manifestations of the acquired immunodeficiency syndrome (AIDS).

The treatment of the herpes simplex infection of the recurrent type has until recently been very difficult. Now patients with painful recurrent herpes simplex infections of the mouth or genitalia can be treated with acyclovir (200 mg five times daily for 5 days). If frequent recurrences are a problem, acyclovir can be given prophylactically to prevent recurrences (200 mg three times daily). Unfortunately, once the drug is stopped, the viral infection tends to reappear.

Herpes Zoster. Herpes zoster infections are caused by a DNA virus whose primary infection in the human produces chickenpox. In adults, especially the elderly, this latent virus can be reactivated, producing a very characteristic, highly painful viral infection involving several dermatomes (Color Plate: Fig. 17.7–5A*). The individual lesions are characterized by grouped vesicles on an erythematous base. In the elderly, this infection can produce a great deal of debility secondary to the pain. Postherpetic neuralgia appears to increase in severity and duration with each decade of life. A herpes zoster infection in patients with Hodgkin disease or other diseases associated with T cell defects may become disseminated all over the body and involve the lungs (Hecht pneumonia). It may also be associated with a high degree of mortality. Herpes zoster infections can be treated with acyclovir (1 to 2 g per day). In addition, elderly patients may be treated with a burst of prednisone (40 to 60 mg daily) completely tapered over a 4-week period in order to minimize the complications of postherpetic neuralgia. The postherpetic neuralgia may respond to Tegretol (400 to 1200 mg per day). This drug must be used with caution because of associated bone marrow depression.

---

*Color Plate: Fig. 17.7–5A to P appears between pages 1190 and 1191.

DRUG REACTIONS

Adverse cutaneous reactions to drugs are frequently encountered and can be difficult to assess in patients receiving numerous medications. There are many different types of drug-induced rashes, both immunologic and nonimmunologic. The characteristic morphology can sometimes aid the physician in determining the causative agent. Some of the more common types of drug eruptions include morbilliform eruptions, urticaria, erythema multiforme, photosensitivity reactions, vasculitis, and fixed drug eruptions.

The drug that is responsible for an adverse reaction is frequently one that has been instituted within several days to weeks before the development of the eruption. Occasionally, however, it may have been taken by a patient for years without incident. Certain medications, such as the nonsteroidal anti-inflammatory drugs and some antibiotics, are more likely offenders than others.

The best treatment for a drug rash is the discontinuation of the offending agent. It may take 1 to 2 weeks after stopping a medication for the eruption to resolve. Topical and systemic antipruritic agents can give symptomatic relief to a patient while the rash is resolving. Anaphylactic reactions with immediate onset of generalized pruritus, urticaria, and wheezing should be treated with subcutaneous epinephrine and intramuscular diphenhydramine. Systemic steroids are sometimes used to treat severe morbilliform reactions, vasculitis, erythema multiforme, erythroderma, and toxic epidermal necrolysis.

CUTANEOUS MALIGNANCIES

Basal Cell Carcinoma

The most common cutaneous malignancy is the basal cell carcinoma. These tumors are seen primarily in Caucasians and are most often located on the face and other sun-exposed areas. A basal cell carcinoma usually begins as a pearly papule with telangiectasia, with or without central ulceration. These tumors gradually enlarge and if left untreated, can be locally destructive, but they rarely metastasize. The diagnosis should be confirmed by a biopsy. Numerous treatments are available for basal cell carcinomas, including excision, cryosurgery, electrodesiccation curettage, and laser therapy. Location and size of the tumor will help determine the preferred modality.

Squamous Cell Carcinoma

The next most frequently encountered cutaneous malignancy is squamous cell carcinoma. Sun exposure, radiographic therapy, and chronic ingestion of arsenicals will increase the risk of developing squamous cell carcinomas. Squamous cell carcinomas may also develop in old scars or chronic dermatoses. Most often a squamous cell carcinoma will arise from an actinic keratosis, a precancerous lesion occurring on skin that has been exposed to excessive amounts of solar radiation. Fair-skinned Caucasians are especially prone to the development of squamous cell carcinomas. This tumor usually presents as a slowly enlarging, indurated nodule with a central crust or ulceration. The surface may also be verrucous. Although squamous cell carcinomas tend to remain localized to the skin, they have a higher rate of metastasis than do basal cell carcinomas. After biopsy confirmation of a squamous cell carcinoma, the treatment of choice in most cases is surgical excision.

Malignant Melanoma

Malignant melanoma is a life-threatening malignancy of the melanocytic cells. Although malignant melanoma was once considered an uncommon tumor, the incidence is rising significantly. Melanoma is most frequently seen in fair-skinned individuals and is uncommon in the black population. When it does occur in blacks, melanoma is most likely to involve the palms, soles, or nails. Sun exposure and a positive family history of malignant melanoma are risk factors for the development of melanoma. There is some evi-

dence that one or more severe sunburns at a young age may increase one's risk of developing a melanoma during one's lifetime.

Malignant melanomas may arise de novo, from a preexisting nevus, or from a lentigo maligna (an irregularly shaped and variably pigmented macule usually located on the face). Changes in a mole that suggest the development of a malignant melanoma include variegation in color (both increased or decreased pigmentation or erythema), ill-defined borders with pseudopodic extensions, size greater than 6 mm, ulceration, bleeding, or the development of nodules (Color Plate: Fig. 17.7–5B).

A recently defined syndrome, the dysplastic nevus syndrome, is associated with an increased risk for the development of malignant melanoma. The syndrome may be familial or sporadic. Patients with the dysplastic nevus syndrome have many atypical-appearing moles usually involving the upper trunk. The clinical appearance of the dysplastic nevus includes a size usually between 6 and 10 mm in diameter, variegation of color, and ill-defined borders. Biopsy of a lesion reveals characteristic changes with atypia and a lymphocytic response. Patients with the dysplastic nevus syndrome require close follow-up for the possible future development of melanomas arising from the dysplastic nevi.

Treatment of a malignant melanoma depends primarily on the thickness of the melanoma as well as the location but usually involves wide excision with or without lymph node dissection. The prognosis varies primarily with thickness and location of the melanoma. The cure rate for a melanoma less than 0.85 mm in thickness is extremely high. This underscores the importance of early recognition and removal of malignant pigmented lesions.

ECZEMA (DERMATITIS)

Eczema is defined as a cutaneous response to various noxious stimuli. Three stages are recognized: acute, subacute, and chronic. An acute eczematous reaction is characterized by patches of erythema, edema, and vesiculation producing weeping of the skin. Histologically, intraepidermal vesicle formation is seen (spongiosis). Subacute eczema is characterized by erythema and slight scale formation. Vesiculation is absent. In chronic eczema, the erythema and edema are minimal; instead, the skin demonstrates thickening with increased prominence of the normal skin markings (lichenification). There are many different types of eczema. Among the more common are primary irritant dermatitis and allergic contact dermatitis.

Primary Irritant Dermatitis

Primary irritant dermatitis results from the application of harsh chemicals, such as alkalies, acids, or solvents, to the skin. The severity of this type of eczematous reaction depends on the concentration of the irritant. All patients exposed to the proper concentration of these irritants will develop an eczematous disease response. The clinical appearance ranges from an acute weeping dermatitis to a chronic eruption with erythema, scaling, lichenification, and fissuring of the skin. Treatment consists of avoidance of the irritant and application of topical steroids when indicated for relief of pruritus and inflammation.

Allergic Contact Dermatitis[4]

Allergic contact dermatitis, in contrast to primary irritant dermatitis, occurs in only a small percentage of individuals. This eczematous disease response results from the patient's developing an allergic cell-mediated reaction to a particular agent. This is a T cell–mediated inflammatory response. The five most common allergens encountered in clinical practice are *Rhus* (poison ivy, oak, or sumac), paraphenylenediamine, nickel compounds, rubber compounds, and the dichromates. In addition to these common substances, persons are subjected every day to hundreds of chemicals that, in some individuals, can produce an allergic contact dermatitis. Physicians practicing in industrial medicine are primarily con-

cerned with primary irritants and allergic contact dermatitis. Treatment of a mild allergic contact dermatitis includes cool compresses if the eruption is acute and weeping, followed by topical steroids. More severe cases are treated with a 3-week tapering course of oral steroids.

Atopic Eczema

Atopic eczema is an extremely common disorder in which there is frequently a positive family history of atopic eczema, asthma, or hay fever. Three stages of atopic eczema are recognized: infantile, juvenile, and adult. Infantile eczema is characterized by the development, between the third and sixth months of life, of an acute eczematous dermatitis predominantly involving the face and, at times, the extensor surfaces of the body. Juvenile eczema is characterized by the development, during the first and second decades of life, of a chronic, eczematous eruption characterized by intense pruritus, scale formation, and lichenification involving predominantly the flexural areas (popliteal and antecubital spaces) of the body. The adult form of eczema may be localized as highly pruritic, coin-shaped patches (nummular eczema) or may involve predominantly the hands (chronic hand eczema).

Patients with atopic eczema frequently have concomitant asthma and hay fever. These patients inherit skin that in contrast to normal skin responds to pruritogenic agents with a prolonged itch sensation and responds to repeated mild trauma (scratching) with the development of eczema. It appears certain that the eczematous lesions are the direct result of scratching of the skin. For example, patients with atopic eczema who are placed in a plaster cast demonstrate sparing of the covered area from the eczematous response.

The course of the disease is characterized by exacerbations and remissions. On infrequent occasions, an acute exacerbation of the eczema may result in the development of an exfoliative erythroderma. In addition, some atopic eczema patients demonstrate an increased propensity to develop recurrent *S. aureus* infections (impetigo, furuncles, boils), ciral infections (warts, recurrent herpes simplex infections), and widespread fungal infections (*Trichophyton rubrum* and mucocutaneous candidiasis). These complications appear to be related to a mild, transient defect in neutrophil chemotaxis and T cell-mediated immune responses. These patients frequently demonstrate elevated serum IgE levels, such as 40,000 IU (normal is approximately 400 IU). Some of these patients have undoubtedly been described under the heading of the hyper-IgE syndrome. Further studies indicate that these patients have an abnormal immune response characterized by high titer IgE anti–*S. aureus* antibodies.

The treatment of the cutaneous features of atopic eczema is directed at reducing the intense pruritus that is so characteristic of this disease process. This can be done by having the patient avoid rough clothing (wool, coarse silk), apply wet compresses to the skin, use antihistamines that are mild antipruritic agents, and apply topical steroids in the form of emollient creams or ointments. Topical steroids are both anti-inflammatory and antipruritic. Secondary infection caused by *S. aureus* should be treated with erythromycin or a penicillinase-resistant penicillin. On rare occasions, exfoliative erythroderma develops and hospitalization is required. Treatment of exfoliative erythroderma includes sedation, continuous wet dressings, and the application of topical steroid creams. Only on unusual occasions should short "bursts" of oral steroids be employed in the treatment of atopic eczema.

PSORIASIS

Psoriasis is an autosomal dominant inheritable disease of epidermal proliferation demonstrating incomplete penetrance. Approximately 30 percent of patients with psoriasis will give a positive family history. Psoriasis is characterized by erythematous, papulosquamous lesions of various sizes and shapes, displaying a silvery, loosely adherent scale (Color Plate: Fig. 17.7–5C). If the scale is removed, minute bleeding points are seen (Auspitz sign). The disease may exist as isolated, indolent patches; as generalized small lesions (guttate); as large, extensive silvery plaques; and as erythroderma. Nail involvement is characterized by subungual hyperkeratosis, onycholysis, yellowish discoloration of the nail bed (small psoriatic plaques), and pitting of the nails. Psoriatic lesions may be initiated by trauma of the skin (Koebner phenomenon). Streptococcal throat infections are associated with flare-ups of guttate psoriasis.

Psoriasis is a disease of abnormal regulation of keratinization in which there is a hyperproliferative state. The disease may be controlled, but not cured, by using topical steroids in the form of creams, ointments, or steroid-impregnated tapes. Coal tar and short-wave (UV-B) ultraviolet light (Goeckerman regimen) and PUVA therapy (the use of a combination of oral psoralens [8-methoxypsoralen] and long-wave ultraviolet light [UV-A]) are also frequently effective therapeutic approaches. In unusual instances when confronted with an exfoliative erythroderma, generalized pustular psoriasis or severe arthritis, methotrexate (25 to 50 mg intramuscularly once weekly or 2.5 to 5 mg every 12 hours for three treatments once weekly) is employed. Caution must be used when employing long-term methotrexate therapy because of the possible development of cirrhosis of the liver. Periodic liver biopsies must be performed.

SEBORRHEIC DERMATITIS

Seborrheic dermatitis (dandruff) is a very common inflammatory dermatosis of the scalp characterized by erythema and greasy scale formation. Other areas of involvement may include the eyebrows, nasolabial folds, sternum, and axillary and pubic areas. This inheritable dermatosis responds rapidly to the use of medicated shampoos (selenium sulfide or tar) and topical steroid preparations. Low-potency steroid cream (1 percent hydrocortisone) is effective for managing eyebrow and nasolabial fold involvement. It must be emphasized that fluorinated steroids should never be employed on a long-term basis to treat facial lesions because of the risk of steroid-induced atrophy and telangiectasia.

ACNE ROSACEA

Acne rosacea is a common, inflammatory dermatosis characterized by erythematous papules and pustules involving primarily the malar eminences and the nose. It generally occurs in patients between 40 and 50 years of age. The disease produces a generalized flushing of the central portion of the face with prominent telangiectasia. In severe forms, scarring and disfiguring enlargement of the nose occur (rhinophyma). This condition responds to long-term, low-dose tetracycline therapy (250 to 500 mg per day).

URTICARIA

Urticaria is an exceedingly common condition. It has been estimated that between 20 and 30 percent of the general population will experience at least one episode of urticaria during their lifetime. Urticaria ranges from erythematous, pea-sized, edematous papules to large circinate lesions with erythematous borders and cleared centers that can cover the entire body. Involvement of the lips, tongue, and epiglottis (angioneurotic edema) can be life threatening. Individual urticarial lesions generally are transient, lasting less than 24 hours.

Urticaria results from the release of histamine and other vasoactive substances from mast cells and circulating basophils. Mast cells degranulate, releasing histamine in response to nonimmunologic as well as immunologic factors. For example, mast cell degranulation may be induced by various drugs (including morphine and codeine); by eating lobsters, crayfish, and other shellfish; and by bacterial toxins. Mast cell degranulation may also occur on an immunologic basis and is generally considered to be a type I immunologic reaction. Two IgE molecules bound to the cell surface of

the mast cell or basophil are cross-linked by binding to the antigen, resulting in the release of histamine.

The causes of urticaria include (1) drugs, of which penicillin is the most common cause of acute urticaria (small traces of penicillin in milk products are an occasional cause of chronic urticaria); (2) food additives, such as tartrazine and sulfites; (3) foods such as shellfish; (4) infections, such as intestinal parasites, chronic sinusitis, or urinary tract infections; (5) internal malignancies; (6) insect bites and stings, especially flea bites in sensitive individuals and jellyfish stings; (7) inhalants, especially pollens; (8) physical urticarias induced by heat, cold, pressure, and rarely ultraviolent light; and (9) connective tissue diseases.

The treatment of urticaria involves identifying, if possible, the etiologic agent. Chronic urticaria, defined as persistent urticaria of greater than 2 to 3 months' duration, demands a thorough physical examination and appropriate laboratory tests directed toward a search for a systemic cause. Unfortunately, in the majority of cases it is not possible to determine the underlying cause of urticaria, and symptomatic treatment is used. It must be emphasized that when the individual urticarial lesion persists for greater than 24 hours a biopsy should be done to rule out the presence of urticarial vasculitis.

Symptomatically, the urticaria can be treated with H1 blockers (e.g., diphenhydramine, hydroxyzine) alone or together with an H2 blocker (cimetidine). Topically, these patients can be treated with colloidal oatmeal baths or a menthol- and/or phenol-containing lotion or cream. On unusual occasions, a short burst of steroids may be required, beginning with 30 to 40 mg of prednisone or its equivalent per day with tapering over a 2-week period.

Erythema Multiforme

Erythema multiforme is an inflammatory dermatosis similar in presentation to urticaria, except that the individual lesions persist for prolonged periods of time. The lesions consist of erythematous, edematous papules, nodules, and plaques that may be localized or involve large areas of the body. Frequently, individual lesions may demonstrate a bull's-eye or target appearance (Color Plate: Fig. 17.7–5D). Others may demonstrate blister formation (see section on bullous diseases).

In recent years, it has been recognized that recurrent erythema multiforme is frequently seen in association with a recurrent herpes simplex infection. These lesions are associated with circulating immune complexes and the presence of immunoreactants in and about the diseased blood vessels; recently, antigens related to the herpes simplex virus have been detected in involved blood vessels.

On occasion, erythema multiforme may predominantly involve mucous membranes (eyes, nose, mouth, urethra, or vagina). Severe denuding occurs, resulting in significant morbidity. This variant is termed the "Stevens-Johnson syndrome." In addition to the infectious cause of erythema multiforme, erythema multiforme has been associated with various drugs including phenacetin, penicillin, sulfonamides, mercury, arsenic, dilantin, and barbiturates.

The treatment of erythema multiforme involves investigation for an underlying cause. All drugs that are not absolutely necessary must be discontinued. In general, the minor forms of erythema multiforme do not require therapy. Prophylactic treatment of the recurrent herpes simplex infections with acyclovir usually results in a disappearance of the recurrent erythema multiforme. At times, the Stevens-Johnson syndrome may require hospitalization and the administration of parenteral fluids and systemic steroids.

ACNE

Acne vulgaris is a very common dermatosis affecting virtually all adolescents. The primary lesions are comedones, erythematous papules, pustules, and in severe cases, cysts (Color Plate: Fig. 17.7–5E). These lesions most frequently involve the face, neck, and less commonly, the back, chest, and upper arms. The disease process is usually self-limited, beginning at the time of puberty and ending generally by the time that the adolescent reaches adulthood. Acne can produce both physical and emotional scars in young people at a vulnerable time in their lives.

The exact pathogenesis appears to be complex. It is clear that the initial events involve the blockage of the hair follicle of the pilosebaceous unit. With the blockage of a pilosebaceous follicle, the contents of the sebaceous glands build up and, at times, can be seen as small whiteheads in the skin. Saprophytic bacteria on the skin such as *Propionibacterium acnes*, which contain lipases, are capable of hydrolyzing the fatty acids into free fatty acids and glycerol. The integrity of the pilosebaceous unit appears to be altered, and it is thought that the free fatty acids, which are capable of inducing an inflammatory response, leak into the surrounding tissue and induce the characteristic inflammation. If severe enough, this inflammation can result in scar formation. Severe cystic acne rarely may be associated with systemic features such as fever, malaise, myalgias, and arthralgias. This form of cystic acne is termed "acne fulminans."

Acne vulgaris occurs in areas of the body that have the highest concentration of sebaceous glands. The sebaceous gland appears to have extreme sensitivity to small quantities of androgens. The characteristic flare of acne at the time of menses is thought to result from androgen-like hormones secreted by the ovaries during ovulation. Estrogens, on the other hand, suppress the sebaceous gland and diminish the acne.

Therapy for acne is directed at several areas. Attempts should be made to remove the blockage from the pilosebaceous hair follicle using a variety of available peeling agents that contain such chemicals as sulfur, resorcinol, vitamin A, or benzoyl peroxide. Blackheads and whiteheads can also be manually removed by a dermatologist employing a small comedone extractor. Tetracycline (250 to 1.0 g per day) has been found to be very effective in the control of acne. The exact mechanism of action of tetracycline is unknown. Whether it acts on the sebaceous gland itself or on the saprophytic bacteria is a moot point. The tetracycline results in a marked alteration in the sebum; the free fatty acid content is diminished.

Although the tetracycline and the peeling agents are successful in controlling approximately 95 percent of acne patients, approximately 5 percent of acne patients develop a severe, aggressively scarring, cystic acne. Recently, a new drug, a vitamin A derivative, 13-*cis*-retinoic acid, had been successfully employed in the treatment of these patients. This drug has demonstrated a dramatic effect on cystic acne patients and is associated with an approximately 85 percent cure rate. This drug is given in a dosage of 1 to 2 mg/kg per day for 16 to 20 weeks. The exact mechanism of action of the 13-*cis*-retinoic acid is unknown. The sebaceous gland, however, undergoes an involution with a subsequent decrease in the production of sebum. 13-*cis*-Retinoic acid is a highly teratogenic drug and must not be employed in women during pregnancy.

BULLOUS DISEASES

The bullous diseases are an uncommon group of skin conditions associated with much morbidity. They are classified as being either intraepidermal or subepidermal depending on the microscopic localization of the split (see Table 17.7–7).

Pemphigus

The pemphigus diseases, which include pemphigus vulgaris, pemphigus foliaceus, pemphigus vegetans, and fogo selvagem (an endemic pemphigus foliaceus found in South America), are examples of intraepidermal blistering diseases. Pemphigus vulgaris is the most severe bullous disease. In the presteroid and preantibiotic era, pemphigus vulgaris was associated with a 50 percent mortality within 12 months of the onset of the disease. It appears to occur with an increased frequently in Jews and has been associated with

TABLE 17.7–7. BULLOUS SKIN DISEASES

Disease	Site of Blister Formation	Pattern and Immunoglobulin Isotypes	Serum Autoantibodies	Clinical Findings
Pemphigus	Intraepidermal	Linear IgG	Yes (90%)	Flaccid bullae on mucous membranes and skin; positive Nikolsky sign
Staphylococcal scalded skin syndrome	High intraepidermal	None	No	Loss of sheets of skin; positive Nikolsky sign; usually a benign disease
Bullous pemphigoid	Subepidermal	Linear IgG	Yes (80%)	Tense blisters especially in flexural areas; negative Nikolsky sign; mucous membranes usually spared
Benign mucous membrane pemphigoid	Subepidermal	Linear IgG	Yes (10%)	Erosions and scarring on mucous membranes of eyes, mouth, and sometimes vagina; 15% have cutaneous blisters as well
Herpes gestationis	Subepidermal	Linear IgG (25%)	Yes (25%)	Tense blisters, usually on an erythematous or urticarial base
Dermatitis herpetiformis	Subepidermal	Granular IgA (~100%)	No	Grouped vesicles on extensor areas of body
Chronic bullous disease of childhood (linear IgA dermatosis of childhood)	Subepidermal	Linear IgA	Yes (occasionally)	Tense bullae, frequently grouped; distributed over lower trunk, buttocks, thighs, and genital areas
Epidermolysis bullosa acquisita	Subepidermal	Linear IgG	Yes (occasionally)	Tense bullae in areas of trauma, e.g., arms, extensor limbs
Bullous erythema multiforme	Subepidermal	None	No	Typical bull's-eye lesions surrounded by tense bullae; may be hemorrhagic
Drug-induced toxic epidermal necrolysis	Subepidermal	None	No	Erythema with flaccid bullae and shedding of skin; positive Nikolsky sign in areas of erythema

the HLA-DRw4 phenotype. Pemphigus is characterized by flaccid blister formation involving the skin and mucous membranes. These flaccid blisters arise on noninflamed skin. The application of a shearing force to the skin results in either new blister formation or denuding of the skin (Nikolsky sign). Widespread denuding of the skin may occur, and the mucous membranes of the mouth, eyes, and vagina may demonstrate a similar sloughing.

Recent studies have documented that pemphigus vulgaris is an autoimmune disease in which the patient produces predominantly an IgG autoantibody directed against a cell surface autoantigen on the keratinocytes. Subsequent to the binding of the antibody to this antigen, the antigen-antibody complex is internalized, and proteolytic enzymes are synthesized by the keratinocyte. The proteolytic enzyme or enzymes produce dissolution of the intercellular substance, completely destroying the normal keratinocyte-to-keratinocyte adhesion. This produces a separation of these cells, resulting in blister formation.

Pemphigus vulgaris is treated with high doses of systemic steroids (prednisone, 60 to 100 mg per day), immunosuppressive agents (Imuran, 150 mg/day, cyclophosphamide, 100 to 150 mg/day), or a combination of systemic steroids and an immunosuppressive agent. Today, the mortality over a 5- to 10-year period is approximately 8 percent. Although the mortality from pemphigus vulgaris has been markedly reduced, this blistering disease and the side effects from prolonged steroids produce much morbidity.

Scalded Skin Syndrome
The scalded skin syndrome is another example of an intraepidermal blistering disease. This is a relatively benign condition characterized by staphylococcal infection in infancy and early childhood with mucopurulent rhinorrhea, conjunctivitis, and mild to moderate toxemia. Flaccid intraepidermal blisters form with loss of sheets of epidermis following minimal shearing pressure (Nikolsky sign). The disease is short lived and recovery is complete. Group two, phage 71 S. aureus is cultured from the nose or conjunctiva.

The disease is produced by a low-molecular-weight protein (25,000 daltons) termed "exfoliatin." This protein is produced by S. aureus and is capable of destroying normal cell keratinocyte integrity, producing an intraepidermal blister formation. However, with the initial infection, the host responds by producing an antitoxin antibody, and thus, subsequent S. aureus phage 71 infections are generally not associated with this cutaneous syndrome.

Bullous Pemphigoid
Bullous pemphigoid is a subepidermal blistering disease occurring most frequently in the elderly. It is characterized by tense blister formation generally occurring in the flexural areas (axillary and inguinal regions). Widespread blistering can occur with subsequent denuding. Unlike pemphigus vulgaris, however, this condition is not associated with significant mortality.

Bullous pemphigoid is an autoantibody disease in which the patient makes an IgG autoantibody directed against an autoantigen localized to the basement membrane zone. Deposition of the antibody at the dermal-epidermal junction is associated with deposition of various complement components. An inflammatory process develops and subsequently, the integrity of the epidermal-dermal junction is disrupted and a blister is formed.

The disease process responds to high doses of prednisone (60 mg per day) and/or Imuran (100 to 150 mg/day).

Benign Mucous Membrane Pemphigoid
Benign mucous membrane pemphigoid is closely related to bullous pemphigoid. Patients with this disorder develop subepidermal blisters with subsequent scarring on mucous membranes of the eyes, mouth and, on rare occasions, the vagina. This disease is thought to be an autoantibody disease in which an IgG autoantibody is directed against an autoantigen localized to the mucous membrane–basement membrane zone. Direct immunofluorescent studies have frequently demonstrated the deposition of immunoglobulin and various complement components at the site of patho-

logic findings. Approximately 15 percent of patients with benign mucous membrane pemphigoid will also demonstrate the presence of subepidermal blisters on the skin. The treatment of this condition, which if untreated can result in blindness in one or both eyes in 20 percent of the cases, is systemic steroids (prednisone, 40 to 60 mg per day) and/or immunosuppressive agents (cyclophosphamide, 25 to 50 mg daily).

Herpes Gestationis

Herpes gestationis is a subepidermal blistering disease of pregnancy that also appears to be closely related to bullous pemphigoid. During the second and third trimesters of pregnancy, these women develop an intensely pruritic, subepidermal blistering disease characterized by tense blisters on erythematous macules, papules, and urticaria-like lesions. This disease process appears to be the result of an avid complement-fixing IgG autoantibody directed against an antigen along the basement membrane zone. Infants born of these affected mothers transiently demonstrate the subepidermal blistering formation. When direct immunofluorescence studies are performed on these neonates, the deposition of complement components is demonstrated along the skin–basement membrane zone.

The treatment of these pregnant mothers is symptomatic. Topical steroids and antihistamines (diphenhydramine) are employed. On unusual occasions, patients require 20 to 40 mg of prednisone daily in order to control blister formation. After the pregnancy, the disease generally completely remits. It may recur with subsequent pregnancies or with the institution of estrogen-type birth control pills.

Dermatitis Herpetiformis

Dermatitis herpetiformis is a chronic, intensely pruritic, subepidermal, blistering disease characterized by grouped vesicles on an inflammatory base and generally localized to extensor areas of the body (buttocks, back, elbows, and knees). Patients are generally middle-aged to elderly. This disease process is associated with granular deposition of IgA along the dermal-epidermal junction. In addition, approximately 80 percent of dermatitis herpetiformis patients will demonstrate a patchy duodenal jejunal atrophy indistinguishable from adult celiac disease (gluten-sensitive enteropathy). As in celiac disease, a gluten-free diet will result in the disappearance of the skin disease, and with reinstitution of a gluten diet, the skin disease will recur. The exact relationship between adult celiac disease and dermatitis herpetiformis is not clear. Both conditions are associated with an increased frequency of the HLA-B8 and DR3 phenotypes. The skin lesions of dermatitis herpetiformis, but not the gut lesions, respond to diaminodiphenylsulfone (Dapsone, 50 to 100 mg daily). When using Dapsone, the patient should first be checked for glucose-6-phosphate dehydrogenase deficiency, and bimonthly blood counts should be obtained and monitored for potential bone marrow suppression.

Chronic Bullous Disease of Childhood

Chronic bullous disease of childhood appears to represent several different entities including bullous pemphigoid and dermatitis herpetiformis. Some patients described under the heading of "bullous disease of childhood" have an IgA autoantibody disease in which the autoantibody is directed against an antigen at the dermal-epidermal junction. Subsequent blister formation follows. Unlike dermatitis herpetiformis, these patients do not have a gastroenteropathy or demonstrate an increased frequency of the HLA-B8 or DR3 phenotypes. Their skin disease, however, does respond to diaminodiphenylsulfone or sulfapyridine. This disease is usually self-limited, resolving around the time of puberty.

Epidermolysis Bullosa Acquisita

Epidermolysis bullosa acquisita is a rare subepidermal blistering disease of variable severity in which the patient makes an autoantibody directed against the subbasal, lamina-anchoring fibril zone of the basement membrane located high in the papillary portion of the dermis. This autoantibody disease is characterized by tense subepidermal blisters involving predominantly the extensor surfaces of the hands and, at times, the mucous membranes, especially of the mouth. These tense blisters generally occur on a noninflammatory base and resolve with scarring and milia formation. This autoantibody disease responds poorly to high doses of corticosteroids and immunosuppressive agents.

Bullous Erythema Multiforme

Erythema multiforme can result in destruction of the dermal–epidermal junction by an intense inflammatory infiltrate producing subepidermal blister formation. This disease process is unassociated with autoantibody formation. This condition may be seen as part of a drug reaction, as a complication of vaccination, as an infection, or as part of a graft-versus-host reaction. The application of shearing forces to the skin produces Nikolsky sign and denuding of large areas of skin. A severe variant of bullous erythema multiforme is Stevens-Johnson syndrome, in which patients have severe involvement of the mucous membranes of the mouth and eyes. Bullous erythema multiforme, especially the Stevens-Johnson variant, is a very serious, life-threatening disease process requiring large doses of systemic steroids (several hundred milligrams of prednisone per day) and fluid and electrolyte management as for burn patients.

Toxic Epidermal Necrolysis

Toxic epidermal necrolysis is usually seen in adults and is drug induced (Color Plate: Fig. 17.7–5F). Patients develop a widespread morbilliform or macular erythematous eruption that is followed by the development of flaccid bullae in areas of erythema where there is a positive Nikolsky sign. Large sheets of skin may be shed. The blister formation is secondary to necrosis of the basal cells and is in a subepidermal location. The mucous membranes are characteristically involved. This is a serious disease with a fairly high mortality. Treatment is largely supportive, and the use of systemic steroids remains controversial.

CUTANEOUS MANIFESTATIONS OF SYSTEMIC DISEASE[2,5]

CONNECTIVE TISSUE DISEASES

Lupus Erythematosus

Skin lesions occur in approximately 25 percent of patients with systemic lupus erythematosus. The most common cutaneous manifestation is an erythematous, coin-shaped (discoid) lesion demonstrating atrophy, telangiectasia, and an adherent scale with follicular plugging (Color Plate: 17.7–5G). Discoid lesions may be seen in patients who have no systemic disease (benign, cutaneous lupus) or in patients with systemic illness. Whether or not a discoid lupus lesion is associated with benign or systemic disease can be ascertained only by a history and physical examination and appropriate serologic testing. Cutaneous lupus lesions usually occur on light-exposed areas and commonly involve the central portion of the face, producing the characteristic butterfly dermatitis on the malar eminences and the nose (Color Plate: Fig. 17.7–5H). Lupus lesions can also involve the scalp, producing a permanent, scarring alopecia.

In addition to the classic discoid lupus lesions, the lupus patients possessing anti-Ro(SS-A) antibodies frequently present with widespread annular, polycyclic, intensely photosensitive cutaneous lupus lesions (Color Plate: Fig. 17.7–5I). These patients usually have only mild systemic disease, which has been termed "subacute cutaneous lupus erythematosus." Lupus patients also frequently have periungual erythema and splinter hemorrhages suggestive of an underlying vasculitis. These cutaneous lupus lesions frequently respond to topical steroids and hydroxychloroquine (200 mg per day). The lesions of subacute cutaneous lupus erythematosus also respond to diaminodiphenylsulfone (50 to 100 mg daily).

Dermatomyositis

Patients with dermatomyositis characteristically develop an erythematous, violaceous, edematous eruption over both upper eyelids (heliotrope). In addition, a highly pruritic and frequently photosensitive erythematous, scaly eruption may be present in a generalized or photo distribution. This may at times be indistinguishable from a lupus rash. Hypopigmentation and hyperpigmentation, with atrophy and telangiectasia (poikiloderma), may also be seen. Dermatomyositis patients frequently have periungual erythema and the presence of very characteristic erythematous, edematous, maculopapular lesions over the dorsal surfaces of the metacarpophalangeal and proximal interphalangeal joints of the hands (Gottron papules) (Color Plate: Fig. 17.7–5J).

Systemic Sclerosis

Systemic sclerosis is characterized by a bound-down thickened skin, waxy in appearance, involving predominantly the acral areas (hands, feet, and face) (Color Plate: Fig. 17.7–5K). These lesions are associated with atrophy, resorption of the distal portions of the finger, and Raynaud phenomenon. Similar sclerosis may be found over widespread areas of the body. There may be involvement of other organ systems including the heart, lungs, kidneys, and gastrointestinal tract. A benign form of scleroderma called "morphea" is characterized by isolated, round, sclerotic plaques. Unlike systemic sclerosis, morphea lesions are generally not associated with systemic involvement.

The CRST syndrome is a variant of scleroderma characterized by calcinosis, Raynaud phenomenon, acral sclerosis, and telangiectasia (Color Plate: Fig. 17.7–5L). There is usually minimal visceral involvement in these patients. These patients frequently possess anticentromere antibodies in their serum. Eosinophilic fasciitis (Shulman disease) is a peculiar sclerotic process, characteristically following strenuous exercise, in which the skin becomes thickened and bound-down. These patients, unlike scleroderma patients, usually lack Raynaud phenomenon. Deep biopsies of skin in these patients' involved areas demonstrate various numbers of eosinophils in the subcutaneous and fascial tissues.

D-Penicillamine has recently been shown to be effective in the treatment of some patients with systemic sclerosis. The drug is given initially at a dose of 250 mg per day for several months and then raised to 500 mg per day and finally, after the passage of several months, raised to 750 mg daily. Unfortunately, this drug is associated with toxicity and the induction of other autoimmune diseases, such as lupus erythematosus, myasthenia gravis, and nephritis, and no controlled studies have been conducted. Oral steroids (prednisone, 40 to 60 mg/day) have been shown to be effective in treating some patients with eosinophilic fasciitis.

Relapsing Polychondritis

Relapsing polychondritis is a chronic, inflammatory disease of cartilage. These patients frequently have erythematous, edematous, painful ears (Color Plate: Fig. 17.7–5M). The cartilage of the nose and trachea may also be involved. The condition responds to high doses of prednisone (40 to 60 mg/day) or diaminodiphenylsulfone (50 to 100 mg daily).

Vasculitis

The cutaneous manifestations of vasculitis are complex. They depend on the skin level of blood vessel involvement and the intensity of the inflammatory insult. Vasculitis can manifest itself as small petechial lesions, purpuric erythematous papules, urticarial lesions, bullae, pustules, and ulcers (Color Plate: Fig. 17.7–5N). Splinter hemorrhages in the nails, periungual telangiectasia, and small linear infarcts are also commonly seen as cutaneous manifestations of vasculitis. Cutaneous vasculitis may represent septic embolization (subacute bacterial endocarditis, gonococcus cutaneous arthritis syndrome), connective tissue disease (lupus erythematosus, scleroderma), or the manifestations of a systemic vasculitis such as polyarteritis nodosa and Wegener granulomatosis. Vasculitic lesions generally respond to high doses of corticosteroids (pred-

nisone, 40 to 60 mg/day) and immunosuppressive agents (Cytoxan, 1 to 2 mg/kg per day).

TABLE 17.7–8. CARCINOMAS MOST LIKELY TO METASTASIZE TO SKIN

• Breast	• Kidney
• Stomach	• Ovary
• Lung	• Colon
• Uterus	• Bladder

MALIGNANCY

The frequency of metastasis to the skin ranges between 1 and 5 percent. The carcinomas with the most frequent cutaneous metastases are breast, stomach, lung, uterus, and kidney. Certain skin areas are more susceptible to metastasis. For example, the scalp is a common site for metastases from the breast, lung, and genitourinary tract; the umbilicus for neoplasms in the gastrointestinal tract; the chest for mammary carcinoma; and the lower abdomen and external genitalia for urinary tract malignancies.

The cutaneous manifestations of metastatic carcinoma generally are subcutaneous or intradermal hard nodules that vary in color. Ulceration may occur. Any skin nodule or tumor that is atypical for known dermatologic disorders should be considered to be a possible metastasis, and a biopsy specimen should be obtained. Certain malignancies are more likely to metastasize to the skin than others (Table 17.7–8).

Some malignancies can produce a fairly characteristic clinical picture when they metastasize (Table 17.7–9). There are also many nonspecific cutaneous findings that may be associated with underlying malignancies (Table 17.7–10). Some of these disorders, such as extensive warts or acanthosis nigricans, have a very low association with internal malignancy and are more likely to be seen in healthy individuals. On the other hand, the disorder known as *hypertrichosis lanuginosum acquisita*, in which patients experience a generalized growth of fine pale lanugo hairs, is nearly always associated with an underlying malignancy.

Mycosis fungoides is a systemic lymphoma beginning in the skin. It may begin as isolated, eczematous patches (parapsoriasis) and evolve over many years (generally 10 years or more) into nodules or tumors (Color Plate: Fig. 17.7–5O). Systemic involvement may occur at this time. At times the mycosis fungoides may progress to the development of a generalized exfoliative erythroderma (Sézary syndrome).

TABLE 17.7–9. CHARACTERISTIC PRESENTATION OF SOME CUTANEOUS METASTASES

Primary Carcinoma	Cutaneous Metastasis
Breast carcinoma	Carcinoma erysipelas—cellulitis-like plaque
Paget disease of breast and extramammary Paget disease	Eczematous, weeping crusted lesions
Malignant melanoma	Diffuse hyperpigmentation
Small-cell carcinoma (others as well)	Cushing syndrome with hyperpigmentation (secondary to ACTH and MSH-like activity)
Carcinoid	Flushing
Bronchogenic carcinoma	Clubbing of fingers
Esophageal carcinoma	Palmoplantar hyperkeratosis
Lymphoma, leukemia	Exfoliative erythroderma

TABLE 17.7–10. NONSPECIFIC CUTANEOUS SIGNS AND SYMPTOMS THAT MAY BE ASSOCIATED WITH UNDERLYING MALIGNANCY

- Generalized pruritus
- Acquired ichthyosis
- Superficial thrombophlebitis
- Leukocytoelastic vasculitis
- Hypertrichosis lanuginosum acquisita (generalized growth of fine, pale hairs)
- Multiple eruptive seborrheic keratoses (Leser-Trelat sign)
- Acanthosis nigricans
- Multiple recalcitrant warts

SARCOID

Sarcoid is a systemic granulomatous disease of unknown etiology. Cutaneous lesions specific for sarcoid occur in approximately 25 percent of patients. Sarcoidal lesions exist as papules, nodules, plaques, subcutaneous tumors, or a generalized scaling erythema (Color Plate: Fig. 17.7–5P). The lesions may be translucent and red-brown or violaceous; less commonly there may be prominent telangiectasia (angiolupoid). If one presses a glass slide against the sarcoid lesion (diascopy), a yellow-brown color may be detected.

In addition to these cutaneous sarcoid lesions, erythema nodosum (multiple, tender, erythematous nodules over the anterior surface of the lower extremities) is seen in approximately 20 percent of patients with sarcoidosis. Erythema nodosum is a nonspecific manifestation of sarcoid and can also be seen in association with other disorders, for example, drug reactions, use of birth control pills, deep fungal infections, streptococcal infections, and tuberculosis.

BLOOD VESSELS

Alterations in blood vessels may provide important clues to systemic disease. Alterations in the hemoglobin may produce very dramatic color changes on the skin. Examples include the pallor of anemia and the plethora of polycythemia vera, the characteristic cherry-red coloration of carbon monoxide poisoning, and the cyanosis associated with cardiopulmonary diseases.

Telangiectasias (dilated capillaries, venules, and arterioles) are commonly seen in connective tissue diseases, especially around the base of the nails (periungual telangiectasia). Spider angiomas are characterized by a central, slightly elevated pulsating arteriole surrounded by radiating telangiectasias. If the central arteriole is compressed, the radiating telangiectasias blanch. These lesions are generally seen over the upper half of the body, and they can be seen in cirrhosis or pregnancy as well as without associated systemic disease. Osler-Rendu-Weber disease, an autosomal dominant disease, is characterized by telangiectatic vascular lesions on the mucous membranes, palms, soles, nails, and ears. Melena, epistaxis, and on unusual occasions, arteriovenous pulmonary fistulas producing cyanosis and clubbing are the result of these lesions.

Kaposi sarcoma is an example of a blood vessel tumor. Excluding the AIDS population, Kaposi sarcoma characteristically begins as purplish macules, papules, and nodules, predominantly on the lower extremities and especially involving the feet and toes of elderly individuals. These nodules may subsequently ulcerate. Lymphedema of the legs is frequently present. The disease is slowly progressive, and these patients usually do not die from the Kaposi sarcoma. In AIDS patients, however, this blood vessel tumor is seen in younger patients and is recognized as a generalized fulminant disease involving many organs of the body.[7]

GASTROINTESTINAL DISEASES

There are a number of gastrointestinal diseases associated with prominent cutaneous manifestations. The Peutz-Jeghers syndrome is characterized by small intestinal polyps that may lead to intussusception and melena. The cutaneous hallmarks of this syndrome are distinctive, macular, hyperpigmented areas on the mucous membranes of the lips. Gardner syndrome is an autosomal dominant disease characterized by premalignant colonic polyps. The cutaneous hallmarks of this syndrome are large epidermal inclusion cysts found predominantly on the face and scarring fibromas. Ulcerative colitis and regional enteritis may be associated with the development of erythema nodosum lesions over the anterior surface of the lower legs. In addition, these two conditions may also be associated with pyoderma gangrenosum. Pyoderma gangrenosum is a rapidly destructive ulcerating cutaneous disease that initially begins as an erythematous papule or pustule that rapidly ulcerates, producing a progressively enlarging ulceration with characteristic purplish undermined edges. The area of ulceration can reach huge proportions (25 to 30 cm) in 6 to 8 weeks. High doses of corticosteroids (prednisone, 100 mg daily) as well as pulse intravenous methylprednisone (1 g/day for 3 successive days) has been shown to be effective in treating some of these patients. Cirrhosis is manifested on the skin by spider angiomas, palmar erythema, and gynecomastia. In approximately 80 percent of cirrhosis patients, the nails become totally white (Terry sign).

ENDOCRINE DISEASES

Cutaneous manifestations of endocrine diseases are important diagnostic features of these diseases (Table 17.7–11). Hypopituitarism following a postpartum hemorrhage (Sheehan syndrome), pituitary tumors, or surgery is associated with pallor as a consequence of decreased melanin pigmentation secondary to the loss of melanocyte-stimulating hormone (MSH).

Excessive secretion of growth hormone produces gigantism in children before the epiphyses have closed and acromegaly in adults.

TABLE 17.7–11. CUTANEOUS MANIFESTATIONS OF ENDOCRINE DISORDERS

Endocrine Disorder	Cutaneous Findings
Hypopituitarism	Pallor secondary to decreased MSH activity
Hyperpituitarism (increased growth hormone)	Gigantism in children Acromegaly in adults
Hyperthyroidism	Warm, moist, fine skin, fine hair, pretibial myxedema, exophthalmos
Hypothyroidism	Dry, rough skin, puffy face, coarse features, coarse hair
Addison disease	Diffuse hyperpigmentation (especially on extensor surfaces and areas of friction)
Cushing disease	Plethoric facies, telangiectasias, purple striae, buffalo hump, supraclavicular fat pads, acne, increased susceptibility to fungal infections
Diabetes mellitus	Increased susceptibility to *S. aureus* and *Candida* infections, necrobiosis lipoidica diabeticorum (atrophic, yellow plaques on anterior shins), neurotropic ulcers

In acromegaly, the skin is thickened, skin tags are often present, and ridges and furrows are formed over the face and scalp (cutis verticis gyrata). The lips are thick. The nose enlarges. The jaw becomes prominent, and the hands become broad.

Hyperthyroidism is characterized by warm, moist, fine skin. Onycholysis (the separation of the nail plate from the nail bed) is also frequently present. The hair is fine and is generally not capable of retaining a permanent hair wave. Vitiligo and prematurely gray hair also develop in many patients with autoimmune thyroid disease. In some hyperthyroid patients, a very peculiar, diffuse, and at times erythematous thickening of the pretibial areas (pretibial myxedema) occurs, associated with increased mucin deposition in the skin. This "peau d'orange" change in the skin resembles the peel of an orange. Hypothyroidism is associated with very dry, roughened skin. The facial expression is often flat and edematous, especially in the infraorbital areas. The hair is coarse and rough.

Adrenal insufficiency (Addison disease) is associated with diffuse hyperpigmentation which is produced by an increased secretion of β-MSH and ACTH from the pituitary. This increased pigmentation is most prominent in exposed areas of the body, recent scars, and areas of friction such as the knuckles, knees, elbows, and belt line. Vitiligo is also present in approximately 10 to 15 percent of patients with Addison disease. Adrenal hyperfunction (Cushing syndrome) is associated with a characteristic, round, plethoric face with prominent telangiectasia. Supraclavicular fat pads and a characteristic buffalo hump over the upper portion of the thoracic spine develop. Striae are very common in the axillary and inguinal regions as well as over the abdomen. Acne lesions and ecchymoses may be prominent. These patients also frequently develop superficial fungal infections (tinea versicolor, *Trichophyton rubrum*). The adrenogenital syndrome results from the excessive secretion of adrenal hormones with androgenic activity. In the female, this may be associated with the development of hirsutism with a male distribution, clitoral enlargement, acne vulgaris including deep, cystic, and pustular acne, increased muscle tone and mass, and the features of a male habitus.

Diabetes mellitus is associated with increased susceptibility to *Candida albicans* infections in the genital region and an increased susceptibility to *S. aureus* cutaneous infections (boils, furuncles, folliculitis). Necrobiosis lipoidica diabeticorum is a complication of diabetes mellitus characterized by sharply demarcated plaques with a thin atrophic surface and prominent telangiectasia. The color of the plaque is a characteristic red-brown-yellow. These lesions usually occur over the anterior surfaces of the lower extremities but can occur infrequently at other sites. Necrobiosis lipoidica diabeticorum may precede the onset of diabetes but generally develops after the patient has had diabetes for several years.

Glucagon-secreting islet cell tumors of the pancreas are often accompanied by a characteristic necrolytic migratory erythema.

METABOLIC DISEASES

The hyperlipidemias are frequently associated with cutaneous manifestations. Cutaneous manifestations are characterized by a variety of cutaneous xanthomas (tendinous, tuberous, or eruptive). Tendinous xanthomas are firm nodules localized predominantly on the tendons of the hands, knees, ankles, and elbows. The tendinous xanthomas are associated with familial hypercholesterolemia. Tuberous xanthomas are large, lipid nodules in the dermis and subcutaneous tissue. These lesions can be found in association with either increased serum cholesterol or increased triglyceride levels. Eruptive xanthomas are small, red-yellow papular lesions arising on an erythematous base and appearing in crops. They develop primarily on the arms, buttocks, and backs of the thighs. Eruptive xanthomas always signal extremely high serum triglyceride levels. When the triglyceride levels return to normal levels, the eruptive xanthomas disappear.

Porphyria cutanea tarda is a disorder of porphyrin metabolism that is usually acquired but may be inherited as an autosomal dominant disease. Defects in porphyrin metabolism lead to increased excretion of urinary porphyrins, primarily uroporphyrin. Clinically, these patients demonstrate vesicles, bullae, erosions, and milia on the dorsal areas of the hands (Color Plate: Fig. 17.7–5Q). These changes are caused by both sun exposure and trauma. Hypertrichosis of the cheeks and forehead is also a frequent finding. Porphyria cutanea tarda may be precipitated by ethanol and estrogens. Treatment consists of either phlebotomies or low-dose chloroquine therapy (125 mg orally twice weekly).

REFERENCES

1. Arndt KA (ed): Manual of Dermatologic Therapeutics, 3d ed. Boston, Little, Brown, 1983
2. Braverman IM: Skin Signs of Systemic Disease. 2d ed. Philadelphia, WB Saunders, 1981
3. Diaz LA, Anhalt GJ, et al: Autoimmune cutaneous diseases. In Rose N (ed): The Autoimmune Diseases. New York, Academic Press, 1985, p 443
4. Fisher AA: Contact Dermatitis, 3d ed. Philadelphia, Lea & Febiger, 1986
5. Fitzpatrick TB, Eisen AZ, et al (eds): Dermatology In General Medicine, 3d ed. New York, McGraw-Hill, 1987
6. Moschella SL, Hurley HJ (eds): Dermatology, 2d ed. Philadelphia, WB Saunders, 1985
7. Penneys NS, Hicks B: Unusual cutaneous lesions associated with acquired immunodeficiency syndrome. J Am Acad Dermatol 13:845, 1985

REFERENCE VALUES FOR LABORATORY PROCEDURES

Robert C. Rock
and Robert E. Miller

DEFINITIONS

The phrase "references values" is preferable to that of "normal range" in defining limits for interpreting quantitative laboratory tests. The reference values for a procedure are defined in terms of both a population of presumably healthy (or, at least, asymptomatic) individuals and the particular analytical technology employed.[5] The term "normal range" is misleading, as the results of most laboratory procedures do not follow gaussian or "normal" distributions in nondiseased subjects, and individuals whose test results are outside the normal range are not necessarily "abnormal."[4]

SOURCES OF VARIANCE

Meaningful comparison of a test result for an individual patient with published reference values requires an awareness of the biologic and analytical variances that affect all laboratory tests. *Biologic* variability includes both *intraindividual* differences, caused by effects of posture, diet, and circadian rhythms, and *interindividual* differences among "healthy" subjects or patients. Interindividual variability is a particular problem when evaluating a "borderline" test result for a single patient. Published listings of reference values—such as the following—have been defined using large, often heterogeneous, groups of subjects and reflect principally interindividual variability. *Analytical* variability includes that associated with the collection and handling of specimens, with test interferences due to drugs and endogenous metabolites, with methodologic differences between laboratories, and with the day-to-day imprecision within any laboratory. Although automation and improved analytical methods have reduced within-laboratory variability and interferences caused by drugs and endogenous metabolites, caution must still be used when interpreting results reported for the same procedure performed in different laboratories.

OPERATING CHARACTERISTICS OF LABORATORY TESTS

The concepts of *sensivity, specificity,* and *predictive values* of diagnostic procedures are discussed in Section 1. Of particular importance in the interpretation of laboratory procedures is the effect of the *prevalence* of clinically significant abnormalities in the population tested, as well as the effect of the reference values used. For example, a test with 95 percent specificity, that is, a false-positive rate of 5 percent, and comparable sensitivity applied to a population with a 1 percent prevalence of disease will produce almost five false-positive results for every true-positive one.[3,7] Use of different reference values or "cutoff" points for a test may significantly alter the sensitivity, specificity, and predictive value of the test; hence reference values must be selected appropriately in light of the biologic and analytical variability of the procedure and of the consequences to diagnosis and patient management of false-positive and false-negative results.

CLINICAL USE OF LABORATORY TESTS AND TEST PERFORMANCE

The original use of laboratory tests was to confirm a clinical diagnosis or evaluate alternative diagnoses. The recent trend toward "screening" (detection of disease in asymptomatic subjects) has increased the need for more sensitive tests, that is, with fewer false-negative results, for initial evaluation of patients, and for more *specific* tests, that is, with fewer false-positive results, for follow-up and definitive diagnosis. Additionally the growing use of laboratory tests to monitor known conditions has placed renewed emphasis upon improved analytical precision of test methods so that small but clinically significant changes in test results can be detected.

ORGANIZATION OF THE TABLE

Reference values are arranged in sections by type of specimen, and alphabetically by procedure within each section. Comments are included where different methods in common use may yield different reference values, for tests that show significant analytic variability or methodologic interferences, and for tests in which there are large sources of biologic variability, for example, effects of fasting, diurnal variation, or pregnancy. Conversion factors *from* conventional units *to* those recommended by the Système Internationale d'Unités (SI units) for major chemical and hematologic procedures are indicated in parentheses.[1,2,6]

REFERENCES

1. Beeler MF: Editorial: SI units and the AJCP. Am J Clin Pathol 87:140, 1987
2. Friedman RB, Anderson RE, et al: Effects of disease on clinical laboratory tests. Clin Chem 26:1D, 1980
3. Galen RS, Gambino SR: Beyond Normality: The Predictive Value and Efficiency of Medical Diagnoses. New York, John Wiley & Sons, 1975
4. Murphy EA, Abby H: The normal range—A common misuse. J Chronic Dis 20:79, 1967
5. Sunderman FW Jr: Current concepts of "normal values, reference values and discrimination values" in clinical chemistry. Clin Chem 21:1873, 1975
6. The SI for the Health Professions. Geneva: World Health Organization, 1977
7. Vecchio TJ: Predictive value of a single diagnostic test in unselected populations. N Engl J Med 274:1171, 1966

BLOOD, PLASMA, OR SERUM

Determination	Reference Values	Comments, SI Units
5'-Nucleotidase, serum	0–17 U/L	
Acetone, serum, qualitative	Negative	
Acid hemolysis test (Ham)	No hemolysis	
Acid phosphatase, prostatic, serum	0.2–0.8 U/L	
Activated partial thromboplastin time (APTT)	21–31 sec	
Adrenocorticotropin (ACTH), plasma	20–100 pg/ml	(0.2202, pmol/L)
Alanine aminotransferase (ALT or SGPT)	Adults: 0–30 IU/L (37C); Infants: 0–54 IU/L (37C)	
Albumin, serum	3.2–5.3 g/dl	(10, g/L)
Aldolase	Adults: 0–8 IU/L; Children: <16 IU/L; Newborns: <32 IU/L	
Aldosterone, plasma (RIA)	Adult females: 0–41.8 ng/dl; Adult males: 7.5–22.7 ng/dl	Normal sodium diet
Alkaline phosphatase, leukocyte	30–130 computed score	
Alkaline phosphatase, serum	Adults: 30–120 IU/L; Infants: 150–420 IU/L; Children: 100–320 IU/L; Adolescent females: 100–320 IU/L; Adolescent males: 100–390 IU/L	
Alphafetoprotein, serum (tumor marker)	<10 ng/ml	
Ammonia, plasma	<50 μmol/L	
Amylase, serum	Adults: 40–200 IU/L (37C); Newborns: 10–110 IU/L (37C)	
Androstenedione, plasma (RIA)	Adult females: 74–230 ng/dl; Adult males: 69–149 ng/dl	
Anion gap	4–20 mEq/L	1, mmol/L
Antithrombin III	70–120% of control	
Arylsulfatase	>5 U/ml	
Aspartate aminotransferase (AST or SGOT)	Adults: 0–35 IU/L (37C); Infants: 20–65 IU/L (37C)	
Bicarbonate	20–24 mmol/L	Calculated result (blood gases)
Bilirubin, direct (conjugated)	0.1–0.4 mg/dl	(17.1, μmol/L)
Bilirubin, total	Adults: 0.3–1.2 mg/dl; Cord blood: <1.8 mg/dl; Infants (<24 hr): <6 mg/dl; (24–48 hr): <8 mg/dl; (3–7 days): <12 mg/dl; (7–30 days): <7 mg/dl; (>30 days): 0.3–1.2 mg/dl	
Bleeding time, Ivy	<6 min	
Bleeding time, template (Simplate_TM)	3.5–10.5 min	
Bromide	750–1500 mg/L	
C-reactive protein	Negative	

BLOOD, PLASMA, OR SERUM (Continued)

Determination	Reference Values	Comments, SI Units
Cholesterol and triglycerides, serum	(see table below)	(0.02586, mmol/L); use of oral contraceptives significantly raises triglyceride and total serum cholesterol levels

	95th Percentile Limits (mg/dl)			
	Total Serum Cholesterol		Serum Triglycerides	
Age	Females	Males	Females	Males
0–4 yr	200	203	112	99
5–9 yr	205	203	105	101
10–14 yr	201	202	131	125
15–19 yr	200	197	124	148
20–24 yr	216	218	131	201
25–29 yr	222	244	144	249
30–34 yr	230	254	150	266
35–39 yr	242	270	176	321
40–44 yr	252	268	191	320
45–49 yr	265	276	214	327
50–54 yr	285	277	233	320
55–59 yr	300	276	262	286
60–64 yr	297	276	239	291
65–69 yr	303	274	243	267
70–74 yr	293	269	231	258
75–79 yr	291	261	242	267
80+ yr	279	275	242	255

Determination	Reference Values	Comments, SI Units
Cholinesterase, erythrocyte	3590–6666 U/dl RBC	
Clot retraction, qualitative	Begins in 30–60 min; complete in 24 hr	
CO$_2$, total	Adults: 24–30 mEq/L; Children: 20–24 mEq/L	(1, mmol/L)
Coagulation time (Lee-White)	3–10 min	Whole blood (37C)
Compound S, plasma (11-deoxycortisol)	<1 μg/dl	Baseline value
Copper, serum	Females: 85–155 μg/dl; Males: 70–140 μg/dl	Lower in infants, children
Cortisol, plasma (RIA)	8 AM: 8–18 μg/dl; Pre-ACTH: 8–18 μg/dl; Post-ACTH: 16–36 μg/dl	Higher in infants
Creatine kinase (CK), serum	Adult females: 0–136 U/L (37C); Adult males: 0–160 U/L (37C)	
Creatine kinase isoenzyme MB	CK-MB: 0–9 μg/L; % Index: 0–3%	Use index when total CK is greater than 1000 U/L
Creatinine clearance	Adult females: 105–132 ml/min; Adult males: 110–150 ml/min	Per 1/73 m² body surface area
Creatinine, serum	Adult females: 0.5–1.1 mg/dl; Adult males: 0.6–1.2 mg/dl; Cord blood: 0.6–1.2 mg/dl; Newborns (1–4 days): 0.3–1.0 mg/dl; Infants: 0.2–0.4 mg/dl; Children: 0.3–0.7 mg/dl; Adolescents: 0.5–1.0 mg/dl	(88.4, μmol/L)

Calcium, ionized, whole blood	1.07–1.25 mmol/L	Corrected to pH 7.40
Calcium, serum	9.0–10.5 mg/dl *Adults:* 9.0–10.5 mg/dl *Children:* 8.0–10.5 mg/dl *Term infants* (< *1 wk):* 7.0–12.0 mg/dl *Premature* (< *1 wk):* 6.0–10.0 mg/dl	(0.2495, mmol/L)
Carbon dioxide, serum (*See* CO_2, *total*)		
Carbon dioxide tension, arterial	35–45 mm Hg	(0.1333, kPa)
Carboxyhemoglobin, blood	*Nonsmokers:* 0–2% total Hgb *Smokers:* 2–10% total Hgb *Toxic levels:* 20–60% total Hgb *Lethal levels:* >60% total Hgb	
Carcinoembryonic antigen (CEA), plasma	<3 ng/ml	May be increased in smokers
Carotene, serum	50–250 μg/dl	Lower in infants, children
Ceruloplasmin, serum	18–45 mg/dl	
Chloride	*Adults:* 96–109 mEq/L *Children:* 99–111 mEq/L	(1, mmol/L)
Cholesterol, serum, total		(0.02586, mmol/L)

Age	*Percentile Limits (mg/dl)* "Moderate" Risk (>75th)	"High" Risk (>90th)
2–19 yr	>170	>185
20–29 yr	>200	>200
30–39 yr	>220	>240
>40 yr	>240	>260

A 1985 NIH Consensus Conference statement concluded that there is increased risk of coronary heart disease in both men and women with total cholesterol values above the 75th percentile of usual population reference values

Cholesterol, HDL	*Females:* >40 mg/dl *Males:* >30 mg/dl	10th percentile limits
Cholesterol, LDL		(0.02586, mmol/L)

	Percentile Limits (mg/dl)			
	Females		Males	
Age	75th	90th	75th	90th
10–20 yr	110	130	110	125
20–24 yr	120	140	120	140
25–29 yr	125	150	140	160
30–34 yr	130	150	145	165
35–39 yr	140	160	155	175
40–44 yr	145	165	160	175
45–49 yr	150	175	165	185
50–54 yr	160	185	165	185
55–59 yr	170	200	170	190
60–64 yr	170	190	165	190
65–69 yr	185	205	170	200
70+ yr	170	190	165	180

Cryofibrinogen	Negative	
Cryoglobulins	Negative	
Dehydroepiandrosterone, plasma	*Females:* 535 ± 160 ng/dl *Males:* 555 ± 180 ng/dl *Prepubertal:* 40 ± 30 ng/dl	Mean ± SD Mean ± SD Mean ± SD
Dehydroepiandrosterone sulfate	*Females:* 82–338 μg/dl (premenopausal) *Males:* 200–335 μg/dl	
Differential count (*See Leukocyte differential count*)		
Eosinophil count, blood		

Age	Absolute Count (per mm³)
0–1 mo	200–660
1–3 mo	140–550
3–6 mo	150–480
6 mo–4 yr	150–440
4–8 yr	150–430
8–14 yr	110–320
14–21 yr	110–320
Adults	120–300

Erythrocyte (red blood cell) count		(1, 10^{12}/L)

Age	Females × 10^6/mm³	Males × 10^6/mm³
0–1 day	3.9–5.5	3.9–5.5
1–3 days	4.0–6.6	4.0–6.6
3–7 days	3.9–6.3	3.9–6.3
7–14 days	3.6–6.2	3.6–6.2
14 days–1 mo	3.0–5.4	3.0–5.4
1–2 mo	2.7–4.9	2.7–4.9
2–6 mo	3.1–4.5	3.1–4.5
6 mo–2 yr	3.7–5.3	3.7–5.3
3–5 yr	3.9–5.3	3.9–5.3
6–12 yr	4.0–5.2	4.2–5.2
13–18 yr	4.1–5.1	4.5–5.3
Adults	4.0–5.2	4.5–5.9

From National Center for Health Statistics (NHANES I & II), DHHS Publications, PHS 82-1670 and PHS 83-1682.

Erythrocyte sedimentation rate (ESR) (*See Sedimentation rate, erythrocyte*)		
Estradiol 17-β, plasma	*Females:* 25–300 pg/ml *Males:* 20–90 pg/ml	
Euglobulin lysis	2 hr or greater	
Factor IX activity	>60% of control	
Factor VIII activity	>60% of control	
Fatty acids, free, plasma	0.19–0.90 mEq/L	
Ferritin, serum	*Adult females:* 10–110 ng/ml *Adult males:* 30–265 ng/ml	(1, μg/L)
Fibrin degradation products (FDP)	1:25 suspicious, 1:50 positive	
Fibrogen, plasma	150–400 mg/dl	(0.01, g/L)
Folate, red blood cell	150–600 ng/ml RBC	(2.266, nmol/L)

(continued)

BLOOD, PLASMA, OR SERUM (Continued)

Determination	Reference Values	Comments, SI Units
Follicle-stimulating hormone (FSH), serum	Adult females (except midcycle): 1.5–16.0 mIU/ml	
	Females (prepubertal): 0–5.0 mIU/ml	
	Males (adult): 2.0–17.2 mIU/ml	
	Males (prepubertal): 0–5.0 mIU/ml	
Free testosterone, serum (RIA) (See Testosterone, free, serum [EIA])		
Gamma globulin	0.7–1.7 mg/dl	Higher in infants, children
	4.3–12.3% of total protein	
Gamma glutamyl transferase, serum	Females: 7–33 mIU/L	
	Males: 11–51 mIU/L	
Gastrin, serum	0–100 pg/ml	
Globulin, serum	1.7–4.4 g/dl	
Glucose, serum (fasting)	70–115 mg/dl	(0.05551, mmol/L)
Glucose-6-phosphate dehydrogenase	7.4–9.4 U/g Hgb	
Glycosylated hemoglobin	4.9–7.7% of total Hgb	
Ham test	No hemolysis	
Haptoglobin, serum	100–300 mg/dl	
hCG (Human chorionic gonadotropin—tumor marker)	<3 mIU/ml	
Hematocrit (See Packed cell volume [PCV])		
Hemoglobin		(10, g/L)

Age	Females (g/dl)	Males (g/dl)
Birth–2 mo	14.1–20.1	14.1–20.1
2–6 mo	9.0–20.0	9.0–20.0
6 mo–4 yr	11.6–13.6	11.6–13.6
5–8 yr	11.7–13.8	11.7–13.8
9–14 yr	12.4–14.8	12.4–14.8
15–21 yr	12.4–14.8	13.2–15.6
Adults	12.0–15.0	13.9–16.3

Determination	Reference Values	Comments, SI Units
Hemoglobin A_{1c}	4.9–7.7% of total Hgb	
Hemoglobin A_2	2.4–3.4% of total Hgb	
Hemoglobin C in hemoglobin C trait	36–50% of total Hgb	
Hemoglobin F	<1% of total Hgb in adults	
Hemoglobin S in sickle cell trait	30–43% of total Hgb	
Hemoglobin, plasma	0–75 mg/L	
Hexokinase, erythrocyte	Under 4 yr: 17.7 ± 2.1 U/dl RBC; Over 4 yr: 14.9 ± 2.1 U/dl RBC	
Hempexin	Neonates: 6.5–25 mg/dl; 1–12 mo: 10–70 mg/dl; 1–12 yr: 40–70 mg/dl; Adults: 50–100 mg/dl	Newborns higher, children lower (0.1791, µmol/L)
Iron	65–175 µg/dl	See Transferrin
Iron binding capacity	Total: 250–410 µg/dl; Saturation: 20–55%	

BLOOD, PLASMA, OR SERUM (Continued)

Determination	Reference Values	Comments, SI Units
Mean corpuscular volume (MCV), erythrocyte		(1, fl)

Age	fl
0–1 day	98–118
1–3 days	95–121
3 days–1 mo	86–124
1–2 mo	77–115
2–6 mo	74–108
6 mo–2 yr	70–86
2–6 yr	75–87
6–12 yr	77–95
12–18 yr	78–100
Adults	80–100

Determination	Reference Values	Comments, SI Units
Methemalbumin	Negative	
Methemoglobin	0–1.5% of total Hgb	
5'-Nucleotidase, serum	0–17 U/L	
Osmolality, serum	285–295 mosm/kg of serum water	(1, mmol/kg)
Osmotic fragility screen	Hemolysis begins at 0.45% NaCl; is marked at 0.35% NaCl	
Oxygen tension, arterial (P_{O_2})	75–100 mm Hg	(0.1333, kPa)
Packed cell volume (Hct)		(0.01)

Age	Females (%)	Males (%)
0–1 day	42–60	42–60
1–3 days	45–67	45–67
3–7 days	42–66	42–66
7–14 days	39–62	39–62
14 days–1 mo	31–55	31–55
1–2 mo	28–42	28–42
2–6 mo	29–41	29–41
6 mo–2 yr	33–39	33–39
2–6 yr	34–40	34–40
6–12 yr	35–45	35–45
12–18 yr	36–46	37–49
Adults	36–46	41–53

White subjects; values for blacks are about 1.5% lower.

Determination	Reference Values	Comments, SI Units
Partial thromboplastin time	60–100 sec	(nonactivated)
pH, arterial, plasma or blood	7.35–7.45	
Phosphatase, acid, prostatic, serum	0.2–0.8 U/L	
Phosphatase, alkaline, serum. (See Alkaline phosphatase, serum)		
Phosphate, inorganic, serum	Adults (16+ yr): 3.0–4.5 mg/dl; Children (0–15 yr): 3.2–6.3 mg/dl	(0.3229, mmol/L)
Phospholipids, serum	125–300 mg/dl	
Plasma hemoglobin	0–75 mg/L	As lecithin
Platelets	150–400 × 10³/mm³	(1, 10⁹/L)
Potassium	3.5–5.0 mEq/L	Up to 6 mEq/L in newborns (1, mmol/L)
17-OH-Progesterone, plasma (RIA)	Females (luteal): 150–386 ng/dl; Females (follicular): 15–102 ng/dl; Males: 36–154 ng/dl	

Lactic acid, arterial	0.5–1.6 mmol/L	
Lactic acid, venous	0.5–2.2 mmol/L	
Lactate dehydrogenase (LDH), serum	Total: 0–200 IU/L (37C)	Higher in newborns
	Fractions:	
	LDH1: 17–27% of total LDH	
	LDH2: 28–38% of total LDH	
	LDH3: 19–27% of total LDH	
	LDH4: 5–16% of total LDH	
	LDH5: 5–16% of total LDH	
Lee-White clotting time	3–10 min	
Leucine aminopeptidase, serum	8–22 mIU/ml (25C)	
Leukocyte (white blood cell) count	(0.001, 10⁹/L)	

Age	Mean × 10^3/mm^3	Range × 10^3/mm^3
0–1 mo	11.0	9.0–30.0
1–3 mo	10.0	5.0–19.5
3–6 mo	9.5	5.7–17.7
6 mo–2 yr	9.5	6.0–17.5
2–4 yr	10.6	6.0–17.0
4–8 yr	9.1	5.5–15.5
8–14 yr	8.1	4.5–13.5
14–21 yr	8.0	4.5–13.0
Adults	8.0	4.5–11.0

Values are for white male and female subjects; counts for black adults and older black children are approximately 500 to 1000/mm³ lower than for whites

Leukocyte differential count	100 cell count with normal total WBC	
	Band neutrophils: 0–6%	
	Segmented neutrophils: 31–76%	
	Lymphocytes: 24–44%	
	Monocytes: 2–11%	
	Eosinophils: 0–5%	
	Basophils: 0–2%	
Lipase, serum	0–1 Cherry–Crandell U/L (37C)	
Luteinizing hormone (LH), serum	Adult females: 3.9–18.0 mIU/ml	Except midcycle
	Adult males: 2.0–22.6 mIU/ml	
	Prepubertal: 0–5.0 mIU/ml	
Magnesium, serum	1.5–2.0 mEq/L	(0.5, mmol/L)
Mean corpuscular hemoglobin (MCH), erythrocyte		(1, pg)

Age	pg
0–3 days	31.0–37.9
3 days–1 mo	28.0–40.0
1–2 mo	26.0–34.0
2–6 mo	25.0–35.0
6–2 yr	23.0–31.0
2–6 yr	24.0–30.0
6–12 yr	25.0–33.0
12–18 yr	25.0–35.0
Adults	26.0–34.0

Mean corpuscular hemoglobin conc. (MCHC), erythrocyte	(10, g/L)

Age	%
0–1 day	30–36
1–3 days	29–37
3–14 days	28–38
14 days–2 mo	29–37
2 mo–2 yr	30–36
2 yr–Adults	31–37

Progesterone, plasma (RIA)	Females (follicular): 19–43 ng/dl	
	Females (luteal): 237–2425 ng/dl	
	Females (prepubertal): 11–35 ng/dl	
	Males (adult): 25–45 ng/dl	
	Males (prepubertal): 12–32 ng/dl	
Prolactin, serum	0–25 ng/ml	Newborn levels tenfold greater
Prostate-specific antigen (PSA)	0–2.8 ng/ml	Postprostatectomy <0.2 ng/ml
Prostatic acid phosphatase, serum	0.2–0.8 U/L	
Protein, serum	Total: 0–2 yr: 3.7–8.8 g/dl	(10, g/L)
	2+ yr: 6.0–8.0 g/dl	
	Albumin: 3.2–5.3 g/dl	
	Globulin: 1.7–4.4 g/dl	
	Electrophoresis:	
	Albumin: 3.1–5.4 g/dl	
	Globulin:	
	alpha-1: 0.1–0.4 g/dl	
	alpha-2: 0.4–1.1 g/dl	
	beta: 0.5–1.2 g/dl	
	gamma: 0.75–1.7 g/dl	
Prothrombin consumption	>35 sec	
Prothrombin time (PT)	10.9–12.5 sec	
Protoporphyrin, erythrocyte	21–61 µg/dl RBC	
Pyruvate kinase, erythrocyte	138–260 U/dl RBC	
Pyruvic acid	0.3–0.9 mg/dl	
Red blood cell (RBC) count (See Erythrocyte count)		

	Supine	Standing
Renin, plasma	±1 SE; varies with hydration and method	
Normal sodium diet	1.6 ± 1.5 ng/ml/h	4.5 ± 2.0
Low sodium diet	3.2 ± 1.1	9.9 ± 4.3

Reticulocyte count	0.5–1.5% of erythrocytes	(0.001)
Reticulocyte count, absolute	10,000–75,000/mm³	(0.001, 10⁹/L)
Sedimentation rate, erythrocyte (Westergren)	Adult females (< 50 yr): 0–15 mm/hr	
	Adult females (> 50 yr): 0–30 mm/hr	
	Adult males (< 50 yr): 0–15 mm/hr	
	Adult males (> 50 yr): 0–20 mm/hr	
	Children: 0–10 mm/hr	
Sedimentation rate, erythrocyte (Wintrobe)	Adult females: 0–20 mm/hr	May be increased in pregnancy and anemia
	Adult males: 0–10 mm/hr	
SGPT (See Alanine aminotransferase)		
Sodium, serum	135–148 mEq/L	(1, mmol/L)
Sucrose hemolysis test	Negative	
Testosterone, free, serum (RIA)	Females: 0.2–0.73 ng/dl	
	Females (3rd week): 0.3–1.12 ng/dl	
	Males: 1.4–5.79 ng/dl	
	Prepubertal: 0.06–0.38 ng/dl	

(continued)

BLOOD, PLASMA, OR SERUM (Continued)

Determination	Reference Values			Comments, SI Units	
Testosterone, plasma (RIA)		Total (ng/dl)	Free + Bound	% Free + Bound	
	Females	15–95	1–11	6–21	
	Males	260–1120	75–390	15–55	
Testosterone, serum		Total (ng/dl)		Free (ng/dl)	
	Females	20–80		0.3–1.9	
	Males	300–1200		9–30	

Thromboplastin time (See Activated partial thromboplastin time; Partial thromboplastin time)

Determination	Reference Values	Comments, SI Units
Thyroid function tests		
Thyroxine (T₄), serum	Total: 5–12 µg/dl; Free: 0.8–2.4 ng/dl	12.87, nmol/L
Thyroid stimulating hormone (TSH), serum	Basal: 0.5–5 µU/ml; 30 minutes post TRH: 6–20 µU/ml	
Triiodothyronine (T₃), serum	90–200 ng/dl	0.01536, nmol/L
Reverse T₃ (rT₃), serum	13–52 ng/dl	
Thyroid binding globulin (TBG)	17–32 µg/dl	As T₄ binding capacity
T₃ resin uptake (T₃U)	25–35%	
Free thyroxine index (FTI)	1.3–3.5	Varies with T₄ and T₃U ranges
Transferrin	20–400 mg/dl	Transferrin × 1.25 = TIBC
Triglycerides. (See Cholesterol and triglycerides, serum)		
Urea nitrogen, serum	12–25 mg/dl	(0.357, mmol/l urea)
Uric acid, serum	Adult females: 2.6–6.0 mg/dl; Adult males: 3.5–7.2 mg/dl; Children: 2.0–5.5 mg/dl	
Viscosity, plasma, relative	1.6–1.9	
Viscosity, serum, relative	1.4–1.8	
Viscosity, whole blood		Varies with PCV
Vitamin A, serum	20–80 µg/dl	
Vitamin B₁₂, serum	200–1000 pg/ml	(0.7378, pmol/L)
Vitamin C	0.2–2.0 mg/dl	
Vitamin D, 1, 25-dihydroxy, serum	20–76 pg/ml	
Vitamin D, 25-OH, serum	10–55 ng/ml	
Vitamin E, serum	5–20 µg/ml	
Zinc, plasma	55–150 µg/dl	

IMMUNOLOGY (Continued)

Determination	Reference Values	Comments, SI Units
CH₅₀	75–160 U/ml	

IgG subclasses, serum

Age	G1 (mg/dl)	G2 (mg/dl)	G3 (mg/dl)	G4 (mg/dl)
Birth–8 mo	140–620	25–170	4–90	2–35
9 mo–2 yr	230–710	30–330	6–98	2–65
3–4 yr	280–880	50–440	6–110	2–115
5–6 yr	290–820	60–500	8–130	2–120
7–8 yr	300–1120	60–500	12–130	2–120
9–14 yr	300–1300	70–500	12–130	2–120
Adults	470–1300	115–750	20–130	2–165

Immune complexes — <12 µg equivalents/ml

Immunoglobulins

Age	IgG (mg/dl)	IgA (mg/dl)	IgM (mg/dl)
Newborns	636–1606	1–4	6–25
1–3 mo	176–906	1–53	17–105
4–6 mo	172–814	4–84	27–108
7–9 mo	217–904	11–90	34–126
10–12 mo	294–1069	16–84	41–149
1 yr	345–1213	14–106	43–173
2 yr	424–1051	14–123	48–168
3 y	441–1135	22–159	47–200
4–5 yr	463–1236	25–154	43–196
6–8 yr	633–1280	33–202	48–207
9–10 yr	608–1572	45–236	52–242
Adults	639–1349	70–312	56–352

Determination	Reference Values	Comments, SI Units
Rheumatoid factor (latex fixation)	0	Titer ≥20 may be significant for rheumatoid arthritis
Rheumatoid factor screen	Negative	
Rheumaton titer	0	
T lymphocytes	Total T cells (Tt): 50–80% of lymphocytes; T helper: 34–56% of lymphocytes; T suppressor: 18–32% of lymphocytes; T helper/T suppressor ratio (Th/Ts): 1.1–2.5	
T and B lymphocytes	Total T cells: 50–80% of lymphocytes; Total B cells: 5–20% of lymphocytes; Natural killer (NK) cells: 3–21% lymphocytes	
Total hemolytic complement (CH₅₀)	75–160 U/ml	

TOXICOLOGY AND THERAPEUTIC DRUG MONITORING

Determination	Reference Values	Comments, SI Units
Acetaminophen	5–20 mg/L	Hepatotoxicity likely with levels above 200 mg/L 4 hr after ingestion (6.62, µmol/L)

IMMUNOLOGY

Test	Value	Comments
Anti-DNA antibody (Double stranded)	Negative	Significant for SLE when ANA is also positive
Anti-ENA antibodies (RNP & Sm)	Negative	Anti-Sm highly correlated with SLE
Anti-ENA antibodies (RO[SS-A] & La [SS-B])	Negative	
Antigastric antibody	0	3+ undiluted is significant; if 1:4 dilution, 3+ is highly significant
Anti-Jo-1	Negative	Correlated with polymyositis
Antismooth muscle antibodies	0	Significant titer 1:40
Antiadrenal antibody	0	3+ undiluted is significant; if 1:4 dilution, 3+ is highly significant
Antihyaluronidase titer (AHT)	0	≥ fourfold rise at weekly intervals is significant
Antimitochondrial antibodies	0	Significant titer 1:10
Antinuclear antibody screen	0	Significant titer 1:160
Antistreptolysin-O screen and titer	0	Significant if fourfold or greater rise in titer can be demonstrated at weekly intervals
Antithyroid antibodies	Microsomal: 0	Borderline titer 1:80; Significant titer 1:160–640; >640 very significant titer
	Thyroglobulin: 0	Borderline titer 1:400; Significant titer 1:1600–6400; >6400 very significant titer

C3 and C4 complement

Age	C3 (mg/dl)	C4 (mg/dl)
Newborns	57–116	7–23
1–4 mo	53–149	7–28
4–6 mo	62–175	7–42
7–9 mo	75–166	10–37
10–12 mo	73–180	12–39
1–2 yr	84–174	12–40
2–3 yr	81–170	9–34
3–4 yr	77–171	10–36
4–5 yr	86–166	13–32
6–8 yr	88–155	12–32
9–10 yr	89–195	10–40
Adults	83–177	15–45

Antiarrhythmic agents

Drug	Value	Comments
Disopyramide (Norpace)	2–5 mg/L	Toxicity >7 mg/L
Lidocaine	1.5–5.0 mg/L	Toxicity >8 mg/L
N-acetyl-procainamide (NAPA)	6–20 mg/L	N-acetylated metabolite has antiarrhythmic activity
Procainamide	4–10 mg/L	
Procainamide + NAPA	10–30 mg/L	Toxicity >40 mg/L
Quinidine	2–5 mg/L	Toxicity >8 mg/L

Antibiotics

Values are "peak" concentrations, with "trough" levels in parentheses

Amikacin	20–35 µg/ml (5–10)
Cefotaxime	20–60 µg/ml
Chloramphenicol	10–20 µg/ml
5-Fluorocytosine	50–100 µg/ml
Gentamicin	4–10 µg/ml (<2)
Kanamycin	15–35 µg/ml (5–10)
Piperacillin	50–150 µg/ml
Sulfonamide	50–100 µg/ml
Ticarcillin	50–200 µg/ml
Tobramycin	4–10 µg/ml (<2)
Vancomycin	10–40 µg/ml

Antidepressant drugs

Drug	Value	Comments
Amitriptyline	(none)	Toxicity >500 µg/L
Amitriptyline + Nortriptyline	120–250 µg/L	Toxicity >1000 µg/L; Range is the sum of amitriptyline and its N-demethlyated metabolite, nortriptyline
Nortriptyline	50–150 µg/L	Toxicity >500 µg/L
Desipramine	75–160 µg/L	Toxicity >500 µg/L
Imipramine	(none)	Toxicity >500 µg/L
Imipramine + Desipramine	120–250 µg/L	Toxicity >1000 µg/L; Range is the sum of imipramine and its N-demethylated metabolite, desipramine

Antiepileptic agents

Drug	Value	Comments
Lithium	0.8–1.5 mEq/L	Toxicity >2 mEq/L (1, mmol/L)
Carbamazepine (Tegretol)	8–12 mg/L	Toxicity >15 mg/L
Ethosuximide (Zarontin)	40–100 mg/L	Toxicity >150 mg/L
Pentobarbital	1–5 mg/L	Toxicity >10 mg/L
Phenobarbital (Luminal)	15–40 mg/L	Toxicity >50 mg/L
Phenytoin (Dilantin)	10–20 mg/L	Toxicity >30 mg/L
Primidone (Mysoline)	8–12 mg/L	Toxicity >15 mg/L; Metabolized to phenobarbital

Cyclosporine

100–200 µg/L — Toxicity >200 mg/L

Digoxin

0.8–2.1 ng/ml — Toxicity >2.5 ng/ml; Expected serum values: 0.8–1.6 ng/ml (0.25 mg/day oral dose) and 1.1–1.9 ng/ml (0.50 mg/day oral dose) (0.0072, mmol/L)

Salicylate

Anti-inflammatory	100–300 mg/L	
Usual therapeutic	20–100 mg/L	

Theophylline (aminophylline), serum

5–20 mg/L

Thiocyanate, plasma

<120 mg/L — Toxicity >25 mg/L

(continued)

URINE

Determination	Reference Values	Comments, SI Units
URINE		
Aldosterone, (RIA)	2–26 µg/24 hr	
Alpha amino nitrogen	64–199 mg/24 hr	Normal sodium diet / Not over 1.5% of total nitrogen
δ-aminolevulinic acid	1.3–7.0 mg/24 hr	
Amylase	1–18 U/hr at 37C	
Calcium	<250 mg/24 hr	Normal diet

Catecholamines	Supine (pg/ml)	Sitting (pg/ml)	Standing (pg/ml)
Norepinephrine	110–410	120–680	125–700
Epinephrine	<50	<60	<90
Dopamine	<30	<30	<30
Total	120–450	140–730	150–750

Determination	Reference Values	Comments, SI Units
Copper	15–50 µg/24 hr	
Cortisol secretion rate	12 ± 2 mg/m³/24 hr	
Creatine	Adult females: 0–80 mg/24 hr; Adult males: 0–40 mg/24 hr	
Creatinine	15–25 mg/kg/24 hr	
Dehydroisoandrosterone	<15% of total 17-ketosteroids	
Delta aminolevulinic acid	1.3–7.0 mg/24 hr	
Glucose, reducing substances	<250 mg/24 hr	
Hemoglobin/myoglobin	None	
Hemosiderin	0	
Homogentisic acid	0	
Homovanillic acid (HVA)	0–10 mg/24 hr	(2.759, µmol/day)
17-Hydroxycorticosteroids	Adult females: 2–8 mg/24 hr; Adult males: 3–9 mg/24 hr	
5-HIAA (hydroxyindoleacetic acid)		
Qualitative	None	
Quantitative	0–5.7 mg/24 hr	
17-Ketosteroids	Adult females: 4–13 mg/24 hr; Adult males: 6–18 mg/24 hr	

Metanephrines	Adults: 0–1.60 mg/24 hr
	0.21–1.28 mg/g creatinine
	Infants and children:
	  1–12 mo: 0.001–4.6 mg/g creatinine
	  1–2 yr: 0.27–5.88 mg/g creatinine
	  2–5 yr: 0.35–2.99 mg/g creatinine
	  5–10 yr: 0.43–2.70 mg/g creatinine
	  10–15 yr: 0.001–1.87 mg/g creatinine	

Osmolality	40–1400 mosm/kg	(1, mmol/kg)
Oxalate, quantitative	8–40 mg/24 hr	
Phenylalanine	0–4 mg/dl	
Phenylpyruvic acid	None	
Porphobilinogen		
Qualitative	None	
Quantitative	0–0.1 mg/dl	
Porphyins (total)	22–88 µg/L	
Potassium	53–91 mEq/24 hr	Varies with diet

Determination	Reference Values	Comments, SI Units
URINE (Continued)		
Protein, quantitative	25–100 mg/24 hr	Varies with diet
Sodium	40–156 mEq/24 hr	
Specific gravity	1.003–1.030	
Tetrahydro-compound S	<0.3 mg/dl	
Urea clearance, maximal	60–100 ml/min	Per 1.73 m² body surface
Uric acid	0.2–0.5 g/24 hr	Normal diet
Urobilinogen, quantitative	Up to 1 Ehrlich U/hr; 0–4 mg/24 hr	
VMA (Vanillylmandelic acid)	2–10 mg/24 hr	
SEMEN		
Fructose	Positive	
Morphology	>70% of normal forms	
Motility	>60% or more motile	
Motility grade	4–5	
Total volume	1.5–5.0 ml	
CEREBROSPINAL FLUID		
Electrophoresis	Predominantly albumin	
Glucose	50–75 mg/dl; 60–70% of blood levels	
IgG	Children (<14 yr): ≤8.2% of CSF total protein Adults: ≤14% of CSF total protein	
IgG index	0.2–0.8	>0.8 indicates IgG synthesis within CNS
Lactic acid	0.6–2.2 mmol/L	
Protein	15–45 mg/dl	Up to 70 mg/dl in children and the elderly (0.01, g/L)
VDRL	Nonreactive	
AMNIOTIC FLUID		
Creatinine	Mature: >2 mg/dl	If maternal creatinine normal
Lecithin/sphingomyelin ratio	Mature: >2.0 Indeterminate: 1.5–2.0 Immature: <1.5	
Phosphatidyl glycerol (PG)	Mature: positive	
FECES		
Bulk	100–200 g/24 hr	
Dry matter	23–32 g/24 hr	
Fat, total	≤6 g/24 hr (6% of dietary intake)	
Nitrogen, total	≤2 g/24 hr (10% of dietary intake)	

Page entries in **boldface** indicate tables.

Page entries in **boldface** indicate tables.

Page entries in **boldface** indicate tables.